Textbook
of Medical–Surgical
Nursing

Lillian Sholtis Brunner
R.N., M.S.N., Sc.D., F.A.A.N.

Board of Overseers, School of Nursing,
University of Pennsylvania, Philadelphia, Pennsylvania

Consultant in Nursing, Schools of Nursing: Presbyterian–
University of Pennsylvania Medical Center, Philadelphia, Pennsylvania,
and The Bryn Mawr Hospital, Bryn Mawr, Pennsylvania

Formerly Assistant Professor of Surgical Nursing,
Yale University School of Nursing, New Haven, Connecticut

Doris Smith Suddarth
R.N., B.S.N.E., M.S.N.

Formerly Consultant in Health Occupations, Job Corps Health Office,
U.S. Department of Labor, Washington, D.C.

Formerly Coordinator of the Curriculum, Alexandria Hospital School
of Nursing, Alexandria, Virginia

With special assistance from
Brenda G. Bare, R.N., M.S.N.

With 32 contributors

J. B. Lippincott Company Philadelphia
London   Mexico City   New York   St. Louis   São Paulo   Sydney

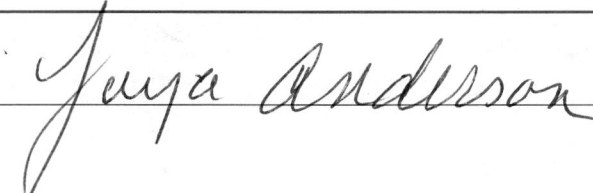

Tanya Anderson

Textbook of
Medical-Surgical
Nursing

Fifth Edition

Sponsoring Editor: Diana Intenzo
Manuscript Editor: Kathleen P. Dunn
Indexer: Angela Holt
Designer and Art Director: Tracy Baldwin
Production Supervisor: J. Corey Gray
Compositor: Tapsco, Inc.
Printer/Binder: The Murray Printing Company

5th Edition

6 5

Library of Congress Cataloging in Publication Data
Main entry under title:

Textbook of medical-surgical nursing.

   Rev. ed. of: Textbook of medical-surgical nursing
Lillian Sholtis Brunner, Doris Smith Suddarth. 4th ed.
c1980.
   Bibliography: p.
   Includes index.
   1. Nursing. 2. Surgical nursing. I. Brunner,
Lillian Sholtis. II. Suddarth, Doris Smith. III. Brunner,
Lillian Sholtis. Textbook of medical–surgical nursing.

[DNLM: 1. Nursing care. 2. Surgical nursing. WY 150
B897t]

RT41.T46   1982   610.73   83–17601
ISBN 0–397–54419–7

The authors and publisher have exerted every effort to ensure
that drug selection and dosage set forth in this text are in accord
with current recommendations and practice at the time of
publication. However, in view of ongoing research, changes in
government regulations, and the constant flow of information
relating to drug therapy and drug reactions, the reader is urged
to check the package insert for each drug for any change in
indications and dosage and for added warnings and precautions.
This is particularly important when the recommended agent is a
new or infrequently employed drug.

It is assumed that nursing practice is performed to comply with
the professional nurse practice act.

Contributors

Abass Alavi, M.D.

Assistant Professor of Nuclear Medicine, Department of Radiology, Hospital of the University of Pennsylvania, Philadelphia, Pennsylvania

Chapter 18: Diagnostic Radiology, Radiotherapy, and Nuclear Medicine

Caroline Stokes Bagley, R.N., M.S.N.

Assistant Professor of Nursing, School of Nursing, The Catholic University of America, Washington, D.C.

Chapter 17: Oncology: Nursing the Patient With Cancer

Brenda G. Bare, R.N., M.S.N.

Curriculum Coordinator, Alexandria Hospital School of Nursing, Alexandria, Virginia

Unit I (Chapters 1–3): Health Maintenance and Health Needs

Winnie F. Barnard, R.N., B.S.

Nursing Coordinator, Clinical Nephrology, Georgetown University Medical Center, Washington, D.C.

Section on "Dialysis" and "Acute Renal Failure" in Chapter 44: Management of Patients With Renal and Urinary Disorders

Elizabeth W. Bayley, R.N., M.S., C.C.R.N.

Assistant Professor, Burn, Emergency and Trauma Nursing, Graduate Nursing Program, Widener University, Chester, Pennsylvania

Chapter 53: Management of the Burn Patient

James F. Elam, PH.D.

Clinical Biochemist, Pathology Department, Alexandria Hospital, Alexandria, Virginia

Appendix: Diagnostic Studies and Their Meanings

Ronald J. Glasser, M.D.

Department of Pediatrics, St. Louis Park Medical Center, Minneapolis, Minnesota

Chapter 49: The Immune System and Immunopathology

Harold A. Goldstein, M.D.

Assistant Professor of Radiology, Division of Nuclear Medicine, Department of Radiology, Hospital of the University of Pennsylvania, Philadelphia, Pennsylvania

Chapter 18: Diagnostic Radiology, Radiotherapy, and Nuclear Medicine

Rosalind W. Harper, R.N., M.N.

Clinical Specialist, Critical Care, Oregon Health Sciences University Hospital, Portland, Oregon

Chapter 25: Respiratory Intensive Care

Lois M. Hoskins, R.N., PH.D.

Associate Professor of Nursing, School of Nursing, The Catholic University of America, Washington, D.C.

Chapter 7: Homeostasis and Pathophysiologic Processes
Chapter 8: Stress and Adaptation

Donna D. Ignatavicius, R.N., B.S.N., M.S.

Instructor, University of Maryland School of Nursing, Baltimore, Maryland

Chapter 51: Management of Patients With Connective Tissue Disorders

Louise M. Juliani, R.N., M.S.N.

Assistant Professor—Professionalism and Management, College of Nursing, University of North Dakota, Grand Forks, North Dakota

Unit XI (Chapters 42–44): Renal and Urinary Problems

Anne Keane, R.N., ED.D.

Associate Professor of Nursing, and Director of Adult Health and Illness Master's Program, University of Pennsylvania, Philadelphia, Pennsylvania

Unit IX (Chapters 34–38): Digestive and Gastrointestinal Problems

Silvia Prodan Lange, R.N., M.N., C.S.

Clinical Specialist, Department of Psychiatry, Pacific Medical Center, San Francisco; and Clinical Teaching Assistant, School of Nursing, University of San Francisco, California

Chapter 12: Illness as a Human Experience

Dorothy B. Liddel, R.N., M.S.N.

Instructor, Medical and Surgical Nursing, Alexandria Hospital School of Nursing, Alexandria, Virginia

Unit XVI (Chapters 59–62): Musculoskeletal and Locomotion Problems

Margo McCaffery, R.N., M.S.

Consultant in the Nursing Care of Patients with Pain, Santa Monica, California; and Assistant Clinical Professor, Nursing, University of California, Los Angeles, California

Chapter 16: The Person Experiencing Pain

Edwina A. McConnell, R.N., M.S.

Consultant, Medical–Surgical Nursing, Nursing Management; and Part-time Staff Nurse, Madison, Wisconsin

Unit XI (Chapters 42–44): Renal and Urinary Problems
Chapter 48: Management of the Male Patient With Disorders Related to the Reproductive System

Diane Deegan McCrann, R.N., M.S.N.

Adult Nurse Practitioner; Instructor, College of Nursing, Villanova University, Villanova, Pennsylvania

Chapter 4: Clinical Interviewing: The Health History
Chapter 5: Physical Assessment

Josephine Messer, R.N., M.S.

Assistant Professor, Department of Nursing, Monmouth College, West Long Branch, New Jersey

Chapter 13: Human Sexuality

Ruth Mrozek, R.N., M.S.

HSRO Coordinator, Veterans Administration Medical Center, Pittsburgh, Pennsylvania

Chapter 6: Documentation of Nursing Practice: Problem-Oriented Recording

Rita Nemchik, R.N., M.S.

Director, Center for Continuing Education, University of Pennsylvania School of Nursing, Philadelphia, Pennsylvania

Chapter 40: Assessment and Management of Patients With Diabetes Mellitus

Paul Oberkircher, M.D.

Chief, Radiology Department, Paoli Memorial Hospital, Paoli, Pennsylvania

Chapter 18: Diagnostic Radiology, Radiotherapy, and Nuclear Medicine

Melvyn P. Richter, M.D.

Director, Department of Radiation Therapy, Fox Chase Cancer Center, American Oncologic Hospital, Philadelphia, Pennsylvania

Chapter 18: Diagnostic Radiology, Radiotherapy, and Nuclear Medicine

Wanda Roberts, R.N., M.N.

Assistant Professor, Department of Physiological Nursing, and Education Coordinator, Burn Center, University of Washington, Seattle, Washington

Chapter 32: Assessment and Management of Patients With Vascular Disorders and Problems of Peripheral Circulation

Joanna Schnaidt Rokosky, R.N., B.S.N., M.N.

Formerly Assistant Professor, Department of Physiological Nursing, School of Nursing, University of Washington, Seattle, Washington

Chapter 9: Fluids and Electrolytes: Balance and Disturbances
Chapter 33: Assessment and Management of Patients With Hematologic Disorders

Mona B. Shevlin, P.A., Ph.D.

Licensed Psychologist; Professor, The Catholic University of America, Washington, D.C.; and Director, Counseling Center for Greater Washington, McLean, Virginia

Chapter 11: Developmental Concepts of the Adult Life Cycle

Suzanne C. O'Connell Smeltzer, R.N., Ed.D.

Assistant Professor, Adult Health and Illness Section, University of Pennsylvania School of Nursing, Philadelphia, Pennsylvania

Chapter 39: Assessment and Management of Patients With Hepatic and Biliary Disorders
Chapter 41: Assessment and Management of Patients With Endocrine Disorders

Loretta Spittle, R.N., M.S.

Coordinator, Critical Care Nurse Internship Program, Alexandria Hospital, Alexandria, Virginia

Chapter 31: Management of Patients With Cardiac Disorders

Sandra L. Underhill, R.N., M.N.

Lecturer, Department of Physiological Nursing, University of Washington, Seattle, Washington

Chapter 27: Assessment of Cardiovascular Function

Kyriake Valassi, Ph.D.

Professor, Nutritional Biochemistry, The Catholic University of America, Washington, D.C.

Chapter 10: Nutritional Considerations in Health Care

Susan L. Woods, R.N., M.N.

Associate Professor, Department of Physiological Nursing, University of Washington School of Nursing, Seattle, Washington

Chapter 28: Electrocardiograms and Heart Arrhythmias
Chapter 29: Management of the Patient in the Cardiac Care Unit

Karen S. Wulff, R.N., M.N., C.C.R.N.

Assistant Administrator, University Hospital, Clinical Faculty Member, School of Nursing, University of Washington, Seattle, Washington

Chapter 30: Management of the Cardiovascular Surgery Patient

Preface

Significant advances continue to be made in the understanding of human behavior, biological and physical sciences, and technology. The traditional role of the nurse in providing nurture, comfort, and care continues to broaden as it encompasses health maintenance and encourages strategies for self-care. The nurse serves as the patient's advisor, counselor, advocate, and educator in helping him to cope with his health and illness problems.

Since "nursing is the diagnosis and treatment of human responses to actual or potential health problems,"* the authors believe that the basic approach in wholistic patient care is the application of the nursing process. This includes assessment, formulating the nursing diagnosis, planning to achieve specific goals, using nursing interventions based on scientific principles, and finally, evaluation that is systematically measured against patient objectives. The nursing process has been applied to selected clinical patterns throughout this book, broader or more detailed application being curtailed by space (book pages) constraints.

The traditional and current purpose of this book is to provide principles and concepts of medical and surgical nursing that will help the student to think, listen, reflect, and grow in understanding and practice of the best possible care of patients with these conditions. To understand the meaning of health, one must also understand physiologic and psychological dysfunctioning (disease) of a part, or *in toto,* and its effect on the whole human being. This knowledge is essential in gathering the nursing data base, assessing response to therapy, and achieving and evaluating improvement in health status. And although "old" diseases have theoretically been conquered, new epidemics arising from opportunistic organisms influenced by environmental changes are a reality in every health care setting. These problems have been addressed.

More specifically, the chapter on stress and adaptation has been strengthened and enlarged to include not only the physiologic parameters of stress but self-regulation of stress that is essential in developing coping behaviors of patients and nurses.

Since human sexuality plays a role in personality development and well-being, a chapter relating to the dimensions of sexuality, problems of sexual dysfunction, and factors limiting sexual expression has been added. The effects of specific illnesses on sexuality are found throughout the book.

"Developmental Concepts of the Adult Life Cycle" is a new chapter that portrays the differences between and changes within individuals with the passage of time. Nursing cognizance of these variations is essential in meeting human needs.

There are increasing numbers of persons over age 65. The problems of management of individuals (and their families) with chronic disease and their maintenance of optimum function (rather than just curing illness) are included where appropriate in the clinical discussions.

Patient education sections have been strengthened. Patients/clients must understand cause and effect, treatment strategies, and the reduction of risk factors if health is to be attained. Specific instruction helps to promote the patient's adherence to achieving his goals. Also, there is recognition of the patient's potential by building on his strengths rather than focusing on his weaknesses.

There has been a consistent effort to appraise research developments and innovations in nursing practice and apply these findings to nursing practice/patient care. Immunologic-related problems are receiving increasing attention, as are connective tissue disorders. These are addresssed as separate but related entities.

The many changes and additions have been made possible by utilizing the talents of recognized nursing colleagues. Hence, the authorship has been expanded to give a balanced presentation of the burgeoning number of diagnostic and treatment modalities and nursing options, each with its strengths and areas of applicability. We are grateful to these contributors for their cooperation and participation, and for sharing their expertise.

As we approach the 21st century, the science of nuring is changing, yet the art of nursing prevails.

* Nursing: A Social Policy Statement.

LSB and DSS

Acknowledgments

William P. Argy, M.D., Professor of Medicine and Associate Director, Division of Nephrology, Georgetown University School of Medicine, Washington, D.C.

Stephen J. Bednar, M.D., Assistant Professor of Medicine, Georgetown University Medical Center, Washington, D.C.

Thomas E. Bressi, M.D., Attending Surgeon, The Bryn Mawr Hospital, Bryn Mawr, Pennsylvania

Ruth T. Burns, R.N., B.S.N., Supervisor, Surgery, Memorial Hospital Medical Center of Long Beach, Long Beach, California

Eileen Conroy, R.N., M.N., Supervisor, Surgery, Memorial Hospital Medical Center of Long Beach, Long Beach, California

Jane B. Dengler, R.N., M.Ed., M.S.N., Associate Director, Nursing Service, The Bryn Mawr Hospital, Bryn Mawr, Pennsylvania

Mervyn L. Elgart, M.D., Professor and Chairman, Department of Dermatology, George Washington University Medical Center, Washington, D.C.

Mary Lou Frain, R.N., B.S., Assistant Director, Nursing Service, Presbyterian–University of Pennsylvania Medical Center, Philadelphia, Pennsylvania

Mary C. Fraser, R.N., M.A., Epidemiology Research Nurse, Cancer Nursing Service/Environmental Epidemiology Branch, National Institutes of Health and National Cancer Institute, Bethesda, Maryland

George W. Gregory, III, M.D., Surgeon, Department of Surgery, Section of Cardiac Surgery, The Reading Hospital and Medical Center, Reading, Pennsylvania

Rosalind W. Harper, R.N., M.S., Associate Director of Nursing Education and Research, The Oregon Health Sciences University, Portland, Oregon

Kay Kern, R.N., M.S.N., Supervisor, Surgery, Memorial Hospital Medical Center of Long Beach, Long Beach, California

James H. Knepshield, M.D., Co-Director, Hemodialysis and Transplantation Service, Georgetown University Medical Center, Washington, D.C.

Etta J. Liberi, R.N., B.S.N., M.S., Director, School of Practical Nursing, Presbyterian–University of Pennsylvania Medical Center, Philadelphia, Pennsylvania

Mary Ann Morgan, R.N., B.S.N., M.S.N., Director, School of Nursing, Presbyterian–University of Pennsylvania Medical Center, Philadelphia, Pennsylvania

Alfred Munzer, M.D., Director, Critical Care, Washington Adventist Hospital, Takoma Park, Maryland

Mary Gill Nolan, R.N., M.N., Vice President/Patient Care Services, Memorial Hospital Medical Center of Long Beach, Long Beach, California

Lynne Oland, M.S.N., Doctoral Student, Physiology, University of North Carolina, Chapel Hill, North Carolina

Sandra B. Painter, R.N., M.S.N., Director of Nursing Service, Presbyterian–University of Pennsylvania Medical Center, Philadelphia, Pennsylvania

B. Warren Pechan, M.D., Assistant Professor of Surgery, Division of Transplantation, Division of Urology, Georgetown University School of Medicine, Washington, D.C.

Donald M. Poretz, M.D., Chief of Infectious Diseases, The Fairfax Hospital, Falls Church, Virginia

Beth Proukou, R.N., B.S.N., Assistant Director, Nursing Service, Presbyterian–University of Pennsylvania Medical Center, Philadelphia, Pennsylvania

Mary F. Rieser, R.N., M.S., Director of Staff Development, Division of Nursing, Hospital of the University of Pennsylvania, Philadelphia, Pennsylvania

John W. Rose, M.D., Medical Staff Fellow, Neuroimmunology Branch, National Institutes of Health, Bethesda, Maryland

Thomas E. Sanchez, M.D., Medical Staff Fellow, Surgical Neurology Branch, National Institutes of Health, Bethesda, Maryland

Gary J. Starecheski, B.Sc., Assistant Director of Pharmacy, and Hospice Pharmacist, The Bryn Mawr Hospital, Bryn Mawr, Pennsylvania

Linda Steichen, R. N., Supervisor, Post Anesthesia Recovery, Memorial Hospital Medical Center of Long Beach, Long Beach, California

Marguerite Trevor, R.N., M.N., Perioperative Educator, Surgery–Post Anesthesia Recovery, Memorial Hospital Medical Center of Long Beach, Long Beach, California

Reuben R. Wolfert, B.S., M.A., Director of Pharmacy, The Bryn Mawr Hospital, Bryn Mawr, Pennsylvania

Research/Library

Albert M. Berkowitz, Chief of Reference Services Division, National Library of Medicine, Bethesda, Maryland

Ann Campisi, Library Assistant, Medical/Nursing Library, Presbyterian–University of Pennsylvania Medical Center, Philadelphia, Pennsylvania

Patricia A. Connors, Librarian, Medical/Nursing Library, Presbyterian–University of Pennsylvania Medical Center, Philadelphia, Pennsylvania

Martin M. Cummings, M.D., Director, National Library of Medicine, Bethesda, Maryland

Eileen Daget, Librarian, Medical Library, The Bryn Mawr Hospital, Bryn Mawr, Pennsylvania

Leslie D. Gundry, Chief Medical Librarian, Medical Library, The Bryn Mawr Hospital, Bryn Mawr, Pennsylvania

Alexander G. Kulchar, Medical Librarian, Medical Library, The Bryn Mawr Hospital, Bryn Mawr, Pennsylvania

Doris Mohn, Librarian, Medical Library, The Bryn Mawr Hospital, Bryn Mawr, Pennsylvania

Alice Makov, Reference: User Education, Scott Memorial Library, The Thomas Jefferson University, Philadelphia, Pennsylvania

Jacqueline van de Kamp, Technical Information Specialist, National Library of Medicine, Bethesda, Maryland

Reference Librarians and Reference Technicians, National Library of Medicine, Bethesda, Maryland

We acknowledge the following persons with special appreciation:

Diana Intenzo, our Executive Editor, for her vision, dedication, and determination to produce the "best" that is humanly possible

Jeanne Wallace, for her quiet and painstaking editorial assistance

Tracy Baldwin and Lynn Klein, for their insightful talents and artistic expertise

Kathleen Dunn, for masterfully adhering to the production time-schedule while overseeing the production phases of this book and yet maintaining tactful finesse and graciousness in all author contact

Mary Murphy, for her many kindnesses and courtesies

Barton H. Lippincott, Edward B. Hutton, and *John Connolly* for their enthusiasm and personal commitment to our books

Of course, our deepest tributes and sincerest appreciations are reserved for those who mean the most to us, our husbands, Mat and Hilton.

Contents

▷ Unit X
Metabolic and
Endocrine Problems   847

39 Assessment and Management of Patients With Hepatic and Biliary Disorders   849

40 Assessment and Management of Patients With Diabetes Mellitus   883

41 Assessment and Management of Patients With Endocrine Disorders   918

▷ Unit XI
Renal and
Urinary Problems   953

42 Assessment of Renal and Urinary Function   955

43 Management of Patients With Renal and Urinary Dysfunction   970

44 Management of Patients With Renal and Urinary Disorders   994

▷ Unit XII
Sexual and
Reproductive Problems   1021

45 Management During the Reproductive Cycle   1023

46 Management of Patients With Gynecologic Disorders   1042

47 Assessment and Management of Patients With Breast Disorders   1065

Textbook
of Medical–Surgical
Nursing

Unit I

Health Maintenance and Health Needs

1

Nursing in Today's World: Concepts and Implementation

▷ Nursing Defined

To clearly articulate a universally accepted definition of nursing has been the goal of many nursing leaders for decades. Such a definition of nursing remains as elusive today as it was over a century ago, when the era of modern nursing began. Over the years many definitions of nursing have evolved that have been attempts to describe the roles and functions of the nurse. These definitions have described the services provided by the nurse, the setting within which the profession of nursing functions, the characteristics of the person who is the recipient of nursing care, and those attributes that distinguish nursing from other service-oriented disciplines in the health care delivery system. However, a definition that is descriptive of nursing in large, urban medical centers as well as in the remote areas of Appalachia and in the aerospace program has not yet been clearly articulated.

Since the time of Florence Nightingale, who wrote in 1858 that the real goal of nursing was "to put the patient in the best condition for nature to act upon him," nursing leaders have defined nursing as both an art and a science. In the earlier years, they tended to emphasize the nursing services that are directed toward the care of the sick. More recently, they have stressed the maintenance and promotion of health as well as the prevention of illness.

One of the classic definitions of nursing, as formulated by Virginia Henderson (1966), delineates the unique function of the nurse as follows:

> to assist the individual, sick or well, in the performance of those activities contributing to health or its recovery (or to peaceful death) that he would perform unaided if he had the necessary strength, will or knowledge. And to do this in such a way as to help him gain independence as rapidly as possible.*

* Henderson V. The Nature of Nursing. New York, Macmillan, 1966.

Review of the literature since the time of Henderson's definition of nursing reveals a multitude of attempts at further defining the unique function of the nurse—unique with regard to the functions of other health care disciplines. Most of these formulations have attempted to define nursing as a profession directed toward meeting both the health and illness needs of "man," who is viewed holistically as having physical as well as emotional, psychological, intellectual, social, and spiritual needs. One such definition of nursing is that presented by Yura and Walsh (1978).

> Nursing is an encounter with a client and his family in which the nurse observes, supports, communicates, ministers, and teaches; she contributes to the maintenance of optimum health, and provides care during illness until the client is able to assume responsibility for the fulfillment of his own basic human needs; when necessary, she provides compassionate assistance with dying.*

Because of the diversity of definitions of nursing that exist in the literature, individual nurses and groups of nurses are left with the choices of subscribing to one of these definitions, of combining components of several definitions, or of developing their own definition. In selecting a definition, the nurse must give consideration to the nurse practice act of the state within which she practices nursing and to the guidelines established by the International Council of Nurses (ICN) and the American Nurses' Association (ANA) in their respective codes for nurses. Whatever the choice, the selected definition should reflect a view of man as an integrated whole—a biopsychosocial being. With such a view, the holistic concept of health is then seen as including physical, emotional, psychological, intellectual, social, and spiritual aspects of human functioning that are interrelated, interdependent, and of equal importance.

- Nursing then can be defined as a service-oriented health profession that is directed toward assisting the individual to meet his health and illness needs relative to all aspects of his functioning capacity.
- The goal of nursing can be defined as the promotion, maintenance, and restoration of health, with concern for the biological and psychosocial factors of health and illness, and with respect for the needs and rights of the person to whom nursing care is rendered.

▷ Conceptual Models in Nursing

If nurses are to accomplish the goals of nursing as defined by nursing leaders, nursing must have a body of theoretical knowledge upon which to base its practice. Great strides toward "theory building" in nursing have been made in recent years.

In the past, nursing has utilized theories from various biopsychosocial sciences. Only within the past several decades have nurses made concerted efforts toward identifying

---

* Yura H and Walsh WB. The Nursing Process, 3rd ed. Appleton–Century–Crofts, 1978.

a circumscribed body of knowledge that is unique to nursing and that can serve as the theoretical basis for the practice of nursing. Such a theoretical basis, when more fully developed, will consist of scientifically derived general principles that will serve to describe, explain, and predict the practice of nursing. Nursing theories will provide a guide for viewing nursing holistically and for determining the probable results of nursing actions in advance of their implementation. However, only as theories of nursing evolve and mature and as they are tested and retested will a general theory of nursing develop.

Much of the progress that has been accomplished in the pursuit of a scientific theory of nursing has been in the areas of concept formalization and model construction. Because nursing is a practice-oriented discipline, concepts of nursing have been evolving over the years. However, only in recent years have nurses attempted to articulate these concepts, to propose that they be used as the framework for nursing practice, and to test and validate them. Many concepts that have their foundations in the biopsychosocial sciences have been found to be particularly applicable to nursing and now serve as useful components of frameworks for nursing practice.

Several of the broad concepts that have been utilized extensively as frameworks for nursing curricula and for nursing practice throughout the country include (1) the wellness–illness continuum, (2) developmental processes throughout the life cycle, and (3) stress adaptation.

The *wellness–illness continuum* provides a means by which the nurse focuses on the patient's positive health attributes and characteristics within the dimensions of his illness or potential illness situation. The individual is recognized as a holistic being who is in interaction with his internal and external environment. With such a focus and view of the individual, the nurse then utilizes the nursing process to assist the patient to use his attributes in attaining and maintaining the highest level of wellness that is possible within his physical and psychosocial limitations. Dunn's concept of high-level wellness serves as the basis for this framework for nursing.

The *developmental processes* approach to nursing provides a frame of reference that emphasizes the complexity of variables that are involved in each of the developmental stages of the life cycle. Such a framework provides direction for the nurse in assisting the patient to accomplish his developmental tasks as they are affected by his state of health and wellness. The theories of Havighurst, Erikson, and Piaget serve as the bases for the developmental processes approach to nursing. Havighurst's developmental tasks emphasize the effects of physical and social developmental changes and events on the individual; Erikson's eight stages of human development emphasize the successful completion of psychosocial tasks necessary for attaining and maintaining one's identity; Piaget's stages of cognitive development emphasize development of cognitive abilities and related sensorimotor skills.

The *stress-adaptation framework* emphasizes the role of the nurse in assessing the patient's behavioral responses to the demands of his internal and external environment.

Nursing interventions are then directed toward assisting the patient to strive toward adaptive behavior that promotes health and prevents illness. The general adaptation syndrome (GAS) as described by Selye and the fight-or-flight syndrome as described by Cannon serve as the bases for the stress-adaptation framework.

These broad concepts and other related concepts, while serving as useful frameworks for nursing practice, are not in and of themselves unique to nursing. Therefore, nursing leaders have attempted to develop, more fully, concepts that are inherent within nursing itself and to construct models that describe the relationships between these concepts and their subconcepts. Four such conceptual models of nursing are the *life processes model* developed by Rogers (1970), the *self-care model* as advocated by Orem (1971), the *adaptation model* as formulated by Roy (1974), and the behavioral systems model developed by Johnson (1980).

These are certainly not the only conceptual models of nursing that have been developed, nor is it the intent of the authors to suggest that nurses should subscribe to any one of these models, forsaking other models that may also serve as valuable frameworks for the practice of nursing. However, it is the intent of the authors to present these models as *examples* of contemporary models of nursing, with the hope that they will generate interest, enthusiasm, and inquiry into the present status and future potential of conceptual frameworks of nursing and the state of theory building in nursing.

Life Processes Model

The life processes model of nursing focuses on the wholeness of the human organism in the person who is the recipient of nursing care. It is Rogers's belief that the purpose of the scientific body of knowledge of nursing is to describe, explain, and make predictions about mankind. Such knowledge leads to the evolution of theories that serve to guide nursing practice. Rogers identified fundamental human attributes that constitute the following basic assumptions upon which nursing science is built:

1. Man is a unified whole possessing his own integrity and manifesting characteristics that are more than and different from the sum of his parts.
2. Man and the environment are continuously exchanging matter and energy with one another.
3. The life process evolves irreversibly and unidirectionally along the space–time continuum.
4. Pattern and organization identify man and reflect his innovative wholeness.
5. Man is characterized by the capacity for abstraction and imagery, language and thought, sensation and emotion.

The qualities of the life processes as described in these assumptions include: wholeness, openness, unidirectionality, pattern and organization, and sentience and thought. The underlying principles describe man as a dynamic entity who interacts mutually and simultaneously with his environment. The changes that occur during this interaction are irreversible, nonrepeatable, and rhythmical, increasing in complexity and proceeding by the continual repatterning of man and his environment.

- With such a view of man, the goal of nursing becomes that of promoting the person's interaction with his environment in such a way that the maximum state of health that is possible is realized by the utilization of the individual's own energies and potential.

This holistic concept of human functioning serves as the basis for making predictions about nursing intervention. Data gathered for making nursing diagnoses are derived from the total pattern of events that have influenced the extent to which man is achieving his maximum health potential. These data then serve as the basis for the establishment of short-term and long-term health goals for the individual, his family, and society, and for the implementation of nursing actions directed toward the achievement of these goals. These nursing actions are aimed at helping the individual to repattern his relationship with himself and his environment so that his maximum health potential can be attained. Such a conceptual model of nursing as proposed by Rogers contributes to the pursuit of a scientific theory of nursing. Testing, retesting, and validation of the model will no doubt serve to further the science of nursing.

Self-care Model

Orem has developed a concept of nursing that places emphasis on the person's need for self-care—those activities that an individual practices for the purpose of maintaining life, health, and well-being. It is the concern of nursing to provide for and manage the person's self-care actions in an attempt to promote life and health and to assist him to recover from disease and injury or to cope with their effects. The need for nursing exists when an adult is unable to satisfactorily meet his self-care demands, or when a parent is unable to meet these demands for his child.

- Nursing is responsible for assisting the person to overcome those circumstances that interfere with self-care and that cause self-care limitations and deficits.

There are two broad categories of self-care demands: universal self-care demands and health-deviation self-care demands. *Universal self-care demands* are those that are required of all individuals in order to maintain integrated human functioning. *Health-deviation self-care demands* are those that occur as a result of disease, injury, disfigurement, or disability and that require that changes be made in the person's routine of self-care, depending upon the nature and extent of the demands. Self-care activity is deliberate action. It is goal-directed, self-initiated, and self-directed and is affected by the person's values and goals.

Orem identifies three systems of nursing activities that are designed to meet the individual's self-care requirements, according to the extent to which self-care action is disrupted: the wholly compensatory system, the partly compensatory system, and the supportive–educative system. The *wholly compensatory system* is utilized when the individual is unable to assume an active role in his care and the nurse assists him by acting for and doing for him. The *partly compensatory system* is utilized when the nurse and the individual participate in accomplishing therapeutic self-care actions. The major responsibility for the performance of these actions may be assumed by the nurse or by the individual, depending upon his physical or medically prescribed limitations, his knowledge and skills, and his psychological readiness to accomplish such activities. The *supportive–educative system* is utilized when the individual is capable of performing, or learning to perform, those measures that are necessary to accomplish his self-care demands, but for which he needs assistance in the form of support, guidance, and teaching.

Thus, as the health status of the individual changes, his needs for nursing activity may demand a change in the nursing system that is appropriate to meet his needs. Such a conceptual model of nursing can serve as a framework for guiding and directing nursing care. Currently the framework is used within various nursing education and nursing service settings. However, further validation of the concept is necessary for the continuation of nursing's pursuit of a sound theoretical base.

Adaptation Model

The adaptation model of nursing developed by Roy is a systems model that incorporates interactionist concepts. *Adaptation* is defined as the process of change, a universal phenomenon of man. Within the model, man is viewed as a biopsychosocial being who is in constant interaction with his environment—an interaction that requires man to make continual adaptations. The capacity for adaptation depends upon the stimuli to which he is exposed and the level of his adaptation. The adaptive level is determined by the effect of three classes of stimuli: focal stimuli, or those stimuli with which the person is immediately confronted; contextual stimuli, which include all other stimuli that are present; and residual stimuli, or stimuli that the person has experienced in the past, such as beliefs, attitudes, and traits. Humans have four modes of adaptation: physiologic, self-concept, role function, and interdependence relations. Thus, adaptive or positive responses to stimuli serve to maintain the total integrity of the individual.

- The role of nursing is that of promoting adaptation in all four modes during health and illness through utilization of the four components of the nursing process: assessing, planning, implementing, and evaluating.

During the assessment phase of the nursing process, the individual's position on the health–illness continuum is identified and the effectiveness of his ability to cope with the stimuli with which he is confronted is evaluated. The planning phase of the nursing process involves the establishment of goals for changing maladaptive behavior to adaptive behavior. Then, the nursing process is completed by the implementation and evaluation of a plan of nursing action directed toward promoting adaptation. The adaptation model of nursing is currently in operation in several schools of nursing and nursing service departments within hospital settings. However, it continues to require further validation as a framework for the practice of nursing.

Behavioral Systems Model

The behavioral systems model for nursing developed by Johnson describes man as a behavioral system that continually strives to maintain balance through adjustments and adaptations to his ever-changing internal and external environment. His behavior is orderly, purposeful, and predictable, and most of the time it is functionally efficient and effective. The behavioral system has seven subsystems (affiliative, dependency, ingestive, eliminative, sexual, aggressive, and achievement), each of which has a specialized task or function that promotes integrated performance of the system as a whole.

The need for nursing arises when the balance of the system is disturbed or is likely to be disturbed sufficiently to warrant external assistance. Nursing is viewed as an external regulatory force directed toward preventing disturbance in the system and preserving or restoring optimal organization and integration of the patient's behavior. The goal of nursing is to assist the patient to modify his behavioral patterns in such a way that he is able to meet the demands of the elements in his life that are not subject to modification.

During the assessment phase of the nursing process, the patient's ability to adapt to his actual or perceived threat without resultant instability is identified. In cases where instability exists or is expected, an in-depth assessment of the involved subsystems is performed. Identification and validation of dysfunctional behaviors lead to the development of nursing diagnoses. Nursing intervention is then directed toward the promotion of regularity in the patient's behavior so that balance is maintained or attained in each subsystem. The nursing process is completed when expected behavioral outcomes have been measured and the plan of care has been revised as necessary to further promote stability of the behavioral system, adjustment to the situation, and adaptation to stress.

The behavioral systems model has been used in various settings to provide direction for nursing practice, education, and research. However, the empirical and theoretical knowledge base for the model needs further development, and the model requires further testing and validation.

Comments

These are but four of the available models of nursing that can serve as frameworks for nursing practice. Educators throughout the country are utilizing these models, adapting them to meet their own individual needs, following other models of nursing, or developing new models. A curriculum based on a conceptual model provides the student and the graduate with a framework for nursing practice within which the nurse can function while providing nursing care and can be guided in furthering her nursing education experiences. It is the hope of the authors that students and graduates who utilize any of the various nursing models can appropriately incorporate into their own frameworks of nursing practice the information about health, illness, and specific disease entities included in this book. Only with an acute appreciation for the physiologic as well as the psychosocial needs of the individual who has a right to health but who experiences the threat of illness can practitioners of nursing fulfill the expectations that are centered in them by society and by the nursing profession.

▷ Nursing and the Health Care Delivery System

Health Defined

The nursing profession exists to meet the health needs of the people. Hence, as health needs change, so must health care. Unprecedented changes have occurred in the structure of our society, in life-styles, and in scientific and technological advances. These changes have altered the pattern of disease and the traditional therapeutic approaches as well as the concept of health care and the expectations that society has of the health professions. Today health is considered more than a basic human right; it has become a matter of public concern, national priority, and political action.

Our health system has traditionally been a disease-oriented system. However, the current trend is to emphasize health and its promotion. Health has been defined by the World Health Organization (WHO) as a "state of complete physical, mental, and social well being and not merely the absence of disease and infirmity."* However, such a definition of health does not allow for any variation in the degrees of wellness or of illness. The concept of a health–illness continuum (as first described by Dunn [1961]) has markedly affected the purposes of the health professions. By viewing health and illness on a graduated continuum, a person is seen as having neither complete health nor complete illness. Instead, a person's state of health is ever changing and has the potential for ranging from high-level wellness to extremely poor health with imminent death. Thus, a person is viewed as simultaneously possessing degrees of both health and illness. A person who has a chronic illness cannot meet the expectations of health as defined by the WHO definition of health. However, according to the health–illness continuum, the person with a chronic illness can attain a high level of wellness if he is successful in meeting his health potential within the limits of his chronic illness.

During the past 50 years, the health problems of the American people have changed significantly. The majority of such problems are no longer infectious and acute but instead are chronic in nature. Almost 50% of the U.S. population have one or more chronic conditions. With this change in the health status of the American people has come an increasing emphasis on health, health promotion, and self-care. Emphasis has shifted from a focus on cure to a

* Preamble of the Constitution of the World Health Organization

focus on prevention and health maintenance. The result has been the evolution of a wide range of health promotion techniques and programs, including multiphasic screening, lifetime health monitoring programs, environmental and mental health programs, accident prevention, and nutrition and health education. A growing interest in self-care is evidenced by the myriad of health and medical care publications, conferences, and workshops designed for the lay public. Organized self-care education programs emphasize health promotion, disease prevention, management of illness, self-medication, and utilization of the professional health care system. In addition, over 500,000 mutual aid groups exist for the purpose of developing and sharing self-care skills with peers who have common chronic disease or disability problems.

Special efforts are being made by health care professionals to reach and motivate members of various cultural and socioeconomic groups concerning life-style and health practices. The main thrust is to design a health care delivery system that makes comprehensive health care available to all the people at a tolerable cost. Of course, this type of health care has broad political and sociological implications as organizers, consumers, politicians, and health care providers become involved in the planning.

Concept of Promotion of Wellness and Health Maintenance

Health workers need to gain a vision of the concept of wellness, of what society could accomplish if it were freed from the burdens of illness. Each individual should be approached in terms of what his potential state of health should and could be. Inherent in this concept is the understanding that health has to be developed, maintained, and cherished by a continuum of effort. After all, it is not a static state of being; instead, it requires that energy be expended toward an ever-reaching higher potential.

It was suggested in the early 1970s (Hoffman, 1972) that "the next major advance in the health of this nation will come through health education, not through more doctors or more hospitals or new discoveries. . . . We must persuade the American people that next to genetics the single most important factor in health is life-style. That even more important than environmental pollution is personal pollution." This suggestion still holds true. Stress, improper diet, lack of exercise, smoking, drugs, accidents, and a lack of cleanliness are all related to this concept of how life-style affects health. Health workers, then, should be concerned with changing behavior in order to promote health. The goal is to motivate people so that they themselves will make improvements in the way they live; in other words, prompt them toward health behavior changes.

The Health Care Delivery System
The Changing Scene
The health care delivery system is rapidly changing as society's health needs and expectations change. A multitude of societal and legislative factors are significant motivators

of the changing patterns of health care. Changes in the population in general are affecting the need for and the delivery of health care. It is estimated that by the year 2000 there will be over 300 million people in the United States. This population expansion has in part been attributed to improved public health services and improved nutrition. Not only is the population increasing, but also the composition of the population is changing. With the decline in birth rate since the mid-1950s and the increase in life span that has resulted from improved medical care, there are fewer school-age children and more senior citizens. Likewise, the mobility of the population is changing. The advent of sophisticated transportation systems has allowed for extreme mobility. The majority of the population reside in highly congested urban areas. Along with this trend toward urbanization, there has been a steady migration of minority groups to the inner cities and a migration of middle-class persons to suburban areas. Because of such population changes, the need for health care for specific age groups and for persons within specific geographic localities is altering the effectiveness of the traditional means of providing health care and is necessitating far-reaching changes in the overall health care delivery system.

Technological advances have occurred in greater numbers during the past several decades than in all other epochs of human civilization. This is an era of sophisticated electronic machines, which have revolutionized the labor force by accomplishing many tasks that previously were accomplished by humans. This is also an era of sophisticated communication systems by which most parts of the world are connected. A variety of systems have been devised for storing, retrieving, and disseminating information. Such scientific and technological advances are themselves precipitating rapid change as well as rapid obsolescence.

Public Concern for Quality Care
The general public has become increasingly interested in and knowledgeable about health care and health maintenance. This interest and knowledge have been stimulated by television, newspapers, nonprofessional magazines, and other communications media. The public has become more health conscious and has in general begun to subscribe strongly to the belief that health and health care constitute a basic right, not a privilege for a chosen few. Members of the health care professions have become increasingly aware of the public's beliefs about health and health care. One indication of such awareness is the Patient's Bill of Rights prepared by the American Hospital Association in 1973, which is directed toward the promotion of more effective patient care and patient satisfaction (Chart 1-1).

The National League for Nursing (NLN) has also issued a statement on patients' rights, which "specifies ways in which a respect for patients' rights and a commitment to safeguarding them can be incorporated into nursing education programs and upheld and reinforced by those in nursing service. In many cases, nurses can directly involve themselves in assuring specific rights; in others, they can make their influence felt indirectly" (Chart 1-2).

Awareness of the public's beliefs and concerns about

health and health care has also been acknowledged by Congress. Comprehensive health planning legislation was enacted during the 1960s. The National Health Planning and Resources Act of 1974 emphasized the need for planning and providing quality health care for all Americans by means of coordinated health services, manpower, and facilities at the national, state, and local levels. Medically underserved populations are the target for primary care services provided for by this act. The establishment of Professional Standards Review Organizations (PSROs) was provided for in the 1972 Amendments to the Social Security Act (Public Law 92–603) in an attempt to provide for quality assurance, which assures accountability in improving the quality of health service delivery and in decreasing unnecessary health resource utilization. These amendments require that PSROs be established in local areas for the purpose of review of health services covered under the Medicare, Medicaid, and Maternal and Child Health programs. These PSROs provide an opportunity for all health care professionals to demonstrate professional accountability to the clients that they serve.

Primary Care and HMOs
Despite the societal changes that demand alterations in the health care delivery system, and despite the interest and efforts of public and private sectors of society, the health care delivery system remains fragmented. Duplication of services exists, and there is minimal coordination of the efforts of various members of the health care delivery team. The goal of comprehensive, individualized health care has not been met. However, continued efforts are being made in this regard. Significant strides have been made toward the implementation of the concept of primary health care and the establishment of health maintenance organizations (HMOs). Primary health care refers to comprehensive first-contact general health care that is designed to provide care to individuals and their families. It differs from secondary care, which is usually provided in a hospital setting or by specialists, and from tertiary care, which is designed to meet the complex needs of persons with complicated problems. Primary health care provides both physical and psychosocial services that are preventive, supportive, and restorative in nature. Care is individualized and provides an entire family the opportunity to have a long-term relationship with a small group of health care professionals and the availability of specialized support services. HMOs provide a means for the delivery of primary health care with emphasis on the adequacy of distribution and the quality of the care provided. They are prepaid group health practice systems designed to deliver comprehensive health care services to a defined group of enrolled individuals. HMOs are based on the holistic concept of care—providing ambulatory and inpatient facilities that meet the health care needs of the whole person. The goal of HMOs is to give comprehensive health care that is of the best quality and quantity for the money available while eliminating fragmentation and duplication of services.

Studies have shown that HMOs are cost-effective and that the quality of care provided by these health care delivery systems is equal to and possibly superior to the care

---

Chart 1-1
AHA's Patient's Bill of Rights

---

1. The patient has the right to considerate and respectful care.

2. The patient has the right to obtain from his physician complete current information concerning his diagnosis, treatment, and prognosis in terms the patient can be reasonably expected to understand. When it is not medically advisable to give such information to the patient, the information should be made available to an appropriate person in his behalf. He has the right to know, by name, the physician responsible for coordinating his care.

3. The patient has the right to receive from his physician information necessary to give informed consent prior to the start of any procedure and/or treatment. Except in emergencies, such information for informed consent should include but not necessarily be limited to the specific procedure and/or treatment, the medically significant risks involved, and the probable duration of incapacitation. Where medically significant alternatives for care or treatment exist, or when the patient requests information concerning medical alternatives, the patient has the right to such information. The patient also has the right to know the name of the person responsible for the procedures and/or treatment.

4. The patient has the right to refuse treatment to the extent permitted by law and to be informed of the medical consequences of his action.

5. The patient has the right to every consideration of his privacy concerning his own medical care program. Case discussion, consultation, examination, and treatment are confidential and should be conducted discreetly. Those not directly involved in his care must have the permission of the patient to be present.

6. The patient has the right to expect that all communications

and records pertaining to his care should be treated as confidential.

7. The patient has the right to expect that within its capacity a hospital must make reasonable response to the request of a patient for services. The hospital must provide evaluation, service, and/or referral as indicated by the urgency of the case. When medically permissible, a patient may be transferred to another facility only after he has received complete information and explanation concerning the needs for and alternatives to such a transfer. The institution to which the patient is to be transferred must first have accepted the patient for transfer.

8. The patient has the right to obtain information as to any relationship of his hospital to other health care and educational institutions insofar as his care is concerned. The patient has the right to obtain information as to the existence of any professional relationships among individuals, by name, who are treating him.

9. The patient has the right to be advised if the hospital proposes to engage in or perform human experimentation affecting his care or treatment. The patient has the right to refuse to participate in such research projects.

10. The patient has the right to expect reasonable continuity of care. He has the right to know in advance what appointment times and physicians are available and where. The patient has the right to expect that the hospital will provide a mechanism whereby he is informed by his physician or a delegate of the physician of the patient's continuing health care requirements following discharge.

11. The patient has the right to examine and receive an explanation of his bill regardless of source of payment.

12. The patient has the right to know what hospital rules and regulations apply to his conduct as a patient.

(Reprinted with the permission of the American Hospital Association.)

---

provided elsewhere in the same communities. However, for HMOs to become a stronger alternative to traditional health care delivery systems, they must become more numerous and widespread throughout the country.

The Future

What the future will bring for the health care delivery system is uncertain. Whether or not national health insurance will ever become a reality is questionable. If such legislation were passed, it would be aimed not only at the financing of health services, but also at the delivery, control, and evaluation of such services. The supporters of national health insurance believe that it would provide a means for furthering the concepts of health promotion, maintenance, and restoration.

▷ ## The Nurse as a Health Care Provider

Professional nursing is changing and adapting to meet changing health needs and expectations. One such adaptation can be noted in the expanded role of the nurse. The expanded roles in nursing have been a response to the need to improve the distribution of health care services and to decrease the cost of medical care. The nurse who functions in an expanded role provides direct care to patients through either independent practice, team or interdependent practice, or practice within a health care agency or with a physician. Specialization has evolved within the expanded roles of nursing, a result of the recent explosion of technology.

Chart 1-2
NLN's Statement on Patients' Rights

According to the NLN statement, nurses have a responsibility to uphold the following rights of patients:

- to health care that is accessible and that meets professional standards, regardless of the setting.
- to courteous and individualized health care that is equitable, humane and given without discrimination as to race, color, creed, sex, national origin, source of payment, or ethical or political beliefs.
- to information about their diagnosis, prognosis, and treatment—including alternatives to care and risks involved—in terms they and their families can readily understand, so that they can give their informed consent.
- to informed participation in all decisions concerning their health care.
- to information about the qualifications, names, and titles of personnel responsible for providing their health care.
- to refuse observation by those not directly involved in their care.
- to privacy during interview, examination, and treatment.

- to privacy in communicating and visiting with persons of their choice.
- to refuse treatment, medications, or participation in research and experimentation, without punitive action being taken against them.
- to coordination and continuity of health care.
- to appropriate instruction or education from health care personnel so that they can achieve an optimal level of wellness and an understanding of their basic health needs.
- to confidentiality of all records (except as otherwise provided for by law or third-party payer contracts) and all communications, written or oral, between patients and health care providers.
- to access to all health records pertaining to them, and the right to challenge and correct their records for accuracy, and the right to transfer all such records in the case of continuing care.
- to information on the charges for services, including the right to challenge these.
- to be fully informed as to all their rights in all health care settings.

(From National League for Nursing: Nursing's Role in Patients' Rights. New York, The League, 1977. Used with permission.)

Nurses now receive advanced education in such specialties as intensive care, coronary care, respiratory care, neonatal intensive care, renal dialysis care, and transplant care, to name just a few. With the expanded role of the nurse, various titles have emerged that attempt to specify the functions as well as the educational preparation of nurses. A few of these titles are clinical nurse specialist, nurse practitioner, and independent nurse practitioner.

Clinical nurse specialists are nurses prepared at the master's level who are proficient in a specialized area of nursing and who utilize this expertise to provide direct nursing care to patients and consultation services, guidance, and teaching to other nurses.

Nurse practitioners are nurses who have advanced skills in history taking and physical examination, which are utilized to assess the physical and psychosocial health and illness needs of individuals, families, or groups. These nurses have expertise in nursing practice and utilize a broad range of competencies to plan and implement direct and indirect nursing care with consideration for coordination of care with other health professionals.

Independent nurse practitioners have departed from the traditional role of the nurse within the health care delivery system and have developed private practices. The main focus of these nurses is on health maintenance through primary health care that is peripheral to the traditional illness-focused system. These nurses provide services in their offices and in clients' homes for the purpose of health assessment, counseling, teaching, and making referrals to other health professionals and agencies. The boundaries of the independent practitioner role are determined by state nurse-practice acts.

In general, then, initial care, ambulatory health care, and anticipatory guidance are all becoming increasingly important in nursing practice. These expanding roles will enable the nurse to function interdependently with other health care professionals and will help to establish more of a collegial relationship between physician and nurse.

Since nursing services are being given outside the hospital as well as within the hospital, nurses have a choice of practicing in a multiplicity of health delivery settings: acute medical centers, ambulatory care settings, clinics, outpatient departments, neighborhood health centers, independent or group nursing practices, or health maintenance organizations. The expanding scope of nursing practice will require expert skills in interviewing, in observing, in physical assessment and examination, in practicing new clinical techniques, in understanding behavioral patterns, in gathering data, and in solving problems for individuals, families, and groups. In addition, the nurse will be more concerned with decision making and evaluation of the outcomes of care. In order to acquire the necessary clinical expertise, the nurse will be responsible for self-development and continuing education during her professional lifetime.

▷ Roles of the Nurse

The professional nurse within both institutional and community health care settings assumes various roles. These may be defined as the practitioner role, the leadership role, and the research role. However, although each role carries specific responsibilities, various aspects of each role interrelate with one another and are found in all nursing positions. Accomplishment of each of these roles is designed to meet the immediate and future health care and nursing needs of the patients who are the recipients of nursing care.

Practitioner Role

The practitioner role of the nurse involves those actions that the nurse accomplishes when assuming responsibility that is primarily directed toward meeting the health care and nursing needs of individual patients, their families, and "significant others." This role is the dominant role of nurses in primary, secondary, and tertiary health care settings. It is a role that can only be achieved through utilization of the nursing process, the fundamental process of all nursing actions.

Because the nursing process serves as the basis of nursing, and because the teaching–learning process is a significant, integral part of the nursing process, Chapters 2 and 3 have been devoted to the study of these two interrelated processes. Careful study of these chapters will enable the nurse to develop expertise in the practitioner role of nursing.

Leadership Role

The leadership role of the nurse has traditionally been perceived as a specialized role assumed by only those nurses who have titles that suggest leadership and who are the leaders of large groups of nurses, related health care professionals, or patients. However, the definition of nursing leadership developed by Yura, Ozimek, and Walsh (1976) gives a broader scope to the concept and identifies leadership as a role that is inherent within all nursing positions. The leadership role of the nurse involves those actions that the nurse accomplishes when assuming responsibility for affecting the actions of others that are directed toward goal determination and achievement. Nursing leadership is a process that involves four behavioral components: deciding, relating, influencing, and facilitating. Each of these components is directed toward change and the ultimate outcome of goal achievement. Basic to the entire process is communication, the effectiveness of which determines the accomplishment of the process. Thus, the leadership process in nursing can be said to be an interpersonal process in which the nurse as a leader utilizes interpersonal relations to effect change in the behavior of those to whom she relates.

The leadership role that a nurse assumes may or may not involve a large number of people. The nurse utilizes the leadership process in a variety of circumstances: when assisting a single patient or his family to make changes in their health-related behaviors, when assisting groups or communities to alter their health practices, and when assisting groups of nurses or other health care professionals to affect the actions of patients, groups of patients, or communities with regard to the achievement of desirable health behaviors. The nurse may even be in a position to use the leadership process for assisting specific sectors of the public or the public in general to alter health-related behaviors through such means as legislation, campaigns, health-oriented public service programs, and the like. Thus, the potential scope of the leadership role of the nurse is vast.

Each nurse assumes a leadership role whether she is focusing her practice on one single patient, groups of nurses or other health care professionals, communities, or the public in general. The role is a significant one that goes hand in hand with and complements the practitioner role of the nurse.

Within an acute care hospital facility, where the nurse is involved in actuating her practitioner role for a single patient or a small group of patients, the role of the nurse as a leader may be rather subtle. She may serve primarily as the patient's advocate, anticipating and meeting the needs that he is unable to meet for himself. She must not only be acutely aware of the patient's needs but be able to communicate his needs to other health care professionals involved in his care and to coordinate the efforts of all of these persons in an effort to promote goal achievement.

Outside the hospital setting the persons served by nurses are more independent and more capable of making decisions about their health and the health behaviors they will strive to achieve. For this reason, the leadership role of the nurse in such a setting may be less subtle than in the hospital setting. The leadership skills utilized by the nurse are the same as those used within the hospital setting, but they must be adapted to the environmental variables that affect the patient population, specifically those variables that affect their health needs and how they can be met. Environmental variables such as cultural values, attitudes, resources, and the influence of community leaders are just a few of the factors that must be considered by the nurse when attempting to effect changes in the health behaviors of persons within a community.

Research Role

The research role of the nurse has traditionally been assumed only by academicians, nurse scientists, graduate nursing students, and researchers from other disciplines. It has only been recently that nurses in general have recognized the acute need for nursing research. Likewise, nurses have just begun to appreciate the significant contributions that can be made to nursing research by nurses without advanced degrees.

The primary task of nursing research is to develop nursing theories that will serve as the scientific basis for the practice of nursing. Further studies are needed to determine the actual effects of nursing intervention and nursing care. Without such research efforts the science of nursing will not grow, and a scientifically based rationale for making changes in nursing practice will not be generated.

It is the responsibility of all nurses to become involved in nursing research—to accept their research role. Nurses who have preparation in research methodology can use their research knowledge and skills to initiate and implement timely studies of nursing. This is not to say that nurses who do not initiate and implement studies of nursing do not play a significant role in nursing research. Every nurse has valuable contributions to make to nursing research and a responsibility to make these contributions. All nurses must constantly be on the alert for nursing problems and important questions about the practice of nursing, which can serve as the basis for the articulation of researchable problem areas. Those nurses directly involved in giving patient care are often in the best position to identify such problems and questions. Their clinical insights are invaluable. Nurses also have a responsibility to become actively involved in ongoing research studies. This participation may involve facilitating the data collection process or it may involve the actual collection of data. Interpreting the study to other health care professionals or to patients and their families is often of invaluable assistance to the nurse who is conducting the study.

Above all, nurses must use research findings in their nursing practice. Research for the sake of research is meaningless. Only with the utilization of research findings in clinical nursing practice will the science of nursing be furthered. Research findings can only be substantiated through utilization and validation. Nurses must be continually aware of studies that are directly related to their own area of clinical practice. The findings of these studies must then be employed in an attempt to improve patient care and to validate the findings themselves. The attitude of every health care agency and every nursing unit within such an agency should be one of interest in the progress of nursing research and one of enthusiasm in the implementation of research findings. It must also be remembered that communication of research findings is imperative. When findings of studies are not made available to other nurses, the impact of the findings on nursing practice is diminished.

Thus, research is an inherent part of nursing. The future of nursing science depends upon the active involvement of nurses in the implementation and utilization of nursing research. Nurses must cultivate their curiosity about nursing practice and their belief in the worth of the practice of nursing by accepting their research role and responsibility. Only with the questioning mind of nurses can nursing research be generated. The scientific basis of nursing depends upon the research efforts of all nurses, practitioners and researchers alike.

▷ The Patient/Client: Consumer and Recipient of Health Care

The term "patient," which is derived from the Latin verb meaning *to suffer,* has traditionally been used to describe those persons who are recipients of nursing care. The connotation commonly attached to the word is one of dependence. For this reason many nurses prefer to use the term "client," which is derived from the Latin verb meaning *to lean* and which connotes alliance and interdependence. For the purposes of this book the term "patient" will be utilized throughout, but with appreciation for each nurse's prerogative to choose the term that seems more suitable.

The Patient's Problems

The central figure in health care services is, of course, the patient. Although the patient reports to the hospital or health facility with a health problem or problems (increasing numbers of patients have multiple disease disorders), he also comes as an individual, a member of a family, and a citizen of the community. Undoubtedly, he is laden with a number of personal concerns that have been amplified and compounded by the alteration in his health status. Confronting him, perhaps, are problems that he feels are inescapable and insurmountable; problems that demand a solution but are incapable of solution; problems for which he feels solely responsible and that he is reluctant to share. He may be wholly absorbed in problems that are of minor consequence while dismissing others that truly are of paramount importance. One of the nurse's important functions is to help him to sort out his problems, reduce them to their essentials, place them in proper perspective, and cope with them effectively.

Troublesome Symptoms as Problems

From the standpoint of the symptomatic patient, the most important problem confronting him is his major symptom. If he is gasping for breath, his most pressing need is to be relieved of his respiratory distress. Dyspnea is his primary problem. To evaluate this symptom and to alleviate it effectively, the nurse must understand correctly the pathologic physiology underlying the patient's dyspnea. Is it caused by pulmonary congestion? by pneumonia? by pleurisy? or by asthma? Does the patient have respiratory obstruction? Should he be placed in an orthopneic position? or in low Fowler's position? or should he lie flat? Should he be receiving oxygen? Is he is need of tracheal suction? Is endotracheal intubation likely to be required? Should a sedative be administered, or is such medication strictly contraindicated in this patient? Close scrutiny of the patient might convince the nurse that his breathing, although abnormally rapid and deep, is not attended by discomfort and does not involve undue effort. In other words, this particular patient may not be dyspneic but may be hyperpneic. Hyperpnea is a different symptom altogether, and the problems it entails are quite different from those of dyspnea. Is this a case of hysterical hyperventilation? or diabetic acidosis? Or has this patient been poisoned? On the appropriate answers to these and a host of other pertinent questions may hinge the correctness of diagnosis, the effectiveness of nursing intervention, and, in many instances, the very survival of the patient.

Every step in the care of the patient represents a team effort, and a key member of the health team charged with this responsibility is the professional nurse. Among the most important of her contributions to this joint effort are her clinical observations. To what extent these observations are

Table 1-1
Death Rates for 15 Leading Causes of Death: United States, 1981

Rank*	Cause of Death (Ninth Revision International Classification of Diseases, 1975)	Death Rate	Percent of Total Deaths
—	All causes	866.4	100.0
1	Diseases of heart	330.6	38.2
2	Malignant neoplasms, including neoplasms of lymphatic and hematopoietic tissues	184.3	21.3
3	Cerebrovascular diseases	71.7	8.3
4	Accidents and adverse effects	44.5	5.1
—	Motor vehicle accidents	22.8	2.6
—	All other accidents and adverse effects	21.7	2.5
5	Chronic obstructive pulmonary diseases and allied conditions	26.1	3.0
6	Pneumonia and influenza	23.7	2.7
7	Diabetes mellitus	15.2	1.7
8	Chronic liver disease and cirrhosis	12.9	1.5
9	Atherosclerosis	12.5	1.4
10	Suicide	12.3	1.4
11	Homicide and legal intervention	10.7	1.2
12	Certain conditions originating in the perinatal period	9.2	1.1
13	Nephritis, nephrotic syndrome, and nephrosis	7.6	0.9
14	Congenital anomalies	5.8	0.7
15	Septicemia	4.4	0.5
—	All other causes	94.9	10.9

* Based on a 10-percent sample of deaths. Rates per 100,000 population.
(From Annual summary of births, deaths, marriages, and divorces: United States, 1981. Monthly Vital Statistics Report, National Center for Health Statistics, 1982.)

significant, informative, and helpful depends on how well the nurse knows and understands symptoms. Confronted with a symptom, the nurse must be able to recognize it as a deviation from the normal. She should also be aware of the patterns of illness in the community and the characteristics of the population being served. Table 1-1 specifies the leading causes of death in the U.S. and hence indicates the most common clinical problems that will be encountered in nursing practice.

The Patient's Basic Needs

Certain basic needs are common to all human beings and demand satisfaction accordingly. Such needs are dealt with on the basis of priority, meaning that certain needs are more pressing than others. However, once an essential need is met, a person moves to a need on a higher level. Approaching needs according to priority reflects Maslow's hierarchy of needs, in which human needs may be ranked as follows: physiologic needs; safety and security; belongingness and affection; esteem and self-respect; and self-actualization, which includes self-fulfillment, desire to know and understand, and aesthetic needs.* Lower-level needs always remain, but because there is a reduction in need tension, the person is able to move to higher-level needs. A person's

* Maslow AH. Motivation and Personality, New York, Harper, 1954.

pursuit of higher-level needs indicates that he is moving toward psychological health and well-being.

Physiologic Needs

These needs predominate in the motivation of human behavior and drive the mechanisms that maintain *homeostasis*—the constancy of the internal environment of an organism (see Chap. 7). They involve the regulation of respiratory, nutritive, and excretory functions, as well as maintenance of the water content of tissues, adjustments of body temperature, and the operation of numerous protective mechanisms. Also included as physiologic needs are the need for rest and sleep, and the avoidance of pain. Sex is considered a basic motive, but not essential for survival.

These physiologic needs are powerful; unless satisfied, they dominate the conscious mind. For example, if a patient is obliged to restrict his fluid intake for therapeutic reasons, thirst will absorb his thoughts. He may discuss nothing but drinking, complain incessantly of thirst, and repeatedly question his nurse and physician as to when fluids will be forthcoming. During this period he is not likely to be too concerned about the aesthetic features of his environment. As soon as his thirst is quenched, he becomes aware of other needs; now he may be disturbed by the absence of privacy.

Safety Needs and Security Needs

If the physiologic needs are satisfied, the concern for safety and security emerges—psychological as well as physical safety. The normal adult is able to protect himself and usually does not feel endangered. He is relatively "safe" from death. His job is "safe." His insurance program and his savings account furnish a sense of economic security.

Illness naturally poses a threat. The sick person may be apprehensive in response to the many different persons with unfamiliar functions who enter his room. Diagnostic tests and therapeutic procedures may contribute to his fears. He wants to feel safe and secure. Although he may not express his feelings in these terms, he wants the health team to be aware of his insecurity. To help protect the patient from danger the nurse must know the nature of his illness and be cognizant of any possible complications. If complications should occur, she should be able to provide intelligent care. The nurse's role in promoting the psychological safety of the patient is discussed in Chapter 12.

Need for Belongingness and Affection

Once the patient's physiologic and safety needs have been satisfied, his need for belongingness and affection will become apparent. Every person, sick or well, desires the companionship and recognition of others. A sick person wants and needs his family or, in their absence, friends. Thus, any signs of friendliness are usually appreciated. The wise nurse is constantly aware of this need and of its importance in relation to the patient's morale. One way to achieve this end is to help the family members to feel that they have a definite contribution to make to the patient's recovery. Assessment and interpretation of the patient's behavior are essential for identification of indicators of his unmet need for belongingness and affection. He may be quiet, uncomplaining, and eager to please. Or, he may demand attention by constantly making requests, asking questions, and being generally disruptive. By accurately interpreting such behaviors, the nurse can intervene in ways that will promote the patient's feeling of acceptance and belonging. Mutual goal setting is important in assuring the patient and his family that they are important members of the health team.

Need for Esteem and Self-respect

Man is by nature a social being, abhorring isolation. Illness removes him from his relatively convivial world and transplants him into a strange environment, an environment that is entirely unsought and unfamiliar, one in which he feels incompetent and alone. Previously an actively contributing member of society, he now must accept a position of dependency. This patient needs to preserve his self-esteem. He needs to be recognized as an individual, a distinct personality. The professional nurse, imbued with the concept of the individual worth and the dignity of man, sees to it that this need is fulfilled. She takes time to listen to the patient. To the extent that he desires it and opportunity permits, she joins him in conversation. She exhibits interest in all matters that seem important to him—her attentiveness, thoughtfulness, and kindliness conveying the conviction that he is held in esteem and that his needs and problems are recognized.

Unmet esteem and self-respect needs are exhibited by feelings of dependency and lack of confidence, competence, and ability. Patient education that focuses on the patient's acquisition of skills and knowledge is helpful in increasing the patient's self-esteem and self-respect.

Need for Self-actualization

Maslow estimated that only about 1% of the adult population ever reach the level of self-actualization. Self-actualization may not be possible for persons in poverty-stricken or emotionally deprived environments. Additionally, many people are satisfied with meeting lower-level needs and do not strive for self-actualization.

Need for Self-fulfillment. Once the patient's physiologic needs have been compensated and he is feeling secure, esteemed, and wanted, his creative impulses may now emerge. During the course of a short hospital stay this need is not likely to be frustrated. However, the patient with a long-term illness must be assured an opportunity to express himself creatively and to feel useful.

Need to Know and Understand. This need is a strong drive. The intelligent person seeks information, organizes it, analyzes it, and searches for its meaning. In general, patients want to know what is in store for them, and they are thwarted by explanations that are too brief or vague. Many patients know a surprising amount about the bodily functions. However, while some of their information may be factual, some of it is likely to be erroneous, and correction or clarification is usually necessary. Their instruction is the responsibility of the nurse, and the teaching of patients is one of the most responsible functions of her profession. To teach correctly and effectively the nurse must have a thorough knowledge of the subject, be skilled in communication, and be cognizant of the basic mechanisms of learning. The explanations, while simple for the sake of comprehension, at the same time must be meaningful if they are to be accepted. The patient's physical and emotional status, his intelligence, his experience as a patient, and his awareness of the situation, as well as the urgency of his need to know and understand must be given consideration. The nurse must also consider the possible implications of her intended remarks and guard with equal care against inaccuracies on her part and misunderstandings on the part of the patient.

Aesthetic Needs. These needs vary in importance from individual to individual, but for all patients the most salutary environment is one that is orderly and one in which there is beauty. The patient with highly developed aesthetic sensibilities will be distressed by unpleasant sights, sounds, odors, and disarray. He may crave flowers, books, or music—amenities that, when supplied, add immeasurably to his well-being.

Comments

In concluding this discussion, it may be pointed out that most of the needs of the average individual, ill or well, can be satisfied only in part. Moreover, the nurse, whose responsibility and privilege it is to help the patient meet his needs and resolve his problems, must recognize the fact that some problems can be neither eliminated nor solved. In relation to the patient with such a problem, the nurse's role is to help him to make a mature, objective, and compensatory adjustment to its continued existence or to its imperfect solution, if this solution is the best that can be achieved.

▷ Approach to the Patient

As nursing searches for ways of fulfilling patient needs, it has devised various methods of approaching the patient. During the 1950s and 1960s the concept of team nursing came to the fore. In recent years, however, questions have been raised concerning the effectiveness of team nursing, and a different approach in the form of primary nursing has been advocated and implemented in many hospital settings. Some studies have shown that primary nursing, when compared to team nursing, significantly increases the quality of patient care and is more cost-effective. However, more research is needed to substantiate these findings.

Primary Nursing

Primary nursing, not to be confused with primary health care, which deals with first-contact general health care, refers to comprehensive care that is provided with continuity. Individualized total care is provided to the patient by the same nurse from the time of the patient's admission until his discharge. This type of nursing care eliminates the fragmented care that has typified team nursing and serves to accomplish a goal for which nurses have recognized a need for years: it allows the nurse to once again give direct patient care rather than manage and supervise the functions of others who care for the patient. In essence, it allows the nurse the opportunity to implement her practitioner role and her leadership role within the framework of rendering direct patient care.

The focus of primary nursing is the patient. The primary nurse accepts total responsibility for quality nursing care for the patient. This nursing care is directed toward meeting his total, individualized nursing needs—his biopsychosocial needs. The primary nurse is responsible and accountable for involving the patient and his family directly in all facets of his care. The primary nurse has autonomy that allows her to make decisions with the patient and his family concerning his care. Thus, the primary nurse is a facilitator of family-centered as well as patient-centered nursing care. All communications with other members of the health team regarding the patient and his health care are made by the primary nurse. This allows the nurse to provide for continuity of care and to promote collaborative efforts directed toward the assurance of quality care. It provides the other health care professionals with the opportunity to communicate directly with the nurse who is responsible for the patient's care.

Ideally, the number of patients for whom the nurse is the primary nurse is limited to three or four. However, this number may range from one to ten depending on the extent of the nursing needs of the patients. The nurse meets the patient as soon as possible after his admission to the health care facility. This allows her to begin to establish a relationship with the patient, which will continue until discharge and, in some cases, after discharge. It allows the patient to identify with the nurse who will be responsible for his care on a continuous basis. Each day that the primary nurse works she cares for the patient. She is aware of problems and needs as they arise, and she assumes the responsibility for securing the means to solve the problems and to meet the needs. Prior to the patient's discharge to another health care facility or to his home, the primary nurse assumes the responsibility for making the appropriate referrals and for assuring that all relevant information is provided to those persons who will be involved in his care. Throughout the entire admission the nurse continually strives to involve the patient's family in his care and in the preparations that are made for his discharge.

During the times when the primary nurse is not scheduled to work, she is assisted by an associate nurse, or co-nurse. This associate nurse implements the nursing care plan and provides feedback to the primary nurse that is invaluable in evaluation of the care plan. However, it remains the responsibility of the primary nurse to make sure that the patient's needs are met and that continuity of care is not lost when she is not present to render the care herself.

Within the concept of primary nursing, the head nurse (or patient care supervisor) functions as a consultant for the primary nurses, and she strives toward providing opportunities for these nurses to continually improve their clinical expertise. The head nurse initiates the nurse–patient relationship by assigning the primary nurse to her designated patients. This is done with knowledge of the primary nurse's capabilities and her particular areas of nursing expertise. The head nurse then serves as a resource person for the primary nurse when she is confronted with patient problems or needs that she is unable to resolve. Periodic evaluation of the primary nurse's performance is the responsibility of the head nurse. Frequent interaction with the primary nurse and her patients gives the head nurse much information that can be used positively in assisting the primary nurse to utilize her capabilities to their utmost and to make strides toward overcoming her limitations. The head nurse also functions as a primary nurse for a small group of patients. By assuming such responsibility, she is allowed to utilize her clinical expertise in giving direct patient care and to serve as a role model for her primary nurses.

Practical nurses, nursing assistants, and nursing students assist within the primary nursing framework. The responsibility for maintaining continuity of total individualized nursing care remains with the primary nurse. However, when direct patient care is not given by the primary nurse, other members of the health team assume this responsibility. They implement the plan of care developed by the primary nurse and consult with the primary nurse when changes in the plan of care seem warranted. In such instances the primary nurse serves as a valuable consultant and teacher for associate nurses and other personnel. Nursing care conferences provide a means for the exchange of information. In these conferences the quality of care rendered to the patient is the focus, and continuity of individualized total patient care is the goal.

Primary nursing has been designed to increase the accountability and responsibility of the nurse to the patient.

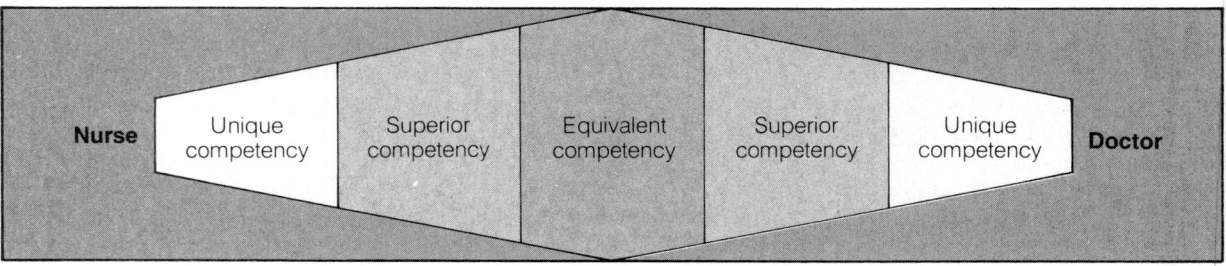

Figure 1-1. Task-oriented relationships between doctors and nurses in the care of patients in terms of the relative competencies of each. The area of equivalent competency applies to tasks for which either a doctor or nurse would be qualified. Superior competency implies that both doctor and nurse have a measure of competency to perform a particular task or exercise a particular judgment, but that education and experience renders one superior to the other. Unique competency refers to activities that only members of one discipline or subdiscipline are qualified to carry out. In any particular situation, the health professional most qualified available at that moment is the one to assume responsibility. For the same problem, under certain circumstances, this may prove to be a nurse, under different circumstances, a physician, depending on individual qualifications and availability. (Redrawn from Engel GL: The biopsychosocial model and the education of health professions. Ann NY Acad Sci, vol 310, 1978.)

Studies conducted at selected hospitals that have implemented primary nursing reveal that primary nurses recognize greater enrichment from their jobs because of the high degree of autonomy, identity, significance, and variety afforded them by the primary nursing system of delivering care.

▷ Summary

Throughout this chapter, the evolution of the profession of nursing has been explored. Many references have been made to the significance of nurses as members of the health team. Over the years nurses have striven to change their role from one of subservience to other members of the health team, particularly the physician, to one that is collegial. As nursing practitioners and researchers make advances in the area of concept formalization and theory building, the unique competencies of the profession of nursing become more clearly articulated. It becomes increasingly more evident that nursing provides certain health care services that are unique to this profession. However, nursing continues to recognize the importance of collaboration with other health care disciplines in meeting all of the health care needs of patients. The diagram prepared by Engel (Fig. 1-1) that depicts the task-oriented relationships between nurses and physicians in terms of equivalent, superior, and unique competencies suggests that nursing is realizing its goal of attaining a collegial relationship with physicians.

▷ Bibliography

Books

Aiken LH. Nursing in the 1980s. Crises, Opportunities, Challenges. Philadelphia, JB Lippincott, 1982.

DeYoung L. Dynamics of Nursing. St Louis, CV Mosby, 1981.

Dunn HL. High-Level Wellness. Arlington, Virginia, RW Beatty, 1961.

Hegyvary ST. The Change to Primary Nursing. A Cross-cultural View of Professional Nursing Practice. St Louis, CV Mosby, 1981.

Henderson V. The Nature of Nursing. New York, Macmillan, 1966.

Johnson DE. The behavioral system model in nursing. In Riehl JP and Roy C. Conceptual Models for Nursing Practice. New York, Appleton–Century–Crofts, 1980.

King IM. A Theory for Nursing. Systems, Concepts, Process. New York, John Wiley & Sons, 1981.

Maslow AH. Motivation and Personality. New York, Harper & Brothers, 1970.

Nightingale F. Notes on Nursing: What It Is, and What It Is Not. New York, D Appleton, 1860.

Nursing. A Social Policy Statement. Kansas City, Missouri, American Nurses' Association, 1980.

The Nursing Theories Conference Group. Nursing Theories. The Base for Professional Nursing Practice. Englewood Cliffs, New Jersey, Prentice–Hall, 1980.

Orem DE. Nursing: Concepts of Practice. New York, McGraw–Hill, 1971.

Riehl JP and Roy C. Conceptual Models for Nursing Practice. New York, Appleton–Century–Crofts, 1980.

Rogers ME. An Introduction to the Theoretical Basis of Nursing. Philadelphia, FA Davis, 1970.

Yura H, Ozimek D, and Walsh MB. Nursing Leadership: Theory and Process. New York, Appleton–Century–Crofts, 1976.

Articles
Theories and Concepts of Nursing

Anna DJ et al. Implementing Orem's conceptual framework. J Nurs Adm 1978 Nov; 8(11):8–11.

Bromley B. Applying Orem's self-care theory in enterostomal therapy. Am J Nurs 1980 Feb; 80(2):245–249.

Craig SL. Theory development and its relevance for nursing. J Adv Nurs 1980 July; 5(4):349–355.

Crawford G, Dufault K, and Rudy E. Evolving issues in theory development. Nurs Outlook 1979 May; 27(5):346–351.

Fawcett J. A framework for analysis and evaluation of conceptual models of nursing. Nurse Educ 1980 Nov/Dec; 5(6):10–14.

Feldman HR. Nursing research in the 1980s: Issues and implications. Adv Nurs Sci 1978 Oct; 1(1):85–92.

Flaskerud JH and Halloran EJ. Areas of agreement in nursing theory development. Adv Nurs Sci 1980 Oct; 3(1):1–10.

Leininger M. Caring: A central focus of nursing and health care services. Nurs Health Care 1980 Oct; 1(3):135–144.

Mastal MF, Hammond H, and Roverts MP. Theory into hospital practice: A pilot implementation. J Nurs Adm 1982 June; 12(6):9–15.

McFarlane EA. Nursing theory: The comparison of four theoretical proposals. J Adv Nurs 1980 Jan; 5(1):3–19.

Rawls AC. Evaluation of the Johnson behavioral model in clinical practice. Image 1980 Feb; 12(1):13–16.

Smith FT. Florence Nightingale: Early feminist. Am J Nurs 1981 May; 81(5):1020–1024.

Weatherston L. Theory of nursing: Creating effective care. J Adv Nurs 1979 May; 4(3):365–375.

Whelton BJ. An operationalization of Martha Rogers' theory throughout the nursing process. Int J Nurs Stud 1979; 16(1):1–10.

Roles of Nurses

Blount M et al. Extending the influence of the clinical nurse specialist. Nurs Admin Q 1981 Fall; 6(1):53–63.

Choi MW. Nurses as co-providers of primary health care. Nurs Outlook 1981 Sept; 29(9):519–521.

Henderson VV. Implementing the clinical nurse specialist role. Nurs Manage 1981 Nov; 12(11):55–58.

Kendrick VM. Nurse practitioner in a VNA. Am J Nurs 1981 July; 81(7):1360–1362.

Little M. Nurse practitioner/physician relationships. Am J Nurs 1980 Sept; 80(9):1642–1645.

Manley MV. Clinical privileges for nonhospital-based nurses. Am J Nurs 1981 Oct; 81(10):1822–1825.

Mentick JL, Trolinger J, and O'Hara–Devereaux M. Nurse practitioners in primary care. Fam Community Health 1980 Aug; 3(2):35–48.

Murphy JF and Schmitz M. The clinical nurse specialist: Implementing the role in a hospital setting. J Nurs Adm 1979 Jan; 9(1):29–31.

Niessner P. The clinical specialist's contribution to quality nursing care. Nurs Leadership 1979 Mar; 2(1):21–30.

Steel JE. Putting joint practice into practice. Am J Nurs 1981 May; 81(5):964–967.

Weiland AP. Clinical nurse specialist: The task behind the title. Virginia Nurse 1979 Spring; 47(1):45–47.

Primary Nursing

Betz M, Dickerson T, and Wyatt D. Cost and quality: Primary and team nursing compared. Nurs Health Care 1980 Oct; 1(3):150–157.

Ciske KL. Accountability—the essence of primary nursing. Am J Nurs 1979 May; 79(5):890–894.

Clifford JC. Primary nursing: A contemporary model for delivery of care. Am J Hosp Pharm 1980 Aug; 37(8):1089–1091.

Flynn KT. Modes of delivery of patient care: Primary or team nursing. Hosp Top 1979 Nov/Dec; 57(6):34–40.

Joiner C, Johnson V, and Corkrean M. Is primary nursing the answer? Nurs Admin Q 1981 Spring; 5(3):69–76.

Leininger M. Changing foci in American nursing education: Primary and transcultural nursing care. J Adv Nurs 1978 Mar; 3(2):155–166.

Nodolny MD. Primary nursing care. Hosp Top 1979 July/Aug; 57(4):10–14.

Previte VJ. Continuing care in a primary nursing setting: Role of a clinical specialist. Int Nurs Rev 1979 Mar/Apr; 26(2):53–56.

vanServellen GM. Primary nursing: Variations in practice. J Nurs Adm 1981 Sept; 11(9):40–46.

Walborn KA. A nursing model for the hospice: Primary and self-care nursing. Nurs Clin North Am 1980 Mar; 15(1):205–217.

Wobbe RR. Primary versus team nursing. Superv Nurse 1978 Mar; 9(3):34–37.

Health, Health Belief Model, Health Promotion

Becker MH. The health belief model and sick role behavior. Health Ed Monographs 1974 Winter; 2:409–419.

Becker MH, Drachman RH, and Kirscht JP. A new approach to explaining sick-role behavior in low-income populations. Am J Public Health 1974 Mar; 64(3):205–216.

Chamblee RF and Evans MC. New dimensions in cause of death statistics. Am J Pub Health 1982 Nov; 72(11):1265–1270.

Curtin LL. Is there a right to health care? Am J Nurs 1980 Mar; 80(3):462–465.

Dwore RB and Kreuter MW. Update: Reinforcing the case for health promotion. Fam Community Health 1980 Feb; 2(3):103–119.

Hoffman CA. The house of medicine. JAMA 1972 July 31; 221(5):483–485.

McIntyre MK. Consumers learn to monitor their own health. Top Clin Nurs 1980 July; 2(2):34–44.

Mitchell FH and Mitchell CC. Entering the 1980s: The health care system and primary care. Fam Community Health 1980 Aug; 3(2):105–113.

Nixon JE. The right to health care: Reflections and implications for nursing administration. Nurs Admin Q 1982 Summer; 6(4):1–7.

Health Maintenance Organizations

Foley ME. Health maintenance organizations. Imprint 1980 Feb; 27(1):33, 61.

Haendel AR, Sinclair LC, and D'Erasmo MJ. Health maintenance organizations. Nurse Pract 1978 Nov/Dec; 3(6):24–41.

Saward EW and Fleming S. Health maintenance organizations. Sci Am 1980 Oct; 243(10):47–53.

2

The Nursing Process

The nursing process has been accepted as the essence of nursing. It is a deliberate, problem-solving approach to meeting the health care and nursing needs of patients. Although the steps of the nursing process have been delineated in various ways by many nursing leaders, the commonalities found in all definitions are: assessment, planning, implementation, and evaluation. These fundamental components can be used to define the nursing process as follows:

1. Systematic assessment of the patient's problems for the purpose of establishing nursing diagnoses
2. Development of a plan of care to solve the problems
3. Implementation of the plan of care or supervision of the implementation of the plan of care by others
4. Evaluation of the effectiveness of the plan of care in resolving the assessed problems

• Thus, the nursing process is a data-collecting, decision-making process that incorporates evaluation and subsequent modification as feedback mechanisms that promote the ultimate resolution of the patient's nursing problems.

Division of the nursing process into four distinct components or steps serves to emphasize the critical nursing actions that must be accomplished when the nurse assumes responsibility for resolving the patient's nursing problems. However, the nurse must remember that the process as a whole is cyclic, the steps being interrelated, interdependent, and recurrent (Fig. 2-1).

▷ Assessment

The assessment component of the nursing process begins with the nurse's first encounter with the patient. It involves the systematic collection of data about the patient's actual and potential health needs and the utilization of these data to formulate nursing diagnoses.

- The nursing diagnoses then become the basis for the nursing care plan.

Sensitive and continuous nursing assessment is essential in order to maintain an awareness of the patient's needs and the effectiveness of the nursing care that he receives.

History Taking

Assessment of the patient's actual and potential health needs is accomplished by means of the nursing history and the physical examination of the patient. The nursing history is carried out for the purpose of determining the patient's state of wellness or illness and is best accomplished as part of a planned interview.

The interview is a dialogue between the patient and the nurse and is a very personal experience. Interviewing is an art that requires wisdom, judgment, tact, and experience. It involves the sensitive direction of a conversation with a patient in order to obtain information about him. The nurse's approach to the patient will largely determine the amount and quality of information that is received. Achieving a relationship of mutual trust and respect requires the ability to communicate a sincere interest in the patient. The patient should be made as comfortable as possible and afforded privacy for the interview.

The principles involved in interviewing a patient are:

1. Listening and questioning
2. Observing and interpreting
3. Synthesizing
4. Incorporating what is learned into a plan of care

To learn about a patient, one must talk little and listen a lot. Listen to the patient with "hearing ears." What is he saying? Because an ill person is so suggestible, do not put words in his mouth. Let him tell his story in his own way. Although many topics may be brought up, look for the main area of concern. Give the patient time, without interruptions, to tell why he is seeking help. Be attentive not only to his verbal expression but also to his nonverbal behavior, which may be exhibited in such subtle forms as gestures, posture, and facial expressions. Anxiety is present in almost every patient; it may be well concealed, but it is there. Anticipate the patient's anxieties and try to relieve them during the interview. All inquiries should be relevant. The patient has the right to expect something from each interview. He should especially be made to feel that he is being understood.

The use of a nursing history guide may help the nurse to obtain pertinent information and to facilitate the course of the interview. A variety of nursing history guides have

Nursing Process

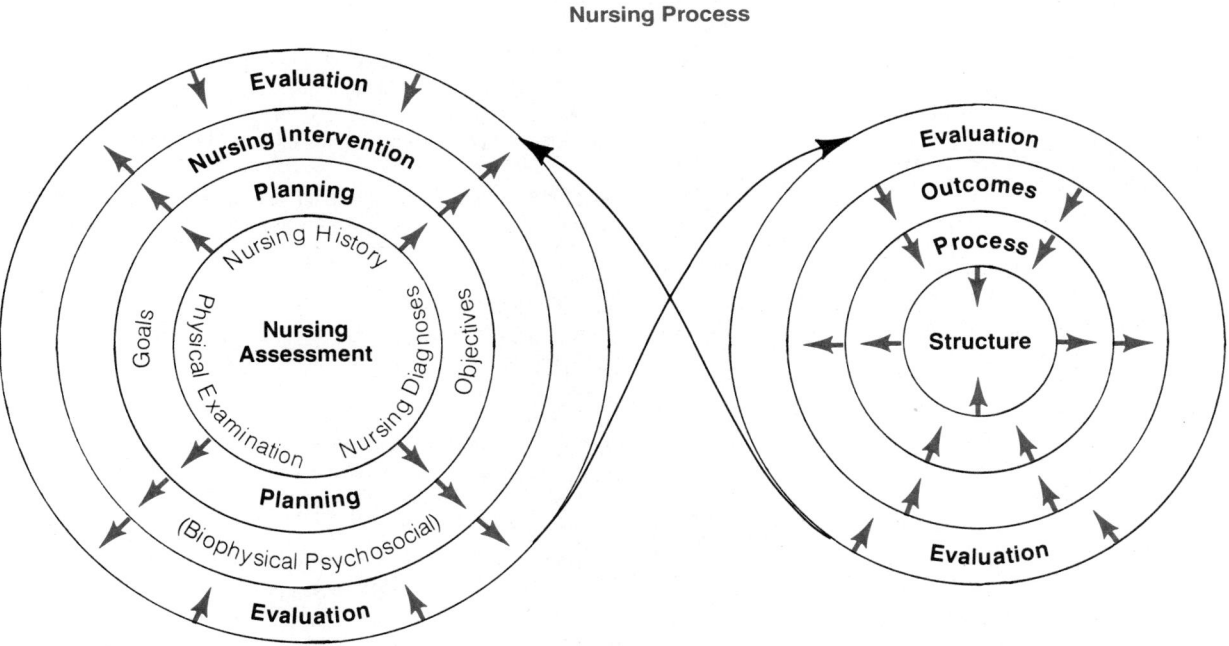

Figure 2-1. The nursing process is depicted schematically in the circle on the left. Starting from the innermost circle, nursing assessment, the process moves outward through the taking of the nursing history, the making of nursing diagnoses, planning, the setting of goals and objectives, and actual nursing intervention, and arrives at the ongoing process of evaluation. To show the consistent role of evaluation, the right circle indicates a gearlike activity: (1) structure—the organizational pattern within which the nursing process takes place and which involves personnel, environment, and facilities; (2) process—the providing of care, including the interaction that takes place between the patient recipient and the care provider; and (3) the final outcome—the condition of the patient/client following this process.

been developed by individual nurses and committees of nurses. Many health care agencies have developed guides that are specifically directed toward obtaining the information that is most essential for their particular patients. Guides that are standard for a particular health care agency tend to reflect the agency's specific philosophy and concept of man, nursing, and health. These nursing history guides are just that—guides. They are designed to guide the interview but must be adapted to the individual responses, problems, and needs of the patient. As the nurse gains expertise in conducting a nursing history, she should strive toward developing her own format, one that allows for adaptability and flexibility while still obtaining the essential information. This essential information must reflect an assessment of the total patient with regard to his basic human needs and his state of wellness or illness. A variety of models can serve as the framework for the assessment of basic needs. Maslow's hierarchy of needs and Erikson's eight ages of man are two examples of frameworks that provide bases for the assessment of the total needs of the client—his physical, psychological, emotional, intellectual, developmental, social, cultural, and spiritual needs. The questions in Chart 2-1 are offered as guidelines for interviewing, but the questions actually asked are determined by the reaction of the individual patient.

In some instances it may be appropriate for the patient to fill out the nursing history form. If this technique of history taking is utilized, it remains the responsibility of the nurse to verify and clarify the information provided by the patient and to seek any additional information that is necessary to identify the patient's nursing needs. Throughout the interview the nurse has the opportunity to interact with the patient not only for the purpose of data collection but also for the purpose of conveying interest, support, and understanding to the patient. For a more detailed discussion of the concepts and techniques of clinical interviewing, see Chapter 4.

The Physical Examination

The physical examination of the patient may be carried out prior to, during, or following the nursing history, depending upon the patient's physical and emotional state, his response to his illness and hospitalization, and the immediate priorities of his illness situation. The purpose of the physical examination is to identify those parameters of physical functioning that indicate that a nursing need exists. The ex-

---

Chart 2-1
Suggestions for Interviewing Patients

Guiding Principle: At the beginning of the interview, focus on what is most troublesome to the patient: What are his symptoms or complaints? Why is he seeking help now?

What brought you to the hospital?
What is causing you the most discomfort?
When did the symptoms appear?
Describe your life situation at the time of the onset of your illness.
Do you believe you are getting better or worse? (the directional trend: improvement or deterioration)
What do you think made you sick?
What do you do for yourself at home when you are sick?
How has this illness affected your way of life? For how long?
What factors aggravate or help your condition?
Are you taking any medications?
Do you have any allergies? (food, drugs)
Do you have any elimination (bowel or urinary) problems?
What is your greatest concern?
Are you being informed about tests and treatment?

Guiding Principle: Learn about the patient's background and experience in order to determine his needs.*

Where is your home?
Do you have a family?
What family member do you usually turn to for help?

What type of work do you do? or, if someone else is the provider, what type of work does he do?
Has your illness interfered with your work?
What activities, hobbies, and forms of recreation do you enjoy?

Guiding Principle: Ascertain what can be done to support the patient and help him make the best use of his resources. What are his defects? strengths? limitations?

What are your food preferences? dislikes?
What are your sleeping habits?
  Regular retiring time?
    Do you like a night light?
    How many pillows do you use?
What are your elimination habits (bowel and urinary)?
Do you have any limitations of seeing? hearing? walking?
What personal preferences do you have?
  Sleep late?
  Ice water or tap water to drink?
Would it be helpful to have a family member or friend stay with you?
What annoys you most about being in the hospital?
What do you miss the most in the hospital?
How long do you think you will stay?
What could the nursing staff do that would be most helpful to you?

* Social, cultural, developmental, and educational levels, and the patient's readiness to learn can be assessed throughout the interview. Clues to the patient's financial status are obtained from his belongings, room, data on the chart, etc.

amination is designed to determine the patient's physical alterations and limitations and also to determine his assets, which may serve to complement his limitations.

- To accomplish the purposes of the physical examination, the nurse must be skilled in the techniques of inspection, palpation, percussion, and auscultation; she must also have a sound basic knowledge of anatomy and physiology and of the symptomatology of the disease process with which the patient presents.

Because the physical examination is such an important part of the assessment component of the nursing process and because it involves specific technical skills that must be learned and continuously refined, Chapter 5 is devoted to the study of the physical examination. This chapter requires careful study, for the nurse must learn to observe with "seeing" eyes, hear with "hearing" ears, feel with "feeling" hands, and interpret the findings of the examination. Significant observations that should be made with each clinical condition appear in the appropriate chapter in which the specific condition is discussed.

Other Components of the Data Base

Following the nursing history and the physical examination, the nurse seeks additional relevant information from the patient's family or significant others, from other members of the health team, and from the patient's health record or chart. Depending upon the patient's immediate illness needs, this information may have been obtained prior to the nursing history and the physical examination. Whatever the sequence of events, the nurse utilizes all available sources of pertinent data to complete the nursing assessment. It is paramount that she study the patient's health record to determine the problem that caused the patient to seek help.

A tentative medical diagnosis has usually been formulated by the physician upon the patient's admission to the hospital. It is absolutely essential to understand the pathophysiological processes underlying this diagnosis. "Therapeutic conversation" is no substitute for knowing the effects of altered physiology, rationale of treatment, and potential complications. This knowledge helps the nurse to anticipate problems that may evolve, to formulate a nursing approach to their solution, and to participate with other members of the health team in providing coordinated health care.

Nursing Diagnosis

The assessment component of the nursing process is concluded with the formulation of the nursing diagnoses. As soon as possible after the completion of the nursing history and the physical examination, the nurse organizes, analyzes, synthesizes, and summarizes the data collected and determines the patient's need for nursing care.

- Those actual or potential health problems that are amenable to resolution by nursing actions are identified as nursing diagnoses.

Nursing, unlike medicine, does not yet have a standard taxonomy of diagnostic labels that convey the same meaning to all nurses. Until recent years, nursing literature has contained little substantive work on the classification of nursing diagnoses. The 1970s brought a surge of professional activity aimed at making nursing diagnosis a function for which the nurse is held legally responsible and accountable. A large number of nurse practice acts were revised to include nursing diagnosis as a nursing function. Nursing diagnosis was included in the ANA Standards of Nursing Practice (1973) and in the standards developed by many nursing specialty organizations.

The five National Conferences on the Classification of Nursing Diagnoses held in the 1970s and the early 1980s have provided an impetus for the identification and classification of nursing diagnoses according to symptomatology. At the fifth conference, held in 1982, a major step was taken toward coordinating the work of developing nursing diagnoses—a new organization, the North American Nursing Diagnosis Association, was created. The diagnostic categories identified by the conference groups are gaining general acceptance by nurses but require further validation and expansion. They are neither complete nor mutually exclusive. More research is needed to determine the predictive and prognostic attributes of the diagnostic labels. Hopefully, in the future, nursing diagnosis will attain its potential of decreasing the ambiguity about the role of the nurse so that a more clearly defined scope of nursing practice will evolve. A list of accepted nursing diagnoses from the fifth National Conference on the Classification of Nursing Diagnoses is shown in Chart 2-2.

In spite of the need for research on the diagnostic process itself and on the diagnostic nomenclature, the term "nursing diagnosis" will be used in sections of this book where the authors have applied the nursing process to specific illness conditions. The term "nursing diagnosis/patient problem" will be used together. However, both nurses and nursing students who are assuming the practitioner role of nursing have a unique opportunity to use currently accepted nursing diagnoses and to develop additional diagnoses that describe actual or potential health problems that are amenable to nursing care. Only through clinical use of nursing diagnostic labels can these labels be validated and expanded.

When developing the nursing diagnoses for a particular patient, the nurse must first identify the commonalities among the assessment data collected. These common features lead to the categorization of related data that reveal the existence of a problem and the need for nursing intervention. *The patient's nursing problem is then defined as the nursing diagnosis.*

It must be remembered that nursing diagnoses are *not* medical diagnoses; they are *not* medical treatments prescribed by the physician; they are *not* diagnostic studies; they are *not* the equipment utilized to implement medical therapy; and they are *not* the problems that the nurse experiences while caring for the patient. They *are* the patient's actual or potential health problems that are amenable to resolution by nursing actions. Nursing diagnoses that are succinctly stated in terms of the specific problems of the patient will guide the nurse in the development of the nursing care plan.

Chart 2-2
Accepted Nursing Diagnoses from the 5th National Conference on the Classification of Nursing Diagnoses

Activity intolerance	Nutrition, Alteration in, Potential for more than body requirements
Airway clearance, Ineffective	Oral mucous membrane, Alteration in
Anxiety	Parenting, Alteration in, Actual
Bowel elimination, Alteration in, Constipation	Parenting, Alteration in, Potential
Bowel elimination, Alteration in, Diarrhea	Powerlessness
Bowel elimination, Alteration in, Incontinence	Rape-trauma syndrome
Breathing patterns, Ineffective	Self-care deficit: Total
Cardiac output, Alteration in, Decreased	Feeding
Comfort, Alteration in, Pain	Bathing/hygiene
Communication, Impaired verbal	Dressing/grooming
Coping, Ineffective individual	Toileting
Coping, Ineffective family, Compromised	Self-concept, Disturbance in
Coping, Ineffective family, Disabling	Sensory perceptual alteration: Visual
Coping, Family, Potential for growth	Auditory
Diversional activity deficit	Kinesthetic
Family processes, Alteration in	Gustatory
Fear (specify)	Tactile
Fluid volume deficit, Actual	Olfactory
Fluid volume deficit, Potential	Sexual dysfunction
Fluid volume excess	Skin integrity, Impairment in, Actual
Gas exchange, Impaired	Skin integrity, Impairment in, Potential
Grieving, Anticipatory	Sleep pattern disturbance
Grieving, Dysfunctional	Social isolation
Health maintenance, Alteration in	Spiritual distress
Home maintenance management, Impaired	Thought processes, Alteration in
Injury, Potential for (specify): Poisoning	Tissue perfusion, Alteration in: Cerebral
Suffocation	Cardiopulmonary
Trauma	Renal
Knowledge deficit (specify)	Gastrointestinal
Mobility, Impaired physical	Peripheral
Noncompliance (specify)	Urinary elimination, Alteration in patterns of
Nutrition, Alteration in, Less than body requirements	Violence, Potential for
Nutrition, Alteration in, More than body requirements	

In order to give additional meaning to the diagnosis, the characteristics and the etiology of the problem must be identified and included as a part of the diagnosis. Consider this clinical example:

Assessment of a patient with a medical diagnosis of diabetes mellitus reveals that the patient does not comply with his dietary regimen. He has the financial means necessary for purchasing the foods included in his diet, he has the home facilities required for preparing his foods, and he expresses a sincere desire to comply with his diet. However, he does not have an understanding of the food exchange system that is necessary for meal planning.

For this patient, the nursing diagnosis of "nonadherence" would give little guidance to the nurse in establishing a plan of care to meet the patient's needs. However, a more specific diagnosis of "nonadherence to dietary regimen related to lack of understanding of the diabetic exchange system" provides the nurse with information about the characteristics and cause of the problem. With such a diagnosis, the nurse is then ready to plan nursing care measures directed toward resolution of the problem.

▷ Planning

Once the nursing diagnoses have been identified, the planning component of the nursing process follows. This phase involves:

1. The assignment of priorities to the nursing diagnoses
2. The specification of short-term, intermediate, and long-term goals of nursing action

3. The identification of specific nursing interventions appropriate for attaining the goals
4. The documentation of the nursing diagnoses, goals, nursing interventions, and expected outcomes on the nursing care plan

Also, during this phase of the nursing process it is the responsibility of the nurse to communicate to the appropriate persons any assessment data indicative of health needs that can best be met by other members of the health team.

Setting Priorities
The assignment of priorities to the nursing diagnoses should be a joint effort by the nurse and the patient or his family members. Any disagreement about the priorities should be resolved in a way that is mutually acceptable. Consideration must be given to the urgency of the problems, the most critical problems receiving the highest priorities. Maslow's hierarchy of needs provides a useful framework for the determination of priority problems. The use of this hierarchy requires that high priorities be given to physical needs. Subsequent to the resolution of physical needs, priorities are reassigned according to the urgency of needs at other levels of the hierarchy (see p. 13).

Establishing Goals for Nursing Action
After the priorities of the nursing diagnoses have been established, the short-term, intermediate, and long-term goals and the nursing actions appropriate for attainment of the goals are identified. The patient and his family should be included in the establishment of the short-term, intermediate, and long-term goals of the nursing actions. The short-term goals are those that are of immediate concern and that can be reached in a short period of time. The intermediate and long-term goals require a longer period of time for their accomplishment and usually involve prevention of complications and further health problems, health education, and rehabilitation. For example, goals for an uncontrolled diabetic patient with a nursing diagnosis of "nonadherence to dietary regimen related to lack of understanding of the diabetic exchange system" may be stated as follows:

Short-term goal:	oral intake and tolerance of 1500-calorie diabetic diet spaced in three meals and one snack
Intermediate goal:	planning of meals for 1 week based on diabetic exchange system
Long-term goal:	adherence to prescribed diabetic diet

The patient and his family should be included whenever possible in the decisions about the nursing interventions to meet the goals. Involvement of the patient and his family in the planning of nursing interventions promotes their cooperation in the implementation of nursing care. The identification of appropriate nursing interventions and their related goals depends upon the nurse's recognition of the strengths and potential of the patient and his family; her understanding of the pathophysiologic alterations that

he experiences; and her sensitivity to his emotional, psychological, and intellectual response to his illness state. Likewise, the nurse's knowledge of nursing, her clinical experience, and her awareness of available supporting resources influence the validity of the nursing interventions that she identifies as appropriate for resolving the patient's problems.

Establishing Expected Outcomes
Expected outcomes of the nursing interventions should be stated in terms of the patient's behaviors, and they should be realistic and measurable. Standard outcome criteria established by the health care agency for the target population applicable to the patient should be utilized whenever possible. However, it may be necessary to adapt these outcome criteria so that they are realistic in terms of the specific patient's potential for resolution of his problems. The critical time period within which the outcomes should be demonstrated by the patient are also identified.

- The outcomes that define the expected behavior of the patient will serve as the basis for evaluation of the effectiveness of the nursing interventions.
- The critical time periods provide a time frame for determining the effectiveness of the nursing interventions and the existence of a need for additional or altered nursing care.

Team Planning
Ideally, the accomplishment of all aspects of the planning phase of the nursing process is a group effort. The nurse collaborates with other members of the nursing team, with the patient and his family, and with appropriate resource persons from the health care agency and community agencies.

In planning with other members of the nursing team, the nurse recognizes that each team member has a role that is supported and respected. Of course, the physician initiates the medical regimen and is a valuable counselor, teacher, and resource person. A nurse clinical-specialist, when available, can make a significant contribution.

Because the plan revolves around a patient, he should have a part in it. The ultimate goal is to help the patient help himself. This means the patient is accepted as a worthy individual and his right to self-determination is respected. Since the plan is oriented in terms of the patient's goals and capabilities, he has every right to express his feelings and voice his opinions about his care. He should be kept informed about his current health status (when feasible), any change in plans, the roles of health care personnel, and the resources available to him.

It is also important to remember that the patient is part of a family. The family members have needs that arise from the patient's illness. They may be included in the planning by questioning them about the patient's reactions and informing them about the nursing care plan and the expected results of treatment. The family may also make pertinent observations and offer effective suggestions.

Another aspect of care planning takes into account the fact that the patient comes from the community. Community agencies have an interest in the patient and are involved in planning. This means that the nurse must be aware of the community services that may be offered a patient following discharge from the hospital. These agencies can be informed of the goal to be reached, and decisions can then be made regarding the type of services that will be needed. Many communities have a directory listing all community resources available. These include community health and visiting nursing services, homemaking services, meals on wheels, social and recreational services, etc. A knowledge of these resources and the method of referral is of inestimable value in helping to cope with long-term health needs.

Formulating the Nursing Care Plan

The entire planning phase of the nursing process culminates in the formulation of the patient's nursing care plan by the professional nurse. The nursing care plan serves to communicate the following information to all members of the nursing team:

1. The nursing diagnoses and their priorities
2. The goals of the nursing interventions
3. The nursing interventions, which are expressed in the form of nursing orders
4. The outcome criteria, which identify the expected behavioral outcomes for the patient
5. The critical time period within which each outcome must be met

The information incorporated into the nursing care plan should be written in a concise, systematic manner that facilitates its use by all nursing personnel. Space must be provided in the care plan for documentation of the patient's response to the nursing interventions—the outcomes. It must be remembered that the care plan is subject to change as the patient's problems change, as the priorities of the problems shift, as resolution of problems occurs, and as additional information about the patient's state of health is collected. As the nursing interventions are implemented, the patient's responses are evaluated and documented, and the care plan is changed accordingly. A well-developed, continuously updated nursing care plan is the patient's greatest assurance that his nursing problems will be resolved and that his basic needs will be met. (For a sample nursing care plan, see Chart 2-3.)

▷ Implementation

The implementation phase of the nursing process follows the formulation of the nursing care plan. Implementation refers to carrying out the proposed plan of care. The nurse assumes responsibility for the implementation but includes the patient and his family and other members of the nursing team and the health team as appropriate. The activities of all persons involved in implementation are coordinated by the nurse.

- The nursing care plan serves as the basis for implementation.
- The short-term, intermediate, and long-term goals are utilized as a focus for the implementation of the designed nursing interventions.

- While implementing nursing care, the nurse continually assesses the patient and his response to the nursing care.
- Alterations are made in the care plan as the patient's condition, problems, and responses change and as reassignment of priorities is required.

Implementation includes all of the nursing interventions that are directed toward resolution of the patient's nursing problems and meeting his health needs. Some of these needs have already been discussed (p. 13). Needs specific to certain conditions are presented in the chapter in which the particular condition is discussed.

General Categories of Nursing Interventions

Included among nursing interventions are hygienic care; promotion of physical and psychological comfort; support of respiratory and elimination functions; facilitation of the ingestion of food, fluids, and nutrients; environmental management; health teaching; promotion of a therapeutic relationship; and a host of therapeutic nursing activities. The nurse uses judgment in the selection of nursing interventions that are based on physiologic principles.

Knowledge of physiology must be constantly sought, integrated, and applied. Consider this clinical example:

A patient with bronchiectasis is exhausted from repeated episodes of unproductive coughing. Traditionally, the doctor would be notified and a medication for cough given. The more self-directing nurse, using nursing abilities based on an understanding of altered pathophysiology, will listen to the patient's lungs with a stethoscope, locate the area of congestion, position him for drainage, and then assist him to assume the posture that will help him cough up the mucus. The physician is also notified and his medical regimen for the patient is followed.

- All nursing interventions are patient-focused and goal-directed. They are based on scientific principles and are implemented with compassion, surety, and a willingness to understand the patient's problems.

Delegating Nursing Actions

The nurse may delegate certain specific actions to other members of the nursing team. When delegating, the nurse must know the capabilities and limitations of the members of the nursing team, select the most appropriate person to implement the actions, and supervise the performance of the actions. The nursing team member should be provided with all of the information that she needs to effectively perform the actions in such a way that the patient remains the focus of the actions at all times.

Many members of the nursing team and the health team may become involved in the patient's care. In order to provide for coordination and continuity of care, information about the patient's response to his care and any changes that must be made in the plan of care must be communicated verbally and in writing to the appropriate persons. Continual updating of the care plan is of paramount importance in assuring coordination and continuity.

Recording Outcomes

The implementation phase of the nursing process is concluded when the nursing interventions have been completed and when the patient's responses to them have been recorded. Recordings should be made concisely, precisely, and objectively. The recordings should:

- Be related to the nursing diagnoses
- Describe the nursing interventions and the patient's responses to the interventions, and
- Include any additional pertinent data

Only with accurate recording can evaluation be carried out. Documentation of information provides the basis for the measurement of the patient's behavioral response to the nursing interventions—his accomplishment of the defined outcome criteria.

▷ Evaluation

Evaluation is the final component of the nursing process and is directed toward determining the patient's response to the nursing interventions and the extent to which the goals have been achieved. The nursing care plan provides the basis for evaluation; the nursing diagnoses, goals, nursing interventions, and outcome criteria provide the specific guidelines that dictate the focus of the evaluation.

Evaluation will answer the following questions:

- Were the nursing diagnoses accurate?
- Did the patient meet the outcome criteria?
- Did the patient meet the criteria within the critical time periods?
- Have the patient's nursing problems been resolved?
- Have the patient's nursing needs been met?
- Should the nursing interventions be retained, altered, or discontinued?
- Have new problems evolved for which nursing interventions have not been planned or implemented?
- What factors influenced the achievement or lack of achievement of the goals?
- Do priorities need to be reassigned?
- Should changes be made in the goals and outcome criteria?

Objective data that answer these questions must be collected from all available sources (*i.e.,* patient, family or significant others, nursing and other health team members). These data should be available in the patient's record and should be substantiated by direct observation of the patient.

Quality Assurance

Evaluation has traditionally been the most neglected component of the nursing process. However, during the past decade the increased emphasis placed on professional accountability and the advent of quality assurance programs have tended to focus much attention on evaluation. Quality assurance programs are now required for reimbursement of services and for JCAH (Joint Commission of American Hospitals) accreditation of hospitals.

- The concept of quality assurance refers to the accountability of the health professions to society for the quality, quantity, and costs of the health services provided.

The impetus for the establishment of quality assurance programs by the health professions was provided by the enactment of the Social Security Amendments of 1972, which provided for the creation of Professional Standards Review Organizations (PSROs) as a system for evaluating the quality of health care delivered. PSROs are based on the concept of peer review, which allows the specific profession to establish its own norms, standards, and criteria for review and to carry out the review process. Nursing, as a nonphysician health care profession, has accepted its responsibility for implementation of peer review and thus for accountability for the quality of the nursing care provided. Nurses have recognized their accountability to their patients, their employing institutions, their colleagues and subordinates, other members of the health care team, and the nursing profession.

Quality assurance programs in nursing are viewed as evaluation systems composed of three dimensions: structure, process, and outcome (see Fig. 2-1).

The *structural dimension* focuses on the organization within which nursing care is provided.

The *process dimension* focuses on the actual performance of the tasks, functions, and activities of nursing care.

The *outcome dimension* focuses on patient welfare, the end results of the care provided to the patient.

Evaluation of structure, process, and outcome are all important and are interrelated, each influencing the other. However, outcomes that provide clinical evidence of the results of care are the ultimate validators of the care rendered. Outcomes focus the attention of the practitioner on the response of the patient to the care that he received. The aim of quality assurance in nursing is to provide a means of improving nursing care where deficits exist.

Outcome Criteria

Goals for accountability and quality assurance in nursing are being realized. The American Nurses' Association has developed basic standards that provide a general model for nursing practice by which the quality of nursing practice may be evaluated. Record-keeping has been revised to provide a problem-oriented approach to documentation of data. The Problem-Oriented Medical Record (POMR) focuses attention on the patient and his problems and allows for the systematic documentation of data by various health team members. The use of outcome criteria as validators of the nursing process has become an accepted trend. Nurses in various health care settings have developed outcome criteria for specific patient populations. Likewise, the American Nurses' Association has developed outcome criteria that have served as guidelines and as prototypes for criteria utilized in various health care agencies. The nursing audit has become an accepted method for comparing results of the actual nursing performance with the established criteria. Nursing audit may involve concurrent review or retrospec-

(Text continues on page 28)

Chart 2-3
Example of a Nursing Care Plan

Mr. George Clark, a 40-year-old attorney, was admitted to the nursing unit from his physician's office. An upper GI series performed the previous day had revealed a duodenal ulcer. A brief hospitalization was planned for initiation of therapy. Upon admission, Mr. Clark expressed anxiety about the fact that the hospitalization was interfering with his work schedule and that he had an important court case to prepare. Nursing history revealed that for several months Mr. Clark had experienced midepigastric pain, which he described as "burning and gnawing." The pain was worse immediately before meals and was relieved by food. He occasionally took antacids but stated he was unable to remember to take them on a regular schedule. He had not noticed blood in his stools. He described his life-style as "busy—sometimes hectic," with a rigorous work schedule and a busy home life in which he and his wife shared the responsibility for raising two teenage sons. He indicated that he smokes two packs of cigarettes per day, drinks three to five cups of coffee daily, and drinks alcohol at social occasions. His vital signs upon admission were BP 136/75, P 92, R 22, T 37.2°C (99°F). The physician's orders upon admission included: regular diet; Amphogel—30 ml every 2 hours; cimetidine (Tagamet)—300 mg with meals and at bedtime; and all stools to lab for occult blood.

Nursing Diagnoses

Pain related to gastric acidity and mucosal erosion
Emotional stress related to role responsibilities at work and home
Potential nonadherence to therapeutic regimen

Goals

Short-term:
Relief of pain

Intermediate:
Begins making alterations in life-style to decrease stress

Long-term:
Alters life-style to reduce emotional and environmental stressors
Adherence to therapeutic regimen

Nursing Interventions	Outcome Criteria	Critical Time*	Outcome
Relieve pain and discomfort, and promote healing:			
Establish q 2 hr schedule for self-administration of Amphojel	Administers Amphojel to self q 2 hr	24 hr	Amphojel administered by patient every 2 hr while awake; patient requested additional supply of Amphojel at appropriate time
	Free from pain	24 hr	Denied pain after 24 hr of medication therapy
Observe for constipation as a side-effect of Amphojel	Absence of constipation	24 hr	Normal bowel movement 24 hr and 48 hr after admission
Observe for side-effects of Tagamet: diarrhea, muscle pain, dizziness, rash, bradycardia	Absence of side-effects of Tagamet	48 hr	No evidence of side-effects of Tagamet after 48 hr
Encourage well-balanced diet that does not cause pain or distress	Adequate intake of nutrients from basic four food groups	48 hr	Intake of adequate amounts of foods from basic four food groups 24 hr after admission
	Avoids foods and fluids that cause pain	24 hr	Continues to drink two cups of coffee daily
	Eats meals at regular times	24 hr	Complains of abdominal distention after meals; distress relieved when meal pattern is changed to six small meals daily

(continued)

Chart 2-3
Example of a Nursing Care Plan (continued)

Nursing Interventions	Outcome Criteria	Critical Time*	Outcome
Assess for signs and symptoms of complications: TPR, BP q 4 hr	Vital signs within normal limits	24 hr	Vital signs stable 24 hr after admission: T 36.8°C–37°C P 74/min–86/min R 14/min–20/min, normal depth BP 118/70–128/74
	Absence of blood in stools	24 hr	Stools negative for occult blood
Promote atmosphere conducive to physical and mental rest: Encourage alternation of periods of rest and activity	Alternates periods of rest and activity	24 hr	Rests in bed 1 hr in morning and 2 hr in afternoon; disconnects phone during rest periods Awake at intervals during night; 8 hr of uninterrupted sleep at night after initiation of 30 mg Dalmane at bedtime
Encourage limitation of visitors and interactions that are stress producing	Limits visitors to family and few friends for short intervals	24 hr	Wife and sons visit 2 hr in afternoon and 2 hr in evening; patient requested friends to postpone visits until after discharge
	Avoids stress-producing interactions	24 hr	Wife and sons aware of need to decrease stress—they apprise patient of happenings at home and avoid discussion of stress-producing topics
Assist patient to alter life-style to decrease stress: Discuss relationship between emotional stress and physiologic functioning	Describes excessive stress as a precursor to alteration in physiologic functioning	48 hr	Accurately described relationship between excessive stress and ulcer formation
Encourage patient to identify stress-producing stimuli	Identifies factors in life-style that produce stress	48 hr	Identified the following stressors: Self-imposed demands of job—inability to delegate responsibilities to others Excessive involvement in sons' school and sports activities and in community-service organizations
Encourage patient to identify life-style adjustments necessary to reduce stress	Identifies life-style adjustments necessary to reduce stress	48 hr	Identifed ways to share work responsibilities with coworkers Identified need to decrease work hours from 12 to 8 or 9 daily and to decrease weekend work hours Identified ways to become a less active participant in sons' sports activities Identified need to decrease involvement in community organizations
	Discusses life-style adjustments with family	48 hr	Family supportive of planned life-style adjustments
Promote adherence to therapeutic regimen	(See teaching plan, p. 34)		

* These times have not been standardized but are individualized according to the patient's needs.

tive review of the patient's record. While the patient is in a health care agency, there can be a concurrent review of the patient's record by a nursing group to evaluate whether or not quality care has been given. This provides the opportunity to make changes. There can be a retrospective review of the patient's record (after he leaves the health care agency), which provides another method of evaluation. However, this method of evaluation does not provide an opportunity to make changes for the specific patient who is evaluated.

All methods utilized to accomplish the evaluation component of the nursing process are directly related to the nursing care plan. Evaluation of the patient's response to nursing interventions is accomplished by comparing the patient's behavioral outcomes with the established outcome criteria. This information then serves as a basis for modification of the nursing care plan.

Evaluation should include self-assessment by the nurse. This can be done through courses of study, programmed learning, reading professional literature, etc. Concurrently, the nurse reviews her own nursing care. She studies the patient's care plan to decide how many correct decisions were made in nursing assessment, planning, and implementation, as compared with ineffective decisions, and how effective the nursing care is, as measured by valid outcome criteria.

However, it is not enough to evaluate only the effectiveness of the nursing care. An important phase of evaluation is "What should be done to improve the nursing care?" Other nursing interventions may have to be tried. Goals may have to be redesigned. Priorities may have to be reassigned. Outcome criteria may have to be made more realistic. There must be a continuous and thorough scrutiny of the care provided. Then changes are made, plans altered, and a course of action initiated that will be most supportive to the patient.

Thus, the steps of the nursing process are cyclic and recurrent. Each step is ongoing and is related to all other steps. Continuous evaluation provides the means for maintaining the viability of the entire nursing process and for demonstrating accountability for the quality of nursing care rendered.

For an overall view of the steps of the nursing process, see Chart 2-4.

Chart 2-4
Steps of the Nursing Process

Assessment

1. Conduct the nursing history.
2. Perform the physical examination.
3. Interview the patient's family or significant others.
4. Study the health record.
5. Formulate the nursing diagnoses.
   a. Organize, analyze, synthesize, and summarize the collected data.
   b. Identify the patient's nursing problems.
   c. Identify the defining characteristics of the nursing problems.
   d. Identify the etiology of the nursing problems.
   e. State nursing diagnoses concisely and precisely.

Planning

1. Assign priority to the nursing diagnoses.
2. Specify the goals.
   a. Develop short-term, intermediate, and long-term goals.
   b. State the goals in realistic and measurable terms.
3. Identify nursing interventions appropriate for goal attainment.
4. Establish outcome criteria.
   a. Make sure that the outcomes are realistic and measurable.
   b. Identify critical times for the attainment of outcomes.
5. Develop the written nursing care plan.
   a. Include nursing diagnoses, goals, nursing interventions, and outcome criteria.
   b. Write all entries precisely, concisely, and systematically.
   c. Keep the plan current and flexible to meet the patient's changing problems and needs.
6. Involve the patient, his family or significant others, nursing team members, and other health team members in all aspects of planning.

Implementation

1. Put the nursing care plan into action.
2. Coordinate the activities of the patient, his family or significant others, nursing team members, and other health team members.
3. Record the patient's responses to the nursing actions.

Evaluation

1. Collect objective data.
2. Compare the patient's behavioral outcomes to the outcome criteria. Determine the extent to which the goals were achieved.
3. Include the patient, his family or significant others, nursing team members, and other health team members in the evaluation.
4. Identify alterations that need to be made in the nursing diagnoses, goals, nursing interventions, and outcome criteria.
5. Continue all steps of the nursing process: assessing, planning, implementing, evaluating.

▷ Bibliography

Books

American Nurses' Association. Guidelines for Review of Nursing Care at the Local Level. Washington, DC, US Government Printing Office, 1976.

Carlson JH, Craft CA, and McGuire AD. Nursing Diagnosis. Philadelphia, WB Saunders, 1982.

Duke University Hospital Nursing Services. Quality Assurance: Guidelines for Nursing Care. Philadelphia, JB Lippincott, 1980.

Erikson EH. Childhood and Society. New York, WW Norton, 1963.

Gordon M. Nursing Diagnosis. Process and Application. New York, McGraw-Hill, 1982.

Griffith JW and Christensen PJ. Nursing Process. Application of Theories, Frameworks, and Models. St Louis, CV Mosby, 1982.

Kim MJ and Moritz DA. Classification of Nursing Diagnoses. Proceedings of the Third and Fourth National Conferences. New York, McGraw-Hill, 1982.

Murchison I, Nichols TS, and Hanson R. Legal Accountability in the Nursing Process. St Louis, CV Mosby, 1982.

Yura H and Walsh MB. The Nursing Process, 4th ed. East Norwalk, Connecticut, Appleton-Century-Crofts, 1983.

Yura H and Walsh MB (eds). Human Needs II and the Nursing Process. East Norwalk, Connecticut, Appleton-Century-Crofts, 1982.

Yura H and Walsh MB (eds). Human Needs III and the Nursing Process. East Norwalk, Connecticut, Appleton-Century-Crofts, 1983.

Articles

Bailey K and Swenson-Feldman E. An innovative approach to the nursing process. Nurs Admin Q 1982 Spring; 6(3):71–76.

Barba M, Bennett B, and Shaw WJ. The evaluation of patient care through use of ANA's standards of nursing practice. Superv Nurse 1978 Jan; 9(1):42–54.

Beck J. The standards as a guide for nursing care plans. Oncol Nurs Forum 1980 Winter; 7(1):28–30.

Betz M. From whence accountability? Nurs Health Care 1981 Nov; 2(9):482–486.

Blake BLK. Quality assurance: An ethical responsibility. Superv Nurse 1981 Feb; 12(2):32–38.

Bruce G et al: Implementation of ANA's quality assurance program for clients with end-stage renal disease. Adv Nurs Sci 1980 Jan; 2(2):79–95.

Bruce JA. Implementation of nursing diagnoses. Nurs Clin North Am 1979 Sept; 14(3):509–515.

Connolly ML. Organize your workday for more effective discharge planning. Nursing '81 1981 July; 11(7):44–47.

Dossey B and Guzzetta CE. Nursing diagnosis. Nursing '81 1981 June; 11(6):34–38.

Given B, Given CW, and Simoni LE. Relationships of processes of care to patient outcomes. Nurs Res 1979 Mar–Apr; 28(2):85–93.

Gleet CJ and Tatro S. Nursing diagnoses for healthy individuals. Nurs Health Care 1981 Oct; 2(8):456–457.

Gordon M, Sweeney MA, and McKeehan K. Development of nursing diagnoses. Am J Nurs 1980 Apr; 80(4):669.

Gordon M, Sweeney MA, and McKeehan K. Nursing diagnosis: Looking at its use in the clinical area. Am J Nurs 1980 Apr; 80(4):672–674.

Gray JW and Aldred H. Care plans in long-term facilities. Am J Nurs 1980 Nov; 80(11):2054–2057.

Harvey BL. Your patient's discharge plan. Nursing '81 1981 July; 11(7):48–51.

Howe MJ. Developing instruments for measurement of criteria: A clinical nursing practice perspective. Nurs Res 1980 Mar–Apr; 29(2):100–108.

Huckabay LMD and Neal MC. The nursing care plan problem. J Nurs Adm 1979 Dec; 9(12):36–42.

Inzer F and Aspinall MJ. Evaluating patient outcomes. Nurs Outlook 1981 Mar; 29(3):178–181.

Jacoby MK and Adams DJ. Teaching assessment of client functioning. Nurs Outlook 1981 Apr; 29(4):248–250.

Leslie FM. Nursing diagnosis: Use in long-term care. Am J Nurs 1981 May; 81(5):1012–1014.

Lunney M. Nursing diagnoses: Refining the system: Am J Nurs 1982 Mar; 82(3):456–459.

Mallick MJ. Patient assessment—based on data, not intuition. Nurs Outlook 1981 Oct; 29(10):600–605.

Manthey M. Nursing care plans. Nurs Manage 1981 Sept; 12(9):28–31.

McCarthy MM. The nursing process: Application of current thinking in clinical problem solving. J Adv Nurs 1981 May; 6(3):173–177.

Pilette PC. Caution: Objectivity and specialization may be hazardous to your humanity. Am J Nurs 1980 Sept; 80(9):1588–1590.

Popkiss SA. Diagnosing your patient's strengths. Nursing '81 1981 July; 11(7):34–37.

Price MR. Nursing diagnosis: Making a concept come alive. Am J Nurs 1980 Apr; 80(4):668–674.

Roeder MA. Patient care plans and the evaluation of nursing process. Superv Nurse 1980 June; 11(6):57–58.

Snyder PJ. Goal setting. Superv Nurse 1979 Sept; 10(9):61–64.

Trussell PM and Strand N. A comparison of concurrent and retrospective audits on the same patients. J Nurs Adm 1978 May; 8(5):33–38.

Walker L and Nicholson R. Criteria for evaluating nursing process models. Nurse Educ 1980 Sept/Oct; 5(5):8–9.

3

Patient Education/ Health Teaching

▷ Health Education Today

Perhaps one of the greatest challenges facing members of the nursing profession today is that of meeting the health education needs of the American public. In this respect, nurses are becoming increasingly sensitive to and conscious of their role as teachers. Health education is considered to be an independent function of nursing practice and a primary responsibility of the nursing profession. Many state nurse practice acts include teaching as a function of nursing.

- Health education is an essential component of nursing care and is directed toward promotion, maintenance, and restoration of health and toward adaptation to residual effects of illness.

The emphasis that has been placed on the need for health education during recent years perhaps stems in part from the belief of many health care leaders that the American public has the right to expect and receive comprehensive health care, including health education. It also reflects the emergence of a better informed American public, who are asking more significant questions about health, health care, and the services offered by the health care delivery system. Because of the emphasis that the American culture places on health and the responsibility of each individual for the maintenance and promotion of his own health, it is the obligation of the members of the health care delivery system and, specifically, of nurses to make health education available to the American public.

One of the largest groups of people in need of health education today are those persons with chronic illnesses. The number of people in this category is continually rising. It is the belief of many health care leaders that persons with chronic illness are entitled to as much health care information as they can handle in order that they may actively participate in and assume the responsibility for much of their own care. Health education can aid the individual in adapting to his illness, in cooperating with his prescribed therapy, and in learning to solve problems when confronted with new situations. Health education can prevent rehospitalization for the same condition, a frequent result when a person does not understand how to care for his chronic condition.

- The goal of health education is teaching people to live life to its healthiest—that is, to strive toward achieving one's maximum health potential.

Every contact that a nurse has with a patient should be considered an opportunity for patient teaching. It is the patient's right to decide whether or not he will learn, but it is the nurse's responsibility to present him with the information that he needs in order to make the decision and to motivate him to appreciate the need for learning.

▷ Adherence to the Therapeutic Regimen

Inherent within the area of patient teaching is the concern for the promotion of the patient's adherence to his therapeutic regimen. The term "compliance" is often used to describe this behavior. However, this term suggests that the patient's role is passive. The term "adherence" implies that the patient assumes an active role in altering his health behaviors.

Adherence to a therapeutic regimen requires that the patient make one or more changes in his life-style. The patient may need to take medications, adhere to a diet, restrict his activities, observe himself for signs and symptoms of illness, practice specific hygienic measures, seek periodic evaluation of his health status, and attend to a host of other therapeutic and preventive measures. The fact that many patients do not adhere to their prescribed regimens cannot be ignored or minimized. The rates of patient adherence to therapeutic and preventive regimens are generally very low, especially when the regimens are complex or of long duration. The characteristics of nonadherent patients and their reasons for not adhering to their prescribed therapy have been the subjects of many studies. For the most part, the findings of these studies have been inconclusive. No one factor has been found to be the predominant cause of nonadherence. Instead, it seems that a wide range of variables interacting with one another influence the degree of adherence.

The factors influencing adherence include:

- Demographic variables, such as age, sex, race, socioeconomic status, and education
- Illness variables, such as the severity of the illness and the relief of symptoms afforded by the therapy
- Psychosocial variables, such as intelligence, attitudes toward health professionals, and acceptance or denial of illness

Knowledge alone concerning health and health promotion and illness and illness prevention has not been found to be a sufficient stimulus to motivate total adherence. However, it has been found that some degree of adherence in some patients is obviously enhanced by the use of teaching programs and by methods directed toward stimulating motivation to adhere to a regimen. The problem of nonadherence to therapeutic regimens is a substantial one that needs to be remedied in order to assist patients to adequately participate in self-care and to successfully achieve their maximum health potential.

The role of the nurse in teaching and directing patients toward adherence behavior is a significant one. It is the responsibility of the nurse to assess all variables that may have an effect upon the patient's adherence and to use this information when developing and implementing the patient's teaching plan.

▷ The Nature of Teaching and Learning

When learning is defined as the acquiring of knowledge, attitudes, or skills, and teaching is defined as helping another person to learn, it becomes evident that the teaching–learning process is an active one. It requires the active involvement of both the teacher and the learner in the effort to reach the desired outcome—change in behavior. The teacher does not give knowledge to the learner but instead serves as a facilitator of learning. In general, there is a lack of knowledge about how learning occurs and is affected by teaching. No single theory of learning suffices to explain how learning occurs. However, some specific principles of learning and some guidelines for teaching have been identified.

Learning Readiness

There are many variables, both internal and external, that affect the learner and the learning situation. One of the most significant of these factors is the learner's readiness to learn—his physical, emotional, and experiential readiness to learn.

Physical readiness is of vital importance because until a patient is physically capable of learning, attempts at teaching and learning may be both futile and frustrating. A patient who is experiencing acute pain is unable to focus his attention away from the pain long enough to concentrate on learning. Likewise, a patient who is short of breath will concentrate his energies on breathing rather than on learning.

- Utilizing Maslow's hierarchy of needs is helpful in considering the concept of physical readiness for learning.

Emotional readiness involves the patient's motivation to learn. Until the person has begun to accept his illness or to accept the fact that illness is a threat to him, he may not be motivated to learn. If his therapeutic regimen is not acceptable to him or is in conflict with his life-style, he may consciously avoid learning. Until he recognizes the need to learn and his own ability to learn, teaching efforts may be thwarted. However, it is not always wise to wait for the patient to become emotionally ready to learn—this time may never come unless efforts are made by the nurse to stimulate the patient's motivation to learn. Illness and the threat of illness are usually accompanied by anxiety and stress. The nurse who recognizes the patient's reactions to his illness or threatened illness can use simple explanations and instructions to alleviate his anxieties and to further motivate him to learn. It must be remembered that since learning involves changes in behavior, it normally produces mild anxiety. Such anxiety is often a useful motivating factor.

- Emotional readiness can be promoted by creating a warm, accepting, positive atmosphere and by establishing realistic learning goals with the patient so that he can realize success and a feeling of accomplishment, which in themselves are motivators of learning.

Feedback about progress also serves to motivate learning. Such feedback should be presented in the form of positive reinforcement when the patient is successful and in the form of constructive criticism when he is unsuccessful.

Experiential readiness to learn refers to the patient's past experiences which enable him to learn what is being taught. Previous educational experiences and life experiences in general are significant determinants of the patient's approach to learning. A person who has had little or no formal education may not be able to understand the instructional materials presented to him—although this is not always true. The person who has experienced difficulty in learning in the past may be hesitant to make new attempts to learn. Many behaviors required for meeting one's maximum health potential require a rather extensive background of knowledge, physical skills, and attitudes. If the person does not have this background upon which to build, learning may be very difficult and very slow for him. For example, until a patient understands the basics of normal nutrition he may not be able to understand the restrictions of a special diet. Also, a person who is not future-oriented will be unable to appreciate many aspects of preventive health teaching. And a person who does not view the desired learning as meaningful to himself and his life-style will reject teaching efforts.

Thus, experiential readiness is closely related to emotional readiness, since motivation tends to be stimulated by one's appreciation for the need to learn and by those learning tasks that are familiar, interesting, and meaningful.

- Prior to initiating a teaching–learning program, the nurse must assess the patient's physical and emotional readiness to learn as well as his level of attainment of those behaviors that are prerequisites to learning what is being taught. This information then becomes the basis for the goals to be established, goals that in themselves can motivate the patient to learn.
- Involvement of the patient in the establishment of goals that are mutually acceptable to him and to the nurse serves the purpose of encouraging the patient to be actively involved in the learning process and to share the responsibility for his learning progress.

The Learning Atmosphere

Although a teacher is not always necessary, most patients who are attempting to learn new or altered health behaviors will need the services of a nurse–teacher at least part of the time. The interpersonal interaction between the patient and the nurse who is attempting to meet the patient's learning needs may be formal or informal, depending upon the method and techniques of teaching that are found to be most appropriate for the individual patient.

The nurse facilitates learning by manipulating those external variables that affect the patient's learning. For example, the physical environment should be such that it is conducive to learning. That is, the room temperature, lighting, noise levels, and the like should be appropriate to the learning situation. Also, the time selected for teaching should be suited to the patient's needs. Scheduling a teaching session at a time of day when the patient is fatigued, when he is anticipating diagnostic or therapeutic procedures about which he is anxious, or when he has visitors does not provide a conducive learning environment. Timing of teaching may also be determined by visits of the family members, if they are to be included in the teaching plan.

Teaching Techniques

The nurse also facilitates learning by selecting teaching techniques and methods that are most appropriate to meet the individual patient's needs.

The lecture or explanation method of teaching is commonly used but should always be accompanied by discussion. The discussion is important, since it affords the patient an opportunity to express his feelings and concerns, to ask questions, and to receive clarification of any misinformation or misunderstandings that he may have.

Group teaching is appropriate for some patients because it allows them not only to receive the information that is needed but also to experience security through being a member of a group. Patients with similar problems or learning needs have the opportunity to identify with each other and thus to gain moral support and encouragement. However, it must be remembered that all patients do not relate well in groups and therefore may not benefit from such experiences.

Demonstration and practice are often essential ingredients of the patient's teaching program, especially when skills are to be learned. The nurse first demonstrates the skill to the patient and then allows him ample opportunity to practice the skill. When special equipment is necessary to perform the skill, such as insulin syringes, colostomy bags, dressings, and the like, it is important that the nurse provide the patient with the same equipment that he will be using after he leaves the hospital. Learning to perform a skill with one kind of equipment and then having to change to a different kind of equipment is more than can be expected of most patients.

Teaching aids are available to supplement the abilities of the nurse to help the patient to learn. These include books, pamphlets, pictures, films, slides, tapes, models, and programmed instruction. Such teaching aids are invaluable when utilized appropriately. It is the responsibility of the nurse to carefully review all such aids before presenting them to patients in order to be sure that they are designed to meet the individual patient's learning needs.

Reinforcement and follow-up are also important factors to consider, since learning takes time. The patient must be allowed ample time to learn and to have his learning reinforced. A single teaching session is never adequate. Followup sessions are imperative in order to promote the patient's confidence in his ability to follow through with what he has learned. Such sessions also give the nurse the opportunity to evaluate the patient's progress and to plan for additional teaching sessions as required. It is also important to realize that the patient may not be able to transfer what he has learned in the hospital to his home setting. Thus, arrangements for follow-up after discharge are often essential for assuring that the full benefits of the hospital teaching program have been realized.

▷ The Nursing Process in Patient Teaching

The teaching–learning process is an integral part of the nursing process. With a focus on learning and with regard for the principles of teaching and learning, the steps of the nursing process—assessment, planning, implementation, and evaluation—are utilized for the purpose of meeting the teaching and learning needs of the patient and his family.

Assessment

Assessment in the teaching–learning process is comparable to that component of the nursing process. It is directed toward the systematic collection of data about the patient's learning needs and readiness to learn and about the family's learning needs. All internal and external variables that affect the patient's readiness to learn are assessed. A learning assessment guide may be helpful in obtaining pertinent information about the patient's need to learn and his readiness to learn. Some of the learning assessment guides available are very general and are directed toward the assessment of general health information. Others are specific to common medication regimens or disease processes. An example is the *Diabetes Mellitus Assessment Guides* published by the American Diabetes Association, North Carolina affiliate, Inc. These assessment guides are designed for the assessment of the diabetic's learning needs with regard to all aspects of the diabetic regimen. Such guides serve to facilitate the assessment but must be adapted to the individual responses, problems, and needs of the patient. As soon as possible after completing the assessment, the nurse organizes, analyzes, synthesizes, and summarizes the data collected and determines the patient's need for teaching. Nursing diagnoses that specifically relate to the patient's learning needs are then succinctly stated and serve to guide the nurse in the development of the teaching plan.

Planning

Once the nursing diagnoses related to the patient's need for learning have been identified, the planning component of the teaching–learning process follows. This plan follows the same sequence utilized in the nursing process:

1. Assigning priorities to the diagnoses
2. Specifying the short-term intermediate, and long-term goals of learning

3. Identifying specific teaching strategies appropriate for attaining the goals
4. Documenting the diagnoses, goals, teaching strategies, and expected outcomes on the teaching plan

As in the nursing process, the assignment of priorities to the diagnoses should be a joint effort by the nurse and the patient or his family members. Consideration must be given to the urgency of the patient's learning needs, the most critical needs receiving the highest priority.

After the priorities of the diagnoses have been established, the short-term, intermediate, and long-term goals and the teaching strategies appropriate for attaining the goals are identified. Studies have indicated that teaching is most effective when the patient's goals and the nurse's goals are in agreement. Goal-directed learning should begin with the establishment of goals that are appropriate to the situation and that are realistic in terms of the patient's ability to achieve them. Goals should be individualized according to the needs of the patient, specifically the needs perceived by the patient, and must be acceptable to the nurse, the patient, and the family. Involving the patient and his family in goal establishment and subsequent planning of teaching strategies promotes their cooperation in the implementation of the teaching plan.

Expected outcomes of the teaching strategies are stated in terms of the patient's behaviors. Every effort is made to develop outcome criteria that are realistic and measurable. The critical time period within which the outcomes should be demonstrated by the patient are also identified. The outcome criteria and the critical time periods will serve as a basis for evaluation of the effectiveness of the teaching strategies.

During the planning phase, the nurse gives consideration to the sequence in which the subject matter will be presented to the patient when each of the teaching strategies is implemented. An outline is often helpful for arranging subject matter and for ensuring that all necessary information is included. Also during this time, the nurse selects and secures the appropriate teaching aids to be used in implementing the teaching strategies.

The entire planning phase of the teaching–learning process is concluded with the formulation of the patient's teaching plan by the nurse. This teaching plan communicates the following information to all members of the nursing team.

1. The nursing diagnoses that specifically relate to the patient's learning needs and the priorities of these diagnoses
2. The goals of the teaching strategies
3. The teaching strategies, which are expressed in the form of teaching orders
4. The outcome criteria, which identify the expected behavioral outcomes for the patient
5. The critical time period within which the outcome must be met
6. The patient's behavioral responses (must be documented on the teaching plan)

The same rules that apply to writing and revising the nursing care plan apply to the teaching plan. (For a sample teaching plan, see Chart 3-1. Note that it is not different from but is simply a continuation of the nursing care plan.)

Implementation

The implementation phase of the teaching–learning process follows the formulation of the teaching plan. The patient, his family, and other members of the nursing team and the health team are included in the implementation. The activities of all of these persons are coordinated by the nurse, and the teaching plan serves as the basis for implementation.

- It is important to remain flexible during the implementation phase of the teaching–learning process and to continuously assess the patient's reponses to the teaching strategies and to make alterations in the teaching plan as necessary.

It is highly desirable that the nurse utilize her creativity to the fullest to promote and sustain the patient's motivation to learn; she should anticipate teaching needs that may arise after the patient's discharge from the hospital that are not foreseen by the patient while he is still in the hospital. Then,

---

Chart 3-1
Example of a Teaching Plan*

Assessment of Mr. Clark's teaching and learning needs revealed the following:

Basic knowledge about the relationship between emotional stress and physiologic functioning
Use of stimulants that promote excessive gastric secretions (*i.e.,* coffee, tobacco, alcohol)
Irregularity of meals
Previous nonadherence to regular schedule of taking antacids
Life-style conducive to excessive stress

Nursing Diagnosis

Potential nonadherence to therapeutic regimen related to knowledge deficit and life-style

Goals

Short-term:
Adheres to medication and diet therapies

Intermediate:
Discontinues use of substances that promote excessive gastric secretions

Long-term:
Alters life-style to reduce emotional and environmental stressors

Teaching Strategies	Outcome Criteria	Critical Time†	Outcome
Explain and discuss the following topics with patient and wife:			
• Schedule of antacid therapy	Takes antacid q 2–4 hr while awake	During and after hospitalization	Accurately explained reasons for necessity of regularity of antacids and meals and for avoidance of gastric irritants
• Regularity of meals	Adheres to regular meal schedule		Identified ways to promote regularity of meals and antacid regimen within work and home schedule
			Wife supportive of meal-regularity plans

(continued)

and only then, can she assist the patient in transferring knowledge from the hospital to his home. The implementation phase is concluded when the teaching strategies have been completed and when the patient's responses to the actions have been recorded. This record serves as the basis for the evaluation of the patient's accomplishment of the defined outcome criteria.

Evaluation

Evaluation is the final component of the teaching–learning process and is directed toward the determination of the patient's response to the teaching strategies and the extent to which the goals have been achieved. Evaluation for the teaching–learning process will answer the same question as that used for the nursing process but with specific regard to teaching and learning. An important phase in evaluation remains: "What should be done to improve the teaching?" Answers to this question will dictate changes that must be made in the teaching plan.

It should never be assumed that an individual has learned because he has been taught. Learning does not automatically follow teaching. A variety of measurement tech-

---

Chart 3-1
Example of a Teaching Plan* (continued)

Teaching Strategies	Outcome Criteria	Critical Time†	Outcome
• Avoidance of foods and fluids that cause pain or distress	Avoids foods and fluids that cause pain or distress Avoids extemes of temperature of foods and fluids Eliminates use of coffee		Substituted decaffeinated coffee for regular coffee 2 days after admission
• Avoidance of tobacco	Stops smoking	During and after hospitalization	Decreased smoking to ½ pack per day 48 hr after admission; contacted Smoke-Enders about participation in program
• Signs and symptoms of ulcer recurrence	Identifies signs and symptoms of ulcer recurrence	48 hr	Identified signs and symptoms accurately
Discuss necessity for life-style alterations with patient and wife	Decreases daily and weekend work hours Plans for daily periods of rest and relaxation Decreases active responsibilities related to sons' sports schedules—initiates sharing of responsibilities with other parents Decreases active involvement in community organizations—initiates sharing of responsibility with other members	During and after hospitalization	Patient and wife working together to begin life-style alterations compatible with stress reduction; sons included in plans Patient and wife listed desirable schedule of daily and weekend activities, incorporating plans for designated periods of rest and relaxation; aware of desirability of flexibility of schedule
Notify physician's office nurse of patient's need for reinforcement of teaching plan	Demonstrates adherence to therapeutic regimen, inclusive of medication and diet therapy and life-style alterations	First physician visit after discharge	

* For background information, see nursing care plan example (Chart 2-3), page 26.
† These times have not been standardized but are individualized according to the patient's needs.

niques can be used to measure changes in behavior that give evidence of learning. These include direct observation of behavior, using rating scales, checklists, or anecdotal notes to document the behaviors, and indirect measures, such as oral questioning and written tests. Measurement of actual behavior (direct measurement) is the most accurate and appropriate technique in many patient teaching situations. However, it should be supplemented with indirect measurements whenever possible. When more than one measurement technique is employed, the reliability of the resultant data is enhanced since each individual measurement technique carries with it a potential source of error.

The use of measurement techniques is only the beginning of evaluation. It is followed by the interpretation of the data and the making of value judgments about learning and teaching. Such evaluation should be done periodically throughout the teaching–learning program, at its conclusion, and at varying periods subsequent to the program. Evaluation of learning after hospitalization is highly desirable but is not always feasible in terms of time, economics, and nursing personnel required for such evaluation. However, coordination of efforts and sharing of information between hospital-based and community-based nursing personnel serves to facilitate such posthospital evaluation.

- It should always be remembered that evaluation is not the end step in the teaching–learning process. The information gathered during evaluation should be utilized to redirect teaching actions with the goal of improving the patient's responses and outcomes that result from the teaching actions.

As in the nursing process, the steps of the teaching–learning process are cyclic and recurrent. Each step is ongoing and is related to all other steps. Continuous evaluation

---

Chart 3-2
A Guide to Patient Teaching

Assessment

1. Assess the patient's readiness for health education.
    a. What are his health beliefs and behaviors?
    b. What psychosocial adaptation is he making?
    c. Is he ready to learn?
        Is he able to learn these behaviors?
        What additional information about him is needed?
        What are his expectations?
2. Formulate the nursing diagnoses that relate to the patient's learning needs.
    a. Organize, analyze, synthesize, and summarize the collected data.
    b. Identify the patient's learning problems, their characteristics, and etiology.
    c. State nursing diagnoses concisely and precisely.

Planning

1. Assign priority to the nursing diagnoses that relate to the patient's learning needs.
2. Specify the short-term, intermediate, and long-term nurse–patient established learning goals.
3. Identify teaching strategies appropriate for goal attainment.
4. Establish outcome criteria.
5. Develop the written teaching plan.
    a. Include diagnoses, goals, teaching strategies, and outcome criteria.
    b. Put the information to be taught in logical sequence.
    c. Write down the key points.
    d. Select appropriate teaching aids.
    e. Keep the plan current and flexible to meet the patient's changing learning needs.

6. Involve the patient, his family or significant others, nursing team members, and other health team members in all aspects of planning.

Implementation

1. Put the teaching plan into action.
2. Know the material to be presented.
3. Use language the patient can understand.
4. Use appropriate teaching aids.
5. Use the same equipment that the patient will utilize after discharge.
6. Encourage the patient to actively participate in learning.
7. Record the patient's responses to the teaching actions.

Evaluation

1. Collect objective data.
    a. Observe the patient.
    b. Ask questions to determine if he understands.
    c. Use rating scales, checklists, anecdotal notes, and written tests when appropriate.
2. Compare the patient's behavioral outcomes to the outcome criteria. Determine the extent to which the goals were achieved.
3. Include the patient, his family or significant others, nursing team members, and other health team members in the evaluation.
4. Identify alterations that need to be made in the teaching plan.
5. Make referrals to appropriate sources or agencies for reinforcement of learning after discharge.
6. Continue all steps of the teaching process: assessing, planning, implementing, evaluating.

provides the means for maintaining the viability of the entire teaching–learning process and for demonstrating accountability for the quality of the teaching provided.

Chart 3-2 is intended to assist in the nurse's utilization of the teaching–learning process.

▷ Bibliography
Books

Bille DA. Practical Approaches to Patient Teaching. Boston, Little, Brown & Co, 1981.

Redman BK. The Process of Patient Teaching in Nursing. St Louis, CV Mosby, 1980.

Squyres WD. Patient Education: An Inquiry into the State of the Art. New York, Springer, 1980.

Articles
General

Arvidson E et al. A health education model for ambulatory care. J Nurs Adm 1979 Mar; 9(3):16–21.

Cannon C and Magargal P. Patient education: The challenge, the opportunity. The Dean's List 1982 Feb.

Chaisson GM. Patient education: Whose responsibility is it and who should be doing it? Nurs Admin Q 1980 Winter; 4(2):1–11.

Evans LK. Health education from a group perspective. Top Clin Nurs 1980 July; 2(2):45–55.

George G. If patient teaching tries your patience, try this plan. Nursing '82 1982 May; 12(5):50–55.

Huckabay LMD. A strategy for patient teaching. Nurs Admin Q 1980 Winter; 4(2):47–54.

Jenny J. A strategy for patient teaching. J Adv Nurs 1978 July; 3(4):341–348.

McCaughrin WC. Patient understanding: The key to quality patient education. QRB 1981 May; 7(5):2–4.

Milazzo V. A study of the difference in health knowledge gained through formal and informal teaching. Heart Lung 1980 Nov–Dec; 9(6):1079–1082.

Nowakowski L. Health promotion/self-care programs for the community. Top Clin Nurs 1980 July; 2(2):21–27.

Rickel L. Why patient education? Oncol Nurs Forum 1981 Spring; 8(2):26–27.

Taylor AG, Skelton JA, and Czykowski RW. Do patients understand patient-education brochures? Nurs Health Care 1982 June; 3(6):305–310.

Adherence to Therapeutic Regimens

Becker MH and Maiman LA. Strategies for enhancing patient compliance. J Community Health 1980 Winter; 6(2):113–135.

Falvo DR. Improving patient compliance. QRB 1981 May; 7(5):5–8.

Haynes RB. Strategies for enhancing patient compliance. Drug Ther 1982 Jan; 12(1):147–154.

Ozuma J. Compliance with therapeutic regimens: Issues, answers, and research questions. J Neurosurg Nurs 1981 Feb; 13(1):1–6.

Stanitis MA and Ryan J. Noncompliance—an unacceptable diagnosis? Am J Nurs 1982 June; 82(6):941–942.

Unit II

Health Assessment of the Client/Patient

4

Clinical Interviewing: The Health History

The clinical interview is one of the most important facets of the nurse–patient relationship. It is through this process that the quality of the relationship is established, information sufficient to provide a thorough assessment of the patient's health status is obtained, and the foundation for nursing diagnosis is made. Behaviors appropriate to the interview and the techniques required to elicit appropriate information are not part of our everyday social lives. These behaviors and techniques must be learned. Interviewing skills require careful development and are refined through experience.

▷ The Role of the Nurse

The role of the nurse in the provision of health care is a dynamically changing one. The scope of nursing practice now includes not only those functions for which the nurse has traditionally been prepared, but a breadth of activities once reserved for physicians and other members of the health care team. In order to facilitate the nursing process, nurses are now employing skills that include gathering the patient data base and performing a physical examination. The concept that only the physician diagnoses patient problems and plans appropriate interventions has also changed.

Intrinsic to the concept of the health care team is the interdependence of health professionals, including physicians, nurses, nutritionists, social workers, and others, each maximizing his or her skills in contributing to the resolution of patient problems. Traditionally, nursing assessments and nursing histories have been present in a variety of styles, lengths, and focuses. Institutions and agencies developed tools that addressed their particular philosophies and concerns, and these tools often appeared in the patient's record as isolated data sheets. Rarely were such assessments reviewed by physicians and other members of the health team and incorporated into a total plan of care.

▷ The Health History

Throughout the nursing assessment, and particularly in the nursing history, interest is centered on the individual's psychosocial and cultural patterns. The interpersonal and physical environments, as well as the individual's life-style and activities of daily living, are explored in depth. Currently, however, many nurses are responsible for gathering a data base that includes a detailed history of the individual's current health problems, his past medical history, his family history, and a review of body systems. These areas, which constitute the focus of a medical history, were previously explored by the physician. The inclusion of these categories within the context of the nursing history has resulted in a total health profile that focuses on health as well as illness and is more appropriately called a health history, rather than a medical or a nursing history. The format of the health history is a combination of the traditional medical history and the nursing assessment. Both the review of systems and patient profile are expanded to include individual and family relationships, life-style patterns, health practices, and coping strategies. These components of the health history are the backbone of the nursing assessment and can easily be adapted to address the philosophy of nursing at a particular institution or agency and the needs of a particular patient population.

The consolidation of the medical history format and the nursing history format within one health history avoids a duplication of information, minimizes efforts on the part of the patient to provide this information, and encourages collaborative effort between the nurse and physician, who may choose to share in the collection and interpretation of the data base.

In order to contribute significantly to the health history, it is necessary for the nurse to be cognizant of (1) ethical considerations in data collection, (2) communication skills and techniques of the interviewing process, and (3) the content of the health history.

▷ Ethical Considerations in Data Collection

Whenever information is elicited from an individual, that individual has the right to know why the information is sought and how this information will be used. For this reason, the nurse not only identifies herself and her role, but explains in detail what a health history is, how the information is elicited, and how this information will be used.

It is important that the individual be fully informed of all aspects of the data collection process and that his decision to participate be freely made. A private setting for the interview promotes an atmosphere of trust between the individual and the nurse and encourages open, honest communication.

Following the interview, the nurse selectively records data that is pertinent to the individual's health status on the health history form. Isolated personal facts or highly sensitive information (arrest record, illegal drug use) are not initially entered in the health record but are discussed with the head nurse, supervisor, or physician. Occasionally, individuals share very confidential matters with the nurse, and the responsibility for the disposition of such information is best shared.

When the interview is completed and the data recorded, the written record is secured from the public and from those health professionals not directly involved in the care of the individual. This is another method of ensuring confidentiality and maintaining a high standard of nursing care and professional conduct.

▷ Basic Guidelines for the Interviewer

- The interviewer approaches the patient as a unique individual. The interviewer puts the individual at ease and provides for his comfort.

The individual who seeks health care for a specific problem is almost invariably anxious. He does not fully understand the significance of his symptoms. Anxiety is compounded by fears related to potential disruption of the person's life-style and perhaps by apprehension about the costs of health care. Given this set of circumstances, the individual feels helpless, for he perceives that the outcome with respect to both his health and his economic well-being lies in the hands of others.

To minimize the patient's anxieties, the nurse introduces herself to the patient, defines her role on the health care team, and explains what the health history is. The nurse further explains that the health history will be used to identify areas of concern to the patient and the nurse regarding the health status of the patient. The individual is reassured that all the information shared is confidential and that only health professionals directly involved in his care will have access to that information.

The nurse ensures a private setting for the interview. If visitors are present, they are asked to leave, firmly but politely, since the patient may find it difficult to communicate when visitors (even close relatives) are present. If, on the other hand, the individual expresses a desire to have a family member present during the interview, this is acceptable and may generate additional information that the patient might otherwise forget or be unable to share. Distractions, such as those caused by radios or television sets, are excluded from the environment.

The interview is conducted with due consideration for the individual's comfort and self-respect. Before beginning, the nurse sees that the individual is comfortable. If the interview is taking place in a hospital room, the nurse asks the patient if he would like another pillow or would prefer to be seated in a chair rather than in bed. The patient who is short of breath may be more comfortable in a sitting position than he would be if supine. If the patient is in pain or in urgent need of going to the bathroom, his discomfort is attended to before the interview begins.

- The interviewer permits the individual to express himself fully.

The goal of the clinical interview is to obtain all of the facts that will ultimately influence both the nursing diagnoses and the plan of care. When pursuing this objective, one constantly strives to assert the least amount of authority necessary to obtain information in the time allotted. This is best achieved in an atmosphere that encourages spontaneity on the part of the individual. Such spontaneity is influenced by the physical setting and by the behavior of the nurse. Even the simple act of the nurse's sitting during the interview conveys an important message to the patient.

It is therefore the nurse's role to facilitate spontaneous behavior and an unrestricted description of the problem as the patient perceives it. Nonverbal communication on the part of the nurse is a critical element in promoting full expression by the patient. The nurse may actively encourage the individual to elaborate or continue by a nod of the head or by repeating the last few words if the patient appears hesitant. A puzzled look will encourage the patient to clarify apparent inconsistencies in the story.

Questions posed are frequently open-ended. "How can we help you?" "Tell me about it." "How did it feel?" are all appropriate questions. "Was it a sharp pain?" "Did it happen only on weekdays?" are inappropriate questions. Such questions presume the answer. Although one certainly wishes to obtain this information, it is sought in a more open-ended way. Otherwise, the patient attempts to "help" the nurse by providing the answer he thinks the nurse wants to hear.

However, the use of open-ended questions is not a useful technique to be employed throughout the entire interview. In order to refine the details that are important to the analysis of symptoms, some degree of direct questioning is necessary. Such questions provide the patient with options for his response. For example, the question "Does the pain have any relationship to meals?" gives the individual the option of answering yes or no. Similarly, the question "Does the pain come before the meal, during the meal, or after the meal?" gives the individual the opportunity to select from among several options. This more direct line of questioning is deferred until later in the interview when the patient has had an opportunity to express himself as fully as possible and his urge to "help" the nurse has been submerged by a well-developed sense of trust and confidence.

It is not assumed that the approach to every patient will be the same. Clearly, the nurse will have to be more directive with certain patients. The sophistication that allows modulation of the interview technique comes only with experience.

- The interviewer uses a health history form to guide the interview and adjusts the sequence of questions to coincide with the flow of conversation.

The health history form is a tool designed to assist the nurse in the collection of data relevant to the individual's health status. For this reason, the form is not memorized or rigidly adhered to at the expense of the individual. For example, if the individual is sharing information about a particular problem and the nurse interrupts to ask direct questions about occupation, education, or family relationships, the flow of information may be broken, and important facts overlooked.

It is also essential to "listen" to the individual as he answers the questions. Brief note-taking during the interview is acceptable, but when overdone is highly distracting to the individual being interviewed. It also limits eye contact and conveys an impersonal message.

- The interviewer demonstrates an understanding of the nature and intensity of the individual's problem.

The interviewing process does not consist entirely of questions and answers. The manner in which the nurse responds nonverbally to the individual, and her ability to listen convey a genuine willingness to understand the meaning of the individual's concerns. Such behavior is often very reassuring to the individual, and thus, the mode of the interview moves from inquiring to therapeutic.

When the patient becomes silent during the interview, he may be emotionally overcome or may be attempting to formulate an accurate description of events. Such silences need not be intruded upon by the nurse. Nor are tearful episodes interrupted. One resists the urge to tell the patient that matters are going to be all right or to provide similar verbal reassurances. Things may not be all right, and the reassurance may appear false. Moreover, the nurse has much to learn by exploring the individual's fears and anxieties. Sometimes open-ended statements, such as "You look sad," or "You seem frightened," will encourage the individual to elaborate upon his feelings and at the same time convey the nurse's empathy.

The nurse also makes every attempt to convey an understanding of and a respect for the individual's beliefs and attitudes. This is done in spite of the fact that such beliefs and attitudes may differ sharply from those held by the nurse. There is no place in the interview for a comment such as "You don't really believe that, do you?" If the individual does not believe it, it is unlikely that he would state it candidly to the health professional conducting the interview. A nonjudgmental attitude is especially necessary when dealing with matters related to sexuality, drug and alcohol use, and cultural patterns.

- The interviewer takes into account the individual's cultural background.

Cultural attitudes about family relationships and the role of women are accepted at face value, just as attitudes toward pain, illness, and hospitalization are accepted. These beliefs and attitudes are derived from personal experiences, which vary according to the individual's cultural background.

- The interviewer is aware of his or her own feelings and attitudes.

Patient behavior that the nurse might find offensive in herself, her family, or her friends may arouse hostility, anger, anxiety, or even, at times, revulsion. The professional cannot allow this to be conveyed to the patient. Quite unconsciously, the nurse might convey irritation, boredom, or disbelief. Similarly, the nurse may be acutely uncomfortable when dealing with individuals who have certain kinds of illnesses, because of her own fears. The nurse's own ethical and moral sense may make it difficult to develop relationships with alcoholic or drug-dependent patients. It is a frequent failing of health professionals to view self-inflicted illness with disdain, hostility, and anger. Feelings are intensified when the patient is acutely intoxicated, and the nurse may return hostility for hostility. The first step in dealing effectively with such patients is to understand the inner compulsions that cause the interviewer to reject the patient.

- The interviewer is attuned to nonverbal communication and learns to recognize gestures that convey defensiveness, hostility, confidence, impatience, etc.

The nurse learns to respond to body language the same way she responds to the spoken word. Much has been written about body language, and a quick perusal of an illustrated book on this subject is highly informative. Frequently, the body language and the patient's verbal expression are at variance. Often, this is obvious—as when the patient describes a seemingly happy event yet appears to be on the verge of tears. The interviewer might respond to such inconsistencies by drawing them to the patient's attention.

- The interviewer communicates in a manner that is consistent with the individual's level of understanding.

This is especially true in regard to the patient's educational background. The nurse is an intelligent person selected from the population for advanced education by virtue of capacities and opportunities not possessed by a large segment of the population. Her use of the English language is sophisticated, and she also possesses a health care vocabulary that is foreign to the majority of the population. Questions are phrased in such a way that they are easily understood by the patient, and counseling is done using as few technical terms as possible. If the patient does not understand the language being used, it is unlikely that he will interrupt for clarification, largely out of fear that he will appear ignorant. Careful questioning may reveal the level of the patient's understanding of an issue that has just been discussed.

A second factor influencing the patient's level of understanding is cultural background. The Puerto Rican mother, for example, has a different perception of personal health than does a mother born and raised in an American suburb. Pregnancy is not something for which she would seek care and attention until labor begins. Thus, she would not understand the need for prenatal care as advocated by health professionals. Nor would a woman from a culture in which obesity is a way of life and admired by men understand the need for diet and weight control. Similarly, Oriental women, not accustomed to complaining of pain, even when severe, would not appreciate the advantages of taking analgesics. All such differences in outlook must be taken into account when dealing with members of other cultures.

Even differences in the life experiences of those who are well educated and from the same cultural background must be considered. An only child of an urban or suburban family may be ill-equipped to deal with the problems of being a mother, in contrast to a woman from a rural society who was reared in a family of eight or ten children. In large families, older children participate in rearing the young.

- The interviewer terminates the interview in an appropriate manner that summarizes the information obtained and ensures that the individual has understood major points discussed.

Before ending the interview, the nurse inquires whether the individual has any questions. The nurse specifically searches for areas of misunderstanding by briefly summarizing the individual's responses. This gives the individual the opportunity to correct misinformation and also to add facts that he may have forgotten to mention earlier.

▷ Content of the Interview

When the patient is seen for the first time by the health team (except in the emergency care situation), the first requisite is to obtain a *data base*. The nurse may be responsible for all or a part of that data base, but in either case the nurse must be familiar with all of its facets. The data base contains the following components:

1. Biographical data
2. Informant
3. Chief complaint
4. History of present illness (or present health concern)
5. Past medical history
6. Review of systems
7. Family history
8. Patient profile
9. Physical examination
10. Radiologic and laboratory information
11. Problem formulation (medical and nursing diagnoses)

Biographical Data
Biographical or introductory identifying information helps to put much of the history in context. This information includes the name, address, age, and sex of the individual, as well as his marital status, occupation, and ethnic origins. Some people prefer a full patient profile at this juncture, but most believe a full profile to be inappropriate until the interviewer has obtained the trust and confidence of the patient. Moreover, a patient in pain, or with an equally urgent problem for which he seeks attention, is unlikely to put a great deal of confidence in an interviewer who is more concerned with the details of his marital status than with quickly addressing the problem for which the patient seeks help.

The Informant
The informant may not always be the patient, as is the case if the patient is a child or an elderly person, or is unconscious, in a coma, or suffering a severe psychiatric disturbance. The interviewer assesses the reliability of the informant and the usefulness of the information provided. For

example, hysterical or depressed patients are unlikely to provide a reliable data base, while patients who abuse drugs and alcohol are likely to use denial as part of their operating mechanism. It is reasonable for the interviewer to make such judgments (based on the context of the entire interview) and to incorporate them in the record.

Chief Complaint

The chief complaint is the issue that brings the patient to seek help. Asking questions such as "What brings you to the clinic today?" or "Why have you been admitted to the hospital?" usually elicits the chief complaint. Frequently, the patient appears without a specific complaint, seeking an ongoing relationship with a health team or requesting a "checkup." If this is the case, it is noted in lieu of a chief complaint. Once the patient has expressed his concern, his exact words are transposed to the record in quotation marks. However, a statement such as "Doctor Smith sent me," is not a chief complaint. Although such information can be included as part of the introductory patient profile, the patient should be asked why he sought Dr. Smith's attention, and this reason should be entered as the chief complaint. If the patient has been admitted for a special purpose, it is so stated (*e.g.*, "for cholecystectomy").

Frequently, the patient will have more than one problem and, therefore, more than one complaint. These are listed in terms of the patient's priorities and then explored through the present illness as separate entities, if they represent separate problems, or as a single present illness if they are multiple manifestations of one cohesive problem.

History of Present Illness (HPI)

Exploration of the facts related to a present illness frequently requires substantial knowledge of the pathophysiology and natural history of disease. If one does not know, for example, the manifestations of an acute myocardial infarction, it is difficult to subtly extract information that will ultimately lead to the diagnosis. The history of any illness is the single most important factor in enabling the health professional to arrive at a diagnosis. The physical examination is helpful but usually reveals manifestations that are an expected consequence of the story that has unfolded. Occasionally, laboratory and radiologic information can be singularly helpful; only rarely do they establish the diagnosis. On the other hand, judicious selection of laboratory and radiologic inquiry demands a careful history.

The "present illness" may well be but one episode in a sequence that is contained within a single disease process. An episode of insulin shock, for example, is only one of an ordered series of occurrences that define the natural history of diabetes. In such an instance, the entire course of the diabetic illness is unfolded in order to put the current complaint in context. Although the episode of insulin shock gains prominence in the delineation of the story, the description of it is obtained in the context of the natural history of the disease and communicated to the record in a similar manner. After all the facts have been obtained from the patient, the details of the present illness, or health concern, from onset until the time of contact with the health team, are constructed. These facts are recorded in *chronological order,* beginning with, for example, "The patient was in

good health until . . ." or "The patient first experienced nausea 2 months prior to admission 1/4/84."

The history of the present illness is a compact, complete story, rather than a statement of numerous disconnected facts. It includes such information as the date and manner (sudden, gradual) of the onset of the problem, the setting in which the problem developed (at home, at work, after an argument), manifestations of the problem, and the course of the illness or problem. The course of the illness or problem includes self-treatment, medical interventions, progress and effects of treatment, and the patient's perceptions of the cause or meaning of the problem.

Specific symptoms (pain, headache, fever, change in bowel habits) are delineated in detail. Critical to the analysis of a symptom is its location and radiation (if pain), quality, severity, and duration. The interviewer also pursues the persistence or intermittence of the symptom, factors that aggravate or alleviate it, and any associated manifestations that the patient may be aware of.

Associated manifestations are symptoms that occur simultaneously with the chief complaint. The presence or absence of associated symptoms may shed light on the origin or extent of the patient's problem, as well as the diagnosis. These symptoms are referred to as significant positive or negative findings and are derived from a review of systems directly related to the chief complaint. For instance, if the patient is complaining of a vague symptom, such as fatigue or weight loss, all body systems are reviewed and included in the history of the present illness. If, on the other hand, the patient's chief complaint is chest pain, only the cardiopulmonary and gastrointestinal systems would be included in the history of present illness. In either situation, both positive and negative findings are recorded.

Past Medical History

A detailed summary of the patient's past medical history is a valuable component of the data base. After obtaining a statement about the patient's general health in the past, the nurse proceeds in an orderly fashion to inquire about the patient's immunization status and any known allergies to drugs or other substances. The dates of immunization, along with the type of allergy and adverse reactions, are recorded. The patient is asked to provide information about his last physical examination, chest x-ray study, ECG, eye examination, hearing examination, dental checkup, and Pap smear (if female). The patient is then interviewed about previous illnesses. Negative as well as positive responses are recorded. Dates, or the age of the patient at the time of illness, as well as the names of the physician and hospital, the diagnosis, and the treatment are also recorded. A history of the following areas is elicited:

- Childhood illness—rubeola, rubella, polio, whooping cough, mumps, chickenpox, scarlet fever, rheumatic fever, strep throat
- Adult illnesses
- Psychiatric illnesses
- Injuries—burns, fractures, head injuries
- Hospitalizations
- Operations
- Current medications—prescription, over-the-counter, home remedies

If a particular hospitalization or major medical intervention is related to the present illness, it need not be repeated; rather, the nurse makes a reference such as "see history of present illness" or "see HPI" on the data sheet.

Family History

The age and health status, or the age and cause of death, of first-order relatives (parents, siblings, spouse, children) and second-order relatives (grandparents, cousins) are elicited to identify diseases that may be hereditary, communicable, or possibly environmental. The nurse specifically inquires about such conditions as cancer, hypertension, heart disease, diabetes, epilepsy, mental illness, tuberculosis, kidney disease, arthritis, allergies, asthma, alcoholism, and obesity. One of the easiest methods of recording such data is the family tree (Fig. 4-1).

Review of Systems

This section of the history includes a complete inventory of major body organ systems in terms of the presence or absence of symptoms past or present. It serves as a check and balance to prevent the interviewer from overlooking any relevant data. Negative as well as positive responses are recorded. If the patient responds positively, that symptom is analyzed according to the process outlined under the history of present illness. Illnesses that have been previously described in the history of the present illness or the past medical history need not be repeated. Reference is made to the appropriate location of relevant information. The system review includes an overview of general health as well as symptoms related to each body system. A review of systems can be organized in a formal checklist, which becomes a part of the health history. Some of these forms are commercially available and others are prepared by health teams in a manner appropriate to team goals and functions. One asset of the checklist process is that it is easily audited and less subject to error than is relying on

the memory of the interviewer, who must obtain detailed information relevant to each organ system. One such format is outlined in Chart 4-1.

Patient Profile

The patient profile is an amplification of the biographical data that is elicited at the beginning of the interview. A complete composite, or profile, of the individual is critical to an analysis of his problem, his capacity to deal with that problem, and the health team's capacity to provide assistance.

The focus of the information elicited at this point in the interview is highly personal and subjective. During this stage of the interview, the nurse encourages the patient's open and uninhibited expression of feelings, values, and personal experiences. Usually, the nurse begins with general open-ended questions and then moves to direct questioning when specific facts are needed. The patient is often less anxious when the interview progresses from information that is less personal (birthplace, occupation, education) to information that is more personal (sexuality, body image, coping abilities).

A general patient profile consists of six content areas:

- Past development
- Education and occupation
- Environment (physical, spiritual, interpersonal)
- Life-style (patterns and habits)
- Self-concept
- Stress response

The patient profile is outlined in Chart 4-2.

Past Development. The patient profile begins with a brief life history. Questions about the patient's place of birth and places where he has lived in the past assist the patient in focusing on the earlier years of his life. Personal experiences during childhood or adolescence that have special significance to the individual may be elicited by asking,

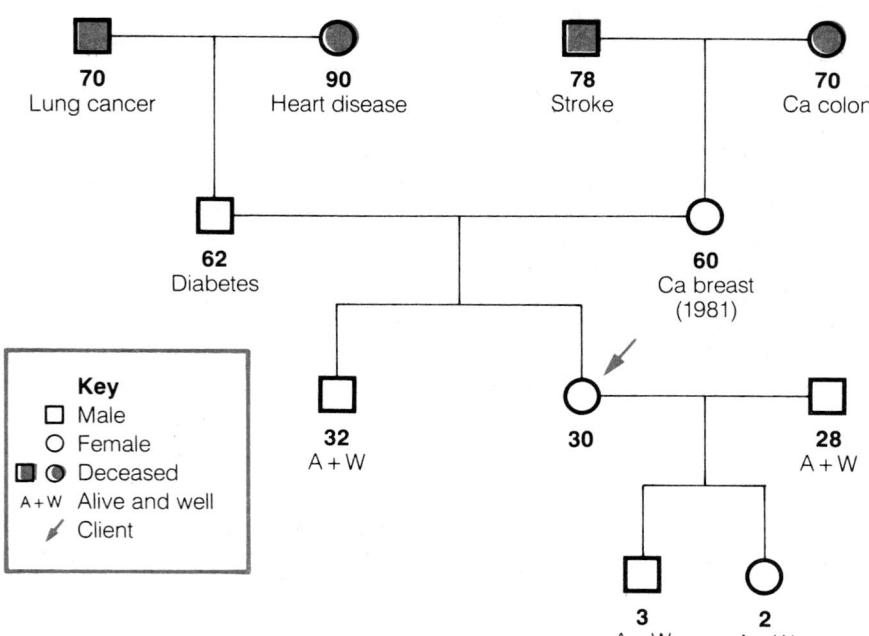

Figure 4-1. Sample recording of family history as a "family tree." Grandparents, parents, siblings, spouse, and children are identified.

"Was there anything that you experienced as a child or adolescent that would be helpful for me to know about?" The interviewer's intent is to encourage the individual to make a quick review of his earlier life, highlighting an event or circumstance of particular significance. Sometimes the individual will not be able to recall anything that he feels is meaningful to share with the nurse. On the other hand, the individual may take the opportunity to share such information as a personal achievement, a failure, a developmental crisis, an instance of physical or emotional abuse, or a valued loss.

Education and Occupation.   Questions related to economic status and educational preparation can be threatening to the individual and are approached indirectly through a focus on his current occupation. If the individual is employed, a statement such as "Tell me about your job" often elicits information about his role, job tasks, and satisfaction with the position. It may be necessary to interject direct questions related to past employment and career goals if the individual does not initially provide this information.

Asking the person "What kind of educational requirements were necessary to attain your present job?" is a more sensitive approach to educational background than "Did you graduate from high school?". It is rarely necessary to know the actual numerical value of the individual's salary; the information needed is whether his income is sufficient to meet his expenses and support the life-style to which he is accustomed. Questions such as "Do you have any financial concerns at this time?" or "Sometimes there just doesn't seem to be enough money to make ends meet. Are you finding this true?" may be helpful. Inquiry about the individual's insurance coverage and plans for health care payment are also appropriate.

Environment.   The person's physical environment and its potential hazards, his spiritual awareness, cultural background, interpersonal relationships, and support system are included in the concept of environment.

Physical Environment.   The type of housing (apartment, duplex, single family) in which the person lives, its location, and information related to safety and comfort within the person's home and neighborhood is elicited. The nurse attempts to identify environmental hazards, such as isolation, inadequate protection, potential fire risks, pollution (noise, air, water), and inadequate sanitation facilities.

Spiritual Environment.   To be thoughtful or contemplative about one's existence, to accept challenges in one's life, and to seek and find answers to personal questions is to be "spiritual." For many persons, this spirituality is expressed through identification with a particular religion. Like cultural influences, spiritual values and beliefs direct the individual's behavior and his approach to health problems and the health care system in general. An individual's spirituality is often challenged during the experience of an illness or a developmental crisis. The individual may experience considerable turmoil about the meaning of this problem or crisis in his life. He is challenged to new perceptions and spiritual growth, and he may find this difficult. A brief spiritual assessment by the nurse is important; it focuses on three areas:

- The extent to which religion is a part of the individual's life
- Religious beliefs related to the individual's perception of health and illness
- Religious practices

The following questions can be used in a spiritual assessment:
- Is religion or God important to you?
    If yes, In what way?
    If no, What is the most important thing in your life?
- Are there any religious practices that are important to you?
- Do you have any spiritual concerns because of your present health problem?

Interpersonal Environment.   This aspect embraces cultural influences, relationships with family and friends, and the presence or absence of a support system.
1. Ethnic background. The beliefs and practices that have been shared from generation to generation are known as cultural or ethnic patterns. They are expressed through language, dress, dietary choices, role behaviors, perceptions of health and illness, and in health related behaviors. The influence of these beliefs and customs on the individual's experience with a health problem and his relationship with the health care team cannot be underestimated. For this reason, an individual's ethnic identity (cultural and social) as well as his racial identity (biological) are determined. The following questions may assist the nurse in obtaining relevant information:
   - Where did your parents or ancestors come from? When?
   - What language do you speak at home?
   - Are there certain customs or values that are important to you?
   - Is there anything special you do to keep in good health?
   - Do you have any specific practices for treating illness?
2. Family relationships and support system. An assessment of family structure (members, ages, roles), patterns of communication, and the presence or absence of a support system is an integral part of the patient profile. Although the traditional "family" is recognized as a mother, father, and children, it is important to keep in mind that there are many different types of living arrangements within our society. "Family" may be interpreted to mean two or more people bound by emotional ties or commitments. Such an open definition of "family" encompasses the couple who live together but are not married, the college student whose dormitory companions provide a "family" structure, or the single person who lives alone but has significant relationships and a support system.

Life-style.   This section of the patient profile provides the nurse with the opportunity to gain information about health related behaviors. These behaviors include patterns

(Text continues on page 51)

Chart 4-1
Review of Systems

Positive responses are circled and described in detail. Negative responses are underlined to indicate the absence of the symptom.

General	Usual weight	Weakness
	Weight change	Fatigue
	Appetite change	Fever
	Night sweats	
Skin	Rash	Pruritus
	Color change	Growths or masses
	Dryness	Hair changes
	Nail changes	
Head	Headache	Dizziness
	Trauma	
Eyes	Vision (near and far)	Blurring
	Glasses or contacts	Pain
	Photophobia	Infection
	Diplopia	Itching
Ears	Hearing	Hygiene practices
	Pain	Tinnitus
	Infection	Vertigo
	Excessive cerumen	
Nose and Sinuses	Discharge	Epistaxis
	Allergies	Pain
	Obstruction	Frequent colds
Mouth and Throat	Sore throats	Dentures or partial plate
	Difficulty swallowing	Hoarseness
	Taste	Lesions (lips, tongue, mucosa)
	Gums	Hygiene practices
	Dentition	
Neck	Stiffness	Limited motion
	Swelling	"Swollen glands"
	Pain	Thyroid disease
Breasts	Pain	Nipple discharge
	Swelling	Dimpling
	Self-examination practices	
Respiratory	Cough	Sputum (color, quantity)
	Shortness of breath (SOB)	Asthma
	Hemoptysis	Recurrent upper respiratory infection (URI)
	Wheezing	

(continued)

Chart 4-1
Review of Systems (continued)

Cardiovascular	Shortness of breath (SOB) Dyspnea on exertion (DOE) Orthopnea Chest pain Palpitations Paroxysmal nocturnal dyspnea (PND)	Phlebitis Coldness or numbness of extremities Edema Varicosities Claudication
Gastrointestinal	Anorexia Nausea Vomiting Indigestion Diarrhea Pain Constipation	Hematemesis Melena Jaundice Food intolerance Change in bowel pattern Hemorrhoids
Genitourinary	Nocturia Incontinence Infection Urgency	Dysuria Dribbling Frequency Hematuria
Genito-reproductive	Female Menses (menarche, cycle, duration, amount, cramps, intermittent bleeding, last menstrual period [LMP]) Number of pregnancies, live births, abortions (G__P__Ab__) If menopausal: age of menses cessation, symptoms of menopause, postmenopausal bleeding	Vaginal discharge Dyspareunia Contraception Pruritus Social (venereal) disease
	Male Pain Discharge Swelling	Sores Social (venereal) disease Contraception practices
Musculoskeletal	Muscular pain or cramps Pain, swelling, or redness of joints Back pain or history of injury	Limitation of movement Ability to perform ADL
Endocrine	Heat or cold intolerance Excessive sweating Changes in hair pattern	Excessive thirst, hunger, or urination
Neurologic	Syncope Seizures Paralysis Weakness Dizziness Vertigo	Numbness or tingling Problems with speech or gait Tremors Memory loss Loss of sensation
Hematologic	Blood transfusions Anemia Easy bruising or bleeding	

Chart 4-2
Patient Profile

Past Development	Place of birth
	Places lived
	Significant childhood/adolescent experiences
Education and Occupation	Jobs held in past
	Current position/job
	Length of time at position
	Educational preparation
	Work satisfaction and career goals
	Financial resources
	Insurance coverage
Environment	Physical
	Living arrangements (type of housing, neighborhood, presence of hazards)
	Spiritual
	Extent to which religion is a part of individual's life
	Religious beliefs related to perception of health and illness
	Religious practices
	Interpersonal
	Ethnic background (language spoken, customs and values held, folk practices used to maintain health or to cure illness)
	Family relationships (family structure, roles, communication patterns, support system)
	Friendships (quality of relationship)
Life-style	Patterns
	Sleep (time individual retires, hours per night, comfort measures, awakens rested?)
	Exercise (type, frequency, time spent)
	Nutrition (24-hour diet recall, idiosyncrasies, restrictions)
	Recreation (type of activity, time spent)
	Habits
	Caffeine (coffee, tea, cola, chocolate)—kind, amount
	Smoking (cigarette, pipe, cigar, marijuana)—kind, amount per day, number of years, desire to quit
	Alcohol—kind, amount, pattern over past year
Self-concept	View of self in present
	View of self in future
	Body image (level of satisfaction, concerns)
	Sexuality—Perception of self as a man or woman
	Quality of sexual relationships
	Concerns related to sexuality or sexual functioning
Stress Response	Major concerns or problems at present
	Past experiences with similar problems
	Past coping patterns and outcomes
	Present coping strategies and anticipated outcomes
	Individual's expectations of family/friends and health team in problem resolution

of sleep, exercise, nutrition, and recreation, as well as personal habits of smoking and the use of alcohol and caffeine. Most persons have little difficulty sharing particulars about their sleeping patterns or recreational choices. On the other hand, many persons are quite sensitive to questions about their smoking and alcohol use. The individual may fear the nurse's scrutiny and thus may minimize the extent of his habit. For this reason, the nurse may be able to elicit more information by asking "What kind of alcohol do you enjoy drinking at a party?" rather than "Do you drink?". Describing the individual as a "social drinker" is vague and not recommended. Instead, the nurse identifies specifically the type of alcohol and the amount ingested per day or per week (*e.g.,* 1 pint whiskey daily × 2 years).

When the nurse suspects that alcohol abuse may be a problem, additional information may be obtained by asking "Has anyone ever said that drinking might be causing a problem for you?" or "Have you ever considered cutting down your alcohol intake?". In a similar fashion, the nurse elicits information related to smoking and caffeine consumption.

Self-concept. The self-concept is a product of relevant experiences with others and is the result of others' reactions to the "self." It is the impression one has of oneself, the product of years of input and interpretation by the individual. Sometimes the interviewer can assess the individual's self-concept by asking him about his view of the present ("How do you feel about your life in general?") and his outlook for the future ("What will your life be like in the future?" or "How do you see yourself in a few years?").

Health concerns may threaten the way an individual perceives himself. His body image, the mental picture he has of himself, is vulnerable during normal developmental crises (adolescence, pregnancy, aging) and also as a result of certain medical and surgical interventions. Simply being hospitalized can alter an individual's perception of himself. Suddenly he sees himself as weak, helpless, and impotent. Surgical alterations such as a colostomy or a mastectomy pose an even greater threat to body image. It is therefore important for the nurse to be aware of the individual's perceptions of himself and his body. The following questions may elicit useful information:

- What do you like most about yourself?
- What would you change about yourself if you could?
- Do you have any particular concerns about your body?

Sexuality. No area of assessment is more personal than a sexual history. Because of anxiety on the part of the interviewer, this area of the patient profile is often overlooked or inadequately assessed. A lack of knowledge related to sexuality and anxiety about her own sexuality may hinder the nurse's effectiveness. The nurse may be perplexed about how or when to elicit this information in a sensitive way.

This assessment can be approached at the end of the interview along with the interpersonal or life-style assessment, or it can be a part of the genitourinary history within the review of systems. The nurse may find it easier to approach a discussion of sexuality following a discussion of menstruation, for instance. A similar discussion with the male patient would follow questions related to the urinary system.

It is advisable to begin the assessment with a general question that takes into consideration the developmental stage of the individual and the presence or absence of intimate relationships. For instance, when discussing sexuality with an adolescent, one or two of the following questions may be helpful:

- Do you have a special friend, a close relationship right now? Tell me about this closeness.
- Some teenagers are interested in having a sexual relationship at this age . . . how do you feel about that?

Such questions may lead to a discussion of concerns related to sexual expression, to the quality of a relationship, or to questions about contraception.

Whether the individual is young or old, the nurse determines whether he is sexually active before exploring issues related to sexual identity, contraception, or the quality of the sexual relationship. The nurse is careful to avoid making assumptions related to fidelity, heterosexuality, or sexual practices. Questions are worded in such a way that the individual feels free to discuss his sexuality as a single person or as a homosexual. Direct questions are usually less threatening when prefaced with such statements as "Most people feel that . . ." or "Many people worry about . . ." This suggests the normalcy of such feelings or behavior and encourages the individual to share information that he might otherwise leave out because he feels that his behavior or feelings are objectionable or different.

The needs of the individual direct the flow of the interview at all times. If the individual is abrupt with his responses and indicates that he does not wish to carry the discussion any further, the nurse proceeds to another part of the data collection. By introducing the subject of sexuality, however, the nurse has indicated to the individual that a discussion of sexual concerns is acceptable and that she will be approachable in the future. (See also Chap. 13, *Human Sexuality.*)

Stress Response. Every individual handles a stressful event in a manner that is intended to eliminate or minimize the stress. The individual's adaptive ability hinges on his capacity to cope effectively with the stressful situation. Exploring past coping patterns, as well as perceptions of current stresses and anticipated outcomes, assists the nurse in identifying the individual's overall ability to handle stress. It is especially important to identify expectations that the individual may have of his family, friends, and the health care team in helping him resolve his problems.

As was previously mentioned, the patient profile section of the data base constitutes the major component of the nursing assessment and represents the nursing profession's strongest contribution to the data base. The education of the nurse and the focus of nursing practice clearly demonstrate this. The extent of the patient profile is usually determined by the individual's needs and the philosophy of nursing at a particular institution or agency. For all patients, however, a general assessment of the categories outlined provides a significant composite profile of the individual. Such a profile is appropriate whether the health problem is acute or chronic and whether the setting is an inpatient or outpatient one.

Health concerns that usually are not complex (earache, tonsillectomy) and can be resolved in a short period of time usually do not require the depth or detail that is required when one is confronted with an individual who is experiencing a major illness or health concern. Additional assessments that go beyond the general patient profile may be employed when the individual's health problems are acute and complex or when the illness is chronic in nature. Specific interviewing tools have been developed by nurses to address areas of family assessment, spiritual assessment, sexuality assessment, and psychological assessment. The reader is referred to articles and books listed in the bibliography for additional learning.

The Remainder of the Data Base

Following a health history, a physical examination is performed. This is discussed in depth in Chapter 5. Based on the information elicited from the history and the physical examination, radiologic and laboratory tests may be indicated. Problem formulation, or statements of medical and nursing diagnoses, and a plan for the management of these problems are included in a discussion of the problem-oriented record in Chapter 6.

Summary

The process of eliciting a health history is a highly complex one that requires new knowledge and understanding, clinical laboratory learning, and reinforcement in the practice setting. There is no one way to approach an individual, or to elicit a health history. The nurse is encouraged to develop a style of interviewing that complements her personality and a health history format that is flexible, to accommodate the practice setting and the individual's needs. The health history format and interviewing techniques outlined in this chapter are presented as guidelines for the nurse in her acquisition of the initial components of the data base.

▷ **Bibliography**

Books

Bernstein L and Bernstein RS. Interviewing: A Guide for Health Professionals, 3rd ed. New York, Appleton–Century–Crofts, 1980.

Gillies DA and Alyn IB. Patient Assessment and Management by the Nurse Practitioner. Philadelphia, WB Saunders, 1976.

Grimes J and Iannopollo E. Health Assessment in Nursing Practice. Belmont, California, Wadsworth Health Sciences Division, 1982.

Hillman RS et al. Clinical Skills: Interviewing, History Taking and Physical Diagnosis. New York, McGraw-Hill, 1981.

Malasanos L et al. Health Assessment. St Louis, CV Mosby, 1981.

Rudy EB and Gray VR. Handbook of Health Assessment. Bowie, Maryland, Robert J. Brady, 1981.

Sana JM and Judge AD (eds). Physical Appraisal Methods in Nursing Practice. Boston, Little, Brown & Co, 1975.

Sherman JL Jr and Fields SK. Guide to Patient Evaluation. Garden City, New York, Medical Examination, 1982.

Articles

Mallick MJ. Patient assessment—based on data, not intuition. Nurs Outlook 1981 Oct; 29(10):800–805.

Mengel A. Getting the most from patient interviews. Nursing '82 1982 Nov; 12(11):46–49.

Minor HE and Macauley CA. The nurse as admission evaluator. Am J Nurs 1981 Jan; 81(1):118.

Schneggenberger C. History taking skills. How do you rate? Nursing '79 1979 Mar; 9(3):97–101.

5

Physical Assessment

Physical assessment, or the physical examination, is an integral part of the nursing assessment. This portion of the data collection process is usually performed following the health history.

In order to facilitate the physical examination, the examiner performs the assessments in a well-lighted, warm area. The patient is undressed and draped appropriately so that only the area to be examined is exposed. The physical and psychological comfort of the patient are considered at all times. For this reason, procedures and their rationale are fully explained. If a particular maneuver is apt to cause discomfort, an explanation of what to expect precedes that part of the examination. The examiner's hands are washed prior to and immediately following the examination. Fingernails are kept short to avoid injuring the patient.

The key to obtaining appropriate data in the least possible amount of time is an organized and systematic examination. Such an approach refines physical assessment skills and encourages cooperation and trust on the part of the patient.

The patient's health history provides the examiner with a complete health profile that guides all aspects of the physical examination. It helps to focus on body organs and systems that are of particular concern to the patient.

The basic tools of the physical examination are the human senses of vision, hearing, touch, and smell. These human tools may be augmented by special man-made tools (*e.g.,* the stethoscope, the ophthalmoscope) to permit a better definition of visual and acoustic details, but these man-made tools should be recognized for what they are: extensions of the human senses. One may hear it implied that some of these tools are sophisticated devices that require divine knowledge for their use; in fact, they are simple instruments that anyone can learn to use, and use well. Sophistication comes with the interpretation of what is seen and heard.

▷ The Process of Physical Examination

Four fundamental processes are employed in the examination of the patient: *inspection, palpation, percussion,* and *auscultation.*

Inspection

The first fundamental process is inspection. The power to observe is one that must be cultivated. General inspection is carried out at the first moment of contact with the patient. The examiner introduces herself to the patient, perhaps shakes hands with him, and exchanges the first words of communication. Many impressions register in this exchange, and numerous valuable observations can be made. The patient is old or young (how old?—how young?—appropriate to his/her stated age?); the patient is thin or fat; the patient is anxious, or perhaps depressed; the patient is normal in body habitus or perhaps deformed in some way (what way?—how different from expected normal?).

Two commonly used phrases are too frequently used as excuses for insufficient attention to the details of observation. *"The patient looks sick."* In what way does the patient look sick? Is he pale, is his skin clammy; is the patient grimacing in pain; is the patient dyspneic; is the skin jaundiced or cyanotic; does the patient have edema? What specific physical features or behavioral manifestations convey that he is "sick"? *"The patient appears chronically ill."* In what way does the patient appear chronically ill? Does he appear to have lost weight? Patients who lose weight secondary to malignancy or other muscle-wasting disease appear different from those who are merely thin. The distribution of their weight loss takes a different form. Does the skin have the appearance of chronic illness? That is, is it pale, or does it give the appearance of dehydration or loss of subcutaneous tissue? These are important observations that health professionals frequently fail to note on the record.

Among general observations that should be noted in the initial examination of the patient are posture and stature, body movements, nutrition, speech pattern, and body temperature.

Posture and Stature. The posture that a patient assumes can often reveal much about his illness. Patients with the dyspnea of cardiac disease prefer to sit and may complain of "smothering" if forced to lie down for even brief periods of time. Persons with emphysema not only sit upright, but assume a posture that is quite characteristic. They thrust their arms forward and laterally onto the edge of the bed ("tripod position") in order to place accessory muscles of respiration at an optimum mechanical advantage for respiratory assistance. Patients with abdominal pain owing to peritonitis prefer to lie perfectly still. Even slight jarring of the bed by the examiner will incite agonizing accentuation of pain. On the other hand, patients with abdominal pain owing to renal or biliary colic are exceedingly restless. They may writhe in the bed or even rise to pace the room. Patients with meningeal irritation associated with headache cannot flex the head or the legs without aggravating their pain.

Body Movements. Abnormalities of body movement may be of two general kinds: generalized discontinuity of voluntary or involuntary movement, or asymmetry of movement. In the former category are included tremors of a wide variety, some of which may occur at rest (Parkinson's disease), while others are incited only on voluntary movement (cerebellar ataxia). Other tremors may exist both during rest and activity (delirium tremens of the alcoholic, thyrotoxicosis). Some voluntary or involuntary movements are fine, others quite coarse. At the extreme are the convulsive movements of epilepsy or tetanus and the gross choreiform movements of patients with rheumatic fever or Huntington's disease.

Asymmetry of movement is seen in patients with disease of the central nervous system (CNS), principally in those who have had cerebral vascular accidents. The patient may manifest drooping of one side of the face or be incapable of normal movement of the right or left upper and lower extremities. Strength is impaired on the involved side, and the patient walks with a foot-dragging gait.

Nutrition. States of nutrition are important to note. Obesity may be generalized as a function of excessive intake of calories or may be specifically localized to the trunk in patients with endocrine disorders (Cushing's disease) or those who have been taking steroid drugs for long periods of time. Loss of weight may be generalized as a function of caloric deprivation or may be reflected more strikingly in loss of muscle mass in patients whose diseases interfere with protein building.

Speech Pattern. Speech may be slurred owing to CNS disease or because of incapacity to articulate owing to damage to cranial nerves. Damage to the recurrent laryngeal nerve will produce hoarseness, as will those diseases that produce edema or swelling of the vocal cords. Speech may be halting or interrupted in flow in some CNS disorders (multiple sclerosis).

Body Temperature. The recording of body temperature is a part of every physical examination. Fever is an increase in body temperature above normal. A normal oral temperature for most persons is an average of 37.0° C (98.6° F). It should be recognized that there is some variation from 37.0° C (98.6° F) that is still within the range of normal. Some persons are quite normal at 36.6° C (98° F) and others at 37.3° C (99° F). Children playing hard during summer months quite regularly run temperatures as high as 37.7° C (100° F), and occasionally higher, but this should subside quite promptly with rest. Moreover, it should be recognized that there is a normal diurnal variation of a degree or two in body temperature throughout the day. Most persons achieve their low early in the morning. Body temperature rises during the day to 37.3° C (99° F) or 37.5° C (99.5° F) and then subsides through the night.

Palpation

Palpation is a vital part of the physical examination. Many structures of the body, although not visible, are accessible by the hand and may, in a way, be "felt." Examples include blood vessels, lymph nodes, the thyroid, the organs of the abdomen and pelvis, and the rectum.

Sounds generated within the body, if within specified frequency ranges, also may be "felt." Thus, certain murmurs generated in the heart or within blood vessels (thrills) may be detected. Thrills cause a sensation to the hand much like the purring of a cat. Voice sounds are transmitted along the bronchi to the periphery of the lung. These may be perceived by touch and will be altered by certain disease states within the lung. The phenomenon is called *tactile fremitus* and is useful in assessing diseases of the chest.

Percussion

The technique of percussion translates the application of physical force into sound. It is a difficult art to perfect, but one capable of yielding much information about disease processes in the chest and abdomen. The principle is to set the chest wall or abdominal wall into vibration by striking it with a firm object. The sound produced is reflective of the density of the underlying structure. Certain densities produce sounds that can be identified as percussion notes. These sounds, listed in a sequence that proceeds from the least to the most dense, are called *tympany, hyperresonance, resonance, dullness,* and *flatness.* The pitch of the sound progresses through a series, from lowest for tympany to highest for flatness; the duration of the sound ranges from long to short.

Tympany is the drumlike sound produced by percussing the air-filled stomach. *Resonance* is the sound elicited over air-filled lungs. *Hyperresonance* is audible while percussing over inflated lung tissue of the patient with emphysema. Percussion of the liver produces a dull sound, while percussion of the thigh results in flatness.

The procedure (for right-handed persons; hands should be reversed if the examiner is left-handed) is conducted as follows (Fig. 5-1): Place the distal phalanx of the left middle finger firmly against the chest wall. The other fingers should be held away from the chest wall, since any pressure they might exert against the thorax would tend to mute or dampen the sound produced. The right hand now becomes the striking object. The middle finger of the right hand is used to strike the terminal phalanx of the middle finger of the left hand just behind the nail bed. If done sharply, a brief resonant tone will be produced. The motion of the right hand should be dominantly a wrist action. The forearm itself should be held steady. The clarity of the sound produced is dependent on the brevity of the action. The intensity is a function of the force used.

Percussion gives one the capacity to assess such normal anatomical details as the degree to which the diaphragm descends during inspiration. The sound over lung tissue is normally resonant; the sound over the diaphragm is dull. One may percuss the border of the heart. One may determine the level of pleural effusion or the location of pneumonic consolidation or atelectasis of a lobe of the lung. Further application of the technique is discussed under examination of the thorax and abdomen.

Auscultation

Sound is produced within the body either by the movement of air through hollow structures or by the forces set up by

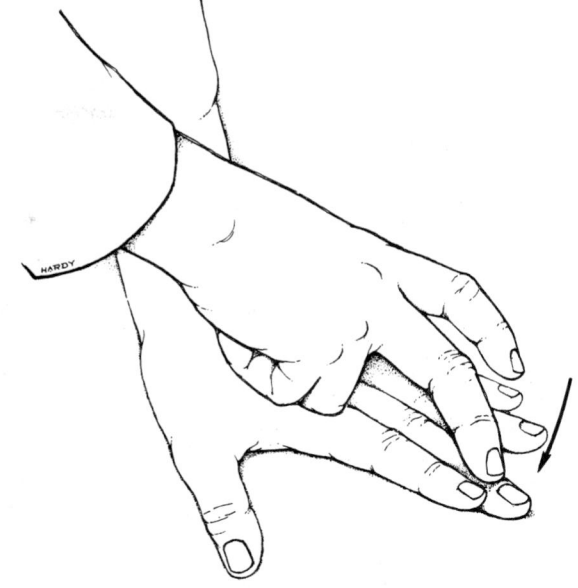

Figure 5-1. Percussion technique. The middle finger of the right hand strikes the terminal phalanx of the middle finger of the left hand. Care should be taken that only the terminal part of the middle finger of the left hand is in contact with the area to be percussed. The middle finger of the right hand should be held rigidly. It is properly a wrist action, and the intensity and clarity of the note will be a function of the quickness with which it is performed.

the movement of columns of fluid that set solid structures in motion. Examples of acoustical phenomena of clinical importance include the movement of air through the trachea and bronchi (breath sounds), the movement of air past functioning vocal cords (spoken voice), the movement of air through the intestines (bowel sounds), the movement of blood through vascular structures that provide critical resistance to flow (murmurs), and the impedance to flowing blood provided by closed valves and the heart wall (heart sounds). Physiologic sounds may be normal (*e.g.,* first and second heart sounds) or pathologic (*e.g.,* murmurs in diastole produced in the heart, or crackles in the lung). Some normal sounds may be distorted by pathology of structures through which the sound must travel (*e.g.,* changes in the character of breath sounds as they travel through the consolidated lung of lobar pneumonia).

Sound produced within the body, if of sufficient amplitude, will set in vibration all structures between the origin of the sound and the body surface. Sound vibration emanating from the body surface may be captured directly by the examiner's ear, or more appropriately, by the stethoscope, an instrument devised as an extension of the human ear.

Although the stethoscope does not have the capacity to amplify sound, it does channel it, thereby making physiologic sound more readily available for our critical evaluation. Two end-pieces are available for the stethoscope—the *bell* and the *diaphragm.* Many stethoscopes come with both pieces built into a single head. Alternating between the pieces becomes a matter of turning the head of the stethoscope or flipping a switch. The bell is a small disc mounted on a conical base; it is attached to a larger disc, the diaphragm. The bell is better suited for the transmission of very-low-frequency sounds. It is important to place the bell so that the entire surface of the disc rests lightly on the skin surface, to avoid flattening the skin and reducing audible vibratory sensations. The diaphragm, the larger disc, is more appropriately constructed for the reception of high-frequency sounds. It is placed firmly against the skin for optimal transmission of sound.

The head of the stethoscope is held between the index and middle fingers to provide a firm contact with the skin surface. Care is taken to avoid touching the tubing or rubbing other surfaces (hair, clothing) during auscultation. This minimizes extraneous noises that could confuse the examiner. The ear-pieces of the stethoscope should fit snugly into the ear canals, and the tubing should not be more than 20 cm in length. Dual tubing transmits sound more faithfully than single tubing.

Sound produced by the body has the features of sound produced in any other manner. That is, it is characterized by intensity, frequency, and quality. The intensity, or loudness, associated with physiologic sound is low. Rarely may sounds of the body, except for speech, be heard without direct application of the ear or the stethoscope to the body surface. With respect to frequency, or pitch, it may be said that physiologic sound is in reality "noise," in that most sounds consist of a frequency spectrum as opposed to single-frequency sounds that we associate with music or the tuning fork. The frequency spectrum may be quite low, yielding a rumbling noise, or comparatively high, producing a harsh or blowing sound. The third feature of sound is quality. This relates to overtones and is the characteristic of sound that allows one to differentiate sound produced by the piano from that produced by the violin. Sound quality enables the examiner to distinguish between the musical quality of high-pitched wheezing (sibilant rhonchi) and the low-pitched rumbling of a diastolic murmur.

The fundamental processes of inspection, palpation, percussion, and auscultation will now be discussed with respect to the various organ systems and parts of the body to which they may be applied.

▷ Examination of the Skin

Assessment of the skin is an integral part of every physical examination and includes all body surfaces, mucous membranes, and the nails. The skin is a reflection of the individual's overall health, and alterations often correspond to disease in other organ systems. A brief survey of the skin is normally conducted at the beginning of the physical examination, and then more fully as each part of the body is examined in sequence. Inspection and palpation constitute the chief techniques of the skin assessment.

A thorough examination of the skin includes an assessment of color, lesions, vascularity, temperature, texture, mobility, and the presence of edema. Skin color varies from individual to individual and ranges from ivory to deep brown. The skin of exposed portions of the body, especially in sunny, warm climates, tends to be more pigmented than that of the rest of the body. The vasodilative effects of fever, sunburn, and inflammation produce a pink or reddish hue in the skin. Pallor is an absence of or decrease in normal skin tones and vascularity and is best observed in the conjuctivae. The bluish hue of cyanosis indicates cellular hypoxia and is easily observed in the nail beds, lips, and mucous membranes. Jaundice, a yellowing of the skin, is directly related to elevations in serum bilirubin and is often noted in the sclerae and mucous membranes.

Assessing color changes in the dark-skinned or black individual may be difficult. Additional lighting may be helpful during inspection. The overall surface of dark skin normally has a reddish base or undertone; the buccal mucosa, tongue, lips, and nails have a pink color. Erythema is often visible as a purplish grey cast to the skin. Dark-skinned individuals normally have yellow conjunctivae; thus, it may be necessary to inspect the hard palate for the yellowing hue of jaundice. Rashes are more easily identified by palpation. Differences in skin texture are detected and borders of the rash defined.

The presence of any eruptions or lesions on the skin is noted. Careful observation of the eruption or lesion helps to identify the type of dermatosis (abnormal skin condition) and indicates whether the lesion is primary or secondary (see Chap. 52, p. 1162). At the same time, the anatomical distribution of the eruption is noted, since certain diseases affect certain sites of the body and are distributed in characteristic patterns and shapes. To determine the extent of the distribution, the left and right sides of the body are compared while the color and shape of the lesion are noted. Following observation, the lesions are palpated to determine their texture and to see if they are hard or soft or filled with fluid. A metric ruler is used to measure the size of the lesions so that any further extension can be compared with this initial baseline measurement. The dermatosis is then documented clearly and in detail, using precise terminology.

It is essential for the examiner to use precise and accurate terminology in any verbal and written communication about the status of the skin. This facilitates the ultimate identification and diagnosis of local and systemic diseases, and requires memorization and the reinforcement of clinical experience.

Once the color of the skin has been inspected and lesions noted, an assessment of vascular changes in the skin is carried out. A description of vascular changes includes location, distribution, color, size, and the presence of pulsations. Common vascular changes include petechiae, ecchymosis, telangiectasia, angiomas, and venous stars.

Skin moisture, temperature, and texture are assessed primarily by palpation. The elasticity (turgor) of the skin, which lessens in normal aging, may be a factor in assessing the hydration status of a patient.

A brief inspection of the nails includes observation of configuration, color, and consistency. Many of the alterations seen in the nail or nail bed reflect local or systemic abnormalities in progress, or are the result of past events. Transverse depressions (Beau's lines) in the nails may reflect retarded growth of the nail matrix secondary to severe illness or, more commonly, are the result of local trauma. Ridging, hypertrophy, and other changes may also be visible with local trauma. Inflammation of the skin around the nail (paronychia) is usually accompanied by tenderness and erythema. The angle between the normal nail and its base is 160 degrees. When palpated, the base of the nail is usually firm. Clubbing is manifested by a straightening of the normal angle (180 degrees or greater) and a softening of the nail base. This softening is perceived as spongelike when palpated.

▷ Examination of the Head and Neck

In examining the head and the sensory organs contained within it, inspection is the principal process employed. Palpation is used to some extent and auscultation to a very limited degree.

Examination of the Head
Head Size.   The head is inspected for its size and shape. A grossly small head is called *microcephaly* and is always associated with mental retardation. Enlargement of the head may occur for one of several common reasons. In infancy, when the fontanelles are open and increased intracranial pressure allows separation of the bony components of the calvarium, an enlarged head may be due to hydrocephalus secondary to stenosis of the aqueduct or to overproduction of cerebrospinal fluid. Enlargement of the head in adult life is less common but may be seen in overproduction of growth hormone, an entity known as *acromegaly.* This disease is associated with broadening of the nose and marked enlargement of the jaw, the hands, and the feet. Enlargement of the frontal part of the skull may also be seen in *Paget's disease* of the bone. This is associated with bowing of the legs and other skeletal deformities.

Hair and Scalp.   The hair and scalp are examined routinely. First, the quantity and distribution of the hair are observed. Then, using both hands simultaneously, the examiner palpates the entire scalp surface for irregularities, lesions, or tenderness.

The most common abnormality encountered is *seborrhea,* commonly known as dandruff. Baldness is common in men, rare in women. It is almost universally congenital, even when occurring at a young age. A history of male baldness on either side of the family predisposes any young person to early loss of hair.

Face.   A great deal can be learned by inspection of the face. The diseases that present with characteristic facial alteration are legion. This accounts for the common capacity of trained health professionals to recognize diseases in the public at large. A partial list of disease entities associated with stereotypical facial change includes myxedema, thyrotoxicosis, acromegaly, scleroderma, discoid lupus erythematosus, Cushing's disease, carcinoid syndrome, and mongolism.

Examination of the Nose and Sinuses
The nose and sinuses are examined by inspection and palpation. For a routine examination, only a simple light source is necessary. A penlight is inexpensive and readily available. A more thorough examination requires the use of a nasal speculum.

The external nose is inspected for lesions, asymmetry, or inflammation. The patient is instructed to tilt his head backward while the examiner gently pushes the tip of the nose upward. The penlight is then used to examine the internal structures of the nose. The mucosa is inspected for color, swelling, exudate, or bleeding. The nasal mucosa is normally more red than oral mucosa, but may appear swollen and hyperemic in the presence of the common cold. Allergic rhinitis, on the other hand, is suspected when the mucosa appears pale and swollen.

The septum is then inspected for deviation, perforation, or bleeding. A slight degree of septal deviation is present in most individuals. Actual displacement of the cartilage into either vestibule may produce nasal obstruction, but such deviation is usually asymptomatic.

With the patient's head in a tilted position, the examiner attempts to visualize the inferior and middle turbinates. With chronic rhinitis, nasal polyps may develop between the inferior and middle turbinates and are distinguished by their grey appearance. Unlike the turbinates, they are gelatinous in nature and freely movable.

The frontal and maxillary sinuses are palpated for tenderness. Using the thumbs, the examiner applies gentle pressure in an upward fashion at the supraorbital ridges (frontal sinuses) and in the cheek area adjacent to the nose (maxillary sinuses). Tenderness in either area suggests inflammation.

Examination of the Oral Cavity
Examination of the oral cavity includes an assessment of both the internal and external structures of the mouth and throat. Removal of dentures and partial plates is necessary to ensure a thorough inspection of the gums. In general, the examination can be accomplished with the use of a bright light source (penlight) and a tongue depressor. If a suspicious lesion is observed, a finger cot or unsterile glove is used to palpate the abnormality. The examination begins with inspection of the lips for color, moisture, and the presence of ulcerations or fissures. The patient is instructed to open his mouth wide as a tongue blade is inserted into the mouth to expose the buccal mucosa for an assessment of color and lesions. The Stensen's duct of each parotid gland may be visible as a small red dot in the buccal mucosa next to the upper molars.

Any inflammation, bleeding, retraction of the gums, or poor dentition is noted. The odor of the breath is also noted. The hard palate is examined, as well as the dorsum of the tongue. A thin, white coat and the large, vallate papillae in V-formation on the distal tongue are normal findings. The patient is instructed to protrude his tongue and move it laterally. This provides the examiner with an opportunity to estimate the tongue's size as well as its symmetry and strength (cranial nerve XII). Further inspection of the ventral surface of the tongue and the floor of the mouth is accomplished by having the patient touch the tip of his tongue to his palate. Any lesions of the mucosa or any abnormalities involving the frenulum or superficial veins are noted. This is a common area for oral cancer, which presents as a white or red plaque, an indurated ulcer, or a warty growth.

A tongue blade can be used to depress the tongue for adequate visualization of the pharynx, but is not always necessary. The patient is instructed to open his mouth wide and take a deep breath. Often this will flatten the posterior tongue and briefly expose a full view of the anterior and posterior pillars, the tonsils, uvula, and posterior pharynx. These structures are inspected for color, symmetry, and evidence of exudate, ulceration, or enlargement. Normally, the uvula and soft palate rise with a deep inspiration or "ah," and indicate an intact vagus nerve (cranial nerve X). If a tongue blade is used to visualize the pharynx, it is pressed firmly beyond the midpoint of the tongue. Proper placement avoids a gagging response and minimizes the patient's aversion to future oral examinations.

Examination of the Neck

The neck is examined by inspection, palpation, and auscultation. It should first be observed for any obvious masses or asymmetry. The neck is inspected for evidence of masses, asymmetry, limitation of motion, or abnormal pulsations. This is performed with the patient in a sitting position with his chin raised and his neck slightly extended.

Lymph Nodes. The head and neck region is palpated for the presence of enlarged lymph nodes (lymphadenopathy). The palmar surfaces of the fingertips are used to exert firm, gentle pressure in a rotary motion at each anatomical site. The lymph node groupings are examined in sequence, beginning with the preauricular nodes and proceeding to the posterior auricular and occipital regions. The tonsillar, submaxillary, and submental regions are palpated before the superficial cervical, deep cervical, and posterior cervical chains are examined. The examination concludes with palpation of the supraclavicular regions. Generally, the lymph nodes are not palpable. When palpable, the lymph nodes are noted for their location, size, consistency, mobility, and the presence or absence of tenderness. Inflamed nodes may be moderately enlarged and are commonly tender but usually movable. The nodes of tuberculosis may become fixed to deep structures or to the skin. The nodes of malignancy are often quite hard, tend to coalesce or "mat," and are frequently fixed to subcutaneous tissue.

Trachea. The position and mobility of the trachea are usually noted by direct palpation. This is done by placing the thumb and index finger of one hand on either side of the trachea just above the sternal notch. The trachea is highly sensitive, and palpating too firmly may incite a coughing or gagging response. The trachea is normally midline as it enters the thoracic inlet behind the sternum, but may be deviated by masses in the neck or mediastinum. Pleural or pulmonary disorders may also result in displacement of the trachea.

Thyroid. Inspection and palpation of the thyroid gland are done routinely on all patients. This examination can be difficult; the identification of specific anatomical landmarks is required to ensure an accurate assessment. The lower neck region between the sternocleidomastoid muscles is inspected for anterior swelling or asymmetry. The patient is instructed to extend his neck slightly and swallow. Thyroid tissue rises normally with swallowing. The thyroid is then palpated for size, shape, consistency, symmetry, and the presence of tenderness.

The examiner may perform this portion of the examination from an anterior or a posterior position. For the beginning examiner, the thyroid is most effectively palpated from the rear, with both hands encircling the patient's neck (Fig. 5-2). The thumbs are rested on the nape of the patient's neck, while the index and middle fingers palpate for the thyroid isthmus and the anterior surfaces of the lateral lobes. When felt, the isthmus is perceived as firm and of a rubber-band consistency. The left lobe is examined by positioning the patient with his neck flexed slightly forward and to the left. The thyroid cartilage is then displaced to the left with the fingers of the right hand. This maneuver displaces the left lobe deep into the sternocleidomastoid muscle, where it can be more easily palpated. The left lobe is then palpated by placing the left thumb deep into the posterior area of the sternocleidomastoid muscle, while the index and middle fingers exert opposing pressure in the anterior portion of the muscle. Having the patient swallow during the maneuver may assist the examiner to locate the thyroid as it ascends in the neck. The procedure is reversed for an examination of the right lobe. The isthmus is the only portion of the thyroid that is normally felt. If a patient has a very thin neck, occasionally two thin, smooth, nontender lobes may also be appreciated.

If the thyroid gland is enlarged by palpation, auscultation over both lobes with the diaphragm of the stethoscope is necessary. Auscultation will identify the localized audible vibration of a bruit. This is an abnormal finding and necessitates referral to a physician. The presence of tenderness, enlargement, or nodularity within the thyroid also requires additional evaluation by a physician.

Veins and Arteries. A discussion of the veins and arteries of the neck is included under the assessment of the cardiovascular system.

Examination of the Eye

Examination of the eye is an essential component of the physical examination, not only because of the importance of the function of the eye to the well-being of the patient, but also because the eye is reflective of many facets of the general state of health. The retina, which may be viewed with the ophthalmoscope, is the only site in the human body where a vascular bed may be examined directly. Diseases such as hypertension and diabetes, both exceedingly common in the population, produce changes that are readily observable. The pupil may be said to be a window to the human microcirculation.

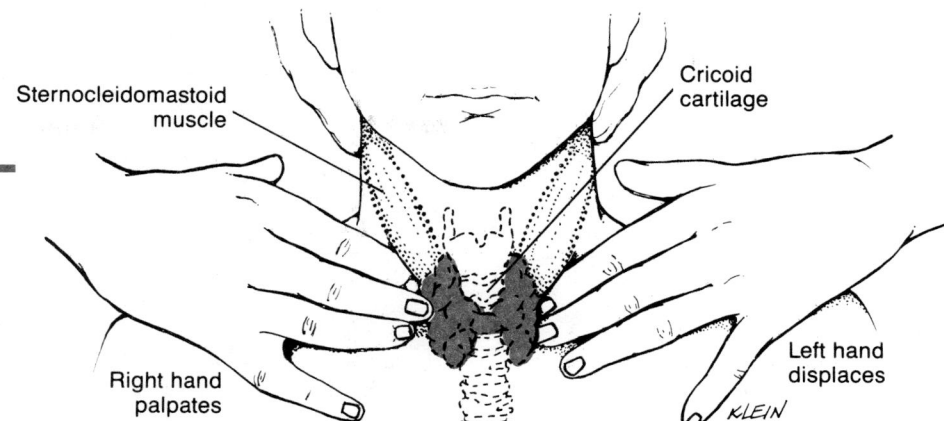

Sternocleidomastoid
muscle

Cricoid
cartilage

Left hand
displaces

Right hand
palpates

KLEIN

Figure 5-2. Technique for palpation of the thyroid gland. The isthmus of the thyroid may be felt in the midline, approximately 1 cm below the cricoid cartilage. The gland is felt laterally beneath the tendinous insertion of the sternocleidomastoid muscle. (Adapted from Bates B: A Guide to Physical Examination, 3rd ed. p. 94. Philadelphia, JB Lippincott, 1983.)

Visual Acuity.   Formal testing of visual acuity is a part of the data base of every patient. Testing of visual acuity is accomplished by means of an eye chart placed 6 meters (20 feet) from the patient. If space is lacking, an inverted eye chart may be placed directly behind the patient's head, and a mirror placed 3 meters (10 feet) from the patient. The patient is instructed to cover one eye with a card, to keep both eyes open, and to read each line of the chart until he is no longer able to distinguish the details for a given size of print. If the patient wears glasses, his acuity should be assessed with and without corrective lenses.

Illiteracy may be circumvented by the use of charts that display the letter "E" in four different positions. This enables one to assess the vision of children as young as 5 years of age.

Visual acuity is expressed in a ratio that relates what the patient *should* see at 20 feet to what the patient *can* see at 20 feet. Acuity of 20/50 means that the patient can see at 20 feet what he should see at 50 feet; 20/200, the boundary of legal blindness, indicates that the patient can see at 20 feet what he should be able to see at 200 feet. Such patients can only discern with accuracy the large letter at the top of the chart. The patient whose visual acuity is less than 20/20 when corrected by his or her own glasses should be referred to an ophthalmologist.

Near vision is not routinely assessed unless the patient is complaining of difficulty in reading at close range or is over age 40. After age 40, the lens may become rigid and incapable of accommodating its shape to close-range vision. This condition is known as *presbyopia*. Having a patient read newsprint at a distance of 12 inches provides a gross screening for this disorder. Patients who experience difficulty with this examination are referred to an ophthalmologist.

External Evaluation of the Eye.   The external structures of the eye are assessed primarily by inspection and include the eyebrow, eyelid, eyelashes, lacrimal apparatus, conjunctiva, cornea, anterior chamber, iris, and pupil. The examination begins with an assessment of the position and alignment of the eyes. The eyebrows are observed for the quantity and distribution of the hair. The positioning of the

lids in relationship to the eyeballs is noted. With the eyes open, no sclera should be visible above the corneas. *Ptosis* (drooping of the lid) may be due to lid edema, muscle weakness, congenital defect, or involvement of the third cranial nerve. The lids are also inspected for color, swelling, lesions, and the presence and direction of eyelash growth. Common abnormalities of the lids are discussed in Chapter 54.

The region of the lacrimal gland in the upper lateral orbit is inspected. If enlargement is suspected, the upper lid can be everted to expose the lacrimal gland for further inspection. Next, the lacrimal apparatus is inspected for swelling. Nasolacrimal duct obstruction or inflammation can often be identified by pressing on the medial aspect of the lower lid just inside the orbital rim. Palpate for tenderness and watch for regurgitation of fluid from the puncta.

Inspection of the sclera and bulbar conjunctiva is performed concurrently. Separation of the lids is done by placing the index finger on the patient's upper orbital rim and the thumb on the lower rim. As the lids are separated, instruct the patient to look up, down, and to each side. Small capillaries are normally visible in the conjunctiva, and the white, fibrous sclera is normally clearly visible. In black-skinned individuals, however, the sclera is often yellowish and is a normal finding, not be be confused with jaundice. The palpebral conjunctiva of the lower lid is readily inspected by having the patient look upward while the lower lid is gently everted.

Utilizing oblique lighting (penlight), the examiner inspects the cornea and anterior chamber for opacities. Normally, the cornea is smooth and transparent. Irregularities are often detected by defects in the light reflection through the cornea. Shadows cast on the iris may be indicative of a corneal lesion or forward displacement of the anterior chamber. The iris is inspected for continuity and unusual markings.

The pupils are normally round, regular, equal in diameter, and equivalently reactive to light. Although a small percentage of the population may have unequal pupils that may be considered normal, the phenomenon is sufficiently unusual that it should lead to thorough examination in order

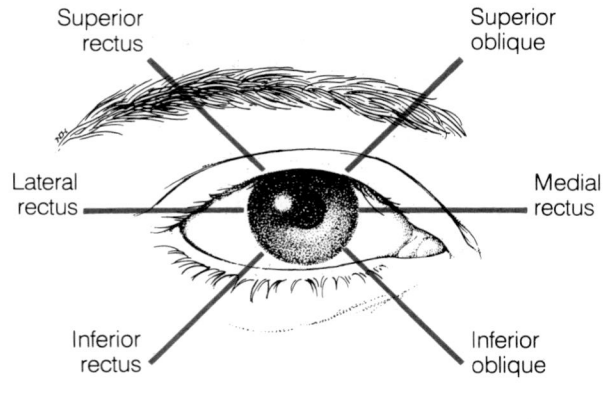

Superior rectus

Superior oblique

Lateral rectus

Medial rectus

Inferior rectus

Inferior oblique

Figure 5-3. The right eye. The function of each eye muscle is tested by having the patient move his eye in the six cardinal positions of gaze.

to ascertain that the inequality is not due to CNS disease. When confronted with light, the normal pupil promptly constricts in a regular concentric fashion. The unstimulated opposite pupil constricts as well. This pupillary reaction is assessed by instructing the patient to focus on a distant object while the examiner shines a bright light on each pupil, in turn.

Constriction of the stimulated pupil is called the *direct light reflex,* whereas constriction of the opposite pupil is termed *consensual light reflex.* Exploration of this phenomenon allows one to separate damage to the optic nerve from blindness owing to more central disease. Direct light stimulation of the nerve-damaged eye results in neither a direct nor a consensual light reflex. Stimulation of the uninvolved eye, however, results in consensual constriction of the pupil of the damaged eye, since the consensual reflex is not dependent upon transmission through the optic nerve.

Pupillary reaction to accommodation is best observed by asking the patient to focus on an object in the distance and then at the examiner's finger, which is positioned 7.5 cm to 12.5 cm (3 inches to 5 inches) from the patient's nose. A normal response is constriction of the pupils as the eyes converge and focus on the examiner's finger.

Autonomic disease owing to central nervous system syphilis or to diabetes may result in a pupil that is incapable of responding to light but retains its capacity to respond to accommodation. Such a pupil is known as an *Argyll Robertson pupil.*

Ocular Tension. An increase in intraocular tension is the cardinal manifestation of glaucoma, a disease responsible for more than one fifth of the blindness seen in the United States. A gross determination of intraocular pressure can be made by applying gentle finger pressure over the sclera of the closed eye. The tips of both forefingers are placed on the closed upper lid. One finger gently presses inward while the adjacent finger senses the amount of pressure exerted against it. Some examiners then compare the tension "felt" or perceived in the patient's eye to their own.

At best, this maneuver is a gross estimation, and when a more accurate measurement must be relied upon, tonometry is indicated (see Chap. 54).

Assessment of Extraocular Muscles. Synergistic action of six small muscles attached to each eye, innervated by three of the cranial nerves, results in parallel gaze. Although the mechanism by which this takes place is highly complex, and analysis of abnormality requires physician consultation, this assessment can be easily done by the nurse.

Parallel alignment of the eyes may be easily detected by shining a light directly into the face while the patient is staring at the light source. The light should be reflected from the pupils of both eyes identically. Central positioning of the light reflex from one pupil associated with asymmetry in the other indicates disturbance in parallax vision. In spite of normal alignment of both eyes when they function together, the tendency of either eye to drift to the nasal or temporal side (and the necessity to involuntarily compensate for this with effort) may be assessed by the *cover test.* One eye is covered by a card or by the hand of the examiner, and the patient is asked to focus the free eye on a stationary object. He is instructed to keep the covered eye open. The card or hand is abruptly removed from the covered eye, and it is this eye to which the examiner devotes his attention. If the eye, when uncovered, has drifted to the temporal side, it will snap back into alignment when the cover is removed. Conversely, if it has drifted to the nasal side, the reverse phenomenon will occur. The tendency of an eye to drift, when covered, to the temporal side is called an *exophoria;* a tendency of an eye to drift to the nasal side is called an *esophoria.*

Integrity of the nervous control of the muscles of the eye may be assessed by directing the patient to move his eyes in the six cardinal positions of gaze (Fig. 5-3) while following an object. The object is moved laterally to either side along the horizontal axis and then along two oblique axes, each of which makes a 60-degree angle with the horizontal. Each of the cardinal positions of gaze represents the function of one of the six extraocular muscles attached to each eye. If *diplopia,* or double vision, develops during the transition to any one of the cardinal positions of gaze, the examiner has an indication that one or more of the extraocular muscles are failing to function properly.

When extraocular movements are checked, the eye is observed for *nystagmus.* Nystagmus is an irregular jerking movement of the eyes in the process of transferring gaze to a lateral position. Nystagmus has two components: a quick component in one or the other direction, and a slower subsequent component that brings the eye back to the intended position. However, nystagmus on extreme lateral gaze is a normal finding and can be avoided by not placing the object too far laterally beyond binocular gaze. A number of conditions cause nystagmus; many of these are benign, whereas others may reflect severe pathology.

Assessment of Field of Vision. Although the visual field may be assessed with a high degree of precision by an ophthalmologist, a rough estimate may be made in the office or at the patient's bedside when the examiner is concerned with the gross disturbance of the visual field. Such a circumstance may arise, for example, in assessing the patient with a cerebrovascular accident. Such patients commonly lose one quarter or one half of the visual fields of both eyes.

A simple and reliable method of testing the fullness of the visual field is direct confrontation. The examiner and patient sit directly facing each other at a distance of 60 cm (2 feet). The patient is instructed to cover one eye with a card while looking directly at the examiner's nose. The examiner covers her eye as a method of comparison. If the patient has covered his left eye, for instance, the examiner covers her right eye. The examiner then takes an object (pen, finger) in her right hand and moves it along a plane halfway between the examiner and the patient. The nasal, temporal, upward, and downward fields are assessed by bringing the object into view from various peripheral points. During each maneuver, the patient informs the examiner the moment he is able to see the object. In order to test the nasal fields of gaze for the same eye, the examiner switches the object from the right hand to the left hand. The entire procedure is reversed for an assessment of the fields of the left eye. When confrontation testing reveals decreases in visual fields or "blind spots," the patient is referred immediately to an ophthalmologist for further evaluation.

Ophthalmoscopy. The internal eye is referred to as the fundus and comprises the retina, optic disc, macula, and retinal vessels. It is visualized with the aid of an instrument called an ophthalmoscope. With practice and repetition, the nurse can become proficient in the use of the ophthalmoscope. The ophthalmoscope is an instrument that projects light through a prism and bends the light at 90 degrees, allowing the observer to view the retina through a lens in such a way that the line of vision is parallel to the bent ray of light. A number of lenses are available and are arranged on a wheel so that they may be chosen by rotating the wheel with the index finger without interrupting the inspection. The standard ophthalmoscope contains an array of gadgetry that includes grids, slits, filters, and the like—none of which are particularly useful. The small, unfiltered aperture is appropriate and most useful for standard ophthalmoscopy.

In order to avoid a confrontation of noses, the right eye of the patient is examined with the right eye of the examiner, the left eye of the patient with the left eye of the examiner (See Fig. 5-4 A). The room is darkened so that the pupil will be dilated. The patient is instructed to hold the eyes still and focus on a real or imaginary distant object. The ophthalmoscope is gripped firmly in the hand, with the index finger resting on the lens wheel. The head of the ophthalmoscope is braced within the angle made by the brow and the nose. The lens chosen for initial inspection should be the one labeled zero unless the examiner is knowingly correcting his or her own defect in visual acuity. If the examiner wears glasses, it may be better to remove the glasses and become familiar with which lens is analogous to zero for the examiner with 20/20 vision; or, the examiner may prefer to keep the glasses on and utilize a zero lens setting. Provided that the patient has 20/20 vision, the zero lens should enable the examiner to obtain a precise focus on the retina. If the retina is out of focus, the lens

wheel is rotated until it is brought into focus. The choice of a lens labeled with a red numeral implies that one is focusing further away than normal; the choice of a lens labeled with a black numeral implies that one is focusing nearer to the examiner. The examiner will choose lenses among the red series for patients who are *hyperopic* (farsighted), and lenses in the black series for patients who are *myopic* (nearsighted).

With the room in darkness, the patient appropriately gazing into the distance, and the ophthalmoscope properly positioned within the cradle of the brow and nose, the examiner may now approach the patient. The examiner stands approximately 37.5 cm (15 inches) from the patient and about 15 degrees lateral to the patient's gaze. When the light is focused on the pupil, the retina will glow red through the dilated pupil opening. This is known as the *red reflex.* The examiner then approaches the patient until her forehead touches her left hand, which she has placed on the patient's forehead (Fig. 5-4A). At this point, provided that the proper lens has been selected, the retina should be in focus, and the venules and arterioles that course through the retina are readily apparent (Fig. 5-4 B). In scanning the surface of the retina, it is important that the examiner hold the scope firmly and move her head rather than the instrument.

The examiner should first focus on the optic disc. In the event that the disc is not in view when the retina is first visualized, the veins that are within the field of vision should be followed down their tributaries toward the disc from which the arterioles emerge and the venules enter. This is analogous to following the limbs of a tree until one sees the trunk. The optic disc is examined for size, shape, color, and the sharpness of its margin. The disc is circular and yellowish pink in color. The margin is sharp and occasionally surrounded by a rim of dark pigment (choroidal crescent). One must become familiar with what is regarded as a normal size. In the center of the disc there is frequently a small physiologic cup into which the central vein of the retina recedes. To accurately focus on the base of this cup, one may have to choose another lens in the direction of the red sequence. A deep cup is seen in glaucoma. Edema of the optic disc with concomitant blurring of the disc margin is seen with increases in cerebrospinal fluid pressure. The disc becomes pink, and accurate focus may require shifting to a lens in the direction of the black sequence. This is termed *papilledema. Optic atrophy* is characterized by extreme pallor of the disc and reduction of its size.

The remainder of the retina is now examined. Abnormalities may be precisely located for other observers by using a standard nomenclature that makes reference to an imaginary clock face, and by referring to the diameter of the disc to delineate distance. Thus, a hemorrhage may be noted to be one half of the disc diameter in size, located two disc diameters away from the disc margin at 2 o'clock. Another observer is then able to replicate this finding.

The examiner now follows each of the major vessels from the margin of the disc. The arterioles are lighter in color and narrower than the venules. Under normal circumstances, arterioles are two thirds to four fifths the diameter of veins. The walls of the vessels are essentially transparent,

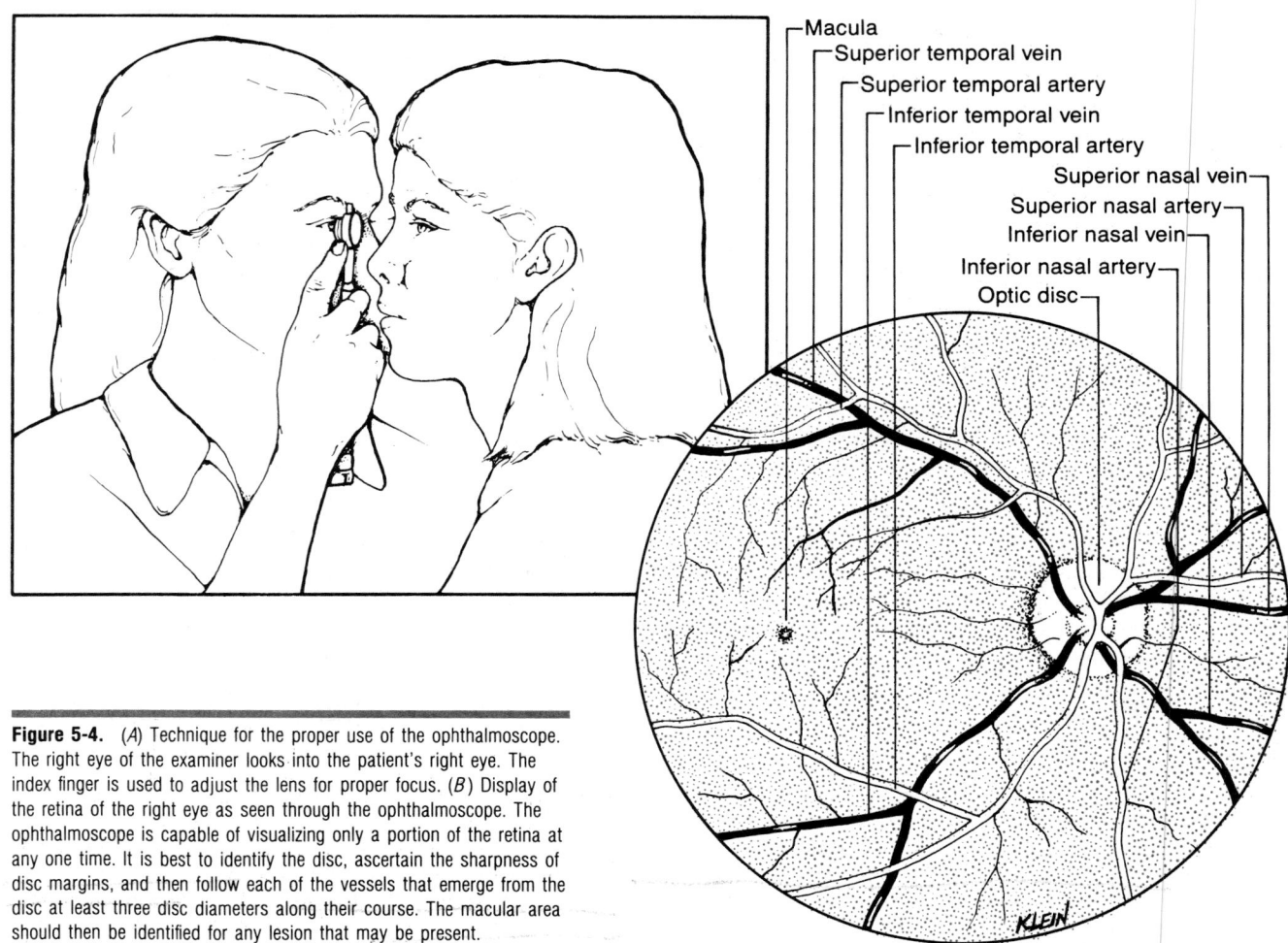

Macula
Superior temporal vein
Superior temporal artery
Inferior temporal vein
Inferior temporal artery
Superior nasal vein
Superior nasal artery
Inferior nasal vein
Inferior nasal artery
Optic disc

Figure 5-4. (*A*) Technique for the proper use of the ophthalmoscope. The right eye of the examiner looks into the patient's right eye. The index finger is used to adjust the lens for proper focus. (*B*) Display of the retina of the right eye as seen through the ophthalmoscope. The ophthalmoscope is capable of visualizing only a portion of the retina at any one time. It is best to identify the disc, ascertain the sharpness of disc margins, and then follow each of the vessels that emerge from the disc at least three disc diameters along their course. The macular area should then be identified for any lesion that may be present.

and what is being observed is the blood column itself. The size and character of the arteriovenous crossings is noted, as well as any lesions in the retina. The retinal changes associated with hypertension and diabetes are quite distinctive and are discussed in Chapters 32 and 40 respectively.

Lastly, the macular area of the retina is visualized by having the patient look directly at the light source. This causes the patient slight discomfort and tearing, and provides the examiner with only a brief second or two during which to inspect the small, circular, red area of the macula. The glistening reflection of its center is called the *fovea centralis retinae*. Any edema, hemorrhages, or lesions are noted and brought to the attention of an ophthalmologist.

All of the techniques that have been discussed for the examination of the eye will not be performed on every patient. Routinely, one inspects the conjunctiva, the cornea, and the pupil and assesses extraocular motion. Ophthalmoscopic examination is a part of every reasonably complete physical examination. Although visual acuity is a part of the data base, it need not be assessed more often than once every year or two, except in elderly individuals.

Examination of the Ear

Examination of the ear is done primarily by inspection and palpation and involves an assessment of the external and middle ear. Auditory acuity is also a vital part of this exam and is included in every physical examination.

Auditory Acuity. A gross estimation of the patient's hearing is effectively screened by assessing the patient's ability to hear a whisper or the ticking of a watch. One ear is tested at a time. In order to exclude the opposite ear from the testing, the examiner cups the opposite auricle with the palm of the hand and produces a masking sound by moving the hand to and fro. At a distance of 1 foot to 2 feet from the unoccluded ear and out of visual range of the patient, the examiner whispers three or four numbers. A soft whisper can be produced if the examiner begins to whisper after a full exhale. In a quiet room, the patient with normal acuity can correctly repeat the numbers whispered. This procedure is done for each ear. If a ticking watch is used, the examiner holds the watch at a distance of 7.5 cm (3 inches) from the auricle. Because the watch produces a higher-pitched sound than the whispered voice, it is less reliable and is not used as the sole means of assessing auditory acuity.

Hearing normally occurs over two pathways. The sounds that are transmitted by way of the air-filled external and middle ear travel by way of *air conduction*. The sounds transmitted through bone directly to the inner ear travel by means of *bone conduction*. In the normal individual, air conduction is the more efficient pathway.

Hearing loss may be one of two types. The first type is a conductive loss and usually results from external (cerumen impaction) or middle ear disorders (otitis media, perforated tympanic membrane). In such instances, the transmission of sound by air to the inner ear, where it is converted to a neural impulse, is blocked. The second type of loss is a sensorineural, or perceptive, loss and involves damage to the eighth cranial nerve. These losses may be distinguished through the use of a tuning fork specifically selected for frequencies within the conversational voice range (512 or 1024 cycles per second).

The *Weber test* uses bone conduction to test lateralization of sound. The tuning fork is set in motion by grasping it firmly by its stem and tapping it lightly between the index finger and thumb. The surface of a knuckle can also be used. It is then placed on the top of the patient's head or in the middle of the forehead. The patient is asked if he can hear a sound. Where does he perceive the sound (one ear? both ears?)? If there is a conductive deficit (cerumen plug, otitis media) in one ear, the sound will be heard better in the poor ear. This is because obstruction in the ear canal or middle ear obliterates the room noise, thus enhancing bone conduction. However, if a sensorineural loss exists (cranial nerve VIII), the sound will not be perceived in the ear with the deficit. Instead, the sound lateralizes to the good ear.

In the *Rinne test,* the base of a vibrating tuning fork is placed on the mastoid process of the temporal bone until the patient can no longer hear it. The examiner quickly places the vibrating fork 2.5 cm (1 inch) from the opening of the auditory canal. Under normal circumstances, the patient will continue to perceive the sound, demonstrating that air conduction lasts longer than bone conduction (AC > BC).

In conductive hearing loss, however, bone conduction exceeds air conduction. That is, once bone conduction through the temporal bone has died out, the patient is unable to hear the fork through the usual conductive mechanism. In contradistinction, nerve deafness permits sound to be conducted by air better than by bone, although both are conducted poorly, and all sound may be perceived to be distant and faint. Use of the Weber and Rinne tests in concert enables one to distinguish conductive loss from nerve loss when hearing is impaired. These tests are not necessarily a part of the usual physical examination, but will be useful if the patient reports hearing deficit or if the examiner detects an inability of the patient to perceive such sounds as a ticking watch or a whispered voice.

External Ear. Inspection of the external ear is a simple procedure and is often overlooked. The auricle and surrounding tissues are carefully inspected for deformities, lesions, or discharges. Movement of the auricle, specifically the tragus, does not normally elicit pain. If this maneuver is painful, suspect acute external otitis. Tenderness in the area of the mastoid may indicate mastoiditis or inflammation of the posterior auricular node. Occasionally, sebaceous cysts and tophi (subcutaneous uric acid deposits) may be present on the pinna. A flaky scaliness on or behind the auricle usually indicates seborrheic dermatitis and may be present on the scalp and facial structures as well.

Otoscopic Examination. Proper inspection of the ear canal and eardrum (tympanic membrane) requires that the canal be free of cerumen. If the membrane cannot be visualized because of wax, the ear canal may be gently irrigated with warm tap water. In the event that firmly adherent cerumen is present, a small amount of mineral oil or an analogous commercial preparation may have to be instilled within the ear canal and the patient instructed to return for subsequent removal of the wax and inspection of the ear. The use of a cerumen spoon for wax removal is reserved for physicians and nurses with specialized training because of the danger of perforation of the tympanic membrane. Cerumen buildup demands attention because it is a common cause of hearing deficit and local irritation.

To examine the ear canal and tympanic membrane, the patient's head is tipped away from the examiner. The auricle is grasped firmly and pulled upward, backward, and slightly outward (Fig. 5-5). This straightens the canal for better visualization. The largest speculum that the canal will accommodate is selected and is guided gently down into the canal and slightly forward. The distal portion of the canal is bony and covered by a sensitive layer of epithelium. Here the pressure of the speculum may be painful.

Any discharge, inflammation, or foreign body in the ear canal is noted. The tympanic membrane is pearl grey and positioned obliquely at the base of the ear canal (Fig. 5-6). The examiner identifies its landmarks: the *pars tensa* and cone of light, the umbo, the manubrium of the malleus, and its short process, if visible. A slow movement of the speculum allows further visualization of the malleolar folds and periphery. The position and color of the membrane, as well as any unusual markings or deviation in the cone of light, are noted.

A "retracted eardrum" occurs when there is increased pressure (blocked Eustachian tube) in the middle ear. This is apparent as the malleus appears shorter and angled backward and as the short process becomes more prominent. Often, the cone of light is broken or absent. Occasionally, air bubbles or a fluid level line may be visible through the tympanic membrane, which suggest serous otitis media. Several dilated blood vessels along the manubrium is a normal finding, not to be confused with the generalized hyperemic membrane of purulent otitis media. All abnormalities are brought to the attention of a physician.

▷ Examination of the Thorax and Lungs

Examination of the thorax and lungs employs the skills of inspection, palpation, percussion, and auscultation. When these techniques are properly employed and the results log-

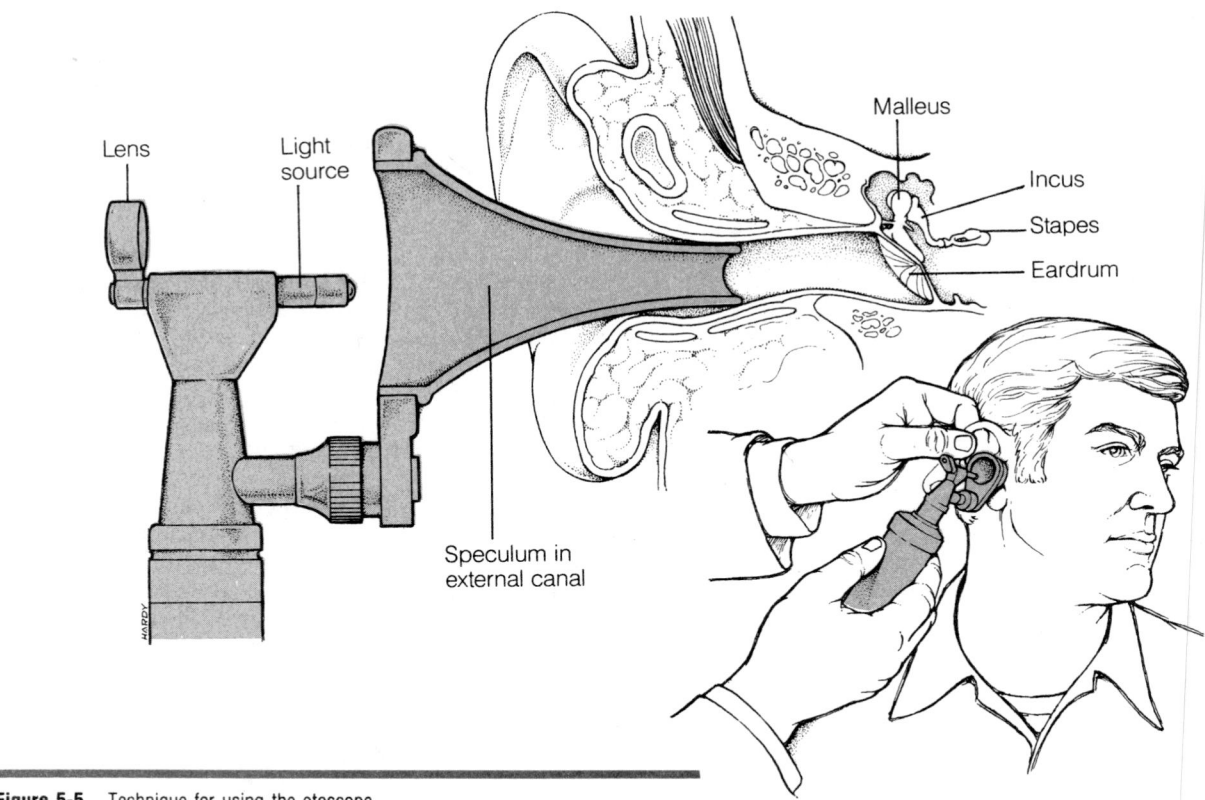

Figure 5-5. Technique for using the otoscope.

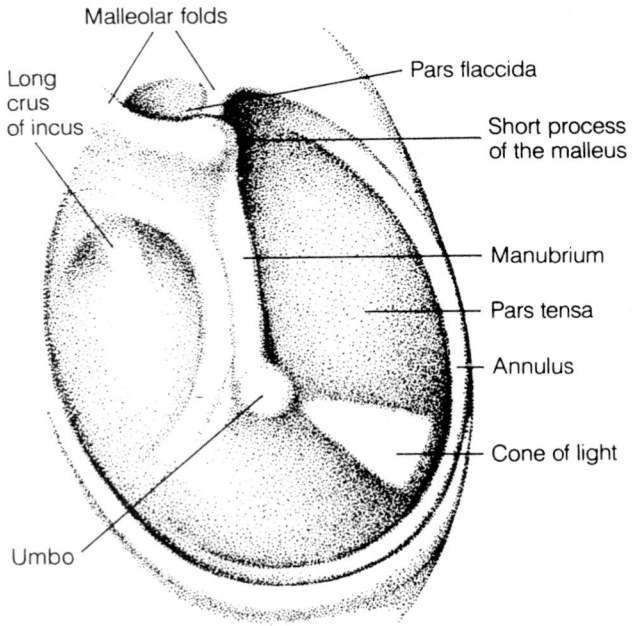

Figure 5-6. Display of the right eardrum as it would be visualized through the otoscope.

ically interpreted, much can be learned that will escape the x-ray film and other diagnostic aids.

Critical to practice in the health professions is the capacity to communicate to others, through the written or the spoken word, precisely what we have found. It is thus necessary to develop a common language. It is inefficient to draw a picture of the thorax each time we wish to display the location of critical findings. Rather, it is customary to refer to distance from known anatomical landmarks or from imaginary lines in common usage.

With respect to the thorax, location may be defined both horizontally and vertically. Horizontal reference is made in terms of the rib or the interspace overlying the examiner's findings (Fig. 5-7). On the anterior surface, identifying the specific rib is facilitated by locating the angle at which the manubrium joins the body of the sternum in the midline. The second rib joins the sternum at this prominent landmark. Other ribs may be identified by counting down from the second rib. The interspaces are referred to in terms of the rib immediately above the interspace. Thus, the fifth intercostal space is the space below the fifth rib. It is in this interspace that the male nipple and the impulse of the heart may be seen in normal persons.

Location of ribs on the posterior surface of the thorax is more difficult. The first step is to identify the spinous process. This may be accomplished by finding the most prominent of the spinous processes, the seventh cervical vertebra (*vertebra prominens*). When the neck is slightly flexed, the seventh cervical spinous process stands out. Others may then be identified by counting down.

To identify thoracic findings in terms of vertical location, reference is made to several imaginary lines (Fig. 5-8). The *midsternal line* is drawn down through the center of the sternum. The *midclavicular line* is an imaginary line drawn from the middle of the clavicle. The point of maximum impulse of the heart most generally lies along this line on the left thorax. When the arm is abducted from the body at 90 degrees, imaginary vertical lines may be drawn from the anterior axillary fold, from the middle of the axilla, and from the posterior axillary fold. These lines are called respectively the *anterior axillary line*, the *midaxillary line*, and the *posterior axillary line*. A line drawn vertically through the superior and inferior poles of the scapula is called the *scapular line*, and a line drawn down the center of the vertebral column is called the *vertebral line*.

It is apparent that the examiner can easily be understood when referring to a heart sound in the sixth left intercostal space at the anterior axillary line. Similarly, one may describe an area of dullness extending from the vertebral to the scapular line between the seventh and tenth ribs on the right without equivocation or confusion.

Topographically, the lobes of the lung may be located on the surface of the chest wall in the following manner (Fig. 5-9). The line between the upper and lower lobes on the left begins at the fourth thoracic spinous process posteriorly, proceeds around to cross the fifth rib in the midaxillary line, and meets the sixth rib at the sternum. This line on the right divides the right middle lobe from the right lower lobe. The line dividing the right upper lobe from the middle lobe is an incomplete one that begins at the fifth rib in the midaxillary line, where it intersects the line between the upper and lower lobes and traverses horizontally to the sternum. Thus, the upper lobes are dominant on the anterior surface of the thorax; the lower lobes are dominant on the posterior surface. There is no presentation of the middle lobe on the posterior surface of the chest.

Inspection of the Thorax

Inspection of the thorax reveals much about musculoskeletal structure, nutrition, and the status of the respiratory system. The skin over the thorax is observed for color and turgor and for evidence of loss of subcutaneous tissue. The musculature of the thorax may reflect recent weight loss. Asymmetry, if present, is noted.

Breathing Patterns. Noting the manner in which the patient breathes is of particular importance. Normally, the ribs articulate with the spine at a 45-degree angle. The act of breathing elevates the ribs, thrusting the sternum forward and up. The interspaces widen, and the angle that the ribs make with the spine more nearly approaches a 60-degree angle. Patients with emphysema have excessive residual volume; that is, they cannot expel the usual volume of air from the lungs during expiration. Because of the large residual volume, the ribs make a less acute angle with the spine, and the sternum is thrust forward excessively, even during expiration. This has the effect of *increasing the anteroposterior diameter* of the thorax.

Normally, the anteroposterior diameter, in proportion to the lateral diameter, is 1:2. In the emphysema patient, the ribs are more widely spaced, and the interspaces tend to bulge on expiration. As a result of overinflation of the lungs, not only is the capacity of the thorax to expand limited, but the diaphragm is depressed, limiting vertical fill-

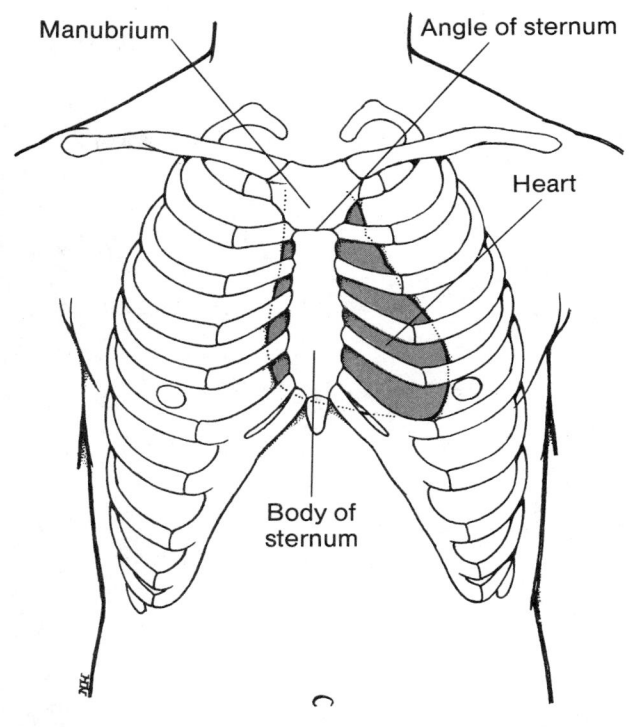

Figure 5-7. Topography of the anterior thorax.

ing. Consequently, the patient must bring into play accessory muscles of respiration, such as the sternocleidomastoids. The appearance of the patient with emphysema is thus quite characteristic and allows the observer to diagnose the disease easily, even from a distance.

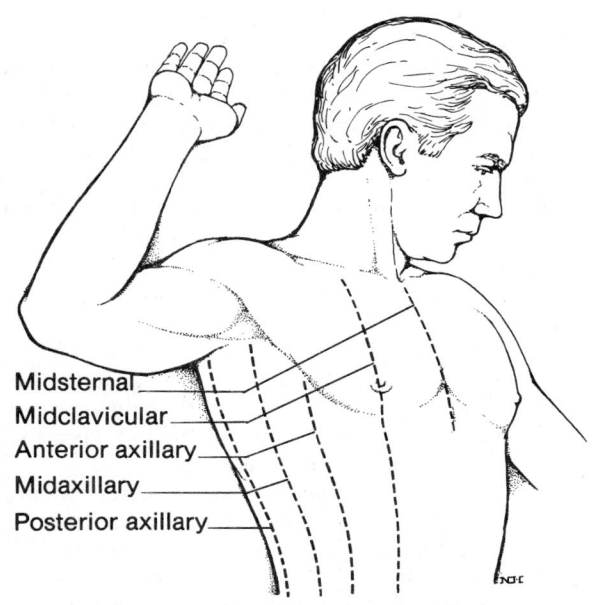

Figure 5-8. Imaginary "longitudinal lines" that permit verbal reference to the location of abnormalities over the chest wall.

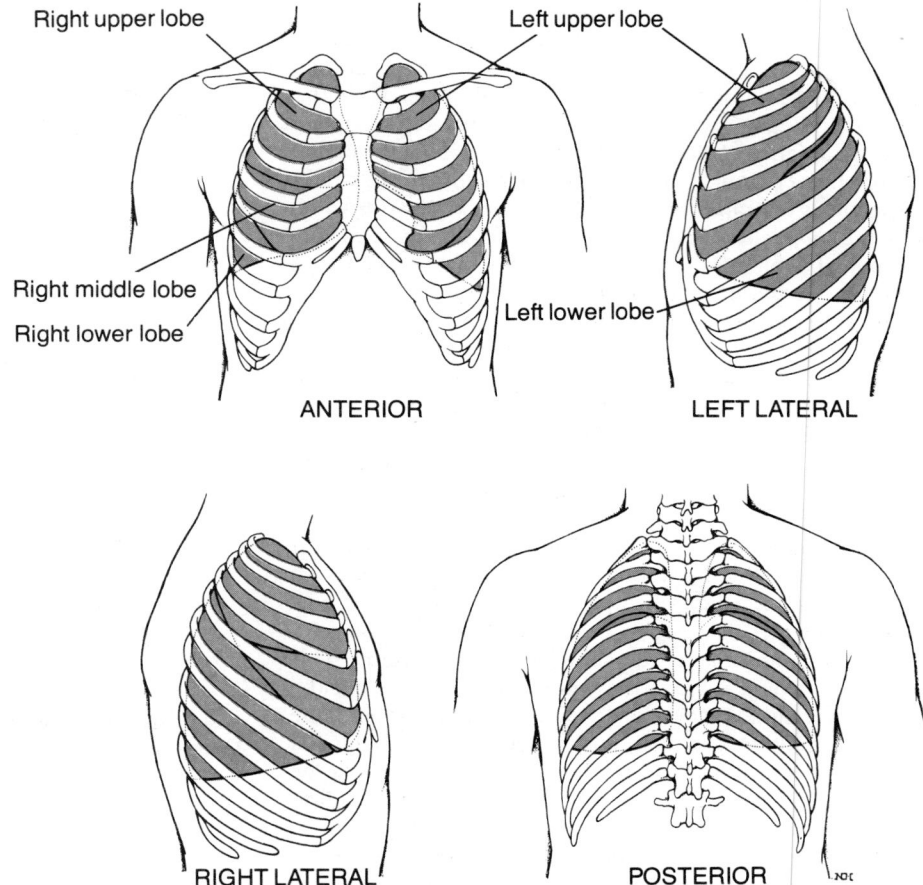

Figure 5-9. Topographical relationship of the ribs to the lobes of the lung.

Observation of the rate and depth of respiration is also important. In the adult, the normal respiratory rate is approximately 16 to 18 per minute; it is regular in depth and rhythm. An increase in the rate of respiration is called *tachypnea;* an increase in depth is called *hyperpnea.* An increase in both rate and depth is referred to as *hyperventilation.* At the extreme of hyperventilation is the marked increase in rate and depth, associated with severe acidosis of diabetic or renal origin, that is called *Kussmaul* respiration. In the critically ill patient, alternating episodes of apnea (cessation of breathing) and hyperpnea may occur. This cyclic phenomenon is referred to as *Cheyne–Stokes breathing.*

The inspiratory phase of respiration is the only one requiring energy in normal physiology. Expiration is passive. Inspiration occupies the first third of the respiratory cycle, expiration the latter two thirds. With rapid breathing, inspiration and expiration are nearly equal.

In thin persons, it is quite normal to note a slight retraction of the intercostal spaces during quiet breathing. Bulging during expiration implies obstruction of expiratory air flow, as in emphysema. Marked retraction of inspiration, particularly if asymmetrical, implies blockage of a branch of the respiratory tree. Asymmetrical bulging of the interspaces, on one side or the other, is created by an increase in pressure within the hemithorax. This may be a result of

air trapped under pressure within the pleural cavity where it does not belong (pneumothorax), or the pressure of fluid within the pleural space (pleural effusion).

The severe pain associated with pleurisy causes intercostal muscle spasm and a "lag" in respiration on the involved side.

Certain patterns of respiration are characteristic of specific disease states. Although the nurse need not recognize the specific pattern or be acquainted with the association of a certain pattern with a disease state, she is expected to be able to describe abnormal patterns of rhythmicity.

Palpation of the Thorax

Following inspection, the thorax is palpated for tenderness, masses, lesions, respiratory excursion, and vocal fremitus. If the patient has reported an area of pain, or if lesions are apparent, direct palpation with the fingertips (for skin lesions and subcutaneous masses) or with the ball of the hand (for deeper masses or generalized flank or rib discomfort) is done.

Respiratory Excursion.   Respiratory excursion is an estimation of thoracic expansion and may reveal significant data about the symmetry of breathing. Differences in expansion are more readily detectable on the anterior thorax, where a fuller range of motion occurs during respiration. The examiner's thumbs are placed along each costal margin, below the xiphoid process, while the hands rest along the lateral rib cage. Sliding the thumbs medially about 2.5 cm (1 inch) raises a small skin fold between the thumbs. The patient is instructed to inhale deeply while the examiner observes the movement of the thumbs during inspiration and expiration. This movement is normally symmetrical. A posterior assessment is done by placing the thumbs adjacent to the spinal column at the level of the tenth ribs. The hands lightly grasp the lateral rib cage. Again, a medial motion of the thumbs raises a skin fold, and the patient is instructed to take a full inspiration and expiration. The examiner observes for normal flattening of the skin fold and feels the symmetrical movement of the thorax. Respiratory lag or impairment is often the result of pleurisy, fractured ribs, or trauma to the chest wall.

Tactile Fremitus. Sound generated by the larynx travels distally along the bronchial tree to set the chest wall in resonant motion. This is especially true of consonant sounds. The capacity to feel sound on the chest wall is called *vocal* or *tactile fremitus.*

There is a wide variation in normal fremitus. It is obviously influenced by the thickness of the chest wall, most especially if that thickness is muscular, although the increase in subcutaneous tissue associated with obesity has some influence. Lower-pitched sounds travel better through the normal lung and incite the chest wall to greater vibration. Thus, fremitus is more pronounced in men than in women because of the deeper male voice.

Normally, fremitus is most pronounced where the large bronchi are closest to the chest wall and least palpable as the examiner progresses from the major bronchi to the distant lung fields. Therefore, it is most palpable in the upper thorax anteriorly and posteriorly. To elicit tactile fremitus, the examiner instructs the patient to repeat the words "ninety-nine" or "one, two, three" with each movement of the examiner's hands. The vibrations are perceived by placing the palmar surfaces of the fingers and hands, or the ulnar aspect of the extended hands, on the thorax. To facilitate comparison, only one hand is used as the examiner moves in sequence down the thorax. Corresponding areas of the thorax are compared (Fig. 5-10). Bony areas are not tested.

The physics of sound transmission through the lung requires explanation. Air does not conduct sound well; solid substance (tissue) does, provided that it has elasticity and is not conglomerated into a nonresonant mass. Thus, an increase in solid tissue per unit volume of lung will enhance fremitus. An increase in air per unit volume of lung will impede sound. Patients with emphysema will exhibit almost no tactile fremitus. A patient with consolidation of a lobe of the lung owing to pneumonia will have an increase in tactile fremitus over the distribution of the projection of that lobe on the surface of the chest wall. Air in the pleural space will not conduct sound.

Percussion of the Thorax

Percussion of the thorax is highly informative. This technique sets the chest wall and underlying structures in motion, producing audible and tactile vibrations. The examiner uses percussion to determine whether underlying tissues are filled with air, fluid, or solid material. One also uses this

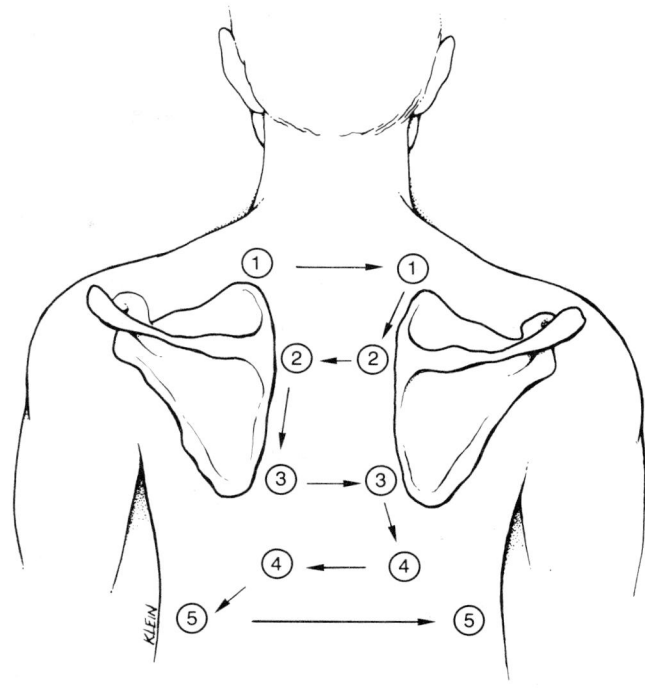

Figure 5-10. Palpation: tactile fremitus. Numbers and arrows indicate sequence of examination. (Adapted from Bates B: A Guide to Physical Examination, 3rd ed, p. 138. Philadelphia, JB Lippincott, 1983.)

technique to estimate the size and location of certain structures within the thorax (diaphragm, heart, liver).

The examination is usually initiated with percussion of the posterior thorax. Ideally, the patient is in a sitting position with his head flexed forward and his arms crossed on his lap. This position separates the scapulae widely and exposes more lung area for assessment. The procedure is as follows. The examiner percusses across each shoulder top, locating the 5-cm width of resonance overlying the lung apices (Fig. 5-11). She then proceeds down the posterior thorax, percussing symmetrical areas at 5-cm to 6-cm intervals. It is important to parallel the middle finger firmly against the chest wall between the interspaces prior to striking it with the middle finger of the opposite hand. Percussion over the scapulae or rib surfaces yields a dull sound and only confuses findings. Percussion over the anterior chest is performed with the patient in an upright position with shoulders arched backward and arms at the side. The examiner begins in the supraclavicular area and proceeds downward, from interspace to interspace. In the female patient, it is often necessary to displace the breasts for an adequate examination. Dullness noted to the left of the sternum between the third and fifth interspaces is the heart and is a normal finding. Similarly, there is a normal span of liver dullness in the right thorax from the fifth interspace to the right costal margin at the midclavicular line.

The lateral walls are examined by having the patient alternately raise an arm and rest the hand on his head while the examiner percusses from the axilla down to the costal

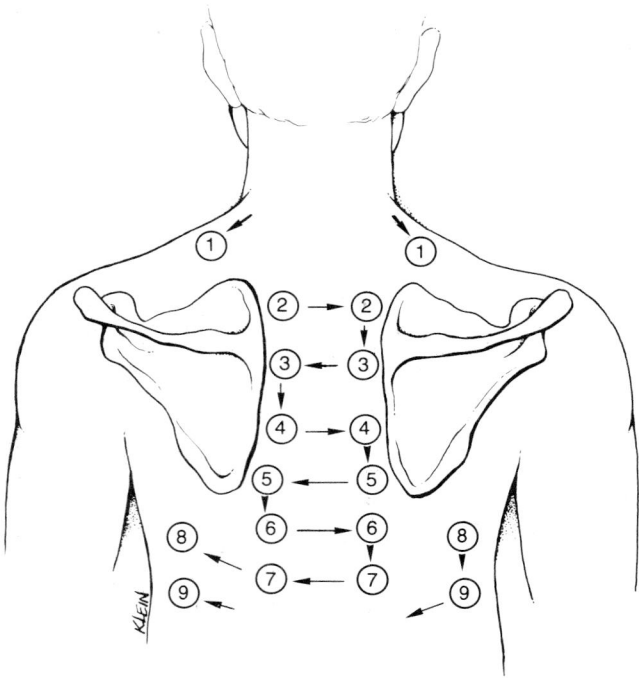

Figure 5-11. Percussion of the posterior thorax. With the patient in a sitting position, symmetrical areas of the lungs are percussed at 5-cm intervals. This progression starts at the apex of each lung and concludes with percussion of each lateral chest wall. (Adapted from Bates B: A Guide to Physical Examination, ed 3, p. 142. Philadelphia, JB Lippincott, 1983.)

margin. The anterior and lateral thorax can be examined with the patient in a supine position. If the patient is too ill, or unable to sit up, percussion of the posterior thorax is done with the patient rolled on his side.

Indication of Disease. Dullness over the lung is a function of increased density of the lung, and will be seen in those circumstances that lead to an increased transmission of sound (*i.e.,* consolidation and compression atelectasis). On the other hand, pleural effusion and obstructive atelectasis, though they do not conduct sound, are nevertheless detected by dullness on percussion. Pneumothorax produces a tympanic, or drumlike, sound, whereas emphysema is perceived as hyperresonant.

Diaphragmatic Excursion. The normal resonance of the lung stops at the diaphragm, where it becomes dull. The position of the diaphragm is different during inspiration than it is during expiration. For assessment of size and position, the patient is instructed to take a deep breath and hold it while the maximum descent of the diaphragm is percussed. This is done along the midscapular lines bilaterally. The point at which the percussion note changes from resonance to dullness is noted. If desired, this point can be marked with a pen. The patient is then instructed to exhale fully and hold it while the examiner again percusses downward to the dullness of the diaphragm. This location is marked. The distance between the two markings indicates the range of motion of the diaphragm.

Maximum excursion of the diaphragm may amount to as much as 8 cm or 10 cm (3 or 4 inches) in healthy, tall, young men. For most persons, it is usually 5 cm to 7 cm (2 to 2¾ inches). The diaphragm is 2 cm (¾ inch) or so higher on the right than on the left. This is because of the spatial relationships of the heart and the liver above and below the left and right segments of the diaphragm respectively. A decreased diaphragmatic excursion may be apparent in patients with pleurisy and emphysema. An increase in intra-abdominal pressure, such as occurs in pregnancy or ascites, may account for a diaphragm that is positioned high in the thorax.

Auscultation of the Thorax

Auscultation is useful in assessing the flow of air through the bronchial tree and in evaluating the presence of fluid or solid obstruction in the lung structures. To determine the condition of the lungs, the examiner auscultates for normal breath sounds, adventitious sounds, and voice sounds.

A thorough examination includes auscultation of the anterior, posterior, and lateral thorax and is performed as follows. The diaphragm of the stethoscope is placed firmly against the chest wall as the patient breathes slowly and deeply through his mouth. Corresponding areas of the chest are auscultated in a systematic fashion from the apices to the bases and along the midaxillary lines. The sequence of auscultation and the positioning of the patient are similar to those used for percussion. It is often necessary to listen to two full inspirations and expirations at each anatomical location to ensure valid interpretation of the sound heard. Deep breathing may result in symptoms of hyperventilation (*e.g.,* lightheadedness) and can be avoided by having the patient rest and breathe normally once or twice during the examination.

Breath Sounds. Normal breath sounds are distinguished by their location over a specific area of the lung and are identified as *vesicular* and *bronchial* (tubular) breath sounds. Vesicular sounds are audible as quiet, low-pitched sounds that have a long inspiratory phase and a short expiratory phase. They are heard normally throughout the entire lung field, except over the upper sternum and between the scapulae, where they are replaced with bronchial breath sounds. Bronchial breath sounds are usually louder and higher pitched than vesicular sounds. In comparison, the expiratory phase is longer than the inspiratory phase. If bronchial sounds are audible elsewhere in the lung, this is an indication of pathology and necessitates physician consultation.

The quality and intensity of breath sounds are determined during auscultation. When air flow is decreased by bronchial obstruction (atelectasis) or when fluid (pleural effusion) or tissue (obesity) separates the air passages from the stethoscope, breath sounds are diminished or absent. For example, the breath sounds of the patient with emphysema are faint and often completely absent.

When heard, the expiratory phase is prolonged and may exhibit a high-pitched whistling tone called *wheezing.* This same sound is also heard in asthma and in any process associated with marked bronchoconstriction.

Adventitious Sounds. The presence of an abnormal condition that affects the bronchial tree and alveoli may produce additional or adventitious sounds. The terminology used to describe these abnormal sounds is changing. For this reason, verbal and written communication regarding the presence of adventitious sounds is sometimes confusing. The current view is as follows.

Adventitious sounds are divided into two categories: discrete, noncontinuous sounds and continuous musical sounds. The duration of the sound is the important distinction to make in identifying the sound as noncontinuous or continuous. *Crackles* (rales, crepitations) are discrete, noncontinuous sounds that are a result of the delayed reopening of deflated airways. *Fine crackles* are usually audible at the end of inspiration and originate from the alveoli. Their sound can be recreated by rubbing several pieces of hair next to one's ear. *Coarse crackles* have a gross, moist sound. They are produced in the large bronchi and are audible in early-to-mid inspiration. Crackles may or may not be cleared by coughing. Crackles are a reflection of underlying inflammation or congestion and are often present in such conditions as pneumonia, bronchitis, congestive heart failure, and pulmonary fibrosis.

Wheezes (rhonchi) are continuous musical sounds that are longer in duration than crackles. They may be audible during inspiration, expiration, or both. These sounds result from the passage of air through narrowed or partially obstructed passages. Obstruction is often due to the presence of secretions or swelling, and hence wheezes may clear with coughing. When the sounds originate in the smaller bronchi and bronchioles, they may be high-pitched, sibilant, and musical. Obstruction in the larger bronchi or trachea, on the other hand, produces sounds that are lower-pitched; and sonorous. Wheezes are commonly heard in patients with asthma and emphysema.

Inflammation of pleural surfaces induces a crackling, grating sound that is usually heard in both inspiration and expiration. The sound is called a *friction rub.* It seems to be quite "close" to the ear and is enhanced by applying pressure with the head of the stethoscope. The sound is imitated by rubbing the thumb and index finger together near the ear. The grating sound of a friction rub is not altered by coughing. If audible only during inspiration, it may be difficult to distinguish from crackles, which may be multiple and so frequent that a continuous sound is perceived.

Voice Sounds. The sound heard through the stethoscope as the patient vocalizes is known as *vocal resonance.* The vibrations produced in the larynx are transmitted to the chest wall as they pass through the bronchi and alveolar tissue. During the process, the sounds are diminished in intensity and altered so that syllables are not distinguishable. The spoken voice is usually assessed by having the patient repeat the phrase "ninety-nine" while the examiner listens with the stethoscope in corresponding areas of the chest from the apices to the bases.

If the vocal resonance is increased in intensity and clarity, *bronchophony* is said to be present. In consolidation, the syllables may become clearly distinguishable, and the voice assumes a bleating quality, termed *egophony.* Egophony is best appreciated by having the patient repeat the letter "e." The distortion produced by consolidation transforms the sound into a clearly heard "a" rather than "e."

Bronchophony and egophony have precisely the same connotation as bronchial breathing and an increase in tactile fremitus. Where one abnormality is detected, so should the others be. A change in tactile fremitus is more subtle and can be missed, but bronchial breathing and bronchophony present loudly and clearly to the examiner.

A very subtle finding, heard only in the presence of rather dense consolidation is the phenomenon of *whispered pectoriloquy.* Transmission of high-frequency components of sound is so enhanced that even whispered words are heard, a circumstance not noted in normal physiology. The implication is the same as that of *egophony.*

A routine assessment of the thorax and lungs includes the following: inspection of the thorax and respirations, percussion of the posterior thorax, and auscultation of the thorax for breath sounds and the presence of adventitious sounds. Unless some facet of the history of a prior observation in the physical examination leads the examiner to pursue additional information about respiratory status, palpation for fremitus and auscultation of voice sounds are omitted.

▷ Examination of the Breast

Examination of the female breast is conducted during any general physical or gynecologic examination, or whenever the patient presents with suspicion, complaint, or fear of breast disease.

The patient is disrobed to the waist and initially is seated in a comfortable position facing the examiner with her hands in her lap.

Inspection

The breasts are inspected for size and symmetry. A slight difference in the sizes of the two breasts is common and is generally a normal finding. The skin is inspected for color, thickening or edema, and venous pattern. Erythema may indicate local inflammation or superficial lymphatic invasion by a neoplasm. Likewise, an increased venous pattern may signal the accessory blood supply of a growing neoplasm. Lymphatic blockage by tumor cells may create edema and pitting of the skin and give the skin surface an orange peel (peau d'orange) appearance.

The nipples, although variable from patient to patient, are normally similar in size and shape. A slight inversion of one or both nipples is not uncommon and is only a significant finding when of recent origin. The position of the nipples is observed for symmetry. The presence of ulceration, rashes, or nipple discharge is an abnormal finding that requires the attention of a physician. In order to elicit a dimpling or retraction that may otherwise go undetected, the examiner instructs the patient to raise both arms overhead. This maneuver normally elevates both breasts equally. Next, the patient is instructed to place the palms of both hands together, pushing forcibly. This facilitates contraction of the pectoral muscles and normally does not alter the breast contour or nipple direction. Any dimpling or retrac-

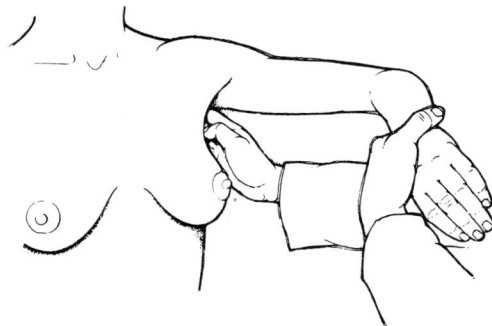

A. Palpation of axillae. Positioning of patient.

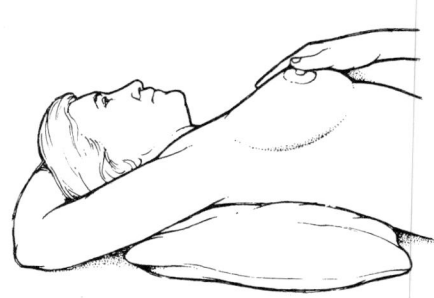

B. Palpation of breast. The patient's shoulder is elevated on a small pillow.

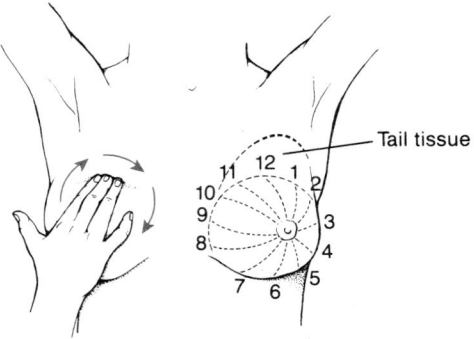

C. The entire surface of the breast, including the tail, is palpated in a clockwise fashion.

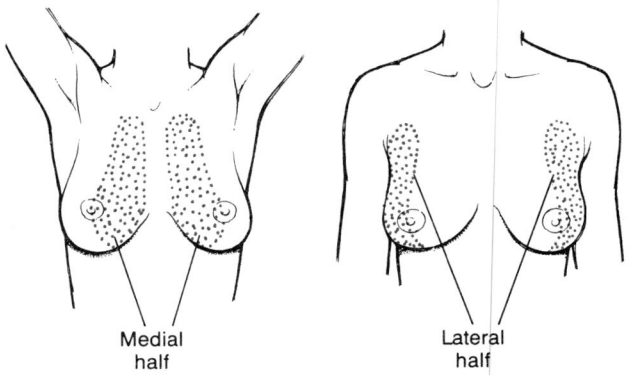

D. The medial half of the breast is examined with the patient's arm overhead, the lateral half with the arm at the side.

Figure 5-12. Breast examination. Palpation of the axilla and the breast.

tion of the breast during these movements is highly suggestive of an underlying malignancy. Lastly, the clavicular and axillary regions are inspected for signs of discoloration, swelling, or lesions.

Palpation

Palpation of the axillae and clavicular areas is easily performed with the patient in a sitting position. To examine axillary lymph nodes, the patient's arm is gently abducted from the thorax by the examiner's hand. The patient's left forearm is grasped and supported with the examiner's left hand (Fig. 5-12A). The right hand is then free to palpate the axilla, noting the presence or absence of nodes that may be lying against the thoracic wall. The fingertips are used to gently palpate the areas of the central, lateral, subscapular, and pectoral nodes. Normally, these lymph nodes are not palpable. If enlarged, note their size, location, mobility, consistency, and tenderness. The arm is put through a full range of motion in order to uncover any nodes or mass lesions that may be hidden under the pectoralis muscle or under subcutaneous fat. The procedure is reversed to examine the right axilla. In a similar fashion, the supraclavicular and infraclavicular areas are palpated.

The patient is now assisted to a supine position on the examining table. Prior to palpation of the breast, the shoulder is elevated on a small pillow in order to balance the breast on the chest wall (Fig. 5-12B). Otherwise, a mass may be missed in the thick tissue if the breast is allowed to fall to the side.

Light palpation in an orderly fashion includes the entire surface of the breast, including the breast tail. The examiner may choose to proceed in a clockwise direction following imaginary concentric circles from the outer limits of the breast toward the nipple. Another acceptable method is to palpate from each "number" on the face of the clock toward the nipple in a clockwise fashion (Fig. 5-12C).

When the medial half of the breast is palpated, the arm may be actively or passively moved above the head in order to tense the pectoralis muscles and provide a flatter surface. When the lateral half of the breast is palpated, the arm is brought back to the patient's side (Fig. 5-12D). The examiner may do this by simple manipulation of a relaxed elbow. A prolongation or "tail" of breast tissue may extend toward the axilla along the pectoralis tendon toward its insertion. This breast tissue also requires palpation and is not to be mistaken for pathology.

During palpation, the consistency of the tissue and the presence of tenderness or masses are noted. If a mass is felt, it is described by its location (*e.g.,* left breast, 2 cm from nipple at 2 o'clock), size, shape, consistency, delimitation, mobility, and presence of tenderness.

Lastly, the areola around the nipple is gently compressed to determine the presence or absence of abnormal secretion.

The breast tissue of the adolescent is firm and lobular, while the postmenopausal woman often has breast tissue that feels stringy and granular in texture. During pregnancy and lactation, the breasts are larger and firmer, and the lobules are more distinct. Cysts are a common finding in menstruating women and are usually well defined and freely movable. Premenstrually, they may be larger and more tender. Malignancies, on the other hand, tend to be hard, poorly defined, fixed to the skin or underlying tissues, and often nontender. Any abnormalities detected during inspection and palpation require additional evaluation by the physician.

Teaching breast self-examination is an important aspect of health maintenance and is easily incorporated into this section of the physical examination (see Fig. 47-1).

The Male Breast. Examination of the male breast and axillae is not to be overlooked. The nipple and areola are inspected for masses, lesions, or discharge. The areola is palpated for masses. Gynecomastia is differentiated from the soft, fatty enlargement of obesity by the firm enlargement of glandular tissue beneath and immediately surrounding the areola. The same procedure for inspection and palpation of the female axillae is employed during an assessment of the male axillae.

▷ Examination of the Cardiovascular System

For convenience, all facets of the cardiovascular examination are discussed under one heading, although it is recognized that different portions of the examination will be done at different times during the evaluation of the patient because it is more convenient to do so.

Examination of the Pulse

In examining the pulse, one is interested not only in the obvious information to be determined from rate and rhythm, but in the configuration of the pulse wave and in the quality of the vessel itself.

The normal pulse *rate* varies from a low of 50 in healthy, athletic, young adults to rates well in excess of 100 following exercise or during times of excitement. Anxiety frequently elevates the pulse rate during the physical examination. If the rate appears higher than expected, it is appropriate to reassess it near the end of the physical examination, at a time when the examiner has established better rapport with the patient.

Equally important in assessing the pulse is notation of the *rhythm.* Minor variations in the regularity of the pulse are normal. The pulse rate, particulary in young persons,

increases during inspiration and slows during expiration. This is called *sinus arrhythmia.*

An irregular pulse palpated in the peripheral arteries is usually indicative of missed beats. Disturbance of rhythm (arrhythmias) often result in what is commonly referred to as a "pulse deficit." Because of the irregularity, the actual heart rate (apical pulse) is not palpated peripherally. The difference between the apical rate and peripheral rate is the pulse deficit. Pulse deficits are frequently seen in such cardiac disorders as atrial fibrillation, atrial flutter, and varying degrees of heart block.

An understanding of the complexity of arrhythmias that may be encountered during the examination requires a sophisticated knowledge of cardiac electrophysiology, knowledge usually possessed by the nurse who specializes in cardiovascular nursing.

The *quality,* or amplitude, of the pulse can be described as normal, diminished, or absent. Some authorities suggest a numerical classification based on a 0 to 4 scale:

> 0—absence of pulsation
> +1—marked impairment of pulsation
> +2—moderate impairment of pulsation
> +3—slight impairment of pulsation
> +4—normal pulsation

Numerical classification is quite subjective; thus, in written communication it is helpful to specify the scale range (*e.g.,* radial +4/+4).

The configuration, or contour, of the pulse frequently conveys important information. In stenosis of the aortic valve, the pulse pressure is narrow and the pulse appears to be feeble. When insufficiency of the aortic valve is present, the rise of the pulse wave is abrupt and its fall is precipitous, giving rise to a "collapsing" pulse. The true configuration of the pulse is best appreciated by palpating over the carotid artery rather than the distal radial artery, since the dramatic characteristics of the pulse wave may be distorted or damped by transmission to smaller vessels.

The condition of the vessel wall is of vital concern, especially in older patients. The pulse rate is usually determined by placing the tips of the index and middle fingers over the radial artery. Once rate and rhythm have been determined, one can assess the quality of the vessel itself. Does it appear to be thickened? Is it tortuous? In order to properly assess the vessel, one must do more than simply compress it. It is necessary to slide the fingers along the vessel and compare it with the feel of the normal vessels.

Arterial pulses are commonly palpated at points where the arteries are near the skin surface and easily compressible against bones or firm musculature. Pulses are detected over the temporal, carotid, brachial, radial, femoral, popliteal, dorsalis pedis, and posterior tibial arteries. For convenience, the radial artery is usually selected for determination of pulse.

Two or three fingertips compress the artery against the distal radius, and the rate, rhythm, quality, contour, and condition of the vessel wall are determined. Similarly, all arterial pulses are located and evaluated as a part of a thorough cardiovascular assessment. A reliable assessment of the pulses of the extremities depends on accurate identi-

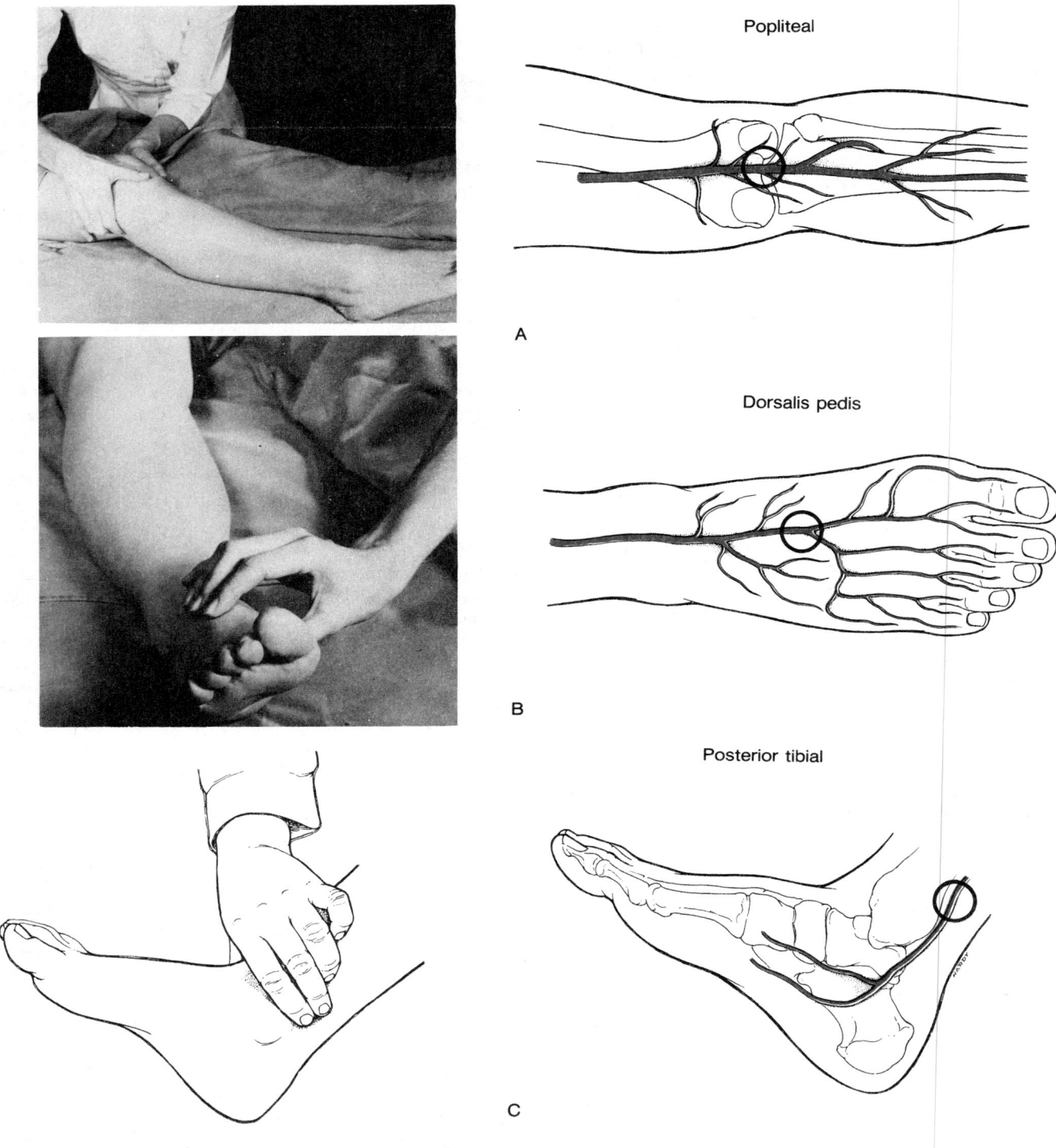

Figure 5-13. (*A*) Popliteal pulse. (*B*) Pedal pulse. (*C*) Posterior tibial pulse. (Photos from Ajemian S: Bypass grafting for femoral artery occlusion. Am J Nurs 67:565.)

fication of the artery location and careful technique (Fig. 5-13). Firm finger pressure can easily obliterate the dorsalis pedis and posterior tibial pulses and confuse the examiner. Light palpation is essential. In approximately 10% of the population, the dorsalis pedis arteries are not palpable. In such circumstances, both are usually absent together, and the posterior tibial arteries alone provide adequate blood supply to the feet.

Examination of Blood Pressure

Blood pressure occurs as a cyclic phenomenon and is measured in millimeters of mercury (mm Hg). The peak of the cycle is called the *systolic pressure;* the low point of the cycle is called the *diastolic pressure.* Blood pressure is usually expressed as the ratio of the systolic pressure over the diastolic pressure, with normal values measuring 120/80 mm Hg.

The difference between systolic and diastolic pressure is called the *pulse pressure.* Normally, this amounts to 40 mm Hg. An increase in blood pressure is called *hypertension;* a decrease is called *hypotension.* The systolic pressure may be elevated alone (*systolic hypertension*) and of necessity results in a widening of the pulse pressure. This happens in atherosclerosis (hardening of the arteries) and in thyrotoxicosis. Elevation of the diastolic pressure is always associated with elevation of the systolic pressure, and the circumstance represents true hypertension. An increase in the diastolic pressure to 95 mm Hg gives rise to concern, particularly in younger patients; an increase in excess of 95 mm Hg in the diastolic pressure constitutes true hypertension and requires investigation and control.

The blood pressure is measured by the use of the sphygmomanometer and the stethoscope. The sphygmomanometer consists of an inflatable cuff and a pressure gauge that communicates with the hollow portion of the cuff. The device is calibrated in such a manner that the pressure that is read from the manometer is quite comparable to the pressure in millimeters of mercury that is being transmitted to the brachial artery. The cuff is wrapped tightly around the upper arm and is infated by a bulb. Pressure on the cuff is increased until the radial pulse disappears. The disappearance of the radial pulse signifies that systolic blood pressure has been exceeded and the brachial artery is occluded. The cuff is then inflated 20 mm Hg to 30 mm Hg above the point at which radial pulsation disappears. If one now slowly lowers the pressure within the cuff by deflating the bulb, there

will come a point at which a pulse will again become discernible in the radial artery. This is the systolic blood pressure. At the same time, a sound is produced within the brachial artery just below the cuff and is audible with the stethoscope. This sound (*Korotkoff sound*) coincides with each pulse beat and will continue to emanate from the brachial artery until the pressure in the cuff has been reduced below diastolic pressure. At that point, the sound ceases. In actual practice, the sound more often becomes muffled (changes character) as diastolic pressure is reached and then disappears at 10 mm Hg to 20 mm Hg below normal diastolic pressure. One is interested in the point at which the sound becomes muffled. If there is any doubt, the blood pressure may be recorded as a tripartite pressure (120/80/60) to imply that the sound became muffled at 80 mm Hg and disappeared at 60 mm Hg.

Accurate recording of the blood pressure depends upon attention to several critical details. The cuff is firmly wrapped around the arm, and the cuff bladder is centered over the brachial artery. The stethoscope is placed directly over the brachial artery, just below the crease of the elbow, the point at which the brachial artery emerges from the two heads of the biceps muscle. An appropriate cuff size is one that is 20% wider than the diameter of the limb. If the cuff is too large for the arm, as in a child, one will underestimate the magnitude of pressure; that is, the pressure obtained will be substantially below true pressure. If the arm is excessively large, as it is in many obese persons, one will overestimate the level of pressure; that is, the patient will appear to be hypertensive when the pressure is, in fact, normal (Fig. 5-14). Special cuffs are manufactured for obese persons and for children.

The measurement of blood pressure is an exercise that a nurse is expected to be able to perform well and reliably. Proper measurement takes practice. Blood pressure in hypertensive persons is usually measured while the patient is lying down, sitting, and then standing. It is measured in

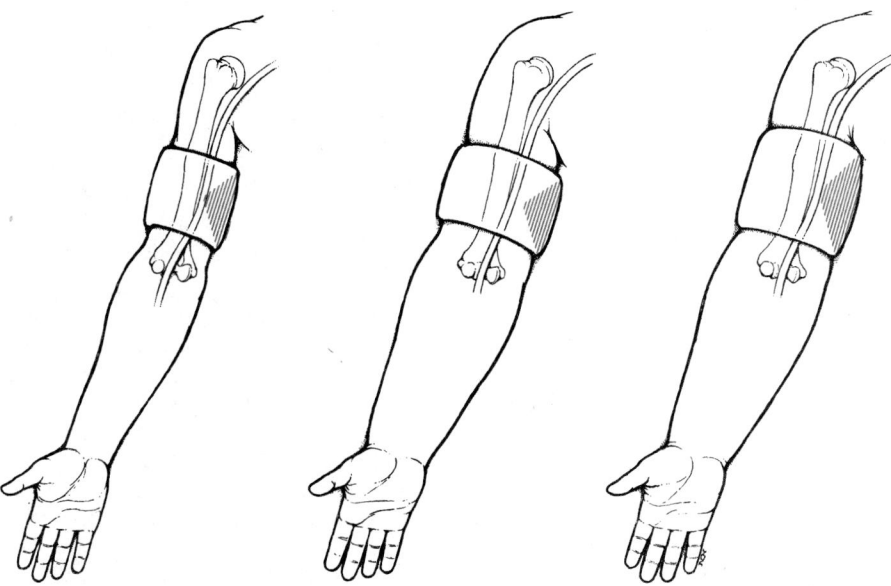

Figure 5-14. Illustration of blood pressure cuff transmission to the brachial artery. Panel to the left represents the normal transmission as it would occur in a normal-sized arm. The center panel demonstrates that with obesity the usual size cuff will not transmit faithfully to the brachial artery without excessive generation of pressure, providing a falsely elevated reading. The panel to the right illustrates the use of a wider ("obesity") cuff in order to obtain accurate readings from persons who are overweight.

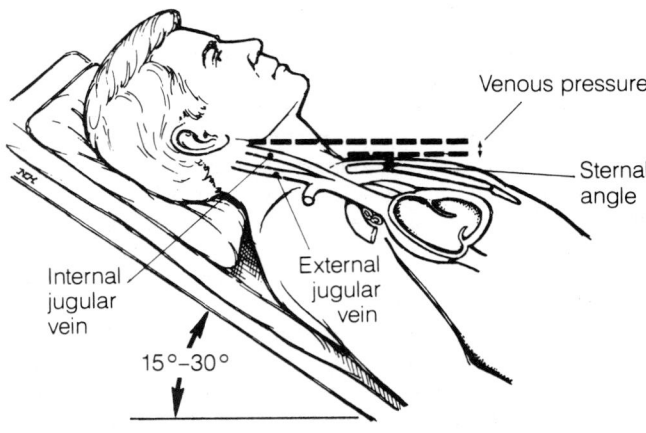

Figure 5-15. An assessment of jugular venous pressure. The highest point at which jugular vein pulsations can be seen is noted. The vertical distance between this point and the sternal angle is measured and recorded as centimeters "above or below" the sternal angle.

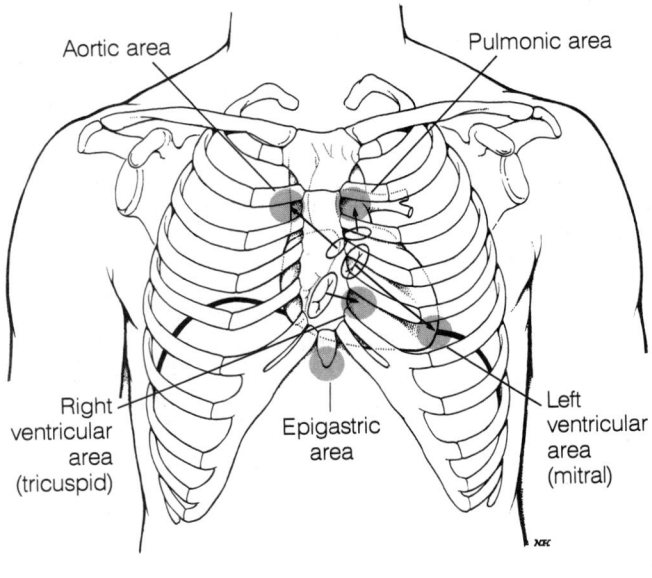

Figure 5-16. Topographical anatomy of the heart as it projects upon the thoracic wall.

both the right and the left arm. Unless there is disease of the vasculature, a difference of no more than 5 mm Hg should be found.

Blood pressure can also be measured in the lower extremities. However, an extra-wide cuff is used.

Inspection and Palpation of the Heart

Inspection of the cardiovascular system involves two important observations. First, the venous system is inspected and any venous pulsations observed; secondly, the *precordium* (surface of the thorax overlying the heart) is inspected for abnormal pulsation.

A gross estimation of right heart function is done by observing the pulsations of the jugular veins of the neck. When visualization of the internal jugular veins is difficult, the pulsations of the external jugular veins are observed for an assessment of central venous pressure. The external jugular veins are more superficial and visible just above the clavicles adjacent to the sternocleidomastoid muscles.

They are frequently distended while the patient lies supine on the examining table or in the bed. As the patient is elevated, however, the distention of the veins will disappear. They are not normally apparent once the angle that the patient makes with the examining table exceeds 30 degrees. For this assessment, the patient is supine, with the head of the bed elevated 15 to 30 degrees. The patient's head is turned slightly away from the side of the neck that is being examined. The examiner first identifies the external jugular vein. If possible, the pulsations of the internal jugular vein are located. The highest point at which these pulsations are seen is noted. The vertical distance between this point and the sternal angle is then measured (Fig. 5-15). This distance is usually recorded in centimeters "above or below" the sternal angle. In general, measurements greater than 3 cm above the sternal angle are considered abnormal.

Obvious distention of the veins with the patient at 45 to 90 degrees (sitting up) implies an abnormal increase in the volume of the venous system secondary to the retention of fluid or obstruction to flow in the superior vena cava. The former circumstance is much more common and is associated with congestive heart failure.

When the neck veins are distended, they easily conduct pulsations that emanate from the heart. They may conduct a wave associated with contraction of the atrium or a wave generated by contraction of the right ventricle that is conveyed through an incompetent tricuspid valve. The former is called an *a-wave;* the latter is called a *v-wave.* Occasionally, in advanced congestive heart failure, these two waves may be seen together in the veins of the neck, even with the patient in the sitting position.

Inspection and palpation of the chest wall is concentrated in five areas (Fig. 5-16):

1. *Aortic area*—second intercostal space to the right of the sternum
2. *Pulmonary area*—second intercostal space to the left of the sternum
3. *Right ventricular or tricuspid area*—fourth and fifth intercostal spaces to the left of the sternum
4. *Left ventricular or apical area*—fifth intercostal space to the left and right of the sternum
5. *Epigastric area*

For the examination, the patient is supine, with his head slightly elevated. Oblique lighting is used to assist the examiner in identifying subtle pulsation. There is a normal impulse that is discrete and well localized directly over the apex of the heart and that may be observed in young persons and in older persons who are thin. This is called the *apical impulse* and is normally located in the left fifth intercostal space in the midclavicular line. In left ventricular hypertrophy, this impulse is broader, more diffuse, and more forceful and may be displaced to the anterior axillary line or even to the midaxillary line.

In a systematic fashion, each area of the precordium is inspected and then palpated. The apical impulse can often be palpated. It is normally felt as a light pulsation, 1 cm to 2 cm in diameter. It is felt at the onset of the first heart sound and lasts only half of systole. The palm of the hand is used initially to locate the apical impulse, and the finger pads are used to describe its size and quality. If the apical impulse is broad and forceful, it is often referred to as a *left ventricular heave* or *lift*. It is so named because it appears to "lift" the hand from the chest wall during palpation.

Murmurs, when they are exceptionally loud, may also be palpated and are felt by the palm of the hand as a "purring" sensation. This phenomenon is called a *thrill* and is always indicative of significant pathology within the heart. Thrills also may be palpated over vessels when there is significant substantial obstruction to blood flow and will occur over the carotid arteries in the presence of narrowing (or stenosis) of the aortic valve.

Percussion of the Heart

In the normal patient, only the left border of the heart is located by percussion. It extends from the sternum to the midclavicular line in the third to fifth intercostal space. The right border lies under the right margin of the sternum, but the sternum is a sounding board and does not permit definition of the border. Enlargement of the heart to either the left or right can usually be noted. In many persons who have very thick chests, are obese, or have emphysema, the heart may lie sufficiently far beneath the thoracic surface so that not even its left border can be noted unless the heart is enlarged.

Unless the examiner detects a displaced apical impulse and suspects cardiac enlargement, percussion is omitted.

Auscultation of the Heart

Before discussing auscultation of the heart, it is necessary to clarify some physical principles as they relate to the production of heart sounds. Let us first review the cardiac cycle.

Cardiac Cycle. The cardiac cycle begins with contraction of the ventricles (Fig. 5-17). As pressure is generated within the ventricles, the mitral and tricuspid valves close, and their leaves balloon into the left and right atria, respectively. Pressure within the ventricles continues to rise until aortic and pulmonic pressures are exceeded, at which point the aortic and pulmonic valves open. The pulmonic valve opens first, since pressure in the pulmonary artery is lower than in the aorta. The period of time between closure of the atrial ventricular valves and the opening of the semi-

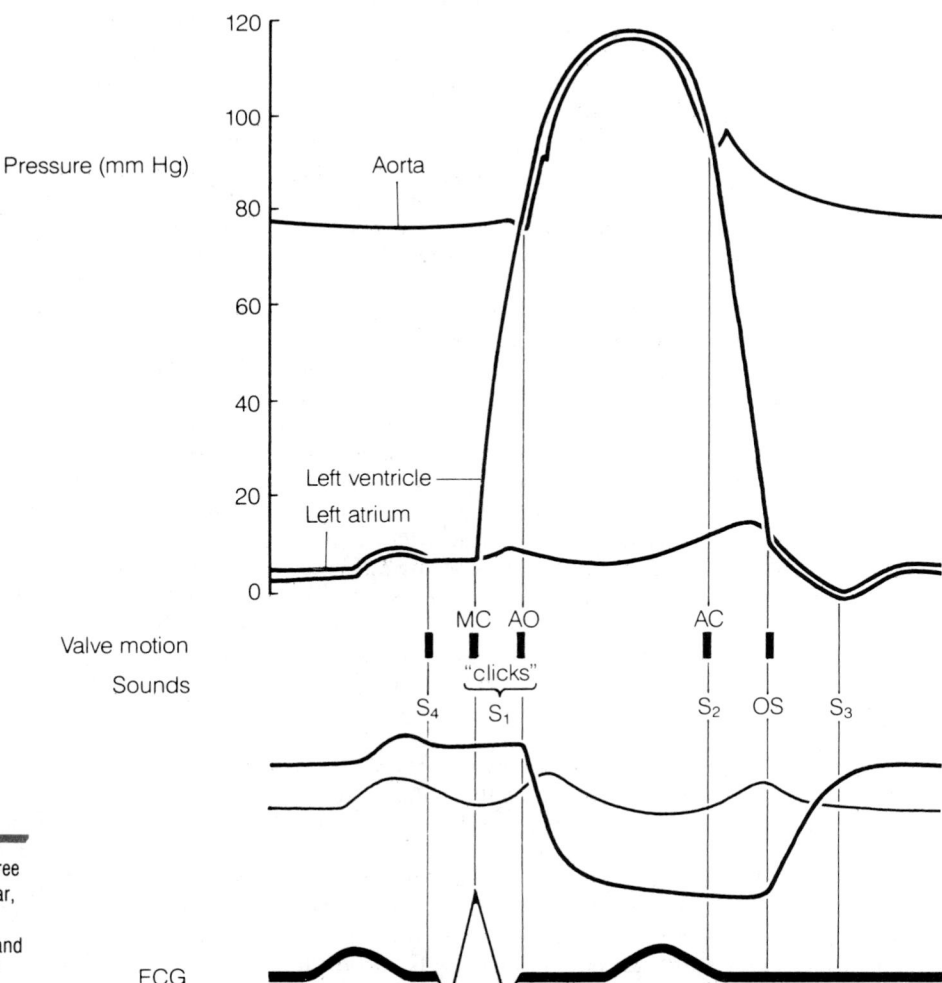

Figure 5-17. Events in the cardiac cycle. Three pressure curves are displayed: aortic, ventricular, and left atrial. Electrocardiographic events precede the mechanical events. Valve closure and opening are indicated, as is the relationship of the cardiac sounds to these events.

lunar valves is called *ventricular contraction*. Opening of the semilunar valves (aortic and pulmonic valves) is the point at which *systole* begins. Systole continues until ventricular energy is spent, aortic and pulmonic pressures exceed pressures within the ventricle, and the semilunar valves close. The aortic valve closes first under normal circumstances, since aortic pressure exceeds pulmonic pressure. Pressure in the ventricle then falls precipitously until it dips below the pressure within the atria, at which time the mitral and tricuspid valves open, and diastole begins. The period of time between the closure of the semilunar valves and the opening of the atrioventricular valves is called *ventricular relaxation*. Once the mitral and tricuspid valves have opened, the ventricles begin to fill. This phase of the cardiac cycle is called *diastole*. Filling is at first rapid, ultimately approaching the plateau. Near the end of diastole, the atria contract against the partially filled ventricle and augment the volume of the ventricular cavities by an additional 10% of volume. Almost immediately thereafter, the mitral and tricuspid valves rebound to a closed position, the ventricles promptly contract, ballooning the valves back into the atria, and the cycle begins again.

Heart Sounds.   Closure of the valves gives rise to "heart sounds" that may be heard on the chest wall. These are called the *transient heart sounds*. In normal physiology, the periods of systole and diastole are silent. Pathology of the ventricle, however, can give rise to transient sounds in systole and diastole that are called *gallops, snaps,* or *clicks*. Significant pathologic narrowing of the valve orifices at times when they should be open or residual gapping of valves at times when they should be closed gives rise to prolonged sounds that are called *murmurs*. Proper identification of normal and abnormal sounds over the precordium is a sophisticated and challenging process, but one with which the nurse can become familiar.

Auscultatory Valve Areas.   Events occurring at each of the four valves are uniquely reflected at specific locations on the chest wall (see Fig. 5-16). These locations do not correspond to the anatomical location of the valve within the chest. Rather, they are reflective of the patterns of radiation of heart sounds toward the chest wall. Sound in vessels through which blood is flowing is always reflected downstream. Events of the mitral valve are usually heard best in the fifth intercostal space at the midclavicular line. This is called the *mitral valve area*. Events occurring at the tricuspid valve are heard best in the fourth intercostal space just to the left of the sternum. This is called the *tricuspid valve area*. The *aortic valve area* is located in the second intercostal space to the right of the sternum, and the *pulmonic valve area* is located in the second intercostal space to the left of the sternum.

Transient Heart Sounds.   The *first heard sound* (S$_1$) is created by the simultaneous closure of the mitral and tricuspid valves. Although heard over the entire precordium, it is heard best in the mitral area. It is increased in intensity when the valve leaflets are made rigid by calcium in rheumatic heart disease and in any circumstance in which ventricular contraction intervenes at a time when the valve is caught wide open. The latter circumstance will occur, for example, when a premature ventricular contraction interrupts the normal cardiac cycle. The first heart sound varies in intensity from beat to beat when atrial contraction is not synchronous with ventricular contraction. This is because the valve may be fully or partially closed on one beat and quite widely patent on the subsequent one as a function of irregular atrial activity. The first heart sound is easily identifiable and serves as the point of reference for the remainder of the cardiac cycle (see Fig. 5-17).

The *second heart sound* (S$_2$) is produced by the closure of the aortic and pulmonic valves. It is quite usual for these valves to close separately, the aortic valve first, followed by the pulmonic valve, and for the resultant sounds to be clearly distinguished as a "split"-second sound. It is even more usual for this split to be accentuated on inspiration and to disappear on expiration as a function of respiratory influence on right ventricular ejection (augmenting it on inspiration, inhibiting it on expiration). The aortic component of the second sound is heard clearly in both the aortic and pulmonic areas and is heard less clearly at the apex. The pulmonic component of the second sound, if present, may only be heard over the pulmonic area. Thus, one may hear a "single"-second heart sound in the aortic area and a split-second heart sound in the pulmonic area.

Gallop Sounds.   Impedance to diastolic filling of the ventricle in certain disease states may give rise to transient vibrations in diastole that are much akin to, though usually softer than, the first and second heart sounds. Heart sounds then come in triplets and have the acoustical effect of a galloping horse; they are therefore called *gallops*. This may occur early in diastole, during the rapid-filling phase of the cardiac cycle, or at the time of atrial contraction. A gallop sound occurring during rapid ventricular filling is called a *third heart sound* (S$_3$) and represents a normal finding in children and young adults. Such a sound is heard in patients who have myocardial disease or in those who are in congestive heart failure and whose ventricles fail to eject all of their blood during systole.

Gallop sounds heard during atrial contraction are called *fourth heart sounds* (S$_4$). An S$_4$ is often heard when the ventricle is hypertrophied and therefore resistant to filling. Such a circumstance may be associated with coronary artery disease, hypertension, or aortic stenosis. On rare occasions, all four heart sounds are heard within a single cardiac cycle, giving rise to what is called a *quadruple rhythm*.

Gallop sounds are very low frequency sounds and may only be heard with the bell of the stethoscope placed very lightly against the chest. They are heard best at the apex, although occasionally when emanating from the right ventricle, they may be heard to the left of the sternum.

Snaps and Clicks.   Stenosis of the mitral valve owing to rheumatic heart disease gives rise to an unusual sound very early in diastole that is high-pitched and best heard along the left sternal border. The sound is caused by high pressure in the left atrium, abruptly displacing a rigid mitral valve. The sound is called an *opening snap*. It occurs too long after the second sound to be mistaken for a split-second sound and too early in diastole to be mistaken for a gallop. It is almost always associated with the murmur of mitral stenosis and is very specific for that disease.

In an analogous manner, stenosis of the aortic valve gives rise to a short, high-pitched sound immediately after the first heart sound that is called an *ejection click*. This is due to very high pressure within the ventricle, displacing a rigid and calcified aortic valve.

Murmurs.   Murmurs are created by the turbulent flow of blood past a critically narrowed valve, by the regurgitant flow of blood through a valve that has failed to close properly, by the flow of blood through a congenital defect within the wall of the ventricle or between the aorta and the pulmonary artery, or by increased flow through a normal structure. Murmurs are characterized and consequently identified by several characteristics, including *timing* in the cardiac cycle, *location* on the chest wall, *intensity, pitch, quality,* and *pattern of radiation.*

The *timing* of the murmur in the cardiac cycle is vital. First of all, the observer determines whether the murmur is occurring in systole or in diastole. Does it begin simultaneously with the first heart sound, or is there some delay between the sound and the beginning of a systolic murmur? Does the murmur run up to (or through) the second heart sound, or is there again delay between the end of the murmur and the occurrence of the second heart sound? Are diastolic murmurs continuous, or do they die out in mid or late diastole?

Location of the murmur is highly critical. The diastolic murmur of *mitral stenosis* is heard only at the apex (mitral area) and may indeed be confined to only a few centimeters of the chest wall. The murmurs of *aortic and pulmonic stenosis,* although usually widely heard, are nevertheless best heard over their respective valve areas. The murmur of *aortic insufficiency* is heard best along the left sternal border, between the third and fourth interspace. (The murmur of *aortic insufficiency* may not be heard at all in the aortic area. This is because the "forward" direction of blood flow for regurgitation at the aortic valve is in the reverse direction.)

The *intensity* of murmurs is conventionally graded from I through VI. The student will have difficulty hearing a grade I murmur. A grade II cardiac murmur should be easily perceived. Murmurs of grades IV or louder are usually associated with thrills that may be palpated on the surface of the chest wall. A grade VI murmur can often be heard with the stethoscope off the chest. A murmur may vary in intensity from its inception to its conclusion. This is very characteristic of certain valvular disorders. The murmur of aortic stenosis, for example, begins sometime after the first heart sound, increases in intensity to midsystole, and then decreases in intensity, stopping prior to the second heart sound. The sound configuration is referred to as "diamond" in shape, and the murmur is referred to as an *ejection murmur* (Fig. 5-18). The midsystolic increase in intensity is characteristic of murmurs that result from ejection through either the aortic or the pulmonic valve. The murmur of mitral insufficiency and the murmur of a ventricular septal defect are, on the other hand, constant in intensity throughout systole. Moreover, they begin simultaneously with the first heart sound and end simultaneously with the second heart sound. These murmurs are referred to as *holosystolic* or *pansystolic.*

The next important quality of a murmur is its *pitch.* The murmur of mitral stenosis is a low, rumbling sound, often heard only with the bell placed lightly on the chest wall. By contrast, the murmur of aortic insufficiency is a very high-

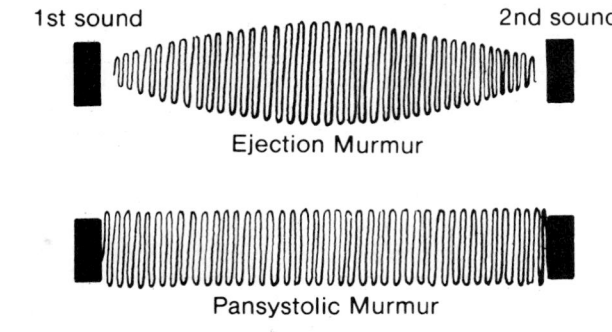

Figure 5-18. Differentiation between ejection murmurs generated at the pulmonic and aortic valves and pansystolic murmurs generated at the mitral and tricuspid valves. Ejection murmurs begin after the first sound, peak in midsystole, and generally conclude before the second sound. Pansystolic murmurs are of equivalent intensity throughout systole, beginning with the first sound and ending with the second sound.

pitched murmur, occasionally "whistling" in character, heard best with the diaphragm. Other murmurs, especially the murmur of aortic stenosis, contain the full spectrum of sound frequency, a characteristic that makes the murmur appear to be very harsh in quality.

The last feature of concern is *radiation* of the murmur. The murmur of mitral insufficiency, best heard at the apex (mitral area), radiates into the axilla. This, of course, reflects the "downstream" nature of its transmission. The murmur of aortic stenosis will, for analogous reasons, radiate into the carotid arteries in the neck. The murmur of pulmonic stenosis, which may sound identical to that of aortic stenosis, will not radiate into the neck; rather, it may radiate into the left shoulder or into the back.

Friction Rub.   In serous pericarditis, a harsh grating sound can be heard both in systole and diastole and is called a *friction rub.* It is caused by the abrasion of the pericardial surfaces during the cardiac cycle. This may be confused with a murmur; care should be taken to identify the sound when appropriate and to distinguish it from murmurs that may be heard in both systole and diastole.

Procedure for Auscultation.   For auscultation, the patient remains supine, and the examining room is as quiet as possible. The right-handed examiner is positioned at the right side of the patient, the left-handed examiner on the left side. Again, a systematic examination is the cornerstone of a thorough assessment.

Using the diaphragm of the stethoscope, the examiner starts at the apical area and progresses upward along the left sternal border to the pulmonic and aortic areas. If desired, the examiner may choose to begin the examination at the aortic and pulmonic areas and progress downward to the apex of the heart. Initially, S_1 is identified and evaluated with respect to its intensity and splitting. It is normally loudest in the apical area and may be split in the tricuspid area. Next, S_2 is identified and its intensity noted. It is loudest in the aortic and pulmonic areas. A physiologic splitting of S_2 is usually audible in the pulmonic area and is accentuated by inspiration. This splitting sound may be perceived as two distinct but close sounds or as one sound that appears flattened or slightly prolonged.

After concentrating on S_1 and S_2, the examiner listens for extra sounds in systole and then in diastole. Sometimes it is useful to ask oneself the following questions: Do I hear snapping or clicking sounds? Do I hear any high-pitched blowing sounds? Is this sound in systole, or diastole, or both? S_3 and S_4 are low-frequency sounds and are auscultated with the bell of the stethoscope placed lightly and completely against the chest. The examiner again proceeds "inch by inch" along the precordium, listening carefully for these sounds. An S_3 sound and mitral murmurs are heard best with the patient on his left side and the stethoscope in the apical area.

If an abnormality is heard, the entire chest surface is reexamined to determine the exact location of the sound and its radiation. Murmurs are described fully by their timing, location, intensity, pitch, quality, and radiation. Once the characteristics of each phase of the cycle have been determined, the relationship of one to another, and the synthesis of events within the cardiac cycle, may be summarized.

Interpretation of Cardiac Sounds

The interpretation of cardiac sounds is a difficult art to acquire. It requires intimate knowledge of cardiac physiology and the pathophysiology of cardiac diseases. However, there are different levels of performance at which the nurse may be expected to function—levels at which auscultation of the heart may be part of her role. The first level of function is simply the recognition that what one is hearing is not normal. There may be a third heart sound; there may be a murmur in systole or diastole; there may be a pericardial friction rub over the midsternum; the second heart sound may be widely split. These findings are to be brought to the attention of a physician and acted upon accordingly. This level of function is useful in screening. It is the kind of activity that one engages in when doing school physicals on normal children or when performing routine physical examinations.

The second level of function employs pattern recognition. The nurse correctly observes the findings and is capable of recognizing the constellation of sounds and its diagnostic significance, if the constellation is a common one. This is the role in which the nurse practitioner has recently been placed.

At its most sophisticated level, cardiac diagnosis can be interpretive. Properly trained nurses can differentiate among arrhythmias and respond accordingly. They can determine the significance of the appearance and disappearance of gallops during treatment of patients who have had myocardial infarctions or are in heart failure. This is the role in which the coronary care nurse and the cardiovascular nurse specialist have been cast. They function with a team of professionals for whom the fine details of cardiovascular diagnosis have become highly tuned, shared skills.

The characteristic features of the most common cardiac abnormalities are outlined in Chapter 27 and will not be discussed here.

As is the case with examination of the chest, physical examination of the cardiovascular system is complex and may be time-consuming. One may ask what constitutes a competent and sufficiently thorough examination. In the absence of cardiac symptoms, one should certainly assess the blood pressure and the pulse rate. Blood pressure may indeed be the most important observation that is made in the examination of any patient, since hypertension is exceedingly common in the population and amenable to adequate control. Inspection of the anterior thorax is easily accomplished, and an apical impulse, if present, should be noted. Percussion of the cardiac border in normal persons is not usually rewarding and only yields valuable information when cardiac hypertrophy is anticipated. The heart is listened to with care in the four principal areas. Any variation from normal mandates further evaluation by a physician.

▷ Examination of the Abdomen

Examination of the abdomen calls for a departure from the usual ordered process of inspection, palpation, percussion, and auscultation. Percussion and palpation alter the frequency of bowel sounds and for that reason are deferred until last. The order then is: inspection, auscultation, percussion, and palpation.

Topography of the Abdomen

The abdomen is conventionally divided into four quadrants by a vertical midline and a horizontal line through the umbilicus (Fig. 5-19). Thus, the liver lies in the right upper quadrant, the spleen in the left upper quadrant, the appendix and cecum in the right lower quadrant, and the sigmoid colon in the left lower quadrant. The midportion of the abdomen above the umbilicus is referred to as the epigastrium, and the midportion of the abdomen below the umbilicus is referred to as the hypogastrium. The antrum of the stomach, the pylorus, and the first third of the duodenum lie in the epigastrium. The bladder and uterus lie in the hypogastrium.

General Approach. Many patients are uncomfortable during the abdominal examination because of pain, embarrassment, or anxiety about the physical examination in general. For these reasons, it is important for the examiner to relax the patient as much as possible by explaining in detail each step of the examination. Preliminary factors to consider are adequate oblique lighting, a warm environment, and proper positioning. The patient is supine, with his head slightly elevated, his knees flexed, and his arms at his side.

Inspection of the Abdomen

Skin. Inspection of the abdomen begins with observation of the skin, which can offer clues to the patient's state of health and past history. For example, the skin over the abdomen provides early evidence of jaundice. With appropriate lighting, jaundice may be as easily discerned on the trunk as it is in the sclerae. Abdominal skin can also reflect the state of hydration of the patient. If the skin "tents" after the abdominal wall is pinched, the patient may be dehydrated. The skin is also observed for scars of previous surgery. Frequently patients neglect to tell the examiner about an

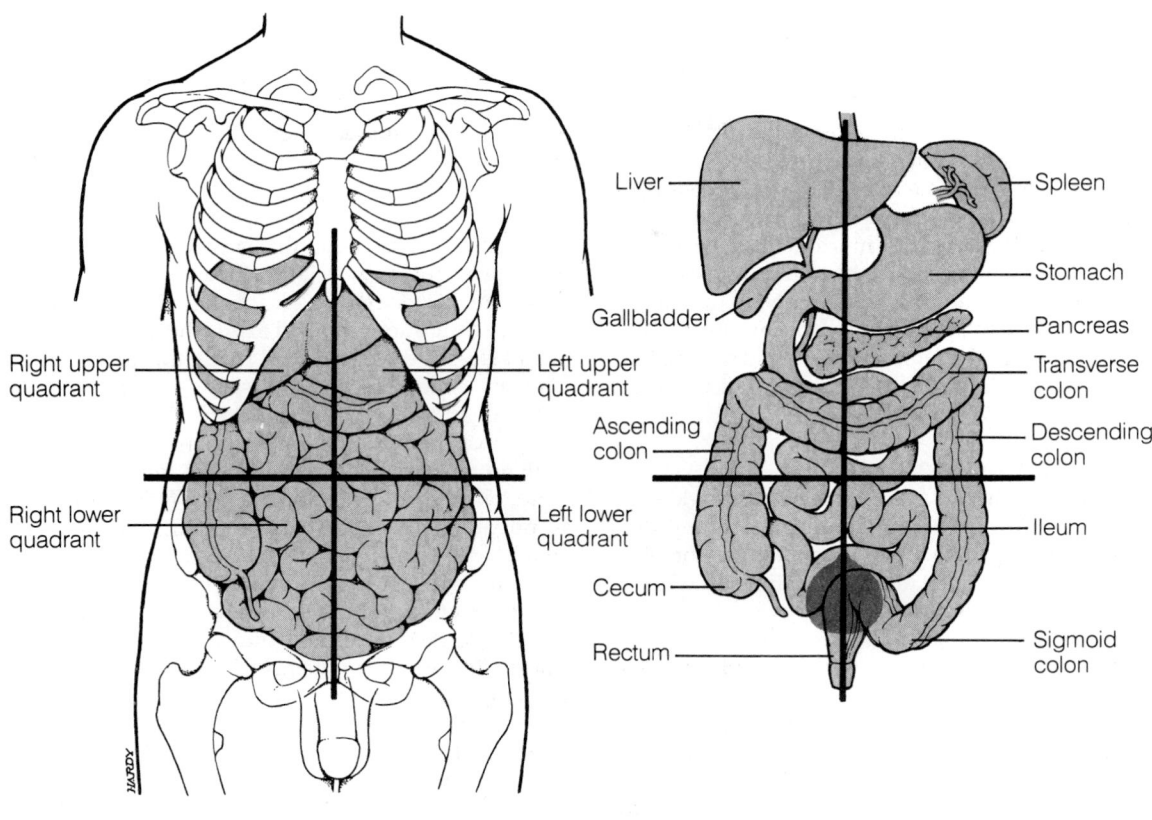

Figure 5-19. Topography of the abdomen as it is related to the location of the abdominal viscera.

appendectomy in the distant past or other surgical procedures that may have occurred in childhood. Such scars as well as other lesions or venous patterns are noted. The contour of the abdomen may be flat, round, protuberant, or scaphoid (concave). Visible masses or asymmetry are noted.

Hernias may be quite visible. Many patients, especially children, have evident umbilical hernias that have no clinical significance. The abdominal contents may herniate through an old scar where muscle layers separated following surgery. Such a hernia may be demonstrated by having the patient lift his head from the bed, thus tensing the abdominal musculature while increasing intra-abdominal pressure. A small bulge reveals the hernia. Inguinal and femoral hernias may also be observed. Inguinal hernias, though rare in women, are exceedingly common in men and are discussed on page 815. Femoral hernias, more common in women, occasionally bulge below the inguinal ligament.

In patients who have bowel obstruction and occasionally in individuals who are thin, one may see peristaltic waves of activity crossing the abdomen. Similarly, the pulsation of the aorta may be visible left of the midline in thin patients and in patients with aortic aneurysms.

Patients with abdominal pain are observed closely. The patient with pain owing to peritonitis will lie quite still and will find that any movement, active or passive, exacerbates the pain and is unbearable. The patient will frequently draw his knees up in a fetal position and lie on his side in a vain attempt to achieve a position of comfort. The patient with abdominal pain that is colicky in nature owing to biliary disease, bowel obstruction, or urinary tract disease is more likely to be restless, writhing in the bed and frequently alternating between a sitting and lying position; he may even occasionally pace the floor.

Auscultation of the Abdomen

There is a wide range of intensity and pitch of bowel sounds that may be considered normal. Bowel sounds are audible as clicks and gurgles; between 5 and 35 occur per minute. The rush of liquid stool across the ileocecal valve into the cecum is clearly audible in the right lower quadrant. This is often the best location for initially auscultating bowel sounds. Using the diaphragm of the stethoscope, the examiner listens in each quadrant for more than a minute before stating that bowel sounds are absent. The absence of bowel sounds accompanies peritoneal irritation or inflammation. The combination of no bowel sounds with other signs of peritonitis is termed *paralytic ileus.*

At the other extreme are the high-pitched, "tinkling" bowel sounds of gatrointestinal obstruction. When obstructed, the bowel fills with air, and peristaltic movement of the tensely distended bowel produces the characteristic high-pitched sound. Both peritonitis (ileus) and bowel obstruction are associated with the absence of defecation or the passing of gas. Therefore, the capacity to have a bowel movement virtually eliminates the possibility that either peritonitis or bowel obstruction exists.

Abdominal murmurs associated with obstructed vessels may also be heard. In patients who have hypertension owing to renal artery stenosis, a systolic murmur may be heard over the flank on the involved side. Severe narrowing of the lower abdominal aorta or the iliac arteries owing to atherosclerosis may also be associated with systolic murmurs. Usually, these will radiate into the femoral vessels and are audible with the diaphragm of the stethoscope as a harsh blowing sound (bruit).

Percussion of the Abdomen
Size of Abdominal Organs. Percussion of the abdomen helps in assessing the distribution of tympany and dullness and specifically delineates the size of abdominal organs, such as the liver, spleen, and bladder. An estimation of liver size is made by percussing upward from tympany of the right upper quadrant until dullness is encountered. Normally, this is noted at the costal margin in the midclavicular line. This point is marked with a pen. Next, the examiner percusses down the midclavicular line, from lung resonance to liver dullness (usually around the sixth or seventh rib). This point of dullness is marked; and the area between the two penmarks is measured. The total span of liver dullness in the midclavicular line ranges from 8 cm (3 inches) in small persons to 12 cm (4¾ inches) in large, muscular men. A liver span in excess of 12 cm implies hepatic enlargement.

Although the spleen lies just under the left costal margin, it usually can be neither felt nor percussed. Occasionally, when the spleen is moderately enlarged, as in infectious mononucleosis, it may be percussed, although not palpated. Percussion over the ninth intercostal space on the left anterior thorax normally produces a tympanic note. However, if the spleen is enlarged, a deep inspiration may push the organ lower in the abdominal cavity, and a dull percussion sound is produced instead of the normal tympany.

A distended bladder may be identified by percussion in the hypogastrium. This is useful in differentiating "overflow" incontinence of a distended and obstructed bladder from incontinence owing to autonomic neuropathy. The nurse may frequently use percussion of the abdomen as a guide in determining whether or not a patient needs to be catheterized.

Palpation of the Abdomen
Technique. Palpation is a useful technique in detecting tenderness, muscle resistance, the outline of organs, and abnormal masses. Light palpation is employed first to detect muscle resistance, tenderness, and superficial masses. The examiner uses the pads of all the fingertips on one hand to lightly depress the abdomen in all four quadrants. Palpable masses, areas of tenderness, or muscle guarding are noted. When the patient is ticklish, the examiner may find it helpful to distract him with conversation. If necessary,

the examiner may place the patient's hand underneath hers until the ticklish episode or "voluntary guarding" is gone. Involuntary guarding, or contraction of the abdominal muscles, may be present in peritoneal inflammation and cannot be controlled by the patient. In such instances, multiple maneuvers by the examiner to relax the abdominal muscles are unsuccessful.

Following light palpation, a deeper palpation is begun. In a systematic fashion, all quadrants are explored. Some examiners prefer to use a bimanual technique for deep palpation. In this technique, one hand is placed upon the other, and while the superior hand exerts the pressure, the inferior hand assesses the abdominal cavity for organs and masses. If a mass is identified, its size, shape, location, mobility, and consistency, as well as the presence of tenderness are noted.

Palpation of the abdomen is approached gently, especially in those patients who have abdominal pain. Furthermore, one begins palpation as far away from the site of pain as possible, moving circumferentially and palpating the painful area last. If the painful area is palpated first, muscle guarding will be induced, preventing the examiner from gaining useful information elsewhere in the abdomen.

Tenderness is usually most exquisite over the area where the patient complains of pain, but it may be elicited elsewhere as well. Quite often, palpation of another part of the abdomen will result in pain perceived in the quadrant in which the disease process is located. For example, palpation anywhere in the abdomen of the patient with appendicitis will elicit pain in the right lower quadrant. Pain, especially the pain of peritonitis, is almost always associated with involuntary muscle guarding, even to the point of rigidity.

Occasionally, pain is not elicited on direct palpation, but may emerge when the hand is abruptly removed from the abdomen. This phenomenon is called *rebound tenderness* and is highly suggestive of peritoneal irritation. Of even greater diagnostic significance is *referred rebound tenderness,* in which the abrupt withdrawal of the hand from the abdomen results in rebound tenderness referred to the site of the disease. An example of this is also noted in appendicitis. One may well be able to palpate the left lower quadrant to a reasonable depth without eliciting pain, but the abrupt withdrawal of the hand results in the perception of severe pain in the right lower quadrant.

Abdominal Organs. The examiner next attempts to palpate body organs. The liver may be palpable in the right upper quadrant, the spleen in the left upper quadrant. A palpable liver presents as a firm, sharp ridge with a smooth surface (Fig. 5-20). Prior percussion informs the examiner of the approximate size of the liver and is useful in interpreting a palpable liver. An example of a normal palpable liver is that which occurs in the patient with emphysema whose diaphragm is depressed, forcing the liver below the right costal margin. When the liver is not palpable, but tenderness is suspected, tapping the lower right thorax briskly may elicit tenderness. The patient's response is then compared by performing a similar maneuver on the left lower thorax.

In the normal individual, the spleen is not palpable. To examine for splenic enlargement, the examiner stands

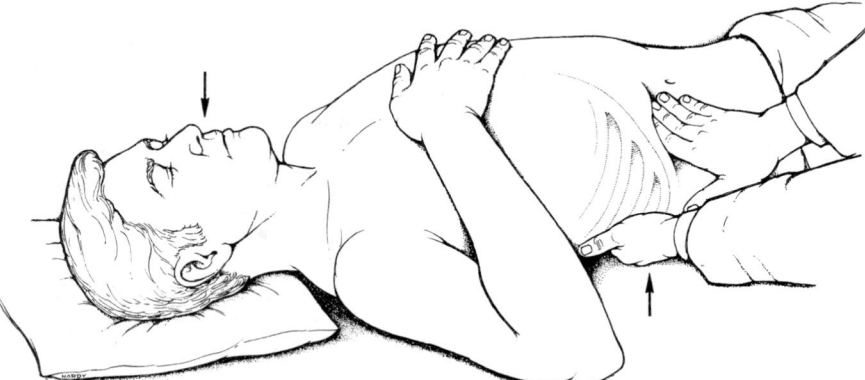

Figure 5-20. Technique for palpation of the liver. As the patient inhales, a palpable liver edge will descend to meet the index finger of the right hand. At the height of inspiration, the examiner releases the pressure of the right hand slightly and tries to feel the liver edge "slip" under the fingertips.

at the patient's right side and reaches across the patient with his left hand to support the left thorax and displace it slightly forward. At the same time, the examiner places her right hand 4 cm to 5 cm below the left costal margin and presses inward and upward toward the location of the spleen. While the patient takes a deep breath, the examiner palpates to feel the tip of the spleen as it is pushed downward by the inspiratory movement. Occasionally, an enlarged spleen cannot be felt with the patient supine and may be appreciated with the patient rolled on his right side.

Palpable organs are characterized by the examiner. Of concern is their size, their consistency, whether or not they are tender, and whether they are regular or irregular in outline. If the liver is enlarged, the degree to which it descends below the right costal margin is recorded in order to provide some impression of its total dimension. The liver of cirrhosis is small and hard in consistency, while the liver of acute viral hepatitis is quite soft, and the edge is easily moved by the hand. The spleen likewise may be very firm, as in Hodgkin's disease, or quite soft, as in infectious mononucleosis. (The spleen may be ruptured by vigorous palpation in infectious mononucleosis.) Tenderness of the liver implies recent acute enlargement with consequent stretching of the liver capsule. The absence of tenderness may imply that the enlargement is chronic. The liver of viral hepatitis is tender; the liver of alcoholic hepatitis demonstrates no tenderness. The examiner should determine whether the liver edge is sharp and smooth or whether it is blunt. He should determine whether the enlarged liver is nodular or whether its surface is smooth. Enlargement or tenderness of the spleen or liver are abnormal findings and require additional evaluation by a physician.

Palpation of the right kidney in the thin individual is possible by "capturing" the kidney bimanually. This is done by placing the left hand under the patient's right flank and the right hand below the right costal margin. Firm pressure of the hands in a squeezing fashion during inspiration may facilitate palpation of the kidney.

The aortic pulsation can be identified as a pulsating sensation to the left of the midline. Deep pressure of the fingertips to the left of the midline usually reveals this pulsation. Pressure on the aorta often elicits tenderness and therefore is done gently. Under normal circumstances, this pulsation is a forward motion and does not expand laterally.

The abdomen is carefully and systematically palpated for masses that do not represent body organs. The examiner begins in one quadrant and proceeds circumferentially and in narrowing, concentric circles. Masses felt are characterized with respect to size, consistency, presence or absence of tenderness, and whether or not they seem uniform and smooth or multinodular.

Hernias. Although many hernias are evident, others, especially those through the inguinal ring, appear only intermittently and with increases in intra-abdominal pressure. The indirect inguinal hernia follows the course of the spermatic cord through the abdominal musculature. One is able to palpate the external inguinal ring in the male patient and determine whether it is normal or whether it is widely patent, permitting descent of intra-abdominal contents into a hernial sac. The technique is as follows (Fig. 5-21).

The patient is examined in a standing position. Short nails and the use of unsterile gloves are recommended. The examiner sits facing the patient and begins by inspecting

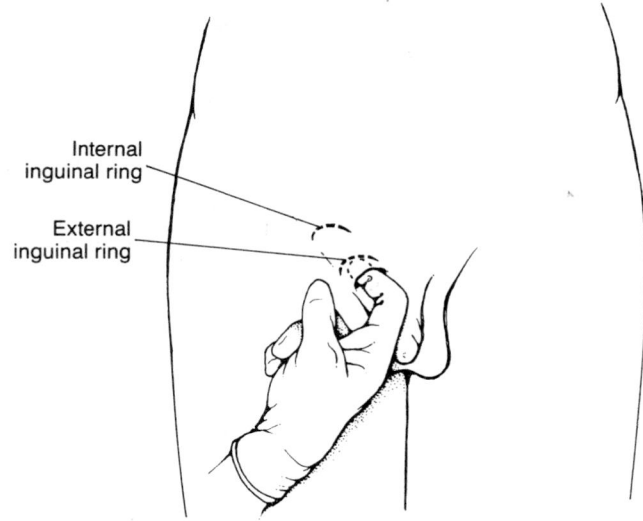

Internal inguinal ring

External inguinal ring

Figure 5-21. Technique for the detection of an indirect inguinal hernia. The spermatic cord lies under the index finger and enters the abdomen at the external inguinal ring.

the inguinal regions for obvious masses. To examine the right inguinal canal the right index finger is placed beside the spermatic cord at the very base of the scrotum, catching a small part of the scrotal fold as the finger ascends. The finger should then be advanced under the skin and subcutaneous tissue of the abdominal wall following the spermatic cord, until the cord is felt to enter the ring of the external oblique muscle. One will feel a small depression that should admit no more than the pad of a fingertip under normal circumstances. This is the inguinal ring. In the presence of a hernia, one may be able to pass the finger through the external oblique muscle toward the internal inguinal ring. In the event that the ring is found to be larger than normal, the examiner should ask the patient to bear down as though he is having a bowel movement (Valsalva maneuver). If a hernia exists, the examiner will feel a sac of peritoneum with or without omentum or bowel emerging through the external inguinal ring to meet the finger. Such a finding requires further evaluation by a physician.

▷ Rectal Examination

The rectal examination is an essential part of the physical assessment of all patients over 40 and is incorporated as a part of the periodic assessment, probably every year or so, of all patients. The examination may be done in one of several positions (Fig. 5-22). In hospitalized patients who are confined to bed, it is most conveniently performed in the left lateral position, with the patient lying on the left side, his right knee drawn up to the level of his chest. In the office the examination may be done with the patient bending over the examining table. Female patients are most conveniently examined in a dorsolithotomy position at the same time that the pelvic examination is being conducted. Further discussion of the examination of the female patient will be deferred until the section on examination of the genital system (see p. 86).

Anal Canal.   The examiner first notes the anus, observing whether external hemorrhoidal tags are present and whether the anus is free of fissures and fistuli. The index finger of the gloved hand is lubricated and inserted slowly into the anal canal. The examiner notes whether good sphincter tone is present, and then slowly advances the index finger along the anal canal and into the rectum. Internal hemorrhoids are not palpable unless they are thrombosed.

Prostate.   The plum-sized, normal prostate usually has a median sulcus (indentation) and is felt on the anterior surface of the rectal wall. On either side of the prostate, the rectal folds fall away. The finger is swept around the rectal mucosa, observing for masses or polyps. Fecal material, which may be mistaken for polypoid masses, may be differentiated by sweeping it away from the rectal mucosa. A prostate that is palpated as firm and smooth, but that bulges into the rectal lumen and lacks a definite median indentation, is common in men over 50 and is referred to as benign prostatic hypertrophy. When the prostate is inflamed, as in prostatitis, it is usually enlarged, boggy, and tender. The prostate is carefully palpated for enlargement or for stony, hard masses, which usually represent malignancy.

Feces.   When the finger is withdrawn, fecal material will usually cling to the glove. This material is examined by appropriate solutions for content that may represent blood.

▷ Examination of the Genitalia

Genital examination is a part of the complete physical examination in all circumstances. Most health professionals understand this basic principle when examining female patients, especially since the advent of the highly efficacious Papanicolaou smear for cancer of the cervix. Too frequently, however, they fail to give the male genitalia the same careful attention.

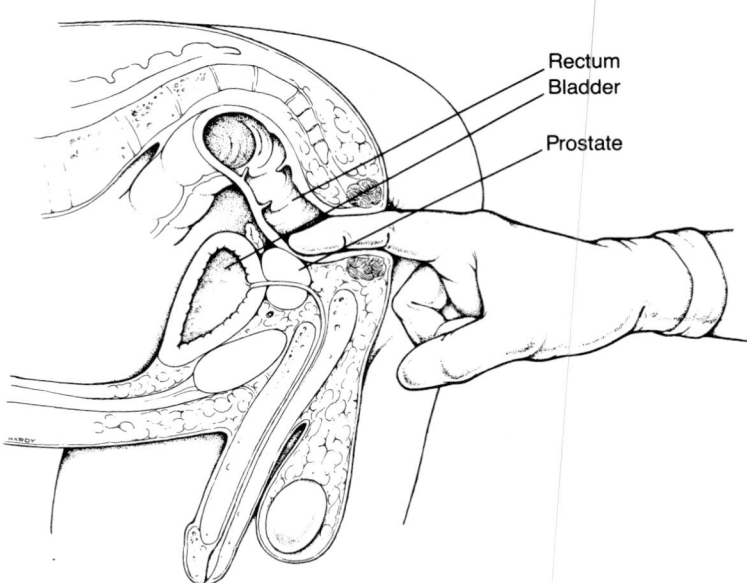

Rectum
Bladder
Prostate

Figure 5-22. Technique for the rectal examination. Following palpation of the prostate gland, the finger is rotated to identify any abnormality of the rectal mucosa that may be reached by the examining finger.

Examination of the Male Genitalia

To ensure the patient's privacy and minimize his embarrassment, the examiner precedes the examination with a brief explanation of "what to expect." Any awkwardness or embarrassment on the part of the examiner can be perceived by the patient and often results in increasing his discomfort. Examination of the male genitalia and hernia assessment are usually done concurrently. An unsterile glove is used during palpation.

The penis is inspected for the location of the urethral opening and for any lesions along the skin of the shaft. An abnormal location of the urethral opening along the dorsal midline of the shaft is called *epispadias;* an abnormal urethral opening along the ventral surface of the shaft is called *hypospadias.* The examiner should observe whether or not the penis has been circumcised. If uncircumcised, the foreskin should be retracted back from the glans penis. Inability of the foreskin to be retracted over the glans is called *phimosis.* Occasionally, inflammation of the foreskin in a retracted position does not allow the foreskin to be drawn forward over the glans. This circumstance is called *paraphimosis.* The glans of the uncircumcised penis should be palpated, especially in older individuals, to determine if any part of it has a firmer consistency than the remainder. This may be indicative of carcinoma of the glans penis. Carcinoma of the circumcised penis does not occur.

The scrotum and its contents also should be examined. Normal testes are of firm consistency and measure 6 cm to 8 cm (2½ to 3 inches) in their longest polar length. Testes of less than 4 cm (1½ inches) in polar length are atrophied or represent abnormal development. The testicles should be palpated for firm masses within their substance. Other masses within the scrotum include the *varicocele* and the *hydrocele.* The varicocele represents enlargement of the plexus of veins that surrounds the spermatic cord and feels like a "bag of worms." The hydrocele is a collection of fluid within a peritoneal remnant lying along the spermatic cord. It often has the consistency of a testicle and may give the appearance of three testicles contained within the scrotum. The hydrocele can be differentiated from other masses within the scrotum by its capacity to transmit light. It is said to *transilluminate.* No other masses in the scrotum have this property.

Examination of the Female Genitalia

The pelvic examination is a facet of physical assessment that may be accomplished by the nurse. Competency can be attained in an environment that fosters practice and clinical supervision.

Although several positions may be used for performing the pelvic examination, the dorsolithotomy position is preferred. If the examiner is required to perform the pelvic assessment in the hospital on a patient who is too ill to be placed on a table equipped with stirrups, the *Sims' position* may be used. In the Sims' position, the patient lies on her left side, with her left arm behind her and her right leg bent at a 90-degree angle. The right labia may be retracted for adequate access to the vagina.

The patient is instructed to void prior to the pelvic examination. The urine may be retained if a urine specimen is part of the total assessment procedure. The patient is then placed on the table in stirrups and encouraged to relax so that her buttocks are presented at the edge of the examination table and her thighs are spread as widely apart as possible. The patient is appropriately draped to avoid embarrassment. The following equipment is necessary: good light source, vaginal speculum, unsterile gloves, lubricant, spatula, cotton-tip applicators, glass slides, fixative solution or spray, and appropriate material for occult blood screening.

When the patient is prepared, the *labia majora* and *minora* are examined. The epidermal tissue of the labia majora, with its hair follicles characteristic of skin, fades to the pink mucous membrane of the vaginal introitus. In the nulliparous woman, the labia minora should come together at the opening of the vagina. In women who have borne children, the labia minora may gape, and vaginal tissue may protrude. The patient is asked to bear down. Birth damage to the anterior vaginal wall may have resulted in incompetency of musculature, so that a bulge representing bladder intrusion into the submucosa of the anterior vaginal wall may be seen. This is called a *cystocele* (Fig. 46-1). Birth trauma may also have affected the posterior vaginal wall, so that a bulge representing the cavity of the rectum may protrude, presenting as a *rectocele* (Fig. 46-2). The cervix or the uterus itself may descend under pressure through the vaginal canal and present itself at the introitus. This is termed *prolapse* of the uterus.

The introitus should be free of hair follicles and of superficial mucosal lesions. The labia minora may be separated by the fingers of the gloved hand and the lower part of the vagina palpated. In virginal women, a *hymen* of variable thickness may be felt circumferentially within a centimeter or two of the vaginal opening. The hymenal ring will usually permit the admission of two fingers, but occasionally is sufficiently restricting so that only one finger may enter the vagina. Rarely, the hymen totally occludes the vaginal entrance. In nonvirginal women, a rim of scar tissue representing the remnants of the hymenal ring may be felt circumferentially around the vagina near its opening. The greater vestibular glands (Bartholin's glands) lie between the labia minora and the remnants of the hymenal ring. These glands frequently become infected in gonococcal disease. Patients may occasionally present with an abscess of one of these glands.

Speculum Examination

Assorted sizes of the bivalved speculum are available in metal or plastic. A metal speculum is warmed with running tap water to make it less uncomfortable when it is inserted. It is not lubricated, since lubrication with commercial jellies may interfere with the examination of the cervical cytology. Two setscrews may be seen on the speculum. One is along the handle and holds the two valves of the speculum together. This one is tightened. The setscrew that holds the thumbrest in place is loosened. The speculum is grasped in the right hand, with the thumb against the back of the thumbrest in order to keep the tips of the valves closed.

The speculum is rotated slightly counterclockwise, and the vaginal orifice is held open by the thumb and the forefinger of the gloved left hand. The speculum is gently inserted into the posterior portion of the introitus and slowly advanced to the top of the vagina (Fig. 5-23). The tip of the speculum may then be elevated and the speculum rotated

to a transverse position. The speculum is then slowly opened to reveal the cervix of the uterus. The cervix having been brought into view, the setscrew of the thumbrest may be tightened to hold the speculum open.

If any purulent material appears at the cervical os, it is cultured with a sterile cotton-tip applicator and immediately

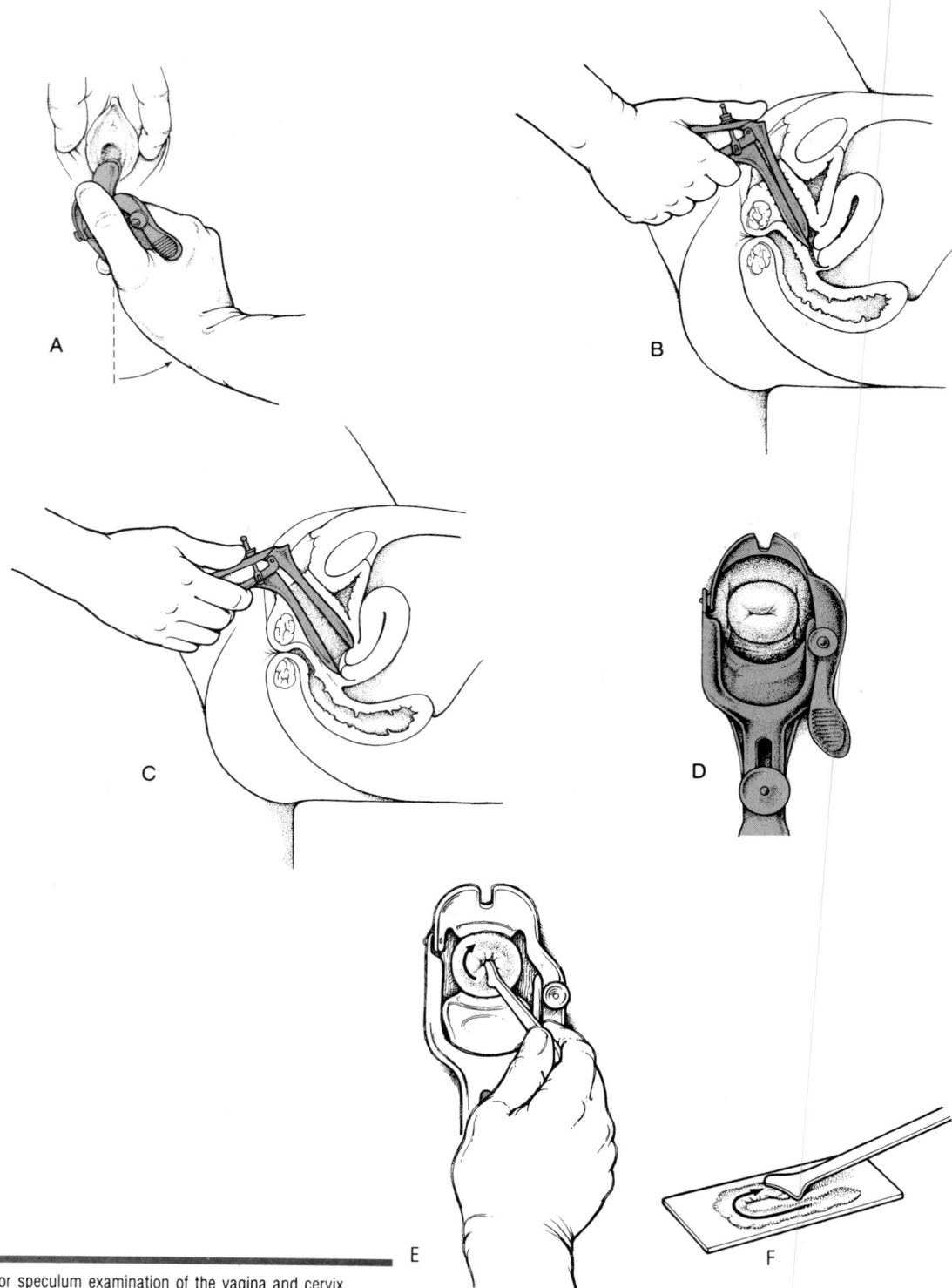

Figure 5-23. Technique for speculum examination of the vagina and cervix.

placed in an appropriate medium for transfer to a laboratory. Some authorities now advocate routine culture for gonococcus in light of the high incidence of the disease in the general population.

The next procedure is the scraping of the cervix for cancer cytology by the *Papanicolaou* method with a wooden spatula constructed for the purpose. The tip of the spatula is placed in the cervical os and the spatula rotated 360 degrees, firmly but nontraumatically (Fig. 5-23 *E, F*). Cellular material clinging to the spatula is then smeared gently on a glass slide, which is promptly placed in fixative solution or sprayed with commercially available fixative material. If desired, additional specimens from the vaginal pool and the endocervical os can be obtained with the use of separate cotton-tip applicators. It is advisable to use two separate slides for these additional specimens and label them accordingly.

All slides are then transmitted to the laboratory along with culture material that may have been extracted from the cervical os.

The cervix is inspected. In nulliparous women, the cervical os is 2 mm to 3 mm in diameter and smooth. Women who have borne children may have a laceration, usually transverse, frequently giving the cervical os a "fishmouth" appearance. Moreover, epithelium from the endocervical canal may have grown out onto the surface of the cervix, appearing as beefy red surface epithelium circumferentially arranged around the os. This is commonly called a *cervical erosion*. Although not always differentiable from a cervical carcinoma, the cervical erosion is, in general, less sharply outlined than malignant tissue. Indeed, malignant change may not be obviously differentiated from the remainder of the cervical mucosa. The presence of endocervical epithelium around the cervical os can lead to chronic infection and discharge from the orifice. Small cysts may appear on the surface of the cervix under these circumstances. These are usually bluish in color and are termed *nabothian cysts*. A polyp of endocervical mucosa may protrude through the os and appears dark red. A carcinoma may appear as a cauliflowerlike growth. It is friable and will bleed easily when traumatized. A bluish color of the cervix is a sign of early pregnancy (*Chadwick's sign*).

The vagina is examined as the speculum is withdrawn. It is smooth in young girls and becomes more thickened after puberty, with many rugae and much redundancy in the epithelium. Vaginal discharge may be present. Discharge owing to bacteria is yellow and has a purulent appearance. Discharge owing to *Trichomonas* is thin and watery, often yellow, and occasionally frothy and malodorous. Discharge due to *Candida* is thick and white and may have a cheesy appearance.

Bimanual Examination

The examiner assumes a standing position for the bimanual examination. This examination is performed with the forefinger and middle finger of the gloved and lubricated hand (Fig. 5-24). These fingers are placed in the vaginal orifice, while the other fingers are held tightly out of the way, with the thumb completely adducted. The fingers are advanced vertically along the vaginal canal, and the vaginal wall is

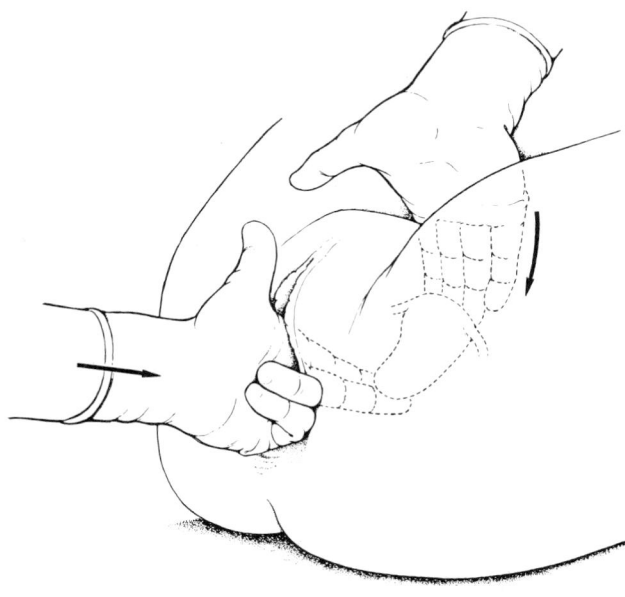

Figure 5-24. Technique for the bimanual examination of the pelvis in the female.

palpated. Firmness of any part of the vaginal wall may represent old scar tissue from birth trauma. Such tissue may be tender. Anterior tenderness or burning may represent urethritis associated with a urinary tract infection.

The cervix is palpated and noted for its consistency, mobility, size, and position. The normal cervix is firm but not hard, and uniformly so. Softening of the cervix and elongation of the cervical canal are seen in early pregnancy. Hardness may reflect invasion by neoplasia. The cervix and uterus are normally freely movable. Fixation in the pelvis may reflect extension of malignancy. The body of the uterus is normally twice the diameter and twice the length of the cervix. The body may be felt on either side of the cervix, curving anteriorly toward the abdominal wall. One out of five women will, however, have a *retroflexed* uterus, which curves posteriorly toward the sacrum.

The opposite hand is now brought into play. This hand is placed halfway between the umbilicus and the pubis and pressed firmly toward the opening of the pelvis. If the uterus is in an appropriate position, movement of the abdominal wall will cause the body of the uterus to descend, and the pear-shaped organ will be freely movable between the abdominal hand and the examining fingers of the pelvic hand. A reasonably accurate impression can be gained of the size, mobility, and regularity of the contour of the uterus.

The right and left parametria are now palpated. The tube and ovary are contained within these structures. The fingers of the pelvic hand are moved first to one side, then to the other, while the abdominal hand is moved correspondingly to either side of the abdomen. The adnexae are trapped between the two examining hands and are palpated for obvious mass, tenderness of adnexal tissue, and mobility of the parametrial contents.

It is common for the ovaries to be slightly tender. Bimanual palpation of the vagina and cul-de-sac is accomplished by placing the index finger in the vagina and the middle finger in the rectum. A gentle movement of these fingers toward each other compresses the posterior vaginal wall and the anterior rectal wall, and assists the examiner in identifying the integrity of these structures. This procedure may give the patient the sensation of moving her bowels. The examiner reassures the patient that although she has the urge to defecate, she is not in fact doing so.

To prevent cross contamination between the vaginal and rectal orifices, the examiner changes his gloves between these examinations.

▷ Rectoabdominal Examination

Examination of the rectum is, of course, a normal part of the physical examination and can be done immediately after the pelvic examination. It may be useful in selected instances to use the rectal approach to palpate the pelvic contents. Examples include young virginal women whose vaginas may not admit the examining fingers, women whose vaginas have been foreshortened by surgery or irradiation, and those who are suspected of having abnormal tissue in the adnexae and uterine ligaments. The gloved finger is inserted into the rectum and the opposite hand used to compress the abdominal wall in a manner analogous to the bimanual examination of the vagina. The uterus is often palpable, and the adnexal structures, which include the ovary and the fallopian tube, may be palpated by moving the finger to the left and right of the cervix.

Upon withdrawal of the finger from the rectum, fecal material clinging to the glove is smeared and stained appropriately for blood, as in any rectal examination.

▷ Neurologic Examination

The neurologic examination is a sophisticated and subtle process, comprising a large number of tests of highly specialized function. Although the neurologic examination is limited in most instances to a simple screening, it is necessary for the examiner to be able to conduct a thorough neurologic assessment when the history or other physical findings warrant it.

A neurologic assessment is divided into five components: cerebral function, cranial nerves, motor system, sensory system, and reflex status. As in other facets of the physical assessment, the neurologic examination follows a logical sequence and is pursued from higher levels of cortical function through to a determination of the integrity of peripheral nerves.

Much of the patient's neurologic function is assessed during the history and during the routine of the earlier parts of the physical examination. One can learn much about speech patterns, mental status, gait, stance, motor power, and coordination. The simple act of shaking a patient's hand as he enters the room conveys an enormous amount of information to the alert observer.

Cerebral Function

Cerebral abnormalities may cause disturbances in communication, in intellectual functioning, and in patterns of emotional behavior. Adequate cerebral functioning is determined by assessing the patient's *mental status.* The examiner observes the patient's appearance and behavior, noting the patient's dress, grooming, and personal hygiene. Observation of posture, gestures, movements, facial expressions, and motor activity often provides important information about the patient's attitude. The manner of speech and the patient's level of consciousness are also observed: Is his speech clear and coherent? Is he alert and responsive, or drowsy and stuporous?

Intellectual function is tested when doubts exist about the patient's intellectual competence. Often, patients in a toxic state or those who have destruction of frontal cortex appear superficially normal until or unless one or more tests of integrative capacity are performed. First, the examiner determines whether the patient is oriented to time, place, and person. Does the patient know what day it is, what year it is, or who is the president of the United States? Is the patient aware of where he is? Is the patient aware of who you are and of his purpose for being in the room? Is the capacity for immediate memory intact? A person with an average IQ is able to repeat seven digits without faltering and is able to recite five digits backward. The examiner might ask the patient to count backward from 100, or to subtract 7 from 100, then 7 from that, then 7 from that, etc. The capacity to interpret well-known proverbs is a test of even higher intellectual function (abstract reasoning). Does the patient know what is meant by "the early bird catches the worm?"

It is important to determine the patient's thought content as it emerges during the course of the interview. Are his thoughts spontaneous, natural, and clear? Are his ideas relevant and coherent? Does he have any fixed ideas, illusions, or preoccupations? What are his insights into these thoughts? Preoccupation with death or morbid events, evidence of hallucinations, and paranoid ideation, are all important and require further evaluation.

An assessment of cerebral functioning also includes the patient's emotional status. Is the patient's affect natural and even, or is he irritable and angry, anxious, apathetic, or euphoric? Does his mood fluctuate normally, or does he unpredictably swing from joy to sadness during the interview? Is his affect appropriate to his words and thought content? Are his verbal communications consistent with his nonverbal communications?

The examiner may now look at more specific areas of higher cortical function. *Agnosia* is the inability to interpret or recognize objects seen through the special senses. The individual may see a pen but not know what it is called or what to do with it. He may even be able to describe it but not to interpret its function. The patient may experience auditory or tactile agnosia, as well as visual agnosia. Each of the dysfunctions implicates a different part of the cortex.

To screen for agnosia, the examiner tests the patient's cortical sensory interpretation. The patient is shown a familiar object and asked to identify it by name. Next, he is confronted with a familiar sound (bell) and asked to identify its source. Tactile interpretation is easily assessed by placing a familiar object (key, coin) in the patient's hand and having him identify it while his eyes are closed.

An assessment of cortical motor integration is carried out by asking the patient to perform a skilled act (throw a ball, move a chair). Successful performance hinges upon the individual's ability to understand the activity desired. He must also have normal motor strength. Failures signal cerebral dysfunction.

Lastly, language function is assessed. The normal person is able to understand and communicate in spoken and written language. Does the patient answer questions relevantly? Can he read a sentence from a newspaper and explain its meaning? Can he write his name or copy a simple figure that the examiner has drawn? A deficiency in language function is called *aphasia*.

Interpretation of neurologic abnormalities is a highly sophisticated and technical process. It is the obligation of the examiner to record and report what is found. Analysis and the conclusions that may be drawn from these findings will usually depend upon the physician's extensive knowledge of neuroanatomy, neurophysiology, and neuropathology.

Examination of the Cranial Nerves

There are 12 pairs of cranial nerves that emerge from the undersurface of the brain. They are designated by the Roman numerals I to XII, according to the order of their placement. The cranial nerves are often assessed during a complete head and neck examination. These nerves, their functions, and the tests for their measurement are outlined in Table 5-1.

Examination of the Motor System

The motor system is quite complex, and the end result of motor function is a synthesis of the integrity of the corticospinal tracts, the extrapyramidal system, and cerebellar function. A motor impulse traverses two neurons. The *upper motor neuron* begins in the cortex of the opposite side of the brain, descends through the internal capsule, crosses to the opposite side in the brain stem, descends through the corticospinal tract, and synapses with the *lower motor neuron* in the cord. The lower motor neuron receives the impulse in the posterior part of the cord and runs to the myoneural junction. The other two systems, the extrapyramidal system and the cerebellar system, act as modifiers.

A thorough examination of the motor system includes an assessment of muscle size, muscle tone, muscle strength, coordination, and balance. The patient is instructed to walk across the room while the examiner notes his posture and gait. The muscles are inspected, and palpated if necessary, for their size and symmetry. Any evidence of atrophy or involuntary movements (tremors, tics) is noted. Muscle tone is evaluated by palpating various muscle groups at rest and during passive movement. The resistance to these movements is noted. Abnormalities in tone include spasticity, rigidity, or flaccidity.

Muscle strength is tested by ascertaining the patient's ability to flex or extend his extremity against resistance. The function of an individual muscle or group of muscles is evaluated by placing the muscle at a disadvantage. The quadriceps, for example, is a powerful muscle responsible for straightening the leg. Once the leg is straightened, it is exceedingly difficult for the examiner to flex the knee. On the other hand, if the knee is flexed, and the patient is asked to straighten the leg against resistance, a more subtle disability can be brought out. It is critically important to compare the two sides if one is looking for minor degrees of disability.

Some authorities advocate the use of a five-point scale for strength of motor power. A five would indicate full power of contraction; a four would indicate fair, but not full, strength; a three would imply just sufficient strength to overcome the force of gravity; a two indicates the ability to move but not to overcome the force of gravity; a one indicates minimal contractile power; a zero implies no contraction whatsoever.

Assessment of motor power can be as restricted or detailed as the examiner wishes. One may quickly test the strength of the proximal muscles of the upper and lower extremities, comparing the two. The motor capacity of the finer muscles that control the function of the hand and of the foot can then be assessed.

Cerebellar influence on the motor system is reflected in balance control and coordination. Coordination in the hands and upper extremities is tested by having the patient perform *rapid, alternating movements* and *point-to-point testing*. First, the patient is instructed to pat his thigh as fast as he can with his hand. Each hand is tested separately. Then, he is instructed to turn his hands from a supine to a prone position as rapidly as possible. Lastly, he is asked to touch each of his fingers with his thumb in a consecutive motion. Speed, symmetry, and degree of difficulty are noted.

Point-to-point testing is accomplished by having the patient touch the examiner's extended finger and then his own nose. This is repeated several times. This assessment is then carried out with the patient's eyes closed.

Coordination in the lower extremities is tested by having the patient run his heel down the anterior surface of his tibia. Each leg is tested in turn. Inability to perform these maneuvers is referred to as *ataxia*. The presence of ataxia or tremors (rhythmic, involuntary movements) during these movements suggests cerebellar disease.

It is not necessary to carry out each of these assessments for coordination. During a routine examination, it is advisable to perform a simple screening of the upper and lower extremities by having the patient perform either rapid, alternating movements or point-to-point testing. When abnormalities are observed, a more thorough examination is indicated.

The *Romberg test* is a screening measurement for balance. The patient stands with his feet together, arms extended in front of him, and eyes closed. The examiner stands close to the patient and reassures him that he will be supported if he begins to lose his balance. Slight swaying is normal. Additional cerebellar tests for balance in the ambulatory patient include hopping in place, alternating knee bends, and heel-to-toe walking.

Table 5-1
Cranial Nerves

Cranial Nerve	Function	Clinical Examination
CN I (olfactory)	Sense of smell	With his eyes closed, the patient identifies familiar odors (coffee, tobacco). Each nostril is tested separately.
CN II (optic)	Visual acuity	Snellen eye chart Visual fields Fundoscopic examination
CN III (oculomotor) CN IV (trochlear) CN VI (abducens)	Extraocular movements Pupillary constriction Lid elevation	Extraocular movement assessment Assessment of size, shape, equality of pupils Direct and indirect light reflex Pupillary accommodation reflex
CN V (trigeminal)	Facial sensation	Have patient close his eyes. Touch cotton to forehead, cheeks, and jaw. Opposite sides of face are compared. Sensitivity to superficial pain is tested by using a safety pin. Alternate between the sharp point and the dull end. Patient reports "sharp" or "dull" with each movement. If responses are incorrect, test for temperature sensation. Test tubes of cold and hot water are used alternately.
	Corneal reflex	While the patient looks up, lightly touch a wisp of cotton against the temporal surface of each cornea. A blink and tearing is a normal response.
	Mastication	Have the patient clench his jaw and move it from side to side. Palpate the masseter and temporal muscles, noting strength and equality.
CN VII (facial)	Facial muscle movement	Observe face for flaccid paralysis (shallow nasolabial folds). Observe for symmetry while the patient performs facial movements: smile, whistle, elevation of eyebrows, frown, tight closure of eyelids against resistance (examiner attempts to open them).
	Taste: anterior $^2/_3$ tongue	Patient extends his tongue. His ability to discriminate between sugar and salt is tested.
CN VIII (acoustic)	Hearing	Whisper or watch-tick test Test for lateralization (Weber) Test for air and bone conduction (Rinne)
CN IX (glossopharyngeal) CN X (vagus)	Taste: posterior $^1/_3$ tongue	Assess patient's ability to discriminate between sugar and salt on posterior $^1/_3$ of the tongue.
	Pharyngeal contraction	Depress a tongue blade on posterior tongue, or stimulate posterior pharynx to elicit gag reflex.
	Symmetrical movement of vocal cords	Note any hoarseness in voice.
	Symmetrical movement of soft palate	Have patient say "ah." Observe symmetrical rise of uvula and soft palate.
CN XI (spinal accessory)	Movement of sternocleido-mastoid and trapezius muscles	Palpate and note the strength of the trapezius muscles while the patient shrugs his shoulders against resistance. Palpate and note the strength of each sternocleidomastoid muscle as the patient turns his head against opposing pressure of the examiner's hand.
CN XII (hypoglossal)	Movement of the tongue	While the patient protrudes his tongue, any deviation or tremors are noted. The strength of the tongue is tested by having the patient move his protruded tongue from side to side against a tongue depressor.

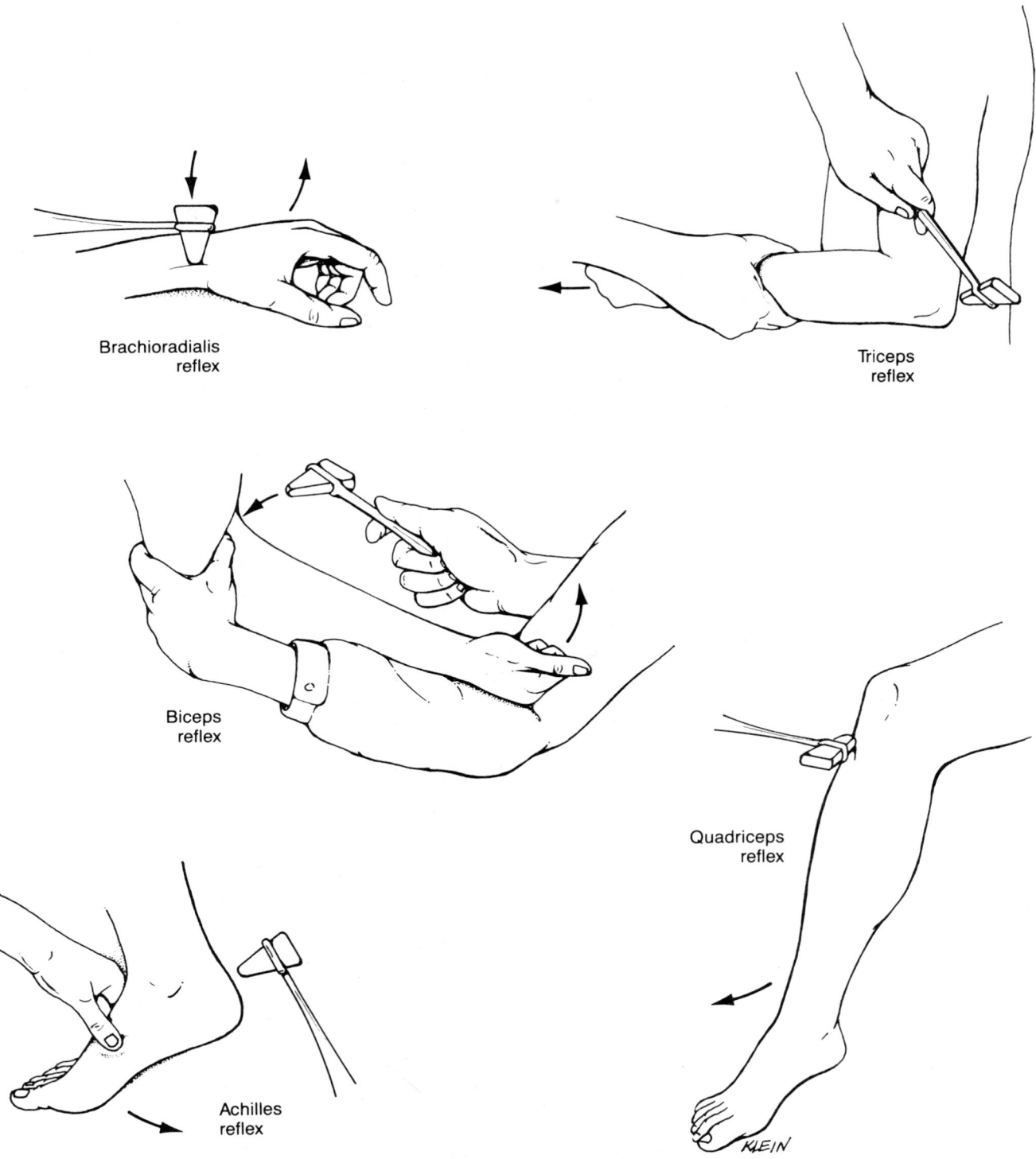

Brachioradialis
reflex

Triceps
reflex

Biceps
reflex

Quadriceps
reflex

Achilles
reflex

KLEIN

Figure 5-25. The proper technique for the elicitation of the major tendon reflexes. The tendon can be struck *directly* with the reflex hammer, or *indirectly* by striking the examiner's thumb, which is placed on the tendon. Arrows indicate the normal extremity motion expected.

Examination of the Reflexes
(See Fig. 5-25.)

The motor reflexes are involuntary contractions of muscles or muscle groups in response to abrupt stretching near the site of the muscle's insertion. The tendon is struck directly with a reflex hammer, or indirectly by striking the examiner's thumb, which is placed firmly against the tendon. In testing the reflexes, we are examining involuntary reflex arcs that depend upon the presence of afferent stretch receptors, spinal synapses, efferent motor fibers, and a variety of modifying influences from higher levels. Common reflexes that may be tested include the biceps, the brachioradialis, the triceps, the patellar, and the ankle (or Achilles) reflex.

A reflex hammer is used to elicit a deep tendon reflex. The stem of the hammer is held loosely between thumb and index finger, allowing a full swinging motion. The wrist motion is similar to that used during percussion. The extremity is positioned so that the tendon is slightly stretched. This requires a sound knowledge of the location of muscles and their tendon attachments. The tendon is then struck briskly and the response compared to the corresponding reflex on the opposite side of the body. Wide variation in reflex response may be considered normal. However, it is more important that the reflexes be symmetrically equivalent. When the comparison is made, both sides should be equivalently relaxed and each tendon struck with equal force.

Valid findings depend upon several factors: proper use of the reflex hammer, proper positioning of the extremity, and a relaxed patient. If the reflexes are symmetrically diminished or absent, the examiner may use a technique called *reinforcement* to increase reflex activity. This involves the isometric contraction of other muscle groups. If lower extremity reflexes are diminished or absent, the patient is instructed to lock his fingers together and pull in opposite directions. Having the patient clench his jaw or press his heel against the floor or examining table may likewise elicit more reliable biceps, triceps, or brachioradialis reflexes.

The absence of reflexes is significant, although ankle jerks (Achilles reflex) may be absent in older people.

Reflex responses are often graded on a 0 to 4+ scale:

    4+—brisk, hyperactive
    3+—more brisk than normal
    2+—normal
    1+—less than normal, slow response
    0 —no response

As was previously mentioned, scale ratings are highly subjective. When used, the findings are recorded as a fraction, indicating the scale range (*e.g.,* 2+/4+). Some examiners prefer to use the terms "present," "absent," and "diminished" when describing reflexes.

The *biceps reflex* is elicited by striking the biceps tendon of the flexed elbow. The examiner supports the forearm with one arm while placing the thumb against the tendon and striking the thumb with the reflex hammer. Note the normal flexion at the elbow and the contraction of the biceps.

To elicit a *triceps reflex,* the patient's arm is flexed at the elbow and positioned in front of the chest. The examiner supports the patient's arm and identifies the triceps tendon by palpating 2.5 cm to 5 cm (1–2 inches) above the elbow. A direct blow on the tendon normally produces contraction of the triceps muscle and extension of the elbow.

With the patient's forearm resting on the lap or across the abdomen, the *brachioradialis reflex* is assessed. A gentle strike of the hammer 2.5 cm to 5 cm (1–2 inches) above the wrist results in flexion and supination of the forearm.

The *patellar reflex* is elicited by striking the patellar tendon just below the patella. The patient may be in a sitting or a lying position. If the patient is supine, the examiner supports the legs to facilitate relaxation of the muscles. Contraction of the quadriceps and knee extension are normal responses.

To facilitate an *ankle reflex,* the foot is dorsiflexed at the ankle and the hammer strikes the stretched Achilles tendon. This reflex normally produces plantar flexion. If the examiner experiences difficulty with the ankle reflex and suspects that the patient is unable to relax, the patient is instructed to kneel on a chair or similar elevated, flat surface. This position places the ankles in dorsiflexion and reduces any muscular tension in the gastrocnemius. The Achilles tendons are struck in turn, and plantar flexion is usually demonstrated.

When reflexes are exceedingly hyperactive, a phenomenon called *clonus* may be elicited. If the foot is abruptly dorsiflexed, it may "chatter" for two or three beats before it settles into a position of rest. Occasionally, in central nervous system disease, this activity will persist, and the foot will not come to rest while the tendon is being stretched, but will persist in repetitive activity. The unsustained clonus associated with normal but hyperactive reflexes is not considered pathologic. Sustained clonus always indicates the presence of nervous system disease and requires evaluation by a physician.

Certain superficial reflexes may be elicited by scratching the skin of the abdominal wall, or the inside of the thigh in men. The former results in involuntary contraction of the abdominal muscles, and the latter results in retraction of the scrotum. Although interesting phenomena, they have little clinical significance.

A well-known reflex, indicative of CNS disease afflicting the corticospinal tracts, is the *Babinski* response. If the lateral aspect of the sole of the foot is stroked, in normal persons, the toes will contract and be drawn tightly together. In persons with CNS disease of the motor system, the toes will fan out and be drawn back. This is normal in newborn infants but represents serious pathology in the adult. There are a variety of described reflexes which convey similar information. Many of them are interesting, but not particularly informative.

Sensory Examination

The sensory system is even more complex than the motor system, because sensory modalities are carried in different tracts, located in different portions of the cord. Remember that the sensory examination is largely subjective and requires the cooperation of the patient. It is recommended that the examiner become familiar with dermatomes that represent the distribution of the peripheral nerves that ramify from the spinal cord. Most sensory deficits result from peripheral neuropathy and will follow anatomical dermatomes. Exceptions to this include major destructive lesions of the brain; loss of sensation, which may affect an entire side of the body; and the neuropathies associated with alcoholism, which occur in a glove and stocking distribution.

Assessment of the sensory system involves tests for tactile sensation, superficial pain, vibration, and proprioception. Throughout the sensory assessment, the patient's eyes are closed. The cooperation of the patient is encouraged by simple directions and reassurance that the examiner will not hurt the patient.

Tactile sensation is assessed by lightly touching a cotton wisp to corresponding areas on each side of the body. The sensitivity of proximal parts of the extremities are compared to distal parts.

Pain and temperature sensation are carried together in the lateral part of the cord. Thus, it is not necessary to test for temperature sense in most circumstances. Superficial pain is assessed by determining the patient's sensitivity to pinprick. The sharp and dull ends of a safety pin are alternately applied to symmetrical areas of the body. The patient is asked to differentiate between a sharp and dull sensation.

The pin is applied with equal intensity at all times, and the two sides are tested symmetrically.

Vibration and proprioception (the subjective sense of joint position) are carried together in the posterior part of the cord. Vibration may be evaluated through the use of a low-frequency (128 cps or 256 cps*) tuning fork. The handle of the vibrating fork is placed against a bony prominence and the patient asked whether or not he feels a buzz. He is instructed to signal the examiner when the buzz ceases. If the patient does not perceive the vibrations at the distal bony prominences, the examiner progresses upward with the tuning fork until the vibrations are felt. As with all measurements of sensitivity, side-to-side comparison is made.

Position sense may be determined by asking the patient to close his eyes and indicate, as the toes are moved, in which direction movement has taken place. Vibration and position sense are often lost together, frequently in circumstances where all others remain intact.

Having tested peripheral sensation, one now asks whether *integration of sensation* in the brain is being carried out properly. This may be done by testing two-point discrimination. That is, if the patient is touched with two sharp objects simultaneously, are they perceived as two, or as one? If a patient is touched simultaneously on opposite sides of the body, he should normally recognize that he has been touched in two places. If he recognizes only one, the one not recognized is said to demonstrate *extinction*. A good test of higher cortical sensory ability is that of *stereognosis*. The patient is instructed to close his eyes and identify a variety of objects (keys, coins, etc.) that are placed in his hand by the examiner.

▷ Examination of the Musculoskeletal System

An examination of the musculoskeletal system ranges from a basic assessment of functional capabilities to sophisticated physical examination maneuvers that facilitate diagnosis of specific muscle and joint disorders. The nurse examiner's assessment is primarily a functional evaluation. Techniques

* cps = cycles per second.

of inspection and palpation are employed to evaluate the patient's posture and gait, joint function, bone stability, muscle integrity and strength, and ability to perform activities of daily living.

The musculoskeletal assessment is commonly integrated into the routine progression of the physical examination. This system relates closely to the neurologic and cardiovascular systems, and thus all three assessments are often carried out together. The basis of the assessment is a comparison of symmetrical regions of the body. The extent of the assessment depends upon the patient's physical complaints, his health history, and any physical clues detected by the examiner that warrant further exploration.

When specific symptoms or physical findings of musculoskeletal dysfunction are apparent, the examination is carried out and carefully documented, and the information is shared with a physician, who may decide that a more extensive examination and diagnostic workup are necessary.

Gait. An assessment of gait is done by having the patient walk normally for a short distance away from the examiner. The examiner observes the gait for smoothness and rhythm. Any unsteadiness or irregular movements are considered abnormal. When a limping motion is noted, it is most likely due to painful weight bearing. In such instances, the patient can usually pinpoint the area of discomfort, thus guiding a further examination. When one extremity is shorter than another, a limp may also be observed as the patient's pelvis drops downward on the affected side with each step. Paralysis in the lower extremities results in a variety of gaits. These gaits are associated with such neurologic disorders as Parkinson's disease, cerebrovascular accident, and cerebral palsy and are discussed in Chapter 56.

Joint Assessment. The joints are evaluated for their size and range of motion, and for the strength of the muscles that flex and extend the joints. The examiner is familiar with the normal range of motion of major joints and focuses on specific joints if functional loss is apparent. Most persons are able to hyperextend all joints. If the maximum extension of a joint still reveals some residual degree of flexion, the range of motion is said to be limited. In the event that joint motion is compromised, or that the joint is painful, the joint is examined for the presence or absence of fluid within its capsule (effusion) and for an increase in temperature that might reflect active inflammation. An effusion is suspected when the joint is swollen in size and the normal landmarks are obliterated. The most common site for joint effusion occurs in the knee. If a small amount of fluid is present in the joint spaces beneath the patella, it may be identified by the following maneuver. The examiner firmly milks the medial and lateral aspects of the extended knee in a downward motion. This displaces any fluid downward. As pressure is exerted against the medial or lateral side, the examiner observes the opposite side for a bulge below the patella. When larger amounts of fluid are present, the patella becomes elevated from the femur during knee extension. If the patella bounces back when tapped firmly against the femur, a "click" may be palpable. This is a test for *ballottement* of the patella. When inflammation or fluid is present in a joint, physician consultation is indicated.

Passive movement of the joint may produce an audible

crunching sound, called *crepitus*. Crepitus may be palpable as well.

Joints and the tissues surrounding them are examined for nodule formation. Rheumatoid arthritis, gout, osteoarthritis, and rheumatic fever all produce characteristic nodules that are diagnostic of the disease. The subcutaneous nodules of rheumatoid arthritis are soft and occur within and along tendons that provide extensor function to the joints. Usually, involvement of the joints assumes a symmetrical pattern. The nodules of gout are hard and lie within and immediately adjacent to the joint capsule itself. Frequently, they rupture, exuding white uric acid crystals onto the skin surface. The nodules of osteoarthritis are hard and painless and represent bony overgrowth that has resulted from destruction of the cartilaginous surface of bone within the joint capsule. These are frequently seen in older adults.

Atrophy of muscle results from disuse as effectively as it does from neurologic damage. Thus, the muscles that provide function to a diseased joint will atrophy when the joint is kept passive to avoid the pain that may arise from moving it. This is dramatically seen in rheumatoid arthritis of the knees, in which the quadriceps muscle may atrophy in a very dramatic way. Often, the size of a diseased joint is exaggerated by the atrophy of muscles proximal and distal to that joint. An assessment of muscle strength is outlined within the neurologic examination (p. 87).

Examination of the Spine.   Inspection of the spine is carried out with the patient's gown open to expose the entire back, buttocks, and legs. The examiner stands behind the patient, noting any differences in the height of the shoulders or iliac crests. The gluteal folds are normally symmetrical. Shoulder and hip symmetry, as well as the straight line of the vertebral column, are inspected with the patient erect and bending forward (flexion).

The normal curvature of the spine is convex through the thoracic portion and concave through the cervical and lumbar portions. The concavity of the lumbar spine is referred to as *lumbar lordosis* and is normal. Excessive curvature of the thoracic spine is called *kyphosis*. Deviation of the spine to the left or right is termed *scoliosis*. Kyphosis and scoliosis may result from damage to the paraspinal musculature in poliomyelitis or from disease of the vertebral column, such as that which may be seen in tuberculosis.

▷ The Physical Examination in Review

Throughout this chapter, the physical examination has been approached by organ systems (*i.e.,* respiratory examination, neurologic examination, and skin assessment). All relevant organ systems are tested in the process, but not necessarily in the sequence described. For example, when the face is examined, it is appropriate at the same time to check for facial asymmetry and, thus, for the integrity of cranial nerve VII; one does not return to this point later, as part of a "neurologic" examination. When systems are combined in this manner, the patient is spared the sequence of sitting up, lying down, sitting up, etc., which would be—to say the least—exhausting.

A "complete" physical examination is not a "routine." Many of the elements previously discussed fall in the category of "subroutines," which are selectively addressed to the patient as a function of his or her particular problem. If, for example, a healthy 20-year-old college student reports for an examination in order to satisfy a requirement to play basketball, and reports no history of neurologic abnormality, the requirements for an adequate survey of the neurologic system are minimal. Conversely, a complaint of transient numbness and diplopia elicits from the examiner a quite complete neurologic investigation. Similarly, a person with pleuritic chest pain receives a much more intensive examination of the chest than the person with, for instance, leg cramps.

The process of physical examination is a thoughtful one. Attempts to elicit physical findings are based upon all the information available at the time the examination is conducted. In general, it is the patient's health history that directs the examiner in efforts to obtain additional data for a complete patient profile.

The process of learning physical examination requires memorization, skill repetition, and reinforcement in a clinical setting. Only after basic physical assessment techniques are mastered and integrated into a complete examination, can the examiner "tailor" the routine screening examination to include thorough assessments of a particular system, including special maneuvers.

▷ Bibliography

Books

Bates B. A Guide to Physical Examination, 3rd ed. Philadelphia, JB Lippincott, 1982.

Bouchier IAD and Morris JS. Clinical Skills: A System of Clinical Examination. Philadelphia, WB Saunders, 1982.

Burnside JW. Physical Diagnosis, 16th ed. Baltimore, Williams & Wilkins, 1981.

DeGowin EL and DeGowin RL. Bedside Diagnostic Examination, 4th ed. New York, Macmillan, 1981.

Delp MH and Manning RT. Major's Physical Diagnosis, 9th ed. Philadelphia, WB Saunders, 1981.

Frantz A. The Well Adult (RN Nursing Assessment Series). Oradell, New Jersey, Medical Economic Books, 1982.

Gillies DA and Alyn IB. Patient Assessment and Management by the Nurse Practitioner. Philadelphia, WB Saunders, 1976.

Hillman RS et al. Clinical Skills: Interviewing, History Taking and Physical Diagnosis. New York, McGraw–Hill, 1981.

Hobson LB. Examination of the Patient: A Text for Nursing and Allied Health Personnel. New York, McGraw–Hill, 1975.

Judge RD, Zuidema GD, and Fitzgerald FT. Clinical Diagnosis, 4th ed. Boston, Little, Brown & Co, 1982.

Malasanos L et al. Health Assessment. St Louis, CV Mosby, 1981.

Perloff JK. Physical Examination of the Heart and Circulation. Philadelphia, WB Saunders, 1982.

Prior JA, Silberstein JS, and Stang JM. Physical Diagnosis, 6th ed. St Louis, CV Mosby, 1981.

Rudy EB and Gray VR. Handbook of Health Assessment. Bowie, Maryland, Robert J. Brady, 1981.

Sana JM and Judge RD. Physical Assessment Skills for Nursing Practice, 2nd ed. Boston, Little, Brown & Co, 1982.

Seedor MM. The Physical Assessment, 2nd ed. New York, Teachers College Press, 1981.

Sherman JL Jr and Fields SK. Guide to Patient Evaluation. Garden City, New York, Medical Examination Pub Co, 1982.

Swartz MH (ed). An Introduction to Physical Diagnosis. New York, Raven Press, 1981.

Walker HK, Hall WD, and Hurst FW. Clinical Methods: The History, Physical and Laboratory Examinations, 2nd ed. Boston, Butterworths, 1980.

Articles

Bauman DJ. Nine ways to improve your cardiovascular examination. Consultant 1979 Nov; 19(11):25–26.

Bluestone R et al. Four diagnosticians show their pearls. Patient Care 1979 Feb 15; 13(3):20–48.

Farrell J. The human side of assessment. Nursing '80 1980 Apr; 10(4):74–75.

Hayden GF. Olfactory diagnosis in medicine. Postgrad Med 1980 Apr; 67(4):110–118.

King RC. A systematic plan for assessing the head and face. RN 1982 Jan; 45(1):55–58.

Prager D. Evaluating the mouth and the hypopharynx during the routine physical examination. CA 1980 Nov/Dec; 30(6):322–323.

Refining the chest examination. Patient Care 1982 Sept 30; 16(16):15–50.

Rubin BA. Black skin. RN 1979 Mar; 42(3):31–35.

6

Documentation of Nursing Practice: Problem-Oriented Recording

The problem-oriented health record system was devised by Lawrence Weed, M.D. over 10 years ago. Since then, many health care delivery systems have incorporated it into their practice settings and many others have adapted it by modifying various components of the system. Dr. Weed's purpose in developing this system of documentation for the patient's health record was to promote a systematic method of organizing all the information needed to accurately diagnose illness and treat patients.

- The problem-oriented system uses the scientific method of problem solving to provide an organized approach to documenting the handling of a patient's problems.

The overall intent of the problem-oriented method of charting is to change the record from a source-oriented document to an integrated patient problem-oriented record that follows the format of a book. The health record starts with a preface, or introduction of the patient (Data Base), proceeds to a table of contents (Patient Problem List), develops the succeeding chapters based on the Problem List (Patient Progress Notes), and finally reaches a conclusion (Discharge Summary).

▷ The Purposes of Patient Health Records

The chief purposes of the health record are to provide a means of communication between the members of the health team participating in patient care and to facilitate coordinated planning and continuity of care. The record fulfills other functions as well: it serves as the business and legal record for the hospital and for the professional staff responsible for the care of patients; it serves as a basis for evaluating the quality of care as well as for reviewing the effective utilization of patient care health practices; and it provides data useful in research, education, and short- and long-range planning.

Nursing care has not always been documented in consistent fashion. The focus in charting has frequently been on recording nursing interventions, such as tasks and routines. These functions are only one component of nursing practice and often represent areas that nurses have delegated to the nonprofessional members of the nursing team. This type of charting effectively demonstrates the traditionally dependent role of nursing practice, which has consisted in following the licensed physician's and dentist's orders for medications and treatments. The areas that reflect the independent functions of nursing practice, such as prevention, health maintenance, restorative nursing measures, and the psychosocial responses of the patient, as well as discharge planning and patient–family teaching, have not been readily documented on the patient's health record. A retrospective review of nurses' charting in any setting illustrates the generalizations nurses have used when charting—for instance, "Good day, up in chair," "Slept well," "No complaints," etc. Very little evidence of patient progress or the effectiveness of the patient care plan was documented.

Today the major frame of reference, or philosophy, of nursing practice is based on the "nursing process," which includes the professional nurse's role in assessing, planning, implementing, and evaluating the patient care given by nurses. This frame of reference for nursing practice, which is analogous to the problem-oriented system of recording, thus makes the nursing process concept attainable and operational in everyday practice.

Although the problem-oriented system does not in itself improve care, it does provide nursing with a tool for documenting nursing practice that is based on scientific method rather than intuition. It also forces the nurse back to the patient's bedside, which enables her to record most effectively all of the parameters she has considered in assessing the patient.

▷ Components of the Problem-Oriented System

The problem-oriented system consists of four components: (1) the data base, (2) the problem list, (3) patient care plans, and (4) progress notes for follow-up on each problem and plan, along with a discharge or transfer summary.

Data Base
The *data base* is a compilation of all of the data obtained on each patient at the time of entry into the health care system. It consists of a complete health history; physical examination; nursing assessment; patient profiles from other sources, such as social worker, pharmacist, nutritionist, dentist, physical therapist, and respiratory therapist; relevant laboratory and radiologic data; and any other data or profiles from other members of the health team involved in the patient's care. The form and content of the data base should be predetermined, and the specified data should be collected for all patients within the institution. Although many disciplines may participate in collecting different parts

of the patient data base, all of the baseline information should be placed together in the same section of the health record.

- The data base should not remain source-oriented, as in the traditional record; nor should the same information be recorded by each discipline. Only new information or additional history or observations should be noted.

When all disciplines are not using the problem-oriented system, it is not always possible to achieve an integrated data base. In this case the nursing department should determine what information is needed about all patients and should seek to avoid duplication of the physician's notes as much as possible.

The nursing assessment, interview, and history or profile of the patient should be obtained on admission or shortly thereafter by the nurse or the nonprofessionals on the nursing team. The general admission information, which serves as the baseline data for nursing, consists of such items as height, weight, temperature, pulse, respiration, and blood pressure. In addition, the patient's diet at home may be included, as well as any assistive devices or prostheses, such as dentures, canes, etc., that the patient has brought with him or that he uses to maintain his independence. Other possible entries include the patient's orientation to his environment; for instance, bed controls, intercom system, bathroom facilities, etc.

The remainder of the nursing assessment or patient's data base must be collected by the professional nurse and could include the patient/family assessment factors found on page 99.

Experience with the problem-oriented system and the nursing process has shown that definite time limits need to be established by the organization so that the patient's problems may be identified as quickly after admission as possible. Many organizations set 8 to 24 hours as the time limit.

After collaborating with the patient in describing the problems he perceives, discussing any additional problems identified from the information given, and selecting only relevant data, the nurse is now ready to record the information on the patient's health record. This information can then be inserted in the section with the physician's history and physical examination; however, if the record is still source-oriented, the data base will be the first sheet in the nursing section and should not be removed or thinned from the record during the patient's stay. The patient's data base for nursing now becomes the introduction or preface to all future patient interactions or responses to treatment.

Patient Problem List
The Patient Problem List now becomes the first page of the record. It serves as the "index" or "table of contents" to the record. For clarification, a *problem* is defined as anything that concerns the patient, endangers his health, requires management, and concerns any member of the health team. Generally, if all professionals are using the problem-oriented system, the primary or responsible physician assumes the responsibility of formulating the patient's problems

from the data base. These problems are numbered and are used by all concerned for making plans and writing titled and numbered progress notes.

Patient problems are classified by field of interest and level of understanding according to the following categories:

- Medical problems
    Diagnosis (*e.g.,* Hodgkin's disease IV B)
    Physiologic finding (*e.g.,* enlarged lymph node)
    Symptom or physical finding (*e.g.,* generalized pruritus)
    Abnormal laboratory finding (*e.g.,* leukocytosis)
- Social problems (*e.g.,* unemployed registered nurse)
- Environmental causes (*i.e.,* health hazards)
    For example, smokes two packs cigarettes/day
- Psychiatric problems
    Diagnosis (*e.g.,* depression)
    Behavioral manifestations (*e.g.,* angry at self)
- Past problems (*i.e.,* from all categories)
    For example, history—abortion, 8 weeks, 1979
    For example, history—appendectomy, 1969

The patient's problems are also classified by status. Active or inactive and resolved problems should all be listed on the "Master Problem List." The Problem List must be modified as the patient changes and as more information is gained. A problem is modified by inserting an arrow, with the date above it, followed by the updated or new diagnosis or by either the word "dropped" or "resolved." For example:

1/20/84—abdominal pain; 1/21/84—partial intestinal obstruction

Minor problems or episodes may be entered as "temporary problems" in the Progress Notes (*e.g.,* patient incident, such as a fall or a headache). When a second progress note is written, it is usually easy to decide if it should be transferred to the Problem List or dropped.

If all professionals are not using the problem-oriented system, the same nurse who collected the Data Base will initiate the patient problem list. The problem is always stated at the nurse's current level of understanding. The nurse is able to list chronic medical problems, past problems, symptoms, physical findings, and abnormal laboratory findings, as well as social, environmental, and psychiatric problems. The nurse does not make a medical diagnosis, but as more information is available from the diagnostic studies and the physician's physical examination, this is used to update the Problem List.

- The most important fact to remember is that if all disciplines are using the system as originally intended, there should be *only one patient problem list.* If each discipline begins to use its own patient problem list, the record is unwieldy and inefficient.

Patient Care Plans

Patient care plans are initiated for each problem that is identified and are keyed by number to the problem list. This is the next step in the scientific method of solving problems,

and when a well-conceived plan is written initially, all that is necessary for long periods of time in the progress notes is a record of the data on observations of the patient in response to the diagnostic or therapeutic treatment prescribed. In many institutions, to facilitate following the plan of care, a card file called a Kardex is used. This does not substitute for documenting the plan in the progress notes, unless the Kardex is considered a permanent part of the health record. More and more institutions are moving toward making the Kardex care plan a permanent part of the record and are recording it in ink rather than in pencil. The Kardex care plan involves all of the professional members of the health team, as required by the patient's problems, so that all members are working together toward the same goal and all of their efforts are congruent.

The plan for each problem should contain three essential components:

1. Directives for the need to collect more data
    (The physician will consider the "rule-outs" or the "possibles," each of which should always be coupled with an action.)
    Example: R/O kidney disease; schedule IVP for Wednesday
    (Nursing will consider the need for more information.)
    Example: Monitor intake and output × 72 hours
2. Directives for management or treatment of the problem
    (The physician will prescribe specific modalities.)
    Example: Aldomet 250 mg, PO, qid
    (Nursing will order specific nursing measures to be taken.)
    Example: BP, lying and standing qid
3. Directives for teaching the patient and one or more family members about his problem, its treatment, and what is expected of him in managing the problem and maintaining an optimum level of health
    (The physician will document what the patient has been told about his illness and what is being planned for him or his family.)
    Example: Patient told that this problem should not interfere with occupation and he should be able to return to work in 3 weeks.
    (The nurse will document whether the patient and his family can repeat or verbalize any instructions given to them.)
    Example: Attended group classes on 3-10; able to answer all questions regarding diet, activity, and medications he will be taking when he returns home.

Whether or not nurses are the only ones implementing the system, they can use the above components in developing their patient care plans. The nurse will need to develop the skill of stating her plans in the form of specific directives in the progress notes, so that they can eventually be transcribed by the unit clerk to the Kardex.

Patient Progress Notes

The progress notes are written in a format that not only relates them clearly and unmistakably to the problem, but also utilizes the scientific method of problem solving on a day-by-day basis (see p. 102). Progress notes are written in a narrative form, using the acronym "SOAPIE."

S: Subjective data (symptoms that the patient describes)

O: Objective data (signs that the professional observes)

A: Assessment (the professional's conclusion about the subjective and objective data)

P: Plan (immediate or future, including patient education)

I: Intervention (nursing action done to, for, or with the patient)

E: Evaluation (patient outcome of nursing process)

Flow sheets are used to follow or monitor a problem that does not lend itself to a single note or requires that multiple parameters be observed and recorded more often than every 6 hours or four times a day; or they may be used for the documentation of nursing and patient activities, such as treatments, daily care, etc.

- The Progress Notes are the most critical part of the problem-oriented system. They are the mechanism that provides a minute-by-minute ongoing assessment of the patient's problem. The progress notes can detect faulty understanding and poor decisions made by the health care provider. They do not improve care, but they can identify inadequate logic in seconds. Progress notes provide the feedback on problem identification and the plans formulated. If all professionals are recording on integrated progress notes, the patient has a greater chance of receiving continuity of care.

The progress notes always begin with the date, time, and problem number and title, and they continue, using the following format:

Subjective Data. The subjective or symptomatic data are obtained from the patient's or family's point of view. When recording subjective data, consider the following: onset (date, time, type), intensity, quality, location, radiation, number of episodes, time of day of episodes, sources of relief (rest, position, medication), precipitating factors, factors that make the problem worse, other associated symptoms existing at the same time, overall course, the degree to which the symptoms have affected the patient's lifestyle, etc.

Objective Data. These include actual clinical observations or laboratory findings appropriate to the problem. When recording objective data, always include the following: location, size, shape, color, temperature, moisture, and consistency. Also, note the presence or absence of swelling, movement, weakness, and associated pain with movement or touch. Many nurses record their nursing actions in this section; others add their immediate interventions to the plan component of the progress notes.

Assessment. This is the portion of the progress notes that deals directly with the subjective and objective data just collected and that presents the health care provider's conclusion, based on that information. If both are consistent with the problem statement, little needs to be said here.

One way of considering assessment in relation to patient progress or regress will be a comparison with the previous documentation, using such terms as "improved," "worse," or "deteriorating," or "same" or "stable." If the problem is a new one, the subjective and objective data should support a new assessment of what is going on with the patient. If the problem statement and the subjective and objective data are not consistent, one can quickly assess the logic or accuracy of the information recorded.

Assessment occurs when the provider records his thinking and conclusions at his level of understanding.

Plan. The original or initial plan, if well thought out and developed, will continue to be followed or will be modified as new information is obtained. The plan will always consider the three areas described earlier: the need for more information, management, and treatment, and patient and family education.

Intervention and Evaluation. Nurses use the same problem-oriented procedure to document their practice. However, there are two components that many nurses have added in order to comply with the requirements of the nursing process and of some regulatory agencies for documenting nursing practice. These components are labeled *I*, for the nursing intervention that was carried out immediately (*e.g.,* raise the head of the bed, notify the physician, etc.), and *E*, for evaluation of the nursing intervention (was it effective or ineffective?) as documented according to patient outcomes. Sometimes the evaluation will appear in the next progress note because more time is needed to observe the patient's response to the nursing intervention.

One can see that when the plan is incorporated in the patient progress notes, it readily becomes a permanent part of the legal record, and the Kardex system reverts to being a tool to facilitate the implementation of the plan.

Discharge or Transfer Summary

The last portion of the record should be a summary of each problem, using the "SOAP" format. The summary should include:

- The cause of the problem
- The status of each problem
- The intervention or management used to handle the problem
- The future plans for following the problem at home, in the office, clinic, or extended care facility
- Agency referrals made
- Instructions and verification of the patient's or family's knowledge of the problem and their responsibility in dealing with it

This summary is vital to the next set of health care providers. It is often done by the physician and includes the contributions made by all of the other health professionals. Even if the physician does include the health team approach in his summary, the nursing and other disciplines involved should include in their discharge summaries the specific goals with which their professions were directly involved.

The transfer summary is most appropriate when the patient is progressing from one level of care to another. An

Chart 6-1
Writing Problem-Oriented Progress Notes

Reminders to Consider Before Writing Problem-Oriented Progress Notes

1. Have the patient's problem list in front of you or open to the problem list on the patient's health record.
2. Think about your patient in light of each problem listed in the active column. Are there any new problems to be added or considered as a result of your observations or interactions with the patient today?
3. Read the immediately previous notes so that you will not unnecessarily repeat information already recorded and so that you will be aware of plans that are in progress.
4. Decide which are the most important problems for you to discuss; always consider life-threatening or major problems first (*e.g.*, although a myocardial infarction may be a very threatening problem, if it is relatively stable or has recently been discussed, the patient's acute anxiety may be a more pertinent topic; it may have a significant impact on his survival).
5. A follow-up note on data-base information or on your plans identified in previous notes may be appropriate if the data is now available, or you might want to comment on the effectiveness or ineffectiveness of your plan (*e.g.*, vital signs, weight, response to treatment or nursing measures, etc.).
6. Always begin your note with the date, time, problem number, and title. List the subjective or objective data, using the factors suggested in this chapter. Record both follow-up data and any new information you have gathered.

7. Write an assessment for each problem considered, stating your thoughts at the level at which you actually understand the information. If you want to write about specific observations or responses to medications or treatments with which you have had little experience, look them up first—you may find valuable information that will help all members of the health team, or you might learn that your idea does not logically follow from the data you have available.
8. Review the plan for each problem listed, or initiate a new plan if you have identified a new problem. Always consider the following three factors:
   a. The need for more information: such as specific observations that might help clarify the problem
   b. Nursing intervention: such as specific nursing measures you can order or initiate to resolve the problem (*e.g.*, have patient turn, cough, and take deep breaths every hour for 24 hours)
   c. Patient or family teaching: what you have told or plan to tell the patient and his family about this problem to increase their understanding of the management
9. Write a progress note when there is something pertinent to say, such as when there has been a change. Some days several notes for the day or for the shift may be indicated, whereas on other days *no* notes will be appropriate for some problems.

Some Don'ts When Recording on the Progress Notes

DON'T include comments on nonproblem item (*e.g.*, bed baths, h.s. care given, doing well, etc.)

DON'T write about things that have already been discussed unless you disagree with the data listed or the conclusions drawn. Be sure to defend your position with exact literature references if you do disagree.

DON'T include comments on normal physiologic functions unless they are pertinent to a particular problem

(*e.g.*, the daily bowel movements should be kept on a routine care flow sheet unless you are discussing a patient who has diarrhea or who has a previously identified problem, such as constipation).

DON'T use the progress notes to record routine tests done or care given (*e.g.*, these can be checked off on the Kardex care plan or considered recorded when the laboratory or x-ray reports come back.)

---

example of this would be the transfer from an intensive care unit to a general patient unit.

▷ Summary

The problem-oriented system makes it possible to document health care practice using the scientific method. It lends itself to computerization, but can be recorded manually. The total concept, when implemented, improves communication among all health professionals. The system promotes the continuing education of each individual member of the health team: the systematic gathering, recording,

and assessment of data; the development and implementation of plans; and the evaluation of results constitute an effective learning process. Above all, the system provides a more meaningful way of reviewing the patient's profile by focusing on the patient and all of the factors that affect his recovery or return to optimum health.

The problem-oriented system is important to nursing practice because it makes the nursing process operational and has the potential of contributing to nursing research by helping to define and evaluate nursing practice.

Points to keep in mind when writing problem-oriented progress notes are summarized in Chart 6-1.

Nursing Assessment

NURSING DATA BASE

White, Susan   11322.1
Dr. Stone   198-74-0360
MTS   1/21/84
59677 25 8-9-59   F.S. Cath.
176 Hollow St. Pgh 15215
HSA 6605-00   198-74-0360
Unemployed R.N.
Parents-Teresa   412-264-7657

GENERAL ADMISSION INFORMATION

DATE: 1/21/84   TIME: 1:00 pm

BASELINE DATA: Height: 163 cm Weight: 49.5 Kg Temp.: 37.6 °C Pulse: 120   Resp.: 22   BP: Ra: 106/70   La: 110/74

PROSTHESES OR ASSISTIVE DEVICES: None

DIET AT HOME: General—when eating

ALLERGIES: "Compazine"   SIGNATURE: R. Jones, R.N.

PATIENT/FAMILY ASSESSMENT

REASON FOR HOSPITALIZATION OR ADMITTING PROBLEM: Nausea, Vomiting, lower abdominal pain with cramping, diarrhea—small amounts of green liquid stool 3-4x day.

DURATION OF THIS PROBLEM: 2 weeks without a normal B.M., poor appetite and weaker past week.

OBSERVATION OF PATIENT'S CONDITION: Very ill young lady with Cushingoid appearance
  Gastrointestinal status: Distended abdomen, mild epigastric tenderness
  Neurologic status: Alert and oriented to time, place, and person; no loss of sensation
  Respiratory status: No difficulty at this time, R. 22
  Skin condition: Skin clear, no petechiae on body; gums-oral mucosa look clear.

CONCURRENT CONDITIONS: "Hodgkin's disease since 1979" Dx 7/79 of Hodgkin's Stage IV B.

PREVIOUS EXPERIENCE WITH HOSPITALIZATIONS: 6th admission here. Rx 8/79 with Exploratory Lap with Splenectomy; 10/80 Radiation Therapy with 4000 Rads to all nodes. 8/81 chemotherapy
MEDICATION: Prednisone 30 mg q.d. with Maalox. Darvon 65mg. Dalmane 30mg. HS PRN.

REACTION TO ALLERGIES: "Compazine makes me hyperactive"

PATTERNS:
  HYGIENE: "Usually shower when I feel good"
  REST/SLEEP: 6-7 hours/night, retires 11-12 midnight, arises 6-7 a.m.
  MEALS/DIET: General, but appetite poor past 2 wks; has been eating soup, cereals, eggs
  ACTIVITY STATUS: Independent in ADL; OOB as tolerated.
  ELIMINATION—BOWEL: Diarrhea 3-4x day- "maybe I am impacted from Vincristine"
             BLADDER: 4-5x day, q.s. no recent change, "occ. nocturia if I can't sleep"
  MENSTRUAL HISTORY: Lmp 1/25/82 No change recently.

HEALTH HAZARD APPRAISAL: BSE q month. To M.D. office q. month, no smoking or alcohol

LIFE STYLE: Prior to 7/79 worked as R.N. in ICU at local hospital. Since 1980 worked only 1 mo. Lives with parents. "Mother fusses over me."

TYPICAL DAY PROFILE: "Up at 7 a.m., bkft with parents, watch T.V., nap, lunch. Sew or knit, frequent visitors. "Boyfriend hasn't given up on me." "Now what!" Anxious and
MENTAL/EMOTIONAL STATUS: "Was doing well until this happened!" teary-eyed. Depressed and angry during interview.

SAFETY APPRAISAL: No problem unless she gets weaker and is unable to get OOB s̄ help.

DISCHARGE PLANNING: Anticipated LOS 1-2 wks if present problem is resolved s̄ surgery and if chemotherapy is completed. Will have to return to clinic each month. Reinforce patient and family as to what to watch for after discharge, if no further relapse.
INFORMANT: Patient, old charts, physician.

SIGNATURE:

(Based on form used by Presbyterian–University Hospital Nursing Service Department, Pittsburgh, Pa.)

Patient Care Plan A

NAME: Susan White

ALLERGIES: Idiosyncrasy to Compazine

Date Ordered	#	Medications	Dosage	Rte.	Time Symbol	Time - Hours	To Be Disc.
1/21	2	Decadron	1mg.	IV	86h	12-6-12-6	
1/21	2	Prednisone	10mg.	P.O	q6h	10-4-10-4	
1/21	2	Maalox	30ml.				
1/25	2	Thorazine	25mg	IM	1/2hr ā Chemo Rx		
1/25	1	Darvon	65mg	PO	q4h	PRN	
1/24	1	Talwin	50mg	IM	q4h	PRN	
1/22	4	Oxaine	5ml.	PO	PRN	Leave at bedside	
1/21	4	Peppermint H₂O	8ml.	PO	PRN		
1/21	3	Valium	5mg.	IM	86h	PRN	
1/21	1	Codeine Sulph.	30mg	IM	q4h	PRN	

Specimens and Cultures	Date Offered	To Be Disc	INIT.	Date To Be Done
Urine R&M	1/21		RJ	
Standing Blood Work				
Routine Blood Work				
CBC & Diff	1/21			1/21
Retic. Platelets	1/21			1/21

Date Ordered	Diagnostic Procedures	Date To Be Done
1/21	Chest X-Ray	7/21
1/21	ECG	7/21
1/21	Flat Plate Abd.	7/21

	Consults	Date Seen
1/21	Surg. CRS Dr. C. Watson	1/21

(Based on form used by Presbyterian–University Hospital Nursing Service Department, Pittsburgh, Pa.)

Patient Care Plan B

Patient Profile

White, Susan   11322.1
Dr. Stone   1   198-74-0360
M+S   1-21-84
56977   25   8-9-59   F   3   Cath
176 Hollow St.   Pgh.   15215
HSA 6605-00   198-74-0360
Unemployed R.N.
Parents-Teresa   412-264-7657

#	PATIENT PROBLEM LIST
1	Abdominal Pain 1/21 partial intestinal obstruction
	a. Nausea and Vomiting
	b. Abdominal cramping
	c. Diarrhea
2	Hodgkins IV B
3	Adaptation to illness
	a. Depression
	b. Anger
4	Esophagitis
5	Cushingoid appearance
6	Allergy or idiosyncrasy to Compazine
7	1979 - Exp. Lap. with Splenectomy

#	DISCHARGE PLANNING:
1	Reinstruct about changes in bowel habits-develop regime & discharge
2	Support patient (ex. concerns over diagnosis) by listening to her. Work with parents to support end-stage disease at home or in hospital. Sacraments of the sick 1/24/84

Tent. Disch. ?2 weeks   Name Susan White

DATE—DIET: 1/2 Liquids as tol.
DATE—ACTIVITY STATUS: 1/21 Bedrest & BRP as tol.
DATE—CARE CATEGORY: 1/21 Partial → Self
PROSTHESES: None
HT. 163 cm   WT. 49.5 kg
DATE—OPERATION:
SAFETY APPRAISAL: Instruct to seek assistance when getting up c̄ I.V.
TPRq 4h. while awake   B/Pq
Assessment Done by   1/21 Ruth Jones

#	Date	Treatments and Nursing Directives	Time
1	1/21	~~Intake and Output~~	
1a	1/21	N G tube to intermittent low suction, cont. irrigation 30ml NSS	9-3-11, 8-10-12 etc.
1a	1/21	Mouth care c̄ baking soda & water pik q4h PRN pc meals	8-12-4-8 etc.
1b	1/21	~~Check for bowel sounds q4h~~	8-12-4-8 etc.
1c	1/21	Observe color, consistency q record on Flow Sheet	
2	1/21	Check for constipation due to chemotherapy side effects daily	
2	1/21	Weigh daily	7:30 A.m.
		Observe Skin for Petechiae and Pruritus	
		Give Premedication 1/2 hr before chemotherapy	
		Urine reductions q.i.d. x48 hrs. than 1x daily	7-11-4-9
3a	1/21	Accept her behavior; let her know you understand	
		She will talk if she trusts you. Pretends sleep when unable to talk	
3b	1/21	Easily recognized-refuses Rx, meds, pulls out NG tube. Knows diagnosis (because she is an RN.) Answer	
		- Sometimes more frightened honestly and keep her informed of Rx, tests, Plans,	
4	1/24	Give oxaine 15 min ac- avoid acidic juices or drinks	
5	1/21	Concerned over body image. Very attractive c̄ Prednisone, Boy- friend still visits-Provide privacy. Help her to look attractive when it is known he is coming. Assess Parents response to her body image change. Explain drug effects.	

Attending Physician   Dr. Stone   Intern Smiley   Room 11322.1

(Based on form used by Presbyterian–University Hospital Nursing Service Department, Pittsburgh, Pa.)

Nurses' Progress Notes

DATE	TIME	PROBLEM	PROGRESS NOTES
1/22/	7-12N	#1 Partial Intestinal Obstruction	S: pain and cramping in abdomen is less today.
			O: Abdomen softer, sluggish peristalsis. N-G tube draining small amount (50-100 ml.) clear yellow liquid. No diarrhea or formed stool.
			A: fecal impaction may be beginning to move
			P: If peristalsis improves, remove N-G tube and start on liquids.
			I: Notified Dr. Smiley. S.S. enema ordered and given.
			E: Enema effectual for return of yellow liquid with many small pieces of hard brown stool.
1/23/	7-12N	#1 Partial Intestinal Obstruction	S: Requesting more to eat than sips of water.
			O: Active bowel sounds, abdomen soft, small formed B.m.
			A: Obstruction resolved. Impaction broken up.
			P: Begin bowel regime to keep stool soft and formed. Instruct patient in importance of having B.m. every day because of constipating effect of chemotherapy.
			I: Dr. Smiley notified. N-G tube removed. Started on liquids as tolerated.
			E: Tolerated liquid lunch; will add more full liquids to evening meal.

Each Progress Note consists of the number and title of problem as stated on the Problem List and any or all of the following components:

S — Subjective Data (Symptoms)
O — Objective Data (Measurable Signs)
A — Assessment (Conclusion)
P — Plan — Immediate or Future
I — Intervention — Nursing Action
E — Evaluation — Effectiveness of Intervention

(Based on form used by Presbyterian–University Hospital Nursing Service Department, Pittsburgh, Pa.)

Special Care Flow Sheet

Define parameters as need for each patient.

NOS._____PROBLEMS_____

DATE 12 **pm.**_____to 12 **pm.**_____

TIME	Blood Pressure	Pulse	Respirations	Temperature	Central Venous Pressure	Urine Volume	Specific Gravity							REMARKS

(Based on form used by Presbyterian–University Hospital Nursing Service Department, Pittsburgh, Pa.)

Discharge Summary

DATE	REMARKS
2/3/84	**#1** Partial Intestinal Obstruction S: "No discomfort. BMs are soft and moving regularly." O: Soft abdomen. No diarrhea. A: Obstruction due to impaction relieved through scheduled bowel regulation program. P: Continue daily pericolace; reemphasize to patient the importance of keeping her stool soft and moving daily because of side effect of medication, Vincristine. To notify M.D. if laxative needed. **#2** Hodgkins IV B S: Understands diagnosis of Hodgkins IV B O: A: End stage of disease progressing P: Worked with parents to accept progression of disease and the minimal response to chemotherapy. Taught them what to expect such as edema, ascites, further weakness, etc. To avoid bruising, since platelets are up.
2/3/84	**#3** Adaptation to Illness S: Still angry about having disease; has not been able to accept condition. O: Lashes out at parents, crying, very frightened of going home. A: Still needs much support to begin to accept living one day at a time. P: Referred her to Visiting Nurse Association in Pittsburgh for Patient/Family Support. **#4** Esophagitis S: No complaints of heartburn any longer. A: Problem resolved at this time. P: Given prescription for Oxaine and instructed to take it if heartburn recurs. **#5** Cushingoid Appearance S: Concerned over physical appearance and what it will do to her relationship with boyfriend and family. O: Moon-shaped face, slight hump on back, beginning to look more and more Cushingoid. Urine reduction negative. A: Steroid dose (Prednisone) will continue to be given, so Patient/Family need to be aware of sign and symptoms of diabetes. P: Continue to encourage her fix herself up with makeup and set her hair, etc. Instructed family in observation of signs and symptoms of diabetes, such as polyuria, polydipsia and polyphagia. Taught her to check urine at least once a day. Instructed family to make as few comments as possible about physical appearance.
2/3/84	Discharged home with parents, *R. Smith. R.N.*

(Based on form used by Presbyterian-University Hospital Nursing Service Department, Pittsburgh, Pa.)

▷ Bibliography

Books

Accreditation Manual for Hospitals. Chicago, Joint Commission on Accreditation of Hospitals, 1982.

Bailey J and Claus K. Decision Making in Nursing: Tools for Change. St Louis, CV Mosby, 1975.

Bullough B (ed). The Law and the Expanding Nursing Role, 2nd ed, pp 81–84. New York, Appleton–Century–Crofts, 1980.

Carnevali D. Nursing Care Planning: Diagnosis and Management, 2nd ed. Philadelphia, JB Lippincott, 1983.

Kim MJ and Moritz DA. Classification of Nursing Diagnoses: Proceedings of the Third and Fourth National Conferences. New York, McGraw–Hill, 1982.

Vaughn–Wrobel B and Henderson B. The Problem-Oriented System in Nursing: A Workbook, 2nd ed. St Louis, CV Mosby, 1982.

Walker JB et al (eds). Dynamics of Problem-Oriented Approaches: Patient Care and Documentation. Philadelphia, JB Lippincott, 1976

Weed L. Medical Records, Medical Education and Patient Care. Cleveland, Case Western Reserve University Press, 1968.

Yura H and Walsh MB. The Nursing Process: Assessing, Planning, Implementing and Evaluating, 3rd ed. New York, Appleton–Century–Crofts, 1978.

Articles

Allen R et al. Validity of problem-oriented record system for evaluating treatment outcome. Psychol Rep 1980 Aug; 47:303–306.

Atwood J and Yarnall SR (eds). Symposium on the problem-oriented record. Nurs Clin North Am 1974 June; 9:entire issue.

Bertucci M et al. Comparative study of progress notes using problem-oriented and traditional methods of charting. Nurs Res 1974 July–Aug; 23:351–354.

Buchanan ME. Methods of data collection. AORN J 1981 Jan; 33(1):137–149.

Hartson D and Hartson KM. The five-minute interview. AORN J 1980 Mar; 31(4):605–608.

Mallick MJ. Patient assessment—based on data, not intuition. Nurs Outlook 1981 Oct; 81:600–605.

Manuel BJ. Two good examples of nurse's notes forms. AORN J 1980 Feb; 31(2):247–252.

McDonelly et al. Problem-oriented nursing care plans. ADJ 1980 Feb; 80:292–297.

Porter A et al. Patient needs on admission. Am J Nurs 1977 Jan; 77:112–113.

Recommended practices for documentation of perioperative nursing care. AORN J 1982 Mar; 35(4):744–748.

Rieder K and Wood M. Problem-orientation: An experimental study to test its heuristic value. Nurs Res 1978 Jan–Feb; 27:25–29.

Woody M and Mallison M. The problem-oriented system for patient-centered care. Am J Nurs 1973 July; 73:1168–1175.

Unit III

Biophysical Concepts Related to Health and Illness

7

Homeostasis and Pathophysiologic Processes

When the body is threatened or suffers an injury, its response may involve functional and structural changes; these changes may be adaptive or maladaptive. The defense mechanisms that the body can mount will determine the difference between adaptation and maladaptation, health and disease. Physiology is the study of the functional activities of the living organism and its parts. *Patho*physiology is the study of *disordered* function of the body. *Mechanisms* are patterns of action performed by different parts of the body to serve a common goal. These mechanisms may be compensatory to restore a lost balance, such as hyperpnea to correct an oxygen deficit and lactic acid excess following running. Or, they may be pathophysiologic, such as failure of the heart, leading to sodium and water retention and high venous pressure, which contribute to further disorder. These mechanisms give rise to signs that may be observed by the nurse or symptoms that may be related by the patient. Based upon these observations and a knowledge of the physiologic processes involved, the nurse can determine the existence of a problem and plan her course of action to treat it.

▷ Dynamic Balance: The Steady State

Physiologic mechanisms must be understood in the context of the body as a whole. Man, as a living system, has both an internal and an external environment. Information and matter are continuously exchanged from one environment to the other. Within the body itself, each organ, tissue, and cell is also a system or subsystem of the whole, each with its own internal and external environment, each exchanging information and matter (Fig. 7-1). The goal of the interaction of the body's subsystems is to produce a dynamic balance or steady state, so that all are in harmony with each other, just as Man, as an individual, seeks harmony with those with whom he interacts. For a better understanding of the concept of steady state, the development of the principles of internal constancy, homeostasis, and adaptation will be described.

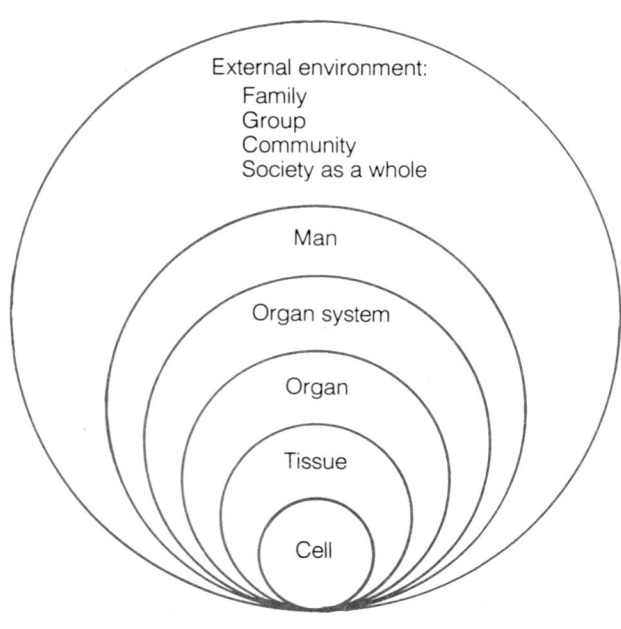

Figure 7-1. Constellation of systems. Each system is a subsystem of the larger system (suprasystem) of which it is a part. In this figure the cell is the smallest system, being a subsystem of all other systems.

Internal Constancy, Homeostasis, and Adaptation

Claude Bernard, a French physiologist in the 19th century, developed the biological principle that for a "free life" there must be a *constancy* or "fixity of the internal milieu," despite changes in the external environment. The internal milieu he addressed was the fluid that bathes the cells, and the constancy was maintained by physiologic and biochemical processes; his principle implied a static process.

Later, Walter B. Cannon coined the term *homeostasis* to describe this constancy; his term introduced a change process into the concept of constancy. Cannon enlarged upon Bernard's work by emphasizing the importance of involuntary neural control of the physiochemical responses to stimuli.

Dubos (1965) took the change or dynamic nature of responses one step further: he stated that there are two complementary concepts, homeostasis and adaptation, both necessary for a successful life. Homeostasis refers to the "necessary adjustments that the body can make rapidly" to maintain its internal composition "within limits precisely defined for each organism." That this means "absolute constancy" is "only a concept of the ideal": there are acceptable ranges of response to stimuli, and the organism chooses among them. *Adaptation,* on the other hand, refers to the responses the individual makes to function adequately under "changed conditions of the environment." Dubos was primarily concerned with man's survival in and adaptation to a changing physical world.

Maintenance of the Steady State

With the application of the theory of general systems to the behavioral sciences, the terms of *steady state* or *dynamic*

equilibrium, which will be used here, describe this condition of internal consistency and harmony with the external environment. The maintenance of the steady state, which is necessary for a condition of health, is under the control of the body's regulatory processes, both voluntary and involuntary. In response to either internal or external stimuli, compensatory mechanisms are put into operation. These mechanisms are adaptive as long as they can maintain a steady state. If the compensatory response is not adequate, a threat to the steady state exists, function will become disordered, and pathophysiologic mechanisms will become operative. The pathophysiologic mechanisms can lead to disease, and they are also active during disease. *Disease* is a threat to the steady state and is defined as any process or event that promotes a change in the internal environment that results in loss or disruption of cell function and thus limits man's freedom to act in the external world.

An analogy can be made to the pendulum of a clock. As it swings to and fro, maintaining correct time, it is in dynamic balance, or a steady state. Someone tips the clock, and the pendulum swings a bit to one side but is still able to maintain reasonably accurate time. The clock is tipped more; now the pendulum swings more to one side than the other, and with each swing the pendulum's own weight increases the erratic movement. The clock's functional ability to provide accurate time is damaged and, if nothing intervenes, may be destroyed altogether.

Nursing Implications

It is important for the nurse to realize that the optimal point of intervention to promote health is during the stage when the individual's own compensatory processes are still functioning. It is therefore imperative to be able to relate the presenting signs and symptoms to the physiology they represent. This makes it possible to identify the individual's position on the continuum of function, from health and compensation to pathophysiology and disease. Thus, if a middle-aged woman presented herself for a checkup, and was found to be overweight, with a blood pressure of 130/85, the nurse would most likely counsel her with respect to diet and activity. She would encourage weight loss; question her intake of salt, which affects her fluid balance, and her intake of caffeine, for its stimulant effect; and discuss ways to decrease the stress in her life. The ultimate goal of her activities would be to control her blood pressure and prevent hypertension.

Another reason for becoming well versed in symptomatology and physiology is that there are many diseases, too numerous to memorize. However, the number of physiologic processes is limited. Having a knowledge of these processes makes it possible to detect the abnormalities or the degree of risk involved and to intervene effectively.

▷ Pathophysiologic Processes at the Cellular Level

The processes described may occur at all levels of the biological organism. (They also occur in society and populations, but this chapter will focus on the physiology of the individual.) If the cell is considered the smallest unit or subsystem (tissues being aggregates of cells, organs aggregates of tissues, etc.), the processes of health and disease, adaptation and maladaptation may all occur at the cellular level. Indeed, pathologic processes are described at the subcellular or molecular level. The cell may then be described as existing on a continuum of function and structure, from the normal cell, to the adapted cell, to the injured or diseased cell, to the dead cell (Fig. 7-2).

Nature of Changes

Changes from one state to another may occur rapidly and may not be readily detectable, because each state does not have distinct or discrete boundaries, and disease represents an extension and distortion of normal processes. For example, tanning of the skin is an adaptive, morphologic response to exposure to the rays of the sun. If the exposure is continued, however, sunburn and injury may occur, and some cells may die, as is evidenced by "peeling."

Earliest changes occur at the molecular or subcellular level and are not easily detectable. Not until steady state functions or structures are altered do changes become apparent. With cell injury some changes may be reversible, whereas others are lethal and lead to death. Also, the adapted state is generally a lower functional level, in that it is maintained by the use of additional energy or reserves, or by a morphologic change of tissue cells into a less specific, or less differentiated, cell type.

Responses to Stimuli/Stressors

Different cells and tissues respond to stimuli with different patterns and rates of response, some being more vulnerable to one type of stimulus or stressor than another. Thus, cardiac muscle cells respond to hypoxia more quickly than smooth muscle cells. The cell involved, its ability to adapt, and its physiologic state are determinants of the response.

Another determinant of the response is the type or nature of the stressor, its duration, and its severity. For example, a drug tolerance to regular small amounts of a barbiturate may develop, but one large dose may result in unconsciousness and death.

Nursing Implications

Organs are capable of a wide range of activity: the heart rate can change from 60 beats/minute to 150 beats/minute, the volume of air breathed can vary from 0.3 liters/minute to 150 liters/minute; thus, the ability of the body to compensate and adapt to differing environmental conditions is remarkable. When injury does occur, it may be reversible up to a point; earliest morphologic changes may be regarded as "fingerprints of disease; when the damage is slight the prints can be erased" (Boyd & Sheldon, 1980). For the health of the patient, it is imperative to detect these early changes.

▷ Control of the Steady State: Control Systems

The concept of the cell on a continuum of function and structure (illustrated in Fig. 7-2) includes the relationship of the "normal cell" and the "adapted cell" to compensatory mechanisms. These mechanisms include the adjustment processes that are continuously occurring in the body to maintain the dynamic balance, or steady state.

Negative Feedback Process

Through the process of negative feedback, deviations from a predetermined set point or range of adaptability are detected, and these trigger a response in which the action offsets the deviation. Blood pressure, acid–base balance, blood glucose level, body temperature, and fluid and electrolyte balance are examples of parameters regulated through such compensatory mechanisms. Each of these parameters has a range for optimal function. If there is either an excess or a deficiency, negative feedback will trigger activity to cause a return to the optimal level.

A familiar illustration of the negative feedback process in a simple control system is the control of room temperature. The door is opened and a cold draft reduces room temperature, which is detected by a thermometer and relayed to a thermostat. The thermostat compares this temperature to a preset reference point. Detecting that the room is cooler, it sends a message to the furnace to fire up, with the effect of heating the room air. The new temperature is fed into the thermostat, and if it is equal to the reference point, the furnace is signaled to shut off. This is *negative feedback,* which is a series of actions in which the goal is to counter the influence of an initiating stimulus or disturbance. It does not change the disturbance, only its effect.

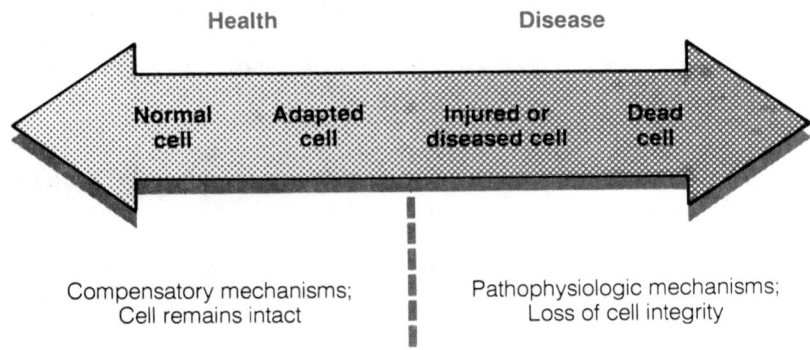

Figure 7-2. The cell on a continuum of function and structure. Changes in the cell are not as easily discerned as the diagram depicts. The point at which compensation is lost and pathophysiology begins is not clearly defined.

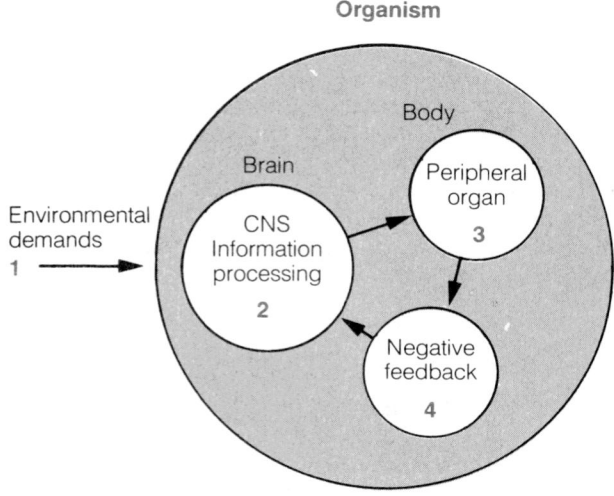

Figure 7-3. Schwartz (1977) Disregulation Model. (Adapted from Schwartz GE. Psychosomatic disorders and biofeedback: A psychobiological model of disregulation. From Psychopathology: Experimental Models by Jack D. Maser and Martin E. P. Seligman. WH Freeman and Company. Copyright © 1977.)

In this case, the door was not closed, but its cooling effect was offset by the heating action of the furnace.

Organs of Homeostasis or Adjustment. Most of the human body's control systems are integrated at the level of the brain in the nervous and endocrine systems. Control activities involve detecting deviations from the predetermined reference point and stimulating compensatory responses in the muscles and glands of the body. The major organs affected are the heart, lungs, kidneys, liver, gastrointestinal tract, and skin. When stimulated, these organs alter the rate of their activity or the amount of secretions they produce. They have been called the organs of homeostasis or adjustment.

Local Responses: Feedback Loops. In addition to the responses controlled by the above system, there are local responses that consist of small feedback loops in a group of cells or tissues. The cells detect a change in their immediate environment and initiate an action to counteract its effect. For example, the accumulation of lactic acid in an exercised muscle will stimulate dilation of blood vessels in the area to increase blood flow and improve the delivery of oxygen and removal of waste products.

The net result of the activities of the control system through feedback loops is a dynamic equilibrium, a steady state achieved by the continuous, variable action of the organs of adjustment along with continuous, small exchanges of chemical substances between cells, interstitial fluid, and blood throughout the body. For example, an increase in the carbon dioxide concentration of the extracellular fluid leads to increased pulmonary ventilation, which in turn decreases the carbon dioxide level. The increased carbon dioxide raises the hydrogen ion concentration of the blood. This is detected by chemosensitive receptors in the respiratory control center of the medulla. This stimulates an increase in the rate of discharge of the inspiratory neurons, which innervates the diaphragm and intercostal muscles and in-

creases the rate of respiration. Excess carbon dioxide is exhaled, the hydrogen ion concentration returns to normal, and the chemically sensitive neurons are no longer stimulated.

Positive Feedback. Before closing this discussion, another type of feedback, positive feedback, should be mentioned. Positive feedback perpetuates the chain of events set in motion by the original disturbance. Compensation does not occur, and the system becomes more out of balance; disorder and disintegration occur. (There are some exceptions to this, the blood clotting mechanisms in humans, for example.)

Disregulation Model

Based upon the concept of negative feedback as a regulatory process in biological control systems, Schwartz (1977) proposed a model to explain the malfunctioning of body tissues leading to disease. When the negative feedback mechanisms are disrupted, or there are excessive environmental demands, the normal adaptive functioning patterns of the body's systems fail; Schwartz called this *disregulation* and named his model the *disregulation model* (Fig. 7-3).

Emphasis is placed upon the brain as the final common pathway for coordinating and regulating bodily processes. Schwartz's model is particularly useful in explaining psychosomatic disorders in which faulty regulation contributes to physiologic malfunction.

The model has four stages, and disregulation can occur in any one or all of them.

Stage 1: Environmental Demands. The individual continually receives demands or input from the external environment. These may be social demands placed upon the organism by other people or physical input, such as changes in the temperature and atmosphere. When the external demands become excessive or unavoidable, the brain may ignore signals being sent to it from within the body: in response to pressure to meet a writing deadline, normal sleeping patterns may be ignored. The negative feedback to the brain may be expressed as headache pain arising from lack of sleep. The goal of the pain mechanism is to get the brain to "turn off." The brain is not functioning properly to meet the individual's sleeping needs. The pressure of external demands may be a factor in numerous disorders: hypertension, gastrointestinal ulcers, migraine, and others.

Stage 2: Information Processing of the Central Nervous System. The brain may have its own internal problem with regulation because of faulty genetic programming or because it has learned to respond inappropriately to stimuli. For example, if the individual in stage one met the deadline and was rewarded for that behavior, this may serve as reinforcement of his inappropriate sleep pattern and become a learned response in similar situations. Another example is that obesity may develop if an individual learns to ignore the signals from the stomach that it is full.

Stage 3: The Peripheral Organ. Even though stage one and stage two are operating appropriately, the peripheral response organ may be at fault. It may be hyporeactive or hyperreactive to the neural stimulation it receives from the brain. Schwartz relates this to the "weak organ" theory of stress. In response to stress, an organ may overreact and become dysfunctional. Thus, one person has a "bad back," another gastrointestinal complaints, and another headaches when overtaxed. That pattern of disorder or disease is likely to continue unless the brain can in some way alter the function of the faulty organ or can itself compensate for it. (The individual must recognize the cause-and-effect relationship.)

Stage 4: Negative Feedback.   In stage four, the negative feedback may be inappropriate and, as a result, the organ involved may lose a protective mechanism. A person with a genetic defect in the system for responding to pain is in danger of injuring himself, because pain sensation is deficient.

When a problem occurs at any one of the stages, it causes a domino chain reaction that affects the others; thus, if the heart rate is faulty, the whole cardiovascular system suffers. It is also possible for more than one stage of the system to be at fault at the same time.

This model is useful for explaining how biofeedback may be used to alter disease processes. Relaxation techniques have been used successfully to lower blood pressure, and control of alpha waves has been used in migraine sufferers. There are many more examples. More study is needed to determine the long-range effects of biofeedback techniques.

▷ Cellular Adaptation and Injury

Cells are complex units dynamically responding to the changing demands and stresses of daily life. They possess a maintenance function and a specialized function: the maintenance function refers to the activities the cell must perform with respect to itself; specialized functions are those that the cell performs in relation to the tissues and organs of which it is a part. Individual cells may cease to function without posing a threat to the organism; however, as the dead cells multiply, the specialized functions are altered and the individual's health is threatened.

Common Adaptations

Cells can adapt to environmental stress by structural and functional changes. A number of these adaptations are common and include hypertrophy, atrophy, hyperplasia, and metaplasia (Table 7-1).

Hypertrophy and Atrophy.   Hypertrophy and atrophy lead to changes in the size of cells and hence the size of the organs they form. Compensatory *hypertrophy* resulting in an enlarged muscle mass commonly occurs in skeletal and cardiac muscle under prolonged, increased workloads. *Atrophy* can be the consequence of a disease, but is more readily associated with aging. There is a decrease in cell and organ size that affects, principally, skeletal muscle, secondary sex organs, the heart, and the brain.

Hyperplasia.   *Hyperplasia* is an increase in the number of new cells in an organ or tissue; as cells multiply, volume increases. It is a mitotic response, but it is reversible when the stimulus is removed. This distinguishes it from neoplasia or malignant growth, which continues after the stimulus is removed. Hyperplasia may occur in response to a body loss or may be hormonally induced.

Metaplasia.   *Metaplasia* is a cell transformation in which a highly specialized cell changes to a less specialized

Table 7-1
Cellular Adaptation

	Change	Stimulus	Example
Hypertrophy	Increase in cell size, leading to increase in organ size	Increased workload	Leg muscles of runner Arm muscles of tennis player Cardiac muscle in person with hypertension
Atrophy	Shrinkage in size of cell, leading to decrease in organ size	Decrease in: 1. Use 2. Blood supply 3. Nutrition 4. Hormonal stimulation 5. Innervation	Secondary sex organs in aging person Extremity immobilized in plaster cast
Hyperplasia	Increase in number of new cells (increase in mitosis)	Hormonal influence Tissue removal or destruction	Breast changes of a girl in puberty or of a pregnant woman Regeneration of liver cells New red blood cells in blood loss
Metaplasia	Transformation of one adult cell type to another (reversible)	Stress applied to highly specialized cell	Changes in epithelial cells lining bronchi in response to smoke irritation (cells become less specialized)

cell. This serves a protective function, because the less specialized cell is more resistant to the stress that stimulated the change. In smokers, the ciliated columnar epithelium lining the bronchi is replaced by squamous epithelium. The squamous cells can survive; however, loss of the cilia and protective mucus can have damaging consequences.

Thus, the adaptations afford the survival of the organism. They reflect changes in the normal cell in response to stress. If the stress continues, the function of the adapted cell may succumb and cell injury will occur.

Injury

Injury is defined as a disorder in steady state regulation; any stressor that alters the ability of the cell or system to maintain the optimal balance of its adjustment processes will lead to injury. Structural and functional damage then occurs, which may be reversible, permitting recovery, or irreversible, leading to death. Homeostatic adjustments are concerned with the small, minute-by-minute changes within the body's systems. With adaptive changes, compensation occurs and a steady state is achieved, although it may be at new levels; with injury, steady state regulation is lost and pathophysiology ensues.

Causes of disorder and injury in the system (cell, tissue, organ, body) may arise from the external or internal environment of the system (Fig. 7-4). Causes may include the following: physical agents, chemical agents, infectious agents, immune mechanisms, genetic defects, hypoxia, and nutritional imbalance.

The most common causes are hypoxia, chemical injury, and infectious agents. An additional factor is that the presence of one injury makes the system more susceptible to another; for example, inadequate oxygenation and nutritional deficiencies make the system vulnerable to infection. These agents act at the cellular level by damaging or destroying the following:

- The integrity of the cell membrane, necessary for ionic balance
- The cell's ability to transform energy (aerobic respiration, production of adenosine triphosphate [ATP])
- The cell's ability to synthesize enzymes and other necessary proteins
- The cell's ability to grow and reproduce (genetic integrity)

Hypoxia

Inadequate cellular oxygenation, *hypoxia,* interferes with the cell's ability to transform energy. Hypoxia may be caused by a decrease in blood supply to an area; by a decrease in the oxygen-carrying capacity of the blood (decreased hemoglobin); by a ventilation–perfusion or respiratory problem, reducing the amount of oxygen available in the blood; or by a problem in the cell's enzyme system, making it unable to utilize the oxygen delivered to it. The usual cause is *ischemia,* or deficient blood supply. This is commonly seen in myocardial cell injury, in which arterial blood flow is decreased because of atherosclerosis. Intravascular clots (thrombi, emboli) interfering with blood supply are the common causes of cerebrovascular accidents. The length of time different tissues can survive without oxygen varies: brain cells may succumb in 3 to 6 minutes (sources vary). If the condition leading to hypoxia is slowly progressive, collateral circulation to the area may develop; however, this mechanism is not highly reliable.

Nutritional Imbalance

Nutritional imbalance refers to a relative or absolute deficiency or excess of one or more essential nutrients. This may be manifested as undernutrition, in which there is an inadequate consumption of food or calories, or in overnutrition, in which there is a caloric excess. Caloric excess to the point of obesity, in which the person is 20% or more above his ideal weight, overloads cells in the body with lipids. By requiring more energy to maintain the extra tissue, obesity places a strain on the body and has been associated with the production of disease, especially pulmonary and cardiovascular disease.

Specific deficiencies arise when an essential nutrient is deficient or when there is a disproportion of nutrients. Protein deficiencies and avitaminosis are examples.

An energy deficit leading to cell injury can occur when there is insufficient glucose or insufficient oxygen to transform the glucose into energy. A lack of insulin may also prevent glucose from entering the cell from the blood. This is the problem in diabetes mellitus, which represents a metabolic disorder, leading to nutritional deficiency.

Diabetes Mellitus. The exact cause of diabetes mellitus is unknown; however, in most cases, it is probably inherited. It most likely involves a combination of the causative factors of injury: genetic defect, diet, and, possibly, destruction of the insulin-producing pancreatic islet cells by a virus. In any event, when there is a lack of insulin, a series of pathophysiologic events occur (Fig. 7-5). Insulin is necessary to transport glucose into the cell. If it is absent, the food eaten is converted to glucose, and the blood sugar

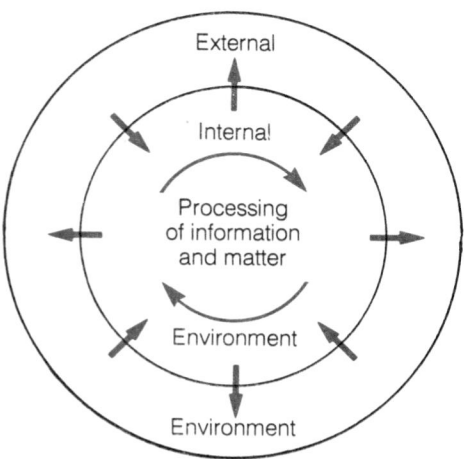

Figure 7-4. Influences leading to disorder may arise from the internal environment and the external environment of the system. Excesses or deficits of information and matter may occur or there may be faulty regulation of processing.

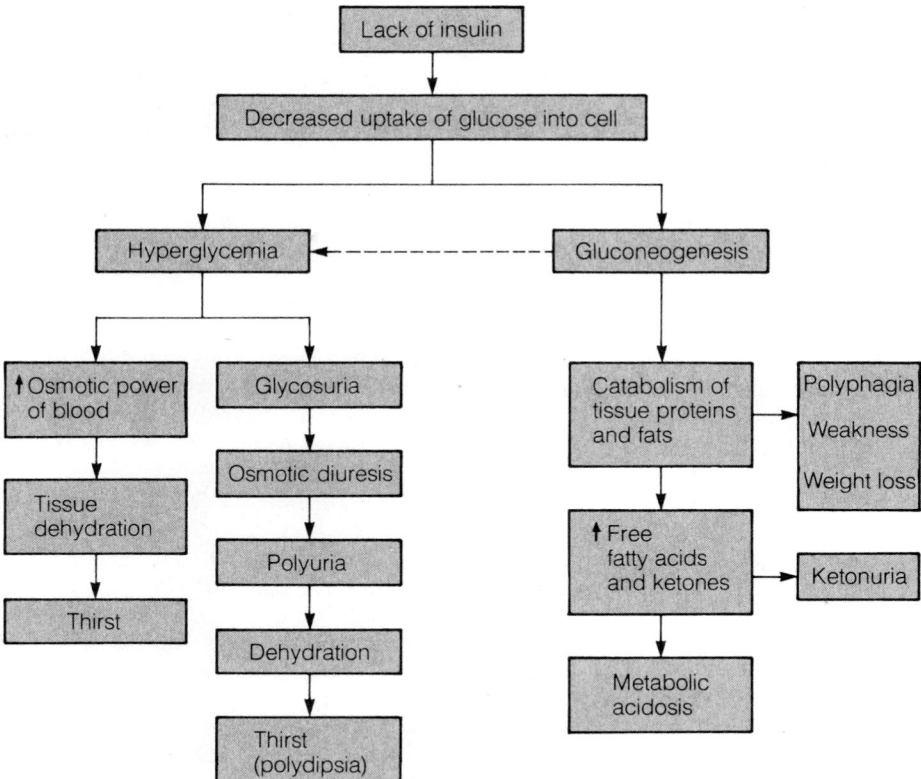

Figure 7-5. Pathophysiology of diabetes mellitus.

rises; because the glucose cannot get into the cell, the body excretes it. Because this hypertonic glucose load must be diluted, fluid is pulled into the circulation from the body. Excessive urination, which occurs to flush out the sugar, leads to excessive thirst. Because the body is literally not being fed, the satiety center sends a hunger signal. At the same time, fatigue and weakness are experienced, and eventually the body looks to its own tissue stores of proteins and fats for energy, and weight loss occurs. The major symptoms are polydipsia (excessive thirst), polyuria (excessive urination), and polyphagia (excessive hunger).

Physical Agents

Physical agents, including extremes of temperature, radiation, electrical shock, and mechanical trauma, may cause injury to the cells or the entire body. The duration of exposure and the intensity of the stressor determine the severity of damage.

Extremes of High Temperature. When temperatures are elevated, irrespective of cause, hypermetabolism occurs: the respiratory rate, heart rate, and basal metabolic rate increase. Eventually, the high temperature causes coagulation of cell proteins, and the cells die. With fever induced by infections; the hypothalamic thermostat may be reset at a higher temperature. Thus, the individual responds to external heat and cold with a new setpoint of perhaps 40° C (104° F), just as he did with the normal setpoint of 37° C (98.6° F). When the fever breaks, the thermostat returns to normal. With fever from heat stroke, the function of the thermoregulatory center breaks down, and temperature soars. It is imperative that the body be cooled rapidly or minor brain damage may occur.

The local response to thermal injury is similar. There is an increase in metabolic activity, and, as heat increases, protein is coagulated, enzyme systems are destroyed, and, in the extreme, charring or carbonization occurs. Burns of the epithelium are classified as partial-thickness burns if epithelializing elements remain to support healing; full-thickness burns lack such elements and must be grafted for healing. The amount of body surface involved determines the prognosis for the patient. If severe, the entire body system becomes involved, and hypermetabolism will develop as a pathophysiologic response.

Extremes of Low Temperature. Extremes of low temperature or cold cause vasoconstriction; blood flow becomes sluggish, and clots may form, leading to ischemic damage in the involved tissues. With still lower temperatures, ice crystals may form, and the cells may burst.

Radiation. Radiant energy may be used for diagnosis and treatment of diseases. In excessive amounts, it causes injury by its ionizing action. Electrical shock may produce burns as a result of the heat generated when electric current travels through the body. It may also stimulate nerves abnormally; for example, fibrillation of the heart may occur.

Mechanical Trauma. Mechanical trauma can result in wounds that disrupt the cells and tissues of the body. The severity of the wound, the blood loss, and the nerve damage are significant factors in the outcome.

Chemical Agents

Chemical injuries may be caused by known poisons, such as lye, which has a corrosive action on epithelial tissue, or by heavy metals, such as mercury, arsenic, and lead, each with its own specific destructive action. Many other chemicals may be toxic in certain amounts, in certain people, and in certain tissues; these include compounds of extrinsic and intrinsic origin. Too much hydrochloric acid (HCl) can damage the stomach lining; large amounts of glucose can cause osmotic shifts, affecting the fluid and electrolyte balance; and too much insulin can cause hypoglycemia and lead to coma. Drugs, including those prescribed by the physician, may cause chemical poisoning. Some individuals are less tolerant of drugs than others and manifest toxic reactions at customary dosages. Aging tends to decrease tolerance to drugs. Polypharmacy, the taking of many drugs at one time, is also associated with the aging population. It is a problem because of the unpredictable effects of the resulting drug combinations.

Alcohol (ethanol) is a chemical irritant, the consumption of which is becoming an increasing problem in society. A pattern of drinking alcohol as a social activity is a growing part of the life-style of young adults; signs of alcohol intoxication are well known. In the body, alcohol is broken down into acetaldehyde, which has a direct toxic effect on liver cells that leads to a variety of liver abnormalities, including cirrhosis in susceptible individuals. Disordered liver cell function leads to complications in other organs of the body.

Infectious Agents

Biological agents known to cause disease in man are viruses, bacteria, rickettsiae, mycoplasmas, fungi, protozoa, and nematodes. The severity of the infectious disease depends on the number of microorganisms entering the body, their virulence, and the host's defenses, such as health, age, and immune defenses. Some bacteria, such as those in tetanus and diphtheria, produce exotoxins that circulate and create cell damage; some, such as the gram-negative bacteria, produce endotoxins when they are killed; and others, such as the tubercle bacillus, induce an immune reaction. Viruses, as the smallest living organisms, survive as parasites of the living cells they invade. Viruses infect specific cells; through a complex mechanism, they replicate within the cells they invade, and then burst out to invade other cells and continue to replicate. An immune response is mounted by the body to eliminate the viruses, and the cells harboring the viruses can be injured in the process.

Typically, an inflammatory response and immune reaction are the pathophysiologic responses of the body to the presence of infection.

Immune Mechanisms

The immune system is an exceedingly complex system; its purpose is to defend the body from invasion by any foreign object or foreign cell type, such as cancerous cells. This is a steady state mechanism, but like other adjustment processes, it can become disordered, and cell injury occurs. Basically, the immune response detects foreign bodies or distinguishes nonself from self and destroys nonself entities. The entrance of an antigen (foreign body) into the body evokes the production of antibodies that attack and destroy the antigen (antigen–antibody reaction). The immune system can be hypoactive or hyperactive. When it is hypoactive, immunodeficiency diseases occur; when it is hyperactive, hypersensitivity disorders arise. In hypersensitivity disorders, the antigen reacts with the cells of immunity (lymphocytes, macrophages, neutrophils, antibodies, or complement) in such a way that "self" or normal cells are injured.

For example, in persons with seasonal allergic rhinitis owing to pollen, the individual hyperreacts to the foreign protein by producing a sensitivity (Fig. 7-6). IgE, the immunoglobulin normally produced as an antibody against such an allergen, is produced in excessive amounts. This antibody attaches to the skin surfaces of the nasal mucosa. When the foreign protein, pollen, is inhaled again, an antigen–antibody reaction occurs at the site. Histamine and other irritating chemical substances are released and cell injury occurs, as is indicated by copious secretions, edema of the mucosa, sneezing because of secretions, and local itching.

Genetic Disorders

Genetic defects as causes of disease are of intense interest as more environmental pollutants are formed and their effects on our genetic structure are studied. Over 2300 inherited traits have been described in human beings (Purtilo, 1978). Many of these produce mutations that have no recognizable effect, such as lack of a single enzyme; others contribute to more gross congenital abnormalities, such as Down's syndrome. Sickle cell disease, the hemophilias, and phenylketonuria are examples of diseases arising from genetic defects.

Cell Death

Any of the injuries discussed can lead to death of the cell. Essentially, the cell membrane becomes impaired, resulting in a nonrestricted flow of ions. Sodium and calcium enter the cell, followed by water, which leads to edema, and energy transformation ceases. Nerve impulses are no longer transmitted; muscles no longer contract. As the cells rupture, lysosomal enzymes escape that destroy tissues; cell death and necrosis occur.

Response to Injury

In response to cell injury initiated by any of the agents previously discussed, there is a local response at the site consisting of inflammation and repair. Recall that with injury the cell membrane is damaged, ionic balance is destroyed, and chemical irritants are released into the tissues. Death of some cells is also apt to occur, so that at one site, following a bee sting for example, some cells are injured and others die.

Inflammation

Three major processes are involved in inflammation:

1. Vasodilation and increased blood flow
2. Increased vascular permeability
3. Leukocytic infiltration into the injured area

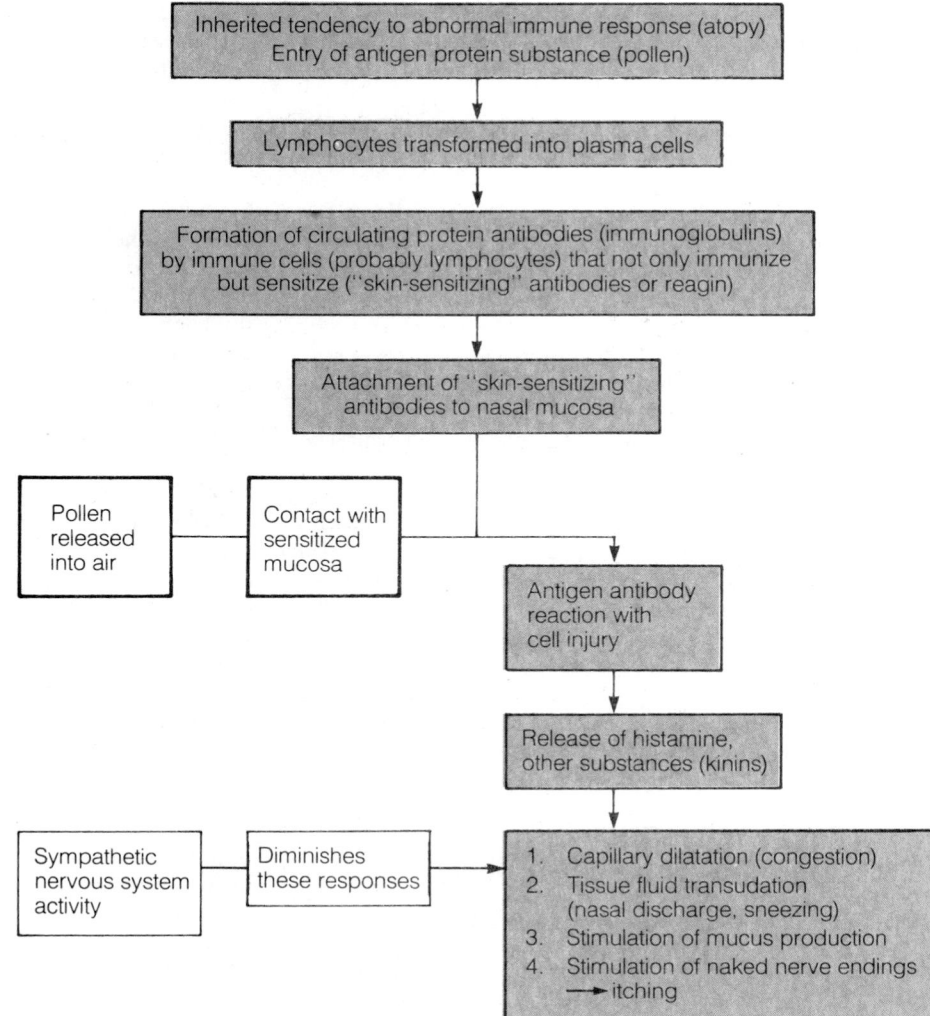

Figure 7-6. Pathophysiology of seasonal allergic rhinitis owing to pollen.

With vasodilation and increased blood flow, *redness* and *heat* develop. Subsequently, the engorgement with blood slows the flow, and fluid escapes into the surrounding tissues, producing *swelling. Pain* and *loss of function* are most likely due to the pressure of the swelling on nerve endings and possibly to the irritation of chemical substances, such as kinins, released from the injured cells.

The five cardinal signs of inflammation are redness, heat, swelling, pain, and loss of function. These appear at the site of the bee sting, for example; they also appear at the sites of a myocardial infarct and of a peptic ulcer. You may observe a miniresponse (hyperemia) by scratching your arm with your fingernail; notice how quickly the response occurs.

Acute inflammation is short-lived, 2 weeks or less, and consists mainly of hyperemic and exudative (pus formation, dead leukocytes, and debris) changes. Chronic inflammation is a sustained reaction that occurs when the offending agent or stimulus persists. In the chronic response, the exudative phase of acute inflammation has subsided, and other cell types, lymphocytes, proliferate.

The local response may be confined to the site, a mosquito bite for example, and only local signs and symptoms may appear. On the other hand, if the injury is more severe, a systemic response may also occur. Fever, increased vital signs, malaise, and leukocytosis are signs of this trend.

Repair

The reparative process begins at approximately the same time as the injury and is indeed interwoven with inflammation. Healing proceeds after the inflammatory debris is removed. Healing may be by *regeneration,* in which there is gradual repair of the defect by proliferation of cells of the same type as those destroyed. Or, it may be by *replacement* with cells of another type, usually connective tissue, resulting in scar formation.

Healing by Regeneration.   The ability of cells to regenerate depends upon whether they are labile, stable, or permanent. *Labile* cells include those that multiply constantly to replace cells worn out by normal physiologic processes; these include epithelial cells of the skin and those lining the GI tract. *Permanent* cells include neurons—the nerve cell bodies, not their axons. Destruction of a neuron is a permanent loss, but axons may regenerate. If normal activity is to return, tissue regeneration must occur in a functional pattern, especially in the growth of several axons. *Stable* cells have a latent ability to regenerate. Under normal physiologic processes, they are not shed and do not need replacement, but if they are damaged or destroyed, they are able to regenerate. These include functional cells of the kidney, liver, pancreas, and other glands of the body.

Healing by Replacement.   Healing may be by primary intention or secondary intention. In *primary intention healing,* the wound is clean and dry, and the edges are approximated, such as may occur in a surgical wound. Little scar formation occurs, and the wound is usually healed in a week. In *secondary intention healing,* the wound or defect is larger and gaping, and has more necrotic material. The wound fills from the bottom upward with granulation tissue. The process of repair takes longer and results in more scar formation with loss of specialized function. Persons who have recovered from myocardial infarcts will have abnormal ECG tracings because the electrical signal cannot be conducted through the connective tissue that replaces the defect.

As has been stated many times in this chapter, the condition of the host, the environment, and the severity of the injury affect the process and outcome, in this case, the process of inflammation and repair.

▷ A Representative Pathophysiologic Process: Hypertensive Heart Disease

Hypertensive heart disease is presented here as a representative pathophysiologic process. Unfortunately, words and figures can only dimly portray the patient's condition, moment by moment or day by day in acute illness, or week by week in chronic illness. The influence of physiologic changes, of social adjustments between patient and health care personnel or family, of unknown or expressed concern and anxiety, and of the patient's total life experience in the development and course of disease is well recognized by the health team. These variables cannot be inserted into a flow diagram—yet, they may be major factors governing the course of the disease.

Mechanisms of Blood Pressure Regulation
A brief summary of selected mechanisms for regulating blood pressure will facilitate the understanding of hypertensive heart disease. The regulation of arterial pressure involves complex nervous and hormonal controls that interrelate to affect the cardiac output and peripheral resistance. This relationship is expressed in the following equation:

Mean Arterial Pressure = Cardiac Output (CO)

$\times$ Total Peripheral Resistance (TPR)

Cardiac output is determined by the stroke volume and the heart rate. Peripheral resistance is determined by the diameter of the arterioles. If the diameter is decreased (vasoconstriction), peripheral resistance increases; if the diameter is increased (vasodilation), peripheral resistance decreases.

Primary regulation of arterial pressure is effected by the baroreceptors in the carotid sinus and aortic arch, which relay impulses to the sympathetic nervous centers in the medulla. These impulses act to inhibit the stimulation of the sympathetic nervous system. When the arterial pressure is increased, the baroreceptor endings are stretched. They fire, inhibiting the sympathetic center. This reduces the discharge of the sympathetic center, with the result that the heart rate is decreased, the arterioles dilate, and the arterial pressure returns to its former level. The reverse happens with a fall in arterial pressure. The baroreceptors control only temporary changes in blood pressure.

One other mechanism, which has a longer-term effect, will be described. Renin, produced by the kidneys when their blood flow is decreased, leads to the formation of angiotensin I, which converts to angiotensin II. Angiotensin II elevates the blood pressure by direct constriction of arterioles. It also indirectly stimulates the release of aldosterone, which leads to renal retention of sodium and water. The latter increases the extracellular fluid volume, which in turn increases the flow returned to the heart, thereby raising the stroke volume and cardiac output. The kidneys also have an intrinsic mechanism to increase sodium and water retention.

When a *persistent* disturbance occurs that causes arteriolar constriction, total peripheral resistance is increased and the mean arterial pressure rises. In the face of the persistent disturbance, cardiac output must increase to maintain balance in the system (see equation). This is necessary in order to overcome the peripheral resistance, so that delivery of oxygen and nutrients to the cells and removal of cellular waste products will be maintained. To increase the cardiac output, the sympathetic nervous system stimulates the heart to beat faster; it also increases the stroke volume by causing a selective vasoconstriction in peripheral organs that returns more blood to the heart. With chronic hypertension, the baroreceptors are reset at a higher level, and they respond as though the new level were normal.

Initially, this mechanism is compensatory. This adaptive mechanism, however, exacts a toll by creating an increased workload for the heart. At the same time, degenerative changes take place in the arterioles that are subjected to continuous high pressure. These changes occur in organs throughout the body, including the heart, which may contribute to a depleted blood supply in the myocardium. To eject blood, the heart must exert enough force to overcome the pressure reflected back to the aortic inlet. In response to this workload, the muscle of the left ventricle hypertrophies. Eventually, it dilates, and the heart becomes enlarged. These two structural changes are adaptive; they improve the stroke volume delivered by the heart. At rest, these compensatory mechanisms may be effective, but on exertion, the heart cannot meet the demands of the body; the patient is easily fatigued and becomes short of breath.

The point at which compensation ends and injury and failure begin is not continuous or discrete. With the increased demands, there are changes in the distribution of blood flow that result in a reduced flow to the kidneys. This stimulates the renin angiotensin–aldosterone mechanism. This mechanism, once compensatory, now aggravates the failing heart by increasing the extracellular fluid volume and the peripheral resistance. The heart becomes engorged with blood that it cannot pump out, and left ventricular heart failure occurs. Failure of the left ventricle has both forward and backward effects. The forward effects are due to low output, which decreases the perfusion of tissues of the body. The decreased perfusion activates sodium and water retention mechanisms in the kidneys and glands, giving positive feedback to the failing heart. The backward effects are due to the decreased emptying of the left ventricle, which raises the end-diastolic pressure. This rise in pressure is reflected back into the left atrium and the pulmonary veins, and congestion occurs in the pulmonary capillaries. Gas exchange is disrupted, and fluid exudes from the capillaries into the alveolar spaces, leading to pulmonary edema. Crackles (rales) will be heard when the lungs are auscultated; severe dyspnea and orthopnea will be present; coughing will occur; and, with pulmonary edema, pink, frothy sputum may be present. Eventually, this backward progression will affect the right heart and lead to right heart failure accompanied by congestion in the veins and organs drained by the venae cavae. The system is in total failure and death is imminent.

The initial disturbance that caused the increased peripheral resistance may be unknown, as is the case in primary or essential hypertension, although a number of agents have been postulated as being contributory. The pathologic mechanism was hypoxia owing to failure of the blood transportation system. In the latter stages, oxygen saturation of the blood was also decreased by the pulmonary edema.

▷ Nursing Implications

In the assessment of the patient who seeks health care, objective signs will be the primary indicators of the physiologic processes that are occurring. Are the heart rate, respiratory rate, and temperature normal? If not, is any change only a temporary one? Are there other indicators of steady state deviation present? What is the blood pressure, height, and weight? Are there any problems in movement or sensation? Does the patient demonstrate any problems in orientation or memory? Are there obvious lesions or deformities present? Further signs of internal processes are indicated in laboratory data, including electrolytes, blood urea nitrogen [BUN], blood sugar, and urinalysis. In making a nursing diagnosis, it is necessary to coordinate the symptoms or complaints expressed by the patient with the physical signs present.

Other chapters of this book will address specific problems and their nursing treatment in greater depth. It has been reiterated many times in this chapter that the state of the host and the environment are two of the three predictors of the health outcome in all situations. These two are directly related to the health patterns of the individual. The nurse has a significant role and responsibility in identifying the health patterns of the individual treated. If those patterns are not achieving balance for the individual physiologically, psychologically, and socially, the nurse is obligated—with the assistance and agreement of the patient—to seek ways to achieve balance. This chapter is physiologically oriented; in that context, the nutritional–metabolic pattern, elimination pattern, activity-exercise pattern, and sleep–rest pattern would be specifically analyzed. However, the way one copes with stress, the way one relates to others, and the values and goals held are interwoven in those "physiologic" patterns. Who you eat with, when you eat, and how much money you have for food are directly related to what you eat and how much. The point is: to evaluate the individual's health patterns and to intervene if a problem exists requires a total assessment of the individual; man functions as a whole.

▷ Bibliography

Books

Anderson WAD, Kissane JM. Pathology (2 vols). St Louis, CV Mosby, 1977.

Boyd W and Sheldon H. Introduction to the Study of Disease. Philadelphia, Lea & Febiger, 1980.

Dorland's Illustrated Medical Dictionary, 26th edition. Philadelphia, WB Saunders Co, 1981.

Freis ED. The Modern Management of Hypertension. Washington, D.C., Veterans Administration, U.S. Government Printing Office, 1973.

Groer ME and Shekleton ME. Basic Pathophysiology, A Conceptual Approach. St Louis, CV Mosby, 1979.

Guyton AC. Medical Physiology. Philadelphia, WB Saunders, 1981.

Miller J. Living Systems. New York, McGraw–Hill, 1980.

Petersdorf RG (ed). Harrison's Principles of Internal Medicine, 10th ed. New York, McGraw–Hill, 1983.

Price SA and Wilson LM. Pathophysiology, Clinical Concepts of Disease Processes, 2nd ed. New York, McGraw–Hill, 1982.

Purtilo DT. A Survey of Human Diseases. Menlo Park, California, Addison–Wesley, 1978.

Robbins SL, Angell M, and Kumar V. Basic Pathology. Philadelphia, WB Saunders, 1981.

Robbins SL and Cotran RS. Pathologic Basis of Disease. Philadelphia, WB Saunders, 1979.

Schottelius BA and Schottelius DD. Textbook of Physiology. St Louis, CV Mosby, 1978.

Vander AJ, Sherman JH, and Luciano DS. Human Physiology, The Mechanisms of Body Function. New York, McGraw–Hill, 1975.

Articles

Hoskins L. The need for nutrition. In Yura H and Walsh M (eds). Human Needs and the Nursing Process. New York, Appleton-Century-Crofts, 1978.

Kilcoyne MM. The developing phase of primary hypertension. Mod Concepts Cardiovas Dis 1980 Apr; 49(4):19–24.

Schwartz GE. Psychosomatic disorders and biofeedback: A psychobiological model of disregulation. In Maser JD and Seligman MEP (eds). Psychopathology: Experimental Models. San Francisco, Freeman, 1977.

Zelis R and Flaim SF. The circulations in congestive heart failure. Mod Concepts Cardiovas Dis 1982 Feb; 51(2):79–84.

8

Stress and Adaptation

Stress is a term that is difficult to define: it is used loosely and means different things to different people. Some use it to describe an *upset feeling* or response; others use it to describe the *source* or *stimulus* for their feeling upset. It has caused enough semantic problems to prompt one investigator to recommend doing away with the term (Mason, 1975). Hans Selye (1976), sometimes called the "father of stress," first stated that "stress is essentially the rate of wear and tear in the body." He later modified that to define stress as the "state manifested by a specific syndrome which consists of all the nonspecifically-induced changes within a biologic system." Selye is an endocrinologist who has made the study of stress his life's work. George Engel (1960), studying psychosomatic illness, defined psychological stress as referring

> to all processes, whether originating in the external environment or within the person, which impose a demand or requirement upon the organism, the resolution or handling of which necessitates work or activity of the mental apparatus before any other system is involved or activated.*

Study in the field of stress and adaptation has been pursued by researchers in different disciplines, according to their individual conceptual views. It can be generalized that studies in physiology have been primarily concerned with the adaptive reactions of the individual to stress, while psychology has been more concerned with the predisposing factors and the precipitating agents to stress. Sociology has investigated the issues of stress and adaptation from the standpoint of families and groups, and the manner in which families and groups influence the individual in stress.

With this background, a number of nurse researchers have proposed models that seek to unify some of the diverse approaches and to study stress and adaptation in man within

* Engel G. Health and disease. Perspectives in Biology 1960 Summer; 3(4):459–485.

a holistic framework (Sutterley & Donnelly, 1982). (A model is a way of organizing reality, what we have seen and experienced, to try to explain relationships and to predict what will occur in similar situations in the future.) A number of nurse theorists have also proposed models for nursing based on the broad theory of adaptation (Roy, 1976; Neuman, 1974; Rogers, 1970).

Holism. The use of a holistic framework grew from the view that the body, mind, and spirit of man are an integral unit. An individual's characteristic behavior patterns reflect this unity. Thus, we can assess the particular behavior patterns of an individual, but we must realize that they reflect the whole person, not just a part. This is a basic concept in nursing.

Historically speaking, the move to holistic health care is recent, having received its impetus in this century largely from investigations in psychosomatic medicine. From ancient times, the mind, body, and spirit were considered separate entities; physicians or "bleeders" and "bile examiners" treated the body; the mind was treated by magicians and occult scientists, and the clergy tended the spirit. It was attractive to attribute disease to a single cause, which, it was thought, could be eradicated. The interrelation of the multitude of factors producing the necessary and sufficient conditions for illness to develop was not a prime consideration. Studies in psychosomatic illness reveal the interaction between mind and body in all aspects of health and illness. Increasingly, it is being realized that emotional stress may contribute to physiologic illness and that physiologic illness contributes to psychologic stress. Indeed, as one experiences joy or sadness, physiologic changes occur as part of that same event.

This chapter describes the process of stress, the adaptive responses to stress, some of the maladaptive outcomes, and the nursing implications associated with the process. The focus is on the individual. To provide a background, some definitions, descriptions, and assumptions are necessary.

▷ Stress and Adaptation Defined

Stress

Stress is a state produced by a change in the environment that is perceived as challenging, threatening, or damaging to the individual's dynamic equilibrium. There is an actual or perceived imbalance in the individual's capability to meet the demands of the new situation. The change or stimulus that evokes this state is the *stressor.* The nature of the stressor is variable: an event or change that will produce stress in one individual will be neutral for another, and an event that may produce stress at one time and place for one individual may not do so for the same individual at another time and place.

Stress is mediated by two factors: the individual's ability to cope and the social support he receives. The desired goal is adaptation or adjustment to the change, so that the individual is again in equilibrium and has the energy and ability to meet new external demands.

Adaptation

Adaptation is a constant, ongoing process that occurs along the time continuum, beginning with birth and ending with death. Also existing along this lifetime continuum is the dimension of health and illness. Health and illness are relative concepts. As the individual traverses the life continuum, he encounters stressors that challenge his ability to meet his needs and maintain equilibrium; successful positive adaptation to these stressors represents health; illness is an unsuccessful or maladaptive outcome. According to Dubos (1965), "Health in the case of human beings means more than a state in which the organism has become physically suited to the surrounding physiochemical conditions through passive mechanisms; it demands that the personality be able to express itself creatively." Dubos described human life as the interplay of three classes of determinants: the universal characteristics of man's nature, "which are inscribed in his flesh and bone"; the conditions of any given situation; and man's ability to make choices and control his own actions.

Because both stress and adaptation may exist at different levels, it is possible to study them at cell, tissue, and organ levels; the biologist's study is mainly concerned with subcellular components or with subsystems of the total body. Stress and adaptation may also be studied in individuals, families, groups, and societies; thus, the sociologist speaks of the adaptation of groups, in the sense that their organization is modified to meet the requirements of the social and physical environment in which they exist. Adaptation is a continuous process of seeking harmony in an environment. The desired end goals of adaptation for any system are growth and reproduction. A major nursing objective is to support and promote the efforts of the individual to achieve a healthy adaptation.

▷ Stressors: The Sources of Stress

All individuals operate at a certain level that may be considered their adaptation level. A certain amount of change is encountered regularly: it is expected, it contributes to growth, and it enhances life. This healthy state can be upset by a number of stressors. This leads to imbalance in the physiologic or psychological state of the individual, resulting in responses that, if prolonged or severe, may lead to illness.

Physiologic Stressors. Sources of stress may be broadly categorized into physiologic stressors and psychosocial stressors. The following agents, catalogued by Robbins and Angell (1976), may be considered as primarily physiologic stressors: chemical agents (drugs, poisons, alcohol), physical agents (heat, cold, radiation, electrical shock, trauma), infectious agents (viruses, bacteria, fungi), faulty immune mechanisms, genetic disorders, nutritional imbalance, and hypoxia. All stressors have both a general effect and a specific effect. The specific effect of these agents and the pathophysiology they incur are the subjects of another chapter; therefore, they will not be described further here. The general effect is the subject of the stress response in this chapter.

Psychosocial Stressors. The list of sources of psychosocial stress is extensive, including much of what might be considered "routine wear and tear." Antonovsky (1979) has described 11 categories of such stressors, which are summarized as follows:

1. *Accidents and the survivors:* The victim, the person responsible for the accident, and the injured persons' loved ones have all encountered a threat, although different in nature.
2. *The experiences of others in our social networks:* We exist in a relationship to others, and whatever happens to them affects us.
3. *Horrors of history:* Auschwitz, Vietnam, Hiroshima.
4. *Intrapsychic, unconscious conflicts and anxieties:* These include the biological drives, such as hunger, thirst, and sex, and also the forces described by Freud.
5. *The fear of aggression, mutilation, and destruction:* The very nature of the need for survival places us in competition for power and a place in society, which arouses an element of fear in us.
6. *The events of history brought into our living room:* Through its dramatizations and live coverage of historical events, the mass media propels the individual and his imagination across time and distance. Unknown events, such as war, starvation, rape, and robbery, become clear and present threats.
7. *The changes of the narrower world in which we live:* The concern here is not only with change, but with the rapidity of change, which Toffler related to in *Future Shock;* this includes demographic, economic, and technological changes.
8. *Phase-specific psychosocial crises:* These include the crises that have been described by Erikson as inherently occurring in the life cycle stages of the human experience.
9. *Other normative life crises—role entries and exits, inadequate socialization, underload and overload:* This category includes all the events that occur as the individual encounters new social roles; as such, it is very broad and incorporates events that have been catalogued by other investigators in life change scales, which will be described later. When the individual moves from one role to another, he will most likely encounter a threat in the form of being inadequately socialized for the change. The concept of overload is commonly accepted as a stressor; however, underload has also been demonstrated to be a stressor.
10. *The inherent conflicts in all social relations:* Antonovsky called these "the internal conflicts of everyday existence that are anchored in the social and cultural organization of every society."
11. *The gap between culturally inculcated goals and socially structured means:* All societies have this potential stressor, a goals–means gap; only a few possess both the means and the wisdom to reach the goal (Antonovsky, 1979).

Life Events and Stress. Relating life events to illness is traced to Adolph Meyer, who in the 1930s used "life charts" of his patients from which he observed a linkage between illnesses and critical life events. Harold Wolff, following this line of research, concluded that people under constant stress had a high incidence of psychosomatic disease. More recently, Holmes and Rahe have developed life events scales that assign numerical values to typical life events. By checking off the number of recent events and deriving a total score, the likelihood of illness can be predicted. The items reflect events that require a change in the individual's life pattern: the variable of change is important because it requires adjustment. Because of methodological problems in the first scale, the Schedule of Recent Events (SRE), it was modified and titled the Recent Life Changes Questionnaire (RLCQ) (Tausig, 1982). The RLCQ contains 118 items that reflect death, birth, marriage, divorce, promotions, demotions, serious arguments, vacations, etc. The events listed include both desirable and undesirable happenings.

The life events studies have attempted to identify the nature of stressful events and assign a normative value to them. From a review of this research, Dohrenwend and Dohrenwend (1980) identified three characteristics that they concluded were most frequently associated with labeling an event stressful: (1) changes in the life pattern or activities of the individual, for better or for worse, (2) undesirability, and (3) upsettingness. This does not rule out other characteristics that may contribute to stress.

The question has been asked: From the standpoint of etiology, which are the more significant—psychosocial stressors or physiologic stressors? In response, Rahe (1975) compared their relative contribution in the manner of "two sliding scales on a slide rule." In some illnesses, such as botulism, the toxin is so powerful that the physical factors scale would be at its upper magnitude in causation and the psychological factors scale would be zero. In illnesses such as low back pain and headache, the converse would be indicated, and psychological factors would have the greater magnitude. Most illnesses fall between these extreme examples, with "substantial etiological input coming from both psychological and physical factors."

Summary. Stressors create a change in the individual's equilibrium. Each individual has a range of adaptability; changes occurring within this range are demands falling within his existing capability. Changes falling outside this range lead to disequilibrium and require readjustment; such readjustment may lead to a new adaptation level, increasing the individual's repertoire of adaptive responses. The stress precipitated will depend on the number of life events or changes occurring simultaneously, the magnitude of the changes, and the quality of the changes. The quality of change will be influenced by the degree of control the individual can exert over what is happening, and whether or not this is a scheduled or expected event.

The sources of stress as described may be discrete events, or they may be the presence of relatively continuous problems. Pearlin and associates (1981) have presented an explanation for how these two major sources of stress, eventful experiences and chronic strain,* operate to pro-

---

* The term *strain* is used by Pearlin to designate "enduring [stressful] problems."

duce stress. This is done in two ways. A seemingly unimportant event may occur that triggers a reaction; the event "functions to bring into focus the unfavorable implications of life problems, and it is the new meaning of old problems that creates distress." In the second way, life events and life strains come together and create new strains or intensify preexisting strains that then evoke stress.

In addition to life events and life strains, there is another step in the etiology of stress that involves the self-concept, particularly mastery and self-esteem (Pearlin et al., 1981). Mastery is concerned with the sense of control an individual has over his own life, and self-esteem refers to a sense of self-worth. When noxious strains persist, unaltered by the individual's efforts, and control is threatened or lost, the self-concept becomes vulnerable. The combination of life events, persistent life strains, and the diminished self-concept leads to stress.

▷ Mediating Resources: Coping and Social Support

The resources commonly used to mediate or intervene in the stress process are of two types: coping and social support. Both resources are used to reduce, avoid, or eliminate stress and the conditions that produce stress. It is important to understand that intervention can occur at several points: prior to the occurrence of a stressful event, after the stressful event but prior to its creating full-blown stress, and during the stress situation itself. In the latter instance, intervention will be most successful if used prior to the individual's loss of self-concept and subsequent defeat. Specific nursing implications are suggested here; education to promote healthy behaviors to avoid stress and the use of stress management techniques to control stress are expanded later in the chapter. It should be repeated that not all stress is bad; some stress is necessary for growth of adaptive functioning. Selye calls this "good stress" *eustress,* and "bad stress," *distress.*

Coping

Much of the research dealing with coping has been reported by psychologists interested in cognitive processes. The work of Lazarus is prominent in this area. Lazarus identifies stress as a transactive process in which the person and the environment are continually relating to each other, back and forth, each being affected by the other in turn (Folkman and Lazarus, 1980). Thus, the event and the person's reaction to it are continually being altered through two processes that he identified as appraisal and coping.

Appraisal. Appraisal is "the cognitive process through which an event is evaluated with respect to what is at stake (primary appraisal) and what coping resources and options are available (secondary appraisal)." During primary appraisal, the situation may be identified as either nonstressful or stressful. Stressful situations are those in which harm or loss has occurred, those that are threatening in that harm or loss is anticipated, and those that are challenging, in which some opportunity or gain is anticipated. The degree of stress is determined by a comparison of what is at stake

and what the person has to cope with it. Lazarus defined coping as "the cognitive and behavioral efforts made to master, tolerate, or reduce external and internal demands and conflicts among them."

Pattern of Coping. Pearlin and associates (1981) stated that, specifically, such efforts will include strategies to modify the situation that gives rise to stress, to modify the meaning inherent in a situation so that threat is reduced, and to manage the symptoms of stress. Reaction to different stressors under different circumstances will vary; however, over time, an individual will develop a typical pattern of coping behavior. This pattern will be influenced by the individual's personal, cultural, and historical background. Coping is effective if the individual maintains psychological balance without excessive or prolonged neuroendocrine stimulation.

Social Support

There is a considerable body of evidence that indicates that social support is an effective moderator of life stress (Henry & Stephens, 1977). Cobb (1976) defined social support as information belonging to one or more of three classes. The first class of information leads the subject to believe that he is cared for and loved. This appears most often in a relationship between two people in which mutual trust and attachment are expressed by helping one another meet their needs. Such expressions, sometimes called *emotional support,* are most commonly thought of in the marital relationship, but also occur between a nurse and patient.

The second class of information leads the subject to believe that he is esteemed and valued. This is most effective when it is announced in public and thus demonstrates the favorable position the individual has in the group. It elevates his sense of self-worth; this is called *esteem support.*

The third class of information leads the subject to believe that he belongs to a network of communication and mutual obligation. That is, there is information shared by the members of the network, they all know what it is, and they are all aware that it is shared. This information is of two types. One is communications, which are "the essence of history"—what is going on, who is affected, etc. Another communication in this category is the knowledge that goods and services are available to the members upon demand; for example, an individual can call upon a close friend in an emergency. Cobb emphasizes that social support encourages independent behavior; it does not lead to dependency.

Social support begins in utero; it is fostered through maternal and paternal attachment behavior, and develops through family, peer, and community relationships as the individual grows. A number of sociological and family theories attest to the production of stress and illness when the family structure is disrupted so that there is no stable hierarchy or authority, territorial limits are not well defined, and strong attachment behavior is lacking.

Social Support and Coping

Social support facilitates the coping behaviors of the individual; however, this is conditional on the nature of the social support (Pearlin et al., 1981). Individuals can have extensive relationships and interact frequently, but the necessary support only comes when there is a deeper "level of involvement and concern, not when they merely touch at the surface of each other's lives." The critical qualities within the network are the exchange of intimate communications and the presence of solidarity and trust.

Evidence of the effect of social support was demonstrated in a study by Nuckolls and associates (1972). In a study of pregnant women, they found the rate of complications to be significantly greater in a group of women with a high life change score and low social support compared to a similar group who received high social support. The group with high support had 33% complications, and the group with low support had 91% complications. Norbeck and associates (1981), recognizing the value of social support theory to nursing, have developed a questionnaire to identify the social support systems used by patients.

▷ Manifestations of Stress

To recapitulate, the individual encounters changes in the environment daily; these may be physiologic, psychological, or social in nature. The individual appraises these changes; if they fall within a range for which he possesses the resources to cope, and the demand is not too great (for example, homeostatic changes), they are *perceived* as nonstressors, slight adjustments are made, and the individual remains in equilibrium. If the individual does not possess the resources to cope with the stressors, or the stakes are great, his equilibrium will be disturbed, and a state of stress will exist. The degree of stress produced will depend on the nature, intensity, and duration of the stressor. In turn, the nature of the responses activated will depend on the degree of stress (mild to severe).

Stress Response

Perception of the stressor is coordinated by structures of the brain and may be a conscious or unconscious process. Initially, following perception, there is a global response, a generalized state of anxiety involving psychoneuroendocrine activation. A more specific response develops as the person has more time to appraise the stressor and the resources available to cope with it. Anxiety will change from a diffuse reaction to a specific emotion: joy–sadness, fear–anger, acceptance–distrust, surprise–anticipation; the endocrine responses will become more specific. In all, there will be a more defined pattern of emotional and physiologic responses. Perception and response are intertwined and occur simultaneously; they cannot be singled out, except for the purposes of discussion as presented here. The stress response has both physiologic and emotional components, and manifestations of these are demonstrated in the individual's observable behavior and his self-reports. As the individual copes with the situation, appraisal will continually occur; coping and appraisal become a circular activity providing feedback to the perception of the situation. If the individual is successful in this activity, adaptation will occur; if unsuccessful, a pattern of maladaptive responses to specific situations may develop, or one of the so-called diseases of adaptation may occur. This is also a period when the individual is particularly vulnerable to other stressors. The sequence of processes described are diagrammed in Figure 8-1.

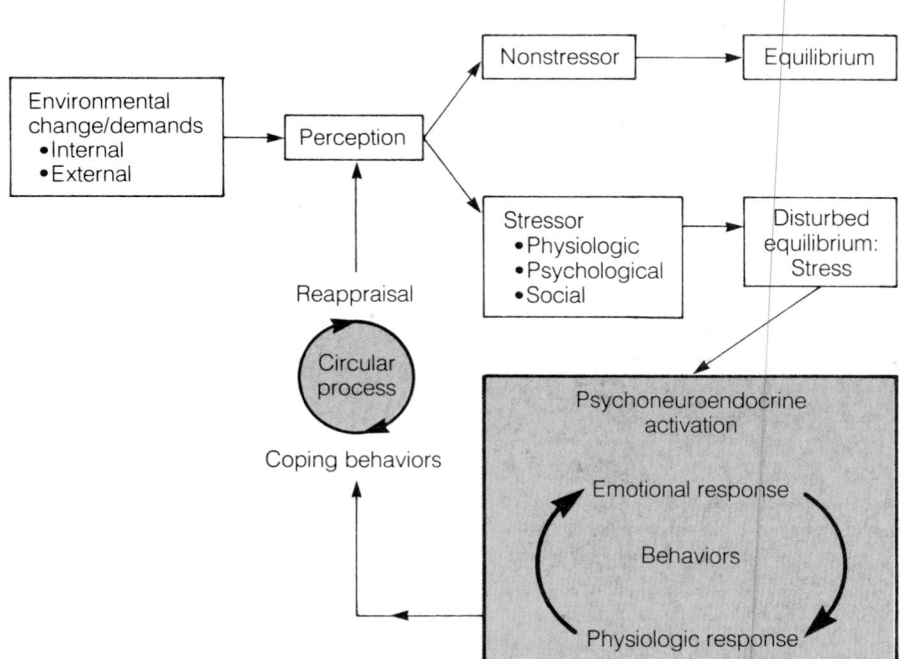

Figure 8-1. The stress process. When an environmental change is perceived by the brain as stressful, psychoneuroendocrine activation occurs, which elicits emotional and physiologic responses in the individual. These are manifested in objective and subjective behaviors. As the individual copes, using his own resources and social supports, reappraisal will recur again and again, providing feedback to the perception of the situation.

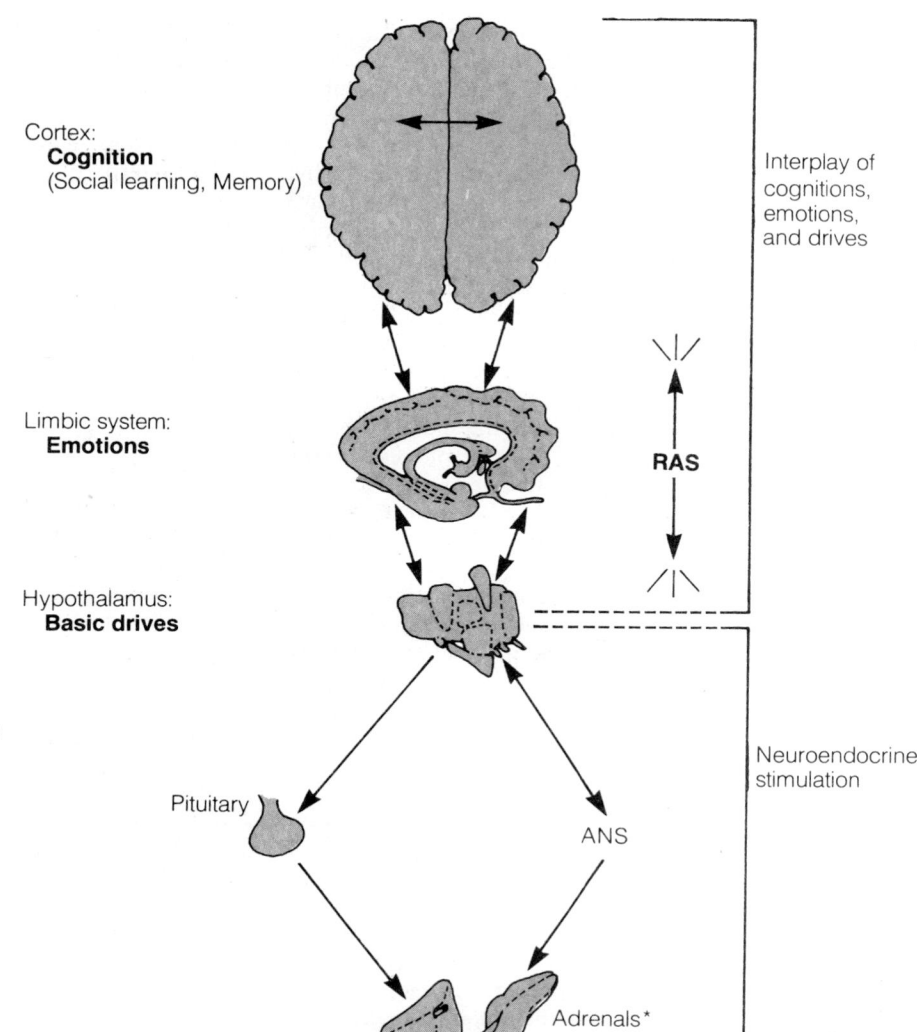

Cortex:
Cognition
(Social learning, Memory)

Limbic system:
Emotions

Hypothalamus:
Basic drives

Interplay of
cognitions,
emotions,
and drives

RAS

Neuroendocrine
stimulation

Pituitary

ANS

Adrenals*

Figure 8-2. In the process of appraisal of environmental change, different levels of the brain are involved. The highest level, the cortex, has evolved more than the other two levels and can exert control over emotional states and basic drives. The lower half of the diagram depicts the response, neuroendocrine stimulation (hypothalamus controls pituitary, autonomic nervous system [ANS]).

* Other glands are also affected by pituitary hormones; however, the adrenal glands play a greater role in stress.

Perception of Stress: Mind–Body Reaction

Psychosocial research has been concerned with the input side of stress: What kinds of life events are stressful, and what resources does the individual have for coping with the stress situation? Physiologic research has dealt with the output side: What neurophysiologic responses occur in stress? How do the two get together? This is not known, but it is speculated that it is the emotional arousal or psychological impact of noxious or stressful agents that leads to the neuroendocrine responses (Mikhail, 1981). In 1831, James Johnson, a London physician, recognized a relationship between the mind and body when he stated:

> A sudden gust of passion, a transient sense of fear, an unexpected piece of intelligence—in short, any strong emotion of mind, will cause the heart to palpitate, the muscles to tremble, the digestive organs to suspend their functions, and the blood to rush in vague and irregular currents through the living machine.*

* Tanner O. Stress, p 10. New York, Time–Life Books, 1976.

The perception of stress involves taking in a sensation and giving meaning to it; cognition implies thinking about it. The perception and cognition of stress are organized in the brain; mind and body are one—emotions have physiologic sequelae, and physiologic illnesses arouse emotions. Restak (1979) compares the brain to "an international casino visited by people from all over the world. Each person comes to the casino with his own currency. In order to gamble, he must change it into the currency of the casino." In similar fashion, all internal and external stimuli coming into the brain must be converted into electrochemical impulses that are the "currency of the brain." Different stimuli are registered in different areas of the brain in different patterns, and the brain interprets these patterns and responds to them. In this way, it controls and regulates the activities of the body.

Interpretation of Stimuli by the Brain

Figure 8-2 presents a model to explain the functional organization of the brain for the interpretation of stimuli. This may be considered a communication and control hierarchy for the pituitary–adrenal system. There are three functional levels: interpretation of basic drive or need states occurs at the lowest level; emotions are interpreted at the intermediate level and cognitions at the highest level.

The hypothalamus sits in the center, surrounded by the limbic system and the cerebral hemispheres. It integrates autonomic mechanisms that maintain the chemical constancy of the internal environment of the body. With the limbic system, the hypothalamus also regulates emotional and instinctual behavior. The hypothalamus is made up of a number of nuclei, and the limbic system contains the amygdala, hippocampus, and septal nuclei, along with other structures. Research supports the concept that these structures each respond differently to stimuli, and each has its characteristic response. The cerebral hemispheres are concerned with cognitive functions: thought processes, learning, and memory. The limbic system has connections with both the cerebral hemispheres and the brainstem. In addition, the reticular formation, which is a network of cells that forms a two-way communication system, extends from the brainstem into the midbrain and limbic system. This network controls the alert or "waking" state of the body; it sends signals that are relayed up to the cortex and relays signals from the cortex downward. Its signals are capable of modifying ongoing input and processing.

Appraisal of Environmental Change

In the process of appraising environmental change to determine the presence of a stressor, cognition, emotion, and drive states interact. Emotions are complex and are described as having both mental and physical components: there is the feeling itself, or affect; there is an awareness of the feeling and possibly its cause, or cognition; there is an urge to take action; and there are physical changes (Ganong, 1979). The cognitive appraisal of the potential stressor contributes to the type of emotional response and its intensity.

Whatever the outcome of the primary appraisal, the response is integrated in the hypothalamus. Either there is no stressor and the hypothalamus continues to maintain a steady state, or there is a stressor and the hypothalamus activates the sympathetic and pituitary adrenal responses.

Evolutionary Theory of Emotion

The adaptation of man has involved the evolution of the brain. This evolution provides a theoretical basis for the development of emotions, and explains the interplay of emotions, thoughts, and behavior (McLean, 1976; Plutchik, 1980). McLean describes a triune brain (Restak, 1979). He calls the oldest and deepest structure of the brain the R-complex and equates this to the reptilian brain, which contains unlearned, preprogrammed sets of behavior. The R-complex behaviors vary for different species. The next layer of structures, the limbic system, is more highly evolved. The addition of this system to the brain of lower animals introduced the emotions of fear and rage, pleasure and pain, and provided some motivation and simple learning to their behavior. Surrounding both of these structures, and still more highly evolved, is the neocortex of humans. This adds cognitive capability and makes learning and memory pos-

sible. Each layer of the brain increases control and adaptability. Generally, thoughts, emotions, and behavior are in harmony; however, they can get out of order and be misinterpreted consciously or unconsciously. For example, you might experience a situation, and each layer of the brain might interpret it differently, resulting in a discrepancy between your feelings and what you say or think or do; your thoughts and feelings may not even relate to the reality of what is occurring around you.

> So programmed are humans by their evolutionary inheritance that extreme fear may lead to a sudden case of diarrhea—according to some scientists, a weight-lightening advantage for a deer or baboon outrunning a leopard, but hardly a convenience for an after-dinner speaker approaching the rostrum or a football player about to take the field.*

Neuroendocrine Response

Two general stereotyped responses to stress are activated— the sympathetic–adrenal medullary response and the pituitary–adrenal cortical response. The first is a neural response, the second a hormonal response; the first acts more rapidly and is shorter-lived than the second. Both are monitored by the hypothalamus. However, certain types of stress can stimulate the sympathetic nervous system (SNS) without the participation of the hypothalamus; for example, in sudden, severe hypotension, the cardiovascular centers of the medulla would integrate the initial response.

Sympathetic–Adrenal Medullary Response: "Fight or Flight."   In emergency situations, the SNS discharges as a unit (Ganong, 1979), releasing norepinephrine at its nerve endings, which are in direct contact with the organs they stimulate. The effect of this discharge prepares the individual to cope with the emergency. This response was first described by Walter B. Cannon, who called it the "fight-or-flight" response, a survival mechanism for our ancestors. Mental activity is increased, and there is a general state of arousal. The heart rate is increased, and blood pressure is raised through vasoconstriction of peripheral circulation: both result in better perfusion of vital organs. Blood glucose is increased and supplies more available energy. The pupils are dilated, and mental activity is excited. Blood vessels of the skin are constricted, to limit bleeding in the event of trauma. Subjectively, the individual is likely to experience cold feet, clammy skin and hands, chills, palpitation, and a knot in the stomach. Typically, the individual appears tense, with the muscles of the neck, upper back, and shoulders tightened; respirations may be rapid and shallow, with the diaphragm tense.

In addition to its direct effect, the SNS stimulates the medulla of the adrenal gland to release epinephrine and norepinephrine into the bloodstream. Their action is similar to that of the SNS and has the effect of sustaining and prolonging those actions. Epinephrine and norepinephrine together also stimulate the nervous system and produce metabolic effects that increase the blood sugar and stimulate

* Tanner O. Stress, p 121. New York, Time–Life Books, 1976.

the metabolic rate (Ganong, 1979). Table 8-1 summarizes the effects of the sympathoadrenal response.

Pituitary–Adrenal Cortical Response. The pituitary–adrenal cortical response is activated by releasing factors secreted by various cells of the hypothalamus. The factor of greatest significance in stress is corticotropin-releasing factor (CRF), which stimulates the pituitary to release adrenocorticotrophic hormone (ACTH). ACTH subsequently stimulates the cortex of the adrenal glands to produce corticoids, mainly glucocorticoids, such as cortisol. ACTH also stimulates the production of mineralocorticoids, such as aldosterone; however, the production of aldosterone is accomplished primarily by the kidney's renin–angiotensin system (RAS). Cortisol stimulates gluconeogenesis, which raises the blood glucose level, making energy available for all the cells of the body. The glucocorticoids also inhibit the inflammatory response to tissue injury and suppress the immune response. These latter effects can be both beneficial and harmful. For example, in the presence of a bacterial infection, glucocorticoids reduce the fever, and the signs and symptoms will disappear; however, the bacteria is unaffected and spreads throughout the body. In suppressing the immune response, glucocorticoids prevent the release of histamine. Therefore, they are of value in relieving the symptoms of allergic reactions, such as swelling, sneezing, itching, and the symptoms of other diseases in which immunity plays a role. The pituitary–adrenal cortical response takes minutes to hours to demonstrate an obvious effect, whereas the sympathoadrenal medullary effect is produced rapidly, within seconds. This response has been called the *Selyean response,* after Hans Selye, whose research is predominantly with adrenocortical effects.

The hormones and catecholamines described above produce the most significant effects in the stress reaction; however, the secretion of other hormones is also affected. ADH, aldosterone, and growth hormone are increased. ADH and aldosterone promote sodium and water retention, which is an adaptive response in the event of hemorrhage or loss of fluids through excessive perspiration. Growth hormone antagonizes the action of insulin and supports the fat-mobilizing effects of epinephrine to help increase the blood glucose. Glucagon is increased in stress (Vander et al., 1975). The evidence for other hormones (such as thyroid hormones, sex hormones, and insulin) is not so clear: the effect is variable, depending on the stressor and situational circumstances (Selye, 1976b).

Table 8-2, from Plutchik (1980), demonstrates the sequence of events that lead to the development of an emo-

Table 8-1
Emergency Situations: Sympathoadrenal Response

Effect	Goal	Mechanism
↑ heart rate ↑ B/P	Better perfusion of vital organs	Increased cardiac output owing to increased myocardial contractility and heart rate; also, increased venous return (peripheral vasoconstriction)
↑ blood glucose	Increased available energy	Increased liver and muscle glycogen breakdown; also, increased breakdown of adipose tissue triglycerides
↑ mental activity	Alert state	Activation of renin–angiotensin system
↑ tension of skeletal muscles	Preparedness for activity, decreased fatigue	Besides excitation of muscles, increased blood is shunted to the muscles from the abdominal viscera.
↑ ventilation (may be rapid and shallow)	Provision of oxygen for energy	
↑ coagulability of blood	Prevention of hemorrhage in event of trauma	Vasoconstriction of surface vessels

Table 8-2
Sequence of Events in the Development of an Emotion

Stimulus Event	Inferred Cognition	Feeling	Behavior	Effect
Threat	"Danger"	Fear, terror	Running or flying away	Protection
Obstacle	"Enemy"	Anger, rage	Biting, hitting	Destruction
Potential mate	"Possess"	Joy, ecstasy	Courting, mating	Reproduction
Loss of valued person	"Isolation"	Sadness, grief	Crying for help	Reintegration
Group member	"Friend"	Acceptance, trust	Grooming, sharing	Affiliation

(From Plutchik R: A general psychoevolutionary theory of emotion. In Plutchik R, Kellerman H [eds]. Emotion, Theory, Research and Experience, Vol 1. New York, Academic Press, 1980.)

tion: the stimulus, what we think it is, the feeling, the behavior, and the effect. Each emotion can also be conceived of as having polar opposites, such as joy–sadness; joy implies possession or gain, while sadness implies loss.

▷ Selye and the General Adaptation Syndrome (GAS)

Because of his profound influence on the scientific development of the study of stress and the manner in which he has popularized the concept, it is important to understand Hans Selye's theory. In 1936, Selye first described a syndrome consisting of enlargement of the adrenal cortex; shrinkage of the thymus, spleen, lymph nodes, and other lymphatic structures; and the appearance of deep, bleeding ulcers in the stomach and duodenum. He identified this as a "nonspecific response" to diverse, noxious stimuli. From this beginning, he developed a theory of adaptation to biological stress, which he named the General Adaptation Syndrome.

Phases of the GAS.   There are three phases in the GAS: the alarm reaction, the stage of resistance, and the stage of exhaustion. During the acute phase, or alarm reaction, the sympathoadrenal and pituitary–adrenal cortical responses are activated. The alarm reaction is defensive and antiinflammatory but self-limited in nature. Because it is impossible to live in a continuous state of alarm (death would ensue), the individual moves into the second stage, resistance. During this stage, adaptation to the noxious stressor occurs. In the first stage, the adrenal cortex, initially enlarged, eventually becomes depleted of its stores (a catabolic stage); in the second stage, resistance develops and the adrenal cortex is replenished (anabolism occurs). If exposure to the same stressor is prolonged, however, the adaptation energy is lost, the signs of the alarm reaction return, and the individual dies. Stages one and two of this syndrome are repeated, in different degrees, throughout life as the individual encounters stressors.

Selye also compared the GAS to the life process. During childhood, the first stage, there have been few encounters with stress to promote the development of adaptive functioning, and the child is vulnerable. During the next stage, adulthood, the individual has encountered a number of life's stressful events and has developed a resistance or adaptation. In the final stage, senility, the accumulation of life's stressors, the wear and tear on the organism, again deplete the individual's ability to adapt, resistance falls, and eventually death ensues (Selye, 1976b).

Local Adaptation Syndrome (LAS).   According to Selye's theory, there is also a local adaptation syndrome. The syndrome includes the inflammatory response and repair processes that occur at the local site of tissue injury. The LAS occurs in small, topical injuries, such as bee stings; in the case of emotional arousal, the cerebral cortex is involved. "Even if the target area is not a small area but instead the cerebral cortex, the general metabolism, or the reticuloendothelial system, there is a primary topical response" (Selye, 1976b). Depending on the severity of the injury,

stimuli is sent to the nervous system to elicit the hypothalamic–pituitary–adrenocortical response; this results in the GAS or systemic stress response. Cortical hormones are released and then superimpose their effect upon the LAS.

Selye emphasized that stress is the nonspecific response common to all stressors, regardless of whether they are physiologic, psychological, or social. The fact that different demands are interpreted by different people as stressors is explained by the many conditioning factors in the individual's environment. Conditioning factors also account for differences in the tolerance of different persons for stress. Some may develop diseases of adaptation, such as hypertension, migraine headaches, etc., while others appear to be unaffected (Selye, 1976b).

Recent Views.   In his early research, Selye used extremes of physical stressors; with newer hormone detection techniques, a variety of stressors of differing intensities have been used, and multihormonal patterns of response are being detected. These indicate that there are different patterns of response to different stimuli, *stimulus specificity,* and that different individuals develop a characteristic pattern of autonomic response that carries over from one type of stress to another, *individual response specificity* (Bootzin and Acocella, 1980). This information has led some to question the nonspecificity theory of Selye (Mikhail, 1981). It has been suggested that the nonspecific response is not elicited by a diverse number of stimuli, but rather by one factor, emotional arousal, and that it is the degree of the arousal that affects the intensity of the hormonal response and thus the manifestations displayed by the individual (Mason, 1975).

Selye (1975) agreed that there are different manifestations; but he stated that these are due to conditioning factors that selectively enhance or inhibit the response. Conditioning factors are internal (such as genetic predisposition, age, and sex) and external (such as drug treatments, diet, and living conditions). The interaction of the agent (with its stressor effect and specific effect) with the individual (characterized by different exogenous and endogenous conditioning) produces different manifestations. "The basic concept of nonspecificity, of the important role played by the hypothalamo–pituitary–adrenocortical axis, and of the stereotyped, nonspecific syndrome remains unaltered" (Selye, 1975).

▷ Maladaptive Responses

The mechanisms identified by Cannon and Selye serve as adaptations to meet threatening situations. These can be both beneficial and harmful. Dubos (1965) stated that these are traits retained from man's evolutionary past that "no longer fit the needs of life in civilized societies." The fight-or-flight response, for example, is an anticipatory response that mobilized the bodily resources of our ancestors to deal with predators and other harsh exigencies of the environment. This same mobilization comes into play in response to emotional stimuli unrelated to danger.

> Whatever the life situation, whether it corresponds to an actual physical danger or merely to an emotional

crisis, the nature and intensity of the anticipatory changes the symbol elicits in the body have remained much the same in modern man as they were in his Paleolithic ancestor.*

When the body has been prepared physiologically to act and does not do so, the result is likely to be frustrating and injurious to the individual's health. For example, consider the father waiting outside the delivery room for his wife to deliver their first baby. He may be as exhausted at the end of labor as the mother. Anxiety prepared him for "fight or flight"; when he could not do either, conflict developed, frustration appeared, tension became obvious, and pacing, perspiration, and other behaviors occurred that used up as much energy as the physical labor. In this case, the father was rewarded—in instances where that might not be true, the conflict and frustration would be intensified.

The fight–flight–rage response stimulates sympathetic adrenal medullary activity. In instances where this is prolonged or excessive, a state of chronic arousal persists, high-renin high blood pressure exists, and arteriosclerotic changes occur that may lead to cardiovascular disease. In the Selyean response, adrenal–cortical hormones are the primary agent. When excessive or prolonged, behavior patterns of withdrawal and depression are seen. Prolonged cortisol production may contribute to failure of the immune response, and infections and tumors may develop. In describing these patterns, Henry and Stephen (1977) stated that the two extremes of behavior in the patterns are essentially those of excessive dominance and excessive subordination. Other patterns of endocrine response can also be related to maladaptation.

Risk-inducing Coping Processes

Lazarus (1980) has indicated that coping itself can add to social, psychological, and physiologic malfunction that increase the risk of illness. One way in which it does this is by direct damage to tissues. For example, the use of alcohol or drugs to alleviate stress may create liver damage; social relationships and psychological welfare may also be affected. Coping by smoking may create lung damage; overeating or undereating may have serious nutritional effects; psychosocial welfare may also be harmed. All of these increase the vulnerability of the body to further disease.

A second way in which coping increases the risk of illness is more indirect and involves the "bodily effects on the internal milieu of the mobilization often required for coping." (Lazarus, 1980). This can best be understood with an example. Type A people are driving, competitive, and achievement-oriented. The pattern they have developed reflects a socialization process that emphasizes the Protestant work ethic. Mobilization of type A behavior requires the increased output of catecholamines, the adrenal–medullary hormones. One might say the life of a type A person is a series of fight-or-flight responses.

A third way in which coping can increase health risk is called palliative by Lazarus. This is typified by the woman who feels a lump in her breast but denies its seriousness

* Dubos R. Man Adapting, p 30. New Haven, Yale University Press, 1965.

and delays seeking medical attention. The intention of palliative coping methods is to control the threat to life, but in the end they increase the risk of developing more severe illnesses because of their delaying action (Lazarus, 1980).

Ego defenses are "basically a coping strategy to deal with conflicts over a particular emotion" (Plutchik, 1980). For example, if you are angry with someone, rather than create a scene that may lead to threats and retaliation, which would endanger your self-concept, you are likely to pick a less dangerous scapegoat or possibly work the anger out in physical exercise. Ego defenses imply an unconscious aspect in that usually the behavior is not the result of a deliberate thinking process, although some of it may be. Continual internal conflict and repression of emotions can lead to psychopathology.

Indices of Stress

Laboratory measurements of indicators of stress have significantly improved since the early experiments in the field and are daily adding to the understanding of this complex process. Among the measures, blood and urine analyses can be used to demonstrate changes in hormonal levels. Reliable measures of stress include blood levels of catecholamines, corticoids, ACTH, and a drop in eosinophils. The blood creatine/creatinine ratio and elevations of cholesterol and free fatty acids can also be measured. Rises in other circulating indicators can be measured, but they are less reliable as stress indicators and the measurements are more difficult to perform (Selye, 1976a).

The electroencephalogram may be used to measure brain activity. Galvanic skin resistance, which measures the electrical conductivity of the skin, may be done. This is primarily a measure of sweat excretion, which rises in stress, and is typically used in lie detector tests. Rises in blood pressure and heart rate can also be measured.

In addition to these measurable signs, there are a number of other indices of stress that may be observed by others or by the individual himself. They are listed in Chart 8-1. Over time, each individual tends to develop a characteristic pattern of behavior in stress that is a warning that the system is out of balance. Researchers have developed many questionnaires to identify the *state* of stress in individuals and also their tendency toward stress, a *trait* of their personality.

Diseases of Adaptation: Maladaptation

The autonomic and endocrine responses to stress serve an adaptive function; their purpose is to restore equilibrium in the individual. They may last minutes, hours, or days; the disturbance they cause is reversible. However, when we speak of "diseases of adaptation," we are speaking of diseases in which the stress response plays the predominant etiologic role, and irreversible pathology may be present. The preceding discussion has identified the mechanisms contributing to the formation of these diseases. Other chapters of the book discuss individual diseases in greater detail.

Selye (1976a) gives the following comprehensive list of disorders:

High blood pressure, diseases of the heart and blood vessels, diseases of the kidney, eclampsia, rheumatic

---

Chart 8-1
Indices of Stress

General irritability, hyperexcitation, or depression
Dryness of the throat and mouth
Overpowering urge to cry or run and hide
Easily fatigued, loss of interest
"Floating anxiety"—do not know exactly why or what
Easily startled
Stuttering or other speech difficulties
Hypermotility: pacing, moving about, cannot sit still
Gastrointestinal signs and symptoms: butterflies in the
    stomach, diarrhea, vomiting
Change in menstrual cycle
Loss of or excessive appetite
Increased use of legally prescribed drugs, such as
    tranquilizers or psychic energizers
Accident proneness
Disturbed behavior
Pounding of the heart
Impulsive behavior, emotional instability
Inability to concentrate
Feelings of unreality, weakness, or dizziness
Tension, alertness
Trembling, nervous tics
Nervous laughter
Grinding of teeth
Insomnia
Perspiring
Increased frequency of urination
Muscle tension and migraine headaches
Pain in the neck or lower back
Increased smoking
Alcohol and drug addiction
Nightmares

(Based on Selye H: Stress in Health and Disease. Woburn,
Butterworths, 1976. Reprinted by permission of the publisher.)

---

and rheumatoid arthritis, inflammatory diseases of the skin and eyes, infections, allergic and hypersensitivity diseases, nervous and mental diseases, sexual derangements, digestive diseases, metabolic diseases, cancer, and diseases of resistance in general.*

Some are due to an "excess of defensive, others to an overabundance of submissive bodily reactions." It is important to retain the holistic concept in considering the multiple factors involved in these diseases. Emotional arousal may lead to the neuroendocrine responses. A pattern of positive feedback may develop that continues to stimulate the production of hormones; the bodily responses feed the emotional arousal, and a vicious cycle ensues. Other reg-

* Selye H. The Stress of Life, pp 169, 170. New York, McGraw–Hill, 1976.

ulatory mechanisms, which have been on the periphery, become involved and contribute to further disturbances.

▷ Stress Reduction

The picture of stress presented here has identified three major factors that influence the development and impact of stress. They include

1. An individual's biological and psychological characteristics
2. The social and environmental context of the life event or situation
3. An individual's coping strategies.

These three factors will be considered in discussing methods that nurses might use for reducing and controlling stress, not only in their patients but also in themselves.

There is a growing emphasis in our society on the quality of life. Inherent in this concept is the promotion of health, the decrease of stress, and the avoidance of illness. With this outlook, health care to prevent illness becomes more significant than cure.

Health Risk Appraisal

Health risk appraisal is an activity designed to promote health by examining the personal habits of the individual and recommending changes where health risk is indicated. Questionnaires typically collect the following types of information:

1. Demographic data: Age, sex, race, ethnic background
2. Personal and family history of certain diseases
3. Life-style factors
   - Eating, sleeping, exercise, smoking, drinking, and driving habits
   - Stressors on the job
   - Role relationships and associated stressors
4. Physical measurements
   - Blood pressure
   - Height, weight
   - Laboratory analyses of blood and urine
5. Membership or nonmembership in a high-risk group, such as a family with a history of cancer

The personal data about the individual are compared with average population risk data, and the risk factors are identified and weighted. The information provided by this analysis includes the following (Doerr & Hutchins, 1981; Goetz & McTyre, 1981):

1. The person's chronological age and risk age
2. The person's compliance age—that is, what he can achieve by making changes in his life-style
3. A list of the person's major health hazards, and suggestions for change

Nursing Implications

Although the collection of data bases like the one just described is a common part of taking a nursing history, the controlled analysis of risk is not customary. The development of a nursing data base that supplies the essential information for making decisions about patient care is a necessity.

Health risk appraisal and patient education to improve health behavior are activities that nurses can perform to prevent health problems and reduce stress. In patients who *already* have health problems, there will be some degree of stress, and the nurse can *anticipate* changes based upon the stress response. For example, the postsurgical patient will have fluid and electrolyte changes corresponding to the general neuroendocrine response. It should be mentioned that this response has a snowballing effect. Although it does not primarily affect the kidney, the vasoconstriction induced as part of the stress response may decrease the flow of blood to the kidney, which stimulates the renin–angiotensin mechanism, leading to an increase in aldosterone with sodium and water retention. Psychosocially, if the individual typically withdraws and becomes nonexpressive in stress situations, that same behavior may be expected here.

Coping Behaviors

It should be remembered that the individual is in constant interaction with his environment, both internal and external. This implies that change is constant, and that change is necessary for optimal psychosocial and physiologic growth. Responding to change requires adaptive energy; the important issue is to regulate the use of energy so that there is an adequate store. This then becomes an issue of regulating one's own actions to reduce stress. The methods described here can be used by the nurse to manage her own stress, and taught or recommended to the patient to manage his stress.

The functions of coping were listed earlier, as follows:

- Modification of the situation giving rise to stress
- Modification of the meaning of the problem to reduce threat
- Control or management of the symptoms produced by the stress

Techniques to reach these goals may include changing jobs if the workplace is the source of excessive stress. Through health appraisals, nurses may identify patient stressors; however, stress control requires self-care and motivation, and therefore the patient must actively and willingly participate in appraising, identifying, and managing his sources of stress. At the same time, sources of strength should be identified and capitalized upon. This helps to improve the self-esteem of the patient and reinforces positive behavior patterns.

Modifications of the meaning of a problem may require taking a longer-range view of a situation, or putting it into perspective. Compulsive behavior, deadlines, and clock watching may need to be re-evaluated.

Controlling the symptoms of stress is important. For one thing, the individual needs to be able to anticipate the development of stress and to know how he typically reacts. Does muscle tension occur? Does he get irritable? What symptoms does he have? These should be signals to alter his activity. It is also important to recognize that stress begets stress. A muscle tension headache or, a more severe example, the presence of a peptic ulcer, adds another stressor to feed into neuroendocrine and cognitive arousal.

Stress-reduction Methods

Numerous methods for reducing stress are available and being publicized. The important point to be remembered is that just as each individual develops a particular pattern of stress response, so will each individual have his preferred method of stress reduction.

Self-regulation of Stress. Sutterley (1982) has described six categories of approaches to self-regulation of stress:

1. Nutrition
2. Exercise, physical activity, recreation
3. Muscle control, kinesiology
4. Meditation, creative imagery
5. Communication, time management
6. Group process, support systems.

Proper nutrition, adequate rest, and regular exercise improve one's well-being and help develop resistance to stressors. Regular exercise assists in weight control, decreases a sense of fatigue and monotony, and increases the exercise tolerance for some patients with angina pectoris and peripheral arterial disease; some studies indicate that it may prevent heart attacks. Regular exercise may help to prevent premature atherosclerosis (Paul, 1979). The need for outside and diversionary activities for everyone has become a fact of life.

Biofeedback. The purpose of biofeedback is to gain some degree of mental control over the autonomic nervous system and possibly decrease blood pressure, control heart rate, and prevent migraine headaches, hyperactive stomachs, etc. Some form of electronic instrumentation is used to monitor a biological function, such as measuring skin conductance with the galvanic skin responder. This information is amplified and sent back to the person, who then tries consciously to alter the machine in some way. For example, by relaxing and decreasing the sweating of his palms, the person attempts to alter the tone of the machine. The activity that produces an altered tone in the machine alters the biological functioning. Through practice and reinforcement, the individual learns how to control the activity without the machine. In Chapter 7, Schwartz's disregulation model, which is a biofeedback model, is described. Schwartz has particularly applied this technique in the treatment of hypertension. Some persons suffering from migraine headaches have developed a technique of "thinking their hands hot," and theoretically have directed the blood-flow from the head to the hands. The long-term efficacy of such techniques is still being tested.

Relaxation Response. Benson (1975) has described what he calls the "relaxation response," which is a calming state opposite to the arousal state of stress. Four elements are necessary to produce the relaxation response: a quiet environment, a comfortable position, a passive attitude, and a mental device or object, such as a word, sound, or phrase to occupy the mind and keep out thoughts. For example, the word "one" could be repeated silently or audibly. By sitting quietly and practicing relaxation 15 to 20 minutes once or twice a day, an individual should be able to achieve positive results in lowering stress levels. Other techniques, such as meditation and yoga, also produce the relaxation response. Still others use the sound of pleasant music or a mountain stream in conjunction with relaxation techniques to help achieve the desired state. Progressive relaxation is another technique that alternately tenses and relaxes muscle groups in a systematic fashion so that the individual can compare the two effects, and ends with a period of complete relaxation.

Other techniques, such as massage, may be used; for example, Longworth (1982) has demonstrated the effectiveness of slow-stroke back massage in patients with high emotional and physiologic arousal.

It is important for the nurse to determine what type of stress reduction activities work best for her and for her patients and to encourage their regular use.

Social Support. The importance of social support as a mediating resource in stress has already been identified. To reinforce that information, the function of social networks includes (Hamburg & Killilea, 1979):

1. The maintenance of positive social identity
2. The provision of emotional support
3. The provision of material aid and tangible services
4. Access to information
5. Access to new social contacts and new social roles.

The emotion—anxiety, fear, guilt—that accompanies stress is unpleasant, and it may continue to grow in a spiraling fashion without intervention. Emotional support from family and significant others provides the individual with love and a sense of sharing the burden. Being able to talk with someone and express one's feelings openly may help one to gain mastery of the situation. Nurses can provide this source of support; however, it is important to identify the individual's social support system and encourage its use. Persons who are loners, or isolated, or who withdraw in times of stress have a high risk of coping failure.

Anxiety may also distort the individual's ability to process information. Perception is narrowed, thoughts may be unclear, and reality may be distorted. For a time, this cognitive blurring is adaptive and allows the individual to tolerate a threat, perhaps some bad news; however, reality must be faced for the longer run. It helps to seek information and advice from others who can assist with analyzing the threat and developing a strategy to manage it. Again, this use of others helps the individual to maintain mastery of a situation and to keep his self-esteem.

There is a growing awareness in the public of the need for support groups. Groups have been formed by parents of children with leukemia, ostomates, mastectomy patients (Reach for Recovery) and other cancer victims, and persons with other serious diseases. There are groups for single parents. Alcoholics Anonymous and spouses of alcoholics, drug addiction groups, and child abuse groups meet for mutual support. Professional, civic, and religious support groups are active in the community. Being a member of a group with similar problems has a releasing effect on the individual that promotes freedom of expression and exchange of ideas. There are also encounter groups, assertiveness training programs, and consciousness raising groups to help people modify their usual behavior.

Human evolution has led to a brain that possesses neural networks characterized by a plasticity that permits behavior to be modified. This flexibility allows man to make choices and thereby exert some control over the strategies they select for survival. The nurse can play a significant role in influencing those choices.

▷ Bibliography

Books

Altman I, Rapoport A, and Wohlwill JF (eds). Human Behavior and Environment, Advances in Theory and Research. New York, Plenum Press, 1980.

Antonovsky A. Health, Stress, and Coping. San Francisco, Jossey–Bass, 1979.

Bakal DA. Psychology & Medicine. New York, Springer, 1979.

Benson H. The Relaxation Response. New York, William Morrow, 1975.

Boddy J. Brain Systems and Psychological Concepts. New York, John Wiley & Sons, 1978.

Bootzin RB and Acocella JR. Abnormal Psychology, Current Perspectives. New York, Random House, 1980.

Dohrenwend BS and Dohrenwend BP (eds). Stressful Life Events: Their Nature and Effects. New York, John Wiley & Sons, 1974.

Dubos R. Man Adapting. New Haven, Yale University Press, 1965.

Ganong WF. Review of Medical Physiology, 9th ed. Los Altos, Lange, 1979.

Garfield CA (ed). Stress and Survival: The Emotional Realities of Life-Threatening Illness. St Louis, CV Mosby, 1979.

Grings WW and Dawson ME. Emotions and Bodily Responses, A Psychophysiological Approach. New York, Academic Press, 1978.

Gunderson EKE and Rahe RH. Life Stress and Illness. Springfield, Illinois, Charles C Thomas, 1974.

Hardy ME. Theoretical Foundations for Nursing. New York, MSS Information Corp, 1973.

Helson H. Adaptation-Level Theory. New York, Harper & Row, 1964.

Henry JP and Stephens PM. Stress, Health and the Social Environment. New York, Springer–Verlag, 1977.

Janis IL. Psychological Stress. New York, John Wiley, 1958.

Kaplan L. Foundation of Human Behavior. New York, Harper & Row, 1965.

Lazarus RS. Patterns of Adjustment, 3rd ed. New York, McGraw–Hill, 1976.

Levi L. Emotions, Their Parameters and Measurement. New York, Raven Press, 1975.

Levine S and Scotch NA. Social Stress. Chicago, Aldine, 1970.

Lidz T. The Family and Human Adaptation, Three Lectures. New York, International Universities, 1963.

Nebraska Symposium on Motivation 1978. Human Emotion. Lincoln, University of Nebraska Press, 1979.

Pelletier KR. Mind as Healer, Mind as Slayer. New York, Dell, 1977.

Restak RM. The Brain: The Last Frontier. New York, Warner Books, 1979.

Robbins SL and Angell M. Basic Pathology. Philadelphia, WB Saunders, 1976.

Roberts SL. Behavioral Concepts and the Critically Ill Patient. Englewood Cliffs, Prentice–Hall, 1976.

Rogers ME. The Theoretical Basis of Nursing. Philadelphia, FA Davis, 1970.

Roy Sr C. Introduction to Nursing, An Adaptation Model. Englewood Cliffs, Prentice–Hall, 1976.

Schontz FC. The Psychological Aspects of Physical Illness and Disability. New York, MacMillan, 1975.

Selye, H. Stress Without Distress. Philadelphia, JB Lippincott, 1974.

Selye H. The Stress of Life. New York, McGraw–Hill, 1976a.

Selye H. Stress in Health and Disease. Boston, Butterworths, 1976b.

Selye H (ed). Selyes' Guide to Stress Research, Vol I. New York, Van Nostrand Reinhold, 1980.

Surgeon General's Report on Health Promotion and Disease Prevention: Healthy People. DHEW (PHS) Pub. #79–55071 A, 1979.

Sutterley DC and Donnelly GF. Coping with Stress. Rockville, Maryland, Aspen Publications, 1982.

Tanner O. Stress. New York, Time–Life Books, 1976.

Vander AJ, Sherman JH, and Luciano DS. Human Physiology, The Mechanisms of Body Function. New York, McGraw–Hill, 1975.

Wolf SW and Goodell H. Harold G. Wolff's Stress and Disease, 2nd ed. Springfield, Illinois, Charles C Thomas, 1968.

Wolff HG, Wolf SG Jr, and Hare CC (eds). Life Stress and Bodily Diseases. Baltimore, Williams & Wilkins, 1950.

Articles

Aiello JR and Thompson DE. Personal space, crowding, and spatial behavior in a cultural context. In Altman I et al. (eds). Human Behavior and Environment. New York, Plenum Press, 1980.

Broussard R. Using relaxation for COPD. Am J Nurs 1979 Nov; 79(10):1962–1963.

Burchfield SR. The stress response: A new perspective. Psychosom Med 1979 Dec; 41(8):661–672.

Burke RJ and Weir T. The type A experience: Occupational and life demands, satisfaction and well-being. J Human Stress 1980 Dec; 6(4):28–38.

Chinn PL. Editorial. Holistic Health. Adv Nurs Sci, 1980 July; 2(4):XIII.

Cobb S. A model for life events and their consequences. In Dohrenwend BS and Dohrenwend BP (eds). Stressful Life Events: Their Nature and Effects. New York, John Wiley & Sons, 1974.

Cobb S. Social support as a moderator of life stress. Psychosom Med 1976 Sept/Oct; 38(5):300–314.

Coping. Top Clin Nurs 1982 July; 4(2):entire volume.

Doerr BT and Hutchins EB. Health risk appraisal: Process, problems and prospects for nursing research and practice. Nurs Res 1981 Sept/Oct; 30(5):299–307.

Dohrenwend BS and Dohrenwend BP. What is a stressful life event. In Selye H (ed). Selye's Guide to Stress Research. New York, Van Nostrand Reinhold, 1980.

Folkman S and Lazarus RS. An analysis of coping in a middle-aged community sample. J Health Soc Behav 1980 Sept; 21(3):219–239.

Frain M and Valiga TM. The multiple dimensions of stress. In Sutterley DC and Donnelly GF. Coping with Stress. Rockville, Maryland, Aspen Publications, 1982.

Frankenhaeuser M and Gardell B. Underload and overload in working life: Outline of a multidisciplinary approach. J Human Stress 1976 Sept; 2(3):35–46.

Gardner R Jr. Attribution of control, essays, and early medical school experience. Psychosom Med 1982 Mar; 44(1):93–109.

Gentry WD et al. Habitual anger-coping styles: I. Effect on mean blood pressure and risk for essential hypertension. Psychosom Med 1982 May; 44(2):195–201.

Goetz AA and McTyre RB. Health risk appraisal: Some methodologic considerations. Nurs Res 1981 Sept/Oct; 30(5):307–313.

Green CP. Assessment of family stress. J Adv Nurs 1982 Jan; 7(1):11–17.

Gross E. Work, organization and stress. In Levine SL and Scotch NA (eds). Social Stress. Chicago, Aldine, 1970.

Guzzetta CE and Forsyth L. Nursing diagnostic pilot study: Psychophysiologic stress. Adv Nurs Sci 1979 Oct; 2(1):27–44.

Hamburg BA and Killilea M. Relation of social support, stress, illness, and use of health services. In Healthy People, The Surgeon General's Report on Health Promotion and Disease Prevention. DHEW (PHS) Pub #79–55071 A, 1979.

Heidt P. Effect of therapeutic touch on anxiety level of hospitalized patients. Nurs Res 1981 Jan/Feb; 30(1):32–37.

Jalowiec A and Powers MJ. Stress and coping in hypertensive and emergency room patients. Nurs Res 1981 Jan/Feb; 30(1):10–15.

Karasek RA et al. Physiology of stress and regeneration in job related cardiovascular illness. J Human Stress 1982 Jan; 8(1):29–38.

Katz JL. Three studies in psychosomatic medicine revisited: A tribute to the psychobiological perspective of Herbert Weiner. Psychosom Med 1982 Mar; 44(1):29–42.

Krantz DS. Cognitive processes and recovery from heart attack: A review and theoretical analysis. J Human Stress 1980 Sept; 6(3):27–38.

Levi L and Kagan A. Psychosocially-induced stress and disease—problems, research strategies and results. In Selye H (ed). Selye's Guide to Stress Research. New York, Van Nostrand Reinhold, 1980.

Longworth JCD. Psychophysiological effects of slow stroke back massage in normotensive females. Adv Nurs Sci 1982 July; 4(4):44–62.

Marcinek MB. Stress in the surgical patient. Am J Nurs 1977 Nov; 77(11):1809–1811.

Mason JW. A historical view of the stress field, part I. J Human Stress 1975 Mar; 1(1):6–12.

Mason JW. A historical view of the stress field, part II. J Human Stress 1975 June; 1(2):22–36.

Mechanic D. Stress, illness, and illness behavior. J Human Stress 1976 June; 2(2):2–6.

Mikhail A. Stress: A psychophysiological conception. J Human Stress 1981 June; 7(2):9–15.

Morris CL. Relaxation therapy in a clinic. Am J Nurs 1979 Nov; 79(10):1958–1959.

Neuman B. The Betty Neuman Model: A total person approach to viewing patient problems. In Riehl JP and Roy C (eds). Conceptual Models for Nursing Practice. New York, Appleton–Century–Crofts, 1974.

O'Flynn–Comiskey AI. The type-A individual. Am J Nurs 1979 Nov; 79(10):1957–1958.

Paul O. The prevention of cardiovascular disease. In Healthy People, The Surgeon General's Report on Health Promotion and Disease Prevention. DHEW (PHS) Pub #79–55071 A, 1979.

Pearlin LI and Schooler C. The structure of coping. J Health Soc Behav 1978 Mar; 19(1):2–21.

Rahe RH. Editorial. J Human Stress 1975 June; 1(2):3.

Richter JM and Sloan R. The relaxation technique. Am J Nurs 1979 Nov; 79(10):1960–1964.

Savitz J and Friedman MI. Diagnosing boredom and confusion. Nurs Res 1981 Jan/Feb; 30(1):16–20.

Schwartz GE. Psychosomatic disorders and biofeedback: A psychobiological model of disregulation. In Maser JD and Seligman MEP (eds). Psychopathology: Experimental Models. San Francisco, Freeman, 1977.

Scott DW, Oberst MT, and Dropkin MJ. A stress-coping model. In

Sutterley DC and Donnelly GF (eds). Coping With Stress. Rockville, Maryland, Aspen Publications, 1982.

Scott R and Howard A. Models of stress. In Levine S and Scotch NA (eds). Social Stress. Chicago, Aldine, 1970.

Selye H. Confusion and controversy in the stress field. J Human Stress 1975 June; 1(2):37–44.

Smith JC and Seidel JM. The factor structure of self-reported physical stress reaction. Biofeedback Self Regul 1982 Mar; 7(1):35–47.

Smith MJT and Selye H. Reducing the negative effects of stress. Am J Nurs 1979 Nov; 79(10):1953–1955.

Sorenson JH and White GF. Natural hazards, a cross-cultural perspective. In Altman I et al. (eds). Human Behavior and Environment, Advances in Theory and Research. New York, Plenum Press, 1980.

Sparacino J. Blood pressure, stress, and mental health. Nurs Res 1982 Jan/Feb; 31(1):89–94.

Stephenson CA. Stress in critically ill patients. Am J Nurs 1977 Nov; 77(11):1806–1809.

Sutterley DC. Stress and health: A survey of self-regulation modalities. In Sutterley DC and Donnelly GF. Coping With Stress. Rockville, Maryland, Aspen Publications, 1982.

Task Force Report. Biofeedback as an adjunct to psychotherapy. Biofeedback Self Regul 1982 Mar; 7(1):1–33.

Tausig M. Measuring life events. J Health Soc Behav 1982 Mar; 23(1):52–64.

Vernikos–Danellis J and Heybach JP. Psychophysiologic mechanisms regulating the hypothalamic–pituitary–adrenal response to stress. In Selye H (ed). Selye's Guide to Stress Research. New York, Van Nostrand Reinhold, 1980.

Vickers RR et al. Type A behavior pattern and coping and defense. Psychosom Med 1981 Oct; 43(5):381–396.

Wilkins WL. Social stress and illness in industrial society. In Gunderson EKE and Rahe RH (eds). Life Stress and Illness. Springfield, Illinois, Charles C Thomas, 1974.

9

Fluids and Electrolytes: Balance and Disturbances

▷ Fluid and Electrolyte Homeostasis

In order for cells to accomplish their numerous physiologic activities, oxygen and nutrients must be continually delivered to the cells and waste products of metabolism continually removed. Cells are bathed in a fluid environment so that water-soluble substances can diffuse in either direction through the cell membrane. From the cell, waste products traverse the interstitial fluid to the vascular system and are circulated to the lungs, liver, or kidneys for detoxification or excretion. Oxygen and metabolic substrates are simultaneously transported within the blood to cells. Therefore, abnormal changes in the volume or content of vascular fluid create cellular dysfunction. Likewise, disordered cell function can rapidly alter the fluid environment. For this reason, diseases of any body system are usually accompanied by fluid–electrolyte and acid–base disturbances.

Body Water

The major contributor to the fluid environment is water, which accounts for 45% to 60% of body weight (Fig. 9-1). Roughly half this water is contained in muscle; the remainder is distributed among bone, blood, skin, and other tissues. Because women have a greater ratio of adipose to muscle tissue than do men, their water content is slightly less. In both sexes, the replacement of muscle by adipose tissue leads to a gradual decline in total body water content during aging.

Approximately 55% of body water is located inside cells and is referred to as intracellular fluid. For a healthy man who weighs 70 kg, total body water is 42 liters, and 25 liters is intracellular.

The remaining 45% of body water is extracellular (*i.e.,* located outside cell membranes). It includes the fluid within blood vessels, the interstitial fluid that surrounds cells, gastrointestinal and other secretions, and the water contained inside solid tissues. Intravascular blood volume approximates 5 liters. Three liters of blood is plasma fluid, and the remainder consists mainly of leukocytes, erythro-

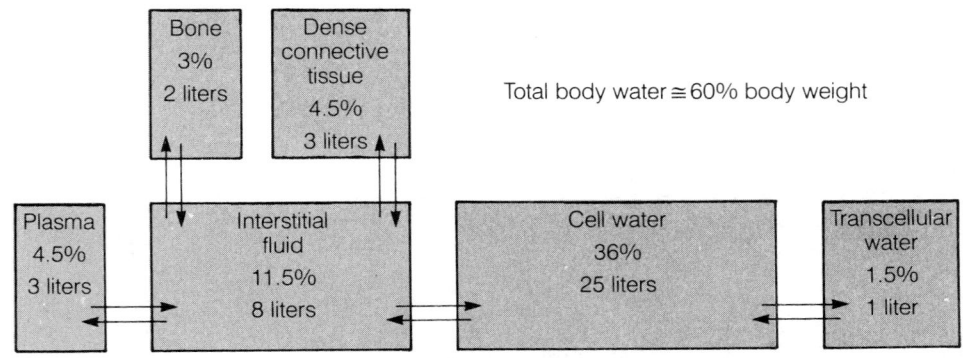

Figure 9-1. Distribution of total body water in an average 70-kg man. The percentages refer to the fraction of the body weight contained in each compartment. (Redrawn from Rose BD: Clinical Physiology of Acid–Base and Electrolyte Disorders, p 16, New York, McGraw-Hill, 1977. Copyright © 1977, McGraw-Hill. Used with the permission of the McGraw-Hill Book Company.)

cytes, and platelets. The interstitial fluid amounts to approximately 8 liters. Transcellular fluids include digestive secretions, perspiration, cerebrospinal fluid, and the secretions of pleural and synovial membranes. The transcellular fluid volume is estimated as 1 liter at any one time, because of the continual reabsorption of much secreted fluid. Approximately 5 liters of water are contained within bone, connective tissue, and other solids.

In summary, extracellular fluid totals 17 liters, as opposed to 25 liters for intracellular fluid. Because the water contained within solid tissue does not readily exchange, this fluid is often ignored in calculations. Therefore, the distribution of body water is usually estimated as one third extracellular and two thirds intracellular.

Intake and Output of Water

On a daily basis, the amount of water consumed must equal that excreted (Table 9-1). Approximately 2600 ml of water are lost from the body every 24 hours. Of this total, urine accounts for 1500 ml, roughly 60 ml per hour. Water content of stool adds another 200 ml. Evaporation of water from the moist surfaces of the skin and respiratory tract contributes

Table 9-1
Typical Daily Water Balance in a Normal Man

Water Intake (ml/day)		Water Output (ml/day)	
Source		**Source**	
Ingested water	1400	Urine	1500
Water content of food	850	Skin	500
		Respiratory tract	400
Water of oxidation	350	Stool	200
Total	2600	Total	2600

(Rose BD: Clinical Physiology of Acid–Base and Electrolyte Disorders, p 34. New York, McGraw-Hill, 1977. Copyright © 1977, McGraw-Hill. Used with permission of the McGraw-Hill Book Company.)

approximately 900 ml. This fluid is called insensible loss and does not include visible perspiration. When profuse perspiration occurs, total water excretion far exceeds 2600 ml. Under normal conditions, water intake matches excretion: 1400 ml are ingested as liquid, 850 ml are contained within food, and 350 ml are produced as cells oxidize nutrients.

Ions and Other Particles

Body water contains cells, cell fragments, and proteins, as well as numerous dissolved substances that interact chemically. Particles that are electrically charged (*i.e.,* contain incomplete orbital electrons) are called *ions.* Substances that can break down or dissociate into ions are referred to as *electrolytes.* Ions are either positively or negatively charged. Positively charged ions are called *cations,* and negatively charged ions are called *anions.* Overall, the sum of the positive charges equals the sum of the negative charges, so that solutions are electrically neutral. Electrolytes in solution are usually expressed as equivalents (Eq) or milliequivalents (mEq), because they chemically combine with each other in proportion to their number of ionic charges or valence.

The total number of ions is equal between the intracellular and extracellular fluid compartments, but the particular ions vary in concentration. Within intracellular fluid, the major positively charged ion is potassium. The major negatively charged ions are phosphate and protein. The major positively charged ion in extracellular fluid is sodium, which is electrically balanced by the negative ions chloride and bicarbonate. The ions in each compartment are listed in Table 9-2.

Methods by Which Normal Fluid and Electrolyte Distribution is Maintained
Diffusion

A variety of processes operate to maintain the normal distribution of ions and fluid. The first of these is *diffusion,* the movement of dissolved particles of gases from an area of higher concentration to an area of lower concentration. Although entirely passive, diffusion is a fundamental means of transporting substances throughout the body. Because this process is slow, the vascular network is arranged to minimize the distance between cells and blood vessels.

Osmosis

When applied to water, the process described above is called *osmosis.* In this case, water moves from a lower concentration of ions (*i.e.,* dilute solution) to a higher concentration of ions (*i.e.,* concentrated solution). As with diffusion, the result is that concentrations of dissolved particles are equalized. Because cell membrane permeability is greater to water than to ions, water movement between fluid compartments is a primary means by which concentrations are kept equal. As a consequence of water movement into or out of cells, the cells swell or shrink.

The two forces that determine the amount of water movement between intracellular and extracellular fluid compartments are hydrostatic pressure and osmotic pressure. *Hydrostatic pressure* refers to the weight of fluid within a column. *Osmotic pressure* measures the amount of water movement that results from the presence of particles in solution. If one fluid compartment containing particles and another without particles are separated by a membrane permeable only to water, the water will move by osmosis toward the compartment containing particles. As water moves into this compartment, hydrostatic pressure is generated, which tends to displace water in the opposite direction. Eventually, the water movement into the particle-containing compartment is equalized by hydrostatic pressure; the pressure measurement at this point is the osmotic pressure of the solution.

Osmotic pressure is measured in terms of osmoles or, within the fluids of the body that are relatively dilute, milliosmoles (1/1000 osmole). An *osmole* is the weight in grams of a substance that dissolves into a standard number of particles. Thus, the tendency of a substance to cause osmosis is described rather than its chemical activity.

Osmolarity and Osmolality. Two additional terms related to the concentration of particles in solution are osmolarity and osmolality. *Osmolarity* refers to the number of particles in the total volume of solution; measurement is in liters. A similar but slightly more precise term is *osmolality,* which means the number of particles per unit weight; osmolality is measured in kilograms. As the concentration of particles contained in a solution increases, the osmolarity or osmolality rises. For clinical purposes, the two terms are often used interchangeably. Osmolality will be used throughout this chapter.

Electrical Forces

Another factor that influences the distribution of water and electrolytes is the electrical charge carried on ions. In general, ions move so as to maintain equal numbers of positive and negative charges on each side of a semipermeable membrane.

Active Transport

All of the processes described thus far have been passive; that is, they have required no energy to sustain them. The

Table 9-2
Ions in Fluid Compartments (Listed in Order of Concentration)

	Intracellular	Extracellular
Cations	Potassium	Sodium
	Magnesium	Calcium
	Sodium	Potassium
	Calcium	Magnesium
Anions	Phosphate	Chloride
	Protein	Bicarbonate
	Sulfate	Protein
	Bicarbonate	Organic Acids
	Chloride	Phosphate
		Sulfate

net result of all these processes is equality of electrical charge and particle concentration between fluid compartments. However, in order for cells to transmit electrical impulses, ion concentrations must differ between the cells' interior and exterior. A high concentration of potassium ions in intracellular fluid and a low concentration within extracellular fluid are accomplished by active transport mechanisms that utilize energy to pump potassium into cells. Active transport similarly extrudes sodium from the cell, so that sodium concentration is low in intracellular fluid and high in extracellular fluid. Because of these concentration differences, an electrical potential is generated at the cell membrane. Neuromuscular transmission of impulses occurs as a result of electrical activity in which sodium rapidly flows into the cell and potassium flows out. These rapid, repetitive ionic shifts, called *action potentials,* are essential to sustain life.

Determination of Serum Osmolality

The result of all these processes is that the osmolality is the same in extracellular and intracellular fluid compartments, although the specific ions that determine osmolality in each compartment differ. The major contributors to osmolality are those ions that are present in the greatest numbers. In extracellular fluid, sodium ions account for most of the positive charge. They are balanced by an equal number of negatively charged ions. Thus, sodium equals roughly half of the total charged particles, and doubling the serum sodium value provides an estimate of serum osmolality. Since the osmolality is equal in both compartments, the serum sodium value also reflects the intracellular osmolality.

Although electrolytes are the major determinants of osmolality, other substances also contribute. The effect of glucose can be ignored as long as the serum glucose value is normal. Plasma proteins account for some of the negative charge that balances sodium. Because the plasma proteins do not move freely across vessel walls, their concentration is higher in the vascular space than in the interstitial space. The result is an osmotic force that pulls fluid into vessels. This pressure exerted by plasma proteins to hold fluid within vessels is known as *colloid osmotic pressure* or *plasma oncotic pressure.*

Isotonic, Hypotonic, and Hypertonic Solutions. When all contributions to osmolality are summed, the total serum osmolality ranges from 275 mOsm/kg to 290 mOsm/kg. Solutions can be categorized according to how their osmolality compares with that of extracellular fluid. When the osmolality is the same as in extracellular fluid, a solution is labeled *isotonic.* Such a solution remains within the extracellular compartment. One third is distributed to the vascular space and two thirds to the interstitial space. A fluid with a lower or higher osmolality is labeled hypotonic or hypertonic, respectively. *Hypotonic* fluids are distributed in proportions of one third to the extracellular compartment and two thirds to the intracellular compartment. They are associated with cell swelling. When *hypertonic* fluids are added to the vascular space, the extracellular osmolality becomes greater than that of intracellular fluid. As a result, water moves from the intracellular to the extracellular compartment, and cells shrink.

Regulation of Volume and Osmolality

Although intake of water and electrolytes may fluctuate on a day-to-day basis, fluid volume and composition remain relatively unchanged in conditions of health. A variety of homeostatic mechanisms maintain the constancy of body fluids despite changing environmental conditions.

Extracellular Volume Regulation

The need for perfusion of body tissues requires a continuous supply of circulating blood. Through several interre-

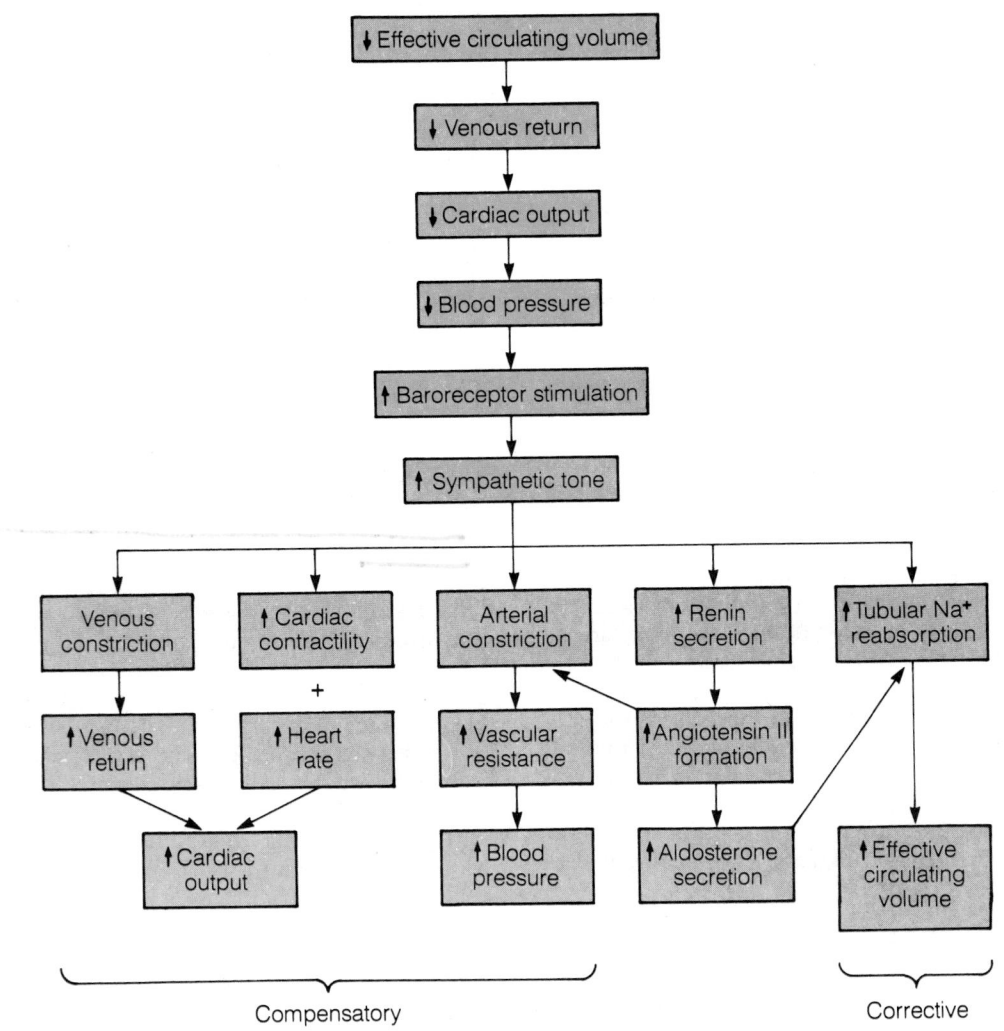

Figure 9-2. Response to decreased extracellular volume. When blood volume decreases, compensatory and corrective activities are initiated by the autonomic nervous system. (Redrawn from Rose BD: Clinical Physiology of Acid–Base and Electrolyte Disorders, p 143, New York, McGraw–Hill, 1977. Copyright © 1977, McGraw–Hill. Used with the permission of the McGraw–Hill Book Company.)

lated activities, the autonomic nervous system maintains blood volume within narrow limits.

Changes in vascular status are sensed by areas of specialized nerve tissue that respond by mechanical stretch to a rise in blood pressure or volume. These receptors are called pressoreceptors or *baroreceptors*. Although baroreceptors are probably located in a variety of areas, those within the carotid arteries and aortic arch are most frequently described. When blood volume is decreased, the stretching of these baroreceptors diminishes, and input to the brain stem is changed. Parasympathetic nervous system activity therefore decreases, and sympathetic nervous system activity increases. Within the heart, sympathetic activity is mediated primarily by epinephrine and increases heart rate and contractility. The vascular response, caused predominantly by norepinephrine, is arterial and venous constriction. This response both accommodates the vascular bed to its smaller volume and contributes the 70% of the blood volume contained within veins. Decreases in blood volume are also relayed to the kidneys, and the enzyme renin is released. Through a series of steps, renin causes secretion of aldosterone, which increases water and sodium reabsorption in isotonic proportions. Thus, an increase in blood volume occurs. These activities are summarized in Figure 9-2.

Increases in blood volume and pressure lead to opposite effects. Parasympathetic activity predominates, and circulating blood volume and pressure are ultimately decreased.

Extracellular Osmolality Regulation

Serum osmolality is regulated by the effects of antidiuretic hormone (ADH), a hormone synthesized in the hypothalamus and stored in the posterior pituitary. Changes in osmolality are sensed by receptors located in the hypothalamus. When osmolality is increased, ADH is released and acts on the distal tubules and collecting ducts of the kidney, so that they become more permeable to water. Thus, more electrolyte-free water is reabsorbed, and urine is excreted in a concentrated form. The sensation of thirst is stimulated in a similar fashion, resulting in increased water intake. As a consequence of both processes, osmolality returns to normal.

ADH is also released when the circulating blood volume is severely decreased. This effect is a late attempt to maintain enough blood volume to perfuse tissues (Fig. 9-3).

When the serum osmolality decreases, the secretion of ADH is reduced. The permeability of the distal tubules and collecting ducts of the kidney is decreased, so that the excess water can be excreted as urine.

▷ Fluid and Electrolyte Disturbances

Disorders of body fluid balance can affect either volume or osmolality. Although disturbances of volume and osmolality can occur simultaneously, they will be discussed separately first.

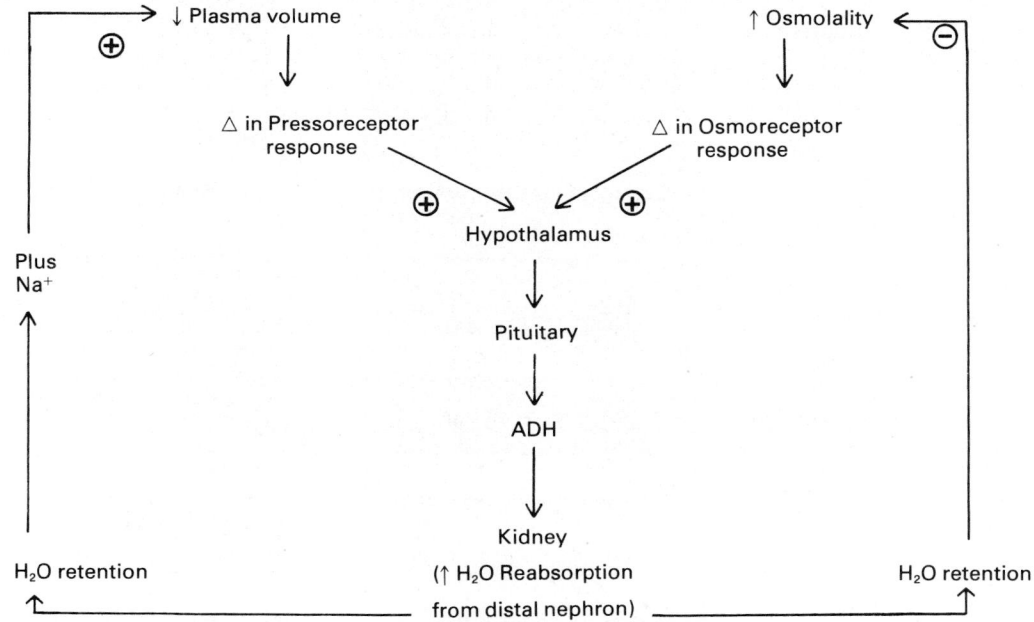

Figure 9-3. ADH-induced water retention. The major stimulus for ADH secretion is increased serum osmolality. A secondary stimulus is a severe decrease in extracellular volume. (From Rokosky JS and Shaver J: Fluid and electrolyte balance. In Underhill SL et al: Cardiac Nursing, p 90. Philadelphia, JB Lippincott, 1982.)

Terminology used to describe alterations in fluid volume or osmolality can be a source of confusion. Synonyms for gains or losses of extracellular fluid volume include saline excess and deficit, isotonic expansion and contraction, extracellular fluid excess and deficit, and hypervolemia and hypovolemia. Synonyms for alterations in serum osmolality include water excess and deficit, intracellular excess and deficit, hyponatremia and hypernatremia, and water intoxication and dehydration.

Extracellular Volume Disturbances

Extracellular Volume Excess (Saline Excess, Isotonic Expansion, Extracellular Fluid Excess, Hypervolemia)

An extracellular volume increase occurs when excessive isotonic fluid is administered or retained. This effect is illustrated in Figure 9-4B, which depicts graphically what happens when 3 liters of isotonic fluid are added. One liter is distributed to the vascular space and two liters to the interstitial space. Because the fluid is isotonic, extracellular osmolality remains the same as intracellular osmolality, and water does not move between the two compartments.

Causes. An extracellular volume excess may be caused by the administration of intravenous fluid at a rate beyond renal capacity for excretion. This risk is greatest in individuals with impaired kidney function or in infants or elderly people. Extracellular volume excess can also result from renal disease that limits sodium and water excretion. Congestive heart failure and cirrhosis of the liver may impair circulation to the kidneys, leading to a compensatory rise in sodium and water reabsorption. Fluid retention following the administration of large doses of corticosteroids results from the increased levels of aldosterone.

Manifestations. Signs of an extracellular volume excess are those of an expanded extracellular volume. When the excess occurs within the vascular space, the effects include elevated blood pressure, fuller pulse, neck vein distention, and increased central venous pressure. The increase in interstitial fluid creates edema. A liter of water weighs 1 kg, or 2.2 pounds. Therefore, rapid weight gain is often an indication of increased extracellular volume. When severe enough, the volume overload may exceed the capacity of the left ventricle to pump it systematically. Consequently, fluid backs up into the lungs, and pulmonary edema results. Because serum osmolality does not change, serum sodium values are unaffected. If the excess develops rapidly, the hematocrit may decrease, because the proportion of red cells to fluid has decreased.

Treatment. An extracellular volume excess is treated according to its severity. Isotonic intravenous fluids, such as 0.9% saline and lactated Ringer's solution, are withheld. In addition, dietary sodium is often limited because it tends to increase water retention. When more severe, diuretics may be required to eliminate the excessive fluid.

Nursing Assessment and Interventions. An important role for the nurse is to determine the degree of risk and, whenever indicated, to assess for extracellular volume excess. Specific assessment measures include obtaining daily weights, keeping intake and output records, and checking for edema in the legs of ambulatory patients or sacrum of patients on bed rest. Girth measurements of the abdomen or extremities are helpful in some instances, because circumference may increase even when pitting edema is not detected. When pulmonary edema is suspected, the lungs should be auscultated for crackles and other abnormal lung sounds.

In addition to administering diuretics and otherwise implementing physician requests, interventions should be initiated to increase patient comfort and level of knowledge about the problem. For example, elevating the backrest usually eases breathing for someone with pulmonary edema. Teaching about the diet helps a patient manage sodium restriction at home.

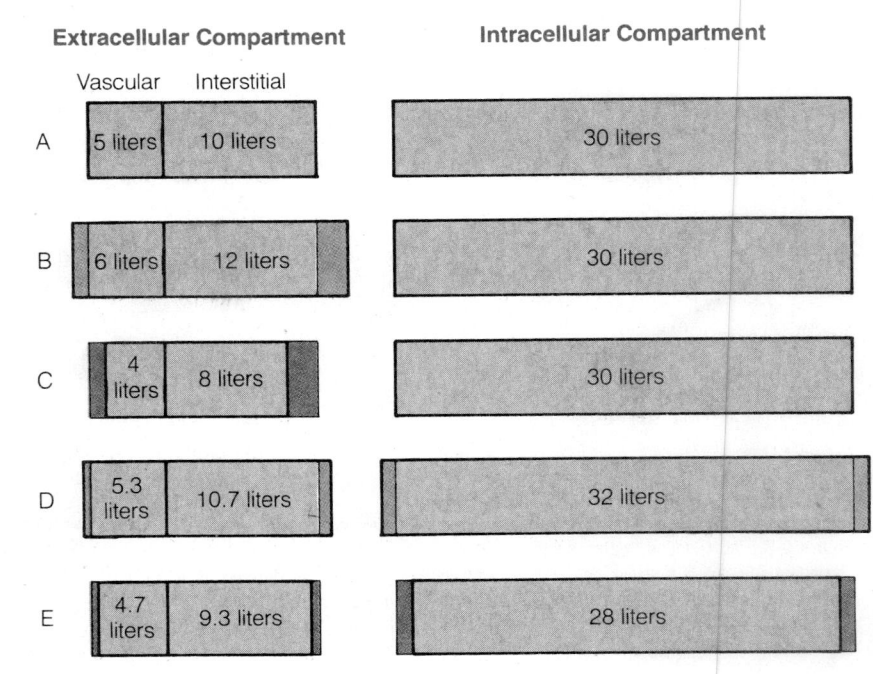

Figure 9-4. (A) Normal fluid distribution approximates ⅓ extracellular (⅓ vascular; ⅔ interstitial) and ⅔ intracellular. For 45 liters, the distribution is 15 liters extracellular (5 liters vascular; 10 liters interstitial) and 30 liters intracellular.
(B) Addition of 3 liters of isotonic fluid; all fluid remains in the extracellular compartment.
(C) Removal of 3 liters of isotonic fluid; all fluid is removed from the extracellular compartment.
(D) Addition of 3 liters of "free" water; 1 liter is added to extracellular compartment and 2 liters to intracellular compartment.
(E) Removal of 3 liters of "free" water; 1 liter is removed from extracellular compartment, and 2 liters are removed from intracellular compartment.

Extracellular Volume Deficit (Saline Deficit, Isotonic Contraction, Extracellular Fluid Deficit, Hypovolemia)

An extracellular volume deficit occurs when isotonic fluid is lost from the body. Figure 9-4C illustrates that when 3 liters of isotonic fluid are removed, 1 liter is lost from the vascular space and 2 liters are lost from the interstitial fluid. Because extracellular osmolality is unchanged, water does not shift between the intracellular and extracellular fluid compartments.

Causes. The most obvious cause of an extracellular volume deficit is blood loss. Bleeding may be readily apparent or occult. Another cause of extracellular volume deficit is excessive elimination by the kidneys. This may occur in some forms of renal failure and is a hazard of diuretic therapy. Instead of being eliminated, extracellular fluid can also be trapped within a body cavity. *Third space accumulation* is the term used to describe this phenomenon, in which abnormal amounts of extracellular fluid are sequestered. Burns, cirrhosis of the liver, and peritonitis are examples of conditions that can cause extracellular fluid to be trapped in this manner.

Clinical Manifestations. Signs of an extracellular volume deficit are those of inadequate vascular volume. A postural blood pressure drop is a key sign. The blood pressure is checked with the patient supine, then repeated in sitting and standing positions. Normally, the sympathetic nervous system counteracts the tendency of gravity to cause pooling of blood in dependent parts. When extracellular volume is decreased, sympathetic tone is inadequate to maintain blood volume, and the blood pressure decreases with upright posture. If changing the position from supine to sitting or standing results in a heart rate increase and either a drop in systolic pressure by 15 mm Hg or a drop in diastolic blood pressure by 10 mm Hg, extracellular volume depletion should be suspected. Other corroborating signs include collapsed neck veins, weight loss, a rise in hematocrit and serum albumin values, and a subnormal central venous pressure reading. When severe, extracellular volume depletion culminates in hypovolemic shock.

Third space losses also cause manifestations of vascular deficit. However, because the fluid is trapped within the body, weight gain and edema may be present simultaneously.

Treatment. The goal of therapy is restoration of blood volume to an adequate circulating level. Isotonic fluids, such as lactated Ringer's solution and 0.9% saline, are administered intravenously. For the patient in shock owing to hemorrhage, blood transfusions are indicated.

Nursing Assessment and Interventions. Patients should be questioned or assessed for a history of bleeding, vomiting, diuresis, or other types of fluid loss. Those patients predicted to be at risk should have frequent postural blood pressure measurements. Additional information may be gained from assessing neck veins, reviewing the hematocrit and serum albumin values, and checking for weight loss. Urine output should also be monitored frequently. As vascular volume drops, the inadequately perfused kidneys are stimulated to reabsorb more sodium and water, and urine output progressively falls.

Positioning is important to maximize cerebral blood flow as well as to maintain adequate circulating volume.

Patients in shock must be positioned flat or with their legs elevated. The Trendelenburg (head-down) position should not be used because it restricts movement of the diaphragm. Persons chronically at risk of extracellular volume deficit, such as those on long-term diuretic therapy, are at risk of fainting when they try to stand. They should be taught to do leg exercises and to get up slowly.

Osmolality Disturbances

In contrast to a gain or loss of isotonic fluid, which affects only the extracellular space, changes in body fluid osmolality affect both the extracellular and intracellular compartments. Whenever osmolality in one compartment is altered, water shifts to balance the osmolality. As a result, osmolality in both compartments becomes equally increased or decreased.

Decreased Serum Osmolality (Water Excess, Intracellular Fluid Excess, Hyponatremia, Water Intoxication)

Figure 9-4D illustrates what happens when 3 liters of electrolyte-free water are added to the extracellular space: 1 liter stays within the extracellular space (one third vascular and two thirds interstitial), and 2 liters move to the intracellular compartment. Both intracellular and extracellular compartments now contain abnormally dilute fluid. The additional fluid in the intracellular compartment causes cells to swell. Because only a small percentage of water remains within the vascular space, manifestations of extracellular volume excess do not occur.

Causes. A decreased serum osmolality can result from excessive ADH secretion by the posterior pituitary, so that more electrolyte-free water is retained by the kidney. Causes of increased ADH secretion include stressful situations, such as pain, trauma, and surgery, and some malignant conditions in which the tumor secretes an ADH-like substance. In most instances, enough water cannot be taken orally to decrease serum osmolality unless renal excretion of electrolyte-free water is impaired. However, rapid infusions of hypotonic fluid can produce this effect.

Clinical Manifestations. Whenever extracellular osmolality decreases, water passively shifts to the intracellular compartment until the intracellular and extracellular osmolalities match. Because the ratio of ions to water has decreased in the extracellular compartment, the serum sodium value drops below normal. As water moves into cells, cell volume increases. The swelling of brain cells leads to neurologic dysfunction. Common symptoms indicating the serum sodium value is under 125 mEq/liter include nausea and malaise. As the condition worsens, changes in mental status, such as confusion and inappropriate behavior, develop, and if not corrected, seizures and coma ultimately result. In general, neurologic dysfunction is most likely to occur when the osmolality disturbance develops rapidly.

Management. The primary way in which a decreased serum osmolality is treated is by restriction of water and other electrolyte-free solutions. Both orally ingested fluids and those that are administered parenterally are severely limited until the serum sodium value returns to normal range. Because brain cells partially adapt to a lowered osmolality over time, hypertonic solutions that draw water out of cells are used only in extreme situations.

Nursing Assessment and Interventions. For patients identified as being at risk, frequent monitoring of serum sodium values is a most important assessment tool. The presence of neurologic symptoms together with a decreased serum sodium value strongly suggests decreased osmolality. In addition to tap water, oral liquids to be restricted include all those that are low in sodium, the major contributor to extracellular osmolality. Examples include coffee, tea, and many juices. IV solutions of 5% dextrose in water are also withheld. Although the dextrose contained in 5% dextrose in water allows the solution to be intravenously administered without bursting red cells, it is rapidly metabolized, leaving only electrolyte-free water.

Increased Serum Osmolality (Water Deficit, Intracellular Fluid Deficit, Hypernatremia, Dehydration)

Figure 9-4E shows that when 3 liters of electrolyte-free water are removed from the body, 1 liter is contributed by the extracellular space (one third vascular and two thirds interstitial) and 2 liters are contributed by the intracellular space. The osmolality in both compartments increases. Within the intracellular compartment, the loss of volume causes cells to shrink. However, the fluid loss from the extracellular compartment is proportionally so small that manifestations of extracellular volume deficit do not occur.

Causes. Normally, an increase in osmolality triggers the sensation of thirst, mediated by the hypothalamus. Water is ingested, and the osmolality returns to normal. If someone is confused, comatose, or otherwise unable to respond to thirst, the serum osmolality will continue to rise. Diabetes insipidus refers to deficient ADH secretion and can be a temporary or permanent result of brain trauma or malignancy. Huge volumes of dilute urine are excreted, and the serum osmolality progressively rises. Copious, dilute urine is also produced in some forms of renal failure because the kidneys are unable to concentrate urine. When high-protein tube feedings are administered, the high osmolar load requires large urine volumes to excrete metabolic end products. If the patient is unable to respond to thirst and if adequate water is not provided, the serum osmolality will rise.

Clinical Manifestations. Movement of water out of the intracellular compartment causes cells to shrink. As brain cells decrease in volume, mental changes occur that are similar to those resulting from a decreased serum osmolality. Serum sodium values rise, indicating that the ratio of particles to water has increased.

Treatment/Management. An increased serum osmolality is treated by the administration of electrolyte-free water until the serum sodium value returns to normal. Correction is gradual to prevent inducing seizures or other neurologic complications.

Nursing Assessment and Interventions. The primary indication of an increased serum osmolality is an increased serum sodium value, which should be routinely monitored in patients believed to be at risk. Evaluation of mental status, intake and output recordings, and urine specific gravity measurements provide corroborating information. Fluids

used to treat an increased serum osmolality include all oral liquids that are sodium-free and 5% dextrose in water given intravenously. Prophylaxis for unconscious or tube-fed patients is possible by calculating water losses and administering enough water for replacement.

Combined Volume and Osmolality Imbalances

Volume and osmolality disturbances frequently coexist. Each is diagnosed and treated separately in the manner previously outlined.

Extracellular Volume Deficit and Osmolality Increase

This combination of problems usually results when transcellular fluids are lost. Although these secretions are components of extracellular fluid, they generally have a lower electrolyte concentration than vascular and interstitial fluids (Table 9-3). Therefore, loss of these fluids in quantity causes the loss of proportionately more water than isotonic fluid, and both an extracellular volume deficit and an increased serum osmolality develop. The extracellular volume deficit is diagnosed by postural blood pressure values and other manifestations of vascular fluid inadequacy. Treatment is by replacement of isotonic fluid. An elevated serum sodium value indicates increased serum osmolality, which is managed by administration of water orally or by 5% dextrose parenterally.

Prophylactic measures can often be initiated to prevent serious deficits from developing. For example, a person suffering from vomiting or diarrhea needs both isotonic and hypotonic fluid replacement. If the person is able to take fluids orally, he should be taught to drink some electrolyte-free liquids, such as weak tea, and some liquids containing sodium, such as meat broth. Similarly, patients on nasogastric suction require intravenous therapy that includes both isotonic and hypotonic fluid. For that reason, hypotonic and isotonic solutions are often alternated.

Extracellular Volume Deficit and Osmolality Decrease

This situation may develop if only hypotonic solutions are used to treat the combination just described. Because the extracellular volume deficit has not been corrected with isotonic fluids, it persists. Eventually, continued replacement with hypotonic fluid causes osmolality to decrease and is manifested by a decreased serum sodium value.

These problems may also result from a significant loss of extracellular volume. Antidiuretic hormone is released as a late compensatory maneuver to increase body fluid. This sequence is seen in severe hypovolemic shock.

Treatment includes correcting the extracellular volume deficit by isotonic fluid replacement and by restricting water and other hypotonic fluids.

Extracellular Volume Excess and Osmolality Decrease

Isotonic fluid retention is a feature of chronic conditions, such as liver and heart failure, in which circulating blood volume is impaired, even though the total extracellular volume is expanded. Eventually, ADH secretion rises as an

Table 9-3
Mean Electrolyte Content of the Transcellular Fluids

Fluid	Na⁺ (mEq/liter)	K⁺ (mEq/liter)	Cl⁻ (mEq/liter)	HCO₃⁻ (mEq/liter)
Saliva	33	20	34	0
Gastric juices*	60	9	84	0
Bile	149	5	101	45
Pancreatic juice	141	5	77	92
Ileal fluid	129	11	116	29
Cecal fluid	80	21	48	22
Cerebrospinal fluid	141	3	127	23
Sweat	45	5	58	0

* The Cl^- concentration exceeds the $Na^+ + K^+$ concentration by 15 mEq/liter in gastric juice. This largely represents the secretion of H^+ by the parietal cells.

(From Rose BD: Clinical Physiology of Acid–Base and Electrolyte Disorders, p 22. New York, McGraw–Hill, 1977. Copyright © 1977, McGraw–Hill. Used with the permission of the McGraw–Hill Book Company.)

attempt to compensate for the inadequate circulating volume. Treatment involves restriction of both isotonic and hypotonic fluids. Because disease is severe at this point, treatment is often only moderately successful.

Extracellular Volume Excess and Osmolality Increase

This combination can result from excessive water restriction in the previous situation or from administration of too much hypertonic solution. Normal osmolality is restored by administration of water or other hypotonic solutions. Isotonic fluids continue to be withheld.

▷ Ionic Disturbances

During the cellular action potential, which allows transmission of electrical impulses, sodium ions flow into the cell and potassium ions move out. Other ions (in particular, calcium) influence the level at which an action potential is triggered. An electrical gradient is generated by the difference between extracellular and intracellular concentrations of ions. Therefore, alterations in the concentration of ions contained within extracellular fluid often lead to changes in the excitability of cells throughout the body.

Potassium

Of the total potassium contained in the body, 98% is contained within cells, and only a small fraction is found within extracellular fluid. As a result, small fluctuations in extracellular potassium values (normal values, 3.0 mEq/liter–5.3 mEq/liter) markedly change the intracellular-to-extracellular potassium gradient and affect neuromuscular transmission. By varying the amount of potassium secreted into urine, the kidneys carefully regulate serum potassium balance. This regulation is important because dietary intake fluctuates from one day to the next. Most foods, except some that are highly refined, contain some potassium. Dietary intake generally ranges from 1875 mg to 5625 mg of potassium per day.

Decreased Serum Potassium: Hypokalemia

Causes. Because potassium is contained in a wide variety of foods, oral intake is rarely inadequate unless there is an increase in renal excretion. Renal elimination is increased by many diuretics and by aldosterone. Vomiting and diarrhea increase potassium loss through the gastrointestinal tract. Hypokalemia can also result from a shift in potassium from extracellular to intracellular fluid without actual elimination from the body. A major cause of this type of shift is alkalosis, which is described later in this chapter.

Clinical Manifestations. Hypokalemia widens the ratio between extracellular and intracellular potassium levels so that it becomes increasingly difficult for cells to reach the threshold at which action potentials can occur. The consequence of this impairment in neuromuscular transmission is the development of weakness in all types of muscle. Skeletal muscle weakness characteristically begins in the legs, then progresses up the trunk. When the serum potassium value drops below 1.5 mEq/liter, involvement of respiratory muscles may lead to apnea. Symptoms owing to weakness of gastrointestinal smooth muscle include anorexia, nausea, vomiting, and constipation. Interference with conduction of electrical impulses within the heart can lead to arrhythmias. A variety of changes in the electrocardiogram pattern may occur, the most characteristic of which is the appearance of U waves (Fig. 9-5). Hypokalemia predisposes to the development of digitalis toxicity. For this reason, patients being treated with both digitalis and a potassium-wasting diuretic are routinely given potassium supplements. Renal function also changes in hypokalemia. The kidneys become less sensitive to ADH, and copious dilute urine is excreted.

Management. If possible, potassium replacement should be accomplished through dietary means. For example, persons receiving potassium-wasting diuretics can be taught to eat foods high in potassium, such as those listed below.

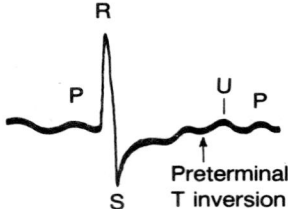

Figure 9-5. Electrocardiogram in hypokalemia. Note increased height of U wave.

Foods High in Potassium

(Over 400 mg [10 mEq] per serving)*

Avocado, ½
Banana, 1 medium
Cantaloupe, 1 cup
Dates, 10 medium
Figs, dried, 5 medium
Fish, lean types, 3 ounces
Grapefruit juice, 1 cup
Honeydew melon, 1 cup
Molasses, 2 Tbsp
Nectarine, 1 large
Orange juice, 1 cup
Potato, baked or boiled, 1 medium
Prunes, 10 medium
Prune juice, ¾ cup
Soybeans, cooked, ½ cup
Tomato juice, canned, low sodium, 1 cup

Salt substitutes are another means of replacement, because potassium is the ion substituted for sodium in these preparations. Pharmacologic replacement can either be oral or intravenous. Before any potassium supplement is administered, adequate urine output must be confirmed. Because oral preparations are bitter-tasting and may cause gastrointestinal irritation, they should be well diluted. Intravenous forms of potassium can cause cardiac arrest if administered too rapidly. For this reason, the potassium is usually diluted to a concentration of no greater than 40 mEq/liter and, in this diluted form, administered at a rate of 16 mEq to 20 mEq per hour.

Increased Serum Potassium: Hyperkalemia

Causes. Renal failure is the most common cause of hyperkalemia. Movement of potassium from the intracellular to extracellular fluid is another cause. A common mechanism is acidosis, which is described later in this chapter. When massive tissue destruction occurs, such as burns, crush injuries, and other types of trauma, large quantities of potassium are released into the extracellular fluid.

* Data from Suitor CW, Hunter MF: Nutrition: Principles and Application in Health Promotion, p 448. Philadelphia, JB Lippincott, 1980.

Clinical Manifestations. Although it seems paradoxical, both hypokalemia and hyperkalemia cause muscle weakness. In the case of hyperkalemia, the difference between extracellular and intracellular potassium concentrations decreases, so that cells are initially able to undergo action potentials more easily. Soon, however, the ability of cells to repolarize is affected, and cells lose their capacity to fire. Skeletal muscle weakness is usually severe once the serum potassium value reaches 8 mEq/liter. Within the heart, transmission of impulses is also affected. Major changes in the electrocardiogram include increased height of T waves, widening of the QRS complex, and, at terminal stages, the appearance of sine waves (Fig. 9-6). Death occurs from ventricular fibrillation or standstill.

Management. How hyperkalemia is treated depends on both cause and severity. Emergency treatment is required when the serum potassium value is greater than 8 mEq/liter or when muscle weakness or electrocardiogram changes appear. In these circumstances, measures are used to temporarily antagonize the effects of potassium or drive it back into cells. Intravenous administration of calcium, glucose, and insulin, or of bicarbonate, accomplishes this effect. These techniques are also valuable when potassium has shifted from the intracellular to the extracellular compartment without exceeding the normal quantity of potassium within the body. When both the intracellular and extracellular concentrations of potassium are elevated, efforts are made to increase potassium excretion. Measures include the administration of cation-exchange resins, such as sodium polystyrene sulfonate (Kayexalate), which allow more potassium to be excreted in stool, and renal dialysis. Persons with persistent hyperkalemia, such as those in chronic renal failure, need to limit dietary intake of potassium. Because potassium is so widely distributed in food, dietary restriction is difficult to achieve. Potassium-containing medications, such as potassium penicillin, must also be avoided. Maintenance of adequate caloric intake and regular exercise within prescribed limits helps prevent tissue catabolism, which may further raise serum potassium levels.

Calcium

Most calcium is contained within bones and teeth, where it provides a strengthening force. However, the small quantity contained within extracellular fluid has numerous important physiologic functions. It affects the threshold at which cellular action potentials can occur and is required

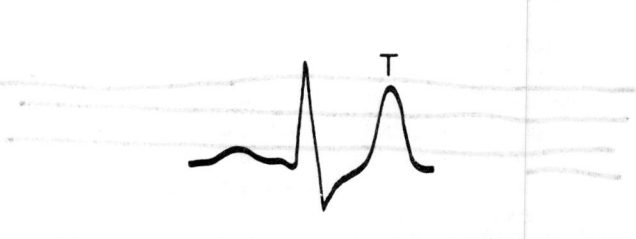

Figure 9-6. Electrocardiogram in hyperkalemia, showing widening QRS complex, decreased amplitude of P wave, and peaked T wave.

for skeletal muscle contraction. In addition, minute quantities of calcium are essential for normal blood clotting.

Slightly less than half the plasma calcium exists in the charged or ionized form that is capable of function. The remainder is bound to plasma protein and, although inactive, is a pool of additional calcium. Unless specialized laboratory equipment is used, serum values reflect both ionized and protein-bound forms. The normal range for total calcium is 8.5 mg/deciliter to 10.5 mg/deciliter. Serum levels usually vary in an opposite direction from those of phosphate: as the serum calcium rises, serum phosphate decreases, and vice versa. The calcium level is largely regulated by the combined actions of parathyroid hormone and vitamin D. When the serum calcium value falls, these substances increase calcium absorption from the gastrointestinal tract and mobilization from bone so that serum levels return to normal. The recommended daily dietary allowance for calcium is 800 mg per day for adults.

Decreased Serum Calcium: Hypocalcemia

Causes.   One cause of hypocalcemia is a deficiency of parathyroid hormone. The four tiny parathyroid glands are situated immediately behind the thyroid gland, and their inadvertent removal is a rare complication of thyroidectomy. Another cause of hypocalcemia is impaired absorption of vitamin D from the gastrointestinal tract. This problem may accompany a variety of disturbances in which absorption of fat-soluble vitamins is impaired. When massive blood transfusions are administered, the citrate contained in the blood to prevent its clotting may bind with calcium and lead to hypocalcemia. Increased binding of calcium to serum protein also results in hypocalcemia. In this case, the serum calcium value is normal, but the active portion is decreased.

Clinical Manifestations.   A decrease in serum calcium alters the threshold at which action potentials occur so that cells can fire more easily. Hypocalcemia thus results in enhanced motor nerve excitability. Symptoms include sensations of numbness or tingling, muscle twitches, cramps, and hyperactive reflexes. Two classic techniques to evoke the hyperactivity of calcium deficit are testing for Chvostek's sign and Trousseau's sign. To test for *Chvostek's sign,* the facial nerve is tapped in front of the ear, and the mouth is observed for twitching. To test for *Trousseau's sign,* a blood pressure cuff is applied to the arm and inflated between diastolic and systolic levels for 3 minutes. A positive response is carpal spasm, an infolding of the hand. When very severe, hypocalcemia may cause tetany, involuntary spasms of skeletal muscle. Effects of severe hypocalcemia ultimately progress to cardiac arrest.

Management.   Patients at risk for hypocalcemia, such as those undergoing thyroidectomy, must be observed carefully and have their serum calcium values monitored. Mild decreases in serum calcium can be corrected by the administration of oral calcium salts or vitamin D. If the calcium deficit is severe enough to cause tetany or cardiovascular problems, cautious intravenous replacement is required. Persons with long-term calcium deficiencies should be taught which foods are high in calcium, such as those listed below.

*Foods High in Calcium**

Dairy Products (alone or as ingredient)

Cheese
Cream
Ice cream
Milk
Yogurt

Other Foods (in large quantity)

Blackstrap molasses
Bok choy
Broccoli
Collards
Kale
Mustard greens
Salmon, canned
Sardines
Tofu
Turnip greens

Increased Serum Calcium: Hypercalcemia

Causes.   Hypercalcemia is a common and serious complication of cancer, particularly when the tumor has invaded bone. Prolonged immobility also results in bone breakdown, causing the serum concentration of calcium to rise. Hyperparathyroidism is yet another mechanism and most commonly results from malignancy of the parathyroid glands.

Clinical Manifestations.   Hypercalcemia alters the electrical threshold of cell membranes, causing action potentials to become more difficult to elicit. Calcium excess thus has a depressant effect on nerve conduction and muscle contraction. Muscle weakness, decreased muscle tone, and gastrointestinal symptoms, such as nausea and anorexia, are common results. Because hypercalcemia accompanies excessive breakdown of bone, pathologic fractures are also a frequent complication. The filtration of high calcium levels through the kidney can lead to the formation of kidney stones and can ultimately impair renal function. Calcium can be deposited in soft tissues as well. Within the heart, effects of hypercalcemia are similar to those of digitalis. Arrhythmias occur and may culminate in cardiac arrest.

Management.   A variety of methods are used to treat hypercalcemia. Both isotonic fluid and diuretics are administered to enhance calcium excretion in the urine. Calcitonin, a calcium-lowering hormone produced by the thyroid gland, is also sometimes administered. Corticosteroids inhibit calcium absorption and shift the calcium to the intracellular space. Sodium bicarbonate causes more calcium to be protein-bound and thus decreases the active portion.

Because calcium and phosphate ions have a reciprocal relationship within extracellular fluid, administration of phosphate lowers the serum calcium level. For long-term treatment, oral preparations of phosphate are used. In

* Data from Suitor CW, Hunter MF: Nutrition: Principles and Application in Health Promotion, p 448. Philadelphia, JB Lippincott, 1980.

emergency situations, intravenous phosphate may be administered. However, phosphate is contraindicated in some instances, the most common of which is chronic renal failure. In this situation, phosphate excretion is impaired, and calcium levels are initially low. As a compensatory response, parathyroid hormone secretion rises, and calcium levels are secondarily increased as well.

Persons with chronic hypercalcemia need to avoid dietary sources of calcium. They should also be taught to keep fluid intake high to minimize the likelihood of calcium stone formation in the kidneys. When hypercalcemia is a result of immobility, measures to promote active weight bearing should be employed. Hypercalcemia potentiates the effects of digitalis. For this reason, administration of digitalis to hypercalcemic patients is hazardous.

Phosphate

The body contains phosphorous ion in the form of numerous phosphate salts. Within cells, phosphate ions provide most of the negative charge to balance the positively charged potassium ions. Intracellular concentrations of phosphate are also essential for many aspects of metabolism, as constituents of enzymes that affect oxygen delivery and energy transfer, and as ingredients of bone. Both intracellular and extracellular concentrations of phosphate help neutralize the acids produced during cell metabolism. Extracellular levels of phosphate rise or fall in an opposite direction from those of calcium so that the product of the two ions remains constant. Regulation of phosphate levels is primarily controlled by vitamin D and parathyroid hormone, both of which stimulate intestinal absorption of phosphate and its release from bone. Parathyroid hormone also increases the excretion of phosphate by the kidneys, a mechanism that helps to raise the serum calcium level on a reciprocal basis. Ordinarily, the enhanced gastrointestinal absorption of phosphate compensates for its increased renal excretion. The normal serum phosphate value ranges from 2.6 mg/deciliter to 4.8 mg/deciliter. A normal balance of phosphate is maintained by a daily intake of approximately 800 mg.

Decreased Serum Phosphate: Hypophosphatemia

Causes. Malnutrition is an important cause of hypophosphatemia. Inadequate phosphorus absorption from the gastrointestinal tract can result from vomiting, diarrhea, or vitamin D deficiency. If ingested in quantity, many antacids bind phosphate and can produce a similar effect. Alcoholism is another important cause, particularly when combined with malnutrition or if alcohol is withdrawn suddenly. Hyperparathyroidism causes excessive phosphate to be excreted in the urine. As a result of the extensive tissue repair that accompanies intravenous hyperalimentation, phosphate is driven into cells, and serum levels may drop.

Clinical Manifestations. Because phosphate is found within all cells, a decrease has widespread effects. Within the central nervous system, dysfunction can range from mental irritability to seizures or coma. Skeletal muscles become weak. Inadequate phosphate within bones can lead to osteomalacia, a form of bone softening. The cellular dys-

function also extends to hematologic cells and can impair oxygenation, blood clotting, and phagocytosis.

Management. Phosphate should be administered prophylactically to patients at risk, such as recipients of intravenous hyperalimentation. Replacement therapy for mild cases of hypophosphatemia can sometimes be accomplished through the diet by having the patient eat foods high in phosphorus, such as those listed below. Pharmacologic replacement can be oral or parenteral.

Foods High in Phosphorus*

Meats
Milk
Foods with phosphate or phosphoric acid added during processing:
    Carbonated beverages made with phosphoric acid
    Cheese, processed types
    Fabricated potato chips (*e.g.,* Pringles)
    Instant pudding
    Processed meats (*e.g.,* bologna, Canadian bacon, hot dogs)
    Refrigerator bakery products
    Salad dressings of many types

Increased Serum Phosphate: Hyperphosphatemia

Causes. Hyperphosphatemia most commonly results from renal failure, since phosphate ions are no longer excreted in the urine. It can also result from hypoparathyroidism. A rare cause is acromegaly, a pituitary condition in which excess bone activity occurs.

Clinical Manifestations. Because of the reciprocal relationship between phosphate and calcium, elevated serum phosphate levels are usually associated with hypocalcemia. All of the manifestations already described for hypocalcemia may thus occur. Phosphate and calcium crystals can also be deposited in the kidneys and soft tissues.

Management. Foods high in phosphate should be avoided. Antacids containing aluminum effectively bind phosphate and permit its excretion in stool. If renal function is adequate, diuretics may help eliminate the excess phosphate. In the case of renal failure, dialysis can be used instead.

Magnesium

Most magnesium is found within cells, where it activates enzymes and plays a role in carbohydrate and protein metabolism. Magnesium has an interdependent relationship with calcium, and an excess or deficit produces many effects similar to calcium excess or deficit. Excretion of magnesium is controlled by the kidneys. Aldosterone increases excretion, while parathyroid hormone decreases excretion. The normal serum value for magnesium is 1.4 mEq/liter to 2.2 mEq/liter. Dietary requirements for magnesium are 350 mg for men and 300 mg for women.

---

* Data from Boykin LS: Nutrition in Nursing, p 163. New York, Medical Examination Publishing Company, 1975; and from Suitor CW, Hunter MF: Nutrition: Principles and Application in Health Promotion, p 313. Philadelphia, JB Lippincott, 1980.

Decreased Serum Magnesium: Hypomagnesemia

Causes. Excessive excretion of magnesium in the urine may result from alcoholism, diuretic therapy, or increased aldosterone levels. Prolonged malnutrition or conditions leading to gastrointestinal malabsorption can also cause magnesium deficiency.

Clinical Manifestations. As with calcium deficiency, magnesium depletion increases the excitability of nerves. Symptoms such as numbness and tingling, muscle cramps, and tetany thus may occur, and Chvostek's and Trousseau's signs can be elicited. It is believed that hypomagnesemia may induce digitalis toxicity, an effect that often occurs in conjunction with potassium depletion. Both calcium and potassium values usually drop as a result of hypomagnesemia.

Management. Foods high in magnesium are listed below. Magnesium sulfate can be administered orally, intramuscularly, or intravenously, depending on the cause and severity of the deficit.

*Foods High in Magnesium**

Bananas
Chocolate
Grapefruit
Green vegetables
Legumes
Nuts
Oranges
Peanut Butter

Increased Serum Magnesium: Hypermagnesemia

Causes. Hypermagnesemia is most frequently a result of kidney failure. When the renal ability to excrete magnesium is impaired, administration of even small amounts of magnesium in the form of antacids or laxatives can cause magnesium excess.

Clinical Manifestations. A moderate elevation of the serum magnesium level may cause hypotension owing to peripheral dilation of blood vessels. As the serum concentration rises further, drowsiness, loss of deep tendon reflexes, coma, and, ultimately, cardiac arrest occur.

Management. Patients in renal failure must limit dietary intake of magnesium and should be taught to avoid magnesium-containing antacids or laxatives. Calcium may be infused to temporarily antagonize the actions of magnesium. Renal dialysis removes magnesium from the serum.

Sodium

Serum sodium values reflect the ratio of sodium and water in extracellular fluid rather than the actual quantity of sodium present. Because excretion and reabsorption of sodium occur together with water, increases or decreases in the content of sodium usually result in a proportionate increase or decrease in extracellular fluid volume. Changes in serum sodium values thus represent alterations in extra-

* Data from Goldberger E: A Primer of Water, Electrolyte and Acid–Base Syndromes, 6th ed, p 359. Philadelphia, Lea & Febiger, 1980.

cellular osmolality, as described earlier in this chapter. The normal range for serum sodium is 135 mEq/liter to 148 mEq/liter.

Chloride

Simultaneous reabsorption and excretion of sodium and chloride preserve the electroneutrality of extracellular fluid. As a result, changes in the chloride concentration usually parallel those of sodium. Gastric fluid, however, contains more chloride per liter than does plasma, so that vomiting or gastrointestinal suction leads to proportionately more chloride than sodium loss. In this situation, chloride is unavailable for reabsorption with sodium, and bicarbonate ion is reabsorbed instead. The result is alkalosis, which is described later under acid–base balance. The normal range for serum chloride is 98 mEq/liter to 106 mEq/liter.

▷ Acid–Base Homeostasis

The acidity of a solution is usually expressed as pH, which is defined as the negative logarithm of the hydrogen ion concentration. Substances that donate hydrogen ions in chemical reactions are *acidic*. Those that accept hydrogen ions are *alkaline* or *basic*. Arterial blood is a slightly alkaline solution with a normal pH range of 7.35 to 7.45. A decrease in the pH below approximately 6.8 or above 7.8 is incompatible with life. Therefore, a variety of homeostatic mechanisms interact to maintain the pH within normal limits.

Normal Acid Production

On a daily basis, an excess of acid is produced that must be neutralized or eliminated in order to maintain an alkaline pH. The bulk of this acid is *carbonic acid*, formed when the carbon in foods is oxidized to yield carbon dioxide. This carbon dioxide combines with water to form carbonic acid, as is illustrated in the following equation:

$$CO_2 + H_2O \rightleftarrows H_2CO_3 \rightleftarrows HCO^- + H^+$$

Carbonic acid is weak, that is, it immediately breaks down to form bicarbonate ion and hydrogen ion. All these reactions are reversible, as is indicated by the arrows in both directions. When carbon dioxide is exhaled by the lungs, the quantity of carbonic acid that can be generated drops. For this reason, carbon dioxide is referred to as an acid, and carbonic acid is described as volatile, since its major ingredient can be exhaled.

A small amount of the acid produced each day is *noncarbonic*. Metabolism of sulfur-containing proteins yields sulfuric acid, and phosphate-containing phospholipids yield phosphoric acid. These acids are nonvolatile, that is, they cannot be excreted by the lungs. Instead, they are excreted exclusively by the kidneys.

Neutralization or Elimination of Body Acid

Acid–base homeostasis is maintained by four interrelated systems: extracellular buffers, the lungs, the kidneys, and cellular buffers. A *buffer* is defined as a chemical that, by being present in a solution, lessens the *pH* change caused by the addition of acid or base. Buffers take up or release hydrogen ions and can be thought of as chemical sponges.

Extracellular Buffers

Quantitatively, the *bicarbonate–carbonic acid* buffer system is the largest in the body. This weak acid and weak base pair combine into different salts when a strong acid or base is added to extracellular fluid. For example, when hydrochloric acid is added to solution, the following reaction ensues:

$$HCl + NaHCO_3 \rightarrow H_2CO_3 + NaCl$$

The strong hydrochloric acid is converted to a neutral salt and carbonic acid. Because the carbonic acid is weak, it immediately breaks down to form carbon dioxide, which is excreted by the lungs. A similar exchange occurs when a strong base, such as sodium hydroxide, is added to extracellular fluid:

$$NaOH + H_2CO_3 \rightarrow NaHCO_3 + H_2O$$

The strong base is thus converted to a weaker one, sodium bicarbonate.

Another buffer is *phosphate,* salts of which can absorb or release hydrogen ions. A strong acid is converted to a weaker form by a phosphate buffer salt, which becomes slightly more acidic:

$$HCl + Na_2HPO_4 \rightarrow NaH_2PO_4$$

The addition of a strong base results in the conversion of the phosphate salt to its slightly alkaline form:

$$NaOH + NaH_2PO_4 \rightarrow Na_2HPO_4 + H_2O$$

Buffering is also effected by *plasma proteins,* which are negatively charged and exist in the form of acid or alkaline salts. They can thus either donate or accept hydrogen ions in a manner similar to that already described for phosphate. All these buffers operate within seconds of the addition of acid or base.

Respiratory Regulation

By altering ventilation, the lungs are able to excrete or retain carbon dioxide and thereby maintain the *pH* within normal limits. When the level of carbon dioxide in arterial blood rises, carbon dioxide diffusion into cerebrospinal fluid influences the cerebral medulla to increase the rate and depth of ventilation. The excess carbon dioxide is thus exhaled. Conversely, decreased levels of carbon dioxide cause a decreased rate and depth of ventilation, again mediated through the medulla. Respiratory adaptation begins within minutes of a change in acid–base status but is limited in its capacity to normalize *pH*.

Renal Regulation

The kidneys' capacity to excrete acid or reabsorb base is virtually unlimited and is accomplished by three mechanisms. The first, *bicarbonate reabsorption,* involves an indirect process whereby sodium and bicarbonate ions are reabsorbed in exchange for hydrogen ions. The hydrogen

ions are reabsorbed to repeat the bicarbonate reabsorption cycle again and again. A second process, the formation of *titratable acid,* refers to the conversion of alkaline phosphate salts to their acidic form, as described earlier. By this mechanism, hydrogen is excreted from the body. Finally, acid is excreted by the *ammonia mechanism.* Ammonia (NH_3) formed by renal cells is changed to ammonium ion (NH_4^+) and is then excreted along with chloride. The renal response to changed acid–base status does not become maximal for several days but can persist indefinitely.

Cellular Buffers

Intracellular buffers contribute to acid–base homeostasis in numerous ways. Buffering by phosphate and protein occurs within cells as well as in extracellular fluid. In addition, the hemoglobin within red blood cells forms a compound with hydrogen ion during its transport by veins to the lungs. Within bones, carbonate (CO_3^{2-}) provides a huge quantity of buffer. When acid is added to plasma, bone carbonate is released into extracellular fluid. In contrast, the administration of base results in increased deposition of carbonate within bone. A final means of cellular buffering involves the exchange of hydrogen and potassium ions between extracellular fluid and cells. In the case of acidosis, hydrogen ions move into cells in exchange for potassium. Alkalosis causes an opposite shift.

Arterial Blood Gas Measurement

The relationships between the *pH* of arterial blood and its content of acid and base are expressed in arterial blood gas measurements. These three components can be viewed as an equation:

$$pH = \frac{PaCO_2}{HCO_3^-}$$

The partial pressure of carbon dioxide is shown by the $PaCO_2$. Because carbonic acid rapidly dissociates into carbon dioxide and water, the $PaCO_2$ value is a good measure of arterial acid quantity. The HCO_3^- value indicates the amount of base present. In order to maintain a normal alkaline *pH*, 20 times more base than acid is present. So long as the base-to-acid ratio remains 20:1, the *pH* does not change. For example, when an increase in body acid is balanced by a proportionate increase in base, the *pH* returns to normal. This process, in which a normal *pH* is achieved by increased acid to balance base, or vice versa, is called *compensation.*

Interpretation of Arterial Blood Gases

Because excretion of carbonic acid is mainly achieved by the lungs, an alteration in $PaCO_2$ reflects a disturbance of respiratory origin. A change in the HCO_3^- value indicates any disorder that is not caused by respiratory dysfunction. Terminology used to describe primary changes in $PaCO_2$ includes respiratory acidosis and alkalosis or carbonic acidosis or alkalosis. The terminology for disorders that are not of respiratory origin is metabolic acidosis and alkalosis or noncarbonic acidosis or alkalosis.

Although certain patient manifestations suggest acidosis or alkalosis, arterial blood gas measurement is the only means by which an acid–base disturbance can be confirmed. The ability to interpret arterial blood gases is therefore an important nursing skill. A sequential method for analyzing blood gases is shown in Chart 9-1.

Arterial Blood Gas Sampling

Specimens for blood gas analysis are usually obtained by arterial puncture. This technique creates the hazards of both hemorrhage and damage to adjacent nerves and should never be attempted without indepth instruction. In addition to the actual technique of drawing arterial blood, obtaining a specimen involves several other aspects. In order to prevent changes in its composition, the specimen is collected in a heparinized syringe, all air is immediately expelled, and it is placed within a container of ice for transport to the laboratory. Firm pressure is applied to the puncture site for at least 5 minutes to prevent hematoma formation. The percentage of oxygen that the patient is breathing and body temperature influence blood gas results and are recorded on the laboratory slip.

▷ Acid–Base Disturbances

Metabolic Disturbances

Metabolic Acidosis

Causes. Many conditions can cause a relative gain in noncarbonic acid. When oxygen is unavailable to cells, as in shock, anaerobic metabolism ensues, and lactic acid is formed as a by-product. Ketoacids are produced when insulin deficiency results in diabetic ketoacidosis. If poisons such as methanol are ingested, various toxic acids accumulate. Severe renal disease may impair the excretion of hydrogen ion. Diarrhea can cause metabolic acidosis because of the loss of bicarbonate ion secreted by the pancreas.

Chart 9-1
Analysis of Arterial Blood Gases

Look at pH. For this maneuver, only a *p*H of 7.4 is considered to be normal, even though the range of normal is actually 7.35 to 7.45.

A *p*H under 7.4 indicates acidemia.
A *p*H over 7.4 indicates alkalemia.

Look at PaCO₂ (range of normal: 35 mm Hg–45 mm Hg). If $PaCO_2$ is normal, there is no primary respiratory problem and no respiratory compensation for a metabolic problem.

Abnormal $PaCO_2$ Values are Interpreted in Relation to *p*H:

↑$PaCO_2$ plus ↓*p*H: acidosis of respiratory origin
↑$PaCO_2$ plus ↑*p*H: respiratory retention of CO_2 to compensate for metabolic alkalosis
↓$PaCO_2$ plus ↑*p*H: alkalosis of respiratory origin
↓$PaCO_2$ plus ↓*p*H: respiratory elimination of CO_2 to compensate for metabolic acidosis

Look at HCO₃⁻ (range of normal: 22 mEq/liter–26 mEq/liter). If HCO_3^- is normal, there is no primary metabolic problem and no metabolic compensation for a respiratory problem.

Abnormal HCO_3^- values are interpreted in relation to *p*H:

↓HCO_3^- plus ↓*p*H: acidosis of metabolic origin
↓HCO_3^- plus ↑*p*H: renal retention of H^+ or elimination of HCO_3^- to compensate for respiratory alkalosis
↑HCO_3^- plus ↑*p*H: alkalosis of metabolic origin
↑HCO_3^- plus ↓*p*H: renal retention of HCO_3^- or elimination of H^+ to compensate for respiratory acidosis

Use Above Findings to Diagnose Acid-Base Status. Possible disorders include compensated or uncompensated respiratory acidosis (synonym, "hypoventilation"), compensated or uncompensated respiratory alkalosis (synonym, "hyperventilation"), compensated or uncompensated metabolic acidosis, and compensated or uncompensated metabolic alkalosis. Simultaneous respiratory and metabolic disorders are also possible. If $PaCO_2$, HCO_3^-, and *p*H are *all* within their normal ranges, acid–base status is normal.

Look at PaO₂ (normal: 80 mm Hg for elderly adults at sea level; 100 mm Hg for young adults at sea level). A PaO_2 below normal for age indicates hypoxemia.

(From Rokosky JS: Assessment of the Individual with Altered Respiratory Function. Nurs Clin North Am 16:198, 1981.)

Clinical Manifestations.   Signs and symptoms result from the response of various tissues to a decreased pH. Early cardiovascular responses include increased blood pressure and heart rate. If the pH drops below 7.15, contractility of the heart decreases, and potentially fatal arrhythmias may develop. Neurologic effects range from lethargy to coma. Hyperkalemia is another result of potassium movement out of cells in exchange for hydrogen. Rapid, deep breathing indicates that respiratory compensation has begun.

When metabolic acidosis is uncompensated, the arterial pH and HCO_3^- values are decreased, but the $PaCO_2$ is normal. As respiratory compensation occurs, the $PaCO_2$ levels drop and the pH moves back up toward normal. However, respiratory compensation cannot completely correct the pH.

Management.   Identification of the underlying mechanisms leading to metabolic acidosis allows the physician to plan specific interventions that will cure the disorder. At the same time, the acidosis itself must be managed to prevent life-threatening reductions in pH. If the pH is maintained over 7.20, severe cardiovascular effects do not usually occur. Raising the pH can be achieved by the intravenous administration of sodium bicarbonate.

As a cellular buffering response, potassium moves out of cells and hydrogen moves in. Acidotic patients thus usually develop hyperkalemia, which is superimposed on their preexisting potassium balance. Management depends on the severity and relationship to pH. Slight hyperkalemia associated with a significant drop in pH does not require immediate intervention. However, the patient with this condition will develop hypokalemia once the pH returns to normal. When hyperkalemia is severe, the effects can be lethal, even if the total body content is normal. This situation is treated by techniques to shift potassium back into cells.

Nursing Assessment and Interventions.   Patients at risk for metabolic acidosis should be assessed for the cardiovascular and neurologic manifestations described earlier. Suspected alterations in acid–base status can only be confirmed by arterial blood gases, however. Persons chronically at risk may benefit from teaching about those situations that predispose them to metabolic acidosis. For example, teaching a diabetic patient that infection increases insulin requirements may help him manage self-care successfully enough to prevent ketoacidosis.

For patients with confirmed metabolic acidosis, much of the care centers around treating the underlying cause and is accomplished in conjunction with the physician. In addition, the nurse should plan care that facilitates respiratory compensation. Positioning to ensure optimal excursion of the thoracic cage is particularly important.

Metabolic Alkalosis

Causes.   Loss of hydrochloric acid from the stomach by vomiting or by gastrointestinal suction is an obvious cause of metabolic alkalosis. If baking soda is ingested in quantity as a home remedy for gastric distress or if more parenteral bicarbonate than is needed to correct metabolic acidosis is administered, metabolic alkalosis will also result.

Metabolic alkalosis is often associated with the concomitant loss of electrolytes and extracellular volume. The kidneys normally respond to an extracellular volume deficit by maximizing the reabsorption of sodium and water. When

chloride ion and extracellular volume are depleted, the reabsorption of sodium becomes more dependent on the secretion of hydrogen or potassium ions. As more hydrogen ion is secreted in exchange for sodium, more bicarbonate is also reabsorbed, and metabolic alkalosis ensues. Hypokalemia causes metabolic alkalosis by a similar mechanism.

Clinical Manifestations.   Metabolic alkalosis increases the amount of extracellular calcium that is bound to protein. As a result, signs and symptoms of hypocalcemia develop. Manifestations of hypokalemia are also common, both because of loss and as a result of cellular buffering. All these signs and symptoms have been described previously.

Uncompensated metabolic alkalosis is diagnosed by increased pH and HCO_3^- values together with a normal $PaCO_2$ value. When the rate and depth of ventilation decrease to compensate, the $PaCO_2$ also drops. Respiratory compensation is never complete.

Management.   In addition to treating other underlying causes, hypochloremia, hypokalemia, and extracellular volume depletion must be corrected. In some situations, these measures do not relieve the alkalosis, and acetazolamide (Diamox) can be administered to increase the renal excretion of bicarbonate.

Cellular buffering compounds hypokalemia caused by the loss of potassium from the body. If considerable potassium has been lost and the pH is markedly increased, these combined effects may result in life-threatening hypokalemia. Simultaneous replacement of potassium and correction of pH are then necessary.

Nursing Assessment and Interventions.   As was already described, the loss of extracellular volume, potassium, or chloride predisposes to the development of metabolic alkalosis. For this reason, patients at risk should be assessed for hypokalemia and extracellular volume deficit as well as for metabolic alkalosis. Laboratory values for chloride and potassium should be closely monitored. Patients at particular risk are those undergoing gastrointestinal suction or receiving diuretic therapy.

When a patient is oxygen deprived, the need to breathe deeply may supersede respiratory compensation for metabolic alkalosis. Thus, patients with metabolic alkalosis should be assessed for hypoxemia and, if necessary, supplemental oxygen should be provided (see Chap. 24).

By teaching, the nurse may prevent metabolic alkalosis from developing in the home setting. For example, the fluid lost by vomiting must be replaced by fluids containing sodium, potassium, and chloride. Among solutions that can be used in the home are salty broth and orange juice. A person who is unable to take liquids for several days should seek medical attention. People should also be taught not to use baking soda as an antacid.

Respiratory Disturbances

Respiratory Acidosis

Causes.   Hypoventilation is a synonym for respiratory acidosis that describes the underlying problem: breathing is inadequate to eliminate carbon dioxide from the arterial blood. Many specific disorders can impair this aspect of lung function. Although any severe lung disease can lead to respiratory acidosis, chronic obstructive pulmonary disease

(COPD) is a particularly common cause. Defective expansion of the chest wall is another mechanism. Paralysis of the diaphragm by spinal cord injury, multiple rib fracture, and congenital abnormalities such as scoliosis are examples of conditions having this effect. Neurologic control of breathing can be temporarily abolished by drug overdose. Hypoventilation can also result from the loss of periodic deep breaths or sighs. Such a loss temporarily accompanies surgical incisions of the chest or upper abdomen.

Clinical Manifestations. The cardiovascular, neurologic, and potassium-related manifestations described under metabolic acidosis are pertinent here as well. Neurologic effects tend to be more pronounced in respiratory acidosis, presumably as a result of rapid carbon dioxide diffusion into cerebrospinal fluid. Headache, blurred vision, and other neurologic findings are often particularly extreme in the morning because less carbon dioxide is eliminated during sleep. When the carbon dioxide value becomes very high, it interferes with alveolar oxygen exchange. In this way, severe respiratory acidosis can cause hypoxemia.

The arterial blood gases for uncompensated respiratory acidosis include decreased pH, increased $PaCO_2$, and normal HCO_3^- values. Renal compensation develops over several days and is represented in the blood gas by an increased HCO_3^-. Renal compensation is highly effective and returns the pH close to normal.

Management. The major goal of therapy is to improve ventilation so that adequate carbon dioxide can be exhaled. Initiating causes for hypoventilation must be identified and treated. Because renal compensation usually restores pH to near-normal levels, chronic respiratory acidosis may not require therapy beyond that for the underlying disorder. In an acute situation, however, mechanical ventilation may be necessary to eliminate the excessive carbon dioxide and to keep the pH within safe limits. Oxygen is administered for severe hypoxemia, and hyperkalemia is managed as described for metabolic acidosis.

Nursing Assessment and Interventions. Situations creating risk for respiratory acidosis must be predicted, and patients at risk must be assessed for hypoventilation. Both rate and depth of ventilation must be observed, since rapid, shallow breathing moves very little air.

Nursing interventions can frequently prevent severe respiratory acidosis. One group of patients at particular risk is surgical patients who have chronic lung disease, are obese, or smoke. Such individuals will benefit from agressive interventions to increase lung expansion, such as frequent deep breathing, use of an incentive spirometer, and ambulation. These same measues are appropriate when respiratory acidosis has been confirmed.

When respiratory acidosis is associated with severe hypoxemia, oxygen therapy is required. COPD may lead to long-standing respiratory acidosis, so that the cerebral medulla is no longer responsive to elevated carbon dioxide levels. Instead, oxygen lack is the only stimulus to ventilation. In this situation, oxygen is administered at low flows so as to maintain this hypoxic drive.

Respiratory Alkalosis

Causes. A synonym for respiratory alkalosis is *hyperventilation,* which means that more carbon dioxide has been exhaled than was produced by body processes. Causes may be of psychological or physiologic origin. Anxiety is a major stimulus to rapid, deep breathing. Many pathophysiologic states are accompanied by anxiety or may in themselves cause hyperventilation. An example is pain. Interference with the neurologic control of ventilation may be caused by drug overdose or may result from damage to the respiratory center in the medulla. When the oxygen content of arterial blood decreases, hyperventilation is an important compensatory mechanism to increase oxygen intake. Finally, respiratory alkalosis may result from mechanical ventilation at too fast a rate.

Clinical Manifestations. A simultaneous increase in the rate and depth of breathing is a major sign. As was described for metabolic alkalosis, changes in serum calcium binding occur and cause manifestations of hypocalcemia. Because carbon dioxide changes are rapidly reflected in cerebrospinal fluid, these effects are usually more pronounced in respiratory alkalosis than in metabolic alkalosis. Feelings of lightheadedness and alterations in consciousness develop for the same reason. Hypokalemia again results from the exchange of potassium and hydrogen between cells and extracellular fluid.

The arterial blood gas values characteristic of uncompensated respiratory alkalosis include an increased pH, decreased $PaCO_2$, and normal HCO_3^-. When renal compensation develops, the HCO_3^- value decreases and the pH moves closer to normal. Renal compensation is highly effective.

Management. Therapy depends on the cause. If the hyperventilation is a physiologic response to hypoxemia, attempts to slow the rate and depth of breathing are inappropriate. Instead, measures should be directed toward correcting the hypoxemia. When hyperventilation is entirely of psychologic origin, it is reasonable to help patients slow their breathing. Occasionally, respiratory alkalosis results from adjusting the settings on a mechanical ventilator in such a way that excessive carbon dioxide is eliminated. This situation is remedied by adjusting the ventilator.

Nursing Assessment and Interventions. Patients with suspected respiratory alkalosis should be thoroughly assessed for hypoxemia, which may be the initiating cause. If hypoxemia is present, provision of oxygen and correction of the underlying physiologic disturbance are activities performed in conjunction with the physician. The nurse should make certain that the patient is positioned optimally for effective ventilation, and she should minimize additional oxygen demands, such as pain or increased body temperature. When respiratory alkalosis appears to have no physiologic benefit, patients should be assisted to slow their breathing. Use of touch, control of pain, and a calm attitude are examples of interventions that may be successful. Sometimes breathing into a paper bag closed around the nose and mouth relieves symptoms.

Summary

By identifying persons at risk, the nurse may be able to plan care that will minimize the development of fluid–electrolyte or acid–base disturbances. Suspected or confirmed disorders are managed in collaboration with the physician. During this time, continued assessment is essential to monitor the effectiveness of therapy. Table 9-4 summarizes these disorders for quick reference.

▷ Fluid and Electrolyte Replacement

Purpose

Most, if not all, disease states alter fluid–electrolyte or acid–base balance. Fluid disturbances range from minimal blood loss following uncomplicated minor surgery to massive loss and complex redistribution of body fluids and electrolytes following major trauma. Similarly, acid–base disturbances may be so minor as to be undetected or may profoundly impair the ability of cells to function. When correction of these imbalances is necessary, the oral route is obviously safest and least invasive. If, however, the alteration is extensive or prolonged or if a person is unable to eat and drink, intravenous therapy is indicated. Despite a wide variation in specific situations requiring such therapy, some major principles guide intravenous fluid replacement. A general description of intravenous solutions, techniques for initiating and maintaining intravenous infusions, and major complications of intravenous therapy constitutes the remainder of this chapter.

Types of Intravenous Solutions

The choice of an intravenous solution depends on the specific purpose for which it is intended. Generally, intravenous fluids are administered to achieve one or more of the following goals:

- To provide water, electrolytes, and nutrients to meet daily requirements
- To replace water and electrolyte deficits
- To provide a medium for intravenous drug administration

Intravenous solutions contain dextrose or electrolytes mixed in various proportions with water. Pure or "free" water can never be administered intravenously because it rapidly enters red blood cells and causes them to burst.

A wide variety of intravenous solutions are commercially available. Differences in brands and their names are less overwhelming if solutions are analyzed according to their makeup rather than memorized by trade name.

Solutions are often categorized as isotonic, hypotonic, or hypertonic, according to whether their total osmolality is the same as, less than, or greater than that of blood. Table 9-5 organizes numerous intravenous solutions into these three categories.

Isotonic Fluids

Fluids that are classified as isotonic have a total osmolality close to that of extracellular fluid and do not cause red blood cells to shrink or swell. The composition of these fluids may or may not approximate that of extracellular fluid, however.

A solution of 5% dextrose in water has a serum os-

molality of 252 mOsm/liter. Once administered, the glucose is rapidly metabolized, and this initially isotonic solution then disperses as a hypotonic fluid, one third extracellular and two thirds intracellular. Therefore, 5% dextrose in water is mainly used to supply water and to correct an increased serum osmolality. One liter of 5% dextrose in water provides less than 200 kilocalories and is a minor source of calories for the body's daily requirements.

Normal saline (0.9% sodium chloride) has a total osmolality of 308 mOsm/liter. Because the osmolality is entirely contributed by electrolytes, the solution remains within the extracellular compartment. For this reason, normal saline is often used to treat an extracellular volume deficit. Although referred to as normal, it contains only sodium and chloride and does not actually simulate extracellular fluid.

Several other solutions contain ions in addition to sodium and chloride and are somewhat more similar to extracellular fluid in composition. Ringer's solution contains potassium and calcium in addition to sodium chloride. Lactated Ringer's solution contains bicarbonate precursors as well. These solutions are marketed, with slight variations, under a variety of different trade names.

Hypotonic Fluids

The general purpose of these solutions is to replace transcellular fluid, because it is hypotonic as compared to plasma. A common situation in which hypotonic fluids are used is for replacement of gastric fluid lost by nasogastric suction or vomiting. Half-strength saline (0.45% sodium chloride) is frequently used. Multiple-electrolyte solutions are also available.

Hypertonic Fluids

When 5% dextrose is added to normal saline or Ringer's solution, the total osmolality exceeds that of extracellular fluid. The dextrose is quickly metabolized, however, and only the isotonic solution remains. Therefore, any effect on the intracellular compartment is temporary. Similarly, 5% dextrose is usually added to hypotonic multiple-electrolyte solutions. Once the dextrose is metabolized, these solutions disperse as hypotonic fluids.

Higher concentrations of dextrose, such as 50% dextrose in water, are given to help meet calorie requirements. These solutions are strongly hypertonic and must be administered into central veins so that they can be diluted by rapid blood flow.

Saline solutions are also available in osmolar concentrations greater than that of extracellular fluid. These solutions draw water from the intracellular compartment to the extracellular compartment and cause cells to shrink. If given rapidly or in quantity, they may cause an extracellular volume excess and precipitate pulmonary edema. As a result, these solutions are given cautiously and usually only when the serum osmolality has decreased to dangerously low levels.

Other Substances Given Intravenously

When someone's gastrointestinal tract cannot accept food, nutritional requirements are often met intravenously. The

(Text continues on page 155)

Table 9-4
Types of Fluid–Electrolyte and Acid–Base Disturbances

Disturbance	Situations Creating Risk	Manifestations	Corrective Therapy
Extracellular volume excess	Excessive isotonic solutions administered intravenously Renal disease Heart failure Cirrhosis of liver Long-term administration of corticosteroids	Rapid weight gain Elevated blood pressure (BP) Full pulse Increased central venous pressure (CVP) Edema Neck vein distention Crackles on lung auscultation Decreased hematocrit	Isotonic fluid restriction Dietary sodium restriction
Extracellular volume deficit	Blood loss Excessive diuresis Fluid sequestration in body cavity (third space)	Decreased postural BP Weight loss Oliguria Decreased CVP Collapsed neck veins Increased hematocrit and albumin values	Isotonic fluid administration
Decreased serum osmolality	Excessive ADH secretion Excessive hypotonic solutions administered intravenously	Nausea Malaise Mental confusion Seizures Decreased serum sodium value	"Free" water restriction
Increased serum osmolality	Inability to respond to thirst No access to water Diabetes insipidus Administration of high-protein tube feedings with inadequate water Prolonged high fever	Nausea Malaise Mental confusion Seizures Increased serum sodium value	"Free" water administration
Extracellular volume deficit and increased serum osmolality	Loss of transcellular fluids by: Vomiting Diarrhea Nasogastric suction Profuse diaphoresis	See *extracellular volume deficit* and *increased serum osmolality.*	
Extracellular volume deficit and decreased serum osmolality	Replacement of transcellular losses exclusively with hypotonic fluid Shock	See *extracellular volume deficit* and *decreased serum osmolality.*	
Extracellular volume excess and decreased serum osmolality	Severe cirrhosis of the liver Severe heart failure	See *extracellular volume excess* and *decreased serum osmolality.*	
Extracellular volume excess and increased serum osmolality	Excessive water restriction in situations of extracellular volume excess and decreased serum osmolality	See *extracellular volume excess* and *increased serum osmolality.*	
Hypokalemia	Potassium-wasting diuretics Hyperaldosteronism Vomiting Diarrhea Alkalosis	Skeletal muscle weakness Respiratory muscle weakness Cardiac arrhythmias U waves on ECG Digitalis toxicity Nausea Vomiting Constipation Polyuria	Potassium administration through dietary or parenteral routes

(continued)

Table 9-4
Types of Fluid–Electrolyte and Acid–Base Disturbances (continued)

Disturbance	Situations Creating Risk	Manifestations	Corrective Therapy
Hyperkalemia	Renal failure Acidosis Massive tissue destruction	Skeletal muscle weakness Cardiac arrhythmias Peaked T waves on ECG	Administration of IV calcium, glucose and insulin, or bicarbonates Cation-exchange resin (Kayexalate) Renal dialysis
Hypocalcemia	Parathyroid removal or deficiency Impaired vitamin D absorption Impaired calcium absorption Hyperphosphatemia Hypomagnesemia Acute pancreatitis Alkalosis	Numbness Tingling Muscle twitches Muscle cramps Tetany	Calcium administration through dietary or parenteral routes Vitamin D administration
Hypercalcemia	Bone metastasis Immobility Hyperparathyroidism Multiple myeloma Sarcoidosis	Skeletal muscle weakness Decreased muscle tone Nausea Anorexia Pathologic fractures Soft tissue calcifications Kidney stones Cardiac arrhythmias Digitalis toxicity	Isotonic fluid administration Diuretic administration Administration of calcitonin, corticosteroids, or phosphate Dietary calcium restriction
Hypophosphatemia	Malnutrition Malabsorption Antacids Alcoholism Hyperparathyroidism Intravenous hyperalimentation Insulin treatment of diabetic ketoacidosis	Mental irritability Seizures Coma Skeletal muscle weakness Osteomalacia Impaired WBC, RBC, and platelet function	Phosphate administration through dietary or parenteral routes
Hyperphosphatemia	Renal failure Hypoparathyroidism Acromegaly	Manifestations of hypocalcemia Kidney stones	Dietary phosphate restriction
Hypomagnesemia	Alcoholism Diuretic therapy Hyperaldosteronism Malabsorption	Manifestations similar to hypocalcemia Decreased serum calcium and potassium values Digitalis toxicity	Magnesium administration through dietary or parenteral routes
Hypermagnesemia	Renal failure	Hypotension Drowsiness Loss or weakness of deep tendon reflexes Coma	Dietary magnesium restriction IV calcium administration
Metabolic acidosis	Shock Diabetic ketoacidosis Toxin ingestion Diarrhea Renal failure	Increased BP (early) Increased pulse (early) Cardiac arrhythmias Lethargy Coma Rapid, deep breathing Hyperkalemia	IV bicarbonate administration

(continued)

Table 9-4
Types of Fluid–Electrolyte and Acid–Base Disturbances (continued)

Disturbance	Situations Creating Risk	Manifestations	Corrective Therapy
		Uncompensated ABG values: $\downarrow pH$, $\downarrow HCO_3^-$, normal $PaCO_2$ Compensated ABG values: $\downarrow pH$, $\downarrow HCO_3^-$, $\downarrow PaCO_2$	
Metabolic alkalosis	Vomiting GI suction Ingestion of baking soda in quantity Hypochloremia Hypokalemia Hyperaldosteronism	Manifestations of hypocalcemia Hypokalemia Slow, shallow breathing Uncompensated ABG values: $\uparrow pH$, $\uparrow HCO_3^-$, normal $PaCO_2$ $\uparrow pH$, $\uparrow HCO_3^-$, $\uparrow PaCO_2$	Isotonic fluid administration Administration of acetazolamide (Diamox)
Respiratory acidosis	Lung parenchymal diseases High spinal cord injury Multiple rib fractures Congenital thoracic cage abnormalities Drug overdose Loss of sigh breaths Shallow breathing from any cause	Increased BP (early) Increased pulse (early) Headache Blurred vision Asterixis Myoclonus Lethargy Coma Cardiac arrhythmias Hyperkalemia Uncompensated ABG values: $\downarrow pH$, normal HCO_3^-, $\uparrow PaCO_2$ Compensated ABG values: $\downarrow pH$, $\uparrow HCO_3^-$, $\uparrow PaCO_2$	Improve depth of ventilation Mechanical ventilation
Respiratory alkalosis	Anxiety Pain Damage to respiratory centers in brain stem Hypoxemia Excessive mechanical ventilation Hyperventilation from any cause	Manifestations of hypocalcemia Lightheadedness Altered consciousness Hypokalemia Uncompensated ABG values: $\uparrow pH$, normal HCO_3^-, $\downarrow PaCO_2$ Compensated ABG values: $\uparrow pH$, $\downarrow HCO_3^-$, $\downarrow PaCO_2$	Oxygen administration if hypoxemic Assistance to slow breathing (if not hypoxemic) Adjustment of mechanical ventilator

parenteral administration of high concentrations of glucose, protein, or fat is discussed in Chapter 36.

Many drugs are also delivered intravenously, either by infusion or directly into the vein. Because intravenous medications circulate rapidly, administration by this route is potentially very hazardous. Administration rates and recommended dilutions for individual drugs are available in specialized texts pertaining to intravenous medications.

▷ Nursing Management of Intravenous Therapy

Venipuncture

The ability to gain access to the venous system is an expected nursing skill in many settings. Components of this responsibility include knowledgeable selection of venipuncture site and type of cannula, and proficiency in the technique of vein entry.

Before proceeding with venipuncture, decisions must be made as to the most appropriate location and type of cannula for a particular patient. Factors influencing these choices include the type of solution to be administered, the expected length of intravenous therapy, the patient's general condition, and the availability of veins. The skill of the person initiating the infusion is also an important consideration.

Choice of Site. Many sites can be used for intravenous therapy, but ease of access and potential hazards vary among them. Veins of the extremities are designated as peripheral locations and are ordinarily the only sites used by nurses. Because they are relatively safe and easy to enter, upper extremity veins are most commonly used. Veins of the arm

Table 9-5
Composition of Some Commonly Used Intravenous Solutions

Solution	Dextrose (mOsm/liter)	Electrolytes (mEq/liter)							Total (mOsm/liter)	mOsm Contributed by Electrolytes†
		Na^+	K^+	Ca^{+2}	Mg^{+2}	Cl^-	HPO_4^{3-}	HCO_3^- *		
Isotonic										
5% dextrose in water (D₅W)	252	—	—	—	—	—	—	—	252	0
Normal saline (0.9% NaCl)	—	154	—	—	—	154	—	—	308	308
2.5% dextrose in half normal saline (D₂.₅/0.45% NaCl)	126	77	—	—	—	77	—	—	280	154
Ringer's solution	—	147	4	5	—	156	—	—	309	309
Lactated Ringer's solution	—	130	4	3	—	109	—	28	272	272
Polysal (Cutter)	—	140	10	5	3	103	—	55	312	312
Hypotonic										
Half normal saline (0.45% NaCl)	—	77	—	—	—	77	—	—	154	154
Normosol-M (Abbott)	—	40	13	—	3	40	—	16	110	110
Hypertonic										
5% dextrose in normal saline (D₅/0.9% NaCl)	252	154	—	—	—	154	—	—	560	308
Ionosol MB with Dextrose 5% (Abbott)	252	25	20	—	3	22	3	23	344	92
Hypertonic saline (3.0% NaCl)	—	513	—	—	—	513	—	—	1026	1026

* HCO_3^- or precursor.
† Glucose is rapidly metabolized and has no sustained effect.

and hand are shown in Figure 9-7. Leg veins should rarely, if ever, be used, because of the high risk of thromboembolism. Central veins frequently cannulated by physicians include the subclavian and internal jugular veins. These larger vessels are possible to enter even when peripheral sites have collapsed, and they allow administration of high-osmolar solutions. However, hazards are much greater, including, for example, inadvertent entry into an artery or the pleural space.

Ideally, both arms and hands should be carefully inspected before a specific venipuncture site is chosen. A location should be selected that does not interfere with mobility. For this reason, the antecubital fossa is avoided, except as a last resort. The most distal site of the arm or hand is generally used first so that subsequent IVs can be moved progressively upward. The vein chosen should be palpated for elasticity and absence of hard knots that may indicate thromboses.

Venipuncture Devices. Three main types of cannulas are available: steel scalp vein needles, indwelling plastic catheters inserted over a steel needle, and indwelling plastic catheters inserted through a steel needle. Scalp vein or butterfly needles are short steel needles with plastic wing han-

dles. These are easy to insert but, because they are small and nonpliable, infiltrate easily (Fig. 9-8). Depending on the brand, short plastic catheters inserted over steel needles are called a variety of names, such as Saf-T-Cath (Deseret Pharmaceutical Inc.), Longdwel (Becton–Dickinson Company), and Angiocath (Inspiron/Bard Company). Insertion requires the additional step of advancing the catheter into the vein following venipuncture (Fig. 9-9). Because they are less likely to infiltrate, these devices are frequently preferred over scalp vein needles. Plastic catheters inserted through a hollow needle are usually called intracatheters. They are available in long lengths and are well suited for placement in central locations. Because insertion requires threading the catheter through the vein for a relatively long distance, these are the most difficult catheters to place (Fig. 9-10).

Informing the Patient. Except in emergency situations, a patient should be prepared in advance for having an intravenous infusion. A brief description of the venipuncture process, information about the expected length of infusion, and restrictions on activities are important topics. An opportunity should also be given for the patient to verbalize concerns. For example, some patients believe they will die if small bubbles in the tubing enter their veins. After acknowledging this fear, the nurse can explain that only large quantities of air administered rapidly are fatal.

Preparation of Site.   Because infection is the major complication of intravenous therapy, strict asepsis is essential during venipuncture. In addition to hand washing and the use of sterile materials, careful preparation of the site is important. The insertion site should be scrubbed with an iodine-containing agent for 60 seconds, working from the center of the field to the periphery. The solution is allowed to remain on the skin for 2 minutes, then removed with alcohol pledgets. For patients allergic to iodine, vigorous swabbing with alcohol is substituted.

Vein Entry.   Guidelines and a suggested sequence for venipuncture are presented in Chart 9-2. For veins that are very small or particularly fragile, modifications in this technique may be necessary. Alternative methods can be found in journal articles or in specialized textbooks of intravenous therapy.

Monitoring Intravenous Therapy

Maintenance of an existing intravenous infusion is a nursing responsibility that demands knowledge of the solutions being administered and principles of flow. In addition, patients must be assessed carefully for both local and systemic complications.

Factors Affecting the Flow of Intravenous Fluids

The flow of an intravenous infusion is subject to the same principles that govern fluid movement in general.

- Flow is directly proportional to the height of the liquid column.

    Raising the height of the infusion container will sometimes improve a sluggish flow.
- Flow is directly proportional to the diameter of the tubing.

    The clamp on IV tubing regulates the flow by changing the tubing diameter. In addition, the flow will be faster through cannulas of large gauge, as opposed to those of small gauge.
- Flow is inversely proportional to the length of the tubing.

    Adding extension tubing to an IV line will decrease the flow.
- Flow is inversely proportional to the viscosity of a fluid.

    Viscous intravenous solutions, like blood, require a larger cannula than do water or saline solutions.

Monitoring the Flow

Because so many factors influence the flow, a solution does not necessarily continue to run at the speed originally set. Therefore, intravenous infusions must be monitored frequently to ascertain that the fluid is flowing at the intended rate. The IV flask or bag should be marked with tape to indicate at a glance whether the correct amount has infused. The flow rate should be calculated when the solution is

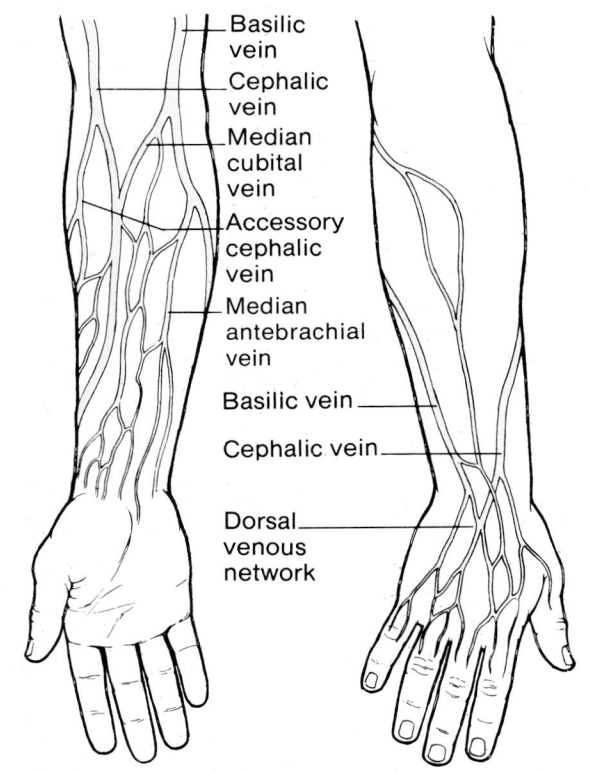

Figure 9-7.   Sites of selection for the insertion of intravenous needles for the parenteral administration of fluids or blood transfusion.

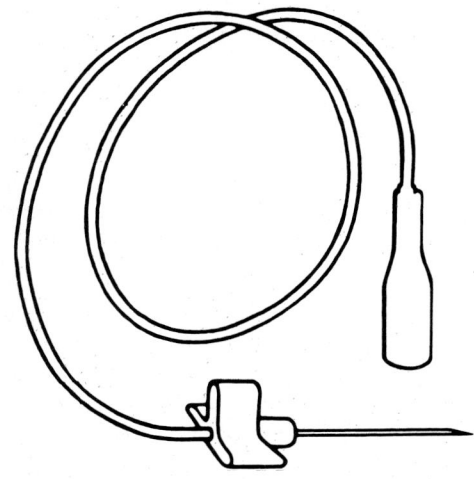

Figure 9-8.   Scalp vein needle. (From Metheny NM and Snively WD: Nurses' Handbook of Fluid Balance, 3rd ed., p 179. Philadelphia, JB Lippincott, 1979.)

originally hung, then rechecked at least hourly. To calculate the flow rate, the number of drops delivered per milliliter must be ascertained. This number varies with equipment

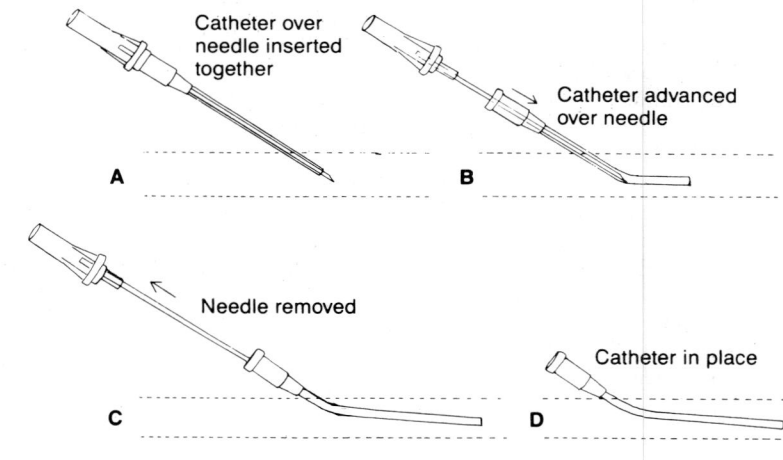

Figure 9-9. Insertion of catheter over a needle. (From Kaye W: Intravenous techniques. In Textbook of Advanced Cardiac Life Support, Chap XII, pp 1–12. Dallas, American Heart Association, 1981. Reprinted by permission of the American Heart Association, Inc.)

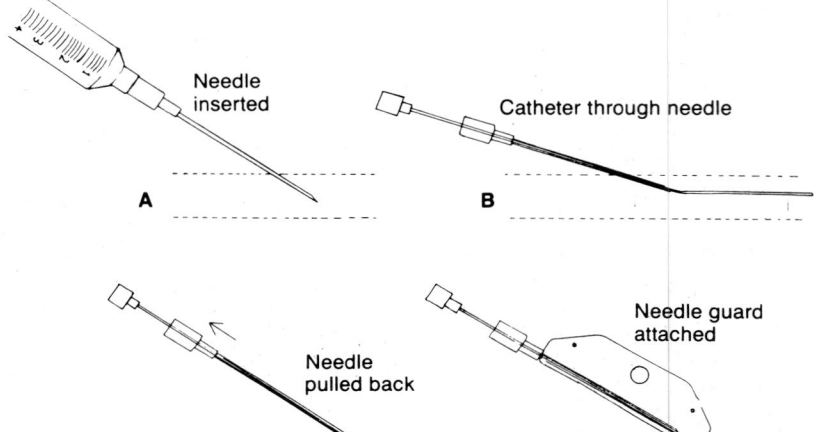

Figure 9-10. Insertion of catheter through a needle. (From Kaye W: Intravenous techniques. In Textbook of Advanced Cardiac Life Support, Chap XII, pp 1–12. Dallas, American Heart Association, 1981. Reprinted by permission of the American Heart Association, Inc.)

and is usually printed on the solution set packaging. A formula that can be used to calculate the drop rate follows:

$$\frac{gtt/ml \ of \ given \ set}{60 \ (min \ in \ hour)} \times total \ hourly \ volume = gtt/min$$

A variety of infusion pumps are available to assist in intravenous fluid delivery. These pumps are particularly useful when potent medications, such as heparin, are being infused. They do not, however, eliminate the need for frequent monitoring of the infusion.

Complications

Overinfusion or Underinfusion

Monitoring the IV rate involves more than keeping the infusion on schedule. Depending on the nature and speed of the fluid being infused and on the patient's underlying conditions, any of the fluid disturbances described in the previous section may develop. For example, an elderly person

deprived of fluids is at high risk for an extracellular volume deficit, because normal compensatory mechanisms for volume change are less efficient in aged individuals. Moreover, slow compensatory responses make these patients equally vulnerable to an extracellular volume excess should intravenous fluids be given too fast. Although maintaining the prescribed rate is one means of preventing complications, patients do not always respond as predicted to the rate that is prescribed. Therefore, repeated assessment for volume and osmolality disturbances is essential. The particular signs and symptoms to watch for are those described in the earlier section on fluid–electrolyte disorders.

Infection

Figure 9-11 illustrates the many sources of microorganism contamination possible with an intravenous infusion. Infection is a major hazard of intravenous therapy that ranges in severity from local involvement of the insertion site to systemic dissemination of organisms via the bloodstream. Mea-

Chart 9-2
Guidelines for Starting an Intravenous Infusion

Nursing Action	Rationale

Preparation

1. Verify order for IV therapy, check solution label, and identify patient.
2. Explain procedure to patient.
3. Wash hands.
4. Choose site.

5. Choose IV cannula.

6. Connect infusion flask or bag and tubing, and run solution through tubing to remove air; cover end of tubing.
7. Raise bed to comfortable working height and position for patient; adjust lighting.

1. Serious errors can be avoided by careful checking.

2. Knowledge increases both patient comfort and cooperation.
3. Asepsis is essential to prevent infection.
4. Careful site selection will increase likelihood of successful venipuncture and preservation of vein.
5. Length and gauge of cannula should be appropriate for both site and purpose of infusion.
6. Equipment must be attached immediately following successful venipuncture to prevent clotting.
7. Proper positioning will increase likelihood of success and provide comfort for patient.

Procedure

1. Apply tourniquet 5 cm to 15 cm (2–6 inches) above injection site; check for radial pulse below tourniquet.

2. Prepare site by scrubbing with iodine-containing solution for 60 seconds in circular motion, moving outward from injection site; allow 2 minutes to dry, then wipe off with alcohol pledget. (If the patient is allergic to iodine, scrub with 70% alcohol.)
3. With hand not holding needle, steady extremity and use finger or thumb to pull skin taut over vessel.
4. Holding needle bevel up and at 45-degree angle, pierce skin to reach but not penetrate vein.
5. Decrease angle of needle until nearly parallel with skin, then enter vein either directly above or from the side.
6. If backflow of blood is visible, straighten angle and advance needle.
   Additional steps for catheter inserted over needle:
   a. Advance needle 0.6 cm (1/4 inch) after successful venipuncture.
   b. Hold needle hub, and slide catheter over the needle into the vein. *Never* re-insert needle into a plastic catheter or pull the catheter back into the needle.
   c. Remove needle, while pressing lightly on the skin over the catheter tip; hold catheter hub in place.
7. Release tourniquet, and attach infusion tubing; open clamp enough to allow drip.
8. Slip a sterile 2 × 2 gauze pad under the catheter hub.
9. Anchor needle firmly in place with a chevron tape.

10. Apply antimicrobial ointment over site and cover with Band-Aid or sterile gauze; tape in place, but do not encircle limb.
11. Tape a small loop of IV tubing onto dressing.

12. Label dressing with type and length of cannula, date, and initials.
13. Calculate drop rate, and regulate flow of infusion.

14. Document site, cannula type, and time in chart.

1. The tourniquet distends the vein and makes it easier to enter; it should never be tight enough to occlude arterial flow.
2. Strict asepsis and careful site preparation is essential to prevent infection.

3. Applying traction to the vein helps to stabilize it.

4. Bevel-up position usually produces less trauma to skin and vein.
5. Two-stage procedure decreases chance of thrusting needle through posterior wall of vein as skin is entered.
6. Backflow may not occur if vein is small; this position decreases chance of puncturing posterior wall of vein.

   a. Advancing the needle slightly makes certain the plastic catheter has entered the vein.
   b. Re-insertion of the needle or pulling the catheter back can sever the catheter, causing catheter embolism.

   c. Slight pressure prevents bleeding before tubing is attached.
7. Infusion must be attached promptly to prevent clotting in cannula.
8. The gauze acts as a sterile field.
9. A stable needle is less likely to become dislodged or to irritate the vein.
10. Antimicrobial ointments somewhat decrease risk of infection; tape encircling extremity can act as tourniquet.
11. The loop decreases the chance of inadvertent cannula removal if the tubing is pulled.
12. Labeling facilitates assessment and safe discontinuation.
13. Infusion must be regulated carefully to prevent overinfusion or underinfusion.
14. Documentation is essential to facilitate care and for legal purposes.

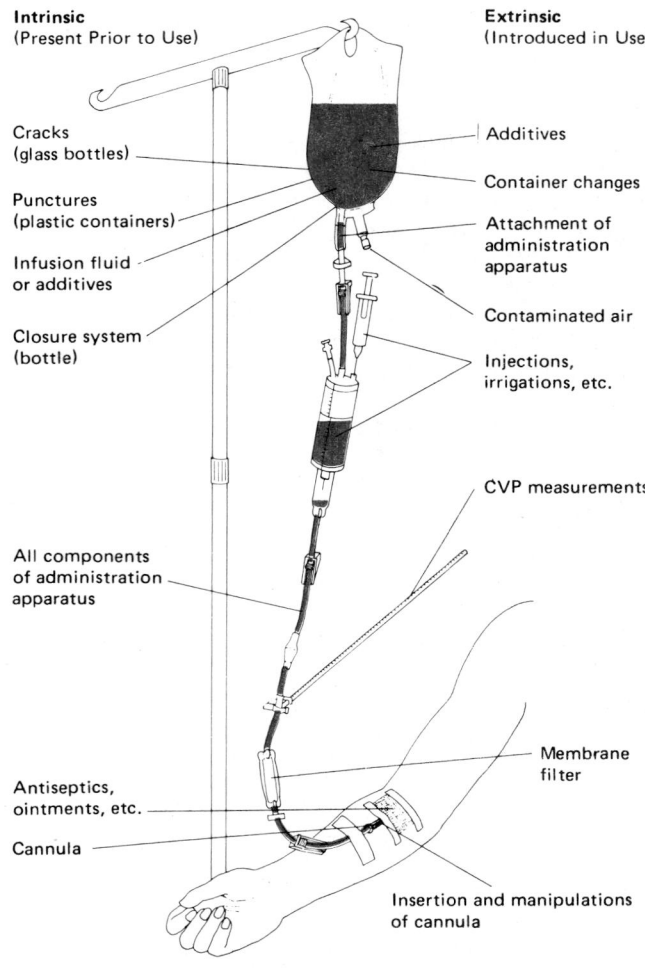

Figure 9-11. Potential mechanisms for contamination of IV infusion systems. (Drawing by NL Gahan from Maki DG: Preventing infection in intravenous therapy. Hospital Practice.)

sures to prevent infection are essential at the time of insertion and throughout the entire period of infusion. Some of these include:

- Careful handwashing before every contact with any part of the infusion system or patient
- Examination of flasks or bags for cracks, leaks, or cloudiness, which may indicate a contaminated solution
- Strict asepsis
- Firm anchoring of the IV cannula to prevent to-and-fro motion
- Daily IV site inspection and replacement of sterile dressing (application of an antimicrobial ointment to the insertion site probably confers a slight additional benefit)
- Removal of the IV cannula at the first sign of local inflammation
- Replacement of the IV cannula every 48 hours if possible
- Replacement of the IV cannula inserted during emer-

gency conditions of questionable asepsis as soon as possible
- Replacement of the flask or bag and the entire administration set every 48 hours, and every 24 hours when blood or lipid products are being infused

Phlebitis and Thrombophlebitis

Two complications that frequently develop at the IV insertion site are venous inflammation, called *phlebitis,* and simultaneous venous inflammation and clot formation, called *thrombophlebitis.* Many factors appear to contribute to these phenomena. Acidic solutions (*e.g.,* dextrose in water) and many medications (*e.g.,* potassium chloride) are highly irritating to the vein. When left in place over 24 hours, plastic catheters are more likely to cause phlebitis than are steel needles. Movement of the catheter within the vein further contributes to venous irritation. Bacterial growth around the catheter tip may be another factor.

In addition to causing local discomfort, which can be severe, phlebitis and thrombophlebitis can also cause systemic complications. The risk of serious infection has been positively correlated with the presence of phlebitis. When thrombophlebitis is present, a portion of the clot can break off and cause pulmonary embolism. This risk is by far greater in the lower extremities and explains why infusions should not be started in the legs.

From the above discussion, it is clear that measures to detect early signs of phlebitis and thrombophlebitis are justified. Daily care of the insertion site allows the area to be closely inspected. The presence of phlebitis can be assumed if the insertion site is red, swollen, or painful to touch. When thrombophlebitis is present, the vein usually feels hard and cordlike. If either sign is present, the infusion must be immediately discontinued. Local application of heat helps to relieve the discomfort in mild cases.

Air Embolism

When introduced into the circulation in large quantity, air impedes the flow of blood and thus acts as an embolus. As a result of reduced blood flow, the patient becomes cyanotic, hypotensive, and unresponsive. The accumulation of air within the right ventricle may lead to a characteristic churning sound called a mill-house murmur. The amount of air needed to cause fatal air embolism in humans is not known and appears to relate to the rate of air administration more than to absolute quantity. When delivered at 70 ml/second to 105 ml/second, 200 ml is estimated to be lethal. An entire IV tubing contains only 5 ml to 10 ml. Therefore, entry of a few air bubbles into a peripheral line does not present a significant hazard. Infusions given under pressure or into central lines are far more likely to be associated with air embolism than are peripheral infusions given by gravity.

Questions are often raised about the amount of air that can safely enter a vein without creating a risk of embolism. Some guidelines for the prevention of emboli are as follows:

- Flush air from tubing before connecting to patient.
- Discontinue or replace infusion before the flask is entirely empty to prevent air in the flask from entering the vein. Because plastic bags collapse as they empty,

they are not a significant source of air. When glass containers empty, however, air collects in the bottle as the solution empties.

- Make certain all connections on the infusion apparatus are tight.
- Keep the regulating clamp on the infusion set no higher than the level of the patient's chest. If the clamp is kept at this level, the hydrostatic pressure within the patient's vein will counteract the pressure of gravity from the administration set.
- If possible, let a loop of tubing drop below the extremity as an added barrier against air entry.
- If air embolism is suspected, immediately clamp the tubing and turn the patient onto the left side in a head-down position. This position slows the flow of air into the vein and allows the air bubble to rise in the right ventricle, so that it does not enter the pulmonary artery. Oxygen should be administered.
- Additional precautions for central lines:

    When the catheter is inserted or while tubing is changed, place the patient in Trendelenburg's position and instruct him to perform Valsalva's maneuver. This maneuver increases intrathoracic pressure and decreases the possibility of air being sucked into the vein.

    Tape all connections to minimize accidental disconnection.

    Check that connections are tight before moving the patient into an upright position.

    Have the patient perform Valsalva's maneuver when the catheter is removed, and cover the site with an occlusive dressing.

Local Infiltration

If the cannula becomes dislodged so that fluid is entering subcutaneous tissue rather than the vein, the infusion must be discontinued and restarted in another location. Infiltration is easily recognized if the insertion area is larger than an identical region in the opposite extremity. However, infiltration is not always so obvious. A common misconception is that a backflow of blood into the tubing proves that the cannula is properly placed within the vein. If the catheter tip has pierced the wall of the vessel, intravenous fluid will seep into tissues as well as flow into the vein. A more reliable means of confirming infiltration is to apply a tourniquet proximal to the infusion site and tighten it enough to restrict venous flow. If the infusion continues to drip despite the venous obstruction, infiltration is present.

Discontinuing an Infusion

The removal of an intravenous cannula is associated with two possible dangers: hemorrhage and catheter embolism. To prevent excessive bleeding, a dry, sterile sponge should be held over the site as the cannula is removed. Firm pressure should then be applied until all bleeding has stopped. If a plastic IV catheter is severed, it can travel to the right ventricle and block the blood flow. To prevent this complication during cannula removal, the type and length of the cannula should be ascertained before the IV is discontinued. Plastic catheters should be withdrawn carefully and their length measured to make certain that no fragment has broken off.

▷ Summary

The administration of intravenous fluids is frequently managed by nurses. Although it is a commonplace and extremely important form of treatment, intravenous therapy is associated with several serious hazards. These potential risks include infection, embolism, and fluid–electrolyte imbalances. By the use of aseptic technique during every contact with the IV apparatus, application of principles of flow, and frequent patient assessment, the nurse can reduce the likelihood of any of these complications.

▷ Bibliography

Books

Collins RD. Illustrated Manual of Fluid and Electrolyte Disorders. Philadelphia, JB Lippincott, 1976.

Davenport HW. The ABC of Acid–Base Chemistry, 5th ed. Chicago, University of Chicago Press, 1969.

Goldberger E. A Primer of Water, Electrolyte and Acid–Base Syndromes, 6th ed. Philadelphia, Lea & Febiger, 1980.

Kinney MR et al. AACN's Clinical Reference for Critical-Care Nursing. New York, McGraw–Hill, 1981.

Kurdi WJ. Modern Intravenous Therapy Procedures. Los Angeles, Medical Education Consultants, 1978.

Maxwell MH and Kleeman CR (eds). Clinical Disorders of Fluid and Electrolyte Metabolism, 3rd ed. New York, McGraw–Hill, 1980.

Metheny NM and Snively WD. Nurses' Handbook of Fluid Balance, 4th ed. Philadelphia, JB Lippincott, 1983.

Mitchell PH and Loustau A. Concepts Basic to Nursing, 3rd ed. New York, McGraw–Hill, 1981.

Plumer A. Principles and Practice of Intravenous Therapy, 2nd ed. Boston, Little, Brown & Co, 1975.

Rose BD. Clinical Physiology of Acid–Base and Electrolyte Disorders. New York, McGraw–Hill, 1977.

Scribner BH. Teaching Syllabus for the Course on Fluid and Electrolyte Balance. Seattle, University of Washington School of Medicine, 1969.

Stroot V, Lee C, and Schaper CA. Fluids and Electrolytes: A Practical Approach, 2nd ed. Philadelphia, FA Davis, 1979.

Suitor CW and Hunter MF. Nutrition: Principles and Application in Health Promotion. Philadelphia, JB Lippincott, 1980.

Trissel LA. Parenteral Drug Information Guide. Washington, DC, American Society of Hospital Pharmacists, 1974.

Widmann FH. Clinical Interpretation of Laboratory Tests, 8th ed. Philadelphia, FA Davis, 1979.

Articles
Fluid–Electrolyte and Acid–Base Balance

Barter FC. Clinical problems of potassium metabolism. 1980; Contrib Nephrol 21:115–122.

Broughton JO. Understanding blood gases. Ohio Medical Products Medical Article Reprint Library, 1979 Aug.

Burch GE and Giles TD. The importance of magnesium deficiency in cardiovascular disease. Am Heart J 1977 Nov; 94(5):649–657.

Cohen JJ. Disorders of potassium balance. Hosp Pract. 1979 Jan; 14(1):119–128.

Elbaum N. Detecting and correcting magnesium imbalance. Nursing '77 1977 Aug; 7(8):34–38.

Felver L. Understanding the electrolyte maze. Am J Nurs 1980 Sept; 80(9):1591–1595.

Gault MH et al. Hypernatremia, azotemia, and dehydration due to high-protein tube feeding. Ann Intern Med 1968; 68:778–791.

Guyton AC et al. An overview of water and electrolyte distribution in the body. Contrib Nephrol 1980; 21:6–9.

Juan D. Hypocalcemia. Arch Intern Med 1979 Oct; 139(10):1166–1171.

Kubo WM and Grant MM. The syndrome of inappropriate secretion of antidiuretic hormone. Heart Lung 1978 May/June; 7(3):469–476.

Max M. Acute hypercalcemic crisis. Heart Lung 1976 July/Aug; 5(4):624–626.

Missri JC and Alexander S. Hyperventilation syndrome. JAMA 1978 Nov 3; 240(11):2093–2096.

O'Dorisio TM. Hypercalcemic crisis. Heart Lung 1978 May/June; 7(3):425–434.

Quinlan M. Solving the mysteries of calcium imbalance: An action guide. RN 1982 Nov; 45(11):50–54.

Randall HT. Fluid, electrolyte, and acid–base balance. Surg Clin North Am 1976 Oct; 56(5):1019–1057.

Roberts W. Principles of fluid and electrolyte balance and imbalance. Contemporary Issues in Critical Care Nurs 1981; 1:1–19.

Robertson GL. Control of the posterior pituitary and antidiuretic hormone secretion. Contrib Nephrol 1980; 21:33–40.

Schrier RW and Berl T. Nonosmolar factors affecting renal water excretion. N Engl J Med 1975 Jan 9; 292(2):81–88.

Skorecki KL and Brenner BM. Body fluid homeostasis in man. Am J Med 1981 Jan; 70(1):77–88.

Tripp A. Hyper and hypocalcemia. Am J Nurs 1976 July; 76(7):1142–1145.

Waites TF. Hyperventilation—chronic and acute. Arch Intern Med 1978 Nov; 138(11):1700–1701.

When potassium therapy is needed. Patient Care 1982 Sept 30; 16(16):63–94.

van Ypersele de Strihou C. Importance of endogenous acid production in the regulation of acid–base equilibrium: The role of the digestive tract. Adv Nephrol 1981; 9:367–385.

Zeluff GW, Suki WN, and Jackson D. Depletion of body phosphate—ubiquitous, subtle, dangerous. Heart Lung 1977 May/June; 6(3):519–525.

Zwillich C, Kryger M, and Weil J. Hypoventilation: Consequences and management. Adv Intern Med 1978; 23:287–306.

Intravenous Therapy

Abbott N, Walrath JM, and Scanlon–Trump C. Infection related to physiologic monitoring: Venous and arterial catheters. Heart Lung 1983 Jan; 12(1):28–34.

Alvaran SB et al. Venous air embolism: Comparative merits of external cardiac massage, intracardiac aspiration, and left lateral decubitus position. Anesth Analg [Cleve] 1978 Mar/Apr; 57(2):166–170.

Band JD and Maki DG. Safety of changing intravenous delivery systems at longer than 24-hour intervals. Ann Intern Med 1979 Aug; 91(2):173–178.

Bartz CC. Phlebitis with intravenous infusion: Influence of *p*H, duration of infusion, and rate of flow. Unpublished masters thesis, Seattle, University of Washington, 1979.

Feliciano DV et al. Major complications of percutaneous subclavian vein catheters. Am J Surg 1979 Dec; 138(6):869–874.

Intravenous admixtures. Am J Nurs 1981 Mar; 81(3):574–575.

Johnson–Early A, Cohen MH, and White KS. Venipuncture and problem veins. Am J Nurs 1981 Sept; 81(9):1636–1640.

Jones BC, Briggs CD, and Norton DA. This new type I.V. dressing can save you time. Nursing '82 1982 Dec; 12(12):70–73.

Kaye W. Catheter- and infusion-related sepsis: The nature of the problem and its prevention. Heart Lung 1982 May/June; 11(3):221–227.

Keithley JK and Fraulina KE. What's behind that IV line? Nursing '82 1982 Mar; 12(3):33–42.

Maki DG. Nosocomial bacteremia. Am J Med 1981 Mar; 70(3):719–732.

Maki DG, Goldman DA, and Rhame FS. Infection control in intravenous therapy. Ann Intern Med 1973 Dec; 79(6):867–887.

McGowan JE. Six guidelines for reducing infections associated with intravenous therapy. Am Surg 1976 Sept; 42(9):713–715.

Millam DA. How to insert an IV. Am J Nurs 1979 July; 79(7):1268–1271.

National Coordinating Committee on Large Volume Parenterals: Recommended standards of practice, policies, and procedures for intravenous therapy. Am J Hosp Pharm 1980; 37:660–663.

Ordway CB. Air embolus via CVP catheter without positive pressure. Ann Surg 1974 Apr; 179:479–481.

Ostrow LS. Air embolism and central venous lines. Am J Nurs 1981 Nov; 81(11):2036–2038.

Pedersen NT and Hessov I. Venous air embolism through infusion sets. Acta Anaesthesiol Scand 1978; 22:117–122.

Peters JL and Armstrong R. Air embolism occurring as a complication of central venous catheterization. Ann Surg 1978; 187–378.

Ross AM. Polyethylene emboli: How many more? Chest 1970; 57:307–308.

Shinozaki T et al. Bacterial contamination of arterial lines. JAMA 1983 Jan 14; 249(2):223–225.

Stratton CW. Infection related to intravenous infusions. Heart Lung 1982 Mar/Apr; 11(2):123–135.

Tully JL et al. Complications of intravenous therapy with steel needles and teflon catheters. Am J Med 1981; 70(3):702–706.

10

Nutritional Considerations in Health Care

▷ The Nurse's Role in Nutritional Care

Nutritional care is an integral part of the maintenance of health and the prevention of disease. If nutritional needs are to be provided, all health professionals must regard nutrition as an important component of care. One of the most effective ways of achieving this goal is through the active participation of nurses on the health care team.

A selective body of knowledge derived from the biological, physical, and psychosocial sciences enables the nurse to assess and evaluate the health status of a client and at the same time identify those problems that are truly nursing concerns.

The nurse's helping relationship with the patient or client is multifaceted and involves mutual participation in assessment, the design of care plans, and the implementation and evaluation of goal-directed activities. The nurse thus has the opportunity to develop a nursing diagnosis related to nutrition because she is in a position to observe the patient's response to diet. She may often plan for home care by arranging counseling sessions with the patient's family members and by suggesting agencies for outside assistance or providing appropriate literature, if available, regarding the details of the diet. In addition, the nurse often helps to maintain lines of communication with various health team members for more effective coordination of activities.

Regardless of diagnosis, the patient should receive a nutritionally adequate diet in order to maintain tissue and body function. Such a diet will speed recovery and build up resistance to infection. Although meeting the patient's nutritional needs requires coordinated effort on the part of the medical and dietary staff, the nurse is the member of the health team who spends considerable time in providing direct services to the patient and establishing a good rapport with him.

▷ The Importance of Nutrition

The quality of nutritional intake has direct effects on physical and mental function. Proper nutrition is conducive to mental efficiency and concentration. On the other hand, nutritional inadequacy during the growth period may result in permanent changes in the size and chemical composition of the brain. All nutrients are involved in maintaining a healthy body: carbohydrates (glucose) are the chief energy source utilized by the cells; protein is needed for muscle building and for enzyme function in oxidizing glucose; and vitamins are necessary for numerous body functions, as is evidenced by the wide range of symptoms related to various vitamin deficiencies (Table 10-1).

Primary and Secondary Nutritional Deficiency

Nutritional deficiency may result from the lack of one or more nutrients in the diet. This type of deficiency is termed *primary*. Underlying reasons for dietary lack may be poor food habits, poverty, ignorance of proper nutritional practices, poor selection of food, lack of food supply, and lack of facilities for preserving and storing food.

Even if the diet is adequate in quantity and quality, other factors may interfere with the utilization of nutrients. This type of deficiency is termed *secondary* or conditioned. The following factors may contribute to secondary nutritional deficiency:

1. Factors that interfere with ingestion: gastrointestinal disturbances, loss of teeth, anorexia, diarrhea
2. Factors that interfere with absorption: achlorhydria, gastrointestinal surgery, biliary disease, frequent use of mineral oil, parasitism
3. Factors that interfere with utilization: liver disease, diabetes mellitus, hypothyroidism, malignancy, alcoholism, antimetabolite and sulfa therapy
4. Factors that increase nutritive requirements: fever, hyperthyroidism, burns, growth, pregnancy, lactation
5. Factors that increase excretion: polyuria, excessive perspiration, diuretic therapy
6. Factors that increase nutrient destruction: lead poisoning, achlorhydria, sulfonamide therapy, frequent use of alkalizers

If no intervention takes place, the effects of nutritional deficiency may become progressive, leading to depletion of body nutrient reserves, anatomical lesions, and chemical and functional changes.

Certain signs and symptoms that suggest possible nutritional deficiency are easy to note because they are specific. However, there are physical signs that have no relation to poor diet and that must be carefully distinguished from nutritional deficiencies. Some of the physical signs may be the result of other factors, such as poor hygiene or exposure to the sun or, possibly, systemic disorders. A physical sign that suggests a nutritional abnormality should be considered a clue rather than a diagnosis and as such should be pursued further. For example, certain signs that may appear to indicate nutritional deficiency may actually reflect other conditions, such as endocrine disorders, infectious disease, or disorders affecting digestion and absorption capacity or excretion or storage of nutrients in the body.

▷ Nutritional Assessment and Counseling

Assessment of nutritional status can be determined by one or more of the following methods:

- Medical and clinical examination
- Anthropometric measurements
- Biochemical tests
- Dietary intake

Clinical Examination

The state of nutrition is easily reflected in a person's appearance. Although the most obvious physical sign of good nutrition is a normal body weight with respect to height, body frame, and age, other tissues can serve as indicators

Table 10-1
Vitamin Deficiency Symptoms

Vitamin A *Retinol*	Night blindness; keratinization of epithelial tissues; xerophthalmia; faulty bone and tooth development
Vitamin D *Calciferol*	Rickets in children; delayed dentition; osteomalacia in adults
Vitamin E *a-tocopherol*	Hemolysis of red blood cells; mild anemia; protection of unsaturated fatty acids
Vitamin K	Prolonged clotting time; hemorrhagic disease in newborn infants; bleeding tendencies in biliary disease or surgical procedures
Thiamin	Poor appetite, atony of the gastrointestinal tract, deficient hydrochloric acid. Mental depression; apathy; beriberi; fatigue; neuritis; paralysis; edema; cardiac failure
Riboflavin	Cracks at corners of lips (cheilosis); scaly desquamation around mouth; glossitis; eye irritation; photophobia; corneal vascularization
Niacin *Nicotinamide* *Nicotinic acid*	Dermatitis (particularly areas exposed to light); neuritis; confusion; scaly skin; pellagra
Pyridoxine (B_6)	Nervous irritability, convulsions; dermatitis; anemia
Folic acid *Folacin*	Megaloblastic anemia; diarrhea; gastrointestinal disturbances
Vitamin B_{12} *Cobalamin*	Pernicious anemia owing to genetic lack of intrinsic factor; neurologic degeneration; lack or deficiency in vegetarians (strict)
Vitamin C *Ascorbic acid*	Scurvy: red, swollen, bleeding gums; poor wound healing, capillary fragility; subcutaneous hemorrhage

of nutritional status; these include the hair, skin, teeth, gums, mucous membranes, mouth and tongue, skeletal muscles, abdomen, lower extremities, and thyroid gland (Table 10-2).

Anthropometric Measurements. The most common anthropometric measurements include height, weight, and the circumferences of the triceps, the subscapular area, and the arm. When anthropometric measurements are gathered as part of data collection, standardized equipment and procedures are used, as well as standard measurement guides. Although such measurements focus on undernutrition, they also detect obesity. (See Table 10-8 for skinfold thickness and arm and muscle circumference, and Table 10-3 for ideal adult weight.)

Biochemical Assessment

Biochemical assessment reflects both the tissue level of a given nutrient and any abnormality of metabolism in the utilization of nutrients. These determinations are made from blood studies (serum protein, serum albumin and globulin, hemoglobin, serum vitamin A, carotene, and vitamin C) and from urine studies (creatinine, thiamine, riboflavin, niacin, and iodine). Some of these tests, while reflecting recent intake of the elements detected, can also identify suboptimum levels when there are no clinical symptoms of deficiency. (Table 10-9 provides a suggested guide for the interpretation of blood data.)

Assessment of Food Intake

The appraisal of food intake considers quantity and quality of diet, and also frequency of consumption of certain food items, in order to determine current or customary intake of nutrients. Commonly used methods of determining individual consumption include the food record and intake estimation by recall. These methods are discussed with the patient and explained during the taking of the diet history.

Food Record. The food record is used most often in nutritional status studies. The person is asked to keep a record of food actually consumed over a period of time, varying from 3 to 7 days. Some instructions are given for accuracy in estimating and describing the specific foods consumed. This method appears to be fairly accurate, depending on the subject's integrity and ability to estimate quantity of food.

24-Hour Recall. The 24-hour recall method is, as the name implies, recall of food intake over a 24-hour period. The subject is asked by the interviewer to recall all food eaten during the previous day and to estimate the quantities of the food consumed. Information obtained by this method is not always representative of usual intake. For this reason, at the end of the interview the subject is asked if the previous day's food intake was a typical one. To obtain supplementary information regarding the typical diet, the interviewer should also ask how frequently foods from certain food groups are eaten.

The dietary and biochemical data for most nutrients provide more information than the clinical examination. The clinical examination is not sensitive enough to detect subclinical deficiencies unless such deficiencies become so advanced that overt signs develop. A low dietary intake of

Table 10-2
Physical Signs Indicative of Nutritional Status

Body Area	Signs of Good Nutrition	Signs of Poor Nutrition
Hair	Shiny, lustrous; firm, healthy scalp	Dull and dry, brittle, depigmented, easily plucked
Face	Skin color uniform; healthy appearance	Skin dark over cheeks and under eyes, skin flaky, face swollen
Eyes	Bright, clear, moist	Eye membranes pale, dry (xerophthalmia); Bitot's spots, increased vascularity, cornea soft (keratomalacia)
Lips	Good color (pink), smooth	Swollen and puffy (cheilosis), angular lesion at corners of mouth (angular fissures)
Tongue	Deep red in appearance, surface papillae present	Smooth appearance, swollen, beefy red, sores, atrophic papillae
Teeth	Straight, no crowding, no cavities, bright	Cavities, mottled appearance (fluorosis), malpositioned
Gums	Firm, good color (pink)	Spongy, bleed easily, marginal redness, recession
Glands	No enlargement of the thyroid	Thyroid enlargement (simple goiter)
Skin	Smooth, good color, moist	Rough, dry, flaky, swollen, pale, pigmented; lack of fat under skin
Nails	Firm, pink	Spoon shaped, ridged
Skeleton	Good posture, no malformation	Poor posture, beading of ribs, bowed legs or knock knees
Muscles	Well developed, firm	Flaccid, poor tone, wasted, underdeveloped
Extremities	No tenderness	Weak and tender; presence of edema
Abdomen	Flat	Swollen
Nervous system	Normal reflexes	Decrease in or loss of ankle and knee reflexes

nutrients over a period of time may lead to low biochemical levels and, without nutritional intervention, may result in characteristic and observable signs and symptoms.

Table 10-3
Ideal Weights Derived From Life Insurance Statistics

1983 Metropolitan Height and Weight Tables*

Men

Height Feet	Inches	Small Frame	Medium Frame	Large Frame
5	2	128–134	131–141	138–150
5	3	130–136	133–143	140–153
5	4	132–138	135–145	142–156
5	5	134–140	137–148	144–160
5	6	136–142	139–151	146–164
5	7	138–145	142–154	149–168
5	8	140–148	145–157	152–172
5	9	142–151	148–160	155–176
5	10	144–154	151–163	158–180
5	11	146–157	154–166	161–184
6	0	149–160	157–170	164–188
6	1	152–164	160–174	168–192
6	2	155–168	164–178	172–197
6	3	158–172	167–182	176–202
6	4	162–176	171–187	181–207

Women

Height Feet	Inches	Small Frame	Medium Frame	Large Frame
4	10	102–111	109–121	118–131
4	11	103–113	111–123	120–134
5	0	104–115	113–126	122–137
5	1	106–118	115–129	125–140
5	2	108–121	118–132	128–143
5	3	111–124	121–135	131–147
5	4	114–127	124–138	134–151
5	5	117–130	127–141	137–155
5	6	120–133	130–144	140–159
5	7	123–136	133–147	143–163
5	8	126–139	136–150	146–167
5	9	129–142	139–153	149–170
5	10	132–145	142–156	152–173
5	11	135–148	145–159	155–176
6	0	138–151	148–162	158–179

To Make an Approximation of Your Frame Size . . .

Extend your arm and bend the forearm upward at a 90 degree angle. Keep fingers straight and turn the inside of your wrist toward your body. If you have a caliper, use it to measure the space between the two prominent bones on *either side* of your elbow. Without a caliper, place thumb and index finger of your other hand on these two bones. Measure the space between your fingers against a ruler or tape measure. Compare it with these tables that list elbow measurements for *medium-framed* men and women. Measurements lower than those listed indicate you have a small frame. Higher measurements indicate a large frame.

Men

Height in 1″ Heels	Elbow Breadth
5′2″–5′3″	2½″–2⅞″
5′4″–5′7″	2⅝″–2⅞″
5′8″–5′11″	2¾″–3″
6′0″–6′3″	2¾″–3⅛″
6′4″	2⅞″–3¼″

Women

Height in 1″ Heels	Elbow Breadth
4′10″–4′11″	2¼″–2½″
5′0″–5′3″	2¼″–2½″
5′4″–5′7″	2⅜″–2⅝″
5′8″–5′11″	2⅜″–2⅝″
6′0″	2½″–2¾″

 * Weights at ages 25–59 based on lowest mortality. Weight in pounds according to frame (in indoor clothing weighing 5 lbs. for men and 3 lbs. for women; shoes with 1″ heels).
 (Revised Height–Weight Tables derived from life-insurance statistics prepared by the Metropolitan Life Insurance Company: men and women. Copyright 1983, Metropolitan Life Insurance Company.)

Evaluating the Dietary Information

Once the dietary information has been obtained, the diet must be evaluated for its nutritive value. The first method is to use acceptable food composition tables, like those issued by the Department of Agriculture. The diet is then calculated in terms of grams and milligrams of specific nutrients. The total nutritive value is then compared with the Recommended Dietary Allowances (RDA) (Table 10-4), and the nutritional evaluation is expressed in terms of percentage of adequacy for each nutrient.

A second method of evaluation is to compare the diet data with recommendations based on foods selected from various food groups for various age levels, such as the "Basic Four Food Groups" or "The Guide to Good Eating" (Table 10-5).

The choice of a method for dietary evaluation depends on the purpose of the assessment. If the health counselor is interested in knowing about the intake of specific nutrients, such as vitamin A, iron, or calcium, then the food record method would be the one to use. The food intake would be analyzed by consulting an official publication listing foods according to composition and nutrient content. This analysis would then be compared with the Recommended Daily Allowances (Table 10-4) and the nutrient intake evaluated in terms of percentage of adequacy in reference to that standard.

Table 10-4
Food and Nutrition Board, National Academy of Sciences–National Research Council Recommended Daily Dietary Allowances,[a] Revised 1980

Designed for the maintenance of good nutrition of practically all healthy people in the U.S.A.

	Age (years)	Weight (kg)	Weight (lb)	Height (cm)	Height (in)	Protein (g)	Vitamin A (µg RE)[b]	Vitamin D (µg)[c]	Vitamin E (mg α-TE)[d]	Vitamin C (mg)	Thiamin (mg)	Riboflavin (mg)	Niacin (mg NE)[e]	Vitamin B-6 (mg)	Folacin[f] (µg)	Vitamin B-12 (µg)	Calcium (mg)	Phosphorus (mg)	Magnesium (mg)	Iron (mg)	Zinc (mg)	Iodine (µg)
Infants	0.0–0.5	6	13	60	24	kg × 2.2	420	10	3	35	0.3	0.4	6	0.3	30	0.5[g]	360	240	50	10	3	40
	0.5–1.0	9	20	71	28	kg × 2.0	400	10	4	35	0.5	0.6	8	0.6	45	1.5	540	360	70	15	5	50
Children	1–3	13	29	90	35	23	400	10	5	45	0.7	0.8	9	0.9	100	2.0	800	800	150	15	10	70
	4–6.	20	44	112	44	30	500	10	6	45	0.9	1.0	11	1.3	200	2.5	800	800	200	10	10	90
	7–10	28	62	132	52	34	700	10	7	45	1.2	1.4	16	1.6	300	3.0	800	800	250	10	10	120
Males	11–14	45	99	157	62	45	1000	10	8	50	1.4	1.6	18	1.8	400	3.0	1200	1200	350	18	15	150
	15–18	66	145	176	69	56	1000	10	10	60	1.4	1.7	18	2.0	400	3.0	1200	1200	400	18	15	150
	19–22	70	154	177	70	56	1000	7.5	10	60	1.5	1.7	19	2.2	400	3.0	800	800	350	10	15	150
	23–50	70	154	178	70	56	1000	5	10	60	1.4	1.6	18	2.2	400	3.0	800	800	350	10	15	150
	51+	70	154	178	70	56	1000	5	10	60	1.2	1.4	16	2.2	400	3.0	800	800	350	10	15	150
Females	11–14	46	101	157	62	46	800	10	8	50	1.1	1.3	15	1.8	400	3.0	1200	1200	300	18	15	150
	15–18	55	120	163	64	46	800	10	8	60	1.1	1.3	14	2.0	400	3.0	1200	1200	300	18	15	150
	19–22	55	120	163	64	44	800	7.5	8	60	1.1	1.3	14	2.0	400	3.0	800	800	300	18	15	150
	23–50	55	120	163	64	44	800	5	8	60	1.0	1.2	13	2.0	400	3.0	800	800	300	18	15	150
	51+	55	120	163	64	44	800	5	8	60	1.0	1.2	13	2.0	400	3.0	800	800	300	10	15	150
Pregnant						+30	+200	+5	+2	+20	+0.4	+0.3	+2	+0.6	+400	+1.0	+400	+400	+150	[h]	+5	+25
Lactating						+20	+400	+5	+3	+40	+0.5	+0.5	+5	+0.5	+100	+1.0	+400	+400	+150	[h]	+10	+50

[a] The allowances are intended to provide for individual variations among most normal persons as they live in the United States under usual environmental stresses. Diets should be based on a variety of common foods in order to provide other nutrients for which human requirements have been less well defined.

[b] Retinol equivalents. 1 retinol equivalent = 1 µg retinol or 6 µg β carotene.

[c] As cholecalciferol. 10 µg cholecalciferol = 400 IU of vitamin D.

[d] α-tocopherol equivalents. 1 mg d-α tocopherol = 1 α-TE.

[e] 1 NE (niacin equivalent) is equal to 1 mg of niacin or 60 mg of dietary tryptophan.

[f] The folacin allowances refer to dietary sources as determined by *Lactobacillus casei* assay after treatment with enzymes (conjugases) to make polyglutamyl forms of the vitamin available to the test organism.

[g] The recommended dietary allowance for vitamin B12 in infants is based on average concentration of the vitamin in human milk. The allowances after weaning are based on energy intake (as recommended by the American Academy of Pediatrics) and consideration of other factors, such as intestinal absorption.

[h] The increased requirement during pregnancy cannot be met by the iron content of habitual American diets nor by the existing iron stores of many women; therefore, the use of 30 mg to 60 mg of supplemental iron is recommended. Iron needs during lactation are not substantially different from those of nonpregnant women, but continued supplementation of the mother for 2 to 3 months after parturition is advisable in order to replenish stores depleted by pregnancy.

Table 10-5
Basic Four Food Groups: The Daily Guide to Good Eating

Food Groups	Recommended Amounts	
Milk Group		8-ounce cups
Milk, cottage cheese, ice cream, yogurt	Children under 9	2 to 3 cups
	Children 9–12	3 to 4 cups
	Adolescents	4 or more cups
	Adults	2 or more cups
	Pregnant women	3 or more cups
	Nursing mothers	4 or more cups
Meat Group	2- to 3-ounce serving; cooked, without bone; 2 servings total	
Lean beef, veal, pork, lamb, poultry, fish		
Alternatives:		
Dried beans, peas, lentils	1-cup serving, cooked	
Peanut butter	4-tablespoons serving	
Eggs	2	
Vegetables, Fruits	½-cup serving, 1 piece fruit; 4 servings total	
Dark green or yellow	1 serving, vitamin A rich	
Citrus fruit or vegetable	1 serving, vitamin C rich—or 2 servings of a fair source	
Other vegetables and fruits	2 or more servings	
Breads and Cereals	4 servings total	
Bread, rolls, biscuits, muffins	1 slice or small piece	
Ready-to-eat cereals	1-ounce serving	
Cooked cereal, cornmeal, grits, macaroni, noodles, rice, spaghetti	½- to ¾-cup serving, cooked	
Miscellaneous Group		
Cream, bacon, butter, margarine, shortening, oil, salad dressing, olives, jam, jelly, sugar, candy, cake, pie, carbonated beverages, relishes, alcoholic beverages, snack foods, pretzels, potato chips, etc.	Provide mostly calories for the day's total intake	

If the purpose of the assessment is to obtain information for diet instruction, then a more appropriate method of data collection would be the 24-hour recall questionnaire. The frequency with which certain foods are consumed can then be compared with the "Basic Four" food groups as a reference for dietary adequacy or excess.

Additional available information, obtained during the interview, should include methods of preparing food, sources available for food (donated foods, food stamps), food buying practices, vitamin and mineral supplements, and income range.

Conducting the Interview

As was indicated in the chapter on interviewing techniques, it is important that the interviewer establish a rapport with the patient in order to promote respect and trust. The success of the interviewer in eliciting pertinent information for dietary assessment depends on the quality of communication established at the outset.

In the initial stages of the interview, the interviewer should introduce and explain the purpose of the interview. The rest of the session should be conducted in a nondirective and exploratory way, allowing the respondent to express his feelings and thoughts. At the same time, the respondent should be encouraged to respond specifically to the questions asked.

The manner in which a question is asked will influence the extent to which the respondent will cooperate. To this end, the interviewer should accept a reply to a question without expressing disapproval, either directly by comment or indirectly by facial expression. For example, if the respondent says, "We eat rattlesnake meat as an appetizer," the reviewer should not express amazement or disgust by making faces or saying anything negative.

Sometimes a series of questions is necessary in order to elicit the information needed. Consider the following exchange:

Interviewer: "What time did you get out of bed yesterday?"

Respondent: "I got up at six o'clock in the morning to prepare breakfast for my husband, and I had a cup of coffee with him."

Interviewer: "Did you put anything in your coffee?"

Respondent: "Only a teaspoon of sugar, nothing else."

Interviewer: "Did you have anything else with your coffee?"

Respondent: "No, not at that time. I had breakfast later, around eight o'clock in the morning."

When attempting to elicit information about the kind and quantity of food eaten at a particular time, the interviewer should not ask a suggestive question, such as "Did you put sugar or cream in your coffee?" Also, assumptions should not be made about the size of servings. Instead, questions should be phrased so that quantities are more clearly determined. For example, to help determine indirectly the size of one hamburger eaten, the following question may be asked: "How many hamburgers were prepared out of the pound of ground meat you said you bought?" Another approach to determining quantities is to use food models of known sizes in estimating portions of meat, cake, or pie or to record quantities in common measurements, such as cups, spoonfuls, etc. (or according to the size of containers, when discussing intake of bottled beverages).

In recording a particular combination dish, such as "Spanish rice" or "stew," ask for the ingredients in the recipe, recording the largest quantities first. Note whether the ingredients were raw or cooked and the number of servings provided by the recipe. When the client has finished listing the foods for the recall questionnaire, it may be helpful to read the list of foods back and ask if anything was forgotten, such as fruit, cake, candy, between-meal snacks, or cocktails.

Assessing Food Consumption

An example of a 24-hour recall form is detailed in Table 10-6. This sample contains dietary information about Mrs. Brown, a 25-year-old housewife, indicating the different kinds of food she consumed, the times during the day when she consumed them, and the quantities she consumed, as measured in household units. An assessment of the adequacy of this diet, using the "Basic Four" food groups as a reference standard, is shown in Table 10-7. The chart indicates that Mrs. Brown's diet is adequate with respect to the bread and cereal group and foods rich in vitamin A, low in food sources of calcium and vitamin C, and only slightly lacking in servings of protein foods.

On the other hand, Mrs. Brown's 24-hour recall record shows an excessive intake of high-calorie foods from the miscellaneous food group. This food consumption practice is reflected in her weight, which is 19% over acceptable normal standards—enough to characterize her as obese.

Planning for Nutritional Care

A plan of action for nutritional care should be based on the results of the dietary assessment and the client's profile. Using the example given previously in Table 10-7, the goal for the nutritional care of Mrs. Brown involves helping her to state clearly and set specific objectives for achieving her goal of weight reduction. Two main objectives derived from the nutritional assessment are:

- Appropriate food selection for a balanced diet
- Appropriate food intake for weight control

To help the client understand why a good diet is necessary to maintain health, the nutritional plan should include a discussion of the nutrient contributions from each of the "Basic Four" food groups and their recommended levels. Specifically, in Mrs. Brown's case, it would be desirable to increase consumption of foods from the milk group and add citrus fruits, in order to achieve an adequate intake of calcium and vitamin C respectively.

Discussing the specific foods in the miscellaneous group that contribute mainly "empty calories" helps to ensure the effectiveness of a weight control plan. The frequent consumption of such foods eventually contributes to overweight.

The initial planning sessions based on clearly defined objectives will help in nutritional counseling and, later, in evaluating progress.

Dietary Counseling Based on Client Needs

Once the dietary evaluation is complete, it is important to discuss the results with the client. The positive aspects of the diet should be stressed and suggestions made for improving intake of foods from the "Basic Four" daily guide.

In the case of Mrs. Brown, to achieve the set objectives, it would be important to involve her in the planning for her diet by assigning her certain activities:

1. Plan meals for a week using as a guide the "Basic Four" food groups for nutritional adequacy.
2. Learn to make appropriate choices from food exchanges considering size of servings within the prescribed calorie levels for weight reduction.
3. Develop skill in planning low-calorie snacks using fruit and low-caloric food.

The instructions should be stated clearly and simply, in terms adapted to the client's educational background. The nutritional counseling may be initiated by the dietitian, while the nurse, as a team member of the health group, can supplement the client's knowledge and offer motivation to follow the prescribed diet.

Various teaching methods can be used to achieve the learning objectives. If programmed instruction is available, this teaching technique can provide general nutritional

Table 10-6
24-Hour Recall Questionnaire for Adults

Name: *Mrs. Brown* Date of recall: *3/4* Day of recall: *Tuesday*

Age: *24 Years* Male _____ Female _✓_ Occupation: *Housewife*

Height (in): *64* Weight (lb): *148* Ideal weight (lb): *124* % of ideal: *119%*

Ingestion Period	Kinds of Foods and Description	Amount in Household Units	Frequency of Consumption of Various Foods	Times per Day-Week-Month		
				×D	×W	×M
6:00 AM	Coffee	1 cup	Milk, whole		4	
	Sugar	1 tsp	Milk, skim			
	Cream	2 tbsp	Yogurt		3	
8:00 AM	Cornflakes	1 cup	Cheese		3	
	Milk, whole	½ cup	Ice cream		5	
			Beef		4	
12:00 NOON	Sandwich		Pork			1
	Bread, white	2 slices	Lamb			1
	Peanut butter	2 tbsp	Fish		1	
	Apple	1 small	Poultry		3	
	Coffee	1 cup	Eggs		5	
	Sugar	1 tsp	Cream	3		
	Cream	2 tbsp	Butter		3	
3:00 PM	Coca-Cola, regular	1 (12-ounce can)	Margarine	3		
	Almond Joy bar	1½ ounces	Oil	1		
			Salad dressings	1		
6:30 PM	Fried filet of sole	3 ounces	Vegetables			
	Green beans	½ cup	Green–yellow	1		
	Boiled potato	1 medium	Citrus fruits		3	
	Lettuce salad	1 cup	Legumes			
	French dressing	2 tbsp	Beans		1	
	Muffin	1 small	Chick peas			1
	Coffee	1 cup	Lentils			
	Sugar	1 tsp	Potatoes	1		
	Cream	2 tbsp	Breads	3		
10:30 PM	Chocolate cake (8″ diam.)	1/16 cake	Pastas		4	
	Coca-Cola, regular	1 (12-ounce can)	Rice			
			Cakes	1		
			Pies		4	
			Candy bars	1		
			Jams—jellies		5	
			Sugar	3		
			Alcoholic beverage			
			Carbonated beverage	3		
			Coffee, tea	3		
			Snack foods	1		
			Vitamin supplement			
			Mineral supplement			

knowledge as part of counseling, while allowing the client to learn at his own pace. If group instruction is used, it can offer an opportunity for several people to share their experiences of a common problem, such as weight reduction, and thereby provide encouragement and a positive outlook for following the dietary program. Individual instruction can then be used to deal with any specific problems the client may have. Such teaching should be coupled with written instructions for an individualized plan, such as a dietary list and charts for plotting the rate of weight loss relevant to the individual client. Additional available literature in the form of leaflets and pamphlets would be very helpful during counseling.

In summary, the nurse plays an important role in providing individualized professional guidance to the person who must adjust daily food consumption to meet health

NOTES Memo

Fri Mar 3 = 230 - 330

Mar - 7 - Tues - 3Pm -
Staff meeting

(IMPORTANT MESSAGE)

FOR_____

DATE_____TIME _____ A.M.
P.M.

M_____

OF_____

PHONE_____
AREA CODE   NUMBER   EXTENSION

TELEPHONED		PLEASE CALL	
CAME TO SEE YOU		WILL CALL AGAIN	
WANTS TO SEE YOU		RUSH	
RETURNED YOUR CALL		SPECIAL ATTENTION	

MESSAGE _____

_____

_____

_____

_____

SIGNED _____

LITHO IN U.S.A.

TOPS (TOPS) FORM 3002S

needs. She may consult with a dietitian or a nutritionist or may refer the client to them. When functioning in a primary health care setting in the community, the nurse should be aware that the client is autonomous and has the power to accept or reject the plan of care. Therefore, it is extremely important to develop skills that will gain the client's co-operation in focusing on the objectives of the plan and carrying out the prescribed regimen.

Evaluating the Counseling Process

The success of nutritional counseling is evaluated in terms of desirable changes in the client's behavior relevant to the objectives of the plan of care. For example, if the client demonstrates knowledge and skill in planning an adequate diet, this accomplishment can be used as one of the points in the evaluation. If Mrs. Brown substitutes fruit for candy bars as snacks in her daily diet, this is an indication that the counseling sessions have been successful. Other criteria may include the quality and quantity of the nutritional knowledge gained by the client as indicated by tests given before and after counseling. Or, the actual loss of weight demonstrated on a weight reduction chart may reflect how successfully this objective has been attained.

Evaluation also leads to reassessment, replanning, or reteaching as the client's situation either changes or shows no improvement. In the latter instance, it would be necessary to revise the plans to reinforce the learning or develop alternative ways of dealing with the situation. Inherent in this approach is an understanding that behavioral changes are made slowly and that the client, as a human being, has rights, values, and an individual life-style.

At the same time that the client's progress is being evaluated, the nurse counselor is evaluating her own effectiveness in accordance with standards of competent professional practice.

▷ Nutrition in Disease

Many disease conditions produce metabolic alterations that result in *negative nitrogen balance*. When these conditions are coupled with anorexia, they can lead to malnutrition. It is known that malnutrition interferes with wound healing, increases susceptibility to infection, and contributes to prolonged bed confinement in the hospital population.

Butterworth cites several examples of nutritional neglect in hospitals. He points out that iatrogenic malnutrition has become a significant factor in determining the outcome of illness in many patients. Among the undesirable practices affecting the nutritional health of hospital patients are:

- Prolonged use of glucose and saline IV therapy
- Withholding of meals because of diagnostic tests
- Use of tube feedings in inadequate amounts and of uncertain composition
- Failure to recognize increased nutritional needs resulting from injury or illness

Many drugs also influence the nutritional status of patients. Some of these medications may have a specific appetite-depressant effect, may irritate the mucosa, or may

Table 10-7
Dietary Adequacy of Food Intake of a 25-Year-Old Housewife, Using the Basic Four Food Groups as a Reference Standard*

Basic Four Group and Miscellaneous Foods	Dietary Adequacy
Milk group	—1½ cups
Meat group	—½ serving
Vegetables, vitamin A rich	OK
Fruits, vitamin C rich	—1 serving
	Vitamin C rich
Bread–cereal group	OK
Miscellaneous foods	Additional calories:
	Sugar
	Cream
	Coca-Cola
	Salad dressing
	Chocolate cake
	Candy bar

* Dietary information derived from Table 10-6, the 24-hour recall questionnaire

cause nausea and vomiting. Others may influence bacterial flora in the intestine or directly affect nutrient absorption, so that secondary malnutrition results.

The body in starvation may convert protein to glucose for energy; the result is persistent loss of muscle tissue. One sensitive indicator of the body's gain or loss of protein is its *nitrogen balance*. An adult is said to be in *nitrogen equilibrium* when the nitrogen intake (from food) equals the nitrogen output (in urine, feces, and perspiration); it is a sign of health. A positive nitrogen balance exists when nitrogen intake exceeds nitrogen output and indicates tissue growth, such as occurs during pregnancy, childhood, recovery from surgery, and rebuilding of wasted tissue. Negative nitrogen balance indicates that tissue is breaking down faster than it is being replaced. It can be brought about by fever, surgery, burns, and other debilitating diseases, as well as by starvation. For instance, each gram of nitrogen loss in excess of intake represents the depletion of 6.25 g of protein or 25 g of muscle tissue. Therefore, a negative nitrogen balance of 10 g per day for 10 days could mean the wasting of 2.5 kg (5.5 pounds) of muscle tissue.

Nutritional Assessment of the Hospitalized Patient

If the hospital has a metabolic nutrition support unit, it is managed by a physician working with a specially trained team consisting of a pharmacist, a nurse clinician, and a dietitian. Nutritional assessment of the hospitalized patient includes the following parameters:

1. Anthropometric measurements
   Weight/height
   Triceps skinfold thickness
   Midarm and arm muscle circumferences

2. Biochemical measurements
   Albumin
   Transferrin
   Total lymphocyte count
   Creatinine/height index
   Urinary tests (sodium, potassium, urea, creatinine)

Weight loss is an extremely important measurement since it reflects inadequate calorie intake. In the semistarved patient, weight loss indicates an increased loss of protein from the body cell mass. With respect to *anthropometric measurements* for protein calorie malnutrition, the best available indicators are triceps skinfold thickness (Figure 10-1), which indicates fat stores, and muscle circumference (Fig. 10-2), which in turn indicates the state of muscle protein (Table 10-8).

Lower serum albumin and *transferrin* levels are useful measures of visceral protein deficits in adults and are expressed as percentages of normal values (Table 10-9). Both are indicators of the degree of malnutrition. Serial measurements of these are used to assess the results of nutritional therapy.

Reduced amounts of *leukocytes* in hospitalized patients who become acutely malnourished as a result of stress and low-calorie feeding are associated with impairment of cellular immunity.

Information about *electrolyte balance* provides an assessment of kidney function as a metabolic response to infused electrolytes. The creatinine/height index calculated over a 24-hour period assesses the metabolically active tissue and indicates the degree of protein depletion, comparing expected body mass for height and actual body cell mass.

The clinical nurse specialist is in a position to take part in nutrition screening by devising her own nutrition record as a tool, if the hospital does not have a separate screening form. Such a brief assessment guide can help to identify patients who need more intensive nutritional evaluation. The findings can then be communicated to the dietitian and the rest of the team for further assessment and for clinical nutrition intervention.

Diagnostic Categories of Malnutrition

After the data for nutritional assessment have been collected, determination of the category of malnutrition that applies to the individual patient becomes the first consideration in order to plan an effective regimen for nutritional support of the hospitalized patient. Table 10-10 indicates nutritional status classification.

Not every patient with an eating problem can be considered a candidate for special nutritional therapy, but the nurse should be on the alert for any secondary nutritional problems that may be dealt with through the nursing care plan. An example of how the nurse can deal with such problems within the framework of the health care team and the Problem Oriented Medical Record system is found in Chart 10-1.

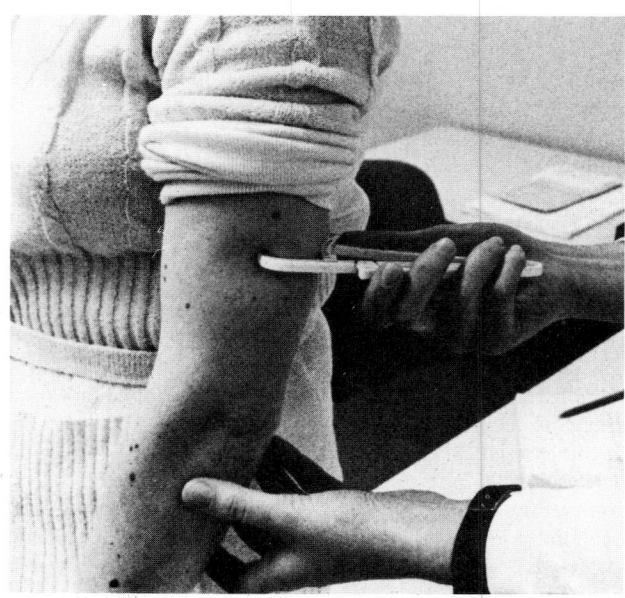

Figure 10-1. Skinfold calipers for measurement of skinfold thickness. (Photo by Doug Herdman/Kettering Medical Center.)

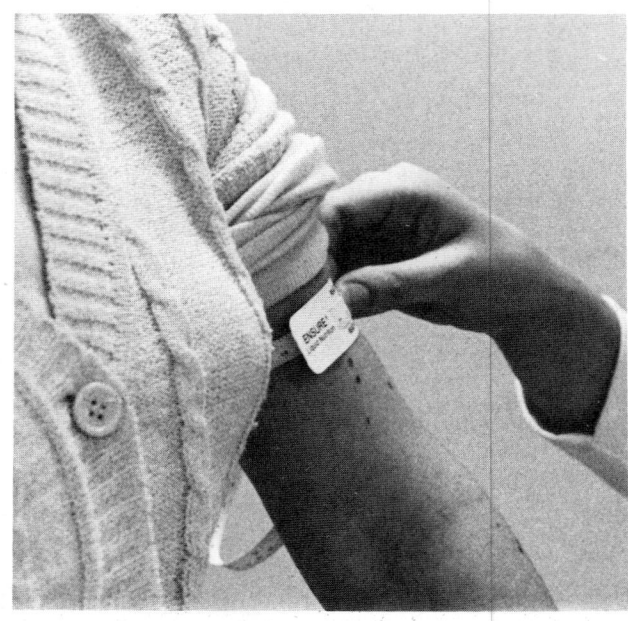

Figure 10-2. Measurement of arm muscle circumference. (Photo by Doug Herdman/Kettering Medical Center.)

Enteral and Parenteral Hyperalimentation

Sometimes patients are so weak that eating sufficient food to meet their hypermetabolic needs is impossible; in these circumstances, enteral and parenteral nutrition are required.

Tube feedings may provide the needed nutritional support when the patient is unable to eat and the digestive tract

Table 10-8
Anthropometric Measurements: Standard Values at Various Deficiency Levels

	(mm) Standard	90% Standard	80% Standard	70% Standard	60% Standard
Triceps Skinfold (Adult)					
Male	12.5	11.3	10.0	8.8	7.5
Female	16.5	14.9	13.2	11.6	9.9
Arm Circumference (Adult)					
Male	29.3	26.3	23.4	20.5	17.6
Female	28.5	25.7	22.8	20.0	17.1
Muscle Circumference (Adult)					
Male	25.3	22.8	20.2	17.7	15.2
Female	23.2	20.9	18.6	16.2	13.9

(Adapted from Butterworth CE and Blackburn GL: Hospital Malnutrition. Nutrition Today 10(2):11–12, Mar/Apr 1975.)

Table 10-9
Suggested Guide to Interpretation of Blood Data*

	Deficient	Low	Acceptable	High
Total plasma protein: g/100 ml	<6.0	6.0–6.4	6.5–6.9	≥7.0
Serum albumin (electrophoretic method): g/100 ml	<2.80	2.80–3.51	3.52–4.24	≥4.25
Serum globulin (percent of serum protein):				
Alpha$_1$			4–7	
Alpha$_2$			9–11	
Beta			11–15	
Gamma			12–16	
Hemoglobin, g/100 ml:				
Men	<12.0	12.0–13.9	14.0–14.9	≥15.0
Women (nonpregnant, nonlactating; ≥13 years)	<10.0	10.0–10.9	11.0–14.4	≥14.5
Children (3–12 years)	<10.0	10.0–10.9	11.0–12.4	≥12.5
Hematocrit (PCV), percent:				
Men	<36	36–41	42–44	≥45
Women (nonpregnant, nonlactating; ≥13 years)	<30	30–37	38–42	≥43
Children (3–12 years)	<30.0	30.0–33.9	34.0–36.9	≥37.0
Plasma ascorbic acid: mg/100 ml	<0.10	0.10–0.19	0.20–0.39	≥0.40
Plasma vitamin A: µg/100 ml	<10	10–19	20–49	≥50
Plasma carotene: µg/100 ml	3	20–39	40–99	≥100
Red cell riboflavin: µg/100 ml—red blood cells	<10.0	10.0–14.9	15.0–19.9	≥20

* Except for the particulates in blood, serum levels of nutrients in children do not differ appreciably beyond infancy from those of adults. Similarly, with the exception of hemoglobin and hematocrit, the serum levels of blood constituents in women of childbearing age are comparable to those of men.
(From Interdepartmental Committee on Nutrition for National Defense. Manual for Nutrition Surveys, 2nd ed.)

is performing well. The route of entry may vary; a small silastic nasogastric tube may be used, or esophagostomy, gastrostomy or jejunostomy tubes may be selected. The feeding may be administered by gravity flow or by a constraint infusion pump.

The rate of flow should be well regulated so as not to exceed 50 ml/hour. It is important to maintain this slow drip in order to prevent dumping symptoms.

The osmolality of the tube formula is also an important consideration in the selection of a tube feeding formula. An

Table 10-10
Nutritional Status Classification

Standards		Mild	Moderate	Severe
Albumin	g%	3.5–3.0	<3.0–2.5	<2.5
Transferrin	mg%	200–180	<180–160	<160
Lymphocyte count		1800–1500	<1500–900	<900
Triceps skinfold	% deficit			
Mid-arm circum.	% deficit	>5%–15%	>15%–30%	>30%
Arm muscle circum.	% deficit			

(Adapted from Kaminski MV and Winborn AL: Nutritional Assessment Guide. Midwest Nutrition, Education and Research Foundation Inc, 1978.)

ideal tube feeding formula should have an osmolality similar to that of blood. This is very important in the initial stages of administration; later, the patient may tolerate a higher osmolality. Some of the elemental formulas have osmolalities ranging from 500 mOsm/kg water to 1000 mOsm/kg water. These can be appropriately diluted before administration.

Formulas can be prepared at home or at the hospital to conform with the patient's nutritional needs.

In recent years, several commercial formulas that fulfill specific patient needs have become available, such as lactose-free, low-residue, or low-sodium defined formulas for special metabolic needs.

The nurse plays an important role in monitoring the tube feedings and assumes the responsibility of observing and recording abnormalities in the administration, as well as any unusual symptoms that might develop.

Total parenteral nutrition (TPN) is indicated when the oral route is unavailable owing to surgery or obstruction, when oral intake is inadequate, and when peripheral infusion of nutrients cannot meet the patient's needs.

The clinical situations for which TPN may be indicated can be summarized as follows; they include circumstances in which:

- The patient is *unable* to ingest any food orally or by tube (major burns, esophageal and gastric carcinoma).
- The patient can and does ingest food (orally or by tube) but *not enough* to maintain an anabolic state (radiation enteritis, malabsorption syndromes, Crohn's disease).
- The patient is able to ingest food orally but *refuses* to do so (e.g., the geriatric postoperative patient, the adolescent with anorexia nervosa, and the psychiatric patient in prolonged depression).
- The patient *should not be fed* orally or by tube feeding (such as those with acute pancreatitis, high enterocutaneous fistula, or chronic diarrhea).
- A patient who is emaciated may require more energy sources as well as electrolytes, vitamins, and minerals. Because of protein wasting, this patient requires a greater supply of protein that he did while in the healthy state. He also may have an impaired metabolism, so that infusion of metabolic end products for oxidation and synthesis is required.

The duration of TPN treatment for any given patient must be determined individually and cannot be prescribed in advance. It depends on the extent and nature of injury or disease, the healing rate, and the previous degree of nitrogen balance.

The TPN mixture for each patient is prescribed by the physician, who is guided by the initial assessment report; he adjusts it as often as necessary to suit the therapeutic regimen and the patient's condition.

Nutritional Requirements in Parenteral Nutrition

Calorie requirements for maintenance are estimated to be 30 cal/kg/day to 35 cal/kg/day, with a nitrogen–calorie ratio

---

Chart 10-1
Applying POMR to a Nutritional Problem

Date: 4/26/84

Problem: Difficulty in mastication and swallowing owing to radiation treatment in the pharyngeal area

S: Mr. R., an elderly man, refuses to eat. He complains of difficulty in masticating and swallowing, and of tasteless food. After one or two bites, he pushes away the tray. He prefers to take a few sips of milk now and then. He feels weak and responds indifferently to his nurse's encouragement to eat.

O: The patient's height is 158 cm (5′6″), his weight on admission was 58 kg (128 lb). His present weight is 52 kg (114 lb). Serum albumin is 2.5 g/100 ml. Hemoglobin is 11 g/100 ml and hematocrit 36%. The prescribed hospital diet is 1800 calories.

A: The radiation treatment has caused soreness and dryness of the mouth and has resulted in "mouth blindness," or lack of taste. Further, inability to accept food has caused a progressive weight loss. The mild degree of malnutrition that has developed has contributed to his weakness and affected his morale.

P: In an attempt to minimize mouth soreness and dryness, discuss and demonstrate mouth care to the patient, and suggest, in consultation with the physician, suitable preparations available for relief of mouth dryness, especially during periods of eating. Subsequently, consult with the dietitian for more acceptable foods for the patient, such as creamy foods and those with gravy, to facilitate swallowing. To improve appetite, substitute foods with aroma to compensate for loss of taste and to stimulate appetite. Between meals provide high-calorie, high-protein beverages taken in small sips, such as milkshakes or other commercial preparations, to increase nutritional intake. Socialize frequently with patient to encourage verbalization of feelings, and involve him in the selection of his menu. Continue to encourage other forms of interaction to keep his morale high.

of 1:300. For anabolic nutrition, the calorie level is approximately 40 cal/kg/day to 45 cal/kg/day, with a nitrogen–calorie ratio of 1:200. This level appears to be adequate for most patients.

Glucose, which is the most physiologic sugar, is given to patients on TPN in solution concentrations of 20% to 40%. Such a concentration is necessary in order to supply the daily requirement of about 3000 calories without fat. For fat-intake needs, *Intralipid,* a fat emulsion, has been approved by FDA and has been used successfully in parenteral nutrition. It contains essential fatty acids. It has been given in about 1.5-mg/kg to 2.5-mg/kg units to patients receiving 2500 to 3500 calories. It must be pointed out that the needs and disease states of the individual patient must be taken into consideration when fat is included in parenteral nutrition.

Nitrogen estimation for nitrogen equilibrium is approximately 8 g/day (1 g nitrogen is approximately 6.25 g protein; therefore, 8 × 6.25 = 50 g protein per day). The positive nitrogen balance in most patients can be achieved with 12 g/day to 13 g/day of nitrogen (12–13 × 6.25 = 75–81 g protein). For patients with burns or sepsis, the amount of protein might be further increased to achieve nitrogen balance. The sources of nitrogen for parenteral nutrition are protein hydrolysates, crystalline amino acids, or whole blood and serum albumin. For TPN, amino acid mixtures are used, in which case the eight essential amino acids should be present in adequate amounts and in proper balance for maintenance needs and protein synthesis.

Vitamins are needed for proper metabolism of amino acids, fats, and carbohydrates. Vitamins in parenteral nutrition are given on the basis of assumptions made from oral requirements previously established. Usually, an injection of 1.4 ml of multivitamin is added to 1 liter of amino acid–glucose solution, and these are given with the solution to patients.

Electrolytes and inorganic trace minerals are also important nutrients. Sodium deficit decreases protein utilization, and potassium is needed for better glucose infusion. Calcium is required for bone mineralization and normal function of the parathyroid gland. Other inorganic elements, such as phosphorous, chloride, acetate, and others, are also included according to the patient's needs.

These solutions are mixed and prepared in the hospital pharmacy under a laminar-flow hood, using aseptic techniques to maintain sterility.

Most of the solutions currently used for TPN in the United States are hyperosmotic. The basic nutrient solution is about six times more concentrated than blood. The route of administration of such concentrated solutions should be via the right subclavian vein or external jugular vein. In that region, high blood flow permits rapid dilution, which minimizes the undesirable effects of phlebitis and thrombosis.

Nursing Roles

Nursing roles in parenteral therapy may be described as follows:

- The hyperalimentation nurse clinician participates in nutritional assessments, follows the patient's progress, and monitors for possible complications.
- The nurse coordinator is trained to assist in catheter insertion and in the safe delivery of solutions.

These are the challenges for nurses working with multidisciplinary teams in a nutritional support service; their participation in education, research, and service in this relatively new modality will help to reduce morbidity and mortality in hospitalized patients. (See also Chap. 36.)

▷ Bibliography

Books

Anderson L et al. Nutrition in Health and Disease, 17th ed, pp 460–465. Philadelphia, JB Lippincott, 1982.

Exchange Lists for Meal Planning, rev ed. New York, American Diabetes Association, 1976.

Green ML and Harry J. Nutrition in Contemporary Nursing Practice, pp 596–600. New York, John Wiley & Sons, 1981.

Robinson EH and Lawler MR. Normal and Therapeutic Nutrition, 16th ed, pp 589–591. New York, Macmillan, 1982.

Suitor CW and Hunter MF. Nutrition. Principles and Application in Health Promotion. Philadelphia, JB Lippincott, 1980.

Weed LL. Medical Records, Medical Education and Patient Care. Cleveland, Case Western Reserve University, 1970.

Articles

Bistrian B. Anthropometric norms used in assessment of hospitalized patients. Am J Clin Nutr 1980 Oct; 33(10):2211–2214.

Blackburn G and Harvey KB. Nutritional assessment as a routine in clinical medicine. Postgrad Med 1982 May; 71(5):46–63.

Blackburn G et al. Nutritional and metabolic assessment of the hospitalized patient. JPEN 1977; 1(1):1–22.

Fagawa–Busby KS et al. Effects of diet temperature on the tolerance of enteral feedings. Nurs Res 1980 Sept–Oct; 29(5):276–280.

Gray GE and Gray LK. Anthropometric measurements and their interpretation: Principles, practices and problems. J Am Diet Assoc 1980 Nov; 77(5)534–539.

Jensen TG. Interpretation of nutritional assessment data. Nutr Supp Serv 1981 Aug; 1(4):14–20.

Kaminski MV. Enteral hyperalimentation: Prevention and treatment of complications. Nutr Supp Serv 1981 Aug; 1(4):29–40.

Keithley J. Proper nutritional assessment can prevent hospital malnutrition. Nursing '79 1979 Feb; 9(2):68–72.

Meng HC. Parenteral nutrition. In Schneider HA, Anderson CE, and Coursin DB (eds). Nutritional Support of Medical Practice, 2nd ed. Hagerstown, Harper & Row, 1983.

Murray RL. Discussion of techniques in anthropometry. Part II. Nutr Supp Serv 1982 Jan; 2(1):11–14.

Newmark SR et al. Home tube feeding for long-term nutritional support. JPEN 1981 Jan–Feb; 5(1):76–79.

Price M. Nursing diagnosis: Making a concept come alive. Am J Nurs 1980 Apr; 80(4):668–671.

Salmond S. How to assess the nutritional status of acutely ill patients. Am J Nurs 1980 May; 80(5)922–924.

Sue MC. Role of supportive health care personnel in nutrition care. Nutr Supp Serv 1981 July; 1(3):21–25.

Unit IV

Psychosocial Concepts Related to Health Care

11

Developmental Concepts of the Adult Life Cycle

During the last 75 years, the major efforts in research, theory building, and life stage development have been focused on and devoted to childhood, adolescence, and old age. The period of early adulthood to middle adulthood has been conspicuously absent in the literature. The time of early adulthood, encompassing the chronological ages of 18 to 35, and the time of middle adulthood, ages 36 to 60, until recently have been relatively uncharted and unexplored aspects of the life span. The main development attributed to this period in life consists of simultaneous processes of change and continuity. This chapter focuses on an overview of early, middle, and late adulthood, stressing aspects of developmental changes, transitions, and tasks, as well as themes and variations of human life.

▷ Stages of Adulthood

Books, monographs, and reports treating the concerns of early and middle adulthood began to appear in 1976. These efforts in research, theory building, and life stage development focused on the divisions of adulthood and the major question of what it means to be an adult. The divisions of adulthood, as developed by theoreticians, have been subdivided into approximately ten stages, as shown in Chart 11-1.

Note that there are overlapping age dates in the various stages; this is due both to differences in theories about stage development and to the difficulty involved in applying specific age classifications to all people.

The major question of what it means to be an adult is divided into several subquestions:

- What are the things that I can expect in my development?
- Is what is happening to me normal?
- Will there be order in my life throughout the adult years as there was during childhood and adolescence?

The issues and essential problems of adult life, as well as the sources of its disappointments, joys, griefs, and fulfillment, are all topics of research and investigation.

Chart 11-1
Stages of Adulthood

1. Early adulthood transition	17 to 22 years
2. Entering the adult world	22 to 28 years
3. Age 30 transition	28 to 33 years
4. Settling down period	33 to 40 years
5. Mid-life transition	35 to 45 years
6. Entering middle adulthood	45 to 50 years
7. Age 50 transition	48 to 55 years
8. Culmination of middle adulthood	55 to 60 years
9. Late adulthood transition	60 to 65 years
10. Late adulthood	65 to 75 years

Interest in adult development was originally prompted by the increasing numbers of people entering this period of life. However, although interest was intensifying, there was also reluctance to explore this phase of life because of anxiety and the fear that deliberate and organized scrutiny would uncover many negative factors. Dread of the process of change, unfulfilled expectations, decline, and decay was ever present.

Early Adulthood Transition (17–22 Years)

The myth that "now that you are 21 you have all the attributes for success" is scary to many young adults. Most people in early adulthood are fearful of leaving the pre-adult world. This age group have been instructed to believe that they must separate from their parents financially, socially, and psychologically, and learn to become independent. Yet, during this period of life, most young adults believe that they will always belong to their parents and that their parents will support them financially, psychologically, and socially, no matter what happens. They believe in their parents' world.

Parents are the bulwark of young adults. Many people in their late teens and early 20s think that only their parents will keep them safe and that their parents represent the only "true" family they will ever have. Often, marriage at this time is a means of breaking away from the parents and gaining greater independence; however, in many cases such marriages result in greater dependence and are likely to fail. Marrying to get away from one's parents is one of the most common unstated reasons for marriage and one of the poorest foundations for its success.

At this time also, the young adult must pull away from adolescent peers and give up hero worship of teachers and adulation of significant others. The relinquishment of these once important experiences and the changes that result may produce a sense of loss, feelings of anxiety, and fear about one's personal future.

Entering the Adult World (22–28 Years)

The chronological age period of 22 to 28, although described as relatively tranquil in comparison to early adulthood transition, is marked by many confrontations with reality and the collapse of childhood myths.

Confronting Childhood Myths. In childhood, it was sufficient to tell adults in authority that one had tried, even if the effort was unsuccessful. The child received positive reinforcement for just making the effort. In adulthood, one must learn that trying is not enough and that it will not suffice to make excuses for one's efforts. Positive reinforcement will not be forthcoming for merely trying. Rewards will be given solely for meeting the standard of what the "prudent man," in whatever state of life, would do.

The adult in this period of life must discard the fallacious thinking that if one does all the right things, one will automatically be rewarded. The individual must realize that following the activity patterns of one's parents does not guarantee success, and that one should not expect or anticipate parental intervention when one's projects are faltering. The idea that parents will always be available to rescue the young adult fosters increasing dependence, which precludes growth toward adult maturity.

One of the most difficult myths to dispel is the belief that there is only one right way to do things. Black-and-white thinking must be shaded with gray in order to begin successful interaction with the adult world. The realization that fair treatment of others does not guarantee fairness in return is not easily accepted by this age group. The idea that a rational approach toward and commitment to important life events will assure the right to prevail must be abandoned. These beliefs, adopted in childhood and reinforced in adolescence, must be challenged and rethought in adulthood.

Rejecting one of the major premises of our society, that working hard will always bring success, is extremely difficult for the young adult, who has grown up hearing this prescription for succeeding in life. On the personal level, the young person must be aware that reliance on self and self-direction must supplant the expectation that his or her spouse or children will provide personal fulfillment. Failure to relinquish this expectation often leads to highly disturbed situations.

Establishing Relationships. The transition into early adulthood has two unique dimensions that must be noted. The first is that during this period many people establish a relationship with a mentor, an older and more experienced person who assists the young person in entering his or her chosen field of work. Initially, the mentor is superior to the young person, but gradually the relationship becomes equalized. Eventually, young adults give up their mentors in much the same way that they gave up their parents.

The second relationship is formed with a special man or woman who brings out the young person's affectionate, romantic, and sexual feelings and simultaneously serves as a critic, guide, and sponsor as the person works toward his or her goal. This special person fulfills a transitional role by helping the young adult to move from dependency on father and mother toward autonomous independence.

Finding Oneself. In addition to the task of confronting childhood myths about how life is managed, this period requires extensive exploration of life structures and the making of tentative commitments that can be modified if necessary. It is a time for broadening one's experience and approaching life with a sense of adventure. However, later in this period some hard life choices must be faced. The person must consider whether or not to marry, whether to seek a job or a career, and how to establish goals to be pursued. During this period, both men and women confront the conflict inherent in trying to meet the contradictory demands of marriage and work. Premature commitments in one or both of these areas are often questioned at this time.

Age 30 Transition (28–33 Years)
The hallmark of the age 30 transition for many people is the growing awareness that if a change is to be made, it must be made soon; otherwise, one will be riveted to commitments made in the 20s, and future possibilities for desired change will be ruled out. This stage of aging is often characterized by a period of depression, which is usually alleviated when the individual develops a different perspective of the world and its inhabitants. It can also be identified as a period of discovery (or rediscovery) of suppressed feelings, interests, aptitudes, talents, and goals that have been ignored or deeply hidden. A realistic understanding of one's strengths, abilities, and liabilities is a formidable task to be undertaken at this time. If the task is successfully completed, the individual becomes aware both of the contradictory feelings competing within himself and of similar feelings that originate in the outside world.

In the age 30 transition, there is a greater sense of urgency. Life is more serious, more restrictive, and more real. For many people, the age of 30 provides a long-awaited second chance to construct a more satisfactory life structure.

Settling Down (33–40 Years)
The transitional period of the late 20s and early 30s is usually followed by a calmer period characterized as "settling down." Settling down is interpreted as that period in life when one takes a hard look at what is really important, becomes serious about a few major goals, and begins to build a life structure around the determined choices. Selecting and purchasing a home at this time fulfills the need of many people to establish roots and become more home-oriented. The need to establish a niche is further extended by a focus on childrearing, which often results in a decline in marital satisfaction. By this time, the romanticism of marriage has lapsed into daily routine.

Consolidating One's Position. In the world of work, advancement becomes a major task. Conflict often occurs because the young person must challenge senior people in the establishment, the very people who have the power to grant or deny the bid for advancement. In this vulnerable position, the young adult often feels both oppressed by others and restrained by internal conflicts and inhibitions. Despite these difficulties, this is a period of extending and attempting to solidify one's position in the work force and at home.

Mid-life Transition (35–45 Years)
The adage that life begins at 40 was heralded as a great positive statement of life; however, most adults secretly believe that life ends at 40 and that this age marks the end of a fulfilling, exciting, and self-directed life. The true feelings of dread about entering middle age have kept this stage of life a well-guarded secret. The mid-life transition is a bridge between early and middle adulthood. It is a point in time when one begins to count the years that are left, rather than all those that are yet to come.

Reappraising the Past. The initial task of this transitional phase is to reappraise the past. The awareness of one's mortality is uppermost in the consciousness. One is confronted with a limited amount of time remaining and a desire to use that time wisely. This is a time when the person's previous life structure comes seriously into question, and answers must be found to questions that assume a new importance:

- How satisfactory is my present life structure—how meaningful to myself, how meaningful to the world?
- How shall that life structure be changed to provide a better basis for the future?

Discarding Illusions. One of the profound discoveries made at this time is the extent to which one's life has been based on illusion. A formidable task that must be undertaken is the process of "de-illusionment"—dealing with the recognition that many long-held and cherished assumptions about oneself and the world are not true. Although indulgence in childhood is encouraged as part of one's imaginative development, as an adult, one is expected to be more realistic and practical. Dispensing with illusions is considered desirable and is anticipated as a natural step in attaining maturity. Moreover, this same term also refers to the process through which a person is stripped of most of his cherished values, beliefs, and opinions about life and people. The result may be feelings either of irreparable loss or of being liberated, so that one may develop more flexible values, beliefs, and opinions. One may be able to look at oneself and others in a more genuine, less idealized manner.

Adapting to Change. As time passes in this life phase, a major task is to modify the life structure of the 30s transition so that it will become appropriate to middle adulthood. External changes at this time, such as distance in the marital relationship (sometimes better, sometimes worse), children grown and leaving home, and parents dead or dependent, have a specific impact on the role expectations of the person as a spouse, family member, son, or daughter.

Changes in an individual's position in the work force have a profound impact on him. As the character of work alters, the individual must change with the innovations or be left behind. World events, social movements, and economic conditions affect each person according to age and period of development.

The internal changes in a person's life structure are significant at this juncture. It is quite common to revise one's social outlook, personal values and goals, and career objectives. Many people describe a feeling of "internal slippage" at this time.

Coming to Terms with Mortality and Creative/Destructive Forces. The mid-life transition activates one's awareness of death and destruction. The individual becomes aware of his mortality as well as of the actual and impending death of significant others; he also realizes that significant persons in his life have acted destructively toward him with both good and bad intentions in mind. He, in turn, has inflicted irrevocable hurt on parents, spouse, lovers, children, friends, and colleagues with the same mixed motivation. In middle adulthood, one becomes painfully aware of the ability to be simultaneously creative and destructive while working toward coexistence of these powerful forces.

Achieving Individualization.   At mid-life, people must come to terms with the synchronous existence of masculine and feminine parts of the self. A man must integrate his powerful need for attachment to others with his antithetical but equally important need for separateness. A woman must integrate her new-found need for separateness and achievement with her lesser need for attachment. As the individualization process occurs, the person becomes a more differentiated and complex human being; most importantly, he develops effective boundaries that link him to the external world with a more satisfying interaction process.

Entering Middle Adulthood (45–50 Years)

Mature adulthood is not a period of stability and certainty, but rather one of change. The changes that occur during this stage of life have no absolute chronological or sequential order, although certain events are biologically, psychologically, and socially determined or expected. The impact of these changes, which often include new sets of relationships, new expectations, and altered or modified evaluations of self, inevitably involves the adult in transitions or turning points. The events of adult life entail either role gains or role losses. Getting married, having a child, acquiring a new home, obtaining a job, and receiving a promotion are usually perceived as role gains. Becoming separated, getting a divorce, being chronically ill, retiring from work, going through menopause, and being widowed are perceived as role losses.

The main themes of adulthood include stress, stock-taking and *locus of control,* shifts in time perspective, changes in biological and psychological functioning, generational roles, and the evolution of careers and activities.

Stress.   The primary source of stress for middle-aged men is their work. For middle-aged women, stress is often a result of their concern for their husbands' work and health; their own health and physical appearance, and the events in the lives of their children are a secondary cause.

Stock-taking, Locus of Control.   Although adults of any age may go through the process of reassessment, the stock-taking of middle age is characterized by a focus on the inner self, a concern with self-development, and a reexamination and reevaluation of competency. The period of "middlescence" often causes people to see their children as capable of getting more enjoyment from sex, love, and life in general than they can; moreover, at the same time, they are aware that their children view them as being on the decline. For some middle-aged people, the position of being "caught between two generations" intensifies a sense of loss and a fear of aging; it also confirms the feeling that they are no longer masters of their fates and their environments.

People inclined toward this view may be described as having an *external locus of control,* in that they feel like puppets on a string, controlled by other people, impersonal social forces, or fate. On the other hand, people with an *internal locus of control* perceive themselves as having power over their own destinies. These are the people who view middle adulthood as a period of maximum capacity that underscores their ability to handle a highly complex environment and more challenging self-goals. For these

people, stock-taking produces a renewed sense of self as they triumph over difficulties and develop new coping skills. For others, however, it is a time of feeling trapped, anxious, or panic-stricken by life events. Many of these people become immobilized and are unable to act, thus sinking into deeper depression.

Shift in Time Perspective.   One of the most startling events in middle age is a shift in time perspective; one starts thinking in terms of the time left to live, rather than the time lived since birth. This awareness of mortality appears to be somewhat more important to men than to women. Men become more conscious of their loss of strength and vitality, more preoccupied with their health, and more fearful that time is running out. Women become more concerned with the health of the significant people in their lives, particularly their spouses. Women may "rehearse for widowhood" by fantasizing about being on their own. However, like men, they become overwhelmingly aware that they have little time left.

The shift in time perspective brings a confrontation with death that is now a personal reality rather than something that happens to other people. An awareness that life in middle age is not progressing as smoothly as was expected may lead middle-aged adults to believe they are abnormal. They often do not realize that other adults experience the same self-doubts, feelings of helplessness, lost hopes, and sense of inadequacy that they are experiencing.

Changes in Biological Functioning.   Although biological decline for most people ordinarily occurs gradually, several minute changes often bring about a major qualitative drop in bodily function by the early 40s. It is necessary to exercise extreme caution when making generalizations about physical changes during the adult years—not only about when they will happen, but whether they will, in fact, occur at all. There is no physical change that can be predicted to happen to all adults. It should be noted that the ages discussed are averages and not absolutes. People deviate widely from these averages at both ends. Some people die of "old age" in their 40s, whereas others live to be well over 100.

Generally, one has reached maximum strength by age 30. After this point in life, there is a slight but steady loss of strength through the adult years. The points of experienced weakness occur more in the back and leg muscles and less in the arm muscles. These weaknesses can be halted by individualized exercise that is undertaken on a regular basis.

The loss of physical attributes takes its greatest toll on people who derive their feelings of worth from their bodies. People who value themselves for their strength or beautiful bodies exhibit psychological patterns of aging as soon as their bodies begin to age significantly. An overemphasis on physical development and beauty in childhood and adolescence can boomerang in maturity and later adult years.

Changes in health during adulthood are not all negative. Middle age does not necessarily bring poor health. Many people live all their adult years without ever being sick or incapacitated in any way. In general, adults can expect fewer acute illnesses, fewer accidents, and more chronic illnesses.

Sensory Acuity.   In the area of the senses, the process of aging starts in infancy. Visual acuity for most people is best at about 20, remains relatively constant to 40, and then, barring gross organic difficulties, begins a slow decline. Hearing, like sight, seems to be at its peak at about 20; from about 20 on, a gradual loss occurs that affects high tones more than low tones and, after age 55, more men than women. Furthermore, after 50 there is a higher incidence of loss of ability to distinguish the finer nuances of taste, although the four basic tastes of sweet, sour, salt, and bitter remain constant. There also appears to be a sharp decrease in the sense of touch after 45.

In the area of sensitivity to pain, there is marked disagreement. Some theorists believe that sensitivity to pain tends to remain steady to approximately age 50 and then declines for different parts of the body, occasioning an increase in pain tolerance. Other theorists believe that the consciousness of pain increases after 50, making older people victims of wide pain sensitivity. The one sense that seems to retain a high level of effectiveness is balance, which is at its best between 40 and 50.

Physical Appearance and Health. One's physical appearance and physical health are probably the most important factors in determining how one approaches everyday life. The influence of physical appearance on physical health can be seen in the attention a person pays to nutrition, exercise, and relaxation. Though there is a minimal amount of physical change throughout early adulthood, middle age is often characterized by dramatic changes in appearance. Probably the most obvious change perceived by others is weight gain. Redistribution of body fat makes the body structure look like a diamond—narrow at both ends and heavy in the middle. The thinning and color change of hair are also noticeable physical changes. Men in their 40s begin to experience hairline recession, reduced hair growth, and ultimate baldness. By the 50s, both women and men are at least gray, if not white-haired. Women begin to experience some hair growth on their upper lips and chins at this time also.

For both men and women, the skin loses elasticity and becomes coarser and darker on the face, arms, and hands. Wrinkles and looseness of the skin also appear. The lower part of the face changes because of alterations in teeth, bone, muscles, and connective tissues. The voice loses timbre and quality and becomes more high-pitched. The physical movements of the body become less graceful owing to joint stiffening and loss of resiliency in the muscles. The cumulative effects of these changes make it painful for the middle-aged adult to look at himself in a mirror.

Psychological Functioning. In the area of psychological functioning, the middle-aged adult recognizes that of all age groups, his is the most powerful. Despite the fact that society is oriented toward youth, it is controlled by the middle-aged. They are the norm-bearers and the policy makers. Furthermore, middle age is generally a period of heightened sensitivity to one's position in a highly complex and confusing social environment. Assessing and reassessing oneself is a major and continual theme throughout this period of life.

Psychologically, the rewards associated with middle age are not as easily discerned as those of early adulthood and old age. In early adulthood, chronological aging (*i.e.,*

getting older) means becoming increasingly eligible for adult rewards, such as more status, power, and attractiveness, whereas advanced old age means receiving rewards for simply surviving; each additional year lived brings a mark of distinction. The middle-aged rely more on the functioning of their bodies, career status, and family cycles to determine their identities than on chronological age. Since changes in these aspects of their lives are not synchronized or predictable, the middle-aged often experience intense conflict and confusion.

Relating to Other Generations. One of the major psychological stresses is the distance the middle-aged experience from both the younger and the older generations. In general, the distance from the young is much greater; younger people can neither understand nor relate to the middle-aged because they lack the necessary life experience. The particular historical events of living create a bond between people who have lived through them together and a distance from those who have not. Although there is also a certain degree of distance between the middle-aged and the elderly, the sense of proximity and identification with them is more intense, because those who are older have experienced what it is like to be middle-aged. There is often a tendency to blur the differences between the middle-aged and the older generation.

Though most middle-aged people have either become or are in the process of becoming aware of the finiteness of time, very few express a desire to be young again. Rather, they wish to have again the vigor and appearance of youth while enjoying the authority and autonomy they have acquired.

A special task of the middle-aged adult is to become more conscious of both the child and the older person within himself and others. Attention to this task allows him to transcend, at least in some degree, the barriers that tend to separate the generations. It is important because one of the major enrichments in life is learning how to be successful in relating in a fully human way to people of all ages.

Relationships between generations are important in all societies. Although most people are aware of profound differences between generations, one can concentrate on increasing positive interaction between them. At each stage of development, people carry within themselves aspects of every generation. However, it is difficult for the child and the adolescent to visualize the "older self" and to develop empathy for persons who are more than 10 years older than they are.

The concept of generation is, for the most part, poorly understood. Members of a given generation are classified at the same age level by contrasting them to both younger and older generations. As years pass, a young adult develops a sense of moving from one generation to the next and of establishing new relationships with the other generations in his world. During adulthood, other persons are roughly the same age if they are not more than 6 or 7 years older or younger. Thus, one's own generation covers a span of some 12 to 15 years. A half generation includes an age spread of from 8 to 15 years in either direction. An older person in a generational relationship maintains an implicit claim to greater authority in the relationship and is often viewed as an older sibling. As the age difference increases to 20 years and beyond, a full generation is marked, and the older person in the relationship carries a parental role. When the age difference is 40 years or more, there is a distance of two generations, and the older person is often viewed as a symbolic grandparent.

A new and troubling change in generational status begins in the late 30s and is usually well-established by the middle 40s. People in their 40s are usually regarded by people in their 20s as a full generation removed and as part of the "establishment." Furthermore, the people in their 40s are often perceived as parental figures and, at a deeper level, as becoming "old," losing their place in society, and having lost their capacity for youthful adventures. More frightening to these people is the growing realization that they are leaving the youthful generation and entering the vaguest and most poorly defined of all generations—"the middle-aged."

Generativity vs. Stagnation.

The theory of the life cycle developed by Erik Erikson encompasses stages from early childhood to late adulthood. The stage that has the most relevance to the middle-aged is that of "generativity versus stagnation." Generativity means the ability to develop authority in younger persons and to establish mutuality with them. It also means offering leadership to younger people while simultaneously treating them as adults and encouraging them to develop greater independence and personal authority. Stagnation refers to the sense of not growing, that is, being static and bogged down in a life that is full of heavy obligations and devoid of self-fulfillment.

The middle-aged person, if generative, is becoming a senior member of the adult world and must learn to relate to persons in their 30s as junior but fully adult members who will succeed him in a few years. He must also be able to relate to people in their 20s as neophytes going through their initial formative period within the adult world.

A formidable but necessary task to be accomplished by the person in middle adulthood is to experience, endure, and fight against stagnation. Stagnation is not purely negative and should not be totally avoided. It is necessary to do battle with stagnation in order to recognize that one's own vulnerability is a source of wisdom that increases one's capacity for sympathy and compassion for others.

Evaluating Past Achievements and Setting New Goals.

Each segment of a person's life is variously mirrored in the relationship of the person to work, family, individual self, social self, life plans, and goals. In general, life has been divided into two halves, with the dividing point at about age 40. By age 40, one has had an opportunity to build a personal life and, ideally, to realize the rewards of youthful endeavors. For most people, the 40s are a period of reexamination. Questions about what has been accomplished, what is yet to be done, and the value of the person's life to the society as well as to others and to himself are posed. The reexamination culminates in coming to terms with the disparity between what a person is and what he had hoped to become.

Irrespective of what answers surface to these profound questions of living, a person must move forward. If one has not been successful in achieving early life goals, this reality must be accepted, and goals to rebuild one's life must be formulated. If one has achieved according to or in excess of expectations of early life goals, the meaning and value of one's success must be considered. A few people may be satisfied with their present lives and may wish to continue as they are for the remainder of the life span. However, despite their satisfactory situations, there will be changes that cannot be anticipated at this point. Many more people experience feelings of entrapment and meaninglessness when they realize that the attainment of their early adulthood goals has not provided the satisfaction they had hoped for. The lives of many people are relatively satisfactory in some respects and disappointing or destructive in others. Whatever the life condition at 40, each person must go through the process of sorting things out, coming to terms with personal limitations, reformulating goals, and moving forward through the life span.

Culminating Events.

Events of marked significance may occur in the late 30s and early 40s: promotion, demotion, firing, establishing a family unit, divorce, personal health breakdown, illness or death of significant others, loss of financial base, acquisition of considerable wealth, and lack of recognition or accolades from the society. Any of these may serve as a culminating event. A culminating event represents a form of success or failure, necessitating movement forward or backward on the path of life. How the person deals with a culminating event dictates chances for the future.

The culminating event frequently makes one aware of the period of mid-life transition. If the precipitating event occurred at another stage of life, it would have different meanings and implications. During middle adulthood, the culminating event must be integrated with life reappraisal. One must look at the event as a factor in the possibilities for a better or worse life in the future. The successful handling of culminating events demands continuous self-renewal and creative involvement in one's own life, as well as in the lives of others.

One of the most important services rendered by members of the helping professions is to assure people who are struggling with the "crises" of middle age and aging that they are not alone in what they are feeling, and that the process of handling culminating events is not outside the range of normal experience.

Age 50 Transition (48–55 Years)

At every point in adult life, crossing the threshold into the next stage represents a loss of youth, diminishing vitality, and, finally, a threat to life itself. Many people use the term "the big O" in referring to the transitions of the 20s, 30s, 40s, 50s, 60s, 70s, 80s, 90s, and 100s. The age 50 transition is considered to include the ages of 48 to 55. This is a time to continue working on the tasks of the mid-life transition while anticipating and planning for the building of a second middle adult structure that will be the medium for completing middle adulthood.

One of the difficult aspects of the age 50 transition is the realization that one is neither young nor old but rather suspended in the middle. At 50, one cannot ignore the graying hair, the wrinkling skin, and the frequent pains, aches, and strained muscles occasioned by activities that in previous years would have caused only minimal physical stress.

One of the worst feelings at this period of transition is the contemplation of long and continuing years of a meaningless existence—a time when youthful passions have ceased, there is little opportunity for creative tasks, and one's contributions to society are minimal. This period evokes strong feelings of self-doubt that intensify as the person realizes he is moving toward being old and begins to fear disintegration, despair, and eventual death. There is often an inner voice that says, "There is little time left to enjoy life—the end is nearly here."

Achieving Immortality. Two of the major tasks in the 50s are defining the ultimate value of life and how one is going to achieve a form of immortality. Successfully resolving these basic needs of life can help to ease the strong feelings of self-doubt, meaninglessness, and despair that so many people experience when entering this period of life. For most people, dealing with a form of immortality translates into a personal decision about the legacy they can or will bequeathe to future generations.

Many people place the highest value on having and raising children and maintaining familial relationships as their most precious gifts to generations to come. Children take the places of their parents in the adult world. Whatever rewards, accomplishments, and satisfactions children receive are also regarded as gifts of the parents. Parents generally feel that parts of them will live on in their children.

Another way of confronting mortality is to bequeathe one's material possessions to charities and worthy causes. People often make sizable contributions to religious groups, colleges, unions, professional organizations, and community projects. These groups reflect continuance and enduring value. The individual's munificence is often accompanied by a pervasive need to guarantee personal immortality by means of a name registered or engraved on a worship bench or plaque.

The legacy of professional and artistic people to future generations can take the form of an enduring product, such as a book, statue, painting, or poem; or perhaps their work will contribute to improved health and better and more comprehensive education for future generations. Whatever the means of attempting to guarantee immortality, be it material possessions, creative products or enterprises, or influences on others, the process must be recognized and implemented for success in the transition of the 50s.

Culmination of Middle Adulthood (55–60 Years)

The end of middle adulthood occurs at approximately 55 to 60 years of age. This period has often been compared to the settling down period of early adulthood. The task of this period is completing middle adulthood and becoming ready for late adulthood. For most people, the decade of the 50s can be a period of great fulfillment if they can resolve the young/old conflict. This conflict suggests that one is both young and old at every age; moreover, the human starts becoming old at birth, yet often remains young in certain respects during old age.

The serenity of ending middle adulthood is achieved when one accepts that there are clearly advantages as well as disadvantages in growing older, just as there were in being young. At this time, the mature adult realizes that when he was young he was lively, growing, heroic, and full of potential but at the same time impulsive, lacking in experience and wisdom, and imperfectly developed. While growing old, he can still be lively and full of potential as well as wise, psychologically and socially powerful, and accomplished.

At the culmination of middle adulthood, one should have struck a balance with the young/old continuum. Once the balance is struck, one can have a solid structure on which to base the use of considerable energy, imagination, and motivation for change. Middle adulthood is the core of the life cycle and the period of intense preparation for what is to come.

Late Adulthood Transition (60–65 Years)

We describe the period of late adulthood transition as the period from ages 60 to 65. It is often marked by the recognition and experience of physical decline. The fact that one becomes more forgetful, takes longer to complete tasks, and has more difficulty getting the body to move heralds the passage from middle to old age. Even if one is in relatively good health and remains physically active, he is constantly reminded of the tentativeness of his condition. Reminders of serious illness and death occur with increasing frequency in the experiences of family and friends. As one approaches 60, it seems that all traces of youth, even the last vestiges remaining from middle age, are about to vanish, leaving only the undetermined vagaries of old age. Not all these aspects of physical and mental change happen to all people, but all are likely to experience some changes and be affected by them.

A major task of the 60s is to maintain youthfulness in a new form appropriate to late adulthood. The process of termination and the modification of the earlier life must take place. As they enter this period, many people have not yet internalized the fact that they will become old; they are aware that old age comes to all people, but somehow believe that this applies to everyone except them. The 60 transition signals the culmination of the strivings of middle age. One must begin to relinquish the role occupied in the center stage of one's world, reduce the heavy responsibilities of middle adulthood, and learn to live in a different relationship with one's society. The gradual loss of recognition, power, and authority can become traumatic.

Probably one of the most difficult changes to accept is the movement of one's generation out of the limelight into a position of subservience. To allow one's children to assume the power and authority of the family is necessary but difficult to accept. In the world of business, similar transitions are also taking place. An older person who has a great deal of authority and the power to make decisions must make way for the middle adult generation, who need to acquire the ultimate power and responsibility. If he tries to hold on to formal authority after 70, he is "out of 'sync' " with his own generation and in conflict with the generation of middle adulthood.

Retirement from formal work endeavors does not mean the end of one's worth; instead, it is an opportunity to continue in valued work that stems from one's own creative energies rather than from societal pressures and financial need. The "work" a retired person chooses may encompass play or, in other words, involve him in his own determined interests for financial gain or personal satisfaction. At this time of life, one should be relatively free from pressures of society and should be able to choose the activities, be they work, play, or a combination of both, that meet one's needs. Thus, the older person should be able to fulfill one of the primary developmental tasks of late adulthood—achieving a balance of involvement with society and self.

Late Adulthood (65–75 Years)

Late adulthood ushers in a period of decline as well as an opportunity for development. The person entering late adulthood senses that he has most probably completed the major part, if not all, of his life work. Whatever he was to do for society has been done, and his choice of a way to guarantee immortality has been made. At this time, the ultimate appraisal of life must be achieved. Finding meaning and value in life as a whole is necessary to avoid bitterness and despair in the final years. In striving to attain personal integrity, the person can come to terms with his own view of death. It is necessary for most human beings to realize that whatever values and expectations they had held dear are not likely to be fully realized. Each person must reconcile the imperfections and elements of destruction in his life. Making peace with oneself and with those who are perceived as having injured one is a necessary task of late adulthood. Most people at this stage of life continue to hold strong convictions but are more realistic about how these convictions can be carried out in daily life.

Late Late Adulthood (80 and Older)

Late late adulthood, the last period of life, encompasses ages 80 and beyond. People who survive beyond 80 generally experience a myriad of infirmities and at least one chronic condition. At this point, signs of aging are more evident than any signs of growth. The scope of life tends to be narrowed, and the individual focuses intently on a few significant relationships—the place where he lives, immediate bodily concerns, and personal comforts. The person has to fight diligently to avoid the feeling that life has no meaning or, worse, that he is simply being tolerated.

All other eras of the life cycle have focused on the development of strategies for a new beginning—a new basis for living. This era focuses on learning how to die, since death is imminent. To continue to live effectively, one must make peace with dying. If one can maintain a personal vitality, engagement in social life will continue. Most important, people at this stage of life can serve as models of wisdom, hope, integrity, and personal nobility. At this time, one reaches an ultimate involvement with self—an awareness that the final task of life is accepting and loving oneself and being ready to move on to the next stage of life, which is death.

▷ **Bibliography**

Books

Barrow GM and Smith PA. Aging, Ageism and Society. New York, West Pub Co, 1979.

Colarusso CA and Nemiroff RA. Adult Development: A New Dimension in Psychodynamic Theory and Practice. New York, Plenum Press, 1981.

Dowd J. Stratification Among the Aged. Monterey, California, Brooks–Cole Pub Co, 1980.

George LK. Role Transitions in Later Life. Monterey, California, Brooks–Cole Pub Co, 1980.

Hultsch DF and Deutsch F. Adult Development and Aging: A Life-Span Perspective. New York, McGraw–Hill, 1981.

Kimmel DC. Adulthood and Aging: An Interdisciplinary Developmental View, 2nd ed. New York, John Wiley & Sons, 1980.

Levinson DJ et al. The Seasons of a Man's Life. New York, Ballantine Books, 1979.

Marshall VW. Last Chapters: A Sociology of Aging and Dying. Monterey, California, Brooks–Cole Pub Co, 1980.

Myerhoff B. Number Our Days. New York, S & S, 1980.

Rogers D (ed). Issues in Life-Span Human Development. Monterey, California, Brooks–Cole Pub Co, 1980.

Rosenfeld JP. Legacy of Aging: Inheritance and Disinheritance in Social Perspective. Norwood, New Jersey, Ablex, 1979.

Sheehy G. Passages: Predictable Crises of Adult Life. New York, EP Dutton & Co, 1976.

Troll LE. Early and Middle Adulthood: The Best is Yet to Be—Maybe. Monterey, California, Brooks–Cole Pub Co, 1975.

Articles

Apolito A. Middle-age crisis: A preventive approach. J Med Soc NJ 1981 Aug; 78(9):603–605.

Bengtson VL and Treas J. Intergenerational relations and mental health. In Birren JE and Sloan RM (eds). Handbook of Mental Health and Aging, pp 400–408. Englewood Cliffs, New Jersey, Prentice–Hall, 1980.

Elwell F and Maltbie-Crannell AD. The impact of role loss upon coping resources and life satisfaction of the elderly. J Gerontol 1981 Mar; 36(2):223–232.

Gould RL. The phases of adult life: A study in developmental psychology. Am J Psychiatry 1972 Nov; 129(5):521–531.

Gutmann D. Female ego styles and generational conflict. In Bardwick JM et al (eds). Feminine Personality and Conflict, pp 77–96. Belmont, California, Brooks–Cole Pub Co, 1970.

Lowenthal MF. Some potentialities of a life-cycle approach to the study of retirement. In Carp FM (ed). Retirement, pp 307–336. New York, Behavioral Publications, 1972.

Lowenthal MF and Weiss L. Intimacy and crises in adulthood. Counseling Psychologist 1976; 6(1):10–15.

Neugarten BL. Adult personality: Toward a psychology of the life cycle, pp 137–147. In Neugarten BL (ed). Middle Age and Aging. Chicago, University of Chicago Press, 1968.

Neugarten BL. The awareness of middle age. In Neugarten BL (ed). Middle Age and Aging, pp 93–98. Chicago, University of Chicago Press, 1968.

Neugarten BL. Adaptation and the life cycle. Counseling Psychologist 1976; 6(1):16–20.

Neugarten BL and Garron DC. Attitudes of middle-aged persons toward growing older. Geriatrics 1951 Jan; 14(1):21–24.

Neugarten BL and Kraines RJ. Menopausal symptoms in women of various ages. Psychosom Med 1965 May–June; 27(3):266–273.

Neugarten BL, Moore JW, and Lowe JC. Age norms, age constraints, and adult socialization. Am J Sociology 1965 May; 70(6):710–717.

Portnoi VA. The natural history of retirement: Mainly good news. JAMA 1981 May; 245(17):1752–1754.

Rosenfeld JP. Benevolent disinheritance: The kindest cut. Psychology Today 1980 May; 13(12):48–49.

Rotter JB. Generalized expectancies for internal versus external control of reinforcement. Psychological Monographs 1966; 80(#1, Whole No. 609):1–28.

Shainess N. Menopause: Midlife crisis or milestone-maker? J Am Med Wom Assoc 1982 Apr; 37(4):87–90.

Streff MD. Examining family growth and development: A theoretical model. ANS 1981 July; 3(4):61–69.

Susser M. Widowhood: A situational life stress or a stressful life event? Am J Public Health 1981 Aug; 71(8):793–795.

12

Illness as a Human Experience

Most people do not expect to get sick or have life-altering accidents. One of the most prominent hopes among Americans is that they and their families will have long and healthy lives. Yet, at any point along the life continuum they may be faced with difficult and painful changes in their health status. Everyone eventually dies.

The experience of illness precipitates many stressful feelings and reactions. These include frustration, anxiety, anger, denial, shame, grief, and uncertainty. Patients and their families have to adapt to the demands of the different stages of illness. Painful and disturbing symptoms lead to diagnostic tests and medical treatment. There are often dreaded questions about prognosis, body changes, and the reactions of others. Hospitalization is a major stress. Although necessary and often life-saving, it plunges people into an unfamiliar and often frightening environment, where they feel vulnerable and out of control. Acute illness calls for immediate action; chronic illness involves intricate changes in life-styles with uncertain futures.

Sick persons are often sensitive and vulnerable. Their whole lives are changed at least temporarily. They struggle with the resurgence of past experiences as they cope with the present reality and the anticipated future. Issues of mortality, dependency, trust, and identity are raised.

Nurses are central figures in the patient's immediate life. Through sensitive understanding and intelligent action they provide many opportunities for patients to maintain basic security, self-esteem, and integrity. They help patients and familes to cope with the crisis of illness.

Serious illness or injury is always more than just physical pain and inconvenience. An individual's life goals, family, work and income, mobility, body image, and life-style may be drastically altered. Whether the changes are temporary or permanent, the situation may develop into a crisis for the person—a crisis that affects family, friends, and professional helpers. Emotional demands on the nurse are often continuous and draining. Without proper understanding and coping skills, the cumulative effect may be overwhelming and may lead to professional and personal problems.

To be of optimal help to patients, families, staff, and themselves, nurses need to know:

The usual stages of illness and various emotional responses

The major tasks of adapting to significant illness or injury

The typical coping strategies used by patients and families

The psychological and social factors that help or hinder coping

Their own reactions to the various stresses and how to deal with them

▷ Stages of Illness

The transition from health to illness is a complex and highly individualized experience. In addition to restoring physiologic balance, the two main tasks are (1) to modify the body image, concept of self, and relations to other people and work; and (2) to readjust realistically to the limitations imposed by the condition. The two tasks begin in the setting in which the person is being treated for the health problem.

In the cycle of health and illness, most people go through three stages: (1) the transition from health to illness, (2) the period of "accepted" illness, and (3) convalescence. The duration and quality of the experience vary with differences in personality, the specific disorder, and the changes made in the person's life.

First Stage

The development of symptoms usually is accompanied by unpleasant sensations, loss of vigor and stamina, and a decrease in the ability to function. Certain symptoms, such as chest pain, indigestion, and headache, may increase in frequency and intensity. Anxiety is often present and is handled with the individual's usual coping mechanisms. To ward off the prospect of sickness, one person may plunge into activity, keeping late hours with extra work and social activities. Another may become passive and withdrawn, hoping that the vague symptoms will go away. A person may put off seeking medical care for fear of the diagnosis, especially if something serious is suspected, such as cancer. Anxiety, guilt, shame, and denial are prominent during this initial period.

If the symptoms persist, the person seeks medical attention. He may have ambivalent feelings toward examination and diagnostic tests, which are reflected in canceled or missed appointments. He may not follow initial recommendations or take prescribed medication. Some patients go from physician to physician, hoping to learn "what's really the matter" or that a previous diagnosis was inaccurate.

When a person experiences a sudden catastrophe, such as heart attack or stroke, he is instantly shifted from health to illness. His immediate concern is that help will not arrive in time or that the medical strangers on whom he is suddenly so dependent will not be competent. Families experience similar fears but have no time to consider alternatives. Apprehension is expressed through excessive demands, refusal to cooperate or accept the proposed treatment, and suspicion of the motives and methods of those trying to help. To offset this reaction, it is helpful to contact close relatives and the person's own physician, if possible. Calm explanation of the necessary procedures and demonstration of technical skill will convey to patients that they are being cared for adequately.

When patients and families are experiencing shock, disbelief, and denial of the condition, nurses help by listening. In a noncritical way, they do not support the denial, but accept the need to cope with the situation in this way at the present time. They establish themselves as professional persons who want to understand and help. They orient patients to the immediate environment and answer questions to the best of their ability.

Second Stage

The second stage is a shift to the period of accepted illness. The patient recognizes and admits that he is sick and in need of help from others, especially from the medical and nursing staffs. Temporarily, he adopts the patient role. This includes abdication from usual responsibilities and cooperation in the task of getting well. In this stage, patients become preoccupied with themselves, their symptoms, and their treatment; interest in current events and even concern about family and friends may be quite limited. Increased dependency accompanies preoccupation with somatic concerns. This behavior is often described as regressive, since it is a return to earlier forms of acting, feeling, and relating to others.

A certain amount of regression is necessary so that patients can allow themselves to rest in bed, eat specified diets, sleep, and let their bodies heal. People who normally resist being dependent may find this very difficult. They are so threatened that they continue to deny their condition in part or refuse prescribed treatment. They push themselves beyond their physical limits and discontinue treatment prematurely. The other extreme of dependency problems is seen in patients who receive so much gratification from dependency that they attempt to continue it indefinitely; the terms "hospitalitis" and secondary gain refer to this.

When acutely ill, patients need a great deal of help from others. Nursing students are often unduly concerned that patients will become too dependent on them. There must be a realistic evaluation of the stage of illness, the patient's need for dependency, and the need for a trusting, caring person. Nurses who care for the same patients over long periods of time should evaluate their own needs for having others dependent on them. The nurse can help patients move through the stages of illness, so that they become autonomous and able to care for themselves again.

During the stage of accepted illness, the patient may express anger, guilt, and resentment. He may be very critical of care and medical management, attacking the very people he depends on. The most helpful nursing approach is to view this reaction as the individual's attempt to deal with the situation. Nurses try to understand how patients and families feel. They encourage the expression of feelings without passing judgment, moralizing, or arguing.

When sick, patients often feel helpless and hopeless. The nursing staff assumes responsibility for the care of patients and are alert to individual differences and needs. They provide opportunities for the patient to make decisions and assume responsibility whenever indicated. As the patient improves and becomes more assured of the staff's availability, interest, and competence, he is less anxious and more able to relinquish dependency. During this period, the patient may be experiencing an acute sense of loss. The clinical picture is depression with sadness, hopelessness, and anger. He may be mourning the loss of health and vigor, the loss of a body part or function, or changes anticipated in job and family. He may be moving into the emotional reactions to dying (see discussion, pp. 202–203).

Third Stage

The third stage is the convalescent or restitution period. The return of health and physical strength often precedes the patient's feeling and acting "well." Just as a lag usually occurs in the initial stage between the appearance of physical symptoms and the emotional acceptance of illness, a reverse lag occurs in recovery. Getting well implies giving up a dependent, regressive position and resuming adult responsibilities and normal relations with others. Although some people are reluctant to give up the patient role, most are motivated toward health but are afraid or hesitant to try out new skills. This is particularly true if the illness and treatment require major changes in work and family relations.

Nurses help patients in this stage by assuming a role analogous to that of an adequate parent of a teenager. They gradually relax protection and offer guidance, advice, and encouragement to progress. They quietly retire to the sidelines, ready to reassure but encouraging experimentation with new skills. They step in only when gross errors in judgment occur. The patient senses the confidence of the nurse and is reassured by it, especially if ideal or perfect results are not expected.

During the convalescent stage, nurses can stimulate patients to renew their interest in the world, communicate better with family, and make plans for the future. For example, groups of persons with similar conditions, such as stroke or mastectomies, meet in support groups. These members may be called in to talk to the patient both before and after an operation, to convey hope and to give realistic, firsthand information on coping with their common disability. At first, patients may be overwhelmed by anxiety or grief and be unable to use these services. During convalescence, they are reminded and encouraged to avail themselves of this help. It is important to keep individual differences in mind because some patients do not want to affiliate with such groups. The connotation of being different, especially with a stigmatized condition, may be too painful to admit publicly.

▷ Adapting to Illness

Just what is it that patients and families have to cope with when they become sick? The major tasks have been identified by Moos and Tsu as:

1. Dealing with the discomfort, incapacitation, and symptoms of the illness or injury
2. Managing the stress of treatment procedures and hospitalization
3. Developing and maintaining adequate relationships with the medical, nursing, and other care-taking staff
4. Preserving a satisfactory self-image and maintaining a sense of competence and mastery
5. Balancing the disturbing feelings aroused by illness and treatment
6. Maintaining relationships with family and friends despite a changed role identity
7. Preparing for an uncertain future in which further loss, death, or recovery are possibilities

These adaptive tasks often occur simultaneously or recur at different stages of the illness.

The stages of transition from health to illness and back to health are most clearly defined when a person has an acute condition that responds favorably to treatment. A similar series of steps takes place in adapting to a chronic condition. The stages are disbelief, developing awareness, reorganization, and resolution. In a successful adaptation to a chronic illness, the person can comfortably or resignedly regard himself as having a specific condition. He acknowledges and copes with the necessary changes in his life imposed by the condition. Although he may have gone through periods of despair, anger, and self-depreciation, he is able to regard himself as a worthwhile person who happens to need help in some form and degree.

Adaptation to chronic illness is a lengthy and continuous process. The extent of adaptation required depends on the type of illness, the degree of disability, and the patient's unique personality. Some chronic illnesses are relatively stable, with few changes; others have acute remissions and slow degeneration; some are terminal. Unpredictability is a hallmark of chronic illness, in terms of symptoms, effectiveness of treatment, hopes for future remissions and medical breakthroughs, and the reactions of others. Patients are often torn between living within their limitations and pushing for more.

Basic Emotional Needs

Everyone has the same basic emotional needs. These have been variously categorized as the need for love, trust, autonomy, identity, self-esteem, recognition, and security, and are summarized by Schutz as the interpersonal need for inclusion, control, and affection. The nonrealization of a need leads to undesired feelings and behaviors. Feelings such as anxiety, anger, loneliness, and self-doubt are raised.

The interpersonal needs for inclusion, control, and affection are expressed in group as well as one-to-one situations. This is seen in relationships among patients on a ward or unit and within their families. The needs are present in staff relationships and often make the difference in the morale of a unit as well as in how well it is run.

These needs are overlapping and continuous. Inclusion is primarily related to the formation of a relationship, while control and affection are demonstrated within the relationship. Inclusion is feeling "in" or "out"; control is "top" or "bottom"; and affection is "remote" or "close." Generally, people establish equilibrium between themselves and others in these three areas. Sickness with hospitalization disturbs this equilibrium, giving rise to a wide variety of new stresses.

Need for Inclusion

The need for inclusion is defined behaviorally as the need to establish and maintain satisfactory relationships with people with respect to association and interaction. It refers to the establishment and maintenance of a feeling of mutual interest in others. The need for inclusion is the need to feel that the self is significant and worthwhile. Inclusion behavior refers to association between individuals and is indicated by such words as "associate," "interact," "belong," "join," and "communicate." Lack of inclusion is connoted by words such as "excluded," "ignored," "withdrawn," "aloof," or "isolated." The need to be included is shown by the desire to attract attention and interest. The "demanding" patient who frequently signals and monopolizes the staff with extensive conversation may simply be indicating strong needs for inclusion. The nurse who feels personally slighted when a patient ignores her attempts at polite conversation or treats her like a servant rather than a professional person may be demonstrating her own inclusion needs.

The desire for prestige and status is a part of inclusion needs; the individual needs people to pay attention to him, know who he is, and distinguish him from others. Identity is closely related to inclusion. One is known as a distinct individual, who therefore deserves attention. The height of inclusion is to be understood, which implies that someone is interested enough to seek and discover a person's particular characteristics, likes, and dislikes.

When a person enters a hospital situation, his first crisis involves inclusion needs. Will the staff know who he is? Will he be treated like a person and not just another case—"Room 111" or "the new cardiac"? Many routines of hospital admission strip the patient of outward signs of prestige and status. His clothes and belongings, even his dentures, may be taken away. He receives a uniform and, often humiliating, a hospital gown. He may be bombarded by a series of questions relating to the most intimate details of his life. He is expected to join the patient "group" but may be given little explanation or few guidelines about what to do. When it is necessary to place a patient in isolation, attention should be given to his inclusion needs—the nurse becomes a vital link in satisfying them.

Other ways to help a patient with his inclusion needs include giving him a thorough and considerate orientation to his physical surroundings. The nurse can inquire about the patient's questions and expectations related to treatment. She can give some guidelines about the scope of her professional responsibility, explaining that she will be available to help in a variety of ways.

The patient who is withdrawn and avoids association with others may have unmet inclusion needs. He may not talk to his roommates or the nurse and may spend long periods sleeping or with the curtains pulled. A certain amount of regression and isolation is often a necessary part of adaptation to illness and recovery, but extremes over a period of time are significant. Underneath an apparent indifference to others may lie a basic anxiety in relation to people. The patient's worse fear may be that others will ignore him and show no interest in him, although the fear is disguised with a lack of interest in others and a seeming independence. Patients who feel abandoned and isolated from their families and friends, who believe that they are so changed now as to be unacceptable, or who feel rejected and ignored by the medical and nursing staff, may give up the struggle. On the other hand, such patients may get life-saving reassurance and support from the nurse who continues to include them in the human race and communicates her recognition of their individuality and worth.

Part of the decision of where to place a patient is based on the need for inclusion. Will he do better in a room with three other people? How close to the nursing station should he be? Patients who are together for long periods of time, such as in an orthopedic ward or a rehabilitation facility, demonstrate a particularly wide variety of inclusion needs.

Need for Control

The second major need is control. This is the need to establish and maintain a satisfactory relation to others with regard to power, decision making, and authority. It has to do with the feeling of mutual respect for the competence and responsibility of oneself and others. Control needs are suggested by such words as "dominance," "influence," "boss," "rebellion," "submission," "leader," "noncooperation," and "follower." Control represents assumption of power over others and therefore over one's own future, whereas *being* controlled means giving up responsibility for oneself.

When a person comes to a hospital, he struggles with his need for control. In addition to the problems of inclusion, he may find other people making decisions for him that he would ordinarily make for himself—when to get up, what to eat, and when to go to the toilet. The rules of the hospital may take away his usual decision-making capacity. An extreme example of control behavior is the person who completely gives up or abdicates his own responsibility. He is a clinging, helpless patient who seeks direction from everyone about what to do and how to do it. This reinforces his conviction that he is incompetent, irresponsible, and powerless. Behind these beliefs often lie anxiety, hostility, and a lack of trust in others as well as oneself. Nursing interventions that help the patient to assume responsibility early for making decisions about his own care contribute to restoring control.

The other extreme in control behavior is reflected in actions of constant rebellion and domination. Although the patient's overt behavior may be that of a strong, competent, responsible person, his underlying feelings may be those of uncertainty in his own power. He takes every opportunity to disprove these fears and therefore has a great deal of difficulty in accepting the need for dependency in such matters as bed rest or following "doctor's orders." Nurses also need to examine their own needs for power and control in relation to patients, coworkers, and physicians.

Need for Affection

The third major need is that of affection. This represents the need to establish with another person a give-and-take relationship based on mutual liking. Affection is suggested by such words as "love," "like," "emotionally close," "personal," "friendship," and "intimacy." Lack of affection is connoted by "hate," "dislike," and "emotionally distant." The need for affection is usually met by family members, spouses, and close friends. When a person is separated from these sources by illness or hospitalization, the need for affection may not be satisfied. Being emotionally close to another generally results in confiding to that person one's innermost anxieties, wishes, and feelings. In the hospital setting, the patient may turn to the nurse to share these things, especially if the family member is unavailable or too anxious to listen. One difference between a social and a professional relationship is that the former implies mutual need satisfaction, the latter, exclusive attention to the patient's needs. However, the need for affection in both patient and nurse must be considered, particularly when the relationship continues over a period of time.

Self-image and Body Image

The individual has a mental and social picture of himself that is based on multiple experiences in the past, present, and anticipated future. Serious illness and injury abruptly interfere with that self-concept. Adaptation to the changes imposed by illness can affect the person's sense of identity. People often rate themselves as courageous or cowardly in terms of how they handle pain; crying may be a sign of weakness to them. A major disability can be viewed as a limitation to be challenged. Some persons regard themselves as cripples, which emphasizes the disability and is stigmatizing. An important aspect of the total self-image that is often affected by physical illness is body image.

Concept of Body Image

The concept of body image is useful in understanding the many complex reactions of people to changes in health status. Body image may be considered as the total, constantly changing and evolving perception of one's physical self as separate and distinct from all others. This perception is based on inner sensations and functionings as well as on information derived from the external environment. Society prescribes norms of physical appearance and behavior. The perception of body image operates on both conscious and unconscious levels.

Integration of experiences regarding the use of the body takes place over a long period of time. The formative years of childhood are particularly significant in laying down the basic body image and its relation to the personality. While a child is being held, fondled, fed, played with, and toilet-trained, he gradually accumulates related concepts pertaining to ability to use his physical body, pride, and sense of identity. Through sensory impressions, mobility, and touch he experiences pleasure, pain, shame, failure, or pride of accomplishment as he tests out his boundaries and abilities. As the small child becomes aware of his separation

from others, he grows increasingly conscious of his own body, its relation to others, and his ability to control his muscles in the acts of locomotion, bowel and bladder retention and release, motor coordination, and speech. During this period, he begins to master these abilities, and thus acquires pride and self-esteem. If he is not able to gain this mastery, because of loss of self-control and parental over-control, he may develop basic attitudes that lead him to regard his body as inadequate, worthless, and shameful. Illness, with enforced dependency and lack of body control, reactivates in persons of all ages many of these early conflicts and perceptions of body image. Feeling ashamed of a disfigurement or deformity stems from early feelings of smallness, weakness, and ugliness as compared to others. The prominent sociocultural values of youth, physical attractiveness, health, and wholeness are incorporated early and reinforced throughout life.

Threats to Body Image.   Threats to the body image, and hence to self-esteem, are recognizable in many nursing situations. Feelings of shame, inadequacy, and guilt may be precipitated, depending on the patient's definition of the situation. Violation of modesty and invasion of privacy cause anxiety and embarrassment. Exposure of the body during physical examinations and such treatments as enemas and catheterizations may be upsetting, even though expected as part of the therapeutic regimen. Disturbances in usual elimination processes and the need for using a bedpan or talking about bowel and bladder habits threatens self-esteem. This is a major problem for people requiring the type of surgery that produces such drastic changes as a colostomy or ileostomy.

Major changes in the body image are brought about by amputation of any part or by surgery on the face, hands, and reproductive organs—areas particularly related to identity and self-esteem. Other parts of the body may have unconscious symbolic meanings for a person and may cause unexpected reactions to relatively minor external changes.

Besides the sudden changes in body structure and functioning that occur through accident or surgical intervention, subtle changes occur in progressive diseases such as arthritis, obesity, and multiple sclerosis. Even normal changes in the body, such as occur in puberty and pregnancy, pose a problem of altering the body image. During adolescence there is a sensitive, often painful awareness of the body and its many changes. Complexion, weight, and development of primary and secondary sexual chracteristics are closely linked to feelings of worth and sexual desirability.

Changes in the body image may result from such side-effects of medication as development of a moon face, changes in the secondary sex characteristics, and growth of facial hair. The reaction of the body to radiation treatment may further threaten the body image, as may changes in skin color, such as occurs in jaundice.

Changes in medical technology require that nurses meet the challenge of new and different approaches to helping people. A person with chronic kidney damage extends his body image to include the "artificial kidney." Organ transplants are another development that raises questions about body image. What does it mean to a person to have another person's heart beating in his chest? What would it be like to have parts of your own body live on after you are clinically dead?

Nursing Implications. The first step in understanding the concept of body image is to become more aware of one's own attitude toward health, illness, mutilation, disfigurement, and changes in body functioning. Anxiety, revulsion, disgust, and pity are often automatic responses to abnormal body appearance and functioning. To help patients who have these conditions, nurses must come to grips with their own feelings. A patient has a right to expect that nurses will be knowledgeable about his condition, impartial toward it, willing to help him, and concerned about him. A patient often uses the nurse's reactions as a test of whether he is still a worthwhile person in spite of his altered appearance or functioning.

The nurse needs to learn what alteration in the body can mean to the individual patient and what adjustments it will require. Both the patient and his family should be considered, because ideally the adjustment that takes place is mutual. In formulating the nursing care plan for a particular patient, it is useful to include the ability of the family to help the patient cope with changes, orientation to reality, specific problems in coping and methods of coping, and nursing care. The nurse needs to determine how she can support the family and the steps she will take in response to the patient's positive moves. She can anticipate grief, mourning, and anger as reactions to changes in body appearance and functioning. The need for hope and steps toward full rehabilitation must be supported.

Social Adjustments. Even after the patient has begun to alter his body image and feels worthwhile and accepted in the hospital setting, he is faced with adjusting to society. Many conditions of altered appearance and functioning are stigmatizing. Because of their close proximity to illness, nurses may lose sight of the fact that being disfigured or incapacitated still evokes negative responses and rejection by most of the population. Any such stigma implies that the person is not quite normal—that he is a disabled person, rather than a person having a specific disability. The tendency to stereotype denies the person's individuality. A person with an obvious physical disability has a major problem in handling tensions in interpersonal situations. He may be subjected to curiosity and stares. He may be asked intrusive questions about his condition or treated as if he were completely helpless.

If the condition is not readily visible, learning to exercise information control may help one to avoid being stigmatized. For instance, wearing a prosthesis for a mastectomy can keep one's radical surgery from becoming common knowledge. Talking about one's health status, body functioning, and difficulties in adjustment is appropriate with health personnel and close family and friends. With other people, excessive dwelling on these topics may lead to rejection and ostracism.

A person making necessary adjustments to alterations in his body is often faced with physical and social insecurity. A physically normal person has a general idea of how high the bus steps are and is able to read from a menu. However, the person with a physical impairment may have to make constant and vigilant adaptations to his physical world. The person who uses a wheelchair must find a restroom large enough to maneuver in; one with diabetes must calculate his allowed intake at a cocktail party; a person with crutches may find a revolving door almost impossible to manage. Adaptation requires energy, ingenuity, and persistence. Sometimes an individual limits his living space and activities in order to provide more predictable situations. Although this arrangement may be safer, it also limits a person's full participation in life.

Reactions of others toward a person with a disability are ambiguous and conflicting. Acceptance and rejection, sympathy and pity, trust and fear, curiosity and revulsion, valuation and devaluation face him in countless interpersonal situations. He is often unsure of where he stands, particularly with strangers. He is also often unsure of himself, because the process of adaptation and self-acceptance is a shifting one.

Emotional Reactions to Illness and Treatment

Many disturbing feelings are aroused by acute and chronic illness and the treatment they require. Some emotional reactions commonly experienced by patients and their families are anxiety, anger, grief, hope, shame, guilt, courage, pride, despair, love, depression, helplessness, envy, loneliness, and faith. Nursing staff members also experience these feelings. How they are experienced and expressed depends on the basic personality, the perception of the situation, and the amount of support from others. There is no right or wrong way to feel about serious illness. Nurses can anticipate patterns and help patients and families express feelings in a constructive way.

Anxiety

Anxiety is a normal reaction to stress and threat. It is an emotional reaction to the perception of danger, real or imagined, that is experienced physiologically, psychologically, and behaviorally. Anxiety and fear are often used synonymously; however, fear generally refers to a specific threat, anxiety to a nonspecific one. A person experiencing anxiety may feel uneasy and apprehensive, and may have a vague sense of dread. Feelings of helplessness and inadequacy may be present along with a sense of alienation and insecurity. The intensity of these feelings may range from mild to severe enough to cause panic, and the intensity may be increased or diminished by interpersonal means.

Anxiety is caused by a threat to the functioning of the organism—either to physical survival or to the integrity of the psychosocial self (self-image). Often, the threat affects both of these areas: a person who is anxious because of acute pain may also be anxious in response to his feelings about his levels of courage and dependency. Illness and hospitalization include the following anxiety-precipitating threats: general threat to life, health, and body integrity; exposure and embarrassment; discomfort from pain, cold, fatigue, and changes in diet; deprivation of sexual satisfaction; restriction of movement; isolation; interruption or loss of one's means of livelihood; precipitation of a financial crisis; dislike, rejection, or ridicule from others as the result of the condition; inconsistent and unpredictable behavior of the authority figures on whom one's welfare depends; frustration of goals and expectations; confusion and uncertainty about the present and the future; separation from family and friends.

Physiologic reactions to anxiety are primarily reactions of the autonomic nervous system and are defensive in nature. They include increases in pulse and respiratory rates; shifts in blood pressure and temperature; relaxation of the smooth muscles in the bladder and bowel; cold, clammy skin; increased perspiration; dilated pupils; and dry mouth. The bodily responses to mild anxiety initially promote learning and the ability to function, but as the reaction increases in severity, learning decreases, perception is reduced or distorted, and the ability to concentrate is greatly diminished. Nurses must be able to evaluate the level of anxiety in a patient so that they can be effective in reducing it. An extremely anxious person is suffering and is very uncomfortable. He has difficulty giving or receiving information of any kind. As far as health matters are concerned, he learns little and magnifies or distorts what he hears.

Characteristic manifestations of anxiety reflect a person's individuality. They include withdrawal, muteness, hyperactivity, swearing, talking and joking excessively, striking out verbally or physically, fantasizing, complaining, and crying. The specific means of coping with anxiety, whether successful or not, varies with individuals and with the situation. One disadvantage of enforced immobility and isolation is that a person who is used to active approaches in handling anxiety is deprived of his usual means of coping and so must develop alternative channels.

Nursing Interventions.   Nursing intervention in anxiety has four aspects:

1. Recognition that the patient is anxious. The nurse is aware of situations that can potentially precipitate anxiety and is alerted to physiologic, emotional, and behavioral clues.
2. The nurse verbally encourages the patient to recognize and express his feelings of anxiety.
3. If the source of the anxiety is external, such as poor orientation to the ward or disturbing noises and sights, the nurse may take steps to change these conditions or, if this is impossible, help the patient to understand and cope with his reactions. She encourages the patient to share his immediate experience by open-ended statements, such as "Tell me what happened" or "What was going on?" Patients often need help in describing their reactions and thoughts. To ask initially "Why are you anxious?" may or may not result in the information. The person may be too afraid or unsure to tell you, he may not know why he is anxious, or he may resent the inquisition.
4. The nurse helps the patient to cope with what is now a specific threat. He may be helped to reevaluate the situation and his reaction to it. Many times just the sharing of a feeling reduces its intensity. The nurse asks the patient what he usually does to handle anxious feelings and helps him to use similar or other means. The

physical presence of the nurse may help, as well as the appropriate use of touch, physical care, and tone of voice.

The apprehension of patients recovering from surgery may be demonstrated by their anxiety about whether the operation was a success and whether they will survive the bewildering, painful, often uncertain postoperative period. The expert physical nursing care given in the recovery room or intensive care unit must take into consideration the patient's fears resulting from isolation; the weird noises and equipment attached to all parts of the body; the blinking, beeping monitor signaling the body's functioning; and the periods of disorientation and loss of physical and emotional control. In this tense situation the nurse must be constantly aware of her own behavioral manifestations of anxiety.

Illness and its treatment precipitate anxiety. For many people, early conflicts are revived. There is often a great deal of uncertainty about the future. Nurses' sometimes are powerless to decrease the patient's anxiety at all, but they can avoid adding to it. For some patients, the thought of getting well and leaving the hospital produces anxiety. The nurses can be helpful to these people by encouraging them to mobilize their strengths and by encouraging decision making and the reacquisition of responsibility.

Nursing in almost all areas is a profession that deals continually with anxiety. The intimate association with life, death, and all the stages in between arouse within the nurse conscious and unconscious fears about her own vulnerability. Recognition, achievement, and attention are all important; she must be able to say that she did all that was possible. There are emotional "high-risk" situations in nursing, such as the intensive care unit and the emergency room, in which the nurse's understanding and management of her own anxiety as well as that of patients and their families is vital.

Anger and Hostility

In addition to anxiety, expressions of anger are common in nursing situations. Conflict and frustration often precipitate aggression, a complex reaction of feelings and behavior that varies in intensity, duration, and expression. Words such as "irritated," "sullen," "unfriendly," "hostile," "assertive," "belligerent," "defiant," "uncooperative," "resentful," "enraged," "furious," and "indignant" describe various forms of aggressiveness. Anger, the general term for this emotion, is one way of handling anxiety, particularly in response to real or perceived threat, insult, or injury. To be a patient means to be sick, helpless, controlled by others, and assaulted—however therapeutically—by needles, catheters, enemas, and surgical procedures. Being told to wait for medication angers many patients who are in pain. Being awakened in the middle of the night to cough and take deep breaths taxes anyone's patience. Hospital rules such as lights out and restrictions on visitors may arouse feelings of anger. When a patient is new to the hospital or clinic, he is often uncertain and anxious about his diagnosis, treatment, and prognosis; as a defense, he may flare up at the nurse or withdraw in sullen noncommunicativeness. Expressions of anger may decrease markedly as the element of the unknown is reduced and the patient becomes more familiar with his surroundings, the personnel, and the treatment program. On the other hand, anger may increase if the threat grows and the patient's needs are not met adequately.

A person who has been angry, unhappy, and chronically dissatisfied with himself and others brings this behavior with him to the clinical setting. He may be argumentative, demanding, unappreciative, sarcastic, and unwilling to go along with nursing care. Extreme overfriendliness, ingratiation, and refusal to make any decision concerning one's care are also expressions of aggression. Occasionally, a patient is aggressive to the point of violence—throwing his dinner tray, shouting, cursing, doing or threatening to do physical harm. Nonverbal expressions of anger—glaring eyes, clenched fist, a sneer—can be nearly as eloquent.

Aggressive behavior that is ascribable to a toxic condition is acceptable; the patient can be excused because he was delirious or "not in his right mind." The continuously hostile patient who is fully conscious and in control is much harder to understand and deal with. The expression of anger in the clinical situation may reflect the person's best manner of coping with perceived threats. Anger may be an attempt to relieve feelings of helplessness and dependency. In other situations, anger is part of the grief process or emergence from apathy and depression. A patient's anger may vanish when someone helps him to identify what is frustrating or threatening him and to take steps toward successfully dealing with the threat.

It is not unusual for people to displace feelings of anger—that is, to express them toward someone or something other than the original frustrator. When one believes oneself to be in a vulnerable position, it may not be safe to express dissatisfaction and anger directly. Therefore, one takes it out on somebody less likely to retaliate or less vitally important to one's emotional and physical well-being. A patient may be very angry with his physician but afraid to complain for fear that he will receive less attention. Instead, he bawls out the nurse and later insists that she contact his doctor. Or, the nurse and the physician may have a covert misunderstanding; she finds herself snapping at the aides and being irritable with the patients. Generally, direct expressions of anger are not socially acceptable, and outbursts are followed by guilt, shame, and profuse apologies. Moreover, because of cultural and socioeconomic differences in the expression of anger, the nurse may be bewildered, insulted, and overwhelmed by behavior considered normal and expected by another individual.

The usual social responses to anger are counterattack, withdrawal, or avoidance of the situation. A nurse's initial reaction to an angry patient is to treat him as she would in social circumstances. Many times this is not appropriate from the therapeutic standpoint. The professional nursing responsibility is to try to help this person, even with and in spite of his anger. The nurse does this by first recognizing her own responses to angry behavior. It is not unusual for a nurse to experience feelings of irritation and annoyance. She may be frightened, embarrassed, and hurt. When a patient lashes out verbally, she may feel inadequate and guilty, even if she has acted appropriately. She may feel helpless or immobilized to the extent that she dreads caring for the patient and begins to avoid him whenever possible. This kind of behavior may heighten the patient's frustration by leaving him isolated, helpless, and unable to depend on the nursing staff to meet his physical and emotional needs. Thus, a vicious circle is established.

Nursing Interventions. Therapeutic responses to angry patients are based on the attempt to understand the person and his situation. The nurse is aware of her own reaction to the patient and attempts to help him sort out the issues involved. She enables the patient to maintain his dignity, pride, and self-esteem. She sets limits on his behavior so that he does not hurt himself or others and helps him to find more appropriate means of expressing his feelings. Although she may feel angry or frightened in reaction to the behavior, she uses her feelings for further problem solving, instead of giving way to retaliation or withdrawal. Helpful questions in arriving at a nursing care plan for patients who are angry and hostile include the following: When does the patient get angry and how does he show it? Does his anger interfere with his receiving the care he needs? Why does his behavior bother me? How do I react? Does he get angry with other people too? Is there someone who does get along with him? What does that person do that is different? Does the patient's hostility serve a useful purpose? How much of this behavior reflects his usual way of reacting to people? How much is he willing to change? What realistic goals shall we work toward? Are there any other resources—physician, family, psychiatric nursing consultant, psychiatrist, occupational therapist, or other patients—that we could call in? If the patient stops expressing anger, will he develop more destructive patterns?

Learning to work therapeutically with angry, hostile patients is a challenging and rewarding part of nursing. Patients who disguise temporary fear and shame with anger appreciate the nurse who stands by them in the crisis without condemnation, rejection, or retaliation. Patients who have made a lifelong adjustment by means of hostile attack are also grateful, although they may never express it directly, to the nurse who refuses to be alienated and who applies herself to understanding and caring for them.

Grief and Mourning

Grief is a complex of emotional responses to the anticipated or actual loss of someone or something valued. The loss may be that of a relative or friend, a part of the body, a job, health, or life. Feelings of anxiety, helplessness, hopelessness, guilt, anger, depression, remorse, sadness, and loneliness are part of grief. Mourning refers to the processes that follow the loss and ultimately result in overcoming the grief. There are many cultural factors involved in the specific way in which grief and mourning take place, from the extremes of stoic acceptance to elaborate and ritualistic weeping, keening, and public display.

The intensity of grief and mourning depends on the significance and extent of the loss to the person. It is generally greater if the loss, especially through death, comes suddenly. If the survivor has been particularly dependent upon the deceased person, or if in any way he was responsible for the death, grief is intensified. A person who is very sensitive to separation as a result of early separations may be deeply affected. Ambivalence (mixed feelings) is present in all significant relationships. If the ambivalence is marked, grief may be particularly intense. Guilt and irrational ideas about the causation of the death may prevent a person from facing himself and mourning effectively.

The stages of mourning are similar to the stages of adaptation to illness—shock and disbelief, awareness, and restitution. Upon recognition of a loss, people often experience a sinking feeling, tightness in the throat, loss of appetite, fatigue, tension, and acute anxiety. The sensorium is altered, and there is a feeling of unreality and distance from people. There is a preoccupation with the deceased or lost object and a state of readiness for its return. Feelings of guilt may be present, and there may be soul-searching and remorse about things that could have been done differently. The grieving person's relationships with other people lack warmth and are characterized by irritation and the desire not to be bothered. He is likely to slow up activities, neglect personal care, and be restlessly and purposelessly active. He may develop symptoms similar to those of the deceased one. Sometimes the shock of the loss is accepted intellectually and the person goes through the motions of making arrangements and caring for others. His emotional reaction is cut off in his attempt to protect himself from the pain of the loss.

In the stage of developing awareness, the person experiences pain, anguish, emptiness, and acute sadness. Crying or the desire to cry is common and often elicits support from others. Many people cannot allow themselves to cry in public and need privacy to handle their grief.

In the stage of restitution, the physical reality of the loss is emphasized. In the case of death, the funeral makes this fact unavoidable. In the case of an amputation, the sight of the stump and the first attempt of using a prosthesis underline the reality. The mourner begins a long process of coping with the absence of the loved person or object. There may be repetitive talk about the person or object and there is a tendency to idealize them, so that only pleasant memories are reinforced. Gradually, this assists in the task of achieving emotional detachment. As dependence on the lost object decreases, the person begins to develop new interests and invests energy in other people. He is able to remember the relationship more realistically, with its good and bad aspects, and can talk about it without emotional dependence on the memory of the relationship.

Nursing Interventions.   Nursing interventions to help patients and families with the experience of grief and mourning include anticipating reactions to loss, supporting the usual coping mechanisms, and allowing the expression of feelings. The nurse provides privacy and availability. When a body part or function is lost, the nurse designs specific nursing care and controls the environment to prevent additional loss of self-esteem. The presence and willingness of nurses to participate in the painful experiences that accompany grief help to prevent feelings of total abandonment. By being aware of the usual patterns of grief and mourning, nurses can recognize maladaptive patterns and help evaluate the need for other types of therapeutic intervention, such as psychotherapy.

Hope

Hope is a complex human experience that has a relationship to health. It is a mixture of feelings and thoughts that center on the fundamental belief that there are solutions to significant human needs and problems. Most people have hoped for and expected a long and healthy life for themselves and significant others. Serious illness and injury raise questions of vulnerability and uncertainty about the future.

The purpose of hope is to ward off despair, which is characterized by mental anguish, disorganization, helplessness, and hopelessness. Loss of hope leads to giving-up behavior that leads to physical and emotional disequilibrium. Death may result from the loss of the will to live or through suicide. Hope is a catalyst that activates the motivational system. It is reinforced by other people who give support and encouragement to continue the struggle. When patients see "the light at the end of the tunnel," they can persist in moving toward future goals of improved functioning. Even with patients who are dying, hope for relief of suffering and meaningful living in the present are important aspects that can be reinforced with nursing care.

Nursing Interventions.   To help patients and families maintain or restore hope, nurses contribute to a hopeful atmosphere that comes from themselves, other staff members, patients, and the physical environment. This is possible if individuals have faced and explored their views of the meaning of life, illness, and death. Feelings of hope, hopelessness, and helplessness are found in all nursing situations. Even while helping others with these feelings, nurses must deal with similar shifts in their own experience of hope. If they feel hopeless, they talk about feelings with others to get encouragement and a clearer picture of the reality of the situation. When hopes for the recovery of a patient are disappointed, staff members, along with families, feel bewildered, angry, and grief stricken.

Role Changes

When people get sick, their role identities change. This affects the ways in which others interact with them and relate to them; relationships with family and friends must be reestablished and maintained.

Some of the most important role changes are those that take place in the family when parents are no longer able to carry out their usual activities with their children. There may be role reversals, with children caring for their parents. In the usual life cycle, aging parents become increasingly dependent on their middle-aged children for help and direction; serious illness makes this even more evident.

Role changes in terms of occupational functioning may be drastically altered. When physicians and nurses become patients, they often find it very difficult to accept the patient role; staff members also have difficulty seeing them in a new light. This is true of persons who are considered "V.I.P.s." They may demand and get deferential treatment, which at times is detrimental to their best interests as well as disruptive to the unit. Many people base their sense of self-worth on the ability to work and be productive. If forced to convalesce or retire because of illness, individuals tend to feel lost and bereft of important links with others. Vocational rehabilitation is an important part of health planning for patients who must make major alterations.

A difficult role for a patient to deal with and others to react to is that of a terminally ill patient, a dying person. For many people, this is an unfamiliar and frightening aspect of life. They do not know what is expected of them, what to talk about, and how to carry on in light of the poor prognosis. Health professionals may withdraw from patients once it is clear that they are not going to recover. Nurses play an important part in helping patients and families go through this period.

Persons with chronic illness struggle with the role of being impaired. They want to be as normal as possible, yet sometimes the conditions of illness interfere with this to a large degree. They must continually make decisions about how to act and what to tell others. This is especially true in social situations; some people simply withdraw and cut themselves off from others, which leads to loneliness and depression.

▷ Coping Strategies

Patients, families, and staff strive to adapt to serious illness in many ways. These coping skills are generally the approaches that were used in other difficult periods. Moos and Tsu described these as coping skills that can be learned and practiced. Although divided into seven categories, the skills are often used in different combinations and vary in appropriateness and helpfulness. At different stages of illness, one or more of the coping skills may predominate.

Denial

Denial involves denying or minimizing the seriousness of the crisis, as well as isolating or dissociating feelings connected with the condition. This approach downplays the symptoms as evidence of illness or disregards the seriousness of the diagnosis. The first reaction to loss is shock and disbelief. Denial or numbing of feelings gives one time to absorb the meaning and protects one from being overwhelmed by feelings. Denial and isolation are ego defense mechanisms that protect against anxiety by distorting reality. Generally, the increase or persistence of symptoms forces the person to abandon the denial in time.

As a coping skill, denying or minimizing the problem helps to maintain psychological equilibrium. It can be harmful when it leads to such things as missing appointments, signing out of the hospital, and refusing appropriate treatment. Inappropriate cheerfulness and lack of concern about symptoms may indicate denial. If anxiety, depression, and anger are not expressed in situations where they are expected, the patient may be using denial for self-protection. However, sometimes patients act this way to protect others. This happens when patients are aware they are dying but

perceive that the family would be more comfortable if the mutual deception was continued. They may be able to talk about fears and feelings with the staff, thereby lessening isolation.

Denial mechanisms operate in families as they try to protect themselves from recognizing the severity of the situation. Even when imminent death is discussed, the family may deny this is possible and act (or fail to act) accordingly.

Nursing Interventions. In dealing with denial of illness as a nursing problem, nurses assess the extent to which the denial is harmful and the ways in which it is beneficial. Generally, the defense of denial is not challenged directly, because such action tends to reinforce the position or leaves the person without necessary ego protection. The nurse does not support or encourage the denial and remains available. When patients can relinquish denial, they need help in dealing with the difficult aspects of reality that they were attempting to ward off.

Denial is a coping skill that nurses use to handle their own feelings about illness, radical surgery, and death. Along with other health professionals, they may need this defense to keep working in high-risk areas. When nurses can talk about their feelings with others, they develop more realistic ways of dealing with the stresses and thus are better equipped to help patients and families face their difficult problems.

Seeking Information

This coping skill involves (1) seeking relevant information that can relieve anxiety caused by misconceptions and uncertainty, and (2) using one's intellectual resources effectively. Patients and families are often relieved by information about the illness, its treatment, and the course the illness is expected to take. This provides a framework in which plans can be made and effective action taken. They are encouraged by hearing about successful treatment of others with the same condition. Worrying is decreased when correct facts and clarification of misconceptions and fears are supplied. Giving a time dimension in which certain reactions are anticipated helps to decrease feelings of helplessness. Informed patients are better able to participate in their own treatment.

Requesting Emotional Support

This skill involves requesting reassurance and emotional support from family, friends, and medical/nursing staff while maintaining a sense of personal competence. Patients are often frightened and anxious. They may feel very much alone. A valuable coping skill is being able to reach out for or receive the concern of others. This maintains hope through encouragement. Whether limitations are temporary or permanent, people need to have a sense of mastery over other functions.

Patients can be encouraged by other people with similar conditions. Support groups for patients and families are helpful in encouraging the expression of feelings, sharing practical problems, and passing along effective ways of coping. Patients are reassured by being told that their cooperation with the health team is helpful in fighting together against the difficult illness.

Sometimes, physicians and nurses use shaming and guilt-provoking tactics to get patients to adhere to treatment programs. These are generally ineffective and lead to the patient's being all the more demoralized or seeking health treatment elsewhere.

Learning Self-care

Learning illness-related procedures confirms personal ability and effectiveness. Individuals can learn to care for themselves even in the aftermath of catastrophic illness and injury. Helplessness is decreased because the sense of pride in accomplishments helps to restore or maintain self-esteem. Family members can often learn how to help a loved one during acute as well as chronic illness. Being able to do something often relieves anxiety and guilt. Patient teaching is an important aspect of nursing care.

Setting Concrete, Limited Goals

The overall tasks of adaptation to serious illness seem overwhelming, yet they can be done. Breaking down the components into small, manageable goals will eventually lead to greater risks and success. Motivation is maintained. The feelings of helplessness are decreased as patients experience the impact of action on outcome. Instead of just worrying about results and the future, the person takes action that is effective. Principles of learning are important in accomplishing the eventual long-term goals.

Rehearsing Alternative Outcomes

There are usually multiple alternatives in most situations. Recognizing this helps a person to feel less trapped and helpless. This is accomplished through mental preparation and discussion with others. Exploring options with the nurse and one's family helps to expand the reality base on which to make decisions. Anticipatory planning reduces helplessness by rehearsing "what will happen if. . . ."

This coping skill is often used in conjunction with information seeking. It helps to decrease anxiety by preparing for the future. Recalling how one has been able to manage other difficulties bolsters confidence.

When there is a choice of several treatment modalities, talking over the alternatives is a vital part of including the patient in self-determination. Health professionals do not always know what is best. They can give information based on knowledge and past experience; the patient and family are left with the final decision. Patients may have definite ideas about what they want done in the final stages of life.

This coping skill is very important for patients with altered body parts and functions. They may need to rehearse what to do in a variety of social situations. They use the staff as sounding boards. Groups of patients and other individuals may be helped by role playing situations.

Finding Meaning in Illness

Illness *is* a human experience. Many people have found that serious illness was a turning point in their lives. This may reflect either a spiritual orientation or a philosophical approach to life. Patients find encouragement in the belief that their suffering may have some meaning or be helpful to others. They may participate in research projects or training programs to this end. Sensitive, poignant accounts of illness have been written by patients, families, and staff that convey hope and inspiration. Plays, movies, and television dramas have made it possible for millions of people to share in some of the finest moments of human caring, courage, and compassion.

Families may be brought together by illness in a painful but very meaningful way. People experience a sense of their basic worth as well as that of others. Many survivors of serious illness interviewed by Smith reported that they had experienced a change in values and priorities, greater concern for others, and a heightened appreciation for the beauty of nature. After serious illness, people may find meaning in helping others through support groups or political action, or by entering one of the health professions.

Factors That Help or Hinder Coping

Serious physical illness is a potential life crisis for the individual and family. Crisis is that state in which the person feels that obstacles to important life goals are insurmountable and that the usual means of problem solving are not sufficient. New approaches are needed. Successful mastery leads to greater self-integration, understanding, and trust in others.

Stressors that disturb equilibrium are divided into biological and psychosocial stressors. These are most often intertwined, since one system affects the other. The *biologic stressors* include illness and injury. Not only is the degree of impairment important but so is the meaning of the condition to the individual. Lack of sleep, poor nutrition, dehydration, drugs, and pain are biological stressors that hinder coping with ongoing and new difficulties.

Psychosocial stressors include interpersonal problems with family and significant others, occupational situations, finances, living circumstances, and legal problems. The person's maturational age, especially childhood, adolescence, and aging, specifically affects the impact of illness. Sometimes, psychosocial issues drop away in importance in the face of acute illness and possible death. In many instances, the coping abilities are stretched even more as new problems are created by the illness.

The *personal characteristics* of an individual include age, intelligence, basic personality style, religious and philosophical beliefs, and previous experiences in coping with difficulties, especially prior illness. These affect the person's perception of the illness and his resources for handling the problems.

Social and situational supports affect the way in which a person copes with illness. These are primarily interpersonal supports—people that the distressed person turns to.

Close friends and understanding family members may be vital to maximal recovery. Isolated persons or patients whose family ties are chaotic and disturbed will be under even greater stress with illness. The professional health team is part of the support system. Because nurses are so close and necessary to the ongoing care of patients, they become vital supports during the uncertainty of illness and treatment. They are sensitive to the patient's need for additional help and are instrumental in arranging for this support from family, clergy, other patients, psychiatric and psychological therapists, and social service agencies.

The *physical environment* may help or hinder coping. The problems of sensory overload, sensory deprivation, and isolation, along with the unfamiliar and frightening aspects of the hospital, all contribute to problems of adjustment. Sometimes, although little can be done about these problems, just recognizing that they cause stress can be reassuring to patients and families.

The patient's *basic coping mechanisms* may be altered because of the circumstances of the illness. Pain, fatigue, and immobility interfere with action methods of tension release. Important persons to whom the patient usually turns may not be available, and impaired mobility may restrict his ability to visit them. Generally, the families of seriously ill patients are also very anxious, which leaves them less able to respond to their loved one. An intensification of usual coping patterns may be seen in disturbed communication, behavior, and ways of interacting with others. Common patterns of disturbed behavior resulting from efforts to cope include excessive withdrawal, making demands, disorientation, depression, and manipulative behavior.

▷ Assessing Psychosocial Needs

Nurses encounter sick people at many stages of illness and treatment. They often see only a small part of the picture. When dealing with acute illness, they see patients and families in the crisis situation without knowing much about what preceded or followed the condition. Strauss regards sick persons as having at least three biographies that have meaning in their illness; they are (1) the person's chronological experience with the illness, (2) treatment experiences with prior medical aid (legitimate or not), and (3) the social biography of the person's life history with family, friends, work colleagues, and strangers. Staff members often know very little about these biographies, although they may affect treatment and recovery in definite ways.

Psychosocial History

A *psychosocial history* is the organized assessment of the important events of a person's life; it is sometimes referred to as a *case history.* The psychosocial history is a specific biography of the individual from before birth (heritage and heredity) through the important developmental stages to the present. The anticipated future is also part of the material. The psychosocial history touches on the turning points—the important milestones. Significant illnesses, physical and mental, experienced by the patient and family

members have an important impact on the immediate situation.

The specific psychosocial history is obtained through initial interviewing and from additional contacts. Nurses should be familiar with the elements of a psychosocial assessment. It describes patients in the context of their lives and identifies major problems and assets. Nurses can obtain and use this information while they are providing other nursing care for patients. The nurse talks with patients in a goal-directed way to determine areas in which help is needed.

In many instances, these are action interviews. The contacts continue over the period of illness; the time spent corresponds to the needs of the patient. Critically ill patients will not be able to communicate much more than immediate needs. It is not necessary to get all this information at one time. As the nurse–patient relationship develops, patients feel more confident in talking about matters of serious concern to them. This is particularly true if the listener is interested, compassionate, and nonjudgmental. Nurses also talk with and assess the psychosocial needs of the family members. In the uncertainty and stress of illness, many persons want and need to talk with their professional helpers.

Mental Status Examination

In addition to the psychosocial history, nurses pay attention to the current mental status of the patient. The mental status examination assesses the ways in which a person is thinking, feeling, and acting. It is both a descriptive inventory of behavior and a method of organizing and recording observations of behavior. Problems are identified, and working diagnoses determine the treatment plan. Many of the aspects of the mental status examination are expressed in ongoing speech and behavior. Specific questions are necessary during a formal examination or when clarification, update, or additional information is needed. Patients with serious physical illness often show dramatic shifts in mental status when recovering from surgery or when delirious. The patient with a history of mental illness may decompensate during the stress of illness. Confusion may escalate to extreme behavior unless it is recognized and treated along with the medical condition. Families may need reassurance about the changes in the psychological state of their loved ones.

▷ Aspects of Communication

Acute and chronic physical illness pose many problems to patients and their families. Nurses communicate with them to (1) identify health needs, (2) clarify misconceptions, and (3) help them verbalize fears and other reactions. Anxiety is lessened or channeled through sharing. Nurses are concerned with the impact of illness on the person's life. They are aware of the need to provide privacy while talking with the patient about his conditions in order to help him.

The basic nurse–patient relationship takes into account the physician, the family, other patients, the rest of the health team, and society at large. The relationship is established and maintained by the communication process—a complex, dynamic exchange of verbal and nonverbal messages.

Communication is based on mutually intelligible symbols. To be understood, a person must have a knowledge of himself and his needs, an ability to speak the language and express himself clearly, and a familiarity with the usual conventions of the situation. To understand others, he must be able to observe and evaluate behavior. To make oneself understandable and to understand others is vital to the establishment of relationships. The patient whose English is inept or who speaks a foreign language, or whose ability to express himself is markedly impaired through physical or psychological causes, poses a challenge to the nurse.

The process of communication may be considered to consist of four segments: (1) *I* (2) *am communicating something* (3) *to you* (4) *in this situation.* Breakdowns in communication can be pinpointed by identifying the segment in which the interference it taking place.

The sender of the message, the *I,* is affected by such factors as age, sex, socioeconomic status, marital status, occupation, intelligence, physical condition (especially as related to the nervous system and the organs of communication), personality, and current emotional status.

The message, *am communicating something,* consists of both verbal and nonverbal elements that may be complementary or incongruous. The patient who says, "Oh, I'm fine. Nothing is the matter," while restlessly moving about, wringing his hands, and sighing, frequently illustrates the latter.

The receiver of the communication, *to you,* is influenced by the same factors as the sender with respect to behavior. The ability to hear or "read" a patient's behavior depends largely upon the ability to listen openly and sensitively. The presence of stereotypes, misconceptions, and anxiety may prevent the nurse from correctly identifying the message from a particular patient.

The context of the communication, *in this situation,* refers to the sociocultural status of the patient, the context of illness, the social order of the hospital, and immediate environmental aspects. The importance of understanding the cultural background and the values of patients has gained recognition in all areas of nursing. When patients enter the hospital world, they may be overwhelmed and bewildered by the change in their status and role. The nurse plays a vital part in orienting patients to their new position. She also needs to acquaint them with the scope of her professional services. Many people do not know that the nurse is prepared and eager to help with a wide variety of health needs. In addition to performing the traditional services related to physical needs, she offers help as a health teacher, a rehabilitation worker, a communications link with other professional services, and, in some instances, a psychotherapeutic counselor.

A person in the first stages of adapting to illness, who is taking the defensive measure of denying his illness, does not seek or welcome accurate information about his condition or treatment. A nurse who attempts to do effective health teaching will find her efforts of little avail at this time. The behavior of the patient, the questions he asks or avoids,

and his reactions to the changes in his health status all give clues to his readiness and needs. In turn, the patient is also very sensitive to the reactions of the medical and nursing staff and seeks to interpret nonverbal messages with regard to his prognosis, especially when it is not favorable.

The expressive function of the nurse involves helping the patient to maintain equilibrium and motivation and supporting his attempts to cope with the experience of illness and treatment, by providing direct gratifications that reduce his tension level. The provision of physical comfort and care is combined with such interpersonal activities as explaining, reassuring, understanding, protecting, and simply being with the patient. When a patient is acutely ill, communication generally takes place on a primitive, chiefly nonverbal level. A touch, a soft but reassuring tone of voice, and the presence of the nurse may convey to the patient that he is not alone and that he is being cared for. When it is anticipated that a patient will experience a direct interference with communication patterns as a result of treatment, it is vital to set up a system of communication in advance. One patient reported: "The worst part about my laryngectomy was that I couldn't tell anyone what I needed—but the magic slate helped."

An important part of the development of interpersonal and communication tools is the nurse's understanding of herself, her interpersonal needs, and her usual patterns of communication. As she becomes more aware of her own needs, she is better able to identify those of her patients and to know when her own perceptions and reactions are preventing her from accurately assessing the situation. This is particularly true when the patient's behavior is frustrating, puzzling, hostile, or demanding. The nurse must be able to evaluate her own responses so that she does not retaliate with anger or rejection. The situations that lead to feelings of helplessness and hopelessness must be talked about and shared so that the nurse can maintain her own equilibrium and give optimal nursing care to patients with incurable, repulsive, or terminal conditions. The nurse's awareness of her own need for approval and recognition plays an important part in her reactions to patient behavior and to the behavior of co-workers, supervisors, and the medical staff.

▷ Reactions of Nurses to Illness

Nurses have many personal emotional reactions to patients and families in the crisis of physical illness. Some common responses are frustration, anxiety, anger, hope, guilt, compassion, helplessness, love, hopelessness, disgust, envy, and pride. These are stimulated by the combination of the personal characteristics of the nurse, the professional tasks and obligations involved, and the intricacies of the patient's illness and personality. Nurses not only react emotionally to patients and families, but also have important emotional interactions with other members of the health team. Illness in a patient may evoke emotional responses based on personal experiences or the experiences of close family members.

Nurses are faced with difficulties in adjusting to the many changes in the health status of their patients. This is particularly true with "difficult" patients, those who are not responding to treatment, and dying patients. A high-risk factor is involved in working in settings such as the emergency unit, intensive care unit, premature nursery, and medical units, where a high percentage of patients die. Nurses have to struggle with conflicts between the idealism instilled in nursing school and the reality of the usual work situation. Even when they recognize psychosocial needs, many nurses feel overwhelmed in helping patients; or, there is "no time." Yet, the ultimate recovery and maximal functioning of patients with serious illnesses depend on their ability to deal with multifaceted problems. Sensitive attention to the emotional needs of patients and families helps make hospitalization and treatment smoother, enhances health teaching, and contributes to the quality of life.

It is important for nurses to be aware of their emotional reactions to clinical situations so that they do not become overstressed and unable to cope. When this happens, they experience the phenomenon known as "burnout," which results in personal distress, in indifference to the suffering of others, and often in the decision to leave the job or profession. Nurses who are aware of their many reactions are better able to help others.

▷ "Problem Patients"

Many patients cope with the difficult and often frightening tasks of adaptation to illness. Some inspire with their courage and dignity. Others simply do the best they can in the immediate situation and over the long period in which they convalesce and learn to live with a chronic illness.

Some patients stand out as not dealing with their illness and treatment in the usually expected ways. They may be called "difficult," "management problems," or, in exasperation, "impossible" or "crocks." These labels indicate the breakdown of usually effective coping patterns in both the staff and the patient. The staff need to talk together about the situation. Consultation is often indicated—with a psychiatrist, a consultation-liaison team, or a psychiatric nursing clinical specialist. These persons can help by clarifying the factors, suggesting alternative approaches, giving reassurance to the staff and patient, providing short-term psychotherapy, and evaluating the need for psychoactive drugs. The principle underlying these approaches is that problem patients are patients with problems.

Problems With Cognition, Affect, and Behavior

According to Groves and Kucharski of Massachusetts General Hospital, problems of patients can be classified in three groups, although there is often overlap. These groups are:

1. *Problems of cognition*—delirium, denial, psychosis, failure to process information
2. *Problems of affect*—anxiety, hostility, depression, apathy
3. *Problems of behavior*—noncompliance, withdrawal, dependency, aggressiveness, manipulation

Cognition refers to the ways in which people process information—their ways of thinking, and hence of responding. Perception, memory, understanding, and judgment are involved. Medical–surgical problems often affect these processes. This is seen particularly in *delirium* and *dementia*. The therapeutic approach consists largely in recognizing the nature of the impairment. When the source is identified, steps can be taken. This can include clarifying the medical treatment, changing the environment, and readjusting the medication regimen.

Disturbances of affect (emotions) become problems in a medical–surgical situation when they are overwhelming or inappropriate. Disturbed behavior may result as an exacerbation of a previous mental illness or in response to the immediate situation, illness, or treatment. Excessive anxiety comes from many sources. The therapeutic approach consists in recognizing the causes of the disturbed feelings and helping to restore control. This is done by talking with patients and families about the situation, making necessary changes, and prescribing medication if needed.

Disturbed behavior is directly related to disturbed cognition and overwhelming affects. Severe depression is very distressing to the patient and interferes with healing. It can also precede suicidal behavior. Misinterpretation of the environment leads to panic and aggressive behavior. Patients signal their unmet needs by such behavior as signing out of the hospital, refusing medical treatment, using drugs and alcohol on the unit, and inappropriate sexual behavior.

Extreme dependency leads to difficult patient–staff interactions. This is shown through clinging, demanding behavior in which the patient begs for reassurance yet is unrelieved by it. There may be ongoing demands for services and for pain medication beyond the expected need. Dependent patients are often manipulative and play staff members off against one another. They show anger and hostility both directly and covertly. Nurses feel frustrated, angry, and hopeless in working with these patients.

Nursing Interventions. The therapeutic approach to patients showing disturbed behavior begins with an assessment of the situation from the standpoint of both the staff and the patient. Clear communication is vital. Necessary limits are spelled out. Generally, longstanding personality styles and defenses are not challenged in the midst of a physical illness. The staff are encouraged to meet needs as much as possible and to allow the patient to exert interpersonal control and distance without being punished or abandoned. During the crisis of illness, psychoactive medication, such as tranquilizers and anti-anxiety agents, can be used to help patients manage disturbed feelings and behavior.

A way of understanding and dealing with problem behavior is through learning theory. Behavior that is learned and continued is behavior that is reinforced—rewarded. There is a system of rewards and punishments (even if not acknowledged) in all social systems, including that of the hospital. Patients bring their learned behavior patterns and react to the new interpersonal environment accordingly.

If patients' behavior tags them as "difficult," nurses should study the situation to identify (1) what constitutes the maladaptive behavior and how this interferes with care, progress, and rehabilitation; (2) how and by whom the behavior is reinforced; and (3) how the environment and reinforcers can be changed so that the behavior changes. This is the approach to behavior modification. Nurses should examine their own behavior to see if they are inadvertently playing a part in continuing the situation. Nursing behavior can influence patient behavior in either positive or negative directions. Positive reinforcers include spending time, smiling, showing interest in the conversation, providing food, giving prn medication, giving backrubs, and granting extra privileges.

Psychosomatic Interactions

Knowledge about the relationship between emotions and physical reactions is increasing. This is a highly complex and little understood matter that the mass media have simplified to the point where the terms "psychosomatic," "neurotic," "imaginary," "faking," "malingering," "psychogenic," and "somatopsychic" are used loosely and create confusion.

Anxiety is experienced as both emotional and physiologic reactions. Many people seek treatment for symptoms that are due to chronic, continued anxiety. The anxiety may represent a reaction to reality factors in the present, such as a job or a marriage, or to long-standing conflicts over sexuality, dependency, aggression, and other factors.

Psychosomatic Illness. Anxiety reactions in which the symptoms center around one organ system are described in the nomenclature as *psychophysiologic reactions* having autonomic and visceral responses (*e.g.,* "psychophysiologic reaction, cardiovascular," if the symptoms are predominantly cardiac in nature). Any organ system can be affected. When actual structural changes do occur, the condition is described as a *psychosomatic illness* that has resulted from a combination of emotional and physiologic factors. Common conditions that are generally considered to involve psychosomatic factors are peptic ulcer, chronic ulcerative colitis, hyperthyroidism, bronchial asthma, essential hypertension, and neurodermatitis. The frequency and severity of these illnesses point to the need for greater understanding of the relationship between mind and body.

Hypochondriasis. Another manifestation of underlying emotional conflict that expresses itself in physical symptoms is *hypochondriasis*. A hypochondriacal patient may be totally absorbed in his body and its functioning, and presents endless complaints and reports. Hypochondriasis may be used as a means of attempting to meet long-standing dependency needs. The nurse must evaluate her reactions to such a patient's complaints and demands. Frustration and anger are common responses to this type of patient. The hardworking nurse often resents someone who avoids adult responsibility so easily. Expressing this anger directly to the patient is not helpful, since he is struggling to maintain some kind of equilibrium. Not recognizing her own anger could result in the nurse's avoiding the patient and not caring for his realistic needs. If the nurse goes overboard and attempts to meet all of the patient's unsatisfied dependency

needs, she soon finds that the patient is insatiable—a bottomless pit. Finding a reasonable middle ground is a challenge in working with these patients. Very little is known about successful nursing approaches to hypochondriacal patients. Excessive preoccupation with one's body, accompanied by unusual ideation, may be a sign of more severe emotional disorders, such as psychotic depression or schizophrenia. Through proper assessment of needs and evaluation of behavior, the nurse may help plan for more appropriate treatment.

Conversion Reactions. Another group of physical reactions that have an emotional basis are *conversion reactions*. Conversion is an ego defense mechanism in which anxiety is eliminated or reduced by the production of a physical symptom. This symptom may be directly related to the emotional conflict; the hand that would strike out is paralyzed; the eyes that would look at the forbidden become blind. In most instances, the conflict and the symbolic meaning of the symptom are complex, disguised, and difficult to unravel. These patients come into a medical–surgical setting for differential diagnosis. A conversion reaction may develop after an organic illness has occurred, which tends to prolong the secondary gains of dependency and security.

Generally, the symptoms of conversion reactions simulate disturbances in the voluntary nervous system or in the organs of the special senses. Disturbances of sensation and motion are the most common. Sensation changes include anesthesia, paresthesia, and pain. Loss of hearing and sight are much more common than loss of the other special senses. Disturbances of motion include paralysis, usually of the extremities or speech mechanism, and uncontrolled movements, such as tics and nonorganic convulsions. If the symptom is diagnosed as a conversion reaction, the treatment is generally best directed by a psychiatrist. The nurse can help greatly by accurately observing the patient's behavior, including his reaction to other people. She must keep in mind that symptom formation in a person with a conversion reaction occurs on an unconscious level—the patient is not faking, and his symptoms are not imaginary. This is his way of coping with situations at the present time; with professional help he may be able to find more adequate ways of doing so.

Disturbances in Orientation. Disturbances in orientation occur frequently in patients on medical–surgical services. Acute brain syndrome, which may be a reaction to anesthesia, infection, surgical or metabolic disturbances, overdose of drugs or alcohol, or assault of the brain, as in head injury, often produce delirium. *Delirium* is a state of altered consciousness or awareness manifested by disorientation and confusion. It is induced by interference with the metabolic processes of the brain and is generally acute in onset and reversible. The first signs are restlessness, anxiety, and suspicion, which quickly mount to agitation, excitement, and confusion. The patient often begins to hallucinate and experience delusions. These distortions of reality are extremely frightening, and the desperate behavior of the person experiencing them necessitates skilled nursing action. Patients recovering from cardiac surgery, in particular, often become delirious. It is necessary to reduce the terror and extreme anxiety of these patients not only for emotional reasons, but also to prevent overloading the body with more stress.

Nursing care for a delirious patient includes continual reorientation, a calm voice, and adequate lighting through the night. If possible, the same nurses should attend the patient much of the time, since they repeatedly demonstrate by familiar words and action that he is safe and cared for. It often helps to tell the patient that you know he is very frightened, but that the things he is experiencing are a reaction to his illness that will go away. Hallucinations caused by organic processes are often vivid and threatening. Along with visual hallucinations, the patient may experience tactile hallucinations in which he feels he is being touched or bugs are crawling on him.

Acute brain syndrome is treated by alleviating the causative agents, and the nurse must be aware that proper hydration, nutrition, and medication are directed toward this end. Restraints may be necessary to keep the patient in bed, but they may also frighten and irritate him. The nurse must be aware of his distortion of reality and poor judgment in order to protect him from injuring himself or others. Patients have walked out of unprotected windows while delirious.

Following an episode of delirium, a person may experience anxiety and shame over his behavior when not in full control. He may fear that he has acted inappropriately, hurt someone, or said vulgar or obscene things. He may be afraid of having told confidences and secrets about himself. If the patient gives evidence of such concern, the nurse can encourage him to talk about his fears and then reassure him that his behavior was understandable in the situation and that his confidence will not be betrayed. This is a potentially shameful situation in which the rights, dignity, and privacy of the patient must be protected.

Chronic brain syndrome may result from damage to brain tissue sustained by the causes of acute brain syndrome, or from long-term infections, such as syphilis; heavy metal intoxication; circulatory disturbances, such as cerebral arteriosclerosis; convulsive disorders; disturbances of growth, metabolism, or nutrition; intracranial neoplasm; prenatal factors; and diseases of unknown etiology, such as multiple sclerosis. The behavior common to people with these conditions is described as *dementia,* and it represents chronic, irreversible brain damage with deterioration of intellectual capacities owing to structural changes. Both delirium and dementia are characterized by loss of abilities—defects in memory, orientation (of time, place, and person), and judgment. In planning nursing care and long-term treatment, the individual's strengths must be evaluated along with his limitations. Environmental manipulation and simplification may help him to live his life to the fullest.

▷ Dying and Death

The style in which a person dies is individual, just as his life was. One of the major problems in understanding death is that, in our culture, it is a taboo and unfamiliar experience.

Dying takes place in hospitals or nursing homes rather than as part of the life cycle at home. Death is a strange new experience that does not affect most persons until their adult years. Many nursing students come into contact with death for the first time during the medical–surgical clinical experience.

For most people, just the thought of death is frightening and even impossible. Regardless of religious beliefs, it is difficult to imagine oneself not existing in the world. Nurses are deeply committed to life and health. The dying patient is in direct opposition to that commitment. Sometime the medical and nursing staff react to dying patients as if they represent a failure of their skill and care. Although nothing can be done to reverse the ultimate process, dying patients and their families can be helped during the final days.

People face death in many ways. According to Kübler–Ross, the emotional responses of a person facing death can be traced through five stages: denial and isolation, anger, bargaining, depression, and acceptance. These five stages do not always occur in sequence; they may be mixed or overlapping. Patients and their families move back and forth through the experience and may be at different stages at a given time.

Denial and Isolation

Recognition and acceptance of the fact that death is to be faced shortly is difficult; the common reaction is to insulate oneself until other defenses are marshaled. Denial permits hope to exist. Often, patients are ready to accept the fact that they are dying, but the family continues to express denial. This delays communication of concerns. Denial and isolation are interrupted when the patient begins to think about unfinished business—personal affairs, finances, arrangements for spouse, children, and others.

Anger

The next emotion expressed is anger. The question "Why me?" does not require an answer, but the patient is helped if the nurse is present to offer support and to listen. The behavior of patients in this stage is difficult because nothing can be done that seems to please. Nurses can expect this expression of anger and should not take it personally. Patients often want to express their sense of outrage and helplessness. When feelings have been vented, they are able to move on.

Bargaining

Bargaining is a phase of coping during which the dying person attempts to negotiate a trade. Usually, it involves a deal with God, the physician, or the nurse: "If I can live long enough to attend my son's wedding, I'll be ready to die." If at all possible, patients should be granted their requests.

Depression

The full impact of the inevitable is apparent to patients in this stage. Defense mechanisms are no longer effective; sadness and anguish are felt and expressed. By crying they also elicit the support of loved ones and nurses. The resolution of this phase leads quietly into the final stage.

Acceptance

This is a time of relative peace. The patient seems to want to review the past and contemplate the unknown future. Often, patients do not talk a great deal but want others nearby. If pain is relieved, the person who has accepted death often wants to be comforted by having contact with those who are meaningful.

Nursing Interventions

To give maximal help to the dying, nurses should examine their own feelings about death. An underlying principle in nursing is that patients are individuals to be treated with respect and dignity regardless of their background or condition. However, studies have shown that social values determine reactions to the dying person. Such factors as age, attractiveness, socioeconomic status, and former accomplishments affect whether the patient is cared for or abandoned while dying. Many times, nurses become the most important link with life for dying patients. They promote physical comfort and emotional support. It is an emotional strain to attend people who are dying. Nurses assigned to areas in which death is a common occurrence need to share their feelings and reactions with others, to obtain needed support.

▷ Bibliography

Books

Aguilera DC and Messick JM. Crisis Intervention: Theory and Methodology, 3rd ed. St Louis, CV Mosby, 1978.

Barton D (ed). Dying and Death, A Clinical Guide for Caregivers. Baltimore, Wilkins & Wilkins, 1977.

Bermosk LS and Corsini RJ (eds.). Critical Incidents in Nursing. Philadelphia, WB Saunders, 1973.

Burkhalter PK. Nursing Care of the Alcoholic and Drug Abuser. New York, McGraw-Hill, 1975.

Carlson C and Blackwell B (eds). Behavioral Concepts and Nursing Intervention, 2nd ed. Philadelphia, JB Lippincott, 1978.

Faguet RA (ed). Contemporary Models in Liaison Psychiatry. New York, Spectrum Publications, 1978.

Gallon RL. The Psychosomatic Approach to Illness. New York, Elsevier Biomedical, 1982.

Garfield CA. Psychosocial Care of the Dying Patient. New York, McGraw-Hill, 1978.

Glickman LS. Psychiatric Consultation in the General Hospital. New York, Marcel Dekker, 1980.

Haber J et al. Comprehensive Psychiatric Nursing. New York, McGraw-Hill, 1982.

Hackett TP and Cassem NH (eds). Massachusetts General Hospital Handbook of General Hospital Psychiatry. St Louis, CV Mosby, 1978.

Infante MS (ed). Crisis Theory: A Framework for Nursing Practice. Reston, Virginia, Reston Pub Co, 1982.

Kastenbaum RJ et al. Old, Sick, and Helpless. Cambridge, Ballinger, 1981.

Kenner CV, Guzzetta CE, and Dossey BM. Critical Care Nursing: Body-Mind-Spirit. Boston, Little, Brown, & Co, 1981.

Kübler-Ross E. On Death and Dying. New York, Macmillan, 1969.

Lambert VA and Lambert CE. The Impact of Physical Illness and Related Mental Health Concepts. Englewood Cliffs, New Jersey, Prentice-Hall, 1979.

Lipp MR. Respectful Treatment: The Human Side of Medical Care. Hagerstown, Maryland, Harper & Row, 1977.

Marshall GN. Facing Death and Grief. Buffalo, Prometheus Books, 1981.

Miller JF. Coping with Chronic Illness: Overcoming Powerlessness. Philadelphia, FA Davis, 1983.

Millon T et al (eds). Handbook of Clinical Health Psychology. New York, Plenum Press, 1982.

Moos R (ed). Coping with Physical Illness. New York, Plenum Medical Book Company, 1977.

Norris CM (ed). Concept Clarification in Nursing. Rockville, Maryland, Aspen Systems Corp, 1982.

Roberts S. Behavioral Concepts and the Critically Ill Patient. Englewood Cliffs, New Jersey, Prentice-Hall, 1976.

Roberts S. Behavioral Concepts and Nursing Throughout the Life Span. Englewood Cliffs, New Jersey, Prentice-Hall, 1978.

Robinson J (ed). Using Crisis Intervention Wisely. Horsham, Pennsylvania, Nursing '79 Books, Intermed Communications, 1979.

Rosenbaum CP and Beebe JE III. Psychiatric Treatment: Clinic, Crisis, and Consultation. New York, McGraw-Hill, 1975.

Schutz W. The Interpersonal Underworld (FIRO). Palo Alto, Science and Behavior Books, 1966.

Selzer R. Letters to a Young Doctor. New York, Simon & Schuster, 1982.

Siegler M and Osmond H. Patienthood. New York, Macmillan, 1979.

Simons RC and Pardes H (eds). Understanding Human Behavior in Health and Illness. Baltimore, Williams & Wilkins, 1981.

Strauss A. Chronic Illness and the Quality of Life. St Louis, CV Mosby, 1975.

Wilkes E. The Dying Patient: The Medical Management of Incurable and Terminal Illness. Ridgewood, George A Boyden and Son, 1982.

Wilson HS and Kneisl CR. Psychiatric Nursing. Menlo Park, Addison-Wesley, 1979.

Wittkower ED and Warnes H (eds). Psychosomatic Medicine; Its Clinical Applications. Hagerstown, Maryland, Harper & Row, 1977.

Wolanin MO and Phillips LD. Confusion, Prevention and Care. St Louis, CV Mosby, 1981.

Woods NF. Human Sexuality in Health and Illness, 2nd ed. St Louis, CV Mosby, 1979.

Articles

Asdalen SP and Stroebel-Kahn F. Coping with quadriplegia. Am J Nurs 1981 Aug; 81(8):1471–1478.

Baldee KS et al. Stress identification and coping patterns in patients on hemodialysis. Nurs Res 1982 Mar/Apr; 31(2):107–112.

Bandman EL and Bandman B. The nurse's role in protecting the patient's right to live or die. Adv Nurs Sci 1979 Apr; 1(3):21–35.

Billings CV. Emotional first aid. Am J Nurs 1980 Nov; 80(11):2006–2009.

Blum J. When you face the alcoholic patient. Nursing 1981 Feb; 11(2):71–73.

Boyajian A. Fighting despair. Am J Nurs 1978 Jan; 78(1):76–77.

Carper BA. The ethics of caring. Adv Nurs Sci 1979 Apr; 1:11–19.

Cohen S. Mental status assessment. Am J Nurs 1981 Aug; 81(8):1493–1518.

Derrick FH. How open heart surgery feels. Am J Nurs 1979 Feb; 79(2):276–285.

Doyen L. Primary anorexia nervosa: A review and critique of selected papers. JPWMHS 1982 June; 20(6):12–17.

Dracup KA and Melsis AI. Compliance: An interactionist approach. Nurs Res 1982 Jan/Feb; 31(1):31–36.

Duldt BW. Anger: An occupational hazard for nurses. Nurs Outlook 1981 Sept; 29(9):510–518.

Duldt BW. Anger: An alienating communication hazard for nurses. Nurs Outlook 1981 Nov; 29(11):640–644.

Duldt BW. Helping nurses to cope with the anger/dismay syndrome. Nurs Outlook 1982 Mar; 30(3):168–174.

Elaine B et al. Helping the nurse who misuses drugs. Am J Nurs 1974 Sept; 74(9):1665–1671.

Fitzsimon V. When the older patient's apathetic. Nursing '82 1982 Apr; 12(4):53–57.

Forsyth DM. The hardest job of all. Nursing '82 1982 Apr; 12(4):86–91.

Fultz JM et al. When a narcotic addict is hospitalized. Am J Nurs 1980 Mar; 80(3):478–481.

Gault P. Plan for a patchwork of problems when your patient is elderly. Nursing '82 1982 Jan; 12(1):50–54.

Grossniklaus DM. Nursing interventions in anorexia nervosa. Perspect Psychiatr Care 1980 Jan/Feb; 18(1):11–16.

Groves C et al. Nursing Grand Rounds: I.C.U. psychosis; helping your patient return to reality. Nursing '82 1982 Jan; 12(1):58–63.

Hagerty BK. Denial isn't all that bad. Nursing '80 1980 Oct; 10(10):58–60.

Hein EC and Leavitt MB. Providing emotional support to patients. Nursing '82 1982 June; 12(6):127–129.

Heinemann E and Estes N. Assessing alcoholic patients. Am J Nurs 1976 May; 76(5):786–789.

Henrich AP and Bernheim KF. Responding to patients' concerns. Nurs Outlook 1981 July; 29(7):428–433.

Huttman BR. No code? Slow code? Show code?. Am J Nurs 1982 Jan; 82(1):133–136.

Jacox AK. Assessing pain. Am J Nurs 1979 May; 79(5):895–900.

Jalowiec A and Powers MJ. Stress and coping in hypertensive and emergency room patients. Nurs Res 1981 Jan/Feb; 30(1):10–15.

Jefferson LV and Ensor BE. Confronting a chemically-impaired colleague. Am J Nurs 1982 Apr; 82(4):574–577.

Kawasaki G et al. Solving the very big problems of the morbidly obese. Nursing '80 1980 Nov; 10(11):40–43.

Kimball CP (ed). Symposium on liaison psychiatry. Psychiatr Clin North Am 1979 Aug; 2(2):181–413.

Krouse HJ and Krouse JH. Cancer as crisis; the critical elements of adjustment. Nurs Res 1982 Mar/Apr; 31(2):96–101.

Kubricht D and Clark JA. Foreign patients: A system of providing care. Nurs Outlook 1982 Jan; 67(1):55–57.

Kurose K et al. A standard care plan for alcoholism. Am J Nurs 1981 May; 81(5):1001–1006.

Lemandri BJ and Boyle DW. Instilling hope. Am J Nurs 1978 Jan; 78(1):79–80.

Leporati NC and Chychula LH. How you can really help drug-abusing patients. Nursing '82 1982 June; 12(6):46–49.

Levinson ML. Obesity and Health. Prev Med 1977 Mar; 6(2):172–180.

Lindenmuth JA et al. Sensory overload. Am J Nurs 1980 Aug; 80(8):1456–1458.

McHugh et al. Preparatory information: What helps and why. Am J Nurs 1982 May; 82(5):780–782.

Meissner J. Measuring patient stress with the hospital stress rating scale. Nursing '80 1980 Aug; 10(8):70–71.

Meissner JE. Uncovering your patient's hidden psychosocial problems. Nursing '80 1980 May; 10(5):78–79.

Mishel M. The measurement of uncertainty in illness. Nurs Res 1982 Sept/Oct; 30(5):258–263.

Nicksig E. Problem patients or problem nurses? Nurs Outlook 1981 May; 29(5):317–319.

Norris CM. The work of getting well. Am J Nurs 1969 Oct; 69(10):2118–2121.

Parker KP. Anxiety and complications in patients on hemodialysis. Nurs Res 1981 Nov/Dec; 30(6):334–336.

Pilette PC. Caution: Objectivity and specialization may be hazardous to your humanity. Am J Nurs 1980 Sept; 80(9):1588–1590.

Popkess SA. Diagnosing your patient's strengths. Nursing '81 1981 July; 11(7):34–37.

Programmed Instruction: Helping depressed patients in general nursing practice. Am J Nurs 1977 June; 77(6):PI 1–32.

Richardson B. A tool for assessing the real world of diabetic noncompliance. Nursing '82 1982 Jan; 12(1):68–73.

Richardson JI. The manipulative patient spells trouble. Nursing '81 1981 Jan; 11(1):48–51.

Richardson K. Hope and flexibility: Your keys to helping OBS patients. Nursing '82 1982 June; 12(6):65–69.

Roberts CS. Symposium on Patient Compliance: Identifying the real patient problems. Nurs Clin North Am 1982 Sept; 17(3):481–489.

Rodgers JA. Women and the fear of being envied. Nurs Outlook 1982 June; 30(6):344–347.

Rosenbaum MS. Depression: what to do, what to say. Nursing '80 1980 Aug; 10(8):64–66.

Ross WD et al. The biopsychosocial approach: Clinical examples from a consultation-liaison service. Psychosomatics 1982 Feb; 23(2):141–151.

Savitz J and Frideman MI. Diagnosing boredom and confusion. Nurs Res 1981 Jan/Feb; 30(1):16–20.

Self PR and Viau JJ. 4 steps for helping a patient alleviate anger. Nursing '80 1980 Dec; 10(12):66.

Smith DW. Survivors of serious illness. Am J Nurs 1979 Mar; 79(3):441–446.

Snyder JC and Wilson MF. Elements of a psychosocial assessment. Am J Nurs 1977 Feb; 77(2):235–239.

Sparachine J et al. Psychological correlates of blood pressure: A closer examination of hostility, anxiety, and engagement. Nurs Res 1982 May/June; 31(3):143–149.

Stanitis MA and Ryan J. Noncompliance; an unacceptable diagnosis? Am J Nurs 1982 June; 82(6):941–942.

Stoller EP. Effect of experience on nurses' responses to dying and death in the hospital setting. Nurs Res 1980 Jan/Feb; 29(1):35–38.

Strain JJ (ed). The medically ill patient. Psychiatr Clin North Am 1981 Aug; 4(2):199–201.

Strauch B et al. Nursing Grand Rounds: Caring enough to give your patient control. Nursing '80 1980 Aug; 10(8):64–66.

Strauss AL et al. Patients' work in the technologized hospital. Nurs Outlook 1981 July; 29(7):404–412.

Taylor P and Gideon M. Cardiac arrest: A crisis for all people. Nursing '80 1980 Sept; 10(9):42–45.

Taylor PB and Gideon MD. Holding out hope to your dying patient. Nursing '82 1982 Feb; 12(2):42–45.

Weiss SJ. The language of touch. Nurs Res 1979 Mar/Apr; 28(2):76–78.

White JH. Symposium on Obesity: An overview of obesity: Its significance to nursing: Definition, prevalence, etiologic concerns, and treatment strategies. Nurs Clin North Am 1982 June; 17(2):191–198.

White JH et al. When your client has a weight problem: Nursing assessment. Am J Nurs 1981 Mar; 81(3):550–553.

Whitney FW. How to work with a crock. Am J Nurs 1981 Jan; 81(1):87–91.

13

Human Sexuality

▷ The Delivery of Sexual Health Care

To effectively deliver sexual health care, the nurse must balance rational scientific data with a humanistic client-centered approach. Three basic requirements are needed to help the nurse separate her sexual self from that of the patient: an adequate knowledge base, critical sexual self-assessment, and a person-centered approach.

An Adequate Knowledge Base. Acquisition of knowledge about sexuality is a lifelong process. In the past decade, sexuality has been redefined in a holistic perspective and has become recognized as an important component of the total person interacting with the environment. In order to distinguish between healthy and unhealthy responses, the nurse must have an understanding of psychosexual development, sexual growth and reproduction, variations in sexual behavior, sexual responses in health and illness, and the impact of life events on sexuality.

Sexual Self-awareness. A critical sexual self-assessment is a desensitization process leading to a greater self-awareness. It includes an acknowledgment of one's own sexuality, as well as an understanding and acceptance of personal attitudes, values, and beliefs. Attitudes stem from religious teachings, cultural mores, familial beliefs, myths, and social taboos; they may interfere with the acquisition of knowledge, objective listening, and proper patient management.

A variety of tools can be utilized for a critical sexual self-assessment. Attitude questionnaires listing issues (*i.e.,* contraception, abortion), behaviors (*i.e.,* masturbation, homosexuality), and life-styles (*i.e.,* open marriage, cohabitation, and personal reactions) can provide the nurse with insight for determining personal attitudes and identifying strengths and limitations in sexual aspects of clinical practice.

Once the attitude is acknowledged, it can be further clarified through introspection, peer group discussions, value clarification exercises, and role playing. A log book with care plans and process recordings can reveal the inability to intervene appropriately owing to conflict. Conflicts may arise from the care of an individual whose behavior attitudes and values differ from that of the nurse.

Person-centered Approach. A *person-centered approach* is appropriate for dealing with sexual problems to ensure recognition of individual differences and to help patients in making their own informed choices. Acceptance of the sexual assessment, sex education, anticipatory guidance, and sexual counseling are based on the individual's perception of sexuality.

Caution and tolerance, as well as effective communication, are necessary to adapt the nursing process to sexual health care. The nurse and the patient may experience varying degrees of comfort when discussing sexuality.

▷ The Role of the Nurse

The role of the nurse in the delivery of sexual health care is to provide a therapeutic environment conducive to sexual health. When acting as a sex educator and counselor, the nurse can assist the patient to acquire knowledge, validate normalcy, and prepare for changes in sexuality throughout the life cycle, in both health and illness. The nurse utilizing the nursing process is able to carry out a meaningful assessment, identify problem areas, plan, implement, coordinate referral sources, and evaluate effectiveness of care.

▷ Sexual Development

Sexual development begins at conception. Females carry X chromosome in the egg, and a male sperm carries X or Y. Thus, the male sperm determines genetic sex. X paired with X equals a female embryo; when X is paired with Y in the presence of androgens, a male embryo develops. All embryos are female until the sixth week of life, when androgens stimulate the growth of male sexual development in the XY fetus. Deviations in early sexual development can occur from chromosomal error or hormonal disturbances. After birth, sexual development is influenced by the behavior of other people through the socialization process.

Basic to our development as sexual human beings is our personal sense of maleness or femaleness and the way we perceive and express it. To provide clarity and consistency, several related terms are defined.

Biological sex is defined as the basic anatomical and reproductive differences between males and females. The components are chromosomal differentiation, hormonal secretions, differentiation of internal sex organs, and external genitalia.

Gender is a behavioral term, a psychological phenomenon. The two components are biological sex and gender identity.

Gender identity refers to the degree to which an individual perceives being a male or a female. To a great extent, this perception is culturally determined. The core of juvenile gender identity is established by 18 months. At the time of puberty, hormonal influences on pubertal morphology, eroticism, and body image lead to the development of adult gender identity. Gender identity becomes relatively immutable by the end of adolescence (Money and Ehrhardt, 1972).

Gender role refers to the way in which an individual expresses gender identity. It is learned behavior through imitation of the same sex parent and complimentation of the opposite sex parent. It is influenced by the complex interaction of parental rewards and punishments. Gender role continues to be defined throughout the life cycle.

Traditionally, in our Western culture, masculinity and femininity referred to restrictive sex-role stereotyped behavior. "Masculine" was defined in terms of strong, aggressive, logical, and independent characteristics. "Feminine" was defined in terms of weak, submissive, dependent, and emotional characteristics. Gender roles have changed, as is seen in the emergence of the contemporary woman. Gender is now viewed on a continuum, so that having characteristics traditionally identified as male traits does not necessarily make an individual less feminine, and vice versa. The term *androgenous* (unisex) refers to both masculine and feminine characteristics, providing more options for individuals and ultimately greater equality between sexes (Bem, 1974).

Sexual preference refers to choice of sexual partner: heterosexual (opposite sex), homosexual (same sex), bisexual (both sexes).

In order to provide anticipatory guidance throughout the life cycle, the nurse should be familiar with psychosexual development: developmental tasks, sexual growth, sexual behaviors, and common sexual concerns, problems, and areas of intervention.

Table 13-1 is a summary of psychosexual development and should be used only as a guideline for obtaining assessment data. The framework utilized has been provided by Erikson; however, in all cases, individual differences should be considered (Erikson, 1963).

▷ Human Sexual Response Patterns

The findings of Masters' and Johnson's research indicated that the human sexual response could be described as a cycle with four stages (Masters and Johnson, 1966). These stages follow a consistent pattern of progression, from excitement to plateau, then to orgasm and resolution. Two basic physiologic responses are responsible for the sexual response cycle: vasocongestion and myotonia.

Vasocongestion is the filling of blood vessels of the genitals and specific body regions, causing enlargement and color changes. *Myotonia* is increased muscle tension, voluntary and involuntary. Both are a result of sexual stimulation, begin during excitement, become more pronounced and reach a peak at orgasm, and subside during resolution.

Sexual desire preceding excitement is controlled by the limbic system in the brain and is greatly influenced by the hormone testosterone. Therefore, anything that inhibits testosterone production may inhibit sexual desire. Stress causes a decrease in testosterone levels; consequently, an individual who perceives a threat, pain, or fear is not likely to experience sexual desire (Kaplan, 1974).

(Text continues on page 212)

Table 13-1
Summary of Stages of Psychosexual Development and Related Nursing Intervention

Developmental Tasks	Sexual Growth	Sexual Behaviors	Sexual Concerns and Problems	Intervention
Developmental Stage: Infancy (0–18 months) **Developmental Crisis: Trust vs. Mistrust**				
Develops a need for affection and to return affection	Sensitivity to a warm, loving environment	Cuddling, hugging, kissing	Touch deprivation	Reinforce the importance of close physical contact and related problems.
	Oral sensitivity, lips, tongue, mouth (oral stage)	Sucking	Oral deprivation (early weaning)	Explain the significance of early weaning and related problems: thumb sucking, emotional difficulty.
Begins to interpret expectations of significant others	Genital sensitivity; erectile potential in males; orgasmic potential in males and females	Stimulation of genitals by self or others; erections in males; primitive orgasms	Parental concern Parental fear	Clarify parental attitudes and beliefs toward self. Explain the primitive nature of the response: higher brain centers not well developed. Reinforce that behavior is normal and cannot harm the infant.
Develops a communication system	Feels good/bad about body parts and functions	Labels body parts based on parental values, voice inflections	Body image	Stress the importance of relating to infant's body in a positive way.
Establishes separateness and becomes social; can differentiate between strange and familiar people	Distinguish between self and others Reinforcement of gender identity	Begins to show maleness or femaleness Identify with same sex parent	Blurred identity, restrictive sex role, stereotyping, coding (pink for girls, blue for boys), limiting play objects	Infant needs close contact with a person to develop gender identity. Sex-role stereotyping can be avoided by focusing on the infant as an individual.
Developmental Stage: Toddler (18 months–3 years) **Developmental Crisis: Autonomy vs. Shame, Doubt**				
Begins to demonstrate toilet training	Learns control of bowel and bladder (anal stage)	Sensual pleasure derived from elimination	Strict toilet training	Relate problems identified with strict toilet training: compulsive behavior, castration anxiety. Provide alternative methods of toilet training.
Begins to participate as a family member	Development of core of gender identity	Imitates behavior of parent of same sex	Anxiety about acceptable behavior for males and females	Avoid sex role stereotyping by providing options: dress, playthings, focus on individual child.
Communicates with others outside family	Learns differences between male and female bodies	Shows an interest in bodies of other children	Parental concern	Clarify attitudes, values, and beliefs.
	Establishes concept of body image	Labels body parts and may ask questions	Poor self-image; may view sexual organs as ''dirty''	Provide vocabulary that emphasizes acceptance of body: genitals, reproduction, elimination.

(continued)

Table 13-1
Summary of Stages of Psychosexual Development and Related Nursing Intervention (continued)

Developmental Tasks	Sexual Growth	Sexual Behaviors	Sexual Concerns and Problems	Intervention
Developmental Stage: Toddler (18 months–3 years) **Developmental Crisis: Autonomy vs. Shame, Doubt** *(continued)*				
Develops autonomous behavior	Genital sensitivity Erection potential Orgasmic potential	Sensual, erotic behaviors; masturbation patterns of self-pleasure, toys, objects	Parental concern	Emphasize normal part of sexual development. Clarify values, attitudes and beliefs.
Developmental Stage: Preschool (4–6 years) **Developmental Crisis: Initiative vs. Guilt**				
Participates actively as a family member	Oedipal attachment to opposite sex parent: complementation—learns what to expect from opposite parent; identification with same sex parent; learns sex roles	Physically affectionate; interested in parents' bodies; fantasizes about parents; may dress in parents' clothing	Excessive attachment to parent; seductive behavior of parent toward child; hostility of same sex parent	Provide alternatives for seductive parent in a nonthreatening manner. Refer parents to parenting class (avoid confusing messages for child). Sexual variations may be related to seductive parent. Refer for counseling.
Responds to expectations of others; begins to understand and establish a sense of morality	Sexual curiosity; penis and clitoris become chief areas of erotic pleasure (phallic stage); capacity to perceive sexual odors	Self-play increases; "plays doctor," touches and sees other children's bodies; asks questions in regard to genitals, reproduction	Parental concern; child may learn to suppress sexual feelings and behavior in order to be accepted by others.	Overreaction leads to guilt; anticipate sexual curiosity; stress importance of answering questions in a nonjudgmental manner. Use penis, vagina as appropriate terminology.
Developmental Stage: School Age (6–12 years) **Developmental Crisis: Industry vs. Inferiority**				
Decreases dependency on family for total love and support; begins to understand peer relationships	Close contact with same sex peers; development of friendships	Homosexual experiences part of same sex relationships; also, sex play with opposite sex common	Parental overreaction; guilty child	Reassure parents that this is a normal part of psychosexual growth and development. Validate normalcy.
	Curiosity about sex (no latency)	Discussion of sex with peers	Confusing or frightening information	Clarify myths, giving accurate information regarding reproduction.
	Orgasm potential (males and females); some girls begin menarche	Mutual masturbation, self-stimulation	Fear owing to lack of information	

(continued)

Table 13-1
Summary of Stages of Psychosexual Development and Related Nursing Intervention (continued)

Developmental Tasks	Sexual Growth	Sexual Behaviors	Sexual Concerns and Problems	Intervention
Developmental Stage: School Age (6–12 years) **Developmental Crisis: Industry vs. Inferiority** *(continued)*				
Acknowledges body changes	Increasing self-awareness; interest in body growth	Comparison of body growth with peers	Concerns over body growth	Elicit sexual history in a comfortable, confidential manner: What do you know about having babies? When you have questions about sex, who do you ask? Do you have questions about sex? Have you noticed changes in your body? How do you feel about changes in your body?
Relates to social, religious, or familial values, attitudes, and beliefs	Learns internal sexual value system; learns self-control	Learns to be secretive; may use slang for shock value	Testing behavior limits; obsessive, anti-social behavior; repression	Refer for counseling, family therapy. Limits of parents to restrict may lead to low self-esteem. No limits delay internal value-system formation.
	Understands concepts of masculinity and femininity	Continues to define sex role in activities inside and outside family	Strict sex-role stereotyping by parents: male may be discouraged from developing "female" skills; females may be discouraged from sports activities	Provide alternatives to limitations of sex-role stereotyping. Focus on preferences of the individual child.
Developmental Stage: Early Adolescence (12–15 years) and Late Adolescence (15–18 years) **Developmental Crisis: Identity Formation vs. Identity Diffusion**				
Acknowledges and accepts physical changes and body image	Female: menarche; development of breasts; distribution of fat to hips and thighs; increased size of uterus; pubic hair growth Male: ejaculation; testicular enlargement; growth of pubic hair and facial hair; voice change and nocturnal emissions	Comparison of body changes with same sex peers; sexual fantasies related to body	Anxiety over change in body image; embarrassment	Discuss relationship of body image and sexual growth and how these changes perceived by the individual are a reflection of self-image. Adolescents have the pain and pleasure of observing the whole process.

(continued)

Table 13-1
Summary of Stages of Psychosexual Development and Related Nursing Intervention (continued)

Developmental Tasks	Sexual Growth	Sexual Behaviors	Sexual Concerns and Problems	Intervention
Developmental Stage: Early Adolescence (12–15 years) and Late Adolescence (15–18 years) **Developmental Crisis: Identity Formation vs. Identity Diffusion** *(continued)*				
Develops close peer relationships with both sexes; develops deep personal relationship with opposite sex	Learns intimacy, heterosexual relationships; develops "crushes"	Heterosexual encounters: kissing, petting, mutual masturbation; heterosexual fantasies. One half of teenagers will have intercourse.	Performance; orgasm; virginity; anxiety.	Provide direct and confidential approach in eliciting sexual history: Are you sexually active? Frequency? How do you feel about it? Provide birth control counseling, STD risk-reduction counseling, Pap testing, BSE, TSE.
			Compulsive, mechanical masturbation	May represent escape from another problem: provide sex counseling.
Attains a male or female role	Increased awareness of sexual feelings integrated in self	Males group together in sports; females group together	Sexual variations may surface: homosexuality, transsexuality, bisexuality	Provide role clarification: What do you think it means to be a man or a woman? Validate normalcy. Refer to sex counseling if problems exist.
Seeks more of a peer relationship with parents	Express feelings about sexual self	Responds to parental limitations	Parental concern, communication breakdown; guilt	Communication is essential. Parents fail to take "crush" seriously. Problems related to double standard may surface. Restrictive limitations impede development.
Developmental Stage: Young Adult (20–45 years) **Developmental Crisis: Intimacy vs. Self-isolation**				
Stabilizes self-image	Acceptance of one's body; pregnancy	Comfortable nude with intimate others	Male: anxiety over penis size Female: anxiety over breast size. Both: self-consciousness; shame	Stress the fact that size of breasts or penis has little to do with sexual gratification. Negative body image may interfere with the establishment of sexual relationships.
Establishes sexual behavior patterns	Mature concept of sexual self; gender role continues to be defined; sexual orientation and sexual life-style established	Heterosexual adjustment— bisexuality, homosexuality, celibacy, masturbation, cohabitation, monogamy, marriage, extramarital sex	Ambivalence to gender role, identity, sexual orientation, "homosexual panic," feelings of being trapped by sex orientation	Elicit sexual history: How do you feel about gender identity, role, and orientation? Explore feelings about sex partner. Regardless of expression, intimacy vs. isolation should be evaluated. Validate normalcy.
	Learns to give and receive pleasure	Experimentation with different forms of sexual expression	Boredom; fear of experimentation; inability to communicate sexual needs to partner; lack of information	Explain sexual response cycle. Discuss patterns of sexual behavior. Identify areas of concern. Possible referrals.

(continued)

Table 13-1
Summary of Stages of Psychosexual Development and Related Nursing Intervention (continued)

Developmental Tasks	Sexual Growth	Sexual Behaviors	Sexual Concerns and Problems	Intervention

Developmental Stage: Young Adult (20–45 years)
Developmental Crisis: Intimacy vs. Self-isolation *(continued)*

Developmental Tasks	Sexual Growth	Sexual Behaviors	Sexual Concerns and Problems	Intervention
Determines desire for having family; protects reproductive integrity	Makes decisions about childbearing	Reproduction control; maintains integrity of sex organs; Pap screening, BSE, TSE-STD risk-reducing behaviors	Unwanted pregnancy; fear of physical exam—pelvic; lack of information regarding STDs or birth control	Elicit sexual history and birth control method, and provide alternatives. Explore feelings about childbearing, STD counseling, and risk reduction.
Formulates life philosophy and develops ethical standards	Develops sexual value system	Behavior reflects individual values, attitudes, and beliefs.	Sexual needs are not met owing to strict, inflexible beliefs.	Values clarification is needed: absolutistic—sexuality for reproduction; hedonistic—pleasure; relativistic—acts judged on the basis of their effects.

Developmental Stage: Middle Age (45–65 years)
Developmental Crisis: Generativity vs. Self-absorption/Stagnation

Developmental Tasks	Sexual Growth	Sexual Behaviors	Sexual Concerns and Problems	Intervention
Acknowledges and accepts physical and emotional changes	Declining hormonal production: menopause—vaginal atrophy and loss of vaginal mucosa; vasomotor symptoms—hot flashes, irritability, fatigue, external genitalia, and breast tissue changes; male climacteric—slower to attain erection, sustained shorter, and ejaculatory force lessens	Focus on quality of sexual encounter vs. quantity; frequency may decline; intercourse expression of love and trust; reaffirmation of self-concept	Anxiety about losing youthfulness, vitality, sex appeal, and fear of loss of partner; may stop sexual activity owing to dyspareunia caused by lack of vaginal secretions; self-image crisis; depression and denial; male concern: losing vigor and virility.	Give anticipatory guidance. Explain changes in sexual response with aging. Postmenopausal women: recommend vaginal lubricant. Regular sexual activity will increase capacity for sexual performance.
Adjusts to independence of grown children	Adjusts to "empty nest"; redefines sex roles	Spends time reestablishing primary relationship; develops and cultivates new joint activities; relinquishes control of children	Attempts to continue to control offspring	Focus on maintenance of relationship with spouse or intimate other.

(continued)

Table 13-1
Summary of Stages of Psychosexual Development and Related Nursing Intervention (continued)

Developmental Tasks	Sexual Growth	Sexual Behaviors	Sexual Concerns and Problems	Intervention
Developmental Stage: Later Maturity (65+) **Developmental Crisis: Ego Integrity vs. Despair**				
Continues close, loving relationship with spouse	Accepts slowed sexual response cycle; development of alternative ways to achieve sexual satisfaction	Adjusts sexual activities; appropriate time may be AM, when less fatigued; oral or manual stimulation; fantasy; emphasis on sensual touching, holding, kissing	Conforms to prevailing societal myth of sex for procreation; lack of information; rigid stereotyped image of what older person should be	Sexual need for intimacy and sexual expression does not change with age. Explain physical changes in sexual response with aging.
Copes with illness or death of spouse or friend	Learns new social patterns; develops alternative ways to achieve sexual satisfaction	Cohabitation; homosexual or lesbian relationship; masturbation; heterosexual relationship; remarriage	Guilt; anxiety; depression; isolation; avoidance of sex altogether	Elicit sexual history: Are you sexually active? Assess sexual patterns and satisfaction. Values clarification needed. Give patient permission for sexual behavior.
Maintains an interdependent relationship with children	Maintaining control of developing relationships	Continues to meet sexual needs	Lack of privacy in environment; children's reactions: anxiety, jealousy, anger	Assist client in maintaining independence. Some grown children fear exploitation of parents. Some are "will watchers." Recommend premarital legal planning.

Excitement

Sexual excitement may be stimulated by external stimuli (visual, auditory, tactile, and olfactory) or by internal stimuli (fantasy and memory).

Female Response. In the female, the first sign of excitement begins with vaginal lubrication owing to transudation of fluid from engorged vessels through the vaginal wall. The inner two thirds of the vagina lengthen and widen; the walls become dark purple and smooth. The uterus begins to be pulled upward in the lower abdomen. Labia majora become thin and flattened in a nulliparous woman. In a multiparous woman, the labia majora swell with blood, double in size, and hang, owing to increased vascularization occurring with pregnancy. The labia minora swell and become engorged with blood, eventually serving to lengthen the vagina.

The nipples become erect owing to involuntary contraction of muscle fibers in the areola. Venous blood trapped in the breasts causes an increase in size. The clitoris enlarges as it fills with blood. This process of tumescence is very similar to penile enlargement, although it occurs not nearly as quickly as it does in the penis.

In older women, the clitoris maintains its high degree of sensitivity. The vagina's ability to expand decreases. The walls become thin and smooth; consequently, there is less protection for the bladder and urethra during intercourse, predisposing the aging female to cystitis. Lubrication may be slower in developing or may be diminished, causing *dyspareunia* (painful intercourse).Water-soluble lubricant will help alleviate this symptom.

Male Response. During the excitement phase, the penis becomes tumescent (erect). This process takes from several seconds to several minutes. The scrotum tenses and thickens; at the same time, the testes elevate toward the perineum as the muscles associated with the spermatic cords contract.

In both men (25%) and women (74%), a skin flush causing a maculopapular sex flush owing to superficial vasocongestive reaction in skin occurs late in excitement or early in plateau. The blood pressure and heart rate begin to accelerate.

Older men experience a slowing of the sexual response. If an older individual is slow to reach erection, he can stimulate his partner and continue to maintain high levels of excitement. Erection takes two to three times longer in men over 50 years of age, and full erection may not be attained until orgasm. In both older men and women, vasocongestive and myotonic responses diminish, causing associated color changes to be less apparent.

Plateau

The length of plateau depends on the effectiveness of the stimulation, the age of the individual, and the desire to attain orgasm. If there are any negative stimuli perceived by males or females, resolution can occur without orgasm. During plateau, muscular tension, heart rate, and blood pressure increase.

Female Response. The outer third of the vagina becomes distended and shortened, with the engorged labia minora forming the orgasmic platform. The clitoris retracts under the clitoral hood but maintains a high degree of sensitivity. The Bartholin's glands secrete a small amount of mucoid substance.

In older women, the engorgement of labia and ballooning of the vagina is decreased, but constriction responses assisting in the formation of the orgasmic platform continue.

Male Response. The penis increases in diameter, and the glans may darken. The testes elevate tightly against the perineum and increase in size owing to vasocongestion. Pre-ejaculatory fluid is secreted from the Cowper's glands.

In both males and females, myotonia increases, resulting in voluntary and involuntary contractions of arms, legs, neck, face, rectum, and buttocks. Carpopedal spasms of hands and feet may occur. Females may contract pubococcygeal muscles (Kegel exercises) to enhance sexual pleasure.

In older men, testicular elevation and scrotum changes diminish. Ejaculatory control increases; however, if erection is partially lost, there may be difficulty in attaining a full erection again, and resolution may occur without orgasm.

Orgasmic Phase

During orgasm, vasocongestion and myotonia reach a peak and are released during involuntary contractions throughout the body. Both male and female orgasms may be described as occurring in stages.

Female Response. Female orgasm begins with intense sensual awareness of the clitoris and pelvis. In the second stage, there is a suffusion of warmth generating from the pelvic area throughout the entire body. In the third and final stage, involuntary rhythmic contractions of the orgasmic platform and the uterus occur, causing a throbbing sensation.

The female orgasmic response is highly variable from individual to individual, as well as from orgasm to orgasm in the same woman. Recent research has indicated that some women ejaculate. The Grafenberg spot, a dime-sized area on the anterior surface of the vaginal wall, secretes a prostaticlike fluid during orgasm with stimulation (Addiego, 1981).

Multiple orgasms occur when sexual tensions do not fall below the plateau phase and stimulation is continued.

Status orgasmus occurs when orgasmic levels can be maintained from 20 seconds to a minute.

Male Response. Male orgasmic response is described in two stages. In the first stage, the prostate seminal vesicles and ampulae contract rhythmically, expelling seminal fluid into the prostatic portion of the urethra and causing a feeling of ejaculatory inevitability.

In the second stage, semen flows into the distended urethral meatus by a series of rhythmic contractions. The male is aware of urethral contractions, as well as fluid volume.

In both males and females, there are generalized muscular contractions of face, thighs, buttocks, and anal sphincter. Vital signs reach their peak: respiration—40/minute; heart rate—110 to 180; blood pressure increases—30 mm Hg to 100 mm Hg systolic, 20 mm Hg to 50 mm Hg diastolic.

The orgasm decreases in duration in the older man and woman. In women, the number of contractions of both the orgasmic platform and the uterus decrease. In men, a single-stage expulsion of seminal fluid occurs, and ejaculatory emission and force decrease.

Resolution

Resolution is characterized by the release of muscular tension and the return of organs to the unstimulated state. There is a physiologic retreat through plateau, and excitement that can take from 10 to 15 minutes. If orgasm has not been achieved, resolution may take all day; however, this causes no harm to the individual. Superimposed on the resolution phase for the male is a mandatory refractory period in which the male cannot attain another erection.

In both the aging male and female, resolution occurs more rapidly. In the aging male, the mandatory refractory period is lengthened.

▷ Deviations From Health and Effects on Sexuality

Deviations from sexual health occur as a result of the complex interaction between the individual and the environment. A holistic approach requires that biological, psychological, and environmental variables be evaluated to achieve an accurate assessment of the individual's level of sexual health.

Kaplan estimates that 3% to 20% of sexual dysfunction or inadequate sexual response is due to purely organic etiology (Kaplan, 1974). Biological variables include anatomical or physiologic disruptions that inhibit any or all of the phases of the human sexual response cycle. The desire phase (libido) of the human sexual response is affected by pain, fatigue, and depression, as well as damage to higher brain centers, specifically the limbic cortex. Any condition that alters the necessary hormonal environment (*i.e.,* blood-level androgens) will influence sexual desire.

Myotonia and vasocongestion may be impaired by disease or trauma that affects the autonomic nervous system and the cardiovascular system. Trauma, surgery, and acute and chronic illness all affect the human sexual response, either directly or indirectly.

Medications prescribed as part of the therapeutic regimen can affect sexual desire, vasocongestion, and myotonia by interfering with hormonal, neurologic, or circulatory mechanisms.

The majority of sexual dysfunctions are due to psychological etiology. These include both intrapersonal and interpersonal factors. Intrapersonal factors include development, thought content and process, mood and affect, and body image. Interpersonal variables include communication, patterns of sexual expression, physical attraction to the sex partner, and conflicts with the sex partner (values, attitudes and beliefs, sex role, and preference). Problems arising from psychological variables can be precipitated by illness or can occur in healthy individuals. They affect the human sexual response by decreasing libido, inhibiting myotonia, or vasocongestion, together or separately.

Environmental variables having a negative effect on sexual functioning can arise from life-style changes, life cycle changes, or life events. The hospitalized, institutionalized, or socially isolated individual may have difficulty in meeting sexual needs. An older adult living with grown children in an environment shared with grandchildren may have limits placed on healthy sexual expression.

Death of a spouse or divorce may force an older adult to develop new patterns of sexual expression. Failure to adapt may cause an individual to repress, avoid, or withdraw from sex altogether.

The combination of physical, psychological, and environmental variables is seen in patients in the health care setting. The therapeutic intervention is based on the identification of problems arising from the interaction of these variables.

▷ Sexual Assessment

A sexual assessment is initiated by collecting subjective and objective data. Essential information from medical and sexual histories, physical examination, and laboratory findings all make significant contributions to the data base.

Sexual History

The sexual history is a tool that enables the nurse to discuss sexual matters openly and gives the patient permission to express sexual concerns to an informed professional. This information can be obtained in conjunction with the medical history after the obstetrical or genitourinary history is completed. By incorporating the sexual history into the general medical history, the nurse is able to move from areas of lesser sensitivity to areas of greater sensitivity after establishing initial rapport.

The interviewing style should be nonjudgmental. If the patient perceives negative verbal or nonverbal communication, sensitive information is likely to be censored. Language used during the interview should be appropriate to the person's age and background. Ambiguity should be avoided by not using euphemisms, which are inaccurate and imprecise and will inevitably lead to confusion (*i.e.,* a couple can make love without having intercourse, can have intercourse without sleeping together, and can sleep to-gether without making love). Open-ended questions may be preferable as discussion starters. For example, when interviewing an adolescent, "How did you learn about masturbation?" is more appropriate than "Do you masturbate?"

Patients may experience considerable anxiety, guilt, and embarrassment during the sexual assessment. Therefore, the environment in which the interview takes place is extremely important. Comfort and privacy *without* interruption, as well as verbal and nonverbal assurances of confidentiality, are essential to establishing and maintaining rapport. Relevant assessment data for the adult include the areas listed in Chart 13-1.

The sexual history of the adult can be initiated by the general open-ended question "Are you sexually active?" If the answer is no, the nurse should explore:

- Sexual experiences in the past and why they were discontinued
- Level of satisfaction with the present status

The person may be satisfied with the present status but still may have concerns about sexual attitudes or behaviors of family and friends. An invitation to ask questions about

---

Chart 13-1
Components of the Sexual Assessment

A. Identification data:

Age	Marital status
Education	Income
Date of birth	Employment

B. Chief complaint

C. Past medical history:

General health	Psychiatric illness
Adult medical illness	Injuries
Surgical procedures	Hospitalizations
Current medications	

D. Habits

Diet	Exercise
Use of alcohol/drugs	Sleep

E. Family history

F. Personal and social history:

Past development	Ethnic background
Urban or rural background	Family
Church	Current life situation

G. Obstetrical history:
Genitourinary history

H. Sexual history

I. Physical examination

any aspect of sexuality is appropriate at this time. The nurse may provide anticipatory guidance or information related to the patient's developmental stage. Also, information about medications and illnesses and their effects on sexual functioning should be explored.

If the patient is sexually active, and if the setting and situation are appropriate, the nurse may explore six areas:

1. Variety and frequency of sexual activity (includes choice of sex partner and degree of sex drive)
2. Current satisfaction with present sexual functioning (which includes sufficient stimulation and lubrication for the female, the ability to obtain an erection and control ejaculation in the male, and the ability of either party to have a satisfying orgasm without pain)
3. Partner function and satisfaction (which include all aspects of sexual and social compatibility)
4. Marital or relationship history
5. The effects of life events (*i.e.,* rape, death of spouse, aging, medication, illness, contraception) on sexual functioning
6. Invitation for giving information regarding sexual concerns

A more detailed history is required when the patient identifies a problem. This should include information about:

1. Early sexual development (*i.e.,* parental, peer, and religious influences on values, attitudes, and beliefs)
2. Adolescent sexual development and experiences (*i.e.,* puberty, masturbation, nocturnal emissions, menstruation, first intercourse, and sexual fantasies)
3. Premarital and postmarital sexual history (*i.e.,* dating, nonmarital sexual relationships, sexual techniques used, frequency of nonmarital sex, and frequency of marital sex and any changes)
4. History of the present problem (*i.e.,* onset, duration, severity, contributing factors and alleviating factors)

This information should be recorded in the patient's own words (Leiblum and Rosen, 1980).

Sexual history taking becomes a dynamic process in which there is an exchange of information between the person and the nurse. It provides the opportunity to clarify myths and explore areas of concern that the person may not have had permission to discuss in the past.

Physical Examination

Similarly, the physical examination affords the nurse an opportunity to provide role modeling and sex education, thus creating a therapeutic milieu.

During the physical assessment, a female patient can be taught breast self-examination (BSE), Kegel exercises, purpose of Pap screening, effective contraception, and behaviors that reduce the risk of contracting sexually transmitted disease. The male patient can be taught testicular self-examination (TSE), sexually transmitted disease risk reduction, contraception, and breast examination.

The attitude of the practitioner doing the physical examination is of the utmost importance. Concerned practitioners may make the process of the physical examination a wholesome, positive experience, taking care to afford comfort and privacy, and explaining all procedures with sensitivity.

People at risk for sexual problems are those who (1) are unaware of the effects of life cycle changes on sexuality, particularly at adolescence and middle age; (2) have communication or behavioral problems; (3) experience traumatic life events (*i.e.,* rape, death of a spouse); (4) have changes in self-image (*i.e.,* surgery); (5) have anatomical or physiologic disruptions (*i.e.,* trauma); (6) are taking pharmacologic agents that affect sexuality; and (7) have changes in life-style (*i.e.,* hospitalized person).

Anon describes a four-level treatment model for sexual therapy that can be adapted to nursing practice (1974).

1. The first level is *permission* and basically involves validating normalcy. Receiving permission for thoughts, fantasies, sexual behavior, etc. may prevent an individual from developing a significant problem and can also relieve guilt. This is primarily preventive intervention.
2. *Limited information* is the second level and provides information specific to the individual's needs. It can be preventive or therapeutic. An example is provision of anticipatory guidance to the adolescent to dispel misinformation and myths regarding sexually transmittable disease. The foregoing could then be reinforced by teaching sexually transmitted disease (STD) risk-reduction behaviors.
3. The third level of intervention is giving *specific suggestions,* or a description of a therapeutic technique. The specific suggestion of using a water-soluble lubricant for a postmenopausal woman with atrophic vaginitis is an appropriate nursing intervention.
4. Occasionally in clinical practice, the nurse identifies a person who may require *intensive therapy,* as in the case of someone who has behavior or communication problems resulting in a sexual dysfunction. The nurse can identify referral sources by contacting the American Association of Sex Educators, Counselors and Therapists (AASECT), Washington D.C., for the names of qualified professionals in the area.

▷ Interventions for Specific Health Problems Affecting Sexuality

Body Image Changes and Sexuality

In understanding the effects of illness on sexuality, one must understand (1) the effects of illness on body image, (2) common coping mechanisms, and (3) the influence of the specific pathologic process on the human sexual response.

Body image, which is the self-perception of the body, begins in early childhood and continues to evolve throughout the life span. It is interwoven with sexual identity, sexual role, and patterns of sexual functioning.

In our society, we see idealized standards of the perfect body and face for men and women. A high value is placed on physical appearance. Conflict arises when self-image does not conform with idealized image. When there is a loss or disfigurement of body structure or function, self-perception, environmental interaction, and interpersonal relationships change.

Moving from levels of health to illness can threaten a person's sense of normalcy, causing lowered self-esteem, a negative self-image, and insecurity. The result can be disturbances of mood and affect. Depression is commonly seen in individuals with changes in body image, and is recognized as part of the grieving process. Dependency occurring as an adjustment to the sick role can be accompanied with feelings of powerlessness and loss of control, influencing sexual adequacy. Prolonged denial or guilt can prevent an individual from revising his self-image to a more positive one.

Performance anxiety occurs when an individual perceives the body change as having a negative impact on sexual role, identity, or functioning. Traditional male and female stereotyped roles may be incompatible with altered body structure or function. Traditional patterns of sexual functioning may no longer be possible. Myths, misinformation, and negative attitudes and values can prohibit an individual from finding new sexual expression, a change often required for those with altered body structure or function.

The severity of the reaction to altered body image is also influenced by the visibility of the affected part, the meaning or symbolism attached to it, and the individual's perception of the way others view the change. Usually, the more visible the part, the more severe the emotional reactions. If the body part is strongly correlated with sexual identity (*i.e.,* the heart for the male; the uterus or breast for the female), the impact on self-image may be profound. A person who perceives one's sexual partner as reacting to the altered body image with disgust may fear rejection. The result may be avoidance of sex, withdrawal, and self-imposed isolation.

The relationship between sexual partners is the most important factor in sexual functioning after illness. In a marital relationship, an unexplained decrease in sexual activity owing to illness, lack of communication, or negative body image usually results in conflict, frustration, and irritability. The sexual partner may withdraw affection for fear that sexual intercourse may harm the patient. Anger and hostility can occur if this is not communicated.

Assessment of patients with body image changes includes evaluating the effects on self-concept and self-esteem; the impact on sex role, sexual identity, sexual functioning, and sexual relationships; and the person's coping mechanisms.

General goals of intervention include allowing the patient to ventilate negative feelings, clarifying misinformation and myths with the patient and spouse separately and together, encouraging recognition of sexual attributes and capabilities, and widening sexual repertoire through permission and education.

Two major conditions that cause changes in self-image are myocardial infarction (MI) and mastectomy.

Myocardial Infarction

The patient who has a myocardial infarction is at risk for sexual dysfunction because of perceived body image changes. Fear of sudden death, fear of impotence, feelings of emasculation, increased dependency on the sick role, and decreased general activity may prevent a patient from returning to pre-infarct levels of sexual functioning.

The actual incidence of sudden death during intercourse post-MI is very low, although it is slightly higher with an unfamiliar partner in a stressful environment (*i.e.,* extramarital affair). The body's energy expenditure during intercourse is equated to that required to walk up two flights of stairs. Depending on the extent of cardiac damage, most post-MI patients can resume normal sexual activity after exercise tolerance is assessed and results are evaluated—usually in 8 to 12 weeks.

Assessment factors include the usual or preferred type, time, and frequency of sexual activity; alcohol and food consumption associated with sexual activity; previous occurrences of angina; previous symptoms of fatigue; sleeplessness associated with sexual activity; and prescribed medications.

Sexual counseling as a part of cardiac rehabilitation has a significant impact on the frequency and quality of subsequent sexual functioning. After the fear of death has passed, a patient may act out sexually toward the nurse. This situation can be used as an opportunity to begin sexual education and counseling. Permission begins by acknowledging the behavior as normal.

Conjugal counseling is necessary to clarify myths and misinformation. Information regarding the normal sexual response cycle, extent of cardiac damage, and effects on intercourse should be included in the teaching plan.

The environment in which intercourse is initiated should be familiar, avoiding extremes of temperature. Food and alcoholic beverages should not be consumed for at least 3 hours prior to intercourse.

If angina is a concern, a nitroglycerin tablet may be taken before intercourse. The patient's lowered level of activity and assertiveness can be supplemented, for example, by foreplay.

The patient can be informed of self-assessment factors or warning signs to stop intercourse until a physician is consulted. These include angina during or after intercourse, prolonged palpitations 15 minutes after intercourse, sleeplessness or fatigue the following day, and elevated heart rate and respirations that continue 20 minutes after intercourse.

Medications frequently prescribed for the cardiac patient include antihypertensives, antidepressants, tranquilizers, hypnotics, and ganglionic blocking agents. These may cause a decrease in sex drive or libido and impair vasocongestion and myotonia. The patient should be informed of these side-effects.

The patient who experiences sexual dysfunction following an MI (erectile dysfunction, premature ejaculation, orgasmic dysfunction) should be referred for further evaluation. Sexual dysfunction may be a result of impaired vasocongestion owing to cardiovascular assault, prescribed medications, anxiety, depression, fear of failure, or fatigue.

Mastectomy

To many women, breasts are a symbol of femininity and are equated with sexual attractiveness and desirability. The reality of cancer, fear of death, change in body image, and fear of rejection create multiple adjustment problems for a woman undergoing a mastectomy. Denial, depression, and anger are experienced as part of the grieving process. Guilt may also be experienced if the woman views the mastectomy as punishment for sexual activity that she believes is excessive or inappropriate, such as engaging in an extramarital affair. The spouse may also experience guilt if he believes that he may have caused damage to the breast during sexual activity. The quality of the marital relationship before the mastectomy influences the subsequent postoperative relationship.

Supportive sexual counseling and enhancement of communication between partners during hospitalization can have a positive effect on postoperative sexual functioning.

Misinformation and myths can be clarified in preoperative counseling. Permission is given when the nurse validates that the woman's concerns are normal. Reassurance that the mastectomy will not affect the capacity for sexual responsiveness is vital. Assessment factors include the marital relationship, the perceived effect of body image change on sex role and identity, the importance of the breast in sexual arousal during foreplay, the identification of support systems, the ability of the woman to express her sexual needs and concerns, and the sexual history. Using a person-centered approach, the nurse should identify whether the spouse should be included in the initial assessment. If not, counseling the spouse separately is recommended.

In the immediate postoperative period, the spouse may be present, providing additional support. He should also be actively involved in postoperative care to prevent delaying confrontation or prolonged denial. Communication, touching, holding, and caressing should be encouraged early in the postoperative period.

The woman and spouse may fear wound disruption. They should be informed that with proper positioning, intercourse usually can be resumed in 1 week. Male superior and side-by-side positions are usually more comfortable. The use of a prosthesis during sexual activity is discouraged to increase comfort and enhance self-acceptance.

Positive role modeling and additional support can be obtained by referral to "Reach to Recovery." It may also dispel the myth that the mutilation is unique.

A woman who does not have a male partner may feel sexually unattractive and experience low self-esteem similar to that experienced by the married woman. However, she may lack the additional support system available to the married woman. It is especially important that this woman move through the stages of denial and establish a positive self-image early in rehabilitation to avoid feelings of abandonment when she goes home.

Specific suggestions to enhance positive body image include looking in the mirror nude to desensitize reactions and explore feelings about altered body image. This reduces the conflict of imagined body image and real body image. Sensate focus exercises or pleasuring exercises can enhance the establishment of a positive body image. Water play with a shower massage is a nonthreatening, self-pleasuring exercise that can increase sensory discrimination. Touching is also an important part of sensate focus.

Asking the client to draw a picture of herself may assist her in venting feelings of altered body image. The nurse can then provide feedback and stress positive aspects of body and sexual functioning.

Breast self-examination should be taught to the mastectomy patient. Because there is a three times greater chance of developing cancer in the other breast, early detection can decrease the risk of mortality.

Health Problems Affecting Sexuality
Spinal Cord Injuries

Adolescents and young adults are frequently the victims of spinal cord accidents and represent a challenge to the delivery of sexual health care. The majority of these patients are male. The injury and consequential changes in self-esteem, self-image, sexual functioning, and interpersonal relationships pose a serious threat to an individual's physical and psychological well-being. Sexual rehabilitation begins when the threat of death is no longer perceived by the person during hospitalization. It is essential that patients with spinal cord injuries receive information about sexual functioning before going home.

The two variables in planning sexual rehabilitation include the level of the injury and the number of fibers severed (complete or incomplete lesion). Individuals with upper motor neuron lesions usually exhibit increased spasticity, hyperreflexia, and reflexogenic erections. Those with lower motor neuron lesions exhibit flaccidity and hyporeflexia. Psychogenic erections are possible, but are seen less frequently.

Reflexogenic erections can be stimulated by genital manipulation or a full bladder and occur during rapid eye movement (REM) sleep in healthy males. The stimulus is transmitted from the penis to the sacral area of the cord via sympathetic nerves to the pelvis. Women experience reflexogenic vaginal lubrication and pelvic engorgement from the stimulation of perineal structures.

Psychogenic erections are initiated in the higher brain centers and travel via thoracolumbar sympathetic nerves to the genitalia. Psychogenic erections are more common in lower motor neuron lesions, because impulses pass down and leave the cord above the level of the injury. The reflex arc is interrupted, and reflexogenic erections are improbable with complete lower motor neuron lesions. Table 13-2 outlines the effects on the human sexual response in complete upper motor neuron lesions and lower motor lesions. It is essential that the patient have realistic expectations regarding the ability to meet his or her sexual needs.

The following assessment factors provided by Comarr and Gunderson (1975) can be utilized in distinguishing complete or incomplete upper motor neuron lesions from complete or incomplete lower motor neuron lesions after spinal shock subsides:

- *Complete upper motor neuron lesion (UMNL):* No sensation or voluntary control of external rectal sphincter; evidence of external rectal sphincter tone and a positive bulbocavernosus reflex
- *Incomplete upper motor neuron lesion:* Positive light touch sensation or partially diminished responses to

Table 13-2
Complete Lesions and Effects on Human Sexual Response

Phase of Human Sexual Response	Upper Motor Neuron (C$_1$, T$_{12}$)	Lower Motor Neuron (T$_{12}$, S$_4$)
Excitement (psychogenic)	No psychogenic erection No vaginal lubrication Other manifestation activated by fibers above the lesion; change in BP, respirations, pulse Breast changes, sex flush	Psychogenic erection Vaginal lubrication Visual, auditory, olfactory, stimuli; dreams, memory fantasy
Plateau (reflexogenic)	Reflexogenic erection caused by stroking penis, catheter change, full bladder (When lesion is T$_5$ to T$_6$, erection is absent, possibly owing to vascular insufficiency of cord.) Reflexogenic vaginal lubrication and pelvic engorgement with perineal stimulation.	No reflex response Reflexes are interrupted
Orgasm	Ejaculation: rare Orgasms can occur as purely cerebral events	Ejaculation and orgasm occur more frequently Ejaculatory force varies

(Adapted from Geiger RC. Neurophysiology of sexual response in spinal cord injury. In Bullard D and Knight V. Sexuality and Physical Disability. St Louis, CV Mosby, 1981.)

pin prick; the loss of voluntary control of external rectal sphincter; external rectal sphincter tone and a positive bulbocavernosus reflex

- *Complete lower motor neuron lesion (LMNL):* No sensation or voluntary control or tone of the external rectal sphincter and no bulbocavernosus reflex
- *Incomplete lower motor neuron lesion:* Partial sensation; no voluntary control of external rectal sphincter; no sphincter tone or bulbocavernosus reflex

Persons who have incomplete lesions will experience less neurologic deficit and have a greater chance of successful coitus. Individual differences must be considered and should influence the approach to sexual rehabilitation.

A patient with a spinal cord injury may be troubled by many myths regarding his sexuality and sexual functioning after the injury. Counseling begins with validating his concerns as normal and giving information to dispel myths and misinformation. Cultural, religious, and social taboos associated with anal intercourse or oral sex should be discussed. Conjugal counseling is recommended; if the patient objects, the spouse can be counseled separately.

Several principles related to the human sexual response in spinal cord injuries should be incorporated into the teaching plan. Sexual excitement occurring from thoughts, fantasies, or tactile stimulation in areas above the level of the lesion does not result in any genital response, and, conversely, reflexogenic genital responses occur without cognitive awareness.

Even though erections are more frequent in complete upper motor lesions, they may not produce sexual satisfaction. Orgasm, however, may occur as a purely cerebral event without either genital stimulation or manifestation of physical components of the human sexual response. Imagery, autosuggestion, and erotic visual material can enhance the possibility of achieving a "phantom orgasm."

Areas available for tactile stimulation are dependent on the level of the injury. Even though individuals with upper motor neuron lesions manifest similar erectile ability, a larger area is sensitive to tactile stimulation in lower-level injuries. Frequently, areas such as the neck, ears, and breasts, which may previously have been insensitive, become highly sensitive with increased stimulation. Areas of tactile hypersensitivity at the level of the lesion can induce profound sexual pleasure for the person with a spinal cord injury.

Infertility in the male is a common sequel to spinal cord injuries. Fertility in the female is usually not affected. The sensory level of the uterus is at T$_6$, and if the injury is at that level, sensation of labor will be absent.

Problems in meeting sexual needs can arise from the absence of a partner, from an inability to engage in traditional sexual patterns, from sexual inexperience before the injury, and from the perception of oneself as asexual.

Sexual assertiveness training can help alleviate some of these problems. Confidence and skillful communication are essential in establishing a new sexual relationship or altering a familiar one.

A person with spinal cord injury can be encouraged to widen his sexual repertoire with new patterns of sexual functioning. Areas of hypersensitivity may be discovered through different approaches to stimulation. Enhanced communication will assist in expressing what feels good.

An indwelling catheter can be taped in place and left in during intercourse. Spasticity in clients with UMNL can be reduced by administering antispasmodics before intercourse, even though there may be a resultant decrease in sensation.

Even with the most profound disability, patients are capable of expressing their sexuality and with education and training are able to achieve high levels of sexual satisfaction. Sexual rehabilitation depends on self-confidence;

a willing sex partner; and a sensitive, knowledgeable health care team.

Diabetes Mellitus

Diabetes mellitus is a common health problem that causes erectile dysfunction in one half of all diabetic men and orgasmic dysfunction in one third of all diabetic women. In both men and women, there is usually no decrease in sexual desire. There is no clear-cut relationship between control and sexual dysfunction. However, transient impotence can occasionally be reversed with diabetic control. Additional dysfunctions that are seen less frequently are retrograde ejaculation and premature ejaculation in males, and dyspareunia in female diabetics with vaginitis, commonly caused by *Candida albicans.*

The etiology is complex; contributing factors include diabetic neuropathy, microangiopathies of chronic diabetes, decreased androgens, decreased pituitary gonadotropins, testicular atrophy, and candidal vaginitis.

Psychogenic factors include adaptation to a chronic illness, dependency, depression, and low self-esteem, leading to performance anxiety.

The onset of sexual dysfunction usually occurs early in males, but can occur years after the diagnosis. The onset of sexual dysfunction in female diabetics usually occurs 4 to 6 years after the diagnosis (Green, 1979). In both males and females, organic dysfunctions develop gradually, whereas the onset of psychogenic dysfunctions is usually abrupt and can be related to a specific time, event, or person. The absence of a reflexogenic erection without significant change in libido rules out psychogenic etiology.

Fertility problems seen in diabetic men are caused by retrograde ejaculation, ejaculatory dysfunction, and decreased sperm count and volume.

Although usually not infertile, diabetic women have a higher number of stillborns, spontaneous abortions, and high birth weight babies. Ovarian malformations occur in some diabetic women.

Assessment factors include sexual history, detailed physical examination, present coping mechanisms, laboratory tests to determine if there is a fertility or control problem, and the existing marital relationship.

Counseling begins with the sexual history. At this time, myths and misinformation should be dispelled and guilt alleviated if it is present, as is frequently the case. For those who are married, conjugal counseling is recommended. Information about genetic transmission and the impact of the disease on fertility and sexual functioning may be discussed. Techniques to overcome intromission difficulties and to enhance stimulation may be explored if the couple is receptive.

For women with dyspareunia, a water-soluble lubricant can be suggested. In addition, any existing candidal infection should be treated. Women with diabetes could be counseled on wearing cotton underpants, avoiding pantyhose, and inserting plain yogurt in the vagina as an aid to maintaining an acid *p*H to prevent recurrent infections.

The diabetic client who experiences sexual dysfunction owing to psychogenic etiology and who identifies the need for assistance with the problem may be referred for sexual therapy.

Hypertension

Hypertension alone has no documented negative effect on the human sexual response, and no restrictions on sexual activity are necessary.

The silent noncompliance with the therapeutic regimen seen in those who are hypersensitive is frequently attributed to drug-induced sexual dysfunction.

Antihypertensive agents produce vasodilation and decreased cardiac output by acting on the sympathetic nervous system either peripherally or centrally. The effects on the human sexual response include decreased libido, erectile difficulty, retrograde ejaculation, and reduced orgasmic intensity. Several antihypertensives block ovulation and suppress menstruation, causing infertility in females.

A detailed sexual history and physical examination are necessary to determine if the sexual dysfunction is due to the antihypertensive medication, other medication, other organic etiology (*i.e.,* diabetes), or psychological factors. If the onset is related specifically to an increase in dosage or changes of medication with no apparent psychogenic etiology or organic pathology, the dysfunction is likely to be due to medication (Tables 13-3 and 13-4).

A person experiencing sexual dysfunction as a result of antihypertensives should be counseled that the problem is reversible and that alternative medications are available.

Table 13-3

Possible Effects of Antihypertensive Drugs on Sexual Response

Antihypertensive Drug	Possible Adverse Effects On Human Sexual Response
Clonidine (Catapres)	Impotence and retrograde ejaculation in men; orgasmic dysfunction in women
Guanethidine (Ismelin)	Erectile dysfunction; ejaculatory dysfunction in men; orgasmic dysfunction in both men and women
Mecamylamine (Inversine); Trimethaphan camsylate (Arfonad)	Erectile and ejaculatory dysfunction
Methyldopa (Aldomet)	Inhibited libido; erectile and ejaculatory dysfunction
Phenoxybenzamine (Dibenzyline)	Ejaculatory dysfunction
Propranolol (Inderal)	Impotence when given in large doses
Reserpine (Serpasil)	Inhibited libido; ejaculatory dysfunction. In women: blocks ovulation; infertility; pseudopregnancy; lactation
Spironolactone (Aldactone)	Inhibited libido; erectile dysfunction; gynecomastia in men. In women: breast pain; dysmenorrhea; amenorrhea

Table 13-4
Commonly Prescribed Medications That Have Adverse Effects on the Human Sexual Response

Drug	Probable Mechanism of Action
Antidepressants	Central depression; peripheral blockade of nervous innervation of sex glands
Amitriptyline (Elavil)	
Desipramine (Norpramin, Pertofrane)	
Imipramine (Tofranil)	
Nortriptyline (Aventyl)	
Pargyline (Eutonyl)	
Phenelzine sulfate (Nardil)	
Protriptyline (Vivactil)	
Tranylcypromine sulfate (Parnate)	
Antihistamines	Blockade of parasympathetic nervous innervation of sex glands
Chlorpheniramine maleate (Chlor-Trimeton)	
Diphenhydramine (Benadryl)	
Promethazine (Phenergan)	
Antispasmodics	Ganglionic blockage of nervous innervation of sex glands
Glycopyrrolate (Robinul)	
Hexocyclium methylsulfate (Tral)	
Methantheline bromide (Banthine)	
Sedatives and tranquilizers	Central sedation; blockage of autonomic innervation of sex glands; suppression of hypothalamic and pituitary function; tranquilization and relaxation
Benperidol	
Chlordiazepoxide (Librium)	
Chlorpromazine (Thorazine)	
Chlorprothixene (Taractan)	
Diazepam (Valium)	
Mesoridazine (Serentil)	
Phenoxybenzamine (Dibenzyline)	
Prochlorperazine (Compazine)	
Thioridazine (Mellaril)	
Ethyl alcohol	Central depression; suppression of motor activity, diuresis; release of inhibitions; relaxation
Barbiturates	Central depression; suppression of motor activity; hypnosis
Narcotics and psychoactive drugs	Central depression; decreased libido; impaired potency
Amphetamines	
Cocaine	
Sex-hormone preparations	Antiandrogenic effects on sexual function; loss of libido; decreased potency
Cyproterone acetate	
Nandrolone phenpropionate (Durabolin)	
Norethandrolone (Nilevar)	

(Adapted from Woods JS: Drug effects on human sexual behavior. In Woods NF: Human Sexuality in Health and Illness, 2nd ed. St Louis, CV Mosby, 1979.)

It is necessary to point out that adverse reactions on the human sexual response are highly individual.

Stress management techniques, such as deep relaxation, yoga, cardiovascular exercise, and compliance with the therapeutic diet, may decrease the necessity of high doses of antihypertensives and can enhance the sexual response.

Sexual Disorders

Sexual Dysfunction Owing to Psychogenic Etiology

The human sexual response is controlled by the autonomic nervous system with sympathetic and parasympathetic subsystems. Under stress and anxiety, the sympathetic system overpowers the parasympathetic system, making the relaxation required for the sexual response impossible. Vasocongestion and myotonia may be inhibited together or separately. This type of dysfunction results in inadequate sexual responses.

Masters and Johnson estimate that 50% of all couples may require some assistance with sexual dysfunctions (1966). The etiology is complex. Chart 13-2 summarizes the variables of psychogenic etiology. Patients with any of the variables are at risk for sexual dysfunctions.

Sexual dysfunctions are categorized as primary or secondary. An individual who has never experienced an adequate response suffers from a *primary dysfunction. Secondary sexual dysfunction* occurs when an adequate sexual response was achieved at least once in the past. The onset of the dysfunction may be related to a specific time, event, or person.

There are a variety of individual responses within each dysfunction. They can be viewed on a continuum, depending on the frequency and severity of the inadequate response.

Male Sexual Dysfunctions

Erectile dysfunction occurs when the vasocongestion aspects of the sexual response are impaired. Varying responses include the complete inability to attain an erection, a partial erection, or a firm extravaginal erection. The presence of a reflexogenic erection rules out organic etiology.

Premature ejaculation occurs when an individual is unable to voluntarily control the ejaculatory reflex and, once aroused, reaches orgasm before or shortly after intromission. It is the most common dysfunction in the male.

Retarded ejaculation is the involuntary inhibition of the ejaculatory reflex. The varying responses include occasional ejaculation, ejaculation through self-stimulation, or the complete inability to ejaculate under any circumstances.

Female Sexual Dysfunction

Orgasmic dysfunction occurs when involuntary control of the orgasmic reflex leads to the inability to achieve orgasm (similar to retarded ejaculation). Varying responses include the complete inability to achieve orgasm under any circumstances and achievement of orgasm through self- or partner stimulation. The latter response is termed *coital orgasmic inadequacy,* and controversy currently exists about whether it is actually a dysfunction.

Sexual therapy is recommended. Organic etiology is ruled out by laboratory tests and a complete physical examination. The prognosis with therapy varies with the severity of the problem and its underlying etiology. When there is deep-rooted conflict or guilt, psychoanalysis or long-term psychotherapy may be necessary.

Inhibited Sexual Desire

Disorders of sexual desire differ from other sexual dysfunctions in that clients have deeper and more intense anxiety, hostility, and defense patterns (Kaplan, 1979). The result is impairment of libido. Organic etiology includes depres-

---

Chart 13-2
Variables of Psychogenic Etiology in Sexual Dysfunction

Intrapersonal Variables

Development
Conflicted parent–child relationship
Strong negative family attitudes toward sex
Traumatic sexual experience

Self and Body Image
Negative body image
Sexual identity conflict
Sexual role conflict
Sexual preference conflict
Low self-esteem

Mood and Affect
Guilt
Depression
Performance anxiety
Phobias: fear of sex, pregnancy, orgasm, rejection

Thought Content
Misinformation
Myths
Acceptance of negative societal beliefs

Interpersonal Variables

Inability to communicate
Anger or hostility toward partner
Distrust
Lack of physical attraction toward partner
Sex role preference, conflict
Conflicting attitudes, values, and beliefs

(Adapted from Kolodny RC et al. Textbook of Human Sexuality for Nurses. Boston, Little, Brown, & Co, 1979.)

---

sion, stress, medications, illness, and low testosterone levels.

Sexual aversion is the fear of sexual activity, leading to avoidance. The phobia may be accompanied with vasosympathetic responses (diaphoresis, nausea, diarrhea, and palpitations).

Disorders of sexual desire require psychotherapy; the prognosis with brief intensive sexual therapy is poor.

The nurse who identifies an individual who is at risk for sexual dysfunction can utilize the nursing process and plan sex education and counseling to dispel misinformation, myths, and negative attitudes and beliefs.

An explanation of the human sexual response and the need for relaxation, freedom from guilt and anxiety, and the validation of normalcy are preventive nursing interventions for all clients.

When a patient who is dysfunctional is identified, the nurse employs a person-centered approach to determine whether the individual is seeking help for the problem. If so, the person can be referred for sexual therapy. Follow-up on the success of therapy will evaluate the individual's satisfaction with the therapist, therapy, alleviation of the dysfunction, and enhancement of the sexual relationship.

▷ Bibliography

Books
Disability

Bullard D and Knight V. Sexuality and Physical Disability. St Louis, CV Mosby, 1981.

Comfort A. Sexual Consequences of Disability. Philadelphia, George F. Stickly, 1978.

Human Sexuality

Anon JS. Behavioral Treatment of Sexual Problems, Volume I, Brief Therapy. Honolulu, Enabling Systems, Inc, 1974.

Butler R and Lewis MI. Love and Sex After Sixty. New York, Harper & Row, 1976.

Erikson EH. Childhood and Society, ed 2. New York, WW Norton, 1963.

Fogel C and Woods NF. Health Care of Women: A Nursing Perspective, pp 334–360, St. Louis, CV Mosky, 1980.

Garfield LB. For Yourself—The Fulfillment of Female Sexuality. New York, Anchor Press/Doubleday, 1975.

Goffman E. Stigma; Notes on the Management of a Spoiled Identity. Englewood Cliffs, New Jersey, Prentice–Hall, 1963.

Godow AG. Human Sexuality. St Louis, CV Mosby, 1982.

Green R. Human Sexuality—A Health Practitioner's Text, ed 2. Baltimore, William & Wilkins, 1979.

Hogan R. Human Sexuality, A Nursing Perspective. New York, Appleton–Century–Crofts, 1980.

Kaplan HS. The New Sex Therapy. New York, Brunner–Mazel, 1974.

Kaplan HS. Disorders of Sexual Desire, New York, Simon & Schuster, 1979.

Kinsey AC, Pomeroy WB, and Martin CW. Sexual Behavior in the Human Male. Philadelphia, WB Saunders, 1948.

Kolodny R, Masters W, and Johnson V. Textbook of Human Sexuality for Nurses. Boston, Little, Brown, & Co, 1979.

Lions EM. Human Sexuality in Nursing Process, New York, John Wiley & Sons, 1982.

Masters W and Johnson V. Human Sexual Response. Boston, Little, Brown, & Co, 1966.

McCary J. McCary's Human Sexuality, ed 3. New York, D. Van Nostrand, 1978.

Mims F and Swenson M. Sexuality—A Nursing Perspective. New York, McGraw–Hill, 1980.

Money J and Ehrhardt A. Man, Woman, Boy and Girl. Baltimore, The Johns Hopkins University Press, 1972.

Morrison E and Price MU. Values in Sexuality. New York, Hart, 1974.

Rosen R and Rosen LR. Human Sexuality. New York, Alfred A. Knopf, 1981.

Woods N. Human Sexuality in Health and Illness, ed 2. St Louis, CV Mosby, 1979.

Mastectomy

Rollin B. First You Cry. Philadelphia, JB Lippincott, 1976.

Nursing Assessment

Block GJ, Nolan JW, and Demsey MK. Health Assessment for Professional Nursing—A Development Approach. New York, Appleton–Century–Crofts, 1981.

Siemens S and Brandzel R. Sexuality Nursing Assessment and Intervention. Philadelphia, JB Lippincott, 1982.

Articles
Adolescence and Sex

Coleman E. Counseling adolescent males. Personnel & Guidance Journal, 1981 Dec; 60(4):215–218.

Peach EH. Counseling sexually active very young adolescent girls. Matern Child Nurs J 1980 May/June; 5(3):191–195.

Coronary Care

Cole CM et al. Brief sexual counseling during cardiac rehabilitation. Heart Lung 1979 Jan/Feb; 8(1):124–129.

Johnston BL et al. Sexual activity in exercising patients after myocardial infarction and revascularization. Heart Lung 1978 Nov/Dec; 7(6):1026–1031.

Papadopoulos C et al. Sexual concern and needs of the postcoronary patient's wife. Arch Intern Med 1980 Jan; 140(1):38–41.

Scalzi C and Dracup K. Sexual counselling of coronary patients. Heart Lung 1978 Sept/Oct; 7(5):840–845.

Wagner NW and Swarajan ES. Sexual activity and the cardiac patient. In Green R. Human Sexuality—A Health Practitioner's Text, ed 2. Baltimore, William & Wilkins, 1979.

Diabetes Mellitus

Davis H. Sexual dysfunction in diabetes: Psychogenic and physiologic factors. Medical Aspects of Human Sexuality 1978; 12(12):48–65.

Ellenberg M. Sex and the female diabetic. Medical Aspects of Human Sexuality 1977; 11(12):30–31.

Kolodny RC. Sexual dysfunction in diabetic females. Diabetes 1971 Aug; 20(8):557–559.

Kolodny R et al. Sexual dysfunction in diabetic men. In Comfort A. Sexual Consequences of Disability. Philadelphia, George F. Stickley, 1978.

Schiavi RC. Sexuality and medical illness: Specific reference to diabetes mellitus. In Green R. Human Sexuality—A Health Practitioner's Text, ed 2. Baltimore, William & Wilkins, 1979.

Disability

Bogle JE and Shaul S. Body image and the woman with a disability. In Bullard D and Knight V. Sexuality and Physical Disability. St Louis, CV Mosby, 1981.

Comfort A. Sex counseling of the disabled in medical practice. In Comfort A. Sexual Consequences of Disability. Philadelphia, George F. Stickley, 1978.

Hypertension

Saunders J. Hypertension. MAHS 1980 Nov; 14(11):118–119.

Human Sexuality

Addiego F et al. Female ejaculation: A case study, Journal of Sex Research 1981 Feb; 17(1):13–21.

Baxter RT and Linn A. Sex counseling and the SCI patient. Nursing '78 1978 Sept; 8(9):46–52.

Bem S. The measurement of psychological androgyny. J Consult Clin Psychol 1974; 42(2):155–162.

Brooks M. Effects of diabetes on female sexual response. Medical Aspects of Human Sexuality 1977; 11(12):63–64.

Bullough B and Bullough V. Sexuality and the nurse. Imprint 1974 Feb; 21(1):17–18.

Comarr A and Gunderson B. Sexual function in traumatic paraplegia and quadriplegia. Am J Nurs 1975 Feb; 75(2):250–255.

Dresen S. The middle years : The sexually active middle adult. Am J Nurs 1975 June; 75(6):1000–1006.

Jacobson L. Illness and human sexuality. Nurs Outlook 1974 Jan; 22(1):50–53.

Kuczynski HJ. Nursing and medical students' sexual attitudes and knowledge. JOGN 1980 Nov/Dec; 9(6):339–342.

Leiblum S and Rosen R. Guidelines for taking a sexual history. Unpublished paper presented at course on human sexuality, Department of Psychiatry, CMDNJ, Rutgers Medical School, New Jersey, Jan 1980.

Lief H and Payne T. Sexuality—knowledge and attitudes. Am J Nurs 1975 Nov; 75(11):2026–2029.

Malo–Juvevra D. Sex therapy and nursing—do they mix? RN 1975 Mar; 38(3):32–33.

Mims F. Sexual health education and counseling, Nurs Clin North Am 1975 Sept; 10(3):519–528.

Payne T. Sexuality of nurses; correlations of knowledge, attitudes, and behavior. Nurs Res 1976 July–Aug; 25(4):286–292.

Pfeiffer E. Sexuality and the aging patient. In Green R. Human Sexuality—A Health Practitioner's Text, ed 2. Baltimore, William & Wilkins, 1979.

Watts RJ. Factors interfering with sexual functions during chronic illness issues. Mental Health Nursing 1979 Dec; 2(2):68–83.

Wood R and Rose K. Penile implants for potency. Am J Nurs 1978 Feb; 78(2):234–238.

Mastectomy

Frank DI. Sexual counseling to a mastectomy patient. Nursing '81 1981 Jan; 11(1):64–67.

Gaylin J. Emotional pain of mastectomy. Psychology Today 1977 Apr; 10(11):98–99.

Thielen PG. Nursing concerns for patients undergoing mastectomy. Issues in Health Care of Women 1980 May/Aug; 2(3/4):55–65.

Spinal Cord Injury

Bors E and Comarr AE. Neurological disturbances of sexual function, with special reference to 529 patients with spinal cord injury. Urol Surv 1960 Dec; 10(6):191–222.

Cole T. Sexuality and the spinal cord injured. In Green R. Human Sexuality—A Health Practitioner's Text, ed 2. Baltimore, William & Wilkins, 1979.

Comarr A and Gunderson B. Sexual function in traumatic paraplegia and quadriplegia. Am J Nurs 1975 Feb; 75(2):250–255.

Dunn M, Lloyd EE, and Phelps G. Sexual assertiveness in spinal cord injury. In Bullard D and Knight V. Sexuality and Physical Disability. St Louis, CV Mosby, 1981.

Geiger RC. Neurophysiology of sexual response in spinal cord injury. In Bullard D and Knight V. Sexuality and Physical Disability. St Louis, CV Mosby, 1981.

Price S and Stroebel–Kahn F. Coping with quadriplegia. Am J Nurs 1981 Aug; 8(8):1471–1478.

Smith J and Bullough B. Sexuality and the severely disabled person. Am J Nurs 1975 Dec; 75(12):2194–2197.

Unit V

Concepts and Challenges in Patient Management

14

Principles and Practices of Rehabilitation

▷ Philosophy of Rehabilitation

It is never how high one rises that determines one's merit, but rather how far one has come, considering his difficulties.

—Archibald Rutledge

Rehabilitation is a dynamic, active program that enables an ill and disabled person to achieve his greatest possible level of physical, psychological, mental, social, and economic efficiency. How close he comes to achieving this goal determines the degree to which he becomes a socially and economically independent member of society. Rehabilitation has been called the third phase of medicine, the first being prevention, the second diagnosis and treatment, the third convalescence and rehabilitation. Modern rehabilitation is a process whereby a patient adjusts to a handicap by learning how to integrate all of his resources and to concentrate more on existing abilities than on the permanent disabilities he must live with. Genuine adjustment is in great part an inner process, because it involves reorientation of the patient's values.

The first comprehensive program in rehabilitation was started in 1947 at the Bellevue Hospital in New York City by Dr. Howard Rusk. Since then, programs have been developed in most medical centers. Many health facilities have elaborate departments; however, a successful program can be carried out even in a small hospital, with a minimum of personnel and equipment. A positive point of view plus dedication, patience, and willingness to move through the many stages from inactivity to activity must be demonstrated by the patient and all those who work with him in achieving this goal.

Rehabilitation concerns not only the individual; it also concerns the nation. Early in 1962 the Department of Health, Education and Welfare launched a new approach in public welfare that stressed "services instead of support, rehabilitation instead of relief." The promotion of rehabilitation services and the family-centered approach received particular emphasis. The Social and Rehabilitation Service (SRS) created in 1967 within the Department of Health, Education and Welfare combined the programs of the Welfare Administration, the Vocational Rehabilitation Administration, the Medicaid program, and the Mental Retardation Division of the Public Health Service. The Rehabilitation Act of 1973 was a milestone. Under Title V, provisions were made for the disabled in the areas of employment, health care, transportation, housing, education, legal rights, voting, and education. The Rehabilitation Comprehensive Services and Developmental Disabilities Amendment (1978) authorizes independent living services for the severely disabled.

The economic advantage of rehabilitation is readily apparent; instead of an individual receiving welfare aid, he will be rehabilitated into employment. Instead of being dependent on society, he will contribute to it. The effect on the individual is to change him from a hopeless dependent to an active, self-sufficient citizen. But it is even more important that the person is helped to develop a satisfying way of life that preserves the uniqueness of his individuality. He gains inner strength from his own resources that makes it possible for him to partake of the joys and meet the problems of life in a meaningful way.

The trend in rehabilitation is to include not only the physically, mentally, and emotionally handicapped (including those suffering from cancer), but also to take in the aged and those who are disadvantaged because of poverty or social deprivation.

In the hospital setting, the patient and his problems are assessed, mutual goals are set, and a program is set up to enable him to achieve self-sufficiency up to the level of his capabilities and desires. His abilities are stressed, rather than his disabilities. Since each patient has a different level of capability, the program is individualized. The ultimate goal is to obtain optimal function in his daily routine—that is, the activities of daily living. Rehabilitation goals must be realistic, taking into consideration the patient's ability (the most important factor) and then his disability. Through such a program, the patient is motivated and helped to attain social interdependence and vocational reintegration when possible.

▷ The Rehabilitation Team

Rehabilitation is a creative process that requires a team of people working together and contributing specialized services for a common goal. The team members represent a variety of disciplines, each health professional making a unique contribution. They meet in group sessions at frequent intervals to evaluate the patient's progress and collaborate in making plans and necessary program changes.

The *patient* is the key member of the rehabilitation team. He participates in goal setting and in learning and working on his rehabilitation program, so that he can eventually control his own life.

The *rehabilitation nurse* is responsible for developing a patient care plan directed toward defined patient goals and for coordinating the actions of other team members

toward these goals. Additional goals include the prevention of complications and the restoration and maintenance of optimal physical and psychosocial health. The nurse establishes a sustained and supporting relationship with the patient and applies nursing assessment, intervention, and evaluation in skin care, positioning, transfer techniques, bladder and bowel management, nutrition, psychosocial support, and patient and family education. In accordance with the ANA Standards of Rehabilitation Nursing Practice, the functions of rehabilitation nursing may be listed as follows:

- Collecting data on the health status of the patient
- Developing a nursing diagnosis (identifying the problems, limitations, and methods of adaptation to health problems)
- Developing goals for nursing care (the end state toward which nursing action is directed)
- Prescribing action to meet the goals (priority setting, alternative interventions, etc.)
- Implementing the nursing care plan
- Evaluating the nursing care plan in terms of stated goals
- Reassessing and reordering priorities and setting new goals; revising the plan of care*

The *physician* has the responsibility of making the medical diagnosis so that therapy can be directed toward realistic goals; part of this responsibility includes directing the patient's therapeutic program.

The *physiatrist* is a physician-specialist in physical medicine and rehabilitation who is responsible for testing the patient's physical functioning, determining the potential functional goal, and supervising the rehabilitation program.

The *physical therapist* teaches and supervises the patient through a prescribed exercise program designed to strengthen weak muscles and prevent deformities. The physical therapist also teaches new ways of locomotion, transportation, and daily activities.

The *psychologist* assesses the patient's motivation, values, and attitudes toward the disability and also works with the family to help them cope with the problems that have arisen as a result of the patient's condition. The psychologist also helps to ease the stress of staff members involved in patient care.

The *occupational therapist* develops skills to assist the patient in adapting to home and work situations. Practical projects are devised to improve the patient's coordination and maintain his interest.

The *social worker* investigates the patient's background and socioeconomic status and assists the patient and his family in adjusting to the home and social environment.

The *vocational counselor* tests the patient to determine his interests and aptitudes so that vocational training can be instituted. He also helps plan job modifications and advises the patient of employment opportunities.

The *rehabilitation engineer* uses science and technology in designing and constructing devices that help severely and multiply handicapped persons to function de-

---

* Adapted from the American Nurses' Association Division of Medical–Surgical Nursing Practice and the Association of Rehabilitation Nurses: Standards of Rehabilitation Nursing Practice. Kansas City, ANA, 1977.

spite their disabilities. The rehabilitation engineer may also design and fabricate orthoses and prostheses.

The *sex counselor* is trained to diagnose and treat sexual dysfunctions of disabled persons. This role may be assumed by the social worker, nurse, psychologist, or other prepared health professional.

The importance of rehabilitation is often underestimated. Approximately 38 million persons in the United States have some limitation of activity. Many older people (whose numbers are increasing) have disabling conditions requiring rehabilitation services. Every patient, regardless of his problem or diagnosis, has the right to rehabilitation services.

Rehabilitation is an integral part of nursing and *should begin with the initial contact with the patient.* Every major illness carries with it the threat of disability. If the patient is hospitalized with a burn and develops a contracture deformity, his recovery time will be greatly delayed. Disabilities are not static but tend to become worse, and some complications of inactivity can give the patient more pain and discomfort than the initial injury or disease.

Though not all hospitals have departments of physical medicine and rehabilitation, *the principles of rehabilitation are basic to the care of all patients,* and the pages that follow point out how the nurse applies them. Other aspects of rehabilitation are discussed under the appropriate clinical conditions throughout the book.

▷ Psychological Implications of a Disability

A physical disability often has a deep psychological significance to the patient. It has a direct impact on the patient's body image and can cause a state of conflict. Physically, a part of his body has deteriorated. He may have the shattering realization that he can do less than he did formerly. His shape and posture may have changed, as may his state of mind. Even his position in society may be altered, as well as his social interaction with others. He perceives himself as a second-class citizen, a devalued person. In short, he feels that he is different.

Disability may mean hardship or even tragedy to the individual, depending on his premorbid personality, occupation, cultural background, and social status, and on the support he receives from significant others.

A person usually goes through a series of emotional reactions to a newly acquired disability. The first reaction may be confusion, disorganization, and denial. The patient is in a state of conflict and has to cope with problems of forced dependence, loss of self-esteem, and feelings that his personal and family integrity are threatened. The patient may refuse to accept his new limitations and at times has an unjustified overconfidence in speedy recovery. His false hopes lead him to hear only what he wants to hear. He is likely to be self-centered and even childlike in his demands. The mechanism of denial is useful up to a certain point, but eventually the reality of the situation must be accepted.

The patient may progress to a stage of grief and depression in which he appears to mourn for his lost function or missing body part. (Depression may also be caused by sensory deprivation and restricted environmental stimulation.) There may be behavioral changes, particularly regression. This stage of grief appears to be a necessary phase in adapting to the disability. Mourning is part of the process of working through all the meanings of the loss. Therefore, the patient should not merely be encouraged blithely to "cheer up." Such an approach can evoke extreme hostility and provoke behavior that will result in a "problem patient." Listening to the patient talk about his loss is important for healing.

The patient may go through a stage of anger in which he projects blame on others. This behavior frequently alienates the family and health care personnel, who either capitulate to his demands or withdraw from him.

Following the stages of depression, grief, and anger, there is generally a period of adaptation and adjustment. In time, the patient becomes more familiar with his condition and is able to tolerate it better. As he revises his body image and modifies his former picture of himself, he redirects his energies toward coping with his physical functioning.

He is able to accept a degree of dependency and not resent being "waited upon." He begins to realize that hopelessness is futile and knows that he must adapt to the permanent aspects of the disability and modify his goals.

The acceptance of the limitations imposed by the disability and the total investment of the patient in his rehabilitation program is basic to adjustment. It is from this point in rehabilitation that the patient begins to look ahead and to develop realistic goals for his future.

At the same time, it is important to realize that not every patient will progress in orderly fashion through the stages of grieving. Many frequently fluctuate between acceptance and grief, so that angry outbursts and depression may continue long after the usual period of mourning has supposedly passed. Each new situation (going home, starting vocational rehabilitation, entering a new relationship) reminds the patient anew of his limitations, his changed body image, and the reality of the permanence of his situation. Thus, even though the disabled person makes progress and increases his independence, he must continually deal with the grief process and the need to grow throughout his life.

At the other end of the spectrum are those patients who do not accept their disability but instead waste emotional energy in rebelling futilely against unalterable damage. Or, there are those patients who ignore the disability and refuse to put forth any effort to adapt for everyday life. Still others may overreact and build a false reputation for being "cheerful and courageous." Although "ignoring" may seem healthy, often it includes a total rejection of the disability, which keeps the patient from doing the things that will be helpful to him. When a person fails to react at the appropriate time, it may indicate that he is not coping adequately. These patients may require assistance from either a psychologist or a psychiatrist.

In general, the nurse's responsibility is to assess the patient and his family in reacting to his disability and to work with him, always emphasizing his assets and remaining strengths, and at the same time listening to him, encouraging him, and sharing in his satisfactions and triumphs as he progresses in his program. It is through the support and inspiration of the members of the rehabilitation team that the patient becomes all that he is capable of being.

▷ Sexuality and the Disabled

There is a growing recognition of the sexual rights and problems of the disabled. Sexuality involves not only biological sexual activity, but also the individual's concept of his masculinity or her femininity and the way he or she reacts to others and is perceived by them. It takes many forms: caring, reaching out, sharing, and emotional intimacy.

Sexual matters are considered to be in the very private realm, and the patient is apt to be reticent about discussing his feelings. The professional person is focusing so intently on the rehabilitation of the patient (*i.e.,* helping him to gain independence) that there is a tendency to forget that sexuality is part of the patient's personality. Recognizing and dealing with sexual concerns is basic in establishing feelings of self-worth, which are essential to total rehabilitation. Professional personnel, family members, and the community must deal with the reality that disabled persons are sexual human beings with needs for social affiliation and sexual intimacy.

Problems faced by the disabled include limited access to information about sexuality, lack of opportunity to form friendships and loving relationships, impaired self-image and low self-esteem, and lack of social skills.

The sex-related concerns of the patient must be identified through an individual approach. Allow the patient to talk about his anxieties related to sex. The disabled person may need further sex education, communication and assertiveness skills, and the specialized services of a sex counselor/therapist.

The reader is referred to the bibliography at the end of the chapter for additional reading on this subject.

▷ Principles and Practices of Rehabilitation Nursing

The most common complications that threaten a patient with a prolonged illness or disability are contractures, pressure sores, and bladder and bowel problems.

Contractures result when muscles are not used or joints are not put through their full range of motion. The contracture is actually a shortening of the muscle, which leads to deformity. These deformities may be prevented if the causal conditions are understood properly and preventive measures are instituted early.

When tissues do not receive adequate nourishment, circulation, and exercise, they tend to deteriorate and to atrophy. Initiating deliberate and proper measures can combat and prevent tissue damage and pressure sores.

Bladder and bowel difficulties may result from disease, injury, or shock. In many patients, refunctioning can be accomplished through individualized teaching and persistent attention to the establishment of regular function.

The major goals of the nurse in rehabilitation are:

1. To prevent deformities and complications
2. To motivate, teach, and support the patient (and his family when necessary) during the daily activities of living, which include self-care
3. To refer the patient for proper follow-up care and supervision.

Each of these categories will now be discussed in detail.

▷ Prevention of Deformities and Complications

Deformities and complications of illness or injury often can be prevented by proper positioning in bed, frequent changes of position, and exercise.

Positioning

Unless contraindicated, the patient should be turned frequently. The reasons for changing body position are:

- To prevent contractures
- To stimulate circulation and help prevent thrombophlebitis, pressure sores, and edema of the extremities
- To promote lung expansion
- To promote drainage of respiratory secretions
- To relieve pressure on a body area

The most common positions that the patient assumes in bed are the dorsal, or supine; the side lying, or lateral; and the prone positions. The essential principles of body alignment necessary for maintaining these positions follow.

Dorsal or Supine Position
1. The head is in line with the spine, both laterally and anteroposteriorly.
2. The trunk is positioned so that flexion of the hips is minimized.
3. The arms are flexed at the elbow with the hands resting against the lateral abdomen.
4. The legs are extended with a small, firm support under the popliteal area.
5. The heels are suspended in a space between the mattress and the footboard.
6. The toes are pointed straight up.
7. Trochanter rolls are placed under the greater trochanters in the hip joint areas.

Side-lying or Lateral Position
1. The head is in line with the spine.
2. The body is in alignment and is not twisted.
3. The uppermost hip joint is slightly forward and supported in a position of slight abduction by a pillow.
4. A pillow supports the arm, which is flexed at both the elbow and the shoulder joints.

Prone Position (on Abdomen)
1. The head is turned laterally and is in alignment with the rest of the body.
2. The arms are abducted and externally rotated at the shoulder joint; the elbows are flexed.

3. A small, flat support is placed under the pelvis, extending from the level of the umbilicus to the upper third of the thigh.
4. The lower extremities remain in a neutral position.
5. The toes are suspended over the edge of the mattress.

Therapeutic Exercises

Exercise involves the function of muscles, nerves, bones, and joints as well as the cardiovascular and respiratory systems. *Return to function is dependent on the strength of the musculature that controls the joints.* Therapeutic exercises are prescribed by the physician and performed with the assistance and guidance of a physical therapist or nurse. The overall goals are to promote mobility (range of motion), to strengthen and retrain deficient muscles, to restore as much normal movement as possible (in order to prevent deformities), to improve endurance and coordination, and to stimulate the functions of various organs and body systems.

Exercise is also valuable in helping to restore the motivation and well-being of the patient. It can help to lift the mind from pessimism and depression to optimism and good humor. The patient should have a clear understanding of what the exercise is to accomplish. Biofeedback training is being combined with exercise to produce greater strength and active range of motion.

Exercise, when correctly done, assists in (1) maintaining and building muscle strength, (2) maintaining joint function, (3) preventing deformity, (4) stimulating circulation, and (5) building strength and endurance. There are five types of exercise: passive, active assistive, active, resistive, and isometric. The description, purpose, and action of each of these exercises are summarized in Table 14-1.

Table 14-1
Therapeutic Exercises

Exercise	Description	Purposes	Action
Passive	An exercise carried out by the therapist or the nurse without assistance from the patient	To retain as much joint range of motion as possible; to maintain circulation	Stabilize the proximal joint, and support the distal part. Move the joint smoothly, slowly, and gently through its full range of motion. Avoid producing pain.
Active assistive	An exercise carried out by the patient with the assistance of the therapist or the nurse	To encourage normal muscle function	Support the distal part, and encourage the patient to take the joint actively through its range of motion. Give no more assistance than is necessary to accomplish the action. Short periods of activity should be followed by adequate rest periods.
Active	An exercise accomplished by the patient without assistance; activities include turning from side to side, from back to abdomen, and moving up and down in bed	To increase muscle strength	When possible, active exercise should be done against gravity. The joint is moved through full range of motion without assistance. (Make sure that the patient does not substitute another joint movement for the one intended.)
Resistive	An active exercise carried out by the patient working against resistance produced by either manual or mechanical means	To provide resistance in order to increase muscle power	The patient moves the joint through its range of motion while the therapist resists slightly at first and then with progressively increasing resistance. Sandbags and weights can be used and are applied at the distal point of the involved joint. The movements should be done smoothly.
Isometric or muscle setting	Alternately contracting and relaxing a muscle while keeping the part in a fixed position; this exercise is performed by the patient	To maintain strength when a joint is immobilized	Contract or tighten the muscle as much as possible without moving the joint; hold for several seconds, then "let go" and relax. Breathe deeply.

Range of Motion Exercises

Range of motion is the movement of a joint through its full range in all appropriate planes (see Table 14-1). Usually, range of motion testing is done by the physician or physical therapist to determine the movement that exists at the joint areas. Testing helps set positive and realistic goals.

Each joint of the body has a normal range of motion. In many musculoskeletal and neurologic conditions the joints may lose their normal range, stiffen, and produce a permanent disability. If the range of motion is limited, the functions of the joint and of the muscle that moves the joint are impaired. In order to prevent painful deformities, range of motion activities are carried out when permitted, to either maintain or increase the maximal motion of a joint and to prevent deterioration.

These exercises should begin as soon as the patient's clinical condition allows. The range of motion exercises are planned for the individual to accommodate the wide variation in the degrees of motion that persons of varying body build and age groups can attain.

Technique.   The patient must be in a comfortable position, lying supine with his arms to the side and his knees extended. Good body posture is to be maintained in each position assumed during the exercise. The bed should be high enough to permit the nurse to reach effectively the part to be exercised. Unless prescribed otherwise, a joint should be moved through its range of motion about three times, at least once a day. The extremity is held at the joint, and the joint is moved smoothly, slowly, and gently through its range. If the joint is painful, as in arthritis, the extremity may be supported in the muscular area. A joint should not be moved beyond its free range of motion. Therefore, the motion should be stopped at the point of pain. When muscle spasm is present, the joint should be moved slowly and to the point of resistance. Then a gentle, steady pressure is exerted until the muscle relaxes.

When range of motion exercises are performed, consideration must be given to the bones above and below the joint to be moved. For example, when the elbow is taken through its range of motion, the humerus must be stabilized while the radius and the ulna are moved through their range of motion in the elbow joint. (Refer to Charts 14-1 and 14-2 for joint motion and a pictorial review of range of motion exercises. See Chart 14-3 for definitions of terms.)

(*Text continues on page 238*)

Chart 14-1
Range of Motion

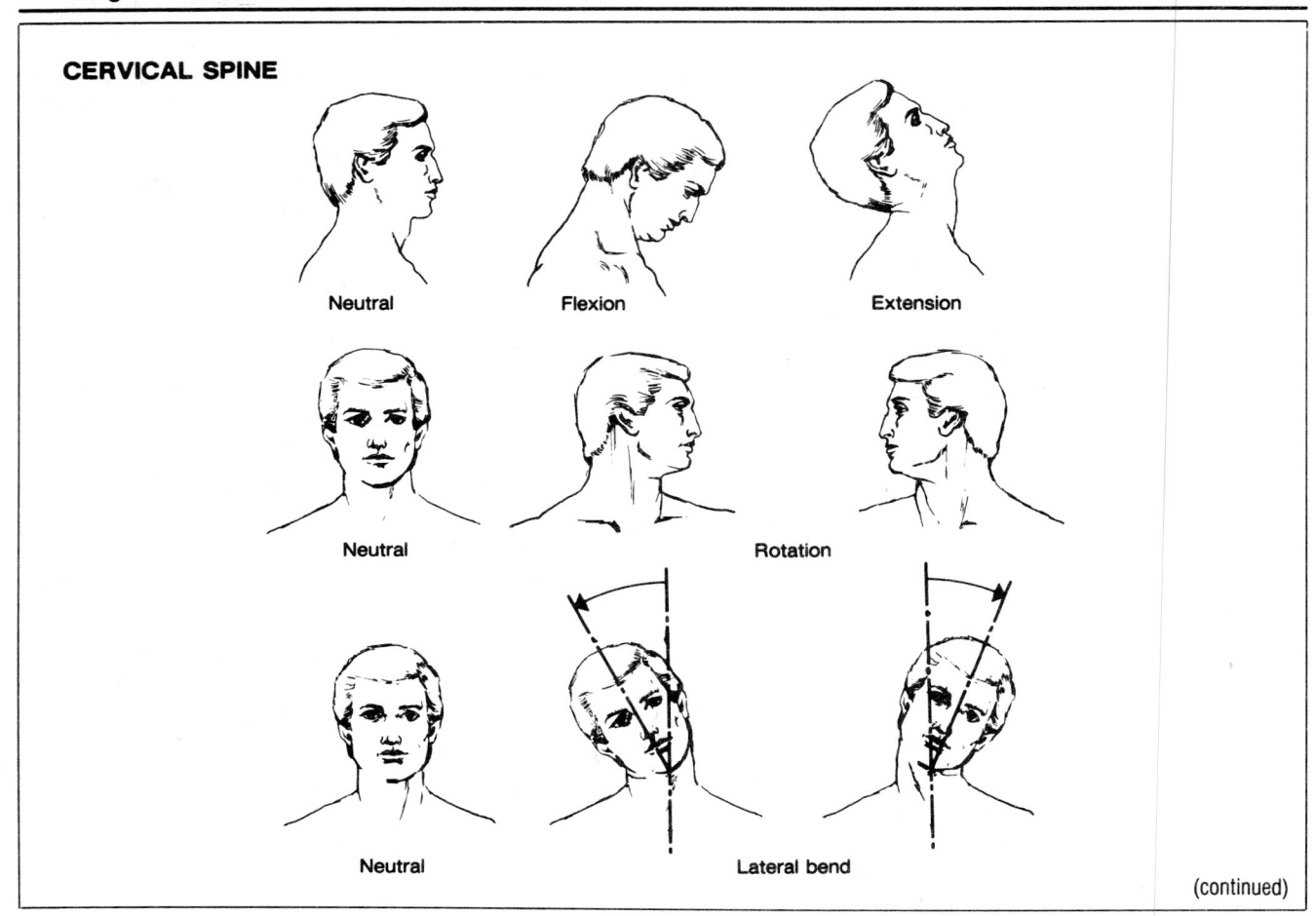

CERVICAL SPINE

Neutral   Flexion   Extension

Neutral   Rotation

Neutral   Lateral bend

(continued)

Chart 14-1
Range of Motion (continued)

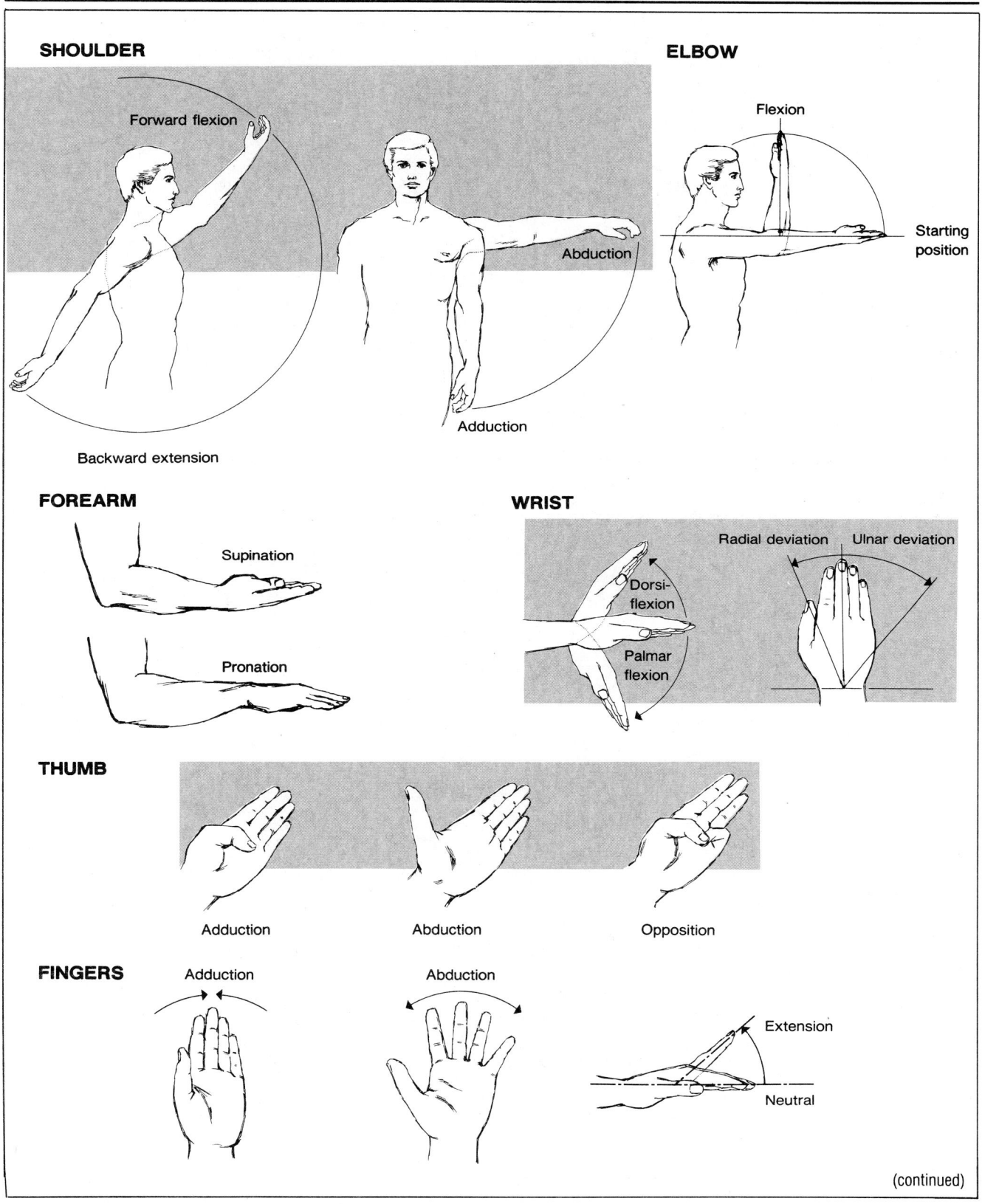

SHOULDER

Forward flexion

Abduction

Adduction

Backward extension

ELBOW

Flexion

Starting position

FOREARM

Supination

Pronation

WRIST

Radial deviation   Ulnar deviation

Dorsi-flexion

Palmar flexion

THUMB

Adduction   Abduction   Opposition

FINGERS

Adduction   Abduction

Extension

Neutral

(continued)

Chart 14-1
Range of Motion (continued)

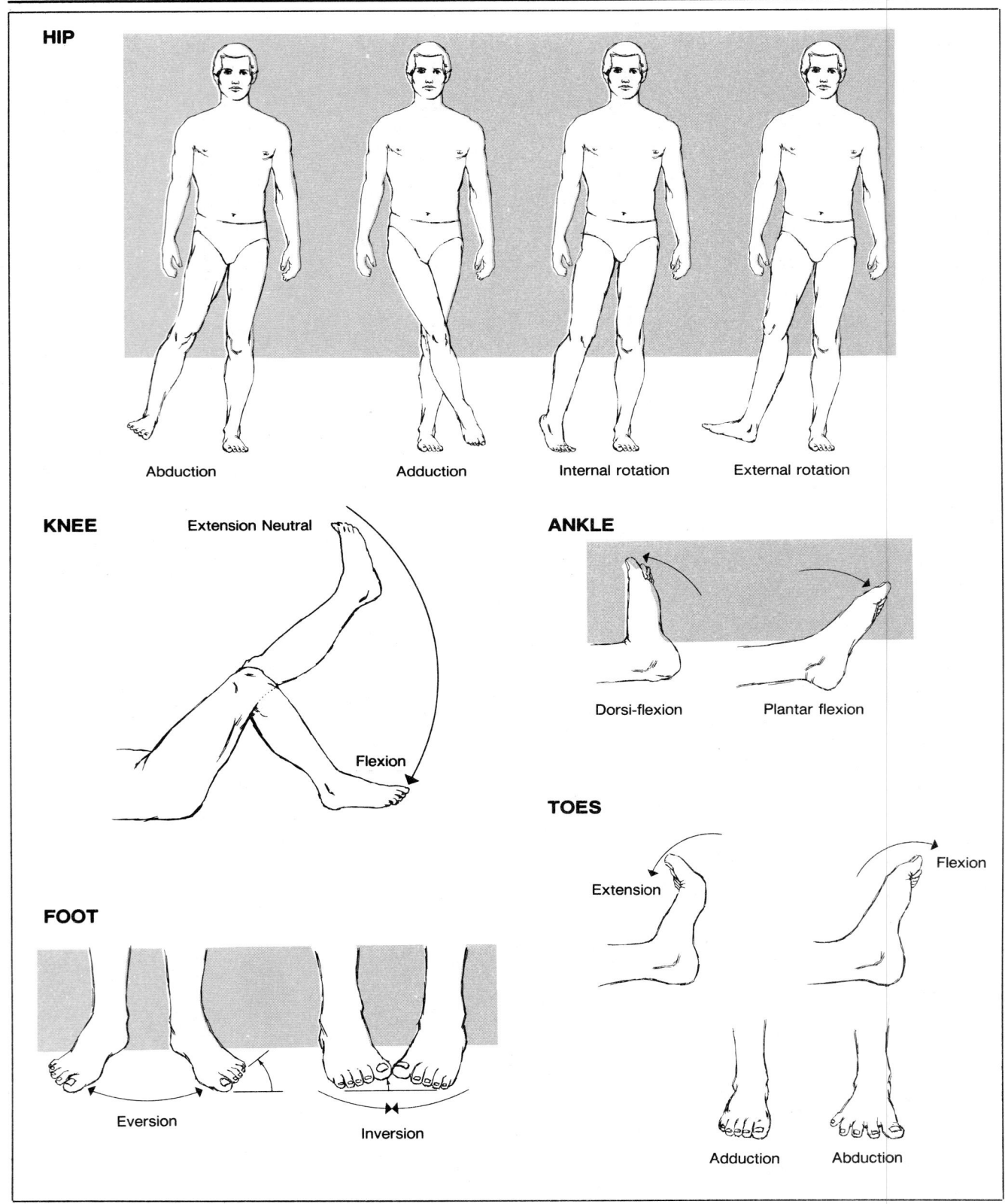

HIP

Abduction   Adduction   Internal rotation   External rotation

KNEE   Extension Neutral

Flexion

ANKLE

Dorsi-flexion   Plantar flexion

TOES

Extension   Flexion

FOOT

Eversion   Inversion

Adduction   Abduction

Chart 14-2
Range of Motion Exercises

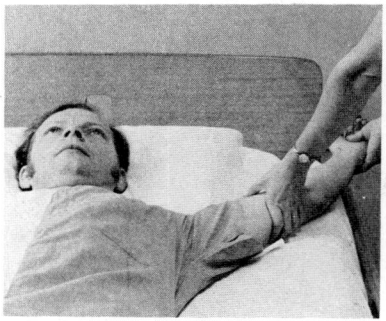

Abduction of shoulder. Move arm from side of body to above the head. Then return arm to side of body or neutral position (adduction).

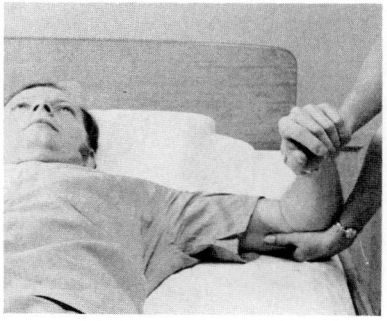

Internal rotation of shoulder. With arm at shoulder height, elbow bent at a 90-degree angle, and palm toward feet, turn upper arm until palm and forearm face backward.

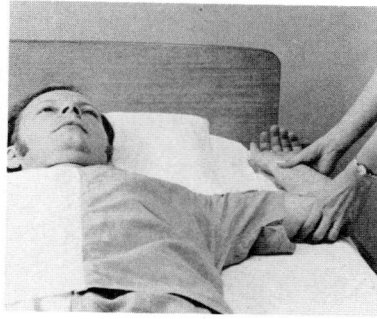

External rotation of shoulder. With arm at shoulder height, elbow bent at 90-degree angle, and palm toward feet, turn upper arm until the palm and forearm face forward.

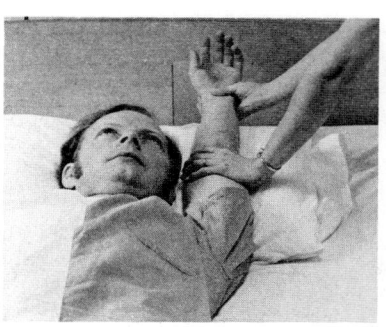

Forward flexion of shoulder. Move arm forward and upward until it is alongside of head.

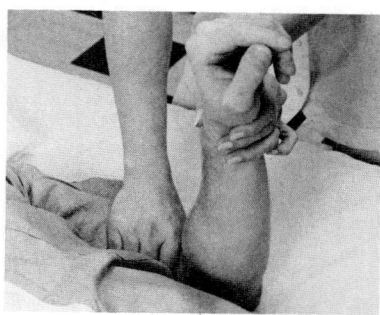

Pronation of forearm. With elbow at waist and arm bent at 90-degree angle, turn hand so that palm is facing down.

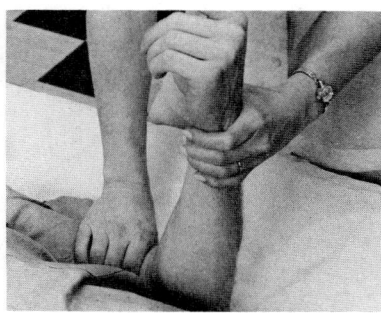

Supination of forearm. With elbow at waist and arm bent at 90-degree angle, turn hand so that palm is facing up.

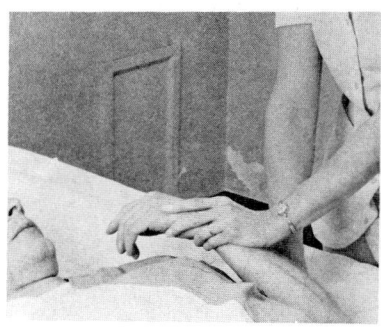

Flexion of elbow. Bend elbow, bringing forearm and hand toward shoulder. Then return forearm and hand to neutral position (arm straight).

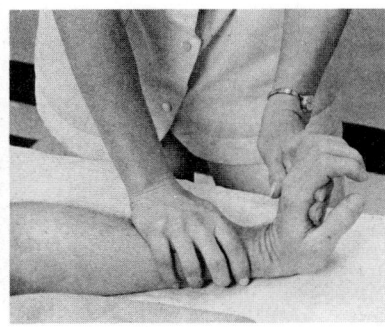

Wrist extension.

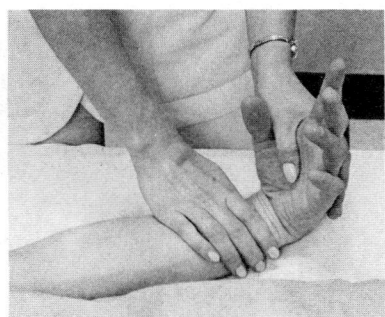

Flexion of wrist. Bend wrist so that palm is toward forearm. Straighten to a neutral position.

(continued)

Chart 14-2
Range of Motion Exercises (continued)

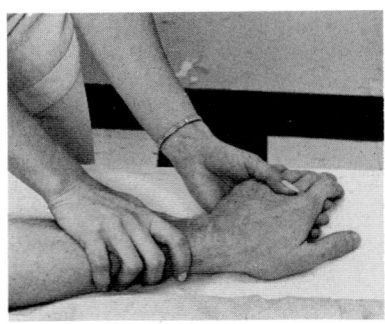

Ulnar deviation. Move hand sideways so that the side of hand on which little finger is located moves toward forearm.

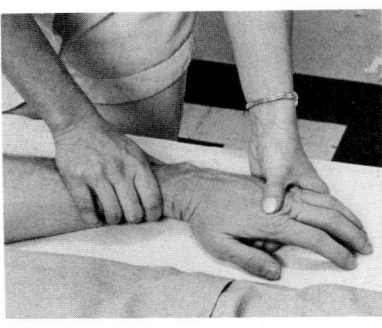

Radial deviation. Move hand sideways so that side of hand on which thumb is located moves toward forearm.

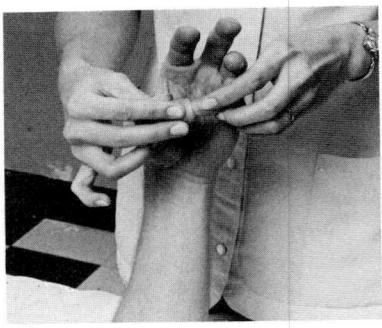

Thumb opposition. Move thumb out and around to touch little finger.

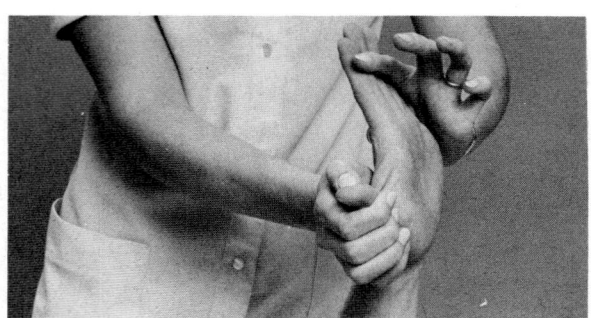

Extension of fingers

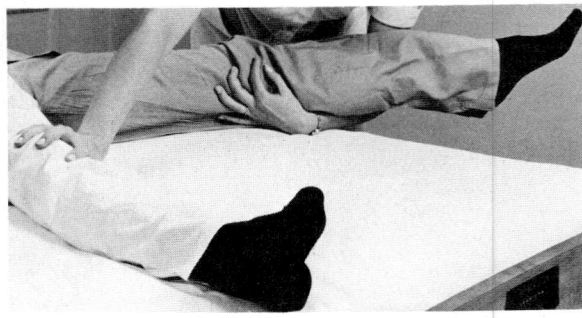

Abduction–adduction of hip. Move leg outward from the body as far as possible. Return leg from abducted position to neutral position and across the other leg as far as possible.

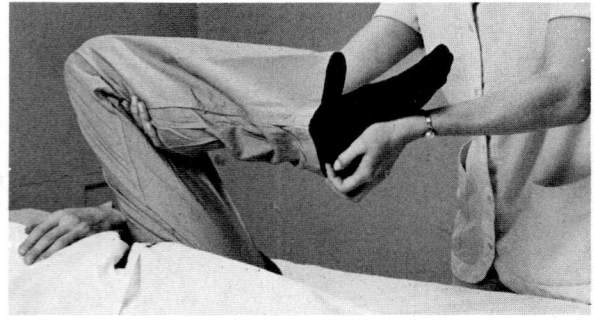

Flexion of hip and flexion of knee. Bend hip by moving the leg forward as far as possible. Return leg from the flexed position to the neutral position.

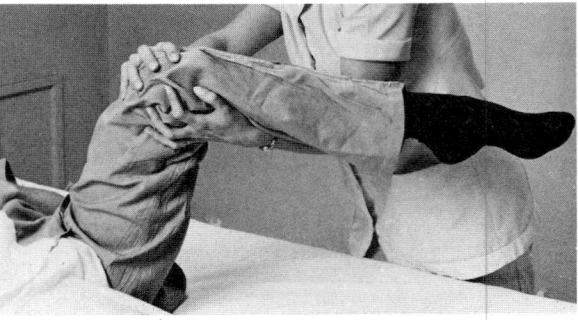

Internal–external rotation of hip. Turn leg in an inward motion so that toes point in. Turn leg in an outward motion so that toes point out.

(continued)

Chart 14-2
Range of Motion Exercises (continued)

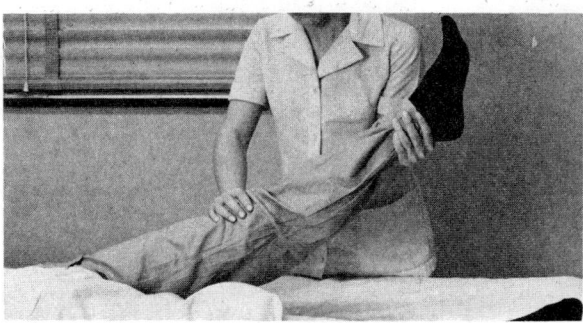

To stretch hamstring muscles, straighten leg and then raise the leg.

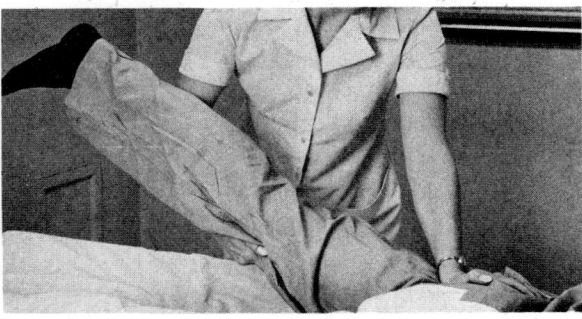

Hyperextension of hip. Place the patient in a prone position, and move leg backward from the body as far as possible.

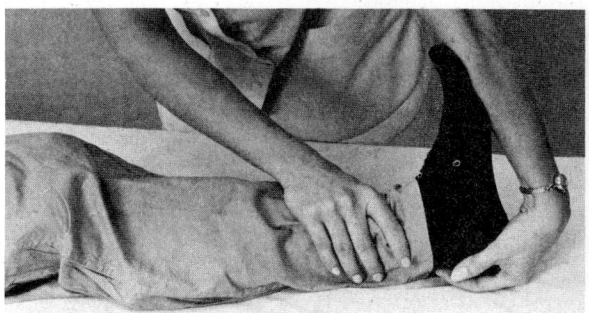

Dorsiflexion of foot. Move foot up and toward the leg. Then move foot down and away from the leg (plantar flexion).

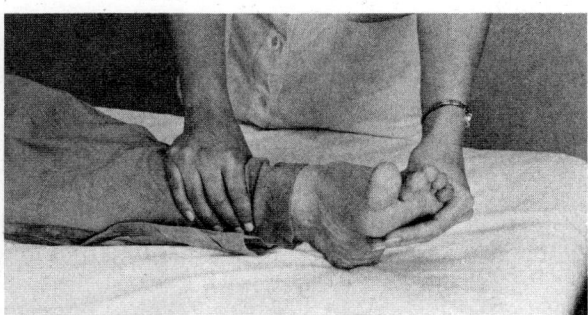

Inversion and eversion of foot. Move foot so that sole is facing outward (eversion). Then move foot so that sole is facing inward (inversion).

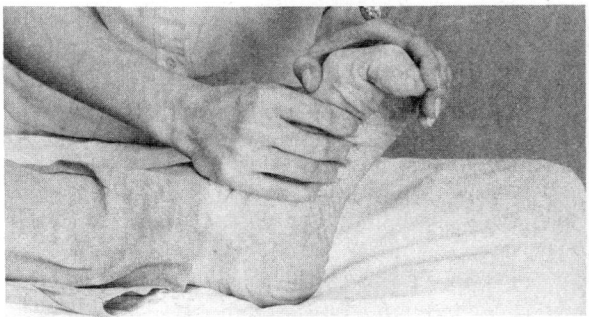

Flexion of toes. Bend the toes toward the ball of foot.

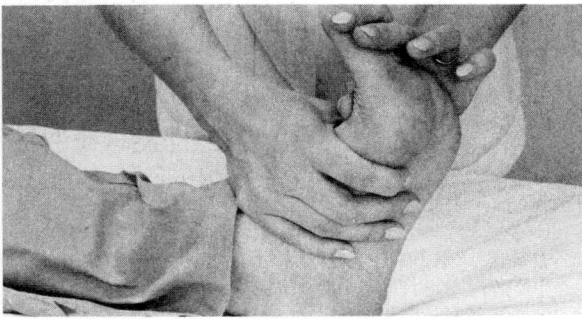

Extension of toes. Straighten toes and pull them toward the leg as far as possible.

Chart 14-3
Definitions

Abduction—movement away from the midline of the body
Adduction—movement toward the midline of the body
Flexion—bending of a joint so that the angle of the joint diminishes
Extension—the return movement from flexion; the joint angle is increased
Inversion—movement that turns the sole of the foot inward
Eversion—movement that turns the sole of the foot outward
Dorsiflexion—movement that flexes or bends the foot toward the leg
Plantar flexion—movement that flexes or bends the foot in the direction of the sole
Pronation—rotation of the forearm so that the palm of the hand is down
Supination—rotation of the forearm so that the palm of the hand is up
Rotation—turning or movement of a part around its axis
  Internal: turning inward, toward the center
  External: turning outward, away from the center

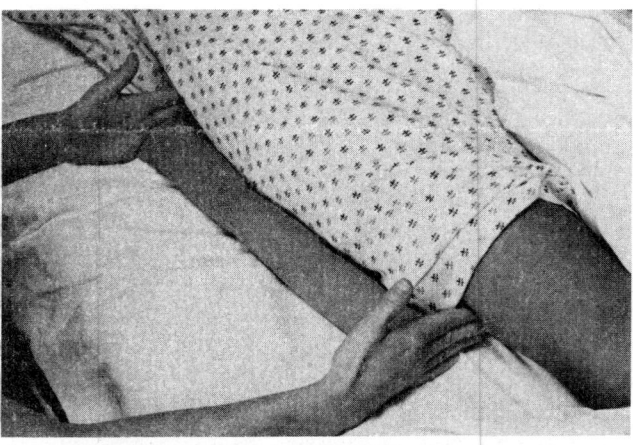

Figure 14-1.   Placement of trochanter roll. (From Farrell J: Illustrated Guide to Orthopedic Nursing. Philadelphia, JB Lippincott, 1982.)

Deterrents to Exercise

Fear and Pain.   The ability of a patient to follow a pattern of exercises may be thwarted by *fear* and *pain.* These produce increased tension and may result in muscle spasm and tightness of joint ligaments. If fear and pain are not relieved, they may lead to stiffness of joints, limitation in range of motion, muscle contractures, and poorly coordinated muscle activity. For example: *pain* in the chest, as observed in chest and breast surgery, cardiac pain, or burns of the thorax, frequently causes many patients to hold the arm close to the body, resting it on the chest or abdominal wall with the elbow flexed. If permitted to continue for prolonged periods of time, this practice may result in tightness of the ligaments around the shoulder and elbow joints; and spasm of the large pectoral muscles and biceps may lead to adaptive shortening, tightening, and contractures of these muscles. The weight of the arm on the chest or the abdomen restricts the expansive motion of the chest wall and muscles of respiration, which leads to inadequate ventilation.

Fear (as observed in patients who have had cardiac, chest, or breast surgery, infections in the lungs, and burns of the chest wall) often causes these patients to assume protective positions that are restrictive in nature and prevent proper physiologic alignment.

Preventing External Rotation of the Hip

Patients who are in bed for periods of time may develop external rotation deformity of the hip. The hip is a ball-and-socket joint and has a tendency to rotate outward when the patient lies on his back. A trochanter roll extending from

the crest of the ilium to the midthigh will prevent this deformity (Fig. 14-1). With correct placement, the trochanter roll serves as a mechanical wedge under the projection of the greater trochanter.

Preventing Footdrop (Plantar Flexion)

Footdrop is a deformity in which the foot is plantar flexed (the ankle bends in the direction of the sole of the foot). If the condition continues without correction, the patient cannot hold the foot in a normal position and will walk on his toes without touching the ground with the heel of his foot. The deformity is caused by contracture of both the gastrocnemius and the soleus muscles. It may also be produced by loss of flexibility of the Achilles tendon.

- Prolonged bed rest, lack of exercise, incorrect positioning in bed, and the weight of the bedding, forcing the toes into plantar flexion, are factors that contribute to footdrop.

To prevent this crippling deformity, a footboard or pillows are used to keep the feet at right angles to the legs when the patient is in a supine position. The feet are positioned so that both plantar surfaces are firmly against the footboard or pillows. A trochanter roll(s) is used to maintain the leg(s) in a neutral position. The patient is encouraged to flex and then to extend (curl and stretch) his feet and toes frequently. The ankles should be moved clockwise and counterclockwise in a rotary motion several times each hour.

Preventing and Treating Pressure Sores

Pathogenesis

Pressure sores (bedsores, decubitus ulcers) are localized areas of infarcted soft tissues produced by pressure. Pressure is exerted on the skin and subcutaneous tissues by the object on which they rest, such as the mattress, chair seat, cast, etc. There is compression of the small nutrient vessels of the skin and underlying tissues, which results in tissue anoxia or ischemia. The cutaneous tissues become broken or destroyed, leading to progressive destruction of underlying soft tissue. Once the skin breaks, an ulcer may form, which may be painful and very slow to heal. Invasion by a profusion of microorganisms (streptococci, staphylococci, *Pseudomonas aeruginosa, Escherichia coli, Proteus* species) and secondary infections is difficult to avoid. There emanates from the lesion an obnoxious-smelling discharge, which is the product of bacterial invasion and tissue breakdown. The lesion, if large enough, permits a continuous loss of serum, which may deplete the circulating blood and the entire body of essential protein constituents. Also, when the ulcer is infected, it may extend deep into the fascia, muscle, and bone, and multiple large sinus tracts may radiate from it. Thus, systemic infection can easily develop, especially from bloodstream invasion by gram-negative bacilli.

Other factors contribute to the development of pressure sores (Chart 14-4). Anemia, whether caused by hemorrhage, nutritional deficiency, or infection, decreases the body's oxygen-carrying ability and predisposes to ulcer formation. Patients with nutritional deficiencies have negative nitrogen, phosphorus, sulfur, and calcium balances, which will produce wasting of tissue and loss of weight. All patients should be screened on admission for susceptibility to pressure sores.

Other metabolic disorders can also contribute to low protein levels. Persons with malabsorption syndrome may develop protein deficiency and severe anemia because of failure to absorb folic acid. Diabetic persons may have a poor quality of tissue, which is easily injured. Many persons have hidden vitamin C deficiencies. In all of these conditions there is evidence of protein depletion (in the form of low serum albumin) that can lead to a pressure sore when illness supervenes.

Motor paralysis with associated muscular atrophy causes

reduction of padding between the overlying skin and the underlying bone, and leads to pressure sores. Paralyzed patients tend to lie in one position, with the body weight concentrated on small areas of skin. This high pressure collapses blood vessels and impedes blood flow, causing a pressure sore to form in a very short time. If the patient has suffered sensory loss, he will not be aware of pain and pressure and will not be aware that the skin is breaking down.

Shearing force is created by the interplay of two other forces: gravitational forces that pull the patient's body toward the foot of the bed, and resting forces created by friction taking place on the skin surface. Shearing forces, by pulling on tissues, stretch and injure tissues and blood vessels. This type of shearing force is applied when the patient is pulled up in bed, is allowed to slump in bed or a chair, or moves up in bed by digging his heels or elbows into the mattress. To prevent this, the patient should be lifted, not dragged up, in bed or on a chair. Sheepskin pads are thought to have shear-resistant properties.

Other causes of pressure sores are edema, which impairs circulation and interferes with the supply of nutrients to the cells, and moisture and friction, which irritate the skin and make it less resistant to injury. Physiologic change in the skin, especially in older patients, because of reduced production of sebum, is another factor.

In summary, the basic causes of pressure sores are pressure (Fig. 14-2), blocking of blood flow, and lack of normal movement.

Assessment of Clinical Manifestations
The first sign of a potential pressure sore is the appearance of erythema (redness) of the skin, which will blanch on pressure. Skin temperature is increased owing to vasodilatation. The redness progresses to a dusky, cyanotic blue-gray appearance, which is the result of skin capillary occlusion and subcutaneous weakening. Blistering and a break in the skin occur, and the early stages of necrosis follow. A small surface sore may overlie a large undermining defect below. This process may involve deeper soft tissues, bursae, muscles, tendons, and even bone or joints. If the ulcer is long-standing and has repeatedly broken down and healed, secondary induration (hardening of tissue) develops and the blood supply to the area is compromised by underlying scar tissue. Deep pockets of infection are often present. These may be covered by a dark crust, which also impedes healing.

▶ **Nursing Assessment**

- Inspect each pressure site for erythema.
    Press on the area. Look for blanching.
    Note how long hyperemia persists following removal of pressure.
- Palpate for warmth.
    Is skin temperature increased?
- Inspect for dry skin, moist skin or a break in the skin.
- Palpate peripheral pulses to evaluate circulatory status.
- Check patient's record for hematocrit, hemoglobin, and serum albumin levels.

Chart 14-4
Risk Factors for Development of Pressure Sores

Prolonged pressure
Immobility, compromised mobility
Loss of protective reflexes, motor or sensory deficit/loss
Shearing forces, friction, trauma
Malnutrition, hypoproteinemia, vitamin deficiencies, anemia
Incontinence
Skin dryness, excessive skin moisture, maceration
Edema, poor skin perfusion
Infection
Advancing age; debilitation
Equipment: traction, casts, restraints, improper bedding and seats

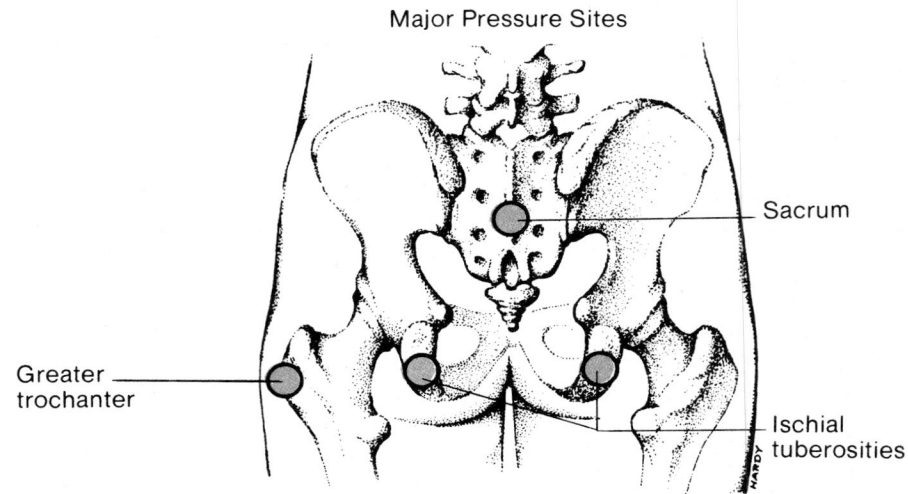

Major Pressure Sites

Sacrum

Greater trochanter

Ischial tuberosities

Figure 14-2. Areas of major pressure sites where pressure sores can develop.

Nursing Diagnosis/Patient Problems

Based on the clinical manifestations, nursing history, risk factors, and diagnostic assessment, the patient's nursing problems include potential alteration in skin integrity related to pressure.

▶ Planning and Nursing Interventions

The goal for the patient and nurse is to prevent the occurrence of a pressure sore. Pressure sores develop with alarming rapidity—within 2 to 4 hours at sites where there is unrelieved pressure. They are a serious complication that may occur in any patient. Their presence greatly prolongs the patient's convalescence and imposes a tremendous physical and economic burden.

The best treatment of pressure sores is prevention. If one bears in mind that the weight-bearing prominences are covered only by skin and small amounts of subcutaneous fat, it is easily seen that the majority of pressure sores are located at such sites: the sacrum and coccygeal areas, greater trochanter, and ischial tuberosities, especially in persons who sit for prolonged periods (see Fig. 14-2). Other bony promontories that are susceptible to pressure sore development are the knees, medial condyle of the tibia, fibular head, malleoli, heels, and elbows.

Goals

The goals of nursing interventions are:

1. To relieve or remove pressure
2. To stimulate the circulation
3. To keep the skin clean and in a healthy condition
4. To ensure nutrition

Relief of Pressure.   The patient needs frequent changes of position and the avoidance of positions that result in excessive pressure. Such measures will prevent prolonged blocking of blood flow, which interferes with skin nutrition. Shifting the weight of the patient lets the blood flow back to the ischemic areas and helps tissue to recover from pressure.

- Thus, the patient should be turned at 1-hour or 2-hour intervals.

He should be positioned on all four sides (laterally, prone, dorsally) in sequence unless contraindicated. In addition to regular turning, there should be small shifts of body weight, such as repositioning an ankle, elbow, or shoulder. The skin should be inspected at each position change and checked for temperature elevation. If redness or heat is noted, keep pressure off the area.

One way to avoid pressure is to use one of the many mechanical devices that have been designed as a means of providing support for specific body areas or for distributing pressure uniformly. An alternating pressure pad mattress covered with 2.5 cm (1″) of thick foam rubber is especially valuable in conditions in which the patient cannot turn. The alternating inflation and deflation of the pad produces constriction followed by dilatation of the superficial blood vessels of the skin. By such action, pressure on any one part is reduced and the blood supply is increased.

For patients susceptible to pressure on bony prominences, there is a variety of pads and supportive devices available that can be placed on top of the mattress. The gel-type flotation pad reduces pressure because the material is similar in consistency to human adipose tissue and "gives" with the patient's weight. Soft, moisture-absorbing padding is also useful since the softness and resilience of padding allows for even distribution of pressure and the dissipation and absorption of moisture, while providing for freedom from wrinkles and friction. Bony prominences may be protected by inserting pieces of gel pads, sheepskin padding, or soft foam rubber beneath the sacrum, the trochanters, heels, elbows, scapulae, and the back of the head when there is pressure on these sites. Large sheepskin pads are said to help distribute pressure over a greater surface area, absorb moisture, allow for air circulation and reduce friction. The patient should not be placed on a poorly ventilated mattress that is covered with plastic or some other impermeable material.

The use of the flotation mattress, or water bed, for treatment of pressure sores has been advocated. As the patient's body sinks into the fluid, additional surface becomes available for weight bearing, thereby further decreasing body weight per unit area. (Pascal's law states that the weight of the body floating on a fluid system is evenly distributed over the entire supporting surface.) Thus, the body weight is lightened and there is less pressure on the body parts. However, shearing forces can be built up on the water bed as the patient's body is suspended on the plastic covering over the surface of the water. The Rehabilitation Engineering Center at Rancho Los Amigos Hospital developed a multifluidic unresisting displacement (MUD) bed, sometimes called a high density fluid support system (HDF). The patient is floated on a bed of high density fluid, a mixture of bentonite clay and barites. Since this fluid is twice as dense as water, there is equal distribution of pressure and reduction of pressure against the total body surface as the patient floats with his body partly in and partly out of the fluid mixture.

Another way to relieve pressure over bony prominences is the bridging technique accomplished through the correct positioning of pillows. Just as a bridge is supported on pillars to allow traffic to move underneath, so can the body be supported by pillows to allow for space between bony prominences and the mattress. For the feet and extremities, a footboard or pillows will support the bedding and thus reduce pressure. To protect the heels, 2.5 cm (1″) of foam rubber may be placed between a well laundered soft sheet and the mattress.

Patients sitting in wheelchairs for prolonged periods should have wheelchair cushions fitted and adjusted on an

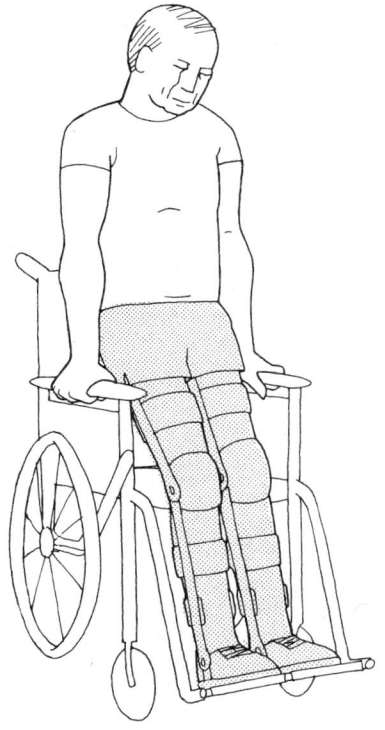

Figure 14-3. Wheelchair push-up to prevent ischial pressure sores. These push-ups should become an automatic routine (every 30 minutes) for the person with paraplegia. He should stay up, out of contact with the seat, for 60 seconds. (Adapted from Hirschberg GG, Lewis L, and Vaughan P: Rehabilitation. Philadelphia, JB Lippincott.)

individualized basis, using pressure measurement techniques as a guide to selection and fitting. The patient should be reminded to shift his weight frequently and raise himself up for a few seconds every half hour while sitting in a chair (Fig. 14-3).

Stimulation of Circulation. Since the stimulation of circulation relieves tissue ischemia, the forerunner of pressure sores, the patient is encouraged to keep active. Active and passive exercises increase muscular, skin, and vascular tone. The patient should be ambulated whenever possible since the level of mobility is an important criterion for prognosis and treatment. (Activity also stimulates the metabolic processes and helps to improve morale.) Gentle skin massage with lotion is useful as another means of stimulating the blood flow in the skin, but only if tissue damage is not present. Circulation is also aided by turning the patient. Turn or, if this is not possible, tilt the patient toward one side and then the other. The use of a rocking bed and a tilt table also aids in stimulating circulation.

Skin Care and General Hygiene. Maceration of the skin by continuous moisture must be prevented by meticulous hygienic measures. The skin should be washed with a mild soap and water and blotted dry with a soft towel. The skin then is lubricated with a bland lotion or a thin layer of silicone cream to keep it soft and pliable. It is desirable that the patient assist in caring for his skin. He should be encouraged to inspect it at frequent intervals for evidence of pressure. He should be taught to use a mirror and inspect posterior areas if he is paraplegic or has other neuromuscular disorders. He should massage and stroke lightly around bony prominences since this promotes venous return, reduces edema, and increases vascular tone. Foreign bodies are kept out of the bed because they serve to irritate the skin. Foundation sheets are tightly stretched to prevent wrinkles.

Nutritional Support. The patient's nutritional status must be adequate and a positive nitrogen balance maintained. Pressure sores develop more quickly and are more resistant to treatment in patients suffering from nutritional disorders. A high protein diet with protein supplements may be helpful. Iron preparations and whole blood transfusions may be necessary since the hemoglobin level is a critical criterion for the development of pressure sores. Vitamin C is necessary for healing and tissue vitality.

▶ **Evaluation**

Expected Outcomes

Prevents pressure sores from occurring

1. Avoids pressure
   a. Changes position every 1 to 2 hours
   b. Changes from supine to side-lying to prone positions
   c. Sleeps in prone position as much as possible
   d. Uses trapeze to raise self off bed at 30-minute intervals while awake
   e. Raises self from seat/wheelchair every 30 minutes
   f. Uses warning system (sensor or timing device) as a reminder to relieve pressure

g. Verbalizes the importance of adequate protein and vitamin C intake
2. Monitors self for signs and symptoms of skin reddening and change in skin temperature
   a. Uses hand mirror to inspect hard-to-see areas
   b. Inspects knees, ankles, elbows, and other accessible areas with each position change

Management

If a pressure sore develops, the objectives of treatment are to continue preventive measures on a more vigorous level (remove the pressure), encourage restoration of circulation and cellular function, and prevent necrosis of deeper structures. The healing of pressure sores requires repair of connective tissue and epithelialization.

The metabolic processes are stimulated by keeping the patient as active as possible. The pressure must be taken off; if the lesion is on the posterior surface, the patient should spend more time in the prone and side-lying positions. The patient is placed on a high-protein, high-vitamin diet to promote healing. These wounds leak body fluids and protein, placing the patient in a catabolic state and predisposing to the serious problem of secondary infection.

Patients who have pressure sores are usually malnourished and tend to have hypoproteinemia and vitamin deficiencies. Protein deficiency must be corrected in order to heal a pressure sore, and carbohydrates are necessary to "spare" proteins and provide an energy source. Extra protein is added to the diet, and the regular diet may have to be supplemented with tube feedings. Wound healing is also dependent on collagen. In turn, ascorbic acid (vitamin C) is necessary for collagen formation. Therefore, patients with pressure sores require additional vitamin C. Supplemental zinc is a stimulant to wound healing in those patients who suffer from a zinc deficiency.

The ulcer must be cleansed daily to clear up sepsis and stimulate the regeneration of epithelium. The ulcer(s) is debrided of necrotic material because devitalized tissue promotes the development of infection, delays granulation, and impedes healing. Dead bone must also be removed. Debridement may be done by surgical dissection or electrocautery. Cultures are obtained of the material deep in the ulcer to determine the resident flora. Usually, in hospitalized patients there is a mixture of gram-positive and gram-negative bacteria. Oxidizing agents (hydrogen peroxide) may be useful in anaerobic infections. Topical cleansing may also be done with solutions of acetic acid, normal saline, half-strength Dakin's solution, etc. If an eschar covers the ulcer, it may be removed to estimate the depth of tissue destruction and to enhance penetration of a topical agent.

After the ulcer is clean, some form of topical therapy may be applied. The large variety of agents available is convincing evidence that the best therapeutic modality for pressure sores has not been found. There are skin barriers, antiseptic plastic sprays, an aerosol spray containing a corticosteroid and an antibiotic, etc. Collagenase therapy uses a local enzymatic debriding agent to digest necrotic tissue and purulent exudates without damaging granulation tissue. This chemical debridement is very effective when used with hydrotherapy to facilitate debridement and promote granulation tissue growth. Usually, this ointment is applied directly to a sterile gauze pad, which is then placed over the wound. A plastic film dressing or a Telfa pad held in place with paper tape is nonirritating to most skin. All excess ointment should be removed from the normal skin. If the wound is infected, a topical antibacterial agent is applied before enzymatic (collagenase) treatment.

Dextranomer (Debrisan) contains dry, porous beads. When placed in a discharging wound, the hydrophilic (water-absorbing) beads absorb proteins, bacteria, fibrin–fibrinogen-split products, and toxins. The flow of debris into the bead layer removes bacteria from the wound surface and allows granulation.

The placement of an absorbable gelatin sponge at the base of the ulcer (changed daily) has also been successful. This pad is a synthetic material with a physical consistency similar to that of human fat tissue. It provides a layer of "artificial fat" over a bony prominence.

Another type of topical preparation is a transparent elastic, self-adhesive film (Op-Site) that is used on either superficial or deep ulcers. The film is similar to skin texture, permeable to air, and waterproof. It is applied to the wound surface and usually left in place 5 to 7 days. The process is repeated until the ulcer heals.

Physical therapy modalities, such as air, sunlight, whirlpool baths, ultraviolet irradiation, and ultrasound, have also been used successfully. Hyperbaric oxygen may promote healing and relieve hypoxia of the wound surface, causing stimulation of capillary regrowth, granulation, and epithelialization.

Surgical intervention is necessary when the ulcer does not respond to conventional treatment. There are many surgical techniques used to resect the lesions and close the defects. Incision and drainage are carried out if the ulcer is not draining properly. Grafting procedures using skin grafts, muscle flaps, or myocutaneous flaps may be necessary for wound closure. Sometimes the ulcer, scar tissue, underlying bursa, and bone must be removed before healing takes place.

Recurrence of pressure sores may be expected and should be watched for and treated immediately.

▷ Supporting the Patient in Daily Self-care

Activities of Daily Living

Activities of daily living (ADL) are those self-care activities that must be accomplished each day in order for the patient to care for his own needs. Indeed, ADL are the key to reentry to home and society. ADL include personal hygiene, dressing, eating, toileting, getting in and out of bed (transfers), using a wheelchair, ambulating (when possible), and performing manual tasks.

- The goal of the patient is to care for himself in his daily routine without depending on others.
- The goal of the nurse is to teach, support, and supervise the patient while he performs these activities.

Activities of Daily Living (ADL) Sheet

| | Evaluation of Patient's Functioning | | |
	Total Assistance	Partial Assistance	Independent

Prescribed Activities

Range of motion

Positioning

Use of tilt table

   Degree

   How long

Exercises

   Breathing

   Balancing

   Crutch training

   Parallel bars

   Steps

Other Information

Appliances or prosthesis

Ambulation

Time permitted up

Bladder/bowel program

Bathing/grooming schedule

Speech problems

Activities being learned

Name:

Diagnosis:

Physician:

Rehabilitation nurse:

Functional Capabilities

1. Flexes neck

2. Raises hand to head

3. Raises hand behind head

4. Reaches out at shoulder level to side (laterally)

5. Pronates/supinates forearm

6. Grasps objects

7. Begins grasp ability

8. Closes fist

9. Opens fist

10. Flexes and extends knee joint

11. Touches floor while seated

12. Crosses leg over opposite knee while sitting (with or without help of hands)

13. Transfers from sitting to standing (with or without holding to support)

14. Walks

Figure 14-4. On the actual record there is sufficient space left under each item for notes.

An ADL program is started as soon as the rehabilitation process starts. The longer a muscle is in disuse, the weaker and more atrophied it becomes. The patient must learn that he will lose what he does not use.

In order to effectively teach a person methods of self-care, he must be motivated. "I would rather do it myself" is a good concept for the patient to develop. The nurse teaches and guides, but the patient must do the work. Since there are individual differences in all persons, self-care techniques need to be flexible and adapted to the patient's needs and mode of living. It is important to remember that there is usually more than one way to accomplish self-care. Since many patients do not perform these commonplace activities easily, a great deal of common sense and a little ingenuity are frequently called for. Often a simple maneuver requires concentration and the exertion of considerable effort.

By using an "Activities of Daily Living (ADL) Sheet" (Fig. 14-4) to evaluate the ability of a patient to perform certain activities, it is possible to determine his limitations. Another advantage of such a guide is that it shows the patient how he is progressing from one time to the next; this may be a valuable morale booster. When a patient's progress can be demonstrated, there is a tendency for such evidence to be a source of motivation. Also, the ADL Sheet keeps the staff informed of the activities that the patient can perform independently and those that will require assistance.

Before initiating an ADL program, the nurse must understand the patient's medical condition, his functional capacity, and his therapeutic goal as well as the details of his care. It is also wise to learn about the patient's family background and educational level in order to know how much support the family can give.

Teaching the Activities of Daily Living

Since there are many ways to teach a task, the following is offered as a guide:

1. Define the goal of the activity; understand the purpose.
2. Ascertain what methods can be used to accomplish the task. (Example: There are several ways of putting on a given garment.)
3. Determine what the patient can do by watching him perform.
4. Ascertain the motions necessary for the accomplishment of the activity.
5. Encourage the patient to exercise the muscles necessary to perform the motions involved in the activity.
6. Select activities that encourage gross functional movements of the upper and lower extremities (*e.g.*, bathing, holding larger objects).
7. Gradually include activities that use finer motions (*e.g.*, buttoning clothes, eating with a spoon).
8. Extend the period of activity as much and as fast as the patient can tolerate.
9. Perform and practice the activity in a real-life situation.
10. Encourage the patient to perform every activity up to his maximal capabilities within the framework of his disability.
11. Support the patient by giving justifiable praise for effort put forth and for acts accomplished.

The ADL Sheet is an information sheet for those who are taking care of the patient. The data on it serve to inform each member of the rehabilitation team what activities the patient can perform. It also serves as an index of progress. For example, after it has been determined that the patient can bathe himself, this information is noted on the ADL Sheet. The nurse who is responsible for the patient reviews this sheet at morning care time and notes what the patient is capable of doing and what activities he is learning. Thus, the patient does not regress, because all members of the rehabilitation team are working toward the same goal.

The ADL Sheet in Figure 14-4 is a guide to the assessment of the functions of the patient. These activities are key goals. If the patient can sit up and raise his hands to his head, he probably can begin to bathe himself. By asking the patient to perform certain motions, the nurse can determine what activities he will be able to do.

Adaptive Equipment (Self-help Devices). Adaptive equipment (self-help devices) includes equipment that can help a patient carry out his daily activities. These may be devised and made by the patient, nurse, or family or purchased ready made. If the patient has difficulty in performing the activity, an adaptation will have to be made. Often, a new method can be learned. If the patient cannot quite reach his head, perhaps he will be able to touch his head by leaning forward. Or, if the method cannot be changed, adaptive equipment (self-help devices) may be used—such as those devised by adding a long handle to a comb, "building up" the handle of a spoon, or making similar modifications. Equipment such as an automatic toothbrush has been found to improve the oral hygiene of those having limited movements of the hands, wrists, and arms. Be alert to "gadgets" coming on the market that may be useful to the handicapped. There are mobility aids and systems for the paralyzed and cerebral palsied; educational aids; occupational and vocational tools; personal aids; and writing, typewriting, and communication aids that have been designed and are in use. There is also a wide selection of electronic assistive devices that help severely disabled persons to function with less dependence on others.

Assisting the Patient With Ambulation
Use of the Tilt Table

Weight bearing on the long bones is essential for normal physiologic functioning. In order to prevent complications of inactivity, the upright position with weight bearing on the long bones is desirable at the earliest possible time. This position prevents decalcification of the bones, thus aiding in the maintenance of normal acid–base balance and the prevention of renal calculi; it also stimulates circulation to the lower extremities.

Some disabilities, such as spinal cord injuries, orthostatic hypotension, brain damage, and those requiring extended periods in the recumbent positions, prevent patients from assuming an upright position by the usual methods. In such instances, a tilt table can be of tremendous use. A tilt table is a board or table that can be tilted gradually from a horizontal to a vertical position, permitting the patient to assume an upright position. It helps the patient with his weight-bearing activities and standing balance, prevents disuse syndrome, and conditions the vascular system. Before the patient is placed on a table, a compression leotard or a snug-fitting abdominal binder and elastic bandages are applied from the toes to the groin. Compression on the abdomen prevents pooling of blood in the splanchnic area and subsequent postural hypotension and inadequate cerebral circulation. Compression applied to the legs restricts the vascular walls of the blood vessels and prevents blood from pooling in the legs and edema from developing.

Tilting the patient from a supine to an upright position causes a decrease in the systolic blood pressure. For this reason, a blood pressure cuff is applied before the table is tilted. The table should be tilted gradually, and someone should stay with the patient throughout this process. If the patient feels dizzy and his blood pressure drops, return him to a flat position. Observe for pallor, diaphoresis, tachycardia, and nausea. These are the signs and symptoms of insufficient cerebral circulation. The tilt of the table is increased by 5- to 10-degree increments. The angle of the tilt is determined by the patient's tolerance and the desired amount of weight bearing. Be careful that the patient does not stand too long, especially if he cannot move his extremities. Prolonged standing may cause pressure ulceration on the bottom of the feet. The feet should be protected with a pair of properly fitted shoes.

Transfer Activities

A transfer is the movement of the patient from one piece of furniture or equipment to another (*i.e.,* from bed to chair or bed to wheelchair).

As soon as the patient is permitted out of bed, transfer activities are started. While still confined to his bed, it is important that the patient practice "push-up" exercises to strengthen the arm and shoulder extensors. It is desirable that the patient be able to raise and move his body in different directions by means of these push-up exercises. A simple, effective procedure follows:

1. Have the patient sit upright in bed.
2. Place a book under each hand.
3. Instruct the patient to push down on the book and thus raise his body weight.

Since the nurse is so frequently concerned with getting weak and incapacitated patients out of bed, it is important to be familiar with the techniques of moving the patient to the edge of the bed, sitting him on the edge of the bed, and assisting him to stand. The steps in each of these maneuvers are listed in Chart 14-5.

Before the patient is taught to transfer, he is evaluated to determine his ability to transfer from one area to another. Always have the patient move toward his stronger side. The nurse demonstrates the technique of transfer and the patient then is ready to practice and perform this activity (Fig. 14-5).

Use of a Transfer or Sliding Board. If the muscles that the patient uses to lift himself off the bed are not strong enough to overcome the resistance of body weight, a polished light-weight board may be used to bridge the gap between the bed and the chair, and the patient slides across on it. This board (or bench) also may be used to transfer the patient from the chair to the toilet or the bathtub.

- Place one side of the transfer board under the patient's buttocks and the other side of the surface to which the transfer is being made (*i.e.,* the chair).
- Instruct him to push up with his hands to shift the buttocks and then to slide across the board to the other surface.

Chart 14-5
Assisting the Patient Out of Bed

Technique for Moving the Patient to the Edge of the Bed

- Move head and shoulders of patient toward the edge of the bed.
- Move feet and legs to the edge of the bed. (The patient is now in a crescent position, which gives good range of motion to the lateral trunk muscles.)
- Place both arms well under the patient's hips. (Before the next maneuver, you should tighten [set] the muscles of your back and abdomen.)
- Straighten your back while moving the patient toward you.

Technique for Sitting Patient on the Edge of the Bed

- Place arm and hand under shoulders of the patient.
- Instruct the patient to push his elbow into the bed while you lift his shoulders with one arm and swing his legs over the edge of the bed with the other. (Gravity pulls the legs downward, which aids in raising the patient's trunk.)

Technique for Assisting Patient to Stand

- Place patient's feet well under him.
- Face the patient while firmly grasping each side of his rib cage with your hands.
- Push your knee against one knee of the patient.
- Rock the patient forward as he comes to a standing position. (Your knee is pushed against the patient's knee as he comes to the standing position.)
- Ensure that the patient's knees are "locked" (full extension) while he is standing. (Locking the knees of the patient is a safety measure for those who are weak or have been in bed for a period of time.)
- Give the patient *enough time* to balance himself.
- Pivot the patient to position him to sit in the chair.

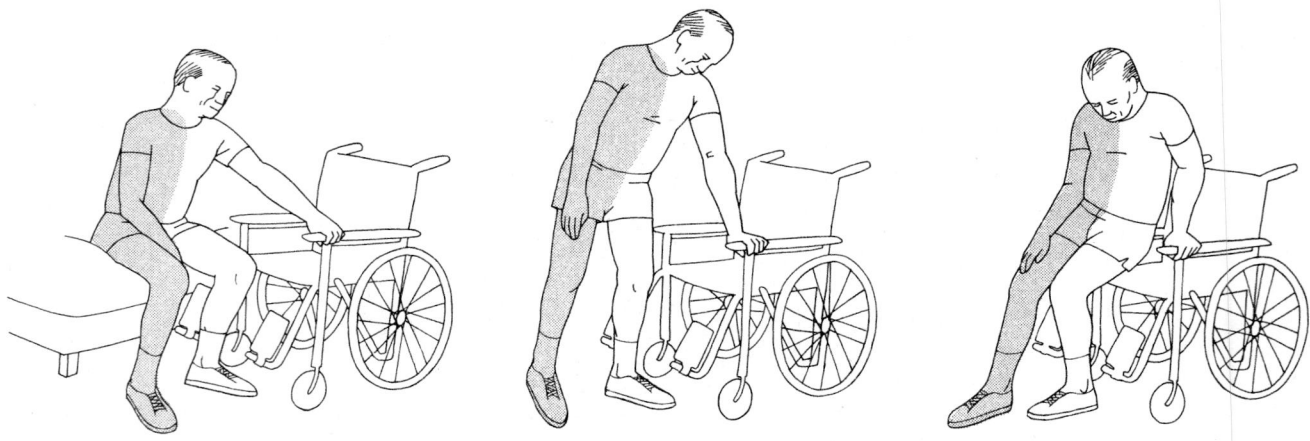

A. Weight-bearing transfer from bed to chair. The patient stands up, pivots until his back is opposite the new seat, and sits down.

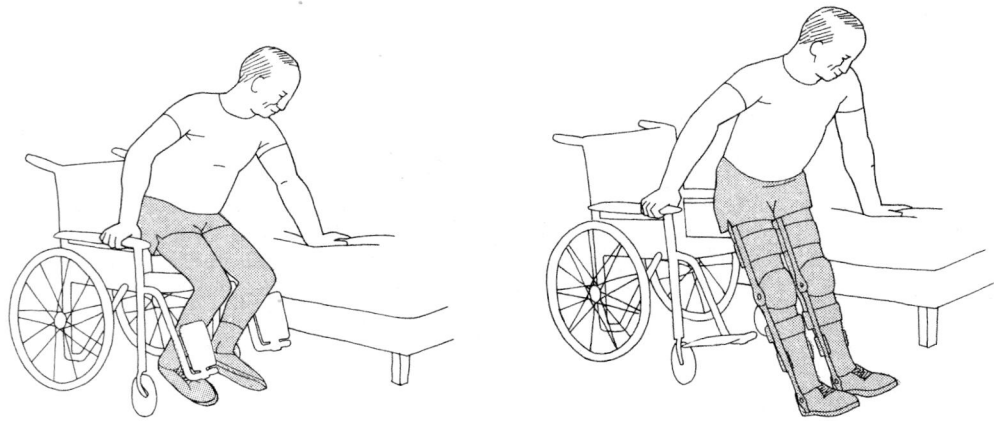

B. (*Left*) Non-weight-bearing transfer from chair to bed. (*Right*) With legs braced.

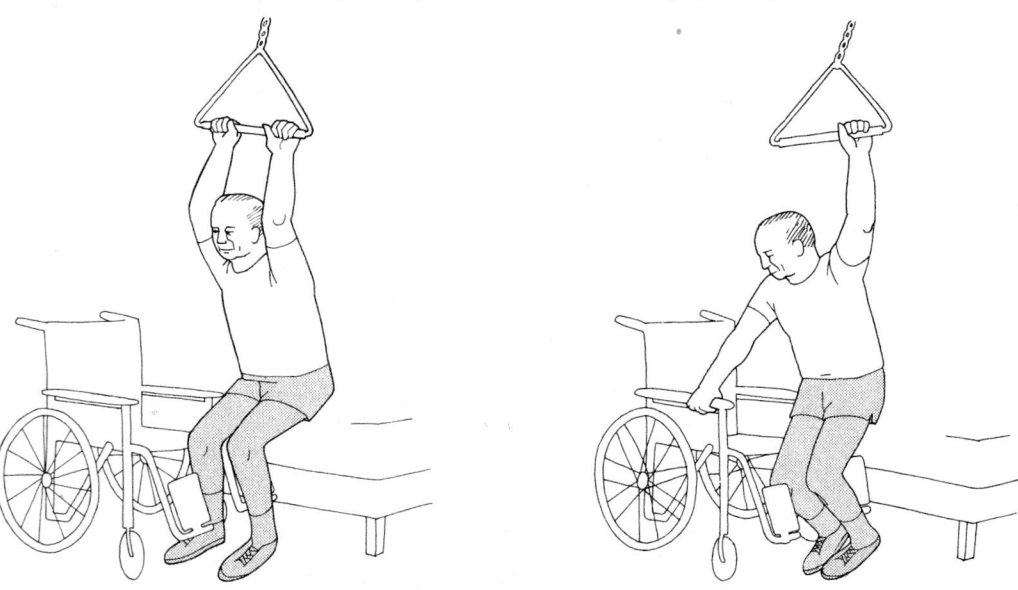

C. (*Left*) Non-weight-bearing transfer, pull-up method (*Right*). Non-weight-bearing transfer, combined method.

Figure 14-5. Methods of transferring the patient from the bed to a wheelchair. The wheelchair is in a locked position. (Redrawn from Hirschberg GG, Lewis L, and Vaughan P: Rehabilitation. Philadelphia, JB Lippincott.

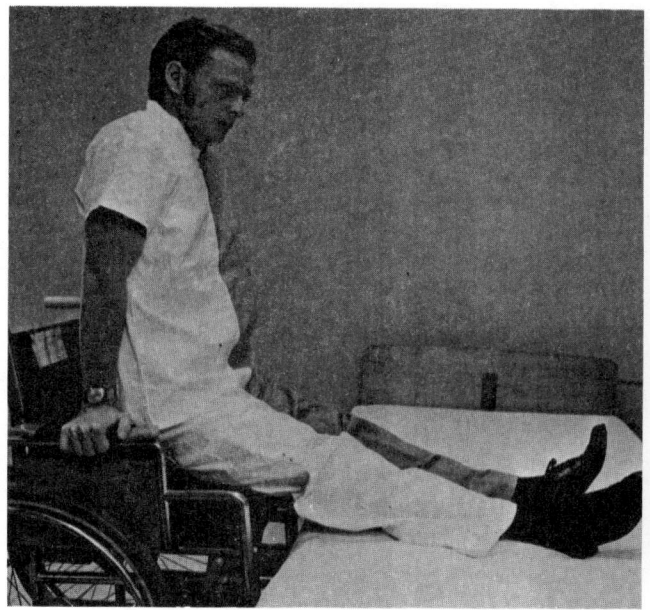 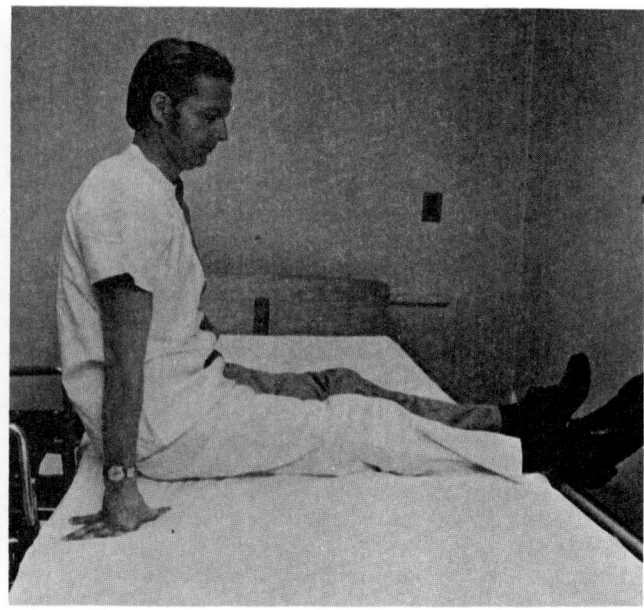

Figure 14-6. Vertical transfer of a paraplegic patient. The wheelchair is placed facing the bed with the wheels locked and the pedals in the "down" position. The patient pushes up on his hands and arms and slides his body forward onto the bed. This is a non-weight-bearing transfer in which the patient is able to transfer on the same level. With conditioning and practice, this transfer can be done to a higher or lower level by the push-up method.

There are other methods of transferring from the bed to the wheelchair when the patient is unable to stand. Figure 14-5 shows the weight-bearing and non-weight-bearing transfers, while Figure 14-6 shows the vertical transfer of a paraplegic patient.

Preparation for Ambulation

Regaining the ability to walk is a prime morale builder. To be prepared for ambulation—whether with braces, cane, or crutches—the patient must be strengthened and conditioned. *Exercise is the foundation of preparation.* By performing mat and parallel-bar exercises, the patient develops balance and coordination and strengthens his muscles. The following are preconditioning exercises that the nurse can teach and supervise.

To strengthen the muscles needed for ambulation, *quadriceps setting* is used. The quadriceps muscles are also guardians of the knee joint. Strengthening of these muscles acts as a deterrent to flexion contractures or instability of the knee. The patient contracts the quadriceps muscle while attempting to push the popliteal area against the mattress and at the same time raising the heel. He maintains the muscle contracture until the count of five and relaxes for the count of five. He should repeat this exercise 10 to 15 times hourly. In *gluteal setting,* he contracts or "pinches" the buttocks together until the count of five, relaxes for the count of five, and repeats.

To strengthen the muscles of the upper extremities, which are used for handling the cane, crutches, or walker employed in early ambulation, *sit-ups* are helpful. While in a sitting position, the patient raises his body from the chair

by pushing his hands against the chair seat (or mattress). He also should be encouraged to do *push-ups* while in a prone position. Teach him to *raise his arms* above his head and lower them in a slow, rhythmical manner while holding traction weights, gradually increasing the poundage of the weights. He can *strengthen his hands* by crumpling newspaper and squeezing a rubber ball. *Pull-ups* on a trapeze, while lifting the body, is another effective conditioner.

Crutch Walking

In the treatment of various forms of arthritis and of most fractures of the lower extremity, and after operations on the leg—especially after amputation—crutches provide a support and balance and a convenient method of getting from one place to another. Since crutch walking is not an inherited skill, it must be taught, and this learning process must begin early. Crutch walking requires a high energy expenditure and considerable cardiovascular stress.

One of the first prerequisites is to develop power in the shoulder girdle and upper extremity muscles, which will bear the patient's weight while he is crutch walking. Exercise to increase the strength and coordination of these muscle groups should be started before the patient is ambulating and then should progress to balancing exercises between parallel bars.

The following muscle groups are important for crutch walking:

- Shoulder depressors—to stabilize the upper extremity and prevent shoulder hiking

- Shoulder adductors—to hold the crutch top against the chest wall
- Arm flexors, extensors, and abductors (at the shoulder)—to move crutches forward, backward, and sideward
- Forearm extensors—to prevent flexion or buckling; important in raising the body for swinging gait
- Wrist extensors—to enable weight bearing on hand pieces
- Finger and thumb flexors—to grasp the hand piece

Of equal importance is psychological preparation, which can be developed long before the physical need is present. The individual needs of each patient must be considered and the methods of approach directed to them. The patient's age, interests, and future intentions, as well as his prognosis, are essential factors.

Measurement for Crutches.   Adjustable crutches are practical because the disease may cause changes in the muscles and the joints, or because the patient may improve and progress to a different crutch base and gait.

To measure a standing patient for crutches, position the patient against the wall with the feet slightly apart and away from the wall. Mark 5 cm (2 inches) out to the side from the tip of the toe. Measure 15 cm (6 inches) straight ahead from the first mark and mark this point. Measure from 5 cm (2 inches) below the axilla to the second mark. This measurement is the approximate crutch length.

If the patient has to be measured while lying down, measure from the anterior fold of the axilla to the sole of the foot, and then add 5 cm (2 inches). Another method is to determine the height of the patient and subtract 40 cm (16 inches).

The hand piece should allow 20 to 30 degrees of flexion at the elbow. The wrist should be extended and the hand dorsiflexed. The patient should wear shoes that fit well and have firm soles. The crutches should be fitted with large rubber suction tips before measuring.

The maintenance of an erect posture is essential to crutch walking. Before trying to use crutches, the patient should learn to stand by a chair on the unaffected leg in order to achieve balance. The nurse explains and demonstrates to the patient how he should manipulate his crutches before he attempts to do so.

Crutch Stance.   The *tripod position* is the basic crutch stance. The crutches rest approximately 20 cm to 25 cm (8–10 inches) in front and to the side of the patient's toes. This gives the strongest and most balanced support. Since, to provide stability, a greater height requires a broader base, a taller patient needs a wider base and a shorter patient a narrower base.

The patient must be taught to support his weight on the hand piece (Fig. 14-7). If the weight is borne on the axilla, the pressure of the crutch can damage the brachial plexus nerves and produce "crutch paralysis." A foam-rubber pad on the underarm piece will relieve pressure on the upper arm and the thoracic cage.

Ability to shift body weight is the next step. The crutch gait selected depends on the nature of the patient's disability. The nurse must know how much (if any) weight can

be placed on the affected side and whether the crutches are being used for balance and support.

Crutch Gaits.   The selection of the crutch gait depends on the type and severity of the disability and on the patient's physical condition, arm and trunk strength, and body balance. The patient should be taught two gaits so that he may change from one to another. Shifting crutch gaits relieves fatigue since each gait requires the use of a different combination of muscles. (If a muscle is forced to contract steadily without relaxing, the circulation of the blood to the part is reduced.) A faster gait can be used for making speed, whereas a slower one is used in crowded places.

All gaits begin in the tripod position. The more common gaits are the 4-point, the 2-point, the 3-point, and the swinging-to and swinging-through gaits. The sequence of movements for each of these gaits is listed in Chart 14-6.

The patient should not practice crutch walking for too long, especially if he has been in bed for a prolonged period. Such signs as sweating or shortness of breath should

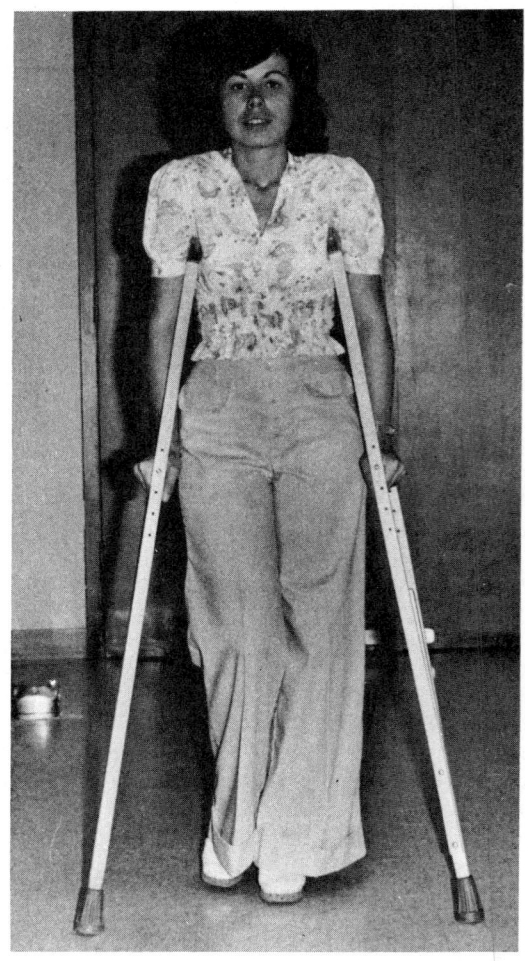

Figure 14-7.   The tripod position for the basic crutch stance. Note that the patient's weight is borne not in the axilla but on the palm of the hand. (Courtesy, National Orthopedic and Rehabilitation Hospital.)

Chart 14-6
Gaits for Crutch Walking

4-point Gait
This gait can be used when supported weight bearing is permitted for both legs. It is safe and gives maximal balance because there are always three points of contact with the floor; thus, it is slow because it requires constant shifting of weight.
Sequence
1. Right crutch
2. Left foot
3. Left crutch
4. Right foot

2-point Gait
This gait is faster since there are only two points of contact with the floor at one time.
Sequence
1. Advance right crutch and left foot.
2. Simultaneously shift weight and advance left crutch and right foot.

3-point Gait
This is a faster gait but requires more strength and balance. The patient must be able to support his entire body weight on his arms.
Sequence
1. Advance the weaker leg and both crutches simultaneously.
2. While putting most of the body weight on the crutches, advance the stronger lower extremity.

Swing-Crutch Gaits

Swing-To Gait
Sequence
1. Bear weight on good leg.
2. Advance both crutches forward simultaneously.
3. While leaning forward, swing the body to a position that is even with the crutches.

Swing-Through Gait
Sequence
1. Advance both crutches forward.
2. Lift both legs off ground and swing forward, landing in advance of the crutches.
3. Bring crutches forward again, rapidly, to prevent being caught off balance.

---

be indications that the lesson on crutches should be stopped and the patient permitted to rest or go back to bed.

Other Crutch-Maneuvering Techniques. Before a patient is sent home on crutches, it is important to ascertain whether or not he can dress himself and whether or not he can get in and out of chairs, on and off the toilet, in and out of doors, up and down stairs and ramps, and in and out of a car, taxi, or public conveyance.

The following procedures should be taught to the patient.

To Sit in a Chair
1. Grasp the crutches at the hand pieces for control.
2. Bend forward slightly while assuming a sitting position.

To Stand Up
1. Move forward to the edge of the chair with the strong leg slightly under the seat.
2. Place both crutches in the hand on the side of the affected extremity.
3. Push down on the hand piece while raising the body to a standing position.

To Go Down Stairs
1. Walk forward as far as possible on the step.
2. Advance crutches to the lower step. The weaker leg is advanced first and then the stronger one. In this way, the stronger extremity shares the work of raising and lowering the body weight with the patient's arms.

To Go Up Stairs
1. Advance the stronger leg first up to the next step.
2. Then advance the crutches and the weaker extremity. (Strong leg goes up first and comes down last.) A memory device for the patient is "up with the good; down with the bad."

Ambulation With a Cane

A cane is used to help the patient walk with greater balance and support and with less fatigue. It also relieves the pressure on weight-bearing joints and prevents undue pressure and use of the unaffected extremity. To fit the patient for a cane, have him flex his elbow at a 30-degree angle and hold the cane 15 cm (6 inches) lateral to the base of his fifth toe. Adjust the cane so that the handle is approximately level with the greater trochanter. An adjustable aluminum cane fitted with a gently flaring tip that has flexible and concentric rings gives optimum stability, functions as a shock absorber, and enables the patient to walk with greater speed and less fatigue.

Cane–Foot Sequence
1. Hold the cane in the hand opposite to the affected extremity (*i.e.,* the cane should be used on the good side).
2. Advance the cane at the same time the affected leg is moved forward.
3. Keep the cane fairly close to the body to prevent leaning, and bear down on the cane when the unaffected extremity begins the swing phase.
4. If for some reason the patient is unable to use the cane in the opposite hand, the cane may be carried on the same side and advanced when the affected leg is advanced.

To Go Up and Down Stairs Using the Cane–Foot Sequence
1. Step up on the unaffected extremity.
2. Then place the cane and affected extremity up on the step.

3. Reverse this procedure for descending steps. (Strong leg goes up first and comes down last).

Assisting With Prosthetic and Orthotic Appliances

A *prosthesis* is an artificial replacement for a missing portion of the body. An *orthosis* (commonly known as a brace) is an orthopedic device or appliance used to provide support and alignment, prevent or correct deformities, and improve the function of the body. The field of orthotics has enlarged to include equipment such as wheelchairs and environmental-control systems (devices and systems to improve the quality of life for the severely disabled). A prosthetist or an orthotist fits these appliances only by prescription of the physician.*

Nursing Interventions

The nurse performs an essential function in the prosthetic phase of the patient's care by helping him to develop an attitude of realistic hopefulness and by preventing deformities, so that the time between the healing of the tissues and the fitting of the prosthesis is kept to a minimum. In the amputation of an extremity, the physical therapist (or the nurse) is responsible for bandaging the stump correctly, so that proper shrinkage and shaping of the stump occurs and the patient can be fitted more effectively with a prosthesis (see p. 1450).

Support and Health Education of the Patient Using Braces

A *brace* is a support that protects weakened muscles; prevents and corrects deformities; immobilizes and protects a diseased or injured joint; protects painful, inflamed, or healing tissue; aids in the control of involuntary muscle movements; improves function; and relieves pain. Thus, braces are supportive, corrective, and protective as well as dynamic (with springs, cables, and elastic bands) and preventive.

Clinical indications for bracing include pain, weakness, or paralysis of a part of the body. The patient is fitted for a brace according to the prescription of the physician. In recent years, synthetics, particularly thermoplastics, have been used in braces. They are functional, lighter, and more cosmetically acceptable to the patient. Velcro straps are also gaining increasing usage.

In caring for a patient wearing a brace, the nurse has the major responsibility of encouraging him to continue under the supervision of a competent therapist or orthotist until he can wear the appliance with ease. This requires time, training, and adjustment. It is also important to encourage the patient to wear the brace as directed and to

---

* Specific prostheses are described later in this book, when the clinical conditions calling for them are discussed (*e.g.,* extremity prostheses for the amputee and a breast prosthesis for the patient who has had a radical mastectomy). Information concerning prosthetic and orthopedic appliances may be obtained also from The American Orthotic and Prosthetic Association, 1440 N Street, N.W., Washington, D.C. 20005.

check to see that it is not applied too tightly and that no skin problems or pressure sores are developing from the brace.

The following are the main points to emphasize in teaching the patient to care for his brace:

1. Place the brace on a table or the floor, or prop it against the wall when it is not in use; hanging may cause distortion of its position.
2. Twisting of the brace may occur with use; check alignment frequently. Look down the full length of the brace. The joints should coincide with the body joints.
3. Before putting a brace on, check carefully for worn areas, missing or loose screws, and the condition of straps and buckles.
4. Pressure areas may occur if metal or plastic rubs the skin. Check the skin for reddened areas immediately after removing the brace.
5. Keep the heels and soles of the shoes in good condition.
6. Clean and dry the brace, when necessary, at night.
7. To clean the plastic parts:
   a. Wipe the plastic parts with a damp cloth.
   b. Do not oil plastic surfaces and joints.
8. To clean the metal parts:
   a. Remove rust or corrosion spots with steel wool.
   b. Clean dirt out of metal joints and locks with a pipe cleaner dipped in a solvent.
   c. Clean the metal parts with a solvent.
   d. Apply a light coat of paste wax to the metal parts to prevent rust.
   e. Put oil in metal joints with an eyedropper or toothpick.
9. Have the brace checked periodically.

Coping With Fatigue

Because it is uncomfortable and tiring to live with a physical handicap, the disabled are vulnerable to fatigue. Physical disabilities have to be faced daily, and frustration brings weariness to mind and body. The fear of falling may be always present, and mobility often remains a minute-by-minute challenge fraught with difficulties. Walking with crutches or braces requires a high expenditure of energy.

The following may be useful in teaching patients how to reduce their energy output, thus conserving their strength to achieve a meaningful life-style.

1. Have well-defined goals and priorities.
   - Keep priorities in order; eliminate nonessential activities.
   - Plan and pace your activities.
     Plan each day.
     Distribute heavy work load throughout week.
     Organize work; have equipment within easy reach.
     Keep work in front of you.
   - Rest before undertaking difficult tasks.
   - Stop before fatigue sets in.
   - Continue with exercise conditioning program to strengthen muscles.

2. Control your environment.
   - Become well organized.
   - Place possessions in same place, so that they can be found with minimum of effort.
   - Place equipment in box/basket (personal care, crafts, work).
   - Use energy conservation and work-simplification techniques.
   - Use adaptive equipment, self-help aids, labor-saving devices.
   - Take safety precautions.
3. Take control of your life.
   - Face the reality of your disability.
   - Emphasize areas of strength.
   - Remain outward looking.
   - Seek inventive ways to tackle problems.
   - Maintain and improve general health.
   - Plan for recreation.

Helping to Overcome Elimination Problems

Urinary and bowel incontinence are frequent problems in the disabled patient. Bladder and bowel control are important functions of the body and are influenced by prescribed social behavior. Incontinence may curtail a person's independence and limit his sense of social acceptance. Patients with various medical and surgical conditions have to be trained to regain control of these functions.

Bladder Training

Incontinence should not be regarded as inevitable in any patient, since bladder training is an available alternative in most instances. This facet of care (bladder training) is a part of nursing function.

True incontinence may be caused by obvious urologic problems or by congenital or acquired neurologic disease. Neurologic incontinence and its management are discussed on pages 975 to 976.

For patients with incontinence from other causes, the key to successful urinary control is:

- Sufficient fluid intake (2500 ml daily)
- Establishment of regular times to void (*i.e.,* a habit pattern)

A schedule is set up with definite times indicated for the patient to try to empty his bladder using either the toilet or commode when possible. The interval between voidings in the early phase of the training period is fairly short (1½ to 2 hours), but as the patient's bladder capacity increases, the interval is lengthened. A suggested procedure is to give a measured amount of fluid every 2 hours. After drinking, the patient waits for 30 minutes and then attempts to void. He gradually lengthens the period between voiding times. (It is best to give larger amounts of fluid during the day and to withhold fluids after 5 PM.)

The patient is encouraged to hold his urine until the specified voiding time. Usually, there is a relationship between drinking, eating, exercising, and voiding, and the alert patient soon can determine his own intake schedule.

Have the patient keep a written voiding schedule, which will give a continuous record of the time and amounts of fluid ingested and the time and amount of each voiding. Regularity is the key to success. To assist in the act of voiding, the patient should either stand or sit with the thighs flexed and the feet and the back supported. Increasing intra-abdominal pressure by massage over the bladder or by leaning forward while sitting will help to initiate evacuation of the bladder.

For the confused elderly patient, watch and determine when he is incontinent, and take him to the bathroom before involuntary voiding occurs. Create an environment that keeps sensory monotony to a minimum. Orient the patient to time and place. Extend his social environment beyond the confines of his room and try to increase the number of his social contacts. An alarm clock may be set at regular intervals throughout the day and several times during the night to remind the patient to void. The patient must approve of the program and have a sincere desire to establish control. It may take several weeks to accomplish this end; patience and persistence on the part of both nurse and patient plus expressions of approval for even slight gains are necessary. It is also important to encourage the patient to continue with self-care and the exercise and occupational therapy programs—boredom and frustration can lead to incontinence. Encourage the patient to make decisions and do meaningful tasks. Have the patient wear his own clothing, since this enhances his self-esteem and dignity and is a strong deterrent to regressive behavior. The use of a diaper at any time is discouraged, because its psychological effect is one of regression rather than progression.

Bowel Training

The objectives of a bowel training program are to develop regular bowel habits and to prevent fecal incontinence, impaction, and irregularity.

- The first essential step in bowel training that requires reflex assistance is the establishment of regularity, a specific and definite time for bowel evacuation.

Any attempts at evacuation should be made within 15 minutes of the same time daily. An active aid to bowel evacuation is the stimulation of peristalsis and the gastrocolic and duodenocolic reflexes. Therefore, the patient should establish his bowel evacuation time after a regularly scheduled meal. One of the best times is after breakfast. However, if the patient has a previously established habit pattern, it should be followed.

Physical activity is another helpful aid to peristaltic activity and bowel movement. Unless contraindicated by other existing conditions, the diet should include adequate intake of fiber (vegetables, fruit, bran, cereals) to prevent hard stools and stimulate peristalsis, and a fluid intake between 2 liters and 4 liters (2.1–4.2 quarts) daily. Prune juice or fig juice (120 ml) taken 30 minutes before a meal once daily is helpful when constipation is a problem.

The reflex habit should be established by regularity early in the course of the patient's illness. It may be aided by mechanical means. About 30 minutes before the scheduled bowel time, a glycerin suppository is inserted into the rectum in order to stimulate the anorectal reflex. After the scheduled interval, the patient is encouraged to attempt to have a bowel movement. If at all possible, he should assume the normal position for defecation. Instruct him to bear down and to contract his abdominal muscles. If need be, he can lean forward to increase intra-abdominal pressure. The patient may be taught to apply pressure to the abdominal wall to assist with defecation.

After this routine is well established, mechanical stimulation with the suppository probably will not be necessary, and in a few weeks the patient will be having regular daily bowel movements.

▷ Promoting Continuity of Patient Care

The objective of a referral system is to maintain continuity of care when the patient is transferred from the health care facility to his home or an extended care facility. It is ideal to begin formulating a plan for discharge when the patient is first admitted to the hospital. The patient's functional potential is estimated by the rehabilitation team, and discharge plans are made with this in mind.

Frequently, the community health nurse is the case finder whose astute observations make the rehabilitation services possible for the patient. By visiting the patient in the hospital, the community health nurse is able to see what adjustments will have to be made in the home. It may be necessary to help the family select, improvise, or borrow needed equipment from another agency. Plan with the patient ways and methods of coping with problems that may arise. Prior to discharge, the patient may experience "separation anxiety" as he realizes that he is leaving the protected environment of the hospital. Give him increased support and encouragement to ease him through this phase.

The patient's support system (family, friends) is assessed and every effort is made for successful home placement. The family will need to know as much about the patient's condition and care as possible so that they will not fear his return home. Their attitude toward the patient, his disability, and his return home, should be assessed. After the patient comes home, the community health nurse makes sure that he does not "lose ground" and that he is able to maintain the independence that he gained in the hospital.

Not all families can be expected to carry on the arduous programs of exercise and physical training that a patient may need or have the resources or stability to care for a severely disabled member. Even a stable family may be overwhelmed by the physical, emotional, economic, and energy drains of disabling disease. The family may require family therapy to allow them to discuss and explore their feelings and attitudes (rejection, aversion, avoidance) toward the disabled family member.

The ADL Sheet is sent home with the patient so that the community nurse knows exactly what activities the patient can perform. The nurse continues to reinforce the teaching that has been done and helps the patient to achieve attainable goals. The degree to which he adapts to his home and community environment depends on the confidence and self-esteem developed during his rehabilitation program and on the acceptance and reactions of his family, employer, and community members.

There is a growing trend toward independent living by severely disabled people. Skill training in attendant management, financial management, and mobility skills may be necessary for the severely disabled person to achieve personal self-determination. The U.S. Department of Housing and Urban Development has a new office of Independent Living with a concern for special housing.

If the patient is transferred to an extended care facility, his ADL Sheet goes with him to orient the staff to activities that he can perform independently. The staff continue to encourage the family to visit, to be involved, and to take the patient home on weekends and holidays if possible.

The Rehabilitation Services Administration provides services whereby disabled persons or those disadvantaged by advanced age or other conditions obtain the help they need to engage in gainful employment. These services are provided by state agencies and include diagnostic, medical, surgical, psychiatric, and hospital services, and assistance in securing prosthetic appliances. There is a counseling, training, placement, and follow-up service available to help the patient to select and attain a vocational objective.

A selected list of agencies and organizations, both governmental and voluntary, that work with or for patients needing rehabilitation services is listed in the *Directory of National Information Sources on Handicapping Conditions and Related Services,* which can be obtained from the Superintendent of Documents, Government Printing Office, Washington, D.C. 20402. This directory contains abstracts and addresses of organizations and federal agencies offering services, information, and resources to handicapped individuals.

▷ Bibliography

Books

Abreu BC. Physical Disabilities Manual. New York, Raven Press, 1981.

Barton A and Barton M. The Management and Prevention of Pressure Sores. Boston, Faber and Faber, 1981.

Basmajian JV. Therapeutic Exercise, 3rd ed. Baltimore, Williams & Wilkins, 1980.

Bishop DS (ed). Behavioral Problems and the Disabled. Baltimore, Williams & Wilkins, 1980.

Boller F and Frank E. Sexual Dysfunction in Neurological Disorders. New York, Raven Press, 1982.

Bolton B and Cook DW. Rehabilitation Client Assessment. Baltimore, University Park Press, 1980.

Bowe F. Comeback. (Six Remarkable People Who Triumphed Over Disability). New York, Harper & Row, 1981.

Bower FL and Brown MS (eds). Nursing and the Concept of Loss. New York, John Wiley & Sons, 1980.

Bullard DG and Knight SE (eds). Sexuality and Physical Disability. St Louis, CV Mosby, 1981.

Constantian MB. Pressure Ulcers. Boston, Little, Brown & Co, 1980.

Eisenberg M, Griggins C, and Duval RJ. Disabled People as Second-class Citizens. New York, Springer, 1982.

Hogan R. Human Sexuality. A Nursing Perspective. New York, Appleton–Century–Crofts, 1980.

Horsley JA et al. Preventing Decubitus Ulcers. New York, Grune & Stratton, 1981.

Ince LP (ed). Behavioral Psychology in Rehabilitation Medicine: Clinical Applications. Baltimore, Williams & Wilkins, 1980.

Johnson WR and Kempton W. Sex Education and Counseling of Special Groups. Springfield, Charles C Thomas, 1981.

Kimball CP. The Biopsychosocial Approach to the Patient. Baltimore, Williams & Wilkins, 1981.

Lindemann JE. Psychological and Behavioral Aspects of Physical Disability: A Manual for Health Practitioners. New York, Plenum Press, 1981.

Lion EM. Human Sexuality in Nursing Process. New York, John Wiley & Sons, 1982.

Logigian MK (ed). Adult Rehabilitation: A Team Approach for Therapists. Boston, Little, Brown & Co, 1982.

Nursing Photobook. Providing Early Mobility. Horsham, Intermed Communications, 1980.

Palmer ML and Toms JE. Manual for Functional Training. Philadelphia, FA Davis, 1980.

Power PW and Dell Orto AE. Role of the Family in the Rehabilitation of the Physically Disabled. Baltimore, University Park Press, 1980.

Redford JB. Orthotics Etcetera, 2nd ed. Baltimore, Williams & Wilkins, 1980.

Rosenbaum EH and Rosenbaum I. Going Home: A Home-care Training Program. Palo Alto, Bull Pub Co, 1980.

Seligman G. Group Psychotherapy and Counseling with Special Populations. Baltimore, University Park Press, 1982.

Sha'ked A. Human Sexuality in Rehabilitation Medicine. Baltimore, Williams & Wilkins, 1981.

Simpson JEP and Levitt R. Going Home. New York, Churchill Livingstone, 1981.

Sine RD et al. Basic Rehabilitation Techniques, 2nd ed. Rockville, Aspen Systems Corp, 1981.

Turner A (ed). The Practice of Occupational Therapy. New York, Churchill Livingstone, 1981.

Van Etten G, Arkell C, and Van Etten C. The Severely and Profoundly Handicapped. St Louis, CV Mosby, 1980.

von Eschenbach AC and Rodriguez DB. Sexual Rehabilitation of the Urologic Cancer Patient. Boston, GK Hall, 1981.

Washburn KB. Physical Medicine and Rehabilitation: Essentials of Primary Care, 2nd ed. Garden City, Medical Examination Publishing, 1981.

Wright GN. Total Rehabilitation. Boston, Little, Brown & Co, 1980.

Articles
Pressure Sores

Antypas PG. Management of pressure sores. Curr Probl Surg 1980 Apr; 17(4):229–244.

Baek SM et al. The gluteus maximus myocutaneous flap in the management of pressure sores. Ann Plast Surg 1980 Dec; 5(6):471–476.

Daltrey DC, Rhodes B, and Chattwood JG. Investigation into the microbial flora of healing and non-healing decubitus ulcers. J Clin Pathol 1981 July; 34(7):701–705.

Elliott TM. Pressure ulceration. Am Fam Physician 1982 Feb; 25(2):171–180.

Eltora I. Hyperbaric oxygen in the management of pressure sores in patients with injuries to the spinal cord. J Dermatol Surg Oncol 1981 Sept; 7(9):737–740.

Feustel DE. Pressure sore prevention. Nursing '82 1982 Apr; 12(4):78–83.

Gerber RM and Van Ort SR. Topical application of insulin to pressure sores: A questionable therapy. Am J Nurs 1981 June; 81(6):1159.

Judd CO. Selected topical agents in the treatment of pressure sores. Can Nurse 1981 July–Aug; 77(7):32–33.

Kerr JC, Stinson SM, and Shannon ML. Pressure sores: Distinguishing fact from fiction. Can Nurse 1981 July–Aug; 77(3):23–28.

Klein RM and Fowler RS. Pressure relief training device: The microcalculator. Arch Phys Med Rehabil 1981 Oct; 62(10):500–501.

Kucan JO et al. Comparison of silver sulfadiazine, povidone-iodine and physiologic saline in the treatment of chronic pressure sores. J Am Geriatr Soc 1981 May; 29(5):232–235.

Morley M. 16 steps to better decubitus ulcer care. Can Nurse 1981 July–Aug; 77(3):29–33.

Newman P and Davis NH. Thermography as a predictor of sacral pressure sores. Age Ageing 1981 Feb; 10(1):14–18.

Parish LC and Witkowski JA. The use of Dextranomer in decubitus ulcers: A histopathologic evaluation. Int J Dermatol 1981 Jan–Feb; 20(1):62–64.

Revler JB and Cooney TG. The pressure sore: Pathophysiology and principles of management. Ann Intern Med 1981 May; 94(5):661–666.

Torrance C. Pressure sores. 4. Mechanical devices. Nurs Times 1981 Apr 16; 77(16 Suppl):13–16.

Torrance C. Pressure sores. 5. Topical applications and wound agents. Nurs Times 1981 May 7; 77(19 Suppl):17–20.

Torrance C. Pressure sores. 6. Physical methods. Nurs Times 1981 June 17–23; 77(25 Suppl):21–24.

Principles and Philosophy of Rehabilitation

Alexy WD. Coping with loss: The principal theme postulate. Rehabil Lit 1980 Mar–Apr; 41(3–4):66–71.

Allen SR and Moschak V. Step by step. Nursing '81 1981 Aug; 11(8):56–57.

Basmajian JV. Biofeedback in rehabilitation: A review of principles. Arch Phys Med Rehabil 1981 Oct; 62(10):469–475.

Fisher SV and Patterson RP. Energy cost of ambulation with crutches. Arch Phys Med Rehabil 1981 June; 62(6):250–256.

Patterson R and Fisher SV. Cardiovascular stress of crutch walking. Arch Phys Med Rehabil 1981 June; 62(6):257–260.

Poole J and Parkinson M. Bilateral shoulder disarticulation: Equipment used to facilitate independence. Am J Occup Ther 1980 June; 34(6):397–399.

Rothberg JS. The rehabilitation team: Future direction. Arch Phys Med Rehabil 1981 Aug; 62(8):407–410.

Smidt GL and Mommens MA. System of reporting and comparing influence of ambulatory aids on gait. Phys Ther 1980 May; 60(5):551–558.

Versluys HP. Physical rehabilitation and family dynamics. Rehabil Lit 1980 Mar–Apr; 41(3–4):58–65.

Ziegler JC. Physical reconditioning—for the convalescent patient. Nursing '80 1980 Aug; 10(8):67–69.

Zola IK. Communication barriers between the "able-bodied" and "the handicapped." Arch Phys Med Rehabil 1981 Aug; 62(8):355–359.

Sexuality and Rehabilitation

Chigier E. Sexuality of physically disabled people. Clin Obstet Gynaecol 1980 Aug; 7(2):325–343.

Greengross W. Sex and physical disability. Br J Med 1981 Oct 24; 283(6299):1089.

Miller S, Szasz G, and Anderson L. Sexual health care clinician in an acute spinal cord injury unit. Arch Phys Med Rehabil 1981 July; 62(7):315–320.

Health Care of the Older Adult

Geriatrics, the care of the aged, is currently receiving specific emphasis in the nursing curriculum. This specialty has as its prime concern the health and the well-being of a large and important segment of the patient population, and it deals with problems of therapy and rehabilitation that are inherently and uniquely complex. Thus, the whole field of *gerontology,* the study of the aging process and its effects on older persons, becomes more important with each passing day.

Aging is a normal process of time-related change that occurs throughout life. It involves all aspects of the organism and is largely characterized by a decline in functional efficiency and decreased capacity to compensate and recover from stress. It does not necessarily occur in an interrelated or synchronous manner, but it does involve physiologic, psychological, and social changes that interact to influence behavior and adaptation. Old age is a normal part of human development and is the final phase of the life cycle. Aging is not something that happens to the other person but is a unique and highly personal experience that affects everyone who lives long enough. Successful adaptation to the aging process probably correlates with the person's previous ability to cope and adapt to change. Other influences include environmental factors, education, and sociocultural determinants as well as the health status of the entire body.

In the past, society tended to shrug off the problems of the aged, possibly because the signs of aging are visible and may stimulate anxiety in younger persons concerning their own mortality. Also, there has been some reluctance to invest too much time and effort in the aged because they are at the end of their life span. However, as the debilitating effects of disease, disability, and various social problems are reduced and eliminated, it becomes a challenge to visualize those normal developmental processes that continue into old age: creativity, life experience, perspective, and judgment.

As a result of current research and observation, new concepts have developed with respect to the quantity and quality of human life. The current generation is described as the generation of the "active elderly." Scientific progress points to projections of greater life expectancies and to a vastly improved quality of life in the years to come. This *quality* of a person's life should be the special concern of those in the helping professions: physicians, psychiatrists, psychologists, social workers, clergymen, and nurses.

▷ Developmental Theories and Themes of Aging

Certain theoretical models of human development help to point out important turning points during the late years of the life cycle. The theories concerning the life cycle incorporate the social, psychological, and biological factors of developmental growth and relate them to age to identify milestones and time development.

The theories of Buhler, Jung, and Erikson, which are considered to be three of the most prominent theories of adult development, have as a common theme the goal of personal resolution in the second half of life.

Buhler's theories were based on a collection of 400 biographies and autobiographies collected in the 1930s in Vienna; Buhler developed a methodology for analyzing these biographies to reveal an orderly progression of phases based on changes in events, attitudes, and accomplishments during the life cycle.

Buhler perceived the period between 45 and 65 as the period of self-assessment of the results of striving for goals determined in early life stages. The period from 65 on is one of awareness of the experience of fulfillment or failure, and the remaining years are spent in either a continuance of previous activities or a return to the need-satisfying orientations of childhood. The conclusion from Buhler's studies is that the individual's assessment of whether he did or did not reach fulfillment was a more critical factor in how well he adjusted to old age than biological decline and insecurity. A person's own sense of having realized his goals and reached a sense of fulfillment may be the crucial final result of lifelong goal setting and striving.

Jung saw no clear sense of meaning or purpose in old age in our society. He stated that although many people reach old age with unsatisfied demands, it is "fatal" for such persons to look back. It is essential that they have a goal in the future, in order to live the second half of life with as much purpose as the first. Jung suggested that in the second half of life the individual direct his attention inward, so that through an intensive inner exploration he may find a meaning and totality in life that makes the acceptance of death possible.

Erikson developed the concept of the eight ages of man, each representing crucial turning points in the life span that stretches from birth to death. Erikson's theory was more fully explored by Peck in an attempt to define more precisely the crucial issues of middle age and old age. According to this expanded theory, the years between 40 and 50 challenge those values that a person places on physical power in favor of the values placed on wisdom. People who cling to their waning physical powers become more and more depressed, but persons who shift to using their mental

abilities as a primary resource appear to age more successfully. At this point in their lives, if men and women redefine themselves as individuals and companions, with less stress on the sexual element, then interpersonal relationships may take on a greater depth of understanding and enhance their marital union. People in their 40s must make a shift in emotional openness. They must reach out to possible friends to supplant the loss of children leaving home, parents dying, or old friends leaving or dying.

As people move along the life span toward old age, there are three central issues to challenge them. First, to develop varied interests so that when they retire or when their children leave home they can engage in meaningful activities that offer a sense of satisfaction. Older people also need to find comfort in human relations to transcend the illness and pain of their fragile bodies. Finally, the old person must be able to find a gratifying meaning for life in the future potential of his family, his ideas, his creations, or future generations in general.

The theorists view the first part of life as growth and expansion, and the latter part of life as inner withdrawal and contraction. The tasks of later life involve finding meaning and wholeness in life and considerations about oncoming death. It appears that a person's own sense of having realized, or not having realized, chosen goals will be more critical in determining how successfully he adapts to aging than biological decline and personal insecurity. (See also Chap. 11.)

Kinds of Aging
Biological Aging. Aging occurs with such changes as whitening of the hair, wrinkling of the skin, and decline in eye focus and high-register hearing. The most serious change for most people is their heightened vulnerability to and lessened ability to recuperate from various illnesses. Biological aging, for each individual, depends on a combination of factors, including genetic inheritance, finances, and good health. However, biological aging is secondary to other problems in its impact on most people.

Psychological Aging. Psychological aging refers to a role that the individual assigns to himself as he reaches a certain chronological age. The two major threats felt by the older person are the deterioration of his concept of self, which results in loss of self-esteem, and extensive and continual grief over frequently occurring losses. People spend their lives attempting to enhance their self-concepts while simultaneously attempting to deter actions by themselves and others that would erode this concept.

The plight of the aged in a youth-oriented society continues to receive attention, and the process of gerontological counseling is now recognized as a specialized form of helping. Individually designed adaptive responses are the helping person's most effective tools.

Older persons are not (as stereotyping would lead us to believe) incapable, inactive, and deficient in intellect and sexual function. They do not spend their time complaining, reminiscing, talking of illnesses, and attending funerals.

The older person should be encouraged to see himself as in a dynamic period of growth rather than in a period of rapid deterioration. Perceiving self with an ongoing, con-

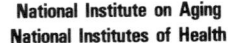

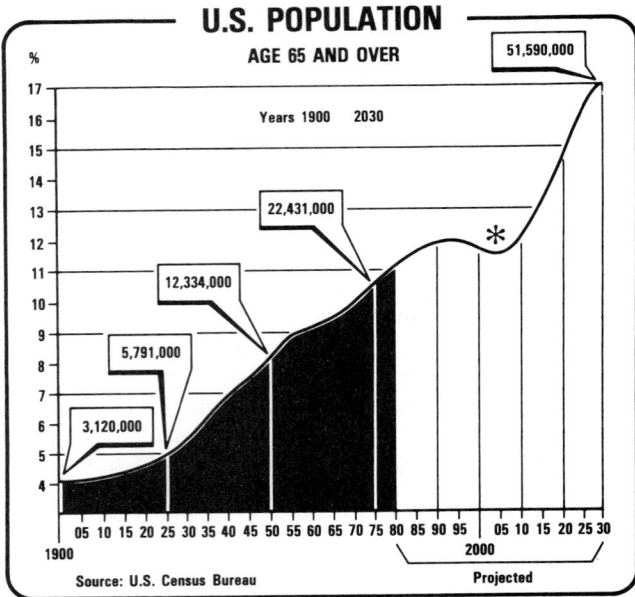

* Decrease due to lowered birth rate during depression of 1930's.

Figure 15-1. Age gauge—chart shows the percentage of the American population 65 and older from 1900; with predictions for 1980 to 2030. (From National Institute on Aging, National Institutes of Health.)

tinuous potential permits the older person to reflect, not ruminate, on the past while continuing to cultivate a hopeful vision for the future.

The sense of psychological loss intensifies as the older person ages and vitality decreases, while vulnerability increases. Many older people become enraged at the helplessness they feel in the face of seemingly uncontrollable events, including the apparent attempts of other people to crush their individuality.

The older person, for the most part, wishes to be treated as a person of worth and dignity. He does not wish to be tolerated, indulged, patronized, or perceived as a pet. People working with and caring for the elderly should not consider them "cute little old ladies" or "dear little old men." Listening attentively, focusing the patients' attention on the here and now, and discussing with them their plans for the future will underscore the feeling that they are being related to as people, each unique and distinct from the other.

Sociogenic Aging. Society imposes roles on people as they reach a certain chronological age. Older persons are seen by many people in our society as either *nonpeople* or *expendable people,* merely because they have lived longer. One of the major difficulties for older people is that their perceptions of themselves reflect the way society has viewed them and the manner in which they themselves have internalized these roles.

A significant amount of current research indicates that a large proportion of mental and attitudinal changes in old

people do not arise from biological effects but rather from societal prescribed role definitions. Older people have been told by our society that they are supposed to be physically, socially, sexually, and intellectually infirm—slow in comprehending events going on around them and rigid in their ways of thinking and behaving.

Our society devalues people once they leave the ranks of the "employed." Yet society automatically retires a worker at the magical age of 70 years. Because educational institutions historically have prepared people to fill work-oriented roles, society tends to classify the elderly as "nonpeople" when they reach retirement. Society also seems to take the attitude that older people should run away and hide until they die. It is important to note that the combination of psychological and sociogenic aging causes more debilitation than biological aging for many people.

▷ Profile of the Aging American

The age "65" generally is thought of as the beginning of old age, but this figure has been rather arbitrarily selected for social (retirement) and legislative (Social Security) purposes. Some specialists in the field of gerontology refer to the "young old" as those in the 65 to 74 age group, while the term "old old" is reserved for those over 75.

At present, over 11% of the population in the United States is over 65 years of age, and demographic projections suggest that the elderly may constitute about 13% to 21% of the population by the year 2030 (Fig. 15-1). People over age 65 are the fastest growing age group in this country and their numbers are expected to continue growing into the 21st century at a faster pace than the rest of the population. The projected life span average from birth for the female is 75.3 years and for the male, 67.6 years. Each day there is a net increase of more than 1400 persons of age 65 and over, and the number of older persons in the United States is already larger than the population of 22 states. The older a person is, the greater the probability of his living longer. The forces producing this phenomenon include medical advances that have reduced maternal and infant mortality and have enabled more people to live to old age.

The elderly population has become older. An analysis of the statistics reveals that those over 75 are the fastest growing segment of the senior citizen group. Although the numbers of people 60 years old and over have increased nearly 7 times since 1900, the 75-and-over age group has experienced a tenfold increase, and the 85-plus group has grown by about 17 times.

There are more older women among elderly people in general owing to the longer life span of women. Most women are usually younger than their husbands and often outlive them by several years. Widows constitute 23% of women 60 to 64 years of age, whereas among those 70 to 75 years and older, the figure jumps to 70%. Most elderly widows live alone, one fourth of their number subsisting on incomes below the federal government's poverty index.

Medical advances also have made an impact on blacks and other nonwhite races. Life expectancy in these groups has nearly doubled. The nonwhite elderly population is expected to grow about 300% by 2035, thereby increasing this proportion of the elderly population from one tenth to one sixth.

The popular picture of old people as frail, institutionalized beings is grossly misleading. Over 95% of older Americans live in the normal community, not in institutions, and an increasing number of these elderly people live alone. According to the latest statistics, the proportion of those living alone has increased from one sixth of all non-institutionalized elderly persons in 1960 to one fourth. Again, this trend is most noticeable among elderly women and has resulted mainly because of the increased number of widows and the availability of greater financial security (supplemental Social Security income) and more and better coverage under private pension plans and health care support programs (Medicare).

Impact and Implications for Health Care

Persons in the 75-year-old and older group require additional resources to handle some of the unique physical and emotional problems that occur more frequently in this age group as a result of chronic disease and impairment. Members of the "old-old" group have more problems than do the "young old." Persons 75 and older spend an average of four and a half times as many days in short-stay hospitals as the national average and 70% more than persons who are 65 to 74 years of age. Three fourths of all nursing home residents are 75 or older and over one third are 85 and older. Thus, there is greater demand for health practitioners, facilities, and supportive services for those over 75.

The social and economic backgrounds of many members of the "old-old" group differ from those of elderly citizens in the "young-old" group. Many were immigrants who had little formal education and worked throughout their lives for relatively low salaries. In the future, more older persons will have been born in this country, will be much better educated, will have worked at higher paying occupations, and will benefit from a variety of economic and retirement plans. And they will be more accustomed to regarding social services and supports as rights. The changing needs of the nation's population will have a definite impact on the health care professions.

Economic Factors Affecting Older People

Level of income undoubtedly affects quality of living as well as health. Currently, 1 of every 13 couples in which the husband is over 65 receives an income of less than $5000. At the other end of the income scale, one of every three elderly couples has an income of $15,000 or more. However, the income of elderly persons living alone or with nonrelatives falls toward the lower income scale. About 15% of persons over 65 have incomes below the poverty level. Among elderly whites, one of every eight (13%) is poor, but about one third of elderly blacks and elderly persons of other races are considered poor.

Thus, the older members of the population are essentially part of a low-income group, primarily because of fixed income and inflation. Most older people are not sharing in the increasing standard of living made possible by the economy that they helped to build. In part, compulsory retirement plans prevent most old people from working regularly, and when they do work they earn less than younger people. Older consumers spend proportionately more of their incomes on food, housing, household operation, and health care than their younger counterparts. They spend proportionately less than younger persons on transportation, clothing, household furnishings, and recreation. It is not that they need so much less; they simply cannot afford a better standard of living.

Health care costs are a large item in the budgets of elderly people. Not only do their health care needs increase just as their incomes are reduced by retirement, but also their needs change, for they now require long-term care as a result of the prevalence of chronic conditions, diseases, and impairments. Currently, the health care costs of the elderly account for over 30% of the nation's spending for health services.

Current population trends, marked by an increasing number of older people, call for major adjustments in our socioeconomic planning.

Housing for the Aged

Since a place to live is a basic human need, and since it is desirable that older people live independently as long as possible, there is a growing trend toward providing housing especially designed for older Americans. The Housing Assistance Administration of the Department of Housing and Urban Development is providing housing units for the older members of the population. The buildings are planned and designed to prevent accidents; they are easy to maintain, modest in size, and within walking distance of varied facilities. The Rent Supplement Program allows older citizens with low incomes to live in decent housing by providing them with rent supplements. This is of special interest to community health nurses as well as allied health workers who are engaged in helping the aged solve their problems.

Since elderly people have a difficult time adapting to a changing environment, it is helpful if their dwelling can be adapted to their needs. For people in their 70s, such safety measures as adequate illumination, nonslip flooring, and grab bars in strategic places are especially important. Single-level living quarters may also be desirable. The very old may also need facilities offering group dining and nursing and medical services.

▷ Physiologic Changes That Occur With Age

The process of aging varies with each individual, since hereditary and environmental factors influence longevity. Intensive and systematic study of aging, both experimentally and clinically, has revealed certain facts about the aging process. Aging occurs on all levels of bodily function: cellular, organic, and systemic. At least in laboratory settings, it appears that cells have a definite life span; they do not divide indefinitely but demonstrate a decreasing capacity for cellular division with age. Also, the cells of elderly persons may not perform as well as those of the young. Some of the research at the cellular level indicates that body cells may age and die because they lack the ability to repair damage that they sustain as a result of their own metabolic processes or as a result of adverse environmental effects.

Grossly speaking, *loss of cells and loss of physiologic reserve make up the dominant processes of aging.* This loss of reserve capacity may occur in many organ systems because of a gradual loss of functional units, a gradual impairment of the remaining units, decreased coordination of functional units, or a combination of these factors.

There are wide differences in aging; different organ systems are affected at different rates, even in the same individual. However, the overall effect of aging is seen in altered body functions—usually in the direction of deterioration.

Changes in Homeostasis

Homeostasis is the body's ability to maintain a stable internal environment (see Chap. 7). The complex mechanism of homeostasis regulates fluid and electrolyte balance, blood pressure, temperature, and food intake. Man is dependent upon the functional integrity of the cell and the stability of the internal environment. If the homeostatic mechanisms are functioning properly, the body is able to adapt or react to stress. However, with aging these mechanisms become less efficient and reserve power is lost. The body usually can function adequately at rest and during short periods of moderate activity, but when external stresses such as trauma or infection occur, there is little or no reserve capacity. This in turn makes the person more vulnerable to disease. Breakdown of bodily function can follow. Recovery is also affected since more time is required for the body to return to normal after illness. Thus, to cope with these physiologic changes, the older person must make adjustments in living by reducing the level of activity.

Changes in the Nervous System

The nervous system is extremely vulnerable to the aging process, as is seen in the progressive loss of cells that occurs with advancing years. There are approximately half as many brain cells in the frontal area of the brain at age 80 as at 40, with a resulting decrease in brain weight. (However, the reserve capacity of the brain generally can compensate for this deficiency.) The steady loss of neurons begins surprisingly early in life and affects both the brain and spinal cord. There is progressive atrophy of the convolutions (gyri) of the brain surface and consequent widening and deepening of the spaces (sulci) between the convolutions. There is also a decrease in the blood flow to the brain. Both the physiologic changes in the brain and the reduced blood supply may be related to personality changes sometimes encountered in the elderly. This may account for the fact that as we grow older there is a tendency to become slightly forgetful (particularly short-term memory), to respond more slowly, to awaken earlier in the morning, and, perhaps, to become more inflexible. More time is frequently needed for decision making. However, there is generally little decline in intelligence test scores up to age 75, although there is a decline in speed of response. Tests have shown that persons with advanced education and ability usually show little or no intellectual deterioration with age as long as there is no time pressure. Many older people remain creative late into life.

Changes in the Special Senses

The aging process produces varying degrees of impairment in hearing, vision, smell, taste, and pain perception, as well as diminished sensations of touch and a slowing of reflexes.

A decrease in the sense of smell and in the number of taste buds at times contributes to a loss of appetite; diminished sensitivity to thirst needs can lead to dehydration and confused behavior as a result of fluid imbalance.

Hearing impairment, which usually is first noticed in the higher frequencies, can result in impairment of speech discrimination and a loss of the full sense of background noises. Since sensory stimulation helps to maintain orientation to one's surroundings, these losses in sensory perception can contribute to the withdrawal and social isolation of some persons.

Vision is affected by a decrease in visual acuity (ability to discriminate fine detail) and accommodation to glare and by a marked diminution of night vision and the peripheral field of vision. This can be particularly frustrating, because reading and television viewing are favorite activities of many older persons who are unable to engage in more strenuous pursuits. The implications for nursing are many; it is necessary to provide increased illumination without glare, use night lights, and employ caution in moving elderly patients from lighted rooms to darkened rooms so as to allow time for adjustment from day to night vision. The major ophthalmologic problems in older people include presbyopia (difficulty in seeing clearly at close range), lacrimal disturbances, cataract, macular degeneration, glaucoma, diabetic retinopathy, and retinal detachment. Newer methods of diagnostic instrumentation and medical and surgical therapy have improved the opportunities for visual rehabilitation.

Pain Perception and Temperature Regulation. Perception of some types of pain decreases, and referral of pain from one part of the body to another seems to become more common with advancing age. In fact, the elderly can be free of pain in some acute disorders, such as myocardial infarction, pneumonia, appendicitis, and peritonitis.

The temperature-regulating mechanisms are less reliable and the heat-generating activities are reduced. In the presence of infection, the aged person may show a *decrease* or little change in body temperature rather than a definite elevation. Therefore, one must watch for changes in facial appearance and small increases in respiratory rate as possible signs of infection in the aging person.

Cardiovascular Changes

In older people, the heart is able to pump effectively under normal circumstances, but because it lacks much of its physiologic reserve, it reacts poorly to sudden stress, such as blood loss, excessive parenteral fluids, or sudden effort. When normal homeostasis is upset, congestive heart failure, arrhythmias, and myocardial ischemia may develop.

The signs of arteriosclerosis become clinically recognizable when it has reached an advanced stage in the elderly. The arteries of old people show progressive chemical and anatomical changes, with an increase in cholesterol, other lipids, and calcium. The elastic fibers progressively straighten, fray, split, and fragment. Poor circulation owing to hardening of the arteries is a cause of many of the ills of the aged. Although blood pressure in the aged may fluctuate, arterial hypertension is indicated when *persistent* elevations of both systolic and diastolic values are present.

Respiratory Changes

Most of the changes that occur in pulmonary function in the aged result from loss of elastic tissue surrounding the alveoli and alveolar ducts and from changes in the anteroposterior diameter of the chest owing to rib and vertebral calcification. There are also changes in the tissues of the lung and a decline in its functional capacity, size, and structure, as well as weakening of the respiratory muscles. Vital capacity becomes reduced while there is a concurrent increase in residual volume. Changes in the pulmonary vasculature also occur. However, ventilation usually remains adequate to meet the demands of ordinary activity. Normally, elderly people should be free from chronic respiratory symptoms and infection, as long as their health status is normal.

Changes in Kidney Function

Kidney function declines with age because of a reduction in the number of glomeruli and diminished filtration and tubular function. The blood flow to the kidney is reduced as a result of decreased cardiac output and increased peripheral resistance. Because of these changes, the kidney becomes a less effective waste-disposal system and loses its efficiency in homeostatic control. However, its initial reserve capacity is so great that under normal circumstances it continues to function adequately throughout life.

Metabolic Changes

As the body ages, the basal metabolic rate slows and the quantity of oxygen used by the tissues is reduced. As metabolic processes change, the glucose tolerance curve tends toward that of the diabetic. If normal standards for glucose tolerance tests were applied to the aged, 50% of this population would be classified as diabetics. Therefore, the usefulness of conventionally interpreted glucose tolerance tests for the aged is in doubt, except for those with long-standing diabetes. Special tables to aid in interpreting glucose tolerance tests in older patients are available.

Gastrointestinal Changes.   In some older persons, gastrointestinal function is impeded by a combination of factors, including loss of teeth or inadequately fitting dentures, an impaired swallowing mechanism, or diminishing gastric and enzyme secretions. Absorption of nutrients and minerals may also be lessened and gastrointestinal motility reduced. One chronic complaint frequently encountered in the elderly is constipation, but the usual causes are lack of fiber and bulk and poor bowel habits rather than a "sluggish bowel."

Musculoskeletal Changes

Generally, there is a slow and steady atrophy of muscle that results in muscle wasting, particularly of the trunk and extremities. With loss of muscle power there is a decrease in strength, endurance, and agility. Bones gradually lose calcium and become more porous and lighter. Because bones become more brittle, falls are especially dangerous in the elderly. Ligaments calcify and ossify, and joints become stiffened from erosions of cartilaginous joint surfaces. Changes in the lining of joint cavities can produce degenerative changes. Such changes contribute to reduction in height and sometimes to a stooped posture and a limited ability to "get around." However, many disabilities occurring from muscular insufficiency can be prevented and corrected. Life-long exercise programs can help to minimize age-related musculoskeletal changes. Since lack of activity aggravates disability from musculoskeletal changes, the aged need to be encouraged to be physically active within the level of their ability and to maintain optimum nutrition, particularly with respect to an adequate intake of protein, calcium, and vitamins.

Skin and Connective Tissue Changes

The skin is among the first structures to show the most obvious changes associated with aging. As a person ages, there is loss of subcutaneous supporting tissue and resultant thinning of the skin. With the loss of subcutaneous fat, the skin assumes the characteristic appearance of aging—folds, lines, wrinkles, and slackness. Thinning and loss of the hair occur, as well as variations in pigmentation of the skin and hair. Purpura and ecchymoses may appear because of the greater fragility of the dermal and subcutaneous vessels and loss of subcutaneous tissues supporting the skin capillaries. Minor trauma can easily cause bruising.

The dermis becomes relatively dehydrated and loses strength and elasticity. The skin in general is prone to excess dryness and itching. The diminished capillary bed and atrophying glands are one cause of the elderly person's inability to cope with cold, heat, and soap.

As a protective measure, older people should avoid overexposure to the sun, which tends to accelerate aging of the skin and increases the tendency to skin cancer. Older people should also protect themselves against minor trauma since the skin gradually loses its ability to heal, particularly in diabetics and those with impaired circulation owing to atherosclerosis in the lower extremities.

Reproductive Changes and Changes in Sexual Activity

Physiologic changes occurring with menopause can affect sexual function and activity in older women. Atrophy of the vaginal canal and diminished vaginal secretions can lead to local irritation, bleeding, and pain with sexual activity. This problem is treatable. In older men, there may be diminished and delayed ability to achieve a full penile erection and a reduction in the frequency of ejaculation. These physiologic changes are frequently associated with psychological changes.

Although there may be an overall decline in sexual activity with advancing age, substantial numbers of older people continue to desire and engage in sexual activity. Sexual desires and capabilities, though modified, may remain sufficiently intact to function in late life. Studies have suggested that continued sexual activity in the aged is dependent upon previous sexual behavior and experience and the availability of a partner. The fact that the majority of aged women are widows may have something to do with the seeming decline in sexual interest in older women.

▷ Preventive Care and Health Maintenance for the Aged

Preventive health care in the elderly is most important because people in this age group have less resilience and suffer more deleterious consequences from any breakdown in homeostasis. Preventive care in the elderly means maintaining health and function, detecting disease at an early stage, and preventing the deterioration of an existing condition.

People who care for and about the aged must have a positive feeling about the health potential of these elderly patients. (One has to be "tough" to reach old age.) Older persons must be educated about health conservation. Of course, the ideal practice would be to detect disease and provide remedial care in the pregeriatric years in order to prevent disabling diseases. Nurse practitioners who have special abilities, education, and interest in geriatrics are making great strides in promoting the health care of the elderly.

Health Appraisal

Elderly persons as a whole are less likely to present themselves for physical examination because they may be inclined to overlook serious symptoms as mere signs of "old age." In addition, lack of mobility and money, a decreased sensitivity to some types of pain, and depression are factors leading to self-neglect.

Varied health assessment techniques can be implemented to help detect and identify elderly people at risk. One such assessment approach uses an automated health screening program. The medical history is combined with certain physiologic parameters to obtain a health profile. This system uses automated procedures, computer analyses, and read-out results to obtain health information. With this method, the state of wellness is assessed and the probability of the presence of one or more diseases and patterns of change is identified. This is correlated with the findings from the physical examination. In part because the natural history of disease is altered in old age, many physical problems do not become obvious until they are considerably advanced.

Many authorities believe that a comprehensive physical examination, including blood examinations, urinalysis, and stool test, should be carried out annually. Of special importance is the ECG, which shows heart abnormalities often unappreciated by the elderly patient. Equally important is a chest x-ray, which can provide evidence of congestive heart failure, chronic lung disease, tuberculosis, cancer, the size of the heart, and changes in large blood vessels and bony structures of the chest. Pulmonary function tests are used to evaluate the effects of such diseases as emphysema. The Papanicolaou smear to detect cancer of the cervix is important in elderly women, as is the tonometer test for glaucoma. It is wise to monitor the weight of older people since subtle weight losses can herald the presence of cancer. Hearing and vision should be tested and corrected, as sensory deprivation can cause a downhill course.

Assessment of health habits is necessary as a basis for health counseling. Positive measures for maintaining health include weight control, exercise, proper nutrition, avoidance of cigarette smoking, and the promotion of accident prevention. All of these appear to contribute to longevity and improved quality of life.

Nutritional Support

Dietary inadequacies in the elderly result from such factors as poor nutritional habits, economic constraints, and underlying disease conditions. Nutrition can have a tremendous impact on health maintenance and disease prevention as well as on the treatment of disease. In general, the nutritional requirements of the elderly appear to be similar to those of other mature adults, except that calorie intake should generally be reduced. The calorie requirement decreases about one third because lean body mass, metabolic rate, and physical activity decline with age. The calorie intake is adjusted on an individual basis to maintain normal weight and to prevent overweight and underweight. However, there is some evidence that the overall mortality rate is lowest among elderly people who are mildly or moderately overweight.

Older people are vulnerable to low nutrient intake. Dietary studies show that calcium, thiamine, ascorbic acid, and vitamin A are the nutrients most commonly lacking in the diets of the aged.

With aging there is a decrease in the amount of body protein, which largely reflects the decrease in skeletal muscle mass. Some researchers recommend that the protein content of the diet should be more than 10% (and possibly 12% to 14%) of the calorie total. Though total body protein breakdown and synthesis decrease with age and one might expect that the protein needs of the elderly would be reduced, there is not enough information concerning the amino acid requirements of the elderly. Physical and psychological stress may result in negative nitrogen balance. Problems of malabsorption and metabolic changes may reduce the efficiency of utilization of nitrogen. For these reasons, the amount of protein should be individually assessed. One gram of protein per kilogram of ideal weight has been recommended as a desirable standard for protein intake for older people.

There is some disagreement over what constitutes an appropriate intake of vitamins for the elderly. The few studies available do not suggest that higher requirements exist in the aged, but the elderly may respond to vitamin supplementation because their vitamin intake is generally low.

Among the minerals, calcium intake especially may have to be supplemented. The high incidence of osteoporosis in older women seems to be age related.

The addition of a moderate amount of fiber to the diet may alleviate constipation and flatulence, which are common complaints in this age group.

Other factors contributing to nutritional deficiencies are social isolation, lack of interest in cooking and eating, and problems in food shopping. Weak and shaky hands can make some types of cooking hazardous. Eating is a social occasion, and many of life's enjoyable moments are associated with food. When the social element is removed and the person lives alone, there is a temptation to stop eating regular meals. Many depend to an undesirable extent on foods and snacks that are inexpensive and can be prepared with the least effort. Persons living at poverty levels cannot afford to buy the protective foods that are needed. Therefore, the proportion of carbohydrates in the diet may be excessively high, as in the "tea-toast" regimen, and the protein consumption far below the minimum requirements.

Loss of interest in food is also prompted by physiologic changes, such as decreased production of saliva and an inability to chew properly because of poorly fitting dentures or the loss of teeth. By the age of 75, 66% of Americans have lost their teeth. People with poorly fitting dentures or no teeth at all tend to eat soft foods, particularly starches and sweets.

Other reasons for loss of appetite in many older people include the loss of taste buds (up to 50%) and a diminished ability to smell. Difficulty in swallowing is also seen.

Appetite can be improved by beginning the meal with appetite stimulants, such as fruit juices and soups made from meat extract. Frequent nutritious small feedings can also help to increase food intake in the anorectic patient. When counseling the patient on diet modifications and working out a dietary regimen related to a specific disorder, the nurse should consider the patient's lifelong food habits. The mere fact that the patient is old does not necessarily mean that food must be soft and bland. It is important that the food be served attractively and be as palatable as possible.

The benefit of eating in a social setting is important to physical and mental well-being. Therefore, the patient should be encouraged to eat with others, attend church dinners and "pot-luck" occasions, and share hostess duties with others. The federal government is subsidizing a program to provide meals for the elderly in a social setting. The nurse can direct persons to these centers for senior citizens that serve hot lunches. "Meals on Wheels" is primarily for the homebound.

Exercise

Activity is one key to the prevention of premature aging. Many of the health problems of the aged arise from a lack of conditioning and a diminished response to stress. Inactivity is a serious threat to the aged, and weakness or stiffness of major postural muscles ultimately causes problems in mobility. Exercise maintains muscular tone throughout the body and is effective in the prevention of and rehabilitation following cardiovascular disease. Exercise training improves functional capabilities, increases vitality, and has psychological benefits. However, there is no evidence that it increases life expectancy.

The goal of physical training for the aged is to extend their active, productive years. A systematic program of exercise that emphasizes the relaxation and stretching of tight muscles as well as the strengthening of weak muscles constitutes a helpful reconditioning plan. Usually, the older person should start with relaxation exercises and then progress to limbering exercises before undertaking the strengthening exercises. For older people, the exercise is not re-

peated more than two to three times to avoid stiffening of joints. The program is gradually increased in intensity. An individualized and supervised program can be applied to the bedridden as well as to the ambulatory patient.

The President's Council on Physical Fitness and Sports and the Administration on Aging have published an exercise program for older Americans titled "The Fitness Challenge in the Later Years,"* which presents graded exercise programs that give a balanced workout, utilizing all major muscle groups.

Accident Prevention

About 22,000 persons 65 years old and over die each year from accidental injuries. Nurses are all too familiar with the frail aged person who is admitted to the hospital with a fractured hip that leads to prolonged incapacity, pressure sores, indwelling catheter, depression, and death. For the elderly person, a fall can literally be the "beginning of the end." National Safety Council figures show that persons over 65 account for 24% of all accidental deaths. For persons over 65 who are hospitalized for accidental injuries, the average stay is 13.5 days, whereas the average is 8 days for other age groups.

Most accidents involving older people occur in the home, and falls are the most common type of accidents. The following suggestions may help older persons to avoid accidents:

1. All stairs should have handrails.
2. Grab bars should be installed next to the bathtub, the shower, and the toilet.
3. Shoes should fit, and the laces must be tied securely; loose slippers are a hazard.
4. Personal belongings and other frequently used items should be stored at a level that is between the hip and the eyes, in order to avoid climbing or bending.
5. Older pedestrians must be reminded to be cautious since their hearing and vision are often impaired.

Plans should be made to deal with emergencies for those living alone and for the handicapped. A buddy system in which telephone contact is made daily is useful, since elderly persons are prone to "drop attacks" and may lie on the floor unattended for long periods of time. Emergency numbers should be written in large letters and placed in a conspicuous place or tape recorded for persons with visual impairment.

▷ Health Problems of the Aged

Disease and Aging

As was indicated earlier, the aged are particularly vulnerable to disease because of such factors as their decreased physiologic reserve, a less flexible homeostatic mechanism, and lessened defense mechanisms of the body. Chronic diseases have been called "the companions of the aged," and most persons over 65 are affected by at least one chronic disease.

* Consumer Information Center, Dept. 151 K, Pueblo, Colorado 81009, No. 151 K; $3.50.

The major disorders of old age include heart disease, malignancy, cerebrovascular disease (mainly senile dementia and stroke), influenza, and pneumonia. Coronary heart disease is the most frequently seen cardiac condition. Cancer of the alimentary tract, especially of the colon, is also common. Sometimes cancers progress more slowly in the aged.

Disease in the aged does not always present with classic signs and symptoms. The usual clinical manifestations may be absent, attenuated, or disguised, and atypical signs and symptoms may be present. Complaints may be overlooked and attributed to aging and senility. Although older people have reduced physiologic reserve, some of the diseases of the aged are curable, or preventable, and the progress of others can be slowed. It is necessary to distinguish disease caused by physical insults and time-related changes from those caused by the effects of socioeconomic adversities and personal crises.

Many of the disabilities associated with old age develop as a result of degenerative vascular disease, namely arteriosclerosis. Multiple small thromboses of the arteries in the cerebral cortex are responsible for the mental deterioration of some so-called "senile" patients. When such occlusions occur, the patient may no longer be able to integrate thoughts or observations and may lose the ability to recall recent events, becoming increasingly irritable and exhibiting signs that in many respects seem to represent a reversion to childhood. The patient may also become less responsive to the environment. On the other hand, an older person may suffer immediate death or serious disability if a sudden occlusion develops in a large arteriosclerotic artery in the brain or if a cerebral hemorrhage occurs. Another complication of arteriosclerosis is occlusive vascular disease of the lower extremities, resulting in intermittent claudication and, possibly, gangrene, which can sometimes necessitate amputation of one or both extremities.

Arteriosclerosis is apt to involve the coronary arteries of the heart and those supplying the kidney. Therefore, the elderly patient is unusually subject to cardiac disorders, such as angina, acute coronary insufficiency, acute myocardial infarction, arrhythmias, and heart failure, which may seriously limit the capacity for physical exertion and can produce transient ischemic episodes and falls. The impairment of kidney function brings with it the ultimate prospect of chronic renal failure.

Gastrointestinal disturbances commonly occur in the older age groups because of neoplastic disease, reduction of the blood supply to the gastrointestinal tract, neuromuscular degenerative changes, alterations of the intestinal linings, and loss of secretions. If impaired peristalsis of the esophagus occurs (owing to diminished muscle and nerve function), swallowing will become difficult and may possibly lead to aspiration pneumonia.

- Because of swallowing difficulties that can occur with age, it is necessary to elevate the head of the bed while feeding an elderly patient who cannot sit up.

Abdominal emergencies, such as internal bleeding or intestinal obstruction, do not always occur with classic symptoms in the elderly. Fainting may signal occult gastrointestinal bleeding. An intestinal obstruction may be silent but is always a serious event. In general, gastrointestinal disturbances create problems in nutritional management and symptomatic therapy.

A respiratory infection in the older person is an *acute emergency* and is complicated by the patient's inability to cough up secretions because of a lack of sufficient expulsive power. Patients with chronic obstructive pulmonary disease often develop respiratory complications following illness, surgery, or trauma.

- Confusion is often the first sign of respiratory infection in the elderly.
- Sedatives or tranquilizers should be given with caution because they make the patient vulnerable to ventilatory failure and suppress the cough reflex.
- Elderly patients with even "minor" respiratory infections require vigorous treatment.

Other frequently occurring disorders in the aged include atrophic and ulcerative lesions of the skin and mucous membranes and enlargement of the prostate gland with urinary obstruction. Description of these and other degenerative disorders are included in the appropriate sections of this text.

Falls in the Elderly

Persons aged 65 or older account for 24% of all accidental deaths in the United States, and falls lead the list of major causes. For an aging person, a fall may be a frightening experience that can lead to immobilization and possibly to pneumonia and complete loss of the ability to walk. Falls by the elderly may result from age-related physiologic decline in postural control (particularly swaying) and deterioration of the central nervous system or from lightheadedness, postural hypotension, heart block, and arrhythmias. Many times, falls occur when an elderly person hurries in response to the need to void or defecate.

Special danger arises from osteoporosis, a condition in which the bones lose calcium and thus become thin and brittle. This condition renders an elderly person susceptible to major fractures. (Hip fracture, Colles' fracture, and compression fractures of the spine are common in older people.) The joints are very often affected by degenerative (hypertrophic) arthritis, causing pain and limiting the motion of the back and of the weight-bearing joints. The eroded joint can "give in," causing the patient to fall.

- A fracture should be suspected in any elderly person who falls.

To reduce the frequency of falls among hospitalized older people, the following measures have been recommended:*

1. Implementing a treatment and rehabilitation program
2. Assessing patient dexterity and carrying out frequent monitoring during the first week of hospitalization, the time period when many falls occur

---

* From Sehested P and Severin–Nielsen T: Falls by hospitalized elderly patients: Causes, prevention. Geriatrics 1978 Apr; 32:101–108.

3. Placing the incapacitated or hemiplegic patient in a wheelchair equipped with a seat belt, pillow, and stable-mounted table

4. Keeping corridors free of furniture and service equipment

5. Having patient wear nonskid shoes

6. Stabilizing bed tables, placing them in easy reach, and immobilizing them when in use

7. Using low beds with low bedrails for confused and restless bed patients

8. Using stable chairs with arms and a seat height suitable for rising and sitting

9. Instructing patients to arise slowly when experiencing a sudden need to void or defecate

10. Using a television camera for continued monitoring of areas where there are restless bed patients, etc., for the recognition and prevention of dangerous situations.

Mental Health of the Aged

The basic psychological needs of all people include respect, security, and self-esteem, as well as a need to feel appreciated and valued by others. These psychological needs are threatened during times of stress and crisis. For the aged, illness makes it more difficult to fulfill these needs. Even in the absence of serious illness, the elderly person is vulnerable to emotional and mental stress because of the sense of loss that can come from the death of friends and family members as well as from retirement, somatic changes, and failing health and mental faculties. Failure to adapt during any time of the life cycle can result in physical and emotional illness.

Although most people maintain their intellectual competence, the incidence of psychiatric and cognitive disorders increases with age; some of these are residuals of lifelong conflicts that never were resolved. Of the elderly living in the community, an estimated 15% to 25% have moderate to severe psychiatric impairment. More than half of those living in nursing homes suffer from senile dementia. Many display signs of regression or turn to alcohol or drugs in reaction to pain, grief, and despondency. Other mental disorders that make their appearance late in life include depression, senile dementia, and persistent paranoid state. Psychiatric symptoms in the elderly may also be the result of metabolic, toxic, infectious, cardiopulmonary, or drug-induced disorders. Even a sudden environmental change or hospitalization can produce confusion in a previously alert elderly person or can convert a mildly confused patient into a psychotic one. Unfortunately, psychiatric problems are often overlooked and mental changes are mistakenly regarded as part of the aging process.

Depression

Depression is the most common emotional disorder in the aged; approximately one million older Americans suffer from this affective disorder. (Depression may also be attributable to biochemical or endogenous factors.) Depression and grief are common in the aged since losses are inevitable. The accumulation of many losses—losses of people, of things, and of hope—may deplete the individual's inner resources and the ability to cope. Depression resulting from losses can easily be overlooked and may be mistaken for physical or organic mental illness. The patient may exhibit anger, denial, withdrawal, or other maladaptive responses that move him further away from reality. He may become overly helpless or dependent. Physical complaints may serve to mask true feelings. Depression in the aged is usually manifested by feelings of apathy, quietness, and emptiness, which may be mistaken for "senile" changes. In any depression, especially when associated with guilt, there is a risk of suicide. Suicide in old age is allied to physical disease, social isolation, and grief and is more prevalent among men, especially white men in their 80s.

Treatment.   There is a natural tendency for depressive illness to improve. The treatment of depression should be as vigorous in the aged as in the young. Antidepressant drugs are usually prescribed with smaller starting doses and smaller dosage increments. In depressions resulting mainly from losses, the therapeutic approach is one of empathy; offering a sympathetic ear and an understanding heart can help the patient to see that depression is the outcome of human problems. Sometimes treatment focuses on assisting the patient to complete the grieving process. Referral to community resources, such as the community mental health service, can be very beneficial. But services cannot substitute for emotional ties with people. The presence of a confidant and personal contacts serve to increase the confidence and self-esteem of the patient. The seriously depressed patient may require hospitalization, especially if there are suicidal tendencies.

Senile Dementia (Chronic Organic Brain Syndrome)

The term *dementia* refers to signs and symptoms of intellectual dysfunction owing to differing etiologies and varying pathophysiologic mechanisms that can occur alone and in combination. It is believed to result from diffuse impairment of brain tissue. The most common long-term disorders of cognitive functioning (attention, learning, memory) in the elderly are seen in senile dementia (often called Alzheimer's disease). Other conditions resulting in dementia include Pick's disease and Jakob–Creutzfeldt disease.

Senile dementia generally refers to a disturbance of mental status or mental deterioration occurring after the age of 65, but a similar or identical conditon may also begin earlier in life. There are neuropathologic changes associated with changes in the patient's cognitive function, which may include loss of neurons, neurofibrillary tangles, granulovascular changes, and neuritic (senile) plaques in the brain. The patient usually experiences gradual deterioration of memory, which at first may be minor and almost imperceptible and is often overlooked and mistakenly thought to be the result of physical illness or emotional upset. Gradually, there is impairment of intellectual function and judgment, disorientation, and shallow or labile affect. Behavioral changes, such as irritability, anger, restlessness, agitation, and depression, are sometimes seen and may be a reaction to senile dementia or the result of loss of cerebral function. In time the individual's ability to carry out self-care activities, to relate to others, and to cope with environmental situations is affected. Varying patterns in the sequence of changes and in the rate of change occur from patient to patient.

Senile dementia is devastating to the human personality and is a source of anguish and frustration to the patient and loved ones. Senile dementia and related disorders are associated with a high mortality rate and significantly shortened life expectancy. It is perhaps the fifth greatest killer in the United States, since death can result from pneumonia, "benign neglect," and the effects of multiple medications that contribute to cardiovascular and neurologic problems, malnutrition, and dehydration.

Management of the Dementias

The goal of treatment is to relieve some of the psychosocial stresses and to improve the general health of the patient. Unfortunately, there is no treatment to halt the progressive deterioration of brain function. Patients with mild or moderate involvement may be well aware of their intellectual deficiencies and react to their personality loss with anxiety. Drug therapy (antianxiety agents; antidepressants) may be prescribed to handle behavioral disturbances and to improve the patient's subjective feelings. Medication can improve sleeping patterns.

The patient requires understanding support from family and health care personnel. Negative feelings and rejection can precipitate more anxiety, depression, and bizarre behavior and further accentuate feelings of insecurity and worthlessness and loss of self-esteem.

A major objective is to keep the patient functioning as long as possible. A greater sense of security can be promoted with an orderly and rather ritualistic existence. Memory aids (lists of daily activities, labeled items) may help in day-to-day living, with emphasis placed on "now." Senile behavior is neither endorsed nor encouraged. Caring persons can help the patient to continue social contacts as long as possible. When the problems become too difficult for the family to manage, the patient may be placed in an extended care facility. The nursing approach to the confused patient is summarized in Chart 15-1, and the reader is referred to a psychiatric nursing textbook for other appropriate nursing interventions. The community services and facilities that may be helpful are listed in Chart 15-2.

Acute Brain Syndrome (Delirium or Acute Confusional States)

Acute brain syndrome is a temporary psychiatric state caused by a physiologic or an anatomical insult to brain tissue. The disorders have a relatively sudden onset and are potentially reversible. They are associated with acute physical illness or physiologic disturbances, cardiac and circulatory problems, neurologic conditions, cerebrovascular disorders, dehydration, electrolyte imbalance, alcohol or drug toxicity, and a wide variety of infections. A reduction of cognitive function and delirium are usually present.

- An underlying physical cause should be suspected in any patient who has *sudden* changes in intellectual function.

In the management of acute brain syndrome, the basic disease must be treated or the etiologic toxic agent must be removed. Specific treatment is aimed at alleviating or curing the condition that underlies the confusion: antimicrobials for infection; removal of drugs; correction of fluid, electrolyte, and metabolic imbalances; removal of fecal impaction; correction of heart failure; treatment of stroke. Appropriate medication, such as the phenothiazines, which exert much of their calming action on the lower brain centers, may be administered. The nursing approaches that may be beneficial to the confused elderly patient are found in Chart 15-1.

▷ Management of the Elderly Patient

Geriatric nursing is a growing challenge in today's world. As more and more elderly people become part of the nurse's clientele, all of the nurse's scientific and humanistic resources are tapped. Not only are there multiple medical problems and nursing needs that must be managed simultaneously, but psychological and socioeconomic problems must be attended to as well. In general, an elderly patient requires 20% more time in nursing care and general assistance than a younger patient. When one approaches a frail, older person with multiple diseases that require several modes of treatment, more than the usual degree of assessment, clinical judgment, and nursing proficiency is required. Gerontological nursing requires an understanding of the human condition enhanced by compassion, patience, and respect. At the same time, great rewards can be gained by interacting with and learning from people who have accumulated a lifetime of experience by successfully adapting to and coping with major social, economic, and personal crises. The underlying principle in approaching the elderly patient is to recognize and respect the individuality and uniqueness of the person.

Nursing Assessment

With a view to understanding the total person, the nurse assesses the patient and seeks information for developing a nursing care plan; she then initiates the plan and evaluates its effectiveness. Knowing the patient's early history can help in developing nursing interventions and prevention strategies. One of the best ways of gathering data is to take the history and then engage in conversation with the patient. The goal is to answer the question *"What are the assets and limitations of this patient?"*

The nurse should be seated near the patient in order to maintain eye contact and should speak slowly and clearly in simple sentences. Hearing the life history is a process that takes time. The older patient usually has a slower response time, so the nursing interveiw should be slow and relaxed. In addition to the patient's responses, nonverbal clues, such as facial expression and posture ("body language"), should be noted. Touching the patient can be reassuring.

The following list of questions is offered as a guide in the nursing assessment of elderly patients.

Physiologic Assessment
How does the patient describe the activities of a "typical" day?
How effective is the patient at self-care?

Chart 15-1
Nursing Approach to the "Confused" Elderly Person

A. Changes in mental status may be the first sign of illness in the elderly.
   1. Expect an underlying physical cause in any patient who has *sudden* changes in intellectual functioning.
   2. Confusion and disorientation may be first sign of infection (*e.g.*, pneumonia), cardiac failure, coronary occlusion, electrolyte imbalance, stroke, dehydration, anemia, malignancy.

B. Aging is not synonymous with senility—senile dementia is a *degenerative* disease of the elderly.

C. Determine when and how the confusion developed.
   1. When was the patient last clear mentally?
      a. Are there any other symptoms? urinary frequency? cough? pain?
      b. What medications are being taken? (Ask to see them.)
   2. Assess the patient.

   Physical Status
      a. Observe respirations and pulse; take temperature.
      b. Check the state of hydration—tongue, tissue turgor.
      c. Examine for peripheral edema.
      d. Look for alterations in color.
      e. Check for evidence of injury.

   Mental Status
      a. Where are you now?
      b. What is today's date? day of month? year?
      c. How old are you?
      d. When is your birthday?
      e. Where do you live?

D. A new environment may bring on confused or "senile" behavior without physiologic causes.
   1. Be optimistic about this turn of events; act on the assumption that this behavior is temporary.
   2. Accept the person as he is, without judgment or criticism.
   3. Maintain eye contact.
   4. Pay attention to what the patient is saying—often a person who is considered confused is only transiently so and much of what he is saying makes sense.
   5. Pick out "meaningful" comments and continue talking with him.
   6. Explain the patient's situation to him repeatedly.
   7. Make short, frequent contacts.
   8. Call the person by name each time a contact is made; touch the patient when you speak to him.
      a. Talk directly to him.
      b. Answer questions in simple, short sentences.
   9. Show the person your name tag.
   10. Convey a therapeutic attitude—listening, smiling, talking, and touching.

E. Provide sufficient sensory input that is recognized as friendly.
   1. Keep the patient oriented with respect to time and place.
      a. Remind him of time, date, and place each morning and whenever necessary.
      b. Keep a calendar and clock, both with easily readable numbers, within his range of vision.
   2. Encourage family to bring in pictures, family album, etc. since familiar objects promote a sense of continuity, aid memory, and provide security and comfort.
   3. Use pictures, music, color, indoor gardens, etc. to enhance the environment.
   4. Read newspaper headlines. Discuss current events.
   5. Take the patient outdoors.
   6. Give the patient something to occupy his hands and mind.
   7. Keep the room well lighted to reduce confusion and fear; use nightlights to reduce risk of "sundowning" (worsening of a condition at night).
   8. Maintain a calm environment. Remove unduly stressful stimuli.
   9. Arrange for visits from others to counteract isolation.
      a. Have family sit by bed so that patient can see and touch them.
      b. Utilize services of a volunteer if no family is available.

F. Respect the patient's territorial rights.
   1. Do not move his personal belongings.
   2. Avoid changing rooms.
   3. Have the patient's personal belongings where he can see and use them.

G. Encourage the patient to assume a *well* and *active* role.
   1. Encourage him to dress in clean, attractive clothing *daily*—the wearing of nightwear confuses the concept of day and night (suggest up-to-date clothing as gifts).
   2. See that he wears shoes—not slippers.
   3. Encourage the patient to *walk* and not use the wheelchair, which limits his environment.
   4. Encourage the patient to eat at a table and not at the bedside.
   5. See that he wears his glasses, hearing aid, dentures, or other prostheses.
   6. Be sure he is drinking adequate fluids.

H. Attempt to alleviate the patient's anxiety and restlessness.
   1. Try "laying on of hands"—touching, stroking, hugging; many aged persons have no one to touch them.
   2. Use warm baths, warm milk, back massage, and understanding and compassion as therapeutic modalities.
   3. Give the patient gentle and constant reassurance.

I. Avoid endorsing senile behavior.
   1. Do not agree with confused statements.
   2. Avoid letting the patient "ramble." Direct him back to reality.
   3. Be consistent. Each member of the health care team should know the nursing objectives and use the same approach.
   4. Schedule the patient's daily activities and adhere to the schedule to promote security.

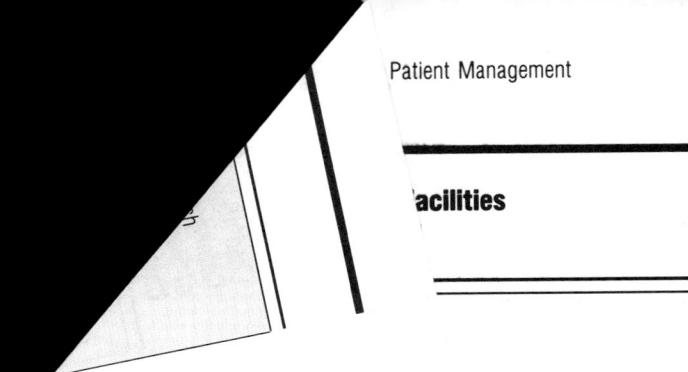

...acilities

Homemakers
Companions
Social workers
Clergymen
Protective and legal services
Programs (VISTA, Senior Aide, SCORE, Peace Corps, Foster Grandparents, Greenthumb, etc.)
Voluntary agencies
Departments of welfare and public assistance
Information and referral services
Screening and evaluation centers
Foster home care
Community mental health centers
Day care and day hospitals
Community senior citizens centers

(From Plutzky M: Principles of psychiatric management of chronic brain syndrome. Geriatrics, *29*:124, 1974. Reproduced with permission of the author from Geriatrics, Volume 29, Number 8, Page 124. Copyright The New York Times Media Company, Inc.)

How much physical capacity does the patient have?
How much muscle strength and coordination does the patient have?
How well does the patient see and hear?
What are the patient's usual eating, sleeping, elimination, and activity patterns? What constitutes a "normal" bowel movement?
What will the patient have to do to regain or maintain functioning ability?

Socioeconomic Assessment
What is the patient's background? early history?
How many person-to-person contacts does the patient have in a day?
What is the family structure?
What family members are living?
Who visits the patient?
What is the patient's religion?
What are the patient's living arrangements?
Are the patient's activities limited because of transportation problems? high-crime environment?
Is the patient economically self-sufficient?
How much independence does the patient possess?
Does the patient participate in any phase of community life?

How can the environment be adjusted to maintain independence?

Psychological Assessment
Is the patient alert and optimistic in outlook?
What does the patient identify as his major concerns and problems?
What are the patient's attitudes toward aging?
What are the patient's attitudes toward himself/herself? Is there a feeling of being needed? useful?
What psychological defenses does the patient use?
What are the patient's activities, interests, and hobbies?
What ego strengths did the patient use in the past?
What are the patient's plans and hopes?

All of these factors affect the patient's reaction to illness and hospitalization. The more the nurse knows about the patient, the more effective is the care given. Since the older patient has more complicated problems and less flexibility for solving them, the nurse may be the only one to whom the patient can turn for help to identify, face, and solve the problems.

Psychosocial Considerations

A newly admitted patient should be made to feel welcome and at home and should be introduced to nearby patients if circumstances allow. At this early meeting, the nurse can observe any incapacities, such as difficulty in hearing, tremor of an extremity, problems in mobility, etc. In elderly patients more than in younger patients, a sudden change from accustomed surroundings to the impersonal routine of a hospital can produce a feeling of insecurity and emotional stress. The understanding nurse can do much to help the patient over this hump of transition between home and institution. Placing the patient near another patient provides an opportunity to talk to someone and helps in making the necessary adjustments to the hospital environment. Touching the patient's hand or shoulder when giving explanations is especially helpful in promoting acceptance, relaxation, and confidence. Many older people have lost all of their social contacts, and the nurse may be the only "caring" person.

Sometimes the transition to a new environment may bring on temporary states of anxiety, confusion, regression, and disorientation. Senile behavior may be exhibited without physiologic cause. The patient may be misjudged as being senile when the real causes are fear, depression, and a feeling of hopeless inadequacy. When symptoms and behavior of senility occur, such as confusion, incontinence, etc., act on the assumption that they are temporary. The nursing approach should be a positive one, conveying the idea that the problem can be altered.

In order to reduce psychic stress, changes should be kept to a minimum. The same personnel should care for the patient whenever possible. The environment should be kept simple and predictable, and a few of the patient's possessions should be kept in plain sight. *Normal routine* should be written on the nursing care plan and adhered to so as to provide reassurance. Since it is sometimes difficult for the elderly to recall names, places, and recent events, especially in an anxiety-provoking situation, such as hospitalization, the nurse should identify herself by name with each contact. To minimize the confusion that often occurs with hospitalization, the patient's family and friends are encouraged to maintain contact and visit frequently.

Like everyone else, older persons respond to suggestions. It is helpful to remind the patient of past successes and to note that each period of life also has its unique problems, benefits, and gratifications. Accepting the patient as he is gives him the assurance that there are caring persons who will help when needed. The demonstration of respect and friendship will do much to enhance self-esteem and mobilize personal resources for self-help.

The elderly fear loneliness and dependency with all of their attendant pains and anguish. As soon as the patient enters the hospital, references and plans should be made concerning discharge from the hospital. This dispels much of the ever-present fear of invalidism, dependency, and death. *All nursing activities are directed toward restoration of the ability for self-care.*

The successful nurse recognizes differences in older people early. Some may be old and physically frail but mentally alert and fresh in spirit. Very readily, one may detect an inherent sense of humor, a philosophical frame of mind, or a thwarted and depressed personality. Often, the patient's temperament will direct the course of progress. Keen observation of these manifestations will present a challenge to the nurse in developing the plan of care.

A fixed routine provides a sense of security for some elderly persons. To know that a certain activity takes place at a certain time provides a schedule that can be anticipated and planned for. The nurse can further convey a feeling of acceptance by remembering the patient's desires and idiosyncrasies, even when they seem trivial.

Before procedures or examinations are done or the siderails put into place, explanations should be offered in order to eliminate fears and tensions. Since older people object to being hurried, sufficient time should be allowed in preparing for a treatment. Every effort should be made to help the older patient feel confidence in those responsible for giving care.

Drug Therapy for the Elderly

Elderly people use more drugs than any other age group, averaging more than 13 prescriptions and renewals a year. One of every four prescriptions is dispensed to a person over 65. Small wonder that the aged are apt to have more adverse drug reactions and interactions than younger people. One study reported that 59% of the elderly outpatient population with chronic illness made errors in self-administration of prescribed medications, and 25% committed potentially serious errors.

Physiologic Considerations

There is great variability in the absorption, distribution, metabolism, and excretion of drugs in older patients owing in part to a reduced capacity of the liver and kidneys to metabolize and excrete the drugs and to lowered levels of circulatory and nervous system efficiency in coping with the effect of certain drugs. Many drugs and their metabolites are excreted by the kidney. However, in the elderly patient, both glomerular and tubular functions are reduced.

- Those administering medications to the elderly must be aware of the commonly used drugs that are primarily removed from the body by renal excretion. An estimate of renal function should be made before such drugs are given.
- At the same time, it is important to realize that decline in cardiac output may decrease the delivery rate to the target organ or storage tissue.
- Changes in the gastrointestinal system may also affect drug therapy. In some elderly patients, a reduced number of mucosal cells and a slowing of gastric motility can prevent the drug from reaching therapeutic plasma and tissue concentrations, and delayed gastric emptying has undesirable effects on drugs that are acid-labile or are metabolized by the stomach mucosa. Alterations in intestinal motility and activity thus change the drug's contact time with the absorptive surface of the mucosa.
- As a result of a slowing metabolism, the drug levels may increase in the tissues and plasma, leading to a prolongation of drug action.

Because some or all of the organ systems may be marginally operational, older patients are apt to show paradoxical or unusual responses to drugs and to develop toxic reactions and their complications. In addition, the elderly have multiple medical problems requiring multiple drug treatment. Table 15-1 lists examples of diseases that may affect drug responses through pharmacokinetic alterations.

Nutritional Considerations

In any drug regimen for the elderly, one must bear in mind that drugs are capable of altering the patient's nutritional status, which may already be compromised by a marginal diet and chronic disease and its treatment. Drugs can depress the appetite, cause nausea, irritate the stomach, and decrease absorption of nutrients, in addition to altering the electrolyte balance and carbohydrate and fat metabolism. A few examples of drugs that are capable of altering the nutritional status are the antacids (producing thiamine deficiency), cathartics (diminished absorption), corticosteroids (lower serum calcium by reducing its absorption), aspirin (associated with folate deficiency), and phenothiazines and tricyclic depressants (increased food intake and weight gain).

Possible Drug Side-effects

The drugs commonly used by elderly persons are capable of producing potentially serious problems.

- Since sedatives and hypnotics can lead to confusion, delusion, hallucinations, falls, habituation, agitation, and possibly noisy behavior, such drugs should be given in smaller doses. Caution should also be taken when opiates are administered since they act as respiratory depressants.
- Before a prescribed opiate is given, the respiratory rate should be counted; if the rate drops below 10 per min-

Table 15-1
Examples of Diseases or Conditions That May Affect Drug Response Through Pharmacokinetic Alterations*

Disease/Condition	Effect
Absorption	
Pyloric stenosis	A decreased gastric emptying rate may result in failure to achieve adequate drug concentrations.
Gastric ulcer	
Vagotomy (surgical or chemical)	
Diabetic gastroparesis	
Severe malabsorption syndrome	Drug absorption may be decreased.
Achlorhydria ·	The absorption of certain basic drugs which require a low gastric pH for complete dissolution may be reduced.
Distribution	
Congestive heart failure	Drugs may be inadequately distributed to other parts of body exposing the regional priorities systems, i.e., heart and brain, to excessive drug concentrations (*e.g.,* lidocaine, procainamide, theophylline).
Hypoalbuminemia	For highly albumin-bound drugs, low serum albumin concentrations may lead to clinical toxicity if the concentration of unbound pharmacologically active drug in the plasma remains increased (*e.g.,* prednisone, phenytoin, phenylbutazone).
Amputations	Failure to take into account the lost muscle mass in the amputee may lead to toxicity with drugs that preferentially distribute into lean body tissue (*e.g.,* digoxin, gentamicin, kanamycin).
Renal Excretion	
Kidney dysfunction	Drugs which are largely excreted unchanged in the urine can accumulate to toxic levels if no precautions are taken to reduce the dose and/or administer less frequently. Since the relative degree of glomerular and tubular dysfunction will often vary with the cause of nephropathy, the frequently observed linear relationship between creatinine and drug clearances may not apply for drugs which are primarily secreted by the tubules.

(continued)

---

ute, the drug should be withheld. Because of the addicting nature of these drugs, no opiate should be given for longer than 72 hours unless specifically prescribed.

- The side-effects of commonly used pain relievers must be taken into account when older patients are concerned. Although salicylates are well tolerated, they can produce salicylism, electrolyte depletion, and possibly serious bleeding from prolonged prothrombin time. Phenacetin, a frequently used over-the-counter pain reliever, may be nephrotoxic and habit-forming.
- If tranquilizers are used for older patients, it is important to note that some (the phenothiazines) can cause hypotension, cerebral depression, and worsening of the agitated state. The minor tranquilizers meprobamate and chlordiazepoxide are useful in alleviating symptoms of anxiety in the ambulatory patient and in calming agitation. However, these drugs have a narrow therapeutic range, so that they may worsen the agitation and produce uninhibited aggressive states in some patients.

- Central nervous system stimulants may be prescribed with the hope of relieving depression, apathy, and lethargy. However, these drugs are given in small dosages since they have a tendency to exaggerate confusion and accentuate paranoia in some patients who have chronic brain disorder. The tricyclic antidepressants may cause cardiac tachyarrhythmias and conduction disturbances.
- Since the heart conduction system, in general, is less effective in older patients, even small doses of digitalis can cause arrhythmias and gastrointestinal and mental symptoms that develop without warning. Digitalis is also not as well tolerated because of less effective kidney function, a decrease in myocardial potassium, and a reduction in body weight. As a result, supplementary potassium and careful dosage maintenance are required.
- Digoxin has a potentially fatal myocardial impact. Diuretics are commonly prescribed for heart failure and can produce debilitating volume and electrolyte depletion.

Table 15-1
Examples of Diseases or Conditions That May Affect Drug Response Through Pharmacokinetic Alterations* (continued)

Disease/Condition	Effect
Renal Excretion	
Congestive heart failure	A significant reduction in cardiac output can result in large decreases in renal blood flow and, to a lesser extent, glomerular filtration rate. Maintenance doses of drugs which are excreted via the kidney may have to be reduced.
Drug Metabolism	
Liver Disease—because the pathophysiology of acute and chronic liver disease is very different, it is evident that their effect on drug metabolism may also differ.	
Acute liver disease—there is primarily hepatocellular necrosis with subsequent decreased activity of drug metabolizing enzymes. Hepatic blood flow is generally regarded as normal, and serum albumin concentration is usually unchanged.	The capacity to metabolize drugs may be significantly impaired during an acute bout of hepatitis (viral). Furthermore, there is no correlation between conventional liver function tests and the prolongation of drug half-life. Complete recovery from viral hepatitis is usually followed by a corresponding recovery of drug metabolizing capability.
Chronic liver disease—there is often replacement of functional tissue by fibrosis, reduced liver blood flow, and decreased serum albumin concentrations. The activity of the drug metabolizing enzymes may be normal or decreased depending upon the degree of compensatory hepatocellular hyperplasia.	The capacity to metabolize drugs may be significantly impaired in chronic liver disease. However, much variability in drug metabolism rates may be seen because of the heterogeneity of the disease. Again there is often no relationship between drug metabolizing ability and the common biochemical tests of liver function. In any form of liver disease, the administration of drugs whose major means of elimination is by hepatic metabolism dictates that frequent clinical and laboratory assessments are necessary for adjusting dosage regimens.
Congestive Heart Failure	In patients with a low cardiac output, proportional reductions in liver blood flow can be anticipated. Furthermore, in right-sided heart failure, the increased right auricular pressure is readily transmitted to the hepatic veins resulting in liver congestion with possible centrizonal liver cell necrosis. Dosage regimens for drugs which are cleared from the plasma principally by hepatic metabolism may have to be decreased.

* (From Reichel W: Clinical Aspects of Aging. Baltimore, Williams & Wilkins, 1978.)

In teaching the patient about the medication regimen, speak slowly and clearly since he may have a hearing, seeing, or memory loss. Tell the patient what each medication is used for and what its side-effects are. Then write out the drug regimen.

The patient often feels that unless a drug has been prescribed, adequate treatment has not been given. As with other age groups, this type of thinking must be corrected. Reinforce the concept that health maintenance includes proper nutrition, a daily program of activity, and periodic health checkups. Drugs are no substitute for caring persons and sound health practices. Patient compliance will be improved when the drug regimen is kept as simple as possible and when the patient is made a partner in the drug-taking regimen.

The patient should not be "fed" medication, but should be encouraged to take it himself. It is also a good idea to give the patient a sip of water before a pill or capsule is swallowed to prevent it from sticking in the throat. Finally, if a patient has a history of suicide threats or attempts, the nurse must be sure that the medication (pill or capsule) is actually swallowed and not retained between the cheeks and the gums or teeth.

General Nursing Interventions

Temperature Regulation

As a person ages, the body becomes less efficient in temperature regulation. In general, older people cannot tolerate a cold environment and are very susceptible to hypothermia. The nursing approach is to palpate the skin for warmth, particularly the extremities, and to make sure that the environmental temperature is adequate. Extra blankets may be added for warmth. Conversely, older persons with cardiovascular disease are prone to develop heat stroke. Efforts are directed to maintain heat and humidity at comfortable levels by fans, air conditioning, and humidifiers or dehumidifiers during hot weather.

Hygienic Care

With aging, the skin becomes thin and inelastic, predisposing the elderly patient to pressure sores. Pressure is the underlying cause of all pressure sores, and because the older patient is sometimes content to lie in bed without moving, the nurse must encourage the patient to turn and move frequently and to engage in graduated activity. The prevention of pressure sores is discussed on page 238.

In the aged, there is reduction of sebum, sweat, and the water-binding capacity of the skin, resulting in a tendency of the skin surface to crack. Rather than avoid bathing, the patient should be advised to lubricate the skin with an ointment (Aquaphor) that traps the moisture. At the same time, special attention must be given to the removal of soapy water from the skin. The danger of residual soap and consequent lysis of the skin is greatest between the toes and fingers and in areas where there are folds. Bathing in hot water and using detergent soaps or bubble baths are to be avoided since these substances aggravate dryness. Senile pruritus is a result of atrophic changes in the epidermis and dermal appendages. The management of pruritus is discussed on page 1168.

Foot Care

For elderly people, foot care is essential in order to maintain mobility, physical well-being, and independence. Common foot disorders of this age group include calluses, bunions, toenail problems, corns, and fungus infections. The feet of older people have survived a lifetime of use, misuse, and trauma. As musculoskeletal problems develop, biomechanical changes occur. All of these are compounded by diabetes, edema, and peripheral vascular ischemia, which increase the patient's susceptibility to infection.

Patient assessment includes attention to possible foot problems as indicated by the patient's complaints and to any signs of abnormality that may suggest possible underlying systemic disorders. The skin is one of the first structures to show degeneration changes associated with aging. The following are offered as guidelines for assessing the lower extremities and feet:

- Is the skin of the extremities thin and shiny?
- Is there loss of hair on the toes? on the front of the legs?
- Are there complaints of pain? paresthesia?
    - Is pain intensified at night? relieved by walking?
    - Is there pain on rest?
- Is there brownish pigmentation? skin erosion? rubor?
- Is the skin mottled?
- Is the extremity cool?
- Does the patient complain of numbness? tingling? burning?
- Are the pulses weak, decreased, or absent?

Care of the Toenails. Thickened and deformed toenails in the elderly occur as a result of vascular insufficiency, nutritional changes, and trauma to the nail matrix. Before the toenails are trimmed, the feet should be soaked in tepid water for 10 or 15 minutes. Soaking softens the nail plate, loosens subungual debris, decreases the possibility of bacterial infection, and helps to relax the patient. The feet are dried by blotting them with a towel instead of wiping them vigorously since friction can injure skin that is delicate, atrophic, or ischemic.

- Sit facing the patient. (The patient's feet should be placed on a footrest.)
- Observe the nails, skin temperature, texture, and color, and look especially for breaks in the skin and signs of infection, redness, and edema.
- Locate the nail and differentiate the nail from the nail bed; a curette can be used for this. (The growth pattern of some nail plates is altered, so it is frequently difficult to distinguish the nail plate from the nail bed.)
- Apply antiseptic solution to the areas around the toenails before cutting the nails. Frequently, the nails are so thick that thinning is required before cutting is possible. This is accomplished by rubbing an emery board across the nail surface.
- To cut the toenails, use only the tip of sterile nail nippers, starting at one corner and taking small "bites" across the entire nail plate. Follow the contour of the nail plate. Little or no force should be necessary.
- Cut the nail so that it rests freely and without pressure on the nail bed. It should be cut even with the end of the toe, and the edges should be smoothed with an emery board.
- Use a curette to carefully debride around and under the nail plate. Debriding removes subungual debris, which may be causing discomfort.
- Apply an antiseptic to the nail plates and toes that have been treated, in order to prevent infection.
- Avoid cutting nails if force is required, if a toe is exuding purulent material or is gangrenous, or if a subungual neoplasm is suspected.
- The feet of the diabetic patient should be treated with special care, preferably by a podiatrist.

Oral and Dental Care

Loss of teeth in the aged usually occurs from degeneration of the periodontal structures: gingivae, alveolar bone, and periodontal membrane. Half of the elderly have no natural teeth. Although a good percentage of these people have dentures, many do not wear them or wear them infrequently for a variety of reasons, including traumatic ulcers and the need for refitting or replacement. Many mistakenly believe that there is no need for dental consultation after the teeth have been removed and replaced by dentures.

Dry mouth, abnormal taste, and burning sensations (from atrophy of taste buds, dehydration, reduced salivary flow, iron and vitamin B complex deficiencies, and low estrogen levels) are common complaints. All of these may result in poor eating habits, which further produce degeneration of oral tissues.

The components of dental care for the aging patient (gerodontics) include eating a proper diet, maintaining healthy oral and denture-bearing structures, being motivated to seek proper care, and having adequate dental services available. The objectives of dental care are to preserve the remaining teeth and to carry out reconstructive procedures, modifying and adding to existing appliances and designing and fitting partial or complete sets of dentures.

If an elderly person has not worn dentures for a long time, it may be wise not to secure dentures but to make sure that the diet has all of the proper nutrients, since adequate nutrition is fundamental to the health of the oral structures.

Receding gums and denture movement accentuate the spaces between the teeth. Tooth brushing will not remove retained food particles, and toothpicks and dental floss will be required. An electric toothbrush or Water Pic is helpful in carrying out an effective oral hygiene program, especially in patients who have tremors, paralysis, or other physical impairments. Persons with decreased salivary flow resulting in cracked lips and fissures of the tongue should be encouraged to drink more water and to use soothing mouthwashes. Unfortunately, not much can be done to correct the problem, since the salivary glands may have undergone regressive changes.

The dentures should be regarded as prostheses. The person with dentures requires a nonabrasive denture-cleaning paste and denture brush. Particles of food that harbor bacteria or yeast can become lodged in the mouth area that is covered by the dentures. Dentures should be stored in fresh water at night.

For the patient who is confined to bed, mouth care should be supervised by the nurse. By carefully evaluating the condition of the mouth, the nurse is able to meet the patient's nutritional needs more effectively, to request dental attention when necessary, and to prevent infections. Any areas of chronic irritation, ulceration, whitening, and thickening should be referred for evaluation by the dentist.

Elimination Problems

Many elderly people become very concerned about bowel elimination and have problems with constipation because of altered gastrointestinal motility, decreased mucus secretion, and changes in muscle tone and elasticity of the colon, as well as changes in diet.

Problems of constipation and bowel incontinence often can be reduced through systematic habit training. While the patient is in the hospital, a bedside commode is easier to use and is more acceptable than a bedpan. Indwelling catheters should not be used to treat urinary incontinence; evidence shows that catheterization is a means of introducing organisms into the urinary tract. The cause of urinary incontinence should be determined. If no pathologic problem can be found, fear, social withdrawal, and loneliness may be factors.

- Experience in long-term care facilities has shown that systematic bladder and bowel training programs, combined with exercises, ambulation, and social activities, can produce significant decreases in the frequency of incontinence.

Sensory Impairments

Approximately 30% of all older persons have hearing loss, which is understandably the most difficult sensory loss for the elderly. Perhaps only one ear is involved or only certain ranges of sound may not be detectable. Whatever the difficulty, simple gestures and signals by the nurse may be understood clearly. Most patients who have diminished hearing are reluctant to call attention to it; therefore, it is up to the nurse to take the initiative in discovering this or any other handicap. The nursing approach to the individual with a hearing loss is discussed on page 1264.

Further, *visual impairment* may predispose the patient to accidents. Grab rails in the bathroom should be available, and all rooms should be well lighted, especially the path from bed to bathroom at night. The bed should be equipped with siderails to remind the patient to remain in bed at night. Siderails can also be held onto when the patient is raising himself to a sitting position and when turning over in bed.

Appearance

An attractive appearance is a great morale booster; to look well implies that one feels well. Since older people at times neglect their appearance, they need to be encouraged to look their best.

Both men and women enjoy nice clothes or a bit of color to brighten their appearance. Even some conservative men seem to like bright-colored pajamas. A small flower on the lapel of a man's bathrobe will brighten his spirits. A shave and a haircut do for a man what lipstick does for most women. Almost everyone finds the fragrance of certain dusting powders and colognes refreshing. This has special appeal when the scent is in keeping with the individual's personality. Surely the nurse will be able to find at least one thing that will help immeasurably to cheer an older patient.

Physical Activity/Rehabilitation

The goal of rehabilitation of the elderly patient is to reestablish self-care and, if possible, to improve ambulatory capacity. An exercise program in accordance with the patient's exercise tolerance is necessary to achieve this goal.

Walking activities should be encouraged as soon as the patient is able. Instruction in the proper use of aids, such as a walker, crutches, or a cane, must be given to the patient, as well as reasons for why it is important to maintain proper body posture and how to achieve it.

The dangers of prolonged bed rest, even prolonged sitting, are numerous and should be avoided even when the patient objects to a change. The rocking chair is more helpful than a straight or an overstuffed chair since it enables all but the most feeble to exercise with dignity at any time. Use of the calf and forearm muscles encourages venous return and increases cardiac output. Pulmonary ventilation is increased and hypostatic pulmonary congestion is discouraged. From the psychological point of view, rocking is socially acceptable; in such a chair, one can participate in home activities and be an integral part of the family.

Recreation

In the words of Piersol and Bortz, "The society which fosters research to save human life cannot escape responsibility for the life thus extended. It is for science not only to add years to life, but more important, to add life to the years."

Recreation is more than just having fun; it is fundamental to physical and mental well-being. No matter how old or disabled one becomes, the desire for the dignity that comes only through purposeful activity is never lost.

As soon as the patient is capable of participating in any type of group activity or is willing to undertake some project on an individual basis, such activity should be planned. The nurse can enlist the help of other personnel, such as occupational therapists and volunteer aides, and of members of the family in organizing activities designed to occupy the patient's time pleasantly, maintain his enthusiasm, and keep him in possession of his faculties and aware of his own personal worth. If a project is successful in this respect, one of the most important goals in the therapeutic process will have been accomplished.

No plan for rehabilitation will be successful unless it is continued beyond the walls of the hospital. Continuity of care can be planned with the community health nurse and other community agencies as well as the patient's own family. In many instances, the geriatric patient does not have a family that he can return to. Real adjustments may have to be made. The smoother the transfer, the more graceful will be the resumption of normal living for the elderly person.

The Family

The idea that older people are rejected by their families is an exaggeration. Old people are not usually ignored by their families nor estranged from their children. Many live within a day's journey of a family member. The cooperation of the family should be enlisted as early as possible in the management of the patient in order to assure convalescent care and protection against possible complications and further recurrences of the disease. Providing information on aging is helpful to families in promoting understanding, support, and improved relationships with older family members.

A developmental crisis occurs when the mental or physical health of an aged parent begins to decline. The inability of the parent to live independently places new demands on adult children who are faced with making a critical decision at this turning point in their own lives. As the shift in roles occurs, there may be feelings of guilt and anger, unresolved conflicts, financial strain, and social pressures. The nurse must recognize and understand that the family is likely to have ambivalent feelings about caring for the parent. Alternative options that the family may consider are provision of support services, such as homemaker services and Meals on Wheels; visits by the community health nurse; and more frequent contacts by the family to assist the patient to continue living in the present setting. If the patient cannot continue to be independent, an extended care facility or retirement home may be the answer. Or the children may have the parent live with one of them, although potential areas of conflict may arise with respect to lack of space and privacy, entertainment of friends (both of adult children and parents), expenses, recreation, vacation, child rearing, and management of household tasks. Such conflicts should be anticipated, identified, and discussed, and steps should be taken to resolve these problems at an early date. The nurse can assist in providing the therapeutic climate in which the family can ventilate their feelings, reduce anxiety and guilt, explore options, and establish priorities. Nursing management of the elderly patient is summarized in Chart 15-3.

▷ The Elderly Patient Undergoing Surgery

Surgery imposes physical and psychological stress, but because of advances in evaluation techniques, surgical procedures, anesthetic techniques, and monitoring capabilities, older patients tolerate elective surgery surprisingly well. The principle to be kept in mind during preoperative evaluation, surgery, and postoperative care is that the aged patient has *less physiologic reserve* (the ability of an organ to return to normal after a disturbance in its equilibrium) than younger patients. The special requirements for optimum results following surgery on an elderly patient include: (1) skillful preoperative evaluation and treatment; (2) experienced and careful anesthesia and surgery; and (3) meticulous and competent postoperative management. The hazards of surgery for the aged are proportional to the number and severity of coexisting diseases and the nature and duration of the operative procedure.

Psychological Considerations

Confidence will be strengthened if the geriatric patient fully realizes that the contemplated operation is less hazardous than the disease it is expected to remedy. Years of living have a tendency to broaden the patient's ability to adjust to crises. On the other hand, one must not assume that the patient is unconcerned or values life less than a younger patient. In old age, one is more conscious of the shortness of the remaining years. The patient may require repeated explanation, clarification, and positive reassurance. The objective is to secure the patient's *active* cooperation; if this is to be achieved, a kindly, considerate approach is basic. The psychological preparation consists of giving simple and straightforward information about what can be expected before and after surgery.

Preoperative Assessment

A careful preoperative evaluation is done in order to assess the patient's physical status and his ability to adapt to operative stress and to correct, as far as possible, existing defects. All medication that the patient is taking should be brought into the hospital and reviewed since some drugs interact with anesthetic agents and can produce dangerous side-effects.

Specific instructions are given in deep breathing and movement of the extremities, and the reasons why these actions are to the patient's advantage are presented.

Preparation for surgery demands a meticulous evaluation of the cardiovascular, respiratory, and renal systems as well as the nutritional and hydration status of the patient. Although the patient may be admitted for one specific problem, frequently there are several degenerative diseases affecting vital systems. Ideally, all deficiencies should be corrected before the patient is taken to the operating room; in reality, some compromises are necessary. After data gathering and assessment are completed, the anesthesia plan, surgical procedure, and postoperative activities are discussed by appropriate members of the health team.

Cardiovascular Function Assessment. Cardiovascular diseases are the most common abnormalities in the elderly

Chart 15-3
Summary of the Principles Underlying the Nursing Management of the Elderly Patient

1. Growth and adaptation continue to occur when the individual's strengths and potential are recognized and reinforced.

2. Nursing care must be individualized, taking into consideration the patient's past experiences, needs, and individual goals.

3. Realistic and attainable goals, which are understood by the patient, are set up to help establish a sense of accomplishment and purpose.
   - Engage in mutual goal setting when possible; preserve a reason for living.
   - Keep communicating to the patient the planned goals of care.
   - Support the patient's belief in his/her own inner resources.

4. The patient should be an active participant in the plan of care.
   - Learn something about the patient before the initial encounter; find out the patient's strengths.
   - Consult the patient's preferences.
   - Concentrate on what the patient can do.
   - Ask the patient's opinions.
   - Encourage the patient to make choices and decisions.
   - Avoid making decisions for the patient; this promotes low self-esteem, dependency, and depression.
   - Support the patient during periods of anxiety. Direct attention to the gains being made.
   - Urge the patient to remain active.

5. Nursing activities should be done *with* the patient rather than *for* the patient.

6. Necessary modifications and compromises imposed by the physiologic limits of aging must be reflected in the medical and nursing management of the patient.

7. The individuality of the patient should be encouraged—to preserve identity and sense of control.
   - Encourage the patient to have and use personal possessions that help to bridge the gap between past and present.
   - Respect the patient's right to self-direction.
   - Give the patient *time* to express his or her feelings.
   - Help the patient to retain the social graces.
   - Help the patient to cope with thoughts of death.

8. Elderly persons should be kept in the mainstream of life to prevent physical, emotional, and mental deterioration.
   - Avoid removing the element of challenge. Encourage contact with others.
   - Work out a "buddy system" to prevent loneliness and isolation.
   - Stimulate mental acuity and sensory input.
   - Encourage physical activity.
   - Share your world with the patient.
   - Remember the patient's preferences; accept his or her idiosyncracies.
   - Provide opportunities for the patient to do some tasks of daily living (water plants; wash own stockings).
   - Provide meaningful diversional activity.
   - Give the patient something to look forward to.

9. The patient's potentialities should be utilized.
   - Select activities that are in keeping with lifelong interests.
   - Do not attempt to alter lifelong character and behavior patterns.
   - Give the patient time to listen, to learn, and to adapt.
   - Help the patient to learn new ways to maintain independence.

surgical patient. The status of the heart's pumping action and the adequacy of the blood vessels are determined, and baseline electrocardiograms are obtained. An effort is made to determine the level of the patient's normal activity and then to evaluate cardiovascular reserve. The cardiovascular response to stress may be assessed before and after exercise.

In the presence of atherosclerosis, the heart, brain, and kidneys are very sensitive to the further reduction of perfusion and oxygenation that anesthesia may produce. The ECG will demonstrate evidences of hypertrophy and conduction abnormalities. Cardiac arrhythmias can often be controlled and congestive heart failure improved, but other manifestations of arteriosclerosis are altered very little by preoperative treatment. Coronary artery disease is considered the most serious heart disease of this age group; its presence increases the operative risk. Medical treatment of anginal symptoms should precede surgery.

The presence of arrhythmias, congestive heart failure, coronary insufficiency, and severe diastolic hypertension increases the mortality rate. If the patient is in congestive heart failure, careful adjustment of digitalis levels, administration of diuretics (with care taken not to dehydrate the patient), sodium restriction, and bed rest are indicated before surgery. As with other patients, tranquilizing drugs, reserpine, propranolol, and monoamine-oxidase inhibitors are preferably discontinued 10 days before the operation. (Under stress, these agents may produce alterations in cardiovascular responses.) If the patient is hypertensive, the blood pressure is controlled before elective surgery and, if possible, is maintained below 160/100 mm Hg.

Peripheral Vascular Assessment. Varying degrees of arterial insufficiency and tissue ischemia are present in the aged. Easy fatigability and numbness of an extremity on exercise, with relief on rest, are common. The peripheral pulses, including the temporal, carotid, brachial, radial, femoral, popliteal, dorsalis pedis, and posterior tibial pulses, should be evaluated and appropriate ones marked before surgery.

Making sure that the patient avoids positions that permit venous stasis or pressure on the blood vessels is a nursing responsibility. Thus, the patient should be instructed to avoid crossing his legs while sitting. The head and foot of the bed must not be elevated at the same time since this position encourages venous stagnation in the pelvic veins. Elastic stockings, if worn throughout the hospital stay, help to keep venous blood in the deeper circulation. Sitting in a chair with the feet hanging down should be discouraged. Since activity improves circulation, the patient should be ambulated as much as possible.

Respiratory Assessment. Although there is some degree of impaired pulmonary function in all postoperative patients, the elderly are at special risk for pulmonary complications because of changes in the lungs and chest owing to aging. The lungs of the elderly lose some of their elastic recoil, and chest compliance is reduced. There is a progressive decrease in vital capacity.

Preoperative assessment includes history, physical examination, chest x-ray, pulmonary function studies, and arterial blood gas analysis. Graded stress testing is directed toward eliciting stress responses. If dyspnea develops, it must be determined whether shortness of breath is the result of a cardiac problem, underlying pulmonary disease, or both.

While caring for the patient, look at the nature and quality of respirations, shortness of breath, coughing and sputum production, and smoking habits. Infection, abnormal states of hydration, and retained secretions are risk factors that respond to therapy before surgery.

- After the operation, the nursing actions are directed toward ensuring adequate hydration, checking for evidence of retained secretions by means of auscultation of the chest, promoting frequent deep breathing and coughing to prevent pulmonary complications, and encouraging early ambulation.

Renal Function Assessment. Disorders of renal function and urinary disturbances are common in the elderly. Between the ages of 50 and 80, the average urea clearance declines 50%. A serum creatinine test and blood urea nitrogen test are done preoperatively to identify renal impairment so that suitable measures can be taken to prevent renal failure. Other tests are done as indicated. In the male, urethral stricture and urethritis, and prostatic hyperplasia and prostatitis are frequently observed urinary problems. It is wise to have the elderly male patient practice using the urinal while lying in bed in the preoperative period since voiding during the postoperative period may be a real problem.

Fluid, Electrolyte, and Nutritional Management

Electrolyte and fluid deficits should be restored before surgery is undertaken. Serum potassium levels are evaluated since a low potassium level increases susceptibility to possible ventricular arrhythmias and digitalis intoxication. When an older patient is given a transfusion, the central

venous pressure should be monitored. The urinary output also serves as a guide in the correction of dehydration states.

The patient may suffer from nutritional deficiency resulting from chronic illness, socioeconomic factors, and poor dietary habits. The goal of nutritional support is to supply the necessary calories and protein to meet metabolic demands and prevent nitrogen loss. Supportive feedings, including oral, hyperalimentation, and tube feedings, are given as necessary. The patient's weight, fluid, and electrolyte balance as well as renal and hepatic functions are monitored.

Preoperative Medication

The purposes of preoperative medications are to calm the patient and to depress secretions. Since drug sensitivity is usually increased in elderly individuals, a conservative approach is used and smaller dosages generally are given. Preoperative medication may not be given at all to the acutely ill or debilitated patient. The preoperative medication may be given to the aged patient earlier on the morning of surgery because of delayed absorption.

Anesthesia

The anesthesia chosen depends on the patient's physiologic status, the length of the operation, and the experience and preference of the anesthesiologist. The arterial partial pressure of oxygen may be temporarily lowered during induction, intubation, and extubation, causing arrhythmias in the elderly. All inhalational anesthetics are potential respiratory and myocardial depressants.

Regional anesthesia, especially spinal anesthesia, is useful for patients undergoing transurethral resection, inguinal herniorrhaphy, and orthopedic procedures and for poor-risk patients who would poorly tolerate inhalation anesthesia. It must be remembered that even though the blood vessels of the elderly patient may be quite inelastic, a profound drop in blood pressure may occur.

If the drop in blood pressure is sudden and prolonged, it may lead to circulatory insufficiency. This in turn may cause cerebral ischemia and thrombosis, followed by embolism, infarction, and anoxemia. To maintain blood pressure at a normal level is of utmost importance in these patients.

It is well to remember that excessive or over-rapid infusions may cause pulmonary edema.

Postoperative Management

The immediate postoperative care is the same as that for any patient, but additional support is given to any impaired function of the cardiovascular, pulmonary, and renal systems.

- Since the possibility of shock is greater in the older patient, it is necessary to monitor the pulse, respiratory rate, blood pressure, and urinary output (and central venous pressure and blood gas determinations if indicated) and to watch for deviation from baseline readings.

Transfer of the patient from the operating room table to the bed is done *slowly* and carefully while monitoring the effects of this action on the blood pressure and assessing for evidence of hypoxia. Special attention is given to keeping the patient warm since body temperature in the elderly is labile. Position should be changed frequently not only for comfort, since lying in one position can be painful, but also to avoid pulmonary and circulatory complications.

Prevention of Complications

Since the patient has a lesser margin of reserve, it is important that complications be prevented, for one postoperative complication can lead to another. The system that is most defective usually fails first. The aged cannot tolerate prolonged periods of stress.

Shock.   Shock causes death more frequently among patients over 60 than among younger patients. An older person cannot tolerate a reduction of blood volume or hypotension for even a short period of time, especially since the heart and blood vessels do not constrict as readily. An added problem for the patient who has sclerotic and narrowed arteries and develops hypotension from shock is a serious reduction in the perfusion of coronary or cerebral vessels. Therefore, the blood pressure must be maintained as close as possible to the patient's normal blood pressure. The urinary output, an indication of adequate blood volume and perfusion, should be between 15 ml and 25 ml per hour.

In treating shock with fluid replacement, it is important to monitor the patient's central venous pressure to prevent overloading of the circulation, which places an unnecessary burden on the heart.

For the treatment of shock, see pages 403–407.

Postoperative Respiratory Complications.   The most frequent respiratory complication of the aged is pneumonia. Decreased lung expansion, weakness, relative fixity of the rib cage, and drug depression of cough reflexes contribute to such complications.

- Measures to prevent respiratory complications include frequent turning, early ambulation, use of small doses of analgesia, removal of tracheobronchial secretions, and breathing exercises.

Yawning is an effective way to prevent or correct atelectasis. Taking a deep breath and holding it as long as possible helps to increase ventilation. If the tracheobronchial tree cannot be cleared by suction and aspiration, a tracheostomy may be necessary.

Gastrointestinal Distention and Ileus.   Gastrointestinal distention and ileus (cessation of intestinal motor action) is encountered following extensive trauma and intra-abdominal operations as well as in systemic and abdominal disease states. Retroperitoneal hemorrhage, intra-abdominal hemorrhage, lack of muscle tone of the large bowel, and fecal impaction can produce ileus, as can the use of narcotics, which can reduce peristalsis. A common cause of postoperative distention is retention of swallowed air in the gastrointestinal tract.

- To prevent postoperative distention, a nasogastric tube may be introduced into the gastric lumen. Management of ileus usually requires decompression by intubation into the small bowel. Keep in mind that an indwelling nasogastric tube in an older patient can cause erosion and perforation of the esophagus and can prevent bronchial secretions from being raised. In addition, nasogastric suction is not well tolerated in the elderly.

In older people, the sluggish peristalsis in the colon sometimes results in incomplete evacuation and therefore in retention of fecal material in the sigmoid colon and the rectum. The absorption of fluid produces a hard fecal mass that is irritating to the intestine and often produces frequent small stools, a sort of pseudodiarrhea. Digital examination reveals a hard mass of fecal material in the rectum. When the mass is broken up by the finger and by enemas, the symptoms are relieved.

Hydration.   Hydration and replacement of electrolyte losses following surgery are the same as for any surgical patient. Substantial amounts of potassium are lost immediately after the operation from fever, acidosis, or breakdown of tissue. Certain considerations should be noted when parenteral infusions are given to elderly patients.

- After the first few postoperative hours, the patient's head and shoulders are raised during replacement therapy in order to reduce the pressure in the pulmonary circuit and avoid pulmonary edema.
- Since an older person's heart and circulatory system cannot stand overloading, infusions and transfusions are given slowly. If there is any question, central venous pressure monitoring will reveal circulatory overloading if it is present.
- Usually, the older patient needs to be encouraged to drink enough fluids. An output of 1 liter or more indicates that intake is sufficient. Obviously, the recording of intake and output is important.

Management of Postoperative Pain.   Postoperative pain relief may be achieved with fairly small amounts of narcotic drugs, such as codeine. The side-effects of narcotics—depressed ventilation and diminished circulation—are dangerous. Enough drug should be given to reduce the pain, but not enough to make it difficult for the patient to perform the required exercises. Moving about is much more desirable than being in a prolonged stuporous condition from oversedation. A certain degree of relaxation can also be achieved with reassurance.

Exercise and Ambulation.   Activity in bed as well as out of bed is essential to recovery.

- Bed exercises include turning from side to side, flexing and extending the legs and the arms, deep breathing, and deliberate coughing.
- In getting out of bed, the patient should turn to his operated side and bend his knees upward. As he swings his feet over the side of the bed, the nurse can assist him to a sitting position.
- Sitting positions that promote venous stasis in the lower extremities are to be avoided. *Ambulation means that the patient walks, not sits in a chair.*

Patients with preexisting cardiovascular and pulmonary conditions should be watched carefully because overexertion may cause a breakdown of these functions. As the period out of bed is gradually increased, the stability of the vital signs serves as a measure of the patient's reaction to exercise and ambulation activities.

Convalescence

Convalescence in the elderly may be difficult because strength is regained slowly. Above all, the older patient needs a great deal of patience. Some authorities advocate that 1 day be allowed for each decade of one's age for convalescence from acute illness. Patients often find this difficult to accept.

Every attempt should be made to maintain an interest in people and to prevent psychological withdrawal. A major concern for the patient and the family is how care will be provided following discharge from the hospital. Of course, this challenge should be addressed by all concerned upon admission. The patient may be fearful of returning home alone, yet the children may not have room to accommodate another person in the house. If the patient must remain alone, there is a problem of increased isolation owing to lessened activity following surgery.

The older patient must be encouraged to become proficient in self-care in order to become self-sufficient as quickly as possible. Thus, the nurse must refrain from becoming overprotective when caring for an elderly patient, but at the same time should provide necessary emotional support as plans are made for the future.

▷ Bibliography

Books

Birren JE and Sloane RB. Handbook of Mental Health and Aging. Englewood Cliffs, New Jersey, Prentice–Hall, 1980.

Blazer DG. Depression in Late Life. St Louis, CV Mosby, 1982.

Burnside IM (ed). Psychosocial Nursing. Care of the Aged. New York, McGraw–Hill, 1980.

Burnside IM (ed). Nursing and the Aged. New York, McGraw–Hill, 1981.

Butler RN and Lewis MJ. Aging and Mental Health, 3rd ed. St Louis, CV Mosby, 1982.

Comfort A. Practice of Geriatric Psychiatry. New York, Elsevier, 1980.

Croft LH. Sexuality in Later Life: A Counseling Guide for Physicians. Boston, Wright, 1982.

Ebersole P and Hess P. Toward Healthy Aging: Human Needs and Nursing Response. St Louis, CV Mosby, 1981.

Eyde DR and Rich JA. Psychological Distress in Aging. Gaithersburg, Maryland, Aspen Systems Corp, 1982.

Fish AA. A New Look at Senility. Springfield, Illinois, Charles C Thomas, 1981.

Forbes EJ and Fitzsimons VM. The Older Adult. A Process for Wellness. St Louis, CV Mosby, 1981.

Futrell M et al. Primary Health Care of the Older Adult. North Scituate, Duxbury Press, 1980.

Geist H. The Psychological Aspects of the Aging Process with Sociological Implications. Huntington, New York, Robert E Krieger, 1981.

Harris DK and Cole WE. Sociology of Aging. Boston, Houghton Mifflin, 1980.

Hendricks JC and Hendricks CD. Aging in Mass Society. Cambridge, Winthrop, 1981.

Hodkinson HM. An Outline of Geriatrics, 2nd ed. New York, Academic Press, 1981.

Hogstel MO. Nursing Care of the Older Adult. New York, John Wiley & Sons, 1981.

Hoyer S. The Aging Brain. New York, Springer–Verlag, 1982.

Johnson WR and Kempton N. Sex Education and Counseling of Special Groups: The Mentally and Physically Disabled, Ill and Elderly. Springfield, Illinois, Charles C Thomas, 1981.

Kane RA and Kane RL. Assessing the Elderly. Lexington, Lexington Books, 1981.

Keller A and Ahmed PI. Aging. New York, Elsevier, 1982.

Koft TH. Long-term Care: An Approach to Serving the Frail Elderly. Boston, Little, Brown & Co, 1982.

Levenson AJ and Hall RCW. Neuropsychiatric Manifestations of Physical Disease in the Elderly. New York, Raven Press, 1981.

Mezey MD, Rauckhorst LH, and Stokes SA. Health Assessment of the Older Individual. New York, Springer, 1980.

Moment GB. Nutritional Approaches to Aging Research. Boca Raton, CRC Press, 1982.

Murray R, Huelskoetter MM, and O'Driscoll D. The Nursing Process in Later Maturity. Englewood Cliffs, New Jersey, Prentice–Hall, 1980.

Neuhaus RH and Neuhaus RH. Successful Aging. New York, John Wiley & Sons, 1982.

O'Hara–Devereaux M et al. Eldercare, A Practical Guide to Clinical Geriatrics. New York, Grune & Stratton, 1980.

Pegels CC. Health Care of the Elderly. Gaithersburg, Maryland, Aspen Systems Corp, 1981.

Poe WD and Holloway RA. Drugs and the Aged. New York, McGraw–Hill, 1980.

Rowe JW and Besdine RW. Health and Disease in Old Age. Boston, Little, Brown & Co, 1982.

Schaie KW and Geiwitz J. Adult Development and Aging. Boston, Little, Brown & Co, 1982.

Slade WR Jr (ed). Geriatric Neurology. Selected Topics. Mt Kisco, Futura, 1981.

Smith EL and Serfass RC (eds). Exercise and Aging: The Scientific Basis. Hillside, New Jersey, Enslow, 1981.

Smith I. Medical Care for the Elderly. New York, SP Medical and Scientific Books, 1982.

Watson WH. Aging and Social Behavior: An Introduction to Social Gerontology. Monterey, Wadsworth Health Sciences Div, 1982.

Weber GH (ed.) Assisting the Elderly in Long-term Care. Springfield, Illinois, Charles C Thomas, 1981.

Wells T. Aging and Health Promotion. Gaithersburg, Maryland, Aspen Systems Corp, 1981.

Wolanin MO and Phillips LRF. Confusion: Prevention and Care. St Louis, CV Mosby, 1981.

Articles

Bailey PA. Physical assessment of the elderly. Top Clin Nurs 1981 Apr; 3(1):15–19.

Barrowclough F. Do they really need all those drugs? Nurs Mirror 1982 Nov 10; 155(19):22–24.

Barrowclough F and Pegg M. Drugs in the later years of life. Nurs Mirror 1982 Nov 10; 155(19):25–26.

Beaton SR. Reminiscence in old age. Nurs Forum 1980; 19(3):271–283.

Blazer D. Diagnosing organic mental disorders in the elderly. Am Fam Physician 1982 May; 25(5):139–145.

Breuer JM. A handbook of assistive devices for the handicapped elderly. Phys Occ Ther Geriatrics 1981 Winter; 1(2):1–77.

Brewer GK. Promoting healthful aging through strengthening family ties. Top Clin Nurs 1981 Apr; 3(1):45–50.

Cohen S and Bunke E. Programmed Instruction: Sensory changes in the elderly. Am J Nurs 1981 Oct; 81(10):1851–1880.

Eliopoulos C. Chronic care and the elderly: Impact on the client, the family and the nurse. Top Clin Nurs 1981 Apr; 3(1):71–83.

Evashwick C, Conrad D, and Lee F. Factors related to utilization of dental service by the elderly. Am J Public Health 1982 Oct; 72(10):1129–1135.

Exercise: Getting the elderly going. Patient Care 1982 Oct 15; 16(17):67–110.

Hays A. Caring for the hospitalized elderly. Am J Nurs 1982 June; 82(6):930–931.

Heller BR and Gaynor EB. Hearing loss and aural rehabilitation of the elderly. Top Clin Nurs 1981 Apr; 3(1):21–29.

Irvine PW. The hearing-impaired elderly patient. Postgrad Med 1982 Oct; 72(4):115–118.

Lancaster J. Maximizing psychological adaptation in an aging population. Top Clin Nurs 1981 Apr; 3(1):31–43.

Lundin DV. Teaching the elderly proper drug use. Postgrad Med 1981 Apr; 69(4):169–170.

Marcinek MA. The right to die: In support of passive euthanasia. Nurs Forum 1981; 20(20):129–137.

Moyer NC. Health promotion and the assessment of health habits in the elderly. Top Clin Nurs 1981 Apr; 3(1):51–58.

Patel KP. A prescribing dilemma. Nurs Mirror 1982 Nov 10; 155(19):26–30.

Rabins PV, Mace NW, and Lucas MJ. The impact of dementia on the family. JAMA 1982 July 16; 248(3):333–345.

Ramos LY. Oral hygiene for the elderly. Am J Nurs 1981 Aug; 81(8):1468–1469.

Reiff TR. The essentials of a geriatric evaluation. Geriatrics 1980 May; 35(5):59–68.

Richardson K. Hope and flexibility: Your keys to helping OBS patients. Nursing '82 1982 June; 12(6):64–69.

Towns JE. How to understand and communicate with a person in sorrow. Nurs Forum 1980; 19(3):301–309.

Towsley MM. The use of family therapy in terminal illness and death. J Psychosocial Nurs and Ment Health Serv 1982 Jan; 20(1):17–22.

Walker JI. Dementia: Positive steps to help maintain function. Postgrad Med 1982 July; 72(1):167.

Yoselle H. Sexuality in the later years. Top Clin Nurs 1981 Apr; 3(1):59–70.

Agencies
Governmental

National Institute of Mental Health, Special Mental Health Program Division, Center for Studies of Mental Health of the Aging, 5600 Fishers Lane, Rockville, MD 20857

National Institute on Aging, National Institutes of Health, Bldg 31, 9000 Rockville Pike, Bethesda, MD 20205

U.S. Department of Health and Human Services, Office of Human Development Services, Administration on Aging, North Building, 330 Independence Avenue, S.W., Washington, D.C. 20201

Voluntary

Action for Independent Maturity, 1909 K Street, N.W., Washington, D.C. 20049

Alzheimer's Disease Society, 32 Broadway, New York, NY 10004

American Association of Retired Persons, 1909 K Street, N.W., Washington, D.C. 20049

American Geriatrics Society, Ten Columbus Circle, New York, NY 10019

American Podiatry Association, 20 Chevy Chase Circle, N.W., Washington, D.C. 20015

Gerontological Society of America, 1835 K Street, Suite 305, Washington, D.C. 20006

Gray Panthers, 3635 Chestnut Street, Philadelphia, PA 19104

Legal Services for the Elderly, 132 W. 43rd Street, 3rd Floor, New York, NY 10036

National Alliance of Senior Citizens, 101 Park Washington Court, Falls Church, VA 22046

National Council of Senior Citizens, 925 15th Street, N.W., Washington, D.C. 20005

National Council on the Aging, 600 Maryland Avenue, S.W., Washington, D.C. 20024

National Geriatrics Society, 212 W. Wisconsin Avenue, 3rd Floor, Milwaukee, WI 53203

National Institute on Aging, Work and Retirement, % National Council on Aging, 600 Maryland Avenue, S.W., Washington, D.C. 20024

National Safety Council, 444 N. Michigan Avenue, Chicago, IL 60611

16

The Person Experiencing Pain

Pain disables and distresses more people than any single disease entity. It is probably the most common and compelling reason why a person seeks medical assistance. Most of the medical–surgical problems included in this book are associated with pain, resulting either from the disease process, diagnostic tests, or therapeutic procedures.

Ironically, little is known about pain. *Algology*—the study of pain—is a new science. Most experts consider pain a mysterious phenomenon that defies precise definition. At the very least, it appears to have three components: (1) a stimulus, physical or mental; (2) a bodily sensation of hurting; and (3) the reaction of the person experiencing it.

The nurse spends more time with the patient with pain than any other member of the health team and therefore has the opportunity to make a significant contribution toward increasing the patient's comfort and relieving pain. The physician must seek to verify the patient's complaint of pain by establishing the cause and treating it. The nurse, in addition to assisting the physician with this goal, also makes a major contribution to palliative pain relief—relief of pain that does not necessarily involve curing the cause of the pain.

In actual clinical practice, when direct care is given to a patient with pain, it is virtually essential that the nurse adopt the patient's point of view about his pain. Unless he is a malingerer, who consciously lies, the patient does not doubt that he has pain. A cardinal rule in the care of patients with pain is that *all pain is real,* regardless of its cause— even when the cause remains unknown. Therefore, the nurse's verification of pain is based simply upon the patient's indication that it exists.

Within this context, *the nursing definition of pain may be stated as whatever bodily hurt the patient says he has, existing whenever he says it does.* This definition encompasses two important points that are ultimately relevant to assessment, intervention, and evaluation.

First, the nurse believes the patient when he indicates that he has pain. It is important to avoid making the erroneous judgment that the patient does not have pain because no physical origin can be identified. Although some painful sensations are initiated by or sustained by the individual's mental or psychological state, he actually feels a sensation of pain; he is not merely thinking or imagining that he has pain. Further, painful states initiated by psychological states, such as anxiety, are usually accompanied by physical changes, like decreased blood flow or muscle tension. Most painful sensations are the result of two sets of stimuli: (1) physical and (2) mental or emotional. Therefore, the assessment of pain involves obtaining information about both the physical and the mental or emotional causes of pain. Nursing intervention involves attempting to reduce the physical or emotional causes of pain.

The second point to keep in mind is that what the patient "says" about his pain need not be limited to verbal statements. Some patients cannot or will not verbalize. Therefore, the nurse is responsible for eliciting information from the patient and for observing the many nonverbal behaviors that indicate the presence of the pain sensation and all that the patient experiences in relation to his pain.

Some patients deny pain, and they pose a different assessment problem. While it is important to believe the patient who admits he has pain, it is equally important to be alert to patients who deny pain when they do in fact "hurt." A very common reason is fear of becoming addicted to narcotics. If the nurse suspects pain in a patient who denies it, she should explore with the patient her reason for suspecting pain, such as the fact that the disease is usually painful or that the patient frowns when he moves. The nurse should also explore with the patient any reason that may cause him to deny pain, such as fear of addiction or further treatment.

▷ Nursing Assessment

Assessment of the patient experiencing pain involves:

- Recognizing whether the pain is acute or chronic
- Identifying the phases of the experience
- Observing the patient's behavioral responses
- Identifying the factors that influence the pain and the patient's response to it

A thorough assessment is of the utmost importance. To help the patient with his pain, the nurse must know that pain is occurring and how it is affecting the patient. This is not always obvious. There may be a language barrier, or the patient may try to hide his pain. Or, the patient may exhibit minimal responses to pain and, therefore, may appear not to experience pain.

Differences Between Acute and Chronic Pain

Pain specialists agree that there are two types of pain—acute and chronic. The differences between acute and chronic pain have implications for both assessment and intervention.

The terms *acute* and *chronic* are temporal classifications of pain, that is, they have to do with the duration of pain. Quite simply, acute pain is of brief duration and chronic pain is prolonged. Acute does not necessarily mean severe; acute pain may range in intensity from mild to severe.

Acute Pain. *Acute pain,* which is a very common daily occurrence, is usually defined as an episode of pain that lasts from a split second to about 6 months. Classically, organic disease or injury is present, although healing may also be accompanied by acute pain. As the healing process progresses, the pain subsides and gradually disappears.

Injuries or diseases that cause acute pain may require treatment or may heal spontaneously. For example, a prick of the finger may heal rapidly, the pain subsiding quickly, perhaps within a few minutes. In the case of a more drastic condition, such as appendicitis, surgery may be necessary. In these cases, the pain decreases with healing of the injury or surgical trauma.

Chronic Pain. *Chronic pain* is sometimes defined simply as pain that lasts for 6 months or longer. Six months is a rather arbitrary period of time for differentiating between acute and chronic pain. An episode of pain may assume the characteristics of chronic pain long before 6 months has elapsed, or some types of pain may remain primarily acute in nature for longer than 6 months. Nevertheless, after 6 months, the majority of pain experiences are characterized by some of the major problems associated with chronic pain.

The following are four common types of chronic pain, that is, prolonged pain experiences: (1) recurrent acute pain, (2) pain with obvious ongoing peripheral pathology, (3) chronic benign pain that may have peripheral or central pathology, and (4) chronic intractable benign pain syndrome.

Recurrent acute pain is intermittent pain. The patient has fairly well-defined episodes of pain interspersed with pain-free intervals. However, these episodes may recur over a period of years. Thus, this is sometimes considered a type of chronic pain. Examples of recurrent acute pain are migraines, sickle cell crises, and exacerbations of rheumatoid arthritis.

Pain with ongoing peripheral pathology may be of limited or unlimited duration. An example of time-limited pain with obvious ongoing peripheral pathology is the pain related to cancer. The pain may be of limited duration because the patient is eventually relieved after months of painful treatments, or the patient may die from the disease. In either case, the pain is not expected to last indefinitely. An example of pain with ongoing peripheral pathology and unlimited duration is pain associated with degenerative arthritis.

Chronic benign pain (CBP) may be due to peripheral or central (brain and spinal cord) pathology. The pathology is often unclear, but it is not life-threatening, as in cancer. (Benign means nonmalignant). An example of CBP with central pathology is post-stroke syndrome following a brain infarct. Tic douloureux is an example of central and peripheral pathology. Low back pain, a very common example of CBP, may be due to peripheral pathology, such as ischemic muscles, or central pathology, such as emotions causing muscle tension. As long as the patient functions well in daily life in spite of his pain, he usually remains classified in this category of CBP.

Chronic intractable benign pain syndrome (CIBPS) has the same characteristics as CBP, but the patient copes poorly. For example, the patient with low back pain may begin to use his pain to avoid dealing with marital or employment problems. Eventually, he may cope poorly with his job or marriage.

▷ Phases of the Pain Experience

The patient may experience any or all of the three phases of a pain experience:

1. The anticipation of pain
2. The sensation of pain
3. The aftermath of pain

Each of these phases must be assessed because each requires nursing intervention, not just the phase during which pain is sensed. Even the patient who has relatively persistent and chronic pain may experience modified forms of these phases as the pain waxes and wanes in intensity.

The anticipation of pain is sometimes more difficult for the patient to bear than the actual sensation of pain. In addition, what happens, or fails to happen, during the anticipation phase profoundly affects the patient's response to the sensation of pain.

Of the three phases, the most frequently overlooked is probably the aftermath. However, close observation may reveal any number of behavioral responses indicating such feelings as fear, embarrassment, or guilt. These feelings may last from hours to months following the cessation of the pain sensation.

▷ Behavioral Responses

The patient's responses during any of the three phases of pain experience may be any one or a combination of a large number of possible reactions. These may include physiologic manifestations, verbal statements, vocal behaviors, facial expressions, body movements, physical contact with others, or alterations in response to the surrounding environment. These behaviors vary greatly from one person to another and may differ within the same person from one time to the next.

When the nurse observes the patient's behavioral response, the purpose is to identify the following:

1. The phase of pain the patient is experiencing (*i.e.,* anticipation, sensation, or aftermath).
2. The intensity of the patient's pain. Whenever possible, it is helpful to ask the patient to rate his pain on a verbal or numerical scale (*e.g.,* none, slight, moderate, severe, or very severe; or 0 to 10: 0 = no pain, 10 = worst possible pain).
3. The patient's tolerance for this particular painful sensation. Pain tolerance may be defined as the maximum intensity or duration of pain the person is willing to endure.
4. Characteristics of the painful sensation. These include location (see Fig. 16-1 for areas to which pain in various organs may be referred), duration, rhythmicity (periods of waxing and waning of the intensity or existence of pain), and quality (*e.g.,* pricking, burning, aching).
5. Effects of pain on activities of daily living (*e.g.,* sleep, appetite, concentration, interactions with others, and physical movement). (Acute pain is usually associated with anxiety, chronic pain with depression.)
6. What the patient believes will help him with his pain. Many patients have definite ideas about what will increase or decrease the intensity of their pain or what will make it more tolerable.
7. The patient's concern about his pain. This may include a wide variety of items, such as financial burdens, prognosis, interference with role performance, and body image changes.

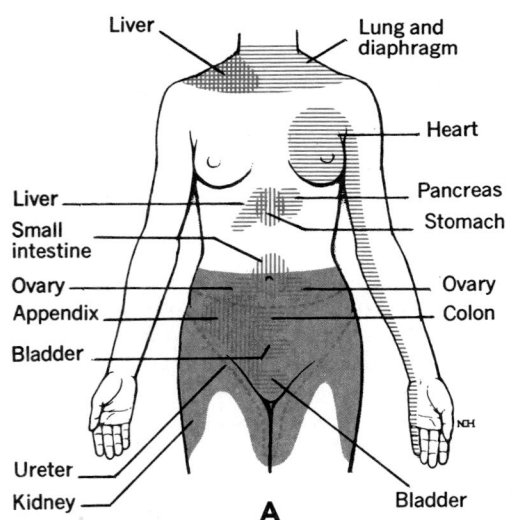
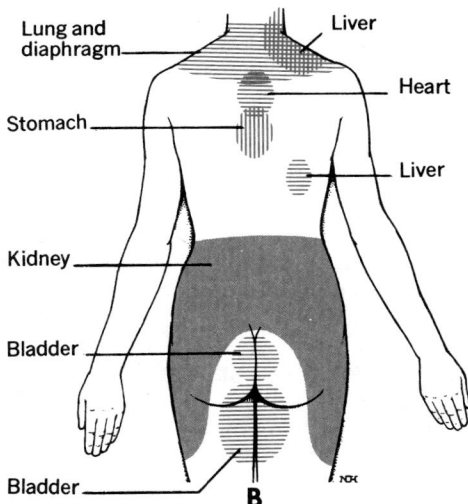

Figure 16-1.   Referred pain. (*A*) Anterior view. (*B*) Posterior view. (From Chaffee EE and Greisheimer EM: Basic Physiology and Anatomy, 3rd ed. Philadelphia, JB Lippincott.)

Adaptation of Responses to Pain

Assessment of physiologic and behavioral indications of pain sometimes is difficult, if not impossible, during periods of adaptation. During this time, observable clues to the existence and nature of pain may be absent or minimal. An understanding of adaptation in contrast to the acute pain model will help prevent the erroneous judgment that a patient has no pain simply because "he doesn't act as though he has pain" (Fig. 16-2).

Without realizing it, most members of the health team appear to be prejudiced in favor of the acute pain model. It is not unusual for the nurse or physician to doubt the statement of a calm patient who says, "I have severe pain in my right leg." One mistakenly tends to expect *all* patients with pain to exhibit at least some of the behavioral responses associated with acute pain. Such responses may be phys-

iologic in that there is an increase in pulse and respiratory rates and the occurrence of pallor and perspiration. The patient in acute pain may also cry, moan, frown, immobilize a body part, clench his fist, or withdraw.

The responses a particular patient makes to the sudden onset of acute pain are not necessarily the ones he makes when pain lasts more than a few minutes or when it becomes chronic. Obviously, the body is unable to sustain an intense physiologic reaction to pain for weeks or years, or even several hours.

Other behavioral manifestations of pain may also change drastically. The fatigue of being in pain may leave the patient too exhausted to moan or cry. He may sleep even with severe pain. Or, the patient may appear relaxed and involved in activities because he has become a master of the art of distracting himself from pain. It is unfortunate

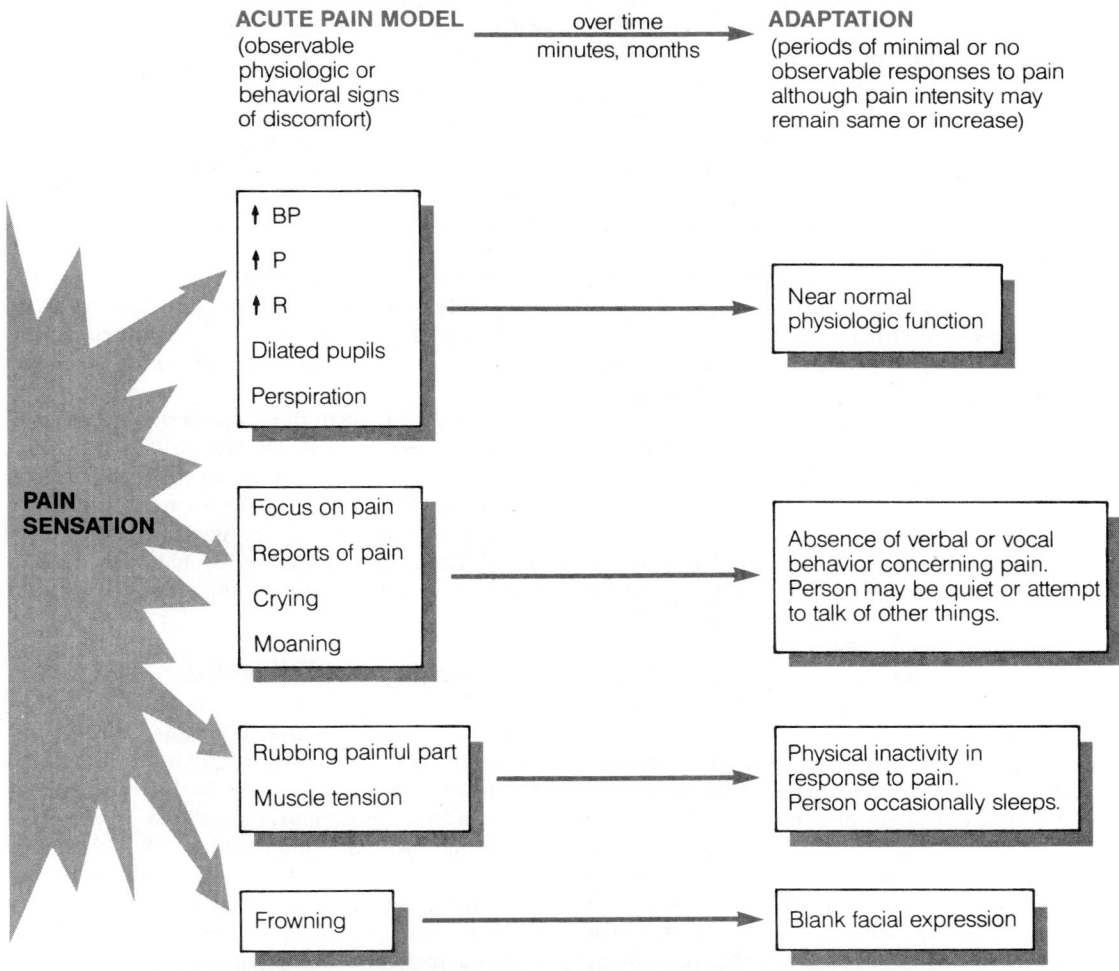

Figure 16-2. Examples of adaptation of responses to pain.

when the patient who has succeeded in minimizing the effect of chronic pain on his life is then doubted by others. His is a bitter victory.

Regardless of the type of adjustment made by the patient with chronic pain, pain over an extended period of time often produces behaviors typical of a disability. To some extent, the patient usually is unable to continue the activities and interpersonal relationships he engaged in before pain began. This may range from merely having to curtail his participation in some vigorous sport to being unable to take care of his personal needs, such as undressing.

Assessing the Harmful Effects of Pain

Special emphasis should be placed on assessing the harmful effects of pain. Frequently, the initial effect of a painful sensation is that of a helpful warning signal. Pain warns us that injury has occurred and that efforts must be taken to treat the injury or prevent further injury. After this initial warning signal, the existence of pain becomes a distressing and often harmful experience. Prolonged or chronic pain may prevent rehabilitation from an illness, or the pain itself may become a disability. Prolonged pain may result eventually in depression, perpetual fatigue owing to the inability to sleep well, weight gain, problems with concentration, job loss, and divorce or other interpersonal problems.

Acute pain may result in problems that retard recovery from the acute illness associated with the pain. Acute pain may disturb the amount and quality of sleep, decrease appetite, reduce fluid intake, and cause nausea and vomiting. For years, the value of rest and nutrition have been recognized as important factors in recovery from illness. When pain interferes with sleep and nutritional intake, the patient is deprived of his natural resources for getting well. In addition, the nausea, vomiting, or decreased fluid intake is a potential threat to fluid and electrolyte balance.

Assessing the existence of pain, its nature, and its distressing and harmful effects requires that the nurse ask specific questions and make careful observations. Global questions are not sufficient. For many reasons, patients tend to give incomplete and inaccurate reports of their pain experience unless the nurse asks for details.

Assessment Tools

The initial assessment of pain may be accomplished using the assessment tool in Figure 16-3. If identification of the location of pain is difficult, the drawings in Figure 16-4 may also be used. Once completed, these forms may become a part of the health record. As the nurse gains experience in the assessment of pain, it may become apparent that the tool needs to be expanded.

To the extent possible, the information on the assessment tool should come from the patient. The health record and the patient's family may supplement the information obtained from the patient. However, remember that only the patient can feel the sensation of pain. Therefore, he is the only one who can rate it. Any verbal or numerical scale can be used as long as the same scale is used with that patient each time. The scale suggested on the assessment tool is 0 to 10 (0 = no pain, 10 = worst possible pain).

Preexisting Factors Influencing the Pain Experience

All aspects of the patient's pain experience are subject to the influence of a large number of factors. These factors may increase or decrease the perceived intensity of pain, increase or decrease the patient's tolerance for pain, and elicit one particular set of behavioral responses rather than other possible reactions.

Some are situational, arising from the immediate circumstances. Others, discussed here, were already a part of the patient's physical and emotional makeup prior to the onset of pain. This section will dwell on only a few of these preexisting factors that both influence the patient's pain experience *and* interfere with the nurse's understanding of it.

Neurophysiologic Mechanisms of Pain

Specific neuroanatomical structures are involved in the transformation of a stimulus into a sensation perceived as painful by the patient. Unfortunately, this fact tends to leave the erroneous impression that there is a direct and invariant relationship between a stimulus and the occurrence of pain. As a result, the nurse may expect all patients exposed to the same stimulus (*e.g.,* appendectomy) to experience the same intensity of pain. This is *not* true. Comparable lesions in different patients do not produce the same sensations of pain. If the nurse does not realize this, she may believe that the patient has pain when he does not or that he has no pain or only slight pain when he is actually experiencing severe pain.

There is lack of agreement about the neurologic mechanisms that underlie a sensation of pain. Currently, the three theories most frequently considered are (1) the specificity theory, (2) the pattern theory, and (3) the gate control theory.

These theories are not mutually exclusive, and none is considered entirely accurate or comprehensive. However, each makes a contribution to our understanding of what causes a person to perceive pain following a specific stimulus.

The gate control theory provides a particularly helpful basis for beginning to appreciate the individuality of the pain experience. It suggests that the existence and intensity of pain is dependent on various neurologic activities that include the transmission of signals from the cortex and thalamus. These structures send signals that involve the individual's memories and feelings along with cultural influences.

Endorphins and Enkephalins

The term *endorphin* is a combination of two words: endogenous and morphine. It means morphine within. Recently, it has been discovered that the human body manufactures its own supply of endorphins and enkephalins, another morphinelike substance. (*Endorphin* and *enkephalin* are sometimes used interchangeably.) When the body releases these substances, one effect is pain relief.

Endorphins and enkephalins probably relieve pain by the same mechanism as morphine and other narcotics, but this mechanism remains unclear. In brief, endorphins or enkephalins probably inhibit the transmission of impulses

Pain Assessment

Name _____ Room _____

Age _____ Diagnosis _____

Primary nurse _____ Doctor _____

Date first seen _____

Medications for pain _____

Location
Have patient point to or trace the area of pain. _____

_____

Quality
Have patient describe pain in his words. _____

Intensity
Rate pain on a 0 to 10 scale: At present _____

1 hour after medication _____

Worst it gets _____

Best it gets _____

Onset
When did the pain start? _____

What time of day does it occur? _____

How often does it appear? _____

How long does it last? _____

Patient's view of pain
What makes the pain better? _____

What makes the pain worse? _____

Any associated symptoms? _____

What has helped control pain in the past? _____

What is the pain preventing the patient from doing that he would like to do?_____

Plan:

_____

_____

_____

_____

_____

Figure 16-3. Pain assessment tool. (Reprinted with permission from the March issue of Nursing '81. Copyright © 1981, Intermed Communications, Inc., Springhouse, PA 19477. All rights reserved.)

Part 1. Where is Your Pain?

Please mark, on the drawings below, the areas where you feel pain. Put E if external, or I if internal, near the areas that you mark. Put EI if both external and internal.

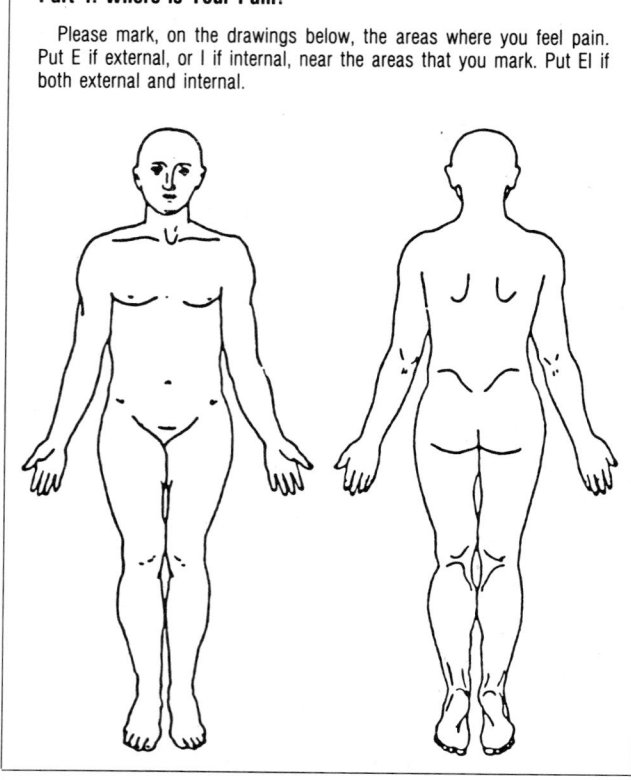

Figure 16-4. Location of pain. The above drawing is taken from the McGill–Melzack Pain Questionnaire. Use of a figure drawing to identify location of pain is helpful if there is more than one site of pain or if location is difficult to describe with words alone. The patient may mark the figures, or the nurse may ask the patient to point to the area(s) of pain on his own body; the nurse then marks the figures accordingly. (From Melzack R: The McGill pain questionnaire: Major properties and scoring methods. Pain 1:277–299, p 280)

that would eventually be felt as painful. Endorphins and enkephalins are peptides that are found in heavy concentrations in the central nervous system.

The fact that these substances exist in the body has several possible implications in clinical practice. First, it helps explain why different people feel different amounts of pain from comparable stimuli. There are probably constitutional differences in endorphin levels as well as certain situational factors, such as anxiety, that influence endorphin levels. Obviously, people with more endorphin feel less pain, and those with less endorphin feel more pain.

Second, certain techniques may relieve pain at least in part because they cause the release of endorphins. Preliminary studies have suggested that placebos, acupuncture, and transcutaneous electric nerve stimulation may cause the release of endorphins.

Third, other methods of pain relief, such as mental imagery, may help the individual release his own endorphins.

Cultural Influences

Early in childhood a person begins to learn what those around him expect and accept with respect to painful ex-

periences. For example, the person may learn that an injury sustained while he is engaging in a sport is not expected to hurt as much as a comparable injury caused by an unexpected accident. Or, he may simply learn that the latter warrants a greater expression of pain than the former. From all of his experiences with stimuli he begins to learn from others what stimuli are supposed to be painful and what kind of behavioral responses he should make. The people in his culture teach him this by their behavior toward him. They may ignore, punish, or praise him, depending on his behavior and their beliefs. Since these beliefs vary from one culture to another, it is apparent that patients reporting the same intensity of pain will not necessarily respond to it in the same ways.

The individual learns the culture's expectations about pain throughout his life and later in life is rarely affected by consistent exposure to the opposing values of other cultures. Consequently, a person tends to grow up believing that his perceptions of and reactions to pain are the only correct and normal ones.

Consider what may happen when a nurse from one culture cares for a patient with pain who comes from another culture. The expectations of the nurse's culture may include avoiding expressions of pain, such as crying and moaning; seeking immediate relief from pain; giving efficient descriptions of the pain; and having confidence in the health professions. This nurse may tend to ignore or be skeptical of the patient whose cultural experiences have taught him to moan and complain about pain, to refuse pain relief measures that do not cure the cause of the pain, to use adjectives like "unbearable" in describing his pain, and to be somewhat distrustful of the physician's ability. A patient with still another cultural background may behave differently, or he may behave similarly but for different reasons.

Many other attitudes and behaviors—a patient's preference for having visitors or being alone, or his attitude toward his diagnosis—may vary from one culture to another. Recognizing the values of one's own culture and learning how these values differ from those of other cultures helps immeasurably in overcoming the tendency to evaluate behavior on the basis of one's personal cultural expectations. A nurse with this outlook will have a greater understanding of what the patient is experiencing. Assessment is far more accurate when it takes into account the wide range of possible attitudes and behavioral responses, and interventions for pain relief are more effective when the nurse is able to respond to the patient's particular beliefs and values.

One word of caution to the nurse who embarks upon further study of the expectations that different cultures have in relation to painful experiences. Because of the research design, much of the written material on this fascinating subject tends to identify certain characteristics according to particular sociocultural groups. This may mislead the nurse by seeming to suggest that a patient can be stereotyped according to his cultural membership. Each patient's personal experiences vary too much for this to be true. It is more productive to use this information for identifying those questions that the nurse must ask about every patient. For example, determining whether a patient wants to be alone with his pain, and why, is far more helpful in planning individualized care than identifying the patient's membership in a sociocultural group and then assuming that his preferences will correspond to those of that group.

Past Experience With Pain

It is tempting and seemingly logical to expect that a person who has had multiple or prolonged experiences with pain will be less anxious and more tolerant of pain than a person who has not experienced much pain. Occasionally, this may be observed, but for the majority of patients, the reverse is true.

Probably the more experience the patient has with pain, the more frightened he will be about subsequent painful events. He may also tend to be less willing to tolerate pain, that is, to want relief from the pain sooner and at lower levels of intensity. This is understandable if we realize that, unfortunately, most patients with pain receive unsatisfactory pain relief from time to time. Thus, the patient with repeated pain experiences may learn to fear the escalation of pain and the possibility that he will not receive relief. Further, quite simply, once a patient experiences severe pain, he knows just how bad pain can become. On the other hand, the patient who has never experienced severe pain actually does not know what to be afraid of!

Sometimes the effect of past experience with pain is a result of an accumulation of many separate painful events throughout the patient's life. For other patients, past painful experiences may have been more or less constant, as in prolonged or chronic and persistent pain. The patient who feels pain for months or years may suffer additional effects from this type of past experience with pain. Notably, the patient's personality may undergo a change. He may become quite irritable, withdrawn, and depressed, and others may find him unpleasant to be around.

The undesirable effects that may result from past experiences point up the need for the nurse to be attentive to all of the patient's experiences with pain. If the patient's pain is regularly relieved, promptly and adequately, perhaps he will be less fearful of future pain and more able to tolerate it.

▷ Nursing Intervention

Basic Care Plan

Once information about the patient is organized, it provides a basis for designing individualized nursing care. *First, the nurse plans to alter factors that influence the nature of the pain sensation and factors that increase the intensity of the patient's behavioral responses to the pain experience.* Of course, some influencing factors cannot or should not be altered. For example, if one factor that causes a painful sensation is pressure from an inoperable malignancy, then it may be impossible to alter this factor. The malignancy simply cannot be removed. However, in some cases positioning, drug therapy, or radiation may decrease the pressure. An example of a factor that both should not and essentially cannot be altered is the influence of the patient's cultural expectations on his behavioral responses to pain.

Since it may not be possible or desirable to alter some of the patient's responses to his pain experience, *the second part of the nurse's plan of care includes determining appropriate responses to the patient's behaviors and attitudes regarding pain.* For example, the patient's cultural and personal experiences may have taught him that the preferred and natural response to pain experiences is not to share his feelings and sensations with anyone. Another patient may feel quite the opposite, wanting to describe his feelings and pain in detail. Appropriate and helpful nursing approaches to these two patients will differ markedly.

After examining what can be done to assist the particular patient with his pain experience, *the third phase of the nurse's plan is to select appropriate goals for nursing intervention.* Whenever possible, these goals are shared with the patient. For a few patients, the goal may be total elimination of the painful sensation. For most patients, this is rarely realistic. Other goals may include a decrease in intensity, duration, or frequency of pain and a decrease in the extent to which pain has a detrimental effect upon the patient. For example, pain may decrease appetite or interfere with sleep and thereby retard recovery from an acute illness. Thus, goals may be a good night's sleep and increased intake of nourishing food. Prolonged pain may decrease the quality of life by interfering with work or interpersonal relationships. Thus, a goal may be to decrease time off from work.

These goals may be accomplished by pharmacologic or nonpharmacologic, noninvasive means. In the acute stages of illness, the patient may be a passive recipient of pain relief measures, but when the patient has the mental and physical energy, he may learn self-management techniques for pain relief, such as relaxation or imagery. Hence, as the patient progresses through the stages of recovery, a goal may be to decrease reliance on medication for pain relief and increase the patient's use of self-management and noninvasive pain relief measures.

Managing Anxiety Related to Pain

It is well known that anxiety may have a profound influence upon the sensation of pain. For that reason, whether or not anxiety is desirable and what should be done about it will be considered in some detail in the following discussion of the three phases of the pain experience—anticipation, sensation of pain, and aftermath.

Anticipation Phase. During the anticipation phase of the pain experience, it may be desirable for the patient to have a moderate amount of anxiety about the impending pain so that he will be motivated to find methods of coping with it. This degree of anxiety is manifested by the patient's worrying about his anticipated pain some of the time but not all of the time. Usually, this anxiety can be produced by informing the patient about when his pain will occur, where it will occur, how intense it will be, and how long it will last. The nurse then channels this anxiety into helping the patient learn a variety of pain relief measures (see pp. 287–291).

During the anticipatory phase of pain, teaching the patient about the nature of the impending painful experience and what he can do to obtain relief usually minimizes the anxiety he will have when he actually feels the pain sensation. With this approach, the patient knows that he can do something about the pain when it occurs. Hence, anticipation of pain is less likely to increase anxiety as much as it would if the patient had no knowledge of what to do about the pain. Learning about pain relief measures probably gives the patient a sense of control over sensations of pain. This control seems to affect the patient's appraisal of the threat of pain—he views pain as less threatening.

One of two extremes of reaction sometimes occurs when a patient is taught about a future painful event: intense anxiety or no anxiety. The nurse may employ desensitization, a form of behavior therapy, as a method of presenting information to the highly anxious patient.

To use desensitization, the nurse first constructs a hierarchy of stimuli that are frightening to the patient. She then provides a relaxing and pleasurable environment for the patient, begins talking with him about the least frightening stimulus, and progresses up the hierarchy until the patient shows signs of anxiety. At this point, she reverts to a less frightening stimulus. This process is repeated at intervals until the patient's anxiety about the most frightening stimulus decreases to a moderate level.

Other anxiety-reducing techniques that may also be effective involve administering tranquilizing drugs, focusing the patient's attention on one specific problem, or eliminating a source of anxiety, for instance, by helping an anxious relative to become less anxious. In some instances, it may be necessary to postpone a painful event until the patient's anxiety can be decreased.

The person who shows little or no anxiety about impending pain may simply know from his past experiences that he has a high tolerance for pain. But some patients who show low anxiety or no anxiety are denying the fact that they may have pain. When pain actually occurs, these patients tend to be quite anxious and to have considerable difficulty in coping with pain. What can be done to assist these patients prior to the painful event is largely unknown. We do not yet know with certainty whether it is better to continue to give them information or to give them no information. When giving the patient specific information about pain does not produce seemingly appropriate anxiety, further information probably should be brief, essential, and general. Emphasis should be placed on pain relief measures.

Preferably, when the nurse suspects that the patient's lack of anxiety reflects an effort to deny information he receives about pain, she explores with the patient whether he wants more information about either pain or its relief. At this point in our knowledge, it appears that his decision should be respected. However, the patient should be closely observed for a marked increase in anxiety as the time approaches for the painful event to occur. The previous suggestions regarding interactions with patients with moderate and severe anxiety can then be employed, depending on the level of anxiety noted.

At times, the nurse may be tempted not to tell a patient that he may experience pain or that the pain may be much greater than he seems to think. She may reason that such knowledge will make him anxious. Indeed, she may be correct. The prospect of pain usually arouses some anxiety in the patient. The nurse must appreciate the necessity of this anxiety and help the patient to use it in a constructive manner—learning about pain relief. If the patient is to learn

ways of increasing his ability to cope with pain, he must first know that pain may occur. Failure to forewarn the patient of pain is probably a mistake *unless* one of the following conditions exists: (1) previous experience shows that forewarning this patient produces such a high level of uncontrollable anxiety that the patient is unable to take positive steps toward learning to handle his pain; (2) the patient specifically requests that he not be forewarned, and this request has been thoroughly explored with the patient; or (3) previous experience shows that teaching this patient about pain and its relief damages his coping mechanism of denial and that he has no other effective mechanism for coping with stress.

What the nurse tells the patient about the pain relief measures available and their effectiveness may also be relevant to the anxiety component of the patient's pain experience. The nurse may prevent an increase in anxiety by explaining briefly to the patient the general type of pain relief he can expect from each pain relief measure. For example, if the patient expects distraction or morphine to eliminate his pain totally, his anxiety may increase when this does not happen. These pain relief measures along with many others do not usually eliminate the sensation of pain and may not even reduce its intensity. Instead, they tend to increase the patient's tolerance for pain or render pain much less bothersome to the patient.

The Sensation of Pain. During the time when pain sensations are felt by the patient, it is desirable to reduce the patient's anxiety to as low a level as possible. When the patient is anxious about his pain, there is a tendency for him to perceive a greater intensity of pain or to be less tolerant of the pain. This in turn produces greater anxiety. Thus, a spiraling process is initiated in which the patient becomes more anxious and experiences greater pain or becomes progressively less tolerant of pain.

Obviously, it is extremely important to interrupt this process as soon as possible. Low levels of anxiety or pain are easier to reduce or control than are higher levels. *Consequently, pain relief measures should be utilized before pain becomes severe.* Many patients have the impression that they should not employ pain relief measures until pain approaches or exceeds the maximum level they are able to tolerate. It is advisable to explain to all patients that pain relief or pain control is more successful if they employ pain relief measures before pain becomes unbearable.

Anxiety during the anticipatory and sensation phases of the pain experience may be managed effectively by nursing activities related to establishing a relationship with the patient with pain and by patient teaching (see p. 287). Almost all nursing interventions for pain relief contribute in some way toward utilizing anxiety or decreasing anxiety.

Aftermath. During the aftermath phase of pain, when the pain sensation subsides, it is hoped that the patient's anxiety also will subside. When this does not happen, certain techniques that help the patient to assimilate the pain experience are useful nursing interventions (see Table 16-1, p. 288).

For many patients, the experience of pain continues after the sensation of pain ceases or subsides. Some patients continue to fear pain simply because they do not know that there is no longer any danger that pain will occur. Conveying to the patient that the source of noxious stimuli has been removed or decreased helps prevent him from anxiously expecting pain to continue or to occur again shortly.

Most patients do not seem simply to forget about a painful experience as soon as pain is no longer felt or anticipated. The patient may be disturbed about his behavioral responses to the pain experience or he may be concerned about how others view his responses. He may have unclear and somewhat frightening ideas about the cause of his pain or the treatment for it. His general sense of personal safety and control may be shaken by his having felt more intense pain than he had ever imagined was possible. The patient who is relieved of chronic pain actually may experience an identity crisis, fearing what he will be like without his pain. In the aftermath phase, the patient also may suddenly begin trembling or perspiring. He may have nausea, vomiting, or chills. Some patients have nightmares about a painful experience for weeks and months after it is over. Obviously, the care of the patient with pain, especially the management of anxiety, extends beyond the anticipation and sensation phases of pain.

▷ Noninvasive Pain Relief Measures

Perhaps because of the lack of either knowledge or time, many patients and health team members tend to regard analgesics as the major method of pain relief. However, there are many nursing activities that can be used to assist the patient with his pain experience. Table 16-1 outlines various categories of such nursing activities, including:

- Establishing a relationship with the patient
- Teaching the patient about pain and its relief
- Using the patient–group situation
- Managing other people who come in contact with the patient
- Using cutaneous stimulation
- Providing distraction from pain
- Promoting relaxation
- Using guided imagery
- Administering pharmacologic agents
- Decreasing noxious stimuli
- Utilizing the assistance of other professionals
- Being with the patient
- Conveying to the patient that the source of noxious stimuli has been removed or decreased
- Assisting with the assimilation of the painful experience

The purpose of the table is merely to introduce the nurse to the variety of nursing activities that may be used to help patients with their pain experiences. This brief synopsis is *not* intended to provide a basis of knowledge sufficient to prepare the nurse to use all of these measures in the actual care of patients. For help in acquiring this knowledge, the nurse is referred to the source footnoted at the bottom of the table. Through reading and practice, the nurse may easily learn to use these activities with patients.

Some of the noninvasive nursing activities listed in Table 16-1 will be discussed here in more detail. "Noninvasive" simply means that no physical or bodily intrusion is involved. Usually, noninvasive methods of pain relief entail very low risks, compared with analgesics. Although noninvasive pain relief measures are not necessarily a substitute for analgesics, for brief episodes of pain lasting only seconds or minutes, a noninvasive technique may be all that is necessary or appropriate. In other instances, especially when there is severe pain that lasts for hours or days, the use of some noninvasive techniques along with medications may be the most effective way to relieve pain.

Nurse–Patient Relationship and Teaching

The two pain relief measures basic to all others are the nurse–patient relationship and patient teaching about pain and its relief. These activities may actually produce pain relief in the absence of any other pain relief measures. Certainly, each may enhance the effectiveness of all other pain relief measures used with the patient. Certain aspects of the relationship and teaching serve to reduce the patient's anxiety about pain, and, as was indicated earlier, reducing anxiety commonly results in pain relief, either by decreasing the intensity of pain or by rendering the pain more tolerable to the patient.

Trust is also an extremely important aspect of the nurse–patient relationship. Conveying to the patient that his complaints about pain are believed can help reduce his anxiety. Some patients spend considerable time and energy trying to convince others that they have pain. Perhaps their pain is doubted because no cause can be found for it or because their behavior is not "typical" for what the health team expects. To say to a patient, "I know you have pain (or discomfort); I only want to understand it better," often will set the patient's mind at rest. Occasionally, a patient who has feared that no one will believe him will become tearful with gratitude and relief when he knows that he can trust the nurse and that she believes him.

As quickly as possible upon encountering a patient with pain, the nurse must convey to the patient that she cares about helping him to obtain pain relief. Often, the patient does not know where to turn for help in relieving the pain. Indeed, sociologists have noted that seldom is anyone on the health team explicitly held responsible for providing pain relief. However, when the nurse says very simply, "Let me know when you begin to hurt so I can help you do something about it," she quickly conveys to the patient that she cares and in some way assumes responsibility for helping with his pain.

The nurse also provides vital information, through patient teaching, about how pain can be controlled. The patient needs to know, for example, that pain should be reported in the early stages before it becomes severe. Too often the patient waits as long as he can endure the pain before reporting it. At that point, the pain may be intense and his anxiety may be very high. It is much easier to prevent severe pain and panic than to relieve them once they exist.

Cutaneous Stimulation

According to the gate control theory, stimulation of large-diameter nerve fibers in the skin may reduce the intensity of pain. Skin stimulation may also cause the release of endorphins. Cutaneous stimulation can be accomplished in

Table 16-1
Nursing Activities to Assist the Patient With His Pain Experience

Category of Nursing Activity	Explanation	Example of Nursing Activity
1. Establishing a relationship with the patient with pain	Interacting with the patient as a total person, believing what he says he experiences, and respecting his reactions and attitudes regarding pain (see text)	Telling the patient you believe what he says about his pain experience
2. Teaching the patient about pain and its relief	Using a variety of the patient's sensory modalities for the purpose of conveying to him information about his pain experience (see text)	Explaining the quality and location of impending pain by applying pressure and pulling the skin in the area where the patient will have an incision
3. Using the patient–group situation	Using the principles of small group functioning to teach the patient and his family about the patient's pain experience	The nurse, two female patients with arthritis, and their husbands discussing modifications in home-making activities following discharge from the hospital
4. Managing other people who come in contact with the patient	Assisting other people to reach their maximum potential for helping the patient with his pain experience	Talking alone with a patient's wife who shows marked anxiety in the presence of her husband when he complains of his undiagnosed abdominal pain
5. Using cutaneous stimulation	Using various qualities, locations, durations, and intensities of stimuli in contact with the skin (see text)	Applying a hand-held vibrator to the scalp and back of the neck to relieve headache
6. Providing distraction from pain	Obtaining the patient's response to and participation in stimuli through the major sensory modalities (see text)	Helping the patient to use "he-who" breathing during a painful dressing change
7. Promoting relaxation	Using a variety of techniques to assist the patient to avoid fatigue and to achieve skeletal muscle relaxation	Helping the patient learn to use slow, rhythmic breathing

(continued)

an almost infinite variety of ways. In devising methods of cutaneous stimulation for pain relief, the nurse considers which quality of stimulation is to be used and the location, duration, and intensity of stimulation. Unfortunately, the approach is one of trial and error, but common sense often is an effective guide.

Various qualities of cutaneous stimulation are easily available at low cost. Some may require a physician's request or may be contraindicated, but usually some type of stimulation will be permissible. Different types of skin sensations may be elicited when the following measures are applied: pressure, vibration, heat, cold, bathing, lotion, menthol cream, and transcutaneous electric nerve stimulation (TENS). Although TENS is not as readily available as the other measures, it has proven to be very helpful in both acute and chronic pain relief, and its use is becoming more widespread. It consists of a battery-operated unit with electrodes that are applied to the skin to produce a tingling, vibrating, or buzzing sensation in the area of pain (Fig. 16-5).

Local application of cold to a painful part is an underused but often highly effective method of relieving pain. Compared to local applications of heat, cold relieves pain faster and has a longer carryover effect. Contrary to popular belief, cold does not necessarily cause muscle contraction. In fact, cold slows the conduction of impulses that maintain muscle tone and may thus cause muscle relaxation. Therefore, cold is not only indicated to decrease bleeding and swelling of a new injury but also may be continued simply for pain relief.

When cutaneous stimulation is employed, it is applied to different areas of the body. Usually, stimulating the skin on or near the pain site is suitable. In other instances, direct stimulation over the pain site must be avoided because it elicits more pain. If stimulation of the skin near the pain site is ineffective or painful, the side of the body opposite the painful area may be stimulated for pain relief. This is called *contralateral stimulation*. For example, the pain of "tennis elbow" on the left side may be relieved as well or better by applying menthol cream to the right elbow rather

Table 16-1
Nursing Activities to Assist the Patient With His Pain Experience (continued)

Category of Nursing Activity	Explanation	Example of Nursing Activity
8. Using guided imagery	Assisting the patient to imagine a pleasant event as a substitute for the pain experience or to imagine a means of ridding his body of the pain (see text)	Helping the patient imagine that he is ridding himself of pain as he exhales slowly
9. Administering pharmacologic agents	Giving to the patient and explaining the effects of medications with pain-relieving potential; assisting the physician in determining the patient's need for analgesics (see text)	Administering analgesics on a preventive basis
10. Decreasing noxious stimuli	Using a variety of techniques to reduce the transmission of pain signals to the cortex of the brain	Splinting an abdominal incision during coughing and deep breathing
11. Utilizing the assistance of professionals	Assisting the patient, his family, and his physician to identify the need for additional help in dealing with pain; assisting the patient and his family to obtain this help and to utilize it to their best advantage	Suggesting to the patient that his clergyman may be able to counsel him about his concern (reduce his anxiety) that his pain is punishment for a sin
12. Being with the patient	Identifying and responding to the patient who would benefit from the mere presence of the nurse or someone else	Getting a hospital volunteer to sit at the bedside of the patient who does not want to be alone with his pain experience
13. Conveying that the source of noxious stimuli has been removed or decreased	Conveying to the patient, when appropriate, that something has been done to diminish or eliminate a cause of his pain (see text)	Telling the patient that the needle for his lumbar puncture has just been removed and all that remains is to cleanse his back
14. Assisting with the assimilation of the painful experience	Identifying the patient's need for and assisting him with the intellectual and emotional incorporation of a painful experience (see text)	Discussing with the patient what sensations he felt and what he was thinking while experiencing his myocardial infarction on the previous day

(Adapted from McCaffery M: Nursing Management of the Patient with Pain, 2nd ed. Philadelphia, JB Lippincott, 1979.)

than the left. This is especially helpful to remember when the site of pain is difficult to stimulate directly, such as when a thick cast has been applied over a painful area or when the entire limb is injured or burned.

The intensity of stimulation is generally moderate. Mild stimulation tends to be ticklish or annoying, whereas intense stimulation may cause pain.

In general, the duration of cutaneous stimulation and the intervals between applications of it vary considerably. Some patients experience pain relief for hours or days following cutaneous stimulation. Others obtain relief only while stimulation is being applied. For these patients, use of a menthol cream or a TENS unit is an efficient means of providing continuous stimulation without hampering activity. It takes only a few minutes to apply, but the stimulation lasts for hours. The TENS unit may be worn 24 hours a day.

Distraction

Distraction, or focusing the patient's attention away from his painful sensations, may be an effective method of pain relief. In some instances, it may decrease the perceived intensity of pain, but usually it increases tolerance for pain, making pain less bothersome. Pain tends to draw attention to itself; but if the person is made less aware of pain or pays less attention to it, he naturally will be less bothered by pain and more tolerant of it.

There are many degrees and types of distraction, ranging from simply avoiding monotony to the use of highly complicated physical and mental activity. When environmental stimuli are deficient in amount, patterning, or variation, the person's centrally regulated thresholds for sensation tend to be lowered. This apparently allows the person to utilize more of the available input. Consequently, he is more sensitive to input such as pain.

If the patient with pain is experiencing some form of sensory restriction, pain relief may result when the nurse provides compensating environmental stimuli. This is a very mild form of distraction that focuses the patient's attention away from his painful sensations. The nurse simply is arranging an environment that is more "normal" for the pa-

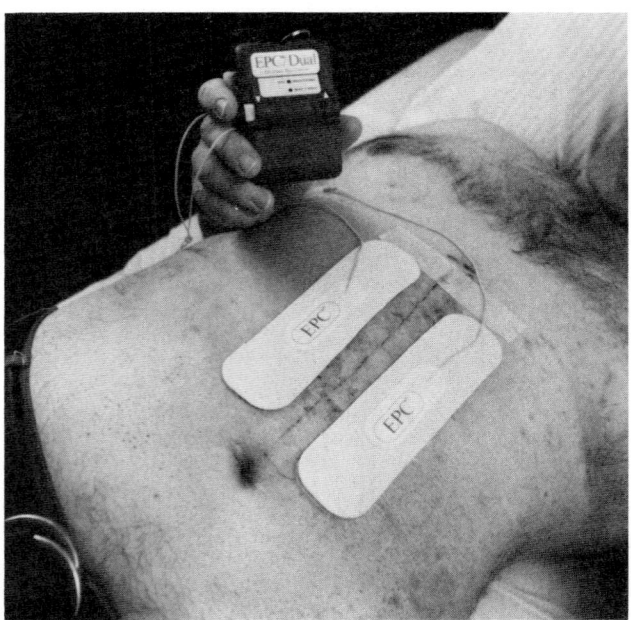

Figure 16-5. Transcutaneous electric nerve stimulation (TENS) being used for relief of incisional pain postoperatively. (From Melzack R: The McGill pain questionnaire: Major properties and scoring methods. Pain 1:277–299, p 280.)

tient. The distraction may merely involve minimizing strange noises, making brief but frequent visits to the patient, bringing him a snack, or teaching him physical exercises appropriate to his condition. The latter is a particularly effective method of reducing the effects of sensory restriction.

More deliberate and intense forms of sensory input may be necessary to distract the patient from brief episodes of increased pain, such as bone marrow aspiration or wound debridement, or longer periods of moderate to severe intensities of pain. Some patients are able to utilize distraction for hours.

The value of distraction techniques for pain relief sometimes is misunderstood by the health team. A common misconception is that the patient who can be distracted from his pain does not have as much pain as he seems to want others to believe. For example, the nurse may erroneously assume that the patient has no pain simply because he is laughing and talking with visitors. However, distraction is a powerful method of pain relief. Doubting the patient's pain because he uses distraction effectively may produce the unfortunate result of causing the patient to stop using the distraction.

The effectiveness of distraction depends on the degree to which the patient makes an effort to receive and create sensory input other than pain. As a general rule, pain relief is increased in direct relation to the patient's active participation, the number of sensory modalities used, and the patient's interest in the stimuli. Therefore, seeing, hearing, and keeping a box score of a baseball game will distract the patient from his pain more than would only one or two of these activities. Involving the sensory modalities of seeing,

hearing, and movement is more effective than using only one or two modalities. If the patient prefers baseball to football, stimuli related to baseball will distract him from pain more than stimuli associated with football.

Increasing the complexity of the distractor as pain increases will work, however, only up to a certain level of pain intensity. With severe pain, the patient is unable to concentrate well enough to engage in highly complicated mental or physical activities.

Many patients devise their own distraction strategies. The patient may hum, mentally calculate math problems, or choose an absorbing television program. The nurse may support these efforts and assist the patient to elaborate on them.

Under conditions of brief, severe pain, it may be necessary to teach the patient a distraction strategy. A technique that may be taught quickly, even to patients who are debilitated, fatigued, sedated, or in severe pain, is to combine rhythmic rubbing with visual concentration. The patient is asked to open his eyes, stare at a specific spot on the wall or ceiling, and rub a part of his body. The rubbing may be done initially by the nurse. Then the nurse may take the patient's hand and guide him in doing the rubbing. Rubbing with a firm, circular motion on bare skin seems to be effective. The rubbing and staring involve a steady source of sensory input through visual and tactile-kinesthetic modalities along with a focus of rhythm. If this is not distracting enough, the patient can be instructed to add another activity, such as breathing in and out slowly. The patient may chant silently to himself, "Breathe in slowly, breathe out slowly." Sensory input through several modalities combined with rhythm and a focus on breathing are common characteristics of successful distraction techniques.

Another distraction technique that is very useful with patients who are fatigued or sedated, or when pain lasts longer than several minutes, is "active listening." The patient may use a tape recorder with an earphone or headset, select a cassette of fast music, and listen to the music, while keeping time by tapping his finger or nodding his head. For visual input, he can focus on an object or close his eyes and imagine something about the music, such as dancing to the music. When the pain increases, the patient can increase the volume; when pain decreases, he decreases the volume. For example, a burned patient undergoing a painful dressing change might use this method of distraction to make the painful experience more tolerable.

Relaxation

Skeletal muscle relaxation may reduce the intensity of pain or increase pain tolerance. Often, however, it is combined with other pain relief measures, such as analgesics or a heating pad, to enhance their effectiveness. Many people learn relaxation techniques for the purpose of dealing with life stresses. Community agencies offer adult education programs in transcendental meditation, yoga, hypnosis, music therapy, and a variety of other potentially relaxing activities. If a patient already knows a technique for relaxing, the nurse may need only suggest that he use it in the presence of pain or to prevent an increase in pain.

Almost all patients with chronic pain need to learn some method of relaxing and to employ it on a regular basis several times a day. In most patients, chronic pain causes fatigue and muscle tension. Regular periods of relaxation are needed to combat this. Sometimes muscle tension contributes directly to increasing pain.

A simple relaxation technique for patients with acute or chronic pain consists of abdominal breathing at a slow, rhythmic rate. The patient may close his eyes and picture the air entering and leaving his lungs as he performs this activity. He begins with a slow, deep breath. Then he begins to breathe slowly and comfortably (not too deeply) at about 6 to 9 breaths per minute. The patient can maintain a constant rhythm by counting silently and slowly to himself as he inhales ("in, 2, 3") and as he exhales ("out, 2, 3"). The patient concludes this relaxation technique by taking another deep breath. When the nurse is teaching this technique to the patient, it is helpful to count out loud for him at first. Initially the patient may benefit from keeping his eyes open and watching the nurse breathe in coordination with him.

Slow, rhythmic breathing may also be used as a distraction technique. It may not be relaxing to the patient until he has practiced it and become skillful in using it.

A quick and easy method of helping the tense patient with severe pain to relax is to give the following instructions: "Clench your fists; breathe in deeply and hold it a moment. As you breathe out, feel yourself go limp. Now start yawning."

Guided Imagery

Therapeutic *guided imagery* may be defined as the use of one's imagination in an especially designed manner to achieve a specific positive effect. In this instance, the effects desired are relaxation and pain relief. Imagery of various types is capable of altering body functions over which we seem to have no direct or conscious control. Most people have experienced this in the form of increased cardiac rate (pounding heart) or perspiration when a distressing mental image comes to mind just before falling asleep. Although images of this sort seem to provoke a stress response, certain other images seem to evoke relaxation responses or pain relief. A considerable amount of the nurse's time usually is required to teach and explain the technique of guided imagery. The patient, too, must invest time and energy in practicing it. For these reasons, guided imagery most often is taught to patients with chronic pain, although it is effective with acute pain as well. To learn to use guided imagery, the patient must be able to concentrate, use his imagination, and follow directions. Therefore, this technique is not appropriate for the patient with brain damage. Also, it is not advisable to try to teach it when the patient is fatigued, sedated, or in severe pain. One simple form of therapeutic guided imagery for relaxation and pain relief consists of combining the slow rhythmic breathing described as a relaxation technique with a mental image of relaxation and comfort. With eyes closed, the patient imagines that each time he exhales slowly he is breathing out muscle tension and discomfort, leaving behind a relaxed and comfortable body. Another variation involves suggesting that the patient imagine a ball of healing energy, like a white light, either on his chest or in his lungs. Each time he inhales, he can imagine that the air sends the ball of healing energy to the area of discomfort. Each time he exhales, he can imagine that the ball floats away from his body, carrying with it the pain and tension. It enters the body again immediately, in a purified state, and can be circulated to the area of discomfort again.

Usually, the patient is asked to practice guided imagery for about 5 minutes, three times a day. Several days of practice may elapse before the patient finds that he can reduce the intensity of pain through this technique. Pain relief can continue for hours after the imagery is used. Most patients begin to experience the relaxing effects of guided imagery the first time they try it.

▷ Medications for Pain Relief

Whether pain is acute or chronic, certain guidelines are useful when medications are indicated for the relief of pain. Usually, medications are most effective when a preventive approach is used and when the dose and interval between doses is individualized to meet the patient's needs. The only safe and effective way to administer narcotics is to observe the individual's response.

Preventive Approach

Using a preventive approach to pain relief means that medications (analgesics in particular) are given before the pain occurs, if it can be predicted, or at least before it reaches a severe intensity. If the patient's pain is expected to occur daily for a great portion of the 24-hour period, a regular schedule around the clock may be indicated. Even if the analgesic is prescribed prn, the nurse can administer the analgesic on a preventive basis as long as the prescribed interval between doses is observed. This is preferable to the usual approach to a prn request, which may require that the patient have pain and ask for his medication, rather than the analgesic being offered before it is needed.

A preventive approach has many advantages. It usually takes a smaller dose to alleviate mild pain or prevent the occurrence of pain than it does to relieve severe pain. Thus, a preventive approach may result in a lower total 24-hour dose. This helps prevent tolerance to analgesics and decreases the severity of side-effects such as sedation and constipation. Further, pain relief can be more complete with a preventive approach. For example, there need not be any peaks of severe pain and the patient spends less time in pain. On a prn approach to pain relief, the patient usually experiences pain, obtains his analgesic, and waits for it to take effect. Within a 24-hour period, this may result in his spending a total of several hours in pain.

It is also felt that better pain control achieved with a preventive approach will reduce the likelihood of the patient's craving the drug. Some health team members seem to feel that the frugal use of narcotics will help prevent addiction in the patient with acute pain. However, there is no basis for this belief. Certainly, a patient who is in pain and has his analgesic withheld is more likely to crave the medication than the patient whose pain is relieved before it becomes distressing to him.

Individualized Doses

Individualizing the dose and the interval between doses is necessary because patients metabolize and absorb medications at different rates, and because adjustments are required for varying intensities of pain. It should not be at all surprising that a certain dosage of a narcotic given at specified intervals would be effective for one patient but totally inappropriate for another. However, too often analgesics, especially narcotics, are prescribed and given in a very standardized and inflexible manner. The nurse must remember that there are no magic numbers for milligrams or for hours between doses. For example, when a patient metabolizes 100 mg of meperidine IM in 2 hours, it should be understood that this is a well documented physiologic phenomenon, not a drug abuse problem.

Because of the fear of creating addiction or causing respiratory depression, there is a trend toward underusing narcotics in the treatment of acute pain or prolonged pain in the terminally ill. The result is much needless suffering. Even prolonged administration of a narcotic is associated with less than 3% incidence of addiction. Further, small doses are not necessarily safe doses. Patients receiving 25 mg to 50 mg of meperidine IM have experienced life-threatening respiratory depression, while other patients have not exhibited any sedation or respiratory depression after taking 200 mg of meperidine IM.

Therefore, it is mandatory for purposes of safety and pain relief that the effects of narcotics be observed, especially when a narcotic is given for the first time to a patient or when a change is made in dosage or frequency. A simple way to make these observations is to maintain a flow sheet, noting time and date, pain rating (scale of 0–10), the pain relief measure, side-effects, and patient activity. At regular intervals, such as every hour following an IM injection, the patient can be asked to rate his pain on a scale of 0 to 10. Respiratory rate can also be noted, along with any other physiologic changes of concern. For example, when a postoperative patient is given the first dose of meperidine, 75 mg IM, a pain rating and respiratory rate, along with other relevant physiologic parameters, should be noted. If 1 hour later the pain rating has not decreased; the patient is reasonably alert; and the respiratory status, blood pressure, and pulse rate are satisfactory, some change in analgesia is indicated. The meperidine dose is safe for this patient but does not relieve the pain. Another dose of meperidine might be given.

Routes of Administration for Moderate to Severe Pain

For moderate to severe pain, the most common routes of administration of a narcotic are the intramuscular or subcutaneous routes. However, there are alternatives to this. If the patient is not permitted any oral intake or is vomiting, the IV or rectal routes may be indicated. Postoperative pain,

for example, has been effectively relieved with rectal suppositories of 10 mg of oxymorphone (Numorphan; two suppositories, totaling 10 mg, provide analgesia equivalent to that of 10 mg of morphine IM or 75 mg of meperidine IM). The rectal route may be indicated for patients with bleeding problems, such as hemophilia.

Intravenous narcotics may be administered by "push" (or "slow push," *e.g.*, over a 5- to 10-minute period) or by continuous drip using an infusion pump. The latter provides a more steady level of analgesia and is indicated when pain is to be controlled over a 24-hour period, such as postoperatively for the first day or so, or in a patient with prolonged cancer pain who cannot take medication by mouth. Preliminary studies show that the majority of patients do not absorb meperidine IM well during the first 8 hours postoperatively and that the IV route may be much safer and more effective in relieving pain.

If the patient can take medication by mouth, this route is preferred to all others since it is easy, noninvasive, and not painful, as are injections. Severe pain can be relieved with oral narcotics *if* the doses are high enough. Certainly, patients with prolonged pain should receive analgesics orally rather than by injection if at all possible. Many narcotics can be given effectively by mouth for severe pain. Oral doses of narcotics that are equal to 10 mg of morphine IM or 75 mg of meperidine IM are: 10 mg to 20 mg of methadone; 30 mg to 60 mg of morphine; and 4 mg to 8 mg of hydromorphone (Dilaudid). In terminally ill patients with prolonged pain, doses may gradually become much higher owing to increased pain or tolerance to analgesia. In the majority of these patients, the higher doses provide additional pain relief (*i.e.*, there is no ceiling on the analgesia of the powerful narcotics), and the higher doses are not lethal (the patient is tolerant to respiratory depression and sedation as well as analgesia).

"Brompton's" was once a very popular oral substance for pain relief in terminally ill patients. It is a liquid that may contain any combination of several ingredients, such as a narcotic, an antiemetic, a central nervous system stimulant, alcohol, and a flavoring agent. Experience has shown that such combinations of ingredients are not the best choice for all patients and that the effectiveness of this mixture was related more closely to how it was given than to what was in it. It was given around the clock on a preventive basis. The value of this approach is discussed above.

Drug Preferences

With both acute and chronic pain, it is wise to use aspirin, acetaminophen (*e.g.*, Tylenol, Datril), or the more potent nonsteroidal anti-inflammatory drugs (NSAID), such as ibuprofen (Motrin) to the extent possible. These drugs provide non-narcotic analgesia without the unpleasant sedation and constipation that so often accompany narcotics. Furthermore, when narcotics are necessary, it is logical to give the non-narcotic analgesic concurrently because the effect decreases the dosage of narcotic needed. Also, aspirin, acetaminophen, and NSAID produce analgesia by action at the peripheral nervous system level to relieve pain, whereas narcotics act primarily at the central nervous system level.

For the patient who has chronic pain, whether it is of malignant or benign origin, the use of tricyclic antidepressants may be considered. Usually, they are not appropriate for acute pain. However, patients with chronic pain almost always are depressed. These drugs have an antidepressant effect after about 14 days. Since they have a sedative effect and the total daily dose may be given at bedtime, they assist in relieving sleep disturbances. Recently, it has been discovered that tricyclic antidepressants probably have an analgesic effect after 10 days of regular administration. Thus, the patient may benefit from a certain level of non-narcotic analgesia.

Probably the most commonly prescribed injectable narcotic is meperidine. However, there are several indications that this practice should be reconsidered. Meperidine is short-acting and very irritating to the tissues, meaning that pain control may require frequent (every 2–3 hours) injections of an irritating substance. Further, meperidine is more toxic than was previously recognized. Neuropsychiatric effects, such as disorientation, bizarre feelings, and hallucinations, are relatively intense with parenteral meperidine. Owing to accumulation of the metabolite normeperidine, multiple doses of meperidine, especially in patients with renal failure, can result in excitatory effects, such as twitches, irritability, and seizures. None of these problems have been observed with morphine, which is an acceptable alternative to meperidine.

Another potential problem is the common practice of giving so-called potentiators with narcotics. Those most frequently prescribed for parenteral administration are probably promethazine (Phenergan) and hydroxyzine (Vistaril). Studies and clinical practice have shown that promethazine is highly sedating; it is not a potentiator of narcotic analgesia but instead is a potentiator of respiratory depression and hypotension, and it may even increase the perceived intensity of pain. Hydroxyzine, by contrast, may have some analgesic properties but is extremely irritating and painful when given intramuscularly. It must be given by the Z-track method (also, see p. 706). Actually, there probably are no potentiators of narcotic analgesia. Quite simply, most of the time analgesia is best achieved with drugs known to be analgesics—the narcotics and non-narcotics.

▷ Special Facilities*

Over the last decade, many pain clinics have been established in the United States to help patients with chronic pain. They tend to utilize a multidisciplinary approach and to offer a variety of perspectives on the relief of pain. Therapy may include biofeedback, acupuncture, nerve blocks,

* For information on obtaining directories of pain clinics, listing the locations of and services offered by pain clinics, write: Committee on Pain Therapy, American Society of Anesthesiologists, 515 Busse Hwy., Park Ridge, IL 60068 *or* Medical World News, 1221 Avenue of the Americas, New York, NY 10020.

For assistance in locating hospice programs throughout the United States, write: National Hospice Organization, 1311 Dolly Madison Blvd., McLean, VA 22101.

hypnosis, autogenic training, group therapy, medication, physical therapy, nutritional counseling, and many others. Not all pain centers offer the same approaches to pain relief. Some clinics or centers treat the patient on an outpatient basis, whereas others admit the patient to a pain control unit (PCU).

When the patient is not able to obtain satisfactory pain relief, the physician may refer him to a pain center for evaluation and treatment. Unfortunately, there are not nearly enough pain centers to care for all the patients with chronic pain. The waiting lists at such clinics often are quite long.

Hospice programs have been developed in many areas to give care and symptomatic relief to the dying patient. Pain control is one of their primary goals. Again, there are not enough of these agencies to care for all of the patients who need them.

▷ Evaluating the Effectiveness of Pain Relief Measures

To determine objectively the effectiveness of nursing activities designed to help the patient with his pain experience, the patient's behavioral responses prior to intervention are compared with those that follow intervention. After the nurse intervenes, she once again assesses the patient's behavioral responses, much as she did in her initial assessment. This assessment is repeated at appropriate intervals following the intervention.

Evaluation

The *comparison* of these assessments reveals the effectiveness of the pain relief measures. This provides a basis for continuing or modifying nursing intervention.

The expected outcome of nursing intervention for pain relief is usually one or more of the following three possibilities, each having many possible manifestations:

1. A decrease in the intensity of pain, manifested by such patient behaviors as the following:
   a. Rates pain at a lower intensity (on a scale of 0–10) following intervention
   b. Rates pain at a lower intensity for longer periods of time
2. An increase in the patient's tolerance for pain, manifested by such behaviors as the following:
   a. Says the pain does not bother him as much as it did prior to intervention
   b. Says he pays less attention to the pain
   c. Spends less time talking about pain
3. Increase in ability to function or in quality of life, manifested by such behaviors as the following:
   a. Is alert and pain free enough to engage in activities important to recovery (*e.g.,* drinking fluids, coughing, ambulating)
   b. Sleeps all night
   c. Increases the amount of time spent out of bed
   d. Increases the amount of time spent at work

Chart 16-1
Nursing Process Guidelines to Management of the Patient With Pain

Assessment

A. Assess the patient's behavioral responses to the pain experience.

1. Identify whether the pain is acute or chronic.
2. Identify the phase or phases (anticipation, presence, aftermath) the patient experiences.
3. During each phase of the pain experience, observe all of the patient's behavioral responses, using the following as a guide:
    a. Physiologic manifestations
    b. Verbal statements
    c. Vocal behaviors
    d. Facial expressions
    e. Body movements
    f. Physical contact with others
    g. Alterations in response to the surrounding environment
    h. Adaptation of physiologic or behavioral responses
4. Use the patient's behavioral responses to determine the following:
    a. Severity of pain
    b. Tolerance for pain
    c. Characteristics such as location, duration, rhythmicity, and quality
    d. Harmful effects of pain upon recovery
    e. What the patient believes will help him with his pain
    f. The patient's concerns about his pain
    g. Any pattern in the patient's behaviors (*i.e.,* behaviors the patient tends to exhibit repeatedly)

B. Assess factors that influence each of the following:

1. The presence of each phase of the pain experience
2. The nature of the painful sensation(s)
3. The patient's behavioral responses, including his concerns and beliefs

Analysis

Organize the most pertinent findings of the assessment of the patient.
1. Identify the phases of the patient's pain experience and the nature of the pain sensation(s), and identify those factors that influence the existence of the phases of the pain experience and the nature of the pain sensation(s).

2. Describe the patient's behavioral responses to each phase of the pain experience, and identify those factors that help to explain why the patient behaves as he does.
3. Formulate nursing diagnosis/patient problem.

Planning and Implementation

Plan and implement nursing intervention to assist the patient with his pain experience.
1. Identify realistic goals for nursing intervention.
2. Use the following categories of nursing activities as a guide to selecting and implementing nursing measures that will alter factors that influence the patient's experiences and behaviors during each phase of his pain and that are appropriate responses to the patient's behaviors:
    a. Establishing a relationship with the patient with pain
    b. Teaching the patient about pain and its relief
    c. Using the patient–group situation
    d. Managing other people who come in contact with the patient
    e. Using cutaneous stimulation
    f. Providing distraction from pain
    g. Promoting relaxation
    h. Using guided imagery
    i. Administering pharmacologic agents
    j. Decreasing noxious stimuli
    k. Utilizing the assistance of other professionals
    l. Being with the patient
    m. Conveying that the source of noxious stimuli has been removed or decreased
    n. Assisting with assimilation of the painful experience
3. Select a variety of nursing activities, remembering that establishing a relationship with the patient with pain and teaching him about pain are basic to the effectiveness of all other pain relief measures.

Evaluation

Evaluate the effectiveness of nursing intervention.
1. Compare the patient's behavioral responses prior to intervention with his responses following intervention.
2. Modify nursing intervention in accordance with the results of the evaluation and the patient's changing status.

▷ Bibliography

Ajemian I and Mount BM (eds). The R.V.H. Manual on Palliative/Hospice Care. New York, Arno Press, 1980.

Bonica JJ and Albe–Fessard DG (eds). Advances in Pain Research and Therapy, vol 1. New York, Raven Press, 1976.

Bonica JJ, Liebeskind JC, and Albe–Fessard DG (eds). Advances in Pain Research and Therapy, vol 3. New York, Raven Press, 1979.

Bonica JJ and Ventafridda V (eds). Advances in Pain Research and Therapy, vol 2. New York, Raven Press, 1979.

Bresler DE. Free Yourself from Pain. New York, Simon & Schuster, 1979.

Cohen KP. Hospice: Prescription for Terminal Care. Germantown, Maryland, Aspen Systems Corp, 1979.

Crue BL Jr (ed). Chronic Pain: Further Observations from City of Hope National Medical Center, New York, SP Medical & Scientific Books, 1979.

Davitz L and Davitz J. Inferences of Patients' Pain and Psychological Distress. New York, Springer, 1980.

McCaffery M. Nursing Management of the Patient with Pain, 2nd ed. Philadelphia, JB Lippincott, 1979.

O'Connor AB (ed). Nursing: Patients in Pain. New York, American Journal of Nursing, 1979.

Physicians' Referral Directory of Comprehensive U.S. Pain Clinics. New York, McGraw–Hill, 1980.

Reynolds MA. Pain: Deliberative Nursing Interventions. New York, Grune & Stratton, 1981.

Roy R and Funks E (eds). Chronic Pain: Psychosocial Factors in Rehabilitation. Baltimore, Williams & Wilkins, 1982.

Saunders CM (ed). The Management of Terminal Disease. Chicago, An Edward Arnold Publication distributed by Year Book Medical Publishers, 1978.

Smith WL, Merskey H, and Gross SC (eds). Pain: Meaning and Management. New York, SP Medical & Scientific Books, 1980.

Sternbach RA (ed). The Psychology of Pain. New York, Raven Press, 1978.

Swerdlow M (ed). The Therapy of Pain. Philadelphia, JB Lippincott, 1981.

Wolf ZR (ed). Pain Management. Topics in Clinical Nursing, vol 2. Germantown, Maryland, Aspen, 1980.

Zborowski M. People in Pain. San Francisco, Jossey–Bass, 1969.

Articles

Agnew DC, Crue BL, Pinsky JJ. A taxonomy for diagnosis and information storage for patients with chronic pain. Bull. Los Angeles Neurological Societies 1979; 44:84–86.

Angell M. The quality of mercy. N Engl J Med 1982 Jan 14; 306:98–99.

Austin KL, Stapleton JV, and Mather LE. Multiple intramuscular injections: A major source of variability in analgesic response to meperidine. Pain 1980 Feb; 8(1):47–62.

Banyard SG. New drug-free technique cuts postop pain. RN 1982 Apr; 45(4):31–33.

Barber J and Gitelson J. Cancer pain: Psychological management using hypnosis. CA—A Cancer J Clinicians 1980 May/June; 30:130–136.

Booker JE. Pain—it's all in your patient's head (or is it?) Nursing '82 1982 Mar; 12(3):47–51.

Boyer MW. Continuous drip morphine. Am J Nurs 1982 Apr; 82(4):602–604.

Bussey JG and Jackson A. TENS for post surgical analgesia. Contemporary Surgery 1981 Mar; 18:35–41.

Cohen FL. Postsurgical pain relief: Patients' status and nurses' medication choices. Pain 1980 Oct; 9(2):265–274.

Coyle N. Analgesics at the bedside. Am J Nurs 1979 Sept; 79:1554–1557.

Davis AJ. Teaching your patients to use electricity to ward off pain. RN 1978 Feb; 41:43–45.

Dolan MB. Controlling pain in a personal way. Nursing '82 1982 Jan; 12:144.

Donovan MI. Relaxation with guided imagery: A useful technique. Cancer Nursing 1980 Feb; 3:27–32.

Frank RM. Pain management and the appropriate use of analgesics. Cancer Nursing 1980 Apr; 3:155–157.

Gever LN. From arthritis pain to dysmenorrhea: A new indication for prostaglandin inhibitors. Nursing '80 1980 Apr; 10:81.

Goodwin JS, Goodwin JM, and Vogel AV. Placebo misuse. Nursing '82 1982 Feb; 12:82–83.

Heidrich G and Perry S. Helping the patient in pain. Am J Nurs 1982 Dec; 12(12):1828–1833.

Holderby RA. Conscious suggestion: Using talk to manage pain. Nursing '81 1981 May; 11:44–46.

Holmes AH. Morphine IV infusion for chronic pain. Drug Intell Clin Pharm 1978 Sept; 12:556–557.

Jordan A. Self-help pain control: An information handout for patients using pain medication. Oncology Nurs Forum 1982 Winter; 9:55–57.

Krieger DT. Endorphins and enkaphalins. Disease-a-Month 1982 July; 28(10):1–53.

Levin RF. Choice of injection site, locus of control, and the perception of momentary pain. Image 1982 Feb/Mar; 14(1):26–32.

Lipman AG. Drug therapy in cancer pain. Cancer Nursing 1980 Feb; 3:39–46.

Mar DD. The "simple" analgesics. Am J Nurs 1981 June; 81:1206–1208.

Mar DD. The narcotic analgesics. Am J Nurs 1981 July; 81:1364–1365.

Marks RM and Sachar EJ. Undertreatment of medical inpatients with narcotic analgesics. Ann Intern Med 1973 Feb; 78:173–181.

Maxwell MB. How to use methadone for the cancer patient's pain. Am J Nurs 1980 Sept; 80:1606–1609.

McCaffery M. Current misconceptions about the relief of acute pain. In Crue BL Jr (ed). Chronic Pain: Further Observations from City of Hope National Medical Center. New York, SP Medical & Scientific Books, 1979.

McCaffery M. Understanding your patient's pain. Nursing '80 1980 Sept; 10:26–31.

McCaffery M. Patients shouldn't have to suffer: How to relieve pain with injectable narcotics. Nursing '80 1980 Oct; 10:34–39.

McCaffery M. How to relieve your patient's pain fast and effectively with oral analgesics. Nursing '80 1980 Nov; 10:58–63.

McCaffery M. Relieving pain with noninvasive techniques. Nursing '80 1980 Dec; 10:55–57.

McCaffery M. When your patient's still in pain don't just do something: Sit there. Nursing '81 1981 June; 11:58–62.

McCaffery M. Large doses are safer than you think. Nurs Life 1981 Nov/Dec; 1:41–42.

McCaffery M. Would you administer placebos for pain? Nursing '82 1982 Feb; 12(2):80–85.

McGuire L. A short, simple tool for assessing your patient's pain. Nursing '81 1981 Mar; 11:48–49.

McGuire L. Continuous morphine infusion. Nursing '81 1981 Oct; 11:10.

McGuire L and Dizard S. Managing pain—in the young patient. Nursing '82 1982 Aug; 12(8):52–55.

Meissner JE. McGill–Melzack Pain Questionnaire. Nursing '80 1980 Jan; 10:50–51.

Miller RR and Jick H. Clinical effects of meperidine in hospitalized medical patients. J Clin Pharmacol 1978 Apr; 18:180–189.

Panayotoff K. Managing pain . . . in the elderly patient. Nursing '82 1982 Aug; 12(8):53–57.

Rodman MJ. The year's new drugs. RN 1980 Jan; 43:97–106.

Rodman MJ. Drug therapy today: How to coax maximum pain relief from standard drugs. RN 1980 Sept; 43:83–92.

Rogers AG. Pharmacology of analgesics. J Neurosurg Nurs 1978 Dec; 10:180–184.

Rogers AG. 21 problems in pain control—and ways to solve them. Your Patient & Cancer 1981 Sept; 65–75.

Shimomura SK and Harris S. Pain management of sickle cell patients. Pharmacol Ther Forum 1978 Dec; 26:1–2.

Stapleton JV, Austin KL, and Mather LE. A pharmacokinetic approach to postoperative pain: Continuous infusion of pethidine. Anaesth Intensive Care 1979 Feb; 7:25–32.

Szeto HH et al. Accumulation of normeperidine, an active metabolite of meperidine, in patients with renal failure or cancer. Ann Intern Med 1977 June; 86:738–741.

Waterson M. Hot & cold therapy. Nursing '78 1978 Oct; 8:46–49.

West A. Understanding endorphins: Our natural pain relief system. Nursing '81 1981 Feb; 11:50–53.

Wood CA, Bailey LR, and Yates JW. Advanced cancer pain management in a community setting. Oncology Nurs Forum 1982 Winter; 9:32–36.

Wright Z. From I.V. to P.O.: Titrating your patient's pain medication. Nursing '81 1981 July; 11:39–43.

Wright Z. Continuous narcotic infusion. Nursing '81 1981 Dec; 11:4–5.

17

Oncology: Nursing the Patient With Cancer

Cancer nursing is an all-inclusive area of practice that covers all age groups and nursing specialties and is carried out in a variety of health care settings, including the home, community, acute care institutions, and rehabilitation centers. However, only within the last decade has the field of cancer nursing, or oncology nursing, emerged as a specialty. Like other specialties in nursing that developed with advances in medicine, cancer nursing has paralleled the development of medical oncology and the major therapeutic advances that have occurred in the care of the person with cancer.

The scope, responsibilities, and goals of cancer nursing are as diverse and complex as those of any nursing specialty. There is a special challenge inherent in caring for people with cancer. The nurse must be equipped to support the individual and his family through a wide range of difficulties marked by physical, emotional, social, cultural, and spiritual upheavals. In order to accomplish the desired outcomes, the nurse must first identify her own reactions to cancer and realistically set goals that can be attained. The fact that the word *cancer* is perceived as synonomous with death and pain in our society is significant. The nurse has the responsibility to realistically support those in her care. Chart 17-1 delineates major areas of responsibility for the nurse caring for the patient with cancer.

Cancer nursing demands an organized and systematic approach to patient care that is guided by standards of practice. These standards of practice provide the framework for establishing the mechanisms of evaluation. The nursing process is the means by which this framework is put into action. The components of assessing, planning, implementing, and evaluating are seen as the key parts in this process. In addition, the nursing process provides a reliable way for the nurse to determine her knowledge level in designing care for this group of patients. In each situation the nurse not only assesses the patient's knowledge level, makes appropriate diagnoses, plans, intervenes, and evaluates, but also applies the same process to herself to assure that her level of preparation is sufficient to guide the patients and their families.

Chart 17-1

Responsibilities of the Nurse Caring for the Cancer Patient and His Family

- Support the idea that cancer is a chronic illness that has acute exacerbations rather than one that is solely synonymous with death and suffering.
- Assess own level of knowledge relative to the pathophysiology of the disease process.
- Make use of current research findings and practices in the care of the cancer patient and his family
- Identify persons at high risk for the development of cancer.
- Assess the nursing care needs of the person with cancer.
- Assess the learning needs, desires, and capabilities of the person with cancer.
- Assess the social support networks available to the person.
- Identify nursing problems of the person and his family.
- Plan appropriate interventions with the person and his family.
- Assist the person to identify his strengths and limitations.
- Assist the person to design short-term and long-term goals for care.
- Implement a nursing plan that interfaces with the medical care regimen and that is consistent with the established goals.
- Collaborate with members of a multidisciplinary team to foster continuity of care.
- Evaluate the goals and resultant outcomes of care with the patient, his family, and the members of the multidisciplinary team.
- Reassess and redesign the direction of the care as determined by the evaluation.

▷ Pathophysiology of the Malignant Process

Cancer should be regarded as a disease process that begins when abnormal cells are derived from normal body cells by some poorly understood mechanism of change. As the disease progresses, these abnormal cells proliferate, still within a local area. However, a stage is then reached in which the cells acquire invasive characteristics and changes occur in surrounding tissues. The cells infiltrate these tissues and gain access to lymph and blood vessels whence they are transported to form *metastases* (cancer spread) in other parts of the body.

Although the disease process can be described in the general terms used above, it should be noted that cancer is not a single disease with one cause; rather it is a group of distinct diseases with different causes, manifestations, treatments, and prognoses.

In order to understand the pathophysiology of cancer, as well as the rationale for choosing a specific therapeutic modality, let us take a brief look at the structure and function of the normal cell and relate these phenomena to the aberrant behavior of the cancer cell.

Cell Structure, Growth, and Function

The basic unit of independent life is the cell, from which the organism as a whole is formed. The living cell is capable of many functions: (1) The cell membrane is selectively permeable to electrolytes, water, nutrients, and various chemical compounds. (2) Various organelles of the cell, such as the mitochondria, convert energy in chemical bonds to carry out cellular activity. (3) Enzymatic processes, such as chemical synthesis or degradation of molecules, occur within the cell. (4) Cells are capable of reproduction (cell cycle). (5) Nuclear DNA affects cellular control, development, and differentiation. (6) Cells can defend against changes in the environment or forces that threaten cellular integrity.

Like the cell, the entire human body has mechanisms for each of these six functions, except that specialization of function and control systems are more highly developed. Yet all of this must spring from the information present in code form in the nucleic acids of the cell nucleus—and that from a single cell, the fertilized egg. The variations of the basic ideas of cell biology are rich and complex, and what follows is but a faint indication of the whole.

A summary of cell substructures and their functions may be found in Chart 17-2.

Control of Cellular Biochemical Events: Role of Nucleic Acids

The control and direction of chemical events provide order and continuity in the life of the cell. Proteins are the bricks of the cellular house, or the catalysts, organizers, and controllers of chemical reactions. They are formed by the combined action of nucleic acids in the nucleus (DNA) and in the cytoplasm (RNA) on amino acids. All of the information needed for the biochemical life of the cell in space and in time is found in the genes of the chromosomes, and this information is transformed into protein molecules.

The answers to a few basic questions will shed some light on the process: What is deoxyribonucleic acid (DNA)? In what sense is it an information data bank? How is a readout (formation of protein) of the information accomplished? DNA is formed from three molecules: phosphate, a five-carbon sugar called deoxyribose, and a variety of purines and pyrimidines (called bases). These are arranged in long strands, the elements being repeated along the strands (Fig. 17-1). The backbone of each strand consists of phosphate sugar linkage. The strands occur in pairs and are twisted together to the right in corkscrew fashion to form a helix. The bases are the purines adenine and guanine and the pyrimidines thymine and cytosine, which are arranged in specific sequences and pairs. The specific arrangement of the bases constitutes the code for the formation of proteins.

Most of the information concerning the role of DNA in heredity and in protein synthesis comes from the study of the DNA strands (prokaryocytes) in viruses and bacteria, in

copy

Chart 17-2
Cell Structure and Function

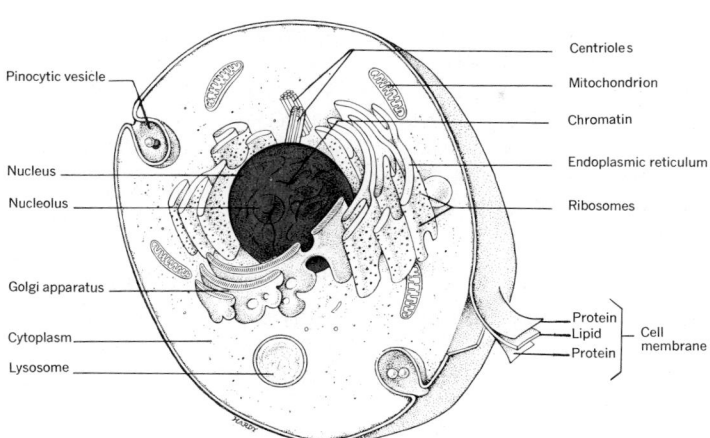

Pinocytic vesicle

Nucleus

Nucleolus

Golgi apparatus

Cytoplasm

Lysosome

Centrioles

Mitochondrion

Chromatin

Endoplasmic reticulum

Ribosomes

Protein
Lipid ⎤ Cell
Protein ⎦ membrane

Cell Membrane

A mosaic of lipids and globular proteins that acts as a boundary between the cell and the environment. It also provides for two-way transport of chemical substances by the following means:

1. Diffusion from an area of high concentration to one of low concentration
2. Specific "carrier proteins" or enzymes that pick up the transported molecules at specific points and move them through the membrane
3. "Carrier proteins" that utilize chemical energy to transport molecules against a chemical gradient (potassium into the cell, sodium out of the cell)
4. Infoldings of the cell that engulf substances, creating pockets that then reopen inward or outward (pinocytosis)

The cell membranes also act as "recognizers" of foreign substances by means of immunoglobulins that cast the cell and combine with antigens to initiate the series of chemical responses called antigen–antibody reactions, which are important to immunity.

Mitochondrion

The mitochondrion is an organelle ("little organ") with enzymes arranged on shelves (cristae) formed from covering membrane. It functions as a means for transferring chemical energy in hydrogen bonds in foodstuffs to adenosine triphosphate (ATP), a common source of energy for cell activities such as transport of molecules, contraction of protein molecules (muscle), and synthesis of chemical compounds. The hydrogen combines with oxygen to form water, and the carbon from which the hydrogen is taken is finally converted into carbon dioxide. The ATP as it releases its energy is converted into *adenosine monophosphate* (AMP), which is ready to again accept hydrogen bond energy to form ATP. Mitochondria, then, capture chemical energy to do chemical work by means of oxidative metabolism.

Endoplasmic Reticulum

A variable network of tubular or vesicular (bubble-shaped) protein structures that are the sites of synthesis of various molecules needed by the cells. Smooth, or agranular, endoplasmic reticulum is involved in lipid synthesis (especially triglycerides), conjugation of bile pigments, conversion of glycogen to glucose (glycogenolysis), and drug detoxification. Granular endoplasmic reticulum is studded with ribosomes composed of ribonucleic acids, and is important in protein synthesis.

Golgi Apparatus

A variable structure, loosely organized; probably another form of the endoplasmic reticulum associated with the formation of secretory molecules (usually arranged in granules), such as the digestive enzymes of the pancreas and the small bowel that are released from the cell. Other digestive enzymes remain in the cell as packets surrounded by a layer of lipoprotein. The function of these packets, called lysosomes, is to digest foreign substances (bacteria) in the cell, or the cell itself in case of cell death (cytolysis).

Structures Specialized for a Particular Cell

microtubules   Protein structures of cilia or sperm that provide motion

myofibrils   Protein structures that shorten and lengthen, as in muscle

Centrioles

A complex of short rods forming a hollow cylinder, generally found near the nucleus. During cell division these migrate to opposite sides of the nucleus and act as a center for the formation and organization of microtubules that make up the spindle and aster of the metaphase portion of mitosis. They may also produce cilia and flagella.

(continued)

Chart 17-2
Cell Structure and Function (continued)

Nucleus

A cell organelle containing deoxyribonucleic acid (DNA), and separated from the cytoplasm by a membrane derived from endoplasmic reticulum. Because of its intense staining properties, DNA is called *chromatin* and may be dispersed or formed into knots or, during cell division, organized into rodlike units called *chromosomes*, which in turn have subunits called *genes*. Genes control the synthesis of protein in cells according to the information contained in the DNA strands. Thus, the nucleus contains the data bank and control system that direct the unfolding biochemical events that constitute the life of the cell.

Nucleolus

A substructure of the nucleus, present in variable numbers, that contains fibrous structures and ribonucleic acid, a component in the sequences of chemical events that originate in the nucleus and end with the formation of protein in the cytoplasm.

Products of Cell Activity

Lipid droplets formed in the cell or, in the case of the intestine, absorbed. Granules, probably enzymes, or histamine in macrophages, etc. Glycogen, or cell starch. Small filaments.

Water and Soluble Substances

Sodium, potassium, urea, glucose, protein molecules, anions, in great numbers.

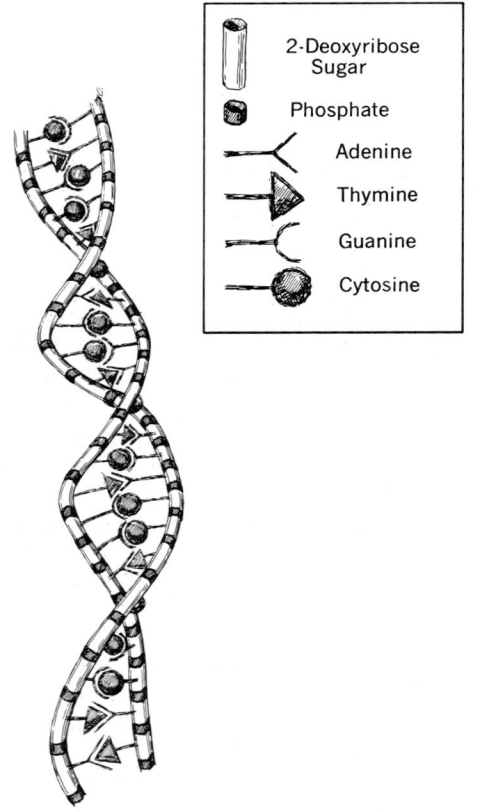

2-Deoxyribose Sugar

Phosphate

Adenine

Thymine

Guanine

Cytosine

Figure 17-1. Schematic representation of the spiral ladder arrangement of repeating nucleotide units found in the DNA molecule. It is thought that anywhere from 500 to 1000 of these rungs make up a single gene, and that there are over 1000 genes in a single chromosome. (From Chaffee EE and Greisheimer EM: Basic Physiology and Anatomy. Philadelphia, JB Lippincott.)

which each chromosome is a single circular strand of DNA with a molecular weight of about one million. Probably this information is true for the human complex chromosomes with strands whose molecular weight approaches one billion. The following discussion refers to prokaryocyte material.

Three bases (a triplet) constitute the unit of the code system (codon). Twenty amino acids are coded, and each has more than one triplet; three codons are used to determine the length of the protein chain and to signal the start or stop of the protein synthesis. DNA must express its code through ribonucleic acid (RNA) contained in the nucleoli and in the cytoplasm. RNA, like DNA, is a helix made up of a sugar, phosphate, and bases, except that the 5-carbon sugar is ribose and the pyrimidine uracil is used instead of thymine. In addition, RNA is a single rather than a double strand. RNA occurs in three forms: messenger RNA, ribosome RNA, and transfer RNA, each with its own function.

A skeleton of the theory of protein synthesis goes something like this:

A DNA helix partially untwists, exposing a section called a gene, which controls the formation for a specific protein. Molecules of ribose, phosphate, and particular bases line up against corresponding units in the DNA, and an enzyme RNA polymerase joins these units together to form messenger RNA. Messenger RNA, now carrying the code, moves to the cytoplasm where it attaches to ribosome RNA. This attachment permits the messenger RNA to accept alignment of amino acids in the sequence determined by the code. The amino acids are brought to the ribosome RNA by transfer RNA that is specific for the amino acid. When all the amino acids are lined up, enzymes join them together, and the protein chain is formed. Thousands of forms of messenger RNA occur, about 60 of transfer RNA, and a few of ribosome RNA.

The twisting and untwisting of DNA, the length of the sequence, and the signals to start and stop synthesis are factors involved in the process. DNA can also reproduce itself via the enzyme DNA polymerase.

During cell reproduction, either for growth or replacement, the DNA is duplicated; the DNA strands are untwisted, replicated, and parcelled into two groups, each containing identical genetic material, the latter process being called *mitosis*. The result is two cells with identical structure and heredity, each cell containing the DNA structure possessed originally by the fertilized ovum. Sex cells (ova or spermatozoa), when dividing, parcel out only one half of the genetic material to each of the resulting cells (reduction division, or meiosis). Fertilization of the ovum restores the full complement of DNA (46 chromosomes), but they are of differing heredity, since genetic material from two separate individuals is combined.

The Cell Cycle

The completed division of a cell is called a *cell cycle*. Cells in tissues are divided into three populations: (1) continuously dividing cells (bone marrow stem cells, crypt cells of the small intestine), (2) nondividing cells (neurons), and (3) resting cells (liver, thyroid gland) that are capable, when appropriately stimulated, of reproducing.

The reference event in the cell cycle is *mitosis*, when the chromosomes are dividing into two portions and are pulled by contracting microtubules (asters) into daughter cells; the cycle extends from mid-mitosis to mid-mitosis of the daughter cells. With respect to DNA, the cycle is marked by two events: the unseen synthesis of DNA (S period of time), and the seen mitosis; the remaining periods are resting periods as far as DNA replication or distribution is concerned. These phases may be identified as follows: S (DNA synthesis), G_0 (resting phase), G_1 (early protein synthesis), G_2 (RNA synthesis and expanded protein synthesis) and M (metaphase). In cells of the human colon, the time of S is 25 hours; of G_1, 15 hours; of G_2, 3 hours; and of M, 1 hour.

Cancer, DNA, and the Cell Cycle

There is a relationship between cancer, DNA, and the cell cycle. Cancer may be considered an unfortunate change in replication structure or control (mutation). Several possible mechanisms have been studied: (1) incorporation of viral DNA into the genetic structure; (2) changes in DNA repair mechanisms; and (3) changes in DNA structure caused by radiation, drugs, metabolic diseases, or recurrent cell injury. These cells with altered DNA enter the active cell cycle and, released from physiologic controls, reproduce endlessly.

Principle of Cancer Therapy

The aim of cancer therapy is to destroy all of the cancer cells while avoiding normal cell damage. The cell in active division, particularly during DNA synthesis or replication, is most sensitive to the toxic effect of chemicals and radiation (x-ray beam, radioactive isotopes, or radium). Development of antitumor drugs has been directed toward either DNA structure or synthesis, or toward protein synthesis, because a change in either will prevent cell duplication.

During chemotherapy, any normal cells in the S portion of the cycle (DNA synthesis) are vulnerable, along with the cancer cells. If large numbers of cancer cells are in the S phase, and but few normal cells, then chemotherapy may result in satisfactory tumor destruction. Agents directed toward RNA and protein synthesis (antibiotics and alkylating agents) are nonspecific in that all cells are active in these chemical activities. Obviously, the normally continuously dividing cells (bone marrow stem cells, gastrointestinal cells) are exceptionally sensitive to the action of anticancer agents, and thus the side-effects of anemia, diminished white cell count, and diarrhea are explained.

One of the main thrusts of current research is the search for chemical agents that synchronize cancer cell division so that all are in the S phase; then, antitumor treatment would be maximally effective. The need to localize anticancer drugs to the tumor as much as possible is obvious.

The unfolding of the DNA-protein synthesis story and the framework of the cell cycle have yielded a good theoretical basis for the development of new agents, particularly those that focus on single anatomical targets or chemical events.

▷ Classification of Cysts and Tumors

Cysts

A *cyst* is an abnormal collection of fluid within a definite sac or wall. Cysts may form in several different ways. When the outlet to a gland becomes blocked and the gland continues to secrete, a *retention cyst* is formed. Remnants of fetal organs secrete a fluid that can form cysts (called *epidermoid cysts*), often of considerable size, especially when springing from the pelvic organs of the female. An extravasation of blood in the tissues may become surrounded by a definite wall and form an *extravasation cyst*.

Cysts may be formed by parasites, especially the *Taenia echinococcus (Echinococcus granulosus)* or dog tapeworm. These cysts, spoken of as *hydatid cysts*, are often of considerable size and are usually found in the liver.

Cysts of several types should be removed when possible, because occasionally they change into malignant growths. They often become infected, at which time incision and drainage are necessary.

Tumors

A *tumor* is a new growth of tissue (neoplasm) in which the multiplication of cells is progressive and uncontrolled. According to gross appearance, a tumor may be described as *exophytic*, that is, growing away from the surface; *verrucous*, growing along the surface; or *infiltrative*, invading the tissue right from the beginning.

Benign or Nonmalignant Tumors

Some tumors are surrounded by a definite capsule and remain localized in the tissue from which they spring. They

Table 17-1
Comparison of Benign and Malignant Cells

	Benign	Malignant
Cell type	Adult	Young
Mitotic action	Slight	Usually considerable
Parent resemblance; morphology	Close resemblance to tissue of origin	Cells tend to be anaplastic—less differentiated than normal cells from which they derive
Encapsulation	Often present	Never present
Growth rate	Slow expansion	Rapid infiltration
Spread	Never occurs; remains localized	Forms secondary growths by metastasis through both lymph and blood stream
Recurrence	Does not tend to recur when removed	Tends to recur when removed, because of infiltration
Tissue destruction	Harms the host only by pressure of growth on surrounding structures	Causes loss of weight and strength, anemia, cachexia, and eventually death

disturb their host only by exerting pressure on the surrounding structures or by robbing the normal tissues of their blood supply. These tumors usually grow rather slowly, and once removed they do not tend to recur. Such tumors are spoken of as *benign* or *nonmalignant*.

Malignant Tumors

Other neoplasms are not surrounded by a capsule, but grow by invasion into the tissues surrounding them; these are *malignant tumors.* Such tumors invade the blood vessels or the lymphatics and extend rapidly along these open channels. Often the tumor cells are broken off and carried by the blood and the lymph to other parts of the body, where they set up a secondary growth.

Secondary growths are looked for at the nearest lymph filter, the lymph nodes. Here cells are caught and may begin to form an independent tumor like the parent or primary growth. Thus, in every patient with cancer of the breast, the axilla is examined carefully for enlarged lymph nodes, because it is known that the lymph flow from the breast is through the axillary lymph nodes.

Tumor cells that invade the blood vessels are carried to organs where the venous blood passes through a capillary bed; thus, we see secondary tumors appearing in the lung from a cancer of the breast or in the liver when the cells are carried by the portal venous system from a tumor in the abdomen. This property of tumors is called *metastasis,* and the new or secondary growth is called a *metastatic growth.* The cells of these secondary tumors grow rapidly and under the microscope resemble the rapidly growing cells found in the embryo. They invade the surrounding tissues in such a manner that it is nearly impossible to remove all the tumor cells and, therefore, they often recur after the main body of the tumor has been removed.

The rapid growth of the tumor and its secondary growths saps the vitality of its host, with the result that there is a rapid loss of weight and strength. These tumors bleed easily, producing a loss of the red cells in the blood—an anemia. The patient finally becomes thin, pale, and weak, a shadow of his former self. This condition is spoken of as *cachexia.* The course of the disease frequently ends in death.

Since a tumor that is at first benign may take on malignant characteristics, in most instances it is beneficial to remove all tumors as soon as they are discovered. For a comparison of the characteristics of benign and malignant tumors see Table 17-1.

Subdivisions According to Tissue Type

Neoplasms are subdivided further according to the kind of tissue of which they are formed (Table 17-2). In embryonic life there are three divisions of tissue from which all others are formed: (1) endoderm, (2) mesoderm, and (3) ectoderm.

Endoderm is the tissue from which the lining membranes (mucosa) of the respiratory tract, the gastrointestinal tract, and the genitourinary tract are formed.

Mesoderm is the tissue from which muscles, bones, fascia, and connective tissue are formed.

Ectoderm is the tissue from which come the skin cells and the cells composing hair follicles, sweat glands, and the entire nervous system.

Complex Tissues.   Some tumors, thought to result from embryologic maldevelopment, contain more than one of the embryonal tissues. Tumors containing two of the tissues, called *teratomas* or *dermoids,* are not infrequently seen in operations on the ovary or the testicle. They may contain bone, teeth, and muscle—all of which arise from the mesoderm—and hair, skin, and subcutaneous glands, all of which develop from the ectoderm.

New growths often are composed of more than one tissue and are named accordingly—fibroadenoma, fibrolipoma, osteosarcoma, and so forth.

▷ Incidence of Various Malignancies

The importance of malignant growth to the nursing and the medical professions can be understood if some of the facts concerning its incidence are reviewed. It is estimated that in the United States malignancy exacts a toll of 430,000 lives annually, ranking second as the principle cause of death, being exceeded only by heart disease. One out of five deaths that occur in adults is caused by malignancy. It is estimated that more than 139,000 cancer patients might have been *copy*

saved in 1982, for example, had they recognized early symptoms and sought prompt treatment. At present only one in three cancer victims is saved, although one in two could be saved if diagnosed early enough and given better treatment. Cancer affects men and women of all ages and of all races; no organ of the body is exempt (Fig. 17-2).

▷ Cancer Causes, Prevention, and Control

Emphasis on cancer prevention and control began with the implementation of the National Cancer Act of 1971. The stated goal was to use research to develop means of reducing morbidity and mortality from cancer by:

- Preventing as many cancers as possible
- Providing maximum palliation to patients not cured
- Rehabilitating treated patients to as normal a state as possible

Since 1971, continued progress has been made in the prevention and control of cancer, largely because of several factors, including the following: people in general are more concerned with their own health; the National Cancer Institute has shifted some of its emphasis to prevention; the American Society of Preventive Oncology was formed in 1976; cancer centers around the country emphasize prevention; and special projects, such as the Breast Cancer Detection Demonstration Project, have been conducted. The most important reason, however, seems to be that prevention of cancer, or any disease, for that matter, makes sense. Formerly, attention was focused on interrupting the disease process itself. It is now generally accepted that through modification of individual behavioral and environmental factors, the development of some cancers can be prevented. The most striking example of this, of course, is the relationship between smoking and lung cancer.

It is therefore imperative that nurses use a variety of means to increase public awareness of those factors that have an impact on the prevention and control of cancers. This can be accomplished through health education, health maintenance programs, dissemination of significant research findings, and generally by supporting the concepts inherent in prevention and control. In order to achieve these outcomes, knowledge of causative factors, signs, symptoms, and risk factors is essential. The major warning signs of cancer are effectively presented in the following format:

C—Change in bowel or bladder habits
A—A sore that does not heal
U—Unusual bleeding or discharge
T—Thickening or lump in breast or elsewhere
I —Indigestion or difficulty in swallowing
O—Obvious change in wart or mole
N—Nagging cough or hoarseness

Causative factors are generally grouped under four headings: (1) physical, (2) chemical, (3) genetic, and (4) viral.

Table 17-2
Classification of Tumor Cells

Origin of Cell	Benign	Malignant
Epithelium:		
Skin epithelium	Papilloma	Cancer—carcinoma
Gland epithelium	Wart (verruca)	
	Polyp	Basal cell carcinoma
	Adenoma	Adenocarcinoma
Endothelial Tissue:		
Blood vessels		Endothelioma
	Hemangioma	Hemangiosarcoma
	Glomus tumor	Hemangioendo-thelioma
	Hemangiopericytoma	Malignant hemangio-pericytoma
Lymph vessels	Lymphangioma	Lymphangiosarcoma
Lymphoid tissue		Lymphosarcoma
Connective Tissue:		
Fibrous tissue	Fibroma	Fibrosarcoma
Adipose tissue	Lipoma	Liposarcoma
Cartilage	Chondroma	Chondrosarcoma
	Osteochondroma	Primary
	Chondroblastoma	Secondary
	Enchondroma	
Bone	Osteoma	Osteosarcoma
	Osteoid osteoma	
	Osteoblastoma	
Marrow elements: Hematopoietic cells		Plasma cell myeloma
		Ewing's sarcoma
		Reticulum cell sarcoma
Muscle tissue:	Myoma	Myosarcoma
Smooth muscle	Leiomyoma	Leiomyosarcoma
Striated muscle	Rhabdomyoma	Rhabdomyosarcoma
Nerve tissue:		
Nerve fibers	Neuroma	Neurogenic sarcoma
Ganglion cells	Ganglioneuroma	Neuroblastoma
Glial cells	Glioma*	Glioblastoma
Meninges	Meningioma	
Pigmented neoplasm	Nevus—mole	Malignant melanoma
Notochord		Chordoma
Uncertain origin	Giant cell tumor	Giant cell tumor
		Adamantinoma

* Many classify glioma as malignant

Physical Causes
Physical factors associated with cancer include exposure to radiation and physical irritation. *Radiation-induced cancers* primarily result from exposure to ultraviolet and ionizing radiation. The major source of ultraviolet radiation is excessive exposure to sunlight. It is known that excessive exposure, especially in fair-skinned persons, increases the risk of squamous cell carcinoma, basal cell carcinoma, and

1982 Estimated cancer incidence by site and sex*

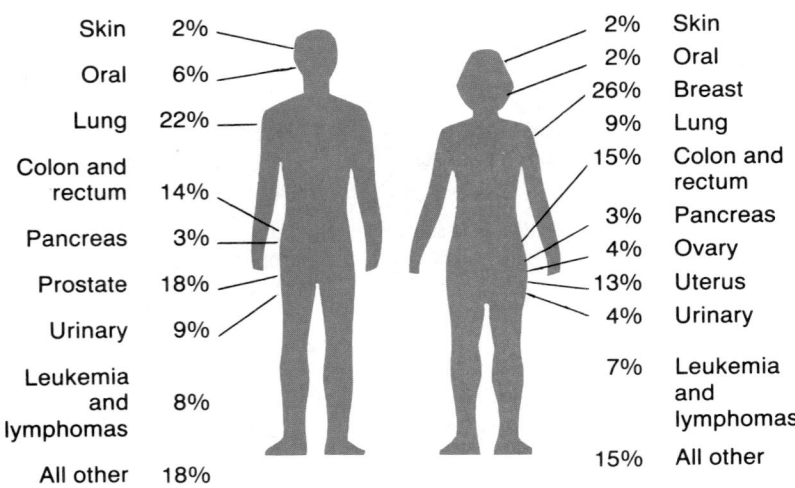

Skin	2%		2%	Skin
Oral	6%		2%	Oral
Lung	22%		26%	Breast
Colon and rectum	14%		9%	Lung
Pancreas	3%		15%	Colon and rectum
Prostate	18%		3%	Pancreas
Urinary	9%		4%	Ovary
Leukemia and lymphomas	8%		13%	Uterus
All other	18%		4%	Urinary
			7%	Leukemia and lymphomas
			15%	All other

*Excluding non-melanoma skin cancer and carcinoma in situ.

1982 Estimated cancer deaths by site and sex

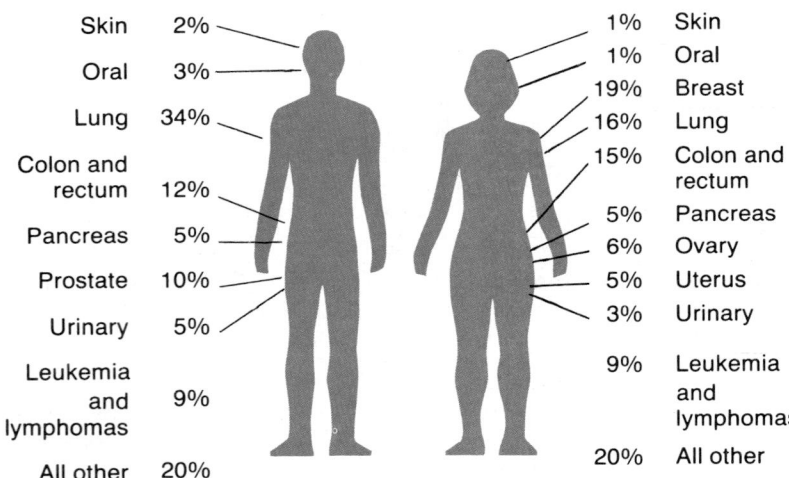

Skin	2%		1%	Skin
Oral	3%		1%	Oral
Lung	34%		19%	Breast
Colon and rectum	12%		16%	Lung
Pancreas	5%		15%	Colon and rectum
Prostate	10%		5%	Pancreas
Urinary	5%		6%	Ovary
Leukemia and lymphomas	9%		5%	Uterus
All other	20%		3%	Urinary
			9%	Leukemia and lymphomas
			20%	All other

Figure 17-2. Estimated cancer incidence and death by site and sex. (Courtesy, American Cancer Society)

melanoma. Ionizing radiation may result from diagnostic procedures or treatment modalities or from radiation found in nuclear power plants and in various occupational settings. Exact dose response levels are not known, making it difficult to determine a safe minimal exposure. Certainly, it is known that some factors, such as the individual's health status, his hormonal and immunological competency, and environmental factors, as well as the site of exposure influence the response to radiation exposure. It remains to be discovered just what the exact mechanism is in this aspect of oncogenesis. It is the responsibility of health care professionals in general to be aware of the potential hazards involved in radiation exposure and to advise persons about the best way to minimize exposure and protect themselves from untoward effects. (See Chapter 18 for a more detailed discussion of radiation.)

Physical irritants such as implanted cellophane, nylon, polyvinyl, and other inert substances have been shown to cause sarcomas in experimental animals. Research efforts seem to indicate that it is the presence of the object, not the chemical composition of the substance, that is the carcinogenic agent. Research continues in this area.

Chemical Carcinogens

Through the years, various chemical compounds have been linked to cancer, including aromatic polycyclic hydrocarbons (coal tar), aromatic amines, aminostilbenes, urethane, and such metals as nickel, iron, beryllium, chromium, arsenic, asbestos, azo dyes, nitroso-amines, and lactones. Other chemical carcinogens include agricultural insecticides, herbicides, fertilizers, and preservatives.

Food Additives and Cancer. Although nitrites are used as food additives in many countries, they are thought to react with amines to form carcinogens. Legislative controls are necessary to reduce or limit the use of such carcinogenic compounds in food processing.

Industrial Environments. In certain "dirty" industries, conditions exist that seem to be conducive to the development of cancer. This is particularly apparent in chemical plants and asbestos processing companies, where the incidence of lung, liver, and bladder cancer is higher than in clean industries.

Pharmaceutical Products. Certain cancers are seen today in patients who received certain medications, such as arsenical preparations, 20 years ago. Stilbestrol, a medication given to selected pregnant women approximately 20 years ago, has been under study as a carcinogen because, upon reaching puberty, some of the female offspring of the women who received this drug have developed vaginal adenosis, a precursor of vaginal carcinoma.

Smoking and Cancer. Cigarette smoking has not only been implicated as a cause of lung cancer but also has been associated with cancer of the mouth, pharynx, esophagus, proximal end of the stomach, and urinary bladder. Smoking less may help an individual to increase his chances of not getting cancer.

Alcohol and Cancer. Alcohol is known to promote the development of cancer. In addition, persons who combine smoking with drinking alcohol have an increased risk of cancer occurring in the mouth, larynx, and esophagus, where the two substances interact. It should be noted, however, that the risk of cancer is increased in heavy drinkers even if they are nonsmokers. This phenomenon may be due to alcohol acting both as a co-carcinogen and as a primary carcinogen or to the alterations that result from malnutrition or other health problems associated with heavy drinking and smoking.

Genetic Factors

Although more knowledge is being gained about the genetic aspects of cancer, not enough is known at present to include it as a part of active cancer prevention. However, there seems to be a genetic predisposition or familial tendency toward acquiring cancer. Persons whose immediate family members have cancer of the breast, stomach, colon, uterus, or lung are more likely to develop a similar cancer.

In addition, familial-linked cancers tend to be characterized by an earlier age of onset and a higher incidence of bilateral disease (breast cancer, pheochromocytomas, and Wilms' tumors). In addition, when people with a family history of cancer are compared with those who do not have such a history, autosomal dominant inheritance patterns are noted as well as a general increased risk of other cancers. It is imperative that these cancer-prone families be identified and their risks addressed. This is a fertile area for nursing research and subsequent intervention.

Viral Causes

Although viruses may indeed play a role in oncogenesis, definitive evidence linking the two has not yet been demonstrated. One theory proposes that the virus becomes incorporated into the genetic makeup of the cell. Once this occurs there is alteration in subsequent generations of that cell, possibly leading to cancer. An example of this mechanism is seen in the Epstein–Barr virus, which is linked to the development of Burkitt's lymphoma in the tropical areas of Africa and Southern China. Why the incidence of this disease is low in countries such as the United States is not totally understood. Possible factors may be the status of the individual's immune system and the general diseases to which he is exposed; in Africa there is an abundance of diseases such as malaria and schistosomiasis. Other possible viral-linked cancers are cervical cancer, which evidence indicates may be associated with the herpes simplex virus, and Hodgkin's disease. Further research is needed in each of these areas.

Other Causes

It should be evident that clear-cut answers to the causes of cancer remain somewhat elusive. The causes of many very common cancers have not been definitely identified. Dietary factors may play a significant role in the development of some cancers, such as those of the colon, breast, and stomach. However, research in this area is hampered by the complex nature of ascertaining the direct cause and effect of foodstuffs ingested by individuals over time. Psychological stress is another area that is receiving increased attention as at least a co-causative factor in the development of cancer. Finally, the broad area encompassed by immunology must continue to be studied extensively. Only continued research will provide answers to the question "What are the causes of cancer?"

▷ Dimensions of Cancer Therapy

Treatment for cancer has been and will continue to be a very complex undertaking. Single-modality therapy is being replaced with combination or *adjuvant therapy,* in which two or more treatment modalities (surgery, radiation therapy, chemotherapy, hormonal therapy, or immunotherapy) may be combined, or two or more forms of a single modality may be used. For example, in chemotherapy, two or more agents that have similar end effects on cells but different mechanisms of action and resultant toxicities may be chosen. The rationale behind this type of therapy lies in the ability of the treatment regimen to interrupt the normal life cycle of the cancer cells from as many vantage points as possible, thereby killing the greatest number of cells. The consequences of this approach also involve normal cells. Chemotherapeutic agents are generally not cell-selective in the sense of discriminating between normal and abnormal cells. However, many agents are significantly more toxic to cancer cells than to normal cells. The agents have their greatest effect on the more rapidly proliferating cells, which include the cancer cells and cells of the bone marrow, mu-

---

Chart 17-3
The TNM System

T—Primary Tumor
N—Regional Lymph Nodes
M—Distant Metastasis

This classification is extended by the following designations:

Tumor
TO—No tumor clinically
TIS—Carcinoma *in situ*
T1, T2, T3, T4—Ascending degrees of increase in tumor
    size and involvement

Nodes
NO—No regional lymph node involvement assessed
    clinically
NX—Regional lymph nodes cannot be assessed clinically
N1, N2, N3, N4—Ascending degrees of nodal involvement

Metastasis
MO—No evidence of distant metastasis
M1, M2, M3, M4—Ascending degrees of metastatic
    involvement of the host

TNM assignments may be grouped into a small number of
clinical stages. Stage-grouping by site is recommended on
the basis of field trials.

(American Cancer Society)

---

cous membranes, skin, and hair. Each individual's response to therapy must be closely monitored to ascertain the occurrence of dangerous toxicities. When chemotherapy is combined with another modality, such as radiation therapy, the toxic effects can be magnified even more. Additional attention must be given to sequencing and dosing when one or more approaches are used.

Adjuvant therapy for cancer provides the most comprehensive approach to the management of the individual with cancer. The most appropriate combination of treatment modalities is determined by a multidisciplinary team often consisting of the patient's own physician, a medical or surgical oncologist, a radiation oncologist, a nurse oncologist, a pharmacist, a rehabilitation therapist, and perhaps research team members. These health professionals design the most appropriate and effective therapeutic regimens for the patient. The options are then presented to the patient and his family for consideration. Throughout this process the nurse is intimately involved and serves as the patient's advocate. The nurse assists the patient and his family with questions that may arise about the treatment options and is also in a position to act as liaison between the patient and his family and members of the multidisciplinary treatment team. In order to be capable of serving in these roles, the nurse must have a thorough understanding of the rationale for the treatment options and of the goals of each modality.

Surgery for Cancer

Surgical removal of the entire cancer remains the best and most frequently used modality of treatment. However, the surgical approach may be selected for a variety of reasons. Surgery may be selected as the primary method of treatment, or it may be diagnostic, prophylactic, palliative, or reconstructive in purpose.

Surgery as Primary Treatment. When surgery is used as the primary approach in the treatment of cancer, the goal is to remove the entire tumor (or as much as is feasible, a procedure often called *debulking*) and any involved surrounding tissue, including regional lymph nodes. Contrary to the design of surgical therapy in the past, the goal is not to excise all possible tumor cells. It is now recognized that the growth and dissemination of cancer cells have often produced distant micrometastases by the time the patient seeks treatment. Therefore, attempting to remove wide margins of tissue in the hopes of "getting all the cancer cells" is often not realistic. This reality substantiates the need for a coordinated multidisciplinary approach to cancer therapy. Once the surgery has been completed, one or more additional modalities may be chosen to increase the likelihood of cancer cell destruction. There are, however, cancers that when treated surgically in the very early stages are considered to be curable (*e.g.,* skin cancers, testicular cancers).

Diagnostic Surgery. Diagnostic surgery is usually performed to obtain a *biopsy,* the excision of a piece of tissue from a suspicious growth. The three most common biopsy methods are the *excisional, incisional,* and *needle* methods.

The *excisional method* is most frequently used for biopsies of the skin, the upper respiratory tract, and the upper and lower portions of the gastrointestinal tract, in which removal of the entire tumor is often possible. This approach not only provides the pathologist with the entire specimen, but decreases the chance of cellular seeding of the tumor. The *incisional method* is used if the tumor mass is too large to be removed. It is imperative that the biopsy be representative of the tumor mass so that the pathologist can provide an accurate diagnosis. Both of these approaches are often endoscopic procedures.

Surgical incision may also be done for the purpose of *staging,* which is a means of determining the extensiveness of the cancer. This is a crucial aspect of the diagnostic process. Treatment regimens, options presented to patients, and prognostic factors are based upon accurate staging. A system called the TNM system has been developed by the American Joint Committee for Cancer Staging and End Results Reporting. The TNM system is a method of categorizing the primary lesion and the extent of involvement. The *T* describes the growth of the primary tumor; the *N* describes the spread to regional lymph nodes; and the *M* describes the distant metastases. Each component of the TNM system is subcategorized to provide for more discrete descriptions of the extent of disease. Chart 17-3 describes the TNM system in greater detail.

It should be noted that other classification systems are used for the staging of diseases such as malignant melanoma, Hodgkin's disease, and lymphomas. A description of each of these systems is beyond the scope of this chapter.

Needle biopsy is performed if a suspicious mass is discovered. There are several advantages and disadvantages to this technique. The procedure itself is fast, inexpensive, and easy to perform and causes the patient only temporary discomfort. Generally, with the equipment in current use, the degree to which the surrounding tissue is disturbed is kept to a minimum, thus decreasing the likelihood of tumor seeding. Even with the most skilled cytologists, there is always the chance of missing the tumor or obtaining a biopsy from such a small area that a full description of the cellular types is not possible. This type of procedure is frequently used for lesions of the lung, breast, liver, and kidney. (A biopsy should never be performed for a suspected lesion of the testes. In that situation, orchiectomy is the primary treatment of all suspected tumors.)

The choice of biopsy to be performed takes into account many factors. Of greatest importance is the type of treatment to consider if a diagnosis of cancer is confirmed. The proposed surgical area includes the area of biopsy so that any cells that might have been dislodged during the procedure are excised at the time of surgery. In addition, the condition of the patient is considered. Assessment of his nutritional, respiratory, renal, and hepatic systems is essential in determining the most appropriate method of treatment. If the biopsy procedure will require general anesthesia, and subsequent surgery is likely, the effects of total anesthesia on the individual are considered. The patient and his family should be given an opportunity to discuss the available options before definitive plans are made. The nurse, as the patient's advocate, serves as a liaison between the patient and the physician in order to facilitate this process. Time should be set aside so that interruptions are at a minimum and all participants are as relaxed as possible. Time for questions and for "thinking" through all that has been discussed should be provided.

Prophylactic Surgery. Prophylactic surgery involves the removal of lesions that are apt to develop into cancer if they are left in the body. An example is the removal of small tumors (polyps) that often grow in the colon. Recently, more aggressive surgical procedures have been performed as prophylactic measures. The two most common are colectomies and mastectomies in individuals who are at a significantly high risk owing to personal and family history. Since the long-term physiologic and psychological effects are not currently known, these therapeutic approaches should be offered selectively to patients. Appropriate preoperative information and counseling, as well as long-term follow-up, should be available.

Palliative Surgery. When cure of the cancer is no longer a realistic goal, the emphasis on the therapeutic regimen shifts from one that is curative to one that is intended to provide the patient with as much comfort as possible, so that he can live a satisfying and productive life for as long as is feasible. Whether the period of time involved is extremely short or is extensive, the major issue is the quality of life—with quality defined by the patient and his family.

Palliative surgery, then, is performed in an attempt to relieve complications of cancer, such as ulcerations, ob-structions, hemorrhage, pain, or infection. This type of surgery includes nerve blocks and cordotomies designed to relieve intractable pain; tumor resection, to relieve obstruction that may occur if a segment of bowel is obstructed (this may result in ostomies, depending upon the extent of invasion); and simple mastectomies for ulcerative breast disease. The nurse must recognize the goal of this therapy and provide appropriate counseling and referrals for patients and their families. Surgical intervention is not the only modality used for palliation. Radiation therapy is frequently used to shrink the tumor, slow its growth, and relieve pain. In addition, various chemotherapeutic and hormonal regimens can be prescribed. Finally, surgical removal of hormone-producing glands that might enhance tumor growth is often performed. These glands include the pituitary, adrenals, ovaries, and testes.

Reconstructive Surgery. This type of surgery may follow curative or radical surgery and is carried out in an attempt to produce a better return of function or a better cosmetic effect. It may be done in one operation or in stages. Presurgery counseling and evaluation are recommended. The surgeon who does the reconstructive surgery should be called in preoperatively. Often, the woman who is to have breast reconstruction done will see the surgeon before hospitalization for a mastectomy. This approach provides the woman something positive to focus on, at a time when thoughts of mutilation and death may be paramount. The physician performing the reconstructive surgery also benefits from seeing the way the woman's breasts appear normally and from establishing rapport with her. The nurse must be cognizant of the woman's sexual needs and the impact that an altered body image may have on her sexuality. Providing the woman and her family with opportunities to discuss these issues is imperative. This is only one example of reconstructive surgery. The needs of individuals in general must be accurately assessed and validated in each situation.

Immunotherapy

Immunotherapy has emerged as an additional treatment modality for the individual with cancer. Generally, this form of therapy is an adjuvant to the three other primary modes (surgery, chemotherapy, and radiation).

The concept of immunotherapy dates back to ancient times. However, not until the last several decades has immunotherapy received a great deal of attention as a treatment modality. Like many new approaches to cancer therapy, it was initially viewed as the hope for the future. Unfortunately, interest in and efficacy of this approach has waxed and waned. There are many reasons for these fluxes. What was initially thought to be simply a matter of dealing with a suppressed immune system has turned out to be a very complex network of events. Cancer is thought to be immunosuppressive, thus accounting for the view that if the cause of the suppression can be reduced or removed and the immune system stimulated, then the cancer can be eradicated. In theory, this approach has merit; what is not discussed is how the cancer developed in the first place. Was it immunosuppression that initially allowed the cancer to occur, or did the cancer cause the immunosuppression? If one considers the latter explanation, one must ask what was it that prevented the immune system from recognizing the cancer cells as foreign invaders. The failure of the body's immune system to recognize the cancer cells as foreign is the key to understanding the concepts of immunotherapy. The work continues as attempts are made to identify antigens that are specific to the surface of the tumor cell in the hope of developing tumor-specific antibodies that will combat them. Such work is being done currently with monoclonal antibodies, highly specific antibodies, which it is hoped can be used in the future to enhance the diagnosis and treatment of cancer.

In addition, much attention has been given to the nonspecific approach to immunotherapy. Interferon and BCG are two examples that fall into this category. The mechanism of action is a general stimulation of the individual's immune system rather than an attempt to attack the specific tumor. Outcomes of these approaches have been variable and need additional research to determine how useful they will be in the future.

Chemotherapy

Historically, cancer chemotherapy was introduced in the 1940s with the advent of the androgens, estrogens, and nitrogen mustard. Although during the 50s and 60s new agents were constantly being developed, in the 70s a leveling off occurred. It is hoped that the 80s will bring a new surge in the discovery and clinical application of additional agents.

The increase in the number of chemotherapeutic agents was accompanied by a more sophisticated approach to the treatment regimen. Attitudes toward chemotherapy have also become more positive. No longer is it viewed as a modality of last resort. Instead, it is considered to be an integral part of cancer therapy as a whole. The practitioner is now able to define the exact purpose for which he chooses chemotherapy, that is, for the purpose of cure, remission, or palliation. Responses that can be elicited in certain neoplastic diseases by the use of specific chemotherapeutic agents are outlined in Table 17-3. In addition, chemotherapy may be selected as the sole therapeutic modality or as an adjuvant to surgery, radiation, or immunotherapy. As with any modality, the choices must be made with extreme care and with the individual patient in mind. Certainly, one advantage of chemotherapy is that it is a systemic method— the only major one available. It therefore represents the best defense against disseminated disease. (Although immunotherapy is recognized as being systemic, to date it does not represent a major force in therapy.) As was indicated earlier, chemotherapy generally does not discriminate between normal body cells and cancer cells. The choice of agents is crucial in order to maximize the therapeutic effects while minimizing the toxic effects.

The overall goal of therapy is to attack the cancer cells during their most vulnerable phases. The fact that cells at any given time are at various stages in their developmental cycle provides the framework upon which many current chemotherapy regimens are built. In order to kill as many cells as possible, drugs with differing specificities are combined. Cycles of administration are also timed so as to allow

these drugs to attack newly proliferating cells. Specific determinations that must be made before chemotherapeutic agents are prescribed include the following:

1. What is the nature of the tumor?
2. Is this therapy to be used as an adjuvant to some other method of cancer treatment, or is it considered after other methods have failed?
3. How effective is each drug for this particular patient?
4. What is the appropriate dosage in relation to the patient's weight and height, in view of the narrow margin between therapeutic dose and toxic level?
5. How much time should be allowed between series of dosages so that normal tissue can recover from toxic effects?
6. What are the side-effects, particularly the extent of damage to bone marrow, which reduces the number of white cells, red cells, and platelets?
7. Has liver function been affected, since these drugs are metabolized in the liver?
8. Has kidney function been affected, since chemotherapeutic agents are excreted via the kidneys?
9. What other agents can be used simultaneously or sequentially to produce maximum effectiveness?

Classification of Agents Used in Cancer Chemotherapy

Classification of drugs used in the treatment for cancer is based on their mechanism of action. The primary categories are alkylating agents, antimetabolites, antibiotics, hormones, plant alkaloids, and miscellaneous and investigational drugs. It should be noted that classification systems do differ and that the following discussion represents the most frequently used methods.

Polyfunctional Alkylating Agents. These agents evolved out of the development of chemical warfare, specifically the agent sulfur mustard. This group can be subdivided into classic alkylating agents, the nitrosoureas, antibiotics (which will be addressed separately), and a miscellaneous alkylatinglike category. The major focus of action seems to be on the agents' ability to interrupt the process of DNA replication. Ultimately, this affects the integrity of the cell, preventing growth and therefore producing cell death. For this reason, alkylating agents are generally considered cell-cycle nonspecific. Their effect is not restricted to the cancer cell, but also affects rapidly proliferating cells of the gastrointestinal tract, respiratory system, bone marrow, skin, and gonadal tissue. Side-effects and toxicities that result can be directly attributed to the systems most affected (*e.g.,* severe nausea, vomiting, diarrhea, stomatitis, and depression of the bone marrow).

Antimetabolites. Antimetabolites are generally considered cell-cycle specific because their major focus of action occurs during the S phase. The actual mechanism of action involves inhibition of enzymes that contribute to the synthesis of nucleic acid. These agents accomplish this by falsely substituting these synthetic agents (folic acid, purine, and pyrimidine antagonists) into the metabolic pathways. Signs and symptoms of toxicity are similar to those of the alkylating agents.

Antibiotics. These drugs are products of microbial fermentation and inhibit RNA and DNA synthesis. Generally,

(Text continues on page 311)

Table 17-3
Responses of Neoplastic Diseases to Chemotherapy

Response, Type of Cancer	Useful Drugs [C]* [CR]†	Percent Response Rate	Survival of Responders (Percent)
Prolonged Survival or Cure			
Gestational trophoblastic tumors	Methotrexate, Dactinomycin, Vinblastine	70 CR†	Cured
Burkitt's tumor	Cyclophosphamide	50 CR	Cured
Testicular tumors:			
Seminoma	Cyclophosphamide, Radiotherapy	45 CR, 45 PR	30 Cured
Other	Chlorambucil, Methotrexate, Bleomycin, Dactinomycin, Mithramycin, cis-Platinum (II) diamminedichloride, Vinblastine, cis, Platinum [C]*	90 CR	(15–30 prolonged remission)
Wilms' tumor	Dactinomycin with surgery & radiotherapy, Vincristine [C]*	30–40 CR 80–90	Cured Cured (early stage)
Neuroblastoma	Cyclophosphamide, Adriamycin, Procarbazine, Vincristine [C]*	>50 5–80	(advanced stage) long-term survival depending on stage
Acute lymphoblastic leukemia	6-Mercaptopurine, Methotrexate, Daunorubicin, Prednisone, L-Asparaginase, 1,3-bis (β-Chloroethyl)-1-nitrosourea, Vincristine [C]*	90 CR	50 cured
Lymphosarcoma (children)	Same as acute lymphoblastic leukemia [C]*	>90	Definite increase
Hodgkin's disease Stages IIB, IIIB, & IV	Nitrogen mustard (Mustargen), Adriamycin, Bleomycin, Prednisone, 5-(3,3-Dimethyl-1-triazene)-imidazole-4-carboxamide, Procarbazine, Vincristine, Vinblastine [C]*	65–85 CR	50–70 Cured
Palliation and Prolongation of Life			
Prostate carcinoma	Estrogens, castration	70	Some increase
Breast carcinoma	Alkylating agents, 5-Fluorouracil, Methotrexate, Adriamycin, Androgens, Estrogens, Prednisone, Nafoxidine, Tamoxifen, Vincristine [C]*	60–80	Increase
Acute myeloblastic leukemia	Arabinosylcytosine & 6-Thioguanine, Daunorubicin, Prednisone [C]*	65	Increase
Chronic lymphocytic leukemia	Alkylating agents, Prednisone	50	Probable increase
Lymphosarcoma (adults)	Alkylating agents, Nitrosoureas, Prednisone [C]*	50	Probable increase
Osteogenic sarcoma	Methotrexate-Citrovorum factor (calcium leucovorin), Adriamycin [C]	20	Increase (advanced stage) Marked increase with adjuvant Rx (early stage)
Lung, small cell	Cyclophosphamide, Adriamycin, Vincristine, Prednisone	70–80	Increase 12–14 months
Palliation With Uncertain Prolongation of Life			
Chronic granulocytic leukemia	Alkylating agents, 6-Mercaptopurine, Hydroxyurea	90	3 years
Multiple myeloma	Alkylating agents, Prednisone, 1,3-bis (β-Chloroethyl)-1-nitrosourea, Vincristine [C]*	60	

(continued)

Table 17-3
Responses of Neoplastic Diseases to Chemotherapy (continued)

Response, Type of Cancer	Useful Drugs [C]* [CR]†	Percent Response Rate	Survival of Responders (Percent)
Palliation With Uncertain Prolongation of Life *(continued)*			
Ovary	Alkylating agents, cis-Platinum (II) diamminedichloride	30–40	
Endometrium	Progestins	25	
Uncertain Palliation			
Lung	Alkylating agents	30–40	Brief responses
Head and neck	Alkylating agents, Methotrexate-Citrovorum factor (calcium leucovorin), Bleomycin, cis-Platinum (II) diamminedichloride	20–30	Brief responses
Large bowel	Arabinosylcytosine, 5-Fluorouracil, Mitomycin C 1-(β-Chloroethyl)-3-(4-methylcyclohexyl)-1-nitrosourea [C]*	15–20	
Stomach	Arabinosylcytosine, 5-Fluorouracil, Mitomycin C [C]*	30	
Pancreas	5-Fluorouracil, Adriamycin, mitomycin (islet cell: Streptozotocin)	<10 (80—in treatment of hypoglycemia)	
Liver	5-Fluorouracil	<10	
Cervix	Alkylating agents, Bleomycin	20	
Melanoma	Alkylating agents, 5-(3,3-Dimethyl-1-triazene)-imidazole-4-carboxamide, Vinblastine	20	
Adrenal cortex	o,p′-Dichloro-diphenyldichloroethane	Relief of Cushingoid syndrome	
Soft tissue sarcoma	Methotrexate-Citrovorum factor (calcium leucovorin), Adriamycin	20	
Local Chemotherapy			
Intracavitary injection for recurrent effusion	Alkylating agents, 5-Fluorouracil, Quinacrine, tetracycline	50—effusions controlled	
Intrathecal injection for meningeal leukemia	Arabinosylcytosine, Methotrexate	80—improvement for 2 months (also part of combination therapy for acute leukemia)	
Extracorporeal perfusion for cancer of extremities	Alkylating agents	Irregular and uncertain	
Continuous infusion for cancer of head and neck, liver and pelvis	5-Fluorouracil, Methotrexate-Citrovorum factor (calcium leucovorin)	Irregular and uncertain	

  * [C] Combination chemotherapy shown to be effective
  † [CR] Complete response; others, partial response (From Krakoff IH. Cancer chemotherapeutic agents. CA—A Cancer Journal for Clinicians 31(3), May–June 1981, American Cancer Society.)

this group of drugs is cell-cycle nonspecific. Toxicities include those seen with the alkylating agents; in addition, cardiac toxicity is seen in high doses with some agents. Finally, many of these drugs are vesicants, causing severe tissue reactions if extravasation occurs.

Hormones. Alteration of the endocrine environment is a major goal in the chemotherapy of certain types of neoplastic disease. Alteration of the environment is accomplished by surgical removal of a tissue that is known to stimulate tumor growth or by the administration of substances that in effect block or inhibit the hormonal action. Some of the major hormonal agents that fall under this heading are the estrogens, progestins, androgens, corticosteroids, and antiestrogens. Surgical procedures that are performed include adrenalectomy, oophorectomy, orchiectomy and hypophysectomy. Many of these agents have few if any side-effects or toxic effects. However, a significant number can cause alterations in the individual's sexuality by resulting in significant changes in body image.

Plant Alkaloids. The vinca alkaloids, vincristine and vinblastine, come from the periwinkle plant. These agents seem to affect the action of the microtubular proteins necessary for the mitotic phase of cell development. It is also speculated that they might interfere with the synthesis of proteins and nucleic acid. For these reasons, the plant alkaloids are considered cell-cycle specific. A major toxic ef-

fect of this c
dose that can b
bone marrow d
vasation will caus

Miscellaneous
placed in this catego
tion have either not be
they cannot be placed i
ples of drugs in this categ
used in lymphoblastic leu
like the antimetabolites and
carbazine, an S-phase specific a
Hodgkin's disease.

Investigational Drugs and Cl. ₃ in this category are those whose safety an ve not been determined in humans. These drug ₃ undergone significant testing in animals and have shown promise as potential antineoplastic agents in man. Before the drug can be approved it must go through several phases of clinical trials.

A complete listing of agents that cause myelosuppression is provided in Table 17-4. See also Fig. 17-3.

Methods of Administration

Cancer chemotherapeutic drugs may be given orally, intravenously, intramuscularly, or intra-arterially, depending on the drug and the carcinoma. High concentrations of drugs

Table 17-4
Incidence and Chronology of Marrow Suppression by Cancer Chemotherapeutic Agents

Drug Class	Examples	Marrow Suppression	Nadir Day	Significant Marrow Suppression	Other Dose-limiting Toxicity
I. Alkylating Agents	Nitrogen mustard Melphalan Cyclophosphamide (CTX) Chlorambucil	Yes	6–8	4–10 days	Nausea and vomiting Cystitis (CTX)
II. Antimetabolites	Methotrexate	Yes	6–9	4–12 days	Stomatitis, renal and hepatic abnormalities
	5-Fluorouracil 6-Mercaptopurine Cytosine arabinoside				
III. Antibiotics	Adriamycin (AD) Actinomycin	Yes	10–14	4–7 days	AD-cardiac toxicity[2] BLM-pulmonary toxicity,[2] dermatitis, fever
	Bleomycin (BLM)[1]	No	—	—	
IV. Natural Products (Plant Alkaloids)	Vinblastine	Yes	4–7	3–10 days	Neurotoxicity
	Vincristine[1]	No	—	—	
V. Other Compounds	DTIC (Dacarbazine)[1]	Occasional	—	—	Nausea and vomiting, flu syndrome
	Steroids[1]	No	—	—	STZ-nephrotoxicity
	Nitrosoureas-BCNU, CCNU, MeCCNU[2]	Yes	20–25	10–40 days	
	Streptozotocin (STZ)[1]	No	—	—	

[1] Nonmarrow suppressive at therapeutic doses
[2] Maximum cumulative dose limited
(From Lokich JJ: Managing chemotherapy—induced marrow suppression in cancer. Hospital Practice 11:63, Aug 1976.)

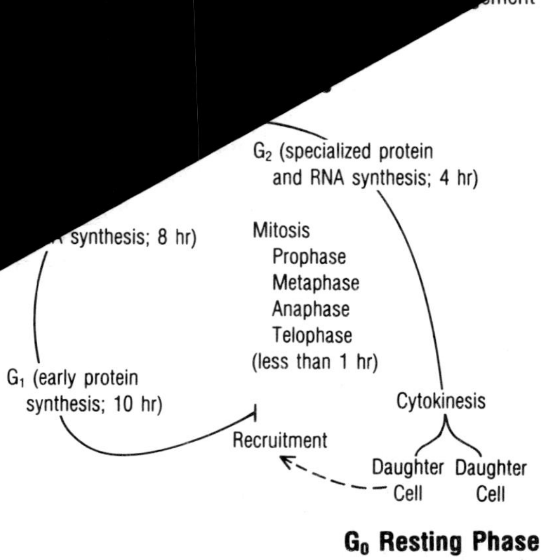

Cell Cycle Nonspecific Agents

1. Alkylating agents: mechlorethamine, melphalan, busulfan, chlorambucil, cyclophosphamide (also S phase)
2. Antibiotics: doxorubicin, dactinomycin
3. Miscellaneous: dacarbazine, cisplatin
4. Nitrosoureas (also G_0 phase)

S Phase Antimetabolites

Methotrexate
Cytarabine
Fluorouracil
Azacytidine
Mercaptopurine
Thioguanine
Hydroxyurea
Procarbazine
Steroids? (Also G_1)
Cyclophosphamide ?

G_2 Phase

Bleomycin

Mitosis

Vincristine
Vinblastine
Etoposide

G_0 Phase

Carmustine
Lomustine
Semustine

Labels within figure:

G_2 (specialized protein and RNA synthesis; 4 hr)

synthesis; 8 hr)

Mitosis
Prophase
Metaphase
Anaphase
Telophase
(less than 1 hr)

G_1 (early protein synthesis; 10 hr)

Cytokinesis

Recruitment

Daughter Cell   Daughter Cell

G_0 Resting Phase

Figure 17-3. Activity of various chemotherapeutic agents in relation to phases of the cell cycle. Drugs listed in Table 17-4, in terms of their marrow-suppressive properties and chronology of associated nadirs, are identified in the schematic diagram above in terms of where, during the cell cycle, they exert their distinctive tumor-killing effect. Actually, all the drugs are active during the entire cycle, but the antimetabolites are particularly effective during the period when a large proportion of tumor cells are in the S phase; similarly, the plant alkaloids are relatively most effective during metaphase. Neither of these drug classes is as effective (on a relative dose basis) as the alkylating agents during the resting phase (G_0). Duration of phases for cell cycle reflect an average. (Adapted from Dorr RT and Fritz WL: Cancer Chemotherapy Handbook, 1980, and from Smith and Thier, Pathophysiology, 1981.)

can be introduced into an organ by injecting them directly into the organ's blood supply. Another method used to deliver large doses of drugs involves administering them to an isolated extremity or region of the body, a process called *regional perfusion*. With both of these methods, the doses administered are greater than could be tolerated by the entire body. Special preparation is necessary for the patient receiving either direct intra-arterial chemotherapy or regional perfusion. Both of these techniques require surgical procedures.

Regional Perfusion. Care of the patient receiving chemotherapeutic drugs by regional perfusion calls for special nursing management before, during, and after the procedure.

Patient Preparation. The patient is weighed on admission and before surgery because the amounts of chemotherapeutic drug and heparin given are calculated on the basis of kilograms of body weight. Blood, urine, and x-ray studies are also done. Preparation of the patient for surgery includes answering his many questions. It is the physician's responsibility to inform the patient of what can be expected of this therapy, including side-effects, so that informed consent may be obtained.

Procedure. In the operating room, the tumor-bearing area is excluded from the general circulation for a set period of time, and a prescribed amount of drug is perfused into the isolated area. A catheter is placed in the desired artery under aseptic conditions and is then attached to intravenous tubing and the perfusion bag. The perfusion is controlled by an infusion pump or an arterial pressure cuff. During the procedure, tourniquets or ligatures are used in an effort to prevent seepage of the drug into the systemic circulation.

Obviously, it is easier to prevent leakage into the systemic circulation when an extremity is involved than when the torso is perfused.

For percutaneous introduction of the catheter into a major artery, it is necessary to use fluoroscopic guidance. This method has the chief advantage of not requiring major surgery, and it can be repeated at intervals. The vessels usually perfused for a lesion in the lower extremity are the iliac, femoral, and popliteal arteries and veins. For upper extremity perfusion, the axillary artery and vein are injected, whereas the abdominal aorta and the vena cava are used in pelvic perfusion (Figs. 17-4 and 17-5).

In patients requiring liver perfusion, a Teflon catheter is placed in the hepatic artery and attached to a portable pump. Such therapy can continue for the desired number of days even after the patient leaves the hospital. In this instance, a self-contained pump is worn beneath the clothing, as a hearing aid would be.

Regional infusions may be used for head and neck cancer, gastric tumors, or cancer of the liver. Usually this procedure is reserved for patients who have had maximum radiation therapy and all the surgery possible. The same side-effects that may occur with systemic chemotherapy may also occur with regional perfusion, since some of the medication does seep into the general circulation.

Nursing Management. The treatment plan should be explained to the patient, with the realization that this patient has probably already experienced many forms of therapy for the malignancy. Thus, there is a need for support, understanding, and reinforcement of hope.

Following the administration of the chemotherapeutic agent, blood tests are done frequently to check on bone

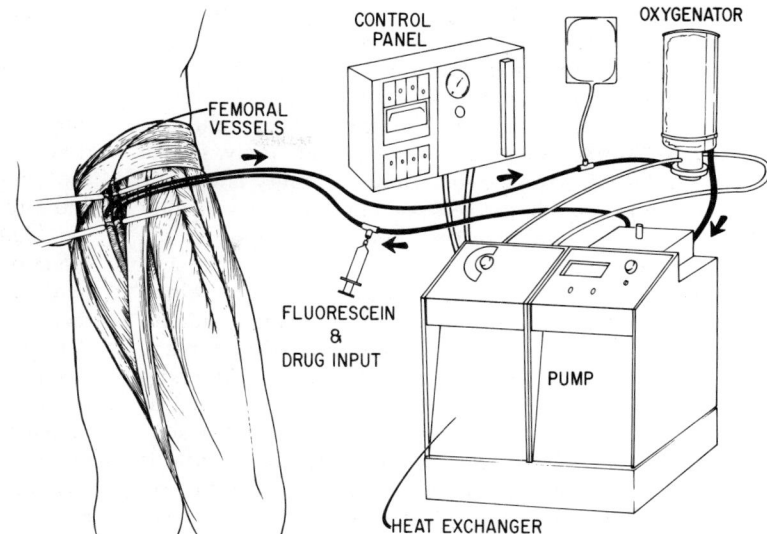

Figure 17-4. This diagram shows equipment used in the operating room to perfuse a lower extremity. The appropriate vessels are exposed, the patient is systemically heparinized, and the vessels are cannulated. Tubing is connected to a pump oxygenator. The extremity is placed on bypass after the tourniquet is applied above the cannula insertion site. Whole blood initiates the process of priming the pump and starting the infusion. Arrows indicate the direction of drug input and fluorescein. The dye, fluorescein, is used to demonstrate extent of perfusion when the extremity is viewed in the dark using a Wood's lamp. (Illustration courtesy Peter R. Jochimsen, M.D.)

marrow depression. Tissue in the local area is observed frequently for any reaction, such as erythema, mild edema, blistering, and petechiae. Any noticeable change is documented, with a full description. Pain usually is not a problem, but if it is present, it may indicate severe injury to normal tissue.

The patient should be encouraged to attend to mouth hygiene. If mouth ulcers, mucositis, tissue sloughing, and swallowing problems develop, special mouth care is given by the nurse.

A tracheostomy set is kept nearby in the event of respiratory difficulties. Oropharyngeal secretions may have to be aspirated. An accurate record of intake and output is kept and a high-calorie diet is offered. If mouth lesions and swallowing problems occur, the diet is modified so that the patient may continue to receive adequate nutriments in softer form (baby foods may be convenient). Nasogastric feedings may be needed if mouth problems interfere with proper diet maintenance.

If the infusion has to be discontinued temporarily because white blood cell or platelet counts fall below a certain level, the patency of the tubing is maintained by flushing with heparinized solution.

The patient who has had an aortic perfusion should be observed for signs of malaise, nausea, vomiting, rising temperature, blood pressure, and pulse (note signs indicative of a hypotensive reaction). Fluids are given intravenously for the first 48 hours; the patient's total intake and output are recorded accurately. The patient is turned frequently, because pressure areas develop easily. These patients require emotional support; for those having surgery, the principles of effective postoperative care are followed.

Nursing Care of Patients Receiving Chemotherapeutic Agents

Anticipatory Nursing. Knowledge of the expected drug action and the signs of toxicity enables the nurse to assess the patient's reactions to the chemotherapeutic

agents. It is understood that these signs may occur in different intensities in different patients and that they may vary with different drugs. The evaluation of the therapeutic effectiveness of a drug requires an understanding not only of drug action but of anticipated effect. It is important to know whether these effects will be immediate or delayed. The nurse will initiate those activities that will prevent or minimize adverse reactions wherever possible.

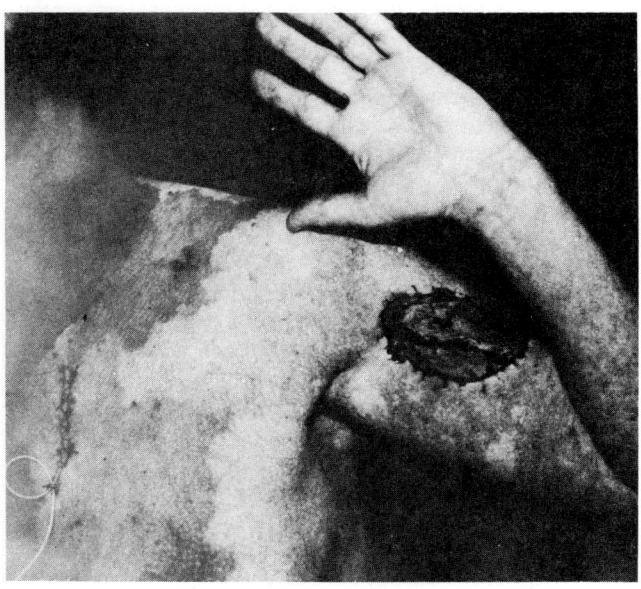

Figure 17-5. Note on the left that an arterial line is placed in the thyrocervical trunk in such a fashion that a chemotherapeutic drug may be given to the left upper extremity. This photograph was taken in the dark after fluorescein was injected into the arterial line. The light areas demonstrate the areas being infused by the drug, whereas the darker areas show that no drug is present. This patient had an excision on the upper arm for recurrent malignant melanoma. (Illustration courtesy Peter R. Jochimsen, M.D.)

Safer Drug Administration. When the drug used is a chemical that may cause tissue damage if extravasated, it is desirable to use discrimination in selecting a vein for administration of the chemotherapeutic agent and extreme caution while administering it. The area chosen should be one that will allow the needle to be secured safely, so that it will not be easily dislodged if the extremity is moved. Some advocate using larger vessels in preference to smaller veins in order to minimize the chemical irritation of the interior surface of the vein.

When injecting the medication directly into a vein is contraindicated, an infusion may be used prior to administering the drug, or a Y-tube (or side arm of IV tubing) may be used. It is advisable to avoid administering the drug into an extremity that has had other pathology, such as lymph node dissection, hematoma, scarring, or sclerosis.

When an infusion is started, the "butterfly" needle is preferred (p. 156). A single puncture of the skin and vessel is desirable, since repeated punctures may initiate a hematoma or further traumatize the area.

While the chemotherapeutic agent is being administered, the patient should be observed and instructed to report and describe any discomforts. If problems occur, it may be necessary to terminate the procedure and restart the medication at another site.

Extravasation. Extravasation (escape of infusion fluids into the tissues) may occur even if the aforementioned precautions are followed. The local signs include a reddened, mottled, or swollen area. The result may be tissue breakdown, possible necrosis, and pain.

If extravasation is suspected, the IV should be discontinued immediately. Procedures for treatment of extravasation vary from agency to agency. Commonly, ice is immediately placed over the site of infiltration. Additional methods may include infiltrating the site with cortisone or isotonic saline, or, in some instances, injecting the specific antidote; for example, the specific antidote sodium thiosulfate is injected when extravasation of mustargen occurs. It is the responsibility of the nurse to know which drugs are vesicants and what the agency's protocol specifies in the event of extravasation.

Even when the IV is quickly discontinued and appropriate intervention instituted, phlebitis and necrosis may occur. Pain at the site may pose an additional source of discomfort and concern for the patient. Supportive nursing intervention may include applying compresses to the affected part and administering appropriate analgesics. Unfortunately, in some extravasated areas necrosis may be so severe that surgical intervention is required.

Nutrition. The patient's nutritional state may be endangered because of nausea, vomiting, and anorexia. Electrolyte depletion and loss of necessary nutrients may disturb cellular function at a time when the patient's metabolic requirements are urgent. Various dietary supports may be provided. By catering to individual preferences and providing snacks, supplements, and frequent small feedings, the nurse can encourage the patient to maintain an adequate dietary intake. A frequent check of weight may reveal changes owing to impaired nutrition.

Prevention of Infection. Infection can pose a significant threat to the person with cancer because of alterations that result from therapy. However, the effects can be mitigated by good preventive nursing care. Potential sources of infection include intravenous lines, catheters, and alterations in the integrity of the skin and mucous membranes. Prevention is the key, and this is accomplished by accurate and astute nursing assessment.

Mouth Care. Although stomatitis cannot be prevented, infection owing to stomatitis can be avoided through meticulous mouth care. Generally, research to date has shown that consistent and regular mouth care is more important than the specific methods employed. It is essential, then, for the nurse to take a detailed history from each patient prior to the institution of therapy. Past and present oral and dental problems should be identified and appropriate intervention planned before therapy is instituted. Once a baseline for oral status is established, reassessment should take place twice daily so that potential problem areas can be identified and appropriate measures instituted. The lips, tongue, and mucous membranes are assessed for color and moisture and to see if they are intact. Odor, the collection of foodstuffs, swollen glandular areas, the amount of saliva present, and any change in taste and ease of swallowing should also be evaluated. A regimen that includes brushing the teeth after meals and before bed, plus frequent rinsing of the mouth, should be instituted before complications arise. Establishing good habits early in the treatment process will help foster oral health during the treatment cycle. Applying solutions such as lemon juice, mineral oil, or glycerin are not recommended because these substances have a tendency to coat organisms rather than remove them; they also decrease saliva and change the pH of the mouth. Dryness of the mouth, a frequent complication in patients who breathe through their mouths or are heavy smokers, can be treated with substances that act much like artificial saliva. New products have recently come on the market and should be considered when appropriate.

Finally, nystatin popsicles (antifungal agent) can be used instead of the oral suspension of nystatin. Not only is the cold soothing, but more nystatin is released than with the oral suspension, and the substance is in contact with the mucosa for a longer time.

The patient should be counseled against eating spicy food that could aggravate an already painful mouth. Ill-fitting dentures should be adjusted to prevent irritation. Alcoholic beverages will need to be diluted and smoking discouraged to reduce the severity of oral symptoms. One way of bypassing the discomfort of eating with a painful mouth is to suggest that the patient use a mouthwash or a rinse of lidocaine (Xylocaine) at mealtime to anesthetize the oral mucosa.

Psychosocial Needs. Perhaps the greatest psychosocial need arising from the use of chemotherapeutic agents is the patient's need to regain an acceptable self-concept and body image. As a result of the effect of these drugs on the hair follicles, the patient may develop alopecia. With the loss of hair, patients may become so depressed that they refuse to interact with others and may even have difficulty looking at themselves. The nurse can be very helpful in these instances by stressing the temporary aspect of the problem and the fact that there will be regrowth of hair. A wig may be the answer for the female patient. In place of a wig, attractive scarves and roller caps can be used to deemphasize this problem. For men, attractive hairpieces are available.

Learning about the effects of various antineoplastic drugs will enable the nurse to recognize that certain patient reactions, such as depression, malaise, euphoria, etc., may be due to the medications. The patient may feel somewhat reassured to know that such feelings are not psychotic and that they may disappear once the drug treatment is terminated.

Attitude.   Some amount of toxicity is expected for a portion of the chemotherapy cycle. It must be remembered that the goal of chemotherapy is to maximize the potential benefits of the drugs and minimize the toxicity. Therefore, it is imperative to sort out one's own feelings toward this mode of therapy and the discomforts it causes. The personal attitude conveyed to the patient and family is of the utmost importance and will affect the caliber of nursing care that the nurse will be capable of giving.

It is hoped that the patient may experience a decrease in pain, an eventual increase in the feeling of well-being, a more hopeful attitude, and, ultimately, prolongation of life. The nurse should continually exert conscious efforts to broaden personal perspectives in order to act more effectively through attitude as well as through knowledge and skill to administer quality nursing care to patients receiving drugs for the treatment of cancer.

Reverse Isolation Unit

The care of a patient whose immune defenses have been reduced by chemotherapy presents a nursing challenge. Such a patient requires strict aseptic precautions, physical barrier isolation, and antibiotic prophylaxis. At the National Institutes of Health, a laminar air-flow room (LAFR) module has been developed for the purpose of providing reverse-isolation for the infection-prone patient who is undergoing intensive intravenous chemotherapy. A barrier is set up within which the patient is free from contact with exogenous organisms, and the possibility of infection is thus reduced.

The continuous air flow (100 feet per minute) prevents airborne organisms from moving against the flow of air toward the patient. The nurse or visitor may stand outside the isolation area and not infect the patient. Personnel who enter the unit must wear a sterile gown, cap, mask, gloves, and shoe covers. This unit allows the patient more freedom and a more normal environment than the previously limiting "life island."

▷ Nursing Care of the Cancer Patient

The nursing management of the patient with cancer is multifaceted and requires the coordinated efforts of a multidisciplinary team. The function of this team is to provide the patient and his family with optimum care and support throughout the cancer experience. Through accurate and thorough assessment of the needs of the patient and his family, complex care decisions can be made. The nurse is a prime force in this process because of her intimate contact with the patient and her role as liaison between the patient, his family, and others who provide services essential to his care.

Illness can pose a crisis for anyone. A diagnosis of cancer causes tremendous disruption in all facets of an individual's life. It is the nurse's responsibility to be acutely aware of the impact that a diagnosis of this magnitude has on the individual and his family. In order to do this, one must establish a relationship with the patient and family, which can be maintained throughout the cancer experience. Many oncology units provide continuity of care by assigning a team of nurses to follow a patient from the time of his initial hospitalization throughout subsequent admissions. Regardless of the method used to deliver care, the goal must be to provide continuity. The nurse can attain this goal through an organized approach to care and by communicating her knowledge to other members of the health care team.

The special needs of cancer patients can be grouped into major categories—physiologic, psychological, sociocultural, and spiritual—and related to the general needs for information, protection, nutrition, elimination, sexuality, mobility, comfort, and the maintenance of other physiologic functions. Many of these needs can be fulfilled as indicated in Chart 17-4.

It should be recognized that just as the well person does not have deficits in all need categories at any one time, neither does the cancer patient. In order to plan care for these individuals, the nurse must address those needs that are most severely compromised. This is best accomplished with the assistance of the patient, his family, and appropriate members of the multidisciplinary team.

▷ Psychological Aspects of Nursing the Cancer Patient

The Optimistic Psychosocial Approach

Because there are so many kinds of cancer (over 100), the diagnosis of cancer need not indicate a fatal outcome. Many forms of cancer are curable; many others achieve "cure" status if they are treated early.

It is generally held, in the field of oncology, that the patient has a right to know the diagnosis and participate in all decisions relative to his care. However, there are numerous factors to be considered in this regard, as will be discussed in the next section.

The manner in which a patient accepts the information that he has cancer often depends on his philosophy of life and his views of life and death. The greatest support may be spiritual consolation. Therefore, the nurse should arrange to have available those spiritual resources that are most likely to meet the patient's individual needs.

(Text continues on page 318)

Chart 17-4
Care of the Patient With Cancer

Assessment

Assess, monitor, and evaluate the following:

1. The patient's awareness of the disease process and how well he understands the diagnostic and therapeutic procedures, their risks, side-effects, and expected outcomes
2. The patient's nutritional status as reflected in his eating patterns; the amount of fluid and food intake; the presence or absence of problems such as anorexia, nausea, vomiting, diarrhea, and constipation; the effects of stomatitis; immobility; swallowing difficulties; etc.
3. The patient's elimination patterns, including intake and output, and the use of laxatives, antidiarrheal and antiemetic medications
4. The presence of infection or the possibility of infection as a result of mouth problems (stomatitis), catheters, wounds, or reduced immunity
5. Signs of bleeding in the urine, stools, sputum, and ecchymotic areas
6. Energy levels, activity levels, and sleeping patterns
7. The presence or absence of pain and or discomfort, what drugs or analgesics have been prescribed or are preferred, other means of pain control, and usual coping mechanisms and support systems.

Planning Goals and Nursing Interventions

A. To control the carcinogenic growth
  1. Prepare the patient for surgery, radiotherapy, or chemotherapy or immunotherapy.
     a. Assist with diagnostic tests to determine if metastasis has occurred.
     b. Combat local and systemic infections.
     c. Correct existing anemia and electrolyte imbalance.
     d. Give the patient psychological support.
        (1) Explain the treatment to help the patient mobilize his intellectual functions and defenses to cope with the anticipated stress.
        (2) Offer reassurance and support.
        (3) Listen to and support the patient as he displays his anxieties.
  2. Assist with the treatment as prescribed.
     a. Surgical treatment
     b. Radiotherapy
     c. Chemotherapy
     d. Immunotherapy
B. To recognize the possibility of complications contributing to the patient's discomfort and illness and to initiate preventive and treatment measures
  1. Radiation sickness
     a. Administer vitamin B as prescribed.
     b. Give sedatives, antihistamines, and antiemetic drugs.

c. Offer small, frequent feedings of high-caloric, high-protein foods.
d. Increase fluid intake.
e. Report patient's reactions.
2. Diarrhea
   a. Give low-residue or bland diet.
   b. Use anodyne suppositories.
   c. Instill oil enemas to soothe rectal mucosa.
   d. Give antidiarrhea medications as prescribed.
3. Skin reaction
   a. Observe the skin for erythema.
   b. Apply oil or bland cream to radiation site.
   c. Protect skin from sunlight, heat, trauma, and tight clothing.
   d. Avoid irritation with soap and water.
   e. Observe for telangiectasis (a permanent, weblike dilatation of capillaries and small arteries).
4. Bone marrow depression
   a. Report results of laboratory evaluation.
   b. Observe for evidences of bleeding.
   c. Protect the patient from infection.
   d. Offer medicated mouthwashes to soothe oral mucosa.
5. Infection
   a. Take temperature at regular intervals since fever in patients with cancer usually indicates infection.
   b. Observe patient with hematologic malignancies and those receiving chemotherapy for symptoms of infection owing to granulocytopenia, lymphopenia.
   c. Give antibiotics as prescribed; Most infections in cancer patients are caused by gram-negative bacilli.
   d. Give fever sponges and apply cold compresses to head, encourage fluids, and administer antipyretic drugs to promote comfort.
6. Hemorrhage
   a. Evaluate the patient with terminal cancer for possibility of
      (1) Thrombocytopenia
      (2) Defects in platelet function
      (3) Necrosis and sloughing of tumor
      (4) Ulceration or invasion and rupture of vessels
   b. Give platelet transfusion or whole blood transfusions as indicated.
   c. Administer anticoagulants (heparin) as indicated.
7. Anemia
   a. Evaluate patient for weakness and symptoms of anemia owing to
      (1) Blood loss
      (2) Hemolysis
      (3) Myelophthisis (wasting of spinal cord)
      (4) Inadequate erythropoiesis

(continued)

Chart 17-4
Care of the Patient With Cancer (continued)

Planning Goals and Nursing Interventions *(continued)*

    b. Prepare patient for transfusion of whole blood or packed cells to maintain hemoglobin above 8 g.

  8. Malnutrition
    a. Assess patient for body wasting and anorexia.
    b. Correct electrolyte imbalance.
    c. Utilize vitamin supplements.
    d. Administer infusions of protein hydrolysates, glucose, and vitamins as directed.

C. To relieve the patient's pain
  1. Develop an understanding of the patient's emotional makeup, his relation to his family, and the projected emotional climate at home.
  2. Evaluate the quality, intensity, and duration of pain as well as the patient's response to pain.
  3. Establish the specific source of pain, since all of the patient's symptoms are not necessarily caused by cancer.
  4. Promote the general comfort of the patient (*i.e.,* turning, moving, ambulating).
  5. Determine the physical resources available at home.
  6. Administer agents to relieve pain when indicated.
    a. Use specific drugs for the relief of nausea and vomiting.
    b. Give ataractic agents for the relief of fear and apprehension.
    c. Utilize hot and cold compresses if indicated.
    d. Give sedative and hypnotic drugs to induce sleep.
    e. Apply local anesthetics if the situation warrants.
    f. Administer muscle relaxant drugs and antispasmodics; use non-narcotic drugs when possible; use the smallest amount of narcotic possible.
    g. Give analgesic drugs for more intense pain.
    h. Use tranquilizers to provide a sense of well-being.
  7. Assist with surgical treatment for the relief of pain.
    a. Prepare for alcohol injections to block nerve pathways for sensory benefit.
    b. Prepare patient for treatment of accessible painful nodule(s).
      (1) Excision
      (2) Injection with alkylating agent
      (3) Anesthetic infiltration or neurosurgical interruption of sensory supply
    c. Prepare for localized radiotherapy for deep lesions.
    d. Prepare for presacral neurectomy when visceral pain is predominant.
    e. Prepare for cordotomy when pain is intractable.
  8. Assure patient that severe pain will be alleviated.
  9. See Chapter 16 for additional therapeutic and psychosocial concepts of pain control.

D. To control malodor
  1. Remove the odor at its source.
  2. Encourage good personal hygiene.
  3. Give normal saline irrigations (if indicated) to external lesions.
  4. Administer prescribed vaginal irrigations when discharging vaginal lesions are present.
  5. Keep perineal area shaved if malodorous discharge is present.
  6. Change perineal pads frequently; remove and wrap in paper and place in covered container *outside* the patient's room.

E. To control the bleeding
  1. Observe for increasing pulse rate.
  2. Observe for amount and color of blood.
  3. Apply digital pressure if site is accessible.
  4. Utilize vaginal or rectal packing as indicated.
  5. Prepare patient for cauterization and ligation of exposed vessels if indicated.

F. To care for bladder frequency and incontinence
  1. Initiate a bladder control program.
  2. Keep an accurate intake and output record.
  3. Give meticulous skin care to perineal area.
  4. Watch for formation of a vesicovaginal or rectovaginal fistula.
  5. Insert an indwelling catheter if all other measures fail.

G. To prevent constipation
  1. Encourage fluids and regular meals.
  2. Place patient on prune juice and glycerin suppository regimen.

H. To reduce edema owing to blocking of lymphatic vessels
  1. Encourage motion and exercise.
  2. Elevate edematous extremity.
  3. Utilize nursing measures to prevent pressure sores.
    a. Relieve the pressure.
    b. Encourage circulation to the part.
    c. Put extremities through range of motion exercises.

I. To assist the patient to cope with his situation
  1. Help the patient to feel that he is understood.
  2. Help the patient to work out his feelings.
  3. Accept the psychological defense mechanisms that he uses.
  4. Recognize that the patient's loss of resources leads to helplessness, fear, and anger.
  5. Encourage the patient to talk about his *feelings* and his situation.
  6. Develop a supportive relationship with the patient.
  7. Utilize all measures to keep the patient's ego intact.
    a. Encourage him to make decisions and choices.
    b. Answer his questions.

(continued)

Chart 17-4
Care of the Patient With Cancer (continued)

Planning Goals and Nursing Interventions *(continued)*

   c.　Listen to him.
   d.　Provide a daily schedule for the patient, including short, daily rest periods.
   e.　Encourage him to keep active and to have interesting pursuits.
  8.　Help restore patient's self-esteem and purpose by offering help when needed and accepting irrational expectations and hostility.
  9.　Demonstrate concern for a suffering human by giving expert care and contributing something to his welfare.

J.　To maintain the patient at optimal physical and emotional condition
  1.　Give a high-caloric, high-protein diet (gavage feedings if indicated).
  2.　Keep caloric intake up with between-meal feedings.
  3.　Give supplementary vitamins and hematinics.
  4.　Administer blood transfusions as prescribed.
  5.　Encourage regular rest periods and arrange for periods in the outdoors.
  6.　Keep the patient as active as possible to build up endurance and avoid debilitation.
  7.　Support the patient during his anxiety and stress.

  8.　Maintain a cheerful and optimistic attitude.
  9.　Encourage verbalization.
 10.　Do little "extras" for the patient.
 11.　Include the family in the patient's care.

Evaluation

Expected Outcomes
1.　Adheres to the therapeutic regimen based on an understanding of the disease process and the rationale for treatment
2.　Maintains optimum state of nutrition by including foods high in essential nutrients, using food supplements to enhance nutritional intake, and avoiding foods contraindicated by the therapeutic regimen
3.　Achieves regularity in elimination of body wastes
4.　Protects self from infection and injury through appropriate mouth care and catheter care, and by checking for possible bleeding
5.　Alters life-style to compensate for decreased activity level, and uses suitable means to enhance and maintain physical strength
6.　Uses available therapies and coping strategies to achieve comfort.

Once the diagnosis of cancer has been established, a very effective and comfortable way of accepting the illness is to live wholly for the present. Projecting thoughts to the future adds doubts and fears; planning and living each day as it comes can provide a sense of achievement. The patient from this point of reference realizes he is still here and acquires a feeling of extension of life. The opposite is true if the reference point is projected to a year from now, for his future then seems shortened and limited. Even dividing one's time into blocks of days walled in by visits to the physician can be helpful. These units of time are quantities that can be appreciated and coped with by the patient.

It is hoped that the prospect of a breakthrough in treatment is closer with each passing day. Countless hours spent in study and analysis are added daily to hundreds of thousands of dollars spent on research. Tomorrow could be the day when significant contributions will be made in the treatment of many kinds of cancer.

In modern cancer therapy the possibility exists that extensive surgery and irradiation therapy may produce changes that are disfiguring or multilating and not easily borne by the patient. The problems thus created may be almost overwhelming. They begin before operation, when the question is raised as to how much the patient should be told about the details of his disease and his operation; they must be handled differently for each patient.

Since surgery or other treatments for cancer interrupt the patient's life-style, it is important to assist him in adapting to a change in his mode of living. How he adapts depends upon the values he places on his behavior, his self-image, and his attitudes toward particular body parts and social and sexual interaction. Cancer and cancer treatment can seriously disrupt the patient's adaptive process, resulting in depression until new methods of coping with an altered life-style are found and coping skills developed.

The adaptation that has to be made must begin in the preoperative period. To this end, the patient participates in the plan of treatment so that, in a sense, he has a real part in all that is done for, by, and with him. Patients are particularly in need of support and reassurance in order to establish confidence in the skill of the surgeon and the hospital environment. When the patient approaches surgery with a sense of hopefulness and expectation, excellent results can be anticipated from a psychological point of view. If, however, surgery is approached with the conviction that the operation is going to be painful, disfiguring, and mutilating, it is almost to be expected that depression and a marked sense of weakness will become apparent postoperatively. The postoperative symptoms of depression may take the form of sleep disturbance, loss of appetite, and other manifestations that may persist for an indefinite period. In their depression, patients may think that the attitudes of nurses, physicians, and attendants show hostility.

A patient who has not taken part in the planning process may experience feelings of dejection accompanied by a sense of helplessness. Such anxiety often makes the patient turn to other people for help, advice, consolation, and reassurance. This state is usually temporary, and the nurse, who is closest to the patient, can be of invaluable aid during this period of rehabilitation. Kindness, warmth, and understanding provide the security the patient needs.

The nurse, of all health personnel, has the most sustained and intimate contact with the patient during hospitalization and thus is the person to whom the patient turns most often for understanding and support during the early postoperative period. If the nurse is able to meet these needs, not only will the pressure and the anxiety be alleviated, but also the patient's perception of the hospital experience will be modified.

In summary, the psychology of the cancer patient is the psychology of a person who is facing a fundamental struggle with security and self-value. Such problems can be met best by working with professional persons. The nurse is in a very advantageous position to aid the patient in efforts to overcome depression and anxiety and to resume normal function after surgery.

Gravity of Prognosis

What is in the mind of a patient suffering from a potentially fatal disease? What are his hopes and fears? How nearly does he suspect intuitively the truth of the situation, and, if he knows the truth, by what psychological mechanisms is he saved from despair? How specifically and in what detail should he be informed regarding his illness and its probable outcome? If he demands an accurate appraisal of his status and a true estimate as to the prognosis, ought not this be supplied? What is his family to be told? What are the responsibilities of the nurse with respect to the transmission of diagnostic and prognostic information to the patient's family?

These and similar questions regularly confront physicians and nurses responsible for the care of the seriously ill. Some of them may be answered without equivocation, with a reasonable degree of certainty and without important reservations, while others, depending on the personal philosophy of the physician, on the family, and on the status of a particular patient, may be answered in generalizations that, although basically valid, are open to a variety of interpretations.

First, with respect to the nurse–patient and the nurse–family relationship, it may be stated that whatever information is to be supplied concerning the diagnosis, whether or not it has been definitely established, never should be volunteered to the patient or his family by the nurse, except as planned in mutual discussions with the patient's physician. By the same token, whatever prognostications are offered by the nurse should be as specific as the physician's, and no more. Finally, any remarks of the nurse's that have a bearing on the possible implications of the diagnosis, prognosis, or treatment should be made advisedly, in the light of the physician's known views and intentions. This admonition deserves considerable emphasis, for nothing is more destructive of confidence and morale than an impression of inconsistency, and nothing is more threatening to therapeutic success than confusion and distrust in the mind of the patient. Obviously, all of the statements and actions of the nurse should be calculated to convey a sense of truth-

fulness and even guarded optimism; no matter how grave the situation or depressing the outlook, the nurse can lend a great deal of encouragement without exceeding either the bounds of reality or professional responsibilities.

Normally, protective psychological mechanisms operate in patients with lethal disease, apparently to excellent effect, for many such patients do not become acutely anxious or profoundly depressed, even when it is seemingly obvious that a fatal outcome is imminent. The precise nature of these mechanisms presumably differs according to the individual and the situation. A conversion of the patient's will to live to a complete acceptance of the idea of death, even a desire for death, may be one aspect of this process of psychological adaptation in patients with prolonged and painful illnesses, although in most instances there is no sign of a death wish. On the contrary, the evidence suggests that the desire to live persists with great tenacity, ideas of death apparently being altogether excluded from awareness.

It is not often that the physician or the nurse must decide how much of the tragic truth to tell; they seldom are asked. An occasional patient does persist in his direct questioning, apparently with logical reason, perhaps related to his business plans or obligations to his family. Under these circumstances some physicians may feel justified in offering a complete evaluation of the case in detail and stating their conclusions in definite terms. The usual experience, that is, a frank discussion, does not often result in total decompensation, and should always be accompanied by compassionate support.

Members of the patient's family and those of his associates who require explicit information, of course, must be made aware of the complete situation, and at least one member of the immediate family should be advised from the outset regarding all possible developments. If this is done, candid discussions concerning prognoses with the victims of hopeless disease are rarely justified. Optimism is to be strengthened, not destroyed, if the humane objective of patient care is to be served completely.

Esthetic Factors

Facial tumors are often unsightly, causing the patient to feel very sensitive about his appearance. Such lesions should be covered, if possible, and other features of the patient accented to detract attention from the tumor site. This can be done by careful grooming, attractive garments, etc. Bright lights in a room should be replaced by softer lights, inasmuch as shades of light and dark can tone down unsightly areas. The nurse can use her ingenuity in helping this individual to bear his burden more easily.

One of the most unpleasant features of cancer in exposed areas on the body is the foul odor that appears sooner or later as a result of the sloughing of tissues. Every effort should be made to keep the patient and his room clean. Dressings should be changed frequently, removed quickly from the patient's room, and deposited in a metal-covered container until they are sent to the incinerator. Bedclothes and the patient's clothing should be changed when soiled. The use of absorbent pads may help when drainage is present. The room should be ventilated properly.

If deodorants are necessary, several of the essential oils, such as oil of geranium, oil of eucalyptus, or oil of orange, may be used. Neutroleum alpha is lasting and not unpleasant when 1 or 2 drops are applied to the dressing or the bedclothing. Powdered charcoal in the dressing or potassium permanganate solution 1:2,000 as an irrigation often helps. Activated zinc peroxide is also effective in cleansing and deodorizing these wounds. Commercially prepared products can be disseminated from a bottle with a wick, by spray, or by means of an electric deodorizer to absorb odors. These are quite successful.

The nurse should try to maintain a rational psychological approach toward death. Often, the nurse is the person to whom the patient turns when he wants to talk about himself, his fears, his hopes, etc. To be able to listen and to offer encouragement are extremely important assets. Many times a patient demonstrates hostility and rebellion. The nurse, by remaining tolerant, offers the patient understanding in spite of his unpleasant actions. This approach will eventually uncover the reasons for the patient's outbursts and will help him to resolve his feelings. (See Psychological Aspects of Nursing the Cancer Patient, p. 315.)

Occupational and Recreational Therapy

Statistics reveal that the home is best suited for the care of the cancer patient for several reasons. The environment is familiar, and friends and family are at hand. Many times, the patient can perform some household duties, and this promotes feelings of usefulness. It is also easier to pursue hobbies, such as caring for tropical fish, developing a miniature garden, etc. In addition, the financial burden on the family is reduced. At the same time, the family has the responsibility for the patient's care and knows what is happening to him, which often is not the case when he is in an institution.

For the patient who does not have a home, the next best available environment should be sought. The nurse with sympathetic understanding can help the patient to make contact with the proper agencies for the adjustment of any social and economic problems.

For an overall view of caring for the patient with advanced cancer, see Chart 17-4.

The Hospice

The concept of the hospice originated in Great Britain but is growing in popularity in this country. The underlying purpose of the hospice is to provide a unit that serves only terminally ill patients, whether it be near or apart from a general hospital. Rooms are decorated in pleasant colors and furnished in a homelike manner. The philosophy of care is designed to promote comfort, and time is provided by those in attendance to talk to and listen to the patient and his family. Pain medications are given in pleasant-tasting concoctions, and special requests are honored if possible.

Each patient decides, with the support of the staff and his clergyman, whether he wishes to be at home or in the hospice. If he prefers his home, a member of the staff will visit the home daily to support and comfort him and his family. If he elects the hospice, he is never left alone when members of the family are not with him. Hospice care does not terminate with the patient's death. Support for the family is continued through a bereavement program.

▷ Nursing Care of the Patient With Advanced Cancer

Some authorities claim that the most important aspect of the care of the terminal patient is good nursing management. Frequent changes of bed linen, cleanliness, and keeping the patient warm are all comfort measures that can relieve a great deal of pain. During this care probably the most common emergency that the nurse should anticipate is hemorrhage, which is due to erosion of blood vessels by the malignancy itself, secondary necrosis, or the sloughing of tissue following irradiation. In some instances, the nurse can control bleeding by digital pressure. In cases of hemorrhage that cannot be controlled by local measures, the patient should be kept quiet in the recumbent position and the physician notified. The nurse should have the necessary equipment available for treating shock and hemorrhage (see pp. 403, 407).

Ambulation

The patient is kept ambulatory as long as possible; however, the nurse must recognize when it is undesirable for him to get out of bed. In this instance, simple exercises or passive range of motion may be indicated.

Pain

Medications are used to control pain so that it is not a persistent and continuous symptom. This means finding an analgesic in a dose suitable to relieve pain, and then giving the analgesic on a regular schedule (not p.r.n.) so that pain does not reemerge. The same criterion applies to the administration of sedatives, antidepressants, and tranquilizers.

▷ Bibliography

Books
Cancer

Bandman EL and Bandman B. Bioethics and Human Rights. Boston, Little, Brown & Co, 1978.

Baserga R. Cell Proliferation, Cancer, and Cancer Therapy. New York, Annals of the New York Academy of Sciences, 1982.

Beauchamp TL and Childress JE. Principles of Biomedical Ethics. New York, Oxford University Press, 1979.

Bellanti JA. Immunology II. Philadelphia, WB Saunders, 1978.

Blumberg B et al. Coping with Cancer. Bethesda, Maryland, U.S. Department of Health and Human Services, Public Health Service, National Institutes of Health, 1980.

Bouchard–Kurtz R and Speese–Owens N. Nursing Care of the Cancer Patient, 4th ed. St Louis, CV Mosby, 1981.

The Breast Cancer Digest. Bethesda, Maryland, U.S. Department of Health, Education and Welfare, Public Health Service, National Institutes of Health, National Cancer Institute, DHEW Publication No. (NIH) 79–1691, 1979.

Burkhalter PK and Donley DL. Dynamics of Oncology Nursing. New York, McGraw-Hill, 1978.

Cassileth BR ed. The Cancer Patient: Social and Medical Aspects of Care. Philadelphia, Lea & Febiger, 1979.

Cohen J, Cullen JW, and Martin LR (eds). Psychosocial Aspects of Cancer. New York, Raven Press, 1982.

Cullen JW et al. (eds). Cancer: The Behavioral Dimensions. New York, Raven Press, 1976.

DeVita VT, Hellman S, and Rosenberg SA. Cancer: Principles and Practice of Oncology. Philadelphia, JB Lippincott, 1982.

Dodd MJ. Oncology Nursing Care Studies. Garden City, New York, Medical Examination, 1978.

Doll R and Peto R. The Causes of Cancer. New York, Oxford University Press, 1981.

Donovan MI. Cancer Care: A Guide for Patient Education. New York, Appleton–Century–Crofts, 1981.

Dorr RT and Fritz WL. Cancer Chemotherapy Handbook. New York, Elsevier North Holland, 1980.

Fraumeni JF. Epidemiological studies of cancer. In Griffin AC and Shaw CR (eds), Carcinogens: Identification and Mechanisms of Action, pp 51–63. New York, Raven Press, 1979.

Goldberg JG. Psychotherapeutic Treatment of Cancer Patients. New York, The Free Press, 1981.

Haskell CM (ed). Cancer Treatment. Philadelphia, WB Saunders, 1980.

Holland JF and Frei E. Cancer Medicine, 2nd ed. Philadelphia, Lea & Febiger, 1982.

Horton J and Hill GF. Clinical Oncology. Philadelphia, WB Saunders, 1977.

Kruse LC et al. Cancer: Pathophysiology, Etiology and Management. St Louis, CV Mosby, 1979.

Laskey KS and Ignoffo RJ. Manual of Oncology Therapeutics. St Louis, CV Mosby, 1981.

Lockich JJ. Primer of Cancer Management. Boston, GK Hall & Co, 1978.

Marino LB. Cancer Nursing. St Louis, CV Mosby, 1981.

Mettlin C and Murphy GP (ed). Progress in Cancer Control. New York, Alan R Liss, 1981.

Mulvihill JJ, Miller RW, and Fraumeni JF. Progress in Human Cancer Research and Therapy, Vol 3, Genetics of Human Cancer. New York, Raven Press, 1977.

Polit D and Hungler B. Nursing Research: Principles and Methods, 2nd ed. Philadelphia, JB Lippincott, 1983.

Saunders DC, Summers DH, and Teller N. Hospice: The Living Idea. Philadelphia, WB Saunders, 1981.

Schottenfeld D and Fraumeni JF. Cancer Epidemiology and Prevention. Philadelphia, WB Saunders, 1982.

See-Lasley K and Ignoffo RJ. Manual of Oncology Therapeutics. St Louis, CV Mosby, 1981.

Tache J, Selye H, and Day SB. Cancer, Stress, and Death. New York, Plenum Medical Book Co, 1979.

Vredevoe DL et al. Concepts of Oncology Nursing. Englewood Cliffs, New Jersey, Prentice–Hall, 1981.

Werner–Beland JA. Grief Responses to Long Term Illness and Disability. Reston, Virginia, Reston Publishing, 1980.

Whelan E. Preventing Cancer. New York, WW Norton, 1978.

Winick M (ed). Nutrition and Cancer. New York, John Wiley & Sons, 1977.

Yura H and Walsh M (ed). Human Needs and the Nursing Process. New York, Appleton–Century–Crofts, 1982.

Articles
Cancer Prevention

Avellanet C. Cancer prevention: Cancer risk factors. Cancer Nursing 1982 Aug; 5(4):295–311.

The Breast Cancer Detection Demonstration Projects: Five-Year Summary Report. CA–A Cancer Journal for Clinicians 1982 July/Aug; 32(4):entire issue.

Fraser MC. The role of the nurse in the prevention and early detection of malignant melanoma. Cancer Nursing Oct; 5(5):351–360.

Gianella A. Cancer prevention: Carcinogenesis, I. Cancer Nursing 1982 Apr; 5(2):133–151.

Gianella A. Cancer prevention: Carcinogenesis, II. Cancer Nursing 1982 June; 5(3):221–233.

Hallal JC. The relationship of health beliefs, health locus of control and self concept to the practice of BSE. Nurs Res 1982 May/June; 31(3):137–142.

Reif AE. The causes of cancer. Am Sci 1981 July/Aug; 69(4):437–447.

Schulmeister L. Screening for skin cancer. Nursing '81 1981 Oct; 11(10):42–45.

Scurry MT and Levin EM. Psychosocial factors related to the incidence of cancer. Int J Psychiatry Med 1978/1979; 9(2):159–178.

Stromborg M. Screening for early detection. Am J Nurs 1981 Sept; 81(9):52–56.

Chemotherapy

Cancer chemotherapy. Med Lett Drugs Ther 1980 Nov; 22(24) Issue 571:101–106.

Dodd MJ and Mood DW. Chemotherapy: Helping patients to know the drugs they are receiving and their possible side effects. Cancer Nursing 1981 Aug; 4(4):311–318.

Fox LS. Granulocytopenia in the adult cancer patient. Cancer Nursing 1981 Dec; 4(6):459–466.

Fredette SL and Gloriant FS. Nursing diagnosis in cancer chemotherapy in theory and practice. Am J Nurs 1981 Nov; 81(11):2013–2022.

Garvey EC and Manganaro M. Nursing implications of hepatic artery infusion. Cancer Nursing 1982 Feb; 5(1):51–56.

Gross J, Johnson BL, and Bertino JR. Possible hazards of working with cytotoxic agents: A review of the literature. Oncology Nurs Forum 1981 Fall; 8(4):10–12.

Hunt JM, Anderson JE, and Smith IE. Scalp hypothermia to prevent adriamycin-induced hair loss. Cancer Nursing 1982 Feb; 4(1):25–31.

Johnson BL and Gross J. Handling methotrexate—a safety problem? Am J Nurs 1982 Oct; 82(10):1531.

Johnston S and Patt YZ. Intraarterial chemotherapy. Nursing '81 1981 Nov; 11(11):108–112.

Kaempfer SH. The effects of cancer chemotherapy on reproduction: A review of the literature. Oncology Nurs Forum 1981 Winter; 8(1):11–18.

Kennedy M et al. Chemotherapy related to nausea and vomiting: A survey to identify problems and interventions. Oncology Nurs Forum 1981 Winter; 8(1):19–22.

Krakoff KM. Cancer chemotherapeutic agents. CA—A Cancer Journal for Clinicians 1981 May/June; 31(3):130–140.

Kreamer KM. Anaphylaxis resulting from chemotherapy. Oncology Nurs Forum 1981 Fall; 8(4):13–16.

Reich SD. Lung toxicity of anticancer drugs. Cancer Nursing 1981 Feb; 4(1):59–60.

Reich SD. Tamoxifen: A brief review. Cancer Nursing 1981 Aug; 4(4):319–320.

Reich SD. Predictive tests of human tumor responsiveness to chemotherapy. Cancer Nursing 1981 Oct; 4(5):419–421.

Reich SD. Antineoplastic agents as potential carcinogens: Are nurses and pharmacists at risk? Cancer Nursing 1981 Dec; 4(6):500–502.

Reich SD. Mitomycin C: A brief review. Cancer Nursing 1982 Apr; 5(2):152–154.

Rose–Williamson KR. Cisplatin: Delivering a safe infusion. Am J Nurs 1981 Feb; 81(2):320–323.

Spross J. Issues in chemotherapy administration. Oncology Nurs Forum 1982 Winter; 9(1):50–54.

Todres R and Wojtiuk R. The cancer patient's view of chemotherapy. Cancer Nursing 1979 Aug; 3(4):283–286.

Trester AK. Nursing management of patients receiving cancer chemotherapy. Cancer Nursing 1982 June; 5(3):201–210.

Vizel M and Oster W. Ocular side effects of cancer chemotherapy. Cancer 1982 May; 49(10):1999–2002.

Weiss RB and Trush DM. A review of the pulmonary toxicity of cancer chemotherapeutic agents. Oncology Nurs Forum 1982 Winter; 9(1):16–21.

Wroblewski SS and Wroblewski SH. Caring for the patient with chemotherapy-induced thrombocytopenia. Am J Nurs 1981 Apr; 81(4):746–749.

General

Aiken S. Family structure and utilization of cancer support groups. Oncology Nurs Forum 1982 Winter; 9(1):22–26.

Bean G et al. Coping mechanisms of cancer patients: A study of 33 patients receiving chemotherapy. CA—A Cancer Journal for Clinicians 1980 Sept/Oct; 30(5):256–259.

Bubela N. Technical and psychological problems and concerns arising from the outpatient treatment of cancer with direct intraarterial infusion. Cancer Nursing 1981 Aug; 4(4):305–309.

Carroll RM. Stress and cancer: Etiological significance and implications. Cancer Nursing 1981 Dec; 4(6):467–474.

Daeffler R. Oral hygiene measures for patients with cancer, I. Cancer Nursing 1980 Oct; 3(5):347–356.

Daeffler R. Oral hygiene measures for patients with cancer, II. Cancer Nursing 1980 Dec; 3(6):427–432.

Daeffler R. Oral hygiene measures for patients with cancer, III. Cancer Nursing 1981 Feb; 4(1):29–35.

Dansak DA and Cordes RS. Cancer: Denial or suppression. Int J Psychiatry Med 1978/1979; 9(3/4):257–262.

Derogatis L and Kourlesis SM. An approach to evaluation of sexual problems in the cancer patient. CA—A Cancer Journal for Clinicians 1981 Jan/Feb; 31(1):46–50.

Doogan R. Hypercalcemia of malignancy. Cancer Nursing 1981 Aug; 4(4):299–304.

Edstrom S and Miller MW. Preparing the family to care for the patient at home: A home care course. Cancer Nursing 1981 Apr; 4(1):49–52.

Frytak S. Is THC an effective antiemetic for cancer patients? Opinion I. CA—A Cancer Journal for Clinicians 1980 Sept/Oct; 30(5):278–282.

Holden C. Cancer and the mind: How are they connected? Science 1978 June 23; 200(4348):1363–1369.

Holland JC. Why patients seek unproven cancer remedies: A psychological perspective. CA—A Cancer Journal for Clinicians 1982 Jan/Feb; 32(1):10–14.

Hubbard SM. Clinical research and cancer nursing. Oncology Nurs Forum 1981 Fall; 8(4):17–23.

Johnson JL and Norby PA. We can weekend: A program for cancer families. Cancer Nursing 1981 Feb; 4(1):23–28.

Johnston JD. Infrequent infections associated with Hickman catheters. Cancer Nursing 1982 Apr; 5(2):125–129.

Kennedy M et al. Chemotherapy related nausea and vomiting: A survey to identify problems and interventions. Oncology Nurs Forum 1981 Winter; 8(1):19–22.

Lerner IS. Laetrile: A lesson in cancer quackery. CA—A Cancer Journal for Clinicians 1981 Mar/Apr; 31(2):91–95.

Lynch HT et al. Hereditary cancer: Ascertainment and management. CA—A Cancer Journal for Clinicians 1979 July/Aug; 29(4):216–232.

Mashberg A, Garfinkel L, Harris S. Alcohol as a primary risk factor in oral squamous carcinoma. CA—A Cancer Journal for Clinicians 1981 May/June; 31(3):146–155.

Mulvihill JJ. Prevention in familial breast cancer: Counseling and prophylactic mastectomy. Prev Med 1982 Sept; 11(5):500–511.

Sallan SE and Cronin CM. Is THC an effective antiemetic for cancer patients? Opinion II. CA—A Cancer Journal for Clinicians 1980 Sept/Oct; 30(5):283–294.

Wegmann JA and Ogrin GM. Oncology nursing conflict: A case presentation of holistic care and the family crisis. Cancer Nursing 1981 Feb; 4(1):43–48.

Nursing Management

Anderson JL. Nursing management of the cancer patient in pain: A review of the literature. Cancer Nursing 1982 Feb; 5(1):33–39.

Beck S. Impact of a systematic oral care protocol on stomatitis after chemotherapy. Cancer Nursing 1979 June; 2(3):185–199.

Craytor JK, Brown JK, and Morrow GR. Assessing learning needs of nurses who care for persons with cancer. Cancer Nursing 1978 June; 1(3):211–220.

Craytor JK and Fass ML. Changing nurses' perceptions of cancer and cancer care. Cancer Nursing 1982 Feb; 5(1):43–49.

Daeffler R. Oral hygiene measures for patients with cancer. Cancer Nursing 1981 Apr; 4(2):29–35.

Feustel DE. Pressure sore prevention: Aye, there's the rub. Nursing '82 1982 Apr; 12(4):78–85.

Gargaro WJ. Turning off life support. Cancer Nursing 1981 Oct; 4(5):395–396.

Grove ME, Ilstrup D, and Ahmann DL. Skills needed by family members to maintain the care of an advanced cancer patient. Cancer Nursing 1981 Oct; 4(5):371–375.

Israel MJ and Mood DW. Three media presentations for patients receiving radiation therapy. Cancer Nursing 1982 Feb; 5(1):57–63.

Kelly PP and Tinsley C. Planning care for the patient receiving external radiation. Am J Nurs 1981 Feb; 81(2):338–342.

Krouse HJ and Krouse JH. Cancer as crisis: The critical elements of adjustment. Nurs Res 1982 Mar/Apr; 31(2):96–101.

Lamb MA and Woods NF. Sexuality and the cancer patient. Cancer Nursing 1981 Apr; 4(2):137–144.

Lauer P, Murphy SP, and Powers MJ. Learning needs of cancer patients: A comparison of nurse and patient perceptions. Nurs Res 1982 Jan/Feb; 31(1):11–16.

Leutzinger R and Judson AL. Drawing blood from a Hickman catheter. Nursing '81 1981 Dec; 11(12):65–69.

Lewis FM. Experienced personal control and quality of life in late-stage cancer patients. Nurs Res 1982 Mar/Apr; 31(2):113–119.

Lynch HT et al. Hereditary cancer: Ascertainment and management. CA—A Cancer Journal for Clinicians 1979 July/Aug; 29(4):216–232.

Maxwell MB. Cancer, hypoalbuminemia, and nutrition. Cancer Nursing 1981 Dec; 4(6):451–458.

Maxwell MB. Pedal edema in the cancer patient. Am J Nurs 1982 Aug; 82(8):1225–1228.

Maxwell MB. The use of social networks to help cancer patients maximize support. Cancer Nursing 1982 Aug; 5(4):275–281.

McCabe SV. An overview of hospice care. Cancer Nursing 1982 Apr; 5(2):103–108.

McCray ND. Assessment tools: Oncology patient assessment tool. Oncology Nurs Forum 1979 Fall; 6(4):15–18.

McDevitt B. Standards of clinical nursing practice: The side effects of chemotherapy in the treatment of leukemia. Cancer Nursing 1982 Aug; 5(4):317–323.

McElroy AM. Burnout—a review of the literature and application to cancer nursing. Cancer Nursing 1982 June; 5(3):211–217.

Moetzinger CA and Dauber LG. The management of the patient with breast cancer. Cancer Nursing 1982 Aug; 5(4):287–292.

Moritz DA. Nursing histories—a guide yes. A form no! Oncology Nurs Forum 19791 Fall; 6(4):18–19.

Ryan LS. Nursing assessment of the ambulatory patient with brain metastases. Cancer Nursing 1981 Aug; 4(4):281–291.

Scogna DM and Schoenberger CS. Biological response modifiers: An overview and nursing implications. Oncology Nurs Forum 1982 Winter; 9(1):45–49.

Stein KZ. Classifying cancer client needs for community health nursing intervention. Cancer Nursing 1982 Aug; 5(4):283–286.

Varricchio CG. The patient on radiation therapy. Am J Nurs 1981 Feb; 81(2):334–337.

Welch D. Nursing the patient with advanced liver metastasis. Cancer Nursing 1979 Aug; 2(4):297–304.

Welch D, Fullo S, and Nelson E. The development of a specialized nursing assessment tool for nurses. Oncology Nurs Forum 1982 Winter; 9(1):37–44.

Whitman H, Donovan CT, and Spross J. Ethical issues in cancer nursing. Oncology Nurs Forum 1980 Fall; 7(4):37–47.

Wilcox PM. Benign breast disorders. Am J Nurs 1981 Sept; 81(9):1644–1651.

Miscellaneous

American Cancer Society: Proceeding of the National Conference on Cancer Prevention and Detection. Illinois, American Cancer Society, 1980.

CA—A Cancer Journal for Clinicians, published bimonthly by the American Cancer Society.

Outcome Standards for Cancer Patients. Oncology Nursing Society 1978 July.

Patient/Family Resources

American Cancer Society, 777 Third Avenue, New York, New York 10017

Make Today Count: Check your local area

National Cancer Institute, Office of Cancer Communications, Bethesda, Maryland 20205

Salsbury KH and Johnson EL, The Indispensable Cancer Handbook. New York, Seaview Books, 1981.

We Can Do, PO Box 731, Arcadia, CA 91006 (ATT: Norman Cousins)

Diagnostic Radiology, Radiotherapy, and Nuclear Medicine

Generally, radiation is used in medicine in three ways—for diagnosis, therapy, and research. For any of these, the available radiation sources can be listed simply as roentgenographic and fluoroscopic machines (x-rays), natural and artificial radioactive isotopes, and the high energy particle machines.

Radiation is effective in destroying cancer cells and preventing their spread. In the individual whose malignancy has spread to such an extent that other forms of treatment are ineffective, radiation may be used as a palliative measure to keep the patient comfortable.

Instruction concerning the nature of radiation is essential in order to reduce fears and to promote the safety of all persons who come in contact with it.

▷ The Physics of Radiation

Radioactivity

Everything in our universe, including man, has been subjected to radiation since the universe was formed. This ever present radiation, called natural background, is a normal part of nature's balance and presents no hazard to ordinary living. Scientists discovered x-rays in 1895 and 1 year later identified radioactivity. Ever since, significant progress has been made in the field of radiation physics.

The elements of the nucleus of an atom achieve stability because of the effect of neutrons on protons. However, in the heavier elements, this becomes increasingly difficult, and such atoms are said to be unstable. In order to become more stable, nuclei give up energy in the form of rays or particles—alpha (α), beta (β), and gamma (γ). Such disintegration is referred to as *radioactivity*.

The units of measurement used in calculating the amount of activity in a radioactive sample are listed in Chart 18-1.

Radioisotopes

The atoms of each chemical element have the same number of protons, so that each atom of the element has the same

---

Chart 18-1
Units to Measure Amount of Activity

Curie (Ci)	the basic measure or unit to measure the amount of activity in a radioactive sample
Millicurie (mCi)	one thousandth of a curie
Microcurie (μ)	one millionth of a curie
Picocurie (pCi)	one trillionth of a curie

Units to Measure Amount of Radiation to Which a Given Substance is Exposed or Absorbed

Roentgen (R)	a standard unit of *exposure* (applicable to x-ray and gamma rays)
Milliroentgen (mR)	one thousandth of a roentgen
Rad	a unit to measure adsorbed dose (1 rad—amount of radiation required to deposit 100 ergs of energy per gram of irradiated material)
Rem	a unit of measure of radiation dose equivalent that takes into account the relative biological effectiveness ("roentgen equivalent man")

---

physical and chemical properties. However, a different form of the same chemical element, called an isotope, may exist. An *isotope* is an element whose nucleus contains a constant number of protons but has a differing number of neutrons, which has the effect of changing its weight. To indicate an isotope, the total number of neutrons and protons is appended; for example, in cobalt-59 (^{59}Co), the isotope of cobalt has a total of 59 protons and neutrons. The optimal ratio between protons and neutrons in a chemical element is one that is stable—^{59}Co is an example. By using nuclear reactors and high speed particle accelerators, it is possible to bombard a stable isotope such as ^{59}Co with additional neutrons. When ^{59}Co absorbs an extra neutron, an unstable or radioactive isotope is formed, ^{60}Co. This isotope has valuable medical uses.

Most radioisotopes emit *particulate radiation* (small fragments of the nucleus having mass and size) and *electromagnetic radiation* ("rays" that have no mass). The basic radiation type is presented by *alpha* and *beta* particles, which are actually parts of radioactive atoms; these break away and travel at high speeds and with great energies.

X-ray is a good example of electromagnetic radiation, one of the basic types. It is made up of rays, or waves, of very high electric energy traveling at very high speeds. When electromagnetic radiation arises from natural or artificially created radioactive isotopes, instead of an x-ray machine, it is called *gamma radiation.*

All four of these types of radiation (α, β, γ, X) act on living tissue by ionization or, in other words, by alteration of atoms in the chemical systems of the cell. If the level of radiation and its resulting intracellular ionization is low enough, no irreversible damage is done to the cell or organism as a whole. However, if the level is high enough, the cell may be altered or even destroyed. When such ionization occurs in the cells of the gonads, genetic mutations may result. Radiation effect is cumulative; the ionization that occurs in cells is not reversible.

The different kinds of rays are capable of different degrees of penetration (Fig. 18-1). Alpha rays can be stopped by a sheet of paper, and most beta rays are hindered by a thin sheet of metal. In tissue, beta rays have a range of up to 15 mm. Gamma rays are the most penetrating of the three; they can penetrate the human body and can cause hazards to others near the patient.

- To summarize, the amount of damage or destruction to tissue varies with the type of radiation, the dosage and intensity of radiation, and the nature of the site to be irradiated.

Radioactive Decay or Disintegration
The rate at which atoms emit their radiation (disintegrate or decay) varies from isotope to isotope. The decay rate or *half-life* is the time (hours, days, months, or years) required for one half of the atoms of a particular radioactive material to decay or be reduced to half of its initial activity. For example, iodine-131 (^{131}I) has a half-life of slightly more than 8 days, whereas radium-226 has a half-life of over 1600 years. When a radioactive agent is administered in an unsealed form to a patient, another factor besides the physical half-life of the radioactive element will play a role in how long radioactivity will be retained in the patient. This is the "biological half-life," which depends on how the body handles injected material. The combination of physical and biological half-lives determines the overall effective half-life of the isotope. Isotopes of longer life are implanted in the patient in sealed containers and then removed for use at another time. An example of this is cobalt-60, which has a half-life of about 5 years.

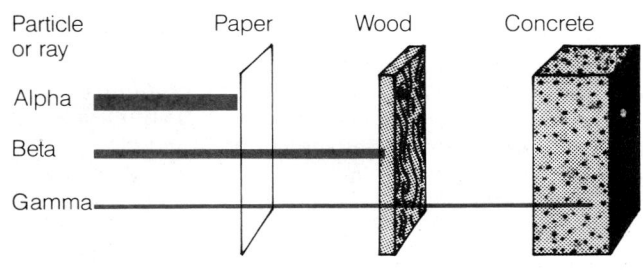

Figure 18-1. Relative penetration of alpha, beta, and gamma radiation. (U.S. Atomic Energy Commission)

▷ Biological Aspects and Clinical Application

Effect of Radiation on Tissue

Ionizing radiation is harmful to living tissue; therefore, good judgment is required to weigh the benefit of radiation exposure versus the risk of tissue damage. Factors that influence such risk are:

1. The dose rate—a prescribed dose causes less tissue destruction if given in small amounts over a long period of time than when given all at once.
2. Area of body exposure—the larger the area exposed, the greater the effect.
3. Cell susceptibility—rapidly dividing cells with no specialized function are more sensitive than nondividing cells and highly differentiated cells (*e.g.,* lymphocytes and germ cells are more sensitive than nerve or muscle cells).
4. Biological variability—some individuals are more susceptible to radiation than others; for example, the healthy person is more responsive than the malnourished person. Noteworthy also is that those skin cells that are more radioresistant are cured of cancer when sufficient radiation is used.

The fact that the injury extends to all components of the exposed tissue and affects most severely the cells that are growing fastest, that is, those engaged in tissue regeneration and repair, accounts for the slow healing and extensive scarring that are characteristic of radiation damage.

The *skin* is especially vulnerable to radiation injury by virtue of its exposed location. Healing is likely to be protracted, and permanent changes caused by radiation are unusually extensive. Therefore, proper skin care for the patient undergoing radiation therapy is essential.

Bone marrow is one of the most radiosensitive of normal tissues, and damage to the marrow is potentially the most lethal of the complications of excessive irradiation. Interruption of marrow function results, in 7 to 8 days, in a fall in circulating platelets to thrombocytopenic levels, giving rise to a hemorrhagic diathesis for which a platelet transfusion may be given. Agranulocytosis develops in about 2 days, causing a heightened susceptibility to bacterial infection that may prove to be as hazardous as thrombocytopenia. Fortunately, antibiotic therapy affords some protection against sepsis in these patients.

Radiation cataracts have been described after excessive exposure of the *eyes* to neutron or x-radiation, and diffuse, incapacitating fibrosis of the *lungs* may follow injudicious irradiation of the thorax. Damage to the *fetus in utero,* with production of congenital malformations, is apt to occur as a result of irradiation during the period from the second to the sixth week of gestation.

Short-Term Effects. If a person has had a major portion of the body exposed to large doses of radiation (over 100 rems) in a short period of time, the symptoms of radiation syndrome will be apparent (Table 18-1). This is manifested in four stages: (1) prodromal—nausea, vomiting, and malaise; (2) latent—symptoms subside; (3) illness—general malaise, epilation, hemorrhage (purpura, petechiae, nose-bleeds, etc.), pallor, diarrhea, inflammation of mouth and throat; and (4) recovery or death.

Long-Term Effects. The long-term effects of radiation are an area of public health concern because of the possible involvement of large numbers of people who may be exposed to low levels of radiation over a long period of time. The classic example is the experience of the women employed in the early 1920s to paint watch and clock dials with luminizing (radium-containing) paints. Years later, bone sarcomas resulted from the carcinogenic effect of the radium. Another example is the Hiroshima survivors who continue to show the effects of low levels of radiation.

When the gonads are exposed to radiation, the long-term effects may not be apparent in the individual but may appear in his progeny. Genetic mutations can be transmitted to subsequent generations. Among the most serious of the late consequences of irradiation damage is the increased susceptibility to malignant metaplasia and the development of cancer at sites of earlier irradiation. Evidence cited in support of this relationship refers to the increased incidence of carcinoma of skin, bone, and lung after latent periods of 20 years and longer following irradiation of those sites. Further support has been adduced from the relatively high incidence of carcinoma of the thyroid 7 years and longer following low-dosage irradiation of the thymus in childhood, and from the increased incidence of leukemia following total body irradiation at any age.

Evidence for long-range damage from irradiation in the form of gene mutations in exposed germ plasm is derived almost entirely from observations on insects and small animals and is based on analogy. Statistical arguments and analogies aside, the potential capacity of radiation to produce gene mutations can scarcely be discounted; the existence of the threat cannot be denied. Accordingly, precautions against unnecessary or excessive exposure to radiation are appropriate, and every available safeguard against radiation damage is definitely indicated.

▷ Radiation Detection, Control, and Precautions

Radiation Detection and Control

Although radiations are very powerful, they cannot be directly seen, heard, smelled, tasted, felt, or in any other way detected by ordinary human senses. However, their characteristic ability to ionize matter through which they pass makes it possible to detect and measure them. Instruments have been developed that record the number of rays or particles of radiation that pass through the detecting unit in a given period of time. These instruments, such as Geiger counters, detect radioactivity and measure its general strength.

Radiation has the additional property of affecting the emulsion of photographic film as light does in a camera. Film badges can be worn while working with or near radiation. When the film from the badge, is developed, the extent of exposure can be determined. This knowledge of total radiation exposure is very important. Within certain limits, cells live quite well while being constantly exposed—there is always a low, continuous radiation back-

Table 18-1
Summary of Clinical Effects of Acute Ionizing Radiation Doses*

| Range | 0 to 100 rems subclinical range | 100 to 1000 rems therapeutic range | | | Over 1000 rems lethal range | |
		100 to 200 rems	200 to 600 rems	600 to 1000 rems	1000 to 5000 rems	Over 5000 rems
Range		Clinical surveillance	Therapy effective	Therapy promising	Therapy palliative	
Incidence of Vomiting	None	100 rems: 5% 200 rems: 50%	300 rems: 100%	100%	100%	
Delay Time	—	3 hours	2 hours	1 hour	30 minutes	
Leading Organ	None	Hematopoietic tissue			Gastrointestinal tract	Central nervous system
Characteristic Signs	None	Moderate leukopenia	Severe leukopenia, purpura, hemorrhage, infection, epilation above 300 rems		Diarrhea, fever, disturbance of electrolyte balance	Convulsions, tremor, ataxia, lethargy
Critical Period Postexposure	—	—	4 to 6 weeks		5 to 14 days	1 to 48 hours
Therapy	Reassurance	Reassurance, hematologic surveillance	Blood transfusion, antibiotics	Consider bone marrow transplantation	Maintenance of electrolyte balance	Sedatives
Prognosis	Excellent	Excellent	Good	Guarded	Hopeless	
Convalescent Period	None	Several weeks	1 to 12 months	Long	—	
Incidence of Death	None	None	0% to 80% (variable)	80% to 100% (variable)	90% to 100%	
Death Occurs Within	—	—	2 months		2 weeks	2 days
Causes of Death	—	—	Hemorrhage, infection		Circulatory collapse	Respiratory, failure, brain edema

* From U.S. Dept. of Defense: The Effects of Nuclear Weapons, p. 591, Washington, D.C., Supt. of Documents.

ground. At the other extreme, too much radiation exposure can cause physical damage and death.

In this country, and in much of the world, laws require that radiation sources and devices be used only by persons who are trained in their theory and operation and who agree to abide by specified standards and limits. Such standards, if properly observed, should enable anyone to work with or near radiation throughout his life without noticeable physical damage, shortening of life expectancy, or genetic harm to future generations. Detailed specific dosage and exposure limits need not concern the nurse who is not working directly in a radiology department, so long as the precautions are carefully followed as outlined by the hospital radiologist for any particular patient involving radiation. Exposure ordinarily will be only occasional and, assuming proper precautions, very slight. However, for patients being treated by means of nuclear medicine, the precautions are more exacting, as is indicated in Charts 18-2 through 18-4, at the end of this chapter.

Prevention of Radiation Damage

Improvements in equipment for diagnostic radiology are clearly desirable and are constantly in progress. Policies have been recommended, more rigid than those of the past, regarding the extent to which diagnostic x-ray examinations should be carried out and the frequency with which they should be repeated. Examinations for possible pregnancy or for purposes of pelvimetry, for example, are discouraged, as are all x-ray studies that are undertaken in the absence of disease. Perhaps the most important aspect of any program that might be designed for the prevention of radiation damage concerns the education of practitioners who work with radiologic apparatus but are untrained in radiology.

Finally, it should be emphasized that the benefits of radiation therapy should never be denied to a patient with a radiosensitive neoplasm because of considerations regarding long-range radiologic safety. As a result of intensive publicity regarding the dangers of radioactive fallout and the complications of radiation damage in general, anxiety over the potential complications of radiotherapy, including x-ray irradiation and the use of radioisotopes, is prevalent among the uninformed public. The nurse is very likely to be in a position to allay such fears in the minds of many patients for whom irradiation has been recommended but who are inclined to refuse it on the grounds of its inherent risks.

Roentgenologic Precautions

The safety of the patient, the therapist, the nurse, the x-ray technician, and any other personnel who might be present during radiography, fluoroscopy, or radiotherapy demands strict observance of certain precautions, including the following:

- No one should be in the room with a patient who is undergoing x-ray therapy or roentgenography.
- The fluoroscopic equipment and technique should be such as to prevent the leakage of radiation.
- Each individual in the fluoroscopic room should protect himself from scattered radiation by wearing a lead apron and, if indicated, lead-impregnated gloves.
- Complete protection of the patient's gonads during radiography and x-ray therapy should be assured by means of appropriate lead shielding.
- The symbol indicating the presence of radioactive material should be displayed in a prominent place as a means of warning all personnel of the need for caution.

The nurse should be familiar with these stipulations and their purpose so that they may be clearly explained to the patient.

When a patient is receiving x-ray therapy, he ought to know why he seems to be left alone when receiving treatment and that a technician is always nearby and can see him through a window or via TV monitoring. Also, the patient should know that there is an intercommunication system that allows him to talk to the technician. It is well to remember that external radiation will never cause any patient to become radioactive himself. He cannot possibly present any radiation hazard to himself, other patients, or the nurse.

▷ Diagnostic Radiology

Diagnostic radiology has assumed an ever increasing role in the overall management of patients. Disease or injury often causes alterations in the function and structure of tissue that may be detected roentgenographically. Therefore, evaluation of the patient frequently requires a roentgenographic examination.

Basic procedures that are employed in various x-ray studies are of immediate concern to the nurse. In certain examinations the nurse is a direct participant and can influence the success or failure of the examination by the manner in which certain preliminary preparative measures are carried out. For example, the nurse can prepare the patient by allaying any suspected fears and by making sure that the patient receives the proper medication at the proper time prior to the examination. The nurse's familiarity with diagnostic roentgenology in general and her appreciation of the objectives of specific tests are essential to understanding patients and their problems.

It is important to understand not only the diagnostic capabilities of the roentgenographic examination, but also the exposure factors and economic considerations involved. A major goal of modern radiology is to minimize exposure of the population to diagnostic radiation. Employing proper safeguards in the use of radiation equipment is one means of accomplishing this end.

Certain basic considerations should be discussed concerning radiation dose and its beneficial and potentially harmful effects. Frequently, patients ask the nurse questions such as "Am I getting too much x-ray?" In general, diagnostic doses of radiation are relatively insignificant, although exposure of the gonads must be considered. Although a single exposure during one examination on one patient is little cause for concern, continued or cumulative radiation exposure can be hazardous and can have far-reaching implications if the exposure occurs during the reproductive years. Certainly, the scientific data gathered from animal experiments support the basis for this concern. The logical conclusion, therefore, is to minimize exposure to radiation whenever possible and to consider all untoward effects. For example, in view of the known fact that the fetus is extremely sensitive to radiation, it may be wise, when doing a nonemergency roentgenographic workup on a female patient of childbearing age, to carry out the procedure during the patient's menstrual period to assure that the patient is not pregnant.

In the final analysis, responsible medical judgment must balance the potential benefits versus the potential risks of any roentgenologic examination. Any examination done unnecessarily should be considered as "too much x-ray"— yet no examination important to the diagnostic or therapeutic management of the patient should be withheld.

Nature of the X-ray Image—Concept of X-ray

As was noted earlier, x-rays are one part of a spectrum of electromagnetic radiation. The rays are produced in a cathode ray tube in which electrons are boiled off a heated filament and accelerated across a potential difference to the anode, the target. When the electrons strike the target, energy, including x-ray energy, is produced. The x-ray beam is passed from the target through a collimator (Fig. 18-2), thereby reducing unnecessary radiation to the patient. The beam penetrates the patient and then emerges, striking the film cassette holder or fluoroscopic screen. A roentgenographic image is produced on an x-ray film. (Similarly, in fluoroscopy the image produced on the fluorescing screen during fluoroscopy is transmitted by the use of mirrors or a television screen for direct vision.)

Roentgenographic Film

X-ray film is composed of a clear plastic base, coated on both sides with an emulsion layer containing silver halide. The silver halide emulsion is sensitive to light and x-rays. During exposure of the film to x-rays and during the process and development procedure, there is a physicochemical alteration of the silver halide emulsion. The blackening of the film producing the intelligible image is caused by the effects on the silver halide of the amounts of radiant energy that reach the film through the object examined.

Differential Absorption

The amount of radiant energy reaching the film cassette is in large part affected by the differential absorption characteristics of tissue. Basically there are four radiographic densities: air, fat, soft tissue, and bone. Absorption is dependent, in turn, upon the tissue density and volume irradiated. A given thickness of bone will absorb more than the same thickness of muscle (soft tissue), and a given thickness of fat will absorb more than a similar volume of air. It is this characteristic that allows demarcation of anatomical structures within the body.

In order to achieve the necessary degree of inequality in density where no such inequality exists (as is the case with vessels in soft tissue or with the lumen of the bowel), it may be necessary to introduce either an artificial high-density "contrast medium" or a natural low-density contrast agent, such as air. This will delineate the lumen of any tube or hollow viscus containing the contrast agent, thereby improving radiographic contrast and diagnostic capability. The roentgenographic study of the gastrointestinal tract, the gallbladder, the bronchi, the kidneys, the spinal canal, the genitourinary tract and blood vessels, etc., depend in each case on the ingestion or the injection of an appropriate contrast agent.

Tomography. Another type of radiographic examination is tomography, also known as body section radiography, planigraphy, or laminography. These terms all refer to a method of radiographic examination in which it is possible to examine a single layer or plane of tissue by blurring out the planes of tissue both above and below the area of interest. This is accomplished by simultaneous motion of the x-ray tube and film cassette in geometric relation to the plane to be examined. Geometrically, the plane of focus represents the fulcrum of the motion of the tube and film, that is, the only area not in motion, with respect to the tube and film. This procedure is frequently helpful in blurring out any overlying, confusing edges. Multiple views of a body region focused at successively deeper layers visualize clearly some structures that would otherwise be obscured.

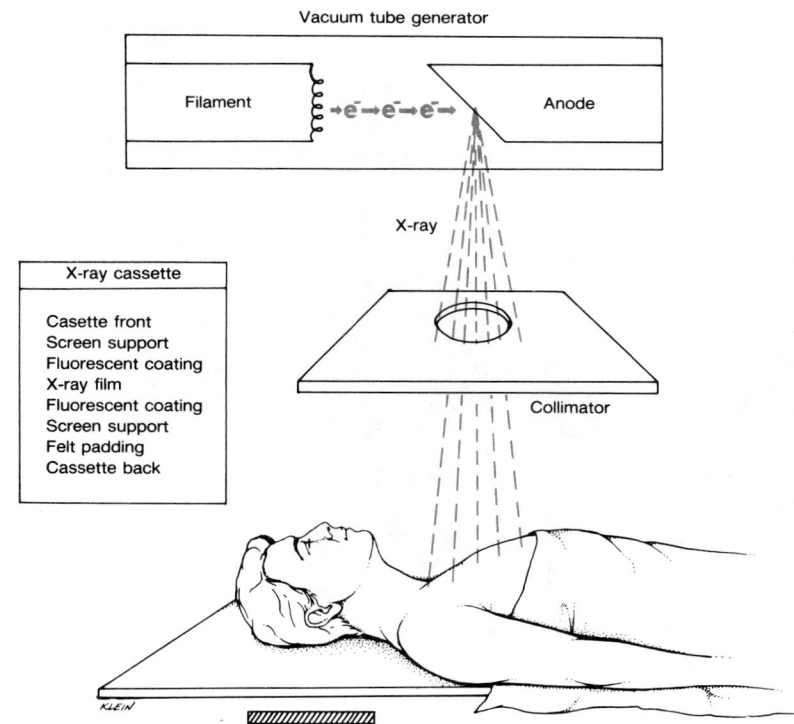

Figure 18-2. Production of x-ray and roentgenogram. Insert shows makeup of typical film cassette.

For example, a tumor partially obstructing a bronchial lumen or an area of bone destruction in the vertebral column may be more clearly visualized by this technique.

Roentgenographic Examination of the Chest

The chest roentgenographic examination is extremely important in diagnosing pulmonary disease and in evaluating abnormalities of the mediastinum, including the heart and the bony thorax. The chest roentgenogram is not only helpful in the workup of the patient at the time of the examination, but also serves as a normal baseline or as a record of the stage or progression of disease. Even though chest radiography may frequently demonstrate lesions not detectable by other means, it is not meant to supplant clinical history and physical examination.

Routine examination of the chest basically includes posteroanterior (PA) and lateral projections (Fig. 18-3). These are usually taken with the tube-film at a distance of 6 feet. It is desirable to have the patient inhale deeply or moderately at the time of examination in order to reduce distortion and allow for magnification of the image.

A wealth of information is obtainable from a chest roentgenogram. Since direct measurement of thoracic structures may be obtained, the lung and pulmonary vessels can be well visualized as can the trachea and proximal bronchi by virtue of their air-containing lumen. The heart and its chambers can be clearly seen, especially when barium is present in the esophagus, allowing the posterior surface of the heart to be outlined. While soft tissue and osseous thorax can be noted, mediastinal structures may not be seen as distinct entities because of a lack of inherent contrast within the mediastinum. However, a pathologic process such as neoplasm or bronchogenic cyst may be visualized by virtue of the displacement of normal structures from their usual location.

Special views, including oblique or apical lordotic positions, may be obtained to further evaluate a suspected abnormality. Chest tomography can help outline detailed anatomy of the lung and its vascular structures or demonstrate a cavity in a tuberculous parenchymal lesion. Fluoroscopy is occasionally helpful in evaluating the chest, particularly in differentiating vascular from nonvascular structures and in assessing diaphragmatic motion or the location of a lesion. Fluoroscopic controls can also be used in bronchography in which the bronchial tree is studied by introducing opaque material into the desired bronchus or bronchi. This is usually done to detail the anatomy of the bronchial tree and to outline the extent of known disease, such as bronchiectasis, or to determine the presence of suspected disease, such as lung tumor.

Roentgenographic Examination of the Abdomen

Abdominal x-rays are most frequently taken in the anteroposterior position. Frequently, this view (often referred to as a "scout roentgenogram") is accompanied by an erect anteroposterior view of the abdomen (Fig. 18-4). In certain situations in which the patient cannot stand, a special view, such as the decubitus view, is obtained. This view is taken with the patient lying on his side with the film cassette placed behind and the x-ray beam directed through the body on a horizontal plane. Another possible view is the direct lateral view, which is used in certain instances, such as in suspected cases of calcified abdominal aortic aneurysm.

A variety of conditions can be ascertained through abdominal x-ray, including bowel obstruction, collection of intra-abdominal fluids (such as ascites or abscess), calculi

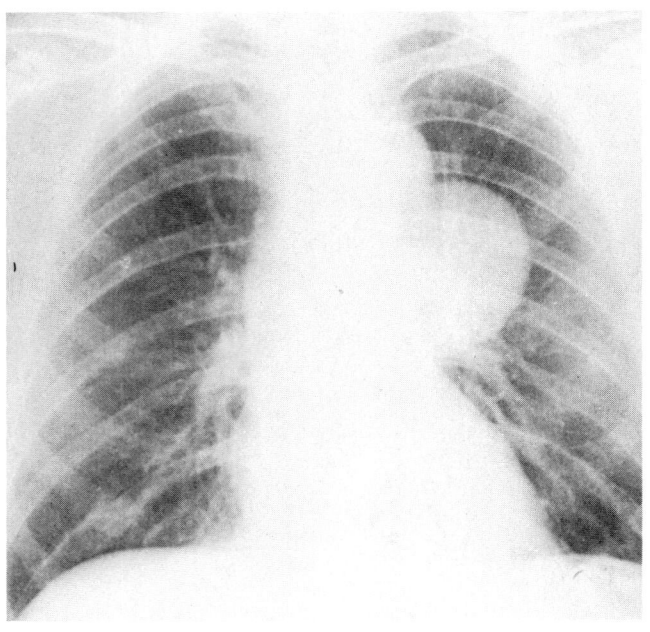
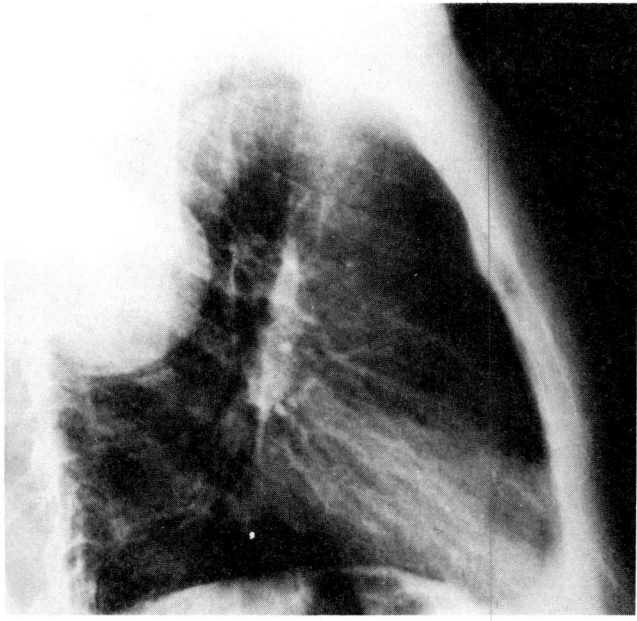

Figure 18-3. PA (posteroanterior) and lateral roentgenograms demonstrate large mass in posterior left chest representing "cannonball" metastasis from primary liposarcoma arising in left thigh.

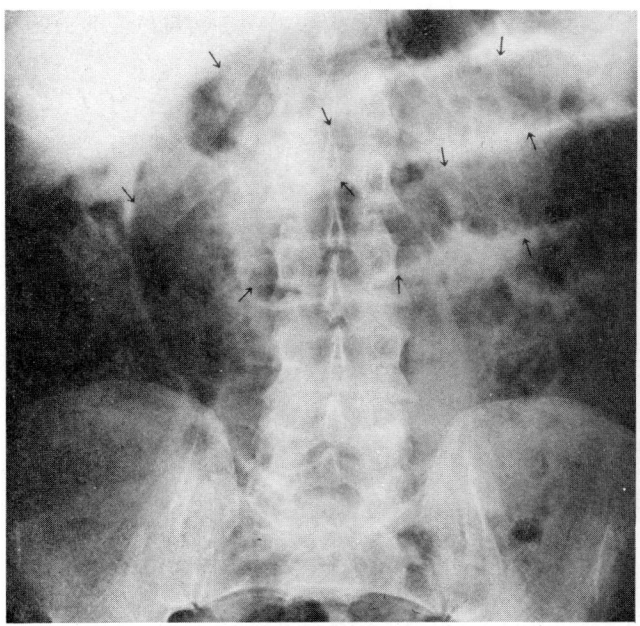 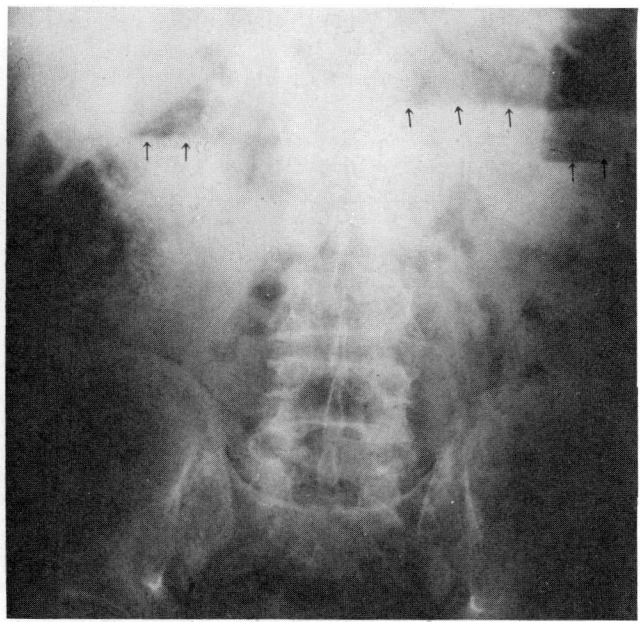

Figure 18-4. Supine and erect roentgenograms of abdomen demonstrate multiple dilated air-fluid filled loops of small bowel, consistent with the diagnosis of small bowel obstruction. Arrows indicate loops.

of the gallbladder or urinary tract, and other pathologic in-tra-abdominal calcifications. Abdominal organs viewed in-clude the liver, kidney, and spleen. The pancreas, on the other hand, is a difficult organ to visualize by routine roent-genogram. Therefore, pancreatic pathology is usually de-tected only by displacement of normal structures.

Contrast agents are particularly useful in evaluating the function and anatomical detail within the lumen of abdom-inal structures in the biliary system and in the gastrointes-tinal and genitourinary tracts. For example, opaque contrast material can help to outline nonopaque gallstones or di-agnose a nonfunctioning gallbladder. An ulcer will be seen as a persistent collection of contrast material. The bowel wall surrounding the ulcer may also be visualized indicating the benign or malignant nature of the ulcer.

The examination of the retroperitoneum, particularly the pancreas, has always been a difficult area to visualize roentgenographically because of the lack of natural contrast substances, either air or fat. Ultrasound and computed body tomography have been particularly helpful in this difficult area.

Skeletal Roentgenograms

Skeletal problems, particularly fractures, are well visualized roentgenographically, as is the process of fracture healing. However, the soft tissues of the joints, including cartilage, are not visualized normally without the use of a contrast medium, which is injected into the joint to outline these structures. This latter technique is called *arthrography*.

Roentgenograms of the skeleton may be helpful in es-tablishing or excluding the diagnosis of nutritional and en-docrine disorders that are complicated by derangements of protein metabolism or calcium and phosphorus deposition.

Abnormal radiolucency of the bones indicating deminer-alization of the skeleton is a characteristic, for example, of rickets, hyperparathyroidism, and myelomatosis. The var-ious types of arthritis often demonstrate roentgenographic changes sufficiently characteristic to allow differentiation. Paget's disease (a congenital disorder) and osteoporosis appear as regions of increased bone density. Furthermore, chronic lead intoxication or hypervitaminosis A may be es-tablished by skeletal roentgenograms. Lymphomas and me-tastasizing carcinomas or sarcomas may often manifest themselves in the skeletal system in the form of osteolytic or osteoblastic lesions. The most common sites of metastatic disease within the skeleton are those areas with active bone marrow and, therefore, relatively high blood perfusion, in-cluding the skull, pelvis, and vertebrae.

Computerized Tomography

The detail and inner structure of an object can be mathe-matically reconstructed from the information obtained from numerous projections taken from multiple angles. This technique has been used in astronomy, electron micros-copy, and computerized tomography.

In computerized tomography (CT) two processes are involved: (1) various views are taken in a single plane, and (2) the data acquired are computed and presented as a rec-ognizable cross-sectional image.

The image results from an x-ray beam passing through the body at many angles. Readings of the attenuation of the x-ray beam are recorded by detectors and stored in the com-puter. This data is then computed (reconstructed) into the image by using complex mathematical equations. The gray scale or brightness of each portion of the cross-sectional image is related to its degree of x-ray absorption. The image

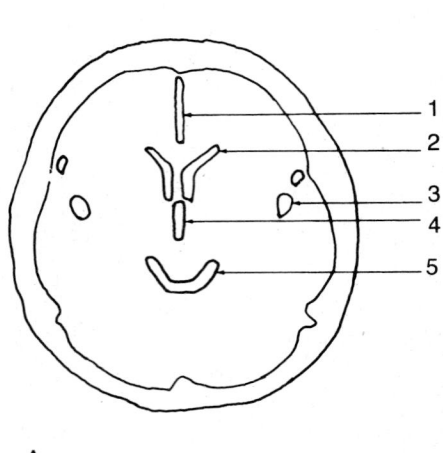 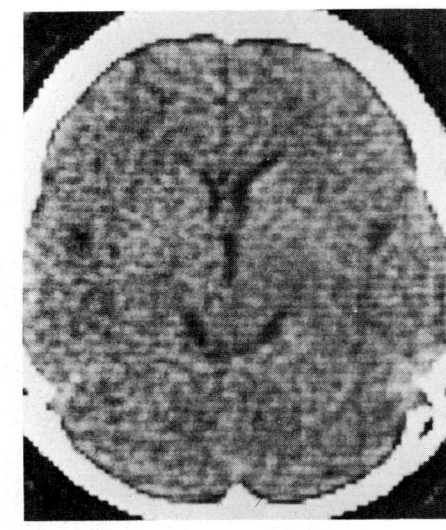 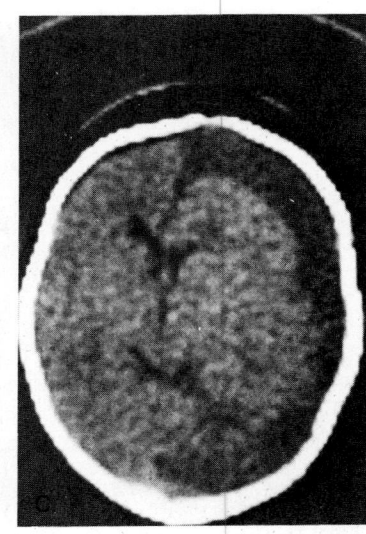

Figure 18-5. CT scans. (Figures courtesy Robert A. Zimmerman, M.D., Hospital of the University of Pennsylvania)

(*A*) Line drawing of *B*. 1—interhemispheric fissure between frontal lobes of brain; 2—frontal horns; 3—temporal horn; 4—third ventricle; 5—fourth ventricle.

(*B*) CT of brain through level of frontal horns. See *A* for detailed anatomy.

(*C*) CT of brain following head trauma. Note radiolucent area (blacker area) surrounding the brain on the right. This represents a chronic subdural hygroma from previous bleeding after trauma. Note the shift of the midline of the brain to the left. The ventricular system is dilated (compare with *B*).

is displayed on an oscilloscope or a television monitor and can be permanently recorded on x-ray or polaroid film.

Machines are currently available that can literally scan "head to toe." Scan time ranges from 2 to 18 seconds. Slice width is measured in millimeters.

Head scans are used in the evaluation of most cranial problems, including brain tumors, intracranial hemorrhage and ischemic disease, infection, hydrocephalus, demyelinating diseases, congenital abnormalities, and various eye, ear, nose, and throat diseases. Figure 18-5 shows the contrast between a normal CT of the head and one taken of a patient who has suffered severe head trauma. CT has been a key factor in decreasing mortality and morbidity in head trauma.

When the patient is undergoing CT examination of the head and body, contrast material is frequently used to increase diagnostic accuracy and to characterize certain lesions. The patients should, therefore, take nothing by mouth, since nausea and vomiting occur in a small number of patients with use of intravenous contrast material. An understanding of the patient's sensitivity to contrast material is essential; risk of the use of such material is small (less than 0.05%) but does include anaphylactoid reaction, development of renal insufficiency (contrast material is contraindicated in suspected plasma cell myeloma), hypotension, and congestive heart failure. Patients who are aged or diabetic, or who suffer from known liver or renal disease are likely to have a higher incidence of complications. CT facilities need to be prepared to handle cardiorespiratory and neurologic emergencies. To repeat, these contrast materials are not without risk. An accurate medical and allergy history of the patient is essential.

Scanning can be done on nearly any part of the body, including the lungs and pleura, mediastinum, liver, gallbladder and biliary tree, pancreas, spleen, urinary tract and adrenals, retroperitoneum, pelvis, and extremities. Figure 18-6 shows a pancreatic pseudocyst demonstrated by CT.

CT of the spine has proven useful for the diagnosis of spinal cord lesions and may obviate the need for myelography in selected patients with a diagnosis of lumbar disc herniation.

CT has already had a profound effect on the practice of medicine and will probably have an even greater impact in the future. It has decreased the number of tests needed, reduced hospital inpatient time, replaced more invasive modalities, and decreased the need for both exploratory surgery and hospitalization.

Invasive Radiology

An area of diagnostic radiology in which nursing care has an important role is interventional radiology. This new aspect of radiology includes many invasive procedures: percutaneous biopsy with guidance by CT and ultrasound, transhepatic cholangiography, catheter drainage of abscess, and balloon dilatation of narrowed or obstructed arteries (transluminal angioplasty). Nursing support is essential in these procedures, since these patients are at more risk and are frequently quite ill.

Arteriography (opacification of arteries by injection of radiopaque contrast medium via percutaneous catheter) continues to provide essential information to the vascular surgeon. Clinicians and researchers are constantly searching for ways to increase the information from the studies at less

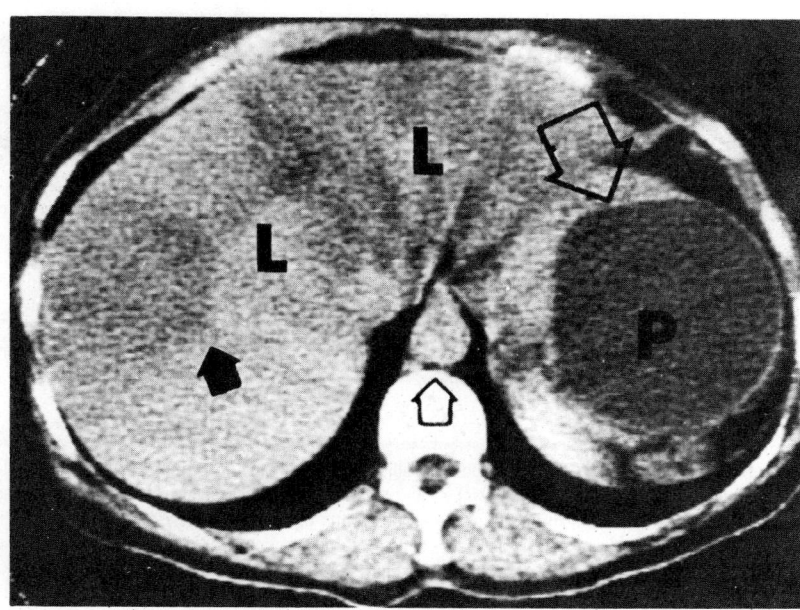

Figure 18-6. CT of body demonstrating pancreatic pseudocyst. Note well circumscribed radiolucent (blacker) pseudocyst (P) on the patient's left side (scans of the body are viewed from the patient's feet). Solid black arrow points to radiolucent areas in the liver (L), which are fatty infiltrations due to cirrhosis. Outlined arrow placed on the lumbar vertebral body points to the upper abdominal aorta.

risk, discomfort, and cost to the patient. A promising recent advance is *digital subtraction angiography.* Specially designed computer programs are used to analyze the filmed image of the artery, correct for magnification and distortion, and calculate the desired measurements. This new development shows promise of a safer, less costly study that may be used to screen patients who are in the early stages of vascular disease.

Diagnostic Ultrasound

Ultrasound (high-frequency sound above the hearing range) has become established as a diagnostic modality with a wide variety of uses in clinical medicine. The high-frequency sound is generated by a transducer (crystal) and converted into a molecular beam that then enters the body. A small percentage of the beam is reflected back to the transducer from tissue interfaces of different densities. The greater the difference in the tissue densities at the interface, the greater the amount of sound reflected back to the transducer.

The reflected sound wave bounces back to the transducer, which records how long it took to come back and how much of the original sound wave came back. By timing the wave, an accurate depth measurement can be made.

As the transducer is drawn over the skin surface, it generates a two-dimensional cross-sectional image of that part of the body. The echoes come from various tissue interfaces both outside and inside the underlying organs. The depth recording and the intensity recording of these echoes produce a cross-sectional image showing the outlines and internal structures of organs based on their sound reflection properties.

Because fluid is homogeneous, there are no internal echoes in fluid. Ultrasound, therefore, is a very sensitive instrument for distinguishing solid from cystic structures.

Because of the great differences that exist between the density of soft tissue and that of air or bone interfaces, ultrasound does not penetrate air or bone. Barium also reflects the sound wave. This is why ultrasound has little application in chest studies and why preparation of the patient is important in abdominal work.

- When ultrasound of the abdomen is scheduled, the patient should be in a fasting state and possibly prepared with an anti-gas agent, such as simethicone.
- Ultrasound should be done before any contemplated barium studies, such as UGI or BE (upper GI or barium enema).
- Good hydration is important since sound is transmitted best in well-hydrated patients.

Ultrasound has wide application, including the brain, thyroid, neck, heart, chest (for pleural effusions), liver, gallbladder and ducts, pancreas, retroperitoneum, aorta, and kidney and pelvis. Ultrasound is frequently preferred as the initial diagnostic study of an abdominal mass. Figure 18-7 illustrates ultrasound scans of a normal gallbladder and one with gallstones.

▷ Radiation Therapy

Principles and Purpose of Radiation Therapy

Radiation therapy is a medical specialty devoted to the management and treatment of cancer by means of ionizing radiations. Ionizing radiations are electromagnetic waves that are generated by either radioisotopes, such as cobalt, radium, and cesium, or by electromechanical devices, such as linear accelerators and betatrons. Charged particles may also be used, and machines are now available for the medical application of neutron, proton, and pi meson beams. X-ray treatments may be delivered by *external beam* (cobalt machine, linear accelerator) (Fig. 18-8), by *intracavitary* means (within a cavity; *i.e.,* intrauterine and vaginal), or by *interstitial* means (within tissue; *i.e.,* radioactive implants). Frequently, combinations of external and internal treatments are used in an attempt to cure local or regional disease or to palliate symptoms and signs of advanced disease, such as pain, bleeding, and obstruction.

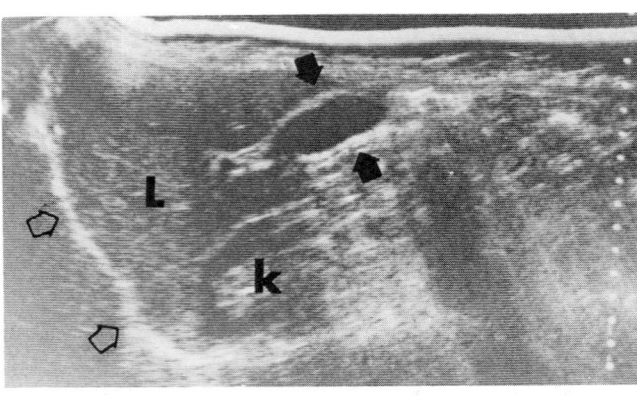
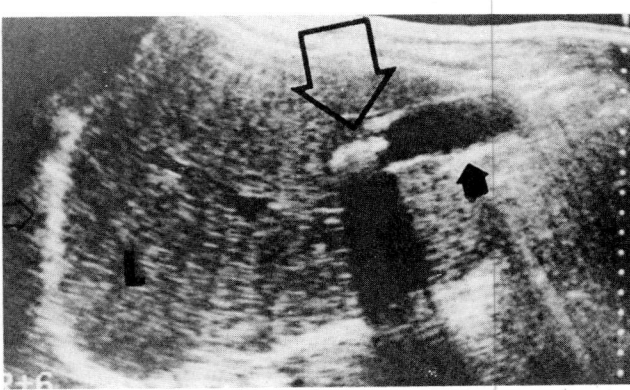

A

B

Figure 18-7. (*A*) Ultrasound scan of normal gallbladder. Longitudinal (sagittal) section to the right of the midline. Tubular, echo-free area (solid black arrows) is normal gallbladder in its usual relationship to the liver (L) and right kidney (K). Outlined arrows point to the dense echoes of the right diaphragm. (*B*) Gallstones. Longitudinal (sagittal) section to the right of the midline. Note the gallbladder (solid black arrow), with dense echoes and acoustic shadowing in the superior aspect (large outlined arrow) indicating presence of gallstones. Liver (L) and right diaphragm (small outlined arrow) are also seen.

A common characteristic of all malignant cells is their capacity for unlimited proliferation. The rate at which this occurs varies with the tumor type. Ionizing radiation interferes nonspecifically with cellular division, and if enough lethal radiation damage has been deposited within the cell, the cell will be unable to reproduce itself successfully. However, cell death may not occur immediately. It may be delayed for a number of cellular divisions, extending from hours to months. This accounts for the fact that tumors treated by radiation therapy may take extended periods of time to regress. Malignant cells generally have the same capacity to repair radiation damage as do normal cells, but they cannot repopulate as efficiently. This difference makes possible the x-ray eradication of tumors with the preservation of adjacent normal tissues. The radiation therapist attempts to increase the therapeutic ratio between normal tissue tolerance and tumor kill by a variety of means, including (1) the skillful placement of radiotherapy fields of treatment, (2) radiation dose schedules (fractionation), and (3) the combined use of irradiation with surgery and chemotherapy.

While tumors cause problems by replacing normal tissues, malignant tumors have the additional ability to *metastasize* by disseminating through the bloodstream and the lymphatic system. Knowledge of the potential pattern of spread of a specific tumor enables the radiation therapist and other members of the cancer treatment team to plan specific therapy. If radiation treatments are elected, the radiation therapist will design treatment portals to encompass these sites. Different doses will be utilized depending on the type of tumor treated and the extent of gross and microscopic disease.

Radiation therapy may be used in conjunction with surgery, either preoperatively or postoperatively, with or without chemotherapy. In preoperative radiation, the objectives are (1) to reduce the possibility of local recurrence by destroying the peripheral, better oxygenated malignant cells that will not be removed by surgery; (2) to reduce tumor bulk and volume, thereby facilitating surgery; and (3) possibly to decrease the likelihood of metastatic spread at the time of surgery. Postoperative irradiation may be used when there is residual tumor or a high likelihood of local recurrence. Such irradiation may include the original tumor volume and adjacent lymph-node-bearing areas. The timing of the irradiation in relation to surgery, either before or after, depends on the specific clinical situation and is determined in advance of treatment by the radiation therapist in conjunction with the surgeon and medical oncologist.

Figure 18-8. Clinac 6X, 6-million electron volt (MeV) linear accelerator for radiotherapy. (Courtesy, Varian)

In modern radiation therapy, a *treatment simulator* is utilized to determine the *treatment portals,* that is, the specific area of treatment. A simulator not only has the same mechanical characteristics and beam geometry of the treatment unit, but also can take high-quality diagnostic x-ray films utilizing fluoroscopic guidance. From these planning films, a formal treatment plan is developed by the radiation therapist in conjunction with a radiation physicist and a radiation dosimetrist. In this fashion, exact measurements can be made and exact doses can be determined for the target volume.

Initiation of Therapy

Once radiation portals and dosage have been determined, the patient begins the course of radiation therapy, which may be brief or protracted. Small lesions, such as superficial skin cancers, may be treated for cure by utilizing very high radiation doses over a brief period. Extensive deep-seated lesions, however, will require a radiation program extending over weeks to months. Administering the total planned dose by lesser daily increments is called *fractionation* and is utilized by the radiation therapist to preserve the integrity of the normal adjacent tissues. The traditional radiotherapy program is given Monday through Friday, 5 days a week, with daily fraction sizes varying usually from 150 rad to 300 rad tumor dose. The *rad* is a unit of absorbed dose in tissue corresponding to 100 ergs per gram of tissue. During the course of therapy, the radiation therapist and the nurse regularly monitor the patient's tolerance of the program and the response of the disease.

Delivering high doses of irradiation to deep-seated tumors while shielding critical structures, such as the spinal cord, heart, kidneys, and bowel, has accounted in large part for the recent progress in cancer management. Such diseases as Hodgkin's disease, cervical and uterine cancer, seminomas and pediatric tumors (such as Wilm's tumor), and rhabdomyosarcoma have a high likelihood of cure with radiation alone or with radiation in combination with surgery and chemotherapy. High-energy treatment machines (*supervoltage*) deposit their maximum dose deep within tissue, thereby reducing to a minimum the severe skin reactions seen with low-energy equipment (*orthovoltage*) used in the past. Orthovoltage deposits its maximum energy in the skin and subcutaneous tissues, limiting the total dose that can be delivered to a deep-seated tumor, and is therefore no longer used in curative radiotherapy. Another advance, collimation of the beam, limits the unwanted scatter to normal, uninvolved tissues and thus increases the patient's tolerance of the radiation treatment.

Side-effects of Radiation Therapy

The side-effects of the treatment depend greatly on the volumes of normal tissue that must of necessity be included in the radiation field. With early, confined disease, the radiation may be restricted to the tumor and a small amount of normal neighboring tissue. In this situation, radiation side-effects may be minimal. With more advanced disease, large volumes are treated and side-effects increase proportionately. Daily dose and total dose also play a role here; as each increases, the acute and chronic reactions may increase.

Nursing Support

Physical and Psychological Preparation

As a key member of the cancer management team, the nurse helps to prepare the patient for the emotional stress of radiation treatment by anticipating and relieving common apprehensions and managing common side-effects. For the patient who has a malignancy, radiation therapy may be misinterpreted as representing terminal care. The nurse should be aware of this apprehension and direct the assessment and nursing plan accordingly, recognizing that radiation therapy is often curative and frequently capable of extending the quality of meaningful life. The nurse and physician should confer about how the purpose of the treatment may best be explained to the patient and the family.

There are certain similarities between a diagnostic x-ray study and an x-ray therapy session. For one thing, the patient must remain still and in some instances must be immobilized with external devices to prevent movement. The treatment period is relatively brief—2 to 3 minutes—and the patient feels no special sensation during treatment. During the actual treatment, all personnel leave the room to avoid exposure to the radiation. Being left alone in a room with huge radiation equipment may frighten the patient unless reassurance and explanation are given by the nurse prior to the session. It is equally important to reassure the patient that the treatment will not make him radioactive unless radioactive material has been taken internally or has been placed in body cavities or tissues (*e.g.,* intrauterine radium in uterine and cervical malignancy).

It may be necessary for the radiation therapist to mark the exact area of treatment on the skin. Pen markings or, preferably, permanent, inconspicuous tattoo dots may be placed at the edges and center of the treatment area. Such marks should be preserved and care taken to see that they are not washed off by the patient or nurse unless permission is given by the radiotherapist.

Occasionally, the treatment course may be altered from the initial plan. Such a change may prove unsettling to the patient. Again, the nurse will be crucial here in helping the patient and the family to understand the reasons for the change.

Skin Reactions

The skin in areas that are being treated may become tender and reddened. Advise the patient not to apply ointments, lotions, cosmetics, or powders to these sites because they may increase the irritation. Likewise, discourage vigorous drying or the use of tight-fitting garments. The region should be kept dry and open to the air as much as possible. *Cornstarch* acts as an excellent drying agent and does not increase the radiation reaction. Even long after a course of radiation therapy, the patient should be cautioned against undue irritation to the area from friction and excessive exposure to sunlight.

Systemic Reactions

Individual response to radiation therapy varies. The side-effects one encounters depend on the nature and extent of the illness and on the area of treatment. The patient is encouraged to report all symptoms to the medical team. Most physical reactions to radiation are temporary and can be alleviated by nursing care and medication.

Adequate *nutrition* is essential during the course of treatment. Since patients frequently experience anorexia (loss of appetite), a balanced diet and vitamin supplements are needed. Persons undergoing treatment to the head and neck region and chest may experience pharyngitis or esophagitis. For these patients, soft or pureed foods and high-calorie liquids are beneficial. Hyperalimentation may be required on a temporary basis to maintain the patient in positive nitrogen balance.

Thick, tenacious sputum; loss of taste; and *dry mouth* are frequent side-effects (often long-lasting) when the upper aerodigestive tract is irradiated. Frequent irrigation of the oral cavity with a dilute saline or bicarbonate solution, particularly after meals, is recommended.

Nausea and *vomiting* are usually experienced only by patients undergoing large-volume irradiation to the upper and midabdomen. It is rarely experienced by those whose radiation portals are away from these sites. Antiemetics, such as phenothiazine compounds; the careful selection of fluids and foods palatable to the patient; frequent, small meals; and the constant reassurance of the nursing team may greatly improve this condition.

Diarrhea and *abdominal cramping* may be experienced by patients receiving pelvic and lower abdominal irradiation. Maintaining fluid balance, using a low-fiber diet, and judiciously administering antispasmodic drugs may greatly alleviate this side-effect.

Increased *urinary frequency, urgency,* and *dysuria* are symptoms of acute radiation cystitis that may be experienced by persons undergoing pelvic irradiation. After infection has been excluded, antispasmodics and local urinary tract anesthetics are usually beneficial.

Weakness and *fatigue* often result from a protracted course of radiation therapy. This fatigue may be temporary, lasting from a few weeks to months. During this period normal activity should be interspersed with time for rest and relaxation. The nurse can often help the patient through these difficult days by showing an understanding of why the patient feels discouraged and listless.

Hair loss owing to irradiation is produced only within the treated area and nowhere else. Should the scalp not be in the portal, balding will not occur. Hair loss may not be permanent, and hair may begin to grow back within 3 months of the completion of the program.

In summary, the nurse is a crucial part of the cancer management team. Knowledge of the realities of the treatment program will help to allay the fears and apprehensions of the patient, and nursing support will facilitate the patient's progress through therapy. The better the communication between the radiation therapist, nurse, and patient, the more successful will be the outcome of the treatment program.

▷ Nuclear Medicine

Basic Concepts

Nuclear medicine has progressed from a minor subspecialty under the jurisdiction of other branches of medicine to a separate specialty with its own training program and specialty board. This rapid growth has occurred mainly because of the development of improved imaging devices and better radiopharmaceuticals. Nuclear medicine procedures are simple to perform, their adverse effects on the patient are minimal, and they yield valuable information. Frequently, nuclear medicine procedures lessen the need for more invasive or more complex diagnostic studies or therapies. All medical personnel dealing directly with patients should have at least a limited acquaintance with radiopharmaceuticals, the instruments involved, and the results to be expected from nuclear medicine procedures. Although this section deals mainly with imaging techniques employed in nuclear medicine, there is a brief discussion of nonimaging *in-vivo* examinations, therapeutic uses of radioactive isotopes, and radiation precautions.

Radiopharmaceuticals

The radiopharmaceutical contains a radionuclide (radioactive element) incorporated into a compound that is used either to localize an organ or a system in the body for a diagnostic purpose, or to irradiate an organ or a system for therapeutic purposes. Also, radiopharmaceuticals are used in studies that are performed on body constituents in a test tube. Because these agents are used only in very minute quantities, no pharmacological response is noted with these chemicals. The radioactive atom disintegrates and in so doing emits energy. The two types of energy are *particulate* radiation, such as alpha or beta particles (nonpenetrating radiation), or *electromagnetic* radiation, such as gamma rays or x-rays (penetrating radiation). The electromagnetic radiation is employed in diagnostic tests, whereas particulate radiation is utilized for internal therapy.

The majority of radionuclides utilized clinically are obtained from nuclear reactors or cyclotrons and have short half-lives. Radionuclides with very short half-lives (less than 2 hours) have limited use because of rapid decay of activity. Radionuclides with very long half-lives (months or longer), because of both significant radiation exposure to the patient and environmental hazards, have been replaced by radionuclides with relatively short half-lives.

In the majority of cases, the radionuclide is only a part of the pharmaceutical, serving as the "tag" to make measurement or detection possible. In these instances, the chemical and biological behavior of the material labeled determines its use in the procedure. Mechanisms of localization include the following: active transport (thyroid scanning with radioiodine), phagocytosis (liver scanning with tagged colloidal particles), sequestration (spleen scanning with red blood cells), capillary blockage (lung scanning with labeled macroaggregated albumin), simple or exchange diffusion (bone scanning with tagged phosphonates), and compartmental localization (cardiac scanning with labeled red blood cells).

Of all the radionuclides available to nuclear medicine laboratories, technetium (^{99m}Tc) is most commonly used in the practice of nuclear medicine today. Preference for ^{99m}Tc is based on a short half-life (6 hours), lack of particle emission, excellent imaging characteristics, reasonable cost, and ease of availability.

Iodine-131 (^{131}I) is another commonly used radiopharmaceutical. Before any ^{131}I-tagged agent is used, the patient's thyroid should be blocked by administering 10 drops of Lugol's solution several hours before the agent is given, and it is advisable to continue this once daily for a couple of days (except in thyroid studies). Radioactive forms of thallium, xenon, gallium, krypton, indium, and phosphorus are other commonly used labels.

Instrumentation

Basically two types of instruments are used in nuclear medicine laboratories.

1. Instruments employed in performing *in-vivo* tests, in which a radiation detection device is used to measure radioactivity in different organs from outside the patient
2. Instruments used in performing *in-vitro* tests, in which radiopharmaceuticals are added to a sample of the patient's blood constituents or urine, etc. to determine the amount of specific substance present

The scintillation counter is the detector most widely employed in everyday clinical nuclear medicine in both types of instruments. The instruments currently available for *in-vivo* procedures include three major categories: (1) stationary probes, (2) scanners, and (3) cameras.

Using modern instruments and available radiopharmaceuticals, most nuclear medicine procedures are completed in less than 1 hour, although there may a delay in the onset of imaging after the radiopharmaceutical has been administered to allow for maximum localization of the drug.

Specific Organ Scanning

The Thyroid

Because of the early availability of radioiodine, the thyroid gland was one of the first organs studied with radionuclides. A large number of thyroid tests (both *in-vivo* and *in-vitro*) are now available to the clinician.

Thyroid Uptake Studies. This test is based on the ability of the thyroid gland to trap and retain iodine. External detection systems can be employed to determine the percentage uptake of iodine at a specific time. Most laboratory personnel ask patients to fast overnight.

Prior to performing the procedure, medical personnel should question the patient concerning:

1. Any previous studies with radiographic iodinated contrast media (*e.g.,* intravenous pyelogram, oral cholecystogram), topical application of iodine-containing compounds (*e.g.,* Betadine), oral ingestion of iodides and medications that contain iodine (*e.g.,* cough medication). All of these agents increase the body's iodide pool and hence decrease tracer uptake in the thyroid gland.
2. Prior use of antithyroid drugs (propylthiouracil and methimazole), which interfere with thyroid function
3. Administration of thyroid preparations, such as thyroid extracts and synthetic thyroid preparations, which again interfere with entrapment of the administered tracer dose

In most laboratories, the uptake of iodine at 2 to 4 hours and 24 hours is routinely measured and expressed as per-

centage thyroidal uptake compared with total administered dose. This test is more reliable in hyperthyroidism than in hypothyroidism and should be used in combination with other tests of thyroid function to provide an accurate diagnosis of many diseases of the thyroid.

Thyroid Scanning. The thyroid gland traps and retains the iodine for a sufficient period of time to allow excellent pictures of the gland to be obtained by scintillation techniques. [131]I was the first radiopharmaceutical used to scan the thyroid gland. However, in recent years it has been replaced in many laboratories by ^{99m}Tc pertechnetate, which is trapped like iodine but not organified into the thyroid hormones. As with thyroid-uptake determination, antithyroid medications, exogenous iodine, or certain drugs may prevent satisfactory concentration of radioiodine and ^{99m}Tc by the thyroid gland. Recently, ^{123}I has become available as the preferable agent for thyroid studies. This radionuclide does not emit beta rays and produces a lower radiation exposure with excellent imaging properties and hence is superior to ^{131}I for diagnostic studies.

The normal thyroid gland varies in shape. In the majority of individuals, the two lobes of the thyroid gland are attached in the middle by a bridge of activity called the isthmus. Abnormal scans usually exhibit change in thyroidal size, shape, and position as well as function. Hyperfunctioning areas are generally referred to as "hot" nodules, whereas hypofunctioning areas are called "cold" nodules. The scan is helpful in the evaluation of thyroid nodules, carcinomas, and masses in the tongue, neck, and mediastinum.

The Respiratory System

Since the introduction of the perfusion lung scan in 1963, lung scanning has been used very extensively in the examination of patients with pulmonary disease, especially pulmonary embolism. Perfusion lung scan is performed by IV injection of particles larger than 10 microns in size. These particles are trapped in the arterioles or capillaries of the lung in the first pass. A satisfactory study is obtained very shortly after the introduction of these particles.

Perfusion lung scanning is usually performed using ^{99m}Tc-MAA (macroaggregated albumin). When ^{131}I-MAA is used, Lugol's solution must be given to the patient several hours prior to the scanning to reduce radiation to the thyroid gland.

A chest x-ray should be obtained immediately before or after lung scan for comparison. Scans in pulmonary embolism will reveal areas of absent perfusion, which appear normal on the corresponding chest x-ray. In patients with abnormal chest x-rays owing to pneumonia, tuberculosis, and other pulmonary diseases, perfusion lung scans will reveal defects that should not be misinterpreted as pulmonary embolism. Repeating lung scans 7 to 10 days after the initial diagnosis of pulmonary embolism is of importance in the follow-up of these patients, since most of these clots start to resolve after they have lodged in pulmonary arteries. Patients with emphysema may also show areas of defect on perfusion lung scans. However, many of these patients have normal chest x-rays, and it is necessary to obtain another radioisotopic study using Xenon-133 (^{133}Xe) to further substantiate this diagnosis. The latter study involves inhalation of ^{133}Xe that has been introduced into a closed system, such as a respirometer. In this study, areas of emphysema will be seen as regions of poor ventilation and slow washout. In patients with pulmonary embolism, ventilation to the areas of embolism is intact. In patients undergoing pneumonectomy, the ventilation perfusion lung scan is useful to quantitate lung perfusion and function preoperatively.

Myocardial Imaging

In recent years the application of radioisotopic techniques has significantly improved our capabilities in the evaluation of patients with cardiovascular disorders. After the intravenous injection of ^{99m}Tc pertechnetate or other ^{99m}Tc-tagged compounds, transit of activity through the major venous system, right heart, lung, left heart, and aorta and its branches can be evaluated. With a similar technique, cardiac shunts can be noninvasively detected and quantified.

If sufficient time (approximately 20 minutes) is allowed to elapse after intravenous injections of nonradioactive pyrophosphate and ^{99m}Tc pertechnetate, the patient's red blood cells will become a radiotracer. With the aid of an electrocardiograph attached to a scintillation camera and a computer, it is possible to obtain images of the blood pool of the heart throughout the cardiac cycle (gated cardiac blood pool studies). From these images one can observe the cardiac wall motion in normal and pathologic states. Also, ejection fraction (percent of blood ejected between end-diastole and end-systole) during cardiac contraction can be calculated from this information. These studies may also be combined with exercise to evaluate cardiac reserve and function.

The introduction of myocardial imaging agents enables one to visualize abnormalities in the myocardium. For example, thallium-201 is injected intravenously, and its uptake by the myocardium reflects perfusion in different parts of the heart. Multiple images are obtained in different projections to evaluate separate parts of the heart. The major use of these techniques has been in the evaluation of coronary artery insufficiency. In a normal person, the distribution of these agents during rest and exercise appears homogeneous, with no areas of defect. In patients with coronary artery insufficiency, the scans appear abnormal or normal in the resting studies, depending on the degree of narrowing of the coronary arteries. However, when these agents are injected after exercise, the majority of patients with coronary artery insufficiency demonstrate areas of decreased perfusion in the myocardium. This test is being used as a complementary examination to the exercise ECG in many cardiac units. Thallium images are obtained very soon after the administration of the radionuclide, and then again 4 hours later. Thallium scanning has also been applied to the early detection of myocardial infarction.

Another major group of radiopharmaceuticals that has been used for the early diagnosis of myocardial infarction is the bone-seeking agents (see bone section, p. 340). Although ^{99m}Tc pyrophosphate has been the agent most commonly used for this purpose, any of the ^{99m}Tc-tagged phosphates appear to be satisfactory. The area of infarction and the surrounding regions reveal uptake of these agents.

Maximal results are obtained when the study is performed 1 day to 1 week after the onset of symptoms. Imaging is performed 1½ to 3 hours after the intravenous injection of ^{99m}Tc-tagged phosphate. This uptake has been attributed to calcific deposits in these areas. With the introduction of portable scintillation cameras, it is possible to obtain these studies at the bedside with minimal discomfort to the patient.

Recently, a nonimaging device, the cardiac probe, has become available. The cardiac probe allows multiple repeat studies of ejection fraction. Since this is a portable instrument, studies can be done at the bedside.

In many patients, these studies reduce the need for cardiac catheterization. In addition, these studies may be repeated with minimal discomfort and risk, whereas repetition of invasive cardiac studies would be unacceptable.

Liver Scans

Liver scanning can be divided into two general categories: scanning for demonstration of anatomical changes and scanning for the evaluation of biliary patency. In order to outline the liver, particles that are phagocytized by the reticuloendothelial system (RES) of the liver are used. ^{99m}Tc sulfur colloid has been used most extensively. Scans are obtained about 10 minutes after intravenous injection of the particles. No preparation is needed for this study. When ^{99m}Tc sulfur colloid is used as a scanning agent, the spleen also appears on the scan. Normally, the distribution of the activity is homogeneous throughout the organ. The liver is a plastic organ that may vary in dimensions. In patients with metastasis, areas of decreased activity appear superimposed on a field of normal liver activity. However, defects in the liver are nonspecific and can be seen in any disease state, such as abscesses or cysts. A nonhomogeneous pattern of liver activity is observed in diseases of hepatic dysfunction, such as cirrhosis.

Evaluation of the Biliary Tract

For evaluation of the biliary tract, ^{99m}Tc-labeled iminodiacetic acids (HIDA, PIPIDA, DISIDA) are the radiopharmaceuticals of choice. ^{131}I rose bengal also may be used. Lugol's solution, however, should be given before the study with iodine. The radiopharmaceuticals are cleared by the hepatocytes and are excreted through the biliary tract into the gastrointestinal tract. The major indication is abdominal pain suspected of originating in the gallbladder. The ^{99m}Tc-tagged agents are injected intravenously, and images are obtained for 1 hour. If the gallbladder is not visualized by this time, follow-up images at 2 or 4 hours should be obtained. Visualization of the gallbladder at 1 hour excludes the diagnosis of acute cholecystitis. Delayed visualization of the gallbladder is consistent with acute or chronic cholecystitis. Additionally, the study may be used to evaluate postoperative biliary drainage and leaks, as well as biliary enteric reflux. The ^{131}I rose bengal is still used in neonates with jaundice being evaluated for biliary atresia.

The Spleen

In the past, red cells damaged by heat or chemicals and tagged with radioactive chromium or mercury were used for spleen scans. However, currently, ^{99m}Tc sulfur colloid, which is picked up by the RES, is preferably utilized for this purpose. Both the spleen and liver are visualized in the scans. The normal spleen has an ovoid or comma shape. Scanning is helpful in the evaluation of splenic size, shape, and position. This technique has also been used in the detection of intrasplenic space-occupying lesions, such as malignancy, hematoma owing to trauma, infarction, and lacerations and rupture. Accessory spleens are easily located by this procedure.

The Pancreas

Although rarely done today, pancreas scanning has been useful for the detection of carcinoma of the pancreas. The agent used for this study is selenomethionine (^{75}Se), a radiolabeled amino acid that is incorporated by the pancreas. The normal pancreas appears in a variety of shapes with no defect in the scan. Areas of abnormality are devoid of activity. These defects are nonspecific, and half of them result from diseases other than carcinoma.

Gastrointestinal (GI) Bleeding

Bleeding in the gastrointestinal tract is a serious medical condition. Diagnosis of the active bleeding site is often difficult even with sophisticated invasive diagnostic techniques, such as arteriography and endoscopy. The GI bleeding scan is performed using ^{99m}Tc sulfur colloid, the radiopharmaceutical used in routine liver and spleen scanning. The patient is injected intravenously, and sequential images are obtained of the abdomen. The study is usually completed in 20 to 30 minutes. The site of bleeding appears as a focus of increased radioactivity. ^{99m}Tc-labeled blood cells are also used in detecting gastrointestinal bleeding. The radionuclide technique not only detects arterial bleeding, which may be revealed by arteriography, but also bleeding from a venous site, which is not seen with arteriography. The GI bleeding study may also detect slower bleeding than that found with arteriography.

Gastric Emptying

The ability to measure the emptying of the stomach's contents is useful in assessing the involvement of some systemic diseases. The liquid and solid components of a meal empty at different rates. Each phase may be labeled with a radiotracer for monitoring. Orange juice may be labeled with ^{99m}Tc sulfur colloid or indium-111 (^{111}In) DTPA. Egg whites cooked with ^{99m}Tc sulfur colloid are used for the solid meal. Other solid meals may include chicken liver, porridge, and hamburger.

The study is usually performed in a fasting patient. One to two hours are necessary to evaluate gastric emptying in most patients, although some are followed longer. If the patient vomits during or after the study, before there has been complete emptying of the stomach, the vomitus must be considered radioactive.

The Kidney

Two types of agents are used to evaluate the kidneys in nuclear medicine. The first group consists of radiopharmaceuticals that bind to the kidney for several hours and outline the renal parenchyma (parenchymal agents). ^{99m}Tc-tagged chemicals, such as ^{99m}Tc iron-ascorbate DTPA (diethylenetriamine-pentacetic acid), ^{99m}Tc dimercaptosuccinate (DMSA), and ^{99m}Tc glucoheptone (GH), are examples. The second group includes functional agents, of which ^{131}I hippuran and ^{99m}Tc DTPA have been used widely in nuclear medicine. These radiopharmaceuticals are excreted by the parenchyma and outline the draining system. With ^{99m}Tc-tagged parenchymal agents, scans are usually obtained 1 to 3 hours after injection. With ^{131}I hippuran and ^{99m}Tc DTPA, the images are obtained immediately after intravenous injection of these agents. Prior to the use of radiohippuran to lower the radiation burden, Lugol's solution should be administered to the patient. Scans with ^{99m}Tc-tagged parenchymal agents show uniform uptake in the kidney. Areas of abnormality, such as carcinoma and cysts, appear without activity. Normal hippuran and DTPA studies show uniform, progressive, symmetrical accumulation of tracer in the kidney, and later in the pelvis, ureters, and bladder. When kidney function is impaired, there is delay in the appearance of this agent in the kidney area, and sometimes delayed scans are obtained in 24 hours to complete these studies. Hippuran and DTPA studies are useful in the detection of obstruction of the ureter. Hippuran has been used for evaluation of renal hypertension.

Voiding Cystourethrogram

To evaluate the reflux of urine from the bladder into the ureters and kidneys, a radionuclide voiding cystourethrogram (VCUG) may be performed. In the direct method, a catheter is placed in the urethra and a ^{99m}Tc-labeled radiopharmaceutical is flowed into the bladder until maximum distention is achieved. The patient then voids into a bedpan while being monitored with the scintillation camera. In the indirect method, ^{99m}Tc DTPA is intravenously injected. When maximum bladder distention is perceived by the patient, the patient voids into the bedpan while being monitored with the scintillation camera. This study does not give the anatomical information of a roentgenographic study, but does provide useful information with only 1% to 2% of the radiation exposure of the roentgenographic technique.

Nervous System

Brain studies are based on the fact that intracranial lesions alter the blood-brain barrier; this allows the administered radiopharmaceutical to localize in or around the lesion. This study is mainly useful in the detection and localization of cerebral vascular disease and infection, as well as primary or secondary brain tumors. ^{99m}Tc-tagged radiopharmaceuticals (GH, DTPA) are the agents of choice today in many laboratories. If ^{99m}Tc pertechnetate is used, perchlorate solution should be given to the patient 20 to 30 minutes prior to administration of ^{99m}Tc to block choroid plexus uptake, which may interfere with interpretation of the scans. In many laboratories, after a rapid bolus IV injection of ^{99m}Tc radiopharmaceutical, multiple serial pictures of cerebral perfusion are obtained. These can add to the information obtained from static scans, which are usually done 1 to 2 hours after introduction of the agent.

Normally, there should be no activity in the cerebral

hemispheres. In patients with brain tumor or stroke, the area of the lesion appears radioactive when compared with the normal brain. In patients with brain tumor, lesions are usually seen whenever the first scan is obtained. However, in patients with stroke, the scan done immediately after the event is usually normal, but in 7 to 10 days most of these patients will show areas of irregular radionuclide uptake on their brain scans. Encephalitis is diagnosed early by the brain scan.

Skeletal System

The localization of bone-seeking agents such as calcium, strontium, and fluorine, and recently ^{99m}Tc-tagged agents has been noted in almost all osseous lesions, including malignancy, osteomyelitis, and healing fractures. This has been attributed to reactive bone formation around bony lesions. When ^{99m}Tc-tagged agents are used, patients are scanned 2 to 4 hours after injection, and no preparation is necessary except to ask the patient to void before the scan, because these agents are cleared by the kidneys into the bladder. The normal bone scan demonstrates a uniform pattern of uptake in the spine, ribs, and other flat bones. Regions of active growth, such as ends of long bones, show increased activity. Areas of abnormality usually appear more active than normal background. The extent of primary bone malignancies (*i.e.,* osteosarcoma, Ewing's sarcoma) may be easily assessed by the bone scan. In patients with malignancy, metastasis to the bone, if present, is clearly indicated on bone scans. Bone scans are the most sensitive means of detecting early lesions in the bones. This is especially important when routine roentgenograms are negative.

Osteomyelitis may have a variable bone scan picture early in the disease process, but will usually be increased days to weeks before the onset of roentgenographic changes. The earlier diagnosis reduces morbidity. The bone scan is also useful in locating stress fractures and nondisplaced traumatic fractures, and in evaluating fracture healing in nonunion.

The bone scan is also of value in assessing joint pain. Abnormalities are seen in rheumatoid arthritis, septic arthritis, gouty arthritis, and sacroiliitis.

Soft Tissue

The localization of infections is a challenging task. Gallium-67 (^{67}Ga) citrate and ^{111}In-labeled leukocytes may be used to locate an infectious focus. In the ^{67}Ga study, the patient is injected intravenously with the radiopharmaceutical and is imaged at 6 hours (optional), 24 hours, and 48 hours, postinjection. Additional images may be needed at 72 or 96 hours postinjection. Usually, a laxative is given before imaging because of excretion of the radiopharmaceutical into the large intestines. Gallium is localized not only in infections, but also in many malignancies and sarcoid. The study utilizing ^{111}In-labeled leukocytes begins with a sterile phlebotomy of the patient. The patient's leukocytes are then recovered and incubated with ^{111}In. The ^{111}In leukocytes are then reinjected into the patient. Twenty-four hours later, an image is obtained. The ^{111}In leukocyte study, which is currently investigational, lacks the interference of the gastrointestinal tract, which occasionally may produce confusing images in the ^{67}Ga study.

Nuclear Magnetic Resonance and Positron-Emission Tomography

Nuclear Magnetic Resonance

Nuclear magnetic resonance (NMR) is a technique that responds not only to gross anatomical features (like x-ray of bony structures) but also to differences in chemical composition (specifically to the myriad compounds of hydrogen found in living tissues).

An NMR is an immense doughnut-shaped electromagnet that can enclose a patient's entire body or a small area of the body. Within this magnetic field, hydrogen nuclei align themselves in wobbling, parallel ranks. Then, by being irradiated with a short, magnetic pulse (4–15 megaherz), the nuclei are pushed over on their sides. Upon the subsidence of the pulse, nuclei return to their positions and, in this process, re-radiate some of the energies they had absorbed. This electromagnetic echo is picked up by sensitive receivers. Computers analyze the signals and display a cross-sectional image of the area under study.

Since bone is invisible by NMR, the modality is particularly effective for such areas as base of the skull and interior of the spine, as well as the inner walls of blood vessels. Cancer tissue shows up well, so that images of these abnormal cells can indicate whether the tumor is growing or regressing. NMR has the capacity to evaluate moving fluid, and hence will have an impact on the diagnosis of vascular diseases, hemorrhage into cerebrospinal fluid, and increasing intracranial pressure.

The chief advantage of NMR is that the patient is not exposed to radiation or an invasive procedure. The chief disadvantage is that the NMR produces only static images.

Positron-Emission Tomography

Positron-emission tomography (PET) is another new diagnostic aid that shows sequential changes in the metabolic activity of any desired cross section of the human body. PET imaging relies on injection of radioactive compound related to blood glucose. The PET scanner is an array of gamma-ray detectors converted to a computer that analyzes signals and displays areas of high-glucose concentration on a color video screen.

PET is used in studying metabolism in such organs as the pancreas, liver, lungs, and heart. It also appears to be very effective in diagnosing brain disorders.

Nonimaging *In-vivo* Studies

Measurement of Red Cell Mass

Measurement of red cell mass involves labeling of the patient's own red blood cells with chromium-51 (^{51}Cr) sodium chromate. Ten to 15 milliliters of the patient's blood are withdrawn and added to a solution of Acid Citrate Dextrose (as an anticoagulant). The radioactive ^{51}Cr is added to this combination, and the content of the vial is kept at room temperature for a period of 30 minutes. During this time, chromate penetrates the red cell membrane and binds to hemoglobin. This phenomenon only takes place when the valence of the chromium is +6. When ascorbic acid is added at the end of 30 minutes, the untagged chromium is converted to chromium with a +3 valence. A small fraction of this preparation is kept as a standard and the remainder is injected into the patient. After 10 to 15 minutes, a blood sample is withdrawn, and radioactivity in the sample and the standard is measured. From these counts, the red cell mass is calculated from the following basic formula:

Red Cell Mass

$$= \frac{\text{Total Radioactivity of Tagged RBCs Injected}}{\text{Radioactivity/ml of RBCs After Mixing}}$$

Plasma Volume

For this purpose, an already prepared solution of ^{131}I or ^{123}I albumin is used. A sample of this solution is injected intravenously, and a fraction is kept as a standard for later calculation. Fifteen minutes later a blood sample is withdrawn and the plasma volume is calculated according to the following formula:

$$\text{Plasma Volume} = \frac{\text{Radioactivity of Injected Tracer}}{\text{Radioactivity/ml Plasma After Mixing}}$$

The plasma volume also can be measured, indirectly, after red cell mass is calculated from the ^{51}Cr-tagged red blood cells as described above. With this approach, the patient's hematocrit is used to calculate the plasma volume.

Measurement of Total Blood Volume

The total blood volume can be measured by using both the tagged red blood cells and the radioiodinated albumin combined. However, for the sake of simplicity, the whole blood volume is commonly calculated indirectly by adding the red cell mass (using ^{51}Cr) and the plasma volume that has been estimated by taking the peripheral hematocrit into consideration.

Red Cell Survival and Sequestration

The measurement of the life span of red blood cells is important in some hematologic disorders when shortened survival of the cells is suspected. In this study a sample of the patient's own cells is tagged with ^{51}Cr sodium chromate in the manner similar to that described for red cell mass determination. The entire preparation is injected into the patient. Blood samples are drawn from the patient, then three times a week for 2 weeks, and, if needed, twice a week for the third and fourth week. From these samples, the half-time survival of the red cells is calculated. The normal red cells survive approximately 120 days (half-life, 60 days) within circulation. Because of elution of ^{51}Cr from the red cells, the normal survival time value obtained with the ^{51}Cr technique is approximately half of this number (half-life of 28 to 30 days).

In patients with shortened red cell survival (hemolytic anemia), the half-time calculated by this technique is less than normal. The degree to which the spleen is responsible for the destruction of red blood cells is often important in the management of patients with hemolytic anemias. If evidence is found for excessive trapping of the red cells by the spleen, surgical removal of this organ should be considered to reduce the red cell destruction. Such evidence can be obtained by external monitoring over the splenic and cardiac areas after the patient has received ^{51}Cr-tagged red blood cells. From the ratios of the values obtained in these areas, red cell sequestration can be determined.

Schilling Test

In patients who lack intrinsic factor in their gastric juice, which is essential for the absorption of vitamin B_{12}, radioactive cobalt-57 (^{57}Co) cyanocobalamin is important in diagnosis. A fasting patient is given a small, oral dose of ^{57}Co-labeled vitamin B_{12}, and the collection of urine is immediately started. One hour later, 1 mg of nonradioactive vitamin B_{12} is injected intramuscularly for the purpose of saturating the tissue-binding sites, thereby reducing the degree of removal by the liver or other organs of the radiolabeled vitamin B_{12}. The 24-hour urine content of the radioactivity is measured, and the percentage of the administered dose that was excreted in the urine is calculated. This measurement is only valid if all the urine is collected for this period. Normal individuals excrete between 8% to 40% of the injected activity. Patients with pernicious anemia excrete 0% to 3% of the radioactivity in 24 hours. In some patients, the diagnosis of intrinsic-factor deficiency can be further confirmed by adding this factor to the radioactive vitamin B_{12} in the second stage of this examination. When the study is repeated with intrinsic factor, the absorption of vitamin B_{12} approaches the normal range.

In patients with an absorptive defect in the small intestine, the addition of intrinsic factor does not correct the percentage of activity in the urine. In some patients the test is repeated after antibiotic therapy to determine if bacterial overgrowth is the cause of the B_{12} deficiency.

A dual isotope technique has been developed using ^{57}Cr cyanocobalamin with intrinsic factor and ^{58}Co cyanocobalamin without intrinsic factor. This allows the first two steps of the Schilling test to be performed simultaneously, decreasing the time of the study.

Treatment With Radionuclides

Because of their versatility, radioactive agents can be administered by different routes for the treatment of various disorders. The major disorders that benefit from these

---

Chart 18-2
Large Amounts of Radioactive Materials

Precautions

Notify the radiology department radioisotope section immediately:

In case of any doubt as to safe procedure
In case of any emergency
If any unexpected complications arise
In case of death:
    Before postmortem care is given
    Before an autopsy is performed
    Before the body is released
During Day: Call Radioisotope Section, Radiology Department
During Night: Call Radiologist on CALL.

Chart 18-3
General Rules for Radiation Protection

To Be Observed By All Personnel

Extent of Hazard

1. The degree of possible hazard associated with a patient who has received radioactive isotopes will depend on the amount and kind of radioactive material administered, where and how it was given, and how long a time has elapsed since its administration.

2. The amounts of radioisotopes contained in patients after treatment or diagnostic study is completed can be classified as follows:

	Half-life Greater Than 15 Hours	Half-life Less Than 15 Hours
Small Amount	Less than 0.2 mCi	Less than 10 mCi
Moderate Amount	0.2 to 5 mCi	More than 10 mCi
Large Amount	More than 5 mCi	

Identification of Patients Who Have Received Radioisotopes

1. Small Amounts
   a. Patients may contain small amounts of radioisotopes after diagnostic studies. For these patients, the Doctor's Progress Sheet in the patient's Hospital Chart is marked to indicate the amount and type of radioactive material administered.
   b. Patients who contain small amounts of radioactive material can be given normal hospital care and attention without any appreciable hazard to personnel.
2. Moderate and Large Amounts
   Patients containing radioactive materials in moderate to large amounts may present a radiation hazard unless certain simple precautions are followed. Patients may be treated with systemic radionuclides, that is, materials administered as solutions (such as iodine-131, colloidal gold-198, or phosphorus-32) or encapsulated radionuclides (such as radium-226, radon-222, cesium-137, iodine-125, californium-252, gold-198 seeds, or iridium-192). To make sure that these patients are identified, the Doctor's Order Sheet is marked to indicate the amount and type of radioactive material administered. In addition, in order to

provide instructions for the safe care of these patients, the following steps are taken:
   a. An appropriate Precaution Sheet, listing special rules to be observed, is inserted into the Hospital Chart.
   b. For patients who contain *moderate or large amounts* of radionuclides, the Hospital Chart is marked with an appropriate label showing the standard radiation symbol. A label is placed on the chart cover and on the Precaution Sheet.
   c. All patients who contain *large amounts* of radioactive material will have a wrist band attached to them by the doctor who administers the radionuclide. The band will indicate the date and the nature and amount of radioactivity.
   d. A precaution tag will be attached to the bed of each patient containing a *large amount* of radioactive material.
   - WHEN YOU SEE THE RADIOACTIVE LABEL ON A CHART, ON A PATIENT, OR ON A PATIENT'S BED, IT IS YOUR RESPONSIBILITY TO LOOK FOR, READ, AND FOLLOW INSTRUCTIONS GIVEN ON THE PRECAUTION SHEET.

Radioactive Excreta

1. There will be some radioactivity in the excreta of all patients who have received radioactive materials except for those instances in which the radioactive material is encapsulated.
   - In all cases other than these exceptions, contamination should be avoided by wearing rubber gloves when handling the patient's excreta, vomitus, or body fluids. If linens become wet with patient excreta, notify the Nuclear Medicine Section, Radiology Department.
2. In some instances it will be necessary to save patients' excreta in containers provided by the Radiology Department. In these cases, special instructions will be issued. When feasible, the patient should be encouraged to collect his own urine.

Discharge of Patients Who Have Received Radioactive Materials From the Hospital

No patient who has received a large amount of radioactive material may be discharged from the Hospital before the time

(continued)

---

agents include (1) hyperthyroidism, (2) thyroid cancer, (3) polycythemia vera, and (4) malignant effusion of the pleural and peritoneal cavities. The radioactive isotopes used generally emit beta rays, which are more destructive than gamma rays.

Hyperthyroidism

^{131}I (sodium iodide) is mainly used for the treatment of hyperthyroidism and thyroid cancer. In patients with hyperthyroidism, usually a relatively small dose of this radionuclide results in the cure of the majority of these patients.

Chart 18-3
General Rules for Radiation Protection (continued)

Death of Patients Containing Radioactive Materials *(continued)*

and date indicated on the Precaution Sheet. Additional special arrangements must be made with the Radiation Health Physicist for patients being treated with iodine-125.

Death of Patients Containing Radioactive Materials

1. If a patient containing more than 5 millicuries of systemic radioactive material dies in the hospital, the physician signing the death certificate should note from the wrist band and the Hospital Chart that the patient contains radioactivity and inform the pathologist of this fact. The Nuclear Medicine Section of the Radiology Department should also be notified.
2. If a patient containing any encapsulated radioactive material dies, the Radiation Health Physicist must be notified.
3. Is there is no autopsy, and the body contains more than 30 millicuries of systemic radioactivity, the physician signing the death certificate should notify the Nuclear Medicine Section, Radiology Department, so that the proper Statement to the funeral director can be prepared.
4. If there is an autopsy, and the body contains more than 5 millicuries of systemic radioactivity, it may be necessary for the pathologist to take special precautions while performing the autopsy.

Special Medical Procedures

Special medical procedures may be necessary with patients containing radioactive materials which may involve the removal of body fluids containing radioactivity. In such cases, advice on the radiation safety of the procedure should be obtained from the Nuclear Medicine Section, Radiology Department.

Emergency Surgery

If emergency surgery is required for a patient containing a *large amount* of systemic radioactivity, the Nuclear Medicine Section, Radiology Department should be notified.

(Courtesy, Hospital of the University of Pennsylvania)

Admission of Patients Who Will Be Treated With Encapsulated Radionuclides

Because of the radiation hazard involved in admitting patients for treatment with certain radionuclides, the following procedures are advised.

1. The physician should notify the Admissions Office in advance when admitting patients.
2. The admission clerk must assign a patient scheduled to receive an encapsulated radionuclide application to a private room.
3. The admission clerk must assign a patient scheduled to receive a dose of iodine-131 greater than 8mCi to a private room.
4. For a patient scheduled to receive a californium-252 application, the admission clerk will attempt to assign the patient to a private room having as many outside walls as possible.
5. Physicians in charge will confirm BEFORE the radioactive application is made that the patient's accommodations are such that no radiation hazard will exist.

Monitoring of Vicinity

The vicinity of patients treated with large amounts of radioactivity will be carefully monitored with a suitable radiation-detecting instrument to ensure that no member of the general population is likely to receive a dose in excess of 100 millirems. Reports of the survey will be attached to the patient's chart and a copy will be sent to the Radiation Survey Office. After the patient is discharged, a survey will be made by the Radiology Department to ensure that no radiation hazard remains.

Visitor Limitations

Unless precautions to the contrary are posted, there are no limitations for visitors to patients containing radioactive materials.

Radiation Hazards

When there is any doubt as to whether an unusual situation exists that may constitute a radiation hazard with systemic radionuclides, call the doctor responsible in the Nuclear Medicine Section, Radiology Department. Regarding patients being treated with encapsulated radionuclides, call the Radiation Therapy Physics Section.

In some patients who are resistant to single-dose treatment, two or more administrations may be necessary to obtain a satisfactory result. In many patients, hypothyroidism, requiring thyroid replacement, may develop months to years after treatment.

Thyroid Cancer

Radioisotope treatment of patients with thyroid cancer usually follows surgical removal of the cancer and part or most of the thyroid gland. In these patients the radionuclide is administered in two stages. The first stage involves the ad-

Chart 18-4
Radiation Precautions: Special Instructions

For Nurses and Patient-Care Attendants

1. It is very important to provide the patient who contains radioactivity with proper nursing care and at the same time to limit radiation exposure to as low a level as is reasonable. To do this, read and observe all General Rules in this section and consult the PRECAUTION SHEET that is in the patient's Hospital Chart.

2. There is no appreciable hazard to hospital personnel from radiation in the vicinity of the patient except for patients who have received large amounts (see pp. 341–343) of radioactive materials. Do not stay in the immediate vicinity (within 3 feet) of patients who have received large amounts of radioactivity longer than is necessary to give proper care and attention. The hazard is very slight, however. A nurse could stand continuously at the bedside of a typical patient being treated with radium for 10 hours before her radiation exposure would exceed the Dose Limiting Recommendations of the National Committee on Radiation Protection for the average dose for occasionally exposed individuals for 1 year. It should be noted that the radiation exposure diminishes rapidly as the distance from the patient is increased. At a distance of 3 feet from the patient, it would require 40 hours to exceed the recommended annual limit. Any nurse who is exposed frequently to radiation would be considered to be a Radiation Worker and should be monitored continuously by the Radiation Safety Office.

   - Special instructions limiting the time a nurse may spend near a patient should be issued when necessary.

3. Body fluids and excreta of patients who have received radioactive nuclides (except encapsulated sources) should be assumed to be radioactive.

   - Avoid direct contact with patient's blood, urine, vomitus and other body fluids. Wear rubber gloves if such contact is anticipated.
   - If bed clothing or patient's clothing becomes wet from body fluids and hence contaminated with radioactivity, notify the Nuclear Medicine Section, Radiology Department, and save for radioactive monitoring by the Nuclear Medicine Section, Radiology Department.

   - If dressings covering the site of administration of gold-198 become stained, notify the Nuclear Medicine Section, Radiology Department.
   - Wash hands after bathing patient. Wear rubber gloves when giving patient other personal attention. Patients who have received large amounts of iodine-131 should not be bathed until 24 hours after the time of administration of the radioactivity.
   - Bedpans should be handled with rubber gloves and thoroughly flushed before returning to general use. For patients who have received large amounts of iodine-131, the bedpan should be flushed out thoroughly after every use and the same bedpan should be reserved for the same patient during his hospitalization.
   - If a spill of any type occurs, mop up immediately. Save all liquids and the mop used. Notify the Nuclear Medicine Section, Radiology Department, immediately so that measurements can be made to evaluate any possible hazard.

4. Needles, seeds, or capsules containing radioisotopes in patients who are being treated with encapsulated sources of radioactivity may sometimes become dislodged or displaced. If there is any indication that this has happened, notify the Radiotherapy Physics Section, immediately. These sources can be handled safely with tongs or forceps but should never be picked up or touched directly.

5. If a patient who contains more than 5 millicuries of systemic radioactivity dies, notify the Nuclear Medicine Section, Department of Radiology. If a patient containing encapsulated radionuclides dies, notify the Radiotherapy Physics Section. Observe all General and Special Rules in this section while preparing the patient for the morgue. Clearly mark the tags that are to be placed on the cadaver, the shroud, and the icebox door with "CAUTION—RADIOACTIVITY."

(Courtesy, Hospital of the University of Pennsylvania)

ministration of enough radioactivity to irradiate the remaining functioning thyroid gland and render the patient hypothyroid. This is usually accomplished by a relatively large dose of ^{131}I. The second stage is accomplished by the administration of another large dose while the patient has become significantly hypothyroid. The second dose is used to destroy the cancer cells in the original site as well as in metastatic sites.

- The urine of cancer patients who have been treated with a large dose of ^{131}I contains a significant amount of radioactivity for several days and should be handled carefully to minimize radiation exposure and to prevent contamination.

Polycythemia Vera

Patients with polycythemia vera may benefit from the intravenous administration of ^{32}P sodium phosphate. A small dose of the agent is administered, and the desired effect (gradual decline of red cell production) is usually observed several weeks later. Since ^{32}P emits only beta rays, these patients are not a source of radiation to others.

Malignant Effusions

Intracavitary administration of radioactive agents is useful only for the treatment of malignant effusions in the pleural and peritoneal cavities. The radiation from ^{32}P is pure beta radiation and is confined to only the patient's body. ^{32}P may reduce the production of the effusions. It is administered in the nuclear medicine laboratory after a secure catheter or needle is in place.

- These patients should be watched very carefully for leakage of fluid from the site of administration or other areas for several days. Any leakage should be reported immediately to the staff of the nuclear medicine laboratory and the radiation safety office of the institution.

Radiation Protection and the Care of Patients Who Have Received Radioactive Materials

We have always been exposed to small but definite amounts of radiation (called background radiation) from the radioactivity in natural materials, from our own bodies, and from cosmic rays from outer space. In addition to background radiation, most of us are exposed to radiation from medical diagnostic x-ray examinations, nuclear weapon testing fallout, radium dial wristwatches, and so forth. Some of us are further exposed to radiation because of the nature of our work.

This section contains suggestions and guidelines for controlling radiation exposures and reducing hazards from the use of radioactive isotopes in the hospital environment. When radioactive materials are properly controlled, the risks from radiation exposure are very small. However, without control, these materials may be dangerous to patients, health care personnel, and the public.

Because radiation cannot be seen or felt, it is extremely important that common-sense rules of radiation safety always be observed by personnel working near sources of radiation. The best way to ensure proper patient care and, at the same time, to keep radiation exposure of personnel at safe, low levels is to understand and carefully observe the guidelines outlined in this section. It is the responsibility of all personnel who may be exposed to radiation in every institution to follow such precautions. The precautions that apply to large amounts of radioactive materials,

general rules for radiation protection, and specific instructions for nurses and health care personnel are summarized in Charts 18-2 through 18-4.

▷ Bibliography

Books
Diagnostic Radiology

Alavi A and Arger PH. Abdomen, Multiple Imaging Procedures. New York, Grune & Stratton, 1980.

Athanasoulis C (ed). Interventional Radiology. Philadelphia, WB Saunders, 1982.

Coulam CM. Physical Basics of Medical Imaging. New York, Appleton–Century–Crofts, 1981.

Dalinka MK. Comprehensive Manual of Radiology. New York, Springer–Verlag, 1980.

Erhlich RA and Given EDM. Patient Care in Radiography. St Louis, CV Mosby, 1981.

Ring E. Interventional Radiology. Boston, Little, Brown & Co, 1981.

Wilson G (ed). Current Radiology, Vol. 3. New York, John Wiley & Sons, 1982.

Radiotherapy

Fletcher GH. Textbook of Radiotherapy. 3rd ed. Philadelphia. Lea & Febiger, 1980.

Hall EJ. Radiobiology for the Radiologist, 2nd ed. Hagerstown, Maryland, Harper & Row, 1978.

Moss WT, Brand WN, and Battifora H. Radiation Oncology. Rationale, Technique, Results, 5th ed. St Louis, CV Mosby, 1979.

Nuclear Medicine

Baum S et al. Atlas of Nuclear Medicine Imaging. New York, Appleton–Century–Crofts, 1981.

Kirchmer PT (ed). Nuclear Medicine Review Syllabus. New York, Society of Nuclear Medicine, 1978.

Martin P. Clinical Nuclear Medicine. Garden City, New York, Medical Examination, 1981.

Articles

Jankowski CB. Radiation emergency. Am J Nurs 1982 Jan; 82(1):90–96, 97–98.

Kelly PP and Tinsley C. Planning care for the patient receiving external radiation. Am J Nurs 1981 Feb; 81(2):338–342.

Varricchio CG. The patient on radiation therapy. Am J Nurs 1981 Feb; 81(2):334–337.

Whalen JP and Balter S. Radiation risks associated with diagnostic radiology. Disease-a-Month 1982 Mar; 28(6):1–96.

Unit VI

Perioperative Management of the Surgical Patient

▷ Perioperative Nursing

Perioperative nursing is the term used to describe the wide variety of nursing functions associated with the patient's surgical experience. The word "perioperative" is an encompassing term that incorporates the three phases of the surgical experience—namely, preoperative, intraoperative, and postoperative. Each of these phases begins and ends at a particular time in the sequence of events that constitute the surgical experience, and each includes a wide range of behaviors and nursing activities that the nurse performs using the nursing process as reflected in the standards of practice (see the chart on p. 348).

The *preoperative phase* of the perioperative nursing role begins when the decision for surgical intervention is made and ends with the transference of the patient to the operating room table. The scope of nursing activities during this time can be as broad as establishing a baseline assessment of the patient, in the clinical setting, or at home; carrying out a preoperative interview; and preparing the patient for the anesthetic he is to receive and the surgery he is to undergo. Or it may be as limited as doing a preoperative patient assessment in the holding area or surgical suite.

The nursing functions included in the *intraoperative phase* of the perioperative role begin when the patient is admitted or transferred to the Surgery Department and end when he is admitted to the recovery area. In this phase, the scope of nursing activity can be as broad as starting the IV, administering IV medications, and carrying out the full scope of physiologic monitoring throughout a surgical procedure, as well as providing for the patient's safety. Or it can be as limited as holding the patient's hand during general anesthesia induction, acting in the role of scrub nurse, or assisting in positioning the patient on the operating room table using basic principles of body alignment.

The *postoperative phase* of the perioperative nursing role begins with the admission of the patient to the recovery area and ends with a follow-up evaluation in the clinical setting or at home. The scope of nursing activities during this period may be as broad as assessing the postoperative status of the patient in terms of the effects of the anesthetic agents and the impact of surgery on body image or role function, as well as evaluating the family's perception of the surgery. Or it can be as limited as communicating pertinent information about the patient's surgery to personnel in the recovery area or surgical nursing unit.

Each segment is reviewed in more detail in this unit. Where pertinent and possible, the nursing process of assessment, planning, intervention, and evaluation is described. (This is also outlined on pp. 376–377.)

Examples of Nursing Activities in the Perioperative Role

Preoperative Phase

Preoperative Assessment

Home/clinic
1. initiates initial preoperative assessment
2. plans teaching methods appropriate to patient's needs
3. involves family in interview

Surgical unit
1. completes preoperative assessment
2. coordinates patient teaching with other nursing staff
3. explains phases in perioperative period and expectations
4. develops a plan of care

Surgical site
1. assesses patient's level of consciousness
2. reviews chart
3. identifies patient
4. verifies surgical site

Planning

determines a plan of care

Psychological Support
1. tells patient what is happening
2. determines psychological status
3. gives prior warning of noxious stimuli
4. stands near/touches patient during procedures/induction
5. communicates patient's emotional status to other appropriate members of the health care team

Intraoperative Phase

Maintenance of Safety
1. assures that the sponge, needle, and instrument counts are correct
2. positions the patient
   a. functional alignment
   b. exposure of surgical site
   c. maintenance of position throughout procedure
3. applies grounding device to patient
4. provides physical support

Physiological Monitoring
1. calculates effects on patient of excessive fluid loss
2. distinguishes normal from abnormal cardiopulmonary data
3. reports changes in patient's pulse, respirations, temperature, and blood pressure

Psychological Monitoring (Prior to Induction and If Patient is Conscious)
1. provides emotional support to patient
2. continues to assess patient's emotional status
3. communicates patient's emotional status to other appropriate members of the health care team

Nursing Management
1. provides physical safety for the patient
2. maintains aseptic, controlled environment
3. effectively manages human resources

Postoperative Phase

Communication of Intraoperative Information
1. gives patient's name
2. states type of surgery performed
3. provides contributing intraoperative factors, i.e., drain, catheters
4. states physical limitations
5. states impairments resulting from surgery
6. reports patient's preoperative level of consciousness
7. communicates necessary equipment needs

Postoperative Evaluation

Recovery area
determines patient's immediate response to surgical intervention

Surgical unit
1. evaluates effectiveness of nursing care in the OR
2. determines patient's level of satisfaction with care given during perioperative period
3. evaluates products used on patient in the OR
4. determines patient's psychological status
5. assists with discharge planning

Home/clinic
1. seeks patient's perception of surgery in terms of the effects of anesthetic agents, impact on body image, distortion, immobilization
2. determines family's perception of surgery

(From: Operating room nursing: Perioperative role. AORN Journal, 27: May 1978).

19

Preoperative Nursing Management

▷ Nursing Process Overview

▶ Assessment

As indicated in the pages that follow, assessment of the surgical patient involves an evaluation of a wide range of physical and psychological factors. A great number of parameters are taken into account in the overall assessment of the patient, and a variety of patient problems or nursing diagnoses can be anticipated or identified on the basis of the data that is gathered.

Patient Problems/Nursing Diagnoses

Based on the data acquired from the health history, including clinical manifestations and diagnostic assessment, the major problems that may exist for the surgical patient include insufficient or inadequate information related to the anesthetic agent; worry, depression, and fear related to the diagnosis and outcome of surgery, including postoperative pain; concomitant risk factors related to previous life-style and history (*i.e.,* weight problems, smoking history, allergy history); and concern about acquiring an injury or infection related to hospital conditions (nosocomial infections) or other adverse outcomes.

▶ Planning and Implementation

Goals

The patient's major goals are:

1. Correction or treatment of a physical problem that requires surgical intervention
2. Relief of anxiety, worry, and depression
3. Acceptance of and preparation for surgical intervention
4. Acceptance and tolerance of the preanesthetic medications and anesthetic agents
5. Avoidance of injury, nosocomial infections, and complications

The major nursing goals are to:

1. Assist the patient in understanding the physical and psychosocial aspects of the surgical experience
2. Acquaint the patient and his family with the environment, protocols, and expectations as surgery is anticipated
3. Teach the patient certain procedures that will help in reducing postoperative complications and in increasing comfort and enhancing recovery
4. Prepare the patient physically and psychologically for the anesthetic and operative procedure
5. Collaborate with other members of the health team in coordinating all preoperative preparations

▶ Evaluation

Expected Outcomes

1. Is surgically treated for an anatomical/physiologic dysfunction (primarily a physician's responsibility). All nursing goals are directed toward assisting in the achievement of this goal.
2. Is relieved of anxiety, worry, and depression
   a. Verbalizes relief about "bills and cost" after talking with social worker
   b. Tells mate that he is looking forward to having the "problem" corrected
   c. Relaxes quietly after being visited by health team members
3. Accepts and prepares for surgical intervention
   a. Verbalizes need for an operation
   b. Participates willingly in preoperative preparation
   c. Queries staff regarding last-minute concerns
   d. Requests a visit with clergyman
   e. Describes the kind of exercises he is expected to do postanesthetically
   f. Reviews information regarding postoperative care
   g. Relates positively to family members regarding the coming operation
4. Accepts and tolerates the preanesthetic and anesthetic agents with the least difficulty and complications
   a. Responds willingly to questions
   b. Queries the anesthesiologist about concerns relating to types of anesthesia and induction
   c. Accepts the preanesthetic medication
   d. Verbalizes an understanding of the purpose of the preanesthetic medication
   e. Remains in bed; tells the nurse why the side rails are in place
   f. Relaxes and closes eyes during transportation to operating floor
5. Avoids injury, nosocomial infections, and complications
   a. Understands that family cannot visit if they have upper respiratory infections
   b. Registers normal vital signs
   c. Presents intact skin—no cuts, abrasions
   d. Has an empty bladder prior to leaving for the operating room
   e. Reports no subjective feelings indicative of imminent upper respiratory infection

▷ Psychosocial Nursing Assessment

Any kind of surgical procedure is always preceded by some type of emotional reaction in a patient, whether it is obvious or hidden, normal or abnormal. For example, preoperative anxiety is an anticipatory response to an experience that the patient may view as a threat to his customary role in life, his body integrity, or even life itself. The extent of the patient's reaction is based on many factors, including the discomforts and sacrifices he anticipates—whether physical, financial, psychological, spiritual, or social—and the surgical outcome he imagines. Will the operation improve his present condition? Will he be disabled? Is this just a temporary measure in a chronic condition?

An important part of the social assessment is to determine the role of the patient's family or significant persons who are meaningful to him. The value and reliance of all available support systems is also determined. Other pertinent findings are the usual functional level and typical daily activities of the patient, which will assist in his care and future rehabilitation plans.

Preoperative Anxiety and Nursing Interventions

From the psychological point of view, it is known that a mind that is not at peace directly influences the functioning of the body. Therefore, it is imperative to know what anxieties the patient is experiencing. By taking a careful nursing history, the nurse will elicit patient concerns that can have a direct bearing on the course of his surgical experience. Undoubtedly, a patient facing surgery is beset by fears: fears of the unknown, of death, of anesthesia, of cancer. Add to this worries about the possible loss of a job, the need to support a family, or the possibility of permanent incapacity and one can get a sense of the enormous emotional strain created by the prospect of surgery. Emotional upsets are more apparent in illness. Consequently, the nurse will be more tolerant and understanding.

Fear is expressed in different ways by different individuals. For example, fear may be expressed indirectly by the patient who asks a lot of questions, repeating them constantly even though answers were given previously. For another person, the reaction may be withdrawal—deliberately avoiding communication, perhaps by concentrating on a book. Still others may talk incessantly about trivialities. Often such behavior ends abruptly as the patient turns to the nurse and says, "I guess you can tell I'm a bit nervous about my operation." The need to keep the outlet of communication open is never greater than at this time. To belittle the patient's fears by saying, "Oh, there's nothing to be afraid of," immediately closes the door and causes the patient to lapse into his own less effective means of coping with his worries.

Such breakdowns in satisfactory interrelations leave the patient upset, bewildered, and even unable to follow simple directions. Often in the course of conversation, something that was mentioned by a nurse or a physician becomes exaggerated out of all proportion to its importance. For example, if an operation is postponed because of a filled schedule, and the patient is merely told that "something had come up," he may begin to worry that the reason for the delay is a deterioration in his condition.

Let us examine the causes of fear that a preoperative patient may experience.

Fear of anesthesia was justified years ago, when little was known about the control and the effect of anesthetic agents. But with refined methods, tested drugs, and skilled anesthesiologists, the hazards are minimized. The ease with which a patient accepts an anesthetic today is attributed to the adequate physical and mental preparation that he receives. The price of poor preparation is a difficult period of induction, followed by an unpleasant emergence from the anesthetic agent. The nurse in daily association with each patient can do much to dispel false conceptions and misinformation. In instances in which the anesthesiologist and the operating room nurse visit the patient the day before surgery, real confidence is established, and the patient accepts the anesthetic more readily and is less fearful, because the number of unknowns has been reduced.

Often the fear of the anesthetic is secondary to the *fear of pain or of death*. Will I feel the knife? What if the anesthesia wears off? The patient needs reassurance that the anesthesiologist will be in constant attendance to take care of these problems. Some surgeons will not operate on a patient who is convinced that he will die. This is a real fear, and it cannot be dismissed lightly. Good rapport between patient and nurse, together with tact on the nurse's part, may bring him to a realization that his fear is magnified. It will help him greatly if those responsible for his care build up his confidence.

The *fear of the unknown* is the worst of all. This fear stems partly from a belief on the patient's part that he is not being told "everything" about his diagnosis or illness. Therefore, the more understanding one has of the probabilities for the future, the better is the adjustment. The nurse can do much to allay the anxieties of the patient and induce a certain peace of mind. A patient frequently expresses fears and misgivings to the nurse but hides them from the surgeon. In such circumstances the nurse communicates these evidences of anxiety privately to the surgeon.

This particular fear of the unknown may be alleviated if the patient has had positive experience in the past with an operation. By comparing that experience with the anticipated one, the patient may reveal fears that are no longer justified.

The *fear of destruction of body image* occurs frequently because surgery in many instances has become more radical. Then too, there is greater emphasis today on youth, the body beautiful, and more revealing clothing, as is verified by magazine and television advertising. Consequently, any surgical encroachment on the body is viewed with distress by many patients, including the scar of a surgical incision.

Fear of separation from former activities, family, and friends may compound the concerns and anxieties of the preoperative patient.

In addition to the above fears, the average patient has many other *worries*. He may have financial problems, family responsibilities, and employment obligations; in addition to these, he may fear a poor prognosis or the probability of a handicap in the future. These problems can be investi-

gated by the nurse. If the difficulty is of such a nature that a medical social worker can give assistance, the aid of such a person is enlisted. If the worry stems from fear of what the prognosis is likely to be, the physician is informed.

When some of these fears have been expressed, brought to light, and examined in their proper perspective, it is possible and even essential to get the patient to reveal what the operation means to him. Have him express his thoughts about the importance and the meaning of this surgery for the immediate future as well as the more distant future. Most fears are manifestations of concern over losing control over one's person, either physically or socially. The patient may be concerned about losing some of his independence, his integrity, and his control over his effectiveness in coping with his environment. The nurse may be in a position to elicit these concerns from the patient. The importance of adequate lines of communication between surgeon and nurse as they work together to prepare the patient for surgery must be emphasized here.

Psychological preparation for subsequent stress includes permitting the patient some degree of worrying. This is more desirable than having little or no anticipatory fear. Moderately fear-arousing information allows the patient to increase his tolerance for stress by developing effective ways of coping with his problems. Absence of worry will deprive the patient of the motivation to prepare himself psychologically for a stressful experience, with the result that when a crisis develops, he will have a low tolerance for stress.

The significance of *spiritual therapy* must not be forgotten. Regardless of the religious affiliation of the patient, the nurse recognizes that faith in a Higher Power can be as therapeutic as medication. Every attempt must be made to help the patient obtain the fullest spiritual help that he requests. This may be accomplished by participating in prayer, by reading passages from the Scriptures, or by calling a clergyman. Faith has great sustaining power; thus, the beliefs of each individual patient should be respected and supported.

The interval of time preparatory to surgery in some instances may become very extended. *Recreation and diversion* can be provided by such activities as reading, listening to the radio, watching television, engaging in handcrafts and games, and so forth. The nurse can arrange for individuals with similar interests to meet. Many times patients can help one another.

Perhaps the most valuable facility at the disposal of the nurse is the ability to *listen* to the patient, especially during the nursing history. By engaging in conversation and using the principles of tactful interviewing (see Chap. 4), the nurse can acquire invaluable bits of information. An unhurried, understanding, and kind nurse invites confidence on the part of the patient.

Every patient should be treated as an individual who has fears and hopes quite distinct from the fears or hopes of the next person. Understanding and helping one patient may require a completely different approach from that used with another. Providing time to answer questions and offering psychological support will ensure a smoother postoperative course for the surgical patient. He will sleep better, recall fewer fearful images, experience less postoperative urinary retention, and need less anesthetic and pain medication. He will recover more rapidly and be discharged from the hospital sooner.

Denial of Anxiety.   The preceding discussion of preoperative anxiety emphasizes the most common problems of the patient facing an operation. The opposite reaction of denying anxiety can also provide obstacles to effective treatment, such as in the case of a person who notices abnormal signs or symptoms but puts off seeking treatment. Denial is a reaction noted in many persons when they are suddenly confronted with potentially shocking information. Usually this reaction does not last longer than a few days or a few weeks, but nevertheless such denial and delay may have serious consequences. This is an area where the nurse's responsibility extends outward in all contacts with members of the community. Any questionable abnormal finding relating to one's body should be checked as soon as possible by a knowledgeable person in the health field.

▷ General Physical Assessment

Before treatment is initiated, a nursing history is taken and the patient is given a physical examination, during which time vital signs are noted and a data base is established for future comparisons. Many diagnostic tests may be performed, such as blood analyses, roentgenographic studies, endoscopies, tissue biopsies, and stool and urine studies. In all of these tests the nurse is in a position to assist the patient in understanding the need for the diagnostic studies. There is also an opportunity during the physical examination to note significant physical findings, such as a rash or pressure sores, that may be contributing to the patient's condition.

These preliminary contacts with the staff during the nursing history, examination, and diagnostic tests provide the patient with an opportunity to ask questions and to get acquainted with those who will be caring for him. In their efforts to establish rapport with the patient, the physician and nurse must respect the patient's feelings and needs.

Assessment of Nutritional Status

Assessment of nutritional needs are determined by measuring the patient's height and weight, triceps skin fold, upper arm circumference, serum protein levels, and nitrogen balance.

Proteins and Vitamins.   Replacement of deficits is especially true with respect to protein and calorie malnutrition, since protein is essential for tissue repair. Protein deficiency may result from anorexia concomitant with the aging process, chronic debilitating illness, cancer, or frequent vomiting. Or, it may be caused by poor food habits and a diet in which meats and eggs are almost absent. Proteins may also be lost in severe burns and through draining abscesses or wounds.

Protein replacement is a slow process and may take several days or weeks. The replacement may be accomplished by means of (1) a diet high in protein (meat, milk, eggs and cheese), carbohydrates, and calories but low in fat; (2) supplementary liquid feedings, such as milk enriched with skim milk powder; or (3) protein hydrolysates

given orally or by infusion. Hypertonic parenteral therapy may be given through a polyethylene tubing placed percutaneously in a large-bore vein, such as the subclavian (using a cutdown) (See Hyperalimentation, p. 780.)

Vitamins are required for specific purposes. Thiamine (vitamin B₁) is necessary for oxidizing carbohydrates and maintaining normal gastrointestinal function. A deficiency in vitamin B₁ is noted in chronic gastrointestinal and liver diseases. Ascorbic acid (vitamin C) is required for wound healing and synthesis of collagen. Vitamin K is necessary for blood clotting and prothrombin production. These vitamins may be given orally or parenterally.

Loss of body fluids results in electrolyte imbalances. The replacement of these fluids is discussed in Chapter 9. The nurse records all intake and output and keeps a daily record of the patient's weight. Periodic evaluations are made to note the patient's progress and readiness for surgery. Dental caries and poor mouth hygiene may contribute to general debilitation and should be corrected (Chap. 34).

A nursing goal and challenge is to encourage the patient to eat by serving him attractive and palatable meals made up of small, manageable servings. If the patient is on parenteral/enteral therapy or is given gastrostomy feedings or infusions, he may need diversion and encouragement. The method of giving fluids depends on the type of replacement therapy. If a nasogastric tube is being used, liquids will be taken more readily if the patient is in a sitting position. If gastrostomy feedings are used, an upright or Fowler's position is effective.

Dehydration, hypovolemia, and electrolyte imbalances are common and should be carefully substantiated. The degree of severity is often difficult to determine. When a patient is being prepared for surgery, often additional time is needed to replace deficits in order to get him in the best possible condition.

Obesity.   If the patient is overweight and if preoperative time permits, physicians will insist that a prescribed and systematic program of weight reduction be undertaken in order that the surgical risk may be lessened. Obesity increases the seriousness of complications to a great extent. During surgery, fatty tissues are not highly resistant to infection; the surgeon faces increased technical and mechanical problems, and therefore dehiscence and wound infections are more common. The obese patient is difficult to care for because of his weight; he breathes poorly when lying on his side and thus is subject to hypoventilation and postoperative pulmonary complications, distention, and phlebitis. In addition, cardiovascular, endocrine, hepatic, and biliary diseases are more common in obese patients. It has been estimated that for each 30 pounds of excess weight, about 25 additional miles of blood vessels are needed. The increased demands on the heart are obvious.

Addiction to Narcotics, Drugs, or Alcohol.   Individuals who have an addiction to drugs or alcohol frequently attempt to hide the habit. Often a variety of infections and trauma sites on the body can be noted. This person requires meticulous attention, patience, and a degree of skepticism when listening to answers.

The acutely intoxicated person is susceptible to injury. If surgery is required, local or regional block anesthesia is used for minor surgery; for more extensive injury, surgery is postponed if possible. Otherwise, the stomach must be intubated and aspirated before general anesthesia is administered in order to prevent vomiting and aspiration.

The person with a history of chronic alcoholism often suffers from malnutrition and other systemic problems; therefore, the surgical risk is increased. In view of this, delirium tremens may be anticipated on the second or third day postoperatively; it is associated with a significant mortality rate.

Assessment of Respiratory Status

The goal for potential surgical patients is to have optimum respiratory function. All patients are urged to stop smoking 4 to 6 weeks before an operation; those undergoing upper abdominal and chest surgery are taught breathing exercises and how to use an incentive spirometer.

Since it is necessary to maintain adequate ventilation during all phases of surgical treatment, surgery is usually contraindicated when the patient has a respiratory infection. Respiratory difficulties increase the possibility of atelectasis, bronchopneumonia, and respiratory failure when anesthetics are superimposed. Patients with pulmonary problems are evaluated by testing pulmonary function and determining blood gas values to note the extent of respiratory insufficiency. Antibiotics may be given for infections.

Assessment of Cardiovascular Status

The goal in preparing any patient for surgery is to have a well-functioning cardiovascular system to meet the oxygen, fluid, and nutritional needs throughout the perioperative period.

Since the margin of safety is lessened when a patient exhibits signs of cardiovascular disease, this condition demands greater than usual diligence during all phases of management and care. Depending on the severity of symptoms, surgery may be deferred until maximal benefits have been obtained from medical treatment. At times, surgical treatment can be modified to meet the likely tolerance of the patient. For example, in an obese patient with acute obstructive cholecystitis and possible diabetes and coronary artery disease, simple gallbladder drainage with removal of calculi may be done rather than a more extensive operation.

Of particular significance in the patient with cardiovascular disease is the necessity to avoid sudden changes of position, prolonged immobilization, hypotension or hypoxia, and overloading of the body with fluids or blood.

Assessment of Hepatic and Renal Function

The goal is to have maximum functioning of the liver and urinary systems so that drugs, anesthetic agents, and body waste and toxins are adequately removed from the body.

The *liver* is important in the biotransformation of anesthetic compounds. Therefore, any disease of the liver has an effect on anesthetic intake. Acute liver disease is associated with a high surgical death rate; hence, preoperative improvement in liver function is desired. Careful assessment is made utilizing various liver function tests (see Chap. 39).

The *kidney* is involved in the excretion of anesthetic drugs and their metabolites. Acid–base and water metabolism are also important considerations in anesthetic admin-

istration. Surgery is contraindicated when a patient has acute nephritis, acute renal insufficiency with oliguria or anuria, or other acute renal problems, unless the surgery is a life-saving measure or is necessary to improve urinary function, as in an obstructive uropathy.

Assessment of Endocrine Function

In uncontrolled diabetes, the chief life-threatening hazard is that of hypoglycemia, which may develop during anesthesia or postoperatively. It results from inadequate intake of carbohydrates or from insulin overdosage. Other hazards that threaten but occur less rapidly are acidosis and glucosuria. In general, the surgical risk of the patient with controlled diabetes is not greater than that of the nondiabetic patient (see Chap. 40).

Assessment of Immunologic Function

An important nursing goal is to determine the presence of an allergy history, including previous allergic reactions. Particularly significant is the notation of sensitivities to certain drugs and past adverse reactions to these medications. Obtain a list of offending agents and document how the allergy was manifested. Also, ask about blood transfusion reactions in the past. Record any affirmative response. Current pharmacotherapy also is recorded. A history of bronchial asthma is reported to the anesthesiologist.

Immunosuppression is now common with steroid therapy, renal transplantation, cancer radiotherapy, and chemotherapy. The mildest symptoms or slightest temperature elevation need to be investigated. Because these patients will not tolerate breaks in technique, great care is taken in practicing meticulous asepsis.

Assessment of Effects of Aging

The goal here is to be aware that the usual norms for a healthy adult need to be modified for those at either end of the aging scale.

It is important for the nurse to remember that in the older person, reactions to injury are less pronounced and slower in appearing. The aged do not tolerate dehydration well. The possibility of long-established diabetes, anemia, obesity, hypoproteinemia, etc. must be considered. Certain drugs are dangerous because they are poorly tolerated. Morphine and the barbiturates are likely to cause confusion and disorientation, even excitement and apprehension. Some drugs have a cumulative effect. Sleeping and eating habits and the use of alcohol and laxatives, as well as the nightly "sleeping" medicine, must not be dismissed as unimportant (see below).

Assessment of Prior Drug Therapy

Attention is given to the history of drug usage by the patient. Potent medications have an effect on physiologic functions; interactions of such drugs with anesthetic agents have caused serious problems, such as arterial hypotension and circulatory collapse or depression.

The potential effects of prior drug therapy are evaluated by the anesthesiologist, who considers the length of time the patient has used the drugs, his condition, and the nature of the proposed surgery. Drugs that cause particular concern are:

Adrenal steroids—It is not advisable to discontinue corticosteroids before surgery. Because the sudden termination of therapy may cause cardiovascular collapse if steroid therapy has been used for a chronic problem over a period of time, it is usually advisable to give a "burst" of high-dose steroid immediately before and after surgery.

Diuretics—In particular, the thiazide drugs may cause excessive respiratory depression during anesthesia; this results from an electrolyte imbalance.

Phenothiazines—These drugs may increase the hypotensive action of anesthetics.

Antidepressants—In particular, monoamine oxidase (MAO) inhibitors increase the hypotensive effects of anesthetics.

Insulin—Interaction between anesthetics and insulin must be considered when a diabetic patient is undergoing surgery.

Antibiotics—"Mycin" drugs such as neomycin, kanamycin, and, less frequently, streptomycin, may present problems; when these drugs are combined with a curariform muscle relaxant, nerve transmission is interrupted and apnea owing to respiratory paralysis may result. Dripps and his colleagues call attention to the possibility of respiratory insufficiency "occurring most often in patients with peritonitis when (antibiotics) irrigation is done at wound closure—respiratory difficulty may occur in the recovery room."* For the reasons cited, it is imperative that the patient's drug history be assessed by the nurse and anesthesiologist.

Risk-Factor Summary

The optimum goal is to have as many positive factors as possible. Every attempt is made to stabilize those conditions that otherwise hinder a smooth recovery. When balance is lost in favor of negative factors, the risks increase, as do postoperative complications (see Chart 19-1).

▷ Operative Permit (Informed Consent)

Before the surgeon has the right to operate, it is necessary to obtain a voluntary and informed consent from the patient. Such written permission protects the patient against unsanctioned surgery and protects the surgeon against claims of an unauthorized operation. In the best interests of all parties concerned, sound medicolegal principles are followed.

Prior to signing the permit, the surgeon should inform the patient in clear and simple terms, by means of diagrams or models if necessary, what the surgery will entail. He should also inform the patient of possible complications, disfigurement, disability, and removal of body parts, as well as what to expect in the early and late postoperative periods. Permission should be repeated for each operation, for each procedure in which it is necessary to enter a body cavity (cystoscopy, paracentesis, etc.), and when general anesthesia is given, as for a closed reduction of a fracture.

* Dripps RD et al: Introduction to Anesthesia, 5th ed, p. 32. Philadelphia, WB Saunders, 1977.

Chart 19-1
Risks Factors for Any Surgical Procedure

Systemic Factors
  Hypovolemia
  Dehydration or electrolyte imbalance
  Nutritional deficits
  Extremes of age
  Infection and sepsis
  Toxic conditions
  Immunologic abnormalities
Pulmonary Disease
Renal Disease
Hepatic Disease
Pregnancy—because of
  Diminished maternal physiologic reserve
  Fetal susceptibility to disease
Cardiovascular Disease
  Coronary artery disease
  Cardiac failure
  Arrhythmias
  Hypertension
  Prosthetic heart valve
  Thromboembolism
  Hemorrhagic diathesis
  Cerebrovascular disease
Endocrine Dysfunction
  Diabetes mellitus
  Adrenal corticosteroid conditions
  Thyroid malfunction

The patient may sign his own permit for operation if he is of age and is mentally capable. If he is a minor or is unconscious or irresponsible, permission must be obtained from a responsible family member. If he is an emancipated minor (married or independently earning his own living), he may sign his own permit. Bear in mind that state regulations and hospital policy must be followed. In an emergency, it may be necessary for the surgeon to operate as a lifesaving measure without the patient's informed consent. However, every effort should be made to contact the patient's family. In such a situation, contact can be made by telephone or telegram.

No patient should be forced to sign an operative permit. Refusing to have an operation is a person's privilege. However, such information must be relayed to the surgeon so that other arrangements can be made; for instance, additional explanations may be offered to the patient and his family or the operation may be rescheduled at a more suitable time.

* The informed consent is placed in a prominent place on the patient's chart and accompanies the patient to the operating room.

Table 19-1
Categories of Contemplated Surgery Based on Urgency

Classification	Indication for Surgery	Examples
I. *Emergency*—Requires immediate attention	Without delay	Extensive burns Major bone fractures Fractured skull Gunshot wounds Stab wounds Bladder or intestinal obstruction Severe bleeding Serious eye injuries
II. *Urgent*—Requires prompt attention	Within 24–28 hr	Acute gallbladder infection Kidney or ureteral stones Bleeding hemorrhoids or uterine tumors Cancer
III. *Required*—Requires operation	Plan hospital admission within a few weeks or months	Eye cataracts Thyroid operations Tonsillectomy Gallbladder problems without acute inflammation Prostatic hypertrophy without bladder obstruction Spinal fusion Bone deformities
IV. *Elective*—Should be operated on	Failure to have surgery is not catastrophic	Repair of scars Simple hernia Vaginal repair Superficial cysts
V. *Optional*—The decision rests with the patient	Personal preference	Cosmetic surgery

▷ Preoperative Nursing Intervention

The twin goals of preoperative care are:

- To present the patient in the best possible physical and psychosocial condition for his operation
- To initiate every effort that will eliminate or reduce postoperative discomforts and complications

The planning, preparation, and care of the patient before an operation are guided by an understanding that he is a unique, multifaceted individual. The length of time that the patient spends in the hospital before surgery is reduced to the barest minimum, not only for reasons of economy, but also to reduce the likelihood of nosocomial hospital-acquired infections.

Surgeons and hospitals differ in the details of preparation for an operation, but the goals remain the same: to make the patient as clean as possible, externally and internally, and to cause the least possible amount of physical and mental exhaustion for the patient in the process.

The rationale for preoperative procedures is obvious. All sources of infection must be eliminated, hence the scrupulous cleanliness of the operative site. The intestines and the bladder must be empty to prevent their contents from being discharged involuntarily while the patient is under the influence of the anesthetic and to prevent them from being inadvertently incised, as sometimes occurs in an abdominal operation when these organs are distended. This is especially true of the bladder and explains why it is so important that it be emptied before a patient is sent to the operating room for a laparotomy.

Any preparation of the patient before an operation is to be carried out in the most efficient and skillful way.

- Approach the patient with an air of decision and interest in his well-being; to do so will gain his confidence—lost confidence is not easily regained.
- Determine exactly what procedures are to be performed and proceed with them in a systematic manner.
- Explain what you are about to do so that the patient is prepared for each step.
- Always work quietly, thoroughly, and neatly; bustle, confusion, and noise will only disturb and unsettle the patient.

During this period of planning and intervention, from the time of admission to the actual operation, one of the most important responsibilities of the nurse is to observe the patient very closely for any unfavorable signs. Any sneezing, sniffling, and coughing must be reported, since operating on a patient with such symptoms may lead to postoperative pulmonary complications.

Nutrition and Fluids

When the operation is scheduled for the morning, the meal on the preceding evening may be an ordinary light diet. Water may be given freely up to 4 hours before operation. In dehydrated patients, and especially in older ones, fluids by mouth often are encouraged before an operation. In addition, fluids may be administered by vein, especially in patients to whom fluids cannot be given by mouth. If the operation is scheduled to take place after noon and does not involve any part of the gastrointestinal tract, the patient may be given a soft diet for breakfast. Most often, oral intake of food or water is withheld beginning at midnight of the day of operation. The goal in withholding food before surgery is to prevent aspiration.

Aspiration occurs when food or fluid is regurgitated from the stomach and inhaled into the pulmonary system. Such inhaled material acts as a foreign substance, is irritating, and causes an inflammatory reaction, and at the same time interferes with and even intercepts adequate air exchange.

The mortality rate is high (60%–70%), and it is a serious problem. To prevent aspiration, food and fluid intake is restricted for 12 hours preoperatively. If obstruction is suspected, a nasogastric tube is positioned.

Intestinal Preparation

A warm cleansing enema may be given the evening before an operation and may be repeated if ineffectual. Unless the condition of the patient presents some contraindication, the toilet, and not the bedpan, is used in evacuating the enema.

Preoperative Skin Preparation

The goal of preoperative skin care is to render the skin as free as possible of microorganisms without causing damage to its physical and physiologic integrity.

When there is time, such as in surgery of a nonemergency nature, the patient may use a soap containing a detergent-germicide to cleanse the skin area for several days before surgery in order to reduce the number of skin organisms.

Prior to surgery, the patients should take a warm, relaxing bath or shower, using Betadine soap. Although it is preferable that this be done on the day of surgery, the time schedule may require that the shower be taken the night before. The purpose for recommending that the cleansing shower be taken as close to surgery as possible is to reduce the risk of skin contamination of the surgical wound. A shampoo the day before operation is advisable unless the condition of the patient does not make it feasible.

It is preferred that the skin at and around the operative site NOT be shaved. However, the use of a depilatory to remove skin hair is acceptable. If the hair on the skin is shaved, the skin may be injured by the razor and become a portal of entry for bacteria; this injured tissue may act as a substrate for bacterial growth. In addition, *the longer the interval between the shave and the operation, the higher the rate of postoperative wound infection.* Skin that is well

cleansed but unshaven is less often implicated in wound infections than shaved skin. Some surgeons prefer that hair be removed in and around the operative site. One approach is to use electrical clippers to remove hair to within 1 mm to 2 mm of the skin; in this way, skin is not abraded.

If hospital protocol requires that the skin be shaved, the patient is told about the shaving procedure, placed in a comfortable position, and not exposed unduly. Any adhesive or grease may be readily removed with a sponge moistened in benzene or ether, if the odor and cold temperature are not objectionable to the patient. A sharp razor is used and a thorough shave given to a wide area, including the operative site and the surrounding region, to reduce sources of contamination. Preparation of specific operative sites is illustrated in Chart 19-2.

Skin shaving may be done by a special "prep" team, by the nurse assigned to the patient, or by a member of the operating room team. Disposable "prep" trays guarantee individualized equipment.

Scratches should be avoided, and any skin eruptions should be reported because they are potential sites of infection.

Depilatory Cream. Chemical compounds (creams to remove hair) are safe for preparing the skin of the surgical patient. If there is question about the possibility of an allergic reaction, a test patch can be tried first. As an economy measure, long hairs may be cut before the cream is applied in order to reduce the amount of cream used.

The depilatory cream usually comes in a collapsible tube and is expressed on the body surface. The cream is spread in a smooth layer of about 1.25 cm (½ inch) in depth over the entire operative site. A wooden tongue blade or a gloved hand can be used to apply the cream. After the cream has been allowed to remain on the skin for 10 minutes, it is scraped off gently with the tongue blade or multiple moistened gauze sponges. When all cream and hair have been removed, the skin is then washed with soap and water and patted dry.

There are several advantages in using a depilatory cream for preoperative skin preparation. The end result is a clean, smooth, and intact skin. Scrapes, abrasions, cuts, and inadequate hair removal are eliminated. It is more comfortable for the patient, since he is less apprehensive and often finds this method relaxing. There is even the possibility of the patient's preparing himself in selected operative procedures. Depilatory creams are more effective and safer for use on uncooperative or agitated patients. This method is no more expensive than other methods. A disadvantage is that a few patients have had some transient skin reactions involving the rectal and scrotal areas.

▷ Preoperative Patient Education

The goal of preoperative teaching is to familiarize the patient with the expected postoperative outcomes, such as the following:

1. Facilitation of the recuperative period
2. Attainment of a sense of well-being with minimal fear of the unknown

3. Decreased need for analgesics
4. Absence of complications
5. Decreased time of hospitalization

The value of preoperative instruction to the patient has long been recognized. However, each patient should be taught as an individual, in terms of his anxieties, needs, and hopes. The background information of one patient is usually very different from that of the next patient. Once these differences are recognized and particular needs are assessed, a program of instruction can be planned and then implemented at the proper time. If the patient is taught essential information several days before he needs it, he may not remember what he was told. If he is instructed too close to the time of surgery, he may not be in prime learning condition because of the effect of the preanesthetic medication.

If instruction is offered at a time when the patient is most receptive and can participate in the learning process, the chances are that he will retain more of the information. In actuality, instruction is spaced over a period of time to allow the patient to assimilate information and to ask questions as they arise. Frequently, teaching sessions are combined with various preparation procedures to allow for an easy flow of information. In essence, the nurse must make a judgment about how much the patient wants and needs to know. In some instances, too much explanation can be worse than not enough.

Limiting teaching to a description of the various steps of a procedure is not as helpful as telling the patient what sensations he will experience. For example, telling the patient that preoperative medication will relax him before the operation is not as effective as informing him that the medication will make him feel light-headed and sleepy. Once he knows what to expect, he will anticipate these reactions, which in turn will cause him to attain a higher degree of relaxation than might otherwise be expected.

Deep Breathing and Coughing

One goal of the nurse caring for a preoperative patient is to promote lung ventilation and blood oxygenation following general anesthesia. This is done by demonstrating to the patient how to take a deep, slow breath (maximal sustained inspiration, MSI) and how to exhale slowly. The patient is placed in a sitting position to provide maximum lung expansion. After practicing deep breathing several times, he is instructed to breathe deeply, exhale through his mouth, take a short breath, and cough from deep in the lungs (Chart 19-3, A and B). If there is to be a thoracic or abdominal incision, the nurse can demonstrate how the incision line can be splinted so that pressure is minimized and pain is controlled. For an abdominal or chest incision, the patient can put the palms of his hands together, interlacing his fingers snugly. Placing the hands across the incisional site acts as an effective splint when he coughs. Of course he needs to know that medications will be given to control pain. The goal in promoting coughing is to mobilize secretions so that they can be removed. When a deep breath is taken before coughing, the cough reflex is stimulated. If coughing is not encouraged, hypostatic pneumonia and other lung complications may occur.

Turning and Active Body Movement

The goals of promoting deliberate body movement postoperatively are to have the patient improve his circulation, to prevent venous stasis, and to contribute to optimal respiratory exchange.

The patient is shown how to turn from side to side and how to assume Sims' lateral position. This position will be used postoperatively (even before he is conscious) and assumed every second hour.

Exercises of the extremities include extension and flexion of the knee and hip joints (similar to bicycle riding while lying on the side). The foot is rotated as though tracing the largest possible circle with the great toe (Chart 19-3, C and D). The elbow and shoulder are also put through the range of motion. At first the patient will be assisted and reminded to do these exercises, but later he is encouraged to do them himself.

The nurse is reminded to use proper body mechanics and to instruct the patient to do the same. When he is placed in any position, the body is to be maintained in proper alignment. Muscle tone is maintained so that ambulation will be made easier.

Pain Control and Medications

The patient is told that he will receive a preanesthetic medication to help him relax and perhaps feel sleepy. He is also informed that it may make him thirsty. Postoperatively, he can expect medications to keep him comfortable but not to prevent him from regaining activity and maintaining an adequate air exchange.

Prophylactic antibiotics may be prescribed in specific instances. Frequently, the cephalosporins are chosen because these agents have a low toxicity and wide spectrum of action.

Other Information

The patient feels more at ease when he knows at what point postoperatively he can expect a visit from his family or friends. It helps him to know that his family will be kept informed regarding the acute phases of his surgical experience. He also appreciates knowing that a spiritual adviser of his preference will be available if he so desires.

If the patient knows beforehand that he will be on assisted breathing and that drainage tubes will be in place along with any special equipment required, he is more likely to accept these accoutrements postoperatively without too much concern.

▷ Immediate Preoperative Preparation

The patient is brought to the operating room about 30 to 60 minutes before the anesthesia is to be started. Prior to this the nurse clothes the patient in the regulation short gown, leaving it untied and open in the back. In the case of a female patient, long hair is plaited in two braids, any hairpins are removed, and the head and the hair are entirely covered with a disposable paper cap. The mouth must be

(Text continues on page 361)

Chart 19-2
Preoperative Skin Preparation

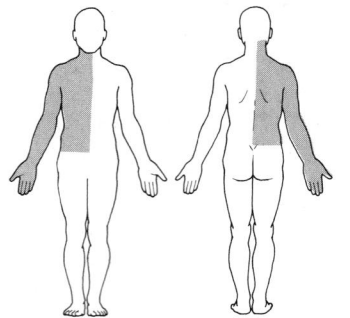

Shoulder prep. Shave fingertips to hairline, midline chest to midline spine on operative side and to iliac crest, including axilla.

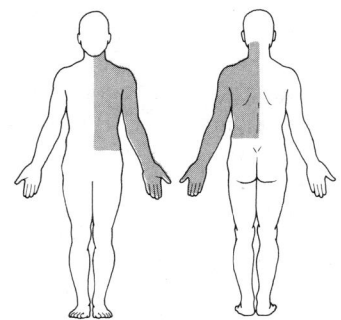

Upper arm prep. Shave fingertips to neckline (hairline), on operative side from midline chest to midline spine on operative side from axilla to iliac crest. Trim and clean fingernails. Use brush on hand and nails.

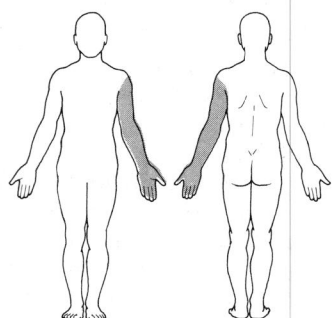

Hand prep. Shave fingertips to shoulder. Trim and clean fingernails. Use brush on hand and nails.

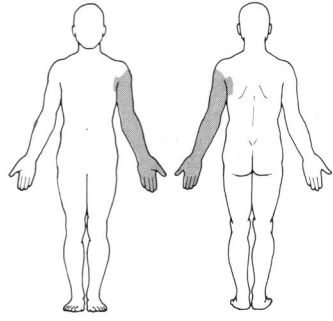

Forearm and elbow prep. Shave from fingernails to shoulder including axilla. Trim and clean fingernails. Use brush on hand and nails.

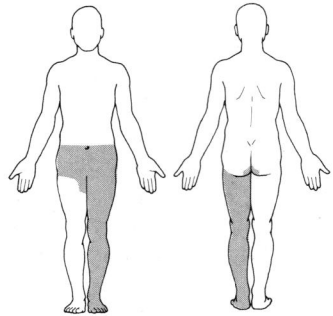

Saphenous vein ligation prep. Shave from umbilicus to toes of affected leg, or both legs. Include pubis and perineal area. Prep entire leg posteriorly.

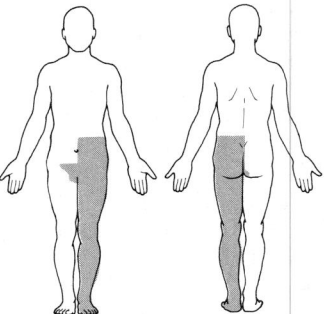

Thigh prep. Shave from toes to 3 inches above the umbilicus, midline front and back. Complete pubic shave. Clean and trim toenails. Use brush on foot and nails.

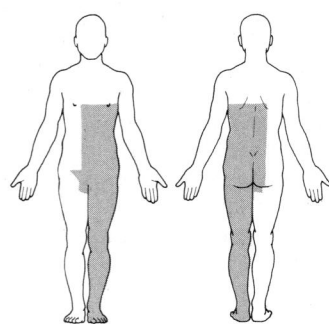

Hip prep. Shave toes to nipple line and at least 3 inches beyond midline back and front. Complete pubic shave. Clean and trim toenails. Use brush on foot and nails. Hip fractures—all preps done in the operating room.

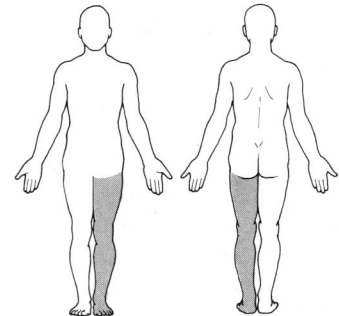

Knee and lower leg prep. Shave entire leg, toes to groin. Clean and trim toenails. Use brush on foot and nails.

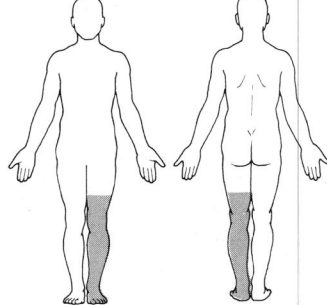

Ankle and foot prep. Shave entire leg, toes to 3 inches above the knee. Clean and trim toenails. Use brush on foot and nails.

(From Committee on Control of Surgical Infections of the Committee on Pre- and Postoperative Care, American College of Surgeons: Manual on Control of Infection in Surgical Patients, Philadelphia, JB Lippincott, 1977).

(continued)

Chart 19-2
Preoperative Skin Preparation (continued)

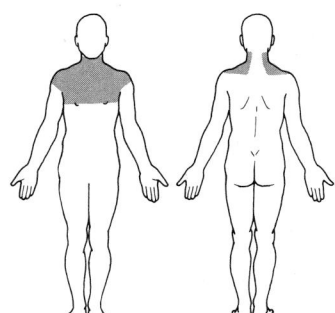

Thyroid prep. Shave from chin line to nipples, including axillary region. Extend to back of neck and upper shoulder as sketched.

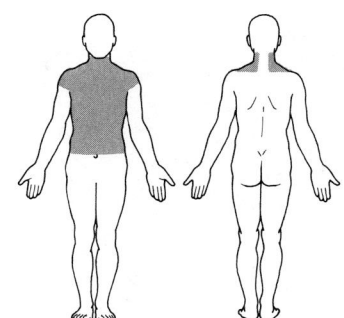

Parathyroid prep (as for sternal splitting). Shave from chin line to umbilicus, shoulder to shoulder in the front. Extend to back of neck and upper shoulder in back as shown. Prep laterally for chest tubes if so prescribed.

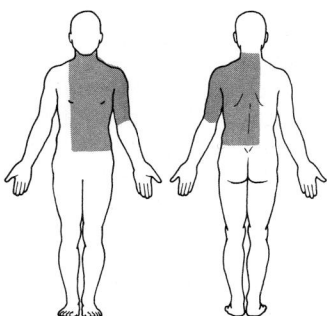

Thoracotomy prep. Shave from chin line to iliac crest, from nipple on unaffected side to at least 2 inches beyond the midline in back. Include axilla and entire arm to elbow.

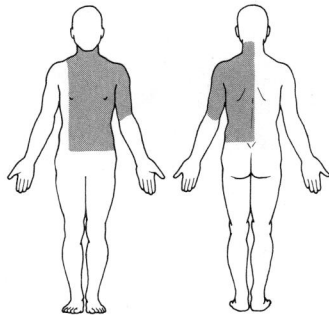

Mastectomy prep. Shave from upper neck to iliac crest, from nipple line on unaffected side to midline of back (affected side). Prep axilla and entire arm to elbow on affected side.

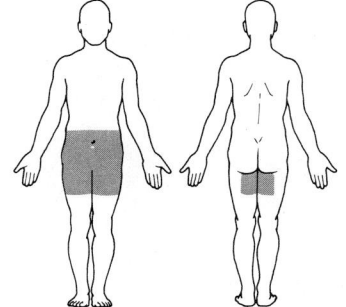

Lower abdominal prep (as for hernia, femoral vein ligation, femoral embolectomy). Shave from 2 inches above the umbilicus to mid-thigh, including the pubic area. Femoral ligation—shave to midline of thigh posteriorly. Hernia and embolectomy—shave to costal margin and down to knee as prescribed.

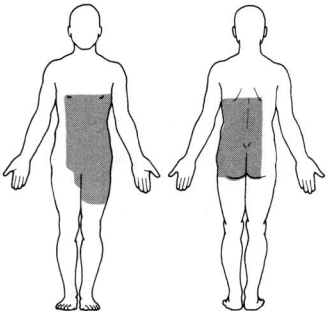

Flank prep (as for renal procedures, adrenalectomy, sympathectomy). Shave from nipple line to pubis and 3 inches beyond the midline in back. Shave pubic area. Shave upper thigh on the affected side.

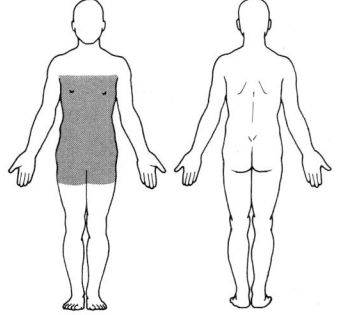

Abdominal prep. Shave from 3 inches above the nipple line to upper thighs, including pubis.

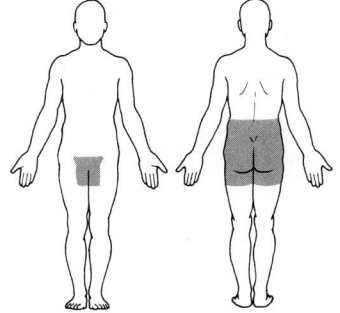

Perineal prep (as for hemorrhoidectomy, fistula-in-ano). Shave pubis, perineum, and perianal area. Shave from the waist in back to at least 3 inches below the groin.

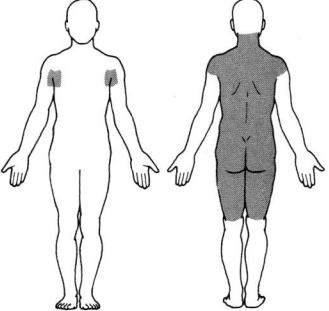

Spine prep. Shave entire back, including shoulders and neck, to hairline and down to knees and to both sides, including axillae.

Chart 19-3
Preoperative Patient Instruction

A. DIAPHRAGMATIC BREATHING

Diaphragmatic breathing refers to a flattening of the dome of the diaphragm during inspiration with resulting enlargement of the upper abdomen as air rushes in. During expiration, the abdominal muscles contract.

1. Practice in the same position you would assume in bed following surgery: a semi-Fowler's position, propped in bed with the back and shoulders well supported with pillows.
2. With the hands in a loose-fist position, allow the hands to rest lightly on the front of the lower ribs—fingernails against lower chest to feel the movement (*A*).
3. Breathe out gently and fully as the ribs sink down and inward toward midline.
4. Then take a deep breath through your nose and mouth, letting the abdomen rise as the lungs fill with air.
5. Hold this breath for a count of five.
6. Exhale and let out *all* the air through the nose and mouth.
7. Repeat 15 times with a short rest after each group of five.
8. Practice this twice a day preoperatively.

B. COUGHING

1. Lean forward slightly from a sitting position in bed, interlace the fingers together, and place the hands across the incisional site to act as a splint when coughing (*B*).
2. Breathe with the diaphragm as described in *A*.
3. With the mouth slightly open, breathe in fully.
4. "Hack" out sharply for three short breaths.
5. Then, keeping the mouth open, take in a quick deep breath and immediately give a strong cough once or twice. This will help clear secretions from the chest. It may cause some discomfort but will not harm incision.

C. LEG EXERCISES

1. Lie in a semi-Fowler's position and perform the following simple exercises to improve circulation.
2. Bend the knee and raise the foot—hold it a few seconds, then extend the leg and lower it to the bed (*C*).
3. Do this about five times with one leg, then repeat with the other leg.
4. Then trace circles with the feet by bending them down, in toward each other, up, and then out (*D*).
5. Repeat these five times.

D. TURNING TO THE SIDE

1. Turn on your side with the uppermost leg flexed most and supported on a pillow.
2. Grasp the side rail as an aid to maneuver to the side.
3. Practice diaphragmatic breathing and coughing while on your side.

E. GETTING OUT OF BED

1. Turn on your side.
2. Push yourself up with one hand as you swing your legs out of bed.

F. USING THE URINAL (FOR MALE PATIENT)

When in bed for a period of time, have the nurse explain the method for using the urinal in bed.

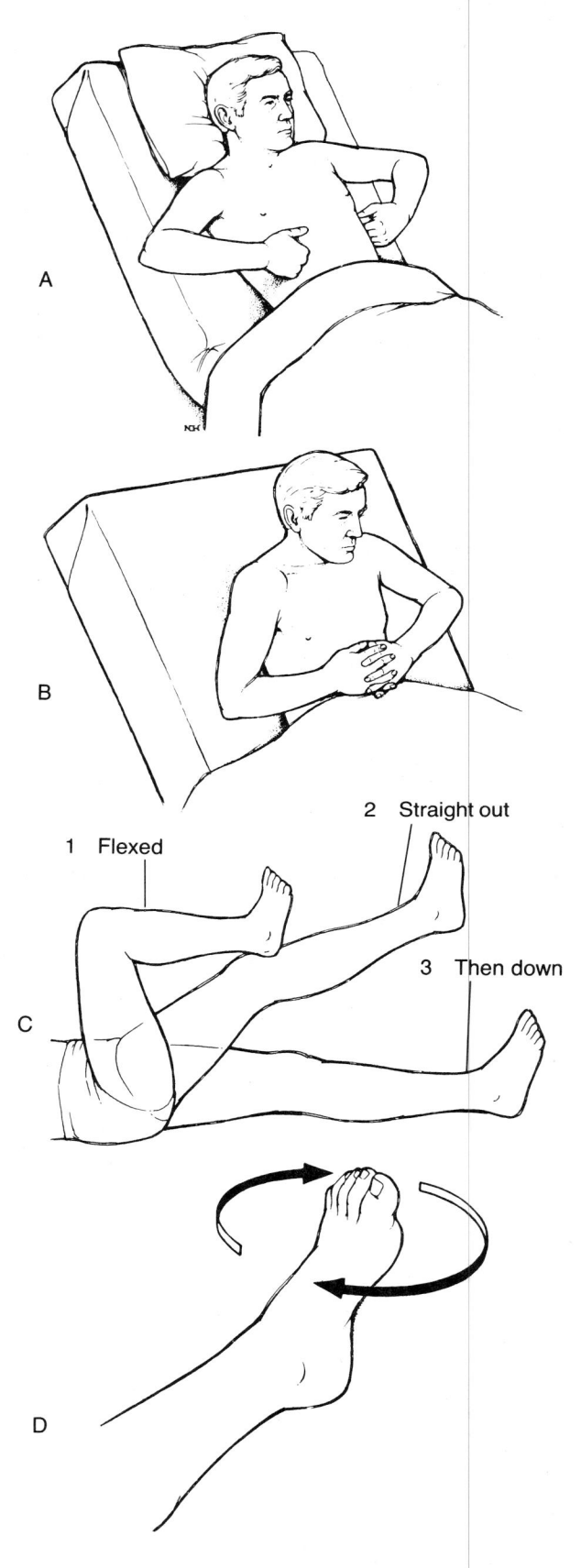

A

B

1 Flexed 2 Straight out

3 Then down

C

D

inspected and all dentures or plates, chewing gum, etc. removed. If these items were left in the mouth, they could easily fall to the back of the throat during induction of anesthesia and cause respiratory obstruction.

Jewelry is not to be worn to the operating room; even wedding rings should be taken off. If a patient has any real objection to the removal of a ring, a narrow tape may be tied to the ring and then fastened securely around the patient's wrist. All articles of value, including dentures and prosthetic devices are labeled clearly with the patient's name and stored in a safe place according to local hospital policy.

All patients (except those with urologic problems) should void immediately before being sent to the operating room. The bladder must be empty, but catheterization should not be resorted to, except in an emergency or when it is desirable to have an indwelling catheter in place to ensure an empty bladder. In this instance, such a catheter would be connected to a closed drainage system. The urine voided is measured, and the amount and the time of voiding are recorded on the preoperative check slip.

For patients with vascular problems that could lead to deep vein thrombosis, elastic stockings may be applied and the legs elevated. However, controversy has developed over these practices, some studies supporting them and others indicating no beneficial effects.*

Preanesthetic Medication—Pharmacokinetics

The main purpose of preanesthetic medication is to reduce the patient's anxiety so that induction and maintenance of anesthesia will be smooth. Atropine is given to decrease secretions and vagally mediated reflex bradycardia. As with other management modalities, medication is prescribed on an individual basis to meet the needs of the particular patient.

Barbiturates. For sedation, *barbiturates* are commonly used, mainly pentobarbital (Nembutal) and secobarbital (Seconal Sodium). However, it is worth noting that studies have shown that the reassuring visit of the anesthesiologist and operating room nurse prior to the operation has a more calming effect than the barbiturates. Nonetheless, the night before surgery, a hypnotic is usually given to allay insomnia, which is brought about by new and different surroundings, apprehension over pending surgery, and disturbing hospital sounds.

Opiates. Drugs such as morphine and meperidine (Demerol) may be prescribed before an operation to reduce the amount of general anesthetic required. These drugs can also be used to produce analgesia in patients who have pain before the operation. At the same time it is important to realize that analgesic doses may depress respiration and the cough reflex and present an increased risk of respiratory acidosis and aspiration pneumonitis. Full doses may cause hypotension, nausea, vomiting, constipation, and abdominal distention.

Anticholinergics. Drugs of this type may be prescribed to reduce respiratory tract secretions and to prevent or treat

severe reflex slowing of the heart during anesthesia. It is given also to counteract secretions that are anticipated with anesthetic induction and intubation. Atropine is the most popular of the medications prescribed. This drug is not given to patients with glaucoma, thyrotoxicosis, or some forms of tachycardia.

Because the belladonna alkaloids (atropine and scopolamine) have varying effects on pulse rate, as well as other shortcomings, a quaternary ammonium compound, glycopyrrolate (Robinul), is an anticholinergic drug that is gaining in popularity because it is twice as potent as an antisialogogue (reducing secretions) and acts three times as long.

Timing of Administration of Drugs. Because preanesthetic medications should be given from 45 to 75 minutes before anesthesia is begun, it is most important that the nurse give this medication precisely at the prescribed time; otherwise, its effect will have worn off or—it will not have begun to act when anesthesia is started.

After the preanesthetic medication is given, the patient is kept in bed because he will begin to feel light-headed and drowsy. (If the patient is unattended, the side rails are placed in position.) If he receives atropine or Robinul, he may be told it will make his mouth dry. During this time, the nurse observes the patient for any untoward reaction to the medications. His environment is kept quiet to assist in relaxing him.

Very frequently, operations are delayed or schedules changed, and it becomes impossible to request that a medication be given at a specific time. In these situations the preoperative medication is prescribed "on call from operating room." Although this is far from ideal and should be avoided whenever possible, the nurse can help by having the medication ready to give and by administering it as soon as the patient is called for. It usually takes 15 to 20 minutes to get a patient ready for the operating room. If the nurse gives the medication before attending to the other details of preparing the patient, he will have at least partial benefit from the preoperative medication and will have a smoother and more pleasant anesthetic and operative course.

Preoperative Record

Chart 19-4 presents a preoperative check list . The completed chart accompanies the patient to the operating room. The informed consent is also attached, as are all laboratory reports and nurses' records. Any unusual last-minute observations that may have a bearing on the anesthesia or surgery are to be placed to the front of the chart in a prominent place.

Transportation to the Presurgical Suite

The patient is transferred to the holding area or presurgical suite in bed or on a previously prepared stretcher. The stretcher should be as comfortable as possible, with a sufficient number of blankets to ensure against chilling from drafty corridors. A small pillow at the head usually is acceptable. The top covers of the stretcher should be long enough to tuck in at both the patient's feet and shoulders. Preferably, the nurse who has cared for the patient up to this time should accompany him to the operating room. An attendant always remains with the patient in the holding

* Rosengarten DS et al: The failure of compression stockings (Turbigrip) to prevent deep venous thrombosis after operation. Br J Surg Apr; 57:296–299.

Chart 19-4
Preoperative Check List*

(Check prior to medicating patient)

1. Surgery consent(s) signed? _____

   a. Name plate impression on consent sheets? _____

2. Special permits signed? _____

   a. Sterilization Consent _____

3. Identa-bands-3 on chart for baby/for Caesarean Sections? _____

4. History and physical reports on chart? _____

5. Laboratory reports on chart: Max 5 days past

   CBC _____ Urinalysis _____

6. Preoperative medication given and charted? _____

7. Hairnets, clips, ornaments, makeup, and jewelry removed? _____
   (wedding rings may be taped on)

8. Contact lens(es) removed? _____

9. Dentures removed? _____

10. List other prostheses removed: _____

11. Underclothing and/or sanitary belt removed? _____

12. Morning TPR charted? _____

13. Identa-band legible and in proper place? _____

14. Patient identification plate on chart? _____

15. Voided? _____ Time: _____

16. Instruct family where to wait for information _____

17. Pre-op teaching _____

18. Valuables secured? _____

19. Any special problems or precautions? _____
   (deafness, language barrier, allergies)

20. Special Orders: _____

Date _____ Time _____

   Signature of nurse releasing patient: _____

   * Memorial Hospital Medical Center, Long Beach, California

---

area until relieved by one of the anesthesiologists. The chart is given to the anesthesiologist or an operating room nurse; it never is left with the patient.

It is important that someone be with the preoperative patient at all times. Even though he has had preoperative medication, appears to be dozing, and seems to be secure on the stretcher with a strap in place, he should not be left alone. It is desirable to have the patient brought directly to a preoperative holding room or induction room, where he is greeted by name and made to feel that he is in safe hands.

The area must be quiet if the preoperative medication is to have maximal effect. The patient should not hear undesirable sounds or conversations that might be misinterpreted or exaggerated.

It is assumed that preoperative preparation has covered every contingency before the patient comes to the operating room. However, as the patient waits with his eyes closed, he is often reviewing some personal thoughts; a question or concern about a particular thing may occur to him and may assume an exaggerated importance. Someone should be available to answer or attempt to find the answer to his question.

Reassurance is given not only verbally but also by facial expression, manner, and a touch or warm grasp of the hand. It is important for the patient to have the security of seeing a familiar face—the nurse who helped to prepare him before he was sent to the operating floor, or the anesthesiologist who visited with him the day before and discussed anesthetic management.

▷ Attending to the Patient's Family

Most hospitals have a special waiting room where the family can wait while the patient is having surgery. This room may be equipped with comfortable chairs, television, telephones, and facilities for light refreshment. Volunteers may remain with the family, serve them coffee, boost their morale, and even keep them informed of the patient's progress. After surgery, the surgeon may meet the family here, join them for coffee, and report his findings.

The family never should judge the seriousness of an operation by the length of time the patient is in the operating room. He may be in surgery much longer than the actual operating time for several reasons:

1. It is customary to send for the patient some time in advance of the actual operating time.
2. Anesthesiologists often make additional preparations that may take from ½ to 1 hour.
3. Occasionally, the surgeon takes longer than he expected with the preceding case, hence delaying the time of beginning the next operation.
4. After surgery, the patient is taken to the recovery room to ensure satisfactory emergence from the anesthetic.

Those waiting to see the patient after the operation should be forewarned that the patient may be returned to his room with a variety of equipment in place, including blood transfusion lines, suction bottles, nasal tube, airway and oxygen lines, tracheostomy tube, monitoring equipment, etc. Family members need to know how they can support the patient preoperatively and in the recovery room. If the prognosis for the patient is more negative than positive, it is not within the prerogative of the nurse to relay this information to the family, even when the odds appear in the patient's favor.

▷ Bibliography

See Bibliography at end of Chapter 21.

20

Intraoperative Nursing Management

▷ The Patient Undergoing Anesthesia

The Anesthesiologist and the Patient

The surgical patient usually is interested in and concerned about the anesthesia that he is to receive. He has heard friends or relatives discuss the subject on the basis of personal experience or hearsay, and not infrequently has formed opinions as to the merits or demerits of various methods in use. Therefore, it is helpful for the anesthesiologist to visit the patient in his room before the operation and to point out that the purpose of the visit is to allay any fears that may exist in the patient's mind. Choice of anesthetic agent is discussed, and the patient has an opportunity to disclose idiosyncrasies as well as types of medications he is currently taking that may affect the choice of an agent (see p. 353).

During this essential visit, the anesthesiologist determines the condition of the patient's lungs and inquires about any pre-existing pulmonary infections and the extent to which the patient smokes. The patient's general physical condition must also be ascertained because this may affect the management of anesthesia (Table 20-1).

The preoperative visit from the anesthesiologist builds up confidence and enables the patient to recognize a familiar face as he is being wheeled into the operating suite. Uncertainty and anxiety are relieved to a certain degree, and a smoother course can be anticipated.

In the anesthetizing room the patient is transferred to the operating table and a last-minute check of his condition is made; blood pressure and pulse and respiratory rates in particular are noted. Induction of the anesthetic is usually done in the operating room.

An anesthesiologist is specifically trained in the art and the science of anesthesiology. After consulting with the surgeon, he usually selects the anesthesia and deals with any technical problems relating to the administration of the anesthetic agent and supervision of the patient's condition during the operation. Such "sharing" of responsibility obviously benefits the patient.

Table 20-1
Classification of Physical Status for Anesthesia Prior to Surgery

Classification	Description	Example
I. Good	No organic disease, no systemic disturbance	Uncomplicated hernias, fractures
II. Fair	Mild to moderate systemic disturbance	Mild cardiac (I and II), mild diabetes
III. Poor	Severe systemic disturbance	Poorly controlled diabetes, pulmonary complications, moderate cardiac (III)
IV. Serious	Systemic disease threatening life	Severe renal disease, severe cardiac disease (IV), decompensation
V. Moribund	Little chance of survival but submitting to operation in desperation	Massive pulmonary embolus, ruptured abdominal aneurysm with profound shock
E. Emergency	Any of the above when surgery is done in an emergency situation	Hitherto uncomplicated hernia that is now strangulated and associated with nausea and vomiting; designation 1(E)
		If classification is III and, an emergency, the designation is 3(E).

(From American Society of Anesthesiology, Inc.: Codes for the Collection and Tabulation of Data Relating to Anesthesia, Inhalation Therapy and Therapeutic Diagnostic Blocks.)

During the course of surgery, the anesthesiologist monitors the patient's blood pressure, pulse, and respirations as well as the electrocardiogram, tidal volume, blood gas levels, blood pH, alveolar gas concentrations, and body temperature. Monitoring by electroencephalograph may be required in some instances. Should the body's physiologic mechanisms become incapable of maintaining these functions within safe limits, the anesthesiologist would then resort to the use of devices that ventilate the patient's lungs and circulate and aerate his blood.

Types of Anesthesia

Anesthesia produces a state of narcosis, analgesia, relaxation, and reflex loss. Inhalation anesthesia is the most popular because of its controllability. The intake and elimination of the agent is in large measure affected by pulmonary ventilation. Greater depth or plane of anesthesia requires greater concentration of the agent and vice versa.

Anesthetics are divided into two classes according to whether they suspend sensation in (1) the whole body (general anesthesia) or in (2) parts of the body (local, regional, epidural, or spinal anesthesia).

General anesthesia can be obtained by inhalation or by intravenous or rectal techniques.

Liquid anesthetics produce anesthesia when their vapors are inhaled. Included in this group are ethyl ether, halothane, trichloroethylene, and enflurane. All are given with oxygen and usually with nitrous oxide as well (Table 20-2).

Gas anesthetics are administered by inhalation, always in combination with oxygen. This group of anesthetics includes nitrous oxide and cyclopropane (Table 20-3).

The substances, when inhaled, enter the blood through the pulmonary capillaries and, when in sufficient concentration, act on the cerebral centers in such a manner as to produce loss of consciousness and of sensation. When ad-ministration of the anesthetic is discontinued, the vapor or gas is eliminated by way of the lungs.

Physiologic and Physical Factors

General anesthetics produce anesthesia because they are delivered to the brain at high partial pressure. Relatively large amounts of anesthetic must be given during induction and the early maintenance phases because the anesthetic is recirculated and deposited in body tissues. As these depots become saturated, smaller amounts of the anesthetic agent are required to maintain anesthesia, since equilibrium or near equilibrium has been achieved between brain, blood, and other tissues. It is apparent that anything that diminishes peripheral blood flow, such as vasoconstriction or a condition of shock, may cause only small amounts of anesthetic to be required. Conversely, when peripheral blood flow is unusually high, as in the muscularly active or apprehensive patient, the brain receives a smaller quantity of anesthetic, with the result that induction is slower, and larger than usual quantities of anesthetic are required.

Methods of Administration. Liquid anesthetics may be given by mixing the vapors with oxygen or nitrous oxide-oxygen and then having the patient inhale the mixture. The vapor is conducted to the patient by a tube and a mask.

The endotracheal technique for administering anesthetics consists of introducing a soft rubber or plastic tube into the trachea, either by exposing the larynx with a laryngoscope or by passing the tube "blindly." It may be inserted through either nose or mouth (Fig. 20-1).

Stages of Inhalation Anesthesia

Anesthesia generally is described as consisting of four stages, each of which presents a definite group of signs and symptoms. Generally, these stages are seen best when ether is the anesthetic used. When narcotics and neuromuscular blockers (relaxants) are given, several of these stages are absent.

Table 20-2
Volatile Liquids as Agents of General Anesthesia

Agent	Administration	Advantages	Disadvantages	Implications
1. Diethyl ether	Open-drop; inhalation	Excellent relaxant Wide margin of safety Inexpensive Relatively nontoxic Used for all types of surgery	Explosive Slow induction: 10 minutes Long recovery; not eliminated for approximately 8 hours Irritating to skin, eyes May cause metabolic acidosis Causes nausea and vomiting Flammable	Protect eyes by keeping them closed. Expect nausea and vomiting—turn head to side to prevent aspiration of vomitus. Practice safeguards in view of flammability.
2. Halothane (Fluothane)	Inhalation; special vaporizer	Not explosive or flammable Induction rapid and smooth Useful in almost every type of surgery Low incidence of postoperative nausea and vomiting	Requires skillful administration to prevent overdosage May cause liver damage May produce hypotension Requires special vaporizer for administration	In addition to observing pulse and respiration postoperatively, it is important that blood pressure be determined frequently.
3. Methoxyflurane (Penthrane)	Inhalation; special vaporizer	Nonflammable Seldom causes postoperative nausea and vomiting Analgesic action continues several hours after surgery Excellent muscle relaxation	Requires skillful administration Renal damage may occur Unpleasant odor	Prolonged postoperative depressant action calls for careful observation by recovery room personnel.
4. Enflurane (Ethrane)	Inhalation	Rapid induction and recovery Potent analgesic Nonflammable and nonexplosive	Respiratory depression may develop rapidly along with EEG abnormalities Not compatible with epinephrine	Observe for possible respiratory depression. Administration with epinephrine may cause ventricular fibrillation.
5. Isoflurane (Forane)	Inhalation	Rapid induction and recovery Muscle relaxants are markedly potentiated	This is a profound respiratory depressant.	Respiration must be monitored closely and supported when necessary.

Table 20-3
Gases as Agents of General Anesthesia

Agent	Administration	Advantages	Disadvantages	Implications
1. Nitrous oxide (N_2O)	Inhalation (semi-closed method)	Induction and recovery rapid Nonflammable Useful with oxygen for short procedures Useful with other agents for all types of surgery	Poor relaxant Weak anesthetic May produce hypoxia	Most useful in conjunction with other agents. Observe precautions with "other agents."
2. Cyclopropane (C_3H_6)	Inhalation (closed method)	Good relaxant Useful in all types of surgery Rapid induction and emergence Wide margin of safety Pleasant	Explosive Powerful depressant; therefore should be administered skillfully Frequently produces disturbances in heart rhythm May cause bronchospasm and acidosis	Employ precautions against explosions. Because cyclopropane may be followed by hypotension, it is important to observe blood pressure postoperatively.

Intranasal intubation

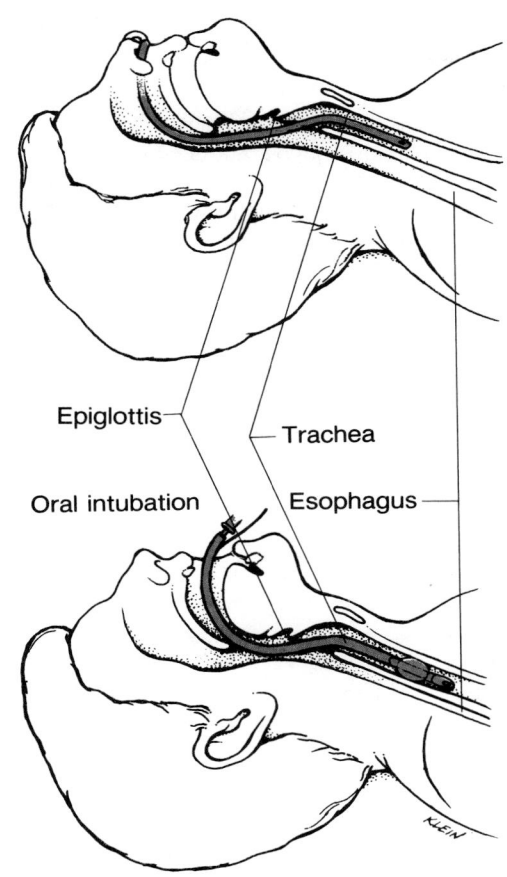

Epiglottis

Trachea

Oral intubation   Esophagus

Figure 20-1. Endotracheal anesthesia. (*Top*) Nasal endotracheal catheter in proper position. (*Bottom*) Oral endotracheal intubation; tube in position with cuff inflated. For both methods, the neck is hyperextended to permit the airway to be open.

Stage I: Beginning Anesthesia. As the patient breathes in the anesthetic mixture, a feeling of warmth steals over his body, dizziness is experienced, and a feeling of detachment develops. He experiences a ringing, roaring, or buzzing in his ears and, though still conscious, is aware that he is unable to move his extremities easily. During this stage, noises are exaggerated; even low voices or minor sounds appear distressingly loud and unreal. For this reason, unnecessary noise or motion must be prevented when anesthesia is started.

Stage II: Excitement. This stage—characterized variously by struggling, shouting, talking, singing, laughing, or even crying—frequently may be avoided by judicious suggestion before anesthesia is begun and by the smooth and rapid administration of the anesthetic. The pupils become dilated but contract if exposed to light; the pulse rate is rapid and respiration irregular.

Because of the uncontrolled movements of the patient during this stage, the anesthesiologist always should be at-

tended by someone ready to help restrain the patient. A strap is in place across the thighs of each patient, and the hands are fixed to an intravenous armboard. Also, the patient lies on a conduction strap for the purpose of avoiding burns during use of diathermy, ECG leads, etc. The patient should not be touched except for purposes of restraint, and under no circumstances should there be palpation of the operative site.

Stage III: Surgical Anesthesia. Surgical anesthesia is reached by continued administration of the vapor or gas. The patient is unconscious, lying quietly on the table. The pupils are small but retain contractile power on exposure to light. Respiration is regular, pulse rate is about normal and of good volume, and the skin is pink or slightly flushed. By proper administration of the anesthetic, this stage may be maintained for hours in one of several planes (1, 2, 3, 4), depending upon the depth of anesthesia needed.

Stage IV: Danger. This stage is reached when too much anesthesia has been given. Respiration becomes shallow, the pulse weak and thready; the pupils become widely dilated and no longer contract when exposed to light. Cyanosis develops and, unless prompt action is taken, death follows rapidly. If this stage should develop. the anesthetic is discontinued immediately and artificial respiration is given. Stimulants, although rarely used, may be administered for circulation if an overdosage of anesthetic has been given. Narcotic antagonists can be used if these agents are at fault.

During smooth administration of an anesthesic, there is, of course, no sharp division between the various stages. The patient passes gradually from one stage to another, and it is only by close observation of the signs exhibited by the patient that an anesthesiologist can control the situation. The condition of the pupils, the blood pressure, and the respiratory and cardiac rates are probably the most reliable guides to the patient's condition.

Other Physiologic Changes

The administration of an anesthetic is attended by other physiologic activities that have not been mentioned. Some anesthetics, especially ether, produce hypersecretion of mucus and saliva. This may be minimized by the preoperative administration of atropine. Vomiting or regurgitation occurs frequently, especially when the patient comes to the operating room with a full stomach. If gagging occurs, the patient's head is turned to the side, the head of the table is lowered, and a basin is provided to collect the vomitus. Suction apparatus should always be available.

During anesthesia, the patient's temperature may fall, and therefore every precaution must be taken against chilling. Warm, cotton blankets should be available. Glucose metabolism is much reduced, and as a result, acidosis may develop.

In addition to the dangers of the anesthetic itself, the anesthesiologist must guard against asphyxia. This may be caused by foreign bodies in the mouth, spasm of the vocal cords, swallowing of the tongue, or aspiration of vomitus, saliva, or blood. These complications are avoided by the use of an endotracheal tube with an inflated cuff.

Neuromuscular Blockers (Muscle Relaxants)

Neuromuscular blockers are agents that block transmission of nerve impulses at the neuromuscular junction of skeletal muscles. Goals in using muscle relaxants are to relax muscles in abdominal and thoracic surgery, relax eye muscles in certain kinds of eye surgery, facilitate endotracheal intubation, treat laryngospasm, and assist in mechanical ventilation.

Purified curare was the first widely used muscle relaxant; tubocurarine was isolated as the active principle. After that, succinylcholine was introduced because it acts more rapidly than curare. Several other agents have since been added (Table 20-4). The ideal muscle relaxant should:

1. Be nondepolarizing with an onset time and duration of action similar to that of succinylcholine but without its problems

2. Have its duration of action between succinylcholine and pancuronium
3. Lack cumulative and cardiovascular effects
4. Be metabolized and not dependent upon the kidney for its elimination

Intravenous Barbiturate Anesthesia

General anesthesia also can be produced by the intravenous injection of various substances, such as thiopental (Table 20-5). A short-acting barbiturate, thiopental sodium (Pentothal) is the most commonly used anesthetic for this purpose. This substance leads to unconsciousness within 30 seconds.

Advantages.   The onset of anesthesia is pleasant; there is none of the buzzing, roaring, or dizziness known to follow administration of an inhalation anesthetic. For this reason, induction of anesthesia with an intravenous agent is pre-

Table 20-4
Muscle Relaxants

Muscle Relaxant	Action	Advantages	Disadvantages.	Uses and Comments
Tubocurarine chloride (d-Tubocurarine chloride; Curare)	Peaks at 30–60 min	50%–70% excreted unchanged in 3–6 hr	Histaminelike reaction Hypotension Increased airway resistance Skin erythema	Contraindicated with history of allergy, asthma
Gallamine (Flaxedil)	1/5 as potent as curare Lasts 25% shorter than curare Blocks vagal ganglia in heart	All excreted unchanged	Tachycardia	Used well with cyclopropane or halothane
Pancuronium bromide (Pavulon)	Similar to curare but 5 times more potent Duration, 60–85 min	Safe; stable Good muscle relaxant Reversible by neostigmine and atropine		Excellent for situations requiring complete relaxation Avoid with myasthenia gravis or renal disease Avoid with patients sensitive to bromide

Depolarizing Neuromuscular Blocking Agents

These mimic the action of acetylcholine at the neuromuscular junction.
Acetylcholine is discharged almost immediately upon release → repolarization of muscle takes place. When depolarizing neuromuscular blocking agents are used, skeletal muscle depolarizes.

Succinylcholine (Anectine; Sucostrin)	Onset is rapid: 3–5 min	Ideal for endotracheal intubation, fracture reduction; treatment of laryngospasm	Contraindicated for patients with low pseudocholinesterase On second IV injection, bradycardia and various arrhythmias May cause fasciculations of the muscles—pain	Treat laryngospasm Treat toxic reaction to local anesthetic drugs Treat status asthmaticus
Decamethonium bromide (Syncurine)	Onset: 30–40 sec Duration: 15–20 min	Excreted unchanged by kidney	Some fasciculation of muscle: jaw masseter muscles; posterior calf muscles Difficult to reverse its action	Produces depolarization of end-plate region

Table 20-5
Intravenous Anesthetic Agents

Agent	Administration	Advantages	Disadvantages	Implications
Barbiturates				
Thiopental sodium (Pentothal)	Intravenous injection (or rectal)	Rapid induction Nonexplosive Requires little equipment Low incidence of postoperative nausea and vomiting	Powerful depressant of breathing Poor relaxant Sometimes produces coughing, sneezing, and laryngospasm Not useful for children because of small veins	Requires intelligent and close observation because of potency and rapidity of drug action.
Narcotics				
Meperidine hydrochloride (Demerol)	Intravenously Subcutaneously Intramuscularly	Prompt onset Because of spasmolytic effect, it is drug of choice for surgery of bile duct, distal colon, and rectum; easily detoxified and excreted	May slow rate of respirations Adverse reactions: dizziness, nausea, and vomiting	In some patients, histamine may be released; treatment is diphenhydramine (Benadryl).
Morphine (high doses)	Intravenously	Not a myocardial depressant	Can depress arterial blood pressure by decreasing systemic vascular resistance Does not provide good amnesia Does not give adequate muscular relaxation	Orthostatic hypotension may occur after morphine.

NOTE: *Neuroleptoanalgesia* refers to a combination of short-acting synthetic narcotic agent (fentanyl) and a butyrophenone (droperidol). Patient becomes very drowsy; responds to voice command, although analgesia is profound.
Of significance: The combination produces peripheral vasodilation followed by a decrease in arterial blood pressure. If administered rapidly, it may cause skeletal muscular rigidity and possibly respiratory impairment.

Agent	Administration	Advantages	Disadvantages	Implications
Fentanyl (Sublimaze; related chemically to meperidine)	Intravenously	75–100 times more potent than morphine and about 25% of duration of morphine (IV) Little effect on cardiovascular system	In very high dosage, an alpha-adrenergic blocking effect	Short duration of action is due to its more rapid redistribution and more active metabolism by liver than other narcotics.

NOTE: *Dissociative*—when under analgesia, the patient does not appear to be asleep or anesthetized, but rather dissociated from his surroundings.

Agent	Administration	Advantages	Disadvantages	Implications
Ketamine (Ketalar; Ketaject)	Intravenously Also, intramuscularly	Rapid induction and short action; often used to supplement nitrous oxide Useful where hypotension may be hazardous; can be administered as analgesic or anesthetic	May cause elevated blood pressure and depressed respirations Patient may experience hallucinations Vomiting and aspiration may occur	Avoid verbal, visual, or tactile stimulation since this may trigger psychic aberration. Droperidol or diazepam may eliminate such psychic emergence phenomena. Observe for signs of respiratory depression. Keep resuscitative equipment nearby.

(continued)

Table 20-5
Intravenous Anesthetic Agents (continued)

Agent	Administration	Advantages	Disadvantages	Implications
Tranquilizers				
Benzodiazepines Diazepam (Valium) Chlordiazepoxide (Librium)	Intravenously Orally Intramuscularly	Preoperative sedation Intraoperative tranquilization during regional anesthesia Production of hypnosis during anesthetic induction	Absorbed unpredictably when given intramuscularly	IV administration may produce thrombophlebitis (central vein therefore is preferred).
Droperidol (Inapsine)	Intravenously	Long duration of action	Weak antihistaminic action and alpha-adrenergic blocking action; inhibition of basic ganglionic dopaminergic pathways—may lead to extrapyramidal rigidity resembling parkinsonism	Major tranquilizer Keep IV fluids and vasopressors available for hypotension.

ferred by patients who have experienced various methods. The duration of action is brief, and the patient awakens with little nausea or vomiting. Thiopental often is given with other anesthetic agents in prolonged procedures.

Intravenous anesthesia has the advantage of being non-explosive, of requiring little equipment, and of being easy to administer. The low incidence of postoperative nausea and vomiting makes the method useful in eye surgery, in which retching endangers vision in the operated eye. It is useful for short procedures, but is used less often for abdominal surgery. It is not indicated for children, who have small veins and who are more susceptible to respiratory obstruction. The reasons in both instances are apparent.

Disadvantages. Thiopental is a powerful depressant of breathing, and its chief danger lies in this characteristic. It should be administered by skilled anesthesiologists and nurse anesthetists, and only when some method of giving oxygen is available immediately should trouble arise. Sneezing, coughing, and laryngospasm are sometimes noted.

Spinal Anesthesia

It must never be forgotten that the patient under spinal, regional, or local anesthesia is awake and aware of his surroundings. Careless conversation, unnecessary noise, unpleasant odors—all are noticed by the patient on the operating table and reflect discredit on the operating room staff. Quiet must be insisted upon. The diagnosis must not be made aloud if the patient is not to be made aware of it at this time.

Anesthesia of the lower extremities, abdomen, and even of the chest may be induced by the introduction of anesthetic drugs into the subarachnoid space. A spinal puncture is made, with sterile precautions, and the drug is injected in solution through the needle. As soon as the in-

jection has been made, the patient is placed on his back. If a relatively high level of block is desired, the head and the shoulders are lowered, depending on the height of anesthesia desired. The spread of the anesthetic agent and the level of anesthesia depend on the amount of fluid injected, the rapidity with which it is injected, the positioning of the patient after the injection, and the specific gravity of the agent. If the specific gravity of the agent is greater than cerebrospinal fluid (CSF), *hyperbaric,* the drug moves to the dependent position of the subarachnoid space; if *hypobaric,* the drug moves away from the dependent portion. These boundaries can obviously be controlled by the anesthesiologist.

In a few minutes anesthesia and paralysis appear, first of the toes and the perineum and then gradually of the legs and the abdomen. The drugs generally used are procaine, tetracaine (Pontocaine), and lidocaine (Xylocaine) (Table 20-6).

Nausea, vomiting, and pain may occur during surgery under spinal anesthesia. As a rule, these reactions result from traction on various structures, particularly those within the abdominal cavity. Such reactions may be avoided by the simultaneous intravenous administration of a weak solution of thiopental and inhalation of nitrous oxide.

When the anesthetic drug reaches the upper thoracic and cervical cord in high concentration, a temporary, partial, or complete respiratory paralysis may occur. This complication is treated by maintaining artificial respiration until the effects of the drug on the respiratory nerves have worn off.

Such postoperative complications as headache, paralysis, or meningitis may occur; the latter two now are extremely rare. Several factors are involved in the incidence of headache: the size of the spinal needle used, the leakage

Table 20-6
Spinal Anesthetic Agents

Agent	Advantages of Spinal Anesthesia (Includes All Agents)	Disadvantages of Spinal Anesthesia (Includes All Agents)
Procaine (Novocain) Tetracaine (Pontocaine) Xylocaine (Lidocaine)	Easily administered by a physician Inexpensive Minimum of equipment required Rapid onset Excellent muscular relaxation	Blood pressure may fall rapidly unless watched carefully and treated with such drugs as ephedrine, etc. If the spinal anesthesia ascends to the chest, there may be respiratory difficulties. Occasionally, postoperative complications occur, such as headache; rarely, meningitis or paralysis.

of fluid from the subarachnoid space through the puncture site, and the degree of the patient's hydration. Any measure that can increase cerebrospinal pressure is helpful in relieving headache. These include keeping the patient flat and quiet, providing body hydration, applying a tight abdominal binder, and injecting fluid into the epidural space.

Nursing Assessment After Spinal Anesthesia. In addition to taking the blood pressure, the nurse observes these patients closely and records the time when motion and sensation return in the legs and the toes. When there is complete return of sensation in the toes (in response to pinprick), the patient may be considered to have recovered from the effects of the spinal drug.

"Serial" or Continuous Spinal Anesthesia. The tip of a plastic catheter may be left in the subarachnoid space during operation, so that more anesthetic may be injected as needed. Greater control of dosage is afforded by this technique. However, there is greater potential for postanesthetic headache because of the large-gauge needle used.

Epidural or Peridural Anesthesia. This anesthesia is obtained by the injection of a local anesthetic into the spinal canal in the space surrounding the dura mater. Interest in this approach has increased because of a desire to find a method of anesthesia without undesirable neurologic sequelae, notably headache, that occasionally result from subarachnoid injection.

Advantages of epidural anesthesia appear to be the absence of neurologic complications and slightly less disturbance of blood pressure. One disadvantage lies in the greater technical problem of introducing the anesthetic into the epidural rather than the subarachnoid space. Another is that the level of anesthesia is less controllable.

Regional Anesthesia

Regional anesthesia is a form of local anesthesia in which an anesthetic agent is injected into or around nerves so that the area supplied by these nerves is anesthetized. The effect depends on the type of nerve involved. Motor fibers are the largest and have the thickest myelin sheath. Sympathetic fibers are the smallest and have a minimal covering. Sensory fibers are intermediary. Thus, a local anesthetic blocks motor nerves least readily and sympathetic nerves most readily. An anesthetic cannot be regarded as having "worn off" until all three systems (motor, sensory, and autonomic) are no longer affected by the anesthetic. There are many types of

regional anesthesia, depending on the various nerve groups that are injected.

Brachial Plexus Block. A brachial plexus block produces anesthesia of the arm.

Paravertebral Anesthesia. Paravertebral anesthesia produces anesthesia of the nerve supplying the chest, abdominal wall, and the extremities.

Transsacral (Caudal) Block. A transsacral block produces anesthesia of the perineum and, occasionally, the lower abdomen.

Local Infiltration Anesthesia

Infiltration anesthesia is the injection of a solution containing the local anesthetic into the tissues through which the incision is to pass. Often it is combined with a local regional block by injection of nerves immediately supplying that area. Local anesthesia is popular for several reasons:

1. It is simple, economical, and nonexplosive. The amount of equipment is minimal. Postoperative care is lessened.
2. Undesirable effects of general anesthesia are avoided.
3. It is ideal for short and superficial operations.

In operations on the abdominal viscera, complete anesthesia is not obtained by infiltration or local block of the anterior abdominal wall, because the viscera are supplied by nerves that have not been affected by the anesthetic. For this reason, a separate injection must be made into the region of the splanchnic nerves, which supply the abdominal organs, except those of the pelvis. This injection may be made from the back (posterior-splanchnic anesthesia), or anteriorly, after the abdomen is opened.

Local anesthesia is often administered in combination with epinephrine. Epinephrine causes constriction of blood vessels, which prevents rapid absorption of the anesthetic drug and thus prolongs its local action; absorption into the bloodstream, which could cause convulsions, is also prevented. Different types of local anesthetic agents are listed in Table 20-7.

Contraindications. Local anesthesia is the anesthesia of choice in any operation which it can be used. However, it is contraindicated for operations upon highly nervous, apprehensive patients. The emotional trauma experienced by these individuals during local anesthesia may be harmful. A patient who begs to be put to sleep rarely does well under local anesthesia.

For some kinds of operations, local anesthesia is impractical because of the number of injections and the amount of anesthetic required, for example, in a radical mastectomy.

Technique. The technique for the introduction of local infiltration requires few materials. Usually, the following are all that are needed:

1. Solution of local anesthetic in various concentrations (0.5%–2%)
2. Sterile container
3. Sterile syringes and needles to fit
4. Sterile sponges and drape

The skin is prepared as for any operation, and a small-gauge needle is used to inject a little of the anesthetic into the skin layers. This produces blanching or a wheal. The anesthetic then is carried ahead of the needle in the skin until an area as long as the proposed incision is anesthetized. A larger, longer needle then is used to infiltrate deeper tissues with the anesthetic. The action of the drug is almost immediate, so that the operation may begin as soon as the injection is finished. Anesthesia lasts anywhere from ¾ hour to 3 hours, depending on the anesthetic and the use of epinephrine.

▷ Artificial Hypotension During Operation

There are times during surgery when it is desirable to lower blood pressure in order to reduce bleeding at the operative site, since this allows for more rapid surgery with less blood loss. In such operations as brain surgery, radical neck dissection, and radical pelvic surgery, artificially induced hypotension has been used.

Deliberate hypotension is accomplished by inhalation or intravenous injection of drugs that affect the sympathetic nervous system and peripheral smooth muscle. Halothane is the inhalational anesthetic agent commonly used. This anesthetic is supplemented with other measures to lower blood pressure, such as a head-up position, positive pressure applied to the airway, and administration of a ganglionic blocking drug, such as pentolinium (Ansolysen) or sodium nitroprusside.

Table 20-7
Local Anesthetic Agents

Agent	Administration and Action	Advantages	Disadvantages	Implications and Use
Amides				
Lidocaine (Xylocaine) and mepivacaine (Carbocaine)	Topical or injection	Rapid Longer duration of action (compared with procaine) Free from local irritative effect	Occasional idiosyncrasy	Useful topically for cystoscopy Injected for use in dental work and surgery Watch for untoward reactions—drowsiness, depressed respirations.
Bupivacaine (Marcaine)	Infiltration Peripheral nerve block Epidural	Duration is 2–3 times longer than lidocaine or mepivacaine	Use cautiously in persons with known drug allergies or sensitivities	A period of analgesia persists after return of sensation; therefore, need for strong analgesics is reduced.
Etidocaine (Duranest)	Infiltration Block			Greater potency and longer action than lidocaine
Esters				
Procaine (Novocain)	Subcutaneously, intramuscularly, intravenously, or spinal	Low toxicity Inexpensive	Some idiosyncrasies Skin rash Poor stability	Watch for reaction; BP, bradycardia, weak pulse. Usually given with epinephrine, causing vasoconstriction, thereby slowing absorption and prolonging nerve-deadening effect
Tetracaine (Pontocaine)	Topical Infiltration Nerve block	Same as procaine	Same as procaine	More than 10 times as potent as procaine Usually given with epinephrine

▷ Malignant Hyperthermia During General Anesthesia

Instances of severe hyperthermia during surgery have been reported in which the temperature has reached over 43.3° C (110° F). The mortality rate is approximately 60% to 70%. Reasons for the phenomenon are related to a biochemical disturbance in skeletal muscle involving calcium distribution. However, careful monitoring can anticipate and sometimes minimize the increase in temperature. When hyperthermia occurs, the anesthetic is discontinued and the operation is halted.

Measures to combat the temperature rise include use of a hypothermia blanket, infusion of iced saline solution, and administration of high concentrations of oxygen and sodium bicarbonate to combat metabolic acidosis. These methods require monitoring: electrocardiogram, temperature probe, placement of arterial and central venous lines, and bladder catheterization.

▷ Position on Operating Table

The position in which the patient is placed on the operating table depends on the operation to be performed as well as the physical condition of the patient (Fig. 20-2). Factors to consider include the following:

1. The patient should be in as comfortable a position as possible, whether asleep or awake.
2. The operative area must be adequately exposed.
3. Circulation should not be obstructed by an awkward position or undue pressure on a part.
4. There should be no interference with the patient's respiration as a result of pressure of the arms on the chest or constriction of the neck or chest caused by a gown.
5. Nerves must be protected from undue pressure. Improper positioning of the arms, hands, legs, or feet may cause serious injury or paralysis. Shoulder braces must be well padded to prevent irreparable nerve injury, especially when the Trendelenburg position is necessary.
6. Concerns for the patient as an individual must be practiced, particularly with the very thin, the elderly, or the obese patient.
7. Every patient needs *gentle* restraint before induction, in case of excitement.

Dorsal Recumbent Position.   The usual position is flat on the back; one arm is at the side of the table, with the hand placed palm down; the other is carefully positioned on an armboard for intravenous infusion (Fig. 20-2). This position is used for most abdominal operations, except for those upon the gallbladder and the pelvis and for the operations described below.

Trendelenburg Position.   This position usually is employed for operations on the lower abdomen and the pelvis in order to obtain good exposure by displacing the intestines into the upper abdomen. In this position the head and body are lowered so that the plane of the body meets the horizontal at an angle. The knees are flexed by "breaking"

the table, and the patient is held in position by padded shoulder braces (Fig. 20-2).

Lithotomy Position.   In this position the patient is lying on his back with the legs and thighs flexed at right angles. The position is maintained by placing the feet in stirrups. Nearly all perineal, rectal, and vaginal operations require this posture (Fig. 20-2).

For Kidney Operations.   The patient is placed on his well side in Sims's position with an air pillow 12.5 cm to 15 cm (5 or 6 inches) thick under the loin, or he is placed on a table with a kidney or back lift (Fig. 20-2).

For Chest and Abdominothoracic Operations.   The position varies with the operation to be performed. The surgeon and the anesthesiologist place the patient on the operating table in the proper position.

Operations on the Neck.   Such operations, for example, those involving the thyroid, are performed with the patient on his back, the neck extended somewhat by a pillow beneath the shoulders and the head and chest elevated, in order to reduce venous pressure.

Operations on the Skull and the Brain.   Such procedures demand special positions and apparatus, usually adjusted by the surgeon.

▷ Intraoperative Nursing

(Also see Chart 20-1, Nursing Process, p. 376.)

The center of attention and activity in the operating room is the patient who is undergoing a surgical procedure for the repair, correction, or relief of a physical problem. The immediate concern from the time the patient arrives in the operating room through the period when the anesthesia is being administered is the psychological reactions of the patient.

Throughout the surgical experience, the nurse functions as the patient's chief advocate. The "caring" and concern of nursing management extends from the time when the patient is prepared for and instructed about the forthcoming operation, through the more immediate preoperative period, into the operative phase and the recovery from anesthesia, and on through convalescence. Throughout this continuum, *priority is given to the patient, his safety, his understanding of the care he is receiving, and the biophysical and psychosocial needs he is experiencing.* Because the operation is usually a unique experience in the patient's life, he needs the security of knowing that someone is protecting his best interests at this time, especially when he is unable to make decisions for himself.

When a patient arrives in the operating room, essentially three different groups are preparing for his care: (1) the anesthesiologist and those assistants who administer the anesthetic agent and place the patient in the proper position on the operating table; (2) the surgeon and those assistants who scrub and perform the operation; and (3) the intraoperative nurses who manage the operating room, are responsible for the safety and well-being of the patient, and coordinate the many activities of the operating personnel and also provide care through enacting "scrub nurse" and circulating activities during the operation (Fig. 20-3). Dur-

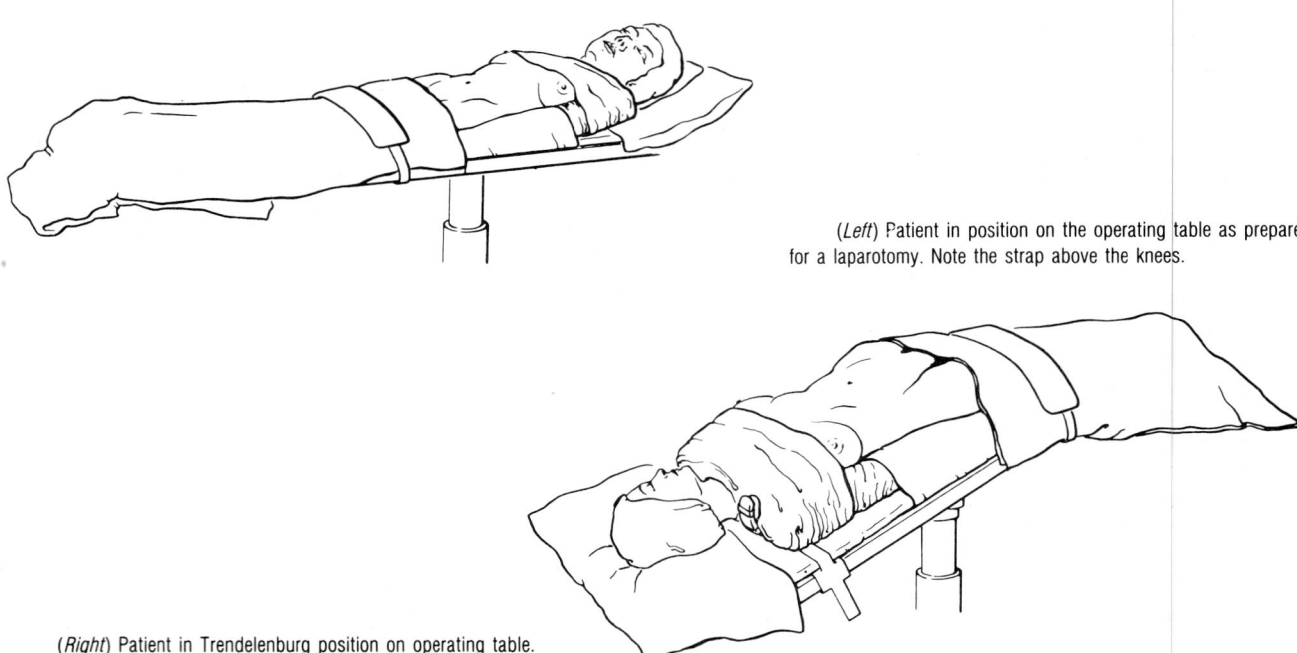

(*Left*) Patient in position on the operating table as prepared for a laparotomy. Note the strap above the knees.

(*Right*) Patient in Trendelenburg position on operating table. Note padded shoulder braces in place. Be sure that brace does not press on brachial plexus.

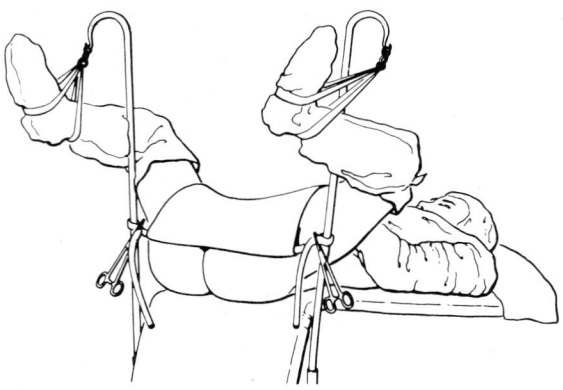

(*Left*) Patient in lithotomy position. Note that the hips extend over the edge of the table.

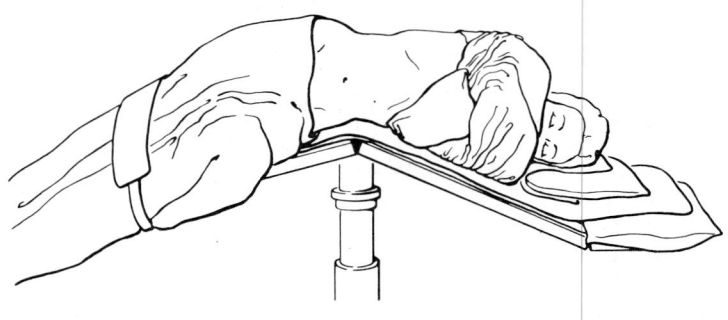

(*Right*) Patient on operating table for kidney operation, lying on his well side. Table is broken to spread apart space between the lower ribs and the pelvis. The upper leg is extended; the lower leg is flexed at the knee and the hip joints; a pillow is placed between the legs. Note the sandbag, which helps to support the patient's chest.

Figure 20-2.   Positions on the operating table.

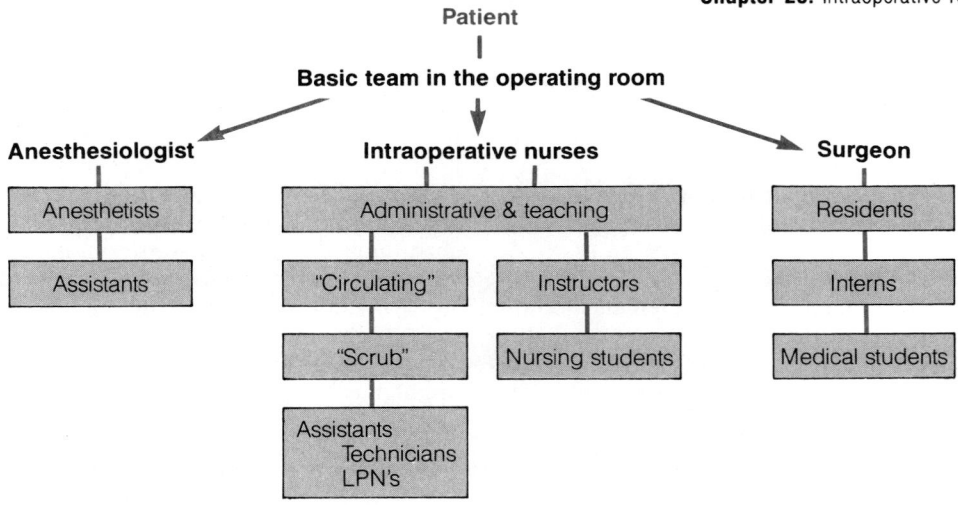

Figure 20-3. Basic operating room team.

ing the course of the operation, information about the patient must be shared by the anesthesiologist, the nurse, and the surgeon, in order to assure optimum patient care. In addition, any pertinent developments, such as undue hemorrhage; unexpected findings; fluid and electrolyte problems; shock; or respiratory difficulties, that are related to patient care in the recovery room must be noted and documented.

▷ Principles of Perioperative Asepsis

As was indicated earlier, in all phases of the surgical experience, the main priority for all personnel is prevention of patient complications, which includes protection of the patient from infection. Inherent in this goal is strict adherence to the principles of asepsis.

The successful practice of aseptic surgery requires the strict observance of rigorous standards for *preoperative* sterilization of surgical materials and of precautions against infection, both *during* the course of the operation and *after* the operation, when the wound must be guarded until such time as it is healed.

To provide the best possible conditions for performing a surgical operation, the operating room is placed in a section of the hospital where it is free from such hazards as contaminating particles, dust, other pollutants, radiation, noise, etc. Strict building codes must be set and adhered to in the selection of materials for construction and in determining room size and air circulation patterns. Electrical hazards, conductivity checks, emergency exit clearances, and storage of equipment and anesthetic gases are checked periodically by the state and the Joint Commission for the Accreditation of Hospitals.

In surgical practice, asepsis prevents the contamination of surgical wounds. Although postoperative wound infection may be caused by natural skin flora or a previously existing infection, it is the responsibility of the personnel in the operating room to utilize aseptic principles to min-

imize this risk. These principles are described and illustrated in detail in the pages that follow, in terms of the various protocols and practices to be carried out.

Protocols
Preoperative
Prior to the operation, all surgical material must be sterilized; this includes any instruments, needles, sutures, dressings, gloves, covers, etc. that may come in contact with the wound and exposed tissues. In addition, the surgeon, the surgical assistants, and the nurses must prepare themselves by scrubbing their hands and arms with soap and water ("scrubbing") and donning long-sleeved, sterile gowns and gloves (described on, pp. 378–380). Head and hair are covered with a cap, and a mask is worn over the nose and mouth to minimize the possibility of bacteria from the upper respiratory tract entering the wound. The patient's skin, over an area considerably larger than that requiring exposure during the course of the operation, also requires meticulous cleansing followed by the application of an antiseptic agent. The rest of the patient's body is covered with sterile drapes.

Intraoperative
During the operation, none of the personnel who have scrubbed touch anything that has not been sterilized. Nonscrubbed personnel refrain from touching or contaminating anything that is sterile.

Postoperative
After the operation, the wound is protected from possible contamination by means of sterile dressings and by the use of sterile saline and antiseptics when the wound is cleansed and the dressings changed. Particular care is taken to protect the unhealed wound from coming in contact with anything that is not sterile. In wounds that become infected, it may be necessary to remove and destroy microorganisms that are already in the tissues by removing or "debriding" devitalized tissues. To prevent subsequent infection from

without, rigid aseptic technique must be followed during the course of treatment.

When infection has already developed in tissues, antimicrobials specific for the offending organism are prescribed, and heat is applied or drainage established to assist the body in eliminating the offending organisms.

Environmental Controls

In addition to the above protocols, the implementation of aseptic principles requires meticulous housekeeping in the operating room. Floors and horizontal surfaces are cleaned frequently with detergent soap and water or detergent germicide, and sterilizing equipment is inspected regularly to assure optimum operation and performance. Although sterilization of linens is no longer done on the operating room floor (it may be done in central supply service, or prepackaged sterilized items may be used), instruments are cleaned and sterilized in a unit close to the operating room. Peel-apart, individually wrapped, sterile items are used to provide additional individual items as needed.

Many operating rooms are equipped with laminar air-flow systems that filter out a high percentage of dust and bacteria. Originally designed for spacecraft, these systems use high-efficiency particulate air (HEPA) filters to remove

---

Chart 20-1
The Nursing Process Utilized in the Operating Room

Assessment—The Nurse

A. Utilize data from patient and the patient record to identify variables that can affect care and that serve as guidelines for developing an individualized plan of patient care.
1. Identify patient.
2. Validate necessary data with patient per department policy.
3. Review patient record for:
   a. Correct informed surgical consent
   b. Completed records for health history and physical examination
   c. Results of diagnostic studies
   d. Nursing history and nursing assessment
4. Complete immediate preoperative nursing assessment.
   a. Physiologic status (*e.g.,* health–illness level, level of consciousness, etc.)
   b. Psychosocial status (*e.g.,* expressions of concern, anxiety level, verbal communication problems, coping mechanisms, etc.)
   c. Physical status (*e.g.,* operative site, skin condition and effectiveness of preparation, shave or depilatory; immobile joints, etc.)

Planning—The Nurse

A. Interpret common variables and incorporate them into the plan of care.
1. Age, size, sex, surgical procedure, type of anesthesia planned, surgeon, anesthesiologist, and team members
2. Availability of necessary equipment specific to procedure and surgeon
3. Need for nonroutine drugs, blood, instruments, etc.
4. Readiness of room for patient; completeness of physical setup; completeness of instrument, suture, and dressing setups

B. Identify aspects of the operating room environment that may negatively affect the patient.
1. Physical:
   a. Room temperature and humidity
   b. Electrical hazards
   c. Potential contaminants (dust, blood and discharge stains on floor, or furniture; uncovered hair, faulty personnel attire, jewelry worn by personnel, "dirty" footwear)
   d. Unnecessary traffic
2. Psychosocial:
   a. Noise
   b. Lack of recognition as a person
   c. Sense of abandonment—unchaperoned in waiting area
   d. Social "chit-chat"

Intervention

A. Provide nursing care based on priority of patient needs.
1. Set up and maintain suction in working order.
2. Set up invasive monitoring equipment.
3. Assist with line insertion (arterial, Swan-Ganz, CVP, IV).
4. Initiate appropriate physical comfort measures for patient.
5. Position patient correctly for anesthesia and surgical procedures; maintain functional body alignment.
6. Follow steps in surgical procedure.
   a. Scrub and circulate competently.
   b. Respond to needs of patient by anticipating what supplies and equipment are required before it is requested.
7. Follow established procedures, for example (not all-inclusive):
   a. Care and use of blood and blood products
   b. Care and handling of specimens, tissue, and cultures

(continued)

more than 99% of airborne particles measuring 0.3 microns or more. Laminar flow also changes air more effectively— about 200 times an hour as compared with air conditioning, which exchanges air 12 times per hour.

Unfortunately, in spite of all these precautions, postoperative wound infections may occasionally occur during an operation, appearing days or weeks later in the form of an incisional infection or abscess.

- Constant surveillance and conscientiousness in carrying out aseptic practices must be stressed continually, since errors and misjudgments can occur as a result of human failure.

Principles Regarding Health and Operating Room Attire

Good health is essential for any person in the operating room. Colds, sore throats, and infected fingers are distinct sources of pathogenic organisms and must be reported. A series of wound infections in postoperative patients were traced in one instance to a mild throat infection in an operating room nurse. Therefore, the importance of reporting any seemingly slight ailment without delay can be readily understood.

Clothing.   Street clothes are never worn in the operating room. Only approved, clean, operating room attire is

---

Chart 20-1
The Nursing Process Utilized in the Operating Room (continued)

Intervention *(continued)*

    c. Antiseptic skin preparation
    d. Donning gown—self; holding gown for surgeon
    e. Open and closed gloving
    f. Counts: sponge, instrument, needle, special
    g. Septic case technique
    h. Urinary catheter management
    i. Drainage/dressing management
  8. Communicate adverse situations to surgeon, anesthesiologist, or charge nurse, or act appropriately to control or reverse the situation.
  9. Use supplies judiciously for cost-effectiveness.
 10. Assist the surgeon and anesthesiologist in implementing their plans of care.

B. Coordinate activities of significant others involved in patient care (list not all-inclusive).
  1. X-ray, laboratory, recovery or intensive care unit, surgical floor
  2. Technicians—cast, laboratory, etc.
  3. Pharmacist
  4. Ancillary operating room personnel and nonprofessional staff

C. Inform patient regarding his intraoperative experience.
  1. Describe any sensory stimulation he will experience.
  2. Use common, basic communication skills to reduce anxiety in the patient, for example (list not all-inclusive:
    a. Touch
    b. Eye contact
    c. Assuring the patient you will be with him in the operating room.
    d. Realistic verbal reassurance

D. Act as the patient's advocate.
  1. Provide physical privacy.
  2. Maintain confidentiality.
  3. Act to provide physical safety and comfort.

E. Operate and troubleshoot all equipment commonly used in the operating room and assigned specialty service (including autoclaves).

F. Participate in patient care conferences.

G. Document all observations and appropriate actions on the required forms, including patient's record.

H. Communicate, orally and in writing, with the recovery room and outpatient surgical nursing staff (as pertinent) regarding the health status of the patient on transfer from the operating room.

Evaluation

A. Evaluate the condition of the patient immediately prior to his discharge from the operating room, for example:
  1. Respiratory condition: breathing easily (on his own or assisted)
  2. Skin condition: color good; absence of abrasions, burns, bruises
  3. Functioning of invasive tubing: IV, drains, catheters, nasogastric—no kinks or obstruction, functioning normally, etc.
  4. Grounding pad site: good condition
  5. Dressings: adequate for drainage, fastened securely, not too tight, etc.

B. Participate in the identification of unsafe patient care practices and intervene appropriately.

C. Participate in evaluating the safety of the environment; for example, equipment, cleanliness, etc.

D. Report and document any adverse behavior or problem.

E. Demonstrate understanding of principles of asepsis and technical nursing practices.

F. Accept legal responsibilities inherent in perioperative nursing.

(Adapted from procedure and practices at Memorial Hospital Medical Center of Long Beach, California.)

permitted. Likewise, OR attire is not worn out of the operating room. Written policies describe the practice that all persons are required to follow. Dressing rooms are located near the operating suite and are reached from an outer corridor. Clothing is changed in the dressing room before entering and upon leaving the operating room.

Close-fitting cotton dresses, pants suits, and jumpsuits are available in a variety of styles. When pants are worn, the ankles should have close-fitting cuffs (drawstring or knitted) to contain organisms shed from the perineum and legs. Shirts and waist drawstrings should be tucked inside the pants to prevent any accidental contact with sterile areas and again to contain skin sheddings. Fresh OR attire is put on each time the person enters the operating room; when this clothing is removed, it is bagged and sent to the hospital laundry.

Mask.   Masks are worn at all times in the operating room for the purpose of minimizing airborne contamination. Droplets containing microorganisms from the oropharynx and nasopharynx must be contained and filtered.

Therefore, the mask must not leak air. At the same time, it should not interfere with breathing or hinder speech or vision, and must be compact and comfortable. Forced expiration, such as that produced by talking, laughing, sneezing, and coughing, should be avoided, since it deposits additional organisms on the mask. Many effective disposable masks are available that have high filtration efficiency: 95+%. Tests prove their superiority over gauze masks. Masks are changed at a minimum between patients and are not to be worn outside the Surgery Department.

Since the mask loses much of its effectiveness when it becomes moistened, it is changed between operations and more often if necessary. The mask is either on or off; it must not be allowed to hang around the neck. When the mask is removed, only the strings are handled in order to prevent contamination of the hands. Mask strings are tied snugly; top strings are tied at the back of the head, and bottom strings are tied at the back of the neck.

Headgear.   Headgear should completely cover the hair (head and neckline including beard), so that single strands

---

Chart 20-2
Guidelines: "Scrubbing" for an Operation

Action	*Rationale*
1. The nails are kept short and free of nail polish; special attention is given to the subungual space (beneath nail) with a sterile nail cleaner early in the scrub.	1. Scrubbing can cause nail polish to chip and peel; this would produce nicks in which microbes could breed.
2. A soft but firm-bristled brush or one of the numerous polyurethane disposable sponges that are impregnated with soap is used for scrubbing.	2. The brush or special sponge facilitates removal of dead skin, soil, and resident organisms.
3. There are many acceptable antiseptic detergents, such as the iodophors.	3. Broad-spectrum microbicidal solution is preferred where gram-negative nosocomial infections predominate.

4. Hands and arms must be well lathered and rinsed frequently. No chemical agent can be relied upon as a substitute for conscientious mechanical cleansing of the skin.	4. Microbes are removed by two actions:
	   a. Physical mechanical separation
	   b. Chemical antisepsis from action of antimicrobial solution

5. The duration of the scrub may be determined by setting a time limit for the conscientious scrubbing of one part after another in a prescribed manner, or by counting a certain number of strokes per part. A practical, reliable, and effective procedure should be followed. Because the moisture and warmth present under surgical gloves provide an ideal growing medium for bacteria, it is essential that a prescribed scrub be done between operations.	5. Individual conscientious attention to detail is important. Hospital policy is followed.
6. Following the scrub, hands and arms are rinsed thoroughly; soap and brush are left in sink or discarded in appropriate container. The elbow or the knee is used to turn the water off. Hands are held higher than the elbows and away from the body.	6. Holding hands higher than the elbows and away from the body allows water to run off at the elbow and prevents contaminated water (from above the elbow) from running down to the scrubbed hands.
7. When drying hands, care is taken to prevent the towel from touching the scrub dress or suit. One hand, then the arm, are dried with a towel, proceeding from fingertips to elbow; the other hand and arm are dried in similar fashion using a dry segment of the towel.	7. Proceeding from the fingertips to the elbow will prevent above-elbow sources of contamination from affecting scrubbed hands and lower arms.

Chart 20-3
Gowning

After the hands and arms are scrubbed using an antiseptic detergent, a sterile gown and gloves are put on. These are worn to allow the wearer to participate in or observe the surgical operation while maintaining a state of asepsis in as practical a way as possible.

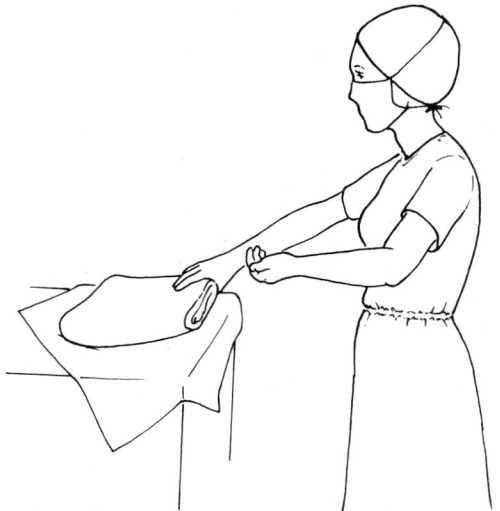

1. The sterile gown may be obtained from an open pack, or it may be handed by someone already scrubbed.

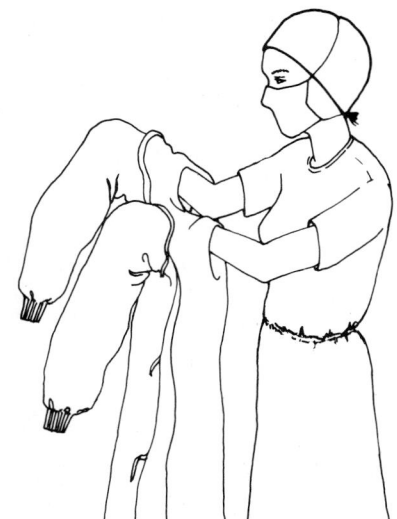

2. Since gowns are folded inside out (to eliminate the need to touch the outside of the garment), the gown can be held by the neckband and allowed to unfold from the extended hands. As the gown unfolds, the armholes should face the wearer. The hands are held upward and slipped into the armholes—but only as far as the sleeve cuff.

3. The circulating nurse can assist by reaching inside the gown and pulling the sleeves over the hands. (Sleeves are pulled to the hands, not over them, when the "closed glove technique" is to be used. See page 380.)

4. To secure the gown, the tapes at the back are tied. If the gown has tapes at the waist, the circulating nurse reaches for the ends of the tapes without touching the gown, draws the tapes back, and ties them. (Gowns may be fastened with Velcro, which eliminates the need for tapes.)

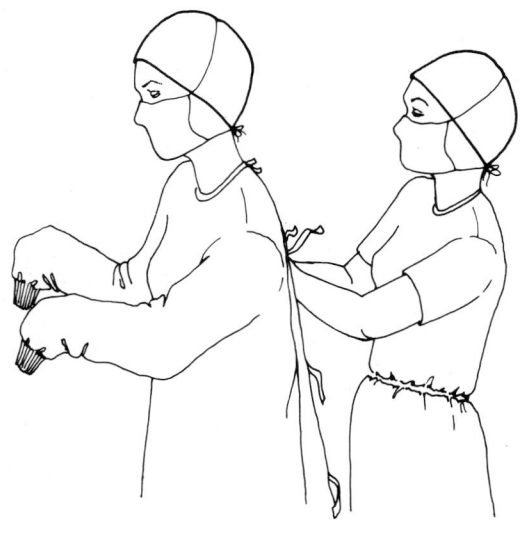

Note: A gown is sterile only as long as it is dry and not torn. If it is wet from perspiration or from any other cause, it must be considered contaminated.

Chart 20-4
Putting on Sterile Gloves: Closed Method

When the gown is donned, the hands are slid into the sleeve only as far as the cuff seam, which is then grasped by the thumb and index finger through the fabric.

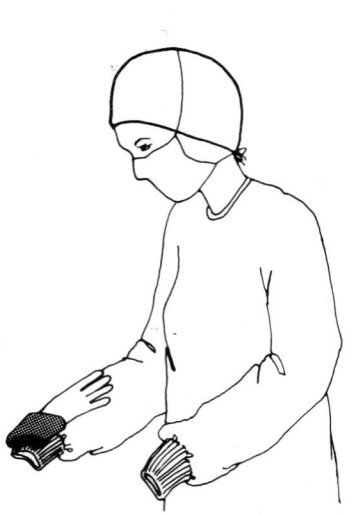

1. One glove is grasped (while the hand is still inside the sleeve) and placed thumbside down on the palmside of the other arm, with glove fingers pointing toward the shoulder. (Glove cuff lies over gown cuff.)*

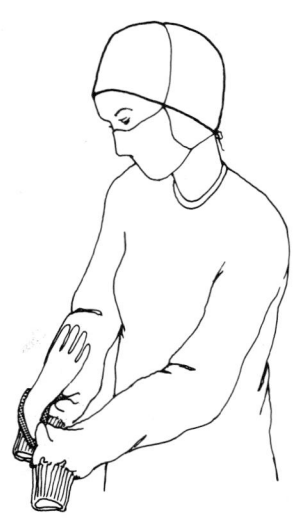

2. The wrist edge of the glove that is against the sleeve is grasped with the finger that holds the seam, and the uppermost glove wrist edge is grasped with the sleeve-covered fingers of the other hand.

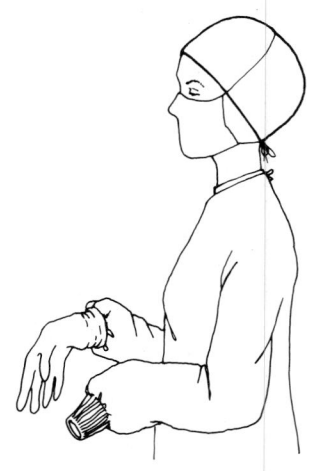

3. The glove wrist is pulled over the gown cuff, care being taken not to fold the gown cuff back or to expose the fingers inside it.

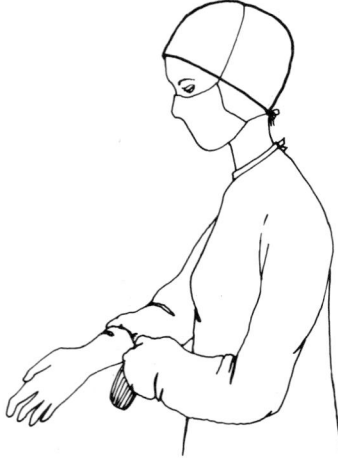

4. As cuff is drawn onto the wrist, the fingers are directed into cots in the glove, and the glove is adjusted to the hand.

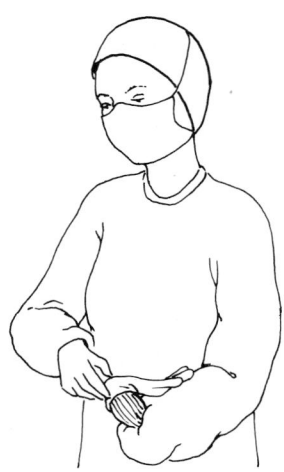

5. The second glove is put on in the same manner, using the newly gloved hand to hold the glove.

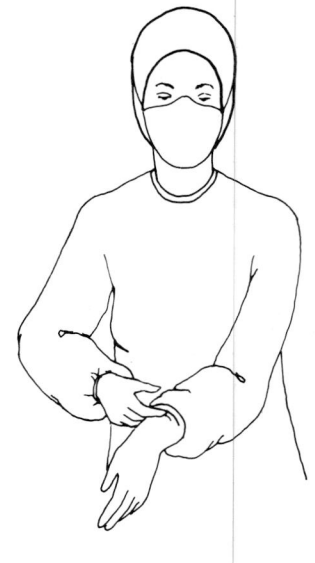

* Shaded or crosshatched areas of the glove (representing the inside of glove) are considered unsterile.

Chart 20-5
Putting on Sterile Gloves: Open Method

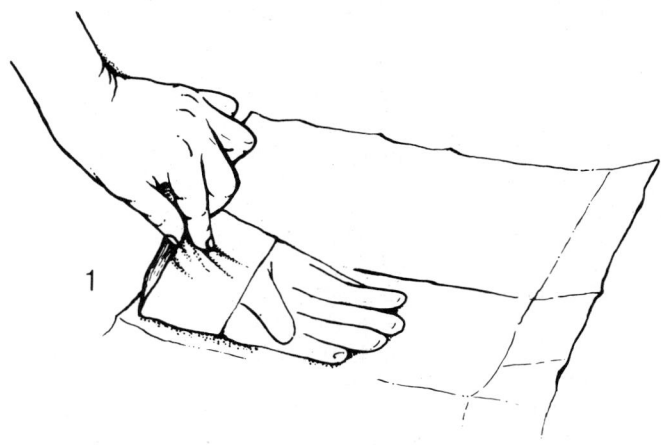

1. When the right glove is put on first, the cuff is grasped on the inside by the left hand.

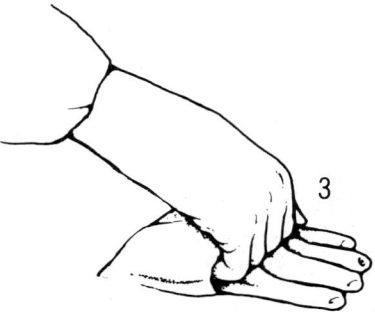

2. The right hand is inserted into the glove, which is then pulled into place with the left hand (the cuff is left in a turned-down position). The grasp is then released.

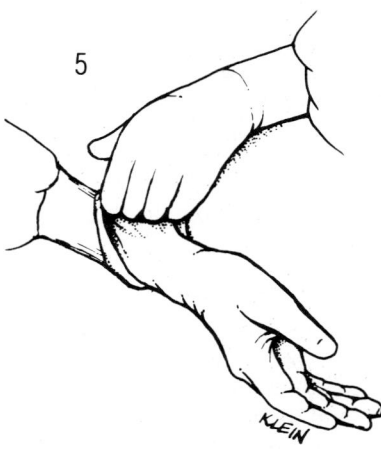

3. Now the right gloved hand can pick up the left glove by inserting the fingers under its cuff. (The outside is the sterile side.)

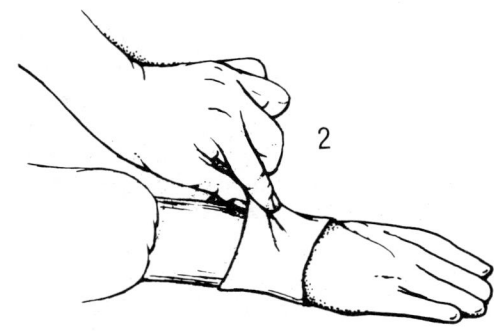

4. The left hand is inserted into the left glove and the glove is pulled into place. The cuff is left in a turned-down position.

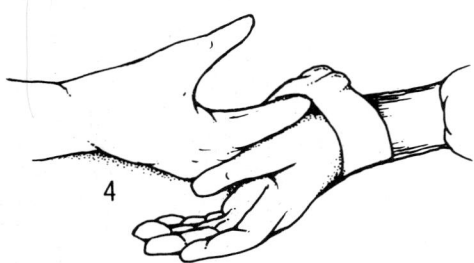

5. After folding the gown cuff snugly to the wrist, and while holding this fold in place with the sterile right gloved thumb, the fingers can safely pull the sterile glove cuff over the gown cuff.

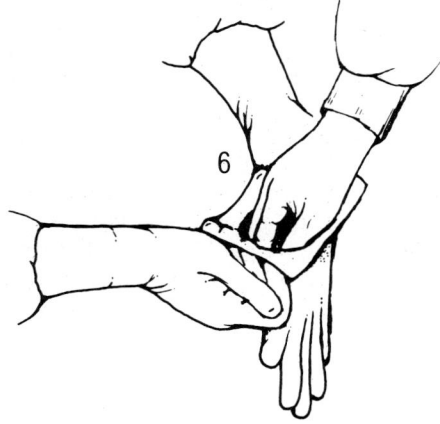

Another method: The scrubbed nurse holds the glove open for the person donning the gloves. The glove is held with the thumb facing the recipient. The top of the glove is spread wide so that the hand can be thrust into the glove without touching the person holding the glove. The glove cuff is pulled up over the gown cuff.

of hair, bobbypins, clips, or particles of dandruff or dust do not fall on sterile fields. The styles of headgear available are disposable, lint-free, and clothlike.

Shoes. Shoes should be comfortable and supportive; clogs, tennis shoes, sandals, and boots are not permitted because they are unsafe and difficult to clean. Shoes are covered with disposable or canvas shoe covers. Conductive covers establish an electrical ground for the wearer. The black strips provided with some conductive shoe covers should be placed inside the shoe in contact with the sole of the foot. Shoe covers are worn one time only and are removed upon leaving the restricted area. Conductometers are usually located at the entrance to the operating room area.

Intraoperative Nursing Functions

(See also Chart 20-1, Nursing Process Utilized in the Operating Room, pp. 376–378.)

Frequently, nursing function in the operating room is described in terms of "circulating" and "scrub" activities.

The *"circulating" nurse* manages the operating room and protects the safety and health needs of the patient by controlling the activities and state of the environment, ensuring cleanliness, proper temperature, humidity, lighting, safety of equipment, and availability of supplies and materials. It is also the responsibility of the circulating nurse to observe and check the patient throughout the operative procedure to ensure that his needs are provided for and his rights upheld. It is also necessary to coordinate the activities of related personnel (laboratory, x-ray, medical, etc.) and to monitor aseptic practices in order to avoid breakdowns in technique.

"Scrub" activities include "scrubbing" for the operation (Charts 20-2 through 20-5); setting up the sterile tables; preparing sutures, ligatures, and special equipment; assisting the surgeon and the surgical assistants during the operation by anticipating the required instruments, sponges, drains, etc.; and keeping the time the patient is under anesthesia and the time the wound is open to a minimum. Toward the end of the operation, equipment and materials must be checked to ensure that all needles, sponges, and instruments are accounted for. In addition, specimens must be labeled and sent to the laboratory. The entire process requires a thorough understanding of the principles of asepsis, anatomy, and tissue care; an awareness of the objectives of the surgery; the knowledge and skill to anticipate needs and work as a skilled member of a team; and the ability to handle any emergency situation in the operating room.

Basic Rules of Surgical Asepsis

General

- Sterile surfaces or articles may touch other sterile surfaces or articles and remain sterile; unsterile contact at ~ny point renders a sterile area contaminated.
- ~ is any doubt about the sterility of an article or ~nsidered unsterile.
- ~ile for one patient (an opened sterile ~ile supplies) can be used for this

patient only. Unused sterile supplies must be discarded or resterilized if they are to be used again.

Personnel

- Scrubbed personnel remain in the area of the operation; if a "scrubbed" person leaves the room, that person's "sterile" status is lost. To return to the operation, this person is required to go through the procedure of scrubbing, gowning, and gloving.
- Only a small part of a "scrubbed" person's body is considered sterile: from front waist to the shoulder area; forearms and gloves.
- Therefore, the gloved hands must be kept in front and above the waistline.
- In some clinics, a special wraparound gown is worn, which extends the sterile area.
- The "circulator" and any unscrubbed personnel remain on the periphery of the surgical operating area at a safe distance in order not to contaminate any sterile area.

Draping

- During draping of a table or patient, the sterile drape is held well above the surface to be covered and is positioned from front to back.
- Only the top of the patient or table that is draped is considered sterile; drapes hanging over the edge are not regarded as sterile.
- Sterile drapes are to be kept in position by the use of clips or adherent material; drapes are not to be moved during the operation. A tear or puncture of the drape permitting access to an unsterile surface underneath renders the area unsterile. Such a drape must be replaced.

Delivery of Sterile Supplies

- Packages are wrapped or sealed in such a way that they can be opened easily without risk of contaminating contents.
- Sterile supplies, including solutions, are delivered to a sterile field or handed to a "scrubbed" person in such a way that sterility of the object or fluid remains intact.
- Edges of wrappers covering sterile supplies or outer lips of bottles or flasks containing sterile solutions are not considered sterile.
- The unsterile arm of the "circulator" must not extend over a sterile area. Sterile articles are to be dropped at a reasonable distance from the edge of the sterile area.

Fluids

- Sterile fluids are poured from a point high enough to prevent accidental touching of the sterile receiving cup or basin, but not so high as to produce splashing (this may cause fluid to touch an unsterile surface and then flow back into the receptacle, causing contamination).

▷ **Bibliography**

See Bibliography at the end of Chapter 21.

Postoperative Nursing Management

The goals of nursing care in the postoperative period are directed toward the reestablishment of the patient's physiologic equilibrium and the prevention of pain and complications. Careful assessment and immediate intervention will assist the patient in planning his return to normal function as quickly, safely, and comfortably as possible.

Considerable effort is expended on *anticipation* and *prevention* of difficulties in the postoperative period. The nursing care of the patient after operation is second in importance only to the operation itself.

▷ Removing the Patient From the Operating Table

The patient is moved from the operating table to the bed or the stretcher with the least possible delay and exposure. The site of the operation should be kept in mind every time a newly operated patient is moved. Many wounds are closed under considerable tension, and every effort should be made not to place any further strain on the sutures. Thus, in thyroid operations, the patient's head is not allowed to hyperextend; in breast amputations, the arm of the operated side is held close to the body; in nephrectomy, the patient is not allowed to lie on the affected side.

Serious arterial hypotension may occur when a patient is moved from one position to another, such as from a lithotomy position to a horizontal position, from a lateral to a supine position, or from a prone to a supine position. Even moving the anesthetized patient to the stretcher can precipitate this problem. Thus, the patient must be moved slowly and carefully.

As soon as the patient is placed on the stretcher or bed, he is covered with lightweight blankets that have been arranged previously on the stretcher. The wet and soiled gown should be removed, a dry gown applied, and the bedding tucked in along the sides as well as at the bottom. On the stretcher the patient is held with straps above the knees and the elbows. The straps serve the double purpose of securing the blankets and of restraining the patient, should he pass through a stage of excitement as he recovers from the anesthetic. Side rails are raised to the position affording protection.

Transferring the Patient

Transfer of the postoperative patient from surgery to the recovery room is the responsibility of the anesthesiologist, with a member of the surgical team in attendance. Additional assistance may be provided by a nurse assigned to this particular patient. Transfer of the patient is done expeditiously, with special attention paid in transit to comfort, safety, and general condition. Various tubes and receptacles are handled carefully for optimum function.

▷ Recovery Room

The recovery room is a unit usually located adjacent to the operating rooms. Patients who are still under anesthesia or are recovering from it are placed in this unit for easy access to (1) nurses who are especially prepared in caring for the immediate postoperative patient, (2) anesthesiologists and surgeons, and (3) special equipment, medications, and replacement fluids. In this setting, the newly operated patient is given the best care available by those best qualified to give it.

The room should be quiet, neat and clean, and free of unnecessary equipment. It should also have (1) walls and ceiling painted in soft, pleasing colors; (2) indirect lighting; (3) soundproof ceiling; (4) equipment that controls or eliminates noise (*e.g.,* synthetic emesis basins, rubber bumpers on beds and tables); and (5) isolated quarters (glass encased) for noisy patients. These seemingly luxurious features may be added at little extra cost, yet psychologically they are of real value to the patient.

Equipment includes every type of breathing aid: oxygen, laryngoscopes, tracheotomy sets, bronchial instruments, catheters, mechanical ventilators, and suction equipment; another necessity is equipment for meeting circulatory needs, such as blood pressure apparatus, parenteral equipment, universal donor blood, plasma expanders, intravenous trays and cutdown trays, cardiac arrest equipment, defibrillator, venous catheters, and tourniquets. Surgical dressing materials, narcotics, and emergency drugs should also be available, as well as catheterization sets and drainage equipment. In addition, monitoring devices may be at hand to provide an accurate and instant appraisal of the patient's condition.

The recovery bed should be one that affords easy access to the patient, is safe and easily movable, can readily be placed in shock position, and possesses features that facilitate care, such as available receptacles for intravenous poles, side guards, wheel brakes, and chart storage rack.

The temperature of the room should be about 20° C to 22.2° C (68° F–70° F) with good ventilation.

A patient remains in this unit until he has fully recovered from the anesthetic agent, that is, has a stable blood pressure, good air passage, and a reasonable degree of consciousness.

▷ Immediate Postoperative Nursing Care

The recovery room nurse who receives the patient reviews the following with the physician: (1) the patient's general condition—age, airway, blood pressure, pulse, and respiration; (2) the operation performed; (3) the kind of anesthetic used; (4) any untoward problem(s) that occurred in the operating room that may have a bearing on postoperative care (*e.g.,* extensive hemorrhage, shock, cardiac arrest); (5) any pathology encountered (if malignancy, whether the patient or his family have been informed); (6) any tubing, drains, catheters, infusions, or other supportive aids that may have been instituted in the operating room; (7) complications to anticipate; (8) special symptoms to watch for; (9) immediate postoperative directives (in writing); and (10) anything special the surgeon or anesthesiologist wishes to be notified about.

Postanesthesia Recovery Room Scoring Guide

Many hospitals use a scoring system to determine the patient's general condition and his readiness to be released from the recovery room. As the patient progresses through the recovery period, his physical signs are observed and evaluated by means of an objective scoring guide, which provides a set of criteria useful to the recovery room staff in assessing the patient's condition following surgery and anesthesia. This evaluation system, a modification of the Apgar score, makes possible a more objective evaluation of the patient's physical condition in the recovery area.

The patient's score is taken at stated intervals, such as every 15 or 30 minutes, and totaled on the official scorecard (Chart 21-1). A patient with a total score of less than 7 must remain in the recovery room until his condition improves or he is transferred to an intensive care area.

Respiratory Considerations

- *The chief immediate postoperative hazards are those of shock and hypoxemia due to respiratory difficulties.*

Shock can be avoided largely by the timely administration of intravenous fluids and blood and by appropriate drugs. The *respiratory difficulties* may be treated as they arise, or better, the patient can be treated so that they do not arise. These disturbances are confined almost entirely to those patients who are under prolonged or deep anesthesia. Patients given local anesthesia or nitrous oxide usually are "awake" a few minutes after leaving the operating room. However, those patients who have experienced prolonged anesthesia usually are completely unconscious, with all muscles relaxed. This relaxation extends to the muscles of the pharynx; therefore, when the patient lies on his back the lower jaw and the tongue fall backward, and the air passages close more or less completely (Fig. 21-1*A*). Signs of this difficulty include choking, noisy and irregular respirations, and, in a short time, a blue duskiness (cyanosis) of the skin.

- The treatment of hypopharyngeal obstruction involves tilting the head back and pushing forward on the angle of the lower jaw, as if to push the lower teeth in front of the upper teeth (Fig. 21-1*B, C*).

Chart 21-1
Post-Anesthesia Recovery Room Scoring Card

Patient: Smith, Raymond
Room: B 1083
Date: 3/7/

POST-ANESTHESIA RECOVERY ROOM
SCORING CARD

Final Score: 10
Physician: Dr. J. Evans
Nurse: Mrs. Peggy Fay, R.N.

Physical Signs →	ACTIVITY		RESPIRATION		CIRCULATION		CONSCIOUSNESS		COLOR		TOTAL SCORE
TIME ↓	Score	Comment	Score	Comment	Score	Comment	Score	Comment	Score	Comment	
Admission A.M. 11:15 P.M.	1	Spinal anesth.	1	chest & abdom. pain	1		1	Semi-conscious	1		5
½ Hour A.M. 11:45 P.M.	1		1		2		1		1	slight pallor	6
½ Hour A.M. P.M.											
Dismissal A.M. 12:15 P.M.	2		2		2		2	alert verbally responsive	2	color improved	10
FINAL SCORE A.M. P.M.	2		2		2		2		2		10

PHYSICAL SIGNS AND CRITERIA FOR THEIR ASSESSMENT

1. ACTIVITY
Muscle activity is assessed by observing the ability of the patient to move his extremities spontaneously or on command.
   Score: 2—able to move all extremities
   1—able to move 2 extremities
   0—not able to control any extremity

2. RESPIRATION
Respiratory efficiency evaluated in a form that permits accurate and objective assessment without complicated physical tests
   Score: 2—able to breathe deeply and cough
   1—limited respiratory effort (dyspnea or splinting)
   0—no spontaneous respiratory effort

3. CIRCULATION
Use changes in arterial blood pressure from preanesthetic level

   Score: 2—systolic arterial pressure between plus or minus 20% of preanesthetic level (Rica-Rocci method)
   1—systolic arterial pressure between plus or minus 20% to 50% of preanesthetic level
   0—systolic arterial pressure between plus or minus 50% or more of the preanesthetic level

4. CONSCIOUSNESS
Determination of the patient's level of consciousness.
   Score: 2—full alertness seen in patient's ability to answer questions and acknowledge his/her location
   1—aroused when called by name
   0—failure to elicit a response upon auditory
Physical stimulation should not be considered reliable since even a decerebrated patient might react to it.

5. COLOR
   Score: 2—normal skin color and appearance
   1—any alteration in skin color: pale, dusky, blotchy, jaundiced, etc.
   0—frank cyanosis

* (Adapted from Fay MR: Introduction to Recovery Room Nursing, pp 11, 29. Denver, Association of OR Nurses)

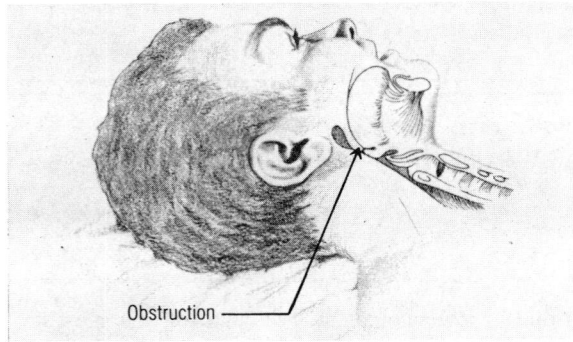

Figure 21-1. Treatment of hypopharyngeal obstruction. (Reprinted with permission from Nursing Update, May 1972.)

A. Hypopharyngeal obstruction always occurs when the neck is flexed and almost always when the head is in the midposition.

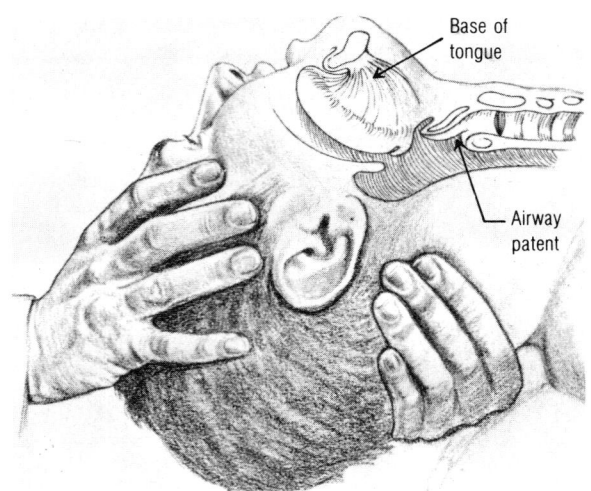

B. Tilting the head back to stretch the anterior neck structure will cause the base of the tongue to be lifted off the posterior pharyngeal wall.

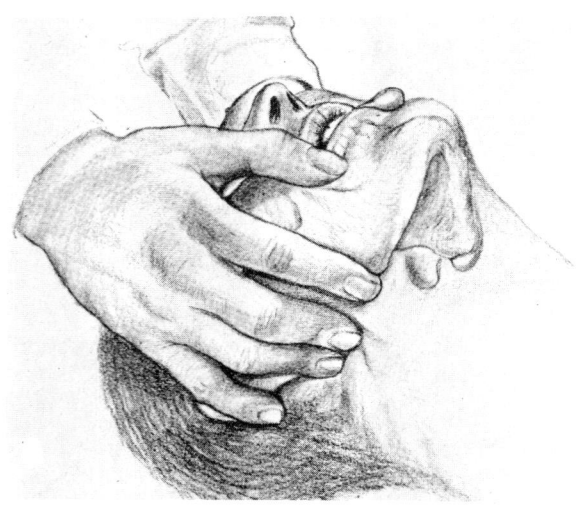

C. Opening the mouth is necessary to correct valvelike obstruction of the nasal passage during expiration, which occurs in about 30% of unconscious patients. Open the patient's mouth (separate lips and teeth) and move the lower jaw forward so that the lower teeth are in front of the upper teeth. To regain backward tilt of the neck, lift with both hands at the ascending rami of the mandible.

This maneuver pulls the tongue forward and opens the air passages. At times it may be necessary to grasp the tongue between layers of gauze and pull it forward for a time. This maneuver prevents respiratory obstruction and is continued when necessary until the patient has regained reflex functions sufficiently to carry on normal respiration.

Often the anesthesiologist leaves a hard rubber or plastic "airway" in the mouth (Fig. 21-2) or a rubber nasal catheter in the nose. Either device can be used to maintain a patent airway. Such a device should not be removed until there are signs, such as gagging, that reflex action is returning.

Occasionally, a patient may be brought to the recovery room with an endotracheal tube still in place and may require continued mechanical ventilation. The nurse will then assist in the preparation of the respirator and in the weaning and extubation procedures.

Not infrequently, respiratory difficulty is produced by an excessive secretion of mucus. Turning the head to the side allows the collected fluid to escape from the side of the mouth. If the patient's teeth are clenched, his mouth may be opened by the method described in Figure 21-3*A*. If vomiting occurs, the head should be turned to the side and the vomitus collected in the emesis basin. The face should be wiped with gauze or paper wipes.

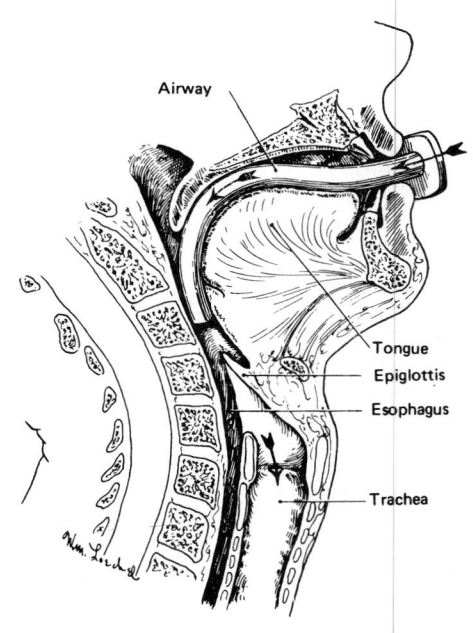

Figure 21-2. Diagrammatic view showing a method by which an "airway" prevents respiratory difficulty after anesthesia. The airway passes over the base of the tongue and delivers air into the pharynx in the region of the epiglottis. Patients are often brought from the operating room with an airway in place. This should remain in place until the patient recovers sufficiently to breathe normally. Usually, as the patient regains consciousness, the airway causes irritation; then it should be removed.

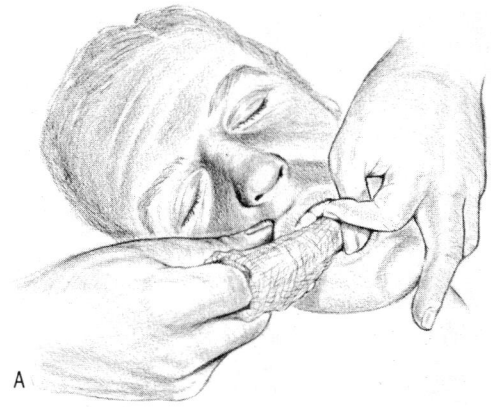 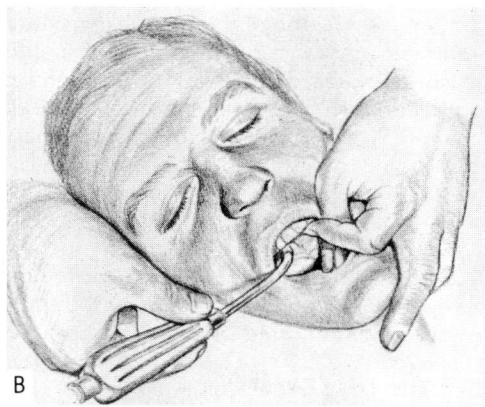

Figure 21-3. (*A*) To maintain a patent airway, it may be necessary to clear the upper airway manually or with suction. If the teeth are clenched, place your thumb against the lower teeth and your index finger against the upper teeth; open the mouth by crossing the thumb and index finger for better leverage. If the teeth are tightly clenched, insert the tip of your index finger behind the last molar and pry open. Circumstances may permit only manual clearing, as illustrated. When possible, use mechanical suction (*B*) or catheter. Suction equipment powerful enough to clear semi-solid materials from the pharynx should produce a negative pressure of at least 300 mm Hg when occluded and a flow of at least 30 liters per minute when open. (Reprinted with permission from Nursing Update, May 1972.)

Mucus or vomitus obstructing the pharynx or the trachea should be aspirated with a pharyngeal suction tip (Fig. 21-3*B*) or a nasal catheter introduced into the nasopharynx or the oropharynx. In most recovery rooms, wall suction or suction machines are available for this purpose. The catheter can be passed into the nasopharynx or the oropharynx at a safe distance of 15 cm to 20 cm (6–8 inches) if secretions are obtained at this level.

- The only sure way of knowing whether a patient is breathing or not is to place the palm of the hand over the patient's nose and mouth in order to feel the exhaled breath. Movements of the thorax and the diaphragm do not necessarily mean that a patient is breathing.

Other Considerations

The function of the recovery room nurse cannot be limited to bedside procedures, safety measures, and the relief of pain; an understanding of the significance of psychological support is also important. If the nurse has never seen the patient before, a definite handicap is immediately presented. The nurse who knows the patient and accompanies him through the immediate preoperative and operative experiences is in a unique position to offer valuable support. In the absence of such continuous care by one nurse, pertinent nurses' notes on the chart help the recovery room nurse to recognize the particular needs of each individual patient.

▷ Goals of Postoperative Nursing Care

The major goal of postoperative nursing care is to assist the patient to return to normal function as rapidly, safely, and comfortably as possible. The specific objectives related to this goal may be listed as follows:

1. To assist the patient in maintaining optimum respiratory function
2. To assess the cardiovascular status of the patient and correct any deviations
3. To promote the comfort and safety of the patient
4. To promote homeostasis through maintenance of fluid and electrolyte balance, proper nutrition, and adequate elimination
5. To enhance wound healing and avoid or control infection
6. To encourage activity through early exercises, ambulation, and rehabilitation
7. To minister to the psychosocial well-being of the patient and his family
8. To document all phases of the nursing process and report pertinent data

1. *To assist the patient in maintaining optimum respiratory function*

Maintaining a patent airway is discussed in the section immediately preceding this.

Positioning. Until the patient regains consciousness, the bed is kept flat. Unless contraindicated, the unconscious patient is positioned on his side with a pillow at his back and with his chin extended to minimize any danger of aspiration. His knees are flexed to reduce strain on abdominal sutures.

Clearing the Airway. If the patient vomits, he should be turned on his side, and the nature and amount of the vomitus should be recorded. At the end of the vomiting episode, the patient's lips and mouth should be wiped with paper tissues and gauze. To relieve thirst, his lips should be moistened.

If frequent aspiration of the nasopharynx and oropharynx is indicated, a clean aspirating catheter should be used and a basin of water kept nearby to flush and clean the catheter. Caution is necessary in suctioning the throat of a patient who has had a tonsillectomy, since the operative area may become irritated, causing bleeding and added discomfort.

Coughing is encouraged to dislodge mucous plugs; careful splinting of abdominal or thoracic incision sites is helpful in helping the patient overcome the feeling that the wound might break open. It is important to remember that coughing is contraindicated in patients who have had eye or plastic surgery.

Promoting Lung Expansion. To encourage lung expansion and exchange of gas, a variety of measures may be followed. For example, having the patient yawn or take sustained maximal inspirations (SMI) will create a negative intrathoracic pressure of minus 40 mm Hg and will expand lung volume to total capacity. During this maneuver, right atrial and pulmonary artery pressures decrease while venous return and cardiac output (CO) increase.

Incentive Spirometry. This is a method by which the patient performs SMI and at the same time sees the results of his efforts as registered on the spirometer equipment. Such motivation hopefully encourages the patient to continue to take deep breaths in order to maximize voluntary lung expansion (Fig. 21-4). The patient needs to be taught how to use the device.

An example of this type of equipment is the Spirocare Incentive Breathing Exerciser, an electric device that functions on a feedback system. When the patient is inhaling, the digital electronic circuitry approximates the patient's breathing performance. An automatic record is made of the number of patient maneuvers and the Exerciser is set for the preselected patient target. This number is illuminated on the panel, showing the patient very vividly what his breathing goal is. When he inhales, the lower registers are the first to light up; subsequent higher numbers are illuminated until the prescribed goal is reached. The combined features of the equipment offer the following advantages:

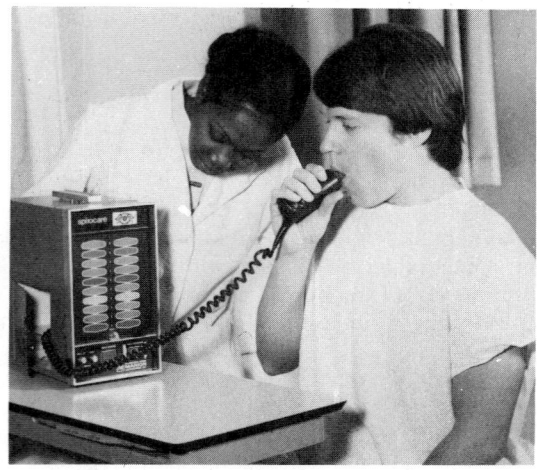

Figure 21-4. Incentive spirometry.

(1) the patient is encouraged to actively participate in his own treatment; (2) it assures that the maneuver will be physiologically appropriate and repeated; (3) it makes a record of the frequency of performance, which provides data for assessment by the nurse, physician, and respiratory therapist; (4) it is a prophylactic device, thereby helping to prevent complication; and (5) it is cost-effective.

Intermittent Positive Pressure Breathing (IPPB). IPPB therapy has been used extensively as a means of promoting lung expansion. However, its effectiveness in reducing postoperative pulmonary complications continues to be scrutinized. Often when it is used, the patient is not instructed to hold his breath at the end of inspiration, and he may not be encouraged to cough following the treatment. These oversights defeat the purpose of IPPB. In addition, when used improperly, IPPB may cause air swallowing, with resultant gastric dilatation and further ventilatory compromise. Similarly, the use of the *blow bottles* technique is being studied for its actual effectiveness in reducing postoperative pulmonary complications. When used correctly— that is, when the patient takes sustained deep breaths and then slowly blows the air out—a slight increase in functional residual capacity is achieved. Unfortunately, the patient usually blows out with greater attention to expiration than inspiration, which leads to rapid reduction in lung volume and results in closure of airways.

Rebreathing Carbon Dioxide. Another less frequently used method for stimulating deep respirations is to have the patient inhale carbon dioxide. This may be accomplished by means of a face mask attached to a gas tank or simply by instructing the patient to blow in and out of a paper bag. Most studies indicate that the tidal volume is not increased to total lung capacity and that hypoxemia will be produced with dead space rebreathing. Because of this, the actual volume of carbon dioxide rebreathing is questionable and may even be hazardous in patients with cardiorespiratory diseases.

Doxapram. Finally, in patients *unable* to cooperate in incentive breathing exercises, doxapram may be helpful; this is a selective respiratory stimulant given intravenously to stimulate carotid chemoreceptors, which then mediate increases in the rate and depth of ventilation. (See Respiratory Complications, p. 409.)

Expected Patient Outcome: Maintains optimal respiratory function

- Shows evidence of normal parameters of respiratory function (clear breath sounds, regular rhythm and rate of respirations, normal arterial blood gases, normal chest x-rays)
- Performs deep-breathing exercises
- Uses incentive spirometer as directed

2. To assess the cardiovascular status of the patient and correct any deviations

The basic consideration in assessing cardiovascular function is monitoring the patient for signs of shock and hemorrhage. The chief guides are the patient's appearance and determinations of pulse, respiration, blood pressure, temperature, central venous pressure (CVP), and blood gas. CVP and blood gas readings are monitored if required by the patient's condition. The pulse and respiration should be noted at frequent intervals for the first 2 hours, and every ½ hour for the next 2 hours. Thereafter, they may be taken less frequently if they remain stable. The blood pressure is taken as often as indicated.

- A temperature over 37.7° C (100° F) or under 36.1° C (97° F), respirations over 30 or under 16, and a systolic blood pressure under 90 are usually considered reportable at once.

However, the patient's preoperative or baseline blood pressure should be known in order to make effective postoperative comparisons.

- A blood pressure that shows a downward trend of 5 mm Hg to 10 mm Hg at each reading should also alert the nurse to a problem.

The general condition of the patient is assessed and recorded, including whether his color is good or cyanotic, his skin cold and clammy or warm and moist, or if there is excessive mucus in the throat and in the nostrils.

Expected Patient Outcomes: (1) Maintains integrity of cardiovascular functioning. (2) Attains preoperative levels of the following parameters:

- Blood pressure, pulse, respirations, and temperature
- Central venous pressure
- Peripheral pulses
- Skin color and temperature

3. To promote the comfort and safety of the patient

A patient coming out of anesthesia may display restless behavior. If it is at all possible, he should not be restrained, but he must be protected from injuring himself or interfering with IV therapy since an infusion is usually running. If the arm is splinted, the needle will not be dislodged. However, the patient can pull the needle out with his free hand.

If the patient has been placed between blankets, they should be removed on complete recovery from the anesthesia—when the temperature, pulse, and respirations are within normal limits. Or the blankets may be removed when they are the cause of excessive perspiration. Recovery beds are made in such a manner that the patient is left between sheets when blankets are withdrawn. Cool sheets usually are a gratifying change and often very soothing. However, care must be taken that the patient is not chilled. Remember that patients who have been anesthetized are susceptible to chills and drafts. Remember also that the obese patient perspires profusely and so loses fluid and salt much more rapidly than the patient who is of normal weight.

Hampered by dressings, splints, or drainage apparatus, the patient very frequently is quite unable to shift his position. Lying constantly in the same position may lead to pressure sores or hypostatic pneumonia, to mention only two of the more serious resulting complications.

- The helpless patient must be turned from side to side at least every 2 hours, and his position must be changed as soon as he becomes uncomfortable.

Simple comfort measures include turning a pillow from side to side so that the patient can rest against a cool surface and providing proper support for the arms and hands, as well as for the feet, so that the patient can stretch his foot muscles and spread his toes.

It is comforting and soothing to the patient coming out of anesthesia to have cool cloths applied to his forehead. Moistening the patient's lips with a cool gauze sponge when water by mouth is *not* permitted may also be comforting. When convenient, a soothing back rub with lotion or alcohol is appreciated.

- The extremities may be stroked very lightly with alcohol. *They never should be rubbed vigorously.* To do so may dislodge a thrombus and result in embolism and death.

Restlessness and Discomfort. Restlessness is a postoperative symptom that should not be passed over lightly. The most common cause probably is general discomfort from the operation owing to the patient's lying in one position on the operating table, the surgeon's handling of tissues, and the body's reaction to recovering from the anesthetic. These discomforts may be relieved by giving the prescribed postoperative sedation and changing the patient's position frequently. At the same time, the nurse will assess other possible contributing causes, such as tight drainage-soaked bandages. Reinforcing or changing the dressing completely will make the patient more comfortable. Urinary output is noted and the patient is observed for urinary retention. Overdistention of the bladder is to be avoided. If possible, the patient should be helped to assume as normal a position as possible for voiding. Various techniques are tried to encourage voiding before resorting to catheterization.

Flatulence and hiccups are other causes of discomfort. Their recognition and treatment are discussed on page 394. Probably the most serious cause of restlessness is hemorrhage. This is discussed on page 407.

Pain. Many psychological factors (motivational, affective, cognitive, and emotional) influence the patient's total pain experience. Recent findings have led to a better understanding of how one's perception, learning, personality, ethnic and cultural factors, and even environment can affect anxiety, depression, and pain significance. The degree and severity of postoperative pain depends on the physiologic and psychological makeup of the person, the subsequent tolerance level, the incision site and the nature of the operation, the extent of surgical trauma, and the kind of anesthetic agent and how it was administered.

The preoperative preparation, including informing the patient what to expect and providing reassurance and psychological support, is a significant factor in decreasing anxiety, apprehension, and even the pain experienced in the postoperative period.

In regard to the need for narcotics, about one third of patients complain of severe pain, one third of moderate pain, and one third of little or no pain. The latter does not mean that these patients have no pain, but they appear to activate psychodynamic mechanisms that impair the registering of pain ("gate closing" theory and impaired nociceptive transmission). It is interesting to note that one third of patients will receive relief from a placebo. Elderly persons react less to postoperative pain than young adults.

Morphine or meperidine hydrochloride (Demerol) often is prescribed for pain and immediate postoperative restlessness. The time of administration frequently is left to the judgment of the nurse, but one should realize that pain in the first 24 hours after an operation requires relief by narcotics, and these drugs should not be denied when the patient is in pain. Complete pain relief in the operative region is seldom attainable; however, changing the patient's position, washing his face, and rubbing his back with a soothing lotion may be useful in assuaging general discomfort temporarily and rendering the hypodermic medication more effectual when it is given.

Expected Patient Outcome: Attains comfort and safety

- Rests at long intervals
- Experiences pain relief through use of analgesics
- Responds appropriately to stimuli
- Attains normal sensorium

4. *To promote homeostasis through maintenance of fluid and electrolyte balance, proper nutrition, and adequate elimination*

Fluid Balance.   Any drainage apparatus, such as nasogastric tube, cholecystostomy or choledochostomy tubes, catheters, enterostomy drains, and chest tubes, should be attached when drainage is to be collected. In case of underwater drainage tubes, such as those used after thoracotomy, clamps should be available to occlude the tube in order to prevent air from entering the chest if the drainage receptacle is accidentally disturbed or the apparatus disconnected.

If permissible, the patient should be offered water in small quantities when nausea ceases. If small amounts are retained by the patient, the quantity given at one time may be increased gradually. Water is best either hot or cold; otherwise, it is likely to cause nausea. There are times when a large glass of water will do a patient no harm, even when he is nauseated, but this never should be given unless prescribed. At times, patients ask for cracked ice, and usually it does no harm when given in small amounts. If orders are that the patient is to have nothing by mouth, cracked ice wrapped in a piece of gauze is refreshing and soothing to the lips.

Diet.   Following surgery, the more rapidly the patient can accept his usual diet, the more quickly will his normal gastrointestinal function resume. The best method for the postoperative patient to take food is by mouth. This stimulates digestive juices and promotes gastric function and intestinal peristalsis. Exercise in bed or early ambulation also assists the digestive process and prevents such problems as distention "gas pains" and constipation. Chewing of food prevents parotitis (inflammation of the parotid glands), a formerly common postoperative problem that occurred in dehydrated patients who also practiced poor mouth hygiene.

The return to a normal dietary pattern should proceed at the pace set by the individual patient. Of course, the nature of surgery and the type of anesthesia directly affect the rate of return. Once the patient has completely recovered from the effects of anesthesia and is no longer nauseated, steps may be taken to restore his normal diet.

Liquids are usually the first substances desired and tolerated by the patient after operation. Water, fruit juices, and tea with lemon and sugar may be given in increasing amounts if vomiting does not occur. The fluids administered should be cool, not ice cold or tepid. Since fluids supply relatively few calories and are tolerated well, gelatin, junket, custard and even buttered toast, milk, and creamed soups may be added gradually. As soon as the patient tolerates soft foods well, solid food may be given.

A well-balanced diet should be provided and should include foods that have been selected and preferred by the patient. Usually it takes 2 to 3 days for appetite to return, so that attractive trays are a therapeutic consideration.

- When surgery has been done on the gastrointestinal tract, fluids and food are not given until peristalsis returns.

The nurse can determine when peristaltic bowel sounds return by listening to the abdomen with a stethoscope. This activity of bowel sounds is reported so that the proper diet modification can be prescribed.

Usually, a nasogastric or gastrointestinal tube is in place for the first 24 to 48 hours following gastrointestinal surgery. Such decompression tubes remove flatus and secretions. Attention is given to the maintenance of proper fluid and electrolyte balance, and an attempt is made with parenteral fluids and perhaps even hyperalimentation to achieve this nutritional level (see Chap. 36, p. 780).

When nothing is given by mouth postoperatively, conscientious mouth hygiene is required.

Urination.   The length of time a patient may be permitted to go without voiding after operation varies considerably with the type of operation performed. Following gynecologic and abdominal operations, catheterization may be required at the end of 8 or 10 hours (sometimes sooner), whereas after other operations it may be put off for 16 to 18 hours.

- Generally speaking, every effort must be made to avoid the use of a catheter.

All known methods to aid the patient in voiding should be tried—letting water run, applying heat, etc. A patient should never be given a cold bedpan. When a patient complains of not being able to use the bedpan, it may be permissible to use a commode rather than resort to catheterization. Male patients sometimes are permitted to sit up or stand beside the bed, but safeguards should be taken to prevent any accidents due to the patient's falling or fainting.

- All urine, whether voided or catheterized, must be measured and the amount noted on the nurse's record.
- An intake and output chart should be kept on all patients following urologic or complex operative procedures and on all aged persons.

Defecation.   Each defecation is recorded. If the bowels do not move spontaneously every other day, a cleansing enema usually is given. As a rule, cathartics are not given to postoperative patients, especially if the operation has been on the abdomen.

Expected Patient Outcome: Attains fluid and electrolyte balance, proper nutrition, and adequate elimination

- Increases fluid intake gradually
- Maintains adequate urinary output
- Resumes normal dietary patterns as appropriate
- Attains active bowel function as indicated by bowel sounds
- Voids adequately without use of catheter

5. *To enhance wound healing and avoid or control infection*

Dressings are inspected periodically to detect signs of undue hemorrhage or abnormal drainage. For incisions on the anterior part of the body, the posterior area is checked for signs of bleeding, since gravity assists in permitting seepage to accumulate in an area quite removed from the incision. Dressings should be reinforced, if necessary, and the time noted on the nurses' record.

Dressings and care of the incision are discussed further on pages 400–401.

Nosocomial Infections. Between 10% and 15% of surgical patients will develop nosocomial (hospital-acquired) infections. Most of these will be in one of four anatomical sites: surgical wound, urinary tract, bloodstream, and respiratory tract. These occur for several reasons:

- Intact skin and mucous membranes have been invaded by tubes and catheters, by the disease process, or by the surgical operation.
- The effects of anesthesia and surgery reduce the resistance of the body.
- The patient environment is made up of many persons who have complicating and often chronic medical problems; consequently, the patient is predisposed to infection.
- The organisms that are found in hospital infections are widespread and resistive: *Staphylococcus aureus, Escherichia coli, Serratia marcescens, Pseudomonas, Klebsiella pneumoniae, Enterobacteriaceae,* and *Proteus.*
- Poor handwashing practices and careless techniques are used.

Each hospital must make an all-out effort to control infections by an intensive education program that reaches every employee. Usually an active Infection Control Committee (including an epidemiologist) can be effective in establishing policies and procedures, and monitoring practice. Conscientious handwashing is essential for every person who comes in contact with patients and moves from one patient to the next. Judicious control of upper respiratory infections and skin lesions must be practiced. A most common cause of infections is contamination related to intravenous infusions (see p. 158 for methods of control). Effective postanesthetic recovery with good cough reflex, frequent turning, and deep breathing by the patient will prevent secretions from being retained and possibly causing atelectasis, lung congestion, and pneumonia. Sterilization of all needles, cannulae, etc., including equipment used in respiratory management, will prevent transmission of pathogenic organisms. Antibiotics are to be prescribed prophylactically when infected areas are encountered, and antimicrobials are to be specifically prescribed for identified organisms in established infections. The nurse plays a key role in infection control by practicing flawless technique and by conscientiously monitoring others.

Expected Patient Outcome: Attains skin integrity

- Is free from redness, warmth, and swelling at incisional area
- Shows evidence of minimal or no drainage
- Applies cocoa butter or other soothing ointments as prescribed
- Identifies initial symptoms of hematoma, injury, and infection
- Changes dressing if necessary

6. *To encourage activity through early exercises, ambulation, and rehabilitation*

Positioning.   Following surgery, the patient may be placed in a variety of positions (depending on the nature of the operation) to promote comfort and ease pain.

Dorsal Position.   The patient lies on his back without elevation of the head. In most cases this is the position in which the patient is placed immediately after operation. The head usually is turned to one side to facilitate easy evacuation of vomitus and to prevent its aspiration into the lungs. Bed covers should not restrict the movement of the toes and the feet of the patient.

This position may be employed to advantage many times when the necessity for drainage does not require the Fowler position. It is believed that when the patient is flat in bed, respiration often is more free and turning is easier, advantages that are important in the prevention of respiratory complications.

Sims' or Lateral Position.   The patient lies on either side with the upper arm forward. The under leg is slightly flexed, while the upper leg is flexed at the thigh and the knee. The head is supported on a pillow, and a second pillow is placed longitudinally under the flexed knee. This position is used when it is desirable to have the patient change position frequently, to aid in the drainage of cavities, such as chest and abdomen, and to prevent postoperative pulmonary, respiratory, and circulatory complications.

Fowler Position.   Of all the positions prescribed for a patient, perhaps the most common, as well as the most difficult to maintain, is the Fowler position. The difficulty in most instances lies in trying to make the patient fit the bed rather than having the bed conform to the needs of the patient. The patient's trunk is raised to form an angle of from 60 to 70 degrees with the horizontal plane. This is a comfortable sitting position. Patients with abdominal drainage usually are put in a Fowler position as soon as they have recovered consciousness, but great caution must be observed in raising the bed.

- It is not unusual for a patient to feel faint after the head of the bed is raised; for this reason, a close watch must be kept on pulse rate and color. If the patient complains of any dizziness, the bed must be slowly lowered.

However, if the condition of the patient is good, the head of the bed may be raised within 1 to 2 hours.

The nurse must determine whether the patient is in correct position and comfortable. Often, very short people are most uncomfortable in the ordinary hospital bed and must be supported by pillows. It is advisable to place a support against the feet to prevent the patient from slipping down in bed, to prevent foot drop, and to make the patient feel more secure.

It is the nurse's responsibility to see that the Fowler position is maintained at all times. No matter how correctly placed or how well supported by pillows the patient is, he will slip down in the course of time. Thus, it will be necessary to move the patient up in bed frequently and to readjust the pillows.

Jackknife, or Semi-Fowler Position. This position is one used to relieve tension following the repair of inguinal or abdominal hernia. It is achieved by raising the head of the patient about 25 cm to 30 cm (10–12 inches) and flexing the knees.

Ambulation. Most surgical patients are allowed and encouraged to be out of bed within 24 to 48 hours after operation.

- The advantage of early ambulation is that it reduces postoperative complications such as atelectasis, hypostatic pneumonia, gastrointestinal discomfort, and circulatory problems.

Atelectasis and hypostatic pneumonia are relatively infrequent when the patient is ambulatory, since ambulation increases respiratory exchange and aids in preventing stasis of bronchial secretions within the lung. Ambulation also reduces the possibility of postoperative distention because it helps to increase the tone of the gastrointestinal tract and the abdominal wall. Therefore, frequent enemas are unnecessary.

Thrombophlebitis or phlebothrombosis are less frequent because ambulation, by increasing the rate of circulation in the extremities, prevents stasis of venous blood. Clinical as well as experimental evidence shows that the rate of healing in abdominal wounds is more rapid when ambulation is started early, and the occurrence of postoperative evisceration in a series of cases actually was less frequent when patients were allowed to be out of bed soon after operation. Statistics also indicate that pain is decreased when early ambulation is allowed. Comparative records show that the pulse rate and the temperature return to normal sooner when the patient attempts to regain his normal preoperative activity as quickly as possible. Finally, there are the further advantages to the patient of a shorter stay in the hospital, with the consequent lower expense.

However, early ambulation should not be overdone. The condition of the patient must be the deciding factor, and a progression of steps must be followed in getting the patient out of bed.

1. First of all, the patient must be placed almost upright in bed until all suggestion of dizziness has passed. This position can be obtained by raising the head of the bed.
2. Then, he may be placed completely upright and turned so that his legs hang over the edge of the bed.
3. After this preparation, the patient may be helped to stand beside his bed.

When the patient has become accustomed to the upright position, he may start to walk. The nurse should be at his side to give support, both physical and moral. Care must be taken not to tire the patient, and the extent of the first few periods of ambulation will vary with the type of operation and the physical condition and age of the patient.

Bed Exercises. When early ambulation is not feasible because of circumstances already mentioned, *bed exercises* may achieve the same desirable results to some extent. General exercises should begin as soon after operation as possible—preferably within the first 24 hours—and they should be done under supervision to ensure their adequacy. These exercises are done to promote circulation and prevent the development of contractures and other deformities as well as to permit the patient the fullest return of his physiologic functions. Such exercises include:

1. Deep-breathing exercises for complete lung expansion
2. Arm exercises through full range of motion, with specific attention to abduction and external rotation of the shoulder
3. Hand and finger exercises
4. Foot exercises to prevent foot drop and toe deformities and to aid in maintaining good circulation. A plastic ball under the covers may be a help in reminding the patient to exercise his leg muscles. Grasping the ball with the toes contracts calf muscles, stimulates circulation, and reduces venous stasis.
5. Exercises to prepare the patient for ambulation activities
6. Abdominal and gluteal contraction exercises

Expected Patient Outcome: Resumes mobility

- Alternates periods of rest and activity
- Increases ambulation progressively
- Resumes normal activities within prescribed time frame

7. *To minister to the psychosocial well-being of the patient and his family*

Almost all postoperative surgical patients need psychological support during the immediate postoperative period. When the patient's condition permits, a close member of his family may see him for a few moments. Thus, the family is reassured, and the patient feels more secure.

The questions posed by an awakening patient often indicate his deep feelings and thoughts. Perhaps he shows concern about the outcome of the operation or about his future—whatever his expression, the nurse should be in a position to answer his query reassuringly without going into a discussion of details. The immediate postoperative period is not the time for discussion of operative findings or prognosis. On the other hand, these questions ought not to be dismissed lightly, for they may offer clues that suggest the method to select in directing future treatment and rehabilitation.

Expected Patient Outcome: Attains/maintains psychosocial well-being

- Participates in self-care activities
- Takes time for attractive grooming
- Talks positively about future plans
- Asks questions relative to resuming sexual relations
- Expresses happiness in seeing friends and family

8. *To document all phases of the nursing process and to record and report pertinent data*

The determination of the significance of the signs and symptoms noted in assessing the patient is a matter of judgment. When viewed in isolation, one sign may be of little importance, but in the broader context it may be the missing link in a very important total evaluation.

There are a few general rules that may be of some assistance in guiding the nurse to make accurate value judgments. Of course, any severe symptom always is important.

- Any apparently slight symptom that tends to recur repeatedly or to increase in severity should be regarded as significant—for example, hiccups may or may not be of importance, depending on their duration.
- A symptom seemingly may be of no consequence in itself but when associated with other definite changes may foretell danger. For example, a repeated sigh means nothing, but, when accompanied by great restlessness, increasing pallor, rising pulse rate, etc., it becomes one of the clinical signs of dangerous hemorrhage.
- Any progressive and steady changes for the worse in the general condition of the patient, even with no outstanding symptoms evident, is of the gravest importance.
- The patient's complaints and statements never should be passed over without investigation.

Recording information accurately and concisely not only informs all medical and nursing personnel of the patient's condition, but also satisfies medicolegal requirements.

If a physician is to be notified for any reason, all necessary information should be at hand before the telephone is picked up, including the latest vital signs and monitor readings. It is also advisable to take the patient's chart, including nursing records, to the telephone in order to refer to them should questions arise.

▷ Postoperative Discomforts

Vomiting—Aspiration

In past years, vomiting was a common and expected postoperative occurrence, particularly following the use of ether as an anesthetic agent. However, with the advent of other anesthetic agents and antiemetic drugs, vomiting has become a less common postoperative phenomenon, although inadequate ventilation during anesthesia can increase the incidence of vomiting. Also, the vomiting that occurs as the patient comes out of anesthesia is frequently an attempt to relieve the stomach of the mucus and saliva swallowed during the anesthetic period.

Other causes of postoperative vomiting include an accumulation of fluid in the stomach, inflation of the stomach, and the ingestion of food and fluid before peristalsis returns. Psychological factors also may play a role; if the patient expects to vomit postoperatively, he usually will. Thus, helpful preoperative instruction can reduce the probability of vomiting after surgery.

When vomiting is likely because of the nature of surgery, a nasogastric tube is passed beforehand and remains in place throughout the operative procedure and the immediate postoperative period. Otherwise, simple symptomatic therapy is usually all that is required. Many authorities believe that most antiemetic drugs (usually derivatives of phenothiazine) promote more undesirable effects, such as hypotension and respiratory depression. If a medication is required, short-acting barbiturates are often prescribed.

- The most important nursing intervention required when vomiting occurs is to prevent aspiration of vomitus, which can cause asphyxiation and death (see pp. 409–411, 505).

Such precautions are also necessary even before the patient begins to vomit. After the airway is removed, the patient is usually turned to the side-lying position to provide effective drainage from the throat and to help prevent the tongue from slipping backwards and irritating the pharynx or possibly obstructing the airway.

- Following the slightest indication of nausea, the patient is turned completely on his side to increase mouth drainage.

If the patient is in a prone position, such as is generally used for children following tonsillectomy, adequate mouth drainage is provided by the position itself. However, to facilitate breathing, a pillow may be placed under the abdomen to permit the chest to expand.

Vomiting requires no special treatment beyond washing out the mouth and withholding fluids for a few hours. The main danger, as was already indicated, is from aspiration of the vomitus.

Under emergency conditions, since a patient who is brought to the operating room may have food in the stomach, some anesthesiologists administer preoperative oral antacids to counteract the acid-aspiration syndrome. Otherwise, if acid from the vomitus is inhaled into the lungs, it causes an asthmalike attack, with severe bronchial spasms and wheezing. Patients can subsequently develop pneumonitis and pulmonary edema and become extremely hypoxic.

Increasing medical attention is being paid to silent regurgitation of gastric contents since it occurs more frequently than realized. The importance of pH in the etiology of acid aspiration is being studied, as is the value of administering an H_2-receptor antagonist, such as cimetidine, preoperatively.

Abdominal Distention

Postoperative distention of the abdomen is another common occurrence. The trauma to the abdominal contents by manipulation during the operation produces a loss of normal peristalsis for 24 to 48 hours, depending on the type and the extent of the operation. Even though nothing is given by mouth, swallowed air and gastrointestinal secretions enter the stomach and the intestines, and if not propelled by peristaltic activity, they collect in the intestinal coils producing distention and causing the patient to complain of fullness or pain in the abdomen. Most often, the gas collects in the colon; hence, a rectal tube may be expected to give relief (Fig. 21-5).

After major abdominal surgery, distention may be avoided by having the patient turn, exercise, and move frequently and by using a gastric or an intestinal tube, whereby the air that is swallowed (swallowed air provides most of the gas that produces distention) may be aspirated from the stomach and the upper intestine. Certain patients swallow air as a part of an anxiety reaction. If these characteristics can be recognized, the nasogastric tube may be used for a longer time than usual, until full peristaltic activity (passage of flatus) is resumed.

Thirst

Thirst is a troublesome symptom after many general anesthetics, and even after some cases of local anesthesia. It stems largely from the dryness of the mouth and the pharynx caused by the inhibition of mucous secretion after the usual preoperative medication of atropine. Many patients operated on under local anesthesia complain of thirst during the operation. In addition, there is a considerable loss of body fluids owing to perspiration, increased mucous secretion in the lungs, and loss of blood, so that the factor of fluid imbalance also contributes to thirst. To combat the loss of fluids, solutions are given into the vein for the first few hours after operation. Even though an adequate amount of fluid is taken by this method, often it does not relieve the thirst.

Since a sticky, dry mouth demands moisture, fluids may be given to most patients as soon as the postoperative nausea and vomiting have passed. Sips of water or hot tea with lemon juice help to dissolve the mucus better than cold water. Ice chips seem to increase thirst and leave the mouth more parched. As soon as the patient can take water by mouth in sufficient quantities, parenteral administration is discontinued.

Hiccup (Singultus)

Hiccup occurs occasionally after abdominal operations. Often it occurs in mild transitory attacks that cease spontaneously or with very simple treatment. When hiccups persist, they may produce considerable distress and serious effects, such as vomiting, acid–base and fluid imbalance, malnutrition, exhaustion, and possibly wound dehiscence.

Hiccup is produced by intermittent spasms of the diaphragm and is manifested by a coarse sound (an audible "hic"), a result of the vibration of the closed vocal cords as the air rushes suddenly into the lungs. The cause of the diaphragmatic spasm may be any irritation of the phrenic nerve from its center in the spinal cord to its terminal ramifications on the undersurface of the diaphragm. This irritation may be (1) direct—such as a stimulation of the nerve itself by a distended stomach, peritonitis or subdiaphragmatic abscess, abdominal distention, pleurisy, or tumors in the chest pressing on the nerves; (2) indirect—such as from toxemia or uremia that stimulates the center; or (3) reflexive in nature—such as irritation from a drainage tube, exposure to cold, drinking very hot or very cold fluids, or obstruction of the intestines.

Treatment. The multitude of remedies suggested for the relief of this condition is proof that no one treatment is effective in every case. The best remedy, of course, is removal of the cause, which in some cases is simple—for example, gastric lavage for gastric distention, shortening or removal of drainage tubes causing irritation. At other times the removal of the cause is almost impossible; then attention must directed toward the treatment of the hiccup itself. Probably the most efficient of the older and simpler remedies is to hold the breath while taking large swallows of cold water.

After studying the problem, a group of anesthesiologists have recommended treatment ranging from the simplest to the most drastic until relief is obtained. Their suggestions, in order, are:

1. Finger pressure on the eyeballs, applied through closed lids for several minutes
2. Induced vomiting
3. Gastric lavage

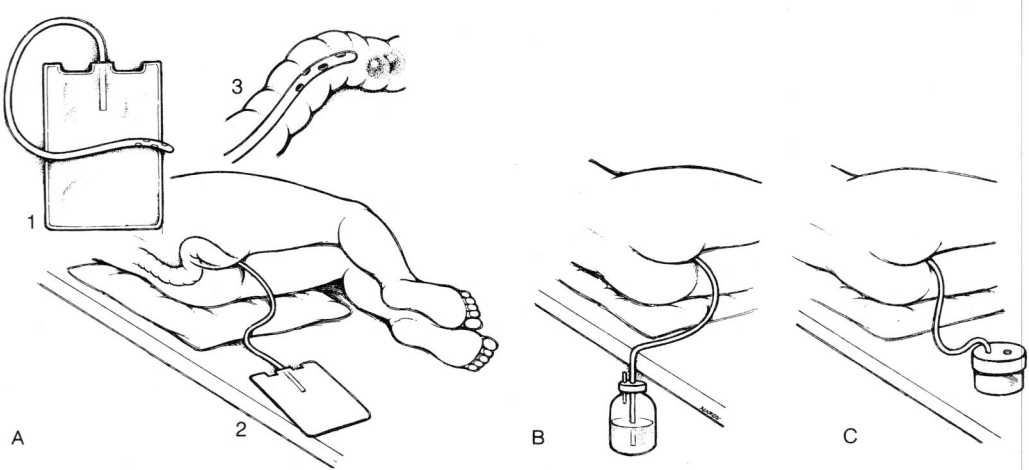

Figure 21-5. Rectal intubation. (*A*) 1—rectal tube attached to plastic bag; 2—tube in place, patient lying on left side; 3—enlargement of lower colon showing gas bubbles that will be tapped by rectal tube. (*B*) Tubing connected to a water bottle with vent. (*C*) Tubing connected to a plastic receptacle.

4. Intravenous injection of atropine
5. Inhalation of carbon dioxide (by breathing in and out of a paper bag or by mechanical means)
6. A phrenic nerve block (should the above measures not work)
7. A phrenic nerve crush as a final resort

Phenothiazine drugs, especially thorazine, have been helpful on occasion. It has also been suggested that an interruption of the reflex arc that results in the intermittent spasm of the diaphragm may be accomplished by the introduction of a rubber catheter 7.5 cm to 11 cm (3–4½ inches) long into the pharynx. The catheter may be introduced either through the nose or through the mouth to tickle the pharynx (Fig. 21-6).

Constipation
The causes of constipation after operation may be minor or serious. The irritation and the trauma to the bowel at the

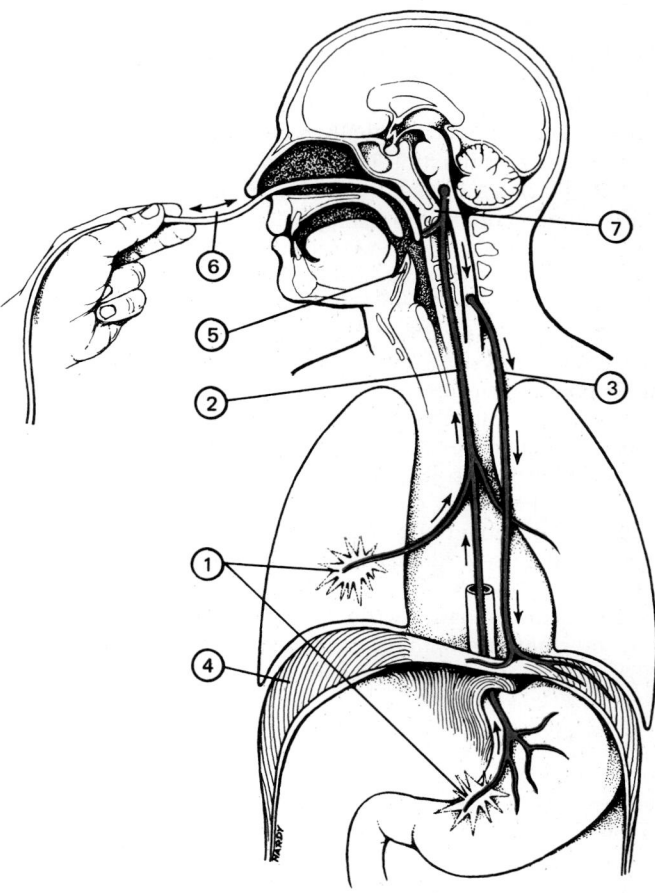

Figure 21-6. Controlling hiccups. Irritations in chest or abdomen (1) are transmitted by the vagus nerve (2). The reflex arc is completed by the transmission of the impulses to the diaphragm by the phrenic nerve (3). This causes contraction of the diaphragm (4) resulting in sudden intake of breath, which in turn is suddenly interrupted by rapid closure of the glottis (5). This is the hiccup.
Introduction of the No. 16 Fr catheter into the nasopharynx about 7.5 cm to 10 cm (3–4 inches) (6) stimulates the pharyngeal branches of the vagus nerve (7) and interrupts the reflex arc, stopping the hiccups.

time of the operation may inhibit intestinal movement for several days, but usually peristaltic function returns after the third day, following the combined effect of early ambulation, perhaps a simple enema, and an increase in diet. Local inflammation, peritonitis, or abscess may cause constipation, in which case treatment of the causal condition is indicated.

• Constipation has been described as a constant symptom of complete intestinal obstruction.

It must be borne in mind, also, that many people are constipated habitually and often give a history of having taken some form of laxative drug every day for years. Attempts should be made to correct their bowel habits as soon as is practical. However, in some instances, especially with elderly patients, these attempts may not be feasible. Liquid petrolatum (paraffin oil) or enemas usually are effective in evacuating the lower blowel.

• Cathartic drugs should never be given, except when prescribed by the physician.

Fecal Impaction.   An avoidable cause of postoperative constipation is fecal impaction. This complication is a result of neglect and never should occur. Early ambulation and regard for proper fluids and diet can prevent this problem in the majority of patients. Those affected usually are individuals past middle age, weakened somewhat by operation, whose bowel movements have been small in amount for several days. Enemas appear to be fairly effective, but distention usually continues, accompanied by general and local abdominal discomfort. The patient often states that he feels that the bowel wants to move but that movement gives no relief. Diarrhea may occur and persist, owing to irritation of the upper rectum and the sigmoid by dammed-up fecal material. The diagnosis is made easily by inserting the gloved finger into the rectum and palpating a hard fecal mass.

Treatment.   The treatment of the condition is to remove the impaction. Enemas of 180 ml (6 oz) of liquid petrolatum (oil enema) often are effective in softening the mass and helping in its discharge. The harder masses may not be moved by this treatment. In these patients, the impaction may be broken up with the gloved finger, or by injecting from 30 ml to 60 ml (1 oz–2 oz) of hydrogen peroxide into the rectum. The foaming action of the drug tends to break up the fecal masses, which then may be evacuated.

Diarrhea
After operation, diarrhea is rare. When it does occur, the patient may have five to ten liquid stools a day, each small in amount. This should be reported at once. Fecal impaction seems to be the most frequent cause of this complication in the aged.

Local irritation, such as a pelvic abscess, is the most frequent cause of diarrhea after operations in which peritonitis was found. Insertion of a gloved finger into the rectum will reveal a tender mass bulging into the rectum. Surgical drainage usually is required, although at times these abscesses rupture spontaneously and drain into the rectum.

▷ Care of the Wound

A *wound* may be described as a disruption in the continuity of cells; it follows, then, that *wound healing* is the restoration of that continuity.

When wounds occur, a variety of effects may result: (1) immediate loss of all or part of organ functioning, (2) sympathetic stress response, (3) hemorrhage and blood clotting, (4) bacterial contamination (when the bacterial count approaches $10^3/cm^3$, the body's defense is usually effective; a septic wound usually contains bacteria within the range of $10^7/cm^3$–$10^9/cm^3$), and (5) death of cells. Careful asepsis is the most important factor in keeping these effects to a minimum and promoting the successful care of wounds.

Wound Classification

Wounds are classified as (1) incised, (2) contused, (3) lacerated, or (4) puncture wounds, according to the manner in which they were made.

Incised wounds are made by a clean cut with a sharp instrument, for example, those made by the surgeon in every operation. Clean wounds (those made aseptically) are usually closed by sutures after all bleeding vessels have been ligated carefully.

Contused wounds are made by blunt force and are characterized by considerable injury of the soft parts, hemorrhage, and swelling.

Lacerated wounds are those with jagged, irregular edges, such as would be made by glass, barbed wire, etc.

Puncture wounds result in small openings in the skin, for example, those made by bullets or knife stabs.

When wounds are potentially infected, they cannot be closed until every effort has been made to remove all devitalized tissue and infection. Therefore, a formal operation is performed for the purpose of cutting out the infected and devitalized tissue. This operation is called *debridement.* Often a small drain is inserted before the wound is sutured to prevent lymph and blood from collecting and retarding the healing process.

Physiology of Wound Healing

Various continuous and overlapping cellular processes contribute to the restoration of a wound: cell regeneration, cell proliferation, and collagen production. The response of tissue to injury goes through several phases: inflammatory, proliferative, and maturation (Table 21-1).

Inflammatory Phase. Vascular and cellular responses occur immediately when tissue is cut or injured. Vasoconstriction of vessels occurs with a deposition of a fibrinoplatelet clot in an attempt to control bleeding. This lasts from 5 to 10 minutes and is followed by vasodilatation of the venules. Microcirculation loses its tonus since norepinephrine is destroyed by the intracellular enzymes. Also, histamine and serotonin are released, which act directly on microcirculation.

When there is damage to microcirculation, blood elements such as antibodies, plasma proteins, electrolytes, complement, and water permeate the vascular space for 2 to 3 days, causing edema, warmth, redness, and pain.

Polymorphonuclear granulocytes and erythrocytes are the first leukocytes to appear. If there is no infection, they decline in numbers; monocytes that transform to macrophages engulf the debris and transport it from the area. Antigen–antibodies also appear.

Basal cells at wound edges undergo mitosis, and the resulting daughter cells migrate. With this activity, proteolytic enzymes are secreted, which dissolve the base of blood clots. The gap between both sides of the wound are progressively filled and eventually meet in 24 to 48 hours. At this point, cell migration is replaced by cell mitosis.

Proliferative Phase. Fibroblasts multiply and form a lattice framework for migrating cells. Epithelial cells form buds at the edges of the wound; these buds develop into capillaries, the nutritional source for the new granulation tissue.

Collagen is the prime component of replaced connective tissue. Fibroblasts initiate the synthesis of collagen and mucopolysaccharides. In a 2- to 4-week period, amino acid chains collect into fibers of increasing length and diameter; these become a well-structured pattern of packed bundles. The synthesis of collagen causes capillaries to reduce in number. Thereafter, collagen decreases in an attempt to balance the amount of collagen that is destroyed. Such synthesis and lysis results in increased tensile strength. However, after 2 weeks, the wound is only 3% to 5% of the original skin strength. By the end of a month, only 35% to 59% of wound strength has been reached. Never more than 70% to 80% of strength is regained.

Table 21-1
Phases of Wound Healing

Phase	Also Referred to As	Length of Time
Inflammatory	Lag Exudative	1–4 days
Proliferative	Fibroblastic Connective tissue	5–20 days
Maturation	Differentiation Resorptive Remodeling Plateau	21 days to months and even years

Maturation Phase. At this time (3 weeks after injury) fibroblasts begin to leave the wound. The scar appears large, but collagen fibrils reorganize into tighter positions. This, along with dehydration, reduces the scar but increases its strength. Such wound maturation continues and reaches maximum strength in 10 or 12 weeks, but it never reaches the original strength of the prewound tissue.

Forms of Healing

In the surgical management of wound healing, wounds are described as healing by first, second, or third intention.

Healing by First Intention (Primary Union). Wounds made aseptically, with a minimum of tissue destruction and properly coapted, as with sutures, heal with very little tissue reaction "by first intention" (Fig. 21-7A). When wounds heal by first intention, granulation tissue is not visible and scar formation is minimal.

Healing by Second Intention (Granulation). In wounds in which pus formation (suppuration) has occurred or in which the edges have not been approximated, the process of repair is less simple and is delayed longer. When an abscess is incised, it collapses partly, but the dead and the dying cells forming its walls are still being thrown out into the cavity. For this reason, rubber tubes, rubber tissue, or gauze packing often is inserted into the abscess pocket to allow the pus to escape easily. Gradually, the necrotic material disintegrates and escapes, and the abscess cavity fills with a red, soft, sensitive tissue that bleeds very easily. It is composed of minute, thin-walled capillaries, growing off from the parent vessels, each bud surrounded by cells that later form connective tissue. These buds, called granulations, enlarge until they fill the area left by the destroyed tissue (Fig. 21-7B). The cells surrounding the capillaries change their round shape; they become long and thin, intertwining with each other to form a *scar* or *cicatrix*. Healing is complete when skin cells (epithelium) grow over these granulations. This method of repair is called *healing by granulation,* and it takes place whenever pus is formed or when loss of tissue has occurred for any reason.

Healing by Third Intention (Secondary Suture). If a deep wound either has not been sutured early or breaks down and then is resutured later, two apposing granulation surfaces are brought together. This results in a deeper and wider scar (Fig. 21-7C).

General Factors That Affect Wound Healing

In the operating room, tissues that are handled with care will repair more rapidly than those handled roughly. Keeping the wound free from starch or talcum powder (from gloves) is also important, since foreign bodies will adversely affect the healing process.

Numerous factors can impair wound healing, such as age, edema, certain drugs that may mask the presence of infection (steroids) or cause hemorrhage (anticoagulants), and overactivity on the part of the patient, which may prevent the wound edges from approximating and thus delay wound repair.

Systemic disorders such as hemorrhagic shock and septicemia along with their sequelae of acidosis and hypoxia are depressants of cell function that directly affect wound

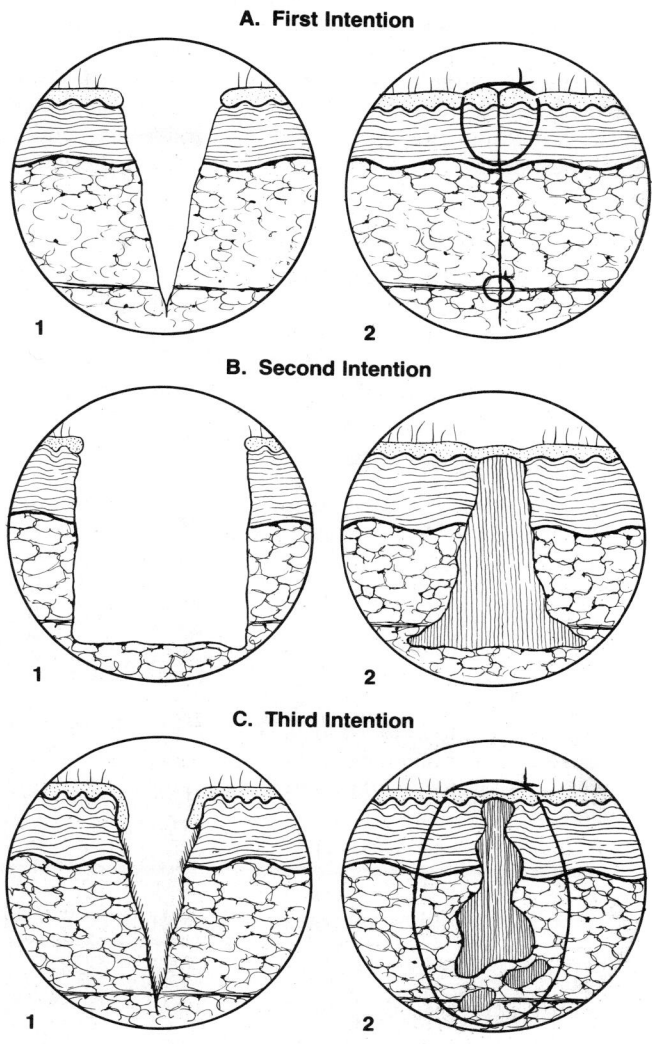

A. First Intention

B. Second Intention

C. Third Intention

Figure 21-7. Schematic representation of healing by first, second, and third intention. When a clean incision through epidermis, dermis, and subcutaneous tissue (A, 1) is closed immediately and heals without complication, a minimal quantity of scar tissue unites the edges firmly (A, 2). In open wounds with tissue loss (B, 1), wound contraction and epithelialization are the major factors in wound closure. The epithelial surface lacks a normal epidermal–dermal junction and can be unstable; the scar is large and wedge shaped (B, 2). When a wound remains open for a few days and is closed secondarily (C, 1), the initial scar is larger than in primarily healed wounds (C, 2). Within a few days, however, third intention wounds epithelialize and eventually may remodel to resemble primary wounds. (From Hardy JD: Rhoads Textbook of Surgery, 5th ed. Philadelphia, JB Lippincott.)

healing. Renal failure and hepatic disease also inhibit tissue repair, as do immunosuppressive therapy and cancer chemotherapy.

Broad-spectrum or specific antibiotics can be effective if given immediately before surgery to patients with specific pathology or bacterial contamination. The use of antibiotics in the wound area shortly after it is closed is not effective because of intravascular coagulation. If sepsis occurs, specific cultures are done to determine the antibiotic to which the bacteria are most sensitive.

Local factors also may affect wound healing, such as poor dressing technique, in which saturated dressings are not changed frequently enough, or a dressing that is too small is applied, permitting bacterial contamination to take place. A dressing also may be too tight and hence reduce the blood supply to the part. (See section on dressings, p. 399.)

Nursing Management and Its Effect on Wound Healing

As a wound moves through the phases of healing, many elements, such as adequate nutrition, cleanliness, rest, and position, determine how quickly the process occurs. These factors are initiated and influenced by nursing intervention. (Also see Chart 21-2.)

Inflammatory Phase

Hemostasis. Following surgery or injury, the control of bleeding is essential before healing takes place. Accumulations of blood create dead space as well as dead cells that must be removed. Thus, an area that becomes a culture medium for infection is created. Bleeding may require that the patient be returned to the operating room so that the incision site can be reopened and the vessels ligated.

Hypovolemia. Insufficient blood volume leads to vasoconstriction and reduced oxygen in a wound. Volume deficit (circulatory impairment) must be monitored and corrected (central venous pressure and pulmonary artery wedge pressure). Replacement of fluids with colloid or crystalloid solution is necessary to control this deficit.

Tissue Oxygenation. Adequate pulmonary and cardiovascular function will supply the microenvironment of a surgical wound with sufficient oxygen. Nursing measures such as requiring the patient to achieve SMI postoperatively and controlled coughing are encouraged to remove accumulated lung secretions. Drains and portable suction may facilitate removing collections of drainage. Such accumulations can cause growth of microorganisms because of the rich culture medium, and can also cause skin necrosis.

Prevention of Wound Stressors. Heavy coughing, the Valsalva maneuver, or vomiting can produce tension on an abdominal wound. A more desirable nursing intervention is to encourage frequent turning, ambulation, and the use of antiemetic medications.

Optimum Nutrition. With large wounds, metabolic disturbances can occur owing to stress responses. Insulin secretion may be inhibited and blood glucose may rise. Careful monitoring of blood glucose levels will serve to indicate insulin deficits. Protein–calorie depletion, a common occurrence, must also be corrected. Often this requires parenteral nutritional therapy (see p. 780) to maintain a positive nitrogen balance. At times, following parenteral nutrition, a dry skin or alopecia may occur, which is suggestive of fat deficiency. This can be replaced by administering fat emulsion or by cutaneous application of sunflowerseed oil.

Chart 21-2
Effective Methods of Lowering Incidence of Wound Infection

Method	*Rationale*
Preoperative	
Shorter preoperative hospitalization	Reduces exposure of patient to nosocomial infections.
Treatment of coexistent infections	Infections, such as respiratory, can initiate pulmonary complications.
Limited shaving of skin hairs	The fewer nicks and cuts in the skin, the less opportunity for infection.
Shorter time between shaving and operation	The longer the time between shaving and the operation, the greater the incidence of infection.
Thorough cleansing of operative site—Betadine shower the evening before and repeated preoperative cleansing with antiseptic detergents	Resident bacteria and skin contaminants are reduced to a minimum.
Intraoperative	
Flawless aseptic technique	Any breaks in technique can initiate infection by introducing contaminants.
Powder or talcum washed off sterile gloves	Foreign particles in a wound, such as talcum or starch, will adversely affect the healing process.
Bleeding controlled with meticulous hemostasis	Bacterial infection is enhanced with ferric iron.
Drains eliminated in clean wounds	Drains are associated with higher wound infection rates.
Closure delayed in contaminated wounds	Permits healing from the base of wound to exterior—otherwise, pocket of infection may develop.

Vitamins A and C supplements can be given postoperatively to those showing nutritional deficits, such as the elderly person who lives alone and lacks well-balanced meals.

Resting of the part or organ (depending on its location and function) also favors healing, as does adequate circulation of blood to and from tissues in order to supply nutrients, leukocytes, antibodies, and other requirements, and to remove the products of tissue metabolism.

Fibroplastic Phase

Maintaining Wound Stability.   This is enhanced by many practices that are initiated postoperatively: reducing preoperative hospitalization, shaving the area immediately preoperatively (if shaving must be done), requiring preoperative showering with detergent-germicide, and administering prophylactic antibiotics when there appears to be risk of possible wound infection.

High-risk patients need to be monitored more closely: the overweight patient, those diabetic patients who are insulin-dependent, and suppressed individuals who are on (or have recently taken) steroids or cytotoxic agents.

If a patient develops a temperature elevation between the fourth and seventh day, a wound infection is suspected. Special monitoring ensues to verify this suspicion.

When there is the potential for wound infection, open packing using fine mesh gauze is effective. Such packing is removed and replaced three times a day until the wound edges are close to approximation.

The Purposes of an Effective Dressing

A dressing is applied to a wound for one or more of the following reasons: (1) to provide proper environment for wound healing; (2) to absorb drainage; (3) to splint or immobilize the wound; (4) to protect the wound and new epithelial tissue from mechanical injury; (5) to prevent adherence of dressing to the wound owing to ingrowth of new tissue; (6) to protect the wound from bacterial contamination and soil from feces, vomitus, and urine; (7) to promote hemostasis, as in a pressure dressing; (8) to maintain proper moisture conditions at wound surface; and (9) to provide mental and physical comfort for the patient.

Whenever possible or feasible, some surgeons prefer to eliminate dressings, either shortly after surgery or within the immediate postoperative period. Examples of circumstances in which dressings are not necessary are facial lacerations, pedicle flap (see skin grafts, p. 1189), or skin grafts on a smooth surface.

When the initial dressing on a clean, dry incision is removed, often it is not replaced. Generally, initial dressings on clean, dry incisions are left in place until the sutures are removed, and if a dressing is replaced at all, its purpose is more esthetic than useful.

The apparent advantages of not using any dressings are these: (1) eliminates the conditions necessary for growth of organisms (warmth, moisture, and darkness), (2) allows for better observation and early detection of wound difficulties, (3) facilitates bathing, (4) tends to minimize the operative procedure, (5) avoids adhesive-tape reaction, (6) appears to be more comfortable for the patient and facilitates his activity, and (7) is economical.

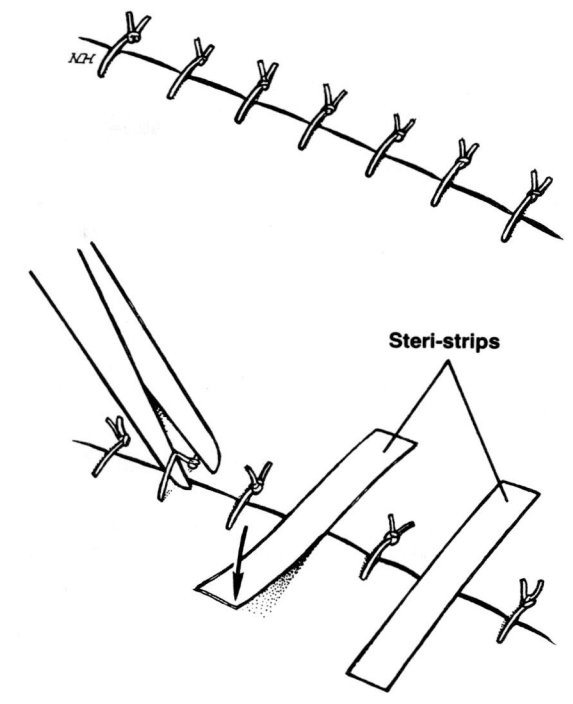

Figure 21-8.   Steri-strips.

The suture line is gently cleansed and swabbed with half-strength hydrogen peroxide every 4 hours until drainage ceases. When sutures are removed (before seventh day), center sutures are removed first and replaced with steri-strips to keep the tender incision line reinforced (Fig. 21-8). Thereafter, the incision line may be swabbed with tincture of benzoin for protection until complete healing has taken place.

Substitute materials, such as sprayed plastic dressings, can also be used, and they seem to provide satisfactory service for clean and dry incisions. This dressing usually lasts from 5 to 7 days. Depending on the product, it either peels off or can be wiped off with a dissolvent. On clean, dry wounds it seems superfluous to be concerned with the ability of the dressing to absorb secretions, since there are practically no secretions to be absorbed. Texture, comfort, and perhaps screening ability against microorganisms (although this latter is a doubtful prerequisite) are more important in such dressings.

Products such as polyethyl glycol (liquid) and hydron (powder) are being investigated as spray-type plastic wound coverings that are flexible and transparent and that allow fluid to be transmitted through the dressing.

In spite of the advantages of not using a dressing, most surgeons prefer to apply a dressing at the time of operation and a second dressing between 4 and 6 days later, after the removal of sutures. Stitches (black silk, nylon, or fine wire) or metal skin clips used to approximate the skin edges are of little value after the sixth or seventh day and are therefore removed.

The dressings are purely protective from a functional point of view, and they give the patient a sense of security that is not present if wounds are treated without dressings.

Surgical Dressing Technique

Because of the dangers of contamination and spread of infection, the most desirable and safe technique is to use a sterile dressing pack for each patient. A surgical dressing cart may be used as a stock table to hold the individually wrapped sterile supplies, including individual flasks of antiseptic solution.

Nursing Responsibility. The nurse should be available to assist the physician in the changing of dressings for several reasons:

1. The "team" working together assures the patient of expert care.
2. The nurse, as a colleague, is better informed concerning the patient and therefore can provide more knowledgeable care.
3. The nurse can ensure the proper disposal of contaminated articles.
4. Although all initial postoperative dressings are done by the surgeon, subsequent applications may be done by the nurse.
5. The condition of surgical dressings should be noted on the patient's chart as carefully as any medication or treatment, and pertinent observations should be documented by the nurse.

Preparation of the Patient. The patient is told that his dressing is to be changed and that it is a simple procedure associated with little discomfort. The dressing change should be scheduled for a suitable time. *Dressings should not be done at mealtime.* If the patient is in an open unit, the curtains are drawn to ensure privacy and to accommodate the patient's sense of modesty. In this regard, the patient should not be exposed unduly. When the dressing has a foul odor or the patient is unusually squeamish, it is better to take the patient to the treatment room, away from other patients. At no time should the incision be referred to as a "scar," since for some patients the term has ugly or undesirable connotations.

Removal of Adhesive. The adhesive is removed by pulling it parallel with the skin surface and not at right angles (Fig. 21-9). Nonirritating solvents available in aerosol containers aid in removing adhesive tapes painlessly and quickly.

The old dressing and the pledgets used in cleaning the wound are removed by means of a forceps and are then deposited in a waterproof bag for easy disposal by burning. Such dressings are never touched by ungloved hands because of the danger of transmitting pathogenic organisms. After instruments are used in the changing of dressings, they are placed in a receptacle such as an emesis basin, not on surfaces where contamination of clean areas is possible. If instruments are disposable, they are discarded in the proper receptacle.

A Simple Dressing. For the routine dressing, an individual sterile pack usually contains scissors, forceps, hemostat, and grooved director or probe, as well as cotton balls, dressings, and perhaps a solution container. When the tray has been properly opened, the person changing the dressing grasps a cotton ball with a forceps and holds it over the emesis basin as the assistant pours a small quantity of the desired antiseptic. After the wound and surrounding

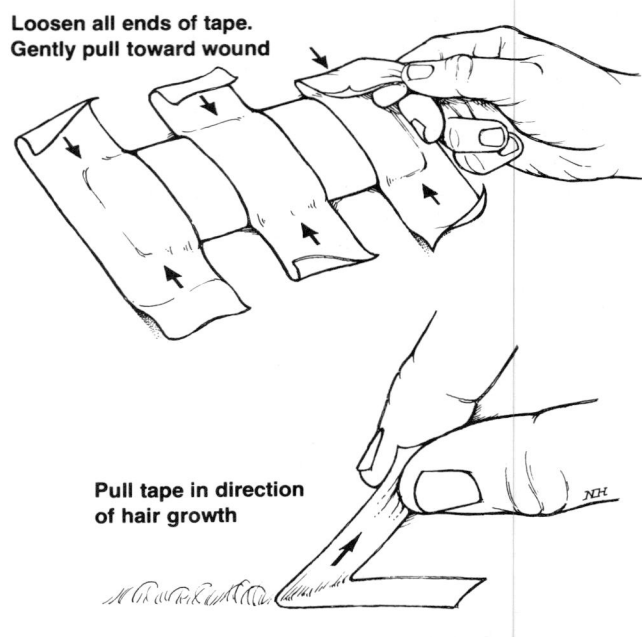

Loosen all ends of tape. Gently pull toward wound

Pull tape in direction of hair growth

Figure 21-9. Removing adhesive tape.

skin are cleansed with an antiseptic, the sutures are removed, a new dressing is applied, and tape is used to keep it in place (see p. 401).

Surgical tape is available for patients who are allergic to the rubber base in the usual adhesive tape. 3M brand Micropore surgical tape is porous in structure and thus permits ventilation and prevents maceration. Tension sutures are allowed to remain in place for a longer period of time in some instances.

- *If there is any doubt about the sterility of an instrument or a dressing, it is considered unsterile.*
- *In no circumstances should the nurse touch soiled dressings with ungloved hands.*

The Dressing of Draining Wounds. It may be necessary to dress draining wounds within 24 hours of the operation. Nothing causes a patient more unnecessary discomfort than a dressing saturated with drainage fluids. It dries on the edges and becomes stiff and scratchy, and the odor frequently is very offensive if not actually nauseating. The nurse may relieve such a situation by changing the outer layers of the dressing at frequent intervals between dressings.

When it is necessary to dress the wound daily, adhesive strips fastened with either tapes or laces (Montgomery straps, Fig. 21-10) are more convenient than simple adhesive strips. These should not be applied so tightly that the dressings beneath are unable to retain drainage.

When the edges of the wound gape and the gauze is adhering to the tissues, the patient may be spared considerable pain if the dressings are moistened with peroxide of hydrogen. For this purpose, a syringe and a basin containing the solution must be provided along with a waste pan to prevent the solution from soiling the bed.

When *drainage tubes* are being shortened, the nurse

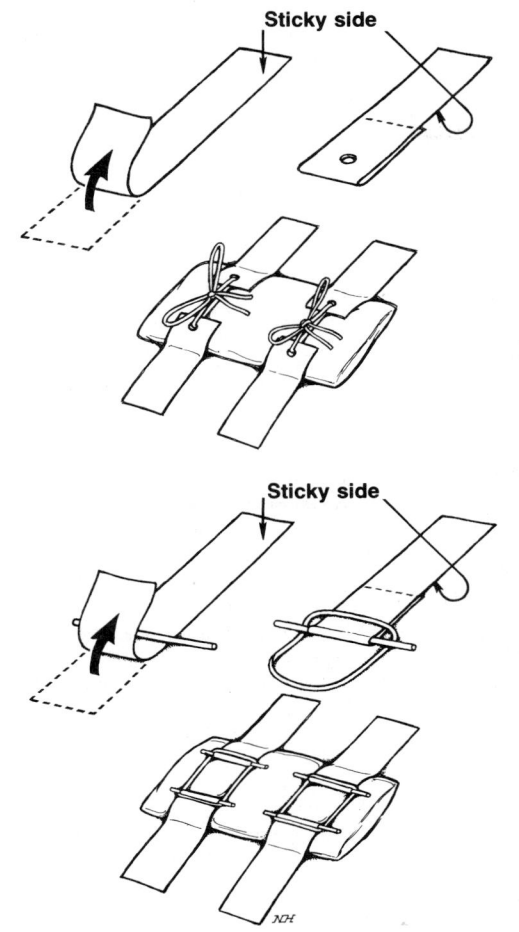

Figure 21-10. Montgomery straps.

should have a sterile safety pin (or Klip) ready to insert in the new tube end. If the tubes are removed, the surgeon frequently inserts a piece of rubber tissue or packing to prevent the drainage tract from closing too quickly.

The drainage from an infected wound frequently proves to be irritating to the surrounding skin. Often this situation may be avoided by the use of a protective ointment or dressing. Petrolatum gauze, nitrofurazone (Furacin roll), and zinc oxide ointments are effective preparations.

When the discharge from the wound contains any digestive enzymes, as in pancreatic or intestinal fistulae and ileostomy or cecostomy wounds, more active measures to protect the skin must be taken. In some cases, the enzyme-containing secretion may be aspirated by constant portable suction (see below). In others, the skin surrounding the wound may be protected by such adhering ointments as zinc oxide ointment or by a creamy paste mixture of aluminum hydroxide gel and kaolin (Protogel) or of magnesium and aluminum hydroxides (Maalox), which both soothe the skin and neutralize the enzymes in the secretions. These must be applied to an absolutely dry skin surface.

When a drainage tube is attached to drainage tubing and a bag or bottle, it is necessary to check the tubing fre-quently for kinking, coiling, and looping that could restrict the flow of drainage.

Portable Wound Suction. The principle involved in portable wound suction is the use of gentle, constant suction to effect drainage of serosanguineous fluid and to collapse the skin flaps against the underlying tissue. The apparatus is equipped with small, multiple, perforated, inert polyethylene tubes. Such tubes are inserted in the drainage areas in the operating room, and the wound is completely closed (Fig. 21-11). An electric suction machine may be connected to the device or operated as an independent unit, depending on the nature of the suction required and whether drip irrigation is to be used.

Portable suction has several advantages over conventional wound suctioning. It is silent, saves space, and is disposable. It is light in weight and permits the patient to ambulate. And, it is inexpensive.

The Completion of a Dressing. Dressings are held in place by adhesive that comes in many types and widths. If the patient is sensitive to the adhesive material, hypoallergenic tape should be used.

The correct way to apply tape is to place the tape at the center of the dressing and then press the tape down on both sides, applying tension evenly away from the midline (Fig. 21-12). Unfortunately, the wrong method of applying tape is more common—fixing one end of the tape to the skin and then pulling it tight over the dressing, often wrinkling and pulling the skin in the process. The resulting continuous and forceful traction produces a shearing effect, causing the epidermal layer to slip sideways and become prematurely separated from the deeper dermal layers.

A commercial silicone aerosol is available that can be sprayed over the adhesive used to hold dressings in place; the silicone waterproofs the dressing so that the patient can bathe or swim, and isolates the area from contamination. The spray is odorless, colorless, nonstaining, noninflammatory, heat stable, and also hypoallergenic.

Elastic adhesive bandage (Elastoplast, Microfoam-3M) is preferable for holding dressings in place over mobile areas, such as the neck or the extremities, or where pressure is required. When the dressing is completed, the soiled dressings are wrapped in a waterproof bag and deposited in the large, covered utility can to await its removal to the incinerator.

▷ Postoperative Complications

The danger inherent in surgery involves not only the risk of the operative procedure, but also the very definite hazard of postoperative complications that may prolong convalescence or even adversely affect the surgical outcome. The nurse plays an important part in the prevention of these complications and in their early treatment, should they arise. The signs and symptoms of the more common postoperative complications are discussed below. In each instance the most effective method of prevention and the usual treatment are emphasized.

It should be borne in mind constantly that attention must be paid to the patient as an individual as well as to his particular surgical condition.

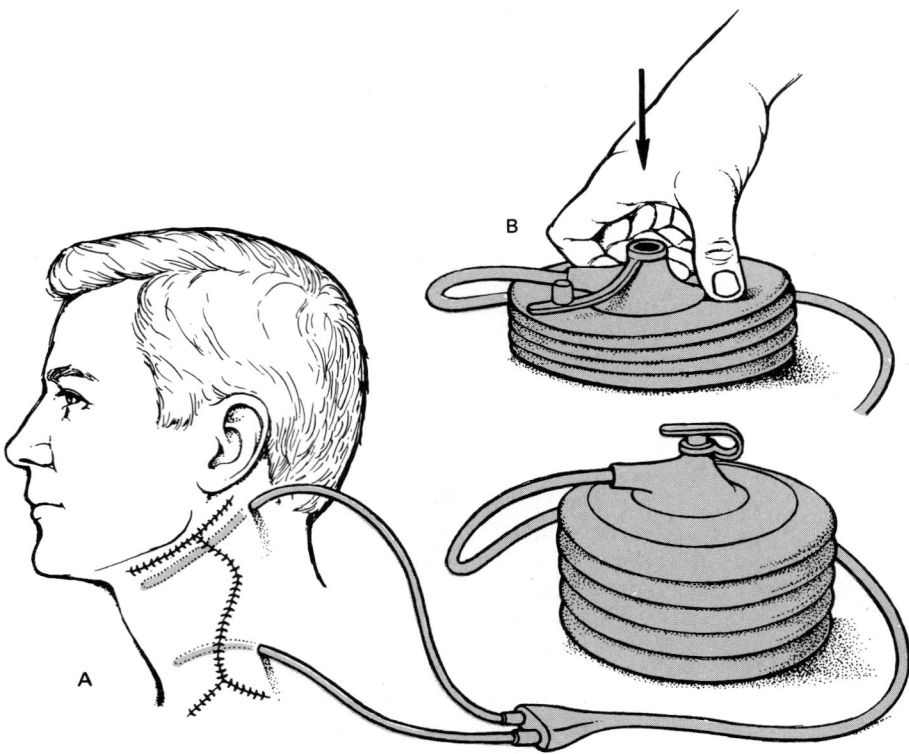

Figure 21-11. Portable wound suction. (*A*) Two perforated catheters are draining the incisional area following a radical neck dissection. By means of a Y-tube, drainage is drawn into a portable wound suction receptacle. When full, open top plug of receptacle and empty. (*B*) To reestablish negative pressure, compress receptacle as indicated and replace plug; suction drainage will resume.

Shock

One of the most serious postoperative complications is shock, which may be described as failure to provide adequate cellular oxygenation accompanied by failure to remove the waste products of metabolism. Shock can occur in association with many kinds of major illness—hemorrhage, trauma, burns, infection, and heart disease—and results from a failure of three aspects of circulation—the heart pump, peripheral resistance, and blood volume. Thus, while there are many kinds of shock, the basic definition centers on an inadequate blood flow to vital organs or the inability of the tissues of these organs to utilize oxygen and other nutrients.

Shock may be classified as hypovolemic, cardiogenic, neurogenic, or septic. The changes involved in each type are summarized in Table 21-2.

Catecholamines (epinephrine and norepinephrine) are elevated during shock and appear to be the dominant hormones in severe shock. Their effect is to constrict arterioles in the skin, subcutaneous tissue, and kidneys; they dilate arterioles of skeletal muscles and liver. Heart output is increased by increasing heart rates and increasing myocardial contractility. The great veins are constricted, thereby increasing venous return. Shock stimulates corticotropin (ACTH) release from the pituitary and thereby increases plasma levels of glucocorticoids. Mineralocorticoids are elevated mostly because of increased activity in the renin–angiotensin systems. Glucagon is released and antidiuretic hormone (ADH) is released. Endorphins are released in conjunction with the release of corticotropin. Endorphins act like opiates, which may contribute to low blood pressure.

The effect of high levels of epinephrine, cortisol, and glucagon and lower levels of insulin (insulin does rise, but not as greatly as the antagonists) stimulate catabolism. There is decreased oxygen utilization owing to decreased cardiac output and insulin insufficiency. See Figure 21-13, in Chart 21-3, for microcirculatory changes in shock.

Hypovolemic Shock. Hypovolemic shock is caused by decreased fluid volume owing to loss of blood, plasma, or water. Fluid volume is frequently decreased after surgery for a number of reasons. At times, more blood is lost at operation than is realized. In addition, the handling of body tissues may cause local trauma and loss of blood and plasma from the circulation, thereby creating a decrease in the circulating blood volume. Hypovolemic shock is characterized by a fall in venous pressure, a rise in peripheral resistance, and tachycardia. (For additional symptoms see Table 21-3.)

Cardiogenic Shock. This type of shock results from cardiac failure or an interference with heart function (poor heart-pump function, causing diminished cardiac output), as in myocardial infarction, arrhythmias, tamponade, pulmonary embolism, advanced (late) hypovolemia, or epidural and general anesthesia. The signs are increased pressure in the venous bed and an increase in peripheral resistance.

Neurogenic Shock. Neurogenic shock occurs as a result of a failure of arterial resistance (such as may be caused by spinal anesthesia, quadriplegia). It is characterized by a fall in blood pressure owing to pooling of blood in dilated capacitance vessels (those with the ability to change volume capacity). Heart activity increases and thus maintains a normal output (stroke volume); this helps in filling the dilated vascular system as it attempts to preserve perfusion pressure.

Septic Shock. Septic shock results most frequently from gram-negative septicemia (infection, peritonitis, etc.). At first, the patient exhibits a fever; rapid, strong pulse; rapid respirations; and normal or slightly decreased blood pressure. Skin is flushed, warm, and dry. However, if infection continues untreated, hypovolemic shock develops. These two phases may be referred to as hyperdynamic septic shock, and the latter (which is similar to hypovolemic shock) as hypodynamic shock. Hypovolemia develops along with depressed cardiac function.

Clinical Manifestations

Even though shock can result from widely different causes (trauma, systemic infection, or cardiac dysfunction), clinical manifestations are generally similar.

- The classical signs of shock are pallor; cool, moist skin; rapid breathing; ischemia of the eyelids, lips, gums, and tongue; a weak, thready pulse; small pulse pres-

Table 21-2
Cardiopulmonary Responses in Severe Forms of Shock

	Pulmonary Arterial Wedge Pressure	Systemic Vascular Resistance	Cardiac Output	Oxygen Consumption
Hypovolemic shock	↓	↑	↓	↓
Hyperdynamic septic shock	±	↓	↑	±
Hypodynamic septic shock	↓	↑	↓	↓
Cardiogenic shock	↑	↑	↓	↓
Neurogenic shock	↓	↓	±	↓

↓ = depressed; ↑ = elevated; ± = may be depressed, elevated, or normal.
(From Dunphy JE and Way LW: Current Surgical Diagnosis and Treatment. Los Altos, California, Lange Medical Publishers, 1981.)

sure; and usually a low blood pressure and concentrated urine.

Medical and Nursing Assessment of the Patient in Shock

Before treatment can be instituted promptly and intelligently, the *goal* in initial assessment is to determine the cause of volume loss and the status of the airway. Such an assessment includes the following.

1. Respirations. Hyperventilation is an early sign of septic shock.

2. Skin. A cold, pale, moist skin indicates vasoconstriction with increased arteriolar resistance and is suggestive of hypovolemic shock. Warm, red skin indicates a decrease in arteriolar resistance and may be seen in septic and neurogenic shock.

3. Pulse and Blood Pressure. Alone, these signs may not be reliable guides to the severity of shock, but their progressive pattern is significant. That is, if each 5- to 15-minute interval shows a fall in pulse and blood pressure, then such signs are indicative of shock. A pulse of 80 per minute and a blood pressure of 120/80 are normal. When systolic pressure is between 90 mm Hg and 60 mm Hg (in the normotensive individual), shock is well advanced. (For the hypertensive person, 30 mm Hg below the base-line systolic pressure is a sign of shock.)

4. Urinary Output. Since the output of urine is one of the most valuable indices of adequacy of vital organ perfusion, an indwelling catheter is recommended for any patient susceptible to shock. A drop in renal artery pressure and flow produces renal artery vasoconstriction and results in decreased glomerular filtration and decreased urine output. Normal urine flow is 50 ml per hour. An output of 30 ml per hour or less (oliguria or anuria) is suggestive of cardiac failure or inadequate volume replacement.

5. Central Venous Pressure. CVP places a value on the volume of blood returning to the heart and the ability

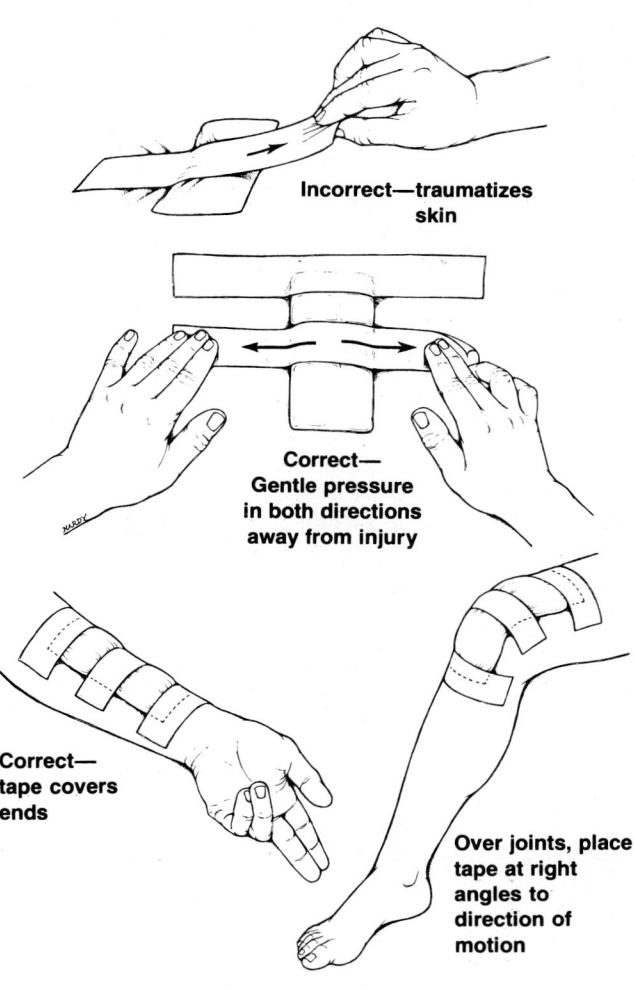

Incorrect—traumatizes skin

Correct— Gentle pressure in both directions away from injury

Correct— tape covers ends

Over joints, place tape at right angles to direction of motion

Figure 21-12. Application of adhesive tape.

Chart 21-3
Pathophysiology of Shock

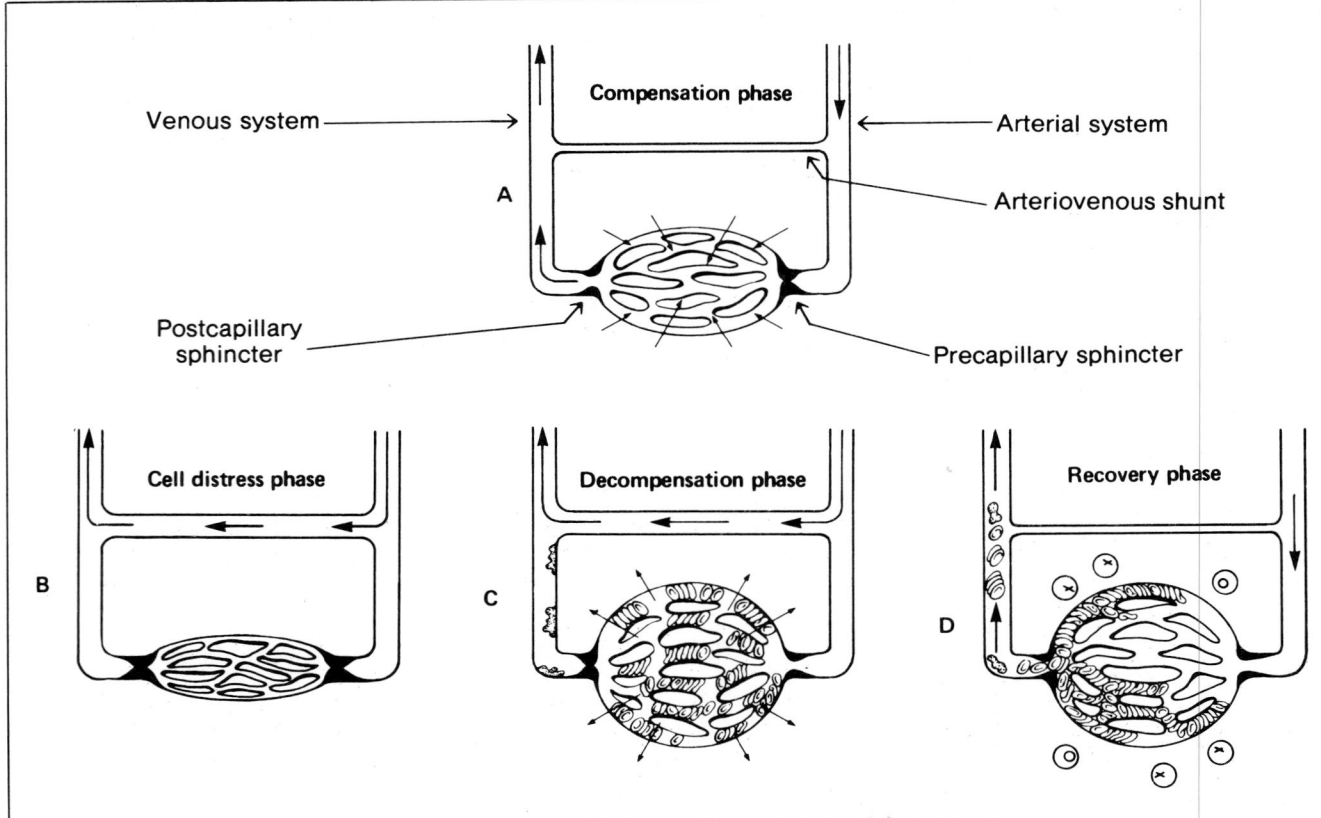

Figure 21-13. Microcirculatory changes in shock. (A) Compensation phase. (B) Cell distress phase. (C) Decompensation phase. (D) Recovery phase. (From Dunphy JE and Way LW: Current Diagnosis and Treatment. Los Altos, California, Lange Medical Publishers.)

When the body sustains an insult, such as hemorrhage, extensive burns, or heart failure, a compensatory reaction occurs. The adrenal medulla releases catecholamines to constrict arterioles and venules in the major organs of the body (kidneys, liver, intestines, etc.) so that more blood is diverted to the brain and heart.

Pathophysiologic Consequences of Shock

The greatest impact of all types of shock is exerted on the microcirculation (arterioles, capillaries, venules—microvasculature), which reacts to shock in a series of steps. The first phase involves a response to the hypovolemia, as is seen in the contraction of the precapillary arteriole sphincters (Fig. 21-13A). This causes capillary pressure to fall, with the result that fluid moves into the vascular spaces and increases the blood volume. By such compensatory action, blood volume returns to normal and the precapillary sphincters relax. However, if shock is more prolonged, recovery is prevented and the next phase, cell distress, is entered (Fig. 21-13B). In this phase, arteriovenous shunts open and divert arterial flow directly back

into the venous system. Meanwhile, the cells in the bypassed segment of microcirculation rely on anaerobic metabolism for energy. Glucose and oxygen are reduced markedly for the cells, and waste products such as lactate increase. Histamine is released and the postcapillary sphincter closes. Capillary flow is slowed considerably and the bed constricts with very few capillaries remaining open. In the decompensation phase (Fig. 21-13C), just before the death of the cell, acidosis (decreasing serum pH) causes the precapillary sphincter to open. Fluid and protein are lost in the interstitial space and the capillary expands with agglutinated red blood cells (sludge). White cells and platelets gather in the venules where acidosis is most profound. Arteriovenous circulation continues to supply essential oxygen to the vital areas of heart and brain. In the recovery phase (Fig. 21-13D), if the blood volume is restored during the decompensation phase before the effects on microcirculation are still reversible, badly damaged cells can be repaired. Cell aggregates can be filtered out by the lungs and into the systemic circulation. However, if there is an overabundance of dead cells, secondary morbidity results.

Table 21-3
Classification and Symptoms of Hypovolemic Shock

	Mild	Moderate	Severe
Percent of blood volume loss	Up to 20%	20% to 40%	40% or more
Decreased perfusion	Skin, fat, skeletal muscle, bone	Liver, intestine, kidneys	Brain, heart
Pulse	Rapid	Rapid—weaker, thready	Very rapid—irregular
Respirations	Deep and rapid	Shallow and rapid	Even more shallow and rapid
Blood pressure	120/80	60–90 mm Hg systolic	Under 60 mm Hg systolic
Skin	Cool, pale	Cold, pale, moist	Cold, clammy, cyanotic lips and nails
Urinary output	Above 50 ml/hr	10 ml/hr–25 ml/hr	10 ml or less/hr → anuria
Level of consciousness	Anxious but oriented and alert	Restless, mentally "fuzzy," vertigo	Lethargic → comatose

Table 21-4
Normal Values

Measurements	Normal Value
Pulse	80/minute
Blood pressure (arterial)	120/80
Urine flow	50 ml/hr
Central venous pressure	5 cm–12 cm (H_2O)
PAP	10 mm Hg–20 mm Hg
PWP	14 mm Hg–18 mm Hg
Arterial blood gases	
PO_2	100 mm
PCO_2	40 mm Hg
*p*H	7.4
Arterial blood lactate	12 mg/100 ml
Hematocrit	35%–45%

of both chambers in the right heart to propel blood. It is a valuable guide to vascular volume replacement when other parameters are also considered: vital signs, cardiopulmonary status, etc. Average CVP is 5 cm to 12 cm water. Several readings are taken to determine the range; a reading near zero may indicate hypovolemia (if patient improves with rapid IV infusion, the patient was hypovolemic). Readings over 15 cm of water may suggest hypervolemia, vasoconstriction, or congestive heart failure.

Left atrial pressure readings are even more useful. Some intensive care units are equipped to measure pulmonary artery pressure (PAP) and pulmonary wedge pressure (PWP), which is left atrial pressure. These are more accurate in indicating the heart's pumping ability. (See Chap. 27, pp. 562–563.)

6. Arterial Blood Gases. The partial pressures of oxygen (PO_2) and carbon dioxide (PCO_2) are useful indices in providing therapy. An arterial oxygen tension below 60 mm Hg indicates a marginal respiratory reserve (see Table 21-4 for normal values). A PCO_2 over 45 mm Hg indicates serious hypoventilation. In shock, PCO_2 is usually within normal limits.

7. Serum Lactate. In 1964 Peretz showed the close correlation (in a person in shock) between arterial blood lactate levels and survival. Later a correlation was shown between lactate elevation and oxygen debt; the higher the lactate level (normal level is 12 mg/100 ml), the greater the oxygen need.

8. Hematocrit. Hematocrit is useful in determining the kind of fluid to use in replacement. (Such a study must be repeated, since a few hours are required to reflect correctly the amount of blood loss.) If the hematocrit is over 55, plasma and saline are given. If the hematocrit is 20 or less, blood is needed. The maximal oxygen-carrying capacity is best when the hematocrit is between 35 and 45.

9. Levels of Consciousness. Consciousness levels may range from alert in mild shock to mental cloudiness in moderate shock. As the condition worsens, the patient becomes lethargic and reacts only to noxious stimuli. Irreversible shock is noted when the patient fails to react to stimuli.

Therapeutic and Nursing Management of Shock

Prevention. The best treatment for shock is prophylaxis. This consists of adequate preparation of the patient, mental as well as physical, and anticipation of any complication that may arise during or after operation. Thus, special equipment for the treatment of shock must be on hand (Chart 21-4). The proper type of anesthesia should be cho-

Chart 21-4
Equipment Needed to Treat Shock

For blood studies:
Prothrombin time
Type and cross match
Hemoglobin
Hematocrit
*p*H
BUN
Serum electrolytes
Lactic acid levels

Sphygmomanometer—stethoscope
Indwelling catheter; urinometer
Suction equipment
Nasal oxygen equipment
CVP tray; Swan-Ganz tray
Defibrillator
IV cannula
Ringer's lactate solution

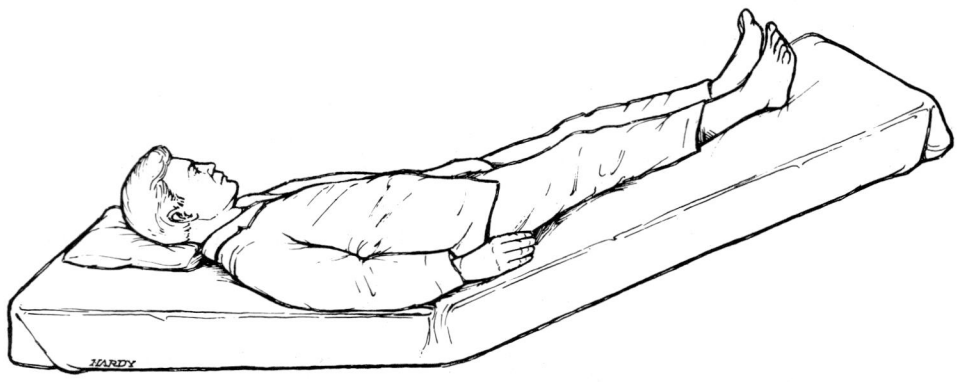

Figure 21-14. Proper positioning of the patient who shows signs of shock. The lower extremities are elevated to an angle of approximately 20 degrees; knees are straight, trunk horizontal, and head slightly elevated.

sen after careful consideration of the patient and his disease. Blood and plasma should be available if indicated. Blood loss should be accurately measured or intelligently estimated.

- If the amount of blood loss exceeds 500 ml, replacement is usually indicated.

Obviously, the individual patient and the particular circumstances must be considered in determining replacement therapy. An older, malnourished person is more likely to require this therapy than a patient whose health is generally good.

Operative trauma should be kept at a minimum as the first step in avoiding shock. After operation, factors that may promote shock are to be prevented. Pain is controlled by making the patient as comfortable as possible and by using narcotics judiciously. Exposure should be avoided, and lightweight, unheated covers should be used to prevent vasodilation. In the recovery room the patient can be watched and cared for by nurses trained especially in the recovery of patients from anesthesia. In addition, a quiet room helps to reduce mental trauma. Any moving of the patient is done gently. He is placed in the dorsal recumbent position to facilitate circulation. Monitoring of vital signs is continued until the patient's recovery indicates that shock is unlikely.

Treatment. (See also *Emergency Treatment of Shock,* Chap. 61.) The patient is kept warm, but overheating is avoided to prevent cutaneous vessels from dilating and depriving vital organs of blood. An infusion of Ringer's lactate solution is started. The patient is placed flat in bed with his legs elevated as in Figure 21-14. (Avoid the Trendelenburg position.) The patient's respiratory and circulatory status is monitored constantly: respiration, pulse, blood pressure, skin, urinary output, level of consciousness, CVP (PAP, PWP, and CO if available).

The basic approach to the treatment of shock is to determine its cause and correct it if possible.

1. The first objective of treatment is to ensure the adequacy of the airway. When the patient is ventilating adequately, blood gas determinations are made to determine adequacy of pulmonary function, and the patient is given oxygen by intubation or nasal cannula (Chart 21-5).

2. The second objective is to restore blood volume. Of the total blood volume, under normal conditions, 20% is in the capillaries, 10% in the arterial system, and the balance in the veins and heart. In shock, there is dilatation of the capillary beds, so that a considerable volume of blood can be accommodated.

Chart 21-5
Indications for Intubation and Mechanical Ventilation

Indications for Intubation*

Unable to maintain airway
Inadequate ventilation on face mask with 40% O_2
Respiratory rate > 35/min
PO_2 < 70 mm Hg†
PCO_2 > 45 mm Hg†
Vital capacity 15 ml/kg
Maximum inspiratory force weaker than −25 cm H_2O

Criteria for Extubation‡

Able to maintain airway
Adequate ventilation on T piece with 30% oxygen
Respiratory rate < 20/min
PO_2 > 70 mm Hg
PCO_2 < 45 mm Hg
Vital capacity > 10 ml/kg
Maximum inspiratory force stronger than −25 cm H_2O

* The trends of these values are more important than the absolute numbers themselves.
† These values presuppose normal pre-existing pulmonary functions.
‡ In the usual case, ALL of these criteria should be met before extubation.

(From Dunphy JE and Way LW: Current Surgical Diagnosis and Treatment, 5th ed, p 179. Los Altos, California Lange Medical Publishers, 1981.)

Two kinds of fluids are used: crystalloids and colloids. *Crystalloids* are electrolyte solutions that diffuse into interstitial spaces. An example is lactated Ringer's injection, a buffering solution, in which lactate is metabolized and excess hydrogen ions are neutralized.

Three parts crystalloids are lost to extravascular space for every one part that remains in the vascular system. This means that for every 2000 ml given, 500 ml increase the vascular volume. For hemorrhagic shock, crystalloids are given initially to lower blood viscosity and aid in microcirculation. After blood typing and cross matching are done, blood is given to bring oxygen to the tissues.

Colloids are blood, plasma, serum albumin, and plasma substitutes, such as dextran: these remain in the intravascular compartment. Blood of the same type as the patient's should be administered in preference to the generally used O-Rh-negative blood. Burn shock requires large amounts of colloid replacement.

3. The third objective is to administer vasodilators. Vasopressors are not used for the patient in shock because they tend to intensify vasoconstriction in the microcirculatory beds. Prolonged use may cause irreversible damage in the tissues of the kidneys, lungs, liver, and gastrointestinal tract.

Vasodilators are given to reduce peripheral resistance, which in turn decreases the work of the heart and increases cardiac output and tissue perfusion. The drug usually used is sodium nitroprusside (Nipride), which stimulates myocardial contractility and lowers peripheral resistance. Some clinics advocate the use of steroids, others use combinations of pharmacotherapeutic agents. Some authorities believe that hypovolemic shock should not be treated with vasoactive drugs. Their effect is to increase vascular resistance and decrease tissue perfusion, thus aggravating the effects of shock.

Nursing management requires constant monitoring of the blood pressure when vasodilators are used. The patient is kept flat during their administration. If the systolic blood pressure falls below 70, the drug is stopped and fluids are increased.

4. The fourth objective is to provide psychological support and minimize the patient's energy expenditure. Promote rest for the patient and assess his reactions to treatment. Offer support and reassurance to relieve apprehension. Administer sedatives cautiously as prescribed for pain, so that circulation is not further depressed. Keep the patient warm, because hypothermia increases hemoglobin saturation but decreases tissue oxygenation. However, proper balance must be maintained, because hypothermia also affects peripheral circulation. Turn the patient every 2 hours and encourage deep breathing to promote optimum cardiopulmonary function. Exercises and gentle massage help to prevent pressure sores.

5. The fifth objective is to prevent complications. Observe all parameters and monitor the patient closely in the 24-hour period following shock, since complications may develop. Peripheral and pulmonary edema owing to fluid overload is the most common complication that results from administering fluids faster than the body can accommodate them (see p. 642, pulmonary edema).

Hemorrhage

Classification

Hemorrhage is classified as (1) *primary,* when it occurs at the time of the operation; (2) *intermediary,* when it occurs within the first few hours after an operation, because of the return of blood pressure to its normal level and the consequent washing out of the insecure clots from untied vessels; and (3) *secondary,* when it occurs some time after the operation, as a result of the slipping of a ligature because of infection, insecure tying, or erosion of a vessel by a drainage tube.

A further classification frequently is made according to the kind of vessel that is bleeding. *Capillary* hemorrhage is characterized by a slow, general ooze; *venous* hemorrhage bubbles out quickly and is dark in color; *arterial* hemorrhage is bright in color and appears in spurts with each heartbeat.

When the hemorrhage is on the surface and can be seen, it is spoken of as *evident;* when it cannot be seen, as in the peritoneal cavity, it is spoken of as *concealed.*

Clinical Manifestations

Hemorrhage presents a more or less well-defined syndrome, depending on the amount of blood lost and the rapidity of its escape. The patient is apprehensive and restless, and moves continually; he is thirsty; and the skin is cold, moist, and pale. The pulse rate increases, the temperature falls, respirations are rapid and deep, often of the gasping type spoken of as "air hunger." As the hemorrhage progresses, cardiac output decreases, arterial and venous blood pressure and the hemoglobin of the blood fall rapidly, the lips and the conjunctivae become pallid, spots appear before the eyes, a ringing is heard in the ears, and the patient grows weaker but remains conscious until near death.

Management

Often the signs of hemorrhage after an operation are masked by the effects of the anesthetic or shock; therefore, the treatment of the patient is in a general way almost identical to that described for shock, viz, (1) place the patient in shock position (see Fig. 21-14) and (2) administer morphine to keep the patient quiet. The wound always should be inspected to find the site of the bleeding if possible. A sterile gauze pad and a snug bandage are indicated, as well as elevation of the part, arm, or leg.

- Giving a transfusion of blood and determining the cause of hemorrhage are the most logical therapeutic measures.
- In giving fluids by vein in cases of hemorrhage, remember that too large a quantity of fluid or too rapid administration may raise the blood pressure enough to start the bleeding again, unless the hemorrhage has been well controlled.

Femoral Phlebitis or Thrombosis

Pathophysiology

Femoral phlebitis or thrombosis occurs most frequently after operations upon the lower abdomen or in the course of septic diseases such as peritonitis and ruptured ulcer. A mild to severe inflammation of the vein occurs in association with a clotting of blood. The complication may result from a number of causes, including injury to the vein by tight straps or leg-holders at the time of operation, pressure from a blanket-roll under the knees, concentration of blood by loss of fluid or dehydration, or, more commonly, the slowing of the blood flow in the extremity owing to a lowered metabolism and depression of the circulation after operation. It is probable that several of these factors may act together to produce thrombosis. The left leg is affected more frequently.

The first symptom may be a pain or a cramp in the calf (Fig. 21-15). Pressure here gives pain, and a day or so later a painful swelling of the entire leg occurs, often associated with a slight fever and sometimes with chills and perspiration. The swelling is due to a soft edema that pits easily on pressure. There is marked tenderness over the anteromedial surface of the thigh.

A milder form of the same disease is termed *phlebothrombosis,* to indicate intravascular clotting without marked inflammation of the vein. The clotting occurs usually in the veins of the calf, often with few symptoms except slight soreness of the calf. The danger from this type of thrombosis is that the clot may be dislodged and produce an embolus. It is believed that most pulmonary emboli arise from this source (see Fig. 21-15).

Medical and Nursing Management

The treatments of thrombophlebitis or phlebothrombosis may be considered as (1) preventive and (2) active.

Prevention.   Efforts directed toward preventing the formation of a thrombus include such measures as adequate administration of fluids after operation to prevent blood concentration, leg exercises, elastic stockings (see below), and early ambulation to prevent stagnation of the blood in the veins of the lower extremity. Some clinics use low-dose heparin prophylactically to prevent deep vein thrombosis and major pulmonary embolism following general surgical operations. This method has not yet been generally accepted.

Leg exercises can be taught before surgery (see p. 357). If the patient recognizes their significance in preventing circulatory complications, he will often initiate his own exercises. To avoid thrombus formation, leg straps should not be fastened in the recovery room, particularly with stretchers that are equipped with side rails. Not only are the straps restrictive, but they can constrict and impair circulation.

Another important nursing measure is to avoid the use of blanket-rolls, pillow-rolls, or any form of elevation that can constrict vessels under the knees. Even the practice of "dangling" (having the patient sit on the edge of the bed with his legs hanging over the side) can be dangerous and is not recommended because pressure under the knees can impede circulation.

Active Treatment.   Some surgeons believe that ligation of the femoral veins is an important therapeutic method. The rationale behind this method of therapy is to prevent pulmonary embolism by eliminating the cause (thrombi

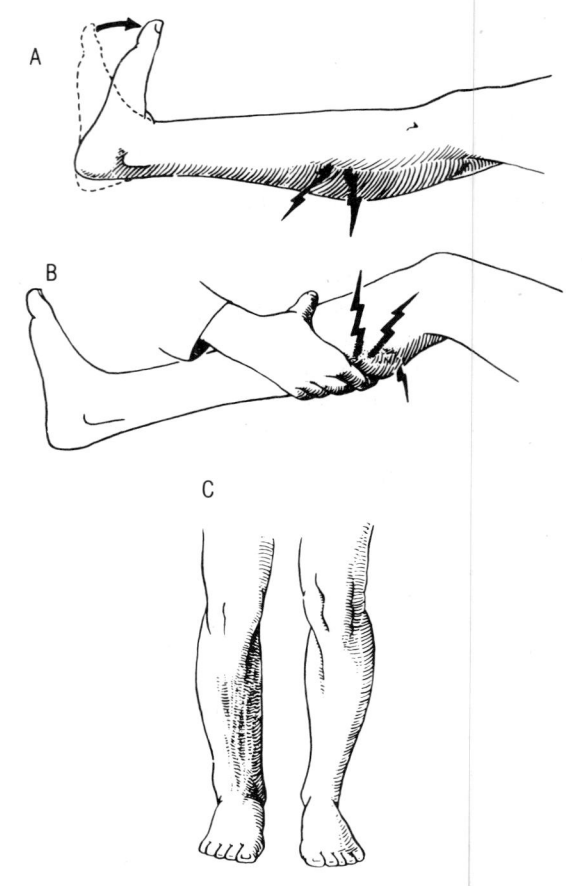

Figure 21-15.   Nursing assessment of signs and symptoms of phlebothrombosis. Signs of phlebothrombosis of the calf muscle veins: (*A*) Homans' sign, pain in the calf on dorsiflexion of the foot with the leg in extension. (*B*) Tenderness of the calf muscles on gentle compression. (*C*) Slight swelling about the ankle and prominence of the veins. (From Gius JA: Fundamentals of General Surgery. Chicago, Year Book Medical Publishers.)

that could become detached from femoral veins and circulate in the blood).

Anticoagulant therapy has taken a prominent place in the prophylaxis and the treatment of phlebitis and phlebothrombosis. Heparin, given intravenously by the drip method or subcutaneously in an oily menstruum, reduces the coagulability of the blood rapidly and is used most often when an immediate effect is desired. Repeated checks of the coagulation time of the blood are necessary to control its administration. Dicumarol or drugs with a similar action are used for the same purpose. It is given by mouth and does not become effective for about 24 hours. Daily dosage is controlled by daily estimations of the prothrombin time of the blood (see also p. 702).

Wrapping the legs from toes to groin with elastic stockings has been practiced both as a prophylactic and as an active treatment of phlebitis and thrombosis. These stockings prevent swelling and stagnation of venous blood in the legs and do much to relieve pain in the phlebitic extremity. However, to be effective, elastic stockings must be used in combination with leg elevation and leg exercises. Early ambulation is helpful, but the nurse also needs to be aware of the problem that can result when a patient with a protuberant abdomen walks a few steps and then sits with legs dependent; namely, the pressure of the abdomen can obstruct venous flow. Several recent research studies have questioned the value of elastic stockings, suggesting an actual danger when they are not applied correctly. Some clinics now do not advocate the use of elastic stockings for any surgical patient.

Pulmonary Embolism

An *embolus* is a foreign body in the bloodstream, formed by a blood clot that becomes dislodged from its original site and is carried along in the blood.

When the clot is carried to the heart, it is forced by the blood into the pulmonary artery, where it plugs the main artery or one of its branches. The symptoms produced may be among the most sudden and startling in surgical practice. A patient experiencing an apparently normal convalescence suddenly cries out with sharp, stabbing pains in the chest and becomes breathless, cyanotic, and anxious. The pupils dilate, cold perspiration appears, the pulse becomes rapid and irregular, then imperceptible, and death usually results. If death does not occur within 30 minutes, there is a chance of recovery.

Fortunately, pulmonary embolism is usually a less dramatic event than that described above and may be heralded by no more than mild dyspnea, arrhythmia, or seemingly innocent chest pain. Keen alertness on the part of the nurse is necessary to detect these subtle emboli in order that treatment may be initiated and further embolization avoided.

- Thus, one of the many reasons for getting the patient out of bed as soon after surgery as possible is to avoid a pulmonary embolism.

(See pp. 530–532 for therapeutic and nursing management.)

Respiratory Complications

Respiratory complications are among the most frequent and serious problems with which the surgical team has to deal.

Experience has shown that such complications may be avoided in large measure by careful preoperative observation and teaching and by taking every precaution during and after the operation. It is well known that those patients who have some respiratory disease before operation are more apt to develop serious complications after operation. Therefore, only emergency operations are performed when acute disease of the respiratory tract exists. The nurse may aid by reporting any symptom, such as cough, sneezing, inflamed conjunctivae, and nasal discharge, to the surgeon before the operation.

During and immediately after the operation, every effort should be made to prevent chilling. Aspiration of the nasopharynx in the recovery room removes secretions that would otherwise cause respiratory problems in the postoperative period. Occasionally, when secretions form that

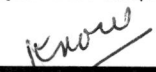

Chart 21-6
Risk Factors Affecting Postoperative Pulmonary Complications

Type of surgery—Greater incidence following all forms of abdominal surgery when compared with peripheral surgery

Location of incision—The closer the incision to the diaphragm, the higher the incidence of pulmonary complications

Preoperative respiratory problems

Age—Greater risk over age 40 than under age 40

Sepsis

Obesity—Weight greater than 110% of ideal body weight

Prolonged bed rest

Duration of operation—Over 3 hours

Aspiration

Dehydration

Malnutrition

Hypotension and shock

cannot be coughed up by the patient, aspiration may be carried out through a bronchoscope, and, in very debilitated patients in whom retained secretions are a complicating factor, a tracheostomy may be performed so that aspiration of the trachea is done directly through the tube as necessary.

Following upper abdominal surgery, total lung capacity (TLC) is reduced, for the following reasons:

1. Deep breathing may be quite painful.
2. Abdominal excursions with respiration normally are twice those of the chest cage. After surgery, they are greatly inhibited.
3. Spontaneous deep breaths are abolished (normally taken every 5 to 10 minutes).
4. Sigh mechanism is also abolished.

Complications are described briefly here and in more detail in Chapters 24 and 25.

Atelectasis. When the mucus plug closes one of the bronchi entirely, there is a collapse of the pulmonary tissue beyond, and a massive *atelectasis* is said to result (Fig. 21-16). (See also p. 451.) The principal factors predisposing to postoperative atelectasis are diagrammed in Figure 21-16.

Bronchitis. This pulmonary complication may appear at any time after operation, usually within the first 5 to 6 days. The symptoms vary according to the disease. A simple bronchitis is characterized by a cough that produces considerable mucopus, but without marked temperature or pulse elevation.

Bronchopneumonia. Bronchopneumonia is perhaps the second most frequent pulmonary complication. Besides a productive cough, there may be considerable temperature elevation, with an increase in the pulse and the respiratory rates.

Lobar Pneumonia. Lobar pneumonia is a less frequent

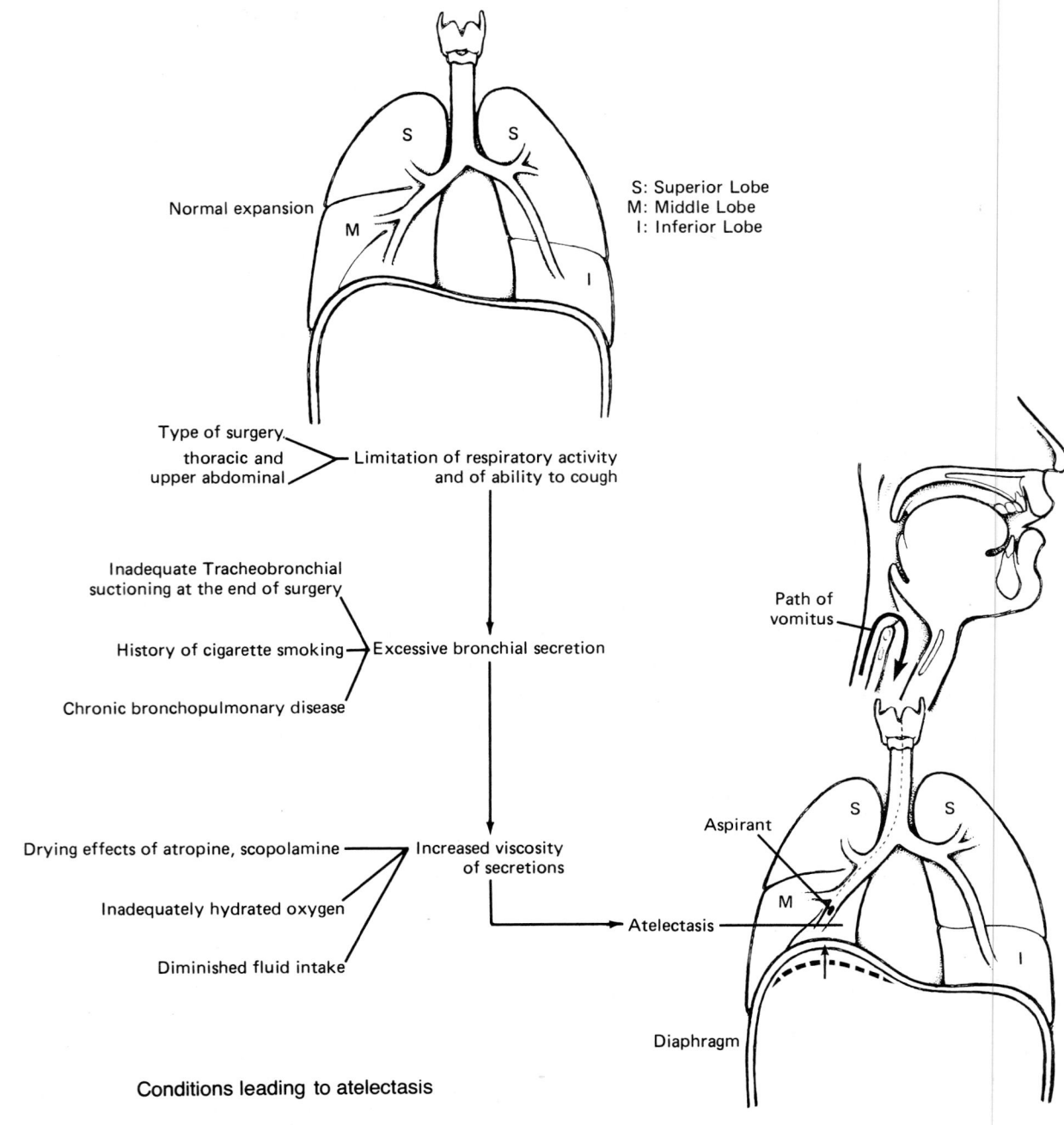

Figure 21-16. Atelectasis.

complication after operation. Usually, it begins with a chill, followed by high temperature, pulse, and respiration. There may be little or no cough, but the respiratory embarrassment, the flushed cheeks, and the evident illness of the patient make a combination of clinical signs that is distinctive. The disease runs its usual course with the added complication of the operative wound.

Hypostatic Pulmonary Congestion. Hypostatic pulmonary congestion is a condition that may develop in old or very weak patients. Its cause is a weakened heart and

vascular system that permit a stagnation of secretions at the bases of both lungs. It occurs most frequently, perhaps, in elderly patients who are not mobilized effectively. The symptoms frequently are not marked for a time—perhaps a slight elevation of temperature, pulse, and respiratory rate, and also a slight cough. However, physical examination reveals dullness and crackles at the base of the lungs. If the condition goes untreated, the outcome may be fatal.

Pleurisy. Pleurisy is not an uncommon occurrence after operation. Its chief symptom is an acute, knifelike pain in the chest on the affected side that is particularly excruciating when the patient takes a deep breath. Also, there usually is some slight temperature and pulse rise, and respirations are rapid and more shallow than normal.

Medical and Nursing Management of Pulmonary Complications

Awareness of the many possible respiratory complications enables the nurse to initiate the many preventive measures cited in the previous discussion (pp. 357, 360). Timely recognition of signs and symptoms allows the nurse to direct efforts to combating specific respiratory difficulties. Not only is the first postoperative day one of concern, but the first postoperative week of the patient's recovery requires close observation and careful management. The early signs of elevations in temperature, pulse, and respiration are significant. Chest pain, dyspnea, and cough may or may not accompany these elevations; however, the patient may seem to be restless and apprehensive. Such indications are important and should be reported and documented.

Measures to Promote the Full Aeration of the Lung. The prophylactic treatment of these conditions includes measures to promote full aeration of the lungs. The nurse should instruct the patient to take at least 10 deep inhalations every hour. Frequently, the patient blows into the incentive spirometer in an effort to expand the lungs fully (see p. 388 for fuller discussion). Turning the patient from side to side sometimes results in coughing, with expulsion of a mucus plug, and recovery. At times mucus may be removed by aspiration through a bronchoscope.

The increased metabolism, more complete pulmonary aeration, and the general improvement of all body functions incidental to getting the patient up out of bed have led many surgeons to regard ambulation as one of the best prophylactic measures against pulmonary complications. When the wound or condition otherwise permits, the patient is usually allowed to get up on the first or second day after operation, and even on the day of surgery. This practice is especially valuable in preventing pulmonary complications in older patients.

Indications for Specific Measures. A most effective method of treating *bronchitis* is the inhalation of cool mist or steam, which may be administered by electric vaporizers. The apparatus must be kept filled with water, and precautions must be taken to prevent the patient from being burned.

In *lobar* and *bronchopneumonia,* the patient is encouraged to take fluids; expectorant and antibiotic drugs also are given. Distention is watched for and prevented, if possible, so as to avoid added respiratory or cardiac embarrassment.

For *pleurisy,* analgesics, hot or cold applications, or, if necessary, a procaine intercostal block may be administered to provide symptomatic relief. A search is made to detect any possible underlying disease (pneumonia, infarction).

Pleurisy with effusion may result secondary to a primary pleurisy. In these patients aspiration of the pleural space is frequently necessary.

Many times the pulmonary complication of *hypostatic pulmonary congestion* becomes more serious than the original surgical condition, in which case the prime objective of therapeutic management is to treat the hypostatic pneumonia.

Because of reduced aeration in many of the pulmonary complications, which means that less oxygen reaches the blood, many clinics employ oxygen therapy in treatment. Principles and management are presented on pages 454–456.

Urinary Problems

Urinary Retention

Urinary retention may follow any operation, but it occurs most frequently after operations on the rectum, the anus, and the vagina, and after herniorrhaphies and operations on the lower abdomen. The cause is thought to be a spasm of the bladder sphincter.

Nursing Management. Quite often, patients are unable to void while lying in bed but, when allowed to sit or stand up, do so without difficulty. When standing does not interfere with the operative result, male patients may be allowed to stand by the side of the bed or female patients to sit on the edge of the bed with their feet on a chair or a stool. However, many patients cannot be permitted this activity, and other means of encouraging urination must be tried. Some people cannot void with another person in the room. These patients should be left alone for a time after being provided with a warm bedpan or urinal.

Frequently, the sound or the sight of running water may relax the spasm of the bladder sphincter. Using a bedpan containing warm water or irrigating the perineum with warm water frequently initiates urination for female patients. A small, warm enema often is of value in such a situation. If the retention of urine continues for some hours, the patient complains of considerable pain in the lower abdomen, and the bladder frequently can be palpated and seen in outline distending the lower anterior abdominal wall.

When all conservative measures have failed, catheterization must be resorted to. If the patient has voided just before operation, this procedure may be delayed in most cases for 12 to 18 hours. There are two reasons for wishing to avoid catheterization: (1) there is the possibility of infecting the bladder and producing a cystitis, and (2) experience has shown that once a patient has been catheterized, frequently subsequent catheterizations may be needed.

Many patients may exhibit a palpable bladder, with lower abdominal discomfort, and still void small amounts of urine at frequent intervals. The alert nurse does not mistake this for normal functioning of the bladder. This voiding of 30 ml to 60 ml (1 oz–2 oz) of urine at intervals of 15 to 30 minutes is, rather, a sign of an overdistended bladder, the very distention being sufficient to allow the escape of small amounts of urine at intervals. The condition usually is spoken of as the "overflow of retention." A catheter usually relieves the patient by draining from 600 ml to 900 ml (20 oz–30 oz) of urine from the bladder. "Incontinence of retention" may be evidenced by a constant dribble of urine, yet the bladder remains overdistended. Because distention injures the bladder, catheterization is indicated. There often is a definite psychic element in urinary retention.

At times, following extensive surgery, the surgeon may anticipate voiding difficulties and insert an indwelling catheter before the patient emerges from anesthesia. Usually, the surgeon desires to be notified if an amount less than 30 ml of urine per hour is collected in the calibrated receptacle.

Urinary Incontinence

Incontinence of urine is a frequent complication in the aged, either after operation or after shocking injuries. It is probably due to weakness with loss of tone of the bladder sphincter. This symptom frequently disappears as the patient gains in strength and normal muscular tone is regained.

Treatment.   See page 251 for bladder training, which is helpful for patients with urinary incontinence.

Urinary Infection

See discussion in Chapter 43.

Gastrointestinal Complications

Nutritional Considerations

Surgery of the gastrointestinal tract frequently disrupts the normal physiologic processes of digestion and absorption. Complications arising from this disruption may take several forms, depending on the location and extent of surgery. For example, oral surgery may present problems of chewing and swallowing, requiring that diet be modified to accommodate the difficulty. Other surgical procedures, such as gastrectomy, small bowel resection, ileostomy, colostomy, etc., have a more drastic effect on the gastrointestinal system and require more extensive dietary considerations, as indicated in Table 21-5.

Intestinal Obstruction

Intestinal obstruction is a complication that may follow abdominal operations. It occurs most often after operations on the lower abdomen and the pelvis, and especially after operations in which drainage has been necessary. The symptoms usually appear between the third and fifth days but may occur at any time, even years after the operation. The cause is some obstruction of the intestinal current—frequently a loop of intestine that has become kinked from inflammatory adhesions or is involved with peritonitis or generalized irritation of the peritoneal surface.

Usually, there is no temperature or pulse elevation. At first the pains are localized, a point which should be noted by the nurse, because the localization of the early pains represents in a general way the loop of intestine that is just above the obstruction.

Usually, the patient continues to have abdominal pains, with shorter and shorter intervals between. When a stethoscope is placed on the abdomen, sounds may be heard that give evidence of extremely active intestinal movements, especially during an attack of pain. The intestinal contents, being unable to move forward, distend the intestinal coils, are carried backward to the stomach, and are vomited. Thus,

Table 21-5
Dietary Support of Common Complications in Surgical Treatment

Procedure	Complications	Dietary Support
Radical oropharyngeal surgery	Difficulty in mastication and swallowing	*Diet:* Liquid consistency—tube feedings *Fluid by mouth:* Fruit juices as tolerated Coffee, tea, gelatin, ice cream
Gastrectomy	*Small pouch:* "Dumping syndrome" Epigastric fullness, distention; pallor, sweating, tachycardia, hypotension, diarrhea	Low carbohydrate Moderate fat High protein Small, frequent feedings Periodic injections of vitamin B_{12}
Small bowel resection	Poor absorption Weight loss (absorptive capacity improves with time)	*Immediate support after surgery:* Long-term parenteral nutrition *Later:* oral intake of high protein, high-calorie, low-fat diet Medium chain triglycerides
Ileostomy Colostomy	Initial loss of water and electrolytes	Daily replacement of electrolytes, full liquid diet, high in protein
Bypass surgery	For relief of pain and obstruction Malabsorption syndrome Maldigestion, diarrhea	Feedings by natural route High protein, high vitamin C Adequate vitamins and minerals

(From Valassi K: Nutritional management of cancer patients in a variety of therapeutic regimens. Arch Phys Med Rehab, Vol 58.)

vomiting and increasing distention gradually become more prominent symptoms. Hiccup often precedes the vomiting in many patients. The bowels do not move, and enemas return nearly clear, showing that a very small amount of the intestinal contents has reached the large bowel. Unless the obstruction is relieved, the patient continues to vomit, distention becomes more pronounced, the pulse becomes rapid, and the end is a toxic death.

Treatment. Sometimes the distention of the intestine above the obstruction can be prevented by the use of constant-suction drainage with the Miller–Abbott, Harris, or Cantor tubes or simple nasogastric tube, in which case the inflammatory reaction of the bowel at the site of the obstruction may subside and the obstruction is relieved. However, at times it is necessary to relieve the obstructed intestine by operation. In addition, intravenous infusions of prescribed solutions usually are given. (See the section on intestinal obstruction for a more complete discussion of the treatment and postoperative care, pp. 837–839.)

Wound Complications

Hematoma (Hemorrhage)
The nurse should know the location of the patient's incision so that the dressings may be inspected for hemorrhage at intervals during the first 24 hours after operation. Any undue amount of bleeding is reported. At times, concealed bleeding occurs in the wound, beneath the skin. This hemorrhage usually stops spontaneously but results in clot formation within the wound. If the clot is small, it will be absorbed and need not be treated. When the clot is large, the wound usually bulges somewhat, and healing will be delayed unless it is removed. After several stitches are removed, the clot is evacuated, after which the wound is packed lightly with gauze. Healing occurs usually by granulation, or a secondary closure may be performed.

Infection (Wound Sepsis)
Staphylococcus aureus accounts for many postoperative wound infections. Other infections may result from *Escherichia coli, Proteus vulgaris, Aerobacter aerogenes,* and *Pseudomonas aeruginosa,* and, occasionally, from other organisms (see Nosocomial Infections, p. 1501). The most important area of prevention lies in meticulous wound management and surgical technique. In addition, housekeeping cleanliness and environmental disinfection are important. When the inflammatory process occurs, it usually begins to show symptoms in 36 to 48 hours. The patient's pulse rate and temperature increase, and the wound usually becomes somewhat tender, swollen, and warm. At times, when the infection is deep, there may be no local signs. When a diagnosis of wound infection is made, the surgeon usually removes one stitch or more and, under aseptic precautions, separates the wound edges with a pair of blunt scissors or a hemostat. Once the infection is opened, a drain of rubber or gauze is inserted. In addition, many surgeons require some form of warm antiseptic solution with which to flush the wound. The surgeon may take a culture of the infected wound and prescribe specific antibiotics. It may be necessary to continue hot, wet dressings if so prescribed (Chart 21-7).

Disruption, Evisceration, or Dehiscence
This complication is especially serious in the case of abdominal wounds. It results from sutures giving way and from infection, and, more frequently, after marked distention or cough. It may also occur because of increasing age

---

Chart 21-7
Risk Factors Contributing to Wound Sepsis

Local	General
Wound contamination	Debilitation
Foreign body	Dehydration
Faulty suturing technique	Malnutrition
Devitalized tissue	Anemia
Hematoma	Advanced age
"Dead" space	Extreme obesity
	Shock
	Length of preoperative hospitalization
	Length of operation
	Associated diseases (*i.e.,* diabetes mellitus)

---

and the presence of pulmonary or cardiovascular disease in abdominal surgical patients.

The earliest sign is usually a gush of serosanguineous peritoneal fluid from the wound. The rupture of the wound may occur suddenly, coils of intestine escaping onto the abdominal wall. Such a catastrophe causes considerable pain and often is associated with vomiting. Frequently, the patient says that "something gave way." When the wound edges part slowly, the intestines may protrude gradually or not at all, and the presenting symptom may be the sudden drainage of a large amount of peritoneal fluid into the dressings.

- When disruption of a wound occurs, the surgeon is notified at once. The protruding coils of intestine should be covered with sterile dressings moistened with sterile saline.

An abdominal (scultetus) binder, properly applied, is an excellent prophylactic measure against an accident of this kind, and often it is used along with the primary dressing, especially for operations on individuals with weak or pendulous abdominal walls. It is often used also as a firm binder when rupture of a wound has occurred. Vitamin deficiency or lowered serum protein or chloride may require correction.

Keloid
Not infrequently in an otherwise normal wound, the scar develops a tendency to excessive growth. Sometimes the entire scar is affected; at other times the condition is segmented. This keloid tendency is unexplainable, unpredictable, and unavoidable in some individuals.

Much investigation has been done along the lines of prevention and cure. Careful closure of the wound, complete hemostasis, pressure support without undue tension on the suture lines—all are reputed to combat this distressing wound complication.

Postoperative Psychosis

Postoperative psychosis (mental aberrations) may be physiologic or psychologic in origin. Cerebral anoxia, thromboembolism, and fluid–electrolyte imbalances are recognized physical factors in postoperative central nervous system impairment. Emotional factors such as fear, pain, and disorientation can contribute to postoperative depression and anxiety.

The individuals most susceptible to psychologic disturbances are older patients and those in the lower socioeconomic levels. Disfiguring surgery or operations for cancer also predispose to intense emotional problems. Dressings that obscure vision or confinement in a body cast can result in behavioral changes because of the reduced sensory input.

The highest incidence of psychotic sequelae appears to occur in those individuals who have had open-heart surgery. Several factors seem significantly related to neurologic damage: age (the older, the more likely), length of extracorporeal circulation (the longer, the greater the likelihood), mean arterial pressure of less than 50 mm Hg during perfusion, and the possibility of air emboli. Even sensory-overload of the intensive care unit is believed to contribute to postcardiotomy delirium.

Nursing Intervention—Preoperative and Postoperative

The patient should be thoroughly informed before the operation about what to expect after surgery. Frequent contact provides reassurance to the patient and allows the nurse to gain significant information about the patient's psychological status as she assesses his responses and thoughts. The judicious use of narcotics can also reduce confusion and disorientation.

Orienting the patient to time, day, and place can help him to accept unfamiliar surroundings. Studies have indicated that thorough preoperative briefing of the patient and his family can usually counteract many of the potential postoperative psychological stresses. In addition, a positive attitude conveyed by all personnel who come in contact with the patient will foster positive feelings in the patient.

For overt psychosis, the patient may require major tranquilizers. Since postoperative psychosis does occur, it is helpful when discussing this with patients to indicate that it is transient. If a patient has illusions or hallucinations, it is often reassuring to him to know that these aberrations are occasionally experienced and do not reflect on his sanity.

Restraint.   In the postoperative care of these patients, it is wise for the nurse to explain the necessity for the patient's remaining in bed until the surgeon permits him to get up. Often, patients prefer to get out of bed to void or to get a drink of water rather than bother the nurse. This may lead to serious complications that a few words of explanation can prevent. However, some patients, especially older patients and those who are disoriented, may find it impossible to grasp. For such patients, the simplest form of restraint is the use of a bed with side rails or side protection. This permits the patient to move about in bed but prevents him from getting out of bed easily and injuring himself.

The room should be lighted to reduce the incidence of visual hallucinations. It is desirable to have a family member stay with the patient as much as possible, since the presence of another person has a reassuring and quieting effect.

To protect both patient and nurse, it often becomes necessary to apply some form of restraint in cases of delirium. The psychological effect of being restrained can be severe; therefore, any form of restraint should be applied *only as a last resort.* All other means of making the patient quiet should be tried first. If possible, he should be isolated from other patients. Any potentially harmful article in his vicinity should be removed.

When restraints are used, the patient should be in a comfortable and natural position, and care should be taken that the part is not so constricted as to interfere with the circulation. Restraint to the chest should be avoided, if possible. The appearance of cyanosis of the hand or foot indicates that the appliance is too tight. The appliances should be padded carefully and placed so as to prevent chafing or pressure sores. The skin underneath them should be inspected frequently, bathed carefully, and massaged at least every 2 or 3 hours. Even though restraints are applied, the patient never should be left unwatched. Any patient requiring restraint should have constant and careful nursing attention.

Delirium

Postoperative delirium occurs occasionally in several groups of patients. The most common types of delirium are toxic, traumatic, and alcoholic (delirium tremens).

Toxic.   Toxic delirium occurs in conjunction with the signs and the symptoms of a general toxemia. This patient is very ill, usually with a high temperature and pulse rate. The face is flushed, and the eyes are bright and roving. The patient moves incessantly, often attempting to get out of bed and disarranging the bedclothes continually. A marked degree of mental confusion is present. These states are seen most often in patients with general peritonitis or other septic conditions.

In such patients, elimination is promoted by encouraging the intake of fluids, and the causative condition is treated by antimicrobial therapy. At times, however, the outcome is fatal.

Traumatic.   Traumatic delirium is a mental state resulting from sudden trauma of any sort, especially in highly nervous people. The malady may take the form of wild, maniacal excitement, simple confusion with hallucinations and delusions, or depression. Sedative drugs—chloral hydrate, paraldehyde, and morphine—are used in treatment. Usually, the state begins and ends suddenly.

Delirium Tremens.   Individuals who have used alcohol habitually over a long period of time are poor surgical risks. Not only is their resistance lower than normal, but the effects of alcohol have most likely damaged practically every organ. In addition, these patients take anesthesia poorly.

After operation, the patient may do well for a few days, but the prolonged abstinence from alcohol causes him to become restless, nervous, and irritated easily by little things. His facial expression may change entirely. He sleeps poorly and often is disturbed by unreal dreams. When approached by the doctor or the nurse, he appears to awake suddenly, asks "Who are you?" and, when he is told where he is, will appear to be fairly normal for a short time. These symptoms should be watched for in patients who have been alcoholics, because active treatment at this stage may avoid the more violent delirium.

Active delirium tremens may come on suddenly or gradually. After a period of restless, nervous semidelirium, the patient finally loses entire control of his mental functions and "horrors reign supreme." His mind is a chaos of everchanging ideas. He talks incessantly and tries to get out of bed to get away from the hallucinations of fear and persecution that torment him continually. If attempts are made to restrain him, he may fight maniacally and often will injure himself and others. In this stage the patient is obviously sick. He is sleepless, perspires freely, and displays a marked tremor in his extremities. Finally, after many hours of torture, the patient becomes stuporous.

Treatment and Nursing Management. When possible, the treatment of these patients should begin 2 or 3 days before operation with a most thorough elimination from the kidneys, the bowels, and the skin. These measures should be continued after operation, especially if any of the early signs of the condition develop. Sedative drugs or tranquilizers should be given to keep the patient quiet. The chief cause of the symptoms in chronic alcoholics has been shown to be a depletion of the carbohydrate stores of the body and an inadequate ingestion of vitamins. Therefore, glucose is given intravenously, and vitamins are administered in concentrated form by mouth and by injection.

▷ Bibliography

Books

American College of Surgeons Committee on Preoperative and Postoperative Care Manual of Preoperative and Postoperative Care. Philadelphia, WB Saunders, 1977.

Beal JM. Critical Care for Surgical Patients. New York, Macmillan, 1982.

Condon RE and DeCosse JJ. Surgical Care: A Physiological Approach to Clinical Management. Philadelphia, Lea & Febiger, 1980.

Condon RE and Gorbach SL. Surgical Infections: Selective Antibiotic Therapy. Baltimore, Williams & Wilkins, 1981.

Condon RE and Nyhus LM (eds). Manual of Surgical Therapeutics, 5th ed. Boston, Little, Brown & Co, 1981.

Deitel M (ed). Nutrition in Clinical Surgery. Baltimore, Williams & Wilkins, 1980.

Dineen P and Gavin H-S. The Surgical Wound. Philadelphia, Lea & Febiger, 1981.

Drain CB and Shipley SB. The Recovery Room. Philadelphia, WB Saunders, 1979.

Dunphy JE and Way LW. Current Surgical Diagnosis and Treatment, 5th ed. Los Altos, California, Lange Medical Publishers, 1981.

Eiseman B. Prognosis of Surgical Disease. Philadelphia, WB Saunders, 1980.

Gruendemann BJ and Meeker MH. Alexander's Care of the Patient in Surgery. St Louis, CV Mosby, 1983.

Hardy JD. Critical Surgical Illness, 2nd ed. Philadelphia, WB Saunders, 1980.

Hardy JD (ed). Hardy's Textbook of Surgery. Philadelphia, JB Lippincott Co, 1983.

Hardy JD. Complications in Surgery and Their Management. Philadelphia, WB Saunders, 1981.

Hunt TK. Wound Healing and Wound Infections. New York, Appleton–Century–Crofts, 1980.

Hunt TK and Dunphy JE. Fundamentals of Wound Management. New York, Appleton–Century–Crofts, 1979.

Israel JS and DeKornfeld TJ. Recovery Room Care. Springfield, Illinois, Charles C Thomas, 1981.

Jordan GL et al. Advances in Surgery. Chicago, Year Book Medical Publishers, 1980.

Kneedler J and Dodge GH. Perioperative Nursing Care. St Louis, CV Mosby, 1983.

LeMaitre GD and Finnegan JA. The Patient in Surgery, 4th ed. Philadelphia, WB Saunders, 1980.

Liechty RD and Soper RT. Synopsis of Surgery, 4th ed. St Louis, CV Mosby, 1980.

Margand PMS, Brooks CG Jr, and Hunter JW II. Preoperative Pulmonary Preparation. A Clinical Guide. Baltimore, Williams & Wilkins, 1981.

Metzger RS and Robertson PA. Intraoperative Learning. Denver, AORN Association, 1977.

Millar S (ed). Methods in Critical Care. The AACN Manual by the American Association of Critical Care Nurses. Philadelphia, WB Saunders, 1980.

Nursing Photobook. Caring for Surgical Patients. Springhouse, Pennsylvania, Intermed Communications, 1982.

Nursing Photobook. Controlling Infection. Springhouse, Pennsylvania, Intermed Communications, 1982.

Nyhus LM. Surgery Annual 1982. New York, Appleton–Century–Crofts, 1982.

Ravitch NM and Steichan FM (eds). Current Problems in Surgery. Chicago, Year Book Medical Publishers, 1981.

Rosoff AJ. Informed Consent. A Guide for Health Care Providers. Rockville, Maryland, Aspen Systems, 1981.

Sabiston DC. Davis–Christopher Textbook of Surgery, 12th ed. Philadelphia, WB Saunders, 1981.

Sager DP and Bomar SK. Intravenous Medications. Philadelphia, JB Lippincott, 1980.

Schwartz SI and Shires T. Principles of Surgery, 3rd ed. New York, McGraw–Hill, 1979.

Zollinger RM and Zollinger RM Jr. Atlas of Surgical Operations. New York, Macmillan, 1982.

Anesthesia

Artresio JF and Yao FSF. Fundamentals of Clinical Anesthesiology. Philadelphia, JB Lippincott, 1983.

Eckenhoff JE. Controversy in Anesthesiology. Philadelphia, WB Saunders, 1979.

Lichtiger M and Moya F. Introduction to the Practice of Anesthesia, 2nd ed. Hagerstown, Maryland, Harper & Row, 1978.

Savarese JJ and Lowenstein E. Anesthesia, Chap 9, pp 155–187. In Nardi GJ and Zuidema GD. Surgery, 4th ed. Boston, Little, Brown & Co, 1982.

Vandam LD (ed). To Make the Patient Ready for Anesthesia: Medical Care of the Surgical Patient. Menlo Park, Addison–Wesley, 1980.

Shock

Perry AG and Potter PA. Shock: Comprehensive Nursing Management. St Louis, CV Mosby, 1982.

Articles
Perioperative

Committee on Nursing Practice. Standards of Perioperative Nursing Practice. Using the revised standards. AORN J 1982 Sept; 36(3):363–377.

Keithley JK and Tasic PW. A unified approach to assessment of the surgical patient. Am J Nurs 1982 Apr; 82(4):612–614.

Koehler JS. Perioperative nursing can be cost effective. AORN J 1980 Dec; 32(6):1068–1076.

Larke GA. Perioperative charting; OR nursing on display. AORN J 1980 Feb; 31(8):194–198.

O'Connor RJ. Informed consent: Legal, behavioral, and educational issues. Patient Counselling and Health Education 1981 Second Quart; 3(2):49–56.

Pesetski JD. A practical guide for perioperative practice. AORN J 1980 Dec; 32(6):1049–1058.

Recommended practices for documentation of perioperative nursing care. AORN J 1982 Mar; 35(4):744–748.

Statements of basic competence for perioperative nurses. AORN J 1982 Apr; 35(5):882–884.

General

Geldbach PL, Klein WF, and Moore RC. Quality control circles solving OR problems. AORN J 1981 Dec; 34(6):1029–1035.

Heaman DJ and Mattle LF. Adolescent emergence excitement. AORN J 1982 Feb; 35(2):230–242.

Mattia MA. Hazards in the hospital environment. Anesthesia gases and methylmethacrylate. Am J Nurs 1983 Jan; 83(1):73–77.

Redmond C. Student nurses in the recovery room. AORN J 1981 Sept; 34(3):534–538.

Roberto N. Advising patients on sex after surgery. AORN J 1980 July; 32(1):55–61.

Schneider M. The recovery room is special procedures unit. AORN J 1981 Sept; 34(3):490–498.

Smith RF. Microbiological safety index. AORN J 1982 Aug; 36(2):311–316.

Wardell B. A standard care plan for the operating room. AORN J 1982 Aug; 36(2):279–287.

Preoperative

Abbott NK, Biala G, and Pollock W. The impact of preoperative assessment on intraoperative nurse performance. AORN J 1983 Jan; 37(1):43–58.

Axford R and Cutchen L. Using nursing research to improve preoperative care. J Nurs Adm 1977 Dec; 7(12):16–20.

Cruse PJE. Preparing the patient for operation. American College of Surgeons Bulletin 1981 May; pp 16–25.

Ennis CE and Andrassy RJ. Nutritional management of the surgical patient. AORN J 1980 June; 31(6):1217–1224.

Fernsebner B. Antimicrobial therapy for surgical patients. AORN J 1982 Sept 36(3):479–486.

Fuller BF. Hemostasis: A balanced system. AORN J 1981 Aug; 34(2):225–230.

Kaul AF et al. Agents and techniques for disinfection of skin. J Enterost Ther 1981 Sept–Oct; 8(5):19–22.

Matheny N. Preoperative fluid balance assessment. AORN J 1981 Jan; 33(1):51–56.

McClurg E. Developing an effective patient teaching program. AORN J 1981 Sept; 34(3):474–487.

Merrell S. A teaching plan for surgical skin preparation. AORN J 1982 June; 35(7):1372–1378.

Mullen JL. Consequences of malnutrition in the surgical patient. Surg Clin North Am 1981 June; 61(3):465–487.

O'Connor RJ. Informed consent: Legal, behavioral, and educational issues. Patient Counselling and Health Education. 1981 Second Quart; 3(2):49–56.

Parker CB. Endoscopic movies for patient teaching. AORN J 1981 Aug; 34(2):254–259.

Phippen ML. Nursing assessment of preoperative anxiety. AORN J 1980 May; 31(6):1019–1026.

Proposed recommended practices for preoperative skin preparation of patients. AORN J 1982 Apr; 35(4):918–923.

Robbins JA and Mushlin AI. Preoperative evaluation of the healthy patient. Med Clin North Am 1979 Nov; 63(6):1145–1156.

Shapiro M. Preoperative prophylactic use of antibiotics in surgery: Principles and practice. Infect Control 1982 Jan–Feb; 3(1):30–40.

Stein TP and Buzby GP. Protein metabolism in surgical patients. Surg Clin North Am 1981 June; 61(3):519–527.

Stotts N. Nutritional assessment before surgery. AORN J 1982 Feb; 35(2):207–214.

Wicklund S. Special Report: Drug management and elective surgery. Nurses' Drug Alert 1983 Jan; 7(1):4–6.

Anesthesia

Dryden GE. Intubation anesthesia equipment should be aseptic for each use. Part 4, pp 73–83. In Eckenhoff JE. Controversy in Anesthesiology. Philadelphia, WB Saunders, 1979.

Fernsebner B. A protocol for malignant hyperthermia. AORN J 1980 Apr; 31(8):814–818.

Hamilton WK and Feeley TW. A need for aseptic inhalation anesthesia equipment for each case is unproven, pp 84–89. In Eckenhoff JE. Controversy in Anesthesiology. Philadelphia, WB Saunders, 1979.

Manchikanti L, Kraus JW, and Edds SP. Cimetidine and related drugs in anesthesia. Anesth Analg 1982 July; 61(7):595–608.

Nisson RL and Yonkers AJ. Malignant hyperthermia. Laryngoscope 1982 Oct; 92(10):1183–1186.

Sterilization of anesthetic equipment, pp 90–91 (editorial comment). In Eckenhoff JE. Controversy in Anesthesiology. Philadelphia, WB Saunders, 1979.

Wetchler BV. Anesthesia for outpatient surgery. AORN J 1981 Aug; 43(2):282–296.

Intraoperative

AORN Standards of Practice. Denver, Colorado, AORN, 1978.

Aseptic barrier materials for surgical drapes. AORN J 1982 Apr; 35(5):906–911.

Beck WC. Alcohol foam for hand disinfection. AORN J 1980 Dec; 32(6):1087–1088.

Beck WC. Aseptic barriers in surgery. Arch Surg 1981 Feb; 116(2):240–244.

Belkin NL. Evaluating surgical gowning, draping fabrics. AORN J 1981 Sept; 34(3):499–571.

Burus LA. Ambulatory surgery growing at a rapid pace. AORN J 1982 Feb; 35(2):260–270.

Can OR garb be stylish and functional? AORN J 1980 Sept; 32(3):423–444.

Darden ML. Blood loss determination. AORN J 1981 June; 33(7):1368–1380.

Defective spore strips cause misleading results. AORN J 1981 Aug; 34(2):245–246.

Dineen P and Poncy M. Testing an externally powderless surgical glove. AORN J 1980 Oct; 32(4):633–645.

Elwyn DH, Kinney JM, and Askonazi J. Energy expenditure in surgical patients. Surg Clin North Am 1981 June; 61(3):545–556.

Hazzard ME. Linking the OR to curriculum goals. AORN J 1980 Nov; 32(5):807–817.

Hercules P. OR experience teaches continuity of care. AORN J 1980 Nov; 32(5):799–806.

McDonald NE. Patient representatives come to the operating room. AORN J 1981 Aug; 34(2):332–340.

McNameer C and McLean B. Nerve palsies: The preventable sort. Can Nurse 1980 July–Aug; 76(7):38–40.

Merrill S. A teaching plan for positioning. AORN J 1982 Jan; 35(1):63–66.

Preston CA, Ivancevich JM, and Matteson MT. Stress and the OR nurse. AORN J 1981 Mar; 33(4):662–671.

Proposed recommended practices for OR sanitation. AORN J 1981 June; 33(7):1262–1266.

Recommended practices for traffic patterns in the surgical suite. AORN J 1982 Mar; 35(4):750–758.

Standards of administrative nursing practice: OR. AORN J 1981 Aug; 34(2):268–280.

Surgical sepsis a delicate balance. AORN J 1982 Mar; 35(4):786–789.

Surgical suite is no place for jewelry, watches, or nail polish. AORN J 1981 June; 33(7):1294–1295.

Postoperative Problems

Albanese AJ and Riley JM. Caring for the intubated patient. RN 1980 Apr; 43(4):38–43, 98–100.

Allen P. Applying standards to practice. AORN J 1980 Apr; 31(5):805–813.

Armstrong ME. Current concepts in pain. AORN J 1980 Sept; 32(3):383–390.

Banyard SG. New drug-free technique cuts postoperative pain. RN 1982 Apr; 45(4):31–33.

Bauman B. Update your technique for changing dressings dry to dry. Nursing '82 1982 Jan; 12(1):64–67.

Boguslawski M. Therapeutic touch: A facilitator of pain relief. Top Clin Nurs 1980 Apr; 2(1):27–37.

Lidocaine may prevent postoperative laryngospasm. AORN J 1980 Jan; 31(1):76.

Lipman TO. How would you treat a man in need of postoperative nutritional support? Drug Therapy 1982 Aug; 12(8):111–114.

Love–Mignogna S. Taping and splinting. Nursing '80 1980 Apr; 10(4):88–92.

McConnell E. Toward complication-free recoveries for your surgical patients. RN 1980 June; 43(6):31–33, 75–100.

McDonnell DE. How to relieve pain with injectable narcotics. Nursing '80 1980 Oct; 10(10):34–39.

Moss G. Postoperative ileus is an avoidable complication. Surg Gynecol Obstet 1978 Jan; 148(1):81–82.

Myers AM. Evaluation of the hemorrhage-prone patient. Postgrad Med 1980 Apr; 67(4):161–170.

Regan WA. Is RR (recovery room) nurse liable for patient injury in understaffed unit? AORN J 1980 Sept; 32(3):465–468.

Risser NL. Preoperative and postoperative care to prevent pulmonary complications. Heart Lung 1980 Jan/Feb; 9(1):57–67.

Robusto N. Advising patients on sex after surgery. AORN J 1980 July; 32(1):55–61.

Sandroff R. The potent placebo. RN 1980 Apr; 43(4):35–37, 88–96.

Standards of Nursing Practice: Recovery room. AORN J 1980 Apr; 31(5):800–804.

Sweeney SS. OR observations: Key to post-op pain. AORN J 1980 Sept; 32(3):391–392.

Wells N. The effect of relaxation on postoperative muscle tension and pain. Nurs Res 1982 July/Aug; 31(4):236–238.

Wyman JB and Wick MR. The vomiting patient. Am Fam Physician 1980 Feb; 21(2):139–143.

Wound Care

Alexander JW. The role of host defense mechanisms in surgical infections. Surg Clin North Am 1980 Feb 60(1):107–116.

Altemeir WA. Perspectives in surgical infections. Surg Clin North Am 1980 Feb; 60(1):5–13.

Beck WC. Aseptic barriers in surgery: Their present status. Arch Surg 1981 Feb; 116(2):240–244.

Besst JA and Wallace HJ. Wound healing—intraoperative factors. Nurs Clin North Am 1979 Dec; 14(4):701–712.

Brachman PS et al. Nosocomial surgical infections: Incidence and cost. Surg Clin North Am 1980 Feb; 60(1):15–25.

Bruno P. The nature of wound healing. Nurs Clin North Am 1979 Dec; 14(4):667–682.

Burn ED. Promoting healing of bone tissue. AORN J 1982 May; 35(6):1186–1191.

Cooper DM and Schumann D. Postsurgical nursing intervention as an adjunct to wound healing. Nurs Clin North Am 1979 Dec; 14(4):713–726.

Cruse PJ and Foord R. The epidemiology of wound infections. A ten-year prospective study of 62,939 wounds. Surg Clin North Am 1980 Feb; 60(1):27–40.

Flynn ME and Rovee DT. Wound healing mechanisms. Am J Nurs 1982 Oct; 82(10):1544–1550.

Frogge MH. Promoting wound healing in the irradiated patient. AORN J 1982 May; 35(6):1088–1093.

Groszek DM. Promoting wound healing in the obese patient. AORN J 1982 May; 35(6):1132–1138.

Keethley JK. Wound healing in malnourished patients. AORN J 1982 May; 35(6):1094–1099.

Kottra CJ. Wound healing in the immunosuppressed host. AORN J 1982 May; 35(6):1142–1148.

Lyons RJ. Promoting healing of skin flaps and grafts. AORN J 1982 May; 35(6):1174–1183.

Mackey C and Hopefl AW. Keeping infections down when risks go up. Nursing '80 1980 June; 10(6):69–78.

Meakins JL et al. The surgical intensive care unit: Current concepts in infection. Surg Clin North Am 1980 Feb; 60(1):117–132.

Miles SAA. The inflammatory response in relation to local infections. Surg Clin North Am 1980 Feb; 60(1):93–100.

Nichols RL. Postoperative wound infection. N Engl J Med 1982 Dec 30; 307(27):1701–1702.

Nichols RL. Techniques known to prevent post-operative wound infection. Infect Control 1982 Jan–Feb; 3(1):34–37.

Query: Electrical clippers use. AORN J 1982 May; 35(6):1064.

Rhoads JE. The impact of nutrition on infection. Surg Clin North Am 1980 Feb; 80(1):41–47.

Schumann D. The nature of wound healing. AORN J 1982 May; 35(6):1068–1077.

Simmons RL. Wound infection: A review of diagnosis and treating. Infect Control 1982 Jan–Feb; 3(1):44–51.

Winters B. Promoting wound healing in the diabetic patient. AORN J 1982 May; 35(6):1083–1087.

Yordan EL Jr and Bernhard LA. The surgeon's role in wound healing. AORN J 1982 May; 35(6):1078–1082.

Infection

Axnick KJ. Infection control consideration in the care of the immuno-suppressed patient. Crit Care Quart 1980 Dec; 3(3):79–88.

Craven DE. Antimicrobial therapy of bacterial nosocomial infections. Crit Care Quart 1980 Dec; 3(3):89–108.

Fischer JE. Relevance of nutrition to infection and sepsis. Contemporary Surgery 1980 Aug; 17(2):50–64.

Garver JS. Isolation techniques in critical care units. Crit Care Quart 1980 Dec; 3(3):29–41.

Hopkins CC. Identification of infection problems in intensive care units. Crit Care Quart 1980 Dec; 3(3):1–9.

Oakes CA. Lower respiratory tract infections. Crit Care Quart 1980 Dec; 3(3):57–62.

O'Donnell J. Antibiotic prophylaxis in surgical infection. Heart Lung 1983 Jan; 12(1):20–22.

Presswood GM. Collection, transport, and interpretation of microbiologic specimens. Crit Care Quart 1980 Dec; 3(3):11–27.

Reinarz JA. Nosocomial infections. Clin Symp 1978; 30(6):2–32.

Underwood MA. Urinary tract infections. Crit Care Quart 1980 Dec; 3(3):63–70.

Shock

Barrows JJ. Shock demands drugs. Nursing '82 1982 Feb; 12(2):34–41.

Eckridge RA. Septic shock. Crit Care Quart 1980 Mar; 2(4):55–75.

Guglielmo J. Evaluation of the use of corticosteroids (for shock). Crit Care Quart 1980 Mar; 2(4):37–42.

Lamb LS. Think you know septic shock? Nursing '82 1982 Jan; 12(1):34–43.

Meador B. Cardiogenic shock. RN 1982 July; 45(4):38–42.

Park GD. Cardiogenic shock. Crit Care Quart 1980 Mar; 2(4):43–54.

Plachetka JR. Sympathomimetic pharmacology (treating shock). Crit Care Quart 1980 Mar; 2(4):27–35.

Programmed Instruction: Nursing care of patients in shock. Part I. Am J Nurs 1982 June; 82(6):943–964.

Programmed Instruction: Nursing care of patients in shock. Part II. Am J Nurs 1982 Sept; 82(9):1401–1422.

Programmed Instruction: Nursing care of patients in shock. Part III. Am J Nurs 1982 Nov; 82(11):1723–1746.

Purcell JA. Shock drugs. Standardized guidelines. Am J Nurs 1982 June; 82(6):965–974.

Robinson WA. Fluid therapy in hemorrhagic shock. Crit Care Quart 1980 Mar; 2(4):1–13.

Unit VII

Problems Affecting Oxygen–Carbon Dioxide Exchange and Respiration

22

Management of Patients With Conditions of the Upper Respiratory Airway

▷ Problems of the Nose

Epistaxis (Nosebleed)

Pathophysiology. A hemorrhage from the nose, referred to as *epistaxis,* is caused by the rupture of tiny, distended vessels in the mucous membrane of any area of the nose. Rarely does epistaxis originate in the densely vascular tissue over the turbinates. Most commonly, the site is the anterior septum, where three major blood vessels enter the nasal cavity: (1) the anterior ethmoidal artery on the forward part of the roof, (2) the sphenopalatine artery in the posterosuperior region, and (3) the internal maxillary branches (the plexus of veins located at the back of lateral wall under inferior turbinate).

Epistaxis may result from injury or disease, although the usual cause of small nosebleeds is "picking" of the nose. Other local causes are deviated septum, perforated septum, cancer, and trauma. Epistaxis may also occur as a symptom of acute rheumatic fever, acute sinusitis, arterial hypertension, and hemorrhagic diseases.

Emergency Therapy. In providing emergency care, remember that cessation of bleeding is aided by having the patient sit upright and by promoting vasoconstriction in the nasal mucous membrane. The patient should breathe through his mouth, refrain from talking, and compress the soft outer portion of the nose against the midline septum for 5 or 10 minutes continuously. Saturating a piece of cotton with a local vasoconstricting drug such as Neo-Synephrine and then inserting the cotton into the nostril may be helpful.

Instruct the patient not to blow his nose during or after a nosebleed. Provide tissues and an emesis basin into which he can expectorate any blood that collects in the nasopharynx. Should these measures fail, the problem should be reported to the physician, who may control the epistaxis by applying aqueous epinephrine 1:1000 to a cotton pledget, inserting it in the nostril near the bleeding source, and applying pressure. The physician may then cauterize the site (if the bleeding point is visible) using an electric cautery

Anatomy of the Upper Respiratory Tract

Nose

The nose has two passages, called *nares*, separated in the middle by the septum. These passages open externally through the anterior nostrils and posteriorly into the nasopharynx. Between these two openings the air passages expand into broad chambers, on the lateral walls of which are three turbinate bones and into which open the paranasal sinuses, cavities within the hollow bones that surround the nasal passages.

Paranasal Sinuses

The paranasal sinuses include the frontal sinuses, located in the lower forehead between and above the eyes; the ethmoidal group of sinuses, both anterior and posterior, extending along the roof of the nostrils; the sphenoid sinuses, opening at the rear; and, located on either side of the nose, the maxillary sinuses (Fig. 22-1). The same type of ciliated epithelium that lines the nasal passages also lines these paranasal sinuses.

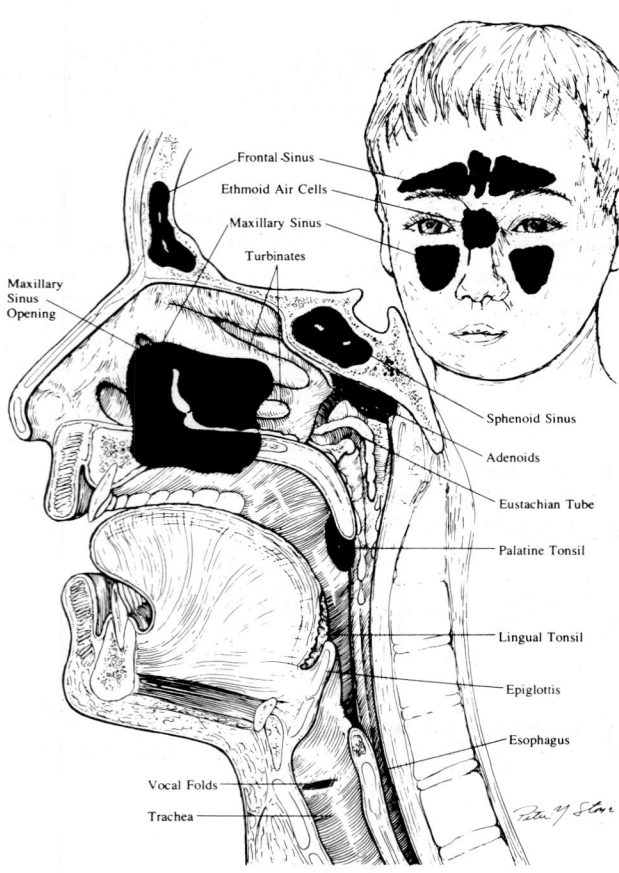

Figure 22-1. Anatomical features of the upper respiratory tract. (From Patient Education Chart material courtesy of and available from *Medical Times*, 80 Shore Road, Port Washington, N.Y. 11050.)

A prominent function of the sinuses is to help give resonance and timber to speech. One notes how "nasal" the voice is when an individual has a head cold and sinusitis.

Turbinate Bones (Conchae)

The turbinate bones, or conchae (the name suggested by their shell-like appearance), are adapted by shape and position to increase the mucous membrane surface of the nasal passages and to obstruct slightly the current of air flowing through them (Fig. 22-1). The sense organs of smell are located in the olfactory membrane, which covers the roof of the nose and the superior turbinate bones.

The current of air entering the anterior nostrils is deflected upward to the roof of the nose and follows a circuitous route before it reaches the nasopharynx. On its way, it comes into contact with a large surface of moist, warm mucous membrane that catches practically all of the dust and germs in the inhaled air. This air is moistened and warmed to body temperature and brought into contact with sensitive nerves. Some of these nerves detect odors, and others provoke sneezing to expel irritating dust.

Pharynx

The pharynx, or throat, is limited below by the larynx and the upper end of the esophagus. Its upper extension is the nasopharynx, into which open the posterior nostrils and the eustachian tubes from the middle ears. The nose and the nasopharynx are lined with the same type of ciliated epithelium as that which lines the trachea and bronchial tree; but the pharynx, which serves as both a respiratory and an alimentary passage, is lined with squamous (flat-celled) epithelium.

Tonsils and Adenoids

The tonsils are two almond-shaped bodies, one on each side at the back of the throat. The adenoid, or pharyngeal tonsil, is located in the roof of the nasopharynx. The tonsils and the adenoids constitute only two of a ring of similar masses of lymphoid tissue that completely encircles the throat. These organs are important links in the chain of lymph nodes guarding the body from invasion by organisms entering the nose and the throat.

Larynx

The larynx is a cartilaginous epithelium-lined structure forming the upper extremity of the trachea. The vocal cords, controlled by muscular attachments, are mounted in its lumen. Over it, preventing the entry of ingested food or liquid, is attached a valve flap called the *epiglottis*. The whole function of the larynx is to permit vocalization. It is the "voice box."

(after injection of a local anesthetic) or a chemical agent such as a silver nitrate stick, a chromic acid bead, or trichloroacetic acid.

Subsequent Therapy. For subsequent therapy, the objectives are to ease pain, identify the bleeding site, and control bleeding.

To Ease Pain. It may be necessary to administer morphine (very judiciously), if pain is troublesome. Another method may be to apply cotton pledgets saturated with a solution of cocaine and epinephrine in order to shrink nasal mucosa and provide comfort.

To Identify the Bleeding Site. Identifying the bleeding site may prove difficult; perhaps only the bleeding area can be determined. A light source whose rays are parallel to the line of vision, such as a concave head mirror, may be used to view deep, narrow spaces of the nasal cavity. If bleeding is occurring from the posterior regions, drug-moistened cotton pledgets may be inserted into the nostril to reduce the blood flow and improve the view. Suction can remove excess blood and clots from the field of inspection. The search may shift from the anteroinferior quadrant to the anterosuperior, then to the posterosuperior, and finally to the posteroinferior area. The field can be kept clear by using suction and by shifting the cotton tampons. However, only about 60% of the total nasal cavity can actually be seen.

To Control Bleeding. When the origin of the bleeding cannot be found, the nose is sprayed with a topical anesthetic and a decongestant and then packed with gauze impregnated with petrolatum. A postnasal packing may be inserted with a balloon-inflated catheter or by the methods shown in Figure 22-2. Pressure may be increased by moistening the gauze. The packing can be kept in place for 48 hours or up to 5 to 6 days if necessary.

Rhinitis

Pathophysiology. *Rhinitis* is an inflammatory lesion involving the mucous membrane of the nose. It is sometimes a manifestation of allergy (p. 1122), in which instance the condition is referred to as "allergic rhinitis," but usually

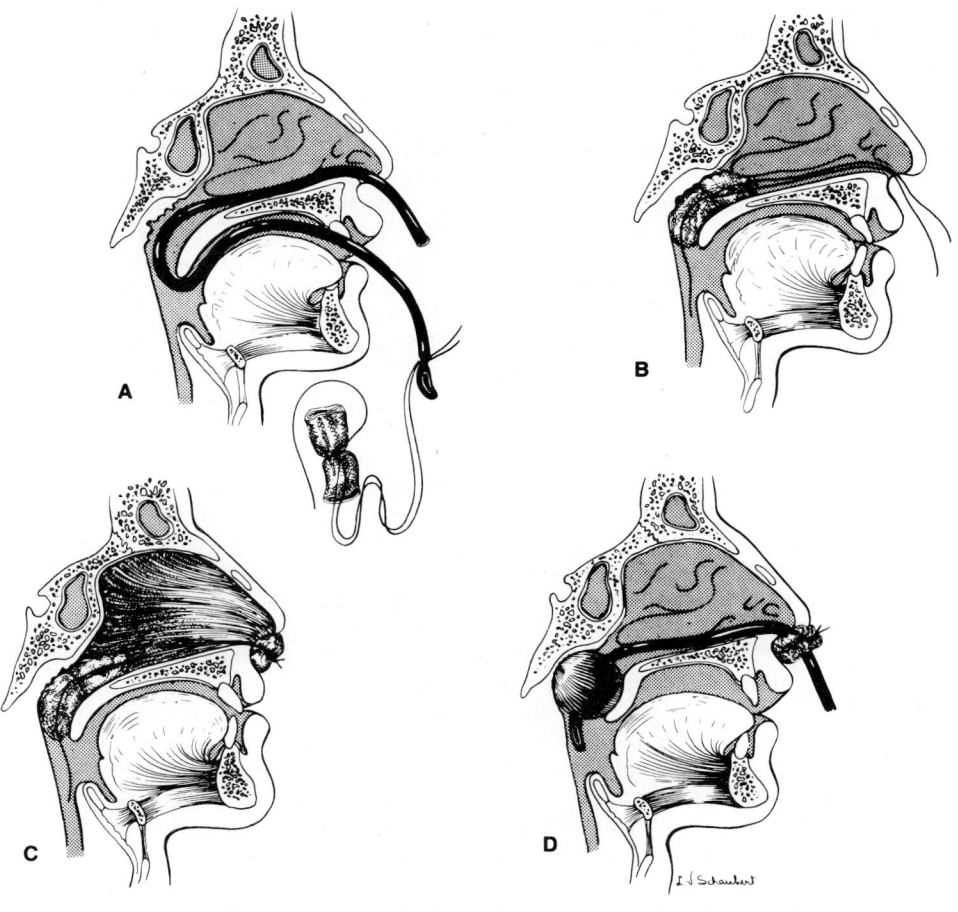

Figure 22-2. Packing to control bleeding from the posterior nose. (*A*) Catheter inserted and pack attached. (*B*) Pack drawn into position as catheter is removed. (*C*) Strip tied over a bolster to hold pack in place with anterior pack installed "accordion pleating" style. (*D*) Alternative method using balloon catheter instead of gauze pack. (Reproduced, with permission, from Dunphy JE and Way LW (eds). Current Surgical Diagnosis & Treatment, 5th ed. Copyright © 1981 by Lange Medical Publications, Los Altos, California.)

it is due to an infection. The most common variety of infection causing viral rhinitis is "coryza" (the common cold). Rhinitis also is encountered with regularity in the early stages of measles and other specific viral infections. Bacterial rhinitis is usually caused by a gram-positive bacterium and is characterized by a purulent nasal discharge. The infection is often secondary to a viral upper respiratory infection. If untreated, rhinitis can lead to sinusitis, otitis media, bronchitis, and pneumonia.

In acute rhinitis, the nasal mucous membrane becomes congested, swollen, and edematous for a short period of time and then quickly returns to normal. After repeated attacks, however, particularly in cases that originate as a result of chronic sinusitis, this swelling becomes obstinate, and the patient has a "chronic catarrh." Persons with this problem say that they are "subject to colds." The fact is that, excluding the recurring attacks of allergic rhinitis, their attacks are acute exacerbations of the same "cold."

If continued, chronic rhinitis leads to the deposition of abnormally large amounts of connective tissue in the nasal mucous membrane, which greatly thickens it and, in addition to hypertrophy, causes the formation of spurs and polyps on the nasal septum. Wasting or atrophy of the mucous membrane, the cartilage, and the bones lining the nasal passages eventually may occur, with the result that these passages become large, empty caverns, in which an abundant exudate builds up on the walls, giving off a disagreeable odor. This condition is called *ozena* or atrophic rhinitis.

Therapy and Nursing Interventions. In acute viral rhinitis, symptomatic treatment includes topical or systemic vasocontricting medications to relieve nasal obstruction, analgesics for headache, and rest to alleviate general discomfort. Adults are advised to avoid crowds.

The patient is cautioned against blowing his nose too frequently or too hard. He should blow his nose by opening his mouth slightly and blowing through both nostrils to equalize the pressure.

Nasal Obstruction

The passage of air through the nostrils is frequently obstructed by a deflection of the nasal septum, hypertrophy of the turbinate bones, or the pressure of polyps—grapelike swellings that arise from the mucous membrane of the sinuses, especially the ethmoids. This obstruction also may lead to a condition of chronic infection of the nose and results in frequent attacks of nasopharyngitis. Very frequently, the infection extends to the sinuses of the nose (mucous-lined cavities filled with air that drain normally into the nose). When sinusitis develops and the drainage from these cavities is obstructed by deformity or swelling within the nose, pain is experienced in the region of the affected sinus.

Management. The treatment of this condition requires the removal of the nasal obstruction, followed by measures to overcome whatever chronic infection exists. In many patients the underlying nasal allergy is the lesion requiring treatment. At times it is necessary to drain the nasal sinuses by a radical operation. The operations performed depend on the type of nasal obstruction found. Usually, they are performed with local anesthesia.

If a deflection of the septum is the cause of the obstruction, the surgeon makes an incision into the mucous membrane and, after raising it from the bone, removes the deflected bone and cartilage with bone forceps. The mucosa then is allowed to fall back in place and is held there by tight packing. Generally, the packing used is soaked in liquid petrolatum to facilitate its removal in 24 to 36 hours. This operation is called a *submucous resection* or septoplasty.

Nasal polyps are removed by clipping them at their base with a wire snare. Hypertrophied turbinates may be treated by astringent applications to shrink them close to the side of the nose.

After these procedures, the head of the bed is elevated to promote drainage and to help in alleviating the patient's discomfort owing to edema. Frequent oral hygiene care should be given because the patient breathes through his mouth.

Fractures of the Nose

Fractures of the nose usually result from direct violence. As a rule, no serious consequences result, but the deformity that may follow often gives rise to obstruction of the nasal air passages and to facial disfigurement.

Assessment and Clinical Manifestations. The nose should be examined internally to rule out the possibility that the injury may be complicated by a fracture of the nasal septum and submucosal septal hematoma. If hematoma develops and is not drained, it may eventually become an abscess with a dissolution of the septal cartilage. The familiar saddle deformity of the nose results.

Immediately after the injury there is usually considerable bleeding from the nose externally and internally into the pharynx. There is marked swelling of the soft tissues adjacent to the nose and, frequently, a definite deformity.

If there is clear fluid draining from either nostril, it suggests a fracture of the cribriform plate with leakage of cerebrospinal fluid (CSF). Since CSF contains sugar, it can easily be differentiated from nasal mucus by using a dipstick (Dextrostix).

Management and Nursing Interventions. As a rule, the bleeding can be controlled by the application of cold compresses. A roentgenogram is helpful in determining the displacement of the fractured bones and in ruling out an extension of the fracture into the skull. With the application of local anesthesia to the nose or with intravenous anesthesia, it is usually possible to bring displaced fragments into alignment and then hold them by intranasal packing or external splints. The important points in the reduction of the fracture are to reform the nasal passages and to realign the bones so as to prevent a disfiguring deformity. After reduction, the swelling that occurs may be decreased by the application of ice compresses with the patient in the sitting position.

Plastic Surgery of the Nose

The nose is such a prominent organ of the face that its deformity may cause the patient considerable embarrassment. The deformity may result from congenital causes, from disease, or from injury.

Deformities resulting from congenital causes often may be corrected by simple operations (rhinoplasty) in which the nose is straightened or lengthened by either removing offending bone or supplying new tissue (usually, costal cartilage). The incisions are so placed as to be inconspicuous. In deformities resulting from injury or disease, various types of plastic surgery may be employed. Skin, tube, or sliding grafts may be used to cover the defects left by scars, malignancy, or injuries. In some instances, especially in older people with malignancy, artificial appliances may be modeled and held in place with the rims of glasses. (See Reconstructive Surgery, p. 1188.)

Nursing Management.   Before surgery, a photograph of the patient's face and nose may be taken to serve as a permanent record and to be used as an aid in determining goals of treatment.

After operation, the patient usually is placed flat on his back with the head slightly elevated. Ice compresses are used frequently to reduce bleeding, swelling, and pain. A splint may be taped to the nose, and in some instances, pressure dressings may be placed over the eyes.

- Hemorrhage is the chief postoperative complication.

It must be remembered that the spitting up or the vomiting of blood that has run back into the pharynx is as much a symptom of nasal hemorrhage as is the flow at the nares. Frequent swallowing, followed by belching, often is indicative of bleeding that results in an accumulation of blood in the stomach.

In patients for whom local anesthesia has been used, the blood sometimes trickles down the throat, but the patient is not sufficiently aware of it to show a swallowing reflex.

- If the bleeding is excessive or continuous, or if any of the constitutional signs of hemorrhage appear, the surgeon should be called and the following items made available: fresh packing, a light, a head mirror, a nasal speculum, and packing forceps.

Patients may have a liquid diet on the day of operation and whatever they prefer after that. Sedatives often are necessary on the day and the night of operation, but after that there is little need for them. The patient is warned that he will be tempted to blow his nose because of a full feeling caused by the packing. He is cautioned against blowing his nose until the surgeon grants permission. Packing is removed usually after 24 hours.

Convalescence and Patient Education.   Swelling and discoloration may be noticed for a few days but will subside by the end of the first week. Usually, normal activities may be resumed after 2 weeks. During that time, heavy weights should not be lifted.

The patient is urged to have follow-up visits with the surgeon and to avoid any pressure on the nose for a few weeks, such as may be caused by eyeglasses. If the patient wears contact lenses, he should consult the surgeon as to when he may resume wearing them.*

▷ Specific Infections of the Upper Respiratory Tract

Common Cold

The phrase "common cold" is a general term that patients use in different ways, usually when referring to symptoms of upper respiratory infection.

Clinical Manifestations and Pathophysiology.   These symptoms are nasal discharge and obstruction, sore throat, sneezing, malaise, fever, chills, and often headache and muscle aching. As the cold progresses, cough usually appears. Most specifically, the term *cold* refers to afebrile, infectious, acute coryza. More broadly, the word refers to acute upper respiratory infection, whereas terms such as *rhinitis, pharyngitis, laryngitis, chest cold,* etc. distinguish the sites of the major symptoms.

The symptoms last 5 days to 2 weeks. If there is significant fever or more severe constitutional problems with the respiratory symptoms, it is no longer a common cold but one of the other acute upper respiratory infections. Many different viruses (over 100) are known to produce the symptoms of the common cold, and about 10% of colds seem to be associated simultaneously with more than one virus. Also, allergic conditions affecting the nose can mimic the symptoms of a cold.

Community Health and Social Significance.   Colds are highly contagious since patients shed virus for about 2 days before the symptoms appear and during the first part of their symptomatic phase. Colds prevail among 15% of the work population at any time during the winter and account for almost half of all work absences and one quarter of the total time lost from work.

Three waves of colds appear yearly in the United States—in the fall just after the opening of school, in mid-winter, and in spring. Immunity after recovery is variable, depending on many factors, including natural host resistance and the specific virus that caused the cold in the first place. The major complication of a cold is the secondary bacterial infection that can affect the ears, nose, sinuses, bronchi, or lungs.

Management.   Management of the common cold consists of adequate fluid intake, rest, prevention of chilling, aqueous nasal decongestants, vitamin C, bronchodilators, and expectorants as needed. Warm salt water gargles soothe the sore throat, and aspirin relieves the general constitutional symptoms. Antibiotics are not indicated in the uncomplicated common cold.

* An excellent pamphlet for patient education is "Facts About Plastic Surgery of the Nose," American Academy of Facial Plastic and Reconstruction Surgery, Inc., 70 West Hubbard Street, Suite 202, Chicago, Illinois 60610.

Using disposable tissues and disposing of them hygienically, covering the mouth when coughing, and avoiding crowds are important measures in preventing the spread of an upper respiratory infection.

Herpes Simplex Infection

The herpes simplex virus most commonly produces the familiar *herpes labialis* (cold sore, fever blister, or canker). Small vesicles, single or clustered, may erupt on the lips, the tongue, the cheeks, and the pharynx. These soon rupture, forming sore, shallow ulcers that are covered with a gray membrane.

Herpes infections appear often in association with other febrile infections, such as streptococcus pneumonia, meningococcic meningitis, and malaria. The virus remains latent in cells of the lips or nose and is activated by febrile illnesses. The herpes virus does not yield in the slightest to any of the chemotherapeutic agents that have become available to date. Analgesics and codeine are helpful in relieving pain and discomfort. Topical anesthetics, such as lidocaine (Xylocaine Viscous) or dyclonine (Dyclone), give a measure of relief for oral pain. Acyclovir may also give some relief. Applications of drying lotions or liquids may help to dry the lesions.

Sinusitis

The sinuses are involved in a high proportion of upper respiratory tract infections. If their openings into the nasal passages are clear, the infections within them recover promptly; but if their drainage is obstructed by a deflected septum or by hypertrophied turbinates, spurs, or polyps, sinusitis may persist as a smoldering secondary infection or it may flare up into an acute suppurative process.

Acute Sinusitis
Assessment and Clinical Manifestations. Acute sinusitis may be localized in one sinus or may involve several (see Fig. 22-1). If all are involved, the condition is called *pansinusitis.* The most prominent symptom of acute sinusitis is pain. Since the location of the pain is diagnostically important, it should be noted and documented by the nurse. In *frontal sinusitis,* the patient complains of frontal headache; in *ethmoidal sinusitis,* the pain is usually in or about the eyes; in *maxillary sinusitis,* pain may be referred to the brow but usually is lateral to the nose and sometimes is accompanied by aching of the upper teeth of the corresponding side; in *sphenoidal sinusitis,* occipital headache may result. Aside from being located in a specific area, pain also may be referred, for example, to the forehead. Nasal congestion and discharge are usually, but not necessarily, present. The patient feels generally miserable, quite apart from pain. Fever, however, if present at all, is usually mild. This may be the case even in the presence of an acute suppurative infection, or "empyema," of a sinus. *Hemophilus influenzae* is the most common bacteria cultured from the sinus; there is low correlation between nasal and sinus cultures.

• The most dangerous variety of sinusitis is empyema of a frontal sinus, because it may rupture posteriorly, producing a brain abscess.

A careful history and diagnostic assessment is done to rule out other local or systemic disorders, such as tumor, fistula, allergy, and viral infections.

Treatment and Nursing Interventions. The goals of treatment are relief of pain, shrinkage of nasal mucosa, and control of infection. These are initiated by administering codeine, meperidine (Demerol), or occasionally morphine. Aspirin is not sufficiently effective. Bed rest is recommended, and the establishment of free drainage of the sinuses is involved. Hot wet packs applied to the face over the involved sinus area 4 times a day will hasten resolution of the infection. Often this can be accomplished by nasal instillations or sprays of phenylephrine hydrochloride (Neo-Synephrine, 0.25%) or by oral decongestants such as pseudoephedrine or a similar vasoconstrictor drug. Depending on the type of infecting organism and the extent of the infection, the patient may be instructed to apply local therapy of this sort at intervals of 1 to 4 hours until drainage is established. Antibiotics may be prescribed; the use of penicillin usually speeds recovery and definitely diminishes the chance of complications that can follow the extension of a bacterial sinusitis. If allergy is suspected as the basis of the inflammatory process, one of the antihistaminic agents (*e.g.,* tripelennamine [Pyribenzamine]) in oral doses may be beneficial, at least symptomatically, in very early stages.

Chronic Sinusitis
Pathophysiology and Manifestations. Chronic sinusitis usually manifests itself by persistent nasal obstruction owing to discharge and edema of the nasal mucous membrane. The patient experiences cough, because of the constant dripping of the discharge backward into the nasopharynx, and headaches, which are apt to be most pronounced on awakening in the morning. Fatigue is also common, as are dullness and nasal stuffiness.

Management. Treatment of chronic sinusitis includes measures to facilitate drainage, antibacterial therapy, and antiallergic measures. Increased humidity, steam inhalations, increased fluid intake, and local heat applications will assist in promoting drainage. Local use of vasoconstricting drugs in the form of sprays or nose drops may be tried.

• However, overuse or prolonged use of vasoconstrictive nasal drugs may aggravate rhinitis and sinusitis by causing rebound congestion, which leads to further overuse.

Oily nose drops are to be avoided. Sterile Ringer's solution used with a nasal douche can be obtained in any drugstore and is a soothing method of cleansing the nose. Structural deformities that obstruct the ostia of the sinus may require surgical attention: polyps may require excision or cauterization; a deflected septum may have to be removed or a narrowed ostium widened.

For drainage of the maxillary sinus, the incision is made along the upper gum line above the canine teeth (Caldwell–

Luc operation). To drain the frontal sinus, an incision is made through the inner third of the eyebrow. A recent increasingly popular surgical approach is an incision made above the brow line. After exploring the entire sinus, diseased tissue is removed and the sinus obliterated with abdominal fat.

Some victims of severe chronic sinusitis obtain relief only by moving to a dry climate.

Prevention of Upper Respiratory Infections

The prevention of most upper respiratory tract infections is difficult, since their causes are legion. The responsible pathogen usually cannot be identified, and vaccines are unavailable except in rare instances. Allergies, pathology of the septum and the turbinate, emotional problems, and various systemic illnesses may be predisposing factors in isolated cases.

The following hygienic measures tend to support the body's defenses and reduce susceptibility to respiratory infections:

- Practice good health measures—nutritious diet, appropriate exercise, adequate rest and sleep.
- Avoid excesses in alcohol and smoking.
- Correct air dryness by proper home humidification, especially during cold weather.
- Avoid air contaminants (dust, chemicals) when possible.
- Avoid unnecessary chilling of the skin, especially the feet; chilling lowers resistance.
- Obtain influenza vaccination if and when directed by a physician.

▷ Problems of the Pharynx and the Tonsils

Acute Pharyngitis

Acute pharyngitis, caused by several viruses and bacteria, is a febrile inflammation of the throat. The pharyngeal membrane becomes fiery red; the lymphoid follicles of the throat and the tonsils become swollen and flecked with exudate; and the cervical lymph nodes may become tender and enlarged. Uncomplicated viral infections usually subside promptly, within 3 to 10 days after the onset. But pharyngitis caused by certain of the more virulent bacteria, such as group A streptococcus, or hemolytic *Staphylococcus aureus,* is a more severe illness during the acute stage and far more important because of the incidence of dangerous complications. These complications include sinusitis, otitis media, mastoiditis, cervical adenitis, rheumatic fever, and nephritis. A throat culture is the chief means of determining the causative organism (Fig. 22-3). When this is obtained, proper therapy can be prescribed. Note that if one member of a family has a proved streptococcal infection, all other family members, whether symptomatic or not, should also

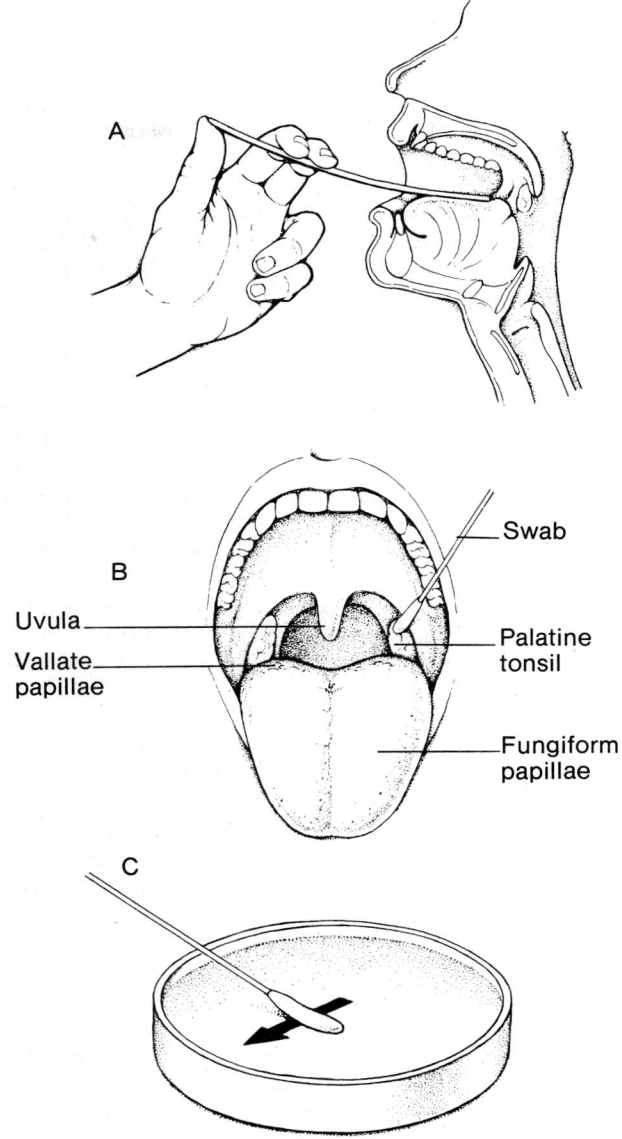

Figure 22-3. Taking a throat culture. When obtaining a throat culture from a patient who "gags," it is helpful to have him close his eyes. Since anticipation is lessened, the culture can be obtained with only a slight gag. (*A*) Grasp the tongue blade so that the thumb pushes the end upward (as a fulcrum) while the fingers push the middle section downward. (*B*) Vigorously rub a cotton or dacron swab over each tonsillar area and the posterior pharynx. (*C*) Streak the swab on a blood agar plate and place in an incubator for 24 hours. A gross reading of the plate can then be made.

have throat cultures done. Those with positive cultures are treated with penicillin.

Nursing Management.   The patient is kept in bed during the febrile stage of illness. When he is ambulatory he needs periods of rest. Medical asepsis must be observed to prevent the spread of infection. The skin should be examined once or twice daily for possible rash, because acute pharyngitis may precede some other communicable disease.

Aside from throat cultures, it may be necessary to secure nasal swabbings and blood cultures for further laboratory investigation to determine the nature of the causative organism.

Warm saline gargles or irrigations are employed, depending on the severity of the lesion and the degree of pain. Recognizing that the benefits of this treatment depend on the degree of heat that is applied, the nurse ensures that the temperature of the solution is sufficiently high to be effective, that is, approaching the limits of tolerance, which vary with each patient, usually between 40.6° C to 43.3° C (105° F–110° F). A throat irrigation, properly performed, is an effective means of reducing spasm in the pharyngeal muscles and relieving soreness of the throat. However, unless the purpose of the procedure, and its technique, are understood clearly by the patient, the results may be less than satisfactory. If throat irrigation is a new experience for the patient, the nurse should explain the procedure and its purpose before commencing.

Symptomatic relief in patients with severe sore throat also may be afforded by applying an ice collar and administering analgesic drugs, for example, aspirin or acetaminophen given at 3- to 6-hour intervals and, if required, codeine sulfate, 3 or 4 times daily. Antitussive medication, in the form of codeine or hydrocodone bitartrate (Hycodan), may be required to control a persistent and painful cough that often accompanies acute pharyngitis. One of the barbiturates, for example, pentobarbital (Nembutal), may be prescribed for the patient as a soporific at bedtime.

If a bacterial etiology is suspected or demonstrated, treatment may include the administration of antimicrobial agents. For group A streptococcus, penicillin is the drug of choice. For those who are sensitive to penicillin and resistent to tetracycline (one fifth of group A streptococci and most *Staphylococcus aureus* organisms are resistant to tetracycline), erythromycin is the drug of choice. Antibiotics are administered at least 10 days for an optimal rate of eradication of group A streptococci from the oropharynx.

A liquid or a soft diet is provided during the acute stage of the disease, depending on the patient's appetite and the degree of discomfort caused by swallowing. Occasionally, the throat is so sore that liquids cannot be taken in adequate amounts by mouth; in this situation, IV fluids are administered. Otherwise, the patient is encouraged to drink to the limit of tolerance, the minimum intake during the febrile stage exceeding, if possible, 2500 ml each day. Often, the patient can achieve this goal more easily if the rationale of therapy is explained adequately to him. His personal tastes (in liquids) should be considered and indulged when possible.

Mouth care may add greatly to the patient's comfort and may aid in preventing the development of fissures of the lips and pyoderma about the mouth when bacterial infection is present.

Convalescence and Patient Education. Resumption of activity should be permitted gradually. Unusually conservative management is indicated in patients with hemolytic streptococcus infection in view of the possible development of complications such as nephritis and rheumatic fever, which may have their onset 2 or 3 weeks after the pharyngitis has subsided. Local extension of an apparently quiescent pharyngitis may develop in the form of sinusitis, otitis media, mastoiditis, or cervical adenitis. Daily assessment of morning and evening temperatures should be continued until convalescence is complete, and the patient or his family should be familiarized with symptoms that deserve investigation because they could lead to possible complications.

Chronic Pharyngitis

Incidence, Pathophysiology, and Manifestations. This disease is common in adults who work in dusty surroundings, use the voice to excess, and suffer from chronic cough. Its incidence also is high among habitual users of alcohol and tobacco.

Three types of chronic pharyngitis are recognized: (1) hypertrophic, characterized by general thickening and congestion of the pharyngeal mucous membrane; (2) atrophic, probably a late stage of type one (the membrane is thin, whitish, glistening, and, at times, wrinkled); and (3) chronic granular ("clergyman's sore throat"), with numerous swollen lymph follicles on the pharyngeal wall.

Patients with chronic pharyngitis complain of a constant sense of irritation or fullness in the throat, of mucus, which collects in the throat and can be expelled by coughing; and of difficulty in swallowing.

Management and Patient Education. The treatment of chronic pharyngitis consists of avoiding alcohol and tobacco, resting the voice, and correcting any upper respiratory, pulmonary, or cardiac condition that might be responsible for a chronic cough.

Nasal congestion may be relieved by nasal instillations or sprays containing ephedrine sulfate, phenylephrine hydrochloride (Neo-Synephrine), or tuaminoheptane sulfate (Tuamine) in saline, and, in the early stages, if there is a history of allergy, one of the antihistaminic drugs, such as tripelennamine (Pyribenzamine), every 4 to 6 hours by mouth. The attendant malaise is controlled effectively by aspirin or acetaminophen. Contact with others should be avoided, at least until the fever has subsided completely, in order to prevent the infection from spreading.

Diseases of the Tonsils and the Adenoids

Tonsils

The tonsils are a pair of lymphatic tissue structures, one of which is situated on each side of the oropharynx; they frequently serve as the seat of acute infection.

Chronic tonsillitis occurs less commonly and may be mistaken for other disorders, such as allergy, asthma, and sinusitis. A thorough physical examination is given and a careful history is taken to rule out related or systemic conditions. A culture of the organisms at the tonsillar site is done to determine the presence of bacterial infection. Medical therapy with appropriate antibiotics is initiated.

Tonsillectomy is usually not done unless medical treatment is unsuccessful and there is severe hypertrophy or peritonsillar abscess that occludes the pharynx, making swallowing difficult and endangering the airway. Enlargement of the tonsils is per se rarely an indication for their removal; most children have normally large tonsils, which decrease in size as the child grows older.

Despite the continuing debate over the effectiveness of many tonsillectomies, the operation is still the most common nondiagnostic surgical procedure done in the United States.

Adenoids

The adenoids consist of an abnormally large lymphoid tissue mass near the center of the posterior wall of the nasopharynx. Unusually enlarged adenoids may cause nasal obstruction. As a chronic problem, adenoid hypertrophy may cause mouth-breathing, earache, draining ears, frequent head colds, bronchitis, fetid breath, voice impairment, snoring, and noisy respiration. Infection of the adenoids frequently accompanies acute tonsillitis.

Extension of the infection to the middle ears by way of the eustachian tubes may result in acute otitis media, the potential complications of which include spontaneous rupture of the eardrums and further extension into the mastoid cells, causing acute mastoiditis. Or the infection may reside in the middle ear as a chronic, low-grade smoldering process that eventually may lead to permanent deafness. Consequently, if adenoiditis is not controlled by antibiotics, and there are recurrent episodes of suppurative otitis media that are causing a hearing loss, it is important for the patient to have a comprehensive audiometric examination (p. 1260). If there is conductive hearing loss, an adenoidectomy may diminish the frequency of otitis media.

Tonsillectomy and Adenoidectomy

Tonsillectomy or adenoidectomy is done only if the patient has had repeated bouts of tonsillitis; hypertrophy of the tonsils and adenoids that border on obstruction; repeated attacks of purulent otitis media; suspected hearing loss due to serous otitis media that has occurred in association with enlarged tonsils and adenoids; and some conditions, such as an exacerbation of asthma, arthritis, or rheumatic fever. These operations should not be done during an acute infection or if the patient has leukemia, aplastic anemia, or hemophilia.

Postoperative Management and Nursing Interventions. Continuous nursing care is required in the immediate postoperative and recovery period because of the significant risk of hemorrhage. For the patient undergoing general anesthesia, atropine is usually given to decrease the amount of mucous secretion. After the operation, the most comfortable position is prone with the head turned to the side to allow for drainage from the mouth and pharynx. The inserted airway is not removed until the patient demonstrates that his swallowing reflex has returned. An ice collar is applied to the neck, and a basin and tissues are provided for the expectoration of blood and mucus.

Bleeding may be bright red if the patient spits the blood out at once. Often, however, the blood is swallowed and immediately becomes brown in color owing to the action of the acid gastric juice.

If the patient vomits large amounts of altered blood or spits bright blood at frequent intervals, or if the pulse rate and temperature rise and the patient is restless, the surgeon is notified immediately and the following items made available: a light, a head mirror, gauze, curved hemostats, and a waste basin.

Occasionally, it may be necessary to suture or ligate the bleeding vessel. In such cases the patient must be taken to the operating room and given anesthesia.

If there is no bleeding, water and cracked ice may be given the patient as soon as desired. The patient is instructed to refrain from too much talking and coughing, because this can produce throat pain. Alkaline mouthwashes may be useful in coping with the thick mucus that may be present after a tonsillectomy.

A liquid or semiliquid diet is given for several days, excluding orange or lemon juice and other acids. Ice cream, ice sherbet, gelatin desserts, custards, and junkets are very acceptable foods.

Codeine is usually prescribed for pain; however, aspirin is contraindicated because it tends to increase bleeding.

Patient Education. The patient may be discharged from the hospital on the day after the operation, but he should convalesce at home for several days. This means getting plenty of rest, eating soft food, drinking fluids, and resuming activity gradually. Any bleeding should be reported to the physician; delayed hemorrhage may occur up to a week after operation.

Peritonsillar Abscess (Quinsy)

Assessment and Clinical Manifestations. *Peritonsillar abscess,* or quinsy, is an abscess that develops above the tonsil in the tissues of the anterior pillar and soft palate. As a rule, it is secondary to a tonsillar infection. The usual symptoms of an infection are present, together with such local symptoms as difficulty in swallowing (dysphagia), thickening of the voice, drooling, and local pain. An examination shows marked swelling of the soft palate, often to the extent of half-occluding the orifice from the mouth into the pharynx.

Management. A considerable measure of relief may be obtained by throat irrigations or the frequent use of mouthwashes or gargles, using saline or alkaline solutions at a temperature of 40.6° C to 43.3° C (105° F–110° F). This treatment hastens the pointing of the process.

The abscess should be evacuated as soon as possible. The mucous membrane over the swelling first is sprayed with topical anesthetic and then injected with local anesthesia; after a small incision has been made, the points of a blunt hemostat are forced into the abscess pocket and opened as they are withdrawn. This operation is performed best with the patient in the sitting position, since this will make it easier for him to expectorate the pus and blood that accumulate in the pharynx. Almost immediate relief is experienced. After-treatment includes warm gargles at intervals of 1 or 2 hours for 24 to 36 hours.

Some laryngologists advocate bilateral tonsillectomy for acute peritonsillar abscess; they claim that this is necessary to prevent recurrences and eliminate unsuspected asymptomatic pockets of infection.

Antibiotics, usually penicillin, are extremely effective in the control of the infection in peritonsillar abscess. Given early in the course of the disease, the abscess may be aborted, and incision can be avoided. If antibiotics are not given until later, the abscess must be drained, but improvement in the inflammatory reaction is rapid.

▷ Problems of the Larynx

The larynx, or voice box, serves as a passageway for air between the pharynx and the trachea. Because of its unique structure, the larynx also acts as a guard at the entrance of the trachea (windpipe), controlling air flow and preventing anything other than air from entering the lower passages. When a foreign body touches the sensitive laryngeal mucosa, the cough reflex is triggered. Exhalation of air through the larynx enables it to become an organ of speech, sounds being created as a result of vocal cord vibrations. Speech patterns are produced with the aid of the pharynx, palate, teeth, tongue, and lips. The larynx may be viewed directly with a laryngoscope (or laryngeal telescope) or indirectly with a laryngeal mirror (Fig. 22-4).

Laryngitis

Assessment and Clinical Manifestations. Inflammation of the larynx often occurs as a result of voice abuse or as a part of an upper respiratory infection. It may also be caused by an isolated infection involving only the vocal cords.

Acute laryngitis is manifested by hoarseness or complete loss of the voice (aphonia) and by severe cough.

Chronic laryngitis, marked by persistent hoarseness, may follow repeated attacks of acute laryngitis. It is sometimes a complication of chronic sinusitis and chronic bronchitis. The condition also may be induced by the frequent inhalation of irritating gases, the excessive use of tobacco or alcohol, or the habitual overuse of the voice, as in the case of public speakers. Laryngoscopic examination of the

patient with chronic laryngitis is always indicated in order to eliminate the possibility of tuberculosis or tumor of the larynx.

Treatment. For acute laryngitis, the treatment is bed rest, steam or aerosol therapy, and abstinence from talking and smoking. If the laryngitis is part of a more extensive respiratory infection owing to a bacterial organism, or if it is severe, appropriate antibacterial chemotherapy should be instituted.

For chronic laryngitis, the treatment of the condition is rest of the voice, elimination of any primary respiratory tract infection that may be present, and restriction of smoking.

Laryngeal Obstruction

Edema of the larynx (or glottis) is a serious, often fatal, condition. The larynx is a stiff box that will not stretch, and the space within it between the vocal cords, through which the air must pass, is narrow. Swelling of the laryngeal mucous membrane, therefore, may close this orifice tightly, leading to suffocation. Edema of the glottis occurs rarely in patients with acute laryngitis, occasionally in patients with urticaria, and more frequently in severe inflammations of the throat—for example, erysipelas and scarlet fever. It is an occasional cause of death in severe anaphylaxis (angioneurotic edema).

When caused by an allergic reaction, treatment includes applying an ice pack to the neck and administering epinephrine, 1:1000 subcutaneously, or adrenal corticosteroid.

Foreign bodies frequently are aspirated into the pharynx, the larynx, or the trachea, and cause a two-fold problem. First, they obstruct the air passages and cause difficulty in breathing, which may lead to asphyxia; later they may be drawn farther down, entering the bronchi or one of their branches and causing symptoms of irritation, such as a croupy cough, bloody or mucous expectoration, and paroxysms of dyspnea. The physical signs and roentgenograms confirm the diagnosis.

In emergencies, when the signs of asphyxia are evident, immediate treatment is necessary. Frequently, if the foreign body has lodged in the pharynx, it may be dislodged by the finger. If the obstruction is in the larynx or the trachea, the

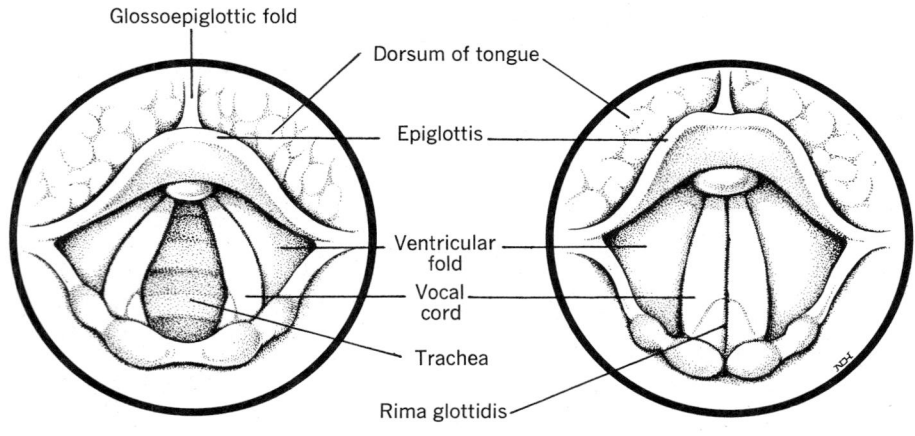

Glossoepiglottic fold
Dorsum of tongue
Epiglottis
Ventricular fold
Vocal cord
Trachea
Rima glottidis

Figure 22-4. Interior of the larynx, as seen with laryngoscope: *left,* rima glottidis wide open; *right,* rima closed. (From Chaffee EE and Greisheimer IM: Basic Physiology and Anatomy, 3rd ed. Philadelphia, JB Lippincott.)

abdominal thrust maneuver may be tried. If all efforts are unsuccessful, an immediate tracheotomy may be necessary.

- To perform the abdominal thrust maneuver, stand behind the person who is choking and place both arms around his waist, with one hand grasping the other wrist. Then quickly and forcefully apply pressure against the victim's diaphragm, pressing slightly upward, just below the ribs. The pressure will compress the lungs and expel the aspirated object.

Cancer of the Larynx

If detected early, cancer of the larynx is readily curable. It occurs about 8 times more frequently in males than in females and most commonly in men from 50 to 65 years of age. It represents about 3% to 5% of all cancers.

In the United States, approximately 9000 new cases are discovered each year, and 3000 persons with cancer of the larynx will die annually. Factors that contribute to laryngeal cancer are irritants such as cigarette smoke, alcohol, vocal straining, chronic laryngitis, noxious fumes, and family predisposition (Fig. 22-5).

▶ **Assessment**

Clinical Manifestations. A malignant growth may occur on the vocal cords (intrinsic) or on another part of the larynx (extrinsic). Hoarseness is noted early in the patient with intrinsic cancer since accurate approximation of the cords during phonation is interrupted by the presence of

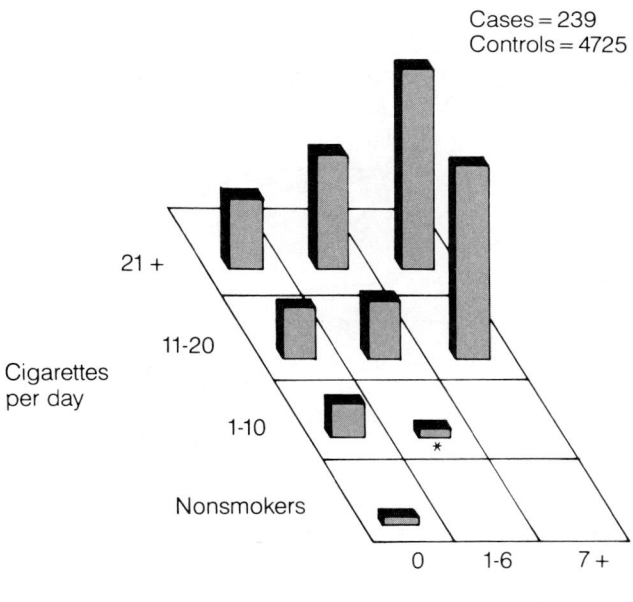

*not significant

Figure 22-5. Relative risks of larynx cancer for males by daily consumption of alcohol and cigarettes. (From McCoy DG, Hecht SS, and Wynder EL: The roles of tobacco, alcohol, and diet in the etiology of upper alimentary and respiratory tract cancers. Preventive Medicine 9(5):622–629, Sept 1980.)

the tumor. Affected voice sounds are not early signs of extrinsic or supraglottic cancer; however, the patient may complain of pain and burning in the throat when drinking hot liquids and citrus juices. Later a lump may be felt in the neck. Subsequently, too, dysphagia (swallowing difficulty), dyspnea, hoarseness, and foul breath may be noticed. Enlarged cervical nodes, weight loss, general debility, and the discomfort of pain radiating to the ear may all be suggestive of metastasis.

Direct laryngoscopic examination may be necessary if the larynx cannot be completely visualized; it is also used for biopsy of the tumor. The growth may involve any of the three areas (glottis, supraglottis, or subglottis) and varies in appearance. The precise involvement is determined since this affects the treatment.

Mobility of the vocal cords is assessed; if normal movement is limited, the growth may affect muscle, other tissue, and even the airway. The lymph nodes of the neck and the thyroid gland are palpated to determine spread of the malignancy.

Scanning and laryngograms of the larynx are effective in determining the extent of tumor growth.

Patient Problems/Nursing Diagnoses

Based on the clinical manifestations and diagnostic assessment, the patient's major nursing problems include voice changes related to impingement by the tumor on the vocal cords; subsequent problems with swallowing related to spread of the malignancy to the pharynx; anxiety and perhaps depression related to the diagnosis of cancer; voice loss related to the involvement of the glottis and surgical removal of the larynx; communication problems related to the laryngectomy and voice rehabilitation efforts.

▶ **Planning and Implementation**

Goals

The patient's goals are improvement of his vocal problem, ability to communicate, elimination or control of the malignancy, avoidance of complications, and adherence to the therapeutic program.

The major goals of treatment are:

1. Improvement of the quality of life
2. Halting the progression of the disease process
3. Rehabilitation of the patient following radiation or surgery for optimum ability to communicate
4. Monitoring the patient thereafter for evidence of recurrence or metastasis

The therapeutic approach includes (1) psychological support, (2) preparation for surgery, (3) meticulous postoperative care, (4) speech rehabilitation, (5) self-care of tracheostomy, and (6) understanding of hygienic measures and emergency care.

Management

Treatment varies with the extent of the malignancy. Precise determination of the exact location and involvement of the malignancy is done by indirect and direct laryngoscopy, biopsy, and x-ray before specific treatment by radiation or surgery is prescribed.

1. Radiation. Good results have been produced by radiation therapy in patients in whom only one cord was affected and was normally mobile (*i.e.,* moved with phonation). In addition, these patients retain a practically normal voice. A few may develop chondritis or stenosis; a small number may later require laryngectomy.

2. Partial Laryngectomy (Laryngofissure, Thyrotomy). This is recommended in the early stages, especially in intrinsic cancer of the larynx (limited to the vocal cords), and has a cure rate of more than 80%. In this operation, the thyroid cartilage of the larynx is split in the midline of the neck, and the portion of the vocal cord that is involved with tumor growth is removed. Sometimes a tracheostomy tube (see p. 491) is left in the trachea when the wound is closed; it is usually removed after a few days.

3. Supraglottic (Horizontal) Laryngectomy. This procedure is used in the management of certain extrinsic tumors. After adequate resection, sufficient normal larynx is left so that the cords remain intact and their function is maintained. During surgery a radical neck dissection is also done on the involved side. Postoperatively, the patient may experience some difficulty in swallowing for the first 2 weeks. The chief advantage of this operation, of course, is that it preserves the voice. The major problem is that there may be local recurrence; therefore, patients have to be selected carefully.

4. Total Laryngectomy. For extrinsic cancer of the larynx (extension beyond the vocal cords), the entire larynx is removed; this includes the thyroid cartilage, the vocal cords, and the epiglottis. Many surgeons recommend that a neck dissection be performed on the same side as the lesion even though no lymph nodes are palpable. The rationale for this approach is that as many as 35% of patients have had metastases to the cervical lymph nodes. Obviously, the problem is more complex when a lesion involves midline structures or both cords. With or without neck dissection, a total laryngectomy requires a permanent tracheal stoma (Fig. 22-6). This is done to prevent aspiration of food and fluid into the lower respiratory tract, since the larynx that provides the protective sphincter is no longer present.

5. Total Laryngectomy With Laryngoplasty. In this delicate three-stage procedure (Assai operation), a dermal tube is fashioned from the upper end of the trachea into the hypopharynx. By closing the permanent tracheostomy opening with his finger, the patient can exhale air up through the dermal tube and into the pharyngeal cavity. The sound produced is transformed into speech that is almost normal and far superior to esophageal speech.

Nursing Interventions

Preparation for Surgery. To plan appropriate nursing care, it is important to consult with the surgeon regarding the nature of the surgery recommended for a particular pa-

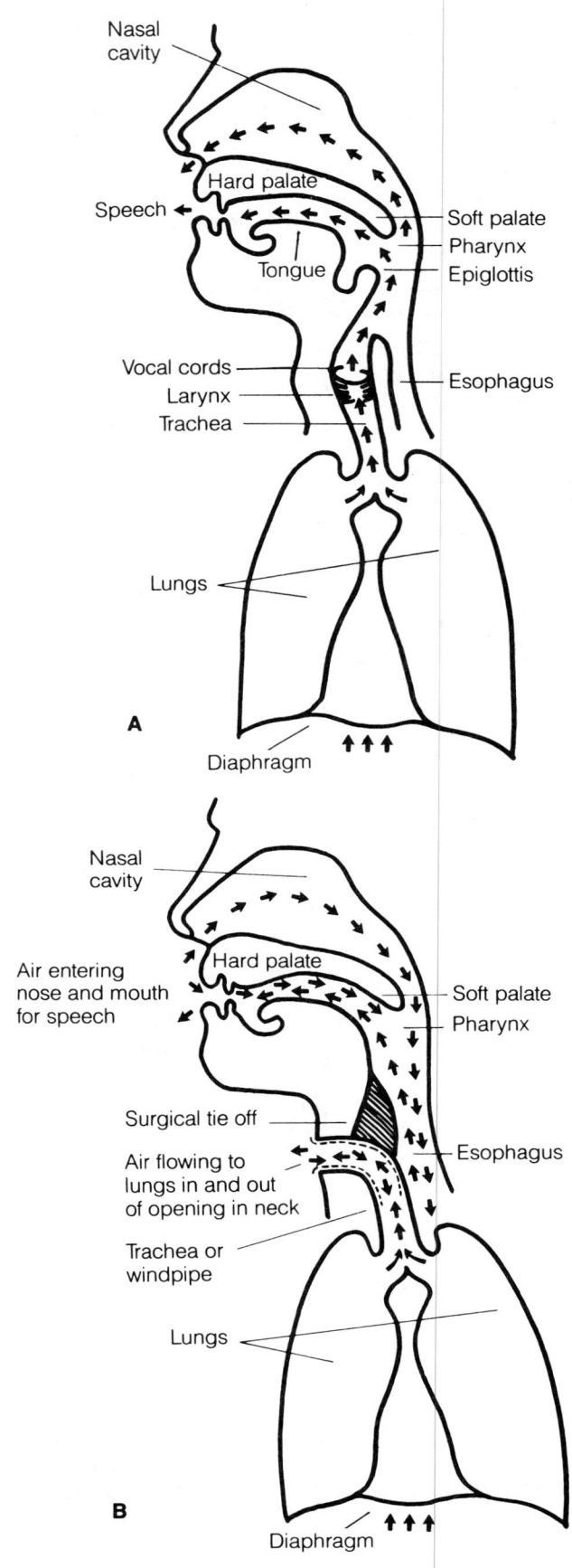

Figure 22-6. Diagram showing direction of air flow before (*A*) and after (*B*) a total laryngectomy. (American Cancer Society)

tient. Some patients experience loss of speech, whereas others do not. Thus, the nursing care plan is based on the surgical plan of therapy.

Since surgery of the larynx is done most commonly for a tumor that may be malignant, the nurse is faced with a patient who is worried for many reasons: Will the surgeon be able to remove all of the tumor? Is it cancer? Will I die? Will I choke? Will I ever speak again? Therefore, the psychological preparation of the patient is as important as the physical. If the patient is going to have a complete laryngectomy, he should know that he will lose his natural voice completely and that, with training, there are ways in which he can carry on a fairly normal conversation. (He also will not be able to sing, laugh, or whistle.) Until he receives this training, the patient needs to know that the nurse can be reached by the call light and that he can communicate in the immediate postoperative phase by writing.

The physician describes the nature of the surgery and tells the patient that he will lose his ability to vocalize speech. He should be reassured that much can be done for him through a rehabilitation program, and he should be referred to a speech pathologist before surgery.

Thorough mouth hygiene prior to surgery is imperative. Usually, antibiotics are prescribed to reduce further the possibility of infection. In men, preoperative shaving includes the beard and the hair on the neck and the chest down to the nipple line.

Postoperative Nursing Management. If a laryngofissure has been performed, a tracheostomy tube will be in place for 2 or 3 days (see p. 491). The physician may insert a nasogastric tube, and feedings are given under the same precautions that prevail in gastrostomy feedings (see p. 775). Intravenous therapy may be given concurrently. Oral feedings often are started on the first day after operation if acceptable to the patient. Speaking is deferred until the physician permits whispering (2 to 3 days). This is followed by gradual resumption of the use of the voice.

If the patient has had a total laryngectomy, a laryngectomy tube will most likely be in place. (In some clinics a laryngectomy tube is not used, in others it is used temporarily, and in many it is used permanently.) The laryngectomy tube (which is shorter than a tracheostomy tube but has a larger diameter) is the only airway the patient has. The care of this tube is the same as for a tracheostomy tube (see p. 493).

Respiratory effectiveness is promoted by positioning the patient in the semi-Fowler to Fowler position following recovery from anesthesia. The patient is observed for restlessness, labored breathing, apprehension, and increased pulse rate, since these suggest respiratory or circulatory problems. Medications that depress respirations are to be avoided. Like other surgical patients, the laryngectomy patient needs to be turned and reminded to cough and take deep breaths. Early ambulation, also, will help in preventing atelectasis and pneumonia.

Wound drains that may be in place assist in removal of fluid and air from the dead space. Portable suction may also be used. Drainage is observed, measured, and recorded; when drainage amounts to less than 50 ml/day to 60 ml/day, drains usually are removed.

The stoma is kept clean by daily cleansing with saline solution or diluted hydrogen peroxide; antibiotic ointment may then be applied around the stoma and suture line.

Vitamins may be given as supplemental feedings, and infusions often are necessary to keep up fluid, electrolyte, and nutritional balance. Since a "magic slate" is often used for communication, it is well to remember which hand the patient uses for writing so that the opposite arm will be used for intravenous feedings. When notes are the means of communication, they should be destroyed to assure the patient's privacy. If the patient is not able to write, flash cards can be used. The phone to the patient's room may be disconnected since he is unable to talk.

Nutrition is maintained by means of a tube passed through a cervical pharyngostomy or by nasogastric catheter. Usually, a nasogastric catheter is passed by the physician after operation, and liquid feedings are given. Thereafter, the nurse is permitted to remove and pass this tube because there is no possibility of its getting into the trachea, the trachea now being sutured permanently to the skin as a tracheostomy. After a few days the patient can be taught to pass his own feeding tube. Good mouth hygiene must be followed rigidly. After about 7 days, when the incision has healed, the surgeon may allow the patient to begin oral feedings. Then he begins to develop his ability to belch. About an hour after he has eaten, the nurse can remind him to belch. Later this conscious action is transformed into simple explosions of air from the esophagus for speech purposes. At this point the speech pathologist works with him in an attempt to make his speech intelligible and as close to normal as is possible.

- Through the postoperative period, be alert for the possible serious complication of rupture of the carotid artery, particularly if wound infection is present. Should this occur, apply direct pressure over the artery, summon assistance, and provide psychological support to the patient until the vessel can be ligated.

The laryngectomy tube may be removed when the stoma is well healed, usually within 3 to 6 weeks after the operation.

Laryngectomy Patient Education
Speech Rehabilitation. The patient should be reassured that much can be done for him through a rehabilitation program. Ideally, the speech pathologist sees the patient before the operation, in order to counsel him and to enlarge upon what the physician has told him. The speech pathologist reassures the patient that with speech therapy the sound source can be replaced with either laryngeal or esophageal speech or by using one of the different types of artificial larynxes.

The partially laryngectomized patient has little difficulty, because in a matter of a few days his voice will improve. However, the completely laryngectomized patient often is depressed and needs encouragement. The rehabilitative management of this patient requires a team that includes the surgeon, the nurse, the patient's family, persons who have had laryngectomies (Fig. 22-7), and the speech pathologist.

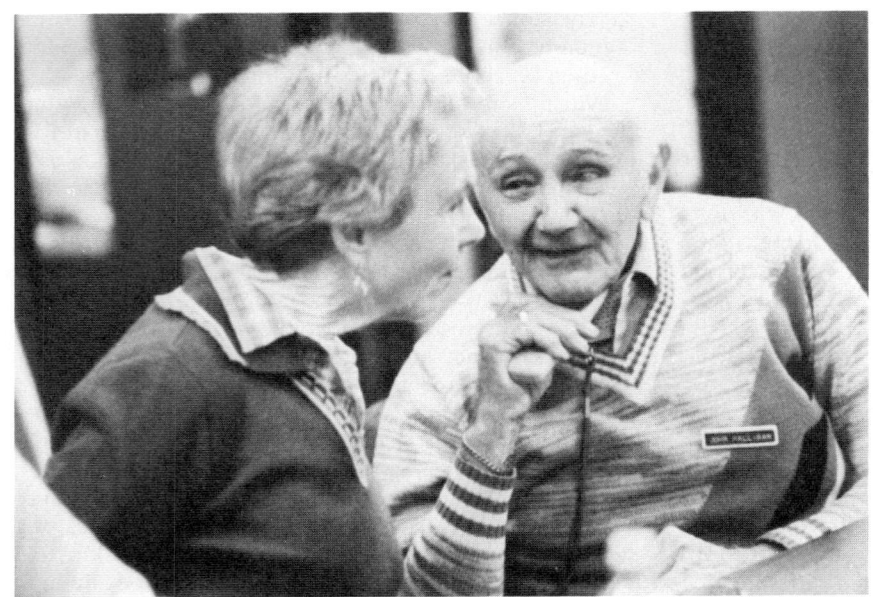

Figure 22-7. A special kind of caller. During recovery, a former laryngectomee may visit the "new" laryngectomee. This caller will use esophageal speech and answer questions written by the patient. Such contact with a former patient has been very effective in encouraging the new patient when he needs it most. (From American Cancer Society, New Jersey Division, Inc. Middlesex County Unit, and Larynx Visitation Program.)

There are two methods of learning to speak after a laryngectomy. The first method relies on laryngeal or esophageal speech. The patient takes air into his mouth, and then by compression of the lips or by strong articulation of "plosive" speech sounds such as "p," "t," or "k," he can aircharge, or inflate, his esophagus. By lip compression or the plosive sound method, the air is sent posteriorly toward the esophagus. As air gets into the upper part of the esophagus, the increased pressure at that point will be released and will produce a vibration or tone. This tone is made at the narrowing between the pharynx and esophagus. The resultant voice sounds low pitched because the neoglottis from which the sounds are now emitted is indeed different from the normal vocal cords. In a few months the new speech becomes automatic and the individual does not have to think about getting an adequate air charge before talking.

Another method of vocalization after a laryngectomy is by means of an artificial larynx. Most laryngectomees are able to learn the esophageal method of voice production. However, if the patient is unable to attain esophageal speech owing to various reasons (advanced emphysema, asthma, stenosis of the esophagus, hearing loss, etc.), an artificial larynx can be used. A variety of artificial larynxes are available. One type consists of a vibrator powered by batteries, which is placed against the side of the neck. When it is turned on, the air inside the mouth is vibrated and the patient articulates in a somewhat normal fashion.

Another device, also battery-powered, utilizes a plastic tube that is inserted into the side and well to the back of the mouth, providing a continuous sound source in the mouth. The individual merely articulates this sound, shaping it in a normal manner to form audible speech.

The International Association of Laryngectomees is a voluntary organization that sponsors "Lost Chord" or "New Voice" clubs to encourage and give opportunities for laryngectomized persons to learn to speak again.

Tracheostomy and Stomal Care. The nurse conveys optimism to the patient, assuring him that he will be able to carry on most of his preoperative activities. The patient needs specific information about what to expect from his tracheostomy (see p. 491). He will frequently cough up rather large amounts of mucus through this opening. Because the air passes directly into the trachea without being warmed and moistened by the respiratory mucosa, the tracheobronchial tree compensates by secreting excessive amounts of mucus. Therefore, the patient will have frequent coughing episodes, and he may be somewhat troubled by the brassy sounding, mucus-producing cough. However, he should be assured that these problems diminish in time as the tracheobronchial mucosa adapts to the patient's altered physiology.

When the patient coughs, the orifice should be wiped clean and cleared of mucus. In addition, the skin around the stoma should be washed twice daily. If crusting occurs, the skin around the stoma can be lubricated with an ointment (prescribed by the physician) and the crusts removed with sterile tweezers. It is necessary that a bib be worn in front of the tracheostomy to keep the mucus from soiling the clothing. The bib may be a simple gauze dressing taped over the neck or one made of other porous fabric.

One of the most important factors in decreasing cough and mucus production as well as crusting around the stoma is to provide adequate humidification of the environment. Mechanical humidifiers and cool mist or steam vaporizers are excellent sources of humidification and are absolutely essential for the patient's comfort. Some system of humidification should be set up in the home *before the patient is discharged from the hospital.* An air-conditioned atmosphere may be distressing to the newly laryngectomized patient, since the air may be too cool or too dry and thus too irritating.

Changes in Taste and Smell. The patient can expect to have a diminished sense of taste and smell for a period after the operation. Because he is breathing directly into the trachea, air is not passing through the nose to the olfactory end organs. Because taste and smell are so closely connected, his taste sensations are altered. However, in time the individual usually accommodates to this problem and his olfactory sensation adapts to meet his needs.

Hygienic and Recreational Measures. Special precautions need to be taken in a shower to prevent water from entering the stoma. Wearing a loose-fitting plastic bib or simply holding one's hand over the opening is effective. However, swimming is not recommended, because the laryngectomee can drown without getting his face wet. Barbers and beauticians need to be cautioned so that hair sprays, loose hair, and powder do not get near the stoma, since they could cause blockage, irritation, and possibly infection.

Recreation and exercise are important. Golf, bowling, bridge, spectator activities, and walking can be enjoyed safely. Moderation in order to prevent fatigue is important because, when tired, the laryngectomee has more difficulty speaking with his new voice. At such times he can easily become discouraged and depressed.

Follow-up and Emergency Care. It is important for the laryngectomee to visit his physician regularly for physical examinations and for advice concerning any problems relating to his convalescent program. He should also carry proper identification, such as a card, to alert a first-aider to the special requirements of resuscitation should this need arise. On the back of the card can be included the name of a responsible person to notify in the event of emergency.

▶ **Evaluation**

Expected Outcomes

1. Improves vocal problems
   a. No longer smokes
   b. Relates the significance of good hygienic measures in keeping mouth and stoma clean
   c. Practices the directives of the speech therapist
   d. Communicates with spouse utilizing each newly learned speech technique
   e. Verbalizes how the vocal problem can be improved with adherence to the therapeutic plan, eventually mastering his very own program, whether it is "belch" or a mechanical device
2. Is able to communicate
   a. Uses magic slate until physician permits whispering
   b. Tells what alternatives are available when voice is not audible: call bell, flash cards, sign language, lip reading, computer aids
   c. Relates what alternatives there are in selecting the right therapy for himself: "belched" speech, artificial larynx
   d. Invites spouse to participate in "New Voice" Club activities
3. Eliminates or controls the malignancy
   a. Submits to laryngectomy or other required laryngeal surgery
   b. No longer smokes
   c. Verbalizes intent to avoid hazardous situations: aerosolized sprays, burning plastic, smoke-filled rooms
   d. Recounts danger signs of cancer: changes in bladder or bowel habits, a sore that will not heal, etc.
4. Adheres to the therapeutic program
   a. Demonstrates good understanding of hygienic principles when caring for stoma
   b. Uses a check-off chart to change laryngeal dressings and clean stomal area; self-care
   c. Practices recommended speech therapy in addition to keeping appointments with speech therapist
   d. Involves spouse with above activities and plans how to increase the humidity in their living quarters
   e. Verbalizes understanding of symptoms that require medical attention
5. Avoids complications
   a. Demonstrates practical and meticulous technique involved in cleaning and changing laryngostomy tube
   b. Covers stomal opening securely when shaving or showering
   c. Relates how an air-conditioned atmosphere may be distressing during his convalescent period: too cool, too dry, too irritating
   d. Makes appointment to have follow-up checks with a clinical nurse specialist/speech therapist/physician
   e. Carries a card indicating procedures to follow in event of an emergency, including who to summon for assistance

▷ **Bibliography**

Books

Chang WHJ. Fundamentals of Plastic and Reconstructive Surgery. Baltimore, Williams & Wilkins, 1980.
DeWeese D and Saunders WH. Textbook of Otolaryngology, 6th ed. St Louis, CV Mosby, 1982.
Lesavoy MA. Reconstruction of the Head and Neck. Baltimore, Williams & Wilkins, 1980.
Paparella MM. 1981 Yearbook of Otolaryngology. Chicago, Year Book Medical Publishers, 1981.
Snow JB Jr (ed). Controversy in Otolaryngology. Philadelphia, WB Saunders, 1980.
Wood RD II and Northern JL. Manual of Otolaryngology. A Symptom-Oriented Text. Baltimore, Williams & Wilkins, 1979.

Articles

Nose

Beekhuis GJ. Silastic alar-columellar prosthesis in conjunction with rhinoplasty. Arch Otolaryngol 1982 Aug; 108(7):429–432.
Boster SR and Martinez SA. Acute upper airway obstruction in the adult. I. Causative disease processes. Postgrad Med 1982 Dec; 72(6):50–57.
Boster SR and Martinez SA. Acute upper airway obstruction in the adult. 2. Causative events. Postgrad Med 1982 Dec; 72(6):61–67.
Goode RL. Magnetic intranasal splints. Arch Otolaryngol 1982 May; 108(5):319.
Hayden GF. Olfactory diagnosis in medicine. Postgrad Med 1980 Apr; 67(4):110–118.
Intranasal corticosteroid aerosols—noninfectious rhinitis. Med Lett Drugs Ther 1981 Nov 27; 23(24):101–102.

Johnson JT. Epistaxis management. Postgrad Med 1981 Nov; 70(5):231–235.

Kveton JF, Pillsbury HC, and Sasaki CT. Nasal obstruction (adenoiditis vs adenoid hypertrophy). Arch Otolaryngol 1982 May; 108(5):315–318.

Lavie P et al. Excessive daytime sleepiness and insomnia (association with deviated nasal septum and nocturnal breathing disorders). Arch Otolaryngol 1982 June; 108(6):373–377.

Malkiewicz J. Examining the nose. RN 1982 Apr; 45(4):55–57.

Nasal hyperthermia may help cold symptoms. AORN J 1980 Jan; 31(1):72.

Newman RK and Johnson JT. Nasal airway obstruction. Postgrad Med 1980 Aug; 68(2):184–191.

Stewart TW Jr. Vasomotor rhinitis. Postgrad Med 1980 Jan; 67(1):171–178.

Tag AR. Toxic shock syndrome: Otolaryngologic presentations (nasal and sinus packing). Laryngoscope 1982 Sept 12; 92(9):1070–1072.

Thomas JR, Mechlin DC, and Templer J. Skin grafts (nose). Arch Otolaryngol 1982 July; 108(7):437–438.

Sinuses and Throat

Current care for pharyngitis. Patient Care 1980 Dec 15; 14(21):50–92.

Current care for sinusitis. Patient Care 1980 Dec 15; 14(21):97–111.

Neel HB and McDonald TJ. Chronic sinusitis. Postgrad Med 1981 Mar; 69(3):109–113.

Neel HB and McDonald TJ. Tonsillectomy and adenoidectomy. Postgrad Med 1981 Sept; 70(3):107–112.

Stewart TW Jr. Common otolaryngologic problems of flying. Am Fam Physician 1979 Feb; 19(2):113–119.

Tonsillectomy justified for severe recurrent throat infections. AORN J 1981 Jan; 33(1):97.

Head and Neck

Alexander MV, Zajtchuk JT, and Henderson RL. Hypothyroidism and wound healing (occurrence after head and neck radiation and surgery). Arch Otolaryngol 1982 May; 108(5):289.

Dropkin MJ. Development of a self-care teaching program for postoperative head and neck patients. Can Nursing 1981 Apr; 4(2):103–106.

Gillis TM. A comparison of combined modalities and single modality in the management of advanced head and neck tumors. Laryngoscope 1982 Sept; 92(9):993–998.

Wood BG. Principles of surgical management of midfacial carcinoma. Laryngoscope 1982 Oct; 92(10):1154–1156.

Larynx

Baker BM and Cunningham CA. Vocal rehabilitation of the patient with a laryngectomy. Part I. Pre- and postoperative counseling. Oncol Nurs Forum 1980; 7(4):23–27.

Baker BM and Cunningham CA. Vocal rehabilitation of the patient with a laryngectomy. Part II. Assessment for vocal rehabilitation. Oncol Nurs Forum 1980; 7(4):28–33.

Baker BM and Cunningham CA. Vocal rehabilitation of the patient with a laryngectomy. Part III. Specific techniques in laryngectomee vocal rehabilitation. Oncol Nurs Forum 1980; 7(4):33–36.

Beukelman DR et al. Objective assessment of laryngectomized patients with surgical reconstruction. Arch Otolaryngol 1980 Nov; 106(11):715–718.

Bradenburg JH. Vocal rehabilitation after laryngectomy. Arch Otolaryngol 1980 Nov; 106(11):688–690.

Johnson JT, Newman RK, and Olson JE. Persistent hoarseness. Postgrad Med 1980 May; 67(5):122–216.

Knapp BA and Panje WR. A voice button for laryngectomees. AORN J 1982 Aug; 36(2):183–192.

Lidocaine may prevent post-op laryngospasm. AORN J 1980 Jan; 31(1):76.

Markus JF and Konrad HR. The right-angle laryngeal telescope in undergraduate medical education. Arch Otolaryngol 1982 June; 108(6):344–346.

McCormick GP et al. Artificial speech devices. Am J Nurs 1982 Jan; 82(1):121–122.

McLoy DG, Hecht SS, and Wynder EL. The roles of tobacco, alcohol, and diet in the etiology of upper alimentary and respiratory tract cancer. Prev Med 1980 Sept; 9(5):622–629.

More laryngectomy patients speaking due to advances. AORN J 1982 Jan; 35(1):75–78.

Pilcher L. Carbon dioxide lasers in laryngeal surgery. AORN J 1981 June; 33(7):1402–1407.

Scully PA and Stratton CJ. Argon laser use in papillomas of the larynx. Laryngoscope 1982 Oct; 92(10):1164–1167.

Shapiro MJ and Ramanathan VR. Trachea stoma vent voice prosthesis. Laryngoscope 1982 Oct; 92(10):1126–1129.

Smith's total laryngectomy. Nurs Times 1980 Oct 23; 76(43):1884–1885.

Ward S. Rigid endoscopy of the respiratory tract. AORN J 1981 Dec; 34(6):1058–1074.

Weinberg B. Airway resistance of the voice button. Arch Otolaryngol 1982 Aug; 108(8):498–500.

Agency

International Association of Laryngectomees, % American Cancer Society, 777 Third Ave., New York, New York 10017

23

Assessment of Respiratory Function

▷ Physiologic Overview

The cells of the body derive their necessary energy from the oxidation of carbohydrates, fats, and proteins. For this process, as for any type of combustion, oxygen is required. Certain vital tissues, such as those of the brain and the heart, cannot survive for long without a continuing supply of oxygen. As a result of oxidation in the body tissues, carbon dioxide is produced and must be removed from the cells to prevent buildup of acid waste products.

Oxygen is supplied to cells and carbon dioxide is removed from cells via circulating blood. No cell is far removed from a capillary, the thin walls of which present little resistance to the passage of dissolved gases. The concentration of oxygen in the tissues, where it is being consumed by cellular metabolism, is lower than it is in the blood within the capillaries. As a result, oxygen diffuses from the capillary blood, through the capillary wall into the interstitial fluid, and then through the membrane of the tissue cell into the cell sap, where it can be used by the mitochondria for cellular respiration. The movement of carbon dioxide proceeds in the opposite direction, from cell to blood. This movement also occurs by diffusion, since carbon dioxide concentration inside the cell is greater, owing to metabolism, than it is in the blood passing through the tissue capillary. An average resting adult utilizes approximately 250 ml O_2/min and produces approximately 200 ml CO_2/min. With strenuous exercise, these values may increase up to tenfold. As a result of the exchange of O_2 and CO_2 in tissue capillaries, arterial blood loses about 25% of its oxygen, whereas carbon dioxide content is increased about 15%.

After these capillary exchanges, blood enters the veins (where it is called venous blood) and travels to the lung capillaries. The oxygen concentration in blood within lung capillaries is lower than it is in the lung gas spaces. As a result, oxygen diffuses from the gas spaces into the blood. Carbon dioxide, since its concentration in the blood is higher than it is in the gas spaces of the lung, diffuses from the blood into the lung gas. Movement of fresh air in and out of the airways (called ventilation) intermittently replenishes the oxygen in and removes the carbon dioxide from the gas within airspaces of the lung. This overall process by which exchanges take place between atmospheric air and the cells of the body is called respiration.

Anatomy of the Lung

The lungs are elastic structures enclosed in the thorax, an airtight chamber with distensible walls. Ventilation involves movements of the walls of the thorax and of its floor, the diaphragm. The effect of these movements is to alternately increase and decrease the capacity of the chest. When the capacity of the chest is increased, air enters through the trachea, because of the lowered pressure within, and inflates the lungs. When the chest wall and diaphragm return to their previous positions, the elastic lungs recoil and force the air out via the bronchi and trachea.

The outer surfaces of the lungs are enclosed by a smooth, slippery membrane, the *pleura,* which also extends to cover the interior wall of the thorax and the superior surface of the diaphragm. The pleura is termed *parietal pleura* where it lines the thorax, and *visceral pleura* where it covers the lungs. Between the two pleural surfaces is a small amount of fluid that lubricates the surfaces and allows them to slide freely during ventilation.

The *mediastinum* is the wall that divides the thoracic cavity into two halves. It is composed of two layers of pleura between which lie all of the thoracic structures except the lungs.

Each lung is divided into lobes. The left lung consists of upper and lower lobes, whereas the right lung has upper, middle, and lower lobes. Each lobe is further subdivided into two to five segments. Lobes of the lungs are separated by fissures, which are extensions of the pleura. A schematic diagram of the airways and the lobes of the lungs is shown in Figure 23-1.

The airways through which gases enter and leave the alveoli are called *bronchioles*. The bronchioles join to form larger and larger bronchi and eventually form one main bronchus for each lung. The two primary bronchi then unite to form the trachea, which is continuous with the oropharynx and the mouth. The walls of the airways contain smooth muscle, which can, upon contraction or relaxation, cause a change in the caliber of the airway. These smooth muscles are innervated by both the parasympathetic and sympathetic nervous systems. The airways also contain bronchial glands, which secrete mucus into the lumen. The bronchi and bronchioles are lined with cells whose luminal surfaces are covered with short "hairs" called *cilia*. These cilia maintain a constant whipping motion that serves to propel mucus and substances from the inside of the lungs toward the mouth.

The human lung is made up of a large number (300 million) of tiny air sacs, which are called *alveoli*. They are scarcely visible to the naked eye (approximately ¼ mm in diameter). Their elastic walls are lined by a single layer of epithelial cells and contain a network of pulmonary capillaries. Certain cells in the walls of the alveoli secrete a lipid-

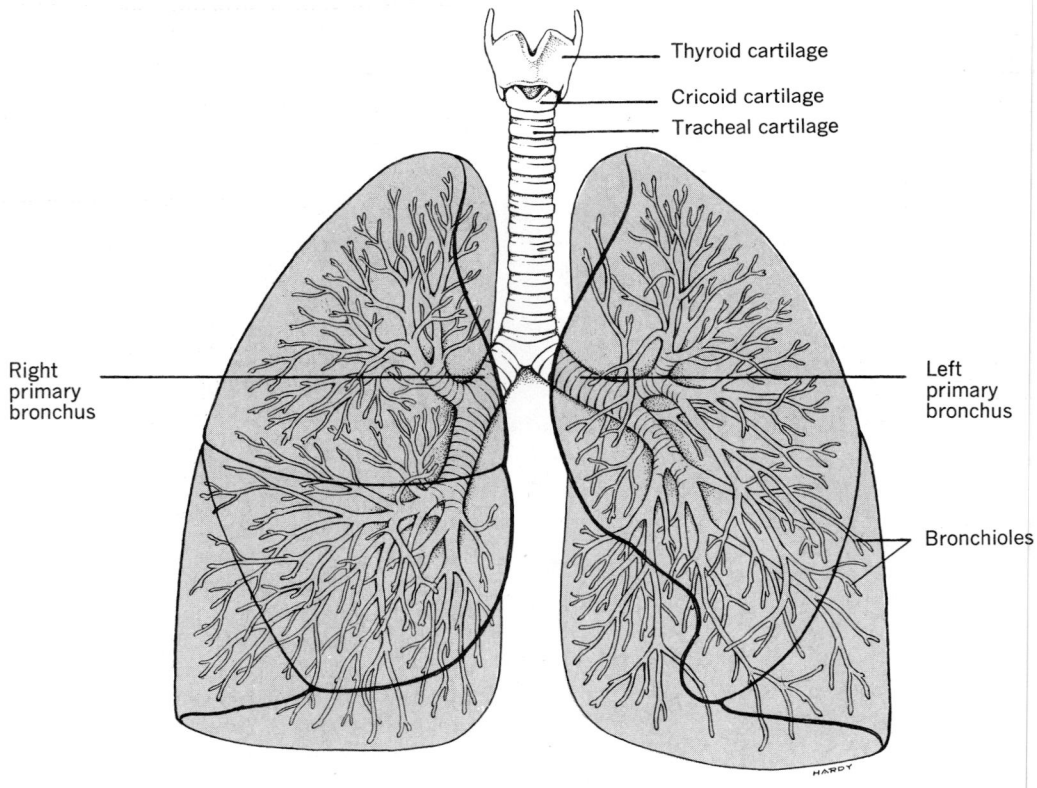

Figure 23-1.   Larynx, trachea, and bronchial tree (anterior view). (From Chaffee EE and Greisheimer EM: Basic Physiology and Anatomy, 3rd ed. Philadelphia, JB Lippincott.)

containing material onto the surface of each alveolus. This thin layer of lipid-rich material is called the *alveolar surfactant*. So numerous are these alveoli that if their surfaces were united to form one sheet, it would cover an area of over 90 square yards.

Mechanics of Ventilation

During inspiration, air flows from the environment into the trachea, bronchi, bronchioles, and alveoli. During expiration, alveolar gas travels the same route in reverse.

The physical factors that govern airflow into and out of the lungs are collectively referred to as the mechanics of ventilation. Air flows from a region of higher pressure to a region of lower pressure. During inspiration, contraction of the diaphragm and other muscles of respiration enlarges the thoracic cavity and thereby lowers the pressure inside the thorax to a level below that of atmospheric pressure. Therefore, air is drawn through the trachea and bronchi into the alveoli.

During normal expiration, the muscles of respiration relax and the thoracic cavity decreases in size. The alveolar pressure now exceeds atmospheric pressure, and air flows from the lungs into the atmosphere.

The rate of inspiratory or expiratory airflow is equal to the pressure gradient between the atmosphere and the alveoli divided by the airflow resistance of the airways:

$$\text{Flow} = \Delta\text{ Pressure/Resistance}$$

Resistance is determined chiefly by the radius of the airway through which the air is flowing. Any process that changes bronchial diameter will therefore affect airway resistance and alter the rate of airflow for a given pressure gradient during respiration. Common factors that may alter bronchial diameter include contraction of bronchial smooth muscle, as in asthma; thickening of bronchial mucosa, as in chronic bronchitis; or obstruction of the airway owing to mucus, tumor, or a foreign body. Loss of lung elasticity, such as is seen in emphysema, may also alter bronchial diameter since the lung connective tissue encircles the airways and helps to keep them open during both inspiration and expiration. With increased resistance, greater than normal respiratory effort is required by the patient to achieve normal levels of ventilation.

The pressure gradient between the thoracic cavity and the atmosphere causes airflow in and out of the lungs and also stretches the lung tissue itself. The pressure required to stretch the lung is determined by the properties of its elastic tissue. A measure of how easily lungs can be stretched is called *lung compliance*. Compliance is usually measured under static conditions.

A compliant lung (high compliance) distends easily when pressure is applied, whereas a noncompliant lung (low compliance) requires greater than normal pressure to distend it. The major factors that determine lung compliance are connective tissue (collagen and elastin) and the surface tension in the alveoli. The surface tension at the surface of the alveoli is normally maintained at a low level by the presence of the alveolar lining material (lung surfactant). Increased connective tissue or increased alveolar surface tension results in low compliance. In respiratory distress syndrome of the newborn (hyaline membrane dis-

ease), there is a surfactant deficiency and lungs are stiff (low compliance). In pulmonary fibrosis, connective tissue proliferates and compliance is decreased. Lungs with low compliance require a greater than normal energy expenditure to achieve normal levels of ventilation.

Pulmonary Circulation

Almost the entire cardiac output ordinarily passes through capillaries of the lung and is capable of exchanging gases with the alveoli. Pulmonary artery pressure is normally about 25 mm Hg systolic, compared with 120 mm Hg in the systemic arteries. Since flow in the pulmonary and systemic circuits is almost the same, the resistance to blood flow in the pulmonary vasculature is roughly one fifth of that in the systemic circulation. In an upright individual, blood flow to the top of the lungs (apex) is somewhat less than that to the base of the lungs, because of the effects of gravity.

A small percentage of the cardiac output even in normal people bypasses alveoli, does not participate in gas exchange, and returns to the left heart, where it mixes with oxygenated blood. This fraction of the cardiac output that bypasses ventilated alveoli is referred to as venous admixture and constitutes a right-to-left shunt.

The pulmonary capillary bed has an important metabolic role, which includes the regulation of the concentration of many vasoactive compounds present in the blood. The lung removes and inactivates serotonin and norepinephrine (potent vasoconstrictors) from the circulating blood. The pulmonary endothelium is selective since compounds with similar structure, such as histamine and epinephrine, are not removed from the blood. The lung converts angiotensin I (an inactive compound) to angiotensin II by the action of converting enzyme located on the pulmonary capillary endothelium. Bradykinin may be inactivated by the same enzyme. These metabolic functions of the capillary endothelium are not unique to the lung and may occur in other capillary beds. However, because of the vast pulmonary capillary endothelial surface area and because all of the cardiac output goes to the lungs, the lung becomes most important for these metabolic processes.

The lung has mechanisms that help to match blood flow to ventilation. With decreased ventilation to a region of the lung, the oxygen concentration in those alveoli decreases. The resulting hypoxia causes local blood vessels to constrict, which diminishes the blood flow to the region. In this way, blood flow and ventilation become better matched. With decreased perfusion to a region of the lung, the carbon dioxide concentration in the alveoli decreases. The hypocapnea causes local bronchi to constrict, which diminishes ventilation to the region and helps to match regional ventilation to blood flow.

▷ Diagnostic Assessment of Respiratory Function

Aside from the general physical examination of the chest, which was discussed in Chapter 5, a wide range of diagnostic studies, described in the following pages, may be conducted in patients with thoracic conditions.

Radiographic Examinations of the Chest

Normal pulmonary tissue is radiolucent; therefore, densities produced by tumors, foreign bodies, etc. can be detected by means of radiographic examination. A chest x-ray may reveal extensive pathology in the lungs in the absence of symptoms. Radiographs are usually taken after full inspiration (deep breath) since the lungs are best demonstrated when they are well aerated. Also, the diaphragm is at its lowest level and the largest expanse of lung is visible. Radiographs taken on expiration may accentuate an otherwise unnoticed pneumothorax or obstruction of a major artery.

Tomography (Planigraphy). Tomography provides films of sections of the lungs at different planes within the thorax. It gives detailed analysis of pulmonary parenchyma and mediastinum and is valuable in demonstrating the presence of solid lesions, calcification, or cavitation within a lesion.

Computed Tomography. Computed tomography is an imaging method in which the lungs are scanned in successive layers by a narrow beam x-ray. A computer printout may be obtained of the absorption values of the tissues in the plane that is being scanned. It has the capability to demonstrate the chest in cross sections and to distinguish small differences in tissue density, thus demonstrating lesions that cannot be detected by conventional radiology. It may be used to define pulmonary nodules, small tumors adjacent to pleural surfaces that are not visible on routine chest x-rays, and to demonstrate mediastinal abnormalities and hilar adenopathy, which are difficult to visualize with other techniques (see p. 331).

Positron Emission Tomography (PET). PET uses high-energy physics and sophisticated computer techniques to study the way cells function in a living person. The patient inhales or is injected with a short-lived radioactive version of an element that occurs naturally in the body (oxygen, nitrogen, carbon, fluorine). The radioisotope emits subatomic particles called *positrons* (a positively charged electron). When a positron encounters an electron, which it does just after emission, both are destroyed and two gamma rays are released. These bursts of energy are recorded by the PET scanner, and its computer determines where in the body the radioactive material is located. PET is particularly useful for quantitative measurements of regional pulmonary perfusion and for studying ventilation–perfusion relationships (see p. 340).

Fluoroscopy. Fluoroscopy is helpful in evaluating a lesion that has been previously identified by x-ray, to see if it is pulsatile. It is also useful in the study of pulmonary dynamics (the motion of pulmonary structures; diaphragmatic motion) and in detecting regional variations in ventilation.

Barium Swallow. A barium swallow outlines the esophagus and reveals displacement of the esophagus and encroachment on its lumen by cardiac, pulmonary, and mediastinal abnormalities.

Bronchography. A bronchogram provides an outline of the bronchial tree or selected areas after a radiopaque medium that coats the bronchial mucosa has been instilled directly into the trachea, bronchi and the entire bronchial tree. This is a diagnostic test for any disease that alters the caliber or patency of the bronchial tree or causes displacement there. It reveals anomalies of the bronchial tree and is important in the diagnosis of bronchiectasis, since involved segments cannot always be outlined by other methods.

The procedure must be carried out while the patient is in a fasting state to reduce the possibility of aspiration of gastric contents. Preoperative medication may include atropine to decrease secretions and vagally mediated reflex bradycardia, and diazepam (Valium) for sedation.

A topical anesthetic is sprayed into the nose, and in the mouth and posterior pharynx to prevent gagging and coughing when the tube is passed. The contrast medium may be instilled by dripping it over the glottis, by slowly injecting it through a tube in the trachea, or by injecting it through a needle inserted percutaneously into the trachea below the glottis.

Nursing Support. After such a roentgenogram, food and fluids are withheld until the patient demonstrates he has a cough reflex. Once the cough reflex has returned, the patient should be encouraged to cough and clear the bronchial tree. Postural drainage may be required. A slight temperature elevation is common following this procedure.

Angiographic Studies of the Pulmonary Vessels

Pulmonary angiography is the rapid injection of a radiopaque medium into the vasculature of the lungs for radiographic study of pulmonary vessels. It can be performed by venous injection into one or both arms (simultaneously) or femoral vein, through a needle or catheter, by introducing a catheter into the main pulmonary artery or its branches, or by introducing a catheter into the great veins or heart proximal to the pulmonary artery.

These procedures include pulmonary angiography, angiocardiography, aortography, bronchial arteriography, superior vena cava angiography, and azygography. Pulmonary angiography is most commonly used to investigate thromboembolic disease of the lungs and congenital abnormalities of the pulmonary vascular tree and to detect abnormal vasculature arising from tumors.

Endoscopic Procedures

Bronchoscopy. Bronchoscopy is the direct inspection and examination of the larynx, trachea, and bronchi through either a flexible fiberoptic bronchoscope or a rigid bronchoscope. In current practice the two devices are often used interchangeably.

The *diagnostic purposes* of bronchoscopy are (1) to examine tissues or collected secretions; (2) to determine the location and extent of pathologic process, and biopsy for diagnosis (by biting forceps, curettage, or brush biopsy); (3) to determine whether a tumor can be resected surgically; and (4) to diagnose bleeding sites (source of hemoptysis).

Therapeutically, bronchoscopy is used to (1) remove foreign bodies from the tracheobronchial tree, (2) remove secretions obstructing the tracheobronchial tree when the patient is unable to clear them, (3) provide postoperative treatment in atelectasis, and (4) fulgurate and excise lesions.

The *fiberoptic bronchoscope* is a thin, flexible bronchoscope that can be directed into the segmental bronchi (Fig. 23-2). Because of its smaller size, flexibility, and excellent optical system, it allows increased visualization of the peripheral airways and is ideal for diagnosing pulmonary lesions. Cytologic examinations can be performed without surgical intervention. Fiberoptic bronchoscopy is better tolerated by patients than rigid bronchoscopy, allows biopsy of previously inaccessible tumors, is safer in the very ill, and can be performed at the bedside or through endotracheal or tracheostomy tubes for patients on ventilators in whom it is desirable to ensure airway patency. Fiberoptic bronchoscopy allows direct intubation of the right upper lobe, which is impossible with the rigid bronchoscope.

The *rigid bronchoscope* is a hollow, metallic tube with a light at its end and is used mainly for the removal of foreign bodies, for suctioning thick secretions, for investigating the source of massive hemoptysis, or for endobronchial surgical procedures (Fig. 23-3).

Possible complications of bronchoscopy include reaction to the local anesthetic, infection, aspiration, bronchospasm, hypoxemia, pneumothorax, and bleeding.

Nursing Interventions.   An informed consent is obtained before the procedure. Food and fluids are withheld for 6 hours before the test to reduce the risk of aspiration when reflexes are blocked. The patient is told what to expect, in order to reduce fear and correct misapprehensions. Preoperative medications (usually atropine and a sedative or narcotic) are given to inhibit vagal stimulation (thereby guarding against bradycardia, arrhythmias, hypotension), suppress the cough reflex, sedate the patient, and relieve anxiety.

- *Caution:* Sedation given to patients with respiratory insufficiency may precipitate respiratory arrest.

Contact lenses, dentures, and other prostheses are removed. The examination is usually done under local anesthesia, but general anesthesia may be given, especially when the rigid bronchoscope is used.

If local anesthesia is used, the pharynx is sprayed with a topical anesthetic (lidocaine [Xylocaine]), and the solution is dropped on the epiglottis and vocal cords and into the trachea to reduce the cough reflex and pain. Diazepam (Valium) may be administered intravenously for additional sedation and for amnesia.

Following the procedure, the patient is given nothing by mouth until the cough reflex returns, as the preoperative sedation and local anesthesia impair the protective laryngeal reflex and swallowing for several hours. Once the patient demonstrates that he can cough, cracked ice may be given, and eventually fluids. Watch for confusion and lethargy in the elderly, possibly owing to large doses of lidocaine given during the procedure. Difficulty in breathing is looked for and reported promptly. The patient should also be observed for evidence of cyanosis, hypotension, tachycardia, arrhythmias, hemoptysis, and dyspnea.

Esophagoscopy.   Esophagoscopy is the viewing of the interior of the esophagus through a lighted tube. It is used in removing foreign bodies; in inspecting lesions of the esophagus, such as ulcers, diverticuli, and tumors; and often in making a positive diagnosis by removing small bits of tissue for microscopic examination (biopsy). The care before and after the procedure is the same as for bronchoscopy.

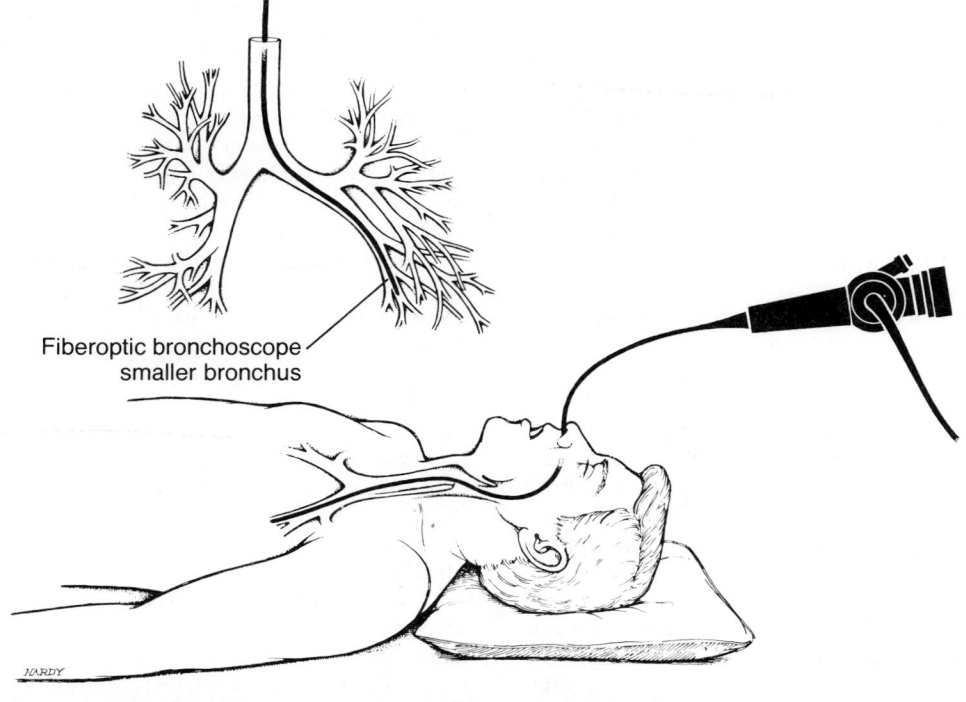

Fiberoptic bronchoscope
smaller bronchus

Figure 23-2.   Fiberoptic bronchoscopy.

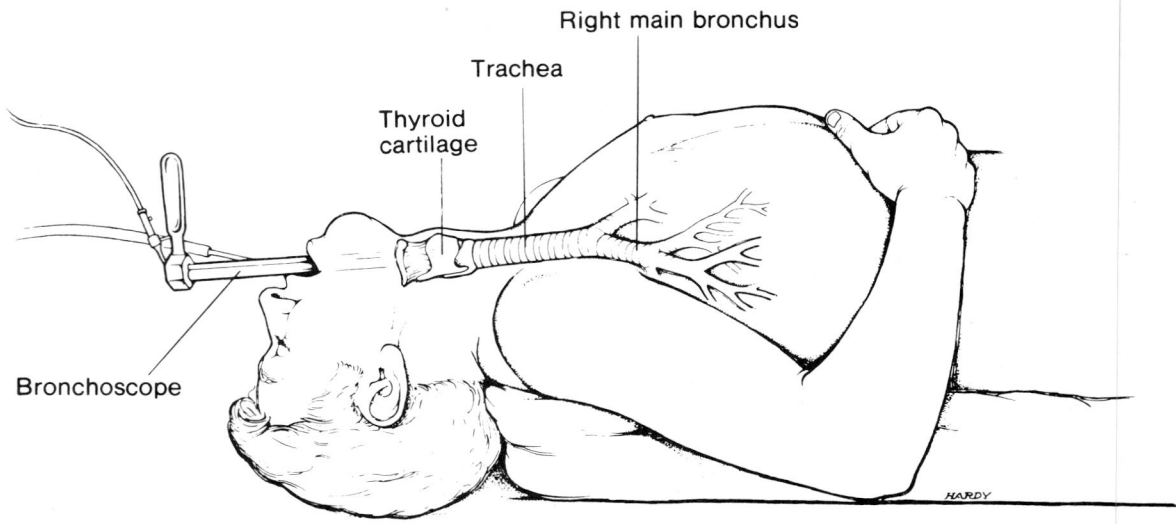

Figure 23-3. Introduction of the rigid bronchoscope.

Thoracoscopy. *Thoracoscopy* (pleuroscopy) is a diagnostic procedure in which the pleural cavity is examined with an endoscope. A small incision is made into the pleural cavity in an intercostal space, the location depending on clinical and radiologic findings. After aspiration of fluid present in the pleural cavity, the fiberoptic mediastinoscope is inserted into the pleural cavity and an inspection is made of its surface. Lesions can be biopsied under direct vision. Following the procedure, a chest tube is inserted and the pleural cavity is drained by underwater-seal drainage.

Mediastinoscopy. See page 447.

Sputum Studies

Sputum may be obtained for study to identify pathogenic organisms and to determine whether malignant cells are present. It may also be used to assess for hypersensitivity states (in which there is an increase of eosinophils). Periodic sputum examinations may be necessary for patients receiving antibiotics, steroids, and immunosuppressive drugs for prolonged periods, since these agents give rise to opportunistic infections. In general, sputum cultures are used in diagnosis, for drug sensitivity testing, and as a guide in treatment. Sputum can be obtained by expectoration. If the patient cannot raise the sputum spontaneously, he can often be induced to cough deeply by breathing an irritating aerosol of supersaturated saline, propylene glycol, or some other agent delivered with an ultrasonic nebulizer. Other methods of collecting sputum specimens include endotracheal aspiration (p. 462); bronchoscopic removal (p. 440); bronchial brushing (p. 447); transtracheal aspiration (p. 442); or gastric aspiration, usually for tuberculosis organisms (p. 1507). Generally, the deepest specimens are most often obtained in the early morning.

The patient is instructed to clear his nose and throat and rinse his mouth in order to decrease contamination of the sputum. He then takes a few deep breaths; coughs (rather than spits), using his diaphragm; and expectorates into a sterile container.

The specimen should be sent to the laboratory immediately; allowing it to stand for several hours in a warm room will result in the overgrowth of contaminant organisms and may make culture more difficult (especially for *Mycobacterium tuberculosis*).

Often a qualitative study is done to determine whether the secretions are saliva, mucus, or pus. Usually, they separate into layers that are seen readily when a conical, glass container is used. A yellow-green color of the material expectorated usually implies infection (*i.e.,* bronchitis or pneumonia).

For quantitative studies, the patient is given a special container in which to expectorate. This is weighed at the end of 24 hours, and the amount and the character of the contents are described and recorded. Such a specimen is disposed of by wrapping it in paper and sending it to the incinerator. To prevent odors, all sputum containers should be covered. Malodorous, discarded mouth wipes should be removed and good room ventilation assured. Of course, frequent oral hygiene is a nursing priority for these patients.

Transtracheal aspiration of sputum is accomplished by transtracheal puncture through the cricothyroid membrane and by the introduction of a fine catheter through the needle into the trachea (Fig. 23-4). The needle is withdrawn, leaving the catheter in place. Sterile saline (2 ml–5 ml) is injected into the catheter to loosen secretions and induce coughing. Then material is aspirated back through the catheter into a syringe. The contents of the syringe are expressed into a sterile culture tube. The catheter is withdrawn and pressure is applied over the puncture site 5 to 10 minutes to minimize bleeding and subcutaneous emphysema.

This technique may also be used to promote coughing and sputum production in thoracotomy patients and in those patients with an absent cough reflex. In this instance, the catheter may be left in place for periodic instillation of saline to induce coughing.

Transtracheal aspiration bypasses the oropharynx and

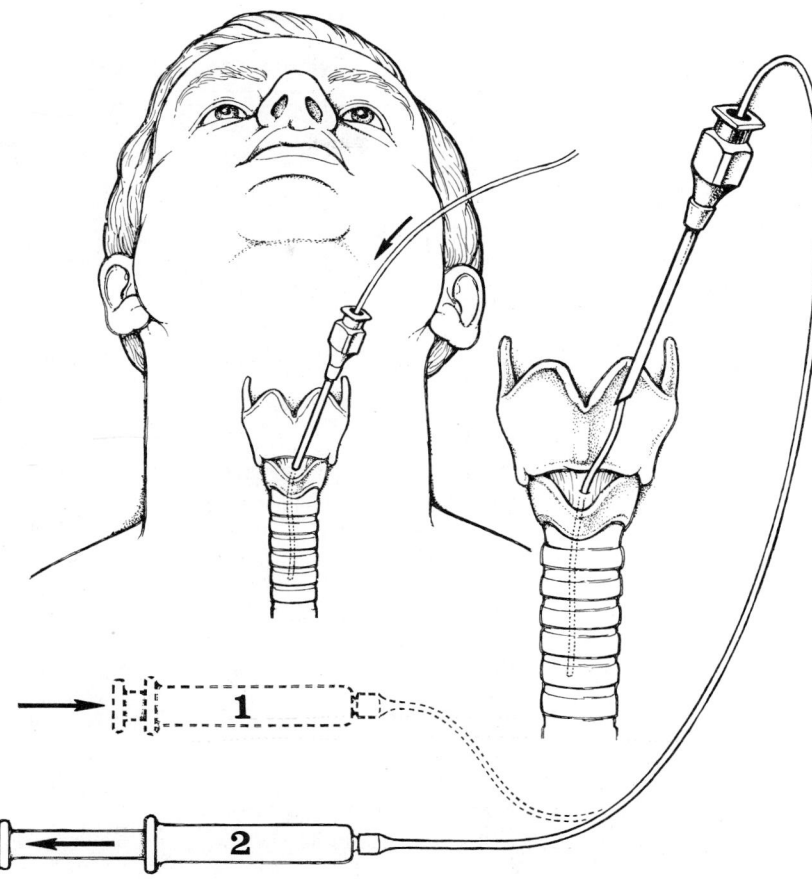

Figure 23-4. After the catheter is positioned into the trachea, the needle is withdrawn, leaving the catheter in place. Sterile saline (2 ml–5 ml) is injected into the catheter (*1*) to loosen secretions and induce coughing. Then the material is aspirated back through the catheter into a syringe (*2*).

thus avoids specimen contamination by mouth flora, particularly anaerobes. It is of special value to the immunocompromised patient with pneumonia who does not produce sputum.

The patient is observed for several hours following the procedure. Possible complications include intratracheal bleeding, hypoxemia, cardiac arrhythmias, pneumomediastinum, and subcutaneous emphysema.

Examination of Pleural Fluid (Thoracentesis)

A thin layer of pleural fluid normally remains in the pleural space. A sample of this fluid can be obtained by thoracentesis or by tube thoracotomy. *Thoracentesis* is the aspiration of pleural fluid for diagnostic or therapeutic purposes (Fig. 23-5). Frequently, a needle biopsy of the pleura is taken at the same time. Guidelines for assisting the patient undergoing a thoracentesis are presented in Chart 23-1. Studies on pleural fluid include gram-stain culture and sensitivity, acid-fast staining and culture, differential cell count, cytology, *p*H, specific gravity, total protein, and lactic dehydrogenase (LDH).

Pleural Biopsy

Pleural biopsy is accomplished via (1) needle biopsy of the pleura or (2) pleuroscopy, which is a visual exploration of the pleural space through a fiberoptic bronchoscope inserted into the pleural space. Pleural biopsy is done when

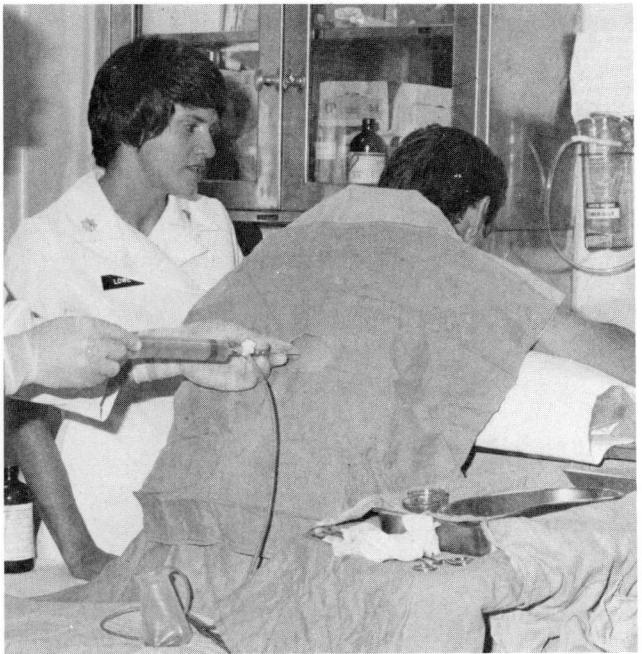

Figure 23-5. The patient is having a diagnostic thoracentesis performed. (Courtesy, Walter Reed Army Medical Center, Washington, D.C.)

Chart 23-1
Guidelines for Assisting the Patient Having a Thoracentesis

A thoracentesis (aspiration of fluid or air from the pleural space) is done on patients with various clinical problems. It may be a diagnostic or therapeutic procedure for:

1. Removal of fluid and air from the pleural cavity
2. Diagnostic aspiration of pleural fluid
3. Pleural biopsy
4. Instillation of medication into pleural space

The responsibilities of the nurse in relation to the patient having a thoracentesis and the rationale of her participation are summarized below.

Nursing Activities	*Amplification/Rationale*
1. Ascertain in advance whether chest roentgenograms have been prescribed and completed and consent form has been signed.	1. Posteroanterior and lateral chest x-rays are used to localize fluid and air in the pleural cavity and to aid in determining the puncture site. Ultrasound scanning may be done when fluid is loculated (pocket of pleural fluid) to help select the best site for needle aspiration.
2. Determine whether the patient is allergic to the local anesthetic agent to be used. Give sedation if prescribed.	

3. Inform the patient about the procedure and indicate how he can be helpful. Explain:
  a. The nature of the procedure
  b. The importance of remaining immobile
  c. Pressure sensations to be experienced
  d. That no discomfort is anticipated after the procedure
	3. An explanation helps to orient the patient to the procedure, assists him to mobilize his resources, and gives him an opportunity to ask questions and verbalize anxiety.

4. Make the patient comfortable with adequate supports. If possible, place him upright and in one of the following positions:
  a. Sitting on the edge of the bed with the feet supported and his arms and head on a padded over-the-bed table
  b. Straddling a chair with his arms and head resting on the back of the chair
  c. Lying on his unaffected side with the bed elevated 30° to 45° if he is unable to assume a sitting position
	4. The upright position facilitates the removal of fluid that usually localizes at the base of the chest. A position of comfort helps the patient to relax.

5. Support and reassure the patient during the procedure.
  a. Prepare the patient for cold sensation of skin germicide solution and of pressure sensation from infiltration of local anesthetic agent.
  b. Encourage the patient to refrain from coughing.
	5. Sudden and unexpected movement by the patient can cause trauma to the visceral pleura with resultant trauma to the lung.

(continued)

there is pleural exudate of undetermined etiology and when there is need for pathologic tissue staining or tissue culture for tuberculosis and fungi.

Pulmonary Function Tests

Pulmonary function tests are done to detect abnormalities in respiratory function and to determine the extent of the abnormality. Such tests include measurements of lung volumes, ventilatory function, diffusing capacity, gas exchange, lung compliance, airway resistance, and distribution of gases in the lung.

The newer tests include more sophisticated measurements. Pulmonary function tests are useful in following the course of a patient with established respiratory disease and assessing response to therapy. They are useful as screening tests in potentially hazardous industries, such as coal mining and those that involve exposure to asbestos and other noxious fumes, dusts, or gases. Preoperatively, they are useful for patients scheduled for thoracic and upper abdominal surgery, patients with a history of smoking and cough, obese individuals, persons over 70 years of age, and patients with pulmonary disease.

Chart 23-1
Guidelines for Assisting the Patient Having a Thoracentesis (continued)

Nursing Activities (continued)	**Amplification/Rationale** (continued)
6. Expose the entire chest. The site for aspiration is determined from chest x-rays and by percussion. If fluid is in the pleural cavity, the thoracentesis site is determined by chest x-ray, ultrasound scanning, and physical findings, with attention to site of maximal dullness on percussion.	6. If air is in the pleural cavity, the thoracentesis site is usually in the 2nd or 3rd intercostal space in the midclavicular line. Air rises in the thorax because the density of the air is much less than the density of liquid.
7. The procedure is done under aseptic conditions. After the skin is cleansed, a local anesthetic is injected slowly with a small-caliber needle into the intercostal space by the physician.	7. An intradermal wheal is raised slowly; rapid injection causes pain. The parietal pleura is very sensitive and should be well infiltrated with anesthetic before the thoracentesis needle is passed through it. To minimize intercostal artery laceration, the needle is inserted into the intercostal space just above the lower rib.
8. The physician advances the thoracentesis needle with the syringe attached. When the pleural space is reached, suction may be applied with the syringe.	
a. A 20-ml syringe with a three-way adapter (stopcock) is attached to the needle (one end of the adapter is attached to the needle and the other to the tubing leading to a receptacle that receives the fluid being aspirated).	a. When a large quantity of fluid is withdrawn, a three-way adapter serves to keep air from entering the pleural cavity.
b. If a considerable quantity of fluid is removed, the needle is held in place on the chest wall with a small hemostat.	b. The hemostat steadies the needle on the chest wall. Sudden pleuritic chest pain or shoulder pain may indicate that the visceral or diaphragmatic pleurae are being irritated by the needle point.
9. After the needle is withdrawn, pressure is applied over the puncture site and a small, sterile dressing is fixed in place.	
10. The patient is placed on bed rest. A chest x-ray is usually obtained following thoracentesis.	10. Chest x-ray verifies that there is no pneumothorax.
11. Record the total amount of fluid withdrawn and the nature of the fluid, its color, and its viscosity. If requested, prepare samples of fluid for laboratory evaluation. A small amount of heparin may be needed for several of the specimen containers in order to prevent coagulation. A specimen container with formalin may be needed if a pleural biopsy is to be obtained.	11. The fluid may be clear, serous, bloody, purulent, etc.
12. Evaluate the patient at intervals for increasing respiratory rate; faintness; vertigo; tightness in chest; uncontrollable cough; blood-tinged, frothy mucus; a rapid pulse, and signs of hypoxemia.	12. Pneumothorax, tension pneumothorax, subcutaneous emphysema, or pyogenic infection may result from a thoracentesis. Pulmonary edema or cardiac distress can be produced by a sudden shift in mediastinal contents when large amounts of fluid are aspirated.

Most pulmonary function tests require some type of spirometer that has a volume-collecting device attached to a recorder that demonstrates volume and time simultaneously. Pulmonary function testing is moving in the direction of computerization; some systems have the capabilities of performing over 100 tests. Smaller hospitals, by using a data transmitter, can send test information to a larger medical facility's computer for analysis.

A number of function tests are carried out since no single measurement can be done to evaluate pulmonary function. Usually, test results are interpreted on the basis of degree of deviation from normal, taking into consideration the patient's height, weight, age, and sex. Normal values have been established on nomograms, which are available in manufacturer's handbooks or with pulmonary function equipment.

Since there is a wide range of normal values, pulmonary function tests may not detect early localized changes. The patient with respiratory symptoms (dyspnea, wheezing, cough, sputum production) should undergo a complete diagnostic evaluation, even though the results of pulmonary function tests are "normal."

Pulmonary function testing by telephone is now available for patients living in remote areas who are unable to make the trip to a medical center. Using transmitters, display monitors, and processing and receiving units, a patient may undergo a battery of ventilation measurements and lung volume studies. A respiratory therapist or allied health person helps the patient through the tests at the remote site while a pulmonary specialist interprets the data at a central location. Such a central outreach program is accessible, reduces the patient's travel time and costs, offers the expertise of a pulmonary specialist in communities that do not have this advantage, and provides the patient and local hospital with the best equipment available.

Table 23-1 lists and describes the most frequently used pulmonary function tests.

Arterial Blood Gas Studies

Measurements of blood pH and of arterial oxygen and carbon dioxide tensions are made when managing patients with respiratory problems and in adjusting oxygen therapy as needed. Arterial blood gas studies aid in assessing the degree to which the lungs are able to provide adequate oxygen and remove carbon dioxide, and the degree to which the kidneys are able to reabsorb or excrete bicarbonate ions to maintain normal body pH. Serial blood gas analysis is also a sensitive indicator of whether or not the lung has been damaged following chest trauma. (See p. 482 for a discussion of arterial blood gas measurement and the technique of arterial puncture.)

Radioisotope Diagnostic Procedures (Lung Scan)

A *perfusion lung scan* is done by injecting a radiopharmaceutical (technetium) into a peripheral vein and then taking a scan of the chest and body to detect radiation. The isotope particles pass through the right heart and are distributed into the lungs in amounts proportional to the regional blood flow, making it possible to trace and measure the blood perfusion through the lung. This procedure is used clinically to measure the integrity of the pulmonary vessels relative to blood flow and to evaluate blood flow abnormalities as seen in pulmonary emboli (see p. 337). Inform the patient that the imaging time is 20 to 40 minutes, that he will lie under the camera, and that a mask will be fitted over his nose and mouth during the test.

A *ventilation scan* is done after the perfusion scan. The patient takes a deep breath of a mixture of oxygen and radioactive gas (xenon; krypton), which diffuses throughout the lungs. A scan is done to detect ventilation abnormalities, especially in patients who have regional differences in ventilation (*e.g.,* emphysema).

Table 23-1
Ventilatory Function Tests

Description	Term Used	Symbol	Remarks
The maximum volume of air exhaled from the point of maximum inspiration	Vital capacity	VC	Slow vital capacity may be normal or reduced in COPD* patients.
Vital capacity performed with a maximally forced expiratory effort	Forced vital capacity	FVC	Forced vital capacity is often reduced in COPD owing to air trapping.
Volume of air exhaled in the specified time during the performance of forced vital capacity	Forced expiratory volume (qualified by subscript indicating the time interval in seconds)	FEV_t, usually FEV_1	A valuable clue to the severity of the expiratory airway obstruction.
FEV_t expressed as a percentage of the forced vital capacity	Ratio of timed forced expiratory volume to forced vital capacity	$FEV_t/FVC\%$, usually $FEV_1/FVC\%$	Another way of expressing the presence or absence of airway obstruction.
Mean forced expiratory flow between 200 ml and 1200 ml of the FVC	Forced expiratory flow	$FEF_{200-1200}$	Formerly called maximum expiratory flow rate (MEFR). An indicator of large airway obstruction.
Mean forced expiratory flow during the middle half of the FVC	Forced mid-expiratory flow	$FEF_{25\%-75\%}$	Formerly called maximum and mid-expiratory flow rate. Slowed in small airway obstruction.
Mean forced expiratory flow during the terminal portion of the FVC	Forced end-expiratory flow	$FEF_{75\%-85\%}$	Slowed in obstruction of smallest airways.
Volume of air expired in a specified period during repetitive maximal effort	Maximal voluntary ventilation	MVV	Formerly called maximum breathing capacity. An important factor in exercise tolerance.

* Chronic obstructive pulmonary disease.
(From American Lung Association: Chronic Obstructive Pulmonary Disease, 5th ed. New York, 1981.)

The *gallium scan* is a radioisotope lung scan used to detect inflammatory conditions of the lungs.

Lung Biopsy Procedures

When the chest x-ray is inconclusive or reveals pulmonary density (indicating an infiltrate; lesion), it is desirable to examine lung tissue to establish the nature of the lesion. There are several nonoperative lung biopsy techniques that are being used because they yield accurate information with low morbidity: (1) transcatheter bronchial brushing, (2) percutaneous (through the skin) needle biopsy, or (3) transbronchial lung biopsy.

In *transcatheter bronchial brushing* a fiberoptic bronchoscope is introduced into the bronchus under fluoroscopic monitoring. A small brush is attached to the end of a flexible wire, which is inserted through the fiberscope. Under the direct vision, the area under suspicion is brushed back and forth, causing cells to slough off and adhere to the brush. The catheter may be irrigated with saline to secure material for additional studies. The brush is removed from the bronchoscope and a microscopic slide is made. Sometimes the brush is cut off and sent to the laboratory for pathologic tests.

This procedure is useful for cytologic evaluations of lung lesions and for the identification of pathogenic organisms (*Nocardia, Aspergillus, Pneumocystis carinii,* and other pathogens). It is especially useful in the immunologically compromised patient.

Nursing support for this procedure includes reinforcing the patient's understanding and seeing that the consent form has been signed. Following the procedure, the patient may have a mild sore throat and transient hemoptysis. Fluids and food are withheld for several hours following the procedure. Possible complications include anesthetic reactions, laryngospasm, hemoptysis, and rarely, pneumothorax.

Another method of bronchial brushing involves the introduction of the catheter through the transcricothyroid membrane by needle puncture. Following this procedure the patient is instructed to hold his thumb over the puncture site while coughing to prevent air from leaking into the surrounding tissues.

Percutaneous needle biopsy may be accomplished with a cutting needle or by aspiration with a spinal-type needle that provides a tissue specimen for histologic study. A *transbronchial lung biopsy* uses cutting forceps introduced by fiberoptic bronchoscope. This study is indicated when a lung lesion is suspected and routine sputum samples and bronchoscopic washings are negative.

Meperidine may be given before the procedure. The skin over the biopsy site is cleansed and anesthetized, and a small incision is made. The biopsy needle is inserted through the skin into the pleura while the patient holds his breath in midexpiration. Under fluoroscopic monitoring, the needle is guided into the periphery of the lesion and the mass is biopsied. Possible complications include pneumothorax, pulmonary hemorrhage, and empyema.

Lymph Node Biopsy

The scalene lymph nodes are enmeshed in the deep cervical pad of fat overlying the scalenus anterior muscle. They drain the lungs and mediastinum and may show histologic changes owing to intrathoracic disease. When these nodes are palpable on physical examination, a biopsy may be in order. A biopsy of these nodes may be done to detect lymph node spread of pulmonary disease and to establish a diagnosis or prognosis in such diseases as Hodgkin's disease, sarcoidosis, fungal disease, tuberculosis, and carcinoma.

Mediastinoscopy is the endoscopic examination of the mediastinum for exploration and biopsy of mediastinal lymph nodes that drain the lungs, without requiring a thoracotomy. Biopsy is usually done through a suprasternal incision. Mediastinoscopy is carried out to detect mediastinal involvement of pulmonary malignancy and to obtain tissue for diagnostic studies of other conditions (*e.g.,* sarcoidosis).

An *anterior mediastinotomy* is thought to provide better exposure and diagnostic possibilities than a mediastinoscopy. An incision is made in the area of the 2nd or 3rd costal cartilage. The mediastinum is explored, and biopsies are done on any lymph nodes found. Chest tube drainage is required after the procedure. This diagnostic modality is particularly valuable to determine whether or not a pulmonary lesion is resectable.

▷ Assessment of Respiratory Symptoms

The major symptoms of respiratory disease are cough, sputum production, chest pain, hemoptysis, wheezing, and dyspnea. The constitutional symptoms of bronchopulmonary disease are anorexia, fever, weight loss, fatigue, malaise, weakness, and sweating. These clinical manifestations are related to the duration and severity of the disease. When data on patients with these symptoms are collected, analyzed, and interpreted, it is important to determine body location, quality, quantity, chronology, and factors aggravating or alleviating the problem.

Cough

Cough results from irritation of the mucous membranes anywhere in the respiratory tract. The stimulus producing a cough may arise from an infectious process or from an airborne irritant, such as smoke, smog, dust, or a gas. "The cough reflex is the watchdog of the lungs" and is the patient's chief protection against the accumulation of secretions in the bronchi and bronchioles.

On the other hand, the presence of cough may indicate serious pulmonary disease. Of equal importance is the type of cough. A dry, irritative cough is characteristic of upper respiratory infection of viral etiology. Laryngotracheitis causes an irritative, high-pitched cough. Tracheal lesions produce a brassy cough. An acute dry cough often occurs in the early stages of virus infections that involve both upper and lower respiratory tracts. A severe or *changing* cough may indicate bronchogenic carcinoma. Pleuritic chest pain accompanying coughing may indicate pleural or chest wall (musculoskeletal) involvement.

Nursing Assessment. Evaluate the character of the cough. Is it dry? hacking? brassy? wheezing? loose? severe?

Note the time of coughing. Coughing at night may herald the onset of left-sided heart failure or bronchial asthma. A cough in the morning with sputum production is indicative of bronchitis. A cough that worsens when the patient is supine may indicate a postnasal drip (sinusitis). Coughing after food intake may indicate aspirated material in the tracheobronchial tree. A cough of recent onset is usually from an acute infectious process.

Sputum Production

A patient who coughs long enough will almost invariably produce sputum. Violent coughing results in bronchial spasm, obstruction, and further irritation of the bronchi and may result in syncope. A severe, repeated, or uncontrolled cough that is nonproductive is potentially harmful. Sputum production is the reaction of the lungs to any constantly recurring irritant. It may also be associated with a nasal discharge. If there is a profuse amount of purulent sputum (thick yellow or green) or a change in color of the sputum, the patient probably has a bacterial infection. Rusty sputum indicates the presence of bacterial pneumonia, if the patient has not received antibiotics. A thin, mucoid sputum frequently results from viral bronchitis. A gradual increase of sputum over a period of time may reveal the presence of chronic bronchitis or bronchiectasis. Pink-tinged mucoid sputum is suggestive of a lung tumor, whereas profuse, frothy, pink material, often welling up into the throat, may indicate pulmonary edema. Malodorous sputum and bad breath point to the presence of lung abscess, bronchiectasis, or an infection caused by fusospirochetal or other anaerobic organisms.

Nursing Management. If the sputum is too thick to raise, it is necessary to decrease its viscosity by increasing its water content through adequate hydration (drinking water) and inhalation of aerosolized solutions. These may be delivered via any type of nebulizer. Methods of assisting the patient to cough productively are discussed on page 461.

Smoking is definitely contraindicated since it interferes with ciliary action, increases bronchial secretions, causes inflammation and hyperplasia of the mucous membranes, and reduces production of surfactant. Thus, bronchial drainage is impaired. If smoking is stopped, sputum volume will decrease and resistance to bronchial infections will improve.

The patient's appetite may be depressed because of the odor of the sputum and the taste it leaves in the mouth. Adequate mouth hygiene, proper environment, and wise selection of food will stimulate appetite. After the patient's mouth is carefully cleansed and rinsed, sputum cups and emesis basins should be removed before the next meal arrives. Serving citrus juices at the beginning of the meal will make the mouth feel better and will help to make the patient more receptive to the rest of the meal.

Dyspnea

Dyspnea (difficult or labored breathing) is a symptom common to many pulmonary and heart conditions, particularly when there is increased lung rigidity and airway resistance.

The right ventricle of the heart will ultimately be affected by lung disease since it must pump blood through the lungs. Sudden dyspnea in a healthy person may indicate pneumothorax (air in the pleural cavity). Sudden shortness of breath in an ill or postoperative patient may denote pulmonary embolism. Orthopnea (inability to breathe except in an upright position) is characteristic of cardiogenic pulmonary congestion. Shortness of breath with an expiratory wheeze is seen in chronic obstructive pulmonary disease (asthma, bronchitis, emphysema). Noisy breathing may result from a narrowing of the airway or localized obstruction of a major bronchus by a tumor or foreign body. The presence of both inspiratory and expiratory wheezing usually signifies asthma, if the patient is not in congestive heart failure. Shortness of breath is quite commonly related to tension and anxiety. In general, the acute diseases of the lungs produce a more severe grade of dyspnea than do the chronic diseases.

Nursing Assessment. Determine the circumstances that produce the patient's dyspnea. How much exertion triggers shortness of breath? Is there an associated cough? Is dyspnea related to other symptoms? What was the mode of onset: sudden or gradual? At what time of day or night is it obvious? Is it worse when the patient is flat in bed? Does it occur at rest? with exercise? walking (how far?)? climbing stairs? running?

The treatment of dyspnea depends on the success with which its cause can be alleviated. Relief of the symptom is sometimes achieved by placing the patient at rest with his head elevated and, in severe cases, by administering oxygen.

Chest Pain

Chest pain associated with pulmonary conditions may be sharp, stabbing, and intermittent, or dull, aching, and persistent. The pain usually is felt on the side where the pathology is located, but it may be referred elsewhere, for example, to the neck, the back, or the abdomen. Chest pain is experienced by many patients with pneumonia, pulmonary embolism with lung infarction, and pleurisy and is a late symptom of bronchogenic carcinoma. In carcinoma the pain may be dull and persistent because of invasion into the chest wall, mediastinum, or spine.

Lung disease does not always produce thoracic pain since the lungs and the visceral pleural covering lack sensory nerves and are insensitive to pain stimuli. But the parietal pleura has a rich supply of sensory nerves that are stimulated by inflammation and stretching of the membrane. Pleuritic pain owing to irritation of the parietal pleura is sharp and seems to "catch" on inspiration; patients say it is "like the stabbing of a knife." They are more comfortable when they lie on the affected side, a posture that tends to "splint" the chest wall, restrict the expansions and contractions of the lung, and reduce the friction between the injured or diseased pleurae on that side. Pain associated with cough may be lessened by manual splinting of the rib cage, as is illustrated in Figure 24-5 (p. 463).

Nursing Assessment. Assess the quality, intensity, and radiation of pain. Look for factors that precipitate it. Determine whether there is a relationship between pain and the patient's posture. Also, evaluate the inspiratory and expiratory phase of respiration and its effect on pain. (See guidelines, pages 552–553.)

Analgesic medications are effective in relieving chest pain, but care must be taken not to depress the respiratory center or a productive cough. For relief of extreme pain, a regional anesthetic block may be done by injecting procaine along the intercostal nerves that supply the painful area.

Hemoptysis

Hemoptysis (expectoration of blood from the respiratory tract) is a symptom of pulmonary or cardiac disorders. It varies from blood-stained sputum to a large, sudden hemorrhage and always merits investigation. The most common causes are (1) pulmonary infection (bronchitis, bronchiectasis, tuberculosis), (2) carcinoma of the lung, (3) abnormalities of the heart or blood vessels, (4) pulmonary artery–vein abnormalities, and (5) pulmonary emboli and infarction. The onset of hemoptysis is usually sudden and may be intermittent or continuous. Several investigations are usually done to determine the cause: blood examination, chest angiography, chest x-ray, and bronchoscopy. A careful history and physical examination are necessary to establish a diagnosis of the underlying disease, irrespective of whether the bleeding produced a fleck of blood in the sputum or a massive hemorrhage. The amount of blood produced is not necessarily in positive correlation with the seriousness of the cause.

Nursing Assessment. Determine first where the blood is coming from. Has it come from the gums, nasopharynx, lungs, or stomach? The nurse may be the only witness to the episode. The following points should be borne in mind in making and recording observations. In patients whose bloody sputum originates from the nose or the nasopharynx, expectoration is usually preceded by considerable sniffing, and blood may appear in the nares. Blood from the lung is usually bright red, frothy, and mixed with sputum. Initial symptoms include a tickling sensation in the throat, a salty taste, a burning or bubbling sensation in the chest, and perhaps chest pain, in which case the patient tends to splint the bleeding side. The term *hemoptysis* is reserved for the coughing of blood arising from a pulmonary hemorrhage. This blood has an alkaline *p*H (greater than 7.0).

In contrast, if the hemorrhage is in the stomach, the blood is vomited (*hematemesis*) rather than coughed up. Blood that has been in contact with gastric juice is sometimes so dark that it is referred to as "coffee-ground" material. This blood has an acid *p*H (less than 7.0).

Management. A patient who has experienced a hemoptysis, whatever its cause, should be placed immediately at complete bed rest. He should be placed on his affected side (if known) to minimize aspiration into the uninvolved lung. The patient is given the prescribed sedative for relief of anxiety. He may need to cough up blood that has accumulated in his dependent lung, but severe coughing is controlled with medication. Since hemoptysis is one of the most frightening of all symptoms, the nurse should spend time

with the patient, giving him support and confidence. A calm approach is the first step of therapy.

If there is a sudden increase in bleeding, endotracheal intubation is carried out quickly to control the airway, as death may occur from airway obstruction. Equipment for performing an immediate laryngoscopy and bronchoscopy should be in readiness for the removal of blood clots and identification of the bleeding site. If the patient shows the initial signs of asphyxia, a balloon embolectomy catheter may be placed in the bronchus and the balloon inflated to occlude the bleeding site. Surgical intervention may eventually become necessary. Vital signs are supported with intravenous fluids, blood transfusions, and supplemental oxygen.

Clubbing of the Fingers

Clubbing of the fingers as a sign of lung disease is found in patients with chronic hypoxic conditions, chronic lung infections (bronchiectasis), and malignancies of the lung. This finding may be initially manifested as sponginess of the nailbed and loss of the nailbed angle. (See p. 57 for assessment.)

Collection of Fluid and Air in the Pleural Cavity

Hydrothorax is a collection of watery fluid in the pleural cavity (pleural effusion), which may occur in such conditions as cardiac or renal failure, hepatic or pancreatic disease, lung and pleural tumors, etc. The presence of fluid may cause respiratory difficulties and require aspiration (thoracentesis). (See p. 514 for the management of pleural effusion.)

Pneumothorax (air in the pleural cavity) may occur spontaneously from rupture of a lung bleb or bulla (see below); it may occur after thoracentesis, pleural biopsy, or percutaneous needle biopsy. It may be secondary to infection or result from high positive end-expiratory pressure of a ventilator. Or it may arise from trauma, the air entering the pleural cavity through a resulting wound, or from the injured lung.

Hemothorax (blood in the pleural cavity) also accompanies chest trauma. Aspiration of the air and blood permits reexpansion of the lung and a return to a more physiologic state. (Pneumothorax and hemothorax owing to chest injuries are discussed on p. 539.)

Spontaneous pneumothorax is the spontaneous appearance of air in the pleural cavity as a result of rupture of the visceral pleura or of emphysematous blebs or bullae. It may occur in healthy adolescents and young adults without pulmonary disease as well as in older persons with chronic pulmonary disease. The patient complains of sudden chest pain and mild to severe dyspnea.

Treatment depends on the etiology of the pneumothorax and on its size and duration. If the pneumothorax is small and the patient is relatively asymptomatic, no intervention is required. However, a larger area will require that the air be removed via thoracentesis. If a significant air leak occurs, it may be necessary to insert into the pleural cavity a chest catheter that is attached to some type of drainage system. Occasionally, a thoracotomy and pleural abrasion are indicated in selected cases of spontaneous pneumothorax, especially for a recurrent condition. Recurrence is a problem with spontaneous pneumothorax and may affect either side of the chest.

In some instances of spontaneous pneumothorax, it is possible to treat the patient on an outpatient basis by means of an intercostal drainage tube and a flutter valve. A No. 16 French catheter or No. 12 Argyle chest tube is inserted into the 2nd intercostal space anteriorly for men and in the 5th intercostal space for women (for cosmetic reasons). The chest catheter may be attached to underwater drainage temporarily and the patient is observed for a few hours. A chest x-ray is obtained. If the lung shows adequate reexpansion, the underwater drainage is discontinued and a disposable flutter valve (Heimlich) is connected to the chest tube. The valve permits the pleural cavity to be drained without suction (Fig. 23-6). Immediate ambulation is possible, and the patient is permitted to return home. The patient is encouraged to cough and to perform the Valsalva maneuver (exhale forcibly against the closed glottis), which will increase intrathoracic pressure and aid in the expulsion of air. As soon as the lung expansion is complete, the chest tube is removed (3–4 days) and the patient is encouraged to return to normal activity. This type of treatment offers a substantial savings in cost.

Chylothorax

Chylothorax is the presence of chyle in the pleural cavity. (Chyle, a milky fluid consisting of lymph and emulsified fat, is absorbed from food following digestion and enters the venous system via the thoracic duct.)

Chylothorax may occur as a result of malignancies of the lung and mediastinum or may follow blunt or penetrating chest trauma. There are even instances on record of chylothorax occurring as a result of yawning or stretching. Thoracic surgical procedures may also cause chylous pleural effusions. (The thoracic duct is vulnerable to traumatic injury during surgical procedures on the heart and great vessels and resection of the left lung, since it crosses to the left of the spine between the 5th and 7th thoracic vertebrae). Usually, symptoms occur after a relatively large amount of chyle collects intrapleurally and causes dyspnea. The roent-

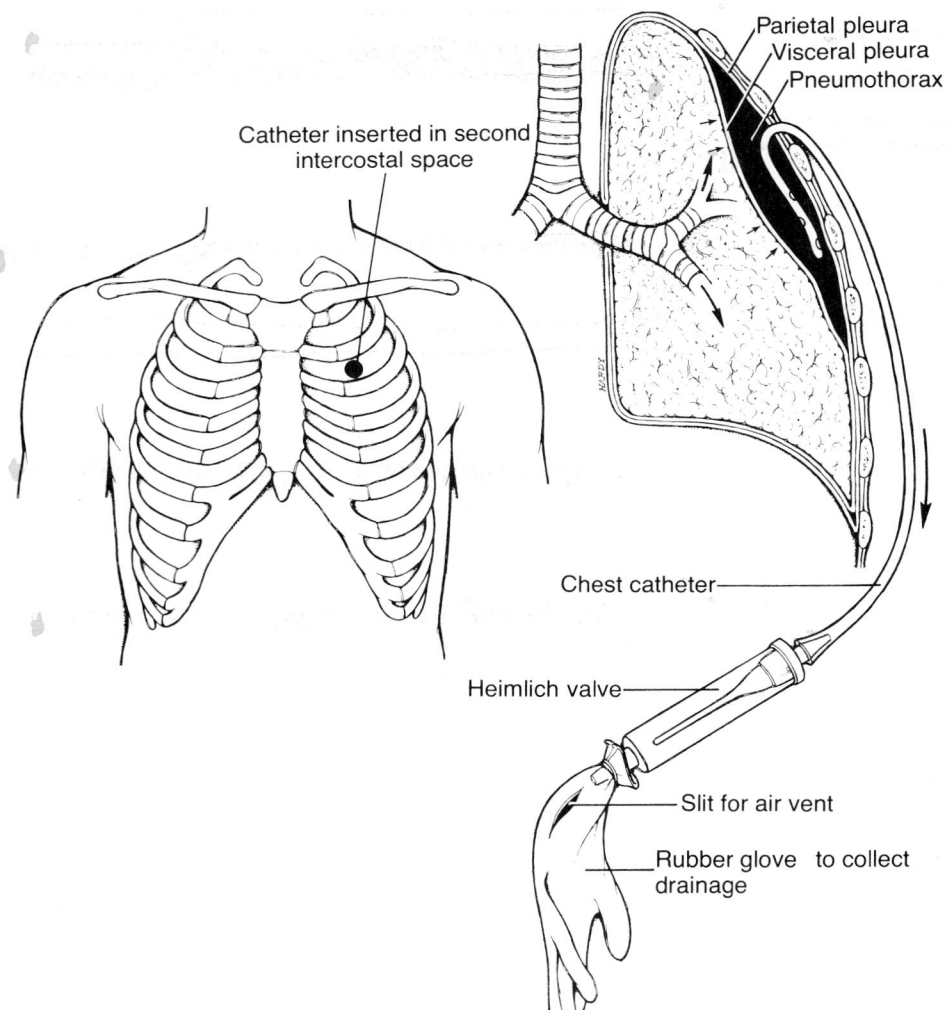

Figure 23-6. Ambulatory treatment of spontaneous pneumothorax.

genographic and clinical findings are similar to those of pleural effusion. A definite diagnosis is made when milky, white fluid is removed either by thoracentesis or tube thoracostomy.

The objectives of therapy are to reduce chyle formation and reexpand the lung. Reduction of lymph flow is achieved by reducing the patient's activities and maintaining him on intravenous hyperalimentation to decrease the volume of chyle. Pulmonary reexpansion is achieved by repeated thoracenteses or closed tube thoracostomy.

Atelectasis

Atelectasis refers to the collapse of a lobule or larger lung unit (Fig. 23-7). It may be caused by obstruction of a bronchus, the effect of which is to impede the passage of air to and from the alveoli communicating with it. The alveolar air thus trapped soon becomes absorbed into the bloodstream, and, all external communication having been blocked, its replacement from the outside air is impossible. The net result is that the portion of lung so isolated becomes airless: it shrinks in size, causing the remainder of the lung to overexpand (compensatory emphysema). Bronchial obstruction capable of causing atelectasis may follow inhalation of a foregn body. It may result from a plug of thick exudate that is not, or cannot be, expelled by coughing. Also, the supine position, splinting of respiratory function owing to pain, respiratory depression from narcotics and relaxants, and abdominal distention increase the potential of airway closure.

- Atelectasis owing to bronchial obstruction by secretions is the usual mechanism producing the "massive collapse" occasionally observed postoperatively and in debilitated bedridden patients.

In these people there is likely to be long, continued respiratory depression, together with inadequate depth of respiratory excursion and perhaps unusually profuse or poorly expectorated bronchial secretions. Tumors of the bronchi often make their presence known first by an atelectasis resulting from their obstructive growth.

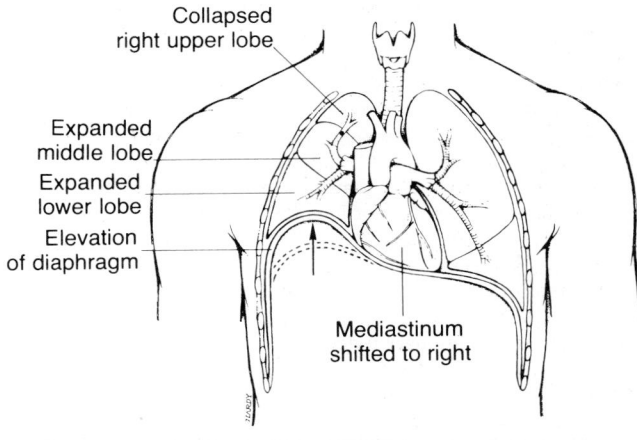

Collapsed right upper lobe

Expanded middle lobe

Expanded lower lobe

Elevation of diaphragm

Mediastinum shifted to right

Figure 23-7. Atelectasis. (Also see Fig. 21-16, p. 410.)

Atelectasis may result from pressure on the lung tissue, which restricts normal lung expansion on inspiration. Such pressure may be produced by a variety of causes: fluid accumulation within the thorax (pleural effusion), air in the pleural space (pneumothorax), an extremely large heart, a pericardium distended with fluid (pericardial effusion), tumor growth within the thorax, or an elevated diaphragm that is displaced upward as the result of abdominal pressure. Under such circumstances there is crowding of the intrathoracic contents, and since the spongy lung tissue is most compressible, the lung collapses without resistance. Where it is compressed it becomes airless, or atelectatic, and the efficiency of pulmonary function is reduced accordingly.

- Atelectasis caused by pressure is encountered most often in patients with pleural effusion owing to cardiac failure, or pleural infection.

Assessment and Clinical Manifestations. If collapse occurs suddenly, and if sufficient lung tissue is involved, the following may be anticipated: marked dyspnea, cyanosis, prostration, and pleural pain, which usually is referred to the lower chest. Fever commonly occurs. Tachycardia and dyspnea are unusually prominent. The patient characteristically sits bolt upright in bed, appears anxious and cyanotic, and has difficulty in breathing. The chest wall on the affected side moves little, if at all, whereas on the opposite side the excursion appears excessive. Lungs that have collapsed because of the obstruction of a bronchus should be reexpanded as rapidly as possible to avoid the common complications of pneumonia or lung abscess.

Management and Nursing Interventions. The goal is to improve ventilation and remove secretions. If atelectasis has resulted from a pleural effusion or pressure pneumothorax, the fluid or air may be removed by needle aspiration. If bronchial obstruction is the cause, it must be removed in order to permit air to enter the lung again. Methods to accomplish this include aspirating secretions, encouraging the patient to cough, and using an aerosol ultrasonic nebulizer, followed by postural drainage and chest percussion. The patient should be turned frequently in an effort to stimulate coughing. If possible, he should be assisted out of bed and walked to assist in mobilizing and in expelling secretions. If these methods fail to remove the obstruction, a bronchoscopy is done. It may be necessary to use endotracheal intubation and mechanical ventilation for a few days.

Prevention. All stuporous, debilitated, and sedated patients should be turned frequently in bed, a procedure that affords increased respiratory excursion on the uppermost side. Encouragement of coughing and deep breathing (at least every 2 hours) is important in preventing and treating atelectasis. The use of incentive spirometry or voluntary deep breathing enhances large-volume inhalation; this emphasis on inspiration is necessary to decrease the potential for airway closure. Judicious use of nasopharyngeal and nasotracheal suction is also helpful in stimulating patients to cough, thereby removing tenacious secretions. (See p. 409 for a discussion of postoperative atelectasis.)

▷ ## Self-care and Prevention of Respiratory Disease

Cigarette smoking; exposure to environmental air pollution; occupational exposure to dust, fumes, and gases; and respiratory tract infections play a role in the development of respiratory disease.

Cigarette smoking is the most important risk factor for diseases of the lung, especially lung cancer, emphysema, and chronic bronchitis. According to the Surgeon General's Report entitled "The Health Consequences of Smoking" (1982), cigarette smokers have overall mortality rates substantially greater than those of nonsmokers. The lighted cigarette generates about 4000 compounds that can be separated into gas and particulate phases. Carbon monoxide (the gas phase), nicotine, and tar (the particulate phase) are the most likely contributors to the health hazards of smoking. It is generally accepted that most cases of bronchogenic carcinoma are attributable to inhalation of carcinogenic pollutants (smoke, environmental toxins) by a susceptible host. The inhalation of cigarette smoke impairs alveolar macrophage function and reduces ciliary action. This results in a reduction in the tracheobronchial mucociliary clearance—the mechanism that normally removes particles from the respiratory tract. Inhalation of cigarette smoke also produces an increase in airway resistance.

There appear to be negative health effects from "passive smoking"—the inhalation by the nonsmoker of fumes from nearby cigarettes, pipes, and cigars. Passive smoking may be hazardous to persons allergic to tobacco smoke or with respiratory disease. In addition, an estimated 2 million Americans are sensitive to tobacco smoke and suffer smoke-caused asthma attacks. Research also indicates that respiratory illness is twice as common in young children whose parents smoke at home as it is in children with nonsmoking parents.

Air pollution presents its own hazard to health. The air may be polluted by hundreds of substances, but in the United States the five "criteria pollutants" that are generally monitored are carbon monoxide (CO); sulfur dioxide (SO_2); total suspended particulate (TSP); ozone, or photochemical oxidants (O_3); and nitrogen dioxide (NO_2). The major pollution problems are from air pollutants emitted from motor vehicles and heat or power generators. When the air is significantly polluted, it is known to increase morbidity and mortality in patients with chronic pulmonary disease.

Exposure to environmental toxic factors (industrial asbestos and agricultural chemicals) may lead to significant respiratory impairment. The pneumoconioses are almost entirely preventable by the maintenance of a safe working environment. The risk of developing occupational lung disease is increased by smoking.

Acute illnesses in early childhood may be associated with an increased frequency of cough and chronic pulmonary disease in early adult life. Also, children with asthma may bring to adulthood a slightly impaired respiratory function, which worsens if they smoke.

The preservation of pulmonary function and the prevention of respiratory disease can best be accomplished by the total elimination of smoking, maintenance of clean environmental air, and prompt treatment of respiratory tract infection.

▷ ## Bibliography

Books

Crompton GK. Diagnosis and Management of Respiratory Diseases. Oxford, Blackwell Scientific Publications, 1980.

Cumming G and Semple SJ. Disorders of the Respiratory System. Oxford, Blackwell Scientific Publications, 1980.

Fishman AP. Assessment of Pulmonary Function. New York, McGraw-Hill, 1980.

Flenley DC. Respiratory Medicine. New York, Macmillan, 1981.

Guenter CA and Welch MH (eds). Pulmonary Medicine, 2nd ed. Philadelphia, JB Lippincott, 1982.

Harper RW. A Guide to Respiratory Care. Philadelphia, JB Lippincott, 1981.

Hunsinger DL et al. Respiratory Technology Procedure and Equipment Manual. Reston, Reston Publishing, 1980.

Kiss GT. Diagnosis and Management of Pulmonary Disease in Primary Practice. Menlo Park, Addison-Wesley, 1982.

Kryger MH. Pathophysiology of Respiration. New York, John Wiley & Sons, 1981.

Manini JJ. Respiratory Medicine and Intensive Care for the House Officer. Baltimore, Williams & Wilkins, 1981.

Putman C. Diagnostic Imaging in Pulmonary Disease. New York, Appleton-Century-Crofts, 1981.

Rarey KP and Youtsey JW. Respiratory Patient Care. Englewood Cliffs, New Jersey, Prentice-Hall, 1981.

Sproule BJ, Lynne-Davies P, and King EG. Fundamentals of Respiratory Disease. New York, Churchill Livingstone, 1981.

Traver GA (ed). Respiratory Nursing. New York, John Wiley & Sons, 1982.

Williams MH. Essentials of Pulmonary Medicine. Philadelphia, WB Saunders, 1982.

Articles

Cannon WB, Mark JBD, and Jamplis RW. Pneumothorax: A therapeutic update. Am J Surg 1981 July; 142(1):26–29.

Chalon J et al. Routine cytodiagnosis of pulmonary malignancies. Arch Pathol Lab Med 1981 Jan; 105(1):11–14.

Chusid EL. Diagnostic procedures in bronchopulmonary disease. Hosp Pract 1981 July; 16(7):99–108.

Ferris EJ. Pulmonary hemorrhage. Chest 1981 Dec; 80(6):710–714.

Hollen EM, Toomey IV, and Given S. Bronchoscopy. Nursing '82 1982 June; 12(6):120–122.

Husband J. Diagnostic techniques: Their strengths and weaknesses. Br J Cancer 1980 Apr; 41(Suppl 4):21–29.

Lipscomb DJ, Flower CDR, and Hadfield JW. Ultrasound of the pleura: An assessment of its clinical value. Clin Radiol 1981 May; 32(3):289–290.

Mackenzie JW. Diagnostic thoracoscopy. In Sabiston DC Jr. Davis-Christopher Textbook of Surgery, pp. 2056–2059. WB Saunders, 1981.

Messenger MA. Pulmonary function tests. The telephone connection. Respir Ther 1982 Jan-Feb; 12(1):27–29.

Milhorn HT Jr. Understanding arterial blood gases. Am Fam Physician 1980 Mar; 21(3):112–120.

Proto AV et al. The chest radiologic workup—special studies. Basics of RD 1980 Sept; 9(1):1–6.

Sahn SA. Pleural manifestations of pulmonary disease. Hosp Pract 1981 Mar; 16(3):73–89.

Schechler DC and Acinapura AJ. Pulmonary diagnostic invasive procedures. Part II. NY State J Med 1980 Oct; 80(11):1702–1711.

Share BL and Stehlin CS. What those breath sounds are telling you to do. RN 1981 Dec; 44(12):48–49.

Siegelman SS et al. CT of the solitary pulmonary nodule. AJR 1980 July; 135(1):1–13.

Steiger Z, Chaudhry S, and Wilson RF. The use of anterior mediastinotomy to assess intrathoracic lesions. Am Surg 1981 June; 47(6):251–253.

Stevens RP, Lillington GA, and Parsons GH. Fiberoptic bronchoscopy in the intensive care unit. Heart Lung 1981 Nov–Dec; 10(6):1037–1045.

Toben BP and Kelly JJ. Flexible fiberoptic bronchoscopy. Respir Ther 1981 May–June; 11(3):73–78.

Agencies
Governmental

National Heart, Lung and Blood Institute, National Institutes of Health, Bethesda, Maryland 20205

Voluntary

American Association for Respiratory Therapy, 7411 Hines Place, Suite 101, Dallas, Texas 75235

American Lung Association, 1740 Broadway, New York, New York 10019

American Thoracic Society, 1740 Broadway, New York, New York 10019

24

Management of Patients With Impaired Respiratory Function

▷ Special Management in Respiratory Conditions

A wide variety of treatment modalities can be used in caring for patients with different types of respiratory conditions. The most common modalities include oxygen therapy; nebulizer therapy; hyperinflation maneuvers; and chest physical therapy, such as postural drainage, percussion and vibration, breathing exercises, and physical conditioning. Other respiratory treatment modalities are discussed in Chapter 25.

Oxygen Therapy

Oxygen therapy is the administration of oxygen at a concentration of pressure greater than that found in the environmental atmosphere. It is particularly useful in the treatment of hypoxemic states that result in inadequate transport of oxygen by the blood. The goal in oxygen therapy is to treat the hypoxemia while decreasing the work of breathing and the stress on the myocardium. Oxygen transport to the tissues depends on many factors: cardiac output, arterial oxygen content, adequate concentration of hemoglobin, and metabolic requirements. All of these must be considered when oxygen therapy is contemplated. (Respiratory physiology and oxygen transport are discussed in Chapter 23.)

Patient Assessment. A change in the patient's respiration is often evidence of the need for oxygen therapy. Other clinical signs of hypoxemia include changes in mental status (progressing through impaired judgment, agitation, confusion, obtundity, coma), dyspnea, increase in blood pressure, changes in heart rate, arrhythmias, cyanosis (late), and cool extremities. Cyanosis is not considered to be an adequate clinical guide to hypoxia, as it is seen only with severe hypoxemia. It may not be seen if the patient is anemic or if cyanosis is due to superficial peripheral vasoconstriction.

The signs and symptoms of oxygen need may depend on how suddenly this need develops. With rapidly developing hypoxia there are changes in the central nervous system since the higher centers are more sensitive to oxygen deprivation. The clinical picture may resemble that of drunkenness, the patient exhibiting similar signs of incoordination and impaired judgment. Longstanding hypoxia (as seen in chronic obstructive pulmonary disease and chronic congestive heart failure) may produce fatigue, drowsiness, apathy, inattentiveness, and delayed reaction time. The need for oxygen is assessed by arterial blood gas analysis (p. 482) as well as by clinical evaluation.

Precautions. Excessive oxygen may produce toxic effects on the lungs and central nervous system or result in depression of ventilation in certain conditions, namely chronic obstructive pulmonary disease (pp. 519–527). In these patients the stimulus for respiration is a decrease in blood oxygen rather than an elevation in carbon dioxide levels. Thus, sudden administration of a high concentration of oxygen will remove the respiratory drive that has been created largely by the patient's chronic low oxygen tension. This can cause a progressive increase in arterial PCO_2, ultimately leading to death from carbon dioxide narcosis (see pp. 486–488). Therefore, oxygen should be administered with care and its effects on each patient should be carefully assessed.

As a general rule, with pulmonary patients, oxygen therapy should only be given to raise the arterial PO_2 to 60 mm Hg. At this level the blood is 80% to 90% saturated, and higher PO_2 values will not add further significant amounts of oxygen to the red cells or plasma. Instead of helping, increased amounts of oxygen may possibly suppress ventilation.

With the use of oxygen, by any method, the patient should be assessed frequently for signs of oxygen need: mental aberration, disturbed consciousness, abnormal color, perspiration, changes in blood pressure, and increasing heart and respiratory rates.

Other precautions to be taken with oxygen involve the careful handling of oxygen equipment. Since oxygen supports combustion, there is always danger of fire when oxygen is used. Thus, "No Smoking" signs must be posted when oxygen is in use. It is also important to realize that the oxygen therapy equipment is a potential source of bacterial cross infection. Thus, the breathing circuits should be changed and sterilized daily.

Methods of Oxygen Administration

Oxygen is dispensed from a cylinder or from a piped-in system. A reduction gauge is necessary to reduce the pressure to a working level, and a flow meter regulates the control of oxygen in liters per minute. Oxygen is moistened by passing it through a humidification system to prevent the mucous membranes of the respiratory tree from becoming dry.

Oxygen may be administered by a variety of means: nasal cannula (or prongs), oropharyngeal catheter, and various types of face masks. It may also be applied directly to the endotracheal or tracheal tube via a T-piece or hyper-inflation bag. The method selected depends on the concentration of oxygen required. The appropriate form of oxygen therapy is best determined after obtaining arterial blood gases, which will indicate the patient's oxygenation status and acid–base balance.

The *nasal cannula* is used when the patient requires a low-to-medium concentration of oxygen for which precise accuracy is not essential. This method is relatively simple to use and allows the patient to move about in bed, talk, cough, and eat without interruption of oxygen flow. Flow rates in excess of 6 liters per minute may lead to air swallowing and may cause irritation to the nasal and pharyngeal mucosa.

The *oropharyngeal catheter* is employed for short-term use to administer moderate to moderately high concentrations of oxygen. To insert the catheter, measure the distance from the external nares to the tip of the ear lobe. Lubricate the catheter with a water-soluble lubricant and pass it through the nose into the oropharynx. Look into the oropharynx (using a tongue depressor and flashlight) to check on the position of the catheter. Pull the catheter back slightly until the tip is not visible. It should not extend beyond the uvula in order to prevent gastric distention. Be sure the patient is not coughing, gagging, or swallowing air during this procedure. Secure the catheter to the bridge of the nose or face with hypoallergenic tape. Change the catheter every 8 to 12 hours and place it in alternate nostrils to prevent catheter encrustation and ulceration of the nasal mucosa. This method of oxygen administration can lead to discomfort and irritation of the nasal mucosa and is rarely used. When nasal oxygen is administered (either by cannula or oropharyngeal catheter), the percentage of oxygen reaching the lungs varies with the depth and rate of respiration.

A *face mask* is used when high concentrations of oxygen are required in the acute phase of certain diseases. A rebreathing bag permits the patient to inhale a high concentration of oxygen from a reservoir bag. Perforations on both sides of the mask serve as exhalation ports. The mask must fit snugly to ensure an airtight seal between the face and the mask. The mask is placed on the patient's face and the liter flow adjusted (as prescribed) so that the rebreathing bag will not collapse during the inspiratory cycle. With a well-fitting rebreathing bag that is adjusted correctly, inspired oxygen concentrations of 30% to 60% can be achieved.

The disadvantages of a face mask are the mechanical restrictions it imposes on eating, drinking, and talking. There is also a certain amount of discomfort associated with the use of a mask for any length of time.

The *venturi mask* is a face mask designed to administer precisely controlled oxygen concentrations. It is so constructed that there is a constant flow of room air blended with a fixed concentration of oxygen. It is used primarily for patients with chronic obstructive pulmonary disease. The venturi mask, which employs the principle of air entrainment, provides a high air flow with controlled oxygen enrichment, allowing a fixed low-oxygen concentration with a flow-rate surplus according to the patient's needs. Excess gas leaves the mask through the perforated cuff, carrying with it the expired carbon dioxide. It allows inhalation of a constant oxygen concentration regardless of the depth or rate of respiration.

The patient's skin should be checked for irritation, and the mask should fit snugly enough to prevent oxygen flow into the eyes. The mask must be removed in order that the patient may eat, drink, take medications, etc., and it becomes uncomfortable after prolonged use.

The *aerosol mask* provides oxygen in approximate concentrations of 35% or greater with high humidity by administering aerosol mist that is either heated or unheated.

Hyperinflation Maneuvers

A mechanical aid to lung expansion is a device that motivates the patient to breathe deeply (incentive spirometer) or helps the patient to inflate his lungs (IPPB). Two methods are frequently used to encourage hyperinflation: *incentive spirometry* and *intermittent positive pressure breathing (IPPB)*.

Incentive Spirometer

The incentive spirometer is a piece of equipment that gives visual feedback to guide the patient to inhale slowly and deeply to maximize lung inflation (Fig. 24-1). It is used in the prevention and treatment of atelectasis, especially in the postoperative patient. The patient is placed in a sitting or semi-Fowler's position, since the diaphragmatic excursion is greater with this posture. However, this treatment may be done with the patient in any position. The tidal volume of the spirometer is set according to the manufacturer's instruction (often 500 ml to start). The purpose of the device is to measure a gradually increasing tidal volume as the patient takes deeper and deeper breaths. The patient takes a deep breath from the mouthpiece, pauses at peak inflation, then relaxes and exhales. To avoid fatigue he

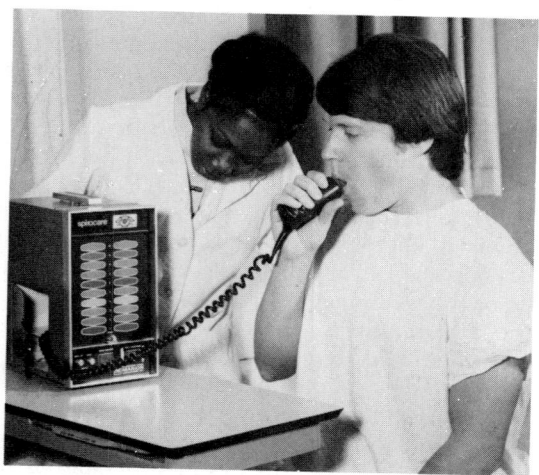

re 24-1. The incentive spirometer stimulates the patient to achieve inspiration. The advantages of this type of therapy are that no ... are necessary, most models are relatively inexpensive, and ...dependently, since the control mechanism is built in.

should take several normal breaths before attempting another with the incentive spirometer. The tidal volume is periodically increased as tolerated. The patient is encouraged to cough after a deep breath since deep lung inflation may loosen secretions so that they can be expectorated. A counter on the incentive spirometer indicates the number of breaths the patient has taken. Ten breaths per hour while the patient is awake is a frequent goal.

Intermittent Positive Pressure Breathing.   IPPB is the breathing of air or oxygen (or a combination of both) at a pressure higher than atmosphere to produce flow of air into the lungs during inhalation. It is used in patients unable to take spontaneous deep breaths. IPPB is prescribed as a mode of delivering aerosolized medications when simpler approaches prove suboptimal in some patients.

Chest Physical Therapy

Chest physical therapy includes postural drainage, encouragement of effective coughing, breathing exercises/breathing retraining, and chest percussion and vibration. The goals of chest physical therapy are to aid in the removal of bronchial secretions, to improve ventilation, and to increase the efficiency of the respiratory musculature.

Postural Drainage (Segmented Bronchial Drainage)

Postural drainage is the use of specific positions so that the force of gravity can assist in the removal of bronchial secretions. The secretions drain from the affected bronchioles into the bronchi and trachea and are removed by means of coughing or suctioning. It is used to prevent or relieve bronchial obstruction owing to secretions.

Because the patient is usually in an upright position, secretions are likely to accumulate in the lower part of the lung. When postural drainage is used, the patient is positioned sequentially in different postures (Fig. 24-2), so that the force of gravity helps to drain secretions from the smaller bronchial airways to the main bronchi and trachea. The secretions are then removed by coughing. Inhalation of the prescribed bronchodilators before postural drainage assists in draining the bronchial tree.

Postural drainage exercises can be directed at any of the segments (bilateral) of the lung. Usually, the lower and middle lobe bronchi empty more effectively when the head is down; the upper lobe bronchi empty more effectively when the head is up. Frequently, the patient is placed in five positions, one for drainage of each lobe: head down, prone, right and left lateral, and sitting upright.

Nursing Implications.   The nurse should be aware of the patient's diagnosis as well as the lung lobes or segments involved, the cardiac status, and any structural deformities of the chest wall and spine. To determine the area(s) needing drainage and the effectiveness of treatment, the chest should be auscultated before and after the procedure. This gives immediate feedback on the effectiveness of treatment.

Postural drainage is usually done two to four times daily, before meals (to prevent nausea, vomiting, and aspiration), and at bedtime. If prescribed, bronchodilators,

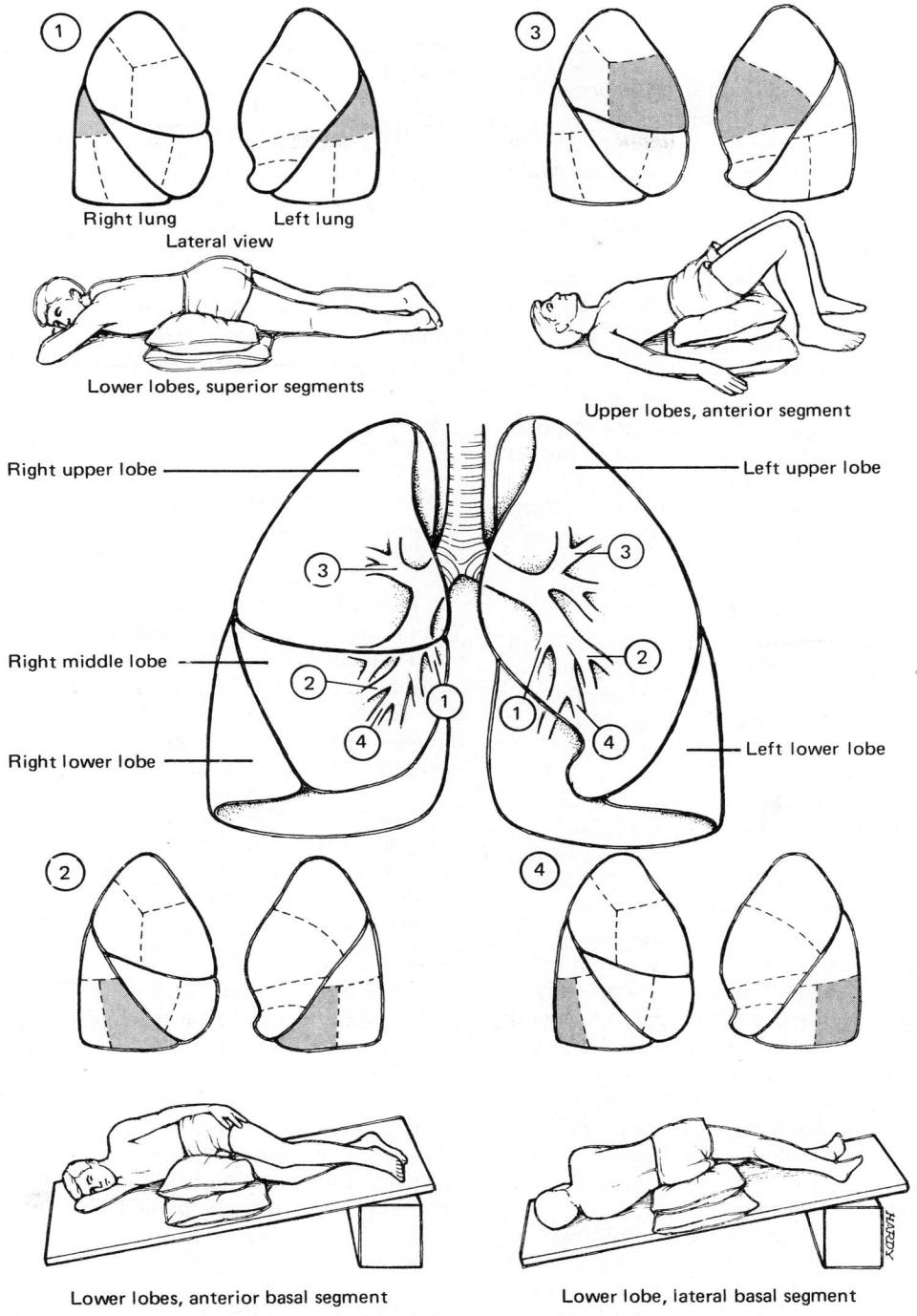

Right lung   Left lung
Lateral view
Lower lobes, superior segments

Upper lobes, anterior segment

Right upper lobe ———————————— Left upper lobe

Right middle lobe ——

Right lower lobe ——— Left lower lobe

Lower lobes, anterior basal segment

Lower lobe, lateral basal segment

Figure 24-2. Postural drainage.

water, or saline may be nebulized and inhaled before postural drainage to reduce bronchospasm, decrease thickness of mucus and sputum, and combat edema of the bronchial walls. The patient should be made as comfortable as possible in each position, and an emesis basin or sputum cup and paper tissues should be available. The patient is instructed to remain in each position for 5 to 10 minutes and to breathe in slowly through his nose and then breathe out slowly through pursed lips to help widen the airways, so that secretions can be drained while the various positions are assumed. If he cannot tolerate the position, he should be helped to assume a modified posture. When the patient changes positions, he is instructed to cough to remove secretions as follows:

1. Assume a sitting position and bend slightly forward, as the upright position permits a stronger cough.
2. Keep the knees and hips flexed to promote relaxation and lessen the strain on the abdominal muscles while coughing.
3. Inhale slowly through the nose and exhale through pursed lips several times.
4. Cough twice during each exhalation while contracting (pulling in) the abdomen sharply with each cough.

The secretions may need to be suctioned mechanically if the patient is unable to cough.

It may also be necessary to use chest percussion and vibration to loosen bronchial secretions and mucus plugs that adhere to the bronchioles and bronchi and to propel sputum in the direction of gravity drainage.

Following the procedure, the amount, color, viscosity, and character of the ejected sputum is noted; the patient's color and pulse are evaluated the first few times the exercises are performed. It may be necessary to administer oxygen during postural drainage.

If the sputum is foul-smelling, this procedure should be carried out in a room away from other patients, and deodorizers should be used. After postural drainage, the patient may find it refreshing to brush his teeth and use a mouthwash before resting in bed.

Chest Percussion and Vibration

To aid in the loosening and removal of thicker secretions, the chest may be tapped (percussion) and vibrated by the therapist or nurse. Percussion and vibration help to dislodge mucus adhering to the bronchioles and bronchi.

Percussion is carried out by cupping the hands and lightly striking the chest wall over the lung segment to be drained in a rhythmical fashion. The wrists are alternately flexed and extended so that the chest is cupped or clapped in a painless manner. A linen towel may be placed over the segment of the chest that is being cupped to prevent skin irritation and redness from direct contact. The patient uses diaphragmatic breathing during this procedure to promote relaxation (see Breathing Retraining). As a precaution, percussion over the sternum, spine, liver, kidneys, spleen, or breasts (in female should be avoided).

Vibration is the technique of applying manual compression and tremor to the chest wall during the exhalation phase of respiration. This maneuver helps to increase the velocity of the expired tidal volume from the small airways, thus freeing the mucus. After three or four vibrations the patient is encouraged to cough, using his abdominal muscles. (Contracting the abdominal muscles increases cough effectiveness.) A scheduled program of coughing and clearing sputum, together with hydration, will reduce sputum in the majority of patients. The number of the percussion and vibration cycle is repeated depending on the patient's tolerance and clinical response; the ___ to 30 minutes.

___ and vibration, changes in breath sounds are evaluated. (Percussion and vibration of the patient on a mechanical ventilator are discussed on p. 504.)

Breathing Retraining

Breathing retraining (breathing exercises) are exercises and breathing practices that are designed and carried out to achieve a more efficient and controlled ventilation, to decrease the work of breathing, and to correct respiratory deficits.

These exercises have a number of purposes: to promote maximum alveolar inflation; promote muscle relaxation; relieve anxiety; eliminate useless, uncoordinated patterns of respiratory muscle activity; slow the respiratory rate; and decrease the work of breathing. Slow, relaxed, and rhythmical breathing also helps to control the anxiety that is present when the patient is dyspneic. Breathing exercises may be practiced in several positions, since air distribution and pulmonary circulation vary according to the position of the chest.

Instructions to the Patient

Tell the patient to breath slowly and rhythmically in a relaxed manner in order to permit more complete exhalation and emptying of the lungs. Instruct him to always inhale through the nose since this filters, humidifies, and warms the air. If the patient becomes short of breath, have him stop until his breathing pattern comes under control.

Diaphragmatic Breathing

The *goal* of diaphragmatic breathing is to strengthen and increase the use of the diaphragm during breathing. Diaphragmatic breathing can become automatic with sufficient practice and concentration.

The patient is instructed as follows:

1. Place one hand on the stomach (just below the ribs) and the other hand on the middle of the chest. This increases awareness of the diaphragm and its function in breathing.
2. Breathe in slowly and deeply through the nose, letting the abdomen protrude as far as it will.
3. Breathe out through pursed lips while tightening (contracting) the abdominal muscles. Press firmly inward and upward on the abdomen while breathing out.
4. Repeat for 1 minute; follow by a rest period of 2 minutes. Work up to 30 minutes, several times a day.

Pursed Lip Breathing

Pursed lip breathing (positive pressure breathing), which improves oxygen transport, helps to induce a slow, deep breathing pattern and assists the patient to control his breathing, even during periods of physical stress. This type of breathing helps prevent alveolar collapse owing to loss of lung elasticity in emphysema.

The *goal* of pursed lip breathing is to train the muscles of expiration so as to prolong exhalation and increase airway pressure during expiration, thus lessening the amount of airway trapping and resistance.

The patient is instructed as follows:

1. Inhale through the nose while counting to 3, and exhale slowly and evenly against pursed lips while tightening the abdominal muscles. (Pursing the lips increases intratracheal pressure; exhaling through the mouth offers less resistance to expired air.)
2. Count to 7 while prolonging expiration through pursed lips.
3. Sit in a chair; fold arms over the abdomen.
   Inhale through the nose (count to 3); exhale slowly through pursed lips while bending forward; count to 7.
4. While walking
   a. Inhale while walking two steps.
   b. Exhale through pursed lips while walking four or five steps.

Many patients will require additional oxygen, using a low flow technique, while doing breathing exercises.

▷ The Patient Undergoing Thoracic Surgery

Operative Procedures

See Figure 24-3.

Lobectomy. When the pathology is limited to one area of a lung, a lobectomy (removal of a lobe of a lung) is done. This operation, which is more common than pneumonectomy, may be carried out for bronchogenic carcinoma, giant emphysematous blebs or bullae, benign tumors, metastatic malignant tumors, bronchiectasis, and fungus infections.

A thoracotomy incision is used, its exact location depending on the lobe to be resected. When the pleura is entered, the involved lung collapses and the lobar vessels and the bronchus are ligated and divided. After the lobe is removed, the remaining lobes of the lung are reexpanded. Frequently, two chest catheters are inserted for drainage

(Fig. 24-4). The upper tube is for the removal of air; the lower one is for drainage of fluid. Frequently, only one well-placed catheter is needed. The chest tube is connected to a chest drainage apparatus for several days.

Pneumonectomy. The removal of an entire lung (pneumonectomy) is done chiefly for cancer when the lesion cannot be removed by a lesser procedure. It also may be performed for lung abscesses, bronchiectasis, or extensive unilateral tuberculosis. The removal of the right lung is more dangerous than the removal of the left since the right lung has a larger vascular bed and its removal imposes a greater physiologic burden.

A posterolateral or anterolateral thoracotomy incision is made, sometimes with resection of a rib. The pulmonary artery and the pulmonary veins are ligated and severed.

The main bronchus is divided and the lung removed. The bronchial stump is stapled and usually no drains are used because the accumulation of fluid in the empty hemithorax is the desired end result.

Segmentectomy (Segmental Resection). Some lesions are confined to a segment of lung. Bronchopulmonary segments are subdivisions of the lung that function as individual units. They are held together by delicate connective tissue; disease processes may be limited to a single segment. Care is used to preserve as much healthy and functional lung tissue as possible, especially in patients who already have a limited cardiorespiratory reserve. Single segments can be removed from any lobe, but the right middle lobe, since it has only two small segments, invariably is removed entirely. On the left side, corresponding to a middle lobe, is a "lingular" segment of the upper lobe. This can be removed as a single segment or by *lingulectomy*. This segment is frequently involved in bronchiectasis.

Wedge Resection. A wedge resection of a small, well-circumscribed lesion may be done without regard for the location of the intersegmental planes. The pleural cavity usually is drained because of the possibility of an air or blood leak. This procedure is done for random lung biopsy and for the excision of small peripheral nodules.

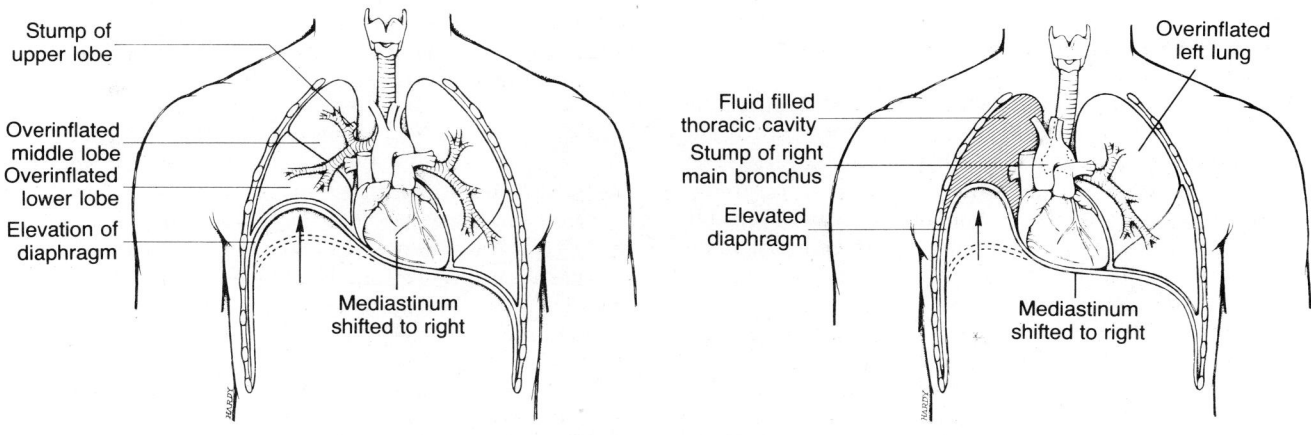

Figure 24-3. Operative procedures. (*Left*) Lobectomy. (*Right*) Pneumonectomy.

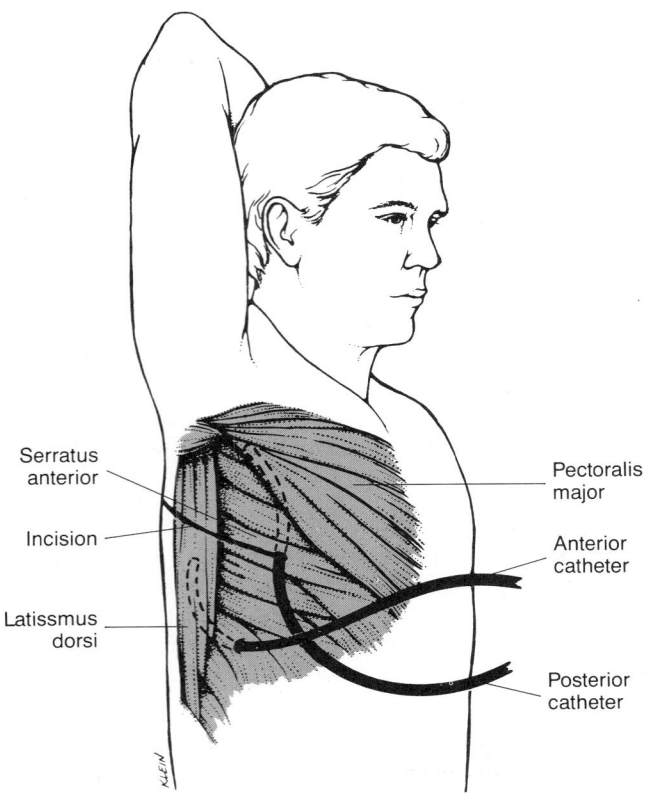

Serratus anterior

Incision

Latissmus dorsi

Pectoralis major

Anterior catheter

Posterior catheter

Figure 24-4. Postoperative drainage of the chest. The upper drainage tube is used for the escape of air from leaks in the resected lung. The tip is anchored in the parietal pleura near the apex and brought out through the anterior end of the incision. The lower tube is usually for serosanguineous drainage.

Bronchoplastic or Sleeve Resection.   Bronchoplastic resection is a procedure in which only one lobar bronchus together with a part of the right or left bronchus is excised. The distal bronchus is reanastomosed to the proximal bronchus or trachea.

▶ Preoperative Assessment

A patient undergoing thoracic surgery requires meticulous assessment and management because not only are these operations wide in scope, but the patient may have obstructive pulmonary disease with compromised breathing. The details of preoperative management may be of greater importance than those in other surgical procedures, since chest operations are of greater magnitude and may present a narrower margin of safety.

Fortunately, the lungs have a large functional reserve. Newer techniques of anesthesia, respiratory therapy, skillful ⋯ and intensive postoperative care have made possible ⋯ re extensive thoracic surgery.

⋯ bjectives of preoperative care are (1) to ascertain ⋯'s functional reserve to determine if he can sur-

vive the operation, and (2) to ensure the optimal condition of the patient for surgery.

Diagnostic Evaluation.   A battery of preoperative tests is done to determine the preoperative status of the patient and to assess his physical assets and liabilities. The initial investigation starts with the history and physical examination—the foundation of preoperative evaluation. The general appearance of the patient, his behavior, and his mental alertness will indicate whether a significant surgical risk is involved.

The decision to perform any pulmonary resection is based on the patient's cardiovascular status and pulmonary reserve. Pulmonary function studies (especially lung volume and vital capacity) are done to determine whether the contemplated resection will leave sufficient functioning lung tissue. Arterial blood gases are assessed to provide a more complete picture of the functional capacity of the lung. Exercise tolerance tests have predictive value. Such tests are especially important in determining whether the patient who is a candidate for pneumonectomy can tolerate whole lung removal.

Preoperative studies are done to provide a baseline for comparison during the postoperative period and to reveal any unsuspected abnormalities. These studies include chest x-rays, ECG (for arteriosclerotic heart disease, conduction defects), BUN and serum creatinine (renal function), glucose tolerance or blood sugar (diabetes), assessment of blood electrolytes, serum protein studies, and blood volume determinations.

Nursing Assessment

Chest auscultation should give an estimate of the intensity of breath sounds in the different regions of the lungs (see Chap. 5). When the chest is auscultated, it is important to note whether breath sounds are normal, indicating a free flow of air in and out of the lungs. (In the emphysematous patient, the breath sounds may be markedly decreased or even absent upon auscultation.) Crackles, wheezes, and hyperresonance are noted, along with decreased diaphragmatic motion. Unilateral diminished breath sounds and rhonchi can be the result of occlusion of the bronchi by mucous plugs. Evidence of retained secretions may be evaluated during auscultation by asking the patient to cough and noting any signs of rhonchi or wheezing. The nursing assessment may also include the following:

- What signs and symptoms are present—cough, expectoration (amount), hemoptysis, chest pain, dyspnea?
- What is the smoking history? How long has the patient been smoking? How much is he currently smoking?
- What is the patient's cardiopulmonary tolerance while resting, eating, bathing, walking?
- What is his breathing pattern? How much exertion is required to produce dyspnea?
- What is the physiologic age of the patient—for example, general appearance, mental alertness, behavior, degree of nutrition?
- What other medical conditions exist; allergies, etc.?
- What are his personal preferences and dislikes?

Patient Problems/Nursing Diagnoses

Based on the clinical manifestations and diagnostic assessment data, the patient's major nursing problems include possible breathing problems related to existing impaired lung function and deficit in pulmonary function from tumor removal; pain and discomfort related to painful incision, protective splinting, coughing, and the presence of chest tubes; possible musculoskeletal disability related to consequences of thoracic surgery; and anxiety related to outcome of procedure, fear of recurrent disease, and possible permanent limitations on life-style.

▶ Preoperative Nursing Interventions

Improvement of Ventilation and Respiratory Function

An important preoperative objective is to improve alveolar ventilation and to reduce the presence of respiratory secretions as much as possible. To achieve this goal, the therapeutic regimen includes *cessation of smoking,* which is a bronchial irritant; fluid intake and humidification to loosen secretions; bronchodilators for relief of bronchospasm; and postural drainage and chest percussion following administration of bronchodilators for clearance of secretions. The volume of sputum is measured daily in patients who expectorate large volumes of secretions. Such measurements are carried out to determine if the amount is decreasing. Antimicrobials are given for infection. Normally, a person inhales to his total lung capacity several times each hour. Deep inspiration is painful following thoracic surgery, and atelectatic complications follow abnormal patterns of breathing. To prevent this, the use of the incentive spirometer to maximize voluntary lung inflation is carried out, and the use of the ultrasonic nebulizer for humidification and mobilization of secretions is taught and performed both in side-lying and sitting positions.

Preoperative Patient Teaching

The patient is informed of what to expect in the postoperative period; that is, the possible presence of chest tube(s) and drainage bottles, the usual postoperative administration of oxygen to facilitate breathing, and the possible use of a ventilator. The importance of frequent turning to promote drainage of lung secretions is explained.

Since a coughing schedule will be necessary in the postoperative period to bring up secretions, the patient should be instructed in the technique of coughing and warned that the coughing routine may prove to be uncomfortable. He is taught to splint his incision with his hands, a pillow, or a folded towel.

Coughing Technique
1. Sit the patient upright with knees flexed and body bent slightly forward.
2. Splint the incision with your (nurse's) hands; later the patient should splint the painful area with firm hand pressure or support it with a pillow or rolled blanket while coughing.

3. Tell the patient to take three short breaths followed by a deep inspiration (inhaling slowly and evenly through the nose).
4. Then instruct him to contract (pull in) the abdominal muscles and cough twice forcefully, with his mouth open and tongue out.
5. If the patient is unable to sit, have him lie on his side with his hips and knees flexed.

Huffing Technique

"Huffing" is the expulsion of air through an open glottis and may be helpful for the patient with diminished expiratory flow rates or for the patient in severe pain who refuses to cough.

1. Show the patient how to take a deep diaphragmatic breath and exhale forcefully against his hand. Explain that he should exhale forcefully in a quick, distinct pant, or "huff."
2. Have the patient practice doing small "huffs" and progress to one strong "huff" as he exhales.
3. This type of forceful exhalation stimulates pulmonary expansion and assists in alveolar inflation.

Psychological Support

Usually, several days are allotted to the preoperative phase, which provides time for the nurse to talk with the patient. By listening, the nurse may be able to discover how the patient really feels about his illness and the proposed treatment, and to what extent he is motivated to get back to normal activity. He may reveal significant reactions: the fear of hemorrhage because of bloody sputum, the discomfort of a chronic cough and chest pain, the fear of death because of dyspnea and tumor—all contribute to his psychological status.

The nurse may help the patient to overcome many of his fears and to mobilize his intellectual functions in order to cope with the stress of surgery. This is done by correcting any false impressions, by offering reassurance about the capability of the surgical team, by reassuring the patient that his incision will "hold," and by dealing honestly with questions about pain and discomfort and their treatment. The management and control of pain should begin before surgery by informing the patient that he, himself, can overcome many postoperative problems by following certain routines related to deep breathing, coughing, turning, and moving.

▶ Planning and Implementation

Regardless of the surgical procedure, certain objectives and problems are common to all patients undergoing thoracic surgery.

Goals

The goals of the patient are:

1. Improvement of breathing
2. Relief of pain and discomfort
3. Absence of disability of affected shoulder and arm
4. Relief of anxiety

After the operation, the major nursing objective is to restore normal cardiopulmonary function as quickly as possible. This is accomplished by (1) maintaining a patent airway, (2) providing for maximum expansion of the remaining lung tissue, (3) recognizing early signs and symptoms of untoward complications, and (4) providing supportive and rehabilitative measures.

Maintenance of a Patent Airway

Every means possible must be utilized to maintain a patent airway. First, secretions must be suctioned from the tracheobronchial tree before the endotracheal tube is removed. In fact, all secretions should be aspirated by suctioning until the patient can cough up secretions effectively. Endotracheal secretions are present in excessive amounts in post-thoracotomy patients owing to trauma to the tracheobronchial tree during operation, diminished lung ventilation, and diminished cough reflex. Excessive secretions will produce airway obstruction, causing air in the alveoli distal to the obstruction to become absorbed and the lung to collapse. Atelectasis, pneumonia, and respiratory failure may follow.

Technique for Endotracheal Suctioning
(Sterile technique is to be used. This procedure should be learned under expert clinical supervision.)

1. Place the patient in a sitting or semi-Fowler's position. Attach the sterile catheter to a "Y" or "T" tube that has been connected to a suction device.
2. Oxygenate the patient several minutes before each suctioning procedure.
3. Give the patient a gauze square, and instruct him to pull his tongue outward; this tilts the epiglottis forward. If the patient cannot comply, have another person do this.
4. Pass a lubricated (with water-soluble gel) catheter through the nostril to the pharynx. Check the position of the tip of the catheter; it should be in the lower pharynx.
5. Instruct the patient to take a deep breath. This opens the epiglottis and helps the catheter to move in the direction of the negative pressure generated by inspiration.
6. Advance the catheter into the trachea only during inspiration.
7. Apply suction intermittently by closing the open end of the "Y" or "T" catheter with the finger and slowly rotating the catheter between the thumb and forefinger.
8. Avoid prolonging suction more than 5 to 10 seconds, since cardiac arrest may ensue in patients with borderline oxygenation.
9. While the catheter is being withdrawn, apply gentle suction to clear the tracheal walls of secretions.
10. Ventilate the patient with oxygen for several minutes before a second passage of the catheter (if a second aspiration is necessary). Check the pulse rate.

Most postoperative thoracotomy patients are given humidified oxygen because of the hypoxemia secondary to abnormal shunting. The patient's ventilation mechanism is impaired primarily because of pain and splinting of the operative side. This can lead to as much as a 30% reduction in vital capacity. Thus, mechanical ventilation is frequently used until the patient can support adequate ventilation. The arterial blood gases as well as clinical assessment are parameters used to determine the need for ventilator support. The management of the patient requiring mechanical ventilation is discussed on pages 495 to 504.

Continuing Nursing Assessment and Monitoring

The blood pressure, pulse, and respiration are monitored every 15 minutes and more frequently as indicated. The character and depth of the respiration and the patient's color serve as important criteria in evaluating whether the lungs are being adequately expanded. The heart rate and rhythm are monitored by auscultation and electrocardiography, as major arrhythmic episodes are common after thoracic and cardiac surgery. Arrhythmias can occur at any time but frequently are seen between the 2nd and 6th postoperative day. The rate of occurrence of arrhythmias increases with patients over 50 years of age and with those undergoing pneumonectomy or esophageal surgery. Antiarrhythmic measures (propranolol; cardiac pacing; countershock) are started immediately when necessary.

An arterial line is maintained to facilitate frequent monitoring of blood gases, serum electrolytes, hemoglobin and hematocrit values, and arterial pressure. Central venous pressure is monitored for the early recognition of hypovolemia.

Coughing Technique

The patient must be encouraged to cough effectively, since ineffective coughing will result in exhaustion and retention of secretions, which can lead to atelectasis and pneumonia. To be effective, the cough should be low-pitched, deep, and controlled. Since it is difficult to cough in a supine position, the patient should be helped to a sitting position on the edge of the bed, with his feet resting on a chair. Coughing should be carried out at least every hour (as described on p. 458) during the first 24 hours and when necessary thereafter. If audible crackles are present, it may be necessary to use chest percussion with the cough routine until the lungs are clear. To lessen incisional pain during coughing, the nurse should support the incision firmly over the operated side and against the opposite chest (Fig. 24-5).

After helping the patient to cough, the nurse should listen to both lungs, both anteriorly and posteriorly, with a stethoscope to determine whether there are any changes in breath sounds, since diminished sounds may indicate collapsed or hypoventilated alveoli. The use of an incentive spirometer stimulates deep and sustained inspiration. Aerosol therapy may be used to reduce the viscosity of the secretions and to prevent excessive drying of secretions.

Control of Pain

Pain following a thoracotomy may be severe, depending on the type of incision and the patient's reaction to and ability to cope with pain. Deep inspiration is very painful following thoracotomy. Pain can lead to postoperative complications if it reduces the patient's ability to breathe deeply and

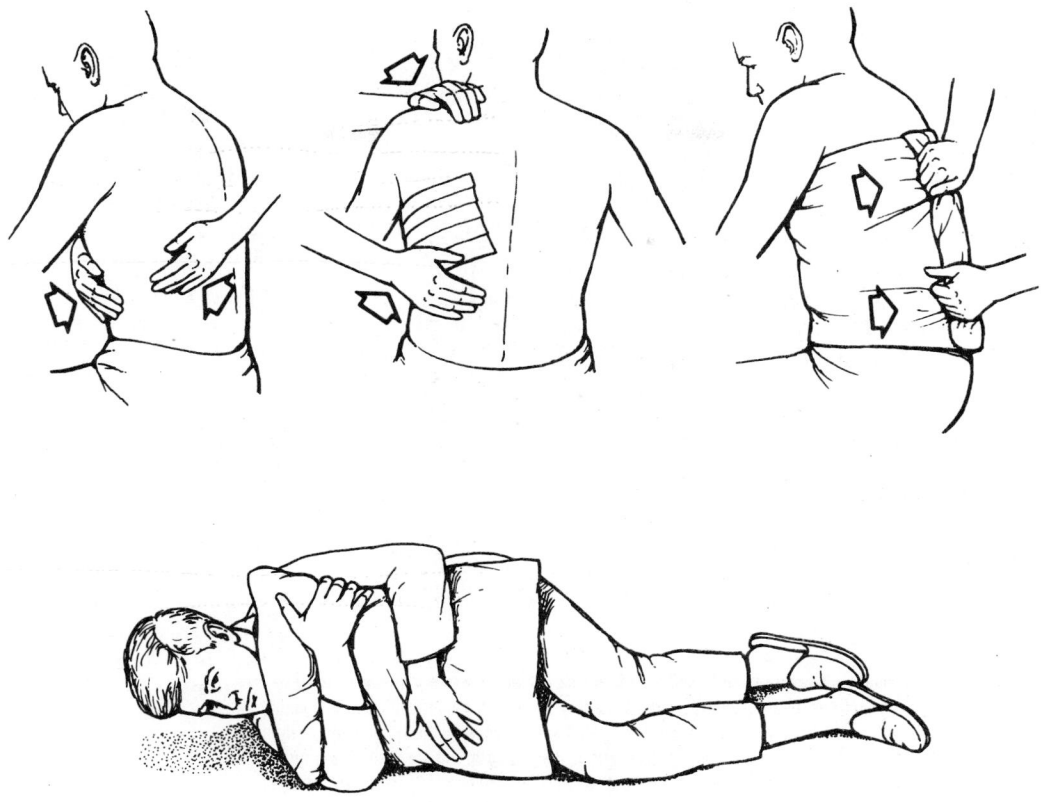

Figure 24-5. Techniques for support of incision while patient with thoracic surgery coughs. (*Top left*) The nurse's hands should support the chest incision anteriorly and posteriorly. The patient is instructed to take several deep breaths, inhale, and then cough forcibly. (*Top middle*) With one hand, exert downward pressure on the shoulder of the affected side while firmly supporting beneath the wound with the other hand. The patient is instructed to take several deep breaths, inhale, and then cough forcibly.

cough, and if it further limits chest excursions so that effective ventilation is decreased. Immediately after the surgical procedure and before the incision is closed, the surgeon may do a nerve block with a long-acting local anesthetic, which can reduce postoperative pain and improve pulmonary function. Small, intravenous doses of a narcotic are given and are titrated to relieve pain while still allowing the patient to cooperate in deep breathing, coughing, and mobilization efforts. However, it is important to avoid depressing the respiratory system with too much narcotic, since the patient should not be so somnolent that he does not cough.

- A word of warning: do not confuse the restlessness of hypoxia with restlessness owing to pain. Dyspnea, restlessness, increasing respiratory rate, increasing blood pressure, and tachycardia are warning signs of impending respiratory insufficiency.

Positioning the Patient

When the patient is oriented and his blood pressure is stabilized, the head of the bed is elevated 30 to 40 degrees during the immediate postoperative period. This facilitates optional ventilation and helps residual air to rise in the upper portion of pleural space, where it can be removed via the upper chest tube.

The surgeon is consulted concerning individual patient positioning. The patient with limited respiratory reserve may not be able to turn on the unoperated side, as this may limit ventilation of the operated side. Vary the position from horizontal to semi-upright, as remaining in one position tends to promote the retention of secretions in the dependent portion of the lungs. Following a pneumonectomy, the operated side should be dependent so that fluid in the pleural space remains below the level of the bronchial stump.

Turning Procedure
1. Instruct the patient to bend his knees and use his feet to push.
2. Have the patient shift his hips and shoulders to the opposite side of the bed while pushing with his feet.
3. Bring the patient's arm over his chest, pointing it in the direction toward which he is being turned, and have him grasp the side rail with his hand.

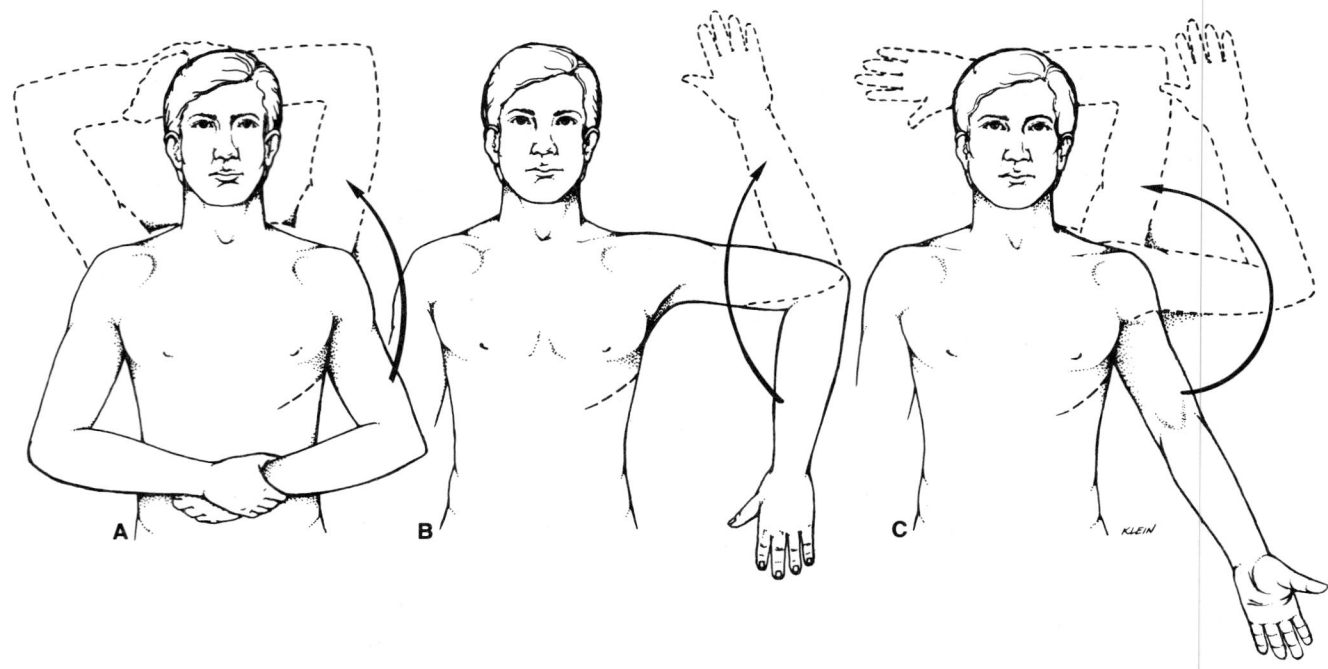

Figure 24-6. Arm and shoulder exercises are done following thoracic surgery to restore movement, prevent painful stiffening of the shoulder, and improve muscle power. (*A*) Hold hand of the affected side with the other hand, palms facing in. Raise the arms forward, upward, and then overhead, while taking a deep breath. Exhale while lowering the arms. Repeat five times. (*B*) Raise arm sideward, upward, and downward in a waving motion. (*C*) Place arm at side. Raise arm sideward, upward, and over the head. Both exercises can also be done while lying in bed.

4. Turn patient in "log roll" fashion to prevent twisting at the waist and possible pulling of the incision, which could be painful.

Ambulation.   If shock has not occurred and the patient does not have heart disease or a limited cardiovascular reserve, he may get out of bed on the evening of the day after surgery, upon the physician's request. Since the chest tube is well secured, this activity need not be restricted. Postural and breathing exercises are started as prescribed in order to produce better lung ventilation, restore motion and muscle tonus in the shoulder girdle and trunk, and maintain normal posture (Fig. 24-6 and Table 24-1). Chest x-rays are taken frequently to ensure full expansion of the patient's lungs and to rule out any unwanted collections of air or fluid.

Fluids and Nutrition

During the operation or immediately after, the patient usually receives a blood transfusion, followed by an intra-

Table 24-1
Skeletal Exercises Designed to Restore Function Following Thoracic Surgery

Muscle Affected by Thoracotomy	Function	Activities to Restore Function
Trapezius	Promotes arm extension, abduction, and reach extension	Extend the arm up and back, out to the side and back, down at the side and back.
Rhomboideus major	Adducts and slightly elevates scapula	Place hands in small of back. Push elbows as far back as possible.
Latissimus dorsi	Depresses the shoulder	Sit erect in an armchair; place the hands on the arms of the chair directly opposite either side of the body. Press down on hands, consciously pulling the abdomen in and stretching up from the waist. Inhale while raising the body until the elbows are extended completely. Hold this position a moment, and begin exhaling while lowering the body slowly to the original position.
Serratus anterior	Rotates scapula and fixes it against the rib cage	Reach over head and "push" in an upward and outward motion.

venous infusion to "keep the vein open" until the blood volume can be reassessed. The rate of administration is slow (10 ml/hour), especially when there is evidence of limited cardiopulmonary reserve and when the pulmonary vascular bed has been greatly reduced, as in pneumonectomy.

- *Caution: Pulmonary edema owing to overinfusion is a real danger.* The early symptoms of such a complication are cyanosis, dyspnea, crackles, and bubbling sounds in the chest, as well as frothy sputum. This constitutes an emergency and is to be reported immediately.

Chest Drainage

The normal breathing mechanism operates on the principle of negative pressure (the pressure in the chest cavity is lower than the pressure of the outside air, causing air to move into the lungs during inspiration). Whenever the chest is opened, from any cause, there is a loss of negative pressure, which can result in the collapse of the lung. The collection of air, fluid, or other substances in the chest can compromise cardiopulmonary function and even cause collapse of the lung. Pathologic substances that collect in the pleural space include fibrin, or clotted blood; liquids (serous fluids, blood, pus, chyle); and gases (air from the lung, tracheobronchial tree, or esophagus).

Surgical incision of the chest wall almost always causes some degree of pneumothorax. Air and fluid collect in the intrapleural space, restricting lung expansion and reducing air exchange. It is necessary to keep the pleural space evacuated postoperatively and to maintain negative pressure within this potential space. Therefore, during or immediately after thoracic surgery, chest catheters are positioned strategically in the pleural space (see Fig. 24-4), sutured to the skin, and connected to some type of drainage apparatus in order to remove the residual air and drainage fluid from the pleural or mediastinal space. This assists in the reexpansion of remaining lung tissue.

A chest drainage system must be capable of removing whatever collects in the pleural space so that a normal pleural space and normal cardiopulmonary function may be restored and maintained. There are many types of commercial chest drainage systems in use, most of which use the water-seal principle (see below). (However, the conventional water-seal chest drainage is less expensive and has the advantage of identifying precisely the time at which the air leak stops, thereby accelerating the time when the chest tube can be removed.) The chest catheter is attached to a bottle, using a one-way valve principle. Water acts as a seal and permits air and fluid to drain from the chest, but air cannot reenter the submerged tip of the tube. The care of the patient with water-seal chest drainage is discussed in Chart 24-1.

Principles of Chest Drainage

Chest drainage can be categorized into three types of mechanical systems (Fig. 24-7).

The Single-Bottle Water-Seal System.   The end of the drainage tube from the patient's chest is covered by a layer of water, which permits drainage of air and fluid from the pleural space, but does not allow air to move back into the chest. Functionally, drainage depends on gravity, on the mechanics of respiration, and, if desired, on suction by the addition of *controlled* vacuum.

The tube from the patient extends approximately 2.5 cm (1 inch) below the level of the water in the container. There is a vent for the escape of any air that might be leaking from the lung. The water level fluctuates as the patient breathes; it goes up when the patient inhales and down when the patient exhales. At the end of the drainage tube, bubbling may or may not be visible. Bubbling can mean either persistent leakage of air from the lung or other tissues or a leak in the system.

The Two-Bottle System.   The two-bottle system consists of the same water-seal chamber plus a fluid collection bottle. Drainage is similar to that of a single unit, except that when pleural fluid drains, the underwater seal system is not affected by the volume of drainage.

Effective drainage depends on gravity or on the amount of suction added to the system. When vacuum (suction) is added to the system from a vacuum source, such as wall suction, the connection is made at the vent stem of the underwater-seal bottle. The amount of suction applied to the system is regulated by the wall gauge.

The Three-Bottle System.   This system is similar in all respects to the two-bottle system, except for the addition of a third bottle to control the amount of suction applied. The amount of suction is determined by the depth to which the tip of the venting glass tube is submerged. (For example, submersion to 10 cm below the surface of the water will equal 10 cm of water suction applied to the patient.)

In the three-bottle system (as in the other two), drainage depends on gravity or the amount of suction applied. The amount of suction in this system is controlled by the manometer bottle. The mechanical suction motor or wall suction creates and maintains a negative pressure throughout the entire closed drainage system.

The manometer bottle regulates the amount of vacuum in the system. This bottle contains three tubes: (1) a short tube above the water level comes from the water-seal bottle; (2) another short tube leads to the vacuum or to suction motor or wall suction; and (3) the third tube is a long tube (standpipe) that extends below the water level in the bottle and is open to the atmosphere outside the bottle. This is the tube that regulates the amount of vacuum in the system. This is regulated by the depth to which this tube is submerged—the usual depth is 20 cm (7.6 inches).

When the vacuum in the system becomes greater than the depth to which the tube is submerged, outside air is sucked into the system. This results in constant bubbling in the manometer (or pressure-regulator) bottle, which indicates that the system is functioning properly.

- *Note:* When the motor is off or the wall vacuum is turned off, the drainage system should be open to the atmosphere so that intrapleural air can escape from the system. This can be done by detaching the tubing from the suction port to provide a vent.

(Text continues on page 468)

Chart 24-1
Guidelines to the Nurse's Role in the Management of the Patient With Water-Seal Chest Drainage*

An intrapleural drainage tube is used after most intrathoracic procedures. One or more chest catheters are held in the pleural space by suture to the chest wall and are attached to a drainage system. The purposes are:

1. To remove solids, liquids, and gas from the pleural space or thoracic cavity and the mediastinal space
2. To bring about reexpansion of the lung and restore normal cardiorespiratory function after surgery, trauma, or medical conditions

Procedure

Nursing Action	*Rationale/Amplification*
1. Attach the drainage tube from the pleural space to the tubing that leads to a long tube with end submerged in sterile normal saline.	1. Water-seal drainage provides for the escape of air and fluid into a drainage bottle. The water acts as a seal and keeps the air from being drawn back into the pleural space.
2. Tape the places where the tubing is connected, if needed. Some connectors hold without taping.	2. Taping the connecting points of the tubing will make certain that the tubing remains airtight to reestablish negative (intrapleural) pressure.
a. The tube should be approximately 2.5 cm (1 inch) below the water level.	a. If the tube is submerged too deep below the water level, a higher intrapleural pressure is required to expel air.
b. The short tube is left open to the atmosphere.	b. Venting the short glass tube lets air escape from the bottle.
3. Mark the original fluid level with tape on the outside of the drainage bottle. Mark hourly/daily increments (date and time) at the drainage level.	3. This marking will show the amount of fluid loss and how fast fluid is collecting in the drainage bottle. It serves as a basis for blood replacement, if the fluid is blood. Grossly bloody drainage will appear in the bottle in the immediate postoperative period and if excessive may require reoperation. Drainage usually declines progressively in the first 24 hours.
4. Ensure that the tubing is not looping or interfering with the movements of the patient.	4. Kinking, looping, or pressure on the drainage tubing can produce back pressure, and may thus possibly force drainage back into the pleural space or impede drainage from the pleural space.
5. Encourage the patient to assume a position of comfort. Encourage good body alignment. When the patient is in the lateral position, place a rolled towel under the tubing to protect it from the weight of the patient's body. Encourage the patient to change position frequently.	5. The patient's position should be changed frequently to promote drainage, and the body should be kept in good alignment to prevent postural deformities and contractures. Proper positioning helps breathing and promotes better air exchange. Pain medication may be needed to enhance comfort and deep breathing.
6. Put the arm and shoulder of the affected side through range of motion exercises several times daily. Some pain medication may be necessary.	6. Exercise helps to avoid ankylosis of the shoulder and assists in lessening postoperative pain and discomfort.
7. "Milk" the tubing in the direction of the drainage bottle hourly.	7. "Milking" the tubing prevents it from becoming plugged with clots and fibrin. Constant attention to maintaining the patency of the tube facilitates prompt expansion of the lung and minimizes complications.
8. Make sure there is fluctuation ("tidaling") of the fluid level in the long glass tube.	8. Fluctuation of the water level in the tube shows that there is effective communication between the pleural cavity and the drainage bottle, provides a valuable indication of the patency of the drainage system, and is a gauge of intrapleural pressure.

(continued)

Chart 24-1
Guidelines to the Nurse's Role in the Management of the Patient With Water-Seal Chest Drainage* (continued)

Procedure *(continued)*

Nursing Action *(continued)*

9. Fluctuations of fluid in the tubing will stop when:
   a. The lung has reexpanded
   b. The tubing is obstructed by blood clots or fibrin
   c. A dependent loop develops
   d. Suction motor or wall suction is not working properly

10. Watch for leaks of air in the drainage system as indicated by constant bubbling in the water-seal bottle.
    a. Report excessive bubbling in the water-seal chamber immediately.
    b. "Milking" of chest tubes in patients with air leaks should only be done if requested by the surgeon.

11. Observe and report immediately signs of rapid, shallow breathing; cyanosis; pressure in the chest; subcutaneous emphysema; or symptoms of hemorrhage.

12. Encourage the patient to breathe deeply and cough at frequent intervals. If there are signs of incisional pain, adequate pain medication is indicated.

13. Stabilize the drainage bottle on the floor or in a special holder.
    Caution visitors and personnel against handling equipment or displacing the drainage bottle.

14. If the patient has to be transported to another area, place the drainage bottle below the chest level (as close to the floor as possible), if he is lying on a stretcher. If the tube becomes disconnected, cut off the contaminated tips of the chest tube and tubing, insert a sterile connector in the chest tube and tubing, and reattach to the drainage system.

15. When assisting the surgeon in removing the tube:
    a. Instruct the patient to perform the Valsalva maneuver (forcible exhalation against a closed glottis, holding one's breath).
    b. The chest tube is clamped and quickly removed.
    c. Simultaneously, a small bandage is applied and made airtight with petrolatum gauze covered by 4″ × 4″ gauze and thoroughly covered and sealed with adhesive tape.

Rationale/Amplification *(continued)*

10. Leaking and trapping of air in the pleural space can result in tension pneumothorax.

11. Many clinical conditions may cause these signs and symptoms, including tension pneumothorax, mediastinal shift, hemorrhage, severe incisional pain, pulmonary embolus, and cardiac tamponade. Surgical intervention may be necessary.

12. Deep breathing and coughing help to raise the intrapleural pressure, which allows emptying of any accumulation in the pleural space and removes secretions from the tracheobronchial tree, so that the lung expands and atelectasis is prevented.

13. If any part of the apparatus is damaged, the closed system of drainage will be destroyed and the patient will be endangered by atmospheric pressure in the pleural space and resultant collapse of the lung. The drainage system must be kept airtight to reestablish negative intrapleural pressure.

14. The drainage apparatus must be kept at a level lower than the patient's chest to prevent backflow of fluid into the pleural space.

15. The chest tube is removed as directed when the lung is reexpanded (usually 24 hours to several days). During removal of the tube the chief priorities are prevention of entrance of air into the pleural cavity as the tube is withdrawn and prevention of infection.

* There are numerous commercial disposable chest drainage devices available that use the water-seal principle.

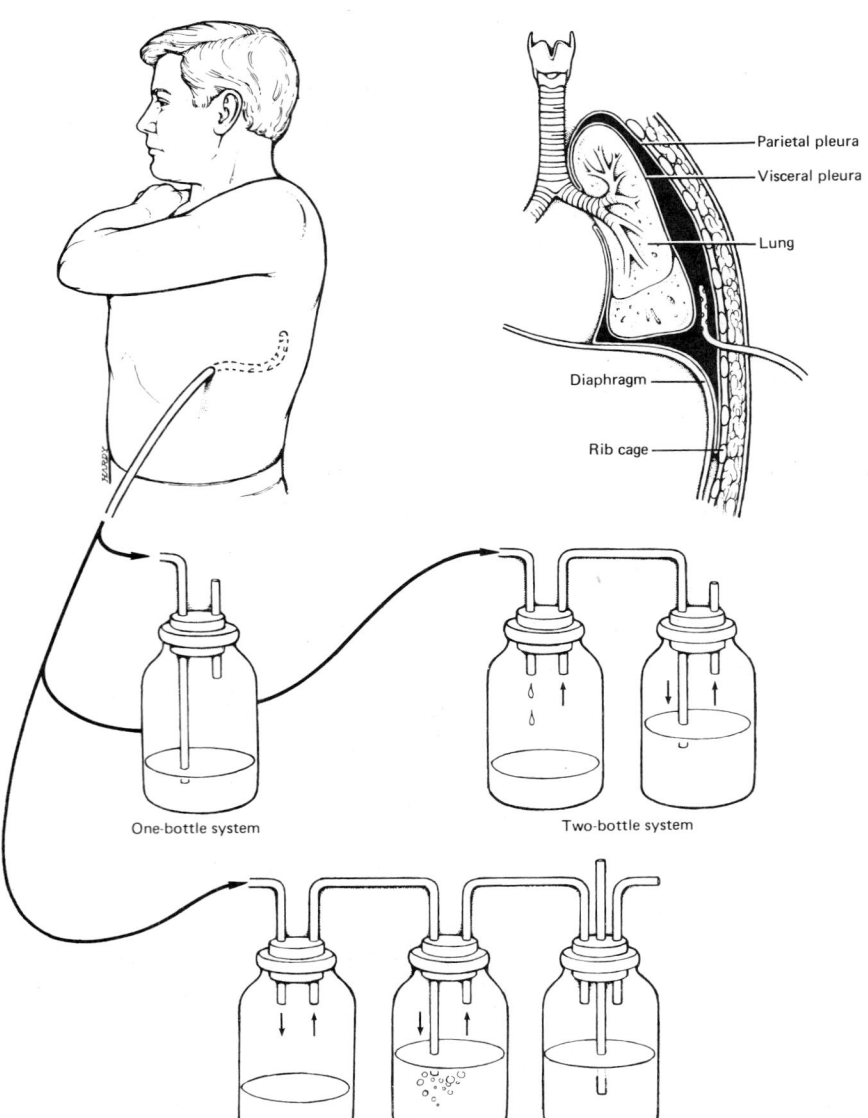

One-bottle system

Two-bottle system

Three-bottle system

Figure 24-7. One-, two-, and three-bottle chest drainage systems.

Parietal pleura

Visceral pleura

Lung

Diaphragm

Rib cage

▶ Evaluation

Expected Outcomes

1. Improves breathing
   a. Demonstrates low-pitched, deep, and controlled coughing to allow maximal lung expansion
   b. Uses incentive spirometer hourly while awake
   c. Demonstrates a respiratory rate within normal range; no periods of dyspnea
2. Is relieved of pain and discomfort
   a. Asks for pain medication, but verbalizes he expects some discomfort while deep breathing and coughing
   b. Splints incision with hands during coughing
   c. Uses controlled breathing during painful procedures, after coughing, etc.
3. Improves musculoskeletal functioning of affected arm and shoulder

   a. Extends his arm and reaches behind his head 3 times daily, increasing the repetition of the activity
   b. Stands in front of a mirror to check posture
4. Copes with anxiety
   a. Discusses his fears and expectations with health care professional
   b. Reads written instructions about posthospital management
   c. Listens to explanations
   d. Can relate goals of treatment and personal responsibility in achieving them
   e. Is willing to talk to social worker about future occupational counseling, etc.

Complications of Thoracic Surgery

Complications following thoracic surgery include cardiac arrhythmias, hemorrhage, respiratory insufficiency and fail-

(Text continues on page 471)

Chart 24-2
Assisting the Patient Undergoing Thoracic Surgery

The Challenge: Meticulous attention must be given to the preoperative and postoperative care of patients undergoing thoracic surgery, because these operations are wide in scope, obstructive pulmonary disease may be present, and the margin of safety is apt to be narrow.

Preoperative Goal: To ensure optimal patient condition for surgery

A. Determine the preoperative status of the patient, his physical assets, and his liabilities.
  1. Assist the patient undergoing diagnostic studies.
     a. History and physical examination
     b. Chest roentgenogram
     c. Pulmonary function studies (p. 444)—to ascertain if patient will have adequately functioning lung tissue after the operation
     d. Special diagnostic studies as required
     e. Baseline studies to ascertain any unsuspected abnormalities and to serve as a baseline reference during the postoperative period when indicated.
       (1) ECG—to disclose presence of arteriosclerotic heart disease or conduction defect
       (2) Blood urea nitrogen, serum creatinine—to obtain a "rough" measurement of renal function
       (3) Blood sugar or glucose tolerance—to detect unrecognized diabetes
       (4) Blood electrolytes, serum protein studies, and blood volume determinations as indicated
       (5) Arterial blood gas studies—to determine presence of hypoxemia/hypercapnia.
  2. Nursing assessment of the patient.
     a. What signs and symptoms are present—cough, expectoration, hemoptysis, chest pain?
     b. What is his smoking history—how long and how much? How much is he presently smoking?
     c. What is the patient's cardiopulmonary tolerance while bathing, eating, walking, etc.?
     d. What is the "physiologic age" of the patient—general appearance, mental alertness, behavior, degree of nutrition?
     e. What other medical conditions exist?
     f. What is his breathing pattern?
     g. How much exertion is required to produce dyspnea?
     h. What are his personal preferences and dislikes?

B. Improve alveolar ventilation and overall respiratory functions.
  1. Encourage the patient to stop smoking, since this increases bronchial irritation.
  2. Employ all measures to minimize pulmonary secretions.
     a. Measure sputum daily in patients with large volume of secretions to determine whether volume of secretions is decreasing.
     b. Instruct the patient to cough against a closed glottis to increase intrapulmonary pressure.
     c. Humidify the air to loosen secretions.
     d. Administer bronchodilators for bronchospasm.
     e. Give antibiotics for infection.
     f. Encourage deep breathing with the use of incentive spirometer.
     g. Employ IPPB therapy to improve pulmonary ventilation.
     h. Carry out postural drainage on patients with increased mucus production.
     i. Teach diaphragmatic breathing preoperatively.
     j. Set up a schedule of breathing exercises that encourage the use of abdominal muscles (p. 458).

C. Evaluate cardiovascular and pulmonary status so that complications may be anticipated and prevented.
  1. Study the results of diagnostic tests to learn of existing deviations from normal.
  2. Observe the patient and his reactions to various activities of daily living.
  3. Give cardiac drugs to patients in congestive heart failure.
  4. Correct anemia, dehydration, and hypoproteinemia—intravenous infusions, tube feedings, blood transfusions as indicated.

D. Prepare the patient for the surgical experience by reassurance, explanation, and skillful preoperative nursing care.
  1. Orient the patient to events in the postoperative period.
     a. Cough and breathing routine
     b. Presence of chest tube and drainage bottles
     c. Oxygen therapy; ventilator therapy
     d. Measures used to control discomfort
     e. Leg exercises; range of motion exercises for affected shoulder
     f. Coping measures (deep-breathing, turning, analgesics) for postoperative discomfort
  2. Encourage expression of psychologic and safety needs.
  3. See that consent form has been signed.

Postoperative Goal: To restore normal cardiopulmonary function as quickly as possible

A. Maintain an open airway.

B. Maintain constant nursing surveillance of the patient.
  1. Take blood pressure, pulse, respirations every 15 minutes or more frequently, as indicated; extend time interval according to the patient's clinical status.
  2. Evaluate character of respirations and patient's color.
  3. Evaluate character of drainage from the chest drainage bottles.
  4. Elevate the head of the bed to a 30- to 40-degree angle when the patient is oriented and his blood pressure is stabilized.

C. Aspirate all secretions with suctioning until patient is able to raise secretions effectively. (Endotracheal secretions are present in excessive amounts in post-thoracotomy patients owing to trauma to the tracheobronchial tree during operation, diminished lung ventilation, and cough reflex.)
  1. Carry out tracheal aspiration on "wet" semicomatose patients to prevent atelectasis.

(continued)

2. Indications for tracheal aspirations are determined by chest auscultation. (See p. 462 for technique of tracheal aspiration.)

3. Look for changes in the color and consistency of aspirates or sputum. Colorless fluid sputum is not unusual; opacification or coloring of sputum may indicate dehydration or infection.

D. Monitor the patient's ECG, since cardiac arrhythmias are more frequently seen after thoracic surgery (especially atrial fibrillation and atrial flutter). A patient with total pneumonectomy is especially prone to cardiac irregularity.

E. Give oxygen in the immediate postoperative period to assure maximum oxygenation—respirations are still depressed, and residual secretions in the peripheral respiratory passages may partially block gas exchange. Monitoring by means of arterial blood gas analysis is usually done.

F. Encourage deep-breathing exercises/sighing to achieve maximal lung inflation and to open closed airways.

G. Give aerosol therapy to reduce viscosity of secretions.

H. Listen to both sides of the chest with a stethoscope to determine if there are any changes in breath sounds.
   1. Are breath sounds normal, indicating free flow of air in and out of lungs?
   2. Are breath sounds distant? wheezing? crackles present?

I. Encourage and promote an effective cough routine.
   1. Sit patient on side of bed with feet supported on a chair if his condition permits.
   2. Support the chest firmly over the operated side and against opposite chest to lessen incisional pain (see Fig. 24-7).
   3. Instruct the patient to cough against a closed glottis (pull in the abdominal muscles) to increase intrapulmonary pressure.
   4. Assist the patient to cough at least every 1 to 2 hours during the first 24 hours and when necessary thereafter.

J. Maintain surveillance and careful management of the chest drainage system.*
   1. Monitor the chest drainage system, which is used to eliminate any residual air or fluid following thoracotomy.
   2. Check amount and character of drainage immediately after the operation and at necessary intervals thereafter—drainage should progressively decrease after first 12 hours.
   3. Persistence of bloody drainage indicates bleeding. Prepare for blood replacement and possible reoperation to achieve hemostasis.
   4. See Chart 24-1 for summary of the nurse's role in the management of the patient with water-seal drainage.

K. Provide intelligent pain relief, since pain limits chest excursions and thereby decreases ventilation.

1. Severity of pain varies with type of incision and the patient's reaction to and ability to cope with pain.
2. Narcotics and analgesics may assist patient to cough more effectively.
3. Narcotics and analgesics may make some patients too somnolent to cough.
4. Watch for signs of respiratory depression.
5. Assist patient having an intercostal nerve block for pain control.

L. Record hourly urinary output; the patient should excrete at least 30 ml of urine hourly after surgery.

M. Administer blood and parenteral fluids at a slower rate after thoracic surgery—Pulmonary edema owing to transfusion overload is an ever-present threat; following pneumonectomy, the pulmonary vascular system has been greatly reduced.

N. Maintain care in positioning the postoperative thoracotomy patient.
   1. Position patient flat in bed at intervals unless this produces dyspnea.
   2. Position patient in a semi-Fowler's position to permit residual air to rise to upper portion of pleural space and be removed via the upper chest catheter.
   3. Patients with limited respiratory reserve may not be able to turn on unoperated side, since this may limit ventilation of the operated side.

O. Anticipate and forestall complications.
   1. Hemorrhage
   2. Cardiac arrhythmias and cardiac complications
   3. Respiratory complications
   4. Pneumonitis; atelectasis
   5. Renal failure
   6. Pulmonary edema
   7. Gastric distention (Utilize nasogastric tube during the first 24 hours as directed.)

P. Restore normal range of motion and function of shoulder and trunk.
   1. Teach breathing exercises to mobilize thorax (p. 458).
   2. Encourage skeletal exercises to promote abduction and mobilization of shoulder.
   3. Ambulate as soon as pulmonary and circulatory systems are compensated.
   4. Encourage progressive activities according to development of fatigue.

Q. Patient Teaching Aspects
   1. There will be some intercostal pain for a period of time, which can be relieved by local heat and oral analgesia.
   2. Weakness and fatigability are common during the first 3 weeks following a thoracotomy.
   3. Range of motion exercises for the arm and shoulder on the affected side should be carried out several times daily to prevent "frozen shoulder."

* A patient with a pneumonectomy usually does not have water-seal chest drainage, since it is desirable that the pleural space fill with an effusion, which eventually obliterates this space. Some surgeons do use a "modified" water-seal system.

ure, persisent air leak, and bronchopulmonary fistula. Atelectasis related to retained secretions, blocked airway passages, airway closure, and altered surfactant is a threat. Gastric distention may occur. There appears to be an increased potential for myocardial infarction and congestive heart failure. Postpneumonectomy space infection can follow lung resection, occurring weeks to years after operation.

Rehabilitation

Rehabilitation begins preoperatively. The goal is to help the patient to return to the highest possible functional capacity. Because large shoulder girdle muscles are transected during thoracotomy, the arm and shoulder must be mobilized by full range of motion of the shoulder (see Fig. 24-6 and Table 24-1). The patient is taught to extend his arm (stretch and reach) and then reach behind his head. This accelerates recovery of muscle function affected by incision, pain, and "splinting," and reduces long-term pain and discomfort, particularly the development of adhesions. All joints should be stretched and flexed. The patient is encouraged to assume a functional erect position to restore normal posture. Other rehabilitation measures include breathing exercises and breathing retraining to improve the efficiency of pulmonary function.

Discharge Planning and Patient Education

The patient is advised of the following:

1. Be aware that:
   a. There is some intercostal pain for a period of time, which can be relieved by local heat and oral analgesia.
   b. Weakness and fatigability are common the first 3 weeks following thoracotomy. Alternate walking and other activities with frequent, short rest periods.
2. Continue with deep-breathing exercises for the first few weeks at home.
3. Practice good body alignment, preferably in front of a full-length mirror.
4. Practice exercises that were done while in the hospital.
   a. Range of motion exercises for the arm and shoulder should be done several times daily to prevent ankylosis of the shoulder ("frozen shoulder").
5. Avoid lifting more than 20 pounds until complete healing has taken place; the chest muscles may be weaker than normal for 3 to 6 months following surgery.
6. Walk at a moderate pace, and gradually extend walking time and distance. Be persistent.
7. Stop any activity immediately that causes undue fatigue, increased shortness of breath, or chest pain.
8. Because all or part of one lung has been removed, stay away from respiratory irritants (smoke, fumes, high air pollution).
   a. Avoid anything that may cause spasms of coughing.
   b. Sit in nonsmoking areas in public places.
9. Have an annual influenza injection if prescribed.
10. Report for follow-up care by the surgeon or clinic as necessary.

Summary

See Chart 24-2 for a summary of the nursing management of the patient undergoing thoracic surgery.

▷ Bibliography

Books

Aberman A and Logan AG (eds). Emergency Management of the Critically Ill. Chicago, Year Book Medical Publishers, 1980.

Brody JS and Snider GL (eds). Current Topics in the Management of Respiratory Diseases. New York, Churchill Livingstone, 1981.

Crompton GK. Diagnosis and Management of Respiratory Diseases. Oxford, Blackwell Scientific Publications, 1980.

Cumming G and Semple SJ. Disorders of the Respiratory System, 2nd ed. Oxford, Blackwell Scientific Publications, 1980.

DeVita VT Jr, Hellman S, and Rosenberg SAA. Cancer: Principles and Practice of Oncology. Philadelphia, JB Lippincott, 1982.

Emerson P. Thoracic Medicine. Boston, Butterworths, 1981.

Forgacs P. Problems in Respiratory Medicine. Lancaster, MTP Press, 1981.

Gothard JWW and Branthwaite MA. Anaesthesia for Thoracic Surgery. Boston, Blackwell Scientific Publications, 1982.

Grenard S and Traverse N. Introduction to Respiratory Therapy, 3rd ed. Chicago, Year Book Medical Publishers, 1981.

Guenter CA and Welch MH (eds). Pulmonary Medicine, 2nd ed. Philadelphia, JB Lippincott, 1982.

Harper RW. A Guide to Respiratory Care. Physiology and Clinical Applications. Philadelphia, JB Lippincott, 1981.

Margand PMS, Brooks CG Jr, and Hunter JW. Preoperative Pulmonary Preparation. A Clinical Guide. Baltimore, Williams & Wilkins, 1981.

Rarey K and Youtsey JW. Respiratory Patient Care. Englewood Cliffs, Prentice–Hall, 1981.

Roe BB. Perioperative Management in Cardiothoracic Surgery. Boston, Little, Brown & Co, 1981.

Scadding JG, Cumming G, and Thurlbeck WM. Scientific Foundations of Respiratory Medicine. Philadelphia, WB Saunders, 1981.

Sproule BJ, Lynne–Davies P, and King EG. Fundamentals of Respiratory Disease. New York, Churchill Livingstone, 1981.

Stringer LW. Emergency Treatment of Acute Respiratory Diseases, 3rd ed. Bowie, Maryland, Robert J Brady, 1982.

Traver GA. Respiratory Nursing: The Science and the Art. New York, John Wiley & Sons, 1982.

Williams MH. Essentials of Pulmonary Medicine. Philadelphia, WB Saunders, 1982.

Woolf CR. The Clinical Core of Respiratory Medicine. Philadelphia, JB Lippincott, 1981.

Articles
Therapeutics

Berdan–Ramberg M. Redefining chest physical therapy. Respir Ther 1981 Jan–Feb; 11(1):29–35.

Ellmyer P and Thomas NJ. A guide to your patient's safe home use of oxygen. Nursing '82 1982 Jan; 12(1):55–57.

Gale GD and Sanders DE. Incentive spirometry: Its value after cardiac surgery. Can Anaesth Soc J 1980 Sept; 27(5):475–480.

Hammon WE and Martin RJ. Chest physical therapy for acute atelectasis. Phys Ther 1981 Feb; 61(2):217–220.

Holody B and Goldberg HS. The effects of mechanical vibration physiotherapy on arterial oxygenation in acutely ill patients with atelectasis or pneumonia. Am Rev Respir Dis 1981 Oct; 124(4):372–375.

Kigin CM. Chest physical therapy for the postoperative or traumatic injury patient. Phys Ther 1981 Dec; 61(12):1724–1736.

Pontoppidan H. Mechanical aids to lung expansion in non-intubated surgical patients. Am Rev Respir Dis 1980 Nov; 122(5, Part 2):109–119.

Snider GL and Rinaldo JE. Oxygen therapy. Am Rev Respir Dis 1980 Nov; 122(5, Part 2):29–36.

Turton CWG. Pleural effusions. Br J Hosp Med 1980 Mar; 23(3):239–240;244;246,247 passim.

Weaver TE. New life for lungs—through incentive spirometry. Nursing '81 1981 Feb; 11(2):54–58.

Thoracic Surgery

Bartlett RH. Postoperative pulmonary prophylaxis. Chest 1982 Jan; 81(1):1–3.

Connolly JE. Thoracotomy and pulmonary resection. Surg Clin North Am 1980 Dec; 60(6):1481–1496.

Erickson R. Chest tubes: They're really not that complicated. Nursing '81 1981 May; 11(5):34–43.

Erickson R. Solving chest tube problems. Nursing '81 1981 June; 11(6):62–68.

Katz LE. Postoperative complications of thoracic surgery: Their recognition and treatment. AANA J 1980 June; 48(3):222–229.

Lockwood P, Lloyd M–H, and Williams GV. The value of a wide range of tests in the assessment of lung function in carcinoma of the bronchus. Br J Dis Chest 1980 July; 74(3):253–258.

Paul WL and Downs JB. Postoperative atelectasis. Arch Surg 1981 July; 116(7):861–863.

Skinner DB and Myerowitz PD. Recent advances in the management of thoracic surgical infections. Ann Thorac Surg 1981 Feb; 31(2):191–198.

Agencies
Governmental

National Heart, Lung and Blood Institute, National Institutes of Health, Bethesda, Maryland 20205

Voluntary

American Association for Respiratory Therapy, 7411 Hines Place, Suite 101, Dallas, Texas 75235

American Lung Association, 1740 Broadway, New York, New York 10019

American Thoracic Society, 1740 Broadway, New York, New York 10019

25

Respiratory Intensive Care

A large percentage of patients requiring intensive care need airway assistance and ventilation. The purpose of this chapter is to expand the nurse's understanding of these acute problems in order to provide optimum care to these critically ill persons. Detailed descriptions of techniques of respiratory care are included as well as the underlying factors that predispose patients to these problems.

First, however, it is necessary to gain an understanding of the basic terminology and concepts encountered in respiratory care.

▷ Terminology and Physiologic Concepts Related to Respiratory Care

Mechanics of Ventilation
Ventilation in its simplest definition is the movement of air in and out of the lungs by means of inspiration and expiration.

Inspiration.   Air flows from the atmosphere to the lungs in response to pressure gradients. As air is breathed in, the diaphragm and external intercostal muscles contract, causing the intrapleural pressure to become more subatmospheric or negative. This negative pressure expands the alveoli, which in turn causes atmospheric air to flow into the lungs. When equilibrium between the airway pressure and intrapleural pressure is achieved, the flow of air stops.

Expiration.   Normally, expiration is passive. When the inspiratory muscles relax, the contraction of the lungs squeezes air out of them. When the pressure gradient between the alveolar and intrapleural pressure is gone, the flow of air stops.

Tidal Volume and Dead Space
Tidal volume is the volume of air that is inspired during normal respiration. It is usually equal to 7 to 8 ml/kg of body weight. Part of the tidal volume enters the alveoli, and the rest stays in the conducting airways. Dead space is the

term applied to the volume of air in the conducting airways (nose, mouth, pharynx, larynx, trachea, and the bronchus down to the terminal bronchioles). The portion of the tidal volume that occupies the dead space cannot take part in oxygen uptake or carbon dioxide elimination.

If the blood supply to some alveoli stops for some reason or other, the gas occupying those alveoli cannot participate in gas exchange. These alveoli, then, function as dead space. To distinguish between the two types of dead space, the first is called *anatomical dead space* and the second *physiologic dead space*. In a normal adult the anatomical dead space is approximately 150 ml and the physiologic dead space is insignificant.

Alveolar Ventilation

When the anatomical dead space volume is subtracted from the tidal volume, the remaining volume is the alveolar ventilation. Alveolar ventilation is extremely important because it represents that portion of the tidal volume that is used for the exchange of oxygen and carbon dioxide in the alveoli. Because carbon dioxide diffuses across the alveolar-capillary membrane very rapidly, its concentration is the most sensitive indicator of the adequacy of alveolar ventilation. The usual measurement of carbon dioxide concentration is the partial pressure of carbon dioxide in arterial blood ($PaCO_2$). When the amount of carbon dioxide produced by body cells remains constant, the alveolar ventilation volume varies inversely with the $PaCO_2$. Thus, if alveolar ventilation decreases, the $PaCO_2$ increases proportionally. When the $PaCO_2$ rises above 40 mm Hg, alveolar hypoventilation is indicated. Conversely, when the volume of alveolar ventilation increases and the $PaCO_2$ falls below 40 mm Hg, hyperventilation is indicated. Clinically, a $PaCO_2$ range of 30 mm Hg to 50 mm Hg is often considered therapeutically acceptable for seriously ill patients.

Minute Ventilation

The volume of air expired through the nose and mouth each minute is referred to as *minute ventilation*. Minute ventilation is subdivided into alveolar ventilation and dead space ventilation, the normal distribution being two thirds to the alveoli and one third to dead space.

Vital Capacity

Vital capacity is the *maximum* volume of gas that can be expelled from the lungs by a forceful expiratory effort following a *maximum* inspiration. To measure the vital capacity, the patient is asked to inhale maximally and exhale *fully* through a gas meter (respirometer). The normal vital capacity is about 70 ml/kg of body weight.

Vital capacity is decreased in most lung diseases, abdominal distention, obesity, muscle weakness, and chest trauma and following upper abdominal or thoracic surgery.

Inspiratory Force

Deep breaths may be decreased or eliminated by central nervous system depression, disease, or drugs; when this occurs, vital capacity is not a useful measurement because a conscious cooperative effort is required for the test. In the unconscious or uncooperative patient the measurement of inspiratory force is substituted for vital capacity. *Inspiratory*

force is the maximum negative pressure that the patient can exert against an occluded airway. The normal inspiratory force is −100 cm H_2O.

Functional Residual Capacity (FRC)

Functional residual capacity is the volume of gas left in the lungs at the end of a normal expiration. It is usually approximately 2.5 liters. The actual volume depends on age, height, weight, sex, and body build. FRC is less in the supine than in the erect position and decreases even more in the head down position. In acute respiratory failure it is markedly diminished. Emphysematous patients, on the other hand, have increased FRC.

Closing Capacity

Small airways (0.5 mm to 0.9 mm in diameter) are easily collapsible. They are kept open by the pull of fibrous tissues attached to their outer surfaces, and this mechanism works only if the volume of the lung is above a certain value. If the lung volume is less than this, the airways close (collapse).

The volume of the lung at which a significant number of small airways close is known as the *closing capacity*. In a healthy young adult it is about 2 liters, and since the lung volume at the end of a normal expiration (FRC) is about 2.5 liters, the small airways always remain open.

With advancing age, the closing capacity gradually increases and may exceed the functional residual capacity. When this happens, significant numbers of small airways close at the end of a normal expiration, and some alveoli may be poorly ventilated. In respiratory distress syndome, extensive small airway closure occurs, leading to hypoxia.

Compliance

Compliance of the lung is the change in lung volume per unit change in pressure. It is a measure of the stiffness of the lung. The lower the compliance, the smaller the change in lung volume per unit change in pressure owing to increased stiffness of the lung.

The pressure change is the difference in pressure between the alveoli and the pleura at the beginning and end of inspiration. Pleural pressure is not routinely measured in clinical practice, and consequently compliance of the lung itself cannot be calculated. However, the combined compliance of the lung and the chest wall is easy to calculate. Acute changes in the compliance of the chest wall are uncommon and when they occur the reason is generally obvious (*e.g.,* tight chest bandage). Changes in the compliance of the lung and chest wall, therefore, usually reflect changes in the compliance of the lung. The greater the stiffness, the greater the pressure required to ventilate the lungs and the lower the compliance. As the condition of the lung improves, the compliance increases and the pressure required to ventilate the lung decreases.

Diffusion

Diffusion is the physical process by which gases move across the alveolar membrane. Gases move from a region of high pressure (tension) to a region of low pressure. Oxygen tension is about 104 mm Hg in the alveoli and 40 mm Hg in venous blood. Oxygen, therefore, moves from the alveoli into the blood. Carbon dioxide tension is about 40 mm Hg in the alveoli and about 45 mm Hg in venous blood. Carbon dioxide, therefore, moves from the venous blood into the alveoli.

Perfusion

Perfusion is the filling of the pulmonary capillaries with venous blood that has returned to the heart from the general circulation. The blood is pumped into the lungs by the right ventricle through the pulmonary artery. The pulmonary artery divides into the right and left branches to supply the two lungs. These two branches divide further to supply all parts of each lung.

The systolic and diastolic blood pressures in the pulmonary artery are about 22 mm Hg and 8 mm Hg respectively. Compared with 120 mm Hg and 80 mm Hg in the aorta, the pulmonary artery pressure is low. Consequently, in an erect position, the pulmonary artery pressure is not enough to supply blood to the apex of the lung against the force of gravity. Thus, when a person is in an erect position, the lung may be divided into three sections: an upper part with poor blood supply, a lower part with maximum blood supply, and the section in between the two with an intermediate supply of blood. When an individual turns to one side, more blood passes to the dependent lung.

Perfusion is also influenced by alveolar pressure. The pulmonary capillaries are sandwiched between adjacent alveoli. If the alveolar pressure is sufficiently high, the capillaries will be squeezed. Depending on the pressure, some capillaries will be completely collapsed, whereas others will be narrowed.

Pulmonary artery pressure, gravity, and alveolar pressure determine the patterns of perfusion. In lung disease these factors vary and the perfusion of the lung may become very abnormal.

Shunting

Normally about 2% of the blood pumped by the right ventricle does not perfuse the alveolar capillaries. This blood, which cannot participate in gas exchange with alveolar gas, is called *shunted blood*. It drains into the left heart through the bronchial, pleural, and thebesian veins. In some pathologic states of the heart and great vessels (ventricular septal defect, patent ductus arteriosus) and lung diseases (pulmonary edema, atelectasis) the amount of blood shunted exceeds the normal 2%.

The shunted blood, which contains the same amount of oxygen as venous blood, mixes with the blood returning from the alveoli to produce arterial blood. The oxygen content of the arterial blood depends on both the oxygen content and the volume of each fraction. Severe hypoxia results when the amount of blood shunted exceeds 20%. The hypoxia is not significantly improved by breathing even 100% oxygen because the oxygen does not come in contact with the shunted blood.

Distribution of Ventilation and Perfusion

Ventilation is the flow of gas in and out of the lung, and perfusion is the filling of the alveolar capillaries with blood. We have seen how the pulmonary artery pressure, gravity, and alveolar pressure lead to uneven perfusions of the lung.

Now we will discuss some of the factors leading to uneven ventilation of the lung and mismatching of ventilation and perfusion. The main factors controlling the distribution of ventilation are:

1. Patency of the airways
2. Local changes in compliance within the lung
3. Gravity

Any factor that reduces the airway caliber (mucosal edema, inflammation, secretion, bronchospasm) will raise the resistance to airflow and decrease the ventilation of the corresponding alveoli. Similarly, any area in which the local compliance has decreased (*i.e.,* that portion of the lung has become more stiff) will receive less ventilation than the surrounding more expandable portions of the lung.

The effect of gravity on ventilation is complex. Because of the consistency of the lung, its weight is distributed within the chest cavity in such a manner that the intrapleural pressure is less negative at the bottom (−2.5 cm of H_2O) than at the top of the lung (−10 cm of H_2O) in the erect position. The pressure within the airways is, however, the same in all parts of the lung. Consequently, the alveoli at the apex are larger than the alveoli at the base of the lung. When one applies these facts to the pressure-volume relationship of the lung, it becomes clear why, in the early phase of inspiration, more of the tidal volume is distributed to the basal region of the lung. The basal region of the erect lung, therefore, receives more blood and air than the apex.

For optimum gas exchange the perfusion of each alveolus must be matched by optimum ventilation. In addition to the pressure-volume relationship of the lung, there are other mechanisms, such as changes in caliber of airways or capillaries, that ensure that ventilation and perfusion are properly matched in the normal lung.

Mismatching of ventilation and perfusion leads to hypoxia. It appears to be the main cause of hypoxia following thoracic or abdominal surgery and most types of respiratory failure. Its effects are similar to those of shunts, except that breathing 100% oxygen eliminates hypoxia owing to mismatched ventilation and perfusion.

Partial Pressure

Partial pressure is the pressure exerted by each type of gas in a mixture of gases. The partial pressure of a gas is proportional to the concentration of that gas in the mixture. The total pressure exerted by the gaseous mixture is equal to the sum of the partial pressures.

The air we breathe is a gaseous mixture consisting mainly of nitrogen (78.62%) and oxygen (20.84%), with traces of carbon dioxide (.04%), water vapor (.05%), helium, argon, etc. The atmospheric pressure at sea level is about 760 mm Hg (mm Hg = torr). From this datum we may calculate the partial pressure of nitrogen and oxygen. Partial pressure of nitrogen is 79% of 760 (.79 × 760) = 600 torr, and that of oxygen is 21% of 760 (.21 × 760) = 160 torr.

The following is a reference list of expressions related to partial pressure:

P = pressure
PO_2—partial pressure of oxygen
PCO_2—partial pressure of carbon dioxide

P_AO_2—partial pressure of alveolar oxygen
P_ACO_2—partial pressure of alveolar carbon dioxide
P_aO_2—partial pressure of arterial oxygen
P_aCO_2—partial pressure of arterial carbon dioxide
P_vO_2—partial pressure of venous oxygen
P_vCO_2—partial pressure of venous carbon dioxide
P_{50}—oxygen tension at 50% hemoglobin concentration
torr—mm Hg

Once the air enters the trachea it becomes fully saturated with water vapor, which displaces some of the gases in order that the air pressure within the lung may remain equal with the air pressure outside (760 torr). Water vapor exerts a pressure of 47 torr when it fully saturates a mixture of gases at the body temperature of 37° C (98.6° F). Nitrogen and oxygen are therefore now responsible for the remaining 713 torr (760 − 47) pressure. Once this mixture enters the alveoli, it is further diluted by carbon dioxide. In the alveoli, the water vapor continues to exert a pressure of 47 torr. The remaining 713 torr pressure is now exerted as follows: nitrogen, 569 torr (74.9%); oxygen, 104 torr (13.6%); and carbon dioxide, 40 torr (5.3%).

When a gas is exposed to a liquid, the gas will dissolve in the liquid until an equilibrium is reached. The dissolved gas also exerts a partial pressure. At equilibrium, the partial pressure of the gas in the liquid is the same as the partial pressure of the gas in the gaseous mixture. Oxygenation of venous blood in the lung illustrates this point. In the lung, venous blood and alveolar oxygen are separated by a very thin alveolar membrane. Oxygen diffuses across this membrane to dissolve in the blood until the partial pressure of oxygen in the blood is the same as that in the alveoli (104 torr). However, since carbon dioxide is manufactured in the cells, venous blood contains carbon dioxide at a higher partial pressure than that in the alveolar gas. In the lung, carbon dioxide diffuses out of venous blood into the alveolar gas. At equilibrium, the partial pressure of carbon dioxide in the blood and in alveolar gas is the same (40 torr).

The entire sequence of changes in partial pressure readings (in torr) may be summarized as follows:

	Atmospheric Air	Tracheal Air	Alveolar Air
PH_2O	3.7	47.0	47.0
PN_2	597.0	563.4	569.0
PO_2	159.0	149.3	104.0
PCO_2	0.3	0.3	40.0
Total	760.0	760.0	760.0

Bicarbonate. A third component of blood, important in the assessment of respiratory function, is bicarbonate (HCO_3), which acts mainly as a buffer in maintaining acid-base balance as reflected in the blood *p*H (the concentration of hydrogen ions in the blood). Normal blood *p*H has a limited range of 7.38 to 7.44. An excess of hydrogen ions results in a *p*H below 7.38 (acidosis); a deficit of hydrogen ions results in a *p*H above 7.44 (alkalosis). The role of bicarbonate in regulating hydrogen ion concentration can be expressed chemically as:

$$CO_2 \text{ (carbon dioxide)} + H_2O \rightleftharpoons H_2CO_3 \text{ (carbonic acid)}$$
$$\rightleftharpoons H^+ \text{ (hydrogen ions)} + HCO_3^- \text{ (bicarbonate ion)}$$

The relationship of bicarbonate to carbon dioxide can also be ascertained from this formula, and it is this relationship that has a direct bearing on the assessment of respiratory function. In normal blood concentrations, the ratio of bicarbonate to carbonic acid (dissolved carbon dioxide) is 20 to 1. If there is an excess of carbon dioxide owing to poor respiratory function (respiratory acidosis), then the balance between the bicarbonate and carbonic acid is upset, at which point the kidneys, in an attempt to reestablish the correct ratio, will excrete less or no bicarbonate. A more complete explanation of the role of bicarbonate in carbon dioxide transport is found on page 478.

Oxygen Transport

Oxygen and carbon dioxide are carried simultaneously by virtue of their abilities to dissolve in blood or to combine with some of the elements of blood. Oxygen is carried in the blood in two forms: (1) as physically dissolved oxygen in the plasma; (2) in combination with the hemoglobin of the red blood cells. Each 100 ml of arterial blood carries 0.3 ml of O_2 physically dissolved in the plasma and 19 ml of O_2 in combination with hemoglobin. Note that the volume of O_2 carried by hemoglobin is considerably greater than that carried in physical solution.

The volume of oxygen physically dissolved in the plasma varies directly with the P_aO_2. The higher the P_aO_2, the greater the oxygen dissolved. For example, it is found that at a P_aO_2 of 10 mm Hg, 0.03 ml of oxygen is dissolved in 100 ml of plasma. At 20 mm Hg, twice this amount is dissolved in plasma and at 100 mm Hg, ten times this amount. Therefore, the amount of dissolved oxygen is directly proportional to the partial pressure, and this is true no matter how high the oxygen pressure rises. For example, in a hyperbaric chamber in which a subject is breathing oxygen at 3 atmospheres, the P_aO_2 would be 2000 mm Hg. The dissolved oxygen would be 6 ml of oxygen per 100 ml of blood.

The volume of oxygen that combines with hemoglobin also depends on P_aO_2, but only up to a P_aO_2 of about 150 mm Hg. Above this P_aO_2, hemoglobin is 100% saturated, by which we mean that hemoglobin will not combine with any additional oxygen. When hemoglobin is 100% saturated, 1 g of hemoglobin will combine with 1.34 ml of oxygen. Therefore, in a person with 14 g% of hemoglobin, each 100 ml of blood will contain about 19 ml of oxygen associated with hemoglobin. If the P_aO_2 is less than 150 torr, the percentage of hemoglobin saturated with oxygen is lower. For example, at a P_aO_2 of 100 torr (normal value) saturation is 97%, and at a P_aO_2 of 40 torr, the saturation is 70%.

The oxygen dissociation curve of hemoglobin (Fig. 25-1) shows the relationship between the partial pressure of oxygen and the percentage saturation of the hemoglobin more clearly. The unusual shape of the oxygen dissociation curve is a distinct advantage to the patient for several reasons:

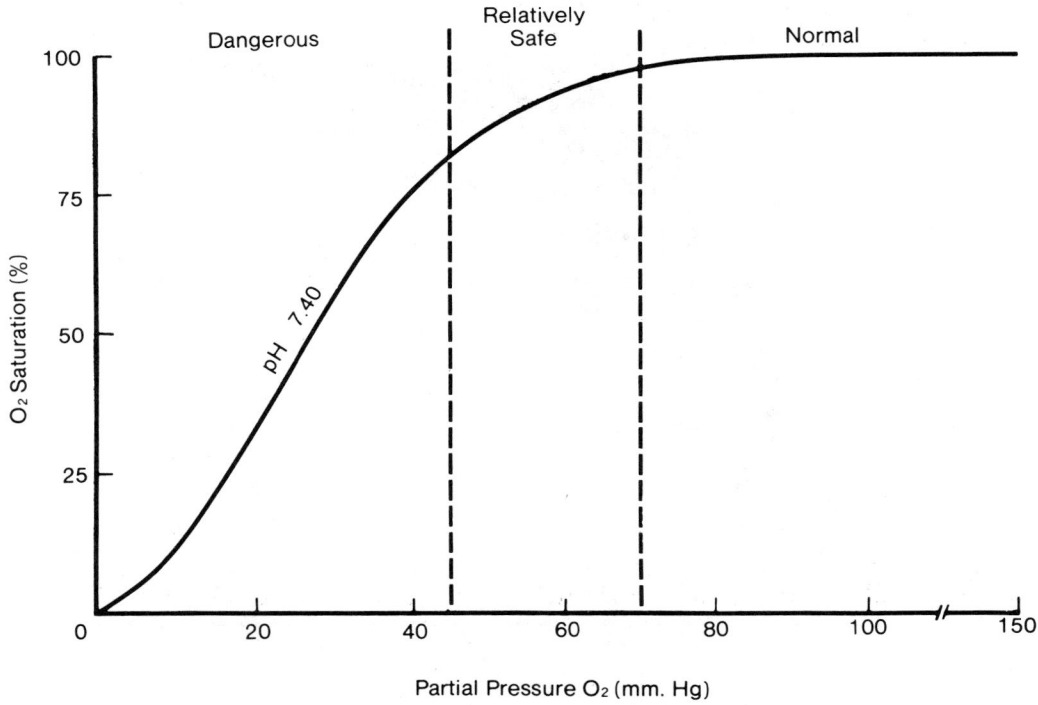

Figure 25-1. Oxygen–hemoglobin dissociation curve showing levels of pH that are normal, relatively safe, and dangerous.

1. If the arterial PO_2 decreases from 100 mm Hg to 80 mm Hg as a result of lung disease or heart disease, the hemoglobin of the arterial blood will still be almost maximally saturated (94%), and the tissues will not suffer from anoxia.
2. When the arterial blood passes into tissue capillaries and is exposed to the tissue tension of oxygen (about 40 mm Hg), hemoglobin gives up large quantities of oxygen for utilization by the tissues.

Oxygen Dissociation Curve

The oxygen dissociation curve indicates the methods used by the body to release oxygen to the tissues so that the oxygen obtained from the lungs is stored and then released to the tissues in amounts sufficient for their needs. The oxygen dissociation curve in Figure 25-1 is marked to show three levels of sufficiency: (1) normal levels—P_aO_2 above 70; (2) relatively safe levels—P_aO_2 45 to 70; and (3) dangerous levels—P_aO_2 below 40.

Figure 25-2 shows that at a normal pH of 7.40, the steep part of the curve is between a P_aO_2 of 40 torr (75% hemoglobin saturation) and 20 torr (33% hemoglobin saturation). P_{50} refers to the oxygen tension (27 torr) at 50% hemoglobin saturation. When we talk about changes in P_aO_2 and saturation, we talk about changes in P_{50}.

The oxygen hemoglobin dissociation curve will shift to either the right or the left, depending on the presence of the following: CO_2; hydrogen ion concentration (acidity); temperature; 2–3 diphosphoglycerate; and steroids.

A rise in these factors will shift the curve to the right, so that more oxygen is then released to the tissues at the same P_aO_2. A reduction in these factors will cause the curve to shift to the left, making the bond between oxygen and hemoglobin stronger, so that less oxygen is given up to the tissues at the same P_aO_2. In the diagram, the normal (middle) curve shows that 75% saturation occurs at a P_aO_2 of 40 torr. If the curve shifts to the right, the same saturation (75%) occurs at the higher P_aO_2 of 57 torr. If the curve shifts to the left, 75% saturation occurs at a P_aO_2 of 25 torr.

Clinical Significance. With a normal hemoglobin of 15 g/100 ml and a P_aO_2 level of 40 torr (oxygen saturation 75%), there is adequate oxygen available for the tissues, but there is no reserve. With a catastrophe (*e.g.,* bronchospasm, aspiration, hypotension, or cardiac arrhythmias), which reduces the intake of oxygen from the lungs, tissue hypoxia would result. The normal value of P_aO_2 is 60 to 80 torr (90% saturation). With this level of oxygenation, there is a 15% margin of excess oxygen available to the tissues.

An important consideration in the transport of oxygen is the cardiac output, which determines the amount of oxygen delivered to the body. Oxygen flux is the term given to the amount of oxygen delivered to the body per minute. For example, in a person with a hemoglobin concentration of 14 g% and hemoglobin saturation of 97%, each 100 ml of arterial blood will contain $(14 \times 1.34 \times .97) = 18.2$ ml of oxygen combined with hemoglobin. Each liter (1000 ml) of blood will contain 182 ml of oxygen. If the cardiac output is 5 liters per minute, the oxygen flux is 910 ml per minute, (182×5). If the cardiac output falls to 2.5 liters per minute, oxygen flux falls to 450 ml. This is why cardiac output measurements are so important. Not all of the oxygen delivered to the body is used up. In fact, only 250 ml of oxygen is

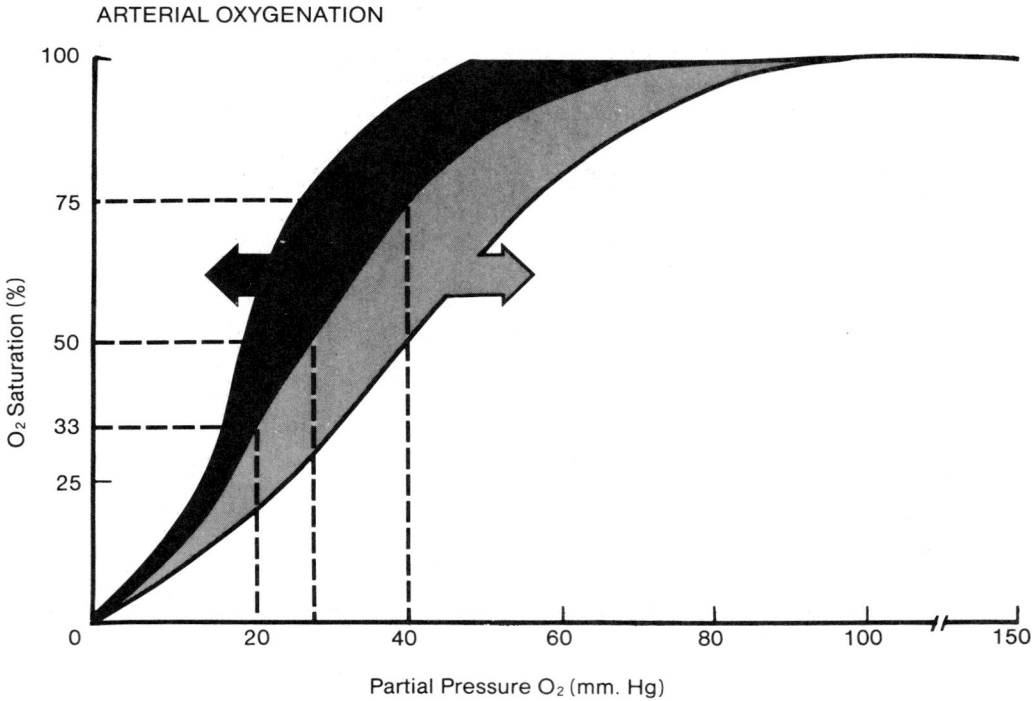

ARTERIAL OXYGENATION

Figure 25-2. Oxygen–hemoglobin affinity. A normal pH shows the steep arc of the curve between a PO_2 of 40 mm Hg (75% saturation) and 20 mm Hg (33% hemoglobin saturation). The diagram shows that at 75% hemoglobin saturation, the PO_2 is 57 mm Hg; when it shifts to the left, the PO_2 in the diagram is 25 mm Hg. P_{50} is normally 27 mm Hg. A shift to the right gives a higher P_{50}, and a shift to the left gives a lower P_{50}. (Adapted from Shapiro B: Clinical Application of Blood Gases. Chicago, Year Book Medical Publishers.)

used up per minute. The rest of the oxygen returns to the right heart, and the PO_2 of venous blood drops to about 40 mm Hg.

Carbon Dioxide Transport

Simultaneously with the diffusion of oxygen from the blood into the tissues, carbon dioxide diffuses in the opposite direction (*e.g.,* from tissue cells to blood) and is transported to the lung for excretion. The amount of carbon dioxide in transit is one of the major determinants of the acid–base balance of the body. Normally, only 6% of the venous CO_2 is removed and enough remains in the arterial side to exert a pressure of 40 torr. (Torr is gas tension in mm Hg.) Most of the carbon dioxide (95%) enters the red blood cells, and the small portion (5%) that remains dissolved in the plasma (PCO_2) is the critical factor that will determine carbon dioxide movement in or out of the blood. The dissolved carbon dioxide takes the form of carbonic acid (H_2CO_3), which is a volatile acid, that is, it undergoes a chemical reaction that changes it from a liquid to a gas (as CO_2), which explains why the blood concentration of carbonic acid (H_2CO_3) is controlled by alveolar ventilation. This is where bicarbonate exerts its influence as a stabilizing force. Note again the relationships of carbonic acid (H_2CO_3), hydrogen ion concentration ($pH^{\pm}$ or pH), and bicarbonate (HCO_3) in the chemical formula

$$CO_2 + H_2O \rightleftharpoons H_2CO_3 \rightleftharpoons H^+ + HCO_3^-$$

The bicarbonate and hemoglobin in the red blood cells allow great quantities of carbon dioxide to be carried in the blood with little or no pH change. This buffering is essential, and it occurs because 30% of carbon dioxide is carried directly on the hemoglobin and 65% is buffered by hemoglobin through the bicarbonate mechanism. The ratio of plasma bicarbonate concentration (primarily controlled by the kidney) to plasma carbonic acid concentration (primarily controlled by the lungs) determines the pH.

Of critical importance is the relationship between the carbon dioxide that is carried as the compound sodium bicarbonate ($NaHCO_3$) and that which is in physical solution in the plasma (PCO_2). The former is referred to as the bound CO_2 and the latter as the dissolved. Under normal conditions, the ratio of the bound to the dissolved CO_2 is remarkably constant at 20:1. Such a ratio is essential to maintain normal acid–base balance of the blood. (The plasma bicarbonate ion concentration is primarily controlled by the renal system, but to a lesser extent is affected by the respiratory system.)

The whole process of oxygen and carbon dioxide transport together with formation of bicarbonate (HCO_3) is summarized as follows:

Tissue Level
1. CO_2 enters the red blood cells, combines with H_2O to form carbonic acid (H_2CO_3).
2. At the same time, hemoglobin releases O_2 to the tissues and becomes reduced hemoglobin (HHb).

3. H_2CO_3 dissociates into H^+ and bicarbonate (HCO_3^-).
4. Reduced hemoglobin (HHb) and HCO_3^- are carried in the venous system to the lungs.

Lung Level
1. Reduced hemoglobin takes up O_2 and gives off H^+.
2. HCO_3^- combines with H^+ to give H_2CO_3.
3. H_2CO_3 dissociates into $H_2O + CO_2$ (expired air).

In summarizing respiratory gas transport, it is important to emphasize that the many processes described do not take place in intermittent stages but occur rapidly, simultaneously, and continuously.

▷ Assessment in Respiratory Intensive Care

Monitoring is a very vital part of respiratory intensive care nursing. Prompt recognition, accurate assessment, and proper management of any adverse changes in the critically ill patient depend entirely on the quality of monitoring. For good reasons, the current trend is toward greater sophistication in monitoring.

There are certain vital signs that should be monitored frequently if not continuously. Blood pressure, heart rate, respiratory rate, and temperature belong to this category. Frequent electrocardiograms are also necessary. Daily chest x-ray is required on all patients on the ventilator. Serum electrolytes, hematocrit, hemoglobin, and white cell count should be checked at frequent intervals. The total daily fluid intake and output and daily weight must be noted to monitor the fluid balance. Certain respiratory and cardiovascular parameters also should be monitored in all critically ill patients (Chart 25-1).

Chest Auscultation

Care of the critically ill patient requires frequent inspection and auscultation of the chest. The important factor to consider is whether breath sounds are present or absent. Presence of normal breath sounds is proof that air is entering the lungs. Absence of breath sounds in areas where they should be heard suggests that although perfusion is present the alveoli are not getting air. Serial auscultation of the chest will allow the nurse to confirm the presence of air exchange, to know when tracheobronchial aspiration is required, and to prevent ventilatory catastrophes. Changes in the aforementioned factors indicate that treatment needs to be modified.

Preparation of the Patient

Careful auscultation of the chest requires some preparation:

- Keep the room as quiet as possible so that distracting noises do not interfere with the sound of the patient's breathing.
- Have the room warm enough to keep the patient from shivering, which can alter the sounds heard from the stethoscope.
- Warm the diaphragm, the large, flat portion of the stethoscope, by holding it in the palm of your hand before placing it directly on the patient's chest.

Chart 25-1
Parameters for Monitoring Respiratory Care

Basic Monitoring	**Fluid Balance**
Blood pressure	Fluid intake
Heart rate	Fluid output
Respiratory rate	Weight
Temperature	
Electrocardiogram	**Blood Tests**
	Electrolytes
Respiratory Parameters	Hemoglobin and hematocrit
Chest auscultation	White cell count
Tidal volume	
Vital capacity	**Urinalysis**
Respiratory force	
Compliance	**Cardiovascular Parameters**
Inspired oxygen concentration	Pulmonary capillary wedge pressure
Alveolar to arterial oxygen tension difference	Cardiac output
Chest X-ray	

- Place the diaphragm firmly on the patient's chest to improve sound transmission, and instruct the patient to breathe deeply and through his mouth so nasal air turbulence will not distort the sounds heard.
- If possible, have the patient in a sitting position with arms relaxed and shoulders rotated slightly forward. This position produces maximal chest expansion while exposing as much lung surface as possible under the stethoscope.
- Begin auscultation at the lung apices, and proceed from the top to the bottom of the lungs, comparing sides of the chest. Listen to one entire breathing cycle at each location. This is important because the duration and quality of the sound may vary with inspiration and expiration.
- Listen to both the anterior and posterior chest. Remember that because of the configuration of the lungs, the anterior and middle or lingular segments of the lungs are heard best anteriorly, while the basal lung segments are more exposed posteriorly.

Breath Sounds and Their Significance
Normal Breath Sounds.   There are three categories of normal breath sounds: (1) vesicular, (2) bronchial or tracheal, and (3) bronchovesicular.

Vesicular breath sounds are heard over most of the lung fields and appear breezy and swishy in character. Inspiration is high-pitched and predominates over expiration. Expiration is low-pitched and both shorter and fainter than inspiration.

Bronchial or tracheal breathing is heard normally over the trachea and main bronchi. Inspiration is louder than expiration and high-pitched. Expiration is of increased duration, so much so that it actually is longer than inspiration. Its pitch is higher and of greater intensity. It has a harsh, tubular quality.

Bronchovesicular breath sounds represent an intermediate stage. They are heard normally in the second interspace anteriorly, in the interscapular area posteriorly, and often at the medial right apex. Inspiration is unchanged from that of vesicular breathing, but expiration is as loud, equal in length, and similar in pitch.

Abnormal Breath Sounds. Crackles are abnormal additional or adventitious sounds and are always pathologic. They may be subdivided into (1) rhonchi—continuous coarse sounds; and (2) moist crackles—interrupted crackling sounds. These abnormal sounds indicate the presence of fluid somewhere in the respiratory tract. The fluid or exudate may result from infection, inflammation, aspiration, edema, or retained secretions.

- The presence of rhonchi implies disease of the larger bronchi. Moist, medium, and fine crackles imply bronchiolar and alveolar disease. Rhonchi are usually heard earlier in inspiration than are crackles, since sound is produced when the column of inspired air meets the exudate at its anatomic location.

Assessment of Lung Volumes

Tidal Volume

The volume of each breath is referred to as the *tidal volume*. The simplest instrument commonly used to measure volumes at the bedside is known as the Wright respirometer (Fig. 25-3).

If the patient is breathing via an endotracheal tube or tracheostomy, the respirometer is directly attached to it and the exhaled volume is read off the dial. In others, the respirometer is attached to a face mask, which is placed to cover the nose and mouth so that it is airtight, and the exhaled volume is measured as before. Hand-held electronic respirometers that provide digital readouts of lung volumes are also available.

The tidal volume may vary from breath to breath. To make the measurement reliable the volumes of several breaths must be measured, and the range of tidal volumes together with the average tidal volume must be noted. The normal tidal volume is 7 to 8 ml per kg body weight. When the tidal volume falls below 5 ml per kg body weight, mechanical ventilation is usually required.

Ventilation Pattern

The normal pattern of ventilation includes approximately 6 to 10 deep breaths or sighs per hour, each considerably larger than tidal volume. If no breaths are larger than tidal volume, alveolar collapse occurs, because not all alveoli are opened with each breath. Alveolar collapse (atelectasis) produces unventilated areas with continued blood flow, and physiologic dead space increases.

Ventilation at low tidal volumes without sighs may produce microatelectasis in as little as 1 hour's time, but periodic deep breaths keep the alveoli open. This is the reason for encouraging postoperative patients to take deep breaths and for using incentive spirometry to increase tidal volume.

Patient Teaching. When teaching a patient to breathe deeply, keep these points in mind:

- Emphasize inspiratory maneuvers. Expiratory maneuvers, such as blow bottles, blow gloves, and coughing, may actually produce alveolar deflation by generating pleural pressures that are higher than airway pressures. Coughing should only be encouraged for patients who have an accumulation of secretions in the airways.
- Emphasize sustained maximal inspirations. Taking a deep breath helps keep pulmonary oxygen levels higher if it is maintained for a few seconds. An incentive spirometer, when used properly, can help prolong alveolar inflation time. If the patient is unable to breathe properly with an incentive spirometer, have him breathe deeply and count to three at end-inspiration with his glottis open.
- Positioning is important. Functional residual capacity is less in a supine position. Have the patient dangle on the side of the bed or sit in a semi-Fowler's position. The patient's upper body must be relaxed to produce maximal chest expansion. Support the patient's arms at his sides or across his abdomen so he is not using his arms to support his position in bed. The knees should be slightly flexed to relax the abdominal muscles.

Respiratory Rate

The normal adult who is resting comfortably breathes at 18 to 20 breaths per minute. Except for occasional sighs, the breathing is reasonably regular.

- Slow breathing is associated with raised intracranial pressure, brain injury, and drug overdose.
- Rapid breathing is commonly seen in pneumonia, pulmonary edema, metabolic acidosis, septicemia, and rib fracture.

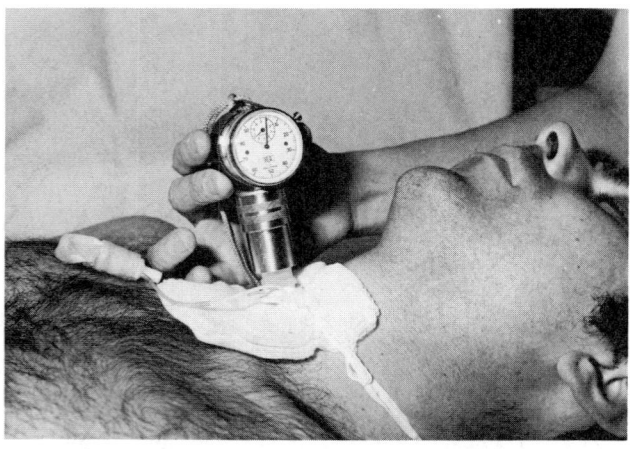

Figure 25-3. The Wright respirometer connected to a tracheostomy tube with the cuff inflated. The small dial measures the tidal volume and vital capacity. The large dial measures the minute volume.

When the rate of breathing falls outside the range of 14 to 25, mechanical ventilation may be necessary. Some patients who are breathing spontaneously may develop respiratory arrest. It is most likely to occur in patients with brain injury or following neurosurgery. Therefore, these patients require continuous monitoring of their respiration. There are instruments now available that will carry out this function.

Minute Ventilation

Tidal volume and respiratory rates alone are unreliable indicators of the adequacy of ventilation because both can vary widely from breath to breath. Together, however, the tidal volume and respiratory rate are important because they determine the minute ventilation, which is useful in the detection of respiratory failure. Minute ventilation is the volume of air expired per minute. It is equal to the product of the tidal volume (V_T) and respiratory rate or frequency (f) according to the equation:

$$\dot{V}E = V_T \times f$$

In practice, the minute ventilation is not calculated but measured directly using a respirometer. Minute ventilation may be decreased by a variety of conditions, including those that:

- Limit neurologic impulses transmitted from the brain to the respiratory muscles, such as spinal cord trauma, cerebrovascular accidents (CVAs), tumors, myasthenia gravis, Guillain–Barré syndrome, and polio.
- Depress respiratory centers in the medulla, as with anesthesia and narcotic sedative overdose
- Affect the lungs by:
    Limiting thoracic movement: kyphoscoliosis
    Limiting lung movement: pleural effusion, pneumothorax
    Reducing functional lung tissue: chronic pulmonary diseases, severe pulmonary edema

When the minute ventilation falls, the amount of alveolar ventilation reaching the lungs must also decrease, and the P_aCO_2 increases.

- Remember, do not rely on visual inspection of the rate and depth of a patient's respiratory excursions to determine the adequacy of ventilation. Respiratory excursions may appear normal or exaggerated, but the patient may actually be moving only enough air to ventilate his dead space.

Alveolar Ventilation

An adequate minute ventilation does not necessarily mean that alveolar ventilation is sufficient. Normally, two thirds of the minute ventilation is used for gas exchange and one third for dead space according to the following equation:

$$\begin{array}{ccccc} \dot{V}E & = & \dot{V}A & + & \dot{V}D \\ \text{ventilation} & & \text{ventilation} & & \text{Dead space} \\ 3/3 & & 2/3 & + & 1/3 \end{array}$$

Rearranging this equation,

$$\begin{array}{ccc} \dot{V}A & = & \dot{V}E - \dot{V}D \\ 2/3 & & 3/3 - 1/3 \end{array}$$

it becomes evident that either a reduction in minute ventilation or an increase in dead space can diminish the volume of alveolar ventilation.

The body tends to keep the arterial PCO_2 at 40 torr (mm Hg) by maintaining the alveolar ventilation, and therefore the CO_2 elimination, reasonably constant. This implies that if the dead space increases, the minute ventilation must increase to compensate for the wasted ventilation of the dead space. If the patient cannot increase minute ventilation, alveolar ventilation falls, carbon dioxide accumulates in the body, and the PCO_2 will increase.

An increase in dead space is usually produced by abnormalities in ventilation and blood flow produced by conditions such as atelectasis, pneumonia, pulmonary edema, and chronic obstructive lung disease.

- A good rule of thumb is to remember that most patients can double their resting minute ventilation in an attempt to maintain an adequate alveolar ventilation when dead space increases. Above this level, they may become too fatigued.

When the minute ventilation exceeds 10 liters per minute, mechanical ventilation is usually required. When a patient is mechanically ventilated, the tidal volume and respiratory rate are chosen to provide a minute ventilation that maintains the arterial PCO_2 at 40 torr. Occasionally a higher or lower PCO_2 is desirable.

Assessment of Breathing Ability

Tests of the patient's breathing ability can be easily assessed at the bedside by measuring the vital capacity, forced expiratory volume, inspiratory force, and compliance. These tests are particularly important for patients at risk of developing pulmonary complications, including those who have undergone chest or abdominal surgery, have experienced prolonged anesthesia, have pre-existing pulmonary disease, or are elderly.

Patients whose chest expansion is limited by external restrictions such as obesity or abdominal distention and who are unable to breathe deeply because of postoperative pain or sedation produce low tidal volumes. Ventilation at low tidal volumes without sigh inflations can produce alveolar collapse. The functional residual capacity falls, lung compliance is reduced, and the patient must breathe faster to maintain the same degree of tissue oxygenation. These events can be exaggerated in patients who have pre-existing pulmonary diseases and in elderly patients whose airways are less compliant owing to earlier closure of small airways during the expiratory cycle.

Vital Capacity

Vital capacity is measured by having the patient inspire maximally and exhale fully through a respirometer. The normal value depends on age, sex, body build, and weight.

- Most patients can generate a vital capacity twice their predicted tidal volume. If the vital capacity is less than 10 ml per kg of body weight, the patient will be too weak to sustain spontaneous ventilation, and respiratory assistance will be required.

When the vital capacity is exhaled at a maximum flow rate, the forced vital capacity (FVC) is measured. Most patients can exhale at least 75% of their vital capacity in 1 second, (forced expiratory volume in 1 second, or FEV_1) and almost all of it in 3 seconds, (FEV_3). A reduction in the FEV_1 suggests abnormal pulmonary air flow. If a patient's FEV_1 and FVC are proportionately reduced, his maximum lung expansion is restricted in some way. If the reduction in FEV_1 greatly exceeds the reduction in FVC, the patient may have some degree of airway obstruction.

Inspiratory Force

Inspiratory force quantitates the effort a patient is making during inspiration. It does not require patient cooperation and hence is useful in the unconscious patient. The equipment needed for this measurement includes (1) a manometer that measures negative pressure and (2) adapters for connection to an anesthetic mask or a cuffed endotracheal tube. The manometer is attached and the airway is completely occluded (Fig. 25-4). This is continued for 10 to 20 seconds while the inspiratory efforts of the patient are registered on the manometer. The normal inspiratory pressure is -100 cm of H_2O. If the negative pressure registered after 15 seconds of occluding the airway is less than -25 cm of H_2O, mechanical ventilation is usually required, because the patient lacks sufficient muscle strength for deep breathing or effective coughing.

Compliance

When a patient is mechanically ventilated, his ease of breathing can be quickly and easily estimated by measuring his compliance. This is accomplished by dividing the tidal volume delivered to the patient by the maximal pressure required to deliver that volume. If the patient is on PEEP (see p. 489), this pressure must be subtracted from the maximum pressure developed during ventilation.

For example, if the tidal volume is 450 ml and the maximum pressure is 15 cm of H_2O, compliance is estimated to be $450 \div 15$ or 30 ml/cm H_2O. But, if 20 cm of water pressure is later required to deliver the same tidal volume, compliance has decreased ($450 \div 20 = 22.5$ ml/cm H_2O).

Because this estimate of compliance is made while air is flowing into the lungs, it reflects changes in air flow resistance as well as lung and chest wall compliance (lung stiffness). Low compliance is a characteristic finding in pneumothorax, hemothorax, pleural effusion, and most acute illnesses of the lung. Compliance is useful in assessing the progress of the disease in respiratory distress syndrome.

- Generally speaking, a rapid reduction in compliance suggests air flow resistance, such as with accumulated secretions. A gradual compliance reduction suggests progressive decreases in lung and chest wall compliance from conditions that restrict lung expansion, such as pleural effusion or atelectasis.

Assessment of Gas Exchange

Arterial Blood Gases

Arterial oxygen and carbon dioxide tensions (P_aO_2, P_aCO_2) and pH must be measured at frequent intervals when managing patients with respiratory problems. The P_aO_2 indicates the degree of oxygenation of the blood, and the P_aCO_2 indicates adequacy of alveolar ventilation. Whenever changes are made in the inspired oxygen concentration, tidal volume, or respiratory rate, arterial blood gases should be measured after allowing 20 to 30 minutes for alveolar and blood gases to equilibrate.

About 3 ml of arterial blood is required for gas analysis. Arterial puncture is performed on areas where good pulses are palpable (*e.g.,* radial, brachial, or femoral artery).

Procedure
- With the left hand, feel along the course of the artery and palpate for pulsation with the middle and index fingers. With the right hand, hold a No. 20 gauge needle and heparinized glass syringe (0.05 ml of 1% sodium heparin for every ml of blood) at a 90-degree angle to the surface. Anchor the wrist to the surface to allow finer control of the needle.
- With the right hand, insert the needle between the closely approximated middle and index fingers of the left hand, aiming at the pulsating artery (Fig. 25-5). It is easier to obtain a sample with a glass syringe, because once the artery is punctured, arterial pressure will push up the plunger of a glass syringe; as a result, air is less likely to enter the sample. After the blood is obtained, apply pressure on the punctured area for 5 minutes to avoid a hematoma.
- Cap the syringe, and place the arterial blood sample in an iced container as it waits analysis. The lower temperature reduces the metabolism and minimizes the alteration of the true values of oxygen, carbon dioxide, and pH.

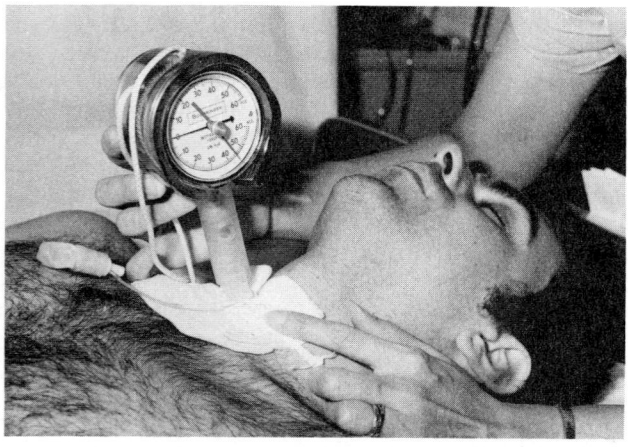

Figure 25-4. Measurement of inspiratory force. The inspiratory force manometer is connected to the tracheostomy tube. The tracheostomy cuff should be inflated. Plug the hole in the connector between the tracheostomy and manometer so that the airway is obstructed on inspiration. Negative inspiratory force is reflected at -45 cm H_2O pressure. Allow the patient to breathe between measurements by unplugging the hole.

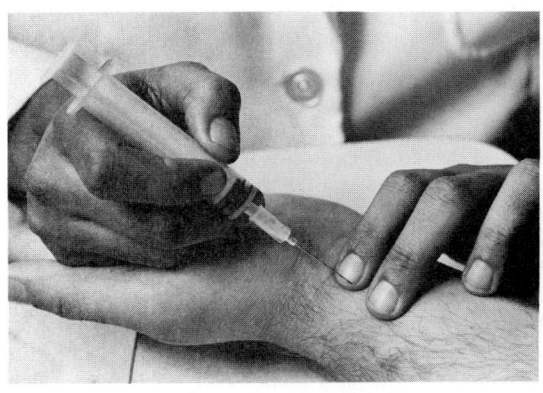

Figure 25-5. Technique of arterial puncture for blood gas analysis.

Precautions
1. Use aseptic technique.
2. Avoid frequent puncture in the same place because of the danger of local aneurysmal dilatation.
3. Do not insert the needle deeper than 0.5 cm (unless necessary), since in most cases this artery is located close to the surface.
4. Know the anatomy in order to avoid trauma to adjacent nerves.
5. Palpate for the presence of the ulnar artery before puncturing the radial artery.

If repeated arterial blood gas determinations are planned, an arterial catheter may be left in the radial artery. However, this may compromise the blood flow through the artery. Before the catheter is inserted, an Allen test (see below) is done to check the adequacy of blood flow through the ulnar artery, so that the perfusion of the hand is not compromised even if the radial artery is blocked. The Allen test is done by causing the hand to blanch and then occluding the radial artery and watching the blood flow to the hand by way of the ulnar artery. This ensures collateral circulation even if thrombosis of the radial artery should occur. It is performed in the following manner:

- If the patient is conscious, ask him to clench his fist while the nurse obliterates the radial and ulnar pulses simultaneously at the wrist. Then ask the patient to unclench his fist and observe the blanching of the palm. Release pressure on the ulnar artery while compressing the radial artery and watch for the return of skin color. If flow through the ulnar artery is good, flushing of the palm will be seen instantaneously.
- If the patient is unconscious, elevate his hand above the heart and squeeze or compress the hand until blanching occurs. Now obliterate the radial and ulnar pulses simultaneously at the wrist. Lower the hand while compressing the radial and ulnar arteries. Then release the pressure on the ulnar artery and watch for the return of skin color as above.

Because indwelling arterial catheters can be used to accurately monitor systolic and diastolic blood pressure,

they are widely used in intensive care units for hemodynamic monitoring as well as arterial gas sampling. Oxygenation can, however, be monitored less invasively using ear oximetry and transcutaneous sensors. An ear oximeter is a device that analyzes light transmission through the pinna of the ear. Oxygen saturations measured by ear oximetry correlate highly with direct measurements of arterial blood saturations. These devices are particularly useful for monitoring PO_2 levels in patients with chronic obstructive lung disease who are susceptible to the development of CO_2 narcosis during oxygen therapy.

Transcutaneous PO_2 measurements are obtained by heating the skin and measuring the PO_2 through cutaneous tissue with an oxygen sensing electrode. In healthy adults, transcutaneous O_2 measurements accurately reflect arterial PO_2 levels. However, both ear oximetry and transcutaneous measurements may correlate poorly with P_aO_2 levels when a patient is hemodynamically compromised, because reductions in cardiac output or poor circulation create venous stasis and oxygen desaturation.

Carbon dioxide can also be monitored less invasively by obtaining expired gas samples and using an infrared CO_2 analyzer or a mass spectrometer to estimate alveolar CO_2 partial pressures. In many instances, end-expired CO_2 partial pressures remain fairly constant in relation to arterial PCO_2 levels and can be used as an ongoing estimate of the P_aCO_2 to detect hypoventilation and assess the patient's tolerance to clinical procedures such as intubation or extubation, and ventilator placement or weaning.

Inspired Oxygen Concentration
The air we breathe contains 21% of oxygen by volume. In other words, the fraction of oxygen in inspired air is 0.21 (fraction = %/100). The fraction of inspired oxygen (F_IO_2) may be increased by adding oxygen to the inspired air (see oxygen therapy for respiratory failure). If the F_IO_2 is not adequate, hypoxia and death will result. Too high an F_IO_2, on the other hand, will lead to needless oxygen toxicity. To ensure that the F_IO_2 is just right, an oxygen analyzer must be used from time to time to measure the concentration of oxygen in the inspired gas.

Alveolar–Arterial Oxygen Tension Difference
The difference in oxygen tension between the alveolar gas (P_AO_2) and arterial blood (P_aO_2) is a measure of the efficiency of the lung as an oxygenator. A sample of arterial blood is easily obtainable to measure the P_aO_2. Unfortunately, a representative sample of alveolar gas cannot be obtained to measure the P_AO_2. However, if the values of the F_IO_2 and P_aCO_2 (CO_2 tension in arterial blood) are known, an acceptable value of P_AO_2 may be calculated from the following formula:

$$P_AO_2 = (713 \times F_IO_2) - P_aCO_2 \times 1.25)$$

Example: If a man breathing room air ($F_IO_2 = 0.21$) has an arterial blood carbon dioxide tension ($P_A{-}CO_2$) of 40 torr (mm Hg), then his P_AO_2 is 99.73 torr.

$$P_{(A-a)}O_2 = P_AO_2 - P_aO_2$$

The normal lung is an efficient oxygenator and the normal range $P_{(A-a)}O_2$ is 5 to 15 torr. Shunts and mismatched ventilation/perfusion renders the lung an inefficient oxygenator. This will become evident by widening of the $P_{(A-a)}O_2$.

Pulmonary Capillary Wedge Pressure (PCW Pressure)

Pulmonary capillary wedge pressure is obtained by using a specially designed cardiac catheter known as the Swan–Ganz catheter. In its simplest design it is a double lumen catheter (Fig. 25-6). The larger of the two lumens is open at both ends and is used for measuring pressures and obtaining pulmonary arterial blood samples. The lumen must be flushed continuously or intermittently with heparinized solution. The other lumen is used to inflate a balloon situated at the tip of the catheter with about 1 ml of air. When the balloon is inflated, it has a diameter of 11 mm to 13 mm, and it surrounds and hides the tip of the catheter.

The catheter is inserted via a large peripheral vein under continuous monitoring of the ECG and the venous pressure through the catheter lumen. When the catheter tip enters the thorax, the venous pressure tracing will show fluctuation with respiration. The balloon is now inflated and the catheter advanced. Blood flow carries the balloon as if it were an embolus and guides the catheter through the right atrium and tricuspid valve into the right ventricle and thence into the pulmonary artery. During insertion the position of the balloon and catheter tip at any moment is reflected in the pressure tracing (Fig. 25-6). The balloon will finally end up (like an embolus) in one of the branches of the pulmonary artery, where it obstructs the flow of blood through that artery; it is now said to be wedged. The pressure recorded is called the pulmonary capillary wedge (PCW) pressure.

The balloon serves three purposes: (1) it guides the catheter; (2) it covers the tip of the catheter and prevents it from irritating the myocardium, which greatly reduces the

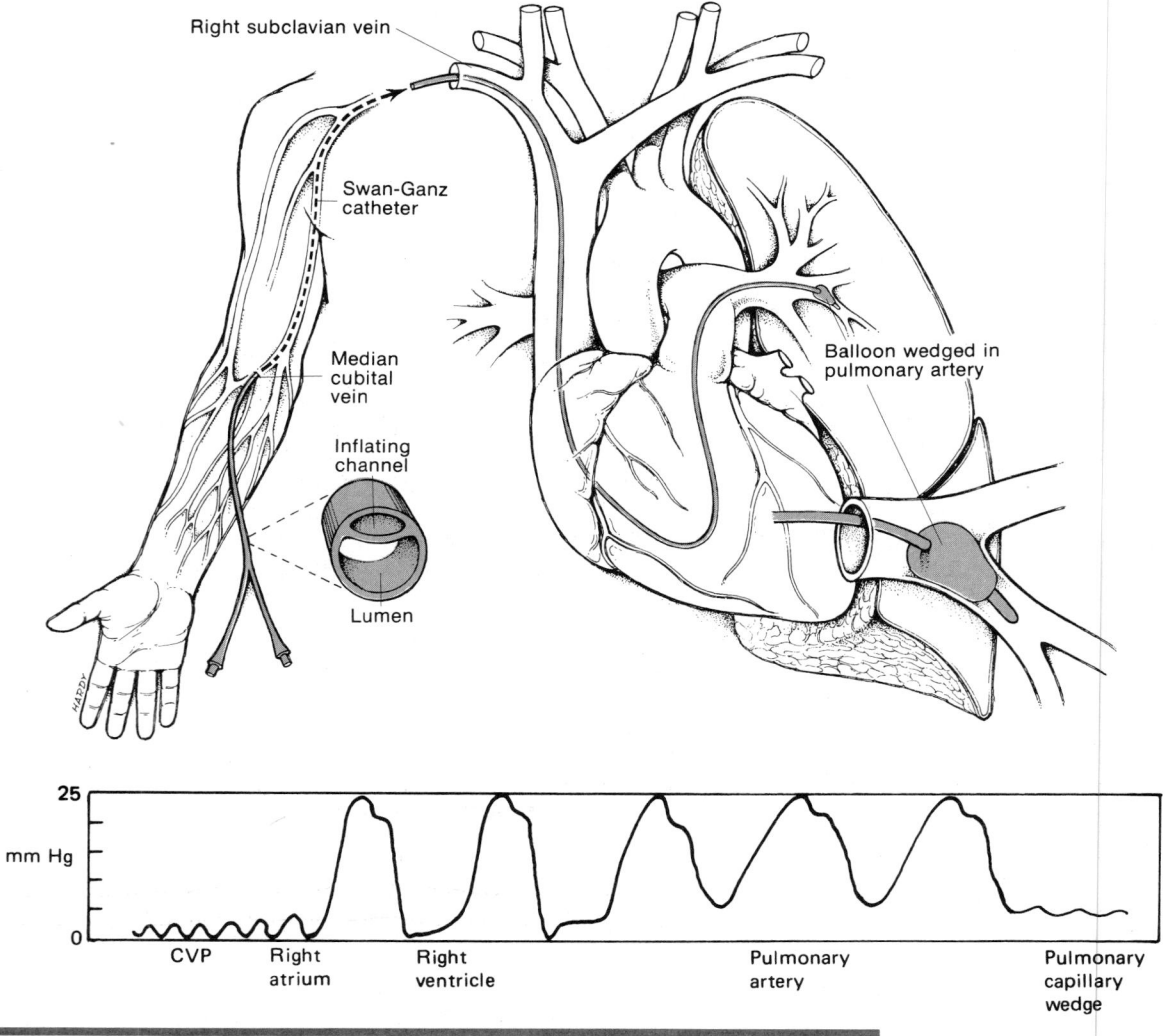

Figure 25-6. Insertion of a Swan-Ganz catheter. The position of the catheter is reflected by the pressure tracings. Capillary wedge pressure is obtained by inflating the balloon.

incidence of arrhythmias; and (3) it is used to obtain the wedge pressure when inflated and the pulmonary artery (PA) pressure when deflated.

To monitor PA and PCW pressures, a monitor with an oscilloscope, transducer and cable, and pressure tubing are required. Transducer domes can be reusable or disposable, and some are available with the necessary stopcocks and tubing already assembled. In the simplest form of pressure monitoring, a pressurized bag of heparinized IV solution is connected to a continuous flush device. One end of the flush device is connected to the Swan–Ganz catheter and the other to the dome of a fluid-filled transducer, which is, in turn, connected by a cable to the monitor. The transducer detects changes in the patient's pressure and converts the signal into an electrical one for display on the monitor oscilloscope. After the catheter is inserted, it is sutured in place and a sterile dressing is applied to the site. Thereafter, the site must be carefully checked for signs of infection.

In order to obtain the proper pulmonary artery waveform, check to be sure that:

- All tubing connections are secured
- Electrical connections between transducer and monitor are tight
- The pressure bag has sufficient fluid in it
- The transducer dome is screwed on finger tight and is devoid of cracks
- There are no air bubbles in the transducer dome or tubing
- The top of the transducer is level with the patient's midchest at approximately the level of the right atrium
- The monitor is properly calibrated, so measurements are accurate
- The head of the patient's bed is in the same position each time measurements are taken

When measuring the PCW pressure, be sure:

- To inflate the balloon slowly with air to avoid rupture
- To stop inflating the balloon as soon as the wedge pressure waveform appears
- Not to introduce more than 1.5 ml of air into the balloon to avoid overinflation
- To avoid keeping the balloon inflated more than 2 respiratory cycles to prevent pulmonary artery perforation
- To read the PCW pressures at end-expiration
- To allow passive deflation of the balloon (Manual air withdrawal can damage the balloon.)
- To keep the balloon deflated when not needed to avoid pulmonary infarction

- After the catheter has been in the patient for some time, it softens and may be carried forward to wedge in a smaller artery, even when the balloon is not inflated. In order to detect this early, monitor the pulmonary arterial tracing continuously. If the tracing disappears, flush the catheter with heparinized solution. If this does not help, withdraw the catheter a few centimeters until the pulmonary arterial tracing reappears.

The PCW pressure is important for two reasons. First, it is one of the factors controlling fluid shift in the lung.

The normal PCW pressure is about 6 mm Hg to 12 mm Hg. If the PCW pressure exceeds 18 mm Hg, pulmonary congestion usually follows because of the movement of fluid out of the capillaries. When the PCW pressure is in excess of 25 mm Hg or 30 mm Hg, pulmonary edema may occur.

The second reason for the importance of the PCW pressure is that it reflects the left atrial pressure and therefore indirectly reflects the left ventricular function. When the PCW pressure is combined with measurements of cardiac output, important conclusions regarding the cardiovascular status may be drawn. If the cardiac output is low and the PCW pressure is high (more than 20 mm Hg), left ventricular failure is indicated (if mitral valve is normal). PCW pressure is also useful in the diagnosis of cardiac tamponade, pulmonary embolism, and acute mitral regurgitation.

Cardiac Output

Cardiac output is the volume of blood delivered to the tissues by the heart every minute. Introduction of the triple-lumen (three-lumen) Swan–Ganz catheter with a thermistor (electronic heat-sensing device) has made cardiac output measurements relatively simple. The third lumen of this type of catheter opens some distance from the tip and is used for measuring central venous pressure (CVP) or administering fluids. The thermistor is situated 4 cm from the tip of the catheter and measures the temperature of the blood that flows by.

When 5 ml or 10 ml of a cold solution are injected through the CVP line of the catheter, the solution mixes with some blood, which is consequently cooled. This cooled blood is ejected into the pulmonary artery, where the temperature drop is detected by the thermistor. The electrical signals arising from the thermistor can be used to trace the curve of this temperature drop on a graph paper (thermodilution curve) and can also be processed by an integrator circuit to yield the cardiac output in digital form.

The cardiac output determines the amount of nutrients delivered to the tissues. We are primarily concerned with oxygen delivered to the tissues. The amount of oxygen present in the cardiac output is known as *oxygen flux*. Oxygen flux depends on the hemoglobin concentration (mg %) and oxygen saturation of hemoglobin (which is determined by the P_aO_2 and P_{50}) and cardiac output.

Cardiac output depends on the cardiac function, tone of the blood vessels, and blood volume. Low blood volume may result from blood loss in accidents, major surgery, hemorrhage from peptic ulcer, esophageal varices, or diverticulitis. Fluid loss seen in intestinal obstruction, peritonitis, severe diarrhea, diabetes, chronic renal failure, dialysis, or injudicious use of diuretics may also lead to low blood volume. Whatever the cause of low blood volume, it leads to low cardiac output.

Poor cardiac function is most frequently due to ischemic heart disease, hypertension, or valvular defects. Hypoxia itself may lead to poor cardiac function and may set up a vicious cycle. When cardiac function is so poor that the cardiac output is inadequate for the needs of the body, cardiac failure is present.

Low cardiac output is often the cause of the patient's being critically ill and is a persistent problem in his management. The use of mechanical ventilators and PEEP (p. 489) may also lead to low cardiac output. Since the output of the right and the left ventricles must be equal, pulmonary perfusion is equal to the cardiac output. When the cardiac output falls, pulmonary perfusion also falls and may lead to hypoxia because of ventilation abnormalities. For these reasons, frequent measurement of cardiac output is very important for the proper management of these patients.

For a summary of the parameters involved in the monitoring of respiratory care, see Chart 25-1.

▷ Causes of Respiratory Failure

Respiratory failure exists whenever the exchange of oxygen for carbon dioxide in the lungs cannot keep up with the rate of oxygen consumption and carbon dioxide production in the cells of the body. This results in a fall in arterial oxygen tension (hypoxemia) and a rise in arterial carbon dioxide tensions (hypercapnia).

One must distinguish between acute respiratory failure and acute exacerbation of chronic respiratory failure. Acute respiratory failure is the respiratory failure appearing in the individual whose lung was structurally and functionally normal before the onset of the present illness. Chronic respiratory failure is the respiratory failure seen in individuals with chronic lung diseases such as chronic bronchitis, emphysema, and black lung disease (coal miner's disease). These patients develop a tolerance to the gradually worsening hypoxia and hypercapnia. Following acute respiratory failure, the lung usually returns to its original state. In chronic respiratory failure the structural damage is irreversible. The principles of management of these two conditions are different; this discussion will be confined to acute respiratory failure.

Causes of acute respiratory failure are numerous and may be subdivided into various categories. One major group includes those diseases in which respiratory failure results from inadequate ventilation; the lung itself remains structurally normal in the early stages. One of the most important causes of inadequate ventilation is upper airway obstruction. Its etiology, diagnosis, and management are discussed on page 489.

Central nervous system depression will also result in inadequate ventilation. The respiratory center, which controls every breath, lies in the lower part of the brain stem (pons and medulla). Drug overdose, head injury, cerebrovascular accidents, brain tumors, encephalitis, meningitis, hypoxia, and hypercapnia are all capable of depressing the respiratory center. In these patients, respiration becomes slow and shallow. Respiratory arrest may occur in severe cases.

The impulses arising in the respiratory center travel in nerves that extend from the brain stem down the spinal cord to receptors in the muscles of respiration. Any disease of the nerves, spinal cord, muscles, or neuromuscular junction involved in respiration would seriously affect ventilation. Polyneuritis, myasthenia gravis, damage to the cervical segment of the spinal cord, and poliomyelitis are examples of such diseases.

Respiratory failure owing to inadequate ventilation should be looked for in the immediate postoperative period, especially following major thoracic or upper abdominal surgery. The reasons for respiratory failure during this period are numerous. The effects of anesthetic drugs (morphine, pentothal, droperidol) are long-lasting. They depress respiration by their own effects or by enhancing the effects of narcotics used for pain control. Pain in the thoracic and abdominal area interferes with deep breathing and coughing. Muscle relaxants (drugs that paralyze muscles) are frequently used during anesthesia. Some patients may have difficulty in breaking down or excreting these drugs, so that their effects last longer than usual, making patients weak in the postoperative period. Ventilation/perfusion abnormality also accounts for respiratory failure following major abdominal and thoracic operations.

Pleural effusion, hemothorax, and pneumothorax are a group of conditions that interfere with ventilation by preventing expansion of the lung. They are usually produced by an underlying lung disease or pleural disease.

Trauma resulting from motor vehicle accidents is a very common cause of acute respiratory failure. In this type of accident, head injury, unconsciousness, and bleeding from nose and mouth lead to upper airway obstruction and respiratory depression. Hemothorax, pneumothorax, and rib fractures may occur and may be responsible for inadequate ventilation. Flail chest may also occur and may lead to respiratory failure.

There are many acute diseases of the lung that may lead to acute respiratory failure. Of these diseases, pneumonia is perhaps the most common. It is usually caused by viral or bacterial activity. Chemical pneumonitis is pneumonia produced by the inhalation of irritant fumes or the aspiration of acidic gastric material. Bronchial asthma, atelectasis, pulmonary embolism, and pulmonary edema are some other conditions that cause acute respiratory failure.

Adult Respiratory Distress Syndrome (RDS)

Most patients in acute respiratory failure get better with the proper management of airway ventilation and oxygenation. However, a small group of patients do not respond to this treatment. They become severely hypoxic (P_aO_2 to 50 mm Hg) in spite of adequate ventilation with 100% oxygen. These symptoms are caused by widespread injury to the alveolar capillary bed. Adult respiratory distress is the name given to this clinical picture.

Clinical Manifestations

The clinical features of the syndrome include initial severe illness with no pulmonary component, followed by a latent period in which pulmonary abnormalities are minimal. There is a subsequent period of progressive respiratory disease with dyspnea and hypoxia. The x-ray will show bilateral involvement of the lungs leading to pulmonary edema.

Adult respiratory distress syndrome frequently results from pneumonia or shock. The pneumonia is usually caused by a virus but may be caused by microorganisms such as bacteria, rickettsia, or leptospira. Chemical pneumonitis, which follows inhalation of noxious fumes or aspiration of acidic gastric material, accounts for some patients' having pneumonia. Shock is usually due to blood loss but may be caused by septicemia.

Motor vehicle accidents or gunshot injuries account for the incidence of shock owing to blood loss. However, blood loss occurring during childbirth, ruptured aortic aneurysm, ruptured esophageal varices, peptic ulceration, and major surgery may also lead to shock. Adult RDS may also follow massive fat embolism, acute pancreatitis, massive blood transfusions, and extracorporeal circulation for open-heart surgery.

Pathophysiology

In spite of the different causes, the clinical picture, pathophysiology, and pathology are similar. RDS appears 6 to 48 hours after the onset of the illness. The patient develops respiratory distress; the rate of breathing increases (tachypnea) and may reach 40 breaths per minute. Each breath is shallow and labored (dyspnea) and may be associated with grunting. Retraction of the intercostal and suprasternal areas is seen during inspiration. Widening of the alae nasi and contractions of the accessory muscles of respiration are other signs of respiratory distress.

Cyanosis appears and fails to respond to oxygen therapy. Evidence of cerebral hypoxia, such as anxiety, confusion, irritability, lack of cooperation, drowsiness, and mental obtundation, may appear. Hypoxia of the heart will result in tachycardia, arrhythmias, and hypotension.

Auscultatory findings are minimal in the early stages, but later bronchial breathing may be heard. In the early stages chest x-ray may show patchy alveolar infiltrates in both lungs, which later become more diffuse.

As was mentioned before, the arterial oxygen tension (P_aO_2) is low (usually around 50 torr) even when the patient is breathing 100% oxygen. In other words, the alveolar to arterial oxygen gradient, $P_{(A-a)}O_2$, is widened. Severe hypoxia is the result of extensive shunting in the lungs. The functional residual capacity (FRC) is markedly diminished.

When the FRC falls below the closing capacity, small airways close and the air in the corresponding alveoli is absorbed, leading to their atelectasis. Oxygen cannot reach the alveolar capillaries, and the blood passing through these capillaries constitutes shunted blood.

Pulmonary edema (fluid in the alveoli) and interstitial edema (fluid in the lung substance) are also seen and contribute to hypoxia. As a result of all of these changes, the lung becomes more stiff (low compliance).

Adult respiratory distress syndrome used to be associated with high mortality. The use of positive end-expiratory pressure (PEEP) has increased the survival rate.

Management of Respiratory Failure

The principles of management of acute respiratory failure are the following:

1. Treat the cause.
2. Maintain a patent airway.
3. Provide adequate ventilation.
4. Provide optimum oxygen.
5. Carry out chest physiotherapy.

Treatment of the cause may involve evacuating the pleural cavity, giving antibiotic treatment for infection, reversing effects of drugs or accelerating their excretion, decreasing raised intracranial pressures, etc. Diseases such as bronchial asthma and pulmonary edema require specific therapy. In some illnesses, such as polyneuritis and poliomyelitis, one has to wait for the illness to resolve.

To maintain a patent airway it may be necessary to intubate the patient or to do a tracheostomy. Once the airway is clear, adequacy of ventilation must be assessed by measuring the respiratory rate, tidal volume, vital capacity, inspiratory force, and arterial carbon dioxide tensions (P_aCO_2). Depending on the results, the patient is allowed to breathe spontaneously or is helped by a ventilator (Table 25-1) and by being monitored in the intensive care unit.

Table 25-1
Indications for Respiratory Support

		Acceptable Range	Chest Physical Therapy Oxygen Close Monitoring	Endotracheal Intubation Tracheostomy Ventilation
Muscle Power	1. Respiratory rate per minute	12–25	25–35	>35
	2. Vital capacity ml/kg (ideal body weight)	70–30	30–15	<15
	3. Inspiratory force in negative cm H_2O	100–50	50–25	<20
Oxygenation	Alveolar to arterial O_2 tension gradient in mm Hg*	50–200	200–350	>450
	pO_2 mm Hg	100–75 air	200–75 (on mask O_2)	<70
Ventilation	pCO_2 mm Hg	35–45	45–60	>60†

(Adapted from Pontoppidan H: Treatment of respiratory failure in nonthoracic trauma. J Trauma 8:940, 1968.)

* After 15 minutes of 100% O_2.

† Except in chronic hypercapnea.

Recognition of Respiratory Complications: Table 25-1 shows objective, practical guidelines used in the bedside evaluation of the patient's respiratory status. *(The trend of change in values is of utmost importance.)* The first column refers to the values of normal acceptable range. The second column lists borderline values where chest physical therapy, oxygen, and close monitoring are essential. The third column lists values that indicate the necessity of intubation, tracheostomy, or ventilation.

Table 25-2
Guidelines for Estimating F_IO_2 in Adults with Low-Flow Oxygen Device

A. Nasal Cannula or Catheter (100% O_2)		B. Oxygen Mask (100% O_2)		C. Mask with Reservoir Bag (100% O_2)	
Flow Rate in Liters	F_IO_2	Flow Rate in Liters	F_IO_2	Flow Rate in Liters	F_IO_2
1 liter	24%	5–6 liters	40%	6 liters	60%
2 liters	28%	6–7 liters	50%	7 liters	70%
3 liters	32%	7–8 liters	60%	8 liters	80%
4 liters	36%			9 liters	90%
5 liters	40%			10 liters	99+%
6 liters	44%				

Note: Normal respiratory pattern is assumed.

With these basic guidelines for the concentration of oxygen administration one is capable of increasing or decreasing the inspired oxygen concentrations within reasonable predictable limits in correlation with the arterial blood gas results.

The arterial oxygen tension (P_aO_2) will show the degree of oxygenation.

Administration of Oxygen

The concentration of oxygen in air is 21%. Another way of expressing the same fact is to say that the fraction of inspired oxygen (F_IO_2) is 0.21. The F_IO_2 may be increased by the addition of oxygen to inspired air. The oxygen must always be humidified to prevent drying of the upper airway or secretions in the airway. Nasal prongs, nasal catheters, or face masks are commonly used to administer oxygen to the spontaneously breathing patient.

With nasal prongs or catheters the F_IO_2 varies between 0.24 to 0.44 (24% to 44%).

The actual F_IO_2 depends on:

1. Flow rate of oxygen
2. Degree of mouth breathing
3. Patency of nasal passages
4. Depth of insertion of nasal catheter

Table 25-2 shows the approximate F_IO_2 obtained with various flow rates of oxygen delivered with nasal prongs or catheters. When blood is taken to measure arterial blood gases, always note the flow rate of oxygen or, better still, measure the F_IO_2 with an oxygen analyzer. It may be necessary to pass a small cannula into the pharynx to obtain a sample of well-mixed inspired gas.

When a higher concentration or a very precise concentration of oxygen needs to be delivered, face masks are preferable. The various types of face masks available include aerosol face masks, venturi face masks, and face masks with reservoir bags that may or may not allow rebreathing. The aerosol face masks are light and acceptable to most patients. They provide an oxygen concentration of 60% to 80% with flow rates of 8 to 10 liters per minute of 100% oxygen. The flow rates must be equal to or greater than the minute ven-

tilation of the patient. Table 25-2 (B) shows the relationship of flow rates to the F_IO_2.

Some masks are fitted with a reservoir bag that fills with oxygen and functions as a reservoir of oxygen. These masks may be provided with valves that keep the exhaled gas from entering the reservoir and thus prevent rebreathing of the exhaled gas. The inspired oxygen concentration is usually above 60% with these masks (Table 25-2 [C]).

The aerosol masks and masks with reservoir bags must fit tightly over the face in order to function properly.

Ventimasks are based on the Venturi principle. These masks are so constructed that as the oxygen flows at a set rate through an orifice it traps and mixes a precise amount of the surrounding air to give the desired oxygen concentration. Masks are available that provide 24%, 26%, 35%, and 40% oxygen. Ventimasks need not fit tightly over the face.

If the patient has an endotracheal tube or a tracheostomy, a T-bar (Briggs adapter) is used for the administration of oxygen (Fig. 25-7). Since the upper airway is bypassed in these patients, the inspired air must be humidified.

The percentage of oxygen inspired by the patient depends on (1) the diluter valve setting of the nebulizer, (2) the output of the nebulizer, (3) the reservoir tube on the expiratory limb, and (4) the inspiratory effort of the patient.

The diluter valve setting puts an upper limit on the inspired oxygen concentration. This concentration may be

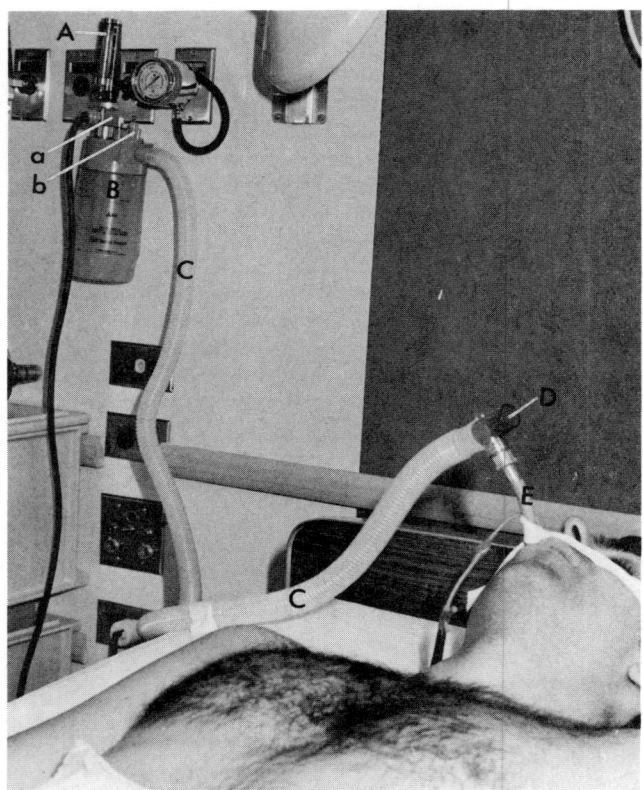

Figure 25-7. The T-bar. Lettered items are as follows: (*A*) Oxygen flow meter. (*B*) Nebulizer—(a) heater, (b) diluter valve. (*C*) Disposable hose. (*D*) T-bar (reservoir tube, 50 ml–200 ml, can be attached at (*D*)). (*E*) Endotracheal tube.

reduced by air pulled in via the expiratory limb during the inspiratory effort of the patient. By increasing the nebulizer outflow and by using a reservoir tube on the expiratory limb, air dilution may be reduced or completely eliminated.

Humidification

The air we breathe contains water in the form of vapor. This is referred to as humidity. The amount of water vapor present in the air at any time varies with the weather conditions and greatly influences our comfort. A given volume of air at a given temperature cannot contain more than a certain amount of water vapor, and when it contains the maximum amount of water vapor, it is said to be 100% saturated.

If the temperature of this sample of air is raised, more water vapor will have to be added to it to saturate it to 100%. Whatever the temperature and percentage saturation of the air we breathe, it is rendered 100% saturated at body temperature when it passes through the nose and reaches the lower part of the trachea.

The oxygen that is commercially available is totally devoid of water vapor (100% dry), and humidifiers are required to provide the water vapor that will make oxygen breathing comfortable and prevent drying up of the respiratory tract and the secretions therein. If the patient is using his own airway, a simple humidifier may be used that will add some water vapor to the oxygen and allow the patient's airway to saturate it to 100%. A simple humidifier is formed by bubbling oxygen through water. Its efficiency is increased by various methods that make the bubbles very small. Many disposable simple humidifiers are available that produce 80% to 100% saturated oxygen at room temperature (100% saturated oxygen at room temperature becomes 37% saturated at body temperature unless more water vapor is added).

A patient breathing via an endotracheal tube or a fresh tracheostomy must be provided with 100% saturated air at body temperature. This may be achieved by heating the water in the humidifier to a temperature above that of the body and letting the humidified oxygen cool to body temperature as it passes through the delivery tube. Many mechanical ventilators use this technique.

Alternatively, a nebulizer may be used to provide humidity. A nebulizer produces small particles of water, some of which evaporate to produce water vapor. Suspension of small particles in gas is referred to as an *aerosol.* There are several types of nebulizers. The Puritan nebulizer is capable of delivering aerosol for a long period. It also traps air that dilutes the oxygen. By adjusting a valve on the nebulizer, it is possible to set the nebulizer to deliver 40%, 60%, 70%, or 100% oxygen. Because of air entrapment, when the nebulizer is set at 40% and 10 liters of 100% oxygen per minute are run through, 40 liters per minute of 40% oxygen with water particles are delivered by the nebulizer.

Positive End-Expiratory Pressure (PEEP)

Positive end-expiratory pressure (PEEP) means the airway pressure remains higher than atmospheric pressure at the end of expiration. Normally, during spontaneous breathing or during mechanical ventilation, at the end of expiration the airway pressure equals the atmospheric pressure (zero end-expiratory pressure). The airway pressure is measured in centimeters of water (cm H_2O). The usual range of PEEP used is 5 cm to 15 cm H_2O. However, higher PEEP values (20 cm–35 cm H_2O) are also used.

PEEP may be applied to a patient on a mechanical ventilator. Such a patient would have positive airway pressure during inspiration and expiration and at the end of expiration. The term "continuous positive pressure ventilation" (CPPV) is sometimes used to describe this situation. When PEEP is applied to a patient who is breathing spontaneously (via his or her own airway, an endotracheal tube, or a tracheostomy), it is called CPAP (continuous positive airway pressure).

However, PEEP can be regulated so that a spontaneously breathing patient on PEEP will have zero airway pressure during the inspiratory phase. The term CPAP cannot strictly be applied to this method. The term sPEEP (spontaneous PEEP) has been used by some to describe the situation.

When PEEP is applied, the FRC is increased, so that small airway closure is prevented. PEEP also splints the airways. With PEEP, shunting is decreased and compliance is improved. The end result is improved oxygenation, as is demonstrated by the decrease in the alveolar to arterial oxygen tension gradient $P_{(A-a)}O_2$. With improved oxygenation the F_IO_2 may be reduced to less toxic levels.

PEEP may produce some undesirable results. A fall in cardiac output may be seen when more than 5 cm of H_2O PEEP are used.

- The amount of oxygen carried to the tissues per minute (oxygen flux) depends as much on the cardiac output as on the degrees of oxygenation. Care must be taken not to compromise oxygen flux by decreasing the cardiac output.

Other complications reported with PEEP include pneumothorax, pneumomediastinum, and interstitial emphysema.

▷ Upper Airway Obstruction

The trachea, larynx, pharynx, nose, and mouth constitute the upper airway. It is vital that this pathway remain patent at all times. The swallowing reflex, the cough reflex, and the tone of the muscles of the pharynx and the larynx ensure that patency is maintained.

However, airway obstruction sometimes does occur. Food particles, vomitus, blood clots, or any other particle that enters the trachea or larynx can obstruct the airway.

Epiglottitis, laryngeal edema, laryngeal carcinoma, and peritonsillar abscess are conditions in which the airway is obstructed by masses arising from the walls of the airway. Thick secretions may also cause airway obstruction. Sometimes obstruction may be produced by collapse of the walls of the airway. Such is the case with retrosternal goiter, enlarged mediastinal lymph nodes, hematomas around the upper airway, and thoracic aneurysm, all of which push upon the wall of the upper airway, leading to its collapse. Upper airway obstruction is very commonly seen in men-

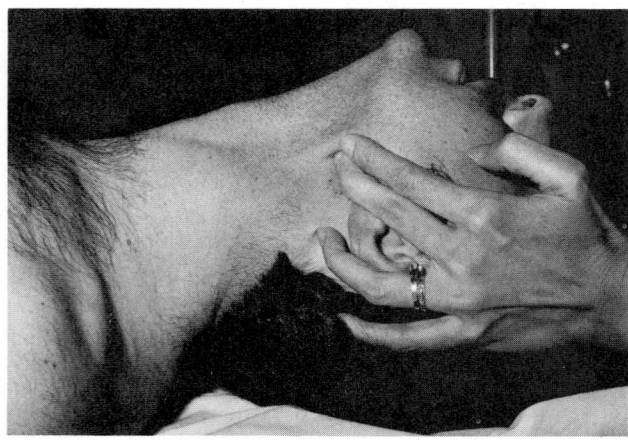

Figure 25-8. To clear upper airway of obstruction, extend the head and push mandible forward.

tally obtunded (unconscious, comatose) patients. These patients lose their protective reflexes as well as the tone of the pharyngeal muscles, with the result that the tongue falls back and obstructs the airway.

Nursing Assessment for Upper Airway Obstruction

Observe the patient for the following signs of upper airway obstruction.

1. Inspiration will cause indrawing of parts of the upper chest, sternum, and intercostal spaces.
2. Exhalation will be characterized by a jerky protrusion and prolonged, somewhat sustained contraction of the abdominal muscles, followed by a brief relaxation before another contraction.
3. Seesaw movement of the chest and abdomen may ensue (combination of 1 and 2 above). (As the inspiratory muscles contract, an inward thoracic depression results while relaxed abdominal muscles are jerkily pushed up. Exhalation is produced by a labored and prolonged abdominal muscle contraction, causing a jerky upward push of the thorax.)
4. Tracheal tug or indrawing of the suprasternal notch may occur.

Management of Upper Airway Obstruction

As soon as upper airway obstruction is diagnosed, measures must be taken to correct it.

- The mouth is opened to see if the tongue has fallen back or if there are secretions, blood clots, or any particles obstructing the airway. Secretions must be suctioned and any particulate matter in the pharynx must be removed immediately with forceps or by suctioning.
- Extension of the head is the simplest way of relieving upper airway obstruction caused by the tongue's falling back. The head must be extended at the atlanto-occipital joint. This will increase the distance between the chin and the cervical spine, which puts the muscles that support the tongue under tension and pulls the tongue forward.
- If simple extension of the head is not adequate to clear

the airway, the mandible should be forced forward. This maneuver is designed to put further tension on the musculature that supports the tongue. It is best executed by standing behind the patient and placing the tips of the index finger and middle finger on each side along the ascending ramus of the mandible. The mandible is lifted upward by exerting pressure on the ascending ramus of the mandible and at the same time tilting the head backward (Fig. 25-8). The fingers and the palm of each hand are applied on each side of the face in order to maintain the extension of the head.

- If this maneuver is not adequate and partial airway obstruction still exists, then an oral airway may have to be inserted or endotracheal intubation done. Unconsciousness and loss of protective airway reflexes require endotracheal intubation to maintain a patent airway and prevent aspiration. Temporary relief is obtained by grasping the tongue with gauze and pulling it forward.
- If assisted ventilation is required, a resuscitator bag and mask are used initially prior to intubation and mechanical ventilation. The mask is sealed onto the patient's face by pressing the mask with the left thumb on the bridge of the nose while the index finger presses around the lips. At the same time the rest of the fingers of the left hand pull on the chin and the angle of the mandible to maintain the head in extension (Fig. 25-9). The right hand inflates the lungs by periodically squeezing the bag.

Endotracheal Intubation

Endotracheal intubation refers to the passing of a tube through the mouth or nose into the trachea. It is done to provide an airway when the patient is having respiratory difficulty that cannot be treated by simpler methods. It is the method of choice in emergency care. Endotracheal intubation can be used as a means of assisting respiration for patients who cannot maintain an adequate airway on their

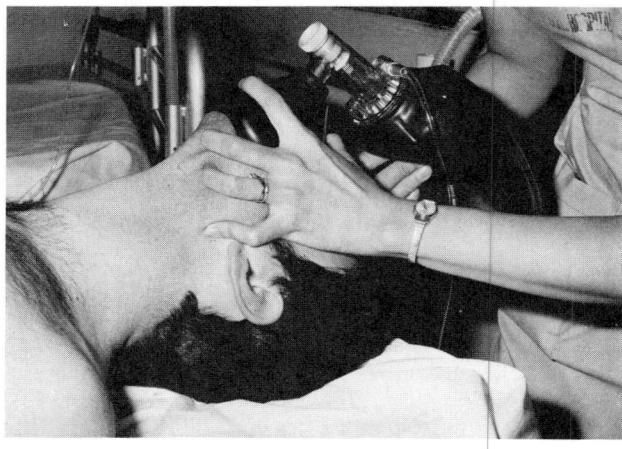

Figure 25-9. Bag and mask ventilation. The head is extended and the mask is sealed to the face by pressing the left thumb on the bridge of the nose and the index finger on the chin. The remaining three fingers pull the chin and mandible upward to maintain the head in extension. The right hand then squeezes the bag.

own (comatose patients; those with upper airway obstruction), and it provides an excellent means for suctioning secretions from the pulmonary tree.

An endotracheal tube usually is passed by means of a laryngoscope. A cuff around the tube is inflated to prevent leakage around the outer part of the tube and to minimize the possibility of subsequent aspiration. (Suctioning of the tracheobronchial secretions is done through the tube.) Warm, humidified oxygen can be introduced through the tube, or the tube may be connected to ventilatory equipment. Endotracheal intubation may be used for up to 72 hours. Then a tracheostomy should be considered.

As in any other treatment modality there are disadvantages associated with endotracheal or tracheostomy tubes. For one thing, the tube causes discomfort. But, more important, the cough reflex is depressed because closure of the glottis is hindered, and this prevents the generation of the high intrathoracic airway pressure necessary to produce an expulsive cough. Secretions tend to become thick and viscid because the warming and humidifying effect of the upper respiratory tract has been bypassed. The swallowing reflexes, composed of the glottic, pharyngeal, and laryngeal reflexes, also are depressed because of prolonged disuse and the mechanical trauma owing to the presence of the endotracheal or tracheostomy tube. Ulceration and stricture of the larynx or trachea may develop. Finally, the patient is not able to talk. For nursing management of the patient on endotracheal intubation see Chart 25-2.

Tracheostomy

A tracheostomy is an operation in which an opening is made into the trachea. When an indwelling tube is inserted into the trachea, the term "tracheostomy" is used. A tracheostomy may be either temporary or permanent.

A tracheostomy is done to bypass an upper airway obstruction, to remove tracheobronchial secretions, to permit the use of mechanical ventilation, to prevent aspiration of oral or gastric secretions in the unconscious or paralyzed patient (by closing off the trachea from the esophagus), and to replace an endotracheal tube. There are many disease processes and emergency conditions that make a tracheostomy necessary.

The procedure is usually done in the operating room or in an intensive care unit, where the patient's ventilation can be well controlled. An opening is made in the 2nd and 3rd tracheal rings. After the trachea is exposed, a cuffed tracheostomy tube of an appropriate size is inserted (Fig. 25-10). The cuff is an inflatable attachment to a tracheostomy or endotracheal tube which is designed to provide the snug fit required for mechanical ventilation.

The tracheostomy tube is held in place by tapes fastened around the patient's neck. Usually, a square of sterile gauze is placed between the tube and the skin before the tape is tied (Fig. 25-10 *B*).

Immediate Postoperative Care. The patient requires continuing nursing monitoring and assessment. The newly made opening must be kept patent by proper suctioning of

---

Chart 25-2
Nursing Management of the Patient Undergoing Endotracheal Intubation

1. Check symmetry of chest expansion.
   a. Auscultate breath sounds of anterior and posterior chest bilaterally.
   b. Do this immediately and then every 30 minutes to 1 hour.

2. Ensure a high humidity.
   a. A visible mist should be seen from the T-bar or inspiratory limb of the respirator.
   b. The oxygen concentration is prescribed by physician depending on arterial blood gas analysis.

3. Secure the tube to the face with tape and mark the proximal end for position maintenance.
   a. Cut proximal end of tube if it is longer than 7.5 cm (3 inches) to prevent kinking.
   b. An oral airway or mouth bite should be in place to stabilize the tube and prevent the patient from biting on the tube.

4. If the cuff is not of the low-pressure type, deflate the cuff every 2 hours.
   a. Thoroughly suction the endotracheal tube and then the oropharynx prior to deflation.
   b. Use sterile suction technique and airway care to prevent iatrogenic contamination and infection.

5. "Sigh" or hyperinflate the patient every hour to open up atelectatic alveoli.
   a. A self-inflating bag is used if the patient is on T-bar or pressure-controlled ventilator.
   b. Volume respirators have a built-in sighing mechanism.
6. Give oral hygiene and suction the oropharynx whenever necessary.
7. To extubate the patient (remove the tube):
   a. Have self-inflating bag and mask ready in case ventilatory assistance is required immediately after extubation.
   b. Suction the tracheobronchial tree and oropharynx before deflating the cuff.
   c. Give oxygen for a few breaths, and then remove the tube.

Care of Patient Following Removal of the Endotracheal Tube

1. Give heated humidity and oxygen via face mask.
2. Monitor respiratory rate and quality of chest excursions. Note stridor, color change, change in mental alertness or personality.
3. Give coughing and deep-breathing exercises for the next few days.

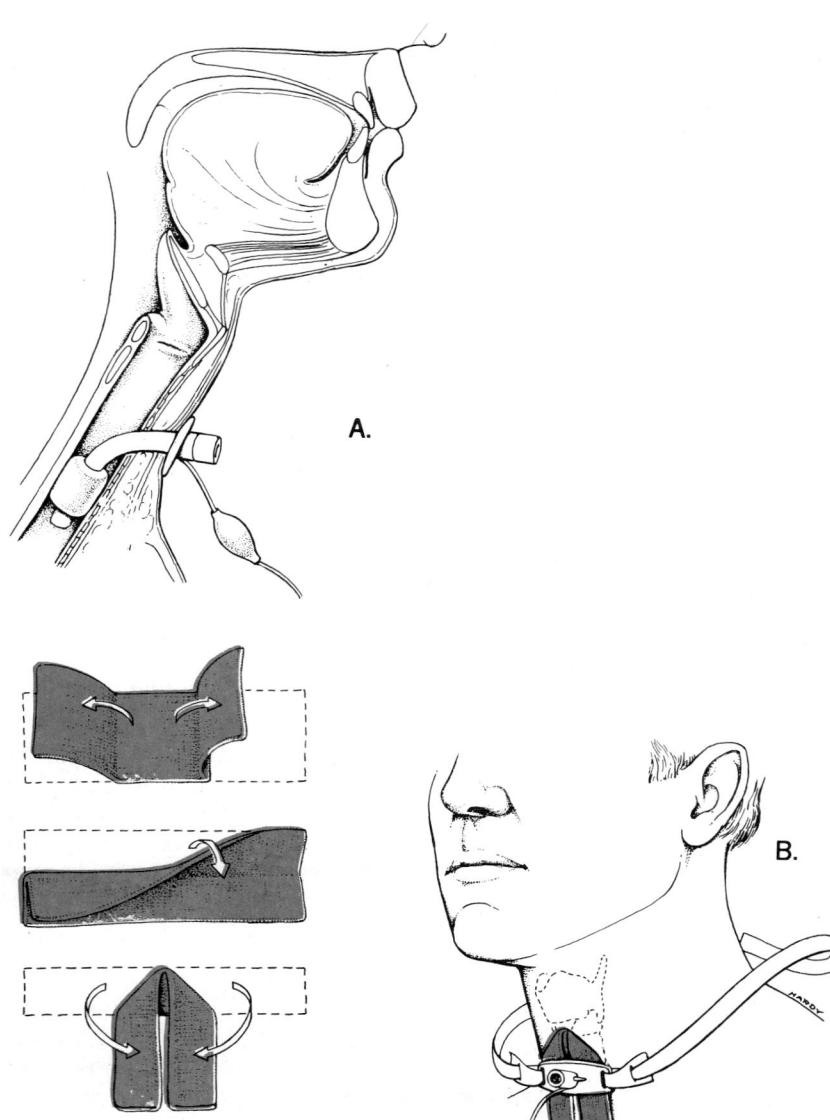

Figure 25-10. (*A*) This drawing shows how the cuff of the tracheostomy tube fits smoothly within the tracheal wall. Pressure should be great enough to ensure a snug fit but not so great as to produce a stenosis. (*B*) The lower illustration shows how to unfold a 3 × 3 gauze square and refold it so that it need not be cut (cut frayed threads could be aspirated) and yet will provide a comfortable neck pad. Change as often as necessary. Note the manner in which the neck twill tapes are fastened to the openings in the neck plate of the tracheostomy tube. This eliminates a knot, which would create pressure on the neck. Twill tape ends should be tied to the side of the neck rather than in back (A knot at the back would not be comfortable to lie on.)

secretions (see below). After the vital signs are stable, the patient may be placed in a semi-Fowler's position to facilitate respiration, promote drainage, minimize edema, and prevent strain on the suture lines. Analgesic and sedative drugs are given with caution since it is undesirable to depress the cough reflex.

Another objective of nursing care is to alleviate the apprehension of the patient. He needs reassurance, for he may have a real fear that he will asphyxiate while he is asleep. Since the patient cannot speak, paper and pencil or a magic slate should be kept near him so that he has a means of communication. A tap bell or other signaling device should be within his reach.

Removal of Secretions; Tracheostomy Suction

When a tracheostomy is present, it is necessary to suction the patient's secretions, since his own cough mechanism is not as effective. Tracheostomy suctioning is performed every 1 to 2 hours or whenever secretions are present. Un-

necessary suctioning can initiate bronchospasm and cause mechanical trauma to the tracheal mucosa.

All equipment that comes into direct contact with the patient's airway must be sterile in order to prevent overwhelming pulmonary and systemic infections. The following equipment is used: (1) suction catheters, (2) gloves, (3) 5-ml to 10-ml syringe, (4) normal saline poured in a cup for irrigation, (5) the patient's own self-inflating bag (hand resuscitator) with supplemental oxygen (the bag should be changed daily to reduce infection), and (6) suction machine.

- Explain the procedure to the patient before beginning and reassure him during suctioning, since he most likely is apprehensive about choking and about his inability to communicate.
- Begin by washing hands thoroughly. Then open sterile package containing catheter and gloves. Connect the catheter end (not tip) to suction tubing before putting

on the gloves. It is all right to touch one end of the catheter with a bare hand, since the catheter end will not enter the patient's airway. Put the glove on the hand that will guide the suction catheter. With the gloved hand, pull the catheter from the package, being careful not to contaminate it. Wet the catheter tip with sterile saline to lubricate it.

- One nurse should suction the patient while a second nurse ventilates and oxygenates him with a self-inflating bag. Before deflating the cuff, suction around the pharynx to remove regurgitated stomach contents or other secretions. Discard the catheter.
- Take patient off the mechanical ventilator or T-bar. The free end of the connection respirator should be anchored to the machine without contamination. Then deflate the cuff.
- Inflate the patient's lungs with the self-inflating bag containing supplemental oxygen to prevent hypoxia and sudden cardiovascular collapse during suctioning. Insert a second sterile catheter deep into the airway.

Then apply suction while gently rotating the catheter out of the bronchial tree. (Suction superficial secretions first.) The aspiration should not exceed 10 to 15 seconds, since the patient can become hypoxic with subsequent arrhythmias and cardiac arrest. Give the patient a breath with the machine or the self-inflating bag with supplemental oxygen after each suction; always inflate the tracheostomy cuff before giving this breath.

- Instill about 2 ml to 3 ml of sterile normal saline into the trachea.
- It is important not to tire the patient. When suction is completed, return the patient to the ventilator. Reinflate the cuff until the air leak disappears. Listen to the breath sounds bilaterally with a stethoscope. Respiration should be quiet and essentially effortless at the end of inspiration. Check exhaled tidal volume and thoracic expansion.

The care of the patient with a tracheostomy is summarized in Chart 25-3.

Chart 25-3
The Care of the Patient With a Tracheostomy

Tracheostomy Care	*Rationale*
A. Tracheostomy cuff 1. Cuffed tube (air injected into cuff) is required during prolonged mechanical ventilation.	1. The purpose of a cuffed tube is to prevent air from leaking during positive pressure ventilation and to prevent tracheal aspiration of gastric contents. A good seal is indicated by the disappearance of any air leakage from the tracheostomy or disappearance of the harsh, gurgling sound of air coming from the throat.

2. Types of cuff:
    a. Low-pressure cuff (preferred)
 	
    b. High-pressure cuff
	2. a. Low-pressure cuffs exert minimal pressure on the tracheal mucosa and thus reduce the danger of tracheal ulceration and stricture. Periodic deflation is not necessary.
	    b. Recommend periodic deflation of high-pressure cuff to allow return of circulation in the tracheal wall.

3. Indications for cuff deflation	3. a. Allowed during spontaneous ventilation if there is no danger of aspiration. b. Periodic deflation for 2 to 3 minutes every 1 to 2 hours if possible during controlled ventilation provided satisfactory air exchange and chest expansion are still present. Deflation is controlled by adjusting the volume and air flow on the ventilator. If the patient has stiff lungs, in spite of respiratory adjustment, air exchange will not be satisfactory with deflated cuff because high airway pressures are needed. Therefore, in these patients, the cuff should be kept inflated.
B. Dressing and skin care 1. Wash hands.	B. The tracheostomy dressing is changed p.r.n. to keep the skin clean and dry. Do not allow moist or soiled dressings to remain on the skin. *(continued)*

Chart 25-3
The Care of the Patient With a Tracheostomy (continued)

Tracheostomy Care *(continued)*	**Rationale** *(continued)*
2. Explain procedure to patient.	2. A patient with a tracheostomy is apprehensive and requires continuing assurance and support.
3. Remove twill tapes (if soiled) by untying.	
4. Hold tube in place and replace tape immediately.	4. Tracheostomy tube can be dislodged by movement or forceful cough. It is difficult to reinsert the tracheostomy tube in a fresh tracheostomy. Airway catastrophe may occur if the tracheostomy tube is dislodged.
5. Clean tracheostomy area with water and peroxide solution.	
6. Place clean twill tapes in position to secure tracheostomy tube. Make a horizontal slit 2.5 cm (1 inch) from end of tape. Insert this end of the tie through the side opening of the outer cannula. The opposite end of the tie can be threaded through the slit end, drawn securely, and fastened at the side of the neck.	
7. Remove soiled dressing and discard.	
8. Put on sterile gloves.	
9. Cleanse wound with sterile applicators or textile cleaners moistened with dilute hydrogen peroxide.	
10. Cleanse entire flange of tracheostomy tube with sterile textile cleaner or sterile applicator moistened with dilute hydrogen peroxide. Do not allow solution to enter tracheostomy.	10. Fluid entering the tracheostomy will irritate the respiratory tract.
11. Use neosporin or betadine ointment on the edge of the tracheostomy wound.	
12. Use sterile tracheostomy dressing from the wrappers, and fit securely under the twill tapes and flange of tracheostomy tube so that the incision is covered (see Fig. 25-11 B).	12. Dressings that will shred are not used around a tracheostomy because of the danger that pieces of material, lint, or thread may get into the tube, and eventually the trachea, causing obstruction or abscess formation. Special dressings that do not have a tendency to shred are used.
C. Changing of tracheostomy tube	
1. Varies from 3 to 5 days.	1. Depends on amount of crust and thickened secretions adhering to the tracheostomy tube.
2. Only a skilled physician should change a fresh tracheostomy.	2. Because airway problems can develop. Original stomal tract may be hard to find.
3. A nurse can change the tracheostomy tube if a patent stomal tract has developed.	
4. Have resuscitation equipment ready.	4. In case airway problems develop in the process of changing.

5. Procedure:
    a. Suction tracheostomy and oropharynx.
    b. Cut off twill ties.
    c. Remove tracheostomy tube.
    d. Insert new tracheostomy tube with obturator following the curvature of the tube until it is set in place.
    e. Remove stylet, inflate cuff, tie twill ties.
    f. Apply tracheostomy dressing.	

The Patient Requiring Mechanical Ventilation

▶ Assessment

A mechanical ventilator is a positive pressure breathing device that can maintain respiration automatically for prolonged periods. It is indicated when the patient is unable to maintain safe levels of arterial carbon dioxide or oxygen by spontaneous breathing.

An outline for assessment of clinical and pulmonary function for patients on mechanical ventilation is presented as follows. It will enable the nurse to intelligently care for the patient and allow early recognition of his problems and progress.

General Assessment

1. Assess the level of responsiveness. Restlessness may indicate early hypoxia, whereas drowsiness may signify increasing PCO$_2$ owing to hypoventilation. Determine whether the drowsiness is due to hypoventilation or to lack of sleep, which is a problem inherent in many intensive care units as a result of frequent interruptions to monitor vital signs, do blood work, and administer medications. A check of arterial blood gases will reveal the presence or absence of increasing PCO$_2$.
2. Determine the degree of respiratory distress. Observe to see the degree of muscle power the patient exerts while breathing.
3. Monitor the patient's temperature. The onset, degree, and pattern of rise in temperature will show the patient's progress and response to therapy. A high temperature causes an increase in oxygen consumption. Very low temperatures may cause some degree of cardiorespiratory depression or arrhythmia.

Assessment of Respiratory Function

1. Check respiratory rate.
2. Note color.
3. Auscultate the chest. (Note air entry and presence or absence of added sounds.)
4. Note bedside pulmonary functions:
   a. Tidal volume
   b. Vital capacity
   c. Minute volume
   d. Inspiratory force
5. Note color, quantity, and consistency of sputum.
6. Note quality of cough effort in its ability to bring up secretions.
7. Provide humidity to the inspired gases. Low humidity will cause drying and inspissation of pulmonary secretions.
8. Know the changes in airway pressure on the machine. Decreased airway pressure may be due to presence of a leak with subsequent low tidal volume. Increased airway pressure may be due to:
   a. Secretions
   b. Airway obstruction
   c. Pulmonary edema
   d. Bronchospasm
   e. Pheumothorax
   f. Flail chest

9. Check chest x-ray evaluation.
10. Check laboratory evaluation.
    a. Culture and sensitivity of tracheobronchial secretions every 3 days
    b. WBC and differential
11. Arterial blood gas assessment: PO$_2$, PCO$_2$, pH, base excess or deficit, Hb or hematocrit.

Assessment of Cardiovascular and Renal Function

1. Systemic BP
2. Heart rate
3. CVP
4. ECG
5. Fluid and electrolyte balance
6. Hypokalemia and hyperkalemia
7. Presence of ostomies
8. Urine output/hour and specific gravity
9. Serum creatinine and BUN
10. Total protein

Assessment of Neurologic Status

1. Motor and sensory function
2. Pupillary size and light reflex

Patient Problems/Nursing Diagnoses

Based on the clinical manifestations, the nursing history and the diagnostic assessment data, the patient's problems include impairment of or potential alteration of respiratory function related to physiologic insult; potential alteration in cerebral and cardiovascular homeostasis related to hypoxia or hypercarbia; potential asynchronism with ventilator related to excessive respiratory secretion, low F$_I$O$_2$, hypercarbia, inadequate minute volume, pulmonary edema, or anxiety; and potential delay in ability to be weaned from ventilator related to physiologic or psychological dependency on ventilatory therapy.

▶ Planning and Implementation

Goals

The major goals for the patient include the following:

1. Improvement of respiratory function while on ventilator
2. Attainment/maintenance of pre-illness level of responsiveness
3. Attainment/maintenance of stability of cardiovascular functioning
4. Adjustment to ventilator with respirations in synchrony with ventilator
5. Achievement of successful weaning from ventilator, cuff, tube, and oxygen

Management and Nursing Interventions. Numerous factors influence the management of the patient on a mechanical ventilator. Table 25-3 and Chart 25-4 present a summary view of factors that must be considered when nursing care is provided.

Adjustment of the Ventilator. The ventilator is adjusted so that the patient is comfortable and "in phase" with the machine (Fig. 25-11). Minimal alteration of the normal cardiovascular and pulmonary dynamics is sought. Arterial blood gases should be satisfactory, and auscultation of the chest should indicate good bilateral gas exchange. The following guidelines are recommended for the initial adjustment of the ventilator for a patient:

1. Set the machine to deliver tidal volume required (10 ml/kg–15 ml/kg).
2. Adjust the machine to deliver 100% inspired oxygen or whatever is necessary to maintain normal P_aO_2 (70 torr–100 torr).
3. Record peak inspiratory pressure.
4. Adjust inspiratory–expiratory ratio. Within the above criteria, make a setting that will provide satisfactory blood gases, with adequate tidal volume and inspiratory–expiratory ratio at the minimum airway pressure.
5. If the patient is not controlled, adjust sensitivity so that the patient can trigger the machine with a minimum effort. Adjust the rate to provide normal PCO_2 (38 torr–42 torr).
6. Record minute volume and measure PCO_2, pH, and PO_2 after 20 minutes of continuous ventilation at 100% inspired O_2 concentration. Estimate inspired O_2 concentration required to maintain PO_2 between 70 mm Hg to 100 mm Hg.
7. After results of arterial blood gases on 100% inspired oxygen are obtained, adjust F_iO_2 accordingly and recheck PO_2. Maintenance F_iO_2 can then be assessed.
8. Added mechanical dead space may be required to maintain normal arterial PCO_2 when large tidal volumes are used.

9. Use 100% F_iO_2 setting to follow progress of pulmonary status. True physiologic shunt can be estimated from the arterial blood gases and an F_iO_2 of 100%.

- Rule out the possibility of an impending catastrophe whenever a patient becomes out of phase with the ventilator. The "out of phase" patient usually has hypoxemia, air leak, obstruction, and inadequate flow rate, minute volume, or inspiratory–expiratory ratios.

If, after life-threatening situations have been corrected, the patient is still out of phase with the ventilator or is breathing too fast, then sedatives and muscle relaxants are given to provide optimum ventilation.

Factors Causing the Patient to "Fight the Ventilator." The patient is in synchrony with the respirator when thoracic air expansion coincides with the inspiratory phase of the machine, and exhalation occurs passively. The patient "fights" the ventilator when he is out of phase with the machine. This is manifested when (1) the patient attempts to breathe in during the ventilator's mechanical expiratory phase; (2) the respirator is triggered faster than 18 times/minute; or (3) there is jerky and increased abdominal muscle effort.

The following factors contribute to this problem: increased secretions, low F_iO_2, hypercarbia, inadequate minute volume, and pulmonary edema. These must be corrected (Table 25-4) before the prescribed sedation or muscle relaxant is given to the patient. Otherwise, the basic problem is masked and the patient will continue to deteriorate.

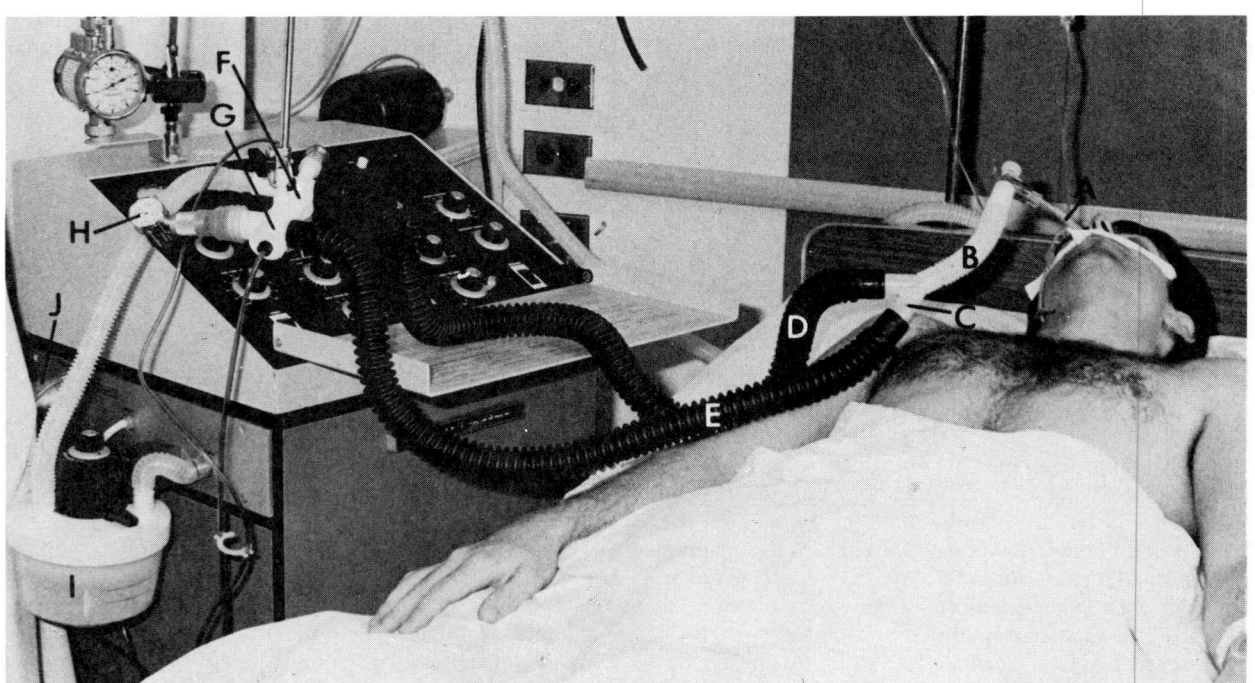

Figure 25-11. Patient on MAI mechanical ventilator. Lettered items are as follows: (A) Endotracheal tube. (B) Mechanical dead space. (C) Y piece. (D) Inspiratory hose. (E) Expiratory hose. (F) Inspiratory valve. (G) Expiratory valve. (H) Wright respirometer. (I) Cascade humidifier. (J) Knob for PEEP (positive end-expiratory pressure.)

Table 25-3
Managing the Patient on a Ventilator

Type of ventilator	1. Volume-controlled ventilator (MAI; Ohio 560, Emerson). Will deliver set tidal volume with varying pressures. 2. Pressure-controlled ventilator. Preset pressure is achieved at varying tidal volumes.	*Sigh (continued)*	2. The sigh is given by machine or manual hand-bag ventilation. 3. Sigh volume is 3 times tidal volume every 5–10 minutes.
Fraction of inspired oxygen (F_iO_2)	Interpretation of PO_2 will depend on the concentration of inspired O_2. Normal values: 1. F_iO_2—room air 21% O_2 PO_2—100 mm Hg or 105 minus half of patient's age 2. F_iO_2 = 100% PO_2 = 500 mm Hg	*Mechanical dead space*	Refers to the volume of tubing from endotracheal or tracheostomy tube connector to the Y piece. *Purpose:* 1. To rebreathe exhaled CO_2. 2. Serves as a pliable connector from tracheostomy tube to Y piece; thus prevents discomfort when patient moves. *Caution:* The volume of mechanical dead space should not be larger than one third of the set tidal volume, especially at 21% of F_iO_2, because hypoxic oxygen concentrations may result owing to exhaled CO_2 dilution. Should not be used to correct metabolic alkalosis.
Tidal volume (V_T)	10–15 ml/kg body weight		
Respiratory rate	10–12/minute		
Sensitivity setting	1. Increased sensitivity indicates that very low negative pressure is required to trigger machine. 2. Do not allow patient to generate more than −2 cm H_2O to trigger the ventilator.		
		Flow rate	*Slow* 1. Opens up more alveoli because of a more even air flow distribution within the respiratory tract. 2. If flow rate is too slow it will prolong inspiration and may hinder venous return.
Type of ventilation	1. Controlled. The machine ventilates the patient according to set tidal volumes and respiratory rate. These patients usually require medication with morphine, curare, or pancuronium. 2. Assist control. The patient triggers the machine.		*High* 1. Shortens inspiratory time. 2. Preferential flow of gases to alveoli with least resistance and may not open atelectatic alveoli at all.
Inspiration to exhalation ratio	1. Should be 1:3, 1:2 or 1:1 (1 second of inspiration to 3 seconds of exhalation, etc.). 2. Inspiration should never be longer than exhalation, because venous return to the right side of the heart occurs on exhalation. Prolonged inspiration prevents venous return and may cause hypotension. 3. Patients with obstructive lung disease need longer exhalation time to keep the bronchi open and allow exit of more air.	*Expiratory retard*	1. Used only when prescribed by physician. 2. Keeps the terminal bronchioles patent, preventing early closure on exhalation; thus, more air can be exhaled.
		Humidity and temperature	1. Heated humidity is provided for all intubated and tracheotomized patients to avoid thick and viscid secretions. 2. Daily clinical evaluation of the viscosity of the patient's secretions provides a guideline for the effectiveness of humidification and nebulization.
Minute volume (V_E)	Tidal volume × respiratory rate/minute. Normal = 6–8 liters/minute.		
Airway pressure	Normal = 15–20 cm/H_2O Low airway pressure is seen with air leak. High airway pressure is seen in: 1. Increased secretions 2. Airway obstruction 3. Bronchospasms 4. Pulmonary edema 5. Pneumothorax 6. Flail chest 7. Patient out of phase with respirator	*Positive end-expiratory pressure*	1. A positive pressure of 5 cm, 10 cm, or 15 cm H_2O is maintained at the end of exhalation instead of a normal 0 cm H_2O pressure. 2. Increases functional residual capacity.
		Synchronization of patient with ventilator	1. Inspiratory and expiratory time of the patient and respirator should be synchronized. 2. Asynchrony (out of phase) with ventilator will result in altered cardiopulmonary hemodynamics and will cause arrhythmias, hypotension, and increased airway pressure.
Sigh	1. The lungs are hyperinflated periodically to open collapsed alveoli.		

Life-threatening problems, of course, require immediate correction (Table 25-5). Thus, the nurse must be constantly on the watch for these difficulties and must be prepared to act.

▶ **Evaluation**

Expected Outcomes

1. Improves respiratory function while on ventilator
   a. Respirations synchronous with ventilator
   b. Arterial blood gases within normal ranges
   c. Respiratory secretions minimal in quantity, thin, and clear
   d. Chest x-ray negative for atelectasis
   e. Attains/maintains normal color of skin and nailbeds
   f. Adequate bilateral gas exchange evidenced by chest auscultation
2. Attains/maintains pre-illness level of responsiveness
   a. Oriented to time, place, and person
   b. Responds appropriately to verbal commands
   c. Communicates appropriately through gestures or written communication
   d. Pupils round, regular, equal, and reactive to light
3. Attains/maintains stability of cardiovascular functioning
   a. Blood pressure normal, at pre-illness range
   b. Pulse rate and rhythm within normal pre-illness range; absence of arrhythmias
   c. Fluid intake and output within normal range
   d. Serum electrolytes normal
4. Adjusts to ventilator with respirations in synchrony with ventilator
   a. Arterial blood gases within normal range
   b. Adequate bilateral gas exchange
   c. Adequate tidal volume and inspiratory–expiratory ratio
   d. Chest expansion coincides with inspiratory phase of ventilation
   e. Cooperates with procedures (*e.g.,* suctioning) that enhance ventilation
   f. Participates appropriately in physical care measures
   g. Rests between procedures

Chart 25-4
Summary: Nursing Management of the Patient on a Mechanical Ventilator

1. A nurse should be in constant attendance while the patient is on a mechanical ventilator.
2. Take vital signs every 5 to 30 minutes: BP, pulse and respirations, CVP, temperature.
3. Auscultate chest frequently (every 15 minutes). Note any change in breath sounds.
4. Aspirate tracheobronchial tree as necessary. Suction around pharynx before cuff deflation. Use sterile technique in airway care and suction. Note added breath sounds and the quality of air exchange before and after tracheobronchial aspiration. Record color and quantity of sputum aspirated.
5. Periodically deflate endotracheal or tracheostomy cuff with high-pressure cuffs. Reinflate cuff with identical volume. At the same time check for air leaks. Stop inflation when significant air leak is gone.
6. Flush arterial line with heparinized saline every hour or maintain a slow, continuous microdrip.
7. Total fluid balance every 8 hours.
8. Record urine specific gravity with hourly urinary output.
9. Give mouth care every 4 to 8 hours to all debilitated and paralyzed patients.
10. In all paralyzed and comatose patients, perform eye care every 12 hours. Use lubricating ointment and tape the eyelids closed.
11. Change respiratory therapy equipment every day.
12. Note end-inspiratory pressure and tidal volume hourly.
13. Empty condensed water from ventilatory tubing p.r.n.
14. Check pressure of humidifier every 2 hours. Be sure a visible mist is produced if nebulizer is used.
15. Record humidifier volume and refill every 8 hours. If refilling is necessary, empty residual water and replace with sterile distilled water. The emptying helps prevent accumulation of pseudomonas, which thrive in warm, moist places.
16. Check temperature of inspired air as often as necessary. Temperature of inspired air should be as close to body temperature as possible in order to provide more humidity. An increase in body temperature will develop if the air is higher than body temperature.
17. Check oxygen lines and flow meters hourly to be sure that they are properly connected and functioning as prescribed.
18. Change patient's position in bed hourly while he is awake, or hourly around the clock if comatose.
19. Coordinate chest physiotherapy with position change, airway suctioning, and IPPB treatments. The frequency of this is to be determined by the clinical status of the patient.
20. Put all joints of comatose or paralyzed patients through a passive full range of motion several times daily. Attention should be directed to the care of the skin of the dependent parts.
21. Assess neurologic signs every hour when indicated.
22. Note amount and quality of drainage in nasogastric tubes and any ostomies.
23. Send all stools to the lab for guaiac test. This is done to evaluate early bleeding owing to stress ulcers.
24. Weigh the patient daily.
25. Help the patient to ambulate as soon as possible.
26. Give diet as tolerated. This will depend on severity of illness.
27. Plan nursing care so that patient has periods of uninterrupted sleep.
28. Notify the physician immediately if a change occurs in the level of responsiveness; also, keep him informed of the occurrence of tachycardia, bradycardia, hypotension, confusion, agitation, tarry stools, arrhythmia, high or low CVP, or labored ventilation.

Table 25-4
Factors That Make the Patient Fight the Ventilator

Problem	Nursing Interventions
1. Increased secretions Volume ventilator—airway pressure is increased but tidal volume is maintained. Pressure ventilator—secretions will make the patient cough or generate increased intrapulmonary pressure, which will oppose the preset pressure on the ventilator; thus, the inspiratory volume is reduced. The reduced tidal volume will promote progressive atelectasis and shunting.	1. Suction as often as necessary. 2. Hourly, hand ventilate with self-inflating bag for 5–10 minutes. 3. Chest physical therapy. 4. Frequent change of position. 5. Adequate humidification and nebulization. 6. For pressure ventilator—adjust flow rate and preset pressure to maintain an adequate chest expansion and satisfactory air entry heard on auscultation. 7. If suctioning of trachea does not improve phasing with ventilator, call the physician.
2. Low F_IO_2—may manifest initially with tachycardia, hyperventilation, or arrhythmias.	1. Measure inspired oxygen concentration and arterial blood gases. 2. Call respiratory therapist to check accuracy of delivered F_IO_2. 3. Call physician for differential diagnosis and management.
3. Hypercarbia—may be manifested initially by hyperventilation, tachycardia, arrhythmias, increased blood pressure, and increasing drowsiness.	1. Measure arterial blood gases. 2. Call respiratory therapist to check mechanical dead space, accuracy of valves, and ventilator performance. 3. Call physician for differential diagnosis and management.
4. Inadequate minute volume $V_E = V_T \times RR$	1. Measure exhaled tidal volume and respiratory rate if minute volume is lower than 6 liters/minute. Increase delivered tidal volumes to 10–15 ml/kg at a rate of 10–12/minute. 2. Call respiratory therapist for accuracy of ventilator performance. 3. Call physician for differential diagnosis and management.

5. Pulmonary edema—may be manifested as follows:
  a. High airway pressure
  b. Poor compliance
  c. Tracheal secretion
    (1) Foamy or pink, frothy secretions
    (2) Abundant watery, and bright red fluid
  d. Engorged neck veins
  e. Dusky, cyanotic color
  f. Chest full of wet crackles
  g. Tachycardia, hypotension
  h. Marked restlessness
	1. 100% F_IO_2.
	2. Hand ventilate with self-inflating bag. Use volume-controlled respirator and PEEP (positive end-expiratory pressure).
	3. Suction trachea.
	4. Elevate head of bed (sitting up position).
	5. Call physician. Give specific drug therapy as directed.

Weaning the Patient From the Ventilator

Weaning takes place in four stages. The patient is gradually weaned from the (1) ventilator, (2) cuff, (3) tube, and (4) oxygen.

Weaning From the Ventilator. Weaning from mechanical ventilation should be done at the earliest possible time consistent with patient safety. It is essential that the decision be made from a physiologic rather than from a mechanical viewpoint. A total understanding of the patient's clinical status is required in making this decision.

Weaning is started when the patient is recovering from the acute stage of his medical and surgical problems and when the etiology of respiratory failure is sufficiently reversed.

The objective measurements of the patient's ventilatory capacities should include the following:

1. An ability to generate a minimum vital capacity of 15 ml/kg body weight, or a vital capacity twice as large as the predicted normal resting tidal volume. The minimum required volume is usually in the range of 1000 ml in a normal adult.

2. An inspiratory force of at least −20 cm water pressure. Occasionally, tidal volume can be used as an added criterion. If tidal volume is used, it must be measured during the patient's quiet respiration. Do not ask the patient to take a deep breath, because the volume thus obtained will be difficult to interpret since it is between his actual tidal volume and vital capacity.

3. A minimum ratio of 2 between the vital capacity and tidal volume is necessary before weaning is attempted.

(Text continues on page 503)

Table 25-5
Life-threatening Problems While on Mechanical Ventilation

Call the physician the moment any life-threatening situation arises following this sequence of priorities:

Priority I. Evaluate the patient's current status and compare it to an earlier observation:

1. Level of responsiveness
2. Degree of distress
3. Color
4. Degree of neck vein distention
5. Chest expansion
6. Abdominal movements

Priority II. Correlate airway pressures on the machine, central venous pressure, pulse rate, and bilateral breath sounds (heard via auscultation).

Priority III. Disconnect patient from the machine and ventilate him with self-inflating bag at high F_iO_2s.

Note: 1. Compliance and chest expansion in relation to amount of inflating pressure
2. Expiratory time
3. Bilateral breath sounds

Priority IV. 1. Pass a catheter through the endotracheal tube and feel for areas of resistance or obstruction.
2. Suction around the pharynx first, then deflate the cuff and note if there is improvement in air exchange with the cuff deflated. (This is true if obstruction is due to the cuff.)

Priority V. If patient is ventilating well on the self-inflating bag, check the machine while another person ventilates the patient by hand.

Problem	Assessment	Nursing Intervention

Airway Leak
 	
1. Patient-connected problem
  a. Inadequate cuff inflation
  b. Inadequate coaptation, or fit, of tracheostomy tube (loose tie around the neck)
  c. Changes in the patient's position can create a leak around tracheostomy.
2. Ventilator-connected problem
  a. Disconnected or loose-fitting ventilator hose and tubes
  b. Malfunction of inspiratory and expiratory valves
  c. Improperly sealed humidifier
	Clinical manifestations depend on amount of leak.
	
	Early Signs
	1. Absent or inadequate chest expansion
	2. Absent or decreased breath sounds
	3. Marked apprehension, if patient is conscious
	4. a. Pressure-controlled ventilator—inspiration is prolonged or continuous
	  b. Volume-controlled ventilator—normal cycle
	5. Zero or markedly reduced airway pressure
	6. Sounding of safety alarm in some machines
	7. Measured exhaled volume is reduced
	
	Late Signs
	1. Arrhythmia 3. Cyanosis
	2. Hypotension 4. Death
		1. Disconnect patient from ventilator.
		2. Inflate patient's chest with self-inflating bag at high F_iO_2s.
		3. Search for source of leak from the patient and from the machine. Once corrected, adequate chest expansion is seen.
		  a. Exhaled volume as measured with Wright respirometer should tally with dialed tidal volume on machine.
		  b. Dialed tidal volume is reduced by 3 ml for every cm H_2O peak airway pressure owing to gas compression in the system.

Airway Obstruction 1. Complete airway obstruction in a patient who is on a ventilator and has no muscle power	Manifestations will vary according to: 1. Pressure-controlled ventilator 2. Volume-controlled ventilator 3. Presence or absence of muscle power 4. Complete or partial airway obstruction 1. Pressure-controlled ventilator: The preset airway pressure is easily reached without any visible chest expansion or any inspiratory or expiratory air exchange on auscultation. Inspiratory time is very short. 2. Volume-controlled ventilator: Acute, high increase in airway pressure occurs without chest expansion or audible air exchange.	1. Disconnect patient from ventilator. Confirm and correct obstruction. 2. Use self-inflating bag; note compliance. 3. Partial obstruction will require greater pressure to expand chest. 4. Complete obstruction makes it impossible to inflate chest or bag. 5. In partial obstruction, exhalation characterized by delayed and reduced bag expansion. 6. Pass catheter down endotracheal or tracheostomy tube, feeling for points of resistance or obstruction. 7. Note improvement in airway pressure and chest expansion while doing the following maneuvers to relieve obstruction:

(continued)

Table 25-5
Life-threatening Problems While on Mechanical Ventilation (continued)

Problem	Assessment	Nursing Intervention
Airway Obstruction *(continued)* 2. Complete airway obstruction in a patient who is on a ventilator and has muscle power	There is no visible muscle effort in chest or abdomen. 1. Same as 1 and 2 when patient has no muscle power. 2. Seesaw movement of chest and abdomen. (During inspiration, the chest is depressed. With expiration there is jerky protrusion and prolonged, sustained contraction of the abdominal muscles followed by a brief relaxation before another protrusion and contraction.) 3. Use of accessory muscles of respiration 4. Extreme anxiety and respiratory distress 5. Initial increase in BP and PR; later, decrease in BP and pulse rate 6. Patient is out of phase with machine.	a. Suction inside tube and around pharynx. Deflate cuff. b. Straighten tube to relieve kinked areas in the pharynx, mouth, or connectors. c. Tilt back head, if patient's head is flexed. d. Adjust tracheostomy tube to fit snugly. (Loose fit will cause air leak and possible obstruction of the lumen against wall.) If patient ventilates well on the self-inflating bag, obstruction may be on the machine. e. Drain condensed water in the loop of ventilator tubing. f. Check valves g. Determine whether the connections are wrong or out of adjustment.

Hemothorax
 	
Blood accumulates in pleural cavity, causing collapse of the lung and hypovolemia or shock.
	1. Auscultation of chest reveals absent breath sounds at bases and midlung fields (on affected side).
	2. Increased airway pressure
	3. Signs of bleeding and hypovolemia (*e.g.,* an increase in pulse rate and a decrease in BP)
	4. Chest x-ray will show density on affected side.
		1. If patient is out of phase with ventilator:
		  a. Disconnect from ventilator
		  b. Ventilate by hand with self-inflating bag at high inspired oxygen concentrations
		  c. Call physician
		2. If patient is synchronous with ventilator, call physician.
		3. In the meantime, differentiate from other life-threatening situations while on ventilator (see pp. 500–503).
		4. Assist with the following:
		  a. Chest tube drainage. The needle trochar is inserted at 5th and 6th intercostal space in the midaxillary line.
		  b. Restore blood volume with blood and fluids.
		  c. Prepare for possible thoracic surgical exploration to ligate bleeder(s).

Tension Pneumothorax Pathophysiology
 	
1. Any direct or indirect communication of a bronchus, bronchiole, or alveolus with the pleural cavity produces a closed pneumothorax.
2. When the visceral pleura acts as a valve, air is permitted to enter the pleural cavity on inspiration but not permitted to escape on exhalation.
3. Successive increments of air build up the intrapleural tension.
4. The progressive buildup of intrapleural tension collapses the lung on the affected side.
	1. Acute onset of respiratory distress while on ventilator
	2. Chest
	  a. Unilateral tension pneumothorax
	    Inspection: unequal chest expansion
	    Auscultation:
	    (1) Unequal breath sounds
	    (2) Absent or distant breath sounds on affected side
	    (3) Inspiration—short, crepitant crackles
	    (4) Exhalation—absent breath sounds or brief, muffled, crepitant crackles
	  b. Bilateral pneumothorax
	    Same chest findings as above but on both sides.	

(continued)

Table 25-5
Life-threatening Problems While on Mechanical Ventilation (continued)

Problem	Assessment	Nursing Intervention
Tension Pneumothorax Pathophysiology *(continued)* 5. The mediastinum shifts to the opposite side. This will *kink* or collapse the great veins and thus will seriously interfere with cardiac filling. 6. Death rapidly follows unless tension pneumothorax is promptly relieved.	3. Rapid progressive increase in airway pressure *Volume ventilator:* increase in airway pressure is shown on manometer. *Pressure ventilator:* reaches the maximum pressure limit with little alveolar expansion. Short inspiratory time. 4. Distended neck veins 5. Increased CVP 6. Hypotension 7. Diagnostic thoracentesis at the 2nd and 3rd intercostal spaces will push out plunger of syringe owing to increased intrathoracic pressure. 8. Chest x-ray: shows pneumothorax and possible displacement of trachea away from the affected side 9. Subcutaneous emphysema	1. Disconnect patient from ventilator. 2. Ventilate patient by hand with self-inflating bag. 3. Call physician. 4. Assist physician with insertion of chest tubes with underwater seal drainage.

Flail Chest (from trauma)	These signs and symptoms will be manifested if the patient is on spontaneous ventilation or on an inadequate pressure-controlled ventilator.
	1. Progressive increase in respiratory distress; increased respiratory rate and reduced tidal volumes
	2. Increase use of all accessory muscles of respiration
	3. a. Inspiration—as chest expands, flail section sinks in, impairing ability to produce negative intrapleural pressure, which is necessary to draw air into the lungs.
	   b. Expiration—flail segment bulges outward, thus impairing ability to exhale.
	   In severe flail chest, air may shift uselessly from side to side.
	4. Accumulation of secretions owing to decreased intrapleural negative pressure, and impaired ability to cough them up.
	5. Rhoncal breath sounds and varying degrees of crackles noted on chest auscultation.
	6. Neck veins engorged
	7. Increased CVP
	8. Cardiac output, BP, and pulse rate initially increased followed by falling BP and pulse rate when the patient can no longer compensate.
	9. Progressive reduction in arterial PO_2
	10. Progressive signs of hypoxemia—restlessness followed by drowsiness leading to coma and death.
		1. Ventilate by hand with self-inflating bag.
		2. Suction secretions.
		3. Call physician.
		4. Attach patient to volume-controlled ventilator.

(continued)

Table 25-5
Life-threatening Problems While on Mechanical Ventilation (continued)

Problem	Assessment	Nursing Intervention
Cardiac Tamponade (Accumulation of excessive fluid in the pericardial space) 1. Increased intrapericardial pressure causes compression of the vena cava and atria and thereby impedes venous return to the heart. 2. Cardiac compression lowers cardiac output. This leads to a fall in BP and a reduction in coronary filling. 3. These are factors that predispose to myocardial hypoxia and failure.	1. Progressively rising venous pressure (CVP). Neck veins distended (pathognomonic) 2. Heart sound distant 3. Quiet fatigue 4. Decreased arterial and pulse pressure 5. Signs of respiratory insufficiency, but mechanical ventilation will aggravate hypotension.	1. Call physician. 2. Assist with pericardiocentesis (p. 653).

When the physician decides that the patient has adequate ventilatory capacity, weaning can be initiated. Baseline measurements are noted: (1) vital capacity, (2) inspiratory force, (3) respiratory rate, (4) resting tidal volume, (5) minute ventilation (f × V_T), (6) arterial blood gases, and (7) F_IO2.

The patient is then attached to a T-bar, on spontaneous ventilation, with warmed and humidified oxygen. The F_IO2 or fraction of inspired oxygen concentration given will depend on the patient's previous satisfactory arterial PO2. Do not wean the patient from oxygen therapy while weaning from mechanical assistance of ventilation. It is unreasonable to expect a patient to assume the work of breathing and, at the same time, to meet the increased cardiovascular demands of decreased inspired oxygen concentrations. During the weaning process the patient must be maintained on the same oxygen therapy, whether he is on the ventilator or off.

F_IO2 can be increased or decreased by either adjusting the flow rate of oxygen, adjusting the diluter valve setting, or adding or reducing a reservoir tube. While the patient is on the T-bar, close monitoring should be done. Psychological support and assurance are necessary.

It is of the utmost importance to follow the trend of the values obtained for the following rather than to rely on isolated measurements: (1) vital capacity, (2) inspiratory force, (3) respiratory rate, (4) resting tidal volume, (5) minute volume, (6) blood gases, and (7) F_IO2.

The second set of blood gases should be drawn 20 minutes after the patient has been on spontaneous ventilation at a constant F_IO2. (It takes 15 to 20 minutes for alveolar arterial equilibration to take place.)

While the patient is on the T-bar he should be observed for signs of hypoxemia or increasing fatigue as manifested by the following: (1) bradycardia, PVCs (premature ventricular contractions), or any sign of increasing cardiac irritability; (2) restlessness; (3) a respiratory rate greater than 35 per minute; and (4) labored respiration. Fatigue or exhaustion is, initially, manifested by an increased respiratory rate associated with a gradual reduction in tidal volume. Later there is a slowing of the respiratory rate.

Serial blood gas analysis and periodic measurements of: (1) inspiratory force, (2) vital capacity, (3) tidal volume, (4) respiratory rate, and (5) minute volume should be continued until they stabilize at satisfactory levels. The frequency of these measurements depends on the patient's clinical progress.

The appearance of signs of exhaustion and hypoxemia correlated with a deterioration of the above measurements suggest the need of immediate ventilatory support. The patient should be placed back on the ventilator each time signs of fatigue or deterioration develop.

Patients who have had short-term ventilatory assistance usually can be extubated within 2 or 3 hours of weaning and allowed spontaneous ventilation via a mask with humidified oxygen. Patients who have had prolonged ventilatory assistance usually require more gradual weaning, which may take several days. They are weaned primarily during the day and placed back on the ventilator at night to sleep.

During the times that the patient is on spontaneous ventilation, the diluter valve, flow rate, and reservoir tube can be adjusted according to the results of the blood gases. IPPB should be given every hour during the day while the patient is on spontaneous ventilation with a T-bar and also after the endotracheal tube has been removed.

Some patients are difficult to wean from mechanical ventilation. A device incorporated into the respirator called "IMV—Intermittent Mandatory Ventilation" will allow the patient to breathe spontaneously as desired, but also delivers a mandatory hyperinflation at regular intervals. IMV is indicated if the patient satisfies all the criteria for weaning but cannot sustain adequate spontaneous ventilation for long periods of time. Upon initiation of IMV the machine is set at a slower rate but larger tidal volume than the patient's spontaneous respiratory activity. It then can be adjusted to maintain satisfactory arterial blood gases.

Following initiation of IMV, serial determinations of the following are made and recorded: (1) respiratory rate, (2) minute volume (V_E), (3) tidal volume (V_T), (4) F_IO2, and (5) arterial blood gases.

If there is no deterioration in these parameters, and as the patient's tidal volume improves, the rate of the ventilator is progressively decreased and the patient is allowed to rely more on spontaneous respiration until weaning is complete.

Successful weaning from the ventilator should be vigorously followed by intensive pulmonary care. Continue (1) oxygen therapy, (2) arterial blood gas evaluation, (3) IPPB, (4) chest physical therapy, and (5) adequate hydration and humidification. Remember that these patients still have minimum pulmonary function and need vigorous supportive therapy before they return to normal.

Weaning From the Cuff. While the patient is on the ventilator, the cuff is kept inflated to avoid aspiration and prevent an air leak and thus to allow adequate chest expansion. Patients with tracheostomies should exercise the larynx by phonation (although no sound or voice comes out) in order to maintain active pharyngeal and laryngeal reflexes. This helps to reduce the chances of aspiration.

Weaning From the Tube. The tracheostomy or endotracheal tube can be removed if the following criteria are present: (1) spontaneous ventilation is adequate; (2) the pharyngeal and laryngeal gag reflexes are active; (3) the patient is maintaining an adequate airway and can swallow, move his jaw, or clench his teeth; and (4) voluntary cough is effective in bringing up secretions. If these are ineffective, the tracheostomy tube is needed so that tracheobronchial secretions can be suctioned. In these patients a fenestrated tracheostomy tube is used in order to minimize resistance to air flow. The presence of an endotracheal or tracheostomy tube prevents closure of the epiglottis, making the cough less forceful.

Before the patient is weaned from the tracheostomy tube, he is given a trial of mouth or nose breathing. This can be accomplished by: (1) changing to a smaller size tube to reduce resistance to air flow while at the same time plugging off the tracheostomy (deflate the cuff) or (2) removing the tracheostomy tube completely.

Weaning From Oxygen. This is the last step. The patient has been weaned from the ventilator, cuff, and tube. His respiratory function has been checked, and oxygen has been given according to the result of the blood gas determinations. The F_IO_2 is then gradually reduced until the PO_2 is in the 70 mm Hg to 100 mg Hg range while the patient is breathing room air. If the PO_2 is less than 70 on room air, supplementary oxygen is recommended.

Evaluation

Expected Outcomes

Achieves successful weaning from ventilator, cuff tube, and oxygen

  a. Gradually assumes work of breathing during ventilator weaning
  b. Maintains cardiovascular stability during weaning
  c. Blood gases within normal range during weaning
  d. Gradually increases length of time off ventilator without respiratory or cardiovascular distress and without anxiety
  e. Chest x-ray negative for aspiration and atelectasis
  f. Pharyngeal and laryngeal gag reflexes active after removal from ventilator

  g. Effective cough after tube removal
  h. Completes weaning from oxygen with ability to maintain PO_2 at 70 mm Hg to 100 mm Hg

▷ Chest Physical Therapy in Intensive Care

The various types of chest physiotherapy include relaxation, breathing exercises, mobilizing and postural exercises, and postural drainage with cupping and chest wall vibrations. These measures may be used to treat both medical and surgical conditions.

The patient is encouraged to breathe deeply and cough effectively. To do so he is taught to relax and avoid splinting while the abdominal and chest wounds are stabilized. The breathing technique should be one of sustained maximum inspiration with slow inspiratory flow, maximum inspiratory volume, and a peak inspiratory hold. The patient should be encouraged to practice for several minutes every hour while awake, for the first 3 to 4 days following surgery.

In both medical and surgical patients, when there is evidence of retained secretions, atelectasis, or pneumonia, postural drainage should be initiated. The patient is positioned so that the drainage of secretions from the affected area is assisted by gravity. As is shown on page 457, there is a drainage position described for each lung segment. The appropriate position is assumed by the patient, and a combination of sustained maximum inspirations, chest wall vibrations upon expiration, or cupping over the affected area are performed. The treatment plan is modified according to the tolerance of the patient and the presence of any medical contraindications.

Alternate Method of Care for Intubated Patients (Bag-Inflation)

The bag-inflation technique requires two persons, one to inflate the patient's lung, and the other to apply chest wall vibrations during exhalation. The procedure is carried out as follows:

- The patient is placed in the side-lying position, and the nurse inflates the patient's lungs with the manual resuscitation bag. The maximum inflation volume should be held at a plateau for a second or so to allow time for poorly ventilated alveoli to fill.

- At the end of the inflation plateau, just as the bag pressure is released, the physical therapist should start to vibrate the chest wall to augment the peak expiratory flow rate and help mobilize secretions. This vibratory compression (produced by molding the hands to the chest wall and tensing the arm and shoulder muscles) is continued to the end of expiration. This helps to dislodge the secretions from the bronchial walls, from which they are expelled by coughing or sterile aspiration.

- Approximately 4 to 6 inflation–expiration cycles are performed, and then the patient is suctioned. However, if secretions are heard at any time, the trachea is suctioned before inflation is started again.

- Each time, after completing this procedure, the therapist listens with a stethoscope while the nurse inflates the lungs. Air entry should be good. The procedure is continued as long as rattling secretions are present and as tolerated by the patient.

- When one side of the chest is clear, the patient is turned and the procedure is repeated on the other side.

This technique should only be carried out by persons skilled in the technique of "bagging," since inability to coordinate the manual ventilation with the patient's own respiratory efforts can result in increased airway pressures, bronchospasm, excessive coughing, and an increased level of agitation in the patient. If the technique results in any of the above, or if the patient is being ventilated with PEEP, or if his condition is unstable, it is advisable to simply "sigh" the patient 5 or 6 times on the mechanical ventilator, following saline instillations and in combination with chest wall vibrations or cupping.

- Caution should be exercised in patients who cannot tolerate vigorous coughing spells, such as those in frank congestive heart failure, those who have recently suffered a myocardial infarction, and those with increased tendency to bronchospasm. Chest physical therapy is also contraindicated in the presence of hypotension, unstable vital signs, medical and surgical catastrophes, and dialysis.

▷ The Clinical Problem of Aspiration

Aspiration is the inhalation of stomach contents; it is a serious complication and may cause death. It can occur when there is loss of protective airway reflexes, such as is seen in patients who are unconscious from drugs, alcohol, stroke, or cardiac arrest, or in instances when a nonfunctioning nasogastric tube allows the gastric contents to drain around the tube and cause silent aspiration.

Massive inhalation of gastric contents, if untreated, will, in a period of several hours, result in the clinical syndrome of tachycardia, dyspnea, cyanosis, hypertension, and finally death. The primary factors responsible for morbidity and mortality after aspiration of gastric contents are the volume of aspirated gastric contents and their character. A full stomach contains solid particles of food. It these are aspirated, the problem then becomes one of mechanical blockage of the airways and secondary infection. A fasting stomach contains gastric juice, which, if aspirated, may prove destructive to the alveoli and capillaries. The presence of fecal contamination (more likely seen in intestinal obstruction) will increase the likelihood of mortality because the endotoxins produced by intestinal organisms may be absorbed systemically, or the thick proteinaceous material found in the intestinal contents may obstruct the airway, leading to atelectasis and secondary bacterial invasion.

Chemical pneumonitis may develop from aspiration and may result in destruction of alveolar–capillary endothelial cells, with a consequent outpouring of protein-rich fluids into the interstitial and intra-alveolar spaces. This results in loss of surfactant, which in turn causes early closure of the airway. Finally, the impaired exchange of oxygen and carbon dioxide causes respiratory failure.

Remember!!!

1. Massive aspiration is fatal.
2. Small, localized aspiration from regurgitation can cause pneumonia and respiratory distress.
3. Silent regurgitation often takes place unobserved and may be more common than we think.

Preventive Measures
When Reflexes are Lacking. Aspiration is likely to occur if the patient cannot adequately coordinate his protective glottic, laryngeal, and cough reflexes. This hazard is increased if the patient has a distended abdomen, is in a supine position, and has his upper extremities immobilized by intravenous infusions or hand restraints. A normal person, when vomiting, can take care of his airway by sitting up or turning on his side and coordinating his breathing, coughing, gag, and glottic reflexes. If these reflexes are active, do not insert an oral airway. If an airway is in place, pull it out the moment the patient gags on it so as not to stimulate the pharyngeal gag reflex and promote vomiting and aspiration. Catheter suction of oral secretions should be executed with minimal pharyngeal stimulation yet at the same time should be effective.

During Tube Feeding. The patient who is receiving tube feedings should be positioned upright during the feeding and for 30 minutes thereafter to allow the stomach to partially empty. Small volumes given under low pressure will help to prevent aspiration.

With Delayed Emptying Time of Stomach. A full stomach may cause aspiration because of increased intragastric or extragastric pressure. The following clinical situations cause delayed emptying time of the stomach and may contribute to aspiration: intestinal obstruction; increased gastric secretions during anxiety, stress, or pain; or abdominal distention because of ileus, ascites, peritonitis, drugs, severe illness, or vaginal delivery.

Following Prolonged Endotracheal Intubation. Prolonged endotracheal intubation or tracheostomy can depress the laryngeal and glottic reflexes because of disuse. Patients with prolonged tracheostomies should be made to phonate and exercise their laryngeal muscles. The pharynx should be suctioned before deflating the cuff to prevent aspiration of regurgitated material. Bear in mind that improperly administered IPPB treatments by mask can distend the stomach and promote aspiration.

▷ Bibliography
Books

Blodgett D. Manual of Respiratory Care Procedures. Philadelphia, JB Lippincott, 1980.
Bushnell SS and Morrison ML. Respiratory Intensive Care Nursing, 2nd ed. Boston, Little, Brown & Co, 1979.
Civetta JM. Intensive Care Therapeutics. New York, Appleton–Century–Crofts, 1980.

Daily EK and Shroeder JS. Techniques in Bedside Hemodynamic Monitoring, 2nd ed. St Louis, CV Mosby, 1981.

Daly BJ. Intensive Care Nursing. Garden City, New York, Medical Examination, 1980.

Emanuelson KL and Densmore MJ. Introduction to Respiratory Therapy. Bethany, Fleschner, 1981.

Grenard S and Traverse N. Introduction to Respiratory Therapy. Chicago, Year Book Medical Publishers, 1981.

Harper RW. A Guide to Respiratory Care: Physiology and Clinical Applications. Philadelphia, JB Lippincott, 1981.

Hunsinger DL et al. Respiratory Technology Procedure and Equipment Manual. Reston, Reston Publishing Co, 1980.

Lehnert BE and Schachter EN. The Pharmacology of Respiratory Care. St Louis, CV Mosby, 1980.

Mackenzie CF et al. Chest Physiotherapy in the Intensive Care Unit. Baltimore, Williams & Wilkins, 1981.

Margand PMS, Brooks CG, and Hunter JW. Preoperative Pulmonary Preparation. Baltimore, Williams & Wilkins, 1981.

Neutze JM et al. Intensive Care of the Heart and Lungs, 3rd ed. St Louis, CV Mosby, 1982.

Rattensborg CC and Via–Reque E. Clinical Use of Mechanical Ventilation. Chicago, Year Book Medical Publishers, 1981.

Shapiro BA. Clinical Application of Blood Gases, 3rd ed. Chicago, Year Book Medical Publishers, 1982.

Shapiro BA, Harrison RA, and Trout CA. Clinical Application of Respiratory Care. Chicago, Year Book Medical Publishers, 1979.

Simon NM (ed). The Psychological Aspects of Intensive Care Nursing. Bowie, Maryland, Robert J Brady, 1980.

Sweetwood HM. Nursing in the Intensive Respiratory Care Unit, 2nd ed. New York, Springer, 1979.

Wade JF. Comprehensive Respiratory Care: Physiology and Technique, 3rd ed. St Louis, CV Mosby, 1982.

West JB (ed). Pulmonary Pathophysiology, 2nd ed. Baltimore, Williams & Wilkins, 1982.

Woolf CR. The Clinical Core of Respiratory Medicine. Philadelphia, JB Lippincott, 1981.

Zagelbaum GL and Paré JAP. Manual of Acute Respiratory Care. Boston, Little, Brown & Co, 1982.

Articles

Albanese AJ and Toplitz AD. A hassle-free guide to suctioning a tracheostomy. RN 1982 Apr; 45(4):24–29.

Brown I. Trach care? Take care—infection's on the prowl. Nursing '82 1982 May; 12(5):44–49.

Cline BA and Fisher ML. ARDS means emergency. Nursing '82 1982 Feb; 12(2):62–67.

Hewlett RS. Respiratory care of the neurological/neurosurgical patient. In Burton GG, Gee GN, and Hodgkin JE (eds). Respiratory Care. Philadelphia, JB Lippincott, 1977.

Hooker CJ. A life-and-breath nursing challenge: Helping patients who must stop smoking. Nursing '81 1981 Nov; 11(11):98–99.

Murphy PA and Schare BL. Timely techniques in caring for the patient with an endotracheal tube. Part 1. Nursing '81 1981 Sept; 11(9):70–73.

Murphy PA and Schare BL. Timely techniques in caring for the patient with an endotracheal tube. Part 2. Nursing '81 1981 Oct; 11(10):65–69.

Petty TL. Adult respiratory distress syndrome. Seminars in Respiratory Medicine 1982 Apr; 3(4):219–224.

Rathlev MC and McNamara MA. Teaching families to give trach care at home. Nursing '82 1982 June; 12(6):70–71.

26

Management of Patients With Conditions of the Chest and Lower Respiratory Tract

▷ Pulmonary Infections

Acute Tracheobronchitis

Acute tracheobronchitis, an acute inflammation of the mucous membranes of the trachea and the bronchial tree, often follows infections of the upper respiratory tract. A patient with a viral infection has a lessened resistance and can readily develop a secondary bacterial infection. Thus, the adequate treatment of upper respiratory infections is one of the major factors in the prevention of acute bronchitis. Aside from infection, inhalation of physical and chemical irritants, gases, or other air contaminants can also cause acute bronchial irritations.

Clinical Manifestations. The patient's symptoms result from the mucopurulent sputum that is secreted by the hyperemic edematous mucosa of the bronchi. The patient has a dry, irritating cough and expectorates a scanty amount of mucoid sputum at first. He complains of sternal soreness from coughing, and has fever, headache, and general malaise. As the infection progresses, the sputum is more profuse and purulent and the cough becomes looser.

Management. The treatment is largely symptomatic. Therefore, the nurse's observations are important in determining the therapeutic plan. The patient is placed on bed rest. Moist heat to the chest will relieve the soreness and pain. Cool vapor therapy or steam inhalations are beneficial in relieving the laryngeal and tracheal irritation. Increasing the vapor pressure (moisture content) in the air will reduce irritation.

Cough depressants should not be given or should be given only with caution when the cough becomes productive. Antihistamines especially may be excessively drying, making secretions more difficult to expectorate. An expectorant such as potassium iodide may be given and the fluid intake increased to "thin" the viscous and tenacious secretions. Antibiotic treatment is indicated when the sputum becomes purulent, as *Streptococcus pneumoniae* and *Haemophilus influenzae* are commonly found to be present.

A primary nursing function is to caution the patient against overexertion, which can induce a relapse or extension of the infection. Aged individuals are prone to develop bronchopneumonia as a complication. They are not always able to cough effectively and therefore tend to retain the mucopurulent exudate. These patients should be turned and should assume the sitting position at frequent intervals. Adequate opportunity for convalescence should be provided after the acute infection subsides, in order to avoid its recurrence.

Pulmonary Infections

Pneumonia

Pneumonia is an inflammatory process of the lung substance that is commonly caused by infectious agents. Pneumonia is the most common infectious cause of death in the U.S. It is classified according to its causative agent, if known: for example, it may be a *bacterial, viral, fungal,* or *lipid pneumonia.* There is also a *chemical* pneumonia, such as that seen after ingestion of kerosene or inhalation of irritating gases. Radiation pneumonitis may follow radiation therapy for breast or lung cancer and usually occurs 6 weeks or more after completion of radiotherapy. *Aspiration* pneumonia is discussed on page 505.

If a substantial portion of one or more lobes is involved, the disease is referred to as *lobar pneumonia. Bronchopneumonia* implies that the pneumonic process is distributed in patchy fashion, having originated in one or more localized areas within the bronchi and extended to the adjacent surrounding lung parenchyma. Of these two types, bronchopneumonia is more common than lobar pneumonia.

In general, persons developing bacterial pneumonia usually have acute or chronic underlying disease that impairs host defenses. More often, pneumonia arises from endogenous flora of the patient whose resistance has been altered or from aspiration of mouth flora. While most viral infections occur in previously healthy persons, when bacterial pneumonia occurs in a healthy person there is usually a history of preceding viral illness. In recent years there has been an increase in the number of patients who have deficient defenses against infections: those on corticosteroids or other immunosuppressive drugs, those on broad-spectrum antimicrobials, those with acquired immune deficiency syndrome, and those requiring the use of life-support technology. These patients who have suppressed immune systems often acquire pneumonia owing to organisms of low virulence. In addition, there are increasing numbers of patients with impaired defenses who develop hospital-acquired pneumonia from gram-negative bacilli (*Klebsiella, Pseudomonas, Escherichia coli, Enterobacteriaceae, Proteus, Serratia*). Also, gram-positive cocci, anaerobes, mycobacteria, nocardial species, viral, chlamydial, fungal, and parasitic agents can cause pneumonia. Commonly encountered pneumonias and their clinical features, treatment, and complications are presented in Table 26-1.

Prevention and Persons at Risk

The nurse should be acquainted with the factors and circumstances that commonly predispose the person to pneumonia in order to identify the high-risk individual and engage in anticipatory and preventive nursing.

- Any condition producing mucus or bronchial obstruction and interfering with normal drainage of the lung (cancer, chronic obstructive pulmonary disease) renders the individual susceptible to pneumonia.
- Immunosuppressed patients are at risk.

Table 26-1
Commonly Encountered Pneumonias

Type (Bacterial)	Organism Responsible	Manifestations
Streptococcal pneumonia	*Streptococcus pneumoniae*	May be history of previous respiratory infection Sudden onset, with shaking and chills Rapidly rising fever; tachypnea Cough, with expectoration of rusty or green (purulent) sputum Pleuritic pain aggravated by cough Chest dull to percussion; crackles, bronchial breath sounds Confusion may be only presenting feature in elderly
Staphylococcal pneumonia	*Staphylococcus aureus*	Often prior history of viral infection Insidious development of cough, with expectoration of yellow, blood-streaked mucus Onset may be sudden if patient is outside hospital Fever Pleuritic chest pain Pulse varies; may be slow in proportion to temperature

- Any patient who is permitted to lie passively in bed for prolonged periods, relatively immobile and breathing shallowly, is highly vulnerable to the risk of bronchopneumonia.
- Any person who has a depressed cough reflex (owing to drugs or weakness) or has aspirated foreign material into the lungs during a period of unconsciousness (head injury, anesthesia) or has an abnormal swallowing mechanism is very likely to develop bronchopneumonia.
- Any hospitalized patient on a nothing-by-mouth regimen or who is receiving antibiotics has increased pharyngeal colonization of organisms and is at risk. In very ill persons, the oropharynx is likely to be colonized by gram-negative bacteria.
- Persons who are intoxicated frequently are particularly susceptible to this infection, since alcohol suppresses the body's reflexes, white cell mobilization, and tracheobronchial ciliary motion.
- Any person scheduled to receive a sedative should be observed for respiratory rate and depth before the drug is given; if respiratory depression is apparent, the drug should not be administered. Respiratory depression predisposes to the pooling of bronchial secretions and subsequent development of pneumonia.
- An important preventive measure is the frequent suctioning of secretions in patients who are unconscious or have poor cough and gag reflexes; this reduces the likelihood that secretions will be aspirated or accumulate in the lungs and induce bronchopneumonia.
- Postoperative pneumonia should be anticipated in the elderly and forestalled by frequent mobilization, coughing, and breathing exercises.
- Routine daily decontamination of respiratory therapy equipment is essential.

Bacterial Pneumonia (*Streptococcus pneumoniae*)

Streptococcus pneumoniae pneumonia is the most common bacterial pneumonia and is most prevalent during the winter and spring months, when upper respiratory infections are most frequent. It may occur as a lobar or bronchopneumonic form in patients of any age. A history of recent respiratory illness can often be elicited.

Streptococcus pneumoniae, the infecting agent that causes the majority of cases of bacterial pneumonia, is a gram-positive, capsulated, nonmotile coccus that resides naturally in the upper respiratory tract. *S. pneumoniae* is commonly referred to as the pneumococcus.

Pathophysiology.   The altered physiology occurring with the pneumonic process is a ventilation problem. The pneumococci gain access to the alveoli where an inflammatory reaction occurs that produces an exudate that pours into the air spaces. White blood cells, mostly neutrophils, also migrate into the alveoli, so that the lung segment assumes a more solid structure as the air-containing spaces become filled. Areas of the lung are not adequately ventilated because of secretions, mucosal edema, and bronchospasm. These conditions cause partial occlusion of the bronchi or alveoli, producing a drop in the alveolar oxygen tension. Venous blood coming into the lungs passes through the underventilated area and goes out of the lung to the left side of the heart without being oxygenated. In essence, the blood is shunted from the right to the left side of the heart. This mixing of oxygenated and unoxygenated blood eventually results in arterial hypoxemia.

Clinical Manifestations.   Classical bacterial (or pneumococcal) pneumonia usually starts with a sudden onset of shaking chill, rapidly rising fever (39.5° C–40.5° C

(Text continues on page 512)

Clinical Features	Treatment	Complications
Herpes simplex lesions often present on face or lips Usually involves one or more lobes	Penicillin G Alternate drug therapy; erythromycin, clindamycin, cephalosporins, other penicillins, trimethoprim-sulfamethoxazole	Shock Pleural effusion Superinfections Pericarditis Otitis media
Frequently seen in hospital setting Staphylococcal pneumonia is a necrotizing infection Treatment must be vigorous and prolonged owing to disease's tendency to destroy the lungs Organism may develop rapid drug resistance Prolonged convalescence usual	Nafcillin, methicillin, clindamycin, vancomycin, cephalothin	Effusion/pneumothorax Lung abscess Empyema Meningitis

(continued)

Table 26-1
Commonly Encountered Pneumonias (continued)

Type (Bacterial)	Organism Responsible	Manifestations
Klebsiella pneumonia	*Klebsiella pneumoniae* (Friedländer's bacillus—encapsulated gram-negative aerobic bacillus)	Onset sudden with high fever, chills, pleuritic pain, hemoptysis Dyspnea, cyanosis Dark brown–red gelatinous sputum expectorated Profound prostration and toxicity
Pseudomonas pneumonia	*Pseudomonas aeruginosa*	Apprehension; confusion Cyanosis; bradycardia Reversal of diurnal temperature curve
Legionnaires' disease	*Legionella pneumophila*	Prodromal period of abdominal pain and diarrhea High fever, chills, cough, chest pain, tachypnea
Pittsburgh pneumonia agent (PPA)	*Legionella micdadei*	Fever, myalgias, nonproductive cough, dyspnea; pleuritic pain may occur. Patchy alveolar infiltrates on chest x-ray
Mycoplasma pneumonia	*Mycoplasma pneumoniae*	Gradual onset; severe headache; irritating, hacking cough producing scanty, mucoid sputum Anorexia; malaise Fever; nasal congestion; sore throat
Viral pneumonia	Influenza viruses Parainfluenza viruses Respiratory syncytial viruses Adenovirus Varicella, rubella, rubeola, herpes simplex, cytomegalovirus, Epstein–Barr virus	Cough Constitutional symptoms may be pronounced (severe headache, anorexia, fever, and myalgia)
Pneumocystis carinii pneumonia	*Pneumocystis carinii*	Insidious onset Increasing dyspnea and nonproductive cough Tachypnea; progresses rapidly to intercostal retraction, nasal flaring, and cyanosis Lowering of arterial oxygen tension Chest x-ray will reveal diffuse, bilateral interstitial pneumonia
Fungal pneumonia	*Aspergillus fumigatus*	Hectic fever, productive cough, chest pain, hemoptysis Chest x-ray reveals broad range of abnormalities from infiltration to consolidation, cavitation, and empyema

Clinical Features	Treatment	Complications
Tends to attack chronically ill, debilitated, alcoholic, and elderly men or those with chronic obstructive pulmonary disease Tissue necrosis occurs rapidly in lungs with cavity formation in some patients May be rapidly fulminating, progressing to fatal outcome High mortality rate	Gentamicin, cefazolin, tobramycin	Multiple lung abscesses with cyst formation Persistent cough with expectoration remains for prolonged period Empyema Pericarditis
Usually acquired in the hospital Susceptible persons: those with preexisting lung disease, cancer (particularly leukemia); those with homograft transplants, burns; debilitated persons; patients receiving prolonged courses of antibiotics and treatment such as tracheostomy, suctioning Respiratory equipment may be contaminated with these organisms	Gentamicin, carbenicillin	Has capacity to invade blood vessel walls, causing hemorrhage and lung infarction High fatality rate
Peak incidence in persons over 50 who are cigarette smokers and have underlying diseases that increase susceptibility to infection	Erythromycin	Respiratory failure
May be hospital-acquired Generally seen in immunocompromised patient	Erythromycin; rifampin; trimethoprim-sulfamethoxazole	Involves multiple lobes; bilateral consolidation common High mortality rate; clinical recovery slow
Occurs most commonly in children and young adults as well as in older adults in community hospital setting Rise in serum-complement-fixing antibodies to the organism	Erythromycin; tetracycline	Persisting cough, meningoencephalitis, polyneuritis, monoarticular arthritis, pericarditis, myocarditis
In majority of patients influenza begins as an acute coryza; others have bronchitis, pleurisy, etc., while still others develop gastrointestinal symptoms Risk of developing influenza related to crowding and close contact of groups of individuals	Treat symptomatically Does not respond to treatment with presently available antimicrobials Prophylactic vaccination recommended for high-risk persons (over 65; chronic cardiac or pulmonary disease, diabetes and other metabolic disorders)	May develop a superimposed bacterial infection Bronchopneumonia Pericarditis; endocarditis
Usually seen in host whose resistance is compromised; seen also in male homosexual population Organism invades lungs of patients who have suppressed immune system (from cancer, leukemia) or following immunosuppressive therapy for cancer, organ transplant, or collagen disease Frequently associated with concurrent infection by viruses, (cytomegalovirus) bacteria, and fungi	Trimethoprim-sulfamethoxazole	Patients are critically ill Prognosis guarded, as it usually is a complication of a severe underlying disorder
Neutropenic individual most susceptible May develop *Aspergillus* as a superinfection	Amphotericin B	High fatality rate Invades blood vessels and destroys lung tissue by direct invasion and vascular infarction

[101° F–105° F]), and stabbing chest pain that is aggravated by respiration and coughing. The patient appears severely ill with marked tachypnea (25–45/minute) accompanied by respiratory grunting, nasal flaring, and the use of accessory muscles of respiration. He often lies on his affected side in an attempt to splint his chest. The pulse is rapid and bounding. The cheeks are flushed, the eyes bright, and the lips and nail beds cyanotic. The patient prefers to be propped up in bed because of his cough, which is short, painful, and incessant. He perspires profusely and is often cyanotic. The sputum is purulent and sometimes blood-tinged or rusty.

Other signs occur in patients who suffer from a condition such as cancer or those who are undergoing treatment with immunosuppressants, which lower their resistance to infection and to organisms heretofore not considered serious pathogens. Such patients present with fever, crackles, and physical signs of lobar consolidation (tactile and vocal fremitus, bronchial breathing, and percussion dullness).

In older patients or those with chronic obstructive pulmonary disease, the symptoms may develop insidiously. Purulent sputum may be the only signal of pneumonia in these patients. It is difficult to detect subtle changes in their conditions as they already have seriously compromised pulmonary function. Assess these patients for unusual behavior, alterations in mental status, prostration, and congestive heart failure. A restless, excited delirium may be exhibited especially in alcoholic patients.

Diagnostic Assessment. Diagnosis is made by history (particularly of recent respiratory infection), physical examination, chest x-ray, blood culture (bloodstream invasion occurs frequently), and sputum examination.

- In order to get a good sample of sputum, have the patient rinse his mouth with water to minimize contamination by normal oral flora. Instruct him to breathe deeply several times and then to cough deeply and expectorate the raised sputum into a sterile container.

Sputum may also be obtained by transtracheal aspiration (p. 442) or fiberoptic bronchoscopy (p. 441) in patients who cannot raise sputum or those who are obtunded, have abnormal host defense mechanisms, or have developed pneumonia after antimicrobial therapy or while hospitalized.

Patient Problems/Nursing Diagnoses

Based on the clinical manifestations and diagnostic assessment data, the patient's major nursing problems include respiratory dysfunction related to infection of the lung parenchyma; complications related to the pneumonic process; and possible nonadherence to a therapeutic and preventive program related to knowledge deficit.

▶ Planning and Implementation

Goals

The goals for the patient are:

1. Improvement of respiratory function
2. Prevention of complications
3. Adherence to the therapeutic and preventive program

Management. The treatment of pneumonia is based on giving an appropriate antibiotic, depending on the results of a carefully done Gram stain. Penicillin G is usually the antibiotic of choice for *S. pneumoniae.* Other effective drugs include erythromycin, clindamycin, the cephalosporins, other penicillins, and trimethoprim-sulfamethoxazole.

Nursing Interventions. The patient is placed on bed rest until infection shows signs of clearing. He is observed carefully and continually until his clinical condition improves. Lethal complications may develop during the first few days of antibiotic treatment. The patient is watched for continuing or recurring fever. Inadequate lung drainage or poor blood supply to the involved lung may reduce the amount of antibiotic agent reaching the invading organism. Resistant or recurring fever may be due to drug allergy (assess for skin rash), drug resistance or slow response of the susceptible organism, super-infection, infected pleural effusion, or pneumonia owing to unusual organisms (such as *Pneumocystis carinii* or fungi).

- Failure of the pneumonia to resolve raises the suspicion of underlying carcinoma of the bronchus.

Elimination and Control of Secretions. Retained secretions interfere with gas exchange and may cause slow resolution (subsidence) of the disease. A high level of fluid intake (within level of cardiac reserve) is encouraged, since adequate hydration thins and loosens pulmonary secretions and also replaces fluid losses owing to fever, diaphoresis, dehydration, and dyspnea. The air is humidified in order to loosen secretions and improve ventilation. A high humidity face mask (using either compressed air or oxygen) delivers warm, humidified air to the tracheobronchial tree and liquefies secretions. The patient is encouraged to cough in the following manner:

1. Inhale slowly through the nose.
2. Exhale and cough forcefully while contracting (holding in) the abdomen. (This tightens the glottis and raises intrapulmonary pressure.)

Chest physiotherapy (percussion and postural drainage) is also important in loosening and mobilizing secretions. The chest is vibrated and clapped and the patient is then placed in the proper position to drain the involved lung. Postural drainage uses the principle of gravity that permits secretions to flow from the smaller bronchi to the larger bronchi to be expectorated or suctioned. If the patient is too weak to cough effectively, the mucus may have to be removed by nasotracheal suctioning or by bronchoscopic aspiration.

Oxygenation. The patient who is hypoxemic should be given oxygen. Arterial blood gas analysis is done to determine oxygen need and evaluate oxygen effectiveness. A high concentration of oxygen is to be avoided in persons with chronic obstructive pulmonary disease since it may worsen alveolar ventilation by removing the patient's only remaining ventilatory drive and lead to respiratory decompensation. Respiratory support measures such as endotracheal intubation, high inspiratory oxygen concentrations, and positive end-expiratory pressure may be required for some patients. These treatment modalities are discussed in Chapter 25.

Pain Relief.   Pleuritic pain may be relieved by codeine or intercostal nerve block. Evaluate the patient's sensorium before administering sedatives or tranquilizers, in order to assess for signs and symptoms of pneumococcal meningitis. Restlessness, confusion, and aggression may well be due to cerebral hypoxemia, in which case sedatives are inappropriate.

Avoid suppressing the cough reflex. However, serious hypoxia may follow paroxysms of coughing, especially in persons with pre-existing heart conditions. Nonproductive paroxysms of coughing may be controlled with codeine. This may, however, be contraindicated in patients with chronic obstructive pulmonary disease (COPD) in whom opiates or other central nervous system depressants cause further hypoventilation.

Abdominal distention may be distressing since the patient may swallow air during intervals of severe dyspnea. It impairs respiratory movement by elevation of the diaphragm. A nasogastric tube may be passed for acute gastric dilation.

Diet.   Initially, the dyspneic patient is anorexic and prefers a liquid diet. With improvement, a normal diet is offered. Persons with congestive heart failure may be on a low sodium diet.

Assessment for Complications.   Patients should respond to treatment within 24 to 48 hours after antibiotic therapy is initiated. Complications of pneumonia include sustained *hypotension and shock* (especially in gram-negative bacterial disease in the elderly). These complications are encountered chiefly in patients who have received no specific treatment, have been treated too little or too late, have received chemotherapy to which the infecting organism is resistant, or are suffering from a pre-existing disease that complicates the pneumonia.

To combat peripheral collapse and maintain arterial blood pressure, a vasopressor agent is given intravenously in the form of a constant infusion and at a rate that is readjusted constantly in accordance with the pressure response. Corticosteroid drugs may be administered parenterally to combat shock and toxicity in patients with pneumonia who are extremely ill and in apparent danger of succumbing to the infection.

Atelectasis (from obstruction of bronchus by accumulated secretions) may occur at any stage of acute pneumonia. Pleural effusion (p. 514) also is fairly common and may signal the beginning of empyema. A diagnostic thoracentesis is usually necessary to evaluate an effusion. A chest tube may be required to control pleural infection by establishing proper drainage of the empyema.

Delirium is another possible complication and is considered a medical emergency when it occurs. It may be caused by hypoxia, meningitis, or the delirium tremens of alcoholism. The patient with delirium is given oxygen, adequate hydration, and mild sedation and is observed constantly. Congestive heart failure, cardiac arrhythmias, pericarditis, and myocarditis are also complications of pneumonia.

Influenza vaccine is recommended yearly to all patients at risk, as pneumonia is a complication of influenza. A summary of the care of the patient with bacterial pneumonia is found in Chart 26-1.

Patient Education.   After the fever subsides, the patient may gradually increase his activities. Fatigue, weakness, and depression may be prolonged after pneumonia. Breathing exercises to clear the lungs and promote full lung expansion are encouraged (p. 458). The patient is instructed to return to the clinic or physician's office for follow-up chest x-rays.

Explain to the patient that it is wise to stop smoking since cigarette smoking destroys tracheobronchial ciliary action, which is the first line of defense of the lungs. It also irritates the mucous cells of the bronchi and inhibits the function of alveolar macrophage (scavenger) cells. Instruct the patient to avoid fatigue, sudden changes in temperature, and excessive alcohol intake, which lowers resistance to pneumonia. Review with the patient the principles of good nutrition and rest, since one episode of pneumonia may make him susceptible to recurring respiratory infections. He should be encouraged to obtain influenza vaccine at the prescribed times, because influenza increases susceptibility to secondary bacterial pneumonia, especially staphylococcus, *Haemophilus influenzae,* and *Streptococcus pneumoniae.*

The patient is encouraged to seek medical advice about receiving vaccine against *Streptococcus pneumoniae* (Pneumovax). This vaccine may be effective against the majority of bacteremic pneumococcal diseases. Because it provides immunity for 3 to 5 years, it is recommended for patients at high risk: those who have had their spleens removed and those with sickle cell disease, chronic lung, cardiac and renal disease, etc.

▶ **Evaluation**

Expected Outcomes

1. Improves respiratory function
   Attains suitable levels of the following parameters:
   (1) Arterial blood gas tension at 60 mm Hg
   (2) Temperature normal
   (3) Pulse and respiration within normal range
   (4) Chest clear upon auscultation
   (5) Keeps a record of fluid intake
2. Is free of complications
   a. Participates in breathing exercises to clear lungs and promote lung expansion
   b. Takes prescribed antimicrobial agent
   c. Cooperates with health care personnel monitoring his condition (vital signs, arterial blood gas analyses, chest x-rays, etc.)
   d. Expectorates secretions
3. Adheres to therapeutic and prevention program
   a. Aware of factors that contribute to development of pneumonia
   b. Talks of joining a support group to stop smoking
   c. Makes an appointment at clinic for follow-up chest x-ray and influenza vaccination

d. Verbalizes that he will cope with fatigue by rest, alternating with increasing activity

(Also, see 1, improves respiratory function, p. 513.)

Atypical Pneumonia Syndromes

Pneumonias association with mycoplasmas, psittacosis, Q fever, Legionnaires' disease, and viruses are included in the atypical pneumonia syndromes (Table 26-1).

Mycoplasma pneumoniae is the most common cause of primary atypical pneumonia. Mycoplasmas are small organisms surrounded by a triple-layered membrane without a cell wall. The organisms grow on a special culture medium but differ from viruses. Mycoplasma pneumonia occurs most frequently in older children and young adults.

It is probably spread by infected respiratory droplets, through person-to-person contact. Often these patients develop positive cold agglutinin titers in their serum, but mycoplasma antibodies can be tested.

The inflammatory infiltrate is primarily interstitial rather than alveolar. It spreads throughout the entire respiratory tract, including the bronchioles. Generally, it has the characteristics of a bronchopneumonia. Earache and bullous myringitis are common.

Clinical Manifestations. Usually, the patient has had an upper respiratory infection, and the onset of his pneumonic symptoms is gradual. The predominant symptoms are a harassing and nonproductive cough, a feeling of tightness in the chest, and generalized aching and prostration, along with tracheal pain when coughing. After a few days, mucoid or mucopurulent sputum is expectorated. The patient complains of headache that is aggravated by the cough.

Planning and Implementation. The goal of nursing care is to promote the patient's rest and comfort. Mycoplasma pneumonia responds to erythromycin and tetracycline. Other atypical pneumonias are viral in origin, and most do not respond to antimicrobials. Warm, moist inhalations are helpful in relieving bronchial irritation. The nursing care and treatment (with the exception of antimicrobial therapy) is the same as that given to the patient who has bacterial pneumonia (pp. 516–517).

Pleurisy

Pleurisy (pleuritis) is inflammation of the visceral and parietal pleurae. When these inflamed membranes rub together during respiration (particularly inspiration), the result is severe, sharp, "knifelike" pain. The pain may become minimal or absent when the breath is held, or it may be localized or radiate to the shoulder or abdomen. Later, as pleural fluid develops, the pain lessens. In the early dry period, the pleural friction rub can be heard with the stethoscope, only to disappear later as fluid appears to separate the roughened pleural surfaces.

Pleurisy may develop with pneumonia or upper respiratory infection, tuberculosis, collagen disease, after trauma to the chest or pulmonary infarction or embolism, in primary and metastatic cancer, in the viral disease known as epidemic pleurodynia, and after thoracotomy.

Careful x-ray and sputum examinations and thoracentesis with pleural fluid examination and possibly pleural biopsy are indicated in order to discover the underlying condition.

Management. The objective of treatment is to discover the underlying condition causing the pleurisy. As the underlying disease is treated (pneumonia, infarction) the pleuritic inflammation usually resolves. At the same time it is necessary to watch for signs of pleural effusion: shortness of breath, pain, and decreased local excursion of the chest wall.

Since this patient has real pain on inspiration, the nurse can offer suggestions to enhance comfort, such as turning frequently on the affected side in order to splint the chest wall; this will lessen the stretch of the pleura. The nurse can also teach the patient to use his hands to splint the rib cage while coughing.

Prescribed analgesics and applications of heat or cold will provide symptomatic relief. Indomethacin, an anti-inflammatory drug, may give pain relief while allowing the patient to cough effectively. If the pain is severe, a procaine intercostal block may be required. Since pain upon breathing produces anxiety, the patient will require support and understanding.

Pleural Effusion

Pleural effusion, a collection of fluid in the pleural space, is rarely a primary disease process but is usually secondary to other diseases. Normally, the pleural space may contain a small amount of fluid (5 ml–15 ml) acting as a lubricant that allows the visceral and parietal surfaces to move without friction.

In certain intrathoracic and systemic diseases, fluid may accumulate in the pleural space to a point where it becomes clinically evident, and it is almost always of pathologic significance. The effusion can be a relatively clear fluid, which may be a transudate or an exudate, or it can be blood, pus, or chyle. A *transudate* (filtrates of plasma that move across intact capillary walls) occurs when factors influencing formation and reabsorption of pleural fluid are altered, usually by imbalances in hydrostatic or oncotic pressures. A transudate indicates that a condition like ascites or a systemic disease like congestive heart failure or renal failure underlies the fluid accumulation. An *exudate* (extravasation of fluid into tissues/cavity) usually results from inflammation by bacterial products or tumors involving the pleural surfaces. In general, the differentiation is made on the basis of protein content and lactic dehydrogenase activity. Pleural effusion may be a complication of tuberculosis, pneumonia, congestive heart failure, pulmonary viral infections, and neoplastic tumors. In fact, 50% of patients with cancer of the lung develop pleural effusion. In approximately one in four patients, pleural effusion is secondary to carcinoma.

Clinical Manifestations. Usually, the clinical manifestations are those caused by the underlying disease; pneumonia will cause fever, chills, and pleuritic chest pain whereas a malignant effusion may result in dyspnea and coughing. A large quantity of pleural effusion will cause shortness of breath with dullness or flatness to percussion over areas of fluid with minimal or absence of breath sounds. Confirmation of the presence of fluid is obtained by chest x-ray, ultrasound, physical examination, and thoracentesis. Tests made of pleural fluid include bacterial cultures, gram stain, acid-fast bacillus stain (for tuberculosis), red cell count, white cell count, chemistry studies (glucose, amylase, lactic dehydrogenase, protein), and pH.

Management. The objectives of treatment are to discover the underlying cause, to prevent fluid collection from recurring, and to relieve discomfort and dyspnea. Specific treatment is directed to the underlying cause (e.g., congestive heart failure, cirrhosis, etc.).

Thoracentesis is done to remove fluid, to collect a specimen for analysis, and to relieve dyspnea. However, if the underlying cause is a malignancy, the effusion may recur within a few days or weeks. Repeated thoracenteses result in pain, depletion of protein and electrolytes, and sometimes pneumothorax. In this event the patient may be treated with chest tube drainage connected to an underwater seal drainage system or suction to evacuate the pleural space and reexpand the lung. Sometimes tetracycline, radioactive isotopes, or cytotoxic or other chemically irritating drugs are instilled in the pleural space to obliterate the pleural space and prevent further accumulation of fluid. After drug instillation, the chest tube is clamped and the patient is assisted to assume various positions to assure uniform drug distribution and to maximize drug contact with the pleural surfaces. The tube is unclamped as prescribed, and chest drainage is usually continued several days longer to prevent reaccumulation of fluid and to facilitate obliteration of the pleural space by formation of adhesions between the visceral and parietal pleurae. Other modalities of treatment for malignant pleural effusions include radiation of the chest wall, surgical pleurectomy, and diuretic therapy.

If the pleural fluid is an exudate, more extensive diagnostic procedures are done in order to determine the cause. Therapy for pleural disease is then instituted.

▷ Lung Abscess

Pathogenesis. A *lung abscess* is a localized, pus-containing necrotic lesion in the lung characterized by cavity formation. It may occur from aspiration of vomitus or infected material (nasotracheal secretions; blood) from the upper respiratory tract. After aspiration, pneumonitis develops, and the area of pneumonia cavitates because the microorganisms have necrotizing potential; hence a lung abscess may develop very rapidly. A lung abscess may also occur secondarily to bronchial obstruction owing to a tumor. Stasis of secretions occurs with infection or necrosis within the tumor mass. Or, it may be a sequela of necrotizing pneumonias, tuberculosis, pulmonary embolism, chest trauma, or bronchial neoplasm.

In the initial stages the cavity in the lung may or may not communicate with a bronchus; eventually, however, it becomes surrounded, or "encapsulated," by a wall of fibrous tissue, except at one or two points where the necrotic process extends until it reaches the lumen of some bron-

chus or the pleural space and thus establishes a communication with the respiratory tract, the pleural cavity, or both. In the first instance, its purulent contents are evacuated continuously in the form of sputum, whereas if a pleural exit is accessible, empyema results; if both types of communication are furnished, the problem becomes one of *bronchopleural fistula*.

Clinical Manifestations. The majority of patients have a cough that produces a small amount of sputum, a low-grade fever, and malaise. In time the sputum becomes copious and often foul-smelling, and at times there is hemoptysis. This occurs frequently when bronchial communication is established and the abscess begins to drain. The patient may complain of a pleuritic type of chest pain. Sometimes the onset is acute, with chills, high fever, cough, and malaise. Physical examination may reveal an area of consolidation and pleural thickening, dullness to percussion, and suppressed breath sounds.

Confirmation of the diagnosis is made by chest roentgenography, sputum culture, and direct visualization with fiberoptic bronchoscopy, which is necessary to rule out the possibility of tumor or a foreign body in the lung.

Preventive Measures for Persons at Risk. The following principles will reduce the risk of suppurative lung disease:

1. Patients who must have teeth extracted while their gums and teeth are infected may be given appropriate antibiotic therapy before any dental manipulations.
2. The patient should be instructed to maintain good dental and oral hygiene, since anaerobic bacteria play a role in the pathogenesis of lung abscess.
3. Appropriate antimicrobial therapy should be given to patients with pneumonia.
4. Bronchoscopy is called for if inhalation of foreign material is suspected.
5. A patient with impaired cough reflexes and loss of glottis closure or one who has swallowing difficulties is apt to aspirate foreign material and hence to develop lung abscess.
6. Other patients at risk are those with an altered state of consciousness from anesthesia, central nervous system disorders (seizures, stroke), drug addiction, alcoholism, or esophageal disease, as well as patients being fed by nasogastric tube.

Management. The *goals of management* are to (1) eradicate the infection and (2) establish adequate drainage of the lung abscess.

Usually, sputum specimens are obtained by transtracheal aspiration since an expectorated sputum specimen will be contaminated by the indigenous flora of the mouth and gingivae. Usually, several species of bacteria are present in a lung abscess. Antimicrobial therapy is given according to sputum culture and sensitivity and is given for an extended period of time. High intravenous doses are generally required, because the antibiotic must penetrate necrotic tissue and abscess fluid.

Provision of adequate drainage of the lung abscess is by postural drainage aided by percussion, coughing, and

(Text continues on page 518)

Chart 26-1
Summary: Guidelines for Caring for the Patient With Bacterial Pneumonia

Goals, Nursing Interventions, and Rationale of Care

I. To assist with collection of laboratory data for the identification of the causative organism:
  A. Bacteriologic study of sputum
    1. Instruct patient to cough productively so that specimens will consist of bronchial secretions.

    Specific antimicrobial therapy depends on the nature and sensitivity of organisms isolated from the culture and the sensitivity tests of the sputum specimen.

    2. If patient is too ill to raise sputum, aspirate trachea with catheter or use transtracheal aspiration.

    Tracheal aspiration can produce a paroxysm of coughing that produces sputum.

    3. Collect sputum in sterile containers.
  B. Hemogram and urinalysis
  C. Bacteriologic study of blood
  D. Posteroanterior and lateral chest x-rays

II. To provide specific therapy to eradicate the organism:

  The therapy of pneumonia depends on laboratory identification of the agent causing the infection and on the drainage of purulent secretions.

  Pneumococci are highly susceptible to the action of penicillin.

  A. Give prescribed antibiotic at correct time intervals.
    1. Penicillin is usually drug of choice.
    2. Erythromycin, clindamycin, etc. can be given if patient is allergic to penicillin.
  B. Observe patient for nausea, vomiting, diarrhea, anal pruritus, skin rash, and soft tissue reactions.

III. To evaluate the patient's response to therapy:
  A. Take TPR and BP at regular 4-hour intervals and more frequently if indicated.

  Lethal complications may develop during the early period of antimicrobial treatment.

  The temperature curve provides an index of the patient's response to therapy and his progress.

    1. Watch for continuing or recurring fever from drug allergy, drug resistance or slow response to therapy, inadequate/inappropriate antimicrobial therapy, superinfection, failure of pneumonia to resolve.

  Hypotension occurring early in the course of the illness may indicate hypoxia or bacteremia.

  Salicylates should be given with caution since they produce a drop in temperature and thus interfere with evaluation of the temperature curve.

  If hypotension is present, there is a decrease in coronary and brain oxygenation, which may produce serious effects.

  B. Evaluate for evidences of peripheral vascular collapse.
    1. Combat shock immediately and vigorously with pressor amines, IV fluids, and blood.
    2. Give penicillin IV if shock is present, as directed.
  C. Assess patient for evidence of delirium.

  Delirium is considered a grave prognostic sign and may be due to hypoxia, hypercapnia, meningitis, or the delirium tremens of alcoholism.

  D. Auscultate chest for crackles, signs of consolidation or pleural effusion.

IV. To provide supportive care and relieve the patient's discomfort:
  A. Assist the patient to cough productively.

  Depression of the cough reflex may produce retention of pulmonary secretions and lead to atelectasis.

    1. Splint the patient's chest while he is coughing.

  Elderly patients have a diminished cough reflex and may require vigorous measures (suctioning, bronchoscopy) for removal of secretions.

    2. Give codeine as prescribed.
    3. Humidify air to loosen secretions and improve ventilation. Encourage high level of fluid intake.

  Adequate hydration thins mucus and serves as an effective expectorant.

    4. Employ postural drainage and percussion to mobilize secretions.

(continued)

Chart 26-1
Summary: Guidelines for Caring for the Patient With Bacterial Pneumonia (continued)

IV. To provide supportive care and relieve the patient's discomfort: *(continued)*

   B. Use measures to reduce pleuritic pain.

Pain and cough result from pleuritic invasion by pneumococci. The discomfort of pleuritic pain can interfere with the mechanics of ventilation. Pleuritic pain causes shallow breathing; the aeration of the pulmonary alveoli is diminished, and this contributes to the development of ventilation–perfusion imbalance and hypoxemia.

      1. Use hot and cold applications as prescribed.
      2. Assist with intercostal nerve block with procaine.
      3. Use analgesics with caution to prevent depression of cough reflex and CNS respiratory drive.
      4. Treat dry cough and laryngospasm with aerosolized water, etc.

   C. Maintain fluid and electrolyte balance.

      1. Offer 2000 ml to 3000 ml of fluids daily.
      2. Administer IV fluids and electrolytes if patient is seriously ill or vomiting.

Fluid loss is high because of fever, dehydration, dyspnea, and diaphoresis.

   D. Give oxygen as indicated for dyspnea, circulatory disturbance, or delirium.

      1. Monitor arterial blood gases to determine oxygen need and evaluate oxygen effectiveness.

Restlessness, confusion, and aggressiveness may be due to cerebral hypoxia.

A patient suffering from pneumonia who has preexisting chronic obstructive pulmonary disease (bronchitis, emphysema) is apt to develop CO_2 narcosis when receiving oxygen. A mechanical ventilator may be required for patients with coexisting chronic ventilatory insufficiency.

V. To be alert for complications:

   A. Pleural effusion; atelectasis
   B. Sustained hypotension and shock
   C. Delayed resolution
   D. Superinfection: bacteremia, pericarditis, meningitis
   E. Toxic delirium (a medical emergency)
   F. Congestive heart failure; arrhythmias
   G. Acute respiratory failure

A significant number of patients with pneumonia develop complications. Patients should respond to treatment within 24 to 48 hours.

VI. To educate the patient concerning prevention of pulmonary disease.

   A. Fatigue, weakness, and depression may be prolonged after pneumonia.
   B. Try to stop smoking.

Cigarette smoking destroys tracheobronchial cilial action, which is the first line of defense of the lungs; smoking also irritates mucous cells of bronchi and inhibits function of alveolar scavenger cells (macrophages).

   C. Keep up natural resistance (adequate rest, good nutrition).

One episode of pneumonia appears to make the individual susceptible to recurring respiratory infections.

   D. Obtain influenza vaccine and pneumococcal vaccine at prescribed times.

Influenza increases susceptibility to secondary bacterial pneumonia.

   E. Avoid overfatigue, chilling, and excessive alcohol intake, which lower resistance to pneumonia.

Colds and upper respiratory tract infections may lead to bacterial invasion of lower respiratory tract.

   F. Report any signs and symptoms of a respiratory infection to the physician.

   G. Urge patients to have follow-up examinations after recovery and dismissal from the hospital.

Pneumonia frequently coexists with other pulmonary pathology, namely, cancer of the lung.

   H. Avoid obliteration of cough reflex and aspiration of secretions.

breathing exercises. Sometimes bronchoscopy is needed to drain the abscess.

A high-protein, high-caloric diet is necessary as chronic infection is associated with a catabolic state, which requires calories and protein to facilitate healing.

After the patient shows signs of improvement as demonstrated by normal temperature, abatement of leukocytosis, and improvement in the chest x-ray (resolution of surrounding infiltrate, diminution in size of cavity, and absence of fluid), the antibiotic is administered orally rather than intravenously. If treatment is stopped too soon, a relapse may occur. The duration of antibiotic therapy may be from 6 to 12 weeks.

Surgical intervention is indicated only when medical therapy has been proved inadequate by failure of the cavity to resolve, by a continuing septic condition, or when major hemoptysis occurs. Pulmonary resection (lobectomy) is the procedure usually performed when there is a thick-walled abscess with purulent drainage. If the patient cannot tolerate thoracic surgery, tube thoracotomy is done. (See p. 460 for care of the patient undergoing thoracic surgery.)

Patient Education.   After surgery there may be a somewhat prolonged period of drainage before the wound closes entirely. It may be necessary to teach a family member to change the simple dressings frequently enough to prevent excoriation of the skin and an offensive odor. If possible, the patient should be placed under the supervision of a community health nurse or some helping agency that will assist the family in meeting any problems that may arise. The patient is encouraged to have patience, since it takes time for chest x-rays to indicate that the condition has cleared. The patient should receive nutritional counseling for attaining and maintaining an optimal state of nutrition.

▷ Empyema

Empyema is a collection of pus in the pleural cavity. At first the pleural fluid is thin, with a low leukocyte count, but frequently it progresses to a fibropurulent stage and finally to a stage where it encloses the lung within a thick exudative membrane.

In most instances empyema is associated with an underlying pulmonary infection. Organisms may invade the pleural space by direct extension or as the result of the rupture of a lung abscess. Empyema may also follow thoracic surgery or penetrating wounds of the chest. The character of the exudate varies according to the infecting organism.

Clinical Manifestations.   The patient has fever, pleural pain, dyspnea, anorexia, and weight loss. Chest auscultation reveals the absence of breath sounds, and there is flatness to chest percussion as well as decreased fremitus (vocal vibration felt by palpation). If the patient has received antibiotic therapy, the clinical manifestations may be altered. The diagnosis is established on the basis of chest x-ray films and thoracentesis.

Management.   The objectives of treatment are to drain the pleural cavity and to achieve full expansion of the lung. This is accomplished by adequate drainage and by appropriate antibiotics selected on the basis of the causative organism. Large doses of the drug are usually given.

Drainage of the pleural fluid or pus depends on the stage of the disease and is accomplished by

1. Needle aspiration (thoracentesis) if the fluid is not too thick,
2. Closed-chest drainage using a large-diameter intercostal tube attached to underwater drainage (p. 465), or
3. Open drainage via rib resection to remove the thickened pleura, pus, and debris and to resect the underlying diseased pulmonary tissue

If the inflammation has been long-standing, an exudate can form over the lung and interfere with its normal expansion. This will have to be removed surgically (decortication). (See p. 461 for the nursing management following thoracotomy.) The drainage tube is left in place until the pus-filled space is obliterated completely; otherwise it will recur. The complete obliteration of the pleural space is checked by x-ray. This process may take a prolonged period of time. Breathing exercises, particularly those emphasizing exhalation against resistance, help to restore normal respiratory function.

▷ Bronchiectasis

Bronchiectasis is a chronic dilatation of the bronchi and bronchioles. Bronchial dilatation may be caused by a variety of causes, including pulmonary infections and obstruction of the bronchus, aspiration of foreign bodies, vomitus, or material from the upper respiratory tract, and extrinsic pressure from tumors, dilated blood vessels, and enlarged lymph nodes. A person may be predisposed to bronchiectasis as a result of respiratory infection in early childhood, measles, influenza, tuberculosis, and IgA deficiency. Following surgery, bronchiectasis may develop when the patient's cough is ineffective, with the result that mucus obstructs the bronchus and leads to atelectasis.

Pathophysiology.   The infection damages the bronchial wall, causing loss of its supporting structure and producing thick sputum that may ultimately obstruct the bronchi. The walls become permanently distended by severe coughing. The infection extends to the peribronchial tissues, so that in the case of saccular bronchiectasis, each dilated tube virtually amounts to a lung abscess, the exudate of which drains freely through the bronchus. The lower lobes are most frequently involved.

The retention of secretions and obstruction ultimately lead to collapse of the distally situated lung (atelectasis). Inflammatory scarring or fibrosis replaces functioning lung tissue. In time the patient develops respiratory insufficiency with decreased vital capacity, decreased ventilation, and an increased ratio of residual volume to total lung capacity. There is impaired mixing of inspired gas (ventilation–perfusion imbalance) and hypoxemia.

Clinical Manifestations.   Characteristic symptoms of bronchiectasis include chronic cough and the production of purulent sputum in copious amounts. A high percentage of patients with this disease experience hemoptysis. Clubbing of the fingers is also very common. The patient is likely to be subject to repeated episodes of pulmonary infection.

Many persons with bronchiectasis pass unrecognized, since their symptoms are mistaken for those of simple chronic bronchitis. A definite clue is offered by the prolonged history of productive cough, with a sputum consistently negative for tubercle bacilli. The diagnosis is established on the basis of bronchography (p. 440) and bronchoscopy (p. 440). These give proof of the presence or absence of bronchial dilatation.

Preventive Measures. All respiratory infections should be promptly treated. Bronchial secretions can be removed (by expectorants, postural drainage, therapeutic bronchoscopy) in order to avoid bronchiectasis. If a child has a prolonged cough and fever, the family should be urged to seek medical treatment. All unconscious persons should be turned (prone position to lateral) to drain all bronchial segments. The educational programs concerning immunization should be continued to prevent pertussis and measles (which may lead to bronchiectasis) so that these severe viral infections will not occur.

Management. The objectives of treatment are to prevent and control infection and to promote bronchial drainage to rid the affected portion of the lung(s) of excessive secretions. Infection is controlled with antibiotics guided by sensitivity studies on organisms cultured from sputum. Patients may be put on a year-round regimen of antibiotics, alternating types of drugs at intervals. Some clinicians use antibiotics throughout the winter or when acute upper respiratory infections occur.

Postural drainage of the bronchial tubes underlies all treatment considerations because draining the bronchiectatic areas by gravity reduces the amount of secretions and the degree of infection. (Sometimes mucopurulent sputum must be removed by bronchoscopy.) The affected chest area may be percussed or "cupped" to assist in raising secretions.

The patient is started out with short periods of postural drainage and the time is increased steadily. Bronchodilators may be given to persons who also have obstructive airway disease. Patients with bronchiectasis almost always have associated bronchitis. Beta-sympathomimetics may be used for bronchodilation and to increase the mucociliary transport of secretions.

To make sputum expectoration easier, the water content of the sputum is increased by aerosolized nebulizer treatments and by an increase in oral fluid intake. A face tent is ideal for providing extra humidification for aerosols. The patient should not smoke since this impairs bronchial drainage by paralyzing ciliary action, increasing bronchial secretions, and causing inflammation of the mucous membranes, resulting in hyperplasia of the mucous glands.

Surgical intervention may be indicated for the patient who continues to expectorate fairly large amounts of sputum and experience repeated bouts of pneumonia and hemoptysis in spite of a good medical regimen, provided the disease involves only one or two areas of the lung that can be removed without producing respiratory insufficiency. The goal of surgical treatment is to conserve normal pulmonary tissue and avoid infectious complications.

All diseased tissue is removed provided that the postoperative lung function will be adequate. It may be necessary to remove a segment of a lobe (segmental resection), a lobe (lobectomy), or an entire lung (pneumonectomy). *Segmental resection* is the removal of an anatomical subdivision of a pulmonary lobe. The chief advantage is that only diseased tissue is removed, with greater conservation of healthy lung tissue. Bronchography aids in the delineation of the segment. The operation is preceded by a period of preparation, which is exceedingly important. The objective is to obtain a dry (as dry as possible) tracheobronchial tree in order to prevent complications (atelectasis, pneumonia, bronchopleural fistula, and empyema). This is accomplished by means of postural drainage or, if the abscess is suitably situated, by direct suction through a bronchoscope. A course of antibacterial therapy may be started.

Following the operation, the care is the same as for any chest surgical patient, as is discussed on pages 461 to 471.

Patient Education. The patient is taught postural drainage exercises. He is encouraged to have regular dental care and to avoid all pulmonary irritants (cigarette smoke, noxious fumes). The patient should monitor his sputum and report any change in character or quantity. A decrease in sputum production is as significant as is an increase. An important preventive aspect is immunization against influenza. Other aspects of health teaching are included under emphysema on page 524.

▷ Chronic Obstructive Pulmonary Disease

Chronic obstructive pulmonary disease (COPD) is a broad classification that includes a group of conditions associated with chronic obstruction of airflow entering or leaving the lungs. *Airway obstruction* is diffuse airway narrowing, causing increased resistance to airflow. Included are chronic bronchitis, emphysema, and asthma. Basically, the person with COPD has (1) excessive secretion of mucus within the airways not owing to specific causes (bronchitis), (2) an increase in the size of the air spaces distal to the terminal bronchioles with loss of alveolar walls and elastic recoil of the lungs (emphysema), and (3) narrowing of the bronchial airways that varies in severity (asthma). As a result there is a subsequent derangement of airway dynamics—for example, loss of elasticity and obstruction to airflow. There is often an overlap of these conditions. Whereas bronchitis and emphysema are discussed in the following pages, asthma is dealt with in Chapter 50, since the triggering device in asthma is allergic in orgin.

Studies support the theory that COPD is a disease of genetic and environmental interaction; cigarette smoking and air pollution may contribute to its development. This is a disease spectrum that may span 20 to 35 years. It appears to begin fairly early in life and is a slowly progressive disorder that is present many years before the onset of clinical symptoms and impairment of pulmonary function.

▷ Chronic Bronchitis

Manifestations and Pathophysiology.   Chronic bronchitis is characterized by excessive mucus secretion, cough, and dyspnea associated with recurring infections of the lower respiratory tract and often with reduced ability to ventilate the lungs. The patient's major problem is the protracted and abundant production of inflammatory exudate that fills and obstructs the bronchioles and is responsible for a persistent, productive cough and shortness of breath. This constant irritation leads to hypertrophy of mucus-secreting glands, goblet cell hyperplasia, and increased mucus production leading to bronchial plugging and bronchial narrowing. Alveoli adjacent to the bronchioles may become damaged and fibrosed. Further bronchial narrowing follows as a result of these fibrotic changes in the airways. In time, irreversible lung changes may occur, with resultant emphysema or bronchiectasis.

A wide range of viral, bacterial, and mycoplasmal infections can produce acute episodes of bronchitis. Bronchitis is encountered in persons who smoke heavily or are exposed to air pollutants that will produce abnormal secretion of mucus with impaired ciliary function. Hereditary factors and reaction to allergens also play a part in its development. Exacerbations of chronic bronchitis are most apt to occur during the winter months. The inhalation of cold air produces bronchospasm in sensitive persons. Progressive bronchitis will almost invariably result in chronic obstructive pulmonary disease.

Preventive Measures.   Because of the disabling nature of chronic bronchitis, every effort should be directed toward its prevention. An important feature is the avoidance of respiratory irritants, particularly tobacco smoke. Persons who are prone to respiratory infections should be immunized against common viral agents with influenza vaccines and with vaccine for *Streptococcus pneumoniae*. All persons with acute upper respiratory infections should receive proper treatment, including antibiotics based on cultures and sensitivity studies at the first sign of purulent sputum.

Management.   The main objectives of treatment are to maintain the patency of the peripheral bronchial tree, to facilitate removal of bronchial exudates, and to prevent disability. Changes in the sputum pattern (nature, color, amount, thickness) and in the cough pattern are important signs to note. Recurrent bacterial infections are treated with antibiotic therapy that is directed by sensitivity studies.

To facilitate the removal of bronchial exudates, bronchodilators are administered to relieve bronchospasm and reduce airway obstruction; thus, gas distribution and alveolar ventilation are improved. Postural drainage and chest percussion following treatments are usually helpful. Water (given orally or parenterally if bronchospasm is severe) is an important part of therapy, since proper hydration helps the patient to bring up secretions. Steroid therapy may be used when the patient fails to respond to more conservative measures. In some instances in which there is an underlying bronchiectasis, postural drainage is most important. The patient must stop smoking, since smoke inhalation causes bronchoconstriction, paralysis of ciliary activity, and inactivation of surfactant. Smokers are also more susceptible to bronchial infection. Basically, the medical treatment, nursing management, and patient education are similar to that for the patient with pulmonary emphysema (p. 524).

▷ Pulmonary Emphysema

Pulmonary emphysema is a complex and destructive lung disease characterized by destruction of the alveoli, enlargement of airspaces, and loss of airway support by the lung parenchyma. It appears to be the end stage of a process that has slowly progressed for many years. In fact, by the time the patient develops symptoms, pulmonary function is often irreversibly impaired. Along with chronic obstructive bronchitis, it is a major cause of disability under Social Security and is the most common respiratory cause of death in the United States.

Cigarette smoking is the major cause of chronic obstructive pulmonary disease (emphysema). However, in a small percentage of patients there is a familial predisposition to emphysema associated with a plasma protein abnormality, a deficiency of alpha$_1$-antitrypsin. The genetically susceptible individual is sensitive to environmental influences (smoking, air pollution, infectious agents, allergens) and, in time, develops chronic obstructive symptoms, namely emphysema. It is imperative that the carriers of this genetic defect be identified to permit genetic counseling and that the environmental factors be modified to delay or prevent overt symptoms of disease.

Pathophysiology

In emphysema the major site of obstruction is the airways where mucus plugging and inflammatory narrowing occur. In later stages the obstruction is caused by loss of the supporting tissues of the airway (elasticity of the lung) with resultant bronchial collapse during expiration. There is dilatation of all of the finer air passages as well as dilatation and coalescence (fusing together) of the alveoli with loss of inherent elasticity and increased dead space. The alveolus is the site in the lung where venous blood and environmental air complete the process of gas exchange. In order for gas exchange to be effective, the alveoli must be adequately ventilated with air. Interference with alveolar ventilation may occur if there is bronchial obstruction or uneven expansion of the lungs with poor air distribution.

The person with emphysema has a chronic obstruction (marked increase in airway resistance) to the inflow and outflow of air from the lungs. The lungs are in a state of chronic hyperexpansion. In order to get air into and out of the lungs, negative pressure is required during inspiration and an adequate level of positive pressure must be attained and maintained during expiration. The rest position is one of inflation. Instead of being an involuntary act, expiration becomes a muscular act. The patient becomes increasingly short of breath, the chest becomes rigid, and the ribs are fixed at their joints. The "barrel chest" of many of these patients is due to loss of lung elasticity in the presence of

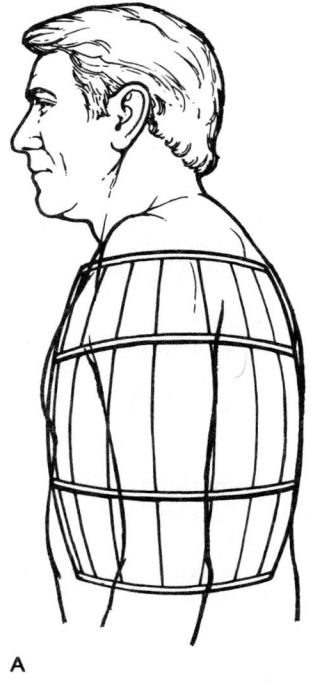
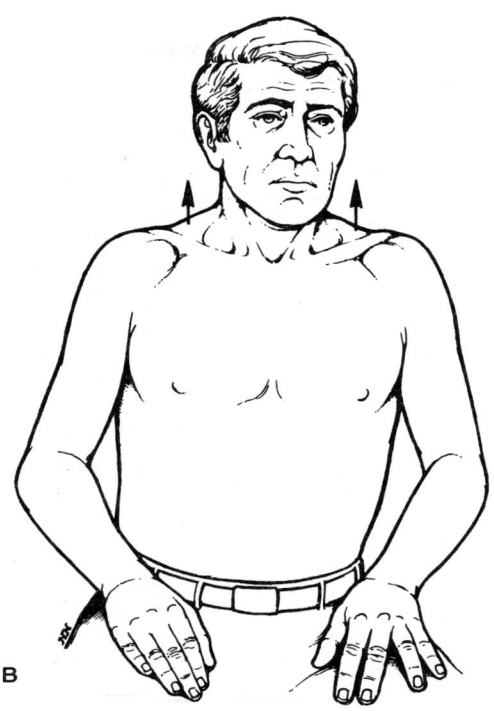

A   B

Figure 26-1. Comparison of typical findings in the patient with pulmonary emphysema. (*A*) The common "barrel chest" condition of the patient with emphysema showing characteristic increase of anteroposterior diameter. (*B*) Another posture of the patient with emphysema showing elevation of shoulder girdle and retraction of the supraclavicular fossae on inspiration.

continued tendency to the chest wall to expand (Fig. 26-1 *A*). In some instances the barrel chest may be due to dorsal kyphosis. Some patients bend forward to breathe, using the accessory muscles of respiration. There is retraction of the supraclavicular fossae on inspiration (Fig. 26-1 *B*). In advanced disease there is also contraction of the abdominal muscles on inspiration. There is a progressive reduction of the vital capacity. Full deflation becomes increasingly difficult and finally impossible. The total vital capacity may be normal, but the 1-second vital capacity is low. The patient moves air more slowly and inefficiently and has to work hard to do it.

The alveolar integrity begins to break down. As the walls of the alveoli are destroyed (a process accelerated by recurrent infections), the internal surface of the lungs, (*i.e.,* the area available for the exchange of oxygen and carbon dioxide between the atmosphere and the blood) continually decreases. In late stages of the disease there is interference with carbon dioxide elimination, and the increased carbon dioxide tension causes a mild to severe *pulmonary acidosis.* There is also impairment of oxygen diffusion with inadequate oxygen saturation of the arterial blood.

As the alveolar walls continue to rupture, the pulmonary capillary bed is reduced. The pulmonary blood flow is speeded and the right ventricle is forced to maintain a higher blood pressure in the pulmonary artery. Thus, right-sided heart failure (cor pulmonale) is one of the compli-

cations of emphysema. The presence of leg edema (dependent edema), distended neck veins, or pain in the region of the liver suggests the development of cardiac failure.

Secretions are increased and retained, since the person is unable to make a forceful cough to expel them. Chronic and acute infections thus take hold in the emphysematous lungs, adding to the air transfer problem.

Classification. There are two main pathologic types of emphysema, which are classified on the basis of the kind of changes taking place in the lung: (1) panlobular (panocinar) and (2) centrilobular (centriacinar).

In the *panlobular (panocinar) type,* there is destruction of the respiratory bronchiole, alveolar duct, and alveoli. All air spaces within the lobule are more or less enlarged. This patient typically has a hyperinflated chest and marked dyspnea on exertion. Sometimes he is referred to as a "pink puffer." This patient remains "pink," or well-oxygenated, until the disease becomes terminal.

In the *centrilobular (centriacinar) form,* the pathologic changes take place mainly in the center of the secondary lobule while the peripheral portions of the acinus are preserved. Frequently, there is a derangement of ventilation/perfusion ratios producing chronic hypoxia, hypercapnia, and polycythemia. This leads to cyanosis, peripheral edema, and respiratory failure. The patient may be called a "blue bloater." In addition to the management outlined on pages 522 to 528, the blue bloater usually receives diuretic therapy for edema. Both types of emphysema may occur in the same patient.

▶ Assessment

Clinical Manifestations. Dyspnea is the presenting symptom in emphysema and has an insidious onset. The patient usually has a history of cigarette smoking and a long history of chronic cough, wheezing, and increasing shortness of breath, especially with respiratory infection. In time even the slightest exertion, such as bending over to tie his shoelaces, produces dyspnea and fatigue (exertional dyspnea). The emphysematous lung is not contracted on expiration, and the bronchioles are not effectively emptied of their secretions.

The patient readily develops inflammatory reactions and infections owing to the pooling of these secretions. After these infections, the patient experiences a prolonged wheezing expiration. Anorexia, weight loss, and weakness are common complaints.

Diagnostic Evaluation. The patient's symptoms and the clinical findings on physical examination provide the initial clues to the individual's problem. Other aids in diagnosis include roentgenography, pulmonary function tests (particularly spirometry) and blood gas studies (to assess ventilatory function and pulmonary gas exchange), and the electrocardiogram to see the cardiac effects.

The nurse's observations, nursing history, and subsequent recording should yield an understanding of the patient and his disease:

- How long has he had respiratory difficulty?
- What are the pulse and the respiratory rates?
- Are the respirations even?
- Does the patient contract his abdominal muscles during inspiration?
- Are the accessory muscles of respiration used?
- Does exertion increase the dyspnea?
- What are the limits to his exercise tolerance?
- Is cyanosis evident?
- Are the patient's neck veins engorged?
- Is he coughing?
- What are the color, amount, and consistency of the sputum?
- What is the status of the patient's sensorium?
- Is there increasing stupor? apprehension?
- At what times during the day does he complain most of fatigue and shortness of breath?
- Have his habits of eating or sleeping been affected?
- What does he know about the disease and his condition?

Patient Problems/Nursing Diagnoses

Based on the clinical manifestations and diagnostic assessment data, the patient's major nursing problems include respiratory impairment related to obstructive lung disease and retained secretions; difficulty with self-care related to dyspnea; fatigue, anorexia, and depression related to hypoxia; and frequent respiratory infections related to nonadherence to the therapeutic program and exposure to pollutants.

▶ Planning and Implementation

Goals

The patient's goals are:

1. Improvement of respiratory function
2. Ability to perform self-care
3. Relief of fatigue, anorexia, and depression
4. Absence of respiratory infections
5. Adherence to the therapeutic program

The major objectives of treatment are to improve the quality of life, to slow the progression of the disease process, and to treat the obstructed airways so as to relieve hypoxia. The therapeutic approach includes (1) treatment measures designed to improve ventilation and decrease the work of breathing, (2) prevention and prompt treatment of infection, (3) use of physical therapy techniques to conserve and increase pulmonary ventilation, (4) maintenance of proper environmental conditions to facilitate breathing, (5) supportive and psychological care, and (6) an ongoing program of patient education (Fig. 26-2).

Measures to Improve Ventilation and Decrease Work of Breathing

Removal of Bronchial Secretions. A major goal in the treatment of emphysema is to diminish the quantity and tenacity of sputum in order to improve pulmonary ventilation and gas exchange. All pulmonary irritants must be eliminated, particularly cigarette smoking, which is the most persistent source of pulmonary irritation. A high fluid intake (2½ to 3 liters or 10 to 12 glasses) daily is encouraged to liquefy secretions. An added reason for encouraging fluid intake is the tendency for the patient to breathe through the mouth, which accelerates water loss.

Inhaling nebulized water is also helpful since it humidifies the bronchial tree, adding water to the sputum and decreasing its viscosity, so that evacuation of sputum is facilitated.

Bronchodilators. Bronchospasm, present in many forms of pulmonary disease, causes reduction of the caliber of the small bronchi, resulting in stasis of secretions and infection. (Bronchospasm is detected by auscultation with a stethoscope.)

Bronchodilators are administered to dilate the airways, because they combat both bronchial mucosal edema and muscular spasm and thus help in reducing airway obstruction and clearing secretions. These include the beta-adrenergic agonists (metaproterenol; isoproterenol) and the methyl xanthines (theophylline; aminophylline), which produce bronchial dilatation by different mechanisms. Bronchodilator drugs may be administered orally, subcutaneously, intravenously, rectally, or via nebulization (conversion into a spray). Nebulized drugs may be delivered by pressurized aerosols, hand-bulb nebulizers, pump-driven nebulizers, or IPPB. These bronchodilators may produce unwanted side-effects, which include tachycardia, cardiac arrhythmias, and central nervous system excitation. The methylxanthines may also produce gastrointestinal disturbances such as nausea and vomiting. Since side-effects are

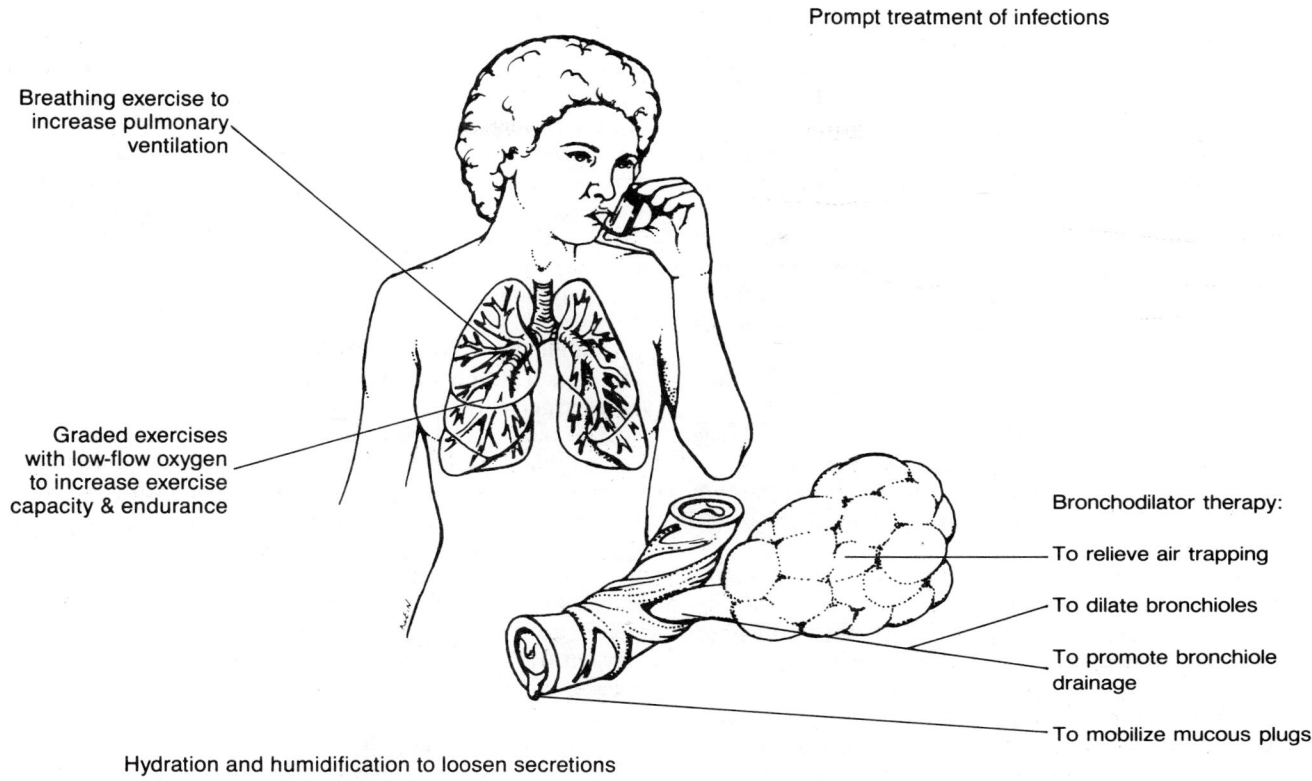

Prompt treatment of infections

Breathing exercise to increase pulmonary ventilation

Graded exercises with low-flow oxygen to increase exercise capacity & endurance

Bronchodilator therapy:

To relieve air trapping

To dilate bronchioles

To promote bronchiole drainage

To mobilize mucous plugs

Hydration and humidification to loosen secretions

Figure 26-2. Supporting the patient with emphysema.

common, the drug dosage is carefully adjusted for each patient, in accordance with his tolerance and clinical response. Nursing assessment is an important guide. The relief of bronchospasm is confirmed by measuring improvement in expiratory flow rates and by assessing whether the patient has a reduction in dyspnea.

Aerosolization (process of dispensing in a fine mist) of saline bronchodilators and mucolytics is frequently used to aid in bronchodilatation. The particle size in the aerosol mist must be small enough to allow the medication to be deposited deep within the tracheobronchial tree.

Nebulized aerosols relieve bronchospasm, decrease mucosal edema, and liquefy bronchial secretions. This facilitates the process of bronchial clearance, helps to control the inflammatory process, and improves ventilatory function. Hand-bulb nebulizers and metered-dose aerosol devices give the patient quick relief. Electrically powered nebulizers and air-powered nebulizers may be useful if the patient has more marked ventilatory impairment. The improvement of the oxygen saturation of the arterial blood and the reduction of its carbon dioxide content assists in relieving the patient's hypoxia and gives considerable relief from constant respiratory fatigue. Nebulizer treatments driven with oxygen must be given with extreme caution in patients who have chronically elevated CO_2 tensions and are breathing on hypoxic stimuli. There appears to be a trend away from the use of IPPB, especially in the home-care setting. Nebulized inhalant treatments should be given before meals to improve lung ventilation and thus reduce the fatigue that accompanies eating. Following inhalation

of bronchodilator aerosols, the patient is advised to inhale moisture to help liquefy secretions. Then expulsive coughing or postural drainage will aid him in expectorating secretions. Help the patient to do this in such a manner that it will not be exhausting to him.

Bronchoscopic removal of secretions may be occasionally necessary for the patient who is unable to cough and raise sputum. For the patient who develops acute respiratory failure (p. 486), endotracheal intubation or tracheostomy is indicated to permit more effective suctioning of secretions, to prevent mucous plugging, and to provide ventilatory assistance.

Prevention and Treatment of Infection

Bronchial infections must be controlled to diminish inflammatory edema and to permit recovery of normal ciliary action. Minor respiratory infections that are of no consequence to the person with normal lungs can produce fatal disturbances of pulmonary function in the person with emphysema. The cough associated with bronchial infection introduces a vicious cycle with further trauma and damage to the lungs, further progression of symptoms, increased bronchospasm, and further increase in susceptibility to bronchial infection. Infection compromises lung function and is a common cause of respiratory failure.

In emphysema, infection does not manifest itself in the same way as it does elsewhere in the body. The patient should be instructed to report to the physician immediately if the sputum becomes discolored, since purulent expectoration or a change in the character or color of the sputum is evidence of infection. He should be taught that any worsening of his symptoms (increased tightness of the chest, increase in dyspnea, and fatigue) is also suggestive of infection and must be reported. Steroids may be given in selected patients with severe disease. Viral infections are hazardous to these patients because they are so often followed by infections owing to *Streptococcus pneumoniae, Haemophilus influenzae,* etc.

The patient is usually placed on antimicrobial therapy: tetracycline, ampicillin, amoxicillin, or trimethoprim with sulfamethoxazole. An antimicrobial regimen is helpful in treating recurrent episodes of purulent bronchitis and appears to shorten the course of fever, cough, etc.

Persons who are prone to respiratory infections should be immunized against influenza and *Streptococcus pneumoniae.* During highly polluted or heavily pollinated days (in the spring) these persons should avoid outdoor exposure since it may increase bronchospasm. Outdoor periods of high temperatures associated with high humidities should likewise be avoided.

Chest Physical Therapy

Chest physical therapy techniques include breathing exercises and general physical conditioning exercises intended to conserve and increase pulmonary ventilation.

Breathing Exercises and Retraining. Most persons with chronic obstructive pulmonary disease breathe shallowly from the upper chest, in a rapid and inefficient manner. This type of upper chest breathing can be changed to the lower costal and diaphragmatic type with breathing exercises and practice. Training in diaphragmatic breathing reduces the respiratory rate, increases tidal volume and alveolar ventilation, and causes a reduction of functional residual capacity.

Pursed-lip breathing slows expiration, prevents collapse of lung units, and helps the patient to control the rate and depth of respiration and to relax, which enables him to gain control of his dyspnea and feelings of panic.

A patient with emphysema has definite periods of the day when his exercise tolerance is decreased. This is especially true on arising in the morning, because bronchial secretions and edema collect in the lungs during the night while he is lying on his back. He often will be unable to shave or to wash. Activities requiring the arms to be supported above the level of the thorax may produce distress. These activities may be tolerated better after the patient has been up and moving around for an hour or more. Because of these limitations, the patient has the right to participate in planning his care with the nurse and in determining the best time for bathing and shaving. A hot beverage on arising will assist him to expectorate and will shorten the period of disability noted on arising.

Another period of increased disability occurs immediately after meals, particularly the evening meal. Fatigue from the day's activities coupled with abdominal distention limits his exercise tolerance. The patient's chief complaint at this time is fatigue. This is another way of saying, "I am dyspneic": dyspnea is the underlying cause of his fatigue.

Exercises and Physical Conditioning. There is a close relationship between physical fitness and respiratory fitness.

Graded exercises and physical conditioning programs employing treadmills, stationary bicycles, measured level walks, etc., have been shown to improve symptoms and to increase work capacity and exercise tolerance. It is useful for the patient to have a physical activity that he can do on a regular sustained basis. A lightweight portable oxygen system is available for the ambulatory patient who requires oxygen therapy during physical activity to improve hypoxia. Many patients can return to work with the benefit of continuous oxygen therapy. This type of rehabilitation improves the quality of life.

Continuous Oxygen Therapy

For certain patients with advanced COPD, continuous low-flow oxygen may be used for hypoxemia with cor pulmonale and secondary erythrocytosis that cannot be corrected by conventional methods. This modality of treatment may alleviate the patient's symptoms and improve the quality of his existence. Oxygen can be supplied to the home by compressed gas, liquid, or concentrator systems. Portable oxygen systems are available that allow the patient to work and travel. Patient teaching is directed at reassurance that oxygen is not "addicting," the precautions involved in using oxygen (no smoking), and the necessity of having regular measurements of arterial blood gases.

Psychosocial Support

Any factor that interferes with normal breathing quite naturally induces anxiety, depression, and changes in behavior. Many persons find the slightest exertion exhausting. Constant shortness of breath and fatigue may render the patient irritable and apprehensive to the point of sheer panic. His enforced inactivity (and reversal of family roles owing to loss of employment), the frustration of having to work to breathe, and the realization that he faces a prolonged, unrelenting disease may cause the patient to react with anger, depression, and demanding behavior. Sexual ability may be compromised, which also diminishes self-esteem.

It is important for the nurse and other health care personnel to adopt a cautiously hopeful and encouraging attitude and keep the patient active up to his level of symptom tolerance. Emphasis should be on controlling his symptoms and increasing self-esteem and sense of mastery and of well-being. Supportive medical and nursing care, ongoing patient teaching, and possibly group therapy sessions help to relieve somewhat an almost overwhelming burden.

Patient Teaching

To help the patient live better, it is essential that he be educated about his disease process. One of the major teaching factors is helping the patient to accept realistic short-term and long-range goals. If he is severely disabled, the objective of treatment is to preserve his present pulmonary function and relieve his symptoms as much as possible. If his disease is mild, the objective is to increase his exercise tolerance and prevent further loss of pulmonary function. The patient has to be told what to expect. He and those caring for him need patience to achieve these goals. Chart 26-2 presents a summary of patient education in emphysema.

Chart 26-2
Patient Education in Emphysema

Teaching the emphysematous patient is one of the most important aspects of his care. The patient becomes an active participant in planning his care and will achieve positive results when he understands the goals of therapy and has guidelines set forth to achieve them.

Goal: To improve the quality of life
I. To delay the progression of the disease process
  A. Avoid exposure to respiratory irritants—cigarette smoke, pollens, fumes, aerosols, dust, cold.
    1. Stop smoking and avoid smoke-filled rooms.
    2. Avoid sweeping, dusting, and exposure to paint, aerosols, bleaches, and other respiratory irritants; use a mask when exposed to dusts.
    3. Keep kitchen ventilated.
    4. Stay indoors with air conditioning when pollution level is high.
    5. Stay out of extremely hot/cold weather to avoid aggravating bronchial obstruction and sputum production.
      a. Try to avoid abrupt changes in environmental temperature.
      b. Keep a warming mask or scarf over nose and mouth to warm inspired air in cold weather.
  B. Prevent and eliminate bronchial infections.
    1. Avoid exposure to persons with respiratory infections; a respiratory infection makes symptoms worse and can produce further irreversible damage.
    2. Avoid crowds and areas with poor ventilation.
    3. Recognize and report evidence of respiratory infection *promptly* to the physician/clinic—chest pain, changes in character of sputum (amount, color, or consistency), increasing difficulty in breathing, sore throat, fever, chills.
    4. Take prescribed antimicrobial at first sign of infection.
      a. Have a home supply available.
      b. Have periodic sputum cultures when receiving long-term antimicrobial therapy.
    5. Take influenza immunization (if not allergic) to decrease likelihood of developing infection.
    6. Use measures to promote oronasal hygiene; use toothbrush, dental floss, mouthwashes properly.
    7. Avoid things to which you are sensitive or allergic.
  C. Reduce bronchial secretions.
    1. Maintain an adequate fluid intake (8–10 glasses daily) to liquefy bronchial secretions so they can be more easily evacuated. Mark down the amount of liquid consumed daily.
    2. Take bronchodilators only as directed.
    3. Follow postural drainage exercises as prescribed.

      a. Stay in each position 5 to 10 minutes.
      b. Use controlled cough after each position.
    4. Use mist therapy to loosen and mobilize retained secretions.
    5. Continue to practice slow, deep breathing with full expiration.
    6. Avoid drugs (cough suppressants, antihistamines, anticholinergics) that suppress cough and dry secretions.
  D. Maintain general health at highest attainable level.
    1. Follow good habits of nutrition—persons with COPD may have loss of muscle mass with poor nutritional status, poor appetite, potassium depletion, sodium retention, and dehydration.
    2. Follow high-protein diet with adequate mineral, vitamin, and fluid intake.
    3. Avoid excessive hot or cold fluids/foods, which may provoke an irritating cough.
    4. Avoid hard-to-chew foods (causes tiring) and gas-producing foods, which cause distention and restrict diaphragmatic movement.
    5. Eat five to six small meals daily to ease shortness of breath during and after meals.
    6. Have rest periods before and after meals if eating produces shortness of breath.
    7. Do not eat when upset or angry.
    8. Avoid potassium depletion—persons with COPD tend to have low potassium levels; also, may be taking diuretics.
      a. Watch for weakness, numbness, tingling of fingers, leg cramps.
      b. Foods high in potassium include bananas, dried fruits, dates, figs, orange juice, grape juice, milk, peaches, potatoes.
    9. Restrict sodium as directed
    10. Use community resources (Meals on Wheels) if energy level is low.
  E. Avoid activities that produce excessive shortness of breath.
    1. Live within the limitations that emphysema imposes.
    2. Learn to relax and work at a slower pace. Obtain vocational counseling to secure a sedentary job if presently working in a demanding manual job.
    3. Avoid overfatigue, which is a factor in producing respiratory distress.
    4. Adjust activities according to individual fatigue patterns.

(continued)

Chart 26-2
Patient Education in Emphysema (continued)

5. Use pursed-lip breathing in a slow and relaxed manner during periods of breathlessness and physical exertion.
6. Try to cope with emotional stress as positively as possible—such stress triggers attacks of dyspnea.
7. Study individual life-style and avoid energy-wasting activities.
8. Exercise to improve physical condition.

F. Understand the importance of preserving existing function.
   1. Become familiar with the nature of the disease and the reasons for the therapeutic regimen.
   2. Accept the fact that therapy and medical supervision must be continued for a lifetime.

II. To increase pulmonary ventilation
   A. Use respiratory therapy treatments consistently and faithfully.
      1. Learn how to assemble and disassemble equipment.
      2. Do the procedure immediately upon arising in the morning and before meals when indicated.
      3. Use nebulizer before events known to precipitate symptoms.
      4. Use the exact amount of medication prescribed by the physician.
      5. Inhale and exhale as evenly as possible during the treatment.
      6. Try to cough *productively* (with controlled coughing) after the treatment.
         a. Breathe slowly and deeply, using diaphragmatic breathing.
         b. Hold breath several seconds.
         c. Cough—two short, forceful coughs with the mouth open; the first cough loosens mucus, and the second cough moves it.

   d. Pause and inhale by sniffing quietly; inhaling vigorously may initiate unproductive coughing, which is energy consuming.
   e. Rest.
   6. Practice oral hygiene after each treatment.
   7. Clean respiratory therapy equipment daily to prevent contamination and secondary infection.
      a. Allow equipment to dry thoroughly before reassembling.
      b. Do not re-use medications/solutions/water left standing in a humidifier/nebulizer.

B. Do breathing exercises to strengthen muscles of expiration, to strengthen and coordinate muscles of breathing, to lessen fatigue, and to help empty lungs more completely.
   1. Learn the importance of slow and relaxed breathing (controlled breathing).
   2. Practice diaphragmatic breathing and pursed-lip breathing (p. 458).
   3. Control your breathing while doing more strenuous work.
      a. Take a slow, fairly deep breath, using your diaphragm.
      b. Perform the activity while exhaling through pursed lips.
   4. Consciously use pursed-lip breathing during episodes of dyspnea and stress.
   5. Rehearse measures to reduce shortness of breath before these episodes occur.
   6. Maintain muscle tone of body by regular exercise.
   7. Follow a daily schedule of graded exercises: walking, riding stationary bicycle. Use supplemental oxygen with graded exercise program if necessary.

The patient should be instructed to avoid excessive heat and cold. Heat increases the body temperature, hence raises the oxygen requirements of the body; cold tends to promote bronchospasm. High altitudes aggravate the hypoxia. Bronchospasm may also be initiated by such air pollutants as fumes, smoke, dust, and even talcum and lint.

Protection of the lung is basic for the preservation of lung function. Patients with emphysema should be informed unequivocally that, for them, smoking is dangerous. Cigarette smoking depresses the function of scavenger cells and affects the ciliary cleansing mechanism of the respiratory tract, the function of which is to keep the breathing passages free of inhaled irritants, bacteria, and other foreign matter. This is one of the major defense mechanisms of the body. When this cleansing mechanism is damaged by smoking, airflow is obstructed and air becomes trapped behind

the obstructed airway. The air sacs greatly distend and the lung capacity is diminished. Cigarette smoking also irritates the goblet cells and mucous glands, causing an increased accumulation of mucus. The mucus accumulation produces more irritation, infection, and damage to the lung capacity. Frequently, the patient is unaware of what is happening until he notices that extra physical effort produces respiratory distress. At this point the damage may be irreversible. Therefore, patients with emphysema should definitely refrain from smoking. There is a wide variety of smoking control strategies, including *prevention,* cessation, and behavioral modification. (Unfortunately, not all patients are capable of stopping smoking completely.)

Patients with emphysema should restrict themselves to a life of moderate activity, ideally in a climate with minimal shifts in temperature and humidity. Stress situations that might trigger a coughing episode or emotional disturbance should be avoided.

▶ Evaluation

Expected Outcomes

1. Improves respiratory function
   a. Stops smoking
   b. Verbalizes that pollens, fumes, gases, dusts, and extremes of temperature and humidity are respiratory irritants to be avoided
   c. Has a check-off system for taking bronchodilators
   d. Demonstrates ability to clean and use respiratory therapy equipment
   e. Coughs less
   f. Uses pursed-lip breathing during periods of stress and dyspnea
   g. Reports that spouse has learned to do percussion/vibration after patient performs postural drainage
   h. Has a check-off system to assure he is drinking eight glasses of fluids/day
   i. Shows signs of decreased respiratory effort
2. Is able to perform self-care
   a. Has a planned schedule so he can pace activities to correlate with his fatigue pattern
   b. Uses controlled breathing while bathing, bending to tie shoes, etc.
   c. Reads articles about energy conservation
3. Is relieved of fatigue, anorexia and depression
   a. Rests before and after meals
   b. Eats six small meals daily to ease shortness of breath
   c. Knows what activities produce shortness of breath/fatigue
   d. Walks and gradually increases walking time and distance to improve physical condition
   e. Plans on joining an emphysema support group
4. Is free of respiratory infection
   a. Knows that the following are early signs of respiratory infection: increasing breathlessness; change in color, amount, and character of sputum; nervousness; irritability; and low-grade fever
   b. Has a supply of prescribed antimicrobials to take at first sign of infection
   c. Verbalizes that he must stay away from people with colds
5. Adheres to therapeutic program
   a. Can explain his disease and what worsens/improves his condition
   b. Verbalizes that he must preserve existing lung function by adhering to his program
   c. Has an appointment for vocational counseling

▷ Pulmonary Heart Disease (Cor Pulmonale)

Cor pulmonale is a condition in which the right ventricle enlarges (with or without failure) as a result of diseases that affect the structure or function of the lung or its vasculature.

Any disease that affects the lungs and has associated hypoxemia may result in cor pulmonale. The most frequent cause is chronic obstructive pulmonary disease (emphysema, chronic bronchitis) in which changes in the airways and retained secretions reduce alveolar ventilation. Other causes are conditions that restrict or compromise ventilatory function, leading to hypoxia or acidosis (deformities of the thoracic cage; massive obesity) or conditions that reduce the pulmonary vascular bed (primary idiopathic pulmonary artery hypertension; pulmonary embolus). Certain disorders of the nervous system, respiratory muscles, chest wall, and pulmonary arterial tree may be responsible for cor pulmonale.

Pathophysiology. Pulmonary disease can produce a chain of events that will in time produce hypertrophy and failure of the right ventricle. Any condition that deprives the lungs of oxygen can cause hypoxemia (decreased arterial oxygen saturation) and hypercapnia (increased carbon dioxide in the blood), resulting in ventilatory insufficiency. Airway hypoxia and hypercapnia cause pulmonary arterial vasoconstriction. There may be associated reduction of the pulmonary vascular bed, as in emphysema or pulmonary emboli. The result is increased resistance in the pulmonary circuit, with a subsequent rise in pulmonary blood pressure (pulmonary hypertension). Pulmonary hypertension is present when the pulmonary arterial pressure at rest exceeds 30 mm Hg systolic, 15 mm Hg mean, or 10 mm Hg diastolic. One sees mean pressures of 45 mm Hg or more in cor pulmonale. Right ventricular hypertrophy may then result and may be followed by right ventricular failure. In short, cor pulmonale results from pulmonary hypertension that causes the right side of the heart to enlarge because of the increased work required to pump blood against high resistance through the pulmonary vascular system.

Clinical Manifestations. Usually, the symptoms of cor pulmonale are those of underlying lung disease. Chronic obstructive pulmonary disease produces shortness of breath and cough. As the right ventricle fails, the patient develops edema of the feet and legs, distended neck veins, an enlarged palpable liver, pleural effusion, ascites, and heart murmur. Headache, confusion, and somnolence may be manifested as a result of carbon dioxide narcosis.

Therapeutic Approach. The objectives of treatment are to improve the patient's ventilation and to treat both the underlying lung disease and the manifestations of heart disease. In chronic obstructive pulmonary disease the airways have to be opened to improve gas exchange. With improved oxygen transport, the reactive pulmonary hypertension that leads to cor pulmonale is relieved. In short, the lung must be treated first. Oxygen is given to reduce pulmonary artery pressure and pulmonary vascular resistance. Although the ideal number of hours per day of oxygen therapy is under study, better survival and greater reduction in pulmonary vascular resistance have been reported with continuous (24 hours/day) oxygen therapy for patients with severe hypoxia. Substantial patient improvement may require 4 to 6 weeks of oxygen therapy. This is usually carried out at home. Assessment of arterial blood gases is necessary to determine adequacy of alveolar ventilation and to monitor low-flow oxygen.

Additional measures include bronchial hygiene and the administration of bronchodilators and chest physical therapy to improve ventilation. If the patient is in respiratory failure, endotracheal intubation and mechanical ventilation may be necessary (p. 495). If the patient is in heart failure, the improvement of hypoxemia and hypercapnia will be necessary to improve cardiac action and output. In addition, he is placed on bed rest, and sodium restriction and diuretic therapy are employed judiciously to reduce peripheral edema (to lower pulmonary artery pressure through a decrease in total blood volume) and the circulatory load on the right heart. Digitalis may be given if the patient has coincident left ventricular failure, a supraventricular arrhythmia, or right ventricular failure that does not respond to other therapy to relieve pulmonary hypertension. It is given with extreme caution, as pulmonary heart disease appears to enhance susceptibility to digitalis toxicity.

ECG monitoring is done when necessary, as there is a high incidence of arrhythmias in these patients. Respiratory infection must be treated, as it commonly precipitates pulmonary heart disease. The patient's prognosis depends on whether or not the hypertensive process is reversible. (The management of the patient with respiratory failure is discussed on p. 487).

Patient Education. There is an interrelationship between smoking, infection, air pollution, and pulmonary heart disease. The patient is counseled to stop smoking and to avoid exposure to air pollutants (*e.g.,* smoke fumes). Respiratory infections should be treated promptly. The family should be counseled that restlessness, depression, and poor sleeping as well as irritable and angry behavior may be encountered and that the improvement should be noted with improvement in arterial blood gas values.

▷ Breathing Disorders During Sleep

Respiratory abnormalities can occur during sleep. Some patients who have adequate blood oxygenation while awake develop hypoxemia while sleeping. *Apnea* is the cessation of airflow at the nose and mouth of more than 15 seconds. *Sleep apnea syndrome,* which is evaluated in a sleep laboratory, is present where there are at least 30 apneic episodes during both rapid eye movement sleep and nonrapid eye movement sleep during 7 hours of nocturnal sleep. Oxygen desaturation is usually evident in apneic episodes.

Sleep apnea may be classified into three types: (1) *central*—simultaneous cessation of both airflow and respiratory movements; (2) *obstructive*—lack of airflow owing to pharyngeal occlusion; and (3) *mixed*—a combination of central and obstructive apnea within one apneic episode.

The patient, usually male, snores loudly, stops breathing up to 15 seconds or more, and then awakens abruptly with a loud snort as his blood oxygen level drops. He may have more than ten apneic episodes per hour to several hundred per night. This can seriously tax the heart and lungs. Increasing age and obesity correlate positively with alterations in breathing and nocturnal oxygen desaturation.

Management is based on whether or not complications are present; life-threatening arrhythmias, chronic cardio-vascular effects, and memory loss and intellectual impairment. If obese, the patient is placed on a weight-reduction program, as most patients with obstructive apnea are obese. Tricyclic antidepressants, respiratory stimulants, and tracheostomy to bypass the obstruction may be modalities of treatment according to the problems of the individual patient. Nocturnal oxygen is beneficial for relieving hypoxemia in some patients. Pacemaker stimulation of the phrenic nerves may be helpful in patients with central sleep apnea.

▷ Pulmonary Embolism

Pulmonary embolism refers to the obstruction of one or more pulmonary arteries by a thrombus (or thrombi) that originates somewhere in the venous system or in the right side of the heart, becomes dislodged, and is carried to the lung. An infarction of lung tissue owing to interruption of the lung's blood supply may result. Pulmonary embolism is a common disorder and is often associated with advanced age and postoperative states. It may occur in an apparently healthy person.

The majority of thrombi originate in the deep veins of the legs. Other sources include the pelvic veins and the right atrium of the heart. Stasis, or slowing of blood flow, owing to damage to the blood vessel wall (particularly the endothelial lining) and changes in the blood coagulation mechanism, are factors favoring venous thrombogenesis.

Pathophysiology

Following a massive embolic obstruction of the pulmonary arteries, there is an increase in alveolar dead space since the area, though continuing to be ventilated, receives little or no blood flow. In addition, a number of vasoactive and bronchoconstrictive substances are released from the clot. These substances compound the ventilation–perfusion imbalance, causing venous admixture and shunting.

The hemodynamic consequences are increased pulmonary vascular resistance owing to reduction in the size of the pulmonary vascular bed, a consequent increase in pulmonary arterial pressure, and, in turn, an increase in right ventricular work to maintain pulmonary blood flow. When the work requirements of the right ventricle exceeds its capacity, right ventricular failure occurs. When this happens there is a decrease in cardiac output followed by a drop in systemic blood pressure and the development of shock.

Preventive Measures/Risk Factors

The ideal method of treatment is prevention. Effort is directed toward preventing venous stasis in patients on bed rest by ambulation or by active and passive leg exercises. When the legs are moved in a "pumping" exercise, the leg muscles assist in increasing venous flow.

Effort is directed toward preventing stasis of blood in the extremities owing to the dependent position of the legs, prolonged sitting, immobility, or constricting clothing. The patient should not be permitted to "dangle" his legs and feet in a dependent position while sitting on the edge of the bed. His feet should be on the floor or on a chair. Instruct the patient to avoid crossing his legs.

Chart 26-3
Pulmonary Embolism: Persons at Risk

The following events and conditions predispose to thrombophlebitis and pulmonary embolism.

Venous Stasis (slowing of blood flow in veins)

Prolonged immobilization
Prolonged periods of sitting/traveling
Varicose veins

Hypercoagulability (owing to release of tissue thromboplastin following injury/surgery)

Injury
Tumor
Increased platelet count (polycythemia; splenectomy)

Venous Endothelial Disease

Thrombophlebitis
Vascular Disease
Foreign bodies (IV/central venous catheters)

Certain Disease States (combination of stasis, coagulation alterations, and venous injury)

Heart disease (especially congestive heart failure)
Trauma (especially fracture of hip, pelvis, spine, lower extremities)
Postoperative state/postpartum period
Diabetes
Chronic obstructive pulmonary disease
Previous pulmonary embolism

Other Predisposing Conditions

Advanced age
Obesity
Pregnancy
Oral contraceptive use
History of preceding thrombophlebitis
Constrictive clothing

Elastic stockings reportedly compress the superficial venous system and increase the velocity of deep venous blood by redirecting the blood through the deep veins; thus, venous stasis is reduced. However, simple leg elevation (above the level of the heart) with flexion at the knees also increases venous flow. Some authorities feel elastic stockings are unnecessary if the legs are elevated.

Have a high index of suspicion for pulmonary embolism in any patient, but particularly those with conditions predisposing to slowing of venous return. Such conditions include trauma to the pelvis (especially surgical) and lower extremities (especially hip fractures), obesity, history of thromboembolic disease, varicose veins, pregnancy,

congestive heart failure, myocardial infarction, and malignant disease; also, postoperative patients and the elderly are more apt to have a slower venous return.

A liberal fluid intake is encouraged since dehydration predisposes to thrombus formation. Intravenous catheters (for parenteral therapy or CVP measurements) should not be left in veins for prolonged periods.

Suppression of platelet function by pharmacologic agents (aspirin; dipyridamole) is being used to prevent platelet aggregation to reduce the likelihood of thromboembolism.

The American Heart Association recommends that patients who are over 40 and hemostatically competent, and who are undergoing major elective abdominothoracic surgery, be given low doses of heparin to diminish postoperative deep thrombus and pulmonary embolism. The heparin is given subcutaneously 2 hours before surgery and continued every 12 hours until the patient is discharged. Low-dose heparin is thought to enhance the activity of antithrombin III, a major plasma inhibitor of clotting factor X_a. (This regimen is not recommended for patients who are experiencing an active thrombotic process or those undergoing major orthopedic surgery, open prostatectomy, or operations on the eye or brain.)

Assessment for Thrombus

The nurse should examine each susceptible patient for a positive Homan's sign, which may or may not indicate impending thrombosis of the leg veins (see pp. 407–408).

1. Position the patient on his back.
2. Lift the leg and dorsiflex the foot.
3. Note if there is pain in the calf during this maneuver (positive Homan's sign); it may indicate deep venous thrombosis.
4. Conduct another clinical assessment by tapping on the anterior tibial crest to see if this elicits pain.
5. Apply a blood pressure cuff around the patient's calf and inflate it. Pain on inflation of the cuff (80 mm Hg–100 mm Hg) is significant, as is tenderness along the course of a vein, pain in the calf or foot area, or edema in the ankle or calf area. It is best to compare both extremities.
6. Look for swelling and palpable veins. Clinical evidence of phlebitis in one leg does not necessarily indicate that this is the site of the embolus; the other leg, even though normal on examination, may be the site.

▶ Assessment

Clinical Manifestations. The symptoms of pulmonary embolism depend on the size of the thrombus and the area of the pulmonary artery occluded. Dyspnea is the one symptom that is usually consistently present with pulmonary embolism. A massive embolism occluding the bifurcation of the pulmonary artery can produce pronounced dyspnea, sudden substernal pain, rapid and weak pulse, shock, syncope, and sudden death.

If one or more branches of the right or left pulmonary arteries are obstructed, the patient experiences dyspnea, mild substernal pain, anxiety, weakness, and tachycardia. Usually, these symptoms are the result of pulmonary infarction. There may also be fever, cough, and hemoptysis. The patient's respiratory rate is accelerated out of proportion to the degree of fever and tachycardia. If the terminal pulmonary arteries are occluded, a pleuritic type of pain develops, together with cough and hemoptysis. Multiple small emboli can lodge in the terminal pulmonary arterioles, producing multiple small infarctions. The clinical picture may simulate that of bronchopneumonia or heart failure. In some instances, the disease presents in an atypical fashion with few signs and symptoms, while in other instances it mimics various cardiopulmonary disorders.

Diagnostic Assessment. A diagnosis of pulmonary infarction may be suspected in patients who have combined symptoms of dyspnea, pleurisy, cough, hemoptysis, tachycardia, pallor, and perhaps signs of shock, especially if phlebitis is present in the legs or if these symptoms occur during the postoperative period.

The chest x-ray may reveal subtle or nonspecific changes. Bronchoconstriction may lead to a focal decrease in breath sounds and wheezing, whereas loss of surfactant may be associated with fine crackles in the affected lung area. Radioisotope lung scanning and pulmonary angiography usually confirm the presence of emboli. Analysis of arterial blood gases and pulmonary function studies are carried out. A phlebogram may be done to detect ''silent'' thrombi in the legs. An electrocardiogram may also reflect changes due to the embolism. However, it is necessary to compare the results with a previous ECG in order to determine whether there is any correlation between the changes and the suspected embolism.

Patient Problems/Nursing Diagnoses

Based on the clinical manifestations and diagnostic assessment data, the patient's major nursing problems include anxiety and discomfort related to dyspnea and chest pain; alteration in respiratory function related to hemodynamic disturbances associated with pulmonary embolism and impairment to the pulmonary vascular bed; potential for alteration in cardiac output related to increased pulmonary resistance and possible right heart failure; and potential for bleeding related to thrombolytic/anticoagulant therapy.

▶ Planning and Implementation

Goals

The major goals for the patient include:

1. Relief of anxiety and discomfort
2. Improvement of respiratory function
3. Improvement in heart action
4. Absence of bleeding

Emergency Treatment

Pulmonary embolism is a true medical emergency; patients tend to deteriorate rapidly. The immediate objective of treatment and care is to stabilize the cardiorespiratory system. The majority of patients who succumb from massive pulmonary embolism do so in the first 2 hours following the embolic event.

- Nasal oxygen is administered immediately to relieve hypoxemia, respiratory distress, and cyanosis.
- An infusion is started to open an intravenous route for drugs/fluids that will be needed.
- Pulmonary angiography, hemodynamic measurements, arterial blood gas determinations, and perfusion lung scans are carried out. A sudden rise in pulmonary resistance increases the work of the right ventricle, which can cause acute right heart failure with cardiogenic shock.
- If the patient has suffered massive embolism and is hypotensive, an indwelling urethral catheter is inserted to monitor urinary volume.
- Hypotension is treated by a slow infusion (IV) of isoproterenol (has a dilating effect on pulmonary vessels and bronchi) or dopamine.
- The ECG is monitored continuously for right ventricular failure, which may have a rapid onset.
- Sodium bicarbonate may be administered to correct metabolic acidosis. Digitalis glycosides, intravenous diuretics, and antiarrhythmic agents are given when appropriate.
- Blood is drawn for serum electrolytes, BUN, CBC, and hematocrit.
- If clinical assessment and arterial blood gases indicate the need, the patient is placed on a volume-controlled ventilator.
- Small doses of intravenous morphine are given to relieve the patient's anxiety, to alleviate chest discomfort, to help him accept the discomfort of the endotracheal tube, and to ease his adaptation to the mechanical ventilator.

Drug Therapy for Pulmonary Embolism

The aim of drug therapy initially is to remove the thrombus/embolus and to restore the circulatory system to normal; then the aim is to prevent recurrence.

There is changing consensus in the management of pulmonary embolism. Although anticoagulant therapy (heparin; warfarin sodium) has traditionally been the primary therapy for the management of acute deep vein thrombosis and pulmonary embolism, thrombolytic therapy (urokinase, streptokinase) lyses thrombi in the deep venous system and emboli in the pulmonary circulation, causing more rapid resolution of the thrombi/emboli and restoring pulmonary circulation to normal. It results in normalization of hemodynamic disturbances with resultant lessening of pulmonary hypertension. Thus, on a long-term basis thrombolytic therapy prevents venous valvular damage (postphlebitic syndrome) and permanent damage to the pulmonary vascular bed, which is often seen in patients treated only with anticoagulants. Thrombolytic therapy also reduces the likelihood of persisting pulmonary hypertension. Since bleeding is an undesirable side-effect, thrombolytic agents are advocated for patients who are suffering from proximal deep vein thrombosis (thrombosis affecting the popliteal vein or deep veins of the thigh and pelvis) and for patients with pulmonary emboli with significant hemodynamic disturbances or where there has been obstruction of blood flow to a lobe or multiple segments.

Before the thrombolytic infusion, a thrombin time (TT), activated partial thromboplastin time (APTT), prothrombin time (PT), hematocrit values, and platelet counts are done. During therapy all but absolutely essential invasive procedures are avoided, with the exception of careful venipuncture with a 22-gauge or 23-gauge needle for therapeutic monitoring. Essential arterial blood gas studies should be performed on an upper extremity with digital compression of the puncture site for at least 30 minutes. The patient is placed on strict bed rest. Pressure dressings are applied to previously involved sites. Vital signs are taken every 4 hours during infusion. No medication should be added to the bottle containing the thrombolytic agents. The TT or APTT is performed 3 to 4 hours after starting the thrombolytic infusion to confirm activation of the fibrinolytic system. In the event of uncontrollable bleeding, the thrombolytic infusion is discontinued. If necessary, fresh whole blood, packed red cells, cryoprecipitate, or frozen plasma is given to replace blood loss and reverse the bleeding tendency.

After completion of the thrombolytic infusion (which varies in duration according to the agent used and condition being treated) the patient is placed on anticoagulants. Anticoagulation slows or stops the underlying thrombotic process, thus preventing recurrence. Heparin is given and controlled according to standard procedures and is followed by warfarin. Anticoagulant therapy and its nursing requirements are discussed on pages 685–689.

Surgical Intervention

If the patient has persistent hypotension, shock, and respiratory distress; if pulmonary artery pressure is greatly elevated; and if angiograms reveal obstruction of a large part of the pulmonary vasculature, embolectomy may be indicated. This requires a thoracotomy with cardiopulmonary bypass technique (discussed in Chap. 30).

Another surgical technique utilized when pulmonary emboli recur, despite adequate medical therapy (or if the patient is intolerant of anticoagulant therapy), is an interruption of the inferior vena cava. This method prevents dislodged thrombi from being swept into the lungs while at the same time permitting adequate blood flow. This can be done by total ligation or the use of teflon clips applied to the vena cava to divide the caval lumen into small channels without occluding caval blood flow. The use of transvenous devices that occlude or filter the blood through the inferior vena cava is a fairly safe procedure for the prevention of recurrent pulmonary embolism. One such technique is the insertion of a prosthetic umbrella device through a cervical incision in the internal jugular vein (Fig. 26-3). The device is advanced through the superior vena cava and the right atrium into the inferior vena cava where it is brought into an open position. The perforated umbrella permits the passage of blood, but prevents the passage of large thrombi.

Following the surgical procedure, the patient's pulmonary artery pressure and urinary output are monitored. The insertion site is monitored for hematoma formation and infection. An adequate blood pressure must be maintained to ensure perfusion of the vital organs. To prevent peripheral venous stasis and lower extremity edema, the foot of

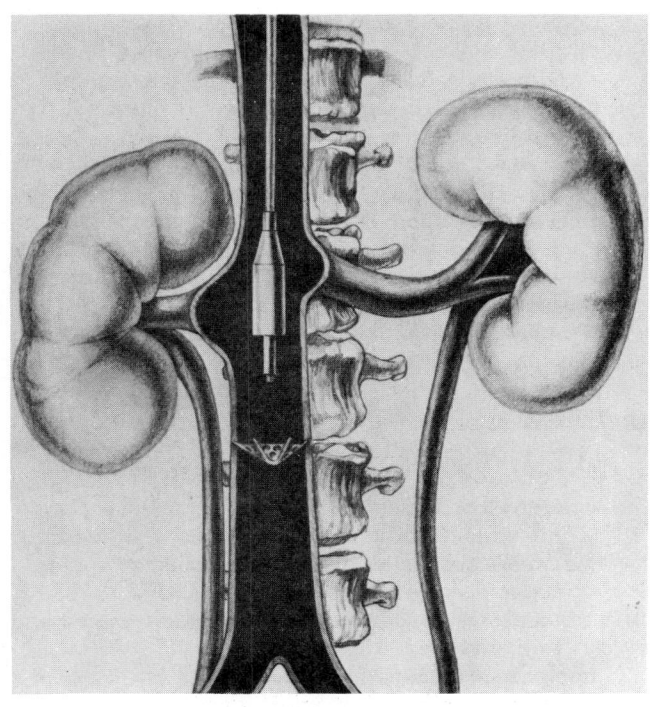

Figure 26-3. Interruption of the inferior vena cava to prevent pulmonary embolism. An umbrella-shaped filter is compressed within an applicator catheter and inserted through an incision in the right internal jugular vein. It is advanced under fluoroscopic control to a position below the renal veins. The filter fixes itself to the wall of the inferior vena cava upon ejection from the applicator, and the applicator is then withdrawn. (Mobin–Uddin Vena Cava Umbrella Filter. Courtesy, Edwards Laboratories Division of American Hospital Supply Corp.)

the bed is elevated. Isometric exercises, elastic stockings, and walking are encouraged when the patient is permitted out of bed. Sitting is discouraged, as hip flexion causes compression of the large veins in the legs.

Transvenous Catheter Embolectomy. A technique has been developed in which a vacuum cupped catheter is introduced transvenously into the affected pulmonary artery. Suction is applied to the end of the embolus and the embolus is aspirated into the cup. The surgeon maintains suction to hold the embolus within the cup, and the entire catheter is withdrawn through the right heart and out the femoral venotomy. An inferior caval filter is often inserted at the same time to protect against a recurrence.

Patient Education

The following patient instructions are intended to help prevent recurrences:

- When taking anticoagulants, look for bruising and bleeding and try to protect yourself from bumping into objects that can cause bruising.
- Use a toothbrush with soft bristles.
- Do not take aspirin or antihistamine drugs while receiving Coumadin. Always check with the physician before taking any medication, including over-the-counter medications.

- Continue to wear antiembolism stockings as long as directed.
- Avoid laxatives, as they affect vitamin K absorption.
- Avoid sitting with your legs crossed or sitting for prolonged periods.
- When traveling, change your position regularly, walk occasionally, and do active exercises of the legs and ankles while sitting. Drink plenty of liquids while traveling to avoid hemoconcentration owing to fluid loss.
- Report dark, tarry stools to the physician/clinic immediately.
- Wear an identification bracelet (or carry a card) stating that anticoagulants are being taken.

▶ Evaluation

Expected Outcomes

1. Is relieved of anxiety and discomfort
   a. Requests medication for pain relief when needed
   b. Experiences relief of chest pain when morphine is taken
   c. Expresses confidence in therapeutic regimen and care-givers
2. Improves respiratory function
   a. Shows no signs of dyspnea or tachypnea
   b. Exhibits normal breath sounds upon auscultation
   c. Has arterial blood gases within normal range
3. Demonstrates improved heart action
   a. Shows no sign of distended neck veins, liver enlargement or peripheral edema
   b. Is free of tachycardia, gallop rhythm, and accentuated pulmonic sounds
   c. Has palpable pedal pulses
   d. Demonstrates normal heart sounds on auscultation
   e. Shows no sign of right ventricular failure on ECG
4. Is free of bleeding
   a. Applies pressure to puncture sites after laboratory tests, etc.
   b. Verbalizes the reason for frequent laboratory evaluations
   c. Shows understanding of self-monitoring for bleeding; says he will report excessive bruising, blood in urine/stools
   d. Wears an identification bracelet stating he is taking anticoagulants

▷ Sarcoidosis

Sarcoidosis is a systemic granulomatous disease of unknown cause. It may involve almost any organ or tissue, but most commonly involves the lungs, lymph nodes, liver, spleen, skin, eyes, phalangeal bones, and parotid glands. The onset usually occurs between the third or fourth decade. Sarcoidosis is fairly common with a worldwide distribution.

Patients with sarcoidosis may have a number of immunologic abnormalities. The first clinical manifestations are usually thoracic, with hilar gland enlargement. The clinical picture includes shortness of breath, cough, vague chest pain, and congestion. The chest x-ray may show hilar adenopathy and disseminated miliary and nodular lesions in the lungs. The granulomas may disappear or gradually convert to fibrous tissue. Extrathoracic involvement includes uveitis, joint pain, fever, and granulomatous lesions of the skin, liver, spleen, kidney, and central nervous system. With multiple organ system involvement, the patient experiences fatigue, fever, anorexia, weight loss, and joint pain.

The diagnosis is confirmed by biopsy of the skin and lymph nodes, which reveal noncaseating granulomas. Pulmonary function tests are abnormal if there is restriction of lung function.

There is no specific treatment, as the natural course of the disease is toward resolution. Corticosteroid therapy may benefit some patients because of its anti-inflammatory effect, thus relieving symptoms and improving organ function. It is useful for patients with ocular and myocardial involvement, extensive pulmonary disease with compromise of pulmonary function, and hypercalcemia. Isoniazid may be given to patients with positive tuberculin tests.

▷ Occupational Lung Diseases

Diseases of the lungs can occur in a variety of occupations as a result of exposure to organic or inorganic (mineral) dusts and noxious gases (fumes and aerosols). The effect of inhaling these materials depends on the composition of the inhaled substance, its antigenic (precipitating an immune response) or irritating properties, the dose inhaled, the length of time inhaled, and the host's response (individual's susceptibility to the irritant). There are a growing number of occupational lung diseases owing to new and untested industrial substances and chemicals (presumed to be harmless). The problem may be compounded by smoking, which appears to have a synergistic effect on occupational lung disease and may increase the risk of lung cancers in people exposed to asbestos.

Preventive Measures and Health Maintenance

First, every effort is made to reduce the exposure of the worker to industrial products. The work environment must be ventilated properly to remove the noxious agent from the worker's breathing zone. Dust control can prevent many of the pneumoconioses and includes ventilation, spraying an area with water to control release of dust, and effective and frequent floor cleaning. Air samples need to be monitored. Toxic substances should be enclosed to reduce their concentration in the air. Workers must wear protective devices (face masks, hoods, industrial respirators) to provide a safe air supply when in a toxic atmosphere. Every employee should be carefully screened and followed, especially the worker at high risk for developing occupational lung disease (hypersensitivity states; asthma). There is a risk of developing serious smoking-related illness (cancer) in industries in which there are unsafe levels of certain gases, dusts, fumes, fluids, and other toxic substances. Ongoing educational programs to teach the worker to bear responsibility for his own health, including smoking cessation and influenza vaccination, have a major role in the prevention of occupational lung disease.

The Pneumoconioses

Pneumoconiosis refers to a nonneoplastic alteration of the lung resulting from exposure to inorganic dust (*e.g.,* "dusty lung"). The most common pneumoconioses are silicosis, asbestosis, and coalworker's pneumoconiosis.

Silicosis. Silicosis is a chronic pulmonary disease caused by inhalation of silica dust (silicon dioxide particles). Since the earth's crust is composed of silica and silicates, exposure is encountered in almost any form of mining (*i.e.,* coal, tin, copper, silver, gold, uranium mining, quarrying (slate, sandstone), or tunneling operations). Stonecutting, the manufacture of abrasives and pottery, and foundry work are other occupations presenting exposure hazards. When the silica particles, which have fibrogenic properties, are inhaled, nodular lesions are produced throughout the lungs. With the passage of time and exposure, the nodules enlarge and coalesce. Dense masses form in the upper portion of the lungs, resulting in loss of pulmonary parenchymal volume. Restrictive lung disease (inability of the lungs to expand fully) and obstructive lung disease from secondary emphysema result. Cavity formation is likely to be the result of superimposed tuberculosis. Exposure of 10 to 20 years is usually required before the disease develops and shortness of breath is manifested. Fibrotic destruction of pulmonary tissue can lead to emphysema, pulmonary hypertension, and cor pulmonale.

There is no specific treatment, and therapy is directed at the complications of silicosis. Preventive measures (p. 532) must be directed at protecting workers from inhaling silica dust. With cavitary lesions or advanced fibrosis, many physicians treat the patient for tuberculosis, even when cultures are negative.

Asbestosis. Asbestosis is a disease characterized by diffuse pulmonary fibrosis owing to the inhalation of asbestos dust. The use of asbestos is almost indispensable in modern industry and there are thousands of applications for its use. Exposure occurs in numerous occupations, including asbestos mining and manufacturing, demolition work, roofing, etc. Materials such as shingles, cement, vinyl asbestos tile, fireproof paint and clothing, brake linings, filters, etc., all contain asbestos. The risk appears to lie in the manufacture, cutting, and demolition of asbestos-containing materials.

The asbestos fibers are inhaled and enter the alveoli, which, in time, are eventually obliterated by fibrous tissue that surrounds the asbestos particles. There is fibrous pleural thickening and pleural plaque formation. The altered physiologic pattern is that of restrictive lung disease with decrease in lung volume, diminished gas transfer, and hypoxemia. The patient has progressive dyspnea, mild to moderate chest pain, anorexia, and weight loss. Cor pulmonale and respiratory failure occur as the disease progresses. A significant proportion of workers exposed to asbestos dust die of lung cancer, especially those who smoke. In addition to lung cancer and asbestosis, exposure to asbestos can produce nonmalignant pleural disease, diffuse malignant mesothelioma, and possibly neoplasms of other tissues. Avoidance, in general, is essential and *asbestos workers should stop smoking.*

There is no effective treatment for asbestosis. Treatment is directed at intercurrent infection and coexisting lung disease. In patients with severe gas transport abnormalities, continuous oxygen therapy may improve exercise tolerance.

Coal Worker's Pneumoconiosis. Coal worker's pneumoconiosis (CWP, "black lung") is a variety of respiratory disease found in coal workers in which there is an accumulation of coal dust in the lungs causing a tissue reaction to its presence. Coal miners are exposed to dusts that are mixtures of coal, kaolin, mica, and silica. The first physiologic reaction to the deposition of coal dust in the alveoli and respiratory bronchioles is an increase of macrophages that engulf (by phagocytosis) the particles and transport them to the terminal bronchioles where they are removed by mucociliary clearance. In time, the clearance mechanisms are unable to handle the excessive dust load, and the macrophages aggregate in the respiratory bronchioles and alveoli. Fibroblasts appear and a network of reticulin is laid down surrounding the dust-laden macrophages. The respiratory bronchioles and the alveoli become clogged with coal dust, dying macrophages, and fibroblasts, which leads to the formation of the coal macule, the primary lesion of CWP. (Macules appear as blackish dots on the lungs.) As the macules enlarge, there is a dilation of the weakening bronchiole with subsequent development of a focal emphysema.

The patient with complicated coal worker's pneumoconiosis has massive lesions of dense fibrotic tissue containing black material. These masses eventually destroy blood vessels and the bronchi of the affected lobe. The patient develops dyspnea, cough, and sputum production with expectoration of varying amounts of black fluid (melanoptosis), particularly if he is a smoker. Eventually cor pulmonale and respiratory failure result. The treatment is symptomatic. (See also treatment of emphysema, p. 522.)

Other Inhalation Disorders

Organic Dust Exposure. The inhalation of organic dusts results in hypersensitivity reactions at the alveolar level. The best known example is *farmer's lung,* which occurs with exposure to moldy hay containing thermophilic actinomycetes (*Microsporum faeni; Thermoactinomyces vulgaris*). This induces an allergic inflammatory reaction with granuloma involving the interstitial tissues of the lung. Within a few hours of heavy exposure, the patient develops chills, fever, malaise, myalgia, arthralgia, chest tightness, dry cough, and dyspnea.

Treatment is directed toward removing the patient from further exposure. Corticosteroids may be administered to decrease systemic toxicity and promote resolution of the pulmonary disease. The patient is treated symptomatically, with oxygen, bronchodilator therapy, and physiologic monitoring as required.

Inhalation of Irritant Gases. The inhalation of gases, aerosols, or fumes is a hazard inherent in many occupations.

The nature of the gas and the duration and intensity of exposure are important factors determining the type of problems that may develop. In an industrial setting, chlorine, ammonia, sulfur dioxide, ozone, nitrogen dioxide, phosgene, and smoke may produce symptoms varying from irritation of the mucosal surfaces to fatal pulmonary injury.

Irritant gases and mists produce injury through asphyxiation, systemic toxicity, immunologic mechanisms, or direct alveolar damage. Inhalation of nitrogen or sulfur dioxide is especially dangerous since these gases may initiate physiologic changes leading to pulmonary edema. In general, the treatment of patients inhaling irritant gases is nonspecific. It involves prompt removal from the agent, maintenance of airway patency, closely monitored oxygenation, prophylactic administration of antibiotics, and the techniques involved in the therapy of respiratory failure.

▷ Tumors of the Chest

A chest tumor may be *primary,* arising within the lung or the mediastinum, or it may represent a metastasis from a primary tumor site elsewhere. Metastatic tumors of the lungs occur frequently, since the bloodstream transports free cancer cells from primary cancers elsewhere in the body. Such tumors grow in and between the alveoli and the bronchi, which they push apart in their growth. This process may occur over a long period of time, causing few or no symptoms.

Primary tumors of the lung may be benign or malignant. Most arise from the bronchial epithelium. Bronchial adenomas are slow growing, usually benign tumors, but they are very vascular and therefore produce symptoms of bleeding and bronchial obstruction. Bronchogenic carcinoma is a malignant tumor arising from the bronchus. Such a tumor is epidermoid, usually located in the larger bronchi, or is an adenocarcinoma, arising further out in the lung. There are also several intermediate or undifferentiated types of lung cancer, identifiable by cell type.

Lung Cancer (Bronchogenic Carcinoma)

Lung cancer is the number one cancer killer among men in the United States and the second most common cause of cancer death in women. Lung cancer is increasing at a greater rate in women than it is in men and will soon exceed breast cancer as the most common cause of cancer death. The survival rate is low, for in approximately 70% of patients, the disease has spread to regional lymphatics and other sites at the time of diagnosis.

It has been suggested that carcinoma tends to arise at sites of previous scarring (tuberculosis; fibrosis) in the lung.

Classification and Staging. The four major cell types of lung cancer (which differ significantly) are epidermoid (squamous cell) carcinoma, small cell (oat cell) carcinoma, adenocarcinoma, and large cell (undifferentiated) carcinoma. Chart 26-4 shows the World Health Organization classification of lung tumors by histologic type. Many tumors contain more than one cell type. The different cell types display different biological behavior and have prognostic

---

Chart 26-4
Histopathologic Types of Lung Tumors

  I. Epidermoid carcinomas
 II. Small cell anaplastic carcinomas
  1. Fusiform cell type
  2. Polygonal cell type
  3. Lymphocyte-like ("oat-cell") type
  4. Others
III. Adenocarcinomas
  1. Bronchogenic
   a. Acinar } with or without
   b. Papillary } mucin formation
  2. Bronchiolo-alveolar
 IV. Large cell carcinomas
  1. Solid tumors with mucin-like content
  2. Solid tumors without mucin-like content
  3. Giant cell carcinomas
  4. "Clear" cell carcinomas
  V. Combined epidermoid and adenocarcinomas
 VI. Carcinoid tumors
VII. Bronchial gland tumors
  1. Cylindromas
  2. Mucoepidermoid tumors
  3. Others
VIII. Papillary tumors of the surface epithelium
  1. Epidermoid
  2. Epidermoid with goblet cells
  3. Others
 IX. "Mixed" tumors and carcinosarcomas
  1. "Mixed" tumors
  2. Carcinosarcomas of embryonal type ("blastomas")
  3. Other carcinosarcomas
  X. Sarcomas
 XI. Unclassified
XII. Mesotheliomas
  1. Localized
  2. Diffuse
XIII. Melanomas

(From Kreyberg L, Liebow AA, and Vehlinger EA: Histological Typing of Lung Tumors. Geneva, World Health Organization, 1967.)

---

significance. Therefore, different approaches to treatment may be indicated by the cell type.

The stage of the tumor refers to the anatomical extent of the tumor and indicates the presence or absence of spread to the regional lymph nodes and the presence or absence of metastases. Staging is accomplished by tissue diagnosis, lymph node biopsy, and mediastinoscopy. Staging is important in determining whether or not tumor resection should be attempted. Prognosis appears most favorable for epidermoid and adenocarcinoma, whereas undifferentiated small cell (oat cell) tumors appear to have a poor prognosis.

Persons at Risk. Bronchogenic cancer is 10 times more common in cigarette smokers than in nonsmokers, the prevalence being related to the length of time and the intensity of smoking. Epidermoid carcinoma, involving the larger bronchi, is thought to be almost entirely associated with heavy (1 pack/day) cigarette smoking. Few cases of this type of cancer have been reported in nonsmokers. Table 26-2 lists the prevalence of the five most common lung cancers in men and women, smokers and those who never smoked, as they presented at Mayo Clinic. For reasons unknown, the incidence of adenocarcinoma is rising faster than that of other types.

Adenocarcinoma of the peripheral bronchi is not associated with any known cause and occurs equally in smokers and nonsmokers. Another risk factor is occupational exposure to asbestos, radioactive dusts, arsenic, and certain plastics alone or in combination with tobacco smoke. It is reported that the risk of lung cancer is 92 times greater for persons exposed to tobacco smoke and asbestos dust. Persons at high risk who insist on continuing to smoke should have regular chest x-rays and sputum examinations in order to increase their chances that lung cancer will be detected while still treatable.

▶ **Assessment**

Clinical Manifestations. Tumors of the bronchopulmonary system may affect the lining of the respiratory tract, lung parenchyma, pleura, or chest wall. The disease begins insidiously (over several decades) and often is asymptomatic until late in its course. The signs and symptoms depend on the location and size of the tumor, the degree of obstruction, and the existence of metastases to regional or distant sites.

The most frequent symptom is cough, probably from irritation by the tumor mass. It is frequently ignored as a "cigarette cough." Starting as a hacking, nonproductive cough, it later progresses to a point where it produces a thick, purulent sputum as secondary infection occurs.

- Thus, a cough that changes in character should arouse suspicion of lung cancer.

A wheeze in the chest (occurs when a bronchus becomes partially obstructed by the tumor) is noted in about 20% of patients. The expectoration of blood-tinged sputum is common, particularly in the morning, and is due to sputum becoming streaked with blood as it passes over the ulcerated tumor surface. In some patients, recurring fever owing to a persisting infection in an area of pneumonitis distal from the tumor is the early symptom. In fact, cancer of the lung should be suspected in persons with repeated unresolved upper respiratory infections. Pain is a late manifestation and is often found to be related to bone metastasis. If the tumor spreads to adjacent structures and regional lymph nodes, the patient may present with chest pain and tightness, hoarseness (involvement of recurrent laryngeal nerve), dysphagia, head and neck edema, and symptoms of pleural or pericardial effusion. The most common sites of metastases are lymph nodes, bone, brain, contralateral lung, and adrenal glands. General symptoms of weakness, anorexia, weight loss, and anemia appear late.

Diagnostic Assessment. If the patient with pulmonary symptoms is a heavy smoker, cancer of the lung can be suspected. Chest x-rays are done to search for pulmonary density, solitary peripheral nodule (coin lesion), atelectasis, and infection. Cytologic examination of fresh sputum obtained by cough or saline washings from a suspected bronchus is done to search for malignant cells. Bronchoscopy with a flexible fiberoptic instrument allows a detailed study of the bronchial segments, identification of the source of malignant cells, and probable extent of anticipated surgery. More recently, fluorescent bronchofibroscopy is being used to detect small, early bronchogenic cancers. Systemically injected hematoporphyrin is absorbed by malignant cells and presents a red fluorescent glow when examined under illumination by violet light.

Lung scans are part of the diagnostic workup. A bone scan or bone marrow study is done for detection of bone metastasis, and liver scanning is used to verify metastatic spread to the liver. Detection of central nervous system metastases is accomplished by brain scanning, computerized tomography, and other neurologic diagnostic procedures. Mediastinoscopy may be used to evaluate tumor

Table 26-2
Occurrence of Five Major Types of Lung Cancers in Smokers and Nonsmokers

| Type | Total | Male | | Female | |
		Smoker	Never Smoker	Smoker	Never Smoker
Epidermoid	992	892	7	80	13
Small cell	640	533	4	100	3
Adenocarcinoma	760	492	39	128	101
Large cell	466	389	16	46	15
Bronchioloalveolar cell	68	35	4	13	16
TOTAL	2926	2341	70	367	148

(From Rosenow EC and Carr DT: Bronchogenic Carcinoma. Reprinted with permission from CA—A Cancer Journal for Clinicians 29:235, 1979. Copyright © American Cancer Society, Inc., 1979.)

spread to hilar lymph nodes of the right lung, and mediastinotomy gives access to the hilar lymphatics of the left lung.

Before surgery, the patient is evaluated to determine whether the tumor is resectable and whether he can tolerate the physiologic impairment resulting from such surgery. Pulmonary function tests combined with split-function perfusion scans are done to determine if the patient will have adequate pulmonary reserve following the procedure. The patient's ability to move air (vital capacity, FEV_1) is important since the ability to generate an effective cough is imperative in the postoperative period.

Patient Problems/Nursing Diagnoses

Based on the clinical manifestations and diagnostic assessment data and in addition to the problems of the patient undergoing thoracic surgery (p. 461), the patient's major nursing problems include possible cough, dyspnea, and chest pain related to airway obstruction; tissue invasion or pulmonary resection; anxiety and depression related to the diagnosis of cancer; and concern about interruption of lifestyle related to impact of disease.

▶ Planning and Implementation

Goals

The goals of the patient are:

1. Relief of cough, dyspnea, and chest pain
2. Ability to cope with anxiety and depression
3. Improvement of the quality of life-style

Management

The objective of management is to provide the maximum likelihood of cure. The treatment depends on the cell type, the stage of the disease (anatomical extent), and the physiologic status (particularly cardiac and pulmonary status) of the patient. In general, treatment may involve surgery, radiotherapy, chemotherapy, and immunotherapy, used separately or in combination.

Surgery. Surgical resection is the preferred method for patients with localized tumors with no evidence of metastatic spread and whose cardiopulmonary function is adequate. (Usually, surgery for small cell cancer of the lung is not advisable because this is a rapidly growing tumor that metastasizes early and widely.) Unfortunately, a large number of patients with bronchogenic cancer are inoperable at the time of diagnosis. The usual operation for small, apparently curable tumor of the lung is lobectomy (removal of a lobe of the lung). An entire lung may be removed (pneumonectomy) in combination with other surgical procedures, such as resection of involved mediastinal lymph nodes. Before surgery, the cardiopulmonary reserve of the patient must be determined. (See pp. 461–471 for the preoperative and postoperative management of the patient undergoing chest surgery.)

Radiation. Radiation therapy may cure a small percentage of patients. It is useful in controlling radio-responsive neoplasms that cannot be resected. The small cell and epidermoid tumors are usually radiation sensitive. It may be used as palliative treatment to decrease tumor size and relieve pressure on vital structures. It can control symptoms of spinal cord metastasis, superior vena cava compression, etc. Also, prophylactic brain irradiation is being carried out on certain patients to kill microscopic metastases to the brain. Respite may be obtained from cough, chest pain, dyspnea, hemoptysis, and bone and liver pain. Relief of symptoms may last from a few weeks to many months and is important in improving the quality of the remaining period of life.

With radiation there is usually toxicity to normal tissue within the radiation field. Complications of radiation therapy include esophagitis, pneumonitis, and radiation lung fibrosis, which may impair ventilatory and diffusion capacity with a significant reduction in pulmonary reserve. Irradiation can also affect the heart in a variety of ways.

Attention should be paid to the patient's nutrition, to signs of anemia, control of infection, and psychological outlook. (See pp. 335–336 for management of the patient receiving radiation therapy.)

Chemotherapy. At the present time chemotherapy is used to manipulate tumor growth patterns, to treat patients with distant metastases, used in combination with surgery or radiation or for patients with small cell cancer of the lung. Combinations of two or more drugs may be more beneficial than single-dose regimens. A large number of drugs are reported to have some activity against lung cancer. Various combinations of doxorubicin hydrochloride (Adriamycin), cyclosphosphamide (Cytoxan), vincristine, cisplatin, and CCNU are being tried. The choice depends on the growth of the tumor cell and the specificity of the drug for a cell cycle phase. These agents are toxic and have a narrow margin of safety. Chemotherapy may give palliation, especially from pain, but does not cure and rarely prolongs life. It is valuable in reducing pressure symptoms of lung cancer and in treating brain, spinal cord, and pericardial metastasis. (See pp. 308–315 for chemotherapy for the patient with cancer.)

Immunotherapy. It has been observed that immunologic responsiveness is suppressed in persons with lung cancer and that this affects their prognosis. Immunotherapy may be tried in an attempt to reverse this immunosuppression. The objective of immunotherapy is to restore or augment the normal mechanisms of host defense against the tumor. A living vaccine (bacille Calmette–Guerin [BCG]) may be introduced into the pleural space (via chest tube or thoracentesis) or by cutaneous immunization to scarification sites in the hope that a local bacterial infection may cause regional activation of the immune system and destroy tumor cells that may have escaped surgical resection. Approximately 14 days following BCG injection, a course of isoniazid is administered to prevent overgrowth of BCG organisms. Levamisole has been used as an immunorestorative agent based on the rationale that manipulation of the patient's immune system will destroy malignant cells. Immunotherapy is monitored by skin tests and lymphocyte culture studies. Although this modality of treatment is in its infancy and the mechanisms of action are poorly understood, there have been clearly detectable benefits in patients with lung cancer.

► **Evaluation**

Expected Outcomes

1. Is relieved of cough, dyspnea, and chest pain
   a. Experiences a decrease in cough, dyspnea, and chest pain
   b. Shows improved activity tolerance
   c. Verbalizes that discomfort has lessened
   d. Verbalizes that treatment (radiation/chemotherapy) may cause some discomfort and side-effects
   (See Evaluation following thoracic surgery, p. 468.)
2. Copes with anxiety and depression
   a. Communicates feelings about lung cancer
   b. Speaks about specific fears
   c. Is able to unburden feelings and conflicts to family/friend
   d. Keeps a written log of feelings about disease
   e. Identifies support systems previously used in times of crisis
   f. Has telephone number of mental health profession(s) if emotional stresses become overwhelming
3. Improves quality of life
   a. Verbalizes feelings about losses and compensatory mechanisms
   b. Discusses the necessity of keeping busy and continuing with usual activities
   c. Identifies hobbies/recreational pursuits he will be able to pursue
   d. Discusses importance of maintaining nutritional status

Tumors of the Mediastinum

Most mediastinal tumors are adjacent to vital structures and have an unpredictable manner of growth. They include neurogenic tumors, thymic tumors, and mesodermal and endocrine tumors. Thymic tumors have the highest percentage of malignancy.

Cysts of the mediastinum usually are small when benign. Dermoid cysts occasionally develop, and these may ulcerate into the air passages.

Manifestations.   Nearly all the symptoms of mediastinal tumors are due to the pressure of the mass against important intrathoracic organs. Among these pressure symptoms are chest pain; bulging of the chest wall; orthopnea (an early sign owing to pressure against the trachea, a main bronchus, the recurrent laryngeal nerve, or the lung); cardiac palpitation, anginal attacks, and various other circulatory disturbances; cyanosis; superior vena caval syndromes (*i.e.,* swelling of the face, the neck, and the upper extremities) and the marked distention of the veins of the neck and the chest wall (evidence of the closure of large veins of the mediastinum by extravascular compression or intravascular invasion); and dysphagia owing to pressure against the esophagus.

Diagnosis.   Roentgenograms are of great value in the diagnosis of mediastinal tumors and cysts. Lateral and oblique films and tomography are used to localize the tumor.

CT scans are used to detect occult thymomas as well as to define a mass lesion.

The biopsy of an enlarged lymph node removed from above the clavicle or one removed during mediastinoscopy may reveal the diagnosis. Blood studies are of value in excluding leukemia, and sputum examinations aid in ruling out tuberculosis.

Management.   Many mediastinal tumors are benign and operable. The location of the tumor in the mediastinum will dictate the type of incision. Most incisions are median sternotomies. The care is the same as for any patient who is undergoing thoracic surgery (pp. 461–471). The major complications, although infrequent, include hemorrhage, phrenic or recurrent laryngeal nerve injury, and infection. If the tumor is malignant and infiltrating, radiotherapy and chemotherapy are the therapeutic modalities used when complete surgical removal is not feasible.

▷ An Aspirated Foreign Body in the Lung

Foreign bodies are frequently aspirated into the lung, especially by children. When this occurs, the object usually lodges in the right main bronchus, because of its more vertical position. However, a foreign body can enter any segment of the lung, depending on the size and character of the object, the position of the person when the aspiration occurs, and whether or not the object could be dislodged by coughing.

The complete closure of the larynx, trachea, or bronchus by a foreign body may result in sudden death. However, the usual result is that the lobes communicating with the occluded bronchus collapse as the air contained in them becomes absorbed into the bloodstream. Sometimes, the foreign object acts as a check valve, allowing air to pass by during inspiration (the bronchial diameter enlarges) but obstructing the exhalation of air during expiration (the bronchial diameter decreases). An inspiratory and expiratory x-ray is helpful in this circumstance, since the lung or the segment beyond the obstruction will not decrease fully during expiration.

A small, solid object such as a pin, a tack, or a tooth in a bronchus causes trouble, not from the obstruction of a bronchus, but from infection. For a short time following the aspiration there may be symptoms of choking, gagging, and coughing. But these symptoms, often mild, abate and for a time become forgotten. For weeks the only suggestion of trouble may be a persistent cough. Such substances as peanuts, grains of corn, etc., on the other hand, produce a severe bronchitis with high irregular fever and all the symptoms and signs of severe pneumonitis. Whether the foreign body is composed of organic or inorganic material, signs of obstructive emphysema, atelectasis, or lung abscess eventually appear.

Management.   The patient is x-rayed to check the presence and position of the foreign body (foreign bodies often shift in position). The prognosis is serious unless the foreign body is removed early, for rarely is it coughed up spontaneously. Therefore, bronchoscopy is indicated when this diagnosis is suspected.

Prevention.   Prevention is extremely important and consists of teaching children not to put small toys, coins, buttons, pencil caps, and such articles in their mouths. Open safety pins should never be put on a pillow near a baby, nor should a child be permitted to play with a button box. Parents require considerable education in such details of child training, and no small part of their responsibility in this regard is the example that they set for their offspring.

▷ Chest Trauma

Injuries to the chest may cause minor or serious disturbances of cardiorespiratory function, depending on which part of the complex mechanism is involved. Thus, a fall against the side of a bathtub may fracture one or two ribs with painful but rather slight disturbance of respiratory function, whereas an automobile accident in which the driver of the car is thrown against the steering wheel may crush the chest, causing cardiac and lung injuries that may be rapidly fatal. In the United States approximately 25% of trauma-related deaths are caused by thoracic injuries alone, and in an additional 50%, chest trauma is a major factor leading to death. *There is frequent association of other injuries, most commonly major fractures, cerebrocranial injuries, and abdominal trauma.* In high-speed accidents there is an abrupt application of a shearing force to the intrathoracic structures as the person rapidly decelerates (a fast-stop situation). This compresses all of the structures within the rib cage, especially the lungs. Other causes of trauma to the chest are falls, crushing injuries, blows to the chest, and knife and gunshot wounds.

The most serious consequences of chest trauma are acute respiratory failure from damage to the chest wall, airways, diaphragm and lungs, and shock owing to large vessel and extrathoracic injuries. Frequently, acute respiratory failure and shock are encountered in combination. This situation is particularly lethal.

Chest injuries may be caused by *nonpenetrating (blunt) trauma,* which does not penetrate but injures by force, and by *penetrating injuries.* Both types of injuries can cause serious respiratory and hemodynamic dysfunction.

Immediate Assessment and Management.   In the treatment of injuries to the chest, efforts are made to correct disturbances of cardiorespiratory function caused by the trauma. The first requirement is to evaluate the patency of the airway by assessing for signs of obstruction, sternal retraction, stridor, wheezing, and cyanosis. Agitation, irrational behavior, and hostility are signs of decreased oxygen delivery to the cerebral cortex. To restore and maintain cardiopulmonary function, an adequate airway is created and ventilation is assured. (This includes stabilizing and reestablishing chest wall integrity, correcting open pneumothorax, decompressing pneumothorax/hemothorax, and eliminating cardiac tamponade.) Hypovolemia and low cardiac output are corrected. These treatment efforts, along with the control of hemorrhage, are usually carried out simultaneously by the emergency department team. The pa-

tient is completely undressed to avoid missing additional injuries. The entire chest is first inspected and palpated. Many injuries involving the chest have associated head and abdominal injuries that require care. Assessment and reassessment are essential to see if the patient is responding to treatment or to detect early signs of a deteriorating condition.

Principles of management are essentially those pertaining to care of the postoperative thoracic patient, discussed on pages 461–471.

Rib Fractures

Rib fractures are the most common chest injury and should be taken seriously, since they may result in underlying lung contusion (p. 540). Such injuries are of special concern in middle-aged and elderly persons who may already have seriously reduced vital capacity. The fifth to the ninth ribs are the ribs most commonly broken. If the rib fragments are driven inward, the jagged edges of the rib(s) may lacerate the lung, spleen, or liver as well as cause hemothorax, pneumothorax, or hemopneumothorax.

If the patient is conscious, he will experience severe pain, tenderness, and muscle spasm over the area of fracture, which is aggravated by coughing, deep breathing, and motion. To reduce the pain the patient will breathe in a shallow manner and will avoid sighs, deep breaths, coughing, and moving. This results in diminished ventilation, collapse of unaerated alveoli, subsequent atelectasis, pneumonitis, and hypoxemia. Because the patient is reluctant to cough, secretions accumulate, which also can lead to atelectasis. Respiratory insufficiency and failure can be the outcome of such a cycle. Following blunt chest trauma, serial analysis of arterial blood gases is a sensitive indicator to determine whether or not the lung has been injured.

Management.   If there are no complications (pneumothorax; hemothorax), the objective is to relieve the pain so that the patient can breathe effectively. Sedation may be given to relieve pain and allow deep breathing and coughing. Using the nurses' hands to support the injured area (or by wrapping a towel around the chest), the patient is encouraged to breathe deeply and cough. Relief of pain can also be achieved by blocking the intercostal nerves that transmit painful sensations from the affected area. Nerve block also abolishes muscle splinting, which limits respiratory excursion. Injections of the intercostal nerve(s) may be made at the lower border of the rib in the region of the intercostal nerve. If necessary, narcotic drugs are used in small, titrated doses and with caution because of their tendency to suppress the cough and depress respiration. Usually, the pain abates in 5 to 7 days and discomfort can be controlled with nonnarcotic analgesia. Most rib fractures heal in 3 to 6 weeks.

Flail Chest

Flail chest is the loss of stability of the chest wall with subsequent respiratory impairment (Fig. 26-4). It is usually the result of multiple rib or sternal fractures. When this happens one portion of the chest wall no longer has a bony

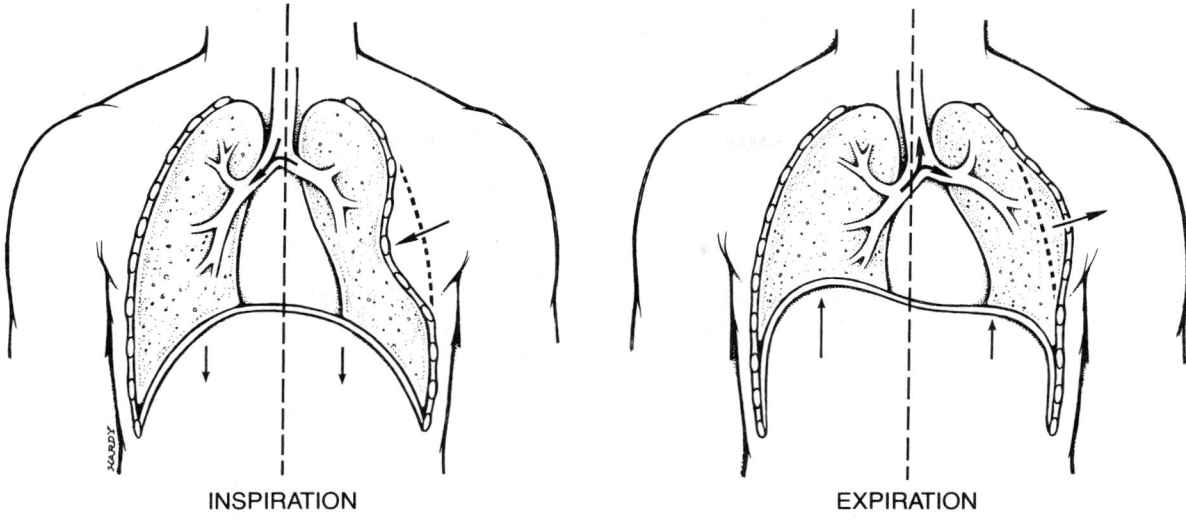

INSPIRATION   EXPIRATION

Figure 26-4. Flail chest and pathophysiologic effects.

connection with the rest of the rib cage. It is usually accompanied by a severe degree of respiratory distress.

Pathophysiology. During inspiration, as the chest expands, the detached part of the chest (flail segment) will show a paradoxical movement in that it is pulled inward during inspiration. This impairs the ability to produce the negative intrapleural pressure required to draw in air. The mediastinum shifts to the normal side. On expiration, since the intrathoracic pressure will exceed atmospheric pressure, the flail segment will bulge outward, impairing the patient's ability to exhale. At the same time, the mediastinum shifts to the injured side. This paradoxical action (air moves between the lungs) results in increased dead space ventilation, retained airway secretions, increasing lung resistance and compliance, and reduction in alveolar ventilation. This parodoxical breathing results in inadequate ventilation; the pulmonary contusion causes hypoxia and combined with pain, hemothorax/pneumothorax; and atelectasis is a major factor in causing respiratory insufficiency.

The diagnosis is made by inspection of the *entire* chest, observing for paradoxical motion, and by palpation of the thorax.

Management. Several modes of therapy are available, depending on the degree of respiratory dysfunction. If only a small segment of the chest is involved, the objectives are to clear the airway (coughing, deep breaths, gentle suctioning) in order to aid in the expansion of the lung, and to relieve pain by intercostal nerve blocks, high thoracic epidural blocks, or careful use of intravenous narcotics.

For mild to moderate flail chest injuries, some clinicians advocate treating the underlying pulmonary contusion with fluid restriction, diuretics, corticosteroids, and albumin while relieving chest pain and by employing pulmonary physiotherapy, combined with close and continuing patient monitoring.

When a severe flail is encountered, endotracheal intubation and mechanical ventilation with a volume-cycled respirator or positive end-expiratory pressure (PEEP) is

used to internally splint the chest wall (internal pneumatic stabilization) and to correct abnormalities in gas exchange. This helps to treat the underlying pulmonary contusion, serves to stabilize the thoracic cage for healing of fractures, and improves alveolar ventilation and intrathoracic volume by decreasing the work of breathing. However, this treatment modality requires long-term endotracheal intubation and ventilator support.

Hemothorax and Pneumothorax

Severe chest injuries usually are accompanied by the collection of blood in the chest cavity (hemothorax) as the result of torn intercostal vessels, lacerations of the lungs, or the escape of air from the injured lung into the pleural cavity (pneumothorax). Often, both blood and air are found in the chest cavity (hemopneumothorax). The lung on that side of the chest is compressed, which interferes with its normal function.

The seriousness of the problem depends on the amount and rate of thoracic bleeding. Needle aspiration (thoracentesis) or chest tube drainage of the blood or air allows decompression of the pleural cavity so that the lung is able to reexpand and again perform its function in respiration. Operative intervention is carried out if bleeding continues at a rate greater than 300 ml/hour for 3 to 4 hours, if the rate of bleeding increases, or if it is not possible to evacuate the blood within the pleural space.

Chest Tube Drainage. A large-diameter intercostal tube (catheter) is usually inserted in the 2nd intercostal space or in the 5th space in the axilla. This usually brings about prompt and effective decompression of the pleural cavity (drainage of blood/air).

Tension Pneumothorax

In some patients, air may be drawn into the pleural space from the lacerated lung or through a small hole in the chest wall. In either case, the air that enters the chest cavity with each inspiration is trapped there: it cannot be expelled through the air passage or small hole in the chest wall.

A tension (pressure) thus is built up within the pleural space, which produces a collapse of the lung and may even push the heart and the great vessels toward the unaffected side of the chest. This not only interferes with respiration, but also disrupts circulatory function, because with increased intrathoracic pressure, venous return to the heart is compromised, causing decreased cardiac output and impairment of peripheral circulation. Diminished cardiac output leads to cardiac arrest. The clinical picture is one of air hunger, agitation, hypotension, and cyanosis.

- *Relief of tension pneumothorax must be looked on as an emergency measure.*

Immediate thoracentesis is done to relieve the positive pressure or "tension" within the chest. If the lung expands and there is no continuing leakage from the lung, further drainage may be unnecessary. If the lung is still leaking, as evidenced by the reaccumulation of an inexhaustible volume of air during the thoracentesis, then constant egress of this air must be provided by a large-bore chest tube with underwater-seal drainage (tube thoracostomy).

In an emergency situation a tension pneumothorax can be quickly converted to a simple pneumothorax by insertion of a large-bore needle into the pleural space, which relieves the pressure and vents the intrathoracic air to the outside. Then a chest tube can be inserted and connected to suction in order to remove the remaining air and fluid and reexpand the lung.

Sucking Wounds of the Chest (Open Pneumothorax)

Open pneumothorax implies an opening in the chest wall large enough to allow air to pass freely in and out of the thoracic cavity with each attempted respiration. Since the rush of air through the hole in the chest wall produces a sucking sound, such injuries are termed "sucking wounds" of the chest. In such patients not only is the lung collapsed, but the structures of the mediastinum (heart and great vessels) are pushed toward the uninjured side with each inspiration and in the opposite direction with expiration. This is termed *mediastinal flutter,* and it produces serious circulatory embarrassment.

- *To stop the flow of air through the opening in the chest wall is a lifesaving measure.*

In such an emergency, anything may be used that is large enough to fill the hole—a towel, a handkerchief, or the heel of the hand, If the patient is conscious, tell him to inhale and strain against a closed glottis. This action assists in the reexpansion of the lung and the ejection of the air from the thorax. In the hospital, the opening is plugged by sealing it with gauze impregnated with petrolatum jelly. A pressure dressing is applied by circumferential strapping. Usually, a chest tube connected to water-seal drainage is inserted to permit egress of air and fluid.

Penetrating Wounds of the Chest

Stab wounds are a common cause of penetrating wounds of the chest, most of which are caused by knives and switch blades, and are frequently associated with alcohol or substance abuse. The appearance of the external wound may be very deceptive, since pneumothorax, hemothorax, and cardiac tamponade along with severe and continuing hemorrhage can occur from any small wound, even one caused by an icepick.

The objective of immediate management is to restore and maintain cardiopulmonary function. After an adequate airway is ensured and ventilation is corrected, the patient is examined for shock and intrathoracic and intra-abdominal injuries. The patient is undressed completely so that additional injuries will not be missed. There is a high risk for associated intra-abdominal injuries with stab wounds below the level of the 5th anterior interspace. Death can result from exsanguinating hemorrhage or intra-abdominal sepsis.

After the status of the peripheral pulses is assessed, an intravenous line is secured. Blood is withdrawn for chemistries, typing, and crossmatching. Simultaneously, a central venous pressure line is established. An indwelling catheter is inserted to monitor urinary volume and to collect a urine sample for laboratory study.

Shock is treated simultaneously with colloid solutions, crystalloids, blood, or vasopressors as indicated by the condition of the patient. Chest x-rays are taken and other diagnostic procedures are carried out (esophagogram, flat plate of the abdomen, arteriogram) as dictated by the needs of the patient.

A chest tube is inserted in the pleural space in most patients with penetrating wounds of the chest in order to achieve rapid and continuing reexpansion of the lungs. Frequently, this will cause a complete evacuation of hemothorax and will decrease the incidence of clotted hemothorax. The chest tube allows early recognition of continuing intrathoracic bleeding, which will make surgical exploration necessary.

If the patient has a penetrating wound of the heart and great vessels and the esophagus and tracheobronchial tree, surgical intervention is required. Associated intra-abdominal wounds also necessitate abdominal exploration.

Pulmonary Contusion

Pulmonary contusion is damage to the lung parenchyma that results in leakage of blood and fluid. It may occur any time when there is rapid compression and decompression of the chest wall (*e.g.,* a steering wheel injury or the blast effect from gunshot wounds).

Pathophysiology. The primary pathologic defect is the abnormal accumulation of fluid in the interstitial and intra-alveolar spaces. It is thought that injury to the lung parenchyma and its capillary network results in a serum protein and plasma leak. The extravascular serum protein exerts an osmotic pressure that enhances loss of fluid from the capillaries. Blood, edema, and cellular debris (from cellular response to injury) enter the lung and accumulate in the bronchioles and alveolar surface, where they interfere with the efficiency of gas exchange. There is an increase in pulmonary vascular resistance and pulmonary artery pressure. The patient experiences systemic hypoxia and carbon dioxide retention. Occasionally, a contused lung occurs on the other side of the point of body impact. This is called a contrecoup contusion.

Clinical Manifestations. Pulmonary contusion may be mild, moderate, or severe. The efficiency of gas exchange is determined by arterial blood gas measurements. The chest x-rays will reveal pulmonary infiltration. The patient experiences tachypnea, tachycardia, crackles on auscultation, pleuritic chest pain, and copious secretions that are sometimes bloody or blood-tinged.

Management. In mild cases of pulmonary contusion, ultrasonic mist nebulization is used to keep the secretions fluid. Postural drainage, physiotherapy, and sterile endotracheal suctioning are used to remove the secretions. Pain is managed by intercostal nerve blocks or by narcotics. Usually, antimicrobial therapy is given, for a damaged lung is susceptible to infection. Oxygen by mask or cannula is usually given for 24 to 36 hours. Fluids are restricted because the injury is thought to be due to an abnormal collection of fluid in the interstices of the lung.

If moderate lung contusion is encountered, in addition to the above symptoms, the patient will have a large amount of mucus, serum, and frank blood in the tracheobronchial tree. He coughs constantly but is unable to clear his secretions. This patient usually requires intubation with a cuffed endotracheal tube and is placed on a ventilator with low-concentration oxygen and positive end-expiratory pressure (PEEP) to maintain the pressure and keep the lungs inflated. Diuretics may be given to reduce edema. A nasogastric tube is passed to relieve gastrointestinal distention. Metabolic acidosis is corrected with intravenous sodium bicarbonate. Frequent cultures are made of tracheobronchial secretions.

A patient with severe pulmonary contusion presents with rapid respirations, tachycardia, cyanosis, agitation, combativeness, and continuous and productive coughing of mucoid, frothy, and bloody secretions. This patient is treated vigorously with endotracheal intubation and ventilatory support, plasma or albumin (to maintain normal oncotic pressure to prevent leakage out of pulmonary capillaries), diuretics, fluid restriction, and perhaps the prophylactic administration of antimicrobials. Whole blood or fresh, frozen plasma may be used to treat hypovolemia. (See also the treatment of adult respiratory distress syndrome in Chap. 25.)

The complications of pulmonary contusion are infections, especially pneumonia in the contused segment, since the extravasation of fluid and blood into the alveolar and interstitial spaces is an excellent culture medium.

Cardiac Tamponade

Cardiac tamponade is the compression of the heart as a result of fluid within the pericardial sac. This is usually caused by blunt or penetrating trauma to the chest. (A penetrating wound of the heart is associated with a high mortality rate.) Cardiac tamponade may also follow diagnostic cardiac catheterization, angiographic procedures, and pace-

maker insertion, which can produce perforations of the heart and great vessels. Pericardial effusion may also develop from metastases to the pericardium from malignant tumors of the breast and lung as well as from lymphomas and leukemias, uremia, and high-dose radiation to the chest.

Pathophysiology. If the fluid formation is slow, the pericardium will distend without producing noticeable clinical symptoms until enough fluid develops to raise the intrapericardial pressure. A rapidly developing effusion interferes with ventricular filling and causes impairment of circulation. Thus, there is a reduced cardiac output and poor venous return to the heart. Circulatory collapse can result.

The symptoms depend on the speed of fluid accumulation. Important signs to watch for are a falling blood pressure, rising venous pressure (distended neck veins), and distant (muffled) heart sounds from impaired diastolic filling of the heart. Pulsus paradoxus (systolic blood pressure drops and fluctuates with respiration) may occur early in the development of cardiac tamponade. The patient may be anxious, confused, and restless, and may have dyspnea, tachypnea, and precordial pain. The central venous pressure is elevated. However, the venous pressure may be low or normal if a large amount of blood has been lost as a result of associated injuries.

Management. The treatment is thoracotomy for penetrating cardiac injuries where cardiorrhaphy (suturing the heart muscle) is done to stop hemorrhage, relieve tamponade, and repair associated lacerations and lesions. (See the care of the patient undergoing heart surgery (Chap. 30) and the patient undergoing chest surgery (Chap. 24.) Pericardiocentesis (needle aspiration of fluid from the periocardium (Chap. 31) may be performed to "buy time" before the patient is taken to surgery. This decompression of the pericardial sac permits effective heart action to be resumed.

Subcutaneous Emphysema

When the lung or the air passages are injured, air may enter the tissue planes and pass for some distance under the skin (*e.g.*, neck, chest). The tissues give a crackling sensation when palpated, and the subcutaneous air produces an alarming appearance as face, neck, body, and scrotum become misshapen by subcutaneous air. Fortunately, subcutaneous emphysema is of itself not a serious complication. The subcutaneous air is spontaneously absorbed, if the underlying air leak is treated or stops spontaneously. Giving the patient inhalations of high concentrations of oxygen will promote the reabsorption of subcutaneous air by washing nitrogen from the blood and improving its diffusion from the subcutaneous tissues back into the circulation. In severe cases, when there is widespread subcutaneous emphysema, a tracheostomy is indicated to insure patency of the airway.

▷ Bibliography
Books

Bloom AL and Thomas DP (eds). Haemostasis and Thrombosis. New York, Churchill Livingstone, 1981.
Borrie J. Management of Thoracic Emergencies, 3rd ed. New York, Appleton–Century–Crofts, 1980.

Carter SK, Glatstein E, and Livingstone RB. Principles of Cancer Treatment. New York, McGraw–Hill, 1982.

Daughtry DC (ed). Thoracic Trauma. Boston, Little, Brown & Co, 1980.

Davies GM. Office Diagnosis and Management of Chronic Obstructive Pulmonary Disease. Philadelphia, Lea & Febiger, 1981.

DeVita VT Jr, Hellman S, and Rosenberg SAA. Cancer: Principles and Practice of Oncology. Philadelphia, JB Lippincott, 1982.

Emanuelsen KL and Densmore MJ. Acute Respiratory Care. Bethany, Fleschner, 1981.

Fishman AP. Update: Pulmonary Diseases and Disorders. New York, McGraw–Hill, 1982.

Guenter CA and Welch MH (eds). Pulmonary Medicine, 2nd ed. Philadelphia, JB Lippincott, 1982.

Hansen HH and Rorth M. Lung Cancer 1980. Princeton, Excerpta Medica, 1980.

Hinshaw HC and Murray JF. Diseases of the Chest, 4th ed. Philadelphia, WB Saunders, 1980.

James DG and Studdy PR. Color Atlas of Respiratory Diseases. Chicago, Year Book Medical Publishers, 1982.

Kiss GT. Diagnosis and Management of Pulmonary Disease in Primary Practice. Menlo Park, Addison–Wesley, 1982.

Lehnert BE and Schachter EN. The Pharmacology of Respiratory Care. St Louis, CV Mosby, 1980.

Livingstone RB (ed). Lung Cancer, Vol 1. Boston, Martinus Nijhoff, 1981.

Miller WC. Chronic Obstructive Pulmonary Disease. Garden City, New York, Medical Examination, 1980.

Mitchell RS and Petty TL (eds). Synopsis of Clinical Pulmonary Disease, 3rd ed. St Louis, CV Mosby, 1982.

Moser KL et al. Better Living and Breathing: A Manual for Patients, 2nd ed. St Louis, CV Mosby, 1980.

Moser KM and Sprag RG. Respiratory Emergencies, 2nd ed. St Louis, CV Mosby, 1982.

Scadding JG and Cumming G (eds). Scientific Foundations of Respiratory Medicine. London, William Heinemann Medical Books, 1981.

Sexton DL. Chronic Obstructive Pulmonary Disease. St Louis, CV Mosby, 1981.

Sharnoff JG. Prevention of Venous Thrombosis and Pulmonary Embolism. Lancaster, MTP Press, 1980.

Traver GA (ed). Respiratory Nursing: The Science and the Art. New York, John Wiley & Sons, 1982.

Trinkle JK and Grover FL. The Management of Thoracic Trauma Victims. Philadelphia, JB Lippincott, 1980.

Articles
Pulmonary Embolism

Dossey B and Passons JM. Pulmonary embolism: Preventing it, treating it. Nursing '81 1981 Mar; 11(3):26–33.

Elliott J. Greater use of fibrinolytic agents urged. JAMA 1980 June 13; 243(22):2275–2276.

Fowler AA and Heyers TM. Thrombolytic therapy for pulmonary embolism and deep venous thrombosis. Postgrad Med 1982 Apr; 71(4):149–158.

Giudice JC, Komansky HJ, and Kaufman J. Pulmonary thromboembolism. New trends in prophylaxis and therapy. Postgrad Med 1980 May; 67(5):81–89.

Glassford DM et al. Pulmonary embolectomy. Ann Thorac Surg 1981 July; 32(1):28–32.

Hockberger RS and Rothstein RJ. Pulmonary embolism. Topics in Emergency Medicine 1980 Apr; 2(1):49–65.

Kim LK et al. Evaluation of a warfarin dosing protocol in treating pulmonary embolism. Am J Hosp Pharm 1981 Oct; 38(1):1520–1521.

Kushner C. A new procedure . . . A sudden complication . . . what's your diagnosis? RN 1981 May; 44(5):53–61, 123.

Lepore AA and Bottino CG. Transvenous filter for pulmonary embolism. NY State J Med 1981 Oct; 81(11):1645–1651.

Menzoian JO et al. Technical modifications in the placement of inferior vena caval filter devices. Am J Surg 1981 Aug; 142(2):216–218.

NIH Concensus Development Conference Summary. Thrombolytic therapy in thrombosis. 1980 Summer; 3(1):entire volume.

Sharma GVRK et al. Effect of thrombolytic therapy on pulmonary-capillary blood volume in patients with pulmonary embolism. N Engl J Med 1980 Oct 9; 303(15):842–845.

Sherry S. Thrombolytic therapy in surgical patients. Curr Surg 1981 Mar–Apr; 38(2):75–79.

Stambaugh RL and Alexander MR. Therapeutic use of thrombolytic agents. Am J Hosp Pharm 1981 June; 38(6):817–824.

Thrombolytic therapy for pulmonary emboli. Drug Ther Bull 1980 June 6; 18(12):45–47.

Wolfe WG and Sabiston DC Jr. Pulmonary embolism. Major Probl Clin Surg 1980; 25:entire volume.

Pulmonary Infections

Ahluwalia MP and Macdonnell KF. Pleural effusions. Compr Ther 1981 June; 7(6):6–13.

Alexander JC and Wolfe WG. Lung abscess and empyema of the thorax. Surg Clin North Am 1980 Aug; 60(4):835–849.

Aronson MD et al. *Legionella micdadei* (Pittsburgh pneumonia agent) infection in nonimmunosuppressed patients with pneumonia. Ann Intern Med 1981 Apr; 94(4, Pt 1):485–486.

Cohen DJ. Lung abscess. Postgrad Med 1982 July; 72(1):215–216.

Delarue NC et al. Lung abscess: Surgical implications. Can J Surg 1980 May; 23(3):297–302.

Estera AS et al. Primary lung abscess. J Thorac Cardiovasc Surg 1980 Feb; 79(2):275–282.

File TM, Tan JS, and Murphy DP. Atypical pneumonia syndrome. Primary Care 1981 Dec; 8(4):673–694.

Frame PT. Acute infectious pneumonia in the adult. Basics of RD. 1982 Jan; 10(3):1–8.

Fraser DW and Broome CV. Pneumococcal vaccine: To use or not. JAMA 1981 Feb 6; 245(5):498–499.

Gerding DN. Etiologic diagnosis of acute pneumonia in adults: A growing challenge. Postgrad Med 1981 Apr; 69(4):136–150.

Harber P and Terry PB. Fatal lung abscesses: Review of 11 years' experience. South Med J 1981 Mar; 74(3):281–283.

Hill CD and Stamm WE. Pneumonia in the elderly: The fatal complication. Geriatrics 1982 Jan; 37(1):40–50.

Mavroudis C et al. Improved survival in management of empyema thoracis. J Thorac Cardiovasc Surg 1981 July; 82(1):49–57.

McHenry MC. The infectious pneumonias. Hosp Pract 1980 Dec; 15(12):41–52.

Mufson MA. Pneumococcal infections. JAMA 1981 Oct 23/30; 246(17):1942–1948.

Palmer DL, Davidson M, and Lusk R. Needle aspiration of the lung in complex pneumonias. Chest 1980 July; 78(1):16–21.

Preheim LC and Sanders WE. Nosocomial pneumonia. Compr Ther 1981 June; 7(6):20–27.

Reynolds HY (ed). Pulmonary infections. Clin Chest Med 1981 Jan; 2(1):entire volume.

Ryan JL. Diagnosis and therapy of community-acquired pneumonias. Med Times 1982 Mar; 110(3):28–31.

Wing EJ, Schafer FJ, and Pasculle AW. Successful treatment of *Legionella micdadei* (Pittsburgh pneumonia agent) pneumonia with erythromycin. Am J Med 1981 Nov; 71(5):836–840.

Winn WC and Myerowitz RL. The pathology of the Legionella pneumonias. Hum Pathol 1981 May; 12(5):401–422.

Winston DJ. *Pneumocystis carinii* pneumonia. Compr Ther 1981 June; 7(6):41–48.

Chronic Obstructive Pulmonary Disease

Braun SR, Fregosi R, and Reddan WG. Exercise training in patients with COPD. Postgrad Med 1982 Apr; 71(4):163–173.

Burki N. Chronic airway obstruction. J Fam Pract 1980 Aug; 11(2):301–305.

Clark SW and Pavia D. Lung mucociliary clearance and the deposition of therapeutic aerosols. Chest 1981 Dec; 80(6, Suppl):entire volume.

Cockroft AE, Saunders MJ, and Berry G. Randomized controlled trial of rehabilitation in chronic respiratory disability. Thorax 1981 Mar; 36(3):200–203.

Craig RJ (ed). Symposium on respiratory care. Nurs Clin North Am 1981 June; 16(2):193–297.

Editorial: The proper use of aerosol bronchodilators. Lancet 1981 Jan 3; 1(8210):23–24.

Hunter AMB, Carey MA, and Larsh HW. The nutritional status of patients with chronic obstructive pulmonary disease. Am Rev Respir Dis 1981 Oct; 124(4):376–381.

Johnston RF and Mondschein FJ. Chronic bronchitis and pulmonary emphysema. Compr Ther 1981 June; 7(6):61–70.

Mangold LA. Emotional support in a pulmonary rehabilitation program. Respir Ther 1981 Jan–Feb; 11(1):55–57.

Mathur PN et al. Effect of digoxin on right ventricular function in severe chronic airflow obstruction. Ann Intern Med 1981 Sept; 95(3):283–288.

Matthay RA (ed). Symposium on chronic obstructive lung diseases. Med Clin North Am 1981 May; 65(3):453–709.

McFadden ER Jr. Aerosolized bronchodilators and steroids in the treatment of airway obstruction in adults. Am Rev Respir Dis 1980 Nov; 122(5, Pt 2):89–96.

McIsaac J. Establishing rapport with the emphysema patient: Prelude to effective teaching. Nurs Admin Q 1980 Winter; 4(2):20–24.

Miller WF. Chronic obstructive pulmonary disease. Hosp Pract 1981 Feb; 16(2):89–106.

Perry JO. Effectiveness of teaching in the rehabilitation of patients with chronic bronchitis and emphysema. Nurs Res 1981 July–Aug; 30(4):219–222.

Petty TL. Home oxygen therapy for COPD. Postgrad Med 1981 Apr; 69(4):102–113.

Snider GL. The pathogenesis of emphysema—twenty years of progress. Am Rev Respir Dis 1981 Sept; 124(3):321–324.

Windsor RA et al. Health promotion and maintenance for patients with chronic obstructive pulmonary disease: A review. J Chronic Dis 1980; 33(1):5–12.

Lung Cancer

Boysen PG et al. Prospective evaluation for pneumonectomy using perfusion scanning: Follow-up beyond one year. Chest 1981 Aug; 80(2):163–166.

Carr DT. Malignant lung disease. Hosp Pract 1981 Jan; 16(1):97–101.

Chaffin P and Reininger S. Bronchogenic carcinoma. A review and study. Nurs Pract 1981 Jan–Feb; 6(1):10–17.

Chaffin P and Reininger S. Bronchogenic carinoma. A review and study. Part 2. Nurs Pract 1981 Mar–Apr; 6(2):14–17, 27.

Clee MD and Sinclair DJM. Assessment of factors influencing the result of sputum cytology in bronchial carcinoma. Thorax 1981 Feb; 36(2):143–146.

Cromartie RS et al. Carcinoma of the lung: A clinical review. Ann Thorac Surg 1980 July; 30(1):30–35.

Eisert DR and Hazra TA. Role of radiation therapy in carcinoma of the lung. JAMA 1982 Jan 15; 247(3):338–340.

Holmes EC. Immune adjuvant therapy in lung cancer. Prog Exp Tumor Res 1980; 25:229–241.

Holmes EC. Surgical adjuvant therapy for lung cancer. Surg Clin North Am 1981 Dec; 61(6):1289–1294.

Livingstone RB. Small cell lung carcinoma—recent advances and current challenges. Recent Results Cancer Res 1981; 76:267–275.

Oldham RK and Greco FA. Small-cell lung cancer. A curable disease. Cancer Chemother Pharmacol 1980 Aug; 4(3):173–177.

Rea HH, Shevland JE, and House AJS. Accuracy of computed tomographic scanning in assessment of the mediastinum in bronchial carcinoma. J Thorac Cardiovasc Surg 1981 June; 81(6):825–829.

Silverman NA and Sabiston DC. Mediastinal masses. Surg Clin North Am 1980 Aug; 60(4):757–777.

Yarbro JW. Lung cancer: Multimodal approach. Front Radiat Ther Oncol 1980; 15:109–120.

Occupational Lung Diseases

Casey KR, Rom WN, and Moatamed F. Asbestos-related diseases. Clin Chest Med 1981 May; 2(2):179–202.

Cenci L. Smoking and the workplace. Bull NY Acad Med 1982 June; 58(5):471–479.

Harber P. Prevention and control of occupational lung disease. Clin Chest Med 1981 Sept; 2(3):343–355.

Summer W and Haponik E. Inhalation of irritant gases. Clin Chest Med 1981 May; 2(2):273–287.

Weiss W. Prevention and control of occupational lung disease. Clin Chest Med 1981 Sept; 2(3):343–355.

Trauma

Carpintero JL et al. Methods of management of flail chest. Intensive Care Medicine 1980 Aug; 6(4):217–221.

Jones KW. Thoracic trauma. Surg Clin North Am 1980 Aug; 60(4):957–981.

Majeski JA. Management of flail chest after blunt trauma. South Med J 1981 July; 74(7):848–849.

Rich W and Reichenberger M. Managing flail chest. Nursing '81 1981 Dec; 11(12):26–31.

Shackford SR, Virgilio RW, and Peters RM. Selective use of ventilator therapy in flail chest injury. J Thorac Cardiovasc Surg 1981 Feb; 81(2):194–201.

Sweetwood H. Cardiac tamponade. RN 1980 Oct; 43(10):35–41.

Worth MH Jr. Managing penetrating chest trauma. Hosp Med 1982 Apr; 18(4):53–68.

Agencies

Governmental

National Heart, Lung and Blood Institute, National Institutes of Health, Bethesda, Maryland 20205

Voluntary

American Association for Respiratory Therapy, 7411 Hines Place, Suite 101, Dallas, Texas 75235

American Lung Association, 1740 Broadway, New York, New York 10019

American Thoracic Society, 1740 Broadway, New York, New York 10019

Unit VIII

Cardiovascular, Circulatory and Hematologic Problems

27

Assessment of Cardiovascular Function

Nursing care is based on data obtained on assessment. A nursing assessment of a patient with heart disease includes taking a history, performing a physical examination, and interpreting basic tests of cardiac functioning. Sound knowledge of cardiac anatomy, physiology, and pathophysiology is necessary for developing assessment skills, planning nursing care, and understanding the purposes of diagnostic tests.

▷ Physiologic Overview

The heart is a hollow, muscular organ located in the center of the thorax where it occupies the space between the lungs and rests upon the diaphragm. It weighs approximately 300 g (10.6 oz), although heart weight and size are influenced by age, sex, body weight, frequency of physical exercise, and heart disease. The function of the heart is to pump blood to the tissues, supplying them with oxygen and other nutrients, and at the same time, removing carbon dioxide and other waste products of metabolism. Actually, there are two pumps within this organ, located on the right and left sides of the heart. The output of the right heart is distributed entirely to the lungs via the pulmonary artery, whereas the output of the left heart is distributed to the remainder of the body via the aorta. These two pumps eject blood simultaneously at approximately the same rate of output.

The pumping action of the heart is accomplished by the rhythmical contraction and relaxation of its muscular wall. During contraction of the muscle (*systole*), the chambers inside the heart become smaller as the blood is ejected. During relaxation of the muscles of the heart wall (*diastole*), the heart chambers fill with blood in preparation for the subsequent ejection. A normal adult heart beats approximately 60 to 80 times per minute, ejects approximately 70 ml from each side per beat, and has a total output of approximately 5 liters/minute.

Cardiac Anatomy

The space in the middle of the chest between the two lungs is called the *mediastinum*. The bulk of the mediastinal space is occupied by the heart, which is encased in a thin, fibrous sac called the *pericardium*. The pericardium is not essential for the proper functioning of the heart, but serves as an envelope to protect its surface. The space between the surface of the heart and the pericardial lining is filled with a very small amount of fluid, which lubricates the surface and tends to reduce friction during cardiac muscle contraction.

Heart Chambers.   The right and left sides of the heart are each composed of two chambers, an *atrium* (pl. atria) and a *ventricle*. The common wall between the right and left chambers is called the *septum*. The ventricles are the chambers that eject blood into the arteries. The functions of the atria are to receive incoming blood from the veins and to act as temporary storage reservoirs for subsequent emptying into the ventricles. The relationship of the four chambers of the heart is shown in Figure 27-1.

The atria and ventricles are easily distinguished by the greater thickness of the muscle that forms the ventricular wall. The left ventricle ejects blood against high systemic pressure, whereas the right ventricle ejects blood against the low-resistance pulmonary vasculature. Therefore, because of the increased work of the left heart, the left ventricular wall is about 2½ times as thick (approximately 1 cm) as the right ventricular wall.

Because of the rotation of the heart within the chest cavity, the right ventricle lies anteriorly (just beneath the sternum), and the left ventricle is situated posteriorly. The left ventricle is responsible for the apex beat or the *point of maximum impulse (PMI)* that is usually apparent on the left side of the chest wall.

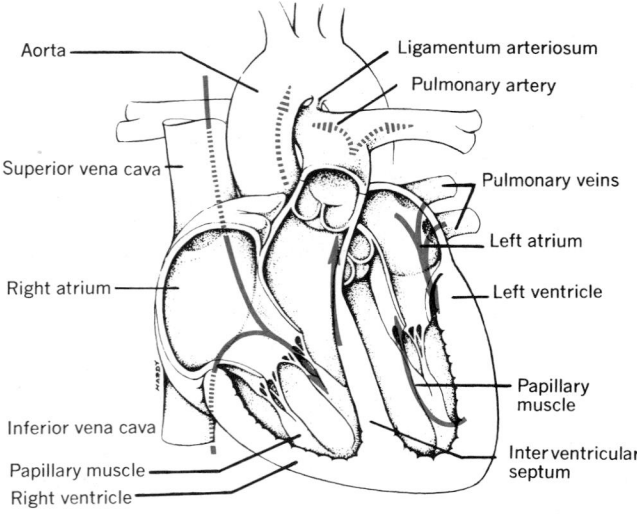

Figure 27-1.   Interior of the heart. Arrows indicate the direction of blood flow. (From Chaffee EE and Greisheimer EM: Basic Physiology and Anatomy. Philadelphia, JB Lippincott.)

Heart Valves.   Heart valves permit blood to flow in only one direction through the heart. Valves, which are composed of thin leaflets of fibrous tissue, open and close passively in response to pressure changes and blood movement. There are two types of valves: *atrioventricular* and *semilunar*.

Atrioventricular Valves.   Valves separating the atria from the ventricles are termed atrioventricular valves. The *tricuspid valve,* so named because it is composed of three leaflets, separates the right atrium from the right ventricle. The *mitral* or *bicuspid valve* (two cusps) lies between the left atrium and left ventricle.

Semilunar Valves.   Semilunar valves are situated between each ventricle and its corresponding artery. The valve between the right ventricle and the pulmonary artery is called the *pulmonic valve;* the valve between the left ventricle and the aorta is called the *aortic valve.* Both of the semilunar valves are normally composed of three cusps. There are no valves between the large veins and the atria.

Papillary Muscles and Chordae Tendineae.   Normally, when the ventricles contract, ventricular pressure tends to push the atrioventricular valve leaflets upward into the atrial cavity. If enough pressure was exerted on the valves, blood would be ejected backward from the ventricles to the atria. *Papillary muscles* and *chordae tendineae* are responsible for maintaining unidirectional blood flow through the atrioventricular valves (from the ventricle to the respective artery). Papillary muscles are muscle bundles that are located on the sides of the ventricular walls. Chordae tendineae are fibrous bands extending from the papillary muscles to the edges of the valve leaflets, acting to tether the free edges of the valves to the ventricular wall. Contraction of the papillary muscles causes the chordae tendineae to become taut. This keeps the valve leaflets closed during systole, preventing backflow of blood. Papillary muscles and chordae tendineae are not necessary for proper functioning of the semilunar valves.

Coronary Arteries.   The heart muscle is metabolically active in that its requirements for oxygen and nutrients are large and continuous. These required substances are supplied to the heart muscle by blood flowing in the coronary arteries (Fig. 27-2). As a manifestation of its large metabolic requirements, the heart uses approximately one half of the oxygen delivered through the coronary arteries in contrast to other organs, which (on the average) use only one quarter of the oxygen delivered to them. The coronary arteries arise from the aorta near its origin at the left ventricle. The wall of the left side of the heart is supplied in large part through the left main coronary artery, which divides into several large branches that run down (left anterior descending coronary artery) and across the left side of the myocardium (circumflex artery). The right heart wall is supplied similarly from a separate *right coronary artery.* Unlike other arteries, the coronary arteries are perfused during diastole.

Cardiac Muscle.   The specialized muscle tissue composing the wall of the heart is called *cardiac muscle.* Microscopically, cardiac muscle resembles striated (skeletal) muscle, which is under conscious control. However, heart muscle is not under conscious control and in that sense resembles smooth (involuntary) muscle. The cardiac muscle fibers are arranged in an interconnected manner (called a syncytium) so that they can contract and relax in coordination. The sequential pattern of contraction and relaxation of individual muscle fibers ensures the rhythmic behavior of the heart muscle as a whole and enables it to function as a pump. The heart muscle itself is called the *myocardium.* The segment of cells on the inner surface of this muscle, which is in contact with the blood, is called the *endocardium,* and the portion of cells on the outer surface of the heart is called the *epicardium.*

Conduction System of the Heart

Specialized cells of the conduction system generate and conduct electrical impulses to myocardial cells, resulting in myocardial contraction. Cardiac muscle cells have an inherent rhythmicity, which is illustrated by the fact that a segment of myocardium removed from the rest of the heart will continue to contract rhythmically if maintained under the proper conditions. The heart rate is determined by the group of myocardial cells with the fastest intrinsic rate. These specialized cells, located at the junction of the superior vena cava and the right atrium, are known as the *sinoatrial (SA) node* and function as the pacemaker for the entire myocardium (Fig. 27-3). The SA node initiates approximately 60 to 100 impulses per minute in a resting normal heart but can change its rate in response to the needs of the body. The electrical signal initiated by the SA node is conducted along the myocardial cells of the atrium to the *atrioventricular (AV) junction.* The AV junction (located in the right atrial wall near the tricuspid valve) is another group of specialized muscle cells similar to the SA node,

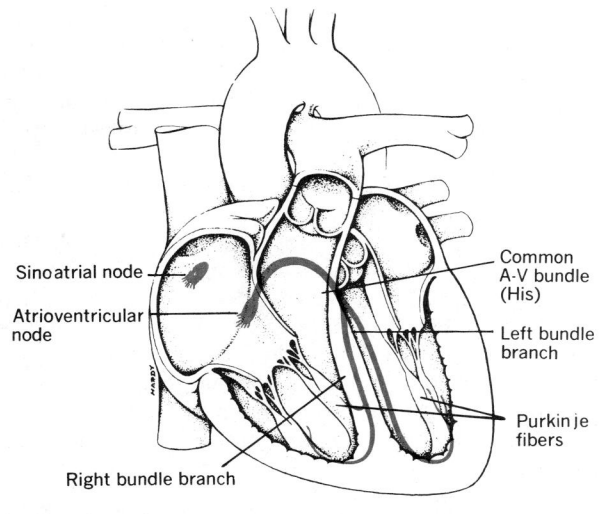

Figure 27-3. Conducting system. Diagram shows relationships of the sinoatrial node, the atrioventricular node, the common atrioventricular bundle and its branches. (From Chaffee EE and Greisheimer EM: Basic Physiology and Anatomy. Philadelphia, JB Lippincott.)

but with an intrinsic rate of about 40 to 60 impulses per minute. The AV junction coordinates the incoming electrical impulses from the atria and relays an electrical impulse to the ventricles. This electrical impulse is conducted away from the AV junction through a bundle of specialized muscle fibers (the *bundle of His*) that travel in the septum separating the left and right ventricles. The His bundle divides into right and left bundle branches near the apex of the heart. The fibers in the right and left bundle branches are called Purkinje fibers. The right bundle fans out into the right ventricular muscle. The left bundle divides again into the left anterior and left posterior bundle branches, which fan out into the left ventricular muscle. Further spread of depolarization through the rest of the myocardium takes place by conduction through the muscle fibers themselves.

If the SA node malfunctions, the AV node generally takes over the pacemaker function of the heart. Should both the SA and AV nodes fail in their pacemaker function, the myocardium will continue to beat at a rate of less than 40 beats per minute, which is the intrinsic pacemaker rate of the electrical impulse of the ventricular myocardial cells.

Cardiac Physiology

Electromechanical Coupling

In the normal cardiac muscle cell, an electrical difference (voltage) exists between the inside and the outside of the cell across its membrane. The inside of the cell is negative relative to the outside of the cell. When the magnitude of this difference is reduced (the inside of the cell becomes less negative), *depolarization* has occurred and contraction of muscle cell results. A cardiac muscle cell is normally depolarized when a neighboring cell is depolarized (although it can also be depolarized by external electrical stim-

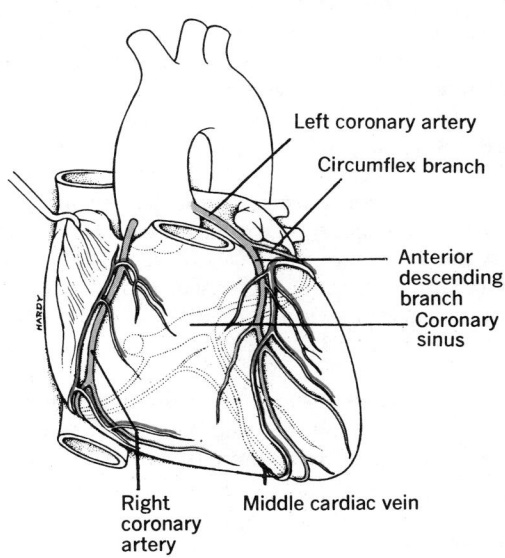

Figure 27-2. Diagram of the coronary arteries arising from the aorta and encircling the heart. The coronary sinus and some of the coronary veins also are shown. (From Chaffee EE and Greisheimer EM: Basic Physiology and Anatomy. Philadelphia, JB Lippincott.)

ulation). Sufficient depolarization of a single specialized conduction system cell will therefore result in depolarization and contraction of the entire myocardium. *Repolarization* occurs as the cell returns to its baseline state (becomes more negative), and corresponds to relaxation of myocardial muscle.

During depolarization the permeability of the cell membranes to certain ions (sodium, chloride, calcium, potassium) changes. One of those changes results in an increased permeability to calcium, allowing for uptake of calcium into the cell. This increase in intracellular calcium concentration leads to shortening of the muscle fibers and development of tension (contraction). After a short period, the membrane voltage returns to its original value, the calcium that had accumulated in its interior is removed, and the cell relaxes. This interaction between changes in membrane voltage and muscle contraction is called *electromechanical coupling*.

Cardiac muscle, unlike skeletal or smooth muscle, has a prolonged refractory period during which it cannot be restimulated to contract. This protects the heart from sustained contraction (tetany), which would result in sudden cardiac death.

Normal electromechanical coupling and contraction of the heart are dependent on the composition of the fluid (extracellular fluid) surrounding the heart muscle cells. The composition of this fluid is in turn influenced by the composition of the blood. A change in blood calcium concentration may therefore alter contraction of the heart muscle fibers. A change in blood potassium concentration is also important since potassium affects the normal electrical voltage of the cell.

Cardiac Hemodynamics

What determines the direction of blood flow from the heart through the circulation and then back to the heart? The important principle is that fluid will flow from a region of higher pressure to a region of lower pressure. The pressures that are responsible for blood flow in the normal circulation are generated by contraction of the ventricular muscle. During contraction, blood is forced from the ventricle into the aorta during the period of time when left ventricular pressure exceeds aortic pressure. When these two pressures become equal, the aortic valve closes and output from the left ventricle ceases. The blood that has entered the aorta increases the pressure in that vessel. This provides a pressure gradient to force blood progressively through the arteries and capillaries and into the veins. The blood returns to the right atrium because pressure in this chamber is lower than pressure in the veins. Similarly, a gradient of pressure is responsible for blood flow from the pulmonary artery through the lung and back to the left atrium. The pressure gradients within the pulmonary circulation are considerably less than those in the systemic circulation because the resistance to flow in the pulmonary vessels is less.

Let us consider the pressure changes that occur in the chambers of the heart during the cardiac cycle, beginning with diastole when the ventricles are relaxed (see Fig. 5-17). During diastole, the atrioventricular valves are open, and blood returning from the veins flows into the atrium and then into the ventricle. Toward the end of this diastolic period, the atrial muscle contracts in response to a signal initiated by the SA node. This contraction raises the pressure inside the atrium and forces an increment of blood into the ventricle. At this point, the ventricles themselves begin to contract in response to propagation of the electrical impulse that began in the SA node some milliseconds previously (systole). During systole, the pressure inside the ventricle rapidly rises, forcing the AV valves to close. The consequence of this action is that no further filling of the ventricle from the atrium can occur, and blood ejected from the ventricle cannot flow back to the atrium. The rapid rise of pressure inside the ventricles forces the pulmonic and aortic valves to open, and blood is ejected into the pulmonary artery and aorta, respectively. The exit of blood is at first rapid, and then, as the pressures in each ventricle and its corresponding artery approach equalization, the flow of blood gradually decreases. At the cessation of systole, the ventricular muscle relaxes and the pressure within the chamber rapidly decreases. This decrease in pressure creates a tendency for blood to come back from the artery into the ventricle, which forces the semilunar valves to close. Simultaneously, as the pressure within the ventricle drops to below atrial pressure, the AV valves open, the ventricles begin to fill, and the entire sequence is repeated. It is important to note that the mechanical events related to filling and ejection by the heart are closely coupled to the corresponding electrical events that cause cardiac contraction and relaxation.

The events just described lead to the repetitive rise and fall of pressures inside the ventricles. The maximum pressure reached is called *systolic pressure* and the minimum pressure is defined as *diastolic pressure*.

Generation of Normal Heart Sounds. The normal heart sounds are produced primarily by closure of the heart valves. The first heart sound, S_1, coincides with closure of the AV valves and is a normal sound. The major component of this sound is the vibration of the leaflets of the mitral and tricuspid valves as they close, although vibration of the myocardial wall may also contribute. It is heard loudest at the apex of the heart. The second heart sound, S_2, also normal, occurs upon closure of the aortic and pulmonic valves. Although these two valves close almost simultaneously, the pulmonic valve usually lags slightly behind. Therefore, under certain circumstances, the two components of the second sound (A_2 and P_2) may be heard separately (split S_2). The S_2 is heard loudest at the base of the heart.

The time between S_1 and S_2 corresponds to systole. This is normally shorter than the time between S_2 and S_1 (diastole). As the heart rate increases, diastole shortens (Fig. 27-4).

Cardiac Output

Cardiac output is the amount of blood pumped by either of the ventricles during a given period of time. The cardiac output of a typical adult is normally about 5 liters/minute but varies greatly, depending on the metabolic needs of the body. Cardiac output equals the stroke volume times the heart rate. *Stroke volume* is the amount of blood ejected

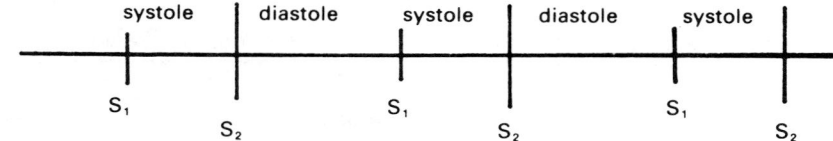

Figure 27-4. The normal heart sounds.

per heartbeat. Cardiac output can be affected, therefore, by changes either in stroke volume or heart rate. The resting heart rate of an average adult is approximately 72 beats/minute and the average stroke volume is about 70 ml/beat.

Control of Heart Rate. Since the function of the heart is to supply blood to all tissues of the body, its output must vary as the metabolic needs of the tissues themselves change. For example, during exercise, the total cardiac output may increase fourfold to 20 liters/minute. This increase is normally accomplished by approximately doubling both the heart rate and the stroke volume. Changes in heart rate are accomplished by reflex controls mediated by the autonomic nervous system, including its sympathetic and parasympathetic divisions. The parasympathetic nerves, which travel to the heart through the vagus nerve, can slow the cardiac rate, whereas sympathetic nerves increase it. These nerves exert their effect on heart rate through their action on the SA node to either decrease or increase its rate of intrinsic depolarization. The balance between these two reflex control systems normally determines the heart rate. The heart rate is also stimulated by an increased level of circulating catecholamines (secreted by the adrenal gland) as well as by the presence of excess thyroid hormone, which produces a catecholamine-like effect.

Control of Stroke Volume. Stroke volume is primarily determined by three factors: (1) intrinsic contractility of the cardiac muscle, (2) the degree of stretch of the cardiac muscle prior to its contraction, and (3) the pressure against which the heart muscle has to eject blood during contraction.

Intrinsic contractility is a term used to denote the force that can be generated by the contracting myocardium under any given condition. It is increased by circulating catecholamines, sympathetic neuronal activity, and certain drugs (such as digitalis). It is depressed by hypoxemia and acidosis. Increased contractility results in increased stroke volume.

The precontraction length of the ventricular muscle fibers is determined by the volume of blood within the ventricle at the end of diastole. This volume, the ventricular end-diastolic volume, is called *preload*. The larger the preload, the greater will be the stroke volume, until a point is reached when the muscle is so stretched it can no longer contract. The relationship between increased stroke volume and increased ventricular end-diastolic volume for a given intrinsic contractility is called Starling's Law of the Heart. This effect is due to a greater initial length, which leads to a greater degree of shortening of cardiac muscle. This results from increased interaction between thick and thin filaments of the sarcomeres (similar to that discussed more fully in the chapter on skeletal muscle physiology).

The pressure against which the left ventricle ejects blood is the pressure in the aorta; right ventricular ejection

works against the pressure in the pulmonary artery. The greater these pressures, the greater will be the tension in the ventricular wall during contraction. This tension is called *afterload*. Increased afterload leads to decreased stroke volume.

The heart can achieve a greatly increased stroke volume, as during exercise, by increasing preload (through increased venous return), by increasing contractility (through sympathetic nervous discharge), and by decreasing afterload (through peripheral vasodilatation with decreased aortic pressure).

The fraction of the end-diastolic volume that is ejected with each stroke is called the *ejection fraction*. With each stroke, 0.56 to 0.78 of the end-diastolic volume is ejected by the normal heart. The ejection fraction can be used as an index of myocardial contractility; it is decreased if contractility is depressed.

▷ Nursing History

Cardiac patients who are acutely ill require a different initial nursing history than do cardiac patients with stable or chronic problems. A patient experiencing an acute myocardial infarction requires immediate, and possibly lifesaving, medical and nursing interventions (for example, relief of chest discomfort and ischemia, or prevention of arrhythmias) rather than an extensive interview. For this patient, a few well-chosen questions regarding chest discomfort, associated symptoms (such as shortness of breath or palpitations), drug allergies, and smoking history should be asked at the same time one is assessing heart rate, rhythm, and blood pressure, and starting an intravenous line. When the patient is more stable, a more extensive history should be obtained.

When caring for an acutely ill cardiac patient, one first must focus on assessment of the heart and cardiac output. Patients with atherosclerotic coronary artery disease commonly experience chest discomfort (angina pectoris or myocardial infarction); shortness of breath, fatigue, and reduced urine output (left ventricular failure with decreased cardiac output); palpitations and dizziness (arrhythmias from ischemia, aneurysm, stress, or electrolyte imbalance); edema and weight gain (right ventricular failure); and postural hypotension with dizziness and lightheadedness (saline depletion from diuretic therapy). Patients with valvular disease may have symptoms of heart failure, arrhythmias, and chest discomfort.

Not all chest discomfort is related to myocardial ischemia. Guidelines are useful in differentiating chest discomfort of serious, life-threatening conditions from those conditions that are less serious or would be treated in a different manner. Table 27-1 summarizes characteristics of angina

Table 27-1

Characteristics of Angina Pectoris, Myocardial Infarction, and Pericarditis

	Location and Radiation	Character and Duration	Precipitating Events
Angina Pectoris	Substernal or retrosternal pain spreading across chest May radiate to *inside* of either arm or to both arms, neck, or jaws	*Pressure;* squeezing, heavy discomfort Usually subsides within 1–10 min	Usually related to exertion, emotion, eating, cold
Myocardial Infarction	Substernal or over precordium May spread widely throughout chest; painful disability of shoulders and hands may be present	Crushing, vise-like, gripping More severe and prolonged than angina May be associated with dizziness, perspiration, and nausea 15%–25% may be silent	Occurs spontaneously Unrelated to emotion, exercise
Pericarditis	Substernal or to left of sternum May be felt in epigastrium May be referred to neck, arms, back	Sharp, intermittent pain; made worse by swallowing, coughing, *rotation of trunk*	Often severe and sudden in onset; pain increases with inspiration and motion of trunk

pectoris, myocardial infarction, and pericarditis. Figure 27-5 illustrates the pain patterns in these conditions. However, there are four important points to remember when evaluating chest discomfort:

- There is little correlation between the severity of the chest discomfort and the gravity of its cause.
- There is poor correlation between the location of chest discomfort and its source.
- The patient may have more than one clinical problem occurring simultaneously.
- In a patient with a history of atherosclerotic coronary artery disease, assume the chest discomfort is secondary to ischemia until proven otherwise.

To facilitate the gathering of subjective information for a cardiovascular nursing history, the patient should be questioned as indicated below. However, it is important to phrase the questions according to the appropriateness of the situation and to pursue logically areas where further clarification is necessary.

1. Breathing
   - Are you ever short of breath?
   - When do you become short of breath?
   - How do you make your breathing better?
   - What makes it worse?
   - How long has breathing been a problem?
   - What activities are necessary for you to do that you are no longer able to do because of your breathing?
   - Are you on any medication to improve your breathing?
   - Does any medication you are taking affect your breathing?
   - What time of day do you prefer to take your medication?

2. Circulation (These symptoms could be examined using the same types of questions listed above.)
   - Chest discomfort*
   - Weight gain or loss
   - Swelling in the hands, feet, or legs (or sacrum if bedridden)
   - Dizziness
   - Fatigue
   - Lightheadedness
   - Palpitations
   - Manifestations of high blood pressure
   - Coldness of hands or feet in warm weather
3. Urination
   - Is the amount of your urine output normal for you?
   - Do you ever get up at night to use the bathroom?
   - How many times?
   - When did you notice the change?
   - Do you take a diuretic?
   - When do you take it?
4. Mentation
   - Do you think as fast as you used to? As clearly?
   - Do you laugh or cry more easily than before?
   - When did you notice the change?
   - Are you taking any medication that might affect your thinking?

When the patient's condition permits, other functional areas should also be assessed.

* Since patients do not always admit to having chest "pain," word equivalents of pain should be used when eliciting the quality of discomfort. Common descriptions used by patients include strangling, constriction, tightness, aching, squeezing, pressing, heaviness, expanding sensation, choking in throat, indigestion, and burning.

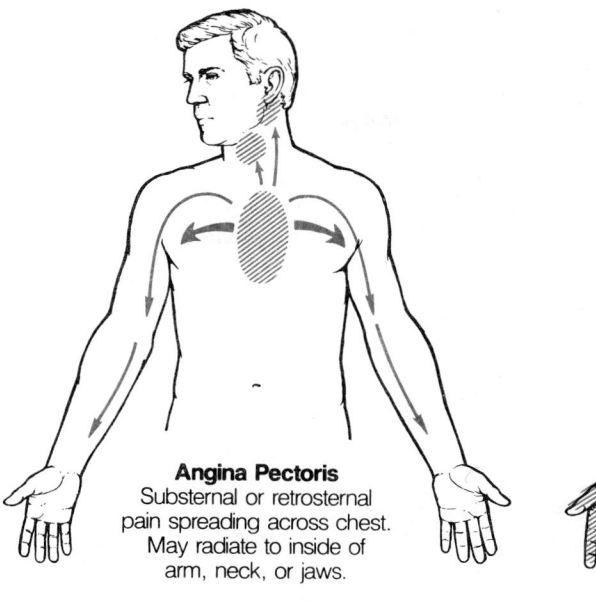

Angina Pectoris
Substernal or retrosternal
pain spreading across chest.
May radiate to inside of
arm, neck, or jaws.

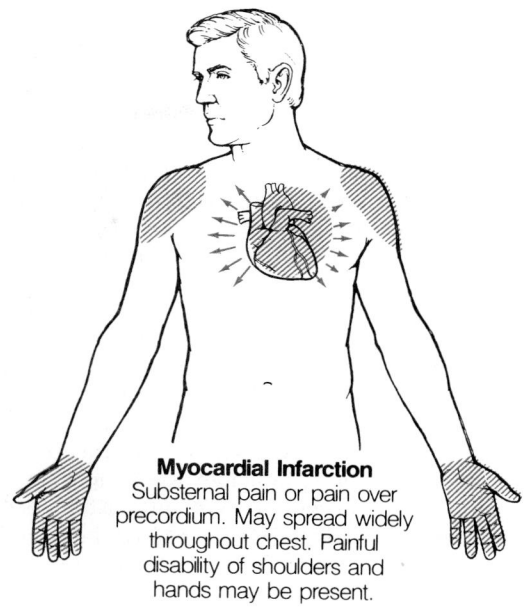

Myocardial Infarction
Substernal pain or pain over
precordium. May spread widely
throughout chest. Painful
disability of shoulders and
hands may be present.

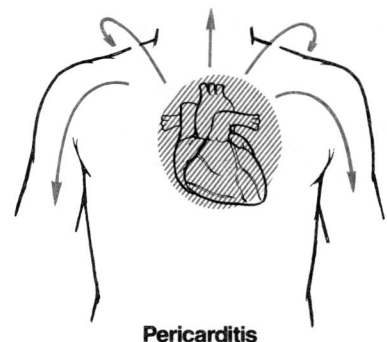

Pericarditis
Substernal pain or pain to the left of sternum. May
be felt in epigastrium and may be referred
to neck, arms, and back.

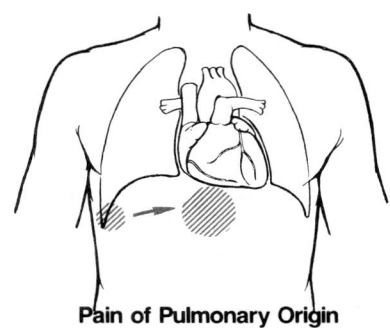

Pain of Pulmonary Origin
Pain arises from inferior portion of pleura.
May be referred to costal margins or upper abdomen.
Patient may be able to localize the pain.

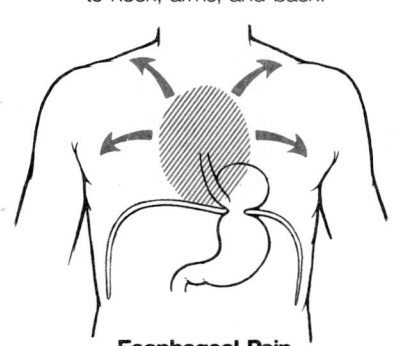

Esophageal Pain
(Hiatus Hernia, Reflux Esophagitis)
Substernal pain. May be projected
around chest to shoulders.

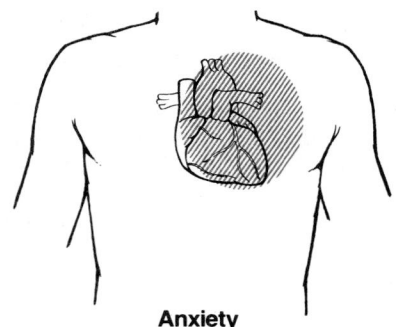

Anxiety
Pain over left chest. May be variable. Does not
radiate. Assess for hyperventilation, sighing
respiration, palpitations. Patient may complain
of numbness and tingling of hands and mouth.

Figure 27-5. Assessment of chest pain.

Information obtained by the nursing history is necessary to plan individualized care while the patient is hospitalized, to aid in discharge planning, and to provide appropriate teaching. Knowing how the patient perceives the effects of the disease process on activities of daily living will help identify specific aims for cardiac rehabilitation or strategies for modifying certain activities to be devised. Since dietary modification (reduction of sodium, saturated fat, or caloric intake) will probably be prescribed, assess the following: food preferences (including cultural or ethnic); eating habits (canned or commercially prepared foods versus fresh foods, and restaurant cooking versus home cooking); who shops for groceries; and who prepares the meals. Knowledge of the patient's financial status assists the nurse in advocating an affordable therapeutic regimen, for example, avoiding an expensive combination of drugs or expensive sustained-release medications when drugs that are as effective and less costly are available. Knowing if any risk factors for coronary artery disease exist will enable the nurse to help the patient modify behaviors that may be contributing to the progression of his heart disease. Refer to Chapter 4 for a more complete description of the nursing history.

▷ Risk Factors in Coronary Artery Disease

The presence of coronary artery disease is associated with one or more characteristic findings that are known as risk factors. Risk factors have been determined on the basis of systematic observations of relationships between certain characteristics and the subsequent development of coronary artery disease. Current research is finding physiologic explanations for these relationships.

Effective patient teaching requires a knowledge base for recognizing the risk factors, applying the criteria for evaluating their importance and interpretating the data from studies that identify risk factors. However, there is not complete agreement about the importance or the effectiveness of modifying risk factors in patients with known coronary artery disease.

Risk factors can be classified in a number of ways. For the purposes of both patient and professional education, the categories used here are unavoidable risk factors, atherogenic personal attributes (for some people, these are also unavoidable), life-style habits, and signs of preclinical cardiovascular disorders.

Unavoidable Risk Factors

Unavoidable risk factors include age, sex, family history of coronary artery disease, and ethnic background. Current research indicates, however, that unavoidable risk factors are often influenced by those that can be avoided, and thereby become modified to some degree.

Age and Sex.　Increasing age is associated with a higher incidence of coronary artery disease. In men, the incidence of coronary disease increases steadily; in women, the incidence increases sharply after menopause, but the incidence in women is still less than in men.

Family History.　A positive family history of coronary artery disease among blood-related family members is a good predictor of coronary artery disease development. Persons with a strong family history should be aware of other risk factors that they can modify that might limit progression of the atherosclerotic process.

Ethnic Background.　Ethnic background may contribute to some risk factor development. For example, high blood pressure is more prevalent in black men than in white men. However, ethnicity, in a broader sense, implies life-styles as well as ethnic origin. Although ethnic origin is not modifiable, the life-styles associated with particular cultures can be altered.

Atherogenic Personal Attributes

Atherogenic personal attributes include elevated serum lipids and lipoproteins, elevated blood pressure, and glucose intolerance. Each of these attributes can usually be modified to some degree.

Elevated Serum Lipids and Lipoproteins.　Elevated serum cholesterol greatly increases the risk of coronary artery disease. Serum cholesterol level is raised by diets high in cholesterol and saturated fats. High-cholesterol, high-saturated fat diets are believed generally to contribute to the atherosclerotic process. However, the degree of dietary contribution of cholesterol and saturated fats remains controversial, as cholesterologenesis is essentially unaffected by diet.

A "normal" serum cholesterol level has not been established, but "norms" for the American society have been and continue to be considerably higher than norms for other cultures, for example, the Japanese culture. The value of serum triglyceride as a predictor of coronary artery disease has been replaced by measurement of serum lipoproteins (combinations of lipids and proteins). Of special importance is serum high-density lipoprotein (HDL) cholesterol. Interestingly, an *elevated* HDL cholesterol is thought to exert a protective effect against atherosclerotic development. The serum HDL level is not affected by diet; it can be increased by physical exercise. Women have higher HDL levels than men.

High Blood Pressure.　High blood pressure is an important coronary artery disease risk factor. It appears to accelerate the atherosclerotic process and precipitates myocardial ischemia, heart failure, and stroke. Current recommendations are to keep the blood pressure as close to 140/90 as possible.

Glucose Intolerance.　Glucose intolerance is evidence of diabetes mellitus, which is known also to occur in people who develop atherosclerotic disease. Recent research has shown that this may be one of the most important risk factors of coronary artery disease in women. It is not, however, a significant risk factor in men. Glucose intolerance is not isolated easily as a risk factor, as most diabetics also have high blood pressure and high serum cholesterol levels, and are overweight.

Life-style Habits

Life-style habits include cigarette smoking, physical inactivity, obesity and weight change, emotional stress, and use of oral contraceptives.

Cigarette Smoking. Cigarette smoking is an important coronary artery disease risk factor in both men and women. It causes more deaths from myocardial infarction and sudden cardiac death than lung cancer or chronic obstructive pulmonary disease. Factors related to the cigarette smoking habit that influence the incidence and mortality rate of coronary artery disease are the number of cigarettes smoked and duration of smoking (expressed in terms of pack-year history*), age at initiation of smoking, and pattern of inhaling. Pipe and cigar smokers usually run less risk of developing coronary artery disease than cigarette smokers because they generally do not inhale. However, if they are reformed cigarette smokers, they usually continue to inhale pipe or cigar smoke. The risk of death from coronary artery disease is reduced when cigarette smoking is stopped, and after 10 years, the risk of mortality from coronary disease approaches that of a nonsmoker.

Physical Inactivity. Most practitioners feel that physical exercise has merit in preventing or minimizing development of coronary artery disease. It has been shown that mortality after myocardial infarction can be reduced in patients participating in cardiac rehabilitation programs. The exact mechanism by which physical activity may protect against coronary artery disease development is not known, but recent data have shown HDL cholesterol levels to be higher among men who are very physically active compared to those who are not.

Obesity and Weight Change. There is an increased risk of coronary artery disease development and mortality in overweight or obese individuals. Obesity is defined as a body-mass index (weight/height^2) greater than 20% above the ideal value. Obesity as an isolated risk factor is difficult to assess, as many obese people also are older and have high blood pressure and elevated serum cholesterol levels. It is also important to note that large weight changes are strongly related to incidence and mortality of coronary disease.

Emotional Stress. Emotional stress is an important coronary artery disease risk factor in both men and women. Even though stress is highly associated with the ''American way of life,'' it must be remembered that stress of one kind or another has been present in almost every situation, and that what is stressful for one individual may not be stressful for another. The difference may be in the manner in which we handle stress, specifically with less than ideal physical activity as an outlet. Although many components of our lifestyle contribute to stress, one of the most researched is the type A personality, characterized by aggressiveness, ambitiousness, competitive drive, preoccupation with deadlines, impatience, and time urgency. Type A personality is a risk factor for coronary artery disease development in both men and women.

Use of Oral Contraceptives. Myocardial infarction among young, healthy women is rare. Use of oral contraceptives (estrogen and progestin) is associated with increased risk of nonfatal and fatal myocardial infarction in young women. The risk from cigarette smoking acts synergistically with the risk from oral contraceptive use, greatly increasing a woman's risk of coronary artery disease development and mortality if she both smokes and uses oral contraceptives.

Signs of Preclinical Cardiovascular Disease

Signs of preclinical cardiovascular disease include electrocardiographic changes of left ventricular hypertrophy (common in the patient with high blood pressure), and nonspecific T wave changes on the resting electrocardiogram. Left ventricular hypertrophy can be modified in the patient with high blood pressure by lowering blood pressure.

Combined Risk Factors

The greater the number of risk factors, the greater the risk of developing coronary artery disease. Combinations of risk factors have a synergistic effect. The American Heart Association's *Coronary Risk Handbook* provides the clinician with a simple method of predicting coronary artery disease risk and is a useful tool for patient involvement in modification of risk.

▷ Physical Assessment

Assessment of physical findings should confirm data obtained in the nursing history. Baseline information is obtained on admission. Until the examiner becomes skilled in physical assessment, the initial findings should be validated by an experienced clinician. In the acutely ill cardiac patient, physical examination is performed with routine vital signs (every 4 hours, or more frequently if indicated). As the patient improves, assessments are done once per shift and progress to once per day until discharge. Because nurses spend 24 hours per day with the patient, they are in the best position to identify any changes that may occur. It is to the patient's benefit to detect changes early, before serious complications develop. The cardiac care unit nurse who telephones the physician to report that the patient ''just does not look good'' lacks the credibility of the nurse who identifies ''a new S_3 gallop, bilateral crackles halfway up the posterior lung fields, and jugular venous distention of 14 cm of water.'' Any changes observed in the assessment should be noted in the chart and reported to the physician.

A cardiac physical assessment should include an evaluation of:

- Patient appearance
- The heart as a pump
- Filling volumes and pressures
- Cardiac output
- Compensatory mechanisms

Factors that reflect a reduced contractility are reduced pulse pressure, cardiac enlargement, and presence of murmurs and gallop rhythms.

Filling volumes and pressures are estimated by the degree of jugular vein distention (JVD) and the presence or absence of crackles, peripheral edema, and postural changes in blood pressure.

---

* Pack-year history equals packs per day times number of years, for example, one pack per day times 10 years is ten pack years.

Cardiac output is reflected by heart rate, pulse pressure, peripheral vascular resistance, urine output, and central nervous system manifestations.

Examples of compensatory mechanisms that help maintain cardiac output are increased filling volumes and elevated heart rate.

The order of examination proceeds logically from head to toe, and with practice can be done in approximately 10 minutes: (1) general appearance, (2) blood pressure, (3) pulse, (4) hand, (5) head and neck, (6) heart, (7) lungs, (8) abdomen, and (9) feet and legs.

Refer to Chapter 5 for a description of physical assessment techniques.

General Appearance

Observe the patient's level of distress. Level of consciousness should be noted and described. Appropriateness of thought content, reflecting the adequacy of cerebral perfusion, is particularly important to evaluate. Family members who are most familiar with the patient can be of help in alerting the examiner to subtle behavioral changes. The nurse should also be aware of the patient's anxiety level, not only to attempt to put him more at ease, but to realize its effects on the cardiovascular system.

Blood Pressure

The technique of blood pressure measurement is described on page 73. Remember the following points:

- Cuff size must be appropriate for the patient.
- Sphygmomanometer should be calibrated correctly.
- Patient's arm should be at heart level.
- Initial recordings are made on both arms, and subsequent measurements are taken on the arm with the highest pressure.
- Position of the patient and site of blood pressure measurement (for example, RA for right arm) is recorded.
- Presence of auscultatory gap is considered, especially in patient with high blood pressure. To avoid obtaining falsely low systolic blood pressures, palpate prior to auscultating the systolic pressure.

Pulse Pressure. Pulse pressure (difference between systolic and diastolic pressures) reflects stroke volume, ejection velocity, and systemic vascular resistance. Use pulse pressure as a noninvasive indicator of the patient's ability to maintain cardiac output. If the pulse pressure in the cardiac patient falls below 30 mm Hg, further assessment of the patient's cardiovascular status may be indicated.

Postural Blood Pressure Changes. Postural (orthostatic) hypotension occurs when the blood pressure drops after an upright posture is assumed and is usually accompanied by dizziness, lightheadedness, or syncope. Although there are many causes of postural hypotension, the three most commonly seen in the cardiac patient are saline depletion, inadequate vasoconstrictor mechanisms, and autonomic insufficiency. Postural changes in blood pressure, along with appropriate history, can help the clinician differentiate between them. Remember the following points:

- Position the patient supine and as flat as symptoms permit for 10 minutes prior to the initial blood pressure and heart rate measurement.

- Always check supine measurements prior to upright measurements.
- Always record both heart rate and blood pressure at each postural change (lying down, sitting, standing).
- Do not remove the blood pressure cuff between position changes, but do check to see that it is still correctly placed.
- Assess postural blood pressure changes with the patient sitting on the edge of the bed with feet dangling, and if necessary, with the patient standing at the side of the bed.
- Wait 1 to 3 minutes after each postural change prior to recording blood pressure and heart rate.
- Be alert for any signs or symptoms of patient distress, and if necessary, return the patient to bed prior to test completion.
- Record any signs or symptoms that accompany the postural change.

Normal postural responses are increased heart rate (to offset reduced stroke volume and maintain cardiac output), a slight to a 15-mm Hg drop in systolic pressure, and a slight drop to an increase of 5 mm Hg to 10 mm Hg diastolic pressure.

Saline depletion should be suspected (in the presence of a history of saline loss, *e.g.,* diuretic therapy) when, in response to sitting or standing, the heart rate increases and *either* the systolic pressure decreases by 15 mm Hg *or* the diastolic blood pressure drops by 10 mm Hg. It is difficult to differentiate saline depletion from inadequate vasoconstrictor mechanisms by postural changes in vital signs alone. With saline depletion, reflexes to maintain cardiac output (increased heart rate and peripheral vasoconstriction) function correctly, but because of lost extracellular fluid volume, the blood pressure falls. With inadequate vasoconstrictor mechanisms, the heart rate again responds appropriately, but because of diminished peripheral vasoconstriction, the blood pressure drops. The following is an example of a postural blood pressure recording showing either saline depletion or inadequate vasoconstrictor mechanisms:

	Blood Pressure	Heart Rate
Lying down	120/70	70
Sitting	100/55	90
Standing	98/52	94

In autonomic insufficiency, the heart rate is unable to increase to compensate for the gravitational effects of upright posture. Peripheral vasoconstriction may be absent or diminished. The presence of autonomic insufficiency does not rule out concurrent saline depletion. The following is an example of autonomic insufficiency as demonstrated by postural blood pressure changes:

	Blood Pressure	Heart Rate
Lying down	150/90	60
Sitting	100/60	60

Radial Pulse

The radial pulse should be assessed for quality and rate. Normally, the upstroke of the pulse wave is rapid and smooth. Small, weak pulses have a diminished pulse pressure, indicative of reduced stroke volume or ejection fraction, or of increased systemic vascular resistance. Large, bounding pulses have increased pulse pressure.

Heart Rate. The heart rate can be determined by counting the radial pulse. If the rhythm is irregular, the pulse should be counted apically and radially for a full minute, and any discrepancy between contractions heard and pulses perfused should be noted. Apical–radial differences commonly occur with atrial fibrillation and premature ventricular contractions. If the difference is very large, it is helpful to have two people count for the same minute.

Hands

In the cardiac patient, the following are the most important findings to note:

- Peripheral cyanosis implies decreased flow rate of blood in the periphery, allowing more time for the hemoglobin molecule to become desaturated. This may occur normally with the peripheral vasoconstriction associated with a cold environment, or pathologically in conditions that reduce blood flow, for example, cardiogenic shock.
- Pallor can denote anemia or an increased systemic vascular resistance.
- Capillary refill time provides an estimate of the rate of peripheral blood flow. Normally, reperfusion occurs almost instantaneously. More sluggish reperfusion indicates a slower peripheral flow rate, for example, in heart failure.
- Hand temperature and moistness is controlled by the autonomic nervous system. Normally, hands are warm and dry. Under stress, they may be cool and moist. In cardiogenic shock, hands become cold and clammy.
- Edema decreases skin mobility.
- Dehydration and aging reduce skin turgor.
- Clubbing of the fingers and toes implies chronic hemoglobin desaturation, as in congenital heart disease.

Head and Neck

Head. In examining the head of a cardiac patient, one needs to be concerned primarily with checking the lips and earlobes for peripheral cyanosis, and the buccal mucosa for central cyanosis. In central cyanosis, hemoglobin does not become fully saturated with oxygen and implies serious heart or lung disease, as in pulmonary edema. Central cyanosis is always accompanied by peripheral cyanosis.

Neck. Jugular vein distention (JVD) is caused by increased filling volume and pressure on the right side of the heart. It is a *late* finding in left ventricular failure. Jugular veins act like manometers and can be used to measure central venous pressure (CVP), which reflects right atrial or right ventricular end-diastolic pressure. To measure jugular vein distention.

- Begin with the patient supine, although the backrest can be elevated for patient comfort.
- Determine heart level by finding the phlebostatic axis

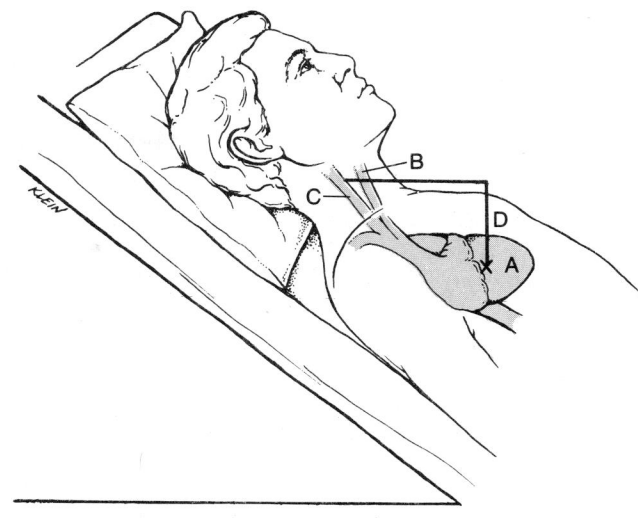

Figure 27-6. Noninvasive determination of central venous pressure. (*A*) Phlebostatic axis. (*B*) Internal jugular vein. (*C*) External jugular vein. (*D*) Vertical distance in centimeters from the meniscus to the phlebostatic axis equals the CVP in cm H_2O.

(4th intercostal space at the sternum, intersecting the mid anterior–posterior line) (Figs. 27-6 and 27-7).
- Locate the neck veins (either the internal or external jugular veins can be used). Blood assumes the level that corresponds to the CVP when the neck veins are occluded by the examiner's fingertip at the angle of the jaw.
- Do not strip the veins first; backfilling of the blood may be prevented by a valve in the jugular vein.
- Position the patient at a backrest angle that will allow the meniscus to be seen below the angle of the jaw.
- Measure the *vertical* distance between the phlebostatic axis and the meniscus with a centimeter ruler. The distance in centimeters corresponds to the CVP (Fig. 27-6, *D*). The normal JVD is 4 cm to 10 cm of water.

Heart

Assessment of the precordium is described on page 74. The cardiac patient is most likely to exhibit the following abnormalities:

- *Abnormal point of maximal impulse (PMI).* Normally, the PMI (the apex beat) is located in the 5th intercostal space, medial to the midclavicular line. Left ventricular enlargement, for example, from left ventricular failure, is evident if the PMI is below the 5th intercostal space or lateral to the mid-clavicular line. When palpated, the PMI should be felt in only one intercostal space. If palpated in two or more adjacent intercostal spaces, left ventricular enlargement can be diagnosed. If two distinctly separate areas with paradoxical movement are seen, a ventricular aneurysm should be suspected.
- *Diastolic filling sounds (S_3 or S_4 gallops).* (See Figs. 27-8 and 27-9.) These sounds are indicative of decreased ventricular compliance, which can be caused by ischemia, heart failure, or hypertensive heart disease. Gallops are heard best with the bell of the stethoscope

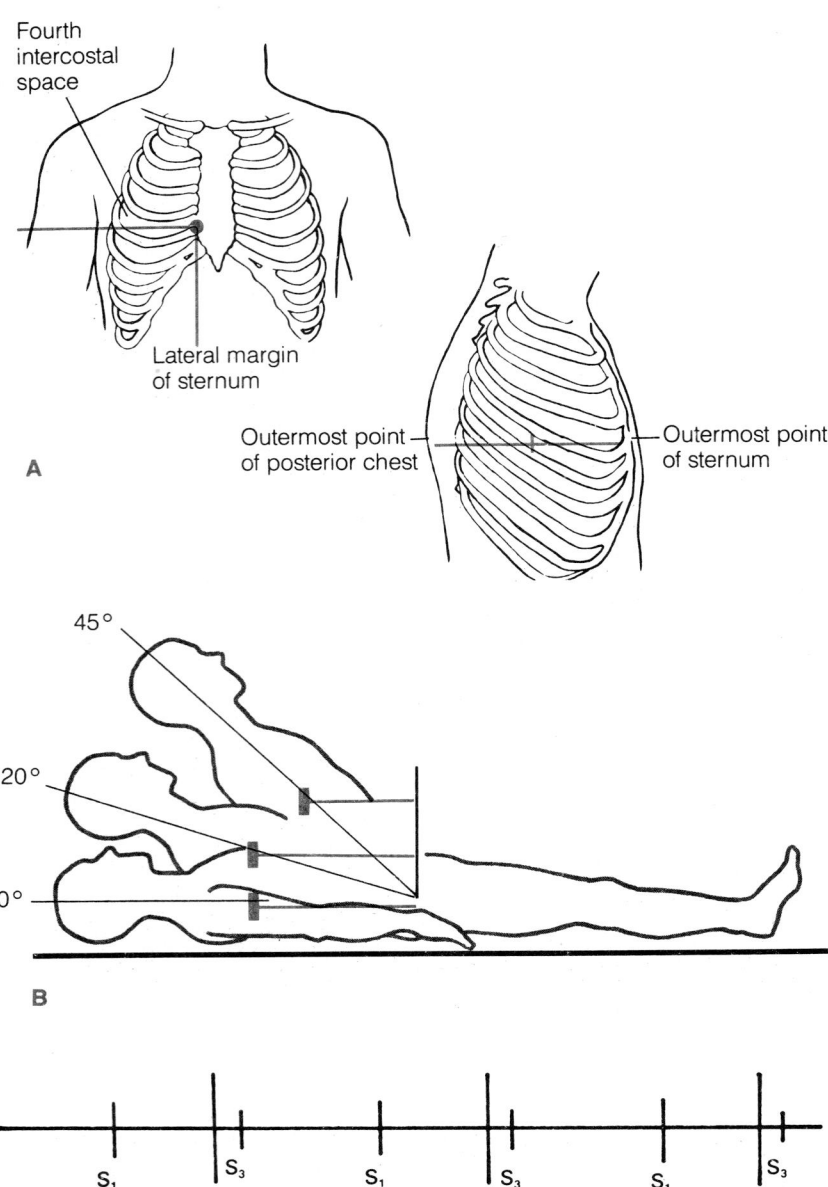

Figure 27-7. The phlebostatic axis and the phlebostatic level. (*A*) The phlebostatic axis is the crossing of two reference lines: (1) a line from the fourth intercostal space at the point where it joins the sternum, drawn out to the side of the body beneath the axilla; (2) a line midpoint between the anterior and posterior surfaces of the chest. (*B*) The phlebostatic level is a horizontal line through the phlebostatic axis. The transducer or the zero mark on the manometer must be level with this axis for accurate measurements. As the patient moves from the flat to erect positions, he moves his chest and therefore the reference level; the phlebostatic level stays horizontal through the same reference point. (After Shinn J et al: Heart Lung, 8(2):324, 1979.)

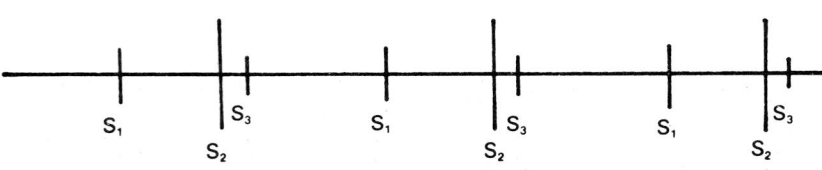

Figure 27-8. An S_3 gallop immediately follows the S_2.

placed over the apex, with the patient in the left lateral position.

- *Systolic murmur.* In the patient with coronary artery disease, the most frequently heard murmur is the holosystolic murmur (cardiac murmur that extends through systole) of mitral regurgitation. Backflow of blood from the left ventricle through the mitral valve occurs if the papillary muscles become ischemic and are no longer able to contract properly. This murmur is loudest at the apex and may be heard with the diaphragm of the stethoscope.

- *Pericardial friction rub.* Transient pericarditis is a common finding in the patient with acute myocardial infarction or may occur as a result of open heart surgery. A pericardial friction rub can be heard using the diaphragm of the stethoscope, with the patient sitting up and leaning foward.

Lungs

Respiratory assessment is described on page 65. Findings frequently exhibited by cardiac patients include:

- *Tachypnea.* Rapid, shallow breathing may be noted in patients who have heart failure or pain, or who are extremely anxious.

- *Cheyne-Stokes respirations.* Patients in severe left ventricular failure may exhibit Cheyne-Stokes breathing. Of particular importance is the duration of the apneic period.

- *Hemoptysis.* Pink, frothy sputum is indicative of acute pulmonary edema.

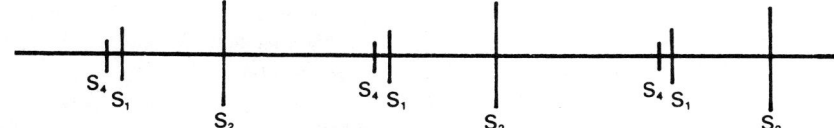

Figure 27-9. An S₄ gallop immediately precedes the S₁.

- *Cough.* A dry, hacking cough from irritation of small airways is common in patients with pulmonary congestion from heart failure.
- *Crackles.* Heart failure, or atelectasis associated with bed rest, splinting from ischemic pain, or the effects of pain medication and sedatives, often results in the development of crackles. Typically, crackles are first noted at the bases (because of gravity's effect on fluid accumulation and decreased ventilation of basilar tissue) but may progress to all portions of the lung fields.
- *Wheezes.* Compression of the small airways by interstitial pulmonary edema may cause wheezing. Beta-blocking agents, such as propranolol, may precipitate airway narrowing, especially in patients with underlying pulmonary disease.

Abdomen

The abdominal examination is described on page 78. For the cardiac patient, two components of the abdominal examination are frequently performed:

- *Determination of liver size.* Liver engorgement occurs because of decreased venous return secondary to right ventricular failure. The liver will be enlarged, firm, nontender, and smooth. Hepatojugular reflux may be demonstrated by pressing firmly over the liver for 30 to 60 seconds and noting a 1-cm rise in JVD.
- *Assessment of bladder distention.* Urine output is an important indicator of cardiac output. In a patient who has not voided or who is unable to void, always assess for bladder distention prior to initiating other measures.

Feet and Legs

Many patients with heart disease have associated peripheral vascular disease, or peripheral edema secondary to right ventricular failure. Therefore, adequacy of peripheral arterial circulation and venous return should be assessed in all cardiac patients. In addition, thrombophlebitis is a complication associated with bed rest and requires careful monitoring. Refer to Chapter 32 for a complete description of these techniques.

▷ Diagnostic Tests and Procedures

Diagnostic tests and procedures are requested to confirm data obtained by interview and examination. Some tests are easy to interpret, while others must be interpreted by expert clinicians. All require that basic explanations be given to patients. Some necessitate special orders prior to the test and special monitoring by the nurse following the procedure.

Laboratory Tests

Laboratory tests may be requested for a variety of reasons: to assist in the diagnosis of acute myocardial infarction (angina pectoris cannot be confirmed by either blood or urine studies); to measure abnormalities in blood chemistries, which could affect the prognosis of a cardiac patient; to assess the degree of the inflammatory process; to screen for risk factors associated with the presence of atherosclerotic coronary artery disease; to determine baseline values prior to therapeutic intervention; to assess drug levels; and to screen generally for any abnormalities. Laboratory studies relating specifically to the cardiac patient are summarized. Because many different methods of measurement are used, refer to individual health care agencies for their normal laboratory values.

Cardiac Enzymes and Isoenzymes

Acute myocardial infarction can be confirmed by the presence of abnormally high levels of enzymes or isoenzymes in the serum. Enzymes are released from all cells as they die and therefore are nonspecific in relation to the particular organ that has been damaged. Certain isoenzymes, however, come only from myocardial cells and specifically reflect death of cardiac muscle. Because different enzymes are released into the blood at varying periods following myocardial infarction, it is crucial to time the drawing of blood in relation to the time of onset of chest discomfort. If drawn too early, enzymes may not yet be elevated; if drawn too late, enzymes may already have returned to baseline. (See Table 27-2 for the time course of cardiac enzymes.) Enzymes used in the diagnosis of acute myocardial infarction are creatine kinase (CK) and its isoenzyme CK-MB, and lactic dehydrogenase (LDH) and its isoenzymes.

Creatine Kinase and Creatine Kinase Isoenzymes. Creatine kinase is regarded as the most sensitive and reliable indicator of all cardiac enzymes. There are three CK isoenzymes: CK-MM (skeletal muscle), CK-MB (heart muscle), and CK-BB (brain tissue). Usually, CK-MB, also known as CK-2, is not present in the serum.

Lactic Dehydrogenase and Lactic Dehydrogenase Isoenzymes. Lactic dehydrogenase is not as reliable an in-

Table 27-2
Time Course of Cardiac Enzymes

Enzyme	Onset	Peak	Return to Normal
CK	3–6 hr	24 hr	72–96 hr
LDH	24 hr	48–72 hr	7–10 days

dicator of acute myocardial damage as CK. However, because it peaks later and is elevated longer than other cardiac enzymes, LDH is a useful diagnostic test in patients who may have sustained acute myocardial infarction but have delayed admission to the hospital. There are five LDH isoenzymes, but only two (LDH_1 and LDH_2) are important in the diagnosis of acute myocardial infarction. Both LDH_1 and LDH_2 predominate in the heart, kidney, and brain, but normally the percentage of LDH_2 compared to LDH_1 is greater. When the percentage of LDH_1 exceeds that of LDH_2, the pattern is said to have "flipped," indicating acute myocardial infarction.

Blood Chemistries

Serum Electrolytes. Serum electrolytes can affect the prognosis of a patient with acute myocardial infarction or any cardiac condition. Serum sodium reflects relative water balance. Serum potassium is an indicator of renal function and may be decreased by diuretic agents. When decreased, potassium causes cardiac irritability and predisposes the patient receiving a digitalis preparation to become digitalis toxic. Elevated serum potassium has a myocardial depressant effect. Calcium is necessary for blood coagulability and neuromuscular excitability.

Blood Urea Nitrogen. Blood urea nitrogen (BUN) is an end product of protein metabolism and is excreted by the kidneys. In the cardiac patient, elevated BUN could reflect reduced renal perfusion (from decreased cardiac output) or saline depletion (from diuretic therapy).

Glucose. Serum glucose is important to measure because many cardiac patients also have diabetes mellitus. Serum glucose may be mildly elevated in stressful situations when endogenous epinephrine is mobilized.

Blood Lipids and Lipoproteins. Cholesterol and triglyceride may be measured to evaluate a person's risk of developing atherosclerotic disease. The patient should be fasting prior to the test. Stress may alter the results.

Blood for lipoproteins also may be drawn to evaluate risk, especially if there is a positive family history of heart disease, or to diagnose a specific lipoprotein abnormality. Decreased levels of high-density lipoprotein (HDL) cholesterol and elevated levels of low-density lipoprotein (LDL) cholesterol increase the risk of development of atherosclerotic coronary artery disease.

Chest X-Ray and Fluoroscopy

A *chest x-ray* is usually requested to determine the size, contour, and position of the heart. It reveals cardiac and pericardial calcifications and demonstrates physiologic alterations in the pulmonary circulation. It does not aid in the diagnosis of acute myocardial infarction, but can confirm the presence of some complications, for example, congestive heart failure. Correct placement of heart catheters, such as pacemakers and pulmonary artery catheters, is also confirmed by chest x-ray.

Fluoroscopy provides visual observation of the heart on a luminescent x-ray screen. It shows heart and vascular pulsations and is useful in the assessment of unusual cardiac contours. Fluoroscopy is a useful tool in the placement and positioning of intravenous pacemaking electrodes and for guiding the catheter in cardiac catheterization.

Electrocardiography

The *electrocardiogram* (ECG) is a visual representation of the electrical activity of the heart as reflected by changes in electrical potential at the skin surface. The ECG is recorded as a tracing on a strip of paper or appears on the screen of an oscilloscope. In order to facilitate the interpretation of the ECG, data about the patient's age, sex, blood pressure, height, weight, symptoms, and medications (especially digitalis and antiarrhythmic drugs) should be noted on the ECG requisition. Electrocardiography is particularly useful in the evaluation of conditions that interfere with normal heart functions, such as disturbances of rate or rhythm, disorders of conduction, enlargement of heart chambers, presence of a myocardial infarction, and electrolyte imbalances. This procedure is discussed in detail in Chapter 28.

Exercise Stress Testing

Exercise stress testing is a noninvasive means of assessing certain aspects of cardiac function. The purposes are to search for ischemic changes in the ECG and to screen for ischemic heart disease, to evaluate patients with chest pain, to assess the results of therapy, and to aid in developing individual physical fitness programs.

Exercise stress testing may be done by having the patient walk on a treadmill, pedal a stationary bicycle, or climb a set of stairs. The patient is exercised by increasing the walking speed and incline of the treadmill or by increasing the load against which the bicycle is pedaled. ECG electrodes are applied to the patient, and tracings are made before, during, and after exercise testing. Blood pressure, skin temperature, physical appearance, and the occurrence or worsening of chest pain are monitored during and following the test.

The patient is instructed to avoid smoking, eating, and drinking for 4 hours prior to the test and to wear comfortable shoes suitable for walking. Women should be told to wear a brassiere that provides adequate support. Following the test the patient should be instructed to rest for a period of time and to avoid stimulants, eating, or extreme temperature changes (*i.e.,* hot or cold showers, going out into the cold).

Vectorcardiography

The vectorcardiogram presents a three-dimensional view of the electrical forces of the heart: horizontal or transverse, frontal, and left sagittal or lateral planes. This diagnostic modality amplifies understanding of the ECG and gives more accurate diagnostic information in certain areas of cardiac diagnosis.

Cardiac Catheterization

Cardiac catheterization is a diagnostic procedure in which a catheter(s) is introduced into the heart and blood vessels in order to (1) measure oxygen concentration (tension), saturation, and pressure in the various heart chambers; (2) detect shunts; (3) provide blood samples for analysis; and (4) determine cardiac output and pulmonary blood flow. Cardiac catheterization is done also to evaluate the patient with chest pain (unstable angina) and to assess heart status before heart surgery. Angiography is usually combined with heart catheterization for coronary artery visualization. During the procedure the patient is monitored electrocardiographically by means of an oscilloscope. Appropriate resuscitative equipment should be readily available when heart catheterization is done.

Angiography is a technique of injecting dye into the vascular system at appropriate sites to outline the heart and blood vessels. It is accompanied by *cineangiograms* (rapidly changing films or movies on an intensified fluoroscopic screen), which record the passage of the contrast media through the vascular tree. This procedure is useful for providing information regarding structural abnormalities such as occlusions, defects, or fistulae or abnormal heart-valve function. Angiography is especially useful in identifying obstructive coronary lesions.

Selective Angiocardiography.

Selective angiocardiography is the injection of a contrast medium through a catheter directly into one of the heart chambers, coronary arteries, or great vessels. The angiocardiogram is recorded by means of a rapid film changer or motion picture camera.

Aortography.

An aortogram is a form of angiography that outlines the lumen of the aorta and the major arteries arising from it. In *thoracic aortography* a contrast medium is used to study the aortic arch and its major branches by means of rapid serial roentgenography. The translumbar or retrograde brachial or femoral approach may be used.

Coronary Arteriography.

In coronary arteriography a radiopaque catheter is introduced into the right brachial artery (via open arteriotomy) or femoral artery (via cutaneous puncture), and is passed into the ascending aorta and manipulated into the appropriate coronary artery under fluoroscopic control. Coronary arteriography is used as an evaluation tool before coronary artery surgery. It is also used to study suspected congenital anomalies of the coronary arteries.

Right-Heart Catheterization.

Right-heart catheterization involves passing a radiopaque catheter from an antecubital or femoral vein into the right atrium, right ventricle, and pulmonary vasculature. This is carried out under direct visualization with a fluoroscope. Pressures within the right atrium are measured and recorded, and blood samples are removed for measurement of the hematocrit and oxygen saturation. The catheter is then passed through the tricuspid valve, and similar tests are performed on the blood within the right ventricle. Finally, the catheter is introduced into the pulmonary artery (*i.e.*, through the pulmonic valve) and as far as possible beyond that point, where "capillary" samples are obtained and "capillary" pressures (also known as wedge pressure) are recorded. Then the catheter is withdrawn.

Right-heart catheterization is considered a relatively safe procedure. Complications, when they do occur, include cardiac arrhythmias, venous spasm, infection of the cutdown site, cardiac perforation, and, rarely, cardiac arrest.

Left-Heart Catheterization.

Left-heart catheterization is usually done by retrograde catheterization of the left ventricle or by transseptal catheterization of the left atrium. In the retrograde technique, the catheter is inserted under direct vision into the right brachial artery (arteriotomy) and advanced under fluoroscopic control down into the ascending aorta and into the left ventricle; or the catheter may be introduced percutaneously by puncture of the femoral artery.

In the transseptal approach the catheter is passed from the right femoral vein (percutaneously or by saphenous vein cutdown) into the right atrium. A long needle is passed up through the catheter and is used to puncture the septum separating the right and left atria. The needle is withdrawn and the catheter is advanced under fluoroscopic control into the left ventricle. In both of these techniques the patient is monitored by electrocardiogram.

Left-heart catheterization gives hemodynamic data (*e.g.*, it permits flow and pressure measurements of the left heart). It is most often performed to evaluate the function of the left ventricular muscle and the mitral and aortic valves or the patency of the coronary arteries. It is used to evaluate patients before and after cardiac surgery. Usually, the right side of the heart is catheterized before the left side is done. Complications include arrhythmias, myocardial infarction, perforation of the heart or great vessels, and systemic embolization.

Following the catheterization, the catheter is slowly withdrawn, the artery is repaired, and the cutdown site is closed and dressed.

Nursing Interventions

Precatheterization nursing responsibilities include the following:

- Prepare the patient to fast after midnight prior to the procedure.
- Prepare the patient for the expected duration of the procedure; warn him that he will be lying on a hard table for about 2 hours.
- Prepare the patient for certain sensations he may experience during the catheterization. Knowing what to expect can help the patient to cope with the experience.

    An occasional thudding sensation (palpitation) may be felt in the chest because of extra systoles that almost always occur, particularly when the catheter tip touches the myocardium.

    When contrast medium is injected into the right heart (during angiography), there may be a strong desire to cough.

    The injection of contrast medium into either side of the heart may produce a feeling of heat, particularly in the head, which leaves in a minute or less.

Postcatheterization nursing interventions include the following:

- Watch the puncture (or cutdown sites) for hematoma formation, and check the peripheral pulses in the affected extremity (dorsalis pedis, posterior tibial pulse in the lower extremity; radial pulse in the upper extremity) every 15 minutes for 1 to 2 hours, then every 1 to 2 hours until stable.

- Evaluate extremity temperature and color, and any patient complaints of pain, numbness, or tingling sensations in the affected extremity to determine signs of arterial insufficiency. Report changes promptly.
- Watch for arrhythmias by observing the cardiac monitor or by listening to the apical heart rate and evaluating the pulse for rhythm changes.
- If protocol requires, see that the patient remains in bed with little movement of the involved extremity until the following morning.
- Report any complaint of chest discomfort immediately.
- Discomfort at the site is not unexpected. Pain medication should be administered as prescribed.

Echocardiography

Ultrasound is acoustic energy propagated at frequencies of more than 1 million cycles per second. In echocardiography, high-frequency sound waves are sent into the heart through the chest wall and are recorded as they return. The ultrasound is generated by a hand-held transducer (a device that converts one form of energy to another form of energy) applied to the front of the chest. An ECG is recorded simultaneously to time events within the cardiac cycle. Motions of the echoes are traced on an oscilloscope and recorded on film. This is the same sonar principle by which submarines detect ships. It is a safe, noninvasive method that gives information similar in many respects to the data obtained with angiocardiography. Echocardiography is especially useful in the diagnosis and differentiation of heart murmurs. An echogram can detect whether the heart is dilated, the walls or septum are thickened, or pericardial effusion is present. It has also been used to study the motion of prosthetic heart valves.

Phonocardiography

Phonocardiography is the graphic recording of heart sounds and pulse waves and their relation to time. It helps to identify, accurately time, and differentiate various sounds and murmurs. It provides a permanent record for future comparison.

Radioisotope Studies

Radioisotope studies are useful for detecting myocardial infarction and decreased myocardial blood flow, and for evaluating left ventricular function. The radioisotopes are injected intravenously, and scans are done using a gamma scintillation camera. (See Chap. 18.)

Myocardial Infarction Imaging. Technetium pyrophosphate (^{99m}Tc) is taken up in areas of myocardial infarction. This technique, known as hot spot identification, is most reliable when the infarction is large.

Myocardial Blood Flow Evaluation. Thallium-201 is used to evaluate blood flow through vessels that are too small to visualize with coronary arteriography. Often this is paired with an exercise stress test to compare changes in myocardial perfusion during exercise and at rest. In this technique, "cold spots" correlating to lack of myocardial perfusion correlate to infarcted areas.

Blood Pool Scanning. The technique of gated cardiac blood pool scanning utilizes a computer to analyze left ventricular function. By comparing the difference in the amount of the radioactive tracer in the end-diastolic volume and the end-systolic volume, the ejection fraction can be calculated. This test can also be used to assess the differences in left ventricular function during rest and exercise.

Hemodynamic Monitoring

Central Venous Pressure Monitoring

Central venous pressure (CVP) is the pressure within the right atrium or in the great veins within the thorax. It represents the filling pressure of the right ventricle and indicates the ability of the right side of the heart to manage a fluid load. It serves as a guide to fluid replacement in seriously ill patients and is a measurement of effective circulating blood volume. CVP may also be used for total parenteral nutrition (hyperalimentation), long-term chemotherapy, and fluid therapy.

CVP reflects right ventricular failure. Most right ventricular failure is secondary to left ventricular failure. Therefore, an elevated CVP is a *late* sign of left ventricular failure.

CVP is a dynamic or changing measurement. The change in CVP correlated with the patient's clinical status is a more useful indication of adequacy of venous blood volume and alterations of cardiovascular function than is a single measurement of CVP. A lowered CVP indicates that the patient is hypovolemic, and this is verified when a rapid intravenous infusion causes the patient to improve. A rising CVP may be due to either hypervolemia or poor cardiac contractility.

The CVP site should be prepared by shaving and cleansing with an antiseptic solution. A local anesthetic may be used. The catheter is threaded through the arm or neck vein into the superior vena cava just above or within the right atrium. Once the CVP catheter is inserted, antiseptic ointment and a dry, sterile dressing are applied. The dressing, intravenous bag, manometer, and tubing are changed every 24 hours.

Vascular pressure is measured by the height of a column of water in a manometer. When measuring CVP, it is crucial that the zero mark on the manometer be placed at the correct position, the phlebostatic axis (see Fig. 27-7). Once this position is located, the chest should be marked with ink. If the phlebostatic axis is used, the CVP can be measured correctly with the patient supine at any backrest position. Normal CVP is 4 cm to 10 cm of water. The most common complications of CVP monitoring are infection and air embolism.

Pulmonary Artery and Pulmonary Artery Wedge Pressure Monitoring

Pulmonary artery pressures reflect left-sided heart pressures and therefore are more useful in assessing left ventricular failure than CVP. Pulmonary artery pressures are monitored only in cardiac care units or other intensive care units and not on general medical–surgical units.

A balloon-tipped, floating catheter is inserted into a large vein that leads into the superior vena cava and right atrium. The balloon is inflated, and the catheter is carried rapidly by the flow of blood through the tricuspid valve, into the right ventricle, out the pulmonic valve, and into a branch of the pulmonary artery. When the catheter reaches a small pulmonary artery, the balloon is deflated and the catheter is secured with sutures.

Pulmonary artery systolic and diastolic pressures are obtained via a transducer and blood pressure monitor. Normal pulmonary artery pressure is 25/9 mm Hg, with a mean pressure of 15 mm Hg. When the balloon is inflated, the catheter is "wedged" in the pulmonary artery. Pressures transmitted to the catheter reflect left ventricular end-diastolic pressure. At end-diastole, when the mitral valve is open, pulmonary artery wedge pressure is the same as the pressure in the left atrium and the left ventricle, *unless* the patient has mitral valve disease or pulmonary hypertension. Pulmonary artery wedge pressure is a mean pressure and is normally 4.5 mm Hg to 13 mm Hg.

Catheter site care is the same as that of a CVP. The catheter flush solution is heparinized normal saline, delivered in small amounts using a pressure bag and flush device. As with the CVP, it is essential to place the transducer at the phlebostatic axis to ensure accurate readings. Measurement of cardiac output can also be obtained by using a pulmonary artery catheter. Complications of pulmonary artery monitoring include infection, pulmonary artery rupture, pulmonary thromboembolism, pulmonary infarction, catheter kinking, arrhythmias, and air embolism.

Systemic Intra-arterial Monitoring

Intra-arterial monitoring is used to obtain direct and continuous blood pressures in critically ill patients with severe high blood pressure or hypotension. Arterial catheters are also useful when obtaining arterial blood gases and serial blood samples. Intra-arterial monitoring is also restricted to critical care units.

Once an arterial site is selected (radial, brachial, femoral, or dorsalis pedis), collateral circulation to the area must be confirmed prior to catheter placement. This can be done by either the Allen test or the ultrasonic Doppler test. (If no collateral circulation existed, and the cannulated artery became occluded, ischemia and infarction of the area distal to the cannulated site could occur.) Site preparation and care is the same as for CVP catheters. The catheter flush solution is the same as for pulmonary artery catheters. A transducer is attached, and pressures are obtained in mm Hg. Complications include local obstruction with distal ischemia, external hemorrhage, massive ecchymosis, dissection, air embolism, blood loss, pain, arteriospasm, or infection.

▷ **Bibliography**

Books

Adolph L and Lorenz R. Enzyme Diagnosis in Diseases of the Heart, Liver and Pancreas. New York, S Karger, 1982.

American Heart Association. Heartbook: A Guide to Prevention and Treatment of Heart Disease. New York, EP Dutton, 1980.

Bates B. A Guide to Physical Examination, 3rd ed. Philadelphia, JB Lippincott, 1983.

Brunwald E. Heart Disease. Philadelphia, WB Saunders, 1980.

Conover MB. Understanding Electrocardiography. St Louis, CV Mosby, 1980.

Fishback FT. Manual of Laboratory Tests. Philadelphia, JB Lippincott, 1980.

Fowler NO. Cardiac Diagnosis and Treatment, 3rd ed. Hagerstown, Maryland, Harper & Row, 1980.

Grossman W. Cardiac Catheterization and Angiography, 2nd ed. Philadelphia, Lea & Febiger, 1980.

Hurst JW et al. The Heart. New York, McGraw–Hill, 1982.

Mangiola S and Ritota MC. Cardiac Arrhythmias. Practical ECG Interpretation, 2nd ed. Philadelphia, JB Lippincott, 1982.

Perloff JA. Physical Examination of the Heart and Circulation. Philadelphia, WB Saunders, 1982.

Underhill SL et al. Cardiac Nursing. Philadelphia, JB Lippincott, 1982.

Articles

Auscultation of the heart. Am J Nurs 1977 Feb; 77(2):1–24.

Bodai BI and Holcroft JW. Use of the pulmonary arterial catheter in the critically ill patient. Heart Lung 1982 Sept–Oct; 11(5):406–416.

Brantigan CO. Hemodynamic monitoring: Interpreting values. Am J Nurs 1982 Jan; 82(1):86–89.

Brown B. Auscultation of heart sounds. Crit Care Update 1981 July; 8(7):26–30.

Cohen JA, Pantaleo N, and Shell WE. What isoenzymes can tell you about your cardiac patient. Nursing '82 1982 Apr; 12(4):46–49.

Finesilver C. Reducing stress in patients having cardiac catheterization. Am J Nurs 1980 Oct; 80(10):1085–1087.

Frank D and Stromberg M. Test your knowledge of chest pain. Nursing '81 1981 Aug; 11(8):89–98.

Gibson K. The type A personality. Cardiovasc Nurs 1980 Sept–Oct; 16(5):25–28.

Humbrecht A and Parys E. How to use heart and breath sounds as part of your nursing care plan. Nursing '82 1982 Apr; 12(4):34–41.

Kannel WB and Dawber TR. Contributors to coronary risk: Ten years later. Heart Lung 1982 Jan–Feb; 11(1):60–64.

Managing an arterial line. Nursing '80 1980 June; 10(6):82–83.

Multiple Risk Factor Intervention Trial Research Group. Multiple risk factor intervention trial. JAMA 1982 Sept 24; 248(12):1465–1477.

Pantaleo N et al. Thallium myocardial scintigraphy and its use in the assessment of coronary artery disease. Heart Lung 1981 Jan–Feb; 10(1):61–71.

Scordo KA. Taming the cardiac monitor. Part 1. Nursing '82 1982 Aug; 12(8):58–64.

Scordo KA. Taming the cardiac monitor. Part 2. Nursing '82 1982 Sept; 12(9):60–68.

Shinn JA, Woods SL, and Huseby JS. Effect of intermittent positive pressure ventilation upon pulmonary artery and pulmonary capillary wedge pressures in acutely ill patients. Heart Lung 1979 Mar–Apr; 8(2):322–327.

Visalli F and Evans P. The Swan–Ganz catheter. Nursing '81 1981 Jan; 11(1):42–47.

Woods SL. Monitoring pulmonary artery pressures. Am J Nurs 1976 Nov; 76(11):1765–1771.

Zeluff GW, Cashion WR, and Jackson D. Evaluation of the coronary arteries and myocardium by radionuclide imaging. Heart Lung 1980 Mar–Apr; 9(2):344–349.

Electrocardiograms and Heart Arrhythmias

The purpose of this chapter is to present basic concepts in electrocardiography and to demonstrate its usefulness in the diagnosis of myocardial infarction (MI), electrolyte imbalances, drug effects and toxicity, and arrhythmias.

▷ Essentials of Electrocardiography

The electrocardiogram (ECG) is a useful test in that it assists in the diagnosis of many diseases and provides vital information about a patient's condition and progress. The ECG is a graphic record of the electrical activity of the heart. Impulse formation and conduction throughout the heart produce weak electrical currents through the entire body. The difference in potential between a positive and a negative area within the body can be measured by a galvanometer, an instrument with a wire between the poles of an electromagnet. As current passes through the wire, the instrument is controlled by the magnetic field. The ECG machine contains a galvanometer that detects changes in surface potential, amplifies the signal, and records these body surface potential changes over time on calibrated moving paper.

Electrical Conduction Through the Heart

The normal electrical impulse of the heart, which inscribes the ECG and causes the heart to contract, begins in the sinoatrial (SA) node, which is located in the superior portion of the right atrium. After beginning in the SA node the impulse travels across the atria so that an atrial contraction occurs. The impulse then arrives at the atrioventricular (AV) node, which lies between the atria and ventricles. The impulse is somewhat delayed in the AV node and then travels down the right and left bundle branches and Purkinje fibers to the ventricular muscle (Fig. 28-1). Then the ventricles contract.

Both the SA and AV nodes are connected to two main nerve systems that control the rate at which the heart beats. The sympathetic nerves cause the heart rate to increase,

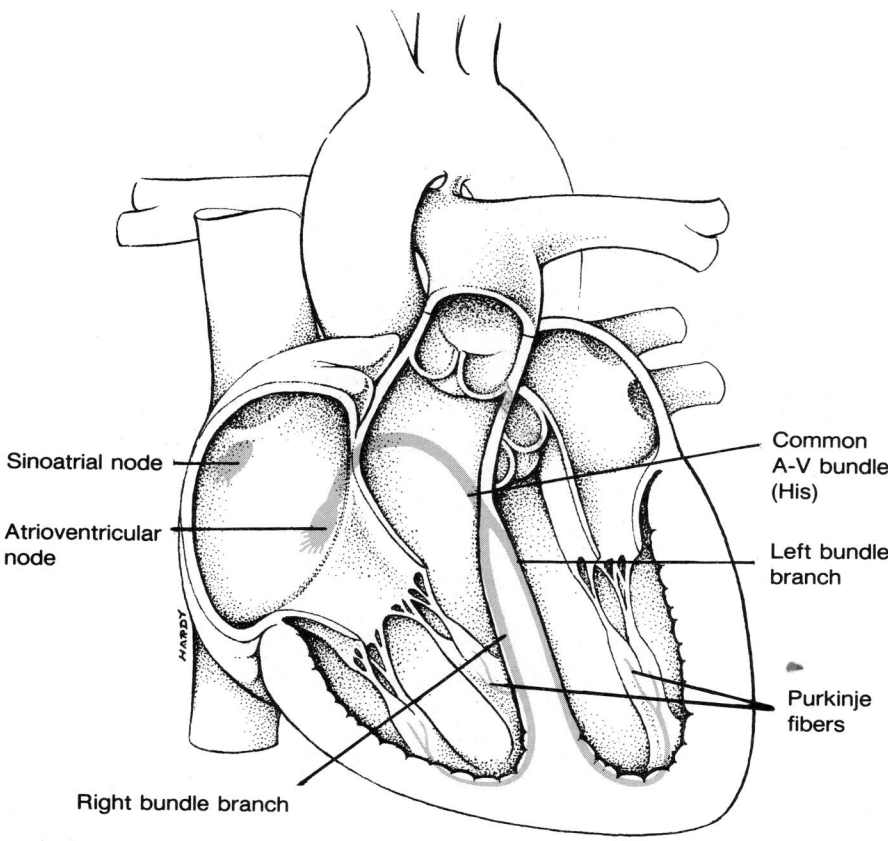

Figure 28-1. Conducting system. Diagram showing relations of the sinoatrial node, the atrioventricular node, the common atrioventricular bundle and its branches. (From Chaffee EE and Greisheimer EM: Basic Physiology and Anatomy, 3rd ed. Philadelphia, JB Lippincott.)

whereas the parasympathetic (vagus nerve) system slows the heart rate.

The 12-Lead ECG

Normally, the ECG consists of 12 leads: three bipolar standard leads (I, II, and III); three unipolar leads (aVR, aVL, aVF); and six unipolar chest leads. The three bipolar leads represent a difference of electric potential between two selected sites. Lead I is the difference of potential between the left arm (LA) and the right arm (RA). Lead II is the difference of potential between the left leg (LL) and the right arm. Lead III is the difference of potential between the left leg and the left arm. Einthoven's triangle (1903) is based on the equation lead II = leads I + III. If leads I, II, and III are bisected by each other, the triaxial reference is produced (Fig. 28-2, A, B). Each of these three leads is 60 degrees apart.

The three augmented unipolar extremity leads are aVR (augmented or increased vector of the right arm), aVL (augmented vector of the left arm), and aVF (augmented vector of the left leg). The unipolar leads represent a difference in potential between one site and the average of the potential of two other sites. Lead aVR is the difference of potential between the right arm and the average of the potential of the left leg and left arm. Lead aVL is the difference

of potential between the left arm and the average of the potential of the left leg and right arm. Lead aVF is the difference of potential between the left leg and the average of potential of the left arm and right arm. The three augmented unipolar leads can be superimposed onto the triaxial reference figure, resulting in a hexaxial reference figure (Fig. 28-2, C, D). Each of these six leads is 30 degrees apart.

The last six leads of the 12-lead ECG are the unipolar precordial (chest) leads and are called "V" leads. The common precordial positions on the chest are shown in Figure 28-3.

Generally, ECG paper moves at a speed of 25 mm/ second. Each small box, horizontally, is equal to 0.04 second. One large box (five small boxes), horizontally, equals 0.20 second; one large box (five small boxes), vertically, is equal to 5 mm. Ten millimeters is equal to 1 millivolt (mV). The ECG is calibrated to 1 mV vertically in order to standardize the ECG (Fig. 28-4).

Waves, Complexes, and Intervals

The ECG is composed of several components or waves, including the P wave, the QRS complex, the T wave, the ST segment, the R interval, and possibly a U wave (usually indicates an abnormality).

The *P wave* represents atrial muscle depolarization. It

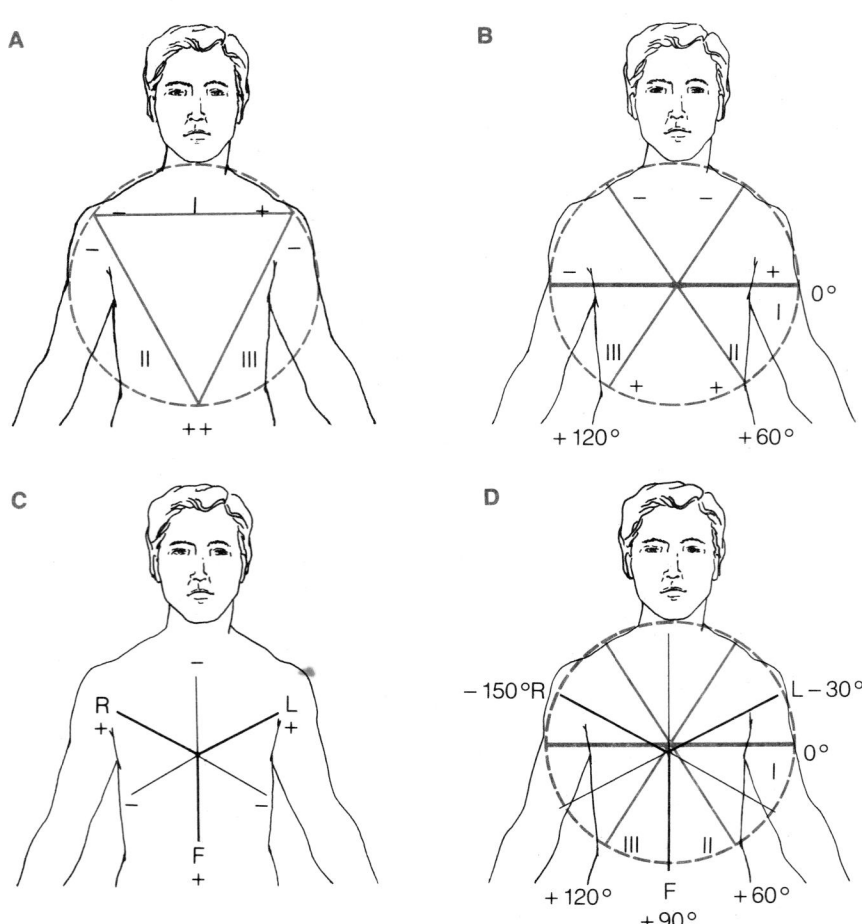

Figure 28-2. (*A*) Bipolar leads (Einthoven's triangle). (*B*) Triaxial reference figure for bipolar leads. (*C*) Augmented unipolar leads; R = aVR, L = aVL, and F = aVF. (*D*) Hexaxial reference figure for bipolar and augmented unipolar leads. (From Underhill SL et al. Cardiac Nursing, p 197. Philadelphia, JB Lippincott, 1982.)

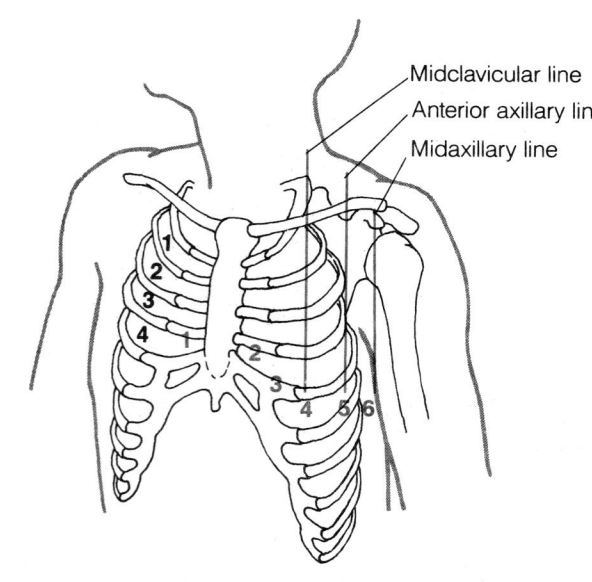

Figure 28-3. Six standard precordial leads—electrode placement: (*1*) Fourth intercostal space, at right side of sternum. (*2*) Fourth intercostal space, at left side of sternum. (*3*) Midway between positions 2 and 4. (*4*) Fifth intercostal space, midclavicular line. (*5*) Same level as #4 in the anterior axillary line. (*6*) Same as #4 and #5 in the midaxillary line. (Adapted from Bernreiter M: Electrocardiography, p 23. Philadelphia, JB Lippincott.)

is normally 2.5 mm or less in height and is 0.11 second or less in duration. The first negative deflection after the P wave is the Q wave, which is less than 0.03 seconds in duration and less than 25% of the R wave amplitude; the first positive deflection after the P wave is the R wave; and the S wave is the first negative deflection after the R wave (see Fig. 28-4).

The *QRS complex* (beginning of Q wave to end of S wave) represents ventricular muscle depolarization. When a wave is less than 5 mm vertically, small letters (q, r, s) are used; when a wave is greater than 5 mm vertically, capital letters (Q, R, S) are used. Not all QRS complexes have all three waveforms.

The *T wave* represents ventricular muscle repolarization. It follows the QRS complex and is usually of the same deflection as the QRS complex. If a U wave is seen, it will follow the T wave. The presence of a U wave may indicate an electrolyte abnormality.

The *ST segment,* which represents early ventricular repolarization of the ventricles, is from the end of the S wave (J joint) to the beginning of the T wave.

The *P-R interval* is measured from the beginning of the P wave to the beginning of the Q wave, or to the beginning of the R wave if no Q wave is present, and represents the time required for the impulse to travel through the atria and conduction system to the Purkinje fibers. In

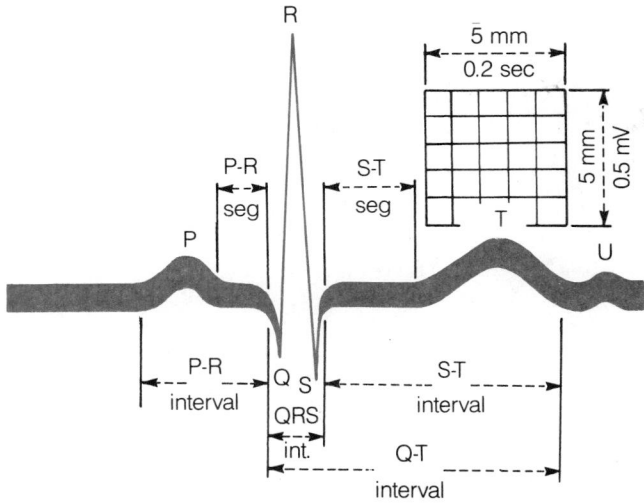

Figure 28-4. Measuring complex components.

adults, the P–R interval normally ranges from 0.12 second to 0.20 second in duration.

The QRS complex is measured from the beginning of the Q wave, or the R wave if no Q wave is present, to the end of the S wave. The QRS complex is normally 0.04 to 0.10 second in duration.

The Q–T interval, which represents electrical systole, is measured from the beginning of the Q wave, or R wave if no Q wave is present, to the end of the T wave. The Q–T interval varies with heart rate, is usually less than half the R–R interval (measured from the beginning of one R wave to the beginning of the next R wave), and usually is 0.32 to 0.40 second in duration if the heart rate is 65 to 95.

Determination of Heart Rate From ECG

Heart rate can be obtained from the ECG strip by several methods. The first, and most accurate, if the rhythm is regular, is to count the number of 0.04-second intervals (0.04 second equals one small box) between two R waves, then divide 1500 by that number. (There are 1500 0.04-second-interval boxes in a 1-minute strip) (Fig. 28-5, *A*).

The second method for computing heart rate, especially useful when the rhythm is irregular, is to count the number of R–R intervals in 6 seconds and multiply that number by 10. The ECG paper is usually marked at 3-second intervals (15 large boxes, horizontally) by a vertical line at the top of the paper (Fig. 28-5, *B*). The R–R intervals are counted, not QRS complexes. If QRS complexes were counted, the computed heart rate might be inaccurately high.

Mean Axis

Impulse formation usually begins in the SA node. Conduction of this impulse throughout the heart results in the propagation of thousands of electrical potentials in many directions in space. Over 80% of these potentials are cancelled out by opposing forces, and only the net result is recorded. The mean vector at a given time in the cardiac cycle represents the sum of electrical potentials as well as the mean magnitude, direction, and polarity. The mean P, QRS, and T vectors can be determined and are usually downward and to the left.

Procedure for Obtaining an Electrocardiogram

To obtain an ECG, the electrodes are placed on the patient as shown in Figure 28-6. With the electrodes in these positions, the first six leads can be obtained. To ensure good contact between the skin and the electrode, the electrodes are placed on a flat surface just above the wrists and ankles,

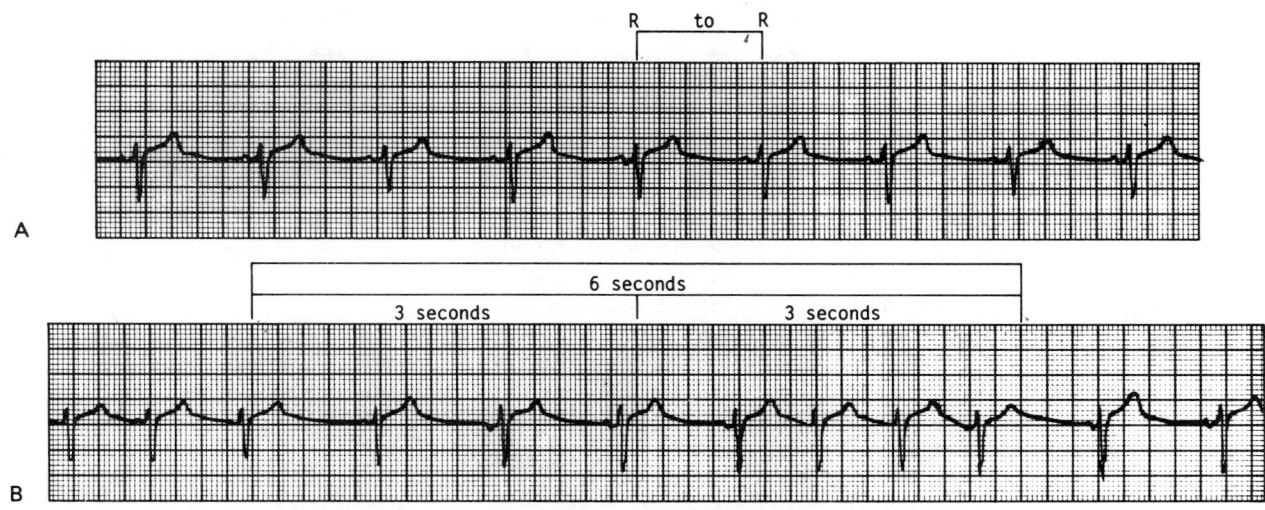

Figure 28-5. (*A*) Heart rate determination for a regular rhythm. There are approximately 25 little boxes between two R waves. 1500 divided by this number equals 60. The heart rate is 60. There are five large boxes between R waves, thus the rate is approximately 60. (*B*) Heart rate determination if the rhythm is irregular. There are approximately seven R–R intervals in 6 seconds. Seven times 10 equals 70. The heart rate is 70. (From Underhill SL et al: Cardiac Nursing, p 201. Philadelphia, JB Lippincott, 1982.)

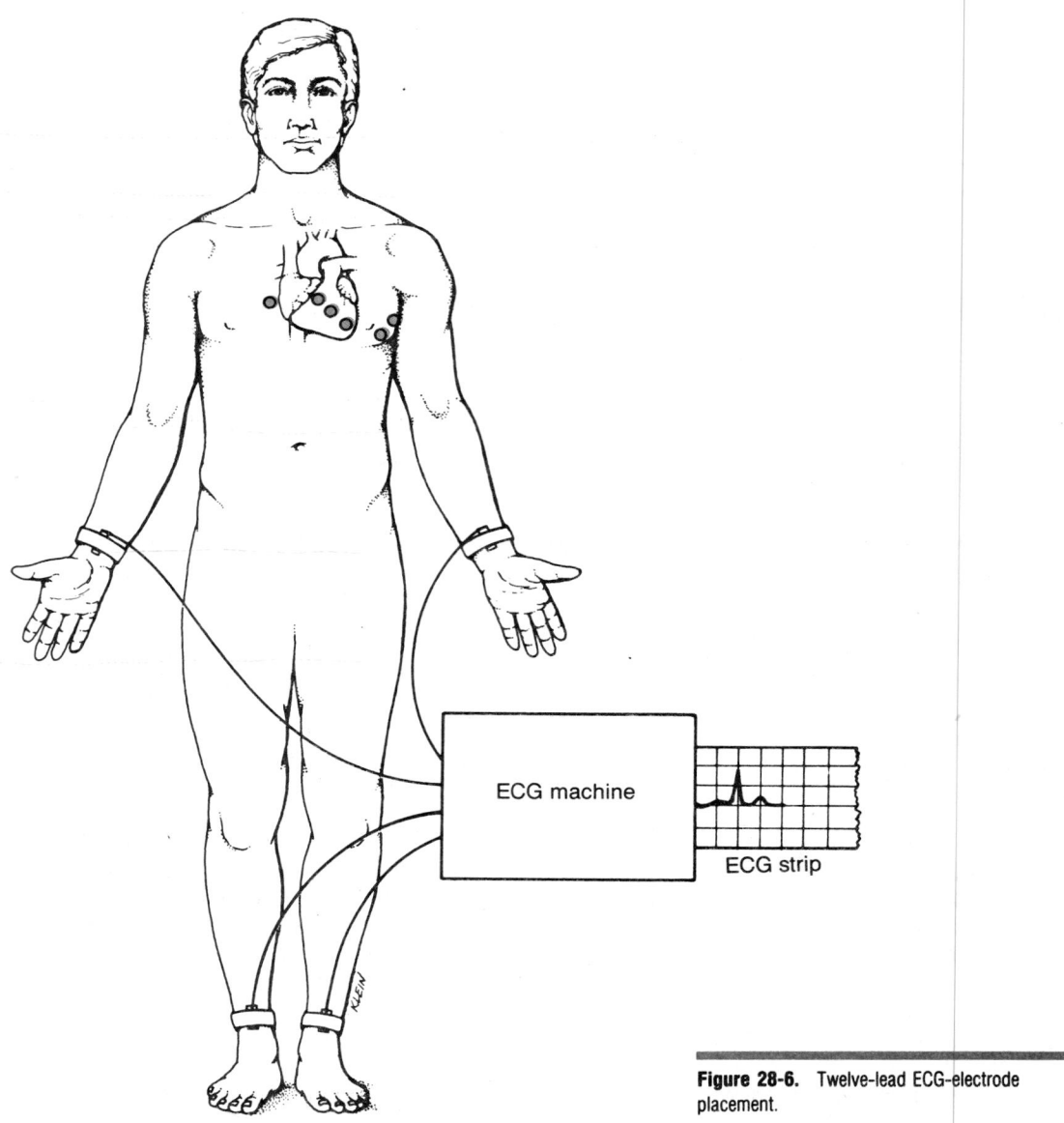

Figure 28-6. Twelve-lead ECG-electrode placement.

and electrode paste or an alcohol sponge is placed under each electrode. The limb straps are adjusted firmly to hold the electrode in place. These straps should not pinch the patient's skin or be so tight as to decrease circulation distal to the strap. The lead selected on the machine is then turned on to record each of the six leads. Next, the six V leads are obtained by moving the chest leads in the six precordial positions. A lead selector switch is turned to "V" to record each of these leads. The arm and leg electrodes must be attached to the patient in order to obtain the V leads. There are some ECG machines that record three or six leads simultaneously.

Each ECG should include the following identifying information:

1. Patient name and identification number
2. Location, date, and time of the recording

3. Patient age, sex, and cardiac medications
4. Race, body build (weight and height measurements), blood pressure, tentative clinical diagnosis, clinical status, and noncardiac medications, such as phenothiazines
5. Any unusual position of the patient during the recording, or the presence of thoracic deformities, amputation, respiratory distress, or muscle tremor

Electrocardiographic Apparatus

In addition to the standard 12-lead ECG, the ECG can be used in other ways. One lead of the ECG can be continuously monitored on an oscilloscope (a fluorescent screen). The waveform from this lead can be written out to provide a permanent record. Continuous ECG monitoring is especially useful in the cardiac care unit to detect arrhythmias.

One lead of the ECG can be monitored by a small tape recorder (Holter Recorder) and recorded on a continuous (1–24 hours) magnetic tape recording. The patient can then be monitored during the day or night to detect arrhythmias or evidence of myocardial ischemia during activities of daily living. The tape recorder weighs approximately 2 pounds and can be carried over the shoulder. The patient keeps a diary of his activity, noting the time of any symptoms, experiences, or any unusual activities performed. The tape recording is then examined (using a specialized instrument called a scanner), analyzed, and interpreted. Evidence obtained in this way is helpful in diagnosing arrhythmias and myocardial ischemia and in evaluating therapy such as antiarrhythmic and antianginal drugs or pacemaker function.

The ECG can also be transmitted by telemetry (telephone lines), thus freeing the patient from a cable connected to the oscilloscope. The ECG signal can then be monitored miles away.

Myocardial Ischemia, Injury, and Infarction
Myocardial Ischemia and Injury. Myocardial ischemia causes the T wave to be larger and inverted owing to altered late repolarization. Possibly, the ischemic region remains depolarized, whereas adjacent areas have returned to the resting state. The change is seen in the leads closest to the involved surface of the heart. Ischemia also causes ST segment changes. If there is epicardial myocardial injury, the injured cells depolarize normally but repolarize more rapidly than do normal cells. Thus, the ST segment is elevated. If the myocardial injury is on the endocardial surface, then the ST segment is depressed (1 mm or more) in the leads where the positive electrode faces the area of injury. With injury, the ST segment depression is horizontal or slopes downward and is 0.08 second in duration.

Myocardial Infarction. Myocardial infarction usually causes abnormal Q waves within 1 to 3 days because of the absence of depolarization current from necrotic tissue, and opposing currents from other parts of the heart. An abnormal Q wave is 0.04 second or longer in duration and is, in depth, 25% of the R wave (provided the R wave itself exceeds 5 mm). Old transmural MI can usually be determined by significant Q waves without ST segment and T wave changes or by reduced voltage of the R wave. In some patients, Q waves disappear. With a transmural MI (involving all three layers of the heart), injury and ischemic changes are also present (Fig. 28-7). The ST segment elevation lasts a few days to 2 weeks. The T wave becomes large and symmetric for 24 hours, then inverts within 1 to 3 days for 1 to 2 weeks. During recovery from an MI, the ST segment often is first to return to normal (1–6 weeks), then the T wave (weeks to months). Q wave alterations are usually permanent (Fig. 28-8).

Electrolyte Imbalance

Electrolyte imbalances also affect the ECG. A discussion of electrolyte balance abnormalities can be found in Chapter 9.

Hypokalemia. Hypokalemia (serum K^+ less than 3.0 mEq/liter) may produce the following changes:

1. U wave equal to or higher than T wave (Fig. 28-9)
2. Diminution of T wave (flat or inverted)
3. Peaked P wave in leads II, III, and aVF
4. ST segment shortening and depression (similar to the effects of digitalis)
5. Ventricular ectopic beats
6. Q–T interval prolonged

The action of digitalis is potentiated by hypokalemia.

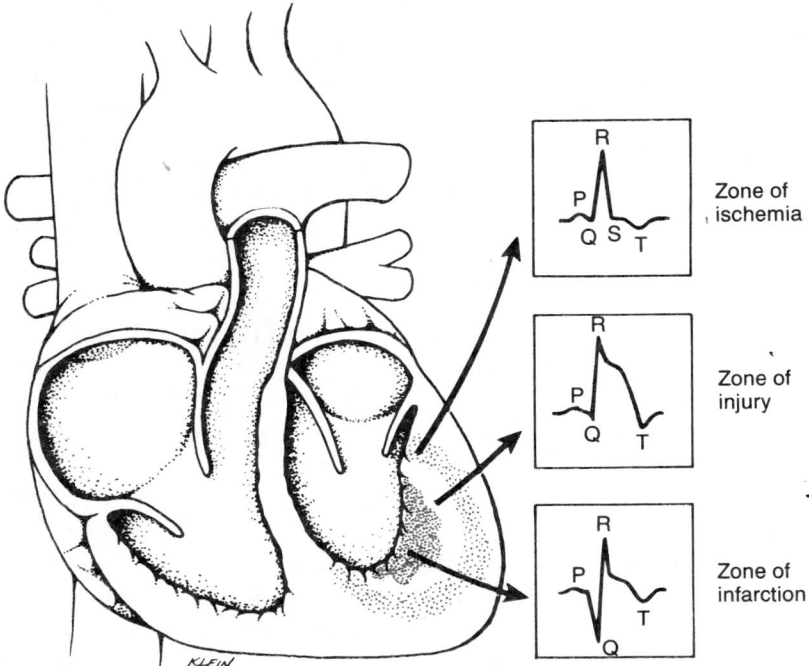

Figure 28-7. Effects of ischemia, injury, and infarction on ECG recording. Ischemia causes inversion of T wave because of altered repolarization. Cardiac muscle injury causes elevation of the ST segment. Infarction causes Q or Q–S waves because of the absence of depolarization current from the dead tissue and opposing currents from other parts of the heart.

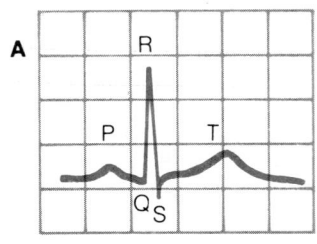

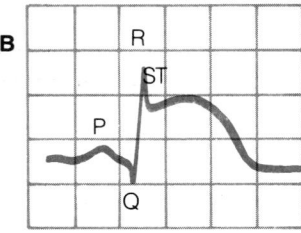

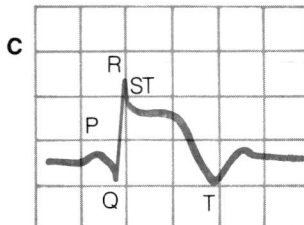

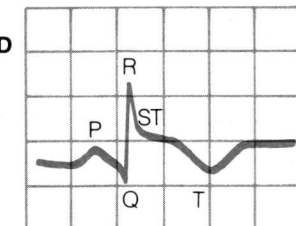

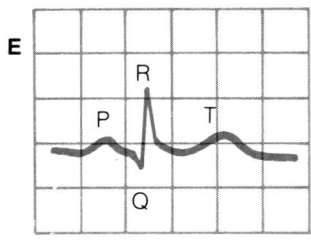

Figure 28-8. ECG interpretation of myocardial infarction. *A.* Normal tracing. *B.* Hours after infarction, the ST segment becomes elevated. *C.* Hours to days later, the T wave inverts and the Q wave may become larger. *D.* Days to weeks later, the ST segment returns to near-normal. *E.* Lastly, the T wave becomes upright again, but the Q wave may remain permanently large.

Hyperkalemia.   Hyperkalemia (serum K^+ greater than 5 mEq/liter) will produce the following changes (Fig. 28-10):

1. Tall, tented, symmetric, narrow T waves (seen best in precordial leads). This requires serum K^+ greater than 6 mEq/liter to 7 mEq/liter.

2. P waves are flat and broad (serum K^+ greater than 7.0 mEq/liter) or disappear completely (serum K^+ greater than 8.8 mEq/liter).

3. Atrioventricular block (usually, first degree)

4. The QRS complex widens (serum K^+ greater than 6.5 mEq/liter) because of wide S waves in the lateral precordium (V_{5-6}). If the cause goes untreated, the patient may progress from sinus bradycardia to first-degree AV block, through junctional and idioventricular rhythms, to ventricular fibrillation or asystole.

5. Shortening of the Q–T interval

Hypocalcemia.   Hypocalcemia (serum Ca^{2+} less than 6.1 mg/100 ml) will produce the following effects (Fig. 28-11):

1. Q–T interval prolonged; increased ST segment duration
2. Flat or inverted T wave
3. Arrhythmias

Hypercalcemia.   Hypercalcemia (serum Ca^{2+} greater than 16 mg/100 ml) may produce these effects, which look like digitalis effect:

1. Q–T interval shortens; ST segments sag and shorten
2. T waves invert
3. Ventricular arrhythmias

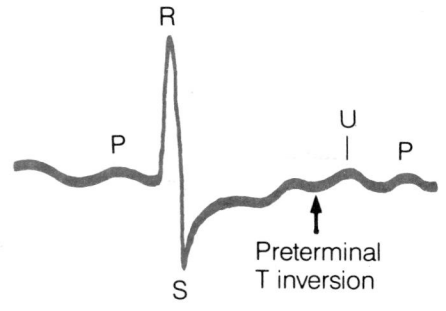

Figure 28-9. ECG of hypokalemia. Hypokalemia is manifested in the ECG by T wave flattening, ST depression, preterminal T wave inversion, and heightening of the U wave.

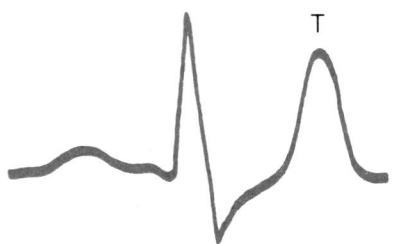

Figure 28-10. ECG of hyperkalemia. The T wave becomes tall, symmetrical, and tent-shaped. There is ST depression, the U wave disappears, the P wave flattens, and both the P–R and QRS intervals prolong.

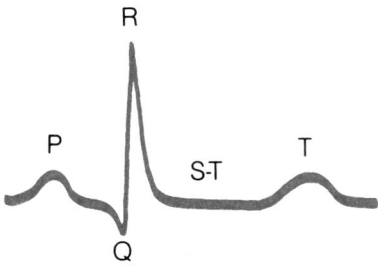

Figure 28-11. ECG of hypocalcemia. Hypocalcemia is manifested by prolonged Q–T interval, prolonged ST segment, and normal T waves.

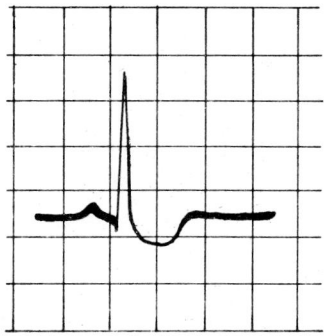

Figure 28-12. Digitalis effect. Notice the rounded, scooped appearance of the ST segment.

The patient with potassium or calcium imbalances may or may not exhibit the ECG changes mentioned. But such changes, if seen, alert the nurse to suspect electrolyte abnormalities, and they must be seen in the context of what is already known about the patient.

Magnesium. Magnesium (Mg^{2+}) concentration in the body does not seem to affect the ECG. Electrocardiographic changes produced by hypocalcemia are augmented if Mg^{2+} concentration is also low, and they tend to be reversed if Mg^{2+} concentrations are increased above normal.

Effects of Drugs on the ECG

Digitalis. Digitalis slows the heart rate (negative chronotropic effect) and decreases AV conduction (negative dromotropic effect). Digitalis also

1. Shortens ventricular activation time
2. Shortens the Q–T interval
3. Depresses the ST segments and makes them sag (Fig. 28-12)
4. In large doses, can decrease the T wave amplitude, cause sinus bradycardia (less than a rate of 50), and prolong the P–R interval greater than 0.24 second
5. In large doses, can cause atrial, junctional, and ventricular extrasystoles (bigeminy) and conduction abnormalities
6. Increases amplitude of U wave

Quinidine and Procainamide. Quinidine and procainamide cause the following effects on the ECG:

1. A slightly prolonged P–R interval
2. A wide QRS complex, thus prolonging the Q–T interval; therapeutic levels can result in a QRS complex of 0.11 second.
3. A depressed, widened, and notched T wave
4. Toxicity can cause SA or AV block, ventricular arrhythmias, and a 50% increase in the QRS complex duration.
5. Inverted T wave

▷ Arrhythmias

An arrhythmia, any cardiac rhythm that is not normal sinus rhythm at a normal rate, can be determined from the ECG. An arrhythmia may result from altered impulse formation or altered impulse conduction or both. The characteristics of normal sinus rhythm (Fig. 28-13) are:

1. Rate: 60 to 100 beats per minute
2. P waves: Precede each QRS complex; P–R interval normal (0.12 second to 0.20 second).
3. QRS complex: Usually has a normal interval (0.04 second to 0.10 second)
4. Conduction: Through the atria, AV node, and ventricles, is usually normal

Arrhythmias Originating in the Sinus Node

Sinus Bradycardia

Sinus bradycardia may be due to vagal stimulation, digitalis intoxication, increased intracranial pressure, or MI involving the SA nodal artery. It is also seen in highly trained athletes, in persons in severe pain, in persons under medication (propranolol, reserpine, methyldopa), in hypoendocrine states (myxedema, Addison's disease, panhypopituitarism), in anorexia nervosa, in hypothermia, and after surgical damage to the SA node.

The following are characteristics of this arrhythmia (Fig. 28-14):

1. Rate: 40 to 60 beats per minute
2. P waves: Precede each QRS complex; P–R interval normal
3. QRS complex: Usually normal
4. Conduction: Usually normal
5. Rhythm: Regular

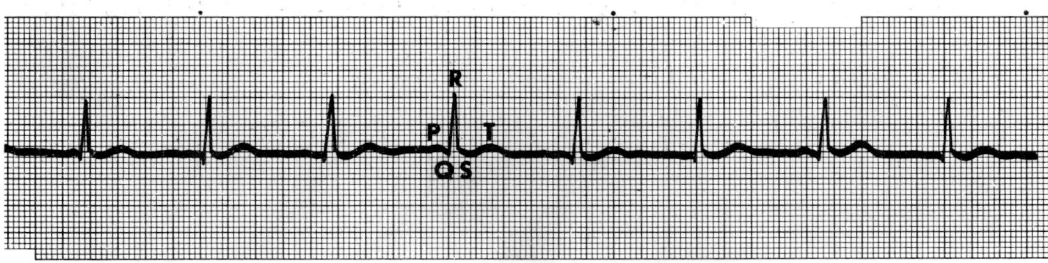

Figure 28-13. Normal electrocardiogram.

All aspects of sinus bradycardia should be the same as those of normal sinus rhythm, except for the rate. If slow heart rate is causing significant hemodynamic changes with resultant syncope (fainting from insufficient flow of blood to the brain), angina, or ectopic arrhythmias, then treatment is directed toward increasing heart rate. If the decrease in heart rate is due to vagal stimulation, attempts should be made to prevent further vagal stimulation. If the patient has digitalis intoxication, then digitalis should be withheld. If atropine does not increase heart rate, then the slow rate is not caused by vagal stimulation.

Sinus Tachycardia

Sinus tachycardia may be caused by fever, acute blood loss, anemia, shock, exercise, congestive heart failure (CHF), pain, hypermetabolic states, anxiety, or sympathomimetic or parasympatholytic drugs. The ECG pattern is as follows (Fig. 28-15):

1. Rate: 100 to 180 beats per minute
2. P waves: Precede each QRS complex; may be buried in the preceding T wave; P–R interval normal
3. QRS complex: Usually has a normal interval
4. Conduction: Usually normal
5. Rhythm: Regular

All aspects of sinus tachycardia should be the same as those of normal sinus rhythm, except for the rate.

Treatment is usually directed at the primary cause. Carotid sinus pressure may be effective in slowing the rate temporarily, and thereby help to rule out other arrhythmias. As heart rate increases, diastolic filling time decreases, resulting in reduced coronary artery filling and in less ventricular diastolic filling (decreased preload).

Sinus Arrhythmia

Sinus arrhythmia is the most frequent heart rhythm and occurs as a normal phenomenon. It commonly occurs in the young or aged, especially with slower heart rates or following enhanced vagal tone from digitalis or morphine. It is absent in the neonate and is commonly found in patients with Cheyne–Stokes respiration. The sinus rate increases with inspiration and decreases with expiration.

This arrhythmia is characterized by the following ECG changes (Fig. 28-16):

1. Rate: 60 to 100 beats per minute
2. P waves: Precede each QRS; P–R interval normal
3. QRS complex: Usually normal
4. Conduction: Usually normal
5. Rhythm: May be related to breathing (rate increases with inspiration and decreases with expiration), or the irregularity may be unrelated to respiration. The irregularity can best be seen by measuring R–R intervals.

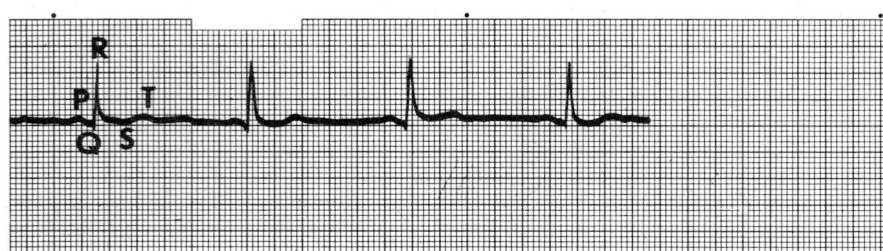

Figure 28-14. Sinus bradycardia.

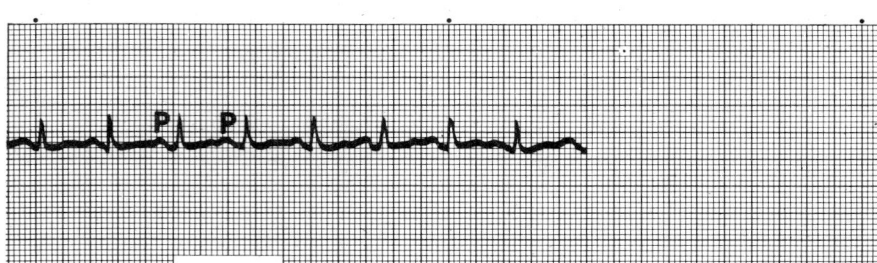

Figure 28-15. Sinus tachycardia.

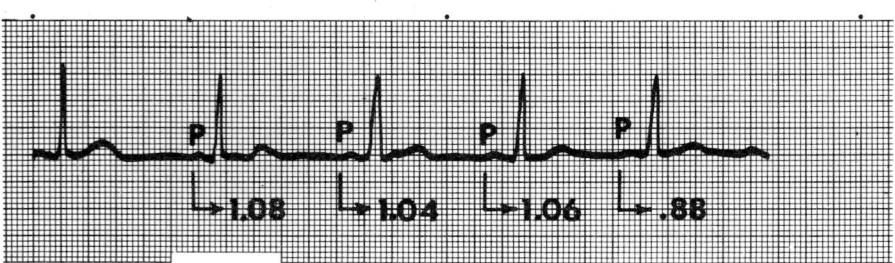

Figure 28-16. Sinus arrhythmia.

Treatment is usually not necessary, but increasing the heart rate with exercise or sympathomimetic drugs will in many cases abolish this arrhythmia.

Sinus Node Arrest

Sinus node arrest can occur from excessive carotid sinus pressure, vagal stimulation, vomiting, straining at stool, involvement of the sinus node or sinus node artery by acute MI, digitalis toxicity, or degenerative forms of fibrosis.

Sinus arrest within normal sinus rhythm has the following characteristics:

1. Ventricular rate: Usually 60 to 100 beats per minute, but frequently in the bradycardia range (fewer than 60 beats per minute)
2. P waves: When P waves are present, the P–R interval is usually normal. If escape beats from the junction or ventricle occur, the P wave may be absent or inverted before or after the QRS complex.
3. QRS complex: Not present during sinus arrest unless escape beats occur
4. Ventricular conduction: Usually normal when it occurs
5. Rhythm: Irregular. Escape beats from the junctional and ventricular areas are common. The variation will be found by measuring the R–R intervals. The P–P intervals will be variable.

Treatment is directed toward normalizing heart rate and eliminating the cause.

Arrhythmias Originating in the Atrial Muscle

Arrhythmias originating in the atrial muscle are the following: premature atrial contractions (PACs); wandering atrial pacemaker (WAP); multifocal atrial tachycardia (MAT); paroxysmal atrial tachycardia (PAT); atrial flutter; atrial fibrillation; atrial flutter–fibrillation.

Premature Atrial Contractions

Premature atrial contractions may be due to atrial muscle irritability caused by caffeine; alcohol; nicotine; stretched atrial myocardium as in congestive heart failure (CHF); stress or anxiety; hypokalemia; atrial ischemia, injury, or infarction; and hypermetabolic states.

Premature atrial contractions have the following characteristics (Fig. 28-17):

1. Rate: 60 to 100 beats per minute
2. P waves: Usually have a configuration different from that of the P waves that originate in the SA node. Another site in the atria has become irritable (enhanced automaticity) and fires before the normal firing time of the SA node. P–R interval may vary from the P–R intervals of impulses originating in the SA node.
3. QRS complex: May be normal, aberrant, or absent. If the ventricles have completed their repolarization phase, they can respond to this early stimulus from the atria.
4. Conduction: Usually normal
5. Rhythm: Regular, except when the PACs occur. The P wave will be early in the cycle and usually will not have a complete compensatory pause. (Time between the preceding complex and the following complex is less than the time for two R–R intervals.)

Premature atrial contractions are frequently seen in normal hearts. The patient may say that his heart skipped a beat. A pulse deficit (the difference between apical and radial pulse rate) may exist. If PACs are infrequent, no treatment is necessary. If they are frequent (more than six per minute) or occur during atrial repolarization, this may herald more serious arrhythmias, such as atrial fibrillation. Again, treatment is directed toward the cause.

Wandering Atrial Pacemaker

Wandering atrial pacemaker occurs when there is variation in the vagal tone at the SA node or when there are changes in sympathetic stimulation. The patient is usually unaware of the arrhythmia. Wandering atrial pacemaker is characterized by the following (Fig. 28-18):

1. Rate: 60 to 100 beats per minute (If the rate is greater than 100, then it is called multifocal atrial tachycardia.)
2. P waves: Will vary from impulse to impulse in size and configuration. Stimulus coming from the SA node or close to it will produce normal-looking P waves. As the pacemaker wanders closer to the AV node, the P waves will become flatter or even inverted. The P–R interval varies, depending on the closeness of the pacemaker to the AV node. At least three different P waves must be seen.
3. QRS complex: Usually normal
4. Conduction: Conduction from the AV node through the ventricles will usually be normal.

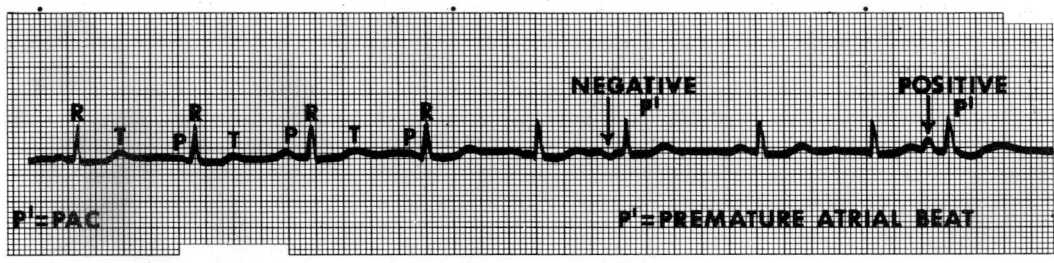

Figure 28-17. Premature atrial contraction.

5. Rhythm: The R–R intervals may vary because of variations in the P–R intervals.

There usually is no need for treatment. Observe for digitalis intoxication. If decreases in heart rate alter cardiac output significantly, then sympathomimetic or parasympatholytic drugs can be used. If the heart rate is over 100 beats per minute (multifocal atrial tachycardia), treatment is directed toward eliminating the cause and decreasing the heart rate with a drug such as propranolol.

Paroxysmal Atrial Tachycardia

Paroxysmal atrial tachycardia is characterized by abrupt onset and abrupt cessation. Rhythm may be triggered by emotions, tobacco, caffeine, fatigue, sympathomimetic drugs, or alcohol. Paroxysmal atrial tachycardia is not usually associated with organic heart disease. The rapid rate may produce angina owing to decreased coronary artery filling. Cardiac output is reduced and congestive heart failure may occur. The patient frequently does not tolerate this rhythm for long periods.

Paroxysmal atrial tachycardia is characterized by the following (Fig. 28-19):

1. Rate: 150 to 250 beats per minute
2. P waves: Ectopic and slightly to grossly normal; may be found in the preceding T wave; P–R interval shortened (less than 0.12 second)
3. QRS complex: Usually normal, but may be distorted if aberrant conduction is present
4. Conduction: Usually normal
5. Rhythm: Regular

The patient may not be aware of paroxysmal atrial tachycardia. Treatment is directed toward eliminating the cause and decreasing the heart rate. Morphine sedation slows the rate without further treatment. Carotid sinus pressure usu-

ally slows the rate or stops the attack and is usually more effective after digitalis or pressors. The use of vasopressors has a reflex effect on the carotid sinus by elevating the blood pressure and thus slowing the heart rate. Short-acting digitalis preparations may be used. Propranolol may be tried if digitalis is unsuccessful. Quinidine may be effective. Cardioversion may be necessary if the patient does not tolerate the fast heart rate.

Atrial Flutter

Atrial flutter (rapid, regular, "fluttering" of the atrium) is usually associated with rheumatic heart disease, atherosclerotic heart disease, thyrotoxicosis, acute cor pulmonale, congestive heart failure, and MI. Any ventricular response of 150 should be suspect for atrial flutter.

Atrial flutter is characterized by the following:

1. Rate: Atrial rate 250 to 350 beats per minute; most commonly 300. The ventricular rate will usually show some degree of block with the ventricle responding in a 2:1 or 4:1 (Fig. 28-20) pattern, rarely 3:1. There may be variations in the block pattern, particularly if treatment has been started.
2. P waves: Characterized by the F waves (flutter waves seen between R waves) occurring in a regular fashion and in a saw-tooth or picket-fence pattern. One F wave usually falls within the QRS-T complex.
3. QRS complex: Usually normal, except where aberrant conduction is present
4. Conduction: Usually normal
5. Rhythm: Usually regular, but irregularities in the block pattern are not uncommon.

Treatment is directed toward eliminating the cause, decreasing the rate of ventricular response, and decreasing atrial myocardial irritability. If quinidine is administered,

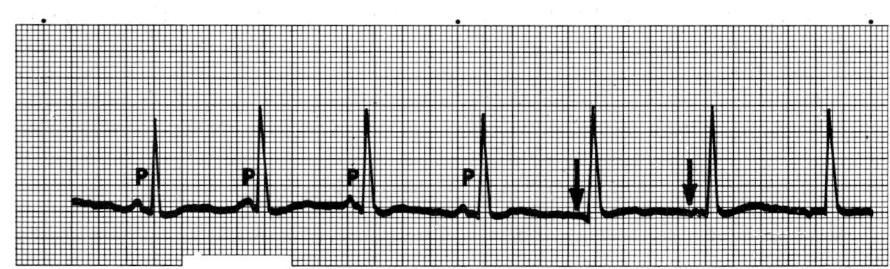

Figure 28-18. Wandering pacemaker.

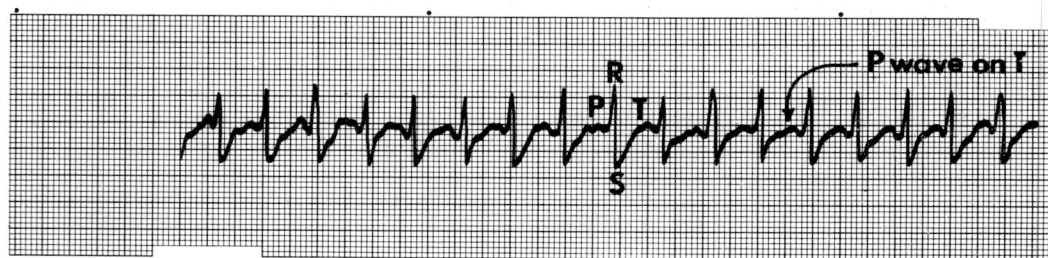

Figure 28-19. Atrial tachycardia.

1:1 conduction could occur unless a negative dromotropic effect is present. Carotid sinus massage may unmask the flutter waves and increase the flutter rate. Cardioversion can usually be achieved with low, direct current shock (10–50 watt-seconds).

Atrial Fibrillation

Atrial fibrillation (disorganized and uncoordinated twitching of atrial musculature) is usually associated with atherosclerotic heart disease, rheumatic heart disease, CHF, thyrotoxicosis, cor pulmonale, and congenital heart disease.

Atrial fibrillation (Fig. 28-21) is characterized by the following:

1. Rate: An atrial rate of 350 to 600 beats per minute; ventricular response usually 120 to 200 beats per minute
2. P waves: No discernible P waves; irregular undulation, termed fibrillary or "f" waves, is seen; P–R interval cannot be measured
3. QRS complex: Usually normal
4. Conduction: Usually normal through the ventricles. Characterized by an irregular ventricular response, because the AV node is incapable of responding to the rapid atrial rate. Impulses that are transmitted cause the ventricles to respond irregularly.
5. Rhythm: Irregular and usually rapid, unless controlled. Irregularity of rhythm is due to concealed conduction within the AV node.

A rapid ventricular response reduces the time for ventricular filling and hence the stroke volume. The atrial kick, which is 25% to 30% of the cardiac output, is also lost. Congestive heart failure frequently follows. Coarse atrial fibrillation (slower atrial rate) is more easily converted than fine atrial fibrillation (faster atrial rate). There is usually a

pulse deficit. Treatment is directed toward eliminating the cause, decreasing the atrial irritability, and decreasing the rate of the ventricular response. In patients with chronic atrial fibrillation, anticoagulant therapy may be used to prevent thromboemboli from forming in the atria.

Sometimes a mixture of atrial flutter and atrial fibrillation is seen, and some call this atrial flutter–fibrillation. Others refer to this as coarse atrial fibrillation. Such an arrhythmia is best classified as atrial fibrillation when the criteria for atrial flutter are not satisfied.

Tachycardia–Bradycardia Syndrome

Tachycardia–bradycardia syndrome is characterized by tachyarrhythmias (paroxysmal atrial fibrillation, flutter, or tachycardia) followed by SA block or sinus arrest, resulting in Stokes–Adams attacks. Clinical correlation with this syndrome has been found with coronary atherosclerosis, amyloidosis, renal insufficiency with azotemia, and trauma following open heart surgery. Some have used the tachycardia-bradycardia syndrome and sick sinus syndrome interchangeably, but this is not totally accurate, because the sick sinus syndrome includes a variety of sinus and atrial arrhythmias and only indicates a "sick" sinus node. In tachycardia–bradycardia syndrome, not only is the sinus node sick, but the impulse formation at the AV node is depressed as well.

Marked bradycardia (heart rate of fewer than 20 beats per minute or prolonged asystole, exceeding 10 seconds) results in cerebral ischemia. Hence, lightheadedness, dizziness, syncope, or convulsions may occur. The tachycardia may cause such symptoms as palpitations, weakness, or chest pain. Treatment is directed toward suppressing the tachycardia with medications (quinidine, procainamide, digitalis, and propranolol) and maintaining an adequate heart rate with a pacemaker.

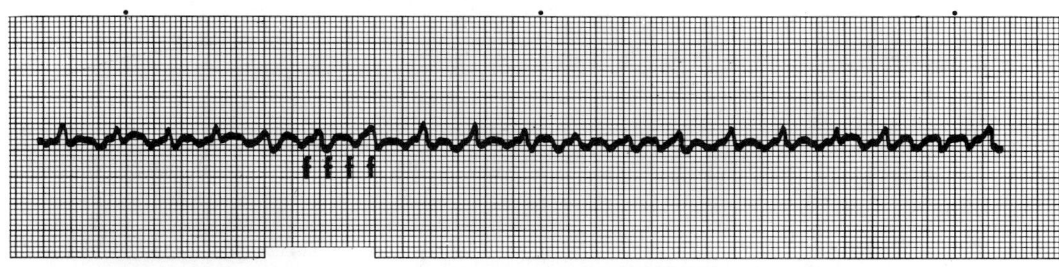

Figure 28-20.   Atrial flutter with 2:1 block.

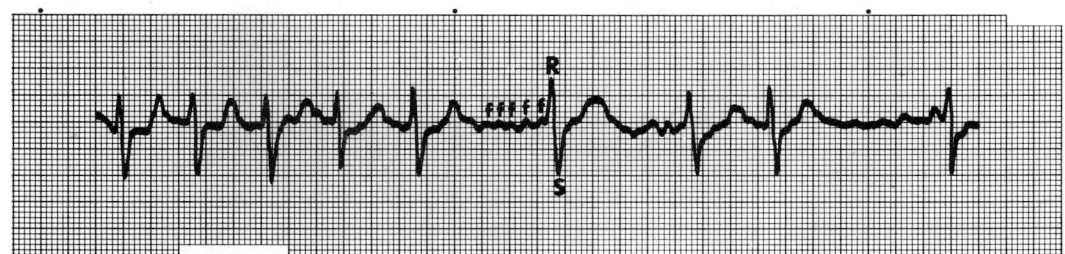

Figure 28-21.   Atrial fibrillation.

Arrhythmias Originating in the Junction

Arrhythmias originating in the junction (area between the atria and ventricles around the AV node) are as follows: junctional rhythm, premature junctional contraction, accelerated junctional tachycardia, and paroxysmal junctional tachycardia.

Junctional Rhythm

A junctional rhythm may occur if there is digitalis intoxication or sinus node disease resulting in a decreased rate of the sinus node. Because the sinus rate is so slow, the junction may compete to be the pacemaker. Junctional rhythm has the following characteristics:

1. Rate: 40 to 60 beats per minute
2. P waves: Usually inverted and may occur before, during, or after the QRS complex, depending on the location of the pacemaker in the junctional tissue. The junctional tissue delays antegrade and retrograde conduction.
3. QRS complex: Normal
4. Conduction: The atria are usually stimulated by the junctional tissue, resulting in an inverted P wave (called retrograde conduction). The conduction from the junctional tissue through the ventricles is usually normal (called antegrade conduction).
5. Rhythm: Usually regular

There is usually no need for treatment, unless a reduction in the heart rate alters cardiac output markedly. If cardiac output decreases so that chest pain, syncope, or arrhythmias occur, sympathomimetic or parasympatholytic drugs may be used. Digitalis should be withheld. Quinidine, procainamide, phenytoin, propranolol, hyperkalemia, and vagal stimulation depress junctional escape centers.

Premature Junctional Contractions

Premature junctional contractions (PJCs) occur because of increased irritability of the junctional tissue. Irritability can be due to digitalis intoxication or to coronary artery disease, resulting in decreased flow through the AV nodal artery. PJCs have the following characteristics:

1. Rate: 60 to 100 beats per minute if the basic rhythm is normal sinus rhythm
2. P waves: May occur before, during, or after the QRS complex, depending on the location of the pacemaker in the junctional tissue. The P–R intervals vary and are shorter than normal (less than 0.12 second).
3. QRS complex: May be normal or aberrant
4. Conduction: The atria are stimulated in a retrograde fashion. The ventricular conduction is usually normal.
5. Rhythm: Regular, except for the premature contraction. The compensatory pause is usually incomplete. Usually, no treatment is indicated. Digitalis should be withheld. If PJCs occur more frequently than six per minute, an antiarrhythmic drug may be prescribed.

Accelerated Junctional Rhythm and Paroxysmal Junctional Tachycardia

In these rhythms, irritability in the junctional area has increased, resulting in a faster rate. Characteristics of accelerated junctional rhythm and paroxysmal junctional tachycardia are as follows:

1. Origin: Junctional tissue
2. Rate: Accelerated junctional rhythm, 60 to 100 beats per minute; paroxysmal junctional tachycardia, 100 to 250 beats per minute.
3. P waves: The position of the P wave in relation to the QRS complex will vary according to the location of the pacemaker in the junctional tissue. The configuration of the P wave will also vary accordingly. If the P wave is seen, it is usually inverted.
4. QRS complex: May be normal or aberrant
5. Conduction: Retrograde to the atria; normal through the ventricles
6. Rhythm: Regular

If the patient is on digitalis, it should be withheld until digitalis intoxication is ruled out, since this is a very common arrhythmia associated with digitalis intoxication. If the patient is not on digitalis, it may be given to increase AV conduction time. If the patient does not tolerate the rate, as demonstrated by signs and symptoms of a decreased cardiac output, then cardioversion may be necessary. This arrhythmia must be documented on the ECG to differentiate from sinus tachycardia or paroxysmal atrial tachycardia. When a rapid junctional rhythm occurs with a bundle branch conduction defect, it is difficult to distinguish this rhythm from ventricular tachycardia.

Arrhythmias Originating in the Ventricular Muscle

Arrhythmias originating in the ventricular muscle are the following: premature ventricular contractions, ventricular bigeminy, accelerated ventricular tachycardia, ventricular tachycardia, ventricular flutter, ventricular fibrillation, and ventricular asystole.

Premature Ventricular Contractions

Premature ventricular contractions (PVCs) are the result of increased automaticity of the ventricular muscle cells. PVCs can be due to digitalis intoxication, hypoxia, myocardial stretch, hypokalemia, fever, acidosis, exercise, or increased circulating catecholamines.

Infrequent PVCs are not serious in themselves. Usually, the patient feels a palpitating sensation, but has no other complaints. However, the concern lies in that these premature contractions may lead to more serious ventricular arrhythmias.

In the patient with acute MI, PVCs are considered serious precursors of ventricular tachycardia and ventricular fibrillation when they (1) occur in increasing number, more than six per minute; (2) are multifocal; (3) occur in pairs or triplets; and (4) come on the T wave (R on T).

PVCs (Fig. 28-22) have the following characteristics:

1. Rate: 60 to 100 beats per minute
2. P wave: May be completely obscured, hidden in the QRS complex of the premature beat. The sinus rhythm is usually uninterrupted, resulting in a complete compensatory pause. If a premature P wave is seen before

the wide QRS complex, the impulse is probably a premature supraventricular beat (an impulse that originates in the atria or junction) with aberration and not a PVC.

3. QRS complex: Usually wide and bizarre. Usually longer than 0.10 second in duration. May have the same focus in the ventricle, or may have a wide variety of configurations if occurring from multiple foci in the ventricles.
4. Conduction: Occasionally retrograde through the junctional tissue and atria
5. Rhythm: Irregular when the premature beat occurs

In order to decrease the myocardial irritability, the cause must be determined and, if possible, corrected. An antiarrhythmic drug may be useful for immediate and possibly long-term therapy.

Ventricular Bigeminy

Ventricular bigeminy is frequently associated with digitalis excess, coronary artery disease, acute MI, and CHF. The term bigeminy refers to a condition in which every other beat is premature.

Ventricular bigeminy (Fig. 28-23) has the following characteristics:

1. Rate: May occur at any heart rate, but rate is usually less than 90 beats per minute
2. P waves: The same as described for PVCs; may be hidden within the QRS complex
3. QRS complex: Every other beat is a PVC with a wide, bizarre QRS complex and a complete compensatory pause.
4. Conduction: The sinus beats are conducted from the sinus node in a normal fashion, but alternating PVCs start in the ventricles and may have retrograde conduction through the junctional tissue and atria.
5. Rhythm: Irregular

If the ectopic beats or normal beat occur every third beat, this is termed trigeminy; every fourth beat, quadrigeminy.

The treatment for ventricular bigeminy is the same as for PVCs. Since the underlying cause of ventricular bigeminy is frequently digitalis toxicity, this should be ruled out or treated if present.

Accelerated Ventricular Rhythm and Ventricular Tachycardia

These arrhythmias are caused by increased myocardial irritability, as are PVCs. They are usually associated with coronary artery disease, atherosclerotic heart disease, and rheumatic heart disease, and may precede ventricular fibrillation. Ventricular tachycardia is extremely dangerous and should be considered an emergency. The patient is generally aware of this rapid rhythm and is quite anxious. Accelerated ventricular rhythm and ventricular tachycardia have the following characteristics (Fig. 28-24):

1. Rate: Accelerated ventricular rhythm 40 to 110 beats per minute; ventricular tachycardia 150 to 200 beats per minute
2. P waves: Usually buried in the QRS complex; if seen, they do not necessarily fall in the normal pattern with the QRS. The ventricular contractions are dissociated from the atrial contractions.
3. QRS complex: Have the same configurations as those of a PVC: wide and bizarre, with T waves in the opposite direction. A ventricular beat may fuse with a normal QRS, resulting in a fusion beat. Three or more PVCs in a row constitute ventricular tachycardia.
4. Conduction: Originates in the ventricle, with possible retrograde conduction to the junctional tissue and atria
5. Rhythm: Usually regular, but irregular ventricular tachycardia are also seen. The ventricular rhythm is rapid. The P waves, if seen, are at a slower rate and are regular.

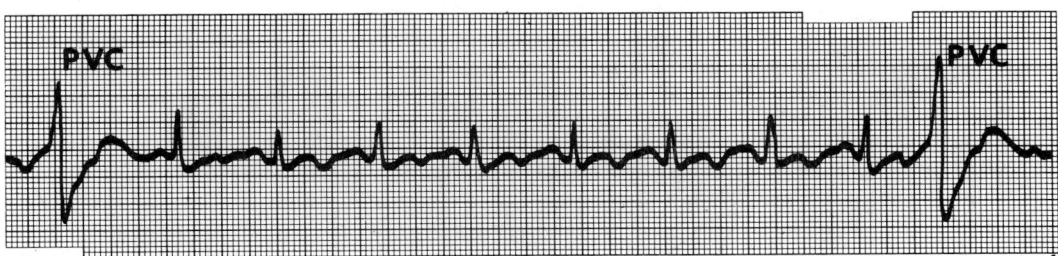

Figure 28-22. Occasional premature ventricular contractions.

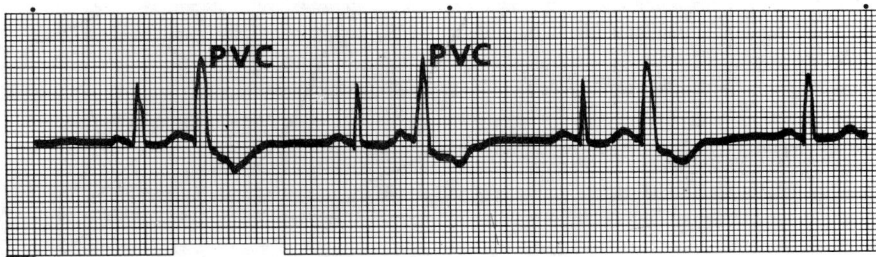

Figure 28-23. Ventricular bigeminy.

There is no association between the atrial rhythm and the ventricular rhythm (AV dissociation).

The patient's tolerance or lack of tolerance of this rapid rhythm will dictate the therapy to be given. The cause of the myocardial irritability must be determined and corrected, if possible. Antiarrhythmic drugs may be used. Cardioversion may be indicated if the reduction in cardiac output is marked.

Cardioversion

Cardioversion is used to terminate arrhythmias that have QRS complexes and is usually an elective procedure. The patient is alert, and informed consent is obtained. The patient is usually given diazepam intravenously prior to cardioversion to promote anesthesia. The amount of voltage used varies from 25 to 400 watt-seconds. Digoxin is usually withheld for 48 hours prior to cardioversion to prevent postcardioversion arrhythmias.

The synchronizer is turned on. The defibrillator is synchronized with a cardiac monitor so that an electrical impulse is discharged during ventricular depolarization (the QRS complex). If the defibrillator were not synchronized, it could discharge during the vulnerable period (T wave) and result in ventricular tachycardia or fibrillation. The synchronizer switch is therefore turned on so that the unit discharges immediately after the onset of the next QRS complex. The "discharge" buttons should be held until the synchronizer fires the defibrillator.

If ventricular fibrillation occurs after cardioversion, the defibrillator must be immediately recharged, the synchronizer turned off, and defibrillation repeated. After use, the defibrillator should be turned off to prevent accidental discharge of the paddles. Oxygen flow should be stopped during precordial shock, if possible, to avoid the hazard of fire.

Indications of a successful response are conversion to sinus rhythm, strong peripheral pulses, and adequate blood pressure. Airway patency should be maintained and the patient's state of consciousness assessed. Vital signs should be obtained at least every 15 minutes for 1 hour, every 30 minutes for 2 hours, then every 4 hours.

Ventricular Flutter

Ventricular flutter has all the characteristics of ventricular tachycardia, but the rate is even faster. The clinical picture is exactly the same as ventricular standstill: the patient may be cyanotic and convulsing; there is no audible heartbeat and no palpable pulse; and the patient is not breathing. This arrhythmia is usually fatal without immediate treatment.

Ventricular flutter (Fig. 28-25) has the following characteristics:

1. Rate: 200 to 400 beats per minute
2. P waves: No visible P waves are seen.
3. QRS complex: Rapid, bizarre, picket-fencelike complexes. T waves are not visible.
4. Conduction: Originates in ventricles. There may be retrograde conduction through the AV node and atria.
5. Rhythm: Not precisely regular

The treatment for ventricular flutter is similar to that for ventricular tachycardia. However, ventricular flutter is a far more acute emergency because the patient is without circulation. This arrhythmia will be fatal unless converted immediately; therefore, no initial attempts are made to convert this arrhythmia with drugs. Precordial shock is the first action to be taken and, in the absence of a physician, may be given immediately by the nursing staff. If a defibrillator is not readily available, external cardiac massage, assisted ventilation, and intravenous supportive drugs should be initiated at once. If the nurse present is having trouble discerning if the arrhythmia is ventricular tachycardia or ventricular flutter, her main concern should be the patient's tolerance of the arrhythmia, and she should treat the arrhythmia as the patient's tolerance indicates.

Ventricular Fibrillation

Ventricular fibrillation is a rapid, ineffective quivering of the ventricles. With this arrhythmia, there is no audible heart-

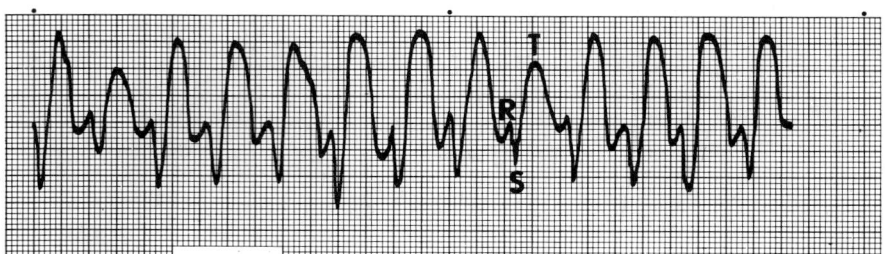

Figure 28-24. Ventricular tachycardia.

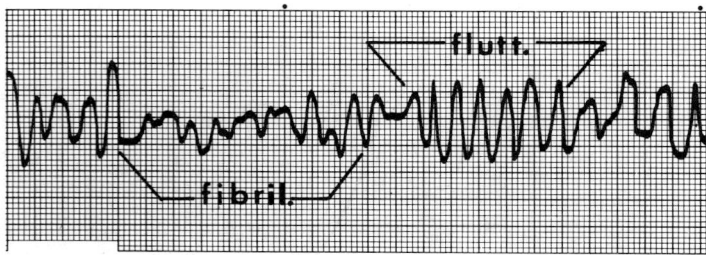

Figure 28-25. Ventricular flutter.

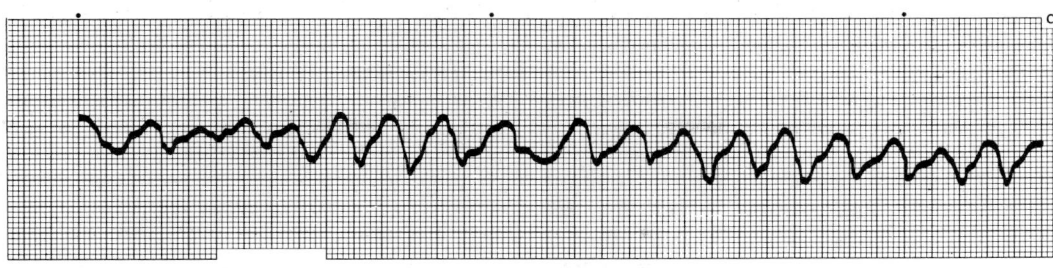

Figure 28-26. Ventricular fibrillation.

beat, no palpable pulse, and no respirations. This pattern is so grossly irregular it can hardly be mistaken for another type of arrhythmia. Malfunction of the monitor may produce such a pattern, but in that case, the clinical picture of the patient would rule out the diagnosis of ventricular fibrillation. Ventricular fibrillation is usually fatal without immediate treatment, since only 5% convert spontaneously.

Ventricular fibrillation (Fig. 28-26) has the following characteristics:

1. Rate: Rapid, uncoordinated, ineffective
2. P waves: Not seen
3. QRS complex: Rapid, irregular undulation without specific pattern (multifocal). The ventricles have only a quivering motion.
4. Conduction: Foci are located in the ventricles, but so many foci are firing at one time that there is no organized conduction: no ventricular contractions occur.
5. Rhythm: Extremely irregular and uncoordinated, without specific pattern

Immediate treatment is defibrillation with 200 to 400 watt-seconds. A synchronized machine will not fire on this disorganized rhythm because there are no predominant waves it can recognize. Defibrillation is used immediately after onset of ventricular fibrillation or of ventricular tachycardia without a peripheral pulse. Defibrillation completely depolarizes all the myocardial cells and terminates the chaotic electrical activity, allowing the SA node to regain control of the heart rhythm unless the myocardium is anoxic or acidotic, in which case this may not be possible.

In defibrillation the electrode paddles are applied to the anterior chest. The standard electrode paddle position for the closed-chest procedure is as follows: one paddle just to the right of the upper sternum below the right clavicle and the other paddle just to the left of the cardiac apex (Fig. 28-27).

In order to reduce skin resistance to current flow and to prevent skin burns, one of the following may be placed between the electrodes and the chest wall: saline-soaked 4-by-4 gauze pads; electrode paste; or defibrillator pads (adhesive pads with electrode gel). Care should be taken to prevent contact between the two areas of conductive material because electrical bridging may occur. If saline-soaked gauze pads are used, cardiac compressions can be resumed after defibrillation without the hands slipping on the chest, a problem that occurs with electrode paste.

- Exert 20 pounds to 25 pounds of pressure on each paddle in order to ensure good skin contact.
- Do not let anyone touch the patient or the bed when the defibrillator is fired.
- Then discharge the defibrillator at 200 to 400 watt-seconds, depending on the weight of the patient.

It is suggested that 3.5 to 6.0 watt-seconds per kg/body weight be used. Defibrillation can occur only if the synchronizer switch is off, because a QRS complex is required for synchronized defibrillation, and ventricular fibrillation

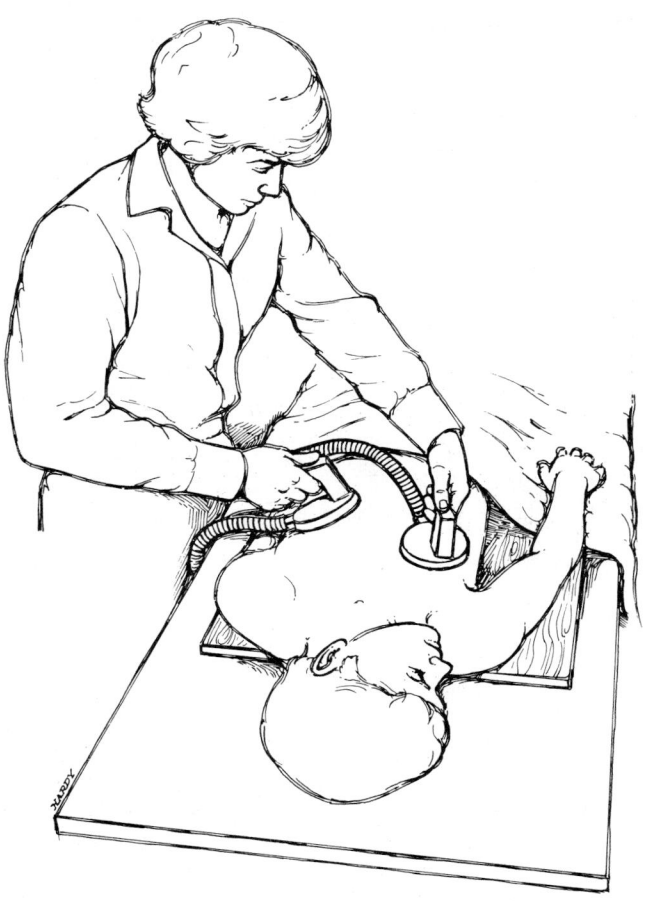

Figure 28-27. Paddle placement in ventricular defibrillation.

has no QRS complexes. After defibrillation, the cardiac monitor and pulse are checked for signs of restored sinus rhythm.

If defibrillation has been unsuccessful, cardiopulmonary resuscitation should be started immediately. Epinephrine and sodium bicarbonate may be used if the fibrillation is fine. Epinephrine may make the fibrillation coarser and thus easier to convert with defibrillation. Blood pressure should be supported, using vasopressors. At no time during the resuscitation should the external cardiac massage and the assisted ventilation be stopped for longer than 5 seconds. (See Chap. 29.)

Ventricular Asystole

In ventricular asystole there are no QRS complexes. There is no heartbeat, no palpable pulse, and no respiration. Ventricular asystole is fatal without immediate treatment. Ventricular asystole has the following characteristics:

1. Rate: None
2. P waves: May see them, but they do not conduct through the AV node and ventricles
3. QRS complex: None
4. Conduction: Possibly, through the atria only
5. Rhythm: None

Cardiopulmonary resuscitation is necessary to keep the patient alive. To decrease any vagal stimuli, 0.5 mg of atropine should be administered intravenously. Epinephrine should be administered and repeated at 5-minute intervals. Sodium bicarbonate should be given. Epinephrine and sodium bicarbonate are not compatible and may not be mixed together. Insertion of a transthoracic or transvenous pacemaker may be necessary. (See Chap. 31.)

▷ Conduction Abnormalities

First-degree AV Block

First-degree AV block is usually associated with organic heart disease or may be due to the effect of digitalis. It is seen frequently in patients with inferior MIs (if the AV nodal artery is involved).

First-degree heart block has the following characteristics (Fig. 28-28):

1. Rate: Variable, usually 60 to 100 beats per minute
2. P waves: Precede each QRS complex. The PR interval is greater than 0.20 second in duration.
3. QRS complexes: Follow each P wave; are usually normal
4. Conduction: Delayed conduction, usually anywhere between the junctional tissue and the Purkinje network, produces a prolonged PR interval. Ventricular conduction is usually normal.
5. Rhythm: Usually regular

This arrhythmia is important, since it may lead to more serious forms of heart block. It is often a warning signal. The patient should be monitored closely for any advancing block.

Second-degree AV Block—Mobitz Type I

Second-degree AV block, Mobitz type I (Wenckebach phenomenon), is usually associated with organic heart disease and is frequently due to digitalis intoxication. This block is frequently seen in association with MI that involves the AV nodal artery.

Second-degree heart block has the following characteristics (Fig. 28-29):

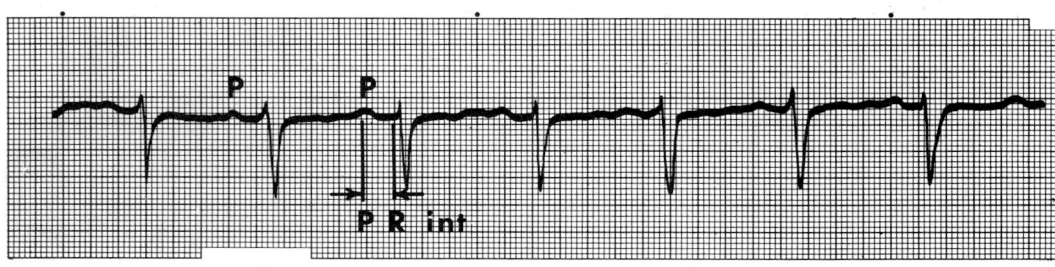

Figure 28-28. First-degree heart block.

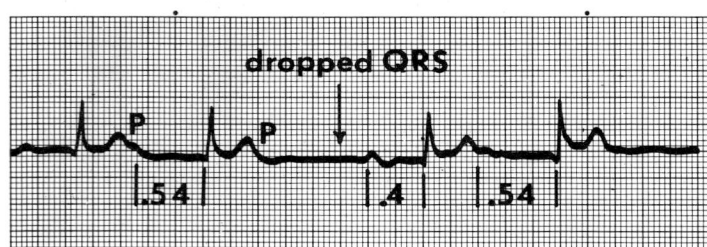

Figure 28-29. Second-degree block, Wenckebach type.

1. Rate: Variable; usually 60 to 100 beats per minute
2. P waves: Precede each QRS complex. The P–R interval becomes increasingly longer until finally a QRS complex is dropped and then the cycle is repeated.
3. QRS complex: Follows most P waves, except when QRS complex is dropped
4. Conduction: The P–R interval becomes increasingly longer until an impulse is not conducted through the ventricles because it is blocked somewhere between the junctional tissue and the Purkinje network.
5. Rhythm: Irregular, since the R–R interval becomes progressively shorter until a QRS complex is dropped.

Digitalis intoxication should be ruled out. Depending on the hemodynamic changes produced, efforts to normalize the heart rate may be necessary.

Second-degree AV Block—Mobitz Type II

Second-degree AV block, Mobitz type II, is also caused by organic heart disease, by MIs involving the AV nodal artery, and by digitalis intoxication. This type of block results in a reduced heart rate and usually a reduced cardiac output. (Cardiac output is the product of stroke volume and heart rate.)

Second-degree heart block has the following characteristics (Fig. 28-30):

1. Rate: 30 to 55 beats per minute. The atrial rate may be two, three, or four times faster than the ventricular rate.
2. P waves: There are two, three, or four P waves for each QRS complex. The PR interval of the conducted beat is usually normal in duration.
3. QRS complex: Usually normal
4. Conduction: One or more of the impulses are not conducted through the ventricles.
5. Rhythm: Usually slow and regular. When an irregularity is seen, it is due to the fact that the block is varying from 2:1 to 3:1 or to some other combination.

Treatment is directed toward increasing the heart rate to maintain a normal cardiac output. Digitalis intoxication should be ruled out and myocardial depressant drugs withheld.

Third-degree AV Block

Third-degree AV block (complete heart block) is also associated with organic heart disease, digitalis intoxication, and MI. The heart rate may be markedly decreased, resulting in a decrease in perfusion to vital organs, such as the brain, heart, kidneys, lungs, and skin.

Complete block—third-degree AV block—has the following characteristics:

1. Origin: Impulses originate in the SA node, but these impulses are not conducted to the Purkinje fibers. They are completely blocked. An escape rhythm from the junctional or ventricular area therefore takes over as the pacemaker.
2. Rate: Atrial rate 60 to 100 beats per minute; ventricular rate 40 to 60 beats per minute if the escape rhythm originated in the junction, 20 to 40 beats per minute if the escape rhythm originated in the ventricle (Fig. 28-31)
3. P waves: The P waves originating from the SA node are seen regularly throughout the rhythm, but they have no association with the QRS complexes.
4. QRS complex: If the escape rhythm originated in the junction, the QRS complexes have a normal supraventricular configuration, but have no association with the P waves. QRS complexes occur regularly. If the escape rhythm originated in the ventricle, the QRS complex is longer than 0.10 second in duration, usually broad and slurred. These QRS complexes have the same configuration as the QRS complex of a PVC.
5. Conduction: The SA node is firing, and P waves can be seen. They are all blocked and not conducted to the

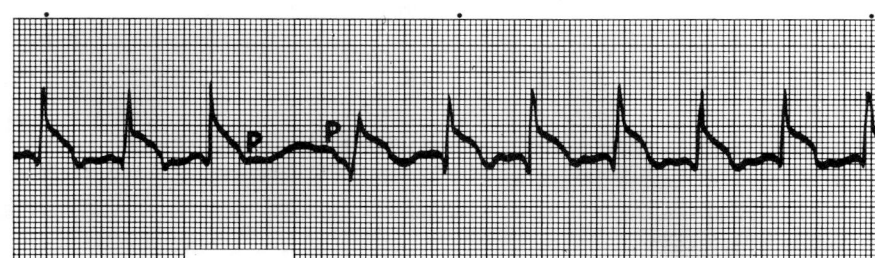

Figure 28-30. Second-degree AV block, Mobitz type II.

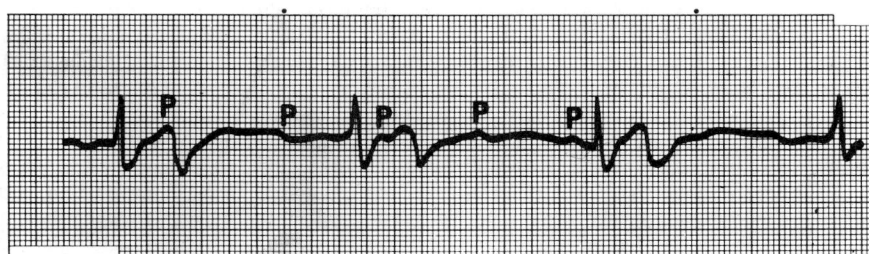

Figure 28-31. Third-degree AV block.

ventricles. Escape rhythms originating in the junction are usually conducted normally through the ventricles. Escape rhythms from the ventricles are ectopic with aberrant configuration.

6. Rhythm: Usually slow but regular

Treatment is directed toward increasing perfusion to vital organs. This may include increasing the rate of escape rhythm: a junctional rhythm can be increased by use of a parasympatholytic (anticholinergic) agent; a ventricular rhythm can be increased by use of a sympathomimetic agent. It may also include insertion of a temporary transvenous pacemaker.

▷ Bibliography
Books

Andreoli KG et al. Comprehensive Cardiac Care, 4th ed. St Louis, CV Mosby, 1979.

Bernreiter M. Electrocardiography. Philadelphia, JB Lippincott, 1963.

Bing OHL. Clinical EKG Guide, 2nd ed. Newtonville, OHL Bing, 1981.

Bishop L. The Wave of Depolarization: A Programmed Course in Electrocardiography. New York, Basic Systems, 1966.

Braun H and Diettert G. ECG Arrhythmia Interpretation: A Programmed Text for Health Personnel. Reston, Reston Publishing, 1979.

Chung E. Electrocardiography, 2nd ed. Hagerstown, Maryland, Harper & Row, 1980.

Chung E. Principles of Cardiac Arrhythmias, 3rd ed. Baltimore, Williams & Wilkins, 1983.

Clark NF. Normal Conduction System and the Electrocardiogram. Philadelphia, FA Davis, 1975.

Conover MH. Cardiac Arrhythmias, 2nd ed. St Louis, CV Mosby, 1978.

Dubin D. Rapid Interpretation of EKG's, 3rd ed. Tampa, Cover, 1974.

Ehrat KS. The Simple Art of EKG Interpretation. Dubuque, Kendall/Hunt, 1978.

Friedman HH. Diagnostic Electrocardiography and Vectorcardiography. New York, McGraw-Hill, 1977.

Goldman MJ. Principles of Clinical Electrocardiography, 10th ed. California, Lange Medical Publications, 1979.

Hurst JW. The Heart. New York, McGraw-Hill, 1982.

Katz AM. Physiology of the Heart. New York, Raven Press, 1977.

Kernicki JG and Weiler KM. Electrocardiography for Nurses. New York, John Wiley & Sons, 1981.

Mangiola S. Self-Assessment in Electrocardiography. Philadelphia, JB Lippincott, 1977.

Marriott HJL. Workshop in Electrocardiography. Florida, Tampa Tracings, 1972.

Marriott HJL. Practical Electrocardiography, 7th ed. Baltimore, Williams & Wilkins, 1983.

Meltzer L, Pinneo R, and Kitchell J: Intensive Coronary Care, 4th ed. Bowie, Maryland, Brady Press, 1983.

Phibbs B. The Cardiac Arrhythmias, 3rd ed. St Louis, CV Mosby, 1978.

Phillips RE and Feeney MK. The Cardiac Rhythms, 2nd ed. Philadelphia, WB Saunders, 1980.

Sharp L and Rabin B. Nursing in the Coronary Care Unit. Philadelphia, JB Lippincott, 1970.

Articles

Estes EH. Electrocardiography and vectorcardiography. In Hurst JW (ed). The Heart, 3rd ed. New York, McGraw-Hill, 1974.

Gallagher JJ et al. The Wolff–Parkinson–White syndrome and the pre-excitation dysrhythmias. Med Clin North Am 1976; 60:114–121.

Hecht HH and Kossman CE. Atrioventricular and intraventricular conduction: Revised nomenclature and concepts. Am J Cardiol 1973 Feb; 31(2):232–244.

Kaplan BM et al. The tachycardia–bradycardia syndrome. Med Clin North Am 1976 Jan; 60(1):81–99.

Kleiger R. Arrhythmias, Part 1. Heart Lung 1977 Jan–Feb; 6(1):60–88.

Kleiger R. Arrhythmias, Part 2. Heart Lung 1977 Mar–Apr; 6(2):249–262.

Marriott HJL and Myerburg RJ. Recognition and treatment of cardiac arrhythmias and conduction disturbances. In Hurst J (ed). The Heart, 4th ed, pp 637–694. New York, McGraw-Hill, 1978.

McNeal GP. Tracing arrhythmias. Am J Nurs 1979 Jan; 79(1):98–100.

Pick A. Digitalis and the electrocardiogram. Circulation 1957 Apr; 15(4):603–608.

Surawicz B. Electrolytes and electrocardiogram. Am J Cardiol 1963 Nov; 12(5):656–622.

Surawicz B et al. Task Force I. Standardization of terminology and interpretation. Am J Cardiol 1978 Jan; 41(1):130–145.

VanderArk CR, Ballantyne F, and Reynolds EW. Electrolytes and the electrocardiogram. Cardiovasc Clin 1973; 5(3):269–294.

Weinberg SL. Ambulatory monitoring of arrhythmias. Cardiovasc Clin 1975; 6(3):121–132.

Woods SL. Arrhythmias complicating myocardial infarction. In Underhill SL et al (eds). Cardiac Nursing, pp 363–377. Philadelphia, JB Lippincott, 1982.

Woods SL. Electrocardiography, vectorcardiography, and polarcardiography. (Polarcardiography section written by E. S. Sivarajan.) In Underhill SL et al (eds). Cardiac Nursing, pp 196–247. Philadelphia, JB Lippincott, 1982.

▷ Additional Reading
Books

Alpert MA. Cardiac Arrhythmias. Chicago, Year Book Medical Publishers, 1980.

Constant J. Learning Electrocardiography: A Complete Course, 2nd ed. Boston, Little, Brown & Co, 1981.

Goldberger AL and Goldberger E. Clinical Electrocardiography, 2nd ed. St Louis, CV Mosby, 1981.

Goldman MJ. Principles of Clinical Electrocardiography, 11th ed. Los Altos, Lange Medical Publications, 1982.

Hampton JR. The E.C.G. Made Easy, 2nd ed. New York, Churchill Livingstone, 1980.

Jones KM and Ochs GM. Interpretation of the Electrocardiogram: A Review for Health Professionals. Norwalk, Connecticut, Appleton–Century–Crofts, 1982.

Kernicki JG and Weiler KM. Electrocardiography for Nurses: Physiological Correlates. New York, John Wiley & Sons, 1981.

Mandel WJ (ed). Cardiac Arrhythmias. Philadelphia, JB Lippincott, 1980.

Mangiola S and Ritota MC. Cardiac Arrhythmias: Practical ECG Interpretation, 2nd ed. Philadelphia, JB Lippincott, 1982.

Marriott HJL and Conover MHB. Advanced Concepts in Arrhythmias. St Louis, CV Mosby, 1983.

Mudge GH Jr. Manual of Electrocardiography. Boston, Little, Brown & Co, 1981.

Phillips RE and Feeney MK. The Cardiac Rhythms: A Systematic Approach to Interpretation, 2nd ed. Philadelphia, WB Saunders, 1980.

Rowlands DJ. Understanding the Electrocardiogram: A New Approach. Edinburgh, Churchill Livingstone, 1980.

Summerall CP III, Mangiaracina J, and McNeely J. Monitoring Heart Rhythm, 2nd ed. New York, John Wiley & Sons, 1982.

Articles

Arcebal AG and Lembers L. Acute myocardial infarction and left bundle branch block. Heart Lung 1981 May–June; 10(3):532–538.

Breu CS and Gawlinski A. A comparative study of the effects of documentation on arrhythmia detection efficiency. Heart Lung 1981 Nov–Dec; 10(6):1058–1062.

Budassi SA. How to calculate a simple electrocardiographic axis. Journal of Emergency Nursing 1982 Nov–Dec; 8(6):322–324.

Duke DM. Intraventricular conduction blocks. Part 1. Introduction and electrocardiographic identification of right and left bundle branch block. Crit Care Nurse 1982 May–June; 2(3):30–39.

Hammond C. ECGs made easier than ever: Lethal strips. RN 1980 Jan; 43(1):54–58, 84.

Haughey BP. Holter monitoring: A method for nursing research. Nurs Res 1983 Jan–Feb; 32(1):59–60.

Jacobs ML and Schamroth L. A study in atrioventricular block. Heart Lung 1982 May–June; 11(3):278–279.

Krasover T. A conceptual approach to the electrocardiogram. Crit Care Nurse 1982 Mar–Apr; 2(2):66–76.

Roffman JA and Feldman A. Ventricular conduction defects: Significance and prognosis. Heart Lung 1980 Jan–Feb; 9(1):111–121.

Shepard N, Vaughan P, and Rice V. A guide to arrhythmia interpretation and management. Home study program. Crit Care Nurse 1982 Sept–Oct; 2(5):58–85.

Worthington L. EKG manifestations of digitalis toxicity. Crit Care Update 1981 Sept; 8(9):5–14.

29

Management of the Patient in the Cardiac Care Unit

▷ The Cardiac Care Unit

The cardiac care unit, or coronary care unit, (CCU) is an area in a hospital that is equipped with special electronic devices used in monitoring patients with actual or potential heart problems. It is staffed by nurses with clinical expertise in cardiovascular nursing. Since the advent of the CCU in the early 1960s, the mortality rate of cardiac patients has dramatically decreased. Some authorities suggest that in myocardial infarction (MI) patients, this decreased mortality rate ranges from 10% to 24%. The main objective of the CCU is to prevent, detect, and treat cardiac arrhythmias, which were originally the leading cause of death of the patient with MI. Additional objectives are to prevent, detect, and treat complications that may occur because of MI. (More information regarding this disease is presented in Chap. 31.)

In order to meet these objectives, the CCU is generally a confined area with limited access from other parts of the hospital. It affords a quiet, temperature-controlled environment, often with private rooms. Resuscitative equipment and electrocardiographic monitoring devices with automatic alarm systems are provided. The basic equipment includes individual oscilloscopes at each patient's bed and a base oscilloscope with multiple channels at the nurses' station that displays the individual patient's electrocardiogram (ECG).

The most important aspect of the CCU, however, is not the equipment but the special nurses who care for the patients in this unusual environment. They must be well prepared to manage, diagnose, and intervene without immediate consultation with physicians, if an emergency occurs. The nurse must be knowledgeable in basic anatomy, physiology, and pathophysiology of the cardiovascular system and must be familiar with the methods and goals of medical therapy and appropriate nursing support. Additional facets of the knowledge base include the ability to assess, diagnose, plan, and evaluate care. The nurse who functions in the CCU is sensitive to the special psychological needs of the patients, the families, and the staff members. The benefits of the care in this specialized unit are directly proportional to the knowledge, skills, and commitment of the nursing staff.

▷ Care of the Patient With Myocardial Infarction

The patient is usually admitted to the CCU for an actual or potential MI. The condition, which is also known as a coronary occlusion or "heart attack," occurs when the coronary arteries that supply blood to the myocardium have such a severely compromised flow that they are unable to maintain the survival of the myocardial muscle. Two coronary arteries originate at the base of the aorta as it leaves the left ventricle. The right coronary artery supplies blood to the right atrium and ventricle and, in the majority of people, to the inferior surface of the left ventricle. The left coronary artery has two main branches. These supply the left atrium and remaining left ventricle and the septum. Coronary artery disease (CAD) occurs when there is partial or total obstruction of these vessels. Atherosclerosis, the leading cause of CAD, is characterized by a narrowing of the lumen of the artery owing to complex deposits known as "atherosclerotic plaques." Obstruction of the vessel occurs, and the portion of the myocardium that it supplies becomes ischemic and finally necrotic. When this tissue death occurs, the normal conduction of electrical activity of the heart may be inhibited and lethal arrhythmias may occur.

Arrhythmias are frequent complications following an MI, and CCUs have been established primarily to monitor the electrical activity of the heart so that irregularities of rhythm can be identified and immediate—often lifesaving—measures instituted. At present, care in the CCU is focused on the prevention, early recognition, and treatment of arrhythmias and the identification and treatment of secondary complications. Arrhythmias are discussed in Chapter 28.

▶ Nursing Assessment

One of the most important aspects of care of the patient on admission to the CCU is the nursing assessment. This serves to establish a baseline of information regarding the present status of the patient, so that any deviations may be immediately noted. The nursing assessment is orderly and inclusive and has as its objective the identification of the priority of needs of the cardiac patient.

Systematic assessment of the patient includes a careful history, particularly as it relates to the description of symptoms: chest pain, dyspnea, palpitations, faintness (syncope), or sweating (diaphoresis). Each symptom must be evaluated with regard to time, duration, and precipitating and relieving factors.

In addition, there are several areas in the physical examination that relate directly to the needs of the patient in CCU. These include the following:

1. Radial Arterial Pulse. Rate, rhythm, and volume are assessed. Many cardiovascular disorders will be reflected here: for example, a rapid, regular but weak pulse indicates low volume and reduced cardiac output; a slow, regular, and strong pulse may indicate heart block; and an irregular pulse indicates cardiac arrhythmia.

2. Jugular Venous Pressure. The assessment of the pressure in this vessel gives a convenient reflection of the pressure in the right side of the heart. Elevation of venous pressure may indicate the failing ability of the heart to pump and empty its contents. The examination is done with the patient at rest, with the head and chest supported at a 45-degree angle. With normal venous pressures, distention of the veins is seen slightly above the clavicle. More extensive venous distention should be noted (Fig. 29-1).

3. Heart Location. The size of the heart may be assessed by identifying its location by means of palpation. The apex beat, often referred to as the point of maximum impulse (PMI), is normally found at the 5th intercostal space in the midclavicular line (Fig. 29-2). A movement to the left and down may indicate left ventricular enlargement.

4. Heart Sounds. Auscultation is the method used to identify the normal heart sounds. A stethoscope of good quality and proper fit is essential for the interpretation of heart sounds. The chest piece must have a bell to identify low-pitched sound and should possess a diaphragm for the auscultation of high-pitched sounds. It is important to apply the bell of the stethoscope lightly to the skin and firmly to the diaphragm in order to hear the sounds correctly. The first heart sound (S_1), heard best over the base and indicating the beginning of systole, should be identified first. The second sound (S_2), heard best at the base of the heart and indicating the beginning of diastole, is identified next (Fig. 29-3). Abnormal sounds are noted. These include the third heart sound (S_3), known as ventricular gallop, and the fourth heart sound (S_4), known as an atrial or presystolic gallop. The S_1 and S_2 together sound like the syllables LUB DUB. The S_1 (LUB) is louder at the apex, the S_2 (DUB) louder at the base. The S_3 sound follows closely after S_2 and has a cadence similar to the word Ken-tuck-y (S_1–S_2–S_3).

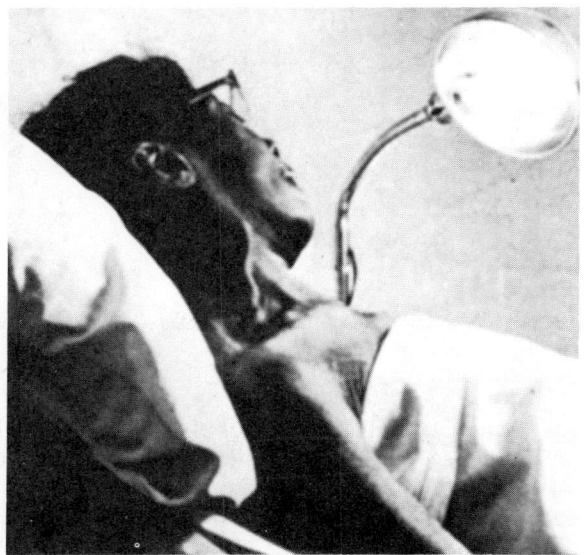

Figure 29-1. This photo illustrates distended neck veins with the patient in a semireclined position, indicating that the heart is incapable of receiving and pumping adequately all the incoming venous blood. (Reproduced with permission of the American Heart Association.)

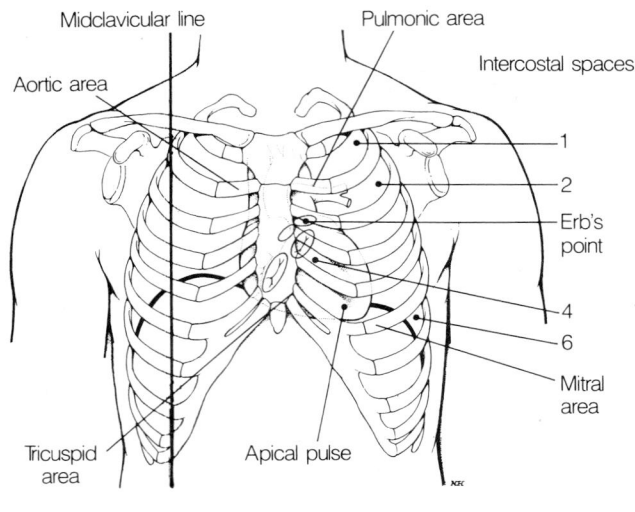

Figure 29-2. The apex beat, often referred to as the point of maximum impulse (PMI), is normally found at the 5th intercostal space in the midclavicular line.

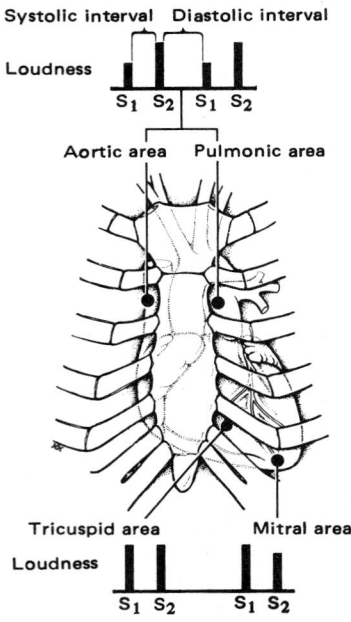

Figure 29-3. Identification of first and second heart sounds.

The S_4 sound precedes the S_1 and has the cadence of the word Ten-nes-see (S_4–S_1–S_2). Other sounds, that is, murmurs, created by blood flowing around an obstruction or flowing backward through an incompetent valve, are noted. All nurses who care for patients in the CCU must become skillful in the identification of heart sounds and murmurs.

5. Edema. The patient should be evaluated for signs of edema caused by the decreasing ability of the heart to work effectively as a pump. This may be noted in the ex-

tremities, particularly at the pretibial area, or in the sacral area. An enlarged liver is also a sign of failing circulatory status and is palpated in the right upper quadrant.

Early assessment of the patient not only serves to establish priorities of needs and provide baseline data for further nursing plans, but also initiates a relationship between the patient and the nurse that can promote confidence in the nursing staff of the CCU.

Patient Problems/Nursing Diagnoses

Based on the data acquired from the health history, including clinical manifestations and diagnostic assessment, the major potential problems of the patient include potential chest discomfort (possibly radiating to arms, neck, jaw, shoulders, and back) related to absent or reduced coronary blood flow; potential arrhythmias and conduction disturbances related to myocardial oxygen needs; potential alterations in breathing patterns (shortness of breath, dyspnea, orthopnea, and paroxysmal nocturnal dyspnea) related to possible left ventricular failure; reduced perfusion to vital organs related to decreased cardiac output; and anxiety and fear of death related to the diagnosis of MI.

▶ Planning and Implementation

Goals

1. Relief of chest pain
2. Avoidance of arrhythmias and respiratory difficulties by maintaining cardiac output to meet oxygen demands
3. Early detection of possible problems through continuous monitoring
4. Reduction of stress and anxiety

Nursing Interventions
Cardiac Monitoring in the CCU. The patient is admitted to the CCU and is attached to a cardiac monitor. The electrodes are placed on the chest according to the lead selected for monitoring.

The electrode site on the skin should be clean (use alcohol), dry (use gauze), and relatively flat. Hair should be shaved and the skin mildly abraded to reduce the resistance. The electrode with electrode paste is then applied to the chest, the alarm limits for heart rate are set (30% above and below the patient's heart rate), the "beeper" in the patient's room is turned off, and the alarm system is activated.

Sources of artifacts in ECG monitoring include involuntary movement, voluntary movement, poor skin preparation, dried out electrodes, and bad grounding. Electrodes are changed often enough (usually about 1 to 3 days) to prevent skin breakdown and to provide artifact-free tracings.

The patient is given a brief explanation of the purpose of ECG monitoring while he is in the CCU and his questions should be answered. The patient's heart rate, rhythm, and conduction must be continuously assessed, since most arrhythmias occur within the first 2 to 3 days after acute MI, and 90% of these patients will have arrhythmias.

Intervention must be directed toward prevention by recognizing and controlling conditions that predispose the patient to arrhythmias. Some of these conditions are hypokalemia, acidosis, hypoxemia, pain, anxiety, fever, and myocardial stretch (caused by congestive heart failure).

- Early identification of arrhythmias and prompt, aggressive treatment are necessary if mortality from MI is to be reduced.

Arrhythmias can result in reduced cardiac output and coronary blood flow, increased myocardial oxygen need, and predisposition to a lethal arrhythmia. The cardiac monitor must be under constant surveillance if arrhythmias are to be detected early and therefore treated early to prevent further problems for the patient (see Chap. 28).

Vital Signs and Intravenous Line.   Blood pressure, pulse, respiration, and temperature (oral or rectal) should be obtained. An intravenous (IV) line (angiocatheter or intracatheter) is established if the patient does not already have one. A scalp-vein needle should be used only temporarily until a more stable IV line can be established, since it is easily dislodged. This IV line is used to give pain medication and emergency cardiac medication. The IV line can be capped and 10 to 100 units heparin in 1 ml of saline injected every 8 hours, and following injection of medication, to maintain patency. Or an IV solution of 5% dextrose and water can be attached and infused at a rate to keep the vein open. A simple explanation of procedures is useful to most patients.

Chest Discomfort and Dyspnea.   If the patient complains of chest discomfort, he should be given analgesic medication. The anxiety associated with pain increases myocardial oxygen demand. In order to decrease myocardial oxygen need, morphine sulfate is given intravenously in small increments of 1 mg to 5 mg. Morphine should not be given to patients who have atrioventricular block or sinus bradycardia, since it has a vagotonic effect. Morphine decreases blood pressure, heart rate, and respiratory rate. If the heart rate is less than 70, meperidine may be the drug of choice. Oxygen at 2 liters to 4 liters per minute by nasal prongs may decrease chest discomfort by increasing oxygen supply to the myocardium. Dyspnea can also cause anxiety and can be relieved by the administration of oxygen. Also, the administration of oxygen may diminish the conversion of ischemic myocardium to necrotic tissue. The magnitude of this benefit is not clear, and the primary physiologic mechanisms remain obscure. Arterial blood gases should be used to evaluate the effectiveness of oxygen therapy and to assess acid–base balance.

Physical rest in bed with the backrest elevated, or in a cardiac chair, will assist in decreasing chest discomfort and dyspnea. The head-up position is beneficial for the following reasons: (1) tidal volume is improved, since there is reduced pressure from abdominal contents on the diaphragm, and thus oxygen exchange is improved; (2) drainage of the upper lobes of the lungs is improved; and (3) venous return to the heart (preload) and cardiac output are reduced, thus reducing the work of the heart.

Other Assessment Parameters.   Throughout this admission procedure, the nurse assesses and documents the patient's cardiovascular, renal, respiratory, neurologic (level of consciousness), and psychological status. These data provide a baseline. If the patient is anxious, myocardial oxygen demand is increased. Explanations of all the activities and equipment will assist in relieving the patient's anxiety. Visits by family or friends may either reduce or cause anxiety. Assessment of the effect of visitors and appropriate intervention is a nursing responsibility. Unit policies should be flexible to provide individual care.

Management.   Generally, medical management includes relief of pain, prevention of ventricular fibrillation and other lethal arrhythmias, prescription for rest and exercise, diet limitations, and the prevention and management of anxiety.

Myocardial Oxygen Needs

The myocardium requires time to recover from the injury of MI. Reduction in myocardial oxygen need will assist the recovery of the myocardium. The size of the infarction is determined by the demand and supply of oxygen to the ischemic and injured zones.

Some ways to decrease the patient's myocardial oxygen need are (1) promote bed rest with progressive mobilization; (2) assist the patient with activities of daily living; and (3) control the environment to minimize stress.

Bed Rest.   Bed rest is important to the healing heart but is not without complications. Immobility has many adverse effects. For the patient with an uncomplicated myocardial infarction, activity progresses from bed rest, to sitting up on the side of the bed with assistance, to sitting in a chair, to walking. The length of time for each activity is increased as tolerated by the patient.

Activities of Daily Living.   Activities of daily living (ADL) can pose a problem to the independent person, because he is now dependent on the nurse for assistance.

It is important to allow the patient as much independence as possible to promote his self-confidence, which in turn facilitates psychological and physiologic recovery. All activities are modified to meet individual needs. Chapter 31 contains principles of rehabilitation after MI.

Diet Considerations.   Most patients are permitted to feed themselves. The diet selected should:

1. Minimize myocardial work, to favor adequate myocardial oxygen balance
2. Maintain normal extracellular volume
3. Minimize patient pain and discomfort

The following dietary principles during the acute phase are recommended by the American Heart Association:

1. Avoid large meals, which potentially increase demand for splanchnic blood flow and thereby increase postprandial cardiac work.
2. Minimize the volume of gastric contents in order to decrease the chance of vomiting and aspiration in the event of cardiac emergencies.
3. Avoid ingestion of myocardial stimulants, such as caffeine or theobromine.
4. Avoid swallowing exceptionally cold or hot food and drink, to help decrease the possibility of cardiac arrhythmias.
5. Avoid as much as possible foods that contribute to constipation and resultant straining with bowel move-

ments, which may predispose a patient to vagal cardiac rhythm changes.

6. Limit foods known to commonly produce excessive gas in the digestive process, such as dried beans, legumes, and apple juice.

7. Offer a diet ample in potassium for all patients except those in renal failure. Most patients on potassium-wasting diuretic therapy will also require supplemental potassium treatment.

Avoiding Valsalva Maneuver. The patient's arms should be supported on the overbed table during the meal to prevent him from doing an unconscious Valsalva maneuver. In a Valsalva maneuver, air is forced over a closed glottis, resulting in increased intrathoracic pressure. This increased intrathoracic pressure may be as high as 80 mm Hg and causes a decreased venous return to the heart (decreased preload) and vagal stimulation, resulting in decreased cardiac output. When the forced air is released, the intrathoracic pressure is decreased, and preload is increased, resulting in an increased workload for the heart. The patient should be instructed to avoid holding his breath, since this can result in a Valsalva maneuver, and to breathe in and out with the mouth open while engaging in any activity that is normally accompanied by a Valsalva maneuver, such as turning or moving up in bed, reaching, vomiting, pulling, defecating, or coughing.

Elimination Considerations. The use of a bedside commode with assistance is less work than the use of a bedpan. The position one assumes using a commode is more natural and allows for appropriate and optimum utilization of the muscles of defecation (abdominal and rectal). Sufficient fluid intake is necessary to prevent constipation. Stool softeners will decrease the need for straining and possibly prevent a Valsalva maneuver.

Hygienic Care. Initially, the patient will need to be bathed (day 1) and then assisted with the bath (days 2 to 5). The patient with an uncomplicated MI usually can take a warm shower after he is discharged from the CCU. A warm shower is preferred over a hot shower, since a hot shower could result in vasodilatation and markedly reduced preload and cardiac output. The patient may need to use a chair in the shower or may need assistance with washing. Discussion of these activities with the patient and physician is necessary to determine their preferences and to develop a workable care plan.

IV Monitoring. With the daily bath, the IV site should be inspected for signs of inflammation (redness, swelling, heat). Findings should be documented on the patient's chart. The site should be cleaned with an antiseptic, and an antibiotic ointment and a dry sterile dressing should be applied. If the site is inflamed, a new IV line should be placed in a different site prior to discontinuing the old line. The IV site is changed at least every 3 days. Also, electrode sites on the chest are assessed daily for skin irritation and washed with soap and water. Different areas of the chest are selected for application of new electrodes.

Reducing Stress. To maintain an environment that reduces stress, one must ensure a calm, quiet, optimistic atmosphere. The staff must demonstrate efficiency and competence in their care. In addition, what is stressful to one individual may not be stressful to another. Thus, each must

be assessed to determine a suitable environment that reduces stress. Antianxiety drugs such as diazepam may also be useful.

▶ **Evaluation**

The expected outcomes for evaluating the care of the patient in the CCU are listed in Chart 29-1, which contains a sample nursing care plan for the patient with an uncomplicated myocardial infarction. Major problems, nursing interventions, and scientific rationale are also delineated. This suggested plan of care must be individualized for each patient and is not meant as a standard care plan to be used on all patients. It is meant to demonstrate the use of the nursing process with a patient having a MI and to provide a guideline for developing an individual plan of care.

Discharge From the CCU

The patient without complications is usually discharged from the CCU after 3 to 5 days. The nasal oxygen and IV line may be discontinued, and the patient is transferred by means of a wheelchair to an intermediate care unit or to a medical unit. This transfer should be anticipated and the rationale explained to the patient and family. The anticipation of transfer may reassure the patient. To provide continuity of care, the unit to which the patient is being transferred is notified of the patient's transfer, and the written plan of care, physician's regimen, and patient's progress are shared.

Post-CCU Care. During the post-CCU phase the risk of complications from MI is markedly reduced. The difference between the intermediate care unit and the medical unit is the intensity and constancy of assessment of cardiac function and potential complications. For example, in the intermediate care area the patient's heart rhythm should be continuously monitored by telemetry; on the medical unit the patient may be monitored, but less frequently. The area designed for intermediate care should be adjacent to or in continuity with the CCU, thus permitting efficient utilization of manpower and physical resources, and facilitating the transfer of patients to this type of care. The number of beds provided for the area should at least equal or exceed by 50% the number in the CCU. Monitoring and resuscitation capability for intermediate care should be identical with that of the CCU. In some institutions the intermediate care unit is not restricted to patients discharged from CCU, but is a place for any patient with cardiovascular disease who may benefit from the monitoring or resuscitative capability of this unit.

The administration of intermediate care should be fully integrated with that of the CCU in order to ensure continuity of optimum management. The training and capabilities of nurses in this unit should be equivalent to that of the CCU nurses. During this phase the patient is allowed to be more independent in activities of daily living.

▷ **Major Complications of Myocardial Infarction**

In addition to arrhythmias, the major complications of MI include congestive heart failure, shock, pulmonary embo-

(Text continues on page 593)

Chart 29-1
Nursing Care of the Patient in the CCU (Uncomplicated Myocardial Infarction)

Nursing Intervention	*Rationale*	*Evaluation Criteria*
Problem 1. Chest Discomfort		
1. Initially assess, document, and report to the physician the following:	1. These data assist in determining the cause and effect of the chest discomfort and provide a baseline so that post-therapy symptoms can be compared.	(For 1 through 6) Patient reports relief of chest discomfort within 15 to 30 minutes Patient appears comfortable:
a. The patient's description of chest discomfort, including location, radiation, duration of pain, and factors that affect it	a. There are many conditions associated with chest discomfort. There are characteristic clinical findings of ischemic pain.	a. Seems restful b. Respiratory rate, cardiac rate, and blood pressure return to prediscomfort level c. Skin warm and dry
b. The effect of chest discomfort on cardiovascular hemodynamic perfusion: to the heart, to the brain, to the kidneys, and to the skin	b. Myocardial infarction decreases myocardial contractility and ventricular compliance and may produce arrhythmias by promoting reentry and increased automaticity. Cardiac output is reduced, resulting in reduced blood pressure and decreased organ perfusion. The heart rate may increase as a compensatory mechanism to maintain cardiac output.	Effects of chest discomfort on cardiovascular hemodynamics detected to maintain within normal limits: a. Heart rate, rhythm, and conduction b. Blood pressure c. Mentation d. Urine output e. Serum BUN and creatinine f. Skin color, temperature, and moisture
2. Obtain a 12-lead ECG recording during pain, as prescribed, to determine extension of infarction or variant angina.	2. An ECG during pain may be useful in the diagnosis of an extension of myocardial ischemia, injury, and infarction, and of variant angina.	
3. Administer oxygen as prescribed.	3. Oxygen may increase the oxygen supply to the myocardium if actual oxygen saturation is less than normal.	
4. Administer narcotic or analgesic medications as prescribed and evaluate the patient's response continuously.	4. Narcotics are useful in alleviating chest discomfort, decreasing anxiety, and increasing sense of well-being. The side-effects of these medications can be dangerous and the patient's status must be assessed.	
5. Ensure physical rest; use of the bedside commode with assistance; backrest elevated to comfort; full liquid diet as tolerated; arms supported during upper extremity activity; use of stool softener to prevent straining at stool. Teach patient to exhale with physical movement to avoid a Valsalva maneuver, and to practice the relaxation response. Visitor privileges are individualized, based on patient response. Provide a restful environment, and allay fears and anxiety by being supportive, calm, and competent.	5. Physical rest reduces myocardial oxygen consumption. Fear and anxiety precipitate the stress response; this results in increased levels of endogenous catecholamines, which increase myocardial oxygen consumption. Also, with increased epinephrine the pain threshold is decreased and pain increases the myocardial oxygen consumption.	
6. Promote the patient's physical comfort by providing individualized basic nursing care.	6. Physical comfort promotes the patient's sense of well-being and reduces anxiety.	

(continued)

Chart 29-1
Nursing Care of the Patient in the CCU (Uncomplicated Myocardial Infarction) (continued)

Nursing Intervention (continued)	*Rationale* (continued)	*Evaluation Criteria* (continued)

Problem 2. Potential Arrhythmias and Conduction Disturbances

Nursing Intervention	Rationale	Evaluation Criteria
1. Same as 3, 5, 6 for Problem 1.	1. Same as 3, 5, 6 for Problem 1.	1, 2. Ideally, normal sinus rhythm without arrhythmia is maintained or restored, or the patient's baseline heart rate, rhythm, and conduction are maintained or restored.
2. Administer prophylactic antiarrhythmic medications as prescribed.		
3. Using a cardiac monitor, continuously assess heart rate, rhythm, and conduction, and document every 4 hours and prior to administration of medications that have a cardiovascular effect. Determine the effect of the arrhythmia on the patient's blood pressure and perfusion to the heart, brain, and kidneys, and report marked changes to the physician.	3. Early detection of arrhythmia allows initiation of therapy and may prevent a lethal arrhythmia. Arrhythmias can result in reduced cardiac output, hypotension, and reduced perfusion to vital organs.	3, 4, 5. Previous heart rate, rhythm, and conduction restored (Chap. 27). All arrhythmias and conduction disturbances are detected as they occur and do not progress to ventricular fibrillation or asystole.
4. Administer antiarrhythmic and other medications as prescribed or according to hospital policy, and evaluate continuously the patient's response to therapy.		
5. Obtain a 12-lead ECG with any marked change in heart rhythm	5. A 12-lead ECG assists in the diagnosis of arrhythmias and conduction disturbances and of further myocardial damage.	
6. Assess patient's status to determine other causes of the arrhythmias or conduction disturbances: a. Perform a cardiovascular assessment. b. Obtain a chest x-ray film.	6. a,b. Data obtained from the history and physical examination and from laboratory studies can assist in the diagnosis of the disease processes (such as left ventricular failure or pulmonary embolism) that can cause arrhythmias by the mechanisms of hypoxemia or myocardial stretch. Also, a chest x-ray film provides information regarding the placement of catheters within the heart. Abnormal placement of a catheter within the heart can cause mechanical irritation of the myocardium and result in arrhythmias.	6. a,b,c. Normal heart and breath sounds without adventitious sounds. Serum potassium remains between 3.6 mEq/liter and 5.5 mEq/liter. Calcium remains between 4.6 mEq/liter and 5.5 mEq/liter. Hemoglobin remains between 12 g/100 ml and 18 g/100 ml. Serum drug levels are within the therapeutic range. Arterial blood gases on room air remain within the normal limits. Chest x-ray film remains within normal limits. Incorrect position of heart catheters is detected early.
c. Obtain venous blood (for electrolytes, hemoglobin, appropriate drug levels) and arterial blood (for blood gases) as prescribed.	c. Electrolyte imbalance (especially potassium or calcium) can cause arrhythmias and conduction disturbances. Reduced hemoglobin decreases the oxygen-carrying capacity of the blood. Hypoxemia, acidosis, alkalosis, and concurrent drug toxicity or subtherapeutic drug levels can cause arrhythmias and conduction disturbances.	

(continued)

Chart 29-1
Nursing Care of the Patient in the CCU (Uncomplicated Myocardial Infarction) (continued)

Nursing Intervention (continued)	*Rationale* (continued)	*Evaluation Criteria* (continued)

Problem 3: Respiratory Difficulties (Shortness of Breath, Dyspnea, Orthopnea)

1. Initially and every 4 hours, and with chest discomfort, assess, document, and report to the physician abnormal heart sounds (particularly S$_3$ and S$_4$ gallops and the holosystolic murmur of left ventricular papillary muscle dysfunction), abnormal breath sounds (particularly crackles), and patient intolerance to specific activities.	1. These data are useful in diagnosing left ventricular failure, Diastolic filling sounds (S$_3$—S$_4$ gallop) result from decreased left ventricular compliance associated with myocardial infarction, Papillary muscle dysfunction (from infarction of the papillary muscle) can result in mitral regurgitation and a reduction in stroke volume, leading to left ventricular failure. The presence of crackles (usually at the lung bases) may indicate pulmonary congestion from increased left heart pressures. The association of symptoms and activity can be used as a guide for activity prescription and a basis for patient teaching.	(For 1 through 4) Patient does not complain of shortness of breath, dyspnea on exertion, orthopnea, or paroxysmal nocturnal dyspnea. Respiratory rate remains less than 20 breaths per minute with physical activity and 16 breaths per minute with rest. Skin color is normal. PaO$_2$ and PaCO$_2$ are within normal range. Heart rate is less than 100 beats per minute with blood pressure within normal limits for this patient. Normal chest film.
2. Same as 5 and 6 for Problem 1.	2. Same as 5 and 6 for Problem 1.	
3. Full liquid diet for 24 hours as prescribed.	3. Digestion requires increased cardiac output, which increases the myocardial oxygen consumption. Full liquid diet facilitates digestion because the need to chew has been eliminated, thus requiring less cardiac demand than eating a regular diet.	
4. Teach patient: a. To adhere to the diet prescribed (for example, explain low sodium, low calories) b. To adhere to activity prescription	4. a. Low-sodium diet may reduce extracellular volume, thus reducing preload and afterload, and thus myocardial oxygen consumption. In the obese patient, weight reduction may decrease cardiac work and improve tidal volume. b. The activity prescription is determined individually to maintain the heart rate and blood pressure within safe limits.	

Problem 4: Reduced Perfusion to Vital Organs Related to Reduced Cardiac Output

1. Initially and every 4 hours, and with chest discomfort, assess, document, and report to the physician the following: a. Hypotension b. Tachycardia and other arrhythmia c. Fatigability d. Mentation changes (use family input) e. Reduced urine output (less than 250 ml per 8 hours) f. Cool, moist, cyanotic extremities	1. These data are useful in determining a low cardiac output state. An ECG with pain may be useful in the diagnosis of an extension of myocardial ischemia, injury, and infarction, and of variant angina.	(For 1 and 2) Blood pressure remains within the individual's normal range. Ideally, normal sinus rhythm without arrhythmia is maintained or patient's baseline rhythm is maintained between 60 and 100 beats per minute without further arrhythmia. No complaints of fatigue with prescribed activity. Remains fully alert and oriented and without personality change.

(continued)

Chart 29-1
Nursing Care of the Patient in the CCU (Uncomplicated Myocardial Infarction) (continued)

Nursing Intervention *(continued)*	***Rationale*** *(continued)*	***Evaluation Criteria*** *(continued)*

Problem 4: Reduced Perfusion to Vital Organs Related to Reduced Cardiac Output *(continued)*

2. Same as 5 and 6 from Problem 1.	2. Same as 5 and 6 from Problem 1.	Urine output is greater than 250 ml per 8-hour tour of duty. Extremities remain warm and dry with normal color.

Problem 5: Anxiety and Fear of Death

1. Assess, document, and report to the physician the patient's and family's level of anxiety and coping mechanisms.	1. These data provide information about the psychological well-being and a baseline so that post-therapy symptoms can be compared. Causes of anxiety are variable and individual, and may include acute illness, hospitalization, pain, disruption of activities of daily living at home and at work, changes in role and self-image owing to chronic illness, and lack of financial support. Because anxious family members can transmit anxiety to the patient, the nurse must also reduce the family's fear and anxiety.	(For 1 through 7) Patient reports less anxiety. Patient and family discuss their anxieties and fears about death. Patient and family appear less anxious. Patient is restful, respiratory rate less than 16 per minute, heart rate less than 100 per minute without ectopic beats, blood pressure within his normal limits, skin warm and dry. Patient participates actively in a progressive rehabilitation program. Patient practices stress-reduction techniques.
2. Same as 5 and 6 from Problem 1.	2. Same as 5 and 6 from Problem 1.	
3. Assess the need for spiritual counseling and refer as appropriate.	3. If a patient finds support in a religion, religious counseling may assist in reducing anxiety and fear.	

4. Allow patient (and family) to express anxiety and fear:
  a. By showing a genuine interest and concern
  b. By providing a conducive atmosphere
  c. By facilitating communication (listening, reflecting, guiding)
  d. By answering questions
	4. Unresolved anxiety (the stress response) increases myocardial oxygen consumption.	

5. Use of flexible visiting hours allows the presence of a supportive family to assist in reducing the patient's level of anxiety.	5. The presence of supportive family members may reduce both patient's and family's anxiety.	
6. Encourage active participation in a hospital cardiac rehabilitation program.	6. Prescribed cardiac rehabilitation may help to eliminate fear of death, may reduce anxiety, and may enhance feelings of well-being.	
7. Teach stress reduction techniques.	7. Stress reduction techniques may help to reduce myocardial oxygen consumption and may enhance feelings of well-being.	

(Adapted from Underhill SL et al: Cardiac Nursing. Philadelphia, JB Lippincott, 1982.)

lism, and heart block. These complications are the result of myocardial ischemia and necrosis.

Congestive Heart Failure

Congestive heart failure (CHF) is the syndrome of physiologic reactions that occurs when the heart ceases to function effectively as a pump to maintain adequate circulation of the blood. In the CCU the major cause of CHF is massive damage to the myocardium following an MI. Many authorities believe that after an MI all patients have a certain amount of CHF, the degree being determined by the size of the infarction. (See Chapter 31 for a discussion of CHF.)

Measurements of circulatory function during an MI have been shown to be valuable in patient monitoring and are commonly utilized in patients with complicated MI. The two most common measurements made are those of pressure and cardiac output. The pressure of blood in the right atrium is assessed by the measurement of central venous pressure (CVP), and in the left atrium by pulmonary artery ("wedge") pressure (Fig. 29-4). Cardiac output may also be determined through the use of a pulmonary artery catheter. Venous pressure and cardiac output can be obtained with the Swan–Ganz catheter (see Chap. 25), which is threaded through the right side of the heart into the pul-

monary artery. The Swan–Ganz catheter can measure the left ventricular end-diastolic pressure (LVEDP) and is the most accurate indicator for the presence of left heart failure. (The major nursing considerations for hemodynamic monitoring related to Swan–Ganz catheterization and central venous pressure are found in Charts 29-2 and 29-3.)

Management.   The treatment of CHF is directed at three main objectives:

1. To provide rest for the heart (to decrease the oxygen need of the heart)
2. To reduce the amount of circulating blood volume (to decrease the oxygen need of the heart)
3. To increase cardiac output by strengthening muscle contraction or decreasing peripheral resistance.

To accomplish these objectives, the patient is placed on bed rest, and the head of the bed is elevated. Diuretic therapy is given (to decrease circulating blood volume), and digitalis is sometimes administered to increase the force of myocardial contractions.

- Patients with MI appear to be sensitive to digitalis and must be monitored for rhythm disturbances when this drug is used.

(Text continues on page 598)

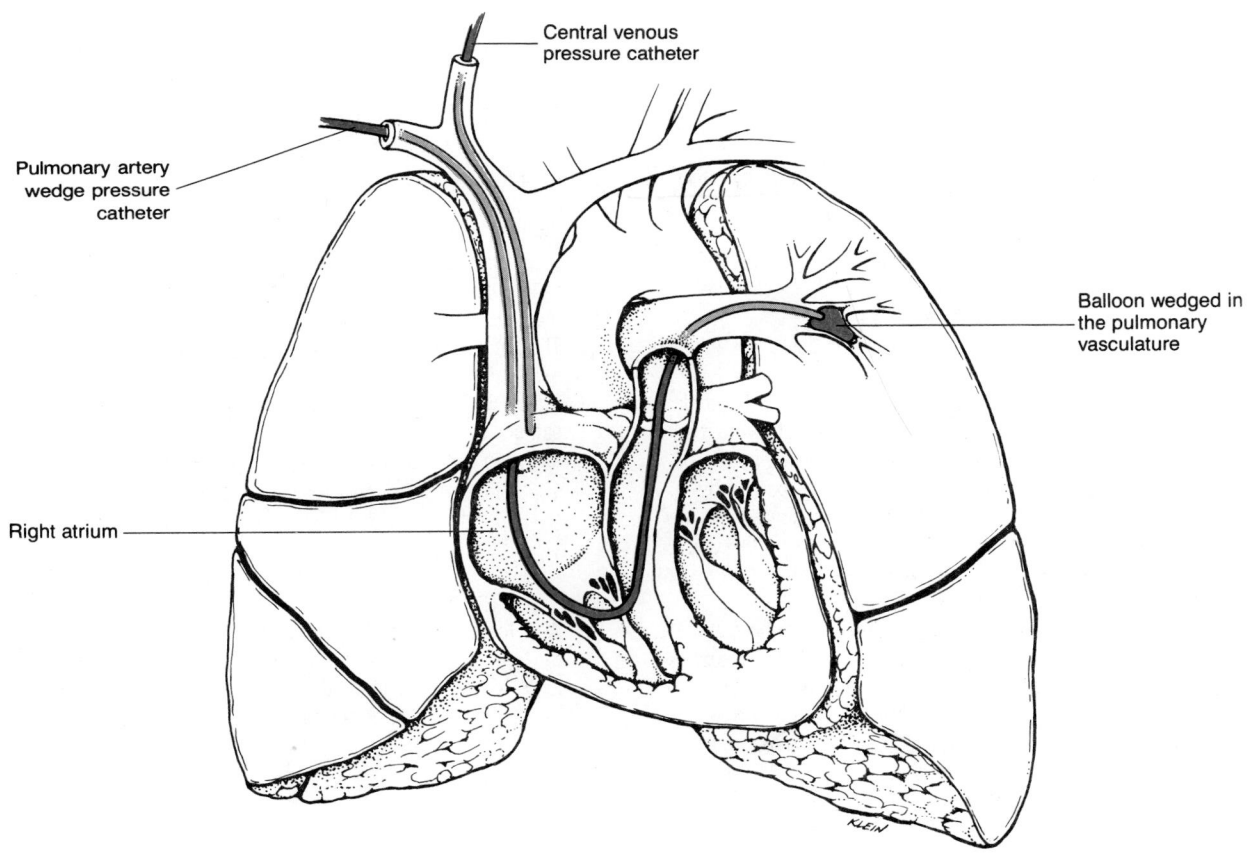

Central venous pressure catheter

Pulmonary artery wedge pressure catheter

Balloon wedged in the pulmonary vasculature

Right atrium

Figure 29-4.   Diagram showing central venous pressure catheter and pulmonary artery (Swan–Ganz) catheter in position: the choice depends on the patient's cardiac status.

Chart 29-2
Guidelines: Hemodynamic Monitoring: Swan–Ganz Catheterization

Nursing Action	*Rationale/Amplification*

Preparatory Phase

1. Explain procedure to patient and family/significant other.

2. Check vital signs and apply ECG electrodes.
3. Place patient in a position of comfort; this is the baseline position.

4. Set up equipment according to manufacturer's directives:
   a. The pulmonary artery catheter requires a transducer; recording, amplifying, and flush systems.

   b. The pressure equipment is calibrated and flushed according to manufacturer's directives.
   c. The balloon is inflated with air and then deflated. or it is inflated with air under sterile water or saline to test for leakage (bubbles).
5. Shave and prepare the skin over insertion site.

1. Tell the patient he may feel the catheter moving through his vein and that this is normal.

3. Note the angle of elevation if patient cannot lie flat, as subsequent pressure readings are taken from this baseline position to ensure consistency.

   a. Monitoring systems may vary greatly. The complexity of equipment requires an understanding of the equipment in use,
      A constant microdrip is maintained, except when reading pressures.
   b. Flushing of the catheter system ensures patency and eliminates air bubbles.
   c. To ensure that the balloon is intact.

Performance Phase *(by the physician)*

1. The Swan–Ganz catheter is inserted through the internal jugular, subclavian, or any easily accessible vein by either percutaneous puncture or venotomy.
2. The catheter is advanced to the superior vena cava. Oscillations of the pressure waveforms will indicate when the tip of the catheter is within the thoracic cavity. The patient may be asked to cough.
3. When the catheter is in the superior vena cava, it is inflated with air and advanced gently.
4. The inflated balloon at the tip of the catheter will be guided by the flowing stream of blood through the right atrium and tricuspid valve into the right ventricle. From this position it finds its way into the main pulmonary artery, carried by blood flow. The catheter tip pressures are recorded continuously by specific pressure wave forms as the catheter advances through the various chambers of the heart.
5. The flowing blood will continue to direct the catheter more distally into the pulmonary tree. When the catheter reaches a pulmonary vessel that is approximately the same size or slightly smaller in diameter than the inflated balloon, it cannot be advanced any further. This is the wedge position, called pulmonary capillary wedge pressure (PCWP) or pulmonary artery wedge pressure (PAWP).

1. The internal jugular vein establishes a short route into the central venous system.

2. Catheter placement may be determined by characteristic wave forms and changes. Coughing will produce deflections in the pressure tracing when the catheter tip is in the thorax.
3. The amount of air to be used is indicated on the catheter.

4. Watch ECG monitor for signs of ventricular irritability as catheter enters the right ventricle. Report any signs of arrhythmia to the physician.

5. With the catheter in the wedge position, the balloon blocks the flow of blood from the right side of the heart toward the lungs, and the resulting capillary wedge pressure is equal to the mean left atrial pressure.

(continued)

Chart 29-2
Guidelines: Hemodynamic Monitoring: Swan–Ganz Catheterization (continued)

Nursing Action (continued)	*Rationale/Amplification (continued)*

Performance Phase *(by the physician) (continued)*

6. The pressure is recorded with the balloon wedged in the pulmonary vascular bed. A mean capillary wedge pressure between 14 mm Hg and 18 mm Hg appears to indicate optimal left ventricular function.

6. Wedge pressure reading provides information about the level of pulmonary congestion and is closely related to left atrial pressure and to left ventricular end-diastolic pressure (in the absence of mitral valve disease). This is a valuable parameter of cardiac function. Filling pressures less than 8 mm Hg to 10 mm Hg in an acutely injured heart are often associated with reduction in cardiac output, hypotension, and tachycardia.

7. The balloon is deflated, causing the catheter to retract spontaneously into a larger pulmonary artery. This gives a continuous pulmonary artery systolic, diastolic, and mean pressure.

7. The normal systolic pulmonary pressure ranges are 15 mm Hg to 25 mm Hg, and the diastolic pulmonary pressure ranges are 8 mm Hg to 12 mm Hg. The normal mean pulmonary artery pressure (average pressure in pulmonary artery throughout the entire cardiac cycle) ranges from 10 mm Hg to 20 mm Hg.

8. The catheter is sutured in place.

8. An antibactericidal ointment may be placed around the site and covered with a sterile dressing.

9. The patency of the catheter is maintained with a low-flow continuous irrigation.

9. A chest x-ray to confirm catheter position and as a baseline for future reference is obtained after Swan–Ganz insertion.

To Obtain a Wedge Pressure Reading

1. Close off the microdrip.

1. The transducer converts the pressure wave into an electronic wave that is displayed on a screen.

2. Inflate the balloon slowly until the contour of the pulmonary arterial pressure changes to that of pulmonary wedge pressure. As soon as a wedge pattern is observed, no more air is introduced. Do not introduce more air into balloon than specified.

2. Pulmonary capillary wedge pressure is only measured intermittently. Do not allow catheter to remain in the wedge position when patient is unattended or when not directly making the measurement.

3. Deflate the balloon as soon as the pressure reading is obtained.

3. Segmental lung infarction may occur if the catheter balloon is left inflated for long periods.

Follow-Up Phase

1. Inspect the insertion site daily.
   Look for signs of infection, swelling, and bleeding.
   Culture the site every 48 hours.

1. A foreign body (catheter) in the vascular system increases the risk of sepsis.

2. Record data and time of dressing change and IV tubing change.

3. Assess the extremity for color, temperature, capillary filling, and sensation.

3. Ischemia (with possible loss of digits) may occur from inadequate arterial flow.

4. Evaluate pulse.

5. Assess for complications: pulmonary embolism, arrhythmias, heart block, damage to tricuspid valve, intracardiac knotting of catheter, thrombophlebitis, infection, balloon rupture, rupture of pulmonary artery.

For Removal of the Catheter

1. Be sure that the balloon is not inflated.

2. The catheter is removed without excessive force or traction; pressure dressing is applied over the site.

2. The site should be checked periodically for bleeding.

Chart 29-3
Guidelines: Hemodynamic Monitoring: Central Venous Pressure

Nursing Action	*Rationale/Amplification*
Preparatory Phase	
1. Assemble equipment according to manufacturer's directions.	
2. Explain that the procedure is similar to an IV and that the patient may move in bed as desired after the passage of the CVP catheter.	2. This helps provide reassurance.
3. Place the patient in a position of comfort. This is the baseline position used for subsequent readings.	3. Serial CVP readings should be made with the patient in the same position. Inaccuracies in CVP readings can be produced by changes in position, coughing, or straining during the reading.
4. Attach manometer to the IV pole. The zero point of the manometer should be on a level with the patient's right atrium. Mark the midaxillary line on the patient with an indelible pencil.	4. The right atrium is at the midaxillary line, which is about ⅓ of the distance from the anterior to the posterior chest wall. The midaxillary line is an external reference point for the zero level of the manometer (which coincides with the level of the right atrium).
5. The CVP catheter is connected to a three-way stopcock, which communicates to an open IV (*e.g.,* saline and heparin) and to a manometer (the measuring device).	5. Or, the CVP catheter may be connected to a transducer and an electrical monitor with either digital or calibrated CVP wave readout.
6. Start the IV flow and fill the manometer 10 cm above anticipated reading (or until the level of 20 cm H_2O is reached). Turn the stopcock and fill the tubing with fluid.	
7. The CVP site is surgically cleansed. CVP catheter (line) is introduced percutaneously or by direct venous cutdown and threaded through an antecubital, subclavian, or internal or external jugular vein into the superior vena cava just before it enters the right atrium.	7. If the catheter is inserted through the subclavian or internal jugular vein, place patient in a head-down position to increase venous filling and reduce risk of air embolism. The correct catheter placement can be confirmed by fluoroscopy or chest x-ray.
8. When the catheter enters the thorax, an inspiratory fall and expiratory rise in venous pressure are observed.	8. The fluid level fluctuates with respiration. It rises sharply with coughing, straining.
9. The patient may be monitored by ECG during catheter insertion.	9. When the tip of the catheter contacts with the wall of the right atrium (or right ventricle), it may produce aberrant impulses and disturb cardiac rhythm.
10. The catheter may be sutured and taped in place. A sterile dressing is applied.	10. Label dressing with time and date of catheter insertion.
11. The infusion is adjusted to flow into the patient's vein by a slow, continuous drip.	11. The infusion may cause a significant increase in venous pressure if permitted to flow too rapidly
To Measure the CVP	
1. Place the patient in the identified comfortable position and confirm the zero point. Intravascular pressures are measured to the atmospheric pressure at the middle of the right atrium; this is the zero point or external reference point.	1. The zero point or baseline for the manometer should be on a level with the patient's right atrium. The middle of the right atrium is the midaxillary line in the 4th intercostal space.
2. Position the zero point of the manometer at the level of the right atrium.	2. All personnel taking the CVP measurement use the same zero point.

(continued)

Chart 29-3
Guidelines: Hemodynamic Monitoring: Central Venous Pressure (continued)

Nursing Action (continued)	*Rationale/Amplification* (continued)

To Measure the CVP *(continued)*

3. Turn the stopcock so that the IV solution flows into the manometer, filling to about the 20-cm to 25-cm level. Then turn stopcock so that solution in manometer flows into patient.

4. Observe the fall in the height of the column of fluid in manometer. Record the level at which the solution stabilizes or stops moving downward. This is the central venous pressure. Record CVP and the position of the patient.

    4. The column of fluid will fall until it meets an equal pressure (i.e., the patient's central venous pressure). The CVP reading is reflected by the height of a column of fluid in the manometer when there is open communication between the catheter and the manometer. The fluid in the manometer will fluctuate slightly with the patient's respirations. This confirms that CVP line is not obstructed by clotted blood.

5. The CVP may range from 5 cm to 12 cm H_2O. (Absolute numerical values have not been agreed upon.)

    5. The change in CVP is a more useful indication of adequacy of venous blood volume and alterations of cardiovascular function. CVP is a dynamic measurement. The normal values may change from patient to patient. The management of the patient is not based on one reading but on repeated serial readings in correlation with patient's clinical status.

6. Assess the patient's clinical condition. Frequent changes in measurements (interpreted within the context of the clinical situation) will serve as a guide to detect whether the heart can handle its fluid load and whether hypovolemia or hypervolemia is present.

    6. CVP is interpreted by considering the patient's entire clinical picture: hourly urine output, heart rate, blood pressure, cardiac output measurements.
       a. A CVP near zero indicates that the patient is hypovolemic (verified if rapid IV infusion causes patient to improve).
       b. A CVP above 15 cm to 20 cm H_2O may be due to either hypervolemia or poor cardiac contractility.

7. Turn the stopcock again to allow IV solution to flow from solution bottle into patient's veins.

    7. When readings are not being made, flow is from a very slow microdrip to the catheter, bypassing the manometer.

Follow-up Phase

1. Observe for complications.
    a. From catheter insertion: pneumothorax; hemothorax; hematoma; cardiac tamponade.
    b. Secondary to presence of indwelling venous catheter: air embolism; catheter embolization; colonization of organisms.
2. Carry out ongoing nursing surveillance of the insertion site and maintain aseptic technique.
    a. Inspect entry site twice daily for signs of local inflammation/phlebitis. Remove catheter immediately if there are any signs of infection.
    b. Change dressings as prescribed.
    c. Label to show date/time of change.
    d. Send the catheter tip for bacteriologic culture when it is removed.

    1. The incidence of complications rises rapidly the longer the CVP catheter is left in place. The patient's complaint of a new or different pain should be assessed and acted upon.

Nursing Alert: A CVP line is a potential source of septicemia.

Oxygen is also usually indicated. Nitroprusside is a vasodilator that is used in several clinical situations; in the CCU it is used most often for left ventricular failure. In a compromised ventricle, nitroprusside improves hemodynamic action by reducing the impedance to left ventricular ejection (afterload), which results in an increase in cardiac output. Also, nitroglycerin may be used to decrease the venous return to the heart (preload) and to decrease the impedance to left ventricular ejection. Some authorities believe that the reduced need for myocardial oxygen may reduce the size of the infarction, and this hypothesis is the subject of extensive clinical investigations.

The nursing responsibility when the patient is receiving nitroprusside or nitroglycerin is directed toward strict monitoring of the circulatory status. Ideally, this is done by observing the internal cardiac pressure readings with a Swan–Ganz catheter and an arterial catheter. When these methods are not available, the standard methods for measuring systemic blood pressure should be used frequently, along with careful assessment of the clinical signs of poor tissue perfusion, such as change in mental status and diminished urinary output. Since these drugs are potent vasodilators, hypotension, with inadequate oxygenation of the tissues, is always a potential problem; the nurse must be aware of this complication.

- Since the use of these drugs is becoming more common in the treatment of CHF as a complication of MI, the nurse must be familiar with the values and problems associated with the use of these drugs and should follow the findings of the clinical results of the testing.

Cardiogenic Shock

Cardiogenic shock (power failure), the end stage of left ventricular dysfunction, occurs when the left ventricle is extensively damaged by MI. The heart muscle loses its contractile power, and the result is a marked reduction in cardiac output with decreased perfusion to vital organs (heart, brain, and kidneys). The degree of pump dysfunction is related to the extent of damage to the heart muscle.

Pathophysiology. The symptoms and signs of cardiogenic shock reflect the circular nature of the pathophysiology of the condition. The damage to the myocardium results in a decrease of the cardiac output, which in turn reduces the arterial blood pressure in the vital organs. Flow to the coronary arteries is reduced, and this results in a decrease in the oxygen supply to the myocardium, which in turn increases ischemia and further reduces the heart's ability to pump. Thus, a "vicious cycle" is set in motion.

- The classic signs of cardiogenic shock are low blood pressure, rapid and weak pulse, signs of cerebral anoxia manifested by confusion and agitation, and decreased urinary output.

Arrhythmias are common and result from a decrease of oxygen to the myocardium. As in CHF, the use of the Swan–Ganz catheter to measure left ventricular pressure is important in assessing the severity of the problem and evaluating management. Continuing elevation of left ventricular end-diastolic pressure (LVEDP) accompanied by a fall in arterial blood pressure indicates the failure of the heart to function as an effective pump.

Management. There are many approaches to the treatment of cardiogenic shock. Any major arrhythmia is corrected, since these may have caused or contributed to the shock. If low intravascular volume is suspected, or found through pressure readings (*i.e.,* hypovolemia), the patient is treated by infusion of volume expanders. If hypoxia is present, oxygen is given, often under positive pressure when regular flow is insufficient to meet tissue demands.

Drug therapy is selected and guided by cardiac output and mean arterial blood pressure. With respect to specific medications, there continues to be controversy about the best approach. One group of drugs used are the catecholamines, which raise the blood pressure and increase the cardiac output. This, however, tends to increase the workload of the heart, and many studies are currently being done to test vasodilator drugs that impede the resistance to the circulation and thereby reduce the workload of the heart. The latter approach is gaining widespread support.

Other therapeutic modalities employed in treating cardiogenic shock involve the use of circulatory assist devices. The most frequently used mechanical support system is the intra-aortic balloon pump (IABP). The IABP uses internal counterpulsation to augment the pumping action of the heart by the regular inflation and deflation of a balloon located in the descending thoracic aorta (Fig. 29-5). The device is connected to a control box that directs its activities by synchronization with the electrocardiogram. Hemodynamic monitoring is also essential to determine the patient's circulatory status during the use of the IABP. The balloon inflates during ventricular diastole and deflates during systole at a rate equal to the heart rate. The IABP augments diastole, which results in increased perfusion of the coronary arteries and myocardium and a decrease in the left ventricular workload. Studies have indicated that prompt use of this method of treatment reduces the mortality rate of patients with cardiogenic shock.

Nursing Implications. Cardiogenic shock, with an untreated mortality rate of over 90%, is described as the most lethal complication of acute MI in the hospitalized patient. The patient with this complication requires constant nursing care and observation. Careful patient assessment, measurement of hemodynamic parameters, and recording of intake and urinary output are essential. The patient must be closely monitored for arrhythmias, which must be corrected immediately.

Other Complications

Pulmonary Embolism. The decreased mobility of the patient and the impaired circulation that follow the MI contribute to the development of intracardiac and intravascular thrombosis. As the patient moves about more, a thrombus may become detached (the detached thrombus is called an embolus) and may be carried to the lungs.

The symptoms of pulmonary embolism include chest pain, cyanosis, shortness of breath, rapid respirations, and hemoptysis. The pulmonary embolus may block the circu-

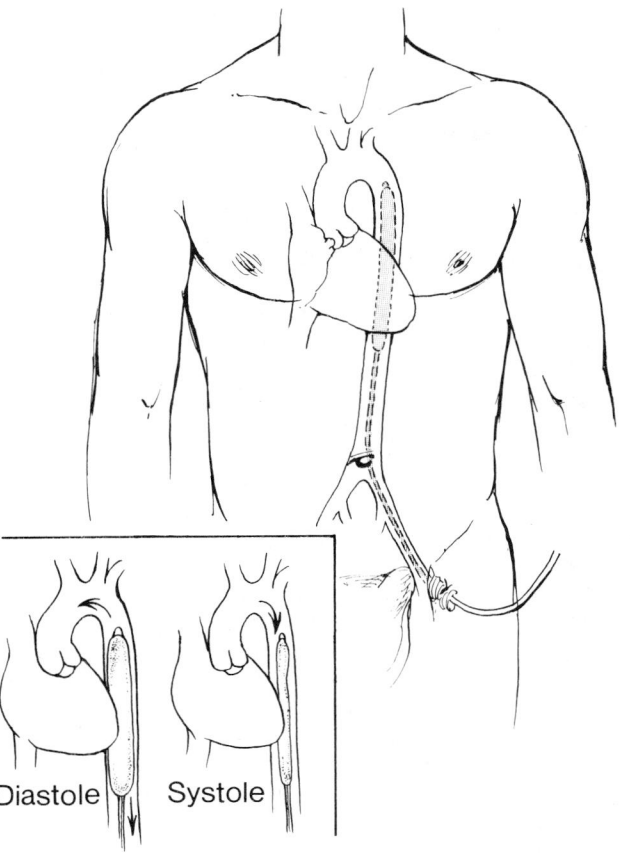

Diastole   Systole

Figure 29-5. The intra-aortic balloon pump augments diastole, which results in increased perfusion of the coronary arteries and myocardium and a decrease in the left ventricular workload.

lation to a part of the lung, producing an area of pulmonary infarction. The pain experienced is usually pleuritic—that is, it increases with respiration and may disappear when the patient holds his breath. Cardiac pain, however, is continuous and usually does not vary with respirations. The treatment of this condition is discussed on pages 530–532.

Systemic embolism may occur from the left ventricle, and the resulting vascular occlusion may present as stroke or renal infarct; it may compromise the blood supply to an extremity. The nurse must be aware of such possible complications and prepared to identify and report signs and symptoms.

Myocardial Rupture. When an infarction extends through much of the cardiac muscle, the heart may rupture, leading to immediate death in most cases. Cardiac rupture, although fairly rare, can occur during the first week following an MI.

Death is caused by cardiac tamponade (the heart is bleeding into its pericardial sac); thus, pericardiocentesis (aspiration of the pericardial cavity) and repair of the myocardium can be lifesaving measures. The clinician detects this condition by noticing a sudden increase in the disten-

tion of the neck veins, a decrease in heart sounds, and a reduction of blood pressure with inspiration. Pericardiocentesis is performed by placing a long No. 18 needle (spinal needle) just to the left of the xyphoid and directing it under the rib cage to the left shoulder (pp. 653–654).

Heart Block. Heart block may follow acute MI as a result of damage to the conduction system, which may interfere with the normal impulse from the atria to the ventricles. This damage may occur above or below the atrioventricular node, the latter being the more serious. When second- or third-degree heart blocks are present, the heart rate is slowed and cardiac output is decreased. This may precipitate CHF, cardiogenic shock, and death.

The usual treatment of choice is artificial pacing (pp. 644–647). Although there continues to be controversy regarding the usefulness of artificial pacing in reducing mortality owing to heart block, this treatment is used more and more. The nurse who functions in the CCU must be prepared to care for patients with pacemakers and must be alert to the most common complication, ventricular arrhythmias resulting in cardiac arrest; emergency equipment must be available.

▷ Emergency Intervention in Cardiac Arrest

A complication of MI that requires immediate action is cardiac arrest. This is a sudden cessation of effective heart action with lack of circulation. In the CCU this is most commonly caused by failure of the electrical conduction system owing to the damaged myocardium. Most often, cardiac arrest in the CCU is preceded by premature ventricular contractions (PVCs) that result in ventricular fibrillation. Ventricular fibrillation is a continuous, ineffective movement of the heart muscle, sometimes described as a "quiver."

Diagnosis must be made immediately so that conversion to effective heart action may be accomplished before irreversible cerebral damage is caused by anoxia. The main symptom is immediate loss of consciousness. Other symptoms include absence of carotid or femoral pulses; absence of audible heart signs; absence of breath sounds; convulsions; dilatation of pupils; and grey, ashen color. In the CCU, the electrocardiographic monitor will show a waving line in ventricular fibrillation or a flat line in ventricular asystole.

In a witnessed cardiac arrest, a precordial thump should be attempted. This sharp, quick single blow to the midportion of the sternum will generate a small electrical stimulus that may restore normal beat. If this is not effective, direct electrical defibrillation is done. If the equipment is not available, or until it is, supportive cardiopulmonary resuscitation (CPR) is started. (Electrical defibrillation is discussed on p. 579.)

Cardiopulmonary Resuscitation

Basic cardiopulmonary resuscitation (CPR) consists of the following ABC sequence: Airway, Breathing, and Circulation. The resuscitation process consists of maintaining an open airway, providing artificial ventilation by means of rescue breathing, and providing artificial circulation by external cardiac compression.

The recommended approach to cardiac arrest in monitored patients is as follows:

1. Give a single precordial thump.
2. Quickly check the monitor for cardiac rhythm, and simultaneously check carotid pulse.
3. If there is ventricular fibrillation or ventricular tachycardia without a pulse, deliver countershock as soon as possible (see pp. 579–580).
4. If the pulse is absent, tilt the head and give four quick, full, long inflations.
5. Check carotid pulse again.
6. If the pulse is absent, begin one-rescuer or two-rescuer CPR (Fig. 29-6).

- **Note:** *It must be emphasized strongly that no time should be lost by waiting to assess the results of the precordial thump or by delivering repeated precordial thumps.*

The first step in CPR is to open an airway. Remove any material from the airway and lift the jaw forward. Insert an oropharyngeal airway if available. Ventilate the patient 12 breaths per minute using direct mouth-to-mouth breathing or by using the bag and mask technique.

The next step after ventilation is external cardiac compression. This must be done with the patient on a firm surface. The heel of one hand is placed on the lower half of the sternum, 3.8 cm (1½ inches) from the tip of the xiphoid and toward the patient's head. Place the other hand on top of the first one. The fingers should not touch the chest wall. Using the body weight while keeping the elbows straight, apply quick, forceful compressions to the lower sternum, 3.8 cm to 5.0 cm (1½–2 inches) toward the spine. Regular compression and release are made 60 times per minute.

When two persons are available, the first person does the cardiac compressions and the second ventilates the patient after five compressions (see Fig. 29-6). If only one person is available, the rate is 2 ventilations to every 15 cardiac compressions.

The decision to terminate resuscitation is based on medical considerations and will take into account the cerebral and cardiac status of the patient.

Following the successful resuscitation of the patient with cardiac arrest, the nurse should carefully monitor the patient's condition, since he is at great risk for another cardiac arrest. Continuation of ECG monitoring is essential and any abnormalities of rhythm must be corrected. Electrolyte and acid–base balances must be established and maintained. Hemodynamic monitoring should be initiated if it was not previously instituted. Selected drugs are used during and after resuscitation (Table 29-1), and these should be immediately available in the CCU.

The nurse who works in the CCU must be aware that patients who witness a cardiac arrest are very distressed by the experience and often exhibit anger or lack of identification with the victim. Both are useful defense mechanisms. Following such an event, there may be an increase in patient requests for sedation, and these should be met, if compatible with the individual patient's total condition.

▷ Psychological Problems in the Cardiac Care Unit

During the Acute Phase

Of great concern to the nurse in the CCU are the psychological problems of the patient with an MI. Problems that are apt to occur early in the hospitalization can be recognized and in some instances prevented. In this regard, the nurse helps the patient and his family to cope with such difficulties. It has been suggested that the typical patient reacts to an MI with a pattern of four basic responses—anxiety, denial, depression, and chronic behavioral traits (Fig. 29-7).

Anxiety.   Anxiety occurs early in the CCU and, in fact, is probably pronounced at the time of admission. Such fears are caused by the prospect of death or by the symptoms that may herald death, such as breathlessness, severe chest pains, and complications of the MI (arrhythmias, cardioversion, or pacemaker insertion). The patient is "scared" and fears death, pain, and the strange environment. Although the patient may appear tense, restless, and watchful, he may or may not voice his feelings and uneasiness. The nurse should explain all interventions to the patient and provide reassurance by accenting positive factors in the situation. Medications for pain relief and sedation are given as frequently as needed.

Denial.   The second predictable psychological reaction is denial, which usually appears on the second or third day of hospitalization and may be either conscious or unconscious. The patient may begin to deny that he ever had a heart attack, or he may say that the diagnosis is incorrect. There is controversy regarding the usefulness of this defense mechanism. Nurses caring for these patients are aware that denial is a common reaction that accounts for the calm nature of the patient, even when his condition is serious. It is not considered helpful to the patient to insist that he is being foolish in his denial. Nonetheless, the nurse should be honest in explaining the patient's condition to him in order to establish the reality of the situation.

Depression.   Depression is the expected response on the third or fourth post-MI day and occurs soon after denial, when the reality of the illness has set in. At this time the patient has often passed the critical stage and is beginning to evaluate the changes in life-style that the illness could cause. Changes in self-concept and self-perception, concerns about earning a living or fulfilling former role requirements, and doubts about the ability to resume the usual activities of living may trouble the patient. It is interesting to note that women experience depression in a less acute manner than male patients. The best approach of the nurse during this period is to listen carefully to the problems ex-

Cardiopulmonary Resuscitation (CPR)

(Basic life support—adult)

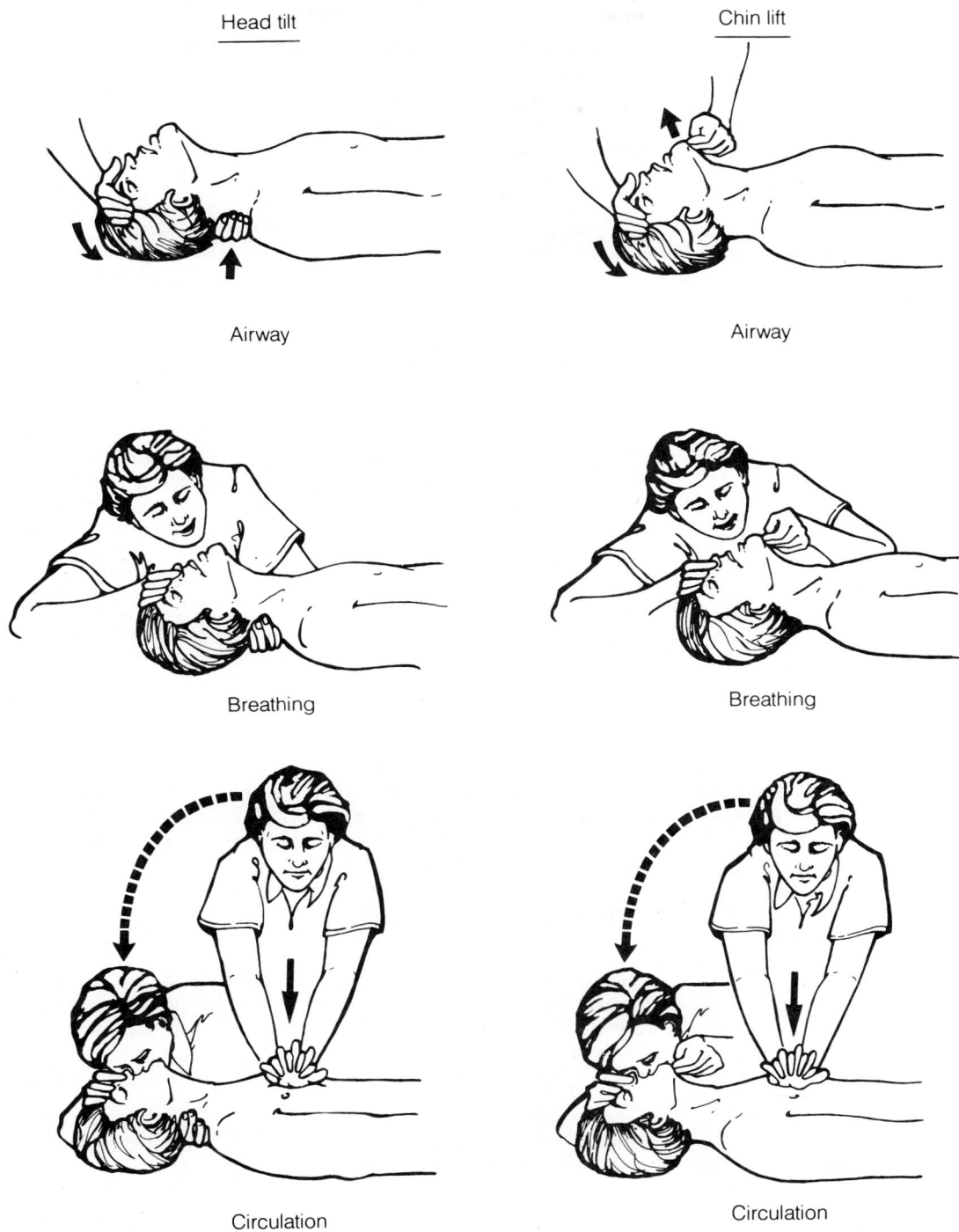

Figure 29-6. Cardiopulmonary resuscitation. (Reprinted from the Supplement to Journal of the American Medical Association, August 1, 1980. Copyright 1980, the American Medical Association. Reprinted with permission from the American Heart Association.)

pressed by the patient and to answer questions and concerns as honestly as possible.

Chronic Behavioral Traits. Following depression, the patient often exhibits chronic traits that may be manifested in behavior problems. One of the more serious problems is the patient who wants to discharge himself from the hospital against the advice of his physician. This may be attributed to the fact that the patient believes he is not seriously ill. He may still be in a denial state and may complain about being in the CCU. Often, "significant others" (wife, clergy, children) may be able to convince the patient that remaining in the unit is in his best interest. Other behavior problems often relate to overt sexual comments or actions directed to the nursing staff by male patients. These expressions may reflect anxiety related to threats to the male role and should be managed with understanding.

Anxiety Related to Transfer

The patient must be prepared for transfer from the specialized care of the CCU to a nursing unit where he will be more independent. The patient-to-nurse ratio in the non-acute setting is much higher, and the patient may feel more

Table 29-1
Essential Drugs Used During Cardiopulmonary Arrest

Drug	Purpose	Dosage	Side-effects and Comments
Oxygen	To correct hypoxemia	4–10 liters/minute	No lung damage when used for less than 24 hours
Sodium bicarbonate (NaHCO$_3$)	To correct metabolic and respiratory acidosis	1 mg/kg intravenously (IV) initially. One half initial dose (0.5 mg/kg) given IV every 10–15 minutes. Analysis of arterial blood gases should guide treatment.	$HCO_3 + H \leftrightarrows H_2CO_3 \leftrightarrows CO_2 + H_2O$ Since CO$_2$ production is increased, adequate ventilation is required. Excessive NaHCO$_3$ leads to metabolic alkalosis with displacement of oxyhemoglobin dissociation curve and consequent impairment of oxygen release to tissues. Hyperosmolality may also develop. Catecholamines and calcium salts should not be added to bicarbonate infusions, because inactivation results. Since bicarbonate has a high pH, avoid mixing any drugs with it.
Epinephrine	To increase perfusion pressure during cardiac compressions To improve the myocardial contractile state To stimulate spontaneous contractions (*e.g.*, in asystole) To increase the vigor of ventricular fibrillation (VF)	0.5 mg–1.0 mg IV or intratracheally (5 ml–10 ml of a 1:10,000 solution). Repeat every 5 minutes as needed. If tracheal and venous routes are not available, the drug may be administered carefully via the intracardiac route.	Epinephrine should not be added directly to a bicarbonate infusion, since catecholamines may be inactivated by alkaline solution.
Atropine	To accelerate cardiac rate by creating a positive chronotrophic effect owing to parasympatholytic action (reduces vagal tone) and by creating a positive dromotropic effect that accelerates AV conduction	0.5 mg IV. Repeat every 5 minutes as needed up to a total of 2 mg.	This increased heart rate may be deleterious in patients with acute MI. Atropine should be given to patients with acute MI only if the bradycardia results in hemodynamic changes.
Lidocaine	To suppress ventricular arrhythmias To elevate the threshold for VF	1 mg/kg IV followed by an infusion of 1 mg/minute–4 mg/minute	Myocardial and circulatory depression. CNS changes: drowsiness, disorientation, decreased hearing ability, paresthesias, muscle twitching, and agitation. Focal and grand mal seizures.

(Adapted from White RD: Essential drugs in emergency cardiac care. In American Heart Association Committee on Emergency Cardiac Care VII, pp 1–13, 1975.)

(continued)

vulnerable. Symptoms of stress may occur, including insomnia, arrhythmias, and possible extension of the infarction. Increased urine catecholamines, suggesting increased stress, have been found in transfer patients. Efforts are currently being made by the nursing staff of the CCU to prepare the patient for transfer. The care of the patient after transfer from the CCU is discussed on pages 633–635.

Related Stress Problems of Nursing Staff

Nurses working in the CCU frequently report high levels of stress. Although many reasons for this reaction have been identified, the chief cause probably is the continual care of critically ill patients who need constant supervision. Other sources of stress that are cited are overwhelming workloads, too much responsibility, poor communication with physicians and staff in other units, limited work area, and inadequate continuing education programs. This high stress level found in the CCU often causes a high "turnover" rate among the nursing staff, which can prove costly to the institution because of the expense involved in preparing a nurse to function in the unit. One of the best methods of dealing with stress in the CCU is recognition of the potential

Table 29-1
Essential Drugs Used During Cardiopulmonary Arrest (continued)

Drug	Purpose	Dosage	Side-effects and Comments
Procainamide	To suppress ventricular arrhythmias; may be effective when lidocaine is not	100 mg IV every 5 minutes at a rate of 20 mg/minute, up to 1 g as needed to control arrhythmia; infusion at 1 mg/minute–4 mg/minute	Hypotension. Widening of QRS complex and lengthening of the P–R and Q–T intervals. AV block and cardiac arrest.
Bretylium tosylate	To elevate the VF To suppress ventricular arrhythmias	For VF, 5 mg/kg undiluted is given rapidly IV. Then defibrillation is attempted. If VF persists, the dose is increased to 10 mg/kg and the shock repeated. For ventricular tachycardia, 500 mg in 50 ml and 5 mg/kg–10 mg/kg IV over 8–10 minutes. The second dose of 5 mg/kg–10 mg/kg can be given in 1–2 hours if arrhythmia persists and if necessary every 6–8 hours. Alternatively, the drug can be administered as a continuous infusion at a rate of 2 mg/minute.	Initial transient increase in arterial pressure and cardiac rate followed by a decrease in both. Cardiac output and preload remain unchanged. Vomiting after rapid injection. Postural hypotension. Contraindicated in digitalis toxicity, except with intractable VF.
Verapamil	To suppress some supraventricular tachyarrhythmias and to slow the ventricular responses in atrial flutter and atrial fibrillation To slow conduction through the AV node	0.075 mg/kg–0.15 mg/kg (maximum: 10 mg) IV over 1–3 minutes. 0.15 mg/kg (maximum: 10 mg) 30 minutes after first dose if necessary. (Total cumulative dose within 30 minutes should not exceed 15 mg.)	Transient hypotension Negatively inotropic Coronary and peripheral vasodilator; contraindicated with use of beta-blocking drug
Calcium chloride	To stimulate spontaneous or more forceful myocardial contractions by creating a positive inotropic effect, by enhancing ventricular excitability; and by prolonging systole	5 mg/kg–7 mg/kg of 10% calcium (Ca^{2+}) chloride solution (3.4 mEq–6.8 mEq). May be repeated every 10 minutes. Ca gluceptate, 5 ml–7 ml (4.5 mEq–6.3 mEq). Ca gluconate, 10 ml–15 ml (4.8 mEq–7.2 mEq).	Calcium and digoxin are synergistic. Calcium and bicarbonate mixed form a precipitate carbonate each should be given separately.
Morphine	To relieve pain To treat pulmonary edema (decreases venous return to the heart)	2 mg–5 mg IV every 5–30 minutes (15 mg in 15 ml IV solution)	Respiratory depression Hypotension

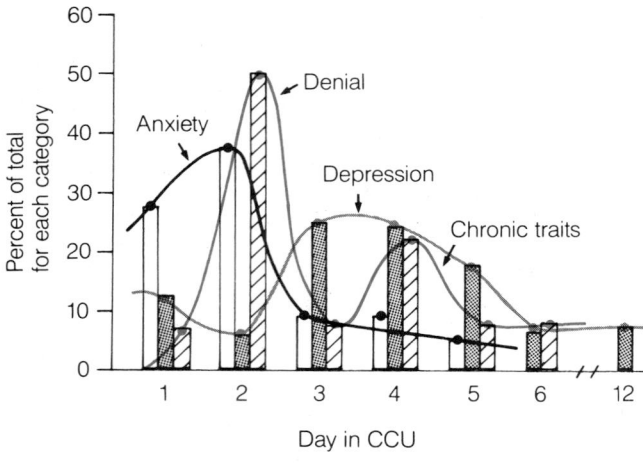

Figure 29-7. Hypothetical schedule of onset of emotional and behavioral reactions of a coronary care unit (CCU) patient. (© Reprinted with permission, American Heart Association.)

sources of stress through open group discussions in unit conferences, inservice education, and other similar activities. Consideration of the emotional needs of the nursing staff is essential for maintaining a therapeutic environment that will ensure good care of the patient with an MI.

▷ **Bibliography**

Books

American Heart Association Subcommittee on Emergency Cardiac Care. A Manual for Instructors of Basic Life Support. Dallas, American Heart Association, 1981.

Bordicks KJ. Patterns of Shock, 2nd ed. New York, Macmillan, 1980.

Diet and Coronary Heart Disease. Dallas, American Heart Association, 1978.

Foster WT. Principles of Acute Coronary Care. New York, Appleton–Century–Crofts, 1976.

Gentry WD and Williams RB. Psychological Aspects of Myocardial Infarction and Coronary Care. St Louis, CV Mosby, 1975.

Hamilton AJ. Selected Subjects for Critical Care Nurses. Missoula, Montana, Mountain Press, 1975.

Holland JM. Cardiovascular Nursing: Prevention, Intervention, and Rehabilitation. Boston, Little, Brown & Co, 1977.

Holloway NM. Nursing the Critically Ill Adult. Menlo Park, Addison–Wesley, 1979.

Let's Plug in the Heart. Buffalo, Graphic Controls, 1979.

McGurn WC. People with Cardiac Problems: Nursing Concepts. Philadelphia, JB Lippincott, 1981.

McIntyre KM and Lewis AJ (eds). Textbook of Advanced Cardiac Life Support. Dallas, American Heart Association, 1981.

Thrombold JC, Monsen ER, and Karkeck JM. Dietary Guidelines for Hospital Cardiac Care Units. Seattle, American Heart Association of Washington, 1976.

Woods SL (ed). Cardiovascular Critical Care Nursing. Contemporary Issues in Critical Care Nursing, Vol 5. New York, Churchill Livingstone, 1983.

Articles

Budassi S. Differential diagnosis of cardiopulmonary arrest. JEN 1981 Mar–Apr; 7(2):79–80.

Coglman MM: Effects of oxygen on ischemic myocardium. Heart Lung 1978 July–Aug; 7(4):635–740.

Delano A et al. Monitoring the acutely ill cardiac patient. Cardiovasc Nurs 1971 Jan–Feb; 7(1):61–64.

Hurst JW, Logue RB, and Walter PF. The clinical recognition and medical management of coronary atherosclerotic heart disease. In The Heart, pp 1252–1260. New York, McGraw–Hill, 1978.

Marriott HJL and Fogg E. Constant monitoring for cardiac dysrhythmias and block. Mod Concepts Cardiovasc Dis 1970 June; 39(6):103–108.

Matheny L. Emergency! First aid for cardiopulmonary arrest. Nursing '82 1982 June; 12(6):34–43.

McNeal GJ. Rectal temperatures in the patient with an acute myocardial infarction. Image 1978 Feb; 10(1):18–23.

McNeer JF et al. Hospital discharge one week after acute myocardial infarction. N Engl J Med 1978 Feb 2; 298(5):229–232.

Patros RJ and Goren CC. The precordial thump: An adjunct to emergency medicine. Heart Lung 1983 Jan; 12(1):61–64.

Pollack–Latham CL (ed). Advances in coronary care. Crit Care Quart 1981 Sept; 4(2):1–103.

Rogers DJ, Branyon ME, and Kinney MR: Care of the cardiac patient. In Andreoli et al (eds). Comprehensive Cardiac Care, 4th ed, pp 280–334. St Louis, CV Mosby, 1979.

Standards and guidelines for cardiopulmonary resuscitation (CPR) and emergency cardiac care (ECC). JAMA 1980 Aug 1; 244(5):453–509.

Sweetwood HM. Oxygen administration in the coronary care unit. Heart Lung 1974 Jan–Feb; 3(1):102–107.

Tuggle DJ. Meeting the emotional needs of survivors of sudden cardiac arrest. Cardiovasc Nurs 1982 Sept–Oct; 18(1):25–30.

Vaughan P and Rice V. Complications of myocardial infarction. Crit Care Nurse 1982 May–June; 2(3):44–51.

Walinsky P. Acute hemodynamic monitoring. Heart Lung 1977 Sept–Oct; 6(5):838–844.

Winslow EH. A symposium on teaching and rehabilitating the cardiac patient. Nurs Clin North Am 1976 June; 11(2):211–383.

Woods SL. Arrhythmias complicating myocardial infarction. In Underhill SL et al. Cardiac Nursing, pp 363–377. Philadelphia, JB Lippincott, 1982.

Woods SL. Diagnosis and treatment of the patient with an uncomplicated myocardial infarction. In Underhill SL et al. Cardiac Nursing, pp 326–377. Philadelphia, JB Lippincott, 1982.

Ziesche S and Franciosa J. Clinical application of sodium nitroprusside. Heart Lung 1977 Jan–Feb; 6(1):99–103.

30

Management of the Cardiovascular Surgery Patient

Since the performance of valvular heart surgery in the 1940s, continued advances in technology associated with cardiac diagnostics, anesthesia, and surgery have made it possible today to perform surgery to correct many congenital heart defects, to bypass blockages in the coronary arteries, to resect arrhythmia foci, and to transplant hearts. In 1978, 95,000 coronary artery bypass graft (CABG) surgeries and 33,000 valve surgeries were performed in the United States. The number of valve surgeries has decreased with the reduced incidence of rheumatic heart disease. The high number of CABG surgeries performed can be attributed to improvements in cardiac cineangiography, cardiopulmonary bypass techniques, and anesthesia techniques.

This chapter will describe the pathology, surgical procedures, and care required by adults with heart disease. Congenital heart defects will not be covered but may be reviewed in a pediatric textbook.

▷ Cardiovascular Procedures

Cardiopulmonary Bypass

Many of the heart surgery procedures are performed while the patient is placed on partial or complete cardiopulmonary bypass (extracorporeal circulation). Any of the heart surgeries that require direct visualization via an incision into the heart (*i.e.,* valve replacements) or that require the heart to be arrested (*i.e.,* CABG) utilize cardiopulmonary bypass. In this procedure, the patient is placed on a machine that consists of a mechanical pump that simulates the pumping action of the left ventricle and an oxygenator that simulates the function of the lungs. The blood is removed from the systemic circulation via cannulas inserted into the inferior and superior venae cavae. By means of the force of gravity or with the aid of a pump, the blood enters the venous reservoir and is then filtered, passed through the oxygenator and heat exchanger, and returned to the patient via a cannula in the ascending aorta or the femoral artery. The oxygenated blood is used by the tissues of the body and then returned to the pump or heart–lung machine, where the process is repeated (Fig. 30-1).

Portions of this chapter originally appeared in *Cardiac Nursing* by Underhill et al., published in 1982 by J. B. Lippincott.

Many surgeons place a cannula vent in the left ventricle with low, intermittent suction to drain any blood returning to the left heart from the pulmonary circulation. Drainage of blood via the vent prevents left ventricular distention, which could lead to increased pulmonary pressures and transcapillary leak of fluids into the lungs.

Although there have been several types of machines, at present the most commonly used are those with the bubble oxygenator or the membrane oxygenator. The bubble oxygenator bubbles oxygen through a long column of blood in a chamber. The blood is foamy when it reaches the top of the chamber and is defoamed when it passes over steel wool or a polypropylene mesh with a silicone antifoam compound on its surface. The membrane oxygenator uses a semipermeable membrane that separates blood from gas-containing oxygen, eliminating direct blood gas interface, which occurs in the bubble oxygenator. Oxygen diffuses across the membrane into the blood in a manner similar to the physiologic process that takes place between the alveoli and capillaries in the lungs.

While some physicians prefer the membrane oxygenator because it eliminates the direct blood gas interface, there seems to be little clinical difference between the bubble and the membrane oxygenators. At present, the bubble oxygenator is more widely used.

A direct complication of extracorporeal circulation that sometimes occurs is aortic dissection resulting from cannulation of the aorta. Secondary complications that can occur include impaired renal function, pulmonary dysfunction, neurologic dysfunction, or postoperative bleeding. These complications result from underlying disease, low blood flow, fluid overload, or inadequate heparinization.

During surgery, the adequacy of tissue perfusion is determined by monitoring the electrocardiogram, arterial blood pressure, left atrial pressure, urine output, and arterial blood gases. Both the anesthesiologist and the pump perfusionist monitor all these parameters.

Mitral Valve Commissurotomy

Mitral valve stenosis is narrowing of the valve orifice secondary to thickening and loss of pliability of the valve leaflets and chordae tendineae. Progressive scarring with deformity and calcification causes fusion of the valve commissures and contraction of the chordae tendineae. The resultant narrowing of the valve orifice impedes the flow of blood through the valve. The left atrium dilates and hypertrophies, and pulmonary pressures increase in some cases, causing high pulmonary vascular resistance and variable degrees of right heart failure.

Mitral stenosis results almost exclusively from rheu-

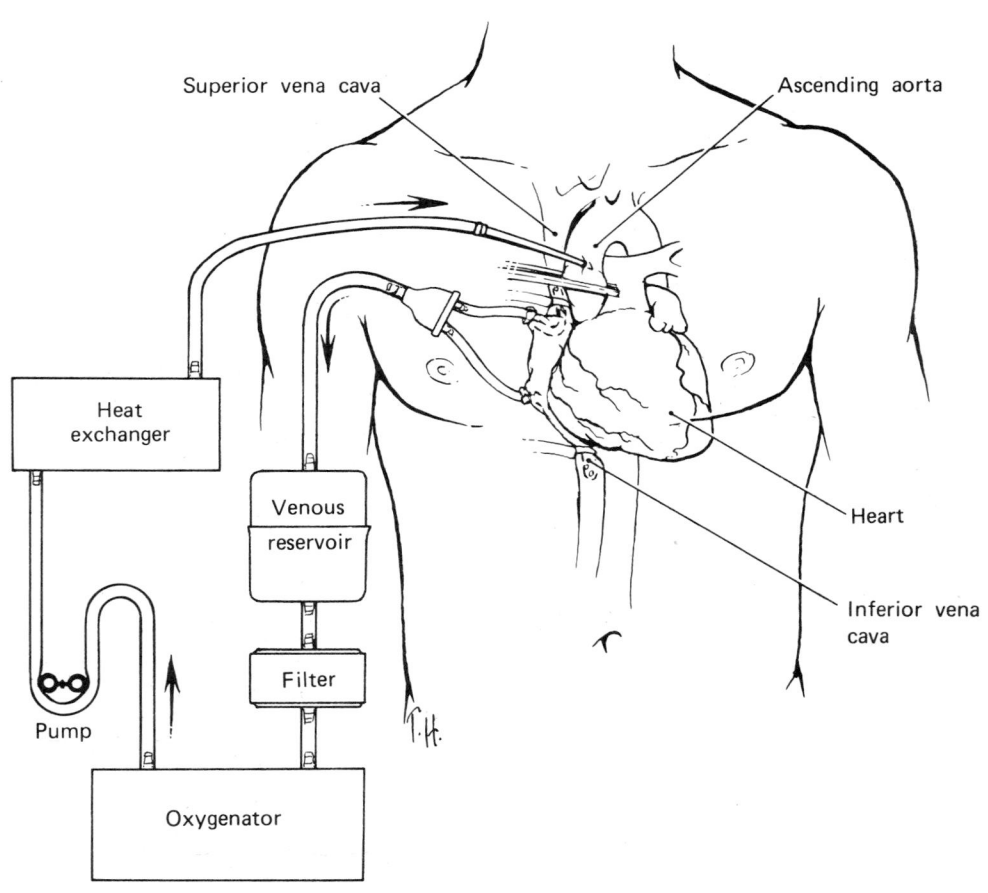

Figure 30-1. Schematic drawing of the heart–lung bypass.

matic endocarditis. Rarely, it results from congenital absence of one of the papillary muscles. Patients with mitral stenosis experience dyspnea associated with the increased pulmonary artery pressures. Some will experience hemoptysis and pulmonary edema. With more advanced disease, patients develop high pulmonary vascular resistance, right heart failure, and low cardiac output. In addition to dyspnea, fatigue, and weakness, these patients frequently have peripheral edema and hepatic engorgement. Most patients with long-standing mitral stenosis also develop atrial fibrillation secondary to dilatation of the left atrium. This irregular rhythm further reduces left ventricular filling and cardiac output because of the loss of atrial contraction in coordination with ventricular filling. Atrial fibrillation and atrial dilatation also allow blood to stagnate in the atrium, forming mural thrombi. Dislodgment of any of these thrombi can cause systemic or pulmonary embolization.

The patient with mitral stenosis can usually be managed with medical therapy initially. The goals of therapy are to reduce pulmonary edema and congestive heart failure, to prevent pulmonary and cardiac infections, to prevent embolization, and to maximize cardiac output by controlling heart rate (see Chap. 31). Patients with progressive symptoms are stabilized medically and then treated surgically. If the valve cusps are still pliable, mitral stenosis can be corrected with a mitral commissurotomy whereby the fused portion of the leaflets of the valve are opened. A pliable valve is determined by the presence of an opening snap on auscultation and the absence of calcification on echocardiography or cinefluorography.

The closed mitral commissurotomy procedure is performed without direct visualization of the mitral valve. The procedure is performed through a right anterolateral thoracotomy. A small incision is made in the left atrium and the mitral valve is dilated by insertion of the surgeon's finger or a metal dilator through the valve. This procedure does not require cardiopulmonary bypass. However, the extracorporeal circulation equipment is prepared and available for use should the commissurotomy fail and valve replacement is required, or should complications occur that require direct visualization and operation on the valve.

Open mitral commissurotomy is performed through a large incision in the left atrium, which provides direct visualization for the procedure. Open commissurotomy requires cardiopulmonary bypass. Some surgeons prefer this technique so they can observe any thrombi in the atrium or any calcium plaques on the valve leaflets. It may also be preferred when it is suspected that the commissurotomy may fail, necessitating valve replacement. Mitral commissurotomy is associated with a low incidence of surgical complication and mortality.

Mitral Valve Replacement or Repair

Mitral insufficiency (regurgitation) results from incomplete closure of the mitral valve. The incomplete closure allows backward flow of blood (regurgitation) from the left ventricle to the atrium during ventricular systole. This regurgitated blood is returned to the left ventricle with the normal amount of circulating blood during atrial systole, thus increasing the volume of blood the left ventricle must han-

dle. This increased blood volume results in dilatation and hypertrophy of both the left atrium and the left ventricle.

Mitral insufficiency is caused by rheumatic or bacterial endocarditis. These infectious processes cause fibrotic and calcific changes that thicken, shorten, and deform the valve cusps in such a way that they do not completely close. Other causes of mitral insufficiency include ischemia or infarction of the papillary muscles, ruptured chordae tendineae secondary to bacterial endocarditis, and congenital deformities.

Patients with mitral insufficiency have chronic pulmonary congestion and symptoms of fatigue, orthopnea, exertional dyspnea, and palpitations. They may develop atrial extrasystoles or atrial fibrillation secondary to dilatation of the left atrium (see Chap. 28). Some patients develop pulmonary edema and hemoptysis, especially if the mitral insufficiency develops suddenly, as from infarcted papillary muscle or ruptured chordae tendineae.

Mitral valve insufficiency is most often treated with drug therapy to increase cardiac contractility, to reduce the pressures the left ventricle must pump against, and to reduce congestive heart failure (see Chap. 31). Surgical treatment is indicated when the patient develops sudden dysfunction and severe failure from ruptured papillary muscle or when the patient with chronic insufficiency develops symptoms (fatigue, palpitations, and dyspnea) during minimal activity.

Whenever possible, the mitral valve is repaired rather than replaced in order to avoid the long-term risks associated with artificial valves. Repair of the mitral valve involves reconstruction of the valve leaflets and annulus. The procedure is called an annuloplasty and usually involves suturing of the valve tissue to a flexible ring (Carpenter's ring).

Should the mitral valve leaflets be calcified and immobile, a valve replacement is performed. This procedure is performed through a median sternotomy incision. The valve, chordae tendineae, and papillary muscles are excised and replaced with an appropriate prosthetic heart valve. The Bjork–Shiley tilting disc valve prosthesis is most often used. Others that may be used include the Starr–Edwards silastic ball valve, the Lillehei–Caster tilting disc valve, and the SJM bileaflet prosthesis. Patients who have any of these valve devices placed are usually maintained on anticoagulant therapy postoperatively to minimize the risk of embolization.

Patients in whom anticoagulant therapy is contraindicated, such as children, young adult females, geriatric patients, and patients with peptic ulcer disease, have biological valves placed. Currently, glutaraldehyde-preserved, stent-mounted, porcine aortic valve xenografts are used (Fig. 30-2).

Patients who have both mitral stenosis and insufficiency may have both a mitral commissurotomy and an annuloplasty done. Some patients require a valve replacement for this mixed stenosis and insufficiency.

Aortic Valve Replacement

Aortic valve replacement is done for patients with aortic insufficiency. Aortic stenosis is narrowing of the valve orifice between the left ventricle and the aorta. Aortic stenosis can result from rheumatic heart disease, congenital bicuspid

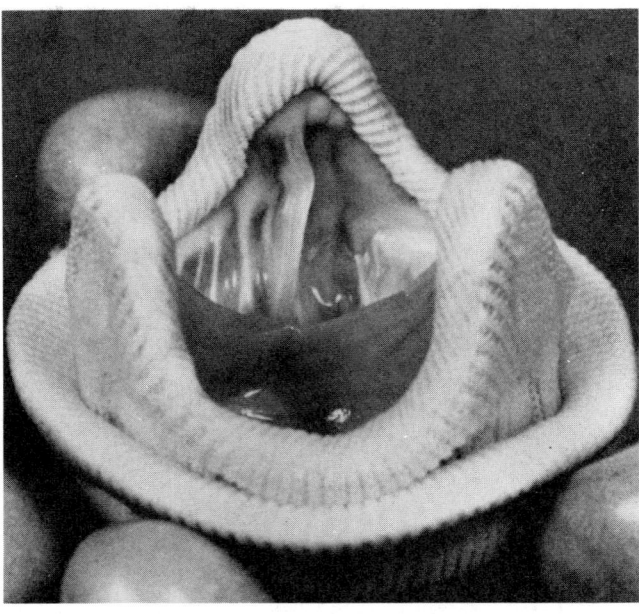

Figure 30-2. Porcine heart valve.

valve, or calcification of unknown origin. Rheumatic changes include thickening and fibrosis of the cusps, fusion of the commissures, and valve calcification.

Aortic stenosis results in left ventricular hypertrophy and decreased ventricular compliance. The high ventricular systolic pressures inhibit the vasoconstriction reflex associated with exercise. The resulting decreased cardiac output reduces cardiac and cerebral perfusion and may cause syncope, angina, and tachyarrhythmias or bradyarrhythmias.

Severe aortic stenotic disease results in left ventricular failure, decreased cardiac output, left atrial failure, pulmonary edema, and eventually right heart failure. Sudden death occurs even in patients who are asymptomatic, probably owing to ventricular fibrillation.

The goal of medical therapy is to reduce congestive failure and angina (see Chap. 31). If patients have heart failure, syncope, or angina, aortic valve replacement is indicated. Some physicians perform aortic valve replacement even on asymptomatic patients because of the risk of sudden death associated with aortic stenosis.

Aortic valve insufficiency is due to incomplete closure of the aortic valve cusps during ventricular diastole. This incomplete closure allows blood to flow backward (regurgitate) from the aorta into the left ventricle. With rheumatic heart disease and bacterial endocarditis, the valve leaflets become thickened and scarred, lose compliance, and eventually become calcified. This process causes deformity that prevents approximation of the valve cusps.

Other causes of aortic insufficiency include congenital bicuspid valves, traumatic tears, dissecting aortic aneurysms, syphilitic aortitis, and cystic medial necrosis. Syphilitic aortitis affects the ascending aorta, causing widening of the aorta and valve orifice. The resultant stress on the aortic valve causes fibrotic changes in the valve cusps, which worsens the insufficiency. The effects of microcysts on the me-

dia of the aorta in cystic medial necrosis can cause dilatation of the aortic root; rupture of the aorta, resulting in an aneurysm; or changes in the connective tissues. These changes distort the aortic valve so that the cusps do not close completely, resulting in insufficiency (regurgitation).

The regurgitation of blood into the left ventricle results in dilatation and hypertrophy of the ventricle. The ventricle pumps more forcefully to expel the blood, and as a result systolic blood pressure is elevated. The elevated systolic pressure triggers a reflex that dilates the peripheral arterioles and decreases peripheral vascular resistance and diastolic blood pressure. Patients with aortic insufficiency characteristically have an elevated systolic blood pressure, a low diastolic blood pressure, and thus a wide pulse pressure. These patients also develop symptoms associated with the increased force of ventricular systole, such as bounding pulse, palpitations, and awareness of pulsations in the neck. Other symptoms include dyspnea with exertion and dizziness with sudden postural change.

Patients who suddenly develop aortic insufficiency without compensatory changes develop heart failure and decreased cardiac output, which can result in death.

The treatment for patients who are symptomatic or for patients who have documented left ventricular hypertrophy and pressure changes is aortic valve replacement. The patient who develops acute aortic insufficiency may require drug therapy to increase cardiac output and to reduce failure prior to emergency aortic valve replacement.

Aortic valve replacement is performed through a median sternotomy incision using total cardiopulmonary bypass. The aortic valve tissue is removed through a transverse incision in the aorta, and a prosthetic valve is sutured in place. Aortic prosthetic devices that are used include the Bjork–Shiley, Lillehei–Caster, SJM, and the Starr–Edwards. These all require prolonged anticoagulant therapy to prevent thromboembolism.

When anticoagulant therapy is contraindicated, a biological valve prosthesis (porcine valve) is used for replacement. These tissue valves are not thrombogenic and do not require anticoagulant therapy, but they may degenerate and necessitate replacement.

Tricuspid Valve Repair or Replacement

Tricuspid valve stenosis is characterized by the same fibrotic and calcific changes as stenosis of the other heart valves. These changes result in narrowing of the valve orifice, which impedes the flow of blood from the right atrium to the right ventricle. The right atrium dilates, and right-sided heart failure leads to venous congestion with cyanosis, hepatomegaly, peripheral edema, and ascites.

Tricuspid stenosis is caused by rheumatic heart disease, bacterial endocarditis, or congenital heart defects. With rheumatic heart disease, the tricuspid valve is frequently both stenotic and insufficient. Most often the mitral valve, and sometimes the aortic valve, have rheumatic disease changes also.

If the stenotic tricuspid valve requires surgical repair, most often a commissurotomy is done. If the valve is both stenotic and insufficient, both a commissurotomy and an annuloplasty may be performed. Replacement of the tricuspid valve is required infrequently. In such cases an artificial or biological prosthesis may be used, depending on the suitability for the individual patient.

Tricuspid insufficiency is incomplete closure of the tricuspid valve during right ventricular systole (incompetence), resulting in backward flow of blood (regurgitation) from the right ventricle to the right atrium. Tricuspid insufficiency is most often a functional disorder caused by failure and dilatation of the heart from severe mitral valve insufficiency. The resulting dilatation of the heart distorts the orifice of the tricuspid valve. Insufficiency may also result from fibrotic and calcific changes caused by rheumatic or bacterial endocarditis.

The symptoms of tricuspid insufficiency are the same as those of tricuspid stenosis. In the symptomatic patient, the treatment is annuloplasty and sometimes valve replacement. If the insufficiency is a functional disorder, the defects in the other heart valves are corrected first.

Tricuspid annuloplasty may be done using a Carpenter flexible ring that is modified to avoid the area of the septal leaflet associated with the atrioventricular node and the His bundle. Another technique used to correct tricuspid insufficiency involves stitching the annulus to narrow the valve (DeVega annuloplasty). Tricuspid valve replacement is performed only on severely deformed, stenotic, and insufficient valves.

Pulmonary Valve Disease

Diseases of the pulmonary valve are uncommon unless associated with congenital heart disease. Such defects are usually diagnosed and treated in the pediatric patient.

Repair of Traumatic Lesions of the Heart

Traumatic lesions of the heart are becoming more common as accidents owing to high-speed transportation increase and crime rates rise. A wide variety of injuries are possible, such as laceration of a coronary artery or rupture of the chordae tendineae, papillary muscles, or valve cusps (blunt, nonpenetrating injuries). Survival from penetrating injuries, such as gunshot or stab wounds, depends largely on the location of the injury, the size of the wound, and the availability of emergency medical and surgical management of cardiac tamponade (acute compression of the heart owing to rapid accumulation of blood in the pericardium) or shock. The particular lesion determines what therapy is required.

Removal of Cardiac Tumors

Cardiac tumors, especially primary tumors, are rare. The most common benign tumor is the myxoma, which is an intercavitary tumor that is formed on a stalk, or pedicle. It is often difficult to diagnose myxomas because of their similarity to thrombi. However, successful removal of these tumors has been achieved. The most common malignant primary tumor of the heart is sarcoma. Secondary malignant tumors of the heart are usually due to metastasis from a primary lesion elsewhere in the body.

Ascending Aorta Repair

Diseases of the ascending aorta, primarily aneurysms, are surgically repaired by cross clamping the area above the

aneurysm, removing the diseased or affected portion, and replacing it with a Teflon or Dacron graft.

Pericardectomy

When inflammation or disease of the pericardium restricts the movement and filling of the heart, the pericardial sac may need to be surgically removed. Some of the causes of pericarditis include infection, connective tissue disorders, hypersensitivity states, neoplasms, and trauma (see Chap. 31).

Constrictive pericarditis restricts filling of the heart and thus reduces venous return and cardiac output. The patient suffers dyspnea and other ill effects of reduced cardiac output.

Pericardectomy is removal of the pericardial sac. The removal is done very gently and slowly. The left ventricle is freed first, so that the increased flow to the right side of the heart is prevented from overloading the lungs and causing pulmonary edema. This method also allows the left ventricle to adjust to the increased blood volume that it will receive as the constriction is removed.

Left Ventricular Aneurysmectomy

An aneurysm is a ballooning enlargement of the ventricle owing to weakening of the ventricular wall. Left ventricular aneurysms occur in 5% to 35% of patients who suffer myocardial infarction secondary to the injury and scarring caused by the infarction. In some cases the presence of an aneurysm may cause the heart to become ineffective as a pump, leading to congestive heart failure, peripheral emboli, and tachyarrhythmias, which can be difficult to treat. Surgical removal of the ballooned portion of the left ventricular wall (aneurysmectomy) may be indicated for the symptomatic patient. Patients often show a marked improvement in cardiac reserve following surgery, and the arrhythmias usually disappear.

Surgical Removal of Arrhythmia Foci and Pathways

Recent advances in direct electrophysiologic study of the heart during surgery has made it possible to locate the origin or pathway of arrhythmias. Direct cardiac mapping has been most successful in the localization of accessory pathways associated with Wolff–Parkinson–White (WPW) syndrome. Direct cardiac mapping can also be used to localize the site of origin of atrial or ventricular arrhythmias and the site of myocardial ischemia and infarction.

Surgical resection of the arrhythmia focus or pathway is indicated if the arrhythmia is life-threatening and is refractory to medical therapy. Preoperatively, complete electrophysiologic study is performed using cardiac catheters to induce arrhythmias and to map and record the activity of the heart.

The surgical procedure is performed through a median sternotomy. Electrodes are placed directly on the heart and a recording is made. In the case of recurrent ventricular tachycardia following myocardial infarction, an aneurysmectomy and CABG procedure are often performed along with the endocardial resection. In WPW syndrome, direct cardiac mapping is performed to locate the accessory pathways. After the pathways are dissected, arrhythmias are induced and further cardiac mapping is performed to exclude the presence of additional accessory pathways. These surgical procedures require use of cardiopulmonary bypass. Perioperative care is the same as for other heart surgery procedures.

Surgical Intervention for Coronary Artery Disease

Coronary artery disease is a narrowing and distortion of the coronary arteries, resulting in decreased blood flow to the myocardium. It is caused by atherosclerosis. The atherosclerotic process causes proliferation of smooth muscle cells and accumulation of lipids in the intima of the artery wall. The cause of this atherosclerosis is not known. Risk factors that have been identified include high blood pressure, hyperlipidemia, smoking, and obesity. Some of the symptoms associated with coronary artery disease are angina, myocardial infarction, and primary ventricular fibrillation.

The choice of medical or surgical intervention for the treatment of patients with coronary artery disease has been the subject of much controversy. Because surgical intervention cannot alter the atherosclerotic disease process, it may not prolong life or reduce the occurrence of myocardial infarction. However, because it reduces angina and increases activity tolerance, surgical intervention is used to improve the quality of life.

Generally, medical therapy is used initially to relieve the pain of angina, to improve the blood and oxygen supply to the myocardium, and to reduce the oxygen needs of the myocardium (see Chap. 31). A criterion generally accepted as rationale for surgical intervention is disabling angina pectoris unrelieved by medical therapy. Because the severity of angina that is disabling can only be determined by the patient, ultimately the decision of whether or not to have surgery must be made by the patient.

The location and amount of stenosis in the coronary arteries, the amount of myocardium served by the stenotic artery, and previous infarction related to an affected artery are all factors considered by the physician when recommending therapy. Patients with greater than 50% stenosis of the left main coronary artery have better prognostic results with surgical intervention. Stenosis of other coronary arteries exceeding 70% occlusion is considered significant disease and may be treated surgically. Generally, unstable angina, postinfarction angina, and myocardial infarction complicated by left ventricular power failure or intractable ventricular arrhythmias are treated surgically. Myocardial revascularization of patients with uncomplicated acute myocardial infarction is done at some centers where physicians believe the surgery will salvage ischemic myocardium.

Coronary artery disease is treated surgically by myocardial revascularization (aortocoronary and internal mammary artery bypass grafting), by heart transplantation, and by coronary transluminal angioplasty (dilatation of diseased coronary arteries with a balloon-tipped catheter). Because the decision of when it is appropriate to use surgical therapy is somewhat controversial, it is imperative that the benefits and risks of the proposed therapy and alternative therapies be explained to the patient and family. The patient must ultimately define what limitations and risks are tolerable and what therapeutic approach is acceptable.

Myocardial Revascularization. Aortocoronary bypass graft surgery connects a segment of a vein or artery between the aortic root and the affected coronary artery at a point distal to the obstruction or stenosis caused by atherosclerosis. Most often a portion of the patient's saphenous vein is used for the graft(s).

Aortocoronary bypass graft surgery is done through a median sternotomy. Most surgeons support the patient on cardiopulmonary bypass so the heart can be arrested and a quiet field provided for anastomosis of the saphenous veins to the coronary arteries.

The segments of saphenous vein are implanted in the aortic root with an end-to-side anastomosis. The veins are placed in a reverse position so that their valves do not interfere with blood flow through the vein (Fig. 30-3).

Direct bypass of the occluded coronary arteries by attachment of a mammary artery distal to the obstruction has also been effective (Fig. 30-4). Some surgeons have had a lower incidence of postoperative occlusion with mammary-artery-to-coronary bypass than with aortocoronary saphenous vein bypass. However, because the mammary artery is of limited length, it can only be used to revascularize the anterior surface of the heart.

Percutaneous Transluminal Coronary Angioplasty. Percutaneous transluminal coronary angioplasty (PTCA) can be performed instead of coronary artery bypass graft (CABG) surgery in some patients with single-vessel coronary artery disease. The procedure is usually performed on patients who have had angina for less than 1 year. Cardiac cineangiography is used to confirm that the patient has a single atherosclerotic lesion in the proximal portion of a single vessel, that it is not calcified, that there is no distal stenosis, and that the lesion is not at a bifurcation.

Percutaneous transluminal coronary angioplasty is done by inserting a balloon-tipped catheter into the diseased coronary artery and reducing the stenosis by inflating the balloon with controlled pressure (Fig. 30-5). The procedure is performed in the cardiac catheterization facility. Preprocedure and postprocedure care is very similar to the care of the cardiac catheterization patient.

Complications of PTCA are abrupt occlusion of the artery through collapse, spasm, or clot; arterial dissection or rupture; or myocardial infarction. The procedure is performed with surgical personnel and an operating room on standby. Should a patient develop any of these complications, emergency CABG surgery is performed.

The patient who has PTCA is hospitalized for only 2 to 4 days and may immediately resume previous activity levels. While the long-term effects of this procedure are not yet fully documented, the advantages of the procedure being less invasive make it preferable to CABG surgery for selected patients.

Heart Transplantation. Heart transplantation is performed for either end-stage coronary artery disease or advanced idiopathic cardiomyopathy. Heart transplantation is currently performed in only a few centers because of the complex surgical and management techniques and because of the infrequency of the procedure. Transplantation is contraindicated in patients with active infection or with donor-specific antibodies. It may be contraindicated for patients

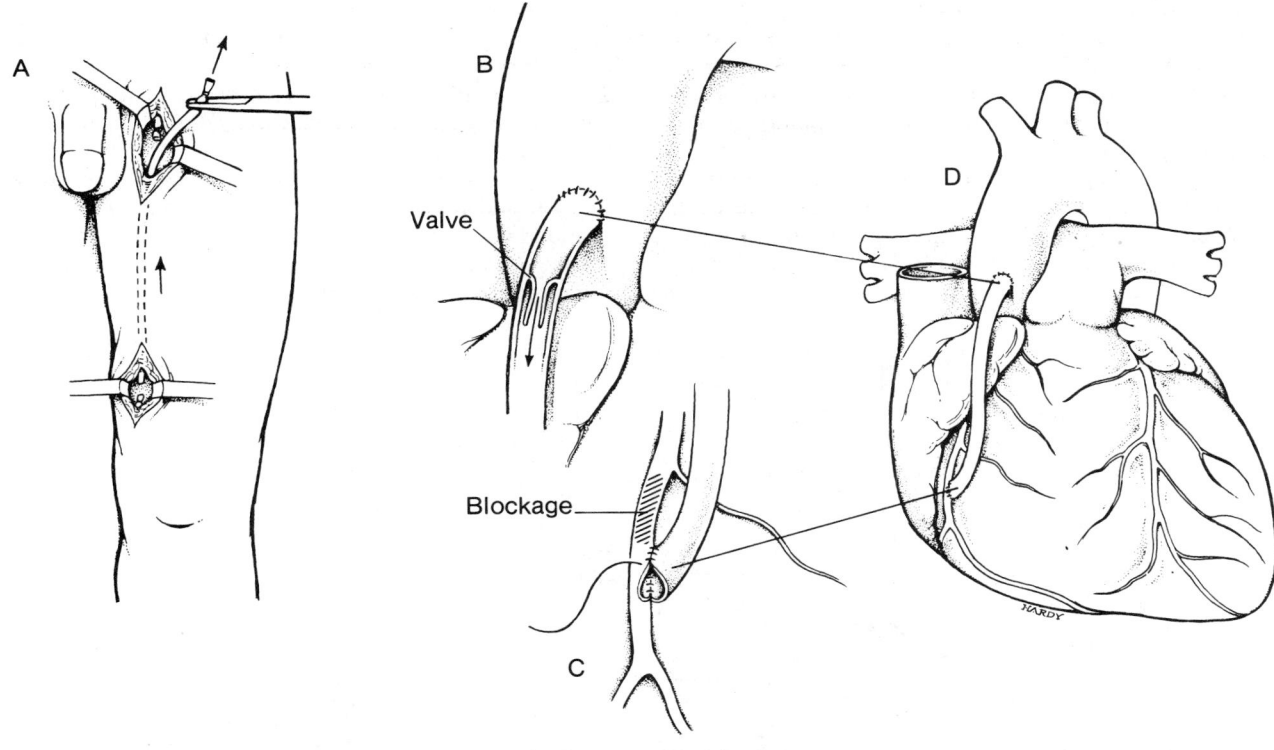

Figure 30-3. Saphenous vein revascularization procedure. (*A*) Saphenous vein is removed from the patient's leg. The vein is reversed so that valves will not interfere with blood flow. (*B*) The distal end of vein is sutured to the ascending aorta. (*C*) At a point distal to the blockage, the vein is sutured to the coronary artery by end-to-end anastomosis. (*D*) The completed bypass reestablishes the flow distal to the blockage.

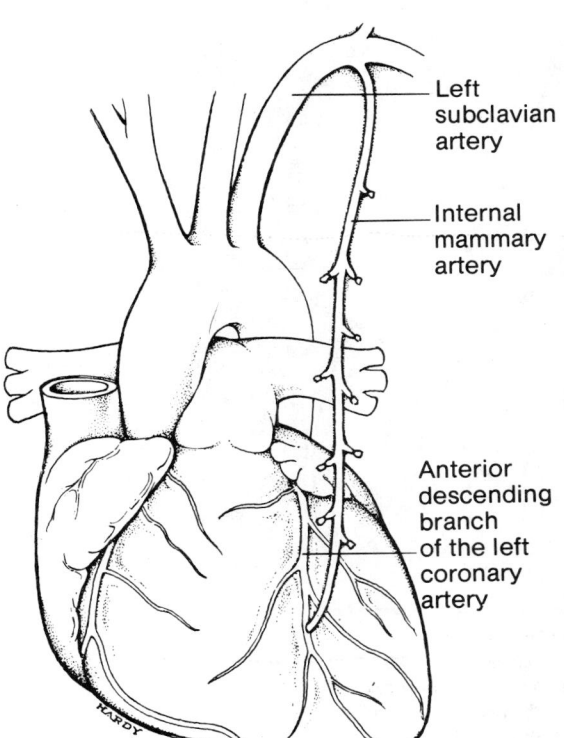

Left subclavian artery

Internal mammary artery

Anterior descending branch of the left coronary artery

Figure 30-4. Mammary artery revascularization procedure, showing mammary artery anastomosis to the anterior descending branch of the left coronary artery.

with other chronic diseases, cachexia, severe pulmonary hypertension, a history of pulmonary infarction, or lymphocyte hyperactivity, or for patients who are over 50 years of age. The patient's emotional acceptance of the transplantation and family support systems are also important for the long recovery period.

The heart is removed from the donor by transecting the great vessels and the atria at a point dorsal to the atrial appendages. In preparing the recipient, many surgeons retain portions of the recipient atria to facilitate anastomosis of the donor heart. First, the atria of the donor heart are sutured to the atria of the patient's heart. Transplantation is completed by connecting the great vessels and then evacuating air from the heart chambers. Transplantation is performed through a median sternotomy. The patient is supported by cardiopulmonary bypass during the transplantation procedure.

The primary focus of postoperative care is to prevent infection and rejection. The patient is kept in protective isolation postoperatively to prevent infection. Immunosuppressive therapy is used to minimize rejection. Atrial electrogram monitoring and endomyocardial biopsy are used

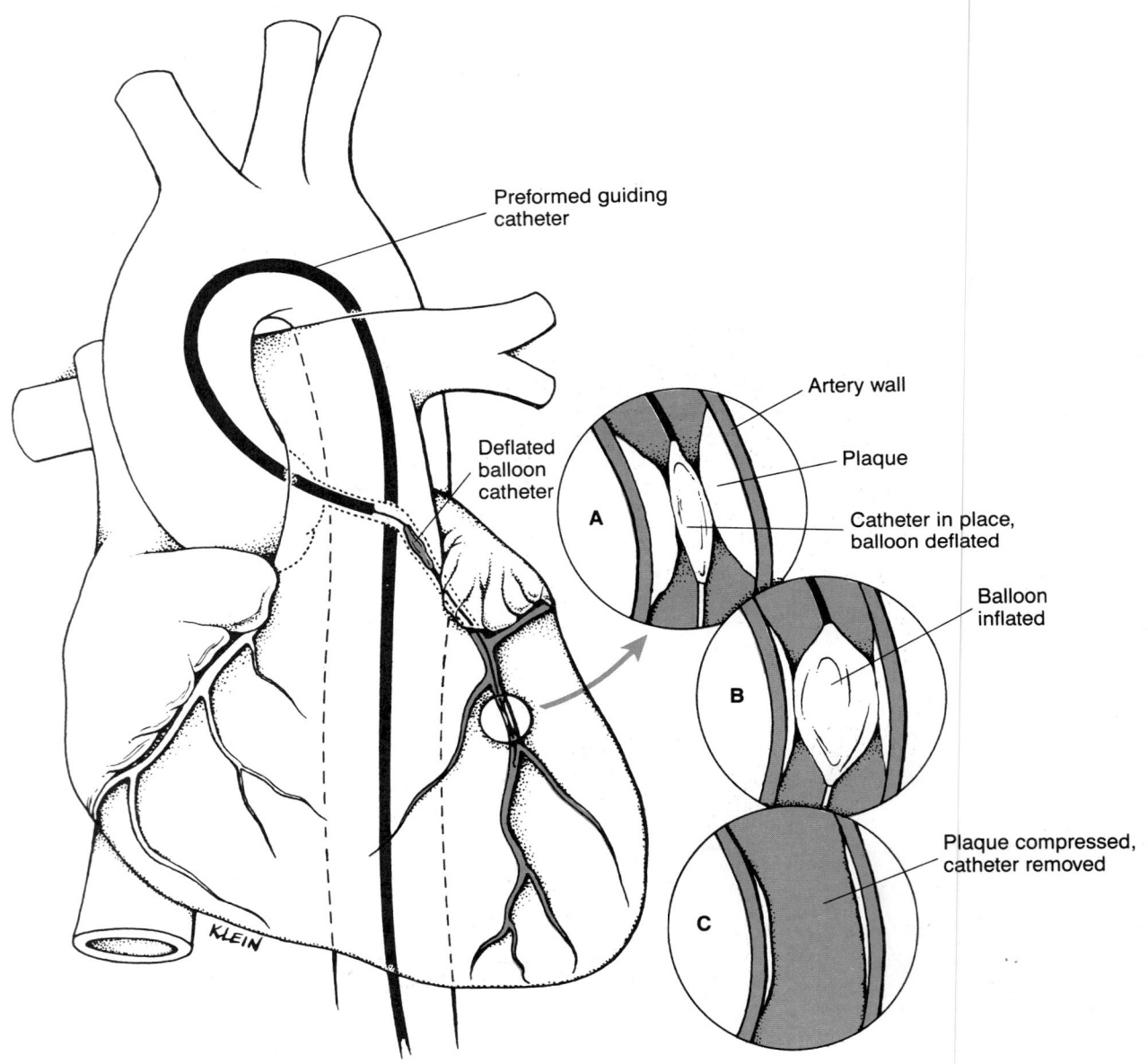

Figure 30-5. Percutaneous transluminal coronary angioplasty is a less invasive procedure than coronary artery bypass surgery in selected patients. (*A*) A balloon-tipped catheter is passed into the affected coronary artery and placed within the atherosclerotic lesion. (*B*) The balloon is then rapidly inflated and deflated with controlled pressure. (*C*) After the plaque is compressed, the catheter is removed, allowing improved blood flow of the vessel. (Redrawn after Purcell JA and Giffin PA: Percutaneous transluminal coronary angioplasty. Am J Nurs 81(9):1620–1626, Sept 1981.)

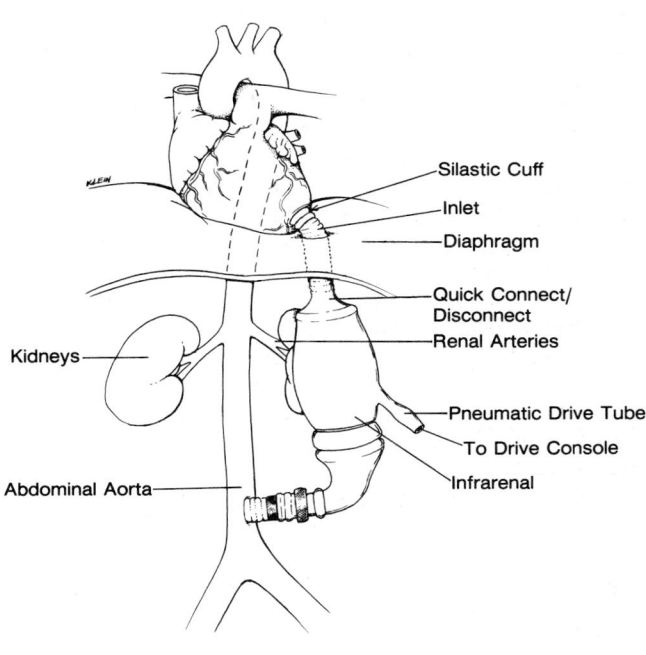

Figure 30-6. Left ventricular assist device.

to assess the effectiveness of therapy and to detect early rejection. Other postoperative care is the same as that described later in the chapter for other heart surgery procedures.

Because of the incidence of heart disease, the complexities of donor heart transplantation, and the limited supply of donor hearts, much research is being done to perfect the total artificial heart. Already, devices are being used to support the damaged heart until it recovers and can completely take over its pumping function. The intra-aortic balloon pump (IABP) has been used most successfully in supporting the damaged heart before and after surgery. It has been less successful in reversing cardiogenic shock. The left heart assist device has also been used to support the pumping function of the heart until it recovers or until a donor heart is available for transplantation (Fig. 30-6).

In some cases, transplantation of both the heart and the lungs is being performed successfully. This procedure is advantageous for the patient whose heart disease has caused pulmonary disease. It is also done for the patient who needs lung transplantation. In these cases, the transplanted heart is needed for early detection of rejection. Changes in the atrial electrogram and the endomyocardial biopsy findings allow early detection and treatment of rejection.

▷ Perioperative Management

The patient who is undergoing heart surgery has many of the same needs and requires the perioperative care de-

scribed for other surgical patients in Chapters 19 to 21. Additionally, because of the intensified fears often associated with heart surgery, the patient (and family) may require more extensive emotional care and teaching. The nature of the surgery and the incidence of postoperative problems also require that the patient receive intensive assessment, monitoring, and physical care.

While the fears of heart surgery patients are the same as those of other surgical patients, the fears are frequently intensified because of the special meaning attached to the heart, the realization of the risk of death associated with heart surgery, the infrequency with which the public encounters persons who have had heart surgery, and the extent to which the patient has been involved in the decision to have surgical or medical therapy for the cardiac condition. The nurse assists the patient in coping with fears in order to reach the goal of a moderate level of anxiety. Emotional care should begin prior to hospitalization and continue through rehabilitation.

A major component of the physical care is timely assessment. Preoperatively, the patient is assessed to determine readiness for surgery and to establish baseline data for reference postoperatively. Immediately after surgery, the patient is managed in a postanesthesia recovery unit or an intensive care unit, where continuous assessment of cardiac function and prompt initiation of therapy are possible. Assessment continues in the rehabilitation phase, where the patient is taught to do self-assessment in order to regulate activity and sometimes adjust medication.

Preoperative Management

The preoperative phase of patient preparation usually begins prior to hospitalization. This phase focuses on stabilizing any other disease conditions and optimizing cardiac function. The patient with diabetes, high blood pressure, chronic obstructive pulmonary disease, or other respiratory, renal, or liver disease has these conditions assessed and medical therapy adjusted to stabilize them. Any sources of possible infection (*i.e.,* periodontal disease, skin lesions, stasis ulcer) should be investigated and treated. Therapy should also be adjusted to control any heart failure, arrhythmias, and fluid or electrolyte imbalances to optimize cardiac function. Special consideration should be given to the anxiety associated with waiting for hospitalization and surgery, and a mild tranquilizer should be prescribed as needed to help control increased heart rate, which may worsen the cardiac condition.

Patient Teaching
Nursing's role with the patient and family begins in the prehospitalization phase of preparation with emotional support and teaching. Establishing rapport, answering questions, listening to fears and concerns, clarifying misconceptions, and informing the patient about what to expect are all interventions the nurse uses to prepare the patient and family emotionally for hospitalization and surgery.

Patient teaching is based on assessed learning needs. Teaching usually includes information about hospitalization, about the surgery (the preoperative care, the length of the surgery, what the patient will feel like, the visiting privileges in the intensive care unit), and about the recovery phase (length of hospitalization, when normal activities, such as housework, shopping, and work, can be resumed). Any changes made in medical therapy and preoperative preparations will need to be explained and reinforced.

Patients should be instructed to avoid aspirin and any drugs containing aspirin for at least 9 days prior to surgery. Aspirin decreases platelet adhesion and may predispose the patient to surgical hemorrhage. Anticoagulant therapy is usually stopped 5 to 7 days before surgery. The patient is also encouraged to stop or reduce smoking a few weeks prior to surgery. If the patient is on digitalis, a short-acting preparation will be prescribed, and sometimes even this is discontinued 36 to 48 hours prior to surgery. Most antiarrhythmics, nitrates, and propranolol will be continued until the night before surgery.

Assessment

The patient with nonacute heart disease will usually be hospitalized only 1 or 2 days prior to surgery. Most of the preoperative medical evaluation is completed before the patient enters the hospital. A new history and physical examination, chest roentgenogram, electrocardiogram (ECG), serum electrolytes, coagulation screen, and typing and crossmatching of blood may be done at this time. These data provide information about other disease conditions and cardiac problems. Nursing intervention focuses primarily on obtaining a baseline assessment of the patient, patient teaching, and continued emotional and physical preparation for surgery.

The preoperative assessment should be thorough and well documented since it provides baseline data for postoperative comparison. The history should include a social assessment of family roles and support systems, and a description of the patient's usual functional level and typical activities. This information will assist with emotional care and rehabilitation planning.

If the preoperative hospitalization period is very short, joint teaching of the patient and family may be more effective. The patient's anxiety increases with the admission process and the immediacy of surgery. Unless the nurse has met the patient before the day of hospitalization, the time may be too short to establish a relationship that contributes to patient learning. Joint teaching capitalizes on the established support relationship of the patient and family to increase learning. Teaching in this phase should be directed primarily by the patient's (and family's) questions. Too much detail may only increase anxiety. The patient may be offered a tour of the intensive care unit, the postanesthesia recovery room, or both. (In some hospitals, the patient will initially go to the postanesthesia unit.) The patient recovering from anesthesia is reassured by having already seen and heard the environment and having met someone from the unit. The patient and family should be informed about some of the tubes that will be present postoperatively and their purposes. Most patients will remain intubated and on mechanical ventilation for 6 to 24 hours postoperatively. They need to be aware that this prevents them from talking, but reassure them that the staff are skilled in other means of communication. They should know to expect several intravenous lines, tubes in the chest, and a urinary catheter.

Explaining the purpose and the approximate time that these will be in place helps to reassure the patient.

The patient's other questions about postoperative care and procedures should be answered. Deep breathing and coughing, using the incentive spirometer or intermittent positive pressure breathing (IPPB), and foot exercises should be explained and practiced by the patient preoperatively. The family's questions at this time will primarily focus on the length of the surgery, who will discuss the results of the procedure with them and when this may occur, where to wait during the surgery, the visiting privileges in the intensive care unit, and how they can support the patient preoperatively and in the intensive care unit.

Psychosocial Support

The nurse helps the patient prepare emotionally by using communication and teaching to induce a moderate level of anxiety. This anxiety enables the patient to cope with the stresses and discomforts postoperatively. The patient in a moderate state of anxiety presents signs of being anxious, but retains the ability to listen and learn. Preoperative intervention with a patient facing heart surgery begins with an assessment of his level of anxiety. If it is low, the patient may be in denial. Allow the patient more controls. If the patient exhibits high anxiety, intervene to lower his anxiety level. Assess the fears that the patient is focusing on and intervene to lessen them. The fears that most patients express are as follows.

1. Fear of the Unknown. This fear is difficult for the patient to express. Not having past experience with heart surgery, the patient does not know enough detail to attach fears to any specific aspect. Instead of specific fears that the patient can identify and begin to cope with, the patient is left with just a generalized dread and anxiety.

Intervention begins with determining other experiences that the patient has had with which details of the impending surgery can be compared. Describe what the patient will feel. If the patient has already had a heart catheterization, compare the similarities and differences between that and the surgery. Also, encourage the patient to talk about any concerns from previous bad experiences.

2. Fear of Pain. The patient may openly express a fear of pain and the inability to tolerate it or may indirectly express this fear by asking many questions about pain, pain medications, and the state of recovering from anesthesia. Encourage the patient to talk about this fear. Make a comparison between the pain experienced with heart surgery and other pain experiences. Inform him about the preoperative sedation, the anesthetic, and the postoperative pain medication. Reassure him that the fear of pain is normal. Admit that he will experience some pain but that he will be closely observed and that the use of medication, positioning, and relaxation will make the pain tolerable.

3. Fear of Body-image Change. Many patients have a fear of the scarring from surgery. This fear is frequently exaggerated by misconceptions from the communications media or imagined distortions owing to lack of knowledge. Patients may talk openly about this fear or express it indirectly through concern about continued love from others or excessive focus on postoperative pain. Discuss this fear with the patient and correct any misconceptions. Assure the patient that the health team members will give consistent descriptions of the incisions and the healing process.

4. Fear of Dying. Some patients share their fear of dying. More only drop clues about their concern, such as questioning their need for teaching about the surgery and postoperative course, asking for reassurance that someone will care for their family the day of surgery, or becoming tearful around their family members or telling them to wait at home on the day of surgery. For those who share this fear openly, reassure them that the fear is normal. Emphasize the postoperative care and routines in teaching since this reassures them indirectly that they will survive the surgery.

For those who only drop clues despite efforts to encourage them to talk about their fear, coach them to express this fear (*i.e.,* "Are you worrying about not making it through surgery? Most people who have heart surgery at least think about the possibility of dying."). Once the fear is expressed, the patient can be helped. By alleviating undue anxiety, emotional preparation of the patient for surgery lessens the chance of preoperative complications, aids in smooth anesthesia induction, and enhances the patient's involvement postoperatively in care and recovery.

Physical Preparation

Physical preparation of the patient usually involves several showers or scrubs with an antiseptic solution. The patient is medicated for sleep the night before surgery and sedated before going to surgery. With few exceptions, almost all cardiac surgical teams use prophylactic antibiotic therapy, and the antibiotics are started preoperatively.

Patients requiring emergency heart surgery may have both heart cineangiography and surgery within hours of the surgical procedure. These patients and their families have little opportunity for teaching and emotional preparation. As a result, specific intervention is usually required postoperatively to help them adjust.

Operative Management

Most of the described surgical procedures are performed through a median sternotomy incision. Because of the possible problems associated with these surgeries, the patient is prepared for continuous monitoring. Electrodes and indwelling catheters and probes are placed prior to the procedure to facilitate assessment of the patient's status and the need for change in therapy. In addition, the patient will be intubated and supported on mechanical ventilation. Intravenous lines will be placed as needed for administration of fluids, medications, and blood products.

Before the chest incision is closed, chest tubes are positioned to evacuate air and drainage from the mediastinum and the thorax. Epicardial pacemaker electrodes are implanted on the surface of the right atrium and sometimes the right ventricle. These epicardial electrodes are used postoperatively to pace the heart or to monitor the heart for arrhythmia differentiation via an atrial lead. Most of the indwelling catheters are retained for continuous monitoring and treatment of the patient in the immediate postoperative period.

In addition to assistance with the surgical, anesthetic, and extracorporeal procedures, the surgical nurses are responsible for the comfort and safety of the patient. Some of their intervention areas include emotional support of the patient (and family), positioning, skin care, and wound care.

Possible intraoperative or postoperative complications include arrhythmias, hemorrhage, myocardial infarction, cerebral vascular accident, embolization, and organ failure secondary to shock, embolus, or adverse drug reactions. Astute patient assessment is critical in preventing these complications or in detecting symptoms and initiating prompt therapy.

Postoperative Management

The immediate postoperative period for the patient who has undergone a cardiovascular operation presents many challenges to the health team. The patient is placed flat in bed and returned to an acute care area. All connections for catheters and tubes are secured. An initial postoperative nursing assessment is made and recorded. The nurse anticipates patient needs and adjusts nursing care accordingly.

The nursing care (Fig. 30-7, Chart 30-1) is directed at the following basic postoperative considerations:

- Providing for adequate tissue oxygenation
- Assessing cardiac output
- Maintaining fluid and electrolyte balance
- Relieving pain
- Maintaining adequate cerebral circulation
- Observing for possible complications

Providing for Adequate Tissue Oxygenation

All body tissues require an adequate supply of oxygen and nutrients for survival. To achieve this end after surgery, endotracheal intubation with ventilator assistance may be left intact from 8 to 48 hours in the postoperative period, depending on the results of blood gas measurements. Studies have shown that patients who are stable following surgery may be extubated as early as 6 hours following surgery, which reduces their anxiety regarding their ability to communicate with the staff. A patient should normally awaken within an hour or two after cardiac surgery. If he does not, the following possibilities should be considered: (1) prolonged drug or anesthetic effect, (2) embolic damage, (3) hypoxia, and (4) previous brain damage. The nurse should assess and maintain the patency of the endotracheal tube by (1) using the sigh mechanism on the ventilator or by manually using the self-inflating bag (Ambu) with 100% oxygen prior to and following suctioning; (2) suctioning frequently to minimize collection of secretions; and (3) observing and reporting blood gas determinations, which are compared with the baseline data.

Since an open airway enhances O_2 and CO_2 exchange, the endotracheal tube must be secured to prevent it from slipping into the right mainstem bronchus and occluding the airway. In addition, suctioning at frequent intervals is essential to remove secretions and mucus plugs. Frequent change of position also provides for optimum pulmonary ventilation and perfusion by allowing the lungs to expand more fully. When the patient's condition stabilizes, his position is changed every 1 to 2 hours and the nurse listens to breath sounds to detect the presence of wheezes and

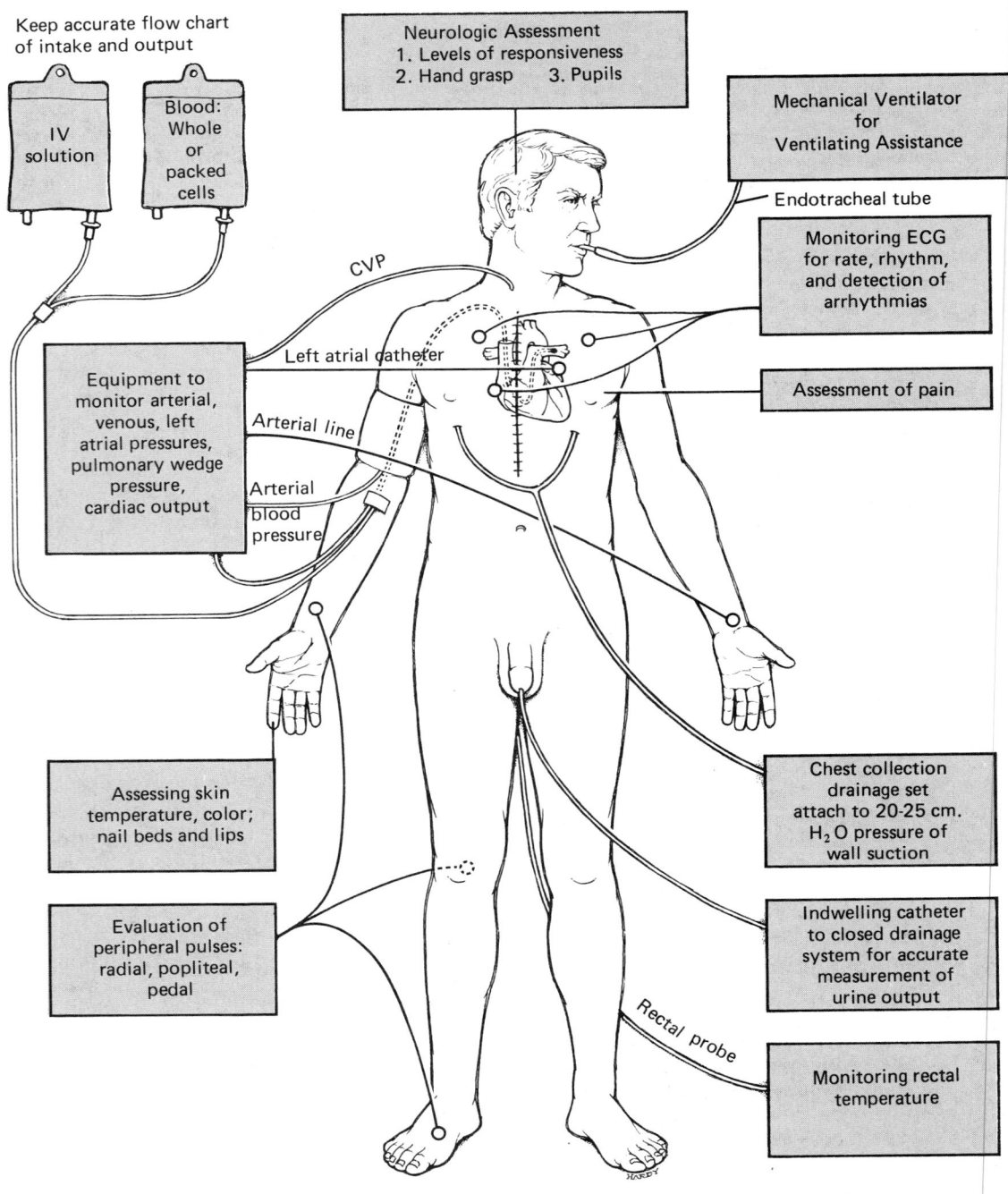

Keep accurate flow chart of intake and output

IV solution

Blood: Whole or packed cells

CVP

Left atrial catheter

Arterial line

Arterial blood pressure

Equipment to monitor arterial, venous, left atrial pressures, pulmonary wedge pressure, cardiac output

Neurologic Assessment
1. Levels of responsiveness
2. Hand grasp   3. Pupils

Mechanical Ventilator for Ventilating Assistance

Endotracheal tube

Monitoring ECG for rate, rhythm, and detection of arrhythmias

Assessment of pain

Assessing skin temperature, color; nail beds and lips

Evaluation of peripheral pulses: radial, popliteal, pedal

Chest collection drainage set attach to 20-25 cm. H_2O pressure of wall suction

Indwelling catheter to closed drainage system for accurate measurement of urine output

Rectal probe

Monitoring rectal temperature

Figure 30-7. Postoperative care of the cardiovascular surgery patient.

fluid in the lungs. Deep breathing and coughing are also encouraged to open the alveolar sacs and provide for increased perfusion. Physical support of the incision is provided when the patient coughs and breathes deeply at regular intervals.

When the patient is ready for extubation, he may gag or "fight" the respirator. Other indications for calling for extubation are an adequate tidal volume, toleration of O_2 with warmed humidification and adequate blood gas determinations. Early extubation is considered when the patient's condition is stable. This means that the patient's pressures are not fluctuating and are within 20% of his preoperative volumes—and hence are high enough to maintain peripheral perfusion as indicated by urinary output, provided that there are no dangerous arrhythmias. With these parameters as guidelines, early extubation has been performed without any adverse effects on the patient's condition or prognosis. During this time the nurse assists with the weaning process and, eventually, the removal of the tube.

(Text continues on page 622)

Chart 30-1
Postoperative Care of the Cardiac Surgery Patient

A. **Nursing Diagnosis:** Potential for development of inadequate ventilation and perfusion related to the trauma of extensive chest surgery

Patient Goal: Adequate ventilation, perfusion, and tissue oxygenation

Nursing Strategies:

1. Provide for tissue oxygenation and assess respiratory status.
   a. Employ assisted or controlled ventilation (see p. 495)—respiratory support is used first 24 hours to provide airway in the event of cardiac arrest, to decrease work of heart, and to maintain effective ventilation.
      (1) Adequacy of ventilation is assessed by patient's clinical status and by direct measurement of tidal volume and arterial blood gases.
      (2) Check endotracheal tube placement.
      (3) Auscultate chest for breath sounds—crackles indicate pulmonary congestion; decreased or absent breath sounds indicate pneumothorax.
      (4) Arterial blood gas analysis (see p. 482) usually performed first hour postoperatively and prn thereafter.
      (5) Sedate patient adequately—to help him tolerate endotracheal tube and cope with ventilatory sensations.
      (6) Utilize chest physiotherapy for patients with lung congestion to prevent retention of secretions and atelectasis.
         (a) Check chest x-ray and auscultate chest to determine problem areas.
         (b) Use percussion and vibrating techniques to loosen secretions.
         (c) Promote coughing, deep breathing, and turning—to keep airway patent, prevent atelectasis, and facilitate lung expansion.
      (7) Suction tracheobronchial secretions carefully (see p. 498)—prolonged aspiration leads to hypoxia and possible cardiac arrest.
      (8) Restrict fluids (per request) for first few days—danger of pulmonary congestion from excessive fluid intake.
      (9) Chest x-ray taken immediately after surgery and daily thereafter—to evaluate state of lung expansion and detect atelectasis; to demonstrate heart size and contour, confirm placement of central line, endotracheal tube, and chest drains.
      (10) See page 503 for weaning process and endotracheal tube removal.

Evaluation:

Expected Outcome: Exhibits adequate ventilation, perfusion, and tissue oxygenation
   a. Airway patent
   b. ABGs within normal range
   c. Endotracheal tube correctly placed, as evidenced by x-ray
   d. Breath sounds clear
   e. Respirations synchronous with ventilator
   f. Tracheobronchial secretions adequately removed by suctioning
   g. Adequacy of color of skin and mucous membranes
   h. Adequacy of temperature of skin
   i. Mental acuity consistent with amount of sedatives and analgesics received

B. **Nursing Diagnosis:** Alteration in cardiac output related to blood loss and compromised myocardial function

Patient Goal: Restoration of cardiac output

Nursing Strategies:

Monitor cardiovascular status to determine effectiveness of cardiac output with hemodynamic monitoring. Serial readings of blood pressure and arterial pressure, heart rate, CVP, and left atrial or pulmonary artery pressure from monitor modules are observed, correlated with patient's condition, and recorded.
   a. Assess arterial pressure every 15 minutes until stable and as directed thereafter—blood pressure is one of the most important physiologic parameters to follow.
      Take direct measurement (arterial line, transducer)—most accurate blood pressure. Extreme vasoconstriction following extracorporeal circulation makes auscultatory blood pressure unobtainable.
   b. Auscultate the heart for evidence of cardiac tamponade (muffled distant heart sounds), precordial rub (pericarditis), arrhythmias.
   c. Check all peripheral pulses (pedal, tibial, radial, brachial, popliteal, femoral, and carotid) as a further check on heart action.
   d. Measure left atrial pressure or pulmonary artery wedge pressure—to determine the left ventricular end-diastolic volume and to assess cardiac output (see p. 594).
      Rising pressures may indicate congestive heart failure or pulmonary edema.
   e. Take central venous pressure readings hourly (see p. 596)—indicate blood volume, vascular tone, and pumping effectiveness of the heart.
      (1) High CVP reading may result from hypervolemia, heart failure, cardiac tamponade. Ventilator may elevate CVP.

(continued)

Chart 30-1
Postoperative Care of the Cardiac Surgery Patient (continued)

Nursing Strategies *(continued)*

    (2) If blood pressure drop is due to low blood volume, CVP will show corresponding drop.

    (3) *Changes* in values are more important than isolated readings.

  f. Watch ECG monitor—cardiac arrhythmias frequently occur after heart surgery.

    (1) Premature ventricular contractions occur most frequently following aortic valve replacement and coronary bypass surgery. May be treated with pacing, lidocaine, potassium.

    (2) Arrhythmias also apt to occur with ischemia, hypoxia, alterations in serum potassium, edema, bleeding, acid–base or electrolyte disturbances, digitalis toxicity, myocardial failure.

    (3) Observe other parameters in correlation with monitor information—a low serum potassium makes the heart susceptible to ventricular arrhythmias.

    (4) See Chapter 28 for discussion of cardiac arrhythmias.

  g. Check cardiac enzymes daily—elevations may indicate myocardial infarction.

  h. Check urine output every ½ to 1 hour (from indwelling catheter)—urine output is an index of cardiac output and renal perfusion.

  i. Continue with ongoing patient assessment.

    (1) Observe buccal mucosa, nail beds, lips, ear lobes, and extremities for duskiness/cyanosis—signs of low cardiac output.

    (2) Feel the skin; cool, moist skin reveals lowered cardiac output. Note temperature and color of extremities.

    (3) Note fullness and tone of superficial veins of feet; evaluate pedal and femoral pulses.

    (4) Assess for venous distention of neck veins or veins of dorsal surface of hands (raised above level of heart)—may signal a changing demand or diminishing capacity of heart.

    (5) Evaluate temperature.

Evaluation:

Expected Outcome: Cardiac output is restored. The following parameters are stable within normal ranges:

  (1) Arterial pressure

  (2) Heart sounds

  (3) Peripheral pulses

  (4) Pulmonary artery wedge pressure

  (5) Central venous pressure

  (6) Cardiac rhythm and rate

  (7) Cardiac enzymes

  (8) Urinary output

C. **Nursing Diagnosis:** Potential for development of fluid and electrolyte imbalance related to alteration in circulating blood volume

Patient Goal: Fluid and electrolyte balance

Nursing Strategies:

1. Maintain fluid and electrolyte balance—adequate circulating blood volume is necessary for optimum cellular activity; metabolic acidosis and electrolyte imbalance can occur after use of pump oxygenator.

  a. Fluids may be limited to avoid overloading.

  b. Keep input and output flow sheet—as a method of determining positive or negative fluid balance and patient's fluid requirements.

    (1) IV fluids (including flush solutions through arterial and venous lines) considered as input.

    (2) Assess hydration status of patient—evaluation of pulmonary wedge, left atrial pressure, and CVP readings; weight, electrolyte levels, hematocrit readings, distention of neck veins, tissue edema, liver size, breath sounds.

    (3) Record urine output every ½ to 1 hour.

    (4) Measure postoperative chest drainage—should not exceed 200 ml/hour for first 4 to 6 hours.

      (a) Watch for sudden cessation of chest drainage—from kinked or blocked chest tube.

      (b) See page 466 for management of patient with water-seal drainage.

2. Be alert to changes in serum electrolytes—a specific concentration of electrolytes is necessary in both extracellular and intracellular body fluids in order to sustain life.

  a. *Hypokalemia* (low potassium)

    (1) May be caused by inadequate intake, diuretics, vomiting, excessive nasogastric drainage, stress from surgery.

    (2) Effects of low potassium—arrhythmias, digitalis toxicity, metabolic alkalosis, weakened myocardium, cardiac arrest.

    (3) Watch for specific ECG changes.

    (4) Give IV potassium replacement as directed.

  b. *Hyperkalemia* (high potassium)

    (1) May be caused by increased intake, red cell breakdown from the pump, acidosis, renal insufficiency, tissue necrosis, and adrenal cortical insufficiency.

    (2) Effects of high potassium—mental confusion, restlessness, nausea, weakness, and paresthesia of extremities.

(continued)

Chart 30-1
Postoperative Care of the Cardiac Surgery Patient (continued)

Nursing Strategies *(continued)*

(3) Be prepared to administer an ion-exchange resin, or sodium polystyrene sulfonate (Kayexalate), which binds the potassium, or give IV sodium bicarbonate or IV insulin and glucose to drive the potassium back into the cells from the extracellular fluid.

c. *Hyponatremia* (low sodium)

(1) May be due to reduction of total body sodium or to an increased water intake, causing a dilution of body sodium.

(2) Assess for weakness, fatigue, confusion, convulsions, and coma.

d. *Hypocalcemia* (low calcium)

(1) May be due to alkalosis (which reduces the amount of Ca^{++} in the extracellular fluid) and multiple blood transfusions.

(2) Signs and symptoms of reduced calcium levels—numbness and tingling in the fingertips, toes, ear, and nose; carpopedal spasm; muscle cramps; and tetany.

(3) Give replacement therapy as directed.

e. *Hypercalcemia* (high calcium)

(1) May cause arrhythmias imitating those caused by digitalis toxicity.

(2) Assess for signs of digitalis toxicity.

(3) Institute treatment as directed—this condition may lead to asystole and death.

Evaluation:

Expected Outcome: Attains fluid and electrolyte balance

a. Electrolytes within normal ranges

b. Blood *p*H 7.35 to 7.45

c. Fluid intake and output balanced

d. Assessment parameters negative for fluid overload and dehydration

D. **Nursing Diagnosis:** Pain related to operative trauma and pleural irritation caused by chest tubes

Patient Goal: Relief of pain

Nursing Strategies:

Relieve patient's pain—cardiac surgical patients experience pain caused by sternotomy incision and irritation of pleura by chest tubes.

a. Record nature, type, location, and duration of pain—pain and anxiety increase pulse rate, oxygen consumption, and cardiac work.

b. Differentiate between incisional pain and anginal pain.

c. Watch for restlessness and apprehension—may be from hypoxia or a low-output state; analgesics or sedatives do not correct this problem.

d. Medicate patient as often as prescribed—to reduce amount of pain and to aid patient in performing deep breathing and coughing exercises more effectively.

(1) Reassure patient that staff understands that treatment is painful and that is is "OK to be angry."

(2) Allow patient to talk about his experience.

Evaluation:

Expected Outcome: Is relieved of pain

a. Receives analgesic as prescribed

b. After analgesic is administered:

Restlessness and complaints of pain decreased

Vital signs stable

Participates in deep breathing and coughing exercises

c. Verbalizes less complaints of pain each day

E. **Nursing Diagnosis:** Potential for alteration in sensorium related to hypoxia

Patient Goal: Stability of neurologic status

Nursing Strategies:

Assess neurologic status—the brain is dependent on a continuous supply of oxygenated blood and must rely on adequate and continuous perfusion by the heart.

a. Hypoperfusion or microemboli (air debris) may produce CNS damage after heart surgery.

b. Observe for symptoms of hypoxia—restlessness, headache, confusion, dyspnea, hypotension, and cyanosis.

c. Assess patient's neurologic status hourly in terms of:

(1) Level of responsiveness

(2) Response to verbal commands and painful stimuli

(3) Pupillary size and reaction to light

(4) Movement of extremities; handgrasp ability

d. Treat postoperative convulsive seizures.

Evaluation:

Expected Outcome: Neurologic status is stable

a. Responds appropriately to verbal commands and painful stimuli

b. Oriented to time, place, and person

c. Pupils equal and reactive to light

d. Moves all extremities on command

e. Strong hand grasp

F. **Additional Nursing Strategies:**

1. Give medications according to therapeutic directives—coronary vasodilators, antibiotics, analgesics, anticoagulants (patients with prosthetic valves).

2. Offer reassurance, orientation to time and place, and attention to patient's needs to avoid postcardiotomy delirium (p. 621).

(continued)

Chart 30-1
Postoperative Care of the Cardiac Surgery Patient (continued)

Complications Following Cardiac Surgery

Nursing Diagnosis: Potential for development of complications related to extensive chest surgery

Patient Goal: Absence of complications

Nursing Strategies:

1. *Hypovolemia* (decreased circulating blood volume)
   a. Low central venous pressure is an indication of hypovolemia.
   b. Assess for arterial hypotension, low CVP, increasing pulse rate, and low left atrial and pulmonary artery wedge pressures.
   c. Prepare to administer blood, IV solutions.

2. *Persistent bleeding*—from cardiac incision, tissue fragility, trauma to tissues, clotting defects; blood clotting disturbances usually transitory following cardiopulmonary bypass; however, a significant platelet deficiency may be present.
   a. Watch for steady and continuous drainage of blood; watch CVP and left atrial pressures.
   b. Treatment: protamine sulfate, vitamin K, or blood components.
   c. Prepare for potential return to surgery for bleeding persisting (over 300 ml per hour) for 4 to 6 hours.

3. *Cardiac tamponade*—results from bleeding into the pericardial sac or accumulation of fluids in the sac, which compresses the heart and prevents adequate filling of the ventricles.
   a. Assess for signs of tamponade—arterial hypotension; rising CVP; rising left atrial pressure; muffled heart sounds; weak, thready pulse; neck vein distention; falling urinary output.
   b. Check for diminished amount of drainage in the chest-collection bottle; may indicate that fluid is accumulating elsewhere.
   c. Prepare for pericardiocentesis (see p. 653).

4. *Cardiac failure* (low-output syndrome)—causes deficient blood perfusion to different organs.
   Observe for falling mean arterial pressure, rising filling pressures (CVP, PCW, or LAP), and increasing tachycardia; patient may exhibit signs of restlessness and agitation, cold and blue extremities, venous distention, labored respirations, tissue edema, and ascites.

5. *Myocardial infarction*
   a. Symptoms may be masked by the usual postoperative discomfort.
      (1) Watch for decreased cardiac output in the presence of normal circulating volume and filling pressure.
      (2) Obtain serial ECGs and isoenzymes to determine extent of myocardial injury.
      (3) Assess pain to differentiate myocardial pain from incisional pain.
   b. Treatment is individualized. Postoperative activity level may be reduced to allow heart adequate time for healing.

6. *Renal failure*—urine output depends on cardiac output, blood volume, state of hydration, and condition of kidneys.
   a. Renal injury may be caused by deficient perfusion, hemolysis, low cardiac output prior to and following open heart surgery; use of vasopressor agents to increase blood pressure.
   b. Measure urine volume; less than 20 ml/hour can indicate decreased renal function.
   c. Carry out specific gravity tests to determine kidneys' ability to concentrate urine in renal tubules.
   d. Watch BUN and serum creatinine levels as well as urine and serum electrolyte levels.
   e. Give rapid-acting diuretics or inotropic drugs (dopamine, dobutamine) to increase cardiac output and renal blood flow.
   f. Prepare patient for peritoneal dialysis or hemodialysis if indicated. (Renal insufficiency may produce serious cardiac arrhythmias.)

7. *Hypotension*—may be caused by inadequate cardiac contractility and reduction in blood volume or by mechanical ventilation (when patient "fights" the ventilator or PEEP is used), all of which can produce a reduction in cardiac output.
   a. Monitor vital signs, left atrial pressure, CVP, and arterial pressure.
   b. Note chest tube drainage—hypotension may be caused by excessive bleeding.
   c. Give blood as directed to maintain left atrial pressure at a level that will provide an adequate circulating volume for good tissue perfusion.

8. *Embolization*—may result from injury to the intima of the blood vessels, dislodgment of a clot from a damaged valve, venous stasis aggravated by certain arrhythmias, loosening of mural thrombi, and coagulation problems.
   a. Common embolic sites are lungs, coronary arteries, mesentery, extremities, kidneys, spleen, and brain.
   b. Symptoms of embolization (vary according to site):
      (1) Midabdominal or midback pain
      (2) Pain, cessation of pulses, blanching, numbness, coldness of extremity

(continued)

Chart 30-1
Postoperative Care of the Cardiac Surgery Patient (continued)

Nursing Strategies *(continued)*

    (3) Chest pain and respiratory distress with pulmonary embolus or myocardial infarction
    (4) One-sided weakness, pupil changes, as in stroke
  c. Initiate preventive measures: antiembolic stockings; omit pressure on popliteal space (leg crossing, raising knee gatch); start passive and active exercises.

9. *Postcardiotomy delirium*—may appear after a brief lucid period.
  a. Psychic disturbances are more frequent after heart operations with extracorporeal circulation than after general surgery.
  b. Signs and symptoms include delirium (impairment of orientation, memory, intellectual function, judgment), transient perceptual distortions, visual and auditory hallucinations, disorientation, and paranoid delusions.
  c. Symptoms may be related to sleep deprivation, increased sensory input, disorientation to night and day, prolonged inability to speak owing to endotracheal intubation, age, preoperative cardiac status, etc.
  d. *Nursing Management*
    (1) Keep patient oriented to time and place; notify patient of procedures and expectations of his cooperation. Give repeated explanations of what is happening.
    (2) Establish rapport with patient preoperatively: have patient visit ICU *before* surgery.
    (3) Encourage family to come in at regular times—helps patient regain sense of reality.
    (4) Plan care to allow rest periods, day–night pattern, and uninterrupted sleep.
    (5) Encourage mobility as soon as possible.
    (6) Keep environment as free as possible of excessive auditory and sensory input. Prevent bodily injury.
    (7) Reassure patient and his family that psychiatric disorders following cardiac surgery are usually transient.
    (8) Remove patient from ICU as soon as possible.
    (9) Allow patient to *ventilate* events of his psychotic episode—helps him deal with and assimilate experience.

10. *Postpericardiotomy syndrome*—a group of symptoms occurring following cardiac and pericardial trauma and myocardial infarction.

  a. Cause is not certain—may be from anticardiac antibodies, viral etiology, etc.
  b. Manifestations—fever, malaise, arthralgias, dyspnea, pericardial effusion, pleural effusion; friction rub.
  c. Treatment is symptomatic (bed rest, aspirin), since condition is self-limiting, but recurrence is not uncommon.

11. *Postperfusion syndrome*
  a. Signs and symptoms—fever, splenomegaly, lymphocytosis.
  b. Draw blood for culture—postperfusion syndrome can mimic bacterial endocarditis or hepatitis.
  c. Treatment is symptomatic, since syndrome is self-limiting.
  d. Reassure patient that this is only a temporary setback in his convalescence.

12. *Febrile complications*—probably from body's reaction to tissue trauma or accumulation of blood and serum in pleural and pericardial spaces.
  a. Control higher degrees of fever by use of hypothermia mattress.
  b. Evaluate for atelectasis, pleural effusion, or pneumonia if fever persists.
  c. Evaluate for urinary tract infection/wound infection.
  d. Bear in mind the possibility of infective endocarditis if fever persists (see p. 649).

13. Hepatitis

Evaluation
Expected Outcome: Is free of complications
  a. The following parameters are stable within normal ranges:
    (1) CVP
    (2) Arterial pressure
    (3) Cardiac rhythm and rate
    (4) Pulmonary artery wedge pressure
    (5) Heart sounds
    (6) Urinary output and specific gravity
    (7) Peripheral pulses
    (8) Respiratory rate, volume, rhythm, and effort
    (9) Cardiac enzymes
    (10) Serum electrolytes
    (11) Temperature
    (12) CBC
  b. Bleeding from operative site decreases appropriately
  c. Neurologic status is stable (see Nursing Diagnosis E, p. 619)
  d. Interacts with family appropriately
  e. Progressively increases activity

Assessing Cardiac Output

In evaluating the patient's cardiac status, the nurse primarily determines the effectiveness of cardiac output through clinical observations and routine measurements. Serial readings of blood pressure, heart rate, central venous pressure, arterial pressure, and left atrial or pulmonary artery pressure from modules are observed and recorded. When inserted in the pulmonary artery the Swan–Ganz catheter (p. 594) indicates left ventricular filling pressure by measuring pulmonary artery pressure (PAP) and pulmonary artery wedge pressure (PWP). At the end of the diastolic phase and before the next systolic contraction occurs, the pulmonary vascular bed, the left atrium, and the left ventricle act for a moment as a single chamber. The changes in the left side of the heart, therefore, are reflected in the mean pulmonary artery and pulmonary artery wedge pressures. Sterility of catheter sites must be scrupulously maintained in order to prevent infection.

Cardiac function is also related to kidney function; therefore, urinary output is measured and recorded. If urine output falls below 30 ml/hour, this may indicate a decrease in cardiac output. Urine specific gravity is also assessed (normally 1.010–1.025), as is urine osmolality. Underhydration may be manifested by low urinary output and a high specific gravity, whereas overhydration is exhibited by high urinary output with low specific gravity.

The growth and function of body cells depend on adequate cardiac output to provide a continuous supply of oxygenated blood to meet the changing demands of the organs and body systems. Since the buccal mucosa, nail beds, lips, and earlobes are sites with rich capillary beds, they should be observed for cyanosis or duskiness as possible signs of reduced heart action. Moist or dry skin may indicate either vasodilation or vasoconstriction respectively. Venous distention of the neck veins or of the dorsal surface of the hand raised to heart level may signal a changing demand or diminishing capacity of the heart. If cardiac output has fallen, the skin becomes cool, moist, and cyanotic or mottled. Peripheral pulses (pedal, tibial, radial) should be routinely palpated as a further check for emboli. If these pulses are absent, which may be due to recent catheterization of that extremity, then the carotid, brachial, popliteal, or femoral pulse is palpated. Irregularities in heart action also serve as important indicators of heart function. When poor perfusion of the heart exists, there may be irregularities in the heart action. The most common arrhythmias encountered during the postoperative period are bradycardias, tachycardias, and ectopic beats. Continuous observation of the monitor for various arrhythmias is an essential part of patient care and management.

Maintaining Fluid and Electrolyte Balance

An adequate circulating blood volume is necessary for optimum cellular activity. In this regard, intake and output should be quickly reviewed and replacement therapy should be instituted early if flow sheets are utilized to determine positive or negative fluid balance. An adult's total body weight is composed of between 50% and 70% fluid. Anything that alters fluid volume or composition can have a marked effect on homeostasis. All intravenous fluids, including flush solutions provided through arterial and venous catheters, as well as through a nasogastric tube, if present, must be considered as intake. The hydration status of the individual may be monitored by means of a number of parameters: pulmonary wedge and left atrial pressure and CVP readings, weight, electrolyte levels, hematocrit readings, distention of neck veins, tissue edema, liver size, and breath sounds (*i.e.,* fine crackles, wheezing).

Chest drainage tubes provide a route for evacuation of blood and air from the pleural cavity. Drainage is usually bloody and copious initially but gradually decreases. Chest drainage tubes should be secured tightly at connection sites and at the skin; the collection device is positioned below chest level in a safe manner (p. 466). The tubes are "milked," or "stripped," at regular intervals to maintain patency. Drainage of blood and fluid to prevent pooling is facilitated by turning the patient from side to side or, alternately, from side to flat in bed to a semi-Fowler's position. An accurate account of chest tube drainage is essential in the immediate postoperative period. Bloody drainage should not exceed 200 ml/hour for the first 4 to 6 hours. Sudden cessation of drainage, on the other hand, may be due to kinked or blocked chest tubes.

Electrolytes are found in both extracellular and intracellular body fluids. A specific concentration is necessary in both compartments in order to sustain life. The nurse should be alert to changes in serum electrolytes, report changes promptly, and institute treatment as prescribed. Especially important are dangerously high or low levels of potassium, sodium, or calcium.

Hypokalemia (low potassium) may be caused by inadequate intake, diuretics, vomiting, diarrhea, excessive nasogastric drainage, and stress owing to surgery—increased aldosterone secretion produces decreased potassium-ion (K^+) and increased sodium-ion (Na^+) retention. The patient must be observed carefully when serum potassium rises or falls outside the normal level ($K^+ = 3.5$–5.0 mEq/liter). Some cardiac surgeons feel that it is important to maintain the K^+ level at 4.5 mEq or higher in order to avoid arrhythmias in the postoperative period. The following effects of low K^+ may be noted: digitalis toxicity, arrhythmias, metabolic alkalosis, a weakened myocardium, and cardiac arrest. One possible specific ECG change is the presence of a U wave that is more than 1 mm high. (A U wave is a positive deflection following the T wave). Additional signs are AV block, flat or inverted T waves, and low voltage. Intravenous potassium replacement should be administered at a rate usually not to exceed 15 to 20 mEq/hour (40–120 mEq is diluted in 1000 ml of IV solution; or a more concentrated solution may be given through a central rather than peripheral catheter, when closely monitored).

Hyperkalemia (high potassium) may be caused by increased intake, red cell breakdown caused by the pump, acidosis, renal insufficiency, tissue necrosis, and adrenal cortical insufficiency. The patient who exhibits symptoms of high K^+ may exhibit mental confusion, restlessness, nausea, weakness, and paresthesia of the extremities. ECG changes specific for hyperkalemia are tall, peaked T waves; increased amplitude; a widening of the QRS complex; and a prolonged Q–T interval. The nurse should be prepared to administer an ion-exchange resin, sodium polystyrene sulfonate (Kayexalate), which binds the potassium, or to give IV sodium bicarbonate or IV insulin and glucose to drive the potassium back into the cells from the extracellular fluid.

Both *hypernatremia* (high sodium) and *hyponatremia* (low sodium) may be seen following cardiac surgery; however, the latter is more commonly observed. Hyponatremia may result from a reduction of total body sodium or an increase in water intake, which causes a dilution of body sodium. The patient must be observed for sodium values outside the normal limits (*i.e.,* $Na^+ = 135–145$ mEq/liter). Replacement of sodium is instituted as directed if there is a true loss from the body. Diuretics are given as directed when reduction in sodium is due to increased water intake. Symptoms of hyponatremia for which the patient is observed are weakness, fatigue, confusion, convulsions, and coma.

Hypocalcemia (low calcium) is caused by (1) alkalosis, which reduces the amount of Ca^{++} in the extracellular fluid, and (2) multiple blood transfusions. When large amounts of citrated blood are given, the level of ionized Ca^{++} is reduced as some of the citrate binds calcium. The calcium level should be checked to see that it is within normal limits ($Ca^{++} = 9.0–11.5$ mg/100 ml). Symptoms exhibited with reduced calcium levels may be (1) numbness and tingling in the fingertips and toes, ears, and nose; (2) carpal pedal spasm; and (3) muscle cramps and tetany. Replacement therapy is indicated immediately.

Hypercalcemia (high calcium) can cause arrhythmias that imitate those caused by digitalis toxicity. Calcium is known to potentiate, or enhance, the action of digitalis. Therefore, the nurse must be alert to signs of digitalis toxicity (p. 638) and must institute treatment for hypercalcemia immediately, since this condition may lead to asystole and death.

Relieving Pain

Deep pain may not be reflected in the immediate area of injury but in a broader, more diffuse area. Patients who have had cardiac surgery experience pain caused by the severance of intercostal nerves along the incision route and irritation of the pleura by the chest catheters. It is essential to observe and listen to the patient for verbal and nonverbal clues of pain. The nurse should accurately record the nature, type, location, and duration of the pain. (Incisional pain must be differentiated from anginal pain.) The patient is medicated as often as prescribed to reduce the amount of pain and to help him perform deep breathing and coughing exercises more successfully. If pain inhibits his performance of these activities, his progress will be jeopardized.

Pain produces tension, which may stimulate the central nervous system to release adrenalin and thus constrict the arterioles. Certain narcotics have a depressant effect on respirations. Morphine sulfate alleviates anxiety and pain and induces sleep, which reduces the metabolic rate and the need for oxygen. Following the administration of narcotics, any observations indicating relief of apprehension and pain are documented in the patient's record.

Maintaining Adequate Cerebral Circulation

The brain is dependent on a continuous supply of oxygenated blood. It does not have the capacity to store oxygen and must rely on adequate continuous perfusion by the heart. Thus, it is important to observe the patient for any symptoms of hypoxia: restlessness, headache, confusion, dyspnea, hypotension, and cyanosis. An assessment of the patient's neurologic status is made hourly in terms of level of consciousness, response to verbal commands and painful stimuli, pupillary size and reaction to light, movement of extremities, hand grasp ability, presence of pedal and popliteal pulses, and temperature and color of extremities. Any indication of a changing status is documented and reported immediately to the surgeon, since it may signal the beginning of a complication in the postoperative period.

▷ Possible Complications Following Cardiovascular Surgery

Hypovolemia. Hypovolemia may be the result of blood loss during the surgical procedure, and although the blood is usually replaced to within 10% of normal, the loss of extracellular fluid volume is more difficult to assess. Nursing management includes observation for signs of hypovolemia: arterial hypotension and low venous pressure (CVP) with an increasing pulse rate, and low left atrial and pulmonary artery wedge pressures. The nurse should be prepared to administer blood to maintain adequate blood balance and additional solutions to replace any deficits in electrolytes and protein.

Persistent Bleeding. Hemorrhage may be the result of tissue fragility, trauma to tissues, or some unexplained clotting defect. Therefore, accurate measurement of blood loss is important. Appropriate treatment may include the administration of protamine sulfate, vitamin K, and blood products (fresh frozen plasma, platelets, or specific blood factors). One may be expected to transfuse until the venous pressure is 12 cm to 15 cm H_2O or the left atrial pressure is 10 mm Hg to 14 mm Hg. All the while, preparations are made for the potential return of the patient to surgery should this be deemed necessary.

Cardiac Tamponade. Cardiac tamponade results from bleeding into the pericardial sac or accumulation of fluids in the sac, which compresses the heart and prevents adequate filling of the ventricles. Nursing management includes observation for signs of tamponade, which is reflected by arterial hypotension accompanied by a rising left atrial pressure; muffled heart sounds; weak, thready pulse; neck vein distention; and falling urinary output. A reduction in the amount of drainage in the chest-collection device may cause one to suspect that the fluid is accumulating elsewhere. A chest x-ray is done to assess fluid accumulation at the mediastinum. Once the nurse is assured that the chest tubes are patent by "milking" or "stripping" them, and has checked to see that they are free from kinking or obstruction, preparation should be made for pericardiocentesis (p. 653).

Cardiac Failure.   The failing heart's diminished pumping action results in an elevated hydrostatic pressure created by the backing up of blood in the vessels (p. 635); fluid is then forced out into the extracellular space. Nursing management includes observation for signs of cardiac failure: (1) a falling mean arterial pressure, (2) a rising venous pressure, and (3) an increasing tachycardia. The patient may exhibit symptoms of restlessness and agitation, peripheral cyanosis, venous distention, labored respirations, tissue edema, and ascites. Diuretic therapy and rapid digitalization may be necessary to avoid acute failure.

Myocardial Infarction.   A myocardial infarction may occur during the postoperative period. However, symptoms may be masked by the usual postoperative discomfort. The patient may be suspected of having sustained an infarction if the mean arterial pressure falls in the presence of normal circulating volume and a normal venous pressure. Nitroglycerin may be used to counteract vasospasm. Serial ECGs may be obtained to determine how serious the injury is. A careful assessment of the pain is made in order to differentiate it from the usual incisional pain, and the patient is medicated cautiously. Shock, if present, should be treated as directed. It may be necessary to reduce the rate at which the patient increases his activity in order to allow the heart adequate time for healing. Other drugs used in the treatment of myocardial infarction, besides nitroglycerin, are phentolamine (Regitine), trimethaphan camsylate (Arfonad), and nitroprusside, when indicated.

Renal Failure.   A low cardiac output prior to and following open heart surgery can cause impairment of renal function. In addition, trauma to blood cells during cardiopulmonary bypass can cause hemolysis of red blood cells. This leads to a buildup of toxic substances owing to the kidney's inability to excrete waste products. Use of vasopressor agents to increase blood pressure can also lead to reduction of the blood flow to the kidneys. Nursing management includes accurate measurement of urine output. An output of less than 20 ml/hour can indicate hypovolemia. Specific gravity tests should be carried out to determine the kidneys' ability to concentrate urine in the renal tubules. Rapid-acting diuretics or inotropic drugs (digitalis, isoproterenol) may be used to increase cardiac output and renal blood flow. The nurse should be aware of the BUN and serum creatinine levels as well as urine and serum electrolytes. It may be necessary to restrict fluids and limit the use of drugs that are normally excreted by the kidneys. The patient may be prepared for peritoneal dialysis or hemodialysis if indicated (pp. 977–984).

Hypotension.   Hypotension may be caused by inadequate cardiac contractility and volume and by mechanical ventilation, when the patient "fights" the respirator or when positive end-expiratory pressure (PEEP) is used, causing a reduction in cardiac output. The circulating blood volume can decrease after the patient has been removed from cardiopulmonary bypass. Normally, as the blood is rewarmed, vasodilation takes place and fluid replacement is instituted to supply an adequate blood volume.

Nursing management includes the monitoring of vital signs: left atrial pressure (LAP), CVP, and pulmonary artery mean and wedge pressures, as well as arterial pressure. It is essential to check tube drainage, since hypotension may be seen when there is excessive drainage from the chest tubes. The nurse may have to give blood as directed in order to maintain left atrial pressure at a level that will provide a blood circulating volume adequate for good tissue perfusion. Symptoms of pulmonary edema may be observed if the left atrial pressure is greatly increased. Knowing what the patient's left atrial pressure should be and assisting in the treatment of low output syndrome are the nurse's responsibilities. An attempt is made to maintain the patient's blood pressure at a desirable level by closely titrating the rate and amount of vasopressor being administered.

Embolization.   The usual embolic sites are the lungs, coronary arteries, mesentery, extremities, kidneys, spleen, and brain. Embolization may result from injury to the intima of the blood vessels, dislodgment of a clot from a damaged valve, venous stasis aggravated by certain arrhythmias, loosening of mural thrombi, and coagulation problems. Air emboli may occur as an effect of cardiopulmonary bypass. Nursing management implies initiating preventive measures early: (1) applying antiembolic stockings, (2) discouraging leg crossing, (3) avoiding use of the knee gatch on the bed, (4) omitting pillows in the popliteal space, and (5) instituting passive exercises followed by active exercises to promote circulation and prevent loss of muscle tone.

Symptoms of embolization, which vary according to site, should be watched for: (1) midabdominal or midback pain; (2) pain, cessation of pulses, blanching, numbness, or coldness of an extremity; (3) chest pain and respiratory distress with pulmonary embolus or myocardial infarction; and (4) one-sided weakness and pupillary changes, such as occur in cerebral vascular accident.

Postperfusion Syndrome.   Postperfusion or postpericardiotomy syndrome occurs in approximately 10% to 40% of patients who undergo cardiac surgery. Its precise etiology is unknown. A common factor appears to be trauma with residual blood in the pericardial sac following surgery. It is characterized by fever, pericardial pain, pleural pain, dyspnea, pleural effusion and pericardial friction, and arthralgia. There may be a combination of these signs and symptoms. Leukocytosis is present along with elevation of the sedimentation rate. These symptoms frequently appear after the patient is discharged from the hospital.

The syndrome must be differentiated from other postoperative complications (incisional pain, myocardial infarction, pulmonary embolus, bacterial endocarditis, pneumonia, or atelectasis). The treatment is dependent on the severity of the symptoms. Salicylates and bed rest usually lead to a dramatic improvement in symptoms. Other symptoms are treated as they occur.

Psychosis.   Psychosis may result from anxiety, sleep deprivation, increased sensory input, and disorientation to night and day when the patient loses track of time. An important finding is that patients who do not or cannot express anxiety before surgery are more prone to develop psychosis in the postoperative period. Psychosis may appear after a brief lucid interval. Characteristic signs of psychosis include: (1) transient perceptual distortions, (2) visual and auditory hallucinations, and (3) disorientation and paranoid delusions. The nurse should be watchful for signs of denial and should provide an opportunity for emotional expression during the preoperative period. Careful explanations of all procedures and of the need for the patient's cooperation help to keep him oriented throughout his postoperative course. Continuity of care, if at all possible, is desirable; a familiar face and a nursing staff with a consistent approach will prove to be assets in the delivery of nursing care. The use of a well-designed and individualized nursing care plan will provide guidelines to assist the nursing team in the coordination of their efforts for the emotional well-being of the patient.

▷ **Bibliography**

Books

Armstrong PW and Baigrie RS. Hemodynamic Monitoring in the Critically Ill. Hagerstown, Maryland, Harper & Row, 1980.

Baue AE and Glenn WWL (eds). Thoracic and Cardiovascular Surgery. Norwalk, Connecticut, Appleton–Century–Crofts, 1982.

Behrendt DM and Austen WG. Patient Care in Cardiac Surgery, 3rd ed. Boston, Little, Brown & Co, 1980.

Braimbridge MV (ed). Postoperative Cardiac Intensive Care, 3rd ed. Boston, Blackwell Scientific, 1981.

Detailed Diagnosis and Surgical Procedures for Patients Discharged From Short Stay Hospitals. United States, 1978. US Department of Health and Human Services, Sept 1980.

Harlan BJ, Starr A, and Harwin FM. Manual of Cardiac Surgery. New York, Springer–Verlag, 1980.

Hudak CN, Lohr T, and Gallo BM. Critical Care Nursing, 3rd ed. Philadelphia, JB Lippincott, 1982.

Hurst JW (ed). The Heart, Arteries, and Veins, 5th ed. New York, McGraw-Hill, 1982.

Ionescu MI. Techniques in Extracorporeal Circulation. Boston, Butterworths, 1981.

Janis IL. Psychological Stress. New York, Academic Press, 1974.

Litwak RS and Jurado RA (eds). Care of the Cardiac Surgical Patient. Norwalk, Connecticut, Appleton–Century–Crofts, 1982.

Miller DW Jr. The Practice of Coronary Artery Bypass Surgery. New York, Plenum, 1977.

Moran JM and Michaelis LL. Symposium on Surgery for the Complications of Myocardial Infarction. New York, Grune & Stratton, 1980.

Munro JL and Shore G. A Colour Atlas of Cardiac Surgery. London, Wolfe Medical Publishers, 1982.

Netter FH. Heart. The Ciba Collection of Medical Illustrations, Vol 5. New Jersey, CIBA Pharmaceutical, 1978.

Neutze JM et al. Intensive Care of the Heart and Lungs, 3rd ed. St Louis, CV Mosby, 1982.

Nursing Photobook. Ensuring Intensive Care. Horsham, Intermed Communications, 1981.

Ream AK and Fogdall RP. Acute Cardiovascular Management: Anaesthesia and Intensive Care. Philadelphia, JB Lippincott, 1982.

Roe BB. Perioperative Management in Cardiothoracic Surgery. Boston, Little, Brown & Co, 1981.

Shinn JA. Cardiac Transplantation and the Artificial Heart, Unit 7, Series 2, Surgical Aspects of Cardiovascular Disease—Nursing Intervention. New York, Appleton–Century–Croft, 1981.

Stack MC. Coronary Artery Bypass Surgery, Unit 5, Series 2, Surgical Aspects of Cardiovascular Disease—Nursing Intervention. New York, Appleton–Century–Croft, 1980.

Underhill SL et al (eds). Cardiac Nursing. Philadelphia, JB Lippincott, 1982.

Articles

Angell WW and Angell JD. Porcine valves. Prog Cardiovasc Dis 1980 Sept/Oct; 23(2):141–166.

Barbarowicz P. A comparison of in-hospital education approaches for coronary bypass patients. Heart Lung 1980 Jan–Feb; 9(1):127–133.

Connors JP and Avioli LV. An update on cardiac surgery. Heart Lung 1981 Mar–Apr; 10(2):323–328

Gallagher JJ et al. Epicardial mapping in the Wolff–Parkinson–White syndrome. Circulation 1978 May; 57(5):854–866.

Grehl TM et al. Heterograft cardiac valve prosthesis: A five-year follow-up. Ann Thorac Surg 1980 Aug; 30(2):173–176.

Gruntzig A, Myler R, and Stertzer S. Percutaneous transluminal coronary angioplasty (PTCA)—present state of the art (abstr). Circulation 1979 Oct; 60(4):Part II, 264.

Isaacson J et al. Post pump psychosis. Crit Care Nurse 1982 Jan–Feb; 2(1):14–16.

Jahnke EJ and Love JW. Bypass of the right and circumflex arteries with the internal mammary artery. J Thorac Cardiovasc Surg 1976 Jan; 71(1):58–63.

Jillings CR. Phases of recovery from open-heart surgery. Heart Lung 1978 Nov–Dec; 7(6):987–994.

Johnston BL et al. Sexual activity in exercising patients after myocardial infarction and revascularization. Heart Lung 1978 Nov–Dec; 7(6):1026–1031.

Jones EL. Coronary artery bypass grafting: Simplification and refinement of surgical technique. Ann Thorac Surg 1980 July; 30(1):84–87.

Josephson ME, Harken AH, and Horowitz LN. Endocardial excision: A new surgical technique for the treatment of recurrent ventricular tachycardia. Circulation 1979 Dec; 60(7):1430–1439.

Lovvorn J. Coronary artery bypass surgery: Helping patients cope with postop problems. Am J Nurs 1982 July; 82(7):1073–1075.

McGoon DC (ed). Cardiac surgery. Cardiovasc Clin 1982; 18(1):1–236 (entire volume).

Miller P and Shada EA. Preoperative information and recovery of open-heart surgery patients. Heart Lung 1978 May–June; 7(3):486–493.

Phillips SJ et al. Emergency coronary artery revascularization: A possible therapy for acute myocardial infarction. Circulation 1979 Aug; 60(2):241–246.

Purcell JA and Giffin PA. Percutaneous transluminal coronary angioplasty. Am J Nurs 1981 Sept; 81(9):1620–1626.

Scordo KA. This procedure called PTCA: Your patient's CABG substitute? Nursing '82 1982 Feb; 12(2):50–55.

Sprengel R. Exciting new alternative to coronary bypass surgery. RN 1981 Dec; 44(12):24–27.

Takardo T, et al. The VA cooperative randomized study of surgery for coronary arterial occlusive disease. II. Subgroup with significant left main lesions. Circulation 1976 Dec; 54(Suppl 3)III:107–117.

Thorpe CJ. A nursing care plan—the adult cardiac surgery patient. Heart Lung 1979 July–Aug; 8(4):690–698.

Williams JB, Karp RB, and Kirklin JW. Considerations in selection and management of patients undergoing valvular replacement with glutaraldehyde-fixed porcine bioprostheses. Ann Thorac Surg 1980 Sept; 30(3):247–258.

Zipes DP and Noble RJ. Assessment of electrical abnormalities. In Hurst JW (ed.) The Heart, Arteries, and Veins, 5th ed, pp. 333–357. New York, McGraw-Hill, 1982.

31

Management of Patients With Cardiac Disorders

▷ Coronary Artery Disease

Coronary Atherosclerosis

The most common heart disorder in the United States is coronary atherosclerosis, a form of arteriosclerosis. This pathologic condition of the coronary arteries is characterized by an abnormal accumulation of lipid substances and fibrous tissue in the vessel wall that leads to changes in arterial structure and function and reduction of blood flow to the myocardium. Causes of atherosclerotic heart disease probably involve alterations in lipid metabolism, blood coagulation, and the biophysical and biochemical properties of the arterial walls.

Pathophysiology.   The functional lesion of atherosclerosis is called the *atheroma*. Atherosclerosis begins when the waxy cholesterol atheroma, which looks like pearly gray mounds of tissue, becomes deposited on the intima of the major arteries. These deposits interfere with the absorption of nutrients by the endothelial cells that compose the vessel lining and obstruct blood flow by protruding into the lumen of the vessel. The vascular endothelium in involved areas becomes necrotic, then scarred, further compromising the lumen and impeding the flow of blood. At sites such as these, where the lumen is narrowed and the wall rough, there is a great tendency for clots to form, which explains the fact that intravascular coagulation, followed by thromboembolic disease, is among the most important complications of atherosclerosis.

Our knowledge of atherogenes is limited. Several theories are purported, but none as yet has been conclusively substantiated. Among suspected mechanisms are thrombus formation on the surface of the plaque followed by fibrous organization of the thrombus, hemorrhage into a plaque, and continuing lipid accumulation. If the fibrous cap of the plaque ruptures, the lipid debris is swept into the bloodstream and obstruction of the arteries and capillaries distal to the ruptured plaque results.

The coronary arteries are particularly susceptible to the effects of atherosclerosis. They twist and turn as they supply the heart, thereby creating angles and nooks ripe for atheroma development.

Clinical Manifestations. Coronary atherosclerosis produces symptoms and complications through narrowing of the arterial lumen and obstruction of blood flow to the myocardium. This impediment to blood flow progresses, to the extreme detriment of the muscle cells that depend for their survival on the native components of blood and on various other constituents that it transports. The major manifestation of ischemia of the myocardium is chest pain. Recurrent chest pain owing to ischemia without irreversible damage to myocardial cells is termed *angina pectoris.* More severe ischemia with cell damage is termed *myocardial infarction.* Irreversibly damaged myocardium undergoes degeneration and is replaced by scar tissue. If the damage to the myocardium is extensive, the heart eventually may fail, that is, it may be unable to support the body's needs for blood by providing an adequate cardiac output.

Other clinical manifestations of coronary artery disease may be ECG changes, ventricular aneurysm, arrhythmias, and sudden death.

Risk Factors and Prevention of Atherosclerotic Heart Disease

Epidemiologic studies and observations reveal that there are risk factors for atherosclerosis that tend to make an individual more prone to develop coronary heart disease. These risk factors include:

Hyperlipidemia
Elevated blood pressure
Cigarette smoking
Elevated blood sugar (diabetes mellitus)
Obesity
Physical inactivity

Positive family history
Stress: type A behavior
Increasing age
Sex, M > F
Use of oral contraceptives

A risk factor may operate independently or in tandem with other risk factors. The more risk factors a person has, the greater is the likelihood of his having coronary artery disease. Persons at risk should have periodic medical examinations, modify their life-styles, and alter their dietary habits.

Hyperlipidemia. The association of elevated blood lipids with coronary artery disease has been established through epidemiologic studies. *Lipids* are a mixed group of biochemical substances that are manufactured endogenously and are also derived from metabolism of exogenous sources. Lipids have a common property of being more soluble in fat or organic solvents than in water. In the blood, the principal lipids are cholesterol, triglycerides (free fatty acids esterified to glycerol), and phospholipids (lipid esters of phosphoric acid). To render them sufficiently water soluble for transport in the blood, the lipids are attached (complexed) to a variety of proteins, the resulting complex being called a lipoprotein.

The lipoproteins can be separated into families either by protein electrophoresis, which causes these electrically charged molecules to migrate in an electrical field, or by high-speed centrifugation, which separates the lipoproteins according to density. Each method employs a different set of names; however, in this discussion the terms that electrophoresis apply to are used, because this assay is available in many clinical laboratories.

Table 31-1 demonstrates the five types of hyperlipidemias and the associated lipoprotein abnormality. Defining

Table 31-1
Primary Hyperlipidemias and Associated Clinical Features

Phenotype	Dominant Lipids	Dominant Lipoproteins	Clinical Features of Elevated Levels
I (rare)	Triglycerides	Chylomicron	Xanthoma Enlarged liver Pancreatitis
II (common)	Cholesterol	Beta	Premature atherosclerosis Xanthoma
III (uncommon)	Cholesterol Triglycerides	Floating beta	Premature atherosclerosis Xanthoma
IV (uncommon)	Triglycerides	Prebeta	Glucose intolerance Hyperuricemia Premature atherosclerosis
V (uncommon)	Triglycerides	Chylomicron Prebeta	Xanthoma Enlarged liver Pancreatitis Glucose intolerance Hyperuricemia Premature atherosclerosis

Table 31-2
Composition of Lipids Present in Plasma

α = *Lipoproteins—high-density lipoproteins (HDL)*

Protein	35%–60%*
Phospholipid	34%–44%
Cholesterol	20%–28%
Triglyceride	17%

β = *Lipoproteins—low-density lipoproteins (LDL)*

Protein	20%–25%
Phospholipid	25%
Cholesterol	46%*
Triglyceride	14%

Very low-density lipoproteins (VLDL)

Protein	10%
Phospholipid	20%
Cholesterol	5%
Triglyceride	65%*

Chylomicrons (nonmigrating)

Protein	2%
Phospholipid	6%–9%
Cholesterol	2%
Triglyceride	85%–95%*

* The highest component in each type of lipid.

the underlying lipid abnormality is essential to assigning dietary control.

For clinical purposes, hyperlipidemia may be suspected if the *fasting* blood cholesterol or triglyceride levels are elevated. Cholesterol and triglycerides are the lipids most frequently associated with coronary heart disease.

Hyperlipidemia may be primary or secondary. Primary hyperlipidemia is generally a hereditary disorder and is the rarest of the phenotypes. The secondary type occurs as a manifestation of numerous other diseases, including hypothyroidism, nephrotic syndrome, diabetes mellitus, and alcoholism. Therapy consists in treating the basic disorder.

Since dietary fat is identified as a significant risk factor in coronary heart disease, the control of fat is an important factor in preventive nutrition.

Dietary fat is regulated by changing either the total amount or the type of fat in the diet or by changing both. Assisting the patient to modify dietary fat intake through effective counseling requires an understanding of the differences between saturated and polyunsaturated fatty acids, cholesterol, medium chain triglycerides, and different other fractions as well as their functions in the human body.

The five types of lipid profiles are indicated in Table 31-1. Proponents of this method view the classification by types as a potentially important key to the prevention and control of coronary heart disease. No single diet or drug will be effective in all conditions in lowering the particular elevated lipid abnormality, but in most people with such

an abnormality the level can be brought within the upper average range.

The compositions of the various types of lipids are indicated in Table 31-2. The α-lipoproteins (HDL) are highest in protein, and the β-lipoproteins (LDL) are highest in cholesterol. The very low density lipoproteins (VLDL) and chylomicrons are higher in triglycerides.

For patients in whom diet alone cannot normalize the specific lipid, there are several medications that have a synergistic effect when taken with the prescribed diet. These are usually grouped into two types: those that decrease lipoprotein synthesis, such as nicotinic acid and clofibrate, and those that increase lipoprotein catabolism, such as cholestyramine, sitosterol, and D-thyroxine. These agents are shown to be biochemically effective in that elevated lipoprotein concentration tends to return toward normal and manifestations of the abnormalities, such as xanthomas (yellow papules in the skin owing to lipid deposits), may disappear. Drug treatment also varies with the type of hyperlipidemia.

The question of the usefulness of diet and drugs in reversing coronary artery disease is still under investigation. A major factor influencing the thoughts of researchers is that lipids are manufactured within the body. Thus, in certain cases dietary control may exercise no influence on serum lipid levels. In summary, it must be said that although dietary control is very controversial, it is indeed widely accepted.

The search for persons who have primary hyperlipidemias assumes importance, because dietary changes effected early in life may well yield a harvest of health. Such measures may constitute a major step toward the positive goal of prevention, as opposed to amelioration, of coronary artery disease.

Behavior Patterns of Coronary Prone Individuals. It is believed that stress and certain behaviors contribute to the pathogenesis of coronary (atherosclerotic) heart disease. Psychobiological and epidemiologic studies have investigated behaviors that characterize the coronary prone person. Individuals who manifest these behaviors (competitive striving for achievement, exaggerated sense of time urgency, aggressiveness and hostility) are classified as type A coronary-prone individuals.* It appears that in addition to reducing other risk factors (smoking, dietary fats) some effort should be made to correct the life-style and alter the behavior and long-term habit structure of this individual.

Angina Pectoris
Pathophysiology
Angina pectoris is a clinical syndrome characterized by paroxysms of pain or a feeling of pressure in the anterior chest. The cause is considered to be insufficient coronary blood flow resulting in inadequate oxygen supply of the myocardium.

Angina is usually caused by atherosclerotic heart disease and almost invariably is associated with a significant

* Glass D: Behavior Patterns, Stress and Coronary Disease. Hillsdale, New Jersey, Lawrence Erlbaum Associates, 1977.

obstruction of a major coronary artery. (The characteristics of the various types of angina are listed in Chart 31-1.)

Any number of factors can produce anginal pain. Physical exertion can precipitate an attack by increasing myocardial oxygen demands. Exposure to cold or even the drinking of iced beverages can cause vasoconstriction and an elevated blood pressure with increased oxygen demand. Eating a heavy meal increases the blood flow to the mesenteric area and places a heavier demand on the heart. Stress and any emotion-provoking situation causing the release of adrenalin and increased blood pressure may accelerate the heart rate, and a bout of anginal pain can result. If blood flow from the left ventricle is obstructed, as in aortic stenosis, the oxygen needs of the myocardium are drastically increased.

Clinical Manifestations

Ischemia of the heart muscle produces *pain* varying in severity from upper substernal pressure to agonizing pain that is accompanied by severe apprehension and a feeling of impending death. The pain is usually felt deep in the chest behind the upper or middle third of the sternum (retrosternal). Although the pain frequently is localized, it may radiate to the neck, jaw, shoulders, and inner aspects of the upper extremities. The patient often experiences a tightness, a choking or strangling sensation that has a viselike, insistent quality. A feeling of weakness or numbness in the arms, wrists, and hands may accompany the pain. Along with the physical pain, the patient also has a sense of impending death, an apprehension that is so characteristic of angina that if it occurs alone, as it sometimes does, it is sufficient for diagnosis.

The diagnosis is often made by an evaluation of the clinical manifestations of pain and the patient's history. In certain types of angina, ECG changes are helpful in making a differential diagnosis of the angina. The patient's response to exertion or stress may also be tested by means of electrocardiographic monitoring while he exercises on a bicycle or treadmill.

▶ Nursing Assessment

If the patient is in the hospital, the nurse should observe and record all facets of his activities with particular regard for those that have been found to precede and precipitate attacks of anginal pain.

> When do attacks tend to occur?
> > Following a meal?
> > After engaging in certain activities?
> > After physical activities in general?
> > After visits from members of the family or others?
> Where is the pain located?
> How does the patient describe the pain?
> Was the onset of pain gradual or sudden?
> How long did it last—seconds? minutes? hours?
> Was the pain steady and unwavering in quality?
> Is the discomfort accompanied by other symptoms, such as excessive perspiration, light-headedness, nausea, palpitation, shortness of breath?
> How many minutes after taking nitroglycerin did the pain last?
> What was the mode of abatement?

Chart 31-1
Types of Angina

Unstable Angina
(preinfarction angina; crescendo angina)

Progressive increase in frequency, intensity, and duration of anginal attacks
Increasing danger of myocardial infarction within 3 to 18 months

Chronic Stable Angina
Predictable, consistent, rarely occurs while at rest

Nocturnal Angina
Pain occurs at night usually during sleep; may be relieved by sitting upright
Commonly due to left ventricular failure

Angina Decubitus
Angina while lying down

Intractable or Refractory Angina
Severe incapacitating angina

Prinzmetal's Angina (Variant; Resting)
Spontaneous type of anginal pain accompanied by ST segment elevation in ECG
Thought to be due to coronary artery spasm
Associated with high risk of infarction

The answers to these questions, ascertained from observation, can form a basis for designing a logical program of prevention.

If a patient senses that an attack is imminent, he should cease all movement, in order to reduce to a minimum the oxygen requirements of the ischemic myocardium. This is done with the hope that oxygen needs can be met by the limited supply available at the moment and the impending attack can thus be averted.

Patient Problems/Nursing Diagnoses

Based on the clinical manifestations, nursing history, and the diagnostic assessment data, the patient's major nursing problems include pain related to myocardial ischemia; anxiety related to fear of death; and potential for complications.

▶ Planning and Implementation

Goals

The major goals for the patient include:

1. Relief of pain
2. Reduction of anxiety
3. Absence of complications

The objectives of treatment are to decrease the oxygen demands of the myocardium and to increase the oxygen supply.

Decreasing Oxygen Demands of the Myocardium. The patient must understand the symptom complex and the need to avoid activities known to cause anginal pain. He needs to become aware of the factors producing this pain: sudden exertion, walking against the wind, exposure to cold, emotional excitement, etc., and he must learn to change, modify, or adapt to these stresses.

There are patients whose attacks occur predominantly in the morning. This idiosyncrasy obviously calls for a change in the schedule of daily activities. As a first step, the patient should plan to rise earlier each morning so that he may complete his shaving, washing, and dressing in a more leisurely fashion. Ideally, he should maintain this unhurried pace throughout the entire day—performing his scheduled tasks and meeting whatever commitments he has without haste or a sense of pressure. Any patient with angina pectoris should be instructed to initiate all movements with deliberation, avoid exposure to cold, avoid tobacco, eat regularly but lightly, and maintain a proper weight. Use of over-the-counter drugs should be discouraged, especially diet pills, nasal decongestants, or others that contain agents that will increase heart rate and blood pressure. Other measures to decrease the oxygen demands of the myocardium may include lowering the patient's blood pressure, correcting valvular disease, and treating hyperthyroidism.

Pharmacologic Therapy: Nitroglycerin. The nitrates are still the mainstay of treatment for angina pectoris. Nitroglycerin is given to reduce myocardial oxygen consumption, which decreases ischemia and relieves anginal pain. Nitroglycerin is a vasoactive drug that acts to dilate both the venous and the arteriolar vascularity and thus has an effect on the peripheral circulation. By increasing the capacity of the venous bed, it causes venous pooling of blood throughout the body. As a result, less blood is returned to the heart and there is a reduction in filling pressure (preload). Nitrates also relax the systemic arteriolar bed and thus cause a fall in blood pressure (decreases afterload). These effects decrease myocardial oxygen requirements, bringing about a more favorable balance between supply and demand.

Nitroglycerin taken sublingually or in the buccal pouch alleviates the pain of ischemia within 3 minutes.

- The patient should be instructed to keep the tongue still and to avoid swallowing saliva until the nitroglycerin tablet is dissolved. If the pain is severe, the tablet can be crushed between the teeth to hasten sublingual absorption.
- As a precaution, the patient should carry the medication at all times in a securely capped dark glass bottle, not in a metal or plastic pillbox.

Nitroglycerin is volatile and is inactivated by heat, moisture, air, light, and time. If the nitroglycerin is fresh, the patient will feel a burning sensation under the tongue and often a feeling of fullness or throbbing in the head. The nitroglycerin supply should be renewed every 6 months.

Instead of following a fixed dosage, the patient regulates drug usage, taking the smallest dose that relieves pain. He is instructed to take the drug in anticipation of any activity that may produce pain. Since nitroglycerin will increase the patient's tolerance for exercise and stress when taken prophylactically (*e.g.,* before exercise, stair climbing, and sexual intercourse), it is best that it be taken *before* the pain develops.

- The patient should note how long it takes for the nitroglycerin to relieve the discomfort. If the pain lasts more than 20 or 30 minutes after the nitroglycerin has been taken, an impending myocardial infarction may be suspected.

Side-effects of nitroglycerin include flushing, throbbing headache, hypotension, and tachycardia. The use of long-acting nitrate preparations is controversial. Isosorbide dinitrate appears to be effective for up to 2 hours if taken sublingually but has an uncertain effect if taken orally.

Topical Nitroglycerin Ointment. Nitroglycerin is also available in a lanolin-petrolatum base, which, when applied to the skin, appears to protect against anginal pain and promote its relief. It is especially useful when patients experience nocturnal angina or are involved in periods of extended activity (*e.g.,* golfing) since it has a prolonged effect of up to 24 hours. The dose is usually increased until headache or an excessive effect on blood pressure or heart rate occurs and then is reduced to the largest dose that does not produce these side-effects. Instructions for application accompany the various products.

Table 31-3 summarizes vasodilators in current use.

Beta-Adrenergic Blockers. If the patient continues to have chest pain despite treatment with nitroglycerin and modification of life-style, the beta-adrenergic blocking agent propranolol hydrochloride (Inderal) is given. This drug appears to reduce myocardial oxygen consumption by blocking the sympathetic impulses to the heart. The result is a reduction in heart rate, blood pressure, and myocardial contractility that establishes a more favorable balance between myocardial oxygen needs and the amount of oxygen available. This helps to control chest pain and allows the patient to work or exercise. Propranolol may be given with sublingual isosorbide dinitrate for anti-anginal and anti-ischemia prophylaxis. Propranolol is cleared by the liver at varying rates, depending on the individual patient. It is usually given at 6-hour intervals. Side-effects include musculoskeletal weakness, hypotension, bradycardia, and mental depression.

When propranolol is started, blood pressure and heart rate should be taken (while the patient is in an upright position) 2 hours after the medication has been administered. If the blood pressure drops significantly, a vasopressor may be needed. If severe bradycardia occurs, atropine is the drug of choice. It is also important to remember that propranolol can precipitate congestive heart failure and asthma.

- Caution the patient not to stop taking propranolol abruptly, since there is evidence that angina may worsen and myocardial infarction may develop if this drug is abruptly discontinued.

Calcium Ion Antagonists. The laboratory investigation of the calcium ion and its role in cardiovascular function has yielded a group of drugs referred to as calcium blockers or antagonists. These drugs possess properties that have

Table 31-3
Commonly Used Vasodilators

Definition: Vasodilators are drugs that relax the smooth muscle of the small arteries and veins.
Action: Arteriolar dilators act as afterload reducing agents.
      Venodilators increase venous capacitance, thus reducing preload.
Special Precaution: Orthostatic or postural hypotension
Dosage Determinant: (1) Severity of signs and symptoms; (2) weight and body build

Vasodilator	Action	Nursing Implications/Precautions
Sodium nitroprusside	Dilates arterioles and venules Increases cardiac output and decreases pulmonary congestion Potent, rapid-acting IV only Short duration	Hypotension is a hazardous side-effect. Releases hydrocyanic acid, which can lead to cyanide poisoning. Serum thiocyanate levels should be drawn if patient is on drug more than a few days.
Phentolamine	Relaxes smooth muscle *directly* Short duration	Excessive hypotension Nausea, vomiting, abdominal pain Tachycardia
Nitrates Isorbide dinitrate	Venodilators, principally Long-acting, hence, good for maintenance therapy	Headaches Postural hypotension
Hydralazine	Relaxes arteriolar smooth muscle Given orally	Vascular headaches Flushing, nausea and vomiting
Prazosin	Equal dilating effect on arteries and veins Oral agent	Polyarthralgia, transient headaches Mild nausea, urinary incontinence, rashes, mental depression, dry mouth, first-dose phenomenon (*e.g.,* transient faintness, dizziness, palpitations and, rarely, syncope occur after taking first dose)

profound effects on myocardial oxygen demands and supply, hence their value in the treatment of angina. Physiologically, the calcium ion performs at the cellular level to influence contraction of all types of muscle tissue and plays a role in the electrical stimulation of the heart.

Calcium ion antagonists increase myocardial oxygen supply by dilating the smooth muscle wall of the coronary arterioles, and decrease myocardial oxygen demands by reducing systemic arterial pressure and thus the work load of the left ventricle.

The two calcium antagonists being used clinically are nifedipine and verapamil. The vasodilating effects of these agents, particularly on the coronary circulation, have made them valuable in angina that results from coronary vasospasm (Prinzmetal's angina). Calcium blockers should be used with great caution in individuals with heart failure because they block the calcium, which supports contractility. Hypotension may occur after IV administration. Other side-effects that may occur are constipation, gastric intolerance, dizziness, or headache associated with dizziness.

Calcium ion antagonists are usually given every 4 to 6 hours. Therapeutic doses vary from one individual to another.

Risk Factor Control.   Several other measures may be necessary in order to decrease the oxygen demands of the myocardium. It is important that the patient stop smoking, since smoking produces tachycardia and raises the blood pressure, thus increasing the work of the heart. Obese individuals should lose weight to reduce cardiac work.

Physical conditioning should be encouraged since it increases exercise capacity and produces a lower heart rate and blood pressure in response to a given exercise. (See page 634 for rehabilitation of the heart patient.)

Surgical Treatment to Increase Oxygen Supply

Angina pectoris may persist for many years in a stable form with brief attacks. However, it is a serious disease. In the unstable stage the episodes of chest pain become more frequent and intense, occurring without apparent provocation. When symptoms cannot be controlled despite an adequate trial of drug therapy, some form of surgical revascularization is considered that can correct the basic problem by bringing a new blood supply to the ischemic myocardium (see page 610).

Percutaneous Transluminal Angioplasty.   The concept of interventional radiology has made possible a less invasive procedure for the revascularization of the coronary arteries. The procedure is referred to as percutaneous transluminal angioplasty (see p. 610).

A balloon-tipped catheter is inserted into the coronary artery and is rapidly inflated and deflated. The purpose of this procedure is to compress the atheroma into the intimal lining of the artery, thereby increasing the blood flow of the same vessel.

Patients eligible for this procedure have atherosclerotic disease affecting only one vessel, have had angina for less than 1 year, and are candidates for surgical revascularization. Because of these rigid criteria, the population that the procedure may benefit is severely limited.

Myocardial infarction is a major complication of this procedure. For this reason it is recommended that this procedure be performed only if a cardiovascular surgical team is on standby.

Patient Education

The education of the patient with angina is designed to acquaint him with the basic nature of his illness and to furnish him with the facts he needs if he is to reorganize his living habits in a way that will reduce the frequency and severity of anginal attacks; delay the progress of the underlying disease, if possible; and help protect him from other complications. The factors outlined in Chart 31-2 are important in the education of the patient with angina pectoris.

▶ Evaluation

Expected Outcomes

1. Is relieved of pain
   (See Chart 31-2, on patient education.)
2. Reduces anxiety
   a. Alters life-style as appropriate
   b. Understands the process of angina
   c. Adheres to medical regimen
   d. Knows to seek medical assistance if pain persists or changes in quality
   e. Avoids being alone during painful episodes
3. Is free of complications
   a. Exhibits normal ECG and level of cardiac enzymes
   b. Is free of signs and symptoms of acute myocardial infarction (see p. 633)

Chart 31-2
Patient Education in Angina

Goal: To improve the quality of life and promote health

Expected Outcomes

I. Prevents an episode of anginal pain
   A. Uses moderation in all activities of life
      1. Participates in a normal daily program of activities that do not produce chest discomfort, shortness of breath, and undue fatigue
      2. Exercises before work, after work, or before meals
      3. Avoids exercises requiring sudden bursts of activity; avoids all isometric exercise
      4. Avoids activities that require heavy effort
      5. Alternates activity with periods of rest. Some fatigue is normal and temporary.
   B. Avoids situations that are emotionally stressful
   C. Avoids overeating
      1. Eats smaller portions
      2. Avoids excessive caffeine intake (coffee, cola drinks), which can increase the heart rate and produce angina
      3. Refrains from engaging in physical exercise for 2 hours after meals
      4. Does not use "diet pills," nasal decongestants, or any over-the-counter medications that can increase the heart rate
   D. Stops smoking, since smoking increases the heart rate, blood pressure, and blood carbon monoxide levels
   E. Avoids cold weather, if possible
      1. Wears scarf over nose/mouth during very cold weather to warm the air

      2. Walks more slowly in cold weather
      3. Dresses warmly in winter
   F. Follows general principles of good hygienic living

II. Copes with an attack of anginal pain
   A. Carries nitroglycerin at all times
      1. Keeps nitroglycerin in a tightly capped, dark-colored glass bottle
      2. Discards the cotton filler/packing
      3. Avoids opening the bottle unnecessarily
      4. Tries to avoid carrying supply right next to body
      5. Discards tablets after 5 months
      6. If tablets are fresh, they should cause a burning sensation when placed under the tongue
   B. Places nitroglycerin under the tongue at first sign of chest discomfort
      1. Does not swallow saliva until the tablet has dissolved
      2. Stops and rests until all pain subsides
      3. States the significance of using the upright position to potentiate the effects of nitroglycerin.
      4. Usually, another nitroglycerin tablet may be taken in 3 to 5 minutes if pain relief is not obtained. If pain persists, calls the physician. If the anginal discomfort is unrelieved by the usual number of nitroglycerin tablets, or if it recurs after a short interval, goes to the nearest emergency facility.
   C. Takes nitroglycerin prophylactically to avoid pain known to occur with certain activities (stair climbing, sexual intercourse)
   D. Is alert for the side-effects of nitroglycerin: headache, flushing, and dizziness

Myocardial Infarction

Myocardial infarction refers to the process by which myocardial tissue is destroyed in regions of the heart that are deprived of an adequate blood supply because of a reduced coronary blood flow. The cause of the reduced blood flow is either a critical narrowing of a coronary artery owing to atherosclerosis or, less commonly, a complete occlusion of an artery owing to embolus or thrombus. Decreased coronary blood flow may also result from shock and hemorrhage. In this situation, there is a profound imbalance between myocardial oxygen supply and demand.

"Coronary occlusion," "heart attack," and "myocardial infarction" are all used synonymously, but the latter is the preferred term. In the United States, well over a million of these attacks occur annually.

The pathophysiology of atherosclerotic heart disease is discussed on page 626. The risk factors are found on pages 554 and 627.

Clinical Manifestations

The patient with myocardial infarction is usually male, is over 40, and has atherosclerosis of the coronary vessels, often with arterial hypertension. However, attacks also occur in women and in younger men in their early 30s or even 20s.

In a typical patient, the pain starts suddenly, usually over the lower sternal region and the upper abdomen, and is continuous, but it may increase steadily in severity until it becomes almost unbearable. It is a heavy, viselike pain, which may radiate to the shoulders and down the arms, usually the left arm. Unlike the pain of true angina, it begins spontaneously (not following effort, emotional upset, etc.), persists for hours or days, and is relieved neither by rest nor by nitroglycerin. The pulse may become very rapid, irregular, and feeble, even imperceptible. Gallop rhythm (accentuated third heart sound making the three heart sounds similar to those of a galloping horse) often develops.

The person with a severe occlusion may be in shock; he appears ashen and breaks out in a clammy sweat. Vomiting is common. In a few hours body temperature rises, blood pressure falls to an unusually low point, the leukocyte count rises to 15,000 or 20,000 cu mm. Changes may be seen in the electrocardiogram within 2 to 12 hours (but may take as long as 72 to 96 hours). These changes reveal not only the presence but also the location of the infarct. Serum enzymes and isoenzymes are elevated and can be correlated with the patient's clinical course (see p. 559). Even if the ECG is normal, elevation of serum enzymes reveals that caution is indicated in the handling of this person.

A significant percentage of patients with acute myocardial infarction diagnosed on the basis of subsequent ECGs deny having experienced any pain or discomfort whatever. These are the so-called silent myocardial infarction patients.

Prognosis

Studies show that the extent of the myocardial damage and the severity of coronary artery obstruction are important predictors of survival. Approximately 70% of patients dying from coronary atherosclerotic heart disease never reach a hospital. The highest mortality occurs during the first hour after onset of symptoms. A large percentage of all *sudden* deaths occur in patients with coronary atherosclerotic heart disease (CAHD). Other patients live a few days and succumb as the result of cardiogenic shock, arrhythmias, congestive heart failure, and other complications.

Of those persons who live long enough to get to a hospital, a much higher percentage survive, especially if an intensive coronary care unit is available. A small infarct may heal, with scar formation, leaving the patient fairly well, but a second occlusion often occurs later, or the patient develops heart failure. In fact, a recurrent infarction within 5 months after recovery from an acute myocardial infarction carries a significant fatality rate. Of those who recover, the majority can return to normal duties.

The most critical period for the patient with a myocardial infarction is the first 48 hours following the attack. The area of infarction can increase in size for several hours or days after the onset of the attack. Cardiogenic shock and ventricular fibrillation are common causes of sudden death during this time period.

The objectives of management are designed to:

- Detect and treat arrhythmias
- Alleviate shock
- Relieve pain
- Rest the myocardium
- Prevent complications
- Achieve physiologic and functional rehabilitation
- Halt the progress of atherosclerosis, the lesion that is basically responsible for the myocardial infarct

Since the patient usually receives this initial care in the cardiac care unit, a detailed discussion will be found on pages 585–599 of Chapter 29, Management of the Patient in the Cardiac Care Unit.

Management Following Discharge From the Cardiac Care Unit

Psychosocial Considerations. Nursing care in the cardiac care unit involves constant surveillance, monitoring, and attention to patient needs. When the patient is transferred from this atmosphere of total dependence to a regular unit, he no longer receives this type of continual care. As a result, he may feel anxious or angry. This anxiety may be manifested by chest pain, headache, dizziness, restlessness, and insomnia. By understanding the patient's feelings and behavior, the nurse can counteract his stress and better plan his care. The patient's negative behavior may derive partly from his incomplete internalization of the education that he received while in the CCU.

- Find out what the patient knows about his condition and correct any misconceptions. Help him to identify his stresses, and encourage him to ventilate and discharge his strong pent-up emotions. Above all, be encouraging and optimistic.

The goal is to assist the patient to develop healthy attitudes toward the illness and to prepare him to manage the self-care that will be required when he returns home.

Physical Considerations. On return from the CCU, physical and emotional rest are still important therapeutic considerations. The patient is usually permitted to ambulate and go to the bathroom. Physical activities are increased gradually, but the patient is instructed to avoid sudden effort, including the Valsalva maneuver (straining). Usually, a fat- and calorie-controlled diet is prescribed; caffeine-containing beverages are discouraged.

The patient's progress is followed with the aid of repeated electrocardiograms and determinations of serum enzymes. Cardiac function is estimated on the basis of symptoms and physical signs. Gradually, self-confidence should be built up and a workable approach to work, recreation, and hobbies should be established that will allow a return to a normal or near-normal life-style.

The patient's prognosis may be jeopardized by the advent, during the initial 2 weeks, of any one of several complications, including arrhythmias, thromboembolism, congestive failure, and myocardial rupture. To be on the alert for any such development is an important nursing responsibility.

Rehabilitation

The goals of rehabilitation for the patient with myocardial infarction are to extend and improve the quality of life. The immediate objectives are to return the patient as rapidly as possible to a normal or near-normal life-style. This includes training the patient for physical activity, educating him and his family, and initiating psychosocial and vocational counseling when necessary.

Actually, cardiac rehabilitation begins as soon as the acute episode occurs. During this stage the nurse can assist the patient toward the realization of his goal of independence, even when he is on strict bed rest. This is achieved by directing his thinking toward the time when he will be active again. The goal here is not to change the patient's life-style but to make necessary modifications. It is best to avoid remonstrating about what the patient should not do. Instead, he should be encouraged to develop short-term and long-range goals based on his needs. It is important to explain the nature of the disease, answer questions honestly, and reassure the patient that most persons return to a useful economic life and resume their usual activities. These are positive approaches in preventing the patient from becoming a cardiac cripple.

There is a divergence of opinion concerning the amount of activity the patient may participate in following a myocardial infarction. Although dangerous complications occur early, the scar formation over the infarcted area is seen at the beginning of the third week. The necrotic debris is resolved by the fourth week, while the development of the scar continues. Thus, there is an area of ischemia in some patients for varying lengths of time, which affects the individual's exercise prescription.

Physical Conditioning. Physical conditioning or exercise training is done to improve cardiac efficiency and enhance the patient's ability to perform work at reduced heart and blood pressure rates. This will reduce the oxygen requirements of the heart and enable the patient to perform more physical activity before developing symptoms of myocardial ischemia (*e.g.,* chest pain, ECG changes). Physical conditioning may be divided into the acute phase, convalescent phase (up to 8 weeks), and maintenance phase (lifelong).

As soon as the patient is *stable* and the physician permits, the arms are put through range of motion exercises. Active motion of the muscles of the shoulder girdle helps to prevent anterior chest wall pain, which may be interpreted as being cardiac in origin. The patient may be able to sit in a chair for 20 to 30 minutes several times a day beginning a few days after admission. As soon as he is able (depending on his signs and symptoms, clinical condition, ECG, serum enzymes) he is encouraged to participate in self-care activities. Early mobilization under supervision is usually permitted after an uncomplicated myocardial infarction. Mobilization begins with walking and progresses to stair climbing. Prolonged immobilization has a deconditioning effect and also contributes to anxiety and depression.

- Evaluate the patient closely and carefully during physical activity for chest pain, dyspnea, weakness, fatigue, and an increase in heart rate of more than 20 beats from baseline or greater than 120 beats per minute.
- Watch also for a fall in systolic blood pressure, the development of an arrhythmia or conduction disturbance, or an increase in ST segment displacement or T wave abnormality on the monitor. If these occur, the activity is stopped immediately and the patient's clinical status is reevaluated.

Isometric exercises are contraindicated because they may impose stress on the left ventricle by raising the blood pressure while at the same time decreasing coronary perfusion. The performance of the Valsalva maneuver (straining) is to be avoided.

A treadmill test with ECG monitoring is done to help in developing guidelines for the design of an appropriate exercise program for the patient. Submaximal testing is done before the patient leaves the hospital and maximal testing before he returns to work. The patient who demonstrates low functional capacity with ischemic ST segment depression and premature ventricular beats will need a different activity program than the patient who has good functional capacity with no significant ECG abnormalities. The level of the patient's physical activity before infarction is also considered.

In general, the activity (walking) is increased in distance and speed. The cardiovascular benefits of exercise depend on whether or not the patient can exercise long enough to reach and maintain the prescribed pulse rate for a period of 15 minutes. (The patient is taught to monitor his pulse during physical activity.)

Several months after myocardial infarction the maintenance phase begins. As a result of physical training, the patient may participate in activities that promote endurance—jogging, running, swimming, cycling. These appear to be useful for heart and lung conditioning. In general, the best type of exercise consists of rhythmic and repetitive movements (calisthenics, walking, running) that require maximal or submaximal effort. Short bursts of intensive effort are to be avoided since they produce a marked rise in blood pressure.

Sexual Activity. Many patients fear that sexual activity will be harmful to their heart condition and will precipitate chest pain.

If the patient can walk vigorously around the block or climb a flight of stairs without symptoms (rapid heart rate, chest pain, etc.) sexual activity may usually be resumed. Some modifications may be necessary—that is, intercourse after a night's sleep and followed by a rest period or the use of more passive positions to decrease cardiac work load. Sexual relations should be avoided after drinking alcohol or ingesting a large meal, if the situation produces anxiety or if abnormal symptoms develop and persist.

Patient Education

Certain general principles for living are usually prescribed at this stage, the character of which must vary widely from patient to patient, owing to marked differences in practical considerations and individual personalities. Questions that will arise may concern such matters as requirements for rest, criteria for controlling activities, and recommendations as to diet and the use of tobacco.

Obesity increases the work of the heart and should be brought under control, speedily and permanently. Arterial hypertension also imposes a myocardial burden and must be treated. Anemia, of course, should be corrected. With respect to smoking, it may be pointed out that most sudden deaths that occur in individuals with a past history of a myocardial infarction are due to cardiac arrhythmias, notably ventricular fibrillation, and that many of the individuals so afflicted are habitually heavy smokers. Smoking increases peripheral and coronary vasoconstriction and may produce a tachycardia. Logically, any individual who has sustained a myocardial infarction is well advised to eliminate the use of tobacco. (See Chart 31-3.)

▷ Cardiac Failure

Pathophysiology

In heart failure, the heart is unable to pump sufficient blood to meet the needs of the tissues for oxygen and nutrients. The cardiac output is frequently lower than normal, although heart failure can occur when there is high cardiac output in conditions when the metabolic requirements of the tissues are abnormally high. There are two predominant patterns of heart failure. The first has low cardiac output as its primary feature. If the low cardiac output develops acutely and is accompanied by low systemic arterial blood pressure, it is termed *cardiogenic shock.* The second pattern, *congestive heart failure,* is characterized by manifestations that are related primarily to retention of fluid in the lungs or peripheral tissues.

The underlying mechanism of heart failure involves the impaired contractile properties of the heart, which lead to a lower than normal cardiac output. The concept of cardiac output is best explained by the equation $CO = HR \times SV$, where cardiac output is a function of heart rate times stroke volume.

Heart rate is a function of the autonomic nervous system. When cardiac output falls, the initial response is that the sympathetic nervous system accelerates the heart rate to maintain adequate cardiac output. When this compensatory mechanism fails to maintain adequate tissue perfusion, the properties of stroke volume compensate.

In heart failure where the primary problem is damaged and inhibited myocardial muscle fibers, stroke volume is impaired. Stroke volume, the amount of blood pumped with each contraction, is dependent upon three factors: preload, contractility, and afterload.

Preload is synonymous with Starling's law of the heart, where the amount of blood filling the heart is directly proportional to pressure created by the length of the stretch of the myocardial fibers. *Contractility* refers to an alteration in the force of contraction that occurs at the cellular level and is unrelated to changes in myocardial fiber length. *Afterload* refers to the amount of pressure the ventricle must create in order to pump blood across the pressure gradient created by the semilunar valves. In heart failure, any one or more of these three factors may be altered such that cardiac output is impaired. The relative ease of determining hemodynamic measurements via invasive monitoring procedures has greatly facilitated differential diagnosis and pharmacologic manipulation of the problem.

Heart failure most commonly occurs with disorders of cardiac muscle that result in decreased contractile properties of the heart. Frequent underlying conditions that lead to disordered muscle function include coronary atherosclerosis, arterial hypertension, and inflammatory or degenerative muscle disease. Coronary atherosclerosis leads to myocardial dysfunction by interfering with the normal blood supply to cardiac muscle. Hypoxia, acidosis (owing to accumulation of lactic acid), and nutrient deprivation of heart muscle result. Myocardial infarction (death of myocardial cells) frequently precedes the development of overt heart failure. Systemic or pulmonary hypertension (increased afterload) increases the work requirement of the heart, and this in turn leads to hypertrophy of myocardial muscle fibers. This effect (*i.e.,* myocardial hypertrophy) can be considered a compensatory mechanism since it increases the contractility of the heart. However, for reasons that are not clear, the hypertrophied cardiac muscle does not function normally, and heart failure may eventually result. Heart failure associated with inflammatory and degenerative diseases of the myocardium is due to direct damage to myocardial fibers with a resultant decrease in contractility.

Heart failure may occur as a result of heart disease that only secondarily affects the myocardium. The mechanisms involved include impediment to flow of blood through the heart (*e.g.,* stenosis of a semilunar valve), inability of the heart to fill with blood (*e.g.,* pericardial tamponade, constrictive pericarditis, or stenosis of AV valves), or abnormal emptying of the heart (*e.g.,* insufficiency of AV valves). Sudden increases in afterload owing to elevated systemic blood pressure ("malignant" hypertension) may result in heart failure in the absence of myocardial hypertrophy.

A number of systemic factors can contribute to the development and severity of heart failure. Increased metabolic rate (*e.g.,* fever, thyrotoxicosis), hypoxia, or anemia require an increased cardiac output to satisfy systemic oxygen demand. Hypoxia or anemia also may decrease the supply of oxygen to the myocardium. Acidosis (respiratory or metabolic) and electrolyte abnormalities may decrease myocardial contractility. Cardiac arrhythmias, which may be present independently or secondary to heart failure itself, decrease the efficiency of overall myocardial function.

Chart 31-3
Patient Education in Myocardial Infarction

A patient with heart disease should learn to regulate his activity according to his individual response.

Goal: To improve the quality of life and promote health

Expected Outcomes

I. Modifies activities during convalescence so that complete recovery is realized
    A. Myocardial healing starts early but is not complete for varying periods; usually 6 to 8 weeks.
    B. A myocardial infarction usually requires some modification of the life-style; adaptation to a heart attack is an ongoing process.
        1. Avoids any activity that produces chest pain, dyspnea, or undue fatigue
        2. Avoids extremes of heat and cold and walking against the wind
        3. Loses weight as directed
        4. Stops smoking
        5. Alternates activity with rest periods. Some fatigue is normal and expected during convalescence.
        6. Uses personal strengths to compensate for limitations
        7. Eats three or four meals daily, each containing the same amount of food
            a. Avoids large meals and hurrying while eating
            b. Restricts caffeine-containing beverages, since caffeine can affect heart rate, rhythm, and blood pressure

        c. Complies with prescribed diet, modifying calories, fat, and sodium as prescribed
        8. Makes every effort to adhere to medical regimen, especially in taking medications
        9. Pursues a pleasurable hobby that affords release of tension
II. Undertakes an *orderly* program of increasing activity and exercise for long-term rehabilitation
    A. Engages in a regimen of physical conditioning with a gradual increase in activity levels
        1. Walks daily, increasing distance and time as prescribed
        2. Monitors pulse during physical activity until the maximal level of activity is attained
        3. Avoids activities that tense the muscles: isometric exercise, weight lifting, any activity that requires sudden bursts of energy
        4. Avoids physical exercise immediately after a meal
        5. Exercises before work, after work, or before retiring
        6. Shortens work hours when first returning to work
    B. Participates in a *daily* program of exercise that develops into a program of regular exercise for a lifetime
    C. Notifies physician when the following symptoms occur:
        1. Chest pressure or pain not relieved in 15 minutes by nitroglycerin (Report to nearest emergency facility.)
        2. Shortness of breath
        3. Fainting
        4. Slow or rapid heartbeat
        5. Swelling of feet and ankles

▶ **Assessment**

Clinical Manifestations. The low output state in heart failure results in widespread manifestations owing to diminished tissue and end-organ perfusion. Some commonly encountered effects related to low perfusion are dizziness, confusion, fatigue, exercise or heat intolerance, cool extremities, and oliguria. Renal perfusion pressure falls, which results in the release of renin from the kidney, which in turn leads to aldosterone secretion, sodium and fluid retention, and increased intravascular volume. The group of manifestations related to low cardiac output are sometimes referred to as "forward heart failure."

The dominant feature in congestive heart failure is increased intravascular volume. In this syndrome, congestion of tissues results from increased arterial and venous pressures owing to decreased cardiac output in the failing heart. Increased pulmonary venous pressure can lead to transudation of fluid from pulmonary capillaries (pulmonary

edema), manifested by cough and shortness of breath. Increased systemic venous pressure can result in generalized peripheral edema and weight gain. This syndrome is sometimes referred to as "backward heart failure." Forward and backward heart failure usually coexist in most patients with heart failure.

The right and left ventricles can fail separately. Since the outputs of the ventricles are coupled, failure of either ventricle may lead to decreased tissue perfusion. The congestive manifestations, however, may differ according to whether right or left ventricular failure exists. Pulmonary congestion predominates when the left ventricle fails, whereas congestion of viscera and peripheral tissue predominates when the right ventricle fails.

Patient Problems/Nursing Diagnoses

Based on the clinical manifestations, nursing history, and diagnostic assessment data, the patient's major nursing problems include decreased mentation related to diminished oxygenation to cerebral tissues; fatigue related to diminished oxygenation to tissues; shortness of breath related to increased circulating blood volume; and increased susceptibility for thromboembolic events related to stasis of peripheral fluid volume.

▶ Planning and Implementation

Goals

The major goals for the patient include:

1. Improved oxygenation to brain and peripheral tissues
2. Decreased total circulating blood volume
3. Decreased susceptibility to thromboembolic events

The basic objectives in the treatment of patients with congestive heart failure are:

1. To promote rest to reduce the work load on the heart
2. To administer pharmacologic agents to increase the force and efficiency of myocardial contraction, which will improve the heart's effectiveness as a pump
3. To eliminate the excessive accumulation of body water by means of diuretic therapy, diet, and rest

Promoting Rest to Reduce Cardiac Work

If the cardiac load is to be decreased, it is essential that the patient have both physical and emotional rest. Rest reduces the work of the heart, increases heart reserve, and reduces the blood pressure. Periods of recumbency also promote diuresis by improving renal perfusion. Rest also decreases the work of the respiratory muscles and oxygen utilization. The heart rate is slowed, which prolongs the diastolic period of recovery and thus improves the efficiency of heart contraction. The patient will be impressed when he hears that each day of complete rest spares the heart approximately 25,000 contractions.

Positioning. The head of the bed may be elevated on 20-cm to 30-cm (8-inch–10-inch) blocks or the patient may be placed in a comfortable armchair. In this position the venous return to the heart (preload) and the lungs is reduced, pulmonary congestion is alleviated, and impingement of the liver on the diaphragm is minimized. The lower arms should be supported with pillows to eliminate the fatigue caused by the constant pull of their weight on the shoulder muscles. The orthopneic patient may sit on the side of his bed with his feet supported on a chair, his head and arms resting on an over-the-bed table, and his lumbosacral spine supported by a pillow. If pulmonary congestion is present, positioning the patient in an armchair is advantageous since this position favors the shift of fluid away from the lungs. Edema, which usually occurs in dependent parts of the body, shifts from the extremities to the sacral areas when the patient is confined to bed.

- Remember that there are dangers inherent in bed rest: pressure sores (especially in edematous patients), phlebothrombosis, and pulmonary embolism. Changes of position, deep breathing, elastic stockings, and leg exercises all help to improve muscle tone, aid in venous return to the heart, and increase the sense of well-being.

Relieving Nighttime Anxiety. Patients in congestive heart failure are very apt to be restless and anxious at night. Raising the head of the bed and keeping a night light on are helpful. The presence of a member of the family provides necessary reassurance to some persons. The patient should be observed for possible respiratory irregularities, such as Cheyne–Stokes respirations, a phenomenon that may occur in cardiac failure. If such a respiratory disturbance is present, it may be worthwhile to test the effect of oxygen inhalations administered (as prescribed) each night just before the hour of sleep. Oxygen may be given during the acute stage to diminish the work of breathing and to increase the comfort of the patient. Small doses of morphine may be prescribed for extreme dyspnea, and chloral hydrate may be given as needed for sleep.

- It should be recalled that the patient with hepatic congestion is unable to detoxify drugs with normal rapidity and should be medicated with caution. As a result of cerebral hypoxia, with superimposed nitrogen retention, the patient may react unfavorably to soporific drugs, becoming confused and increasingly anxious in response to medication. Such a patient should not be restrained; restraints are likely to be resisted, and resistance inevitably increases the cardiac load.

If the patient insists on getting out of bed at night, he should be seated comfortably in an armchair. As his cerebral and systemic circulations improve, the quality of his sleep will improve.

Avoiding Stress. Rest is not possible without relaxation. Emotional stress produces vasoconstriction, elevates the arterial pressure, and speeds the heart. Promoting physical comfort and avoiding situations that tend to promote anxiety and agitation may help the patient to relax. The period of rest is continued for a few days to a few weeks until the congestive heart failure is controlled.

Administering Pharmacologic Therapy

Digitalis. Cardiac glycosides (digitalis), diuretics, and vasodilators form the basis of the pharmacologic treatment of congestive heart failure.

Digitalis increases the force of myocardial contraction and slows the heart rate. Several effects are produced: an increase in cardiac output; a decrease in heart size, venous pressure, and blood volume; and diuresis, which relieves edema. The effect of a given dose of digitalis depends on the state of the myocardium, electrolyte and fluid balance, and renal and hepatic function.

A loading dose of digitalis may be given to induce the full therapeutic effect of the drug. This is usually done in the treatment of more severe forms of congestive heart failure. Otherwise, the patient is started without a loading dose. A maintenance dose is given and continued daily. In either case, the patient is observed closely and given a daily dose just adequate to replace the amount of drug that is destroyed or excreted, in order to maintain the digitalis effect without toxicity. The optimal dosage is the amount that relieves the patient's signs and symptoms of congestive failure or slows the ventricular response therapeutically *without causing toxicity*. The patient is closely observed for relief of his signs and symptoms: lessening dysnpea and orthopnea, decrease in crackles, and relief of peripheral edema.

Digitalis Toxicity.   Anorexia, nausea, and vomiting are early effects of digitalis toxicity. There may be alterations in the heart rhythm, bradycardia, premature ventricular contractions, ventricular bigeminy (coupling of normal and premature beat), and paroxysmal atrial tachycardia.

- The apical heart rate is taken before digitalis is administered. If there is excessive slowing of the heart rate or change in rhythm, the drug is withheld and the physician is notified.
- If prescribed, the serum digitalis level is checked prior to administration of the drug.

Chart 31-4 summarizes the major cardiac glycosides, along with their actions and the nursing surveillance required when these drugs are administered. (For a more detailed discussion of digitalis toxicity, see below.)

Vasodilator Therapy.   Of particular significance in the management of congestive heart failure are the vasoactive drugs. The family of nitrates are popular because, clinically, they are well-tried drugs. The nitrates have a strong dilator effect on the venous bed and lesser dilator effect on the systemic bed. The venous and arterial pooling of blood in the periphery reduces preload and afterload substantially. This allows ventricular function to normalize and hence improves cardiac output. Side-effects are minimal.

Other commonly used vasodilators are summarized in Table 31-3, page 631.

Eliminating Excessive Body Water: Diuretic Therapy

Diuretics are given to promote the excretion of sodium and water through the kidneys. These drugs may not be necessary if the patient responds to restricted activity, digitalis, and a low-sodium diet.

- When diuretics are given they should be administered early in the morning so that the resultant diuresis will not interfere with the patient's nighttime rest.
- An input and output record is kept, since the patient may lose a large volume of fluid after a single dose of a given diuretic.

Chart 31-4
Digitalis and Cardiac Glycoside Preparations

I. Actions of Digitalis

Increases force and velocity of myocardial contractions
  a. Increases cardiac output by enhancing force of contraction of ventricle
  b. Slows heart rate
  c. Decreases heart size
  d. Decreases venous pressure
  e. Promotes diuresis
  f. Slows the ventricular rate in the setting of supraventricular arrhythmias

II. Clinical Uses

1. Congestive heart failure
2. Atrial fibrillation; atrial flutter
3. Supraventricular tachyarrhythmias
4. Before cardiac surgery

III. Preparations

The choice of drug depends on the speed of onset desired, duration of action required, and individual patient response. The recommended dosage varies considerably.

Oral	*Parenteral*
Digitalis	Ouabain
Digitoxin	Deslanoside (Cedilanid-D)
Digoxin	Digitoxin
Lanatoside C	Digoxin (Lanoxin)
Acetyldigitoxin (Acylanid)	
Gitalin (Gitaligin)	

IV. Nursing Considerations and Actions

Special Precaution: The incidence of digitalis toxicity is high. Toxic effects do not always appear in a predictable manner.

1. Watch for toxic effects; *arrhythmias* (most important toxic effect), *anorexia,* nausea, vomiting, bradycardia, headache, malaise.
2. Assess clinical response of patient by relief of symptoms (dyspnea, orthopnea, crackles, hepatomegaly, peripheral edema).
3. Elderly patients may tolerate digitalis therapy poorly; assess for bradycardia, impaired renal function.
4. Monitor serum potassium levels in patients receiving digitalis, especially those receiving both digitalis and diuretics. There is a predisposition to arrhythmias if the state of potassium balance is not evaluated and corrected.
5. Assess for symptoms of electrolyte depletion in patients taking digitalis: lassitude, apathy, mental confusion, anorexia, decreasing urinary output, azotemia.
6. The following factors may increase sensitivity to digitalis: myocardial infarction, potassium depletion, kidney or hepatic disease, diuretic therapy, diarrhea, loss of appetite, advancing age, hypoxia and hypercapnia in pulmonary disease, acidosis, alkalosis.

- As a basis for evaluating the effectiveness of therapy, patients receiving diuretic drugs are weighed daily at the same time. In addition, skin turgor is examined for evidences of edema or dehydration. The pulse rate is also monitored.

The dosage schedule is determined by the patient's daily weight, physical findings, and symptoms. Table 31-4 summarizes the diuretics in common use. Furosemide (La-six) is a particularly useful diuretic in the treatment of heart failure because it dilates the venules, thereby increasing venous capacitance, and in turn reduces preload (venous return to the heart).

Diuretic Side-effects.   Prolonged diuretic therapy may produce *hyponatremia* (deficiency of sodium in the blood), which results in apprehension; weakness; fatigue; malaise; muscle cramps and twitching; and rapid, thready pulse.

Table 31-4
Commonly Used Diuretics

Definition: Diuretics are agents that increase the rate of urine flow.
Action: Dependent upon functionally active kidneys; most diuretics decrease the reabsorption of electrolytes (principally sodium) by the kidneys, promoting water loss as a secondary action.
   In the treatment of hypertension the naturetic (sodium excretion) effect is probably the action of importance.
   In edema states, the salt and water actions are both important.
Special Precaution: Some diuretics may produce electrolyte depletion, including potassium loss, which causes weakness and induces cardiac arrhythmias. Vigorous diuresis can produce hypovolemia.
Dosage Determination: (1) Patient's daily weight; (2) clinical signs and symptoms; (3) physical examination; (4) state of renal function

Diuretic	Action	Nursing Implications
Thiazides and related drugs Chlorothiazide (Diuril) Hydrochlorothiazide (HydroDIURIL, Esidrix, Oretic) Methyclothiazide (Enduron) Polythiazide (Renese) Chlorthalidone (Hygroton) Quinethazone (Hydromox)	Increases renal excretion of sodium (naturesis), potassium, chloride, bicarbonate (alkaline urine) with accompanying "osmotic" water loss Used principally in states of edema and hypertension Most widely used for prolonged administration	Monitor for electrolyte depletion. Watch for signs and symptoms of electrolyte imbalance: hyponatremia, hypokalemia, hypochloremic alkalosis. Adverse reactions may occur, manifested by gastrointestinal, central nervous system, hematologic, and cardiovascular signs and symptoms. Supplementary potassium is usually given with these diuretics.
Potassium-sparing diuretics Spironolactone (Aldactone)	Inhibits action of aldosterone in distal tubule and reduces reabsorption of sodium and chloride Gives gradual diuretic effect Used in treatment of cirrhosis and edema when other diuretics are toxic or ineffective	Monitor for electrolyte depletion. Usually used in combination with thiazide diuretic. Watch for side-effects—skin rash, gynecomastia.
Triamterene (Dyrenium)	Inhibits reabsorption of sodium ions in exchange for potassium and hydrogen ions in distal tubule	Usually used as an adjunct to thiazide therapy. May cause elevation in blood uric acid. Watch for nausea, vomiting, diarrhea, weakness, headache, and skin rash.
Potent diuretics Furosemide (Lasix) Ethacrynic Acid (Edecrin)	Usually reserved for patients who do not respond to classical thiazide diuretics Blocks the reabsorption of sodium and water in proximal renal tubule and interferes with reabsorption of sodium in ascending limb of loop of Henle and in the most proximal portion of the distal tubule Associated with sodium, potassium, chloride, and hydrogen ion loss (acid urine) Have an almost immediate action (within 5 minutes) when given IV	Monitor for electrolyte depletion: may produce *profound diuresis* with hyponatremia, hypokalemia, hypochloremic alkalosis, and circulatory collapse. Potent and rapid-acting. Especially useful in acute pulmonary edema. Watch for nausea, vomiting, diarrhea, skin rash, pruritus, blurring of vision, postural hypotension, vertigo, hearing loss. Furosemide is chemically related to sulfonamides; consider cross allergies. Administer early in the day to avoid nocturia and consequent loss of sleep.

Profuse and repeated diuresis can also lead to *hypokalemia* (potassium depletion). Signs are weak pulse, faint heart sounds, hypotension, muscle flabbiness, diminished tendon reflexes, and generalized weakness. This poses new problems for the cardiac patient, because among the complications of hypokalemia are marked weakening of cardiac contractions and the precipitation of digitalis toxicity in individuals receiving digitalis, both of which increase the likelihood of dangerous arrhythmias.

- Periodic assessment of the electrolytes will alert to hypokalemia and hyponatremia.
- To lessen the risk of hypokalemia and its attendant complications, patients receiving diuretic drugs may be given a potassium supplement (potassium chloride). Bananas, orange juice, dried prunes, raisins, apricots, dates, figs, peaches, and spinach are good dietary sources of potassium.

Other problems associated with diuretic administration are hyperuricemia, volume depletion, hyperglycemia, and diabetes mellitus.

The elderly male patient requires ongoing nursing surveillance inasmuch as the incidence of urethral obstruction owing to prostatic hypertrophy is high in this age group. Signs of bladder distention should be sought regularly by palpation over the bladder.

Providing Dietary Support

The rationale of dietary support is to provide the type of diet that will cause the heart the least possible work effort and muscular strain and to maintain the good nutritional status of the patient, taking into consideration his likes, dislikes, and cultural food habits.

Sodium Ion Manipulation. Restriction of the sodium ion is indicated for the prevention, control, or elimination of edema, such as in hypertension or congestive heart failure. Sodium should be specified in describing the regimen rather than "low salt" or "salt free," and the quantity should be indicated in milligrams. Very often mistakes are made in hospital units because of inconsistencies in the translation of salt to sodium. It is important to realize that salt is not 100% sodium. There are 393 mg, or approximately 400 mg, of sodium in 1 g (1000 mg) of salt.

Although the major source of sodium in the average American diet is salt, many types of natural foods contain varying amounts of sodium. Therefore, even if no salt is added in cooking and if salty foods are avoided, the daily diet may still contain approximately 1000 mg to 2000 mg of sodium.

Other sources of sodium can be found in some processed foods. Added food substances—such as sodium alginate, which improves texture; sodium benzoate, which acts as a preservative; or di-sodium phosphate, which improves cooking quality in certain foods—increase the sodium intake when included in the daily diet. Therefore, patients on low-sodium diets should be advised not to buy processed foods and to check labels carefully for such words as "salt" or "sodium." For diets that call for less than 1000 mg of sodium, low-sodium milk and bread and salt free butter should be considered.

Patients on sodium-restricted diets should also be cautioned against buying nonprescription medications, such as alkalizers, cough syrups, laxatives, sedatives, or salt substitutes, because these products contain sodium or excessive amounts of potassium. Any over-the-counter medication of this type should not be purchased without first consulting the physician.

When diets are very restrictive of both fat and sodium, the patient may find the food unpalatable and may refuse to eat. A variety of flavorings and herb seasonings may be used to improve the taste of the food and encourage the patient to accept the diet. Every effort should be made to take into account the patient's likes and dislikes.

Patient Education

After the patient's congestive failure is under control he is encouraged to gradually resume the activities he was accustomed to prior to his illness, particularly his job. The patient's earlier life-style should be retained if possible. However, some modifications in his habits, work, and interpersonal relationships usually have to be made. Any activity that produces symptoms must be curtailed or other adaptations made. The patient should be helped to identify his emotional stresses and to explore ways in which these may be ventilated and discharged.

All too frequently patients keep returning to the clinic and hospital for recurring episodes of congestive heart failure. Not only does this create psychological, sociological, and financial problems, but the physiologic burden on the patient can be serious. Previously normal organs of the body may ultimately be damaged. Repeated attacks can lead to pulmonary fibrosis, liver cirrhosis, enlargement of the spleen and kidneys, and even brain damage owing to insufficient oxygen during acute episodes. *To ensure that the patient will persevere in his therapy requires patient education, involvement, and cooperation.* Many of the recurrences of congestive heart failure appear to be preventable. These include failure to follow the drug therapy *properly,* dietary indiscretions, inadequate medical follow-up, excessive physical activity, and failure to recognize recurring symptoms. A summary of what the patient should know about his condition is given in Chart 31-5.

It must be emphasized that cough medicines, alkalizers, pain remedies, etc., contain fairly large amounts of sodium. The patient must be warned against using these products and advised to rinse his mouth with clear water when using toothpaste and mouthwashes. In some areas the drinking water has a high sodium content. To find out what this content is, the patient should contact his local health department. As an added precaution for older patients whose eyesight is dimming and whose fingers are less nimble as a result of arthritis, the printing on the drug bottle should be large and easily readable and the bottle should be equipped with an easy-open stopper.

Congestive heart failure can be controlled. The patient must never become lax in following his therapeutic program. Careful follow-up of patients with heart lesions, maintenance of correct weight, sodium restriction, prevention of infection, avoidance of noxious agents such as coffee and tobacco, and avoidance of unregulated or excessive

Chart 31-5
Patient Education in Congestive Heart Failure

A patient with heart disease should learn to regulate his activity according to his individual response.

Goal: To prevent progression of disease and the development of congestive heart failure

Expected Outcomes

I. Lives within the limits of the cardiac reserve
- A. Obtains adequate rest
  1. Has a regular daily rest period
  2. Shortens working hours if possible
  3. Avoids emotional upsets
- B. Accepts the fact that taking digitalis and restricting sodium intake may be a permanent way of life
  1. Takes digitalis daily, exactly as prescribed
     - a. Does not substitute another brand of digitalis for the one prescribed
     - b. Checks own pulse rate daily
     - c. Has a check-off system for assurance that medicine(s) has been taken
  2. Takes diuretic as prescribed
     - a. Weighs at the same time daily to detect any tendency toward fluid accumulation
     - b. Reports weight gain of more than 0.9 kg to 1.4 kg (2–3 pounds) in a few days
     - c. Knows the signs and symptoms of potassium depletion; if taking oral potassium, keeps a check-off system along with diuretic medication
  3. Takes vasodilator as prescribed
     - a. Learns to take own blood pressure at prescribed intervals
     - b. Knows signs and symptoms of orthostatic hypotension

- C. Restricts sodium as directed
  1. Consults the written diet plan and the list of permitted and restricted foods
  2. Examines labels to ascertain sodium content (antacids, laxatives, cough remedies, etc.)
  3. Avoids using salt
  4. Avoids excesses in eating and drinking

- D. Reviews activity program
  1. Increases walking and other activities gradually, provided that they do not cause fatigue and dyspnea
  2. In general, continues at whatever activity level can be maintained without the appearance of symptoms
  3. Avoids extremes of heat and cold, which increase the work of the heart. Air conditioning may be essential in a hot, humid environment.
  4. Keeps regular appointments with physician or clinic

II. Is alert for symptoms that may indicate recurring congestive heart failure
  1. Recalls the symptoms experienced when illness began. Reappearance of previous symptoms may indicate a recurrence.
  2. Reports immediately to the physician or clinic any of the following:
     - a. Gain in weight
     - b. Loss of appetite
     - c. Shortness of breath on activity
     - d. Swelling of ankles, feet, or abdomen
     - e. Persistent cough
     - f. Frequent urination at night

exercise all aid in preventing the onset of congestive heart failure. In patients with valvular heart disease, surgical correction of the defect at the appropriate time may spare the heart and prevent failure.

▶ **Evaluation**

Expected Outcomes

1. Improves oxygenation to brain and peripheral tissues
   a. Is alert and oriented to time, place, and person
   b. Exercises to a point short of fatigue
      (See Chart 31-5.)
2. Decreases total circulating volume
   a. Weighs self daily
   b. Loses weight gradually with health supervision
   c. Measures urinary output
   d. Is free of peripheral edema
   e. Adheres to medication regimen

3. Decreases susceptibility to thromboembolic events
   a. Avoids standing or sitting in one position for long periods of time
   b. Engages extremities in active range of motion if immobile or in bed for long periods of time
   c. Wears support stockings
   d. Avoids tight and restrictive clothing, especially socks and stockings
      (See also Chart 31-5.)

The Patient With Severe or Chronic Congestive Heart Failure

Severe or chronic heart failure that does not yield to conventional measures will require additional treatment, such as the use of vasodilators, to increase cardiac output by dilating peripheral blood vessels and reducing *impedance* (resistance) to left ventricular outflow.

Sodium nitroprusside has a vasodilator effect in both

the arterial and venous vascular beds by relaxing vascular smooth muscle. This results in venous pooling and a reduction in peripheral vascular resistance. It decreases left ventricular filling pressure and increases cardiac output. This aids renal blood flow and thus causes diuresis. Sodium nitroprusside, given by intravenous infusion, is potent and rapid-acting. The flow rate is monitored by an infusion pump or microdrip regulator and is titrated according to the patient's blood pressure response. Ideally, while on this drug, the patient's pulmonary artery pressures and cardiac output are monitored (see pp. 484–485).

- If hypotension occurs, the infusion is stopped, the patient's legs are elevated, and intravenous fluids are given for rapid volume expansion.

Long-acting nitrates (Isorbide dinitrate) act primarily on the veins and help to lower left ventricular end-diastolic pressure and relieve pulmonary congestion. Nitroglycerin ointment appears to have a similar beneficial action. These drugs are discussed on page 630.

Other drugs include phentolamine, which acts chiefly on arterioles to raise cardiac output; orally administered hydralazine, which produces systemic arteriolar dilatation; and prazosin (Minipress), which causes systemic vasodilatation of both the arteriolar and venous systems. These drugs are being used as impedance reduction therapy and to raise cardiac output in ambulatory patients with chronic heart failure.

▷ Acute Pulmonary Edema

Pathophysiology

Pulmonary edema is the abnormal accumulation of fluid in the lungs, either in the interstitial spaces or in the alveoli.

Pulmonary edema represents the ultimate stage of pulmonary congestion, in which fluid has leaked through the capillary walls and is permeating the airways, giving rise to dyspnea of dramatic severity. Pulmonary congestion, it will be recalled, occurs when the pulmonary vascular bed has received more blood from the right ventricle than the left can accommodate and remove. The slightest imbalance between inflow on the right side and outflow on the left side of the heart may have drastic consequences: for example, if with each heartbeat the right ventricle pumps out just one more drop of blood than the left, within the space of only 3 hours the pulmonary blood volume will have expanded 500 ml!

Noncardiac pulmonary edema has a wide variety of causes: toxic inhalants, drug overdose, neurogenic pulmonary edema. Clinical management is directed toward reducing pulmonary blood flow and pulmonary arterial pressure.

The most common cause of pulmonary edema is cardiac disease—atherosclerotic, hypertensive, valvular, myopathic. Most patients with pulmonary edema have chronic heart disease of a type that imposes a strain on the left ventricle, such as arterial hypertension or aortic valve disease. The development of pulmonary edema signifies that cardiac function has become grossly inadequate. There is an elevated left ventricular end-diastolic pressure and a rise

in pulmonary venous pressure. This produces an increase in hydrostatic pressure, which results in transudation of fluid. Impaired lymphatic drainage contributes to the accumulation of fluid in the lung tissues.

The pulmonary capillaries, engorged with an excess of blood that the left ventricle has been incapable of discharging, no longer are able to retain their contents. Fluid, first serous and later bloody, escapes into the adjacent alveoli through the communicating bronchioles and bronchi. It then mixes with air and, churned by respiratory agitation, is expelled from the mouth and nostrils, producing the ominous "death rattle." Because of the fluid buildup, the lungs become stiff and cannot expand, and air cannot enter. The result is severe hypoxia.

However, death from pulmonary edema is by no means inevitable. If appropriate measures are taken, and taken promptly, many attacks can be aborted and many patients can survive this complication to benefit from measures directed against its return. Fortunately, pulmonary edema usually does not develop precipitously but is preceded by the premonitory symptoms of pulmonary congestion. Moreover, even after it has become well established, it usually does not progress to a fatal termination with lightning rapidity; its course may occupy a period of many minutes, even hours, during which time treatment may prove to be effective.

Clinical Manifestations

The typical attack of pulmonary edema occurs at night after the patient has been lying down for a few hours. Recumbency increases the venous return to the heart and favors the resorption of edema fluid from the legs. The circulating blood becomes diluted, and its volume expands. The venous pressure mounts and the right atrium fills with increasing rapidity. There is a corresponding increase in the right ventricular output, which eventually surpasses the output from the left ventricle. The pulmonary vessels become engorged with blood and proceed to leak. Meanwhile, the patient has become increasingly restless, oppressed with anxiety, and unable to sleep.

There is a sudden onset of breathlessness and a fearful sense of suffocation. The patient's hands become cold and moist, the nail beds become cyanotic, and the complexion turns gray. In addition, the pulse is small and rapid and the neck veins are distended. There is incessant coughing, which produces increasing quantities of mucoid sputum. As the pulmonary edema progresses, the patient's anxiety develops into near panic and he becomes confused, then stuporous. He breathes noisily and moistly, nearly suffocated by the blood-tinged, frothy fluid that now is pouring into his bronchi and trachea. He literally is drowning in his own secretions. The situation is precarious and demands immediate action.

Management

The objectives of therapy are to improve ventilation and oxygenation, reduce pulmonary congestion, and increase cardiac output. A combination of the following measures help to implement these objectives.

Positioning.   Proper positioning can help reduce venous return to the heart.

- Place the patient upright, with his legs and feet down. This has the immediate effect of decreasing venous return, lowering the output of the right ventricle, and decongesting the lungs.
- Then place the patient in an upright position in bed (Fig. 31-1).

Oxygenation. Oxygen is administered in high concentration by face mask to relieve hypoxia and dyspnea. It must be given with high enough pressure to overcome the pressure barrier from the edema fluid and to provide oxygenation of the blood. If signs of hypoxemia persist, oxygen is delivered by intermittent or continuous positive pressure. If respiratory failure occurs despite optimal management, endotracheal intubation and mechanical ventilation are required. The use of positive end-expiratory pressure (PEEP) is effective in reducing venous return, lowering pulmonary capillary pressure, and improving oxygenation. Oxygenation is monitored by measurement of arterial blood gases.

Morphine. Morphine is given intravenously in small doses to reduce anxiety and dyspnea and to decrease peripheral resistance so that blood can be redistributed from the pulmonary circulation to the periphery. This action decreases pressure in the pulmonary capillaries and decreases transudation of fluid.

- Morphine is not given if pulmonary edema is caused by cerebral vascular accident or if chronic pulmonary disease or cardiogenic shock is present.
- Watch for excessive respiratory depression and have a morphine antagonist (naloxone hydrochloride [Narcan]) available.

Diuretics. Either furosemide or ethacrynic acid is given intravenously to produce a rapid diuretic effect. In addition, furosemide causes vasodilatation and peripheral venous pooling with a subsequent reduction in venous return that occurs even before the diuretic effect. Thus, dyspnea is rapidly relieved and pulmonary congestion is decreased. Since a large volume of urine will accumulate within minutes after administration of a potent diuretic, an indwelling catheter must be inserted.

- Watch for falling blood pressure, increasing heart rate, and decreasing urinary output; these indicate that the total circulation is not tolerating diuresis.
- Patients with prostatic hypertrophy must be watched for signs of urinary retention.

Aminophylline. When the patient is wheezing and bronchospasm appears to play a significant role, aminophylline may be given to relax bronchospasm.

- Give aminophylline *slowly* by vein, since arrhythmias, syncope, and sudden death may follow too rapid administration.

Rotating Tourniquets. The application of rotating tourniquets (or automatic inflating cuffs) on the extremities decreases venous return and right ventricular output, which aids in decongesting the lungs. The immediate effect is equivalent to removing about 1000 ml of circulating blood. Rotating tourniquets are an adjunct to pharmacologic therapy.

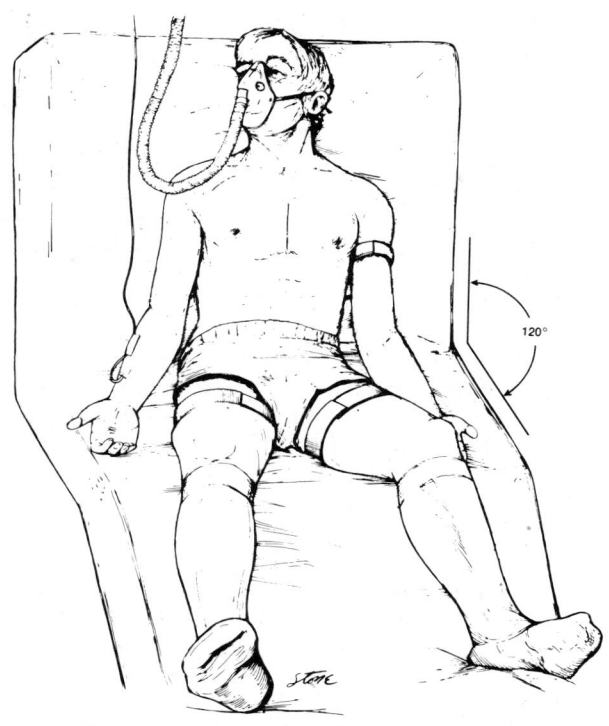

Figure 31-1. The patient with pulmonary edema is placed upright to reduce venous return to the heart. The administration of oxygen improves arterial hypoxemia and cardiac function. The application of rotating tourniquets brings about a rapid decrease in venous return and may result in dramatic clinical improvement. (Courtesy, Am Fam Physician.)

- Tell the patient the purpose of the treatment and that the skin of the extremities may become discolored.
- Take an initial blood pressure reading to serve as a baseline for future comparisons.
- Mark the peripheral pulses, if time permits.
- If tourniquets are used (instead of cuffs), they are positioned over a small towel as high as possible on three extremities. The arterial pulse should not be occluded. One extremity should be free of a tourniquet during each time interval. (A tourniquet is not placed on an extremity in which an IV line is inserted.)
- Release one tourniquet every 15 minutes; then apply a tourniquet to the previously free extremity. The venous outflow in any one extremity may be occluded for 45 minutes and unoccluded for 15 minutes. However, tourniquets may have to be rotated at 5-minute intervals on elderly patients or those with poor circulation in order to prevent gangrene and other complications.
- Rotate the tourniquets in a consistent clockwise pattern.
- Monitor the blood pressure every few minutes, since the use of tourniquets may precipitate hypotension in some patients.
- When the patient's symptoms have been relieved, discontinue the use of the tourniquets by removing them one at a time at 15-minute intervals. Simultaneous removal of all tourniquets could precipitate a recurrence of pulmonary edema.

- Examine each extremity after the tourniquet is removed for color, warmth, and the presence of a palpable pulse.

When an automatic rotating tourniquet machine is used, the cuffs are inflated and deflated automatically in sequence. The nurse follows the protocol of the machine's manufacturer in applying the cuffs, adjusting the pressure, checking for leaks in the system, etc. Clinical assessment of the patient is the same as for manual rotating tourniquets (see above).

Phlebotomy. If the patient is refractory to management, it is sometimes helpful to reduce the venous return to the heart by withdrawing 250 ml to 500 ml of blood from a peripheral vein (a phlebotomy or venesection). Phlebotomy is especially valuable when pulmonary edema has followed overtransfusion or administration of excessive intravenous fluid.

The resulting decrease in venous return is accompanied by a corresponding decline in the right ventricular output. Accordingly, the pulmonary artery pressure drops, the pulmonary vessels become less congested, and the lung capillaries, no longer congested, reabsorb the fluid that has escaped. The edema clears; the immediate danger has passed.

Digitalis. In order to improve the contractile force of the heart and increase the output of the left ventricle, the patient may be given a rapid-acting digitalis preparation. The improved cardiac contractility will increase cardiac output, enhance diuresis, and reduce diastolic pressure in the ventricles. Thus, pulmonary capillary pressure and the transudation of fluid into the alveoli will be reduced.

- Digitalis must be given with extreme caution to patients with acute myocardial infarction, since these patients are sensitive to digitalis and may develop toxic arrhythmias.
- The serum potassium level is measured at intervals because diuresis may have produced hypokalemia. If this occurs, a potassium supplement is given to prevent digitalis toxicity.
- If the patient has been on digitalis, the drug is usually withheld until the possibility of digitalis intoxication is ruled out.

Vasodilator Therapy. Vasodilator drugs have been used to reduce impedance (resistance) to left ventricular ejection of blood. The drug action allows more complete ventricular emptying and increases venous capacity, so that left ventricular filling pressure is reduced and a dramatic decrease in pulmonary congestion may be achieved rapidly. Sodium nitroprusside may be given intravenously by means of carefully monitored infusions. The dosage is titrated to keep the arterial systolic pressure at the prescribed level, and the patient is monitored by measuring pulmonary artery pressures (Swan–Ganz, p. 484) and cardiac output.

Psychological Support. Extreme fear and anxiety are cardinal features of pulmonary edema. These emotions, which are self-perpetuating, make the condition more severe. Reassuring the patient and providing skillful anticipatory nursing are integral parts of the therapy.

Prevention

Like most medical and surgical complications, pulmonary edema is easier to prevent than to treat. To be recognized in its early stages, when the presenting symptoms and signs are solely those of pulmonary congestion, the nurse should auscultate the lung fields daily on susceptible patients. Observation of a dry, hacking cough and the presence of a third heart sound (S_3) is often the earliest indication of pulmonary congestion. The S_3 is best heard at the apex with the patient lying in the left lateral decubitus position.

In an early stage the situation may be corrected by relatively simple measures. These include (1) placing the patient in an upright position, (2) eliminating overexertion and emotional stress to reduce the left ventricular load, and (3) administering morphine to reduce anxiety and dyspnea.

The long-range approach to the prevention of pulmonary edema must be directed at its precursor, namely, pulmonary congestion. See measures to prevent congestive heart failure (p. 640) and the various facets of patient teaching (p. 641).

In addition to these measures, it may be wise for the patient to sleep with the head of his bed elevated on 25-cm (10-inch) blocks. It is especially important to take extreme precautions when giving infusions and transfusions to cardiac patients and elderly persons.

- Intravenous fluids are given at a slower rate, with the patient positioned upright in bed and kept under close nursing surveillance, in order to prevent circulatory overloading, which could precipitate acute pulmonary edema.

Surgical treatment may be necessary to eliminate or to minimize valvular defects that limit the flow of blood into or out of the left ventricle, since such defects impair the cardiac output and predispose the patient to the development of pulmonary congestion and edema.

▷ Dysrhythmias

A dysrhythmia is a clinical disorder of the heartbeat that may include a disturbance of rate, rhythm, or both. Dysrhythmias are derangements of the heart's conduction system and not of heart structure. Dysrhythmias are identified by site of origin and the mechanism involved. For example, a ventricular premature contraction originates at a ventricular site, and the mechanism of disturbance is prematurity of contraction. Dysrhythmias are discussed in detail in Chapter 28.

Pacemaker Therapy

A *pacemaker* is an electronic device that provides repetitive electrical stimuli to the heart muscle for the control of heart rate. It initiates and maintains the heart rate when the natural pacemakers of the heart are unable to do so. Pacemakers are generally used when a patient has an arrhythmia or the forerunner of an arrhythmia that causes failure of cardiac output (such as can be seen in bradycardias, particularly complete heart block, tachyarrhythmias, and arrhythmias following myocardial infarction). Temporary pacing is also done to control the heart rate during open heart surgery or thoracotomy.

Pacemaker Design

Pacemakers consist of two component parts: (1) the electronic pulse generator, which contains the circuitry and batteries that generate the electrical signal; and (2) the pacemaker electrodes (also called leads or wires), which transmit the pacemaker impulses to the heart. The stimuli from the pacemaker travel through a flexible catheter electrode that is threaded through a vein into the right ventricle or introduced by direct penetration of the chest wall. The pulse generator is usually implanted in a subcutaneous pocket in the pectoral or axillary region. Sometimes an abdominal site is selected.

Pacemaker generators are insulated to protect against body moisture and warmth. The pulse generator (or pacemaker) contains its own supply of power, which is provided by battery cells. The main power sources in current use are mercury–zinc batteries (lasting 3 to 4 years), lithium cell units (lasting up to 10 years), and a nuclear-powered pacemaker (^{238}plutonium source) that last 20 years to a lifetime. There are also pacemakers that can be recharged externally. Since pacemakers rely on batteries, battery exhaustion (with the exception of nuclear power and rechargeable batteries) is inevitable. Therefore, the generator that contains the batteries must be replaced periodically.

Types of Pacemakers

The most commonly used pacemaker is the *demand* (synchronous; noncompetitive) pacemaker, which is set for a specific rate and stimulates the heart when normal ventricular depolarization does not occur. It functions only when the natural heart rate goes below a certain level. The *fixed* rate pacemaker (asynchronous; competitive) stimulates the ventricle at a preset constant rate that is independent of the patient's rhythm. It is used infrequently, usually in patients with complete and unvarying heart block.

Temporary Pacemaker Systems. Temporary pacing is usually an emergency procedure and permits the observation of the effects of pacing on heart function so that the optimum pacing rate for the patient can be selected before a permanent pacemaker is implanted. It is used in patients who have suffered myocardial infarction with conduction block, in patients with cardiac arrest with bradycardia and asystole, or in selected postoperative cardiac surgery patients. Temporary pacing may be done for hours, days, or weeks and is continued until the patient improves or a permanent pacemaker is implanted.

Temporary pacing may be carried out either by an endocardial (transvenous) approach or by the transthoracic approach to the myocardium. The transvenous electrode is passed under fluoroscopic guidance through any peripheral vein (antecubital, brachial, jugular, subclavian, femoral) and the catheter tip is positioned in the apex of the right ventricle. The most common complications occurring during pacemaker insertion are ventricular arrhythmia and, much less frequently, cardiac perforation. A defibrillator should be immediately available.

Nursing Management. The pacemaker generator and control unit can be attached around the patient's waist or to his right arm, with plenty of slack available so that the motion of the arm will not dislodge the catheter. No metal parts of the output terminal or pacemaker wires should be exposed. All such bare metal should be scrupulously covered with nonconductive tape in order to prevent accidental ventricular fibrillation from stray currents, which might reach the heart if exposed metal parts were to come in contact with a metal conductor, such as a bedrail. Aberrant current sources (from malfunctioning equipment) can travel over the surface of a damp skin and can also cause ventricular fibrillation. *The patient must be placed in an electrically safe environment.* All monitoring and other electrical equipment should be grounded with three-pronged plugs inserted into a proper outlet.

It is important that the nurse be familiar with the complications of the procedure (p. 646) and with the operating instructions for the pacemaker equipment being used. The vein through which the pacing wire has been inserted is monitored for evidence of phlebitis. In addition, it may be necessary to change the amplitude of the stimulation impulse and adjust the rate of stimulation as an emergency intervention.

Permanent Pacing. For permanent pacing, the endocardial lead is passed transvenously into the right ventricle, and the pulse generator is implanted within the body underneath the skin below the right or left pectoral region or below the clavicle (Fig. 31-2). This is termed an endocardial or transvenous implant. This procedure is usually done under local anesthesia. Another method of permanent pacing is the implantation of the pulse generator in the abdominal wall. The electrode is passed transthoracically to the myocardium, where it is sutured in place. For this method, termed an epicardial or myocardial implant, a thoracotomy is required to provide access to the heart. This procedure is frequently part of an open heart operation. Another electrode is screwed into the myocardium through a small incision in the subxiphoid area with minimal injury to heart muscle. This requires no sutures.

Nursing Management. Following the procedure, the patient is monitored by electrocardiogram. After implantation, the pacemaker rate tends to vary by 2 to 3 pulses and then stabilizes. An intravenous line is kept open to provide a readily accessible vein for drug administration in the event of an arrhythmia and for fluids to combat dehydration. Data about the model, date and time of insertion, location of the pulse generator, stimulation threshold, and pacer rate should be noted on the patient's record and on a card at the head of the bed.

The incision site under the pressure dressing where the pulse generator is implanted is watched for evidences of bleeding, hematoma formation, and infection.

All electrical equipment used in the vicinity of the patient is grounded with three-pronged plugs inserted into a proper outlet. Improperly grounded equipment can generate leakage currents capable of producing ventricular fibrillation. A biomedical engineer, electrician, or other qualified person should make certain that the patient is in an electrically safe environment.

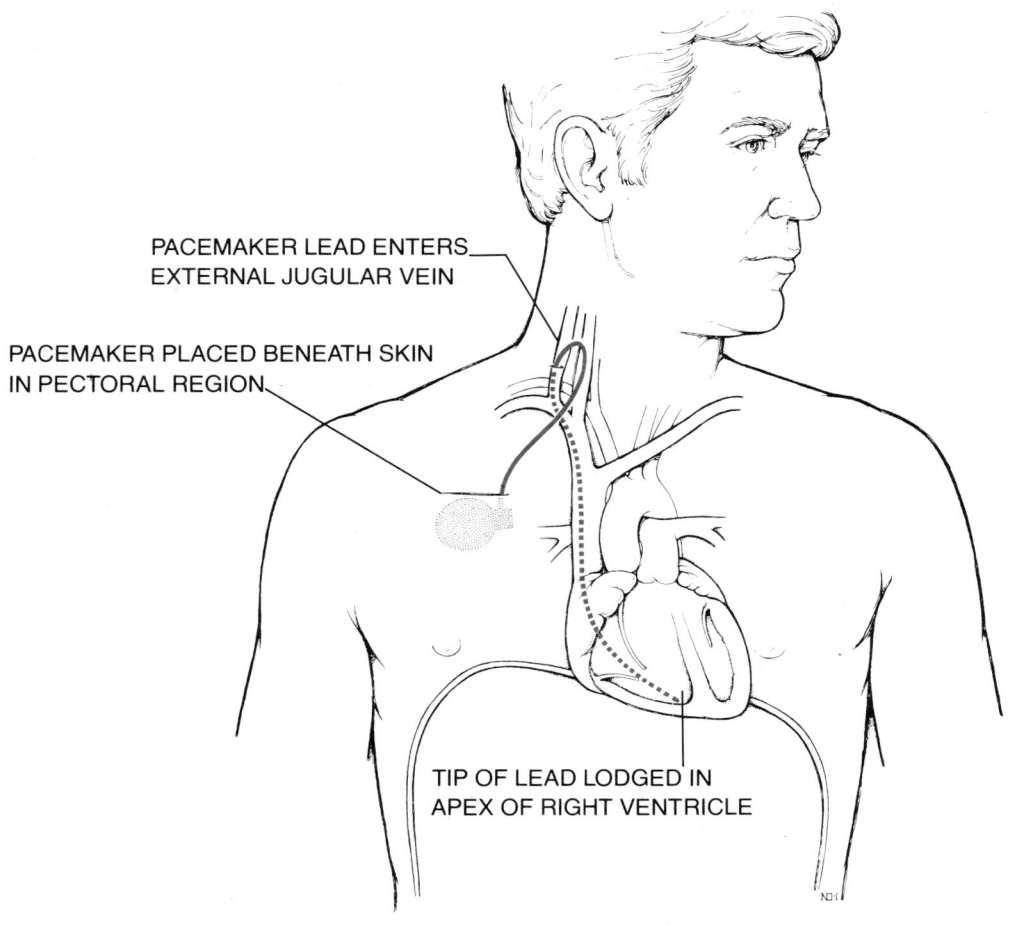

Figure 31-2. Pacemaker therapy.

After permanent pacemaker implantation, the patient initially will be aware of the pulse generator under his skin and will want to touch it frequently. Reassurance should be given that this is no cause for concern. Patients usually feel ambivalent about their pacemakers: they understand their benefits, but feelings of dependence, anxiety over altered life-style, and awareness of changing body image may be troubling. To counter the uneasy feelings it is best to take a positive approach in talking with the patient. The patient will require support and should be informed that the pacemaker will improve his cardiac output and thus give him more energy. (See Chart 31-6 for patient education.)

Complications

Complications associated with implanted pacemakers relate to (1) their presence within the body and (2) improper functioning. The following complications may arise from the presence of the pacemaker:

1. Local infection (sepsis or hematoma formation) may occur at the site of venous cutdown or subcutaneous pacemaker placement.
2. Arrhythmias—ventricular ectopic activity may follow irritation of the ventricular wall by the electrode. (Pacemakers can produce baffling arrhythmias.)
3. Perforation of the myocardium or right ventricle by the catheter may occur.
4. High ventricular threshold—may cause abrupt loss of pacing.

Pacemaker malfunction can arise from failure in one or more components of the pacing system. The majority of pulse generator failures are from depletion of the power supply (*i.e.,* battery failure). The patient should be informed that the battery cells are sealed in the pulse generator. When it is time for a battery change, a new incision is made over the old incision. The old pulse generator is removed, and the new unit is connected to the existing leads and reimplanted in the already existing pocket. This is usually done under local anesthesia. Other complications include fracture (breakage) or dislocation of the electrodes and electronic failure.

Pacemaker Surveillance

Pacemaker clinics have been established to monitor patients and to test pulse generators for warnings of impending pacemaker system failure. Testing of pacemaker pulse amplitude and duration and analysis of pulse contour require amplification equipment. With special equipment, lead fracture

Chart 31-6
Patient Education: The Patient With a Pacemaker

Expected Outcomes

1. Reports to physician/pacemaker clinic periodically as prescribed, so that the rate of the pacemaker and its function can be checked. This is especially important during the first month after implantation.
   a. Adheres to weekly monitoring schedule during the first month after implantation
   b. Checks pulse daily. Reports *immediately* any sudden slowing or increasing of the pulse rate. This may indicate pacemaker malfunction.
   c. Resumes weekly monitoring when battery depletion is anticipated (The time for reimplantation depends on the type in use.)

2. Wears loose-fitting clothing around the area of the pacemaker
   a. Explains the reason for the slight bulge over the pacemaker implant

   b. Notifies physician if the area becomes reddened or painful

3. Studies the manufacturer's instructions and becomes familiar with pacemaker

4. States that physical activity does not usually have to be curtailed, with the exception of heavy contact sports

5. Carries an identification card/bracelet indicating physician's name, type and model number of pacemaker, manufacturer's name, pacemaker rate, and hospital where pacemaker was inserted

6. Avoids being close to microwave ovens, arc welders and large electrical generators, and electric cautery and diathermy equipment (although at this time electrical interference is not a major problem)

7. Shows identification card and requests scanning by a hand scanner when going through weapons detector at airport

8. Verbalizes that hospitalization is necessary periodically for battery changes/pacemaker unit replacement

and insulation disruption can be detected. A 12-lead ECG is done during each patient visit to the clinic.

Another method of follow-up is evaluation by transtelephone monitoring of the transmission of the generator's pulse rate. By means of special equipment the sound tone of the patient's pacemaker is transmitted over the telephone to a receiving system at a pacemaker clinic. The sounds are converted into an electronic signal and permanently recorded on an ECG strip. The pacemaker rate and other data concerning pacemaker function are obtained and evaluated by a cardiologist or a cardiovascular surgeon. This simplifies the diagnosis for a failing generator, provides reassurance, and improves the management of the person who is physically remote from pacemaker testing facilities.

Pacemaker Developments
External and Long-Range Recharging. There is now available an electronic pacemaker whose battery can be recharged externally. Like other pacemakers, the device is implanted under the skin in the chest wall or in the abdomen. Its lead wires (one enclosed inside the other) are threaded through a vein so that one end is in the heart and the other attached to a battery. To recharge the battery the patient dons a lightweight canvas shoulder harness and attaches the charger unit to it over the location of his implanted battery. The charger is linked to a small console that is plugged into an ordinary electric socket. When the unit is turned on, an electromagnetic field is generated that rejuvenates the power cell in the battery through the skin. Recharging the battery takes only about 90 minutes at home each week.

Nuclear-Powered Pacemakers. Nuclear-powered pacemakers are now being implanted in patients in selected centers in this country. The nuclear heart pacer is designed to operate for at least 15 to 20 years. The design of the pacemaker's nuclear power source is based on the principle of thermoelectricity—the direct conversion of heat to electrical energy. When certain metals are joined together, they form a thermocouple that, when heated at one end, will generate an electrical current. The pacemaker's thermocouple is composed of a copper and nickel alloy and a nickel and chromium alloy drawn into wire strands and woven into a glass tape. The heat developed by the decay of the radioisotope nuclear fuel (plutonium-238) is used to heat the wires at one end. The electrical current, as in conventional pacemakers, is fed into a pulse generator that supplies the pacing pulses to the heart via conventional wire electrodes. The radiation exposure to the patient from the nuclear fuel is considered to be within acceptable levels.

Atrioventricular Pacing. Pacemaker technology has fostered the growth of safe and effective pacemaker therapy for many complex cardiologic problems that include not only ventricular pacemakers but atrial pacemakers as well. Both of these types of pacemakers can in specific instances function in the same patient (*i.e.,* atrioventricular sequential pacing).

▷ Cardiac Arrest

Cardiac arrest is defined as the sudden, unexpected cessation of the heartbeat and effective circulation. All heart action may stop, or asynchronized muscular twitchings (ventricular fibrillation) may occur.

There is an immediate loss of consciousness and an

absence of pulses and audible heart sounds. Dilation of the pupils of the eyes begins within 45 seconds. Convulsions may or may not be present.

- There is an interval of approximately 4 minutes between the cessation of circulation and the appearance of irreversible brain damage. This varies with the age of the patient. During this period, the diagnosis of arrest must be made and the circulation must be restored.
- *The most reliable sign of arrest is the absence of a carotid pulsation.* Valuable time should not be wasted taking the blood pressure or listening for the heartbeat.

Details of the resuscitation procedure may be found on pages 599–600.

▷ **Infectious Diseases of the Heart**

Pathophysiology

The endocardium is the endothelial layer of tissue that lines the heart's cavities and covers the flaps of its valves. Of the diseases that affect it, the majority represent various types and stages of inflammation (*i.e., endocarditis* or its aftermath). They include (1) rheumatic endocarditis, one of the many complications of acute rheumatic fever; (2) infective endocarditis, produced by direct bacterial invasion of the endocardium, particularly that portion covering the valve leaflets; and (3) chronic valvular heart disease, based on structural deformities of the heart valves, whether of congenital origin or acquired as a result of either rheumatic or bacterial endocarditis in the past.

When an area of endocardium becomes inflamed, a fibrin clot, called a vegetation, may form. In time this clot becomes converted into a mass of scar tissue. The scarred endocardium becomes thickened, stiffened, contracted, and deformed. A fringe of vegetations ranging along the free margins of the valve flaps, marking the site of earlier erosions, represents the basic lesion of endocarditis and is the forerunner of chronic valvular heart disease.

Two functional disorders of the valves may result from these pathologic changes: stenosis or regurgitation. In stenosis the valvular opening becomes narrowed and does not permit the passage of normal amounts of blood. Regurgitation results from the valves shriveling and producing a wider opening. The valve leaflets can no longer perform their function of closing to prevent a backflow of blood.

Rheumatic Endocarditis

Pathophysiology. Rheumatic fever is a sequel to a Group A streptococcal infection. It is considered a preventable disease. The most prominent symptom of rheumatic fever is polyarthritis, but the most serious damage occurs in the heart, where every structural component is likely to be the site of an inflammatory reaction. The heart damage and the joint lesions are not infectious in origin, in the sense that these tissues are not invaded and directly damaged by destructive organisms; rather, they represent a sensitivity phenomenon occurring in response to the *hemolytic streptococcus.* Blood leukocytes accumulate in the affected tissues and form nodules, which eventually are replaced by scars. The myocardium is certain to be involved in this inflammatory process; that is, *rheumatic myocarditis* develops, which temporarily weakens the contractile power of the heart. The pericardium likewise is affected; that is, *rheumatic pericarditis* also occurs during the acute illness. These myocardial and pericardial complications usually are without serious sequelae; on the other hand, the effects of *rheumatic endocarditis* are permanent and often crippling.

Clinical Manifestations. Rheumatic endocarditis anatomically manifests itself first by tiny translucent vegetations, which resemble beads about the size of the head of a pin, arranged in a row along the free margins of the valve flaps. These tiny beads look harmless enough and may disappear without injuring the valve flaps, but more often they have serious effects. They are the starting point of a process that gradually thickens the flaps, rendering them just a little shorter, just a little thicker than normal, just a little shriveled along their edges—enough to prevent them from closing the orifice of the valve perfectly. The result is leakage, a condition called valvular regurgitation. The most common type of valvular regurgitation is mitral regurgitation.

In other patients the inflamed margins of the valve flaps become adherent, resulting in a narrowed, or "stenotic," valvular orifice. A small percentage of patients with rheumatic fever become critically ill with intractable heart failure, serious arrhythmias, and rheumatic pneumonia. These patients should be treated in an intensive care unit.

Most patients recover with gratifying speed and their recovery ostensibly is complete. However, although free of symptoms, the patient is left with certain permanent residuals that often gradually lead to progressive valvular deformities. The extent of cardiac damage, or even its existence, may not have been apparent on clinical examinations during the acute phase of the disease. Eventually, however, the heart murmurs that are characteristic of valvular stenosis, regurgitation, or both, become audible on auscultation and, in some patients, even detectable as "thrills" on palpation. The myocardium usually can compensate for these valvular defects very well for a time, despite its increased burden. As long as it can do so, the patient remains in apparent good health. However, sooner or later it fails to compensate—and decompensation, when it occurs, is signaled by the manifestations of congestive heart failure, as described on page 636.

Management. The objectives of management are to observe for and control congestive heart failure and pericarditis (which may be life-threatening) and to give symptomatic relief to other manifestations.

The patient with rheumatic endocarditis should be confined to bed as long as he is febrile and has signs of active carditis. He should remain quiet thereafter until the erythrocyte sedimentation rate (a fair though nonspecific index of rheumatic activity) returns to normal. Salicylates are prescribed in large doses to suppress rheumatic activity by controlling toxic manifestations, lessening constitutional symptoms, and improving the well-being of the patient. Corticosteroid therapy is given to the very ill person with carditis. However, treatment has no effect on valvular deformities that may occur.

The patient with rheumatic endocarditis, whose valve function is faulty but whose disease is quiescent, does not require therapy as long as the heart pumps effectively. Nevertheless, the danger exists of recurrent attacks of acute rheumatic fever, of bacterial endocarditis, or embolism from vegetations or mural thrombi in the heart, and of eventual cardiac failure. (The relation between valvular disease and congestive heart failure is discussed on p. 654 and the treatment of heart failure on p. 637.)

Prevention. The prevention of rheumatic fever is accomplished by (1) the prevention of streptococcal infections, especially in susceptible individuals and (2) early and adequate treatment of streptococcal infections in all individuals.

Persons who present a well-documented history of rheumatic fever (or chorea) or who show evidence of rheumatic heart disease should be given continuous prophylaxis with penicillin (or other suitable antibiotic) indefinitely. The patient must recognize and should accept the fact that he is a "rheumatic fever patient," and as such can lead a normal life only if he is willing to submit to certain limitations and inconveniences. In relation to this facet of patient education, the nurse is in a position to play a very important role.

A first-line approach in preventing initial attacks of rheumatic fever is to recognize individuals with streptococcal infections, treat them adequately, and control epidemics in the community. Every nurse should be familiar with the symptoms and signs of streptococcal pharyngitis (see Chart 31-7). *A throat culture is the only method by which diagnosis can be determined.*

Infective Endocarditis

Infective endocarditis (bacterial endocarditis) is an infection of the valves and endothelial surface of the heart caused by direct invasion of bacteria or other organisms, leading to deformity of the valve leaflets. It may be acute, subacute, or chronic. Acute endocarditis usually occurs on normal valves. Causative microorganisms include bacteria (streptococci, enterococci, pneumococci, staphylococci), fungi, and rickettsiae. The subacute form is usually caused by *Streptococcus viridans.*

Etiology. Infective subacute endocarditis usually develops in patients who have a history of valvular heart disease. At great risk are patients with rheumatic heart disease or mitral valve prolapse and individuals who have had prosthetic-valve surgery.

Hospital-acquired endocarditis occurs most often in patients with debilitating disease, those with indwelling catheters, and those on prolonged intravenous or antibiotic therapy. Patients on immunosuppressive drugs or steroids may develop fungal endocarditis. Therefore, infective endocarditis often accompanies medical and surgical therapy and is more common in older persons, probably due to decreased immunologic responses to infection, metabolic alterations arising from changes in the aging body, and increased instrumentation, especially in genitourinary disease. There is a high incidence of staphylococcal endocarditis among drug addicts, the disease occurring for the most part on normal valves.

Chart 31-7
Prevention of Rheumatic Heart Disease

Rheumatic fever is a preventable disease. By eradication of rheumatic fever, the great cardiac crippler—*rheumatic heart disease*—would be virtually eliminated. Through the use of penicillin therapy in patients with streptococcal infections, almost all primary attacks of rheumatic fever could be prevented. The symptoms and signs of streptococcal pharyngitis are:

Fever (38.9° C to 40° C, or 101° F to 104° F)
Chilliness
Sore throat (sudden in onset)
Diffuse redness of throat with exudate on oropharynx (may not appear until after the first day)
Enlarged and tender lymph nodes
Abdominal pain (more common in children)
Acute sinusitis and acute otitis media (may be due to streptococcus)

Clinical Manifestations. The onset of infective endocarditis usually is insidious. The signs and symptoms develop from destruction of heart valves, from embolization of fragments of vegetations, and from toxicity of the infection.

The general manifestations include vague complaints of malaise, anorexia, weight loss, cough, and back and joint pain, which may be mistaken for influenza. Fever is intermittent and may be absent in patients who are receiving antibiotics or corticosteroids or in those who are elderly or have congestive heart failure or uremia. Skin and nail manifestations are observed in some patients. Splinter hemorrhages (linear and hemorrhagic streaks) may be noted under the fingernails and toenails, and petechiae may appear in the conjunctiva and mucous membranes. Hemorrhages with pale centers (Roth's spots) may be seen in the fundi of the eyes from emboli in the nerve fiber layer of the eye. Osler's nodes (painful, raised, tender, red lesions on the pads of fingers and toes) may occur and are thought to be secondary to acute vasculitis from an immunologic reaction. Janeway's lesions are hemorrhagic macular areas found on the palms or soles and are now thought to be a hypersensitivity reaction or deposit of immune complex.

The cardiac manifestations include heart murmurs, which may be absent initially. Changing murmurs may be encountered in the acute form and indicate valvular damage owing to vegetations or to perforation of the valve or of the chordae tendinae. Heart enlargement or evidences of congestive heart failure are also seen.

The central nervous system manifestations include headache, transient cerebral ischemia, focal neurologic lesions, and strokes, which may be caused by emboli involving the cerebral arteries.

Embolization may be a presenting symptom occurring at any time and involving other organ systems. The embolic phenomena may be manifested in the lung (recurrent pneumonia; pulmonary abscesses), kidney (hematuria; renal failure), spleen (left upper quadrant pain), heart (myocardial infarction), brain (stroke), or peripheral vessels.

Management. The objective of treatment is total eradication of the invading organism by adequate doses of an appropriate antimicrobial. The causative organism can be isolated through serial blood cultures. It is treated with a bactericidal (capable of destroying bacteria) agent or other appropriate drug based on proven sensitivity to the causative agent. The antibiotic is usually given parenterally in a continuous intravenous infusion for a period of 4 to 6 weeks. Thus, it is important to note on the nursing care plan the date on which the intravenous needle or cannula was inserted. Bactericidal serum levels of the selected antibiotic are monitored by titering it against the causative organism. If the serum does not demonstrate bactericidal activity, increased dosages of the antibiotic are given or a different antibiotic is tried. There are numerous antimicrobial regimens currently in use, but penicillin is usually the drug of choice.

Blood cultures are taken periodically to monitor the course of therapy. Treatment with amphotericin B and surgery with valve replacement is usually required for the patient with fungal endocarditis.

Evaluation of Therapy. The patient's temperature is monitored at regular intervals, since the course of fever is one determinant of the effectiveness of treatment. However, febrile reactions may also occur as a result of drug therapy. After adequate antimicrobial therapy is initiated, bacteria usually disappear. The patient should demonstrate an improved sense of well-being, better appetite, and decreased lethargy. During this time, the patient requires a great deal of psychosocial support, especially since he feels well but finds himself confined to the hospital with restrictive IV therapy.

Complications. Even though the patient may respond to the antimicrobial therapy, endocarditis can be very destructive to the heart and other organs. Congestive heart failure and cerebral vascular catastrophes may occur before, during, or after therapy. Valve stenosis or regurgitation, myocardial erosion, and mycotic aneurysms are some potential heart complications. A myriad of other organ complications can result from septic or nonseptic emboli, immunologic responses, or hemodynamic deterioration.

Surgery. The advent of surgical valve replacement has favorably changed the prognosis of patients with severely damaged heart valves. Usually, valve excision and replacement are required for (1) patients who develop congestive heart failure as a result of aortic or mitral valve involvement in spite of adequate medical treatment; (2) patients who have more than one serious systemic embolic episode; and (3) persons with uncontrolled infection, recurrent infection, or fungal endocarditis. A large number of patients who have prosthetic valve endocarditis (infected prostheses) will require valve replacement.

Prevention. Infective endocarditis occurs most often in persons with structural abnormalities of the heart and great vessels, especially valvular heart disease. Any procedure that is associated with transient bacteremia may cause bacteria to lodge on damaged or abnormal valves. *Persons at risk are patients with structural abnormalities of the heart and great vessels, those with prosthetic heart valves, or patients with most types of congenital heart disease, rheumatic or other acquired valvular heart disease, and idiopathic hypertrophic or subaortic stenosis.*

Antibiotic prophylaxis (usually penicillin, penicillin plus streptomycin, or penicillin plus gentamicin) is recommended for persons at risk, for the following procedures and circumstances:*

1. Dental procedures causing gingival bleeding
2. Surgery or instrumentation of the respiratory tract (tonsillectomy/adenoidectomy, bronchoscopy) or procedures involving disruption of respiratory mucosa; surgery or instrumentation of the genitourinary tract (especially urethral procedures, including catheterization) or prostatic manipulation; or surgery or instrumentation of the gastrointestinal tract and gallbladder
3. Cardiac surgery in which extracorporeal circulation is utilized, especially replacement of prosthetic valves. These recommendations apply to the recovery period as well.
4. Surgical procedures on infected or contaminated tissues
5. Obstetrical infections (postpartum infection; septic abortion)

Myocarditis

Acute *myocarditis* is an inflammatory process involving the myocardium. The heart is a muscle, hence its efficiency depends on the health of the individual muscle fibers. When the muscle fibers are healthy, the heart can function well in spite of severe valvular injuries; when the muscle fibers are poor, life is in jeopardy.

Pathophysiology. Myocarditis usually results from an infectious process, particularly of viral, bacterial, mycotic, parasitic, protozoal, or spirochetal origin, or it may be produced by hypersensitivity states such as rheumatic fever. Therefore, myocarditis may be seen in patients with acute systemic infections, those receiving immunosuppressive therapy, or those with infective endocarditis.

Myocarditis can cause heart dilatation, mural thrombi, infiltration of circulating blood cells around the coronary vessels and between the muscle fibers, and degeneration of the muscle fibers themselves.

Clinical Manifestations. The symptoms of acute myocarditis depend on the type of infection, the degree of myocardial damage, and the capacity of the myocardium to recover. Symptoms may be mild or absent. The patient may complain of fatigue and dyspnea, palpitations, and occasional precordial discomfort. Clinical examination may reveal cardiac enlargement, faint heart sounds, gallop rhythm, and a systolic murmur. A pericardial friction rub may be heard if the patient has associated pericarditis. Pulsus alternans (a pulse in which there is a regular alternation of weak and strong beats) may be present. Fever and tachy-

---

* From Statement Prepared by the Committee on Prevention of Rheumatic Fever and Bacterial Endocarditis of the American Heart Association: Circulation, 56:139A–143A, July 1977.

cardia are frequently seen and evidences of congestive heart failure usually develop.

Management. The patient is given specific treatment for the underlying cause, if it is known (*e.g.,* penicillin for hemolytic streptococci). He is placed on bed rest to decrease cardiac work, that is, to reduce the heart rate, stroke volume, blood pressure, and heart contractility. Bed rest also helps to decrease residual myocardial damage and the complications of myocarditis. The treatment is essentially the same as that used for congestive heart failure (p. 637). The pulse, heart sounds, and temperature are evaluated to determine whether the disease is subsiding and to assess for the occurrence of congestive heart failure. If an arrhythmia occurs, the patient should be placed in a unit with continuous cardiac monitoring so that personnel and equipment are readily available if a life-threatening arrhythmia occurs.

When there is evidence of congestive heart failure, digitalis is given to slow the heart rate and augment myocardial contractility.

- Patients with myocarditis are sensitive to digitalis. There must be continuing nursing surveillance to assess the patient for digitalis toxicity (arrhythmia, anorexia, nausea, vomiting, bradycardia, headache, malaise).

Elastic stockings and passive and active exercises should be used since embolization from venous thrombosis and mural thrombi can occur.

Patient Education. The prevention of infectious diseases by means of appropriate immunizations and early treatment appears to be important in decreasing the incidence of myocarditis. Following a bout of myocarditis, there is usually some residual heart enlargement. Physical activity is increased slowly, and the patient is instructed to report any symptoms that occur with increasing activity, such as a rapidly beating heart, etc. Competitive sports and alcohol must be avoided.

▷ Cardiomyopathies

Myopathy refers to any disease of muscle. The cardiomyopathies are a group of diseases that affect the structure and function of the myocardium. The term *primary cardiomyopathies* is used if the condition is of unknown etiology. The term *secondary cardiomyopathies* implies that the myocardial involvement results from a known disease that is usually also manifested outside the heart. Arteriosclerotic disease of the coronary arteries, viral infections, alcoholism, neuromuscular disease, connective tissue disease, degenerative changes in the myocardium, metabolic disturbances, malnutrition, vasculitis, pregnancy, toxic agents, drugs, and other causes may all produce heart muscle disease. The manner in which they affect the heart muscle is not known. Explorations based on cellular and enzyme functions, infectious agents, and immunologic causes are being sought.

Clinical Manifestations. Most patients with myocardial disease have signs and symptoms of heart failure: dyspnea on effort, nocturnal dyspnea, cough, expectoration, and weakness. Physical findings reveal manifestations of sys-

temic venous congestion: jugular vein engorgement, pitting edema, hepatic engorgement, tachycardia. Gallop rhythm is one of the identifying marks of myocardial disease. (Gallop rhythm is a tripling or quadrupling of heart sounds, resembling the galloping of a horse.) It may be heard best with the bell of the stethoscope when the patient is in the left lateral decubitus position. The ECG may be normal in patients with heart muscle disease.

Management. Rest (physical and emotional) is an important aspect of management. Rest decreases the cardiac output, arterial blood pressure, and heart size. Sodium restriction, digitalis, diuretics, and vasodilators are other treatment modalities. (See pp. 637–641 for the patient with congestive heart failure.)

▷ Pericarditis

Pericarditis refers to an inflammation of the pericardium, the membranous sac enveloping the heart. It may be a primary illness or may develop in the course of a variety of medical and surgical diseases. The following are some of the causes underlying or associated with pericarditis.

1. Idiopathic or nonspecific causes
2. Infection
   Bacterial (streptococcus, staphylococcus, meningococcus, gonococcus, etc.)
   Viral (coxsackie, influenza, other)
   Mycotic (fungal), rickettsial, parasitic, etc.
3. Disorders of connective tissue—systemic lupus erythematosus, rheumatic fever, rheumatoid arthritis, polyarteritis
4. Hypersensitivity states—immune reactions, drug reactions, serum sickness
5. Diseases of adjacent structures—myocardial infarction, dissecting aneurysm, pleural and pulmonary disease (pneumonia)
6. Neoplastic disease (secondary to metastasis from lung cancer, breast cancer), leukemia; following radiation; primary (mesothelioma)
7. Trauma—chest injury; cardiac surgery; during cardiac catheterization, pacemaker implantation
8. Pericarditis associated with renal disorders (uremia).

Clinical Manifestations. The characteristic symptom of the patient is *pain* and the characteristic sign is a *friction rub.* Pain is almost always present in acute pericarditis and is most common over the precordium. The pain may be felt beneath the clavicle and in the neck and left scapular region. Pericardial pain is aggravated by breathing, turning in bed, and twisting the body; it is relieved by sitting up. In fact, the patient prefers to adopt a forward-leaning or a sitting posture. Dyspnea may occur as the result of restriction of the heart contraction, which leads to a decreased cardiac output. The patient may appear extremely ill. Pericarditis per se often gives rise to no signs other than fever and the production of a friction rub.

Examination for Friction Rub. A pericardial friction rub occurs when the pericardial surfaces lose their lubricating fluid because of inflammation. The rub is audible on auscultation and is synchronous with the heartbeat. A pericardial friction rub is diagnostic of pericarditis and should be searched for diligently.

- Place the diaphragm of the stethoscope tightly against the thorax and listen at the left sternal edge in the 4th intercostal space (Fig. 31-3). This is where the pericardium comes into contact with the left chest wall. A pericardial friction rub has a scratching or leathery sound. The rub is louder at the end of expiration and may be heard best while the patient is sitting.

Nursing Assessment. While observing the patient, try to discover whether or not the pain is influenced by respiratory movements, with or without the actual passage of air; by flexion, extension, or rotation of the spine, including the neck; by movements of the shoulders and arms; by coughing; or by swallowing. Recognizing these relationships may be very helpful in establishing a diagnosis.

Management. The objectives of management are to determine the cause, to administer therapy for the specific cause (when known), and to be on the alert for cardiac tamponade (compression of the heart from fluid in the pericardial sac). The patient is placed on bed rest when cardiac output is impaired, until the fever, chest pain, and friction rub have disappeared.

Meperidine or morphine may be given for pain relief during the acute phase. Salicylates relieve pain and hasten reabsorption of fluid in the patient with rheumatic pericarditis. Corticosteroids are sometimes given to control symptoms, hasten resolution of the inflammatory process in the pericardium, and prevent recurring pericardial effusion.

- Be alert to the possibility of cardiac tamponade. Use nursing assessment skills to anticipate and identify the triad of symptoms—falling arterial pressure, rising venous pressure, and a quiet heart sound.

Patients with infections of the pericardium are treated with the antimicrobial agent of choice based on identification and sensitivity tests. The pericarditis of rheumatic fever may respond to penicillin. Isoniazid, ethambutol, rifampin, and streptomycin in various combinations are used in the treatment of tuberculosis that produces pericarditis. Amphotericin B is used in fungal pericarditis, and adrenal steroids are used in disseminated lupus erythematosus.

As the patient's condition improves, activity may be increased gradually. However, if pain, fever, or friction rub reappear, bed rest must be resumed.

Pericardial Effusion

Pericardial effusion refers to the escape of fluid into the pericardial sac. This may accompany pericarditis and advanced congestive heart failure.

Clinical Manifestations. The characteristic sign of pericardial effusion is an extension of flatness (not dullness) to percussion across the anterior aspect of the chest wall. The patient may complain of a feeling of fullness within the chest or have substernal or an ill-defined pain.

Normally, the pericardial sac contains less than 50 ml of fluid. Pericardial fluid may accumulate slowly without noticeable symptoms. However, a *rapidly* developing effusion can stretch the pericardium to its maximum size and can cause decreased cardiac output and venous return to the heart. The result is *cardiac tamponade* (compression of the heart). (Cardiac tamponade is also discussed under Chest Injuries on p. 541.) Signs include a feeling of precordial oppression, owing to the stretching of the pericardial sac, and shortness of breath; the blood pressure drops and fluctuates. Blood pressure is lowest on inspiration (*pulsus paradoxus*), at which point the pulse may not be perceptible. The venous pressure tends to rise (20 cm or more) or is evidenced by the engorged neck veins and enlarging liver. The heart sounds become feeble in intensity (quiet heart), and there are signs of cardiac enlargement and compression of the left lung posteriorly. (See Fig. 31-4 for assessment of cardiac tamponade owing to pericardial effusion.)

- The important considerations are falling blood pressure, narrowing pulse pressure, rising venous pressure (look at the neck veins), and quiet heart sounds. *This is a life-threatening situation, demanding close and constant observation.*

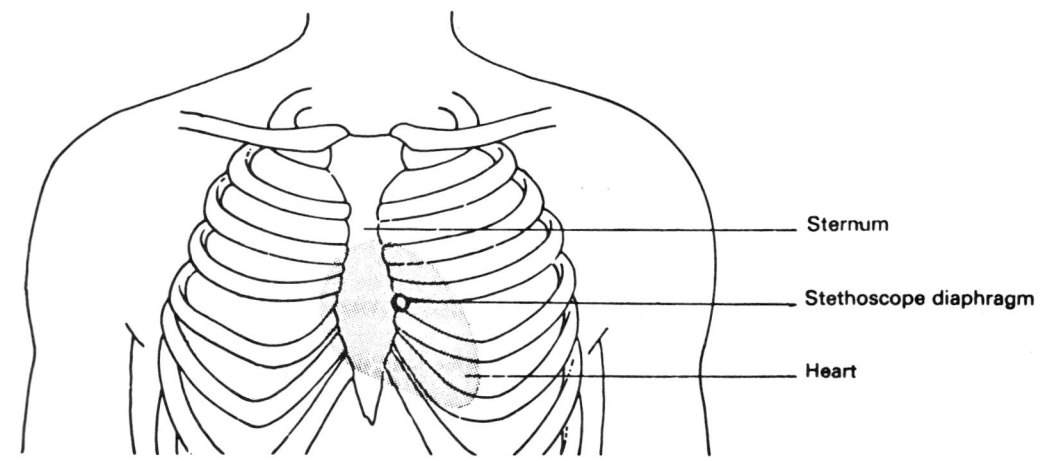

Figure 31-3. Auscultation for pericardial friction rub.

Pericardial Aspiration (Pericardiocentesis)

If the cardiac function becomes seriously impaired, a pericardial aspiration (puncture of the pericardial sac) is performed to remove fluid from the pericardial sac. The major purpose is to relieve cardiac tamponade, which restricts normal heart action.

During the procedure the patient is monitored by ECG, and central venous pressure measurements are made. A defibrillator is turned on, and other emergency resuscitative equipment should be readily available.

The head of the bed is elevated to a 45- to 60-degree angle so that the needle can be inserted into the pericardial sac more easily. A stable large-bore needle is inserted and a slow intravenous drip of saline or glucose is started should it be necessary to administer emergency drugs or blood.

The pericardial aspiration needle is attached to a 50-ml syringe by a three-way stopcock. The V lead (precordial lead wire) of the ECG is attached to the hub of the aspirating needle with alligator clips, because the monitoring of ECG oscillation is useful in determining whether or not the needle has contacted the myocardium. This is evidenced by an elevation of the ST segment or stimulation of premature ventricular contractions.

There are several possible sites for pericardial aspiration (Fig. 31-5). The needle may be inserted in the angle between the left costal margin and the xiphoid, near the cardiac apex, to the left of the 5th or 6th interspace at the sternal margin, or on the right side of the 4th intercostal space. The needle is advanced slowly until fluid is obtained.

A fall in central venous pressure associated with a rise in blood pressure indicates that relief of cardiac tamponade has occurred. The patient almost always feels immediate improvement. If there is a substantial amount of pericardial fluid, a small catheter may be left in place to drain recurrent bleeding or effusion.

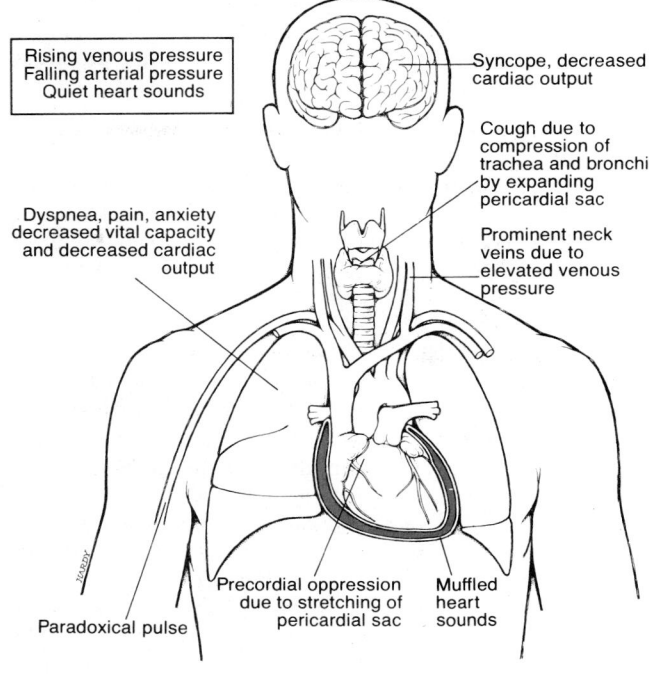

Figure 31-4. Assessment for cardiac tamponade owing to pericardial effusion. Pathophysiologic consequences of cardiac tamponade.

During the procedure it is important to watch for the presence of bloody fluid. Pericardial blood does not clot readily, whereas blood obtained from inadvertent puncture of one of the heart chambers does clot. If blood accumulates rapidly, immediate thoracotomy and cardiorrhaphy (suturing of heart muscle) are indicated.

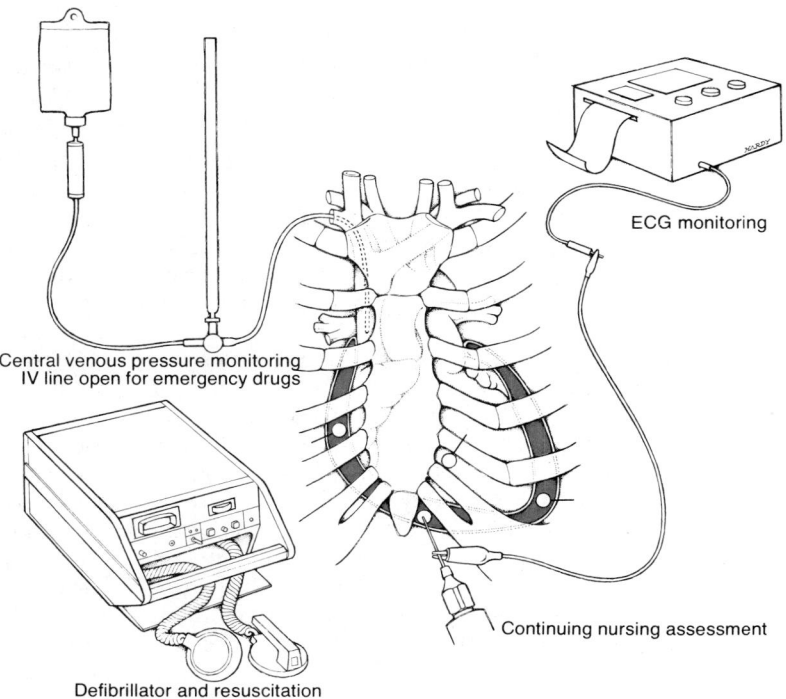

Figure 31-5. Nursing support of the patient undergoing pericardiocentesis. (Small circles indicate sites for pericardial aspiration.)

Pericardial fluid is sent to the laboratory for examination for tumor cells, bacterial culture, chemical and serological analysis, and differential cell count. A hematocrit is done if the fluid is bloody.

- Following pericardiocentesis, the patient will require careful monitoring of the blood pressure, venous pressure, and heart sounds to evaluate for the possible recurrence of cardiac tamponade. A repeated aspiration is then necessary. The patient should be in an intensive care unit. Sometimes cardiac tamponade is treated by open pericardial drainage.

Chronic Constrictive Pericarditis

Chronic constrictive pericarditis is a condition in which there is chronic inflammatory thickening of the pericardium that compresses the heart and prevents it from expanding to normal size. The major hemodynamic deficit results from a restriction of ventricular filling.

Often the adherent pericardium becomes calcified. The heart action is greatly restricted by this tough, unyielding enclosure, and edema, ascites, and hepatic enlargement result. The fixation of the heart to the pericardium may produce a retraction of the chest wall with every beat.

Chronic constrictive pericarditis is caused by long-standing pyogenic infections, postviral infections, tuberculosis, or hemopericardium.

The signs and symptoms are predominantly those of congestive heart failure (p. 636), but dyspnea on effort is the most prominent symptom. Chronic atrial fibrillation is commonly present.

Surgical removal of the tough encasing pericardium (pericardiectomy) is the only treatment of any benefit. The objective of the operation is to release both ventricles from the constrictive and restrictive inflammation. (See pp. 615–623 for the care of the patient after cardiac surgery.)

▷ Acquired Valvular Diseases of the Heart

The function of normal heart valves is to maintain the forward flow of blood from the atria to the ventricles and from the ventricles to the great vessels. Valvular damage may interfere with valvular function by stenosis (narrowing) of the valve or by impaired closure that allows backward leakage of blood (valvular insufficiency, regurgitation, or incompetence).

Acquired valvular heart disease often is a result of previous rheumatic carditis that has damaged one or more of the heart valves. The mitral valve is involved most frequently, followed by the aortic, tricuspid, and pulmonic valves. If the heart muscle remains strong, the circulatory apparatus can adjust itself efficiently even though a valve is injured badly. The details of such adjustment, called *compensatory changes,* include modifications in the rate and character of the heartbeat, changes in the blood, hypertrophy of the myocardium, redistribution of the blood in the body, etc. All of these changes lessen the unfavorable results of the valve defect.

Mitral Valve Prolapse Syndrome

The *mitral valve prolapse syndrome* is a dysfunction of the mitral valve leaflets that renders the mitral valve incompetent with resultant valvular regurgitation. This syndrome may produce no symptoms or it may progress rapidly and result in sudden death. In recent years this syndrome has been diagnosed more frequently, ostensibly as a result of improved diagnostic methods. Many individuals have this syndrome but no symptoms. Often the symptoms are first identified during a physical examination of the heart, which reveals an extra heart sound referred to as a "mitral click." The presence of a click indicates early valvular incompetence with disruption of normal blood flow. The mitral click may deteriorate into a murmur over a period of time as the valve leaflets become progressively more dysfunctional. Concomitant with the progression of the murmur may be signs and symptoms of heart failure as mitral regurgitation ensues.

Medical management is directed at controlling the associated symptoms. Some individuals experience worrisome dysrhythmias and require antidysrhythmic agents. Others may experience mild heart failure and require therapy (see p. 635 for a discussion of heart failure). In advanced stages, mitral valve replacement may be necessary.

Of significant importance is the education of these individuals regarding prophylactic antibiotic therapy prior to invasive procedures that may introduce infectious agents systemically (*e.g.,* dental work, GU/GI procedures, IV therapy, etc.). If in doubt, patients are advised to consult their physician.

Mitral Stenosis

Mitral stenosis is the progressive thickening and contracture of the mitral valve cusps, which causes narrowing of the orifice and progressive obstruction to blood flow. It is by far the most common of the late cardiac lesions produced by rheumatic fever and is considered the typical lesion.

Pathophysiology. In this disorder, acute rheumatic endocarditis has "glued" the mitral valve flaps (commissures) together and, by shortening the chordae tendineae, has pulled the flap edges down almost to the tips of the papillary muscles, greatly narrowing the mitral orifice. Normally, three fingers should pass easily through this orifice, but in well-marked cases of stenosis one can hardly put a lead pencil through it. The left ventricle is not affected, but the left atrium has great difficulty in emptying itself through the narrow orifice into the ventricle. Therefore, it dilates and hypertrophies. Since no valve protects the pulmonary veins from a backward flow from this atrium, the pulmonary circulation becomes markedly congested. As a result of the abnormally high pulmonary arterial pressure that must be maintained by the right ventricle, it is subjected to an unfunctional strain and eventually fails.

Clinical Manifestations. Patients with mitral stenosis are likely to show progressive fatigue as a result of low cardiac output, dyspnea on exertion owing to pulmonary venous hypertension, cough, and repeated respiratory infections. Hemoptysis is another common symptom resulting from pulmonary venous hypertension.

The pulse is weak and often irregular because of atrial fibrillation. Atrial fibrillation results from the dilated and hypertrophied atrium. The dilation and hypertrophy render the atrium electrically unstable, resulting in a permanent atrial dysrhythmia. Diagnostic aids that assist the cardiologist in making an accurate diagnosis are phonocardiography, echocardiography, and cardiac catheterization with angiography to verify the severity of the mitral stenosis.

Management. Antibiotic therapy is instituted to prevent rheumatic recurrences, while developing congestive heart failure is treated with digitalis, sodium restriction, and limitation of activity. Surgical intervention consists of a valvotomy to rupture the fused commissures of the mitral valve or replacement of the mitral valve with a prosthetic valve (see p. 607).

Mitral Insufficiency (Regurgitation)

Mitral insufficiency results when incompetence and distortion of the mitral valve prevent the free margins from coming into apposition during systole. The chordae tendineae may become shortened, preventing complete closure of the leaflets. Valvular movement is more restricted than in mitral stenosis. In about one half of the patients, mitral regurgitation is caused by chronic rheumatic heart disease.

Pathophysiology. Shortening or tearing of one or both of the mitral valve flaps prevents the perfect closure of the mitral orifice, while the powerful left ventricle is forcing the blood into the aorta. Then, at each beat the left ventricle forces some of the blood back into its atrium; this blood is added to the blood that is beginning to flow into this chamber from the lungs. The left atrium must, therefore, dilate and hypertrophy. This backward flow of blood from the ventricle also checks the current of blood flowing under low pressure from the lungs, which, therefore, become congested. This, in turn, throws an extra strain on the right ventricle. Therefore, the result of even a slight mitral leak always involves both lungs and the right ventricle.

Clinical Manifestations. Palpitation of the heart, shortness of breath on exertion, and cough owing to chronic passive pulmonary congestion are common symptoms. The pulse may be regular and of good volume, but frequently it becomes irregular, as a result of either extrasystoles or fibrillation, which may persist indefinitely.

Management. Management is the same as that for congestive heart failure (p. 637). Surgical intervention consists of mitral valve replacement.

Aortic Valve Stenosis

Aortic valve stenosis is the narrowing of the orifice between the left ventricle and the aorta. In adults, aortic valvular stenosis may be congenital, or it may be a result of rheumatic fever or cusp calcification of unknown cause. There is progressive narrowing of the valve orifice over a period of several years to several decades.

Pathophysiology. The obstruction to the aortic outflow places a pressure load on the left ventricle, which shows the strain by a thickening of the muscle wall. The heart muscle increases in size (hypertrophy) in response to all degrees of obstruction, but heart failure occurs when obstruction is severe.

The flaps of the aortic valve fuse and partially close the opening between the heart and the aorta. The left ventricle overcomes this obstruction to circulation by contracting more slowly but with greater energy than normal, forcibly squeezing the blood through the very small orifice. The heart's compensatory mechanisms begin to fail and clinical signs develop.

Clinical Manifestations. In moderate to severe cases of aortic stenosis, the patient first experiences exertional dyspnea, which is a manifestation of left ventricular decompensation with pulmonary congestion. Other signs are dizziness and fainting because of reduced blood volume to the brain. Angina pectoris is a frequent symptom and results from the increased oxygen demands imposed by the increased work of the left ventricle and by myocardial hypertrophy. Blood pressure may be low, and often there is a narrow pulse pressure because of diminished blood flow.

Upon physical examination, a loud, rough systolic murmur may be heard over the aortic area. The sound to listen for is a systolic crescendo–decrescendo murmur, which may radiate into the carotid arteries and to the left ventricular apex. The murmur is low-pitched, rough, rasping, and vibrating. If one rests the hand over the base of the heart, a vibration is felt that is the most intense of all cardiac thrills and resembles the purring of a cat (Fig. 31-6). The purring sound is related to the turbulence caused by the blood flow across a narrowed valve orifice. The evidence of left ventricular hypertrophy may be seen on a 12-lead ECG.

Left-heart catheterization is necessary in order to accurately measure the severity of this valvular abnormality. Pressure tracings are taken from the left ventricle and the base of the aorta. The systolic pressure in the left ventricle is considerably higher than that in the aorta during systole.

Management. A significant risk of sudden death exists for those patients who are treated medically without surgical repair. The uncorrected condition will lead to heart failure and a rapid downhill course. Studies have shown that the average life expectancy is 3 to 4 years from the onset of syncope, 2 to 3 years from the onset of angina, and 18 months to 2 years from the onset of dyspnea and heart failure.

Because the aortic valve cusps fuse and the leaflets become rigid, scarred and, in advanced disease, calcified, it is necessary to repair and restore function through surgery (aortic valve replacement). (See Chap. 30 for the care of the patient undergoing cardiac surgery.)

Aortic Insufficiency (Incompetence; Regurgitation)

Aortic insufficiency is caused by inflammatory lesions that deform the flaps of the aortic valve, preventing them from completely sealing the aortic orifice during diastole and thus allowing a backflow of blood from the aorta into the left ventricle. This valvular defect may follow endocarditis of the rheumatic or bacterial type or may be due to congenital abnormalities or diseases that cause dilatation or tearing of the ascending aorta (syphilitic disease, rheumatoid spondylitis, dissecting aneurysm).

Pathophysiology. Because of the leak in the aortic valve during diastole, some of the blood in the aorta, always under high pressure, hisses back into the left ventricle,

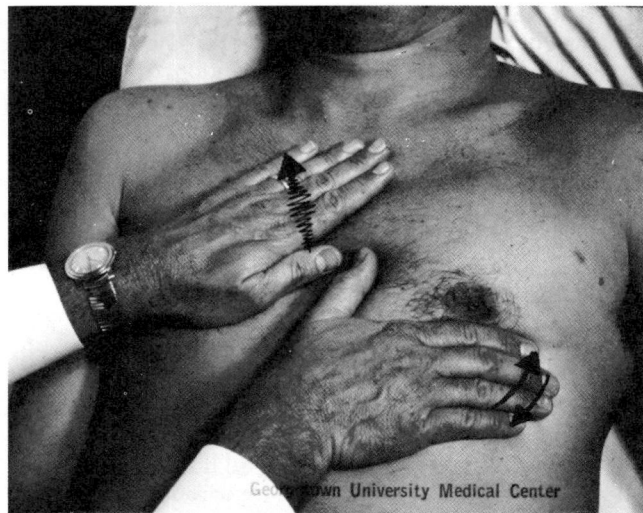

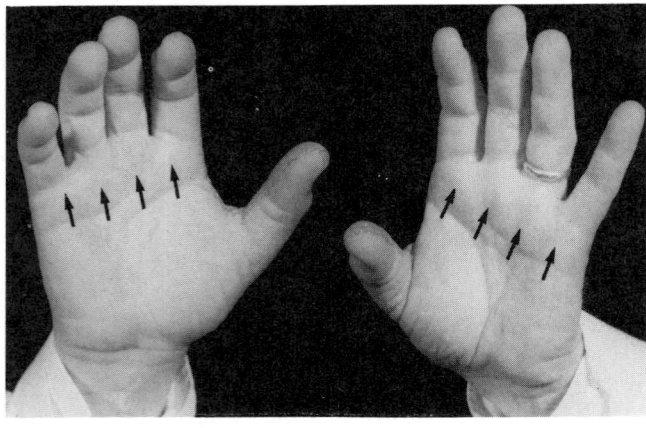

Figure 31-6. Assessing for palpable thrill of aortic stenosis. The thrill is felt at the base of the heart, and its direction is toward the right shoulder and right side of the neck. The vibrations are best detected with the palmar surfaces of the hands. (From Shah PM and Roberts DL: Diagnosis and treatment of aortic valve stenosis. In Harvey WP et al. (eds.): Current Problems in Cardiology. Chicago, Year Book Medical Publishers, 1977. Copyright © 1977 by Year Book.)

which must handle both the blood that the left atrium normally delivers into the ventricle through the mitral orifice and that returning from the aorta. The left ventricle dilates to accommodate this increased volume, hypertrophies in order to expel it, and does so with more than normal force, thus raising the systolic blood pressure. By another reflex, the cardiovascular system tends to become accommodated: the peripheral arterioles become relaxed, so that the peripheral resistance is lessened and the diastolic pressure greatly lowered.

Clinical Manifestations. The disease develops insidiously, and the earliest manifestation is awareness of the increased force of the heartbeat. There may be marked arterial pulsations that are visible or palpable over the precordium. Arterial pulsation in the neck will also be marked,

the head sometimes bobbing in synchrony with the heartbeat. This is a result of the increased force and volume of the blood ejected from the hypertrophied left ventricle. Exertional dyspnea and easy fatigability follow. Signs and symptoms of left ventricular failure (orthopnea, paroxysmal nocturnal dyspnea) occur with moderate to severe regurgitation.

The pulse pressure (the difference between the systolic and diastolic pressure) is considerably widened in these patients. One of the characteristic signs of the disease is the manner in which the pulse strikes the palpating finger with quick, sharp strokes and then suddenly collapses (water-hammer pulse). The nature of the pulse wave is quite unmistakable, since it rises rapidly to a peak and collapses quickly.

Diagnosis. The diagnostic method used is cineangiography, in which an opaque medium is injected into the root of the aorta, usually by way of a catheter passed from the femoral artery. In aortic regurgitation, the opaque liquid can be seen passing into the left ventricle from the aorta.

Compensation may remain excellent for a long time, but when the left ventricle dilates because of weakness, a rapid downhill course is initiated.

Management. A major priority is the prevention of infection of the already deformed aortic leaflets. Antimicrobial prophylaxis is used for all dental procedures, any form of instrumentation, and all surgical procedures involving the genitourinary tract, the lower intestinal tract, the gallbladder, and the drainage of infected material.

Aortic valve replacement is the treatment of choice, but the optimal time for valve replacement remains controversial. (The management of the patient undergoing cardiac surgery is discussed in Chap. 30.)

Tricuspid Lesions

Tricuspid stenosis is the restriction of the tricuspid valve orifice as the result of commissural fusion and fibrosis usually following rheumatic fever. It is commonly associated with diseases of the mitral valve.

Tricuspid insufficiency allows the regurgitation of blood from the right ventricle into the right atrium during ventricular systole.

Clinical Manifestations. The symptoms of tricuspid regurgitation are marked. At each beat the right ventricle forces blood in two directions: through the pulmonary valve (the normal direction), and back through the leaking tricuspid valve into the right atrium. The flow of venous blood from the systemic circulation is impeded, causing signs of general cyanosis and overfilling of all the veins of the body.

A pulse wave similar to that sent by the left ventricle throughout the arterial tree may be transmitted into the larger veins. Therefore, the liver, now swollen to perhaps two or three times its normal size, pulsates. The walls of the stomach, intestines, kidneys, and other abdominal organs, since they are turgid with venous blood, cannot function well and produce symptoms of chronic passive congestion. The legs and the dependent portions of the body become edematous. Fluid collects in the abdominal cavity (ascites) and in the pleural cavities (hydrothorax). If the heart responds to medical or surgical therapy, circulation improves, the congestion of the various organs is relieved, and all symptoms may abate.

Management. The treatment consists of surgical treatment of associated mitral valve disease, tricuspid valvuloplasty, or tricuspid valve replacement.

▷ **Bibliography**

Books

Bigger JT. A Primer on Calcium Ion Antagonists. Whippany, New Jersey, Knoll Pharmaceutical Co, 1981.

Braunwald E (ed). Heart Disease. Philadelphia, WB Saunders, 1980.

Braunwald E et al (eds). Congestive Heart Failure. New York, Grune & Stratton, 1981.

Charles ED and Kronenfeld JJ (eds). Social and Economic Impacts of Coronary Artery Disease. Lexington, DC Heath & Co, 1980.

Chung EK. Cardiac Emergency Care, 2nd ed. Philadelphia, Lea & Febiger, 1980.

Crawford MH. Non-invasive Assessment of Patients with Ischemic Heart Disease. Chicago, Year Book Medical Publishers, 1981.

Dalen JE and Alpert JS. Valvular Heart Disease. Boston, Little, Brown & Co, 1981.

Davies JA and Spillman SJ. Cardiac Rehabilitation for the Patient and Family. Reston, Reston Publishing, 1980.

Diet and Coronary Heart Disease—A Conference Report. London, Butter Information Council, May 1980.

Donoso E. Advances and Controversies in Cardiology, Vol VI. New York, Thieme–Stratton, 1981.

Fowler NO. Cardiac Diagnosis and Treatment, 3rd ed. Hagerstown, Harper & Row, 1980.

Helfant RH. Bellet's Essentials of Cardiac Arrhythmias, 2nd ed. Philadelphia, WB Saunders, 1980.

Hurst JW (ed). The Heart, 5th ed. New York, McGraw–Hill, 1982.

Johnson RA (ed). The Practice of Cardiology, 1st ed. Boston, Little, Brown & Co, 1980.

Kaltenback M (ed). Coronary Heart Disease—Transluminal Coronary Angioplasty and Coronary Fibrinolysis. New York, Springer–Verlag, 1981.

Karliner JS (ed). Coronary Care. New York, Churchill Livingstone, 1981.

Lee WR. Essentials of Clinical Cardiology. Bowie, The Charles Press, 1980.

Long C (ed). Prevention and Rehabilitation in Ischemic Heart Disease. Baltimore, Williams & Wilkins, 1980.

Mandel WJ. Cardiac Arrhythmias. Philadelphia, JB Lippincott, 1980.

Mason DT and Collins JJ (eds). Myocardial Revascularization. New York, Yorke Medical Books, 1981.

Olsen EGJ. The Pathology of the Heart, 2nd ed. London, The MacMillan Press, 1980.

Rapaport E (ed). Current Controversies in Cardiovascular Disease. Philadelphia, WB Saunders, 1980.

Reiffel J et al (eds). Psychosocial Aspects of Cardiovascular Disease. New York, Columbia University Press, 1980.

Samet P and El–Sherif N (eds). Cardiac Pacing, 2nd ed. New York, Grune & Stratton, 1980.

Santamore WP and Bove AA. Coronary Artery Disease. Baltimore, Urban Schwarzenberg, 1982.

Sokolow M and McIlroy MB. Clinical Cardiology, 3rd ed. Los Altos, Lange Medical Publications, 1981.

Weiss GB. New Perspectives on Calcium Antagonists. Bethesda. American Physiological Society, 1981.

Willerson JT. Ischemic Heart Disease: Clinical and Pathophysiological Aspects. New York, Raven Press, 1982.

Articles
Assessment and Diagnosis

Bauman DJ. Creatine phosphokinase isoenzymes and the diagnosis of myocardial infarction. Postgrad Med 1980 Jan; 67(1):103–116.

Cannon C. Hands-on guide to palpation and auscultation. RN 1980 Mar; 43(3):20–27, 76.

Cohen JA et al. A message from the heart: What isoenzymes can tell you about your cardiac patient. Nursing '82 1982 Apr; 12(4):46–49.

Frank–Stromborg M and Stromborg P. Practice guide: Test your knowledge of chest pain. Nursing '81 1981 Aug; 11(8):89–98.

Galen RS. Enzymes in the diagnosis of myocardial infarction. Heart Lung 1981 May–June; 81(3):484–485.

Humbrecht B and VanParys E. From assessment to intervention: How to use heart and breath sounds as part of your nursing care plan. Nursing '82 1982 Apr; 12(4):34–41.

Patient assessment: Abnormalities of the heart beat—a programmed instruction. Am J Nurs 1977 Apr; 77(4):1–26.

Pepler C. Your finger on the pulse: Evaluating what you feel. Nursing '80 1980 Nov; 10(11):32–39.

Roberts R. Diagnostic assessment of myocardial infarction based on lactate dehydrogenase and creatine kinase isoenzymes. Heart Lung 1981 May–June; 81(3):486–503.

Winkel RA. Ambulatory electrocardiography. Mod Concepts Cardiovasc Dis 1980 Feb; 49(2):7–12.

Atherosclerosis, Angina, and Myocardial Infarction

Cantwell R et al. What do you know about cardiac drugs for a code? Nursing '82 1982 Oct; 12(10):34–42.

Chesney MA and Rosenman RH. Type A behavior: Observations on the past decade. Heart Lung 1982 Jan–Feb; 82(1):12–19.

Cowley MJ, Vetrovec GW, and Wolfgang TC. Efficacy of percutaneous transluminal angioplasty: Technique, patient selection, salutory results, limitations and complications. Am Heart J 1981 Mar; 101(3):272–280.

Dehn M. Rehabilitation of the cardiac patient: The effects of exercise. Am J Nurs 1980 Mar; 80(3):435–440.

Devney AM. Rehabilitation of the cardiac patient: Bridging the gap between inhospital and outhospital care. Am J Nurs 1980 Mar; 80(3):446–450.

Fletcher G. Exercise and coronary risk factor modification in the management of atherosclerosis. Heart Lung 1981 Sept–Oct; 81(5):811–813.

Fuller EO. The effect of antianginal drugs on myocardial oxygen consumption. Am J Nurs 1980 Feb; 80(2):250–254.

Hansen MS and Woods SL. Nitroglycerin ointment—where and how to apply it. Am J Nurs 1980 June; 80(6):1122–1124.

Janz N and Lampman RM. Coaching your cardiac patient along the path to recovery. Nursing '81 1981 Dec; 11(12):37–41.

Kennedy GT. Variant angina: Clinical symptoms, pathophysiology, and management. Heart Lung 1981 Nov–Dec; 81(6):1073–1081.

Matheny L. Emergency! First aid for cardiopulmonary arrest. Nursing '82 1982 June; 12(6):34–45.

Matheny LG. Defibrillation: When and how to use it. Nursing '81 1981 June; 11(6):69–72.

McCarthy CL. Percutaneous transluminal coronary angioplasty: Therapeutic intervention in the cardiac catheterization laboratory. Heart Lung 1982 Nov–Dec; 82(6):499–504.

Meador B. Warning signs to watch for in your post-MI patient. RN 1981 July; 44(7):25–31.

Miller Sr P et al. Health beliefs of and adherence to the medical regimen by patients with ischemic heart disease. Heart Lung 1982 July–Aug; 82(4):332–339.

Ott B. Percutaneous transluminal coronary angioplasty and nursing implications. Heart Lung 1982 July–Aug; 82(4):294–298.

Partridge SA. The nurse's role in percutaneous transluminal coronary angioplasty. Heart Lung 1982 Nov–Dec; 82(6):505–511.

Pepine CJ, Margolis JR, and Conti RC. Transluminal coronary angioplasty. JAMA 1980 Oct 24; 244(17):1966–1969.

Purcell JA and Giffin PA. Percutaneous transluminal angioplasty. Am J Nurs 1981 Sept; 81(9):1620–1625.

Purcell JA and Holder CK. Intravenous nitroglycerin. Am J Nurs 1982 Feb; 82(2):254–259.

Rodman MJ. Drug therapy today: Latest thinking on drug therapy post-MI. RN 1981 Jan; 44(1):74, 82–96.

Rodman MJ. Drug therapy today: Latest strategies for post-MI dysrhythmias. RN 1981 Feb; 44(2):63–68.

Taylor PB and Gideon MDD. Cardiac arrest—a crisis for all people. Nursing '80 1980 Sept; 10(9):42–45.

Tannenbaum RP et al. The pain of angina pectoris: How to recognize it: How to manage it. Nursing '81 1981 Sept; 11(9):44–51.

Winslow EH and Weber TM. Rehabilitation of the cardiac patient: Progressive exercise to combat the hazards of bedrest. Am J Nurs 1980 Mar; 80(3):440–445.

Congestive Heart Failure/Pulmonary Edema

Dossey B and Passons JM. Pulmonary embolism—preventing it—treating it. Nursing '81 1981 Mar; 11(3):26–33.

Franciosa JA. The role of vasodilators in managing congestive heart failure. Postgrad Med 1980 Jan; 67(1):87–91, 94–98.

Franciosa JA. Nitroglycerin and nitrates in congestive heart failure. Heart Lung 1980 Sept–Oct; 80(5):873–882.

Giles TD. Principles of vasodilator therapy for left ventricular congestive heart failure. Heart Lung 1980 Mar–Apr; 80(2):271–276.

Heggie J. Pulling your patient through congestive heart failure. RN 1980 Sept; 43(9):31–36, 131–132.

Kirschenbaum HL and Rosenberg JM. What to watch for with digitalis. RN 1981 Nov; 44(11):69–72.

Lapinski ML. Cardiovascular drugs and the elderly population. Heart Lung 1982 Sept–Oct; 82(5):430–433.

Lemberg L. Digitalis in congestive heart failure. Arch Intern Med 1978 Mar; 138(3):451–452.

Lemberg L. Clinical considerations in the use of vasodilators for congestive heart failure. Practical Cardiology 1981 Apr; 7(4):63–73.

Meissner JE and Gever LN. Reducing the risks of digitalis toxicity. Nursing '80 1980 Sept; 10(9):32–38.

Segal BL. New approaches to therapy of acute heart failure. Am Fam Physician 1980 Feb; 21(2):131–135.

Toledo LW. How vasodilators backfire. RN 1982 July; 45(7):40–45.

Endocarditis/Pericarditis

Barry J and Gump D. Endocarditis: An overview. Heart Lung 1982 Mar–Apr; 11(2):138–143.

Brown AK. Pericardial disease. Practitioner 1980 Mar; 224(14):249–252.

Cohen PS, Maguire JH, and Weinstein L. Infective endocarditis caused by gram-negative bacteria: A review of the literature, 1945–1977. Prog Cardiovasc Dis 1980 Jan–Feb; 22(4):205–242.

DeLeon AC Jr. Mitral valve prolapse. Postgrad Med 1980 Jan; 67(1):66–77.

Dormer AE. The management of infective endocarditis. Practitioner 1980 Mar; 224(1341):225–259.

Dracup KA. Managing and understanding the patient with infective endocarditis. Nursing '80 1980 May; 10(5):44–50.

Duffy KF et al. A severe case of viral myocarditis. Am J Nurs 1981 June; 81(6):1148–1151.

Guzman L. Nursing management of the parenteral drug abuser with infective endocarditis. Heart Lung 1981 Mar–Apr; 81(2):289–293.

Haughey CW. Alcoholic cardiomyopathy. Nursing '80 1980 Sept; 10(9):54–58.

Kluge RM. Infections of prosthetic cardiac valves and arterial grafts. Heart Lung 1982 Mar–Apr; 11(2):146–151.

Kotler MN and Segal BL. The inflamed heart: Pericarditis in the elderly. Geriatrics 1980 Jan; 35(1):630–673.

Kovalesky A. Mitral valve prolapse. Nursing '81 1981 Apr; 11(4):58–61.

Simonetti D. Prolapsed mitral valve: Living with chest pain. Am J Nurs 1980 Aug; 80(8):1430–1432.

Stuart EM et al. Nursing rounds: Care of the patient with a mitral commissurotomy. Am J Nurs 1980 Sept; 80(9):1611–1632.

Pacemaker

Beeler B. Infections of permanent transvenous and epicardial pacemakers in adults. Heart Lung 1982 Mar–Apr; 82(2):152–155.

Kronke GM et al. What to do when your patient's pacemaker stops working. Nursing '81 1981 Oct; 11(10):74–78.

32

Assessment and Management of Patients With Vascular Disorders and Problems of Peripheral Circulation

▷ Physiologic Overview

Adequate perfusion, which results in oxygenation and nutrition of body tissues, is dependent, in part, upon a functionally intact cardiovascular system. Efficient pumping action of the heart, patent and responsive blood vessels, and an adequate circulating blood volume are essential for adequate blood flow. Nervous system activity, blood viscosity, and the metabolic needs of tissues influence the rate of blood flow, thereby the adequacy of blood flow.

The peripheral vascular system consists of the systemic circulation and the pulmonary circulation serially connected in a closed system with the right and left heart. The blood vessels provide distensible channels for the transport of blood from the heart to the tissues and back to the heart. Cardiac ventricular contraction supplies the driving force for movement of blood through the vascular systems. *Arteries* distribute oxygenated blood from the left side of the heart to the tissues while the *veins* convey unoxygenated blood from the tissues to the right side of the heart. *Capillary* vessels, located within the tissues, connect the arterial and venous systems and constitute the site of exchange of nutrients and metabolic wastes between the circulation and the tissues. *Arterioles* and *venules* immediately adjacent to the capillaries, together with the capillaries, comprise the *microcirculation*. A schematic representation of the circulation is shown in Figure 32-1.

The *lymphatic* system complements the function of the circulatory system. Lymphatic vessels transport *lymph* (a fluid similar to plasma) and tissue fluids (containing smaller proteins, cells, and cellular debris) from the interstitial space to systemic veins.

Anatomy of the Vascular System
Arteries and Arterioles. *Arteries* are thick-walled structures that carry blood from the heart to the tissues. The

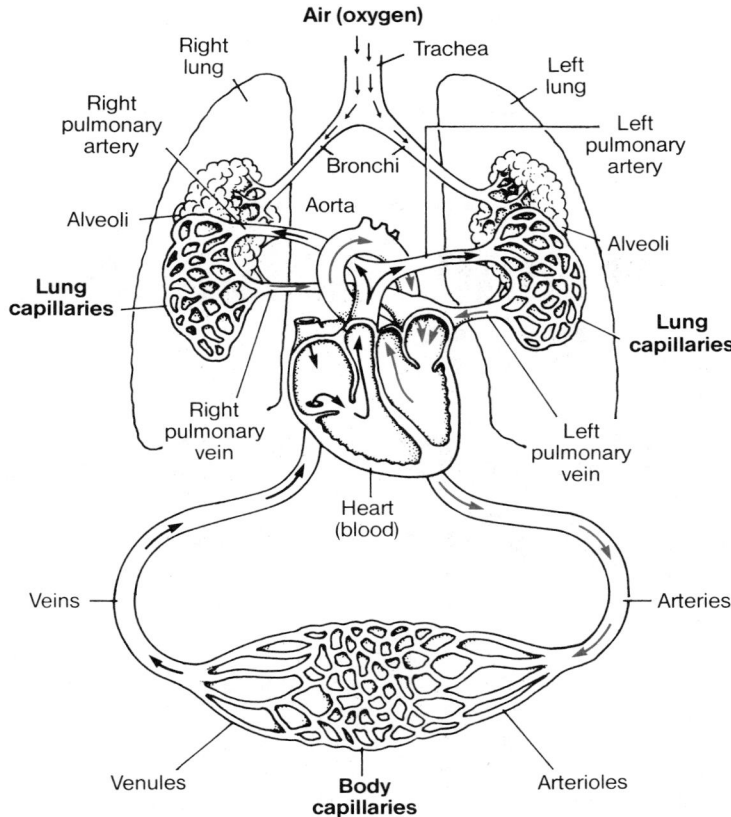

Air (oxygen)

Figure 32-1. Schematic drawing of systemic circulation. (Start at bottom of diagram.) Loaded with carbon dioxide, blood from the body capillaries goes through venules and veins into the right chamber of the heart (black arrows). It is pumped into the two lungs. Having dropped carbon dioxide and picked up oxygen, it goes back to the left chamber of the heart (color arrows). From there it is pumped through the aorta into the body circulation (arteries and arterioles) until it reaches the body capillaries, where it gives up oxygen and picks up carbon dioxide. (National Tuberculosis and Respiratory Disease Association.)

aorta, which has a diameter of approximately 25 mm (1 inch), gives rise to numerous branches, which in turn divide into smaller vessels that approach 4 mm (0.16 inch) in diameter by the time they reach the tissues. Within the tissues, the vessels divide further, diminishing to approximately 30 microns in diameter; these vessels are called *arterioles.*

The walls of the arteries and arterioles are divided into three layers: an inner endothelial cell layer called the *intima,* which is in contact with the blood; a middle layer called the *media;* and an outer layer called the *adventitia.* The intima provides a smooth surface for contact with the flowing blood. The adventitia is a layer of connective tissue that anchors the vessel to its surrounding structures. The media makes up the major portion of the vessel wall. In the aorta and other large arteries of the body, this layer is composed chiefly of elastic and connective tissue fibers that give the vessels considerable strength and allow them to accommodate cardiac stroke volume and maintain an even, steady flow of blood. There is much less elastic tissue in the smaller arteries and arterioles, and the media in these vessels is composed primarily of smooth muscle.

Smooth muscle, by contraction and relaxation, controls vessel diameter. Chemical, hormonal, and nervous system factors influence the activity of smooth muscle. Because arterioles can alter their diameter, thereby offering resistance to blood flow, they are often referred to as resistance vessels. Arterioles regulate the volume and pressure in the arterial system and blood flow to the capillaries.

Because of the large amount of muscle, the wall of the arteries is relatively thick; it accounts for approximately 25% of the total diameter of the artery and approximately 67% of the total diameter of arterioles. The muscle and adventitia of the arterial wall require their own blood supplies to meet metabolic requirements. The blood vessels that supply the wall are the *vasa vasorum.* The intima is thin and is in such close contact with the blood within the vessel that it can receive its nourishment directly from that source.

Capillaries.   Capillary walls lack muscle and adventitia and are composed of a single layer of cells. This thin-walled structure permits rapid and efficient transport of nutrients to the cells and removal of metabolic wastes. The diameter of capillaries ranges from 5 to 10 microns, which requires that red blood cells alter their shape to pass through these vessels. Changes in capillary diameter are passive and are influenced by changes in the resistance of precapillary and postcapillary vessels. A muscular sphincter, called the *precapillary* sphincter, is located at the arteriolar end of the capillary and is responsible, along with the arteriole, for controlling capillary blood flow.

Some capillary beds contain *arteriovenous anastomoses,* through which blood passes directly from the arterial to the venous system. These vessels are believed to regulate heat exchange between the body and the external environment.

The distribution of capillaries throughout the tissues varies with the type of tissue. For example, skeletal tissue, which is metabolically active, has a more dense capillary network than does less active tissue, such as cartilage.

Veins and Venules.   Capillaries join together to form larger vessels called *venules,* which in turn join to form the veins. The venous system is therefore structurally analogous to the arterial system. Venules correspond to arterioles, veins to arteries, and the vena cavae to the aorta. Analogous types of vessels in the arterial and venous systems have approximately the same diameters.

The walls of the veins, in contrast to those of the arteries, are thinner and considerably less muscular. The wall of the average vein amounts to only 10% of the vein diameter, in contrast to 25% in the artery. The wall of a vein, like that of an artery, is composed of three layers.

The thin, less muscular structure of the vein wall allows greater distensibility of these vessels. Greater distensibility permits the "storage" of large volumes of blood in the veins under low pressure. For this reason, veins are referred to as *capacitance vessels.* Approximately 75% of the total blood volume is contained in the veins. The sympathetic nervous system, which innervates the vein musculature, can stimulate venoconstriction, thereby reducing venous volume and increasing the general circulating blood volume.

Some veins, unlike arteries, are equipped with valves. In general, veins that transport blood against the force of gravity, as in the lower extremities, have one-way valves that prevent the distal reflux of blood as it is propelled toward the heart. Valves are composed of endothelial leaflets, the competency of which depends on the integrity of the vein wall.

Lymphatic Vessels.   The lymphatic circulation begins in the tissues and is a one-way system that carries lymph from tissues back to the venous circulation. The lymphatics are thin-walled capillaries similar to the blood capillaries, except that lymphatic vessels are more permeable to large molecules because of wider spaces between endothelial cells and absence of a basement membrane. Peripheral lymphatics join larger lymph vessels and pass through regional lymph nodes before entering the venous system. The lymphatics converge into two main trunks, the thoracic duct and the right lymphatic duct. These ducts empty into the junction of the subclavian and the internal jugular veins. The thoracic duct drains most of the lymph vessels in the body. The right lymphatic duct conveys lymph primarily from the right side of the head, neck, thorax, and upper arms. Like veins, lymphatics contain one-way valves to prevent fluid reflux. Muscular contraction of the lymphatic walls and surrounding tissues aid in the propulsion of lymph toward venous drainage points.

Circulatory Needs of Tissues

The amount of blood flow needed by body tissues is constantly changing. The percentage of the cardiac output received by individual organs or tissues is determined by the metabolic needs of the cells and the function of the tissues (Table 32-1). When metabolic requirements increase, blood vessels dilate to increase the flow of oxygen and nutrients to the tissues. When metabolic needs decrease, vessels constrict and blood flow decreases. Metabolic demands of tissues increase with physical activity or exercise, local heat application, fever, and infection. Reduced metabolic requirements of tissues accompany rest or decreased physical activity, local cold application, and cooling of the body. Failure of blood vessels to dilate in response to the need for increased blood flow will result in tissue ischemia.

As blood passes through tissue capillaries, oxygen is removed and carbon dioxide added. The amount of oxygen extracted by each tissue is different. For example, heart muscle tends to extract about half the oxygen from arterial blood in one passage through its capillary bed, whereas in the kidneys only about 7% of the oxygen is removed as blood passes through the organ. The average amount of oxygen removed collectively by all of the body tissues is about 25%. This means that the blood in the vena cavae contains about 25% less oxygen than aortic blood. This is known as the *systemic arteriovenous oxygen difference.* The systemic arteriovenous oxygen difference increases when the amount of oxygen delivered to the tissues is decreased relative to their metabolic needs. More detailed information about the blood flow and oxygen extraction as blood passes through capillary beds in various tissues is summarized in Table 32-1.

Blood Flow

Blood flow through the cardiovascular system always proceeds in the same direction: left heart to aorta, arteries, arterioles, capillaries, venules, veins, vena cava, and finally to the right heart. The reason for this unidirectional flow is that a pressure difference exists between the arterial and venous systems. Since arterial pressure (approximately 100 mm Hg) is greater than venous pressure (approximately 4 mm Hg), and fluid always flows from an area of high pressure to an area of low pressure, blood flows from the arterial to the venous system.

Although the pressure difference or gradient (ΔP) in the vascular system provides the impetus for propulsion of blood forward, an opposing force to blood flow provided by the blood vessels also exists. This is termed *resistance* (R). Thus, the rate of blood flow is determined by dividing the change in pressure by the resistance.

(1) $$\text{Flow} = \Delta P / R$$

From this equation it is clear that when resistance increases, a greater driving pressure is required in order to maintain the same degree of flow. Physiologically, an increase in driving pressure is accomplished by an increase

Table 32-1
Typical Values for Blood Flow and Oxygen Consumption for Various Organs in the Human

Organ	Organ Weight (kg)	Blood Flow During Rest			Oxygen Usage During Rest			
		Organ Blood Flow (ml/min)	Blood Flow Unit Wt (ml/min/ 100 g)	% Total Cardiac Output	A-V O_2 Difference, (ml/100 ml blood)	Organ O_2 Usage (ml/min)	O_2 Usage Unit Wt (ml/min/ 100 g)	% Total O_2 Usage
Brain	1.4	750	55	14	6.0	45	3.00	18
Heart	0.3	250	80	5	10.0	25	8.00	10
Liver	1.5	1,300	85	23	6.0	75	2.00	30
GI tract	2.5	1,000	40					
Kidneys	0.3	1,200	400	22	1.3	15	5.00	6
Muscle	35.0	1,000	3	18	5.0	50	0.15	20
Skin	2.0	200	10	4	2.5	5	0.20	2
Remainder (skeleton, bone marrow, fat, connective tissue, etc.)	27.0	800	3	14	5.0	35	0.15	14
TOTAL	70 kg	5500 ml/min		100		250		100

(From Folkow B and Neil E: Circulation. New York, Oxford University Press.)

in the force of contraction of the heart. If arterial resistance is chronically elevated, the heart muscle hypertrophies in order to sustain the greater contractile force.

In the majority of blood vessels, flow is *laminar* or streamlined with blood in the center of the vessel moving slightly faster than the blood near the vessel walls. Laminar flow is silent. In some instances, particularly at vessel bifurcations, laminar flow becomes turbulent. Turbulent blood flow creates sounds that can be heard superficially with a stethoscope. The sound created by turbulent blood flow is called *bruit.* Turbulent blood flow may also occur when the velocity of blood flow is high, with decreased blood viscosity, with greater than normal vessel diameter, or when vessels have narrowed or constricted segments.

Blood Pressure.   See page 73 for physiology and measurement.

Capillary Filtration and Reabsorption
Fluid exchange across the capillary wall is continuous. This fluid, which has the same composition as plasma without the proteins, forms the interstitial fluid. The equilibrium between hydrostatic and oncotic forces of the blood and interstitium, as well as capillary permeability, govern the amount and direction of fluid movement across the capillary. Normally, the blood pressure (hydrostatic pressure) at the arterial end of the capillary is relatively high, compared with that at the venous end. This high pressure at the arterial end of the capillaries tends to drive fluid out of the capillaries' blood and into the tissue. The plasma proteins in the capillaries exert an osmotic force (osmotic pressure) that tends to pull fluid back into the capillary from the tissue space, but this osmotic force cannot overcome the high hydrostatic pressure at the arterial end of the capillary. At the venous end of the capillary, however, the osmotic force predominates over the low hydrostatic pressure and there

is a net reabsorption of fluid from the tissue space back into the capillary. Virtually all of the fluid that is filtered at the arterial end of the capillary bed is reabsorbed at the venous end, except for a very small amount. This excess filtered fluid enters the lymphatic circulation. These processes of filtration, reabsorption, and lymph formation aid in the maintenance of tissue fluid volume and in the removal of tissue waste and debris. Capillary permeability, under normal conditions, remains constant.

Under certain abnormal conditions, the filtration of fluid out of the capillaries may greatly exceed the amounts reabsorbed and carried away by the lymphatics. This can result from damage to capillary walls, causing increased permeability, obstruction of lymphatic drainage, elevation of venous pressure, or decrease in plasma protein osmotic force. The accumulation of fluid that results from these processes is known as *edema.*

Hemodynamic Resistance
Peripheral vascular resistance is the opposition to blood flow provided by the blood vessels.

$$(2) \quad R = \frac{8\eta L}{\pi r^4} \quad \text{where}$$

r = radius of the vessel
L = length of the vessel
η = viscosity of the blood
$8/\pi$ = a constant

Inspection of this equation shows that the resistance is proportional to the viscosity of the blood and the length of the vessel, but inversely proportional to the fourth power of the vessel radius.

The most important factor in the vascular system determining the resistance is the vessel radius. Small changes in vessel radius will lead to large changes in resistance. The predominant sites of change in caliber of blood vessels, therefore resistance, are the arterioles and the precapillary sphincter. Total circulatory resistance is termed *systemic vascular resistance.*

Blood viscosity and vessel length, under normal conditions, do not change significantly. Therefore, these factors do not usually play an important role in blood flow. However, a large increase in hematocrit may increase blood viscosity and reduce capillary blood flow.

Peripheral Vascular Regulating Mechanisms

Since the metabolic needs of body tissues, even at rest, are continuously changing, an integrated and coordinated system of regulation is necessary so that blood flow to individual areas is maintained in proportion to the needs of that area. As might be expected, this regulatory mechanism is complex and consists of central nervous system influences, circulating hormones and chemicals, and independent activity of the arterial wall itself.

Sympathetic (adrenergic) nervous system activity, mediated by the hypothalamus, is the most important factor in regulating the caliber, and thus the blood flow, of peripheral blood vessels. Arteries are relatively abundantly innervated by the sympathetic nervous system. Stimulation of the sympathetic nerves causes vasoconstriction. The neurotransmitter responsible for sympathetic vasoconstriction is norepinephrine. Sympathetic activation occurs in response to a number of physiologic and psychological stressors. Removal of sympathetic activity, such as by drugs or sympathectomy, will result in vasodilatation.

Other hormonal substances also affect peripheral vascular resistance. *Epinephrine,* released from the adrenal medulla, acts like norepinephrine in constricting peripheral blood vessels. However, in low concentrations epinephrine causes vasodilation in skeletal muscles, the heart, and the brain. *Angiotensin,* a substance formed from the interaction of renin (synthesized in the kidney) and a circulating serum protein, stimulates arterial constriction. Although the blood concentration of angiotensin is usually small, its vasoconstrictor effects become important in certain pathophysiologic states, such as congestive heart failure and hypovolemia.

Alterations in local blood flow are influenced by a number of circulating substances that have vasoactive properties. Potent vasodilator substances include histamine, bradykinin, and certain muscle metabolites. A reduction in available oxygen and nutrients, and changes in local *p*H also affect local blood flow. Serotonin, a substance liberated from platelets that aggregate at the site of vessel wall damage, constricts arterioles. The application of heat to parts of the surface body will cause local vasodilatation, while the application of cold will cause vasoconstriction.

▷ Pathophysiology of the Vascular System

Reduced blood flow through peripheral blood vessels characterizes all peripheral vascular diseases. The physiologic effects of altered blood flow depend on the extent to which the reduced flow exceeds tissue demands for oxygen and nutrients. If tissue needs are high, even modestly reduced blood flow may be inadequate to maintain tissue integrity, and tissues become *ischemic* (deficient blood flow) and malnourished and will ultimately die if adequate blood flow is not restored.

Heart Failure.   Inadequacy of peripheral blood flow occurs whenever the heart's pumping action becomes inefficient. Left-sided heart failure causes a backup of blood into the lungs and a reduction in forward flow or cardiac output, which results in inadequate arterial blood flow to the tissues. Right-sided heart failure causes systemic venous congestion and a reduction in forward flow.

Alterations in Blood Vessels.   Intact, patent, and responsive blood vessels are also necessary for adequate delivery of oxygen to tissues and removal of metabolic wastes. Arteries can become obstructed by atherosclerotic plaque, thrombus, or emboli. Damage and subsequent obstruction of arteries follow chemical or mechanical trauma and infections or inflammatory processes. A complete arterial obstruction is associated with a greater incidence of tissue necrosis from deficient blood flow than is a partial obstruction. Likewise, a sudden arterial occlusion causes profound and frequently irreversible tissue ischemia and death. When arterial occlusions develop gradually, the opportunity for the growth of new vessels to replace occluded ones (collateral circulation) is greater.

A reduction in venous blood flow can be caused by obstruction of the vein by a thrombus, incompetent venous valves, or a reduction in the effectiveness of the pumping action of surrounding muscles. Blocking of venous blood flow results in an increase in venous pressure, a subsequent rise in capillary hydrostatic pressure, and a net filtration of fluid out of the capillaries, resulting in edema. Edematous tissues cannot receive adequate nutrition from the blood and consequently are more susceptible to breakdown or injury and to infection.

Obstruction of lymphatic vessels also results in edema. Lymphatics can become obstructed by tumor or by damage resulting from mechanical trauma or inflammatory processes.

▷ Assessment of Circulatory Insufficiency of the Extremities

Despite the variety of specific peripheral vascular diseases, all patients with these disorders experience ischemia and therefore will have some of the same symptoms. The type and severity of symptoms present depends, in part, on the type, stage, and extent of the disease process as well as the speed with which the disorder develops. The distinguishing features of arterial and venous insufficiency are presented in Table 32-2.

Pain.   A severe crampy-type pain in extremities following activity or exercise is experienced by patients with peripheral arterial insufficiency. This pain, referred to as *intermittent claudication,* is thought to be due to the accumulation of metabolites in ischemic tissues that produce muscle spasms. When the patient rests, and thereby de-

Table 32-2
Clinical Manifestations of Peripheral Vascular Disease

Arterial Insufficiency *(Embolism)*	Venous Insufficiency *(Thrombosis)*
Acute	
1. Severe, steady pain	1. Steady pain, moderate to severe
2. Cold, pallid extremity	2. Skin warm; may be mottled, pale, or cyanotic
3. Diminution or loss of sensory and motor function	3. No significant neurologic deficit
4. Absent pulsation beyond embolus	4. Pulses present or diminished
5. Veins collapsed	5. Veins full (legs slightly dependent)
6. No swelling (unless ischemia is far advanced)	6. Usually moderate to severe swelling with tenderness over veins and muscles
Chronic	
1. Intermittent claudication progressing to pain at rest with severe ischemia	1. Aching, heavy sensation, muscle cramps
2. Extremity cool, distal pulsations diminished	2. Prominent superficial veins; usually warm feet
3. Delayed healing of minor traumatic lesions	3. Pigmentation and edema, lower leg
4. Atrophy of skin with loss of hair	4. Scaling, thickening, and scarring of skin
5. Pallor—when elevated Rubor—when dependent	5. Ulceration around ankle
6. Ulceration, superficial gangrene	

(From Harvey AM (ed): The Principles and Practice of Medicine, 20th ed. New York, Appleton–Century–Crofts, 1980.)

creases the metabolic needs of the muscles, the pain goes away. The progression of the vascular disease can be monitored by documenting the amount of exercise or the distance a patient can walk before pain occurs. Pain in the extremities when the patient is resting can indicate a severe degree of arterial insufficiency or venous disease.

The site of arterial disease can be deduced from the location of claudication. Calf pain may accompany reduced blood flow through the superficial femoral artery, while pain in the thigh may result from flow obstruction in the pelvic arteries.

Changes in Skin Appearance and Temperature. Adequate blood flow warms the extremities and gives them a rosy coloring. Inadequate blood flow results in cool and pale extremities. Further reduction of blood flow to these tissues, such as would occur with extremity elevation, results in even a whiter or more blanched appearance. A reddish blue discoloration of the extremities (rubor) can also be observed and is indicative of severe peripheral arterial damage where vessels are unable to constrict and remain dilated. *Cyanosis,* a bluish coloring of the skin is manifested when the amount of oxygenated hemoglobin contained in the blood is reduced.

Additional adverse changes seen in the extremities as a result of chronically reduced nutrient supply include loss of hair, brittle nails, dry or scaling skin, atrophy, and ulcerations. Edema may be apparent either bilaterally or unilaterally. Gangrenous changes appear after prolonged severe ischemia and represent tissue death and decay.

Pulses. Determining the presence or absence, as well

as the quality, of peripheral pulses is important in assessing the status of peripheral arterial circulation (Fig. 32-2). Occlusive arterial disease impairs blood flow and can reduce or obliterate palpable pulsations in the extremities. When pulses cannot be reliably palpated, it is sometimes helpful to use a Doppler ultrasound device to detect peripheral flow.

Angiography. Anatomical information about peripheral blood vessels can be obtained through radiographic studies. The procedure involves the injection of contrast medium directly into the vascular system and visualization of the vessels as the radiopaque material flows through them. In this manner, the location of vascular obstructions or aneurysms and the presence of collateral circulation can be demonstrated. Usually, patients experience a temporary feeling of warmth as the contrast medium is injected. Local irritation at the injection site may occur. Infrequently, a patient may have an allergic reaction to the iodine contained in the contrast material. This reaction can appear immediately after the injection or can be delayed until the patient returns to his room. Manifestations may include dyspnea, nausea and vomiting, sweating, tachycardia, and numbness of the extremities. Any such reaction is reported at once. Treatment may include the administration of epinephrine (adrenalin), antihistamines, or steroids.

Patient Problems/Nursing Diagnoses

Based on the clinical manifestations, the nursing history, and the diagnostic assessment data, the patient's major nursing problems include ischemia related to reduced peripheral

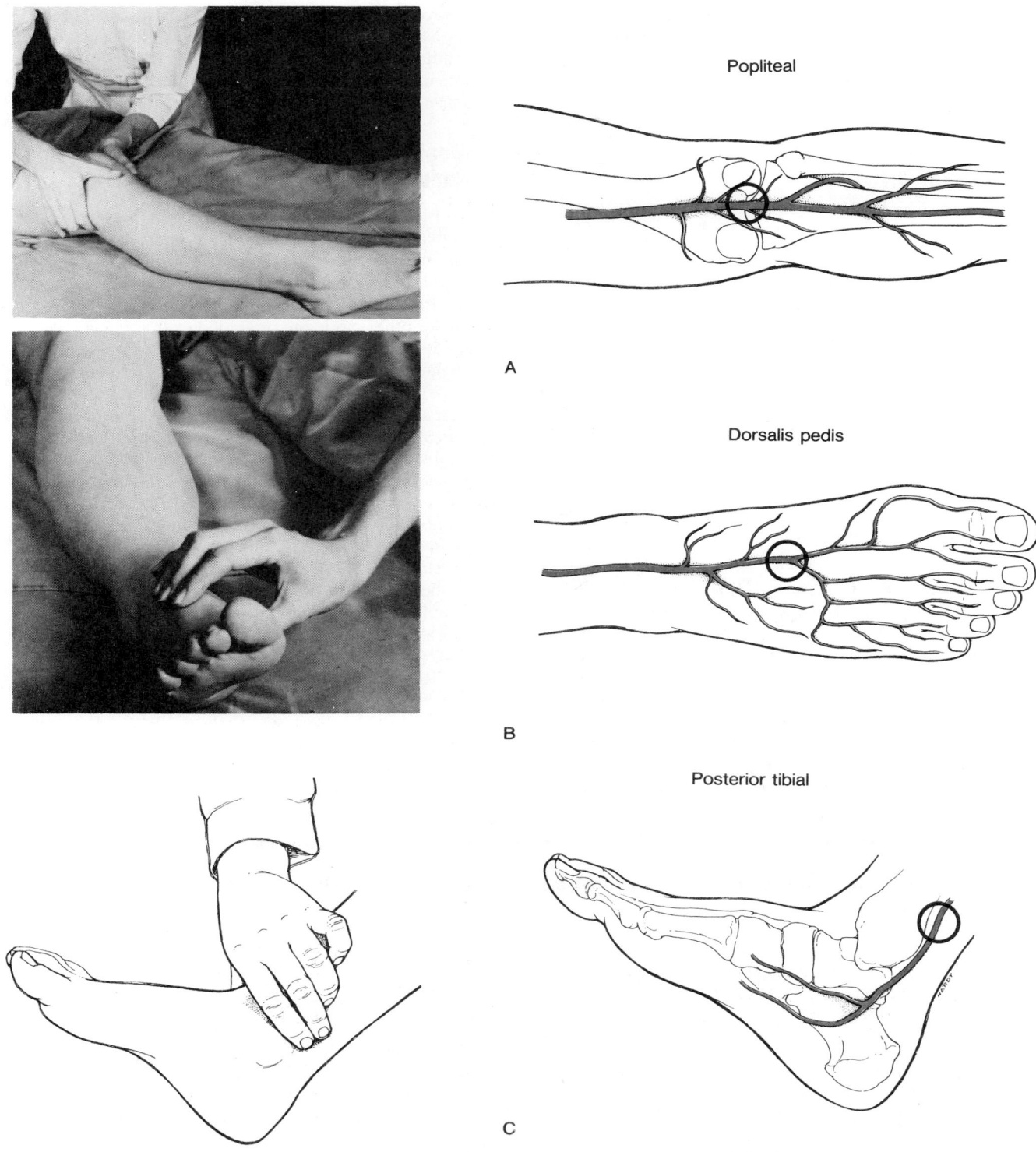

Popliteal

A

Dorsalis pedis

B

Posterior tibial

C

Figure 32-2. Assessing peripheral pulses. (*A*) Popliteal pulse. (*B*) Pedal pulse. (*C*) Posterior tibial pulse. (Photos from Ajemian S: Bypass grafting for femoral artery occlusion. American Journal of Nursing 67:565.)

blood flow; potential impairment of tissue integrity related to ischemia; and potential nonadherence to the rehabilitation program related to knowledge deficit and nonacceptance of necessary life-style changes.

▷ Planning and Nursing Implementation

Goals

The major goals of the patient include:

1. Increased arterial blood supply to the extremities
2. Decreased venous congestion
3. Promotion of vasodilatation
4. Absence of pain
5. Attainment or maintenance of tissue integrity
6. Adherence to the rehabilitation program

Measures used by the patient and members of the health care team to accomplish a single goal must be evaluated in terms of the positive as well as negative effects they may have on the simultaneous achievement of other goals. A summary of the management of patients with peripheral vascular disease is presented in Chart 32-1.

Management of the Patient With Peripheral Vascular Disease

The goals of clinical care for patients with peripheral vascular disease are determined by the major problems experienced by these patients and include (1) increasing arterial blood supply to the tissues, (2) reducing venous congestion, (3) promoting vasodilation and preventing vasoconstriction, (4) relieving pain, (5) preventing injury and infection of tissues, and (6) promoting healing. Measures

used to accomplish a single goal must be evaluated in terms of the positive as well as negative effects they may have on the simultaneous achievement of other therapeutic goals. A summary of the management of patients with peripheral vascular disease is presented in Chart 32-1.

Measures to Increase Arterial Flow and Reduce Venous Congestion

Arterial blood supply to a part can be enhanced when the part is placed below the level of the heart. For the lower extremities, this can be accomplished by elevating the head of the bed on 15-cm (6-inch) blocks or allowing the patient to assume a sitting position with his feet resting on the floor. Walking or other moderate or graded exercises may be recommended to promote blood flow by muscular exercise to encourage the development of collateral circulation. Pain can serve as a guide in determining the amount of exercise a person should engage in. The onset of pain indicates tissues are not receiving adequate oxygen, and the patient should rest before continuing activity.

In patients with venous insufficiency, placing the lower extremities in a dependent position will only worsen the venous pooling associated with this condition. The pull of gravity impedes venous return to the heart and promotes venous stasis. Therefore, individuals with venous insufficiency should elevate their legs above heart level as much as possible. When upright, these patients should avoid standing still or sitting for prolonged periods of time. Walking aids venous return by the activation of the "muscle pump." In bed, patients with venous insufficiency should have the foot of their bed elevated on blocks.

Active postural exercises, such as the *Buerger Allen exercises,* may be prescribed for the patient with circulatory disorders of the lower extremities. The routine involves placing the extremities in three positions: elevation, de-

---

Chart 32-1
Therapeutic Goals and Management of the Patient With Peripheral Vascular Problems

A. Increase arterial blood supply by:
1. Lowering the extremities below the level of the heart
2. Encouraging moderate amount of walking or graded extremity exercises
3. Engaging in active postural exercise (Buerger–Allen exercises)

B. Reduce venous congestion by:
1. Elevating extremities above heart level
2. Avoiding standing or sitting for prolonged periods
3. Walking to activate the "muscle pump"

C. Promote vasodilatation and prevent vascular compression by:
1. Maintaining warm temperature and avoiding chilling
2. Discouraging or, preferably, avoiding smoking
3. Avoiding emotional upsets and stress management
4. Avoiding constricting clothing and accessories

5. Avoiding leg crossing
6. Administering vasodilator drugs
7. Using adrenergic blocking drugs
8. Sympathectomy, as a last measure

D. Relieve pain by:
1. Promoting increased circulation
2. Administering analgesics

E. Prevent injury and infection and promote healing by:
1. Avoiding extremity trauma
2. Wearing protective shoes and padding for pressure areas
3. Attending to meticulous hygiene: bathing with neutral soaps, applying body lotions, carefully trimming nails
4. Avoiding scratching or vigorous rubbing
5. Assuring good nutrition

pendency, then horizontal. The patient lies flat in bed with both legs elevated above the heart for 2 to 3 minutes. Then, sitting on the edge of the bed with the legs relaxed and dependent, the patient exercises the feet and toes (upward and downward, inward and outward) for about 3 minutes. Finally, the patient lies flat with the legs at the same level as the heart and covered for warmth for about 5 minutes. The times for each maneuver may vary. Pain and dramatic color changes indicate the need for termination of the maneuver and rest. This routine may be repeated several times a day.

Not all patients with peripheral vascular disease should exercise. Therefore, before recommending any program to patients it is important to consult with the physician. Patients with leg ulcers, cellulitis, gangrene, or acute thrombotic occlusions require bedrest. These latter conditions can be made worse by activity.

Promotion of Vasodilatation and Prevention of Vascular Compression

Arterial dilation promotes increased blood flow to the extremities and is therefore a desirable goal in patients with peripheral arterial disease. However, in instances where the arteries are severely sclerosed, inelastic, or damaged, dilation is not possible. For this reason, measures to promote vasodilatation, such as drugs or surgery, may only be minimally effective.

Warmth promotes arterial flow by preventing chilling and thus the vasoconstriction associated with cold exposure. Adequate clothing and warm environmental temperatures protect the patient against chilling. If chilling occurs, a warm bath or drink is helpful. When heat is applied directly to ischemic extremities, the temperature of the heat source should not exceed body temperature. Burn injuries can occur at lower temperatures in ischemic extremities as compared to normal limbs. In addition, excess heat may exacerbate the metabolic rate of the extremities and increase the need for oxygen, which cannot be met by the reduced arterial flow through the diseased artery. Therefore, patients are instructed to test the temperature of bath water, hot water bottles, or heating pads before using them, or to avoid them altogether. Application of a heating pad to the abdomen can cause reflex vasodilatation in the extremities and is safer than direct application to affected extremities.

Nicotine causes vasospasm and can thereby dramatically reduce circulation to the extremities. Patients with arterial insufficiency who smoke must be fully informed of the circulatory consequences of this habit and be encouraged to stop completely. Emotional upsets stimulate the sympathetic nervous system, which results in peripheral vasoconstriction. Although emotional stress is unavoidable, it can be minimized to some degree by environmental manipulation and a consistent stress management program. Emotionally charged situations should be avoided. Counseling services or relaxation training may be indicated by individuals unable to cope effectively with situational stressors.

Constricting clothing and accessories such as garters, belts, girdles, and shoe laces will impede circulation to the extremities and promote venous stasis and therefore should be avoided. Likewise, leg crossing should be discouraged since it compresses vessels in the legs.

Relief of Pain

Frequently, the pain associated with peripheral vascular disease is chronic and continuous. It limits activities, affects work and responsibilities, disturbs sleep, and alters one's sense of well-being and optimism. Because of this, patients are often depressed, irritable, and unable to exert the energy necessary to execute prescribed therapies. The latter makes it more difficult to alleviate pain since the best means to do so is through the institution of measures that augment circulation. Analgesics can be helpful in reducing pain to the point where the patient may be more able to participate in the therapies that will increase circulation and ultimately relieve pain more effectively.

Prevention of Tissue Damage and Promotion of Healing

Poorly nourished tissues are more susceptible to damage and bacterial invasion. When lesions develop, healing may be delayed or inhibited owing to the poor blood supply to the area. Infected, nonhealing ulcerations of the extremities can be very debilitating, requiring prolonged, often expensive hospitalization and treatments. Amputation of the extremity may eventually be necessary. Thus, measures to prevent these complications should be of high priority and vigorously implemented.

Trauma to the extremities should be avoided. Sturdy, well-fitting shoes or slippers will prevent foot injuries and blisters. The use of neutral soaps and body lotions prevent drying and cracking of skin. Scratching and vigorous rubbing can abrade skin and create a site for bacterial invasion. Finger and toenails should be carefully trimmed straight across. Protective padding over corns and calluses will prevent breakdown and alleviate pressure. All signs of blisters, ingrown toenails, infection, or other problems should be reported to the health care professionals for treatment and follow-up. Individuals with diminished vision may require assistance in periodically examining the lower extremities for trauma.

Good nutrition will promote healing and prevent tissue breakdown and is included in the overall preventive program for individuals with peripheral vascular disease. Vitamins B and C and adequate protein are necessary. Obesity strains the heart, increases venous congestion, and reduces circulation. A diet low in lipids may be indicated for patients with atherosclerosis, and the physician and dietitian should be consulted.

▷ Evaluation

Expected Outcomes

1. Increases arterial blood supply to extremities
   a. Exhibits extremities warm to touch
   b. Has improved color of extremities (is free of rubor or cyanosis)

   c. Is free of muscle pain with exercise

   d. Demonstrates palpable peripheral pulses

2. Decreases venous congestion

   a. Elevates lower extremities as prescribed

   b. Avoids prolonged standing or sitting

   c. Decreased edema of extremities

3. Promotes vasodilatation

   a. Protects extremities from exposure to cold

   b. Does not smoke

   c. Uses stress management program to minimize emotional upset

   d. Avoids constricting clothing and appliances (*e.g.,* tight seat belts)

   e. Avoids leg-crossing

4. Is free of pain

   a. Utilizes measures to increase arterial blood supply to extremities

   b. Utilizes analgesics as prescribed

5. Attains/maintains tissue integrity

   a. Inspects skin daily for evidence of traumatic injury

   b. Avoids trauma and irritation to skin

   c. Wears protective shoes

   d. Adheres to meticulous hygienic regimen

   e. Eats well-balanced diet that contains adequate protein and vitamins B and C

6. Adheres to the rehabilitation program

   a. Practices frequent position changes as prescribed by physician

   b. Practices postural exercises as prescribed by physician

   c. Takes medications as prescribed

   d. Avoids vasoconstrictors (*e.g.,* clothing, smoking, leg-crossing)

   e. Utilizes measures to prevent trauma

   f. Utilizes stress management program

   g. Accepts condition as chronic but amenable to therapies that will decrease symptomatology

▷ Diseases of the Arteries

Arteriosclerosis and Atherosclerosis

Arteriosclerosis is the most common disease of the arteries; it literally means "hardening of the arteries." It is a diffuse process characterized by fibromuscular or endothelial thickening of the walls of small arteries and arterioles. Atherosclerosis refers to a generalized process characterized by focal changes in the intima of arteries. These changes consist of the accumulation of lipids, calcium, blood components, carbohydrates, and fibrous tissue (atheroma or plaque). Although the pathologic processes of arteriosclerosis and atherosclerosis differ, rarely does one occur without the other, and thus the terms are used interchangeably. Since atherosclerosis is a generalized disease of the arteries, when it is present in the extremities it is usually present elsewhere in the body.

Pathophysiology and Etiology. The most common direct result of atherosclerosis in arteries include narrowing (stenosis) of the lumen, obstruction by thrombosis, aneurysm development, and rupture. Its indirect results are malnutrition and the subsequent fibrosis of the organs that the sclerotic arteries supply with blood. All actively functioning tissue cells require an abundant supply of nutrients and oxygen and are sensitive to any reduction in their supply. If such reductions are severe and permanent, these cells undergo ischemic necrosis and are replaced by fibrous tissue, which requires much less nutrition.

Atherosclerosis primarily affects the main arteries throughout the entire arterial tree in varying degrees, usually in a patchy manner. Branch arteries are affected usually only at their bifurcation.

There are many theories that attempt to explain why and how atherosclerosis develops. However, none of these viewpoints are entirely conclusive, and it may be that there is not a single cause or mechanism for the development of atherosclerosis, but rather that multiple processes are involved.

Morphologically, atherosclerotic lesions are of three types: fatty streaks, fibrous plaque, and complicated lesions. *Fatty streaks* are yellow and smooth, protrude slightly into the lumen of the artery, and are composed of lipids, primarily cholesterol. These lesions have been found in the arteries of persons of all age groups, including infants. It is not clear whether fatty streaks predispose the formation of fibrous plaques nor if they are reversible. They do not usually cause clinical symptoms.

The *fibrous plaque* characteristic of atherosclerosis is composed of smooth muscle cells, collagen fibers, plasma components, and lipids. It is yellowish gray and protrudes to varying degrees into the arterial lumen, at times completely obstructing it. This plaque is believed to be an irreversible lesion.

The *complicated* atherosclerotic lesion is almost always associated with complete occlusion of the artery with subsequent ischemia or infarction of the organ served by the involved vessel. In this lesion, fibrous plaque becomes calcified and ruptures. There is hemorrhage into the plaque or thrombus development (Fig. 32-3).

Gradual narrowing of the arterial lumen as the disease process progresses stimulates the development of collateral circulation (Fig. 32-4). While this vascular "bypass" allows continued perfusion to the tissues beyond the arterial obstruction, it is often inadequate to meet imposed metabolic demands, and ischemia results.

Clinical Manifestations. The clinical symptoms and signs resulting from the atherosclerotic process depend on the organ or tissue affected. Coronary atherosclerosis (heart disease), angina pectoris, and acute myocardial infarction are discussed on pages 626–635. Cerebrovascular disease, including transient cerebral ischemic attacks and stroke, are discussed on pages 1307–1311. For atherosclerosis of the aorta including aneurysm, see page 672. Atherosclerotic lesions of the extremities are discussed below.

Risk Factors. Many factors are associated with the development of atherosclerosis. These factors have been determined from systematic observations of relationships between the development of atherosclerosis and certain characteristics. While it is not completely clear whether modification of these risk factors will prevent the devel-

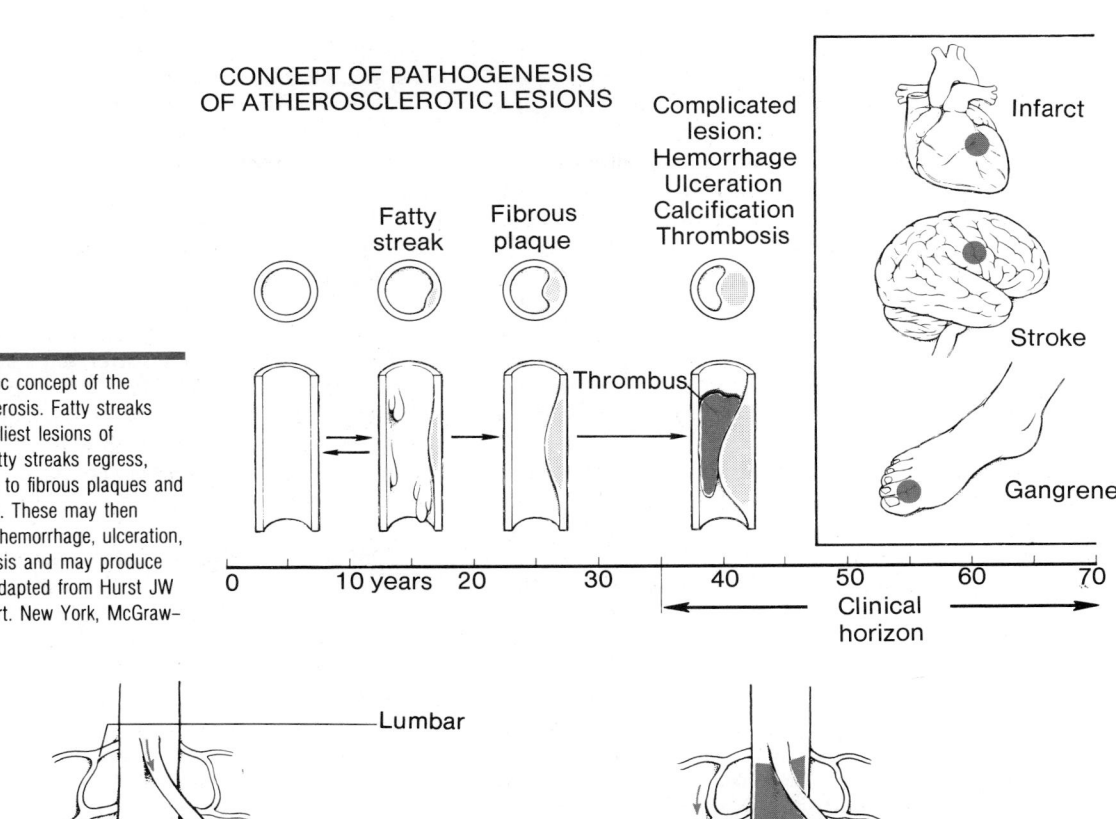

CONCEPT OF PATHOGENESIS
OF ATHEROSCLEROTIC LESIONS

Figure 32-3. Schematic concept of the progression of atherosclerosis. Fatty streaks constitute one of the earliest lesions of atherosclerosis. Many fatty streaks regress, whereas others progress to fibrous plaques and eventually to atheromata. These may then become complicated by hemorrhage, ulceration, calcification, or thrombosis and may produce myocardial infarction. (Adapted from Hurst JW and Logue RB: The Heart. New York, McGraw–Hill.)

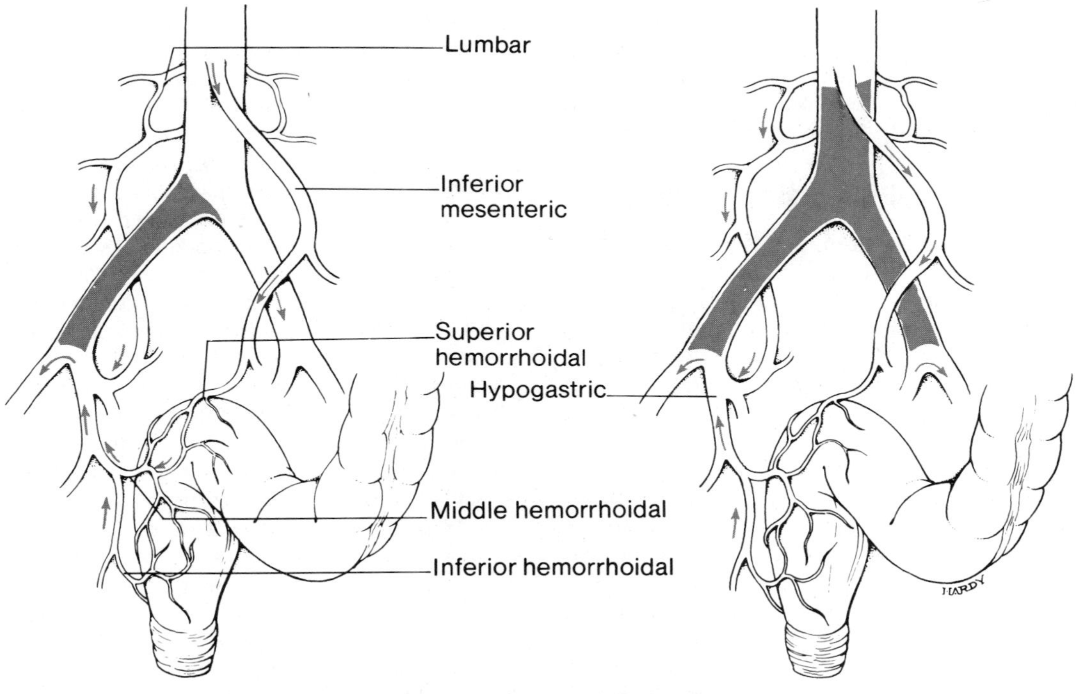

Figure 32-4. Development of collateral channels in response to occlusion of the right common iliac artery and the terminal aortic bifurcation.

opment of cardiovascular disease, there is evidence that the process may be slowed by doing so. Some risk factors, those that are genetically determined, are unavoidable. However, it is believed that genetic factors can be influenced by alteration of other risk factors and thereby can indirectly be modified.

A diet high in fat has been strongly implicated in the causation of atherosclerosis. Approximately 39% of the cal-

ories Americans ingest are derived from fats. Fats are classified according to their chemical structure as *saturated* or *unsaturated*. Saturated fats include fats of animal origin, such as those in meat, milk, butter, and eggs, and also solid vegetable oils. The intake of primarily saturated fats is positively correlated with the elevation of serum cholesterol and triglycerides and with the development of atherosclerotic cardiovascular disease. Serum triglycerides are also found to be elevated in diets high in refined carbohydrates (sugar). On the other hand, unsaturated fats, such as corn oil, cottonseed oil, safflower oil, and the fats in fish, may be capable of reducing blood cholesterol and triglyceride levels. Based on these findings, the American Heart Association recommends that, in order to reduce the risk of cardiovascular disease, individuals should reduce the total amount of fat ingested in the diet and substitute unsaturated fats for the saturated.

Certain drugs are now being used to reduce blood lipid levels in conjunction with dietary modification. Among these are clofibrate, cholestyramine, dextrothyroxine, and large doses of nicotinic acid. Clofibrate is the only lipid-lowering drug in common use in clinical practice. Side-effects continue to be studied.

Other risk factors include cigarette smoking, sedentary activity patterns, emotional stress, obesity, and hormones, particularly estrogen. The presence of hypertension or diabetes seems to accelerate the atherosclerotic process. In addition, many other factors, such as caffeine and alcohol, may contribute in a minor way to the development of the disease.

Despite the fact that no single risk factor has been identified as the major contributor to the development of atherosclerotic cardiovascular disease, it is clear that the greater the number of risk factors, the greater the likelihood of developing the disease. Therefore, the elimination of combined risk factors should be strongly emphasized.

Peripheral Arterial Occlusive Disease

Arterial insufficiency of the extremities is usually found in individuals over 50 years of age and predominantly in the lower extremities. Consequently, the age of onset and severity are influenced by the type and number of atherosclerotic risk factors present. Obstructive lesions are predominantly confined to segments of the arterial system extending from the aorta, below the renal arteries, to the popliteal artery (Fig. 32-5).

Clinical Manifestations. The hallmark and only specific symptom of peripheral arterial insufficiency is *intermittent claudication,* that is, pain or discomfort in the legs (calf, thigh) occurring with exercise and terminating with rest. This pain is insidious in onset and is produced by muscle hypoxia and the accumulation of metabolites. One of the diagnostic features of intermittent claudication is that the amount of activity that produces claudication in an individual on one occasion will produce it again on repeated occasions.

A feeling of coldness or numbness in the extremities may accompany intermittent claudication and is a result of the reduced arterial flow. Upon examination, the extremities may be cool and exhibit pallor on elevation or a ruddy, cyanotic color with dependency. Skin and nail changes, ulcerations, gangrene, and muscle atrophy may be evident. Bruits may be auscultated with a stethoscope (a bruit is the sound produced by turbulent flow of blood through an irregular, stenotic lumen or through a dilated [aneurysm] segment of the vessel). Peripheral pulses may be diminished or absent. The examination of the peripheral pulses is an important part of the examination for arterial occlusive disease and should include the femoral, popliteal, posterior tibialis, and pedal pulses.

Inequality of pulses between extremities or the absence of a normally palpable pulse is a reliable sign of occlusion. The femoral pulse in the groin and the posterior tibialis pulse behind the medial malleolus are most easily found. The popliteal pulse is sometimes difficult to palpate behind the knee in the obese patient, and the pedal artery varies in location on the dorsum of the foot and is normally absent in about 7% of the population (see Fig. 32-2).

Patients with peripheral arterial insufficiency may eventually develop *rest pain,* which is indicative of a severe obstruction of blood flow. The pain is persistent, aching, or boring and is usually present in the distal extremities. Elevation or horizontal placement of the extremity will aggravate the pain, while dependency of the extremity will reduce the pain.

Assessment. The presence, anatomical location, and physiologic extent of arterial occlusive disease are determined by a careful history of the patient's symptoms and physical examination. Observations of extremity color and temperature are made and pulses palpated. The nails may be thickened and opaque, and the skin shiny, atrophic, and dry with sparse hair growth. Arteriography is used to confirm the diagnosis if surgery is contemplated. To determine the qualitative and quantitative aspects of the problem, Doppler ultrasonic flow studies can be done.

The Doppler is an electronic stethoscope through which blood flow can be heard, even at times when pulses are not palpable. In addition, lower extremity blood pressure measurements can be obtained by coupling the Doppler with a standard pneumatic cuff. When comparing leg blood pressures with arm pressures, the patient with arterial occlusive disease of the lower extremities may demonstrate pressure in the legs lower than that in the arms. Additional diagnostic tests for evaluating peripheral arterial occlusive disease include *oscillometry* to measure alterations in pulse volume at different levels of the extremity; an *exercise test* to determine the amount of activity possible prior to the onset of intermittent claudication; *plethysmography,* which monitors changes in the pulse and leg size with each heartbeat; and a *lumbar sympathetic block.* This latter test, used to evaluate peripheral circulation, involves injection of a local anesthetic into the lumbar epidural space to block the sympathetic nerves that go to the legs. Since the sympathetic nerves control the tension in the muscles of the blood vessels, a block of these nerves should produce vasodilation and increased temperature in the legs if the vessels are normal. Atherosclerotic vessels are incapable of vasodilation; hence there is either no increase in temperature in the legs or only a slight one. This test is often used to determine whether or not sympathectomy would be of benefit to the patient with impaired circulation of the legs.

Digital subtraction angiography (DSA) is a radiologic visualization of arterial vessels utilizing computer technology. Usually, angiography requires hospital admission the day before the test and 24 hours after the test. In addition, there are risks of vessel injury and possibly stroke. With DSA no hospitalization is necessary and the risks are less.

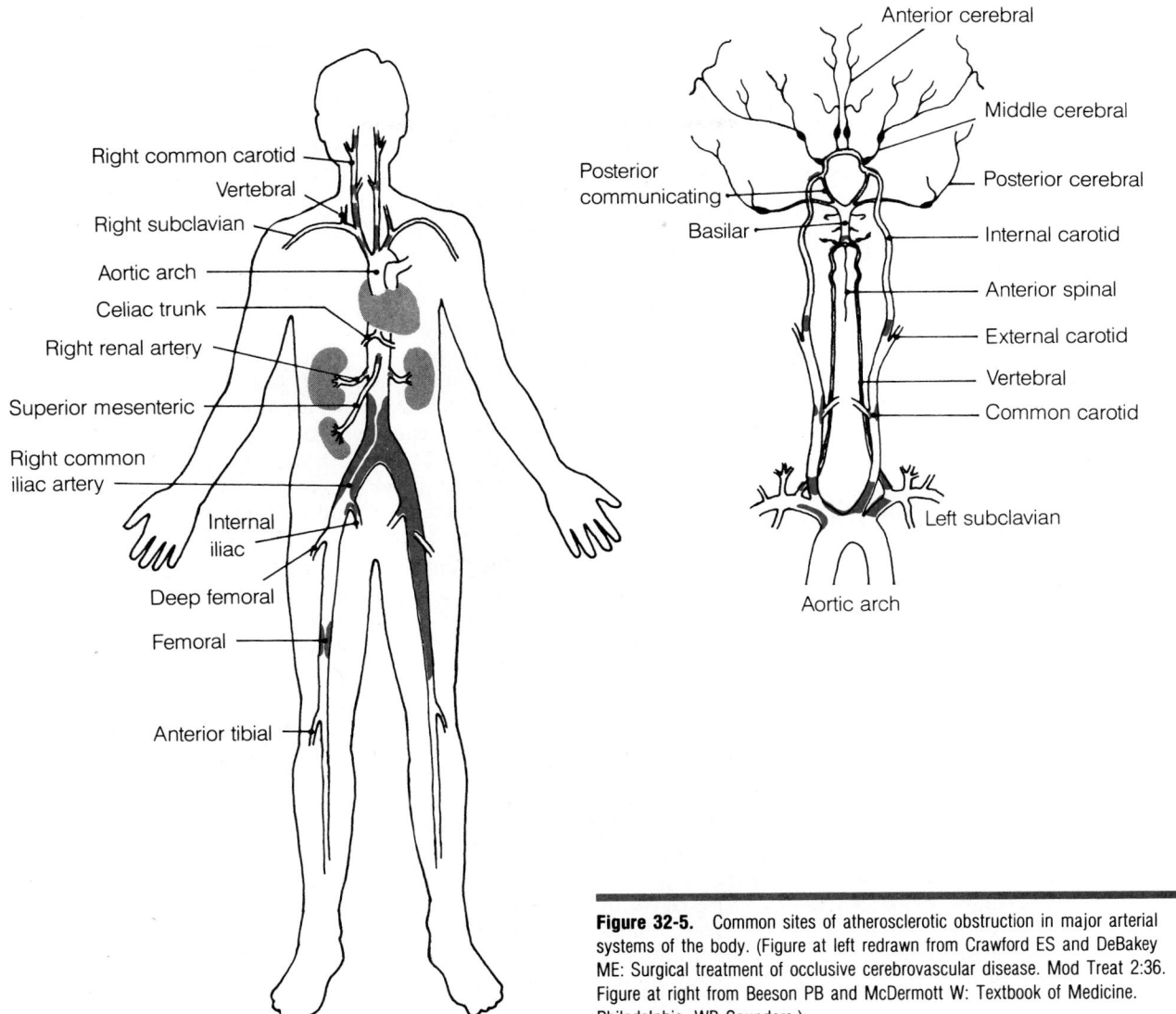

Figure 32-5. Common sites of atherosclerotic obstruction in major arterial systems of the body. (Figure at left redrawn from Crawford ES and DeBakey ME: Surgical treatment of occlusive cerebrovascular disease. Mod Treat 2:36. Figure at right from Beeson PB and McDermott W: Textbook of Medicine. Philadelphia, WB Saunders.)

The patient is not to eat for 2 hours prior to the test; he is requested to hold his breath at the appropriate time and to be still in the supine position on the radiographic table.

Usually, the brachial artery is selected for lidocaine local injection; a small nick is made through which a 16-gauge Angiocath is threaded toward the superior vena cava. Contrast medium is injected when the radiologist has positioned the patient under fluoroscopy for adequate exposure of the desired site. By the use of an image-intensifier video system, vessels are displayed on a TV monitor. By computer, those images not required are subtracted so that the final intense image of the desired area is heightened. The study takes about 30 to 40 minutes; upon completion, the catheter is removed. Pressure is applied to the nick site for several minutes, and thereafter the patient is instructed to increase fluid intake to about 2000 ml in the subsequent 24 hours in order to encourage excretion of the contrast medium. The rare side-effect is an allergic reaction to the iodine in the contrast medium.

Treatment.   The general care measures for patients with peripheral arterial disorders were described earlier in this chapter and are summarized in Chart 32-1. Generally, patients feel better on some type of exercise program. Often, if this program is combined with weight reduction and the cessation of smoking, patients can improve their activity limitations.

In some instances, *sympathectomy* may be beneficial to improve collateral circulation in patients with intermittent claudication. Excision of sympathetic ganglia will release arteriolar constriction and improve peripheral blood flow. In other patients, when intermittent claudication has become gravely disabling, vascular *grafting* or *endarterectomy* may be helpful. In the former procedure, either the diseased segment of artery is removed and a synthetic graft inserted in place of it, or the obstructed segment is left intact and instead "bypassed" by use of a graft. Material used for arterial bypass grafts may be synthetic (*e.g.,* Dacron, Teflon) or autogenous vein grafts (*e.g.,* saphenous vein). When an endarterectomy is performed, the atheromatous obstruction is "shelled out" through an incision into the artery. The artery is then sutured closed to restore vascular integrity.

Nursing Assessment and Interventions. The primary objective in postoperative management of patients who have had these vascular procedures is to maintain adequate circulation through the arterial repair. Extremity pulses should be checked and recorded frequently. Disappearance of a pulse may indicate thrombotic occlusion of the graft, and the surgeon is immediately notified. The color and temperature of the extremity is also monitored and any changes reported. An adequate circulating blood volume should be established and maintained. Continuous monitoring of urine output, central venous pressure, mental status, and pulse rate and volume will permit early recognition and treatment of fluid imbalances. Leg crossing and prolonged extremity dependency should be avoided in order to prevent thrombosis. Leg elevation will reduce edema.

Thromboangiitis Obliterans (Buerger's Disease)

Buerger's disease is characterized by recurring inflammation in the arteries and veins of the lower and upper extremities, and results in thrombus formation and occlusion of the vessels. It is differentiated from other vessel diseases by its microscopic appearance. In contrast to atherosclerosis, Buerger's disease has no lipid aggregates in the intimal coat, has more changes in the adventitia, and results in a thrombosis that contains many more cells. The disease begins in the small arteries and later progresses to the larger vessels. Although this condition is different from atherosclerosis, in older patients, atherosclerosis of the larger vessels may occur following involvement of the smaller vessels.

Etiology and Clinical Manifestations. The cause of Buerger's disease is unknown. It occurs most often in men between the ages of 20 and 35, and it has been reported in all races in many areas of the world. There is considerable evidence that heavy smoking is either an etiologic or aggravating factor. Generally, the lower extremities are affected, but arteries of the upper extremities or viscera are also commonly involved. Superficial thrombophlebitis may be present. Arteriography confirms arterial occlusive disease.

Pain is the outstanding symptom of Buerger's disease. The patient complains of cramps in the feet or legs after exercise (intermittent claudication), which are relieved by inactivity; often there is considerable burning pain that is aggravated by emotional disturbances, smoking, or chilling. Rest pain in the digits, a feeling of coldness, or a sensitivity to cold may be early symptoms. Various types of paresthesias may develop, and pulses may be diminished or absent.

As the disease progresses, definite redness or cyanosis of the part appears when it is dependent. Color changes may affect only one extremity or only certain digits or certain parts of a digit. Ulceration with gangrene may occur.

Management and Nursing Interventions. The treatment of Buerger's disease is essentially the same as that for atherosclerotic peripheral vascular disease. The main ob-

jectives are to improve circulation to the extremities, prevent the spread of the disease, and protect the extremities from trauma and infection. The continuation of smoking is highly detrimental, and patients are advised to stop completely.

Rest, adequate hydration, and scrupulous attention to cleanliness are essential. Daily washing of the feet with bland soap and warm water is desirable. Circumstances predisposing to extremity trauma and infection must be strictly avoided. Shoes and stockings must be fitted accurately, and the feet must be protected adequately from cold. Caustic antiseptics, such as iodine or phenol and its derivatives, should not be applied to the feet if the peripheral circulation is inadequate.

Vasodilators are rarely prescribed, because these drugs only cause dilatation of healthy vessels; therefore, vasodilators may even divert blood away from the partially occluded vessels, which makes the situation worse. Regional sympathetic block or ganglionectomy may be useful in some instances to produce vasodilatation and thereby increase blood flow.

Prognosis. If gangrene of a toe develops as a result of arterial occlusive disease in the leg, it is unlikely that toe amputation or even a transmetatarsal amputation will succeed. Usually a below-knee amputation, or occasionally an above-knee amputation, is necessary. The indications for amputation are worsening gangrene, especially if moist; severe rest pain; or sepsis secondary to gangrene. If any of these are present in a situation where bypass surgery is not feasible, then amputation becomes necessary.

Aortic Diseases

The aorta is the main trunk of the arterial system and is divided into the ascending aorta (5 cm [2 inches] contained in the pericardium), the aortic arch (extending upward, backward, and downward), and the descending aorta. The entire aorta is designated as thoracic above the diaphragm and abdominal below the diaphragm.

Aortitis

Aortitis is inflammation of the aorta, particularly of the aortic arch. Two types are known to occur: Takayasu's disease and syphilitic aortitis. Takayasu's disease, or occlusive thromboaortopathy, is uncommon; syphilitic aortitis is almost never seen today.

Takayasu's Disease. Takayasu's disease is a chronic inflammatory disease of the aortic arch and its branches seen primarily in young or middle-aged females. It results in ischemic symptoms affecting the upper extremity, brain, and eyes. In the early stages, it may respond to corticosteroids.

Syphilitic Aortitis. Syphilitic aortitis, unlike the arteriosclerotic type, usually begins before the age of 50. It starts at the root of the aorta and spreads in the form of a few discrete patches scattered over an otherwise normal intima. In most cases, the inflammatory process produces moderate dilatation of the aorta, but can produce more serious complications, such as aortic insufficiency, aneurysm, or occlusion of the coronary ostia. Symptoms experienced by patients include sensations of substernal oppression or weight, viselike feelings of constriction of the chest, or attacks of agonizing pain. Sudden, short attacks of dyspnea may also occur.

Aortic Aneurysms

Classification of Aneurysms.   An *aneurysm* is a localized sac or dilatation of an artery formed at a weak point in the vessel wall (Fig. 32-6). Very small aneurysms owing to local infection are designated as *mycotic aneurysms*. An aneurysm that is somewhat larger but still limited in extent, projecting from one side of the vessel only, is called a *saccular aneurysm*. If an entire arterial segment becomes dilated, a *fusiform aneurysm* develops. Aneurysms are serious since rupture is always a possible event, leading to hemorrhage and death.

The most common cause of aneurysm is atherosclerosis. However, wall trauma, infection (pyogenic or syphilitic), and congenital defects of the artery wall also give rise to the development of aneurysms.

Aneurysm of the Thoracic Aorta

Approximately 85% of all cases of thoracic aortic aneurysm are caused by atherosclerosis. They most frequently occur in men between the ages of 40 and 70. The thoracic area is the most common site for the development of a dissecting aneurysm. About one third of patients with thoracic aneurysms die from rupture.

Clinical Manifestations.   Symptoms are variable and depend on how rapidly the aneurysm dilates and how the pulsating mass affects surrounding intrathoracic structures. Most are asymptomatic. Pain usually is the most prominent symptom. It is usually constant and boring in character and may only be perceived when the individual is lying in a supine position. Other conspicuous symptoms are *dyspnea,* the result of the pressure of the sac against the trachea, a main bronchus, or the lung itself; *cough,* frequently paroxysmal and with a brassy quality ("goose cough"); *hoarseness,* stridor, weakness of the voice, or complete aphonia (manifestations of pressure against the left recurrent laryngeal nerve); and *dysphagia,* owing to impingement on the esophagus.

Dilated superficial veins on the chest, the neck, or the arms; edematous areas on the chest wall; and cyanosis are often evident when large veins in the chest are compressed by the aneurysm. The pupils of the eyes may be unequal because of pressure against the cervical sympathetic chain. Diagnostic evaluation of a thoracic aortic aneurysm is principally by roentgenoscopy.

Management.   Whether medical or surgical treatment is selected to treat thoracic aortic aneurysms depends on the type of aneurysm present. The goal of surgery is to remove the aneurysm and restore vascular continuity, using a vascular graft (Fig. 32-7). Intensive monitoring is usually required after this type of surgery, and the patient is placed in the critical care unit.

Medical management of the patient involves, in part, strict control of arterial blood pressure and a reduction in pulsatile aortic flow. Systolic pressure is maintained around 100 mm Hg to 120 mm Hg with antihypertensive drugs (*e.g.,*

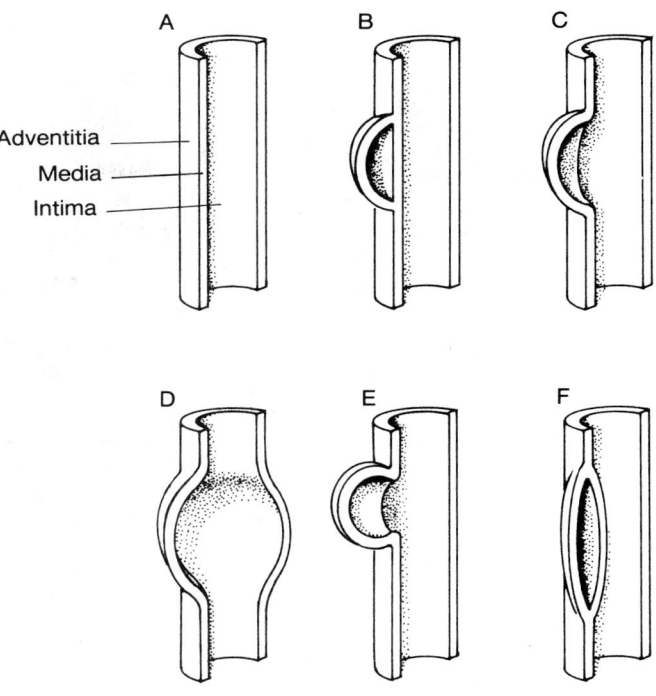

Figure 32-6.   Characteristics of arterial aneurysm. (*A*) Normal artery. (*B*) False aneurysm—actually a pulsating hematoma. The clot and connective tissue are outside the arterial wall. (*C*) True aneurysm. One, two, or all three layers may be involved. (*D*) Fusiform aneurysm—symmetrical, spindle-shaped expansion of entire circumference of involved vessel. (*E*) Saccular aneurysm—a bulbous protrusion of one side of the arterial wall. (*F*) Dissecting aneurysm—this usually is a hematoma that splits the layers of the arterial wall.

reserpine, guanethidine). Pulsatile flow is reduced by medications that reduce cardiac contractility (*e.g.,* propranolol).

Abdominal Aortic Aneurysm

The most common cause of abdominal aortic aneurysm is atherosclerosis; syphilis is present in less than 1% of patients. Four times more men than women are affected and the condition is most prevalent after age 60. Most of these aneurysms occur below the renal arteries. Untreated, the eventual outcome may be rupture and death.

Pathophysiology.   The factor common to all aneurysms is a damaged media in the vessel. This may be caused by congenital weakness, trauma, or disease process. Once an aneurysm develops, the tendency is toward an increase in size.

Clinical Manifestations and Diagnosis.   About two fifths of patients with abdominal aortic aneurysms have symptoms; the remainder are asymptomatic. Some patients complain that they can feel their "heart beating" in their abdomen when lying down. The most common symptom is *abdominal pain,* which may be persistent or intermittent and is often localized in the middle or lower abdomen to the left of the midline. The next most common symptom is *low back pain.* This is a serious symptom that usually signifies rapid expansion or impending rupture of the aneurysm. Less frequently, the patient complains of feeling an abdominal mass or abdominal throbbing. More than half of

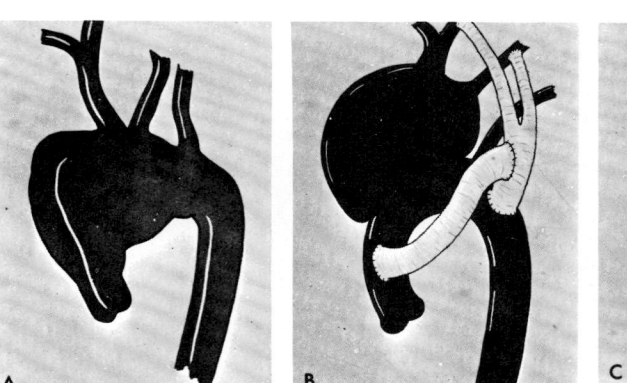
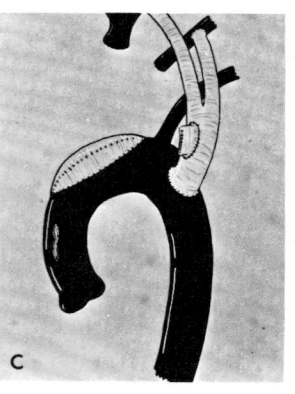
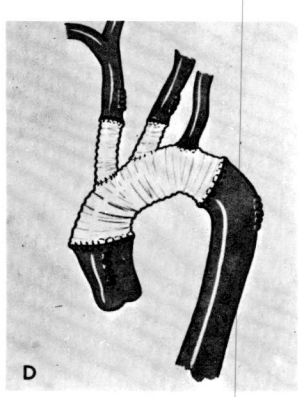

Figure 32-7. (*A*) Location and extent of aortic aneurysm. (*B*) Method of treatment utilizing temporary bypass graft to maintain normal aortic circulation during excision of aneurysm. (*C*) Completed procedure with patch graft angioplasty to repair excised segment of aortic arch and conversion of temporary bypass graft to innominate and left common carotid arteries into the permanent graft. (*D*) Temporary bypass grafts used to maintain normal aortic circulation during excision and graft replacement of aneurysm have been completely removed, and aortic graft has been inserted. (From DeBakey ME: Changing concepts in vascular surgery. Figs 12B, 12E, 13C and 13D, J Cardiovasc Surg 1:3–44.)

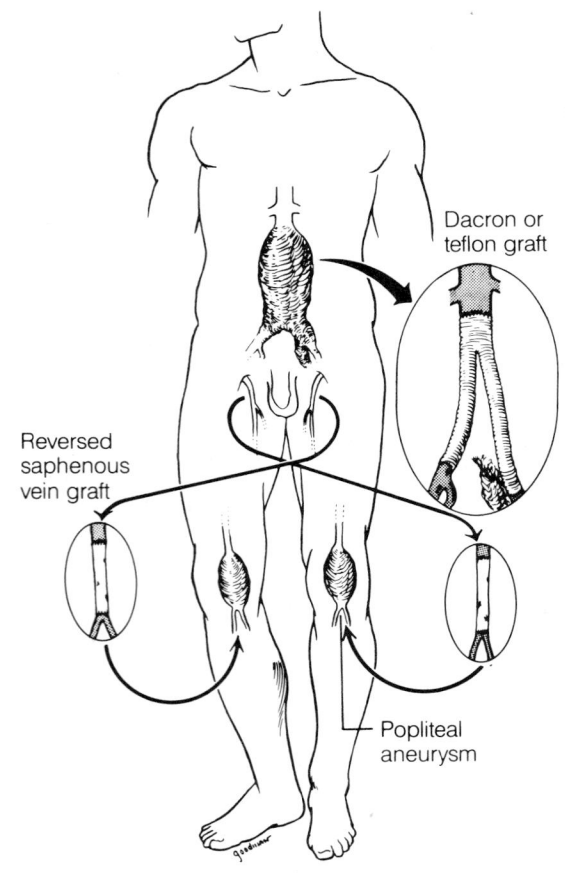

Figure 32-8. Surgical treatment of a patient who had a large abdominal aneurysm involving the iliac arteries plus bilateral symptomatic popliteal aneurysms. These were resected and the abdominal aneurysm was replaced with a Teflon graft. The popliteal aneurysms were replaced by saphenous vein grafts, which appear to function much better at the flexion crease than the synthetic graft. (Hardy JD et al: Aneurysms of the popliteal artery. By permission of Surgery, Gynecology, & Obstetrics, Mar 1975, 140:402.)

these patients exhibit hypertension. An interesting finding is the comparison of blood pressure readings of the thigh and arm. Ordinarily, the systolic blood pressure of the thigh exceeds that of the arm by 15 mm Hg or more. In about three quarters of patients with abdominal aortic aneurysm, the systolic pressure in the thigh is abnormally low in comparison with that in the arm.

A most important diagnostic indication of this type of aneurysm is the presence of a pulsatile abdominal mass. A systolic bruit may be heard over the mass. Confirmation of the aneurysm by abdominal x-ray is possible if the aneurysm is calcified. An abdominal aortogram, ultrasonography, or digital subtraction angiography (DSA) may also be used to define and confirm the presence of the aneurysm.

Management. The likelihood of rupture is significant in patients with an expanding or enlarging abdominal aneurysm. Consequently, surgery is the treatment of choice for abdominal aneurysms greater than 5 cm (2 inches) in diameter or those that are enlarging. This involves resection of the aneurysm and insertion of a bypass (synthetic) graft (Fig. 32-8). Although this is a major operation, elective aneurysm has been reported to have a mortality rate of 5%.

Preoperatively, nursing assessment should be guided by the fact that the aneurysm might rupture, and by the recognition that the patient may have cardiovascular, cerebral, and pulmonary impairment secondary to atherosclerosis. Therefore, the functional capacity of all organ systems should be established. Medical therapies designed to stabilize physiologic function should be promptly implemented. Postoperative care requires intense monitoring of pulmonary, cardiovascular, renal, and neurologic status. After the acute recovery phase, an exercise schedule may be prescribed. Prolonged sitting should be avoided.

Signs of a rupturing abdominal aortic aneurysm include a constant intense back pain, falling blood pressure, decreasing red cell count and increasing white count, plus a soft abdomen. Following a retroperitoneal rupture of an aneurysm, hematomas have been noticed in the scrotum, perineum, or penis. Signs of heart failure or loud bruit may suggest a rupture into the vena cava. Rupture into the peritoneal cavity is rapidly fatal. The overall surgical mortality rate for a ruptured aneurysm is 50% to 75%.

Dissecting Aneurysm of the Aorta

Pathophysiology.   Occasionally, an aorta diseased by arteriosclerosis develops an intimal tear owing to a type of medial degeneration. This entity, which is often associated with hypertension, is three times more common in men than in women and occurs in the age group between 40 and 70. Dissecting aneurysms are extremely dangerous, resulting in death if untreated.

The intimal tear permits blood to dissect its way into the substance of the aortic wall. The result is the formation of a large hematoma in the arterial wall, which may extend for a considerable distance, producing severe and persistent pain. Death is most frequently caused by external rupture of the hematoma.

Clinical Manifestations and Assessment.   The process of dissection leads to shearing and occlusion of the arteries branching from the aorta in the area involved by the process. The tear occurs most commonly in the region of the aortic arch. The dissection of the aorta may progress backward in the direction of the heart, obstructing the opening to the coronary arteries or producing hemopericardium or aortic insufficiency, or it may extend in the opposite direction, causing occlusion of the arteries supplying the gastrointestinal tract, the kidneys, the spinal cord, and even the legs.

The onset of symptoms is usually sudden. Severe and persistent pain, described as "tearing" or "ripping," may be reported in the anterior chest or below the scapulae posteriorly. The patient may manifest pallor, sweating, and tachycardia. Blood pressure may be elevated, unobtainable, or markedly different from one arm to the other. Other symptoms are variable depending on the location and extensiveness of the dissection. Because of the variable clinical picture associated with this condition, early diagnosis is often difficult. Aortography and ultrasound aid in the diagnosis. Medical or surgical treatment of aneurysm again depends on the type present and follows the same general principles as outlined for treatment of thoracic aortic aneurysms (see p. 673).

Other Aneurysms

Aneurysms may also arise in the peripheral vessels, most often as a result of atherosclerosis. These may involve such vessels as the renal artery, the subclavian artery, or (most frequently) the popliteal artery, in the area of the knee. Such aneurysms may be bilateral.

The aneurysm produces a pulsating mass and a disturbance of peripheral circulation distal to it. Pain and swelling develop because of pressure on adjacent nerves and veins. Surgical repair of such aneurysms is now carried out with replacement grafts.

Arterial Embolism

Pathophysiology.   Arterial emboli arise most commonly from thrombi that develop in the chambers of the heart as a result of atrial fibrillation, myocardial infarction, vascular disease, or chronic congestive heart failure. These

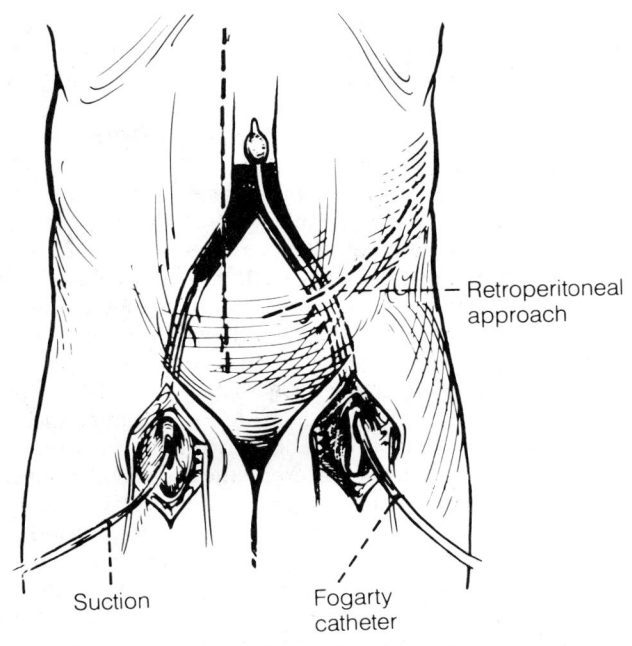

Figure 32-9. Aortic bifurcation embolectomy may be approached directly through the abdomen or in a retrograde fashion via the femoral arteries by suction or Fogarty catheter. (From Rhoads et al: Surgery. Philadelphia, JB Lippincott.)

thrombi may become detached and carried from the left side of the heart into the arterial system, where it can plug an artery that is too small to allow it to pass. Emboli may also develop in advanced aortic atherosclerosis owing to roughening or ulceration of the atheromatous plaques. The sequelae of arterial emboli depend primarily on the size of the embolus, the organ involved, and the state of the collateral vessels. The immediate effect is cessation of distal blood flow. The clot can progress above and below the obstruction. Secondary vasospasm can contribute to the ischemia. Fragmentation of the embolus can occur, resulting in occlusion of more distal vessels.

Emboli tend to lodge at arterial bifurcations and atherosclerotic narrowings. Cerebral, mesenteric, renal, and coronary arteries are often involved, in addition to the large arteries of the extremities.

Clinical Manifestations.   The symptoms of acute arterial embolism in extremities with poor collateral flow are acute, severe pain and a gradual loss of sensory and motor function. Pain may be aggravated by movement of the extremity. Distal pulses are lost, and the extremity becomes pale, mottled, and numb. Superficial veins may be collapsed because of decreased blood flow to the extremity. A sharp line of color and temperature demarcation may occur distal to the site of the occlusion as a result of ischemia.

Management.   Embolectomy is the treatment of choice when a major vessel has been occluded (Fig. 32-9). This procedure involves incising the vessel and removing the clot. The success of surgery in preserving extremity viability depends on the length of time the extremity has been ischemic. After 6 to 10 hours, muscle necrosis develops and the extremity cannot be salvaged. Prior to surgery, the patient should remain on bed rest with the extremity level or slightly (15 degrees) dependent. The affected part is kept at room temperature and protected from trauma. Padded side rails, pillows between the legs, and bed cradles to keep the weight of linen off the extremity are useful.

Medical management of an acute embolic occlusion includes intravenous anticoagulation with heparin, which will prevent propagation of the clot and thus reduce muscle necrosis. Thrombolytic agents such as streptokinase and urokinase may be useful to hasten embolic lysis. The pain associated with vasospasm may be relieved by a small dose of the drug papaverine hydrochloride.

Postoperative Nursing Management. During the postoperative period, every effort is made to encourage movement of the leg in order to stimulate circulation and prevent stasis. Since each patient is different, the nurse collaborates with the surgeon about the appropriate level of activity needed. Anticoagulants may be continued for a period of time after surgery in order to prevent thrombosis of the operated artery and to diminish the development of thrombi at the initiating site. The nurse should frequently assess the surgical wound for evidence of hemorrhage, which can occur when anticoagulants are given.

Arterial Thrombosis

Arterial thrombosis can also acutely occlude an artery. This slowly developing clot usually occurs at the site of damage of the arterial wall, which is most commonly due to atherosclerosis. Thrombi may also develop in an arterial aneurysm. The manifestations of an acute thrombotic arterial occlusion are similar to those described for embolic occlusion. However, treatment is made more difficult with a thrombus because the arterial occlusion has occurred in a degenerated vessel. This requires more extensive reconstructive surgery to restore flow than is required with an embolic event.

Vasospastic Disorders

Raynaud's Disease

Raynaud's disease is a form of intermittent arteriolar vasoconstriction that results in coldness, pain, pallor, and, occasionally, ulceration of the fingertips. The etiology is unknown, although many patients seem to have immunologic disorders. Episodes may be triggered by emotional factors or by unusual sensitivity to cold. It is most common in females between the ages of 16 and 40 years and is seen much more frequently in cold climates and during the winter months. If the degree of vasoconstriction is moderate, there may still be some arterial flow. However, blood flow is relatively stagnant, producing a cyanotic (blue) color in the fingers. If the spasm is severe, the fingers become a deadwhite color. After rewarming, the fingers develop a reactive hyperemia and appear red. Thus, the characteristic color change of Raynaud's phenomenon is described as blue, white, and red. The involvement tends to be bilateral and symmetrical.

The term *Raynaud's phenomenon* is currently used to refer to localized, intermittent episodes of vasoconstriction of small arteries of the extremities, causing color and temperature changes. It is generally unilateral and affects only one or two digits. It is not usually indicative of the status of the entire peripheral vascular system.

The prognosis for Raynaud's disease varies: some patients slowly improve, some grow slowly worse, and others show no change. The vasoconstriction appears to be mediated through the release of catecholamines at the neuroarteriolar junction.

Nursing Management. Avoidance of the particular stimuli that provoke vasoconstriction is the prime objective in controlling Raynaud's disease. An effort should be made to avoid situations that may upset the patient. Since concern over serious complications such as gangrene and amputation are certainly upsetting, the patient should be reassured that serious sequelae are not usual with Raynaud's disease. Smoking should be avoided.

Exposure to cold must be minimized. In areas where the fall and winter months are cold, the patient should remain indoors as much as possible. Sharp objects should be handled carefully to avoid digital injury. Vasodilator drugs, such as reserpine or other rauwolfia derivatives, may be prescribed, although their effectiveness is variable.

Interruption of the sympathetic nerves by removal of the sympathetic ganglia or division of their branches may afford some improvement in patients with Raynaud's disease.

▷ Hypertension

Incidence and Significance

Hypertension can be arbitrarily defined as persistent levels of blood pressure in which the systolic pressure is above 150 mm Hg and the diastolic pressure is above 90 mm Hg. Hypertension is a major cause of heart failure, stroke, and kidney failure. It is called the "silent killer," because the individual is often symptom-free. It has been estimated by the National Heart, Lung and Blood Institute that 50% of persons with hypertension do not know they have it. Once a patient is identified as having hypertension, his blood pressure must be checked frequently, since it is a lifetime condition.

About 20% of the adult population develop hypertension; more than 90% of these have *essential* (primary) hypertension, which has no identifiable medical cause. The remainder develop elevations in blood pressure from some specific etiology, such as renovascular narrowing or parenchyma-renal disease.

Elevated blood pressure is associated with many disease states, such as thyrotoxicosis or preeclampsia, and it is corrected when the basic disease is corrected. Because of the frequency of hypertension, a national program for screening potential hypertensive individuals was launched in 1972 by a special committee under the Department of Health, Education and Welfare (Chart 32-2).

Essential hypertension usually begins as a labile (intermittent) process in the late 30s to early 50s and gradually becomes "fixed." On occasion it appears abruptly and severely and takes an accelerated or "malignant" course that causes rapid deterioration of the patient.

Overstimulation with coffee, tobacco, and stimulatory drugs, as well as emotional disturbances and obesity, play a role, but the disease is strongly familial. It affects more women than men, but men, especially blacks, are less able to tolerate the disease.

Prolonged elevation of blood pressure eventually damages blood vessels throughout the body, most notably in the eyes, heart, kidneys, and brain, so that failing vision, coronary occlusion, congestive heart failure, renal failure, and strokes are the usual consequences of prolonged, uncontrolled hypertension.

Increased peripheral resistance controlled at the arteriolar level is the basic cause for the elevated blood pressure, but the causes of increased resistance are poorly understood. Drug therapy is aimed at reducing peripheral resistance, so as to lower the blood pressure and lessen the stresses on the vascular system.

Pathophysiology of Essential Hypertension

The vasomotor center is situated in the medulla of the brain. Emanating from this vasomotor center are the sympathetic nervous system tracks, which go down the spinal cord and emerge from the spinal column at the sympathetic ganglia in the thorax and abdomen. Stimulation of the vasomotor center sets in motion impulses that travel down through the sympathetic nervous system to the sympathetic ganglia. At this point, the preganglionic neurons release acetylcholine, which stimulates the postganglionic nerve fibers in the blood vessel, where the release of norepinephrine results in constriction of the vessels. Numerous influences may affect the response of the blood vessel to these vasoconstrictor stimuli. Hypertensive individuals are very sensitive to norepinephrine, although it is not known exactly why.

In the hypertensive patient, many factors moderate the vasomotor and vasoconstrictor responses, such as anxiety and fear.

Occurring concurrently with sympathetic nervous system stimulation of the blood vessels in response to emotional stimuli is stimulation of the adrenal gland. The adrenal medulla secretes epinephrine, which causes vasoconstriction. The adrenal cortex secretes cortisol and other steroids, which may enhance the vasoconstrictor response of the blood vessels. Vasoconstriction results in reduced blood flow to the kidney, causing the release of renin. Renin leads to the formation of angiotensin, a potent vasoconstrictor, which in turn stimulates secretion of aldosterone by the adrenal cortex. This latter hormone promotes sodium and water retention by the kidney tubules, causing an increase in intravascular volume. All of these factors tend to perpetuate the hypertensive state.

▶ Assessment

Clinical Manifestations. On physical examination, no abnormalities other than high blood pressure may be found, but there may be changes in the retinae with hemorrhages, exudates, narrowed arterioles, and, in severe cases, papilledema.

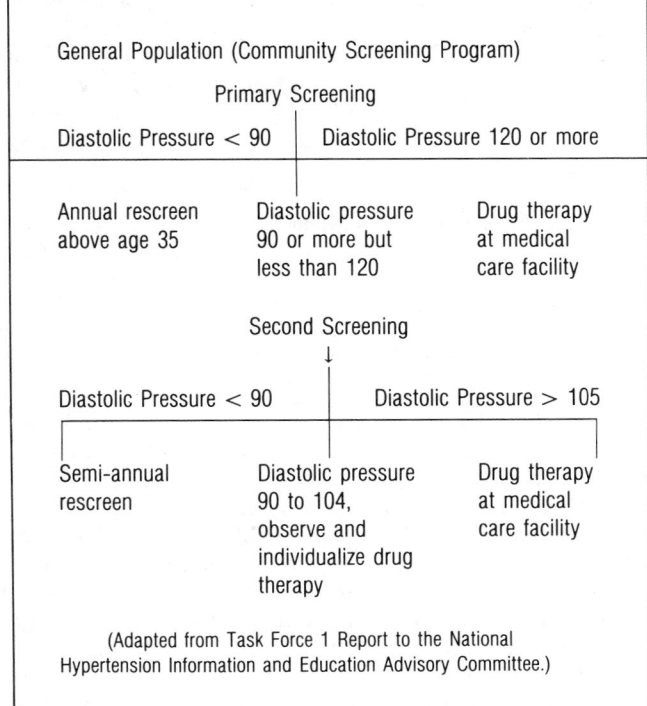

Chart 32-2
Identifying Hypertension in the General Population Based on Diastolic Blood Pressure in mm Hg

General Population (Community Screening Program)

Primary Screening

| Diastolic Pressure < 90 | Diastolic Pressure 120 or more |

| Annual rescreen above age 35 | Diastolic pressure 90 or more but less than 120 | Drug therapy at medical care facility |

Second Screening

| Diastolic Pressure < 90 | Diastolic Pressure > 105 |

| Semi-annual rescreen | Diastolic pressure 90 to 104, observe and individualize drug therapy | Drug therapy at medical care facility |

(Adapted from Task Force 1 Report to the National Hypertension Information and Education Advisory Committee.)

Individuals with hypertension can be asymptomatic and remain so for many years. The appearance of symptoms usually indicates vascular damage, and specific manifestations are related to the organ systems served by the involved vessels. Coronary artery disease with angina is the most common sequela in hypertensive individuals. Left ventricular hypertrophy occurs in response to the increased work load placed on the ventricle to contract against higher systemic pressures. When the heart can no longer sustain the increased work load, left heart failure ensues. Pathologic changes in the kidneys may be manifested as nocturia and azotemia (increased BUN and creatinine). Cerebral vascular involvement may produce a stroke or transient ischemic attack manifested by temporary hemiplegia, blackouts, or alterations in vision. Cerebral infarcts account for 80% of the strokes and transient ischemic attacks in hypertensive individuals.

Diagnostic Evaluation. A thorough history and physical examination are necessary. Eye grounds are checked and laboratory studies are done to determine target organ damage. Left ventricular hypertrophy (LVH) can be assessed by the electrocardiogram; protein in the urine can be detected by urinalysis. Inability to concentrate the urine and an increase in the blood urea nitrogen may also be present. Special studies, such as renograms, intravenous pyelograms, renal arteriograms, split renal function studies, and the determination of renin levels, may also be done to identify patients with renovascular disease. The presence of additional risk factors is sought and evaluated.

Patient Problems/Nursing Diagnoses

Based on the clinical manifestations, the nursing history, and the diagnostic assessment data, the patient's nursing diagnoses include potential development of multisystem alterations in health status related to hypertensive vascular damage; and potential nonadherence to therapeutic regimen related to an inadequate knowledge base or undesirability of regimen.

▶ Planning and Implementation

Goals

The major goals for the patient include:

1. Absence of progression of vascular changes
2. Adherence to the therapeutic regimen

The objective of treatment for hypertension is to lower the blood pressure to as close to normal levels as possible without introducing adverse effects. Adherence to therapy must be maximized in a cost-effective manner.

The major nursing goals to achieve these objectives include counseling and instructing patients about life-style changes, drug protocols, and dietary control, and to promote adherence to the overall therapeutic program through patient education.

Management.   The type of treatment program selected for individual patients is determined by the degree of hypertension, complications present, number and extent of risk factors, and the patient's personal, financial, and physical resources available to adhere to the treatment program. In cases of mild hypertension, conservative medical management may be the most beneficial approach. Individuals are counseled and instructed in ways to change poor health habits. Dietary control of salt and cholesterol, weight reduction, a regular exercise program, abstinence from tobacco, and stress management are addressed, and modifications are realistically planned with the patient.

When the conservative approach is ineffective, or the patient's diastolic blood pressure is consistently greater than 105 mm Hg, drug therapy is usually necessary. The selection of the appropriate drug or combination of drugs for the treatment of hypertension is highly individualized. In the "stepped care" approach, drugs are used that have the potential for the most effectiveness with the least side-effects and the best chance of acceptance by the patient. Table 32-3 describes the various pharmacologic agents used in the treatment of hypertension.

Patient Education.   A lot of energy is required of patients with hypertension to adhere to life-style, diet, and activity restrictions and to take regularly prescribed medications. The effort does not always seem reasonable, particularly when they are symptom-free without medications but experience side-effects with the medications. Much supervision, education, and encouragement are often needed with hypertensive individuals to arrive at an acceptable plan for living with their hypertension and the treatment regimen. Compromises may have to be made on some aspects

of the therapy in order to achieve success in higher priority areas.

A thorough understanding of the disease process of hypertension as well as the effect of medication and health habits on this process is important. The concept of hypertension control versus cure is important to explain. The temporary nature of medication side-effects should be emphasized. Consultation with a dietitian may be useful in exploring the number of possible ways to modify salt and fat intake. Lists of low-salt foods and beverages should be provided. Salt substitutes are readily available and inexpensive. Beverages containing caffeine should be limited to moderate intake. Alcohol may have synergistic effects with the patient's medications, and he or she should be fully informed of this. Support groups for control of weight, smoking, and stress may be beneficial for some patients. Others may need more support from family and friends.

Written information of the expected effects and side-effects of medications is very useful in maintaining a safe self-administration program. When side-effects do occur, patients need to know when and who to contact. In addition, patients should be advised of the possibility of rebound hypertension with sudden discontinuation of antihypertensive medication and of the possibility of sexual dysfunction related to the drugs.

Sometimes the patient is taught to measure blood pressure at home (Fig. 32-10). Some authorities believe that this involves the patient in his own care and emphasizes the fact that failing to take the medication can lead to a rise in blood pressure. It is difficult to convince many patients that the blood pressure is normally variable and does not stay fixed at one number.

▶ Evaluation

Expected Outcomes

1. Exhibits no progression of vascular changes
   a. Maintains blood pressure within acceptable range with medication or diet therapy
   b. Gives no evidence of symptoms of angina
   c. Reveals no ECG changes indicative of left ventricular hypertrophy
   d. Has normal BUN and serum creatinine levels
   e. Exhibits no progression of retinal pathology
   f. Gives no evidence of symptoms of cerebral infarction
2. Adheres to the therapeutic regimen
   a. Explains rationale for all aspects of therapeutic regimen
   b. Includes family in decisions regarding changes in life-style necessitated by therapeutic regimen
   c. Adheres to dietary regimen as prescribed: sodium, cholesterol, and calorie reduction
   d. Loses weight as prescribed
   e. Becomes involved in a regular program of exercise
   f. Takes own blood pressure daily (if appropriate)
   g. Takes medications as prescribed
   h. Reports side-effects of medications to physician prior to altering or discontinuing medications
   i. Abstains from tobacco, caffeine, and alcohol

Table 32-3
Chemotherapy for Hypertension

Purpose: To maintain blood pressure within normal ranges by the simplest and safest means possible with the fewest side-effects for each individual patient

Medication	Major Action	Advantages	Contraindications	Effects and Nursing Considerations
I. Diuretics and related drugs:				
A. Chlorthalidone (Hygroton) Quinethazone (Hydromox) Chlorothiazide (Diuril) Hydrochlorothiazide (Esidrix; HydroDiuril)	At beginning of therapy: Decrease of blood volume, renal blood flow, and cardiac output Depletion of extracellular fluid Negative sodium balance (from natriuresis), mild hypokalemia Directly affects vascular smooth muscle	Effective orally Effective during long-term administration Mild side-effects Enhance other antihypertensive drugs Counter sodium retention effect of other antihypertensive drugs	Gout Known sensitivity to sulfonamide-derived drugs Severely impaired kidney function	Dry mouth, thirst, weakness, drowsiness, lethargy, muscle aches, muscular fatigue, tachycardia, GI disturbance Orthostatic hypotension may be potentiated by alcohol, barbiturates, or narcotics Because thiazides cause sodium loss, patient is instructed to watch for postural hypotension in the summer. (Eating salted pretzels in hot weather may avert this.) Administer supplementary potassium
B. Loop diuretics Furosemide (Lasix) Ethacrynic acid (Edecrin)	Volume depletion Blocks reabsorption of sodium and water in kidney Antagonizes action of aldosterone	Action is rapid Potent-blocks To be used only when thiazides fail	Same as for thiazides	Volume depletion is rapid—profound diuresis Electrolyte depletion—replacement is required Thirst, nausea, vomiting, skin rash, postural hypotension Sweet taste noted; oral and gastric burning
C. Potassium-sparing diuretics Spironolactone (Aldactone) Triamterene (Dyrenium)	Competitive inhibitor of aldosterone Acts on distal tubule independently of aldosterone	Spironolactone effective in treating hypertension accompanying primary aldosteronism Both spironolactone and triamterene retain potassium	Renal disease Azotemia Severe hepatic disease	Drowsiness, lethargy, headache—decrease the dosage Diarrhea and other GI symptoms—give drug after meals Skin eruptions, urticaria Mental confusion, ataxia—perhaps dosage needs to be reduced Gynecomastia (not for triamterene)
II. Reserpine (alkaloid of Rauwolfia serpentina)	Impairs intracellular storage of norepinephrine	Slows pulse, which counteracts tachycardia of hydralazine	History of depression Psychosis Obesity Chronic sinusitis Peptic ulcer	May cause severe depression; report manifestations since this may require that drug be omitted Nasal stuffiness, which may require nasal vasoconstrictor Increases appetite—therefore, suggest stricter diet Recurrence of peptic ulcer

(continued)

Table 32-3
Chemotherapy for Hypertension (continued)

Medication	Major Action	Advantages	Contraindications	Effects and Nursing Considerations
III. Methyldopa (Aldomet)	Dopa—decarboxylase inhibitor	Effective in patients not controlled with thiazide-reserpine (with or without hydralazine) Useful in patients with renal failure Does not decrease cardiac output or renal blood flow Does not induce oliguria	Liver disease	Drowsiness, dizziness Dry mouth; nasal stuffiness (troublesome at first but then tends to disappear) Hemolytic anemia (a hypersensitization reaction)—positive Coombs' test—may not indicate drug discontinuance
IV. Hydralazine hydrochloride (Apresoline)	Decreases peripheral resistance but concurrently elevates cardiac output Acts directly on smooth muscle of blood vessels	Used as a third drug of choice when patient does not respond to thiazide-reserpine, thiazide-methyldopa, thiazide-guanethidine	Angina or coronary artery disease Congestive heart failure Hypersensitivity	Headache, tachycardia, flushing, and dyspnea may occur—can be prevented by pretreating with reserpine Peripheral edema may require diuretics May produce lupus erythematosus-like syndrome
V. Recently approved drugs: Propranolol (Inderal)	Blocks the sympathetic nervous system (beta adrenergic receptors), especially the sympathetics to the heart, producing a slower heart rate and lowered blood pressure	Reduces pulse rate in patients with tachycardia and blood pressure elevation and is useful as an adjunctive drug with those that act at the neuroeffector site of the blood vessel	Bronchial asthma Allergic rhinitis Right ventricular failure owing to pulmonary hypertension Congestive heart failure	Mental depression manifested by insomnia, lassitude, weakness, and fatigue Lightheadedness and occasional nausea, vomiting, and epigastric distress Blood dyscrasias such as agranulocytosis and thrombocytopenic purpura do occur but are uncommon

(continued)

j. Utilizes available community resources for stress management and reduction
k. Explains rationale for continuance of therapeutic regimen, even though symptom-free
l. Keeps follow-up clinic or physician appointments

Hypertensive Emergencies

Occasionally, acute, life-threatening elevations in blood pressure occur that require prompt treatment. Hypertensive emergencies frequently occur in patients whose hypertension has been poorly controlled or in whom medications have been abruptly discontinued. The degree of organ failure present because of the hypertension will determine the rapidity with which the blood pressure must be lowered. The presence of acute left ventricular failure or cerebral dysfunction indicates the need for immediate reduction in blood pressure over the next 24 to 48 hours.

The drugs of choice in hypertensive emergencies are those that have immediate effect. Intravenous nitroprusside has an immediate vasodilating action that is short-lived and

Table 32-3
Chemotherapy for Hypertension (continued)

Medication	Major Action	Advantages	Contraindications	Effects and Nursing Considerations
V. Recently approved drugs: (continued) Prazosin (Minipress)	Peripheral vasodilator acting directly on the blood vessel; similar to hydralazine	Acts directly on the blood vessel and is an effective agent in those patients with adverse reactions to hydralazine	Angina pectoris and coronary artery disease. Induces tachycardia if not preceded by administration of propranolol and a diuretic	Occasional vomiting and diarrhea, urinary frequency, and cardiovascular collapse, especially if given in addition to hydralazine without lowering the dose of the latter. Patients occasionally experience drowsiness, lack of energy, and weakness
Clonidine hydrochloride (Catapres)	Exact mode of action not understood, but acts through the central nervous system, apparently through centrally mediated alpha-adrenergic stimulation in the brain, producing blood pressure reduction	Little or no orthostatic effect. Moderately potent and sometimes is effective when other drugs fail to lower blood pressure	Severe coronary artery disease, pregnancy, children	Most common side-effects are dry mouth, drowsiness, sedation, and occasional headaches and fatigue. Anorexia, malaise, and vomiting with mild disturbance of liver function have been reported. Skin rash, dreams and nightmares, insomnia, and anxiety have been reported but are not common
VI. Guanethidine (Ismelin)	Prevents release of sympathetic transmitter, norepinephrine. It is a depressant of adrenergic activity Depletes tissue stores Causes venous pooling Decreases pulse rate, cardiac output, and renal blood flow	Potency	Pheochromocytoma, because it greatly enhances pressor effect of catecholamines	Severe orthostatic hypotension accentuated by alcohol, exercise, hot weather Warn against suddenly standing or standing for a long time Diarrhea and nausea, nocturia Failure of ejaculation; counsel about possible sexual dysfunction Fatigue and giddiness; blackout

is thus widely used as the initial treatment in crisis. Other drugs used for hypertensive emergencies include reserpine (Serpasil), methyldopa (Aldomet), phentolamine (Regitine), diazoxide (Hyperstat), and hydralazine (Apresoline). Most of these potent drugs are potentiated by diuretics. Extremely close monitoring of the patient's blood pressure and cardiovascular status is required during treatment with these medications. A precipitous drop in blood pressure can occur, and action must be taken immediately to prevent shock.

▷ Vein Disorders

Venous Thrombosis, Thrombophlebitis, Phlebothrombosis, and Deep Vein Thrombosis (DVT)

Although the above terms do not necessarily represent an identical pathology, for clinical purposes they are often used interchangeably.

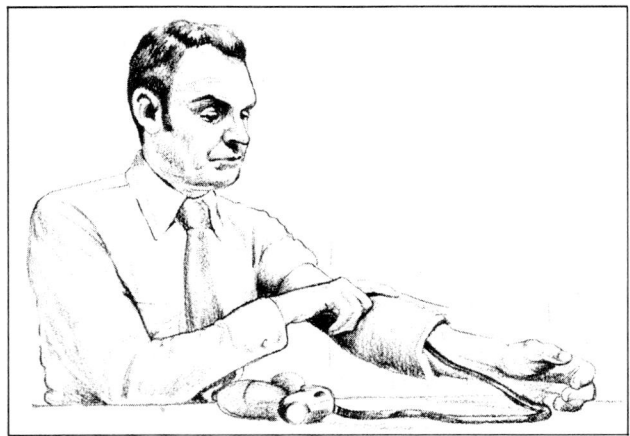

Keep your arm at the level of the heart and fit the cuff closely—but not too tightly—around your upper arm. You won't have to adjust the cuff again; simply slip it on and off at each reading.

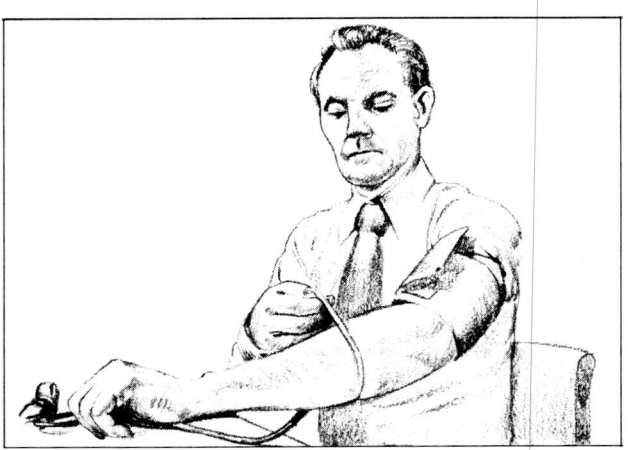

If you are not using a cuff design with the stethoscope sewn into it, you can slip two flat elastic bands up to the elbow and fasten the stethoscope diaphragm under them.

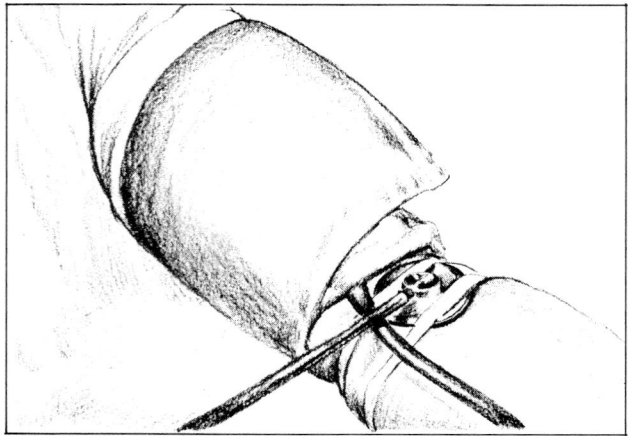

Place the diaphragm as shown, on the front surface of the upper arm directly above the elbow crease. Close the screw valve on the bulb, and squeeze the bulb to inflate the cuff. Listen through the stethoscope; when the cuff squeezes the artery so that the blood flow momentarily stops, you no longer hear the heartbeat. Pump the pressure up 20–30 mm Hg above the last pulse heard.

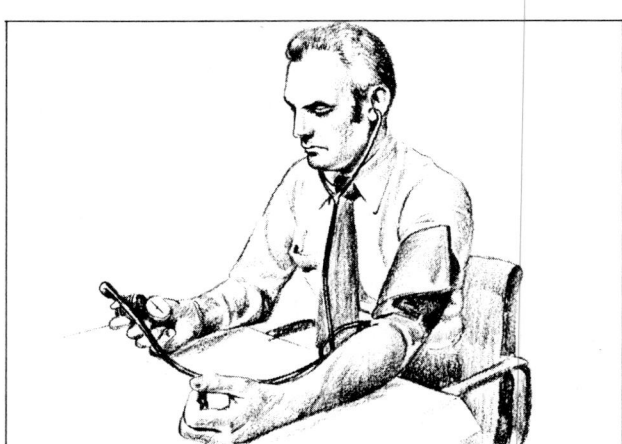

Open the valve slowly to release the cuff pressure, and listen for the first sound of the heart pumping blood through the arteries. At this moment the meter shows the systolic blood pressure. As you reduce the pressure, the pumping sound fades. At the point you no longer hear it, the meter shows the diastolic pressure—the usual pressure on the arteries. Record your pressures immediately.

Figure 32-10. How to measure your own blood pressure at home. Since you must hold the arm you test completely still to avoid driving up the blood pressure, and you need one hand to pump up the cuff and then deflate it, and one to hold the stethoscope bell in place, you may feel that you really need an extra hand. It is possible, however, to take your own blood pressure without that extra hand. (Reproduced with permission of Patient Care magazine. Copyright © 1977, Patient Care Publications, Inc., Darien, CT. All Rights Reserved.)

Pathophysiology and Etiology

Although the exact etiology of *venous thrombosis* remains unclear, three antecedent factors are believed to play a significant role in its development: stasis of blood, injury to the vessel wall, and altered blood coagulation. The presence of at least two factors appears to be necessary for thrombosis to occur. Venous stasis occurs when blood flow is retarded, such as with heart failure or shock; when veins are dilated, such as following drug therapy; and when skeletal muscle contraction is reduced, such as with immobility, extremity paralysis, or anesthesia. Bed rest has been shown to reduce blood flow in the legs at least 50%.

Disruption of the lining of blood vessels creates a site for clot formation. Direct vessel trauma, such as after a fracture or dislocation; diseases of the veins; and chemical irritation of the vein from intravenous drugs or solutions can all damage veins.

Increased coagulability of blood occurs most commonly in patients who have been abruptly withdrawn from anticoagulant medications. Oral contraceptives and a number of blood dyscrasias can also lead to hypercoagulability.

Thrombophlebitis is inflammation of the walls of the veins with formation of a clot. When a clot develops initially in the veins without inflammation, the process is referred to as *phlebothrombosis*. Venous thrombosis can occur in any vein but is most frequent in the veins of the lower extremities. Both superficial and deep veins of the legs may be affected. Of the superficial veins, the saphenous vein is most frequently affected. Of the deep leg veins, the iliofemoral, popliteal, and small calf veins are most often involved.

Venous thrombi are composed of an aggregate of platelets attached to the vein wall and a tail-like appendage containing fibrin, white blood cells, and many red blood cells. The "tail" can grow larger or propagate in the direction of blood flow as successive layering of the clot constituents occurs. The danger associated with a propagating venous thrombosis is that parts of a clot can become detached and produce an embolic occlusion of the pulmonary blood vessels. Fragmentation of the thrombus can occur spontaneously as the clot undergoes natural dissolution, or it can occur in association with elevation in venous pressure, such as occurs with sudden standing or muscular activity after prolonged inactivity. Other complications of venous thrombosis are described in Figure 32-11.

Assessment
Clinical Manifestations. At least one third of all patients with venous thrombosis of the lower extremities have no symptoms. In others, symptoms are variable and not usually specific for thrombophlebitis. However, despite this uncertainty, the presence of clinical signs should always be investigated further.

Obstruction of the *deep* veins of the legs produces edema and swelling of the extremity since the outflow of venous blood is inhibited. The amount of swelling can be determined by measuring extremity circumference at various levels with a tape measure. One extremity is compared to the other at the same level for size differences. Bilateral swelling may be difficult to detect. The skin over the affected leg may become warmer, and superficial veins may become more prominent. Tenderness, which usually occurs later, is produced by inflammation of the vein wall and can be detected by gentle palpation of the limb. *Homan's* sign, or a pain in the calf following sharp dorsiflexion of the foot, is not specific for deep venous thrombosis since it can be elicited in any painful condition of the calf. In some cases, signs of a pulmonary embolus is the first indication of a deep venous thrombosis.

Thrombosis of *superficial* veins produces pain or tenderness, redness, and warmth of the involved area. The risk of dislodgment and embolization of superficial venous thrombi is very low; thus, this condition can be treated at home with rest, extremity elevation, analgesics, and possibly anti-inflammatory agents.

Diagnostic Evaluation. *Phlebography* (venography) involves the injection of a radiographic contrast medium into the venous system through a dorsal foot vein. The di-

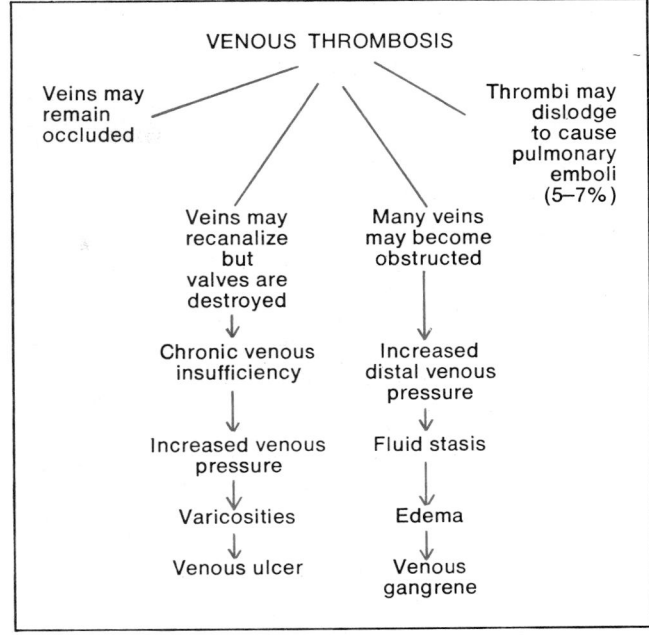

Figure 32-11. The seriousness of venous thrombosis is readily noted.

agnosis is based on the demonstration of an unfilled segment of vein in an otherwise completely filled vein with its connecting collaterals. Injection of the contrast media can cause a brief but painful vein inflammation.

Another method used to measure alterations in the velocity of blood flow in leg veins is an ultrasonic *Doppler flow meter.* When the Doppler probe is placed over veins that are obstructed, the Doppler flow reading will be diminished in comparison to the opposite extremity, or absent. This method is relatively inexpensive, portable, simple, rapid, and noninvasive.

^{125}I-labeled fibrinogen scanning, a recently developed diagnostic method, has provided a sensitive method for

---

Chart 32-3
High Risk for Thrombophlebitis

Bed rest—myocardial infarction, congestive heart failure, sepsis, traction
General surgery—in patients over 40 years old
Leg trauma—especially fractures, casts
Previous venous insufficiency
Obesity
Oral contraceptives
Malignancy

early detection of venous thrombosis. The test relies on the fact that radioactive fibrinogen, when injected intravenously, will concentrate in the forming clot. The level of radioactivity can then be serially measured by an external counter, and the progression of the clot can be monitored.

Preventive Measures

Elastic Stockings.   One approach to prophylaxis is the use of elastic stockings, which are usually prescribed for patients on a regimen of restricted activity, particularly those who are confined to bed. These stockings, by exerting a sustained, evenly distributed pressure over the entire surface of the calves, reduce the caliber of the superficial veins of the lower extremities, resulting in increased flow in the deeper veins. It is important to note that any type of stocking, including the elastic type, can be converted into a tourniquet if applied incorrectly (*i.e.,* rolled tightly at the top). In such instances, the stockings will produce stasis instead of preventing it. Elastic stockings are removed for a brief interval at least twice daily. While they are off, the skin should be inspected for signs of irritation and the calves examined for possible tenderness. Any skin changes or signs of tenderness should be reported.

Recent research studies have questioned the value of using elastic stockings and have indicated that the stockings may be ineffective or provide only modest benefit in some patients. It seems logical that if elastic stockings are used as the only preventive measure without adjunctive therapies, their efficacy would be substantially reduced.

Body Position and Exercise.   When the patient is on bed rest, the feet and lower legs should be elevated periodically above heart level. The superficial and tibial veins empty rapidly in this position and remain collapsed. Active and passive leg exercises, particularly those involving calf muscles, should be performed preoperatively and postoperatively to increase venous flow. Early ambulation is most effective in preventing venous stasis. Deep-breathing exercises are beneficial, since they produce increased negative pressure in the thorax, which assists in emptying the large veins.

Intermittent Venous Compression.   Although not commonly used, intermittent venous compression using pneumatic cuffs or boots may help to prevent deep vein thrombosis. The boot consists of a soft plastic inner boot and an inelastic outer boot, which are attached at the top and heel. The leg appears to float, since pressure is exerted uniformly in all directions. Cyclic inflation and deflation of the boot provides intermittent repetitive compression of the feet and legs. Such compression can be used in the operating room and during the postoperative period until the patient is ambulatory. The boots can be removed and reapplied daily by the nurse to permit skin care. Although intermittent venous compression boots can be worn with comfort for long periods of time, their use is contraindicated in patients with acute thrombophlebitis and suspected deep vein thrombosis.

Nursing Assessment

Careful nursing assessment is invaluable in detecting early signs of venous disorders of the lower extremities. Patients with a history of varicose veins, hypercoagulation, cardiovascular disease, or recent major surgery or injury, and the obese, elderly, and women taking oral contraceptives are in the high-risk group.

- Question the patient about the presence of leg pain, any functional impairment, or edema.
- Inspect the legs from the groin to the feet, noting asymmetry and measuring and recording calf circumference. (One early indication of edema is engorgement of the concavity behind the medial malleolus.)
- Note any increase in temperature in the affected leg. (To determine temperature differences more effectively, cool hands in cold water, dry, and place them simultaneously on both of the patient's ankles and then on the calves.)
- To identify areas of tenderness and any thromboses (as evidenced by cordlike venous segments), palpate the leg carefully using three or four fingers, advancing the hands back and forth from the ankle to the knee and then to the groin.

Management

The objectives of medical treatment are to prevent propagation of the thrombus and the inherent risk of pulmonary embolism and to prevent recurrent thromboemboli.

Therapeutic anticoagulation can accomplish both of these goals. Heparin is administered by intermittent intravenous infusion or by continuous infusion. Drug dosage is regulated by the partial thromboplastin time (PTT).

Heparin is usually continued for 10 to 12 days until organization of the clot has taken place. The patient is then started on oral anticoagulants for long-term prevention.

Many centers use thrombolytic (fibrinolytic) therapy since lysis and digestion of clots take place effectively. Such therapy is given within the first 3 days following acute arterial occlusion. Streptokinase and urokinase are both from biological sources and are about equal in thrombolytic activity. Urokinase is much more expensive than streptokinase. Both agents are contraindicated whenever a strategic hemostatic plug might be affected and dislodged. If bleeding occurs and cannot be stopped, the drug is discontinued. Occasionally, dextran has been used to decrease viscosity and aggregation of blood cells in patients with deep venous thrombosis. Use of this agent is associated with a relatively high incidence of allergic reaction and is therefore not widely used.

Bed rest, elevation of the affected extremity, elastic stockings, and analgesics for pain are adjuncts to anticoagulant therapy. Usually, bedrest is required for 5 to 7 days following a deep venous thrombosis. This is approximately the length of time necessary for inflammatory symptoms to subside and organization of the thrombus to occur. When the patient begins to ambulate, elastic stockings are used. Walking is superior to standing or sitting for long periods. Bed exercises, such as dorsiflexion of the foot against a foot board, are also recommended.

Warm, moist packs to the affected extremity will reduce discomfort associated with deep venous thrombosis. Mild analgesics for pain control will provide additional relief. A summary of the management of thrombophlebitis is presented in Table 32-4.

Surgical Management.   Surgery for deep vein thrombosis is necessary when (1) the patient cannot be given anticoagulants; (2) the danger of pulmonary embolism is extreme; and (3) the venous drainage is so severely compromised that permanent extremity damage will probably result. A thrombectomy is the treatment of choice when surgery is necessary.

Anticoagulant Therapy for Thromboembolism

Anticoagulant therapy is the administration of a medication to delay the clotting time of blood, to prevent the formation of a thrombus in postoperative patients, and to forestall the extension of a thrombus once it has formed. Anticoagulants cannot dissolve a thrombus that has already formed.

Measures for the *prevention* or reduction of blood clotting within the vascular system are indicated in patients with thrombophlebitis, patients suspected of recurrent embolus formation, those with persistent leg edema secondary to heart failure, and the elderly person with a hip fracture who is likely to be immobilized for a considerable time. The usual treatment consists of the single or combined administration of heparin or coumarin derivatives, which reduce the normal activity of the clotting mechanism (Table 32-5).

Administration

Continuous pump infusion is the preferred method for administering heparin (providing there are appropriate facilities and adequate personnel for monitoring). This method is preferred because evidence suggests a lower incidence of hemorrhagic complications. Dosage is calculated on the basis of weight and any possible bleeding tendencies indicated by a pretreatment clotting profile. If renal insufficiency exists, lower doses are required. The nurse should periodically check for kinks or leaks in the tubing and inspect the entire system frequently to ensure that the exact dose is being administered. Periodic coagulation tests and hematocrit evaluations are obtained. Observation of the patient for bleeding gums, ecchymotic areas, or signs of pain should be made and may be indicative of an overdose of anticoagulants.

Intermittent intravenous injection is another means of administering heparin, in this instance as a dilute aqueous solution given every 4 hours. Administration may be facilitated by the use of a "heparin lock"—a small, butterfly-type scalp vein needle with injection site at the end of tubing.

Oral anticoagulants, such as Coumadin, are monitored by the prothrombin time. Adequate anticoagulation is achieved when the prothrombin time is kept at 1½ to 2 times the normal.

Precautions and Nursing Assessment.   *The principal complication of anticoagulant therapy is the occurrence of spontaneous bleeding anywhere in the body.* Bleeding

Table 32-4
Thrombophlebitis

	Superficial	**Deep**
Clinical Manifestations	Local swelling; bumpy and knotty Red, tender, local induration	"Heaviness" on standing Cramping leg pain Swelling: 　Calf vein thrombus—none 　Femoral vein thrombus—mild to moderate 　Ileofemoral vein thrombus—severe Positive Homans' sign
Assessment	Venography—to rule out deep vein thrombosis	Blood flow studies to show inflow, filling and emptying Venography—to determine presence of phlebitis, recanalization, extent of occlusion
Management	Bed rest Warm, moist compresses Legs elevated Then, elastic support after acute stage Heparin, intermittent or continuous Acetaminophen for pain Antibiotics if necessary If deep veins are patent, superficial phlebitic veins may be removed	Bed rest Warm, moist compresses Foot of bed elevated to 15 cm (6 inches) Surgery, possibly, to prevent embolic development

Table 32-5

Comparison of Heparin and Coumarin Derivatives

	Heparin Sodium	**Coumarin Derivatives**
Physiologic Action	Interferes with clotting reaction at many points but primarily acts as an antagonist to thrombin.	Blocks the formation of prothrombin from vitamin K, a conversion normally taking place in the liver
Therapeutic Action		
Advantages	Used for short-term therapy primarily (may also be used for long-term therapy). Action is prompt and predictable. It can be used outside the body as well as inside: it may be used in certain dialysis procedures and in place of sodium citrate in donor blood.	Used for long-term therapy Is given orally and provides efficient absorption from gastrointestinal tract Uniform strength of medication because of synthetic production Less expensive than heparin sodium Control factor better than with heparin sodium Sodium warfarin more completely absorbed than bishydroxycoumarin
Disadvantages	Must be given parenterally, intravenously, or into the fat subcutaneously. A few patients have developed allergic reactions, and transient hair loss or osteoporosis has been reported (after several months of therapy).	Prolonged lag period (2–3 days) before the appearance of its effect Unpredictable duration of anticoagulant action (at times persisting up to 3 weeks)
Administration	Test clotting and prothrombin time first. Clotting times are obtained every 4 to 6 hours, at which time repeat doses of heparin are given. The object is to get the clotting time 2 to 3 times the normal control (first clotting time). *Subcutaneous route*—least recommended because of erratic absorption, possible puncture of vessels, and discomfort. The average therapeutic dose is 20,000 to 30,000 units daily either by *continuous infusion* with an infusion pump or in divided doses by *intermittent IV injection* every 4 to 6 hours. *Prolonged Therapy:* May be given deep subcutaneously (into the fat) in lower abdomen. Use a fine, short, sharp needle (No. 25–27 gauge, 1.27 cm–1.60 cm [0.5–0.62 inches]). Grasp roll of fat gently, and in dartlike fashion insert needle at right angle to the skin surface. Following injection, do not rub site but firmly press site with an alcohol sponge. Each time use a new location on lower abdomen. *Note:* Intramuscular administration of heparin is avoided because of likelihood of local hematomas and tissue irritation.	Test prothrombin clotting time first (see below). Warfarin: Administer initial dose of 15 mg to 25 mg. Give a second dose, somewhat smaller, on following day (10 mg). Adjust subsequent doses on basis of daily prothrombin determinations. Average dose is usually 5 mg/day. Therapeutic level of hypoprothrombinemia may be reached in 3 to 4 days.
Action for Adverse Effects	Discontinue heparin. Protamine sulfate (acts as a base to neutralize acidic heparin). Blood transfusion when hemorrhage is present.	Administer vitamin K preparations: For mild bleeding control: Phytonadione tablets (oral use) (Mephyton) (vitamin K_1) For moderate to severe bleeding control: Phytonadione solution (Aqua-MEPHYTON) IV or IM.

Prothrombin time is measured in seconds or percent of normal.

Normal: 12.5 seconds or 100%

Desired Therapeutic Range: 25 to 30 seconds when the control is 12 seconds (approximately 1½–2½ times the control in seconds). When the prothrombin time is measured in percent of normal, the desired therapeutic range is felt to be 20% to 30%.

from the kidneys will be manifested by microscopic hematuria and is often the first sign of anticoagulant overdose. Bruises, nosebleeds, and bleeding gums are also early signs of bleeding. The effects of heparin can be promptly reversed by the intravenous injection of protamine sulfate. The reversal of the effects of coumarin derivatives is more difficult, but effective measures include administering phytonadione and possibly fresh whole blood or plasma.

Oral anticoagulants interact with many other medications, and close monitoring of patient's drug schedules is necessary. Drugs that potentiate oral anticoagulants are salicylates, anabolic steroids, chloral hydrate, glucagon, chloramphenicol, neomycin, quinidine, and phenylbutazone (Butazolidin). It is advisable to study drug interactions for patients taking specific oral anticoagulants.

Patient Education About Oral Anticoagulants

The patient should be informed about the medication he is taking, its purpose, and the need to take the correct amount at the specific times prescribed. He should also be aware that blood tests are scheduled periodically to determine how the blood is clotting and whether a change in medication dosage is required. Specific teaching directives should include the following points:

- Take the anticoagulant tablet at the same time each day, usually between 8:00 and 9:00 AM.
- Wear or carry identification indicating what anticoagulant is being taken.
- Since other medications affect the way the anticoagulant normally acts, do not take any of the following medications without the physician's consent: vitamins, cold medicines, antibiotics, aspirin, mineral oil, and phenylbutazone (Butazolidin).
- Remember that alcohol may alter the body's response to an anticoagulant.
- Avoid food fads, crash diets, or marked changes in eating habits.
- Do not take Coumadin unless so directed by the physician.
- Do not stop taking Coumadin (when prescribed) unless so directed by the physician or nurse.
- When seeking treatment from another physician, a dentist, or a podiatrist, indicate that an anticoagulant is being taken.
- Contact personal physician prior to dental extraction or elective surgery.
- If any of the following signs appear, report them immediately to the physician:
    Faintness, dizziness, or increased weakness
    Severe headaches or stomach pain
    Red or brown urine
    Any bleeding, such as cuts that do not stop bleeding
    Bruises that increase in size, nosebleeds, or unusual bleeding from any part of the body
    Red or black bowel movements
    Skin rash
    Pregnancy
- Be extra careful to avoid injury that can cause bleeding.

Chart 32-4
Contraindications to Anticoagulant Therapy (Risk Factors)

Lack of patient cooperation
Bleeding from the following tracts:
    Gastrointestinal
    Genitourinary
    Respiratory
Hemorrhagic blood dyscrasias
Aneurysms
Severe trauma
Alcoholism
Compulsive drug use
Recent or impending surgery of:
    Eye
    Spinal cord
    Brain
Severe hepatic or renal disease
Recent cerebrovascular hemorrhage
Infections
Open ulcerative wounds
Occupations that involve a significant hazard of injury

- Women should notify their physicians if they suspect that they are pregnant.

Chronic Venous Insufficiency

Pathophysiology and Clinical Manifestations

Venous insufficiency is a disease state resulting from the incompetency of venous valves in the legs. Both superficial and deep leg veins can be involved. Valvular incompetence can occur whenever there has been a prolonged increase in venous pressure, such as occurs with deep venous thrombosis.

Because the walls of the veins are thinner and more elastic than the arteries, they distend readily when venous pressure is consistently high. In this state, leaflets of the venous valves are stretched and prevented from closing completely, thereby allowing a backflow or reflux of blood in the veins. Venous stasis and edema result.

When the deep veins in the legs have incompetent valves following a thrombus, *postphlebitic syndrome* may develop. This disorder is characterized by chronic venous stasis resulting in edema, altered pigmentation, pain, stasis dermatitis, and stasis ulceration. Superficial veins may be dilated. The disorder is long-standing, difficult to treat, and often disabling.

Stasis ulcers develop as a result of the rupture of small skin veins and subsequent ulcerations. When these vessels rupture, red blood cells escape into surrounding tissues, then degenerate and leave a brownish pigment that stains the tissues. The pigmentation and ulcerations usually occur in the lower part of the extremity in the area of the medial malleolus of the ankle. The skin becomes dry, cracks, and itches. Subcutaneous tissues fibrose and atrophy. The risk of injury and infection of the extremities is increased.

Leg ulcers can be associated with other conditions affecting the circulation of the lower extremities (Fig. 32-12). The potential complications and the principles of care, however, will be similar for all types.

Management and Patient Teaching

Management of the patient with venous insufficiency is directed at reducing venous stasis and preventing ulcerations. Measures that increase venous blood flow are antigravity activities and compression of superficial veins with elastic stockings.

Elevation of the legs above the heart should be performed frequently throughout the day (at least 30 minutes every 2 hours). At night, the patient should sleep with the foot of the bed elevated about 6 inches (15 cm). Prolonged sitting or standing is detrimental, thus walking should be encouraged. When sitting, the patient should avoid placing pressure on the popliteal spaces, such as occurs with leg-crossing, or sitting with the legs dangling over the side of the bed. Constricting garments such as girdles or garters worn above the legs should be avoided.

Elastic compression of the legs reduces pooling of venous blood and enhances venous return to the heart. Thus, elastic hose are recommended for patients with venous insufficiency. The fit of the stocking is important, and it should provide for a greater pressure at the foot and ankle, gradually declining to a lesser pressure at the knee or groin. If the top of the stocking is too tight or a twisting has occurred, a tourniquet effect is created, which worsens venous pooling. Stockings should be applied following a period of leg elevation, when the venous blood volume is at its lowest. The technique for putting on elastic hose is depicted in Figure 32-13.

Extremities with venous insufficiency are conscientiously protected from trauma. The skin is kept clean, dry, and soft. Signs of ulceration are immediately reported to

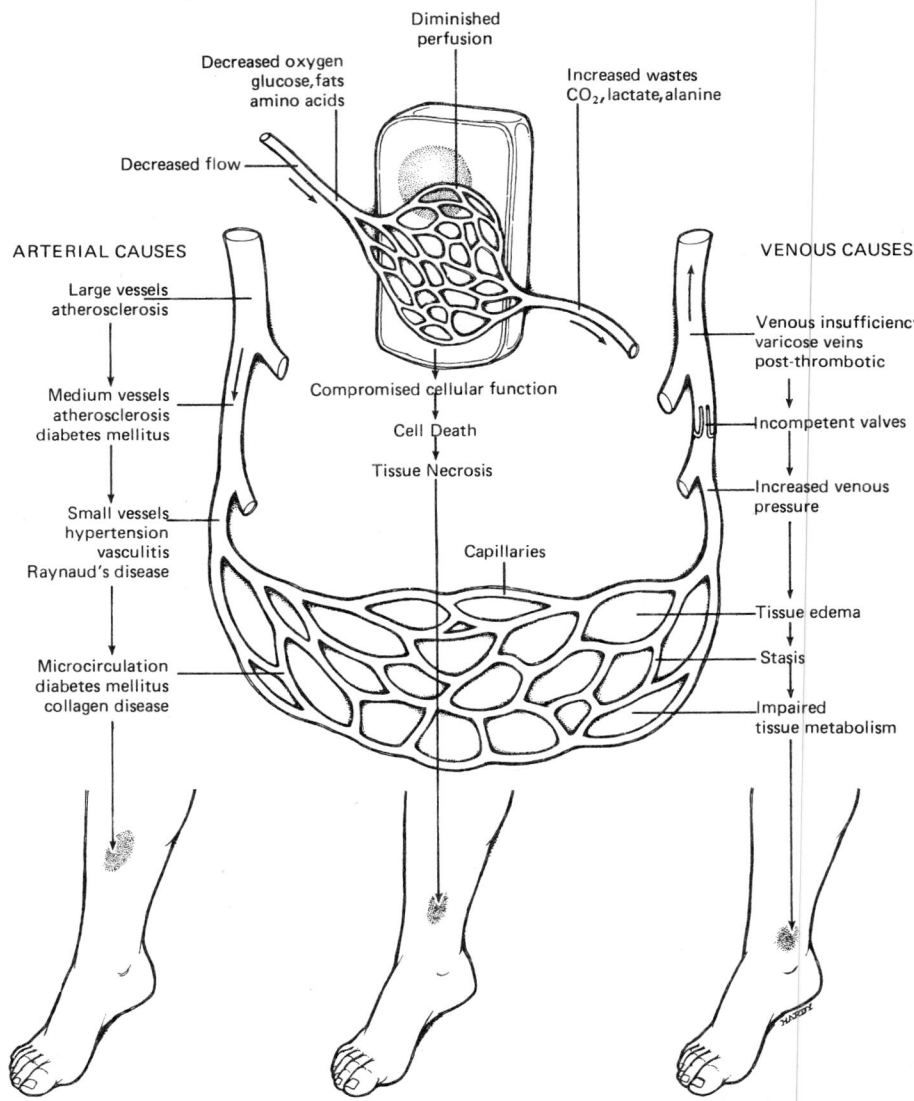

Figure 32-12. Pathophysiology of leg ulcers. On the left some of the conditions are indicated that cause diminished blood flow to peripheral tissue. Oxygen and energy sources are further aggravated by capillary changes brought about by diabetes mellitus and collagen disease. Cellular function is compromised when insufficient oxygen and energy substrates are supplied. Tissue necrosis takes place and results in ulceration. A somewhat similar situation occurs when there is venous insufficiency brought about by a different hemodynamic pattern. Increased venous pressure reduces capillary flow. Edema and stasis result, impairing cellular metabolism and again leading to ulceration.

the health care professional for treatment and follow-up. A variety of topical agents and soaps can be used in conjunction with washing and débridement therapies to promote healing of leg ulcers. The goals of treatment are to remove devitalized tissue and to keep the wound clean and moist while healing takes place. Gentle handling of the affected extremity and protection of granulation tissue are important. Adequate nutrition is essential. In some instances, application of an occlusive dressing to a clean wound is beneficial. Several of these are depicted in Figure 32-14.

Leg Ulcers

A leg ulcer is an excavation of the skin surface that is produced by the sloughing of inflammatory necrotic tissue. The most frequent cause is vascular insufficiency, either venous or arteriolar. It is estimated that of all leg ulcers, postphlebitic and varicose ulcers account for about 70%; the remaining 30%, such as those caused by burns, sickle-cell anemia, and neurogenic disorders, are of nonvenous origin. Venous ulcers usually occur above the medial ankle (malleolus), whereas arterial ulcers occur farther from the ankle and sometimes higher.

The nursing challenge in caring for these persons is great, whether the older person is in the hospital or at home. The physical problem is often a long-term one that causes a substantial drain on the patient's physical, emotional, and economic resources.

Pathophysiology. Inadequate exchange of oxygen and nutrient substrates in the tissue is the metabolic abnormality underlying the development of leg ulcers. When the cellular metabolism cannot maintain energy balance, cell death results (necrosis). Alterations in blood vessels at the arterial, capillary, and venous level may affect cellular processes and lead to the formation of ulcers (see Fig. 32-12).

Assessment and Clinical Manifestations. Because there are many causes of ulcers, it is important that a proper causative diagnosis be made so that appropriate therapy may be prescribed. The medical and nursing history of the person is important in determining venous or arterial insufficiency. Symptoms of aching, fatigue, heaviness, and especially swelling of the leg should be evaluated, and aortic, iliac, femoral, popliteal, and pedal pulses should be carefully checked. Note dependent redness. Look for chronic pitting or nonpitting edema. More conclusive diagnostic aids are Doppler ultrasound studies, arteriography, and venography. Laboratory tests can assist in determining whether infection is the primary cause of the ulcer; cultures may be required.

Management. Goals of therapy can be successfully managed by simple therapy of the ulcer itself:

1. *To control infection:* Since all ulcers are infected, it is necessary to establish dependent drainage. Systemic antimicrobial therapy is used based on appropriate culture and sensitivity determinations. Topical antibiotics have not been as effective as desired.

2. *To promote healing by keeping the wound clean:* Cleansing requires very gentle handling; a mild soap, lukewarm water, and cotton balls are used. Flushing out of necrotic material can be done with hydrogen peroxide. Debriding can be performed using instru-

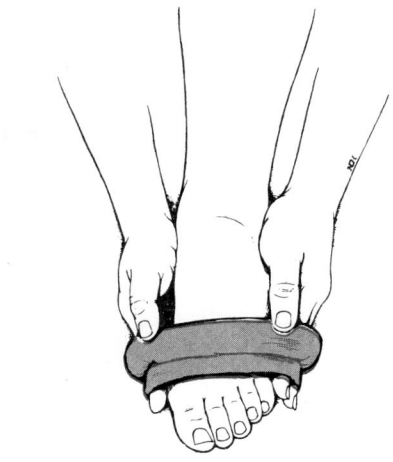

Figure 32-13. A support stocking can be rolled, spread apart, and unrolled as the hands hold it in place—moving from foot to ankle and up the calf. Ideally, the stocking should be put on while the patient is in bed.

ments to cut away devitalized tissue. It can also be done by applying isotonic saline dressings of fine mesh gauze to the ulcer bed. When dry, the dressing is removed along with the debris adhering to the gauze.

Enzymatic debridement may be preferred by some physicians, and enzyme ointments may be used to treat the ulcer. The ointment is placed over the lesion but not over normal surrounding skin. The lesion and ointment are then covered with a saline-soaked sponge that has been thoroughly wrung out. A gauze dressing and a loose bandage are then applied. For the first 3 or 4 days, applications are made every fourth hour, then every eighth hour. When pink granulating tissue develops, saline wet dressings are used.

A newer method of treating ulcers involves the use of dextranomer (Debrisan) beads, small, highly porous spherical beads (0.1 mm to 0.3 mm in diameter) that possess the ability to absorb wound secretions. Bacteria and products of tissue necrosis and protein degradation are actively suctioned into the bead layer, which changes color according to the infecting organism. When the beads are completely saturated they take on a greyish yellow color, at which point their cleansing action stops. When the beads become saturated, they are removed and a fresh layer should be applied.

3. *To provide rest:* If there is arterial insufficiency, blood flow may be improved by elevating the head of the bed on 7.5-cm to 15-cm (3-inch–6-inch) blocks. Note whether such elevation increases dependent edema, since this must be avoided. Supplemental diuretics may be required.

4. *To correct nutritional disturbances:* Nutritional deficiencies must be determined and an adequate diet maintained. Such a diet should include vitamins (particularly vitamin C), protein, and minerals (iron).

5. *To revascularize tissue by arterial reconstruction:* Aortoiliac, aortofemoral, or femoropopliteal revascularization often are effective in correcting arterial insufficiency.

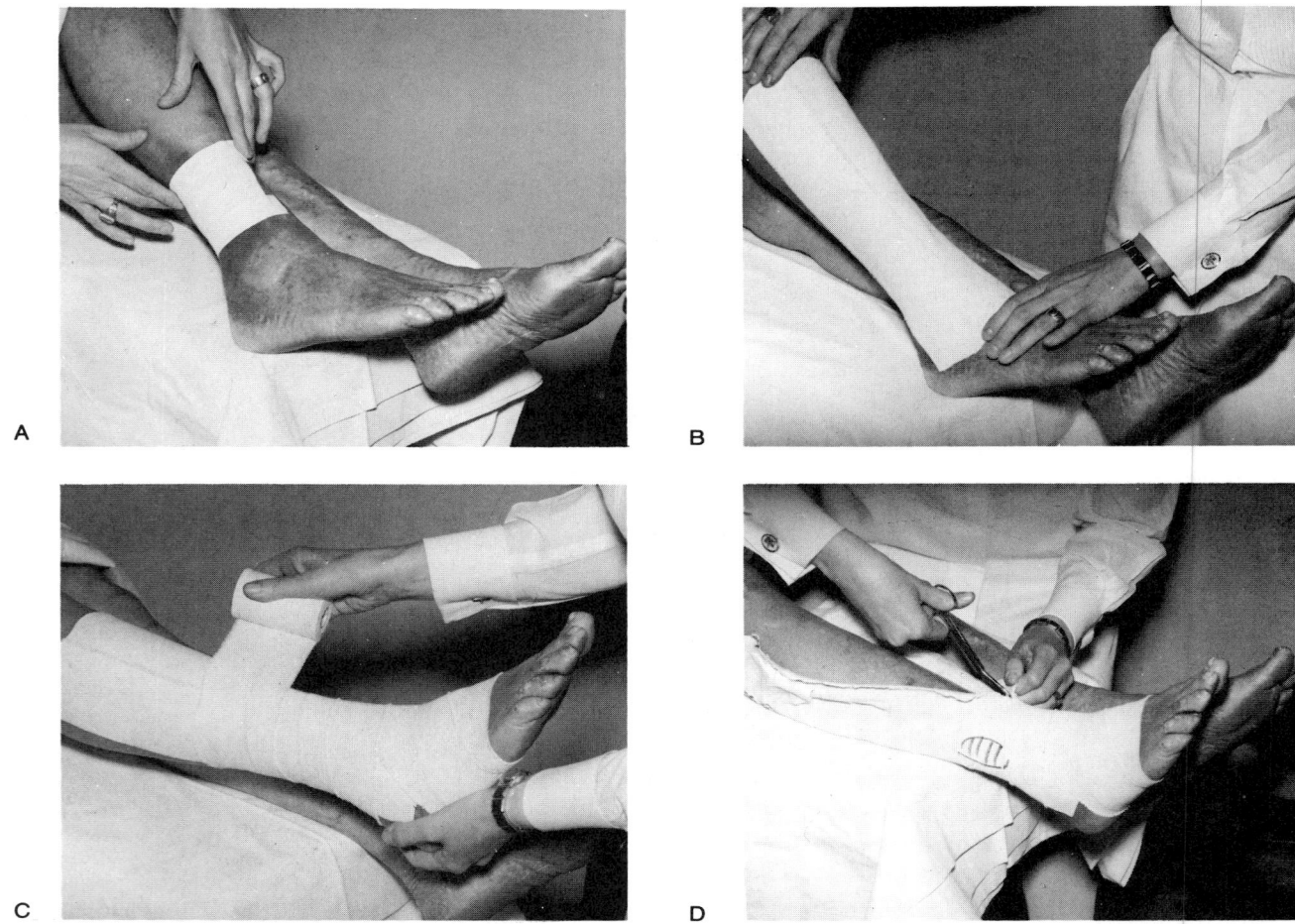

Figure 32-14. Elastoplast bandage. (*A*) After ointment has been applied, ulcer is covered with a Telfa or other nonadherent bandage and secured with hypoallergenic tape if plain adhesive tape irritates the patient's skin. (*B*) Strips of Elastoplast give support and protection. (*C*) Starting with a turn around the foot, bandage is spiraled upward with firm, even pressure and fastened securely below knee. (*D*) After several days, bandages must be removed with special care; even slight trauma could cause injury. (From Wilson S: Chronic leg ulcers. American Journal of Nursing 67:98.)

Varicose Veins

Incidence

Varicose veins (varicosities) are abnormally dilated, tortuous, superficial veins caused by incompetent venous valves (Fig. 32-15). Most commonly, this condition occurs in the lower extremities, in the saphenous veins, or the lower trunk; however, it can occur elsewhere in the body (*e.g.,* esophageal varices) (see p. 869).

It is estimated that varicose veins affect one out of five individuals in the world. The condition is most common in individuals in occupations requiring prolonged standing, such as salespeople, barbers, beauticians, elevator operators, nurses, and dentists. A hereditary weakness of the vein wall may contribute to the development of varicosities, and it is not uncommon to see this condition occur in several members of the same family.

Pathophysiology and Manifestations

Varicose veins may be caused primarily (without involvement of deep veins) or secondarily (resulting from obstruction of deep veins). A reflux of venous blood in the veins results in venous stasis. If only the superficial veins are affected, the individual may have no symptoms, but cosmetically, the appearance of the dilated veins may be unappealing. If symptoms are present, they may take the form of dull aches, muscle cramps, and increased fatigue of muscles in the lower legs.

When deep venous obstruction results in varicose veins, individuals may demonstrate the signs and symptoms of chronic venous insufficiency: edema, pain, pigmentation, and ulcerations. Susceptibility to injury and infection is greater.

Assessment

A common diagnostic test for varicose veins is the *Brodie–Trendelenburg test.* This test will demonstrate backward flow of blood through incompetent valves of the superficial veins and of the branches that communicate with the deep veins of the leg. With the patient lying down, the affected leg is elevated to empty the veins. A tourniquet is then

---

Chart 32-5
Health Teaching: Care of the Feet and Legs for the Person With a
Peripheral Vascular Problem

Cleanliness
1. Wash feet at least once daily.
2. Use warm water and bland soap.
3. Dry feet thoroughly, especially between the toes. Blot and pat with a towel, but do not rub.

Warmth
1. Wear cotton hose, since they are comfortable and absorb moisture.
2. Prevent feet from getting cold; this reduces blood supply.
3. Avoid applying heat to the feet or legs unless approved by a physician or nurse.
4. Avoid swimming in cold water.
5. Avoid sunburn.

Safety
1. Protect feet by performing exercises on level ground.
2. Avoid walking in crowds.
3. Use care in cutting toenails.
    a. First soak feet for 10 minutes in warm water to soften nails.
    b. Cut nails straight across; avoid cutting nails close to flesh.

Comfort Measures
1. Wear shoes that provide adequate toe room, have a good arch, and feel comfortable.
2. Apply powder if feet tend to become moist.
3. Apply a thin coating of lanolin if feet are dry and scaly.

Preventing Constriction of Blood Vessels
1. Avoid circular garters that cut off blood supply to legs and feet.
2. Do not cross legs at knees.
3. Place a pillow at foot end of bed under covers to prevent top bedding from exerting pressure on toes.
4. Apply lamb's wool between toes if they rub each other.

Exercise
Walking stimulates circulation and promotes tissue repair.

Medical Attention
1. Report redness, blistering, swelling, or pain.
2. Report athlete's foot, peeling and itching between toes.
3. Do not use any medication on feet or legs unless prescribed by the physician.

Smoking
Avoid tobacco in any form, since it aggravates peripheral vascular conditions.

---

applied around the upper thigh to occlude the veins, and the patient is asked to stand. If the valves of the communicating veins are incompetent, blood flows into the superficial veins from the deep veins. If, upon release of the tourniquet, blood flows rapidly from above into the superficial veins, the inference is that the valves of the superficial veins are also incompetent. This test is used to determine the type of treatment to be recommended for the varicose veins.

The *Perthes' test* is a diagnostic procedure that easily indicates whether the deeper venous system and communicating veins are competent. A tourniquet is applied just below the knee and the patient is requested to walk. If the varicose veins disappear, the deep system and communicating vessels are competent. If the vessels do not empty and become even more distended on walking, incompetency or obstruction is inferred.

Additional diagnostic tests for the presence of varicose veins are the Doppler flow meter, phlebography, and plethysmography. The *Doppler flow meter* can detect the retrograde flow of blood in the superficial veins with incompetent valves following compression of the leg proximally. *Phlebography* involves the injection of radiographic contrast into the leg veins so that vein anatomy can be visualized during various leg movements. *Plethysmography* allows measurement of changes in venous blood volume.

Preventive Suggestions and Health Teaching

Activities that cause venous stasis should be avoided, such as wearing tight garters or a constricting panty girdle, crossing the legs at the thighs, and sitting or standing for long periods of time. Frequent changes of position, elevating the legs when they are tired, and getting up to walk several minutes of every hour promote circulation. The patient should be encouraged to walk 1 or 2 miles a day if there are no contraindications. Walking up the stairs rather than using the elevator or escalator is helpful in promoting circulation. Swimming is also good exercise for the legs.

Support hose or elastic stockings are useful. The overweight patient should be assisted in a weight-reduction plan.

Surgical Treatment

Surgery for varicose veins requires demonstrated patency of deep veins. Once this is established, *ligation* of the saphenous vein is accomplished under general anesthesia. The vein is ligated high in the groin where the saphenous vein meets the femoral vein. An incision is then made in the ankle, and a metal or plastic wire is passed the full length of the vein, ''stripping'' as it passes (Fig. 32-16). The branches of the saphenous vein break off at their junctions. Pressure and elevation keep bleeding at a minimum during surgery.

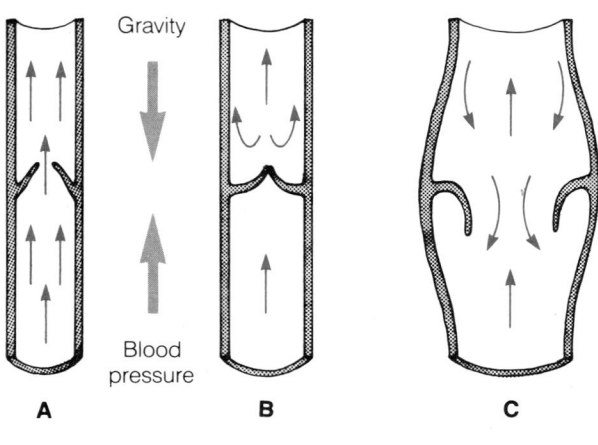

Figure 32-15. (*A, B*) *Competent* valves showing blood flow patterns when the valve is open (*A*) and closed (*B*), allowing blood to flow against gravity. (*C*) With faulty, or *incompetent*, valves, the blood is unable to move toward the heart.

Postoperative Nursing Management. Elastic compression of the leg is maintained continuously for about 1 week after vein stripping. Exercise and movement of the legs and elevation of the foot of the bed are necessary. Walking may be started 24 to 48 hours after surgery. Standing still and sitting are contraindicated.

Analgesics may assist patients to move affected extremities more easily. The bandages are inspected for bleeding, particularly at the groin since the greatest risk of bleeding occurs there. Sensations of "pins and needles" or hypersensitivity to touch in the involved extremity may indicate a temporary or permanent nerve injury resulting from surgery. The saphenous vein and saphenous nerve are in close proximity to each other in the leg.

Patients will require long-term elastic support of the leg after discharge from the hospital, and plans are made to provide adequate supplies. Exercises of the legs will also be necessary, and the development of an individualized plan will require consultation with the patient and physician.

Sclerotherapy. In *sclerotherapy* an irritating chemical, such as 3% sodium tetradecyl sulfate (Sotradecal), is injected into the vein, which irritates the vein wall and produces localized phlebitis and fibrosis, thereby obliterating the vein lumen. This treatment may be done alone for small varicosities or may follow vein ligation or stripping. Sclerosing is a palliative, not curative, treatment. Following injection of the sclerosing agent, elastic compression bandages are applied to the leg. These are worn for approximately 6 weeks. Walking is important for maintenance of blood flow in the extremity and should be emphasized.

If the patient experiences a burning sensation in the injected leg for one or two nights, a mild sedative and walking will relieve the problem. The bandage should be removed for the first time under the direction of the physician.

Because bathing may be a problem during this time, a plastic bag may be placed over the bandaged leg and secured above the bandage to allow the patient to shower.

▷ The Lymphatic System

The lymphatic system consists of a set of vessels that spread throughout most of the body. These vessels start as lymph capillaries that drain tissue spaces. They unite to form the lymph vessels, which in turn pass through the lymph nodes and finally empty into the large thoracic duct that joins the jugular vein on the left side of the neck. *Lymph* is the fluid found in lymph vessels. *Tissue fluids* are found outside of vessels in the cellular interspaces. The lymphatic system of the abdominal cavity maintains a steady flow of digested

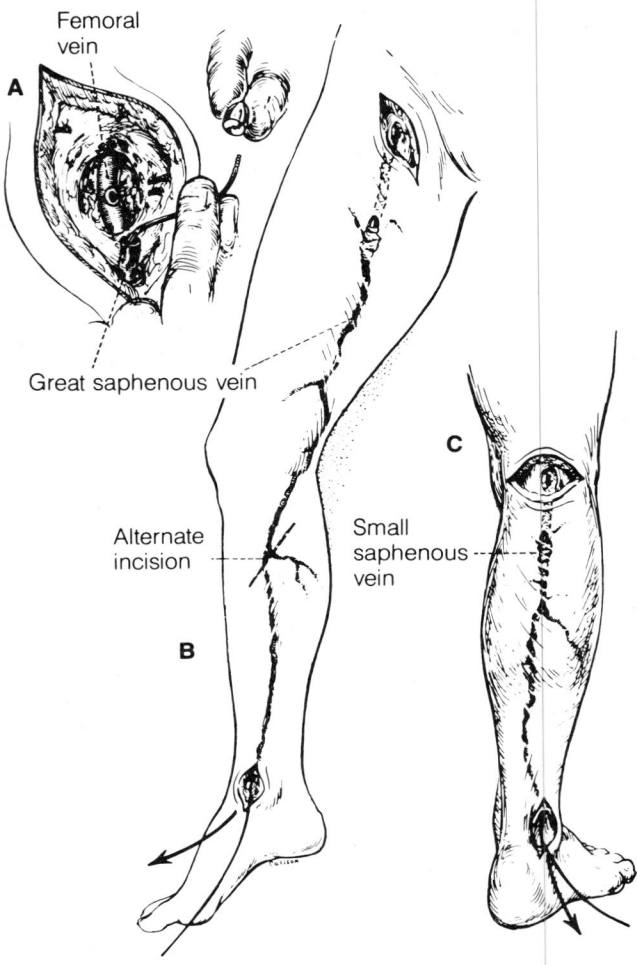

Figure 32-16. Ligation and stripping of the great and the small saphenous veins. (*A*) The tributaries of the saphenous vein have been ligated, and the saphenous vein has been ligated at the saphenofemoral junction. (*B*) Vein stripper has been inserted from the ankle superiorly to the groin. The vein is stripped from above downward. A number of alternate incisions may be needed to remove separate varicose masses. (*C*) The small saphenous vein is stripped from its junction with the popliteal vein to a point posterior to the lateral malleolus. (From Rhoads et al: Surgery. Philadelphia, JB Lippincott.)

fatty food (chyle) from the intestinal mucosa to the thoracic duct. In other parts of the body the lymphatic system's function is regional; the lymphatic vessels of the head, for example, empty into clusters of lymph nodes located in the neck, and those of the extremities into nodes in the axillae and the groin.

Assessment by Lymphangiography

Radiologic visualization of the lymphatic system is possible after the injection of contrast medium directly into lymphatic vessels in the hands and feet. This technique affords a means of detecting lymph node involvement by metastatic carcinoma, lymphoma, or infection in sites that are otherwise inaccessible to the examiner except by the direct surgical approach.

The first step in this procedure is the location of a lymphatic vessel in each foot (or hand) by injecting Evans blue dye intradermally between the first and the second digits. Approximately 15 to 20 minutes later, the skin proximal to the injection site is incised. A blue lymphatic segment is identified, isolated, cannulated with a 25- to 30-gauge needle, and infused very slowly with a contrast medium containing iodine and oil. Appropriate x-ray pictures are taken at the conclusion of the injection, 24 hours later, and periodically thereafter, as indicated.

Apart from its diagnostic value in cases of unsuspected lymph node disease, lymphangiography offers a means of evaluating the presence and the extent of metastases in patients who are known to have cancer. Moreover, since lymphomatous lymph nodes retain the contrast medium for 4 to 6 weeks after the injection, any change in their size that may occur in response to irradiation or chemotherapy can be measured and used as a criterion of therapeutic effect.

Lymphangitis and Lymphadenitis

Lymphangitis is an acute inflammation of the lymphatic channels. It arises most commonly from a focus of infection in an extremity. Usually, it is caused by the streptococcus. The characteristic red streaks that extend up the arm or the leg from an infected wound outline the course of the lymphatics as they drain.

The lymph nodes located along the course of the lymphatic channels also become enlarged, red, and tender (acute lymphadenitis), and can become necrotic and form an abscess (suppurative lymphadenitis). The nodes involved most often are those in the groin, the axilla, or the cervical region.

Because these infections are nearly always caused by organisms that are sensitive to antibiotics, it is unusual to see abscess formation. Recurrent episodes of lymphangitis are often associated with progressive lymphedema.

Lymphedema—Elephantiasis

Lymphedema is a swelling of tissues in the extremities owing to an increased quantity of lymph caused by an obstruction of lymphatics. It is especially marked when the extremity is in a dependent position. The most common type is congenital lymphedema (lymphedema praecox), which is due to hypoplasia of the lymphatic system of the lower extremity. This disorder is usually seen in females and appears first between the ages of 15 and 25.

The obstruction may be in both the lymph nodes and the lymphatic vessels, and at times it is seen in the arm, after a radical mastectomy for carcinoma, and in the leg in association with varicose veins or a chronic phlebitis. In the latter case the lymphatic obstruction usually is due to a chronic lymphangitis. Lymphatic obstruction owing to a parasite (*Filaria*) is seen frequently in the tropics. When chronic swelling is present, there may be frequent bouts of acute infection characterized by high fever and chills. These lead to chronic fibrosis, thickening of the subcutaneous tissues, and hypertrophy of the skin. This condition, in which chronic swelling of the extremity recedes only slightly with elevation, is given the name *elephantiasis*.

Management. Lymphedema is currently managed by three modes of therapy: physical therapy, coumarin, and surgery. Lymphatic fluid can be manually compressed from the soft tissues by squeezing the extremity distally. In this manner, drainage of fluid proximally can be accomplished. Active and passive exercises assist in the movement of lymphatic fluid into the bloodstream. Mechanical pulsatile air pressure devices are also available.

Coumarin and similar types of drugs remove proteins from the interstitial spaces. Removal of protein reduces tissue colloid osmotic pressure and allows the interstitial fluid to move back into the capillaries, thereby reducing lymphedema.

Surgical treatment of lymphedema is performed in order to reduce the size of the extremity and improve its appearance, to reduce the incidence of inflammatory episodes, and to limit secondary skin changes associated with chronic lymphedema. One surgical approach involves the excision of affected subcutaneous tissue and fascia with skin grafting to cover the defect. Another procedure involves the transfer of superficial lymphatics into the deep lymphatic system by a buried dermal flap to provide a conduit for lymphatic drainage.

Diuretics have been used palliatively for lymphedema in conjunction with elevation and elastic compression of the affected extremity. However, the use of diuretics is controversial since their action is not to remove protein.

Postoperatively, the management of skin grafts and of flaps is the same as when these therapies are used for other conditions. Prophylactic antibiotics may be prescribed for 5 to 7 days. Constant elevation of the affected extremity and observations for complications are essential. Complications can include flap necrosis, hematoma or abscess under the flap, and cellulitis.

▷ **Bibliography**
Books

Bergan JJ and Yao JST. Aneurysms. Diagnosis and Treatment. New York, Grune & Stratton, 1982.
Bernhard V and Towne J (eds). Complications in Vascular Surgery. New York, Grune & Stratton, 1980.
Condorelli M (ed). Hypertension. New York, Raven Press, 1982.

Fairbairn JF et al. Peripheral Vascular Diseases, 5th ed. Philadelphia, WB Saunders, 1979.

Friedman SA (ed). Vascular Diseases. Boston, John Wright–PSG, 1982.

Haimovici H. Vascular Emergencies. New York, Appleton–Century–Crofts, 1982.

Hallet J. Manual of Patient Care in Vascular Surgery. Boston, Little, Brown & Co, 1982.

Iwai J (ed). Salt and Hypertension. New York, Igaku Shoin, 1982.

Juergens JL, Spittell JA Jr, and Fairbairn JF II. Allen–Barker–Hines Peripheral Vascular Diseases. Philadelphia, WB Saunders, 1980.

Miller DC and Roon AJ. Diagnosis and Management of Peripheral Vascular Diseases. Menlo Park, California, Addison–Wesley, 1982.

Thompson DA. Cardiovascular Assessment. St Louis. CV Mosby, 1981.

Underhill S et al. Cardiac Nursing, Chaps. 5, 10, 28, 47. Philadelphia, JB Lippincott, 1982.

Articles
General

Atchison JS and Murray J. Post-vascular surgery. Nursing '78 1978 Dec; 8(12):36–39.

Baron HC. Rest pain from ischemia—causes and treatment. Consultant 1980 Aug; 20(8):51–52+.

Bowman ED et al. The role of the nurse in a peripheral vascular laboratory. Point View 1982 Oct 1; 19(4):10–12.

Callow AD. Current status of vascular grafts. Surg Clin North Am 1982 June; 62(3):501–513.

Criss E. Digital subtraction angiography. Am J Nurs 1982 Nov; 82(11):1706–1707.

Cudkowicz L. Current status of thrombolytic therapy. Heart Lung 1978 Jan–Feb; 7(1):97–100.

Datta PK. Ischaemic leg. A case for critical selection—its investigation and surgical management (pictorial). Nurs Mirror 1982 Mar 3; 154(9):34–37.

Deyton D. Antithrombotic therapy. Postgrad Med 1979 Jan; 65(1):135–146.

Doyle JE. Bypass graft surgery. Am J Nurs 1982 Oct; 82(10):1559–1562.

Drury DA. Foot care for the high-risk patient. RN 1982 Nov; 45(11):46–49.

Ekers MA and Satiani B. EAB (extra-anatomic bypass). A new route for vascular rehabilitation. Nursing '82 1982 Nov; 82(11):34–41.

Ells L. We had to help Katie adjust her expectations (amputation). Nursing '82 1982 June; 12(6):60–63.

Gever LN. Streptokinase and urokinase. Nursing '83 1983 Jan; 13(1):76.

Hertzer NR. Surgical management of intermittent claudication. Am Fam Physician 1977 Sept; 16(9):108–116.

Hessler K and Kenny M. Using human umbilical vein grafts. AORN J 1981 Apr; 33(5):862–866.

Hetherington H. Peripheral vascular disease. Nurs Times 1981 Dec 23–Jan 5; 77(52):2241–2245.

Joachim G. How to give a great foot massage. Geriatr Nurs 1983 Jan/Feb; 4(1):28–29.

King SL. Patient care in vascular surgery. AORN J 1981 Apr; 33(5):843–848.

Lawson M et al. Intravenous access by vascular access graft. NITA 1981 Mar/Apr; 4(2):146–147.

Mathewson MA. New uses for old drugs (vasodilators). Crit Care Update 1982 Nov; 9(11):7–13.

Miller KM. Assessing peripheral perfusion. Am J Nurs 1978 Oct; 78(10):1673–1674.

Mistretta CA and Crummy AB. Diagnosis of cardiovascular disease by digital subtraction angiography. Science 1981 Nov 13; 214(4522):761–765.

Pierson S et al. Efficacy of graded elastic compression in the lower leg. JAMA 1983 Jan 14; 249(2):242–243.

Precautions to be taken with fibrinolytic therapy. FDA Drug Bull 1978 Jan–Feb; 8:5.

Rabb D. Peripheral vascular disease. Can Nurse 1982 Sept; 78(8):30–33.

Sauvage LR. Porous fabric arterial prosthesis. AORN J 1981 Apr; 33(5):854–861.

Talkington CM and Thompson JE. Prevention and management of infected prosthesis (vessel grafts). Surg Clin North Am 1982 June; 62(3):515–530.

Whelan TJ Jr. Management of vascular disease of the upper extremity. Surg Clin North Am 1982 June; 62(3):373–389.

Wilson SE et al. Current status of vascular access techniques. Surg Clin North Am 1982 June; 62(3):531–551.

Winston TR, Henly WS, and Geis RC. Surgery for peripheral vascular disease. AORN J 1981 Apr; 33(5):849–853.

Worthington de Toledo L. How vasodilators backfire, RN 1982 July; 45(7):41–45.

Assessment and Diagnosis

Barnes RW. Current status of noninvasive tests in the diagnosis of venous disease. Surg Clin North Am 1982 June; 62(3):489–500.

Bernstein EF and Fronek A. Current status of noninvasive tests in the diagnosis of peripheral arterial disease. Surg Clin North Am 1982 June; 62(3):473–487.

Criss E. Digital subtraction angiography. Am J Nurs 1982 Nov; 82(11):1706–1707.

Hackett C. Neurovascular assessment technique. Nursing '83 1983 Mar; 13(3):40–43.

Hudson B. Sharpen your vascular assessment skills with the Doppler ultrasound stethoscope. Nursing '83 1983 May; 13(5):54–57.

Listening to the limbs—peripheral auscultation. Emergency Medicine 1982 Feb 28; 14(2):34.

MacKinnon JL. Study of Doppler ultrasonic peripheral vascular assessments performed by physical therapists. Phys Ther 1983 Jan; 63(1):30–34.

Mistretta CA and Crummy AB. Diagnosis of cardiovascular disease by digital subtraction angiography. Science 1981 Nov 13; 214(4522):761–765.

Roberts R and Ring EJ. Current status of percutaneous transluminal angioplasty. Surg Clin North Am 1982 June; 62(3):357–372.

Arterial Conditions

Baum PL. Carotid endarterectomy. Nursing '83 1983 Mar; 13(3):50–59.

Bernstein EF and Fronek A. Current status of noninvasive tests in the diagnosis of peripheral arterial disease. Surg Clin North Am 1982 June; 62(3):473–487.

Craven RF and Curry TD. When the diagnosis is Raynaud's. Am J Nurs 1981 May; 81(5):1007–1009.

Czar M et al. Atherosclerotic occlusive arterial disease: Promotion of optimal health. Occup Health Nurs 1981 Dec; 29(12):21–27.

Dendy A. Peripheral arterial disease: Road to rehabilitation. Nurs Mirror 1980 Aug; 151(8):44–45.

Doyle JE. Arterial insufficiency. Nursing '81 1981 Apr; 11(4):74–79.

Ekers MA and Satiani B. EAB: A new route for vascular rehabilitation—extra-anatomic bypass treatment of peripheral vascular disease. Nursing '82 Nov; 12(11):34–41.

Friedman SA. Guide to diagnosis of peripheral arterial disase. Hospital Medicine 1979 Jan; 15(1):87–91+

Jasinkowski N. The unique needs of a distal bypass patient. RN 1982 Mar; 45(3):43–47+.

Logan J and Ziebell E. Axillofemoral artery bypass. Can Nurse 1982 Sept; 78(8):25–29.

Massey EW et al. The two causes of claudication. Emergency Medicine 1981 July; 15(7):92–93+.

Sauvage LR. Porous fabric arterial prosthesis. AORN J 1981 Apr 33(5):854–861.

Smith S. Digital plethysmography for determination of Raynaud's phenomenon and disease (pictorial). CVP 1982 Oct–Nov; 77–79.

Spittell JA. Occlusive peripheral arterial disease. Postgrad Med 1982 Feb; 71(2):137–151.

Hypertension

Barnes G. The nurse's contribution to the Medical Research Council's Trial for mild hypertension. Nurs Times 1981 July 15–21; 77(29):1240–1245.

Caldwell JR. Practical approach to hypertension. I. Diagnostic evaluation. Postgrad Med 1979 May; 65(5):66–77.

Caldwell JR. Practical approach to hypertension. 2. Treatment. Postgrad Med 1979 May; 65(5):81–82.

Chobanian AV. Hypertension. Clin Symp 1982; 34(5):3–32.

Finnerty FA Jr. Hypertension in the elderly. Postgrad Med 1979 May; 65(5):119–125.

Gwen B and Gwen CW. Adherence to hypertensive therapy. Geriatr Nurs 1983 May/June; 4(3):172–175.

Guttman MC and Meyer DL. Social science in hypertension control. Family Community Health 1981 May; 4(5):63–72.

Hill M and Fink JW. In hypertensive emergencies, act quickly. Nursing '83 1983 Feb; 13(2):34–41.

Hill MN and Foster SB. High blood pressure. Nursing '82 1982 Feb; 12(2):72–75.

Kelber Sr MB. Plasma renin activity. Nursing '82 1982 Apr; 12(4):14–144.

Kirschenbaum HL et al. What to watch for with hydralazine and minoxidil—interactions and reactions. RN 1982 Dec; 45(12):42–43.

Loustan A and Blair BJ. A key to compliance—systematic teaching to help hypertensive patients follow through on treatment. Nursing '81 1981 Feb; 11(2):84–87.

Lowther NB and Carter VD. How to increase compliance in hypertensives. Am J Nurs 1981 May; 81(5):963.

Nursing Update. Antihypertensives. Nursing '83 1983 Mar; 13(3):between pp. 64 and 65.

Onesti G. Selection of drugs for hypertensive crisis. Am Fam Physician 1980 Dec; 22(6):141–142.

Pleuss J and Kochar MS. Dietary considerations in hypertension. Postgrad Med 1981 June; 69(6):34–43.

Ram CVS. Diuretics in the management of hypertension. Postgrad Med 1982 Feb; 71(2):155–168.

Relaxation, biofeedback and exercise for the treatment of hypertension. Medical Letter 1978 July 14; 20:62–63.

Semple P. Hypertension, Part I. Nurs Mirror 1980 Oct 2; 151(14):18–21.

Semple P. Hypertension, Part II. Nurs Mirror 1980 Oct 9; 151(15):24–26.

Semple P. Hypertension, Part III. Nurs Mirror 1980 Oct 16; 151(16):30–32.

Sparacino J. Blood pressure, stress, and mental health. Nurs Res 1982 Mar/Apr; 31(2):89–93.

Sparacino J et al. Psychological correlates of blood pressure: A closer examination of hostility, anxiety, and engagement. Nurs Res 1982 May/June; 31(3):143–149.

Stromberg MF and Stromborg P. Test your knowledge of managing the patient with hypertension. Nursing '81 1981 Mar; 11(3):56–59.

Therapy for mild hypertension. JAMA 1983 Jan 21; 249(3):365–367.

Thibodeau JA and Hebert P. Use of nursing model to develop a hypertension protocol. Nurse Pract 1981 Mar–Apr; 6(2):21–27.

Anticoagulant and Thrombolytic Therapy

Cheng TC. Thrombocytopenia associated with minidose heparin therapy. Postgrad Med 1981 Dec; 70(6):73–78.

Gever LN. Streptokinase and urokinase. Nursing '83 1983 Jan; 13(1):76.

Hull R. Adjusted subcutaneous heparin vs warfarin sodium in the long-term treatment of venous thrombosis. N Engl J Med 1982 Jan 28; 306(4):189–194.

Kirschenbaum HL and Rosenberg JM. Coumarin. RN 1982 Oct; 42(10):54–56.

Silverstein A. Neurological complications of anticoagulation therapy. Arch Intern Med 1979 Feb; 139(2):217–219.

Sohn CA. Rescind the risks in administering anticoagulants. Nursing '81 1981 Oct; 11(10):34–41.

Thompson DA. Teaching the client about anticoagulants. Am J Nurs 1983 Feb; 82(2):278–281.

Aneurysm

Baum PL. Abdominal aortic aneurysm? Nursing '82 1982 Dec; 12(12):34–41.

Edwards WS. Thoracoabdominal aortic aneurysms. Surg Clin North Am 1982 June; 62(3):441–448.

Ochsner JL. Management of femoral pseudoaneurysms. Surg Clin North Am 1982 June; 62(3):431–440.

Venous Conditions

Barnes RW. Current status of noninvasive tests in the diagnosis of venous disease. Surg Clin North Am 1982 June; 62(3):489–500.

Bergan JJ, Flinn WR, and Yao JST. Venous reconstructive surgery. Surg Clin North Am 1982 June; 62(3):399–410.

Dale WA. Venous bypass surgery. Surg Clin North Am 1982 June; 62(3):391–398.

Fedullo PF. Deep venous thrombosis in the intensive care unit. Respiratory Therapy 1982 Mar; 12(3):77–80.

Hessler K and Kenny M. Using humans umbilical vein grafts. AORN J 1981 Apr; 33(5):862–866.

Varicose Veins

Hinnant JR and Stallworth JM. Simplified surgery for varicose veins. AORN J 1981 July; 34(1):135–150.

Iveson–Iveson J. Varicose veins: The general etiology, the complications, and the treatment. Nurs Mirror 1981 Sept 2; 153(10):37.

Lofgren KA. Varicose veins: Their symptoms, complications, and management. Postgrad Med 1979 June; 65(6):131.

Leg Ulcers

Antrobus M. Case study—venous ulcers. Nurs Times Community Outlook 1982 Dec 8; 78:346.

Doyle JE. All leg ulcers are not alike: Managing and preventing arterial and venous ulcers. Nursing '83 1983 Jan; 13(1):58–63.

Martin I. Varicose ulcers. Breaking down in vein, Part I. Nurs Mirror 1981 July 29; 153(5):34–35.

Martin I. Varicose ulcers. Breaking down in vein, Part II. Nurs Mirror 1981 Aug 5; 153(6):34–35.

McCulloch JM. Intermittent compression for the treatment of a chronic stasis ulceration: A case report. Phys Ther 1981 Oct; 61(10):1452–1453.

Seville RH et al. Nurs Times 1981 July 15–21; 77(29):1249–1253.

33

Assessment and Management of Patients With Hematologic Disorders

▷ Physiologic Overview

The hematologic system comprises the blood and the sites where blood is produced, including the bone marrow and lymph nodes. The blood is a specialized organ that differs from other organs in that it exists in a fluid state. The fluid consists of cellular components suspended in blood plasma. The blood cells are divided into erythrocytes (red blood cells, normally 5 million per mm^3 of blood) and leukocytes (white blood cells, normally 5,000–10,000 per mm^3 of blood). Thus, there are approximately 500–1000 erythrocytes for each leukocyte. Also suspended in the plasma are small, nonnucleated cell fragments called platelets (normally 150,000–450,000 platelets per mm^3 of blood). These cellular components of blood normally make up 40% to 45% of the blood volume. The fraction of the blood occupied by erythrocytes is called the *hematocrit*. Blood appears as a thick, opaque, red fluid. Its color is imparted by the hemoglobin contained within the red blood cells.

The volume of blood in humans is approximately 7% to 10% of the normal body weight, which represents about 5 liters. The blood is recirculated through the vascular system and serves as a link between body organs, carrying oxygen absorbed from the lungs and nutrients absorbed from the gastrointestinal tract to the body cells for cellular metabolism.

It also carries waste products produced by cellular metabolism to the lungs, skin, liver, and kidneys for subsequent transformation and elimination from the body. The blood also carries hormones, antibodies, and other products of internal secretion to their sites of action or utilization.

In order to perform its functions, blood must remain in its normally fluid state. Because it is fluid, the danger always exists that trauma can lead to loss of blood from the vascular system. To prevent this, the blood has an intricate clotting mechanism that is activated when necessary to seal leaks in the blood vessels. When blood is withdrawn from the body, the clotting system is activated and the blood clots, unless an anticoagulant is present. The liquid portion that remains after the blood has clotted is termed blood *serum.*

Excessive clotting is equally dangerous because it potentially obstructs blood flow to vital tissues. To prevent this complication, the body has a fibrinolytic mechanism that eventually dissolves the clots formed within blood vessels.

Bone Marrow

The bone marrow occupies the interior of spongy bones and the central cavity of the long bones of the skeleton. The marrow accounts for 4% to 5% of the total body weight and therefore constitutes one of the larger organs of the body. The marrow can be either red or yellow. Red marrow is the site of active blood cell production and constitutes the major hematopoietic (blood producing) organ. Yellow marrow, on the other hand, is composed mainly of fat and is not active in the production of blood elements. During childhood, the major portion of the marrow is red. As the individual ages, a large portion of the marrow in the long bones is converted into yellow marrow, but it retains the potential for reversion to hematopoietic tissue if necessary. Red marrow in the adult is confined chiefly to the ribs, vertebral column, and other flat bones.

The marrow is a highly vascularized organ that consists of connective tissue containing free cells. The most primitive of this population of free cells are the stem cells, which are precursors of two different cell lines. The myeloid line includes erythrocytes, several types of leukocytes, and platelets. The lymphoid line differentiates into lymphocytes.

Erythrocytes

The normal red blood cell is a biconcave disc, its configuration resembling that of a soft ball compressed between two fingers. It has a diameter of about 8 microns but is a very flexible cell, so flexible that it is capable of passing easily through capillaries that may be as small as 4 microns in diameter. The volume of a red blood cell is about 90 cubic microns. The red blood cell membrane is so thin that gases such as oxygen and carbon dioxide can easily diffuse across it. Mature red blood cells consist primarily of hemoglobin, which makes up 95% of the cell mass. These cells have no nuclei and have many fewer metabolic enzymes than do most other cells. The presence of a large amount of hemoglobin enables the cell to perform its principal function, the transport of oxygen between lungs and tissues.

The oxygen-carrying pigment hemoglobin is a protein with a molecular weight of 64,000. The molecule is made up of four subunits, each containing a heme moiety attached to a globin chain. Iron is present in the heme portion of the molecule. An important property of the heme moiety is its ability to loosely and reversibly bind to oxygen. When hemoglobin is combined with oxygen, it is called *oxyhemoglobin.* Oxyhemoglobin has a brighter red color than hemoglobin that does not contain oxygen (reduced hemoglobin), so that arterial blood is a brighter red than venous blood. Whole blood normally contains about 15 g of hemoglobin per 100 ml of blood, or 30 μg of hemoglobin per million erythrocytes.

Production of Erythrocytes (Erythropoiesis).   Erythroblasts arise from the primitive stem cells in bone marrow. The erythroblast is a nucleated cell that in the process of maturing within the bone marrow accumulates hemoglobin and gradually loses its nucleus. At this stage, the cell is known as a *reticulocyte.* Further maturation into an erythrocyte entails the loss of dark staining material and a slight shrinkage in size. The mature erythrocyte is then released into the circulation. Under conditions of rapid erythropoiesis, reticulocytes and other immature cells may be released prematurely into the circulation.

Differentiation of the primitive multipotential stem cell of the marrow into an erythroblast is stimulated by erythropoietin, a substance produced mostly by the kidney. Under conditions of prolonged hypoxia, as in the case of individuals dwelling at high altitudes or after severe hemorrhage, erythropoietin levels are increased and red blood cell production is stimulated.

For normal erythrocyte production, the bone marrow requires iron, vitamin B_{12}, folic acid, pyridoxine (vitamin B_6), and other factors. If any of these factors is deficient during erythropoiesis, decreased red blood cell production and anemia result.

Iron Stores and Metabolism.   Total body iron content in the average adult is approximately 3 g, most of which is present in hemoglobin or one of its breakdown products. Normally, about 0.5 mg to 1 mg of iron is absorbed per day from the intestinal tract to replace losses of iron in the feces. Additional amounts of iron, up to 2 mg per day, must be absorbed by the adult female to replace blood lost during menstruation. Iron deficiency in the adult (decreased total body iron content) generally indicates that blood has been lost from the body, for example, by hemorrhage or excessive menstruation.

The concentration of iron in blood is normally about 0.5 μg/ml to 2.0 μg/ml. With iron deficiency, bone marrow iron stores are rapidly depleted, hemoglobin synthesis is depressed, and the red blood cells produced by the marrow are small and low in hemoglobin.

Vitamin B_{12} and Folic Acid Metabolism.   Vitamin B_{12} and folic acid are required for DNA synthesis in many tissues, but deficiencies of either of these vitamins has the greatest effect on erythropoiesis. Vitamin B_{12} or folic acid deficiency is characterized by the production of abnormally large red blood cells (called megaloblasts). Because these cells are abnormal, many are sequestered in the bone marrow and their rate of release is decreased. This condition results in megaloblastic anemia.

Both vitamin B_{12} and folic acid are derived from the diet. Vitamin B_{12} combines with intrinsic factor produced in the stomach. The vitamin B_{12}-intrinsic factor complex is absorbed in the distal ileum. Folic acid is absorbed in the proximal small intestine.

Red Blood Cell Destruction.   The average lifespan of a circulating red blood cell is 120 days. Aged red blood cells are removed from the blood by the reticuloendothelial system, particularly in the liver and the spleen. The reticuloendothelial cells produce a pigment called bilirubin from the hemoglobin that is released from the destroyed red blood cells. Bilirubin is a waste product that is excreted in the bile. The iron, freed from the hemoglobin during bilirubin formation, is carried in plasma bound to the protein called transferrin to the bone marrow, where it is reclaimed for production of new hemoglobin.

Function of Erythrocytes.   The major function of the red blood cells is to transport oxygen from the lungs to the tissues. Erythrocytes are uniquely capable of performing this function because of their high concentration of hemoglobin. If hemoglobin was not present, the oxygen-carrying capacity of blood would be decreased by 99% and would not be sufficient to meet the metabolic needs of the body. An important property of hemoglobin is that it binds oxygen loosely and reversibly. As a result, oxygen readily binds to hemoglobin in the lungs, is carried as oxyhemoglobin in arterial blood, and readily dissociates from hemoglobin in the tissues. In venous blood, hemoglobin combines with hydrogen ions produced by cellular metabolism and thus buffers excess acid.

Leukocytes

Leukocytes are divided into two general categories, granulocytes and mononuclear cells. In normal blood, the total leukocyte count is 5,000 to 10,000 cells per cubic millimeter. Of these, approximately 60% are granulocytes and 40% are mononuclear cells. Leukocytes can be readily differentiated from erythrocytes by the presence of a nucleus, their larger size, and different staining properties.

Granulocytes.   Granulocytes are defined by the presence of granules in their cytoplasm. The diameter of a granulocyte is generally two to three times that of an erythrocyte. Granulocytes are divided into three subgroups, which are characterized by their staining properties as seen on microscopic examination. Eosinophils have bright red granules in their cytoplasm, whereas the granules in basophils stain deep blue. The third, and by far the most numerous, cell in this series is the neutrophil, with granules that show a dull violet hue. The nucleus of the mature granulocyte generally has multiple lobes (usually two to four) connected by thin filaments of nuclear material. Because of their nuclear characteristics, these cells are called polymorphonuclear (PMN) leukocytes. The immature granulocyte has a single-lobed ovoid nucleus and is called a band cell. Ordinarily, band forms account for only a small percentage of circulating granulocytes, although their percentage can increase greatly under conditions in which the rate of production of polymorphonuclear leukocytes is increased. The number of circulating granulocytes found in the healthy individual is maintained relatively constant, but in the presence of infection, large numbers of these cells are rapidly released into the circulation. Granulocyte production from the stem cell pool is thought to be controlled in a manner similar to the regulation of erythrocyte production by erythropoietin.

Mononuclear Leukocytes.   Mononuclear leukocytes (lymphocytes and monocytes) are white blood cells with a single-lobed nucleus and a granule-free cytoplasm. In normal adult blood, lymphocytes account for approximately 30% and monocytes approximately 5% of the total leukocytes. Mature lymphocytes are small cells with scanty cytoplasm. They are produced primarily in the lymph nodes

and in the lymphoid tissue of the intestine, spleen, and thymus gland from precursor cells that originated as marrow stem cells. Monocytes are the largest of the blood leukocytes. They are produced by the bone marrow and give rise to tissue histiocytes, including Kupffer cells of the liver, peritoneal macrophages, alveolar macrophages, and other components of the reticuloendothelial system.

Function of the Leukocytes.   The function of the leukocytes is to protect the body from invasion by bacteria and other foreign entities. The major function of neutrophilic polymorphonuclear leukocytes is to ingest foreign material (phagocytosis). Neutrophils arrive at the site within an hour of the onset of an inflammatory reaction and initiate phagocytosis but are relatively short-lived. The influx of monocytes is later, but these cells continue their phagocytic activities for long periods.

The function of lymphocytes is primarily to produce substances that aid in the attack on foreign material. One group of lymphocytes (T-lymphocytes) kills foreign cells directly or releases a variety of lymphokines, substances that enhance the activity of phagocytic cells. The other group of lymphocytes (B-lymphocytes) produces antibodies, protein molecules that destroy foreign material by several mechanisms.

Eosinophils and basophils function as reservoirs of potent biological materials such as histamine, serotonin, and heparin. Release of these compounds alters the blood supply to tissues, such as occurs during inflammation, and helps to mobilize body defense mechanisms. The increase in the number of eosinophils in allergic states indicates that these cells are involved in the hypersensitivity reaction.

Platelets

Platelets are small particles, 2 to 4 microns in diameter, that are present in the circulating blood plasma. Their number varies normally between 150,000 and 450,000 per cubic millimeter of blood. They are formed from the fragmentation (the pinching off of bits of membrane and cytoplasm) of giant cells of the bone marrow called megakaryocytes. Platelet production is regulated by thrombopoietin.

Platelets play an essential role in the control of bleeding. When vascular injury occurs, platelets collect at the site. Substances released from platelet granules and other blood cells cause the platelets to adhere to each other and form a patch or plug, which temporarily stops bleeding. Additional substances released from platelets activate coagulation factors in the blood plasma.

Blood Coagulation

Blood coagulation is the process whereby the components of the liquid blood are transformed into a semisolid material called a blood clot. The blood clot is made up mainly of blood cells entrapped in a meshwork of fibrin. Fibrin is formed from proteins in the plasma as the result of a complex series of reactions.

Many factors are involved in the reaction cascade that forms fibrin. The clotting factors are listed in Table 33-1, and the extrinsic and intrinsic pathways for fibrin generation are shown diagramatically in Figure 33-1. When tissue is injured, the extrinsic pathway is activated by the release

Table 33-1
Clotting Factors

Official Number	Synonym	Contemporary Version
I	Fibrinogen	I (fibrinogen)
II	Prothrombin	II (prothrombin)
III	Tissue thromboplastin	III (tissue factor)
IV	Calcium	IV (calcium)
V	Labile factor	V (labile factor)
		VI: PF$_3$ (platelet coagulant activities)
		VI: PF$_4$
VII	Stable factor	VII (stable factor)
VIII	Antihemophilic factor	VIII: AHF (antihemophilic factor)
		VIII: VWF (von Willebrand factor)
		VIII: RAg (related-antigen)
IX	Christmas factor	IX (Christmas factor)
X	Stuart–Prower factor	X (Stuart–Prower factor)
XI	Plasma thromboplastin (antecedent)	XI (plasma thromboplastin antecedent)
XII	Hageman factor	XII: HF (Hageman factor)
		XII: PK (Prekallikrein, Fletcher)
		XII: HMWK (high molecular weight kininogen)
XIII	Fibrin stabilizing factor	XIII: fibrin stabilizing factor

The Roman numerals and synonyms designating each clotting factor accepted by the International Committee on Blood Clotting Factors are located in the left-hand columns. Note the absence of factor VI. The version in the right-hand column incorporates more recently recognized clotting factors but is not officially recognized.
(From Green D: General considerations of coagulation proteins. Ann Clin Lab Sci 8(2):95–105, 1978.)

from the tissue of a substance called thromboplastin. As the result of a series of reactions, prothrombin is converted to thrombin, which in turn catalyzes the conversion of fibrinogen to fibrin. Calcium (factor IV) is a necessary cofactor for many of these reactions. Clotting by the intrinsic pathway is activated when the collagen lining blood vessels is exposed. Clotting factors are then sequentially activated until, as with the extrinsic pathway, fibrin is ultimately formed. Although longer, this sequence is probably most often responsible for clotting *in vivo*. The intrinsic pathway is also responsible for initiating the clotting of blood that comes into contact with glass or other foreign surfaces, such as when blood is withdrawn from the body into a test tube. It is for this reason that anticoagulants often must be used when drawing blood for chemical or other tests. The anticoagulants that are often used are either citrate, which binds the plasma calcium, or heparin, which prevents the conversion of prothrombin to thrombin. Citrate cannot be used as an anticoagulant *in vivo* because binding of plasma calcium would cause death. Heparin can be used clinically as an anticoagulant. Coumarins are also used clinically for their anticoagulant action of interfering with the production of several of the plasma coagulating factors.

Clots that form in the body are eventually dissolved by the action of the fibrinolytic system, which consists of plasmin and other proteolytic enzymes. Through the action of this system, clots are dissolved as tissue is repaired, and the vascular system is returned to its normal baseline state.

Blood Plasma

After cellular elements are removed from blood, the remaining liquid portion is called *blood plasma*. It contains ions, proteins, and other substances. If plasma is allowed to clot, the remaining fluid is called *serum*. Serum has essentially the same composition as plasma except that its fibrinogen and several of the clotting factors have been removed.

Plasma Proteins.   Plasma proteins consist largely of albumin and globulins. The globulins in turn consist of alpha, beta, and gamma fractions derived by a laboratory test called serum protein electrophoresis. Each of these groups is made up of distinct proteins. The gamma globulins, which consist largely of antibodies, are called immunoglobulins. These proteins are produced by the lymphocytes and plasma cells. Important proteins in the alpha and beta fractions are the transport globulins and the clotting factors, which are made in the liver. The transport globulins carry various substances in bound form around the circulation. For example, thyroid-binding globulin carries thyroxin, and transferrin carries iron. The clotting factors, including fibrinogen, remain in an inactive form in the blood plasma until activated by the clotting cascade.

Albumin is particularly important for the maintenance of fluid volume within the vascular system. Capillary walls are impermeable to albumin, hence its presence in the plasma creates an osmotic force that keeps fluid within the vascular space. Albumin, which is produced in the liver, has

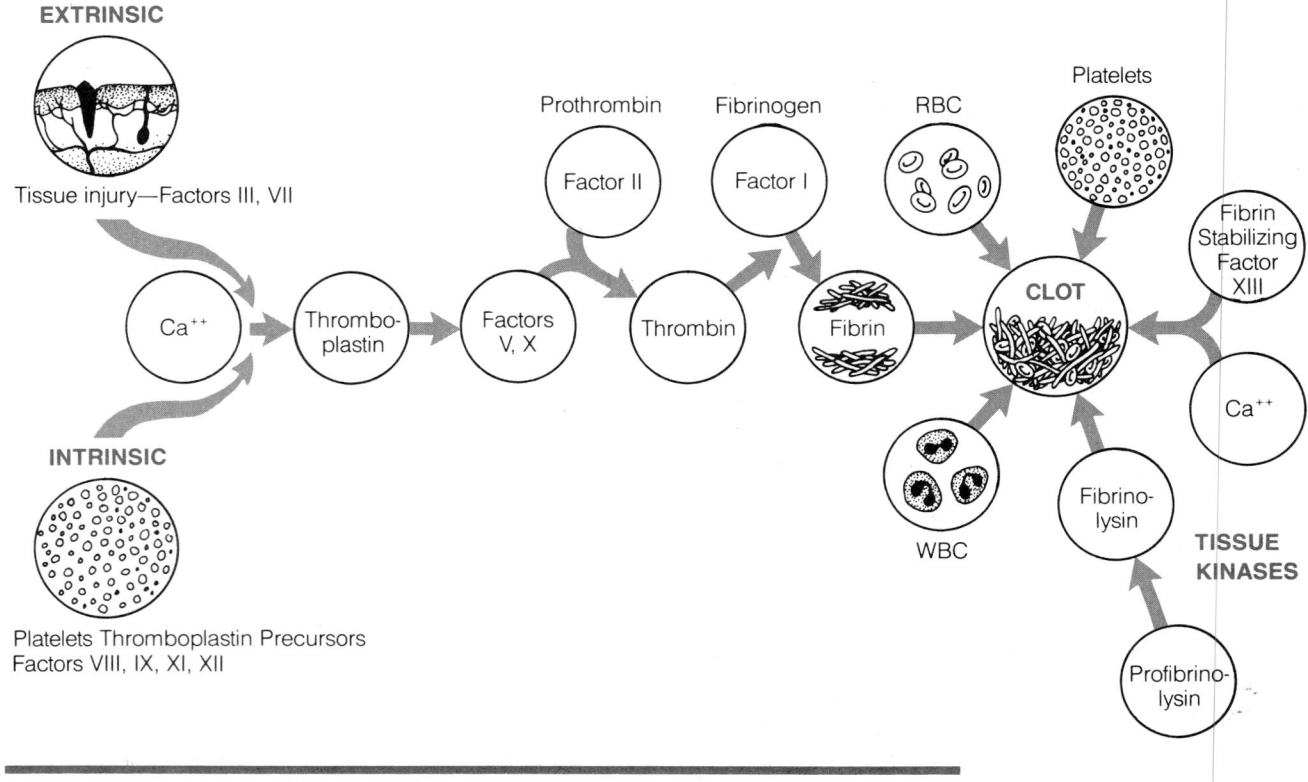

Figure 33-1. The blood-clotting mechanism. The schematic drawing represents the factors essential to change blood into a solid gel. The entire chain reaction in which fibrinogen (a plasma protein) is converted to fibrin (the clot) takes place at the site of vessel damage. (Adapted from Feller I and Archambeault C: Nursing the Burn Patient. Ann Arbor, Michigan, The Institute for Burn Medicine.)

the capacity to bind to a number of substances that are often present in plasma. In this way, it functions as a transport protein for metals, fatty acids, bilirubin, and drugs, among other substances.

Pathophysiology of the Hematologic System

Anemias. A frequent disorder of the hematologic system is a decrease in the number of circulating red blood cells. This condition, called anemia, can result from either underproduction of red blood cells by the bone marrow or increased destruction of circulating red blood cells. Underproduction of red blood cells can be due to a deficiency of cofactors for erythropoiesis, including folic acid, vitamin B_{12} and iron. Red blood cell production may also be reduced if bone marrow is suppressed (by tumor or drugs) or is inadequately stimulated owing to lack of erythropoietin, such as occurs in chronic renal disease. Increased destruction of red blood cells may occur because of an overactive reticuloendothelial system (*e.g.*, hypersplenism) or because the bone marrow produces abnormal red blood cells (*e.g.*, sickle cell anemia). Since the red blood cell and its contained hemoglobin are important for the delivery of oxygen to tissues, anemias may result in tissue hypoxia.

Bleeding Disorders. Bleeding disorders can be attributed to deficiency of either platelets or clotting factors in the circulating blood. Platelet function in the blood plasma can be reduced as the result of bone marrow insufficiency,

increased splenic destruction, or abnormal circulating platelets. Deficiencies of clotting factors are usually due to underproduction of these factors by the liver. Hemophilia is a hereditary disorder that results from deficiency of clotting factors VIII and IX.

▷ Blood Study Procedures

Methods of Obtaining Blood

Venipuncture. Most routine hematologic studies are performed on venous blood, which is usually obtained from an antecubital vein, although occasionally, in very obese persons or those whose veins have been thrombosed by chemotherapy, it may be necessary to puncture one of the veins on the dorsum of the hand.

After a tourniquet has been tied around the upper arm, the arm and hand veins become prominent. The vein chosen for venipuncture should be straight, not tortuous, and should be well fixed in the subcutaneous tissue, so that it does not roll away. The skin below the vein is stretched with one hand while the opposite hand is used to push the needle through the skin and then slowly into the vein. Blood is immediately placed in the collection tube appropriate for the particular test required. The tubes are color coded to specify what, if any, additive they contain. For some tests the blood is allowed to coagulate; for others it

Chart 33-1
Common Problems of Patients With Blood Disorders

The Problem	Nursing Interventions
Fatigue and weakness	Plan nursing care to conserve the patient's strength. Give frequent rest periods. Encourage ambulation activities as tolerated. Avoid disturbing activities and noise. Encourage optimal nutrition.
Hemorrhagic tendencies	Keep the patient at rest during the bleeding episodes. Apply gentle pressure to the bleeding sites. Apply cold compresses to the bleeding sites when indicated. Do not disturb clots. Use small-gauge needles when administering medications by injection. Support the patient during transfusion therapy. Observe for symptoms of internal bleeding. Have a tracheostomy set available for the patient who is bleeding from the mouth or the throat.
Ulcerative lesions of the tongue, gums, or mucous membranes	Avoid irritating foods and beverages. Give frequent oral hygiene with mild, cool mouthwash solutions. Use applicators or soft-bristled toothbrush. Keep the lips lubricated. Give mouth care both before and after meals.
Dyspnea	Elevate the head of the bed. Use pillows to support the patient in the orthopneic position. Administer oxygen when indicated. Prevent unnecessary exertion. Avoid gas-forming foods.
Bone and joint pains	Relieve pressure of bedding by using a cradle. Administer either hot or cold compresses as prescribed. Provide for joint immobilization when prescribed.
Fever	Administer cool sponges. Give antipyretic drugs as prescribed. Encourage fluid intake unless contraindicated. Maintain a cool environmental temperature.
Pruritus or skin eruptions	Keep the patient's fingernails short. Use soap sparingly. Apply emollient lotions in skin care.
Anxiety of the patient and his family	Explain the nature, the discomforts, and the limitations of activity associated with the diagnostic procedures and treatments. Offer the patient the service of listening. Have an empathetic attitude. Promote the patient's relaxation and comfort. Remember the patient's individual preferences. Encourage the family to participate in the patient's care (as desired). Create a comfortable atmosphere for the family to visit with the patient.

is kept fluid by the presence of an anticoagulant in the collection tube.

Finger Puncture. The finger puncture method is used frequently for blood smears and counts. This method utilizes capillary blood, but for practical purposes the results are identical to those obtained with venous blood. Lances of various shapes are available. These make a puncture of 1 mm to 2 mm. Best results are obtained if the patient's hand is warm and if the pulp of the index or middle finger is punctured. The skin should be cleaned with alcohol first and then carefully wiped dry with a lint-free sponge. If any alcohol remains, it will alter red cell morphology. The drops of blood obtained by this method can be gently touched to glass slides or cover slips, for peripheral smears. Capillary blood can also be drawn into calibrated red cell and white cell pipettes and into microhematocrit tubes.

The most common hematologic tests are described in Chart 33-2.

Bone Marrow Aspiration

Bone marrow is usually aspirated from the sternum or iliac crest in adults. Most patients need no more preparation than a careful explanation of the procedure, but for some very anxious patients, meperidine (Demerol) or a minor tranquilizer may be useful. It is always important for the physician

or nurse to describe and explain the procedure as it is being performed. First, the skin area is cleansed as for any minor surgery. Then a small area is anesthetized with lidocaine (Xylocaine), through the skin and subcutaneous tissue to the periosteum of the bone. The bone marrow needle is introduced with a stylet in place, and when the needle is felt to go through the outer cortex of bone and enter the marrow cavity, the stylet is removed, a syringe is attached, and a small volume (0.5 ml) of blood and marrow is aspirated. The actual aspiration always causes brief pain, and the patient should be warned of this.

If a bone marrow biopsy is necessary, it is best performed after the aspiration and with a special needle. Sev-

---

Chart 33-2
Common Hematologic Laboratory Tests

Test	Definition
Complete blood count	Includes enumeration of number of white cells, red cells, and platelets per cubic millimeter of venous blood, as well as a differential count, percentage of each type of nucleated cell in the blood (*i.e.*, percent polymorphonuclears, percent lymphocytes, etc.).
Reticulocyte count	Percentage of young (1–2 days old), nonnucleated erythrocytes in peripheral blood; they are recognized in special stains of blood smears as cells with lacy inclusions, which consist of RNA.
Hemoglobin electrophoresis	A drop of blood placed on a solid medium (paper, starch block, gel, or cellulose acetate) is exposed to a current of electricity while being bathed by a buffer solution. The different hemoglobins (*e.g.*, A, A-2, F, S) travel at varying speeds, depending on their charge. At the end of the procedure, the paper or gel is stained, and the hemoglobins in each sample can be identified.
Sickling test	A drop of blood is mixed with a drop of a reducing agent (sodium metabisulfite). This substance deprives the red cells of oxygen and induces sickling if S hemoglobin is present. Sickling of red cells is observed under the microscope in 30 minutes if the blood was obtained from a person with either sickle trait or sickle cell anemia. Normal blood does not undergo any change.
Leukocyte alkaline phosphatase (LAP)	An enzyme present in high concentrations in granules of neutrophils. A special stain of peripheral blood smears is used to estimate the amount of LAP present per cell. The normal score is 20 to 130. Untreated chronic myelogenous leukemia patients have scores of less than 20, and the test is useful to help diagnose CML. High scores are seen in infection and steroid-induced leukocytosis.
Coombs' test	Determines the presence of gamma globulin (hence, antibodies) on the surface of erythrocytes (direct Coombs' test) or in the plasma (indirect Coombs' test).
Bleeding time	A screening test for disorders of platelet function. It is the time taken for bleeding to cease after a standardized skin wound is produced, usually on the volar surface of the forearm. When it is prolonged, this suggests an inherited or acquired platelet defect, for example, von Willebrand's disease or aspirin ingestion.
Platelet aggregation	A measure of the time and completeness of the formation of platelet aggregates in a sample of plasma, after the addition of an agent such as epinephrine or ADP.
Prothrombin time test	Measures the coagulant activity of the "extrinsic" system, including fibrinogen, prothrombin, and factors V, VII, and X. It is used to monitor Coumadin therapy, as well as for a screening test for liver disease.
Partial thromboplastin time test	A screening test for deficiencies of all plasma coagulation factors except VII and XIII. Is usually abnormally prolonged if levels of factors are less than 30% of normal. It is often used to monitor heparin therapy.

eral types of needles are available, the procedure varying according to the type of needle used. Since these needles are large, the skin should be punctured first with a surgical blade (No. 9 or 11) to make a 3-mm or 4-mm incision. Only the iliac bone is used for this procedure (Fig. 33-2), since the sternum is too thin.

The major hazard of these procedures is a slight risk of hemorrhage. Following bone marrow aspiration, pressure should be applied to the site for several minutes. After a biopsy, pressure is applied to the posterior iliac crest for 60 minutes by the combination of a pressure dressing and having the patient lie recumbent in bed. Most patients have no discomfort after a bone marrow aspiration, but the site of a biopsy may ache for a day or two.

▷ Anemia

Anemia is a laboratory definition that implies a low red cell count and a below normal hemoglobin or hematocrit level. These levels are somewhat arbitrary since there is a range of normal values.

Pathophysiology

The appearance of anemia reflects either marrow failure or excessive red cell loss, or both. Marrow failure (*i.e.,* reduced erythropoiesis) may occur as a result of a nutritional deficiency, toxic exposure, tumor invasion, or, as in many instances, from causes unknown. Red cells may be lost through hemorrhage or hyperhemolysis (increased destruction). In the latter case the problem may be rooted in some red cell defect that is incompatible with normal red cell survival or explainable on the basis of some factor extrinsic to the red cell that promotes red cell destruction.

Red cell lysis occurs mainly within the phagocytic cells of the reticuloendothelial system, notably in the liver and spleen. As a by-product of this process, bilirubin, formed within the phagocyte, enters the bloodstream, and any increase in hemolysis is promptly reflected by an increase in plasma bilirubin. (This concentration normally is 1 mg/100 ml or less; levels above 1.5 mg/100 ml produce visible jaundice of the sclerae.)

If, as happens in certain specific hemolytic disorders, red cells are destroyed within the circulating bloodstream, hemoglobin itself appears in the plasma (hemoglobinemia) and, if its concentration there exceeds the capacity of the plasma haptoglobin to bind it all (*i.e.,* if the amount is more than about 100 mg/100 ml), then this pigment is free to diffuse through the renal glomeruli and into the urine (hemoglobinuria). Thus, the presence or absence of hemoglobinemia and hemoglobinuria provides information about the location of abnormal blood destruction in a patient with hemolysis and can be a clue to the nature of the hemolytic process.

A conclusion as to whether the anemia in a particular patient is caused by hemolysis or by inadequate erythropoiesis usually can be reached on the basis of (1) the reticulocyte count in the circulating blood; (2) the degree to which young red cells are proliferating in the bone marrow and the manner in which they are maturing, as observed on

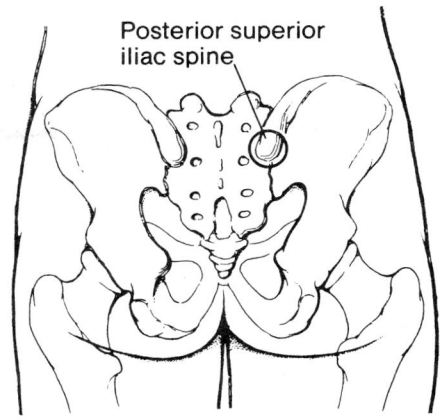

Figure 33-2. Site of bone marrow biopsy.

biopsy; and (3) the presence or absence of hyperbilirubinemia and hemoglobinemia. Moreover, one can actually quantitate erythropoiesis by measuring the rate at which injected radioactive iron is incorporated into circulating erythrocytes, and one can measure the life span of the patient's red cells (ergo, the hemolytic rate) by tagging a portion of these with radioactive chromium, reinjecting them, and following their disappearance from the circulating blood over the course of the ensuing days or weeks. Methods by which one particular type of marrow failure can be distinguished from another type, and one hemolytic disease from another, are specified in relation to each of the conditions discussed.

Clinical Manifestations

Aside from the severity of the anemia, several factors affect the anemic patient and tend to influence the severity and even the presence of his symptoms: (1) the speed with which the anemia has developed, (2) its prior duration (*i.e.,* its chronicity), (3) the metabolic requirements of the particular patient, (4) any other disorders or disabilities with which the patient is currently afflicted, and (5) special complications or concomitant features of the condition that has produced this anemia.

The more rapidly an anemia develops, the more severe its symptoms. An otherwise normal individual can tolerate as much as a 50% gradual reduction in hemoglobin, red count, or hematocrit without pronounced symptoms or significant incapacity, whereas the rapid loss of as little as 30% may precipitate profound vascular collapse in the same individual. A person who has been anemic for a very long period of time, with hemoglobin levels between 9 g/100 ml and 11 g/100 ml, experiences few or no symptoms other than slight tachycardia on exertion; exertional dyspnea is likely to occur below, but not above 7.5 g/100 ml; weakness, only below 6 g/100 ml; dyspnea at rest, below 3 g/100 ml; and cardiac failure, only at the profoundly low level of 2 g/100 ml to 2.5 g/100 ml.

Patients who customarily are very active are more likely to experience symptoms, and symptoms that are more pronounced, than a more sedentary individual. A hypothyroid patient, requiring, as he does, less than the usual amount of oxygen, may be perfectly asymptomatic, without tachycardia or increased cardiac output, at a hemoglobin level of 10 g/100 ml. Contrariwise, at any given level of anemia, patients with underlying heart disease are far more apt to experience angina or symptoms of congestive failure than someone without heart disease.

Finally, as will emerge in the discussions that follow, many anemic disorders are complicated by various other abnormalities—abnormalities that do not depend on the anemia but that are inherently associated with these particular diseases. These abnormalities may give rise to symptoms that completely overshadow those of the anemia, as is exemplified by the painful crises of sickle cell anemia (p. 707).

There are a number of hematologic disorders in which anemia is the presenting problem, or the problem of paramount concern, and which, as a group, exemplify all of the etiologic factors that have been discussed and all of the pathogenic mechanisms that have been formulated to date with respect to anemia.

Classification of Anemias

There are several ways to classify the anemias; the physiologic approach is to determine whether the deficiency in red cells in due to a defect in production of red cells (hypoproliferative anemia) or in survival of the red cells (hemolytic anemia).

In the hypoproliferative anemias, red cells usually survive normally, but the marrow is unable to produce adequate numbers of cells: thus, the reticulocyte count is depressed. This situation can be a result of marrow damage by drugs or chemicals (*e.g.,* chloramphenicol, benzene) or may be due to lack of erythropoietin (as in renal disease) or to lack of iron, vitamin B_{12}, or folic acid.

When hemolysis is the major cause of anemia, the abnormality is usually within the red cell itself (as in sickle cell anemia or G-6-PD [glucose-6-phosphate dehydrogenase] deficiency), in the plasma (as in the immune hemolytic anemias), or in the circulation (as in heart valve hemolysis). In all of these hemolytic anemias, the reticulocyte count is elevated and the indirect bilirubin is high, often enough to cause clinical jaundice.

Hypoproliferative Anemias

Aplastic Anemia

Pathophysiology. *Aplastic anemia* is anemia caused by a decrease in precursor cells in the bone marrow. It may be idiopathic, that is, without apparent cause; result from certain infections; or be caused by drugs, chemicals, or radiation damage. Agents that regularly produce marrow aplasia in sufficient dosage include benzene and benzene derivatives; antitumor agents such as nitrogen mustard and its congeners, the periwinkle alkaloids, etc.; the antimetabolites, including methotrexate and 6-mercaptopurine; and certain toxic materials, such as inorganic arsenic. Other agents occasionally responsible for aplasia or hypoplasia include certain antimicrobials, anticonvulsants, antithyroid drugs, antidiabetic agents, antihistamines, analgesics, sedatives, phenothiazines, insecticides, and heavy metals. The most common offenders in this respect are the antimicrobials chloramphenicol and the organic arsenicals, the anticonvulsants mephenytoin (Mesantoin) and trimethadione (Tridione), the anti-inflammatory analgesic drug phenylbutazone, and gold compounds.

In many situations, aplastic anemia occurs when a drug or chemical is ingested in toxic amounts. However, in a small minority of persons it develops after a drug has been taken in the recommended dosage. These latter cases may be considered a type of idiosyncratic drug reaction in persons who are hypersusceptible for reasons as yet unknown. Provided that their exposure is terminated early (*i.e.,* on the first appearance of reticulocytopenia, anemia, granulocytopenia, or thrombocytopenia), a prompt and complete recovery may be anticipated. (Unfortunately, one cannot be so optimistic in the case of chloramphenicol recipients. Reactions in individuals hypersusceptible to this drug may be completely unrelated to dosage; they may develop without premonitory changes in the hemogram long after the drug has been discontinued and can progress to a complete and fatal aplasia despite all available therapy.)

Whatever the offending drug, if exposure is allowed to continue after signs of hypoplasia have appeared, bone marrow depression almost certainly progresses to the point of complete and irreversible failure—hence, the importance of frequent complete blood counts for every patient receiving a drug or exposed regularly to any chemical that has been implicated in the production of aplastic anemia.

Clinical Manifestations. Since the bone marrow is hypocellular, attempts at marrow aspiration frequently yield only a few drops of blood. A biopsy is usually necessary to demonstrate a severe decrease in normal marrow elements and replacement by fat. The abnormality is probably in the stem cell, the precursor for granulocytes, erythrocytes, and platelets. As a result, pancytopenia (deficiency in all of the cellular elements of the blood) occurs.

The onset of aplastic anemia characteristically is a gradual one, marked by weakness, pallor, breathlessness on exertion, and other manifestations of anemia. A presenting symptom in about a third of the patients is abnormal bleeding owing to thrombocytopenia. When the granulocytic series is involved as well, the patient is likely to present with fever, acute pharyngitis, or some other form of sepsis, in addition to bleeding. Physical signs, save for pallor and skin hemorrhages, are unremarkable. The blood count is marked by variable degrees of pancytopenia. Red cells are normocytic and normochromic, that is, of normal size and color. Frequently, patients have no characteristic physical findings: adenopathy and hepatosplenomegaly are lacking.

As might be expected from a condition that affects all hematopoietic cells, aplastic anemia carries a very poor prognosis. Three methods of treatment are currently employed: bone marrow transplantation, administration of antithymocyte globulin, and androgenic hormone therapy. The goal of bone marrow transplantation is to provide the patient with an undamaged supply of functioning hematopoietic tissue. Successful transplantation requires the ability to match donor and recipient and to prevent complications during the recovery process. Antithymocyte globulin is administered on the premise that the thymus gland has somehow made hematopoietic cells vulnerable to self-destruction on an immunologic basis. Although still investigational, this form of therapy has shown promise. The observation that male hemoglobin values rise with puberty is the rationale for androgen administration. Remission has been achieved for some patients but at the risk of virilization and other complications.

Supportive therapy plays a major role in the management of aplastic anemia. Any offending drug is discontinued. The patient is supported with transfusions of red cells and platelets as necessary to prevent symptoms. Eventually, such patients may develop antibodies to minor red cell antigens and to platelet antigens, so that transfusions no longer raise the counts sufficiently. Death is usually caused by hemorrhage or infection, although modern antibiotics, especially those active against gram-negative bacilli, have been a major advance for these patients. Reverse isolation techniques are used for the patient with pronounced leukopenia. Antibiotics should not be used prophylactically in neutropenic patients, since this favors the emergence of resistant bacteria and fungi.

Preventive Management.   An extremely important area is prevention of drug-induced aplastic anemia. Blood cell counts must be carefully monitored in patients receiving potentially marrow-toxic drugs, such as chloramphenicol. Persons taking toxic drugs on a long-term basis need to appreciate the need for periodic blood studies and to know what symptoms to report.

Patients with diagnosed aplastic anemia are vulnerable to the effects of leukocyte, erythrocyte, and platelet deficiency. They should be assessed carefully for signs of infection, tissue hypoxia, and bleeding. Any wound, abrasion, or ulcer of mucous membrane or skin is a potential site of infection and should be guarded against. Oral hygiene also is very important. Depending on the degree of weakness and fatigue, care should be planned to preserve the patient's energy. When thrombocytopenia is present, minor trauma, including subcutaneous and intramuscular injections, must be avoided. Regular atraumatic bowel movements are important, since hemorrhoids can develop and become infected or bleed.

Red Cell Aplasia

Red cell aplasia is an isolated anemia owing to lack of red cell formation in the marrow. This is a rare disorder in which only the erythroid cells are affected. The marrow is cellular, but the erythroid element is almost absent. There is a severe anemia without granulocytopenia or thrombocytopenia. The condition is sometimes associated with tumors of the thymus or certain drugs, such as phenytoin (Dilantin), or it may arise during the course of a hemolytic anemia. Some patients can be shown to produce an antibody to immature red cells, and this may be the cause of the disease. Treatment measures include red cell replacement, thymectomy, and administration of immunosuppressive drugs, such as corticosteroids and cyclophosphamide.

Myelophthisic Anemias

Myelophthisic anemias are a varied group of anemias that differ as to cause but are similar in that all show partial replacement of normal marrow space by abnormal tissue. This tissue may be fibrous (in myelofibrosis) or it may consist of plasma cells (in multiple myeloma) or metastatic carcinoma cells. A marrow biopsy is often necessary to make the diagnosis. Pancytopenia is present, although usually less severe than in aplastic anemia, but there are also young marrow cells circulating, apparently because there is abnormal release from the damaged marrow. Myeloblasts and nucleated red cells are seen in small numbers. The treatment is that of the primary disease. Androgens occasionally improve the patient's condition.

Anemias in Renal Disease

There is a great deal of variability in the degree of anemia seen in kidney disorders, but in general, patients with a BUN greater than 100 mg/100 ml blood are anemic. The symptoms of anemia often constitute the patient's major problems. The hematocrit usually falls between 20% and 30% and is lower for more severe uremia, although it rarely falls below 15%. The red cells appear normal on peripheral smear.

This anemia is due to both a mild shortening of red cell survival and a deficiency of erythropoietin. Some erythropoietin is evidently produced outside the kidney, since some erythropoiesis does continue, even in anephric patients (those whose kidneys have been removed), and developing red cells can be seen in the bone marrow.

- Patients undergoing chronic hemodialysis lose blood into the artificial kidney and may thus become iron deficient. Folic acid deficiency develops because this vitamin passes into the dialysate.
- Dialysis patients should be treated with iron and folic acid and occasional transfusions.

Androgens have been shown to stimulate enough erythropoiesis to obviate the need for transfusions in some patients. Most patients with uremia can tolerate moderate anemia with few symptoms and should not be transfused unless symptoms are present.

Anemias in Chronic Diseases

Many chronic inflammatory diseases are associated with anemia of a normochromic, normocytic type. These include rheumatoid arthritis, lung abscesses, osteomyelitis, tuberculosis, and many malignancies. The hemoglobin rarely falls below 9 g/100 ml, and the bone marrow has normal cellularity with increased stores of iron. Erythropoietin levels are low, perhaps because of decreased production, and there is a block in the utilization of iron by erythroid cells. Most of these patients are comfortable and do not require treatment for the anemia. With amelioration of the underlying disorder, the marrow iron is used to make red cells, and the hemoglobin rises.

Iron Deficiency Anemia

Iron deficiency anemia is the most common type of anemia in all age groups. It is a condition in which the total body iron content is decreased below a normal level.

Etiology.   The common cause of iron deficiency in men or postmenopausal women is bleeding (*e.g.,* from ulcers, gastritis, or gastrointestinal tumors) or malabsorption, especially after gastric resection. Rarely, iron can be lost in the urine during intravascular hemolysis, as in paroxysmal nocturnal hemoglobinuria or heart valve hemolysis.

Clinical and Laboratory Manifestations. In individuals who are iron deficient, the blood hemoglobin and the red blood cell count are reduced. The hemoglobin is reduced more than is the number of red cells, and for this reason the latter tend to be small and relatively devoid of pigment, that is, "hypochromic." Hypochromia is the hallmark of iron deficiency. The cause of this deficiency is the failure of the patient to ingest, or absorb, sufficient dietary iron to compensate for the iron requirements associated with body growth or for the loss of iron that attends bleeding, whether the bleeding is physiologic (*e.g.*, menstrual) or pathologic.

The patient with iron deficiency presents primarily with the symptoms of anemia. If the deficiency is severe, he may also have a smooth, sore tongue; thin, spoon-shaped fingernails; and pica (a craving to eat unusual substances, such as clay, laundry starch, or ice). All of these symptoms subside after therapy.

The laboratory studies show a hemoglobin that is proportionally lower than the hematocrit and red count, because of the small, poorly hemoglobinized red cells (microcytosis and hypochromia). The white count is usually normal, and the platelet count is variable.

Treatment. It is always important to search for a cause of iron deficiency. This may be a sign of a curable gastrointestinal malignancy or of uterine fibroids or cancer. Except in pregnancy, when the cause is obvious, stool specimens should be tested for occult blood. Several oral iron preparations are available: ferrous sulfate, gluconate, or fumarate are equally effective, but the enteric forms may be poorly absorbed and should be avoided. Usually, three or four doses a day are necessary. Although iron is best absorbed on an empty stomach, taking it with food is usually advised to minimize gastric distress. Patients may be better able to tolerate the therapy if the dose is started at one tablet daily and then raised. They should be warned that iron salts often change the stools to a darker color.

Nursing Interventions. Preventive education is important because iron deficiency anemia is so common in menstruating and pregnant women. Food sources high in iron include organ and other meats, cooked white beans, raisins, and molasses. Taking iron-rich foods with a source of vitamin C enhances absorption.

Iron therapy usually has to be continued for many months to replenish iron stores. In rare cases, intramuscular administration of iron may be necessary; that is, when oral iron is not absorbed or is poorly tolerated or when iron is needed in large amounts. The injection causes some local pain and can stain the skin. A method for parenteral administration of iron preparations follows:

1. Discard needle used to draw medication into syringe; use fresh needle for injection.
2. Use a needle 5 cm (2 inches) long—medication is injected deep into muscle.
3. Retract skin over muscle *laterally* before inserting needle—to prevent leakage and staining of skin.

Occasional febrile or allergic reactions are seen.

Megaloblastic Anemias

The anemias caused by deficiencies of the vitamins B_{12} and folic acid show identical bone marrow and peripheral blood changes. This is because both vitamins are essential for normal DNA synthesis. In each case, the marrow is hyperplastic and the precursor erythroid and myeloid cells are large and bizarre; some are multinucleated. But many of these cells die within the marrow, so that the mature cells, which leave the marrow, are decreased in number. Thus, a pancytopenia develops. In a far advanced situation, the hemoglobin may be as low as 4 g/100 ml to 5 g/100 ml, the white blood count 2,000 to 3,000 per cu mm, and platelets less than 50,000 per cu mm. The red cells are large and the polymorphonuclears are hypersegmented.

Vitamin B_{12} Deficiency

Etiology. A deficiency of vitamin B_{12} can occur in several ways. Inadequate dietary intake is very rare but can develop in strict vegetarians who consume no meat. Faulty absorption from the gastrointestinal tract is more common. An absence of intrinsic factor normally secreted by cells of the stomach is called *pernicious anemia*. This is primarily a disorder of elderly persons and has a familial tendency. The abnormality is in the gastric mucosa: the stomach wall becomes atrophic and fails to secrete intrinsic factor. This substance ordinarily binds with the dietary vitamin B_{12} and travels with it to the ileum, where the vitamin is absorbed. Without intrinsic factor, no orally administered B_{12} can enter the body. Even if adequate vitamin B_{12} and intrinsic factor are present, a deficiency can occur if disease involving the ileum or pancreas impairs absorption.

Clinical Manifestations. After the body stores of vitamin B_{12} are used up, the patient begins to show signs of the anemia. He gradually becomes weak, listless, and pale. The hematologic effects of deficiency are accompanied by effects on other organ systems, particularly the gastrointestinal tract and nervous system. Patients with pernicious anemia develop a smooth, sore, red tongue and mild diarrhea. They may become confused, but more often have paresthesias in the extremities and difficulty keeping their balance because of damage to the spinal cord: they lose position sense. These symptoms are progressive, though the course may be marked by spontaneous partial remissions and exacerbations. Without treatment, patients die after several years, usually from congestive failure secondary to anemia.

Diagnostic Evaluation. One means of determining the cause of vitamin B_{12} deficiency is the Schilling test. The patient is given a small dose of radioactive B_{12} in water to drink, followed by a large, nonradioactive intramuscular dose. When the oral vitamin is absorbed, it will be excreted in the urine; the IM dose helps to flush it into the urine. A 24-hour specimen is collected and measured for radioactivity. If very little has been excreted, the test is repeated several days later (the "second stage"), with a capsule of oral intrinsic factor added to the oral B_{12}. If the patient has pernicious anemia, this time much more radioactivity will be found in the 24-hour urine. If the problem is due to an ileal or pancreatic defect, administration of digestive enzymes will increase absorption and subsequently increase urine radioactivity.

Treatment. Vitamin B_{12} deficiency is treated by replacement. Strict vegetarians can prevent or treat deficiency with oral supplementation with vitamins or fortified soy milk. When, as is much more common, the deficiency is due to defective absorption or absence of intrinsic factor, replacement is by intramuscular injections of vitamin B_{12}.

At first, B_{12} is given daily, but eventually most patients are managed with 100 μg IM monthly. This can produce dramatic recoveries in desperately ill patients. The reticulocyte count rises within a week, and in several weeks the blood counts are all normal. The tongue improves in several days. The neurologic manifestations require more time for recovery, and if there is severe neuropathy, paralysis, or incontinence, the patient may never recover fully.

- Vitamin B_{12} therapy must be continued for the life of the patient who has had pernicious anemia or noncorrectable malabsorption in order to prevent recurrence of the anemia.

Nursing Interventions. These patients may need support during the diagnostic tests and nursing care for several aspects of their disease: anemia, congestive failure, neuropathy. When they are incontinent or paralyzed, care must be taken to prevent pressure sores and contracture deformities. The Schilling test can be useful only if the urine collections are complete; here, the nurse's assistance is essential. The patients must be taught about the chronicity of their disorder and the necessity for monthly injections, even when they are asymptomatic. The gastric atrophy associated with pernicious anemia increases the risk of gastric carcinoma. Therefore, these patients need to understand that ongoing medical follow-up is important.

Folic Acid Deficiency

Folic acid is another vitamin that is necessary for normal red blood cell production. It is stored as different compounds, referred to as folates. The folate stores in the body are much smaller than those of vitamin B_{12}, so it is much more common to see dietary folate deficiency. This occurs in patients who rarely eat uncooked vegetables or fruits (*i.e.,* primarily elderly people living alone or alcoholics). Folic acid requirements are increased in chronic hemolytic anemias and in pregnancy, hence these patients may develop the anemia while ingesting an adequate diet.

- Patients on prolonged intravenous feeding or hyperalimentation may become folate deficient after several months, unless the vitamin is given intramuscularly. Some patients with small bowel diseases may not absorb it normally.

Clinical Manifestations and Laboratory Tests. All of these patients have the characteristic findings of megaloblastic anemia along with a sore tongue. Symptoms of folic acid and vitamin B_{12} deficiencies are quite similar, and the two anemias may coexist. However, the neurologic manifestations of vitamin B_{12} deficiency do not occur with folic acid deficiency and persist if vitamin B_{12} is not replaced. Therefore, careful distinction between the two anemias must be made. Serum levels of both vitamins can be measured.

Management. Treatment is good diet and 1 mg of folic acid a day. This should be given intramuscularly only in patients with malabsorption. With the exception of the vitamins given during pregnancy, most proprietary vitamin preparations do not contain folic acid, hence it must be given as a separate tablet.

Hemolytic Anemias

In hemolytic anemias, the erythrocytes have a shortened life span. The bone marrow is usually able to compensate partially by producing new red cells at three or more times the normal rate. Consequently, all of these anemias have certain laboratory features in common: the reticulocyte count is elevated, the fraction of indirect bilirubin is increased, and the haptoglobin (a binding protein for free hemoglobin) is often low. The bone marrow is hypercellular, with erythroid proliferation. The only truly diagnostic test for hemolysis is the red cell survival study. This is usually only necessary for difficult diagnostic problems. About 20 ml to 30 ml of the patient's blood is removed, incubated with radioactive chromium-51, and then reinjected. The chromium-51 labels the red cells exclusively. After these cells have equilibrated with the circulating blood, small samples are taken at intervals over the next days and weeks, and the radioactivity is measured. A normal chromium-51 survival time is 28 to 35 days. Red cells of patients with severe hemolysis (such as sickle cell anemia) have survivals of 10 days or less.

Inherited Hemolytic Anemias

Hereditary Spherocytosis

Hereditary spherocytosis is a hemolytic anemia characterized by small, sphere-shaped red cells and splenomegaly. This is an uncommon disorder inherited in a dominant fashion.

Clinical Manifestation and Diagnosis. An abnormality of the erythrocyte membrane causes cells to lose membrane as they pass through the spleen and to become spherical in shape. These spheres are relatively rigid and easily destroyed. The peripheral blood contains many of the characteristic small spherical cells, and the patient has an anemia that may be exacerbated during infections, even minor viral illnesses. In addition, the spleen is enlarged. The disorder is usually diagnosed in childhood, but may be missed until adult life, since there are few symptoms.

Management. Splenectomy is the treatment; it does not change the erythrocyte defect but removes the site of membrane loss and hemolysis. After splenectomy (p. 719), the patients have normal hemoglobin levels, only slight shortening of red cell survival, and few spherical cells in the peripheral smear. Patients have a normal life expectancy. The major complications are all prevented by splenectomy: (1) aplastic crises after infection, often with severe anemia; (2) nonhealing leg and ankle ulceration; and (3) gallstones.

Sickle Cell Anemia

Sickle cell anemia is a severe hemolytic anemia resulting from a defective hemoglobin molecule and associated with

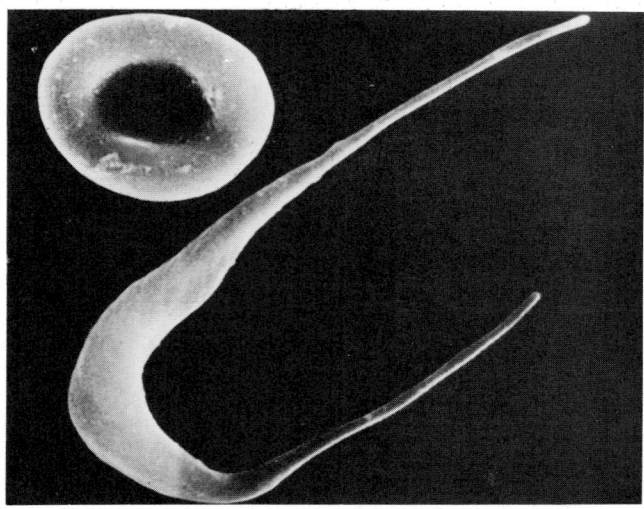

Figure 33-3. Unusual photo of a sickled cell and a normal red blood cell, taken under the auspices of the Comprehensive Sickle Cell Center, University of Miami. (Photo by Dr. Bruce R. Cameron.)

attacks of pain. This disabling disease is found predominantly in Africans and in black Americans, but it also occurs in people from Mediterranean and Arab countries.

Pathophysiology. The defect is a single amino acid substitution in the β chain of hemoglobin. Since normal hemoglobin A contains two α and two β chains, there are two genes for synthesis of each chain. A person with sickle cell trait has inherited only one abnormal gene, hence his red cells can synthesize both normal β chains and β^s chains; thus, he has A and S hemoglobin. If two people with sickle cell trait marry, some of their children may inherit two abnormal genes and will then have only β^s chains and only S hemoglobin; these children have sickle cell anemia.

Clinical Manifestations. The sickle hemoglobin has the unfortunate property of acquiring a crystal-like formation when exposed to low oxygen tension. The oxygen in venous blood is low enough to cause this change; consequently, the cell containing S hemoglobin becomes deformed, rigid, and sickle-shaped when in the venous circulation (Fig. 33-3). These long, rigid cells can become lodged in small vessels, and when they pile up against each other, blood flow to a region or an organ may be slowed. When ischemia or infarction results, the patient may experience pain, swelling, and fever. Such a chain of events is presumed to explain the painful crises of this disease, but what triggers the chain or how to prevent it is not understood.

Diagnostic Evaluation. The diagnosis can be made by hemoglobin electrophoresis or by "sickle prep," in which a drop of blood is mixed with sodium metabisulfite and watched under the microscope for sickling. Sickling in this test occurs whether the patient has sickle trait or sickle cell anemia; only the electrophoresis can make the distinction. The patient with sickle trait has a normal hemoglobin and hematocrit level as well as a normal blood smear; however,

the "sickler" has a low hematocrit and sickled cells on smear.

Sickle Trait. The patient with sickle trait is protected from crises because the hemoglobin A in his cells prevents them from sickling under ordinary circumstances. He has no anemia and looks and feels well. About 8% of black Americans have sickle trait.

Sickle Cell Anemia. Patients with sickle cell anemia are usually diagnosed in childhood, since they are anemic in infancy and begin to have crises at 1 or 2 years of age. Many die in the first years of life, but antibiotics and patient and physician education about this disease have probably improved the outlook in the last 10 to 20 years, and some patients live into the sixth decade. All siblings of a patient with sickle cell anemia should be tested for the disease.

Symptoms. Symptoms are secondary to hemolysis and thrombosis. Patients are always anemic, with hemoglobin values in the 7 to 10 g/100 ml range. Jaundice is characteristic and is usually obvious in the sclerae. The bone marrow expands in childhood in a compensatory effort, sometimes leading to enlargement of the bones of the face and skull. As a result, patients may have prominent foreheads and high cheekbones. The chronic anemia is associated with tachycardia, flow murmurs, and often cardiomegaly. Arrhythmias and heart failure may occur in older patients.

Like patients with spherocytosis, sicklers may develop aplastic crises when infected and may have gallstones and leg ulcers. The latter may be chronic and painful and require grafting. These patients are unusually susceptible to infection, particularly pneumonias and osteomyelitis. Infection has been one of the most common causes of death.

All of the patient's tissues and organs are constantly vulnerable to microcirculatory interruptions by the sickling process and therefore are susceptible to hypoxic damage or true ischemic necrosis at any time. Thrombotic episodes may result in minor pain in an extremity, in severe pain and swelling in a hand or knee, in pain simulating an acute abdominal crisis, or in the sudden appearance of a "stroke," with hemiplegia. These crises are completely unpredictable; they can occur monthly or very rarely and may last for hours, days, or weeks. Certain effects of infarction are permanent, such as hemiplegia, aseptic necrosis of the femoral head, and renal concentrating defects.

Treatment. There is no specific treatment for the hemoglobin abnormality. The disease could be prevented only by intensive genetic counseling of the population at risk, a difficult and controversial task. Crises cannot now be prevented, although researchers are evaluating several chemicals with antisickling properties. However, these are still in the investigational stage. Since infection seems to predispose to crises in children, all infections should be promptly treated or prevented when possible. Since dehydration and hypoxia promote sickling, patients are instructed to avoid high altitudes, anesthesia, or fluid loss. Because of the renal defect, these patients easily become dehydrated. Folic acid therapy is given continuously, since the marrow has an increased requirement.

When sickle crisis occurs, the mainstays of therapy are hydration and analgesia. Increased fluid intake helps to dilute the blood and reverse the agglutination of sickled cells within the small blood vessels. Patients and families can learn to handle minor crises at home, but if there is no relief after several hours, hospital admission may be necessary. The patients often have fever and leukocytosis with crisis, so that infection or appendicitis or cholecystitis may be suspected and must be ruled out. Intravenous fluids (3 liters/day–5 liters/day for adults) are essential. Narcotic analgesics are often necessary because of the severity of pain and should be given in adequate doses. They should never be used chronically, however, for some patients do become addicted.

Transfusions are reserved for particular situations: (1) aplastic crisis, when the patient's hemoglobin falls rapidly; (2) severe painful crisis not responding to any other therapy after several days; (3) as a preoperative measure, to dilute the amount of sickle blood; (4) sometimes during the latter half of pregnancy in an attempt to prevent crises.

Nursing Management. The nurse can help the patient and family to adjust to this chronic disease and to understand the importance of hydration and prevention of infection. When leg ulcers are present, they require careful dressing and protection from trauma and wound contamination. If they fail to heal, grafting may be necessary. Cardiac disease is managed in the same way as for the nonsickler. During crisis, the patient should be kept quiet and allowed to rest undisturbed. Swollen limbs should not be exercised and pain should be relieved. Male patients may develop sudden, painful episodes of priapism (persistent penile erection) and need to know that it is common and has no long-term deleterious effects.

Other Hemoglobinopathies

C Hemoglobin. C hemoglobin is less common among American blacks than S hemoglobin. The C trait is asymptomatic, and homozygous C disease is a mild hemolytic anemia with splenomegaly but no serious complications.

Thalassemia. Thalassemia occurs primarily in people of Greek and Italian extraction. In this disease, A hemoglobin is made in smaller than normal amounts, but there is no abnormal hemoglobin. Thalassemia minor (or trait) has few symptoms. Thalassemia major (Cooley's anemia) is a very severe hemolytic disease, often fatal in childhood. It is rarely encountered in adults.

Glucose-6-Phosphate Dehydrogenase Deficiency

The abnormality in this disorder is in G-6-PD, an enzyme within the red cell that is essential for membrane stability. A few patients have inherited an enzyme so defective that they have a chronic hemolytic anemia. But the most common type of defect results in hemolysis only when the red cells are stressed by certain situations, such as fever or the presence of certain drugs. The disorder came to the attention of researchers during the Second World War, when some soldiers developed hemolysis while taking primaquine, an antimalarial drug. Drugs that are hemolytic for G-6-PD-deficient individuals are antimalarial drugs, sulfonamides, nitrofurantoin, the common coal tar analgesics (including aspirin), the thiazide diuretics, the oral hypoglycemic agents, chloramphenicol, para-aminosalicylic acid (PAS), vitamin K, and, for certain individuals subject

to "favism," the fava bean. Primarily blacks and peoples of Greek or Italian origin are affected. The type of deficiency found in the Mediterranean group is more severe than that in the black group, resulting in greater hemolysis and sometimes in life-threatening anemias. All types are inherited as X-linked defects; thus, many more males are at risk than are females. In this country, about 15% of black males are affected.

Clinical Manifestations. The patients are asymptomatic and have normal hemoglobin levels and reticulocyte counts most of the time. Several days after exposure to an offending drug, they may develop pallor, jaundice, and hemoglobinuria, and the reticulocyte count will rise. Special strains of the peripheral blood may then show Heinz bodies (degraded hemoglobin). Hemolysis continues for a week, and then spontaneously the counts begin to improve, since the new young red cells are resistant to lysis. In the Mediterranean type, this recovery does not occur.

Diagnosis and Management. The diagnosis is made by a screening test or a quantitative assay of G-6-PD. The treatment is removal of the drug. Transfusion is only necessary in the Mediterranean variety. The patient should be educated about his disease and given a list of drugs to avoid. These include sulfonamides, hypoglycemic agents, antimalarials, nitrofurantoin, phenacetin, aspirin (in high doses), and para-aminosalicylic acid.

Acquired Hemolytic Anemias

See Table 33-2.

Immune Hemolytic Anemia

When antibodies combine with red cells they can be either isoantibodies, reacting with foreign cells, as in transfusion reactions or erythroblastosis fetalis, or autoantibodies, which react with the cells of the host. The immune hemolysis that results may be very severe. Antibodies coat the red cells, producing a positive Coombs' test. These cells are then removed by the spleen and the rest of the reticuloendothelial system. Many cells are destroyed, and others return to the circulation as spherocytes with reduced membrane and a shortened survival rate.

In *idiopathic autoimmune hemolytic states,* it is not known what induces the immune system to produce the antibodies. The disease usually begins suddenly, often in persons over 40 years of age. In some cases, the hemolysis is associated with systemic disease (especially systemic lupus erythematosus, chronic lymphatic leukemia, or lymphoma). Other patients, with identical clinical pictures, can be shown to be producing antibodies to a drug (especially penicillin, cephalosporins, or Quinidine). The antibodies or the drug–antibody complexes then attach to red cells, resulting in hemolysis. Patients taking large doses of methyldopa may develop antibodies to their own red cells; only a few of these patients have a significant hemolytic anemia.

Clinical Manifestations. Presentation can be quite variable. A positive Coombs' test may be the only manifestation in mild cases. More often, signs of anemia are present, such as fatigue, dyspnea, palpitations, and jaundice. Occasionally, the anemia is so severe that the patient presents with overwhelming hemolysis and shock.

Table 33-2
Acquired Hemolytic Anemias

Name	Cause	Manifestations and Treatment
Paroxysmal nocturnal hemoglobinuria	Unknown—sometimes occurs after aplastic anemia	Dark urine (hemoglobinuria) especially in morning Sometimes pancytopenia Multiple venous thrombosis No treatment known
Immune hemolytic anemia	Antibodies produced, sometimes secondary to drug (methyldopa [Aldomet], penicillin)	Jaundice, spherocytes Responds to steroids
Microangiopathic hemolytic anemia	RBC damaged during flow through abnormal small blood vessels, as in malignant hypertension	Fragmented RBC seen on smears Treat primary disease
Heart valve hemolysis	RBC damaged by regurgitant flow through incompetent valve prosthesis	Fragmented RBC Treatment: replace valve
Spur cell anemia	Severe liver disease, usually portal hypertension Increased lipid in RBC membrane	Spur-shaped RBC No treatment
Infections	Malaria, *Clostridium welchii*, especially after septic abortion	Hemoglobinuria possible Treat the infection
Hypersplenism	Large spleen from any cause: cirrhosis, lymphomas	Sometimes pancytopenia Treatment: splenectomy

Management.   Any possibly offending drug should be discontinued. The treatment consists of high doses of corticosteroids until hemolysis decreases. Usually after several weeks, the hemoglobin has returned toward normal and the steroid dose can be lowered; in some patients it can be discontinued entirely. In severe cases blood transfusions may be required. Since the antibody may react with all possible donor cells, transfusion requires careful typing and slow, cautious administration.

Splenectomy removes a major site of red cell destruction, hence this operation is often performed if steroids do not produce a remission. If neither corticosteroids nor splenectomy is successful, immunosuppressive drugs may be administered.

▷ Polycythemia

Polycythemia refers to an increased concentration of red cells; it is a term used when the red cell count is greater than 6 million/cu mm or the hemoglobin exceeds 18 g/100 ml. True polycythemia is present when the total body red cell mass is increased. "Relative" polycythemia occurs when the red cell mass is normal but the plasma volume is reduced; this may be produced by diuretic therapy or by unknown factors. Red cell mass can be measured accurately by an isotopic technique.

Secondary Polycythemia.   Secondary polycythemia is due to excessive production of erythropoietin. This may occur in response to a hypoxic stimulus, as in chronic obstructive pulmonary disease or cyanotic heart disease, or in certain hemoglobinopathies in which the hemoglobin has an abnormally high affinity for oxygen (*e.g.,* hemoglobin$_{Chesapeake}$). In some cases of secondary polycythemia, the production of erythropoietin is inappropriate, since there is no hypoxemia: this is the situation in a few patients with renal carcinoma, renal cysts, cerebellar hemangioblastoma, hepatoma, or uterine fibroids.

Polycythemia Vera.   Polycythemia vera, or primary polycythemia, is a proliferative disorder in which all the marrow cells seem to have escaped from the normal control mechanisms. The bone marrow is intensely cellular, and in the peripheral blood, the red count, white count, and platelets are often all elevated. Patients typically have a ruddy complexion and hepatosplenomegaly. The symptoms are referable to the increased blood volume (headache, dizziness, fatigue, and blurred vision) or to decreased blood flow (angina, claudication, thrombophlebitis). Bleeding is also a complication, perhaps because of the engorged capillaries. Another common problem is pruritus.

Management.   The objective of management is to reduce the high blood viscosity. Phlebotomy is an important part of therapy and can be done repeatedly to keep the hemoglobin within normal range. Radioactive phosphorus or chemotherapeutic agents can be used to suppress marrow function but may increase the risk of leukemia. When the patient has an elevated uric acid level, allopurinol is used to prevent gouty attacks. Cyproheptadine may be administered to control pruritus.

▷ Leukopenia and Agranulocytosis

Leukopenia is a condition in which the white cells number fewer than normal. *Agranulocytosis* is a condition in which there is almost complete absence of polymorphonuclear cells. A leukocyte count of fewer than 5000/cu mm or a granulocyte count of fewer than 2000/cu mm is abnormal and may be a signal of a generalized bone marrow disorder, such as megaloblastic anemia, aplasia, metastatic tumor, myelofibrosis, or acute leukemia. Viral infections and overwhelming bacterial sepsis can also cause leukopenia. Most commonly, the etiology is drug toxicity: phenothiazines are implicated most frequently; antithyroid drugs, sulfonamides, phenylbutazone, and chloramphenicol are also contributing factors. The patient is not symptomatic unless infection develops, which usually occurs when the granulocytes are fewer than 1000/cu mm. Fever and severe sore throat with ulcerations are common complaints. Bacteremia may follow soon after.

Management. Any possibly offending drugs are withdrawn. If the granulocyte count is very low, the patient is isolated from hospital personnel and visitors by strict precautions. Cultures of all orifices and blood are essential, and when fever occurs it is treated with broad spectrum antibiotics until the specific organism is known. Good oral hygiene is helpful.

Hot saline irrigations of the throat are employed to keep it clear of necrotic detritus and exudate. Comfort is provided by supplying an ice collar and whatever analgesic, antipyretic, and sedative drugs may be indicated. The essence of treatment, apart from eradicating the infection, is to eliminate, if possible, the factor responsible for the bone marrow depression. Spontaneous restoration of marrow function, except in the case of neoplastic diseases, often occurs in time, that is, within 2 or 3 weeks, if death from infection can be averted.

▷ Hematopoietic Malignancies

Blood-forming tissues are characterized by rapid and continuous turnover of cells. Normally, production of specialized blood cells from stem cell precursors is carefully regulated according to the body's needs. If homeostatic control of production is disrupted, neoplastic proliferation may result. A wide variety of hematopoietic malignancies can develop and are often classified according to the cell line involved. *Leukemia,* literally white blood, is a neoplastic proliferation of white cells. The defect is believed to originate in the hematopoietic stem cell. The *lymphomas* are neoplasms of lymphoid tissue. Hodgkin's disease accounts for 40% of all lymphomas and is believed to result from defective T-lymphocytes. Many other lymphomas are derived from B-lymphocytes. Both Waldenström's macroglobulinemia and multiple myeloma are neoplasms affecting plasma cells produced by B-lymphocytes.

Leukemia

The common feature of the leukemias is an unregulated proliferation or accumulation of white cells in the bone marrow, with replacement of normal marrow elements. There is also proliferation in the liver, spleen, and lymph nodes, and invasion of nonhematologic organs, such as the meninges, gastrointestinal tract, kidney, and skin. The leukemias are often classified according to the cell line involved, as either lymphocytic or myelocytic, and according to the maturity of the malignant cells, as either acute (immature cells) or chronic (differentiated cells). The etiology is unknown, but there is some evidence that genetic influence and viral pathogenesis may be involved. Bone marrow damage with radiation (as in the atomic bomb survivors) or chemicals (benzene) can cause leukemia.

▶ Assessment

Although the clinical picture will vary with the type of leukemia involved, the nursing history may reveal a range of signs and symptoms reported by the patient and noted during the physical examination. Included in the clinical manifestations may be weakness and fatigue, bleeding tendencies, petechiae and ecchymoses, pain, headache, vomiting, fever, and infection. Blood studies may reveal alterations of the white blood cells, anemia, and thrombocytopenia. Specific manifestations are identified under the discussion of each of the types of leukemia, which follow.

Patient Problems/Nursing Diagnoses

Based on the clinical manifestations, the nursing history, and the diagnostic assessment data, the patient's potential problems include weakness and fatigue related to anemia and episodes of bleeding; potential development of infection related to thrombocytopenia; bleeding tendencies related to thrombocytopenia; pain related to proliferation of leukemic cells; and anxiety related to the prognosis of the disease.

▶ Planning and Implementation
Goals

The patient's goals include:

1. Increased strength and endurance
2. Absence of infection
3. Absence of bleeding
4. Relief of pain
5. Ability to cope with the diagnosis and prognosis

Nursing Management. Like other patients with malignant diseases, patients with leukemia are often depressed, frightened, and lonely. A well-informed and sympathetic nurse can contribute immeasurably to their comfort by explaining procedures, anticipating side-effects of drugs, and encouraging patients to participate in the therapeutic regimen. The therapy can become very complex, and too often the patient feels that more is being done "to him" than "for him." The nurse can be a sympathetic listener and help him to mobilize his defenses to cope with his emotional and physical stresses. When a patient is placed in reverse isolation because of granulocytopenia, his sense of rejection is intensified, and nursing personnel must be sensitive to this.

These patients should be approached in the same manner as those with aplastic anemia and should be assessed for thrombocytopenia, granulocytopenia, and anemia. The risk of bleeding correlates well with the level of thrombocytopenia. In addition to having petechiae and ecchymoses, patients may develop major hemorrhages when their platelet counts drop below 20,000. For undetermined reasons, fever or infection also increases the likelihood of bleeding. Any increase in petechiae and any melena, hematuria, or nosebleeds should be reported. Undue trauma or intramuscular injections must be avoided, and acetaminophen, rather than aspirin, should be used for analgesia. Hemorrhage is treated by bed rest and transfusions of red cells and platelets.

Because of the lack of mature and normal granulocytes, these patients are always threatened by infection, the major cause of death in leukemia. The likelihood of infection increases with the degree of neutropenia, so that granulocyte counts under 100/milliliter of blood make the development of systemic infection highly probable. Immune dysfunction compounds the risk of infection. Patients must be systematically assessed for any evidence of infection, such as fever, erythema, or pain. Some typical signs of infection, such as the appearance of exudates, are often not apparent and make the need for careful observation even greater. Frequent oral hygiene may decrease the likelihood of infection originating from the oral cavity. Because of the high risk of infection arising from intravenous cannulas, gloves should be worn to start infusions, daily site care should be provided, and the cannula should be changed every 48 hours. Rectal abscesses are not unusual, hence it is important to ensure normal elimination and avoid rectal thermometers, enemas, or rectal trauma. The urinary tract is another common site for infection. Avoidance of catheterization and, when catheterization is essential, scrupulous asepsis during catheter insertion and maintenance are important.

Anemia results from defective erythropoiesis, accelerated red cell destruction, and episodes of bleeding. If weak and easily fatigued, the patient may need assistance to choose priorities and will need alternate rest and activity periods. Patients must also be assessed for dyspnea, tachycardia, and other evidence of inadequate oxygen supply to vital organs.

Infiltration of abnormal leukocytes into systemic tissues also causes a variety of disabling symptoms. Pain is a common problem owing to infiltration and enlargement of abdominal organs, lymph nodes, bones, and joints. Gastrointestinal involvement may also cause anorexia and increase the risk of hemorrhage. Signs of central nervous system infiltration include headache, confusion, and other manifestations of increased intracranial pressure. Ongoing assessment of every body system will help to identify these

widespread effects so that care can be planned to decrease symptoms as they occur.

Because chemotherapeutic agents destroy rapidly proliferating cells, bone marrow depression, gastrointestinal disturbances, and hair loss (alopecia) are common. Effects on the bone marrow exacerbate the problems of thrombocytopenia, leukopenia, and anemia described above. Gastrointestinal problems include anorexia, nausea, vomiting, diarrhea, and mucosal lesions in the mouth. Because good nutrition is so important for cancer patients, careful timing of drug administration, use of antiemetics, and choice of less irritating foods are essential. Alopecia can sometimes be prevented by the application of a tourniquet to the scalp before chemotherapy. Patients who lose hair may need assistance to obtain a wig for use until the hair grows back. The massive cell destruction resulting from chemotherapy increases uric acid levels and makes patients vulnerable to renal stone formation. Therefore, patients need a high fluid intake. The severity of these toxic effects varies among different agents, and additional side-effects occur as well. Specific drugs must be reviewed carefully before administration.

▶ **Evaluation**

Expected Outcomes

1. Experiences increased strength and endurance
   a. Explains causes for weakness and fatigue
   b. Spaces activities throughout the day
   c. Rests at specified intervals
   d. Makes appropriate alterations in life-style to accommodate decreased physical activity
   e. Shows progression in activity endurance from day to day
2. Is free of infection
   a. Attempts to maintain adequate nutritional intake
   b. Utilizes acceptable method and routine of oral hygiene
   c. Describes signs and symptoms of infection and preventive measures
   d. Avoids those with known infection
   e. Alerts health care personnel of first signs of infection
3. Is free of bleeding
   a. Adheres to therapeutic regimen
   b. Avoids situations that predispose to physical trauma
   c. Uses atraumatic measures of oral hygiene
   d. Monitors urine, stools, and vaginal discharge for evidences of bleeding
   e. Alerts health care personnel at first sign of bleeding
4. Achieves relief of pain
   a. Uses analgesics as prescribed
   b. Positions self to relieve pain related to splenomegaly
   c. Accepts radiation therapy
5. Copes with diagnosis and prognosis
   a. Verbalizes feelings about prognosis to family/support system
   b. Utilizes defense mechanisms appropriately
   c. Sets realistic goals

Acute Myelogenous Leukemia (AML)

This form of leukemia affects the hematopoietic stem cell that differentiates into all myeloid cells: monocytes, granulocytes (basophils, neutrophils, eosinophils), erythrocytes, and platelets. All age groups are affected; incidence rises with age.

Clinical Manifestations. Most of the signs and symptoms evolve from insufficient production of normal blood cells. Vulnerability to infection results from granulocytopenia, weakness and fatigue occur owing to anemia, and bleeding tendencies arise as a result of thrombocytopenia. The proliferation of leukemic cells within organs leads to a variety of additional symptoms: pain from enlarged liver or spleen; lymphadenopathy; headache or vomiting secondary to meningeal leukemia (most common in lymphocytic leukemia); and bone pain from expansion of marrow.

Onset is often insidious, with symptoms occurring over a period of 1 to 6 months. The peripheral blood will show a decrease in both erythrocyte and platelet counts. Although the total leukocyte count can be low, normal, or high, the percentage of normal cells is usually vastly decreased. A bone marrow specimen is diagnostic.

Treatment. Chemotherapy is the major form of therapy and in some instances results in remissions lasting a year or longer. Commonly used drugs include cytosine arabinoside (Cytarabine, Ara-C) and 6-Mercaptopurine (6-MP, Purinethol). Transfusions of red cells and platelets are administered to temporarily provide normal cells. When a tissue match with a close relative can be obtained, bone marrow transplantation is used to provide normal bone marrow after destruction of leukemic marrow by chemotherapy.

Prognosis. At the present time, survival of treated patients averages only 13 months, with death usually a result of infection. Untreated patients survive only about 2 months.

Chronic Myelogenous Leukemia (CML)

This type of leukemia is also believed to be a malignancy of myeloid stem cells. However, more normal cells are present than in the acute form, and therefore the disease is milder. Uncommon before age 20, the incidence of chronic myelogenous leukemia rises with age.

Manifestations. The clinical picture is similar to that of acute myelogenous leukemia, but signs and symptoms are less severe. Onset is typically insidious. Leukocytosis is always present, sometimes at extraordinary levels.

Treatment and Prognosis. The drug of choice for chemotherapy is busulfan (Myleran). The final event in most patients is a transformation into an acute myelogenous leukemia that is usually resistant to all therapy. Overall, patients live for 3 to 4 years. The nursing process is similar to that of acute leukemia (p. 711).

Acute Lymphocytic Leukemia (ALL)

This form of leukemia is believed to be a malignant proliferation of lymphoblasts. Acute lymphocytic leukemia is most common in young children, with a peak incidence at 4 years of age. After age 15, incidence is uncommon.

Manifestations. Lymphocytes proliferate in marrow and peripheral tissue and crowd the development of normal cells. As a result of marrow proliferation of malignant cells, normal hematopoiesis is inhibited, and leukopenia, anemia, and thrombocytopenia develop. Erythrocyte and platelet counts are low, and leukocyte counts may be either low or high but always include immature cells. Manifestations of leukemic cell infiltration into other organs are more common with acute lymphocytic leukemia than with other forms.

Treatment and Prognosis. Therapy for this childhood leukemia has improved to the extent that approximately 50% of children survive at least 5 years. The major form of treatment is chemotherapy with prednisone and one or more other drugs, such as vincristine. Irradiation of the craniospinal region and intrathecal injection of chemotherapeutic drugs help prevent central nervous system recurrence.

Chronic Lymphocytic Leukemia (CLL)

A disease of elderly people, chronic lymphocytic leukemia tends to be a mild disorder that primarily affects persons over age 35.

Manifestations. Many patients are asymptomatic and are diagnosed during physical examination or treatment for another disease. Possible manifestations are those of anemia, infection, or enlargement of lymph nodes and abdominal organs. The erythrocyte and platelet counts may be normal or decreased. Lymphocytosis is always present.

Treatment and Prognosis. If mild, chronic lymphocytic leukemia may require no treatment. When symptoms are severe, chemotherapy with cyclophosphamide (Cytoxan) and chlorambucil (Leukeran) is often used. Highly variable in course, the average survival time is 7 years.

When the patient no longer responds to therapy, he may be hospitalized for supportive care. He has often experienced remissions and exacerbations of his disease, and he has known hope and despair. He is very tired and ill and requires knowledgeable nursing assessment, support, and expert physical care. (See also section on patients with advanced carcinoma, p. 320.)

▷ Malignant Lymphoma

The lymphomas are neoplasms of the cells of the lymphoid system: the lymphocytes and histiocytes. They are often classified according to the degree of cell differentiation and the origin of the predominant malignant cell. These tumors usually start in lymph nodes, but can involve lymphoid tissue in the spleen, the gastrointestinal tract (for example, the tonsils or the wall of the stomach), the liver, or bone marrow. They often spread to all of these areas and to extralymphatic tissues (lungs, kidneys, skin) by the time of death. The etiology of these tumors is unknown.

Hodgkin's Disease

Hodgkin's disease, like other lymphomas, is a malignant disease of unknown etiology that originates in the lymphatic system and involves predominantly the lymph nodes. It is somewhat more common in males and has two peaks of incidence: one in the early 20s and the other after age 50. Because many manifestations are similar to those occurring with infection, an infectious origin for the disease continues to be sought.

The malignant cell of Hodgkin's disease, its pathologic hallmark and its essential diagnostic criterion, is the "Reed–Sternberg cell," a gigantic atypical tumor cell, morphologically unique and of uncertain lineage, which many regard as an aberrant histiocyte.

Patients with Hodgkin's disease are customarily classified into subgroups based on pathologic criteria that reflect the grade of malignancy and suggest the prognosis. *Hodgkin's paragranuloma,* for example, with fewest Reed–Sternberg cells and least disturbance of nodal architecture, carries a much more favorable prognosis than *Hodgkin's sarcoma,* in which the lymph nodes are virtually replaced by tumor cells of the most primitive type. The majority of patients, with so-called *Hodgkin's granuloma* (which includes two conditions currently designated "nodular sclerosis" and "mixed cellularity") are in an intermediate position with respect to the density and destructiveness of tumor cells, therapeutic responsiveness, and overall outlook.

Clinical Manifestations

Hodgkin's disease usually begins as a painless enlargement of the lymph nodes on one side of the neck, which becomes increasingly conspicuous. However, for months generalized pruritus may be the first and only symptom and later is often a most distressing one. The individual nodes remain firm and discrete (that is, they do not soften and do not fuse) and they are seldom tender and painful. Soon the lymph nodes of other regions, usually the other side of the neck, also enlarge in the same manner. The mediastinal and retroperitoneal lymph nodes may also enlarge, causing severe pressure symptoms: pressure against the trachea results in dyspnea; pressure against the esophagus causes dysphagia; pressure on the nerves causes laryngeal paralysis, and brachial, lumbar, or sacral neuralgias; pressure on the veins results in edema of one or both extremities and effusions into the pleura or peritoneum; and pressure on the bile duct causes obstructive jaundice. Later the spleen may become palpable, and the liver may enlarge. In some patients the first nodes to enlarge are those of one axilla or of one groin. Occasionally, the disease starts in mediastinal or peritoneal nodes and may remain limited to them. In still other cases the enlargement of the spleen is the only conspicuous lesion.

Sooner or later a progressive anemia develops. A leukocytosis often is observed with an abnormally high polymorphonuclear count and an elevated eosinophil count. About half of the patients have a slight fever, the temperature seldom rising above 38.3° C (101° F). However, the patients with mediastinal and abdominal involvement present a remarkable intermittent fever. The temperature goes as high as 40.0° C (104° F) for periods of 3 to 14 days, returning to normal within a few weeks. Untreated, this disease is progressive in its course; the patient loses weight and becomes cachectic, the anemia becomes marked, anasarca appears, the blood pressure falls, and in 1 to 3 years death is likely to ensue.

Diagnosis

The diagnosis of Hodgkin's disease hinges on the identification of its characteristic histologic features in an excised lymph node. A diagnosis having been firmly established on the basis of the requisite criteria, it becomes necessary to assess as accurately as possible the total extent of tumor involvement and to define the manner in which it is distributed. In other words, one attempts to pinpoint the location of every tumor lesion inside and outside the lymphatic system and to exclude the presence of a tumor in organs and tissues that are not yet involved. This is a difficult, expensive, and uncertain undertaking but an extremely important one, since these are the very considerations on which treatment is to be based.

Treatment

Current concepts of treatment stem from the following observations and premises:

1. Hodgkin's disease spreads from its original location (usually a single node) by way of the lymphatic channels to contiguous lymph nodes, which in turn become the sites of tumor growth; it rarely skips lymph nodes en route to more distant sites of metastasis.
2. Rarely does Hodgkin's disease spread beyond the lymphatic system to involve other organs and tissues until late in the disease.
3. Hodgkin's disease is completely and permanently eradicated from any site that has received a radiation dose of 3500 to 4500 rads within the space of about 4 weeks. Megavoltage radiation techniques permit the delivery of such a dose to one or more entire lymph node chains.
4. Areas of the body in which the lymph node chains are located can tolerate doses of this magnitude without serious damage (as can the area of the spleen and the oronasopharynx, both of which may become involved in Hodgkin's disease), provided that vital structures such as the lungs, liver, gastrointestinal tract, kidneys, and bone marrow are protected by carefully shaped lead shields.

From the foregoing it is postulated that Hodgkin's disease is potentially curable by radiotherapy, provided it has not extended beyond the lymph node chains, spleen, and oronasopharynx. Failing signs of such extension, patients with this disease should have the benefit of "curative" radiotherapy in which tumoricidal doses are delivered not only to obvious tumor nodes but to all adjacent nodes and lymph node chains as well. Conversely, any sign of spread beyond the treatable areas automatically disqualifies the Hodgkin's patient from such a program, in which case a combination of chemotherapy and palliative radiotherapy would be indicated.

Nursing Management

Radiation therapy often requires many weeks of daily trips to the hospital. The dosage to the tumor and adjacent lymph node areas is generally 4500 rads. Patients develop dysphagia, dry mouth, nausea, skin rashes, and some hair loss. They are helped by such measures as skin creams, oral lidocaine, and antiemetics. A commonly used drug regimen is a combination of nitrogen mustard, vincristine (Oncovin), prednisone, and procarbazine (MOPP). As with any chemotherapy, side-effects include marrow suppression, gastrointestinal disturbances, and alopecia.

Patients with Hodgkin's disease are extremely vulnerable to infection, both as a result of radiation and chemotherapy and as a consequence of defective immune responses caused by the tumor. Temporary or permanent sterility is a risk of radiation therapy, despite careful shielding of reproductive organs.

Staging of Hodgkin's Disease. For the sake of simplicity, uniformity, and convenience in categorizing patients with Hodgkin's disease with respect to the extent and activity of their disease, and hence their eligibility for curative radiotherapy, the disease generally is classified, or "staged," as follows:

Stage I: disease limited to a single node and contiguous structures or, a single extralymphatic organ or site

Stage II: disease involves more than a single node or group of contiguous nodes, but is confined to one side of the diaphragm only

Stage III: disease is present both above and below the diaphragm and may include solitary involvement of the spleen, one extrahepatic site, or both

Stage IV: disease has disseminated diffusely to one or more extrahepatic sites with or without associated lymph node involvement

Stages are further subdivided on the basis of the presence or absence of constitutional symptoms: those without are designated A and those with are designated B. Chemotherapy is often added for stage IIB and for stage IIIA. For stages IIIB and IV, combination chemotherapy is used, and radiation is generally reserved for the palliative treatment of local lesions that are especially damaging or painful. Currently, patients diagnosed at stage IA or IIA have a 5-year survival rate of 90% and can essentially be considered cured. Survival rates progressively decrease with more advanced stages.

Non-Hodgkin's Lymphomas

Lymphocytic lymphomas are more indolent and have a better prognosis than histiocytic lymphomas. Manifestations are similar to those of Hodgkin's disease, but patients with these disorders are more likely to have generalized lymph node disease or extranodal disease when first discovered. If the disease is localized, irradiation is the treatment of choice. Chemotherapy is substituted for generalized involvement. As with Hodgkin's disease, infection is a major problem. Central nervous system involvement is also common.

Mycosis Fungoides

This is a rare lymphoma of the skin. It usually begins as a pruritic, red rash, and months or years later the skin becomes infiltrated with plaques and tumors of lymphoma. The body may be covered with mushroomlike growths varying in size from 1 cm to 5 cm (0.4–6 inches). Eventually, the malignant process reaches nodes, liver, and spleen. Patients are very uncomfortable with the itching and disfigurement of this disease. Treatment with nitrogen mustard (which may be used topically) or irradiation can achieve palliation.

The patient with painful ulcerative lesions will require skilled nursing. A bed cradle should be placed over him to remove the weight of bedding from his painful skin lesions. Bacteriostatic ointment may be prescribed as a preventive measure against secondary infection and to seal off air from open nerve endings. Other aspects of management are similar to those for the patient with Hodgkin's disease.

▷ Multiple Myeloma

Multiple myeloma is a malignant disease of plasma cells that infiltrate bone and soft tissues. This is not classified as a lymphoma. The malignant cell is the plasma cell, the neoplastic proliferation taking place mainly in the bone marrow. Lymph nodes are not involved.

Patients generally present with a normochromic, normocytic anemia; back pain; and sometimes leukopenia or thrombocytopenia, owing to marrow infiltration by malignant plasma cells. The diagnosis of myeloma can be made by aspiration or biopsy of the bone marrow. X-rays showing destructive lesions of many bones are suggestive but not diagnostic for this disease. The malignant plasma cells produce large quantities of abnormal globulins, which appear in the serum electrophoresis as a paraprotein "spike." Fragments of these globulins are excreted in urine as Bence Jones proteins.

Patients may be incapacitated by constant bone pain. Plasma cell tumors can appear in many sites in these patients, including skin, mouth, and pleura; these are often painless. The osteolytic lesions are often associated with hypercalcemia, and bone fractures are common, especially in the vertebrae or ribs.

Management. Phenylalanine mustard (Alkeran), cyclophosphamide, and steroids are the drugs used to decrease the tumor mass and relieve bone pain. They can prolong life from 1 year to 2 or 3 years. Radiation is very useful for palliation of bone pain and for reducing the size of extraskeletal plasma cell tumors. Good hydration is essential in order to prevent renal damage from precipitation of Bence Jones protein in the renal tubules, hypercalcemia, and hyperuricemia. Thus, it is important to assess these patients for signs and symptoms of renal insufficiency. When the patients have severe pain, they need narcotic analgesics and local irradiation, and sometimes back braces to relieve pressure. Pathologic fractures are also possible. It is important to keep the patients as active as possible, since bed rest only increases the likelihood of hypercalcemia. Bacterial infections, especially pneumonia, are common in these patients, since they have impaired capacity for antibody production. Patients with multiple myeloma should not be put on fasting regimens for diagnostic tests since dehydrating procedures can precipitate acute renal failure.

▷ Bleeding Disorders

Pathophysiology

The body is normally protected against excessive and lethal blood loss by numerous complicated and interrelated mechanisms. As indicated in Figure 33-1, hemostasis includes three phases. The first, the *vascular phase,* involves immediate vasoconstriction of injured vessels. This vessel spasm is sufficient to stop capillary bleeding. The second phase, or *platelet phase,* refers to platelet aggregation at the site. These tiny cells are rapidly attracted to the damaged endothelium and form loose plugs. More platelets gather, and eventually these fuse together and contract, forming stable plugs. The platelet plug effectively stops bleeding in small vessels, such as venules, and provides temporary protection in larger injuries. Complete and permanent sealing of vascular wounds is accomplished through the clotting of the blood, which results in the production of an adherent gel-like mass that effectively controls most types of hemorrhage. Initiated through either the intrinsic or extrinsic pathway, a chain reaction occurs in which blood proteins are sequentially activated until factor Xa is formed. At this point, factor Xa interacts with factor V, calcium, and a platelet substance to convert prothrombin to thrombin. This is a very active enzyme, which has several functions: one is to encourage further platelet aggregation; another is to convert fibrinogen to fibrin. Therefore, strands of fibrin begin to form in the vicinity of the platelet plug, reinforcing the plug and producing a larger clot. The fibrin clot is then further stabilized by the formation of bonds between the molecules, catalyzed by another plasma protein, factor XIII. The result is that the damaged vessel is sealed, and blood flow in the area is slowed. Then, tissue repair of the vessel endothelium can proceed. Eventually, much of the fibrin clot will be lysed by another plasma protein system—the plasmin system, which produces fibrinolysis.

Several other homeostatic mechanisms contribute to hemostasis. Hemorrhage from a large, lacerated vessel is retarded as a result of an abrupt lowering of the arterial blood pressure (*i.e.,* "shock"), which reduces the rate of blood flow throughout the body and therefore reduces the rate of its escape. Further protection also may be furnished by compression of the leaking vessel by the swelling mass of blood (hematoma) surrounding the vessel. A final factor of great importance in the prevention of bleeding is the normal resistance of blood vessels to mechanical rupture, whether by the pressure of blood exerted from within the vessel or traumatic pressures exerted from the outside.

Abnormalities that predispose to hemorrhagic diseases can affect vessels, platelets, and any of the plasma coagulation factors, fibrin, or plasmin. Some patients can have defects at several sites simultaneously. Bleeding may be a manifestation of a primary coagulation defect (as in hemophilia), may occur secondary to another disease (as in cirrhosis, uremia, or leukemia), or may even be due to drugs (overdose of Coumadin).

Clinical Manifestations

The symptoms and signs of bleeding disorders vary, depending on the type of defect. A careful history can often give clues to the diagnosis. Abnormalities of the vascular system give rise to local bleeding, usually into the skin. Since platelets are primarily responsible for the cessation of bleeding from small vessels, patients with thrombocytopenia will have petechiae—small red or purple spots, often in clusters, seen on the skin and mucous membranes. Trauma results in excessive bruising but not large, uncontrolled he-

matomas. After cuts or skin puncture, bleeding stops promptly with local pressure and does not recur when pressure is released. In contrast, in hemophilia and abnormalities of other coagulation factors, the platelets function normally so that there are no petechial or superficial hemorrhages. Instead, deep bleeding occurs after minor trauma, such as intramuscular hematomas and hemorrhage into joint spaces. External bleeding recurs several hours after pressure is removed—as, for example, severe bleeding starting several hours after a tooth extraction.

Vascular Disorders

Spontaneous rupture of small vessels that are defective or injured results in leakage of blood into the skin, mucous membranes, and serosal surfaces. The smallest hemorrhages, pinhead in size, are called *petechiae.* Hemorrhages up to 1 cm in diameter are referred to as *purpura,* and larger, blotchy lesions are described as *ecchymoses.*

Vascular dysfunction can be caused by a variety of mechanisms. Alterations in the connective tissue framework supporting blood vessels is believed to explain the bleeding associated with vitamin C deficiency and adrenocortical hormone excess. Vascular injury can also result from systemic diseases such as diabetes mellitus or the action of bacterial toxins. A particularly important cause of vascular injury is immunologically mediated. As a consequence of drug reactions, bacterial infections, allergic disorders, or collagen-vascular diseases, vascular damage occurs. Effects range from minor local injury to widespread thromboses or hemorrhage.

Platelet Defects

The sudden onset of petechiae, purpura, or excessive bruising or bleeding from the nose or gums should stimulate a search for a platelet defect. Deficiencies of platelet number, or thrombocytopenias, are most common, but there are also some rare disorders of platelet function, in which the platelet count is normal but the clinical picture is identical to that in thrombocytopenia. The platelet function disorders can be diagnosed by special tests for platelet factor 3 and platelet adhesiveness and aggregation. The most important functional disorder to remember is that induced by aspirin: even small amounts of aspirin prevent normal platelet aggregation, and the bleeding time test is prolonged for several days after aspirin ingestion. Although this defect does not cause bleeding in most normal people, patients with another coagulation disorder (such as thrombocytopenia or hemophilia) can experience life-threatening hemorrhage after taking aspirin.

Thrombocytopenia

Thrombocytopenia can result either from decreased production of platelets by the marrow or from increased peripheral destruction. Some of the causes are listed in Table 33-3. If the platelet deficiency is secondary to an underlying disease, this can usually be diagnosed from the examination of the patient or the bone marrow. When peripheral destruction is the cause of thrombocytopenia, the marrow shows increased megakaryocytes and normal platelet pro-

Table 33-3
Thrombocytopenias

Cause	Treatment
I. Failure of Production	
Leukemia	Treat the leukemia
Tumor invasion of marrow	
Aplastic anemia	Bone marrow transplant, androgens, antithrombocyte globulin
Megaloblastic anemia	B_{12} or folic acid
Toxins	Discontinue toxin
Drugs: thiazides, chloramphenicol, cytotoxic drugs	Discontinue drug
Infection	Treat infection
II. Increased Destruction	
Owing to antibodies	
ITP	Steroids, splenectomy
Lupus erythematosus	Steroids, immunosuppressive drugs
Malignant lymphoma	Steroids
Drugs: quinine, sulfonamides, alcohol, gold	Discontinue drug
Owing to entrapment in large spleen	
Owing to infections	Splenectomy
Bacteremia	
Postviral infections	Treat infection
III. Increased Utilization	
Disseminated intravascular coagulation	Heparin

duction. Bleeding and petechiae usually do not occur with platelet counts above 50,000/cu mm, although excessive bleeding can follow surgery.

When the platelet count drops below 20,000/cu mm, petechiae appear and there is excessive menstrual bleeding, nosebleeds, and hemorrhage after surgery or dental extractions. When the platelet count is less than 5,000/cu mm, spontaneous fatal central nervous system hemorrhage or gastrointestinal hemorrhage can occur.

Management. The management for secondary thrombocytopenia is usually that of the underlying disease. If platelet production is impaired, platelet transfusions may help to raise platelet counts and stop bleeding or prevent intracranial hemorrhage. If excessive destruction is the problem, transfused platelets will also be destroyed and will not raise the count.

Idiopathic Thrombocytopenic Purpura (ITP)

ITP is a disease of all ages but commonly affects children and young women. Although the precise etiology remains unknown, viral infections sometimes precede the disease in children. Antiplatelet antibodies are produced so that platelet life span is markedly shortened. Occasionally, the antibodies can be demonstrated *in vitro,* but usually the diagnosis is made from the decreased platelet count and survival time and increased bleeding time. Other overt causes of thrombocytopenia must be ruled out. Symptoms

may begin suddenly, with petechiae and mucosal bleeding. The platelet count is generally below 20,000/cu mm. Death may result from intracranial bleeding. There are no physical findings of note other than the hemorrhages.

Management. Corticosteroids are the treatment of choice: the bleeding ceases in 1 to 2 days, and platelet counts rise in a week or so. About three quarters of patients respond to steroids, but many have a relapse when the drug is withdrawn. These patients, as well as the nonresponders, are subjected to splenectomy. Splenectomy produces a lasting remission in most patients, though transient recurrences of thrombocytopenia sometimes occur months or years later. The rare patients who do not respond to splenectomy are sometimes treated with the immunosuppressive drugs azathioprine or cyclophosphamide.

Clotting Factor Defects

Hemophilia

There are two hereditary bleeding disorders that are indistinguishable clinically, but that can be separated by laboratory tests—hemophilia A and hemophilia B. Hemophilia A is due to a deficiency of factor VIII clotting activity, whereas hemophilia B stems from a deficiency of factor IX. Factor VIII deficiency is about five times more common. Both types of hemophilia are inherited as X-linked traits, so that almost all affected individuals are males; their mothers and some of their sisters are carriers but are asymptomatic.

Clinical Manifestations. The disease, which may be very severe, is manifested by large, spreading bruises and bleeding into muscles and joints, even after minimal trauma. Patients often note pain in a joint before swelling and limitation of motion are apparent. Recurrent joint hemorrhages can result in damage so severe that chronic pain or ankylosis (fixation) of the joint occurs. Many of the patients are crippled by the joint damage before they become adults. The disease is recognized in early childhood, usually in the toddler age group.

Prior to the availability of factor VIII concentrates, many patients died of the complications before reaching adulthood. Some hemophiliacs have a milder deficiency, having between 5% and 25% of the normal level of factor VIII or IX. These patients do not experience the painful and disabling muscle and joint hemorrhages, but bleed only after dental extractions or surgery. Nevertheless, such hemorrhages can prove fatal if the cause is not recognized quickly.

Management. In the past, the only treatment was fresh frozen plasma, which had to be given in such large quantities that the patients became volume overloaded. Now factor VIII and IX concentrates are available to all blood banks. Patients are given concentrates when they are actively bleeding or as a prophylactic measure before dental extractions or surgery. Some families are taught how to administer the concentrate at home, at the first sign of bleeding.

A few patients eventually develop antibodies to the concentrates, so that their factor levels cannot be elevated. Treatment of this problem is extremely difficult and often unsuccessful. Epsilon aminocaproic acid (EACA) is an inhibitor of fibrinolytic enzymes. This drug can slow the dissolution of blood clots that do form, and is sometimes used after oral surgery in hemophiliacs.

In terms of general care, patients with hemophilia should never be given aspirin or intramuscular injections. Dental hygiene is very important as a preventive measure, since dental extractions are so hazardous. Splints and other orthopedic devices may be very useful in patients who have suffered joint or muscle hemorrhages.

Von Willebrand's Disease

This is a common bleeding disorder, inherited as a dominant character and affecting males and females equally. It is due to a mild deficiency of factor VIII (15%–50% of normal) associated with an impairment of platelet function. The laboratory tests show normal platelet count, prolonged bleeding time, and slightly prolonged partial thromboplastin time. Patients commonly have nosebleeds, excessively heavy menses, bleeding from cuts, and postoperative bleeding. They do not suffer from massive soft tissue or joint hemorrhages. Both of the defects can be corrected by the administration of cryoprecipitate (any precipitate that results from cooling). (See p. 721.)

Hypoprothrombinemia

Prothrombin, as was previously noted, is essential for the clotting process.

This protein is produced in the liver by a vitamin K dependent chemical process. Vitamin K enters the body from food sources as well as from synthesis by bacteria that reside in the intestine. Normal prothrombin activity in the blood depends on adequate absorption of this vitamin from the gastrointestinal tract and on adequate liver function. Therefore, prothrombin deficiency may arise as a result of diarrhea, from a lack of bile in the gastrointestinal tract (necessary for absorption of fat-soluble vitamin K) owing to biliary tract obstruction, from surgical removal or mucosal damage of a large part of the small intestine, from prolonged antibiotic therapy, or as the result of liver disease.

The principal manifestation of prothrombin deficiency, as observed in patients with hemophilia, is prolonged hemorrhage from blood vessels that are damaged by trauma or disease, which explains the characteristic occurrence of ecchymoses, hematuria, gastrointestinal bleeding, and postoperative hemorrhages.

Coumarin Toxicity. The coumarins are drugs that are often employed medically for the express purpose of inducing a partial depression of prothrombin activity, since the drugs interfere with the action of vitamin K in the liver. Therapy is usually calculated to prolong the prothrombin time by 2 to 2½ times the normal time. In this range, thrombosis is inhibited and thrombophlebitis is prevented. However, if taken in excessive dosages, whether intentionally or mistakenly, or if certain other drugs are administered simultaneously that interfere with metabolism, the complete picture of prothrombin deficiency, with a severe hemorrhagic disorder, may be produced. Among drugs that enhance coumarin-induced anticoagulation are phenylbutazone, indomethacin, chloral hydrate, and salicylates. Other drugs, such as barbiturates, decrease coumarin effects.

Management. Hypoprothrombinemia, if due to vitamin K deficiency, responds to treatment with any of several preparations that are available for oral or parenteral administration. However, when corrective measures are urgently required, particularly in patients with liver disease or coumarin toxicity, the effective treatment requires the direct replacement of prothrombin by means of transfusion, since purified preparations of prothrombin are not yet available.

Liver Disease. The liver cell makes all the plasma protein coagulation factors except factor VIII. Therefore, in severe hepatic disease of any sort, deficiencies of these factors may occur. The prothrombin time and partial thromboplastin time will both be prolonged. If the spleen is enlarged as well (as in cirrhosis), the platelet count may also be depressed. These patients frequently bruise easily and may have life-threatening hemorrhage from peptic ulcers or esophageal varices. Treatment includes fresh frozen plasma, fresh blood, and factor IX complex (Konyne). Vitamin K does not improve the disorder.

Disseminated Intravascular Coagulation (DIC)

Occasionally, widespread clotting in small vessels of the body occurs, leading to consumption of the clotting factors and platelets, so that paradoxically the patient presents with a bleeding disorder characterized by low fibrinogen, prolonged prothrombin time and partial thromboplastin time, low factor VIII, and thrombocytopenia. Such patients may bleed from mucous membranes, venipuncture sites, and the gastrointestinal and urinary tracts. They may also develop renal failure owing to fibrin deposition in small vessels of the kidney. Many serious illnesses may predispose to DIC, including septicemia, premature separation of the placenta in a pregnant woman, metastatic malignancies, hemolytic transfusion reactions, and massive tissue trauma. The best treatment is correction of the underlying disease, but in the meantime intravenous heparin may retard the coagulation process and permit normalization of clotting tests and a decrease in the hemorrhagic manifestations.

▷ Therapeutic Measures in Blood Disorders

Splenectomy

The surgical removal of the spleen is sometimes necessary following trauma to the abdomen. Since the spleen is very vascular, severe hemorrhage can result after splenic rupture. Under such circumstances, splenectomy becomes an emergency procedure.

Splenectomy is also often performed as a treatment for a number of hematologic disorders. An enlarged spleen may be the site of excessive destruction of blood cells, and when this destruction is life-threatening, the operation may prove palliative. This is the case in autoimmune hemolytic anemia or idiopathic thrombocytopenic purpura when these disorders do not respond to corticosteroids. Some patients with severe anemia owing to inherited red cell defects (such as thalassemia or pyruvate kinase deficiency) may benefit from splenectomy. Patients with rheumatoid arthritis may develop splenomegaly with destruction of granulocytes and granulocytopenia; removal of the spleen may improve the blood count and reduce the tendency toward infection.

Very large, bulky, and painful spleens (as may occur in myelofibrosis or chronic myelogenous leukemia) usually do not need to be removed, but when symptoms and blood counts do not respond to drugs, splenectomy can be helpful. Most patients with hereditary spherocytosis are essentially cured of their hemolytic process by splenectomy.

When the spleen is large, the operation can be difficult, but generally there is a very low mortality. Morbidity may result from postoperative atelectasis, pneumonia, abdominal distention, and subphrenic abscess formation. Young patients are at increased risk of pneumococcal infections for several years after splenectomy. Patients with high platelet counts (such as those with myelofibrosis) often are found to have even higher counts after splenectomy—greater than a million—and this can predispose the patient to serious thrombotic or hemorrhagic problems.

Blood Transfusion

Blood Donation

Since blood and blood components are used so frequently, nearly all hospitals now have blood banks, and most large hospitals also have facilities for removal of blood from donors. These donor clinics are often the responsibility of nurses, who must screen prospective donors, supervise the phlebotomies, and care for the health and safety of the donors.

Donor Interviewing

Each prospective donor is examined and interviewed before the donation for his own protection and that of the recipient. The questioning must be tactful but complete, and an experienced interviewer will learn how to ask each question in several ways in order to obtain the most complete answers. Donors should appear to be in good health and should be free of any of the following disqualifying factors:

1. A history of viral hepatitis, recently or at any time in the past, or a history of close contact with a hepatitis or dialysis patient within 6 months
2. A history of receiving a blood transfusion or injection of any fraction of blood other than serum albumin or gamma globulin within 6 months
3. A history of untreated syphilis or malaria, since these can be transmitted by transfusion even years later. If an individual has been free of symptoms and off therapy for 3 years after malaria, he may be a donor.
4. A history of evidence of drug abuse in which drugs were self-injected (since addicts have a high hepatitis carrier rate)
5. A skin infection, because of the possibility of contamination of the phlebotomy needle
6. A history of recent asthma, urticaria, or allergy to drugs because hypersensitivity can be passively transferred to the recipient
7. Pregnancy within 6 months, because of the nutritional demands of pregnancy on the mother
8. A history of tooth extraction or oral surgery within 72 hours, since such procedures are frequently associated with transient bacteremia
9. A history of recent tatoo, because of the higher risk of hepatitis
10. A history of exposure to infectious disease within the past 3 weeks, because of the risk of transmission to the recipient
11. Recent immunizations, because of the risk of transmitting live organisms (2-week waiting period for live, attenuated organisms; 2 months for rubella; 1 year for rabies)
12. Presence of cancer, because of the lack of knowledge about transmission
13. A history of whole blood donation within the past 56 days

Blood donors who pass this screen are then examined with regard to blood pressure, pulse, oral temperature, weight, and hemoglobin level. The latter is often checked via a screening test that only estimates the hemoglobin. Individuals under 17 and over 65 years of age are usually disqualified. Donors are expected to meet the following minimal requirements:

1. The body weight should exceed 50 kg (110 pounds) for a standard 450-ml donation. Donors weighing less than 50 kg (110 pounds) may be bled proportionately less.
2. The oral temperature should not exceed 37.5° C (99.6° F).
3. The pulse rate should be regular and between 50 and 100 beats per minute.

4. The systolic arterial pressure should be between 90 and 180 mm Hg, and the diastolic pressure between 50 and 100 mm Hg.
5. The hemoglobin level in the case of a female should be at least 12.5 g/100 ml; in the case of a male, 13.5 g/100 ml.

Phlebotomy

The donor is placed in a semirecumbent position, the skin over the antecubital fossa is carefully scrubbed with an iodine preparation, a tourniquet is applied, and venipuncture is performed. Withdrawal of 450 ml of blood takes less than 15 minutes. Following removal of the needle, the donor is asked to hold his arm straight up, and firm pressure is applied with sterile gauze for 2 or 3 minutes or until bleeding stops. A firm bandage is then applied. The donor is asked to remain recumbent until he feels able to sit up, usually 1 or 2 minutes. If weakness or faintness is experienced, he should rest for a longer period. After getting up, he is given food and fluids in a reception area and is asked to remain another 15 minutes. Donors should be instructed to leave the dressing on and avoid heavy lifting for several hours, to avoid smoking for 1 hour and alcoholic beverages for 3 hours, to increase fluid intake for 2 days, and to be sure to eat well-balanced meals for 2 weeks. The labels on the blood bag and tubes are checked carefully before and after donation to avoid any error that could prove fatal to a recipient.

Complications

Excessive bleeding at the site of venipuncture is sometimes due to a bleeding disorder in the donor, but more often is the result of a technical error: laceration of the vein, excessive tourniquet pressure, or failure to apply enough pressure following withdrawal of the needle.

Fainting is relatively common and may be related to emotional factors, vasovagal reaction, or prolonged fasting before donation. Sometimes, because of the loss of blood volume, hypotension and syncope occur when the donor assumes an erect position.

- If the donor appears pale or complains of faintness, he should immediately lie down or sit with his head lowered below his knees. The nurse should observe him for another 30 minutes.

Anginal chest pain may be precipitated in patients with unsuspected coronary artery disease.

Convulsions may occur in epileptic patients. Both angina and convulsions require further medical evaluation.

Blood and Blood Components

A unit of blood that has been drawn from a donor consists of approximately 450 ml of whole blood and 63 ml of Citrate Phosphate Dextrose anticoagulant-preservative. The latter serves as the anticoagulant and also provides the red cells with a sugar for metabolism. This blood can be maintained at 1° C to 6° C in the blood bank for 21 days, but after that it is discarded because too many of the red cells are unable to survive *in vivo*. Samples of the unit are always taken immediately after donation so that the blood can be typed and tested for the presence of syphilis, hepatitis, and antibodies. A label on the unit thereafter states the blood type and certifies that the unit is negative for syphilis serology and hepatitis B antigen.

Whole blood is a complex tissue with both cellular and many noncellular plasma components. Recently it has been recognized that whole blood is necessary only in certain clinical situations; many times, component therapy can replace the particular deficiency without subjecting the patient to unnecessary risks, such as circulatory overload. In addition, use of components is more economical, since it makes it possible to meet the needs of more than one patient from a single blood donation. Many blood banks are able to separate whole blood into these fractions, and all of the components are available from the American Red Cross.

Whole Blood. Whole blood may be used to treat acute, massive hemorrhage or hypovolemic shock owing to hemorrhage. It is not indicated for the correction of anemia. Whenever possible, components should be used instead.

Packed Red Cells. Red cells are separated from whole blood by centrifugation or sedimentation; most of the plasma is removed, leaving a hematocrit of approximately 80%. Packed red cells are indicated for transfusions in all anemic patients, in surgical patients before and after operation, and in many cases of acute blood loss. The use of packed cells instead of whole blood reduces the volume load. Thus, this method is safer for patients with incipient congestive failure and reduces the incidence of transfusion reactions owing to plasma factors.

Frozen Red Cells. The method of freezing red cells allows storage for long periods of time—even years—but is expensive. Hence, frozen cells are used only under unusual circumstances, such as for patients with very rare blood types or with antibodies to the common minor antigens.

Platelets. Patients with thrombocytopenia and hemorrhage often require transfusions of large numbers of platelets. Platelets taken from 4 to 8 units of blood are necessary to raise the count of a severely thrombocytopenic patient to a hemostatic level. Therefore, "platelet-rich plasma" with a small volume is used rather than whole blood. Several methods are available for harvesting fresh platelets: (1) Plasma can be removed after centrifugation of a unit of freshly collected whole blood; the plasma is then centrifuged again slowly to separate the platelets. Several such platelet "units" can then be pooled and given to the recipient, who thus receives platelets from several different donors. (2) A single donor can undergo *plasmapheresis*, in which blood is donated, the red cells are separated and returned to the donor immediately, and the plasma is spun down to obtain platelets in a volume of only 10 ml to 20 ml. In this way, multiple units can be donated.

Platelet concentrates are generally kept at room temperature with agitation and are administered within 48 hours of collection to ensure viability. Each unit of platelets will raise the recipient's platelet count by about 10,000 per cubic milliliter. Single donor platelet transfusions are especially valuable for patients who have received many transfusions and have developed antibodies to all except HLA (transplantation antigen) matched blood products.

Granulocytes. Severely granulocytopenic patients with infection can sometimes benefit from transfusions of normal white cells. Large numbers of granulocytes less than 24 hours old must be administered. The donor's white cells are continuously removed as blood is drawn from one vein and constantly returned to another vein. The process requires about 4 hours of donor time, and the donor must be anticoagulated during the procedure.

Plasma. Whole plasma was originally used in the treatment of hypovolemic shock, but now other colloids (such as albumin) or electrolyte solutions (like Ringer's lactate) are usually preferred. Plasma can be used to replace deficient coagulation factors in acquired or inherited bleeding disorders. Only fresh frozen plasma (which can be stored for 12 months) contains all the coagulation factors, including V and VIII. However, fractions of plasma have now been prepared that can replace all the factors, except V, in small volume concentrates. Fresh frozen plasma may be administered to replace clotting factors in patients who are hemorrhaging and being massively transfused with whole blood or packed red cells. It is also used to treat patients with severe liver disease.

Albumin. Plasma albumin is a large protein molecule that usually stays within vessels and is a major contributor to plasma oncotic pressure. This material is used to expand the blood volume of patients in hypovolemic shock and to elevate the level of circulating albumin in patients with hypoalbuminemia. These preparations, in contrast to all other fractions of human blood, cellular or soluble, are subjected to heating at 60° C (140° F) for 10 hours, and therefore can be certified unequivocally as free of all viral contaminants, including the hepatitis virus. Whereas the risk of hepatitis transmission is an important consideration in connection with every other type of transfusion therapy (except gamma globulin), no such complication has ever been known to follow the use of albumin.

Factor VIII Fractions. These components have brought about a revolution in the treatment of patients with classical hemophilia. Whereas previously large volumes of plasma were necessary to treat bleeding episodes in this disease, now the volumes are so small that circulatory overload cannot occur. Cryoprecipitate is made from fresh frozen plasma, and the method of preparation is simple enough for use in most blood banks. Once the precipitate is separated, the rest of the plasma can be used for other purposes. The cryoprecipitate is redissolved in plasma or saline for use in patients who are deficient in fibrinogen, factor VIII, and factor XIII or have von Willebrand's disease. A glycine precipitate is available commercially, as Hemofil.

Prothrombin Complex. This fraction, commercially marketed as Konyne and Proplex, contains prothrombin and factors VII, IX, and X and some factor XI. It is useful for the treatment of bleeding in congenital or acquired deficiencies of these factors. However, the hepatitis hazard is significant with this material.

Transfusion Technique

Administration of blood and blood components demands knowledge of correct techniques for administration and possible complications. After verifying the order and explaining the procedure to the recipient, the nurse must obtain the blood or blood component from the blood bank.

Labels are carefully checked with another nurse. Vital signs should be recorded prior to initiating the transfusion.

Whole blood or packed red cells are generally administered through a 19-gauge or larger needle into a large vein. Special tubing is used that contains a blood filter to screen out fibrin clots and other particulate matter. For the first 15 minutes, the transfusion is run very slowly, at about 20 drops per minute, and the patient is observed carefully for adverse effects. If no ill effects occur during this time, the flow rate is then increased unless the patient is at high risk for overload. The patient must continue to be frequently observed. A summary of major points to consider when administering blood components is listed in Table 33-4.

▶ Assessment

Prior to initiating transfusion therapy it is important to check to see that the blood has been typed and cross matched and that the ABO group and Rh type on the blood containers are in accordance with the compatibility record. The blood should also be checked for the presence of gas bubbles and any abnormal color or cloudiness. Gas bubbles may indicate bacterial growth; abnormal color or cloudiness may be a sign of hemolysis. The labels identifying the number and type of the donor blood and the recipient blood are noted and the identification of the patient confirmed directly by asking him to state his name and indirectly by checking his identification wrist band. At the same time, the patient's chart is checked for blood type and number. The patient's TPR and blood type are taken in order to provide a baseline for comparing vital signs at a later time.

After the blood transfusion is started, the patient should be watched closely for 15 to 30 minutes to assure that no signs of reaction or circulatory overload occur. Monitoring vital signs is carried out at regular intervals as indicated.

Patient Problems

Based on the fact that every patient who receives a blood transfusion is subject to the possible development of complications of transfusion therapy, the patient's major problems include the possible development of circulatory overload, febrile reaction, allergic reaction, hemolytic reaction, delayed hemolytic reaction, and diseases transmitted by the transfusion (*e.g.,* hepatitis, malaria, and syphilis).

▶ Planning and Nursing Implementation

Goals

The major goals of care include avoiding the following possible complications of transfusion therapy:

1. Absence of circulatory overload
2. Absence of febrile reaction
3. Absence of allergic reaction
4. Absence of hemolytic reaction
5. Absence of delayed hemolytic reaction
6. Absence of disease transmitted by blood transfusion

Transfusion Complications

Much has been learned about the cause of transfusion reactions in recent years; hence, many of the adverse effects can be prevented. Nevertheless, transfusion is never without

Table 33-4
Administration of Blood Components

Product	Administration Technique	Major Complications
Packed red cells	Use standard blood filter and make sure cells cover entire surface. Administer only with 0.9% NaCl. Squeeze bag to mix cells every 20 to 30 minutes during administration. Administer 1 unit over 1 to 2 hours. If necessary to help cells infuse, add 50 ml to 100 ml 0.9% NaCl.	Transfusion reactions less frequent than with whole blood
Platelets	Use special nonwettable filter. Administer only with 0.9% NaCl. Administer as rapidly as tolerated, usually 4 units/hour.	Febrile reactions common
Granulocytes	Use standard blood filter. Administer only with 0.9% NaCl. Administer over 2 to 4 hours.	Febrile and allergic reactions common Leukoagglutinin reactions possible, leading to hypotension, anaphylaxis, and respiratory distress
Plasma	Use straight line set. Administer as rapidly as patient tolerates.	Risk of circulatory overload Risk of hepatitis greater than with whole blood (if multiple donors)
Albumin	Undiluted 25% albumin should be administered at 1 ml/minute if patient is normovolemic. Administer as rapidly as possible for patient in hypovolemic shock.	Risk of circulatory overload No risk of hepatitis
Factor VIII	Administer by syringe or component drip set.	Allergic and febrile reactions common Hepatitis risk same as with whole blood
Prothrombin	Administer through straight line set.	Allergic and febrile reactions possible Risk of hepatitis greater than with whole blood

certain risks, and these must be considered before the therapy is initiated.

Circulatory Overloading. In patients with normal blood volume (as in chronic anemia) or increased blood volume (as in renal failure or heart failure), the addition of whole blood or packed cells can precipitate pulmonary edema. Packed red cells are safer to use, and if the rate of administration is sufficiently slow, circulatory overloading may be prevented.

- The signs to look for are dyspnea, orthopnea, cyanosis, or sudden anxiety. If the transfusion is continued, severe dyspnea and coughing of pink, frothy sputum can occur.
- The patient should be placed in an upright position, the blood should be discontinued, and rotating tourniquets should be applied. Phlebotomy or diuretics may be necessary if improvement does not occur rapidly.

Febrile Reactions. Patients may develop a fever during transfusion because of the presence of bacterial pyrogens, sensitivity to leukocytes or platelets, hemolytic episodes, or unknown factors. Owing to the widespread use of disposable transfusion equipment, bacterial pyrogens are rarely a cause. Infrequently, blood can be grossly contaminated with large numbers of microorganisms that survive in the 4° C (39.2° F) storage. If such blood is infused, the patient develops fever and shaking chills within 30 minutes, and shock soon follows. Even when the cause of this reaction is recognized early (by gram stain of the donor blood), the mortality rate is high. Sensitivity to leukocyte or platelet antigens is much more common, especially in previously transfused patients or women who have borne children. The temperature rises during the administration of blood or shortly afterward and is rarely associated with chills, hypotension, or nausea. This type of reaction has a good prognosis, and the treatment is aspirin. Subsequent transfusions should utilize leukocyte-poor blood.

Allergic Reactions. Some patients may develop urticaria (hives) or generalized itching or, rarely, wheezing or anaphylaxis. The cause of these reactions is thought to be sensitivity to a plasma protein in the transfused blood, or passive transfer of antibodies from the donor that react with some antigen (for example, in a drug or food) to which the recipient is exposed. To avoid this, allergic individuals are disqualified as donors. The reactions are usually mild and respond to antihistamines. If severe, parenteral epinephrine is used.

Hemolytic Reactions. The most dangerous type of transfusion reaction occurs when the donor blood is incompatible with that of the recipient. Antibodies in the recipient's plasma rapidly combine with donor erythrocytes, and the cells are hemolyzed either in the circulation or in the reticuloendothelial system. The most rapid hemolysis occurs in ABO incompatibility (*e.g.,* if the donor is group A and the recipient is group O, and therefore has anti-A and anti-B antibodies). Rh incompatibility is often less severe.

- Symptoms consist of chills, low back pain, headache, nausea, or chest tightness, followed by fever and hypotension and vascular collapse. Severe reactions usually start within 10 minutes after the transfusion is begun. Hemoglobinuria (red urine) appears at the next voiding.
- The reaction must be recognized promptly and the transfusion discontinued immediately; the chances of a fatal episode are much reduced if less than 100 ml of incompatible blood are infused.

Treatment is directed toward correcting the hypotension and preventing the renal damage that can follow hemoglobinuria. The patient is supported with intravenous colloid and given mannitol as an osmotic diuretic to maintain a good urine flow. An indwelling catheter may be necessary for accurate measurement of output. If, after 24 hours, urine flow cannot be maintained, mannitol is contraindicated since it can be assumed that acute tubular necrosis has occurred. The management henceforth will be that of the renal disorder and will include fluid restriction and possibly dialysis until spontaneous healing takes place.

Delayed Reactions. Delayed hemolytic reactions occur at about 1 to 2 weeks and are recognized by a gradual fall in hemoglobin level and a positive Coombs' test. There is no hemoglobinuria, and these reactions are not dangerous. However, recognition is important because subsequent transfusions may cause an acute hemolytic reaction.

Serum Hepatitis. Serum hepatitis is an important risk of transfusion therapy, both for whole blood and for most components (see above). Blood obtained from "skid row" paid donors carries a higher risk than that from volunteer donors. Pooled blood products also constitute a significantly higher risk. Tests are currently used to detect hepatitis B virus, but a method for detecting hepatitis nonA–nonB is not yet available. Hepatitis is further discussed on page 861.

Malaria. Malaria is sometimes transmitted in blood donated by asymptomatic individuals who have been exposed to the disease in Southeast Asia. Recipients develop high fever and headache several weeks after the transfusion.

Syphilis. Syphilis is rarely transmitted now because of the serologic tests required on all units of blood and because the organism does not survive refrigeration.

Nursing Interventions in Transfusion Reaction

If it is suspected that a transfusion reaction is occurring because of any of the conditions mentioned above, the nurse should stop the transfusion and call the physician immediately. The following steps are taken in order that a diagnosis may be made regarding the type and severity of the reaction:

- The transfusion set is disconnected, but the intravenous line is kept open with a dextrose or saline solution in case intravenous medication should be needed rapidly.
- *The blood bag and tubing are saved, not thrown away.*

They should be sent to the blood bank for repeat typing and culture.
- The patient's blood is drawn for plasma hemoglobin, culture, and retyping.
- A urine sample is collected as soon as possible and sent to the laboratory for a hemoglobin determination. Subsequent voidings of urine should be observed.
- The blood bank is notified that a suspected transfusion reaction has occurred.

▶ Evaluation

Expected Outcomes

1. Is free of circulatory overload
   Exhibits normal vital signs:
      Breath sounds clear to auscultation
      Respiratory rate 14/minute to 18/minute
      Respirations unlabored
      BP within normal range
2. Is free of febrile reaction
   a. Exhibits normal temperature and pulse rate
   b. Is free of chilling, headache, flushing
3. Is free of allergic reaction
   a. Shows no signs of rash, itching, hives
   b. Has respirations of normal rate and that are unlabored
4. Is free of hemolytic reaction
   a. Exhibits normal vital signs:
      Temperature within normal range
      Pulse rate within normal range
      BP within normal range
      Urine clear, amber
   b. Has no pain in back, head, and chest
5. Is free of delayed hemolytic reaction 5 to 10 days after transfusion
   a. Has normal temperature and hematocrit
   b. Shows no sign of jaundice
6. Is free of disease transmitted by blood transfusion
   Is free of symptoms of disease: hepatitis, malaria, syphilis

Bone Marrow Transplantation

This is an exciting addition to the therapeutic possibilities for hematologic disease. Bone marrow can be aspirated by needle from multiple sites of an anesthetized normal donor and easily transfused intravenously into the recipient. The marrow cells immediately travel to the marrow spaces that have been emptied by disease (*i.e.,* aplastic anemia) or by chemotherapy.

The major barrier to the success of bone marrow transplantation is the antigenic difference between donor and recipient. Thus, transplants between identical twins are almost always successful, and sibling transplants are often successful. If the donor and the patient are not identical in HLA (transplantation antigen) types, pretreatment of the patient with immunosuppression is necessary. Many recipients succumb to graft vs. host disease or severe infections while awaiting the recovery of the transplanted marrow. However, methods of immunosuppression and supportive care have improved greatly over the last few years, and this is currently the best treatment for severe aplastic anemia. Bone marrow transplantation is also used to treat some forms of leukemia.

▷ Bibliography

Books

Boggs DR and Winkelstein A. White Cell Manual, 4th ed. Philadelphia, FA Davis, 1983.

Corbett JV. Laboratory Tests in Nursing Practice. New York, Appleton–Century–Crofts, 1982.

DeVita VT, Hellman S, and Rosenberg SA. Cancer: Principles and Practice of Oncology. Philadelphia, JB Lippincott, 1982.

Gunz F. (ed). Leukemia, 4th ed. New York, Grune & Stratton, 1983.

Harker LA. Hemostasis Manual, 2nd ed. Philadelphia, FA Davis, 1974.

Hilgartner M (ed). Hemophilia in the Child and Adult, New York, Masson, 1982.

Hillman RS and Finch CA. Red Cell Manual, 4th ed. Philadelphia, FA Davis, 1974.

Holland JF and Frei E. Cancer Medicine, 2nd ed. Philadelphia, Lea & Febiger, 1982.

Mollison P. Blood Transfusion in Clinical Medicine, 7th ed. St Louis, CV Mosby, 1983.

Petersdorf RG. (ed). Harrison's Principles of Internal Medicine, 10th ed. New York, McGraw–Hill, 1983.

Price SA and Wilson LM. Pathophysiology: Clinical Concepts of Disease Processes, 2nd ed. New York, McGraw–Hill, 1982.

Robbins SL and Cotran RS. Pathologic Basis of Disease, 2nd ed. Philadelphia, WB Saunders, 1979.

Rubin P. Clinical Oncology, 5th ed. Rochester, American Cancer Society, 1978.

Rutman R and Miller WV. Transfusion Therapy: Principles and Procedures. Rockville, Maryland, Aspen Systems Corp, 1981.

Suitor CW and Hunter MF. Nutrition: Principles and Application in Health Promotion. Philadelphia, JB Lippincott, 1980.

Widmann FK. Clinical Interpretation of Laboratory Tests, 9th ed. Philadelphia, FA Davis, 1983.

Articles
Anemias

Crosby WH. Red cell mass: Its precursors and its perturbations. Hosp Pract 1980 Feb; 15(2):71–81.

Doswell WM. Sickle cell anemia. Nursing '78 1978 Apr; 8(4):65–70.

Forget BG. Hemolytic anemias: Congenital and acquired. Hosp Pract 1980 Apr; 15(4):67–78.

Goldstein M. The aplastic anemias. Hosp Pract 1980 May; 15(5):85–96.

Green JB. Macrocytic anemias. Postgrad Med 1977 June; 61(6):155–161.

Herbert V. The nutritional anemias. Hosp Pract 1980 Mar; 15(3):65–89.

McFarlane J. Sickle cell disorders. Am J Nurs 1977 Dec; 77(12):1948–1954.

Pack B. (ed). Symposium on sickle cell disease. Nurs Clin North Am 1983 Mar; 18(1):129–229.

Bleeding Disorders

Bowie EJ and Owen CA. Hemostatic failure in clinical medicine. Semin Hematol 1977 July; 14(3):341–363.

Jennings BM. Improving your management of DIC. Nursing '79 1979 May; 9(5):60–67.

Rizza CR. Clinical management of haemophilia. Br Med Bull 1977 Sept; 33(3):225–230.

Wheelis RF. Making sense of coagulation tests. Bulletin of the Mason Clinic 1979 Spring; 33(1):1–9.

Wroblewski SS and Wroblewski SH. Caring for the patient with chemotherapy-induced thrombocytopenia. Am J Nurs 1981 Apr; 81(4):746–749.

Blood Transfusion

Blood transfusions: How to administer whole blood and its components. Nursing '80 1980 Mar; 10(3):67–69.

Buickus BA. Administering blood components. Am J Nurs 1979 May; 79(5):937–941.

Cullins LC. Preventing and treating transfusion reactions. Am J Nurs 1979 May; 79(5):935–937.

Emminizer S, Klopp EH, and Haver JM. Autotransfusion: Current status. Heart Lung 1981 Jan/Feb; 10(1):83–87.

Horwitz CA. Blood transfusion therapy. Postgrad Med 1981 Apr; 69(4):155–164.

Kazak A. Processing blood for transfusion. Am J Nurs 1979 May; 79(5):931–934.

McCredie KB. Platelet and granulocyte transfusion therapy. Postgrad Med 1977 Aug; 62(2):151–153.

McCurdy PR. Blood component therapy. Postgrad Med 1977 Aug; 62(2):143–147.

Parker AL. Massive transfusions. Am J Nurs 1979 May; 79(5):944–948.

Rutman R et al. Screening donors and the phlebotomy procedure. Am J Nurs 1979 May; 79(5):926–930.

Sandler SG. Recent advances in the practice and technology of blood transfusion. Primary Care 1980 Sept; 7(3):347–367.

Scarlato M. Blood transfusions today: What you should know and should do. Nursing '78 1978 Feb; 8(2):68–72.

Shafer N, Wilkenfeld M, and Shafer R. Blood transfusion reactions. Leg Med 1980; 207–220.

Thomas SF. Transfusing granulocytes. Am J Nurs 1979 May; 79(5):942–944.

Woods ME and Mazza I. Blood and component therapy. Nurs Clin North Am 1980 Sept; 15(3):629–646.

Leukemia/Lymphoma

Desotell S. A brighter future for leukemia patients. Nursing '77 1977 Jan; 7(1):18–24.

LeBlanc DH. People with Hodgkin's disease: The nursing challenge. Nurs Clin North Am 1978 June; 13(2):281–300.

Markus S. Taking the fear out of bone marrow examinations. Nursing '81 1981 Apr; 11(4):64–67.

Ostchega Y. Preventing and treating cancer chemotherapy's oral complications. Nursing '80 1980 Aug; 10(8):47–52.

Zimmerman S et al. Bone marrow transplantation. Am J Nurs 1977 Aug; 77(8):1311–1315.

Agencies
Governmental

National Heart, Lung and Blood Institute, National Institutes of Health, Bethesda, Md. 20205

Voluntary

American Red Cross, 18th and E Sts., N.W., Washington, D.C. 20006

Center for Sickle Cell Disease, Howard University, 2121 Georgia Ave., N.W., Washington, D.C. 20060

Leukemia Society of America, 211 East 43rd St., New York, New York 10017

National Hemophilia Foundation, 25 West 39th St., New York, New York 10018

American Cancer Society, 777 Third Ave., New York, New York 10017

Unit IX

Digestive and Gastrointestinal Problems

34

Assessment and Management of Patients With Ingestive Problems and Upper Gastrointestinal Disorders

Since the process of ingestion begins with the mastication of food in the mouth, adequate nutrition is related to good dental health and the general condition of the mouth. The presence and condition of the teeth has a direct bearing on nutritional well-being by influencing the type of food ingested and the degree to which food particles are properly mixed with salivary enzymes. Any discomfort in the mouth, owing to lip lesions, inflammation of the buccal mucosa, or other conditions, can have a deleterious effect on food intake. Esophageal problems related to the apparently simple act of swallowing can also adversely affect food and fluid intake, thereby jeopardizing general health and well-being.

Given the close interrelationship between adequate nutritional intake and all of the structures of the upper gastrointestinal tract (lips, mouth, teeth, esophagus), preventive health teaching should place heavy emphasis on helping people to avoid the common discomfort and disorders associated with any of these structures.

▷ Dental Conditions and Care of the Teeth

Care of the Teeth

The nurse, as a proponent of sound health practices, is in a unique position to teach and emphasize the importance of regular, periodic dental examinations. By supporting community dental health programs, by demonstrating proper dental techniques, and by supervising appropriate dental practices, the nurse can facilitate the therapeutic plan and can encourage patient cooperation and persistence with periodontal programs.

▶ **Nursing Assessment**

An evaluation of the patient's current dental health will help identify needed health teaching and possible dental problems. The nurse should ask about the patient's usual routine for cleaning and flossing the teeth and for regular examination and cleaning by a dentist. The nurse questions whether the client has any known dental problems, especially those that interfere with eating, and if he wears dentures or has difficulty in chewing. Since elderly people are more likely to have problems with dental health, the nurse should anticipate this possibility.

The nurse then inspects the teeth and gums, noting the general state of hygiene, including presence of odor, absence of teeth, presence of dental caries, and any obvious malformation of the teeth.

▶ **Planning and Interventions**

Oral Hygiene. Instructing the client about proper dental hygiene is a major component of nursing intervention.

Healthy teeth require conscientious and effective daily cleaning. The purpose of toothbrushing is to mechanically break up the bacterial plaque that collects around teeth. Proper brushing requires a soft, rounded-tip, bristle brush. The bristles of the brush are directed into the gingival sulcus in a horizontal scrubbing motion. Ten strokes are recommended for each surface. Dental floss should also be used every 24 hours to reach those areas between the teeth not accessible to the brush. The floss is inserted between the teeth and moved back and forth in a gentle sawing motion until it reaches under the gum line. Of course, the normal movement of the muscles of mastication and the normal flow of saliva also aid greatly in keeping the teeth clean. Even so, it is necessary to disorganize plaque once during each 24-hour period, preferably before bedtime. This practice prevents decay and periodontal disease.

Since many ill patients do not eat and salivate normally, the natural cleaning process of the teeth is reduced. If a patient is absolutely unable to brush his teeth, as in the case of patients with cerebrovascular disease or those disabled by trauma, then it becomes a nursing responsibility. In any case, merely swabbing the patient's mouth and teeth with glycerin and lemon juice is inadequate, since all it does is coat collections of bacteria without removing them. The *most effective method is,* again, *mechanical cleansing.* It is better to wipe the patient's teeth with a washcloth than to have him swish an antiseptic mouthwash several times and then emit it into the emesis basin. If a toothbrush is used, an electric brush is more effective in cleansing someone else's teeth than the conventional hand toothbrush. While the left hand of the nurse retracts the lips and cheeks, the right hand can direct the electric brush to all surfaces of the patient's teeth. Even the tongue may receive a beneficial light brushing. Once any toothbrush is used, it should be cleaned thoroughly with soap and water and allowed to dry.

▶ **Evaluation**

Evaluation of the teaching efforts of nurses related to dental hygiene can be carried out through observation of proper brushing technique by the patient and through follow-up questioning about the importance of regular dental hygiene. Evaluation of long-term adherence related to dental hygiene is far more difficult. Nurses who see patients on a long-term basis, such as clinic or school nurses, are better able to provide reminders about the importance of regular dental hygiene than are nurses who see patients for short-term, episodic hospital care. Hospital-based nurses can help the patient arrange for postdischarge dental follow-up through the Home Care Department, the Discharge Coordinator, or the local community nurse.

Dental Conditions

Dental Plaque and Caries

At least 95% of Americans sooner or later experience tooth decay. This is an erosive process that results from the action of bacteria on fermentable carbohydrates in the mouth, which in turn produces acids that dissolve tooth enamel. The extent of damage to the teeth depends on several factors, the most significant of which are (1) the presence of dental plaque; (2) the strength of the acids and the ability of the saliva to neutralize them; (3) the length of time the acids are in contact with the teeth; and (4) susceptibility of the teeth to decay. Dental plaque is a gluey, gelatinlike substance that adheres to the teeth and affords protection for the bacteria. The initial action that causes damage to a tooth occurs under dental plaque.

Dental decay begins with a small hole, usually in a fissure or flaw of the enamel, or in an area that is hard to clean. Left unchecked, it penetrates the enamel into the dentin. Because the dentin is not as hard as the enamel, decay progresses somewhat more rapidly and in time reaches the pulp. When the blood, lymph vessels, and nerves are exposed, they become infected, and an abscess may form, either within the tooth or at the tip of the root. Soreness and pain usually accompany the abscess. As the infection increases, the face may become swollen, and there may be pulsating pain. The dentist can determine by x-ray pictures the extent of damage and the type of treatment needed. It may be necessary to extract the tooth.

Measures used in the prevention and control of dental caries include reducing the intake of *sugars* (refined carbohydrates), practicing effective mouth care (as described), and applying fluoride to the teeth, or drinking fluoridated water. This information is especially useful to the nurse practicing in "well baby," adolescent, or maternity clinics, where groups are found with special dental needs.

Fluoridation. Adjusting the fluoride level in the drinking water to an optimal healthful level of one part per million can help to prevent up to two thirds of tooth decay. Such a concentration of fluoride makes tooth enamel more resistant to the acids that are formed in the mouth. When ingested from birth to about 10 years of age, fluoridated water can give permanent protection. Some sections of the western United States have natural fluoridation; other areas of the country have enacted legislation for controlled fluoridation of public water supplies. In these areas, studies have demonstrated a reduction in dental decay. Fluoridation also lessens the possibility of malocclusion and gingival disease.

Most areas of this country, however, do not have fluoridated water, and people must find other ways of receiving the benefits of fluoride. Four other methods are possible: (1) Vitamin preparations can include fluoride. Treatment must start early in life and continue until the age of 10. (2) A concentrated solution can be applied directly to the teeth. This procedure is done by the dentist and has the advantage of providing professional control and also encouraging regular checkups. (3) Sodium fluoride can be added to the water in the home; however, home fluoridators that operate automatically are expensive and may do little good, since children drink most of their daily water supply in school. (4) Sodium fluoride can be provided in tablet or liquid drops as a dietary additive; this, too, is expensive and often impractical.

Technological Advances. Technological advances in recent years have produced several new coatings that bond to the enamel of the tooth and protect it from decay. These composite dental resins consist of an epoxy resin product and a form of acrylic acid, plus reinforcing fillers, such as glass beads or quartz fillers. Dentists can use the new materials to seal pits and fissures when the teeth first grow in, thus preventing decay. The new materials can also be used to restore teeth eroded near the gum, a common site of periodontal disease.

A new translucent tooth-filling material, made by mixing a special aluminosilicate glass powder with a solution of polyacrylic acid, has several advantages over conventional enamel fillings made with phosphoric acid. The polyacrylic acid is much milder than phosphoric acid (which can damage the tooth, if the cavity is not lined before it is filled). Also, the new filling is adhesive, which eliminates the need for extensive drilling to secure the filling.

Dentoalveolar Abscess or Periapical Abscess

This type of abscess results from a suppurative process involving the apical dental periosteum and the alveolar process in the periapical region. It may appear in two forms. The acute form is usually secondary to a suppurative pulpitis that arises from an infection extending from dental caries. The infection of the dental pulp extends through the apical foramen of the tooth to form an abscess about the apex, at its site of implantation in the alveolar bone. The abscess produces a dull, gnawing, continuous pain, often with a surrounding cellulitis and edema of the adjacent facial structures. The gum opposite the apex of the tooth is usually swollen on the cheek side, where the abscess is prone to point. The swelling and cellulitis of the facial structures may make it difficult to open the mouth. In well-developed abscesses there may be a systemic reaction, fever, and malaise.

In the early stages of an infection, a dental surgeon may drill an opening into the pulp chamber to relieve tension and pain and to provide drainage. Usually, the infection has progressed to a periapical abscess, and drainage must be provided by an incision through the gingivae down to the jaw bone. Foul pus escapes under pressure.

Nursing Goals and Interventions

Much dental surgery is done on an out-patient basis. However, when a patient is hospitalized for treatment of dentoalveolar or periapical abscesses, the nursing care needed is that required by the problems generated by an acute localized infection. The general goals are to relieve pain; to combat the infection; and to ensure adequate hydration, nutrition, and rest.

The postoperative care consists of hot saline mouthwashes given at least every 2 hours, except when the patient is asleep. He should be encouraged to expectorate the foul pus that escapes, and a basin should be within easy reach. External heat, in the form of hot compresses or a heating pad, hastens the subsidence of the inflammatory swelling and soreness. In patients with a high fever, an antibiotic (penicillin) is usually administered.

Bed rest and a soft diet are necessary during the acute stage. Analgesic drugs are used as necessary, to relieve pain. The nurse must recognize that the pain and swelling may interfere with an adequate fluid intake, and a special effort must be made to overcome any deficit. After the inflammatory reaction has subsided, the tooth may have to be extracted, or appropriate root canal therapy given.

Chronic dentoalveolar abscess is a slowly progressive infection, with the same mode as the acute form. It differs from the acute form in that the process may progress to a fully formed abscess without the patient's knowing it. The infection eventually leads to a "blind dental abscess" that is really a periapical granuloma. It may enlarge to as much as 1 cm in diameter. It is often discovered in x-ray examination and is treated by extraction or root canal therapy, often with apicoectomy.

Periodontal Disease

Periodontal disease (pyorrhea) is a condition affecting the gums (gingivae) and other supporting structures (bone, cementum, and periodontal membrane). At the onset, there is little discomfort and few other signs of the condition. Later there may be bleeding, infection, gum recession, and loosening of the teeth. As a result, the teeth may fall out or may need to be extracted. It is estimated that one in four persons have the disease at some stage of its development, and up to 90% of all persons in their 40s are affected. Dental authorities suggest that the principal reason why most people, after age 50, require dentures is the effect of this increasingly prevalent disease.

Malocclusion, poor fillings, and inadequate diet are suspected causes of periodontal disease; in addition, improper cleaning and poor mouth hygiene contribute to the problem. Tartar or calculus that cannot be brushed from the teeth tends to build up and requires professional removal twice a year. If this is not done, gums become swollen and tender, infection progresses, and pockets that collect pus and bacteria are formed between the gums and teeth. The protective layer that normally covers the gums is destroyed, exposing the blood vessels, which bleed easily. Bacteria thrive on the nutrients in the blood and tissues that fill and line the space. The bone supporting the teeth is destroyed, and the tooth becomes loose.

Some authorities believe that this condition is frequently associated with other systemic diseases, such as diabetes and certain skin and blood disorders; however, conclusive evidence is lacking. At present, the best advice is to brush the teeth and floss carefully, at least once a day, and to have the teeth cleaned professionally twice a year. Such a cleaning should include the area below the gum line. Poor occlusion should be corrected, crooked teeth straightened, and missing teeth replaced with bridgework or another form of splinting. Not too long ago, such work by an orthodontist was considered a luxury and done only for cosmetic reasons. Today the value of such treatment is seen in the prevention of periodontal disease and other mouth problems. However, because of cost, this type of therapeutic intervention is still generally available only to those with adequate dental health plans.

In the near future, perhaps, three-dimensional photography will assist periodontists in measuring the changes in the shape or elevation of the gum, signs that allow early detection of periodontal disease.

Orthodontal Correction for Malocclusion

Malocclusion is a faulty relationship between the teeth when the jaws are closed. Correction of malocclusion requires three factors: an orthodontist who has special training, a patient who cooperates, and adequate time. Most treatments begin when the patient has shed his last primary tooth and the last permanent successor has erupted, usually around 12 or 13 years of age.

In order to realign the teeth, the orthodontist gradually forces the teeth into a new location by the use of wires or bands. This therapy is commonly known as teeth-straightening. Although the patient may object to the effect of these devices on his appearance, this psychological burden must be overcome if good results are to be achieved in the future. During this time, it is essential that the patient keep his mouth meticulously clean. In the final phase of treatment, a retaining device is worn for several hours each day to support the tissues as they adjust to the new location of the teeth. Encouragement is often necessary for the individual to persist in this most important part of the treatment. When an adolescent undergoing orthodontal correction is admitted to the hospital for some other problem, it may be necessary to remind him to continue wearing the retainer, if it does not interfere with the problem requiring hospitalization.

Braces are also used as part of the means of correcting long or short jaw syndrome. These procedures, called orthognathic surgery, are done when the jaw is either too long or too short for proper mandibular alignment. When the jaw is too long, bony material is extracted; when the jaw is too short, a bone graft or inert material may be inserted. The postoperative care of these patients is similar to that needed by patients with a fractured mandible (see p. 734).

Dental Implants and Transplantation

Successful research is being done involving the transplantation of teeth and the possible "storage" of teeth in a bank. Some researchers have restricted their transplants to undeveloped or "bud" teeth, whereas others are trying to transplant teeth at many stages of development. However, at present, homotransplants (transplanting teeth from one person to another) will have to await additional research to combat the rejection process. Successful autotransplants

(using the patient's own teeth) have been reported. For example, a defective first molar has been replaced successfully by the patient's own third molar.

Teeth made from acrylic and other plastics have been implanted successfully, in several instances. In 1972, Neff, of Georgetown University, reported on an artificial plastic tooth made of Vacalon that, when implanted in baboons, functioned much like a natural tooth. New tissue grew around the implant, and bone grew through the vents in the implant roots, as would occur with natural teeth. Neff's research may lead to the development of similar implants for humans. Also under study is the use of ceramic tooth roots made of high-density alumina (with metallic post and a conventional gold crown).

Implants are not to be considered as fully acceptable alternatives to other forms of dental treatment. Rather they are to be used only when other forms of treatment do not suffice to restore the mouth to its masticatory function. There is an element of unpredictability in the field of oral implants. Therefore, their use should be regarded as a last approach to sound dentistry.

Dental Extraction

A tooth is extracted because it is defective, damaged, or in the path of future orthodontal correction.

Extraction wounds usually heal quickly and without complications if simple precautions are taken. Lessened activity reduces the likelihood of bleeding. Cold applications soon after extraction, such as an ice bag or cold, moist cloth applied to the side of the face for about 15 minutes of every hour for several hours, will relieve discomfort and swelling. Rinsing the mouth is not done the first day, so that the clot will not be disturbed. Thereafter, rinsing and cleansing of the teeth is resumed.

Oozing of blood may be apparent the first day, but if heavier bleeding occurs, place a clean, folded gauze pad directly on the bleeding spot. Instruct the patient to close his teeth tightly over the pad and to apply pressure for about 30 minutes. Repeat, if necessary. If there is prolonged or severe pain, swelling, or bleeding, the dentist should be notified.

Impacted Third Molars. It may be desirable to hospitalize the patient when all four molars are to be extracted at one time. Using endotracheal general anesthesia, the oral surgeon inserts a mouth retractor to provide exposure. Incisions are made laterally in the mandible to approach the impacted tooth. The jaw eventually regenerates bone that has been removed. Closure of the mucous membrane is accomplished with black silk sutures.

Postoperatively, soreness and edema are noticeable, but can be relieved by analgesics and ice packs. Liquids may be offered from a spouted container if the facial muscles are too sensitive to allow the patient to suck from a straw. After the fifth day, stitches are removed and mouthwashes can proceed from saline to sodium peroxyborate monohydrate (Amosan). Brushing of the teeth is resumed when the gums have healed. Any pain or swelling after 1 week should be reported; infection is common, but can be easily treated with drainage, packing, and antibiotics.

Artificial Dentures

It is common practice for people to postpone indefinitely the final decision to obtain artificial dentures, even though there is no possibility of having the few remaining teeth repaired. Hesitant patients may be encouraged to pursue this health need by pointing out to them the positive aspects of obtaining dentures: improved appearance, better nutrition, and reduced likelihood of infection. When dentures have been obtained, patience is required in learning to use them effectively.

Dentures require careful scrubbing, using a good denture brush, mild soap and water, salt, and sodium bicarbonate. The addition of a drop of household chlorine acts as a deodorant and gives a fresher taste. Most dentists recommend that dentures be removed at night, scrubbed, and allowed to soak in a proprietary cleaner. Sodium hypochlorite-phosphate (Mersene) has been shown to be most effective.

Pressure or irritation caused by dentures should be reported to the dentist, who can make the proper adjustment. Uncorrected pressure areas may cause lesions, which in turn may become malignant.

Many persons now prefer to have "immediate dentures." Usually, the back teeth are extracted first, which allows the tissues time to heal. Meanwhile, the artificial teeth are made and are ready for placement immediately after the front teeth have been extracted.

Partial dentures should not be left in place for prolonged periods without being removed for a good cleaning. They are held in place with metal clasps that encircle the teeth. These clasps can be spread: using gentle force with two index fingers, one side can be loosened, and then the other. When reapplied, the cleaned partial dentures usually can be pressed into place.

Nursing Considerations

Nursing activities related to orthodontal corrections, dental implantations and transplantations, extractions, and dentures should begin with an assessment of the information that the client and family possess. Nursing interventions include supplying needed information and correcting misinformation. These activities will permit realistic postprocedure expectations and cooperation in needed self-care activities. Self-care activities can be evaluated by questioning the patient or by having him demonstrate his abilities.

▷ Lesions of the Lips

Actinic Cheilitis. Actinic cheilitis results from the cumulative effect of exposure to sun radiation and may lead to squamous cell carcinoma. It is manifested by whitish hyperkeratosis, fissuring, and erythema. Treatment consists of protecting the lips with a good sunscreen ointment. In some instances, electrosurgery or cryosurgery may be required. Periodic checkups are mandatory to detect possible malignancy. Certain groups of people, such as farmers and very fair people, are especially susceptible to this problem.

Contact Dermatitis. Lipsticks, cosmetics, ointments to prevent chapping, and even toothpaste and chewing gum may be the source of allergens that cause erythema, vesiculation, burning, and itching of the lip. These conditions are treated by eliminating the suspected contactant, applying topical corticosteroid ointment, and using hypoallergenic cosmetics.

General Approach to Care

Lesions of the lips and mouth can have a direct effect on nutritional status. Sores that are painful can be aggravated by the ingestion of juices and spicy or rough foods. While the patient may not be hospitalized for lip or mouth sores, these people are frequently seen in out-patient settings, such as clinics or school health settings, and in in-patient settings in which the person has other major health problems.

▶ Nursing Assessment

An initial approach to the patient with lip or mouth lesions includes taking a nursing history concerning the length of time the lesions have existed, any known precipitating factors, methods of treatment used to date, known associates with similar problems, and a statement of the problem in the patient's words.

The nurse then inspects the lesions, noting their appearance, location, size, and drainage, if any.

▶ Planning and Nursing Interventions

Goals

General nursing goals for these patients are as follows:

1. To identify problem lip and mouth lesions and to arrange for appropriate medical treatment
2. To ameliorate the effects of existing conditions through the use of analgesics; proper hygiene; warm rinses; and soft, nonirritating foods
3. To teach patients how to avoid those situational variables that influence the development of future lesions or that aggravate existing lesions

The observations noted on assessment are clearly charted and also entered on the patient's care plan, along with those problem-solving activities designed to deal with them. A typical approach might be to apply cold soaks to the lips every 3 hours, provide bland liquids and foods, teach the patient how to clean his mouth regularly without irritating his lips, and provide analgesics as needed.

▶ Evaluation

Evaluation of the nursing interventions can be carried out through an assessment of pain relief and maintenance of adequate nutritional status. Since these nursing actions are supportive, as opposed to curative, measures, successful resolution of the lesions may not be an appropriate measure of their usefulness. Evaluation activities also include questions designed to identify whether the person knows how to avoid or deal with future problems of this sort.

▷ Mouth Conditions

Herpes Simplex Infection

The herpes simplex virus most commonly produces the familiar *herpes labialis* (cold sore, fever blister, or canker). The infection may take the form of an acute herpetic gingivostomatitis. The patient frequently experiences a burning sensation 24 to 48 hours before blisters appear. Small vesicles, single or clustered, may erupt on the lips, the tongue, the cheeks, and the pharynx. These soon rupture, forming sore, shallow ulcers that are covered with a gray membrane. Herpes infections appear often in association with other febrile infections, such as streptococcal pneumonia, meningococcic meningitis, and malaria. Some relief is experienced with the application of topical analgesics. Other common therapies include (1) applying spirits of camphor twice a day; (2) applying a moistened styptic stick to the vesicles several times a day; and (3) dusting the lesions with bismuthformic-iodide (BFI) antiseptic powder twice daily.

Some patients may associate herpes simplex with hearsay stories relating this herpes virus to cancer. Although herpes virus 2 has been associated with carcinoma of the cervix in women, there is no documented evidence to show the exact relationship between the two.

Gingivitis

Gingivitis (inflammation of the gums) is the most common disease of oral tissues. At first there is inflammation and slight swelling of the superficial gingivae and interdental papillae. Slight bleeding may occur and prompt the patient to refrain from adequately cleaning his teeth. Such neglect compounds the problem, in that food debris, bacterial plaque, and calculus (tartar) can result in chronic degenerative gingivitis, and, later, in periodontal disease. Good, conscientious mouth hygiene and periodic professional teeth-cleaning can prevent the problem.

Necrotizing Gingivitis (Vincent's Gingivitis, "Trench Mouth")

Necrotizing gingivitis is a pseudomembranous ulceration affecting the edges of the gums, the mucosa of the mouth, the tonsils, and the pharynx. It is thought to be caused by a combination of two organisms, a spirochete and a fusiform bacillus. Smears made from the ulcerations are found to be teeming with the characteristic organisms, and establish the diagnosis. However, the condition may also be due to poor oral hygiene, low tissue resistance, and infection produced by a complex of microorganisms.

The chief symptom is painful, bleeding gums. Swallowing and talking are also painful, especially when infection has spread to the tonsils and pharynx. There may be a mild fever and swelling of the lymph nodes in the neck.

Management.   Goals of nursing care here are similar to those general goals for patients with lip and mouth lesions and are directed toward controlling and treating the infection, reducing fetid breath, making the patient comfortable, and maintaining nutrition. The plan of care includes washing and irrigating the mouth hourly with fluids rich in free oxygen, such as dilute hydrogen peroxide or sodium perborate in a 2% solution, to combat the anaerobic spirochete. Procaine penicillin, given intramuscularly, or potassium phenoxymethyl penicillin (penicillin V), given orally, is effective. Definitive measures such as dental prophylaxis and gingival massage are postponed until the acute inflammation has subsided.

Food should be of liquid or soft consistency to reduce trauma to the gums. Highly seasoned or strongly acid foods should not be served; it is also desirable to avoid smoking and alcohol.

Adolescents are often afflicted with this problem because of poor eating habits, irregularity, and insufficient rest. Patient education is directed toward correcting mouth problems and emphasizing proper oral hygiene to prevent a recurrence.

White Lesions of the Mouth

White lesions of the mouth may be keratotic or nonkeratotic.

White Keratotic Lesions.   These lesions are elevated, have an uneven surface, and are firmly adherent and slow to change.

Focal Keratosis.   These lesions are white patches or plaques that do not fit a disease entity and seem to be caused by irritation. Treatment consists of eliminating the irritant, such as smoking, chewing tobacco, jagged teeth, malocclusions, and biting the cheek or lip. Biopsy may be necessary if the lesion persists.

Lichen Planus.   Lichen planus is a mucocutaneous disease recognized as white papules at the intersection of a network of interlacing lesions. Often the lesions are ulcerated and painful. If asymptomatic, reassurance may be all that is needed. If painful, the diet is limited to soft, bland foods. Small amounts of viscous lidocaine (Xylocaine viscous 2%) held in the mouth for 2 to 3 minutes may relieve soreness while eating. Direct application of triamcinolone acetonide (Kenalog in Orabase) after meals or at bedtime may promote healing. Corticosteroids given systemically or injected intralesionally have been effective. Periodic examinations of chronic lesions are necessary because of their malignancy potential.

White Nonkeratotic Lesions.   These lesions are due to exudative or ulcerative processes, are of short duration, and are fairly easy to remove.

Aphthous Stomatitis (Aphthous Ulcers, Canker Sores). Among the most common lesions of the mouth are recurrent aphthous ulcers (canker sores). Aphthous ulcers are shallow ulcers found in the mucous membrane of the mouth, most often on the inner side of the lips and cheeks, and in the sulcus between the lips and gums. However, they may appear anywhere in the mouth, including on the tongue. The lesions begin with a burning, tingling sensation and slight swelling of the mucous membrane, which soon becomes a shallow ulcer with a whitish center surrounded by a red border. These ulcers are especially painful when eating, and are particularly aggravated by acid or spicy foods. Since these ulcers are tender to pressure, any abrasion of or movement of the skin around the ulcer makes it painful to speak or move any of the facial muscles. The ulcers may be single or multiple, and they often tend to heal at one site and recur elsewhere. The sores may appear at any time in life; most often they begin in childhood or adolescence and may appear as frequently as once a month. In most cases, however, they do not occur more than once a year or so. These ulcers last only a short time—from 10 to 14 days—and eventually heal spontaneously, leaving no scar.

In spite of intense studies, no definite cause can be found for canker sores. An L-form of alpha hemolytic streptococcus has been proposed as the microbial cause. There seem to be definite predisposing factors, such as emotional or mental stress, related to their occurrence. In females, they seem to appear at the time of menstrual periods, and they occur much more frequently among women than men. Fatigue, change in a life situation, and anxiety are other predisposing factors.

Because these studies have uncovered no specific cause, there is no specific treatment for canker sores. Where anxiety is an obvious etiologic factor, tranquilizing drugs may be beneficial. A soft, bland diet may reduce pain. Various antibiotic and steroid preparations applied locally, or injected systemically, offer some relief. Fortunately, these ulcers eventually heal spontaneously in a relatively short time.

Oral Candidiasis (Moniliasis, Thrush). This condition produces white, cheesy plaques that can be rubbed off to leave an erythematous and, often, bleeding base. Predisposing factors may include diabetes mellitus, lymphoma, or other debilitating conditions; corticosteroids; and antibiotics. Treating the basic cause may improve the condition. In addition, nystatin (Mycostatin), taken orally or as an oral suspension, is effective. The suspension is a medicated fluid that should be swished about the mouth vigorously for at least 1 minute. If the condition becomes chronic, it is more difficult to treat and requires persistent attention to basic care.

▷ Disorders of the Salivary Glands

The goals of nursing care for patients with disorders of the salivary glands include the following:

1. To help detect disorders of the glands, such as infection, through history (*e.g.,* of pediatric outbreak of mumps) and through inspection and palpation of enlarged salivary glands (see Fig. 34-1 for location of glands).
2. To anticipate these disorders in clients who are especially susceptible (such as the elderly or the debilitated)
3. To provide supportive care and relief to those patients with symptoms caused by blockage of the glands (such as relief of elevated temperature and pain)

Acute Inflammation—Parotitis

The most common inflammation of the salivary glands is *parotitis* (inflammation of the parotid gland); however, infection can occur in the other glands as well. The essential lesion of mumps (epidemic parotitis) is an inflammation of the salivary gland (usually the parotid) and is primarily a pediatric communicable disease.

Elderly, acutely ill, and debilitated individuals whose salivary glands fail to secrete sufficiently because of general

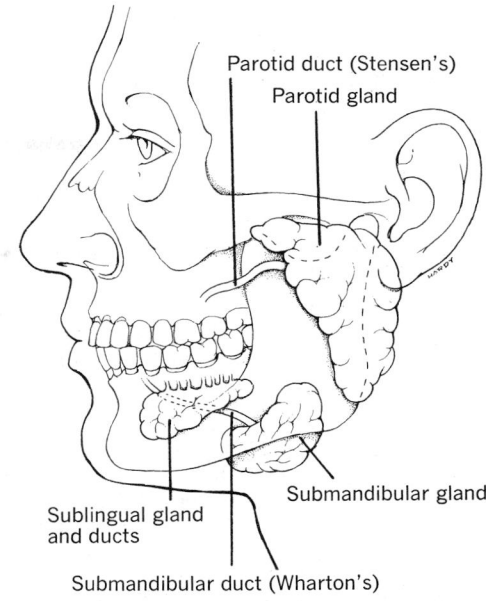

Figure 34-1. The salivary glands and their ducts. (From Chaffee EE and Greisheimer EM: Basic Physiology and Anatomy, 3rd ed. Philadelphia, JB Lippincott.)

dehydration often develop parotitis. The infecting organisms travel from the mouth through the salivary duct. Because older people tend to have parched mouths and do not chew solid foods adequately, they offer poor defense against invasion of the parotid ducts by pathogenic organisms.

The offending organism usually is the staphylococcus (except in mumps). The onset of this complication is sudden, with an exacerbation of the fever and of the symptoms of the primary condition. The gland swells and becomes tense and tender. Pain is felt in the ear, and there is interference with swallowing. The swelling increases rapidly, and the overlying skin soon becomes red and shiny.

Nursing Intervention. In order to prevent postoperative parotitis, patients are advised to have necessary dental work done before surgery. In addition, optimal patient preparation includes maintaining an adequate nutritional and fluid intake along with good mouth hygiene.

After surgery, having the patient chew gum or suck hard candy may prevent obstruction of the salivary gland ducts. At the onset of the swelling, an icebag may be applied over the affected gland, and chemotherapy may be instituted with penicillin or one of the sulfonamides. A suppurating gland may require incision and drainage.

Salivary Calculus (Sialolithiasis)

Salivary stones may develop in the submaxillary gland, following glandular infection or ductal stricture owing to trauma or inflammation. Sialograms (x-ray pictures taken with a radiopaque substance injected into the duct) may be required to show obstruction of the duct by stenosis. Salivary stones are composed mainly of calcium oxalate. If located within the gland, they are irregularly lobulated and vary in diameter from 3 mm to 30 mm. Stones in the duct are small and oval.

Calculi within the salivary gland cause no symptoms unless infection arises; but a calculus that obstructs the gland's duct causes sudden, local, and often colicky pain, which is suddenly relieved by a gush of saliva. This characteristic complaint can be elicited in a nursing history. Where this condition exists, the gland is swollen and quite tender, the stone itself often is palpable, and its shadow may be seen on roentgenograms. The calculus can be extracted fairly easily from the duct in the mouth; sometimes enlarging the orifice permits the stone to pass spontaneously. It may be necessary to remove the gland if there are repeated recurrences of symptoms and calculi in the gland itself.

Tumors of the Salivary Glands

Neoplasms of almost any type develop in salivary glands, but the majority of them are malignant. In 75% of all these patients, tumors develop in one parotid gland. The tumors remain small and quiescent for years, then suddenly begin to increase in size. Neoplasms are diagnosed on the basis of history and physical examination; tests such as needle biopsy are contraindicated. Encouraging results in detection of neoplasms have been reported with radiosialography (scanning with Tc-99m).

The best treatment of a parotid tumor is the early and complete excision of the mass. Fortunately, most of these growths occur superficially, rather than in the deep retromandibular lobe. Partial excision of the gland, along with all of the tumor, combined with careful dissection to preserve the vulnerable facial (7th) nerve, is the common procedure. For more involved tumors, it may be necessary to sacrifice the nerve when a parotidectomy is done. If the tumor is malignant or mixed, irradiation therapy follows surgery. Local recurrences are common; the recurrent growth usually is more malignant than the original one.

In the postoperative period, the nurse should be aware that the patient may have some facial paralysis (if the nerve was not excised), owing to tissue trauma and edema. This will gradually subside.

▷ Fracture of the Mandible, Jaw Repositioning or Reconstruction

Fractures of the mandible may consist of simple fractures without displacement, resulting from a blow on the chin. They may also be the result of planned surgical intervention, as in the correction of long or short jaw syndrome, or they may be very complicated, involving loss of tissue and bone from a severe accident. Mandibular fractures are usually closed fractures. In simple fractures, without loss of teeth, the lower jaw is immobilized by wiring it to the upper jaw. The wires are placed around the teeth in both the upper and lower jaw, on each side of the fracture line. The lower jaw is held tight against the upper jaw by cross-wires or rubber bands placed around the wires about the teeth. This simple form of fixation is used when there are teeth that can be used in the wire fixation. In other cases, in which teeth are missing or bone displacement has occurred, various other forms of fixation can be used. Some of these, such as metal arch bars, are applied in the mouth; other methods are more involved, requiring pins inserted into the bone, with fixation to a plaster head piece. The nursing problem then is one of treating a fracture in the mouth in a patient who cannot open his jaws.

▶ Planning and Implementation

Goals

The goals of nursing care for a patient with a fractured jaw can be divided into short-term and long-term goals.

Short-term Preoperative Goals
1. To prepare the patient psychologically, if possible, for the surgical procedure designed to immobilize his jaw, through a brief explanation of the purpose of the surgery, stressing that breathing and swallowing will be possible postoperatively
2. To stabilize the patient with possible multiple trauma by maintaining the airway, monitoring vital signs, and supporting circulation

Short-term Postoperative Goals
1. To maintain an open airway
2. To maintain jaw immobilization
3. To provide assurance regarding the patient's ability to breathe and swallow
4. To maintain adequate oral hygiene
5. To provide adequate nutrition

Nursing Interventions

Immediately following surgery, the patient should be placed on his side, with his head slightly elevated (Fig. 34-2). The nasogastric suction tube inserted during surgery is connected to low-pressure suction; this removes stomach contents and lessens the danger of aspiration. Antiemetic drugs are also administered. Prevention of vomiting is most desirable. If the patient does vomit, and the wires are cut, surgery and rewiring have to be repeated later. A plier-type of wire cutter (or scissors, if rubber bands are used) should be taped to the head of the bed for emergency use.

Clearing of the nasopharyngeal area can be done with a small catheter inserted through the nasal orifice. The oral cavity can be aspirated by first inserting a tongue blade to move the cheek away from the teeth; the catheter is inserted in an area where teeth are not in close position or where a tooth is missing, or in the space behind the third molar.

Constant attention by the nurse in the postsurgery recovery time is necessary. As the patient regains consciousness, he needs to be reminded again that his jaw is wired but that he can breathe and swallow. As he emerges from anesthesia, his head may be elevated. If an extraoral appliance is used to immobilize the mandible, the patient needs instruction on positioning himself so that he does not roll onto the device. To prevent dry and cracking lips, a lubricant is applied.

Careful attention to the hygiene of the mouth must be insisted upon, using warm alkaline mouthwashes or oxygenating rinses at least every 2 hours, and after each feeding. In addition, the mouth should be inspected at least once or twice daily to ensure thorough cleansing. A flashlight and a tongue blade to retract the cheeks are essential equipment. If permissible, a small, soft toothbrush can be used carefully.

The diet must necessarily be liquid, but sufficient caloric and fluid intake can be given easily to these patients. They can be fed through a straw without much difficulty, and soft foods can generally be given with a spoon. Water should be given after each liquid feeding, followed by a mouthwash.

Usually, the patient is out of bed the first postoperative day, and the length of time for ambulation is gradually increased each day.

▶ Evaluation

Short-term Goals. These evaluation activities must center around the maintenance of an adequate airway and continuance of psychological support. The patient is encouraged to participate as soon as possible in oral hygiene and feeding activities. In this way the nurse can assess the patient's need for further instruction in these important self-care activities.

Long-term Goals (Postoperative and Postdischarge). Long-term nursing goals center around the maintenance of proper jaw fixation, oral hygiene, and adequate nutrition. The patient must assume the primary responsibility for these activities; therefore, adequate predischarge teaching must be done. Because this patient is in the hospital post surgery for a relatively short period of time, teaching should consist both of oral instruction and of printed material that the patient can review at home.

Patient Education. Depending on conditions, including age and the patient's stability, most patients are able to leave the hospital before the wiring is removed. Of prime importance is the proper functioning of the fixation appliance. To ensure this, the patient has to see his physician at certain intervals. At these examinations, the patient's mouth and device are checked for cleanliness, and his general nutritional condition is assessed. This means that he needs to know how to give himself mouth care, how to feed himself, and what kinds of foods to take. If there are any sites of irritation, these need to be reported.

▷ Precancerous Lesions

Leukoplakia buccalis (also called "smoker's patch") and the related *keratosis labialis* are seen in middle-aged adults, more than 80% of whom are men. These conditions are characterized in the early stages by the appearance of one or two small, thin, often crinkled, pearly patches on the mucous membrane of the tongue, the mouth, or both, owing to keratinization of the mucosa and sclerosis of its underlying tissue (Fig. 34-3). In time, most of the tongue and the mouth may become covered by a creamy, white, thick, fissured or papillomatous mucous membrane that desqua-

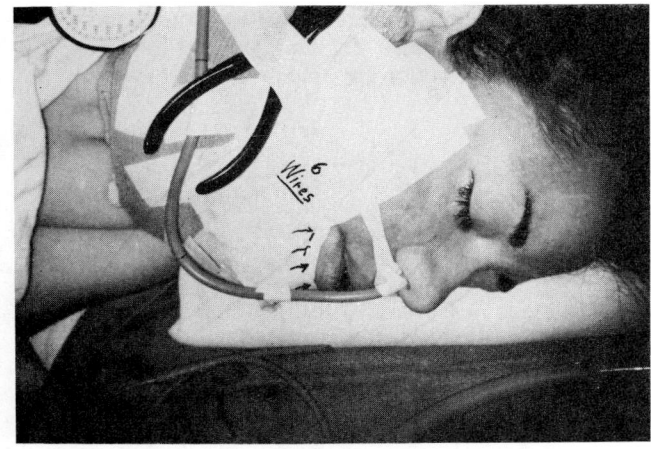

Figure 34-2. This patient, shown in the lateral position in the recovery room, had surgery for mandibular prognathism, necessitating intermaxillary fixation. Note the wire cutter attached to the collar bandage, the bandage marked with the location and number of intermaxillary wires, the Levin tube in place, and a nasopharyngeal tube and suction catheter readily available. Also note the manometer available to ascertain blood pressure. (Marsh Robinson, D.D.S., M.D.)

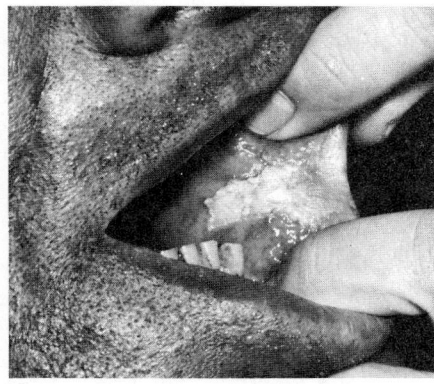

Figure 34-3. Leukoplakia. Note the white patches above and to the right of the teeth.

mates occasionally, leaving a beefy-red base. This condition results from chronic irritation by carious, infected, or poorly repaired teeth; by tobacco; and by highly spiced foods. It will disappear in time after cessation of smoking. Occasionally, it is due to syphilis. Not infrequently, cancers start in the keratinized patches. Detection of these patches through a nursing history and examination is a prime nursing responsibility in this situation.

▷ Oral Cancer

Cancer in the oral cavity, which may occur in any part of the mouth, including the pharynx, is highly curable, if discovered early. However, it accounts for 3% of all cancer deaths in this country. Males are afflicted three and a half times more than females. Of the 8000 oral cancer deaths annually, the distribution by site is estimated as follows:

Lips	3%
Tongue	24%
Salivary gland	8%
Floor of mouth	6%
Other and unspecified sites in mouth	15%
Pharynx	44%

Squamous cell (epidermoid) carcinoma constitutes over 90% of all mouth cancer. The next most common type, adenocarcinoma, arises from the submucous glands. The third grouping includes malignancy of the jaw bone. The cure rate for these cancers is below 30%. However, most oral cancers can be prevented by good dental care and avoidance of smoking. In tobacco chewers, the mucous membrane of the cheek is the most common site of cancer. A jagged tooth and poor dental hygiene may be the cause. Betel and areca nut, mixed with tobacco, used widely for chewing in South India, is believed to be related to that country's high incidence of oral cancer (40% of all cancers).

General Management

Oral cancers are generally treated surgically or with a combination of surgery and radiation. The treatment program is quite rigorous and requires both physical support of the patient and psychological support of the patient and his family. In addition to dealing with the demands of treatment, the patient and his family are dealing with a diagnosis that produces fear that is frequently out of proportion to the actual prognosis. Teaching and other intervention efforts by the nurse must take this into account.

Nursing Goals and Interventions

The general nursing goals for these patients can be divided into three phases: the detection and referral phase, the treatment phase, and the active rehabilitation phase.

Assessment and Referral. The principle nursing activities in this phase include a careful nursing history to detect symptoms requiring medical evaluation. Complaints of sores; lumps; pain in the mouth; stiffness in the neck; and difficulty with swallowing, chewing, or speaking require attention. In addition, the nurse carefully inspects the mouth for sores or other signs of irritation. The nurse also realizes that clients with a history of moderate to heavy drinking or of smoking over a 20-year period, or with poor dental hygiene are at risk for oral cancer. Many nurses participate in community education projects designed to bring this information to clients and to facilitate referral for adequate medical therapy.

Management. The goals in this phase are to prepare the patient physically and psychologically for surgical and perhaps radiation therapy. Whether the intended treatment is curative or palliative will influence the patient's adjustment and the kind of support given. Reassurance and patient education regarding the diagnostic tests and the surgical procedure are major ways of preparing the patient during the treatment phase.

Specific information regarding perioperative care should be given, including information about pain relief, oral hygiene measures, care of drains, nutrition, optimal activity levels, and methods of communication. The patient who knows what to expect postoperatively may be more cooperative. However, the anxious patient can be easily overwhelmed with too much or too specific information. Instruction and discussion by the nurse during this phase is generally given to the patient while family members are present. In this way, clarification and reassurance can be reinforced by informed family members who are the patient's usual source of support.

Active Rehabilitation. This phase begins with an assessment of the physical and emotional deficits caused by the illness or the treatment. Active rehabilitation measures are begun by the nurse during the perioperative period. The goal of these efforts is to help the patient regain as much function as possible, given the limitations of the disease, the treatment, or the individual's capacity. Most nursing intervention measures have some rehabilitative aspect, but some major rehabilitative measures include efforts toward maintaining adequate nutrition and hydration, speech rehabilitation, psychological adjustment to alterations in body image, resocialization activities, and possibly adjustment to further palliative measures.

Cancer of the Lip and Tongue

Cancer of the Lip

This tumor, usually called an epithelioma, occurs most frequently as a chronic ulcer on the lower lip in men. Predisposing factors may be chronic irritation of a warm pipe stem or prolonged exposure to the sun and wind. More significant, however, is the tendency for leukoplakia to progress to an epidermoid lip cancer. A typical lesion is a painless indurated ulcer with raised edges. Any wart or ulcer of the lip that does not heal in 3 weeks should be biopsied.

Small lesions usually are excised liberally; larger lesions involving more than one third of the lip may be treated best by radiotherapy, because of superior cosmetic results. The choice depends on the extent of the lesion, the skill of the surgeon or radiologist, and what is necessary to cure the patient while preserving the best appearance. Fortunately, only about 10% to 15% of lip cancers metastasize. When lymph nodes appear to be involved, a neck dissection is indicated.

Cancer of the Tongue

The tongue is a muscular and highly vascular organ with abundant lymphatic drainage. If cancer of the tongue develops, the constant expansion and contraction of the tongue can easily force small tumor cells into the lymphatic channels and eventually into the regional lymph nodes, where they become embedded. This cancer is most common in men in their later decades of life.

Clinical Manifestations. The early stage of cancer of the anterior undersurface of the lateral aspects of the tongue is usually detected as a small ulcer that has not healed in 3 weeks or as an area of thickening. After several months, the cancer invades the underlying muscle body of the tongue. Pain or soreness of the tongue on eating hot or highly seasoned foods, and limitation of motion, are noticeable. As the growth spreads to neighboring structures, other symptoms develop, such as excessive salivation, slurred speech, blood-tinged sputum, trismus, and pain on swallowing liquids. If untreated, the patient is unable to swallow, and earache, faceache, and toothache become almost constant. Unable to eat or sleep, the patient finally succumbs to hemorrhage (lingual artery), cervical lymph node metastasis, or general debilitation.

Management.   Radiation and surgery are the treatments of choice. Preoperative irradiation is often followed by surgery 4 to 6 weeks later. Enlargement of lymph nodes indicates metastases, necessitating more extensive surgical dissection, combined with radium and x-ray therapy. When the tongue is involved, it is often necessary to perform a *hemiglossectomy* (removal of a lateral segment of the tongue).

Malignancy at the base of the tongue (posterior) produces less obvious symptoms: slight dysphagia, sore throat, salivation, and some blood-tinged sputum. This is a difficult site for effective irradiation, and because of the mutilating effects of total glossectomy, and the likelihood of metastasis, the cure rate of posterior tongue cancer is very low. (For nursing management, see Cancer of the Mouth.)

Cancer of the Mouth

Clinical Manifestations.   Because the mouth is such an accessible and observable site, more intensive professional and patient education programs are needed for early detection of mouth lesions. Any patient with a white, patchy area; sore spot; or ulceration of lips, gums, or mouth that fails to heal in 3 weeks should be urged to see a physician.

Most oral cancers cause no symptoms in the early stages. Often the individual feels a roughened area with his tongue. Since pain is often one of the last symptoms to appear, a painless condition should not prevent further professional examination; swelling, numbness, or loss of feeling in any part of the mouth may also be symptoms.

The patient's first complaint may be the appearance of a lump in the neck, indicating metastatic spread. Pain usually occurs when there is secondary infection or tumor invasion of adjacent tissues. Occasionally, the first complaints are difficulty in chewing, swallowing, or speaking.

Assessment.   Oral exfoliative cytology is a means of screening intraoral lesions. As the first step in the screening process, the patient's mouth is examined carefully. Then the tongue is grasped with a 4 × 4 gauze square and moved gently to expose the suspicious area. With a moistened tongue blade, the lesion is then scraped. If a hyperkeratotic lesion is present, the surface keratin is scraped off so that the deeper epithelial cells are available for the specimen, since these cells are usually involved in early malignant change. The cells are smeared on a glass slide, immersed carefully in alcohol, and sent to the laboratory for cytologic examination.

Adequate examination of the oral cavity requires good lighting, including a head mirror. The use of a wooden tongue blade is helpful in retracting the cheek and holding back the tongue. A finger cot or rubber glove is helpful to the examiner in palpation (see p. 57). Look for white areas (leukoplakia), fissures, ulcers, red areas (erythroplakia), masses, or unusual pigmentation. Biopsy is essential for definitive diagnosis. Exfoliative cytology is an adjunct to biopsy, as are staining techniques (*e.g.,* toluidine blue test).

Management.   Management varies with the nature of the lesion and preference of the physician. Electrocoagulation, radiotherapy, resectional surgery, or combinations of therapy are effective. In more extensive ablative procedures it may be necessary to graft tissue by flap or pedicle grafts (see p. 1189). For even more advanced lesions involving the tongue, mandible, larynx, and neck, the trend is away from extremely radical surgery (which only ends in cosmetic and functional disaster) and toward combining chemotherapy and radiation.

Surgical Intervention.   General preparation for surgery is similar to that described on page 355. Depending on the nature of the operation, the anesthesia may be local or general. The surgery may be confined to the lip, may involve only the tongue, or may include resection of facial tissue and the mandible, with possible dental extraction. If there is metastasis to the lymph nodes of the neck, neck dissection may be necessary.

Postoperative Nursing Interventions

Patent Airway.   In the immediate postoperative period, a priority nursing intervention is to maintain a patent airway. To do this, the patient is placed in a supine position, with the head turned to the side, or in the lateral position, with special emphasis on facilitating drainage from the mouth. If suctioning is required, precautions are necessary to avoid injury to the suture line and sensitive tissues, such as exist in a hemiglossectomy. Perhaps a dental suction tip may be required until such time as the patient is able to take care of his own secretions.

Mouth Hygiene.   To reduce the number of bacteria and to keep the mouth clean are important objectives before, as well as after, surgery or radiation. If the patient is conscious and able to help himself, the nurse can teach him effective mouth care. He may need reminding and proper supplies, including an effective toothbrush or gauze-padded applicator stick, as well as oxygen-releasing and antimicrobial mouth-rinsing solutions. If the patient is a mouth-breather, he needs more mouth attention than the average person. Lanolin applied to dry and cracking lips is also soothing.

Dentures must be removed frequently and cleaned. Before they are replaced, the mouth also should be cleaned. Frequently, care is given to the teeth, but the "furred" or coated tongue is neglected, resulting in bad breath.

Mouth irrigations are given to keep the mouth clean, provide comfort, and assist in the healing process. The prescribed solutions may be normal saline, diluted hydrogen peroxide, sodium bicarbonate solution, or alkaline mouthwash. Gentle lavaging with a catheter inserted between the cheek and teeth loosens mucus and is refreshing. A power spray has the advantage of getting the solution into inaccessible areas.

In the unconscious patient, the nurse is wholly responsible for maintaining good mouth hygiene. The use of a special mouth tray with all necessary applicator sticks, padded tongue depressors, mouthwashes, lubricants, and so forth, encourages frequent mouth attention.

Dry Mouth (Xerostomia) or Excessive Salivation. Dryness of the mouth is a frequent sequela of oral cancer, particularly when the salivary glands have been exposed to radiation or major surgery. It also is noted in patients who are receiving psychopharmacologic agents or in those who are unable to close the mouth, and who become mouth-breathers.

To minimize this problem, the patient is advised to avoid dry, bulky, and irritating foods and fluids as well as alcohol and tobacco. He should also be encouraged to increase his intake of fluids, if not contraindicated. Some degree of relief is obtained through the lubricating action of such substances as petrolatum, mineral oil, and glycerin (cough drops with glycerin). Salivary flow can be stimulated with sugar-free lemon lozenges or sugar-free chewing gum. In a dry environment, the use of humidifiers may also help.

Drooling or excessive salivation may be an annoying problem to the patient in the pre- or post-operative period. The measures taken to control drooling depend on the cause, severity, and relative permanence of the dysfunction. If the problem is moderate to severe but temporary, as may be the case following surgery, mechanical suction devices used with a soft catheter are effective. If drooling is mild, management may be obtained by training the patient to swallow more frequently, by providing emotional reassurance and support, and by using anticholinergic agents (antisialogogues), such as those containing atropine or belladonna (Banthine, Robinul). For more severe drooling, it may be necessary to resort to plastic reconstruction of the oral structures.

Mouth wipes, as well as a paper bag attached to the bed or the bedside stand to receive soiled tissues, always should be on hand. An effective way of holding dressings of the mouth or the lower jaw in place is by the use of a face mask. The strings can be tied at the top of the head.

To combat odors, the physician may prescribe oxidizing agents for a mouthwash, such as potassium permanganate 1:10,000, hydrogen peroxide in half strength, sodium perborate, and so forth. In extensive mouth sores, a power spray can clean wounds effectively, and necrotic tissue can be removed more easily.

Nutritional Needs. The general physical condition of a person often is reflected in his mouth. Therefore, good nutritional levels must be maintained. If the breath has a foul odor, the nurse must encourage and assist the patient with his oral hygiene before and after each feeding. A bad taste in the mouth spoils the taste of food and limits the intake of nourishment.

Individuals with mouth lesions may have feeding problems. The use of a plastic straw or a teaspoon may be effective. The type of feeders employed with children may be of use. Food should be soft or liquid, and nonirritating, that is, not too hot or too cold, and not highly seasoned. It should be served attractively, to tempt the patient to take it. Small, frequent feedings are more desirable than large, less frequent ones. The desires as well as the nutritional needs of the patient should be taken into consideration. If

he is not able to take anything by mouth, it may be necessary to feed him parenterally to maintain fluid and electrolyte balance and to prevent starvation and negative nitrogen balance. Such feeding may be by way of parenteral hyperalimentation (see p. 780), a lateral pharyngostomy stab wound (to prevent nasal discomfort), or nasogastric intubation. The position of the tube can be checked by injecting slowly, drop by drop, 1 ml or 2 ml of saline. If the tube is in the esophagus, as it should be, the patient should have no reaction. If it is in the trachea, he will cough violently. The care of this tube is similar to that of a gastrostomy tube (see p. 775). As the patient progresses to the point where he can insert his own feeding catheter, he should be given time, privacy, assistance, and encouragement. Perhaps a mirror will help.

Psychosocial Concerns. The patient with a mouth or facial problem requires patience and understanding. Quite naturally, he tends to withdraw from people, is self-conscious about mouth odors, and is sensitive about his appearance. The nurse is challenged to communicate with him, encourage his expression of fears and concerns, and offer him support and explanations as necessary. The immediate family needs to be aware of their supporting role and, in turn, should be informed of the plan of therapy for the patient and urged to participate in the plan of care.

Particular areas of patient concern are fear of pain; drooling; and difficulty in communicating, feeding, and swallowing. In addition, he may express a strong desire for solitude and may be self-conscious about his appearance. (The need to remove, temporarily, any large mirrors in the room should be considered by the nurse.) The results of surgery or radiation concern him, especially the fear of disfigurement; if the resection is extensive, the possibility of prosthetics (fitting an artificial part) may be explained.

Environmental Considerations. A therapeutic environment must be maintained by good room ventilation, particularly with the patient who has a malodorous cancer lesion. A room deodorant may be advisable.

Speech Rehabilitation. Surgery for mouth cancer often interferes with speech. Providing the patient with a pad of paper and a pencil or "magic slate," so that he can express his needs and thoughts, may make a tremendous difference in his depressed condition. Often these patients are reluctant to associate with other patients, and prefer to be alone. If there are two or more patients with a similar condition, they can help each other. It is easier for them, and for others, if they have their meals apart from other patients.

The patient's family and friends should be encouraged to visit so that he is aware that others care about him. He can be helped to care for his appearance. With speech training and adjustment to a prosthesis, he will become increasingly aware that the future holds promise for him.

Radium. If radium implants are used, the usual radium precautions are observed. When radium needles are implanted, a thread is attached to each needle. The patient should know upon waking from surgery that these needles will be present and that they are not to be removed. Mouth care in this instance can be given with a power spray. Radium may be implanted in a moulage (molded dental compound), which may be applied to some part of the mouth for a specific length of time. It is usually permissible to remove the mold for meals and at night. When it is reinserted, it is important for the nurse to note that it is in its proper position. (For care of radium, see p. 1059.)

Convalescent and Extended Care in the Home. The posthospital objectives of patient care are similar to those in the hospital. The individual who is recovering from treatment of a mouth condition needs to breathe, to secure nourishment, to avoid infection, and to be alert for adverse signs. The patient, members of his family or the person responsible for his home care, the nurse, and whoever else may be involved, such as a speech therapist, dietitian, psychologist, and so forth, need to prepare an individualized plan. If suctioning the mouth or a tracheostomy tube is required, it is important to determine what equipment is needed and how

to use it, as well as where it can be obtained. Consideration should be given to the humidification and aeration of the room, as well as to measures to control odors. How to prepare foods that are nutritious, properly seasoned, and of the right temperature can be explained. Perhaps it may be more feasible to use commercial baby food than to prepare liquid and soft diets in a blender. The use and care of prostheses must be understood. The importance of cleanliness with dressings and mouth care is reviewed. The person caring for the patient needs to know the signs of obstruction, hemorrhage, infection, depression, and withdrawal, as well as what to do about these problems. Follow-up visits to the clinic or physician are important, to determine progression or regression and to receive any modifications in medication or general care.

Chart 34-1
Nursing Management of the Patient With Oral Cancer

Goals, principles, and interventions

Preoperative Care

A. To provide psychosocial support to the patient with mouth cancer:
   1. Recognize that the patient is unusually concerned about appearance and possible disfigurement following surgery.
   2. Respect his feelings, accept him as a person, and support him as he faces his selected treatment.
   3. Encourage family support; explain that the patient needs encouragement and understanding.
   4. Anticipate the patient's concerns about cancer, effectiveness of treatment, and likelihood of cancer spread.

B. To promote optimum cleanliness of the involved area, in order to minimize postoperative complications owing to infection:
   1. Solicit patient's participation in conscientious mouth hygiene.
   2. Provide materials suitable to the condition; if a soft-bristled toothbrush cannot be used, because "it hurts," suggest a turkish washcloth wrapped around a finger.
   3. Utilize Water-pik or a power spray to loosen adhering particles in the mouth.
   4. Select mouth rinses that are effective, noninjurious, and soothing; some may be too stringent, whereas half-strength hydrogen peroxide may be more bland.
   5. Use oxidizing mouth rinses if the bubbling action can assist in removing necrotic material.
   6. Clean mouth before cleaned dentures are replaced.

C. To promote optimum nutritional condition:
   1. Encourage adequate intake of food and fluids; if anorexia is noted, try to overcome it by serving attractive, small servings frequently.
   2. Provide an environment conducive to relaxation during mealtime.
   3. Supplement the diet with vitamins (particularly vitamin C, to assist in wound healing) and other dietary requirements as needed by the particular patient.
   4. Avoid irritating foods or beverages: too hot, too cold, too bitter, too rough.

D. To prepare patient physically and psychologically for the treatment and its possible after-effects:
   1. If the treatment is radiation, explain what form. *Example:* cobalt exposure, moulage implant, radium needle insertion.
   2. Answer questions regarding effects of radiation. *Example:* loss of hair, visitors permitted during treatment, effect on sterility, skin irritation.
   3. If surgery is the mode of treatment, check with physician as to anticipated surgery and determine what information has been given to the patient. Support this therapeutic plan.
   4. Acquaint patient with what to expect after the operation.
   5. Teach him how he can help himself and those caring for him:
      a. Anticipate voice and communication problems: use of magic slate and other means of communication.
      b. Types of dressings and drainage equipment
      c. How pain can be relieved
      d. How long he will be in the recovery room
      e. Where his family will be

(continued)

Chart 34-1
Nursing Management of the Patient With Oral Cancer (continued)

Postoperative Management

A. To avoid respiratory and circulatory complications:
  1. Maintain a functioning airway by placing patient in a supine position with head turned to side (or lateral position with facilitation of drainage from mouth).
  2. Suction carefully to avoid injury to freshly sutured areas.
  3. Initiate conscientious monitoring of vital signs and patient responses.
  4. Anticipate physical activity on emergence from anesthesia and be prepared to protect patient and operative site.
     a. Use sedation, as judgment dictates.
     b. Prevent patient's hands from pulling out tubes.
     c. Quietly explain where he is and what he can or cannot do.

B. To provide relief from incisional pain:
  1. Administer analgesics and narcotics as prescribed.
  2. Schedule rest periods between necessary activities.
  3. Provide reassurance and supportive care.

C. To maintain cleanliness of mouth during healing phases:
  1. Practice those oral hygienic measures used prior to treatment.
  2. Apply lubricant to dry lips.
  3. Provide increased humidity with humidifier, if environment is dry.
  4. Increase fluid intake, if dry mouth (xerostomia) is a problem.
  5. Suction for drooling or make a gauze wick, which can be placed in the corner of patient's mouth to direct excessive salivation to an emesis basin.
  6. Practice asepsis in changing dressings; be gentle, and remember that the patient can see your facial expressions.

D. To provide adequate nutrition for systemic needs and wound healing:
  1. Utilize parenteral or nasogastric tube feedings as recommended.

  2. Maintain proper fluid intake; monitor fluid output.
  3. Encourage range of motion and other exercises, so that appetite is enhanced and body circulation is stimulated.
  4. Offer small, attractive servings when patient begins oral feedings.
  5. Promote a pleasant environment for eating: radio, clean surroundings, conversation, and perhaps the presence of other similar patients.

E. To encourage optimism by a carefully planned psychosocial program:
  1. Prepare spouse or family for their role in helping the patient.
  2. Stress the positive, and compliment the patient on each step of progress.
  3. Involve the patient in his own care; gradually increase this activity until he can use a mirror and care for himself.
  4. Answer his queries honestly; encourage his questions.

F. To prepare patient for convalescence (speech rehabilitation, extended care, and use of a prosthesis):
  1. Explain the objectives of convalescent care:
     a. Maintain nutrition.
     b. Be fastidious with cleanliness.
     c. Emphasize positive accomplishments.
     d. Develop hobbylike activities.
     e. Encourage seeing friends.
     f. Look forward to getting back to usual work.
     g. Be aware of signs of complications and what to do about them.
     h. Keep follow-up appointments.
  2. Learn how to use and maintain a prosthesis.
  3. Practice the art of communication if speech has been disturbed.
  4. Recognize limitations and how to adjust by using alternative measures.
  5. Return to the physician for annual or semiannual checkups.

Over 90% of recurrences will appear within the first 18 months; therefore, meticulous inspection by the physician every 4 to 6 weeks is essential. Early detection of local recurrences or metastasis, followed by aggressive treatment, can cure as many as 50% of these patients. Follow-up visits become less frequent after 2 years but must be continued for life, because of the frequency of other primary carcinomas. One important part of continuing care is the elimination of alcohol consumption and smoking.

Palliative Patient Care.   Because of further extension of a malignancy by metastasis and necrosis, it may not be possible medically to halt the spread of disease. All efforts are then directed toward the comfort measures—physical, psychological, and spiritual. With the family's help this may be continued in the hospital, a nursing home, a hospice setting, or the patient's own home.

Evaluation

The success of some nursing interventions must be repeatedly evaluated in the immediate postoperative period. These include activities directed toward the maintenance of an open airway, proper suctioning, oral hygiene, pain relief, care of drains, psychological reassurance, and adequate communication. As the patient is able, he is gradually included in care activities. This will provide him an opportunity to learn self-care activities and a period of time to gain confidence in his self-care skills. In addition, family members are encouraged to participate in the patient's care.

Long-term evaluation of nursing interventions can occur when the patient returns for follow-up care. Problems of self-care in the home setting, or difficulty readjusting postsurgically, can be evaluated by the community nurse. Postdischarge plans for this patient are carefully coordinated with the patient and members of the health care team.

▷ Radical Neck Dissection

Malignancies of the head and neck, including cancers of the lips, tongue, gums, palate, tonsils, and of the mucosa of the mouth, pharynx, and larynx, may be treated early by surgery, irradiation, or chemotherapy, with good results. These cancers (stages I and II) are in an area that can be easily seen, making early diagnosis and treatment possible. Most observers agree that such patients do not die from recurrence at the site of the primary growth, but rather from metastasis to the cervical lymph nodes in the neck, which often takes place by way of the lymphatics before the primary lesion has been treated. Only the nodes on one side of the neck are involved, unless the tumor is located at or near the midline, in which case the nodes of both sides of the neck may contain metastatic tumors.

Because radiation does not by itself give good results in controlling the metastatic cancer in the lymph nodes in the neck, an operation called a "radical neck dissection" is performed.

> *Functional neck dissection* is a relatively new approach in which there is complete dissection of the lateral cervical space and the major cervical lymphatics, while at the same time preserving the marginal mandibular and greater auricular nerves, internal jugular vein, carotid artery, and vagus and sympathetic nerves, as well as the phrenic nerve and brachial plexus. Obviously, this approach appears a reasonable alternative to radical radiotherapy and is a preferred alternative to traditional neck dissection in the control of regional metastasis when neck disease is either occult or still confined to mobile lymph nodes.

A *radical neck dissection* involves removal of all the tissue under the skin, from the ramus of the jaw down to the clavicle, and from the midline back to the angle of the jaw, in one mass. This includes removing the sternocleidomastoid muscle and other smaller muscles, as well as the jugular vein in the neck, because the lymphatic nodes are found widely distributed throughout these tissues (Fig. 34-4A). For stages III and IV (more advanced malignancy) a combination of treatment modalities may be used.

During or after the procedure a tracheostomy is often performed. Because there may be profuse drainage of serum and lymph after such an extensive procedure, drainage tubes or portable wound suction are often used in the wound (Fig. 34-4B).

▶ Planning and Implementation

Goals

The nursing goals for patients requiring radical neck dissection include both physical and psychological preparation for major surgery. In addition to the impending physical rigors of this surgery, this patient is aware that his malignancy includes metastasis to his cervical nodes. This information is bound to cause concern and anxiety regarding the postsurgical outcome.

Nursing Interventions

Preoperatively, the principal nursing intervention activities include providing information, assessing coping mechanisms, providing psychological support, and developing initial rapport.

Before the operation, the patient should be informed about the impending surgery, what is to be done in the operating room (amplification of surgeon's explanation) and what the postoperative period will be like. At the same time, the patient can be given an opportunity to express concerns about the upcoming surgery. During this exchange, the nurse has an opportunity to assess the patient's coping abilities, encourage questions, and develop a plan for offering assistance. A sense of mutual understanding and rapport will make the postoperative experience less troublesome for the patient. After the operation, any expressions of concern on the patient's part can guide the nurse in providing additional support. These intervention activities deliberately include supportive family members.

The general postoperative nursing intervention activities are similar to those described on pages 384–393 for the patient who has had extensive neck surgery and therefore may have problems with breathing and swallowing. The specific postoperative physical nursing interventions for this patient include maintenance of a patent airway and continuous assessment of respiratory status; wound care and attention to dressings, including careful observation for hemorrhage; and management of oral hygiene and nutritional needs.

Patent Airway. After the endotracheal tube or airway has been removed and the effects of the anesthesia have worn off, the patient may be placed in a Fowler's position to facilitate breathing and promote comfort. This position also increases lymphatic and venous drainage, facilitates swallowing, and decreases venous pressure on the skin flaps.

Signs of respiratory distress, such as dyspnea, cyanosis, and changes in vital signs, must be watched for, since they may suggest edema, throat irritation from the endotracheal tube, hemorrhage, or inadequate drainage. Temperature is usually taken rectally.

In the immediate postoperative period, the nurse may be able to detect the presence of stridor (coarse, high-pitched sound on inspiration) by listening frequently at the trachea with a stethoscope. In this situation, the physician should be summoned.

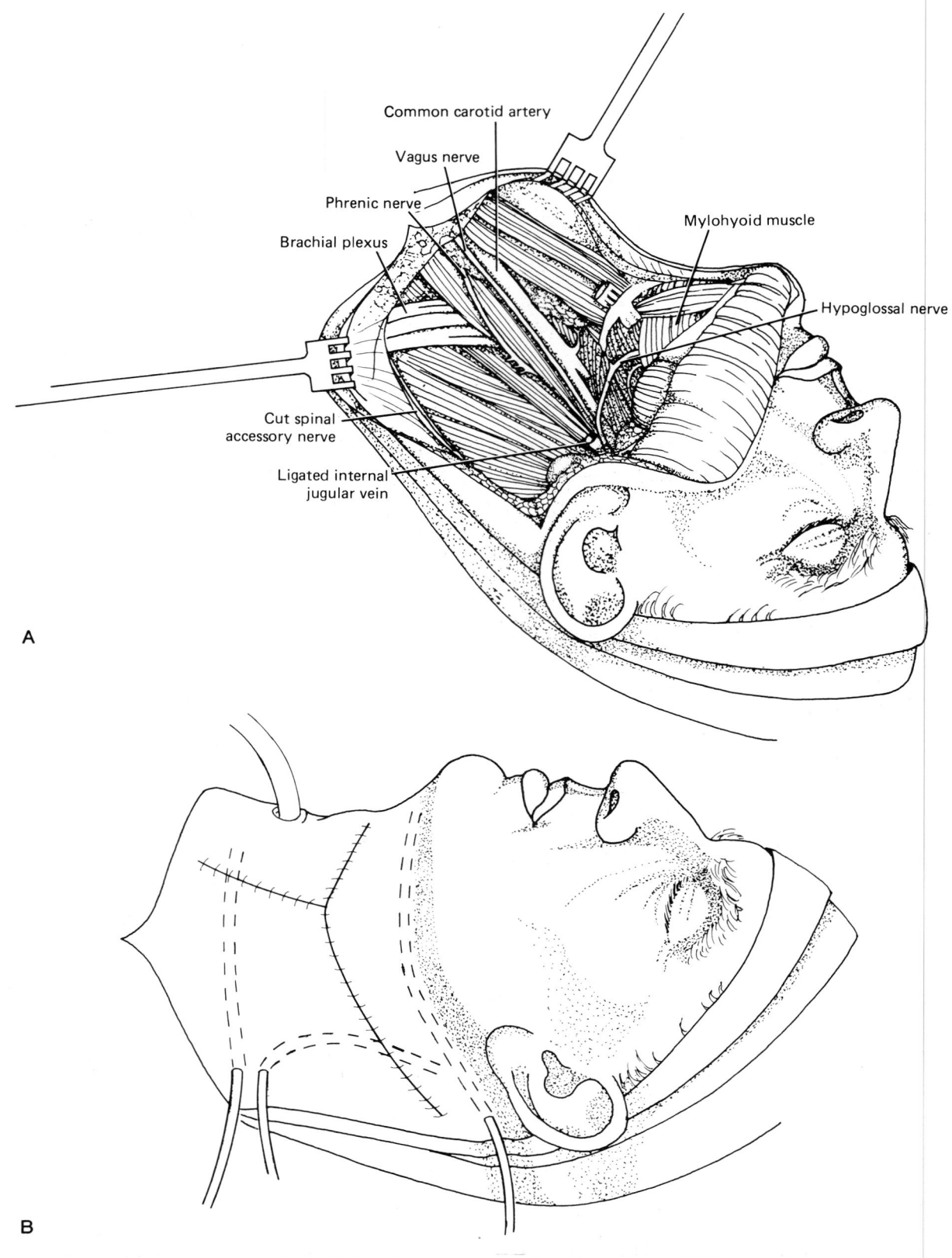

Common carotid artery

Vagus nerve

Phrenic nerve

Brachial plexus

Mylohyoid muscle

Hypoglossal nerve

Cut spinal
accessory nerve

Ligated internal
jugular vein

A

B

Figure 34-4. Radical neck dissection is indicated in the presence of enlarged malignant lesions of the tongue, pharynx, and nasopharynx, or gross metastasis in the neck. (*A*) Skin flaps are raised to expose the superficial structures of the neck. The surgeon then removes all lymph nodes, fat, muscles, areola tissue, and nerves. *Note:* Postoperative deficits are: (1) neck is sunk in to a certain degree, is somewhat stiff, and has a large external scar; (2) the spinal accessory nerve is usually removed, causing the shoulder to drop 1 cm to 2 cm. Rehabilitation efforts gradually minimize the crippling effect. (*B*) This view shows wound closure with portable suction drainage tubes in place. (Redrawn from Conley JJ: Radical neck dissection. Contemporary Surgery, 5:65, Sept 1974.)

Coughing is encouraged, to remove secretions. The patient should assume a sitting position, with the nurse supporting the neck with her hands, so that he may be able to bring up bothersome secretions. If this technique fails, the patient may have to be suctioned. Care must be exerted to protect the suture lines during suctioning. If a tracheostomy tube is in place, suctioning is done through this tube using sterile technique.

Wound Care. With portable wound suction drainage, there is no need for pressure dressings, because the skin flaps are drawn down tightly; approximately 80 ml to 120 ml of serosanguineous secretions are drawn off by a portable suction unit the first day. This amount diminishes thereafter. If portable wound suction is not used, drains may be placed in the wound and pressure dressings applied, to obliterate dead spaces and to provide immobilization. These may need to be reinforced from time to time. Dressings are observed for evidence of hemorrhage and constriction, which may affect respiration. Drains may be removed before the massive dressings are changed in about 5 days. Lighter dressings permit greater freedom of movement. Aeroplast or other antiseptic plastic sprays protect the wound. The patient usually is allowed out of bed the first postoperative day.

Oral Hygiene and Nutrition. Mouth hygiene is necessary and welcomed by this patient. It is done frequently and helps to enhance the appetite. A nasogastric tube may be inserted for feeding purposes or to help decompress the stomach.

Psychosocial Support. The psychological postoperative nursing intervention is directed toward the support of a patient who has had a radical change in body image and who has major concerns regarding his prognosis. Such a patient also has difficulty in communication and is concerned about his continuing ability to breathe and swallow normally. Adjustment to the results of this surgery will take time, and the nurse should enlist the support of family members in encouraging and reassuring the patient.

The person who has had extensive neck surgery often is sensitive about his appearance, either when the operative area is covered by bulky dressings or when an incision line is exposed, as with portable drainage. If the nurse conveys acceptance of the patient and his appearance, and expresses a positive, optimistic attitude, the patient is more likely to be encouraged. In spite of the wide removal of tissue, the cosmetic and functional defects are less than might be expected. The patient also needs an opportunity to voice his concerns regarding the success of the surgery and his prognosis. Most of these individuals are able to maintain and gain weight and are soon restored to economic independence. (When palliative care is necessary, the principles presented on p. 320 can be followed.)

Possible Complications. Because of the extensiveness of the surgery, hemorrhage is a possible complication. Later, postoperative respiratory problems may cause pneumonia, unless the patient is turned and encouraged to breathe deeply. Wound infection has been reduced considerably, with the use of portable wound suction in place of pressure dressings. Neural complications can occur if the cervical plexus or spinal accessory nerves were severed.

Since lower facial paralysis may occur as a result of injury to the facial nerve during the dissection, this should be watched for and reported if noted. Likewise, if the superior laryngeal nerve is damaged, the patient may have difficulty with swallowing liquids and food because of the partial lack of sensation of the glottis.

▶ **Evaluation**

Evaluation of nursing interventions must be continuous and systematic. Long-term evaluation of nursing interventions can begin while the patient is still hospitalized. By including the patient in his care, the nurse can assess his level of knowledge, confidence, and necessary psychomotor skills (*e.g.,* for suctioning). Questioning the patient about the desired frequency of self-care activities will provide an opportunity for needed reinforcement or encouragement. Referral to the community nurse for necessary follow-up or for initial assistance with care permits ongoing evaluation of the patient's progress.

In addition to an evaluation of physical progress, the patient's success with reestablishing an active role in family, community, and work life is assessed. To evaluate this area, the nurse must know the patient's pre-illness participation level and his postoperative expectations. Since this type of surgery is a major event, or crisis, for the family, their adjustment must also be evaluated.

Rehabilitation Following Head and Neck Surgery

Many problems can be avoided with a conscientious exercise program. The purpose of the exercises depicted in Figure 34-5 is to regain maximum shoulder function and neck motion following neck surgery. These exercises are recommended by the physician when it is felt that the neck incision is sufficiently healed. Excision of muscle and nerve results in a weakness of the shoulder that can cause "shoulder drop," with some forward curvature of the shoulder. Exercises will assist the patient in returning to normal activity.

Exercises are done in the morning and evening. At first each exercise is done once; thereafter, it is gradually increased by one, every day, until each is done ten times. Sweeping, smooth motions are used, in a relaxed manner. After each exercise the patient is directed to go limp and relax. Between exercises and when not using the arm or hand, the patient is encouraged to rest the arm and hand on a padded support to keep the shoulder lifted slightly.

▷ Conditions of the Esophagus

The esophagus is the mucus-lined tube that leads from the pharynx through the chest to the stomach.

Difficulty in swallowing (dysphagia) is the most common symptom of esophageal disease. This symptom may range from an uncomfortable feeling that a bolus of food is "caught" in the upper esophagus (before it eventually passes into the stomach) to acute pain on swallowing (odynophagia). Obstruction to the passage of food (both solid and soft) and even liquids may be felt anywhere along the esophagus. Often the patient can indicate if the problem is located in the upper, middle, or lower third of the esophagus.

There are many forms of esophageal pathology, the order of frequency beginning with esophagitis and pro-

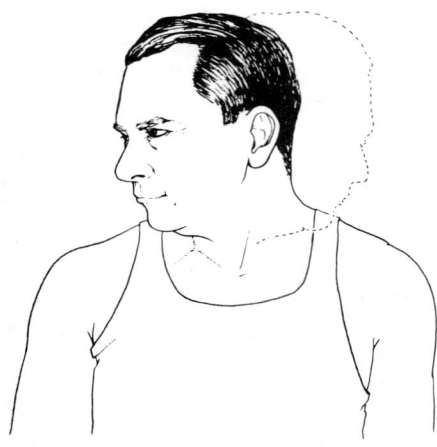

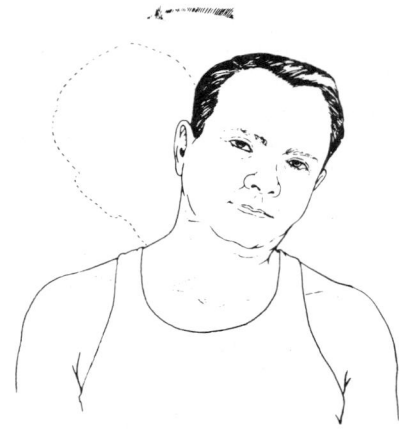

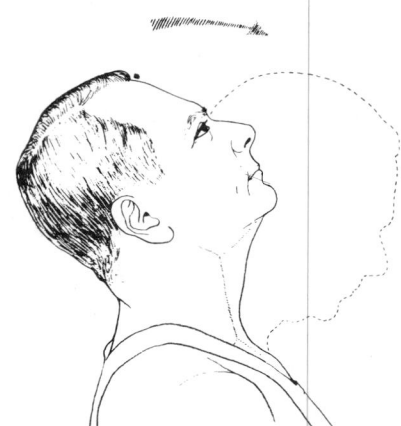

1a. Gently turn head to each side and look as far as possible.

1b. Gently tip right ear toward right shoulder as far as possible. Repeat on left side.

1c. Move chin to chest and then lift head up and back.

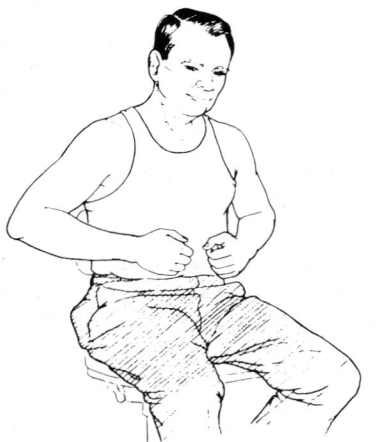

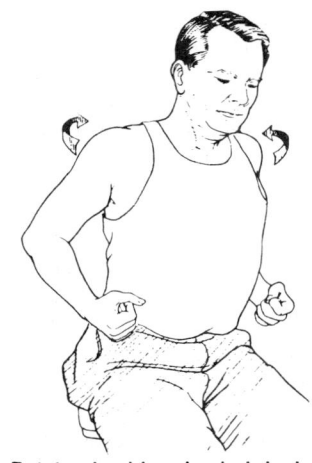

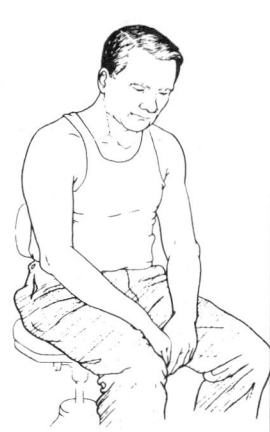

2a. Place hands in front with elbows at right angles away from body.

2b. Rotate shoulders back, bringing elbows to side.

2c. Relax whole body.

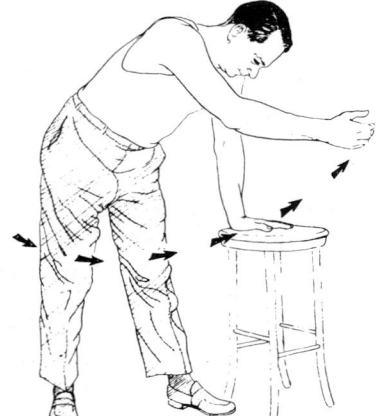

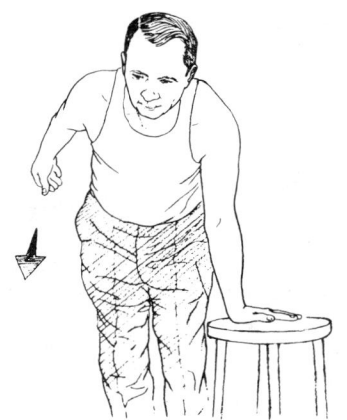

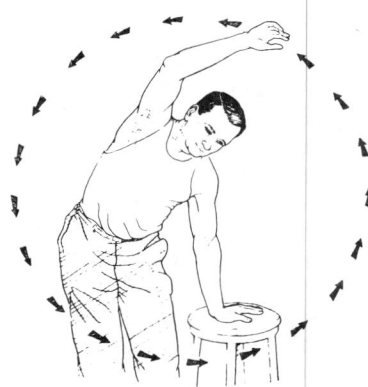

3a. Lean or hold onto low table or chair with hand on the unoperated side. Bend body slightly at waist and swing shoulder and arm from left to right.

3b. Swing shoulder and arm from front to back.

3c. Swing shoulder and arm in a wide circle, gradually bringing arm above head

Figure 34-5.   Rehabilitation exercises following head and neck surgery. The objective is to regain maximum shoulder function and neck motion following neck surgery. (From Exercise for Radical Neck Surgery Patients. Published by Head and Neck Service Department of Surgery, Memorial Hospital, New York, N.Y.)

gressing to malignancy, stricture, obstruction owing to foreign bodies, and diverticula.

General Approach to Care

Nursing Goals and Interventions

The general nursing goals for patients with suspected or known disorders of the esophagus can be divided into three phases: the detection and referral phase, the treatment phase, and the rehabilitative or maintenance phase.

Assessment. The goals of assessment are to identify problems or complaints related to conditions of the esophagus and to facilitate needed medical evaluation or follow-up. These goals are met in several ways: through teaching about the dangers of placing sharp objects in the mouth or of swallowing chemicals or unidentified solutions; through obtaining a careful nursing history and assessment of symptoms; and through encouragement or facilitation of further necessary evaluation.

Certain complaints the client makes should alert the nurse to the presence of possible esophageal disorders. These include decrease or loss of appetite, anorexia, dysphagia, regurgitation, eructation, heartburn, a sensation that food is sticking in the throat, a feeling of early satiety, nausea, vomiting, or weight loss. If the patient admits to any of these complaints, the nurse should question those factors that affect them, such as the time of their occurrence; their relationship to eating; factors that relieve or aggravate them, such as position change, belching, antacids, or vomiting. This history should also include questions about the existence of past or present causative factors, such as infections and chemical, mechanical, or physical irritants. Included also is a history of alcohol and tobacco use.

Management. The goals of treatment are to prepare the patient physically and psychologically for diagnostic tests, treatments, and possible surgical intervention. Reassurance and discussion regarding the purposes and procedures involved are the principal nursing interventions. Some disorders of the esophagus evolve over time, while others are the result of trauma (*e.g.,* chemical burns or perforation). The emotional and physical preparation for the latter group is more difficult owing to the shortened time period and the circumstances of the injury. Evaluation of treatment interventions must be ongoing and directed to whether the patient has enough information to participate in care and diagnostic efforts. If surgery is involved, immediate and long-term evaluation is similar to that of a patient having chest surgery.

Rehabilitation or Maintenance. The goals of rehabilitation must reflect whether surgery or more conservative measures such as diet, positioning, use of antacids, etc., were used in the treatment phase. If the condition is corrected, short-term evaluative measures may be sufficient. If an ongoing condition exists, the nurse must help the patient plan for needed physical and psychological adjustment and for follow-up care. Many elderly patients may be found in the group with ongoing conditions. These patients need support for realistic meal planning, use of medications, and participation in a full life. A multidisciplinary approach is helpful here, including the nutritionist, social worker, nurse, and physician. Postdischarge care includes responsible family members.

Esophageal Trauma

Foreign Bodies. Swallowed foreign bodies—dentures, fishbones, pins, and the like—may injure the esophagus as well as obstruct its lumen. Usually, foreign bodies can be removed with the aid of the esophagoscope. When the foreign body is made of metal (bobby pins, safety pins, needles, jacks, nails, and tacks), it may not be safe to allow the object to make its way slowly through the stomach and intestinal tract. A bar magnet, fastened to a cable, may be maneuvered into place with the aid of fluoroscopy, and the object withdrawn. It is possible for a skilled esophagoscopist to remove open safety pins through the esophagoscope.

If an impacted bolus of meat is lodged in the esophagus, it can usually be dissolved with proteolytic enzymes. The injuries to the esophagus are the more serious part of the problem, because they may lead to deep cervical or mediastinal abscess or to stricture formations. Drainage of such abscesses requires a thoracic exposure.

Chemical Burns. The patient who accidentally or intentionally swallows a strong acid or base (such as lye) is emotionally distraught, as well as in acute physical pain. In these instances, the esophagus is washed with large volumes of water. The patient is treated immediately for shock, pain, and respiratory distress. Attempts should be made to neutralize the chemical.

The acute chemical burn of the esophagus has associated severe burns of the lips, mouth, and pharynx, with pain on swallowing and, sometimes, difficulty in respiration, owing either to edema of the throat or to a collection of mucus in the pharynx. The patient may be profoundly toxic. Esophagoscopy is performed as soon as possible to determine the extent and severity of damage. If the patient is able to swallow, fluids should be given in small quantities. Secretions should be aspirated from the pharynx if respiration is affected. The necessity for high fluid intake may require administration by parenteral means.

Corticosteroid therapy is also administered, to suppress inflammation and to minimize subsequent scar and stricture formation. Antibiotics are given to combat infection and to prevent mediastinitis. A nasogastric tube is passed for feeding purposes and to ensure patency of the esophageal lumen.

About a week after chemical ingestion, passage of a dilating bougie (*bouginage*) may be done daily, beginning with a No. 28 Fr. bougie. When the lumen is "stable," bouginage can be terminated.

Occasionally a patient is admitted after the acute phase has subsided, but multiple stricture levels have formed in the esophagus. These may be dilated by peroral use of bougies; if this is not successful, it may be necessary to try the retrograde bouginage method. A gastrostomy opening is made, and a braided silk string is swallowed. One end is brought out through the gastrostomy opening and the other end through the nose. The two ends are tied together and form a complete loop. Dilatation is obtained by pulling larger and larger bougies upward through the esophagus by means of the string. It is important that this string be left in place at all times. The gastrostomy is kept open by means

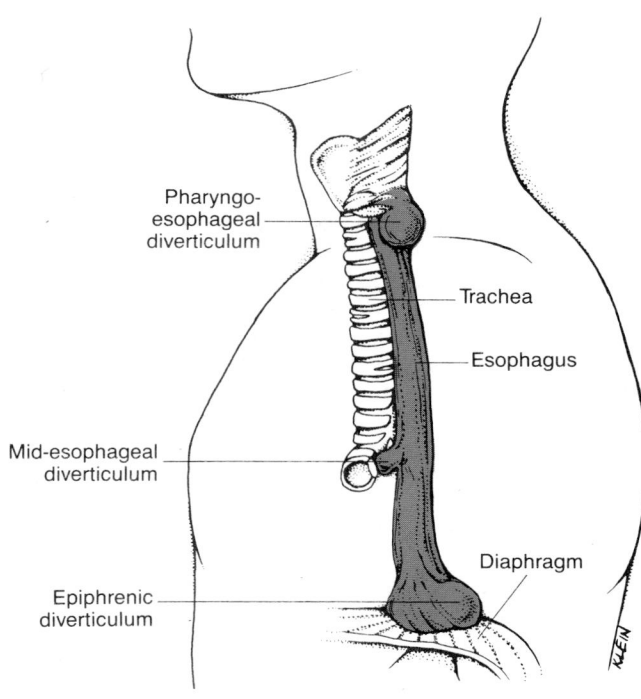

Figure 34-6. Illustration shows possible sites for the occurrence of esophageal diverticula. The site will determine the location of the surgical incision to correct the problem.

of a gastrostomy tube, through which feedings may be given if necessary.

Perforation. The esophagus is not an uncommon site of injury. Perforation may result from stab or bullet wounds of the neck or chest, as well as from accidental puncture by a surgical instrument during examination or dilatation. Spontaneous perforation of the esophagus has been known to occur during vomiting.

The patient experiences spontaneous pain followed by dysphagia. Infection, fever, and leukocytosis may be noted. In some instances, signs of pneumothorax and subcutaneous emphysema are observed. X-ray examination and possible esophagogram are effective in locating the perforation site.

Management. Because of the high risk of infection, broad-spectrum antibiotic therapy is initiated. A nasogastric tube is passed, to provide suction and to reduce the amount of gastric juice that can reflux into the esophagus and mediastinum. Nothing is given by mouth, but nutritional needs are met by intravenous hyperalimentation. Surgery is performed to close the wound, and postoperative nutritional support then becomes a primary concern. Parenteral hyperalimentation is preferred to gastrostomy since the latter might cause reflux into the esophagus. Depending on the incisional site and nature of surgery, the postoperative nursing management will be similar to that for thoracic or abdominal surgical patients.

Esophageal Diverticulum

Pathophysiology. A *diverticulum* of the esophagus is an outpouching or protrusion of mucosa and submucosa through a weakness in the musculature (*pulsion* type). If there is a pulling outward of the esophageal wall from inflamed or scarred peribronchial lymph nodes, the term *traction diverticulum* is used (Fig. 34-6).

Pharyngoesophageal Diverticulum. The most common type of diverticulum, which occurs more frequently in men than in women, is pharyngoesophageal pulsion diverticulum (Zenker's pulsion), which occurs posteriorly through the cricopharyngeal muscle in the midline of the neck. The patient first notices difficulty in swallowing and a fullness in the neck. He may complain of belching, regurgitation of undigested food, and gurgling noises after eating. The diverticulum or pouch becomes filled with food or liquid. When the patient assumes a recumbent position, undigested food is regurgitated and may also cause coughing, owing to irritation of the trachea. Halitosis and a sour taste in the mouth are also common, because of the decomposition of food retained in the diverticulum.

Diagnostic Measures. To determine the exact nature and location of a diverticulum, barium roentgenograms are done. Esophagoscopy usually is contraindicated, because of the danger of perforating the diverticulum, with resulting mediastinitis. The blind passing of a nasal tube should be avoided. The tube should be guided into the stomach under direct vision of a lighted scope. Because this patient is often a victim of unbalanced diet and fluid levels, an evaluation of his nutritional state is done to determine dietary needs.

Management. When a patient has difficulty in swallowing, it is usual to limit the diet to those foods that pass more easily. Blenderized meals supplemented with vitamins are usually prescribed. The nurse arranges for the nutritionist to see this patient and his family to discuss plans for continuing this treatment at home.

Since the condition is progressive, the only means of cure is surgical removal of the diverticulum. Care is taken, surgically, to avoid undue trauma to the common carotid artery and internal jugular veins. The sac is dissected free and amputated flush with the esophageal wall. In addition to a diverticulectomy, a myotomy of the cricopharyngeal muscle is often done, in order to relieve spasticity of the musculature, which otherwise seems to contribute to a continuation of the previous symptoms.

Midesophageal and Epiphrenic Diverticula. The occurrence of diverticula in the midtubular esophagus is less common; symptoms are less acute, and usually the condition does not require surgery.

Epiphrenic diverticula are usually larger pulsion diverticula occurring in the lower esophagus just above the diaphragm, and occasionally higher. They are thought to be related to the improper functioning of the lower esophageal sphincter. Surgery is indicated only if the symptoms are troublesome and growing progressively worse. A transthoracic (thoracotomy) approach is used, which means that pre- and post-operative nursing management is similar to that for chest surgical patients (see pp. 461–471).

After operation, the patient is fed through a nasogastric

tube that usually is inserted at the time of operation. The feedings may include any liquid, but a careful record of their kind, amount, and character must be kept. After each feeding, the tube should be irrigated carefully with water. The wound also must be observed for evidences of leakage from the esophagus and a developing fistula.

If the operative risk is prohibitive, medical and nursing management is similar to that advocated for the peptic ulcer patient; antacids, anticholinergics, and abstinence from coffee, alcohol, and smoking (see p. 792). In addition, reflux is avoided by (1) keeping the head elevated; (2) remaining upright for 2 hours in the postprandial period; (3) avoiding abdominal compression from garments and posture; (4) eating small meals; and (5) reducing, if overweight.

Esophageal Achalasia

Achalasia is the term used to designate functional esophageal obstruction, with a marked dilatation of the esophagus. This is usually associated with a lack of peristaltic activity in the esophagus itself and with a failure of the esophageal sphincter to relax in response to swallowing. Narrowing of the esophagus just above the stomach results in a gradually increasing dilatation of the esophagus in the upper chest, and the symptoms produced are those of difficulty in swallowing, both liquids and solids. The patient has a sensation of food sticking in the lower portion of the esophagus. As the condition progresses, regurgitation of the food is common; this may occur spontaneously or may be brought about by the patient to relieve the discomfort that is produced by the prolonged distention of the esophagus by food that will not pass into the stomach. There may be secondary pulmonary complications owing to spillover of esophageal contents (aspiration pneumonia). The cause of this condition is believed to be a degeneration of the nerves that go to the involuntary muscles of the esophagus. Emotional upsets may aggravate the problem. Achalasia is diagnosed by cineroentgenograms using barium, which show the marked dilatation of the upper esophagus and the narrowing of its lower end. Esophagoscopy is done to rule out carcinoma.

Management. There are differences of opinion as to the best method of treating esophageal achalasia. The conservative approach to treating early achalasia involves stretching the narrowed area of the esophagus via the distention of a bag (Mosher pneumatic) placed in this area through the mouth (Fig. 34-7). Vigorous dilatation produces subxiphoid pain; therefore, an analgesic or tranquilizer is prescribed before the treatment.

Other dilating agents (bouginage), such as French bougies or mercury-weighted dilators, are not effective, since achalasia is not a stricture, but a failure of the inferior esophageal sphincter to relax. Hydrostatic dilatation usually gives good results, but the dilatation required may result in a rupture of the esophagus, in a small number of patients.

In late achalasia or for the more resistant lesions, an *esophagomyotomy* is performed, which is the division of the muscular fibers that enclose the narrowed area of the esophagus, allowing the mucosa to pouch out through the divided area in the muscle layer (Fig. 34-7). This permits food to be swallowed without obstruction, and the operation

is used with very good results. A disadvantage of esophagomyotomy is that about a third of the patients develop reflux of gastric contents into the esophagus. When the above operation is extended to include the cardiac end of the stomach, it is referred to as a *cardiomyotomy.*

It has been claimed by Ellis that surgery is preferred for early achalasia. His study indicates that dilatation is painful, traumatic, and involves a definite risk of rupture of the distal esophagus. In addition, when surgery follows dilatation that has failed, the scarring of the thin esophageal wall caused by the initial procedure makes it difficult to create a relaxed esophageal sphincter.

Diffuse Esophageal Spasm

Diffuse esophageal spasm is a motor disorder of the esophagus diagnosed by esophageal pressure examination. It is usually manifested in old age and may be an early stage of achalasia. There is pain on swallowing (odynophagia), dysphagia, and chest or back pain.

Conservative therapy is to administer sedatives for pain, avoid food and fluids that precipitate symptoms, and eliminate sources of tension. Nitroglycerin or long-acting nitrites sublingually will relieve substernal pain in some patients. Later, it may be necessary to utilize pneumatic dilatation, if manometric studies reveal increased lower esophageal sphincter pressure.

Hiatus Hernia and Reflux Esophagitis
Pathophysiology and Clinical Manifestations. The esophagus enters the abdomen through an opening in the diaphragm, to empty, at its lower end, into the upper part of the stomach. The opening in the diaphragm normally encircles the esophagus tightly; therefore, the stomach lies completely within the abdomen. In a condition known as *hiatus* (or *hiatal*) *hernia,* the opening in the diaphragm through which the esophagus passes becomes enlarged, and part of the upper stomach tends to come up into the lower portion of the thorax. This complication may be present in many patients without any signs or symptoms. It is only when the sphincter of the lower end of the esophagus becomes incompetent and reflux occurs that symptoms develop.

Specific assessment questions are: Where is the pain? When did it start? Does it occur before or after you eat? How long does it last? How frequently does it occur? What aggravates or relieves the pain? What foods seem to aggravate or irritate the problem? Is the pain related to changes in your position? Does sitting upright relieve the pain?

Often there is a feeling of fullness in the lower chest and a splashing sound noted in the substernal area in patients in whom the hiatal hernia is large. In addition, the gastric juice produced by the stomach mucosa tends to be retained in the portion of the stomach above the diaphragm, and for this reason, ulcerations and bleeding may occur. Finally, the erosive action of the gastric juice on the stomach and the lower esophagus may produce a condition known as *esophagitis,* which causes pain and discomfort in the substernal area.

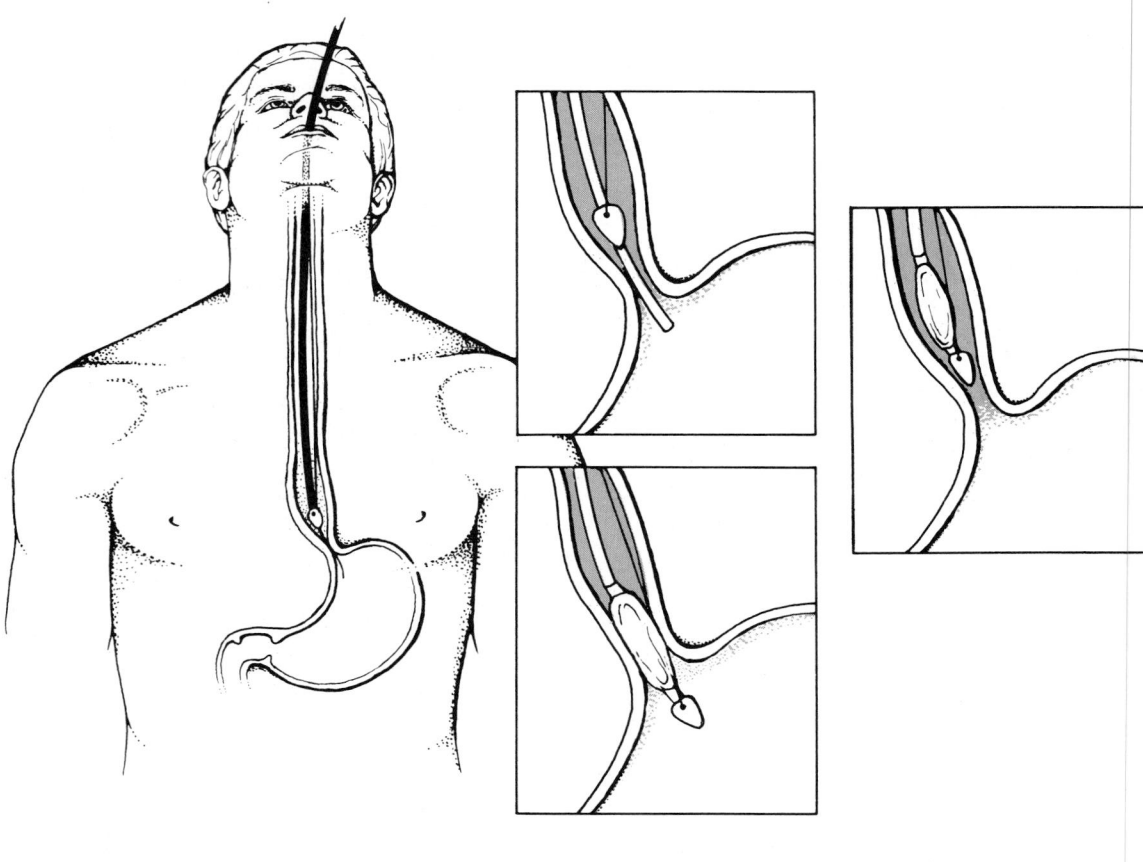

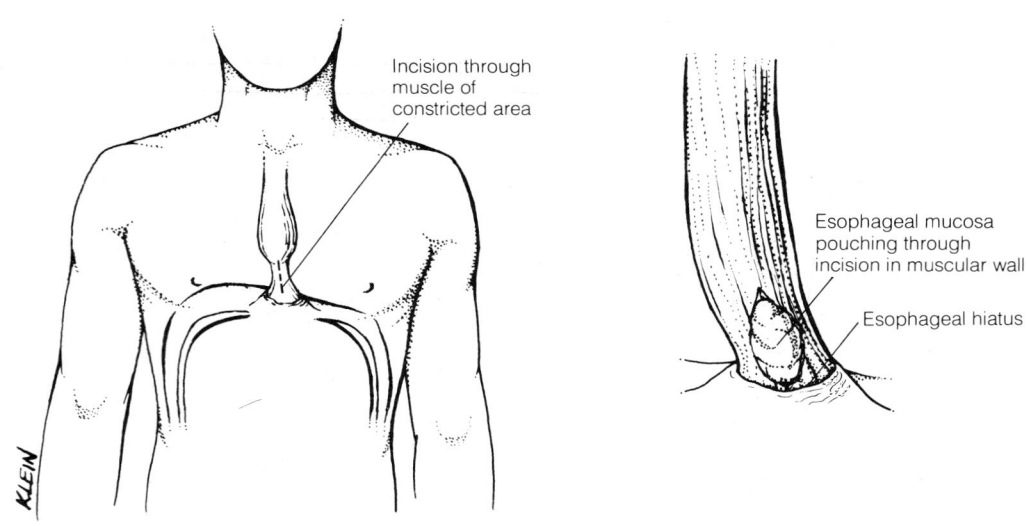

Incision through
muscle of
constricted area

Esophageal mucosa
pouching through
incision in muscular wall

Esophageal hiatus

KLEIN

Figure 34-7. (*Top*) Minor surgical approach. Dilatation of the lower esophagus with rubber balloon technique in cases of cardiospasm (achalasia). The dilator is passed, guided by a previously swallowed thread, into the upper stomach. When the balloon is in proper position, it is distended by pressure sufficient to dilate the narrowed area of the esophagus. (Redrawn from Olsen, Ellis, and Creamer: Achalasia of the cardia. Am J Surg 93:299–307.) (*Bottom*) Major surgical approach. Treatment of achalasia. The esophagus is approached from in front, on the left side. An incision is made through the muscularis of the esophagus sufficiently to allow a pouching of the esophageal mucosa. Separation of the muscular fibers relieves the narrowing at the lower end of the esophagus and permits the patient to swallow normally again.

All of these symptoms produce an uncomfortable, and often very ill, patient if bleeding is a factor.

Management. In those hernias that are found incidentally on x-ray examination and do not produce symptoms, no treatment is necessary. Many of these hernias are of the *sliding* type (axial esophagogastric), in which the stomach tends to extend into the chest when the patient is lying down but slides back into the abdomen when the patient is erect. For this type of hernia, the patient is placed on a strict medical regimen of antacids and advised to avoid lying down after meals (or the head of the bed should be elevated). He should also avoid tight garments and heavy lifting. Weight reduction is adequate treatment for about 90% of patients. For severe heartburn and pain, an oral mucilage preparation (such as Oxaine-M, which contains both an antacid and local anesthetic) may be effective. Some physicians prescribe diazepam (Valium) to be taken several minutes before meals.

When the hernia is of the *rolling* type (concentric, paraesophageal), it is a constant problem and must be corrected surgically. The same is true of sliding hernias in which symptoms occur. To correct the main problem caused by reflux, modern surgical treatment involves wrapping the upper end of the stomach around the esophagus (fundoplication) in order to restore an effective high-pressure barrier to reflux. Other techniques (valvuloplasties) are available, depending on the preference of the surgeon.

Postoperative Nursing Management. The immediate postoperative care of these patients is that used for any thoracotomy or laparotomy. In patients with thoracotomy, a chest tube is often introduced and placed in closed suction. The drain is usually taken out in a day or two, after the lung has completely expanded. The patient is given fluids and food on the second or third day after operation, and gradually increasing amounts of food are given as tolerated. In some individuals, edema at the site where the esophagus passes through the diaphragmatic hiatus may interfere with food intake for a time, but usually this subsides without incidence in 2 or 3 days.

Esophageal Varices

Varices of the lower esophagus are really a secondary manifestation of cirrhosis of the liver. This subject is discussed on page 869.

Cancer of the Esophagus
Incidence and Etiology. About 4% of all cancer deaths in the United States are due to cancer of the esophagus; more than twice as many men as women acquire this condition, usually between the ages of 50 and 70. Chronic trauma, such as that produced by the frequent use of alcohol, tobacco, spicy food, and poor mouth hygiene, appears to be an underlying factor. In the Orient, the drinking of large quantities of very hot tea is suspected of contributing to the high incidence of esophageal malignancy.

Pathophysiology. Unfortunately, the patient may have an advanced ulcerated lesion of the esophagus before symptoms present. Malignancy, usually of the squamous cell epidermoid type, may spread beneath the esophageal mucosa, or it may spread directly into, through, and beyond the muscle layers into the lymphatics. In the latter stages, obstruction of the esophagus is noted, with possible perforation into the mediastinum and erosion into the great vessels.

Nursing Goals and Interventions
The goals of detection and referral, and of treatment and palliation, are appropriate to organize the care of the patient with known or suspected cancer of the esophagus.

Assessment. Unfortunately, when symptoms exist that are related to esophageal cancer, the disease is generally advanced. Symptoms include dysphagia, initially with solid foods and eventually with liquids; a feeling of a lump in the throat; painful swallowing; substernal pain or fullness; and, later, regurgitation of undigested food with foul breath and hiccoughs. The patient is first aware of intermittent and increasing difficulty in swallowing. At first only solid food gives trouble, but as the growth progresses and the obstruction becomes more complete, even liquids cannot pass into the stomach. Regurgitation of food and saliva occurs, hemorrhage may take place, and there is a progressive loss of weight and strength owing to starvation. Later symptoms include substernal pain, hiccough, respiratory difficulty, and foul breath. *The delay between onset of early symptoms and the time when the patient seeks medical advice is often 12 to 18 months.* The nurse insists that anyone with swallowing difficulties be encouraged to see a physician immediately.

Management. The goals include providing physical and psychological support to the patient during diagnostic and treatment procedures. Interventions are similar to those discussed for general conditions of the esophagus. They are directed at maintaining a patent airway and adequate oral hygiene and nutrition, and supporting the patient and family members who are aware of a serious condition.

Palliation. A relatively long-term goal is to assist the patient and family to adjust to the implications of a fatal illness. Interventions include helping them identify their strengths and resources, and identifying appropriate referral agencies, such as the community nurse, hospice agencies, and spiritual counselors.

Assessment and Management
Diagnostic Evaluation. The diagnosis is confirmed by esophagogram, cytologic examination of esophageal washings, barium x-ray studies, and esophagoscopy. Bronchoscopy usually is performed, especially in tumors of the middle and the upper third of the esophagus, to determine whether the trachea has been involved by the tumor and to help in determining whether the lesion can be removed. Mediastinoscopy is used to determine involvement of nodes and other mediastinal structures. Cancer of the lower end of the esophagus may be due to adenocarcinoma of the stomach, extending upward into the esophagus.

Management. The patient may be treated by surgical excision of the lesion, radiation, or a combination of both modalities. Usually, surgery is preferred for lower esophageal tumors, whereas radiation is favored for upper esophageal lesions. With radiation, the lesion may shrink, thereby expanding the lumen and permitting the patient to swallow. Relatively few patients are cured; hence palliative therapy may be required, including combinations of treatment such as gastrostomy, jejunostomy, cervical esophagostomy, dilatation of the stricture, insertion of the intraluminal prosthetic tube, and chemotherapy.

The surgical approach may be through the thorax, or through the abdomen and thorax, depending on the location of the tumor. A common approach for lesions of the lower esophagus is to remove the involved portion of the esophagus and reform the continuity of the gastrointestinal tract by bringing the stomach into the chest and implanting the proximal end of the esophagus into it (esophagogastrostomy). The chest is closed, after a drain is inserted into the pleural cavity and connected to closed suction.

Lesions in the middle and upper thirds of the esophagus, particularly, are often not suitable for surgical excision and, fortunately, occur less frequently. However, some success has been reported with a method in which a tunnel is created beneath the sternum and a resected segment of either jejunum or colon replaces the diseased esophagus. A palliative procedure in which a plastic tube is introduced through a cervical incision has been done with resultant symptomatic relief, improvement in nutrition, and amelioration of psychological symptoms.

Radiation is used before surgery, in some clinics; in others, it is used after surgery. The ideal method of treating this problem has not yet been found; each patient is approached in a way that appears best for him. If the growth is found to be inoperable, either before or at operation, a gastrostomy is performed as a palliative procedure to permit the administration of food and fluids (see p. 775).

Preoperative Nursing Management. The major nursing problems of the patients with an esophageal carcinoma are difficulty in swallowing (dysphagia), malnutrition, and psychological concern and awareness of the seriousness of the condition. Another annoying problem is excess saliva (drooling and spitting). Nursing planning and intervention are directed toward improving the patient's nutritional and physical condition in preparation for surgery or radiation therapy. A weight-gaining program based on a high-caloric and high-protein diet, in liquid or soft form, is advocated, if it can be managed by mouth. If not, then intravenous or parenteral hyperalimentation is initiated.

A common postoperative complication is aspiration pneumonia; the preoperative teaching program must emphasize postanesthetic turning, deep breathing, coughing, and exercises. As part of the effort to prevent pulmonary complications, expectorants and bronchodilators may be prescribed. Good oral hygiene is also encouraged, since regurgitation leaves an unpleasant taste in the mouth.

This patient should be acquainted with the nature of the postoperative equipment that will be used, including closed chest drainage, nasogastric suction, parenteral fluids, and perhaps a gastrostomy tube.

Postoperative Nursing Management. Immediate postoperative care is similar to that provided for patients undergoing thoracic surgery (see p. 461). Following emergence from anesthesia, the patient is placed in a semi-Fowler's position, and later a Fowler's position, to assist in preventing reflux of gastric secretions. He is observed carefully for regurgitation and dyspnea. Temperature is monitored to detect any elevation that may indicate seepage of fluid through the operative site into the mediastinum.

If a prosthetic tube has been inserted or an anastomosis has been done, the patient will have a functioning continuum between the throat and the stomach. He will need encouragement and patience as he begins to swallow small sips of water and, later, pureed small feedings. When he is able to increase food intake to a significant amount, intravenous and parenteral findings are discontinued. If a prosthetic tube (such as a pliable latex tube held open with fine wire coils) is used, it may easily become obstructed if food is not chewed sufficiently. After each meal, he is to remain upright for at least 2 hours to assist in movement of food. The nurse is challenged to encourage this patient to eat, since his appetite is usually poor. Family involvement and home-cooked favorite foods may help the patient to eat. If he complains of gastric distress, antacids may help. When radiation is part of the therapy, the patient's appetite is further depressed.

Often, in either the pre- or post-operative period, an obstructed or nearly obstructed esophagus causes difficulty with excess saliva, so that drooling becomes a problem. This is of concern in an esophagostomy, also. In this situation, the use of small plastic bags fastened to the stoma are helpful in collecting secretions. Or, a wick-type piece of gauze may be placed at the corner of the mouth to direct secretions to a dressing or emesis basin. Of more concern is the possibility of aspiration of saliva into the tracheobronchial tree, with the danger of pneumonia.

When the patient is ready to go home, the family is instructed in how to give nutritional care; what to observe; how to handle signs of complications; how to keep the patient comfortable; and how to obtain needed physical and emotional support.

Prognosis. If the malignancy is detected early, removal is simplified, and the continuity of the digestive system is easily maintained. However, the mortality rate among patients with cancer of the esophagus is high, owing to three factors: (1) Usually, the patients are older persons, in whom the incidence of pulmonary and cardiovascular disorders is high. (2) Before significant symptoms occur, the tumor has already invaded surrounding structures. It is impossible to excise a liberal area of tissue because of the proximity of vital structures. (3) The malignancy tends to spread to nearby lymph nodes, and the unique relation of the esophagus to the heart and lungs makes these organs easily accessible to the extension of the tumor. In several series of operative cases, 45% to 80% showed evidence of metastasis when examined in the operating room.

▷ Bibliography

Articles
Mouth

Aphthous ulcers. Postgrad Med 1981 June; 69(6):158.
Beck S. Impact of a systematic oral care protocol on stomatitis after chemotherapy. Cancer Nursing 1979 June; 2(3):185–199.
Bock J. Herpes: Scourge of the seventies. Can Nurs 1980 Jan; 76(1):22–24.
Couillard–Getreuer DL. Herpes zoster in the immunocompromised patient. Cancer Nursing 1982 Oct; 5(5):361–370.

Dupont JB, Guillamondegui OM, and Jeese RH. Surgical treatment of advanced carcinoma of the base of the tongue. Am J Surg 1978 Oct; 136(4):501–503.

Gannon EP. Giving your patients meticulous mouth care. Nursing '80 1980 Mar; 10(3):70–76.

Heller KS and Shah JP. Carcinoma of the lip. Am J Surg 1979 Oct; 138(4):600–603.

Kempinski C et al. Nursing Grand Rounds: Squamous cell carcinoma—mouth: An experience in primary care. Nursing '79 1979 Oct; 9(10):45–47.

Lieberman ZH, Byrd DL, and Davidson TJ. Immobilization of the mandible in oral cancer therapy. Am J Surg 1979 Oct; 138(4):508–511.

Lynch JM. Helping patients through the recurring nightmare of herpes. Nursing '82 1982 Oct; 12(10):52–57.

McAnally T. Parotitis. Postgrad Med 1982 Feb; 71(2):87–99.

Meissner JE. A simple guide for assessing oral health. Nursing '80 1980 Apr; 10(4):84–85.

Ostchega Y. Preventing . . . and treating . . . cancer chemotherapy's oral complications. Nursing '80 1980 Aug; 10(8):47–52.

Scheiger JL, Lang JW, and Schweiger JW. Oral assessment: How to do it. Am J Nurs 1980 Apr; 80(4):654–657.

Stoehr S. A surgical answer to spastic dysphonia. AORN J 1980 Dec; 32(6):977–982.

Yanachek MP. Growing role for the nurse in oral surgery. AORN J 1979 Aug; 30(8):314–326.

Head and Neck

Aquilar NV, Olson ML, and Shedd DP. Rehabilitation of deglutition problems in patients with head and neck cancer. Am J Surg 1979 Oct; 138(4):501–507.

Bocca E, Pignataro O, and Sasaki CT. Functional neck dissection. Arch Otolaryngol 1980 Sept; 106(9):524–527.

Cornelius J. Screening for head and neck cancers. Nurs Pract 1979 Jan; 4(4):15–19.

Keith CF. Wound management following head and neck surgery. Nurs Clin North Am 1979 Dec; 14(4):761–778.

Larsen GL. Rehabilitation for the patient with head and neck cancer. Am J Nurs 1982 Jan; 82(1):119–121.

Middleton DB and Farrante JA. Periorbital and facial cellulitis. Am Fam Physician 1980 Feb; 21(2):97–103.

Schneider WR. Nutrition in head and neck cancer: Nursing implications. Oncol Nurs Forum 1979 Jan; 6(1):5–11.

Esophagus

Griffith J and Davis J. A 2-year experience with surgical management of carcinoma of the esophagus and gastric cardia. J Thorac Cardiovasc Surg 1980 Mar; 79(3):447–452.

Heck H and Rossi R. Esophageal and gastroesophageal carcinoma: An evolving philosophy of management. Cancer 1980 Oct; 46(10):1873–1878.

Hoffman T et al. Carcinoma of the esophagus. An aggressive one-stage palliative approach. J Thorac Cardiovasc Surg 1981 Jan; 81(1):44–49.

Israel R and Wood J. Esophagitis related to cromolyn. JAMA 1979 Dec 21; 242(25):2758–2759.

Manteuffel SL and McDonough JJ. Esophageal reconstruction with free jejunal grafts. AORN J 1979 Dec; 30(6):1059–1064.

Parker E et al. Carcinoma of the esophagus. Observations of 40 years. Ann Surg 1982 May; 195(5):618–623.

Perro KB, Goetze CM, and Monaghan JJ. Esophageal gastric tube airway. Nursing '80 1980 Aug; 10(8):61–63.

Rajan RK. Esophageal diverticula. Am Fam Physician 1979 Mar; 19(3):119–122.

Schuchmann G et al. Treatment of esophageal carcinoma. A retrospective review. J Thorac Cardiovasc Surg 1980 Jan; 79(1):67–73.

Agencies

American Dental Association, 211 East Chicago Ave., Chicago, Illinois 60611.

35

Assessment of Digestive and Gastrointestinal Function

▷ Physiologic Overview

Anatomy of the Gastrointestinal Tract

The gastrointestinal tract is a tube that is continuous with the external environment at both ends. The pathway extends from the mouth through the esophagus, stomach, and intestines to the anus. The esophagus is located in the mediastinum in the thoracic cavity, anterior to the spine and posterior to the trachea and heart. It is a collapsible tube that becomes distended when food passes through it.

The stomach is situated in the upper portion of the abdomen to the left of the midline, just under the left diaphragm. It is a distensible pouch with a capacity of approximately 1500 ml. The inlet to the stomach is called the esophagogastric junction. It is surrounded by a ring of smooth muscle, called the lower esophageal sphincter, which, on contraction, closes the stomach off from the esophagus. The outlet from the stomach is called the pylorus. Circular smooth muscle in the wall of the pylorus forms the pyloric sphincter and controls the size of the opening between the stomach and small intestine.

The small intestine is the longest segment of the gastrointestinal tract and accounts for about two thirds of the total length. It is folded back and forth upon itself and occupies a major portion of the abdominal cavity. It is divided into three parts; an upper part, called the *duodenum;* the middle part, called the *jejunum;* and the lower part, called the *ileum.* The common bile duct, the conduit for both bile and pancreatic secretions, empties into the duodenum.

The junction between the small and large intestines usually lies in the right lower portion of the abdomen. It is in this area that the vermiform appendix is located. At the junction of the small and large intestines is a valve (ileocecal valve) that functions in a similar fashion to the pyloric and esophagogastric sphincters, mentioned previously. The large intestine consists of an ascending segment on the right side of the abdomen, a transverse segment that extends from right to left in the upper abdomen, and a descending segment on the left side of the abdomen. The terminal portion of the large intestine is the rectum, which is continuous with the anus. The anal outlet is surrounded by the external anal sphincter, which, unlike the other sphincters of the gastrointestinal tract, is composed of striated muscle and is under voluntary control.

Blood Supply to the Gastrointestinal Tract. Since the gastrointestinal tract is so long, its blood supply is from arteries that originate along the entire length of the thoracic and abdominal aorta. Of particular importance are the vessels to the large and small intestines—the superior and inferior mesenteric arteries. These two arteries form small loops, or arcades, which encircle the intestine, supplying its wall with oxygen and nutrients. Blood in the veins that drain the intestine is enriched by nutrients absorbed from the lumen of the gastrointestinal tract. These veins merge with others in the abdomen to form a large vessel called the portal vein, which carries the nutrient-rich blood to the liver. The blood flow to the entire gastrointestinal tract is about 20% of the total cardiac output, and it is significantly increased after eating.

Innervation. The gastrointestinal tract is innervated by both the sympathetic and parasympathetic parts of the autonomic nervous system. The parasympathetic fibers travel in the vagus nerve and in nerves that arise from the sacral segment of the spinal cord. In addition, the upper esophagus and the external anal sphincter are under voluntary control, and are supplied by somatic nerves that arise from the cervical spinal cord and from the sacral spinal cord, respectively.

The Digestive Process

In order to perform their functions, all cells of the body require nutrients, which must be derived from the intake of food that contains protein, fat, carbohydrates, vitamins, and minerals, as well as cellulose fibers and other vegetable matter without nuritional value. This diet provides the energy needs of the body and maintains body weight at approximately constant levels.

The intake of food is a voluntary act that is controlled by conscious sensations of hunger and satiety, modified by learned behavior. These sensations originate in the higher centers of the brain, probably in the hypothalamus. The hypothalamus itself is influenced by visual and olfactory sensations, nervous and hormonal signals originating in the digestive tract, and behavioral patterns.

The primary functions of the gastrointestinal tract are:

1. To break down food particles into their small constituent molecules, for digestion
2. To absorb the small molecules produced by digestion into the bloodstream
3. To eliminate undigested and unabsorbed foodstuffs and other waste products from the body

The pathway that foodstuffs take in the digestive tract begins at the mouth, where they are chewed and swallowed. The bolus of food is then conveyed down through the esophagus into the stomach, where it remains for a variable length of time. It then enters the small intestine, where much of the digestion and absorption of nutrients takes place. The unabsorbed food passes from the small intestine into the colon (also called the large intestine) for further modification and storage prior to elimination (defecation). A schematic diagram of the structures of the gastrointestinal tract is shown in Figure 35-1. The total length of the gastrointestinal pathway, from mouth to anus, is approximately 400 cm to 500 cm.

Large volumes of fluid containing hormones and enzymes are secreted into the gastrointestinal tract in order to aid in the process of digestion, absorption, and elimination. The total secretion into the lumen of the gastrointestinal tract is about 8 liters per day, but less than 200 ml per day of liquid is excreted in the feces. This illustrates the massive absorptive capacity of the gastrointestinal tract.

- Derangements of the absorption function of the digestive system can lead to serious alterations of body fluids.

Gastrointestinal Motility and Secretions

Motility refers to the coordinated contractions of the muscles in the walls of the gastrointestinal tract that propel food and secretions from the mouth toward the anus. These sequential rhythmic contractions are referred to as *peristalsis.* At the same time that the food is being propelled through the gastrointestinal tract, it comes into contact with a wide variety of secretions that aid in breaking down and digesting the food particles (Fig. 35-2).

Oral Digestion. The first secretion encountered is saliva, which is secreted in the mouth by the salivary glands at the rate of about 1.5 liters daily. Saliva contains an enzyme, *ptyalin,* or salivary amylase, which helps in the digestion of starches. It also serves as a solvent for the molecules in the food that stimulate the taste buds. Eating or even the sight, smell, or thought of food can cause reflex salivation. The major function of saliva is to lubricate the food as it is chewed, thereby facilitating swallowing.

Swallowing. Swallowing, the initial act in the propulsion of food, is under voluntary control. It is regulated by a swallowing center in the medulla oblongata of the central nervous system. Voluntary efforts to initiate swallowing are ineffective unless there is something to swallow, such as air, saliva, or food. As the food is swallowed, the epiglottis moves to cover the tracheal opening and thus prevents aspiration of food into the lungs. Swallowing results in the propulsion of the bolus of food into the upper esophagus. The smooth muscle in the wall of the esophagus undergoes rhythmic contractions that move sequentially from above to below and help to propel the bolus of food from the upper esophagus toward the stomach. During this process of esophageal peristalsis, the lower esophageal sphincter, at the junction of the esophagus and the stomach, relaxes and permits the bolus of food to enter the stomach. Subsequently, the lower esophageal sphincter closes tightly to prevent reflux of stomach contents into the esophagus.

- When there is reflux of the acid contents of the stomach into the esophagus, an uncomfortable sensation occurs beneath the sternum. This sensation is commonly called heartburn.

Gastric Action. Within the stomach, food is exposed to gastric juice, the major characteristic of which is its very

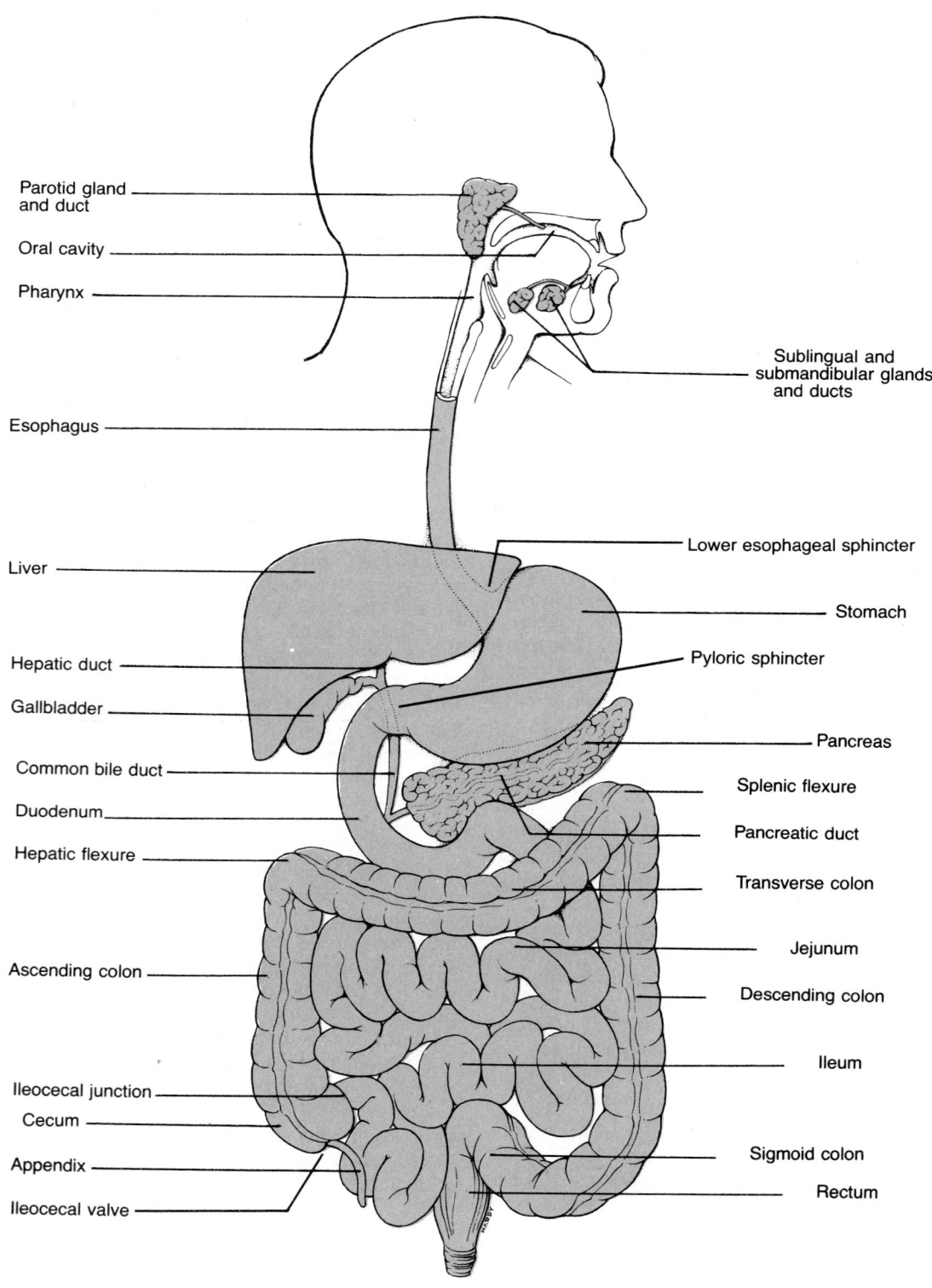

Figure 35-1. Diagram of the digestive system, showing the digestive or alimentary canal and sphincters. (From Chaffee EE and Greisheimer EM: Basic Physiology and Anatomy, 3rd ed. Philadelphia, JB Lippincott.)

acid *p*H. The acidity (*p*H as low as 1) is due to the secretion of *hydrochloric acid* by the glands of the stomach. The volume of gastric secretion is 2.5 liters per day. The function of the highly acidic stomach secretion is to aid in digestion, breaking food down into more absorbable components. The secretion of hydrochloric acid occurs in response to a meal. Between meals, the rate of secretion of acid into the stomach is low.

- Individuals who chronically secrete excessive amounts of gastric acid are susceptible to development of gastric and duodenal ulcers.

The gastric secretions also contain the enzyme *pepsin,* which is an important enzyme for the digestion of proteins (Table 35-1).

Another component of gastric secretions is *intrinsic factor.* This compound is synthesized by cells of the stomach and combines with vitamin B$_{12}$ in the diet, so that the vitamin can be absorbed in the ileum.

- In the absence of intrinsic factor, vitamin B$_{12}$ cannot be absorbed, resulting in pernicious anemia. Research studies have shown that the death of an animal after its stomach is removed is caused by the loss of intrinsic factor.

Peristaltic contractions in the stomach propel its contents toward the pylorus. Large food particles cannot pass through the pyloric sphincter and are churned back into the body of the stomach. In this way, food in the stomach is mechanically agitated and is broken down into smaller particles. Therefore, different types of meals remain in the stomach for times varying from a half hour to several hours, depending on the size of food particles, composition of the meal, and other factors.

Peristalsis in the stomach and contractions of the pyloric sphincter allow the partially digested food to enter the small intestine at a rate that permits efficient absorption of nutrients.

Intestinal Secretions. Secretions in the *duodenum* come from the pancreas, the liver, and the glands in the wall of the intestine itself. The major characteristic of these secretions is their high content of digestive enzymes.

The pancreatic secretion has an alkaline *p*H, owing to a high *bicarbonate* concentration. This serves to neutralize the acid entering the duodenum from the stomach. The pancreas also secretes digestive enzymes, including *trypsin,* which aids in the digestion of protein; *amylase,* which aids in the digestion of starch; and *lipase,* which aids in the digestion of fats.

Bile (secreted by the liver and stored in the gallbladder) contains bile salts, *cholesterol,* and *lecithin,* which emulsify the ingested fats and make them more accessible to digestion and absorption. The bile salts themselves are reabsorbed into the portal blood when they reach the ileum.

Secretions from the intestinal glands consist of mucus, which coats the cells and protects the duodenum from attack by hydrochloric acid; hormones; electrolytes; and enzymes. The total amount of intestinal secretions is approximately

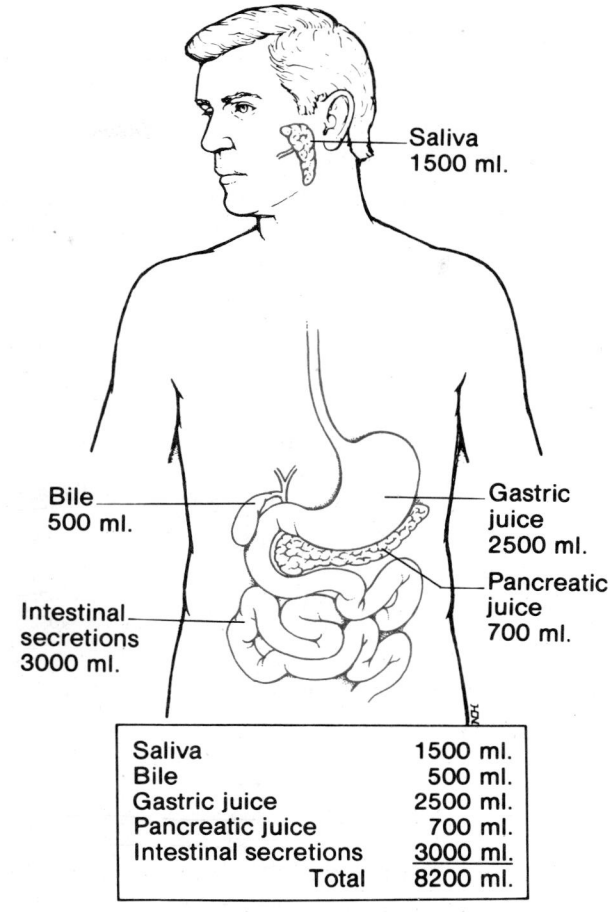

Figure 35-2. Total volume of digestive secretions produced in 24 hours. (Adapted from Bowen A: Intravenous alimentation in surgical patients. Mod Med.)

Saliva	1500 ml.
Bile	500 ml.
Gastric juice	2500 ml.
Pancreatic juice	700 ml.
Intestinal secretions	3000 ml.
Total	8200 ml.

1 liter per day of pancreatic juice, 0.5 liters per day of bile, and 3 liters per day from the glands of the small intestine.

Gastrointestinal Hormones and Bacteria

Hormones. Three major hormones have been found to control the rate of secretion of the gastrointestinal fluids and gastrointestinal motility (Table 35-2).

Gastrin is secreted by the cells of the stomach. It partially regulates the secretion of gastric acid and influences contraction of the lower esophageal and pyloric sphincters. The stimulus to gastrin release is distention of the stomach.

Secretin, secreted by the mucosa in the upper portion of the small intestine, stimulates the secretion of *bicarbonate* in pancreatic juice and inhibits the secretion of gastric acid. The stimulus to the release of secretin is acid entering the small intestine from the stomach.

Cholecystokinin-pancreozymin (CCK-PZ), also released from the cells in the upper small intestine, acts on both the gallbladder and the pancreas. It causes contraction

Table 35-1
The Major Digestive Enzymes

Name of Enzyme	Substrate	Products of Reaction	Source of Enzyme	Site of Action
Action of Enzymes That Digest Carbohydrate				
Salivary amylase (ptyalin)	Starch (amylose) as in grains, potatoes, legumes	Dextrins, maltose, glucose	Secretions from parotid and submaxillary glands (saliva)	Mouth—if chewing is very thorough Some in fundus of stomach if mixing with acidic gastric juice is delayed
Pancreatic amylase	Starch	Dextrins, maltose, glucose	Secretions from pancreas	Small intestine
	Dextrins	Maltose, glucose		
Disaccharidases	Disaccharides	Monosaccharides	Mucosal cells of small intestine	Brush border of intestinal wall
Maltase	Maltose (in corn syrup, beer)	Glucose		
Sucrase	Sucrose (in table sugar, fruits)	Glucose and fructose		
Lactase	Lactose (in milk)	Glucose and galactose		
Action of Enzymes That Digest Protein				
Pepsin (protease)	Protein	Large peptides	Chief cells of gastric mucosa (secreted as the inactive proenzyme pepsinogen*)	Stomach
Trypsin Chymotrypsin Carboxypeptidase	Protein and polypeptides (Polypeptides are primarily from the partial digestion of protein.)	Polypeptides, dipeptides, amino acids	Pancreas (secreted as the inactive proenzymes trypsinogen, chymotrypsinogen, and procarboxypeptidase*)	Lumen of the small intestine
Aminopeptidase	Polypeptides	Smaller peptides, amino acids	Mucosal cells of small intestine	Brush border of small intestine
Dipeptidase	Dipeptides	Amino acids		
Action of Enzymes That Digest Fat (Triglyceride)				
Pharyngeal lipase†	Triglycerides (in foods containing fat, such as meat, butter, nuts, cheese)	Fatty acids, diglycerides, monoglycerides	Mucosa of pharynx	Fundus of stomach
Gastric lipase†	Short-chain triglycerides (dairy fats)	Short-chain fatty acids, diglycerides, monoglycerides	Gastric mucosa	Stomach
Pancreatic lipase	Triglycerides, diglycerides	Diglycerides, monoglycerides, fatty acids (short, long, and medium chain)	Pancreas	Lumen of small intestine

* Activation of proenzymes takes place in the lumen of the intestinal tract
† Not essential for adequate digestion of fat.
(From Suitor CW and Hunter MF. Nutrition: Principles and Application in Health Promotion, p 142. Philadelphia, JB Lippincott, 1980.)

Table 35-2
Hormones That Influence the Functioning of the Gastrointestinal Tract

Hormone	Stimulus for Its Production	Target Glands or Tissues or Organs	Effect on Secretions	Effect on Motility
Gastrin	Myenteric reflexes caused by: Distention of stomach with food	Gastric glands	Increased secretion of gastric juice, which is rich in HCl	Increased motility of stomach; decreases time required for gastric emptying
	Secretagogues: Partially digested protein; caffeine; other substance(s) present in regular and decaffeinated coffee, alcohol; extractives			Relaxation of ileocecal sphincter Excitation of colon Constriction of gastroesophageal sphincter
Enterogastrone (?) (has not been isolated and identified)	Fat in duodenum (?)		Decreased secretion of gastric juice	Decreased gastric motility Relaxation of sphincter of Oddi; increased contraction of gallbladder
Cholecystokinin	Fat in duodenum	Gallbladder	Release of bile into duodenum	
		Pancreas	Increased production of enzyme-rich pancreatic secretions	
		Stomach	May inhibit gastric secretion somewhat	
Secretin	pH of chyme in duodenum below 4–5	Stomach	May inhibit gastric secretion somewhat	Inhibits stomach contractions
		Pancreas	Increased production of bicarbonate-rich pancreatic juice	

(From Suitor CW and Hunter MF. Nutrition: Principles and Application in Health Promotion, p 146. Philadelphia, JB Lippincott, 1980.)

of the gallbladder and release of digestive enzymes from the pancreas. The stimulus to the release of CCK-PZ is the presence of fatty acids and amino acids in the small intestine.

Bacteria. Bacteria are normal components of the contents of the gastrointestinal tract. Their presence is essential for normal gastrointestinal function. Few bacteria are present in the stomach or upper small intestine, probably because they are killed by the acid secretions in the stomach. However, the bacterial population increases in the ileum and becomes a major component of the contents of the large intestine. Bacteria function as an aid to digestion and also synthesize essential nutrients that otherwise might not be available for absorption. The bacterial mass comprises about 10% of the dry weight of the stool.

Digestion and Absorption of Nutrients

Food, ingested in the form of fats, protein, and carbohydrates, is broken down into its constituent nutrients by the process of digestion.

Carbohydrate digestion begins in the mouth with the breakdown of starches by the action of *salivary amylase*. It continues in the esophagus, but is inhibited in the stomach by gastric acid. Continuation of carbohydrate digestion occurs in the duodenum by the action of *pancreatic amylase*. The end result of this process is the liberation of small sugar molecules known as *disaccharides* (*e.g.,* sucrose, maltose, galactose). Enzymes attached to the mucosal cells of the intestine convert the disaccharides into *monosaccharides,* such as glucose and fructose, which are then absorbed into the blood.

- Glucose is the major carbohydrate that the tissue cells utilize as fuel.

Proteins are long chains of amino acids linked together chemically. The hydrochloric acid in the stomach aids in breaking down proteins into smaller particles that are more easily attacked by the digestive enzymes. The process of protein digestion begins in the stomach by the action of pepsin and continues in the duodenum by the action of pancreatic enzymes, such as trypsin. When the proteins are broken down into their constituent amino acids, they are actively absorbed through the mucosal cells of the small intestine into the blood. The tissues utilize amino acids in synthesizing their constituent proteins.

Ingested fats must be dispersed into small droplets (emulsified) so that they can be attacked by digestive enzymes. Emulsification of fats takes place as the result of the churning action in the stomach and duodenum and contact with bile salts. Pancreatic lipase then breaks down the emulsified fats into monoglycerides and fatty acids. These are solubilized as *micelles,* which move to the mucosal surface of the intestine, where they are absorbed. Within the mucosal cells, the fatty acids are recombined into fats, which then enter the lacteals (part of the lymphatic system) and eventually enter the bloodstream. The tissues utilize fats as a fuel; excess fat is stored in the fat cells that are widely distributed throughout the body.

Vitamins in the diet are absorbed essentially unchanged from the gastrointestinal tract. The fat-soluble vitamins A, D, E, and K are absorbed by a mechanism similar to that described above for fats. Vitamin B_{12} is absorbed after combination with intrinsic factor, as previously described.

Minerals in the diet, such as calcium and iron, are absorbed in the small intestine. Calcium absorption requires the presence of vitamin D and is modified by the action of parathyroid hormone.

- Iron in the diet is needed to replace small amounts of iron normally lost by the body, but only a limited fraction of the ingested iron can be absorbed. Therefore, repletion of iron stores of the body by oral therapy, in a patient with iron deficiency, is a long-term process.

Little of the *water and electrolytes* in the diet, and in the 8 liters per day of gastrointestinal secretions, are excreted in the stool.

Intestinal Peristalsis

Peristalsis propels the contents of the small intestine toward the colon. Intense peristaltic waves may be responsible for the gurgling sounds emanating from the gastrointestinal tract at various times. Segmental contractions of the intestinal smooth muscle occur, in addition to its peristaltic contractions. These segmental contractions do not propel contents toward the colon, but rather churn it back and forth, to permit more efficient digestion and absorption. Food leaving the small intestine must pass through the ileocecal valve to enter the colon. This valve is normally closed and helps prevent colonic contents from refluxing back into the small intestine. However, with each peristaltic wave of the small intestine, the valve opens briefly and permits some of the contents to pass through. The first part of a meal usually reaches the ileocecal valve in about 4 hours, and all of the unabsorbed food has entered the colon by 8 or 9 hours after eating.

Motility of the colon consists of relatively weak peristaltic activity that moves the colonic contents slowly, and strong peristaltic rushes that propel the contents for considerable distances. When the contents reach and distend the rectum, an urge to defecate is experienced. Eating stimulates the peristaltic rushes in the colon, resulting in desire to defecate, shortly after a meal. This gastrocolic reflex is the reason that defecation after meals is the rule in children. However, in adults, habit and cultural factors are more important in determining the time for elimination of fecal contents. The first part of a meal reaches the rectum about 12 hours after eating. From the rectum to the anus, transport is much slower, and as much as one fourth of the meal may still be in the rectum 3 days after ingestion. This slow transport of colonic contents allows efficient reabsorption of water and electrolytes.

Defecation

Distention of the rectum reflexly initiates contractions of its musculature and relaxation of the internal anal sphincter, which is ordinarily closed. When the desire to defecate is felt, the external anal sphincter voluntarily relaxes, permitting expulsion of colonic contents. Normally, the external anal sphincter is maintained in a state of tonic contraction. Thus, defecation is seen to be a spinal reflex that can be voluntarily inhibited by keeping the external anal sphincter closed. In this regard, it is similar to micturition. Contraction of abdominal muscles (straining) facilitates emptying of the colon.

- The presence of neurologic lesions that disrupt the innervation of the rectum lessens the effectiveness of reflex evacuation and can lead to abnormal retention of fecal material (fecal impaction).

The average frequency of defecation in humans is once daily, but the range is extremely variable. It is commonly observed that some people defecate several times daily, while others may defecate only a few times per week. More importantly, changes in bowel habits may signify colonic disease. An increase in frequency of defecation is called *diarrhea,* whereas decreased frequency is called *constipation.*

Feces and Flatus.   The feces consist of undigested foodstuffs, inorganic materials, water, and bacteria. Their composition is relatively unaffected by alterations of diet, since a large fraction of the fecal mass is of nondietary origin, derived from the gastrointestinal tract. This is why appreciable amounts of feces continue to be passed despite prolonged starvation. The brown color of the feces is due to breakdown of bile by the intestinal bacteria. With obstruction of the bile ducts, bile is absent from the intestine, and the stools become white (acholic stools). Formation of chemicals, especially indole and skatole, by the intestinal bacteria are responsible in large part for the fecal odor.

The gastrointestinal tract normally contains approximately 150 ml of gas. Gas expelled from the upper gastrointestinal tract (belching) has its origin as swallowed air. Gas expelled from the lower gastrointestinal tract (flatulence) consists of swallowed air, as well as gas produced by bacteria in the colon. The gas in the colon contains methane, hydrogen sulphide, ammonia, and other potentially harmful gases. These gases can be absorbed into the portal circulation and are detoxified by the liver.

- Patients with liver disease are frequently treated with antibiotics to reduce the number of colonic bacteria and thereby inhibit the production of toxic gases.

▷ Pathophysiologic Overview

Abnormalities of the gastrointestinal tract are numerous and exemplify every type of major pathology that can affect other organ systems. Figure 35-3 presents a composite view of the various types of gastrointestinal disorders that may occur. Congenital, inflammatory, infectious, traumatic, and neoplastic lesions have been encountered in every portion, and at every site, along its 7.5-meter (25-foot) length. In common with many other organ systems, it is subject to circulatory disturbances, faulty nervous control, and senescence.

Obstruction of the Gastrointestinal Tract. Various degrees of obstruction to the passage of intestinal contents in the gastrointestinal tract may result from tumors growing into the lumen, twisting or kinking of the intestine, infarction of tissue owing to interruption of the blood supply, aspirated foreign bodies, or other reasons. As a consequence of obstruction, the force of the intestinal contractions is increased, the intestine becomes distended above the point of obstruction, and abdominal pain and bloating result. The peristaltic waves may actually reverse their direction, leading to vomiting. Excessive vomiting may result in the loss of large volumes of fluid from the body, causing *dehydration,* and loss of large amounts of hydrochloric acid, causing *systemic alkalosis.* If the obstruction in the gastrointestinal tract occurs at, or below, the duodenum, biliary material will be in the vomitus, giving the characteristic green color. If the colon is obstructed, the ileocecal valve may become stretched and incompetent, colonic contents can reflux, and the patient may vomit fecal material.

Psychosocial Considerations in Gastrointestinal Disorders

Apart from the many organic diseases to which the gastrointestinal tract is susceptible, there are many extrinsic factors—some related to disease, others not—that can interfere with its normal function and produce symptoms. An anxiety state, for example, often finds its chief expression in indigestion, anorexia, or motor disturbances of the intestines, producing constipation or diarrhea. Students facing examinations or stressed executives facing major decisions can readily be susceptible to gastrointestinal disorders. Also, some psychological problems are thought to have a role in physical dysfunction. For example, personality factors are thought to have an influence in peptic ulcer disease.

In addition to the state of mental health, physical factors such as fatigue and an unbalanced or abruptly changed dietary intake can markedly affect the gastrointestinal tract. In both assessing the patient and instructing him, the nurse should realize that a combination of mental and physical factors affect the status of the gastrointestinal tract.

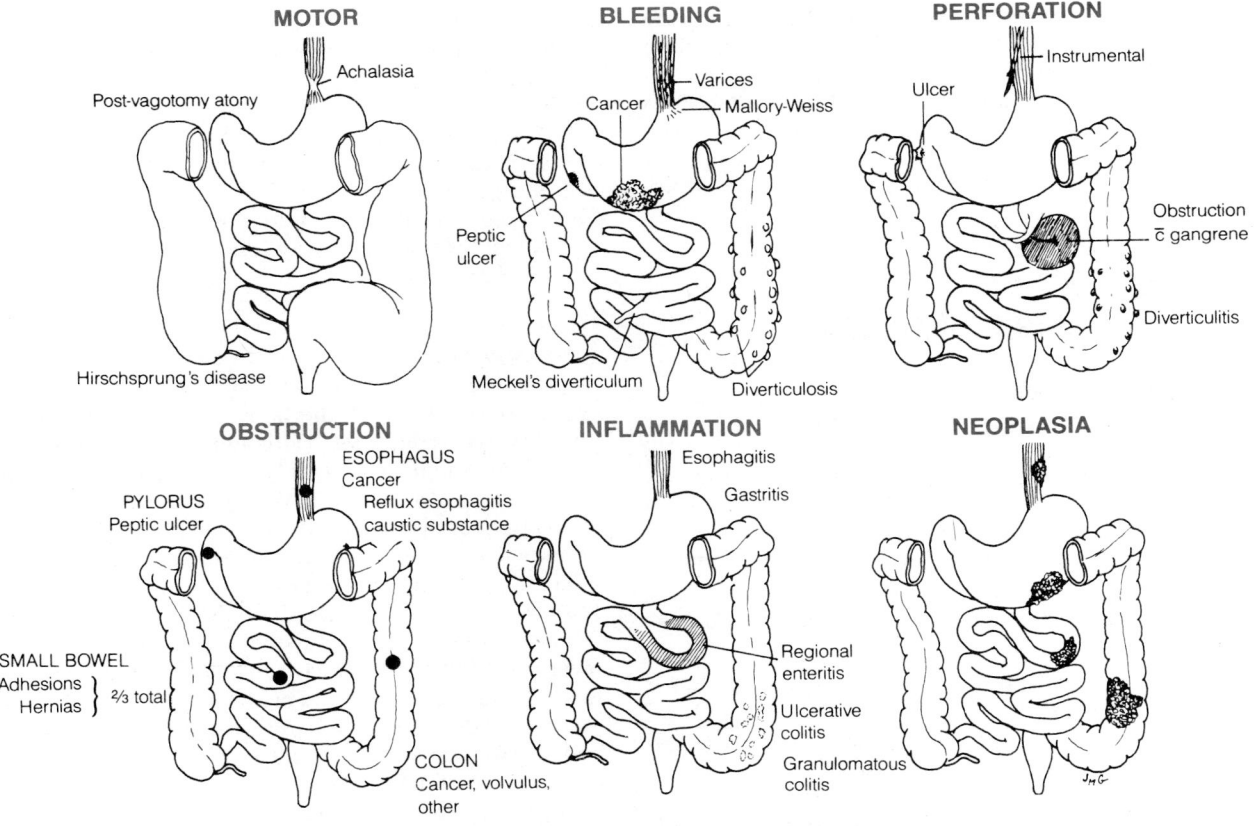

Figure 35-3. Pathophysiology of the gastrointestinal tract can be classified in many ways. The above illustration vividly shows the many conditions that can occur under the six classifications. (From Hardy JD: Rhoads Textbook of Surgery, 5th ed. Philadelphia, JB Lippincott.)

▷ Surgical Considerations

Abdominal Topography

For purposes of convenience in description, the abdomen has been divided into nine regions by imaginary lines, as illustrated in Figure 35-4 (Chart 35-1).

The abdominal cavity normally contains a small amount of fluid that lubricates the peritoneal surfaces. This cavity is lined with a thin, glistening membrane called the *peritoneum,* which covers most of the abdominal organs, forming folds between which the coils of intestine are located. Some organs (such as the liver, pancreas, kidney, and urinary bladder) are not covered completely by peritoneum; hence inflammations of these structures may not always involve the general abdominal cavity but may develop into retroperitoneal extensions or abscesses.

Abdominal Incisions and Surgical Procedures

Incisions

Laparotomy or *abdominal section* are terms used to describe any operation that involves opening the abdominal cavity. The gridiron, or McBurney, incision (see Fig. 35-4 in Chart 35-1) is the simplest. It opens the abdomen through a small wound made by spreading the fibers of the muscles through which it passes. This incision is especially suitable for operations on the appendix, and since it has the advantage of being closed without tension, it makes a firm wound in which hernias rarely form.

More widely useful, however, are the vertical incisions made in the midline or to either side of it. These are made to pass between or through the rectus muscles. Many other types of incisions may be made, depending on the preference of the surgeon.

▷ Assessment of Gastrointestinal Function

Clinical Manifestations of Gastrointestinal Disturbances

Assessment of gastrointestinal function is done to detect suspected problems or to confirm the existence or extent of a problem. The major parts of an assessment are the health history and physical examination, and the diagnostic tests.

Nursing goals for patients requiring gastrointestinal assessments are:

1. To identify potential problems and facilitate referral for further evaluation
2. To provide physical and psychological support to the patient during the diagnostic phase
3. To provide an information base for establishing a nursing care plan and related nursing interventions

The patient's complaints provide a convenient starting point for the health history and permit a focus on issues of concern to him.

Changes in Bowel Habits

Diarrhea. Diarrhea, defined as the presence of more than the usual number of daily bowel movements, or an increase in volume of stool, is a major abnormality of gastrointestinal function. A common mechanism for diarrhea is an increased rate of movement of the contents through the intestine and colon, so that inadequate time is available for absorption of the gastrointestinal secretions, resulting in an increased fluid content of the stool. Inflammation or other diseases of the colonic mucosa can also lead to diarrhea, as can infection from pathogens or parasites or overuse of cathartics. When these occur, water and electrolytes are not sufficiently reabsorbed and increased amounts of fluids or liquid reach the rectum, resulting in increased stool volume. *Steatorrhea,* defined as a large amount of fat in the stools, is commonly due to pancreatic disease. The decreased activity of pancreatic enzymes is responsible for decreased fat digestion. Disease of the biliary tract can also cause steatorrhea, owing to the absence of bile salts. The consequences of diarrhea are loss of potassium, causing electrolyte imbalance; loss of bicarbonate, leading to acidosis; and loss of nutrients, leading to malnutrition.

Constipation. Constipation is the retention of or a delay in expulsion of fecal content from the rectum. In this situation, water is absorbed from the fecal matter, producing stools that are hard and dry and of smaller volume than normal. A variety of factors can produce constipation, such as decreased food or fluid intake, or an intake of primarily low residue foods; decreased exercise or activity patterns; atony of the aged bowel; neuroses; colon or rectal lesions; and intestinal obstructions.

- When evaluating a complaint of either diarrhea or constipation, it is necessary to obtain a history of current and past (or usual) bowel habits, including a description of the content, frequency, and consistency of bowel movements, in addition to their relationship to meals, pain, or activity.

Indigestion

As a result of disturbed nervous control of the stomach, or of disease elsewhere in the body, many persons suffer intensely from "indigestion," although their stomachs appear normal. Abdominal pain is the most common complaint of these patients. This pain is usually in the upper abdomen and is frequently associated with eating, occurring during, or immediately after, a meal. Its character may be described as crampy, or a feeling of fullness, distention, or burning. Fatty foods are apt to cause the most discomfort, probably because they remain in the stomach longest, and because these patients commonly have an abnormal aversion to fatty foods. Coarse vegetables and highly seasoned foods likewise cause considerable distress. Alkalies such as sodium bicarbonate afford only partial relief, or perhaps none at all. The basis for the abdominal distress is obviously the patient's own gastric peristaltic movements. Bowel movements may or may not relieve the pain.

Questions to ask during assessment should be directed toward identifying the offending foods or fluids, the usual interventions tried by the patient, and their effect.

Chart 35-1
Abdominal Incisions and Surgical Procedures

Before studying about patients with specific gastrointestinal problems and operations, the nurse should be familiar with the prefixes denoting abdominal organs and the suffixes used to denote the diseases of or operations on these organs. Suffixes used to denote the names of diseases and operations are:

itis—inflammation of—as *appendicitis*, an inflammation of the appendix
otomy—to make a cut into—as *gastrotomy*, to make an opening into the stomach
ostomy—to make a mouth or opening into—as *cystostomy*, to insert a tube into the urinary bladder
ectomy—to cut or remove—as *salpingectomy*, to remove the fallopian tube
pexy—to sew up in position—as *nephropexy*, to sew the kidney up in position
orrhaphy—to repair a defect—as *herniorrhaphy*, to repair a hernial defect
plasty—to improve by changing the position of the tissue—as *pyloroplasty*, an operation to enlarge the pyloric opening of the stomach

Organs	*Prefix*	*Example*
Stomach	*Gastr*	*Gastritis*—inflammation of stomach
Pylorus	*Pylor*	*Pylorectomy*—removal of pyloric end of stomach
Liver	*Hepa*	*Hepatitis*—inflammation of liver
Gallbladder	*Cholecyst*	*Cholecystitis*—inflammation of gallbladder
Common bile duct	*Choledoch*	*Choledochitis*—inflammation of common bile duct
Small intestine	*Enter*	*Enteritis*—inflammation of intestine
Colon	*Col*	*Colitis*—inflammation of large colon
Appendix	*Appendic*	*Appendicitis*—inflammation of appendix
Loin or abdomen	*Lapar*	*Laparotomy*—incision in the abdomen
Urinary bladder	*Cyst*	*Cystitis*—inflammation of urinary bladder
Fallopian tube	*Salping*	*Salpingitis*—inflammation of fallopian tube
Ovary	*Oophor*	*Oophoritis*—inflammation of ovary
Pelvis of kidney	*Pyel*	*Pyelitis*—inflammation of pelvis of kidney
Kidney	*Nephr*	*Nephritis*—inflammation of kidney

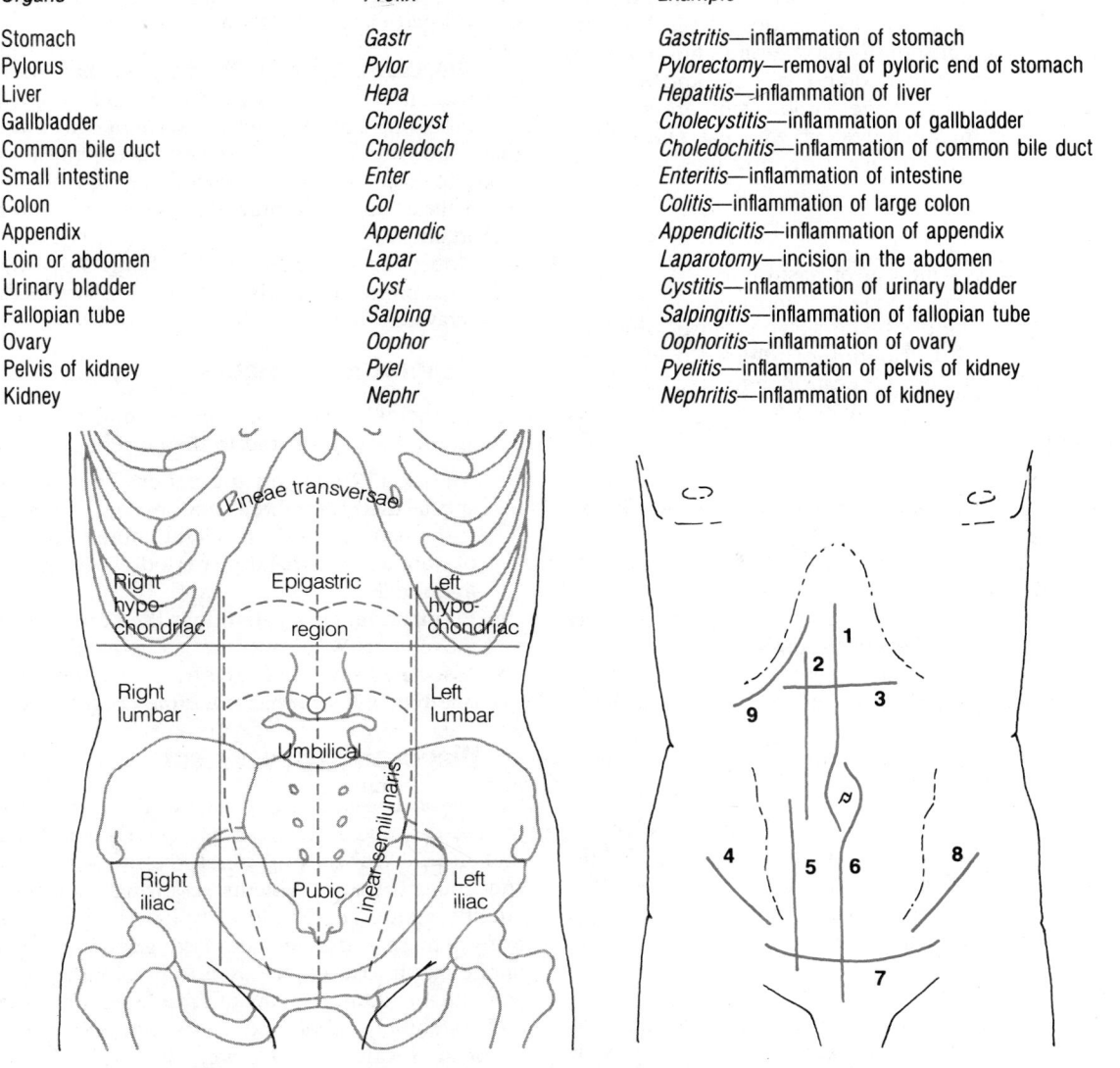

Figure 35-4. (*Left*) Regions of the abdomen. (*Right*) Diagram to show the various abdominal incisions that are used: (1) upper midline incision, (2) upper right rectus incision, (3) transverse incision in the upper abdomen, (4) gridiron incision on the right, (5) lower right rectus incision, (6) lower midline incision, (7) Pfannenstiel incision, (8) left gridiron incision, (9) subcostal incision.

Intestinal "Gas"—Belching and Flatulence

The accumulation of gas in the gastrointestinal tract may result in *belching,* the expulsion of gas from the stomach through the mouth, or *flatulence,* the expulsion of gas from the rectum.

Air that reaches the stomach is quickly expelled, but not necessarily by belching. Periodically, stomach gas moves into the lower esophagus (simple reflux) and then returns to the stomach, owing to a peristaltic contraction of the distal esophagus. Belching occurs when simple reflux is accompanied by contraction of the anterior abdominal muscles. At the first urge to belch, simply swallowing may interrupt the belch.

Usually, gases in the intestine pass into the colon and are released as flatus. Patients often complain of bloating, distention, or being "full of gas."

The so-called *heartburn, acid eructation,* etc., are due to reverse peristalsis, probably gastroesophageal reflux. Questions are aimed at identifying the offending foods or fluids, keeping in mind that some foods are known to be gas-producing, such as cabbage. People who are anxious, who have loose-fitting dentures, or who eat rapidly frequently swallow air, which in turn contributes to intestinal "gas."

Pain

Pain can be a major symptom of gastrointestinal disease. The character, duration, frequency, and time of the pain vary greatly, depending on the underlying cause, which affects the location and distribution of referred pain. Other factors, such as meals, rest, defecation, and vascular disorders, may directly affect pain. Major sites of localization of pain are as follows:

Esophageal: Retrosternal; may radiate to back
Gastric: Epigastric; may radiate to back, especially left subscapular
Duodenal: Epigastric; may radiate to back, especially right subscapular
Gallbladder: Right upper quadrant or epigastric; may radiate to back or right subscapular
Pancreatic: Epigastric; may radiate to back or left lumbar
Appendicular: Periumbilical, later to right lower quadrant
Colonic: Hypogastrium, right or left lower quadrant
Rectal: Pelvic area

Questions to ask are intended to identify the onset, character, severity, duration (constant or intermittent), frequency, and location of the pain, in addition to its relationship to meals and activity. Activities or interventions that relieve or aggravate the pain are also identified.

Vomiting

This is an involuntary act in which violent contractions of the abdominal muscles forcefully expel gastric contents up through the esophagus. It is preceded by closure of the glottis and pylorus, together with relaxation of the gastric wall and cardiac orifice. *Retching* involves these same movements, except that the cardiac orifice remains closed, so that gastric contents are not expelled. Vomiting is usually preceded by *nausea,* an unpleasant sensation suggesting that vomiting is imminent. Such symptoms are associated with gastrointestinal disturbances. Assessment includes determining from the patient any aggravating factors, frequency of vomiting, time of occurrence, and the quantity, odor, color, and taste of the vomited material.

Hematemesis is the vomiting of blood. When this happens soon after hemorrhage, the vomitus is bright red. If blood has been retained in the stomach, digestive processes change the hemoglobin to a brown pigment, which gives the vomitus a coffee-ground appearance. Occasionally, the patient has difficulty in differentiating between hematemesis and hemoptysis (expectoration of blood-tinged sputum), particularly if a coughing paroxysm has preceded it.

Assessment questions are aimed at identifying aggravating factors, the frequency of vomiting; the time of occurrence (especially in relation to eating); the quantity, odor, color, and taste of the vomited material; and the presence of food particles, blood, or mucus.

Anorexia, Dysphagia, and Polyphagia

Anorexia is the lack of appetite for food. *Dysphagia* refers to swallowing difficulty, while *odynophagia* indicates pain on swallowing. *Polyphagia* means excessive eating, or voracious appetite. These are descriptive signs that alone may mean little, but in combination with other symptoms are important.

Questions are aimed at identifying the length of time these symptoms have existed, as well as factors that relieve or aggravate them.

General Assessment

Some general information is also sought, if not already elicited in the history, related to the current complaint.

- Nutrition: When did the patient eat last? Is he on a special diet? Have there been any recent dietary changes? Is the patient's current weight stable? If a loss (or gain) of weight, over what time period? Was the loss (or gain) intended?
- Elimination: How often does the patient have a bowel movement? When was the last movement?
- Associated symptoms: Has the patient been around anyone recently who has the same complaints?

Diagnostic Assessment

Diagnostic assessment of the gastrointestinal tract includes the use of x-rays and ultrasound, and the passage of various oral and anal tubes. In general, the nurse has a supportive and educative role. Patients requiring such tests are frequently anxious, elderly, or debilitated. The preparation for many of these studies includes fasting and the use of laxatives or enemas, measures that are poorly tolerated by weakened patients. In addition, many of these tests require seemingly endless waiting, either for the tests to begin or be completed, or for the results to be known.

Nursing Goals and Interventions

Nursing goals for the patient requiring gastrointestinal diagnostic assessment are to provide for the physical and emotional preparation of the patient.

Nursing interventions to achieve this are: (1) To provide

needed information about the test and those activities required of the patient. This should include both oral and written instructions. In this way, the patient can review what is required of him. (2) To encourage family members, or others, to accompany the patient in need of physical or emotional support during the test.

Short-term evaluation of the above can be done through questioning the patient or family about the purposes and requirements of the test and about their plans to provide needed support.

Roentgenography of the Upper Gastrointestinal Tract

The entire gastrointestinal tract can be delineated by x-rays, following the introduction of barium sulfate or a similar radiopaque liquid as the contrast medium. This material, a tasteless, odorless, nongranular, and completely insoluble (hence, not absorbable) powder, is ingested in the form of a thick or thin aqueous suspension for purposes of upper gastrointestinal tract study ("upper GI series") and is instilled rectally for visualization of the colon ("barium enema").

Patient Preparation.   In preparation for a GI series, the patient is to receive nothing by mouth after midnight prior to the test. A laxative may be prescribed to clean out the intestinal tract. Since smoking can stimulate gastric motility, the patient is discouraged from smoking the morning before the examination.

Procedure.   For purposes of examining the upper gastrointestinal tract, the patient is required to swallow barium under direct fluoroscopic examination.

As the contrast medium descends into the stomach, the position, patency, and caliber of the esophagus are visualized, enabling the examiner to detect or exclude any anatomic or functional derangement of that organ. An important observation can also be made in relation to the heart, namely, observing the presence or the absence of right atrial enlargement. An enlarged right atrium invariably impinges on the esophagus and is revealed by the resulting pressure defect in the esophagus. The roentgenographic appearance of the lower esophagus after a swallow of thick barium suspension also allows for detection of esophageal varices, a manifestation of portal hypertension, as in cirrhosis of the liver.

Fluoroscopic examination next extends to the stomach, as its lumen fills with barium. The motility and the thickness of the gastric wall, and the mucosal pattern are observed for evidence of spasms, ulcerations, malignant infiltrates, and other anatomic abnormalities, including pressure defects from without. The patency of the pyloric valve and the anatomy of the duodenum are also observed, with particular reference to possible ulceration of the mucosa, spasm of the wall, or displacement of the structure as a whole by a tumor in the adjacent area.

During the fluoroscopic examination, roentgenograms are exposed in order to obtain a permanent record of the findings. Additional roentgenograms are taken at intervals, for as long as 24 hours thereafter, as a means of estimating the rate of gastric emptying and the degree of small bowel motility.

Double Contrast Studies.   The double contrast method of examining the upper gastrointestinal tract involves administering a thick barium suspension medium to outline the stomach and esophageal wall. Next, tablets that release carbon dioxide in the presence of water are given. (To reduce these bubbles, simethicone is given.) The primary advantage of this technique is the finer detail that can be shown within the esophagus and stomach, permitting signs of early superficial neoplasms to be noted.

Continuous Infusion Method.   A truly detailed study of the small intestine involves the continuous infusion, through a duodenal tube, of 500 ml to 1000 ml of a thin barium sulfate suspension. This is carried out as a separate procedure. The barium column fills the intestinal loops and is observed continuously by fluoroscope and filmed at frequent intervals as it progresses through the jejunum and the ileum.

Roentgenography of the Colon (Barium Enema)

The purpose of a barium enema is to reveal the presence of polyps, tumors, and other lesions of the large intestine and to demonstrate any abnormal anatomy or malfunction of the bowel.

Patient Preparation.   The preparation of the patient includes those measures necessary to produce an empty and clean lower bowel. Usually, this includes taking nothing by mouth after midnight, cleansing enemas until returns are clear, and perhaps a laxative by mouth/or a rectal suppository.

* If the patient has active inflammatory disease of the colon, only gentle enemas should be used.

Procedure.   In the x-ray department, the radiopaque substance is instilled rectally; it is viewed in the fluoroscope and then filmed. If the patient has been prepared satisfactorily and the colonic contents have been evacuated completely by enemas, the contour of the entire colon, including cecum and appendix (if patent), is clearly visible and the motility of each portion readily observed. The procedure takes about 15 minutes and is followed by an evacuating enema or laxative to facilitate barium removal.

Gastric Analysis

Examination of the gastric juice offers a means of estimating the secretory activity of the gastric mucosa and of ascertaining the presence, or the degree, of gastric retention in patients suspected of having pyloric or duodenal obstruction.

* A diagnosis of pernicious anemia is excluded by the finding of acid.
* A diagnosis of gastric carcinoma may be established by the discovery of cancer cells in the gastric juice.

The fasting patient is intubated through a nostril with a Levin duodenal tube, a small tube with catheter tip marked at points 45 cm, 55 cm, 65 cm, and 75 cm from the distal end. (See p. 770 for nursing management during intubation.)

When the second marker of the Levin tube is at the point of entering the nares, the tip of the tube, 55 cm distant, should be within the stomach. Once in place, the tube is secured to the patient's cheek by means of a small strip of adhesive tape, and the patient is placed in a semireclining

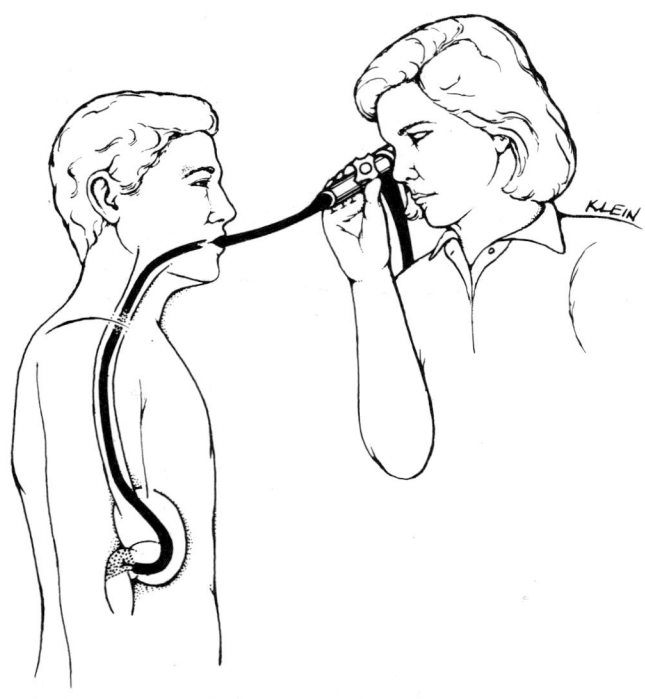

Figure 35-5. Patient undergoing gastroscopy. Note the extreme flexibility of the tube with the patient in the sitting position.

position. If he exhibits any tendency to gag, he is instructed to pant gently with his mouth wide open, the effect of which is to minimize contact between the tube and the soft palate. The entire stomach contents are aspirated by gentle suction into a syringe.

Pentagastrin, histamine, or betazole hydrochloride (Histalog) may be given to stimulate gastric secretions. Pentagastrin is preferred because of the lack of side-effects. If histamine or Histalog is used, the patient is told that he may experience a flushed feeling after the injection of this medication. Also, blood pressure and pulse are frequently monitored to detect hypotension. Emergency medications such as epinephrine and diphenhydramine hydrochloride (Benadryl) are to be kept nearby if required. Specimens are labeled to indicate time before and after histamine injections.

The acidity of the specimen is determined by means of an indicator, such as Töpfer's reagent, by indicator paper, or by a pH meter. Other examinations, in special instances, may include cytologic study by the Papanicolaou technique for the presence or absence of carcinoma cells. Enzyme analysis of the gastric juice is sometimes indicated.

One of the most important items of information to be gained from gastric analysis relates to the ability of the mucosa to secrete hydrochloric acid:

- Patients with pernicious anemia secrete no acid under basal conditions or after stimulation.
- Patients with severe chronic atrophic gastritis secrete little or no acid. Some patients with gastric cancer secrete little or no acid.

- Patients with peptic ulcer invariably secrete some acid; patients with duodenal ulcers usually secrete an excess amount.

Upper Gastrointestinal Fiberoscopy

This procedure allows for direct visualization of the gastric mucosa through a lighted endoscope (gastroscope) and is especially valuable when gastric neoplasm is suspected (Fig. 35-5). Fiberscopes are flexible scopes equipped with fiberoptic lenses. Colored photographs or motion pictures can be taken through them. However, precautions must be taken to protect the scope, since the fiberoptic bundles may be broken if the scope is bent acutely. To prevent the patient from biting the scope, mouth guards are essential.

Patient Preparation. The patient is placed in a fasting state for 6 to 8 hours before the examination. One half hour before the procedure, he is given meperidine hydrochloride (Demerol). Usually, gargling with a local anesthetic, along with the administration of intravenous Valium just before the scope is introduced, will suffice. Sometimes atropine may be helpful in reducing secretions. Glucagon may be given to relax smooth muscle.

Procedure. The patient's lips, oral cavity, and pharynx are sprayed with tetracaine hydrochloride (Pontocaine) or a liquid gargle of ethyl aminobenzoate (Hurricane), after which the gastroscope is passed smoothly and slowly. The fiber gastroscope is almost completely flexible and gives the physician an opportunity to view a large part of the gastric wall. Experienced gastroscopists may recognize a cancer and remove a piece of tissue for microscopic examination. Ulcers and their healing may be identified in response to treatment documented.

Follow-up Care. Following a gastroscopy the patient is instructed not to eat or drink until the gag reflex returns in about 3 or 4 hours; this is done to prevent aspiration into the lungs. Postgastroscopy assessment by the nurse includes observation for signs of perforation, such as pain, unusual discomfort, and an elevated temperature. Minor throat discomfort can be relieved with lozenges, cool saline gargle, and oral analgesic medications.

Anoscopy, Proctoscopy, Sigmoidoscopy, and Colonofiberoscopy

These procedures make use of tubular instruments that incorporate small electric lights that allow the lumen of the lower bowel to be viewed directly. The anoscope is employed to examine the anal canal; proctoscopes and sigmoidoscopes (Fig. 35-6) are used to inspect the rectum and the sigmoid, respectively, for evidence of ulceration, tumors, polyps, or other pathology.

The flexible sigmoidoscope permits an examination of up to 40 cm to 50 cm from the anus, more than the 25 cm that can be seen with the rigid sigmoidoscope. While there is a more proximal distribution of lesions of the colon, polyps and cancer are found more commonly on the left side of the colon. Lefall urges that a flexible sigmoidoscopy be performed at age 50, be repeated in 1 year, and then performed every 3 years after that.

Patient Preparation. Such an examination requires that the lower bowel be clean; therefore, a warm tap-water enema

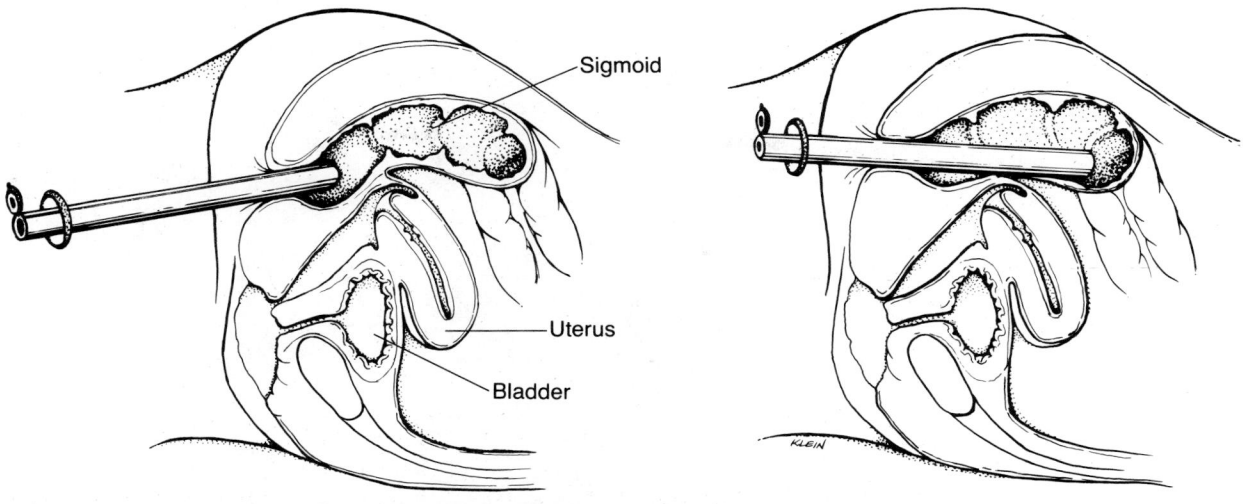

Figure 35-6. Sigmoidoscopy. (*Left*) Direction of motion as the sigmoidoscope, with obturator in place, enters the rectum. (*Right*) The sigmoidoscope reaches the rectosigmoid junction. At this point, the obturator is removed, a light carrier is inserted, and a magnifying lens is attached to aid in visualization.

or Fleet enema is given until clear. It may be necessary for the patient to be on clear liquids the day before the examination. Generally, laxatives are not given.

Procedure.   The patient assumes the knee–chest position, resting on his knees, feet extending over the edge of the bed or the examining table. With knees spread apart to give steady support, the patient leans over and rests the side of his face on the bed or the table, with his forearms on either side of the head and his hands placed, one on top of the other, above the head. His back is now inclined at about a 45-degree angle, and he is in proper position for the introduction of an anoscope, proctoscope, or sigmoidoscope. Maximal convenience and comfort are afforded by a table that has been especially designed for rectal endoscopy—the so-called proctoscopic table, which tilts the patient into the optimal position.

• The patient undergoing a proctosigmoidoscopic examination should be kept informed as to the progress of the examination, and praised for his cooperation. Let him know that he will experience a feeling of pressure and will feel as though he is going to have a bowel movement. Explain that this is from the pressure of the instrument and will last only a brief period of time. It may be necessary to attach suction equipment through the scope to remove any secretion, exudate, blood, or excreta that might be obstructing the area of observation. After each use these tubes must be cleansed thoroughly and the collecting bottles emptied and cleaned likewise. Disposable sigmoidoscopes are now available. While they eliminate the need for cleaning, they must be disposed of safely.

As part of the endoscopic examination, one or more small pieces of tissue may be removed for histologic study, a procedure referred to as a *biopsy*. This is done with small biting forceps introduced through

the instrument. Rectal and sigmoidal polyps, if present, may be removed by means of a wire snare, which is used to grasp the pedicle or stalk, and an electrocoagulating current, used to sever it and to prevent bleeding. It is extremely important that all tissue that is excised by the endoscopist be placed immediately in moist gauze or in an appropriate receptacle, labeled correctly and legibly, and then delivered without delay to the pathology laboratory.

Fiberoptic Colonoscopy

Direct visual inspection of the colon is possible by means of a flexible colonoscope. This procedure is used as a diagnostic aid, and the instrument may be used to remove foreign bodies, polyps, or tissue for biopsy (Fig. 35-7).

Patient Preparation.   The patient is informed about the procedure and requested to cooperate and relax during the examination. In addition, the intestinal tract is emptied by limiting the patient's intake to liquids (perhaps for a 3-day period), cleansing the tract with a laxative for 2 nights, and giving a Fleet enema or saline enema until clear the morning of the test.

Before the examination, Demerol may be administered. During the examination, Valium may be useful in relieving anxiety.

Procedure.   This procedure is performed with the patient lying on his left side with his legs drawn up. Discomfort may result from instilling air to open the colon or from tugging the colon so that the scope can be maneuvered. Complications are rare following this procedure, although perforation or hemorrhage are possible.

Stool Examination

The basic examination of the stool includes an inspection of the specimen for its amount, consistency, and color, and

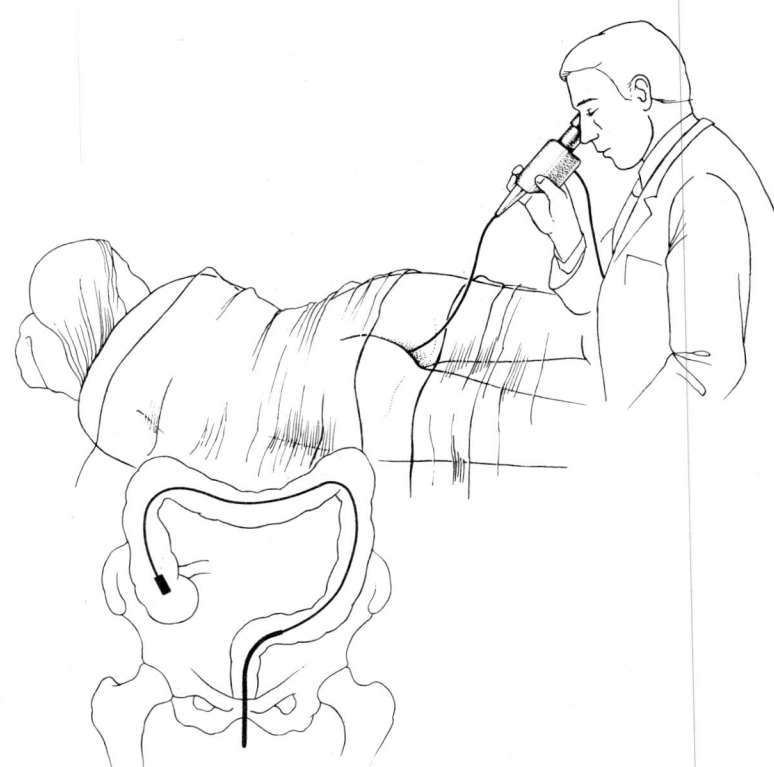

Figure 35-7. Technique of colonoscopy. The patient is turned from one side to the other to take advantage of gravity as the scope is being advanced. Insert shows path of flexible scope from rectum through sigmoid colon and descending, transverse, and ascending colon. If the physician desires to check scope position with fluoroscopy, a lead apron should be donned.

a screening test for occult blood. Special tests indicated in specific cases may include tests for fecal urobilinogen, fat, nitrogen, parasites, food residues, and other substances.

Stool Color.   The color of stools varies from light to dark brown. (Milk-fed infants pass stools that are golden-yellow in color, owing to unchanged bilirubin.) Various foods and medications affect stool color as follows: meat protein produces a dark brown coloration; spinach, a green hue; carrots and beets, red; cocoa, dark red or brown; senna and santonin, a yellowish hue; calomel, green; bismuth, iron, licorice, and charcoal, black; and barium, a milky white appearance.

- Blood in sufficient quantities, if shed into the upper gastrointestinal tract, produces a tarry black color (melena).
- Blood entering the lower portion of the gastrointestinal tract or passing rapidly through it will appear bright or dark red.
- Lower rectal or anal bleeding can be suspected if there is streaking of blood on the surface of the stool or if blood is noted on toilet tissue.

Even considerable quantities of hemoglobin may fail to produce a distinctive color, in which event it is termed "occult blood."

Tests for Occult Blood or to Confirm Melena.   The most common stool tests are based on the benzidine, gum guaiac or the orthotolidin reaction. A form of the guaiac test is the Hemoccult test. A dry paper slide is used, on which the stool specimen is smeared. The slide comes in an envelope that can be mailed, if needed, and examined later.

Stool Consistency and Appearance.   In various disorders the stool assumes a typical appearance:

In *steatorrhea,* the stools are generally bulky, greasy, foamy, and foul in odor; stool color is gray, with a silvery sheen.

With *biliary obstruction,* the stool becomes "acholic" and is light gray or "clay colored," owing to the absence of urobilin.

In *chronic ulcerative colitis,* mucus or pus may be visible on gross inspection of the stool.

Constipation, obstipation, or *fecal impaction* may result in the passage of small, dry, rocky-hard masses called *scybala.* This type of stool may traumatize the rectal mucosa sufficiently to cause hemorrhage, in which case the fecal masses are streaked with red blood.

Ultrasonography

Ultrasonography is a noninvasive diagnostic technique in which sound waves are passed into internal body structures; varying deflections of these sound waves are bounced back, much like a reflection. Reflections, in turn, are displayed on an oscilloscope. Vertical deflections from a horizontal baseline represent the depth of the reflected tissues. When scans are taken from several angles, and a computer is added to the system, a two-dimensional image of the abdominal organs can be produced. Usually, for abdominal examination, a transducer is placed on the abdomen after a coating of lubricant jelly has been applied to the skin.

The chief advantage of the ultrasonography is the spatial reproduction of masses in transverse and longitudinal directions. There is no ionizing radiation or any noticeable biological side-effects in the energy range used for diagnostic purposes. It is relatively inexpensive. This type of diagnostic procedure is useful in studying the liver, pancreas, spleen, gallbladder, and retroperitoneal tissues.

Disadvantages include the following: (1) A high degree of skill is required of the operator. (2) This technique cannot be used when a structure to be examined lies behind bony tissue, which prevents passage of sound waves to deeper structures. (3) Gas in the abdomen or air in the lungs present a problem, since ultrasound is not well transmitted through gas or air.

Computed Body Tomography (CBT Scanning)

CBT is a diagnostic method in which a very narrow beam of x-ray is used to detect the density differences from very small cubes of tissue. These data are computerized and then reconstructed so that transverse cross sections of the body can be shown on a television monitor.

The indications for CBT scanning are diseases of the liver, spleen, kidney, pancreas, and pelvic organs. However, good detail depends on the presence of fat, which means that this diagnostic tool is not useful for very thin, cachectic individuals. Also, since a scanning time of 5 seconds is required, it is impossible to maintain complete stillness (e.g., heartbeat) during the procedure. Therefore, motion artifacts are produced and the results are a less than clear picture. Finally, radiation doses are appreciable.

▷ Bibliography

Books

Abbott MK. Invasive Radiologic Diagnostic Procedures. Philadelphia, FA Davis, 1978.

Bates B. A Guide to Physical Examination, 3rd ed. Philadelphia, JB Lippincott, 1983.

Delp MH and Manning RT. Major's Physical Diagnosis, 9th ed. Philadelphia, WB Saunders, 1981.

Gitnick GL. Practical Diagnosis: Gastrointestinal and Liver Disease. New York, John Wiley & Sons, 1979.

Grimes J and Iannopollo E. Health Assessment in Nursing Practice. Belmont, California, Wadsworth Health Sciences Division, 1982.

Sherman J and Fields S. Guide to Patient Evaluation. Garden City, New York, Medical Examination, 1982.

Sreenivas VI. Acute Disorders of the Abdomen: Diagnosis and Treatment. New York, Springer–Verlag, 1980.

Wolf S. Abdominal Diagnosis. Philadelphia, Lea & Febiger, 1979.

Articles

Beck M. Preparing your patient physically for an esophagogastroduodenoscopy. Nursing '81 1981 Feb; 11(2):15–16.

Beck M. Three more gastrointestinal tests and how to help your patient through each. Nursing '81 1981 May; 11(5):22–24.

Beck M. Two intestinal tests: One oral, one anal. Nursing '81 1981 July; 11(7):22, 24, 27.

Bush W, Mallarkey M, and Webb RL. Adverse reactions to radiographic contrast material. West J Med 1980 Feb; 132(2): 95–98.

Endoscopy and upper GI series. Am Fam Physician 1980 Mar; 21(3):182.

Gilbertson V et al. The earlier detection of colorectal cancers. Cancer 1980 June; 45(6):2899–2901.

Harvey CK. Protecting personnel from diagnostic x-ray. AORN J 1979 Oct; 30(4):612.

Hogan W et al. Endoscopic evaluation of inflammatory bowel disease. Med Clin North Am 1980 Nov; 64:1083–1102.

Lamphier T and Lamphier R. Upper GI hemorrhage: Emergency evaluation and management. Am J Nurs 1981 Oct; 81(10):1814–1817.

Lefall L. Colorectal cancer—prevention and detection. Cancer 1981 Mar; 47(3):1170–1172.

Leicester RJ et al. Flexible fiberoptic sigmoidoscopy as an out-patient procedure. Lancet 1982 Jan 2; 8262(1):34–35.

Liebermann TR and Barnes M. Gastrointestinal fiberoptic endoscopy: Diagnostic and therapeutic aspects. Surg Clin North Am 1979 Oct; 59(5):786–787.

Sterilization or disinfection of flexible fiberoptic endoscopes. AORN J 1979 Aug; 30(2):350–352.

Agency

National Institute of Arthritis, Metabolism and Digestive Diseases. National Institutes of Health, Bethesda, Maryland 20205

36

Gastrointestinal Intubation and Special Nutritional Management

▷ Gastrointestinal Intubation

Gastrointestinal intubation is the insertion of a short or long flexible rubber or plastic tube into the stomach or intestine via the mouth or nose. The purpose may be diagnostic, preventive, or therapeutic. Aspiration (suctioning) through this tube is achieved by various means: suction from a syringe, suction from an electric suction machine, or suction from a built-in wall suction outlet. Any solution to be administered through this tube may be poured from a syringe or delivered by drip regulated by gravity or an electric pump.

Short Tubes

A *nasogastric catheter,* or so-called short tube, is introduced through the nose or the mouth into the stomach. Two such short tubes are the Levin tube and the Salem sump tube.

Levin Tube.   The Levin tube (14 F.), is a single-lumen tube made of plastic or rubber, with holes near its tip. The tube is used to remove fluid and gas from the upper gastrointestinal system or to obtain a specimen of gastric contents for laboratory studies. It may also be the means of administering medications or feeding (gavage) directly into the gastrointestinal tract (Fig. 36-1).

The Levin tube usually has circular marks on the tubing; when the tube has been inserted into the stomach, the section at the patient's nostril is located between the second and third marks. Gas, and the fluids that collect in the stomach, may be removed by aspiration through the tube.

Gastric Sump Tube.   The gastric sump pump (Salem, VENTROL) is a radiopaque, clear plastic, double-lumen nasogastric tube (Fig. 36-2). It is used to decompress the stomach and keep it empty. The inner, smaller tube vents the larger suction–drainage tube to the atmosphere by means of an opening at the distal end of the tube. It is passed the same way as the Levin tube. It can protect gastric suture lines because, when used properly, the sump pump never allows the force of suction at the drainage "eyes," or outlets, to exceed 25 mm Hg, the level of capillary fragility.

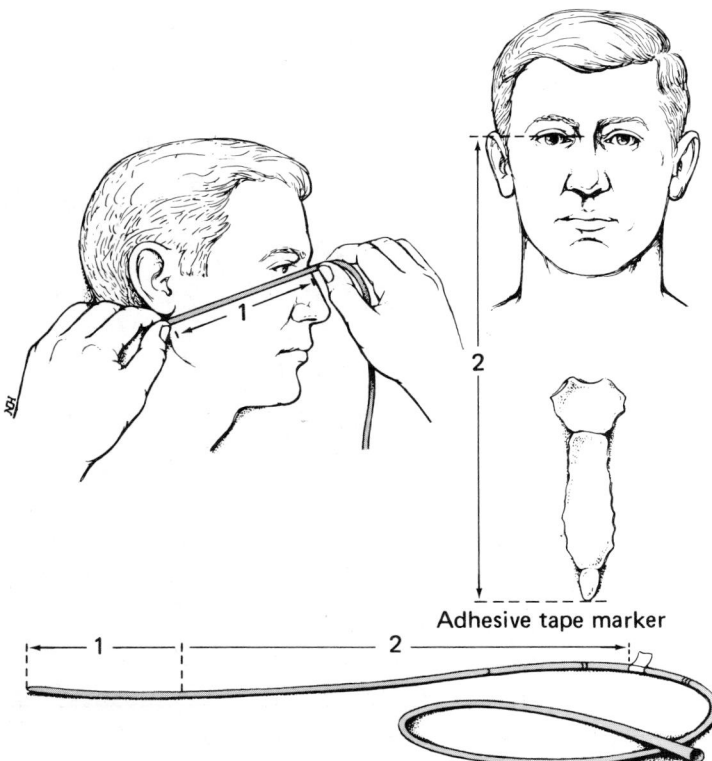

Figure 36-1. To measure the distance a Levin tube is to be passed in a patient to ensure passage into the stomach: (*1*) Measure the distance on the tube from the patient's tragus (ear lobe) to bridge of nose, plus (*2*) the distance from the bridge of the nose to the bottom of the xiphoid process. Mark this distance with a piece of adhesive tape. Note that the Levin tube usually has circular marks on the tubing; when it is in the patient's stomach, it is between the second and third marks.

Adhesive tape marker

This action is controlled by a small vent tube (blue pigtail). Continuous suction is set at a low of 30 mm Hg with the pigtail (usually blue) outlet kept open. If available suction is intermittent, rather than continuous, it may be set at 80 mm Hg to 120 mm Hg. Because of its cyclic setting, by the time suction reaches the gastric mucosa, it will be reduced to about 25 mm Hg.

To prevent reflux of gastric contents through the vent lumen (blue pigtail), the vent lumen is kept above the patient's midline; otherwise it will act as a siphon. Irrigation may be done through either the main lumen or the vent lumen; if the vent lumen is used, irrigation is followed with 10 ml of air, to clear the lumen.

Long Tubes

The *long tubes, or nasoenteric tubes,* are introduced through the nose, esophagus, and stomach into the intestinal tract. They are used to aspirate the intestinal contents to prevent gas and fluid distention of the coils of intestine (decompression).

The long tubes are the Miller–Abbott, the Harris, and the Cantor tubes. These are used in the active treatment of intestinal obstruction of the small intestine. They also are used prophylactically, being inserted the night before an abdominal operation to prevent obstruction after the operation. The intestine is threaded on the tube and so shortened, and held together compactly, making it relatively easier to pack off the intestine at the time of operation on the colon.

Because peristalsis either decreases or stops for 24 to 48 hours after an operation, owing to the effects of anesthesia and of visceral manipulation, nasogastric or nasoenteric suction prevents certain sequelae from developing. Fluids and flatus are evacuated, so that vomiting is prevented and tension reduced along the incision line. Edema, which can cause obstruction, is also reduced. Blood supply to the suture line is enhanced, thereby providing nutrition to the site. Usually, the tubes are allowed to remain in place after operation until peristalsis is resumed, as shown by the passage of gas by rectum.

Miller–Abbott Tube.   This is a double-lumen, No. 16 Fr., 3-meter (10-foot) tube, one lumen of which is used to introduce mercury or to inflate the balloon at the end of the tube; the other lumen, entirely independent, is used for aspiration. Before the tube is inserted, the balloon should be tested and its capacity measured; it is then deflated completely. The tube should be lubricated sparingly, and chilled well, before the tip is inserted through the patient's nose. Markings on the tube indicate the distance it has been passed.

Harris Tube.   This is a single-lumen, mercury-weighted tube of about 1.8 meters (6 feet), with a lumen of 14 Fr. This tube has a metal tip that is introduced first, into the nostril, after having been lubricated. The mercury-weighted bag follows. The weight of the mercury carries the bag by gravity. Since this is a single-lumen tube that is used wholly for suction and irrigation, there is no difficulty in irrigating it. Usually, a Y tube is attached to the end of the tube, so

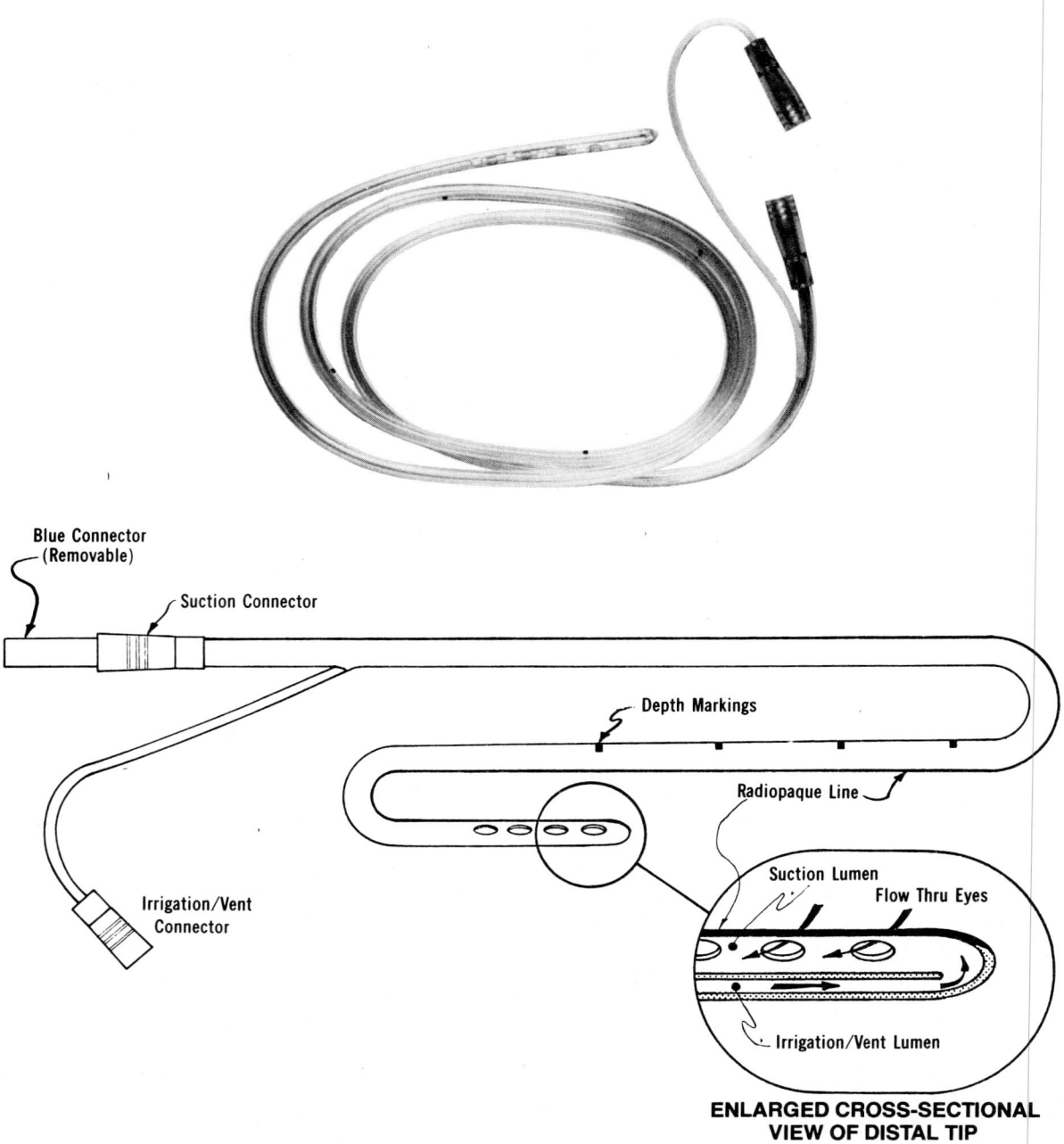

Blue Connector
(Removable)

Suction Connector

Depth Markings

Radiopaque Line

Irrigation/Vent
Connector

Suction Lumen

Flow Thru Eyes

Irrigation/Vent Lumen

ENLARGED CROSS-SECTIONAL
VIEW OF DISTAL TIP

Figure 36-2. The photograph and line drawing are of the VENTROL Levin (Sump) tube. Note the blown-up version showing the direction of flow for suction and irrigation. (National Catheter Co., Argyle, New York)

that the suction apparatus is attached to one side, and an outlet with a clamp is available on the other side for irrigating purposes.

Cantor Tube. The Cantor tube is 3 meters (10 feet) long, and No. 18 Fr. Its distinguishing feature is that it is larger than the other long tubes, and has 4 ml or 5 ml of mercury in the bag at the extreme end of the rubber tubing. Prior to insertion, the bag is wrapped about the tube. After the tube is lubricated, it is passed through the nostril and advanced to the esophagus (Fig. 36-3). The patient is in a sitting position and is offered sips of water to facilitate pas-

sage of the tube. Fluoroscopy is helpful in passing the tube into the duodenum.

Ewald Tube. This is a large-lumen gastric tube that can be passed through the mouth and into the stomach for the purpose of washing out poisons or aspirating large clots, or other substances, from the stomach.

Nursing Management

Goals for the patient requiring nasogastric or nasoenteric tubes are: (1) successful passage of the tube, (2) little or no fear or discomfort related to the presence of the tube,

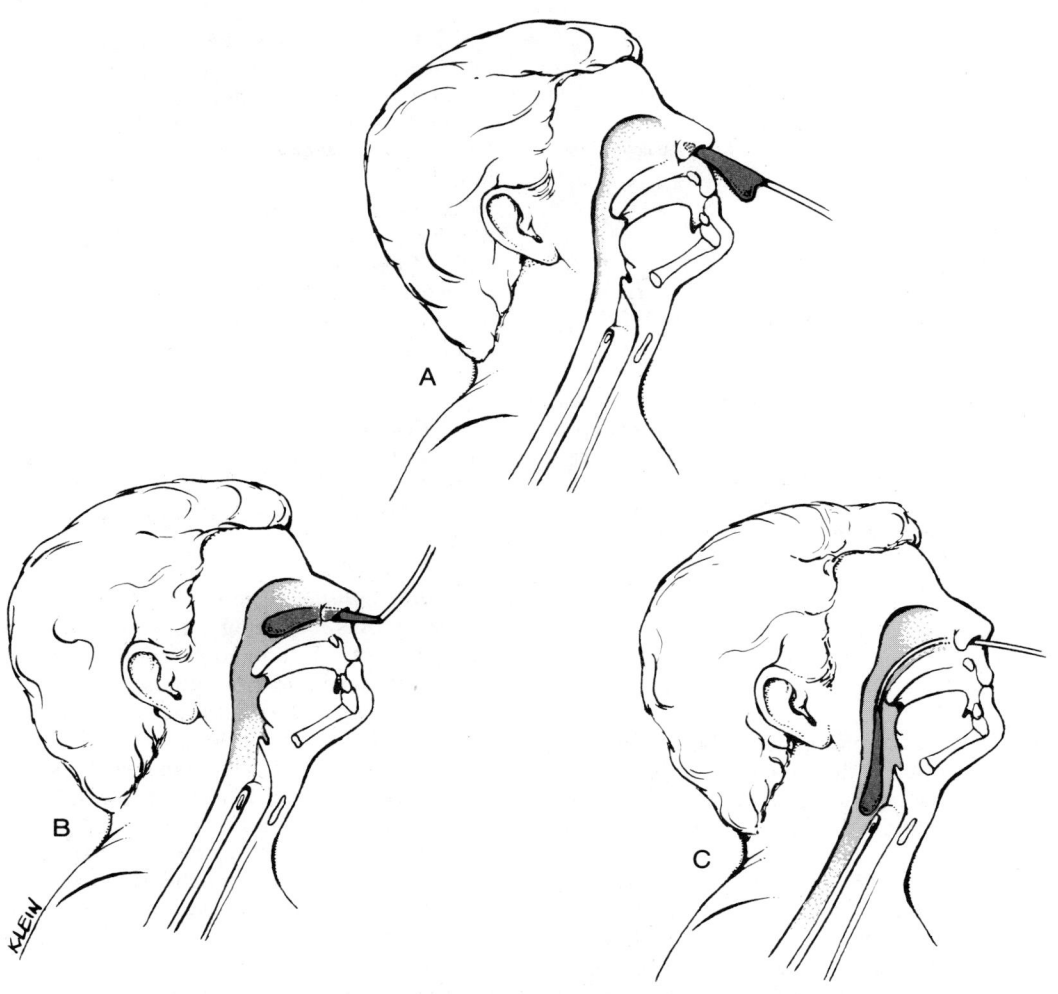

Figure 36-3. Passage of Cantor tube. (*A*) Tube with weighted mercury bag is introduced into the nostril. Note the natural tilt of the tubing. (*B*) After the mercury bag has entered the nostril, the catheter is tilted upward (head can also be tilted slightly upward) to facilitate gravity pull on the weighted bag. (*C*) The weight of the mercury pulls the bag downward. (Redrawn from Hardy JD: Rhoads Textbook of Surgery, 5th ed. Philadelphia, JB Lippincott.)

and (3) no complications related to nasogastric intubation and suction.

Nursing interventions can be organized into the following areas:

- Instruction regarding the purposes of the tube and the procedures required for insertion and advancement
- Insertion and advancement of the tube
- Care of the tube, including attachment, irrigation, and positioning of the patient
- Oral and nasal hygiene

Instruction.   Before the patient is intubated, the nurse explains the purpose of the tube. This information may make the patient more cooperative and tolerant of an initially unpleasant procedure. The general activities related to the passage of the tube are then reviewed, including the fact that the patient may have to breathe through his mouth and that passage of the tube may cause him to gag until the tube has passed his gag reflex.

Insertion of the Tube.   During insertion, the patient usually sits up with a towel spread bib-fashion over his chest. Tissue wipes should be available The patient is screened from other patients, and adequate light is provided. Occasionally, the physician will swab the nostril and spray the oropharynx with tetracaine hydrochloride (Pontocaine) to dull the nasal passage and the gag reflex and to make the procedure more tolerable. Gargling with a liquid anesthetic or holding ice chips in the mouth for a few minutes will have the same effect. Encouraging the patient to breathe through his mouth or pant often helps, as does swallowing water, if permitted.

A rubber nasogastric tube is sterilized and placed in a basin containing cracked ice for about 5 minutes before use, to make the tubing firm, rather than limp. (A plastic tube may need to be warmed to make it more pliable.)

After the end of the tube is lubricated with water-soluble jelly, the patient is instructed to tilt his head back while the tube is introduced through the nostril. When the tip is po-

Incorrect | Correct

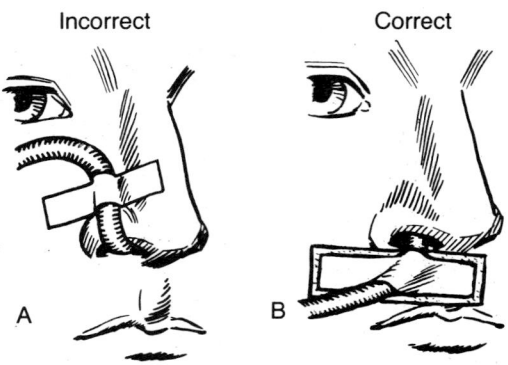

Figure 36-4. Nasogastric tube attachment. (*A*) Excessive pressure by the tube on the ala nasi should be avoided. (*B*) Satisfactory method for securing the tube, which will prevent injury to the nasopharyngeal passages. Method of tube fixation: apply a thin coat of tincture of benzoin to the area under the nose and place a strip of hypoallergenic tape on the prepared area. The nasogastric tube is fixed in position by anchoring it on top of the tape. By using this method, the nares may be cleaned frequently and the tube reanchored, without causing undue discomfort to the patient. (Adapted from Artz CP and Hardy JP: Complications in Surgery and Their Management. Philadelphia, WB Saunders.)

sitioned in the stomach, the nasogastric tube is secured to the nose, forehead, or above the upper lip (Fig. 36-4). In the case of nasoenteric intubation (the passage of a tube to the small or large intestine), the tube is not taped immediately.

Advancement of the Tube.   After the tube has passed through the pyloric sphincter, it may be advanced 5 cm to 7.5 cm (2–3 inches) every hour, so that gravity and peristalsis will aid in the passage of the tube. The patient is generally asked to lie on his right side for 2 hours, on his back for 2 hours, and then on his left side for 2 hours. Ambulation, if possible, also helps to advance the tube.

If the tube is advanced too rapidly, it will curl and kink in the stomach. If the position of the tube must be verified, the diaphragm of a stethoscope may be placed over the xiphoid process, while 5 ml to 10 ml of air are injected into the lumen of the tube, at which time a "whooshing" sound is heard. Another method is to aspirate the tube and check secretions with *p*H paper. If the *p*H is above 7 (alkaline), the tube is in the intestine; if below 7 (acid), the tube is still in the stomach. When the tube has been inserted the required distance, it is secured.

Tube Monitoring.   The nasogastric catheter is attached to the tube leading to the trap bottle, usually by a Y tube. The other end of the Y tube is attached to a small piece of rubber tubing closed by a clamp. Through this tube, irrigations of the nasogastric catheter may be done to ensure its patency. Otherwise, fluid or gas may accumulate, which can result in discomfort, vomiting, or abdominal distention. Repositioning the patient is another way of facilitating drainage. When double-lumen tubes are used, it is wise to note which tube is for irrigation and which for suction. To avoid tension on the tube, the tube line from the nose to the trap bottle is fixed in position on the bed, either with a safety pin threaded through the bed sheet or with adhesive-tape loops, tied or pinned to the bed.

Oral and Nasal Hygiene.   Regular and conscientious oral and nasal hygiene is a vital part of patient care, since the tube may be in place for several days. Applicator sticks dipped in water can be used to clean the nose. This can be followed by cleansing with water-soluble oil. Frequent mouth attention is comforting. If the nasal and pharyngeal mucosa is excessively dry, steam or cool vapor inhalations may be beneficial. Throat lozenges, an ice collar, chewing gum (if permitted), and frequent movement also assist in relieving discomfort. These activities will keep the mucous membranes moist and will help prevent infection of the parotid glands.

Evaluation

Patients undergoing suction decompression are susceptible to a variety of problems, including fluid volume deficit, pulmonary complications, and parotitis, which require careful evaluation.

Fluid Volume Deficit

1. Symptoms indicating a fluid volume deficit include:
   - Dryness of skin and mucous membranes
   - Decreasing urinary output
   - Lethargy and exhaustion
   - Drop in body temperature
2. Assessment of fluid volume deficit involves maintaining an accurate record of the following:
   - Drainage—amount, color, and type, every 8 hours
   - Amount of fluid instilled by irrigation of the nasogastric catheter, and the amount of water taken by mouth. An isotonic solution, such as normal saline, is used for irrigations in order to avoid electrolyte loss through gastric drainage.
   - Amount and character of vomitus, if any
   - Duration of any period in which the suction apparatus did not appear to function
   - Effects produced by the treatment

Pulmonary Complications

1. It has been shown that nasogastric intubation produces a higher incidence of postoperative pulmonary complications by interfering with coughing and clearing of the pharynx.
2. The nurse examines the lung fields regularly, through auscultation, to determine the presence of congestion. In addition, this patient is encouraged to cough and to take deep breaths regularly. The nurse also carefully confirms the proper placement of the tube before instilling any fluids.

Parotitis

1. When administering oral hygiene, the nurse carefully inspects the mucous membranes for signs of irritation or excessive dryness. In addition, she palpates the area around the parotid glands to detect any soreness or lumps, and any skin or mucous membrane irritation or necrosis.
2. The nostrils, oral mucosa, esophagus, and trachea are susceptible to irritation and necrosis. Visible areas are inspected frequently and the adequacy of hydration

assessed. In addition, the patient is assessed for the presence of esophagitis and tracheitis. Symptoms include sore throat and hoarseness.

Removal of Tube. When it is desirable to remove the tube, it is necessary to deflate the balloon and withdraw it, gently and slowly, for about 15 cm to 20 cm (6–8 inches), at intervals of 10 minutes, until the tip reaches the esophagus, when the remainder is withdrawn rapidly from the nostril. If the tube does not come out easily, force should not be used—notify the physician.

As it is withdrawn, the tube is concealed in a towel, because the sight of it may cause the patient to vomit. After removal of the tube, the patient will be grateful for good mouth care.

▷ Nasogastric Tube Feedings

Tube feedings are given to meet nutritional requirements when oral intake is inadequate or not possible. Table 36-1 summarizes the numerous conditions requiring enteral nutrition. Liquid formulas are designed to improve nutritional intake by either oral or tube administration. In the past, hospital tube feedings were based on various combinations of milk and cream. However, many patients showed poor tolerance of such feedings by displaying symptoms of diarrhea, flatulence, fullness, borborygmi, and even nausea and vomiting. This intolerance may be directly related to lactase deficiency. Such a deficiency has been demonstrated in 6% to 20% of white Americans and 60% of black Americans. The result has been modifications in formulas, and reliance on commercially prepared synthetic liquid diets. Such products vary greatly in cost and composition, completeness of nutritional content, presence of "residue," lactose, amino acids, and other nutrients.

Commercial formulas frequently present problems because the composition is "fixed." Some patients may not be able to tolerate certain ingredients, such as sodium, protein, or potassium. "Modular" diets can be prepared commercially, and the critical constituents sodium, potassium, or fat can be added by the dietitian. Attention should be given to including all essential minerals and vitamins. Total intake of calories and nutrients needs to be assessed when there is a reduction in total intake, or excessive dilution, of feedings.

Dehydration and azotemia (an excess of urea and other nitrogenous wastes in the blood) may occur from high-protein mixtures or from those lacking fat. Additional fluid should be given, so that the desired urinary output is maintained and waste products are excreted. Fat, in the form of highly unsaturated vegetable oils, may be added.

Diarrhea may occur if feedings are administered cold or too rapidly, or if the formula is high in osmolality (owing to excessive amounts of sugars, free amino acids, and electrolytes), or if there is bacterial contamination. A point to remember regarding contamination is that adding raw eggs to the mixture may carry a danger of introducing *Salmonella* contaminants.

Many patients are highly resistant to tube feedings, particularly those feedings administered via nasogastric intu-

Table 36-1
Conditions Requiring Enteral Nutrition

Condition or Need	Cause
Preoperative preparation with elemental diet	——
Gastrointestinal problems with elemental diet	Fistulae, short bowel syndrome, Crohn's disease, ulcerative colitis, nonspecific maldigestion or malabsorption
Cancer therapy	Radiation, chemotherapy
Convalescent care	Surgery, injury, severe illness
Coma, semiconsciousness*	Stroke, head injury
Hypermetabolic conditions	Burns, trauma, multiple fractures, sepsis
Alcoholism, chronic depression, anorexia nervosa*	Chronic illness, psychiatric or neurologic disorder
Debilitation*	Senility, disease
Maxillofacial or cervical surgery	Disease or injury
Oropharyngeal or esophageal paralysis*	Disease or injury
Mental retardation*	——

* Some of these patients will be at risk for regurgitating or vomiting and aspirating administered formula. Accordingly, each case must be considered individually.

(From Jensen T. Home enteral nutrition. Dietetic Currents, Ross Timesaver 9:15–20, July–Aug 1982.)

bation. Often a medium- or fine-bore Silastic tube is tolerated better than a plastic or rubber tube. The finer-bore tube, however, requires a finely dispersed formula, to prevent the tube from clogging.

Jensen notes that a wide variety of formulas, containers, feeding tubes and catheters, delivery systems, and pumps are currently available for use in tube or enteral feedings. She identifies the following issues as important when considering the most appropriate formula and delivery system for a given patient: nutrient sources, concentrations, osmolality, viscosity, and mineral content of a given formula, as well as the method and rate of administration, patient dexterity, available storage and refrigerator space, and cost of the formula and supportive equipment.

Some feedings are given as supplements, and others are provided to meet the patient's total nutritional needs. Nutritionists must work closely with physicians and nurses in determining the best formula for the individual patient.

▶ Nursing Assessment

The nurse generally participates in the assessment of patients with suspected nutritional problems. A preliminary assessment should answer the following questions:

1. What is the patient's nutritional status as judged by his current physical appearance; dietary history, including a history of food intolerance; and recent weight loss or gain?
2. Are there any existing chronic illnesses or situations that will increase metabolic demands on the body?
3. Is his fluid and electrolyte balance in order?
4. Is his digestive tract functioning? Does it have good absorptive capacity?
5. Are his kidneys and urinary system adequate?
6. What medications is he on, and what other therapy is he receiving that may affect his digestive intake and digestive system?
7. Does the dietary prescription fulfill his needs?

In addition, a more elaborate assessment is done on those patients who may require extensive nutritional therapy. This is done by a team that includes the nurse, physician, and nutritionist. In addition to the history and physical examination, nutritional assessment consists of recording any weight change, determining serum albumin and transferrin levels, total lymphocyte count, testing for delayed hypersensitivity reaction, and evaluating muscle function.

Patient Problems/Nursing Diagnoses

Based on the clinical manifestations and diagnostic assessment data, the patient's major nursing problems may include an alteration in nutritional status related to inadequate intake of nutrients; potential for development of complications related to tube feedings; and potential nonadherence to tube feeding regimen related to inadequate knowledge or skill or nonacceptance of the need for tube feedings.

▶ Planning and Implementation

Goals

The major goals for the patient include:

1. Attainment and maintenance of nutritional balance
2. Absence of complications related to tube feedings
3. Adherence to the tube feeding regimen

Interventions

The nurse must administer the feedings and teach the patient and his family about the purposes of the feedings, and, if appropriate, how to mix and administer them in preparation for home use. If the patient is alert and sitting, or in a low Fowler's position, and has normal gastric functioning, nasogastric feedings are generally safe. However, rapid release of formula into the small intestine can result in diarrhea, pain, and weakness ("dumping syndrome"). If gastric emptying is delayed or if the formula is administered too rapidly or too frequently, reflux can occur with aspiration of gastric contents. The nurse must therefore carefully monitor the rate of drip and avoid too rapid administration of fluids. Electrical pumps to control the rate and pressure of the delivery of viscous fluids are available. Most of these intravenous pumps are relatively heavy and must be attached to an IV pole. This can limit ambulation; several pumps

designed specifically for enteral tube feedings that are lightweight and easy to handle and that require minimal instruction for use are currently being developed and marketed.

Residual gastric content should be checked before each feeding. (This solution is returned to the patient.) If the amount of aspirated gastric content is greater than 150 ml, the feeding should be delayed and the patient reassessed in 2 hours. If this occurs twice, the physician is notified.

Before and after the administration of tube feedings, about 50 ml of water are administered in order to assure tube patency and to decrease the chance of bacterial growth and tube crusting or occlusion.

Continuous monitoring of the tube-feeding regimen is necessary to determine its effectiveness.

* Assess placement of tubing, position of patient, and flow rate.
* Observe patient's ability to tolerate the formula (assess for feeling of fullness, bloating, urticaria, nausea, vomiting, diarrhea, and constipation).
* Check clinical responses, as noted in laboratory findings: blood urea nitrogen, hemoglobin, serum protein, and hematocrit.
* Assess the patient's general condition by noting the appearance of the skin (turgor, dryness, color) and mucous membranes; urinary output; state of hydration; and weight gain or loss.
* Determine psychosocial adjustment to nasogastric feedings: Is the patient comfortable, tolerant, annoyed, relaxed or tense, troubled?
* Determine patient's and family's need for further teaching about methods of administration, refrigeration, preparation, and ability to obtain formula in a home setting. Printed instructions related to home care are generally available in most hospitals, and the nurse reviews these instructions with the patient and family before discharge.
* Determine whether adequate arrangements have been made for follow-up care in the community setting (*e.g.,* physician, visiting nurse, and nutritionist).

▶ Evaluation

Expected Outcomes

1. Attains/maintains nutritional balance
   a. Has positive nitrogen balance
   b. Hematologic diagnostic studies within normal limits (*i.e.,* BUN, hemoglobin, hematocrit, serum protein)
   c. Attains or maintains desired body weight
   d. Attains or maintains hydration of body tissue
2. Is free of complications related to tube feedings
   a. Tolerates formula used for tube feeding
   b. Has no gastric distention, nausea, vomiting, diarrhea, constipation
   c. Urinary output adequate for excretion of nitrogenous wastes
   d. Shows no signs of aspiration pneumonia or respiratory distress; has normal breath sounds and negative chest x-ray

▷ Gastrostomy

This operation is performed to create an opening into the stomach for the purpose of administering food and fluids. In some instances, it may be used for prolonged nutrition, as in the elderly or debilitated patient. Gastrostomy is preferred to nasogastric feedings in the comatose patient because the cardioesophageal sphincter remains intact. Also, regurgitation may occur in nasogastric feedings, but is less likely in gastrostomy.

When an impermeable stricture of the esophagus exists, the gastrostomy opening may be permanent. The esophageal stricture may be due to scar-tissue contracture. In children, it occurs often as a result of lye burns, and in older people it is usually due to a carcinomatous growth.

Preoperative Preparation

The purpose of the operative procedure should be explained to the patient so that he will have a better understanding of his postoperative course. He needs to know that the purpose of this surgery is to bypass his esophagus, and that liquid feedings will be administered directly into the stomach by means of a rubber or plastic tube or a prosthesis. If the prosthesis is to be permanent, the patient should be aware of it. Psychologically, this is often difficult for the patient to accept; however, when the procedure is being done to relieve discomfort, prolonged vomiting, debilitation, and the inability to eat, it is more acceptable.

Postoperative Care

Postoperative nursing intervention includes providing adequate food and fluids, tube and skin care, psychological support, and teaching about self-care responsibilities.

Food and Fluids. The first fluid nourishment is given by the surgeon soon after surgery. This is usually tap water and 10% glucose. At first only 30 ml to 60 ml (1 oz–2 oz) are given at a time, but the amount is gradually increased. By the second day, from 180 ml to 240 ml (6 oz–8 oz) may be given at one time, provided it is tolerated and if there is no leakage of fluid around the tube. In some clinics, in the early postoperative period the nurse aspirates gastric secretions and reinstills them, after adding enough feeding to bring the volume to the desired total. By this method, gastric dilatation is avoided.

Blended foods are gradually added to clear liquids until a full diet is reached. Powdered feedings that are easily liquefied are commercially available. However, a food blender can be used to liquefy a normal diet, which can then be fed through the tube. Blenderized tube feedings allow the patient to follow his usual diet pattern, which proves to be psychologically more acceptable. In addition, good bowel function is promoted, since the fiber and residue are similar to that of a normal diet. Excessive intake of milk is to be avoided in patients with lactase deficiency.

In preparing the patient for his gastrostomy feeding, assure his privacy by closing the door or drawing the curtains before the gastrostomy tube is uncovered. Check the patency of the tube by administering water at room temperature. Repeat the procedure at the end of the feeding to clear the tube of food particles, which could decompose

if allowed to remain in the tube. The meal should be served at room, or near body, temperature. A funnel or barrel of a syringe is used to introduce the liquid into the catheter. Tilting the receptacle will enable air to escape, rather than being trapped in the stomach (Fig. 36-5). The feeding should be allowed to flow into the stomach by gravity. The rate of flow can be regulated by raising or lowering the receptacle or by using an electric pump. If there seems to be an obstruction, stop the feeding and report the problem.

Record the amount and contents of each feeding, as well as the patient's reaction. Usually 300 ml to 500 ml are given for each meal and should require 10 or 15 minutes to complete. The amount is often determined by the patient's reaction. If he feels "full" it may be desirable to give smaller amounts more frequently. Keeping the head of the bed elevated for at least a half hour after feeding facilitates digestion.

Some patients smell, taste, and chew small amounts of food before taking their tube feedings. This procedure stimulates the flow of salivary and gastric secretions, and it may give the patient some sensation of normal eating. The chewed food is then deposited by the patient into a funnel attached to his gastrostomy tube and not swallowed. This may be a messy process, unacceptable to the patient, or it may be tolerated if privacy is provided. In addition to its effects on digestion, the stimulation of saliva promotes mouth care.

Tube and Skin Care. After 5 or 6 days, the tube may be removed, if loose, and a fresh one inserted after being lubricated with a thin coating of petrolatum. The tube is held in place by a thin strip of adhesive that is first twisted about the tube and then firmly attached to the abdomen. A catheter plug or rubber-tipped hemostat may close the outlet of the tube immediately following a feeding, to prevent leakage. This can also be facilitated by having the patient relax for a short time after his feeding. A small dressing is applied over the tube outlet; the tube is coiled on a dressing and is held in place by Montgomery straps or a firm abdominal binder. Thereafter, the tube should be changed every 2 or 3 days and the patient taught how to do this for himself. Once the opening into the stomach has been established, there is no need for sterile technique in changing and introducing a gastrostomy tube, which may be reinserted only when a feeding is given. However, items are to be thoroughly clean.

The patient can learn how to feed himself and what foods may be taken. Evaluation of the patient's knowledge of tube care and his dexterity in handling the tube and dressing changes begins while the patient is hospitalized. Family members should be included in these activities, as they may have to take an active role in care after discharge.

The skin about a gastrostomy opening requires special care. It may become irritated owing to the enzymatic action of gastric juices that leak around the tube. If uncared for, the skin becomes macerated, red, raw, and painful. Daily washing with soap and water around the tube, and the application of a bland ointment such as zinc oxide or petrolatum, are protective measures.

After several weeks, the tube may be removed and reinserted 10 cm to 15 cm (4–6 inches) for feedings. Between

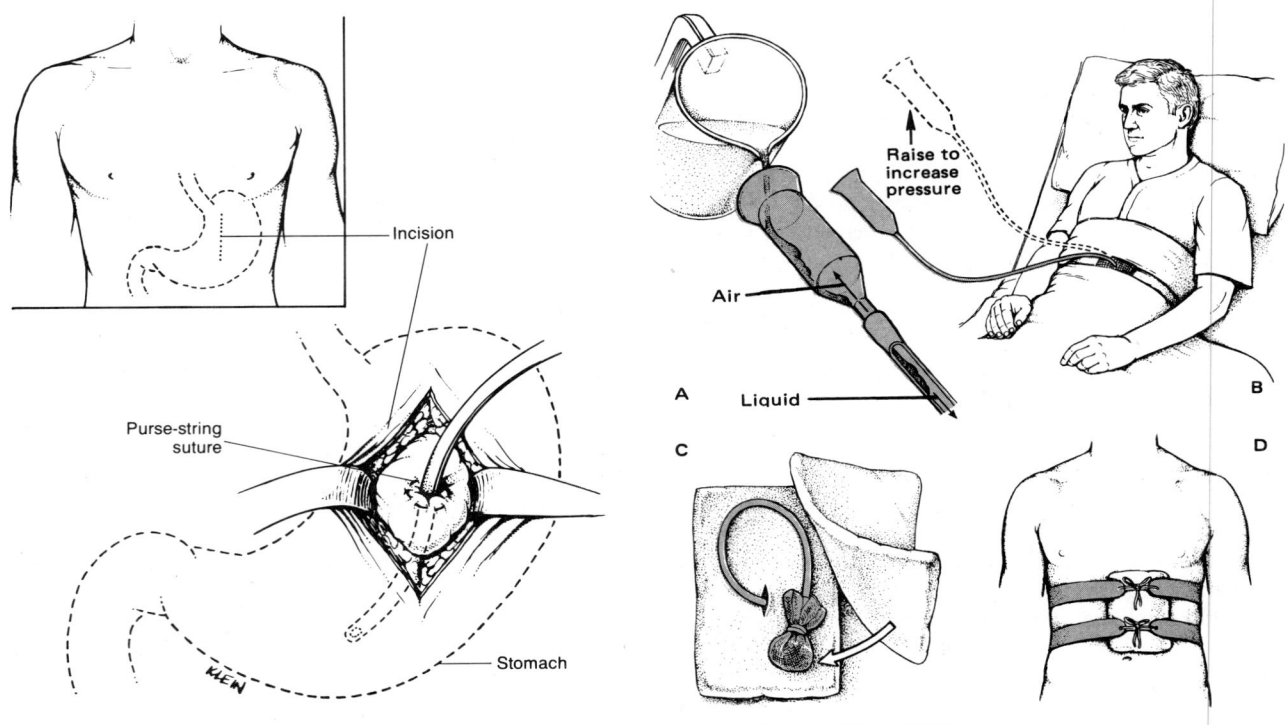

Figure 36-5. The patient with a gastrostomy. (*Left*) The drawing at the top shows the site of incision. A tube is inserted into the anterior gastric wall and held in place with several purse-string sutures, as shown below. (*Right*) Gastrostomy feeding. (*A*) Proper method of tilting the receptacle to permit air to escape. (*B*) Raising the receptacle increases the pressure. (*C*) After the feeding, opening of tube is covered with sterile gauze square held by rubber bands, and tubing is coiled on dressing. (*D*) Tubing is covered with dressing or abdominal pad held with Montgomery straps.

times, the gastrostomy opening may be protected by a small gauze pad, held in place by adhesive.

Skin status is evaluated daily for signs of breakdown, irritation, or excoriation. The patient and family members should be encouraged to participate in this inspection and in hygiene activities.

Psychosocial Considerations

The patient with a gastrostomy has had a major assault on his body image. A normal body function, eating, can no longer be taken for granted. Adjusting to this change takes time and requires family support and acceptance. An evaluation of the existing family support system is necessary, and the nurse may need to provide for postdischarge support through the community nurse or the social service worker. Also, gastrostomy as a therapeutic intervention is only done in the presence of a major, chronic, or perhaps terminal illness, and the stress of the existing illness is bound to be felt in the family system. Calm discussion regarding the purposes and routines of gastrostomy feeding and care can help avoid gastrostomy being an overwhelming situation.

Self-care Responsibility. To enhance self-care, the patient must be instructed properly in posthospital care and encouraged to establish as normal a routine as possible. These goals are achieved through teaching about tube feedings and tube and skin care and through ongoing evaluation

by questioning and return demonstrations. The patient (or other in the home setting) must view himself as capable and responsible for care; know the method and frequency of administration of self-care activities; and have adequate supplies, including the physical, financial, and social resources to maintain care. In addition to individual teaching, the use of printed instruction is necessary as a reinforcement. Adequate provision of needed supervision and support must be arranged.

▷ Enteral Therapy

Enteral tube feedings are delivered to the distal duodenum or proximal jejunum when it is necessary to bypass the esophagus and stomach. Enteral feedings can also be delivered by the following routes: nasoduodenal, esophagostomy, gastrostomy, and needle jejunostomy. Figure 36-6 demonstrates a small feeding tube passed transnasally into the stomach and distal to the pylorus. This approach can be used when it is possible to pass a tube (no esophageal or gastric obstruction) and when the gastrointestinal tract is functioning.

Rombeau and Barot conclude that the cost of enteral feeding by tube is comparable to the cost of purchasing, preparing, and delivering most standard hospital diets, and that it is a safe and effective method of nutrient delivery for extended periods of time. They suggest or propose that the advantages of enteral tube feedings are as follows:

- Intraluminal delivery of nutrients preserves gastrointestinal integrity
- Tube feedings preserve the normal sequence of intestinal and hepatic metabolism prior to nutrient delivery to the arterial circulation
- The intestinal mucosa and liver are important in fat metabolism and are the only sites of lipoprotein synthesis
- Normal insulin–glucagon ratios are maintained with the intestinal administration of carbohydrates

Osmosis and Osmolality.   Solutions that are highly concentrated and foods that have certain characteristics can upset the normal water balance within the body. Fluid balance is maintained by the process of *osmosis*. It is accomplished within the body by moving water through membranes from a dilute solution of lower osmolality to a more concentrated one of higher osmolality until the solutions are nearly of equal osmolality. The osmolality of normal body fluids is approximately 300 mOsm per kg. The body attempts to keep the osmolality of the contents of the stomach and intestines at approximately this level.

The proteins are extremely large particles and therefore have little or no osmotic effect. However, individual amino acids and carbohydrates are smaller particles and therefore have greater osmotic effect. Fats are not water soluble and do not form a solution in water; thus, they have no osmotic effect. Since electrolytes such as sodium and potassium are comparatively small particles, they have a great effect on osmolality, and consequently on tolerance.

Osmolality is an important consideration for patients being fed past the pylorus. When a concentrated solution of high osmolality is taken in large amounts, water will move to the stomach and intestines from fluid surrounding the organs and the vascular compartment. The patient experiences a feeling of fullness, nausea, and diarrhea, which can bring about dehydration, resulting, in some cases, in hypotension and tachycardia. Collectively, these symptoms have been given the name of "dumping syndrome." This problem can generally be alleviated by starting the patient on a more dilute solution and by increasing the concentration over several days.

There is a wide range of tolerance among patients as to the effects of osmolality. Usually, debilitated patients are more sensitive to such disorders. Therefore, the nurse should be knowledgeable about the osmolality of formulas and should observe and prevent such disorders.

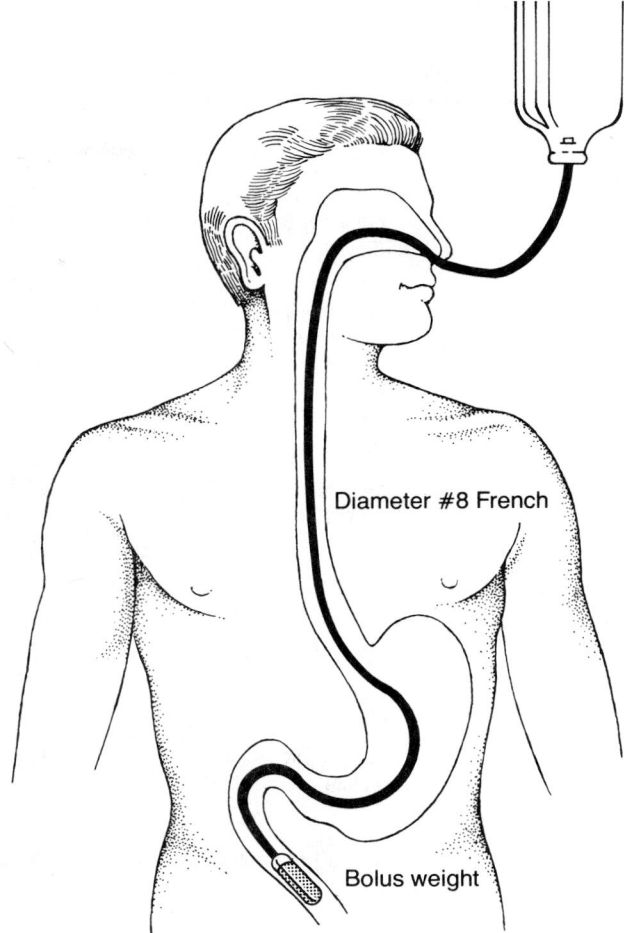

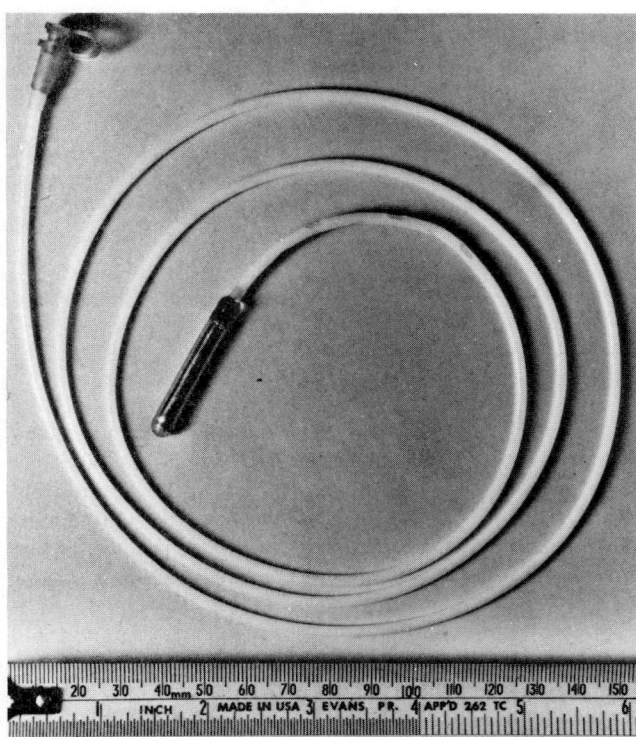

Figure 36-6.   The enteric feeding tube is small in diameter (No. 8 Fr.) and radiopaque, with mercury-filled bolus weight. It is passed easily through the nostril into the stomach and through the pylorus to allow continuous pump tube feeding in the distal duodenum or proximal jejunum. Made of polyurethane, it is sterilized with ethylene oxide. (The above Dubbhoff™ Enteric Feeding tube is a product of Biosearch Medical Products, Inc., Raritan, New Jersey.)

Table 36-2
Nutritionally Complete Liquid Diets*

Protein Source	Product	mOsm/kg	gm/1000 Kcal			
			Protein	Fat	CHO	Lactose
Intact protein	Compleat B (Doyle)	490	40.0	40.0	120.0	24.4
	Sustacal (Mead Johnson)	625	60.3	23.0	137.8	16.7
Protein isolates	Ensure (Ross)	450	35.0	35.0	136.7	0
	Isocal (Mead Johnson)	350	32.5	42.0	125.0	0
	Precision (Doyle)	300	30.0	31.3	150.0	0
	Renu (Organon)	330	33.0	40.0	130.0	0
Protein hydrolysates	Flexical (Mead Johnson)	723	22.4	34.0	154.0	0
Crystalline amino acids	Vivonex (Eaton)	500	20.4	1.4	226.3	0
	Vivonex HN (Eaton)	850	45.6	0.9	202.4	0

* Partial listing only
(From Rombeau J and Barot L. Enteral nutritional therapy. Surg Clin North Am 61:605–620, July 1981.)

Table 36-2 lists some of the commercially available, nutritionally complete liquid diets, including measures of their osmolality, protein, fat, carbohydrate, and lactose content.

Patient Preparation.   A discussion of the goals of care for patients receiving tube feedings, including the passage of the tube, is found on page 770.

Management

When preparing and administering a tube feeding, it is essential that all measures of cleanliness be observed. Temperature of the feeding, volume of the feeding, flow rate, and adequate fluid intake are critically important.

The newer polyurethane or silicone rubber feeding tubes are of small diameter, No. 6 or 8, and have a mercury tip (rather than a weighted mercury-filled bag). A variety of tubes are available (Dobbhoff, Keofeed, MedPro), and each has instructions for ease of passage. Since they are softer, more pliable, and much thinner than the conventional nasogastric tube, they provide greater patient comfort. However, kinking of tubing may present a problem. A guide or other means of stiffening the tube may be recommended to ease its passage. Essentially, such a tube is passed in the same way as a nasogastric tube—that is, with the patient in high Fowler's position. If this is not feasible, place the patient on his right side.

Feedings are administered either by gravity (drip) or by continuous controlled pump that is either volumetric (ml/hour) or peristaltic (drops/hour). With jejunal feedings, continuous pump infusions are usually necessary. While little data are available to compare the effects of jejunal versus gastric tube feedings, Rombeau and Barot report that continuous jejunal infusion of a protein isolate is comparable to both intermittent and continuous gastric feedings in the percentage of kilocalories delivered and the number of days needed to meet full caloric intake.

The pump, preferably, is a small, simple finger-action pump that has a rechargeable battery and permits patient ambulation.* Feedings are lactose-free, with an osmolality of only 300 mOsm/kg; a feeding may be given undiluted and provides 1 calorie/ml. Feeding rates of about 100 ml/hour to 150 ml/hour (2400–3600 calories/day) are effective in inducing positive nitrogen balance and progressive weight gain, without producing abdominal cramps and diarrhea. If the feeding is intermittent, 200 ml to 350 ml are given in 10 to 15 minutes. Additional water after feeding is important to prevent hypertonic dehydration. At the beginning of administration, the feeding should be diluted to at least half the strength, and not more than 50 ml to 100 ml given at a time, or 40 ml/hour to 60 ml/hour in contin-

* IVAC pump Model 530, IVAC Corp., LaJolla, California.

uous drip administration. This gradual administration helps the patient to develop tolerance, especially for hyperosmolar solutions.

Nursing Assessment. An assessment of the nutritional status of the patient is done before enteral tube feedings are begun. In addition to the considerations discussed on page 771, an assessment should also include an evaluation of the patient's and family's need for information about this treatment.

Nursing Implementation

- The patient receiving enteral tube feedings should be in an upright position to avoid aspiration or reflux.
- If the patient is ambulatory, he is encouraged to walk, since movement facilitates absorption of the feeding. A portable pump and infusion standard can be used.
- Fluid balance is carefully recorded to identify decreased intake or excessive diarrhea.
- Fractional urine specimens are evaluated every 6 hours for sugar and acetone.
- Antidiarrheal medications are administered when needed.
- Feedings are delayed for 2 hours if gastric residual is greater than 150 ml. If this amount persists, the physician is notified.
- Weight is checked daily.

- The patient and family members are gradually included in these activities.

Guidelines for the nurse monitoring the management of tube-fed patients include:

- Watch for sudden gain in weight.
- Observe for signs of edema (periorbital or dependent puffiness).
- Observe for signs of dehydration (dry mucous membranes, thirst, decreased urine output).
- Record the actual formula intake by the patient, including incidents of vomiting and diarrhea or distension.
- Note any signs of inability of the patient to communicate.
- Test for urine glucose concentration (report +3 and +4 concentrations).
- Consult daily laboratory tests for blood urea nitrogen and serum electrolytes.
- Check the proper positioning of the tube.
- Watch for possible complications (see Table 36-3 for a summary of complications associated with enteral tube feedings, along with related interventions).
- Evaluate, through questioning and return demonstration, the level of knowledge, dexterity, and confidence of the patient and family in carrying out self-care activities. Determine need for postdischarge follow-up.

Table 36-3
Complications of Tube Feeding

Complication	Therapy
Mechanical	
Nasopharyngeal irritation	Ice chips, topical anesthetics, decongestants
Luminal obstruction	Flush, replace tube
Mucosal erosions	Reposition tube, ice water lavage, remove tube
Tube displacement	Replace tube
Aspiration	Discontinue tube feeding
Gastrointestinal	
Cramping/distention	Change formula if patient is lactose intolerant, reduce infusion rate
Vomiting/diarrhea	Reduce infusion rate, dilute formula, add anti-diarrheal agents
Metabolic	
Hypertonic dehydration	Increase free water
Glucose intolerance	Give insulin, reduce infusion rate
Hyperosmolar nonketotic coma	Discontinue tube feeding
Hepatic encephalopathy	Decrease amount of protein
Renal failure	Decrease phosphate, magnesium, potassium; protein restriction; essential amino acid solution
Cardiac failure	Reduce sodium content, fluid restriction

(From Rombeau J and Barot L. Enteral nutritional therapy. Surg Clin North Am 61:605–620, July 1981.)

Parenteral Hyperalimentation Therapy (Total Parenteral Nutrition—TPN)

When a patient's intake of nutrients is significantly less than that required by the body to meet energy expenditures, a state of *negative nitrogen balance* results. This means that protein utilization is greater than protein intake. Parenteral hyperalimentation is a method of supplying nutrients to the body by the intravenous route. The goals of hyperalimentation are to attain improved nutritional status and weight gain, and to improve healing ability.

Traditional intravenous feedings do not provide sufficient calories or nitrogen to meet the daily requirements of patients. In response, the body begins to convert protein to carbohydrates by the process of gluconeogenesis. However, hyperalimentation intravenous solutions contain water, amino acids, glucose, vitamins, and electrolytes in a concentration sufficient to provide the calories and nitrogen to meet the patient's daily nutritional needs.

The average adult postoperative patient requires approximately 1500 calories a day to spare body protein. If this patient has complications, such as fever, trauma, or hypermetabolic disease, he will require up to 10,000 additional calories daily. The amount of volume necessary to provide these calories would surpass fluid tolerance and lead to pulmonary edema or congestive heart failure. To provide the required calories in small volume, it is necessary to increase the concentration and use an avenue of administration that will rapidly dilute incoming nutrients to the proper levels of body tolerance.

When hypertonic glucose is administered, it satisfies caloric requirements and allows amino acids to be released for protein synthesis, rather than being utilized for energy. Additional potassium is added to provide proper electrolyte balance and to transport glucose and amino acids across the cell membranes. In order to prevent deficiencies and fulfill requirements for tissue synthesis, other elements, such as calcium, phosphorus, magnesium, and sodium chloride, are added.

The pharmacy department may prepare the prescribed nutritional intravenous solutions. These are mixed, utilizing strict aseptic precautions, under a filtered air laminar flow hood. Basically, the solution consists of 25% glucose and synthetic amino acids (FreAmine); this provides the patient with 1000 calories and 6 g of nitrogen per liter. Electrolytes are added as determined by the serum electrolyte needs of the individual patient. Solutions delivered to the unit are refrigerated until needed and then allowed to warm to room temperature. Formulas for local hospital use can be made for individual patients. Commercial preparations (Amigen, Aminosol, FreAmine, Hyprotigen C, and others) are available but also must be modified to meet individual needs.

Clinical Application

Clinical situations in which hyperalimentation is indicated include:

1. Patients whose intake is insufficient to maintain an anabolic state (*e.g.,* severe burns, malnutrition, short-bowel syndrome)

2. Patients unable to ingest food orally or by tube (*e.g.,* paralytic ileus, Crohn's disease with obstruction, postradiation enteritis)
3. Patients who refuse to ingest adequate nutrients (*e.g.,* anorexia nervosa, geriatric postoperative patients)
4. Patients who should not be fed orally or by tube (*e.g.,* acute pancreatitis, high enterocutaneous fistula)
5. Patients who need preoperative and postoperative nutritional support (*e.g.,* bowel surgery)

Certain criteria must be met before a patient receives total parenteral nutrition (*e.g.,* a 10% deficit in body weight; an inability to take oral food or fluids within 7 postoperative days; and hypercatabolic situations, such as major infection with fever).

Method of Administration

Because hyperalimentary solutions have about 5 or 6 times the solute concentration of blood (and exert an osmotic pressure of about 2000 mOsm per liter) they are injurious to the intima of peripheral veins. Therefore, to prevent phlebitis and other venous complications, these solutions are administered into the circulatory system by means of a large-bore needle or catheter inserted into a high-flow large blood vessel. Concentrated solutions are then diluted in this vessel, very rapidly, to isotonic levels.

The preferred route is the subclavian vein, which leads into the superior vena cava. An alternate route is the internal jugular to the superior vena cava. With long-term use, an indwelling catheter is a constant source of potential infection.

Nursing Management

Nursing goals are (1) to maintain the integrity of the system; (2) to avoid contamination and to maintain the sterility and patency of the indwelling catheter; (3) to administer the prescribed infusion at a constant rate over the 24-hour period; (4) to monitor the fluid balance; (5) to carefully assess for potential problems and to initiate preventive measures; (6) to maintain a therapeutic nurse–patient relationship; and (7) to prepare the patient and responsible family members to assume self-care activities if the patient is to be discharged on home hyperalimentation therapy.

Patient Preparation. The procedure is explained to the patient so that he realizes the importance of not touching the area where the catheter is inserted and is aware that he will be able to be ambulatory during the extended time of therapy. For the procedure, the patient is placed supine, in Trendelenburg's position (to produce dilatation of neck and shoulder vessels, which makes entry easier and prevents air embolus). A rolled sheet is placed vertically along the vertebral column, from the neck to the end of the rib cage, in order to hyperextend the shoulders. The area is shaved, if necessary, and the skin prepared with acetone or ether to remove surface oils. Final skin preparation includes scrubbing with tincture of iodine or povidone–iodine solution. The patient is instructed to turn his head facing to the side opposite from the site of venipuncture; he is to remain motionless while the catheter is inserted and the wound dressed, so as to afford maximum accuracy in the placement of the tube.

782

Insertion of the Catheter.
Sterile drapes are applied. Procaine or lidocaine is injected for local anesthesia into the skin and underlying tissues. The target area is the inferior border at midpoint of the clavicle (Fig. 36-7). A No. 14, 5-cm (2-inch) needle on a syringe is inserted and moved

parallel to and beneath the clavicle u⟋ clavian vein. The syringe is then ⟋ (8-inch), 16-gauge radiopaque cathetᴇ the needle into the vein; the needle is witʜ syringe is detached from the needle and the ⟍

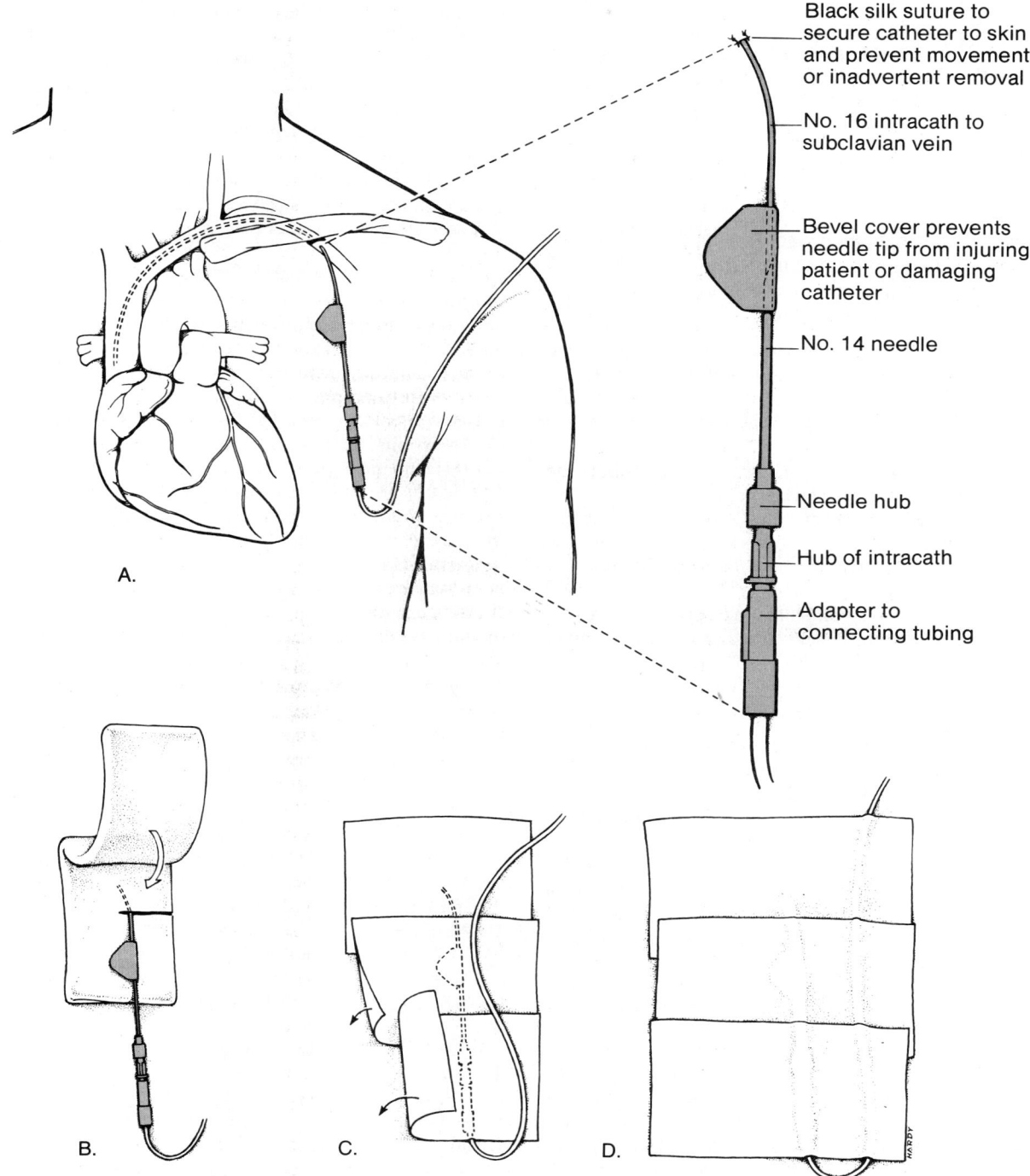

Black silk suture to secure catheter to skin and prevent movement or inadvertent removal

No. 16 intracath to subclavian vein

Bevel cover prevents needle tip from injuring patient or damaging catheter

No. 14 needle

Needle hub

Hub of intracath

Adapter to connecting tubing

A.

B.

C.

D.

Figure 36-7. Hyperalimentation. (*A*) Note insertion of needle into subclavian vein (*B*) A split sterile dressing accommodates intracatheter. Covering this split dressing is another sterile dressing. (*C*) Adhesive dressings complete the occlusive dressing. (*D*) Completed dressing.

erted, the patient may be asked to perform the Valsalva maneuver. (To do this, he is instructed to bear down with his mouth closed. Compression of the abdomen may also accomplish the maneuver.) The Valsalva maneuver is done to produce a positive phase in the central venous pressure in order to lessen the possibility of air being drawn into the circulatory system.

The intracatheter is attached to tubing from a 250-ml flask of 5% dextrose in water. The catheter is usually sutured to the skin. The position of the tip of the catheter may be checked at this point by x-ray to confirm its location before the hyperalimentation solution is administered. Following this, the area is again swabbed with germicide solution, and antibiotic ointment is applied directly to the insertion site. A spray of tincture of benzoin to a liberal area precedes the application of a 5-cm (2-inch) adhesive strip to provide an occlusive dressing.

Nursing Implementation and Evaluation. There are several potential complications related to the insertion of a central venous catheter. The nurse must observe the patient for these problems:

- Pneumothorax, hydrothorax, or hemothorax (related to inadvertent puncture of the pleura and apex of the lung). Observe for symptoms of chest or back pain, cough, dyspnea, shortness of breath, changes in vital signs, and decrease in breath sounds or in lung expansion.
- Subclavian artery or thoracic duct injury (subclavian artery is adjacent to subclavian vein, and thoracic duct empties into left subclavian vein). Observe incision site and dressings for leakage of blood or lymph. Note vital sign change. Observe for asymmetrical swelling or motor asymmetry.
- Motor-sensory deficit (brachial plexus located in region of catheter insertion). Check arm and hand on catheter insertion side.

Maintenance of Fluid and Electrolyte Balance. A continuous, uniform infusion of hyperalimentation fluid over a 24-hour period is desired. An electrical pump (*e.g.,* Imed infusion pump) is used to achieve this, but the nurse is responsible for seeing that the appropriate amount of solution is infused.

The infusion rate is calculated on the basis of amount of fluids prescribed over a 24-hour period. This rate must be maintained *consistently* (*e.g.,* 3000 ml for 24 hours = 125 ml per hour). The rate is checked every 30 minutes. Intravenous alarm controllers may be used. If the rate increases or decreases, the infusion rate may be speeded up or slowed down by not more than 10% of the original rate (unless otherwise requested by physician) in order to compensate.

- If the rate is too rapid, hyperosmolar diuresis occurs (excess sugar will be excreted), and if severe enough may cause intractable seizures, coma, and death. (Fractional urine determinations, using Clinitest tablets or test tapes, may be done every 6 hours to monitor excess excretion of sugar, and specific gravity of the urine may be done every 6 hours to evaluate adequacy of fluid intake.) Symptoms of rapid fluid intake include headache, nausea, fever, chills, and increasing lassitude.

- If the flow goes too slowly, the patient does not get the maximum benefit of calories and nitrogen.

The patient is weighed daily at the same time, under the same conditions, for accurate comparison. Under this regimen, 0.11 kg to 0.45 kg (0.25 lb–1 lb) per day weight gain of lean body tissue can be expected. Accurate input and output records are kept, and if the patient also receives oral nutrients, this is recorded according to caloric count.

Prevention of Infection. The insertion site is to be kept dry under an air-occlusive dressing. Dressings or adhesive are not to be removed for 48 hours. The patient is encouraged to move from side to side or to ambulate as desired. However, he must be reminded not to touch the dressings. If they bother him or cause itching, he is to report this.

Vital signs are checked every 4 hours, and temperature elevations are reported. Special care is given to draining wounds, fistulas, and pressure areas.

Procedure for Dressing Change

Inform the patient that his dressings are to be changed every other day, and have him lie in a low Fowler's position. The nurse and patient may reduce the possibility of airborne contamination by wearing masks. Remove old dressings very carefully, to prevent the catheter from becoming dislodged. Check the area for leakage, kinked catheter, and skin reactions, such as inflammation, pain, or purulence. Using sterile gloves, cleanse the area with acetone, followed by tincture of iodine or thimerosal (Merthiolate), with the aid of a sponge holder and 3 × 3 gauze pledgets. Clean from the center, moving outward. Alcohol may be used in the same manner, to remove iodine. Apply antibiotic ointment to the insertion site and cover with a small dressing, slit to fit around the catheter. Remove the gloves and apply tincture of benzoin to the skin area around the sterile dressing to protect the skin and to facilitate the application of an adhesive tape (Elastoplast) occlusive dressing. Rapidly replace the intravenous tubing, including piggyback lines, to prevent buildup of organisms along the lumen of the inner tubing. Replace the filter, if required. Cover the union of the catheter and tubing to prevent separation and to avoid exposure to air. Secure with adhesive tape.

If the patient has a draining wound, such as a tracheostomy, in the nearby area, additional precautions are taken to keep the wound dry by applying transparent, plastic operating-room adhesive drape over the dressings, to insure waterproofing. Use hypoallergenic adhesive tape if the patient complains of itching from conventional tape. Record the dressing change, and report the condition of the local area as well as the patient's reaction.

Patient Medications and Activity

Administering medications through the main catheter so that they may mix with the nutritional solution is not recommended because of the possibility of incompatibility (insulin is an exception). If incompatible drugs must be given, they should be infused through a peripheral IV line, not by piggyback. Nor should transfusions of blood products be given through the main catheter, since red cells may possibly coat the lumen of the catheter, thereby reducing the flow of solution.

Table 36-4
Prevention and Management of Problems in Parenteral Hyperalimentation

Preventive Measures	Problem Situation	Implication	Nursing Action
Ensure occlusiveness of dressing. Assess status of dressing frequently.	*Dressing loosens* or comes off	Danger of contamination → infection	Reinforce with 5-cm (2-inch) tape. If question of contamination, reapply dressing.
Inspect each flask before using; note expiration date.	*Possible contamination* of solution; cloudy, floating particles	Solution is excellent culture medium Danger of contamination → infection, emboli	Replace flask at once. Send contaminated flask to pharmacy. Cultures are required. Adjust intake and output records.
Frequently examine tissues near insertion site; note patient complaints.	*Swelling* around insertion site; edema of face or neck; pain in shoulder or arm on side of intracatheter	Fluid infiltrating tissues	Slow infusion rate. Check vital signs. Notify physician.
Observe for signs of dyspnea, respiratory difficulty, pulmonary edema, congestive heart failure.	*Engorged veins* of neck, arm, hand on side of intracath	Circulatory overload and inadequate fluid distribution	Check vital signs and report all signs and symptoms to physician. Have resuscitative measures ready. Reassure patient.
Monitor the flow rate frequently (every half hour), so that it is constant.	*Fluid running too rapidly:* nausea, headache, lassitude	Hyperglycemia with glucosuria → cellular osmotic diuresis and extensive dehydration	Check vital signs. Notify physician. Slow infusion to newly calculated flow rate.
Make fractional urine determinations and check urine specific gravity every 6 hours. Observe for signs of hyperglycemia: nausea, headache, lassitude.	Test tapes show glucosuria Patient symptoms: agitation, twitching, convulsions, mental lethargy, semicoma, coma → death	Hypertonic overload → dehydration	Administer insulin, if prescribed (very small doses). Administer IV fluid (isotonic) relatively rapidly.
Check tubing for kinks. Monitor the flow rate frequently (every half hour). Observe for signs of hypoglycemia: general muscular weakness, restlessness, perspiration, vertigo, pallor, trembling, hunger pangs in epigastrium.	*Fluid running too slowly*	Hypoglycemia; patient not receiving adequate nutrition	Recalculate flow rate so that adjustment compensates for slowdown (not to exceed 10% without physician's direction). Avoid too rapid flow rate. Assess patient for symptoms of hypoglycemia.
Monitor flow rate regularly. Assess patient status frequently.	*Infusion runs dry*	Deficient nutrition Possibility of air embolus during flask replacement Backflow of blood into catheter, with possible clot formation and occlusion	Replace with next bottle. Remove air from tubing aseptically or change administration tubing completely.

(continued)

Table 36-4
Prevention and Management of Problems in Parenteral Hyperalimentation (continued)

Preventive Measures	Problem Situation	Implication	Nursing Action
Change catheter dressing with patient in low Fowler's to recumbent position. Change administration tubing rapidly and secure snugly, while patient performs Valsalva maneuver.	*Air embolus*	Segment of vascular system may be blocked, causing circulation cutoff Signs and symptoms: cyanosis; hypotension; rapid, weak pulse; elevated venous pressure; change in heart sounds → coma	Be alert for chest pain or fainting. Listen for air being sucked into catheter during change of tubing. Replace tubing immediately. Place patient on left side in Trendelenburg position. Keep him quiet and reassure him. Take vital signs; notify physician.
Monitor vital signs every 4 hours. Maintain strict aseptic practice at all times.	*Chills or fever*	Allergic reaction Sepsis: wound infection, caused by catheter, tubing, or solution Infection from patient's disease	Notify physician; be prepared to replace nutrient solution with 5% glucose in water. Check temperature every half hour until normal. Be prepared for possible discontinuance of hyperalimentation.
Record daily intake and output, as well as weight.	*No weight gain,* and possibly a weight loss	There must be a reason for this negative outcome; cancer?	Check daily weighing procedure for consistency in conditions.
Change position frequently. Observe for signs of redness over bony areas. Provide good skin care.	*Pressure sores*	Lying in one position too long	Institute appropriate nursing measures to treat reddened area.
Promote active and passive exercises to improve muscle strength.	*Loss of muscle strength*	Lack of exercise	Encourage range of motion exercises at least 3 times daily.
Encourage patient to verbalize feelings.	*Discouraged patient*	Inadequate understanding; lack of support	Provide psychosocial support and encouragement. Explain all aspects of therapy.
Be alert for signs of scaly skin, poor wound healing, increased capillary fragility, alopecia.	*Serum essential fatty acid deficiency*	Fatty acids not available to transport metabolites	Fat emulsions may be given daily to patients who have been on IV hyperalimentation for at least 2 weeks.
Assess patient's electrolyte levels.	*Deficiency or excess of nutritional essentials:* calcium, phosphate, sodium, potassium, magnesium, iron, copper, folic acid, vitamin A, vitamin D	Nutritional imbalance	Alert physician to initiate corrective measures.

- Blood is not aspirated from hyperalimentation tubing for blood studies unless it is a life-saving measure.
- Because of the danger of emboli, a small amount of heparin is flushed into the central venous catheter daily. (Dosage ranges from 800 units to 1000 units.)

Activities and ambulation are encouraged when the patient is physically capable of them. With a plastic catheter in the subclavian vein, the patient has freedom to move his extremities and should be encouraged to keep up good muscle tone. Reinforce the teaching and exercise program initiated in the occupational and physical therapy departments.

Problems and Dangers

Chemical imbalances may occur, which require frequent determinations of serum electrolytes (especially potassium) and glucose. Sepsis is a major problem, hence the special emphasis on strict aseptic technique throughout the procedure. Incompatibility and deterioration of various substances must be kept in mind.

Total intravenous alimentation is complicated and hazardous and should be limited to carefully selected patients. Careful monitoring and conscientious care by experienced physicians and nurses can reduce the risk of many complications.

Table 36-4 offers a summary of problems in parenteral hyperalimentation, along with suggestions for their prevention and management.

Discontinuance of Parenteral Hyperalimentation

Parenteral hyperalimentation is discontinued gradually to allow for adjustment to decreased levels of glucose. Following hypertonic solution, isotonic glucose is administered for several hours to protect against rebound hypoglycemia. Oral carbohydrates will shorten tapering time. Spe-

cific symptoms include weakness, faintness, sweating, shakiness, feeling cold, confusion, and increased heart rate.

Postoperative Hyperalimentation

The benefits of hyperalimentation in the postoperative patient are now being realized in combating the extensive catabolism and negative nitrogen balance that often follow a surgical procedure. A "lag phase" in wound healing is related to a negative nitrogen balance; this is associated with the deposition of immature collagen. By using a triple-lumen esophagogastric aspiration-duodenal feeding tube (Fig. 36-8), such as the G-Moss tube, it is possible to feed the patient and remove all swallowed air to avert postoperative ileus. The length of time the tube is in place varies with the nature of the surgery. In summary, the advantages of hyperalimentation in the immediate postoperative period in certain operative conditions are enhanced wound healing,

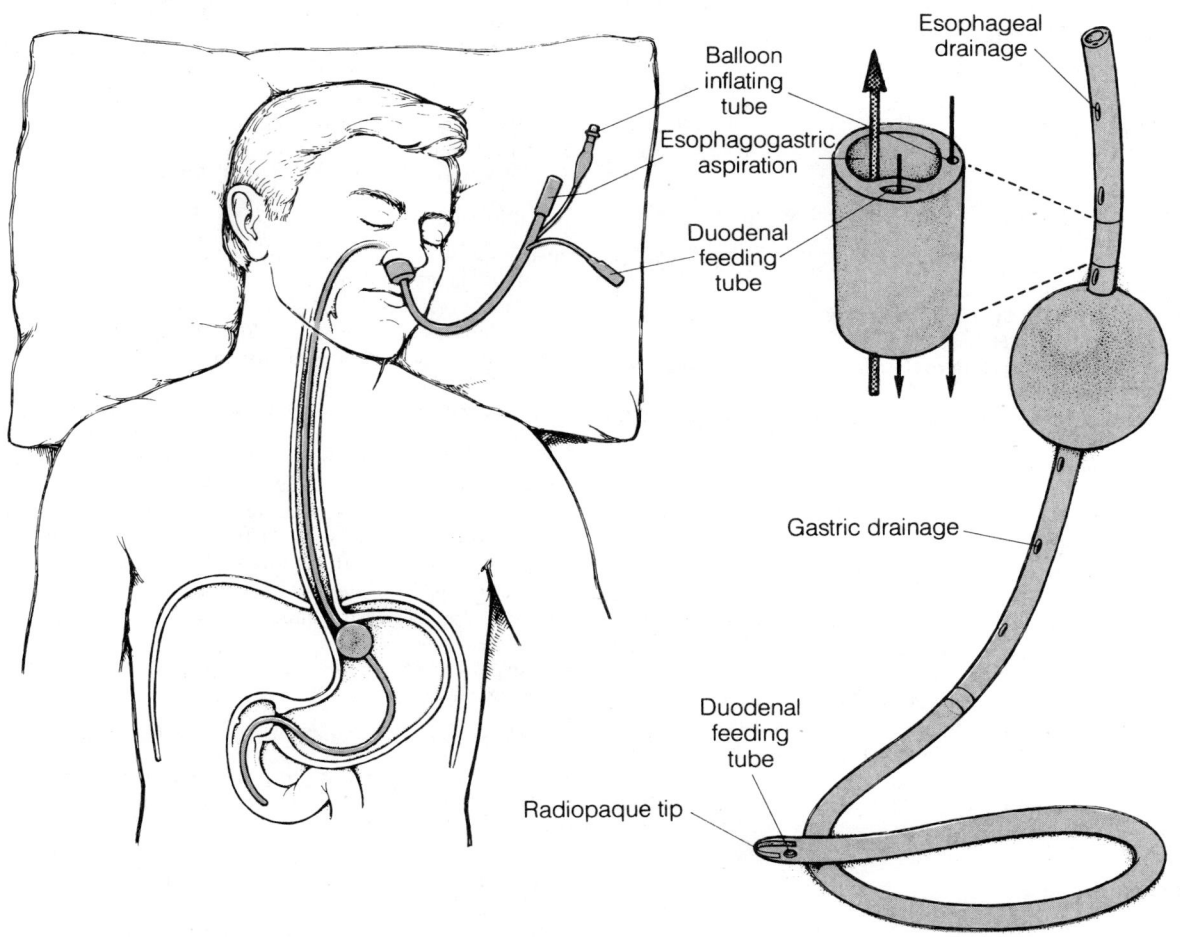

Figure 36-8. Nasogastric decompression and feeding tube has three channels to provide (1) a complete elemental diet fed into the duodenum immediately after surgery (such early feeding speeds recovery); (2) esophageal and gastric aspiration, important in that swallowed air reaching stomach and intestines can cause paralytic ileus; and (3) air to inflate plastic balloon at cardia. (From Moss G: Postsurgical decompression and immediate elemental feeding. Hospital Practice, May 1977, p 74.)

a brighter and more mentally alert postoperative patient, absence of ileus, and earlier discharge from the hospital. Undoubtedly, this procedure will be expanded to include more patients.

Home Hyperalimentation

Successful home hyperalimentation requires teaching the patient and his family specialized skills via an intensive training program and through follow-up supervision in the home. This must be done through a team effort. The financial costs of such programs are less than those incurred in a hospital. Initiation of a home program may be the only way the patient can be discharged. Ability to learn, availability of family interest and support, adequate finances, and the physical plan of the home are factors that must be assessed when the decision for home hyperalimentation is made. Institutions sponsoring home hyperalimentation programs have developed teaching brochures for every aspect of the treatment, including catheter and dressing care, use of the Imed pump for fluid infusions, infusions of fat emulsions, and instillation of heparin flushes.

▷ Bibliography
Books

Cunningham JJ (ed). Controversies in Clinical Nutrition. Philadelphia, GF Stickley, 1980.

Flock M. Nutrition and Diet Therapy in Gastrointestinal Disease. New York, Plenum, 1981.

Given BA and Simmons SJ. Gastroenterology in Clinical Nursing 4th ed. St Louis, CV Mosby, 1983.

Goodhart RS and Shils ME. Modern Nutrition in Health and Disease, 6th ed. Philadelphia, Lea & Febiger, 1981.

Grant JP. Handbook of Total Parenteral Nutrition. Philadelphia, WB Saunders, 1980.

Hodges RE. Nutrition in Medical Practice. Philadelphia, WB Saunders, 1980.

Krause MV and Mahan LK. Food, Nutrition and Diet Therapy, 6th ed. Philadelphia, WB Saunders, 1979.

McLaren DS. Color Atlas of Nutritional Disorders. New York, Year Book Medical Publishers, 1981.

Parenteral/Enteral Hyperalimentation Protocol. Philadelphia, Nutritional Support Service, Hospital of the University of Pennsylvania, 1982.

Silberman H. Parenteral and Enteral Nutrition for the Hospitalized Patient. New York, Appleton-Century-Crofts, 1982.

Suitor CJ and Hunter MF. Nutrition. Philadelphia, JB Lippincott, 1980.

Winick M (ed). Nutrition and the Killer Diseases. New York, Wiley-Interscience, 1981.

Articles
General

Anderson M et al. The double-lumen Hickman catheter. Am J Nurs 1982 Feb; 82(2):272-273.

Bjeletich J and Hickman R. The Hickman indwelling catheter. Am J Nurs 1980 Jan; 80(1):62-65.

Black G et al. Organization and administration of a nutritional support service. Surg Clin North Am 1981 June; 61(3):709-720.

Buzby G and Steinberg J. Nutrition in cancer patients. Surg Clin North Am 1981 June; 61(3):691-700.

Caldwell M and Kennedy-Caldwell C. Normal nutritional requirements. Surg Clin North Am 1981 June; 61(3):489-508.

Elwyn D et al. Energy expenditure in surgical patients. Surg Clin North Am 1981 June; (3):545-556.

Fischer J and Bower R. Nutritional support in liver disease. Surg Clin North Am 1981 June; 61(3):653-660.

Grant J et al. Current techniques of nutritional assessment. Surg Clin North Am 1981 June; 61(3):437-464.

Heymsfield S et al. Nutritional support in cardiac failure. Surg Clin North Am 1981 June; 61(3):635-652.

Kudsk K et al. Nutrition in trauma. Surg Clin North Am 1981 June; 61(3):671-680.

Leutzinger R and Judson A. Drawing blood from a Hickman catheter. Nursing '81 1981 Dec; 11(12):65-69.

Levine G. Nutritional support in gastrointestinal disease. Surg Clin North Am 1981 June; 61(3):701-708.

MacBurney M and Wilmore D. Rational decision making in nutritional care. Surg Clin North Am 1981 June; 61(3):571-582.

McLean A and Meakins J. Nutritional support in sepsis. Surg Clin North Am 1981 June; 61(3):681-690.

Nachlas MN, Crawford DT, and Pearl JM. Current status of jejunoileal bypass in the treatment of morbid obesity. Surg Gynecol Obstet 1980 Feb; 150(2):256-270.

Panel report on nutritional support of patients with gastrointestinal diseases. Am J Clin Nutr 1981 June; 34(6):1206-1212.

Steffee W. Nutritional support in renal failure. Surg Clin North Am 1981 June; 61(3):661-670.

Stein T and Buzby G. Protein metabolism in surgical patients. Surg Clin North Am 1981 June; 61(3):519-528.

Intubation

Bush J. Cervical esophagostomy to provide nutrition. Am J Nurs 1979; Jan; 79(1):107-109.

Carpenter C. Oral rehydration. Is it as good as parenteral therapy? N Engl J Med 1982 May 6; 306(18):1103-1104.

Giving medication through a nasogastric tube. Nursing '80 1980 May; 10(5):70-75.

Grossman MB. Gastrointestinal endoscopy. Clin Symp 1980; 32(3):1-36.

Hanson RL. New approach to measuring adult nasogastric tubes for insertion. Am J Nurs 1980 July; 80(7):1334-1335.

Hoppe M. The new tube feeding sets for your patients are what you feed them. Nursing '80 1980 Mar; 10(3):79-85.

Jensen T. Home enteral nutrition. Dietetic Currents, Ross Timesaver 1982 July-Aug; 9:15-20.

Oral care for nasogastric tube patients. Nursing '79 1979 May; 9(5):98-99.

Walike BC and Walike JW. Relative lactose intolerance. JAMA 1977 Aug 29; 238(9):948-951.

Parenteral Hyperalimentation and Gastrostomy

Burt ME et al. A controlled, prospective randomized trial evaluating the metabolic effects of enteral and parenteral nutrition in the cancer patient. Cancer 1982 Mar 15; 49(6):1092-1105.

Copeland EM, Daly JM, and Dudrick SJ. Intravenous hyperalimentation, bowel rest, and cancer. Crit Care Med 1980 Jan; 8(1):21-28.

Daly J and Long J. Intravenous hyperalimentation: Techniques and potential complications. Surg Clin North Am 1981 June; 61(3):583-592.

Dickinson R et al. Controlled trial of intravenous hyperalimentation and total bowel rest as an adjunct to the routine therapy of acute colitis. Gastroenterology 1980 Dec; 79(6):1199-1204.

Driscoll RH and Rosenberg IH. Total parenteral nutrition in inflammatory bowel disease. Med Clin North Am 1978 Jan; 62(1):185-201.

Erikkson B and Douglass HO Jr. Intravenous hyperalimentation. An adjunct to treatment of malignant disease of upper gastrointestinal tract. JAMA 1980 May 23; 243(20):2049–2052.

Gever MN. Parenteral iron supplements. Nursing '80 1980 Aug; 10(8):60.

Giving parenteral nutrition. In Nursing Photobook: Managing I.V. Therapy, pp 89–109. Horsham PA, Intermed Communications, 1980.

Goodgame JT. A critical assessment of the indications for total parenteral nutrition. Surg Gynecol Obstet 1980 Sept; 151(3):433–441.

Hyperalimentation standards of practice of The National Intravenous Therapy Association, Inc. (NITA). Oncology Nurs Forum 1981; 9(3):36–40.

Ivey MF. The status of parenteral nutrition. Nurs Clin North Am 1979 June; 14(2):285–303.

Lees C et al. Home parenteral nutrition. Surg Clin North Am 1981 June; 61(3):621–34.

Moss G. Postoperative ileus is an avoidable complication. Surg Gynecol Obstet 1979 Jan; 148(1):81–82.

Müller JM et al. Preoperative parenteral feeding in patients with gastrointestinal carcinoma. Lancet 1982 Jan 9; 1(8263):68–71.

Orr G et al. Alternatives to total parenteral nutrition in the critically ill patient. Crit Care Med 1980 Jan; 8(1):29–34.

Persons C. Why risk TPN when tube feeding will do? RN 1981 Jan; 44(1):35–41.

Rombeau J and Barot L. Enteral nutritional therapy. Surg Clin North Am 1981 July 61:(3):605–620.

Steiger E and Grundfest S. A review of home hyperalimentation. Contemporary Surgery 1979 Aug; 15(8):33–40.

Steinberg JJ. Parenteral nutrition before surgery. Lancet 1982 Feb 20; 1(8269):553.

Weser E. Editorial: Total parenteral nutrition and bowel rest in inflammatory disease. Gastroenterology 1980 Dec; 79(6):1337.

Agencies

American Dietetic Association, 430 N. Michigan Ave., Chicago, Illinois 60611

American Institute of Nutrition, 9650 Rockville Pike, Bethesda, Maryland 20014

American Society for Clinical Nutrition, 9650 Rockville Pike, Bethesda, Maryland 20014

National Institute of Arthritis, Metabolism and Digestive Diseases. National Institutes of Health, Bethesda, Maryland 20205

37

Management of Patients With Gastric (and Duodenal) Disorders

▷ Gastritis

Acute Gastritis

Gastritis (inflammation of the stomach) is most often due to a dietary indiscretion. The individual eats too much or too rapidly or eats food that is noxious because it is too highly seasoned or is infected. Other causes of acute gastritis include alcohol, aspirin, uremia, or radiotherapy. Gastritis may also be the first sign of an acute systemic infection.

Pathophysiology and Clinical Manifestations. The gastric mucous membrane becomes edematous and hyperemic and undergoes superficial erosion; it secretes a paucity of gastric juice, containing very little acid but much mucus. The patient may have uncomfortable feelings in his abdomen, with headache, lassitude, nausea, and anorexia, often accompanied by vomiting and hiccupping. Some patients, however, are asymptomatic.

The gastric mucosa is capable of repairing itself after a bout of gastritis. Occasionally, hemorrhage occurs; it may be severe and may require surgical intervention. If the irritating food is not vomited, but reaches the bowel, colic and diarrhea may result. As a rule, the patient is well in about a day, although he may not have much appetite for the next 2 or 3 days.

Nursing goals of care for patients with gastritis are to provide physical support through an acute episode, and in a patient with a chronic or more severe episode, to provide for further referral or emergency care. Later, when the acute episode has passed, the goal is to provide information that will help the patient to avoid a subsequent attack.

Nursing Assessment. A history is important to identify whether known dietary excesses or other indiscretions are associated with the current symptoms, whether others in the patient's environment have similar symptoms, whether the patient is vomiting blood, and whether any known caustic element has been swallowed. The length of time of the current symptoms and any interventions tried by the patient, and their effects, should also be identified.

Management and Nursing Intervention. Management consists of permitting the patient nothing by mouth until acute symptoms subside. When the patient is able to take nourishment by mouth, a bland diet, perhaps supplemented by alkalies, is offered. If the symptoms persist, parenteral administration of fluids may become necessary.

Evaluation of Nursing Interventions. When the acute episode has subsided, the nurse should discuss with the patient the importance of avoiding the causative agent (if known). The nurse should evaluate the patient's knowledge of drugs (*e.g.,* antacids) to be taken in the event of future episodes. If alcohol ingestion is a factor, the nurse should provide information regarding appropriate referral, and if diet is a factor, the nurse should discuss with the patient an acceptable, nonirritating diet. Written instructions regarding drug and diet information are helpful for the patient's review after discharge or treatment.

Corrosive Gastritis. A more severe form of acute gastritis is caused by the ingestion of strong acids or alkalies (corrosive gastritis). Immediate treatment consists of diluting and neutralizing the offender.

- To neutralize acids, use common antacids (milk, aluminum hydroxide, etc.); to neutralize an alkali, use lemon juice or diluted vinegar.
- If corrosion is extensive and severe, avoid emetics and lavage, because of the danger of perforation.

Therapy thereafter is supportive, including nasogastric intubation, analgesics and sedatives, antacids, intravenous fluids, and electrolytes.

It may be necessary to evaluate the situation by fiberoptic endoscopy. Emergency surgery may be required to take care of gangrenous or perforated tissue. Corrosive gastritis can result in scarring and cause pyloric obstruction, which may require gastrojejunostomy or resection.

Chronic Gastritis

Pathophysiology. In patients with chronic gastritis, the mucous membrane of the stomach becomes thickened and its rugae are prominent. As time passes, both the lining and the walls become thinned, and secretion lessens in quantity and in quality, eventually consisting almost entirely of mucus and water.

Causes. One of the important causes of chronic gastritis is chronic uremia. Among the local causes of gastritis are benign and malignant ulcers of the stomach and cirrhosis of the liver complicated by portal hypertension, the latter causing chronic congestion of the stomach wall.

Clinical Manifestations. Symptoms of chronic gastritis vary greatly. The appetite may be poor (anorexia) or too good (bulimia); there is usually some distress ("heartburn") after eating, and often there are eructations of gas. The taste in the mouth is unpleasant; there is usually considerable nausea, and perhaps some vomiting, especially early in the morning. The diagnosis is determined by gastroscopy, upper gastrointestinal x-ray series, and histologic examination.

Management. Treatment is similar to the medical regimen recommended for the patient with peptic ulcer. Patients with diffuse atrophic gastritis may require supplementary vitamin B_{12}.

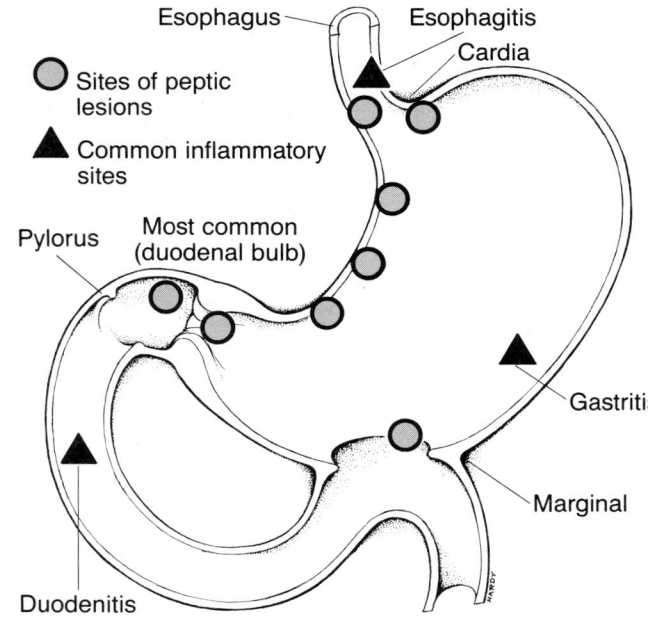

Figure 37-1. "Peptic" lesions may occur in the esophagus (esophagitis), stomach (gastritis), or duodenum (duodenitis). Note peptic ulcer sites and common inflammatory sites.

▷ Peptic Ulcer

A *peptic ulcer* is an excavation formed in the mucosal wall of the stomach, the pylorus, the duodenum, or the esophagus (Fig. 37-1). A peptic ulcer is frequently referred to as a gastric, duodenal, or esophageal ulcer, depending on its location. It is caused by the erosion of a circumscribed area of mucous membrane. This erosion may extend as deeply as the muscle layers or through the muscle to the peritoneum. Peptic ulcers are more apt to be in the duodenum than in the stomach. As a rule, they occur singly, but there may be a number of them present at one time. Chronic gastric ulcers tend to occur in the lesser curvature of the stomach, near the pylorus. See Table 37-1 for a comparison between gastric and duodenal ulcers.

Etiology and Predisposition

Etiology and Incidence. The etiology of peptic ulcer is poorly understood. It is known that peptic ulcers occur only in the areas of the gastrointestinal tract that are exposed to hydrochloric acid and pepsin. The disease occurs with the greatest frequency between the ages of 20 and 60, but is relatively uncommon in women of child-bearing age, although it has been observed in childhood, and even in infancy. More men than women are affected, although there is some evidence that the incidence in women is increasing.

Table 37-1
Comparison Between Duodenal and Gastric Ulcer

	Chronic Duodenal Ulcer	Chronic Gastric Ulcer
Age	Usually 50	Usually 45 and over
Sex	Male–female; 4:1	Male–female; 2:1
Blood Group	Most frequently—O	No differentiation
Social Class	More frequently in those subjected to stress and responsibility: executives, leaders in competitive fields	More common among laboring persons
General Nourishment	Usually well-nourished	Often malnourished
Acid Production: Stomach	Hypersecretion	Normal—hyposecretion
Pain	2–3 hours after a meal; nighttime: often awakened between 1 AM and 2 AM. Ingestion of food relieves pain	Occurs ½ to 1 hour after a meal; nighttime: rarely; relieved by vomiting. Ingestion of food does not help; sometimes pain is increased
Vomiting	Uncommon	Common
Hemorrhage	Melena more common than hematemesis	Hematemesis more common than melena
Malignancy Possibility	Never	Perhaps in less than 10%

After menopause, the incidence of peptic ulcer in women is almost equal to that in men. Since peptic ulcers in the body of the stomach occur without excessive acid secretion, an attempt should be made to differentiate gastric from duodenal ulcers.

It is estimated that 5% to 15% of the population in the United States have ulcers, but only about half of these are recognized. Duodenal ulcer was first recognized around 1900, and the incidence increased until the 1950s. Since then there has been a steady decrease in the United States, but the reason is unclear.

Predisposition.   Attempts continue to be made to delineate the "ulcer personality." Psychoanalysts claim that an ulcer results from repression of strong dependency needs. Others claim that occupational stress, with no opportunity to express hostility, is another strong factor. It seems to develop in persons who are emotionally tense, but whether this is the cause or the effect of the condition is uncertain. Familial tendency also appears as a significant predisposing factor, revealing that 3 times as many ulcer patients have relatives with the same diagnosis. A further hereditary link is noted in the finding that individuals in blood-group O are 35% more susceptible than persons in groups A, B, and AB. Other predisposing factors associated with peptic ulcer include emotional stress, eating hurriedly and irregularly, and smoking excessively. Rarely, ulcers are due to excessive amounts of the hormone gastrin, produced by tumors (gastrinomas—Zollinger–Ellison syndrome).

Pathophysiology

Peptic ulcer occurs in gastroduodenal mucosa because such tissue is unable to withstand the digestive action of gastric acid and pepsin. The erosion is due to an increase in concentration or activity of acid-pepsin, or to a decrease in the normal resistance of the mucosa.

Gastric secretion occurs in three phases: (1) cephalic, (2) gastric, and (3) intestinal. Since these phases are interactive and not independent of one another, a disturbance in any one phase may be ulcerogenic.

Cephalic (Psychic) Phase.   The first phase is initiated by stimuli such as the sight, smell, or taste of food, acting upon cerebral cortical receptors that, in turn, stimulate the vagal nerves. Essentially, an unappetizing meal has little effect on gastric secretion, whereas a more tasty, appealing meal evokes a high secretion. This accounts for the traditional emphasis on serving a bland meal to the peptic ulcer patient. Today many gastroenterologists agree that the bland diet has no significant effect on gastric acidity or ulcer healing. However, excessive vagal activity during the night, when the stomach is empty, is a significant irritant.

Gastric Phase. The gastric phase of gastric secretion is mediated by the hormone *gastrin*. Gastrin, which can be measured by a radioimmunoassay, enters the bloodstream from the antrum and is carried to glands in the fundus and body of the stomach; here it stimulates the production of gastric juice. Gastrin activity may be greater in patients with pyloric stenosis. The antrum of the patient with gastric ulcer contains less gastrin than that of the individual with a duodenal ulcer. Following partial gastrectomy or gastrojejunostomy, if part of the antrum is left in place but no longer is in contact with the acid-secreting portion of the stomach, the antrum continues to release gastrin, because acid no longer bathes the mucosa to inhibit gastrin release. Excess gastrin in the blood can lead to marginal ulcers. Excessive gastrin is also present in Zollinger–Ellison syndrome.

Intestinal Phase. During the intestinal phase a hormone, secretin, is secreted when hydrochloric acid enters the duodenum. Secretin, in turn, stimulates bicarbonate secretion from the pancreas, which neutralizes the acid. Secretin also inhibits the gastric phase of gastric secretion.

Gastric Mucosal Barrier. In man, gastric secretion is a mixture of mucopolysaccharides and mucoproteins secreted continuously by the mucosal glands. This mucus adsorbs pepsin and protects it against acid. Hydrochloric acid is secreted continuously, but secretions increase owing to neurogenic and hormonal mechanisms that are initiated by gastric and intestinal stimuli. If hydrochloric acid were not buffered and neutralized, and if the outer layer of mucosa did not offer protection, hydrochloric acid, along with pepsin, would destroy the stomach. Hydrochloric acid comes into contact with only a small gastric mucosal surface (oxyntic glandular mucosa): it diffuses into it with amazing slowness. This impenetrability of the mucosa is called the *gastric mucosal barrier*. It is the chief defense of the stomach against being digested by its secretions. Other factors that influence mucosal resistance are the blood supply, acid–base balance, integrity of mucosal cells, and epithelial regeneration (Fig. 37-2).

Note then, that a person is likely to develop a peptic ulcer from one of two causes: hypersecretion of acid-pepsin, or a weakened gastric mucosal barrier. Anything that decreases the production of gastric mucus or damages gastric mucosa is ulcerogenic: salicylates, alcohol, and indomethacin fall into this category.

Clinical Manifestations

Symptoms of duodenal ulcer (the most common form of peptic ulcer), may last for a few days, weeks, or months and may even disappear only to reappear, often without an identifiable cause. Exacerbations seem to occur in the spring or fall, but even this pattern is inconsistent. Many individuals have symptomless ulcers, and in 20% to 30%, perforation or hemorrhage may occur without any preceding manifestations.

Pain. As a rule, the patient with duodenal ulcer complains of pain, or a burning, sharply localized sensation in

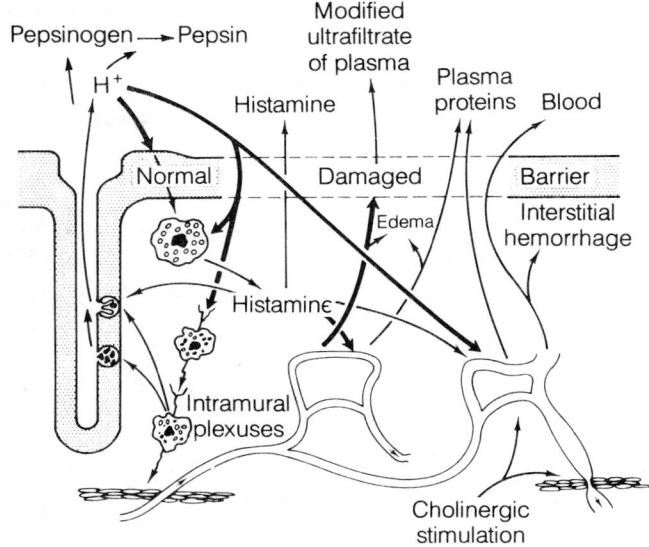

Figure 37-2. Pathophysiologic consequences of the back-diffusion of acid through the broken gastric mucosal barrier. Acid, which diffuses slowly through the normal mucosa, rapidly enters one whose barrier has been broken. Acid destroys mucosal cells and liberates histamine. Histamine stimulates acid secretion, causes vasodilatation, and increases capillary permeability to proteins. The mucosa become edematous, and fluid derived from interstitial fluid is forced through the mucosa. This fluid may contain a large amount of plasma proteins. Acid stimulates the intramural plexuses, and motility of the stomach is increased. It also stimulates pepsin secretion, perhaps by way of histamine liberation and perhaps through its effect on the plexuses. Mucosal capillaries may be destroyed by acid, so that interstitial hemorrhage and frank bleeding occur. Bleeding is more frequent and copious when there is concurrent cholinergic stimulation, probably because contraction of gastric muscle increases venous and capillary pressures. (From Davenport HW: Physiology of the Digestive Tract, 3rd ed. Copyright © 1971 by Year Book Medical Publishers, Inc., Chicago. Used by permission.)

the midepigastrium or in the back. It is believed that the pain occurs when the increased acid content of the stomach and duodenum erodes the lesion and stimulates the exposed nerve endings. Another theory suggests that contact of the lesion with acid stimulates a local reflex mechanism that initiates contraction of the adjacent smooth muscle.

Pain precedes meals from 1 to 3 hours and becomes progressively more severe toward the end of the day. It may also waken the individual between 12 AM and 3 AM. However, there is no pain when the patient awakens in the morning because the flow of gastric acid is at its lowest at this time.

Pain typically is relieved quite promptly by food or alkalies, either of which neutralizes the free acid in contact with the ulcer. If the patient takes neither food nor alkali, the pain gradually wears off as the secretion of acid stops and it empties into the intestine. The character of the pain may be described as a dull, burning sensation; a feeling of emptiness; or a gnawing pain so severe that the patient is in agony. When the ulcer has begun to penetrate into the pancreas, pain in the back may become noticeable.

Some relief is obtained by local pressure on the epigastrium. Sharply localized tenderness can be elicited by

---

Chart 37-1
Risk Factors for Duodenal Ulcer

Family history of peptic ulcer
Emotional stress:
    Anxiety
    Anger
    Resentment
Caffeine-containing beverages:
    Coffee
    Tea
    Cola
Certain drugs:
    Salicylates
    Indomethacin

---

gentle pressure in the epigastrium at, or slightly to the right of, the midline.

Pyrosis (Hypersialorrhea, Heartburn). Some patients experience a burning sensation in the esophagus and stomach, which moves up to the mouth, occasionally with sour eructation. Eructation, or burping, is common when the patient's stomach is empty.

Vomiting. Although rare in uncomplicated duodenal ulcer, vomiting may be a symptom of peptic ulcer. It is due to gastric outlet obstruction caused by either muscular spasm of the pylorus or mechanical obstruction. The latter may be due to scarring or to acute swelling of the inflamed mucous membrane adjacent to the acute ulcer. Vomiting may or may not be preceded by nausea; usually it follows a bout of severe pain, which is relieved by ejection of the acid gastric contents. The vomitus may contain food particles from the previous day.

Constipation and Bleeding. Constipation may be apparent in the patient with duodenal ulcer, probably as a result of diet and medications.

About 20% of individuals who bleed from an acute duodenal ulcer have had no previous digestive complaints; however, they develop symptoms thereafter.

▶ Assessment

The history of the patient serves as an important base for diagnosis (Chart 37-1). The presence of pain that is relieved by food or antacids, and the absence of pain upon arising are highly suggestive of duodenal ulcer. The appearance of blood in the stools is an important diagnostic finding, suggestive of hemorrhage. Stools should be collected daily until the laboratory reports are negative for occult blood.

Diagnosis of duodenal ulcer is most easily made by barium studies of the upper gastrointestinal tract. Gastric secretory studies may be of some value in determining the type of treatment and to check for the possibility of Zollinger–Ellison syndrome. An analysis of the gastric juice, obtained by aspiration of the juice through a tube, is described on page 763. Often, production of acid for the sample is stimulated by injecting pentagastrin. However, gastric secretory studies have largely been replaced by fiberoptic endoscopy for diagnosis and for determining the healing of duodenal ulcer. This is a procedure that augments radiographic studies and permits direct visualization of the duodenal mucosa (see p. 764).

Patient Problems/Nursing Diagnoses

Based on the clinical manifestations, the nursing history, and the diagnostic assessment data, the patient's major nursing problems include pain related to gastric acidity and mucosal erosion; anxiety and emotional stress; potential nonadherence to the therapeutic regimen; and potential development of complications.

▶ Planning and Implementation

Goals

The major goals for the patient include:

1. Relief of pain
2. Reduction of anxiety and emotional stress
3. Compliance with the therapeutic regimen
4. Absence of complications

Goals of nursing care for patients with known or suspected peptic ulcer disease are (1) to identify problems potentially related to peptic ulcer disease, and to facilitate necessary referral for evaluation and care; (2) to provide physical and psychological support for patients during diagnostic and treatment phases; (3) to provide for relief of physical and emotional symptoms; and (4) to promote compliance with the therapeutic regimen.

To assist the patient in meeting his goals, the major objectives of therapy are (1) to control gastric acidity, (2) to reduce emotional and environmental stressors, (3) to heal the ulcer, and (4) to educate the patient concerning his future life-style.

Management

From the beginning, once the diagnosis is established, the patient should be informed that he can learn how to keep his problem under control, but he may expect both remissions and recurrences.

Gastric Secretion. Gastric acidity is controlled by appropriate sedation and by neutralization of the gastric juice, at frequent and regular intervals, with drugs, nonirritating foods, and antacids. Sometimes antispasmodics are given to reduce pylorospasm and intestinal motility. Anticholinergic agents may be prescribed to inhibit gastric secretion. Drugs that block the acid-secreting action of histamine (H_2 blockers)—cimetidine, for example—or that produce an acid-resistant barrier over the ulcer—Sucralfate, for example—have been shown to be effective in healing duodenal ulcers.

Hospitalization, if required at all, can be limited to 2 or 3 days, unless bleeding, obstruction, perforation, or severe nocturnal pain are present.

Rest and Stress Reduction. Reducing environmental stress is a difficult task requiring both physical and mental interventions on the patient's part, and aid and cooperation of family members and significant others. The patient may need help in identifying situations that are stressful or exhausting. A rushed life-style and an irregular schedule may aggravate symptoms and interfere with regular meals taken in relaxed settings and with regular administration of medications. In addition to stress reduction suggestions, the patient may also benefit from suggestions about regular rest periods during the day, at least during the acute phase.

Diet. Since there is little evidence to support the theory that bland diets are more beneficial than regular meals, patients have been encouraged to eat whatever agrees with them. However, there are a few precautions to consider in the early stages of healing. *The objective of the diet for peptic ulcers is to avoid oversecretion and hypermotility in the gastrointestinal tract.* These can be minimized by avoiding extremes of temperature and overstimulation by meat extracts, coffee, alcohol, and seasonings, especially pepper and mustard. In addition, an effort should be made to neutralize the acid by the use of buffering foods such as milk, and by the use of antacids. At first, small, frequent feedings also will be beneficial.

Diet compatibility becomes an individual matter. If the patient tolerates a particular food, he may eat it. If it produces pain, he will avoid it. Milk and cream are no longer considered central to therapy. In fact, diets rich in milk and cream are potentially harmful, over a long period, because they increase serum lipids, a contributing factor in producing atherosclerosis. Skim milk stimulates secretion to some extent; the more effective the neutralization, the more enhanced is the stimulus to new acid secretion. As the patient approaches alkalinity, gastrin release is stimulated and acid secretion is increased.

Unless there are unusual problems, current therapy permits meals of normal size 3 times a day, eaten at the same time each day, with no evening snack—rather than six small meals a day.

Antacids. Antacids continue to be a mainstay of peptic ulcer treatment. The objective is to select the antacid that provides the safest and longest period of acid neutralization. Usually, antacids leave the stomach rapidly, so that frequent doses are required.

Sodium bicarbonate is probably the best neutralizer of acid contents in the stomach, but is not recommended because it is emptied from the stomach too rapidly, and over a period of time can easily lead to alkalosis. The next most effective antacids are calcium-containing compounds; however, they are unpleasant-tasting and constipating. They are in disfavor because calcium produces an increase in serum gastrin and in acid secretion. Taken over a period of time, they can lead to hypercalcemia and impaired renal function. Less effective are the aluminum hydroxide and magnesium hydroxide preparations. However, they are the most effective antacids available.

Most antacids contain mixtures of aluminum and magnesium hydroxide, or magnesium hydroxide, aluminum hydroxide, and calcium carbonate in various combinations and suspensions. Magnesium hydroxide is a good buffering antacid, but used alone may cause diarrhea. Therefore, a preferable combination is magnesium hydroxide with magne-

Chart 37-2
Composition of Common Antacids

Antacid	Contents
Aludrox	Aluminum hydroxide gel, magnesium hydroxide
Amphojel	Aluminum hydroxide gel
A-M-T	Magnesium trisilicate, aluminum hydroxide gel
Camalox	Aluminum and magnesium hydroxide, calcium carbonate
Creamalin	Hexitol stabilized, aluminum hydroxide gel, magnesium hydroxide
Di-Gel	Aluminum hydroxide and magnesium hydroxide, simethicone
Ducon	Aluminum hydroxide and magnesium hydroxide, calcium carbonate
Delcid	Aluminum hydroxide, magnesium hydroxide
Gelusil	Magnesium hydroxide, aluminum hydroxide, simethicone
Gelusil-M	Magnesium trisilicate, aluminum and magnesium hydroxide
Kolantyl Gel	Aluminum hydroxide, magnesium hydroxide
Maalox	Magnesium hydroxide and aluminum hydroxide, simethicone
Malcogel	Magnesium trisilicate, aluminum hydroxide gel
Marblen	Magnesium and calcium carbonates, aluminum hydroxide
Mylanta	Aluminum hydroxide gel, magnesium hydroxide, simethicone
Mylanta-II	Aluminum hydroxide gel, magnesium hydroxide, simethicone
Phosphaljel	Aluminum phosphate gel
Riopan	Magaldrate and simethicone
Robalate	Dihydroxyaluminum aminoacetate
Silain-Gel	Aluminum and magnesium hydroxide, simethicone
Titralac	Calcium carbonate, glycine
Trisogel	Magnesium trisilicate, aluminum hydroxide gel
Wingel	Aluminum and magnesium hydroxide, hexitol stabilized

sium trisilicate (which has less laxative effect) or aluminum hydroxide (more constipating). Aluminum hydroxide gels can bring on hypophosphatemia.

Although no antacid presently available is capable of maintaining a pH of 3.5 or above (required to keep pepsinogen inactive) for longer than 30 to 45 minutes, antacids are capable of preventing rebound hyperacidity and systemic alkalosis.

In the early phase, liquid antacids are taken hourly, 15 ml to 30 ml (1 or 2 tablespoons), beginning 1 hour after breakfast until bedtime (*e.g.,* Gelusil, Mylanta, Maalox, Creamalin, Amphojel). If the patient is awakened at night with epigastric pain, he notes the time, and therafter sets his alarm clock for an hour earlier, to take the antacid (see "Duration of Regimen" for continued pattern of antacid therapy).

- For patients who have an associated heart problem requiring sodium restriction, magaldrate (Riopan) is an anatacid of choice, since it contains practically no sodium. This is especially recommended for elderly patients.

Anticholinergics. As an adjunct to the antacid compounds, an anticholinergic drug is usually given. Anticholinergics are given to block vagal stimulation of parietal cells, so as to reduce acid secretion. Anticholinergics also decrease gastric motor activity, which allows the antacid to remain in the stomach longer, and they are generally administered about a half hour before meals.

Among the antisecretory drugs are atropine, propantheline bromide (Pro-Banthine), methantheline bromide (Banthine), oxyphencyclimine (Daricon), methscopolamine (Pamine), and others. These are usually only recommended for a short period of time, when pain has not been relieved with antacids. They are occasionally used at nighttime with a double dose of antacid, for persistent night pain.

Side-effects of anticholinergic drugs include dryness of the mouth and throat; excessive thirst; difficulty in swallowing; flushed, dry skin; rapid pulse and respiration; dilated pupils; and emotional excitement.

- Anticholinergic medications should not be used by patients with glaucoma, urinary retention, or pyloric obstruction.

Physicians vary in their preference for prescribing anticholinergic drugs. At times such drugs are in favor, and at other times they are not. While these drugs are suggested for patients who suffer from severe, persistent nocturnal pain, they are not recommended for long-term use.

H$_2$ Receptor Antagonist—Cimetidine (Tagamet). Histamine has two receptors for its action: H$_1$ receptor is located on bronchial and nasal mucosa, cardiac tissue, and blood vessels; H$_2$ receptor is found primarily in the stomach. Common antihistamines block the action of H$_1$ receptors but have no effect on H$_2$ receptors in the stomach. Cimetidine, a H$_2$ receptor antagonist, has a dramatic effect on lowering acid secretion in the stomach. A very high dose of the drug reduces acid secretion to an almost unmeasurable level.

Cimetidine is given orally with each meal and at bedtime. It relieves ulcer pain, and thus decreases the need for antacids. Short-term treatment with cimetidine has resulted in complete ulcer healing, but low-dose maintenance therapy may be needed to prevent recurrence. Even though H$_2$ receptors are distributed in body tissue, only gastric receptors appear to be affected by this drug. It is a valuable medication.

Other Drugs. Sucralfate (Carafate) is a recent locally acting drug that has also been shown to have antiulcer properties. Sucralfate forms complexes with proteinaceous exudates, such as albumin and fibrinogen, in the ulcer crater and forms an adherent barrier over the ulcer. This barrier is acid-resistant, as opposed to acid-reducing. The result is that acid is prevented from passing through to the ulcer, but the acid is not appreciably neutralized. Sucralfate is only minimally absorbed from the gastrointestinal tract and does not depend on systemic activity for its antiulcer effects.

Duration of Regimen. The patient should stay on the drug program to ensure complete healing of the ulcer. Since most patients become symptom-free in a week, it becomes a nursing objective to emphasize the importance of following the prescribed regimen so that the breakdown of the healing process and the return of chronic ulcer symptoms are averted. Rest, sedatives, and tranquilizers add to the comfort of the individual and are used as needed. Cimetidine therapy is generally continued for 4 to 6 weeks.

After the first week, the purpose of using antacids switches from that of relieving symptoms to preventing symptoms. If antacid is taken on a fasting stomach, its buffering action is effective for only about 30 minutes, but when taken an hour after a meal, the buffering effect may last 2 to 3 hours. For the 2nd through the 6th weeks, the best plan appears to be to have the patient on regular meals. One hour after each meal, he takes 30 ml of antacid; 3 hours after each meal, he takes another 30 ml of antacid. This medication is also recommended at bedtime. This pattern of therapy concentrates antacid in the stomach and duodenum at those times when the gastric secretion otherwise would be highest, achieving the desired neutralizing effect. The goal is to keep the pH of gastric contents above 4 between meals. At this pH, pepsin becomes relatively inactive.

From the 6th or 7th week to 6 months, antacid is taken about an hour after meals and at bedtime. Thereafter, antacid therapy is usually dropped. If the person experiences a stressful situation or has been indiscrete in his diet and symptoms recur, he may resume antacid therapy until he is symptom-free.

Prognosis

Recurrence of an ulcer is possible and may happen within 2 years in about one third of all patients, although this incidence may be affected with prophylactic use of such drugs as cimetidine. The likelihood of recurrence is lessened if the individual avoids tea; coffee; alcohol; and ulcerogenic drugs, such as salicylates, corticosteroids, and phenylbutazone. If symptoms recur, he is to resume antacid medications hourly. (Antacid tablets may be taken when required during a normal day's activities; however, it is necessary to chew them thoroughly and to recognize that three or four tablets are equal in potency to 1 tablespoon of liquid antacid.) If relief is not obtained, medical advice should be sought.

Patient Education

In order to deal successfully with ulcer disease, the patient must understand his situation and those factors that will help or aggravate his condition. Areas that need consideration and perhaps modification, along with evaluative questions, are the following:

- *Medication:* Does the patient know what medications are to be taken at home, including name, dosage, frequency, and possible side-effects (*e.g.,* cimetidine, antacids, and anticholinergics)? Does the patient know what drugs to avoid (*e.g.,* aspirin, bicarbonate of soda)?
- *Diet:* Does the patient know what particular foods tend to upset him? Does he know that coffee, tea, colas, alcohol, and spices have acid-producing potential? Does he know to take antacids if he overeats or overdrinks? Does he understand the importance of regular meals taken in a relaxed setting?
- *Rest and stress reduction:* Is the patient aware of sources of stress in family and work environments? Has this illness or other situations produced symptoms of stress or poor coping in the family or work setting? Is the patient aware that smoking probably increases the irritation to his ulcer? Can the patient identify rest periods during the day? Can the patient plan for added periods of rest or relaxation after unavoidable periods of stress? Does the patient need extended psychological counseling?
- *Follow-up care:* Does the patient realize that follow-up supervision is necessary for about 1 year? Does he realize that his ulcer could recur? Does he know to seek medical assistance if symptoms recur?

For guidelines of nursing implementation for the patient with a peptic ulcer, see Chart 37-3.

▶ Evaluation

Expected Outcomes

1. Is relieved of pain
   a. Is free of pain between meals
   b. Uses antacids to prevent pain
   c. Avoids foods and fluids that cause pain
   d. Eats meals at regular times
   e. Experiences no side-effects of antacids (diarrhea, constipation, fluid retention)
   f. Uses anticholinergics as prescribed
   g. Has no side-effects of anticholinergics
2. Anxiety and emotional stress are reduced
   a. Uses sedatives and tranquilizers as prescribed
   b. Experiences no side-effects of sedatives and tranquilizers
   c. Identifies situations that produce stress
   d. Identifies life-style adjustments necessary to reduce stress
   e. Alters life-style as appropriate
   f. Involves family in decisions regarding life-style adjustments

3. Adheres to the therapeutic regimen
   a. Alternates periods of rest with activity
   b. Complies with dietary regimen
   c. Complies with medication regimen
   d. Reports symptoms of ulcer recurrence
   e. Keeps follow-up clinic or physician appointments
4. Is free of complications
   a. Is free of bleeding
   b. Has stable vital signs
   c. Maintains hemoglobin and hematocrit within normal ranges
   d. Is free of occult blood in stools
   e. Is free of hematemesis
   f. Has no symptoms of perforation
   g. Experiences no symptoms of pyloric obstruction
   h. Exhibits no symptoms of intractable ulcer
   i. Complies with therapeutic regimen

Complications of Peptic Ulcers

There are four major complications of a peptic ulcer: hemorrhage, perforation, pyloric obstruction, and intractable ulcer.

Hemorrhage. Manifested by hematemesis, melena, or both, hemorrhage is the common complication of peptic ulcer. Occasionally, this appears without any antecedent history of dyspepsia. Early symptoms may be giddiness and faintness; nausea may precede or accompany bleeding. A large amount of blood, even 2000 ml to 3000 ml, may be vomited. The patient may become almost exsanguinated, and rapid blood replacement may be required to save his life. When the hemorrhage is of large proportions, most of the blood is vomited; when small, much or all of the blood may be passed in the stools, which will appear tarry black, owing to the digested hemoglobin.

Management. Since hemorrhage can be massive and fatal, bleeding must be stopped quickly, and the blood replaced.

- Immediate nursing evaluation includes assessment of vital signs. If vital signs are unstable, preparation should be made for a *peripheral line* intravenous infusion (saline, and later blood or blood component) and a *central line* for infusion and measurement of central venous pressure. Also, a large-gauge (18-gauge or larger) angiocatheter may be inserted (to define the bleeding site).
- The laboratory is notified to type and crossmatch 6 units of blood.
- Additional laboratory tests are requested, including hemoglobin and hematocrit evaluations, and chemical tests such as benzidine, guaiac, or orthotoluidine, to detect occult blood that does not alter the gross appearance of the stools, since this type of melena is decidedly more common than gross hemorrhages from the bowel.
- An indwelling urinary catheter is inserted to monitor urinary output. Special diagnostic studies, such as endoscopy (to locate the exact bleeding site), angiography, and barium studies, may be called for.
- A nasogastric tube may be placed in the stomach to determine the presence of fresh blood or "coffee-

Chart 37-3
Guidelines for Nursing Implementation of the Patient With a Peptic Ulcer

Patient Problems/Nursing Diagnoses

1. Pain related to gastric acidity and mucosal erosion
2. Anxiety and emotional stress
3. Potential nonadherence to the therapeutic regimen
4. Potential development of complications

Nursing Goals and Interventions

A. To assure mental and physical rest:
1. Remove or modify sources of stress in patient's environment.
2. Instruct patient and family about the value of rest and relaxation.
3. Explain the need to take such prescribed medications as sedatives and soporific medications to promote relaxation and sleep.
4. Encourage patient to take medications and dietary feedings on time.

B. To relieve pain and discomfort and to promote healing:
Explain the purpose of the drug regimen:
a. H$_2$ receptor antagonists to reduce acid secretion, or other antiulcer drug to neutralize the effects of acid secretion
b. Antacid drugs to neutralize gastric secretions and afford symptomatic relief
c. Anticholinergic drugs to decrease gastric motility and reduce volume of gastric secretions
d. Adequate hydration to relieve side-effects of anticholinergic drugs

C. To rest the motor and secretory activities of the stomach through a therapeutic diet:
Emphasize and explain the rationale for the following:
a. Small, frequent feedings to absorb excess acid

b. Nonstimulating foods to avoid irritation of the gastric mucosa
c. Regular meals taken in a relaxed environment

D. To assist the patient to accept and follow his therapeutic regimen:
1. Teach importance of taking prescribed medication and diet on time.
2. Assist patient to develop insight into causes of his tension and frustration.
3. Implement and reinforce instructions issued by the physician.
4. Teach the importance of moderation and regularity in activities.
5. Encourage the elimination of smoking.
6. Stress the value of psychological counseling for family and patient if needed.

E. To recognize the complications of peptic ulcer:
1. Hemorrhage:
a. Prepare for prompt and rapid transfusion for blood replacement.
b. Administer sedatives to allay anxiety and keep patient at rest.
c. Assist with gastric intubation for aspiration of stomach contents.
d. Evaluate clinical response to blood replacement.
e. Observe continuously to maintain blood pressure at physiologic level.
f. Observe urinary volume.
g. Observe stools for blood; collect stool specimens daily for laboratory analysis.
h. Prepare for surgical intervention, if indicated.
2. Perforation:
a. Assist with transfusion to treat shock.
b. Prepare to institute nasogastric suction to remove gastrointestinal secretions.
c. Give drugs to control pain.
d. Prepare patient for immediate surgery.

ground" material, which can then be removed by suction.
- Antacids may be given via nasogastric tube along with IV cimetidine therapy. The gastric *p*H should be monitored and kept within a 6 to 8 range.
- Some clinics use normal iced saline for lavage to remove blood and clots. Often the No. 18 French tube is too small, and a No. 22 French size is used. The normal saline solution may be taken by mouth and the fluid withdrawn through the tube by suction. Usually, the nasogastric tube is left in place during the cooling procedure. This removes acid, prevents nausea and vomiting, and provides a means of monitoring for further bleeding.

- Whole blood or plasma transfusions are given to keep the circulating blood volume at a safe level. One does not wait for a drop in blood pressure before starting transfusion therapy if there are signs of tachycardia, sweating, and coldness of the extremities.
- The blood pressure and pulse rates are monitored every 15 to 30 minutes when bleeding is suspected, and hemoglobin and hematocrit are frequently checked.
- The color, consistency, and volume of stools and vomitus are observed and recorded.
- Oxygen therapy is given, and the patient is placed in the supine position with his legs elevated. (A full Trendelenburg position is avoided, as this restricts ventilation, causing further hypoxemia.)

- In the event of hypovolemic shock, the procedures outlined on page 405 are carried out.
- When bleeding ceases, hourly antacids and diet as tolerated are given. Anticholinergic medications are postponed, because of masking effects on pulse rate.

Lamphier and Lamphier describe several new nonsurgical approaches for the control of upper gastrointestinal hemorrhage:

- *Intra-arterial vasopressin infusions via pump directly into a bleeding artery:* A repeat arteriogram is needed to evaluate the efficacy of treatment.
- *Selective embolization:* Emboli of autologous blood clots with or without Gelfoam (absorbable gelatin sponge), or a mixture of the patient's own blood, Amicar (epsilon aminocaproic acid), and platelets are forced through a catheter to a point above the bleeding lesion.
- *Endoscopic electrocoagulation of hemorrhage sites:* A coagulation electrode is passed through the biopsy channel of the endoscope, and bleeding sites are electrocoagulated. Cessation of bleeding can be evaluated before the endoscope is removed.

Indications for Surgery. If bleeding recurs in 48 hours after medical therapy has begun, or if more than 5 units of blood are required in 24 hours to maintain blood volume, the patient is likely to be scheduled for surgery. Some clinics have a policy that if a patient with peptic ulcer hemorrhages 3 times, surgery is indicated.

Other determining factors for surgery are the patient's age (if he is over 60, massive hemorrhaging is 3 times more likely to be fatal), a history of chronic duodenal ulcer, and a coincidental gastric ulcer.

The ulcer-bearing area is removed, or the bleeding vessels are ligated. In many patients a procedure is included that is aimed at controlling the underlying ulcer diathesis (*e.g.,* vagotomy and pylorectomy, or gastrectomy).

Perforation. Perforation of a peptic ulcer may occur unexpectedly, without much evidence of preceding indigestion. Perforation into the free peritoneal cavity is an abdominal catastrophe and an indication that surgery may be needed.

The typical history constists of:

- Sudden, severe upper abdominal pain (persisting and increasing in intensity).
- Pain may be referred to the shoulders, especially the right shoulder, owing to irritation of the phrenic nerve in the diaphragm.
- Vomiting and collapse.
- Abdomen extremely tender, and boardlike in rigidity.
- Signs of shock.

Immediate surgical intervention is indicated, because chemical peritonitis develops within a few hours following perforation and is followed by a bacterial peritonitis. Therefore, the perforation must be closed as quickly as possible. In a few patients, it may be deemed safe and advisable that a definitive operation be performed for the ulcer disease, in addition to the perforation being sutured.

Postoperative Management. A nasogastric tube is inserted, and the gastric contents are drained.

- Fluid and electrolyte balance is monitored.
- Patient is assessed for presence of peritonitis or localized infection (increased temperature, abdominal pain, paralytic ileus, increased bowel sounds or absent bowel sounds, abdominal distension). Antibiotic therapy is given parenterally.

Pyloric Obstruction. Pyloric obstruction occurs when the area distal to the pyloric sphincter becomes scarred and stenosed from spasm or edema, or from scar tissue that is formed when the ulcer alternately heals and breaks down. The patient has symptoms of nausea and vomiting, constipation, epigastric fullness, anorexia, and (later) weight loss.

In treating the patient, the first consideration is the relief of the obstruction by gastric decompression. At the same time, attempts are made to confirm that obstruction is the cause of discomfort. This is done by checking the amount of fluid aspirated from the nasogastric tube. A residual of over 200 ml is strongly suggestive of obstruction. Some physicians also utilize the load test, which involves infusing 750 ml of normal saline via the nasogastric tube into the mid-antrum of the stomach. The patient is rotated, to permit normal gastric emptying; 20 minutes later, aspiration is done, and if more than 400 ml is retrieved, obstruction is confirmed.

Before surgery is undertaken, decompression continues, and extracellular fluid volume, as well as electrolyte and metabolic derangements, are corrected. Conscientious daily fluid monitoring is continued. With supportive measures, the patient's condition may improve. It may be feasible to repeat the load test; if negative, medical treatment continues. If positive, surgery, in the form of a vagotomy and antrectomy, may be required. If the patient is severely malnourished during this time, parenteral hyperalimentation may be utilized.

Intractability. An intractable ulcer is one that continues to give problems and is resistant to all forms of treatment. A careful history of the patient includes a thorough review of dietary and drug habits, which could reveal long-term use of caffeine-containing drinks or aspirin-containing medications. The entire gastrointestinal tract is carefully assessed to determine other possible problems, such as hiatus hernia, gallbadder disease, or diverticulitis.

The patient and family are informed of the fact that surgery is no guarantee that an ulcer will not return. The possible postoperative sequelae, such as intolerance to dairy products and sweet foods, are also discussed.

Surgical Treatment

Surgery for ulcer disease is done when medical therapy has not been successful or when complications arise, such as hemorrhage, perforation, or pyloric obstruction. Patients requiring ulcer surgery may have had a long illness, be discouraged, have interruptions in their work role, and experience pressures in their family life.

Assessment and Nursing Implementation. Through a careful nursing history and assessment of the patient, these factors can be elicited and used in developing specific nursing goals. By collaborating with other members of the health team and seeking input from them, the nurse can develop a therapeutic plan of care to assist in resolving the patient's problem and to reduce the chances of recurrences.

1. *Preparing the patient for diagnostic tests:* The patient undergoes laboratory analyses, roentgenologic series, and a general physical examination before surgery is attempted. The nurse prepares the patient for each of these diagnostic measures by explaining their nature and significance to him.
2. *Attending to the patient's fluid and nutritional needs:* The nutritional and fluid needs of the patient are of major importance. In those patients with pyloric obstruction, there usually is prolonged vomiting, with resultant weight and fluid loss. Every effort is made to restore an adequate nutritional level and to maintain an optimal fluid and electrolyte balance.
3. *Clearing and emptying the gastrointestinal tract:* Nasogastric suction often is required to empty the stomach, especially in patients with pyloric obstruction. The tube is inserted before the operation and left in place for operative and postoperative use.

    It is important that the colon be empty when the patient comes to surgery; this is ensured by an enema the day before operation. If gastrointestinal roentgenograms have been made shortly before the day of operation, it is most important that enemas be given to remove the barium that may remain in the colon completely.
4. *Limiting fluid intake:* The patient usually is limited to fluids during the 24-hour period preceding surgery.
5. *Shaving and preparing the skin:* The abdomen should be prepared, from the nipple line to the symphysis, although the incision usually is made in the upper right quadrant or the midline.

Surgical Approaches for Ulcers

Vagotomy and Gastroenterostomy or Pyloroplasty.   A popular method of treating the patient with a recurrent peptic ulcer involves cutting the vagus nerves (vagotomy) and establishing gastric drainage. The drainage operation is necessary because vagotomy is often followed by gastric retention. Since the vagus nerves provide the motor impulses to the gastric musculature, severing the nerves often leads to gastric atony. The drainage operation may be in the form of a gastroenterostomy or a pyloroplasty. The vagotomy divides the nerves that are known to stimulate gastric acid hypersecretion in most cases of duodenal ulcer. The gastric drainage operation not only drains the atonic stomach produced by the vagotomy, but also reduces the stimulation of gastric acid by reducing the formation of gastrin produced in the antral area of the stomach.

Vagotomy and Antrectomy.   Since the ulcers are believed to result from the acid pepsin of the stomach, vagotomy and antrectomy are designed to lower the production of acid by the stomach to a point at which further ulcerations will not occur. This may be done by removing the acid-stimulating mechanism of the stomach, that is, dividing the vagus nerves and removing the antral portion of the stomach (vagotomy and antrectomy).

Partial Gastrectomy and Possible Vagotomy.   A third method is partial gastrectomy, with or without vagotomy. The remaining segment of stomach is anastomosed to the duodenum (Billroth I procedure), or more extensive excision of the stomach may be performed and the remaining segment anastomosed to the jejunum (Billroth II procedure) (Table 37-2).

Proximal Gastric Vagotomy Without Drainage.   A relatively new procedure in the United States (widely done in Great Britain and Europe) is the denervation of the acid-secreting parietal cell mass of the stomach while preserving vagal innervation to the gastric antrum and extragastric abdominal viscera. This procedure (also referred to as highly selective or parietal cell vagotomy) is safe, with few side-effects, such as dumping syndrome. However, it is too early to assess the effect of this operation on long-term recurrence of duodenal ulcers.

Postoperative Care.   Postoperative care is the same as for gastric surgery. See page 801.

Zollinger–Ellison Syndrome (Gastrinoma)

Zollinger–Ellison syndrome should be considered a possibility when a patient presents with several peptic ulcers; it is identified by a triad of findings: hypersecretion of gastric juice, multiple duodenal ulcers (second and third portions), and gastrinomas (islet cell tumors) in the pancreas. The incidence of malignancy is approximately 65%. The huge amounts of secreted hydrochloric acid almost have the effect of the stomach's trying to digest itself. The serum gastrin level is increased. Steatorrhea (unabsorbed fat in the stool) may be evident, because excessive gastric acid inactivates lipase in the intestine, thereby precipitating bile salts and decreasing fat digestion. The result is steatorrhea and diarrhea. Gastrin also decreases water and salt absorption, which in turn leads to diarrhea.

Patient Assessment.   Diarrhea and hypercalcemia are common problems. A nursing assessment frequently reveals that the patient's symptoms are often refractory (unyielding) to large amounts of antacids. He may disclose taking several pints of milk a day with no apparent relief from pain.

Management.   Hypersecretion of acid can be controlled with H_2 receptor blocking agents (cimetidine) while the patient is prepared for surgery. (Long-term use of cimetidine in these patients has not been evaluated yet.) The patient's weight needs to be monitored, and fluid and electrolyte balance must be brought under control. Surgery that is necessary usually includes a gastrectomy (to remove acid-secreting surface) and possibly partial pancreatectomy (to remove tumors). In the postoperative period, dietary instruction is necessary; vitamin B_{12} is given monthly. Careful follow-up monitoring is done to detect metastasis.

Stress Ulcer

Stress ulcer is the term given to a group of duodenal or gastric ulcers that occur following physiologically disturbing conditions.

Pathophysiology and Etiology.   Stressful conditions such as burns, shock, severe sepsis, and multiple organ trauma can initiate the development of such ulcers. Fiberoptic endoscopy within 24 hours of injury reveals shallow erosions of the stomach wall; by 72 hours, multiple gastric

Table 37-2
Gastric Operations for Peptic Ulcers

Operation	Description	Mortality	Recurrence	Advantages	Sequelae
Vagotomy with drainage: pyloroplasty or gastroenterostomy	Vagotomy may be total or partial (preserving hepatic branch of anterior nerves and celiac branch of posterior nerve)	Under 1%	10%–15%	Fairly simple Clinical results: 75%—excellent 10%—fair 10%—poor	Some patients experience problems of fullness after eating (33%), dumping syndrome (10%), diarrhea (10%)
Vagotomy with antrectomy	Resection of vagus nerves and removal of antrum	3.9%	3.3%	Marginal ulceration rate lowest	In some patients, fullness after eating, dumping syndrome, diarrhea, anemia, malabsorption
Partial gastrectomy Billroth I (gastroduodenostomy; anastomosis after resection)	Removal of distal ⅓ to ½ of stomach; anastomosis with duodenum	2%		Restores normal continuity	Dumping syndrome, anemia, malabsorption, and weight loss Billroth I has a 4% marginal ulceration rate
Billroth II (gastrojejunostomy; anastomosis after resection)	Removal of distal segment of stomach and antrum; anastomosis with jejunum				Billroth II has a 2% marginal ulceration rate
Proximal gastric vagotomy without drainage	Denervation of acid-secreting parietal cells but preserving vagal innervation to gastric antrum and extragastric abdominal viscera	Under 1%	1%–9%	No dumping, reflex gastritis, or diarrhea No need for antibiotics, since gastrointestinal tract is not open	Appears to be a safe procedure; needs long-term assessment

erosions are observed. As the stressful condition continues, the ulcers spread. When the patient recovers, the lesions are reversed. This is typical of stress ulceration.

Differences of opinion exist as to the actual causation of mucosal ulceration. Usually, it is preceded by shock; this leads to a decrease in gastric mucosal blood flow and a reflux of duodenal content into the stomach. In addition, large quantities of pepsin are released. The combination of ischemia, acid, and pepsin creates an ideal climate to produce ulceration. When acute stress ulceration is combined with central nervous system trauma, stress ulcers (Cushing's ulcers) are often deeper and more penetrating. Gastric erosions are frequently observed about 72 hours after extensive burns (Curling's ulcers).

Prophylactic Therapy. Antacids are the basis of this mode of treatment. If the patient is acutely ill, antacids may be given through the nasogastric tube. Frequent gastric aspiration is done to check pH, in an attempt to get it to, or above, 3.5. Antacid therapy can also inhibit the activity of proteolytic enzyme pepsin.

Management. Stress ulcers are treated aggressively with antacid therapy and cimetidine therapy. Other methods

of management of upper gastrointestinal hemorrhage are discussed on page 795.

▷ Gastric Cancer

Cancer of the stomach continues to decrease in the United States, for some unexplained reason (a 40% decline in the United States in the past 25 years). However, it is still a serious problem, accounting for 15,000 deaths annually, mostly in persons over 40, and occasionally in younger people. The incidence is 4 times greater in Japan, which has led to mass surveys for earlier diagnosis. Heredity appears to be a factor, as does chronic inflammation of the stomach.

Clinical Manifestations. The early symptoms of this disease are often indefinite, since most of these tumors start on the lesser curvature, where they cause little disturbance to the gastric functions. Later, after they have spread to the cardiac orifice, or especially to the pylorus, the suffering may be distressing; this is due not to the cancer as such, but to disturbance in gastric motility. Weight loss, weakness, anemia, and sometimes icterus appear late in the disease.

Pain, in gastric cancer, as in cancer in almost all other parts of the body, is a late symptom. Whereas pain is a sensitive indicator of disturbed physiology or disease, it is ironic that pain rarely warns the individual who has cancer while there is still an opportunity of curing it. The most important early symptoms of gastric cancer are:

- A progressive loss of appetite
- The appearance of, or change in, gastrointestinal symptoms that have been increasingly apparent for a matter of weeks or months only
- The appearance of blood in the stools
- Vomiting (If the tumor causes obstruction at the cardiac orifice, vomiting or a feeling of fullness will immediately follow a meal. If the tumor is near the pylorus, it eventually obstructs this channel, and vomiting becomes a prominent symptom.)
- Occasional vomiting of coffee-ground vomitus, or signs of blood in the stool

The blood that leaks slowly from the cancer (large hemorrhages are rare in patients with gastric cancer) is altered chemically and forms small clots or precipitates. The patient may not vomit, but traces of blood may be found in the stools when examined in the laboratory.

When gastric juice, obtained by aspiration, reveals no free hydrochloric acid, gastric neoplasm is suspected. Biopsies through the gastroscope are most helpful. Cytologic studies verify the diagnosis. Occasionally, the tumor is palpable, especially if it is located near the pylorus. Since metastasis frequently occurs before warning signs are experienced, roentgenograms, fluoroscopy, and gastroscopy are most valuable in determining the extent of the problem.

Dyspepsia of more than 4 weeks' duration in any person over 40 calls for complete roentgenographic examination of the gastrointestinal tract.

Surgical Management.   There is no successful treatment of gastric carcinoma except removal of the tumor. If the tumor can be removed while it is still localized to the stomach, the patient can be cured. If the tumor has spread beyond the area that can be excised surgically, cure cannot be effected. However, in many of these patients, effective palliation may be obtained by resection of the tumor (see p. 801, "Nursing Care Following Gastric Resection"). If a *radical subtotal gastrectomy* has been performed, the stump of the stomach is anastomosed to the jejunum, as in the gastrectomy for ulcer. When *total gastrectomy* is performed, gastrointestinal continuity is restored by an anastomosis between the ends of the esophagus and jejunum. Palliative, rather than radical, surgery is done if there is metastasis to other vital organs, such as the liver.

▷ # Nursing Management of Patients Undergoing Gastric Surgery

Patient Problems/Nursing Diagnosis

The major nursing problems of patients undergoing surgery for gastric cancer include inadequate knowledge of the surgical procedure and postoperative course; potential development of complications; and potential nonadherence to the therapeutic regimen.

▶ ### Planning and Implementation

Goals

The major goals for the patient include:

1. Understanding of the surgical procedure and postoperative course
2. Absence of complications
3. Adherence to the therapeutic regimen

Goals of nursing care for the patient requiring gastric surgery are:

1. To provide physical and psychological support in the perioperative period
2. To promote understanding of the surgical procedure and the postoperative course, and decrease the likelihood of postoperative complications
3. To promote realistic adherence to the postoperative and posthospitalization regimen

Preoperative Nursing Interventions.   *Preoperative nursing care* includes explaining the surgical procedure to the patient and preparing the patient for what to expect after the operation, such as nasogastric intubation and receiving fluids intravenously. However, if the operation is an emergency, because of hemorrhage, perforation, or acute obstruction, adequate psychological preparation may not be possible. In this event, the nurse caring for the patient in the postoperative period should anticipate his concerns, fears, and queries, and be available for support and explanation.

Partial Gastric Resection

Postoperative nursing strategies following partial resection include the following:

1. *Positioning the patient:* When recovery from anesthesia is complete, the patient is placed in a modified Fowler's position, for comfort and for easy drainage of the stomach.
2. *Avoiding pulmonary complications:* Pain medications are administered as prescribed, so that deep breathing and productive coughing may be effective in preventing pulmonary complications. This will overcome the patient's tendency to take shallow breaths in fear of incisional pain. The patient will be asked to take deep breaths and to cough hourly in the immediate postoperative period. The nurse should listen with a stethoscope for the presence of lung congestion.
3. *Checking nasogastric tube drainage:* Drainage from the nasogastric tube may contain some blood for the first 12 hours, but excessive bleeding should be reported. Since a nasogastric tube is in place and peristalsis has not yet returned, fluids by mouth are withheld. The nurse should evaluate the patient for the return of peristalsis by listening to the lower abdomen with a stethoscope. It is also important to observe for signs of distention (increased girth) and to contact the surgeon for any needed readjustment of the nasogastric tube.

4. *Giving nose and mouth care:* The nostrils can be cleaned with an applicator stick moistened with water, followed by swabbing with another applicator stick dipped in mineral oil. To relieve dryness of the mouth, mouthwashes may be given frequently. Cool water sponges to the lips are preferred to cracked ice chips, since ice often intensifies thirst.

5. *Attending to fluid needs:* Parenteral fluids are given to meet fluid and nutritional needs, as well as to compensate for fluid lost in drainage and vomitus. Fluid input as well as output is recorded.

Following the return of peristalsis and the removal of the nasogastric tube, fluids by mouth may be restricted for several hours, then begun sparingly. Small amounts of water are used at first, after which the amount is gradually increased as tolerated. Cold fluids usually cause distress. Therefore, warm, weak tea with sugar and lemon is preferred.

6. *Providing dietary intake:* Bland foods are gradually added until the patient is able to eat six small meals a day and drink 120 ml of fluid between meals. The key to increasing the dietary content is to offer increments gradually as tolerated and to recognize that each person is different. If regurgitation occurs, the patient may be eating too fast or too much. It also may indicate that edema along the suture line is preventing fluids and food from moving into the intestinal tract. If gastric retention does occur, it may be necessary to reinstitute naogastric suction.

7. *Encouraging ambulation:* Usually on the first postoperative day, the patient is encouraged to get out of bed. Ambulation is then increased daily.

8. *Providing wound care:* Wound dressings may have serosanguineous drainage because of drainage tubes left in the wound. Dressings are reinforced if necessary; however, undue drainage saturation is reported.

Total Resection

Nursing strategies for the patient having a total gastric resection include the care described on page 387 ("Postoperative Abdominal Surgical Care") and page 461 ("Postoperative Chest Surgical Care"), since the chest cavity is usually entered. Nasogastric suction will not involve as much drainage, since the stomach is no longer present to produce secretions or to act as a receptacle. The nasogastric tube is removed as soon as normal bowel sounds are heard. Clear fluids are given hourly and small feedings offered after 2 or 3 days, providing there is no evidence of anastomosis leakage (temperature elevation), edema, or obstruction (regurgitation). If there is regurgitation or an increase in temperature, report it immediately.

For guidelines of nursing implementation for the patient following gastric resection, see Chart 37-4.

Nutritional Management After Gastric Surgery

Often a patient who has had gastric surgery has been undernourished before the operation because of food intolerance or preoperative diagnostic testing. There may be sig-

---

Chart 37-4
Guidelines for Nursing Implementation of the Patient Following Gastric Resection

Major Patient Problems/Nursing Diagnoses

1. Inadequate knowledge of the surgical procedure and postoperative course
2. Potential development of complications
3. Potential nonadherence to the therapeutic regimen

Nursing Goals and Interventions

A. To relieve the patient of pain and discomfort:
1. Promote frequent turning for comfort and for the prevention of pulmonary and vascular complications.
2. Maintain meticulous oral hygiene to counteract mouth dryness.
3. Give analgesics or narcotics for pain control.
4. Administer parenteral antibiotics for prevention of infection.
5. Withhold oral fluids until prescribed (to allow sealing of suture line).
6. Use gastric suction to remove liquids, blood, and gas from stomach.

B. To identify complications that may follow gastric surgery:
1. Shock:
   a. Evaluate drainage from dressing and drainage bottle.
   b. Evaluate blood pressure, pulse, and respiratory rates.
   c. Give blood and fluid replacement at time prescribed.

2. Hemorrhage:
   a. Watch gastric aspirate in drainage bottle for evidence of blood.
   b. Observe the suture line for bleeding.
   c. Evaluate blood pressure, pulse, and respiratory rates.
   d. Prepare patient for blood transfusion, and start replacement if indicated.
   e. If bleeding continues, prepare patient for surgical intervention.

(continued)

Chart 37-4
Guidelines for Nursing Implementation of the Patient Following Gastric Resection (continued)

Nursing Goals and Interventions *(continued)*

3. Pulmonary complications:
   a. Auscultate for clear lung sounds.
   b. Encourage deep breathing and coughing to counteract voluntary diaphragm splinting.
   c. Promote frequent turning and moving to mobilize bronchial secretions.
   d. Ambulate, when prescribed, to increase respiratory exchange.
4. Thrombosis and embolism:
   a. Encourage participation in self-care activities to increase circulation.
   b. Encourge early ambulation to minimize stasis of venous blood.
   c. Use elastic stockings as indicated to prevent venous stasis.
   d. Check dressing and binders for tightness that impairs circulation.
5. Wound evisceration:
   a. Use abdominal binders if prescribed for support.
   b. Prevent distention and wound infection.
   c. Support incision when coughing.
   d. Promote good nutrition.
   e. Inspect dressing frequently.
6. "Dumping syndrome":
   a. Teach patient to avoid eating large meals.
   b. Avoid salty, or highly concentrated carbohydrate foods.
   c. Take fluids between meals.
   d. Avoid liquids with meals.
   e. Eliminate sweets from the diet.
   f. Eat regularly, slowly, and in a relaxed environment.
   g. Lie down after meals.
   h. Take anticholinergic drugs before meals (as directed) to lessen gastrointestinal activity.
7. Leakage from duodenal stump (disruption of duodenum):
   a. Evaluate for pain, elevation of temperature, accelerated pulse rate, abdominal rigidity, and deteriorating clinical course.

   b. Observe for appearance of bile-stained drainage.
   c. Prepare for surgical drainage.
      (1) Obtain drainage equipment.
      (2) Prepare for intravenous infusions and blood transfusions.
      (3) Institute nasogastric suction.
      (4) Protect skin from irritating drainage.
8. Pancreatitis:
   Assess for abdominal pain, rapid pulse, and temperature elevation.
      (1) Establish continuous gastric suction.
      (2) Maintain fluid and blood volume and electrolyte balance.
      (3) Control pain.
      (4) Give medications and antibiotics as prescribed.

C. To promote adequate nutrition:
1. Give intravenous fluids to prevent shock and maintain optimal fluid and electrolyte balance.
2. Give oral fluids when audible bowel sounds are present.
3. Increase fluids according to patient's tolerance.
4. Keep patient on bland diet with vitamin supplements as indicated by his condition.
5. Maintain supplementary iron-vitamin therapy to ensure adequate intake.
6. Avoid foods that may initiate development of "dumping syndrome" (see B, 6).
7. Enteral tube feedings or parenteral hyperalimentation therapy may be necessary.

D. To promote adherence to the therapeutic regimen:
1. Help patient to modify his environmental stresses.
2. Encourage him to remain under medical supervision.
3. Encourage a nutritious diet with a gradual decrease in number of meals to three per day.
4. Weigh regularly.
5. Have yearly hematologic study and medical evaluation for evidences of pernicious anemia.
6. Arrange for psychological counseling if needed.

---

nificant protein deficiency, which may require parenteral nutritional support (see p. 780) for the first 5 or 6 postoperative days. Mouth feeding is resumed as soon as the patient feels hungry and bowel sounds are elicited.

Dysphagia may be noticed in those patients who have had truncal vagotomy, which causes trauma to the lower esophagus. This patient may be more comfortable on a soft diet for the first 10 days to 2 weeks. To encourage the patient to eat, attractive dishes and appetizing food should be served in a pleasant atmosphere. With regard to long-term management of this patient, weight loss is a common prob-

lem owing to diminished food intake, since the patient experiences early fullness that, in turn, curbs his appetite. Anorexia may also be due to the "dumping syndrome," which occurs in about one fifth of individuals, following partial gastrectomy (see "Dumping Syndrome," p. 803).

Appropriate nursing intervention is to suggest the following patient teaching points:

- Fluids should be taken before or between meals, rather than with meals.
- Smaller but more frequent meals should be eaten.

- Meal composition should be more dry than fluid-filled.
- Diets with small-molecule carbohydrates, such as sucrose and glucose, should be avoided, but fat may be consumed to tolerable levels.
- It may be advisable to supplement diet with vitamins and medium-chain triglycerides.

Other dietary deficiencies that the nurse should be aware of include (1) malabsorption of organic iron, which may have to be supplemented with oral or parenteral iron; and (2) low serum level of vitamin B_{12}, which may require supplementation by the intramuscular route.

Postoperative Complications
(For an overall outline of the complications following gastric resection and the related nursing management, see Chart 37-4.)

Shock. Shock has been mentioned as a complication, especially in very ill patients. The restoration of normal temperature and the administration of fluids are the prophylactic measures necessary. For symptoms and treatment of shock, see pages 402–407.

Hemorrhage. Hemorrhage is occasionally a complication after gastric operations. The patient exhibits the usual signs (see p. 407) and may vomit bright red blood in considerable amounts. Since this experience can prove upsetting to the patient, diazepam (Valium) or phenobarbital is effective in lessening patient apprehension. Nasogastric drainage or lavage is also helpful. Adrenalin hydrochloride solution may be given to produce vasoconstriction.

- When hemorrhage occurs, it is important to initiate antishock measures and notify the physician. Blood, blood substitutes, and intravenous equipment are made available.
- Nursing support of the patient is given concurrently with emergency therapy.

Pulmonary Complications. Pulmonary complications frequently follow upper abdominal incisions because of the tendency to shallow respirations. Therefore, the nurse utilizes foresight and initiates appropriate preventive measures to promote optimum oxygen–carbon dioxide exchange and adequate circulation.

Steatorrhea. Steatorrhea (unabsorbed fat in stool) is partially the result of rapid gastric emptying, which prevents adequate mixing with pancreatic and biliary secretions. In mild cases, steatorrhea can be controlled by reducing the intake of fat and taking an antimotility drug.

The Dumping Syndrome. The term *dumping syndrome* designates an unpleasant set of vasomotor and gastrointestinal symptoms that occur after meals in about 10% to 50% of patients who have had gastrointestinal surgery or a form of vagotomy.

Clinical Manifestations. Early symptoms may include a sensation of fullness, weakness, faintness, dizziness, palpitations, and diaphoresis, cramping pains, and diarrhea. Later, there is a rapid elevation of blood glucose followed by a compensatory reaction of insulin secretion. This results in a reactive hypoglycemia, which is also unpleasant for the patient. Symptoms that may occur 10 to 90 minutes after eating are vasomotor and are manifested by pallor, perspiration, palpitations, headache, and feelings of warmth, dizziness, and even drowsiness.

Pathophysiology. The pathophysiology underlying this syndrome is not completely understood, but there may be several causes for its occurrence. One is the mechanical result of surgery in which a small gastric remnant connects into the jejunum through a large opening. Foods that are high in carbohydrates and electrolytes have to be diluted in the jejunum before absorption can take place, yet the passage of food from the stomach remnant into the jejunum is too rapid. The ingestion of fluid at mealtime is another factor that causes the stomach contents to empty rapidly into the jejunum. The symptoms that occur are probably brought about by rapid distention of the jejunal loop anastomosed to the stomach. The hypertonic intestinal contents draw extracellular fluid from the circulating blood volume into the jejunum to dilute the high concentration of electrolytes and sugars.

Nursing Strategies. In anticipation of the possibility of the patient's experiencing the dumping syndrome, nursing intervention is directed toward proper dietary instruction.

- The patient should be positioned in a semirecumbent position during mealtime. Following the meal, he should lie down for 20 to 30 minutes to delay stomach emptying.
- Fluids are discouraged with meals but may be given up to an hour before mealtime or 1 hour following mealtime.
- Fat may be given to tolerance, but carbohydrate intake should be kept low (sucrose and glucose are avoided).
- Antispasmodics also may aid in delaying the emptying of the stomach.

Surgery is resorted to only if absolutely necessary (less than 1% of patients).

Gastritis and Esophagitis. With the removal of the pylorus, which acted as a barrier to the reflux of duodenal contents, a bile reflux gastritis and esophagitis may occur. This is manifested by burning epigastric pain and the vomiting of bilious material. Eating or vomiting does not relieve the situation. Binding agents such as cholestyramine, aluminum hydroxide gel, or metoclopramide hydrochloride (Reglan, Maxeran) have been used with some success.

Bezoars (Phytobezoar). Bezoars are gastrointestinal concretions (hardened particles) of digested plant material (such as skins, seeds, and fibers of fruit and vegetables). The patient complains of a feeling of upper abdominal fullness and a "dragging" sensation. The undigested fibers congeal to form a mass that becomes coated by mucous secretions; this produces a *bezoar*. Bezoars may erode the gastrointestinal mucosa and may cause ulceration, hemorrhage, perforation, or obstruction. Upon x-ray or endoscopy, a freely movable mass is observed. The endoscope can be used to break up the concretion. Restricting cellulose-containing foods (especially citrus fruits, such as oranges) is a good prophylactic measure, as is proper mastication of food.

Vitamin B_{12} Deficiency. Total gastrectomy brings to an abrupt, complete, and final halt the production of "intrinsic factor," the gastric secretion that is required for the absorption of vitamin B_{12} from the gastrointestinal tract (see

p. 755). Therefore, unless this vitamin is supplied by parenteral injection throughout life, the patient inevitably suffers from vitamin B$_{12}$ deficiency, which leads in time to a condition identical to that of a patient with pernicious anemia in relapse. All of the manifestations of pernicious anemia, including macrocytic anemia and combined system disease, may be expected to develop within a period of 5 years or less, to progress in severity thereafter, and, in the absence of therapy, to prove fatal. This complication is avoided by the regular monthly intramuscular injection of 100 μg to 200 μg of vitamin B$_{12}$, a regimen that should be started without delay after gastrectomy.

▶ **Evaluation**

Nursing evaluation of the patient having gastric surgery should be both short-term and long-term in scope. Short-term evaluation can be done through an assessment of the absence of physical complications and through an assessment of the patient's coping behavior.

Short-term Evaluation

- *Stable respiratory status:* Respiratory rate between 14 per minute and 20 per minute; clear breath sounds heard
- *Lack of infection or excessive drainage or hemorrhage:* Vital signs stable; minimal blood in gastric drainage after 12 hours
- *Stable hydration and nutrition:* Adequate intake and output; adequate urinary drainage; gradually tolerating fluids and bland foods; maintaining or possibly gaining weight; absence of dumping syndrome
- *Daily increases in activity and ambulation*
- *Stable psychological coping:* Patient understands the purposes of the surgical procedure and the postoperative course; verbalizes his concerns about the surgical outcome; uses support of family or significant others appropriately

Long-term Evaluation.

This should be directed toward an assessment of the patient's physical and psychological readiness to return to his home and the community. (If the patient has gastric cancer, goals are for maintenance and palliation.) The patient and family will benefit from a team approach to discharge care. The team members include the visiting nurse, physician, nutritionist, and perhaps the social worker. Written instructions about meals, activities, medications, and follow-up care are helpful. The postdischarge plan has to be individualized, and the patient's physical status, resources, and prognosis taken into account. The plan should include the following areas:

- *Nutrition and hydration:* The patient may be on small, frequent feedings or may have progressed to regular meals. Resumption of regular meals may require a period of 6 months. If a major portion of the stomach was removed, the patient may require enteral tube feedings or perhaps parenteral hyperalimentation therapy (see Chap. 36).
- *Activity and rest:* Gradual resumption of activities should be encouraged according to the individual's abilities. This could require a period of at least 3

months but is dependent upon the patient's previous activity schedule. Periods of rest should be encouraged each day.

- *Analgesics:* If the patient requires medication for pain, instructions regarding usage, administration, etc., should be given.
- *Follow-up supervision:* The patient should understand that follow-up care is necessary. Travel arrangements for clinic and office visits may be necessary.
- *Long-term coping:* The need for assistance for the patient and family in coping with the situation should be anticipated. Appropriate community agencies (*e.g.,* church, hospice, home health worker) should be identified and referrals made as needed.

Expected Outcomes

1. Understands the surgical procedure and postoperative course
   a. Expresses concerns about surgery
   b. Discusses feelings about surgery with health team members and family
   c. Discusses the surgical procedure and postoperative course
2. Is free of complications
   a. Maintains respiratory rate 14 per minute to 20 per minute
   b. Demonstrates clear breath sounds
   c. Shows minimal blood in gastric drainage after 12 hours
   d. Has stable vital signs
   e. Attains adequate fluid intake
   f. Maintains adequate urinary output
   g. Increases activity and ambulation daily
   h. Tolerates fluids and bland foods gradually
   i. Maintains/gains weight
   j. Is free of symptoms of dumping syndrome
3. Adheres to therapeutic regimen
   a. Resumes normal activities within 3 months
   b. Alternates periods of rest and activity
   c. Keeps follow-up clinic or physician appointments
   d. Tolerates three regular meals daily within 6 months after surgery

▷ **Bibliography**

Books

Becker HD and Caspary WF. Postgastrectomy and Postvagotomy Syndrome. New York, Springer–Verlag, 1980.

Berk JE. Developments in Digestive Diseases. Philadelphia, Lea & Febiger, 1980.

Bongiovanni G. Manual of Clinical Gastroenterology. New York, McGraw–Hill, 1982.

Given BA and Simmons SJ. Gastroenterology in Clinical Nursing, 3rd ed. St Louis, CV Mosby, 1979.

Greenberger NJ and Winship DH. Gastrointestinal Disorders, 2nd ed. Year Book Medical Publishers, 1981.

Hollender LF and Marrie A. Highly Selective Vagotomy. New York, Masson, 1979.

Spiro HM. Clinical Gastroenterology, 3rd ed. New York, Macmillan, 1982.

Articles
General

Boehmer VW and Turk MF. Caring for the gastroplasty patient. AORN J 1981 Dec; 34(6):1036–1042.

Brian–Caldwell B. Turning an impossible situation into a manageable one (gastric bypass). Nursing '81 1981 Sept; 11(9):52–57.

Burkhart C. Upper GI hemorrhage: The clinical picture. Am J Nurs 1981 Oct; 81(10):1817–1820.

Curtailing a life-threatening crisis–GI bleeding. Nursing '81 1981 Apr; 11(4):70–73.

Lamphier TA and Lamphier RA. Upper GI hemorrhage: Emergency evaluation and management. Am J Nurs 1981 Oct; 81(10):1814–1817.

Petlin AM and Carolan JM. How to stop a GI bleed. RN 1981 Apr; 44(4):43–49.

Rogers K et al. Gastric-juice enzymes—an aid in the diagnosis of gastric cancer? Lancet 1981 May 23; 1(8230):1124–1126.

Simmons S and Given B. Nissen fundoplication for hiatus hernia repair. AORN J 1981 July; 34(1):35–46.

Steinberg JJ. Parenteral nutrition before surgery. Lancet 1982 Feb 20; 1(8269):453.

Tweedle D. Parenteral nutrition before gastrointestinal surgery. Lancet 1982 Mar; 1(1):681–682.

Peptic Ulcer and Gastric Conditions

Babb RR. Cimetidine. Postgrad Med 1980 Dec; 68(6):87–93.

Burkle WS. Tagamet. Nursing '80 1980 Apr; 10(4):86–87.

Cimetidine prophylaxis of gastrointestinal bleeding. JAMA 1980 Sept 12; 244(11):126.

Cimetidine update. Am J Nurs 1981 May; 81(5):1026–1027.

Drug Data: Antacid therapy. Am J Nurs 1981 Apr; 81(4):788–789.

Dyck WP. Cimetidine in the management of peptic ulcer disease. Surg Clin North Am 1979 Oct 59(5):863–868.

Frank–Stromborg M and Stromborg P. Test your knowledge of caring for the patient with peptic ulcer. Nursing '81 1981 May; 11(5):66.

Gastrointestinal stapling safe. AORN J 1980 Jan; 31(1):62–63.

Grossman MI. Editorial: Elevated serum pepsinogen I: A genetic marker for duodenal disease. N Engl J Med 1979 Jan 11; 300(2):89.

Koo J et al. Cimetidine versus surgery for recurrent ulcer after gastric surgery. Ann Surg 1982 Apr; 195(4):406–412.

Leeds AR et al. Pectin in the dumping syndrome: Reduction of symptoms and plasma volume changes. Lancet 1981 May 16; 1(8229):1075–1078.

Mangla JC and Pereira M. Tricyclic antidepressants in the treatment of peptic ulcer disease. Arch Intern Med 1982 Feb; 142(2):273–275.

Marshall JB and Settles RH. Zollinger–Ellison syndrome. Postgrad Med 1980 July; 68(1):38–50.

Morris SJ and Rogers AI. Diarrhea after gastrectomy and vagotomy. Postgrad Med 1979 Jan; 76(1):219–230.

New drugs for ulcers, sucralfate (now) and rantidine (soon). The Harvard Medical School Health Letter 1982 July; 7(9):5.

Rodman MJ. The drug interactions we all overlook (antacids). RN 1980 Oct; 43(10):47–49.

Rotter JT. Duodenal-ulcer disease associated with elevated serum pepsinogen I. N Engl J Med 1979 Jan 11; 300(2):63–65.

Singer JA and Rason GR. Gastric ulcer: The importance of follow-up care. Am J Surg 1979 Sept; 136(3):302–305.

Steinberg WM, Lewis JH, and Katz DM. Antacids inhibit absorption of cimetidine. New Engl J Med 1982 Aug 12; 307(7):400–404.

Sucralfate—a new drug for duodenal ulcer. Med Lett 1982 Jan 8; 24:2–3.

Sucralfate approved for duodenal ulcer. FDA Drug Bull 1982 Apr; 12(1):3–4.

38

Management of Patients With Intestinal Disorders

▷ Constipation

Constipation is a term that describes an abnormal infrequency of defecation, and also abnormal dryness of the stools.

Obstipation (no bowel movements) is indicative of bowel obstruction or adynamic ileus.

Chronic Constipation

Most normal persons have one bowel movement a day. Some, however, go 2, 3, or 4 days without a movement; their stools are normally moist, and they suffer no discomfort. On the other hand, some constipated persons at times have a diarrhea of liquid stools, owing to the irritation caused by the presence in the colon of hard, dry fecal masses. Such stools contain a good deal of mucus, secreted by glands in the colon in response to these irritating masses. In severe constipation, the rectum may become impacted, that is, filled with masses of hard feces that must be removed by the fingers or first softened by instillations of oil before they can be washed out by an enema.

Pathophysiology. There are few organic causes of chronic constipation. The most important of these are cancer of the bowel, morphine addiction, and lead poisoning. Painful hemorrhoids and anal fissures, by inducing rectal spasm, also may lead to temporary constipation. Other factors that predispose to constipation include limitation of muscular exercise, unfamiliar diet, weakness, debility, fatigue, and inability to increase intra-abdominal pressure, as seen in emphysema.

By far the most common type of constipation is functional, rather than organic. Many patients develop a constipation habit because of the careless or neurotic habit of delaying each bowel movement as long as possible. The rectal mucous membrane and musculature become insensitive to the presence of fecal masses, and consequently the stimulus required to produce the necessary peristaltic rush for defecation becomes increasingly greater. The initial effect of this fecal retention, or hoarding, is to produce irritability of the colon, which, at this stage, goes frequently into spasm, especially after meals, giving rise to colicky midabdominal or low abdominal pains. Eventually, after several years, the colon loses muscular tone; it is essentially unresponsive to normal stimuli. At this point, the patient may be said to have *atonic constipation,* whereas in the earlier stage the condition is sometimes referred to as *spastic constipation,* although neither type should be regarded as a separate entity. Atony of the bowel also occurs with aging, and this can be complicated with constant use of laxatives.

Nursing Assessment and Intervention

Goals of nursing care for the patient with constipation are (1) to restore or maintain regular bowel function, and (2) to refer patients with questionable symptoms for further evaluation.

When talking with patients about their bowel habits, it is helpful to keep in mind that some may be embarrassed to discuss such a personal body function. Tact and respect for the reserved patient is generally appreciated. Questions of a more personal matter may be placed later in the history after rapport has been established.

In simple or functional constipation, the role of the nurse is to assist with the reeducation of the patient. The physiology of defecation should be explained carefully, with particular emphasis on the importance of heeding promptly the urge to defecate. Instruct the patient to have a regular time for defecation, preferably after a meal. Thinking about the act of defecation, that is, "autosuggestion," may be an aid in initiating the reflex. A small footstool to promote flexion of the thighs ensures an optimal posture during defecation.

Patients who worry about having a *daily* bowel movement need reassurance. Carefully explain that some healthy persons have a bowel movement three times daily while others do so only two or three times a week. Knowing that some of the food eaten may normally remain in the intestinal tract 48 hours after ingestion will help the patient to understand and accept the fact that a daily bowel evacuation is not always necessary. The use of laxatives should be discontinued. If the feces remain in the rectum too long and become dehydrated and hardened, the patient may be instructed to instill 60 ml to 90 ml (2 oz–3oz) of warm oil

into the rectum at bedtime. A small enema of physiologic saline the next morning should help to alleviate this condition.

Measures helpful in breaking the constipation habit include:

1. Establishing a regular time to go to stool each day
2. Drinking a large glass of prune juice or lemon juice in warm water each morning
3. Taking a bulk-forming laxative that does not irritate the bowel, such as Metamucil: 1 heaping teaspoonful in a glass of water, followed by a second glass of water, once or twice daily
4. Assuring a plentiful daily fluid intake
5. Establishing a regular schedule of physical activity or exercise

The patient must know what constitutes a normal diet and should be aware of the similarities between his prescribed diet and the normal diet. In general, a high-residue, high-fiber diet is prescribed for atonic constipation; a bland or low-residue diet is indicated for the patient with an irritable colon (Table 38-1). Approximately the same amount of food should be eaten at each meal, and 2 liters of fluid ingested daily (or more, if the patient perspires freely).

Evaluation. An evaluation of the patient's success in complying with the suggested bowel regimen can be done through assessing whether the patient has:

- Established a regular time for defecation with regular bowel movements
- Has been successful in avoiding laxatives or has limited himself to bulk-forming laxatives, such as Metamucil
- Has altered his diet to include foods and fluids that promote normal bowel movements
- Has developed a reasonable schedule of physical activity or exercise

Acute Constipation

Acute constipation, in contrast with the chronic variety, always indicates an acute and, frequently, a serious disorder. The symptom may prompt one to think in terms of a laxative, but it must be remembered that acute constipation may be an early symptom of acute appendicitis, and that a laxative given in this condition may well produce perforation of the

Table 38-1
A Suggested Relationship Between Diet and Effect on Intestine

Diet	Movement	Bulk	Consistency	Intralumen Pressure	Susceptibility to Disease
High-residue Bulky Unrefined	Rapid	Large	Soft	Low	Low
Low-residue Concentrated Refined	Slow	Small	Hard	High	High

inflamed appendix. In general, a cathartic should not be given for fever, nausea, or pain merely because the bowels fail to move; and, before such medication is offered, it must be quite clear that no inflammatory disease of the intestinal tract is present.

Enemas are relatively safe as regards the possible perforation of an inflammatory lesion of the bowel, provided that they are administered with extreme caution. Saline solutions, or water alone, may be instilled, but nothing more irritating should be used, and the nurse should be prepared to halt the irrigation at once if pain is induced or increased in the slightest degree.

Complications of Constipation

The maintenance of elimination is basic to the care of every patient. The mechanical difficulties and the physical discomforts associated with defecation and micturition that harass the bed patient are widely known. The effort entailed in defecation is considerable. With the use of a bedpan, the muscular strain is inevitably greater, and when constipation is imposed in addition, the performance of this function can be extremely fatiguing, if not altogether exhausting. This is a serious consideration in the management of patients with congestive heart failure, those who have suffered a recent myocardial infarction and are susceptible to cardiac rupture, and those with arterial hypertension.

To facilitate elimination, the patient should assume the normal position for defecation. In most instances there is less strain if the patient is assisted to a bedside commode. Or the patient may be seated on the bedpan at the side of the bed, with his feet supported on a chair. If he cannot sit up, a small support should be placed under the lumbosacral curve to minimize strain and increase his comfort while using the bedpan.

Straining at stool has a striking effect on the arterial blood pressure (Valsalva maneuver). During the period of active straining, the flow of venous blood in the chest is temporarily impeded, owing to an increase in intrathoracic pressure that tends to collapse the large veins in the chest. The atria and the ventricles receive less blood, and consequently less is delivered by the systolic contractions of the left ventricle; the cardiac output is decreased, and there is a transient drop in arterial pressure. Almost immediately after this period of hypotension, a rise in arterial pressure occurs; the pressure is elevated momentarily to a point far exceeding the original level (the "rebound" phenomenon). In patients with arterial hypertension, this compensatory reaction may be exaggerated greatly, and the peaks of pressure attained may be dangerously high—sufficient, indeed, to rupture a major artery in the brain or elsewhere.

It is not possible to make more than a rough estimate of the frequency with which the act of defecation is the terminal event and brings on death owing to vascular accidents that result from straining at stool. The danger is not sufficiently appreciated, however, particularly in patients with vascular diseases of the type described. Inasmuch as straining is promoted by constipation, the latter cannot be dismissed as altogether inconsequential; on the contrary, it must be concluded that the regularity and the consistency of the stools, as well as the mechanical aspects of defecation, are matters of primary concern.

▷ Diarrhea

Diarrhea is one of the cardinal symptoms of small-bowel disease, although it may also be due to emotional stress; to infections; or to gastric, pancreatic, and large intestine disorders. It is a condition in which there is unusual frequency of bowel movements, as well as changes in the amount, the character, and the consistency of the stools. It is best defined, quantitatively, as more than 200 g of stool per day.

Clinical Manifestations. In acute cases the stools are grayish brown, foul smelling, and filled with undigested particles of food and mucus. The patient complains of abdominal cramps, distention, intestinal rumbling (borborygmus), anorexia, and thirst. Painful spasms (tenesmus) of the anus may attend each defecation.

Nursing Assessment. Diarrhea and its associated symptoms occur in a variety of disorders. The nurse will facilitate the diagnosis in each case by recording discerning observations, including the patient's symptoms, behavior, and remarks. Watery stools are characteristic of small-bowel disease, whereas loose, semisolid stools are associated more often with disorders of the colon. Voluminous, greasy stools suggest intestinal malabsorption, and the presence of mucus and pus in the stools denotes inflammatory enteritis or colitis. Oil droplets in the toilet water are almost always diagnostic of pancreatic insufficiency. Nocturnal diarrhea may be a manifestation of diabetic neuropathy. Questions to ask the patient include:

- Do you have loose stools or more frequent stools? How frequent?
- What do they look like?
- How long have you had this problem? Is this the first time?
- Does this occur during the day only? Just in the morning? Nightly too?
- Is there an urgency about your movements? Signs of incontinency?
- Have you noticed mucus mixed with your stool? Blood, pus, or undigested food?
- Have you traveled recently? Out of the country?

Acute Diarrhea

Pathophysiology. Most acute diarrheas are due to increased secretion of water and electrolytes by the intestinal mucosa. The irritant stimulating the diarrhea may arise from a localized infection or ulceration in the intestinal wall, owing, for example, to carcinoma or diverticulitis. The irritant may be chemical. Castor oil, after it has been acted upon by the digestive juice, is an example of a mild intestinal irritant, as are most of the vegetable cathartics. Certain unripe fruits, which cause crampy diarrhea, likewise belong in this category.

The inflammatory response to these mild irritants is slight; little or no mucous membrane lining is destroyed on exposure to them unless their concentration in the intestinal fluid is excessive. Their chief effect is to produce hyperemia (vascular dilatation, with local increase in blood flow) of the intestinal mucosa and increase in mucous secretion. There also occurs a motor response of hyperperistalsis, which persists until the irritant is excreted. This explains the symptoms of crampy diarrhea.

Infectious Diarrhea. By far the most common intestinal irritants are the products of certain bacteria, whether their growth occurred in the intestine or in the food before it was eaten. In the case of the enteric pathogens, the organisms causing bacillary dysentery, bacterial growth with release of the irritating toxins takes place in the intestine. On the other hand, practically all cases of food poisoning, or ptomaine poisoning, are due to the ingestion of food heavily contaminated and already containing the toxin. *Staphylococcus aureus,* for example, if given an opportunity to grow in food, produces an exotoxin that is extremely irritating to the intestinal tract.

Clinically, except for the presence of diarrhea, there is little similarity between a case of food poisoning owing to the ingestion of food containing bacterial toxins and a case of bacillary dysentery. The diarrhea in food poisoning is explosive in onset, develops within a very few hours following the toxic meal and, except in severe cases, subsides within 1 or 2 days—as soon as the toxin is excreted and the inflammatory response subsides. There is little or no fever, and usually the only associated symptoms are those directly attributable to the diarrhea, namely, dehydration and weakness.

Dysentery owing to the growth of gastrointestinal pathogens within the gastrointestinal tract, on the other hand, develops with a more gradual onset and persists for several days or weeks, with striking constitutional symptoms in addition to the diarrhea.

These clinical differences are quite understandable when it is realized that in the infectious diarrheas, a bacterial invasion of the intestinal mucosa is involved. Then, not only must the bacterial toxins be excreted or destroyed, but also the bacteria themselves must be eradicated, and this takes considerably longer.

▶ Assessment

The diagnosis of an acute diarrhea is based on the course of the disease: the type of onset and progression, the presence or absence of fever, and a study of the stools, which are examined for bacteria as well as for blood and pus. In cases of possible infection, the suspected food is tested by bacteriologic cultures. It is very important to remember that diarrhea often is present in various systemic infections. It may be the initial misleading complaint in certain of the exanthemata before the appearance of the rash, or it may appear as an early symptom of hepatitis. It may complicate or mask such conditions as pneumonia and pyelitis.

▶ Planning and Implementation

Goals

Goals of nursing care for the patient with diarrhea are:

1. Provision of physical support during the acute episode
2. Maintainance of adequate hydration
3. Correction of alterations in fluid and electrolyte balance related to hyperperistalsis

Nursing Intervention. Patients with acute diarrhea are placed on bed rest until the episode has terminated. Fluid and electrolyte replacement, orally or parenterally, is an extremely important measure, symptomatically as well as supportively. During the acute stages the gastrointestinal tract is kept at rest by administering only liquids and foods low in bulk or by withholding oral feeding entirely. Glucose can be absorbed normally in many diarrheas and will reduce water loss. Antidiarrheal agents are often given to delay the passage of food through the intestine, including diphenoxylate hydrochloride (Lomotil), paregoric (Camphorated Tincture of Opium) and codeine. This, however, is controversial in that in some bacterial diseases it may be better not to give an agent that slows intestinal motility. Ready access to a bathroom, privacy, and adequate personal and environmental cleaning after each episode of diarrhea are measures that the patient will appreciate.

Preventive Health Measures. All cases of acute diarrhea should be treated as potentially infectious until they are proved otherwise. If the diarrhea is of infectious origin, those caring for the patient should determine whether there is any diarrhea among the family and neighbors. Ask the patient about recent sources of food and water. By reporting a larger than usual number of cases of diarrhea, the nurse assists in determining whether an epidemic is starting in the community.

Proper precautions to avoid the spread of the disease through contamination of the hands, the clothing, the bed linen, etc., with feces or vomitus, must be taken.

Diarrhea always should be regarded as a potential risk under conditions of crowding; outbreaks occur with particular frequency in institutions such as prisons, boarding schools, army camps, and even hospitals, unless sanitary precautions are observed rigidly and constantly.

Precautions include ensuring that proper storage and refrigeration facilities are available and are used for the handling of all fresh fruits and meats. Meat products should be cooked thoroughly, and all cooked meats should be refrigerated immediately unless they are consumed promptly. Milk and milk products should be refrigerated constantly and protected against exposure. Food items that are particularly prone to infection and provide the best environment for bacterial growth include custards and cream fillings, such as are prepared in éclairs, cream pies, layer cakes, cream puffs, etc. Such materials should be cooked thoroughly and then brought to refrigerator temperature immediately.

Proper housekeeping, especially in kitchen maintenance, is obviously very important in the prevention of epidemic diarrhea. All materials used in the preparation and the serving of food must be cleansed rigorously and kept in immaculate condition. All food handlers should receive detailed instructions in hygienic principles and practices and, upon the development of any illness that is potentially infectious, should be relieved of their duties immediately.

Evaluation. Evaluation activities can be carried out through an assessment of:

- The return of normal peristalsis, as evidenced by normal bowel sounds and the absence of diarrhea without antidiarrheal agents
- Adequate fluid and electrolyte balance, as evidenced by normal tissue turgor; moist mucous membranes; adequate urinary output; absence of fatigue and muscle weakness; normal body temperature; ability to resume

adequate food and fluid intake orally; and an alert, oriented patient.

▷ Diseases of Malabsorption

Digestion is the process whereby nutrients are reduced to appropriate form for intestinal absorption. Intestinal absorption transports nutrients across the mucosa to the portal blood system.

Besides nutrients, the intestinal tract is the recipient of a large volume of fluid and electrolytes. Of about 1500 ml of ingested liquid, plus about 7000 ml from the gastrointestinal tract (salivary, gastric, biliary, pancreatic, and intestinal sources), all but 500 ml are absorbed proximal to the ileocecal valve. Thus, the intestine continually shifts the volume and composition of its contents to fulfill its major function of absorption.

Interruptions in the complex digestive process may occur anywhere to cause *malabsorption.* The chief result of malabsorption is malnutrition manifested by weight loss. Diarrhea is a prominent symptom. Steatorrhea (excessive fat in the feces) is of more specific value in diagnosis.

Malabsorption diseases may be grouped according to the following three classifications: (1) maldigestion, (2) decreased absorption by intestinal mucosa, and (3) a combination of causes (Table 38-2). In addition, certain inflammatory bowel disorders, such as ulcerative colitis and regional enteritis (Crohn's disease), cause increased protein breakdown (catabolism) in the small intestine, with resulting loss of protein into the lumen of the intestine (protein-losing enteropathy).

The Primary Malabsorption States

The above term is applied to three closely related conditions: (1) *tropical sprue,* (2) idiopathic steatorrhea (nontropical sprue), and (3) *celiac disease.*

Pathophysiology and Clinical Manifestations. Tropical and nontropical sprue are diseases of adults; in clinical manifestations and pathologic changes, the two conditions are very similar. However, their geographic incidence and their causes differ, and they respond to different treatments. Celiac disease is limited to childhood but resembles idiopathic steatorrhea in all other respects, and probably represents the juvenile phase of that disease. Other causes are extensive resection of the small bowel and tumor infiltration of the small bowel wall.

The pathologic defect is similar in all three conditions. The principal lesion involves the mucosa of the small intestine, especially the intestinal villae, which become severely blunted or are lost altogether. As a result, the absorptive surface within the small bowel is substantially reduced in area, and food absorption is correspondingly impaired.

The hallmarks of the *malabsorption syndrome,* of whatever cause, are diarrhea or frequent loose, bulky, foul stools that have increased fat content and are often greyish in color; associated weakness, weight loss, and lack of well-being round out the picture.

Patients with the malabsorption syndrome, if untreated,

become weak and emaciated, owing to starvation. Failure to absorb the fat-soluble vitamins A, D, and K causes these patients to develop the corresponding avitaminoses. Manifestations of abnormal bleeding are likely to appear as a result of K deficiency and hypoprothrombinemia (see p. 718). Anemia develops, which is of the macrocytic-type characteristic of folic acid deficiency (see p. 707). Impaired absorption of calcium may be responsible for gradual demineralization of the skeleton and, in the case of children with celiac disease, for the stunting of growth. Moreover, calcium deficiency may lead to extreme neuromuscular hyperirritability, including attacks of hypocalcemic tetany.

Management. Dietary considerations are preeminent, as the basic factor in the pathogenesis of idiopathic steatorrhea and celiac disease is a specific and profound intolerance to a protein substance (gluten) contained in wheat, rye, and barley. A constituent of gluten, *gliadin,* for reasons that are not clear, exerts toxic effects on the mucosa of the small intestine, damaging or destroying its villi and crippling its function. The increased familial incidence of these disorders suggests that a hereditary factor, that is, an inborn error of metabolism, may be involved, and that enzymatic activities governing the digestion of gliadin may be affected. In any case, the elimination of gluten from the patient's diet is followed by striking clinical improvement. His diarrhea ceases and his nutritional status is restored to normal. This gratifying remission may be expected to last as long as the patient remains on a gluten-free diet, and no longer. Unfortunately, the total exclusion of gluten is difficult to accomplish, since this substance is incorporated into many foods as a binder and filler. It is contained in almost every bakery product, "wheat-free" or otherwise, and is an ingredient of other foodstuffs as well, including some brands of ice cream.

The factors primarily responsible for the onset and the progression of tropical sprue have not as yet been clarified. Its clinical course appears to be unaffected by the presence or the absence of gliadin in the diet; hence gliadin intolerance seemingly plays no role in its pathogenesis. Of greatest benefit in this condition is the administration of folic acid, which usually is prescribed until a remission is established, and daily thereafter for a period of 4 to 6 months. Broad-spectrum antibiotics are equally important. The beneficial effects of folic acid in patients with tropical sprue appear with such regularity and on occasion are so striking as to suggest that this particular malabsorption syndrome may be attributable to, as well as productive of, folic acid deficiency.

▷ Appendicitis

The appendix is a small, fingerlike appendage about 10 cm (4 inches) long, attached to the cecum just below the ileocecal valve. No definite function can be assigned to it in man. It fills with food and empties as regularly as does the cecum, of which it is a part. It empties inefficiently, however, and its lumen is very small, so that it is prone to become obstructed and is particularly vulnerable to infection (appendicitis).

Table 38-2
Clinical and Pathophysiologic Aspects of Diseases of Malabsorption and Maldigestion

Diseases of Maldigestion	Physiologic Pathology	Clinical Features
Gastric resection with gastrojejunostomy	Decreased pancreatic stimulation because of duodenal bypass; poor mixing of food, bile, pancreatic enzymes; decreased intrinsic factor; bacterial stasis in afferent loop	Weight loss, moderate steatorrhea, anemia (combination of iron, vitamin B_{12} malabsorption, folate deficiency)
Pancreatic insufficiency (chronic pancreatitis, pancreatic carcinoma, pancreatic resection, cystic fibrosis)	Reduced intraluminal pancreatic enzyme activity, with maldigestion of lipid and protein	History of abdominal pain followed by weight loss; marked steatorrhea, azotorrhea; also frequent glucose intolerance (70% in pancreatic insufficiency)
Ileal dysfunction (resection or disease)	Loss of ileal absorbing surface leads to reduced bile-salt pool size and reduced vitamin B_{12} absorption; bile in colon inhibits fluid absorption	Diarrhea, weight loss with steatorrhea, especially when greater than 100 cm resection, decreased vitamin B_{12} absorption
Stasis syndromes (surgical strictures, blind loops, enteric fistulas, multiple jejunal diverticula, scleroderma)	Overgrowth of intraluminal intestinal bacteria, especially anaerobic organisms, to greater than 10^6 per ml, results in deconjugation of bile salts, resulting in decreased effective bile-salt pool size, also bacterial utilization of vitamin B_{12}	Weight loss, steatorrhea; low vitamin B_{12} absorption; may have low D-xylose absorption
Zollinger–Ellison syndrome	Hyperacidity in duodenum inactivates pancreatic enzymes	Ulcer diathesis, steatorrhea
Lactose intolerance	Deficiency of intestinal lactase results in high concentration of intraluminal lactose with osmotic diarrhea	Affects 70% of U.S. blacks and probably all other non-Caucasian races; varied degrees of diarrhea and cramps after ingestion of lactose-containing foods; positive lactose tolerance test, decreased intestinal lactase
Celiac disease (gluten enteropathy)	Toxic response to a gluten fraction by surface epithelium results in destruction of absorbing surface	Weight loss, diarrhea, bloating, anemia (low iron, folate), osteomalacia, steatorrhea, azotorrhea, low D-xylose absorption; folate and iron malabsorption; diagnostic biopsy change
Tropical sprue	Unknown toxic factor results in mucosal inflammation, partial villous atrophy	Weight loss, diarrhea, anemia (low folate, vitamin B_{12}); steatorrhea; low D-xylose absorption, low vitamin B_{12} absorption; typical but nonspecific biopsy change
Whipple's disease	Bacterial invasion of intestinal mucosa	Arthritis, hyperpigmentation, lymphadenopathy, serous effusions, fever, weight loss; steatorrhea, azotorrhea, diagnostic biopsy change
Certain parasitic diseases (giardiasis strongyloidiasis, coccidiosis, capillariasis)	Damage to, or invasion of, surface mucosa	Diarrhea, weight loss; steatorrhea; organism may be seen on jejunal biopsy or recovered in stool
Immunoglobulinopathy	Decreased local gut defenses, lymphoid hyperplasia, lymphopenia	Frequent association with *Giardia*; hypogammaglobulinemia or isolated IgA deficiency; diagnostic or typical biopsy changes

(From Halsted JA: The Laboratory in Clinical Medicine. Philadelphia, WB Saunders.)

Appendicitis is the most common cause of acute inflammation in the right lower quadrant of the abdominal cavity. About 6% of the population will have appendicitis at some time in their lives; males are affected more than females, and teenagers more than adults.

Clinical Manifestations

Acute appendicitis starts typically with a progressively severe generalized or upper abdominal pain, which, within a few hours, becomes localized in the right lower quadrant of the abdomen. This pain usually is accompanied by a low-

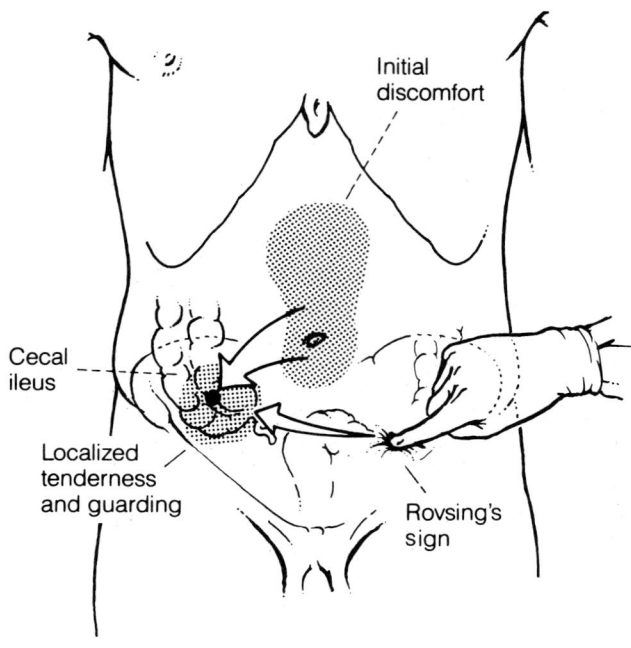

Figure 38-1. This illustrates the area of initial discomfort in appendicitis. As the inflammation progresses, discomfort shifts to the lower right segment of the abdomen. To elicit Rovsing's sign, pressure in the left lower quadrant will intensify pain in the right lower quadrant. (From Gelin LE et al: Abdominal Pain: A Guide to Rapid Diagnosis. Philadelphia, JB Lippincott.)

grade fever, and often by vomiting. At McBurney's point, located halfway between the umbilicus and the anterior spine of the ilium, local tenderness is noted when pressure is applied and there is some rigidity of the lower portion of the right rectus muscle. A moderate leukocytosis is often present. Loss of appetite is common.

Just how much tenderness there will be, how much muscle spasm, whether or not there is constipation or diarrhea, etc., depend not so much on the severity of the appendiceal infection as on the location of the appendix. If the appendix curls around behind the cecum (retrocecal appendix), pain and tenderness may be felt in the lumbar region; if its tip is in the pelvis, these signs may be elicited only on rectal examination. Pain on defecation suggests that its tip is against the rectum; pain on micturition suggests that it is near the bladder or impinges on the ureter. Eventually, the inflamed appendix fills with pus and then is apt to perforate. Once it has ruptured, the pain becomes more diffuse; abdominal distention develops, owing to paralytic ileus, and the condition of the patient worsens.

▶ Assessment

When these symptoms occur in the male, they may be strongly suggestive of acute appendicitis. In the female between 10 and 40 years of age, these manifestations may also suggest a problem with an ovarian cyst, ruptured ovarian follicle or corpus luteum, ruptured ectopic pregnancy, or mittelschmerz (intermenstrual pain).

Upon physical examination, common findings include local and rebound tenderness. Early gentle palpation of the

abdomen reveals diffuse tenderness around the umbilicus and midepigastrium. As the condition progresses, pain shifts to the lower right quadrant. If the patient coughs or the anterior abdominal wall is percussed, pain is enhanced. An interesting Rovsing's sign may be elicited by palpating the left lower quadrant (Fig. 38-1), which, paradoxically, causes pain to be felt by the patient in the right lower quadrant.

The more severe the pain, the more the patient will guard and protect the abdomen, and the greater will be muscular rigidity.

A posture of right hip flexion is a protective maneuver by the patient, suggesting irritation of the psoas muscle (positive psoas sign) by the inflamed appendix. Application of an ice pack (*never of heat*) may provide comfort.

Management.   Operation is always indicated if acute appendicitis is suspected, unless there is good evidence that perforation has occurred recently and that a generalized peritonitis has developed. When the patient is treated conservatively, he is given parenteral electrolyte and amino acid solutions, gastric suction, and antibiotics, in the expectation that the infection will localize and then be susceptible to surgical drainage. As long as the question of operation is undecided, morphine is withheld, even in the face of moderate suffering, because it may mask the patient's symptoms. After the decision has been made, the patient may be sedated comfortably.

▶ Planning and Implementation

Goals

Nursing goals for the patient facing surgery for appendicitis are:

1. To reduce anxiety or stress related to the impending surgery through provision of information about the perioperative period
2. To provide physical support during the perioperative period

Preparation for Operation.   If an operation is necessary, the patient is carefully prepared; an intravenous infusion is started to establish good urinary output and replace existing fluid loss. Aspirin may be prescribed to lower the elevated temperature. Antibiotic therapy is often instituted as a preventive measure against infection. If there is evidence or likelihood of paralytic ileus, a nasogastric tube may be passed. The patient is asked to void, the abdomen is shaved, and the prescribed preoperative medications are given. Usually, an enema is not given, but, if one is requested, it is given low and slowly.

If the patient has been suffering from acute abdominal pain, he may view the operation as a means of relief. This acceptance of surgery makes his anesthetic and postanesthetic course a relatively easy one. The operation may be performed under general or spinal anesthesia. The usual incisions are the McBurney, the muscle-splitting or the gridiron, and the Rockey–Davis (transverse).

Postoperative Nursing Management

Appendectomy Without Drainage.   As soon as the patient recovers from the anesthesia, he should be placed in Fowler's position. Morphine may be given at intervals of 3 or 4 hours. Fluids are usually given as soon as the patient can tolerate them, unless he has been dehydrated. In this case they are given intravenously. Food may be given as desired on the day of operation, if the patient's condition permits. If his temperature is within normal limits and he does not have undue discomfort in the operative area, he may be discharged in 48 hours. The stitches are removed from the incision between the fifth and the seventh days, in the physician's office.

Appendectomy With Drainage. If drainage is required following the appendectomy, there is a possible complication of local or general peritonitis. The patient is placed in Fowler's position as soon as he recovers from the anesthetic, and treatment for peritonitis should be instituted, as described on page 814. These patients are monitored carefully for many days for signs of intestinal obstruction and secondary hemorrhage. Secondary abscesses may form in the pelvis, under the diaphragm, or in the liver. These cause an elevation of temperature and pulse rate, with an increase in the leukocyte count. A fecal fistula, with the discharge of feces through the drainage tract, develops at times. This complication arises most often after the drainage of an appendiceal abscess. Any sign of feces on the dressing should be brought to the attention of the surgeon.

▶ **Evaluation**

Short-term evaluation can be carried out through an assessment of the following:

- Normal body temperature
- Stable vital signs
- Respiratory rate between 14 and 20

- Normal bowel sounds
- Absence of signs of infection, such as inflamed, reddened wound; edema; or drainage from wound
- Adequate intake of food and fluids

Long-term evaluation can be carried out through questioning the patient about his understanding of:

- Any limitations on his return to work or daily activities, or need for altered rest patterns
- Needed follow-up care or supervision (*e.g.*, removal of sutures; wound care and inspection)

Complications

If the appendix can be removed before inflammation has progressed to the point of perforation, there is no further trouble. The abdomen can be closed at once, and the patient can be out of the hospital in a few days. However, if perforation has occurred, the patient may develop generalized peritonitis, or an appendiceal abscess may result, in which case the surrounding loops of bowel become adherent and wall off the spreading peritonitis. For an explanation of nursing management in these instances, see Table 38-3.

▷ Meckel's Diverticulum

Meckel's diverticulum is a congenital abnormality consisting of a blind tube, comparable with the appendix, that usually opens into the distal ileum near the ileocecal valve. A portion of this duct persists as a diverticulum in approximately 2% of the population. It is more common in men than in women.

Table 38-3
Potential Complications Following Appendectomy

Prompt recognition by the nurse and effective management of treatment can prevent prolonged disability for the patient.

Complication	Nursing Assessment and Intervention
Peritonitis	Observe for abdominal tenderness, fever, vomiting, abdominal rigidity, and tachycardia. Employ constant nasogastric suction. Correct dehydration. Give antibiotic agents.
Pelvic or lumbar abscess	Evaluate for anorexia, chills, fever, and diaphoresis. Watch for "diarrhea," which may indicate pelvic abscess. Prepare patient for rectal examination. Prepare patient for operative drainage procedure.
Subphrenic abscess (abscess under the diaphragm)	Assess patient for chills, fever, and diaphoresis. Prepare for x-ray examination. Prepare for surgical drainage of abscess.
Ileus: Paralytic ileus Mechanical ileus	Assess for bowel sounds. Employ nasogastric intubation and suction. Replace fluids and electrolytes by intravenous route. Prepare for operation, if diagnosis of mechanical ileus is established.

The importance of Meckel's diverticulum lies in the fact that its mucosal lining not infrequently may become inflamed and may lead to intestinal obstruction, or it may perforate, causing peritonitis.

The most common symptoms of a diseased Meckel's diverticulum are abdominal pain, typically umbilical in location, or the passage of stools containing blood. The blood is a dark crimson color. (A slowly bleeding gastric or upper intestinal lesion is tarry black; a colonic hemorrhage usually produces bright red bleeding). The treatment is surgical excision of the diverticulum.

▷ Peritonitis

Peritonitis is inflammation of a part or all of the parietal and visceral surfaces of the abdominal cavity. Usually, it is due to bacterial infection, the organisms coming from disease of the gastrointestinal tract, the internal genital organs of the female, and, less often, from outside, by injury or by extension of inflammation from an extraperitoneal organ, such as the kidney. *Inflammation* and *ileus* are the direct effects of this infection. Common causes of peritonitis are presented in Figure 38-2. In addition to these causes, peritonitis is also found associated with continuous ambulatory peritoneal dialysis (see p. 984).

Pathophysiology. Peritonitis is caused by leakage of contents from abdominal organs into the abdominal cavity, usually as a result of inflammation, ischemia, trauma, or tumor perforation, or, in the case of peritoneal dialysis, through the inadvertent introduction of contaminated material. Initially, the material that spills into the abdominal cavity is sterile, (except in the case of peritoneal dialysis), but within hours bacterial contamination occurs. Edema of tissues results, and in a short while exudation develops. Fluid in the peritoneal cavity becomes turbid with increasing amounts of protein, white cells, cellular debris, and blood. The immediate response of the intestinal tract is hypermotility, but this is soon followed by paralytic ileus, with an accumulation of air and fluid in the bowel.

Clinical Manifestations. Symptoms depend on the location and the extent of the inflammation, which is determined by the disease causing the peritonitis. At first a diffuse type of pain is felt. This tends to become constant, localized, and more intense near the site of the process. The affected area of the abdomen becomes extremely tender, and the muscles become rigid. Rebound tenderness and ileus may be present. Usually, nausea and vomiting occur, and peristalsis is diminished. The temperature and the pulse rate increase, and there is almost always an elevation of the leukocyte count. These early clinical manifestations of peritonitis also are the symptoms of the disease causing the condition.

Management and Nursing Intervention. *Objectives of management are to establish and eliminate the cause of peritonitis, correct fluid and electrolyte imbalance, com-*

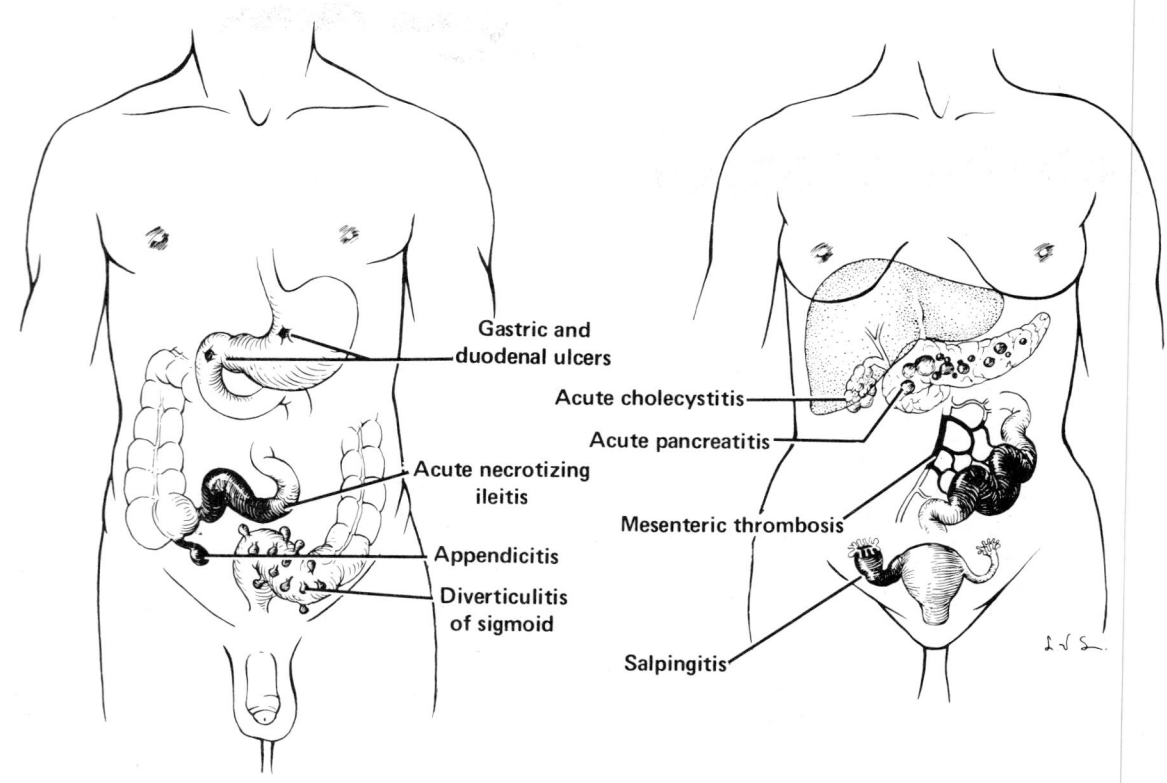

Figure 38-2. Common primary causes of peritonitis. (From Dunphy JE and Way LW: Current Surgical Diagnosis and Treatment. Los Altos, California, Lange Medical Publishers.)

bat infection, and make the patient as comfortable as possible.

Because there often is an outpouring of fluids and electrolytes, it is necessary to prevent hypovolemia, shock, and impaired renal function. In addition to these potential threats, fluid accumulates in the abdominal cavity, exerting pressure against the diaphragm, which, in turn, restricts proper ventilatory function. To avert these life-threatening complications, fluid, colloid, and electrolyte replacement is given high priority. Accurate recording of input and output, including vomitus, assists in calculating fluid replacement. In addition, determination of central venous pressure (see p. 596) may be helpful. A rise in pressure levels to 15 cm or higher may indicate circulatory overload.

Intestinal intubation and suction assist in relieving abdominal distention and help in promoting intestinal function. Oxygen therapy by nasal cannula or mask will promote ventilatory function, but occasionally a tracheostomy and ventilatory assistance may be required. Urinary output is monitored and recorded.

Treatment is directed toward removing the cause: if it is an acutely inflamed appendix, an appendectomy is performed; if it is a ruptured duodenal ulcer, the opening in the duodenum is closed; and so on.

If the cause of the peritonitis is removed at an early stage, the inflammation subsides and the patient recovers. Frequently, however, the inflammation is not localized, and the whole abdominal cavity becomes involved, in which case, the patient is acutely ill. He has severe pain and must be treated compassionately.

Accurate assessment of pain is important. A description of the nature of the pain, its location and shifts in the abdomen, may help ascertain the source of difficulty. Since sepsis is the major cause of death from peritonitis, massive antibiotic therapy is usually initiated early in the treatment. Cultures of peritoneal fluid are taken, but until the laboratory reports are available, large doses of a broad-spectrum antibiotic are given intravenously.

Eventually, unless the cause of peritonitis is eliminated, the patient may succumb to intestinal obstruction. This is brought about by small bowel adhesions and even local abscess formation. If these can be localized, surgical drainage is effective.

Surgical Intervention. "Refunctionalization" may be done surgically. This requires lysis of adhesions, drainage of the abscesses, removal of necrotic tissue, and assurance of continuity of the intestinal tract. Resection and anastomosis may be necessary. Such surgery, along with proper maintenance of nutrition and fluid balance, can assist the patient in recovering.

Postoperative Management. Conscientious and frequent monitoring of cardiac activity, central venous pressure, ventilation, fluid input, and urine output is essential.

Drains are inserted frequently during the operation, and it is essential that the nurse observe and record the character of the drainage. Care must be taken in moving and turning the patient to prevent the drains from being dislodged accidentally.

Evaluation. Signs that the peritonitis is subsiding include a fall in temperature and pulse rate, a softening of the

Table 38-4
Incidence of Hernia

Type	Frequency (Approximate %)
Inguinal, indirect	70
Inguinal, direct	15
Umbilical	5–10
Incisional	5–10
Femoral	5 or less
Others	2 or less

abdomen, a return of peristaltic sounds, passing of flatus, and bowel movements. Food and fluids can then be given by mouth in increasing amounts, and parenteral fluids are reduced.

Two of the most common complications that must be watched for are wound evisceration and abscess formation. Any suggestion from the patient that an area of the abdomen is tender or painful or "feels as if something just gave way" should be reported. The sudden occurrence of serosanguineous wound drainage strongly suggests wound dehiscence (see p. 413).

▷ Abdominal Hernia

A *hernia* ("rupture") is a protrusion of an organ or structure through the wall of the cavity in which it is naturally contained. This definition may apply to any part of the body; for instance, the protrusion of the brain after a subtemporal decompression is called *cerebral hernia*. However, in general, the term is applied to the protrusion of an abdominal viscus through an opening in the abdominal wall.

Indirect inguinal hernia is the most common type of hernia (see Table 38-4). This hernia is due to a weakness of the abdominal wall at the point through which the spermatic cord emerges in the male, and the round ligament in the female. Through this opening the hernia extends down the inguinal canal and often into the scrotum or the labia (Fig. 38-3). It is common in the male, and it may appear at any age.

Inguinal hernia is a major cause of hospitalization, especially among men, in whom it occurs three times more frequently than in women. Most hernias result from congenital or acquired weakness of the abdominal wall, coupled with sustained increased intra-abdominal pressure from coughing or straining, or from an enlarging lesion within the abdomen. Once the hernia occurs, it has a tendency to increase in size.

The hernial sac is formed by an outpouching of the peritoneum and may contain the large or small intestine, omentum, and, occasionally, the bladder. When the hernia first is formed, the sac is filled only when the patient is on his feet, the contents returning to the abdominal cavity as soon as he lies down.

Direct inguinal hernia passes through the posterior inguinal wall. It also is most common in males, more dif-

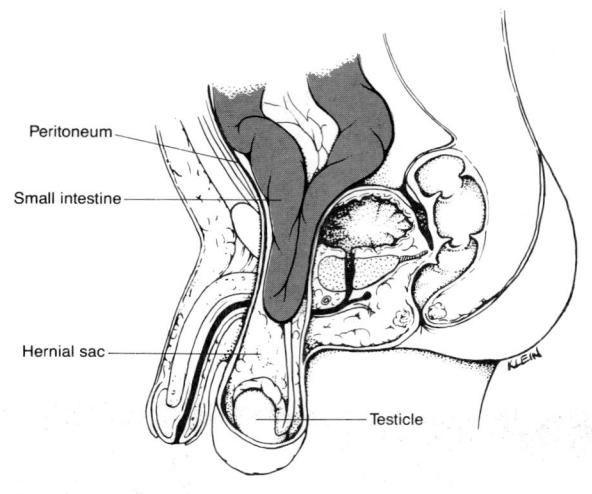

Peritoneum

Small intestine

Hernial sac

Testicle

Figure 38-3. Inguinal hernia. Note that the sac of the hernia is a continuation of the peritoneum of the abdomen and that the hernial contents are intestine, omentum, or other abdominal contents that pass through the hernial opening into the hernial sac.

ficult to repair than indirect inguinal hernia, and often recurs after surgery.

Umbilical hernia results from failure of the umbilical orifice to close. It is most common in obese women and in children, as a protrusion at the umbilicus. This hernia is also seen in patients with cirrhosis and ascites.

Ventral or incisional hernias occur owing to a weakness of the abdominal wall. They are due most frequently to previous operations in which drainage was necessary, complete closure of the tissues being impossible. Weakened by infection, only a slight bulge results at first, but this increases gradually in size until a definite hernial sac is produced.

Femoral hernia appears below the inguinal (Poupart's) ligament (*i.e.,* below the groin) as a round bulge. It is more frequent in women.

A hernia is referred to as *reducible* when the protruding mass can be placed back into the abdominal cavity. This can occur naturally when the patient lies down, or it may require manual reduction (the mass is pushed back into the cavity). As time goes on, adhesions form between the sac and its contents, so that the hernia becomes *irreducible* or *incarcerated.* Such a hernia is one that cannot be reduced and in which the intestinal flow may be obstructed completely.

In a *strangulated hernia* the contents not only are irreducible, but the blood and intestinal flow through the intestine in the hernia is stopped completely. This condition develops when the loop of intestine in the sac becomes twisted or swollen and a constriction is produced at the neck of the sac. The result then is an acute intestinal obstruction, plus the added danger of gangrene of the bowel. The symptoms are pain at the site of strangulation, followed by colicky abdominal pain, vomiting, and swelling of the hernial sac.

Management

Nursing goals are to detect hernias and arrange for adequate referral; to prepare the patient for surgery or, if surgery is unwise or unacceptable, to teach the patient how to care for his hernia (*e.g.,* mechanical reduction, weight loss, perhaps use of a truss); and to teach the patient to detect signs of incarceration or strangulation.

In most instances, the hernia should be repaired by operation; otherwise, it is in continual danger of strangulation. When strangulation occurs, operation becomes imperative and is attended invariably by considerable risk.

Mechanical Reduction. Very often the patient can reduce his own hernia. In order to keep the mass from protruding when a standing position is assumed, a *truss* (a pad made of firm material that is placed over the hernia and held in place with a belt) may be worn. Most authorities agree that a truss creates more problems than it can solve. It may cause skin irritation and lesions, owing to constant rubbing. When improperly fitted it may cause strangulation of the hernia. However, a truss may be recommended (1) for infants, when there is need to wait for a weight gain before surgery or for remission of another problem, such as bronchitis or diaper rash; (2) for adults who have an underlying problem that needs to be resolved first; or (3) when a patient has worn a truss for years, is terrified of the hospital, and will not part with the truss. In this latter instance, the proper fitting of the truss must be done by a qualified person. The Valsalva maneuver can also be used to check for the effectiveness of the truss. Daily bathing and the use of corn starch powder can lessen the possibility of skin irritation. Usually, the truss is worn directly over the hernia and not over clothing, which could cause slipping. It must be emphasized that a *truss does not cure a hernia;* it simply prevents the abdominal contents from entering the hernial sac.

Surgical Repair. The operation involves removal of the hernial sac after it has been dissected free from surrounding structures and the contents have been replaced in the abdominal cavity, and the neck ligated. The muscle and the fascial layers then are sewn together firmly over the hernial orifice to prevent a recurrence. When the tissues are not sufficiently strong, reinforcement can be obtained by overlaying the suture line with synthetic sutures or mesh, which is also sutured in place (hernioplasty). The presence of the mesh stimulates more than the usual amount of fibroblastic activity and thereby enhances the strength of the repair. When a strangulation has occurred, the operation is complicated by an intestinal obstruction and injury to the bowel.

Preoperative Care. In emergency conditions of strangulated or incarcerated hernia, the nurse prepares the patient as in any other acute surgical problem. However, most patients are in good physical condition and are having a herniorrhaphy as elective surgery. The patient may be prompted by the knowledge that an unrepaired hernia may become a serious emergency, or that he may have difficulty securing employment because of this condition.

An important nursing checkpoint is to determine whether the patient has an upper respiratory infection, chronic cough from excessive smoking, or sneezing owing to an allergy. It may be necessary to postpone the operation until a more preferable time, since coughing or sneezing could weaken the postoperative wound, thereby negating the purpose of surgery.

Postoperative Care. The patient may be allowed out of bed the day of, or the day after, surgery. Diet is determined by the desires of the patient, following local or spinal anesthesia. However, if a general anesthesia was used, fluid and food are restricted until peristalsis returns.

Urinary retention is common in the postoperative period; if the patient can get out of bed to void, there usually is no difficulty. In any case, it is necessary to prevent bladder distention; this may require catheterization, if other nursing measures fail.

Following repair of an inguinal hernia, swelling of the scrotum may occur. Because this is extremely painful, the patient is reluctant to move. Elevating the scrotum on a rolled towel and applying small ice bags intermittently are helpful. A narcotic may be given for pain, and antibiotics to prevent epididymitis. A suspensory bandage or jock strap may give support and comfort.

Infection that interferes with healing occurs occasionally. Soreness in the operative region and temperature elevation may suggest such a problem. Systemic antibiotics or local wound treatment with heat application, followed by incision and drainage, may be required.

Should the patient cough or sneeze after the operation, he should be instructed to splint the incision site with his hand, to lessen the pain and also protect the incision site.

For more extensive hernia repair, such as may be required following umbilical or large incisional hernia, nasogastric suction may be used to prevent distention, vomiting, and straining. Mild cathartics may be prescribed to prevent straining during defecation.

Patient Education. Once the hernia is repaired, some surgeons permit the patient to do whatever he wishes, on the premise that he will not engage in painful activity, thereby preventing injury to the incision. If the patient has had local anesthesia, he is allowed more liberties than one who has had general anesthesia.

There may be restrictions on heavy lifting for 2 months; however, some surgeons believe that activities of everyday life help to strengthen the hernia repair. In any event, the nurse may review good body mechanics with the patient before his discharge.

Evaluation. Short-term evaluation of nursing interventions can be carried out through an assessment of the return of peristalsis, adequate urinary output, decrease in scrotal swelling, absence of infection, relief of pain, and avoidance of straining at stool. Long-term evaluation can be carried out through an assessment of the patient's knowledge of the restrictions established.

▷ Regional Enteritis (Crohn's Disease)

Regional enteritis (*Crohn's disease,* granulomatous colitis, granulomatous ileocolitis) is a chronic transmural inflammatory disease of unknown etiology, that may involve any portion of the intestinal tract.

This disease is characterized by inflammatory involvement of segments of the intestine separated by normal intervening areas. Other pathology may include a thickened mesentery and bowel wall and enlarged lymph nodes.

Clinical Manifestations. Symptom onset is usually insidious, but abdominal pain and diarrhea are prominent, and unrelieved by defecation. Scar tissue and formation of granulomas interfere with the ability of the intestine to transport products of the upper intestinal digestion through the constricted lumen, resulting in crampy abdominal pains. Since intestinal peristalsis is stimulated by the eating of food, the crampy pains occur after meals. To avoid these bouts of crampy pain, the patient avoids food or takes it only in amounts and types inadequate for normal nutritional requirements, so that weight loss, malnutrition, and secondary or macrocytic anemia occur. In addition, ulcers form in the lining membrane of the intestine, and other inflammatory changes take place, resulting in a constant irritating discharge that is emptied into the colon from the weeping, swollen intestine. This causes a chronic diarrhea. The end result is a very uncomfortable person who is thin and emaciated from inadequate food intake and constant fluid loss. In some cases, the inflamed intestine may perforate and form intra-abdominal and anal abscesses. Melena may occur, along with malabsorption syndrome. Fever is not a prominent symptom, except when abscesses are present.

Common complications are stricture and fistula formation. Fistulae may extend to the skin or to other loops of bowel; they are apt to occur when a patient has had unrecognized regional enteritis and has undergone an appendectomy.

This disease affects both sexes equally and appears more often in those of Jewish origin. There is a definite familial occurrence. Regional enteritis may occur in any decade of life, but it reaches its highest incidence between the ages of 15 and 35.

Assessment. The most conclusive diagnostic aid is a barium study of the upper gastrointestinal tract that reveals the classic "string sign" on x-ray of the terminal ileum, indicating the constriction of a segment of intestine.

A proctosigmoidoscopic examination is usually done initially to establish whether there is an inflammatory process in the rectosigmoid area. If this area is normal, the diagnosis of ulcerative colitis is ruled out.

Management. In mild episodes, conservative treatment consists of a low-residue, bland diet, with vitamin supplements to improve nutrition. Iron may be prescribed for concomitant anemia. Diarrhea is treated symptomatically. Sedatives may help, and steroids are useful in the treatment of acute attacks but have not been shown to prevent recurrences.

When the symptoms do not respond to these conservative measures, or when massive bleeding occurs, surgical treatment is necessary. This will be determined by the individual case. If the lesion can be delineated to a particular area, it may be resected. Unfortunately, even with surgery, recurrences are common.

▷ Ulcerative Colitis

Ulcerative colitis is an ulcerative and inflammatory disease of the colon and rectum, with rare involvement of the distal ileum.

Pathophysiology

Ulcerative colitis is characterized by multiple ulcerations, diffuse inflammations, and desquamation of the colonic epithelium, with alternating periods of exacerbations and remissions. Most commonly, the disease begins in the rectum and sigmoid and spreads upward, ultimately involving the entire colon. The complications of ulcerative colitis may be local or systemic. Local complications include perforation, hemorrhage, abscess, stricture, and carcinomatous degeneration. Systemic complications include arthritis, erythema nodosum, and nephrolithiasis.

The cause of the disease is unknown. In some patients, an autoimmune mechanism may be responsible. Some authorities consider ulcerative colitis an example of psychosomatic disease, but to date this has not been substantiated. There may be several precipitating factors, the net effect of which is a self-perpetuating destructive infection of the mucosal lining of the large intestine. It is a serious disease, accompanied by systemic complications and a high mortality rate. Eventually, 10% to 15% of the patients develop carcinoma of the colon.

Clinical Manifestations and Assessment

Diarrhea, abdominal pain, and rectal bleeding are the usual symptoms of this condition. In addition, there may be evidence of weight loss, fever and tenesmus, and possibly vomiting. There often is cramping, and the feeling of an urgent need to defecate. Hypocalcemia and iron deficiency frequently develop.

In the diagnosis of chronic ulcerative colitis, dysentery owing to the common intestinal organisms, and especially *Entamoeba histolytica* infection, must be ruled out by careful stool examination. Sigmoidoscopy and barium enema x-ray examination are of value in distinguishing this condition from other diseases of the colon with similar symptoms.

- In acute ulcerative colitis, cathartics are contraindicated when the patient is being prepared for barium enema, since they may cause severe exacerbation of the condition, which may lead to megacolon (excessive dilatation of the colon), perforation, and death. If the patient is required to have this diagnostic test, perhaps a liquid diet for a few days before the x-ray, followed by a gentle tap water enema on the day of examination, is sufficient.

Management and Nursing Implementation

Treatment for chronic ulcerative colitis may be pursued in three areas: medical, surgical, and psychotherapeutic. The objectives of medical therapy are to reduce inflammation and suppress inappropriate immune responses, and also to provide rest for a diseased bowel, so that it may heal. Surgical treatment is designed to remove the source of symptoms, that is, to remove the diseased segments of the intestine and maintain intestinal function through a permanent ileostomy. Psychotherapy is aimed at determining those factors that distress the patient, dealing with these factors, and attempting to resolve conflicts, so that they no longer aggravate the patient.

Surgical management of this condition has improved considerably, and increased knowledge in caring for the patient with an ileostomy has made this approach a reasonably optimistic one. In addition, steroid therapy has alleviated distressing physical symptoms, producing a marked decrease in anxiety and depression in this patient.

The goals of nursing care are to reduce the inflammation of the colon, to provide emotional support and reduce stress, and to provide rest and comfort as required.

Remission of Inflammation. The patient with ulcerative colitis is encouraged to rest after meals, but usually he is not confined to bed unless absolutely necessary. Activity within the limit of his physical capacity is desirable, so that he will not regard himself as an invalid. Toilet facilities and privacy should be available nearby.

Well-balanced, low-residue, high-protein diets with supplemental vitamin therapy and iron replacement are effective in meeting nutritional needs. Fluid and electrolyte imbalance owing to dehydration caused by diarrhea is corrected by intravenous therapy. Any foods that exacerbate diarrhea should be avoided. Milk may contribute to diarrhea if lactose intolerance is present. In addition, cold foods are to be avoided, along with smoking, since both increase intestinal motility.

Sedation and antidiarrheal medications are given to reduce to a minimum the colonic peristalsis, in order to rest the inflamed bowel. Constipation must be watched for, since it may lead to megacolon, with impending perforation. The nurse can be on guard for this possibility by measuring abdominal girth.

Antidiarrheal medications and sedation are continued until the patient's stools approach normal frequency and consistency. Sulfonamides such as sulfasalazine (Azulfidine) or sulfisoxazole (Gantrisin) are often effective in mild or moderate colitis. Antibiotics are used for secondary infections, particularly for purulent complications, such as abscesses, perforation, and peritonitis. Azulfidine is helpful in preventing recurrences.

ACTH and corticosteroids are most effective early in the course of an acute inflammatory phase of this disease, rather than in the chronic phase. A clinical remission is noted in 5 to 10 days, in four fifths of patients treated, as indicated by improved appetite, better mood, a decrease in fever, and an absence of bloody diarrhea. When steroids are reduced or stopped, the symptoms of the disease are likely to return. If steroids are continued, adverse sequelae such as hypertension, fluid retention, subcapsular cataracts, and hirsutism may develop.

Careful assessment and recording of the clinical manifestations as the patient responds to various medications is of high priority among the nurse's responsibilities. It requires an understanding of drug action and potential side-effects.

Reduction of Emotional Stress. Authorities agree that it is unwise to stereotype the patient with ulcerative colitis.

While emotional factors may play a role in this ailment, they need not overshadow its physical basis. It is possible that the disease may be associated with a wide range of psychological symptoms, including emotional immaturity, dependency, ambitiousness, perfectionism, or a combination of these traits. The patient may display evidence of excessive dependency, mood swings, depression, extreme sensitivity, anxiety, and outbursts of aggressive behavior. If this is so, it is important that the nurse recognize that this behavior is not directed at any one individual, but is a means of expressing a need. Obviously, a patient who is suffering a severe debilitating disease, such as ulcerative colitis, will not have the control or stamina of other patients. Therefore, his moods will vary, and his symptoms will fluctuate as his condition improves or deteriorates.

The nurse needs to recognize that the patient's behavior may be affected by innumerable factors aside from any inherent emotional characteristic. Any patient who is suffering from the discomforts of frequent bowel movements and rectal soreness is anxious, discouraged, and depressed. Thus, it is important to develop a relationship with the patient that gives him a feeling that he is receiving support in his attempts to deal with the stresses that have plagued him. Let him know that his complaints are understood, encourage him to talk and ventilate his feelings, and listen to matters that are disturbing to him, even if they seem trivial. Try to direct his attention to himself, and not his intestinal tract.

Education of the patient to accept and learn to live with a chronic disease is an important aspect of treatment. Recognition of the fact that disability is lessened following surgery for ulcerative colitis is an optimistic aspect in treating this patient surgically.

Evaluation.   An evaluation of outcomes can be done through an assessment of success with the following:

Remission of Inflammation

- Adheres to dietary regimen
- Improves appetite
- Alternates periods of rest with periods of activity
- Uses medications as prescribed and without complications
- Is free of bloody diarrhea

Reduction of Emotional Stress

- Discusses feelings about illness with health team members and family
- Alters life-style to cope with stress
- Participates in meaningful diversional and occupational activities

Surgical Treatment and Nursing Management

Approximately 15% to 20% of patients with ulcerative colitis require surgical intervention. Indications for surgery include no improvement and continued deterioration, profuse bleeding, perforation, stricture formation, and indications that carcinoma has developed. The operation of choice is usually a total colectomy (removal of the colon) and ileostomy; any procedure more limited will prove to be of only temporary benefit in most patients.

Preoperative Care.   A period of preparation, with intensive fluid, blood, and protein replacement, is necessary before operation is attempted. Antibiotics are useful adjuncts. If the patient has been on steroids for a long period of time, steroids will probably be continued during the surgical phase, before being gradually tapered. Meanwhile, the patient should be assessed for adrenal insufficiency by observing and recording pulse, blood pressure, urinary output, general appearance, and reaction.

Usually, the patient is on a low-residue diet offered frequently in small feedings. All other preoperative measures are similar to general abdominal surgery. The abdomen is marked for the proper placement of the stoma by the surgeon or the ostomy nurse. Care is taken to see that the ostomy or stoma is conveniently placed. Information about an ileostomy is presented to the patient by means of literature, models, and discussion. The patient should have a fairly good idea of what his surgery is all about and what to expect postoperatively. He may even be encouraged to wear an ileostomy appliance for a day or two before surgery. This will facilitate his adjustment to it after the operation.

Since it is rather difficult to accept an ileostomy, the patient needs all the support possible. It is necessary to help him to develop an outlook that views an ileostomy as a challenge; if accepted with courage, he can master it and proceed to live normally and effectively. Such an outlook is difficult to accept; thus, the task of developing a proper attitude in the patient becomes a major objective for the nurse, who also must have a positive attitude if an optimistic outlook is to be transmitted to the patient. Other patients who have had ileostomies are an excellent source of help to this patient, as are especially trained enterostomal therapists.

Postoperative Care.   The opening of the small intestine on the abdomen (ileostomy) continuously discharges the liquid contents of the small intestine, because the stoma does not have a controlling sphincter. As soon as the operation is completed, a temporary plastic bag with an adhesive facing is placed over the ileostomy and firmly pressed onto surrounding skin. The contents draining from the ileostomy are thus kept from coming into contact with skin and are collected and measured as the bag becomes full. After the ileostomy has had a chance to heal, a permanent appliance is obtained and held in place on the skin with a special cement. The stomal size should be rechecked in 3 weeks, when edema has subsided. The final size and type may be selected in 3 months, after the patient's weight has stabilized and the stoma shrinks to a stable shape.

Because these patients lose much fluid and food in the early postoperative period, an accurate record of fluid intake, urinary output, and fecal discharges is necessary, to help gauge the fluid needs of the patient. Fluids, and a low-residue, high-calorie diet are given until the patient becomes accustomed to the new digestive arrangement.

▷ Ileostomy

Psychosocial Implications

In an ileostomy, the excretory orifice is located on the lower abdomen and must be attended to several times each day.

Table 38-5
Comparison of Regional Enteritis and Ulcerative Colitis

	Regional Enteritis Granulomatous (Transmural) Colitis	Ulcerative Colitis (Mucosal)
I. *Pathology*		
Early	Transmural thickening	Mucosal ulceration
Late	Deep, penetrating granulomas	Mucosal minute ulceration
II. *Clinical manifestations*		
Location	Ileum, right colon (usually)	Rectum, left colon
Bleeding	Usually not, but may occur	Common—severe
Perianal involvement	Common	Rare—mild
Fistulas	Common	Rare
Rectal involvement	About 20%	Almost 100%
Diarrhea	Less severe	Severe
III. *Diagnostic studies*		
X-ray	Reveals skip areas	Diffuse involvement
	Shortening of colon	No shortening of colon
IV. *Therapeutic management*	Steroids, Azulfidine	Steroids, Azulfidine
	Intravenous alimentation	Azulfidine is useful in preventing recurrence
	Partial or complete colectomy, with ileostomy or anastomosis	Proctocolectomy, with ileostomy
	Rectum can be preserved in some patients	
	Recurrence common	Rectum can be preserved in only a few patients "cured" by colectomy
V. *History*	Crippling; indolent	Exacerbations, remissions; may be lethal
		Toxic megacolon

Because of this, the patient understandably may think that everyone is aware of the ileostomy. He may consider the stoma as mutilative, when compared with other abdominal incisions that heal and are hidden. Because there is loss of a body part and a major change in anatomy, the ileostomy patient often goes through the various phases of grieving. The nurse can expect the patient to experience shock, disbelief, denial, rejection, anger, and restitution. Nursing support through these phases is important, and understanding of the patient's emotional outlook in each instance should determine the nurse's approach. For example, any form of teaching is of no avail until the patient has reached the stage of restitution.

Concern over body image may lead to questions related to family relationships, sexual function, and the ability to become pregnant and to deliver normally.

Finally, this patient needs to know that someone understands and cares about him. Sincere friendliness and a nonjudgmental attitude must be exhibited by the nurse. This evident interest will aid in gaining the patient's confidence, so important to therapy and preoperative preparation. Dependency needs are satisfied through good nurse–patient relationships.

Such patients probably are the most challenging of all to the nurse. Their prolonged illness makes them irritable, anxious, and depressed. The nurse can coordinate patient care through nursing conferences attended by consultants such as the physician, psychologist, psychiatrist, social worker, and dietitian. The team approach lends support in approaching a complex nursing problem.

On the other hand, an operation establishing an ileostomy can produce dramatic changes in a patient who has suffered from colitis for several years. Once the misery of the disease is lifted and the patient learns how to take care of the ileostomy, he can become a normal, affable person. But until the patient has progressed to this phase, an empathetic and tolerant approach by the nurse will play an important part in the patient's recovery.

The camaraderie of other ostomates is also a help. A nonprofit health service agency that is dedicated to the rehabilitation of ostomates is the United Ostomy Association, Inc.* This organization gives patients useful information on living with an ostomy, through an educational program of literature, lectures, and exhibits. Local associations provide visiting services by qualified members who give hope, and rehabilitation services, to new ostomy patients. Local hospitals may have an enterostomal therapist on the staff; this is a valuable resource person for the ileostomy patient.

Rehabilitation and Patient Education Following an Ileostomy

There are certain rehabilitation problems unique to the ileostomy patient, one of which is irregularity of bowel evacuation. The patient with an ileostomy cannot establish reg-

* 1111 Wilshire Blvd., Los Angeles, California 90017.

ular bowel habits, because the contents of the ileum are fluid and are discharging continuously. Therefore, the patient must wear an appliance (a vinyl or plastic bag) day and night. The appliance is regarded, then, as an intestinal prosthesis.

Several days after the operation, the ileostomy diameter is carefully measured with a stoma-measuring card (various apertures indicate various sizes) so that a suitable opening in the mounting ring will be available in the permanent appliance. The ring is sealed to the skin with an adhesive disc and permits the patient to carry on normal activities without fear of leakage or odor.

The location and length of the stoma is significant in the management of the ileostomy by the patient. The surgeon places the stoma as close to the midline as possible and in a position where even an obese patient with a protruding abdomen can care for himself readily. Usually, the ileostomy stoma is about 2.5 cm (1 inch) long, which makes it convenient to attach the appliance.

The ileostomy may be noisy at first, owing to edema caused by slight obstruction of tissues. Eventually it will become quieter. A low-fiber diet is followed at first, with strained fruits and vegetables. These foods are important for vitamins A and C. Later there are few dietary restrictions, except for avoiding foods that are high in fiber or hard-to-digest kernels, such as celery, popcorn, corn-on-the-cob, poppy seed or caraway seeds, and coconut. Fluids may be a problem during the summer, when they are lost during perspiration as well as through the ileostomy. Drinks such as Gatorade are helpful in maintaining electrolyte balance. If the effluent (fecal discharge) is too watery, fibrous foods (such as whole grain cereals, fresh fruit skins, beans, corn, and nuts) are restricted. If the effluent is excessively dry, salt intake is increased. An increased intake of water or fluid will not increase the effluent, since excess water is excreted in the urine.

Another possible problem is skin excoriation around the stoma. Not only does the ileostomy drainage contain enzymes that rapidly excoriate the skin, but if cement is used in putting the appliance on, the skin may be irritated when the appliance is removed. To avoid these problems, nystatin powder (Mycostatin) is dusted lightly on the peristomal skin, to prevent irritation and yeast growth.

A regular schedule for changing the appliance before leakage occurs is established. In teaching the patient to use and care for his appliance, stress the following essential points:

To Remove the Appliance

1. Sit or stand in a comfortable position.
2. Fill a container with the prescribed solvent. Apply a few drops of solvent with a medicine dropper between the disc of the appliance and the skin. *Do not pull off the appliance.* As the solvent works, the pouch loosens, and pulling is unnecessary.

Chart 38-1
Phases of the Rehabilitation Process of the Ileostomy Patient

I. Preoperative Phase: The Period Before Surgery

Goal: To reduce fear as much as possible

Implementation:
1. Present precise factual explanations regarding nature of surgery and creation of an ileostomy.
2. Plan to be repetitive in presenting facts.
3. Provide ample opportunity for patient to ask questions of a professional person.
4. Use diagrams, photographs, and appliances to acquaint the patient with an ileostomy.
5. Allow sufficient time to assimilate the prospect of an ileostomy.
6. Recognize the psychological value of having the patient converse with a successful ileostomate.
7. Include the family in spelling out patient needs and in answering his questions.
8. Explore vocational possibilities through the state vocational rehabilitation service, to allow time for processing.

II. Crisis Phase: Immediate Postoperative Period

Goal: To offer support, hope, and a sense of security

Implementation:
1. Provide consistent, effective care to instill confidence in the patient.
2. Exert vigilance in skin care to prevent the discomfort and pain of excoriation.
3. Utilize several approaches in odor control: (a) small doses of bismuth subcarbonate by mouth, (b) adequate appliance hygiene, (c) ventilation and deodorizers in room.
4. Avoid appliance management near mealtime.
5. Accept the patient's feelings (depression, silence, uncooperativeness, and refusal to eat) with understanding.
6. Acquaint the family with the possibility of the patient's exhibiting anxiety by his being demanding or abusive.
7. Avoid having the patient experience an emotional and intellectual vacuum by providing opportunities for verbalization.
8. Provide opportunity for gradual but steady involvement of the patient in handling the appliance.

(continued)

Chart 38-1
Phases of the Rehabilitation Process of the Ileostomy Patient (continued)

III. Recuperative Phase: Increased Responsibility for Self-Care

Goal: To assist patient in accepting self, expressing doubts, and adapting to his total situation

Implementation:
1. Reassure the patient (to offset his doubts) by letting him know that progress is being made toward the goal of making him self-dependent in managing his ileostomy.
2. Encourage the patient to talk about his self-acceptance with a sympathetic social worker or a psychiatric clinical specialist.
3. Develop a united expression of patient acceptance among nurses, family, and friends.
4. Repeat explanations of the surgery performed (if required) and reassure patient that he does not have cancer (if this is the case).
5. Provide an opportunity for family to verbalize concerns.
6. Suggest that it is normal, in recovery, to have occasional pains and upsets.
7. Obtain literature for patient from ileostomy groups.
8. Encourage visits by the dietitian so that he will know when and how to resume a normal diet. Include a family member.
9. Involve him further in self-care so that he continues to move toward independence of others with regard to bowel function.

IV. Transition Phase: Return to Community

Goal: To shift patient's concern from himself to that of himself-in-relation-to-others.

Implementation:
1. Assist the patient in previewing the home situation and seeking out fears and concerns.
2. Suggest discrimination in revealing or concealing his ileostomy from friends and work associates: tell those who would understand, but do not tell those whom he suspects would not understand.

3. Encourage the patient to do more and more for himself, but refrain from letting him feel abandoned.
4. Acquaint the patient thoroughly with his permanent appliance, and plan a routine that can be transferred to his own bathroom.
5. Provide instruction and literature in anticipation of skin problems: prophylaxis is easier than treatment.
6. Plan one or two outings away from the hospital for short times to offset the possible fears of the appliance's falling off or of people staring.
7. Initiate referrals to community nursing agency, an ileostomy patient, and social or vocational agencies, as needed.
8. Encourage discussion of plans to return to usual sexual activities.

V. Posthospital Phase: The First Postoperative Year

Goals: To recover physical well-being and offset physical disability
To perfect self-care, to negate any handicap
To resume social role and complete rehabilitation

Implementation:
1. Instruct patient in the detection of serious difficulties and who to contact for assistance.
2. Direct the patient on how to avoid fluid and electrolyte imbalance, which can be initiated by partial obstruction, a bout of flu, or an accident.
   Report diarrhea of more than 12 hours' duration to the physician.
3. Have patient carry an ID card on which is included a brief description of the method of removing the appliance and giving skin care, and the name and phone of surgeon or hospital to contact in case of emergency.

(Adapted from Lenneberg E and Rowbotham JL: The Ileostomy Patient. Springfield, Illinois, Charles C Thomas.)

To Cleanse the Skin

1. Use a cotton ball soaked in solvent. Wet the skin around the stoma. During the time the skin is being cleansed, a gauze dressing may cover the stoma, or a vaginal tampon can be inserted gently to absorb excess drainage. Avoid rubbing, because solvents are irritating.
2. Wash the skin with a soft cloth moistened with *tepid* water and mild soap, or permit the patient to shower or bathe before putting on the clean appliance. If the patient prefers, he may shower before removing the bag. Micropore tape applied to the sides of the disc will keep it secure during bathing.

To Put on the Appliance

1. When there is no irritation, a disposable plastic bag can be applied directly to the skin, after the cover has been removed from the adherent surface of the bag. Press firmly in place for 30 seconds.
2. When there is skin irritation, after skin cleansing, apply Kenalog spray (antibiotic); blot excess moisture with a cotton pledget and dust lightly with nystatin (Mycostatin) powder.
3. Moisten a Karaya gum washer and apply when it is tacky or "sticky."
4. Press the adhesive disc on the faceplate of the pouch

against the washer. This will allow skin to heal while the appliance is in place.

The amount of time that a person can keep the appliance sealed to his body depends on the location of the stoma and on body structure. Usually, the normal wearing time is 2 to 4 days. The appliance is emptied every 4 to 6 hours, or at the same time the patient empties his bladder. The pouch has an emptying spout at the bottom this is closed with a rubber band or special clip made for this purpose.

The appliance is cleaned and aired according to the manufacturer's directions. Usually, thorough washing with soap and water, using a soft nylon brush, is effective. There are many deodorizers and cleaning aids available that the patient can use. Full-strength distilled vinegar, rather than strong bleaches, is effective for soaking the bag. Commercial liquid deodorizers are also available, and are preferred by some patients. Other deodorants that are inexpensive are pieces of charcoal, or two aspirin tablets crushed and dropped into the bag. Foods such as spinach and parsley act on the intestinal tract as deodorizers, whereas foods that cause odors are cabbage, onions, and fish. Most patients alternate bags and allow the cleaned bag to be exposed to moving fresh air, out of direct sunlight. Bismuth subcarbonate tablets taken by mouth three or four times a day are effective in reducing odor. Some physicians prescribe a stool-thickener, such as diphenoxylate (Lomotil) (by mouth), to assist in odor control.

Finally, the person with an ileostomy is able to resume any activity, sport, or occupation he desires. There are no restrictions on sexual activity or bearing children. The only limitation is the person himself. Most patients do very well in adjusting because of feeling better and being free of pain.

Continent Ileostomy (Kock Pouch)

An interesting variation from the traditional incontinent ileostomy is the continent ileostomy introduced in the late 1960s by Nils Kock, a Swedish surgeon. Although thousands of patients have learned to adapt to the usual ileostomy, there is great appeal in the idea of an ileostomy device that gives patients voluntary control over the emptying from an ileostomy without the cumbersome "bag." Not all patients requiring an ileostomy can benefit from the continent (Kock pouch) type. Patients with regional enteritis are not suitable candidates, because the condition affects the terminal ileum, which is the section used to create the pouch. Eligible candidates are those with chronic ulcerative colitis and multiple or familial polyposis, or patients who have the traditional ileostomy for ulcerative colitis.

Physiologic Adaptation

The amount of effluent from an ileostomy is approximately 1000 ml per 24 hours. In order to accommodate this volume, a receptacle capable of holding 500 ml of fluid would have to be constructed, with the objective of emptying about three times daily. Consideration also needs to be given to reducing pressure at the outlet to prevent the receptable contents from backing up into the proximal small intestine. Kock's method was to split an intestinal segment at its an-

timesenteric border and fold the split segment twice in a special way; thus, the motor activity in different parts of the created pouch counteracted itself, and no raise in intraluminal pressure occurred, despite vigorous motor activity. A nipple valve is constructed at the outlet from the receptacle by purposely creating an intussusception of a part of the terminal segment into the receptacle (see Fig. 38-4C). The creation of this receptacle or reservoir may be done initially when a patient presents for an ileostomy, or it may be constructed from the conventional ileostomy if sufficient ileum is present.

After the diseased colon and terminal ileum have been resected, the continent pouch is constructed. From the resected end, about 45 cm (18 inches) of ileum are freed. The initial 15 cm (6 inches) will eventually be used to create the nipple, which will emerge on the abdomen (about ¼ inch). The next 30 cm (12 inches) are folded in a loop and stitched together (Fig. 38-4A). Then a U-shaped incision is made along the full length of the stitched loop (Fig. 38-4B). The remaining septum (initial suture line) is resutured to bring the raw edges together to form a smooth internal surface for the reservoir.

To create the nipple, the ileum is pulled in on itself (intussuscepted) (Fig. 38-4C) and stitched in place as an opening (stoma) on the abdomen. The edges of the exposed pouch are approximated to form the ileal receptacle or pouch (Fig. 38-4D).

The "valve" is forced to close when pressure is created by feces filling the pouch; the closing of the valve prevents fecal leakage from the stoma. When a catheter is inserted, effluent is released. In the operating room, a catheter is inserted through the nipple valve and is attached, after the operation, to gentle suction, to prevent the pouch from filling until all incision and suture lines heal (about 10 days).

Nursing Management and Patient Education

Preoperative preparation is similar to that for the patient having a traditional ileostomy. Teaching before surgery will relate to managing the drains from the outlet, the nature of drainage, need for nasogastric intubation, parenteral fluids, and perineal packing and care.

After the operation, a catheter will extend from the stoma and will be attached to a closed suction system. This drainage will be maintained for close to 2 weeks. The catheter is irrigated, usually every 2 hours, to assure its patency. About 20 ml to 30 ml of normal saline or sterile water may be introduced gently into the pouch by means of a syringe. Return flow is not aspirated, but permitted to drain by gravity.

Nasogastric suction also is a part of immediate postoperative care, with the tube requiring frequent irrigation, as requested. The purpose of nasogastric suction is to facilitate healing and to relieve pressure on the suture line by preventing a buildup of gastric contents. The patient is on parenteral fluids for 4 to 5 days. Thereafter, sips of clear liquids are offered, and the diet gradually progressed. Nausea and abdominal distention are watched as signs of an obstruction; should they occur, the physician is to be notified.

As with other patients undergoing abdominal surgery, early ambulation is encouraged. Pain medications are given

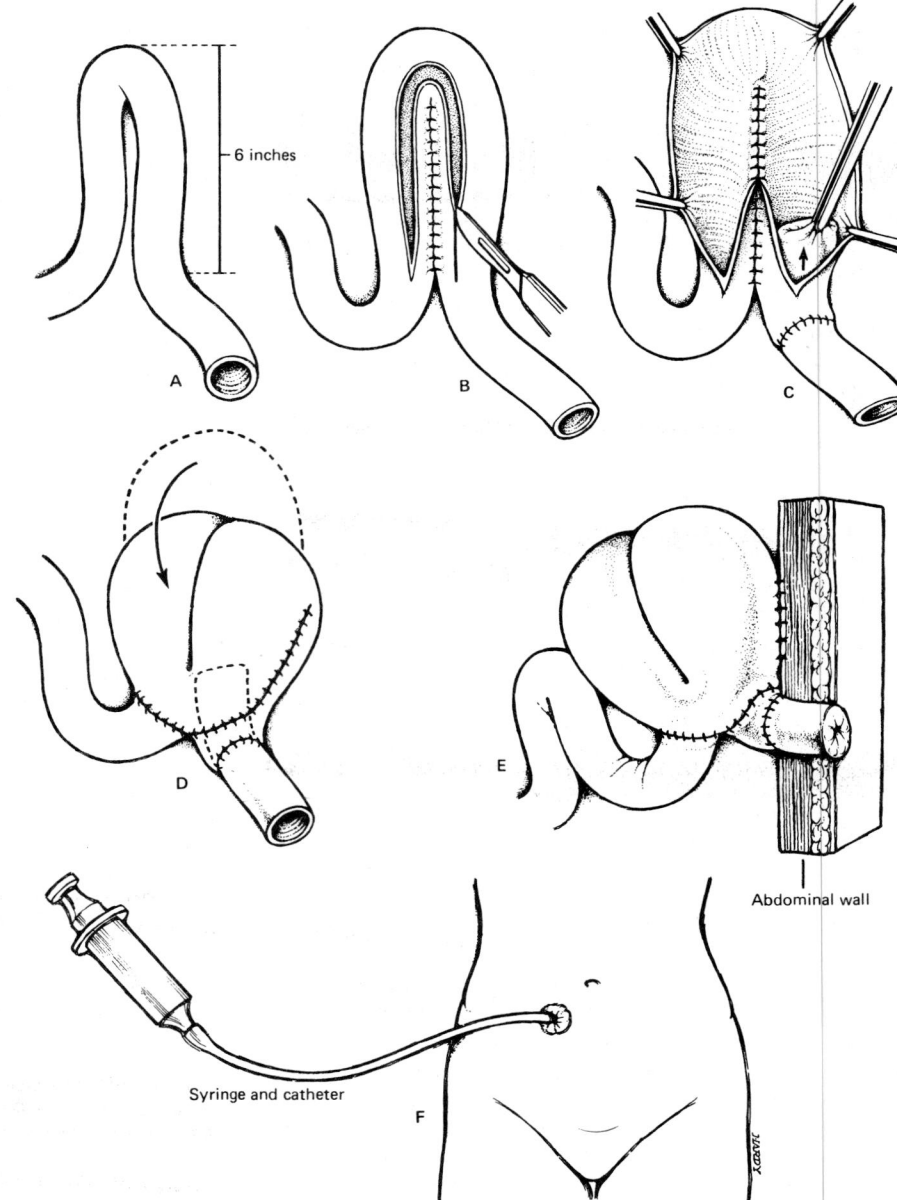

Figure 38-4. Continent ileostomy.

if required. By the end of the first week, rectal packing is removed. Since this procedure may be uncomfortable, the patient may be given a sedative an hour before this dressing is done. Changing the perineal dressings may also be facilitated by moistening the dressings a day before they are removed. After the packing is removed, the perineum is irrigated 2 to 3 times daily until full healing takes place.

In about 10 to 14 days, when the healing process has progressed to the point where the catheter is removed from the stoma, it is time for the patient to learn to manage the drainage of the pouch. The equipment required includes a catheter, tissues, water-soluble lubricant, gauze squares, a syringe, irrigating solution in a bowl, and an emesis or receiving basin.

1. Lubricate the catheter and gently insert about 5 cm (2 inches), at which point some resistance may be felt at the valve or "nipple." When gentle pressure is used, the catheter usually will enter the pouch.

2. If there is much resistance, fill a syringe with 20 ml of air or water and inject the air or water through the catheter, while still exerting some pressure on the catheter. This will permit the catheter to enter into the pouch (Fig. 38-4F).

3. Place the other end of the catheter in a drainage basin, which is placed below the level of stoma, so that gravity will facilitate drainage. Later, of course, drainage can be carried out at the toilet, with drainage delivered into the toilet bowl. Drainage may include flatus as well as effluent.

4. Following drainage, the catheter is removed, and the area around the stoma is gently washed with warm water. Pat dry and apply an absorbent pad over the stoma. Fasten the pad with hypoallergenic tape.

The whole procedure should not require more than 5 to 10 minutes and is done at first every 3 hours. The time between irrigations is gradually lengthened so that it is done about three times daily.

When discharge is thick, water can be injected via the catheter to loosen and soften it. Effluent consistency is affected by food intake. As time goes on, the pouch will stretch, and whereas at first drainage is only about 60 ml to 80 ml, it will eventually increase to accommodate 500 ml to 1000 ml. The gauge to determine frequency of drainage is the sensation of pressure in the pouch.

Continued Patient Education for Home Care

The spouse and family should be familiar with the adjustment that will be necessary when the patient returns home. They need to know why it is necessary for the ileostomate to occupy the bathroom for 10 minutes at certain times of the day, and why he needs certain equipment. Their understanding is necessary to reduce tension—a relaxed patient tends to have fewer problems.

Psychosocial needs of the patient are stressed. For the most part, he is particularly pleased that he will not need to wear an ileostomy bag, and this encourages him to master control over his own pouch.

A successful cover for the stoma for home use consists of a dressing that is absorbent on one side and plasticized on the other. (High-quality disposable diapers can be cut into 7.5 cm × 7.5 cm (3 × 3) squares; this makes an ideal dressing.) The dressing is held in place with tape. To reduce skin excoriation, the tape is placed differently with each application, so that it does not contact the same area of skin each time.

A water-soluble lubricant, rather than petrolatum, should be used. The latter has a tendency to clog the catheter and is difficult to wash from it.

The position to assume in the bathroom is one of individual preference and convenience. The patient may sit on the toilet seat, stand in front of the toilet, or sit on a chair in front of the toilet. It is suggested that an adapter and a length of tubing be available to attach to the catheter so that effluent does not splatter, but drains easily into the toilet bowl.

Encourage experimentation when there are problems with drainage. If the catheter meets resistance when attempts are made to insert it, the patient should be encouraged to relax before draining the pouch and to be sure to lubricate the catheter well. It may be easier for the patient to lie down when the catheter is inserted and then stand up for drainage purposes.

Injection of air or water may help in passing the catheter through the stoma into the pouch. (Skin care, odor, diet, activities, and so forth, are similar to that recommended for other ostomy patients; see p. 820. Also see Table 38-7, p. 833.)

▷ Diverticulosis and Diverticulitis

A *diverticulum* is a saccular dilatation, a blind passage, so to speak, leading from the lumen of the bowel. (An example of this abnormality is Meckel's diverticulum, an outpocketing of the ileum). Diverticula, in fact, may occur anywhere along the course of the gastrointestinal tract, from the esophagus to the rectum. Congenital predisposition is likely. They may be the result of local degeneration and weakening of the muscular wall, or they may be due to increased mechanical pressure from abnormal, high-pressure contractions of the sigmoid colon in response to neurohumoral stimuli. An individual who possesses diverticula is said to have *diverticulosis*. An obstruction of a diverticulum leads to infection and inflammation. This is referred to as *diverticulitis*.

Pathophysiology and Pathogenesis

Diverticulitis usually occurs in patients over 40 years of age. It is by no means rare. It is found in approximately 10% of the United States population, but is more common in those over 50 years. Its incidence is approximately 40% in those over 70 years of age. It has been estimated that approximately one third of the patients with diverticulosis at one time or another experience diverticulitis. Diverticulitis is most common in the sigmoid colon. This condition may occur in acute attacks, or it may persist as a long-continued, smoldering infection. Inflammation of a diverticulum, if its obstruction continues, tends to spread to the surrounding bowel wall, giving rise to irritability and spasticity of the colon. An abscess may develop, leading to peritonitis, and erosion of the blood vessels (arterial) may produce bleeding.

Clinical Manifestation and Diagnostic Evaluation

Constipation from spastic colon syndrome often precedes the development of diverticulosis by many years. Other signs of diverticulosis are bowel irregularity and diarrhea. A moderately severe acute diverticulitis has as its most common symptom crampy pain in the left lower quadrant of the abdomen, and a low grade fever. Following local inflammation of the diverticula, there may be a narrowing of the large bowel, with fibrotic stricture, leading to cramps, narrow stools, and increased constipation. With the development of granulation tissue, occult bleeding may occur, producing iron-deficiency anemia. In addition, weakness and fatigue are evident. If an abscess develops, there is tenderness, a palpable mass, fever, and leukocytosis. If an inflamed diverticulum perforates, abdominal pain results that is localized over the involved segment—usually the sigmoid; local abscess or peritonitis results. With the development of peritonitis, the symptoms of rigidity, abdominal pain, loss of bowel sounds, and shock, develop. Uninflamed or slightly inflamed diverticula may erode areas adjacent to arterial branches, thus causing massive rectal bleeding.

A history generally elicits the two main presenting symptoms of diverticulitis: pain in the lower left quadrant, along with a marked change in bowel habits (diarrhea or constipation). Diagnosis is made on the basis of sigmoidoscopy (direct visualization) and fluoroscopic and x-ray findings with a barium enema.

Management and Patient Education

The goals of nursing care are (1) detection and referral for further evaluation, and (2) patient education regarding current dietary treatment and medications (especially use of stool softeners).

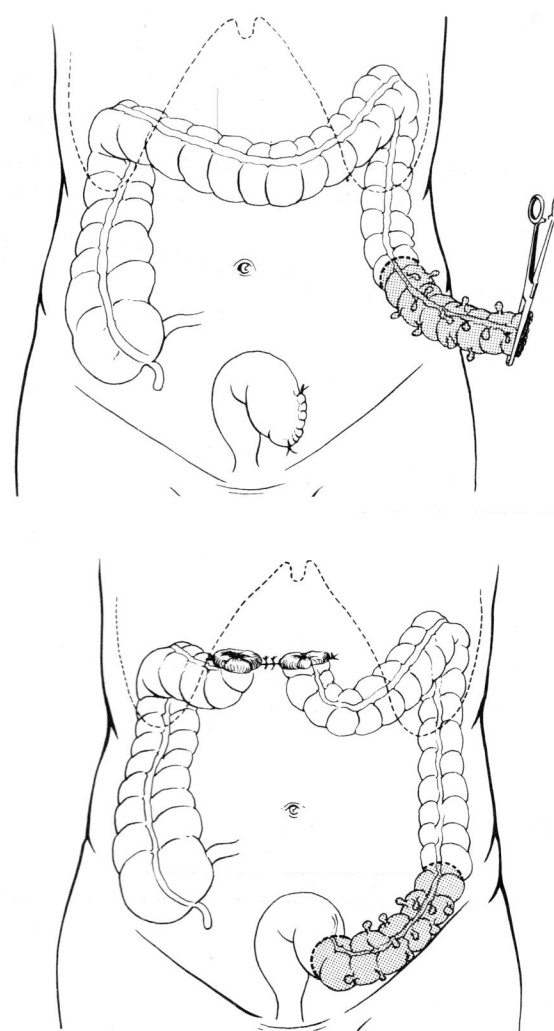

Figure 38-5. (*Top*) Two-stage (Hartmann) resection for diverticulitis of the colon. *Stage I:* The affected segment (shaded) has been divided at its distal end and brought out through the abdominal wall. It will then be removed by transection at its proximal margin (dotted line), leaving a healthy colostomy stoma on the surface of the abdomen. The upper end of the rectosigmoid stump has been sutured closed. Alternatively, it could have been exteriorized without closing it. *Stage II:* The divided ends of the bowel will be mobilized and anastomosed. (*Bottom*) Three-stage procedure for resection of a segment of the colon involved by diverticulitis. *Stage I:* Transverse colostomy. *Stage II:* Resection of the involved segment (shaded) (lines of resection indicated by dotted lines) and anastomosis of healthy ends. *Stage III:* Closure of transverse colostomy. (From Dunphy JE and Way LW (eds): Current Surgical Diagnosis and Treatment, 3rd ed. Los Altos, California, Lange Medical Publishers.)

The patient should understand the nature of his problem and recognize that the objective is to rest the intestinal tract and alleviate constipation. Heretofore, diverticulosis of the colon was considered relatively harmless, but because of the potential for developing complex problems, prevention is now given major emphasis.

There are differences of opinion regarding the proper type of diet for these patients. Some recommend refined, low-roughage foods to avoid irritation. Others suggest a fibrous diet to avoid collection of feces in pouches, with resulting infection. At present, there is a fair amount of clinical evidence that increased dietary fiber appears to improve diverticular disease; however, even though this evidence is persuasive, the value of fiber still has not been demonstrated.

If mastication is a problem, foods should be puréed. For spastic pain, antispasmodics such as propantheline bromide (Pro-Banthine) and oxyphencyclimine (Daricon) are taken before meals and at bedtime. Sedatives and tranquilizers, as well as bowel antimicrobials, may also be required. Stool normalization can be achieved by the use of one or more of the following: bulk preparation, such as Metamucil; stool softener, such as dioctyl sodium sulfosuccinate (Colace); instillation of warm oil into the rectum; and an evacuant suppository, such as Dulcolax. Such a prophylactic plan will reduce the bacterial flora of the bowel, diminish the bulk of the stool, and soften the fecal mass, so that it traverses more easily the area of inflammatory obstruction. During therapy, fluid and nutritional requirements may be met intravenously.

Acute Diverticulitis Without Obstruction

The patient with a mild degree of illness and no fever is placed on bed rest and a soft or liquid diet, along with mineral oil to soften the stools. This may be supplemented with intravenous fluids and electrolytes. If there is distention, nasogastric suction may be initiated. Antibiotics, analgesics, and antispasmodics are usually given. Upon subsidence, the above prophylactic regimen may be followed.

Surgical Treatment

Surgery is considered if obstruction is untreatable medically or if there is perforation or bleeding that recurs. (In 80% of patients, diverticular bleeding stops spontaneously). There are two types of surgery: (1) one-stage resection of the involved sigmoid section, for recurrent attacks, or (2) multiple-staged procedures for complications (obstruction, perforation, fistulae) (Fig. 38-5). Surgery is preceded by barium studies. In preparing the patient for surgery, it is important to avoid irritating the colon, which is already terribly sensitive and susceptible to perforation. A mild saline laxative and carefully administered cleansing enemas may be sufficient.

The surgery performed varies with the operative findings. When possible, the area of diverticulitis is resected and the remaining bowel joined end to end (primary resection and end-to-end anastomosis). A two-stage resection is sometimes done in which the diseased colon is resected, as with a one-stage operation, but no anastomosis is performed, and both ends of the bowel are brought out onto the abdomen as stomata. The "double-barrel" colostomy is then anastomosed at a later procedure (Fig. 38-5). In some patients, such an operation may appear impossible or inadvisable, in which case a colostomy is performed in the right transverse colon. Diverting the fecal flow from the area of diverticulitis allows the inflammatory process to subside, and a later operation removing the colon containing the diverticulitis is done, followed by an anastomosis. When this method of treatment is chosen, the colostomy is only temporary, and after the area of diverticulitis has been removed and the intestinal continuity established by the anastomosis, the colostomy is closed. Thus, this is a three-stage procedure, requiring the care for a colostomy during part of the treatment (see p. 829). A colostomy on the right side of the transverse colon drains liquid or mushy feces and requires that a bag be worn constantly. Irrigations are rarely of value in this type of colostomy, but ordinary cleanliness is obtained by baths or showers, using soap and water to cleanse the skin about the colostomy stoma. (The nursing management of the patient with a colostomy is discussed on p. 831).

▷ Intestinal Polyps

Benign polyps are much more common in the large intestine than in the small intestine. If there are numerous growths, the condition is referred to as *polyposis*—often, apparently, a congenital abnormality. These polyps frequently become cancerous; invariably, in familial polyposis, simple benign polyps infrequently become malignant. Because of the increased evidence that most colorectal cancers arise from preexisting polyps, detection through regular sigmoidoscopy is recommended, along with the removal of all benign polyps and adenomatous lesions.

▷ Cancer of the Colon

Tumors of the small intestine are rare; on the other hand, tumors of the colon are relatively common. In fact, cancer of the colon and rectum is now the most common type of internal cancer in the United States. Over 100,000 Americans are afflicted annually; about half that number die of it annually—although almost three out of four patients might be saved by early diagnosis and prompt treatment. The low 5-year survival rate of 42% is due primarily to late diagnosis.

Pathophysiology and Clinical Manifestations
Cancer of the colon and the rectum always arises from the epithelium lining the intestine. The effects produced depend largely on the location of the cancer.

As in the case of cancer elsewhere in the gastrointestinal tract, the chief symptoms are the passage of blood in the stools, anemia, obstruction, and perforation. A suddenly developing obstruction may be the first symptom of cancer involving the colon anywhere between the cecum and the sigmoid, for in this region, where the bowel contents are liquid, a slowly developing obstruction will not become evident until the lumen is practically closed. Cancer of the sigmoid and the rectum causes earlier symptoms of partial obstruction, with constipation, alternating with diarrhea, lower-abdominal crampy pains, and distention.

- Any patient with a history of unexplained change in bowel habit, with changes in the shape of the stool, or with the passage of blood in the stools should be studied carefully to rule out cancer of the large bowel.

Chart 38-2
Risk Factors for Cancer of the Colon

Age—over 40
Blood in stool
History of rectal polyps
Presence of adenomatous polyps or villous adenomas
Family history of colon cancer or polyposis
Personal history of chronic inflammatory bowel disease

The possibility that a rectal carcinoma exists—detectable, but still asymptomatic and still operable—is one important reason for the inclusion of a rectal examination as part of every routine physical examination (see p. 86). Additional symptoms, often present, are those of progressive weakness, anorexia, weight loss, anemia, and lower abdominal pain.

Diagnostic Assessment.   Along with the abdominal and rectal examination, the most important diagnostic procedures for cancer of the colon are fecal occult blood testing (through the use of commercially available guaiac-impregnated slides) and the sigmoidoscopic examination (see p. 764). Usually, the most conclusive of all tests is the biopsy with colonoscopy (see p. 765).

Management and Nursing Intervention
Nursing goals are (1) to provide early detection and facilitate referral, and (2) to provide physical and emotional support in the perioperative period.

Preparation for Operation.   Usually, a high-caloric, low-residue diet is given for several days before operation, if time and the patient's condition permit. If an emergency does not exist, these patients are prepared for several days by being given intestinal anti-infectives, such as kanamycin, erythromycin, and neomycin. These are given by mouth to reduce the bacterial content of the colon and to soften and decrease the bulk of the contents of the colon. In addition, mechanical cleansing of the bowel may be done by laxatives, enemas, or colonic irrigations.

Careful attention is given to complaints of pain, which are assessed and described as to their nature, location, and duration. The nurse also records fluid losses such as occur with vomiting and diarrhea. This will aid in regulating the fluid intake and maintaining adequate balance. If the hemoglobin is below 12 g, a blood transfusion may be given, since anemia is common. Preoperative nasogastric intubation facilitates the performance of intestinal surgery and minimizes postoperative distention. An indwelling catheter is inserted to ensure that the bladder is empty during surgery. This will aid in keeping postoperative perineal dressings dry. The abdomen and perineum are shaved as described on page 356.

In the event that there is any possibility of a *colostomy* (a temporary or permanent opening of the colon through the abdominal wall), the patient should be informed by the surgeon. This is a life-saving arrangement that is compatible with active participation in social and business life. The nurse is in a position to assist the patient in accepting a colostomy; with courage, optimism, and determination, the patient can adjust to a new life-style, with daily improvement until he has established his individual pattern of management. Members of the health team, the enterostomal therapist, his family, and other ostomates are available to assist and support him.

Operative Treatment. This will depend on the position and the extent of the cancer. When the tumor can be removed, the involved colon is excised for some distance on each side of the growth to remove the tumor and the area of its lymphatic spread (Fig. 38-6). If distant (liver) metastasis has occurred, the tumor may be excised for palliation, but without benefit of cure. The intestine may be reunited by an end-to-end anastomosis of the colon. When the

growth is situated low in the sigmoid or the rectum, the colon is cut above the growth and brought out through the abdominal wall, forming thus an abdominal anus, called a *colostomy*. The growth then is removed from below by a perineal incision (*abdominoperineal resection*, Fig. 38-7).

In the event that the tumor has spread and involves surrounding vital structures, it is considered to be inoperable. When the growth in the rectum or the sigmoid is inoperable, and especially when symptoms of partial or complete obstruction are present, a colostomy may be performed. A loop of the colon, near the junction of the descending colon and the sigmoid, is brought out of the abdomen through a lower left rectus incision and maintained in place by a plastic rod or rubber tube inserted underneath the loop. If the obstruction is complete, the loop may be drained by the insertion of a rubber tube or by the use of a right-angled tube, which

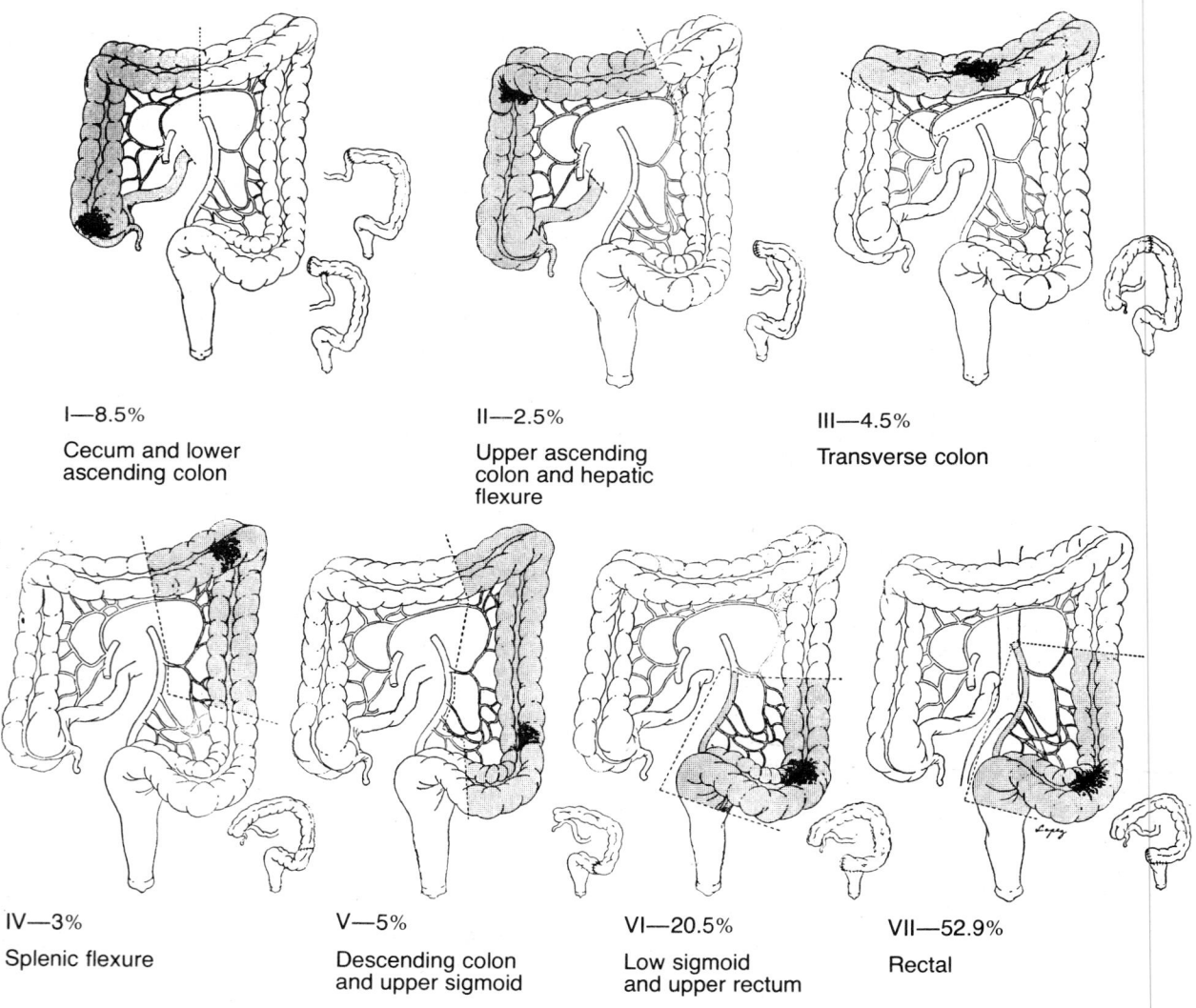

I—8.5%

Cecum and lower ascending colon

II—2.5%

Upper ascending colon and hepatic flexure

III—4.5%

Transverse colon

IV—3%

Splenic flexure

V—5%

Descending colon and upper sigmoid

VI—20.5%

Low sigmoid and upper rectum

VII—52.9%

Rectal

Figure 38-6. This indicates an approximate incidence of cancer of the colon. Also shown are areas where cancer can occur, what area is removed, and (in the very small diagram) how the anastomosis is done. For rectal cancer, an abdominoperineal resection is done with colostomy. (Adapted from American Cancer Society.)

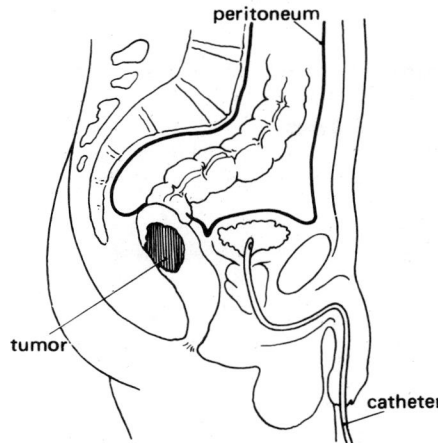

1. Presurgical patient. Note tumor in rectum.

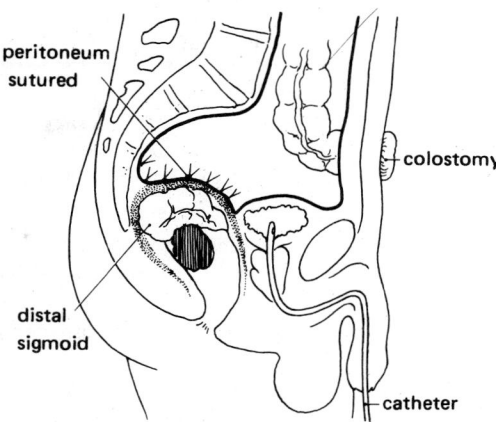

2. At operation, sigmoid is removed and colostomy established. The distal bowel has been dissected free to a point below pelvic peritoneum, which is sutured over the closed end of the distal sigmoid and rectum.

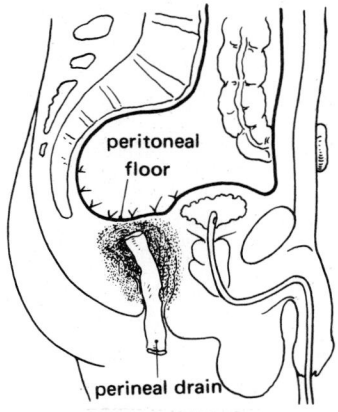

3. Perineal resection includes removal of the rectum and free portion of the sigmoid from below. A drain is inserted in this void.

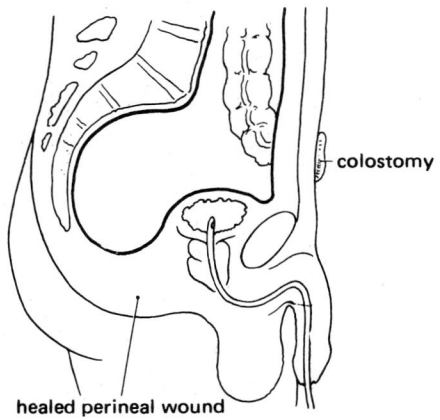

4. The final result after healing. Note healed perineal wound and the permanent colostomy.

Figure 38-7. Abdominoperineal resection for carcinoma of rectum.

is held in the intestine by a purse-string suture. When the obstruction is incomplete, the colostomy loop is allowed to remain unopened for several days to permit the peritoneal cavity to become thoroughly sealed off. During this time the patient is given a liquid diet. The intestine is opened by electrocautery, as hemorrhage is slight after its use. (See Table 38-6 to compare differences and similarities between a colostomy and an ileostomy.)

▷ Care of the Patient With a Colostomy

To give adequate support, care, and instruction to this patient, the nurse must know not only basic information about the patient's physical condition, nutritional status, and the proposed surgery, but also the patient himself. What does he think, feel, express, suppress, desire, fear, etc.? In daily contacts with the patient who has a colostomy, valuable rapport can be established to facilitate his adjustment. The nurse must understand and practice psychology and the principles of learning as they apply to each particular individual. In addition to the shock of the colostomy, the patient is perhaps also dealing with a diagnosis of cancer. These two issues together can tax his coping ability and that of his family.

Patient Problems/Nursing Diagnoses

The major nursing problems for patients facing colostomy for rectal cancer include anxiety related to impending surgery and inadequate knowledge of the surgical procedure and

Table 38-6
Comparison of Colostomy and Ileostomy

Categories	Colostomy	Ileostomy
Definition	A portion of the colon is brought through the abdominal wall, thereby creating a temporary or permanent opening.	A portion of the ileum is brought through the abdominal wall, thereby creating a permanent opening.
Indications	Pathologic conditions involving large bowel, for example: (1) Inflammatory or obstructive processes of the lower intestinal tract (2) Congenital or traumatic disruption of the intestinal tract (3) Cancer of the rectum or sigmoid flexure, where anastomosis is not possible	Pathologic conditions involving small bowel, for example: (1) Ulcerative colitis, in the vast majority of cases (2) Regional enteritis (Crohn's disease)
Purpose	To provide an outlet for intestinal waste products	To serve as an exit for waste products when colon has been removed
Location	Colon	Ileum
Reservoir	Limited	None (except with continent ileostomy [Kock pouch], where capacity can be 500 ml)
Incidence of evacuation	24–48 hours with control measures	Constant (three times/day with continent ileostomy)
Consistency of discharge	Liquid to formed stool	Yellow, green, or brown liquid
Means of control	No voluntary control; potential control with diet or irrigation	No voluntary control; adherent appliance necessary

(Adapted from American Cancer Society: Colostomy and Ileostomy Care. A Guide of Practical Information for Nurses.)

postoperative course; potential development of complications related to the surgical event; and potential nonadherence to the therapeutic regimen related to nonacceptance of the patient's condition.

▶ Planning and Nursing Implementation

Goals

The major goals for the patient include:

1. Ability to cope with the stress of impending surgery
2. Absence of complications
3. Adherence to the therapeutic regimen

Patient Education. Thousands of people who have colostomies are engaged actively in business today. With the improvement of surgical and nursing procedures, and the assistance of patients who have "lived" with their colostomies, it is now possible to give intelligent assistance to the person about to have a colostomy or an ileostomy. Many hospitals have teaching protocols available for guidance with preoperative and postoperative teaching of the colostomy patient. However, the support and the teaching of a patient must be individualized. Therefore, the same approach may not be appropriate for all patients. Before the operation, some may find that a simple line drawing illustrating the nature and the function of the lower intestinal

tract is helpful. By this means, the deviations necessary for the particular situation can be explained. For others, having another patient who has had a colostomy talk to them presents a comfortable opportunity for the expression of fears and doubts. Other patients express a desire for minimal information and should be given only necessary, basic information. The extent of psychological preparation must be approached on a personal basis.

Psychosocial Support. The patient may be anxious, distracted, and grieving over his diagnosis and the impending surgery. The nurse should expect this and include family members and supportive friends in efforts to support the patient's coping behaviors.

The patient needs to know what a colostomy is and how it functions; he should know that it need not hamper his way of living and that with patience, as well as some trial-and-error methods, he will be able to manage, control, and master it. During the interval of preoperative care the nurse should encourage the patient to talk out his concerns and fears; in this way the nurse will be able to direct and help him.

It is well to remember that this is a frightening and difficult experience for the patient. Most likely he has never seen an incision under surgical dressings and, less likely, a colostomy. The shock of this first sight may be minimized if, before the operation, he is shown drawings, a model, and

Chart 38-3
Guidelines to Nursing Management of a Patient Having a Colostomy

Goals/Nursing Interventions	*Rationale/Amplification*

Preoperative

To Reduce Intestinal Flora to as Low a Level as Possible

1. Administer intestinal antiseptics as prescribed—usually given several days before surgery.	1. Usually, sulfa drugs are most effective. Not only is bacterial count reduced, but there is a softening and reduction of colon contents.
2. Give laxatives, enema, or colonic irrigations as prescribed.	2. Promotes intestinal cleansing.

To Promote Patient's Physical and Psychosocial Comfort

1. Assess patient's complaints.	1. Assists in pinpointing source of problem.
2. Support patient's coping mechanism.	2. Permits patient to verbalize feelings, and allows nurse to anticipate his concerns. Respect for patient's privacy must be granted.
3. Ascertain whether a temporary or permanent colostomy is to be performed, and whether surgeon has instructed the patient regarding this plan.	3. An informed patient greatly assists in optimum postoperative care. Patient preparation and acceptance are necessary for successful adjustment to new life-style.

To Maintain Optimum Physiologic Levels of All Bodily Functions

1. Record in descriptive form all intake and output.	1. Fluid losses may occur, owing to vomiting and diarrhea; electrolytes such as potassium, sodium, and chloride need to be replaced.
2. Note hematocrit and hemoglobin levels.	2. If hemoglobin is below 12 g, it may be necessary to transfuse patient.

To Prevent Postoperative Discomfort and Complications

1. Insert a nasogastric tube, as recommended by the physician.	1. Minimizes abdominal distention, and eliminates the discomfort of vomiting.
2. Insert indwelling catheter, if so prescribed.	2. Keeps bladder empty during intestinal surgery, and helps to avoid accidental injury.
3. Perform usual activities related to the immediate preoperative nursing care of this patient.	3. Systematic preparation enhances psychological acceptance of surgery.

Postoperative

To Provide Skilled Nursing Care Through the Immediate Postoperative, Postanesthetic Stage

Follow usual nursing management of patient having abdominal surgery.	See pages 384 and 387.

To Assess Normal and Healthy Status of Colostomy, so That Any Deviation Is Easily Detected

1. Recognize nature of colostomy, so that type and frequency of effluent can be anticipated.	1. Ascending colostomy—fluid feces. Colostomy near hepatic flexure—semifluid feces. Transverse colostomy—mushy feces. Splenic flexure colostomy—semimushy feces. Descending colostomy—solid feces.

(continued)

Chart 38-3
Guidelines to Nursing Management of a Patient Having a Colostomy (continued)

Goals/Nursing Interventions *(continued)*	***Rationale/Amplification*** *(continued)*
Postoperative *(continued)*	
2. Observe stoma and surrounding tissue for adequacy of viability.	2. Mature stoma is deep pink or red; will be moist with mucus. Stoma will feel soft to firm. The nonmature stoma will be friable. Skin margins should approximate to the stoma completely, circumferentially. Peristomal skin should look healthy and similar to that of entire abdomen.
To Anticipate Problems in Caring for the Colostomy—Psychosocial and Physical See page 821, Phases of the Rehabilitation Process of the Ileostomy Patient.	Note the similarities in the care of "ostomy" patients.
To Plan for Colostomy Care Based on the Needs of the Particular Individual 1. Select a method of taking care of the colostomy, and adhere to this method.	1. Consistency is effective in maintaining optimal functioning of colostomy. Patient is less likely to be confused if the method is clearly spelled out.
2. Use available agents that have proven their effectiveness.	2. Karaya comes in various forms and is effective in keeping skin healthy and free from enzymatic action of stomal drainage. Stomahesive (Squibb) is effective when excoriation is present.
3. Soap and water is sometimes irritating to the skin and stoma.	3. May be particularly true of the elderly patient. Oil-based or cream-based soaps could be used, but may prevent adherence of Stomahesive or Karaya ring. Using water without soap to cleanse skin of elderly may be sufficient to maintain hygiene.
To Review and Stress Information Needed When Patient With a Colostomy Goes Home See Regulating the Colostomy, page 832; Choice and Care of Equipment, page 834; Hygienic Measures, page 836; Sexual Activity, page 836; and Selection of Appropriate Diet, page 836. Also review Phases of the Rehabilitation of the Ileostomy Patient, pages 821–822.	

perhaps a picture or two of the anatomy involved. He also needs to know that the reddish appearance and large size of the stoma will diminish in time.

Postoperative Care.   The patient is helped out of bed on the first postoperative day and is encouraged to care for his colostomy from the very first irrigation. The return to normal diet is rapid, and every effort is made to encourage him to live as he did before his operation. Psychologically, this appears to deemphasize the abnormality of the situation.

The colostomy is opened on the second or the third postoperative day by the surgeon, at which time there is often an evacuation of loose stools. In anticipation of this the nurse will have protected the bedding with a plastic sheet covered with a towel and will have an emesis basin positioned at the patient's side.

Regulating the Colostomy

Colostomy Irrigations.   Regulation is effected either by irrigation or by training the bowel to evacuate naturally without irrigations. The choice often depends on the individual and the nature of the colostomy. An ascending colostomy is difficult to control and usually requires daily irrigation. Sigmoidostomy may require irrigation only every 2 or 3 days, if at all.

The stoma on the abdomen does not have voluntary

Table 38-7
Common Intestinal Ostomies

	Ileostomy	Ileal Loop (Urinary Conduit)	Transverse Colostomy	Descending or Sigmoid Colostomy
Intestinal Segment Involved	End of ileum	Loop of ileum is made into a pouch into which transplanted ureters drain urine	Transverse colon	Descending or sigmoid colon
Effluent	Liquid, semi-liquid, soft	Urine only	Soft and, at occasional intervals, fairly firm; softer toward ileum	Descending—fairly firm stool; Sigmoid—even more solid
Odor	Slightly odorous	Nonodorous	Very malodorous	Usually malodorous
Skin Effect	Enzymes highly irritating	Urine is irritating to unprotected skin	Irritating, with continuous discharge	Fairly irritating
Types of Appliance	Open-ended pouch worn at all times; if Kock pouch, no appliance is worn	Open-ended pouch worn at all times	Pouch worn at all times. (Either a large stoma with two openings, or two separate stomas; fecal discharge from one and mucus from the other)	Depends on patient and his control. Some wear no appliance and irrigate regularly. Others wear closed pouch, if effluent is firm; open-ended, if discharge is more liquid continuously

muscular control and may empty at irregular intervals. The time of irrigation should be selected with regard to the schedule the person will pursue after leaving the hospital.

The purpose of irrigating a colostomy is to empty the colon of gas, mucus, and feces so that the patient can go about his social and business activities without fear of fecal drainage. By irrigating the stoma at a *regular* time, there is less gas and retention of irrigating fluids. It is best to irrigate after a meal, since ingestion of food stimulates peristalsis and defecation.

The initial irrigation is usually done on the fourth or fifth postoperative day. There are two methods of irrigating a colostomy: the conventional one, using an enema irrigation procedure, and a second method utilizing a bulb syringe.

Irrigation by Enema. The following equipment is used:

- Irrigating set (2-liter [quart] can or bag, tubing, adapter); catheter, clamp, colostomy irrigator
- Solution at 40.5° C (105° F)
- Petrolatum to lubricate catheter
- Toilet tissue to clean around colostomy before and after irrigation
- Newspaper or paper bag to receive soiled dressings
- A place to set or hang the irrigating container
- Dressings for colostomy following irrigation

The patient may sit in a chair before the toilet in the bathroom. A rubber or plastic sheet can be used as a trough leading to the toilet bowl. Encourage the patient to watch the procedure, and explain each step as it is performed. The catheter, lubricated with petrolatum to reduce friction, is inserted 5 cm to 7.5 cm (2–3 inches) at first, and the solution is allowed to run into the colon. (A Laird or wide cone tip, when plugged into the stoma about 1.2 cm [½ inch], permits irrigation without leakage or the danger of perforation.)

The catheter then can be inserted gently up to 10 cm to 15 cm (4–6 inches). If resistance is met, digital examination may reveal muscle spasm or a mass of stool *Force is contraindicated, since it is possible to perforate the bowel.*

At first, only about 500 ml of solution is given, after which the amount may be increased gradually every day up to 1500 ml. The temperature of the solution is about 40.5° C (105° F), and the irrigating can is placed about 45 cm to 60 cm (18–24 inches) above the level of the colostomy opening. Since distention of the colon is an effective stimulus for bowel evacuation, the irrigating solution should be introduced in such amount, and with such pressure, as to distend the bowel and give the patient a feeling of fullness. If the patient complains of cramps, the level of the can may be lowered to lessen the force of flow. The patient should be taught that the rate of flow of solution varies with the pressure and the caliber of tube. Pressure depends on height; therefore, when increased pressure is desired, the container of solution may be raised, and vice versa. Solutions may be soapy solution, plain water, or saline. The irrigation may be given daily, every other day, or every 3 days, according to the need and preference of the patient. Some patients prefer to take a warm bath after an irrigation. This promotes a feeling of cleanliness and relaxation. During the irrigation, when done at home, it may be pleasant and diverting to have a radio nearby. While waiting for the return flow, it may be an opportune time to read. (The entire procedure usually takes between 45 minutes and 1 hour). Nothing but flatus and a slight amount of mucus should escape from the colostomy between irrigations.

Irrigation by Bulb Syringe.   The second method of colostomy irrigation is the *bulb syringe* method. This type of irrigation stimulates fecal return, rather than washing the feces out. There is no prolonged trapping of water in the colon and no spillage or accidents during the day.

The patient is seated on the toilet. A 250-ml (8-oz) soft rubber bulb syringe is used. The hard nozzle is cut off, and a No. 24 French catheter is attached to the end of the bulb syringe. *No more than 750 ml (24 oz) of water is used.* The bulb syringe method is shown in Figure 38-8.

The patient may massage the lower part of the abdomen to ensure adequate return. The bag is left in place for 15 minutes, after which the stoma is covered with a piece of gauze and held in place by a girdle, elasticized shorts, or an elastic belt. The patient completes the procedure by washing the pitcher and bulb syringe with soapy water.

Other Types of Colostomies

"Wet" Colostomy.   "Wet" colostomies are those through which both urine and feces are excreted, because of transplantation of ureters into the colon. These colostomies are never irrigated, because of the danger that contaminated material will be forced into the ureters and produce infection.

Double-Barrel Colostomy.   In a double-barrel colostomy, there are two openings, the proximal and distal segments of colon. The proximal portion is the functioning colon, whereas the distal end is irrigated only to keep it clean and free of mucus. If there is an obstruction in this section, it may be necessary to siphon the fluid. In case the cancer has not been removed, it is well to irrigate the lower loop, from anus to colostomy, every 2 or 3 days, to remove the irritating mucus that collects.

Care of Perineal Wound

If the malignancy has been removed by the perineal route, the wound is observed carefully for signs of hemorrhage. This wound usually contains a drain or packing that is removed gradually, so that about the seventh day all drains are out. There usually are sloughing bits of tissue that must come away for the following week or 10 days. This process is hastened by the mechanical irrigation of the wound. It is appreciated by the patient if the prescribed medication for pain is administered before the procedure is begun. An irrigating container with normal saline or hydrogen peroxide is effective, particularly since the latter effervesces, thereby promoting mechanical removal of tissue debris. Enzymes (streptokinase or streptodornase) are also effective in liquefying necrotic tissue. This may be done two or three times a day and then gradually less frequently. Observe and record the condition of the perineal wound; note any bleeding, infection, or necrosis. During the procedure it is important to protect the bed with an extra waterproof sheet and absorbent pads, and it may be well to plan the irrigation so that it can be performed before the patient receives morning care.

Changing the patient's position from one side to the other every 2 to 4 hours is desirable, since not only is it uncomfortable to lie in a dorsal recumbent position, but such a position may also interfere with healing by causing wound separation. By the beginning of the second postoperative week, sitz baths may be prescribed, to improve circulation and promote healing and cleanliness. A half-inflated rubber ring is comfortable to sit on.

An indwelling catheter remains in place for several days to prevent urinary retention and pressure on the perineal area. Continuing assessment of the patient's urinary status is maintained to control infection and maintain hydration.

Choice and Care of Equipment

Early in the postoperative care of the patient with a colostomy or ileostomy, the use of a plastic stoma bag is effective in preventing skin irritation and reducing offensive odors. Various types of irrigating sets are available from surgical supply houses.*

Colostomy bags may be worn immediately after irrigation; then a change to a simple dressing may be effective. Patients are instructed in the care and the cleaning of equipment to prolong its life and keep it free of odors. Cleaning by soap or a detergent and water, and exposure to fresh air, usually is sufficient; however, it may still be necessary to deodorize the appliance; liquid deodorizers are available to use in washing and soaking equipment. The other aspect of the problem is the control of odors arising from the body excreta as they collect in the appliance. Inserting readily soluble deodorizing tablets in the appliance or putting a few drops of chlorophyll solution into the bag will help in the control of odors. Powdered charcoal, two crushed aspirin tablets, or a teaspoon of baking soda may be sprinkled into the bag to absorb odors. Also effective are commercially available colostomy deodorants.

As a rule, colostomy bags are not necessary. As soon as the patient has learned a routine for his evacuation, bags may be dispensed with, and a simple dressing of disposable tissue (often covered with Saran wrap) is used, held in place by an elastic belt or girdle. Except for the escape of gas and a slight amount of mucus, nothing comes from the colostomy opening between irrigations; therefore, the inconvenience of a colostomy bag is unnecessary.

---

* Public Law HR-1, Oct. 30, 1972, specifically has included "colostomy bags and supplies directly related to colostomy care" as being covered under Medicare.

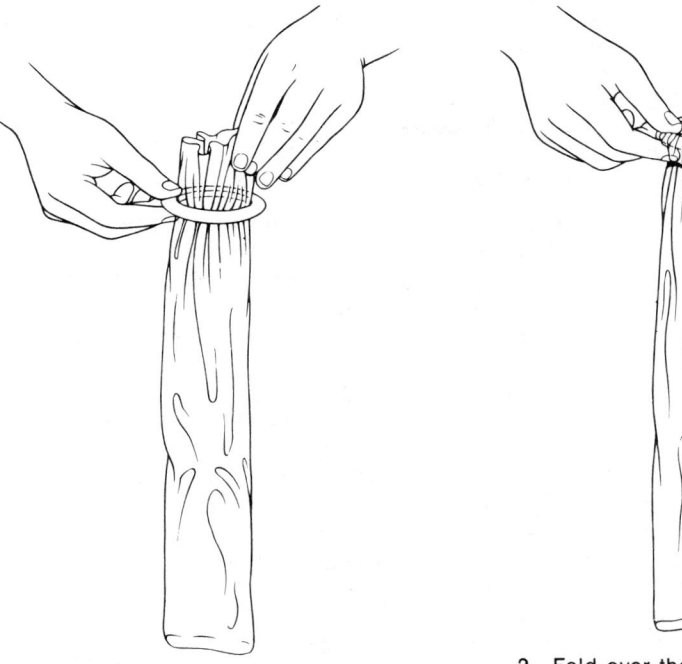

1. Insert one end of drainage sheath through the plastic ring.

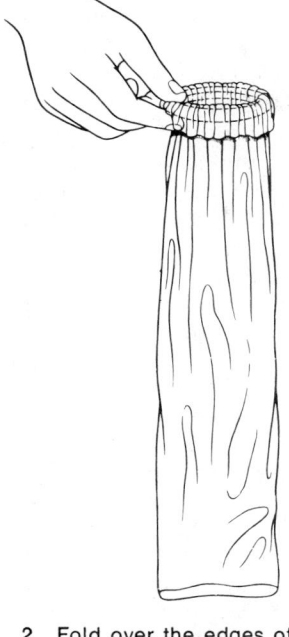

2. Fold over the edges of the sheath and roll around ring securely and evenly.

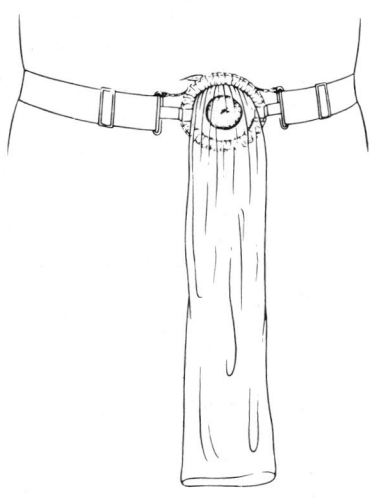

3. The ring with sheath is placed over the stoma, and the belt clips hooked onto the ring. This holds the appliance securely over the opening.

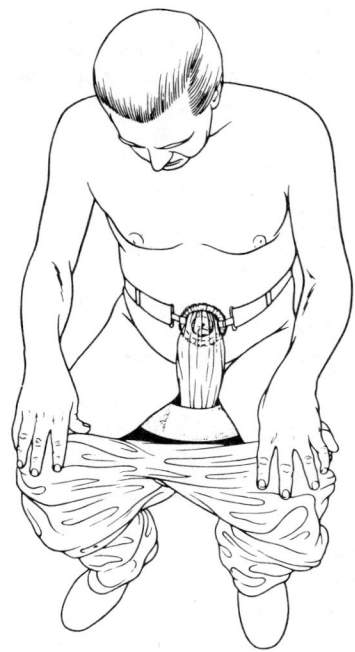

4. After cutting a small hole in the sheath above and to one side of the stoma, the sheath is tucked between the legs so that it leads directly into the toilet.

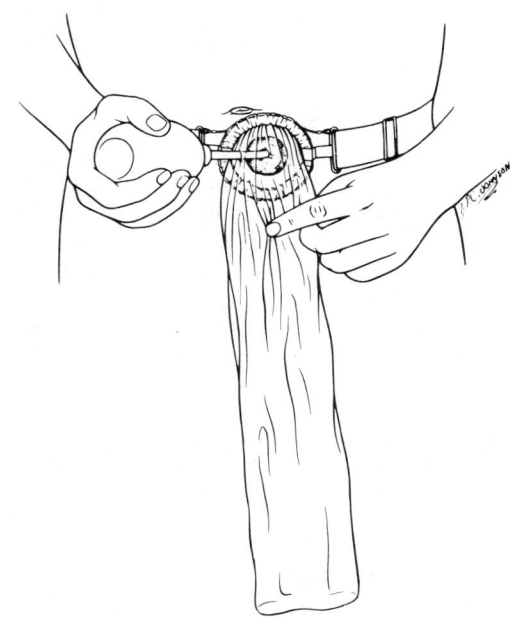

5. Moisten the tip of the syringe with a standard lubricating jelly. Insert the lubricated syringe tip through the hole of the drainage sheath and gently into the stoma about 7.5–12.5 cm. (3–5 inches).

Figure 38-8. The bulb syringe method of colostomy irrigation. (From Postel AH, Grier WRN, and Localio SA: Training the Patient in the Bulb Syringe Method of Colostomy Irrigation. New York, New York University Medical Center.)

Hygienic Measures

Thorough drying after washing with soap and water may be all that is necessary for good skin care. If the skin around the stoma appears red or irritated, the following may be applied, after cleaning and drying the area: triamcinolone acetonide (Kenalog) spray followed by a light dusting of nystatin powder (Mycostatin). Milk of magnesia paste, Maalox, or Gelusil are also soothing and facilitate healing.

Diarrhea and constipation are controlled as described below.

In general, the patient needs to be reminded that good health practices will materially aid his feeling of well-being and his positive adjustment to his colostomy. Diet should be adequate and well-balanced; laxatives are rarely used. Lastly, it is valuable to observe a usual time for doing certain activities (*e.g.,* mealtime, irrigation time, bedtime, and so forth). A regular schedule for meals, irrigation, exercise, and sleep will be helpful in achieving colostomy regularity.

Sexual Activity

The patient should be encouraged to discuss plans to return to his usual sexual activity. Some patients will initiate questions about sexual activity directly, while others will give indirect cues about their concerns. Still others may view this surgery as mutilative and a threat to their sexuality. The nurse needs to assess this and attempt to identify the patient's concerns. If the nurse is uncomfortable with this or if the patient's concerns seem complex, the nurse should seek assistance from an appropriate source, such as the "ostomy nurse," sex educator, or psychiatric clinical specialist.

Selection of Appropriate Diet

Diet is individualized as long as it is well-balanced and does not cause diarrhea or constipation. Since certain foods will produce odors or gas, the patient may wish to avoid them: beans, cabbage, cucumbers, fish, radishes, and onions.

If the patient has problems with diarrhea, the use of paregoric, bismuth subgallate, bismuth subcarbonate, or diphenoxylate with atropine (Lomotil) will control it. For constipation, prune or apple juice or a mild laxative is effective. For dietary support of complications, see Table 38-8.

▶ Evaluation

Expected Outcomes

1. Copes with the stress of impending surgery
   a. Expresses concerns about surgery
   b. Discusses feelings about surgery with health team members and family
   c. Discusses the surgical procedure and postoperative course with an ostomate or an enterostomal therapist (if available)
   d. Expresses feelings about changes in body functioning (*i.e.,* elimination)
   e. Recognizes the need to learn colostomy self-care after surgery
2. Is free of complications
   a. Ingests adequate amount of fluids
   b. Shows balance between urinary output and fluid intake
   c. Tolerates well-balanced diet
   d. Has no constipation and diarrhea
   e. Progresses toward regular schedule of elimination
   f. Demonstrates intact skin around colostomy stoma
   g. Shows signs that incisional wounds are healing without infection
3. Adheres to therapeutic regimen
   a. Establishes a routine for self-care activities
   b. Performs self-care of colostomy (*i.e.,* irrigation, skin care, changing of stoma bag)
   c. Discusses postdischarge self-care activities with family and health team members
   d. Accepts services of visiting nurse, if appropriate
   e. Describes measures to take if diarrhea or constipation occur
   f. Avoids foods that cause diarrhea, constipation, flatus, or odor
   g. Keeps follow-up clinic or physician appointments

Table 38-8
Dietary Support of Common Complications in Surgical Treatment for Cancer

Procedure	Complications	Dietary Support
Small bowel resection	Poor absorption Weight loss Absorptive capacity improves with time	Immediate support after surgery: long-term enteral or parenteral nutrition Later: Oral intake of high-protein, high-caloric, low-fat diet Medium-chain triglycerides
Ileostomy Colostomy	Initial loss of water and electrolytes	Daily replacement of electrolytes, full liquid diet, high in protein
Bypass surgery	For relief of pain and obstruction Malabsorption syndrome Maldigestion, diarrhea	Feedings by natural route High protein, high vitamin C Adequate vitamins and minerals

(Adapted from Valassi K: Nutritional management of cancer patients in a variety of therapeutic regimens. Arch Phys Med Rehabil 58: Sept 1977.)

▷ Intestinal Obstruction

An intestinal obstruction is inability of the intestinal contents to flow normally along the intestinal tract, owing to some hindrance. There are two types of intestinal obstruction:

1. Mechanical (dynamic ileus, organic ileus, spastic ileus), in which there is an intraluminal obstruction or a mural obstruction from pressure on the intestinal walls, and
2. Paralytic ileus (adynamic ileus), in which the intestinal musculature is unable to propel the contents along the bowel. (Stimuli that inhibit intestinal peristalsis are: laparotomy, trauma, infection, mesenteric ischemia, and metabolic disorders.)

An obstruction may be partial or complete. Its seriousness depends on the region of bowel that is affected, the degree to which the lumen is occluded, and, especially, the degree to which the blood circulation in the bowel wall is disturbed. Small bowel obstruction is always serious, because, as a consequence of persistent vomiting, it leads to profound disturbances in the electrolyte balance of the body: first, to alkalosis, from the loss of the gastric hydrochloric acid; then, to profound dehydration and acidosis, owing to the loss of water and sodium from the small intestine. If the obstruction is only partial and develops slowly, the symptoms are relatively mild. Large bowel obstruction, even if complete, is also comparatively undramatic, provided that the blood supply to the colon is not disturbed. However, if the blood supply is cut off, intestinal strangulation (tissue death) occurs, and the patient's life is in jeopardy.

Causes and Pathophysiology. Proximal to the intestinal obstruction there is an accumulation of intestinal contents, fluid, and gas. In the small intestine, distention reduces the absorption of fluids and stimulates gastric secretion. As a result, fluids and electrolytes are lost. With increasing distention, pressure within the intestinal lumen causes a decrease in venous and arteriolar capillary pressure. This, in turn, causes edema, congestion, necrosis, and eventual rupture or perforation of the intestinal wall.

With vomiting, there is a loss of hydrogen ions and potassium from the stomach, producing hypochloremia, hypokalemia, and metabolic alkalosis. When there are acute fluid losses, hypovolemic shock may occur. In the large intestine, dehydration occurs more slowly because there is less fluid loss, owing, primarily, to less fluid intake.

One of every three cases of acute colonic obstruction is due to cancer of the large bowel (see p. 827). Intestinal obstruction very occasionally results from a foreign body lodged in the bowel (i.e., a large fruit stone, a gallstone; a mass of parasitic worms, etc.). In other patients, a stricture of the bowel may result from the contracting scar of an ulcer in its wall.

The intestine may also become pinched in a peritoneal pocket (hernia) or linked by peritoneal adhesions (prime cause of small bowel obstruction), or a loop of intestine may become twisted about itself (volvulus).

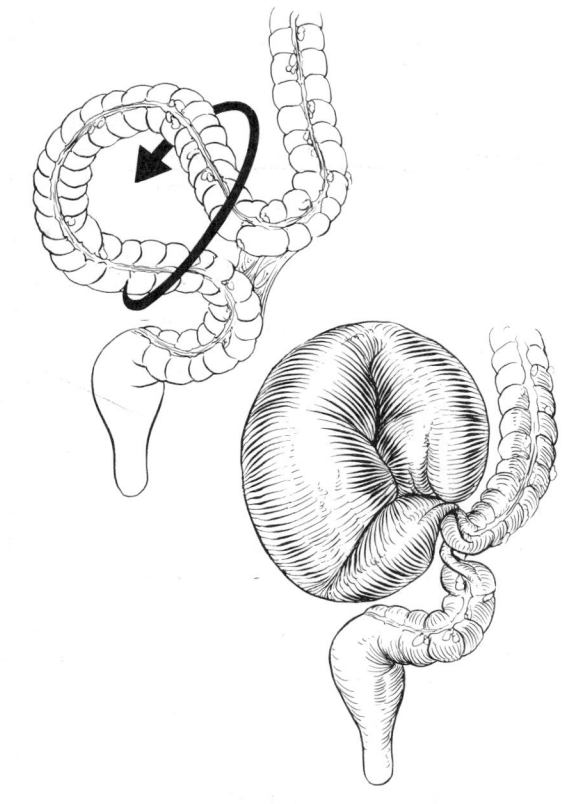

Figure 38-9. Volvulus of the sigmoid colon. The twist is counterclockwise in most cases of sigmoid volvulus. Note the edematous bowel (From Dunphy JE and Way LW (eds): Current Surgical Diagnosis and Treatment. Los Altos, California, Lange Medical Publishers.)

Volvulus (Fig. 38-9) is a life-threatening obstruction, because the intestinal lumen is obstructed both proximally and distally. The accumulation of gas and fluid in the trapped bowel leads to necrosis, perforation, and peritonitis.

Hernia (see pp. 815–816) is one of the most common and important causes of intestinal obstruction (second to small bowel obstruction), and, if strangulated, is a surgical emergency.

Paralytic Ileus

A paralytic ileus is a paralysis of peristaltic movement owing to the effect of trauma or toxins on the nerves that regulate intestinal movement. Functional paralytic ileus following abdominal surgery may last 12 to 36 hours. Because of this, food and fluids are withheld until normal peristalsis returns, as indicated by bowel sounds (heard with the stethoscope) or the passing of flatus. Paralytic ileus may also happen after back injuries, after operation on the kidney, and frequently with peritonitis.

The lack of peristalsis results in a distention of the intestine with gas produced by decomposition of the intestinal contents or by the swallowing of air. Few or no peristaltic sounds can be heard, and the patient may be extremely uncomfortable, if not in marked pain. Relief of the distention associated with paralytic ileus often is obtained by intestinal intubation (see p. 769).

Intussusception

Intussusception is another cause of intestinal obstruction. In this condition, the bowel above a certain point pushes itself into the bowel below that point, much as a telescope is shortened by pushing one section into the next. This occurs through peristalsis. The point at which intussusception most commonly develops is at or near the ileocecal valve. The telescoping, or invagination, also may start at the point of attachment of a tumor in the colon—particularly a pedunculated tumor—as a result of its becoming engaged by a peristaltic wave and propelled along the colon, dragging into the lumen that portion of the wall to which its pedicle is attached.

Postoperative Adhesions

After abdominal operations, there are many areas within the abdomen that may not be completely healed, and loops of intestine may become adherent to these areas. Such inflammatory adhesions usually are only temporary and of no particular importance. However, occasionally these adhesions may produce a kinking of an intestinal loop, which causes obstruction of the intestinal flow. This obstruction usually appears on the third or fourth day after operation, when peristalsis normally is resumed and when food and fluids are being given to the patient for the first time. The symptoms are typical of any intestinal obstruction—crampy abdominal pain, distention, vomiting, etc.

The difficulty usually is relieved by nasoenteric suction. Decompressing the bowel above the site of the obstruction allows the inflammation to subside and relieves the obstruction. When the obstruction cannot be relieved by this conservative means, an operation may be necessary to free the adherent intestine and to permit the intestinal flow to be resumed.

Clinical Manifestations of Intestinal Obstruction

The symptoms of intestinal obstruction depend on what part of the bowel is obstructed.

Small Bowel Obstruction.   The initial symptom is usually pain that is wavelike in character. The patient may pass blood and mucus, but no fecal matter and no flatus. Vomiting occurs. This pattern is often characteristic. If the obstruction is complete, the peristaltic waves become extremely vigorous and assume a reverse direction, the intestinal contents being propelled toward the mouth instead of toward the rectum. If the obstruction is in the ileum, fecal vomiting takes place. First, the patient vomits the stomach contents, then the bile-stained contents of the duodenum and the jejunum and, finally, with each paroxysm of pain, the darker, fecal-like contents of the ileum are ejected. Soon, owing to the loss of water, sodium, and chlorides in the vomitus, the unmistakable signs of dehydration become evident. The patient complains of intense thirst, drowsiness, generalized malaise, and aching. The tongue and the mucous membranes become parched; the face acquires a pinched appearance. The abdomen becomes distended, and, the lower the obstruction in the gastrointestinal tract, the more marked is the disten-

tion. If the situation is allowed to continue uncorrected, shock appears, owing to dehydration and loss of plasma volume. The patient is prostrated; the pulse becomes increasingly weak and rapid; the temperature and the blood pressure are lowered; the skin is pale, cold, and clammy. At this point, death may supervene rapidly.

Large Bowel Obstruction.   Large bowel intestinal obstruction differs clinically from the small bowel type in that the symptoms develop and progress relatively slowly. This difference is due to the fact that the colon is able to absorb its fluid contents, and it can distend to a considerable degree beyond its normal full capacity. In patients with obstruction in the sigmoid or the rectum, constipation may be the only symptom for days. Eventually, the abdomen becomes markedly distended; loops of large bowel become visibly outlined through the abdominal wall, and the patient suffers from crampy lower abdominal pain. Finally, fecal vomiting develops. The terminal features are essentially those of ileum obstruction. In patients with fecal impaction, shock is usually not present.

Nursing Assessment and Interventions

The nurse obtains a patient history relative to the function of the gastrointestinal tract, including descriptive information related to stool passage (constipation, obstipation, diarrhea—and frequency). The patient's appetite is assessed to see if it is normal or if there have been signs of anorexia. The patient is queried with regard to weight gain or loss, vomiting (frequency, amount, and description), and pain (location and description).

The abdomen should be assessed with a stethoscope in order to auscultate audible peristalsis (bowel sounds) and gas movement. Whereas bowel sounds are normally gurgling and swishing in nature, obstructions are reflected in high-pitched peristaltic rushes (sudden intense sounds that reach a crescendo peak and then collapse readily). The girth of the abdomen is also measured and recorded. Although it may be flat at first, as the obstruction continues, distention is noted. For purposes of comparison, the abdomen should be measured with a tape at the same time each day, by the same person. When infection and necrosis are progressing, there is evidence of temperature and pulse elevation and a white blood cell count rapidly rising to 15,000 or 20,000. Tenderness is usually a symptom of strangulation.

Any stool that is passed is to be saved, so that it can be inspected directly and tested for the presence of occult blood.

If the disorder is an incarcerated external hernia, an attempt may be made to reduce it, not by applying pressure to the extruded mass, but simply by having the patient lie flat on his back with knees flexed and an ice compress placed continuously over the mass. This position, and the cold, may cause the edema and swelling of the incarcerated bowel to subside, allowing the loop to escape back through the ring or opening into which it has worked itself.

Fluid, electrolyte, and nutritional needs are evaluated, and met by parenteral therapy. Decompression of the small intestine is accomplished by nasoenteric suction. X-rays, especially survey films of the abdomen and possibly barium studies, in selected instances, may be done to confirm the diagnosis. Preoperative nursing attentions are similar to those followed for major abdominal surgery (see p. 355).

Surgical Intervention

The surgical treatment of intestinal obstruction depends largely on the cause of the obstruction. In the most common causes of obstruction, such as strangulated hernia, obstruction by adhesions, and so forth, the operation consists of repair of the hernia or division of the adhesion to which the intestine is attached. In some hernias, it may be necessary to remove the strangulated portion of bowel and perform an anastomosis. Operation for intestinal obstruction may be simple or complicated, depending on the duration of the obstruction and the condition of the intestine found at operation.

When the large intestine becomes obstructed, usually by cancer, it is frequently necessary to relieve the colonic obstruction before it is possible to resect the cancer itself.

This is done by inserting a large tube into the cecum (cecostomy) or by making an opening in the colon above the site of the obstruction, by bringing a loop of colon up to the skin surface. When this is opened, the obstruction is relieved, and the tumor can be treated at a later time. This operation is called a *loop colostomy* (see p. 828).

Nursing Evaluation. Evaluation of surgical outcomes is similar to that of the patient having intestinal surgery (Chart 38-4). The specific outcome criteria here are return of peristalsis, resolution of abdominal distention, relief of pain, and adequate intake and output.

▷ Anorectal Conditions

Assessment and Clinical Manifestations

Patients with anorectal disorders seek medical help primarily because of pain and rectal bleeding. Other frequent complaints are protrusion of hemorrhoids, anal discharge, itching, and swelling.

Chart 38-4
Summary of the Principles and Objectives of Medical, Surgical, and Nursing Management of the Patient Undergoing Intestinal Surgery

Preoperative Goals

I. To ensure optimal patient condition for surgery:
  A. Give whole blood or packed red cells as prescribed to patient debilitated by bleeding, infection, or a malignant neoplasm.
  B. Correct fluid and electrolyte deficiencies before operation.
    Give intravenous infusions of lactated Ringer's solution, etc., as prescribed prior to surgery, to prevent electrolyte imbalance and diminished renal function during surgery.
  C. Promote the nutrition of the patient.
    1. Correct existing protein deficiencies before operation.
    2. Encourage between-meal feedings.
    3. Give intravenous protein hydrolysates or albumin, if indicated.
  D. Assist in diagnostic examinations to evaluate the patient's pulmonary, cardiac, hepatic, and renal functions.
    1. Evaluate TPR and BP at prescribed intervals.
    2. Give medications and treatments indicated, when heart failure is present.
    3. Support the patient undergoing diagnostic bowel studies.
  E. Insert indwelling catheter immediately before surgery to prevent manipulation and trauma to the bladder.

II. To reduce bacteria in the intestinal tract to prevent postoperative infection:
  A. Employ effective measures to empty the colon.
    1. Give laxatives as prescribed, to cleanse the bowel by catharsis.
    2. Administer enemas and colonic irrigations to rid the bowel of feces and gas.
    3. Offer a low-residue diet to reduce fecal content in lower bowel.
    4. Place patient on liquid diet at the prescribed interval before surgery.
  B. Give antibacterial agents (intestinal antiseptics) to control the bacterial flora of the gastrointestinal tract.
    1. Give drug combinations (usually sulfathalidine and neomycin) as prescribed.
    2. Observe patient for symptoms of pseudomembranous enterocolitis:
      a. Tender, distended abdomen
      b. Vomiting; diarrhea
      c. Fever

III. To decompress gastrointestinal tract through an indwelling tube to minimize vomiting and distention:
  A. Use a Levin tube for stomach and upper small bowel decompression.
  B. Use a Miller–Abbott tube or other prescribed tube for intestinal decompression.

(continued)

Chart 38-4
*Summary of the Principles and Objectives of Medical, Surgical, and Nursing Management
of the Patient Undergoing Intestinal Surgery (continued)*

Postoperative Objectives

IV. To supply fluids and electrolytes and body nutrients to the patient in the immediate postoperative period:
  A. Use an intravenous catheter if IV therapy is to be carried out for more than a few days.
    1. Use arm for placement of intravenous catheter to permit greater patient mobility.
    2. Examine needle site for evidence of thrombophlebitis or chemical phlebitis.
    3. Elevate patient's head and back (after he regains consciousness) while he is receiving intravenous infusions.
  B. Record type of intravenous fluid, starting time, finishing time, amount absorbed, and any untoward reactions.
  C. Employ meticulous oral hygiene measures when patient is not taking fluids by the oral route.
V. To ensure continuing function of the nasogastric or nasoenteric tube so that postoperative aspiration, distention, and ileus are minimized:
  A. Record amount and type of gastrointestinal aspirate.
  B. Watch for symptoms of fluid volume deficit:
    1. Skin dryness
    2. Lethargy
  C. Promote comfort of intubated patient.
    1. Lubricate nares with water-soluble ointment.
    2. Turn the patient frequently.
    3. Humidify the room to decrease dryness of mucous membranes.
    4. Apply cold compresses to neck periodically if patient complains of sore throat.

  D. Remove tube when peristalsis is reestablished (indicated by auscultation, the passage of flatus by rectum, and the clinical symptoms of the patient). (This done at request of the physician.)
VI. To promote the comfort and safety of the patient:
  A. Give analgesic agent according to clinical symptoms and needs of the individual patient.
    1. Assess the patient for hypotension and restlessness.
    2. Use special caution in giving narcotics to elderly patients.
  B. Combat sleeplessness with appropriate nursing measures and prescribed sedative and hypnotics.
  C. Encourage the patient to turn, breathe deeply, and cough, at specified intervals. Auscultate for symptoms of lung congestion.
  D. Change the dressing, when indicated, if patient has a draining wound, ileostomy, or colostomy.
  E. Encourage the patient to ventilate his feelings and anxieties about his condition.
VII. To observe the patient for complications (see Chart 38-5)
VIII. To encourage the patient to have follow-up examinations following surgery:
  A. Inform the patient to expect periodic x-ray examinations of the colon, chest, lumbar spine (especially if patient has cancer).
  B. Reinforce the physician's instructions concerning regular follow-up examinations.
  C. Advise the patient to report any unexplained symptoms or recurring symptoms immediately to his physician.

Bleeding is frequently seen in anorectal disease. (The most common cause of rectal bleeding is hemorrhoids.) The patient's description of the bleeding, as well as the nurse's assessment, assists in establishing the diagnosis. The bleeding may be bright red, but occasionally it is a darker color, owing to its remaining in the rectal ampulla before expulsion, and also from admixture with feces. Bleeding from the anal canal usually has a bright red appearance.

In assessing the patient's symptoms, the nurse should investigate the following:

1. Is there blood coating the stool, or is it mixed with the feces?
2. Is there pain during evacuation? Is there associated abdominal pain?
3. How long does the pain last after evacuation?
4. How does the *patient* describe the pain?
5. Is any protrusion noted from the anus?
6. Is a discharge evident? Mucoid? Purulent? Bloody?

The Rectal Examination and Patient Preparation

Visual inspection and digital examination of the anus and the rectum are indispensable for detecting and identifying lesions involving these structures. Moreover, rectal examination is extremely useful in diagnosing or excluding many intra-abdominal and pelvic conditions, including appendicitis; diverticulitis; salpingitis; tumors of the ovary, the uterus, and the colon; and prostatic lesions of various types.

Rectal examinations may be done with the patient in the knee–chest, Sims's lateral, or inverted position, on a special proctoscopic table. Whatever position is used, the patient is informed of the procedure and how it is to be done. He is draped so that only the rectal area is exposed (see p. 86 for rectal examination technique).

Anorectal Abscess

Anorectal abscess is located in the pararectal spaces. Usually, it is caused by infection of pathogenic microorganisms. Incidence is higher in men than women.

Chart 38-5
Summary of Potential Complications Following Surgery of Small and Large Intestine

Anticipation of and vigilance for complications have first priority in caring for postoperative patients. Prompt recognition and management of these complications can prevent prolonged disability and, in some instances, death.

Complication	Nursing Assessment and Implementation
Paralytic ileus	Initiate or continue nasogastric intubation. Prepare patient for x-ray study. Ensure adequate fluid and electrolyte replacement. Give antibiotics if patient has symptoms of peritonitis.
Mechanical obstruction	Evaluate patient for intermittent colicky pain, nausea, and vomiting. Prepare for intestinal intubation, electrolyte replacement, and reoperation, if patient does not respond to conservative treatment.
Infection: Intraperitoneal infections Abdominal wound infection	Assess for evidence of constant or generalized abdominal pain, rapid pulse, and elevation of temperature. Prepare for tube decompression of bowel. Restore fluid and electrolytes by IV route. Give antibiotics as directed.
Intra-abdominal septic conditions Peritonitis	Evaluate patient for nausea, hiccuping, chills, spiking fever, tachycardia. Give antibiotics as prescribed. Prepare patients for drainage procedure. Institute intravenous fluid and electrolyte therapy. Prepare patient for reoperation if his condition deteriorates.
Abscess formation	Administer antibiotics as directed. Apply hot compresses as prescribed. Prepare for surgical drainage.
Wound complications: Infection	Watch temperature graph for evidences of spiking fever. Observe for redness, tenderness, and pain around wound. Assist in establishing local drainage. Obtain specimen of drainage material for culture and sensitivity studies.
Wound disruption	Watch for sudden appearance of profuse serous drainage from wound. Cover wound area with sterile towels held in place with binder. Prepare patient immediately for surgery.
Anastomotic complications: Dehiscence of anastomosis	Prepare patient for surgery.
Fistulas	Employ bowel decompression. Give parenteral fluids to correct fluid and electrolyte defects.

Management. An abscess may occur in a variety of spaces in and around the rectum. Often it contains a quantity of foul-smelling pus, and is painful. If the abscess is superficial, swelling, redness, and tenderness are observed. A deeper abscess may result in toxic symptoms and even lower abdominal pain, as well as fever. More than half of rectal abscesses will result in fistulas.

Palliative therapy consists of sitz baths and analgesics. Surgical treatment consists of incision and drainage; this may be all that is necessary. When deeper infection exists, with the possibility of a fistula, it is necessary to remove the fistulous tract. This may be done initially, or it may require

a second operation. Often no packing is used; if packing is used, usually the wound is lined with petrolatum gauze. Later, when it is necessary to remove the packing, soaking it first with peroxide of hydrogen is helpful.

These wounds are allowed to heal by granulation. Bowel movements should be formed, rather than liquid or soft. Cathartics or mineral oil are not usually used.

Fistula in Ano

Fistula in ano is a tiny tubular tract that extends into the anal canal from an opening located beside the anus (Fig. 38-10). Pus or stool leak constantly from the cutaneous

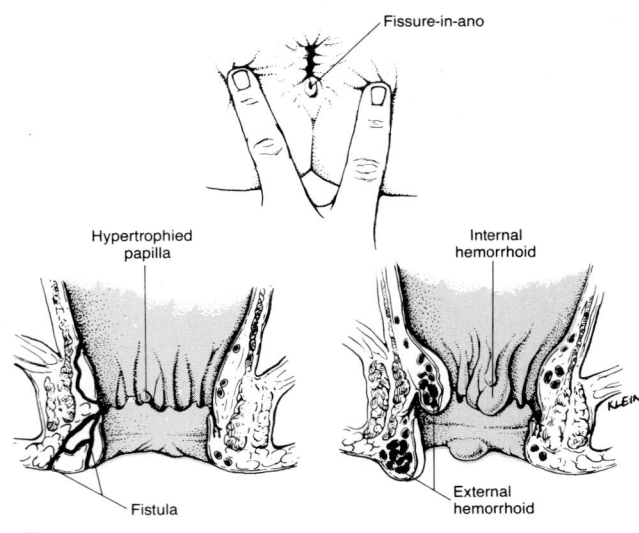

Figure 38-10.   Various types of anal lesions.

opening, making it necessary for the patient to wear a protective pad. This condition may be an early sign of regional enteritis.

Management.   Three or 4 hours before operation, the perineum should be shaved and the lower bowel evacuated thoroughly with several warm soapsuds enemas. The patient should be allowed to evacuate the enemas on a commode. The last enema should return clear and should be evacuated entirely.

For operation, the patient usually is placed in the lithotomy position, and the sinus tract is identified by inserting a probe into it or by injecting the tract with methylene blue solution. The fistula then may be dissected out or laid open by an incision from its rectal opening to its outlet. The wound is packed with gauze.

Postoperative treatment and complications are the same as those described under "The Patient Having Rectal Surgery" (pp. 843–844).

Fissure in Ano

Fissure in ano is a longitudinal ulcer in the anal canal (see Fig. 38-10). It is associated frequently with constipation, and its most pronounced symptom is excruciating pain during defecation.

Management.   Over half of these fissures will heal if treated by conservative measures, and the remainder will require minor surgery. A bland laxative will prevent constipation. A suppository combining an anesthetic with a steroid is comforting. Anal dilatation under anesthesia may be required.

In surgical management, the same preoperative preparation as for fistula in ano is indicated. Several types of operations may be performed: in some cases, the anal sphincter is dilated and the fissure is excised; in others, a part of the external sphincter is divided. This establishes a paralysis of the external sphincter, with consequent relief of spasm, and permits the ulcer to heal. When there is a large, overhanging sentinel hemorrhoid, excision of the ulcer and of the hemorrhoid is performed.

Hemorrhoids

Hemorrhoids are simply varicose veins in the anal canal. They may come and go, and almost everyone has them at some time. They are very common in pregnancy. When they fade away, they may leave a telltale skin tag. They occur in two locations. Those occurring above the internal sphincter are called *internal hemorrhoids,* and those appearing outside the external sphincter are called *external hemorrhoids* (see Fig. 38-10). They cause itching, bleeding at stool, and pain. Internal hemorrhoids prolapse frequently through the sphincter and cause considerable discomfort. If the blood within them clots and becomes infected, they grow painful and are said to be *thrombosed.*

Management.   Hemorrhoid symptoms and discomfort can be relieved by good personal hygiene and by avoiding excessive straining during defecation. A diet that contains fruit and bran may be all the treatment that is necessary; failing this, perhaps a hydrophilic laxative will help.

Many physicians have their preferred medications, which, when injected above the sensitive squamous mucosa through an anoscope, have no direct effect on thrombosed veins, per se, but induce a fibrous reaction. This reaction in submucosal tissues of the upper anal canal and lower rectum tends to draw tissue upward toward its normal site. This method has little effect on advanced hemorrhoids.

A conservative measure is the rubber-band treatment. As the hemorrhoid is visualized through the proctoscope, the upper part above the mucocutaneous line is grasped with an instrument, and a small rubber band is slipped over it. Tissue distal to the rubber band becomes necrotic and is removed. Because of fibrosis, lower anal mucosa is drawn up and adheres to the underlying muscle. While this treatment has been satisfactory in some patients, it has proved painful in others and may cause some secondary hemorrhage.

The most recent treatment is cryosurgical hemorrhoidectomy, which is currently being evaluated for its effectiveness. By freezing the tissues of the hemorrhoid for a sufficient time to cause necrosis, this method acts similarly to the rubber-band method. However, it is painless.

The methods of treating hemorrhoids just described are not effective for advanced thrombosed veins, which are usually treated by surgical hemorrhoidectomy.

The operation usually involves digital dilatation of the rectal sphincter and removal of the hemorrhoids by the use of a clamp and cautery or by ligation and excision. After completion of the operative procedures, a small tube, often covered with petrolatum gauze, may be inserted through the sphincter to permit the escape of flatus and also of blood, if there should be any hemorrhage. Instead of the tube, some surgeons place pieces of Gelfoam or Oxycel gauze over the anal wounds. Dressings, in such cases, are held in place by a T-binder.

Pilonidal Cyst

A *pilonidal cyst* is found in the intergluteal cleft on the posterior surface of the lower sacrum. It is thought by some to be formed by an infolding of epithelial tissue beneath the skin, which may communicate with the skin surface through one or several small sinus openings. Hair frequently is seen protruding from these openings, and this gives the cyst its name—*pilonidal*—a nest of hair. The cysts rarely give symptoms until adolescence or early adult life, when infection produces an irritating drainage or an abscess. This area is easily irritated by perspiration and friction.

Trauma appears to play a part in producing the inflammatory reaction in these cysts.

Management. In the early stages of the inflammation, the infection may be controlled by the antibiotic therapy. Once an abscess has formed, as in cases of a hair-containing sinus, surgery is indicated. When an abscess is present, incision and drainage are performed. Usually, however, because the abscesses tend to recur or form secondary sinuses that cause irritating drainage, radical excision of the cyst is necessary. In patients with hair-containing sinuses without marked inflammatory reaction, operation is necessary, for the same reason. The entire cyst and the secondary sinus tracts are excised. In many patients the resulting defect may be sutured, but in some the defect may be so large that it cannot be closed entirely, and it is allowed to heal by granulation.

The *nursing care* of these patients is relatively simple. In those with abscess, hot, moist applications are used frequently. After excision of the cyst, the care is that of any superficial wound. For the first few days, this patient often is more comfortable lying on his abdomen or side with a pillow between his legs. Most patients may be allowed out of bed soon after operation, and their postoperative care is managed at home.

The Patient Having Rectal Surgery

Patients facing rectal surgery are ordinarily upset and irritable. The nursing approach should focus on the special psychological problems involved. This patient has a special need for privacy. The perineum often is shaved carefully before surgery. This may vary with the nature of the operation. Usually, a lower bowel irrigation is prescribed, which should be given at least 2 hours prior to surgery. The skin area is cleaned as thoroughly as possible.

Postoperative Management
Patient Problems/Nursing Diagnoses. Following rectal surgery, the patient may experience the following problems: potential complications, such as pain; voiding difficulties; hemorrhage; and possible nonadherence to the therapeutic regimen.

Goals. The major goals for the patient include (1) absence of complications, and (2) adherence to the therapeutic regimen.

Absence of Complications. During the first 24 hours after rectal surgery, there may be painful spasms of the sphincter and muscles. Therefore, control of pain is of prime consideration. Liberal use of analgesics during this time may be necessary. After 24 hours have elapsed, topical anesthetic agents may be beneficial for relief of local irritation and soreness.

Voiding may be a problem, owing to a reflex spasm of the sphincter at the outlet of the bladder and a certain amount of muscle-guarding from apprehension and pain. All methods to encourage voluntary micturition should be tried before resorting to catheterization. After rectal operations, patients are usually allowed out of bed to void.

- After hemorrhoidectomy, hemorrhage may occur from the veins that were cut. If a tube has been inserted through the sphincter after operation, evidence of bleeding should be apparent on the dressings. If, however, the patient feels faint, restless, and anxious, and the pulse rate increases, the nurse should recognize internal or concealed hemorrhage and give appropriate treatment until the surgeon arrives.

Hygiene of the perianal area is important for patient comfort. This is accomplished by gentle cleansing with warm water and *drying* with absorbent cotton wipes. The patient should be instructed to avoid rubbing the area with toilet tissue.

To relieve soreness and pain, moist heat is employed in the form of warm compresses and sitz baths three or four times daily, and especially after each bowel movement. Moist heat is soothing and relaxes sphincter spasm. An ice-cap to the head or over the heart helps to prevent the faint feeling experienced by many patients during sitz baths. Wet dressings saturated with equal parts of cold water and witch hazel help relieve edema. Petrolatum should be applied around the anal area when wet compresses are being used continuously, to prevent skin maceration. Instruct the patient to assume a prone position at intervals, since this position promotes dependent drainage of edema fluid.

Medications prescribed may include *suppositories* that contain anesthetics, astringents, antiseptics, tranquilizers, antinauseants, and even bronchodilators. Patients will be more compliant, and less apprehensive and uncomfortable, if the suppository is inserted properly. The most effective position for the patient to assume while the suppository is being inserted is side-lying, with the uppermost leg flexed. The suppository is unwrapped; the buttocks are spread apart with one hand and the suppository inserted with the other. If the suppository was stored in the refrigerator (to prevent melting), it may be warmed to room temperature to lessen irritation of rectal mucosa. Water-soluble suppositories may be lubricated with water or lubricating jelly; however, cocoa butter suppositories are self-lubricating.

The patient may be so fearful of pain that he fails to respond to the signal for defecation and thus develops constipation. Usually, cathartics are avoided. It is better to have a formed stool rather than many liquid or soft ones. The painful sphincter spasm can be relieved at once by a hot sitz bath or hot compresses. Mineral oil may be prescribed. Some surgeons prefer that a warm oil-retention enema be given when the patient feels a desire to defecate; a soapsuds enema given through a well-lubricated catheter may be prescribed if there has been no bowel movement by the third day after operation. The food preferred by the patient is usually given.

The patient may assume any position that is comfortable. The prone position or side-lying position, with a pillow between the knees, is quite comfortable for these patients. A foam cushion or air ring will greatly increase the patient's sitting comfort. Early ambulation is generally encouraged.

Patient Education.   When it is time for the patient to be discharged from the hospital, he should know how to take sitz baths and how to test the temperature of the water. Sitz baths may be given in a bathtub three or four times a day. If this tends to make some postoperative patients weak, sitz baths may be given by employing a dishpan or some large container with enough water to cover the perineum.

The patient is informed about his diet and made aware of the significance of proper eating habits. Also, he ought to know what laxatives he can take safely and why exercise is important. The surgeon usually outlines a schedule in detail to cover the daily routine. This can be reviewed with the patient by the nurse.

Nursing Evaluation.   Patient care outcomes can be evaluated as follows.

Expected Outcomes

1. Is free of complications
   a. Has no pain and discomfort
   b. Has voluntary micturition with emptying of the bladder
   c. Is free of hemorrhage
   d. Experiences no incisional infection
   e. Has normal bowel movements
2. Adheres to the therapeutic regimen
   a. Takes sitz baths as directed
   b. Has adequate intake of food and fluid
   c. Adheres to exercise regimen
   d. Keeps clinic or physician appointments

▷ **Bibliography**

Books

Bongiovanni G. Manual of Clinical Gastroenterology. New York, McGraw–Hill, 1982.

Broadwell DC and Jackson BS. Principles of Ostomy Care. St Louis, CV Mosby, 1981.

Feddian–Green RA and Turcotte JG. Gastrointestinal Hemorrhage. New York, Grune & Stratton, 1980.

Greenberger NJ and Winship DH. Gastrointestinal Disorders, 2nd ed. New York, Year Book Medical Publishers, 1981.

Kirsner JB and Shorter RG. Inflammatory Bowel Disease. Philadelphia, Lea & Febiger, 1980.

Nord JH and Brady PG. Critical Care Gastroenterology. New York, Churchill Livingstone, 1982.

Schachter H and Kirsner JB. Crohn's Disease of the Gastrointestinal Tract. New York, John Wiley & Sons, 1980.

Spiro HM. Clinical Gastroenterology, 3rd ed. New York, Macmillan, 1982.

Articles
General

Beck ML. Guiding your patient a step at a time through a colonoscopy. Nursing '81 1981 June; 11(6):28–30.

Farmer RG. Long-term prognosis of inflammatory bowel disease. Postgrad Med 1981 Oct; 70(4):124–135.

Gordon AM Jr. Enteral nutritional support. Postgrad Med 1981 Nov; 70(5):155–162.

Intestinal bypass patients show long-term complications. AORN J 1982 Jan; 35(1):96–99.

Kornguth ML. Weight problems: Nursing management. Am J Nurs 1981 Mar; 81(3):553–554.

Langford RW. Teenagers and obesity. Am J Nurs 1981 Mar; 81(3):556–559.

Leape LL and Ramenorsky ML. Laparoscopy for questionable appendicitis. Ann Surg 1980 Apr; 191(4):410–413.

Lewis JH, Clement S, and Dobbins WD. Acute colitis. Postgrad Med 1981 Oct; 70(4):145–164.

Mendeloff AI and Halberstam MJ. How to tell ulcerative colitis from Crohn's disease—and how to treat both. Modern Medicine 1980 Dec 15; 48:85–95.

Myers S et al. Quality of life after surgery for Crohn's disease: A psychosocial survey. Gastroenterology 1980 Jan; 78(1):1–6.

Miller BK. Jejunoileal bypass: A drastic weight control measure. Am J Nurs 1981 Mar; 81(3):563–568; 569–572.

Overeaters anonymous and a self-help group. Am J Nurs 1981 Mar; 81(3):560–563.

Pickwickian syndrome. Am J Nurs 1981 Mar; 81(3):555.

Ryan AJ. Validation of appendectomy, can it be done? Postgrad Med 1979 Jan; 65(1):19–21.

Shaw LM. Treating GI reflux with a prosthesis. AORN J 1982 June; 35(7):1303–1308.

Smith DE, Kirchmer NA, and Stewart DR. Use of the barium enema in the diagnosis of acute appendicitis and its complications. Am J Surg 1979 Dec; 138(6):829–834.

Smith GW. Lower GI bleeding in the elderly. Postgrad Med 1980 Mar; 69(3):36–49.

Strauch B et al. Caring enough to give your patient control (Crohn's disease). Nursing '80 1980 Aug; 10(8):54–59.

White JH. Weight problems. Am J Nurs 1981 Mar; 81(3):550–553.

Ileostomy

Akwari OE, Kelly KA, and Phillips SF. Myoelectric and motor patterns of continent pouch and conventional ileostomy. Surg Gynecol Obstet 1980 Mar; 150(3):363–371.

Bromley B. Applying Orem's self-care theory in enterostomal therapy. Am J Nurs 1980 Feb; 80(2):245–249.

Fowler E, Jeter KF, and Schwartz AA. How to cope when your patient has an enterocutaneous fistula. Am J Nurs 1980 Mar; 80(3):426–429.

Gebhart EM. Perioperative care of the ostomy patient. AORN J 1982 Aug; 36(2):296–310.

Lerner J, Harsh J, and Eisenstat TE. Why pre-op stoma planning is a must. RN 1980 Aug; 43(8):48–51.

MacClelland DC. Kock pouch: A new type of ileostomy. AORN J 1980 Aug; 32(2):191–201.

Sachar DB and Present DH. Immunotherapy in inflammatory bowel disease. Med Clin North Am 1978 Jan; 62(1):173–183.

Stark KJ. Nursing care of the Kock pouch patient. AORN J 1980 Aug; 32(2):202–206.

Trainor MA. Acceptance of ostomy and the visitor role in a self-help group for ostomy patients. Nurs Res 1982 Mar/Apr; 31(2):102–106.

Traverso CJ. SOAP noting common stomal problems. Journal of Enterostomy Therapy 1980 Jan–Feb; 7(1):8–11.

Traverso CJ. SOAP noting common stomal problems. Journal of Enterostomy Therapy 1980 Mar–Apr; 7(2):11–12.

Traverso CJ. SOAP noting common stomal problems. Journal of Enterostomy Therapy 1980 May–June; 7(3):8–9.

What's a continent ileostomy? Nursing '81 1981 Nov; 11(11):84–89.

Colon, Colostomy

Arnell IA and Nassberg BR. Administer a barium enema through a colostomy. Nursing '81 1981 Feb; 11(2):81–83.

Bedell K and Kinimaka L. Sexuality in the male following abdominoperineal resection. Journal of Enterostomy Therapy 1980 Mar/Apr; 7(1):114–118.

Bell GA. Closure of colostomy following sigmoid colon resection for perforated diverticulitis. Surg Gynecol Obstet 1980 Jan; 150(1):85–90.

Bille DA. Legal ramifications of the ostomates bill of rights. Journal of Enterostomy Therapy 1980 Jan–Feb; 7(1):12–16.

Boyd JB et al. Operative risk factors of colon resection in the elderly. Ann Surg 1980 Dec; 192(6):743–746.

Burakoff R. An updated look at diverticular disease. Geriatrics. 1981 Mar; 36(3):83–91.

Click C. Chemotherapy and the ostomy patient. Journal of Enterostomy Therapy 1980 Sept–Oct; 7(5):10–12, 16.

Copeland MM. The national large bowel cancer project. A progress report. Cancer 1980 Mar; 45(5 Suppl):1041–1046.

Devroede G et al. Working through history and physical clues to colitis. Patient Care 1980 Apr 30; 14(8):50–107.

Devroede G et al. Confirming the elusive colitis diagnosis. Patient Care 1980 June 15; 14(10):38–81.

Dickinson RJ et al. Controlled trial of intravenous hyperalimentation and total bowel rest as an adjunct to the routine therapy of acute colitis. Gastroenterology 1980 Dec; 79(6):1199–1203.

Editorial: Oral therapy for acute diarrhoea. Lancet 1981 Sept 19; 8247(2):615–617.

Gebhart EM. Perioperative care of the ostomy patient. AORN J 1982 Aug; 36(2):296–310.

Gilbertsen VA et al. The earlier detection of colorectal cancers. A preliminary report of the results of the occult blood study. Cancer 1980 June; 45(11):2899–2901.

Hogan W et al. Endoscopic evaluation of inflammatory bowel disease. Med Clin North Am 1980 Nov; 64(6):1083–1102.

LeFall LD Jr. Colorectal cancer—prevention and detection. Cancer 1981 Mar; 47(5 Suppl):1170–1172.

Leicester R et al. Flexible fibreoptic sigmoidoscopy as an outpatient procedure. Lancet 1982 Jan 2; ( ):34–35.

Minervini S et al. Comparison of three methods of whole bowel irrigation. Am J Surg 1980 Sept; 140(3):400–402.

Rankin G. Crohn's disease. Its recognition and complications. Primary Care 1981 June; 8(2):309–319.

Rusch V and Simonowitz DA. Crohn's disease in the older patient. Surg Gynecol Obstet 1980 Feb; 150(2):184–186.

Sredl D and Wilhite M. The enterostomal therapist—a new breed of nurse. Superv Nurse 1980 Jan; 11(1):51–52.

Strauch B et al. Caring enough to give your patient control (Crohn's disease). Nursing '80 1980 Aug; 10(8):54–59.

Trainor MA. Acceptance of ostomy and the visitor role in a self-help group for ostomy patients. Nurs Res 1982 Mar/Apr; 31(2):102–106.

Visintainer M and Wolfer J. Sex and the colostomy. RN 1979 Jan; 42(1):61–62.

Weser E. Editorial: Total parenteral nutrition and bowel rest in inflammatory bowel disease. Gastroenterology 1980 Dec; 79(6):1337.

Wilpeski MD. Helping the ostomate return to normal life. Nursing '81 1981 Mar; 11(3):62–66.

Rectal Conditions

Abcarian H. Anorectal disorders: When is conservative care enough? Mod Med 1980 Jan 15; 48(2):37–52.

Amin N. Giardiasis. Postgrad Med 1979 Nov; 66(5):151–156.

Buls JG and Goldberg SM. Modern management of hemorrhoids. Surg Clin North Am 1978 June; 58(3):469.

Eckhauser FE, Lindenauer SM, and Morley GW. Pelvic exenteration for advanced rectal carcinoma. Am J Surg 1979 Sept; 138(3):411–414.

Editorial: Piles and their values. Lancet 1981 July 11; 8237(2):77.

Fisher SG. Psychosexual adjustment following total pelvic exenteration. Cancer Nurs 1979 June; 2(3):219–225.

Green JP et al. Anal carcinoma: Current therapeutic concepts. Am J Surg 1980 July; 140(1):151–155.

Slawson M. Thirty-three drugs that discolor urine and/or stools. RN 1980 Jan; 43(1):40–41.

Agencies

Canadian Foundation for Ileitis and Colitis, 294 Spadina Ave., Toronto, Ontario M5T 2E7, Canada

National Foundation for Ileitis and Colitis, Inc., 295 Madison Ave., New York, New York 10017

National Institute of Arthritis, Metabolism and Digestive Diseases, National Institutes of Health, Bethesda, Maryland 20205

United Ostomy Association, 1111 Wilshire Blvd., Los Angeles, California 90017

Unit X

Metabolic and Endocrine Problems

39

Assessment and Management of Patients With Hepatic and Biliary Disorders

▷ Physiologic Overview

The liver, the largest organ of the body, can be considered a chemical factory whose job is to manufacture, accumulate, alter, and excrete a large number of substances involved in metabolism. The location of the liver is essential in this function, since it receives nutrient-rich blood directly from the gastrointestinal tract, and then either stores or transforms these nutrients into chemicals that are used elsewhere in the body for metabolic needs. The liver's role is especially important in the regulation of glucose and protein metabolism. The liver manufactures and secretes bile, which has a major role in the digestion and absorption of fats in the gastrointestinal tract. The liver functions as an organ of excretion by removing waste products from the bloodstream and secreting them into the bile. The bile produced by the liver is stored temporarily in the gallbladder until it is needed for the process of digestion, at which time the gallbladder empties and bile enters the intestine.

Anatomy

The liver is located behind the ribs in the upper right portion of the abdominal cavity. It weighs about 1500 g and is divided into four lobes. Each lobe is surrounded by a thin layer of connective tissue, which extends into the lobe itself and divides the liver mass into small units, called *lobules*. A schematic diagram of the liver and its anatomical relationships is shown in Figure 39-1.

    The circulation of the blood into and out of the liver is of major importance in its function. The blood that perfuses the liver is derived from two sources. Approximately 75% of the blood supply comes from the portal vein, which drains the gastrointestinal tract and is rich in nutrients. The remainder of the blood supply enters by way of the hepatic artery and is rich in oxygen. Terminal branches of these two blood supplies join to form common capillary beds, which constitute the sinusoids of the liver. Liver cells (hepatocytes) are thus bathed by a mixture of venous and arterial blood. The sinusoids empty into a venule that occupies the

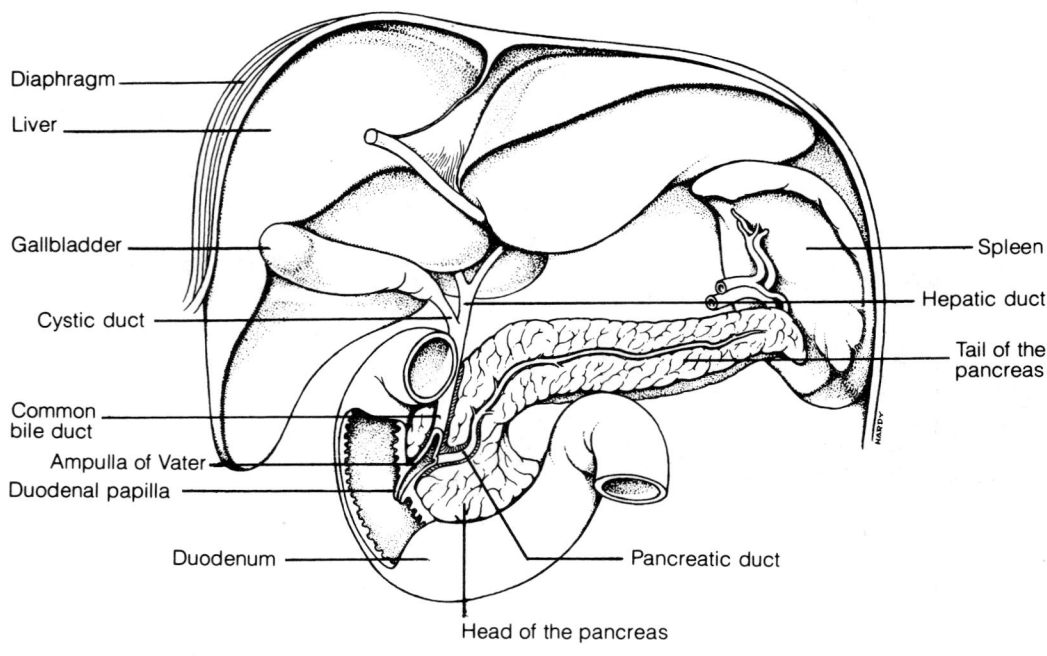

Figure 39-1. Liver and biliary system. (From Chaffee EE and Greisheimer EM: Basic Physiology and Anatomy, 3rd ed. Philadelphia, JB Lippincott.)

center of each liver lobule and is called the *central vein.* The central veins join to form the hepatic vein, which constitutes the venous drainage from the liver and empties into the inferior vena cava, close to the diaphragm. Note that there are two sources of blood flowing into the liver, but there is only one exit pathway.

In addition to hepatocytes, phagocytic cells belonging to the reticuloendothelial system are present in the liver. Other organs that contain reticuloendothelial cells are the spleen, the bone marrow, lymph nodes, and lungs. In the liver, these cells are called *Kupffer cells.* Their main function is to engulf particulate matter in the blood.

The smallest bile ducts, called *canaliculi,* are located between the lobules of the liver. These canaliculi receive secretions from the hepatocytes and carry them to larger bile ducts, which eventually form the *hepatic duct.* The hepatic duct from the liver and the cystic duct from the gallbladder join to form the *common bile duct,* which empties into the small intestine. The flow of bile into the intestine is controlled by the sphincter of Oddi, located at the junction where the common bile duct enters the duodenum.

The gallbladder, a pear-shaped, hollow, saclike organ, about 7.5 cm to 10 cm (3–4 inches) long, lies in a shallow depression on the inferior surface of the liver, to which it is attached by loose connective tissue. The capacity of the gallbladder is 30 ml to 50 ml of bile. Its wall is composed largely of smooth muscle. The gallbladder is connected to the common bile duct by the cystic duct.

Metabolic Functions of the Liver

The liver plays a major role in the regulation of blood glucose concentration. After a meal, glucose is taken up from the portal venous blood by the liver and converted into glycogen, which is stored within the hepatocytes. Subsequently, the glycogen is converted back to glucose and released as needed into the bloodstream, in order to maintain normal levels of blood sugar. Additional glucose can be synthesized by the liver through a process called *gluconeogenesis.* For this process, the liver can utilize amino acids from protein breakdown, or lactate produced by exercising muscles.

Utilization of amino acids for gluconeogenesis results in the formation of ammonia as a by-product. The liver converts this metabolically generated ammonia into urea. Ammonia produced by bacteria in the intestines is also removed from portal blood for urea synthesis. In this way, the liver converts ammonia, a potential toxin, into urea, a harmless compound that can be excreted in the urine.

The liver also plays an important role in protein metabolism. The liver synthesizes almost all of the plasma proteins (except gamma globulin), including albumin, alpha and beta globulins, blood-clotting factors, specific transport proteins, and most of the plasma lipoproteins. Vitamin K is required by the liver for synthesis of prothrombin and some of the other clotting factors. Amino acids serve as the building blocks for protein synthesis.

The liver is also active in fat metabolism. Fatty acids can be broken down for the production of energy and production of ketone bodies (acetoacetic acid, beta-hydroxybutyric acid, and acetone). Ketone bodies are small compounds that can enter the bloodstream and provide a source of energy for muscles and other tissues. Breakdown of fatty acids into ketone bodies occurs predominantly when the availability of glucose for metabolism is limited, as during starvation or in diabetic patients. Fatty acids and their metabolic products are also used for the synthesis of cholesterol, lecithin, lipoproteins, and other complex lipids. Under some conditions, lipids may accumulate in the hepatocytes and result in the abnormal condition called fatty liver.

Vitamins A, B$_{12}$, D, and several of the B complex are stored in large amounts in the liver. Certain metals, such as iron and copper, are also stored within the liver. Because the liver is rich in these substances, liver extracts have been used for therapy of a wide range of nutritional disorders.

Drug Metabolism. Many drugs, such as barbiturates and amphetamines, are metabolized by the liver. Metabolism generally results in loss of activity of the drug, although in some cases activation may occur. One of the important pathways for drug metabolism involves alteration of the drug by the cytochrome P-450 system. Another pathway of importance involves conjugation (binding) of the drug with a variety of compounds, such as glucuronic or acetic acid, to form more soluble substances. The conjugated products may be excreted in the feces or urine, similar to bilirubin excretion.

Bile

Bile is continuously formed by the hepatocytes and collected in the canaliculi and bile ducts. It is composed mainly of water and electrolytes, such as sodium, potassium, calcium, chloride, and bicarbonate, and also contains significant amounts of lecithin, fatty acids, cholesterol, bilirubin, and bile salts. Bile is collected and stored in the gallbladder and is emptied into the intestine when needed for digestion. The functions of bile are excretory, as in the excretion of bilirubin, and as an aid to digestion through the emulsification of fats by bile salts.

Bile Salts. Bile salts are made by the hepatocytes from cholesterol. After conjugation with amino acids (taurine and glycine), they are excreted into the bile. The bile salts, together with cholesterol and lecithin, are required for emulsification of fats in the intestine. This process is necessary for efficient digestion and absorption. Bile salts are then reabsorbed, primarily in the distal ileum, into portal blood for return to the liver and are again excreted into the bile. This pathway from hepatocytes to bile to intestine and back to the hepatocytes is called the *enterohepatic circulation*. Because of the enterohepatic circulation, only a small fraction of the bile salts that enter the intestine is excreted in the feces. This decreases the demand for active synthesis of bile salts by the liver cells.

Bilirubin Excretion

Bilirubin is a pigment derived from the breakdown of hemoglobin by cells of the reticuloendothelial system, including the Kupffer cells of the liver. Hepatocytes remove bilirubin from the blood and chemically modify it through conjugation to glucuronic acid, which makes the bilirubin more soluble in aqueous solutions. The conjugated bilirubin is secreted by the hepatocytes into the adjacent bile canaliculi and is eventually carried in the bile into the duodenum. In the small intestine, bilirubin is converted into urobilinogen, which is in part excreted in the feces and in part absorbed through the intestinal mucosa into the portal blood. Much of this reabsorbed urobilinogen is removed by the hepatocytes and is secreted into the bile once again (enterohepatic circulation). Some of the urobilinogen enters the systemic circulation and is secreted by the kidneys in the urine. Elimination of bilirubin in the bile represents the major route of excretion for this compound. The bilirubin concentration in the blood may be increased either in the presence of liver disease or when the flow of bile is impeded (*e.g.,* with gallstones in the bile ducts). With bile duct obstruction, bilirubin does not enter the intestine and, as a consequence, urobilinogen will be absent from the urine.

Gallbladder

The gallbladder functions as a storage depot for bile. Between meals, when the sphincter of Oddi is closed, bile produced by the hepatocytes enters the gallbladder. During storage, a large portion of the water in bile is absorbed through the walls of the gallbladder, so that gallbladder bile is five to ten times more concentrated than that originally secreted by the liver. When food enters the duodenum, the gallbladder contracts, and the sphincter of Oddi relaxes, allowing the bile to enter the intestine. This response is mediated by secretion of the hormone cholecystokinin-pancreozymin (CCK-PZ) from the intestinal wall.

Pathophysiology

Liver dysfunction results from damage to the liver parenchymal cells, either directly, from primary liver diseases, or indirectly, due to obstruction to bile flow or to derangements of hepatic circulation.

Disease processes that lead to hepatocellular dysfunction may be caused by infectious agents, such as bacteria and viruses, and by anoxia, metabolic disorders, toxins and drugs, nutritional deficiencies, and states of hypersensitivity. Probably the most common cause of parenchymal damage is malnutrition, especially in alcoholism. The response of the parenchymal cells is much the same for most noxious agents: replacement of glycogen by lipids, producing fatty infiltration, with or without cell death or necrosis. This is commonly associated with inflammatory cell infiltration and growth of fibrous tissue. Cell regeneration can occur if the disease process is not too toxic to the cells. The end result of chronic parenchymal disease is the shrunken, fibrotic liver seen in cirrhosis.

Hepatocellular dysfunction is manifested by alteration of the metabolic and excretory functions of the liver. Serum bilirubin concentration rises, leading to jaundice or yellowing of the skin; this results from intrahepatic obstruction of bile channels. Abnormalities of carbohydrate, fat, and protein metabolism occur with liver dysfunction. Abnormal protein metabolism results in decreased serum albumin concentration and edema. Ammonia, a by-product of metabolism, is absorbed from the gastrointestinal tract but is not converted to urea by the damaged liver cells. An increased serum ammonia level may produce signs of central nervous system impairment.

The vascular architecture of the liver may be disturbed,

causing increased portal-vein blood pressure, which results in leakage of fluid into the peritoneal cavity, or ascites, and esophageal varices. The lack of normal production of various blood-clotting factors can lead to bleeding from any site, but the patient is particularly prone to gastrointestinal bleeding.

Gynecomastia and other disturbances of sexual function and sex characteristics may occur due to failure of the liver to normally inactivate estrogens.

Acute liver damage may cause acute liver failure, may be completely reversible, or may progress to chronic disease. The end result of chronic liver damage is cirrhosis, characterized by replacement of parenchymal cells with fibrotic tissue. Liver failure is present when the ability of the liver to carry out its excretory and metabolic functions falls below the needs of the body. Hepatic coma results when liver dysfunction is so severe that the liver is unable to remove end products of metabolism from the bloodstream.

Table 39-1
Liver Function Studies

Test	Normal	Clinical Functions
I. *Pigment studies*		
A. Serum bilirubin, direct	0–0.3 mg/dl	These are measures of ability of liver to conjugate and excrete bilirubin. They are abnormal in liver and biliary tract disease, causing jaundice, clinically.
B. Serum bilirubin, total	0–0.9 mg/dl	
C. Urine bilirubin	0	
D. Urine urobilinogen	0–1.16 mg/24 hr	
E. Fecal urobilinogen (infrequently used)	40–280 mg/24 hr	
II. *Dye clearances*		
A. Bromsulphalein excretion (BSP test)	<5% retention 45 minutes after dye injection of 5 mg/kg body weight	BSP binds to albumin in blood. Liver cells unbind BSP, conjugate it, and excrete it in bile. Normal clearance depends on hepatic blood flow, functioning liver cell mass, and lack of obstruction. Retention is increased in liver cell damage or decreased liver blood flow.
B. Indocyanine green	500–800 ml/sq m body surface/min	Extracted from blood and excreted by liver. Depends on hepatic blood flow, functioning liver cells, and lack of obstruction.
III. *Protein studies*		
A. Total serum protein	7.0–7.5 g%	Proteins are manufactured by the liver. Their levels may be affected in a variety of liver impairments.
B. Serum albumin	3.5–5.5 g%	
C. Serum globulin	1.5–3.0 g%	
D. Serum protein electrophoresis	Albumin 63–69% of total Alpha 1 glob. 3.9–7.3% Alpha 2 glob. 3.9–7.3% Alpha 2 glob. 6.9–11.8% Beta glob. 6.9–11.8% Gamma glob. 9.8–20%	Albumin — Cirrhosis, Chronic hepatitis, Edema, ascites Globulin — Cirrhosis, Liver disease, Chronic obstructive jaundice, Viral hepatitis
IV. *Prothrombin time* Response of prothrombin time to vitamin K	100% return to normal	Prothrombin time may be prolonged in liver disease. It will not return to normal with vitamin K in severe liver cell damage.
V. *Serum alkaline phosphatase*	Varies with method. 2–5 Bodansky units	Manufactured in bones, liver, kidneys, intestine. Excreted through biliary tract. In absence of bone disease, it is a sensitive measure of biliary tract obstruction.

(continued)

▷ Diagnostic Assessment of Hepatic Function

Liver Function Tests. Over 70% of the parenchyma of the liver may be damaged before liver function tests become abnormal. Function is generally measured in terms of serum enzyme activity (*e.g.,* alkaline phosphatase, transaminases, lactic dehydrogenase), clearance of sulfobromophthalein (Bromsulphalein or BSP), and serum concentrations of proteins, bilirubin, ammonia, clotting factors, and lipids. Several of these tests may be helpful for assessment of patients with liver disease; however, the nature and extent of hepatic dysfunction cannot be determined by these tests alone. Many other disorders can influence their results; therefore, the tests are not sensitive indicators of liver dysfunction. A list of the commonly used liver function tests is shown in Table 39-1.

Table 39-1
Liver Function Studies (continued)

Test	Normal	Clinical Functions
VI. *Serum transaminase studies* A. SGOT B. SGPT C. LDH	10–40 units 5–35 units 165–400 units	Based on release of enzymes from damaged liver cells. These enzymes are elevated in liver cell damage.
VII. *Blood ammonia* (arterial)	20–50 mg/dl	Liver converts ammonia to urea. Ammonia level rises in liver failure.
VIII. *Cholesterol* Ester	150–250 mg/dl 60% of total	Elevated in biliary obstruction. Decreased in parenchymal liver disease.
IX. *Radiologic studies* A. Barium study of esophagus B. Plain film of abdomen C. Liver scan with radio-tagged iodinated rose bengal, gold, or technetium D. Cholecystogram and cholangiogram E. Celiac axis arteriography F. Splenoportogram (splenic portal venography)		For varices. Varices in esophagus indicate increased portal pressure. To determine gross liver size. To show size, shape of liver. To show replacement of liver tissue with scars, cysts, or tumor. For gallbladder and bile duct visualization. For liver and pancreas visualization. To determine adequacy of portal blood flow.
X. *Peritoneoscopy or laparoscopy*		Direct visualization of anterior surface of liver, gallbladder, and mesentery through a trocar.
XI. *Liver biopsy* (see p. 854 and Fig. 39-2)		To determine anatomic changes in liver tissue.
XII. *Measurement of portal pressure*		Elevated in cirrhosis of the liver.
XIII. *Esophagoscopy/endoscopy*		To search for esophageal varices and abnormalities.
XIV. *Electroencephalogram*		Abnormal in hepatic coma and impending hepatic coma.
XV. *Ultrasonography*		To show size of abdominal organs and presence of masses.
XVI. *Computed tomography (CT scan)*		To detect hepatic neoplasms; diagnose cysts, abscesses, and hematomas; and distinguish between obstructive and nonobstructive jaundice.
XVII. *Angiography*		Visualizes hepatic circulation and detects presence and nature of hepatic masses.

Liver Biopsy. A procedure that greatly facilitates the diagnosis of most hepatic disorders is the liver biopsy (*i.e.*, the sampling of liver tissue by needle aspiration for the purpose of histologic study). Nursing responsibilities in relation to liver biopsy and the rationale of the nurse's participation in this procedure are summarized in Chart 39-1. A graphic presentation is found in Figure 39-2.

▷ Clinical Manifestations of Hepatic Dysfunction

The complications of liver disease are numerous and varied. In many instances their ultimate effects are incapacitating or lethal; their advent is ominous, and their treatment is notoriously difficult.

Among the most frequent and important of these complications are:

1. Jaundice, resulting from increased bilirubin concentration in the blood
2. Portal hypertension and ascites, resulting from circulatory changes within the diseased liver and producing severe gastrointestinal hemorrhages and excessive Na⁺ and water retention
3. Nutritional deficiencies, attributable to the inability of the malfunctioning liver cells to metabolize certain vitamins, and responsible for impaired central and pe-

---

Chart 39-1
Liver Biopsy and the Role of the Nurse

Nursing Activities	*Rationale*
1. Ascertain in advance that hemostasis tests have been requisitioned, completed, and reported and that compatible donor blood is available.	1. Many patients with liver disease have clotting defects and are prone to bleed abnormally.
2. Measure and record the patient's pulse, respirations, and arterial pressure immediately prior to biopsy.	2. Prebiopsy values provide a basis on which to compare the patient's vital signs and evaluate his status following the procedure.
3. Describe to the patient in advance:	3. Explanations serve to allay his fears, to ensure his cooperation, and to reinforce his instruction.
a. Steps of the procedure	
b. Sensations expected	
c. After effects anticipated	
d. Restrictions of activity to be imposed afterward	
4. Give support to the patient during the procedure.	4. The presence of an understanding nurse enhances comfort and promotes a sense of security.
5. Expose the right side of the patient's upper abdomen (right hypochondriac).	5. The skin at the site of penetration will be cleansed and infiltrated with local anesthetic.
6. Instruct the patient to inhale and exhale deeply several times, finally to exhale, and to hold his breath at the end of expiration (see Fig. 39-2).	6. Holding the breath immobilizes the chest wall and the diaphragm; penetration of the diaphragm thereby is avoided, and the risk of lacerating the liver is minimized.
The physician promptly introduces the biopsy needle by way of the transthoracic (intercostal) or transabdominal (subcostal) route, penetrates the liver, aspirates and withdraws. The entire procedure is completed within 5 to 10 seconds.	
7. Instruct the patient to resume breathing.	
8. Immediately following the biopsy, assist the patient to turn on his right side; place a pillow under his costal margin, and caution him to remain in this position, recumbent and immobile, for several hours.	8. In this position, the liver capsule at the site of penetration is compressed against the chest wall, and the escape of blood or bile through the perforation is impeded.
9. Measure and record the patient's pulse and respiratory rates and his arterial pressure at 10- to 20-minute intervals for the prescribed period of time, or until his status proves to be stable, and his condition is satisfactory. Be alert to and report promptly any increase in pulse rate or any decrease in arterial pressure, any complaint of pain or manifestations of apprehension.	9. These signs may indicate the presence and the progress of hepatic bleeding, severe hemorrhage, or bile peritonitis, the most frequent complications of liver biopsy.

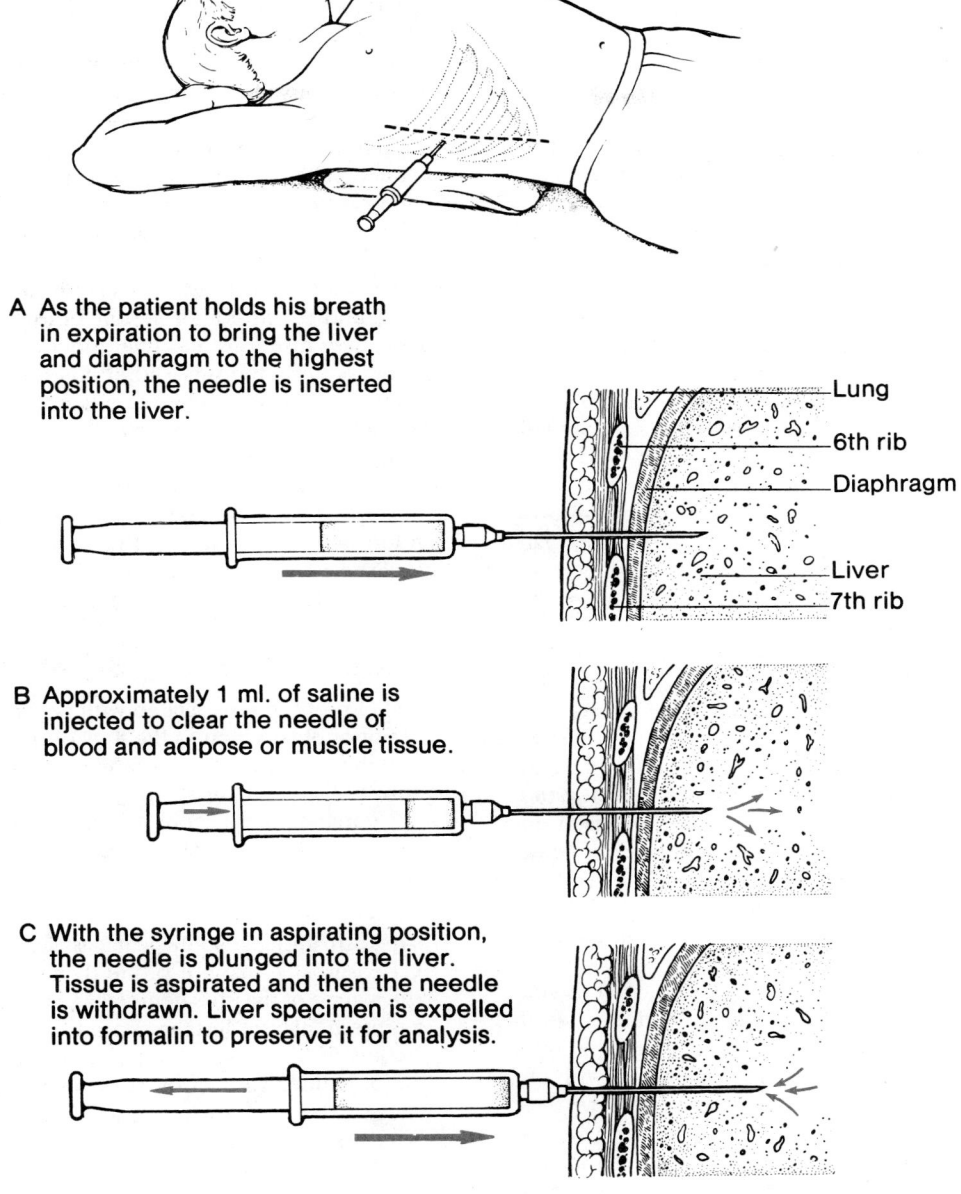

A As the patient holds his breath in expiration to bring the liver and diaphragm to the highest position, the needle is inserted into the liver.

Lung
6th rib
Diaphragm
Liver
7th rib

B Approximately 1 ml. of saline is injected to clear the needle of blood and adipose or muscle tissue.

C With the syringe in aspirating position, the needle is plunged into the liver. Tissue is aspirated and then the needle is withdrawn. Liver specimen is expelled into formalin to preserve it for analysis.

Figure 39-2. Liver biopsy.

ripheral nervous systems and abnormal bleeding tendencies
4. Hepatic coma, reflecting the incomplete metabolism of protein by the diseased liver

Jaundice

When, for any reason, the bilirubin concentration in the blood becomes abnormally increased, all the body tissue, including the sclerae and the skin, become tinged with a yellow or a greenish yellow color. This condition is called *jaundice*. There are several types of jaundice: (1) hemo-

lytic, (2) hepatocellular, (3) obstructive, and (4) jaundice due to hereditary hyperbilirubinemia. Hepatocellular and obstructive jaundice are the two types commonly associated with liver disease.

Hemolytic Jaundice. Hemolytic jaundice is the result of an increased destruction of the red blood cells, the effect of which is to flood the plasma with bilirubin so rapidly that the liver, although functioning normally, cannot excrete the bilirubin as rapidly as it is formed. This is the type of jaundice that is encountered in patients with hemolytic transfusion reactions and other hemolytic disorders. The bilirubin in the blood of these patients is predominantly of the unconjugated, or "free," type. Fecal and urine urobilinogen are increased; on the other hand, the urine is free of bilirubin. Patients with this type of jaundice, unless their hyperbilirubinemia is extreme, do not experience symptoms or complications as a result of the jaundice *per se.* However, very prolonged jaundice, even if mild, predisposes to the formation of "pigment stones" in the gallbladder, and extremely severe jaundice—for example, in patients with levels of free bilirubin above 20 mg to 25 mg per 100 ml—is attended by a definite risk of possible brain stem damage.

Hepatocellular Jaundice. This is jaundice caused by inability of diseased liver cells to clear normal amounts of bilirubin from the blood. The cellular damage may be from infection, such as in hepatitis A, hepatitis B, hepatitis nonA nonB (from virus-infected blood transfusion), or yellow fever virus, or from drug or chemical toxicity (such as carbon tetrachloride, chloroform, phosphorus, arsenicals, certain psychotherapeutic drugs, or ethanol).

Cirrhosis of the liver is a form of hepatocellular disease that may produce jaundice; it is usually, but not always, associated with excessive alcoholic intake. It may be a late result of viral-caused liver cell necrosis. In prolonged obstructive jaundice, cell damage eventually develops, so that both types appear together.

Clinical Manifestations. Patients with hepatocellular jaundice may be mildly or severely ill, with lack of appetite, nausea, loss of vigor and strength, and possible weight loss. In some instances of hepatocellular disease there may be no jaundice clinically. However, the serum bilirubin concentration and urine urobilinogen level may be elevated. In addition, the SGOT* and SGPT† may be increased, indicating cellular necrosis. At onset there may be complaints of headache, chills, and fever, if the cause is infectious. Depending on the cause and extent of the liver cell damage, hepatocellular jaundice may or may not be completely reversible.

Obstructive Jaundice. Obstructive jaundice of the extrahepatic type may be caused by the bile duct's being plugged by a gallstone, by an inflammatory process, by a tumor, or by pressure from an enlarged gland. Or the obstruction may involve the small bile ducts within the liver substance (*i.e.,* intrahepatic obstruction), caused, for example, by pressure on these channels from inflammatory swelling of the liver substance or by an inflammatory exudate within the ducts themselves. Intrahepatic obstruction due to stasis and inspissation of bile within the canaliculi is an occasional occurrence, following the ingestion of certain drugs, which accordingly are referred to as "cholestatic" agents. These include phenothiazines, antithyroid medications, sulfonylureas, tricyclic antidepressants, and nitrofurantoin.

Clinical Manifestations. Whether the obstruction is intrahepatic or extrahepatic, and whatever its cause may be, if bile cannot flow normally into the intestine, but is dammed back in the liver substance, it is reabsorbed into the blood and carried throughout the entire body, staining the skin, the mucous membrane, and the sclerae. It is ex-

creted in the urine, which becomes a deep orange color and foamy in appearance. Because of the decreased amount of bile in the intestinal tract, the stools become light or clay-colored. The skin may itch intensely, requiring repeated starch or oil baths. Dyspepsia, and especially an intolerance to fatty foods, may develop temporarily, due to impairment of fat digestion in the absence of intestinal bile. Here the SGOT and SGPT rise only moderately, but the bilirubin and alkaline phosphatase are elevated.

Hereditary Hyperbilirubinemia. *Gilbert's syndrome* is a familial disorder that is due to a diminution of glucuronyl transferase and an increased unconjugated bilirubin that causes jaundice. Although serum bilirubin levels are increased, liver histology and liver function tests are normal, and there is no hemolysis. Other conditions that are probably caused by inborn errors of biliary metabolism include *Dubin–Johnson syndrome* (chronic idiopathic jaundice, with pigment in the liver) and *Rotor's syndrome* (chronic familial conjugated hyperbilirubinemia without pigment in the liver); "benign" cholestatic jaundice of pregnancy, with retention of conjugated bilirubin, probably secondary to unusual sensitivity to the hormones of pregnancy; and probably also benign recurrent intrahepatic cholestasis.

Portal Hypertension and Ascites

One set of problems associated with hepatic cirrhosis arises as a result of obstruction to the flow of portal venous blood through the liver, the effect of which is to elevate the blood pressure throughout the entire portal venous system. Although portal hypertension is commonly associated with hepatic cirrhosis, it can also occur with noncirrhotic liver disease.

There are two major sequelae of portal hypertension:

1. The formation of esophageal, gastric, and hemorrhoidal varicosities, which are prone to rupture and often are the source of massive hemorrhages from the upper gastrointestinal tract and the rectum (see p. 869). The likelihood of bleeding is increased by the blood-clotting abnormalities frequently present in patients with cirrhosis. The varicosities form because of the elevated pressures transmitted to all of the veins that drain into the portal system.

2. The second important manifestation of portal hypertension is accumulation of fluid (ascites) in the abdominal cavity. As ascites develops, intravascular volume tends to fall, and renin is released by the kidneys. This results in secretion of increased quantities of the hormone aldosterone by the adrenal glands, which, in turn, causes the kidneys to retain sodium and water in an attempt to return intravascular volume to normal. Unfortunately, if portal hypertension continues, fluid retention will contribute to the formation of even more ascites.

Assessment

Ascites can be determined by percussing the abdomen. When fluid has accumulated in the peritoneal cavity, the flanks will bulge when the patient assumes a supine position. The presence of fluid accumulation can be confirmed

---

* SGOT—Transaminase (Aspartate aminotransferase)
† SGPT—Transaminase (Alanine aminotransferase)

either by percussing for shifting dullness (Fig. 39-3, *A, B*) or by detecting a fluid wave (Fig. 39-3, *C*). A fluid wave is likely to be found only when there is a large amount of fluid present. Daily measurement and recording of abdominal girth are indicated to assess the progression of ascites and its response to treatment. The role of dietary modification, drug therapy, paracentesis, and shunting in controlling ascites is discussed below.

Controlling Fluid Retention and Ascites

Nutritional Control.   The goal of treatment for the patient with ascites is a negative sodium balance to reduce fluid retention. Table salt, salty foods, salted butter and margarine, and all the ordinary canned and frozen foods should be avoided. The taste of unsalted foods can be improved by using salt substitutes, such as lemon juice, oregano, and thyme. Commercial substitutes need to be cleared with the physician; for example, those containing ammonia could precipitate hepatic coma. Liberal use should be made of powdered, low-sodium milk and milk products. If water accumulation is not controlled on this regimen, the salt restriction must be more stringent with the daily sodium allowance reduced to 200 mg, and diuretics administered.

Diuretics.   Another method of reducing edema and ascites is to induce diuresis. This involves the reduction of sodium intake to approximately 9 mEq to 22 mEq (200 mg–500 mg) daily; restriction of fluids, if the serum sodium is low; and administration of an oral diuretic drug such as chlorothiazide (Diuril). Spironolactone (Aldactone), an aldosterone-blocking agent, also may be supplied to reinforce the action of these diuretics and to help prevent undue potassium loss. If these medications fail, it may be necessary to use a more potent diuretic, such as furosemide (Lasix). Beyond this, ethacrynic acid (Edecrin) may be prescribed. These latter diuretic medications are used cautiously, since with long-term use they may induce severe sodium depletion (hyponatremia). Ammonium chloride and acetazolamide (Diamox) are contraindicated because of the possibility of precipitating hepatic coma. Daily weight loss should not exceed 0.227 kg (or less than ½ lb) daily.

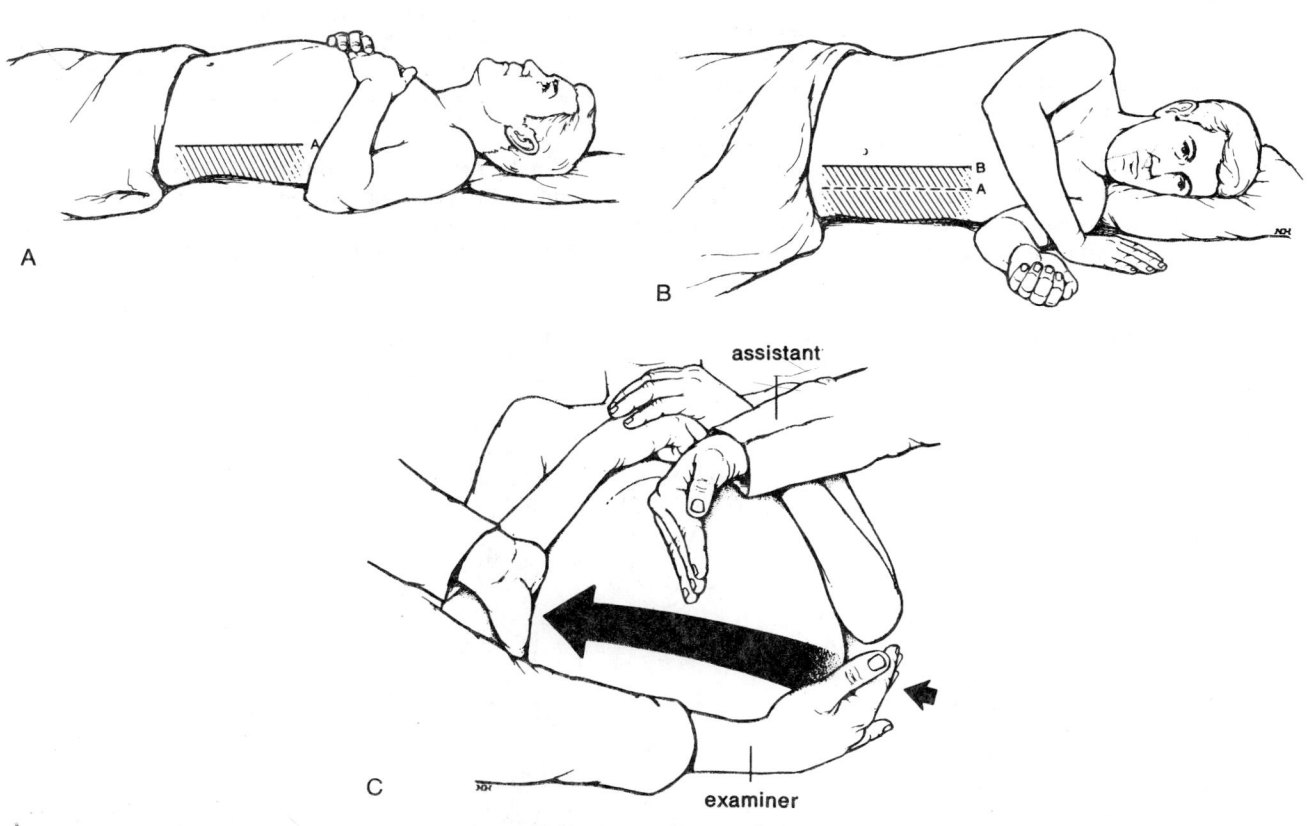

Figure 39-3. Assessing for ascites. (*A*) To percuss for shifting dullness, each flank is percussed, with the patient in a supine position. If fluid is present, dullness will be noted at each flank. The most medial limits of the dullness should be marked as indicated in *A*. The patient should then be shifted to his side. (*B*) Shows what happens to the area of dullness if fluid is present. (*C*) To detect the presence of a fluid wave, the examiner places one hand alongside each flank. A second person then places a hand, ulnar side down, along the patient's midline, and applies light pressure. The examiner then strikes one flank sharply with one hand, while the other hand remains in place to detect any signs of a fluid impulse. The assistant's hand dampens any wave impulses traveling through the abdominal wall. (Copyright © 1974, American Journal of Nursing Company. Reproduced with permission from American Journal of Nursing, 74, No. 9, Sept. 1974.)

Diuretic therapy should be carefully monitored by the nurse to detect possible complications: encephalopathy and electrolyte disturbances. When potassium stores are depleted, the amount of renal ammonia in the systemic circulation increases, which may cause impaired cerebral functioning. Possible electrolyte problems include hypokalemia, hyponatremia, and hypochloremic alkalosis. Careful intake and output documentation, daily assessment of abdominal girth, and daily weighing of the patient are required.

Skin integrity will be affected if meticulous care is not carried out. Pressure over bony prominences and edematous tissue must be relieved by frequently changing body position, or possibly by using an alternating pressure mattress. Lower extremities may have to be elevated and support hose applied. Salt-poor albumin may be given intravenously to temporarily elevate the serum albumin, which increases serum osmotic pressure. This helps reduce edema by causing the ascitic fluid to be drawn back into the bloodstream, from whence it can be eliminated by the kidneys.

Paracentesis

Once considered an acceptable form of treatment for ascites, paracentesis is now utilized primarily for diagnostic examination of ascitic fluid, treatment of massive ascites resistant to other therapy and causing severe problems to the patient, and as a prelude to other procedures, including x-ray, peritoneal dialysis, ascites reinfusion, or surgery.

If paracentesis is warranted (Fig. 39-4), the aspiration is limited to the slow removal of 2 liters to 3 liters, to relieve acute symptoms. Removing large amounts of fluid may cause hypotension, oliguria, and hyponatremia. If fluid in excess of this amount is removed, ascitic fluid tends to form again, drawing fluid from extracellular tissue throughout the body.

Nursing Implementation.   The nurse prepares the patient for paracentesis by providing the necessary information, instructions, and reassurance.

- *Have the patient void as completely as possible just prior to paracentesis, to lessen the danger of inadvertently piercing the bladder.*

Sterile equipment and appropriate collection receptacles are made ready. Preparatory to the procedure, the patient is placed in the upright position on the edge of the bed, fully supported, with his feet resting on a stool and one arm fitted with a sphygmomanometer cuff. The trocar is introduced with aseptic technique through a stab wound in the midline below the umbilicus, and the fluid is drained through an effluent tube into a container.

During the procedure the nurse helps the patient to maintain the proper posture.

- Observe the patient closely for evidence of vascular collapse, such as the appearance of pallor, increase in pulse rate, or decline in blood pressure, the latter having been recorded at frequent intervals from the beginning of the procedure.

When the procedure is concluded, the patient is placed in a comfortable position. The amount of fluid collected is measured, described, and recorded, and samples of the fluid, properly labeled, are sent to appropriate laboratories

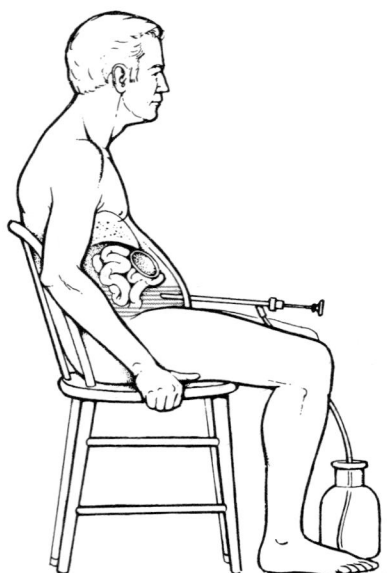

Sitting position is preferred since the intestines will float away from the site of paracentesis

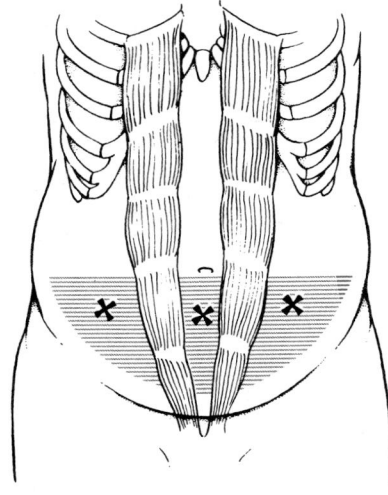

The indicated sites for performing the procedure avoid injury to the deep inferior epigastric vessels

Figure 39-4. The patient undergoing paracentesis.

for examination of the cellular sediment, its specific gravity, protein concentration, and bacterial content.

Shunts

Although surgical bypass procedures, or shunts, may decrease portal hypertension and ascites formation, the high operative mortality in patients with severe liver dysfunction limits surgical shunting as an effective treatment for ascites.

Attempts have been made to treat ascites through reinfusion of ascitic fluid into the general circulation; however, there is risk of infection from such treatment. In addition, this treatment is temporary, and reaccumulation of ascites recurs within 2 months in more than 70% of patients.

The insertion of a LeVeen or peritoneojugular shunt has been successful in reducing ascites. In this method, a perforated silicone tube is directed through a small transverse abdominal incision into the peritoneal cavity (Fig. 39-5). The proximal end of the tube is attached to a valve; from the valve another tube emerges and is threaded subcutaneously to the superior vena cava. When pressure in the abdominal cavity rises to 3 cm H_2O or above, the valve opens, and excess fluid is transported to the superior vena cava. When pressure falls, the valve closes.

In the postoperative period, the patient is monitored closely and the hematocrit is measured every 4 hours. Vascular volume expansion and hemodilution may result from the inflow of ascitic fluid. Excessive hemodilution may be interrupted by placing the patient in a sitting position. A diuretic such as furosemide may be prescribed to avoid the possibility of pulmonary edema. Blood studies include careful monitoring of the coagulation profile, because reabsorption of substances in the ascitic fluid may inhibit clotting and lead to bleeding. Body weight, abdominal girth, and urinary output are recorded every 2 hours. Ordinarily, the hematocrit falls, abdominal girth decreases, weight drops, and urinary output rises.

Following the relief of ascites, dietary considerations will depend on the cardiac status and presence of peripheral edema. These patients require continued care and monitoring, for even though the ascites may be cleared, the liver problem is not improved by the insertion of a peritoneojugular shunt.

Nutritional Deficiencies

Another group of complications that is common to patients with severe chronic liver disease of all types is caused by inadequate intake of proper vitamins. Among the specific deficiency states that occur on this basis are (1) vitamin A deficiency, beriberi, polyneuritis, and Wernicke–Korsakoff psychosis, all attributable to a deficiency of thiamine; (2) skin and mucous membrane lesions characteristic of riboflavin deficiency; (3) "rum fits," which probably are due to pyridoxine deficiency; (4) hypoprothrombinemia (see p. 718), characterized by spontaneous bleeding and ecchymoses, due to vitamin K deficiency; (5) the hemorrhagic lesions of scurvy (*i.e.,* vitamin C deficiency); and (6) the macrocytic anemia of folic acid deficiency.

- The threat of these avitaminoses provides the rationale for supplementing the diet of every patient with chronic

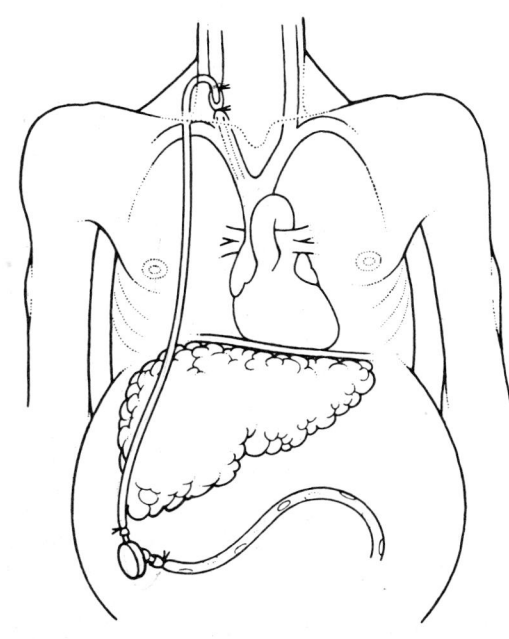

Figure 39-5. This is a diagrammatic illustration of a peritoneojugular shunt for reducing ascites. The valve lies in the lower right side extraperitoneally, and a perforated collecting tube extends into the peritoneal cavity. The venous tube traverses the subcutaneous tissue from the valve to the neck, where it enters the internal jugular vein and extends to the superior vena cava. Note the cachexia (malnutrition) typified by thin arms and evident rib cage. The distended abdomen and enlarged liver are pushing the diaphragm upward, which may exert pressure against the heart and lungs. (From Schiff L and Schiff ER (eds): Diseases of the Liver. JB Lippincott, 1982.)

liver disease (especially when alcoholism is involved) with ample quantities of vitamins A, B complex, C, K, and folic acid.

Hepatic Coma

Hepatic coma, one of the dreaded complications of liver disease, occurs with profound liver failure and results from the accumulation of ammonia and other identified toxic metabolites in the blood. Ammonia accumulates because damaged liver cells fail to detoxify and convert to urea the ammonia that is constantly entering the bloodstream as a result of its absorption from the gastrointestinal tract and its liberation from kidney and muscle cells. The increased ammonia concentration in the blood causes brain dysfunction and damage, resulting in hepatic encephalopathy and hepatic coma.

Assessment and Clinical Manifestations. The earliest symptoms of hepatic coma include minor mental aberrations and motor disturbances. The patient appears to be slightly confused and experiences alterations in mood. He becomes untidy and experiences altered sleep patterns. He tends to sleep during the day and to wander at night. As hepatic coma progresses, he may be difficult to awaken. He may exhibit asterixis or flapping tremor of the hands. Simple tasks, such as handwriting, become difficult. A sample of handwriting, taken daily, may provide graphic evidence of progression of hepatic coma. In the early stages of hepatic coma, the patient's reflexes are hyperactive; with deepening of coma these reflexes disappear and the extremities may become flaccid.

Electroencephalogram (EEG) shows generalized slowing and an increase in amplitude of brain waves, and the appearance of characteristic tri-phasic waves. Except for the triphasic waves, all of the other manifestations noted are also observable in other conditions. Occasionally, fetor hepaticus, a characteristic breath odor like fresh mowed grass, acetone, or old wine, may be noticed. In a more advanced stage there are gross disturbances of consciousness, and the patient is completely disoriented with respect to time and place. With further progression of the disorder, he lapses into frank coma and may have convulsions. Approximately 35% of all patients with cirrhosis of the liver die in hepatic coma.

Aggravating and Precipitating Factors. Circumstances that increase blood ammonia content tend to aggravate or precipitate hepatic coma. The largest source of blood ammonia is the enzymatic and bacterial digestion of dietary and blood proteins in the gastrointestinal tract. Ammonia from these sources is increased as a result of gastrointestinal bleeding, a high-protein diet, bacterial growth in the small and large intestines, and uremia. The ingestion of ammonium salts will also increase blood ammonia. In the presence of alkalosis or hypokalemia, increased amounts of ammonia are absorbed from the gastrointestinal tract and from the renal tubular fluid. On the other hand, blood ammonia is *decreased* by elimination of protein from the diet and by the administration of antibiotics, such as neomycin sulfate, that reduce the number of intestinal bacteria capable of converting urea to ammonia.

Other factors unrelated to increased blood ammonia that may induce hepatic coma in susceptible patients include overdiuresis, dehydration, infections, surgery, fever, and consciousness-altering drugs, such as sedatives, tranquilizers, and narcotics.

Management

- The patient with impending hepatic coma is observed frequently to assess neurologic status. A daily record is kept of handwriting and performance in arithmetic.
- Fluid intake and output and body weight are recorded each day.
- Vital signs are measured and recorded every 4 hours.
- Evidence suggesting pulmonary or other infection is sought frequently and reported promptly if observed.
- Serum ammonia level is monitored daily.
- If it becomes apparent that hepatic coma is impending, the patient's protein intake is reduced sharply or eliminated altogether, for the time being.
- To reduce ammonia absorption from the gastrointestinal tract, a high cleansing enema may be prescribed.
- In addition, an antibiotic drug such as neomycin is given as an intestinal antiseptic.
- Electrolyte status is carefully monitored, and corrected if abnormal.

- Sedative and analgesic drugs, if prescribed at all, are administered to this patient in very conservative doses and under very close observation.

Lactulose (Cephulac) is given to reduce blood ammonia, which probably acts by a combination of mechanisms that promote the excretion of ammonia in the stool: (1) ammonia is kept in the ionized state, resulting in a fall in colon pH—this reverses the normal passage of ammonia from the colon to the blood; (2) catharsis takes place, which decreases the ammonia absorbed from the colon; and (3) the fecal flora is changed to organisms that do not produce ammonia from urea.

Two or three soft stools per day are hoped for; this means lactulose is performing as intended. However, watery diarrheal stools indicate drug overdose. Possible side-effects include intestinal bloating and cramps, which usually disappear in a week. To overcome the sweet taste to which some patients object, lactulose can be diluted with fruit juice. The patient is closely monitored for hypokalemia and dehydration. Other laxatives are not given during lactulose administration, because their effects would disturb dosage regulation. Lactulose enemas have also been used effectively in acute hepatic encephalopathy for patients who are comatose or in whom oral administration is contraindicated or impossible.

Other Manifestations of Liver Dysfunction

Many patients with liver dysfunction develop generalized edema, due to hypoalbuminemia that results from decreased hepatic production of serum albumin. The production of blood-clotting factors by the liver is also reduced, leading to an increased incidence of bruising, nosebleeds, bleeding from wounds, and, as described above, gastrointestinal bleeding. Decreased production of several clotting factors may be due, in part, to deficient absorption of vitamin K from the gastrointestinal tract. This probably is caused by the inability of liver cells to use vitamin K to make prothrombin. Absorption of the other fat-soluble vitamins (vitamins A, D, and E) as well as dietary fats may also be impaired, due to decreased secretion of bile salts into the intestine.

Abnormalities of glucose metabolism also occur; the blood sugar may be abnormally high shortly after a meal (*i.e.*, a diabetic-type glucose tolerance test), but hypoglycemia may occur during fasting because of decreased hepatic glycogen reserves and decreased gluconeogenesis.

- Because of decreased ability to metabolize drugs, usual drug dosages must be reduced for the patient with liver failure.

Decreased metabolism of estrogens can lead to gynecomastia, testicular atrophy, loss of pubic hair in the male, and menstrual irregularities in the female, as well as spider angiomata and reddened palms ("liver palms"). Splenomegaly (enlarged spleen) with possible hypersplenism occurs commonly as a manifestation of portal hypertension.

Patients with liver dysfunction due to biliary obstruction commonly develop severe itching (pruritus) due to retention of bile salts.

▷ Hepatic Disorders

Viral Hepatitis

The increasing incidence of viral hepatitis is a growing public health concern. Although the mortality rate is low, the disease is important because of its ease of transmission, morbidity, and the prolonged loss of time from school or employment that it can cause.

Breakthroughs in better understanding of viral hepatitis in the recent past have been due to recognition in 1968, by Blumberg, that Australian, or Au antigen, was a specific immunologic marker for hepatitis B infection. This led to a series of new designations, and Australian antigen now is referred to as hepatitis B surface antigen: HB_sAg. More recently, a specific antigen for hepatitis A has been identified (HA Ag). Also, tests have been developed to detect anti-HAV, HB_s, and HB_c antibodies, as well as the E-antigen and anti-E-antibody associated with hepatitis B. This means that diagnostic tests, including complement fixation, immune adherence, and radioimmunoassay, are available for recognizing hepatitis A and hepatitis B. The existence of one or more agents capable of producing nonA nonB hepatitis has also been recognized.

Nursing Considerations. The nurse is especially concerned with four major problem areas of viral hepatitis: (1) the care of the patient with hepatitis; (2) the increased risks in hemodialysis units and in individuals using illicit injectable drugs; (3) the fact that many individuals who have the disease are asymptomatic, which may present serious epidemiologic problems; and (4) the apparent health needs of the community required for its elimination. The last category includes the following considerations:

- Proper community and home sanitation
- Conscientious individual hygiene at all times
- Safe practices of food preparation and dispensation
- Effective health supervision in schools, dormitories, barracks, camps
- Continuous health education programs
- Reporting of every case of viral hepatitis to the local health department

For a comparison of the many aspects of the major forms of viral hepatitis, see Table 39-2.

Hepatitis A Virus (HAV)

Hepatitis A, formerly designated infectious hepatitis, is probably an RNA virus of the enterovirus family. The mode of transmission of this disease is the fecal–oral route, primarily through the ingestion of food or liquids infected by the virus. The virus has been found in the stool of infected patients prior to the onset of symptoms, and during the first few days of illness. Typically, a young adult acquires the infection at school and brings it home, where haphazard sanitary habits spread it through the family. It is more prevalent in underdeveloped countries or in instances of overcrowding and poor sanitation. An infected food handler can spread the disease, and people can contract it by consuming water or shellfish from sewage-contaminated waters. It is rarely, if ever, transmitted by blood transfusions. Animal handlers can contract hepatitis A from infected primates.

The incubation period is estimated to be from 1 to 7 weeks, with an average of 30 days. The course of the illness may be prolonged, lasting from 4 to 8 weeks. It generally lasts longer and is more severe in those above age 40.

Assessment and Clinical Manifestations. Most patients are anicteric (without jaundice) and symptomless. When symptoms appear, they are of a mild, flulike upper respiratory infection, with low-grade fever. Anorexia is an early symptom and is often severe. It is thought to result from release of a toxin by the damaged liver or by failure of the damaged liver cells to detoxify an abnormal product. Later, jaundice and dark urine may become apparent. Indigestion is present, in varying degrees, marked by vague epigastric distress, nausea, heartburn, and flatulence. The patient may also develop a strong aversion to the taste of cigarettes or the presence of cigarette smoke and other strong odors. These symptoms tend to clear as soon as the jaundice reaches its peak—perhaps 10 days after its original appearance. The liver and the spleen are often moderately enlarged for a few days after onset; otherwise, apart from jaundice, there are few physical signs to be elicited.

Management. Bed rest during the acute stage and the provision of a diet that is both acceptable and nutritious are part of the treatment and nursing care. During the period of anorexia, the patient should receive frequent small feedings, supplemented, if necessary, by intravenous infusions of glucose. Since this patient would rather not look at food, or eat, it requires gentle persistence and ingenuity to whet his appetite. Optimal food and fluid levels need to be maintained to counteract probable weight loss and prolonged recovery. Even before the icteric phase, however, many patients recover their appetites and thereafter need no reminders to maintain a good diet.

The patient's sense of well being as well as laboratory test results are generally appropriate guides to bed rest and restriction of physical activity. Gradual but progressive ambulation seems to hasten recovery, provided the patient rests after activity and does not ambulate or participate in activities to the point of fatigue.

Prognosis. Recovery from type A hepatitis is the rule; a rare case progresses to acute liver necrosis or fulminant hepatitis, terminating in cirrhosis of the liver, or death. Hepatitis A confers immunity against itself; however, the person may contract other forms of hepatitis. The mortality rate of hepatitis A is approximately 0.5%. No carrier state exists, and no chronic hepatitis is associated with hepatitis A.

Control and Prevention. Ways to reduce the risk of contracting hepatitis A are:

- Good personal hygiene, stressing careful handwashing (after bowel movement and before eating)
- Environmental sanitation—safe food and water supply, as well as effective sewage disposal

Table 39-2
Hepatitis

	Hepatitis A Virus (HAV)	Hepatitis B Virus (HBV)	NonA NonB Hepatitis Virus (NANBH)
Other Names	Type A hepatitis, infectious or epidemic hepatitis; IH virus	Type B hepatitis, serum hepatitis, SH virus, Dane particle	Hepatitis "C", "D"; Type C
Epidemiology			
Cause	Hepatitis A virus	Hepatitis B virus	Another virus
Method of transmission	Fecal-oral route; poor sanitation Person to person Waterborne, foodborne—shellfish Rarely, if at all, by blood transfusion	Parenterally, or by intimate contact with carriers or those with acute disease; male homosexuals. Vertical transmission from mothers to babies. Contaminated instruments, syringes, needles; renal dialysis*	Transfusion of blood and blood products Personnel in renal transplant and dialysis units Parenteral drug abusers Institutions with long-term residents*
Source of virus/ antigen	Blood; feces; saliva	Blood Saliva Semen, vaginal secretions	Appears to be blood-borne
Distribution by age	Young adults (15–29) and middle-aged who have escaped childhood infection	Affects all ages, but mostly young adults	Same as HBV
Incubation period	3–5 weeks Mean: 30 days	2–5 months Mean: 90 days	Variable: 14–115 days Mean: 50 days
Occurrence	Worldwide	Worldwide	Worldwide Accounts for 20% of sporadic cases
Antibody	Anti-HAV Present in convalescent sera and immune serumglobulin (ISG)	Anti-HB$_c$ (core antigen) Anti-HB$_s$ (surface antigen)	—
Immunity	Homologous	Homologous	—
Severity	Most anicteric and asymptomatic	More severe than HAV	Wide spectrum of severity, resembling HAV or HBV. Often prolonged illness—months. May progress to chronic hepatitis.*

(continued)

• Administration of Immune Globulin: Type A hepatitis can be prevented by the administration of globulin intramuscularly during the period of incubation, if this treatment is instituted within a period of 2 to 7 days following exposure. This bolsters the person's own antibody production and provides about 6 to 8 weeks of passive immunity. Immune Globulin may suppress overt symptoms of the disease; the resulting subclinical case of hepatitis A would produce active immunity to subsequent attacks of HAV. Although rare, systemic reactions to Immune Globulin may occur.

Caution is required when anyone who has previously had angioedema, hives, or other allergic reaction is treated with any human immune globulin. Epinephrine should be available for use during systemic or anaphylactic reactions.

Hepatitis B Virus (HBV)

Hepatitis B virus is a double-shelled particle containing DNA. This particle is composed of:

HB$_c$Ag—hepatitis B core antigen (antigenic material in an inner core)

Table 39-2
Hepatitis (continued)

	Hepatitis A Virus (HAV)	Hepatitis B Virus (HBV)	NonA NonB Hepatitis Virus (NANBH)
Nature of Illness			
Signs and symptoms	May occur with or without symptoms: flulike illness Preicteric phase: Headache, malaise, fatigue, anorexia, lassitude, fever Icteric phase: Dark urine, scleral icterus, jaundice, liver tenderness, and perhaps enlargement	May occur without symptoms 1000 IU/liter-serum transaminase level May develop antibodies to virus Similar to HAV, but more severe Fever and respiratory symptoms rare, but may have arthralgias, rash	Similar to HBV Less severe and anicteric
Diagnosis and method	Elevated serum transaminase Complement fixation rate Radioimmunoassay	Check serum for HB$_s$Ag, HB$_e$Ag, anti-HB$_c$, in absence of anti-HB$_s$ } Elevated serum transaminase Radioimmunoassay—hemagglutination	(Obtainable as a panel)
Severity	Usually mild Fatality rate 0%–1%	Variable, may be severe Fatality rate varies: 1%–10%	
Specific treatment	Adequate fluids, rest, nutrition	Same as HAV In research: vaccine antiviral chemotherapy to eliminate chronic HBV carrier state (being tested)	
Prevention			
	Good sanitation Proper personal hygiene Effective sterilization procedures Careful screening of food handlers Immune Globulin given within a few days of exposure	Specific hepatitis B immune globulin (HBIG) probably useful after exposure by ingestion, inoculation, or splash involving hepatitis B surface antigen (HB$_s$Ag) Hepatitis B vaccine recommended for preexposure immunization of those at high risk	Mandatory screening of blood donors: (1) For HB$_s$Ag, 20% (2) For NonA NonB, 80%

* Probably the same, for HBV and NANBH, recent intensive research suggests.

HB$_s$Ag—hepatitis B surface antigen (antigenic material in an outer coat)

HB$_e$Ag—an independent protein circulating in the blood

Each antigen elicits its specific antibody:

anti-HB$_c$—persists throughout the acute phase of illness; may indicate continuing HBV in the liver
anti-HB$_s$—detected during late convalescence; usually indicates recovery and development of immunity
anti-HB$_e$—usually signifies reduced infectivity

HB$_s$Ag can be detected transiently circulating in the blood in 80% to 90% of infected patients. HB$_c$Ag cannot be detected in blood. HB$_s$Ag may be noted in the blood for months and years, which suggests that these individuals may be asymptomatic carriers, if HB$_e$Ag is absent. If it is present, these patients may have chronic hepatitis and may be more infectious.

From the community health point of view, about 15% of American adults are positive for anti-HB$_s$, which indicates that they have had hepatitis B. Anti-HB$_s$ may be positive in as many as two thirds of users of illicit injectable drugs.

Chart 39-2
Hepatitis Glossary

HAV	Hepatitis A virus
HBV	Hepatitis B virus
NANBH	Hepatitis nonA nonB
(nA, nB)	Hepatitis nonA nonB
HB$_s$Ag	Hepatitis B surface antigen; Australian antigen
HB$_c$Ag	Hepatitis B core antigen
HB$_e$Ag	Hepatitis B e-antigen
Anti-HAV	Antibody to hepatitis A virus
Anti-HB$_s$	Antibody to hepatitis B surface antigen
Anti-HB$_c$	Antibody to hepatitis B core antigen
Anti-HB$_e$	Antibody to hepatitis B e-antigen
HBIG	Hepatitis B immunoglobulin
ISG	Immune serum globulin
IG	Immune globulin

Transmission of HBV is primarily through percutaneous and permucosal routes. The virus has been found in blood, saliva, semen, and vaginal secretions and can be transmitted through mucous membranes and breaks in the skin. Therefore, those at risk of developing HBV include the general surgeon, clinical laboratory worker, dentist, nurse, and respiratory therapist. Staff and patients in hemodialysis and oncology units and homosexually active males are also at increased risk. Mandatory screening of blood donors for HB$_s$Ag has greatly reduced the occurrence of hepatitis B following blood transfusion.

Assessment and Clinical Manifestations.   Clinically, the disease closely resembles type A hepatitis. However, the incubation period is relatively much longer: between 2 and 5 months. The mortality is appreciable, ranging from 1% to 10%, depending on the infective dose and the condition of the patient. Symptoms and signs of hepatitis B may be insidious and variable. Fever and respiratory symptoms are rare: some patients have arthralgias and rashes. The patient may lose his appetite and experience dyspepsia, abdominal pain, generalized aching, malaise, and weakness. Jaundice may or may not be evident. If jaundice occurs, it is accompanied by light-colored stools and dark urine. The patient's liver may be tender and enlarged to 12 cm to 14 cm vertically. The spleen is enlarged and palpable in a small number of patients; the posterior cervical nodes may also be enlarged.

Management.   It is important that bed rest be continued until the hepatitis has definitely subsided. Subsequently, the patient's activities should be restricted until the hepatic enlargement and the elevation of serum bilirubin have disappeared. Adequate nutrition should be maintained; proteins are restricted when the liver has a decreased ability to metabolize protein by-products, as demonstrated by symptoms. Other therapeutic measures employed to control the dyspeptic symptoms and general malaise include the use of alkalies, belladonna, and antiemetics. However, all medications should be avoided if emesis is a problem. This patient should be hospitalized and treated with fluid therapy.

Convalescence may be prolonged, complete symptomatic recovery sometimes requiring 3 to 4 months or longer. During this stage, gradual restoration of physical activity is permitted and encouraged, following complete clearing of the jaundice.

Psychosocial considerations are recognized by the nurse, particularly as they apply to isolation and separation procedures. Special planning is required to minimize any alterations in sensory perception. The family must be included in such planning.

Prognosis.   Mortality of HBV has been reported to be as high as 10%. Another 10% of patients who have HBV progress to a carrier state or develop chronic hepatitis.

Control and Prevention.   The goals are (1) to interrupt the chain of transmission, (2) to protect those individuals at high risk through the use of hepatitis B vaccine, and (3) to use passive immunization for unprotected individuals exposed to HBV.

Continued screening of potential blood donors for the presence of HB$_s$Ag will further decrease the risk of transmission by blood transfusion. A reduction in the number of persons acquiring hepatitis B could occur if paid blood donors could be replaced by an all-volunteer donor population. Washed red blood cells appear to reduce the risk of hepatitis transmission. The use of disposable syringes, needles, and lancets reduces the risk of spreading this infection from one patient to another in the process of collecting blood samples or administering parenteral therapy. Good personal hygiene practices are fundamental to infection control. In the laboratory, work areas should be disinfected daily. Gloves are to be worn when handling HB$_s$Ag positive specimens. Eating is prohibited in the laboratory.

Administering medication by individual-dose ampules is essential. Where users of illicit injectable drugs share the same needle, serious outbreaks of hepatitis have occurred.

Hepatitis B Vaccine.   Hepatitis B vaccine has recently become available for prevention of HBV. Its use is recommended for those at high risk of developing hepatitis B, including health care workers exposed to blood, hemodialysis and oncology patients and staff, homosexually active males, and users of illicit injectable drugs. Initial studies have shown that hepatitis B vaccine produces active immunity to HBV in 90% of healthy persons. It provides no protection against other types of hepatitis and does not provide protection to those already exposed to HBV. Side-effects are infrequent. The most common postinjection complaint is soreness and redness at the injection site.

Hepatitis B Immunoglobulin.   Hepatitis B Immune Globulin (HBIG) is recommended for unprotected individuals exposed to HBV through accidental contamination of mucous membranes or breaks in the skin. HBIG is prepared from pooled venous plasma of donors with a high titer of anti-HB$_s$ antibodies and provides passive immunity.

Immune Serum Globulin.   The United States Public Health Service Advisory Committee on Immunization Practices recommends HBIG for a single exposure to blood containing hepatitis B virus, either by accidental inoculation via needle stick or by splashing contaminated material on mucous membranes, such as might occur while pipetting blood or fluid. HBIG is given intramuscularly as soon as possible, but no later than 7 days after exposure. A second dose is given in 25 to 30 days after the first.

Hepatitis nonA nonB

Those varieties of hepatitis that are not identified as hepatitis A or B are classified as nonA nonB hepatitis. Repeated episodes of nonA nonB hepatitis and variations in incubation periods of this form of hepatitis suggest the existence of multiple causative agents. NonA nonB hepatitis is blood-borne, and the possibility of a carrier state is likely. This form of hepatitis is now the major cause of transfusion-related viral hepatitis and is often observed in parenteral drug abusers.

Hepatitis nonA nonB occurs not only in patients, following blood transfusion, and among drug users, but in personnel associated with renal transplantation units and in residents in homes for the mentally retarded. Another community health-related implication is that whereas only about 10% to 20% of posttransfusion hepatitis is type B, 80% to 90% is nonA nonB hepatitis. Commercial blood appears to transmit hepatitis virus much more than blood from volunteer donors.

Incubation time is variable, and severity covers a wide spectrum that most resembles hepatitis B. Most manifestations are anicteric (without jaundice). Illness may be prolonged, lasting several months, and resulting in chronic hepatitis. It is possible that Immune Globulin may offer limited protection against nonA nonB hepatitis.

Toxic Hepatitis and Drug-Induced Hepatitis

Certain chemicals have poisonous effects on the liver, and when taken by mouth or injected parenterally produce acute liver cell necrosis, or *toxic hepatitis.* The chemicals most commonly implicated in this disease are carbon tetrachloride, phosphorus, chloroform, and gold compounds. These are true hepatotoxins.

Many drugs may induce hepatitis, but are sensitizing, rather than toxic. The result, *drug-induced hepatitis,* is similar to acute viral hepatitis; however, parenchymal destruction tends to be more extensive. Some examples of drugs that can lead to hepatitis are cinchophen, isoniazid, halothane, acetaminophen, and certain antibiotics and antimetabolites.

Clinical Manifestations and Management.

Toxic hepatitis resembles viral hepatitis in onset. Obtaining a history of exposure to hepatotoxic chemicals, drugs, or other agents assists in earlier initiation of treatment and removal of the offending agent. Anorexia, nausea, and vomiting are the usual symptoms; jaundice and hepatomegaly are noted on physical assessment. Symptoms are more intense for the more severely poisoned patient.

Recovery from acute toxic hepatitis is rapid if the hep-

atotoxin is identified early and removed or if exposure to the agent has been limited. Recovery, however, is unlikely if there is a prolonged period between exposure and onset of symptoms. There are no effective antidotes. The fever mounts; the patient becomes deeply toxic and prostrated. Vomiting may be persistent, with the vomitus containing blood. Clotting abnormalities may be severe, and hemorrhages may appear under the skin. The severe gastrointestinal symptoms may lead to vascular collapse. Delirium, coma, and convulsions develop, and within a few days the patient usually dies.

There is little to be done by way of treatment, except to provide comfort measures, blood, fluids, and electrolytes. A few patients recover from acute toxic hepatitis only to develop chronic liver disease.

Drug-induced hepatitis may progress to hepatic failure. In the event that the liver heals, there may be scarring, followed by postnecrotic cirrhosis. Manifestations of sensitivity to a drug may occur on the first day of its use or not until several months later, depending on the drug. Usually, the onset is abrupt, with chills, fever, rash, pruritus, arthralgia, anorexia, and nausea. Later, there may be jaundice and dark urine, and an enlarged and tender liver. When the offending drug is withdrawn, symptoms may gradually subside. However, once provoked, reactions may be severe and even fatal, even though the drug is stopped. If fever, rash, or pruritus occur from any medication, it should be stopped immediately.

Concern has been expressed regarding the effect of halothane (Fluothane)—a commonly used, nonexplosive inhalation anesthetic—on the liver. Since it may cause serious, and sometimes fatal, liver damage, precautions should preclude its use in (1) persons with known liver disease; (2) repeated instances, particularly in patients who have had a fever of unknown cause after the first administration of halothane; and (3) patients with evidence of prior sensitization. Such sensitization would have been in evidence during the second postoperative week, with such manifestations as fever, rash, eosinophilia, arthralgia, or jaundice.

Hepatic Cirrhosis

Cirrhosis of the liver refers to scarring of the liver. Three kinds are generally considered:

1. *Laennec's portal cirrhosis* (alcoholic; nutritional), in which the scar tissue characteristically surrounds the portal areas. This is most frequently due to chronic alcoholism and is the most common type of cirrhosis. It is discussed below.
2. *Postnecrotic cirrhosis,* in which there are broad bands of scar tissue, as a late result of a previous acute viral hepatitis.
3. *Biliary cirrhosis,* in which there is pericholangitic, perilobular scarring. This type usually is the result of chronic biliary obstruction and infection (cholangitis) and is much more rare than Laennec's and postnecrotic cirrhosis.

The portion of the liver chiefly involved consists of the portal and the periportal spaces, where the bile canaliculi of each lobule communicate to form the liver bile ducts. These areas become the site of inflammation, and the bile ducts become occluded with inspissated bile and pus. An attempt is made by the liver to form new bile channels; hence, there is an overgrowth of tissue made up largely of disconnected, newly formed bile ducts and surrounded by scar tissue.

Clinical manifestations of this disease include intermittent jaundice and fever and the finding of an enlarged, hard, irregular liver, which eventually becomes atrophic. The treatment is the same as that described for portal cirrhosis, that is, the treatment of any form of chronic liver insufficiency and, when indicated, surgical treatment designed to eradicate the biliary tract infection.

Pathophysiology

The basic mechanism responsible for the development of Laennec's cirrhosis is yet to be described. Cirrhosis occurs with greatest frequency among alcoholics. However, many explain the role of alcohol in the production of cirrhosis on the basis of nutritional deficiency with reduced protein intake, rather than on alcohol toxicity, and certainly some cases of cirrhosis are observed among people who do not drink alcoholic beverages. Nonetheless, several investigators have shown that although nutritional factors are undoubtedly involved, alcohol itself has to be incriminated in the pathogenesis of the alcoholic fatty liver and the associated effects.

Some individuals appear to be more susceptible than others to this disease, whether they are alcoholics, malnourished, or not. Other factors may play a role, such as exposure to certain chemicals (carbon tetrachloride, chlorinated naphthalene, arsenic, or phosphorus) or infectious schistosomiasis. Twice as many men as women are affected, and the majority of patients are between 40 and 60 years of age.

Laennec's cirrhosis is a disease characterized by episodes of necrosis involving the liver cells, sometimes occurring repeatedly throughout the course of the disease. The destroyed liver cells are replaced by scar tissue, the amount of which, in time, may exceed that of the functioning liver tissue. Islands of residual normal tissue and regenerating liver tissue may project from the constricted areas, giving the cirrhotic liver its characteristic hobnail appearance. The disease usually has a particularly insidious onset and a very protracted course, occasionally proceeding over a period of 30 or more years.

▶ Assessment

Clinical Manifestations. (See Fig. 39-6.) Early in the course of cirrhosis, the liver tends to be large and its cells loaded with fat. The liver is firm and has a sharp edge on palpation. Abdominal pain may be present due to recent, rapid enlargement of the liver, producing tension on Glisson's capsule. Later in the course of the disease, the liver decreases in size as scar tissue contracts the liver tissue. The liver edge, if palpable, is nodular.

The late manifestations are due partly to chronic failure of liver function and partly to obstruction of the portal circulation. Practically all the blood from the digestive organs is collected in the portal veins and carried to the liver. Since a cirrhotic liver does not allow the blood free passage, it is dammed back into the spleen and the gastrointestinal tract, with the result that these organs become the seat of chronic passive congestion; that is, they are stagnant with blood, and so cannot function properly. Such patients are apt to have chronic dyspepsia and changes in bowel habit, with constipation or diarrhea. There is gradual weight loss. Fluid may accumulate in the peritoneal cavity, producing ascites. This can be demonstrated through percussion for shifting dullness or a fluid wave (see Fig. 39-3). Splenomegaly may also be present. Spider telangiectases, or dilated superficial arterioles resembling bluish red spiders, are frequently observed on inspection of the face and trunk.

The obstruction to blood flow through the liver resulting from the fibrotic changes also results in the formation of collateral blood vessels in the gastrointestinal system and shunting of blood from the portal vessels into blood vessels with lower pressures. As a result, the cirrhotic patient will often have prominent, distended abdominal blood vessels, which are visible on abdominal inspection (caput medusae), and distended blood vessels throughout the gastrointestinal tract. The esophagus, stomach, and lower rectum are common sites of collateral blood vessels. These distended blood vessels form varices or hemorrhoids, depending on their location. Because these vessels were not intended to carry the high pressure and volume of blood imposed by cirrhosis, they may rupture and bleed. Therefore, assessment must include observation for occult and frank bleeding from the gastrointestinal tract. Approximately 25% of patients develop small hematemesis; others have profuse hemorrhage from the stomach and esophageal varices.

Other late symptoms of cirrhosis are attributable to chronic failure of liver function. The concentration of plasma albumin is lowered, predisposing to the formation of edema. Overproduction of aldosterone occurs in cirrhosis, causing sodium and water retention and potassium excretion. Because of inadequate formation, utilization, and storage of certain vitamins, notably vitamins A, C, and K, signs of their deficiency frequently are encountered—particularly hemorrhagic phenomena associated with vitamin-K deficiency. Chronic gastritis and poor gastrointestinal function, together with the factors of poor diet and impaired liver function, account for the anemia often associated with this disease. The anemia and the patient's poor nutritional status and poor state of health result in severe fatigue, which interferes with the ability to carry out routine daily activities.

Additional clinical manifestations include deterioration of mental function with impending hepatic encephalopathy and hepatic coma. Therefore, neurologic assessment is in order and should include the patient's general behavior, cognitive abilities, orientation to time and place, and speech patterns.

In addition to noting the occurrence of clinical manifestations, the nurse should obtain accurate information about the patient's dietary and alcohol intake. It is also im-

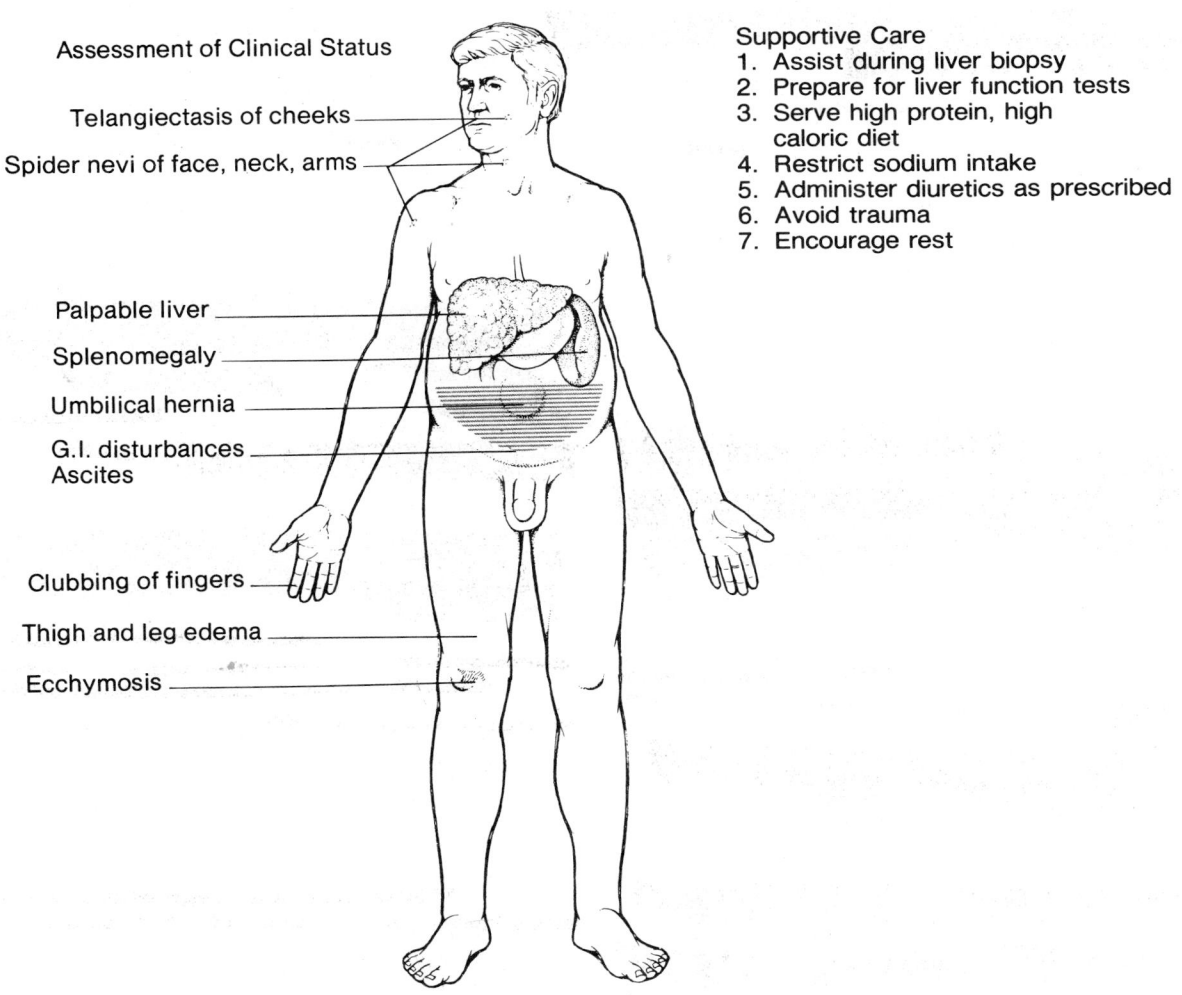

Assessment of Clinical Status

Telangiectasis of cheeks

Spider nevi of face, neck, arms

Palpable liver

Splenomegaly

Umbilical hernia

G.I. disturbances
Ascites

Clubbing of fingers

Thigh and leg edema

Ecchymosis

Supportive Care
1. Assist during liver biopsy
2. Prepare for liver function tests
3. Serve high protein, high caloric diet
4. Restrict sodium intake
5. Administer diuretics as prescribed
6. Avoid trauma
7. Encourage rest

Figure 39-6. Clinical assessment and care of the patient with cirrhosis.

portant to note exposure to toxic agents encountered during work or recreation. Any medications or drugs taken by the patient are recorded and checked for hepatotoxicity. Exposure to general anesthetics that may be hepatotoxic are also noted.

Diagnostic Assessment. The extent of liver disease and the kind of treatment are determined after studying the laboratory findings. Because the liver is a complex, functioning organ, the tests are many (see Table 39-1). The patient needs to know why these tests are being done, why they are important, and how he can cooperate. In severe parenchymal liver dysfunction, serum albumin tends to decrease, and serum globulin rises. Enzyme tests indicate liver cell damage: serum alkaline phosphatase, SGOT, and SGPT levels increase, and serum cholinesterase may decrease. Excretory function is tested by the liver's ability to eliminate sulfobromophthalein (Bromosulphalein) and cardiogreen dye. In cirrhosis, the sulfobromophthalein and cardiogreen are retained. Bilirubin tests are done to measure bile ex-

cretion or bile retention. Photolaparoscopy, in conjunction with biopsy, may be done to permit direct visualization of the liver.

Ultrasound scanning will measure the difference in density of parenchymal cells and scar tissue. Computed tomography (CT scan) and radioisotopic liver scans give information about liver size and hepatic blood flow and obstruction.

Patient Problems/Nursing Diagnoses

Based on the clinical manifestations, history, and diagnostic assessment data, the patient's major nursing problems include the inability to carry out self-care activities related to fatigue, general debility and muscle wasting, and discomfort; inadequate nutritional intake related to chronic gastritis, decreased gastrointestinal motility, and anorexia; altered skin integrity related to edema, jaundice, and compromised immunologic status; potential bleeding related to altered clotting mechanisms and portal hypertension; and altered mental function related to deterioration of liver function and increased serum ammonia level.

▶ Planning and Nursing Implementation

Goals

The goals of the patient are:

1. Increased ability to carry out self-care activities
2. Improved nutritional intake
3. Improved skin integrity
4. Decreased risk of bleeding
5. Improved mental function

To assist in accomplishing these goals, the major objectives of therapy are (1) to promote rest to reduce the demands on the dysfunctional liver, (2) to meet the patient's nutritional needs, (3) to prevent further threats to skin integrity, (4) to minimize risk of bleeding, and (5) to minimize metabolic derangements and limit those factors causing further deterioration of mental function.

Rest.   The patient with active liver disease requires rest and other supportive measures to permit the liver to reestablish its functional ability. The patient's weight and the volume of his fluid intake and output are measured and recorded daily. His position in bed is adjusted for maximal respiratory efficiency, which is especially important if ascites is marked. Oxygen therapy may be required, in liver failure, to oxygenate the weakened cells, lest more die.

Rest permits the liver to restore itself by limiting the demands of the body and increasing the liver's blood supply. Since the patient is more susceptible to infection, efforts to prevent respiratory, circulatory, and vascular disturbances need to be initiated. These measures may help prevent such problems as pneumonia, thrombophlebitis, and pressure sores. When the patient's nutritional status improves and the patient gains strength, he is encouraged to increase his activity gradually. Activity and mild exercise, as well as rest, are planned.

Meeting Nutritional Needs.   The cirrhotic patient who has no ascites or edema and exhibits no signs of impending coma should receive a nutritious, high-protein diet supplemented by vitamins of the B complex and others as indicated (including vitamins A, C, and K, and folic acid). Since proper nutrition is so important, every effort must be made to encourage the patient to eat. This is as important as any medication. Often small, frequent meals can be accepted better than three large meals because of the abdominal pressure exerted by ascites.

Patient preferences are to be considered. Patients with prolonged or severe anorexia, or those who are vomiting or eating poorly for any reason, can be fed by nasogastric tube or parenteral hyperalimentation.

Patients with fatty stools (steatorrhea) should receive water-soluble forms of fat-soluble vitamins—A, D, and E (Aquasol A, D, and E). Folic acid and iron are prescribed, to prevent anemia. If the patient shows signs of impending or advancing coma, a low-protein diet should be given temporarily; too much protein from meats may produce portal systemic encephalopathy (PSE), and too little may cause negative nitrogen and wasting. Suggested protein foods are dairy products (eggs, skim milk), cereal (wheat germ, white rice), and fish (shellfish, salmon, sardines). A high-caloric intake should be maintained, and supplementary vitamins and minerals should be supplied (*e.g.*, oral potassium, if the serum potassium is normal or low, and if renal function is normal). As soon as the situation permits, the protein intake should be restored to normal, or above. Diet therapy is determined on an individualized basis.

Skin Care.   Skin care is observed meticulously, because of the presence of subcutaneous edema, the immobility of the patient, jaundice, and increased susceptibility to skin breakdown and infection. Frequent position changes are necessary to prevent pressure sores. Irritating soaps and use of adhesive tape are avoided to prevent trauma to the skin. Lotion may be soothing to irritated skin; measures are taken to minimize the patient's scratching of the skin.

Prevention of Bleeding.   Because of decreased production of prothrombin and the diseased liver's decreased synthesis of substances used in blood coagulation, hemorrhage is possible. Precautionary measures include protecting the patient with padded side rails, applying pressure to an injection site, and avoiding injury from sharp objects. Observe for melena and check stools for blood, as signs of possible internal bleeding.

Minimizing Mental Dysfunction Due to Portal Systemic Encephalopathy (PSE).   PSE is a possible neurologic syndrome that includes various combinations of myelopathy, chorea-athetosis, dysarthria, and even dementia. It has occurred in postshunt patients and in those with advanced cirrhosis. PSE is mainly caused by ammonia and its effect on cerebral metabolism. Many factors predispose the patient with cirrhosis to PSE; some are unforseeable, but many are avoidable. The nurse is in a position to observe early evidence of this condition and promote early treatment. The nurse also uses strategies to orient the patient to reality.

Patient Education and Posthospital Care.   Before discharge, the patient receives detailed instructions, in part from the nurse, principally relating to dietary habits. Of utmost importance is the exclusion of alcohol from the diet. The patient may need the assistance of a skilled psychiatrist, trusted religious adviser, or Alcoholics Anonymous.

Sodium restriction will continue for a considerable period of time, if not permanently; if this diet is to be followed correctly, the patient will require written instructions.

The success of treatment depends on convincing the patient of the need to adhere willingly and wholeheartedly to the therapeutic plan. This includes rest; probably a change in life-style; an adequate, well-balanced diet; and the elimination of alcohol. The patient is also instructed as to the symptoms of impending encephalopathy, and the possibility of bleeding tendencies and easy susceptibility to infection. Recovery is neither rapid nor easy; there are frequent setbacks and apparent lack of improvement. For many persons, the loss of support given by alcohol is discouraging. The understanding nurse can play a significant role in offering support and encouragement to this patient.

Summary.   For an overall view of the nursing management of the patient with cirrhosis, refer to Chart 39-3.

▶ **Evaluation**

Expected Outcomes

1. Demonstrates ability to perform self-care activities
   a. Plans activities and exercises to allow alternating periods of rest and activity
   b. Reports increased strength and well-being
   c. Displays increased weight gain without increased edema and ascites formation
   d. Participates in hygienic care
2. Increases nutritional intake
   a. Demonstrates intake of appropriate nutrients and avoidance of alcohol as reflected in diet log
   b. Gains weight without increased edema and ascites formation
   c. Reports decrease in gastrointestinal disturbances and anorexia
   d. Identifies foods and fluids that are nutritious and allowed on diet
   e. Identifies foods restricted from diet
   f. Adheres to vitamin therapy regimen
   g. Describes the rationale for small, frequent meals
   h. Excludes alcohol from diet
3. Demonstrates improved skin integrity
   a. Shows intact skin without evidence of breakdown or infection
   b. Achieves decreased edema in extremities and trunk
   c. Demonstrates normal turgor of skin of extremities and trunk
   d. Changes position frequently
   e. Inspects bony prominences daily
   f. Avoids trauma to skin
   g. Reports decreased or absent pruritus
   h. Utilizes lotions to decrease pruritus
4. Experiences decreased risk of bleeding
   a. Is free of ecchymotic areas or hematoma formation
   b. Reports absence of frank bleeding from gastrointestinal tract (*e.g.,* absence of melena and hematemesis)
   c. Reports negative results of test for occult gastrointestinal bleeding
   d. Utilizes measures to prevent trauma (*e.g.,* uses soft toothbrush, blows nose gently, arranges furniture to prevent bumps and falls, avoids straining during defecation)
5. Demonstrates improved mental function
   a. Has serum ammonia level within normal limits
   b. Is oriented to time, place, and person
   c. Demonstrates normal attention span (*e.g.,* is able to complete reading of desired articles, books; able to watch television with interest)
   d. Converses with family and health team members appropriately
   e. Reports urinary and fecal continence

Bleeding Esophageal Varices

Signs of jaundice, ascites, and portal hypertension are manifestations of advanced liver disease. Usually, the patient is a potential bleeder and requires careful monitoring of laboratory blood studies, hematemesis, and melena.

Pathophysiology and Symptoms

Esophageal varices are dilated tortuous veins usually found in the submucosa of the lower esophagus; however, they may extend well up into the esophagus and into the stomach. Such a condition nearly always is caused by portal hypertension, which, in turn, is due to obstruction of the portal venous circulation within the substance of a cirrhotic liver (see p. 865). Hemorrhage from ruptured esophageal varices is the most common single cause of death in patients with cirrhosis. Because of increased obstruction of the portal vein, venous blood from the intestinal tract and spleen seeks an outlet through collateral circulation (new avenues of return to the right atrium). The pathophysiologic effect is increased strain, particularly on the vessels in the submucosal layer of the lower esophagus and upper part of the stomach. These collateral vessels are not very elastic, but rather are tortuous and fragile, and bleed easily. Other lesser causes of varices are abnormalities of the circulation in the splenic vein or superior vena cava, and hepatic venothrombosis.

Bleeding esophageal varices are life-threatening and can result in hemorrhagic shock, producing decreased cerebral, hepatic, and renal perfusion. In turn, there will be an increased nitrogen load from bleeding into the gastrointestinal tract and an increased serum ammonia level. Bleeding esophageal varices should be suspected in the presence of hematemesis and melena, especially in the patient who has been addicted to alcohol. Usually, the dilated veins cause no symptoms unless the mucosa over them becomes ulcerated. Then massive hemorrhage takes place. Factors that contribute to rupture and hemorrhage are muscular strain from lifting heavy objects, straining at stool, sneezing, coughing or vomiting, esophagitis, or irritation of vessels by poorly chewed foods or irritating fluids. Salicylates and any drug that erodes esophageal mucosa or interferes with cell replication may also cause bleeding.

Assessment

The patient's history and physical examination serve as a basis for ascertaining the problem. Neurologic assessment will assist in identifying possible hepatic encephalopathy resulting from the breakdown of blood in the gastrointestinal tract and a rising serum ammonia level. Manifestations range from drowsiness to coma. Portal hypertension may be suspected if dilated abdominal veins and rectal hemorrhoids are detected. Also apparent may be a palpable enlarged spleen (splenomegaly) and ascites. Laboratory tests that may be required are various liver function tests, such as Bromsulphalein retention, serum transaminase, bilirubin, alkaline phosphatase, and serum proteins. Esophagoscopy or endoscopy most clearly clinches the diagnosis, because even the site of hemorrhage may be seen. The site of bleeding must be identified, as one third or more patients bleed from other sources. Gastritis and duodenal ulcer frequently coexist with cirrhosis. Nursing support before and during examination by esophagoscopy or endoscopy can be effec-

(Text continues on page 872)

Chart 39-3
Guidelines of Nursing Management for the Patient With Laennec's Cirrhosis

Problems	Nursing Interventions
Anorexia	Encourage patient to eat meals and supplementary feedings. Offer frequent small feedings. Give attention to esthetic factors and attractive trays at mealtime. Eliminate alcohol.
Nausea and vomiting	Provide oral hygiene before meals. Use an ice collar for nausea. Give tube feedings, as required.
Weight loss and fatigue	Offer continuous encouragement of intake of high-protein, high-calorie diet. Give supplementary vitamins (A, B complex, C, and K). Give parenteral fluids as prescribed. Conserve patient's energy.
Abdominal pain	Assure bed rest to protect liver. Administer antispasmodics and mild sedatives. Encourage patient to eat slowly and chew thoroughly. Observe, record, and report presence and character of pain.
Hematemesis	Be alert for symptoms of anxiety, epigastric fullness, weakness, and restlessness. Observe for presence of bleeding and shock. Record vital signs at frequent intervals. Keep patient quiet and limit activity. Observe during blood transfusions. Assist physician in passage of tube for esophageal balloon tamponade. Measure and record nature, time, and amount of vomitus. Give meticulous oral hygiene. Maintain patient in fasting state, if indicated. Administer vitamin K as prescribed. Stay in constant attendance during episodes of bleeding. Offer cold liquids by mouth when bleeding stops (if prescribed).
Melena	Observe each stool for color, consistency, and amount.
Constipation	Ensure adequate fluid and food intake. Encourage exercises.
Diarrhea	Increase fluid intake. Give medications as prescribed.
Jaundice	Note and record varying degrees of jaundice of the skin and the sclerae. Relieve pruritus with good skin care, bathing without soap, and massage with emollient lotions. Keep patient's fingernails short to prevent skin excoriation from scratching. Give empathetic attention to patient's complaints and problems.
Edema of extremities	Restrict sodium. Administer diuretics as prescribed. Give careful attention and care to skin. Turn and change position frequently. Elevate extremities at intervals. Weigh patient daily. Record intake and output. Carry out passive range of motion exercises. Provide small foam-rubber supports under heels, malleoli, etc. Carefully control rate of flow of intravenous infusions.

(continued)

Chart 39-3
Guidelines of Nursing Management for the Patient With Laennec's Cirrhosis (continued)

Problems	Nursing Interventions

Ascites	Restrict sodium.
	Give diuretics, potassium, and protein supplements as prescribed.
	Record intake and output and daily measurement of abdominal girth.
	Give careful attention to skin.
	Elevate head of bed, to facilitate breathing.
	Give pillow support under costal margin when in side-lying positions.
	Assist patient during paracentesis:
	   1. Have him void before procedure.
	   2. Position correctly and use pillow support.
	   3. Record both the amount and the character of fluid aspirated.
	   4. Protect puncture site with dry dressings.
	   5. Check dressing for fluid seepage and evidence of wound infections.
	Observe for symptoms of impending coma.

Hydrothorax and dyspnea	Elevate head of bed.
	Conserve patient's strength.
	Change position at intervals.
	Assist patient during thoracentesis:
	   1. Support and maintain position during procedure.
	   2. Record both the amount and the character of fluid aspirated.
	   3. Observe for evidence of coughing, increasing dyspnea, or pulse rate.

Fever	Record temperature regularly. Encourage fluid intake. Give cool sponges for elevated temperature. Supply icecap to head as prescribed. Give antibiotics as prescribed. Avoid exposure to infections. Keep patient at rest. Note urinary volume and concentration.
Hemorrhagic manifestations: ecchymosis, epistaxis, petechiae, and bleeding gums	Avoid trauma. Maintain safe environment. Avoid forceful blowing of nose. Prevent trauma to gums from toothbrushing. Encourage intake of foods with high content of vitamin C. Apply cold compresses where indicated. Record location of bleeding sites. Avoid constrictive clothing. Use small-gauge needles for injections.
Increasing stupor: mental changes, lethargy, hallucinations, and hepatic coma	Restrict dietary protein. Give frequent small feeding of carbohydrates. Protect from infection. Keep environment warm and draft-free. Pad the side-rails of the bed. Limit visitors. Provide careful nursing surveillance to ensure patient's safety. Avoid narcotics and barbiturates. Arouse at intervals. Give sensitive nursing care during terminal phase. Check for adequately fitting nasal tubings when nasal oxygen therapy is prescribed.

tive in relieving a stressful experience. Careful monitoring can detect early signs of cardiac arrhythmias, perforation, and hemorrhage. After the examination, fluids are not given until the gag reflex returns. Lozenges and gargles may be offered to relieve throat discomfort.

Portal vein pressure can be measured in the operating room by introducing a needle into the spleen; a manometer reading above 20 ml saline is abnormal. Combined umbilical-portal and hepatic vein catheterization is the most practical method for measuring portal pressure and at the same time permits radiologic study of the hepatic vascular bed. Blood flow studies may also be done, which assists in determining cardiac output.

Splenoportography using sodium diatrizoate is studied in serial or segmental roentgenograms to detect extensive collateral circulation in esophageal vessels, which would be indicative of varices. Other tests are hepatoportography and celiac angiography. These are usually done in the operating room or x-ray department.

Overall nursing assessment includes an evaluation of the emotional concerns of the patient and any physical problems. Vital signs are taken, and the nutritional needs are determined. If the patient was admitted for hemorrhage, the situation becomes an emergency.

Management

The patient with bleeding varices is critically ill, requiring continuous nursing attention. Nursing assessment requires that the extent of bleeding be evaluated and vital signs monitored continuously when hematemesis and melena are present. Signs of potential hypovolemia are to be noted, such as cold, clammy skin; tachycardia; blood pressure drop; restlessness; and increased or shallow peripheral pulse. Blood volume monitoring is accomplished with a central venous pressure (CVP) or arterial catheter. Oxygen is required, to prevent hypoxia and to maintain adequate blood oxygenation. Blood transfusion also may be needed.

Since patients with bleeding esophageal varices are subject to electrolyte imbalance, intravenous fluids are prescribed to restore fluid volume and replace deficient electrolytes. Urinary output is carefully monitored; an indwelling catheter may be indicated.

Nonsurgical Management

Nonoperative treatment is the treatment of choice because of the high mortality of emergency surgery for control of bleeding esophageal varices and because of the poor physical condition of the patient with severe liver dysfunction.

Drug Therapy. Vasopressin (Pitressin) may be the initial mode of therapy because of its constriction of the splanchnic arterial bed and resulting decrease in portal pressure. It may be given intravenously or by intra-arterial infusion. Either method requires monitoring by the nurse. Gastric aspiration and vital signs offer indices of the effectiveness of vasopressin.

- Coronary artery disease in this patient would be a contraindication to the use of vasopressin, since coronary vasoconstriction may promote a myocardial infarction.

Electrolyte evaluation and monitoring of fluid intake and output are necessary, since hyponatremia may occur and vasopressin may have an antidiuretic effect.

Sengstaken–Blakemore Tube. To control the hemorrhage in certain patients, pressure is exerted on the cardiac portion of the stomach and against the bleeding varices by a double-balloon tamponade (Sengstaken–Blakemore tube, SBT) (Fig. 39-7). The three openings are for specific purposes: gastric aspiration, inflation of the gastric balloon, and inflation of the esophageal balloon.

The balloon in the stomach is inflated, and the tube is pulled gently to exert a force against the cardia. Irrigation of the tubing is performed to detect bleeding; if returns are clear, the esophageal balloon is not inflated. If bleeding continues, the esophageal balloon is inflated. The desired pressure in both balloons is 25 mm Hg to 30 mm Hg, as measured by the manometer. After the balloon is inflated, there is a possibility of injury or rupture of the esophagus. Constant nursing surveillance is necessary at this time. Traction is placed on the tube at the site of insertion. A nasogastric tube may be inserted through the other nares to aspirate esophagopharyngeal secretions. This is not necessary in the "Minnesota tube" (Fig. 39-8), because a fourth lumen is included in the outlets to the tamponade tube to provide a direct route for esophageal aspiration.

Usually, a cathartic such as magnesium sulfate is introduced through the tube to eliminate blood in the gastrointestinal tract; otherwise, ammonia absorption could occur, which may lead to hepatic coma and death. Thereafter, neomycin is administered to reduce intestinal bacterial flora, which are a source of ammonia-forming enzymes.

Gastric suction can be provided by connecting the proper catheter outlet to suction. The tubing is irrigated hourly, and drainage will indicate whether bleeding has been controlled. Iced saline lavage or irrigation may be used in the stomach balloon in order to constrict the gastric vessels. In such instances, the nurse will anticipate possible chilling of the patient and provide comfort measures. The pressures on the tubes and traction are released periodically, as prescribed. Balloon tamponade is continued for several days and then cautiously released, followed by removal of the tube if no bleeding recurs.

Although this method has been fairly successful, it is important to note some inherent dangers. If the tube is left in place or inflated too long or at too high a pressure, ulceration and necrosis can develop in the stomach or esophagus. If the tube suddenly ruptures, the result is disastrous—(airway obstruction and aspiration of gastric contents into the lungs). Using a brand-new tested tube that is less than a year old may prevent this calamity. Asphyxiation is another problem, caused by the counterweight pulling the tube into the oropharynx. These potential dangers suggest the need for intensive and intelligent care. The balloon may be deflated for 5 minutes at 8- to 12-hour intervals to prevent erosion and necrosis of the stomach and esophagus.

Nursing comfort measures include frequent mouth and nasal care. For secretions that accumulate in the mouth, tissues should be within easy reach of the patient. The patient who has experienced bleeding esophageal hemorrhage is

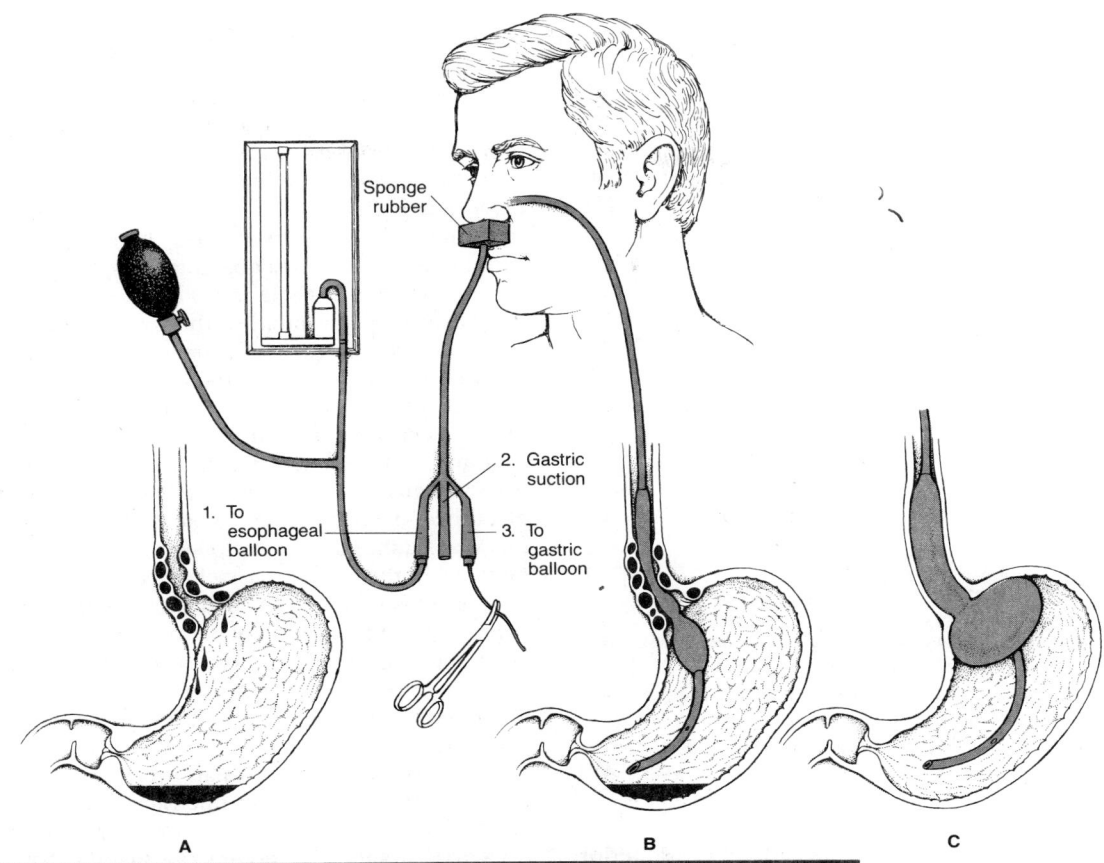

Figure 39-7. Diagram showing esophageal varices and their treatment by a compressing balloon tube (Sengstaken–Blakemore). (*A*) Dilated veins of the lower esophagus. (*B*) The tube is in place in the stomach and the lower esophagus, but is not inflated. (*C*) Inflation of the tube and the compression of the veins that can be obtained by inflation of the balloon.

usually anxious and frightened. The patient is more relaxed if he knows that the nurse is nearby and will respond immediately to his call.

Injection Sclerotherapy. This method of treatment has recently regained favor as a treatment of bleeding esophageal varices in patients who are poor surgical risks. In injection sclerotherapy, a sclerosing agent is injected through a fiberoptic endoscope into the bleeding esophageal varices to promote thrombosis and eventual sclerosis. Although long-term survival following this treatment has yet to be demonstrated, the procedure has successfully treated gastrointestinal hemorrhage. In addition, it has been used as a prophylactic measure to treat esophageal varices before bleeding has occurred. Following treatment, the patient must be observed for bleeding, perforation of the esophagus, and aspiration pneumonia.

Other Measures. Bleeding also is treated by sedation and complete rest of the esophagus (parenteral feedings). Straining and vomiting must be prevented. Gastric suction usually is employed to keep the stomach as empty as possible. The patient complains of severe thirst, which may be relieved by frequent oral hygiene and moist sponges to the lips, if permitted. The nurse keeps close surveillance on the

patient's blood pressure. Vitamin K therapy and multiple blood transfusions often are indicated. A quiet environment and calm reassurance will help to relieve the patient's anxiety.

Surgical Management

Surgical procedures that may be employed for esophageal varices are (1) direct surgical ligation of varices, and (2) portacaval and splenorenal venous shunt operations.

Surgical Bypass Procedures. The most common procedure is to create an anastomosis between the portal vein and the inferior vena cava, which is spoken of as a *portacaval anastomosis* (Fig. 39-9). When portal blood is shunted into the vena cava, the pressure in the portal system is decreased, and consequently the danger of hemorrhage from esophageal and gastric varices is reduced. When the portal vein cannot be used because of thrombosis, or for other reasons, a shunt may be made between the splenic vein and the left renal vein (*splenorenal shunt*) following splenectomy. Some surgeons prefer this shunt to the portacaval shunt, even when the portal vein can be used.

A *mesocaval* shunt is a third type of bypass procedure, in which the inferior vena cava is severed and the proximal

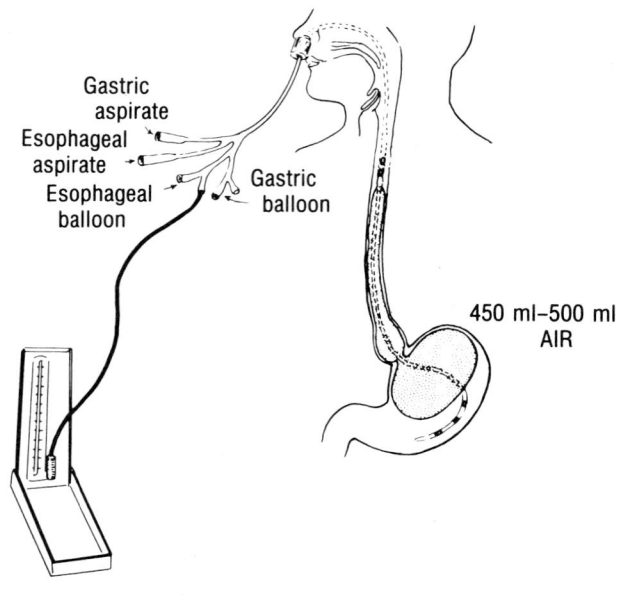

Figure 39-8. This is the Minnesota Four-Lumen Esophagogastric Tamponade Tube for the control of bleeding from esophageal varices. Note that this tube has an additional outlet for aspiration of the esophagus. This safety feature prevents the aspiration of regurgitated gastric juice, blood, and saliva while the gastric balloon is inflated. (Davol, Inc., Cranston, R.I.)

end of the cava is anastomosed to the side of the superior mesenteric vein.

These operations are rather extensive procedures and are not always successful, because of secondary clotting in the veins used for the shunt. Nevertheless, a shunt is the only method by which a lowering of pressure in the portal system may be brought about, and since hemorrhages from the esophageal varices are often fatal, many of these relatively poor-risk patients must be subjected to these attempts to save their lives.

Postoperative Nursing Management. Bleeding anywhere in the body is upsetting and anxiety-provoking, resulting in a crisis situation for the patient and his family. If the patient is an alcoholic, behavioral problems can further complicate the situation. The nurse provides support and pertinent explanations regarding medical and nursing interventions. Monitoring the patient closely will help in detecting and managing complications.

Postoperative care is similar to that for any abdominal operation, but complications may arise, including hemodynamic shock, hepatic encephalopathy, electrolyte imbalance, metabolic and respiratory alkalosis, delirium tremens, and seizures. These procedures do not alter the course of the progressive liver disease, and bleeding may recur as new collateral vessels develop.

Hepatic Tumors

Hepatic tumors generally are cancerous in nature. It has only been in recent years that benign liver tumors have gained any significance, since their incidence has increased with the use of oral contraceptives.

As for cancerous tumors, few cancers originate in the liver. Those that are primary tumors ordinarily occur in patients with cirrhosis, especially of the postnecrotic type. Such a *hepatoma* is generally inoperable, because of rapid extension and metastasis elsewhere. *Cholangiocarcinoma* is a primary malignant tumor, usually arising in normal liver. If found early, there may be cure; however, the likelihood of early detection is small.

Metastases are found in the liver in about one-half of all late cancer cases. The primary growth may be almost anywhere, and since the bloodstream and the lymphatics from the body cavities nearly all reach the liver, malignant tumors anywhere in the trunk are likely to reach this organ eventually. Moreover, the liver apparently is an ideal place for these malignant cells to thrive. Often the first evidence of a cancer in an abdominal organ is the appearance of liver metastases, and, unless exploratory operation or autopsy is performed, the primary growth may never be discovered.

Diagnosis of malignant disease of the liver is made, regardless of the location of the primary tumor, when there is a recent loss of weight, loss of strength, and anemia, the last being the most common early symptoms of any cancer that interferes with nutrition. Abdominal pain may be present and accompanied by rapid enlargement of the liver, which on palpation presents an irregular surface. Jaundice is present only if the larger bile ducts are occluded by the pressure of malignant nodules in the hilum of the liver. Ascites occurs if such nodules obstruct the portal veins, or if tumor tissue is seeded in the peritoneal cavity.

Radiation therapy and chemotherapy have been used in the treatment of malignant disease of the liver with varying degrees of success. Although these therapies may prolong survival of some patients, the major effect is palliative.

Percutaneous biliary or transhepatic drainage has been used recently to bypass biliary ducts obstructed by liver, pancreatic, or bile duct tumors in patients with inoperable tumors or in those considered poor surgical risks. Under fluoroscopy, a catheter is inserted through the abdominal wall, past the obstruction into the duodenum. Percutaneous biliary drainage prolongs survival time and decreases discomfort from jaundice and pruritus.

Surgical Management

Successful hepatic lobectomy for cancer can be done when the primary hepatic tumor is localized or when, in the case of metastasis, the primary site can be completely excised and the metastasis is limited. Metastases to the liver, however, are rarely limited or solitary. Capitalizing on the regenerative capacity of the liver cells, some surgeons have successfully removed 90% of the liver.

Preoperative Evaluation and Preparation. As the patient is being prepared for surgery, his nutritional, fluid, emotional, and physical needs are evaluated and met. Meanwhile, he may be undergoing extensive and exhausting diagnostic studies. The support, explanation, and encouragement by the nurse will help him to achieve the most desirable level for surgery. It may be necessary to prepare the

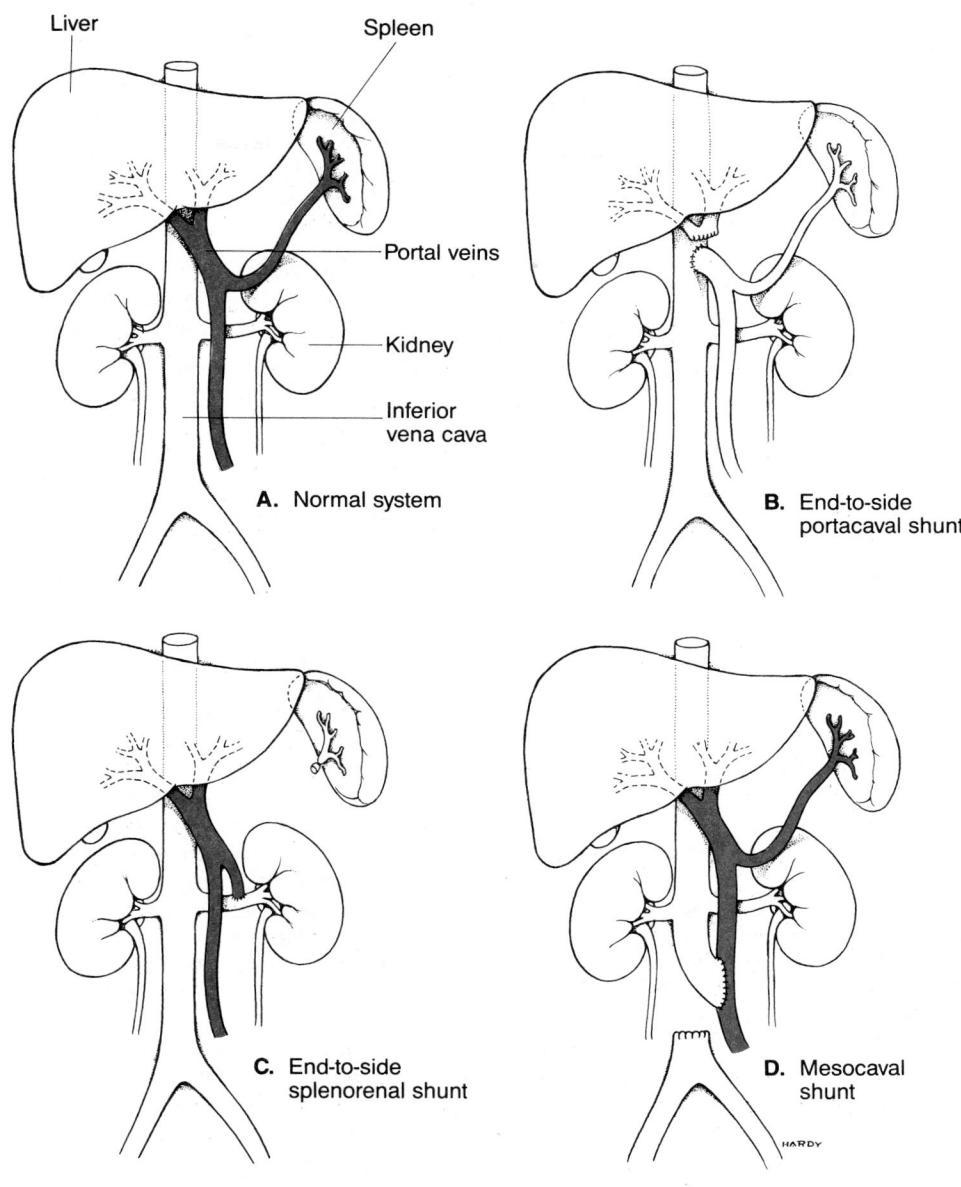

Liver   Spleen

Portal veins

Kidney

Inferior
vena cava

A. Normal system

B. End-to-side
portacaval shunt

C. End-to-side
splenorenal shunt

D. Mesocaval
shunt

HARDY

Figure 39-9. Types of portal-systemic venous shunts.

intestinal tract by way of cathartic, colonic irrigation, and intestinal antibiotics to minimize any possibility of ammonium accumulation and to anticipate the possibility of the intestines being opened at surgery. Specific studies may include liver scanning, liver biopsy, cholangiography, selective hepatic angiography, percutaneous needle biopsy, peritoneoscopy, laparoscopy, ultrasound and CT scans, and blood tests, particularly serum alkaline phosphatase and serum glutamic oxaloacetic acid.

Surgical Intervention. If it is necessary to restrict blood flow from the hepatic artery and portal vein beyond 15 minutes (under normothermic conditions, 15-minute occlusion is permissible), it is likely that hypothermia will be used.

The nurse needs to be cognizant of the anatomy referred to by the surgeon in the care of these patients. The usual true (functional) division of the liver is into two lobes, the larger (by six times) right lobe and the left lobe, with two smaller segments sandwiched between, the caudate and the quadrate (refer to anatomy textbook). Most surgeons prefer the anatomic (surgical) division of the lobes. Here the liver is divided into a right and a left lobe by a lobar fissure that is almost in line with the gallbladder bed and the inferior vena cava on the visceral surface. According to this division, the branching of hepatic vessels and the portal vein lend themselves to a more even segmentation. Obviously, a right-liver lobectomy according to the surgical division is less extensive than it would be in the functional division.

For a right-liver lobectomy or an extended right lobectomy (including medial left lobe), a thoracoabdominal incision is used. A generous abdominal incision is made for a left lobectomy.

Postsurgical Nursing Management. There are potential problems related to cardiopulmonary involvement, portal and general circulation, and respiratory and liver dysfunction. Metabolic abnormalities require careful attention. A constant infusion of 10% glucose may be required in the first 48 hours to prevent a precipitous fall in blood sugar, resulting from decreased gluconeogenesis. Protein synthesis and lipid metabolism are also altered, necessitating infusions of albumin. Extensive blood loss may occur and, as a result, the patient will receive infusions of blood and intravenous fluids. The patient requires constant attention for the first 2 or 3 days, as described for abdominal and thoracic postsurgical nursing care (see pp. 387, 461). Early ambulation is encouraged. Liver regeneration is rapid; in one patient who had a 90% resection of the liver, a normal liver mass was restored in 6 months.

Liver Abscesses

Whenever an infection develops anywhere along the gastrointestinal tract, there is danger the infecting organisms may reach the liver through the biliary system, portal venous system, or hepatic arterial or lymphatic systems. Most bacteria are promptly destroyed, but occasionally some gain a foothold. The bacterial toxins destroy the neighboring liver cells, and the necrotic tissue produced serves as a protective wall for the organisms. Meanwhile, leukocytes migrate into the infected area. The result is an abscess cavity full of a liquid containing living and dead leukocytes, liquefied liver cells, and bacteria. Pyogenic abscesses of this type may be single, or multiple and small. The result is a life-threatening disease. In the past the mortality rate was 100% due to vague clinical symptoms, inadequate diagnostic tools, and inadequate surgical drainage of the abscess.

The clinical picture is one of sepsis with few or no localizing signs. The temperature is increased and may be accompanied by chills. The patient may complain of dull abdominal pain and tenderness in the right upper quadrant of the abdomen. Hepatomegaly, jaundice, and anemia may develop. With the aid of a CT scan and a liver scan for early diagnosis, and surgical drainage of the abscess, mortality has been greatly reduced.

Treatment includes intravenous antibiotic therapy; the specific antibiotic used in treatment depends on the organism identified. Although a protozoan, *Entamoeba histolytica,* is the most common cause of liver abscess. In certain geographic areas, gram-negative bacilli have been implicated with increased frequency. Continuous supportive care is indicated because of the serious condition of the patient.

Hepatic Transplantation

Human liver transplantation has in most instances been done for life-threatening liver disease for which no other form of treatment was available. This includes biliary atresia, liver cirrhosis, and chronic aggressive hepatitis. Hepatic transplantation for treatment of malignant liver neoplasms has been abandoned for the most part because of the incidence of recurrence of malignancy in patients receiving immunosuppressive therapy.

Two types of liver transplantation have been carried out:

1. *Orthotopic*—total replacement of the liver, with anatomical reconstruction of the vasculature, or replacement of the liver with a transplant in the same area of the right upper quadrant. This is the most common procedure as it is technically easier and has been the more successful procedure.
2. *Heterotopic*—placing an auxiliary or second liver in the groin or pelvis.

The main difficulties in hepatic transplantation are technical problems causing obstruction, drug toxicity, immunochemical rejection, hepatic arterial thrombosis, or hepatic abscess. Because hepatic transplantation is performed only for severe liver disease, the patient is a poor surgical risk and frequently has many systemic problems that influence preoperative and postoperative care.

Postoperative Nursing Measures. The patient is maintained in as germ-free an environment as possible, because immunosuppressive drugs reduce the body's natural defense. The patient is monitored constantly for all cardiovascular parameters, as well as arterial pressures, blood gases, and *p*H. Respiratory assistance is provided via a mechanical ventilator. The patient is suctioned as required, and sterile humidification is provided. Rejection signs are monitored through such liver function tests as SGOT, liver scans, bilirubin, and cholangiogram. Coagulation studies indicate the functioning of the transplanted liver. Cultures of urine and blood, and throat swabs are taken frequently.

Hourly progress determines when the patient is ready to be weaned from the ventilator, when he may take oral fluids, and when physical activity may gradually be resumed.

The family members must be informed about the patient's condition at frequent intervals, since extensive care required in the immediate postoperative period minimizes their contact with the patient. Constant emotional support is needed to assist the patient to accept the fact that he has endured surgery and is slowly recovering with a new liver.

The patient and family members will require teaching about immunosuppressive drugs, signs and symptoms of rejection, and the importance of follow-up care. Despite recent advances, the incidence of long-term survival after hepatic transplantation remains low.

▷ Biliary Conditions

Several disorders affect the biliary system and interfere with normal drainage of bile into the duodenum. These disorders include carcinoma that obstructs the biliary tree and infection of the biliary system. However, gallbladder disease with gallstones is the most common disorder of the biliary system. Estimates indicate that approximately 500,000 persons a year in the United States are hospitalized for gallbladder disease and that about two thirds of these are treated surgically. Although not all occurrences of gallbladder infection (*cholecystitis*) are related to gallstones (*cholelithiasis*), 95% of patients with acute cholecystitis have gallstones. On the other hand, a majority of the 15 million Americans with gallstones have no pain and are unaware of the presence of stones.

Cholecystitis

At times the gallbladder may be the seat of an acute infection (cholecystitis) that causes acute pain, tenderness, and rigidity of the upper right abdomen, associated with nausea and vomiting and the usual signs of an acute inflammation. This condition is spoken of as *acute cholecystitis.* If the gallbladder is found to be filled with pus, there is said to be an *empyema* of the gallbladder.

Cholelithiasis

Cholelithiasis (calculi) usually form in the gallbladder from the solid constituents of bile and vary greatly in size, shape, and consistency.

Gallstones are uncommon in children and young adults but become increasingly prevalent after age 40. The incidence of cholelithiasis increases thereafter to such an extent that it has been estimated that by the age of 75, one of every three persons will have gallstones.

Pathophysiology

There are two major types of gallstones: those composed predominantly of pigment and those composed primarily of cholesterol. Pigment stones probably form when unconjugated pigments in the bile precipitate to form stones. The risk of developing such stones is increased in individuals with cirrhosis, hemolysis, and infections of the biliary tree. These stones cannot be dissolved and must be removed surgically.

Cholesterol stones account for most gallbladder disease in the United States. These stones result when bile is supersaturated with cholesterol, which precipitates out of the bile to form stones. This can occur when the liver secretes bile abnormally high in cholesterol and lacks the proper concentration and proportion of bile salts. It appears that cholesterol exists in the bile in a highly supersaturated state, so that it will later precipitate out in the gallbladder if it is not kept in solution by the right mixture of bile salts. This would indicate that the liver is the origin of the disease, rather than the gallbladder itself. Cholesterol is insoluble in water, its solubility depending on bile acids and lecithin (phospholipids). Saturated bile is a prerequisite to gallstone formation (lithogenesis). Evidence suggests there is decreased bile acid synthesis and increased cholesterol synthesis in the liver of gallstone-prone patients. This probably accounts for the increase in biliary cholesterol secretion and the lowered level of bile acids, which are necessary to dissolve cholesterol. The cholesterol-saturated bile, in addition to predisposing to the formation of gallstones, may act as an irritant and produce inflammatory changes in the gallbladder.

Four times more women than men develop cholesterol stones and gallbladder disease; they are usually over 40 years of age, multiparous, and obese. There is increased incidence of stone formation in users of oral contraceptives, estrogens, and clofibrate, which are known to increase biliary cholesterol saturation. In addition, there is increased risk because of malabsorption of bile salts in individuals with gastrointestinal disease or T-tube fistula, or in those who have had ileal resection or bypass.

▶ **Assessment**

Clinical Manifestations. Gallstones may be silent, producing no pain and only mild gastrointestinal symptoms. Such stones may be detected incidentally during surgery or diagnostic evaluation for nonrelated problems.

The patient with gallbladder disease due to gallstones may develop two types of symptoms: those due to disease of the gallbladder itself and those due to obstruction of the bile passages by a gallstone. The symptoms may be acute or chronic. Epigastric distress, such as fullness, abdominal distention, and vague pain in the right upper quadrant of the abdomen, may occur following a meal high in fried or fatty foods.

If a gallstone obstructs the cystic duct, the gallbladder becomes infected and distended. The patient develops a fever and may have a palpable abdominal mass. The patient experiences biliary colic with excruciating upper right abdominal pain that radiates to the back or right shoulder, usually associated with nausea and vomiting. These symptoms are more noticeable several hours after a heavy meal. The patient moves about restlessly, unable to find a comfortable position.

Such a bout of biliary colic is caused by contraction of the gallbladder, which has been stimulated by fat and cannot release bile because of obstruction by the stone, or calculus. When distended, the fundus of the gallbladder comes in contact with the abdominal wall in the region of the right ninth and tenth costal cartilages. This produces marked tenderness in the right upper quadrant upon deep inspiration and prevents full inspiratory excursion. The pain of acute cholecystitis may be so severe that analgesics such as meperidine hydrochloride are required; nitroglycerin has also been used effectively. Morphine sulfate is thought to increase spasm of the sphincter of Oddi and is therefore avoided.

Jaundice occurs in a small percentage of patients with gallbladder disease and usually occurs with obstruction of the common bile duct. Obstruction of the flow of bile into the duodenum results in the following characteristic symptoms: the bile, no longer carried to the duodenum, is absorbed by the blood, giving the skin and mucous membrane a yellow color. This is frequently accompanied by marked itching of the skin.

The excretion of the bile pigments by the kidneys gives the urine a very dark color. The feces, no longer colored with bile pigments, are grayish, like putty, and usually are spoken of as "clay-colored."

Obstruction of bile flow also interferes with absorption of the fat-soluble vitamins A, D, E, and K. Therefore, the patient may exhibit deficiencies of these vitamins if biliary obstruction has been prolonged. Vitamin K deficiency will interfere with normal blood clotting.

If the gallstone is dislodged and no longer obstructs the cystic duct, the gallbladder drains and the inflammatory process subsides after a relatively short time. If the gallstone continues to obstruct the duct, abscess, necrosis, and perforation with generalized peritonitis may result.

Diagnostic Assessment

Abdominal X-ray.   An abdominal x-ray may reveal radiopaque stones containing calcium in the gallbladder. In addition, other changes in the gallbladder may be visualized. This x-ray requires no special preparation of the patient other than an explanation of the procedure.

Cholecystography.   Radiologic examination of the gallbladder is carried out for the detection of gallstones and to estimate the ability of the gallbladder to fill, concentrate its contents, contract, and empty in normal fashion. Very few gallstones are sufficiently radiopaque to be visualized by ordinary roentgenographic technique; they must be demonstrated as negative shadows in a gallbladder filled with a radiopaque substance. To demonstrate this, iodide-containing dye that is excreted into the bile by the liver and concentrated in the gallbladder is administered to the patient, either by mouth or by intravenous injection.

Note: Oral or intravenous cholecystography in the obviously jaundiced patient is a waste of time, since the liver cells will not transport dye to the biliary tract in a jaundiced individual. This is important to the nurse, since the physician's requests may be written before obvious jaundice develops; if jaundice occurs, the nurse can inform the physician of this fact.

Drugs given as contrast media include Telepaque, Cholografin, and Oragrafin.* These preparations are given in oral doses of 2 g to 3 g, 10 to 12 hours before x-ray study. Intravenous cholecystography involves the injection of an iodide approximately 10 minutes prior to roentgenography. During the interval between the administration of the iodide and the x-ray study, the patient is permitted nothing by mouth, lest the gallbladder be stimulated to contract and thereby expel the contrast medium.

A repeat of the oral cholecystogram with a second dose of the contrast medium may be necessary if the gallbladder is not visualized on the first attempt.

Nursing Considerations.   Instructions to patients who are scheduled for x-ray studies of the gallbladder (cholecystogram; gallbladder series) include:

1. One hour or more after the evening meal, and approximately 10 hours before roentgenography, the patient receives tablets or capsules of contrast medium by mouth.
2. These tablets are to be ingested as per directions, together with a volume of water totaling at least 8 ounces.
3. The patient then is to receive nothing by mouth, except water, until bedtime. Thereafter, until the roentgenogram is taken, not even water is permitted. If the patient vomits after the ingestion of the dye, the physician may

---

* Telepaque = iopanoic acid; Cholografin Meglumine = iodipamide meglumine; Oragrafin = sodium ipodate.

---

suggest that the medication be given after nausea subsides, or the test may be postponed.
4. Laxatives are not to be given during this preparation period.
5. A saline enema may be administered early in the morning of the test.
6. Breakfast is omitted.

Procedure.   The right upper abdominal quadrant then is photographed by x-ray. If the gallbladder has filled and concentrated the dye normally, it is seen as a pear-shaped shadow from 5 cm to 7.5 cm (2–3 inches) long, under the right costal margin. If stones are present, there are mottled densities within this shadow corresponding to their outlines. Although not part of the routine cholecystogram, a fatty meal or cholecystokinin may be given to the patient and x-rays repeated to assess emptying of the gallbladder. If the gallbladder is found to fill and empty normally and to contain no stones, it is concluded that no gallbladder disease is present. If gallbladder disease is present, the gallbladder may not be visualized because of obstruction by gallstones. If the gallbladder is visualized, shadows of gallstones may be present.

Percutaneous Transhepatic Cholangiography.   The oral and the intravenous radiographic techniques just described permit the visualization of the gallbladder (and occasionally the larger ducts) only if the liver cells are functioning properly and are capable of excreting the radiopaque dye into the bile. Percutaneous transhepatic cholangiography, which involves the injection of dye directly into the biliary tree itself, is effective, regardless of the state of liver function. Moreover, because of the relatively large concentration of dye that is introduced into the biliary system, all components of the latter, including the hepatic ducts within the liver, the common hepatic duct throughout its length, the cystic duct, and the gallbladder, are delineated with clarity.

This procedure is useful in distinguishing jaundice caused by liver disease (hepatocellular jaundice) from that due to biliary obstruction; for investigating the gastrointestinal symptoms of patients whose gallbladders have been removed; for locating stones within the bile ducts; and in diagnosing cancer involving the biliary system.

Procedure.   The patient, fasting and well sedated, lies supine on the x-ray table. The injection site, usually in the midclavicular line immediately beneath the right costal margin, is disinfected and anesthetized with lidocaine (Xylocaine). A small incision is made at this point and a thin, flexible needle with stylet is inserted cephalad, posteriorly at a 45-degree angle and parallel to the midline. When the needle has penetrated to a depth of approximately 10 cm (4 inches), the stylet is removed and replaced by a plastic connector tube with 50-ml syringe attached. Gentle suction is applied while the needle is slowly withdrawn, until bile appears in the syringe. As much bile as possible is withdrawn, a radiopaque dye is injected, and an x-ray picture taken. Before the needle is removed as much dye and bile as possible are aspirated in order to forestall subsequent leakage into the needle tract and eventually into the peritoneal cavity, thus avoiding the possibility of bile peritonitis.

Endoscopic Retrograde Cholangiopancreatography. A new endoscopic procedure permits direct visualization of structures once available only during laparotomy. Endoscopic retrograde cholangiopancreatography (ERCP) involves insertion of a flexible fiberoptic endoscope into the esophagus to the descending duodenum (Fig. 39-10). The common bile duct and pancreatic duct are cannulated, and contrast material is injected into the ducts, permitting visualization and evaluation of the biliary tree. ERCP also permits direct visualization of these structures and access to the distal common bile duct to retrieve a retained gallstone.

Nursing Considerations. The procedure requires a cooperative patient to permit insertion of the endoscope without damage to the gastrointestinal tract. Prior to the procedure, the patient needs an adequate explanation of the procedure and his role in it. He receives sedation immediately prior to the procedure. During ERCP, the nurse may be called upon to monitor intravenous fluids, administer medications, and position the patient. Following the procedure, the nurse monitors the patient's condition, observing vital signs and checking for signs of perforation or infection. The nurse also monitors the patient for side-effects of any medications received during the procedure and return of the patient's gag reflex following the use of local anesthetics.

Ultrasonography. The use of ultrasound is based on reflected sound waves detected in this noninvasive test. It does not depend on gallbladder or liver function; therefore, it can be used for jaundiced or pregnant patients, or for those allergic to gallbladder contrast medium. Ultrasonography can detect a dilated common bile duct or calculi in the gallbladder. It is reported to detect gallstones with 95% accuracy.

Patient Problems/Nursing Diagnoses

Based on the clinical manifestations and diagnostic assessment data, the major nursing problems of the patient with gallbladder disease include pain related to obstruction of the biliary system, and inflammation and distention of the gallbladder; and dietary intolerance related to inadequate bile secretion. The patient undergoing surgery for treatment of the gallbladder disease also experiences problems related to abdominal surgery, including potential respiratory problems because of the high abdominal incision made for cholecystectomy, and possible complications related to altered biliary drainage.

▶ Planning and Implementation

Goals

The patient's goals are:

1. Relief of pain
2. Relief of dietary intolerance
3. Absence of respiratory complications
4. Absence of complications of altered biliary drainage related to surgical intervention

The major objectives of therapy are to reduce the incidence of acute attacks of gallbladder pain and cholecystitis by supportive and dietary management, and, if possible, to remove the cause of cholecystitis by pharmacotherapy or surgical intervention.

Supportive and Dietary Management. Approximately 80% of patients with acute gallbladder inflammation achieve a remission with rest, intravenous fluids, nasogastric suction, analgesia, and antibiotics. Unless the patient's condition deteriorates, surgical intervention is delayed until the patient's acute symptoms subside and complete evaluation can be carried out.

The diet, immediately after an attack, is usually limited to low-fat liquids. Powdered supplements high in protein and carbohydrate can be stirred into skim milk. The following may then be added as tolerated: cooked fruits, rice or tapioca, lean meats, mashed potatoes, non-gas-forming veg-

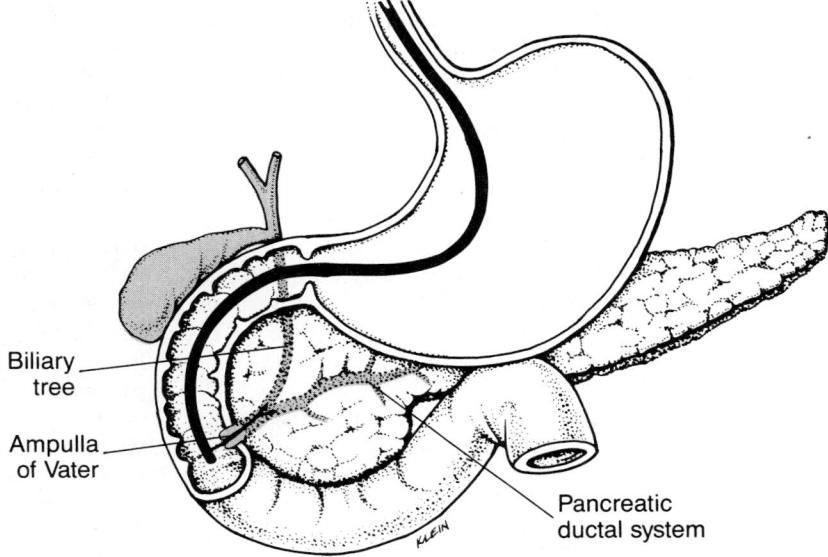

Figure 39-10. Via a side-viewing fiberoptic duodenoscope, the ampulla of Vater is catheterized and the biliary tree injected with contrast material. The pancreatic ductal system is also assessed, if indicated. This procedure is of special value in ampullary or periampullary neoplasms, which may be simultaneously visualized and biopsied. Acute pancreatitis is a contraindication. (Redrawn from Misra PS and Bank S: Gallbladder disease: guide to diagnosis. Hosp Med 1982 Feb; p 136.)

Chart 39-4
Terminology

Cholecystitis—inflammation of the gallbladder
Cholelithiasis—calculi in the gallbladder
Cholecystectomy—removal of the gallbladder
Cholecystostomy—opening and drainage of the
    gallbladder
Choledochotomy—opening into the common duct,
    usually to remove duct stones
Choledocholithiasis—stones in the common duct
Choledocholithotomy—removal of stones in the
    common duct
Choledochoduodenostomy—anastomosis of common
    duct to duodenum
Choledochojejunostomy—anastomosis of common
    duct to jejunum

etables, bread, coffee, or tea. Avoid eggs, cream, pork, fried foods, cheese and rich dressings, gas-forming vegetables, and alcohol. The patient needs to be reminded that fatty foods may bring on an attack.

Dietary management may be the major mode of therapy in those patients who have experienced only dietary intolerance to fatty foods and vague gastrointestinal symptoms.

Pharmacotherapy. Chenodeoxycholic acid (chenodiol or CDCA) has been effective in dissolving about 60% of radiolucent gallstones composed primarily of cholesterol. The mechanism of action seems to be the inhibition of liver synthesis and secretion of cholesterol, thereby desaturating bile. Existing stones can be decreased in size, small ones dissolved, and new stones prevented from forming. The therapy is most effective if the stones are small. The effective dose of chenodiol depends on body weight.

Certain other medications, such as estrogens, oral contraceptives, clofibrate, and dietary cholesterol, may adversely affect the results of treatment with chenodeoxycholic acid. If the patient is taking these drugs, the physician should be made aware of this.

Cholesterol stones may recur in a small percentage of patients after chenodeoxycholic acid is terminated; therefore, a low dose of this drug may be continued to prevent recurrence. Patients' adherence to this mode of therapy requires further study and follow-up.

If acute symptoms of cholecystitis continue or recur, pharmacotherapy is inappropriate as a substitute for surgery, and surgical intervention is indicated.

Surgical Management

Surgical treatment of gallbladder disease and gallstones is necessary for the relief of long-continued symptoms, for the removal of the cause of biliary colic, and for treatment of acute cholecystitis. Surgery may be elective when the patient's symptoms have subsided or may be performed as an emergency procedure if the patient's condition necessitates it.

Preoperative Management. In addition to x-ray studies of the gallbladder, chest x-rays, electrocardiogram, and liver function tests (see Table 39-1) may be performed. Vitamin K may be administered if the patient's prothrombin level is low. If the level is unusually low, a fresh blood transfusion may be given before surgery is done to supply ingredients necessary for blood clotting.

Nutritional requirements are considered; if the patient is not eating properly, it may be necessary to provide intravenous glucose with protein hydrolysate supplements. This will aid wound healing and help prevent liver damage.

Preparation for a gallbladder operation is the same as for any upper abdominal laparotomy. Instruction and explanation are given the day before surgery with regard to turning and deep breathing. Because the abdominal incision is high on the abdomen (subcostal), the patient is often reluctant to move and turn; pneumonia and atelectasis are possible postoperative complications that are to be avoided by breathing deeply and by turning. Since drainage tubes are usually required after operation, the patient should be informed of this, so that he knows what to expect. The patient should also be informed about the likelihood of nasogastric suction during the immediate postoperative period.

Surgical Intervention. Patients usually are placed on the operating table with the upper abdomen raised somewhat by an air pillow or sandbag to make the biliary area more accessible.

Cholecystectomy. In this operation, the gallbladder is removed after ligation of the cystic duct and artery. The operation is performed in most cases of acute and chronic cholecystitis.

Choledochostomy. In this operation, an incision is made into the common duct for removal of stones. After the stones have been evacuated, a tube usually is inserted into the duct for drainage. The gallbladder also contains stones and, as a rule, a cholecystectomy is performed at the same time.

Cholecystostomy. This operation is performed when the patient's condition prevents more extensive surgery or when an acute inflammatory reaction obscures the biliary system. The gallbladder is opened, the stones and the bile or the pus are removed, and a tube is sutured in the opening for drainage. As soon as the patient is returned to bed, the nurse should connect this tube to a drainage bottle placed at the side of the bed. Failure to do this may result in the leakage of bile around the tube and in its escape into the peritoneal cavity. Following recovery from the acute episode, the patient may return to surgery for cholecystectomy.

Postoperative Nursing Management. As soon as the patient has recovered from anesthesia, he is placed in the low Fowler's position. Fluids may be given by vein, and nasogastric suction (tube probably inserted immediately prior to surgery) may be instituted to relieve distention. Water and other fluids may be given in about 24 hours, and a soft diet started later, after bowel sounds return.

The location of the subcostal incision is likely to cause the patient to splint the operative site by inadvertently taking shallow breaths to prevent pain. Since full aeration of the lungs is necessry to prevent respiratory complications, analgesics should be given as prescribed and the patient encouraged to turn, cough, and breathe deeply at frequent intervals.

Drainage. As mentioned before, in patients who have undergone a cholecystostomy or choledochostomy, the drainage tubes must be connected immediately to a drainage receptacle. In addition, tubing should be fastened to the dressings or to the bottom sheet, with enough leeway for the patient to move without dislodging it. The patient must know why he cannot roll onto the tube and that it must remain patent at all times.

Following a cholecystectomy, a drain (Penrose) is placed in the gallbladder bed and brought out through a stab wound. Drainage of blood, serosanguineous fluids, and bile are absorbed by dressings, which are changed as required. Montgomery straps are helpful in maintaining a comfortable dressing.

After a cholecystostomy, a tube is placed in the gallbladder and fixed in position by a purse-string suture. This is connected to a gravity drainage tube and a receptacle.

In a choledochostomy, after the bile duct has been explored, dilated, and relieved of stones, a T tube is positioned in the common duct to permit drainage of bile until edema subsides. This tube is connected to gravity drainage tubing.

Following these surgical procedures, the patient is observed for indications of infection, leakage of bile into the peritoneal cavity, and obstruction of bile drainage. If bile is not draining properly, an obstruction is probably causing bile to be forced back into the liver and bloodstream. Since jaundice may result, the nurse should be particularly observant of the color of the sclerae. The nurse should also note and report right upper quadrant abdominal pain, nausea and vomiting, bile drainage around the T tube, clay-colored stools, and a change in vital signs.

Bile may continue to drain from the drainage tract in considerable quantities for a time, necessitating frequent changes of the outer dressings and protection of the skin from irritation. Skin pastes of zinc oxide, aluminum, or petrolatum prevent the bile from literally digesting the skin.

In order to prevent total loss of bile, the drainage tube or collecting receptacle may be elevated above the level of the abdomen, so that bile drains through the apparatus only if pressure develops in the duct system. The bile collected should be measured and recorded every 24 hours, its color and character being documented. After several days of drainage, the tubes may be clamped for an hour before and after each meal, the purpose being to deliver bile to the duodenum to aid in digestion. Within 7 to 14 days, the drainage tubes are removed from the gallbladder or common bile duct.

Careful Monitoring. In all patients with biliary drainage, the stools should be observed daily and their color recorded. Specimens of both urine and feces may be sent to the laboratory for examination for bile pigments. In this way, it is possible to determine that the bile pigment is disappearing from the blood and is draining again into the duodenum. A careful record of fluid intake and output is kept and totaled for each 24 hours.

Nutritional Needs. The diet of these patients may be low in fats and high in carbohydrates and proteins. The patients themselves usually refuse to eat fatty foods because of the nausea that follows.

Preventing Complications. These patients are especially prone to pulmonary complications, as are all patients with upper abdominal incisions. Thus, they should be taught to take deep breaths every hour to aerate the lungs fully. Other complications, such as thrombophlebitis and pulmonary atelectasis, may be avoided by promoting early ambulation as soon as permissible. Such complications are more likely to occur in the more obese patient. An abdominal binder may help to make the patient comfortable when he first gets out of bed. Since a drainage receptacle is attached when the patient is ambulating, the collecting bag may be placed in a bathrobe pocket or fastened so that it is below the waist or common duct level.

Patient Education. Usually, there are no special dietary instructions, other than to maintain a nutritious diet and avoid excessive fats. Fat restriction usually is lifted in 4 to 6 weeks when biliary ducts dilate to accommodate the volume of bile once held by the gallbladder, and when the ampulla of Vater again functions effectively. After this, when one eats fat, adequate bile will be released into the digestive tract to emulsify the fats and allow their digestion. Prior to this, fats would not be completely or adequately digested in some persons, and flatulence might occur. However, the purpose of gallbladder surgery is to allow for a normal diet, ultimately.

The patient should know what medications are required (vitamins, anticholinergics, and antispasmodics) and why they are given. He also should be aware of symptoms that are reportable to his physician—jaundice, dark urine, pale-colored stools, pruritus, or signs of inflammation, such as pain or fever.

Some patients note "looseness of the bowels," consisting of one to three bowel movements a day—the reason being a continual trickle of bile through the choledocho-duodenal junction following cholecystectomy. Usually, such frequency diminishes over a period of a few weeks to several months. Follow-up visits are essential for this patient.

▶ **Evaluation**

Expected Outcomes

1. Achieves relief of pain
   a. Reports decrease in pain of cholecystitis and cholelithiasis, and absence of postoperative incisional pain
   b. Splints abdominal incision to decrease pain
   c. Avoids foods that cause pain
   d. Uses postoperative analgesia as prescribed
   e. Utilizes appropriate preventive activities when pain-free postoperatively (*e.g.,* turns, coughs, breathes deeply, ambulates)
2. Obtains relief of dietary intolerance
   a. Maintains adequate dietary intake
   b. Avoids foods that cause gastrointestinal symptoms
   c. Reports decreased incidence or absence of nausea, vomiting, diarrhea, flatulence, and abdominal discomfort

3. Is free of respiratory complications
   a. Is free of temperature elevation, cough, and increased respiratory rate
   b. Demonstrates full respiratory excursion with deep inspiration and expiration
   c. Coughs effectively, using pillow to splint abdominal incision
   d. Uses postoperative analgesia as prescribed
   e. Exercises as prescribed (*e.g.,* turns, ambulates)
4. Is free of complications related to altered biliary drainage
   a. Is free of temperature elevation, abdominal pain, change in vital signs, or drainage around drainage tube
   b. Exhibits or reports gradual decrease in bile drainage
   c. Reports skin, mucous membranes, stool, and urine to be of normal color
   d. Demonstrates that skin around T tube or drainage tube is intact and free of excoriation
   e. Identifies signs and symptoms of biliary obstruction to be noted and reported
   f. Has serum bilirubin level within normal range

▷ Bibliography

Books

Koff RS. Liver Disease in Primary Care Medicine. New York, Appleton–Century–Crofts, 1980.

Orr ME, Shinert J, and Gross J. Acute Pancreatic and Hepatic Dysfunction. Bethany, Connecticut, Fleschner, 1981.

Schiff L and Schiff ER. Diseases of the Liver. Philadelphia, JB Lippincott, 1982.

Triger DR. Practical Management of Liver Disease. Boston, Blackwell Scientific Publications, 1981.

Articles
General

Alpert E and Jackson D. Besides the liver, what does the virus of hepatitis attack? Heart Lung 1982 Mar–Apr; 11(2):177–180.

Brown M. New internal bile drain prolongs lives. RN 1982 Jan; 45(1):46–47.

Dougherty WM. Serum bilirubin. Nursing '82 1982 Nov; 12(11):138–139.

Garvey ED and Manganaro M. Nursing implications of hepatic artery infusion. Cancer Nurs 1982 Feb; 5(1):51–55.

Gitnick G. Assessment of liver function. Surg Clin North Am 1982 Feb; 61(1):197–207.

Howard PH, Raebel M, and Hurley DL. The use of antimicrobial agents in patients with hepatic and renal dysfunction. Surg Clin North Am 1982 Apr; 62(2):333–340.

Myers MB. Jaundice. Nurs Pract 1981 Apr; 6(2):8, 10, 12, 27.

Jackson BS and Carlisle PM. How post-op complications can burgeon into crisis. RN 1981 Jan; 44(1):26–32.

Liver Dysfunction

Ali AS and Baig FN. Hepatorenal syndrome. Am Fam Physician 1982 June; 25(6):127–131.

Alcoff J. Viral hepatitis. J Fam Pract 1982 July; 15(1):141–162.

Alpert E and Jackson D. Besides the liver, what does the virus of hepatitis attack? Heart Lung 1982 Mar–Apr; 11(2):177–180.

Bryan JA. Viral hepatitis. 1. Clinical and laboratory aspects and epidemiology. Postgrad Med 1980 Nov; 68(5):66–76.

Bryan JA. Viral hepatitis. 2. Prevention and Control. Postgrad Med 1980 Nov; 68(5):81–86.

Favero MS, Maynard JE, and Leger RT. Prevention and control of infections in specialized areas—viral hepatitis. Crit Care Quart 1980 Dec; 3(3):43–55.

Hepatitis B vaccine. The Medical Letter 1982 Aug 20; 24(616):75–76.

Inactivated hepatitis B virus vaccine. Morbidity and Mortality Weekly Reports 1982 June 25; 32(24):317–328.

Mar DD. New hepatitis B vaccine: A breakthrough in hepatitis prevention. Am J Nurs 1982 Feb; 82(2):306–307.

Misra P. Hepatic encephalopathy. Med Clin North Am 1981 Jan; 65(1):209–226.

Nachbauer CA and Fischer JE. The failing liver. Surg Clin North Am 1981 Feb; 61(1):221–230.

Neuman HH. Hepatitis A, B and N: Some practical aspects. Conn Med 1981 Nov; 45(11):713–715.

Taylor PD. Liver transplantation. Am J Nurs 1981 Sept; 81(9):1672–1673.

Thompson MA. Managing the patient with liver dysfunction. Nursing '81 1981 Nov; 11(11):101–107.

Bleeding Esophageal Varices

Gruber M and Nuwer N. Treating esophageal varices with injection sclerotherapy. Am J Nurs 1982 Aug; 82(8):1214–1216.

Gusberg R. Shunts for variceal hemorrhage: Why? when? what? Surg Clin North Am 1980 Oct; 60(5):1265–1272.

Matory WE, Sedgwick CE, and Rossi RL. Nonshunting procedures in management of bleeding esophageal varices. Surg Clin North Am 1980 Apr; 60(2):281–295.

Sax FL and Cooperman AM. Bleeding esophageal varices. Surg Clin North Am 1981 Feb; 61(1):209–219.

Gallbladder Disease

Beck ML. Preparing your patient physically for an esophagogastroduodenoscopy. Nursing '81 1981 Feb; 11(2):15–16.

Gracie WA and Ransohoff DF. The natural history of silent gallstones. N Engl J Med 1982 Sept; 307(13):798–800.

Jackson BS and Carlisle PM. How post-op complications can burgeon into crisis. RN 1981 Jan; 41(1):26–32.

Misra PS and Bank S. Gallbladder disease: Guide to diagnosis. Hospital Medicine 1982 Feb; 18(2):109–111, 116, 121–125, 128–131, 135, 138.

Pimstone NR and Mok HYI. Current status of medical treatment of gallstones. Surg Clin North Am 1981 Aug; 61(4):865–874.

Rossi RL, Gordon M, and Braasch JW. Intubation techniques in biliary tract surgery. Surg Clin North Am 1980 Apr; 60(2):297–312.

Stiklorius C. Two diagnostic procedures that demand your all-out care. RN 1982 Aug; 42(8):64–65.

Thorpe CJ and Caprini JA. Gallbladder disease: Current trends and treatment. Am J Nurs 1980 Dec; 80(12):2181–2185.

Agencies

American Digestive Disease Society, 7720 Wisconsin Ave., Bethesda, Maryland 20814

Canadian Foundation for Ileitis and Colitis, 294 Spadina Ave. Toronto, Ontario M5T 2E7, Canada

National Foundation for Ileitis and Colitis Inc., 295 Madison Ave., New York, New York 10017

National Institute of Arthritis, Metabolism and Digestive Diseases, National Institutes of Health, Bethesda, Maryland 20205

United Ostomy Association, 1111 Wilshire Blvd., Los Angeles, California 90017

40

Assessment and Management of Patients With Diabetes Mellitus

▷ Overview

Diabetes mellitus is now defined as a genetically heterogenous group of disorders that are characterized by glucose intolerance. Previously defined as a chronic multisystem disorder characterized by hyperglycemia caused by insulin insufficiency or inadequate insulin action, the new definition reflects the latest research findings in epidemiology, genetics, virology, immunology, and biochemistry. This new knowledge has not negated the old definition. Rather, it has pointed out how little we knew about this complex disease. Diabetes is characterized by disorders in the metabolism of carbohydrate, protein, fat, and insulin, as well as the structure and function of blood vessels. These abnormalities account for both the acute as well as the chronic complications of the disease.

Types of Diabetes

New research has indicated more than one cause of diabetes and much diversity of definition, expression, and disease course. In order to develop an international standard for naming, defining, and classifying diabetes according to present day knowledge, the National Institutes of Health convened an international group of experts in 1978. Conditions formerly called diabetes were reclassified in order to:

- Eliminate the confusion of terminology and diagnosis
- Remove the psychological and socioeconomic labels from persons they harm rather than help
- Standardize research reporting
- Assist in more accurate diagnosis

The new classification system was finally adopted by the American, British, Australian, and European diabetes associations in 1979. The major groups are now labelled as follows:

    Type I—Insulin-dependent Diabetes Mellitus (IDDM)
    Type II—Noninsulin-dependent Diabetes Mellitus (NIDDM)

Impaired Glucose Tolerance (IGT)
Gestational Diabetes Mellitus (GDM)
Diabetes mellitus associated with other conditions or syndromes

Table 40-1 summarizes the major categories, current terminology, old labels, and major clinical characteristics. It is important to recognize that this classification is dynamic rather than static in two ways. First, as research findings become available, it appears that there are many differences among individuals within each category. Second, with time, patients may move from one category to another. For example, a gestational diabetic, after delivery, may move into the insulin-dependent (type I) category. These types also differ in their etiology, clinical course, management, and long-term complications.

There may be defects at various cellular levels involving the production and utilization of insulin. These are usually categorized as:

1. Prereceptor causes
   - Defective insulin molecule
   - Incomplete conversion of proinsulin to insulin
   - Circulating insulin antagonists
2. Receptor causes
   - Decreased insulin binding to receptor
3. Postreceptor causes
   - Defect in effector systems distal to receptor binding

Etiology and Incidence

The etiology of the disease is not completely understood, and there are probably multiple etiologies within each type, varying from patient to patient. In type I (insulin-dependent) diabetes, it is felt that genetics and viruses or an autoimmune response, alone or in combination, are involved. However, in type II (noninsulin-dependent) diabetes, genetics and obesity play a more significant role.

Genetic Factors. Diabetes has always been thought of as a genetic or inherited disease. To date, no single mode of inheritance can explain all the types of diabetes adequately. In fact, all of the mendelian modes of inheritance have been proposed. Different types of diabetes may be inherited in different ways in different families—"genetic heterogeneity."

The search for a genetic marker for diabetes has important implications for the understanding of the inheritance of diabetes. Recent work done with the human leukocyte antigen (HLA) system that is used in tissue typing has demonstrated a relationship with some HLA antigens and diabetes. Certain of these antigens are consistently found in insulin-dependent diabetes. Some researchers have observed a relationship between various HLA antigens and those diabetic persons with long-term complications. Although much of this work is still inconclusive, it appears that having certain HLA patterns increases a person's risk for developing diabetes. It may be possible in the future to identify potential diabetic persons by these markers and then attempt to offset the disease itself.

Viral Factors. Although viruses have been associated with diabetes for more than 100 years, it was not until 1965

that viral research increased significantly. The genetic makeup of cells in an individual probably determines whether the virus can attach itself to the cell surface, enter the cell, and change its metabolism.

The characteristically abrupt appearance of insulin-dependent diabetes could be the result of an infection with a diabetogenic virus in a person already genetically predisposed. The infection might cause an autoimmune (antigen–antibody) reaction. Other diseases of self-destruction have been known for some time. For instance, thyroiditis is a disease in which an infection of the thyroid gland causes the body to produce antibodies against its own thyroid gland. As mentioned earlier, islet cell antibodies have been found in at least 50% of all insulin-dependent diabetics.

The evidence for a viral cause of diabetes comes *indirectly* from epidemiologic studies, and more directly and recently from clinical cases. Insulin-dependent diabetes more commonly occurs in late autumn and early spring, typical viral (flu) seasons. Since it occurs abruptly and at a time of year when viral infections are frequent, a diabetogenic virus could cause insulin-dependent diabetes. It is now felt that this type of diabetes in many, if not most, cases is related to an environmental cause (*i.e.,* viruses that perhaps cause an autoimmune destruction of the person's own beta cells).

Some viral strains cause the death of beta cells in genetically susceptible animals. Not until 1979 was there *direct* evidence. A young boy who became comatose after 3 days of a flulike illness died of ketoacidosis. Autopsy showed that many beta cells were destroyed and that Coxsackie B4 virus was located in the islet cells of the pancreas. When the virus was cultured and injected into genetically susceptible animals, it caused a lethal ketoacidosis. In order for insulin-dependent diabetes to develop, at least 90% of the individual's beta cells must stop producing insulin. This could result from one very strong viral attack, or it could be the result of a series of viral infections that eventually destroy the beta cells.

There is apparently no relationship between viruses and the etiology of noninsulin-dependent diabetes. Antibodies against one of the suspected viruses, Coxsackie B4, have been found in the blood of newly diagnosed insulin-dependent diabetics and not in noninsulin-dependent diabetics.

Evidence that suggests a viral cause for insulin-dependent diabetes includes the following:

1. It usually occurs in young people, whose systems are more prone to viral infections.
2. It occurs suddenly, like viral infections.
3. It occurs when viral infections are prevalent.
4. Beta cells are inflamed early in the viral infection.
5. A viral infection develops before the diabetes develops.
6. It often develops in a child with no family history of diabetes.

Since less than 0.2% of the population has insulin-dependent diabetes and it is not known what percentage of these are caused by a virus, it appears that there is much research to be done. There are at least 20 other viruses besides Coxsackie B4 that have been associated with the

Table 40-1
Classification of Diabetes Mellitus and Related Glucose Intolerances

New Category	Old Names	Clinical Characteristics	Nursing Implications
Type I: Insulin-dependent diabetes mellitus (IDDM) (5%–10% of all diabetics)	Juvenile diabetes Juvenile-onset diabetes (JOD) Ketosis-prone diabetes Brittle diabetes	Any age, but usually young Mostly thin at diagnosis	Critical to maintain normal-range blood sugars
		Causes may be genetic or viral but probably involve abnormal immune responses	Potential future vaccine (?) for immunization of susceptible individuals
		Often have islet cell antibodies	
		Little or no endogenous insulin	Essential to monitor status of blood sugar during day for good control
		Need injections to preserve life	Knowledge emphasis on: • Relationship between food and exercise in controlling blood sugar • Adjusting insulin • Interpreting urine and blood tests
			Skills emphasis on: • Insulin administration • Urine/blood testing for sugar • Pump care
		Ketosis-prone	Life-threatening situation, crucial for patient to detect or prevent
			Peer pressure during adolescence and adulthood regarding compliance with diet, insulin, and testing
Type II: Noninsulin-dependent diabetes mellitus (NIDDM) (90%–95% of all diabetics: nonobese—20% of type II; obese—80% of type II)	Adult-onset diabetes Maturity-onset diabetes Ketosis-resistant diabetes Stable diabetes Maturity-onset diabetes of youth (MODY)	Any age, usually over 40 but occasionally under 21	Very important to maintain normal-range blood sugars
		Causes may be genetic or obesity	Weight reduction crucial, but problems with motivation and compliance
		Mostly obese at diagnosis	
		No islet cell antibodies	
		Varying amounts of endogenous insulin, often higher than normal levels present	Monitoring of urine for sugar less reliable with age, since urine sugar threshold changes
		May need insulin to avoid hyperglycemia	Often overused as treatment; if used inappropriately, increases obesity
		Rare ketosis, except in stress or infection	Less life-threatening than type I, but majority of diabetics in this class
Impaired glucose tolerance (IGT)	Asymptomatic diabetes Chemical diabetes Subclinical diabetes Borderline diabetes Latent diabetes	Blood glucose levels between normal and that of diabetes Above-normal susceptibility to atherosclerotic disease Renal and retinal complications usually not significant	Both obese and nonobese should be screened periodically for diabetes, but obese should reduce weight

(continued)

Table 40-1
Classification of Diabetes Mellitus and Related Glucose Intolerances (continued)

New Category	Old Names	Clinical Characteristics	Nursing Implications
Gestational diabetes (GDM)	Gestational diabetes	Begins or is recognized during or after pregnancy Above-normal risk of perinatal complications	Usually highly motivated to maintain normal blood sugars because of baby
		Glucose intolerance transitory, but frequently recurs: • 50% go on to develop overt diabetes within 15 years • 80% go on to develop overt diabetes after 20 years, particularly postmenopausal	Nursing challenge—keep or reduce weight to ideal; may delay onset
Diabetes mellitus associated with other conditions or syndromes	Secondary diabetes	Accompanied by conditions known or suspected to cause the disease: pancreatic or hormonal, drug or chemical toxicity, abnormal insulin receptors, certain genetic syndromes	See above for type I or II
Previous abnormality of glucose tolerance (PrevAGT)	Latent diabetes Prediabetes	Previous history of hyperglycemia Current normal glucose metabolism	Periodic screening of blood glucose, probably yearly after age 40 or if symptoms develop
Potential abnormality of glucose tolerance (PotAGT)	Potential diabetes Prediabetes	No history of glucose intolerance Likely to become diabetic: • Positive family history • Evidence of islet cell antibodies • Mothers of babies over 9 lb at birth • Pima Indians • Obese	Maintain or reduce to ideal weight (same as above—PrevAGT)

development of insulin-dependent diabetes—a fact that can make vaccine development difficult. These viral infections that lead to diabetes might be prevented if the type of virus causing beta cell damage can be isolated and if it can be proven that viruses are more than a minor cause of diabetes.

Combined Factors. Heredity, viruses, and an autoimmune response may contribute, either singly or in combination, to the development of insulin-dependent diabetes. Heredity appears to be the least important contributor. Heredity and obesity contribute to the development of non-insulin-dependent diabetes. Heredity in this type of diabetes is more significant than in the insulin-dependent type.

Although the exact mechanism of inheritance has not yet been explained, blood relatives of known diabetics should maintain life-long vigilance for this condition. Other people susceptible to diabetes include obese persons and mothers who have delivered large babies. These people and

other high-risk individuals (Chart 40-1) should be examined regularly for evidences of diabetes.

Epidemiology. Diabetes mellitus is a long-term illness that afflicts about 5% of Americans. It is estimated that another 5% are undiagnosed. The disease occurs with greater prevalence after the age of 40. It is the third leading cause of death by disease and is increasing at a rate of 6% yearly. Diabetes is the leading cause of new cases of blindness in the United States today. Mortality from diabetes mellitus is primarily from cardiovascular and renal disease. Kidney disease (nephropathy) is 17 times more common among diabetics than nondiabetics. This complication accounts for 50% of the deaths in insulin-dependent diabetics. The incidence of heart disease and stroke is doubled for diabetics. Morbidity is a result of these complications, as well as diabetic neuropathy. Impotence, found in more than one half of all male diabetics, is usually the result of neuropathy.

The economic cost of diabetes, without taking the complications into consideration, is more than 5 billion dollars yearly and is increasing each year.

Pathophysiology

Diabetes mellitus is a disease resulting from a breakdown in the body's ability to produce or utilize insulin. Insulin is a powerful hormone secreted by the beta cells in the islets of Langerhans of the pancreas. It plays a major role in the metabolic processes of the body by controlling the storage and metabolism of ingested metabolic fuels. Following a meal, the secretion of insulin facilitates the uptake, utilization, and storage of glucose, amino acids, and fat. It promotes the storage of glycogen in the liver, the utilization of glucose in the muscles, and the storage of fat in adipose tissues by enhancing the transport of glucose across the cell membrane. Insulin regulates the level of blood glucose, which is formed from ingested carbohydrates or from the conversion of amino acids and fatty acids to glucose by the liver (gluconeogenesis).

In the well person the rate at which insulin is released from the pancreas is proportional to the amount of glucose in the blood. Normally, the beta cells in the pancreas stimulate or withhold insulin secretion minute by minute, according to changing blood glucose levels. In diabetes, insulin is not secreted in proportion to blood glucose levels because of several possible factors: deficiency in the production of insulin by the beta cells; insensitivity of the insulin secretory mechanism of the beta cells; delayed or insufficient release of insulin; or excessive inactivation by chemical inhibitors or "binders" in the circulation.

In some noninsulin-dependent persons with diabetes, however, insulin secretion is increased, resulting in higher circulating insulin levels. Despite the excess insulin present, it is not utilized because of an inadequate number of insulin receptors present on cells. This mechanism has been observed in obese noninsulin-dependent diabetics. With weight loss, the number of insulin receptors on the cells increase, thereby allowing glucose to enter the cell. This may result in a normal glucose tolerance.

An elevated fasting blood glucose level in diabetes reflects decreased uptake of glucose by the tissues or increased gluconeogenesis. If the concentration of glucose in the blood is sufficiently high, the kidney may not reabsorb all of the filtered glucose; the glucose then appears in the urine (glucosuria).

With increased gluconeogenesis (which is in part under the control of the adrenocortical hormones), protein and fats are mobilized, rather than stored or deposited in the cells. When there is deficiency of insulin, muscles cannot utilize glucose. Free fatty acids are then mobilized from adipose tissue cells and broken down by the liver into ketone bodies for energy. Diabetic ketoacidosis is characterized by excessive amounts of ketone bodies in the blood. Patients with diabetic ketoacidosis exhibit hyperventilation and loss of sodium, potassium, chloride, and water from the body. The net metabolic result of acute, uncontrolled diabetes mellitus is loss of fat stores, liver glycogen, cellular

protein, electrolytes, and water. The sequelae of long-term diabetes involves the large vessels in the brain, heart, kidneys, and extremities, and the small vessels in the eyes, kidneys, and nerves. The mechanism is not precisely determined, but several hypotheses have been proposed. An increased thickening of the basement membrane of the small vessels of the body, abnormalities in the sorbitol pathway, duration of the disease, and blood glucose levels that are not maintained in the normal range are all thought to contribute to the long-term complications of this disease.

▷ Assessment

Clinical Manifestations

Insulin-dependent diabetes mellitus (IDDM) usually begins in childhood, but may occur at any age and is not uncommon in adults. Measurable circulating insulin may occur early in the course of the disease, but it soon disappears. In most instances the onset is abrupt, with weight loss, weakness, polyuria (excessive excretion of urine), polydipsia (excessive thirst), and polyphagia (excessive ingestion of food). As insulin production decreases, hyperglycemia develops as a result of the body's inability to use glucose. Hyperglycemia exceeds the renal threshold of glucose due to an exhaustion of the renal reabsorptive capacity. Fluid loss through the kidneys results, producing losses of water, sodium, magnesium, calcium, potassium chloride, and phosphate. Because the body is not able to utilize ingested calories, body tissues are broken down to supply carbohydrate. An increased appetite is seen at first, but the

Table 40-2
Blood Tests for Glucose

Visual (Strip)	Range
Chemstrip bG (Biodynamics)	20–800
Dextrostix (Ames)	0–250
Visidex (Ames)	20–800

Meter	Range
Accu-Chek bG (Biodynamics)	40–400
Dextrometer (Ames)	0–400
Glucometer (Ames)	0–400
Glucoscan II (Lifescan)	50–350
Stat Tek (Biodynamics)	50–800

hearty appetite may soon disappear as the metabolism becomes more unbalanced. Protein and lipid catabolism produce loss of weight and muscular wasting. The patient is prone to develop ketosis (elevated level of ketone bodies in body tissues and fluids). Often the diagnosis is first made when the patient is brought to the hospital in a coma, due to ketoacidosis. Insulin is always required.

Noninsulin-dependent diabetes mellitus (NIDDM) usually occurs after the age of 40. It can occur in younger persons who do not require insulin and who are not prone to developing ketosis. This type of diabetes is referred to as *maturity onset diabetes of the young* (MODY). In general, these patients may never require insulin and are usually adequately managed by diet alone.

The majority (about 80%) of noninsulin-dependent diabetes mellitus patients are overweight when the condition is first discovered. The symptoms may be so minor that the disorder goes undetected for many years, and the diagnosis may be suspected as the result of a routine urinalysis. Frequently, the diabetes is discovered when the patient presents for treatment because of complications: deteriorating vision, pain in the legs, impotence, etc. Often blood glucose tests are normal, with hyperglycemia being seen only postprandially or as a result of a glucose tolerance test.

The onset is insidious and may take years to develop. Fatigue, tendency to drowse after a meal, irritability, nocturia, itching of the skin (especially about the vulva in the female), skin wounds that heal poorly, blurring of vision, and cramps in the muscles are all warning symptoms of noninsulin-dependent diabetes.

The *management* of diabetes in both insulin-dependent and noninsulin-dependent types can be affected by many factors, many of which the diabetic may influence (*e.g.,* dietary intake, weight control, activity) and others that he may not have any control over (*e.g.,* general health, etc.). Treatment is variable throughout the course of the disease and requires constant adjustment. Poorly controlled diabetes (elevated blood glucose levels) over a period of years is usually followed by the accelerated development of neuropathy, retinopathy, and generalized atherosclerosis. Decreased resistance to infection is common only when the

blood glucose levels are consistently elevated. On the other hand, meticulous control of diabetes may postpone, and may prevent, the development of these long-term complications.

Diagnostic Evaluation

Blood Glucose Tests (Diagnostic)
Postprandial Test. The presence of sugar in the urine is a signal of diabetes and calls for an immediate blood glucose test, principally a postprandial (following a meal) blood glucose test or a glucose tolerance test. If the blood glucose is normal, the patient may have a low renal threshold for sugar or may have some other nondiabetic melituria. A postprandial blood glucose test requires that a blood sample be taken 2 hours after the patient has eaten a high-carbohydrate (75 g–100 g) meal. See Table 40-2 for specific diagnostic criteria.

Glucose Tolerance Test. The oral *glucose tolerance test* is the most sensitive test for diabetes. The patient ingests a high-carbohydrate diet (150 g–300 g) for 3 days preceding the test. After an overnight fast, a blood sample is drawn. Then a 75-g carbohydrate load, usually in the form of a carbonated sugar beverage (Glucola), is given to the patient. The patient is instructed to sit quietly during the test and to avoid exercise, tobacco, or any oral intake except water.

Blood samples are usually drawn at ½-, 1-, and 2-hour intervals after glucose ingestions. The following glucose tolerance values are considered normal for adults:

	Venous Whole Blood	Capillary Whole Blood
Fasting	<100 mg/dl	<100 mg/dl
½-, 1-, or 1½-Hour oral Glucose Tolerance Test	<180 mg/dl	<200 mg/dl
2-Hour oral Glucose Tolerance Test	<120 mg/dl	<140 mg/dl

Since advancing age alters the glucose tolerance curve, higher values are permissible in people over 50. Interpretation of these tests must take into account the possibility that preexisting diet, activity, and concurrent medications may cause variation. Laboratory values also may vary according to the methodology used.

An important variable is the dietary preparation for the test by the patient. It may be necessary to give written directions to the patient to ensure the required intake of carbohydrates. The oral glucose tolerance test is usually preferred to the intravenous tolerance test because it is more physiologic (*e.g.,* absorption of ingested glucose by the intestines). There are some who feel that the intravenous glucose tolerance test is more accurate because it eliminates the possibility of inadequate test preparation by the patient.

Medications that affect glucose tolerance should be discontinued about 3 days before the test. Illness or extreme stress will also affect the test results.

Strip Tests. Various strips are currently available for detecting abnormal blood glucose levels. These strips are used in community health screenings for diabetes because they are convenient and inexpensive. At the present time, they can be read visually or with a meter to give a higher degree of accuracy.

A drop of blood is applied to a reagent strip. Specific manufacturer directions should be carefully followed with regard to washing and timing. If the test is carefully done, the depth of the color will be proportional to the glucose concentration. This screening test does not substitute for a reliable laboratory.

Urine Glucose Tests (Diagnostic)

Testing urine for glucose is no longer used to establish the diagnosis of diabetes. Many factors, especially in the adult, may affect the presence or absence of glucose in the urine (*i.e.,* serum or plasma glucose levels, age, and the renal threshold). Aging tends to raise the renal threshold, and although the presence of glucose in the urine may help to confirm the diagnosis of diabetes, its absence does not rule out the possibility of the disorder.

Patient Monitoring for Glucose and Acetone

Urine Testing for Glucose (Monitoring)

The presence of glucose in the urine depends on the serum or plasma glucose level and the renal threshold. When the blood glucose level is higher than the renal threshold for glucose, glucose will be spilled in the urine and can be detected by a variety of tests. In diabetes, glucose may appear in the urine when the blood glucose rises above 160 mg to 180 mg per deciliter.

Glucosuria may appear in the diagnosed diabetic when the patient has an infection, is under stress, is not taking an adequate amount of insulin, is not getting enough exercise, or is not following his meal plan.

A second voided urine specimen is useful when documenting certain points of blood glucose control. The patient is instructed to void and discard the urine. It is discarded because it was excreted by the kidneys over a period of time and retained in the bladder, resulting in a possible mixture of glucose-containing urine and glucose-free urine. After the first specimen has been voided and discarded, the patient waits about 15 to 30 minutes before voiding again. The second specimen will be urine *recently* produced by the kidneys. It can be useful in occasionally documenting hypoglycemia or the need for giving supplemental insulin. However, it does not accurately reflect the *blood* sugar level at that time.

The disadvantages of second voided specimens are the dilution of glucose by drinking liquids between specimens (in order to increase the likelihood of obtaining a second specimen), which may mask glucosuria, and the extra effort and inconvenience to the patient.

Urine testing for glucose is adequate for noninsulin-dependent diabetics since their diabetes is fairly stable. However, such tests do not provide enough accuracy for the insulin-dependent diabetic who must adjust his blood sugar levels based on accurate test results in order to maintain near-normal blood sugar levels. Urine testing for glucose should be performed by insulin-dependent diabetics who cannot, for some reason, use blood sugar testing, since it can approximate levels of blood glucose.

As indicated earlier, urine testing for sugar is also affected by the aging process. Aging raises the renal threshold so that negative tests for urinary glucose may occur when the blood glucose is elevated.

There are several methods of testing urine for glucose. False tests may be obtained if deteriorated reagent tablets or strips are used or if the directions are not followed accurately. Certain drugs taken by the patient can also produce false test results.

Copper Reduction Tests. The *Clinitest* method of testing urine incorporates the idea of copper reduction in detecting glucose. The reagent tablet contains copper sulfate, which will yield an orange color if glucose is present in the urine.

Two-Drop Method. This method allows for an estimated concentration of sugar up to 5% and is more accurate at higher glucose concentrations.

1. Hold dropper vertically and place 2 drops (0.1 ml) of urine in test tube.
2. Rinse the dropper. Add 10 drops (0.5 ml) of water in test tube.
3. Add 1 Clinitest reagent tablet. Do not shake test tube.
4. Wait 15 seconds after boiling stops.
5. Compare color of urine with appropriate color chart. Use only the 2-drop method color scale, which has seven colors, ranging in value from 0% to 5%.

Five-Drop Method

1. Hold dropper vertically and place 5 drops of urine in the test tube.
2. Rinse dropper. Add 10 drops of water in test tube.
3. Add 1 Clinitest tablet in test tube.
   a. Watch while reaction takes place. Do not shake test tube during reaction or for 15 seconds after boiling inside test tube has stopped.
   b. Observe the solution in the test tube *while the reaction takes place and during the 15-second waiting period to detect pass-through color changes caused by glucosuria over 2%.*
      (1) If the solution passes through orange and dark shades of green–brown, it indicates that more than 2% urine sugar is present.
      (2) Record as such without reference to color scale.
4. After 15-second waiting period, shake test tube gently and compare with the color scale for the 5-drop method. Record the results.

Enzyme Methods. *Tes-Tape* and *Diastix* are enzyme-impregnated tapes/strips that are dip methods for testing the urine for glucose. The tape or strip is merely moistened with urine and subsequently indicates the presence or absence of glucose. Timing varies with the type of test, but is very important. The color on the tape/strip is compared to the closest matching color block on the color chart of the product being used. The results are then recorded.

Results for both copper reduction tests and the enzyme methods are recorded in percentages.

Urine Testing for Ketones (Monitoring)

Ketones in the urine signal that diabetic control is deteriorating and that the body has started to break down stored fat for energy. Mobilization of fat results in acetonemia and acetonuria and can be detected by testing the urine for acetone. Tests for ketone bodies are done when there is persistent glucosuria or elevated blood glucose levels, or when the patient is not feeling well.

There are two tests that can be done by the patient to determine the presence of acetone (ketone bodies) in the urine. The *Acetest* uses a chemical reagent that reacts with ketone bodies in the urine to yield a colored product; the depth of color is roughly correlated to the ketone-body concentration.

The *Ketostix* test uses a reagent strip that is dipped in the urine. After the time specified on the product information sheet, a lavender color appears if the urine contains ketones. The depth of color is compared with the color chart.

Keto-Diastix is a combined reagent strip designed for the determination of ketones and glucose in urine. Large amounts of ketones may depress the color development of the glucose test area.

Testing urine for ketones is still very important for those insulin-dependent diabetics who test their blood for glucose, since ketones signal a dangerous condition—ketosis.

Blood Testing for Glucose (Monitoring)

Blood glucose testing on a routine basis by the patient has replaced urine testing as a tool the patient can use to keep his blood sugar in the near-normal range. Blood glucose testing shows the exact amount of glucose in the blood at the time of testing, unlike urine testing, which shows only the percentage of glucose present in the urine when the sample is taken.

A drop of blood is obtained from either the fingertip or earlobe with one of a variety of lancetlike devices. The drop of blood is placed on one of the testing strips (Chem-strip bG or Dextrostix) for 60 seconds. At the end of 60 seconds, the blood is wiped off the Chemstrip bG or washed off the Dextrostix. The results can be read either visually or with an electronic meter. If the visual method is used, the color block on the strip (after an appropriate waiting period) is compared to the color chart on the package. If the meter is used, the strip is inserted into the meter for an exact reading (Fig. 40-1).

While approximating blood glucose visually is accurate enough for many insulin-dependent diabetics, a meter is either preferred or necessary by others. Costs for these methods of monitoring blood glucose must be considered by the patient, as well as the time and commitment on his part.

In general, blood testing is much more expensive than urine testing. Electronic meters cost several hundred dollars in addition to purchasing the other supplies needed daily.

Hemoglobin A₁c (Glycosylated Hemoglobin A₁c). At the present time, this test is done only in a laboratory. It is a blood test that shows the *pattern* of blood glucose levels over a period of time. When blood glucose levels are elevated, a glucose molecule attaches itself to hemoglobin in a red blood cell. The longer the glucose in the blood remains above normal, the more glycosylated hemoglobins form. This complex (the hemoglobin attached to the glucose) is permanent and lasts for the life of the red blood cell, approximately 120 days. If near-normal blood sugars are maintained with only occasional rises in blood glucose, the overall value will not be greatly elevated. However, if the *pattern* of blood glucose values is consistently high, then the test result will also be elevated. The normal values vary from laboratory to laboratory, but a value of 6 to 8 is considered within the "normal" range. Values within the normal range indicate consistently near-normal blood sugars, a goal easier to attain for the insulin-dependent diabetic who monitors his blood glucose level himself, and with the help of multiple insulin injections or insulin pump (continuous subcutaneous insulin injection) therapy.

Patient Problems/Nursing Diagnoses

Based on the clinical manifestations, the nursing history, and the diagnostic assessment data, the patient's major nurs-

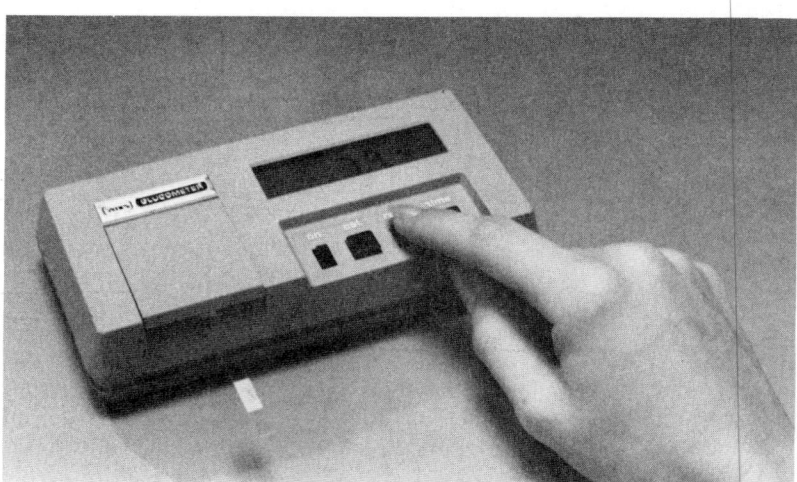

Figure 40-1. An example of a commercially available glucometer which measures electronically the amount of glucose in the blood. (Courtesy Ames Division, Miles Laboratory, Inc.)

ing diagnoses include hyperglycemia related to inadequate metabolism of glucose; potential for development of ketosis/ketoacidosis related to insulin deficiency and faulty fat metabolism; potential for development of hypoglycemia related to imbalance between insulin need and insulin intake; potential development of long-term complications related to persistent hyperglycemia and accelerated atherosclerotic changes of blood vessels (macroangiopathy of the heart and peripheral circulation, nephropathy, retinopathy, peripheral neuropathy, increased susceptibility to infection); and potential nonadherence to the therapeutic regimen related to nonacceptance of disease and regimen or to knowledge deficit (dietary regimen, weight control, insulin therapy, exercise program).

▷ Planning and Implementation

Goals

The major goals for the patient include:

1. Maintenance of normoglycemia with few episodes of hypoglycemia or hyperglycemia
2. Absence of ketosis/ketoacidosis
3. Absence of hypoglycemia
4. Absence/control of long-term complications
5. Adherence to therapeutic regimen

The goals of management are to help the patient to live a comfortable and useful life, to attain and maintain optimal body weight, to correct biochemical and metabolic abnormalities, and to prevent the development or progression of long-term complications through patient education.

Ideally, the well-controlled patient is (1) free of symptoms of hypoglycemia/hyperglycemia; (2) has normoglycemia, with few episodes of hypoglycemia or little or no hyperglycemia; (3) maintains optimum weight; and (4) has little or no glucosuria. The American Diabetes Association has established the following treatment goal for all diabetics: The goals of appropriate therapy for those with diabetes should include a serious effort to achieve levels of blood glucose levels as close to those in the nondiabetic as feasible.

Treatment depends on the type of diabetes. Management is based on dietary control, exercise, and hypoglycemic agents. Chart 40-2 summarizes the differences in the nursing management of patients with insulin-dependent diabetes mellitus and noninsulin-dependent diabetes mellitus. Patient education is the foundation for all nursing management.

Dietary Management in Diabetes Mellitus

Diet and weight control constitute the foundation of diabetes management. Reasonable expectations for the nutritional management of the patient with diabetes are to:

1. Provide all the essential food constituents (vitamins, minerals, etc.)
2. Achieve and maintain ideal weight
3. Meet energy needs
4. Achieve normal-range blood glucose levels
5. Lower blood lipid levels, if elevated

The meals should be measured and spaced at regular intervals. The menu is varied, with emphasis placed on what the patient is allowed rather than on what is forbidden, as well as taking into consideration the patient's food likes/dislikes, life-style, and ethnic and cultural background in the daily selection of food.

Obesity is corrected as soon as possible, since obese people are more resistant to both endogenous and exogenous insulin because of a decreased number of insulin receptors. Many patients who are overweight may achieve normoglycemia, since weight loss restores the number of insulin receptors on the cells. Success with diet for the patient with diabetes can be achieved more readily if the diet is fitted to the person with diabetes, instead of fitting the person to the diet.

Calorie Requirements. The first step in preparing the meal plan is to determine the patient's basic calorie requirements, taking into consideration age, sex, body weight, and degree of activity. There are several methods of assessing calorie needs. A simple method, for instance, in most weight-maintenance diets is to multiply ideal weight by 30 cal/kg to 35 cal/kg. For weight reduction, a 15-cal/kg to 20-cal/kg ideal weight is suitable. Long-term reduction diets can be achieved with caloric levels between 1000 and 1200 calories, for most people. The calorie requirement can be raised to a maintenance level when the patient achieves the desired weight.

The most important objective in dietary treatment of diabetic patients is control of total calorie intake to attain or maintain ideal weight. Success of this measure alone is often associated with reversal of the glucose intolerance. In the instance of a young, underweight patient with insulin-dependent diabetes, priority should be given to providing a diet with enough calories to maintain normal growth and development.

Calorie Distribution. While sources of calories are also to be taken into consideration, there is less emphasis now on restricted carbohydrate levels than in past years. This provides greater flexibility in diet and improves the ability of patients to adhere to an effective program of calorie restriction. Special consideration is also given to the fat content of diabetic diets. The Nutrition Committee of the American Diabetes Association issued a statement in 1971 pointing to the disadvantages of standard diabetic diets that are high in fat. Epidemiologic evidence has been cited suggesting the favorable effects of high-starch, low-fat diabetic diets on both serum triglyceride levels and vascular disease.

The most preferred caloric distribution at present, as recommended by the American Diabetes and the American Dietetic Associations (1979), is as follows: 55% to 60% of calories deriving from carbohydrates, 20% to 30% from fat, and the remaining 12% to 20% from protein, for all caloric levels.

Carbohydrates. Within the established calorie distribution, carbohydrates should be taken in the form of polysaccharides (complex sugars). Approximately 15% to 20% of the carbohydrate should also be derived from disaccharides and monosaccharides in the form of lactose and fructose, from foods such as milk and fruits, respectively. It has been found that increasing the amount of carbohydrate without increasing the total daily number of calories does not

Chart 40-2
Summary: Differences in Nursing Management of Insulin-dependent Diabetes Mellitus and Noninsulin-dependent Diabetes Mellitus

Insulin-dependent Diabetes Mellitus (IDDM)

1. Nursing assessment, diagnosis, and treatment should be focused on the state of insulin dependency. There is a greater need for "normalizing" blood sugars because of longer life ahead and higher risk of serious long-term complications.
2. Etiology is thought to be less genetic and more viral/autoimmune; therefore, the future role of the nurse might be in encouraging susceptible individuals to be immunized.
3. Short-term problems involve balancing (avoiding hypoglycemia and hyperglycemia) and "normalizing" blood sugars, on a daily basis.
4. Obesity is usually not a problem. Diet, exercise, and insulin are the management tools available to the patient. These tools need to be thoroughly understood and used by a motivated patient. Patient gains from following the treatment plan, in an attempt to normalize blood sugars, are not always immediate. In addition, current techniques for attaining normal blood glucose values (multiple injections, insulin pumps, etc.) are still far from perfect. Lifetime motivation for this patient is a nursing challenge.
5. There are long-term problems with serious, expensive complications, that is, retinal, renal, neuropathic, and arterial disease (microvascular and macrovascular complications).
6. Since this type is more life-threatening, nursing tends to focus on the acute problems and neglect the potential long-term patient problems. In addition, dealing effectively with a diabetic who has long-term complications is time consuming and at times difficult because of the presence of many complications at one time with a poor prognosis.
7. Since this group is such a small percentage of the diabetic population, it is often regarded as "interesting" by nurses. If these diabetics pay close daily attention to normalizing blood glucose levels and keep sugars fairly normal, they can avoid hospitalization. Based on nursing research, these diabetics need a reemphasis of knowledge and skills throughout their life. This can have tremendous implications for long-term nursing care, health care costs, patient well-being, and the delay or prevention of long-term complications.

Noninsulin-dependent Diabetes Mellitus (NIDDM)

1. Nursing assessment, diagnosis, and treatment should be focused on maintaining effective insulin levels.
2. More frequent familial patterns of inheritance suggest a strong genetic basis that is influenced by obesity.
3. Short-term problems are related to hyperglycemia and weight control/maintenance. Hyperglycemia related to infection, stress, and surgery may temporarily need to be treated with insulin.
4. Since 80% to 90% are obese, hyperglycemia and glucose intolerance are usually improved and occasionally reversed with weight reduction.
5. Long-term problems are related to obesity/weight reduction and to an increase in arterial disease (macrovascular). Renal and retinal complications (microvascular) are infrequent in this type.
6. Noninsulin-dependent diabetes is not especially life-threatening, but the majority of diabetics fall in this class.

---

increase the insulin needed. Diabetics can tolerate more carbohydrate than was formerly supposed.

Fat. The increase of carbohydrate has been made at the expense of fat, which is presently set at a level of 20% to 30% of caloric intake. The lowering of the proportion of dietary fat may reduce factors predisposing to the development of coronary heart disease, the most important cause of death and debility in the diabetic.

Protein. The protein level of 12% to 20% of calories is considered appropriate.

Fiber. When diabetics, treated with either insulin or oral hypoglycemic agents, were given high-fiber meals, postprandial hyperglycemia was decreased. There is also evidence that the insulin requirement may be reduced. However, the long-term benefits as well as the mechanism of action still remain to be established. It has been hypothesized that added fiber increases the passage of foodstuffs through the intestinal tract, thereby allowing less glucose absorption.

If fiber is added, it should be introduced slowly. High fiber (40 g) intake needs to be maintained from day to day because of possible fluctuations in blood glucose levels. Potential problems with such a high fiber intake may include abdominal fullness, nausea and vomiting, increased flatulence, increased bowel movements, and vitamin/mineral deficiencies.

Dietary Adaptation. Adapting dietary therapy to specific needs of individual patients on the basis of diagnostic tests is essential. If, for instance, a diabetic patient is found to have type IV hyperlipoproteinemia, a lower carbohydrate intake would be beneficial in controlling this type of lipid abnormality. Patients with high levels of triglycerides, however, will benefit from a lowered fat intake (less than 30% of the diet). Diabetics with high cholesterol levels may require even greater reductions of dietary cholesterol and saturated fat. Guidelines for the treatment of hyperlipoproteinemias in diabetes are available.

Exchange Lists. The 1976 revision of the "Exchange Lists for Meal Planning" reflects the most current thinking in the area of nutrition education. Many revisions and additions have been made to the Exchange Lists, based on concern for total caloric intake and modifications of fat and carbohydrate in the diet.

List 1   *Milk exchanges:* The basis of this exchange is nonfat milk. If low-fat or whole milk is used, appropriate fat exchanges must be deducted.

List 2   *Vegetable exchanges:* includes all vegetables except starchy vegetables. Vegetables on list 2 average 25 calories per one-half cup serving. Starchy vegetables appear in the bread exchange.

List 3   *Fruit exchanges:* remain the same as in the old edition.

List 4   *Bread exchanges:* has been expanded to include a wider variety of prepared foods. Those appearing in bold type are of low fat content. Foods such as ice cream and angel food cake were not included because of their sugar and calorie content. Their use should be discussed individually with the patient.

List 5   *Meat exchanges:* includes not only lean meat, but also medium-fat and high-fat meats and differ in calorie content significantly because of the fat content. Other protein-rich foods are included for vegetarians or for those who use them as a meat substitute. Vegetarians should see a nutritionist in order to avoid potential problems.

List 6   *Fat exchanges:* has been revised to show differences in the kind of fat contained in them—saturated or polyunsaturated. Saturated fat has been associated with an increase in blood cholesterol (a possible risk factor in coronary heart disease). The physician may advise a reduction of foods high in this kind of fat. Polyunsaturated fat has been associated with a decrease in blood cholesterol. The physician may advise substituting foods containing this kind of fat whenever possible. A system of bold type is used in the booklet to indicate the low-fat concept.

Each list contains additional information on the vitamin and mineral content of the foods listed. The following foods should not be included in the meal plan: sugar, candy, honey, jam, jelly, cookies, syrup, condensed milk, chewing gum, pies, cakes, and soft drinks with sugar.

The patient should be taught to read labels. Foods that are advertised and labeled as "dietetic," "sugar-free," and "fat-free" often contain high proportions of carbohydrate and should be avoided. In addition, they are very expensive and often not as tasty as the items they are imitating.

The use of alcoholic beverages and sugar substitutes should be discussed with the physician or dietitian for possible inclusion in his meal plan.

The details of these exchange lists are widely available in hospitals, diet manuals, and books on nutrition and diabetes. Several cookbooks for diabetes are available and contain recipes that yield food portions with defined amounts of carbohydrate, fat, and protein, translated into food exchanges per portion. The patient should be cautioned to avoid recipes that contain excessive amounts of sugar.

To be practical and effective, a dietary program must be based on the patient's life-style and appropriate patient motivation coupled with careful dietary instruction and follow-up.

A number of sources of information show popular food exchanges. The H. J. Heinz Company and the Campbell Soup Company have published lists showing the composition of their soups in terms of food exchanges. The local affiliates of the American Diabetes Association also have lists for ethnic and regional foods.

The nurse plays an important role in reinforcing the patient's knowledge and understanding of the importance of diet in diabetes, and the more effective use of the exchange lists. The effect of this counseling is to reinforce the patient's motivation to follow the prescribed dietary regimen.

▶ **Evaluation**

Expected Outcomes

Follows the prescribed dietary regimen:

1. Eats three or more regularly spaced meals each day, timed to coincide with the action of insulin
2. Becomes thoroughly familiar with the food exchange lists
3. Learns how to follow a calculated diet
4. Knows the caloric value of foods frequently eaten
5. Uses household measures or a gram scale until serving sizes can be judged accurately
6. Avoids concentrated carbohydrates
7. Avoids periods of fasting and feasting
8. Keeps weight at optimal level; normalizes body weight
   a. Weighs weekly
   b. Keeps a weight record
9. If taking insulin, eats extra calories when unusual physical activity is anticipated
10. Eats a bedtime snack when taking insulin (if permissible)
11. Avoids foods high in cholesterol

Exercise

Exercise is extremely important in the management of diabetes because of its effects on blood glucose and free fatty acids. Exercise lowers blood glucose by increasing the uptake of glucose by body muscles. It also improves circulation and muscle tone. These effects are useful in the diabetic with regard to losing weight, easing stress or tension, and maintaining a feeling of well-being. Exercise also raises the levels of high-density lipoproteins (HDL), thereby lowering cholesterol and triglyceride levels. This is especially important to the diabetic because of an increased risk for cardiovascular disease.

However, diabetics with blood glucose levels over 300 mg/dl or who have ketones in their urine should not begin exercising until their blood glucose levels are in the normal range. If the diabetic exercises in this situation, the exercise will raise his blood glucose levels by the following mechanism. Exercising with elevated blood glucose levels will cause increased secretions of glucagon, growth hormone, and catecholamines. The liver will then release more glucose, resulting in an increase in blood glucose. Therefore, exercise should not be performed until blood glucose levels are normalized.

The insulin-dependent diabetic should be taught to eat a 10-g carbohydrate snack (a fruit exchange) before engaging in moderate exercise in order to prevent unexpected hypoglycemia. Extra food is required for extra activity and need not be deducted from the regular meal plan. The exact amount of food needed can only be determined through trial and error.

The noninsulin-dependent diabetic who is not taking insulin or an oral agent does not require extra food before exercise. Exercise increases the number of insulin receptors in these patients, and if coupled with weight loss, will further increase the numbers of these receptors. Eventually, the patient's glucose tolerance may return to normal.

Persons with diabetes should be taught to exercise at the same time (preferably when blood sugar levels are at their peak) and in the same amount each day. Regular daily exercise, rather than sporadic exercise, should be encouraged.

Complications of diabetes may change the physiologic response to exercise because of microangiopathy. The ability of blood vessels to dilate is affected, and exercise tolerance is impaired. In addition, capillary permeability to fluids and proteins is increased. Exercise also decreases blood flow to the kidneys. Proteinuria is increased, and these factors may aggravate diabetic nephropathy. Exercise may also aggravate diabetic retinopathy by increasing blood pressure, thereby increasing the risk of a hemorrhage into the vitreous or retina. In patients with ischemic heart disease, there is a risk of triggering angina or a myocardial infarction.

In general, diabetics should discuss an exercise program with their physician. A physical examination and an ECG are indicated for persons over the age of 35.

Insulin Therapy

As stated earlier, insulin is secreted by the beta cells of the islets of Langerhans and works to lower the blood glucose by facilitating the uptake and utilization of glucose by muscle and fat cells and by decreasing the release of glucose from the liver. Since insulin is necessary for the normal metabolism of fat and protein, a lack of insulin causes a breakdown of these stores.

When the patient's body fails to produce enough insulin, and when diet alone cannot control the diabetes, then insulin must be administered. One or more insulin injections each day are usually taken by persons with insulin-dependent diabetes as well as by those with noninsulin-dependent diabetes who cannot be adequately controlled by diet alone or by diet and oral agents.

Obese noninsulin-dependent diabetics who have no complications, few symptoms, and no ketonuria, can usually control their diabetes by means of caloric restriction. However, these same patients, who are usually controlled by diet alone or by diet and an oral hypoglycemic agent, may require insulin temporarily during illness, infection, pregnancy, surgery, or during some other stressful event.

Insulin is extracted from either beef and pork pancreases obtained from animals going to slaughter. There are a number of insulin preparations available, each of which varies in onset of action, time of peak or maximum effect, and duration or length of action (Table 40-3). These preparations are classified into three groups: (1) short-acting insulin; (2) intermediate-acting insulin; and (3) long-acting insulin. In many patients, combinations of short-acting and an intermediate insulin are given to maintain metabolic control. Other combinations are also used with less frequency.

Because of potential shortages of beef and pork sources, research in producing insulin is a critical problem today.

Insulin has also been produced synthetically. It can be done in several ways. It can be made in the laboratory by linking together the amino acids that make up insulin. However, it is impractical because of the expense and the number of materials needed. Another method replaces an amino acid in pork insulin to produce human insulin. It is now being tested for potential use.

Biosynthetic human insulin, Humulin, has also been produced by genetically altered bacteria (*Escherichia coli*). It has been tested in humans and is now available in the United States. One of the proposed advantages of human insulin over animal insulin was the absence of antibodies. However, patients who use human insulin still produce antibodies to it, but at lower levels. It is thought that the production of this low level of antibodies is caused by the route of administration (subcutaneous), which is not physiologic, as well as the kind of insulin that is used. Whether these insulin antibodies are in any way harmful is still undetermined. It is currently being used in patients and is often given to newly diagnosed insulin-dependent patients with diabetes.

Insulin (which is prescribed in units) is available in two concentrations (strengths) that correspond to the number of units of insulin per milliliter of solution: U-40 (40 units per ml) and U-100 (100 units per ml). In the United States, the aim is to have only one strength, U-100, available in all varieties of insulin. The insulin syringe must correlate with the strength of insulin used. For example, U-100 insulin is given with a U-100 syringe.

Table 40-3
Commercial Insulin Preparations

Manufacturer	Product	Available Concentration	Source	Onset (approx.)	Peak (approx.)	Duration (approx.)
Lilly	Regular	U-40 U-100	Beef* Pork* Beef-Pork	15 min–1 hr	2–4 hr	5–7 hr
Squibb	Regular	U-40 U-100	Pork	15 min–1 hr	2–4 hr	5–7 hr
	Regular	U-100	Pork**	15 min–1 hr	2–4 hr	5–7 hr
Nordisk	Velosulin	U-100	Pork**	15 min–1 hr	2–4 hr	5–7 hr
Novo	Actrapid	U-100	Pork**	30 min–1 hr	2½–5 hr	8 hr
Lilly	Semilente	U-40 U-100	Beef-Pork	1–3 hr	2–8 hr	12–16 hr
Squibb	Semilente	U-100	Beef	1–3 hr	2–8 hr	12–16 hr
Novo	Semitard	U-100	Pork**	1½ hr	5–10 hr	16 hr
Novo	Protophane NPH	U-100	Pork**	1–1½ hr	4–12 hr	24 hr
Lilly	NPH	U-40 U-100	Beef* Pork* Beef-Pork	1–3 hr	6–12 hr	24–28 hr
Squibb	NPH	U-40 U-100	Beef	1–3 hr	6–12 hr	24–28 hr
	NPH	U-100	Beef*	1–3 hr	6–12 hr	24–28 hr
Novo	Monotard	U-100	Pork**	2½ hr	7–15 hr	22 hr
Nordisk	Insulatard	U-100	Pork**	2–4 hr	4–12 hr	24–28 hr
Lilly	Lente	U-40 U-100	Beef* Pork* Beef-Pork	1–3 hr	6–12 hr	24–28 hr
Squibb	Lente	U-40 U-100	Beef	1–3 hr	6–12 hr	24–28 hr
	Lente	U-100	Beef**	1–3 hr	6–12 hr	24–28 hr
Novo	Lentard	U-100	Beef-Pork**	2½ hr	7–15 hr	24 hr
Lilly	PZI	U-40 U-100	Beef* Pork* Beef-Pork	4–6 hr	14–24 hr	36+ hr
Squibb	PZI	U-100	Beef	4–6 hr	14–24 hr	36+ hr
Lilly	Ultralente	U-40 U-100	Beef-Pork	4–6 hr	18–24 hr	36+ hr
Squibb	Ultralente	U-100	Beef	4–6 hr	18–24 hr	36+ hr
Novo	Ultratard	U-100	Beef**	4 hr	10–30 hr	36 hr
Nordisk	Mixtard (premixed) Regular—30% NPH—70%	U-100	Pork**	like Regular and NPH when mixed		

* Iletin II (either purified pork or purified beef) available only in U-100
** Purified
N.B. Squibb and Novo recently merged to form Squibb Novo, Inc. The insulins Squibb and Novo have marketed will remain unchanged, but they will be packaged under this new company name.
(From Nemchick R: The news about insulin. RN 1982 Dec; 45(12):52.)

Regulation of Dosage

The dosage of insulin is adjusted according to the levels of glucose, the degree to which glucose is present, and the time when high glucose levels appear in relation to insulin administration and meals. Meals are distributed to conform to insulin peaks and the exercise patterns of the patient. Insulin curves vary from patient to patient, and the response of individual patients may be highly variable.

In the absence of complications, treatment may be started with 10 to 20 units of intermediate-acting insulin, given subcutaneously before breakfast. This dosage is increased gradually, as indicated by the patient's response to the previous dose, until glucosuria is absent and the blood glucose before each meal is near normal. Larger doses may be necessary at the onset, depending on the degree of insulin insufficiency. The meals must coincide with the action of the insulin. During initial regulation, and when insulin requirements are changing rapidly (during an acute illness), it is common practice to give supplemental injections of regular insulin before each meal, depending on the results of a recent test for glucose and the previous response of the patient. Constant monitoring of glucose levels and close attention to insulin dose and food intake are crucial during an acute illness.

There is a narrow margin between the therapeutic and hypoglycemic effects of insulin. It is important that the patient and the nurse know when hypoglycemia is most likely to occur with each type of insulin (see Table 40-3). The patient is instructed to test for sugar before each meal and at bedtime while insulin is being regulated or during periods of illness. The patient may need to keep a record of the results in a notebook and take it to the physician or clinic with each visit so that insulin adjustments can be made, if he is not able to adjust his daily insulin dosage himself.

Health Teaching for Self-injection of Insulin

As soon as the need for insulin has been established, the patient is instructed in the technique of self-injection (Chart 40-3). He should be persuaded to give his own injection as soon as possible. An optimistic but firm approach will offer the patient encouragement. Another family member or friend should also be taught.

Rotation of Sites. Systematic rotation of injection sites (Fig. 40-2) is necessary to prevent scar tissue from forming and to allow for uniform absorption of insulin. To assure a definite rotation schedule, the patient may keep a record of each injection site.

Areas that are about to be exercised (*e.g.,* right arm for playing tennis) should be avoided that day, since injection in that site can result in a more rapid absorption of insulin. Areas with loose skin and a sufficient amount of subcutaneous fat are sites suitable for insulin injection; that is, lateral surface of arms, anterior aspect of the thighs, anterior and lateral aspects of the abdominal wall, and lateral areas of the back, just above the buttock. Each injection should be separated from the previous injection by approximately 2.5 cm (1 inch), and each site should be used no more often than every 3 weeks.

The rate of insulin absorption varies with the site used. Regular insulin is absorbed faster when injected into the deltoid area than into the anterior thigh. Absorption is faster in the thigh and abdomen than in the buttocks. In general, although site rotation is still important, it may be better to rotate within a site and then move onto another site instead of rotating daily from arm to thigh to abdomen, etc.

Some patients do not rotate sites because repeated injections into the same site become less painful. However, lipohypertrophy may occur, and insulin will not be absorbed as well.

Chart 40-3 summarizes the important factors to include in teaching insulin administration.

Problems With Insulin

Local Allergic Reactions. A local allergic reaction in the form of redness, swelling, tenderness, and induration, or a wheal may appear at the site of injection. These reactions usually occur during the beginning stages of therapy and disappear with continued use of insulin. These allergic reactions are becoming less frequent because of the increased purity of insulins. The physician may prescribe an antihistamine to be taken 1 hour before the injection if such a local reaction occurs.

Occasionally, if alcohol is not allowed to dry on the skin before injection, it is carried into the tissues. This results in a localized, reddened area.

Systemic Allergic Reactions. Systemic allergic reactions to insulin range from hives to angioedema and anaphylaxis. The treatment is desensitization, with small volumes of insulin given as desensitizing doses.

Insulin Lipodystrophy. *Lipodystrophy* refers to a localized disturbance of fat metabolism, in the form of either lipoatrophy or lipohypertrophy. These reactions occur at the site of injection and may appear separately, in combination, or in succession, in the same patient. *Insulin-induced atrophy* is loss of subcutaneous fat and appears as slight dimpling or more serious pitting of subcutaneous fat. It occurs most commonly in women and children. The use of U-100 insulin, which is 99% pure, has almost eliminated this disfiguring complication. Lipoatrophy is treated by injection of purified insulin into the periphery of the lipoatrophic area.

Lipohypertrophy is the development of fibrofatty masses at the injection site and occurs more often in children and adult men. It is caused by the prolonged use of the same injection site. If insulin is injected into scarred areas, the absorption is irregular and the action of the insulin unpredictable. This is one reason why the rotation of injection sites is so important. The patient should avoid injecting insulin into these areas until the hypertrophy disappears.

Insulin Edema. A generalized retention of fluid is sometimes seen after diabetic control is suddenly established in a patient who has had prolonged uncontrolled diabetes.

Insulin Resistance. Most diabetics at one time or another have some degree of insulin resistance. This may occur for various reasons, the most common being obesity, which can be overcome by weight loss.

Chart 40-3
Self-Injection of Insulin

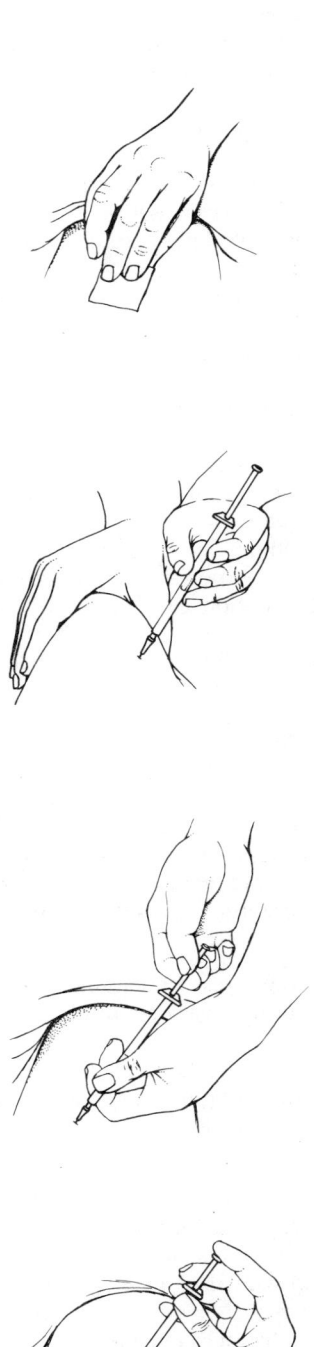

- The technique of filling the syringe is demonstrated, and the skin is disinfected with alcohol.

- The person is instructed to pull the skin taut on the anterior surface of the thigh or to form a skin fold by picking up subcutaneous tissue between the thumb and forefinger. Either of these techniques ensures that the needle tip is inserted into subcutaneous tissue and outside the muscle. The skin should not be pressed tightly together between the fingers, since this is a cause of local induration.
- The person is instructed to insert the needle with a quick thrust into deep subcutaneous tissue.
- When the arm is used as the site of injection, another person may need to assist, or the arm can be stabilized by leaning against a wall or door.

- The person then pulls back slightly on the plunger of the syringe to assure that the needle is not in a blood vessel before the insulin is injected. (If blood appears, the needle should be removed and a new site and a new syringe used.)

- The insulin is then injected. After injecting the insulin, the person holds the alcohol sponge against the needle, while gently withdrawing it, to prevent painful pulling of the skin while the needle is withdrawn.

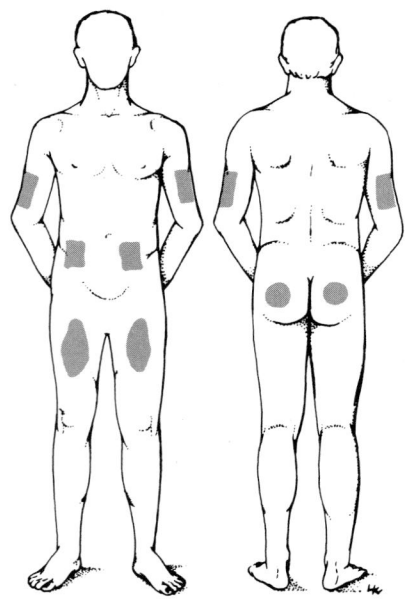

Figure 40-2. Suggested rotation sites for insulin injections to allow for uniform absorption and to prevent insulin lipodystrophy.

True insulin resistance has been defined as a daily requirement of 200 units or more. Some patients need as many as 500 units to 2000 units daily for a certain period of time.

In most insulin-dependent patients with diabetes, immune antibodies develop and bind the insulin, thereby decreasing the insulin available for use. All animal insulins cause antibody production in humans, since these insulins contain different types of amino acids than those found in human insulin.

Some patients develop high levels of antibodies. Many of these patients give a history of interrupted insulin therapy for several months or more. Treatment consists of administering a purer insulin preparation, and occasionally prednisone may be needed. This is usually followed by a dramatic reduction in insulin requirement.

During treatment, U-500 insulin may be needed and is available on special order from the Lilly Company.

In rare instances, insulin may be degraded when given subcutaneously and may need to be given intravenously.

▶ **Evaluation**

Expected Outcomes

Becomes familiar with all aspects of insulin usage:

1. Knows when the prescribed insulin is having its peak action
2. Adjusts insulin dosage according to urine sugar tests, as prescribed
3. Rotates the sites of insulin injections in a systematic manner
4. Keeps the syringe and needle in one particular place

5. Keeps a reserve supply of insulin in the refrigerator; is aware of expiration date on bottle
   a. Keeps bottle in current use at *room temperature*
   b. Avoids injecting cold insulin, because it may contribute to tissue reaction
6. Has an extra insulin syringe available
7. Knows the conditions that produce insulin reactions
   a. Omission of a meal
   b. Unaccustomed or strenuous exercise
   c. Too much insulin
8. Knows the symptoms of an insulin reaction
   a. Any unfamiliar or peculiar sensation
   b. Hunger, perspiration, weakness, tremor, pallor, palpitation, tachycardia
9. Knows how to combat an impending insulin reaction
   a. Eats carbohydrates (orange juice, sugar, candy) when symptoms first occur
   b. Tests urine
   c. Carries extra carbohydrate at all times (sugar lumps, candy)
   d. Eats extra carbohydrate before strenuous exercise and during periods of prolonged exercise, or reduces insulin dosage
   e. Eats a snack at bedtime
10. Keeps a check-off system, to ensure taking insulin
11. Carries diabetic identification card or wears identification bracelet
12. When traveling, carries diabetic supplies in hand luggage

Insulin Delivery Systems

It was not until the early 1960s that plasma insulin levels could be measured, which allowed researchers to see how inadequate conventional insulin therapy was.

In a person with a properly functioning pancreas, the beta cells produce smooth, rapid bursts of insulin secretion with each meal. This secretion of insulin is regulated through:

1. The nervous system (vagus, catecholamines)
2. Gastrointestinal hormones (gastric-inhibitory peptide, etc.)
3. Islet hormonal factors (somatostatin, glucagon) as well as substrate concentrations of glucose and amino acids, which affect the amount and duration of insulin secretion by the pancreas

Insulin-dependent persons with diabetes lack this type of secretion. Insulin injections, at best, can produce only peaks and valleys of insulin levels that are irregular and usually poorly coordinated with rises in blood sugar. The levels that are produced by one or more injections a day can prevent ketoacidosis and hypoglycemia in many patients. However, very few insulin-dependent diabetics can avoid swings of glucose, glucagon, free fatty acids, growth hormone, etc., that are not physiologic. With more and more evidence pointing to "tight control" in preventing or delaying the dreaded long-term vascular complications, and the fact that near-normal blood sugars impart a feeling of well-being and an improvement of growth and development

Chart 40-4
Teaching Insulin Administration

Choosing and Buying the Right Equipment

1. Know the manufacturer, type, and concentration of prescribed insulin.

2. U-80 insulins are no longer available. U-40 insulins will soon be phased out.

3. Any change in insulin should be made cautiously and only under medical supervision. Changes in purity, strength (U-40, U-100), brand (manufacturer), type (Lente, NPH, etc.), or source (beef, pork or beef/pork, biosynthetic human) may result in the need for a change in dosage. When you change to a "purified insulin," a dosage decrease may be necessary. Adjustment may be needed with the first dose or may be needed over a period of several weeks. A small number of patients may require a significant change in dosage.

4. Insulin prices may vary greatly depending on preparation/purity, species source, and concentration.

5. Check insulin expiration dates when purchasing.

6. Store insulin in a cool place. Avoid temperature extremes.

7. Select insulin syringes based on comfort, convenience, and cost.
   - Disposable syringes are usually 1.25 cm (½ inch), 27-gauge, with a lubricated needle.
   - If taking less than 50 units, disposable syringes also come in a ½-ml size that measures up to 50 units.
   - Glass syringes are cheaper but are harder to find and involve time and dexterity in daily cleansing (*e.g.,* arthritic patients).

Before Injection

1. Match the syringe to the insulin concentration to avoid serious problems with either hypoglycemia or hyperglycemia. Use U-100 insulin with a U-100 syringe.

2. Know when insulin works—its onset, peak, and duration—and time snacks, meals, and exercise accordingly.

3. Understand that many diabetics take more than one type of insulin and inject more than once daily in order to achieve near-normal blood sugars.

4. Store insulin being used at a cool room temperature. Extra insulin may be kept in the refrigerator. The most important fact regarding storage is to avoid extremes in temperature.

Injection

1. Choose the right site; choices include arms, thighs, abdomen, and buttocks.

2. Rotate sites to prevent "lipodystrophy"—lumps or indentations that can be caused by repeated injections in one area.

3. Rotate injection sites to help absorption. Injecting in the same site repeatedly often results in a less painful injection *but* poorer absorption. This may account for delayed insulin action, which can cause serious problems.

4. Free injection rotation guides are available from:
   - Monoject, 1831 Olive Street, St. Louis, MO 63103. This guide matches dates of month to sites for either one or two injections per day.
   - Becton–Dickinson Consumer Products, P.O. Box 500, Rochelle Park, NJ 07662. This guide consists of a body map that can be used as an injection log, and a punched out site selector that aids in determining the correct space between sites.

5. Avoid injecting into areas you plan to exercise that day (*e.g.,* avoid right arm if you are a right-handed tennis player). Exercise can cause a more rapid absorption of insulin and cause unexpected hypoglycemia.

After Injection

1. Always be prepared for hypoglycemia; carry hard candy or sugar. Chocolate candy takes longer to absorb because of its fat content.

2. If in doubt about whether person is experiencing hypoglycemia or hyperglycemia, *always* treat for hypoglycemia.

3. Quick-acting, commercially prepared sugar products are available:
   - Glutose (Paddock Laboratories)
   - Monojel (Monoject)

These are to be used if the hypoglycemic person can still swallow.

4. Glucagon (Eli Lilly Company) is a pancreatic hormone that raises blood sugar. It is available only by prescription and is injected subcutaneously, using an insulin syringe. The patient may need to administer it himself if he is vomiting. If unconscious, it should be administered by someone who knows how to give an injection (*i.e.,* a family member, neighbor, friend).

5. Always wear medical identification stating that the person has diabetes and is on insulin. Carrying a card in a wallet is inadequate since emergency personnel may not find it.

in diabetic children, it seemed logical to search for a better insulin delivery system.

Insulin Pump Development

Research on developing means to mechanically duplicate the work of the beta cell began around 1972. If a device could be made small enough, implanted in the patient, and then function as an insulin delivery system, then the diabetic would be the recipient of an artificial beta cell. The ultimate goal then is for the artificial beta cell to be implantable, functional and convenient. However, development of this insulin delivery system has produced two similar, yet dissimilar, products, the "closed"-loop and the "open"-loop systems.

Closed-Loop System.   In 1973, Albisser developed the first insulin delivery system (closed-loop system) at the Hospital for Sick Children in Toronto, Canada. In this system, the patient is connected to the machine via a venous catheter. The closed-loop system (feedback) devices are capable of monitoring glucose concentrations in the blood. The closed loop refers to the closed loop formed by the pancreas that delivers insulin in response to the body's glucose levels. The main components of such a device include a glucose sensor, an insulin pump, and a computer. Intravenous blood glucose levels are continuously monitored by a sensor in the device. The computer determines the insulin rate by means of algorithms, and the insulin pump adjusts itself without any participation on the part of the patient in order to control blood glucose concentrations. It also adjusts the rate of either glucagon or glucose delivery. This is the type of system that could be the diabetic's answer to his beta cell problem. However, two criteria must be met: miniaturization and implantability. The first has been solved, the second has not. One of the current research problems is the immune response to the implanted cell.

These closed-loop systems have been developed and are in use clinically. The first one developed commercially, the Biostator, a bedside device, was done so by Life Science Instruments (a division of Miles Laboratories). It is large, must be connected to the patient intravenously, and is used in large medical centers only.

Open-Loop Systems.   The open-loop systems refer to a lack of a built-in feedback component for blood sugar regulation. In other words, the patient himself is the glucose sensor via his own blood glucose monitoring. These pump systems, continuous subcutaneous insulin infusion (CSII), therefore require continuous dietary compliance and are dependent on the patient for delivery of the appropriate premeal insulin dose, based on the results of his self-glucose monitoring, which is critical to the system's success.

Pump therapy began in France in 1974 with the semiautomatic subcutaneous delivery of regular insulin via an electronically controlled syringe, and spread to Denmark, Germany, and the United Kingdom.

Insulin Pumps in Use.   Basically, those insulin pumps being used today in diabetic persons, outside the hospital, are battery-driven syringes that deliver a basal rate of insulin continuously throughout a 24-hour period (Fig. 40-3). In addition, they have the capability of delivering a pre-meal dose (bolus). The amount of insulin delivered in the 24-hour period is determined by the results of numerous (4–8) blood glucose measurements done by the patient. Both types of doses (basal and pre-meal) are an attempt to maintain blood sugars in the normal range. Insulin physiologically follows a pattern of a low rate of secretion during fasting, which is mimicked by the insulin pump's basal rate, and a high output after meals, which is mimicked by the pre-meal bolus. Algorithms have been developed to allow the pump to deliver small quantities of insulin between meals and through the night with bolus doses at mealtimes. In this way, individual variations in daily living, food intake, and exercise may be considered.

At the present time, the insulin pump used in conjunction with blood glucose monitoring by the patient attempts to mimic the normal insulin function of the pancreas. It must be used only under a physician's direct supervision.

The pump (Fig. 40-3) consists of a case containing a battery (disposable or rechargeable), electronic circuit, motor and gear box, and syringe mover or pump. This is attached to a plastic tubing of varying length, which is then connected to a 27-gauge needle inserted in subcutaneous tissue. Usual sites are either the abdomen or thigh. Pump users keep a needle in place 1 to 3 days before replacing it.

The battery supplies power to the electronic circuit that drives the motor. The motor causes the syringe to empty.

Supplies needed to use the pump include syringes, batteries, infusion sets (catheters), diluent, dilution chart, short-acting (regular) insulin, tape, a carrying case, and blood glucose monitoring equipment. These cost between $10–20 weekly. Third-party reimbursement varies from full coverage of the pump and weekly supplies to partial coverage to none.

At the present time, there are at least six types of pumps being used by more than 6000 insulin-dependent diabetics. They vary in size, manner of operation, and price. The price range for the pump alone is $1000 to $2500.

Candidates for Pump Therapy.   Not all insulin-dependent diabetics are pump candidates. The American Diabetes Association has issued the following guidelines for pump therapy candidates.

Closed-Loop System (Intravenous Delivery in a Hospitalized Setting)

1. Initial treatment of ketoacidosis
2. Maintenance of blood glucose control during surgery and the immediate postoperative period
3. Maintenance of blood glucose control during pregnancy, especially during labor and delivery and periods of ketoacidosis
4. Maintenance of blood glucose control during severe and complicated medical illnesses when conventional insulin treatment is unsatisfactory. Examples of these illnesses would be a myocardial infarction or severe infection. Continuous intravenous delivery could also be advantageous for insulin-dependent patients receiving hyperalimentation or who are under restricted oral intake, such as during treatment of a bleeding peptic ulcer.
5. Treatment of the rare patient with excessive subcuta-

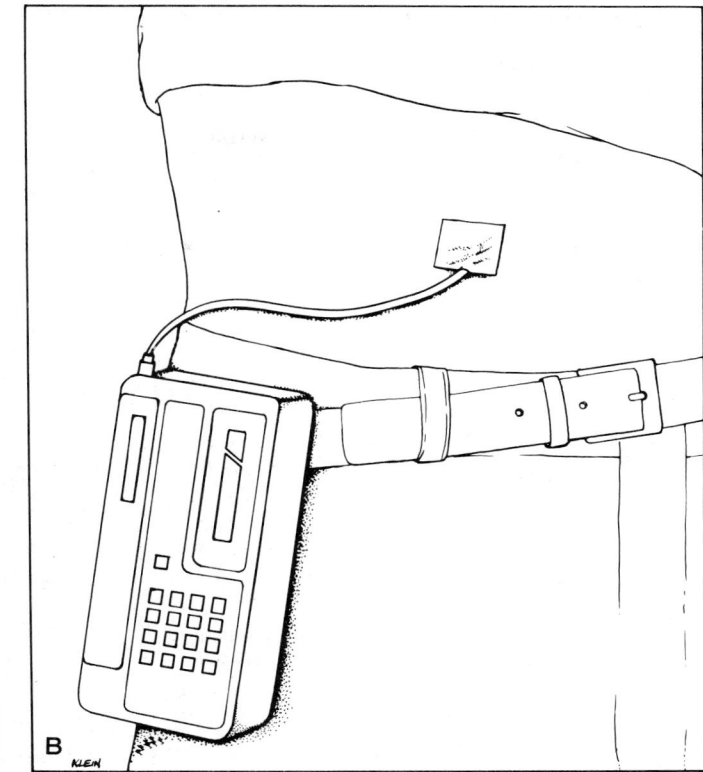

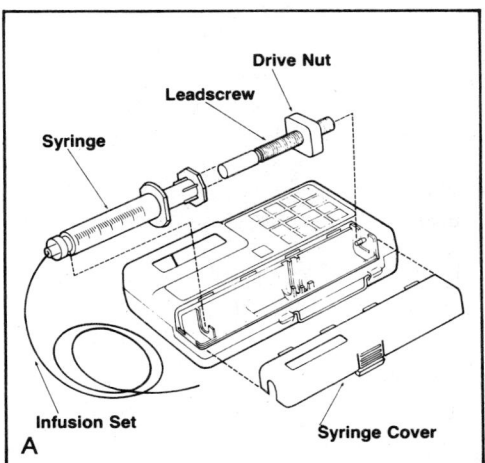

Figure 40-3. Infusion insulin pump. (*A*) Schematic drawing of infusion pump. (Courtesy of Cardiac Pacemakers, Inc., St. Paul, Minnesota.) (*B*) Insulin pump in place.

neous degradation of injected insulin when other measures fail. This situation may necessitate continuous intravenous delivery with a central line at home.

Open-Loop System (Subcutaneous Delivery With a Portable Pump as a Long-term Outpatient Procedure)

1. Failure to achieve an acceptable level of diabetic control in certain type I diabetics with unusual fluctuations in blood glucose levels, despite intensive efforts with proper diet and multiple injections of insulin in single or mixture form
2. Last trimester of pregnancy while hospitalized; still unresolved is whether insulin pump therapy is feasible in pregnant patients with diabetes outside the hospital, where diet and activity are more difficult to control.

Implantable Insulin Pumps.   Implantable pumps at this time are much more experimental than the external pumps. Some of these hockey puck-sized pumps have been implanted experimentally in humans (Minnesota, 1980). Problems related to these pumps involve the insulin reservoir and the membrane of the pump through which the insulin must pass. This pump cannot hold a lifetime supply of insulin, and so it must be filled with an injection from the outside. Another problem is that it cannot deliver an extra dose of insulin at mealtimes, an important advantage in controlling blood sugars. The ideal pump would be one that

adds more insulin automatically as the blood sugar goes up, just like the normal pancreas does. The implantable pump presently in use, with special permission from the U.S. Food and Drug Administration, is limited to persons with some residual insulin function. An improved version of the pump with a magnetically activated valve is being tested in dogs. This type allows the delivery of an extra mealtime dose by holding a magnet over the pump in the chest for a minute or two.

The implantable pump is similar to implantable pumps that, for the last 3 years, have been used to deliver constant doses of either blood-thinning or cancer therapy drugs.

The pump consists of two chambers, one of which holds the insulin, while the other holds a compressible fluorocarbon gas. Once every 2 weeks, the drug reservoir is filled with about 1⅓ ounces of insulin solution, using a syringe with a needle inserted through the skin. The injection of the liquid compresses the fluorocarbon into a liquid, and its gradual expansion over the next 12 to 14 days drives the insulin through a narrow nozzle into a tube.

Chart 40-5 summarizes the health teaching for patients using insulin pumps.

Research in Pancreatic Transplantation
Whole Organ.   Most studies have focused on using pancreatic tissues that consist of both endocrine and exocrine parts. Although with this approach one can avoid isolating human islets from the pancreas, it creates other problems.

Chart 40-5
Health Teaching for Patients Using Insulin Pumps

1. The goal of insulin pump therapy is to achieve better diabetes control, not to provide an easier means of giving insulin.
2. The pump restores to normal, circulating lipids and amino acids as well as the concentrations of anti-insulin hormones.
3. A basal infusion rate of insulin coupled with premeal boluses attempts to mimic the way a healthy pancreas works.
4. The daily insulin dose via the pump is usually lower.
5. Only fast-acting (regular) insulin is used in insulin pumps.
6. Use only the proper syringe for your pump to give the correct flow rate.
7. The life of a disposable battery in the pump varies with the freshness of the battery and the storage conditions. For longest life, batteries should be stored in the refrigerator, but not in the freezer.
8. Use usual techniques of asepsis when inserting the needle. It should be inserted at a 45-degree angle. The needle is then taped as one would tape an intravenous needle. An application of Betadine may be applied to the site.
9. Implantable pumps are now being tested in humans.
10. The diabetic person simply does not put on the pump and achieve good control. It serves as a ''constant'' reminder that he needs to follow the rules of living with diabetes.
11. Emotions about the pump range from utter devotion to tolerance to downright contempt. A patient might experience all or only one. The attitudes about the pump are the result of having a device that improves blood sugars and, therefore, how well one feels. In addition, it requires enormous amounts of motivation, time, energy, and money.
12. Patients complain that the pumps are ''too bulky'' and are a constant reminder that they ''have diabetes.'' Wearing a pump may possibly alter body image or make a patient feel dependent on a mechanical device. The pump is cosmetically unacceptable to many patients. Initially, patients have difficulty sleeping with a pump. This can usually be resolved by the patient within a few days. Care must be taken when toileting and showering, since the pump is not waterproof. Some patients find wearing a pump bothersome during some types of activity (*i.e.*, sexual activity).
13. Few research studies (almost none in nursing) have been conducted about the effects on the person using the pump and his significant others. This is an area of much needed research.
14. Insurance companies may pay for all or part of the cost for meters used in monitoring blood sugar.

For example, the drainage of pancreatic enzymes must be provided for, as well as an adequate supply of blood to the newly transplanted organ. Additional problems include the requirement for immunosuppressive therapy and the accompanying increase in serious infection, a problem in the nondiabetic person but even more so in the person with diabetes. The whole pancreas or segments of the pancreas are currently being transplanted, but usually only in conjunction with a kidney transplant (because of diabetic nephropathy).

Islet Cells. Advantages in using isolated islets include easy manipulation of the cells (because of their small size, they can be injected through a small-gauge needle), easy provision of oxygen and food supply, avoidance of problems with enzymes, and lower incidence of immunogenic problems. This work is currently being done in animals.

Cultured Islet Cells. Culturing islet cells at room temperature prior to transplantation, and injecting antilymphocyte serum to diabetic recipient rats have increased the success rate with islet cells.

Oral Hypoglycemic Agents

(See Table 40-4.)

Oral hypoglycemic agents may be effective for selected, stable, noninsulin-dependent, nonketotic diabetics who cannot be treated by diet alone or who are unable or unwilling to take insulin. These drugs may be useful for the aged; those with poor vision, crippling arthritis of the fingers, and tremor of the hands; and those who for some reason refuse to take insulin. (Insulin is preferable to oral hypoglycemic agents if dietary treatment fails to control diabetes.)

In the United States, the available oral hypoglycemic agents are the sulfonylureas (tolbutamide, chlorpropamide, acetohexamide, and tolazamide). They are thought to exert their primary action by direct stimulation of pancreatic insulin secretion. Therefore, a functioning pancreas is necessary for these drugs to be effective, and they cannot be used in the treatment of patients who are insulin-dependent and ketosis-prone. The sulfonylureas can be divided into short-, intermediate-, and long-acting agents with varying duration of action. Side-effects of these drugs are relatively rare and include hematologic, hepatic, and dermatologic reactions. Hypoglycemia may occur when an excessive dose of a sulfonylurea is used or when meals are omitted or food intake is decreased. Hypoglycemia should be treated as usual, but special emphasis should be given to patients taking Diabinese because of the possibility of prolonged hypoglycemia due to its long-time action. The sulfonylureas also interact with various drugs: sulfonamides, salicylates, phenylbutazones, barbiturates, thiazides, alcohol, catecholamines, etc.

For successful treatment with oral agents, the diet must

Table 40-4
Oral Hypoglycemic Agents

Trade Name	Generic Name	Manufacturer	Duration of Action
First Generation			
Orinase	Tolbutamide	Upjohn	6–12 hr
Dymelor	Acetohexamide	Lilly	12–24 hr
Diabinese	Chlorpropamide	Pfizer	up to 60 hr
Tolinase	Tolazamide	Upjohn	14–24 hr
Second Generation*			
Micronase	Glyburide	Upjohn	12–24 hr
Diabeta	Glyburide	Hoechst	12–24 hr
Glucotrol	Glipizide	Pfizer	10–18 hr

* Currently awaiting approval by FDA for use in the United States, but available for use in Canada, Europe, and elsewhere in the world.

be restricted in total calories and carbohydrates, and the patient's urine and blood glucose values monitored.

- Oral hypoglycemic drugs must be abandoned temporarily in favor of insulin if the patient develops an infection with fever, suffers trauma, or undergoes major surgery.

If, as time goes on, the patient's urine tests and blood glucose values are no longer responsive to oral hypoglycemic therapy, the patient is then treated with insulin. This is referred to as a *secondary failure*. A *primary failure* occurs when the blood glucose level remains high a month after drug use.

A study by the National Institutes of Health, called the University Group Diabetes Program, has given rise to many questions concerning the safety and effectiveness of long-term oral hypoglycemic agents. This study group found a higher death rate from heart disease in their tolbutamide-treated patients than in those treated with a placebo. However, since the tolbutamide-treated patients were older and had more baseline cardiac disease than did the control patients, the conclusions may not be justified.

At the present time, the American Diabetes Association does not feel that the use of oral hypoglycemic agents should be restricted. However, it does recognize that the study's findings confirm the importance of diet in treating noninsulin-dependent diabetic patients. Upon diagnosis, some of the patients who are younger are placed on insulin by physicians who agree with the study.

▶ Evaluation

Expected Outcomes

Takes prescribed oral hypoglycemic medication

1. Adheres faithfully to the prescribed diet
2. Tests urine daily
3. Takes the medication exactly as directed

▷ **Acute Complications of Diabetes**

There are three conditions that can produce coma in the diabetic: hypoglycemia, diabetic ketoacidosis, and hyperosmolar coma.

Hypoglycemia ("Insulin Reactions")

Hypoglycemia (abnormally low blood glucose level) occurs when the blood glucose falls below 50 mg per dl. It can be caused by too much insulin, too little food, or excessive physical activity. Hypoglycemia may occur 1 to 3 hours after regular insulin, 4 to 18 hours after NPH or Lente insulin, and 18 to 30 hours after protamine zinc or ultralente insulin. Most episodes occur before meals, but they may occur at any time of the day or night.

When the blood glucose falls rapidly, the sympathetic nervous system is stimulated to produce adrenalin, causing sweating, tremor, tachycardia, palpitation, and nervousness. When the blood glucose falls slowly, there is depression of the central nervous system, resulting in headache, light-headedness, confusion, emotional changes, memory lapses, numbness of the lips and tongue, slurred speech, incoordination, staggering gait, double vision, drowsiness, convulsions, and eventually, coma. Since the brain depends on glucose for its energy supply, as hypoglycemia progresses, brain function deteriorates. Permanent central nervous system damage may result from prolonged hypoglycemia.

The combination of symptoms varies considerably in different patients and in the same patient at different times.

- Every patient taking insulin should be familiar with the warning symptoms so that he can take sugar promptly.
- Any abnormal behavior in a patient taking insulin should be considered to be due to hypoglycemia and treated as such until proven otherwise.
- Hypoglycemia must be treated promptly, because sustained hypoglycemia can lead to convulsions or coma and death. When the first warning symptoms appear,

Chart 40-6
Guidelines to Follow During Periods of Illness

- Take insulin or oral hypoglycemia agents as usual.
- Insulin-dependent diabetics may even need more insulin to compensate for increased blood glucose levels as a result of the illness.
- Report nausea, vomiting, and diarrhea to your physician, since extreme fluid loss may be dangerous.
- Test blood or urine frequently for glucose. If only blood tests are being done for glucose, test urine for ketones.
- Follow your meal plan. Soft foods and liquids may be substituted for regular food to supply needed calories.
- Keep in touch with your physician.

the patient should take some form of simple, fast-acting sugar orally: orange juice, sugar, hard candy (Lifesavers), or a soft drink containing sugar; if the symptoms persist for 10 to 15 minutes, the snack should be repeated. If it is more than an hour until the next meal, the patient should also eat a complex carbohydrate and protein.

- Every patient taking insulin should always carry candy, a few lumps of sugar, or Glutose or Monojel for the prompt relief of hypoglycemia.

Prevention and Patient Education. Hypoglycemia is prevented by following a regular pattern and timetable for eating, administering insulin, and engaging in daily exercise. Between-meal and bedtime snacks are often needed to counteract the maximum insulin effect. In general, the patient should cover the time of peak activity of insulin by eating a snack and by taking additional food when engaging in an increased level of physical activity. Routine glucose tests are performed so that changing insulin requirements may be anticipated and adjusted.

Because unexpected hypoglycemia may occur, any patient treated with insulin should wear an identification bracelet or tag indicating that he has diabetes.

Some diabetics with autonomic neuropathy or those taking propranolol may not experience symptoms of hypoglycemia. It is very important for these patients to perform blood glucose tests to determine blood glucose levels.

If the patient is unconscious and unable to swallow, glucagon hydrochloride is administered subcutaneously. This hormone, which is made in the alpha cells of the pancreas, causes glycogenolysis in the liver (if hepatic glycogen stores are not depleted). Glucagon raises the blood glucose high enough for most patients to wake up after the first dose and take orange juice or ginger ale by mouth. This additional "sugar" intake is important, because the elevation of blood glucose following glucagon administration is only temporary, and a hypoglycemia relapse is a real and constant danger. Glucagon is packaged as a powder in 1-mg vials and given in the same manner as insulin. It comes with a vial of diluent and once mixed, must be used. Do not use glucagon after the expiration date. It is sold by prescription only and should be part of the emergency supplies kept available by insulin-dependent persons with diabetes. It is useful in patients who receive little or no warning of their attacks and go into hypoglycemia.

If the patient cannot swallow and is unconscious, the intravenous administration of 50 ml of 50% glucose in water is the most effective treatment for hypoglycemia in a hospital and is used when it is available or when a second dose of glucagon is ineffective.

Somogyi Phenomenon. The Somogyi phenomenon is a paradoxical situation in which sudden falls in blood sugar are followed by rebound hyperglycemia. This situation is usually caused by gradual excessive administration of insulin. The underlying mechanism is that the hormonal responses to hypoglycemia counteract the effect of insulin. The patient's condition becomes uncontrollable, because the effect of the administered insulin is antagonized. The situation remains out of control when more insulin is given, and the patient has periods of hyperglycemia interspersed with hypoglycemia. One is alerted to this possibility when there are symptoms of hypoglycemia (irritability, confusion, etc.), with urine tests showing frequent glucosuria. The treatment consists of gradually lowering the amount of insulin until the appropriate dosage is reached.

Diabetic Ketoacidosis and Coma

Diabetic ketoacidosis is due to an absence or inadequate amount of insulin, which results in hyperglycemia and leads to a series of biochemical disorders. The pathophysiology is the result of insulin deficiency affecting many aspects of the metabolism of carbohydrate, protein, and fat. As a result, the amount of glucose entering the cells is reduced, and fat is metabolized instead of carbohydrate. Free fatty acids are mobilized from adipose tissue. Liver oxidases act upon these fatty acids to produce ketone bodies. The ketone bodies escape into the blood, and metabolic acidosis results, with lowering of serum bicarbonate, PCO_2, and pH. The overall clinical picture is one of hyperglycemia, water and electrolyte loss, acidemia, and coma.

Causes. Ketoacidosis may be precipitated by failure to take insulin, by insufficient insulin intake, or by resistance to insulin. It may be caused by infection (of the respiratory tract, urinary tract, gastrointestinal tract, or of the skin), by physiologic stresses such as acute illness, surgery, trauma, pregnancy, and or by emotional stresses that reduce the effectiveness of the available insulin. (Chart 40-6 presents guidelines for persons with diabetes to follow during periods of illness.) Anti-insulin factors (growth hormone, glucagon, cortisol) are released during stress and may play a part in the development of ketoacidosis. Ketoacidosis occurs more commonly in insulin-dependent diabetes. It is a serious complication, with a mortality rate ranging from 5% to 9%.

Clinical Manifestations. The clinical manifestations occur as a result of changes in body fluid, electrolytes, and acid–base status. Early manifestations are polyuria (excessive urination), polyphagia (excessive appetite), and polydipsia (excessive thirst). Osmotic diuresis causes water loss (dehydration) and electrolyte depletion. As the patient becomes more dehydrated, oliguria (diminished urination) develops. Malaise and visual changes may be noted by the patient. Headache, muscle aches, and abdominal pain are frequent complaints, as are nausea, vomiting, and gastric stasis and ileus. If infection has precipitated the ketoacidosis, fever may be present. The patient's respiratory rate increases to compensate for acidosis. Coma and severe acidosis are ushered in with Kussmaul breathing (very deep, but not labored, respirations) and a sweetish odor of the breath, due to acidemia.

The patient is drowsy and soon becomes comatose. The blood glucose is elevated, the serum bicarbonate and the blood *p*H are decreased, the blood urea is increased, and the plasma ketone is strongly positive. The urine is strongly positive for sugar and acetone. The patient's condition is serious at this stage, but recovery can be anticipated after prompt and vigorous treatment with insulin and intravenous fluids.

Management.   The immediate goals in the management of ketoacidosis are (1) to restore normal carbohydrate, protein, and fat metabolism; (2) to reverse hypovolemia; and (3) to correct electrolyte imbalance. A flow sheet is kept of vital signs and ketone measurements, as well as of blood glucose and electrolytes, arterial blood gases, and the medications and treatment given. A rapid physical examination is carried out, to detect evidence of infection, myocardial infarction, stroke, etc.

- An infusion of isotonic or hypotonic saline is started immediately to rehydrate the patient and improve tissue perfusion. The fluid deficit may range between 6 and 10 liters, and the rate of replacement depends on the patient's condition.
- Insulin is given to reduce blood glucose by promoting glucose utilization and to inhibit lipolysis (splitting up of fat), thereby preventing accumulation of ketones in the blood. The insulin regimens in current use are variable both in amounts and route of administration.

Until recently, high doses of insulin were given by intravenous boluses or by the intramuscular or subcutaneous routes, and repeated every 4 hours. It was difficult to maintain steady plasma levels by this protocol.

Low-dose insulin regimens are being used with increasing frequency. Continuous low-dose intravenous therapy with insulin may be given to obtain immediate insulin action and to maintain steady blood levels of insulin. Low-dose insulin is controllable and gives a more predictable response. A constant infusion pump or pediatric drip (with insulin placed in 250 ml of half normal saline) may be used. Albumin or some other colloid may be added to the intravenous solution to prevent insulin from adhering to the infusion bottle and tubing. There are variations in the low-dose insulin regimens, including administration of insulin by intermittent intramuscular injection.

As the blood glucose level declines, glucose is added to the infusion, and the insulin concentration is reduced. There is now danger of hypoglycemia.

- Close monitoring of the patient is essential, since metabolic parameters change and call for continuing assessment of the patient and fluid and electrolyte status. Frequent laboratory determinations of blood glucose, serum ketones, serum bicarbonate, and serum potassium are needed.

At first the patient's serum potassium may be normal or raised, but when the blood glucose level begins to approach normal, hypokalemia threatens the patient. Hypokalemia occurs when serum potassium levels are reduced as a result of potassium "migrating" into the cells along with glucose, under the influence of insulin. Hypokalemia also results when extracellular potassium ions are exchanged for intracellular hydrogen ions, in the correction of acidosis.

- Frequent estimates of serum potassium and ECG monitoring are essential for early recognition of hypokalemia. Potassium replacement is usually started early. Tingling, paresthesia, decreased tendon reflexes, and respiratory depression are clinical manifestations of hypokalemia.

Hypotension that does not respond to intravenous fluids is treated with albumin, plasma, vasopressors, etc. Monitoring of central venous pressure is important, to achieve safe fluid balance, especially in elderly patients or those with myocardial disease. Nasogastric intubation and suctioning relieve vomiting and acute dilatation of the stomach and reduce the possibility of aspiration.

Consciousness should be restored and metabolic disturbances corrected within 12 to 24 hours. After the acute problem is corrected, the patient is regulated as described earlier. The precipitating cause of the coma should be determined to prevent a recurrence.

Prevention.   The patient should be taught and retaught the fundamentals of insulin administration and glucose testing, and the management of diabetes to prevent recurrence of diabetic ketoacidosis.

Hyperosmolar Nonketotic Coma

Hyperosmolar hyperglycemic coma is a syndrome in which hyperglycemia and hyperosmolarity predominate, with possible alterations of the sensorium (sense of awareness). At the same time, ketosis is minimal or absent. This condition occurs most frequently in older people (50 to 70 years) who have had no previous history of diabetes, or only mild maturity-onset diabetes. The acute development of the condition can be traced to some precipitating event, such as an acute illness (pneumonia, myocardial infarction, stroke), ingestion of drugs known to provoke insulin insufficiency (thiazide diuretics, propranolol), and therapeutic procedures (peritoneal dialysis/hemodialysis, hyperalimentation). In the more chronic picture, there is a history of days to weeks of polyuria, with inadequate fluid intake. Upon admission to the hospital, the patient is found to have severe hyperglycemia ("syrupy blood"), profound dehydration, and variable neurologic signs ranging from sleepy confusion to coma.

The basic biochemical effect is lack of effective insulin. The patient's persistent hyperglycemia causes osmotic diuresis, resulting in losses of water and electrolytes. To maintain osmotic equilibrium, water shifts from the intracellular fluid space to the extracellular fluid space. With glucosuria and dehydration, hypernatremia and increasing hyperosmolality occur. The reasons why these patients show minimal ketosis is not clear.

The clinical picture is one of hypotension, dehydration (dry mucous membranes, poor skin turgor), fever, tachycardia, and variable neurologic signs (alteration of sensorium, seizures, hemiparesis, etc.). This is a serious condition with a mortality rate ranging from 5% to 50%.

Management. The objective of management is to correct the volume depletion and hyperosmolar state. Then a search is made for the precipitating cause. Fluid therapy is started with hypotonic saline that is titrated by CVP monitoring. Insulin may be given either by high-dose or low-dose regimen. Potassium chloride is added when the urinary output is adequate and is guided by ECG monitoring. Other therapeutic modalities are determined by the condition of the patient and the results of continuing clinical and laboratory evaluation.

▷ Long-term Complications of Diabetes

There has been a steady decline in deaths due to diabetic ketoacidosis and infection, but an alarming rise in deaths due to cardiovascular and renal complications. Long-term complications are becoming more common as more diabetics live longer with their diabetes.

Atherosclerotic complications, with myocardial infarction, cerebrovascular accidents, uremia, and gangrene cause 70% of deaths among diabetic persons. There is no effective means of preventing or postponing the development of atherosclerosis in diabetics and nondiabetics. However, there is more and more evidence demonstrating that maintenance of blood glucose levels in the normal or near-normal range may delay the long-term complications. Even though much has been written on this subject, we still do not know why it occurs earlier and progresses more rapidly in diabetics.

Vascular Complications

Diabetes mellitus is accompanied by changes in the entire vascular system. With the duration of diabetes, changes develop in the blood vessels that lead to the long-term complications of the disease. The changes that occur in the blood vessels can be categorized into those that involve the large or the small vessels. Complications of the larger vessels (macrovascular disease or macroangiopathy) are cardiovascular in nature and involve the heart and the peripheral circulation, especially the legs. Complications of the smaller vessels (microvascular disease or microangiopathy) involve the eyes, kidneys, and nervous system.

The specific pathologic lesion (microangiopathy) of long-standing diabetes is characterized by thickening of the capillary basement membrane in every organ. The prevalence of microangiopathy parallels the duration of diabetes and its rate of progression and is now thought to be directly related to blood sugar control.

Intracapillary glomerulosclerosis (Kimmelstiel–Wilson syndrome) is the specific renal disease of diabetes and is related to thickening of the capillary basement membrane in the glomerulus. It appears that blood sugars above normal are responsible for the pathologic changes in the kidney. Renal failure is common in diabetics who develop the disease at an early age. (The pathophysiology and treatment of renal failure is discussed in Chap. 44.)

Involvement of the capillaries of the retina may lead to blindness, due to diabetic retinopathy (see below). Microangiopathy of the vessels supplying the skin, peripheral nerves, and walls of the large arteries may be a factor in skin diseases and diabetic neuropathy.

The changes occurring in the larger arteries appear to be the same atherosclerotic changes that occur in nondiabetics as a result of the aging process. However, the changes tend to occur at an earlier age in diabetes. Occlusion of major vessels due to atherosclerosis causes strokes, myocardial infarction, intermittent claudication, and gangrene. Advanced vascular disease in the large and small arteries of the legs is common in diabetes and is often severe enough to lead to gangrene of the affected extremity. Such changes may be extensive enough to result in ossification of the wall of the artery. These changes in the smaller arteries present a serious problem, since an occlusion to one of the large arteries cannot be followed by the formation of adequate collateral circulation.

Nursing Assessment for Impaired Circulation. Clinical manifestations of impaired peripheral arterial circulation include paleness of the lower extremities, reduced pulse volume in the arteries of the lower extremities, blanching and exaggerated pallor of the feet and legs after the legs are elevated for 60 seconds, delayed (greater than 10 seconds) return of color to the feet and legs after the lower extremities are moved from an elevated position to a dependent position, loss of hair over the dorsal surface of the foot, thickened toenails, and brown spots on the skin of the lower extremities.

Diabetic patients who have impaired peripheral circulation are vulnerable to infection and gangrene, which commonly results from trauma. The patient may be unaware that he has somehow injured his leg. Such unawareness of injury is a result of peripheral neuropathy, which commonly accompanies diabetes.

Diabetic Retinopathy

The vision of a diabetic can be affected in many ways. Each part of the eye and the visual system is susceptible to the complications of diabetes. The severity of the problem can range from a change in the eyeglass prescription to total blindness. These changes are extremely important because even the smallest change can affect life-style (*i.e.,* insulin measurement, testing for glucose in blood or urine, driving, etc.).

Types of visual problems in the diabetic may include:

- Refractive changes
- Extraocular muscle palsy
- Corneal problems
- Glaucoma
- Cataracts
- Retinopathy

Vision may be affected by some of these problems, but in general, if the pathology includes the macula and its function, then vision will be decreased.

The eye pathology is referred to as diabetic retinopathy. It causes changes in the small blood vessels in the retina of the eye. The retina is the area of the eye that receives images and sends information about the images to the brain. It is richly supplied with blood vessels of all kinds, small arteries and veins, arterioles, venules, and capillaries. The pathology involves the walls of the blood vessels, most especially the capillaries in the retina.

Diagnostic Evaluation. Retinopathy is frequently seen years after the diagnosis of diabetes and is rarely totally absent in a patient with diabetes who has had the disease for years. Occasionally, it may be the first clinical sign of diabetes—the sign that brings the patient to the physician and eventually leads to the diagnosis of diabetes.

Diagnosis is by direct visualization with an ophthalmoscope or with a technique known as fluorescein angiography. Fluorescein angiography can document the type and activity of the retinopathy. It is a technique in which a dye is injected into an arm vein. The dye is carried to various parts of the body through the blood, but especially through the vessels of the retina of the eye. This technique allows the ophthalmologist, using special instruments, to see the retinal vessels in bright detail and gives useful information that cannot be obtained with just an ophthalmoscope. Photographs of the fundus of the eye are taken through a series of filters that excite and record the fluorescence of the dye. The dye is bound to the blood proteins and first appears in the choroid and then in the arterial branches of the retina. Areas of leakage from the vessels and areas of neovascularization (new vessel formation) are stained with fluorescein.

Side-effects of this diagnostic procedure performed in an outpatient setting may include:

- Nausea during the dye injection
- A yellowish, fluorescent discoloration of the skin and urine that may last 12 to 24 hours
- An occasional allergic reaction, usually hives or itching

However, in general it is a safe diagnostic procedure.

Patients should be told the sequence of procedures as well as:

- The fact that it is a painless procedure
- The potential side-effects
- What type of information the technique can provide
- That the flash of the camera may be slightly uncomfortable for a short period of time

Problems in the blood-retinal barrier are possible before they become clinically visible in the fundus. The pathology increases with the duration of the diabetes and "poor control" of the blood sugar.

Pathology. The pathologic changes in the vessels begin as bulges in the walls of the capillaries (microaneurysms), and eventually fluids leak into the surrounding areas of the retina (Fig. 40-4). If the changes are limited to the retina, it is referred to as background retinopathy. This does not generally interfere with vision and occurs in 50% of all diabetics after 10 to 15 years with diabetes. In some diabetics, this condition progresses to "proliferative retinop-

athy," the stage of new vessel formation (neovascularization) in and around the retina. These vessels branch out and grow into other areas of the eye. These vessels have thin, leaky walls and can cause damage by hemorrhage and scar formation. Unless the macula of the eye is involved, considerable retinopathy can be present before interfering with vision.

Electron microscopy has shown an increased production of basement membrane material as the microaneurysms form. As this material ages, thickening of the basement membrane continues. The wall fragments and the debris leak from the capillary to the surrounding areas. Since the integrity of the basement membrane is impaired, the capillary loses its selective permeability. The capillaries continue to change, losing cells from their walls, and gradually, the lumena of the capillaries are obliterated. This leads to a loss of adequate blood flow in this important area of the eye and to the formation of "shunt" vessels (neovascularization). These defective vessels are grown in an attempt to supply areas of the retina deprived of blood (retinal hypoxia) because of the disease process. If no treatment is instituted at this time, the condition will progress to proliferative retinopathy in which vessels grow into the vitreous humor. These vessels hemorrhage into the vitreous, causing major problems that can lead to severe visual impairment, glaucoma, retinal detachment, and finally blindness.

Nonproliferative (Background) Retinopathy. Classifying retinopathy into nonproliferative and proliferative types is useful in diagnosis, treatment, and counseling. Eighty percent of all cases of retinopathy fall in this group. It is more common in type II diabetics. This aspect of retinopathy waxes and wanes with time. An increase in the number of microaneurysms usually means an increase in the activity of the retinopathy or changes that may lead to reduced vision. The type of pathology seen in the nonproliferative stage include:

- Microaneurysm formation (appear as red spots on fundus)
- Intraretinal hemorrhages
- Venous changes: dilation, beading, or sausaging, and occasional venous loops
- Exudate deposition*
    Hard: glistening yellow fatty deposits in retina
    Soft: "cotton-wool spots"—fluffy, white opacities in the nerve fiber layer of retina; actually, infarcts—areas of ischemia
- Macular edema*

Preproliferative Retinopathy. This stage will soon progress to proliferative retinopathy in 3% to 10% of all diabetic patients. The type of pathology seen in this stage includes:

- Increased venous abnormalities
- "Cotton-wool spots"
- Areas of nonperfusion or capillary closure in the retina
- Large clusters of microaneurysms
- Dot/blot hemorrhages
- Diffuse macular edema

This stage progresses to the next if new vessels increase. The best way to keep track of the activity is to have pho-

* May cause reduced vision.

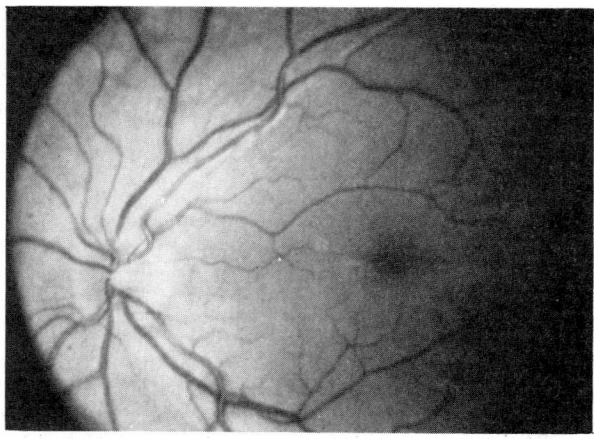

A

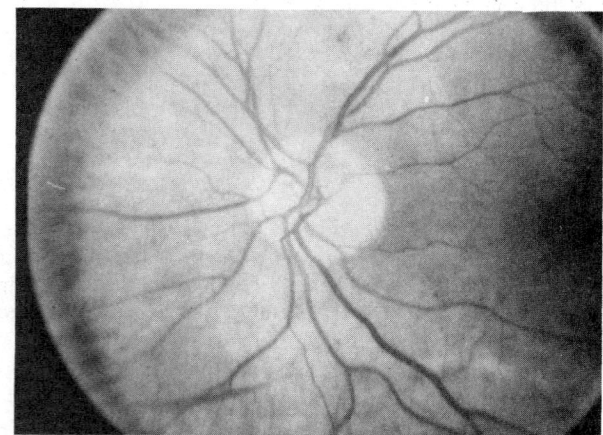

B

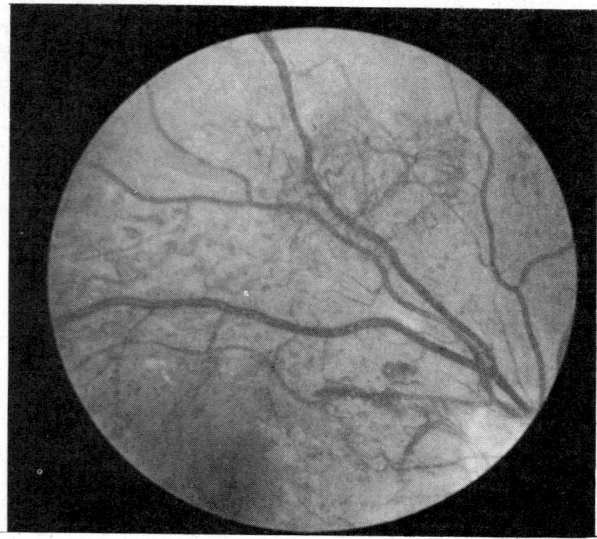

C

tographs taken of the fundus. These can be compared with previous photos to determine if the retinopathy is stable or progressing.

Proliferative Retinopathy. This stage is the most serious. It begins with the appearance of new blood vessels on the optic disc or on the surface of the retina and is associated with generalized retinal ischemia. These vessels are fragile and prone to hemorrhage. These can cause preretinal or vitreous hemorrhages and traction retinal detachments.

Macular Edema. It has just recently been realized that a significant loss of vision can occur as a result of macular edema. In this aspect of the disease, there is a breakdown of the blood-retinal barrier with an accumulation of fluid within the retina. Retinal structures become distorted; damage occurs in the neural part of the retina. At first, this damage is reversible; later it is not. The process occurs slowly, often with no ophthalmologically visible hemorrhages or exudates. The first symptom the patient notices is a distortion of vision, which, if left untreated, progresses to visual impairment.

Neovascularization. This growth of new blood vessels goes against the normal functioning of the eye. Part of the eye, especially the vitreous, which should remain clear if it is to transmit light, becomes clouded with a network of new blood vessels. In addition, the new vessels leak badly and further cloud the vitreous. Fibrous tissue replaces the free blood, and as the vitreous contracts, it pulls the retina from its normal attachment (retinal detachment).

Management

Photocoagulation. The principle of photocoagulation is that strong light energy can be converted into heat energy when it is absorbed by the two pigments in the retina melanin (a natural retinal pigment) and hemoglobin (in the red blood cell of the retinal blood vessels) (Fig. 40-5). The heat energy burns the area being treated and creates a controlled scar.

If the laser treatment is performed early enough, it will usually cause the abnormal vessels to shrink and disappear. The procedure is usually done in a retinal specialist's office with highly specialized equipment. Patients do not experience intense pain, and discomfort varies with the patient.

Vitrectomy. When a major hemorrhage into the vitreous occurs, the vitreous fluid becomes mixed with blood and prevents light from passing through the eye, which can cause blindness. Until 1971 little could be done, even with a laser. To use a laser, it is necessary to see the retina.

A vitrectomy is a surgical procedure that uses an instrument that contains a drill and a suction. It is inserted into the eyeball and is used to remove the hemorrhage,

Figure 40-4. Diabetic retinopathy. (*A*) In the fundus photograph of a normal eye, the light, circular area to the left, over which a number of blood vessels converge, is the optic disc, where the optic nerve meets the back of the eye. To the right of the optic disc is a smaller, dark spot on the photograph, the macula. The macula is the part of the retina on which images in the center of a person's visual field are focused. This part of the retina has a high concentration of light-sensitive cells, called *cones*, which provide sharp, clear color vision in bright light. (*B*) The fundus photograph of a patient with diabetic retinopathy shows neovascularization—growth of a fine network of abnormal new vessels—directly on the optic disc. Small dots on the photograph are microaneurysms, while larger blotches are hemorrhages. One example of a hemorrhage in this photo is an almost horizontal streak on the lower left. (*C*) This fundus photograph showing severe diabetic retinopathy reveals widespread neovascularization, microaneurysms, and hemorrhaging. (Photo: Courtesy National Eye Institute)

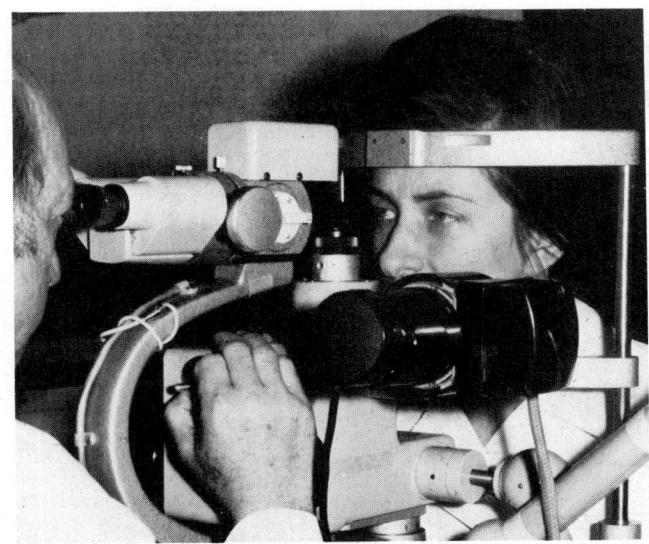
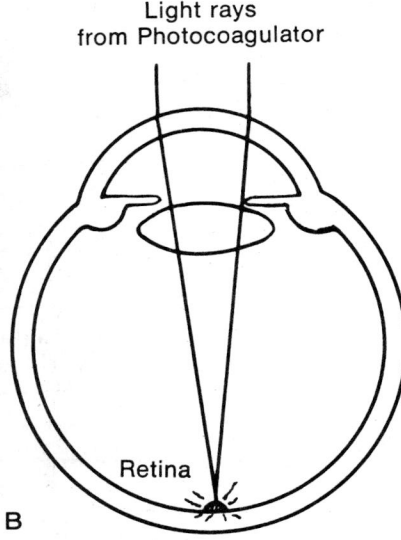

Figure 40-5. Photocoagulation. (*A*) The photograph shows a model receiving treatment with the argon laser, which generates a fine but intense blue–green beam of light. In this therapy the intense beam of light is directed into the eye and focused on a tiny spot in the retina. (Courtesy, Dr. Arnall Patz, Wilmer Eye Institute, Johns Hopkins Hospital, Baltimore, Maryland.) (*B*) Principle underlying photocoagulation. The intense beam of light acts in much the same way as the sun's rays focused through a magnifying glass produce a small burn on a leaf. (Reproduced with permission from American Association of Workers for the Blind, Inc., Blindness Annual.)

replacing it with saline or another liquid. The instrument is then removed and the hole sealed. It can then be determined if laser therapy is needed. Its use is still limited; the procedure is undergoing evaluation in a double blind study being conducted at the National Institutes of Health.

The instrument can also be used to cut the fibrous bands that cause traction on the retina, which might cause retinal detachment.

Only eyes that are severely damaged and in which hemorrhage is not resolving spontaneously are appropriate candidates for the procedure.

Side-effects of the procedure include vitreal and retinal hemorrhages, rubeosis iridis, and neovascularization. It is a procedure not to be taken lightly.

Pituitary Ablation. This surgical procedure had been used in the past for the treatment of proliferative retinopathy. However, today most feel that the benefits are outweighed by the side-effects.

Growth hormone, produced in the anterior pituitary gland, increases the severity of diabetes and retinopathy. Pituitary ablation is done to arrest malignant or accelerated proliferative retinopathy by surgical removal—by cutting the stalk of the gland or by using x-rays or radioactive implants to destroy the gland. As a result of the procedure, the insulin requirement falls, and there is a 50% regression in the eye damage. However, it also results in a functional loss of thyroid, adrenal, and sex hormones. These must be replaced forever. Another result is an increased sensitivity to even small amounts of insulin. Both can create difficult problems for persons with diabetes in addition to his vision problems. Since retinopathy waxes and wanes, the value of a pituitary ablation may not have the consistent effect on vision that once seemed apparent.

Health Teaching

In all forms of therapy for retinopathy, something is destroyed in the process of saving vision. The facts must be presented to the patient and his family as honestly as possible. The course of the retinopathy will be long and stressful. In counseling the patient, it is important to stress:

- That the appearance of retinopathy can be expected after many years of diabetes, and its appearance does not necessarily mean that the diabetes is on a downhill course
- That the odds for maintaining vision is in his favor
- That frequent eye examinations are the best way to preserve vision, because it allows for the detection of any retinopathy

Some additional points to keep in mind when the patient with diabetes has some type of visual impairment are as follows:

- Visual impairment can be a shock to anyone. A person's response to vision loss depends on his personality, self-concept, and coping mechanisms.
- As in any loss, blindness and its acceptance by the patient will occur in stages; some patients may learn to accept blindness in a rather short period of time, while others may never accept it.
- Although retinopathy occurs bilaterally, the severity may differ in each eye.
- Many of the chronic complications of diabetes happen simultaneously. For example, a blind diabetic may also have peripheral neuropathy and may experience impairment of manual dexterity, tactile sensation, and depth perception.

- As in all patients, a thorough assessment of physical status and capability is important not only upon the first contact, but throughout the course of the retinopathy. Areas to be assessed should include:

  Activities of daily living
  Insulin administration
  Urine or blood glucose testing
  Daily foot care
  Meal planning
  Other medications
  Physical activities

Upon being diagnosed as a diabetic, an initial examination by an ophthalmologist is necessary. Thereafter, the diabetic should be examined by an ophthalmologist as follows:

- Type I—5 years after initial examination, then yearly
- Type II—yearly

A good eye examination for a diabetic should include measurement of visual acuity and examination of the retina, optic disc, and blood vessels directly with an ophthalmoscope, preferably with the pupil dilated for a better view of the ocular fundus. For both type I and type II diabetics, the fundus of the eyes should also be examined each time the patient sees his physician for a routine checkup.

Reasons for referral to an ophthalmologist specializing in retinopathy include:

- Neovascularization
- Vitreous hemorrhages
- Decreased visual acuity
- Increased microaneurysms
- Venous dilatation
- Macular exudates
- Cotton-wool spots
- Pregnancy or renal disease
- Poor diabetes control

The Diabetic Neuropathies

Diabetic neuropathy (pathology of the nerves) of the peripheral and autonomic nervous system are common complications of diabetes. Diabetic neuropathy may affect the entire nervous system, but is more readily recognized in the peripheral nerves. The prevalence increases with the age of the patient and the duration of the disease.

Pathology.   The causes for diabetic neuropathy are unknown. The pathogenesis may be due to either a vascular or a metabolic mechanism. There is support for the theory that metabolic aberrations of neurons or their myelin sheaths may be responsible for the nerve damage seen in diabetes. In the poorly controlled diabetic, an enzyme system (the sorbitol pathways) may become overactive during periods of insulin insufficiency, resulting in overproduction of fructose in the myelin sheath, which causes it to rupture, thereby disrupting nerve conduction.

Clinical Manifestations.   Involvement of the autonomic nervous system covers a broad range of functions, including orthostatic hypotension, sexual impotency and retrograde ejaculation, pupillary changes, abnormal sweating, bladder paralysis, and nocturnal diarrhea.

Peripheral neuropathy most commonly manifests itself in the lower extremities. Pain and paresthesia are the outstanding manifestations. The pain has been described as dull or aching, cramping, burning, lancinating, or crushing. The pain is usually intensified at night and may be relieved by pacing the floor, which distinguishes this pain from the pain due to peripheral vascular insufficiency, which is intensified by walking.

The paresthesias have been described as sensations of tingling or burning, or of coldness and numbness. Because of these varied discomforts, it is quite common for the patient to be depressed and irritable and to suffer from anorexia.

Loss of sensation can lead to infection, gangrene, and amputation. The patient may be unaware of a blister, a protruding nail in his shoe, a burn from an electric blanket, etc. Instruction and reinforcement of previous learning about foot care is vital (see discussion below).

Nursing Assessment for Neuropathy of Extremities

- Place the patient in a supine position.
- Shield the patient's view of his feet with one hand, grasp the second toe on the sides with the thumb and forefinger, and move the toe back and forth several times.
- Stop the movement, and ask the patient in which direction the toe is pointed. If his proprioceptive senses (which provide information about position or movement of the body) are functioning adequately, the patient will respond correctly. An incorrect response may be an indication of neuropathy.
- Test also for response to pinprick and light touch, as well as knee and ankle reflexes. Absence of knee or ankle reflexes is significant.

Management.   There is no evidence that treatment will reverse peripheral neuropathy, but some clinicians feel that careful diabetic control may halt or delay its progress.

Foot Care in Diabetes

The feet of the diabetic patient are subject to sepsis and ischemia from deficient nerve function and poor circulation. Diabetic neuropathy may cause pain and paresthesia, but the greatest problem is loss of pain and temperature sensation in the feet.

Without pain perception, repeated trauma to the feet is tolerated until calluses and ulcers form, and the joints become damaged. Because of numbness of the feet, the patient may fail to notice a tack or a stone in his shoe. In addition, burns may occur when the patient is unable to recognize that a heating pad or a footbath is too hot. External heat is the most common single cause of gangrene. In view of these dangers, heat should not be applied below the knee of any diabetic patient.

Vascular involvement of the feet may lead to occlusion of large, medium, and small arteries and cause atrophic changes in the skin. The swelling that results from cellulitis may cause decreased circulation at a time when it needs to be increased. (Occlusive vascular disease can coexist with neuropathy.) If there is no response to antibiotics and debridement, the ischemia may cause gangrene to start in the tips of the toes and then spread slowly up the leg.

Large-vessel insufficiency causes intermittent claudication (pain on walking, relieved by rest), blanching of the feet upon elevation, dusky redness of the feet when dependent, atrophic skin changes, cold feet, and finally pain at rest. Involvement of the autonomic nervous system may lead to an absence of sweating, which causes dry, cracked skin that permits bacteria to enter the foot.

Thus, the triad of neuropathy, vascular disease, and infection leads to gangrene and amputation in older diabetics. In the presence of gangrene, amputation is done at the lowest level that has an adequate blood supply and is free of infection. The care of the patient undergoing amputation of an extremity is discussed on pages 1445–1449.

Management. Diabetic patients who have neuropathy and vascular problems should be under the supervision of a podiatrist. However, often the nurse is the only member of the health care team who is available to provide direct care and guidance. The patient must be taught to wash and examine his feet every day. Unless the nails are thick, the vision poor, or the neuropathy severe, the patient should learn to trim his own nails. (See instructions for cutting toenails, p. 270.)

Assessment by the Nurse

1. Ask the patient if he is a diabetic. Watch particularly for any lesion of the foot that does not heal.
2. Compare the skin color of the foot with the opposite foot and then with the other parts of the body (ankle, leg, hands).
3. Look for a mild cyanotic color in the digital or midtarsal area. This is caused by diminution of the arterial supply to the toes and sluggish venous return.
4. Change the position of the extremity and note the color changes. Pallor on elevation and dusky cyanosis on dependency indicate vascular insufficiency.
5. Feel the temperature of the feet. They should be about equal.
6. Examine the toenails. Thick, dry, and ridged nails may be a clue to circulatory impairment and diabetes.
7. Look for tinea pedis (fungal infection) between the toes and onchomycosis (fungal infection in the nails). Fungal infection of the feet is more serious in the diabetic.
8. Inspect for calluses, corns, blisters, cracks, and abrasions; look between the toes and on the soles of the feet.
9. Palpate the dorsalis pedis and posterior tibial arterial pulses; absence of a discernible pulse or diminution of pulses indicates atherosclerosis.

Infections

There appears to be a correlation between diabetes and susceptibility to infection, perhaps because of depleted host defenses and if glucose concentration in the tissues is greater than normal. High blood glucose may impair the ability of granulocytes to carry out a number of vital functions. Hyperglycemia also depresses leukocyte phagocytosis.

Infections are more serious in the diabetic because resistance to infection is decreased by hyperglycemia, and because diabetes becomes temporarily more severe in the presence of infection. Infections in the diabetic are exacerbated by dehydration, insulin antagonism, impaired phagocytosis, and neuropathy. Infection is a common precipitating cause of acute complications, such as diabetic ketoacidosis.

The extremities may be vulnerable to infection because of diminished arterial circulation, which lowers resistance to bacterial invasion and local injury. Cellulitis may spread rapidly. Fungal infections between the toes may produce fissures that provide further portals of entry for bacteria. Infections of the foot can lead to gangrene, with loss of toes, forefoot, or the foot and lower leg. A diabetic patient with an infected foot generally requires hospitalization. (The prevention of foot problems is discussed on p. 914.)

Dermatologic problems abound in diabetes mellitus. Fungal infections, particularly candidiasis of the skin and vagina, are frequently found in poorly controlled diabetics. The presence of boils or carbuncles and severe pruritus should raise the suspicion of possible diabetes.

The increased prevalence of urinary tract infections in diabetes is related to incomplete emptying of the bladder, due to poor bladder tone, a neurologic complication that may result from diabetic neuropathy, and possibly to an increased frequency of catheterization. Bladder infection produces ascending infections of the urinary tract. Serious complications from renal infection are more frequent in the person with diabetes.

Management. When the blood glucose is elevated, the leukocytes are unable to effectively destroy bacteria. All infections, and especially those associated with leukocytosis and a spreading infection, cause an increased need for insulin. Ketoacidosis may result if the insulin dose is not increased adequately. Testing the urine for sugar and acetone, and frequent blood glucose determinations are necessary to ascertain and compensate for rapidly changing insulin requirements. The cause of the infection should be determined by cultures, so that the appropriate antibiotic may be given.

▷ Evaluation

Expected Outcomes

1. Maintains normoglycemia with few episodes of hypoglycemia or hyperglycemia
   a. Maintains fasting blood sugar range of 130 mg to 140 mg
   b. Maintains urine free of glucose and acetone (no greater than 1+ glucose)
   c. Experiences no symptoms of hyperglycemia
   d. Experiences no symptoms of hypoglycemia
   e. Is aware of the degree of diabetic control (see specific outcomes, Chart 40-7, D).
2. Utilizes measures to prevent ketosis/ketoacidosis
   a. Takes adequate amount of insulin as prescribed
   b. Avoids physiologic and psychological stresses that reduce insulin effectiveness

c. Seeks medical consultation when stresses cannot be avoided

d. Maintains control of diabetes during periods of illness (see specific outcomes, Chart 40-7, H)

3. Utilizes measures to prevent hypoglycemia
   a. Adjusts insulin intake in accordance with exercise
   b. Avoids situations that produce insulin reactions: omission of a meal, unaccustomed or strenuous exercise
   c. Recognizes symptoms of an insulin reaction
   d. Takes precautions to prevent an insulin reaction (see specific outcomes, Chart 40-7, E, 9)

4. Utilizes measures to prevent/control long-term complications
   a. Utilizes measures to prevent/control macroangiopathy of heart and peripheral circulation
      (1) Experiences no symptoms of stroke
      (2) Experiences no symptoms of myocardial infarction
      (3) Experiences no intermittent claudication
      (4) Exhibits no progression of pulse volume deficit in lower extremities
      (5) Avoids tobacco and other vasoconstrictors
      (6) Avoids trauma to lower extremities
   b. Experiences no nephropathy (or no progression of nephropathy)
      (1) Has BUN within normal range
      (2) Has serum creatinine within normal range
      (3) Has serum potassium within normal range
      (4) Excretes adequate urine volume in relation to fluid intake
      (5) Has urine specific gravity within normal range
   c. Utilizes measures to prevent/control retinopathy
      (1) Keeps appointment with ophthalmologist yearly
      (2) Describes the importance of good diabetes control to deter progression of retinopathy
   d. Utilizes measures to prevent/control peripheral neuropathy
      (1) Experiences no pain (or no progression of pain) in lower extremities
      (2) Experiences no paresthesias (or no progression of paresthesias) in lower extremities
      (3) Exhibits presence of knee and ankle reflexes
      (4) Describes the importance of good diabetes control to deter progression of neuropathy
      (5) Practices proper foot care to prevent infection (see specific outcomes, Chart 40-7, G)
   e. Utilizes measures to prevent infection
      (1) Practices proper foot care
      (2) Practices proper skin care
      (3) Describes signs and symptoms of infections of skin, vagina, urinary tract, and respiratory tract

5. Adheres to therapeutic regimen
   a. Describes diabetes and how it affects the body (see specific outcomes, Chart 40-7, A)
   b. Maintains health at an optimal level
   c. Adheres to exercise program (see specific outcomes, Chart 40-7, B)
   d. Follows the prescribed dietary regimen (see specific outcomes, Chart 40-7, C)

e. Utilizes measures to determine degree of control of diabetes (see specific outcomes, Chart 40-7, D)

f. Utilizes proper practices of insulin therapy (see specific outcomes, Chart 40-7, E)

▷ Health Education for Diabetes

Since the responsibility for the management of diabetes rests with the individual, each patient is taught to perform duties usually done by the physician, nurse, dietitian, and laboratory technician. The educational program is started at the time of diagnosis and must be continued throughout the life of the patient. Continuing education reinforces learning and is necessary for better control of the disease and for greater self-reliance of the patient or significant other. A responsible member of the patient's family should be included in the educational program. The community health nurse also has a role. Group instruction may be an effective method of education in diabetic clinics, hospitals, and community health departments.

Realistic educational outcomes for the newly diagnosed patient include understanding of the (1) pathophysiology of diabetes; (2) basic concepts of dietary management; (3) administration of insulin; (4) exercise regimen; (5) urine testing; (6) recall of signs and symptoms of hypoglycemia and hyperglycemia; and (7) basic principles of foot care.

The reader is referred to Chapter 3 for discussion of the principles of health teaching and patient education. A summary of detailed information necessary for the education of diabetic patients is found in Chart 40-7.

▷ The Patient With Diabetes Undergoing Surgery

Because of the possibility of generalized vascular disease, decreased resistance to infection, and changing insulin requirements due to stress, the patient must be followed very closely at the time of surgery. Surgical stress aggravates hyperglycemia because of an increased secretion of epinephrine and glucocorticoids. The metabolic stress of anesthesia also accentuates problems of hyperglycemia and ketosis. In addition, the patient's normal schedule of food intake, which is the foundation of diabetic treatment, is interrupted.

Preoperative Management. In the preoperative period, the aim is to have the diabetes well controlled and to correct any problems of hydration and electrolyte imbalance. The greatest danger is hypoglycemia, since the central nervous system is very sensitive to glucose deprivation and the clinical signs of hypoglycemia are difficult to interpret when the patient is unconscious from anesthesia.

If the patient has been on an oral hypoglycemic agent or long-acting insulin, then regular insulin is substituted a day or two before surgery. The preoperative medication is kept to a minimum, since these patients are susceptible to sedatives and narcotics.

There are a wide variety of protocols for the management of the patient's nutrient and insulin requirements before, during, and after surgery, depending on the degree of

Chart 40-7
Patient Education for Diabetes Mellitus (Expected Outcomes)

The person with diabetes mellitus must accept a major role in the management of his disease. His education must be amplified, reinforced, and updated continuously, since diabetes is a life-long disease.

Objective: To maintain the best possible control of diabetes.

Patient's Expected Outcomes

A. Describes diabetes and how it affects the body
  1. Visits the physician on a regular basis
  2. Studies and reviews available literature from reputable sources
  3. Secures booklets and pamphlets from the American Diabetes Association, Inc., 2 Park Ave., New York, N.Y. 10016
  4. Attends available classes

B. Maintains health at an optimal level
  1. Maintains a consistent daily routine
  2. Gets adequate rest and sleep
  3. Exercises regularly and consistently
    a. Avoids "spurts" of arduous exercise before meals
    b. Exercises after meals
    c. Keeps some form of carbohydrate (sugar, candy, orange juice) available during exercise periods
    d. Takes extra food for extra physical activity
  4. Seeks employment with regular hours when possible; adjusts diet and medication to work schedule
  5. Has teeth and gums checked regularly for periodontal disease

C. Follows the prescribed dietary regimen
  1. Eats three or more regularly spaced meals each day, timed to coincide with the action of insulin
  2. Becomes thoroughly familiar with the food exchange lists
  3. Learns how to follow a calculated diet
  4. Uses household measures or a gram scale until serving sizes can be judged accurately
  5. Avoids concentrated carbohydrates
  6. Avoids periods of fasting and feasting
  7. Keeps weight at optimal level; normalizes body weight
    a. Weighs weekly
    b. Keeps a weight record
  8. If taking insulin, eats extra calories when unusual physical activity is anticipated
  9. Eats a bedtime snack when taking insulin, if prescribed
  10. Avoids foods high in cholesterol

D. Utilizes measures to determine the degree of diabetic control
  1. Tests blood for glucose at specified intervals
  2. Tests urine for ketones when blood sugar evaluations are high or during periods of illness

  3. Knows that acetone in the urine indicates need for *more insulin*
  4. Protects all urine testing equipment from light, moisture, and heat (to prevent false interpretation due to deterioration of test materials)

E. Utilizes proper practices of insulin therapy
  1. Knows when the prescribed insulin is having its peak action
  2. Adjusts insulin dosage according to blood sugar test, as prescribed
  3. Rotates the sites of insulin injections in a systematic manner
  4. Keeps a reserve supply of insulin in the refrigerator; is aware of expiration date on bottle
    a. Keeps bottle in current use at *room temperature*
    b. Avoids injecting cold insulin, because it may contribute to tissue reaction
  5. Has extra syringes available
  6. Avoids conditions that produce insulin reactions
    a. Omission or delay of a meal
    b. Unaccustomed or strenuous exercise
    c. Too much insulin
  7. Recognizes symptoms of an insulin reaction
    a. Any unfamiliar or peculiar sensation
    b. Hunger, perspiration, weakness, tremor, pallor, palpitation, tachycardia
  8. Takes precautions to prevent an insulin reaction
    a. Eats carbohydrates (orange juice, sugar, candy) when symptoms first occur
    b. Tests blood
    c. Carries extra carbohydrate at all times (sugar lumps, candy)
    d. Eats extra carbohydrates before strenuous exercise and during periods of prolonged exercise, or reduces insulin dosage
    e. Eats a snack at bedtime if prescribed
  9. Keeps a check-off system, to ensure taking insulin
  10. Wears identification bracelet or necklace
  11. When traveling, carries diabetic supplies in hand luggage
    a. Has letter from physician confirming diagnosis of diabetes and prescription for extra syringes
    b. Keeps watch at the time-of-departure point until arrival at destination; does not change diabetic regimen en route

F. Takes prescribed oral hypoglycemic medication
  1. Adheres faithfully to the prescribed diet
  2. Tests urine daily
  3. Takes the medication exactly as directed

(continued)

Chart 40-7
Patient Education for Diabetes Mellitus (Expected Outcomes) (continued)

Patient's Expected Outcomes *(continued)*

G. Practices proper foot care to prevent infection
1. Inspects feet carefully and routinely for calluses, corns, blisters, cracks, abrasions, redness, and nail abnormalities
   a. Uses a small mirror to check bottom of each foot (if unable to see foot)
   b. Uses a magnifying glass under good light if eyesight is poor, or has someone else check feet
2. Bathes feet daily in warm (never hot) water
   a. Does not soak the feet for prolonged periods
   b. Dries feet carefully, especially between the toes
3. Massages feet with a lubricating lotion, except between toes
4. Prevents moisture between toes, to avert maceration of skin
   a. Inserts lamb's wool between overlapping toes
   b. Uses powder in the web spaces, especially if feet perspire
5. Wears well-fitting, noncompressive shoes and socks—long enough, wide enough, soft, supple, and low-heeled
   a. Buys shoes in the afternoon—feet are larger in the afternoon than in the morning
   b. Has each foot measured before buying shoes—feet enlarge with age
   c. Has the measurement taken while standing, since foot is larger in the standing position
   d. Does not "break in" shoes all at one time
   e. Checks shoes repeatedly for protruding nails
   f. Avoids rubber- or plastic-soled shoes, which cause feet to perspire and may lead to fungal infections
   g. Avoids working in bedroom slippers or other casual foot attire
6. Goes to a podiatrist on a regular basis if corns, calluses, and ingrown toenails are present
   a. Cuts toenails straight across, to prevent ingrown toenails
      (See p. 270 for instructions for cutting toenails.)
7. Avoids heat, chemicals, and injuries to the feet—does not go barefoot or expose feet to hot water bottles, heating pads, caustic solutions, etc.
   a. Switches off electric blanket before going to bed; wears socks at night to keep feet warm, if necessary

   b. Avoids overheated baths and sitting too close to the fire
8. If an injury occurs to the foot:
   a. Washes the area with mild soap and water
   b. Covers with a dry, sterile dressing, *without* adhesive
   c. Wears white socks; dye in colored socks and wool serves as an irritant when skin is already irritated
   d. Calls the physician
H. Maintains diabetic control during periods of illness
1. Calls physician immediately when any unusual symptoms become evident; does not allow diabetes to get out of control
2. Makes dietary adjustments during illness according to physician's directions
3. Continues taking insulin; physician may increase dosage during illness
4. Monitors blood glucose
5. Tests urine for acetone more frequently; keeps records
6. Describes the conditions that bring about diabetic acidosis
   a. Nausea and vomiting
   b. Failure to increase insulin when blood sugar is increasing
   c. Failure to take insulin
   d. Dietary excesses
   e. Infections
   f. Stress
7. Takes precautions to prevent impending diabetic acidosis
   a. Examines urine for acetone, and reports results to physician
   b. Takes additional insulin as advised by physician
   c. Goes to bed and keeps warm
   d. Alerts someone to be in attendance
   e. Drinks a glass of liquid hourly, if possible
   f. Ensures oral intake of enough calories to prevent sudden drop in blood sugar
I. Follows other health directives
1. Avoids tobacco—nicotine constricts blood vessels, causing reduction in blood flow to feet
2. Reports excessive itching—may indicate elevated blood sugar
3. Takes only medications prescribed by physician—many drugs enhance effect of insulin and oral antidiabetic agents

diabetes, nature of surgery, the degree and persistence of glucosuria, and whether or not ketonuria is present. The key to control is careful monitoring for potentially rapid changes that will affect the patient's metabolic state.

On the morning of surgery, a fasting blood sugar is drawn 1 hour before the operation. Usually, the patient is given an intravenous infusion of 5% or 10% dextrose in water to provide necessary calories and carbohydrate, accompanied by the subcutaneous injection of insulin in a somewhat smaller dose than was required before surgery.

Postoperative Management. During the postoperative period, nutrition is maintained with intravenous dextrose until the patient is able to tolerate food by mouth. The insulin is adjusted on a sliding scale according to the results of the blood tests for glucose. Supplemental doses of regular insulin may be given as required. It is desirable to give insulin subcutaneously, since insulin added to an intravenous solution may adhere to the walls of the bottle and tubing, and IV fluids may be given at different rates, making insulin dosages difficult to adjust.

Following surgery, the diabetes may intensify and become difficult to control. Healing is often delayed due to vascular disease, poor circulation, and altered metabolism. A higher incidence of vascular complications (myocardial infarction; stroke) may occur due to the increased incidence of atherosclerosis in diabetics.

▷ Bibliography

Books

American Diabetes Association. Diabetes in the Family. Bowie, Maryland, Robert J Brady, 1982.

American Diabetes Association and The American Dietetic Association. Exchange List for Meal Planning. New York, 1976.

American Diabetes Association, Inc. and The American Dietetic Association. A Guide for Professionals: The Effective Application of "Exchange Lists for Meal Planning." New York, 1977.

Bennett M. The Peripatetic Diabetic. New York, Hawthorn Books, 1969.

Bernstein R. Diabetes: The Glucograf Method for Normalizing Blood Sugar. New York, Crown Publishers, 1981.

Biermann J and Toohey B. The Diabetic's Sport and Exercise Book: How to Play Your Way to Better Health. Philadelphia, JB Lippincott, 1977.

Biermann J and Toohey B. The Diabetic's Book: All Your Questions Answered. Los Angeles, JP Tarcher, 1981.

Blevins D. The Diabetic and Nursing Care. New York, McGraw-Hill, 1979.

Bowen A. The Diabetic Gourmet. New York, Barnes and Noble Books, 1980.

Bressler R and Johnson D (eds). Management of Diabetes Mellitus. Boston, John Wright–PSG, 1982.

Brothers M. Diabetes: The New Approach. New York, Grosset & Dunlap, 1976.

Christy A and Germann J. Diabetes: Recipes for Health. Bowie, Maryland, Robert J Brady, 1983.

Coustan D and Garvey S. The Baby Team: A Positive Approach to Pregnancy With Diabetes. St Louis, Monoject Division of Sherwood Medical, 1979.

Ellenberg M and Rifkin H. Diabetes Mellitus, 3rd ed. New Hyde Park, Medical Examination, 1983.

Etzwiler D et al (eds). Education and Management of the Patient With Diabetes Mellitus, 2nd ed. Elkhart, Indiana, Ames, 1978.

Guthrie D and Guthrie R (eds). Nursing Management of Diabetes Mellitus, 2nd ed. St Louis, CV Mosby, 1982.

Hamburg B et al (eds). Behavioral and Psychosocial Issues in Diabetes. Proceedings of the National Conference, US Dept. of Health and Human Services, NIH Publication No. 80–1993, 1979.

Kivelowitz T. Diabetes: A Guide to Self-management for Patients and Their Families. Englewood Cliffs, New Jersey, Prentice-Hall, 1981.

Kozak G. Clinical Diabetes Mellitus. Philadelphia, WB Saunders, 1982.

Krall L (ed). Joslin Diabetes Manual, 11th ed. Philadelphia, Lea & Febiger, 1978.

Lodewick P. A Diabetic Doctor Looks at Diabetes: His and Yours. Cambridge, Massachusetts, RMI Corporation, 1982.

Mayer E. Enjoying Food on a Diabetic Diet. New York, Dolphin Books, 1974.

National Diabetes Information Clearinghouse. Diet and Nutrition for People with Diabetes. Bethesda, Maryland, National Diabetes Information Clearinghouse, 1983.

Peterson CM. Take Charge of Your Diabetes: A New Approach to Self-management. Elkhart, Indiana, Ames, 1979.

Podolsky S (ed). Clinical Diabetes: Modern Management. New York, Appleton–Century–Crofts, 1980.

Rifkin H and Raskin P (eds). Diabetes Mellitus, Vol V. Bowie, Maryland, Robert J Brady, 1981.

Sims D (ed). Diabetes: Reach for Health and Freedom. St Louis, CV Mosby, 1980.

Steiner G and Lawrence P (eds). Educating Diabetic Patients. New York, Springer, 1981.

Strauss A and Glaser B. Chronic Illness and the Quality of Life. St Louis, CV Mosby, 1975.

Van Son A (ed). Diabetes and Patient Education: A Daily Nursing Challenge. New York, Appleton–Century–Crofts, 1982.

Articles

Agner E et al. Impaired glucose tolerance and diabetes mellitus in elderly subjects. Diabetes Care 1982 Nov/Dec; 5(6):600–604.

Alogna M. Perception of severity of disease and health locus of control in compliant and noncompliant diabetic patients. Diabetes Care 1980 July/Aug; 3(4):523–524.

Anderson JW and Ward K. Long-term effects of high-carbohydrate, high-fiber diets on glucose and lipid metabolism: A preliminary report on patients with diabetes. Diabetes Care 1978 Mar/Apr; 1(2):77–82.

Barbosa J et al. Long-term, ambulatory, subcutaneous insulin infusion versus multiple daily injections in brittle diabetic patients. Diabetes Care 1981 Mar/Apr; 4(2):269–274.

Baumgardner B et al. An instructional guide for patients placed on an insulin infusion pump. Diabetes Educator 1980 Winter; 6(4):15.

Birch K. Evaluation of hypo-test, a semiquantitative audio urine-glucose analysis for blind diabetic individuals. Diabetes Care 1982 July/Aug; 5(4):430–432.

Blankenship GW and Skyler JS. Diabetic retinopathy: A general survey. Diabetes Care 1978 Mar/Apr; 1(2):127–137.

Bodansky HJ et al. Risk factors associated with severe proliferative retinopathy in insulin-dependent diabetes mellitus. Diabetes Care 1982 Mar/Apr; 5(2):97–100.

Boyles V. Injection aids for blind diabetic patients. Am J Nurs 1977 Sept; 77(9):1456–1458.

Christiansen C and Sachse M. Home blood glucose monitoring: Benefits for the patient and educator. Diabetes Educator 1980 Fall; 6(3):13–21.

Clark AJ et al. A double-blind crossover trial comparing human insulin (recombinant DNA) with animal insulins in the treatment of previously insulin-treated diabetic patients. Diabetes Care 1982 Nov/Dec; 5(Suppl 2):129–134.

Clements R and Vourganti B. Fatal diabetic ketoacidosis: Major causes and approaches to their prevention. Diabetes Care 1978 Sept/Oct; 1(5):314–325.

Colwell J et al. Pathogenesis of atherosclerosis in diabetes mellitus. Diabetes Care 1981 Jan/Feb; 4(1):121–133.

Coughlin WR et al. Diabetic retinopathy. Diabetes Forecast 1978 Nov/Dec; 31(6):26–28.

Danowski T et al. Diabetic complications and their prevention or reversal. Diabetes Care 1980 Jan/Feb; 3(1):94–99.

Davis W et al. Factors affecting the educational diagnosis of diabetic patients. Diabetes Care 1981 Mar/Apr; 4(2):275–278.

De Fronzo R. Glucose intolerance and aging. Diabetes Care 1981 July/Aug; 4(4):493–501.

Doody R and Grose N. The family medical history: Assessing patient understanding of diabetes mellitus. Diabetes Care 1981 Mar/Apr; 4(2):285–288.

Editorial: Glycosylated hemoglobins in diabetes: A reappraisal. Diabetes Care 1979 Sept/Oct; 2(5):451–452.

Ellenberg M. Sex and diabetes: A comparison between men and women. Diabetes Care 1979 Jan/Feb; 2(1):4–8.

Free A and Free H. Urine glucose tests for diabetic patients with impaired vision. Diabetes Care 1978 Jan/Feb; 1(1):14–17.

Gonen B and Rubinstein A. Glycosylated hemoglobins in diabetes: A reappraisal. Diabetes Care 1979 Sept/Oct; 2(5):451–452.

Graber A et al. Planning for sex, marriage, contraception, and pregnancy. Diabetes Care 1978 May/June; 1(3):202–203.

Guthrie D et al. Single-voided vs. double-voided urine testing. Diabetes Care 1979 May/June; 2(3):269–271.

Hauser S and Pollets D. Psychological aspects of diabetes: A critical review. Diabetes Care 1979 Mar/Apr; 2(2):227–232.

Jackson C. Diabetes: How your patient looks at it. Nursing '81 1981 May; 11(5):82–83.

Keeson C et al. Glycosylated hemoglobin in the diagnosis of non-insulin-dependent diabetes mellitus. Diabetes Care 1982 July/Aug; 5(4):395–398.

Keon H and Hanna A. Self-administration of insulin by a hemiplegic individual. Diabetes Care 1980 Nov/Dec; 3(6):705.

Koivisto VA and Felig P. Effects of leg exercise on insulin absorption in diabetic patients. N Engl J Med 1978 Jan 12; 298(2):279–283.

Leichter S et al. Readability of self-care instructional pamphlets for diabetic patients. Diabetes Care 1981 Nov/Dec; 4(6):627–630.

Liang JC and Goldberg MF. Review: Treatment of diabetic retinopathy. Diabetes 1980 Oct; 29(10):841–851.

Madsbad S et al. Influence of smoking on insulin requirement and metabolic status in diabetes mellitus. Diabetes Care 1980 Jan/Feb; 3(1):41–43.

McCarthy J. Diabetic nephropathy. Am J Nurs 1981 Nov; 81(11):2030–2034.

McDermott K, Cooks M, and Peterson CM. Patient determined glycosylated hemoglobin measurements: An aid to patient education. Diabetes Care 1981 July/Aug; 4(4):480–483.

Mecklenburg R et al. Clinical use of the insulin infusion pump in 100 patients with type 1 diabetes. N Engl J Med 1982 Aug 26; 307(9):513–518.

Medalie J. Risk factors other than hyperglycemia in diabetic macrovascular disease. Diabetes Care 1979 Mar/Apr; 2(2):77–84.

Melton LJ et al. Incidence and prevalence of clinical peripheral vascular disease in a population-based cohort of diabetic patients. Diabetes Care 1980 Nov/Dec; 3(6):650–654.

National Diabetes Data Group: Classification of diabetes mellitus and other categories of glucose intolerance. Diabetes 1979 Dec; 28(12):1039–1051.

Nemchik R. Diabetes today: A startling new body of knowledge. RN, 1982 Oct; 45(10):31–37.

Nemchik R. Diabetes today: A very different diet; a new generation of oral drugs. RN 1982 Nov; 45(11):41–45, 97–99.

Nemchik R. Diabetes today: The news about insulin. RN 1982 Dec; 45(12):49–54.

Nuttal FQ and Brunzell JD. Principles of nutrition and dietary recommendations for individual with diabetes mellitus. Diabetes 1979 Nov; 28(11):1027–1030.

Nyberg K. When diabetes complicates your pre- and post-op care. RN 1983 Jan; 46(1):42–47.

Page P et al. Patient recall of self-care recommendations in diabetes. Diabetes Care 1981 Jan/Feb; 4(1):96–98.

Pietri A and Raskin P. Cutaneous complications of chronic continuous subcutaneous insulin infusion therapy. Diabetes Care 1981 Nov–Dec; 4(6):624–626.

Plasse N. Monitoring blood glucose at home: A comparison of three products. Am J Nurs 1981 Nov; 81(11):2028–2029.

Policy Statement. American Diabetes Association. The UGDP controversy. Diabetes Care 1979 Jan/Feb; 2(1):1–3.

Policy Statement. Indications for use of continuous insulin delivery systems and self-measurement of blood glucose. Diabetes Care 1982 Mar/Apr; 5(2):140–141.

Rotter J et al. Diabetes mellitus: The search for genetic markers. Diabetes Care 1979 Mar/Apr; 2(2):215–226.

Sanborn C et al. Shift work: How to adjust patterns of diabetes care. Occup Health Nurs 1982 Dec; 30(12):25–28.

Schade D and Eaton RP. Pathogenesis of diabetic ketoacidosis: A reappraisal. Diabetes Care 1979 May/June; 2(3):296–306.

Schade David et al. Future therapy of the insulin-dependent diabetic patient—the implantable insulin delivery system. Diabetes Care 1981 Mar/Apr; 4(2):319–327.

Schiffrin A and Belmonte MM. Comparison between continuous subcutaneous insulin infusion and multiple injections of insulin: A one-year prospective study. Diabetes 1982 Mar; 31(3):255–264.

Sheppard M and Wright AD. The effect on mortality of low-dose insulin therapy for diabetic ketoacidosis. Diabetes Care 1982 Mar/Apr; 5(2):111–113.

Skyler J. The spectrum of insulin resistance. Diabetes Care 1979 May/June; 2(3):319–322.

Skyler JS. Diabetes and exercise: Clinical implications. Diabetes Care 1979 May/June; 2(3):307–311.

Skyler JS. Complications of diabetes mellitus: Relationship to metabolic dysfunction. Diabetes Care 1979 Nov/Dec; 2(6):499–509.

Skyler J et al. Algorithms for adjustment of insulin dosage by patients who monitor blood glucose. Diabetes Care 1981 Mar/Apr; 4(2):311–318.

Streja D et al. Nutrition therapy in non-insulin-dependent diabetes mellitus. Diabetes Care 1981 Jan/Feb; 4(1):81–84.

Surr CW. New blood-glucose monitoring products (Part 1). Nursing '83 1983 Jan; 13(1):42–45.

Surr CW. New blood-glucose monitoring products (Part 2). Nursing '83 1983 Feb; 13(2):58–62.

Sutherland D et al. Pancreas transplantation—an historical overview and its current status. Diabetes Educator 1982 Spring; 8(1):11–13.

Taub S et al. Gastrointestinal manifestations of diabetes mellitus. Diabetes Care 1979 Sept/Oct; 2(5):437–447.

Taylor A and Cox D. Job stress: Its impact on the diabetic worker. Occup Health Nurs 1982 Dec; 30(12):29–32.

Unger R. Meticulous control of diabetes: Benefits, risks, and precautions. Diabetes 1982 June; 31(6):479–483.

U.S. Department of Health and Human Services and Department of Health, Education and Welfare: Diabetic neuropathies. NIH Publication No. 79–1641, 1979.

Walford S et al. The influence of renal threshold on the interpretation of urine tests for glucose in diabetic patients. Diabetes Care 1980 Nov/Dec; 3(6):672–678.

Manuals

A Handbook for the Visually Impaired Diabetic. Diabetes Association, 345 Union Street, Hackensack, New Jersey 07601 (large print).

Feet First. A booklet about foot care for older people and people who have diabetes. U.S. Dept. of HEW, 1970.

Guide to Good Living. The American Diabetes Association. New York, New York, 1982.

Guidelines for Diabetes Care. American Diabetes Association and American Association of Diabetes Educators, 1981.

Reference Manual for Evaluation of Diabetes Education Programs. American Association of Diabetes Educators, 1982.

Standards and Guidelines for Diabetes Education in Canada. The Professional Health Workers Section, Canadian Diabetes Association, 1981.

Third Annual Report of the National Diabetes Advisory Board. U.S. Department of Health and Human Services, Public Health Service, NIH Publication No. 80–2072, Apr 1980.

The Treatment and Control of Diabetes: A National Plan to Reduce Mortality and Morbidity. A Report of the National Advisory Board, U.S. Department of Health and Human Services, Public Health Service, NIH Publication No. 81–2284, Nov 1980.

Agencies
Voluntary

American Association of Diabetes Educators, North Woodbury Road, Box 56, Pitman, New Jersey 08071

American Diabetes Association, 2 Park Avenue, New York, New York 10016

American Dietetic Association, 620 N. Michigan Avenue, Chicago, Illinois 60611

Joslin Diabetes Foundation, 15 Joslin Road, Boston, Massachusetts 02215

Juvenile Diabetes Foundation, 23 East 26th Street, New York, New York 10010

Government

National Diabetes Data Group, National Institutes of Health, Westwood Building, Bethesda, Maryland 20205

National Diabetes Information Clearinghouse, Box NDIC, Bethesda, Maryland 20205

Selected Resources for the Person With Diabetes With Visual Impairment

American Foundation for the Blind, Inc., 15 West 16th Street, New York, New York 10011; Telephone: 212-924-0420 (Catalog of devices, vision aids, insulin syringes)

Braille Volunteers of Huntington, P.O. Box 9422, Huntington, West Virginia 25704 (Exchange lists in Braille and basic information about diabetes)

Iowa Commission for the Blind, 4th and Ecoway, Des Moines, Iowa 60309 (Exchange lists in large print)

Library of Congress, Division for the Blind and Physically Handicapped, 1291 Taylor Street, N.W., Washington, D.C. 20542; Telephone: 202-882-5500

Meditec, Inc., 9485 East Orchard Drive, Englewood, Colorado 80110 (Insulin gauges for visually handicapped)

New Jersey Affiliate, Inc., American Diabetes Association, 345 Union Street, Hackensack, New Jersey 07601 (*A Handbook for the Visually Impaired Diabetic*—large print)

Office of Vocational Rehabilitation (Check your own state office.)

Seeing Eye Dog, Washington Valley Road, Morristown, New Jersey 07960; Telephone: 201-539-4425

Social Security Administration (Check your local office.)

41

Assessment and Management of Patients With Endocrine Disorders

▷ Physiologic Overview

Endocrine glands, which secrete their products directly into the bloodstream, are clearly differentiated from exocrine glands, such as sweat glands, which secrete through ducts onto epithelial surfaces. The chemical substances secreted by the endocrine glands are called *hormones.* Hormones help to regulate organ function in concert with the nervous system. The dual regulatory system involving rapidly responding nervous activity with more slowly responding hormonal influences permits precise control of body function in the face of varied bodily and environmental changes.

Several different types of hormones are known to exist. These include steroid hormones, such as hydrocortisone; peptide or protein hormones, such as insulin; and amine hormones, such as epinephrine. These different classes of hormones exert their actions on the target tissues by different mechanisms, as discussed below. A schematic diagram of the important endocrine glands is shown in Figure 41-1. Table 41-1 lists the important hormones, their target tissue, and some of their properties.

Certain anatomical features are common to the endocrine glands. The glands are composed of secretory cells arranged in minute clusters (acini). No ducts are present, but the glands are richly vascularized, so that the chemicals they produce can rapidly enter the bloodstream.

The concentration in the bloodstream of most hormones is maintained at a relatively constant level. If the hormone concentration rises, further production of that hormone is inhibited. When the hormone concentration falls, the rate of production of that hormone is stimulated. This mechanism for regulation of hormone concentration in the bloodstream is called *feedback control.* The principle of feedback control is important in the regulation of many biological processes.

Mechanism of Hormone Action. Hormones can alter the function of the target tissue by interacting with chemical receptors located either on the cell membrane or in the interior of the cell. Peptide and protein hormones interact

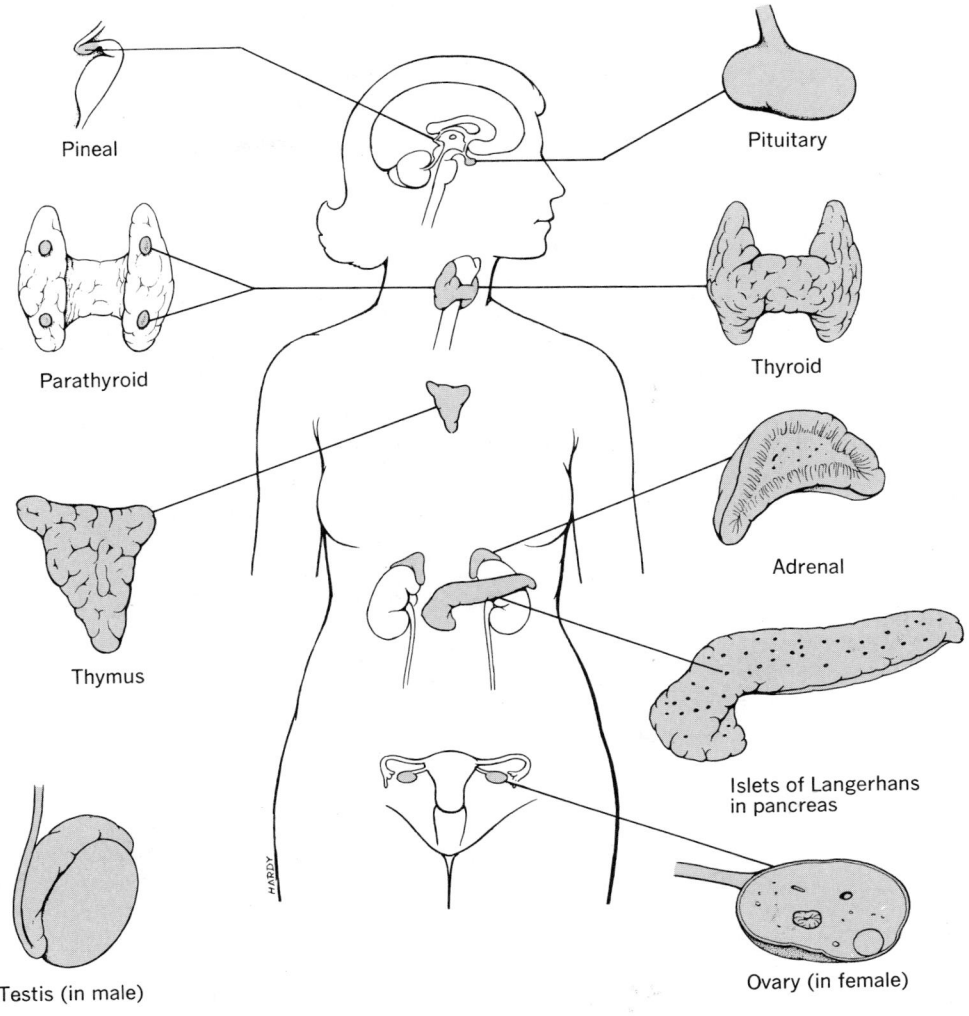

Figure 41-1. General location of the major endocrine glands. (From Chaffee EE and Greisheimer E: Basic Physiology and Anatomy, 4th ed. Philadelphia, JB Lippincott, 1980.)

with receptor sites on the cell surface, which results in the stimulation of intracellular enzyme adenyl cyclase. This in turn results in increased production of cyclic 3':5'-adenosine monophosphate (cyclic AMP). The cyclic AMP inside the cell alters enzyme activity. Thus, cyclic AMP is the "second messenger" that links the peptide hormone at the cell surface to a change in the intracellular environment. Some of the protein and peptide hormones may also act by inducing changes in membrane permeability. These hormones act relatively rapidly, within seconds or minutes. The mechanism of action for amine hormones is similar to that described above for peptide hormones.

Because of their smaller size and higher lipid solubility, steroid hormones penetrate through the cell membranes and interact with intracellular receptors. This steroid-receptor complex modifies cell metabolism by leading to the formation of messenger RNA from DNA. The messenger RNA then stimulates protein synthesis within the cell. Ste-

roid hormones, because they exert their action by the modification of protein synthesis, require several hours in order to exert their effects.

The Pituitary Gland

The pituitary gland, or the hypophysis, has been referred to as the "master gland" of the endocrine system. It secretes hormones that, in turn, control the secretion of hormones by other endocrine glands. The pituitary itself is controlled in large part by the hypothalamus, an adjacent area of the brain. The pituitary gland is a round structure about 1.27 cm (½ inch) in diameter located on the inferior aspect of the brain and connected to the hypothalamus by the pituitary stalk. The pituitary gland is divided into anterior, intermediate, and posterior lobes.

The important hormones secreted by the posterior lobe of the pituitary gland are *vasopressin* (antidiuretic hormone, or ADH) and *oxytocin*. These hormones are synthesized in

Table 41-1
Endocrine System in Summary

Endocrine Gland and Hormone	Principal Site of Action	Principal Processes Affected
Pituitary Gland		
(a) Anterior lobe		
Growth hormone (somatotropin)	General	Growth of bones, muscles, and other organs
Thyrotropin	Thyroid	Growth and secretory activity of thyroid gland
Adrenocorticotropin	Adrenal cortex	Growth and secretory activity of adrenal cortex
Follicle-stimulating	Ovaries	Development of follicles and secretion of estrogen
	Testes	Development of seminiferous tubules, spermatogenesis
Luteinizing or interstitial cell stimulating	Ovaries	Ovulation, formation of corpus luteum, secretion of progesterone
	Testes	Secretion of testosterone
Prolactin or lactogenic (luteotropin)	Mammary glands and ovaries	Secretion of milk; maintenance of corpus luteum
Melanocyte-stimulating	Skin	Pigmentation (?)
(b) Posterior lobe	Kidney	Reabsorption of water; water balance
Antidiuretic (vasopressin)	Arterioles	Blood pressure (?)
Oxytocin	Uterus	Contraction
	Breast	Expression of milk
Pineal Gland		
Melatonin	Gonads (?)	Sexual maturation (?)
Thyroid Gland		
Thyroxine and triiodothyronine	General	Metabolic rate; growth and development; intermediate metabolism
Thyrocalcitonin	Bone	Inhibits bone resorption; lowers blood level of calcium
Parathyroid Glands		
Parathormone	Bone, kidney, intestine	Promotes bone resorption; increased absorption of calcium; raises blood calcium level
Adrenal Glands		
(a) Cortex		
Mineralocorticoids (*e.g.,* aldosterone)	Kidney	Reabsorption of sodium; elimination of potassium
Glucocorticoids (*e.g.,* cortisol)	General	Metabolism of carbohydrate, protein, and fat; response to stress; anti-inflammatory
Sex hormones	General (?)	Preadolescent growth spurt (?)

(continued)

the hypothalamus and travel down the nerve cells that connect the hypothalamus to the posterior pituitary gland, where they are stored. Vasopressin secretion is stimulated by an increase in the osmolality of the blood or by a decrease in blood pressure. The primary function of vasopressin is to control the excretion of water by the kidney. Oxytocin secretion is stimulated during pregnancy and at the time of parturition (childbirth). The primary functions of oxytocin are to facilitate milk ejection during lactation and to increase the force of uterine contractions during parturition. Exogenous oxytocin can be used therapeutically to initiate labor.

The important hormones of the anterior pituitary gland are follicle-stimulating hormones (FSH), luteinizing hormone (LH), prolactin, adrenocorticotropic hormone (ACTH), thyroid-stimulating hormone (TSH), and growth hormone (GH). The secretion of each of these major hormones is controlled by releasing factors (RF) that are secreted by the hypothalamus. These releasing factors reach the anterior pituitary via the bloodstream in a special circulation called the pituitary portal blood system.

The hormones released by the anterior pituitary enter the systemic bloodstream and are transported to their target

Table 41-1
Endocrine System in Summary (continued)

Endocrine Gland and Hormone	Principal Site of Action	Principal Processes Affected
Adrenal Glands (continued)		
(b) Medulla		
Epinephrine	Cardiac muscle, smooth muscle, glands	Emergency functions: same as stimulation of sympathetic system
Norepinephrine	Organs innervated by sympathetic system	Chemical transmitter substance; increases peripheral resistance
Islet Cells of Pancreas		
Insulin	General	Lowers blood sugar; utilization and storage of carbohydrate; decreased gluconeogenesis
Glucagon	Liver	Raises blood sugar; glycogenolysis
Somatostatin	General	Lowers blood sugar by interfering with release of growth hormone and glucagon
Testes		
Testosterone	General	Development of secondary sex characteristics
	Reproductive organs	Development and maintenance; normal function
Ovaries		
Estrogens	General	Development of secondary sex characteristics
	Mammary glands	Development of duct system
	Reproductive organs	Maturation and normal cyclic function
Progesterone	Mammary glands	Development of secretory tissue
	Uterus	Preparation for implantation; maintenance of pregnancy
Gastrointestinal Tract		
Gastrin	Stomach	Production of gastric juice
Enterogastrone	Stomach	Inhibits secretion and motility
Secretin	Liver and pancreas	Production of bile; production of watery pancreatic juice (rich in $NaHCO_3$)
Pancreozymin	Pancreas	Production of pancreatic juice rich in enzymes
Cholecystokinin	Gallbladder	Contraction and emptying

(From Chaffee EE and Greisheimer E: Basic Physiology and Anatomy, 3rd ed. Philadelphia, JB Lippincott.)

organs. TSH, ACTH, FSH, and LH have as their main function the release of hormones from other endocrine glands. Prolactin and growth hormone do not have as their primary effects the release of hormones from other endocrine glands. Prolactin acts on the breast to stimulate milk production. Growth hormone has widespread effects on many target tissues and is discussed below. The other trophic hormones will be discussed in conjunction with their target organs.

Growth Hormone. Growth hormone, also referred to as somatotropin, is a protein hormone that increases protein synthesis in many tissues, increases the breakdown of fatty acids in adipose tissue, and increases the glucose levels in the blood. These actions of somatotropin are essential for normal growth, although other hormones, such as thyroid hormone and insulin, are required as well. The secretion of growth hormone is increased by stress, exercise, and low blood sugar. The half-time of growth hormone activity in the blood is about 20 to 30 minutes. It is largely inactivated in the liver. If secretion of growth hormone is insufficient during childhood, generalized limited growth and dwarfism result. Conversely, oversecretion during childhood results in gigantism, with individuals reaching 7 or even 8 feet in height. Excess growth hormone in adults results in deformities of bone and soft tissue and enlargement of viscera (acromegaly), but no increase in height.

Abnormal Pituitary Function. Abnormalities of pituitary function are due to oversecretion or undersecretion of any of the hormones produced or released by the gland. Abnormalities of the posterior and anterior portions of the gland may occur independently. Oversecretion (hypersecretion) most commonly involves ACTH or growth hormone, resulting in the conditions known as Cushing's disease or acromegaly, respectively. Hyposecretion (undersecretion) commonly involves all of the anterior pituitary hormones and is termed panhypopituitarism. In this condition, the thyroid gland, the adrenal cortex, and the gonads atrophy due to loss of the trophic hormones. The most common disorder related to posterior lobe dysfunction is diabetes insipidus, a condition in which abnormally large volumes of dilute urine are excreted due to deficient production of antidiuretic hormone.

The Thyroid Gland

The thyroid gland is a butterfly-shaped organ located in the lower neck anterior to the trachea. It consists of two lateral lobes connected by an isthmus. The gland is approximately 5 cm long and 3 cm wide and weighs about 30 g. The blood flow to the thyroid, per gram of gland tissue, is very high (about 5 ml/min per gram of thyroid), approximately five times the blood flow to the liver. This indicates the high metabolic activity of the thyroid gland. The thyroid gland produces three different hormones: thyroxine (T_4) and triiodothyronine (T_3) which are referred to collectively as thyroid hormone, and calcitonin.

Thyroid Hormone. Thyroid hormone is composed of two separate hormones made in the thyroid gland, thyroxine and triiodothyronine. These hormones are amino acids that have the unique property of containing iodine molecules bound to the amino acid structure. T_4 contains four iodine atoms in each molecule, while T_3 contains only three. These hormones are synthesized and stored by the cells of the thyroid gland until needed for release into the bloodstream. The hormones are stored bound to a glycoprotein called thyroglobulin.

Iodine Uptake and Metabolism. Iodine is essential to the thyroid gland for synthesis of its hormones. In fact, the major use of iodine in the body is by the thyroid, and the major derangement in iodine deficiency is alteration of thyroid function. Iodine is ingested in the diet and absorbed into the blood in the gastrointestinal tract. The thyroid gland is extremely efficient in taking up iodide from the blood and concentrating it within the cells. There, iodide ions are converted to iodine molecules, which react with tyrosine (one of the common amino acids) to form the thyroid hormones.

Regulation of Thyroid Function. The secretion of thyrotropin, or thyroid-stimulating hormone (TSH), by the pituitary gland controls the rate of thyroid hormone release. In turn, the release of TSH is determined by the level of thyroid hormones in the blood. If thyroid hormone concentration in the blood decreases, release of TSH increases, which causes increased output of T_3 and T_4. This is an ex-

ample of feedback control. Thyrotropin-releasing hormone (TRH), secreted by the hypothalamus, exerts a modulating influence on the release of TSH from the pituitary. Environmental factors, such as a fall in temperature, may lead to increased secretion of TRH and, thereby, result in elevated secretion of thyroid hormones.

Function of Thyroid Hormones. The primary function of the thyroid hormones is to control the cellular metabolic activity. Thyroid hormone action can be evaluated through measurement of the basal metabolic rate (BMR), defined as milliliters of oxygen consumed by the body per minute at rest. In the absence of thyroid secretion, the BMR may decrease by 30% to 40%. Administration of exogenous thyroid hormones can return the BMR to normal. The presence of adequate thyroid hormone is also necessary for normal growth. The thyroid hormones, through their widespread effects on cellular metabolism, influence every major organ system.

Calcitonin. Calcitonin, or thyrocalcitonin, is another important hormone secreted by the thyroid gland. Its secretion is not controlled by TSH. It is secreted by the thyroid gland in response to high plasma levels of calcium, and reduces the plasma level by increasing calcium deposition in bone.

Abnormalities of Thyroid Function. Inadequate secretion of thyroid hormone during fetal and neonatal development will result in stunted physical and mental growth (cretinism), due to general depression of body metabolic activity. In the adult, hypothyroidism (myxedema) is manifested by lethargy, slow mentation, and generalized slowing of body functions. Oversecretion of thyroid hormones (hyperthyroidism) is manifested by greatly increased metabolic rate. Many of the other characteristics of hyperthyroid patients reflects the potentiation of circulating catecholamines (epinephrine and norepinephrine) by excess thyroid hormones. Oversecretion of thyroid hormones is usually associated with an enlarged thyroid gland (goiter). Goiter also commonly occurs in the presence of iodide deficiency. In this latter condition, lack of iodide results in low levels of circulating thyroid hormones, which causes increased release of TSH; the elevated TSH causes overproduction of thyroglobulin and hypertrophy of the thyroid gland.

The Adrenal Glands

There are two adrenal glands in the human, each attached to the upper portion of a kidney. Each adrenal gland is, in reality, two endocrine glands. The adrenal medulla at the center of the gland secretes catecholamines, while the outer portion of the gland, the adrenal cortex, secretes corticosteroids.

Adrenal Medulla. The adrenal medulla functions as part of the autonomic nervous system. Stimulation of preganglionic sympathetic nerve fibers, which travel directly to the cells of the medulla, causes release of the catecholamine hormones, epinephrine or norepinephrine. About 90% of the secretion of the adrenal medulla in man is epinephrine (also called adrenalin). The major effects of epinephrine release are involved in preparation to meet a challenge (fight-or-flight response). Secretion of epinephrine causes decreased blood flow to tissues that are not needed in emergency situations, such as the gastrointestinal tract, and causes increased blood flow to those tissues that are important for effective fight or flight, such as cardiac and skeletal muscle. Catecholamines also induce release of free fatty acids, increase the basal metabolic rate, and elevate the level of blood sugar.

Adrenal Cortex. The three kinds of steroid hormones produced by the adrenal cortex are glucocorticoids, the prototype of which is hydrocortisone; mineralocorticoids, mainly aldosterone; and sex hormones, mainly androgens (male sex hormones).

Glucocorticoids. The glucocorticoids are given their name because they have an important influence on glucose metabolism; increased hydrocortisone secretion results in elevated blood sugar. However, the glucocorticoids have major effects on the metabolism of almost all organs of the body. Glucocorticoids are secreted from the adrenal cortex in response to the release of adrenocorticotrophic hormone (ACTH) from the anterior lobe of the pituitary gland. This system represents another typical example of negative feedback. The presence of glucocorticoids in the blood inhibits the release of corticotropin-releasing factor (CRF) from the hypothalamus, and also inhibits ACTH secretion from the pituitary. The resultant decrease in ACTH secretion causes diminished release of glucocorticoids from the adrenal cortex. A functioning adrenal cortex is necessary for life, although survival is possible by appropriate replacement with exogenous adrenal cortical hormones.

The glucocorticoids are frequently administered for their therapeutic effects. In pharmacologic doses, they inhibit the inflammatory response to tissue injury and suppress allergic manifestations. Toxic effects of glucocorticoids include possible development of diabetes, osteoporosis, peptic ulcer, increased protein breakdown resulting in muscle wasting and poor wound healing, and redistribution of body fat. The presence of large amounts of exogenously administered glucocorticoids in the blood inhibits release of ACTH and endogenous glucocorticoids. Because of this, the adrenal cortex can atrophy. If exogenous glucocorticoid administration is suddenly discontinued, adrenal insufficiency results, due to the inability of the atrophied cortex to adequately respond.

Mineralocorticoids. Mineralocorticoids exert their major effects on electrolyte metabolism. They act principally on renal tubular and gastrointestinal epithelium to cause increased sodium ion absorption in exchange for excretion of potassium or hydrogen ions. Aldosterone secretion is only minimally influenced by ACTH. It is primarily secreted in response to the presence of angiotensin II in the bloodstream. Angiotensin II concentration is increased when renin is released from the kidney in response to decreased perfusion pressure. The resultant increased aldosterone levels promote sodium reabsorption by the kidney and the gastrointestinal tract, which tends to restore blood pressure to normal. The release of aldosterone is also increased by hyperkalemia. Aldosterone is the primary hormone for the long-term regulation of salt balance.

Adrenal Sex Hormones (Androgens). Androgens, the third major type of steroid hormones produced by the adrenal cortex, physiologically exert effects similar to male sex hormones. The adrenal gland may also secrete small amounts of some estrogens, or female sex hormones. Secretion of adrenal androgens is controlled by ACTH. When secreted in normal amounts, the adrenal androgens probably have little effect, but when secreted excessively, as with certain inborn enzyme deficiencies, masculinization may result. This is called the *adrenogenital syndrome.*

The Parathyroid Gland

The parathyroid glands, normally four in number, are situated in the neck, embedded in the posterior aspect of the thyroid gland. These small glands are easily overlooked and can be removed at the time of thyroid surgery unless great care is exercised by the surgeon. Inadvertent surgical removal is the most common cause of hypoparathyroidism.

Parathormone, the protein hormone from the parathyroid glands, regulates calcium and phosphorus metabolism. Increased parathormone results in increased calcium absorption from the kidney, the intestine, and bones, thereby raising the blood-calcium level. Some actions of this hormone are potentiated by the presence of vitamin D. Parathormone also tends to lower the blood phosphorus. Excess parathormone can result in markedly elevated serum Ca^{++}, which constitutes a potentially life-threatening situation. When the product of serum calcium and serum phosphorus becomes high, calcium phosphate may precipitate in various organs of the body and cause tissue calcification.

The output of parathormone is regulated by the serum level of ionized calcium. Increased serum calcium results in decreased parathormone secretion, forming a feedback system.

The Pancreas

The pancreas, located in the upper abdomen, has both exocrine (digestive enzymes) and endocrine gland function. In contrast to endocrine glands, an exocrine gland is one whose secretions travel through a duct to their site of utilization and are not secreted into the bloodstream.

Exocrine Pancreas. The secretions of the exocrine portion of the pancreas are collected in the pancreatic duct, which joins the common bile duct and enters the duodenum at the ampulla of Vater. Surrounding the ampulla is the sphincter of Oddi, which partially controls the rate at which the secretions from both the pancreas and gallbladder enter the duodenum.

The secretions of the exocrine pancreas are digestive enzymes and an electrolyte-rich fluid. The secretions are very alkaline because of their high concentration of sodium bicarbonate, and are capable of neutralizing the highly acid gastric juice that enters the duodenum. The enzyme secretions include *amylase,* which aids in the digestion of carbohydrates; *trypsin,* which aids in the digestion of proteins; and *lipase,* which aids in the digestion of fats. Other enzymes that aid in the breakdown of more complex foodstuffs are also secreted.

The stimulus for secretion of these exocrine pancreatic juices are hormones originating in the gastrointestinal tract. Secretin is the major stimulus for increased bicarbonate secretion from the pancreas, while the major stimulus for digestive enzyme secretion is the hormone cholecystokinin-pancreozymin (CCK-PZ). The vagus nerve also influences exocrine pancreatic secretion.

Endocrine Pancreas.   The islets of Langerhans, the endocrine part of the pancreas, are collections of cells embedded in the pancreatic tissue. They are composed of alpha, beta, and delta cells. The hormone produced by the beta cells is called *insulin;* the alpha cells secrete glucagon, and the delta cells secrete somatostatin. A major action of insulin is to lower blood sugar by permitting entry of the sugar (glucose) into the cells of the liver, muscle, and other tissues where the glucose can be either stored as glycogen or burned for energy. Insulin is also instrumental in promoting the storage of fat in adipose tissue and in the synthesis of proteins in various body tissues. In the absence of insulin, glucose is not able to enter the cells and is excreted in the urine. This condition, called diabetes mellitus, can be diagnosed by high levels of glucose in the blood and urine. In diabetes mellitus, fats and protein can be utilized for energy instead of glucose, with consequent loss of body mass. The rate of insulin secretion from the pancreas is regulated in normal people by the level of sugar in the blood.

The effects of glucagon are chiefly to raise the blood sugar (opposite to those of insulin), primarily by promoting the conversion of glycogen to glucose in the liver. Glucagon is secreted by the pancreas in response to a fall in the level of blood glucose.

Somatostatin, recently discovered, is secreted by the delta cells of the pancreas and exerts a hypoglycemic effect by interfering with release of growth hormone from the pituitary and glucagon from the pancreas, both of which tend to raise blood sugar levels.

Endocrine Control of Carbohydrate Metabolism.   Glucose for body energy needs is derived by metabolism of ingested carbohydrates and also from proteins by the process of gluconeogenesis. Glucose can be stored temporarily in the liver, muscles, and other tissues in the form of glycogen. The endocrine system controls the level of blood glucose by regulating the rate at which glucose is synthesized, stored, and removed into the bloodstream. Through the action of hormones, blood glucose is normally maintained at approximately 100 mg per 100 ml of blood. Insulin is the primary hormone that leads to a lowering of blood glucose. Hormones that act to raise the blood sugar are glucagon, epinephrine, adrenocorticosteroids, growth hormone, and thyroid hormone.

▷ **The Thyroid Gland**

Assessment: Tests of Thyroid Function

The number of tests to determine thyroid function has increased steadily. No tests can be used to the exclusion of others; several may be required to give a composite assessment of thyroid function. In addition, clinical signs and symptoms are evaluated before a diagnosis can be made.

The stimulating effect of the thyroid gland is exerted through the production and distribution of two hormones: levothyroxine (T_4), which maintains body metabolism in a steady state, and triiodothyronine (T_3), which is approximately five times as potent as thyroxine and has a more rapid metabolic action. In testing, reliance is placed on the measurement of the levels of thyroid hormones in the blood.

Serum T_4.   The test most commonly used is the determination of serum T_4 by radioimmunoassay or competitive binding techniques. A blood sample is not affected by exogenous iodine. The range of T_4 in serum is normally between 4.5 μg and 11.5 μg per deciliter. T_4 is bound mainly to thyroxine-binding globulin (TBG) and prealbumin; T_3 is bound less firmly.

Serum binding of thyroid hormone is clinically significant, since anything that interferes with binding may change the total concentration of the hormone measured in the serum. Protein-wasting diseases, such as nephrosis, and the use of androgens, for example, decrease thyroxine-binding globulin and interfere with accurate test results.

Serum T_3.   This test measures free and bound, or total, serum content of triiodothyronine. Its secretion occurs in response to TSH secretion, as does T_4. Although T_3 and T_4 serum levels generally increase or decrease together, T_3 levels appear to be more accurate indicators of hyperthyroidism, which causes a greater rise in T_3 than T_4 levels.

Resin T_3 Uptake.   This test uses a reagent of radioactive triiodothyronine to indirectly measure thyroid hormone levels in the serum by determining the amount of hormone bound to thyroid-binding globulin and the number of available binding sites. Normally, TBG is not fully saturated with thyroid hormone, and additional binding sites are available to combine with radioiodine-labeled triiodothyronine added to the patient's blood specimen. Measurement of the number of free binding sites, therefore, provides an index to the amount of thyroid hormone already present in the patient's circulation. The normal T_3 uptake value is 25% to 35% which indicates that approximately one third of the available sites of TBG are occupied by thyroid hormone. If the number of free or unoccupied binding sites is low, as in hyperthyroidism, the T_3 uptake is greater than 35%. If the number of available sites is high, as occurs in hypothyroidism, the test results are less than 25%.

T_3 uptake is useful in evaluation of thyroid hormone levels in patients who have received diagnostic or therapeutic doses of iodine. The test results may be altered by the use of estrogens, androgens, salicylates, phenytoin, anticoagulants, or steroids.

Thyroid-Stimulating Hormone.   The secretion of T_3 and T_4 by the thyroid gland is under the control of thyroid-stimulating hormone (TSH, thyrotropin) from the pituitary gland. Measurement of serum TSH concentration is valuable in diagnosis and management of thyroid disorders and in differentiation between disorders due to disease of the thyroid gland itself and disorders due to disease of the pituitary or hypothalamus.

Thyrotropin (TSH) Radioimmunoassay.   Thyrotropin can be measured in the serum by radioimmunoassay; this method affords multiple determinations. In patients with primary hypothyroidism, TSH levels are elevated; low levels are seen in hyperthyroid patients.

Thyrotropin-Releasing Hormone (TRH).   The TRH stimulation test provides a direct means of testing pituitary reserve for TSH. The patient fasts overnight. Just before and 30 minutes after administration of TRH, blood specimens are drawn for TSH levels. In hypothyroidism due to primary disease of the thyroid gland, there is an increased serum TSH; in hypothyroidism due to disease of the pituitary or hypothalamus, there is an absent or delayed response to TRH. TRH may be given orally or intravenously. If given intravenously, it may cause the patient to experience the following transient symptoms: nausea, or a desire to urinate.

Protein-Bound Iodine. Protein-bound iodine is a conjugated molecule formed when thyroxine becomes attached to certain plasma-protein components. Thyroid function may be assessed in relation to the concentration of protein-bound iodine (PBI) in the blood. In this test, serum proteins are precipitated, washed, and then measured for iodine content. Normal values range from 4 µg to 8 µg per 100 ml of plasma. Values above 8 µg indicate thyroid overactivity; conversely, concentrations below 4 µg are considered evidence of hypothyroidism.

A disadvantage of this test is the unreliable results that may occur if the patient has taken medications containing iodine.

When a patient is scheduled for thyroid function tests, it is necessary to know beforehand whether he has taken medications with iodine in them, since this will alter the results of some tests. Iodide-containing medications are divided into those containing inorganic iodide, and those containing organic iodide (Table 41-2).

Antiseptics, cough syrups, and nail strengtheners may also serve as sources of iodine. Other medications that may affect thyroid function test values are estrogens, salicylates, cortisone derivatives, antibiotics, and mercurial diuretics. The variety of interfering factors is one reason why this test is becoming outdated.

Radioactive Iodine Uptake (RAI). This test measures the rate of iodine uptake by the thyroid gland. The patient is given a tracer dose of ^{131}I, and a count is made over the thyroid, using a scintillation counter, which detects and counts the gamma rays released from breakdown of ^{131}I in the thyroid. Thyroid activity, divided by the amount of administered activity (expressed as a percentage) is the uptake value. It is a simple test and provides reliable results. It is affected by the patient's intake of iodide or thyroid hormone; therefore, a careful preliminary clinical history is essential in evaluating results. Normal values vary from locality to locality with the intake of iodine (9%–16%, 12%–30%, etc.). Patients with hyperthyroidism accumulate a high proportion of the ^{131}I (in some patients up to 90%), whereas patients with hypothyroidism exhibit a very low uptake. (See also Chap. 18, p. 337.)

Thyroid Scan, Radioscan, or Scintiscan. Similar to the RAI uptake test, in this test a highly focused scintillation detector moves back and forth across the area to be studied in a series of parallel tracks that move progressively downward. At the same time, a printing device records a mark whenever a predetermined number of counts has been received. This produces a visual representation of the localization of radioactivity in the area being scanned. Although ^{131}I has been the most commonly used isotope, ^{125}I, and especially ^{99m}Tc (sodium pertechnetate), are being used because of their physical and biochemical properties, which allows a lower radiation dose to be given to the patient.

Scanning is helpful in determining location, size, shape, and anatomical function of the thyroid gland, particularly when thyroid tissue is substernal or large. Identification of areas of increased function ("hot" areas) or decreased function ("cold" areas) can assist in diagnosis. Although most areas of decreased function are not malignancies, lack of function increases the liklihood of malignancy, particularly if only one nonfunctioning area is present. Scanning of the entire body, to obtain the total body profile, may be carried out in a search for a functioning thyroid metastasis.

Table 41-2
Inorganic and Organic Iodides

Examples of Inorganic Iodides	Examples of Organic Iodides
Lugol's solution	X-ray contrast media: time
Diiodohydroxyquin (Diodoquin)	required for elimination of
Potassium iodide (Quadrinal)	contrast media from body:
Iodochlorhydroxyquin	Gallbladder . . . . months
(Entero-Vioform)	Bronchographic . . . . years
Sodium iodothiouracil (Itrumil)	Myelogram . . . . life
	Pyelogram . . . . rapidly

Hypothyroidism and Myxedema

Hypothyroidism is a condition in which there is a slow progression of thyroid hypofunction, followed by symptoms indicating thyroid failure. This condition is usually referred to as primary hypothyroidism. When the thyroid dysfunction is due to failure of the pituitary gland, the condition is known as secondary hypothyroidism; when failure of the hypothalamus is the underlying cause, the term tertiary hypothyroidism is used. When thyroid deficiency is present at birth, the condition is known as *cretinism*. In such instances, the mother may also suffer from a thyroid deficiency.

The cause of hypothyroidism may be idiopathic or it may result from surgical removal of the thyroid gland, destruction by radioactive iodine, or damage by an autoimmune disease such as Hashimoto's thyroiditis. The patient's metabolism declines proportionately to the reduction in production of thyroid hormone.

Clinical Manifestations

Early symptoms of hypothyroidism are nonspecific, but extreme fatigue makes it difficult for the person to complete a full day's work. Menstrual disturbances such as menorrhagia or amenorrhea occur, in addition to loss of libido. Complaints of hair loss, brittle nails, and dry skin are common, and numbness and tingling of the fingers may occur. On occasion, the voice may become husky, and the patient may complain of hoarseness.

With more severe grades of hypothyroidism, the temperature and the pulse rate become subnormal and the patient begins to gain weight. (Severe hypothyroid patients may be cachectic.) The skin becomes thickened because of an accumulation of mucopolysaccharides in the subcutaneous tissues (the origin of the term *myxedema*). The hair thins and falls out; the expression of the face becomes stolid and masklike.

At first the patient may be irritable and may complain of fatigue, but as the condition progresses, the emotional responses are subdued. The mental process becomes dulled, and the patient appears apathetic. Speech is slow, the tongue enlarges, and hands and feet increase in size. The patient frequently complains of constipation and intolerance to cold. Deafness also may occur. The advanced myxedematous state may produce personality changes.

Myxedema affects women five times more frequently than men and occurs most often between 30 and 60 years of age. It is not without its complications, because there is an associated tendency to the rapid development of atherosclerosis, with all the undesirable features of that disease. The patient with advanced myxedema may be hypothermic and may be abnormally sensitive to sedatives, opiates, and anesthetic agents.

Management

The prime objective is to restore a normal metabolic state by replacing the missing hormone. Synthetic levothyroxine (Synthroid) is the preferred preparation for treating hypothyroidism and suppressing nontoxic goiters. The dosage for hormone replacement is scheduled on the basis of the patient's normal or suppressed serum TSH concentration. Usually, dosage varies from 0.1 mg to 0.2 mg daily. Desiccated thyroid is used less frequently, since it often results in transient elevated serum concentrations of T_3, with occasional symptoms of hyperthyroidism. If replacement therapy is adequate, the symptoms of myxedema disappear, and normal metabolic activity is resumed.

Prevention of chilling is part of the nursing management of these patients, since a person with hypothyroidism cannot generate heat, and thus becomes hypothermic. Adequate hydration, a diet containing fruit and vegetables, and the use of stool softeners are usually necessary to prevent constipation and impaction. However, excess hydration is to be avoided, as the hypothyroid patient may not excrete a fluid load, even after diuretics, thus making dilutional hyponatremia a hazard.

Nursing judgment and selective action are required in caring for patients with myxedema, because of the possibility of several complications:

1. *Severe untreated hypothyroidism is attended by an increased susceptibility to all hypnotic and sedative drugs.* These agents, even in small doses, may induce profound somnolence, lasting far longer than anticipated. Moreover, they are prone to cause respiratory depression, which could easily prove fatal.

   With this in mind, the dosage of any such drug is most conservative (*e.g.,* no more than a half or one third the dosage ordinarily employed in patients of similar age and weight who are not myxedematous). Drugs in this category are not used unless the indications are very specific, and if they are given, the nurse must be unusually alert for signs of impending narcosis or respiratory failure.

2. *Myocardial ischemia or infarction may occur in response to therapy in patients with myxedema.* Any patient who has been myxedematous for a long period of time is almost certain to have elevated serum cholesterol levels, atherosclerosis, and coronary artery disease to some degree. As long as metabolism is subnormal and the tissues, including the myocardium, require relatively little oxygen, a reduction in blood supply is tolerated very well. However, when thyroid hormone is given, the situation changes: the oxygen requirements are greater, but its delivery cannot be speeded up unless, or until, the atherosclerosis improves, which will occur very slowly, if at all. The signal that the oxygen needs of the myocardium are outstripping its blood supply is angina pectoris. Angina or arrhythmias may also occur when thyroid replacement is initiated, because thyroid hormones enhance the cardiovascular effects of catecholamines.

   The nurse must be alert for signs of angina, especially during the early phase of treatment, and if detected, it must be heeded at once in order to avoid a fatal myocardial infarction. Obviously, the administration of thyroid hormone must be discontinued immediately, and later, when it can be resumed safely, substitution therapy should be given, with caution, at a lower level of dosage and under the close observation of the physician and the nurse.

   Elderly arteriosclerotic patients may also become confused and agitated if their metabolic rates are raised too quickly in myxedema.

3. *Myxedema coma may be the final stage of severe, long-standing, untreated hypothyroidism.* Myxedema coma occurs mostly in the elderly, during winter months. Signs include hypotension, bradycardia, hypothermia (even below 37° C, recorded on the average thermometer), and convulsions.

The treatment consists of maintaining vital functions by measuring arterial blood gases to determine carbon dioxide retention and to provide assisted ventilation to combat hypoventilation. Fluids are to be administered cautiously because of the danger of water intoxication. External heat application is discouraged, since it will increase oxygen requirements and may lead to vascular collapse. If hypoglycemia is evident, concentrated glucose may be given, to prevent fluid overload. Thyroid hormone (TH), usually sodium levothyroxine (Synthroid), is given intravenously until consciousness is restored. Then the patient is continued on oral thyroid hormone therapy. Because of an associated adrenocortical insufficiency, steroid therapy may be initiated.

Nursing measures appropriate to the unconscious patient apply, such as frequent turning; prevention of aspiration; and attention to constipation, fecal impaction, or urinary retention (see pp. 1297–1305).

Marked clinical improvement follows the administration of hormone replacement; such medication must be continued for life, although signs of myxedema disappear over a 3- to 12-week period.

Precautions must be taken during the course of therapy because of interaction of thyroid hormones with other drugs. Thyroid hormones may increase blood glucose levels, which may necessitate adjustment in doses of insulin or oral hypoglycemic agents. The effects of thyroid hormone may be increased by phenytoin and tricyclic antidepressants. Thyroid hormones may also increase the pharmacologic effects of digitalis glycosides, anticoagulants, and indomethacin, requiring careful observation and assessment by the nurse for side-effects of these drugs.

The realization that the disorder has led to such severe consequences can cause the patient to feel depressed. In such a situation, conveying a sense of understanding and providing time to ventilate anger and frustration will help the patient adjust to the disorder.

Hyperthyroidism (Graves' Disease)

Spontaneous hyperthyroidism constitutes a well-defined disease entity, variously designated as *Graves' disease, Basedow's disease,* and *exophthalmic goiter.* Its etiology is unknown, but the excessive output of thyroid hormones is thought to be due to abnormal stimulation of the thyroid gland by circulating immunoglobulins. Long-acting thyroid stimulator (LATS) is found in significant concentration in the serum of many of these patients and may be related to a defect in the patient's immune surveillance system. The disorder, which affects women five times more frequently than men, and peaks in incidence in the third and fourth decades, may appear after an emotional shock, stress, or an infection—but the exact significance of these relationships is not understood.

Assessment

Patients with well-developed hyperthyroidism exhibit a characteristic group of symptoms and signs. Their presenting symptom is often nervousness. They are often emotionally hyperexcitable, irritable, and apprehensive; they cannot sit quietly; they suffer from palpitation; and their pulse is abnormally rapid at rest as well as on exertion. They tolerate heat poorly and perspire unusually freely; the skin is flushed continuously, with a characteristic salmon color, and is likely to be warm, soft, and moist. A fine tremor of the hands may be observed. Many patients exhibit bulging eyes (exophthalmos), which produce a startled facial expression.

Other important symptoms include an increased appetite and dietary intake (unless gastrointestinal symptoms develop), progressive loss of weight, abnormal muscular fatigability and weakness, amenorrhea, and changes in bowel habit, either to constipation or diarrhea. The pulse rate of these patients ranges constantly between 90 and 160; the systolic, but characteristically not diastolic, blood pressure is elevated; atrial fibrillation may appear, and cardiac decompensation in the form of congestive heart failure is common, especially in elderly patients.

The thyroid gland invariably is enlarged to some extent. It is soft and may pulsate; a thrill often can be felt and a bruit heard over the thyroid arteries—signs of greatly increased blood flow through the organ.

In the more advanced cases, the diagnosis is established readily on the basis of the symptoms and the tests described previously: an increase in serum thyroxine and an increased ^{131}I uptake by the thyroid, in excess of 50%.

The course of the disease may be mild, characterized by remissions and exacerbations and terminating with spontaneous recovery in the course of a few months or years. On the other hand, it may progress relentlessly, the untreated patient becoming emaciated, intensely nervous, delirious—even disoriented—and the heart eventually "racing itself to death."

Management

As yet, no treatment for hyperthyroidism has been discovered that combats its basic cause. However, reduction of thyroid hyperactivity provides effective symptomatic relief and removes the principal source of its most important complications.

Three forms of treatment are available for treating hyperthyroidism and controlling excessive thyroid activity: (1) pharmacology, employing antithyroid drugs that interfere with the synthesis of thyroid hormones and other agents that control manifestations of hyperthyroidism; (2) radiation, involving the administration of the radioisotope ^{131}I or ^{125}I for destructive effects on the thyroid gland; and (3) surgery, whereby most of the thyroid gland is removed.

Pharmacotherapy. The objective of pharmacotherapy is to inhibit one or more stages in hormone synthesis or hormone release; another goal may be to reduce the amount of thyroid tissue, thereby reducing hormone production.

Antithyroid drugs (thiocarbamides, thioamides) effectively block the utilization of iodine by interfering with the iodination of thyrosine and the coupling of iodothyrosines in the synthesis of thyroid hormones. Since this prevents the synthesis of thyroid hormone, the patient with hyperthyroidism is greatly benefitted. The most commonly used medications are propylthiouracil (Propacil, PTU) or methimazole (Tapazole), until the patient is euthyroid (*i.e.,* neither hyper- nor hypo-thyroid). These drugs block extrathyroidal conversion of thyroxine (T_4) to triiodothyronine (T_3). Since antithyroid drugs do not interfere with release or activity of previously formed thyroid hormones, it may take several weeks to stabilize the patient, at which time the maintenance dose is established, followed by a gradual withdrawal of the medication over the next several months.

Therapy is controlled on the basis of clinical criteria, including changes in pulse rate, pulse pressure, body weight, size of the goiter, and basal metabolic rate. Perhaps up to half of the patients experience prolonged remission of hyperthyroidism after thiocarbamide therapy is withdrawn. Toxic complications of thiocarbamides are relatively uncommon; nevertheless, periodic examinations cannot be neglected, in view of the possibility that drug sensitization, followed by fever, rash, urticaria, or even agranulocytosis and thrombocytopenia, may develop. With any sign of infection, especially pharyngitis and fever, the patient is advised to stop the medication, call the physician, and have hematologic studies performed. Patients on antithyroid drugs are instructed not to use decongestants for nasal stuffiness because they are poorly tolerated. These drugs are contraindicated in late pregnancy as they may produce goiter and cretinism in the fetus.

Thyroid hormone may occasionally be given with antithyroid drugs in an attempt to put the thyroid gland at rest. In this approach, hypothyroidism from excess antithyroid drug is avoided, as is stimulation of the thyroid gland by thyroid-stimulating hormone. Thyroid hormone is available as desiccated thyroid, thyroglobulin (Proloid), and levo-thyroxine sodium (Synthroid). These are slow-acting preparations that take about 10 days to achieve their full effect. Liothyronine sodium (Cytomel) has a more rapid onset and lasts a short time.

Adjunctive Therapy.   Iodine or iodide compounds, once the only therapy available for patients with hyperthyroidism, are no longer used as the sole method of treatment. Such compounds reduce the release of thyroid hormones from the thyroid gland and reduce the vascularity and size of the thyroid. Compounds such as potassium iodide, Lugol's Solution, and saturated solution of potassium iodide (SSKI) are used to prepare the patient for a subtotal thyroidectomy and for patients with thyrotoxic crisis. Reducing glandular vascularity prevents postoperative hemorrhage.

Solutions of iodine and iodide compounds are more palatable in milk or fruit juice and are administered through a straw to prevent staining of the teeth. These compounds reduce the metabolic rate more rapidly than antithyroid drugs, but their action is not as lasting.

- Patients receiving these drugs should be observed for the development of goiter and should be cautioned against use of over-the-counter medications that contain iodides and can increase the response to iodide therapy. Cough medications, expectorants, bronchodilators, and salt substitutes may contain iodide and should be avoided by the patient receiving iodide therapy.

Adrenergic blocking agents may also be used to control the sympathetic nervous system effects that occur in hyperthyroidism. Examples are reserpine, propranolol, and guanethidine, which are useful in controlling nervousness, tachycardia, and tremor.

Radioactive Iodine.   Until recently, radioiodine was considered an ideal form of treatment for diffuse toxic goiter. The eventual occurrence of hypothyroidism, however, is one of the more prominent objections. Practically all of the iodine that enters and is retained in the body becomes concentrated within the thyroid gland. This applies to the radioactive isotopes of iodine as well, providing the basis for a very effective device for the selective inhibition of thyroid activity, namely, by the administration of radioiodine (^{131}I). The objective of this treatment is the irradiation of the gland, which is accomplished without jeopardizing other radiosensitive tissues. Radioactive iodine has been used in toxic adenomas or multinodular goiter, in most varieties of thyrotoxicosis (rarely permanently successful), and is preferred for the treatment of patients beyond the childbearing years with diffuse toxic goiter.

Prior to treatment with radioactive iodine, the patient receives antithyroid drugs for 6 to 18 months. When drugs are given as temporary therapy for the purpose of reducing the production of hormones to normal, radiation or surgical therapy can then be undertaken safely.

Nursing supervision of this patient is primarily a teaching function. The patient is instructed as to what to expect of this tasteless, colorless radioiodine, which is administered by the physician. If the patient is hospitalized during administration of ^{131}I, radiation safety precautions identified by the hospital's radiation safety committee should be followed. Following treatment with ^{131}I, the patient is discharged and usually followed closely until the euthyroid state is reached.

A single dose of the drug is given by mouth (a radioactive "cocktail"), based on 80 to 160 microcuries per gram of estimated thyroid weight. The patient is watched for signs of thyroid storm (see p. 930).

In about 3 to 4 weeks, symptoms of hyperthyroidism subside. If remission is not achieved, the treatment is repeated after several months. Close supervision is required by periodic visits to the physician to ascertain normal rates of function. If hypothyroidism results from gland destruction, thyroid hormones will have to be taken by the patient.

Those caring for the patient need to give reassurance, since patients often overreact to such medications as radioactive drugs, which require special supervision.

Surgical Intervention.   The surgical removal of about five sixths of the thyroid tissue (subtotal thyroidectomy) practically assures a prolonged remission in most patients with exophthalmic goiter. Before surgery, the patient is given propylthiouracil until signs of hyperthyroidism have disappeared. Iodine also is prescribed, either before or after a full remission has been achieved with propylthiouracil. The effect of iodine is to reduce the size and the vascularity of the goiter. It may be given in the form of Lugol's solution, potassium iodide, or hydriodic acid.

- Patients receiving iodine medication must be watched for evidence of iodine toxicity (iodism), the appearance of which is the signal for immediate withdrawal of the drug. Symptoms of iodism include swelling of the buccal mucosa, excessive salivation, coryza, and skin eruptions.

Thyroidectomy for treatment of hyperthyroidism usually is scheduled within a few days after the patient's basal metabolic rate has been reduced to normal.

In appraising the value of surgery, it is considered a less than ideal form of treatment, because there is a possibility of permanent postoperative hypothyroidism, of hypoparathyroidism, and of damage to the recurrent laryngeal nerve. (See p. 931 for pre- and post-operative management of the patient undergoing thyroidectomy.)

Overview of Nursing Management.   The objectives of nursing management are to assist the patient in overcoming his symptoms and to help him return to a euthyroid condition. It is best to maintain a calm manner in approaching the patient, since much of his nervousness and anxiety is beyond his control. Added stress arises from a fear of cancer, which the patient may relate to the weight loss that is a characteristic feature of hyperthyroidism. In the initial nursing assessment, it is desirable to uncover such thoughts and to allay fears that are not justified.

Activities to lessen the irritability of the nervous system resulting from hyperthyroidism may include the following: protecting the patient from stressful experiences, such as upsetting visitors or the presence of annoying or very ill patients; providing a cool and uncluttered environment; and encouraging the patient to enjoy pleasant music, light television entertainment, and interesting and relaxing hobbies.

Hyperthyroidism also affects the gastrointestinal system. The appetite is increased but can be satisfied by providing several well-balanced meals of small size, even up to six meals a day. Proper foods and fluids are given to control diarrhea, which results from increased peristalsis and may result in further weight loss as well as nutritional imbalance. Quiet and pleasant surroundings at mealtime will assist the digestive process. Highly seasoned foods and stimulants such as coffee, tea, cola, and alcohol contribute to reflex diarrhea and are to be discouraged. Alcohol presents an additional problem; if the patient is sensitive to it, drinking without food may cause hypoglycemia.

Eye protection is essential for patients who experience eye changes secondary to hyperthyroidism. Instillation of an ophthalmic medication such as methylcellulose is not only soothing, but protects the exposed cornea. The upward gaze increases prominence of the eyes and may provoke strabismus. Since exophthalmos is thought to be caused by excess fluid in the tissues, it may be helpful if salt and water intake are restricted. Tactfully moving the furniture in the room so that the patient does not see his reflection in a dresser mirror is a thoughtful maneuver. Friends and visitors are advised not to comment on the patient's protruding eyes.

Thyroiditis

Subacute or granulomatous thyroiditis (deQuervain's thyroiditis), an inflammatory disorder of the thyroid gland that predominantly affects women in their 50s, presents as a painful swelling in the anterior neck that lasts 1 or 2 months, then disappears without residual effects. Evidence indicates that this disorder may be due to a viral infection. The thyroid enlarges symmetrically and occasionally is painful. The overlying skin is often reddened and warm. Swallowing may be difficult and uncomfortable. Irritability, nervousness, insomnia, and weight loss—manifestations of hyperthyroidism—are common, and many patients experience chills and fever as well.

The purpose of treatment is to control the inflammation. In general, acetylsalicylic acid (aspirin) controls the symptoms of inflammation in mild cases but should be avoided if symptoms of hyperthyroidism occur, because it displaces thyroid hormone from its binding sites and increases the amount of circulating thyroid hormone. In more severe inflammations, glucocorticoids are effective but do not necessarily influence the underlying cause.

Chronic Thyroiditis (Hashimoto's Thyroiditis). Chronic thyroiditis, which occurs most frequently in women 30 to 50 years of age, has been termed "Hashimoto's disease" depending on the histologic appearance of the inflamed gland. In contrast with acute thyroiditis, the chronic varieties are usually not accompanied by pain, pressure symptoms, or fever, and thyroid activity is apt to be normal or low, rather than increased.

There is evidence to suggest that cell-mediated immunity plays a significant role in the pathogenesis of thyroiditis. A genetic predisposition also seems to be significant in etiology. If untreated, the disease runs a slow, progressive course, leading eventually to myxedema.

The objective of treatment is to reduce the size of the thyroid gland and prevent myxedema. Thyroid hormone therapy is prescribed to reduce thyroid activity and the production of thyroglobulin. If hypothyroid symptoms are present, thyroid hormone is given. Antithyroid drugs may be given if an associated thyrotoxicosis exists. Surgery may be required if pressure symptoms persist.

Thyroid Tumors

Tumors of the thyroid gland are classified on the basis of being benign or malignant, as well as on the presence or absence of associated thyrotoxicosis, and the diffuse or irregular quality of the glandular enlargement. If the enlargement is sufficient to cause a visible swelling in the neck, the tumor is referred to as a "goiter."

All grades of goiter are encountered, from those that are barely visible to those producing an unsightly disfigurement. Some are symmetrical and diffuse, others nodular. Some are accompanied by hyperthyroidism, in which case they are described as "toxic"; others are associated with a euthyroid state and are called "nontoxic" goiters.

Endemic (Iodine-Deficient) Goiter. The most common type of goiter, encountered chiefly in geographic regions where the natural supply of iodine is deficient (*e.g.,* the Great Lakes area of the United States), is the so-called *simple or colloid goiter.* Aside from being caused by an iodine deficiency, simple goiter may also be caused by an intake of large quantities of goitrogenic substances in patients with unusually susceptible glands. These substances include excessive amounts of iodine or of lithium, which is currently used in the treatment of manic-depressive states.

Simple goiter represents a compensatory hypertrophy of the thyroid gland, presumably due to stimulation by the pituitary gland. The pituitary gland produces a hormone controlling thyroid growth, and this production is excessive if there is subnormal thyroid activity, as when insufficient iodine is available for production of the thyroid hormone. Such goiters usually cause no symptoms except for the swelling in the neck, which may result in tracheal compression, when excessive.

Management. Many goiters of this type recede after iodine imbalance is corrected. Supplementary iodine such as saturated solution of potassium iodide (SSKI) is prescribed in order to depress the pituitary's thyroid-stimulating activity.

When surgery is recommended, postoperative complications can be minimized when certain criteria exist: (1) a relatively young person without the complications of concurrent medical illnesses, such as diabetes, heart disease, drug allergies; (2) a preoperative euthyroid state resulting from treatment with antithyroid drugs; (3) proper preoperative iodide administration to reduce the size and vascularity of the goiter; and (4) an experienced surgeon in thyroid surgery.

Patient Teaching. Simple or endemic goiter can be prevented by providing children in iodine-poor districts with iodine compounds. If the mean iodine intake is less than 40 µg per day, the thyroid hypertrophies. The World Health Organization recommends that salt be iodized to a concentration of one part in 100,000, which is adequate for the prevention of endemic goiter. In the United States, salt is iodized to one part in 10,000. The introduction of iodized salt has been the single most effective means of preventing goiter in susceptible populations.

Nodular Goiter. Certain thyroid glands are nodular because of the presence of one or several areas of *hyperplasia* (overgrowth) that appear to develop under conditions similar to those responsible for the colloid or simple goiter. No symptoms may arise as a result of this condition, but, not uncommonly, these nodules slowly increase in size, some descending into the thorax, where they cause local pressure symptoms. Some nodules become malignant and some become associated with a hyperthyroid state. Thus, many nodular thyroids eventually require surgical intervention.

Thyroid Cancer

Cancer of the thyroid is much less prevalent than other forms of cancer. According to the American Cancer Society, approximately 1000 patients die annually of this malignancy. The most common type is papillary adenocarcinoma, which accounts for over half of thyroid malignancy. This neoplasm starts in childhood or early adult life, remains localized, and eventually metastasizes along the lymphatics and lymph nodes if untreated. It appears as an asymptomatic nodule in a normal gland.

An association exists between external radiation of the head and neck in infancy and childhood and subsequent development of thyroid carcinoma. Between 1940 and 1960 radiation therapy was occasionally used to shrink enlarged tonsillar and adenoid tissue, to treat acne, or to reduce an enlarged thymus. Consequently, people who underwent such treatment should consult a physician, request an isotope thyroid scan as part of the evaluation, either submit to surgical thyroidectomy or take thyroid hormones if prescribed for abnormalities of the gland, and continue with annual checkups if all is normal.

Follicular adenocarcinoma appears in later life, usually over age 40, and accounts for about 20% to 25% of thyroid neoplasms. It is encapsulated and feels elastic or rubbery on palpation. This tumor eventually spreads by hematogenous routes to bone, liver, and lung. The prognosis is not as favorable as for papillary adenocarcinoma.

Other types of cancer are medullary (5%), which present as solid, hard nodular tumors, and anaplastic (5%), which are hard, irregular masses that grow quickly and may be painful and tender.

Management. Proper management of thyroid carcinoma is surgical removal. Total or near total thyroidectomy is performed when possible.

Modified neck dissection is done if there is lymph node involvement. Following surgery, ablation procedures are carried out with [131]radioactive iodine to eradicate residual thyroid tissue. Radioactive iodine also maximizes the chance of discovering thyroid metastasis at a later stage if total body scans are carried out.

Following surgery, thyroid hormone is administered in suppressive doses to lower the levels of thyroid-stimulating hormone (TSH) to an euthyroid state.

Patient Teaching. Postoperatively, the patient will require instructions about the need to take exogenous thyroid hormone to prevent the occurrence of hypothyroidism. Later follow-up includes clinical assessment for recurrence of nodules or masses in the neck and signs of hoarseness, dysphagia, or dyspnea. Chest x-rays are done as recommended. Total body scans are advised annually for the first 3 postoperative years and less frequently thereafter. Prior to planned total body scans, thyroid hormones are stopped for about a month preceding the tests.

T_4, TSH levels, serum calcium, and phosphorus are assessed to determine if the thyroid hormone supplementation is adequate and to note whether calcium balance is maintained.

While local and systemic reactions to radiation may occur and may include neutropenia or thrombocytopenia (see p. 716), these complications are rare when ^{131}I is used. Surgery combined with radioiodine produces a higher survival rate than does surgery alone.

Thyroid Storm or Crisis

Thyroid storm, thyrotoxicosis, or *thyrotoxic crisis* is a form of severe hyperthyroidism, usually of abrupt onset and characterized by hyperpyrexia, extreme tachycardia, and altered mental state, which frequently appears as delirium. Thyroid storm is a life-threatening condition and is usually precipitated by stress such as injury, infection, nonthyroid surgery, thyroidectomy, tooth extraction, insulin reaction, diabetic acidosis, pregnancy, digitalis intoxication, abrupt withdrawal of antithyroid drugs, or vigorous palpation of the thyroid. These factors will precipitate thyroid storm in the partially controlled or completely untreated hyperthyroid patient. Patients who are maintained in an euthyroid state through the proper adjustment of an antithyroid drug may go through many of these episodes without a crisis being precipitated.

While thyroid crisis may be difficult to identify, the following signs are suggestive: (1) tachycardia (over 130), (2) temperature above 37.7° C (100° F), (3) exaggerated symptoms of hyperthyroidism, and (4) disturbances of a major system, for example, gastrointestinal (weight loss, diarrhea, abdominal pain), neurologic (psychosis, somnolence, coma), or cardiovascular (edema, chest pain, dyspnea, palpitations).

Untreated thyroid storm is almost always fatal, but with proper treatment, the mortality rate can be reduced substantially.

Management. The immediate objective is to reduce body temperature and heart rate. Measures to reduce the temperature include a hypothermia mattress or blanket, ice packs, a cool environment, and hydrocortisone. Acetaminophen is preferred to salicylates because aspirin displaces T_4 and T_3 from thyroxine-binding globulin, thereby leading to an increase in free thyroid hormones. Humidified oxygen is administered to improve tissue oxygenation, thereby meeting the high metabolic demand. Dextrose-containing intravenous fluids are administered to replace liver glycogen stores that have been decreased in the hyperthyroid patient. Propylthiouracil (PTU) or methimazole is given to interrupt hormonogenesis. Hydrocortisone is prescribed to treat shock or adrenal insufficiency. Iodine is administered to decrease thyroxine output from the thyroid gland. For cardiac problems such as atrial fibrillation, arrhythmias, and congestive heart failure, sympatholytic agents may be given. Propranolol in combination with digitalis has been effective in reducing severe cardiac symptoms.

- The patient with thyroid storm or crisis is critically ill and requires astute observation and aggressive and supportive nursing care during and after the acute stage of illness.

Thyroidectomy

Preoperative Management. Before undergoing surgery for treatment of hyperthyroidism, the patient will be treated with appropriate drug therapy to return his thyroid hormone levels and metabolic rate to normal and to reduce risk of thyroid storm and hemorrhage during the postoperative period. One important approach in the preoperative period is to gain the confidence of the patient and keep him free from worry and anxiety. Some forms of occupational therapy are recommended because they are quieting and relaxing.

The patient with hyperthyroidism often comes from a home made tense and unhappy by his restlessness and nervousness. It is necessary to protect the patient from such unpleasantness and unhappiness in order to avoid precipitating thyroid storm. If there is evidence of nervous upsets when family or friends visit, it may be advisable to limit visiting privileges during the preoperative period.

Nutritional intake is regulated to include adequate carbohydrate and protein foods. A high daily caloric intake is necessary because of the increased metabolic activity and rapid depletion of glycogen reserves. Supplementary vitamins, particularly thiamine chloride and ascorbic acid, are to be provided. Tea, coffee, cola, and other stimulants are to be avoided.

If the patient is to undergo diagnostic testing prior to surgery, he is informed of the purpose of the test and the preoperative preparations in order to reduce anxiety. In addition, a special effort is made to ensure a good night's rest preceding surgery.

Preoperative teaching includes demonstrating to the patient how to support his neck with his hands to prevent stress on the incision, that is, raising his elbows and placing his hands behind his neck will provide support and put much less strain and tension on the neck muscles.

Postoperative Management. The patient is moved and turned carefully so as to support the head and avoid tension on the sutures. The most comfortable position is the semi-Fowler position with the head elevated and supported by pillows. Narcotics are given as prescribed for pain. Occasionally, the patient is given humidified oxygen to facilitate breathing. The nurse should anticipate apprehension in the patient and inform him that oxygen will assist his breathing and help him to feel less tired. Intravenous fluids will be administered during the immediate postoperative period, but water may be given by mouth as soon as nausea ceases. Usually, there is a little difficulty in swallowing; initially, cold fluids and ice may be taken better than other fluids. Often patients prefer a soft diet to a liquid diet.

The surgical dressings should be checked periodically and reinforced when necessary. It is important to remember that when the patient is in the dorsal position, evidence of bleeding should be looked for at the sides and the back of the neck as well as anteriorly. In addition to checking the pulse and the blood pressure for any indication of internal bleeding, it is also important to be on the alert for complaints from the patient of sensation of pressure or fullness at the incision site. Such signs may indicate hemorrhage and should be reported.

The patient is advised to talk as little as possible, but when he does speak, the nurse should note any voice changes that might indicate injury to the recurrent laryngeal nerve that lies just behind the thyroid next to the trachea.

Occasionally, difficulty in respiration occurs, with the development of cyanosis and noisy breathing, as a result of edema of the glottis or an injury to the recurrent laryngeal nerve. This complication requires that an airway be inserted. Therefore, a tracheostomy set is kept at the patient's bedside at all times, and the surgeon is summoned at the first indication of distress.

When the nurse is not in constant attendance, an overbed table may be used to afford easy access to those materials and items that are needed frequently, such as paper wipes, water pitcher and glass, small emesis basin, etc. These are kept within easy reach so that the patient will not need to turn his head in search of them. It is also convenient to use this table when vapor-mist inhalations are given for the relief of excessive mucous secretions.

The patient usually is permitted out of bed on the first postoperative day and has a choice of diet. A well-balanced, high-caloric diet is prescribed to regain any weight loss. Sutures or skin clips usually are removed on the second day. The average patient is ready for discharge from the hospital.

Complications. Hemorrhage, edema of the glottis, and injury to the recurrent laryngeal nerve are complications that have been reviewed previously. Occasionally, in thyroid operations, the parathyroid glands may be injured or removed, producing a disturbance of the calcium metabolism of the body. As the blood calcium falls, there appears a hyperirritability of the nerves, with spasms of the hands and feet and muscular twitchings; this group of symptoms is termed *tetany,* and its appearance should be reported at once since laryngospasm, although rare, may occur. Tetany of this type is usually treated by the administration of calcium gluconate. This calcium abnormality may be temporary following thyroidectomy.

Patient Teaching. The necessity for rest, relaxation, and nutrition is explained to both the patient and his family. Specific instructions are issued regarding follow-up visits to the physician or the clinic, which are inevitably necessary and invariably important. The patient should be permitted to resume his former activities and responsibilities completely once thyrotoxicosis has been eliminated.

Responsibilities and factors relating to the home environment that engender emotional tension often have been implicated as precipitating causes of thyrotoxicosis. The patient's hospitalization affords an opportunity to evaluate these factors and possibly alter the environmental situation. This is the most favorable time for establishing a close rapport with the patient and for supplying whatever psychological support and assistance are needed to promote emotional readjustments.

▷ The Parathyroid Glands

Hyperparathyroidism

Hyperparathyroidism, which is due to overproduction of parathyroid hormone by the parathyroid glands, is characterized by bone calcification and the development of renal stones containing calcium in the kidneys. Secondary hyperparathyroidism with similar manifestations occurs in patients with chronic renal failure and so-called "renal rickets," as a result of phosphorus retention, increased stimulation of the parathyroid glands, and increased parathyroid hormone secretion.

Clinical Manifestations and Diagnosis. These patients may have no symptoms or may experience signs and symptoms resulting from involvement of several body systems. The patient may experience symptoms of apathy, fatigue, muscular weakness, nausea, vomiting, constipation, and cardiac arrhythmias, all attributable to an increased concentration of calcium in the blood. Psychological manifestations may vary from emotional irritability and neurosis to psychoses due to the direct effect of calcium on the brain and nervous system. An increase in calcium produces an increase in the excitation potential of nerve and muscle tissue. Occasionally, the patient may be misdiagnosed as "psychoneurotic."

The formation of stones in one or both kidneys, related to the increased urinary excretion of calcium and phosphorus, is one of the important complications of hyperparathyroidism and occurs in 55% of patients with primary hyperparathyroidism. Renal damage results from the precipitation of calcium phosphate in the renal pelvis and parenchyma, resulting in nephrocalcinosis, obstruction, pyelonephritis, and uremia.

Musculoskeletal symptoms accompanying hyperparathyroidism may result from demineralization of the bones or bone tumors, composed of benign giant cells resulting from overgrowth of osteoclasts. The patient may develop skeletal pain and tenderness, especially of the back and joints; pain on weight-bearing; pathologic fractures; deformities; and shortening of body structure.

The incidence of peptic ulcer and pancreatitis is increased with hyperparathyroidism and may be responsible for many of the gastrointestinal symptoms that occur.

The diagnosis of hyperparathyroidism is established by the clinical picture, by persistently elevated serum calcium, and by skeletal changes detected by x-ray pictures. Only occasionally can a parathyroid tumor be palpated.

Parathyroid hormone assay and urinary and serum levels of calcium and phosphorus are used to establish the diagnosis of parathyroid disease. Sulkowitch's test is a semiquantitative test of the urine for calcium content and can be used as a screening tool. A reagent is added to the urine specimen, and the reaction produced determines the extent of calcium in the urine. A normal reaction is a fine, white cloud of precipitated calcium; hypercalcemia produces a heavy, milky precipitate, and hypocalcemia is indicated by absence of a precipitate.

Management. The insidious onset and chronic nature of hyperparathyroidism, and its diverse and often vague symptoms, may result in depression and frustration of the patient. The family may have considered the patient's illness to be psychosomatic. An awareness of the course of the disorder and an understanding approach by the nurse may help the patient and family to deal with their reactions and feelings.

The treatment of primary hyperparathyroidism is the surgical removal of abnormal parathyroid tissue. In the preoperative period it must be recognized that kidney involvement is possible, since these patients are subject to renal calculi. A fluid intake of 2000 ml or more is encouraged to help prevent calculi formation. Cranberry juice is suggested because it is effective in lowering urinary pH. It can be added to juices and ginger ale for variety. Because of the possibility of stone formation, urine is strained, and any evidence of calculi is saved for laboratory analysis. The patient is observed for other manifestations of renal calculi, such as abdominal pain and hematuria. Thiazide diuretics should not be used in the patient with hyperparathyroidism since they decrease the renal excretion of calcium, thereby causing further elevations in serum calcium levels.

Mobility of the patient, with walking or use of a rocking chair, is encouraged as much as possible because bones subjected to normal stress give up less calcium. Bed rest, on the other hand, increases calcium excretion and predisposes the patient to renal calculi formation.

Nutritional needs are met, but foods high in calcium and phosphorus, such as milk and milk products, are limited. If the patient has a coexisting peptic ulcer, specifically prescribed antacids and protein feedings will be necessary. Since anorexia is common, efforts are made to encourage the patient's appetite. Prune juice, stool softeners, and physical activity, along with increased fluid intake, should offset constipation, a common postoperative problem for this patient.

The nursing management of the patient undergoing parathyroidectomy is essentially the same as that for a thyroidectomy patient (see p. 931). Although not all parathyroid tissue will be removed during surgery in an effort to maintain control of calcium–phosphorus balance, the patient must be watched closely to detect symptoms of tetany, which may be an early postoperative complication.

Although it is rare, acute hypercalcemic crisis can occur in hyperparathyroidism. This occurs with extreme elevation of serum calcium levels. Serum calcium levels over 15 mg/100 ml result in neurologic, cardiovascular, and renal symptoms that can be life-threatening. Treatment includes rehydration with large volumes of intravenous fluids, diuretic agents to promote renal excretion of excess calcium, and phosphate therapy to correct hypophosphatemia and decrease serum calcium levels by promoting calcium deposit in bone and decreasing gastrointestinal absorption of calcium. Cytotoxic agents, calcitonin, and dialysis may be used in emergency situations. The patient in acute hypercalcemic crisis requires close monitoring for complications, deterioration of condition, or reversal of serum calcium levels.

Supportive measures are necessary for the patient and family.

Hypoparathyroidism

The most common cause of hypoparathyroidism is inadequate secretion of parathyroid hormone following interruption of the blood supply or surgical removal of parathyroid gland tissue during thyroidectomy, parathyroidectomy, or radical neck dissection. Atrophy of the parathyroid glands of unknown etiology is a less common cause of hypoparathyroidism.

Pathophysiology. Symptoms of hypoparathyroidism are due to a deficiency of parathormone that results in an elevation of blood phosphate, hyperphosphatemia, and a decrease in the concentration of blood calcium, hypocalcemia. Hypocalcemia results because in the absence of parathormone, there is decreased intestinal absorption of dietary calcium and decreased resorption of calcium from bone and through the renal tubules. Decreased renal excretion of phosphate causes hypophosphaturia, and low serum calcium results in hypocalciuria.

Clinical Manifestations. Hypocalcemia causes irritability of the neuromuscular system and contributes to the chief symptom of hypoparathyroidism, *tetany*—a general muscular hypertonia, with tremor and spasmodic or incoordinated contractions occurring with or without efforts to make voluntary movements. In latent tetany there is numbness, tingling, and cramps in the extremities, with the patient complaining of stiffness in the hands and feet. In overt tetany the signs include bronchospasm, laryngeal spasm, carpopedal spasm (flexion of the elbows and wrists and extension of the carpophalangeal joints—Fig. 41-2), dysphagia, photophobia, cardiac arrhythmias, and convulsions. Other symptoms include anxiety, irritability, depression, and even delirium.

Assessment. Latent tetany is suggested by a positive Trousseau's sign or a positive Chvostek's sign. *Trousseau's sign* is positive when carpopedal spasm is induced by occluding the blood flow to the arm for 3 minutes using a blood pressure cuff. *Chvostek's sign* is positive when a sharp tapping over the facial nerve just in front of the parotid gland and anterior to the ear causes the mouth, nose, and eye to twitch.

The diagnosis is often difficult because of vague symptoms of aches and pains. Therefore, laboratory studies are especially helpful. Tetany develops at serum calcium levels of 5 mg/100 ml to 6 mg/100 ml or below. Serum phosphate levels are increased, and x-ray studies of bone show increased density. Calcification is noticed on x-rays of subcutaneous or paraspinal basal ganglia of the brain.

Management. The objective of therapy is to raise serum calcium to approximately 9 mg/100 ml to 10 mg/100 ml and to eliminate the symptoms of hypoparathyroidism and hypocalcemia. When hypocalcemia and tetany occur following a thyroidectomy, the immediate treatment is to administer calcium gluconate intravenously. If this does not control convulsive tendencies immediately, it may be necessary to administer sedatives such as chloral hydrate or pentobarbital.

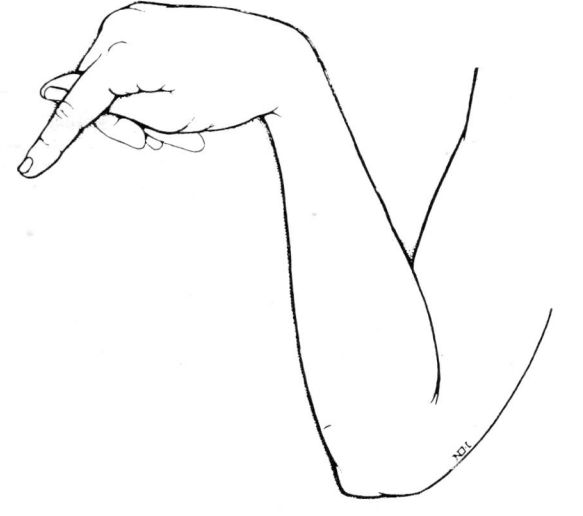

Figure 41-2. Carpopedal spasm.

Parenteral parathyroid hormone can be administered to treat acute hypoparathyroidism with tetany. The high incidence of allergic reactions to injections of parathyroid hormone limits its use to acute episodes of hypocalcemia. The patient receiving parathyroid hormone is monitored closely for changes in serum calcium levels and allergic reactions.

Because of neuromuscular irritability, the patient with hypocalcemia and tetany requires an environment that is free of noise, sudden drafts, bright lights, or sudden movement. If the patient experiences respiratory distress, bronchodilating medications, a tracheostomy, or mechanical ventilation may be necessary.

Nursing management of the patient with possible acute hypoparathyroidism encompasses the following actions:

- The attention of the nurse in the care of postoperative patients having thyroidectomy, parathyroidectomy, and radical neck dissection is directed toward anticipating signs of tetany, convulsions, and respiratory difficulties.
- Calcium gluconate is kept at the bedside with equipment necessary for intravenous administration. If the patient has cardiac problems, is subject to arrhythmias, or is receiving digitalis, then calcium gluconate is administered by slow infusion.
- Calcium and digitalis increase systolic contraction, and furthermore, they potentiate each other. This may produce potentially fatal arrhythmias. Consequently, the cardiac patient requires constant vigilance and undoubtedly should be on continuous cardiac monitoring.

Therapy for the patient with chronic hypoparathyroidism is determined after serum calcium levels are studied. The prescribed diet is high in calcium and low in phosphorus. Although milk, milk products, and egg yolk are high in calcium, they are restricted because they also contain high levels of phosphorus. Spinach is also avoided because it contains oxalate, which would form insoluble calcium substances. Oral tablets of calcium salts, such as calcium gluconate, may supplement the diet. Aluminum hydroxide gel or aluminum carbonate (Gelusil, Amphojel) is also given after meals to bind phosphate and promote its excretion through the GI tract.

Variable dosages of a vitamin D preparation, dihydrotachysterol (AT 10 or Hytakerol), or ergocalciferol (vitamin D_2) or cholecalciferol (vitamin D_3) are usually required and enhance calcium absorption from the GI tract.

The convalescent phase of patient care is the time to instruct the patient in drug and diet therapy. He needs to know why he must maintain a high calcium and low phosphate intake, and what the symptoms of hypocalcemia and hypercalcemia are so that he may immediately contact his physician should these symptoms occur.

▷ The Adrenal Gland

Pheochromocytoma

A *pheochromocytoma* is a tumor, usually benign, originating from the adrenal medulla, and in particular, from the chromaffin cells. In 90% of patients, the tumor arises in the medulla, whereas in about 10% it occurs in the extra-adrenal chromaffin tissue located in or near the aorta, ovaries, spleen, or other organs. It affects people between the ages of 25 and 50 and affects males and females equally. The patient's family should also be screened for this tumor because of the high incidence of pheochromocytoma in family members.

Clinical Manifestations.   Functioning tumors of the adrenal medulla cause arterial hypertension and other cardiovascular disturbances. The nature and severity depend on the relative proportions of epinephrine and norepinephrine secretion.

The hypertension may be intermittent or persistent. If it is of the sustained type, it may be difficult to distinguish from so-called "essential hypertension." In addition to hypertension, the symptoms are essentially the same as those encountered after the administration of epinephrine in large doses, namely, tachycardia, excessive perspiration, tremor, and nervousness. Hyperglycemia may result from conversion of liver and muscle glycogen to glucose by epinephrine secretion.

The clinical picture in the paroxysmal case of pheochromocytoma usually is characterized by acute, unpredictable attacks, lasting only a few seconds or minutes, or several hours, during which the patient feels excessively anxious, tremulous, and weak, and suffers from headache, vertigo, blurring of vision, tinnitus, air hunger, and dyspnea. Other symptoms include polyuria, nausea, vomiting, diarrhea, abdominal pain, and fear. Palpitations and tachycardia are common. Postural hypotension may occur.

Assessment.   Because of mass educational programs stressing the importance of periodic blood pressure determination, the nurse is frequently involved in evaluating patients with hypertension. Of particular concern is the patient who experiences attacks of paroxysmal hypertension.

These episodes or attacks, along with any precipitating factor, are carefully documented. Since paroxysmal hypertension is a frightening experience, the patient should not be left alone. Although fewer than 1% of hypertensive patients have pheochromocytoma, it is important to consider because it is usually curable with surgery.

The diagnosis of pheochromocytoma is suspected if signs of sympathetic overactivity occur in association with marked elevation of blood pressure. Determination of the catecholamines in urine and blood offers the most direct and conclusive test for overactivity of the adrenal medulla. VMA (vanillylmandelic acid) determination in particular is preferable (normal urinary values: 2 to 6 mg/24 hours). In addition, urine collected over a 2- to 3-hour period after a spontaneous or induced attack of hypertension should be assayed for catecholamine content. Coffee, vanilla, certain fruits, vegetables, and drugs are eliminated from the diet before assessment for VMA, as these substances may alter the test results.

Pharmacologic tests may be used for screening purposes, although they are rarely necessary unless clinical symptoms strongly suggest pheochromocytoma and the results of testing of urinary catecholamines are negative. Pharmacologic tests depend on the reaction of the blood pressure to *provocative* drugs and to *adrenergic blocking* drugs. Provocative agents are those that stimulate a sharp rise in arterial pressure, while adrenergic blocking drugs precipitate a definite fall in arterial pressure in patients with this disease. The most commonly used provocative drug is histamine. The test is positive for pheochromocytoma if there is a marked increase in both systolic and diastolic blood pressures within 1 to 4 minutes after the intravenous injection of histamine. Normotensive persons without pheochromocytoma experience a headache, flush, and often a slight fall in blood pressure.

The testing agent of choice among the adrenergic blocking agents is phentolamine (Regitine), which neutralizes the action of epinephrine. Even very small doses of this agent may cause a precipitous fall in the arterial blood pressure of patients with pheochromocytoma. Therefore, norepinephrine (Levophed) or other vasopressors should be available if required to reverse severe hypotension.

The tyramine test depends on direct release of catecholamines from nerve endings. Rapid intravenous administration of tyramine in graded doses up to 2 mg will produce an increase in blood pressure within 45 to 60 seconds and will reach a peak in 1 to 1½ minutes. The response lasts less than 3 minutes. If systolic pressure rises 20 mm Hg to 80 mm Hg and diastolic pressure rises about 40 mm, it is considered positive. If the increase in blood pressure is unusually high or prolonged, phentolamine will reverse it rapidly.

In summary, about 90% of patients with pheochromocytoma can be diagnosed by a single test for urinary norepinephrine and epinephrine or VMA levels. Pharmacologic tests are dangerous but may aid in diagnosing the other 10% of patients with this condition. Histamine and tyramine tests are performed with caution and not in patients with a blood pressure over 170/100. Adrenergic blocking agents should be used in testing only when the blood pressure is high.

Management. The treatment of pheochromocytoma is surgical removal of the tumor, usually with adrenalectomy. Preliminary patient preparation includes effective control of blood pressure and blood volumes. Usually, this is carried out over 10 days to 2 weeks. Alpha-adrenergic blocking agents such as phentolamine or phenoxybenzamine hydrochloride (Dibenzyline) may be used safely without causing undue hypotension. These agents inhibit the effects of catecholamines but do not alter their synthesis or degradation. Beta-adrenergic blocking agents may be used in patients with cardiac arrhythmias or in those not responsive to alpha-adrenergic blocking drugs. Alpha- and beta-adrenergic blocking agents must be used with caution, because patients with pheochromocytoma may be extraordinarily sensitive to them. Still another group of drugs that may be used preoperatively are catecholamine synthesis inhibitors. These are occasionally used when the effects of catecholamines are not reduced by adrenergic blocking agents.

In the postoperative period, monitoring of the patient's vital signs, arterial pressures, ECG, and fluid balance is an important nursing function. In addition, nursing care of a patient undergoing abdominal surgery is indicated. Usually, hypotension is controlled by blood replacement and by use of small amounts of pressor agents. If a bilateral adrenalectomy has been done, corticosteroid replacement is required. The patient is assessed frequently for recurrence of hypertensive episodes and onset of hypotension.

Several days after surgery, 24-hour urine excretion of catecholamines and their metabolites is measured to determine whether surgery has been successful. When levels have returned to normal, the patient may be discharged. Thereafter, periodic checkups are required, especially in young patients or in patients whose families have a history of pheochromocytoma.

Adrenal Cortex

The adrenal cortex is considered necessary for life. Adrenocortical secretions make it possible for the body to adapt to stress of all kinds. How well one adapts to stress varies from individual to individual. Without the adrenal cortex, severe stress will cause peripheral circulatory failure, shock, and prostration. Life would be maintained only with nutritional and electrolyte replacement and replacement of adrenocortical hormones.

Adrenocortical hormones are classified into three groups: mineralocorticoids, glucocorticoids, and sex hormones. *Mineralocorticoids* are concerned with sodium and water retention and potassium excretion. Examples are aldosterone and desoxycorticosterone, a natural precursor of aldosterone. *Glucocorticoids* are concerned with metabolic effects, including carbohydrate metabolism. Examples are cortisol and corticosterone. Glucocorticoids enhance the metabolic breakdown of body proteins and fat to provide fuel during periods of fasting. They antagonize the action of insulin, enhance protein catabolism, and inhibit protein synthesis. They affect defense mechanisms of the body and influence emotional functioning either directly or indirectly. In high concentrations, they suppress inflammation and inhibit scar tissue formation. In adrenal insufficiency, patients may be depressed and upset, whereas with excessive replacement they tend to become euphoric. The *sex hormones* secreted by the adrenal cortex are androgens and estrogens.

Disorders of the adrenal cortex develop as a result of hyposecretion or hypersecretion of the adrenocortical hormones. Adrenal insufficiency may result from disease, atrophy, hemorrhage, or surgical removal of the adrenal gland or glands.

Chronic Primary Adrenocortical Insufficiency (Addison's Disease)

Pathophysiology and Clinical Manifestations. Addison's disease, caused by a deficiency of cortical hormones, results when the adrenal cortex is surgically removed with bilateral adrenalectomy or is destroyed, often as a result of idiopathic atrophy or infections such as tuberculosis or histoplasmosis. The symptoms of adrenocortical insufficiency may also result from sudden cessation of exogenous adrenocortical hormonal therapy, which suppresses the body's normal response to stress and interferes with normal feedback mechanisms. This hormonal deficiency gives rise to a characteristic clinical picture. The chief clinical manifestations include muscular weakness, anorexia, gastrointestinal symptoms, fatigue, emaciation, generalized dark pigmentation of the skin, hypotension, low blood sugar, low blood sodium, and high serum potassium. In severe cases the disturbance of sodium and potassium metabolism may be marked with depletion of the sodium and water through the urine and severe chronic dehydration.

Assessment. Although the clinical manifestations presented appear specific, the onset of Addison's disease usually occurs with nonspecific symptoms. The diagnosis of Addison's disease depends on the proper laboratory tests. Suggestive laboratory findings include a decrease in the concentrations of blood sugar and sodium (hypoglycemia and hyponatremia), an increased concentration of blood potassium (hyperkalemia), and relative lymphocytosis.

The definitive diagnosis depends on the demonstration of low levels of adrenocorticol hormones in the blood or urine. If the adrenal cortex is destroyed, baseline values are low, and ACTH injection fails to cause the normal rise in plasma cortisol and urinary 17-hydroxycorticosteroids. If the adrenal gland is normal but not stimulated properly by the pituitary, a normal response to repeated dosages of exogenous ACTH is seen, but no response follows the administration of metyrapone, which stimulates endogenous ACTH.

As the disease progresses, with acute hypotension developing due to hypocorticism, the patient moves into Addisonian crisis, which is a medical emergency marked by cyanosis, fever, and the classic signs of shock: pallor; apprehension; rapid, weak pulse; rapid respirations; and low blood pressure. In addition, the patient may complain of headache, nausea, abdominal pain, and diarrhea, and show signs of confusion and restlessness. Even slight overexertion, exposure to cold, acute infections, or a decrease in salt intake may lead to circulatory collapse. The stress of

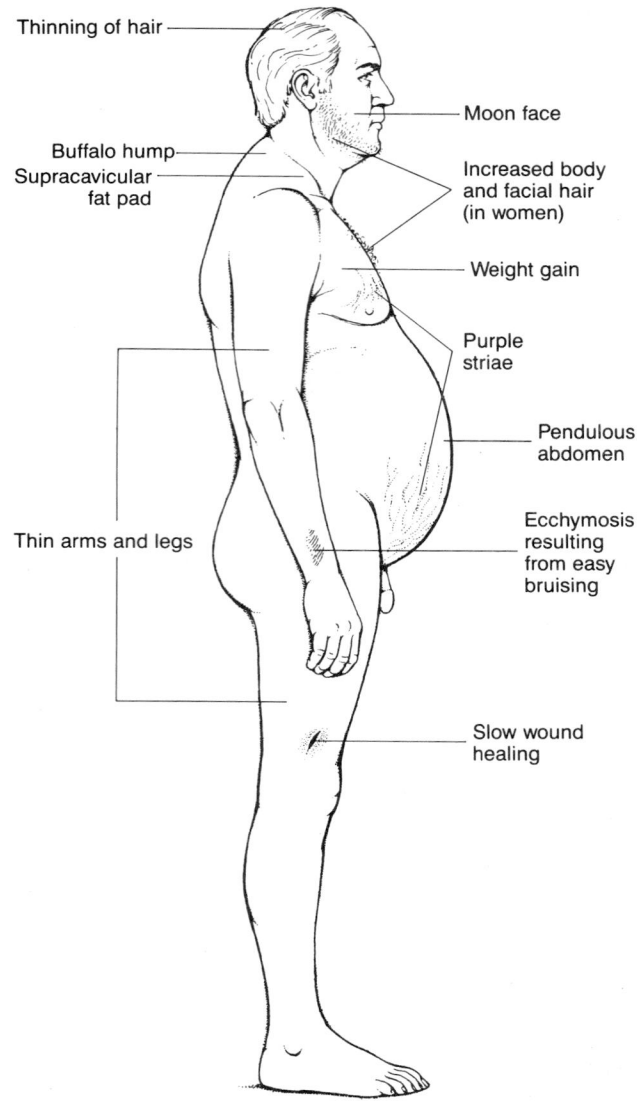

Thinning of hair

Buffalo hump
Supraclavicular
fat pad

Moon face

Increased body
and facial hair
(in women)

Weight gain

Purple
striae

Pendulous
abdomen

Thin arms and legs

Ecchymosis
resulting
from easy
bruising

Slow wound
healing

Figure 41-3. Features of Cushing's syndrome invariably include truncal obesity, thin extremities, moon face, buffalo hump, and supraclavicular fullness. Broad purple striae appear at stretch points, such as the abdomen, hips, and shoulders. Body and facial hair is increased, and thinning of scalp hair may be noted only if androgens are increased.

surgery or dehydration resulting from preparation for diagnostic tests or surgery may precipitate an Addisonian or hypotensive crisis.

Management. Immediate treatment is directed toward combating shock: restoring blood circulation, administering fluids, monitoring vital signs, and positioning the patient in a recumbent position with legs elevated. Emotional support is provided the patient concurrently with physical care. Hydrocortisone is given intravenously and followed with 5% dextrose in normal saline. Vasopressor amines may be required if hypotension persists.

When the patient's condition is stabilized, precautions are taken to avoid stressful conditions, since stress could

precipitate another hypotensive experience. Attempts are made to detect signs of infection or other stress that may have triggered the crisis in the first place. Oral intake may be initiated as soon as tolerated by the patient. Fruit juice and salted broth are given to provide sodium and correct electrolyte imbalance. Gradually, intravenous fluids are decreased as oral fluids are accepted.

During the patient's convalescence, the patient is assessed for symptoms of sodium or potassium imbalance. Vital signs continue to be monitored, and the patient's physical energy and emotional state are assessed. Cortisol (hydrocortisone) continues to be administered to simulate the diurnal pattern of normal secretion: highest levels between 4 and 6 AM, and lowest in the evening.

When the patient is discharged from the hospital, the basal dosage of cortisol is established; however, the patient is instructed to supplement this dosage during stressful conditions. He needs to know the signs of excessive or insufficient amounts, since he will be managing his own health care and medication schedule. The patient is instructed to carry information with him at all times, stating that he is receiving adrenocortical steroids. (See p. 939.)

Cushing's Syndrome

Cushing's syndrome is the opposite of Addison's disease, its clinical characteristics reflecting excessive, rather than deficient, adrenocortical activity. The syndrome may result from excessive administration of cortisone or ACTH, or hyperplasia of the adrenal cortex.

Pathophysiology. The basic lesion responsible for Cushing's syndrome may be a tumor arising in the cortex of one of the adrenal glands or a basophilic adenoma of the pituitary glands (see p. 950) involving an overgrowth of pituitary cells, producing the adrenocorticotrophic hormone (ACTH), which stimulates the adrenal cortex despite adequate amounts of circulating adrenocortical hormones. The normal feedback mechanisms that control the function of the adrenal cortex become ineffective, and the usual diurnal pattern of cortisol is lost. The signs and symptoms of Cushing's syndrome are primarily a result of unregulated secretion of glucocorticoids and androgens or sex hormones, although there may also be altered mineralocorticoid secretion.

▶ **Assessment**
Clinical Manifestations. When overproduction of the adrenal cortical hormone occurs, growth arrest, obesity, and musculoskeletal changes occur.

The classical picture of Cushing's syndrome in the adult shows a characteristic "central type obesity," with a fatty "buffalo hump" in the neck and supraclavicular areas, a heavy trunk, and relatively thin extremities (Fig. 41-3). The skin is thinned, fragile, and easily traumatized; ecchymoses and striae develop. The patient complains of weakness and lassitude. Sleep is disturbed because of altered diurnal secretion of cortisol. Excessive protein catabolism occurs, producing muscle wasting and osteoporosis. Kyphosis, backache, and compression fractures of the vertebrae may result. Retention of sodium and water occurs as a result of increased mineralocorticoid activity contributing to the hypertension and congestive heart failure commonly seen in Cushing's syndrome.

The patient takes on a "moon-faced" appearance and may experience increased oiliness of the skin and acne. There is increased susceptibility to infection. Hyperglycemia or overt diabetes may develop.

In females of all ages, variable elements of virilization are produced. Excess androgens also cause virilism, which is characterized by the appearance of masculine traits and the recession of feminine traits. There is an excessive growth of hair on the face (hirsutism), the breasts atrophy, menses cease, the clitoris enlarges, and the patient's voice deepens. Libido is lost in males and females.

Changes occur in mood and mental activity, with the patient occasionally developing a psychosis. Distress and depression are common and are increased by the magnitude of the physical changes that occur with this syndrome. If the Cushing's syndrome is a consequence of pituitary tumor, visual disturbances may occur.

The patient may also report weight changes, altered sleep patterns, and slow healing of minor cuts and bruises.

Diagnostic Assessment. Diagnostic evaluation of this syndrome includes an increase in blood sodium and blood sugar and a decreased concentration of potassium, a reduction in the number of blood eosinophils, and a disappearance of lymphoid tissue. Diagnostic studies usually include 24-hour urine collection for levels of 17-hydroxycorticosteroids and 17-ketosteroids, the urinary metabolites of cortisol and androgens. In Cushing's syndrome, these levels and plasma cortisol levels are elevated. Several blood specimens may be obtained at different times of the day and analyzed to assess the pattern of cortisol secretion, as the normal diurnal variation in secretion may be lost. Plasma ACTH is elevated when the disorder is caused by pituitary tumor.

Patient Problems/Nursing Diagnoses

Based on the clinical manifestations and diagnostic assessment data, the patient's major nursing problems include inability to carry out self-care activities related to weakness, fatigue, muscle wasting, and altered sleep patterns; altered skin integrity related to edema, impaired healing, and thin and fragile skin; increased susceptibility to injury and infection related to altered protein metabolism and inflammatory response; altered body image related to altered physical appearance; impaired sexual functioning and decrease in activity level; and altered mental function related to mood swings, irritability, and depression.

▶ Planning and Nursing Intervention

Goals

The major goals for the patient include:

1. Increased ability to carry out self-care activities
2. Improved skin integrity
3. Prevention of injury and infection
4. Improved body image
5. Improved mental function

To assist in accomplishing these goals, the major objectives of therapy are to remove the cause of Cushing's syndrome if possible and (1) to promote a balance between rest and exercise, (2) to prevent further threats to skin integrity, (3) to minimize risk of injury and infection, (4) to improve the patient's body image and reduce further alterations in body image, and (5) to eliminate or reduce factors causing deterioration of mental function.

If possible, the cause of Cushing's syndrome is removed. If it is due to externally administered corticoids, it may be necessary to reduce the dosage. On the other hand, this course of action may have to be weighed against the original disorder for which the corticoids were prescribed. For pituitary disorders, hypophysectomy or pituitary irradiation may be required. Adrenalectomy (see p. 938) remains the treatment of choice in cases of adrenal hyperplasia. Rare hyperplasia cases may benefit from a primary therapy directed against the pituitary, for example, patients with large pituitary adenomas or those with mild adrenal hyperfunction. In the latter, slow but successful responses to radiotherapy may be anticipated.

Rest and Activity. Weakness, fatigue, and muscle wasting make it difficult for the patient with Cushing's syndrome to carry out normal activities. Yet moderate activity should be encouraged to prevent complications of immobility and promote increased self-esteem. Insomnia often contributes to the patient's fatigue. Rest periods are planned and spaced throughout the day. Efforts are made to promote a relaxing, quiet environment for rest and sleep.

Skin Care. Meticulous skin care is necessary to avoid traumatizing the patient's fragile skin. Use of adhesive tape is avoided because it can irritate the skin and tear the fragile skin when the tape is removed. The skin and bony prominences are assessed frequently, and the patient is encouraged to change position frequently to prevent skin breakdown.

Prevention of Injury and Infection. A protective environment must be established to prevent falls, fractures, and other injuries to bones and soft tissues. The patient who is very weak may require assistance in ambulating to prevent falls or bumping into sharp corners of furniture. Unnecessary exposure to visitors, staff, or patients with infections is avoided. The patient is assessed frequently for subtle signs of infection since the anti-inflammatory effects of glucocorticoids may mask the common signs of inflammation and infection.

Assistance With Body Image Changes. If removal of the cause of Cushing's syndrome is possible and is carried out, the major physical changes will disappear in time. However, the patient may benefit from discussion of the impact the changes have had on self-concept and relationships with others. The weight gain and edema seen with Cushing's syndrome may be modified by a low-carbohydrate, low-sodium diet. A high protein intake may reduce some of the other bothersome symptoms.

Patient and Family Support. Explanations to the patient and family members about the cause of emotional instability are important in helping them cope with the mood swings, irritability, and depression that may occur. Psychotic behavior may occur in a few patients and should be reported. The patient and family members are encouraged to verbalize the feelings that may occur.

Additionally, the patient is prepared for adrenalectomy if indicated, and postoperative care (see below). Peptic ulcer and diabetes mellitus are common in the patient with Cushing's syndrome; therefore, management includes assessment of stools for blood and urine for glucosuria, and appropriate intervention if indicated.

▶ Evaluation

Expected Outcomes

1. Performs self-care activities
   a. Plans activities and exercises to allow alternating periods of rest and activity
   b. Participates in hygienic care
   c. Reports improved well-being
   d. Sleeps soundly at night and during planned rest periods
   e. Is free of complications of immobility
2. Attains/maintains skin integrity
   a. Has intact skin, without evidence of breakdown or infection
   b. Shows evidence of decreased edema in extremities and trunk
   c. Avoids trauma to skin
   d. Changes position frequently
   e. Inspects bony prominences daily
3. Shows evidence of decreased risk of injury and infection
   a. Is free of fractures or soft tissue injuries
   b. Is free of ecchymotic areas
   c. Utilizes measures to prevent trauma (*e.g.,* seeks assistance when necessary, arranges rugs and furniture to prevent falls and bumps)
   d. Avoids persons with cold or flu symptoms
   e. Experiences no temperature elevation, redness, pain, and other signs of infection and inflammation
4. Achieves an improved body image
   a. Utilizes makeup appropriately and selects clothes that enhance appearance
   b. Socializes with others
   c. Utilizes good grooming (*e.g.,* skin care, hair care)
   d. Is not gaining weight
   e. Adheres to diet (*e.g.,* consumes high-protein, low-carbohydrate, low-sodium diet)
   f. Verbalizes feelings about changes in appearance, sexual function, and activity level
   g. States that physical changes are a result of excessive corticosteroids
5. Exhibits improved mental functioning
   a. Identifies reason for mood changes as excessive corticosteroid level
   b. Verbalizes feelings to nurse and to family
   c. Participates in family activities
   d. Notifies nurse, physician, and family if feelings become overwhelming

Primary Aldosteronism

The principal action of aldosterone is to conserve body sodium. Under the influence of this hormone, the kidneys excrete less sodium and more potassium and hydrogen.

Excessive production of aldosterone, which occurs in some patients with functioning tumors of the adrenal gland, causes a distinctive pattern of biochemical changes and a corresponding set of clinical manifestations that are diagnostic of this condition. Such patients exhibit a profound decline in the blood levels of potassium (hypokalemia) and hydrogen ions (alkalosis), as demonstrated by an increase in its pH and carbon-dioxide combining power. The serum sodium level is normal or elevated depending on the amount of water reabsorbed with the sodium. Hypertension is usually present, although aldosteronism is the primary cause of only 3% of cases of hypertension.

Hypokalemia is responsible for the variable muscle weakness in patients with aldosteronism, as well as an inability on the part of the kidneys to acidify or concentrate the urine. Accordingly, the urine volume is excessive, leading to complaints of polyuria. Serum, by contrast, becomes abnormally concentrated, contributing to excessive thirst (polydipsia) and arterial hypertension. A secondary increase in blood volume and possible direct effects of aldosterone on nerve receptors such as the carotid sinus are other factors producing the hypertension. Hypokalemic alkalosis may decrease the plasma-ionized calcium level and predispose the patient to tetany and paresthesias. Trousseau's and Chvostek's signs can be used to assess neuromuscular irritability before overt paresthesia and tetany occur (see p. 933).

Diagnostic studies reveal, in addition to a high or normal serum sodium level and low serum potassium level, high serum aldosterone levels and low serum renin levels.

Treatment of primary aldosteronism usually involves surgical removal of the adrenal tumor through adrenalectomy.

Adrenalectomy

Adrenalectomy is the treatment of choice in primary Cushing's syndrome and aldosteronism. In addition, it is also used in the treatment of adrenal tumors and for malignancy of the breast and prostate gland.

For Adrenal Tumors. All of the endocrine disturbances associated with a functioning tumor of the adrenal cortex or medulla can be relieved completely, and the patient improved dramatically, by surgical removal of the involved gland. Adrenalectomy is performed through an incision in the loin or the abdomen. In general, the postoperative care resembles that given for any abdominal operation. Following surgery for adrenal cortical tumors, the patient is susceptible to fluctuations in adrenocortical hormones and may require administration of corticosteroids, fluids, and other agents to maintain blood pressure and prevent acute complications. Attention is also directed toward maintenance of a normal serum glucose level with insulin and appropriate intravenous fluids and dietary modifications.

Nursing management in the postoperative period includes frequent assessment of vital signs so that early indications of hemorrhage and possible adrenal crisis may be detected and treated. Stressful situations can be avoided by explaining the treatment, promoting comfort measures, establishing priorities of care, and providing rest periods.

For Malignancy of Breasts or Prostate. (See also pp. 1069 and 1098.)

Certain malignancies, notably those of the breast and the prostate, are affected by the hormones produced by endocrine glands. Thus, ovarian hormones are known to have an effect on carcinoma of the breast, and hormones of the testes on carcinoma of the prostate. In some patients, even after suppression of endocrine stimulation, the hormones are still present, and they have been found to arise from adrenal glands. For this reason, bilateral adrenalectomy may be performed in an effort to control recurrent carcinoma of the breast or the prostate. The adrenals are approached either transabdominally or through the posterior bed of the 12th rib.

Postoperatively, adrenal cortical hormone must be administered in appropriate dosage to overcome the sudden deprivation of those hormones by the operation. The dosage of adrenal cortical hormone may be reduced gradually as the body adjusts itself to its new level of hormone production.

Corticosteroid Therapy

While corticosteroids are used extensively for adrenal insufficiency, they are also widely used in suppressing inflammation, controlling allergic reactions, and reducing the rejection process in transplantation. Such *anti-inflammatory* and *antiallergy* actions make corticosteroids effective in treating rheumatic or connective tissue diseases such as rheumatoid arthritis, and systemic lupus erythematosus. High doses seem to permit individuals to tolerate higher degrees of stress. Such *anti-stress* action may be due to the ability of corticosteroids to aid circulating vasopressor substances in keeping the blood pressure elevated, or it may be due to other effects, such as the maintenance of plasma glucose.

Although the synthetic steroids are safer for some patients because of relative freedom from mineralocorticoid activity, most natural and synthetic corticosteroids produce similar kinds of chronic toxicity (Table 41-3). The size of the dose required to bring about desired anti-inflammatory and antiallergy effects also causes metabolic effects, pituitary gland suppression, and changes in the function of the central nervous system. Such changes may be disabling and even dangerous.

In view of the above, it is obvious that while adrenocorticosteroids are highly effective therapeutically, they may also be very dangerous. Dosages of these medications are frequently altered to allow high concentrations when absolutely necessary and then tapered in an attempt to avoid undesirable effects. This requires that patients be closely observed for side-effects and the dose reduced when high doses are no longer required.

Table 41-3
Commonly Used Steroid Preparations

Commonly Used Name	Other Names
Hydrocortisone	Cortisol, Hydrocortone, Compound F
Cortisone	Cortone, Compound E, Cortogen
DOC	Percorten
Aldosterone	Electrocortin, Aldocorten
Prednisolone	Meticortelone, 1-2 Dehydrocortisol
Prednisone	Meticorten, 1-2 Dehydrocortisone
Methylprednisolone	Medrol
Triamcinolone	Aristocort, Kenacort
Dexamethasone	Decadron, Hexadrol, 9a-Fluoro-16a-methyl-prednisolone
Fludrocortisone	Florinef, F-Cortef, 9a-Fluoro-hydrocortisone

Problems Encountered in Clinical Use

Dosage of corticosteroids is determined by the nature and chronicity of the illness as well as by any other medical problem the patient has. Rheumatoid arthritis and bronchial asthma are chronic disorders that corticosteroids do not cure; however, these drugs may be useful when other measures no longer provide adequate control of symptoms. In such a situation, the adverse effects of steroids are weighed against the current problems of the patient. These drugs may be used for a period of time but then should be gradually reduced as the patient's symptoms subside. The nurse plays an important role in providing encouragement and understanding during the times the patient may feel less comfortable while taking smaller doses.

Acute flare-ups and crises are treated with massive doses of corticosteroids, as in emergency treatment for bronchial obstruction in status asthmaticus, systemic toxicity of an acute rheumatic fever attack, and shock from septicemia caused by gram-negative bacteria. Of course other measures are utilized as required, such as anti-infective agents or drugs, and measures to treat shock.

At times corticosteroids are continued past the acute flare-up stage for the purpose of combating possible complications that are deemed worse than the side-effects of steroids. Systemic lupus erythematosus is an example of such a condition.

A different problem exists when glucocorticosteroids are used in treating eye infections. Outer eye infection can be treated by topical application of eye drops, since these do not cause systemic toxicity. However, long-term application may cause an increase in intraocular pressure, which may lead to glaucoma in some patients. In other individuals, prolonged use of steroids may lead to cataract formation.

Topical administration of steroids in the form of creams, ointments, lotions, and aerosols are especially effective in many dermatologic disorders. It may be more effective in some conditions to use occlusive dressings around the affected part so that maximum absorption of the drug is achieved. Occasionally, intralesional injections are required; however, the adverse effect of the underlying tissues becoming atrophied may occur. Fortunately, such dimpling or atrophy is only temporary.

Undesirable Effects of Corticosteroid Therapy

The likelihood of adverse effects is more likely when steroid therapy is used for long periods of time. In general, such effects are classified as follows (also see Chart 41-1):

1. Metabolic Effects. Changes in the metabolism may occur following large doses of glucocosteroids or mineralocorticoids. Excessive glucocorticoid activity (hypercorticism) causes clinical manifestations of Cushing's syndrome (see p. 936), including the characteristic rounding of the face and an abnormal distribution of body fat.

Because of changes that the steroids make in the metabolism of carbohydrate, protein, and fat, certain other complications may occur. For example, some patients may develop peptic ulcer, diabetes mellitus, or osteoporosis. This does not mean that steroid therapy is to be avoided. It does mean that supportive therapy is required to minimize the threat of these other conditions. For example, it is necessary for the patient with a history of peptic ulcer to continue with antacids and perhaps antispasmodic medications, at the same time recognizing that peptic ulcer pain may not be present as a warning sign during the administration of corticosteroids. For the patient with diabetes, oral hypoglycemia agents should be continued or insulin dosages adjusted as needed. For the patient with osteoporosis, it is helpful to adhere to a high-protein diet and to take calcium salt (a vitamin D supplement), looking out for a possible hypercalciuria. Special efforts are made to prevent an injury that may result in a fracture.

Infection may spread with minimal symptoms, because the patient's defense against invading organisms is lowered by the metabolic effects of the steroid. Viral and fungal infections create further problems because of the difficulty in treating these conditions.

2. Central Nervous System. Euphoria results from the action of corticosteroids on the central nervous system. Since such reaction often creates psychological dependency upon steroids, the patient may resist being removed from these drugs. With prolonged use of corticosteroids, the patient may experience mood swings that include excitement, restlessness, depression, and sleeplessness. Nursing support and understanding are required as the patient moves through these experiences. Any tendency to emotional, psychological, or psychotic difficulties needs to be brought to the attention of the physician before steroids are prescribed.

3. Endocrine Effects. Prolonged steroid therapy has a tendency to suppress certain functions of the anterior portion of the pituitary gland. Hence, growth in children may be halted following long-term treatment with steroids due to adrenal atrophy and suppression of the pituitary's capacity to release ACTH. Although this effect may not be apparent under ordinary circumstances, it is obvious during times of unusual stress. During these periods of acute adrenal insufficiency, massive doses of corticosteroids are required to prevent adrenal collapse.

Dosage Schedule

Attempts have been made to determine the best time to administer pharmacologic doses of steroids. Once the pa-

tient's symptoms have been controlled on a 6-hour or 8-hour program, a switch is made to a once-daily or every-other-day schedule. In keeping with the natural secretion of cortisol, the best time of the day for the total steroid dose is in the early morning from 7 to 8 AM. Large-dose therapy at 8 AM, when the gland is most active, produces maximal suppression of the gland. A large 8 AM dosage is more physiologic, as it allows the body to escape effects of the steroids from 4 PM to 6 AM, when serum levels are normally low—hence minimizing Cushingoid effects. If symptoms of the disease being treated are successfully suppressed, alternative-day therapy is helpful in preventing pituitary–adrenal suppression in patients requiring chronic therapy. Taking the total steroid dose every other day presents some problems in that patients complain of discomfort on the second day. It may be necessary for the nurse to explain to the patient that this regimen may be necessary to prevent toxic reactions.

Withdrawal of Steroids. Corticosteroid dosages are reduced gradually to allow normal adrenal function to return and to prevent steroid-induced adrenal insufficiency. Authorities differ as to the benefits of administering injections of adrenal-stimulating pituitary hormone corticotropin to assist in increasing the rates at which the adrenal glands recover their function.

▷ The Pancreas

Acute Pancreatitis

Several classification systems have been used to categorize the various stages and forms of pancreatitis. One system describes acute pancreatitis as a disease in which structure and function of the pancreas are restored after the acute episode has resolved. In chronic pancreatitis, there are persistent abnormalities in the pancreas even if the initiating cause has been removed.

Another classification system describes forms of acute pancreatitis on the basis of laparotomy or autopsy findings; these are interstitial, hemorrhagic, and necrotic or gangrenous pancreatitis.

Regardless of the classification system used, the patient admitted to the hospital with a diagnosis of pancreatitis is acutely ill and requires skilled nursing and medical care.

Pathophysiology and Etiology

Acute pancreatitis or inflammation of the pancreas is brought about by the digestion of this organ by the very enzymes it produces, principally trypsin. Exactly how this autodigestion gets started is not known with certainty. However, 75% to 85% of patients with acute pancreatitis are found to have either gallstones or a long history of alcohol abuse. Chronic alcohol ingestion produces secretory and eventually structural changes in the pancreas. Gallstones, on the other hand, enter the common bile duct and lodge at the ampulla of Vater, obstructing the flow of pancreatic juice or causing a reflux of bile from the common bile duct into the pancreatic duct, thus activating the powerful pancreatic enzymes within the gland. Normally, these remain in an inactive form until the pancreatic juice reaches the lumen of the duodenum. Spasm and edema of the ampulla of Vater, resulting from duodenitis, can probably produce pancreatitis. Other less common common causes of pancreatitis include bacterial or viral infection, with pancreatitis being a complication of mumps virus. Blunt abdominal trauma, ischemic vascular disease, hyperlipidemia, hyperparathyroidism, and the use of corticosteroids, thiazide diuretics, and oral contraceptives have been associated with an increased incidence of pancreatitis. In addition, there is a small incidence of hereditary pancreatitis.

Chart 41-1
The Patient on Steroid Therapy

Acceptable and Expected Side-effects*

Nature of Effect	Action
Facial mooning (Cushing's syndrome)	May be minimized by restricted caloric intake.
Weight gain	Restrict caloric intake; may require a switch in steroid medication.
	May require diuretics and potassium.
Edema	Prescribe diuretics and potassium.
Potassium loss	May require switch to a fluorinated synthetic.
	Administer potassium supplement.
Acne	Treat with topical medications.
Increased urinary frequency and nocturia	Check for evidence of genitourinary infection or diabetes mellitus; urinalysis.
Insomnia, headache, fatigue	Treat symptomatically.

Undesirable and Unacceptable Side-effects

Nature of Effect	Action (Report to Physician)
Allergic reaction to bovine ACTH or steroid	Withdraw drug promptly.
	Substitute synthetic ACTH or steroid.
Cardiovascular system effect:	
Hypertension	Suggest reduction in dosage of steroids.
Thromboembolic complications	
Arteritis	
Infection	Suggest antimicrobial medications as indicated.
	Suggest local treatment and cleanliness.
Eye complications:	
Glaucoma	Refer to ophthalmologist.
Corneal lesions	
Musculoskeletal effects	Suggest sex hormones—synthetic estrogens or androgens.
	Suggest calcium supplement and vitamin D.
Adrenal insufficiency (after prolonged use) as manifested by peripheral circulatory collapse—in upright position.	Administer hydrocortisone promptly (intravenously) and saline intravenously. The following day, give steroid replacement.

Counseling of Patients on Long-term Steroids

1. Recognize that steroids are valuable and useful medications but if taken longer than 2 weeks, certain side-effects may be noticed.
2. "Acceptable" side-effects may include weight gain (perhaps due to water retention), acne, headaches, fatigue, and increased urinary frequency.
3. "Unacceptable" side-effects that are to be reported to the physician include dizziness when rising from chair or bed (postural hypotension indicative of adrenal insufficiency), nausea, vomiting, thirst, abdominal pain, or pain of any type.
4. Additional side-effects that are reportable are feelings of depression or nervousness, or development of an infection.
5. If the patient has a fall or is in an auto accident, his condition may precipitate adrenal failure. He requires an immediate injection of hydrocortisone phosphate. (Long-term patients should wear a Medic Alert tag and have a kit with hydrocortisone.)

* Although these side-effects may be acceptable in terms of the therapeutic goal and overall consequences, they may be unacceptable to the patient.

Classification of Acute Pancreatitis.

Pancreatitis ranges in severity from a relatively mild, self-limiting disorder to a rapidly fatal disease that does not respond to any treatment. Edema and inflammation usually confined to the pancreas itself are the major events in the more mild form of pancreatitis, which is termed interstitial or edematous pancreatitis. Although this is considered the more mild form of pancreatitis, the patient is acutely ill and at risk of developing shock, fluid and electrolyte disturbances, and sepsis.

Acute hemorrhagic pancreatitis represents a more advanced form of acute interstitial pancreatitis. Enzymatic digestion of the gland is more widespread and complete. The tissue becomes necrotic, and the damage extends to its vascular radicles, so that blood escapes into the substance of the pancreas and beyond into the retroperitoneal tissues. Late complications consist of pancreatic cysts or abscesses. The mortality rate of acute hemorrhagic pancreatitis is 30%.

▶ Assessment

Clinical Manifestations. Severe abdominal pain is the major symptom of pancreatitis that brings the patient to medical attention. Abdominal pain and tenderness, along with back pain, result from irritation and edema of the inflamed pancreas that stimulate the nerve endings. An increase in tension on the pancreatic capsule and obstruction of the pancreatic ducts also contribute to the pain. The abdominal pain may be localized to the epigastrium or may be diffuse and difficult to locate. It is generally more severe after meals and is unrelieved by antacids. Pain may be accompanied by abdominal distention and a poorly defined palpable abdominal mass.

Nausea and vomiting are common in acute pancreatitis. The vomitus is usually gastric in origin but may also be bile stained. Fever, jaundice, mental confusion, and agitation may also occur.

Although hypertension is not rare in acute pancreatitis, hypotension is more ominous and may reflect hypovolemia and shock in acute hemorrhagic pancreatitis. Hypovolemia is due to loss of large amounts of protein-rich fluid into the tissues and peritoneal cavity. The patient may develop tachycardia; cold, clammy skin; and cyanosis in addition to hypotension.

Respiratory distress is a common occurrence, and the patient may develop diffuse pulmonary infiltrates, dyspnea, tachypnea, and arterial hypoxemia.

The diagnosis of acute pancreatitis is based on a history of abdominal pain, the presence of known risk factors, physical examination findings, and selected diagnostic findings.

Diagnostic Assessment

Blood Studies. Serum amylase is the most important aid in diagnosing acute pancreatitis. Peak levels are reached in 24 hours, with a rapid fall to normal levels within 48 to 72 hours. Serum lipase and amylase levels in the urine also become elevated and remain elevated longer than serum amylase. The white blood cell count is usually elevated; hypocalcemia is present in many patients and appears to be correlated with the severity of pancreatitis.

Transient hyperglycemia and glucosuria, and elevated serum bilirubin levels, occur in some patients with acute pancreatitis.

X-Ray Studies. An x-ray of the abdomen and chest is indicated, although its greatest benefit is in differentiating pancreatitis from other disorders causing similar symptoms.

Ultrasonography and Computed Tomography (CT Scan). Although not widely used for diagnostic studies of pancreatitis, these tests are helpful in identifying pancreatic cysts or pseudocysts in acute pancreatitis.

Stools. Usually, the stools of patients suffering with pancreatic disease are bulky, pale, and foul-smelling. Fat content varies between 50% and 90% in pancreatic disease; normally, the content is 20%.

Patient Problems/Nursing Diagnoses

Based on the clinical manifestations and diagnostic assessment data, the major nursing problems of the patient with acute pancreatitis include severe pain and discomfort related to edema and distention of the pancreas and peritoneal irritation; altered fluid and nutritional status due to vomiting, inadequate fluid intake, fever and diaphoresis, and fluid shifts; and respiratory impairment related to severe pain, dyspnea, and pulmonary infiltrates.

▶ Planning and Nursing Intervention

Goals

The major goals for the patient include:

1. Relief of pain and discomfort
2. Improved fluid and nutritional status
3. Improved respiratory function

To assist in accomplishing these goals, the major objectives of therapy are (1) to relieve pain and eliminate causative factors, (2) to provide appropriate fluid and nutrition to meet the patient's requirements, and (3) to improve respiratory function and prevent respiratory complications.

Relief of Pain. Since the pathologic process responsible for pain is autodigestion of the pancreas, the objective of therapy is *to decrease the production of these enzymes.* Oral feedings are interrupted to control the formation and secretion of secretin; the patient is maintained on parenteral fluids and electrolytes. Anticholinergic drugs are administered to block the nerve impulses that stimulate pancreatic secretion, and nasogastric suction is employed. Demerol is given to relieve pain. The acutely ill patient will be maintained on bed rest to decrease the metabolic rate and reduce the secretion of pancreatic and gastric enzymes. The patient and family members are instructed about the relationship of alcohol to the onset of pain and attacks of pancreatitis. Most attacks of acute interstitial pancreatitis are self-limited and may be expected to subside in 3 or 4 days.

Maintenance of Fluid Balance and Nutrition. Nausea, vomiting, gastric suction, movement of fluid from the vascular compartment to the peritoneal cavity, and diaphoresis and fever increase the patient's need for fluid and electrolyte replacement. Intravenous fluids will be administered and may be accompanied by transfusion of blood and albumin to maintain the patient's blood volume. Careful measurement of intake and output is essential to determine changes in the patient's fluid requirements. Changes in vital signs and the appearance of ascites reflect changes in the patient's status and indicate the need for careful evaluation of the patient's fluid requirements. Circulatory collapse and shock are possible complications; therefore, frequent assessment of the patient is indicated, and emergency medications are kept readily available.

If the patient's acute symptoms subside, oral feedings are reintroduced gradually. Between acute attacks, the patient receives a diet high in carbohydrates and low in fat and proteins. Heavy meals are to be avoided, as are alcoholic beverages.

Respiratory Care. The patient is maintained in a semi-Fowler's position to decrease pressure on the diaphragm by a distended abdomen and to increase respiratory expansion. Frequent changes of position are necessary to prevent atelectasis and pooling of respiratory secretions. Anticholinergic medications given, to decrease gastric and pancreatic secretions, also dry the secretions of the respiratory tract, predisposing the patient to obstruction and infection. Pulmonary assessment is essential to observe for any changes in respiratory status. The patient is instructed in techniques of coughing and deep breathing to improve respiratory function.

▶ **Evaluation**

Expected Outcomes

1. Experiences relief of pain and discomfort
   a. Is free of pain and discomfort
   b. Uses anticholinergics as prescribed and appropriately
   c. Avoids alcohol
   d. Utilizes pain medication appropriately without overuse
   e. Reports pain, nausea, and vomiting
2. Attains/maintains adequate fluid and nutritional intake
   a. Has normal skin turgor
   b. Eats foods high in carbohydrates and low in fat and protein
   c. Avoids alcohol
   d. Maintains adequate fluid intake
   e. Has no increase in abdominal girth
   f. Avoids food that causes pain or discomfort
   g. Reports feelings of lightheadedness; diaphoresis; and cold, clammy skin
3. Experiences improved respiratory function
   a. Maintains semi-Fowler's position when in bed
   b. Changes position in bed frequently
   c. Coughs and takes deep breaths at least every hour
   d. Drinks at least 8 glasses of fluids per day to liquify secretions

A summary of nursing management of the patient with acute pancreatitis is provided in Chart 41-2.

Chronic Pancreatitis

After repeated attacks of acute interstitial pancreatitis, or, in some instances, after the prolonged use of alcohol in large amounts, patients may develop progressive chronic fibrosis and inflammation of the pancreatic gland itself, with obstruction of its ducts and destruction of its secreting cells. The incidence of chronic pancreatitis is increased in adult men and is characterized by recurring attacks of severe upper abdominal and back pain, accompanied by vomiting. Attacks often are so painful that narcotics, even in large doses, do not provide relief. As the disease progresses, these patients may become addicted to opiates. Because of the destruction of the gland by fibrosis, the pancreatic secretions may be deficient in amount, or obstruction of the ducts by fibrosis may prevent the pancreatic juice from entering the duodenum and playing its role in digestion. As a result, the digestion of foodstuffs, especially proteins and fats, is disrupted. The stools become frequent, frothy, and foul-smelling, due to the impairment of fat digestion, which results in a stool with a high fat content. This condition is referred to as *steatorrhea*. As the disease progresses, calcification of the gland may occur, and calcium stones may form within the ducts.

Diagnostic Tests. In contrast to the patient with acute pancreatitis, serum amylase levels and white blood count are unremarkable. However, in the late stages of chronic pancreatitis, x-ray of the abdomen may reveal calcification of the pancreas. Ultrasonography or CT scan may be helpful in the presence of pancreatic cyst formation. An abnormal glucose tolerance test, indicative of diabetes, may be present. Endoscopic retrograde cholangiopancreatography (ERCP), described on page 879, may permit evaluation of the pancreas in chronic pancreatitis, although the procedure is contraindicated in acute pancreatitis.

Management. The management of chronic pancreatitis depends on its probable cause in each particular patient. When it develops in association with gallbladder disease, efforts are made to relieve the difficulty by operating on the biliary tract, exploring the common duct, and removing the stones; usually, the gallbladder is removed at the same time. In addition, an attempt is made to improve the drainage of the common bile duct and the pancreatic duct by dividing the sphincter of Oddi, a muscle that is located at the ampulla of Vater (this operation is known as a *sphincterotomy*). Nursing management after such an operation is the same as that indicated for all patients undergoing biliary tract surgery. A T tube usually is placed in the common bile duct, requiring a drainage bottle to collect the bile after the operation.

In the absence of evidence indicating biliary tract disease, the most common cause of chronic pancreatitis is chronic alcoholism. In such patients, the pancreas becomes markedly fibrotic, to the extent that the pancreatic ducts may be obstructed. In some patients the obstruction may be relieved by sphincterotomy, but in others, the obstruction is located in the gland itself and is therefore not amenable to this procedure. Other possible approaches include opening the pancreatic duct and placing the entire gland inside a loop of jejunum; or the tail of the pancreas may be removed and the remaining stump sutured into the end of a loop of jejunum. These somewhat complicated operations are performed with the object of draining the pancreatic juice by way of a route that bypasses the obstruction in the ductal system. Morbidity and mortality following these surgical procedures are high because of the poor physical condition of the patient prior to surgery and the concomitant occurrence of cirrhosis.

(Text continues on page 946)

Chart 41-2
Guidelines for Nursing Goals and Nursing Interventions Management of the Patient With Acute Pancreatitis

Nursing Actions	*Rationale*
A. Relieve pain and discomfort.	A. The agonizing pain is probably due to edema and distention of the capsule, and peritoneal irritation.
1. Give meperidine (Demerol) in fairly high dosages, as indicated by the amount of pain present (unless patient is hypotensive).	1. Meperidine acts by depressing the CNS and thereby increasing the patient's pain threshold. Morphine is not usually given because it has a tendency to produce spasm of the sphincter of Oddi. Control of pain is important because restlessness increases body metabolism, which stimulates the secretion of pancreatic and gastric enzymes. The vagal stimulation to pancreatic secretion is stimulated by pain and anxiety.
2. Assist the patient to assume positions of comfort. Encourage the patient to turn at regularly scheduled intervals. Use pillow supports and foam-rubber pads, as necessary.	2. Frequent turning relieves pressure and aids in preventing pulmonary and vascular complications.
B. Minimize pancreatic secretion.	
1. Give anticholinergic drugs as prescribed.	1. Anticholinergic drugs reduce gastric and pancreatic secretion.
2. Withhold oral intake.	2. The intestinal stimulus to pancreatic secretion is influenced by food and fluid intake.
3. Keep the patient on bed rest.	3. Bed rest decreases body metabolism and thus reduces pancreatic and gastric secretions.
4. Employ continuous nasogastric suction.	4. Nasogastric suction removes gastric contents and prevents gastric secretions from entering the duodenum and stimulating the secretin mechanism. Decompression of the intestines (if intestinal intubation is used) also assists in relieving respiratory distress.
a. Measure gastric secretions at specified intervals.	
b. Observe and chart color and viscosity of gastric secretions.	
c. Ensure that the nasogastric tube is patent, to permit free drainage.	
C. Promote the comfort of the intubated patient.	
1. Use water-soluble lubricant around external nares.	1. To prevent irritation
2. Turn patient at intervals.	2. To relieve pressure of tube on esophageal and gastric mucosa
3. Give oral hygiene and gargling solutions.	3. To relieve dryness and irritation of oropharynx
4. Utilize semi-Fowler's position frequently.	4. To decrease pressure on diaphragm and allow greater lung expansion
D. Give medications as directed.	
1. Give antibiotic drugs only for coexisting infections.	1. Edema, necrosis, hemorrhage, and suppuration are present in varying degrees in acute pancreatitis. These conditions are the results of secondary infection. Pancreatic abscess and bacteremia may also be present.
2. Give insulin as prescribed.	2. To combat hyperglycemia, if present.
E. Prevent serum calcium deficiency.	E. Keep a supply of intravenous calcium gluconate readily available to prevent tetany.

(continued)

Chart 41-2
*Guidelines for Nursing Goals and Nursing Interventions Management of the Patient
With Acute Pancreatitis (continued)*

Nursing Actions *(continued)*	**Rationale** *(continued)*
F. Replace blood and fluid and electrolyte loss.	F. Electrolyte losses occur from nasogastric suctioning, severe diaphoresis, emesis, and as a result of the patient's being in a fasting state.
1. Give plasma, albumin, and blood as prescribed.	1. During acute pancreatitis, plasma may be lost into the abdominal cavity, which diminishes the blood volume.
2. Give intravenous electrolytes (sodium, potassium, chlorides) as prescribed.	2. The amount and type of fluid and electrolyte replacement is determined by the status of the blood pressure, the laboratory evaluations of serum electrolyte and blood urea nitrogen levels, the urinary volume, and the assessment of the patient's condition.
G. Combat shock if present.	G. Extensive acute pancreatitis may cause peripheral vascular collapse and shock. Blood and plasma may be lost into the abdominal cavity, and therefore there is a decreased blood and plasma volume. The toxins from the bacteria of a necrotic pancreas may cause shock.
1. Administer adrenocorticol steroids to those who do not respond to conventional treatment. 2. Evaluate the amount of urinary output. Attempt to maintain this at 50 ml/hour.	
H. Support patient's heart and lungs, to prevent complications. 1. Maintain blood volume with blood transfusions, plasma, albumin, dextran.	1. Patients with hemorrhagic pancreatitis lose large amounts of blood and plasma, which decreases effective circulation and blood volume. Replacement with blood, plasma, albumin, or dextran assists in ensuring effective circulating blood volume. Acute pancreatitis produces retroperitoneal edema, elevation of the diaphragm, pleural effusion, and inadequate lung ventilation. Intra-abdominal infection and labored breathing increase the body's metabolic demand, which further decreases pulmonary reserve and leads to respiratory failure.
2. Guard the patient's cardiopulmonary reserve. a. Evaluate the pulse, respiratory rate, and blood pressure at indicated intervals. b. Give digitalis as prescribed.	
I. Reduce the excessive metabolism of the body. 1. Give antibiotics as prescribed. 2. Place patient in an air-conditioned room. 3. Administer nasal oxygen as required for hypoxia. 4. Utilize a hypothermia blanket if necessary.	I. Pancreatitis produces a severe peritoneal and retroperitoneal reaction that causes fever, tachycardia, and accelerated respirations. Placing the patient in an air-conditioned room and supporting him with oxygen therapy decreases the work load of the respiratory system and the tissue utilization of oxygen. Reduction of fever and pulse rate decrease the metabolic demands of the body.
J. Educate the patient to try to prevent further attacks of pancreatitis. 1. Keep appointments with physician (or clinic) at specified times.	1. Known causes of pancreatitis (gallbladder disease, gastric or duodenal ulcer, etc.) should be searched for and treated.
2. Refrain from alcoholic beverages and avoid excessive use of coffee. 3. Avoid heavy meals. Abstain from eating when nervous or tense.	2. Alcohol and coffee increase pancreatic secretion. 3. Spicy foods and heavy meals are strong gastric stimulants.

Despite these operative procedures the patient is likely to continue having pain and digestive difficulties from the pancreatitis unless he abstains completely from the use of alcohol. This point should be emphasized by the nurse in the course of instructing the patient and the family.

Total pancreatectomy and islet cell autotransplantation have recently been carried out on patients with chronic pancreatitis and pain who did not respond to other treatment. The patient is at risk of hyperglycemia as well as other complications resulting from malnutrition and immobility. Initial success with these procedures has been reported in spite of the high risk of complications.

Pancreatic Cysts

As a result of the local necrosis that occurs at the time of acute pancreatitis, collections of fluid may form in the vicinity of the pancreas. These become walled off by fibrous tissue and are called *pancreatic cysts.* They are the most common type of pancreatic cyst, most other types developing as a result of congenital anomalies.

Pancreatic cysts may attain considerable size. Because of their location behind the posterior peritoneum, when they enlarge, they impinge on and displace the stomach or the colon, which are adjacent. Eventually, through pressure or secondary infection, they produce symptoms, requiring that they be drained.

Management. Drainage into the gastrointestinal tract or through the skin surface of the abdominal wall may be established. In the latter instance, the drainage is likely to be profuse and destructive to tissue because of the enzyme contents. Hence, steps must be taken to protect the skin in areas adjacent to the drainage site to prevent excoriation. Ointments protect the skin, provided that they are applied before excoriation takes place. Another method involves the constant aspiration of digestive juice from the drainage tract by means of a suction apparatus, so that contact with the digestive enzymes is avoided. This method demands a great deal of nursing attention to be sure that the suction tube does not become dislodged from the drainage tract and that the entire apparatus functions properly without interruption.

Pancreatic Tumors

Carcinoma of the Pancreas

Cancer may arise in any portion of the pancreas: in the head, the body, or the tail, producing clinical manifestations that vary, depending on the location of the lesion and whether or not functioning, insulin-secreting pancreatic islet cells are involved. Tumors that originate in the head of the pancreas, the most common location, give rise to a distinctive clinical picture and will be discussed separately. Functioning islet cell tumors, whether benign (adenoma) or malignant (carcinoma) are responsible for the syndrome of hyperinsulinism, and are described on page 947. With these exceptions, carcinoma of the pancreas is notoriously lacking in clear-cut, characteristic symptomatology, and because of its rather nondescript features, patients with this form of cancer usually do not seek medical attention until late in the course of their illness.

Assessment. Common to all types of pancreatic carcinoma are symptoms of rapid, profound, progressive, and inexplicable weight loss, as well as vague, upper or mid-abdominal discomfort that is unrelated to any gastrointestinal function and difficult to describe. Such discomfort radiates as a boring pain in the midback and is unrelated to posture or activity. People with pancreatic carcinoma often find that they get some relief from pain by sitting hunched forward. Since pain is often accentuated by lying supine, a full-length foam-rubber pad placed under the patient has proven beneficial and protects the bony prominences from pressure. A very important clue, when present, is the onset of symptoms of insulin deficiency; glucosuria, hyperglycemia, and abnormal glucose tolerance. Diabetes is sometimes an early sign of carcinoma of the pancreas. Meals often aggravate epigastric pain, which usually occurs weeks before the appearance of jaundice and pruritus. A helpful tool in diagnosis is a gastrointestinal roentgenography series, which may demonstrate deformities in adjacent viscera caused by the impinging pancreatic mass. Ultrasonography, CT scanning, and endoscopic retrograde cannulation of the pancreas (ERCP) are useful in establishing the diagnosis.

Management. Therapy usually is limited to palliative measures. Definitive surgical treatment (*i.e.,* total excision of the lesion) often is not feasible because of the extensive growth when the lesion is finally diagnosed and the probable widespread metastases—especially to the liver, lungs, and bones.

Tumors of the Head of the Pancreas

Assessment. Tumors in this region of the pancreas are detected by the fact that they obstruct the common bile duct where it passes through the head of the pancreas to join the pancreatic duct and empty at the ampulla of Vater into the duodenum. Obstruction to the flow of bile produces jaundice, clay-colored stools, and dark urine. There may be some degree of abdominal discomfort or pain, and pruritus may be noted. Nonspecific symptoms such as anorexia, weight loss, and malaise may or may not be present. If present, suspicion of visceral cancer is heightened.

This disease must be differentiated from the jaundice due to a biliary obstruction caused by a gallstone in the common duct, which usually is intermittent and appears typically in obese individuals, most often women, who have had previous symptoms of gallbladder disease. The tumors producing the obstruction may arise from the pancreas, from the common bile duct, or from the ampulla of Vater.

Management. When these patients come to the hospital, they are in such a poor nutritional and physical state that a fairly long period of preparation is necessary before operation can be attempted. Various liver and pancreatic function studies are carried out, vitamin K is given to restore the blood prothrombin activity, and diets high in protein often are given, with pancreatic enzymes. Blood transfusions frequently are used as well.

Following conventional blood and roentgen studies, more sophisticated diagnostic aids may be used, including duodenography, angiography by the hepatic or celiac artery catheterization, pancreatic scanning, and percutaneous transhepatic cholangiography. However, undoubtedly the most valuable aid is laparotomy with biopsy of the pancreas.

Surgical Management. Many surgeons perform only a biliary-enteric shunt, to relieve the jaundice. This will give some relief and, perhaps, time for a suspicious lesion to eventually prove nonmalignant. Other surgeons perform pancreatoduodenectomy.

Preoperative preparation includes adequate hydration and nutrition, correction of prothrombin deficiency with vitamin K, and treatment of anemia to minimize postoperative complications.

In the operating room, if a tumor is found, it may be removed if it has not invaded many of the important structures adjacent to it (portal vein, superior mesenteric artery). The operation entails removal of the head of the pancreas, the duodenum, and adjacent stomach, and the distal part of the common bile duct (Fig. 41-4). The stomach, the cut end of the pancreas, and the common bile duct then are anastomosed to the jejunum (Fig. 41-4A). This operation, first suggested by Whipple, may be done in either one or two stages. It has resulted in the cure of many patients with cancer of the ampulla and the bile ducts, but unfortunately is only palliative in most cases of carcinoma of the head of the pancreas. When excision of the tumor cannot be performed, the jaundice may be relieved by diverting the bile flow into the jejunum. This is done by anastomosing the jejunum to the gallbladder, a procedure known as cholecystojejunostomy.

Management for Whipple Procedure. The postoperative management of patients who have undergone a Whipple procedure is similar to the management of patients following gastrointestinal and biliary surgery. The psychosocial considerations, however, are more specific and must be properly approached by the nurse. In view of the fact that the patient has undergone major and risky surgery and is severely ill, he most likely will experience bouts of anxiety and depression that will undoubtedly affect his response to therapy.

While many professionals question the justification of the Whipple procedure because of the high mortality rate, this negative thinking must not affect the attitudes of those who are caring for the patient. As in all nursing, the challenge is to promote patient comfort, prevent complications, and assist the patient in returning to and maintaining as normal and comfortable a life as possible (Chart 41-3).

Hyperinsulinism

This disorder results from the overproduction of insulin by the pancreatic islets. Symptoms resemble those of excessive doses of insulin and are attributable to the same mechanism—an abnormal reduction in the concentration of blood sugar. Clinically, it is characterized by episodes during which the patient experiences unusual hunger, nervousness, sweating, headache, and faintness; in severe cases, convulsive seizures and episodes of unconsciousness may occur. The findings at operation or postmortem examination may indicate hyperplasia (overgrowth) of the islets of Langerhans, or a benign or malignant tumor involving the islets and capable of producing large amounts of insulin. Occa-

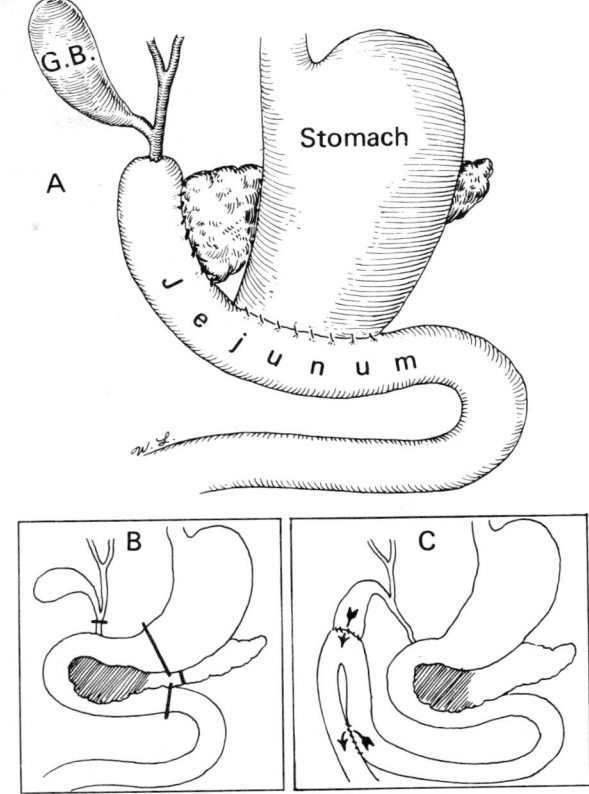

Figure 41-4. Pancreatoduodenectomy (after Whipple). (*B*) Shows lines that indicate removal of head of pancreas, duodenum, and adjacent stomach, and distal segment of common bile duct. (*A*) Indicates the end result for resection of the carcinoma of the head of the pancreas or the ampulla of Vater. The common duct is sutured to the end of the jejunum, and the remaining portion of the pancreas and the end of the stomach are sutured to the side of the jejunum. (*C*) An alternate method of treatment when an inoperable tumor of the head of the pancreas has been found. In such cases the bile may be permitted to flow again into the intestine by anastomosing the jejunum to the gallbladder. In addition, an accessory operation between the loops of jejunum has been performed.

sionally, tumors of nonpancreatic origin produce an insulinlike material that can cause hypoglycemia. This condition occasionally is responsible for convulsions coinciding with decreases in the blood glucose to levels that are inadequate to sustain normal brain function (*i.e.,* below 30 mg/100 ml).

All of the symptoms that accompany spontaneous hypoglycemia are relieved by the oral or parenteral administration of glucose. Surgical removal of the hyperplastic or neoplastic tissue from the pancreas offers the only successful method of treatment. About 15% of people with spontaneous (functional) hypoglycemia eventually develop diabetes mellitus.

Pancreatic Islet Tumors

In the pancreas are located the islets (islands) of Langerhans—small nests of cells that secrete directly into the bloodstream and, therefore, are part of the endocrine system. The secretion, insulin, is involved in the metabolism

Chart 41-3
Nursing Management of the Patient Undergoing a Whipple Procedure

Nursing Goals	*Nursing Interventions*
To facilitate respiratory exchange following prolonged surgery	1. Maintain on ventilator until fully reacted. 2. Give oxygen and monitor arterial pO_2 and pH. 3. Administer IPPB as required. 4. Monitor the endotracheal tube or tracheostomy tube.
To detect adverse signs indicating peripheral vascular collapse, hemorrhage, or other complications	1. Monitor vital signs intensively for the first 48 to 72 hours: temperature, pulse, respiration, blood pressure, and CVP. 2. For hypotension, assist in administration of whole blood and albumin; recognize signs of incompatibility, such as sudden chilling, hives, headache, nausea, vomiting. If these occur, discontinue the transfusion and notify surgeon.
To assess kidney function; renal failure is a common postoperative complication	1. Maintain an hourly record of urinary output. 2. Keep a running account of input.
To relieve pain and discomfort of patient	1. Administer meperidine hydrochloride (Demerol) to increase patient's pain threshold. Morphine is used sparingly because it depresses respiration. 2. Assist the patient in assuming positions of comfort; frequent turning relieves pressure areas and aids in preventing pulmonary and vascular complications.
To overcome prothrombin deficiency and to assist in prevention of postoperative hemorrhage and renal failure	Continue administration of vitamin K as prescribed (begun preoperatively) until oral feedings are resumed.
To prevent chest complications and assist abdominal drainage	Offer incentive spirometry; encourage leg exercises; have patient sit on first day.
To detect untoward signs, as revealed in laboratory reports: 1. Hemoconcentration	1. Note increase in hematocrit, such as $45\% \rightarrow 50\% \rightarrow 55\% \rightarrow 60\%$ This would indicate a significant loss of plasma; be prepared to administer serum albumin.
2. Falling serum calcium level	2. Recognize variations in serum calcium levels; if they are falling, have calcium gluconate available for daily administration with IV therapy
To provide for adequate decompression of afferent jejunal segment	Check for adequate drainage from T tube; prevent kinking of tube.
To prevent dilatation of jejunum (which would exert pressure against anastomoses) and to prevent subdiaphragmatic pressure	Provide suction to the Levin tube; keep nasogastric tube in place until gastrointestinal function is resumed.

(continued)

of sugar. A deficient secretion of insulin produces diabetes mellitus. On the other hand, tumors of these cells produce hypersecretion of insulin and an excessive rate of metabolism of the body's glucose, or sugar. Hypoglycemia, the resulting fall in blood sugar level, produces symptoms of weakness, mental confusion, and even convulsions. These may be relieved almost immediately by taking sugar by mouth or by intravenous glucose. The 5-hour glucose tolerance test is helpful in diagnosing insulinoma, the tumor of the pancreatic islet cells, and in distinguishing it from the more common functional hypoglycemia.

Once the diagnosis of a tumor of the islet cells has been made, surgical treatment with removal of the tumor usually is recommended. The tumors may be benign adenomas or they may be malignant. Complete removal usually results in a most dramatic cure. In some patients, such

Chart 41-3
Nursing Management of the Patient Undergoing a Whipple Procedure (continued)

Nursing Goals (continued)	*Nursing Interventions* (continued)
To maintain comfort of intubated patient and prevent mucous membrane and skin irritation	1. Assist him in receiving cleansing and refreshing mouth care. 2. Apply lubricant to external nares. Provide vapor-mist therapy to increase humidity.
To minimize the possibility of infection or abscess formation	1. Administer antibiotics as prescribed. 2. Maintain aseptic technique in handling wound dressings and drainage, pulmonary secretion aspiration through endotracheal tube, or tracheostomy.
To sustain nutritional requirements of the body and to maintain homeostasis	Assist in replacing fluids and electrolytes when assessment indicates these are lost.
To prevent major gastrointestinal complications: 1. Partial intestinal obstruction; this may cause increased intraluminal pressure, which may disrupt a weak point in the pancreaticojejunal anastomosis. 2. Pancreatic leakage, which in turn may promote paralytic ileus and eventually produce a partial intestinal obstruction.	Withhold oral intake until gastrointestinal function is resumed. Assess bowel sounds and abdominal distention.
To assess the patient's need for insulin	Note any symptoms suggestive of diabetes mellitus (rare unless pancreas is removed): irritability, skin-itching, blurring of vision, hyperglycemia.
To detect early signs of other complications: 1. Infection: subdiaphragmatic abscess, wound abscess, peritonitis 2. Hemorrhage: due to leakage of activated pancreatic juice and digestion of neighboring arteries 3. Jaundice 4. Undigested fat	1. Continue monitoring vital signs until sufficient time for healing has elapsed and until it is determined that all anastomoses are secure and patent. 2. Check stools for blood. Recognize variations in vital signs indicative of hemorrhage. 3. Observe color of sclera; recognize that patient may scratch skin because of itchiness. 4. Observe stools; if frothy and light-colored, it may indicate undigested fat. This may require tablets of pancreatic enzyme to aid in fat digestion.
To prepare patient for convalescence and understanding of posthospital activities, including the importance of consistent follow-up visits	1. Discuss role of pancreas regarding insulin and intestinal digestion and the possible need for continued treatment. 2. If chemotherapy (cancer) is to be used after the operation, stress its need and effects. 3. Remind patient to eat small, frequent meals initially. 4. Encourage family support of the patient. 5. Instruct family in recognizing untoward signs that need to be reported should they occur.

symptoms may not be produced by an actual tumor of the islet cells, but by a simple hypertrophy of this tissue. In such cases a partial *pancreatectomy*—removal of the tail and part of the body of the pancreas—is performed.

Management. In preparing these patients for operation, the nurse must be alert for symptoms of hypoglycemia and be ready to give sugar, usually with orange juice, should they appear. After operation, the nursing management is the same as that following any upper-abdominal operation with special emphasis on observation of serum glucose levels.

Ulcerogenic (Zollinger–Ellison) Tumors

Some tumors of the islets of Langerhans are associated with a hypersecretion of gastric acid that produces ulcers in the stomach, the duodenum, and even the jejunum. The hypersecretion is so great that even after partial gastric resection, enough acid to produce further ulceration may remain. When a marked tendency to develop gastric and duodenal ulcers is noted, an ulcerogenic tumor of the islets of Langerhans is suspected.

These tumors, which may be benign or malignant, are treated, when possible, by excision. Frequently, however, because of extension beyond the pancreas, removal is not possible. In many patients, a total gastrectomy may be necessary to reduce the secretion of gastric acid sufficiently to prevent further ulceration.

▷ The Pituitary Gland

Hypopituitarism

Hypopituitarism is pituitary insufficiency resulting from destruction of the anterior lobe of the pituitary gland. *Panhypopituitarism* (Simmonds' disease) is total absence of all pituitary secretions and is rare.

The total destruction of the pituitary gland by trauma, tumor, or vascular lesion removes every stimulus that is normally received by the thyroid, the gonads, and the adrenal glands. The resulting endocrinopathy is characterized by extreme weight loss, emaciation, atrophy of all endocrine glands and organs, hair loss, impotence, amenorrhea, hypometabolism, and hypoglycemia. Coma and death will ensue without replacement of the missing hormones.

Pituitary Tumors

Tumors of the pituitary gland are of three principal types, representing an overgrowth of (1) eosinophilic cells, (2) basophilic cells, or (3) chromophobic cells (*i.e.,* cells with no affinity for either eosinophilic or basophilic stains).

Eosinophilic tumors, if they develop early enough in life, result in gigantism. The individual thus affected may be over 7 feet tall and large in all proportions, yet so weak and lethargic that he can hardly stand. If the disorder begins during adult life, the excessive skeletal growth occurs only in the feet, the hands, the superciliary ridges, the molar eminences, the nose, and the chin, giving rise to the clinical picture called *acromegaly*. Enlargement, moreover, is not confined to the skeleton, but involves every tissue and organ of the body. Many of these patients suffer from severe headaches and visual disturbances because the tumors exert pressure on the optic nerves. Assessment of central vision and visual fields may reveal loss of color discrimination, diplopia, or blindness of a portion of a field of vision. Decalcification of the skeleton, muscular weakness, and endocrine disturbances, similar to those occurring in patients with hyperthyroidism, also are associated with tumors of this type.

Basophilic tumors give rise to the so-called *Cushing syndrome* (see p. 936), with features largely attributable to hyperadrenalism, including masculinization and amenorrhea in females, truncal obesity, hypertension, osteoporosis, and polycythemia.

Chromophobic tumors, which comprise 90% of pituitary tumors, produce no hormones, but destroy the rest of the pituitary gland, causing hypopituitarism. Patients with this disease are inclined to be obese and somnolent, exhibiting fine, scanty hair; dry, soft skin; pasty complexion; and small bones. They also experience headaches, loss of libido, and visual defects progressing to blindness. Other symptoms include polyuria, polyphagia, a lowering of the basal metabolic rate, and a subnormal body temperature.

See page 1325 for the transsphenoidal approach to the removal of a pituitary tumor and page 1320 for the nursing management of a patient undergoing cranial surgery.

Hypophysectomy

Hypophysectomy, or removal of the pituitary gland, may be done for several reasons, including treatment of primary tumors of the pituitary gland. In diabetic retinopathy (see p. 906) it is used to halt the progress of hemorrhagic retinopathy and avoid blindness. Hypophysectomy is also done as a palliative measure to relieve bone pain secondary to metastasis of malignant lesions of the breast and prostate. Pituitary hormones influence the growth of the normal breast and stimulate the function of the ovaries and the adrenal glands. Hypophysectomy removes the hormonal influences of these glands and reduces stimuli to the continued growth of the neoplasm.

There are several methods of pituitary ablation (removal). It can be done surgically through the transfrontal, subcranial, or oronasal–transsphenoidal approaches (see p. 1325). The pituitary can also be destroyed by irradiation or cryosurgery.

The absence of the pituitary gland alters the function of many parts of the body. Menstruation ceases and infertility occurs after total or nearly total ablation of the pituitary gland. Substitution therapy with adrenal steroids (hydrocortisone) and thyroid hormone may be necessary following destruction or removal of the pituitary gland.

Diabetes Insipidus

Diabetes insipidus is a disorder of the posterior lobe of the pituitary gland due to a deficiency of vasopressin, the antidiuretic hormone (ADH). It is characterized by great thirst (polydipsia) and large volumes of dilute urine. The cause is unknown, although it may be secondary to head trauma, brain neoplasm, or surgical ablation or irradiation of the pituitary gland. Without the action of ADH on the distal nephron of the kidney, an enormous daily output of very dilute, waterlike urine with a specific gravity of 1.001 to 1.005 occurs. The urine contains no abnormal substances, such as sugar and albumin. Because of the intense thirst, the patient tends to drink 4 to 40 liters of fluid daily, with a special craving for cold water.

The primary symptoms may begin at birth. When it occurs in adults, the polyuria may have an insidious onset, although sometimes it occurs suddenly and may be related to an injury.

The disease cannot be controlled by limiting the intake

of fluids. Attempts to do this causes the patient to suffer extremely from an insatiable craving for fluid, and to develop severe dehydration and hypernatremia.

Assessment. The fluid deprivation test is carried out, in which fluids are deprived for 8 to 12 hours or until 3% of the body weight is lost. The patient is weighed frequently during the time fluid is withheld. Plasma and urine osmolality studies are done at the beginning and end of the test. Inability to increase specific gravity and osmolality of the urine are characteristic of diabetes insipidus. The patient with diabetes insipidus will continue to excrete large volumes of urine with low specific gravity and will experience weight loss, rising serum osmolality, and elevated serum sodium levels. The patient's condition needs to be assessed frequently during the test, and the test is terminated if the patient develops problems such as tachycardia, excessive weight loss, or hypotension.

Management. The objectives of therapy are (1) to assure adequate fluid replacement, (2) to replace vasopressin (which is usually a life-long therapeutic program) and (3) to search for and correct the underlying intracranial pathology.

Desmopressin (DDAVP) is a synthetic drug for the treatment of diabetes insipidus and is particularly valuable because its action lasts longer and it has fewer adverse effects than other preparations previously used to treat the disease. It is administered intranasally with the patient sniffing the solution into his nose through a flexible plastic tube. Two administrations daily appear to control the symptoms.

Another form of therapy is the intramuscular administration of antidiuretic hormone, vasopressin tannate in oil, which is given at intervals of 36 to 48 hours, or longer. The effect is a reduction in urinary volume for 24 to 48 hours. The vial of medication should be warmed to make it easier to administer the oil preparation. The injection is given in the evening so that maximum results are obtained during sleep. Abdominal cramps may be a problem with this type of therapy.

The drug lypressin (Diapid Nasal Spray) is absorbed through the nasal mucosa into the blood and is another method of administering vasopressin. Its duration may be too short for patients with severe disease. The patient should be observed for chronic rhinopharyngitis if this modality of treatment is used.

Recently clofibrate, a hypolipidemic agent, has been found to have an antidiuretic effect on patients with diabetes insipidus who have some residual hypothalamic vasopressin. Chlorpropamide (Diabinese) and thiazide diuretics are also used in mild forms of the disease, as they potentiate the action of antidiuretic hormone. The patient receiving chlorpropamide should be warned of the possibility of hypoglycemic reactions.

The patient will require encouragement and support if he is undergoing studies of a possible cranial lesion. The patient and family members are instructed about follow-up care and emergency measures. The patient is also advised to carry information about this disorder and his medications with him at all times.

▷ Bibliography

Books

Brown R (ed). Anesthesia and the Patient with Endocrine Disease. Philadelphia, FA Davis, 1980.

Dillon RG. Handbook of Endocrinology, 2nd ed. Philadelphia, Lea & Febiger, 1980.

Felig P et al. Endocrinology and Metabolism. New York, McGraw-Hill, 1981.

Fregly M and Luttge W. Human Endocrinology. New York, Elsevier, 1982.

Griffen JE. Manual of Clinical Endocrinology. New York, McGraw-Hill, 1980.

Hall R. Fundamentals of Clinical Endocrinology, 3rd ed. New York, Year Book Medical Publishers, 1981.

Hershman JM. Management of Endocrine Disorders. Philadelphia, Lea & Febiger, 1980.

Malseed RT. Pharmacology: Drug Therapy and Nursing Considerations. Philadelphia, JB Lippincott, 1982.

Ryan WG. Endocrine Disorders: A Pathologic Approach. Chicago, Year Book Medical Publishers, 1980.

Vaitukaitis JL. Current Endocrinology. Basic and Clinical Aspects. New York, Elsevier, 1982.

Williams RH. Textbook of Endocrinology. Philadelphia, WB Saunders, 1981.

Articles
Thyroid

Clark F. Thyrotoxicosis. Practitioner 1982 Feb; 226(1364):197–198, 201–204.

Honigman RE. Thyroid function tests. Nursing '82 1982 Apr; 12(4):68–71.

Jenkins EH. Living with thyrotoxicosis. Am J Nurs 1980 May; 80(5):956–958.

Klein I and Levey GS. Thyroid storm. Hospital Medicine 1982 Mar; 19(3):34a–34p.

Martyn PA. If you guessed cardiovascular disease, guess again. Am J Nurs 1982 Aug; 82(8):1238–1241.

Parathyroid

Hoffman JTT and Mewby TB. Hypercalcemia in primary hyperparathyroidism. Nurs Clin North Am 1980 Sept; 15(3):469–480.

Kinder BK et al. Diagnostic and therapeutic approaches to primary hyperparathyroidism. Surg Clin North Am 1980 Oct; 60(5):1285–1295.

O'Riordan JLH. Calcium and the endocrine system. Practitioner 1982 Feb; 226(1264):237–241.

Roberts JW. Symptomatic hyperparathyroidism. Surg Clin North Am 1982 Apr; 62(2):225–228.

Adrenal Glands

Gotch PM. Teaching patients about adrenal corticosteroids. Am J Nurs 1981 Jan; 81(1):78–81.

Jones SG. Adrenal patient—proceed with caution. RN 1982 Jan; 45(1):66–68, 70, 72.

Jones SG. Kid-glove care in pheochromocytoma. RN 1982 Feb; 45(2):66–68, 70, 72, 74.

Jones SG. Bilateral adrenalectomy: Post-op dangers to watch for. RN 1982 Mar; 45(3):66, 68.

Kaktis JV and Pitts LH. Complications associated with use of megadose corticosteroids in head-injured adults. Neurosurg Nurs 1980 Sept; 12(3):166–171.

Sanford SJ. Dysfunction of the adrenal gland: Physiologic considerations and nursing problems. Nurs Clin North Am 1980 Sept; 15(3):481–498.

Pancreas

Beck ML. Preparing your patient physically for an esophagogastroduodenoscopy. Nursing '81 1981 Feb; 11(2):15–16.

Broe PJ, Mehigan DG, and Cameron JL. Pancreatic transplantation. Surg Clin North Am 1981 Feb; 61(1):85–98.

Cooperman AM. Chronic pancreatitis. Surg Clin North Am 1981 Feb; 61(1):71–83.

Dickerman RM and Dunn EL. Splenic, pancreatic, and hepatic injuries. Surg Clin North Am 1981 Feb; 61(1):3–15.

Fankucken EI. Current concepts in pancreatic imaging. Surg Clin North Am 1981 Feb; 61(1):17–45.

Gotch PM. Are you ready for a total pancreatectomy patient? RN 1981 Nov; 44(11):54–57.

Kelber Sr MB. Pancreatic enzymes. Nursing '82 1982 Dec; 12(12):65–67.

Kosel K et al. Total pancreatectomy and islet cell autotransplantation. Am J Nurs 1982 Apr; 82(4):568–571.

Lin RS and Kessler II. A multifactorial model for pancreatic cancer in man. JAMA 1981 Jan 9; 245(1):147–152.

Ranson JNC. Acute pancreatitis—where are we? Surg Clin North Am 1981 Feb; 61(1):55–70.

Ropka ME. Pancreatic insufficiency in the person with cancer. Cancer Nurs 1981 Feb; 4(1):37–41.

Rudick J. Physiology of pancreatic secretion. Surg Clin North Am 1981 Feb; 61(1):47–54.

Stiklorius C. Two diagnostic procedures that demand your all-out care. RN 1982 Aug; 42(8):64–65.

Pituitary Gland

Markowitz S et al. Acute pituitary vascular accident (pituitary apoplexy). Med Clin North Am 1981 Jan; 65(1):105–116.

McInerney M. Prolactin producing pituitary adenomas. J Neurosurg Nurs 1981 Feb; 13(1):15–17.

Smith J. Nursing management of diabetes insipidus. J Neurosurg Nurs 1981 Dec; 13(6):313–317.

Solomon B. The hypothalamus and the pituitary gland: An overview. Nurs Clin North Am 1980 Sept; 15(3):435–451.

Stillman MJ. Transsphenoidal hypophysectomy for pituitary tumors. J Neurosurg Nurs 1981 June; 13(3):117–122.

Unit XI

Renal and Urinary Problems

42

Assessment of Renal and Urinary Function

▷ Physiologic Overview

The kidneys, ureters, bladder, and urethra comprise the urinary system. The kidney's main responsibility is to extract unwanted substances, including water, from the blood. The extracted materials that comprise the urine are transported through the ureters for temporary storage in the urinary bladder. During the act of micturition (urination), the bladder contracts and the urine is expelled from the body through the urethra. The purpose of urine formation is to regulate the water content and electrolyte composition of the body fluids. Although fluid and electrolytes can be lost by other means, such as in sweat or feces, it is the kidneys that have to precisely regulate the internal environment of the body. The renal excretory function is necessary for maintenance of life. However, unlike the cardiovascular and respiratory systems, complete malfunction of the kidneys may not cause death for several days. In addition, with modern medical management it is possible to substitute for certain renal function by means of an artificial kidney.

An important feature of the urinary system is its ability to adapt to wide variations in fluid load based on the personal habits of the individual. Basically, the kidney must be able to excrete that which is ingested into the diet, and not eliminated by other organs. This usually amounts to 1 to 1½ liters of water per day, 6 g to 8 g of salt (sodium chloride) per day, 6 g to 8 g of potassium chloride per day, and 70 mg of acid equivalents per day. In addition, protein is ingested and metabolized by the body into urea and other waste products that must also be excreted in the urine.

Anatomy of the Urinary System

The kidneys are paired organs, each weighing approximately 125 g, located in a position lateral to the bodies of the lower thoracic vertebrae, a few centimeters to the right and left of the midline. They are surrounded by a thin, fibrous tissue known as the capsule. Anteriorly, the kidneys are separated from the abdominal cavity and its contents by layers of peritoneum. Posteriorly, they are shielded by the lower thoracic wall. There is no anatomical difference between the two kidneys other than they are located on opposite sides of the body. The blood supply to each kidney is delivered through the renal artery and drained through the renal vein. The renal arteries arise from the abdominal aorta, and the renal veins carry blood back into the inferior vena cava. The kidneys can efficiently clear the blood of waste materials in part because their total blood flow is great and represents 25% of cardiac output.

Urine is formed within the kidneys in functional units, known as nephrons. The urine formed within these nephrons passes into collecting ducts that join to form the pelvis of each kidney. Each kidney pelvis gives rise to a ureter. The ureter is a long tube (25 cm) with a wall composed largely of smooth muscle. It connects each kidney to the bladder and functions as a conduit for urine.

The urinary bladder is a hollow organ that is situated anteriorly just behind the pubic bone. It acts as a temporary storage reservoir for the urine. The walls of the bladder consist largely of smooth muscle called the detrusor muscle. Contraction of this muscle is mainly responsible for emptying the bladder during urination. The urethra arises from the bladder and runs through the penis in the male and opens just above the vagina in the female. A short distance from its origin, the urethra is encircled by a small bundle of muscle fibers that is called the external urinary sphincter. This sphincter is the major site for control of the initiation of urination.

The Nephron. The kidney is divided into an outer portion called the cortex and an inner portion known as the medulla (Fig. 42-1). In the human, each kidney is composed of approximately 1 million nephrons, the functional unit of the kidney. Each nephron consists of a glomerulus and a tubule (Fig. 42-2), with the glomerulus measuring about 0.2 mm in diameter and the tubule approximately 25 mm

to 45 mm in length. The glomerulus, the beginning of the nephron, is composed of tufts of capillaries that are fed by an afferent arteriole and drained by an efferent arteriole. The latter is a thick-walled muscular vessel (it is not a vein) that helps to maintain a high pressure in the glomerular capillaries. Like capillaries in general, the walls of the glomerular capillaries are composed of a layer of endothelial cells and a basement membrane. On the other side of the basement membrane are the epithelial cells that form the beginning of the tubule. The tubule itself is divided into three parts: a proximal tubule, the loop of Henle, and a distal tubule. The distal tubules coalesce to form collecting ducts that are about 20 mm long and pass through the renal cortex and the medulla to empty into the pelvis of the kidney. The total length of a typical nephron, including the collecting duct, ranges from 45 mm to 65 mm.

Function of the Nephron. The process of urine formation begins as blood flows through the glomerulus. Fluid is filtered through the walls of the glomerular capillary tufts into the proximal tubule. Under normal conditions, approximately 20% of the plasma passing through the glomerulus is filtered into the nephron, amounting to about 180 liters of filtrate per day. The filtrate, very similar to blood plasma without its proteins, consists essentially of water, electrolytes, and other small molecules. Within the tubule and collecting ducts, some of these substances are selectively reabsorbed into the blood. Other substances may actually be secreted into the filtrate as it travels down the tubule. The urine is the remaining fluid (along with its contents) that reaches the pelvis of the kidney. Some substances, such as glucose, are usually completely reabsorbed in the tubule and do not appear in the urine. The processes of reabsorption and secretion in the tubule frequently involve active transport and require the utilization of metabolic energy. The amount of various substances normally

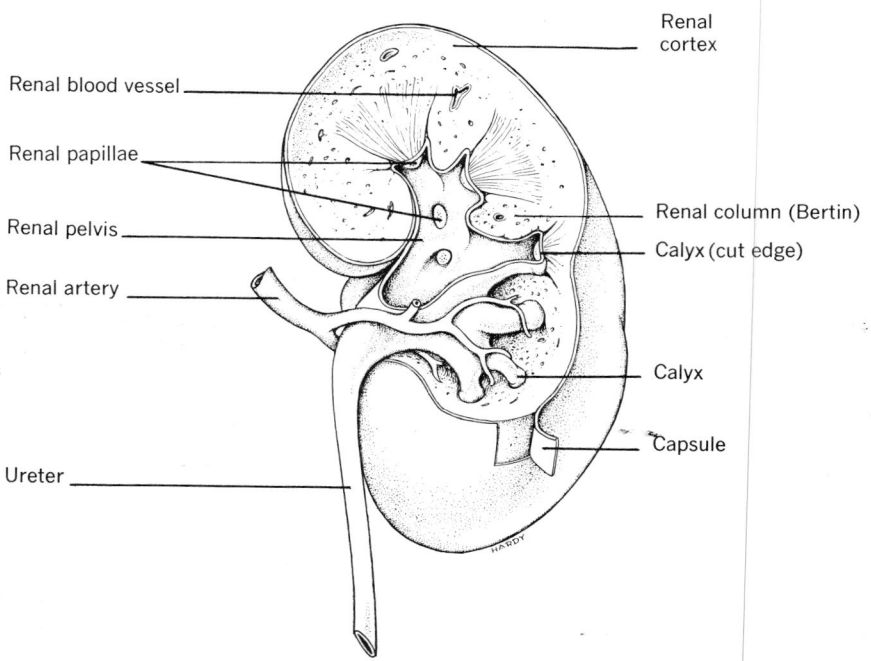

Renal cortex
Renal blood vessel
Renal papillae
Renal pelvis
Renal artery
Renal column (Bertin)
Calyx (cut edge)
Calyx
Capsule
Ureter

Figure 42-1. Diagram of internal structure of kidney, showing relations of renal pelvis and calyces to pyramids in medullary region. (From Chaffee EE and Greisheimer EM: Basic Physiology and Anatomy, 4th ed., Philadelphia, JB Lippincott, 1980.)

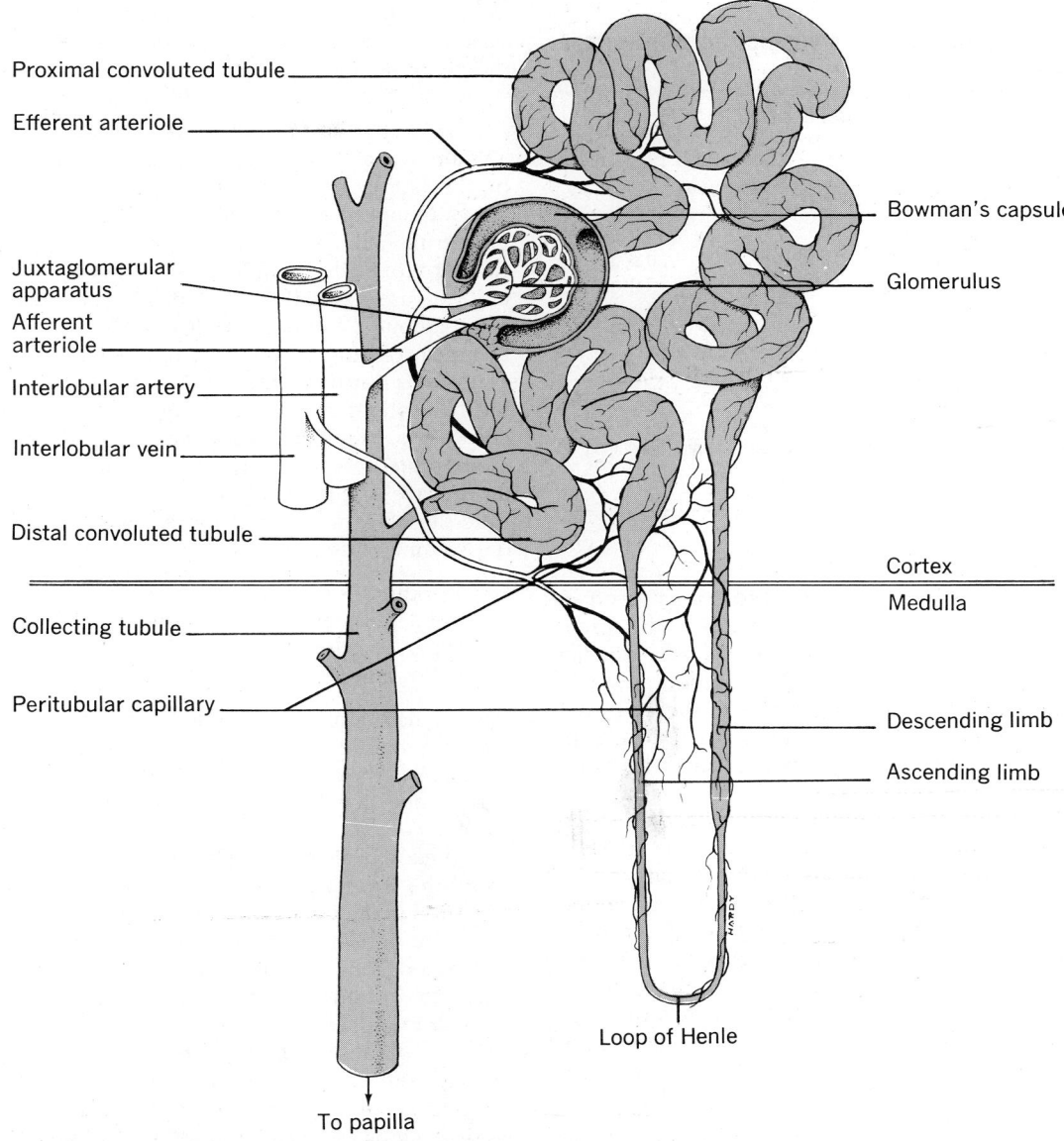

Proximal convoluted tubule

Efferent arteriole

Juxtaglomerular apparatus

Afferent arteriole

Interlobular artery

Interlobular vein

Distal convoluted tubule

Collecting tubule

Peritubular capillary

To papilla

Bowman's capsule

Glomerulus

Cortex

Medulla

Descending limb

Ascending limb

Loop of Henle

Figure 42-2. Diagram of a nephron and its blood supply. Also shown is a collecting tubule that receives urine from neighboring nephron units. Note that the loop of Henle dips into the medullary layer of the kidney. (From Chaffee EE and Greisheimer EM: Basic Physiology and Anatomy, 4th ed. Philadelphia, JB Lippincott, 1980.)

filtered by the glomerulus, reabsorbed by the tubules, and excreted in the urine is shown in Table 42-1.

Urine Composition

The kidney functions as the main excretory organ of the body. It disposes of unwanted materials that are ingested as well as the byproducts of the body's metabolism. In the normal individual, the amounts of these materials excreted per day are exactly equal to the amounts ingested and formed, so that over a period of time, there is no net change in the total body composition.

Urine is composed primarily of water. A normal person ingests approximately 1 to 2 liters of water per day, and normally all but 400 ml to 500 ml of this is excreted in the urine. The remainder is lost from the skin during breathing and in the feces. The second major class of substances excreted in the urine is the electrolytes, including sodium, potassium, chloride, bicarbonate, and other less abundant ions. The average American diet contains about 6 g to 8 g each of sodium chloride (salt) and potassium chloride per day, and nearly all of this disappears in the urine. The third group of substances appearing in the urine is made up of the breakdown products of protein metabolism. The major breakdown product is urea, of which about 25 g are produced and excreted per day. Other products of protein metabolism that must be excreted are creatinine phosphates

Table 42-1

Filtration, Reabsorption, and Excretion of Certain Normal Constituents of Plasma

	Filtered 24 Hr	Reabsorbed 24 Hr	Excreted 24 Hr*
Sodium	540 g	537 g	3.3 g
Chloride	630 g	625 g	5.3 g
Bicarbonate	300 g	300 g	0.3 g
Potassium	28 g	24 g	3.9 g
Glucose	140 g	140 g	0 g
Urea	53 g	28 g	25 g
Creatinine	1.4 g	0 g	1.4 g
Uric acid	8.5 g	7.7 g	0.8 g

* These are typical normal values. Wide variation is found, depending on diet.

and sulphates. Uric acid, formed as a breakdown product of nucleic acid metabolism, is also eliminated in the urine.

It is important to recognize that some substances that are present in high concentrations in the blood are ordinarily not present in the urine. Examples of these are the normal foodstuffs, glucose, and amino acids. These substances are filtered at the glomerulus and normally are completely reabsorbed by active transport in the renal tubule. Glucose will appear in the urine if its blood level is so high that its concentration in the glomerular filtrate exceeds the capacity of the tubules to reabsorb it. In a normal person, the glucose is completely reabsorbed when its concentration in the blood is less than 200 mg/100 ml. In diabetes, in which the blood glucose levels exceed the kidney's reabsorption capacity, glucose will appear in the urine. Protein is also not normally found in the urine. These molecules are not filtered at the glomerulus because of their large size. When protein appears in the urine, it usually signifies damage to the glomeruli, causing them to become "leaky."

Regulation of Acid Excretion

The breakdown of proteins involves the generation of acid compounds, in particular phosphoric and sulfuric acids. In addition, a certain amount of acid material is ingested daily. Unlike CO_2, these are nonvolatile acids and cannot be eliminated by the lung. Since accumulation of these acids in the blood would lower its pH and inhibit cell function, they must be excreted in the urine. A normal person has to excrete approximately 70 mEq of acid each day. The kidney is able to excrete some of this acid directly into the urine to the extent of lowering its pH to 4.5, 1000 times more acidic than blood.

More acid usually needs to be eliminated from the body than can be excreted directly as free acid in the urine. This is accomplished by the renal excretion of acid that is bound to chemical buffers. The acid (H^+) is secreted by the renal tubular cells into the filtrate where it is buffered chiefly by phosphate ions and ammonia (NH_3). Phosphate is present in the glomerular filtrate, and ammonia is produced by the kidney cells and secreted into the tubular fluid. Through the buffering process, the kidney is able to excrete large quantities of acid in a bound form without further lowering the pH of the urine.

Regulation of Electrolyte Excretion

The amount of electrolytes and water that must be excreted by the kidney each day varies greatly, depending on the amounts ingested. The 180 liters of filtrate formed by the glomeruli each day contains about 1100 g of sodium chloride. Approximately 2 liters of water and 6 g to 8 g of sodium chloride are normally excreted per day in the urine. The small amounts excreted relative to the amount filtered reflect reabsorption of sodium from the filtrate into the blood as it travels down the tubules. Water from the filtrate follows the reabsorbed sodium in order to maintain osmotic balance. Thus, over 99% of the water and sodium filtered at the glomerulus is reabsorbed into the blood by the time the urine leaves the body. By regulating the amount of sodium (and therefore water) reabsorbed, the kidney can regulate the volume of body fluids.

- If sodium is excreted in excess of the amount ingested, the patient will become dehydrated.
- If less sodium is excreted than is ingested, the patient will retain fluid.

The regulation of the amount of sodium excreted depends on the hormone, aldosterone, which is synthesized and released from the adrenal gland. In the presence of increased aldosterone in the blood, less sodium is excreted in the urine.

Release of aldosterone from the adrenal gland is largely under the control of angiotensin, a peptide hormone manufactured in the liver and activated in the lung. Angiotensin levels are in turn controlled by the hormone, renin, which is released from cells in the kidneys. This complex system is activated when pressure in the renal arterioles falls below normal levels, as occurs with shock and dehydration. The effect of activation of this system is to increase the retention of water and expansion of intravascular fluid volume.

Another electrolyte whose concentration in the body fluids is regulated by the kidney is potassium, the most abundant intracellular ion. The excretion of potassium by the kidney is increased by increased aldosterone levels in contrast to the effects of aldosterone on sodium excretion.

- Retention of potassium is the most life-threatening effect of renal failure.

Regulation of Water Excretion

Regulation of the amount of water excreted is also an important function of the kidney. With a large water intake, a large volume of dilute urine must be excreted. Conversely, with a low water intake, the urine that is excreted must be concentrated. The relative degree of dilution or concentration of the urine can be measured in terms of its *osmolality*. This term refers to the amount of solid material (electrolytes and other molecules) that is dissolved in the urine. The filtrate in the glomerular capillary normally has the same osmolality as the blood, with a value of approximately 300 mOsm/liter. As the filtrate passes through the tubules and collecting ducts, the osmolality may vary anywhere from 50 mOsm/liter to 1200 mOsm/liter, the maximal diluting and concentrating ability of the kidney.

The osmolality of the urine specimen can be measured. This is a more exact measurement than specific gravity. Osmolality reflects the number of particles of solute in a unit of solution, unlike specific gravity, which reflects both the quantity and the nature of particles. Therefore, protein, glucose, and intravenous contrast medium affect specific gravity more than osmolality. Osmolality is done when a precise measurement of the concentration and diluting ability of the kidney is needed. Normal urine osmolality is 500 mOsm/liter to 800 mOsm/liter. Normal specific gravity is 1.003 to 1.030.

How are water excretion and urine concentration regulated by the kidney? The glomerular filtrate has essentially the same electrolyte composition as the blood plasma without the proteins. Therefore, regulation of urine concentration is carried out in the tubule by varying the amount of water that is reabsorbed in relation to electrolyte reabsorption. The amount of water that is reabsorbed is under the control of antidiuretic hormones (ADH, vasopressin). ADH is a hormone that is secreted by the posterior part of the pituitary gland in response to changes in osmolality of the blood. With decreased water intake, blood osmolality tends to rise and stimulate ADH release. ADH then acts on the kidney in order to cause increased reabsorption of water, thereby restoring the osmolality of the blood back toward normal. With excess water intake, the secretion of ADH by the pituitary is depressed and, therefore, less water is reabsorbed by the kidney tubule. This latter situation leads to increased urine volume and is called diuresis.

- Loss of the ability to concentrate and dilute the urine is the most common early manifestation of kidney disease.

In this condition, a dilute urine of fixed specific gravity (approximately 1.010) or fixed osmolality (approximately 300 mOsm/liter) is excreted.

Renal Clearance

The most commonly used test to evaluate how well the kidney performs its excretory function is termed *clearance*. Clearance of a substance A is given by the following equation: clearance equals (the urine concentration of A) times (the urine volume in a given time) divided by the plasma concentration of A.* For example, if the arterial plasma concentration of a substance is 0.1 mg/ml, the urine concentration of the same substance is 50 mg/ml, and the urine volume is 1.0 ml/min, the clearance of that substance according to the above equation is 500 ml/min. This means that 500 ml of blood is completely cleared of that substance in one minute. In the body, few substances are actually completely cleared from the blood during a single passage through the kidney. In the example given above, if the blood is cleared of only 50% of the substance, urine concentration of the substance would be 25 mg/ml and the

calculated renal clearance would be 250 ml/min. It is possible to measure the renal clearance of any substance, but the one that has proven particularly useful is the creatinine clearance. Creatinine is an endogenous waste product of skeletal muscle that is excreted by glomerular filtration and is not appreciably reabsorbed or secreted by the renal tubules. Therefore, creatinine clearance is a good measure of the glomerular filtration rate (GFR). The normal adult GFR is about 100 ml/min to 120 ml/min.

Storage of Urine and Micturition

Urine formed by the kidney is transported from the renal pelvis through the ureters and into the bladder. This movement is facilitated by peristaltic waves occurring about one to five times per minute and generated by the smooth muscle in the ureter wall. Urine flows into the bladder in spurts synchronous with the peristaltic contractions. There are no sphincters between the bladder and the ureters, although reflux of urine from the bladder in normal subjects is prevented by the unidirectional nature of the peristaltic waves and because each ureter enters the bladder at an oblique angle. However—

- with overdistention of the bladder due to disease, the elevated pressure in the bladder can be transmitted back through the ureters, leading to ureteral distention and possible reflux of urine. This can lead to kidney infection (pyelonephritis) and damage from the elevated pressure (hydronephrosis).

The pressure in the bladder is normally very low, even as the urine accumulates, because the bladder's smooth muscle adapts to the increased stretch as the bladder is slowly filled. The first sensations of bladder filling ordinarily occur when about 100 ml to 150 ml of urine are present in the bladder. In most cases, there is a desire to void when the bladder contains approximately 200 ml to 300 ml. With 400 ml a marked feeling of fullness is usually present.

Voiding of urine is prevented by contraction of the external urethral sphincter. This muscle is under voluntary control and is innervated by nerves from the sacral area of the spinal cord. Voluntary control is a learned behavior that is not present at birth. When there is a desire to urinate, the external urethral sphincter is relaxed, and the detrusor muscle (bladder smooth muscle) contracts and expels the urine from the bladder through the urethra. The pressure generated in the bladder during micturition (urination) is approximately 50 cm to 150 cm of water. Residual urine in the urethra drains by gravity in the female and is expelled by voluntary muscle contractions in the male.

The contraction of the detrusor muscle is regulated by a reflex involving the parasympathetic nervous system. The reflex is integrated in the sacral portion of the spinal tract. The sympathetic nervous system plays no essential part in micturition, but does prevent semen from entering the bladder during ejaculation.

- If the pelvic nerves to the bladder and sphincter are destroyed, voluntary control and reflex urination are abolished and the bladder becomes overdistended with urine. If the spinal pathways from the brain to the urinary system are destroyed (for example, after a spinal cord transection), reflex contraction of the bladder is

---

* Clearance =

$$\frac{\text{(urine concentration of A)} \times \text{(urine volume in a given time)}}{\text{plasma concentration of A}}$$

maintained, but voluntary control over the process is lost. In both of these types of loss of innervation, the muscle of the bladder can contract and expel urine, but the contractions are generally insufficient to empty the bladder completely, and residual urine is left behind.

The most common clinical method used to study bladder function is catheterization—passage of a catheter through the urethra into the bladder. With this technique, it is possible to measure the amount of urine left in the bladder after micturition (residual urine). Normally, this should be no more than 50 ml. However, catheterization is to be avoided whenever possible, because it increases the risk of infection. Another test for bladder dysfunction is to measure the pressure in the bladder after instillation of various volumes of saline. This latter procedure is called a *cystometrogram.*

▷ Renal Pathophysiology

Diseases of the kidney can be classified according to the segment of the nephron that is primarily affected. Glomerulonephritis and the various etiologies of the nephrotic syndrome primarily affect the renal glomerulus. Vascular diseases, infections, and toxins affect primarily the renal tubule, although some element of glomerular dysfunction may coexist. Obstruction to the outflow of urine due to calculi (stones), protein, or other material in the collecting ducts or ureters may eventually lead to damage of the entire nephron. When the degree of kidney damage is severe, renal failure occurs and may result in the condition called *uremia.*

Glomerular Diseases
Nephritic Syndrome.   The nephritic syndrome occurs in response to a group of diseases in which inflammation of the glomerulus (glomerulonephritis) is predominant. The major manifestations are hematuria, proteinuria, sodium and fluid retention, hypertension, and occasionally oliguria. These abnormalities are due to damage to the glomerular capillaries, which permits leakage of red blood cells into the tubular lumen. Glomerulonephritis most commonly results from immune reactions. Common causes are the reaction to some streptococcal infections predominantly in children and the autoimmune diseases, such as Goodpasture's syndrome and lupus erythematosus. Glomerulonephritis may resolve completely, although in some patients renal failure may result.

Nephrotic Syndrome.   The nephrotic syndrome results from a group of glomerular diseases associated with increased permeability of the glomerulus to proteins. Frequently there are no observable alterations of kidney structure by light microscopy. The primary manifestation of the disease is the loss of plasma proteins, particularly albumin, in the urine. Although the liver is capable of increasing its production of albumin manifold, it is unable to keep up with the daily loss of albumin through the kidney; thus, hypoalbuminemia results. The resultant decreased oncotic pressure leads to generalized edema. A tendency to de-

creased circulating blood volume activates the renin-angiotensin system, leading to retention of sodium, which also contributes to the development of edema. Patients with nephrotic syndrome also exhibit an elevated lipid concentration in their blood (lipemia), the cause of which is not known. The nephrotic syndrome can occur with almost any intrinsic renal disease or systemic disease that affects the glomerulus. See page 1002 for further discussion.

Renal Failure
Renal failure is present when the excretion of water, electrolytes, and metabolic waste products is insufficient because of kidney damage that prevents the kidneys from maintaining the normal internal environment of the body. Acute renal failure has a sudden onset and is frequently reversible. Chronic renal failure usually develops gradually but can also occur as a consequence of a preceding acute episode. One normal kidney is generally sufficient for normal urinary function so that renal failure requires bilateral kidney damage. The signs and symptoms of renal failure are in large part a manifestation of the altered fluid and electrolyte balance of the body. The diagnosis is generally made by the finding of *azotemia,* defined as elevation of nitrogenous waste products in the blood. Uremia results when this condition is severe.

Pathogenesis of Renal Failure.   Decreased excretion of metabolic waste products can occur as a result of kidney damage, a decrease in blood flow to the kidney, or acute obstruction to the flow of urine.

- Decreased urine output due to complete urinary obstruction can occur in patients who have an enlarged prostate, stones (calculi) in the ureters or urethra, or infiltrating tumors. Secondary damage to the kidneys and renal failure will result if the obstruction is not relieved promptly.
- Alterations of renal blood flow can occur with hypotension, congestive heart failure, dehydration, or thrombosis of renal arteries. Acute decrease in renal blood flow may lead to secondary renal damage and renal failure. Decreased excretion of waste products due to decreased renal blood flow in the absence of kidney damage is called "prerenal azotemia."
- Acute renal failure due to kidney injury results from acute vasculitis, acute glomerulonephritis, severe ("malignant") hypertension, or, more commonly, acute damage to the renal tubules (acute tubular necrosis, ATN).
- The clinical conditions that may result in ATN include hypotension (shock), exposure to nephrotoxic chemicals, intravascular hemolysis with hemoglobinuria (*e.g.,* due to transfusion reactions, extensive burns, or infusion of water intravenously), or crush injury of an extremity with myoglobinuria.

The etiologies of chronic renal failure include the causes for acute renal failure and include, in addition, chronic infection (pyelonephritis), nephrosclerosis, diabetic nephropathy, collagen diseases, and other chronic, progressive kidney diseases. See page 997 for further discussion.

Uremia

Uremia is a term used to designate the manifestations of chronic renal dysfunction. Uremia is a generalized condition that affects all organ systems of the body.

Fluids and Electrolytes. The fluid and electrolyte abnormalities that occur in renal failure are the consequence of a decreased number of functional nephrons. The fundamental pathophysiologic alteration in kidney function is a decreased overall glomerular filtration rate (GFR) due to a reduced number of filtering glomeruli, leading to decreased clearance of substances that depend on the rate of filtration for their excretion. Decreased glomerular filtration rate can be diagnosed by a decreased insulin, urea, or creatinine clearance. As creatinine clearance decreases, serum creatinine increases. Because of creatinine's constant production, it is the most specific and sensitive indicator of kidney disease. The blood urea nitrogen (BUN) also rises with kidney damage, but its level is also affected by protein intake and tissue breakdown. Uric acid also rises.

In addition to decreased GFR, a decrease in the number of functional nephrons results in decreased modification of the glomerular filtrate by the tubules prior to its excretion as urine. As a result, the urine resembles a filtrate of plasma, having a fixed specific gravity or osmolality. This inability to concentrate or dilute the urine prevents appropriate responses by the kidneys to fluctuations in daily intake of water and electrolytes. Decreased intake of fluid or salt can lead to dehydration or sodium depletion; excess salt or water intake may cause water intoxication or sodium overload. Decreased tubular function also results in inability to excrete increased loads of potassium (K^+) and acid (H^+). With advanced renal disease, the normal production of H^+ by body metabolism or release of K^+ from damaged cells of the body can themselves result in acidosis or hyperkalemia. Decreased excretion of acid results primarily from the inability of the tubules to secrete ammonia (NH_3) and to reabsorb sodium bicarbonate ($NaHCO_3$). There may also be decreased excretion of phosphates and organic acids. Decreased excretion of potassium results from inability of the tubules to secrete this ion into the urine. In addition to the inability to excrete these normal body constituents, the excretion of drugs may be markedly altered, necessitating adjustment of their usual dosages.

Calcium Metabolism and Bone Changes. Disorders of calcium metabolism with secondary bone changes are among the major manifestations of uremia. The primary finding is usually a decreased serum calcium concentration. The pathophysiologic processes leading to hypocalcemia are diverse. The most important factor is probably reciprocal depression of free calcium secondary to the elevation of serum phosphorous due to its decreased excretion in the urine. An additional mechanism for hypocalcemia is decreased conversion of vitamin D to its active form by the damaged kidneys, leading to diminished absorption of calcium from the gastrointestinal tract. Decreased serum calcium secondarily stimulates the parathyroid glands to produce increased parathormone, resulting in the condition called secondary hyperparathyroidism. This condition is manifested by demineralization of bone and formation of bone cysts. The bone changes are worsened as a result of

decreased deposition of calcium due to decreased active vitamin D and increased resorption of calcium due to chronic acidosis. The demineralization of bone leads to frequent fractures and bone pain. The term *renal osteodystrophy* is frequently used to designate the complex bone changes that occur with uremia.

Anemia. Anemia, another common manifestation of uremia, is generally due to decreased rate of production of red blood cells by the bone marrow and increased rates of red blood cell destruction. Decreased erythropoiesis is related to a decreased rate of production of erythropoietin by the kidneys. The red cells in the peripheral blood generally appear to be of normal size (normocytic) and of normal hemoglobin concentration (normochromic). Blood loss due to bleeding from the gastrointestinal tract or other sites may contribute to the anemia.

Cardiovascular Manifestations. Hypertension, frequently associated with chronic renal failure, may be either the cause or the result of renal damage. Primary hypertension leads to kidney damage as a result of atherosclerosis of the renal vasculature manifested by nephrosclerosis. Secondary hypertension occurs due to increased renin production by the diseased kidney, leading to generalized vasoconstriction as well as salt retention with consequent expansion of the vascular volume.

- Patients with compromised excretory function are more prone than normal persons to volume overload since they are less able to compensate for acute increases in water and salt intake.
- Chronic congestive heart failure with pulmonary and peripheral edema frequently occurs as a consequence of hypertensive cardiac disease complicated by the effects of fluid overload and anemia.
- Congestive heart failure results in decreased renal blood flow with elevation of blood urea out of proportion to the degree of kidney damage.

Other Manifestations of Uremia. Among the diverse manifestations of uremia are gastrointestinal symptoms, including anorexia, nausea, vomiting, and hiccoughs; neuromuscular symptoms, including mental clouding, inability to concentrate, drowsiness, lethargy, twitching, convulsions, and tetany (related to the low serum calcium); and dermatologic symptoms, including severe itching and uremic frost (due to the high concentration of urea in sweat). These patients also have altered cellular immunity manifested by decreased delayed hypersensitivity and increased susceptibility to infection probably related to a decreased ability of leukocytes to kill bacteria. The precise mechanism for many of these diverse conditions has not been worked out. However, retention of products normally excreted in the urine, such as ammonia, phenols, and other organic and inorganic compounds, is the probable cause.

Course of Renal Failure

The basic mechanisms underlying the pathophysiologic changes of acute and chronic renal failure are similar. However, their clinical presentations are markedly different. There are two phases of acute renal failure: the oliguric phase and the polyuric phase.

Oliguric Phase. Acute renal failure occurs due to sudden insults to the kidney that result in a decreased rate of urine formation. This is called the oliguric phase of acute renal failure.

- During the oliguric phase, the potential life-threatening complications are related to fluid and electrolyte retention (in particular, hyperkalemia and acidosis).

Polyuric Phase (Diuretic). If the original insult is removed, the recovery process begins with gradually increasing glomerular filtration rate. At this stage, the renal tubular cells may still be unable to reabsorb the water and electrolytes in the increasing volume of glomerular filtrate. As a result, the volume of urine that is excreted is increased above normal, resulting in the polyuric phase of acute renal failure.

- The potential life-threatening complications of the polyuric phase are dehydration and electrolyte depletion.

Complete recovery from acute renal failure, if it occurs, may require several months. Some patients with acute renal failure, despite the removal of the initial insult, will not recover normal renal function and will develop chronic renal failure. More commonly, however, chronic renal failure develops gradually and insidiously. The disease is frequently not discovered until the patient develops symptoms related to fluid and electrolyte abnormalities. At this stage, kidney function has generally decreased by more than 50% and the creatinine concentration in the blood has risen above normal.

▷ Assessment of Urinary Function

Clinical Manifestations of Urinary Dysfunction

The following symptoms and signs are suggestive of urinary tract disease: pain, changes in micturition, and gastrointestinal symptoms.

Pain

Genitourinary pain is not always present in renal disease but is generally seen in the more acute conditions. Pain of renal disease is caused by sudden distention of the renal capsule. Its severity is related to how quickly the distention develops.

Kidney pain may be felt as a dull ache in the costovertebral angle and may spread to the umbilicus. Ureteral pain produces pain in the back, radiating to the abdomen, upper thigh, testis, or labium. Pain in the flank (the side between the ribs and ilium), radiating to the lower abdomen or epigastrium and often associated with nausea, vomiting, and paralytic ileus, may indicate renal colic. Bladder pain (low abdominal pain or pain over the suprapubic area) can be due to an overdistended bladder or bladder infection. Urgency, tenesmus (painful straining), and terminal dysuria are usually present. Pain at the urethral meatus reveals irritation of the bladder neck or a foreign body in the canal, or is from urethritis due to infection or trauma. Severe pain in the scrotal region results from inflammatory swelling of the epididymis or testicle, or torsion of the testicle, while perineal and rectal fullness and pain signal acute prostatitis or prostatic abscess. Back and leg pain may be due to metastases of cancer of the prostate to the pelvic bones. Pain in the penile shaft may originate from urethral problems, while pain in the glans penis is usually due to prostatitis.

Changes in Micturition (Voiding)

Normal micturition is a painless function occurring five to six times daily and occasionally once at night. The average person voids 1200 ml to 1500 ml of urine in 24 hours. This of course is modified by fluid intake, sweating, outside temperature, vomiting, or diarrhea.

Urinary frequency is voiding that occurs more often than usual when compared to the patient's usual pattern or generally accepted norm of once every 3 to 6 hours. It may result from a variety of conditions: infection, diseases of the urinary tract, metabolic disease, hypertension, and certain medications (diuretics).

Urgency (strong desire to void) may be due to inflammatory lesions in the bladder, prostate, or urethra; acute bacterial infections, chronic prostatitis in men; and chronic posterior urethrotrigonitis in women.

Burning on urination is seen in patients with urethral irritation or bladder infection. Urethritis frequently causes burning during the act of voiding, whereas cystitis may produce burning both during and after urination.

Pneumaturia (passage of gas in the urine while voiding) raises the suspicion of sigmoid diverticulitis, or a fistulous connection between the bowel and bladder, rectosigmoid cancer, regional enteritis, or the presence of gasforming urinary tract infections.

Dysuria (painful or difficult voiding) stems from a wide variety of pathologic conditions.

Strangury is slow and painful urination in which only small amounts of urine are voided. Blood staining may be noted. This may be seen in severe cystitis.

Hesitancy (undue delay and difficulty in initiating voiding) may indicate compression of the urethra or neurogenic bladder, or outlet obstruction.

Nocturia (excessive urination at night) suggests decreased renal concentrating ability, heart failure, diabetes mellitus, or poor bladder emptyings.

Urinary incontinence (involuntary loss of urine) may result from injury of the external urinary sphincter, acquired neurogenic disease, and severe urgency from infection.

Stress incontinence (intermittent leakage of urine from sudden strain) is from weakness of the sphincteric mechanism.

Enuresis (involuntary voiding during sleep) is physiologic to the age of 3 years. After this it may be functional or symptomatic of obstructive disease of the lower urinary tract.

Polyuria (large volume of urine voided in a given time) may be due to diabetes mellitus, diabetes insipidus, chronic renal disease, diuretics, and excessive fluid intake.

Oliguria (small volume of urine; output between 100–500 ml/24 hours) and anuria (absence of urine in the bladder; output less than 50 ml/24 hours) indicate a serious renal dysfunction requiring immediate medical intervention. These conditions may occur from shock, trauma, incompatible blood transfusion, drug poisoning, etc.

Hematuria (red blood cells in the urine) is considered a serious sign since it may indicate cancer of the genitourinary tract, acute glomerulonephritis, or renal tuberculosis. The color of bloody urine is dependent upon the *p*H of the urine and the amount of blood present; acid urine is a dark, smoky color, while alkaline urine is red. Hematuria may also be due to systemic causes such as blood dyscrasias, anticoagulant therapy and neoplasms, trauma, and extreme exercise.

Proteinuria (*albuminuria*) (abnormal amounts of protein in the urine) is characteristically seen in all forms of acute and chronic renal disease. Normal urine does not contain persistent protein in significant quantities.

Gastrointestinal Symptoms

Gastrointestinal symptoms may occur with urologic conditions because the gastrointestinal and urinary tracts have common autonomic and sensory innervation and because of renointestinal reflexes. The anatomical relation of the right kidney to the colon, duodenum, head of the pancreas, common bile duct, liver, and gallbladder may also cause gastrointestinal disturbances. The left kidney is also related to the colon (splenic flexure), stomach, pancreas, and spleen. Gastrointestinal symptoms related to urologic conditions include nausea, vomiting, diarrhea, abdominal discomfort, paralytic ileus, and gastrointestinal hemorrhage.

Appendicitis also may be accompanied by urinary symptoms.

Health History and Nursing Assessment

When reviewing a health history it is essential that the patient understands the questions being asked. In discussing problems involving the genitourinary system, the patient may "forget" or deny symptoms because of anxiety or embarrassment. The following information related to urinary function is sought:

- What is the patient's chief concern? Why is he seeking help?
- What is the patient's present and past occupation(s)? (Look for occupational hazards relevant to the urinary tract; contact with chemicals, plastics, pitch, tar, rubber.)
- What is the patient's smoking history?
- What is the past history, especially in relation to urinary problems?
- Is there a family history of renal disease?
- What childhood diseases did the patient have?
- Is there a history of urinary infections?
- Did enuresis extend beyond the usual age (past 3 years old)?
- Is nocturia present or absent? Date of onset?

- Are there any disorders of voiding?
  Dysuria? When does it occur? Where is it felt? Initial or terminal dysuria?
  Hesitancy? Straining? Pain during or after urination?
  Changes in color of urine? Diminished urine output?
  Incontinence? Stress incontinence? Urgency incontinence?
  Any history of hematuria?
- Is pain present?
  Location? Character? Radiation? Duration? Related to voiding? What brings it on? What relieves it?
- Has the patient had fever? Chills? Passage of stones?
- Any history of genital lesions or sexually transmitted diseases?
- For the female patient:
  Number of children? Their ages?
  Forceps deliveries?
  Catheterized? When?
  Any signs of vaginal discharge? Vaginal/vulvar itch or irritation?
- Does the patient have diabetes mellitus? Hypertension? Allergies?
- Has the patient ever been hospitalized with urinary tract infection?
  Before the age of 12?
  Cystoscopy? Indwelling catheter? Kidney x-ray procedures?

The nurse not only elicits information about the patient's physical complaints, but also assesses his psychosocial status and educational needs. The nurse evaluates the patient's anxiety (including perceived threats to body image), support systems, and sociocultural patterns. By putting together the information gathered during the initial and subsequent nursing assessments, the nurse finds valuable clues regarding misunderstandings, lack of knowledge, and needs for patient teaching.

Physical Assessment

By direct palpation it is sometimes possible to determine the size and movability of the kidneys.

- Place one hand on the patient's back so that the fingers are clear of the lower ribs and the other hand (palm down) is located anterior to the kidney with the fingers just above the level of umbilicus.
- Ask the patient to inhale deeply, then push the anterior hand forward.

It may be possible to feel the smooth, rounded lower pole of the kidney; the right is more easily felt than the left because it is somewhat lower than the left.

Renal disease may produce tenderness over the costovertebral angle. (The costovertebral angle lies where the twelfth or bottom rib joins the spine.)

In a rectal examination in the male, the prostate gland may be palpated digitally as a part of the study of urinary difficulty that occurs when there is hyperplasia of the prostate in older men (see p. 1093).

The inguinal area is examined for enlarged nodes, inguinal or femoral hernia, and a varicocele. In women the vulva, urethra, and vagina are examined.

Diagnostic Assessment

Roentgenograms

Roentgenograms are used in a variety of ways to study the urinary tract. The examination usually begins with a plain film of the abdomen or KUB (kidney, ureters, and bladder) to delineate the size, shape, and position of the kidneys, and to reveal any deviations, such as calcifications (stones) in the kidneys or urinary tract, hydronephrosis, cysts, tumors, or kidney displacement by abnormalities in the surrounding tissues.

Infusion Drip Pyelography. Infusion drip pyelography is an intravenous infusion of a large volume of dilute solution of contrast material to produce opacification of the renal parenchyma and complete filling of the urinary tract. This method of examination is especially useful when regular urographic techniques fail to show the drainage structures satisfactorily (*e.g.,* in a patient with an elevated blood urea nitrogen) or when prolonged opacification of the drainage structures is desired so that tomograms (body section radiography) can be made. Films are obtained at specified intervals after the start of the infusion to demonstrate the filled and distended collecting system. The patient preparation is the same as for excretory urography except the patient is not dehydrated. (See below.)

Excretory Urography (Intravenous Urogram or Intravenous Pyelogram). An excretory urogram or intravenous pyelogram (IVP) is the introduction (IV) of a radiopaque contrast medium that concentrates in the urine and thus permits visualization of the kidneys, ureter, and bladder. The contrast medium is cleared from the bloodstream by renal excretion. A *nephrotomogram* (body section roentgenograms that bring into focus the different layers of the kidney and the diffuse structures within each layer) is done as part of the study.

Excretory urography is conducted as part of the initial assessment of any suspected urologic problem, especially in the diagnosis of lesions in the kidneys and ureters. It also provides a rough estimate of renal function. The contrast material, such as sodium diatrizoate or meglumine diatrizoate is given intravenously, after which multiple films are taken serially to visualize drainage structures.

Patient Preparation. The patient may be prepared for the procedure as follows:

1. A laxative may be given the night before the scheduled examination to eliminate feces and gas in the intestinal tract.
2. Liquids may be restricted 8 to 10 hours before the test. However, elderly patients with poor renal reserve or marginal renal function, or patients with multiple myeloma may not tolerate dehydrating procedures and should be given water to drink. Persons with uncontrolled diabetes mellitus may also be sensitive to fluid restriction.

3. The patient should not be overhydrated since this may dilute the contrast material causing inadequate visualization.
4. The patient's history should be checked for any indications of allergies that might cause an adverse reaction to the contrast material.

If the patient has a positive allergic history, a test dose of the contrast material may be injected intradermally. If no skin reaction occurs in 15 minutes, the regular intravenous test dose of contrast material is given. Although rare, as with the administration of any intravenous drug, an anaphylactoid reaction may occur. This reaction may occur even though the skin sensitivity test has been negative.

- All IV urogram rooms should have emergency drugs (epinephrine, corticosteroids, vasopressors, etc.), as well as oxygen, tracheostomy equipment, etc., ready for immediate therapy in case an anaphylactoid reaction occurs.

Retrograde Pyelography. In retrograde pyelography, ureteral catheters are passed up through the ureters into the renal pelvis by means of cystoscopic manipulation. A contrast material is then introduced into the catheters by gravity or syringe. Retrograde pyelography is usually done if intravenous urography provides inadequate visualization of the collecting systems. It is being used less frequently because of improved techniques in excretory urography.

Cystogram. A catheter is inserted into the bladder and contrast material instilled to outline the bladder wall and to evaluate vesicoureteral reflux (backflow of urine from the bladder into one or both ureters). Cystograms are also taken in conjunction with simultaneous pressure recordings inside the bladder.

Cystourethrogram. A cystourethrogram provides visualization of the urethra and bladder either by retrograde injection of the contrast material into the urethra and bladder or by roentgenograms taken while the patient voids the contrast material. In a *voiding cystourethrogram,* the bladder is filled with contrast material and the patient voids while rapid spot films are taken. With the image intensifier, the presence or absence of vesicoureteral reflux or congenital abnormalities of the lower urinary tract can be demonstated. It is also used to investigate the problems of bladder emptying and incontinence.

Renal Angiography. The purpose of this procedure is to visualize the renal arterial supply. A special needle is used to pierce the femoral (or axillary) artery, and a catheter is threaded up through the femoral and iliac arteries into the aorta or renal artery. Contrast material is injected to opacify the renal arterial supply. Angiography evaluates blood flow dynamics, demonstrates abnormal vasculature, and differentiates primarily renal cysts from renal tumors.

Nursing Implications. Before the procedure a cathartic may be prescribed to eliminate fecal material and gas from the colon so that unobstructed x-rays will be visualized. The proposed injection sites (groin for femoral approach or axilla for axillary approach) are shaved. The peripheral pulse sites (radial, femoral, dorsalis pedis) are marked for easy access in postprocedural assessment. The patient is informed that a transient feeling of heat may be sensed along the course of the vessel when the contrast material is injected.

Following the procedure, the vital signs are taken until stable. If the axillary artery was punctured, the blood pressure is taken on the opposite arm. The puncture site is examined for swelling and hematoma development. The peripheral pulses are palpated. The color and temperature of the involved extremity is noted and compared with the uninvolved extremity. Cold compresses may be applied to the puncture site to decrease edema and pain.

Computed Tomography.   Computed tomography is a noninvasive technique that provides an excellent cross-sectional view of the kidney and urinary tract. A computer measures small changes in x-ray absorption and magnifies the differences from tissue to tissue so that a display can be made and read. It provides information on the extension of invasive lesions of the kidney. No special patient preparation is needed. (See p. 331 for a more complete discussion of computed tomography.)

Ultrasonic Scan.   Ultrasound utilizes sound waves that are passed into the body. Organs in the urinary system create characteristic ultrasonic pictures. Abnormalities such as masses, malformations, or obstructions can be identified. This is a noninvasive technique and no special patient preparation is required. There are specially developed devices that permit scanning via the rectum or within the bladder.

Endourology (Urologic Endoscopic Procedures)

The Cystoscopic Examination

A direct method of urethra and bladder study and visualization is the cystoscopic examination. The cystoscope has a self-contained optical lens system that provides a magnified, illuminated view of the bladder. It also has a guide system that allows a ureteral catheter to be passed through the ureter and up into the kidney. The cystoscope can be manipulated to allow complete visualization of the urethra and bladder as well as the ureteral orifices and prostatic urethra. The cystoscope also permits the urologist to obtain a urine specimen from each kidney to evaluate renal function. Cup forceps can be inserted down the cystoscope for biopsy. Calculi may be removed from the urethra, bladder, and ureter via cystoscopy.

With the development of fiber-light illumination and flexible, interchangeable telescopes, there is better visualization. A urethroscopy is performed first. The endoscope is passed under direct vision. After inspection of the urethra, the telescope is changed so that a better view of the bladder may be obtained. Sterile irrigating solution is run in and out of the bladder to distend the bladder and wash away blood clots, thereby allowing better visualization.

The *telescope* with a very small lens is then passed through the cystoscope, enabling the urologist to view the inside of the bladder (Fig. 42-3). The use of a high-intensity light allows for a better view of the bladder and urethra and permits still and motion pictures to be taken of these structures.

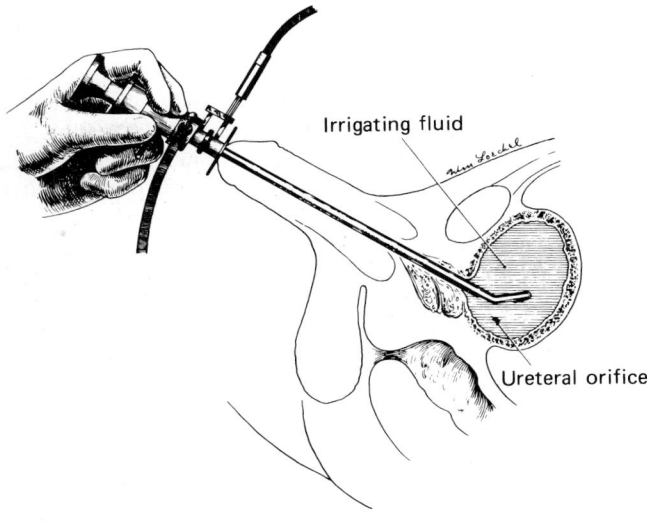

Figure 42-3.   A cystoscope being introduced into the bladder of the male. The upper cord is an electric line for the light at the distal end of the cystoscope. The lower tubing leads from a reservoir of sterile irrigating fluid that is used to inflate the bladder.

Prior to the procedure, a sedative may be given. A local topical anesthetic is instilled into the urethra by the urologist before the cystoscope is inserted. Some patients are given intravenous diazepam (Valium) in combination with topical urethral anesthesia. Occasionally, it may be necessary to use spinal or general anesthesia.

Nursing Intervention.   As with many diagnostic procedures, the nurse explains the meaning of the examination in order to inform the patient and allay his fears. Additional preprocedure preparation usually includes having the patient drink one or two glasses of water before going to the examining department.

Postprocedure management is directed at relieving any possible discomfort resulting from the examination. Some burning upon voiding, blood-tinged urine, and urinary frequency from trauma to the mucous membrane may be expected after cystoscopic examination. Moist heat to the lower abdomen or warm sitz baths are helpful in relieving pain and promoting muscle relaxation. Occasionally, following cystoscopic examination, the patient with obstructive pathology may experience urinary retention as a result of edema caused by the instrumentation. The patient with prostatic hyperplasia should especially be watched for urinary retention. Warm sitz baths and relaxant medications are helpful for relieving retention, but an indwelling catheter may have to be inserted.

Renal and Ureteral Brush Biopsy

Brush biopsy techniques provide specific information when abnormal x-ray findings of the ureter or renal pelvis raise some uncertainty as to whether the defect is a tumor, a stone, a blood clot, or an artifact. First, a cystoscopic examination is conducted. Then a ureteral catheter is introduced, followed by a biopsy brush that is passed through the catheter. The suspected lesion is brushed back and forth in order to obtain cells and surface tissue fragments for histologic analysis.

Following the procedure, the patient may be given an intravenous infusion to help clear the kidneys and prevent clot formation. Urine may show blood (usually clearing in 24 to 48 hours) from oozing at the brushing site. Postoperative renal colic occasionally occurs and responds to analgesics.

Renal endoscopy or nephroscopy is the introduction of a fiberscope into the renal pelvis during an open renal operation (pyelotomy), or percutaneously to view the interior of the renal pelvis, remove calculi, biopsy small lesions, and diagnose renal hematuria and selected renal tumors.

Needle Biopsy of the Kidney

Needle biopsy of the kidney is performed by percutaneous needle biopsy through renal tissue or by open biopsy through a small flank incision. It is useful in evaluating the course of renal disease and in securing specimens for electron and immunofluorescent microscopy, particularly for glomerular disease. Before the biopsy is carried out, an entire battery of coagulation studies are conducted to identify any patient at risk for postbiopsy bleeding.

The patient may be placed on a fasting regimen 6 to 8 hours before the test. An intravenous line is established. A urine specimen is obtained and saved for comparison with the postbiopsy specimen. Inform the patient that he will be asked to hold his breath (to stop movement of the kidney) during insertion of the renal biopsy needle.

The procedure is carried out as follows: The sedated patient is placed in a prone position with a sandbag under the abdomen. A local anesthetic agent is infiltrated into the skin at the biopsy site. The biopsy needle is introduced just inside the renal capsule of the outer quadrant of the kidney. The location of the needle may be identified through fluoroscopy or by ultrasound, in which a special probe is used. Open biopsy may be done through a small flank incision.

Postbiopsy Nursing Management.   After the specimen is obtained, pressure is applied to the kidney. To provide maximum quiet rest and to minimize bleeding, the patient may be kept in a prone position immediately following biopsy. He is kept supine as long as directed.

The nurse must be watchful for hematuria, which may appear soon after biopsy. The kidney is a highly vascular organ, and approximately one fourth of the entire cardiac output passes through it in about 1 minute. The passage of the biopsy needle lacerates the kidney capsule, and bleeding can occur in the perirenal space. Usually, the bleeding subsides on its own, but a large amount of blood can accumulate in this space in a short period of time without noticeable signs until cardiovascular collapse is evident.

- To detect early signs of bleeding it is important that the vital signs be taken every 5 to 15 minutes for the first hour and then with decreasing frequency as indicated.
- Signs suggestive of bleeding include a rise or fall in blood pressure, anorexia, vomiting, and the development of a dull, aching discomfort in the abdomen.
- Any signs of backache, shoulder pain, or dysuria are to be reported.

Flank pain may occur but usually represents bleeding into the muscle rather than around the kidney. Colicky pain similar to that of ureteral colic may develop when a clot is present in the ureter and may cause excruciating, sharp flank pain that radiates to the groin.

All urine voided by the patient is scrutinized for evidences of bleeding and compared with the prebiopsy specimen and subsequent voiding samples. If bleeding persists, as indicated by an enlarging hematoma, avoid palpating or manipulating the abdomen. A hematocrit and hemoglobin study is done within 8 hours to assess for anemia. Usually, the fluid level is kept at 3000 ml daily unless the patient has renal insufficiency. If bleeding occurs, the patient is prepared for blood transfusion and surgical intervention for control of hemorrhage, which may necessitate surgical drainage or nephrectomy (removal of kidney).

Patient Education

The nurse should keep in mind that a delayed hemorrhage can occur a number of days after biopsy. Instruct the patient to avoid strenuous activity, strenuous sports, and heavy lifting for at least 2 weeks. The physician or clinic are to be notified if any of the following occur: flank pain, hematuria, light-headedness and fainting, rapid pulse, or any other signs and symptoms of bleeding.

Radioisotope Studies

Radioisotope studies are noninvasive procedures that do not interfere with normal physiologic processes and require no specific patient preparation. Radiopharmaceuticals (^{99}Tc-labeled compound or ^{131}I-hippurate) are injected intravenously. Studies are obtained with a scintillation camera placed posterior to the kidney with the patient in a supine, prone, or sitting position. The resultant image (called a scan) indicates the distribution of the radiopharmaceutical within the kidney. (It shows a dot image on film.) See also page 339.

The Tc scan provides information about kidney perfusion and sometimes is used instead of an intravenous urogram when renal function is poor. The hippurate scan provides information about kidney function.

Urodynamic Measurements.   Urodynamic measurements provide physiologic and structural tests to evaluate bladder and urethral function by measuring the (1) rate of urine flow, (2) bladder pressures during voiding and at rest, (3) internal urethral resistance, and (4) bladder contraction and relaxation. Bioengineering approaches are combined with computer technology to study pressures (abdominal, vesical, detrusor), sphincter activity, bladder innervation, muscle tone, and sacral reflex.

The following are the most frequently performed urodynamic measurements:

Uroflowmetry (flow rate) is the record of the volume of urine passing through the urethra per time unit (ml/second).

A *cystometrogram* is a graphic recording of the pressures exerted at varying phases of filling of the urinary bladder. Intermittent filling of the bladder can be recorded and compared to changes in intravesical pressures. The patient is asked to void, and the physician observes the time it takes to initiate voiding; the size, force, and continuity of the urinary stream; the degree of straining, hesitancy; etc. The patient is then placed in a lithotomy position, and a retention catheter is passed through the urethra and into the bladder. The residual volume is measured and the catheter left in place. The urethral catheter is connected to a water manometer, and water is allowed to flow into the bladder, usually at the rate of 1 ml per second. The patient informs the examiner when he feels the first desire to void and again when the bladder feels full. The degree of bladder filling at these points is recorded. The pressures above the zero level at the symphysis pubis are measured, and the pressures and volumes within the bladder are plotted and recorded.

The *urethral pressure profile* measures urethral resistance along the length of the urethra. Gas and fluid are instilled through a catheter that is withdrawn while the pressures along the urethral wall are obtained.

A *cystourethrogram* is visualization of the urethra and bladder either by retrograde injection or by voiding of contrast material.

When using a *voiding cystourethrogram,* the bladder is filled with contrast medium, and the patient voids while rapid spot films are taken. The presence or absence of vesicoureteral reflux or congenital abnormalities in the lower urinary tract can be demonstrated. The voiding cystourethrogram is also used to investigate difficulty in bladder emptying and incontinence.

Electromyography uses the placement of electrodes in the pelvic floor/musculature or anal sphincter to evaluate neuromuscular function of the lower tract.

Urinalysis

Urinalysis provides a wealth of important clinical information and is regarded as an indispensable part of every clinical study. Urine examination of every patient includes the observation and evaluation of:

1. Urine color and clarity
2. Urine odor
3. Measurement of urine acidity and specific gravity
4. Tests for the presence of protein, glucose, and ketone bodies in the urine (proteinuria, glucosuria, and ketonuria, respectively)
5. Microscopic examination of the urine sediment after centrifuging for the detection of red blood cells (hematuria), white blood cells, casts (cylindruria), crystals (crystalluria), pus (pyuria), and bacteria (bacteriuria)

Numerous additional tests are applicable in special situations.

Collection of Urine Samples

All urine tests are performed ideally on fresh specimens, preferably the first voiding of the day since this specimen is most concentrated and more likely to reveal abnormalities. Random specimens are satisfactory for most analyses provided that they have been collected in clean containers and have been adequately protected against bacterial and chemical deterioration. Urine should not be left standing at room temperature since it becomes alkaline due to contamination of urea-splitting bacteria from the environment. All specimens should be refrigerated as soon as possible after they are voided. Microscopic examination should be done within a half hour after collection, because allowing the specimen to stand causes dissolution of cellular elements and bacterial overgrowth unless the specimen is obtained by sterile methods. Urine cultures should be processed immediately. If this is not possible, they should be stored at 4° C (39° F). *Urine specimens should be collected from the patient by means of the clean-catch midstream technique using a wide-mouthed container* (see below and Fig. 42-4).

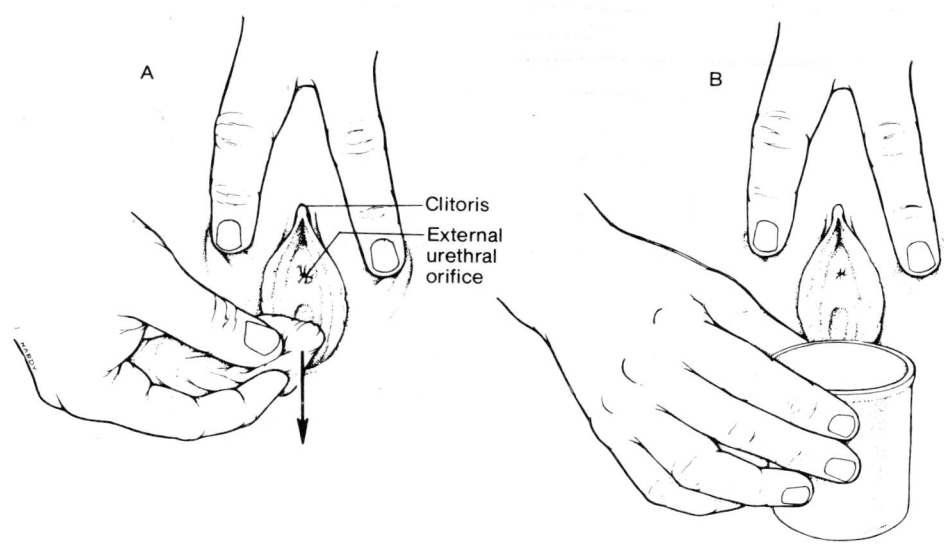

Figure 42-4. Obtaining a clean-catch midstream urine specimen in the female. (*A*) Instruct the patient to hold the labia apart and wash from high up front toward the back with gauze soaked in soap. (*B*) The collection cup is held so that it does not touch the body, and the sample is obtained only while the patient is voiding with the labia held apart.

24-Hour Urine Collections

Many quantitative analytic tests are carried out on specimens that represent the patient's urinary output over a 24-hour period. The procedure is as follows:

Instruct the patient to empty his bladder at a specified time (such as 8:00 AM). This urine is discarded. Collect all urine voided during the next 24 hours. The last specimen is collected and saved 24 hours after the collection was started (*i.e.,* 8:00 AM).

The patient's bladder should be empty when the test starts and empty when it ends. The urine is collected in a clean container. Depending on the test to be performed, a preservative may have been added or the urine may need to be refrigerated. Failure to transfer one specimen voided during the test period invalidates the test. A successful collection requires the complete understanding and cooperation on the part of the patient and all unit personnel concerned with the patient's care.

Clean-Catch Midstream Urine Specimens

Urine specimens voided in the usual manner are practically useless for bacteriologic study because of inevitable contamination by organisms residing in the vicinity of the urethral meatus. Such contamination can be avoided by catheterizing the urinary bladder. However, since the dangers of catheterization are known, especially the production of chronic pyelonephritis, this procedure is no longer recommended except for specific indications. Reliable bacteriologic studies are possible without catheterization, utilizing the so-called clean-catch midstream technique.

Instructions to the Male Patient

- Expose the glans and cleanse the area around the meatus with soap. Remove all soap with water-soaked pledgets.
- Do not collect the first portion of the voiding; discard it.
- Collect the next portion by voiding into a sterile wide-

Table 42-2
Tests of Renal Function

1. There is no single test of renal function; renal function is variable from time to time.
2. The rate of change of renal function is more important than the result of a single test.

Test	Purpose/Rationale	Test Protocol

Renal Concentration Test
  Specific gravity
  Refractive index
  Osmolality of urine
	Evaluates the ability to concentrate solutes in the urine.
	Concentration ability is lost early in kidney disease; hence, this test detects early defects in renal function
		Fluids may be withheld 12 to 24 hours to evaluate the concentrating ability of the tubules under controlled conditions. Specific gravity measurements of urine are taken at specific times to determine urine concentration

Phenolsulfonphthalein Excretion Test (PSP)	A diagnostic agent (phenolsulfonphthalein) is given to determine the functional capacity of the kidney. (PSP test can also be used as a measure to assess residual urine.) Delayed excretion is seen in renal disease, cardiac failure, primary vascular disease.	Encourage fluids 1 to 1½ hours before the test. Phenolsulfonphthalein is given IV. 1. Record exact time dye is administered. 2. Collect urine in 15 minutes, 30 minutes, and 1 hour.
Creatinine Clearance* (Endogenous creatinine clearance)	Provides a reasonable approximation of rate of glomerular filtration. Measures volume of blood cleared of creatinine in 1 minute. Most sensitive indication of early renal disease. Useful to follow progress of patient's renal status.	Collect all urine over 24-hour period. Draw one sample of blood within the period.
Serum Creatinine	A test of renal function reflecting the balance between production and filtration by renal glomerulus. Most sensitive measure of renal function.	Do test on blood serum.
Serum Urea Nitrogen (Blood Urea Nitrogen—BUN)	Serves as index of renal excretory capacity. Serum urea nitrogen is dependent on the body's urea production and on urine flow. (Urea is the nitrogenous end product of protein metabolism.) Affected by protein intake, tissue breakdown.	Do test on blood serum.

* Clearance is the amount of blood cleansed of a constituent per unit of time.

mouthed bottle or large-caliber tube that is protected by a sterile closure.

- Do not collect the last few drops of urine since prostatic secretions may be introduced into the urine at the end of the urinary stream.

Instructions to the Female Patient

- Separate the labia to expose the urethral orifice (see Fig. 42-4).
- Cleanse around the urinary meatus with sponges soaked in liquid soap.
- Wipe the perineum from the front to the back.
- Remove all soap with water-soaked pledgets, wiping from front to back.
- Keep the labia separated and void forcibly, but do not collect the first portion of the voiding. (The distal portion of the urethral orifice is colonized by bacteria; the initial voiding washes away the urethral contaminants.)
- Collect the midstream portion of the urinary flow, making sure that the container does not come in contact with the genitalia.

Renal Function Tests

Renal function tests are used to evaluate the severity of kidney disease and to follow the patient's clinical progress. These tests also give information concerning the kidneys' effectiveness in carrying out their excretory function. Renal function may be within normal limits until about 50% of renal function has been lost. Best results are obtained by combining a number of clinical tests. Table 42-2 lists the more common tests of renal function.

▷ Bibliography

Books

Alken C-E, Sokeland J, and Engel RME. Urology. Guide for Diagnosis and Therapy. New York, Georg Thieme, 1982.

Antonovych TT and Mostofi FK. Atlas of Kidney Biopsies. Washington, DC, Armed Forces Institute of Pathology, 1980.

Blandy J. Lecture Notes on Urology. Boston, Blackwell Scientific Publications, 1982.

Brenner BM and Rector FC Jr. The Kidney, Vols 1 and 2, 2nd ed. Philadelphia, WB Saunders, 1981.

Fischback F. A Manual of Laboratory Diagnostic Tests. Philadelphia, JB Lippincott, 1980.

Larson E, Lindbloom L, and Davis KB. Development of the Clinical Nephrology Practitioner. St Louis, CV Mosby, 1982.

Lerner J and Khan Z. Mosby's Manual of Urologic Nursing. St Louis, CV Mosby, 1982.

McConnell EA and Zimmerman MF. Care of Patients with Urologic Problems. Philadelphia, JB Lippincott, 1982.

Mitchell JP. Endoscopic Operative Urology. Boston, Wright PSG, 1981.

Schrier RW. Manual of Nephrology. Boston, Little, Brown & Co, 1981.

Schulman CC. Advances in Diagnostic Urology. New York, Springer–Verlag, 1981.

Articles
Assessment/Diagnostic Studies

Boh DM and VanSon AR. The water-load test. Am J Nurs 1982 Jan; 82(1):112–113.

Clayman RV et al. Nephroscopy: advances and adjuncts. Urol Clin North Am 1982 Feb; 9(1):51–63.

Constantinou CE. Principles and methods of clinical urodynamic investigations. Critical Reviews in Biomedical Engineering 1982 Feb; 7(3):229–264.

Maree SM. Assessing the excretory system. AORN J 1981 Mar; 33(4):734–756.

McConnell EA. Urinalysis: A common test, but never routine. Nursing '82 1982 Feb; 12(2):108–111.

Werner JR and Bartone FF. Urodynamic assessment of the urologic patient. Nebr Med J 1981 Nov; 66(11):242–244.

Zinner NR and Sterling AM. Female incontinence. Prog Clin Biol Res 1981; 78:1–407 (entire volume).

Agencies
Governmental

National Institute of Arthritis, Metabolism and Digestive Diseases, National Institutes of Health, Bethesda, Md. 20205

Voluntary

National Kidney Foundation, 116 E 27th St., New York, N.Y. 10016

United Ostomy Association, 1111 Wilshire Blvd., Los Angeles, Calif. 90017

43

Management of Patients With Renal and Urinary Dysfunction

▷ Psychosocial Considerations

Conditions of the genitourinary tract may precipitate emotional stresses and problems related to feelings of guilt and embarrassment when the external genitalia are examined and treated. Problems of incontinence may cause disgust and feelings of helplessness. Some patients are constantly uneasy over the possibility of an "accident," although others appear careless and indifferent.

Operations on the male organs of reproduction can pose a threat to the masculinity of the patient, no matter what his age. Although many men may hide their fears of impotency by blaming "prostate trouble," many male sexual problems (difficulties in erection, premature ejaculation, etc.) are psychological in origin and related to a variety of causes—fear, guilt, aversion to partner, fatigue. Because of hidden fears, a male patient may react with anger and hostility to those caring for him, or his anger may turn inward and produce more than the usual amount of pain. Patients with urinary infections sometimes become depressed when they undergo prolonged periods of treatment. Anxiety in any stressful situation can produce urinary frequency and urgency.

The urologic patient, as any other patient, needs to feel respected as an individual and understood. He wants his questions answered, his fears allayed, and his discomfort relieved. Reassurance is a part of nursing, and these patients may require more than the usual amount of reassurance, support, and acceptance.

▷ Fluid and Electrolyte Imbalance

Assessment

A major problem for patients with renal disorders is the maintenance of fluid and electrolyte balance. The nurse must be skilled and conscientious in observing the clinical condition of the patient, and in recording the data gathered.

Every patient with a urologic disorder has a fluid intake-output chart on which is recorded all fluid intake, whether by ingestion or by parenteral administration. The volume of urine excreted also is recorded. In addition, temperatures are recorded every 4 hours, and the weight once daily. All these records provide invaluable assistance in determining how much fluid the patient should receive.

The nurse should also be alert to a host of signs and symptoms pertaining to body fluid disturbances (see Chap. 9 and also pp. 958–959). For example, the following symptoms are prone to occur in patients with renal disease:

1. Acute weight loss (in excess of 5%), a drop in body temperature, dryness of skin and mucous membranes, longitudinal wrinkles or furrows of tongue, and oliguria or anuria—could indicate volume deficit of extracellular fluid
2. Acute weight gain (in excess of 5%), edema, moist crackles in lungs, puffy eyelids, and shortness of breath—could indicate volume excess of extracellular fluid
3. Abdominal cramps, apprehension, convulsions, fingerprinting on sternum, and oliguria or anuria—could indicate sodium deficit of extracellular fluid
4. Dry, sticky mucous membranes, flushed skin, oliguria, or anuria, thirst, and rough and dry tongue—could indicate sodium excess of extracellular fluid
5. Anorexia; gaseous distention of intestines; silent intestinal ileus; weakness; and soft, flabby muscles—could indicate potassium deficit of extracellular fluid
6. Diarrhea, intestinal colic, irritability, and nausea—could indicate potassium excess of extracellular fluid
7. Abdominal cramps, carpopedal spasm, muscle cramps, tetany, and tingling of ends of fingers—could indicate calcium deficit of extracellular fluid
8. Deep bone pain; flank pain; and muscle hypotonicity—could indicate calcium excess of extracellular fluid
9. Deep, rapid breathing (Kussmaul); shortness of breath on exertion; stupor; and weakness—could indicate primary base bicarbonate deficit of extracellular fluid
10. Depressed respiration, muscle hypertonicity, and tetany—could indicate primary base bicarbonate excess of extracellular fluid
11. Chronic weight loss; emotional depression; pallor; ready fatigue; and soft, flabby muscles—could indicate protein deficit of extracellular fluid
12. Positive Chvostek's sign, convulsions, disorientation, hyperactive deep reflexes, and tremor—could indicate magnesium deficit of extracellular fluid

The nurse must possess a thorough understanding of the patient's gains and losses of body fluids and must share this information with other members of the team caring for the patient. When supervising intravenous therapy, the nurse adjusts the flow rate in accordance with the physician's request.

Repeated blood examinations are essential for maintaining surveillance of electrolyte balance. The nurse usually has the responsibility of preparing the patient for these somewhat unpleasant venipunctures by explaining that the studies are essential for the best possible care.

▷ Maintaining Adequate Urinary Drainage

In the patient with urologic disease, as in any other patient (or any normal individual, for that matter) urinary excretion of waste materials is imperative. The composition of the body fluids is determined not so much by what the patient ingests as by what the kidneys keep. In health, the kidneys are amazingly efficient, excreting the materials that are not needed and retaining those that are. But in the patient with damaged kidneys, all therapeutic efforts are directed toward seeing that the homeostatic capabilities of the kidneys are not exceeded.

When drainage of the urinary system becomes necessary, catheters are inserted directly into the bladder, the ureters, or the kidney pelves. Catheters must be chosen for the purpose in mind. They come in various sizes, shapes, and lengths and may have one or more openings placed in various positions near the tip. A catheter may be constructed of hard or soft rubber, woven fabric, silicone, metal, glass, or plastic. The tip may be opened or closed and may have a mushroom shape, such as the Pezzer catheter; a winged shape, such as the Malecot catheter; or may simply be round and blunt.

Catheterization

Principles of Management

There are times when the catheter is a lifesaving instrument, as is the case when the patient is unable to void. At other times, catheterization may be necessary to determine the amount of residual urine in the bladder after the patient has voided, to bypass an obstruction that blocks the flow of urine, or to provide postoperative drainage following an operation on the bladder or a prostatectomy.

- No patient should be catheterized unless absolutely necessary since catheterization can lead to urinary tract infection.

Urinary tract infections appear to be responsible for 35% of all hospital-acquired infections; most of these follow instrumentation of the urinary tract, mainly catheterization. The pathogens responsible for catheter-associated urinary tract infections include *Escherichia coli, Klebsiella, Proteus, Pseudomonas, Enterobacter, Serratia,* and *Candida.* Many of these are part of the patient's endogenous bowel flora or are acquired by cross contamination by patients or hospital personnel or by exposure to nonsterile equipment.

Microorganisms may gain access to the urinary tract by three main pathways: (1) through introduction from the urethra into the bladder at the time of catheterization; (2) from the thin film of urethral fluid outside of the catheter at the catheter–mucosa interface; and (3) by migration to the bladder along the internal lumen of the catheter after contamination (most common).

To safeguard the patient, the following points of care are essential in urethral catheter management:

- Strict surgical asepsis is employed.
- The urethra is adequately cleansed.
- The catheter should be smaller than the external urinary meatus to help minimize trauma and allow secretions to drain out alongside the catheter.
- The catheter is well lubricated with an appropriate antimicrobial lubricant.
- The catheter is passed gently and skillfully.
- The catheter is removed as soon as possible.

Nursing Care of the Patient With an Indwelling Catheter and a Closed Urinary Drainage System. When an indwelling catheter is necessary, a closed drainage system is essential. (A closed drainage system is one that is closed to outside air.) Such a system may consist of an indwelling catheter, a connecting tube, and a collecting bag emptied by a drainage valve. Or it may consist of a triple-lumen indwelling urethral catheter attached to a closed sterile drainage system. The three-way catheter allows urinary drainage through one channel, inflation of the bag with water or air through the second channel, and a continuous irrigation of the bladder with antibacterial solution through the third channel.

▶ **Assessment**

The patient who has an indwelling catheter should be observed for signs and symptoms of urinary tract infection: cloudy urine, hematuria, fever, chills, anorexia, and malaise. The area around the urethral orifice should be observed for suppurative drainage and excoriation. Frequent urine cultures (daily or every other day) provide the most accurate means for assessment of infection.

Nursing assessment also includes observation of the drainage system to assure that the system constantly provides for adequate drainage of urine. The catheter itself is observed to make sure that it is properly anchored to prevent pressure on the urethra at the penoscrotal junction in the male patient, and tension and traction of the bladder in both male and female patients. An accurate record of the patient's fluid intake and urine output provides additional information about the adequacy of urine elimination.

Patient Problems/Nursing Diagnoses

The patient's major nursing problems include potential for development of urinary tract infection related to catheter-induced pathogenic microorganisms and inadequate drainage of urine; potential for trauma to urethra or bladder related to improper positioning of the external portion of the catheter; and possible nonadherence to catheter-care regimen.

▶ **Planning and Nursing Implementation**

Goals

The major goals for the patient include:

1. Absence of urinary tract infection
2. Absence of trauma to urethra and bladder
3. Adherence to regimen for catheter care

Nursing Interventions

Certain principles of care should be followed when managing a closed urinary drainage system:

- In order to prevent contamination of a closed system, the tubing should not be disconnected, nor should any part of the collecting bag or drainage tube be contaminated.
- The bag should not be raised above the level of the patient's bladder since this will cause reflux of contaminated urine into the patient's bladder from the bag. Urine flow must be downhill.
- Columns of urine should not be allowed to collect in the tubing since a free flow of urine must be maintained to prevent infection. Improper drainage occurs when the tubing is kinked or twisted, allowing pools of drainage to collect in the loops of the tubing.
- The drainage bag should not be allowed to touch the floor. The bag and collecting tubing must be changed if contamination occurs, if the urine flow becomes obstructed, or if the junctions start to leak.
- The bag should be drained at least every 8 hours and more frequently if there is a large volume of urine, to lessen the risk of bacterial proliferation.
- Care should be taken to see that the drainage tube (valve/spout) is not contaminated. Each patient should have his own urine receptacle in which to empty the bag.

The catheter acts as a foreign body in the urethra and produces a reaction in the urethral mucosa with some urethral discharge. Formerly, frequent cleansing of the meatal catheter junction and applications of antimicrobial solutions were recommended to block the pathway of bacteria entering the bladder and to reduce the number of bacteria on the meatal surface. Studies suggest that current methods of meatal care should be discouraged, as catheter manipulation during cleansing may be causing increasing rates of infection. Gentle washing with nonantiseptic soap during the daily bath is warranted to remove gross debris and obvious encrustations from the external catheter surface. The catheter is anchored as securely as possible to prevent to-and-fro movement in the urethra. Suppurative drainage and encrustation occur at the exit of any tube. Encrustation arising from urinary salts may enter the bladder when the catheter is removed and may serve as a nucleus for stone formation. There appears to be significantly less encrustation associated with silicone catheters. The introduction of 10 ml of 10% povidone-iodine into the drain spout three times daily after draining the collecting bag has been shown to block the entry of bacteria in the collecting spout.

A liberal fluid intake must be ensured in order to produce mechanical flushing and to dilute urinary elements producing encrustation. (The intake must be within limits of the patient's cardiac reserve.) Keeping the urine acid helps to prevent tube obstruction and encrustation of urinary sand and calculus deposits. Oral intake of ascorbic acid and potassium acid phosphate, and an acid ash diet help to acidify urine.

Urine cultures should be monitored daily or every other day as a means of surveying for infection. Many catheters have an aspiration (puncture) port from which a specimen can be obtained.

Measures must be taken to prevent cross contamination since many urinary tract infections are due to extrinsically acquired organisms transmitted by cross contamination. Patients at risk are women, elderly debilitated patients, and those who are critically ill.

- There must be renewed emphasis on *handwashing* between patients and before and after handling any part of the catheter or drainage system.
- Catheterized patients with bacteria in the urine should not be in the same room with noninfected catheterized patients. It is best to assign only one patient with an indwelling catheter to a room.

Anchoring the Indwelling Catheter. The catheter must be properly secured to prevent movement and traction on the urethra. In the male patient, the catheter is taped horizontally to the thigh (Fig. 43-1) or to the abdomen to prevent pressure on the urethra at the penoscrotal junction, which can eventually lead to the formation of a urethrocutaneous fistula.

In the female patient, the drainage tubing attached to the catheter is taped to the thigh to prevent tension and traction on the bladder.

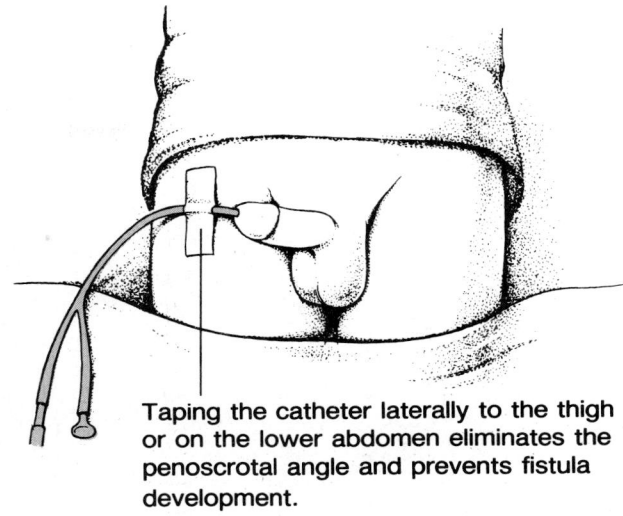

Taping the catheter laterally to the thigh or on the lower abdomen eliminates the penoscrotal angle and prevents fistula development.

Figure 43-1. The catheter is taped to the thigh or to the abdomen in the male patient.

▶ Evaluation

Expected Outcomes

1. Is free of urinary tract infection
   a. Excretes urine that is clear and yellow or amber, with a specific gravity of 1.005 to 1.025
   b. Has a negative urine culture for microorganisms
   c. Has a normal temperature
   d. Demonstrates adequate fluid intake and urine output
   e. Does not have excessive drainage or excoriation around urethral orifice
2. Is free of trauma to urethra and bladder after catheter is removed
   a. Is free of pain or discomfort on voiding
   b. Eliminates 200 ml to 400 ml of urine with each voiding
   c. Shows no signs of urinary incontinence
3. Adheres to regimen for catheter care and participates in care of catheter as able
   a. Cleans around meatal-catheter junction daily
   b. Avoids kinking or twisting drainage tubing
   c. Maintains position of drainage bag below the level of the bladder
   d. Checks drainage tube periodically for free flow of urine
   e. Maintains proper anchorage of catheter to thigh

▷ Suprapubic Bladder Aspiration

Suprapubic bladder aspiration is a method of establishing drainage from the bladder by inserting a catheter or tube through the suprapubic area into the bladder by either a stab incision or puncture with a needle or trocar. It is used as a temporary measure to divert the flow of urine from the urethra when the urethral route is impassable (urethral injuries; strictures; prostatic obstruction) following gynecologic operations, when bladder dysfunction is apt to occur

(vaginal hysterectomy, vaginal repair surgery), and after pelvic fractures.

The patient lies supine. The bladder is distended with sterile saline solution via a urethral catheter (which is then removed), or the patient is given fluids before the procedure (oral or intravenous). Distention of the bladder makes the bladder easier to locate by the suprapubic route.

The suprapubic area is surgically prepared and the puncture site located approximately 5 cm above the symphysis. The procedure may be accomplished by open operation (incision of the bladder) or by puncture with a trocar/cannula assembly. The trocar/cannula is passed in a slightly caudal direction, and entrance into the bladder is verified by reflux of urine through a hole in the trocar/cannula. A catheter is threaded through the cannula into the bladder (Fig. 43-2). The cannula is withdrawn, leaving the catheter in place. The catheter is secured with sutures, tape, or a body-seal system, and the area around the catheter is covered with a sterile dressing. The drainage tubing is attached to a closed sterile system and the tubing secured to the lateral abdomen with tape to prevent undue tension on the catheter.

Suprapubic bladder drainage may be maintained continuously for several weeks. If a trial of voiding is requested, the catheter is clamped for 4 hours, during which time the patient attempts to void. After the patient voids, the catheter is unclamped and the residual urine measured. Usually, if the amount of residual urine is less than 100 ml on two separate occasions (morning and evening), the catheter may be removed. However, if the patient complains of pain or discomfort, the catheter is usually left open.

Usually, patients with suprapubic drainage are able to void sooner after surgery than those with urethral catheters. Suprapubic drainage is also considered to be more comfortable than an indwelling catheter, provides greater patient mobility, allows measurement of residual volume without urethral instrumentation, and presents less of a risk for bladder infection. The suprapubic catheter is removed upon request, and a sterile dressing is placed over the site.

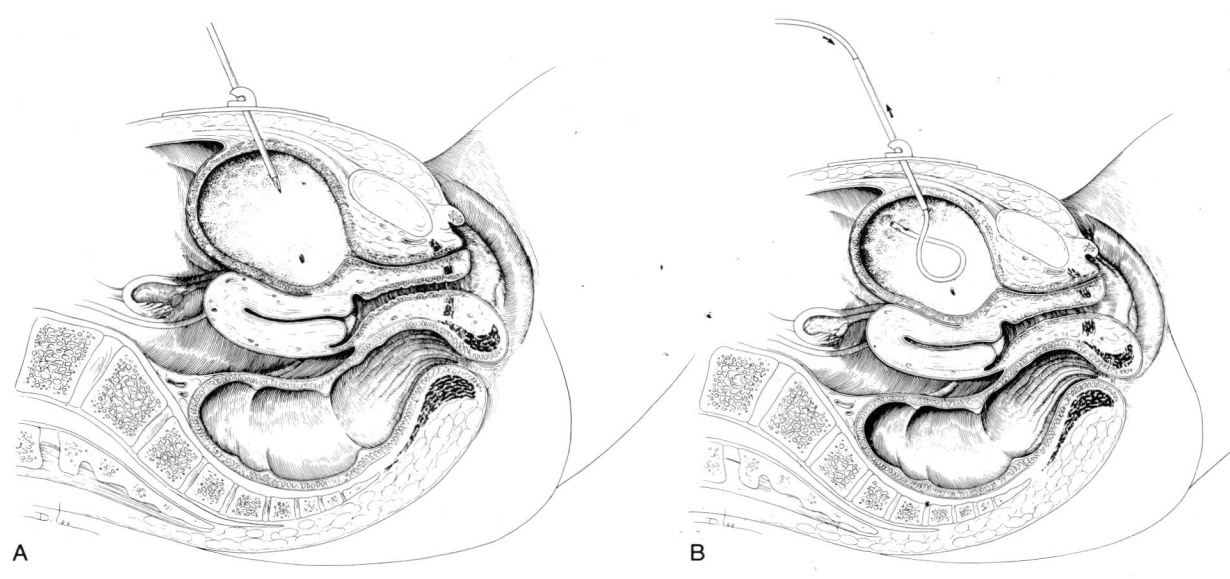

A   B

Figure 43-2. (*A*) A SILASTIC® Cystocath® Suprapubic Drainage System (Reif Design). Using steady pressure, the trocar-cannula is passed in a slightly caudal direction until entrance into the bladder is felt: The trocar-cannula is shown in its correct bladder entry position. The position can be verified by reflux of urine up through the trocar-cannula. (*B*) The silicone drainage catheter is inserted through the cannula and well into the bladder. The catheter is inserted before the bladder is completely decompressed. When removing the cannula, the catheter should be held fairly straight so that it will not accidentally get caught on the rim of the cannula as the cannula is withdrawn. This will prevent the inadvertent withdrawal of the catheter from the bladder while the cannula is removed. (Courtesy, Dow Corning Corporation.)

▷ Urinary Retention

Urinary retention (both acute and chronic) refers to the inability to urinate despite a desire to do so. Chronic retention will often lead to overflow incontinence (due to pressure of retained urine in the bladder) or residual urine. *Residual urine* is the term applied to urine that remains in the bladder after voiding.

The problem of retention may arise in any postoperative patient, particularly those who have undergone surgery on the perineal or anal regions resulting in reflex spasm of the sphincters. It may also occur in the acutely ill, the elderly, or the bedridden. Urinary retention may be due to anxiety, prostatic enlargement, urethral pathology (infection, tumor, calculus), trauma, neurogenic bladder dysfunction, and other conditions. Certain medications cause retention. These include anticholinergics–antispasmodics, such as atropine; antidepressant–antipsychotic agents, such as phenothiazine; antihistamine preparations, such as pseudoephedrine hydrochloride (Sudafed); beta-adrenergic blockers, such as propranolol, and antihypertensive agents, such as hydralazine.

Complications that arise from retention include infection (which may readily develop as a result of overdistension of the bladder) or even impaired renal function, especially if obstructive uropathy (pathologic change in urinary tract due to obstruction) is present.

Nursing Assessment

The signs and symptoms of urinary retention may easily be overlooked unless there is a conscious effort to check their presence.

- Determine the time of the last voiding.
- Is the patient passing small amounts of urine frequently?
- Is the patient dribbling?
- Is the patient complaining of pain or discomfort in the lower abdomen? (Note, however, that discomfort may be relatively mild if the bladder distends slowly.)
- Check for signs of a rounded swelling arising out of the pelvis, which could indicate retention.
- Palpate the suprapubic area for an oval-shaped mass.

Goals and Interventions

The goal of nursing management is to prevent overdistension of the bladder with resultant infection and to treat the underlying cause. Nursing measures to encourage voiding include providing privacy, helping the patient to the bathroom or commode in order to provide a more natural setting for voiding, or allowing the male patient to stand beside the bed while using the urinal, since most men find this position more comfortable and natural for urination. Additional measures include providing a source of warmth to relax the sphincters (*i.e.*, sitz baths, warm compresses to the perineum, showers), giving the patient hot tea to drink, and offering psychological reassurance and support.

Following surgical procedures, the prescribed analgesic should be administered because pain in the incisional area can make voiding difficult. When the patient cannot void, careful catheterization is resorted to in order to decompress the bladder before overdistention occurs. In the case of prostatic obstruction, attempts at catheterization (by the urologist) may not be successful, requiring that a suprapubic cystostomy be done.

Urinary Incontinence

If urinary incontinence (involuntary loss of urine) results from an inflammatory condition (cystitis), it will probably be temporary in nature. However, if it results from a serious neurologic condition (paraplegia), it could easily be a permanent problem.

Stress incontinence is the involuntary loss of urine through an intact urethra as a result of a sudden increase in intra-abdominal pressure. It is seen mostly in women and is due to congenital conditions (exstrophy of the bladder, ectopic ureter) or to obstetrical injury, lesions of the bladder neck, extrinsic pelvic disease, fistulae, detrusor dysfunction, and a variety of other conditions.

The therapy for this type of incontinence is usually surgical correction. There are a wide range of surgical procedures: vaginal repair, abdominal suspension of the bladder, elevation of the bladder neck, etc. A modified artificial sphincter that uses a silicone-rubber balloon as a self-regulating pressure mechanism is being used to provide urethral closing. Another method of controlling stress incontinence is through the application of electronic stimulation to the pelvic floor by means of a miniature pulse generator with electrodes mounted on an intra-anal plug.

Management.   Most patients with urinary incontinence can be conditioned to gain urinary control through systematic habit training or the establishment of an automatic bladder. Such a program requires more nursing time than changing the patient's wet bed, but it is most rewarding to see a patient lose his fear of embarrassment as progress is made in rehabilitation. The rehabilitation of the patient with urinary incontinence is discussed on page 251.

▷ Neurogenic Bladder

Neurogenic bladder refers to a bladder disturbance that results from a lesion of the nervous system. It may be caused by spinal cord injury or tumor, certain neurologic diseases (multiple sclerosis), congenital anomalies (spina bifida, myelomeningocele), and infection.

There are two types of neurogenic bladders: spastic and flaccid. The spastic (reflex or automatic) bladder disorder is caused by any lesion of the cord above the voiding reflex arc (upper motor neuron lesion). The result is a loss of conscious sensation and cerebral motor control. There is reduced bladder capacity and marked hypertrophy of the bladder wall. As a result, the bladder behaves in a reflex fashion with minimal or no controlling influence to regulate its activity.

The flaccid (atonic, nonreflex, or autonomous) neurogenic bladder is caused by a lower motor neuron lesion, most commonly due to trauma. The bladder continues to fill and becomes greatly distended. The bladder muscle does not contract forcefully at any time. Sensory loss may accompany a flaccid bladder, and the patient is unaware of discomfort. Overdistention causes damage to the bladder musculature, infection due to stagnant urine, and infection of the kidneys by back pressure of urine.

The major complication of neurogenic bladder is infection that results from stasis of urine and subsequent catheterization. Hypertrophy of the bladder walls also results, ultimately leading to vesicoureteral reflux and hydronephrosis. Urolithiasis may develop from urinary stasis and infection and from demineralization of bone from the patient's being on prolonged bed rest. Renal failure is the major cause of death of patients with neurologic impairment of the bladder.

Nursing Goals and Interventions

The care of the patient with neurogenic bladder is a major challenge to the nurse. There are several long-term objectives to attain: (1) to prevent overdistention of the bladder, (2) to empty the bladder regularly and completely, (3) to maintain urine sterility with no stone formation, and (4) to maintain adequate bladder capacity without ureterovesical reflux.

The immediate management of the patient with a neurogenic bladder consists of catheterizing the patient intermittently or inserting a three-way catheter with closed drainage to avoid overdistention. In intermittent catheterization, the bladder is catheterized at designated intervals (4, 6, or 8 hours) with a small catheter. This intermittent emptying approximates physiologic bladder function and circumvents complications usually encountered with an indwelling catheter; however, strict asepsis is necessary. An hourly fluid intake and output record is kept to assess individual output patterns. The patient may be taught self-catheterization (see p. 976).

If continuous catheterization and drainage are used in a male patient, the catheter is taped to the abdomen to avoid the sharp angulation of the catheter and prevent pressure at the penoscrotal angle.

With the use of either intermittent or continuous catheterization, a liberal fluid intake is encouraged to reduce the urinary bacterial count, reduce stasis, decrease the concentration of calcium in the urine, and minimize the precipitation of urinary crystals and subsequent stone formation. The patient is kept as mobile as possible and is up on the tilt table or wheelchair or prepared for ambulation. The diet is low in calcium to prevent calculosis (presence of calculi).

Diagnostic Studies.   As soon as the patient's condition permits, evaluation studies are performed to assess for bladder and bladder neck problems. The initial studies provide a baseline against which later changes can be measured. Serial studies of BUN, creatinine clearance, and serum creatinine are done to determine the status of renal function. A cystogram determines the presence of vesicoureteral reflux. A urethrogram may be done to detect the presence of urethral complications. Pressure and flow studies as well as an IV urogram are also carried out. A cystoscopic examination may be requested to assess loss of muscle fibers and elastic tissues and to provide an opportunity for biopsy if necessary.

Treatment of Chronic Phase. The problems of patients with neurogenic bladder disease vary considerably from patient to patient. It is difficult to assess what the rehabilitation potential and eventual urologic disability may be.

If possible, the objective is to develop effective spontaneous reflex voiding, which is accomplished in the following manner:

- Ask the patient to drink a measured amount of fluid from 8 AM to 10 PM; no fluids (except sips) are taken after 10 PM to avoid bladder overdistention.
- At a specific time(s) the patient attempts to void by applying pressure over the bladder, by tapping the abdomen, or by stretching the anal sphincter with a finger to trigger the bladder.
- Immediately following the voiding attempt, catheterize the patient to determine the amount of residual urine. Measure all urine voided and catheterized.
- Palpate the bladder at repeated intervals to determine whether the bladder is being emptied.
- Caution the patient to be alert for any signs that indicate a full bladder: perspiration, coldness of hands or feet, feelings of anxiety, etc.
- The intervals between catheterization are lengthened and the patient's program is moved forward as less and less residual urine is measured. Catheterization is usually discontinued when the volume of residual urine is at an acceptable level compatible with urine sterility and radiologic normalcy of the upper urinary tract.

Flaccid Bladder

A patient with a flaccid bladder may be placed on the same type of bladder routine as outlined above. A 2-hour voiding schedule is established to prevent overdistention. Parasympathomimetic drugs (bethanechol [Urecholine]) may help to increase the contraction of the detrusor muscle. This approach may be very effective, especially for a hypotonic bladder in which there is no significant obstruction of the bladder outlet.

Patients can also be taught to perform self-catheterization at intervals until spontaneous complete emptying of the bladder is achieved. Although intermittent catheterization may have to be carried out for a prolonged period of time, it appears to be a safe and successful method of managing patients who have neurogenic bladders.

Sometimes it is not possible for the patient to achieve reflex bladder control or self-catheterization. The male patient then may use a condom-collecting device if the bladder empties well and no residual urine remains. The female patient may need to wear pads or waterproof pants. Surgical intervention may be carried out to correct bladder neck contractures or vesicoureteral reflux or to perform some type of urinary diversion procedure.

Intermittent Self-catheterization

Intermittent self-catheterization provides periodic drainage of urine from the bladder. It is the treatment of choice following spinal cord injury. Aseptic techniques are required during the hospital training period, but the patient may use a "clean" (nonsterile) technique at home. Self-catheterization promotes independence, results in fewer complications, and permits more normal sexual relations. The objectives are to decrease the morbidity associated with the long-term use of an indwelling catheter and to achieve a catheter-free status if possible.

The main teaching emphasis must be placed on the importance of frequent catheterization and the emptying of the bladder at the prescribed time irrespective of the circumstances. An overdistended bladder slows the circulation of blood through the bladder walls and weakens its resistance to infection.

The female patient will require a mirror to help locate the urinary meatus. She is taught to catheterize herself by inserting a catheter 7.5 cm (3 inches) into the urethra in a downward and backward direction. The male patient is taught to lubricate the catheter and retract the foreskin of the penis with one hand while grasping the penis and holding it at a right angle to the body. (This maneuver straightens the urethra and makes it easier to insert the catheter.) The catheter is inserted 15 cm to 25 cm (6–10 inches) until the urine begins to flow. After the catheter is removed, it is washed in soapy water (if available), rinsed and wrapped in a paper towel, plastic bag, or case, depending on what is available. A patient following this routine should be seen by a urologist at regular intervals to prevent complications, such as reflux, hydronephrosis, and external sphincter spasm.

▷ Dialysis

Dialysis refers to the diffusion of solute molecules through a semipermeable membrane, passing from the side of higher concentration to that of lower concentration. Fluids pass through the semipermeable membrane by means of osmosis, or external pressure applied to the membrane. If the patient with renal failure does not respond to medical treatment, some method of dialysis is performed to remove the waste products. The purpose of dialysis is to maintain the life and well-being of the patient until kidney function can be restored, if possible. Methods of therapy include *peritoneal dialysis* and *hemodialysis*.

Dialysis is used in renal failure to remove toxic substances and body wastes normally excreted by healthy kidneys, and in the management of patients with intractable edema, hepatic coma, hyperkalemia, hypertension, and uremia. The main indications for *acute dialysis* are a high and rising level of serum potassium, fluid overload (or impending pulmonary edema), pronounced acidosis, pericarditis, and severe mental confusion. In renal failure, the reasons for initiating chronic dialysis are nausea and vomiting with anorexia, mental confusion, chronic high potassium, fluid overload (in the presence of diuretics and fluid restriction), and a general lack of well-being.

Peritoneal Dialysis.   In this therapy, the surface of the peritoneum, which amounts to approximately 22,000 sq cm, acts as the diffusing surface. An appropriate sterile dialyzing fluid (dialysate) is introduced into the peritoneal cavity at intervals. Urea is cleared at the rate of approximately 15 ml/min to 20 ml/min. Creatinine is cleared somewhat more slowly. With the development of nonirritating silicone catheters and improvements in commercial dialyzing solution, peritoneal dialysis is fairly easy to perform. Besides the indications mentioned, peritoneal dialysis is occasionally used as a means of treating peritonitis (inflammation of the peritoneum). Antibiotics are added to the dialysate in order to come in direct contact with the infected site. It is also occasionally used as a means of lavage in abdominal trauma.

Peritoneal dialysis can be carried out a few days after abdominal surgery.

It usually takes 36 to 48 hours to achieve with peritoneal dialysis what hemodialysis accomplishes in 6 to 8 hours. Peritoneal dialysis can be intermittent (several times per week, from 6–48 hours) or continuous (hourly exchanges).

With the development of a permanent access device to the peritoneal cavity (surgically implantable silastic catheter), automated closed-cycle peritoneal dialysis machines, and plastic bags to hold the dialysate, this procedure is being done in the home for long-term therapy of patients with chronic renal failure. (The role of the nurse in assisting the patient undergoing peritoneal dialysis is outlined in Chart 43-1.)

Chart 43-1
The Role of the Nurse Assisting the Patient Undergoing Peritoneal Dialysis—Guidelines for Nursing Management

Peritoneal dialysis is a substitute for kidney function during renal failure. The peritoneum is used as a dialyzing membrane.

Goals:

1. Aid in the removal of toxic substances and metabolic wastes.
2. Establish electrolyte balance.
3. Remove excessive body fluid.
4. Assist in regulating the fluid balance of the body.
5. Control blood pressure.
6. Control severe, intractable heart failure when diuretics no longer promote elimination of water and sodium.

Nursing Action	*Rationale*
1. Prepare the patient physically and emotionally for the procedure.	1. Nursing support is offered by explaining procedure mechanics to the patient and his family, providing opportunities for the patient to ask questions, allowing him to verbalize his feelings, and giving appropriate physical care.
2. See that the consent form has been signed.	
3. Weigh the patient before dialysis and every 24 hours thereafter, preferably on an in-bed scale.	3. The weight at the beginning of the procedure serves as a baseline of information. Checking the patient's weight daily is helpful in assessing the state of hydration.
4. Take temperature, pulse, respiration, and blood pressure readings prior to dialysis.	4. A knowledge of vital signs at the beginning of dialysis is necessary for comparing subsequent changes in vital signs.
5. Have the patient empty his bladder.	5. If the bladder is empty, there is less likelihood of perforating it when the trocar is introduced into the peritoneum.
6. Assist with insertion of a central venous pressure catheter if needed. ECG monitoring may also be employed.	6. Central venous pressure measurements may be carried out to assess fluid volume changes. Cardiac arrhythmias may occur due to serum potassium changes and vagal stimulation.
7. Flush the tubing with dialysis solution.	7. The tubing is flushed to prevent air from entering the peritoneal cavity. Air causes abdominal discomfort and drainage difficulties.
8. Make the patient comfortable in a supine position.	

(continued)

Chart 43-1
The Role of the Nurse Assisting the Patient Undergoing Peritoneal Dialysis—
Guidelines for Nursing Management (continued)

Nursing Action *(continued)*

9. The following is a brief description of the method of insertion of a temporary peritoneal catheter (trocar), which is done under strict asepsis by the physician.
    a. The abdomen is prepared surgically, and the skin and subcutaneous tissues are infiltrated with a local anesthetic.
    b. A small midline stab wound is made 3 cm to 5 cm below the umbilicus.
    c. The trocar is inserted through the incision with the stylet in place, or a thin stylet cannula may be inserted percutaneously.
    d. The patient is requested to raise his head from the pillow after the trocar is introduced.

    e. When the peritoneum is punctured, the trocar is directed toward the left side of the pelvis. The stylet is removed, and the catheter is inserted through the trocar and maneuvered into position.
    Dialysis fluid is allowed to run through the catheter while it is being positioned.

    f. After the trocar is removed, the skin may be closed with a purse-string suture. (This is not always done.) A sterile dressing is placed around the catheter.

10. Attach the catheter connector to the administration set, which has been previously connected to the container of dialysis solution (warmed to body temperature, 37° C).

11. Drugs (heparin, potassium, antibiotics, etc.) are added to the dialysate after it is taken from the warmer.

12. Permit the dialyzing solution to flow unrestricted into the peritoneal cavity (usually takes 5–10 minutes for completion). (If patient experiences pain, slow down the infusion.)

13. Allow the fluid to remain in the peritoneal cavity for the prescribed time period (15 minutes to 4 hours).

14. Unclamp the outflow tube. Drainage should take approximately 10 to 30 minutes, although the time varies with each patient. Prepare the next exchange at the end of the drainage period.

Rationale *(continued)*

a. Surgical preparation of the skin minimizes or eliminates surface bacteria and decreases the possibility of wound contamination and infection.
b. The midline area is relatively avascular.

d. This maneuver tightens the abdominal muscles and permits easier penetration of the trocar without danger of injury to the intra-abdominal organs.

This prevents the omentum from adhering to the catheter, impeding its advancement or occluding its opening.
f. The catheter is attached to the skin to prevent loss of the catheter in the abdomen.

10. The solution is warmed to body temperature for patient comfort and to prevent abdominal pain. Heating also causes dilation of the peritoneal vessels and increases urea clearance.

11. The addition of heparin prevents fibrin clots from occluding the catheter. Potassium chloride is added as requested, unless the patient has hyperkalemia. Antibiotics are added for treatment of peritonitis.

12. The inflow solution should flow in a steady stream. If the fluid cannot flow in a steady stream, the catheter may need to be repositioned, since its tip may be buried in the omentum, or it may be occluded by a blood clot. Flushing may help.

13. In order for potassium, urea, and other waste materials to be removed, the solution must remain in the peritoneal cavity for the prescribed time (dwell or equilibration time). The maximum concentration gradient takes place in the first 5 to 10 minutes for small molecules, such as urea and creatinine.

14. The abdomen is drained by a siphon effect through a closed system. Gravity drainage should occur fairly rapidly, and steady streams of fluid should be observed entering the drainage container. The drainage usually has no color or is straw-colored.

(continued)

Chart 43-1
The Role of the Nurse Assisting the Patient Undergoing Peritoneal Dialysis—
Guidelines for Nursing Management (continued)

Nursing Action (continued)	**Rationale** (continued)
15. If the fluid is not draining properly, move the patient from side to side to facilitate the removal of peritoneal drainage. The head of the bed may also be elevated. *Never push in the catheter*. Ascertain if the catheter is patent. Check for closed clamp, kinked tubing, or air lock.	15. If the drainage stops, or starts to drip before the dialyzing fluid has been adequately drained, it may indicate that the catheter tip is buried in the omentum. Rotating the patient may be helpful (or it may be necessary for the physician to reposition the catheter). Pushing in the catheter introduces bacteria into the peritoneal cavity.
16. When the outflow drainage ceases to run in a steady stream, and most or more of the infused dialysate is returned, clamp off the drainage tubing and infuse the next exchange, using strict aseptic technique.	
17. Take blood pressure and pulse every 15 minutes during the first exchange, and every hour thereafter. Monitor the heart rate for signs of arrhythmia.	17. A drop in blood pressure may indicate excessive fluid loss due to the glucose concentrations of the dialyzing solutions. Changes in vital signs may indicate impending shock or overhydration.
18. Take the patient's temperature every 4 hours (especially after catheter removal).	18. An infection may become evident after dialysis has been discontinued.
19. The procedure is repeated until the blood chemistry levels improve. The usual time is 36 to 48 hours; depending on the patient's condition, he will receive 24 to 48 exchanges. In acute conditions, catheters are usually removed within 48 to 72 hours. A new trocar is inserted for the next treatment.	19. The duration of the dialysis depends on the severity of the condition and on the size and weight of the patient.
20. Keep an exact record of the patient's fluid balance during the treatment.	20. Complications (circulatory collapse, hypotension, dehydration, shock, and death) may occur if the patient loses too much fluid through peritoneal drainage. Large fluid losses around the catheter may be missed unless the dressings are checked carefully.
a. Know the status of the patient's loss or gain of fluid at the end of each exchange; check dressing for leakage, and weigh on gram scale if significant.	
b. The fluid balance should be about even or should show slight fluid loss or gain, depending on the patient's fluid status.	
21. Promote patient comfort during dialysis.	21. The dialysis period is lengthy, and the patient becomes fatigued.
a. Provide frequent back care and massage of pressure areas.	
b. Rotate from side to side.	
c. Elevate head of bed at intervals.	
d. Allow patient to sit in chair for brief periods if condition permits. (Only with surgically implanted catheter.) (With trocar, patient is on strict bed rest.)	
22. Observe the following.	
a. Respiratory difficulty	a. This is caused by pressure from the fluid in the peritoneal cavity and the upward displacement of the diaphragm, producing shallow respirations.
(1) Slow the inflow rate.	
(2) Make sure tubing is not kinked.	
(3) Prevent air from entering the peritoneal cavity by keeping the drip chamber of the tubing three fourths full of fluid.	(3) In severe respiratory difficulty, the fluid from the peritoneal cavity should be drained immediately and the physician notified.

(continued)

Chart 43-1
The Role of the Nurse Assisting the Patient Undergoing Peritoneal Dialysis—
Guidelines for Nursing Management *(continued)*

Nursing Action *(continued)*	**Rationale** *(continued)*
(4) Elevate head of the bed; encourage coughing and breathing exercises. (5) Turn patient from side to side.	
b. Abdominal pain Encourage patient to move about.	b. Pain may be caused by the dialyzing solution's not being at body temperature, incomplete drainage of the solution, chemical irritation, irritation by the catheter, peritonitis, or air pressing on the diaphragm and causing referred shoulder pain.
c. Leakage (1) Change the dressings frequently on the trocar, being careful not to dislodge the catheter. (2) Use sterile, plastic drapes to prevent contamination.	c. Leakage around the catheter predisposes to peritonitis.
23. Keep accurate records: a. Exact time of beginning and end of each exchange; starting and finishing time of drainage b. Amount and type of solution infused and drained c. Fluid balance (accumulative) d. Number of exchanges e. Medications added to dialyzing solution f. Pre- and post-dialysis weight, plus daily weight g. Level of responsiveness at beginning, throughout, and end of treatment h. Assessment of vital signs and patient's condition	

Complications

1. Peritonitis	1. Peritonitis is the most common complication. Antibiotics may be added to the dialysate and also are given systemically.
a. Watch for nausea and vomiting, anorexia, abdominal pain, tenderness, rigidity, and cloudy dialysate drainage. b. Send specimen of dialysate for WBC and full set of cultures.	
2. Bleeding	2. A small amount of bleeding around a new catheter is not significant if it does not persist. During the first few exchanges, the blood-tinged fluid from subcutaneous bleeding is not uncommon. Small amounts of heparin may be added to inflow solution to prevent the catheter from becoming clogged. A hematocrit of the drainage fluid may be taken to help determine the amount of bleeding.
3. Constipation	3. Inactivity, decreased nutrition, phosphate binders, and the presence of fluid in the abdomen tend to cause constipation.
4. Low serum albumin	4. Small amounts of albumin are lost with each exchange, resulting in a lowered serum albumin. Edema may occur with possible hypotension.

Hemodialysis

Hemodialysis is a process in which the uremic toxins and accumulated waste products are removed from the blood. This type of therapy is used for patients who are acutely ill and require short-term dialysis (days to weeks) or for patients with end-stage renal disease (ESRD), who require long-term therapy. A synthetic, semipermeable membrane replaces the renal glomeruli and tubules and acts as the filter for the impaired kidneys. For patients with chronic renal failure, hemodialysis provides reasonable rehabilitation and life expectancy. However, hemodialysis does not cure renal disease and is not able to compensate for losses of the kidneys' endocrine or metabolic activities. The patient must be given dialysis treatment for the rest of his life (usually three times a week for 4 hours per treatment) or until he receives a successful kidney transplant. Patients are placed on chronic dialysis when they need dialysis therapy in order to live.

The requirements for hemodialysis for a patient with end-stage renal failure are (1) access to the patient's circulation, (2) a dialyzer with a semipermeable membrane (the artificial kidney), and (3) an appropriate dialysate bath.

Access to the Patient's Circulation

Access to the patient's circulation is achieved through an arteriovenous (A–V) *shunt* (external silastic tubing placed in an adjacent artery and vein), a *fistula* (internal access using the patient's own vessels), or a *graft* (internal access using a foreign material).

A–V Shunt. The A–V shunt can be placed wherever an artery and vein are close together. Usually, the silastic tubing is placed in the radial artery and the adjacent vein, but the ankle can also be used. The shunt was the original vascular access for chronic dialysis, but now it is used only temporarily, (while the patient awaits maturation of a fistula or graft) or as an immediate access to treat acute renal failure.

The use of the femoral and subclavian catheters has greatly reduced the use of the A–V shunt. With the shunt, the tubing from the artery and vein exits the skin and joins with a connecting piece to form a closed arc for the blood to flow between dialyses. When dialysis is performed, the connector is removed and the tubing coming from the artery is inserted into tubing *going to* the artificial kidney. Tubing *from the* artificial kidney is inserted into the venous segment of the shunt. The blood then can pass from the patient's vascular system, through the artificial kidney filtering system, and back again into the patient's blood vessel (vein). The blood is traveling via a blood pump from 200 ml/min to 300 ml/min, depending on the patient's size, the condition of the blood vessels being used, and the overall condition of the patient's vascular system.

The shunt is cleaned before each dialysis with antiseptic solution, after which a dry sterile dressing is applied and secured with a stretchable gauze bandage. The patient is instructed to observe the shunt several times a day for evidence of clotting and to avoid wearing a watch or jewelry or carrying a handbag over the shunt arm. While the shunt provides ready access to the patient's circulation, the shunt itself has a limited life span due to infection or clotting. It could separate at the connection site, producing hemorrhage and possibly death. It is also a visible reminder to the patient of his disability.

Fistula. The fistula is created surgically by the anastomosis of an artery to a vein, either side to side or end to side. The fistula takes 2 to 6 weeks to mature before it should be used. This gives time for healing to take place and for the venous segment of the fistula to dilate. The fistula needs to dilate in order to accommodate two large-bore (14-gauge or 16-gauge) needles. The needles can be inserted into the vessel to obtain blood flow adequate to pass through the dialyzer. The arterial segment of the fistula is used for arterial flow and the venous segment for retransfusion of the dialyzed blood. The fistula has greatly reduced the problems of infection and clotting.

Graft. The graft is created by suturing a piece of bovine carotid artery, Gore–Tex material (heterograft), or umbilical cord graft into the patient's own vessel (Fig. 43-3). This is done to provide an already developed segment in which to place the needles for dialysis. Usually, the graft is created when the patient's own vessels are not suitable to be used for a fistula. Grafts are usually placed in the forearm, upper arm, or upper thigh. Patients with compromised vascular systems, such as those with diabetes, often need to have a graft in order to have hemodialysis.

Patients undergoing venipuncture three times a week with large-bone needles often cannot adjust to "being stuck," even though lidocaine (Xylocaine) is usually used to anesthetize the area. In these instances, the patient may desire peritoneal dialysis.

Underlying Principles of Dialysis

The objectives of hemodialysis are to extract toxic nitrogenous substances from the blood and to remove excess water. Heparinized blood passes, by means of a blood pump, through the artificial kidney machine to the semipermeable membrane or artificial kidney, and the dialysate bath flows on the other side of the membrane. The toxins and wastes in the blood are removed by diffusion, moving from an area of greater concentration in the blood to an area of lesser concentration in the dialysate. The blood and dialysate do not mix. The dialysate is composed of all the important electrolytes in their ideal extracellular concentrations. The electrolytes in the blood can be brought under control by proper adjustment of the dialysate bath. (Small pores in the semipermeable membrane do not allow the loss of red blood cells and proteins.)

Excess water is removed from the blood by osmosis. The removal of water can be controlled by creating a desired pressure gradient (ultrafiltration). The body's buffer system is maintained by the addition of acetate, which is diffused from the dialysate into the patient and metabolizes to form bicarbonate. Purified blood is returned to the body through one of the patient's veins. At the end of the dialysis treatment, the majority of poisonous wastes have been removed, electrolyte and water balance has been restored, and the buffer system has been replenished.

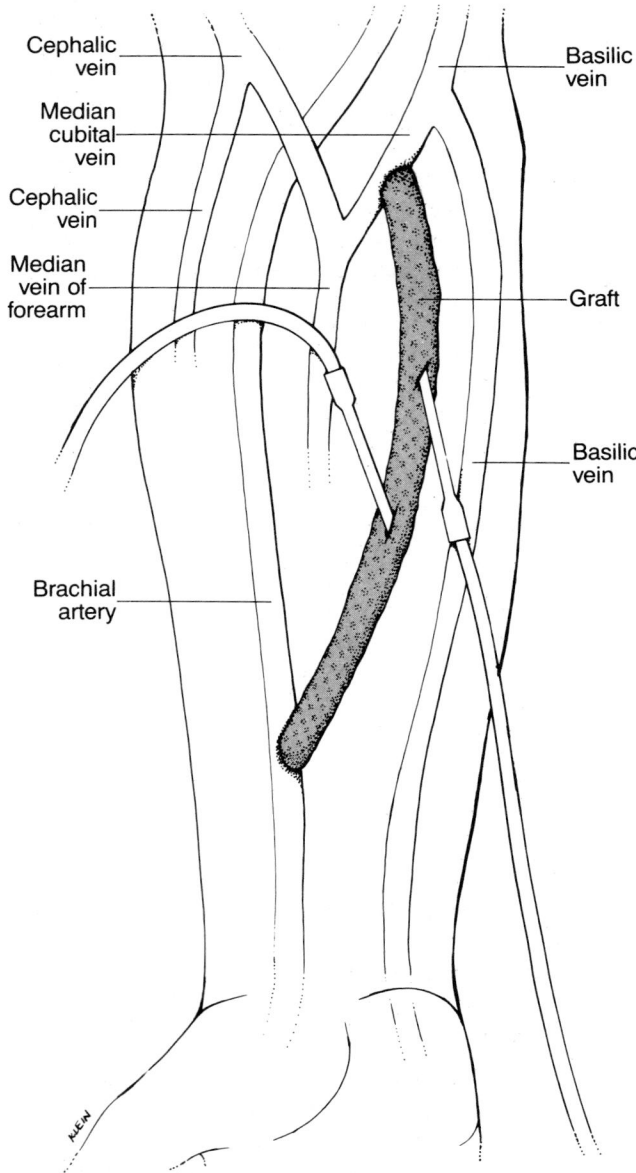

Cephalic
vein

Median
cubital
vein

Cephalic
vein

Median
vein of
forearm

Brachial
artery

Basilic
vein

Graft

Basilic
vein

Figure 43-3. Drawing of a graft (vascular access) used for hemodialysis.

During dialysis, the patient, the dialyzer, and the dialysate bath require constant monitoring to detect the numerous complications that can arise during dialysis—hepatitis, air embolism, inadequate or excessive ultrafiltration, blood leaks, infection, shunt or fistula complications, etc. The nurse in the dialysis unit has an important role in monitoring and supporting the patient and in carrying out a continuing program of patient assessment and education (Fig. 43-4).

Dialyzers and Dialysate Bath. There have been unprecedented developments in dialyzers and technology for treatment of end-stage renal disease, but most dialyzers conform to one of the following types: the coil dialyzer, the flat plate dialyzer, and the hollow fiber artificial kidney.

Management of the Patient on Long-Term Hemodialysis

An optimum dietary program is most important for patients on hemodialysis because of the effects of uremia (wasting, poor dietary intake, the reduced palatability of the restricted diet, the loss of nutrients during dialysis, and any concurrent illnesses).

- The diet of the patient usually involves some adjustment or restriction of protein, sodium, potassium, or fluid intake. Protein intake must be of high biological quality, consisting of complete amino acid composition, (eggs, meat, milk, fish) to prevent poor protein utilization and to maintain positive nitrogen balance and replace amino acids lost during dialysis. If many water-soluble nutrients and metabolites have been removed from the tissues as a result of the effects of dialysis, the patient may require additional vitamins and minerals. After dialysis procedures are initiated, the patient's clinical condition usually improves, and there is usually a diminished need for stringent dietary restrictions.

Many drugs are excreted wholly or in part by the kidneys. Patients requiring drug therapy (cardiac glycosides, antibiotics, antiarrhythmic agents, antihypertensive agents) are monitored closely to ensure that blood and tissue levels of these drugs are maintained without toxic accumulation. This type of information is kept in mind when the patient asks, "Is it all right to take this medicine for a headache?"

Complications

Although hemodialysis can prolong life indefinitely, it does not halt the natural course of the underlying kidney disease, nor does it completely control uremia. The patient is subjected to a number of problems and complications. The leading cause of death among patients undergoing chronic hemodialysis is arteriosclerotic cardiovascular disease—an important factor in limiting survival. Disturbances of lipid metabolism (hypertriglyceridemia) appear to be accentuated by hemodialysis. Congestive heart failure, coronary heart disease and anginal pain, stroke, and peripheral vascular insufficiency may incapacitate the patient. Anemia and fatigue contribute to diminished physical and emotional well-being with attendant lack of energy and drive, and loss of interest. Gastric ulcers and other gastrointestinal problems occur from the physiologic stress of chronic illness, medication, etc. Disturbed calcium metabolism leads to renal osteodystrophy that produces bone pain and fractures. Other problems include fluid overload associated with congestive heart failure, malnutrition, and disequilibrium syndrome from rapid fluid and electrolyte changes. Patients with virtually no renal function have been maintained for a number of years by intermittent hemodialysis. For some, a successful kidney transplant would eliminate the need for chronic, long-term hemodialysis treatment.

Long-term therapy presents a problem for the patient (and for society) as to cost and reimbursement. With im-

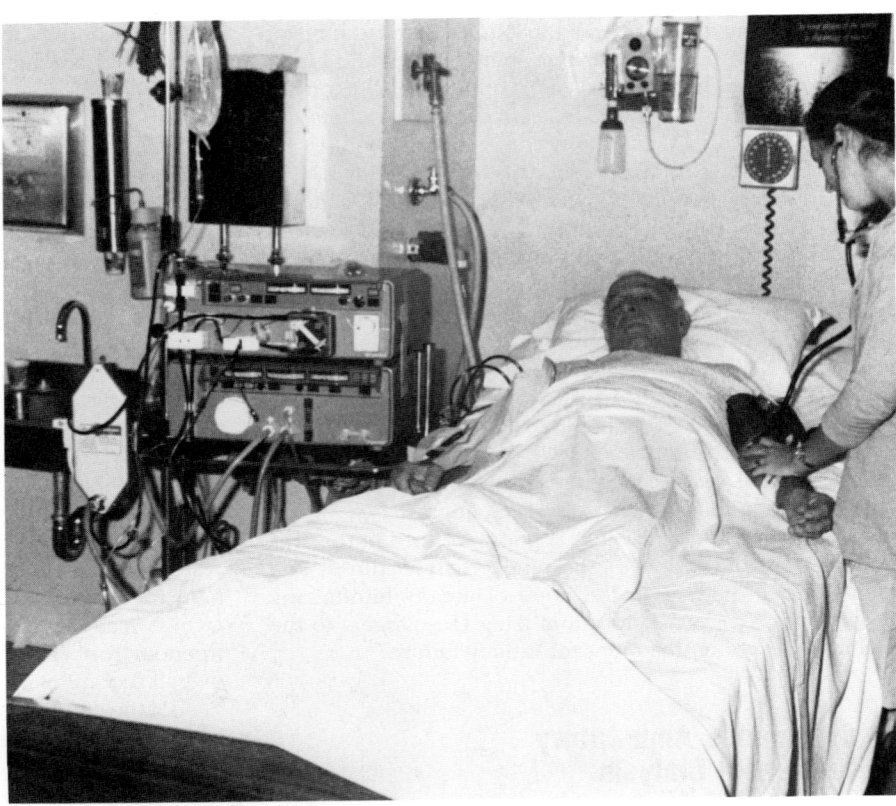

Figure 43-4. Hemodialysis (HD) patient assisted by nurse. (Courtesy, Georgetown University Hospital.)

proved techniques and a greater number of patients on treatment, the cost of chronic dialysis is an area that will have major focus and is of great concern.

Psychosocial Considerations

Persons undergoing long-term hemodialysis are concerned with very real problems. Unpalatable meals (from restrictions on sodium and potassium) and living with thirst imposed by a restricted fluid intake added to a regimented and complicated life-style can be very demoralizing. Generally, the patient's medical status is unpredictable and his life is disrupted; he often has financial problems, difficulty in holding a job, waning sexual desires and impotence, depression from living the life of a chronically ill person, and fear of dying. Younger persons worry about marriage, having children, and the burden that they bring to their families.

Dialysis imposes an altered life-style on the family. The amount of time required for dialysis decreases social activities and can create conflict, frustration, guilt, and depression in the family. Frequently, the patient's family and friends regard him as a "marginal person" with a limited life expectancy. It may be difficult for the patient, spouse, and family to express anger and negative feelings.

The nurse can support the family by letting them know that feelings of anger and dismay are normal emotional reactions in this situation. It also helps to provide verbal and written instructions and to inform them of resources that are available for help. The family should be involved in treatment and decision making.

It is a small wonder that the suicide rate among dialysis patients is high. To avoid such drastic outcomes and to provide an outlet for frustrations, the patient should be given a chance to express any feelings of anger and concern over the limitations imposed by the disease and treatment, as well as possible financial problems, job insecurity, pain, and discomfort.

If anger is not expressed, there is always the danger that it will be directed inward and lead to depression. It also can be projected outward to other people, thereby complicating an already tenuous family situation. The patient needs a close relationship with someone to whom he can turn in times of stress and discouragement. Some patients will use the mental mechanism of denial to deal with the overwhelming array of medical problems (infections, hypertension, anemia, neuropathy, etc.). The nurse can help by doing everything possible to support the patient in coping with these ever present problems and fears.

Home Dialysis

For selected patients, hemodialysis is carried out in the home with equipment similar to that used in the hospital. However, not all people are candidates, since this procedure requires a highly motivated patient who is willing to take responsibility for his dialysis procedure and to be able to adjust each treatment to meet his body's changing needs.

The patient with kidney failure and the family member who will act as helper must undergo a training program to learn how to prepare, operate, and disassemble the dialysis machine; maintain and clean the equipment; administer drugs (heparin) into the machine lines; and handle emergency problems (hemodialysis coil rupture, shock, convulsions). The home is surveyed to see if electrical outlets and plumbing facilities are adequate. The emphasis is on letting the patient assume primary responsibility for the treatment and carry on with normal daily activities. When a home dialysis service is not feasible, the patient may be referred to a limited-care dialysis center outside the hospital.

Federal Assistance. In 1973 the Social Security Administration, through Medicare, became the third-party payer for the dialysis and transplant costs of 95% of those patients on dialysis. In 1977 the federal government spent over 594 million dollars in providing dialysis and transplantation for 33,000 patients. By 1988 it is estimated that a minimumn of 2 billion dollars will be spent for over 70,000 end-stage renal disease patients. As of 1982, over 66,000 persons were end-stage renal disease patients.

In the meantime, research is going forward in the area of "the wearable kidney," shortened dialysis times, and computerized dialysis, in the hope of greatly minimizing the patient's treatment and minimizing the dangers to the patient undergoing treatment for kidney failure.

Continuous Ambulatory Peritoneal Dialysis

Continuous Ambulatory Peritoneal Dialysis (CAPD) has emerged as a new technique for patients with end-stage renal disease who want to take an active part in their treatment. CAPD is recommended for selected patients and is not generally considered appropriate for all patients requiring chronic dialysis. While some patients perform hemodialysis at home, most patients must travel to a hemodialysis center for treatment, although some areas of the country have provided intermittent peritoneal dialysis (IPD) at home for many years.

CAPD is a form of peritoneal dialysis with important differences for the patient. It is peritoneal dialysis performed at home by the patient. (Sometimes a family member is trained to perform the exchanges for the patient.) The technique can be adjusted to the individual patient's capacity to learn and the patient's physiologic requirements for dialysis.

Traditional peritoneal dialysis, like hemodialysis, requires machines and sometimes relies on skilled nurses and technicians to perform the procedure. Treatments are also intermittent, necessitating repeated sessions usually lasting from 12 to 48 hours, during which time the patient is attached to a machine. In contrast, CAPD is continuous, machine-free, and self-administered.

The CAPD technique was first introduced in 1975, but was not in wide use until 1980. Initially, glass bottles were used to deliver the fluid, which required that the tubing be disconnected each time the exchange was performed. In 1978 approval of the flexible plastic container by the Food and Drug Administration (FDA) allowed the bag and tubing to remain attached with each exchange. (The bag is folded and tucked beneath the clothing during the dialysis dwell time—the time between exchanges.) This provides the patient great freedom, but even more important, it reduces the number of connections and disconnections at the catheter end of the tubing, thereby reducing the accompanying risk of contamination and peritonitis. Three important aspects that brought CAPD into wide use are (1) the use of the plastic container (bag) for the dialysate, (2) the fact that the administration tubing remained attached to the catheter during and between exchanges, and (3) the use of an infection-free, permanent abdominal catheter.

In addition, the use of the titanium connector eliminated the possibility of the catheter and tubing becoming accidentally disconnected. The success of CAPD often depends upon the maintenance of the permanent catheter placed in the peritoneal cavity. Catheter problems can arise and include one-way obstruction, dislodgment from the pelvis, omental wrapping, dialysate leak, exit-site infection, fibrin-clot formation, and bacterial/fungal contamination.

Patients choose CAPD to gain freedom from a machine, to have control over their daily activities, to avoid dietary restrictions, to have greater fluid intake, to elevate the serum hematocrit, to have blood pressure under greater control (which may be from decreased plasma volume), to have freedom from venipuncture, and hopefully to gain a general overall feeling of well-being.

Of the patients currently on CAPD, about one third who have never been on prior therapy chose CAPD. The remaining patients had been on hemodialysis. Patients are encouraged to move from one therapy to another, and all dialysis patients are encouraged to consider transplantation at any time during their treatment.

How It Works. Approximately 2 liters of sterile dialyzing solution is infused through the abdominal catheter into the peritoneal cavity. This is done by attaching the solution container (flexible plastic bag) to the catheter via a solution transfer set (connecting tubing or administration set) and raising the container to above shoulder level (Fig. 43-5). The solution flows into the abdominal cavity via gravity. Once the container is empty, it is rolled up and placed under the patient's clothing (Fig. 43-6). While the patient goes about everyday activities, toxic wastes and excess water pass from his bloodstream through the network of tiny blood vessels in the peritoneal membrane into the solution. (Diffusion and osmosis are the principles involved, as in hemodialysis and IPD). Once the dwell time has been complete, the plastic container is unrolled and lowered to below the abdomen, allowing the dialyzing solution and excess fluid to drain from the abdominal cavity back into the container. The solution and container are discarded, and a new container of solution is attached (exchange) and the fresh fluid infused. An exchange is performed usually four times a day (maybe as many as six times a day or as few as three). The fluid then is changed four times a day. This technique is continuous, 24 hours a day, 7 days a week. The patient performs the exchanges at intervals spread throughout the day (*e.g.,* at 8 AM, noon, 5 PM, and 10 PM) and sleeps during the night. No exchange is performed at night. Each exchange usually takes from 30 to 40 minutes to perform. This consists of a 20-minute drain period, a 5- or 10-minute exchange period, and a 5- or 10-minute period of infusion.

Principles. CAPD, being a continuous treatment, produces a steady state of blood values of the nitrogenous waste

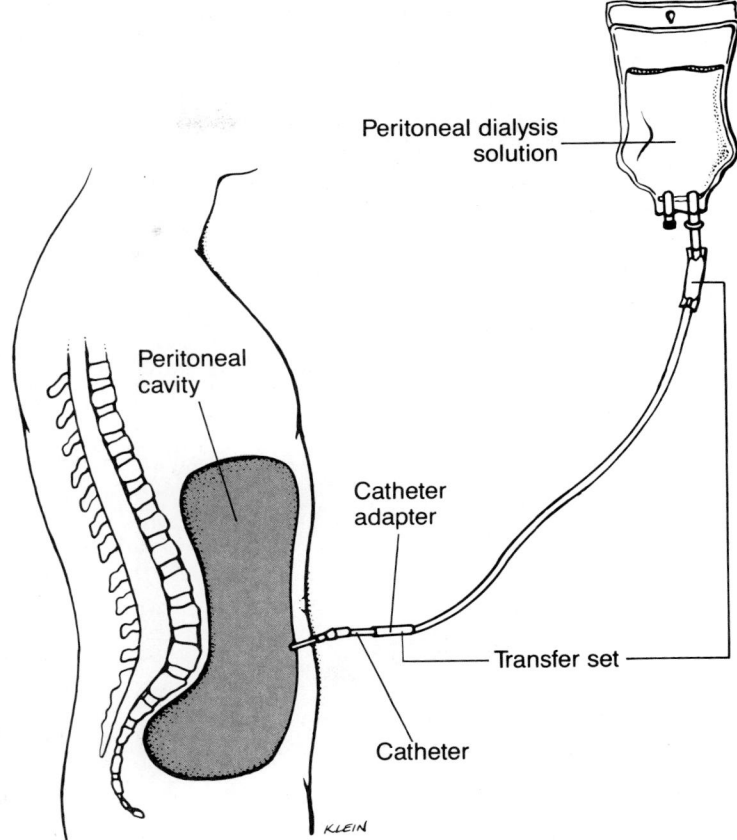

Figure 43-5. Drawing of Continuous Ambulatory Peritoneal Dialysis (CAPD) fluid infusing into peritoneal cavity. (Redrawn after CAPD: A new alternative in dialysis. Reprinted with permission of National Kidney Foundation, Inc., 1980.)

products. The precise blood levels depend on the residual kidney function, the daily dialysate volume, and, of course, on the rate of production of the waste products. There are less fluctuations in the serum chemistries on CAPD, as the dialysis is constantly in progress. The serum electrolytes usually stay in the normal range.

The length of time that the dialysate stays in the peritoneal cavity has a positive effect on clearance of middle-sized molecules. It is thought that these middle molecules may be significant uremic toxins. The clearance of these molecules is greatly enhanced by CAPD as compared to hemodialysis or IPD.

Low molecular weight substances, such as urea, diffuse more rapidly than middle-size molecules in both forms of dialysis, but they are removed more slowly during CAPD than during hemodialysis.

The removal of excess water during peritoneal dialysis is achieved by the addition of hypertonic glucose to the dialysate, creating an osmotic gradient. The flexible plastic bag can expand to twice its size during the drain period to accommodate the removal of excess body fluid as well as the removal of the dialysate from the abdominal cavity.

Complications

CAPD is not without complications. Most complications are minor in nature, but several, if left unattended, can have serious consequences for the patient. Abdominal hernias may develop during CAPD, probably as a result of contin-

uously raised intra-abdominal pressure. Older patients with or without previous surgical scars are prone to develop this complication. The types of hernias that have developed during CAPD include incisional, inguinal, diaphragmatic, and umbilical. The persistently raised intra-abdominal pressure can cause worsening of symptoms of hiatus hernia and hemorrhoids. Large numbers of patients choosing CAPD are in the older age group, in which cardiac and cerebral complications are often more prevalent. Hypertriglyceridemia, frequently found in patients on CAPD, raises the possibility that this therapy may accelerate atherogenesis. It does not seem to have an aggravating influence on atherogenic factors related to lipoproteins, namely decreased HDL cholesterol and elevated LDL cholesterol levels. In fact, in some patients, concentration of HDL cholesterol increased, thereby providing a beneficial effect. Other complications include obesity, low back pain, anorexia due to a constant sweet taste from the glucose, and inability to eat because of the presence of fluid in the abdomen.

Peritonitis. Peritonitis is the most common complication and also the most serious complication. Most peritonitis episodes are due to accidental contamination caused by *Staphylococcus epidermidis*. Fortunately, these episodes result in mild symptoms and have a good prognosis. Peritonitis due to *Staphylococcus aureus* produces a higher morbidity, has a more serious prognosis, and runs a longer course. Gram-negative organisms may originate in the bowel, particularly when there is more than one organism

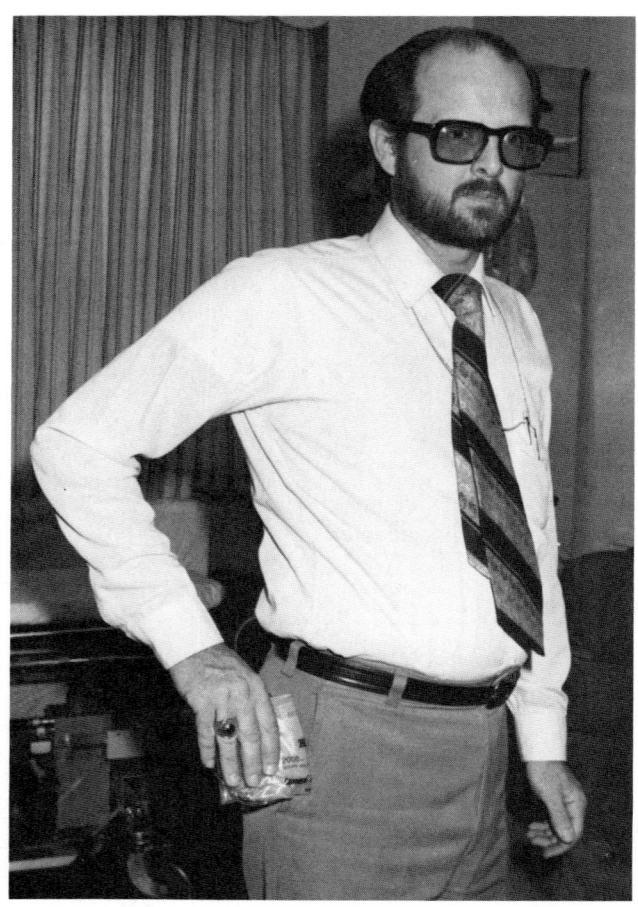

Figure 43-6. Continuous Ambulatory Peritoneal Dialysis (CAPD) patient tucking away bag and tubing. (Courtesy, Georgetown University Hospital.)

in the peritoneal fluid, and especially when the organisms are anaerobic.

Peritonitis is treated in the hospital if the patient is not well enough to do his own exchanges. The patient is usually put on IPD for 48 hours or more while receiving parenteral antibiotic therapy. If the symptoms are minor and the patient feels well enough, he can be treated as an outpatient. Antibiotics are usually added to the dialysate and are also taken orally for 10 days. The infection usually clears in 2 to 4 days. Careful culture techniques are important for the treatment of the organism by the correct antibiotic.

With a persistent catheter exit-site infection (usually *Staphylococcus aureus*), treatment is difficult without the removal of the permanent catheter. If removal is delayed, often these patients will develop peritonitis with the same organism found at the exit site.

Patients with fungal peritonitis need to have the peritoneal catheter removed in order to clear the infection. Peritonitis with three positive peritoneal fluid cultures also necessitates catheter removal.

Usually, after the catheter is removed the patient is maintained on hemodialysis for about 1 month before a new catheter is inserted.

Technical Complications. The CAPD technique depends on reliable materials. Many technical problems can arise. Early dialysate leaks are sometimes noted immediately following catheter insertion. Dialysate usually leaks through the incision and exit site. Patients who are predisposed to this complication usually have loose abdominal walls, or have had previous multiple pregnancies, or are receiving medium- to high-dose systemic corticosteroids at the time of catheter insertion. Usually, the leak stops spontaneously if dialysis is withheld for several days to give the incision and exit site enough time to heal. During this period, it is important to avoid or minimize factors that might delay healing, such as undue abdominal muscle activity and straining during bowel movement.

Late leaks can occur spontaneously months or years after catheter placement. These leaks may occur through the exit site or into the abdominal wall.

Bleeding. A bloody effluent (drainage) may be observed occasionally, especially in young, menstruating females. In most cases, no cause can be found for the bleeding. Catheter displacement from the pelvis has occasionally been associated with the bleeding. Some patients have had bloody effluent following an enema or from minor trauma. Invariably, bleeding stops after a day or two and requires no specific intervention. More frequent exchanges during this time may prevent plugging of the catheter by blood clots.

Selection of Patients for CAPD

For new patients with end-stage renal disease, the patient's preference, and desire to be involved in his treatment become very important criteria in selecting the appropriate therapy. When deciding on the treatment modality, it is important to take into consideration the patient's family support system, as well as his ability to perform self-dialysis.

For patients who are already on chronic hemodialysis, CAPD is indicated for those who have problems with their present treatment modality, such as vascular access, excessive thirst, severe hypertension, postdialysis headaches, and severe anemia requiring frequent transfusion, as well as for those in-center dialysis patients who would like to do their dialysis at home.

CAPD is the treatment of choice for most *home* dialysis patients.

Patients awaiting a kidney transplant can be safely maintained on CAPD, and peritoneal dialysis can be the treatment of choice during rejection episodes.

Diabetic persons with end-stage renal disease may be a group in whom CAPD may be an *absolute* indication. The excellent control of hypertension, the control of uremia, and the satisfactory control of glycemia by intraperitoneal administration of insulin may arrest the diabetic complications.

Patients who want control over their lives and are willing to be compliant in their care do well on CAPD. Almost half of all new end-stage renal disease patients are choosing CAPD for their form of therapy.

As of late 1982, approximately 6500 patients were on CAPD in the United States. This is 10% of all patients with end-stage renal disease, and this figure is expected to increase with improvements in bag and tubing connections and with favorable federal reimbursement programs.

Contraindications for CAPD. Contraindications for CAPD include poor clearance of solutes, due either to adhesions from previous operations or to systemic inflammatory disease. These may be the only *absolute* contraindications, but others include recurrent chronic backache with preexisting disc disease (which could be aggravated by the continuous pressure of dialysis fluid in the abdomen). The presence of a colostomy, ileostomy, nephrostomy, or ileal conduit may increase the risk of peritonitis, and such patients should probably not be treated with CAPD. Patients receiving immunosuppressive treatment with corticosteroids or other agents of medium- to high-dose therapy may have increased complications from poor healing of catheter exit site(s). Whether or not these patients are prone to peritonitis is a controversial issue. Systemic lupus erythematosus patients on low-dose steroid treatment seem to do well on CAPD. Patients with chronic obstructive pulmonary disease may not be candidates for CAPD.

Patient motivation is certainly one of the most important factors in the success of CAPD. Patients developing frequent peritonitis episodes are usually less motivated and more depressed, and may have suffered major life crises, such as loss of job, accidents, divorce, or deaths.

Patients with arthritis or poor hand strength have difficulty performing the exchange and should probably not go on CAPD. Blind or partially blind patients can be trained to perform CAPD, so sight is not a prerequisite.

Older patients generally do well on CAPD, but some older patients who live alone tend to become further isolated. They miss the socialization of the dialysis center. Some older patients who might be experiencing signs of aging have difficulty discerning when a problem is a problem. On the other hand, patients in their 20s often interfere with their treatment by wanting too much control over it and end up taking medications that have not been prescribed, and worrying needlessly about small details. Sometimes this group just cannot relax long enough to allow the therapy to work for them. This group is also very angry that their lives have been interrupted by renal failure, and this anger may prevent them from doing well on CAPD.

Diet Considerations. The liberalized diet for persons on CAPD is one of the most attractive aspects to most patients in choosing CAPD. Usually, potassium, sodium, and fluids are not restricted. Because of protein loss with continuous peritoneal dialysis, the patients are instructed to eat a high-protein, well-balanced diet. Patients are also encouraged to eat bran daily to help prevent constipation. Often patients gain from 3 to 5 pounds within a month after being on CAPD, so they are asked to keep carbohydrate ingestion to a minimum in order not to gain an excessive amount of weight.

The patients usually lose about 2 liters of fluid over and above the 8 liters of dialysate infused into the abdomen during a 24-hour period. This provides ample room for a normal fluid intake, even in an anephric patient. The fluid loss and blood pressure can be controlled by the selection of glucose concentration of the dialysate. Glucose solutions of 1.5%, 2.5%, and 4.25% are available in several sizes, from 500 ml to 3000 ml, thus allowing the dialysate selection to fit the patient's tolerance, size, and physiologic needs. Usually, the patient is instructed in making these choices for himself in the home setting.

Patient Education

Patients can be taught to do CAPD as inpatients or outpatients. If they are medically stable and have transportation to and from the training facility, they can be taught as outpatients. They can continue to work and be supported by in-center hemodialysis during the training period. Usually, the training period takes 10 days to 2 weeks. If the patient is an inpatient or comes daily to the training facility, the training period can be shortened.

During the training period, patients are taught very basic anatomy and physiology about their kidneys, the disease process, the exact exchange procedure, any expected or unexpected complications and the appropriate way to react, the measurement of vital signs (in particular, accurate blood pressure measurement), catheter care, proper handwashing, and, most importantly, when and whom to call with a problem. The dietitian and social worker meet with the patient during the training period and at intervals afterward.

The patient is taught according to his own learning ability and learning level, but is taught as much as he can handle without feeling uncomfortable. Patients do not have to be educated to learn CAPD, but they must have the ability to learn.

The primary nurse training the patient, as well as all of the CAPD nurses, become very well acquainted with the patient and his family. After the patient goes home, the nurses keep in close touch with him by telephone. Patients depend on being able to check with the nurses to see if they are making the right choices as to dialysate or control of blood pressure or to simply discuss a problem. They are seen by the CAPD team as outpatients once a month or more if needed. The patient's exchange procedure is checked at that time to see that he is using good aseptic technique. Patients fall easily into bad habits or make changes in the procedure. The patient's administration tubing is changed by the CAPD nurses every 4 to 8 weeks. Infrequent tubing changes decrease the chance of possible contamination. Blood chemistries are followed closely to make certain the therapy is adequate treatment for the patient.

The dedication and competence of the nursing team is in direct correlation with a successful CAPD program and a healthy, happy CAPD patient.

Body Image Concerns. Even though CAPD has given the end-stage renal disease patients more freedom and control over their treatment, it is not without its problems. The patients often speak of an altered body image due to the abdominal catheter and the presence of the bag and tubing. Where to "wear" and hide the bag and tubing can be a problem. The patients often say their waist size increases from 1 to 2 inches (or more) with the presence of fluid in the abdomen and that this affects their clothing selection as well as their feeling of "being fat." Sexual activity can be altered; the patient and his partner may be reluctant to engage in sexual activities partly due to the presence of the catheter being psychologically "in the way" of natural per-

Chart 43-2
Hemodialysis Compared to CAPD

Hemodialysis	CAPD
Advantages	
1. Widely available	1. Liberal diet permitted
2. More normal:	2. Simplicity
Total protein	3. Easier than home
Albumin	hemodialysis
Serum calcium	4. More normal:
3. Perhaps more normal:	Potassium
Serum triglyceride	Bicarbonate
	Hematocrit
	5. Probably better
	preserved HDL
	6. Blood pressure under
	good control
	7. Usually no fluid
	restriction
Disadvantages	
Possibility of:	Possibility of:
1. Vascular access	1. Abdominal catheter
2. Machine-dependent	2. Time commitment
3. Hemorrhage	3. Peritonitis
4. Air emboli	4. Protein washout
5. Hepatitis	
6. Diet restriction	
7. Fluid restriction	
8. Less blood pressure	
control	

formance. There is significant concern whether the presence of the 2 liters of dialysate, peritoneal catheter, and empty bag interferes with the sexual function and body image of these patients, especially females.

Sometimes body image is so altered that the patient does not want to look at or care for the catheter for days or weeks. Talking with other patients who have a positive attitude may help. Some patients seem to have no psychological problems with the catheter; they think of it as their lifeline and are quite glad to have it as a life-sustaining device. Patients sometimes say they feel they are doing exchanges all day long and have no free time, particularly in the beginning. They may experience depression over going home, as they feel overwhelmed with the responsibility of self-care.

CAPD is not for everyone with end-stage renal disease, but it is a viable form of therapy for a select group of patients (perhaps 15%–25% of all end-stage renal disease patients) who not only want to do self-care, but experience a feeling of independence from a machine and its accompanying rigid schedule. If patients are compliant, willing to do the exchange as taught, and able to fit the therapy into their own routines, they can live relatively normal lives and feel a measure of accomplishment and success with CAPD. Often patients relate that they "feel better" on CAPD, have more energy, and feel more like they did before they had renal failure. Some of these feelings may be due to an improved physiologic state, but also to a much improved self-image. It would be wrong to encourage all patients to seek CAPD. Instead, the patient should be assisted to find the therapy most suitable for his particular life-style and with which he can best reach an optimal state of well-being. (Chart 43-2 presents the advantages and disadvantages of hemodialysis and CAPD.)

Continuous Cycler Peritoneal Dialysis

Continuous Cycler Peritoneal Dialysis (CCPD) is a combination of overnight intermittent peritoneal dialysis with a prolonged dwell during the day.

The patient is connected to a cycler machine every evening and receives three to five 2-liter exchanges during the night; in the morning he caps off his catheter after infusing 1 to 2 liters of fresh dialysate. This dialysate stays in the abdominal cavity until the patient is ready to attach himself again to the cycler machine at bedtime. The patient is able to sleep because the machine is very quiet, and extra long tubing from the machine allows the patient to move while asleep.

Most proponents of this technique feel it decreases the infection rate and permits the patient to be free of exchanges throughout the day, enabling him to work more freely and carry out his activities of daily living.

▷ The Patient Undergoing Kidney Surgery

Preoperative Nursing Management

All operations on the kidney should be attempted only after a period of study and preparation. *Every effort is made to ensure that renal function is as good as possible.* This is the major preoperative goal. Patients with preexisting renal disease tend to have a higher incidence of compromised renal function. Fluids are encouraged in liberal amounts to promote increased excretion of waste products before surgery. Since kidney infection may be present preoperatively, a wide-spectrum antimicrobial is given to avoid the hazards of bacteremia. A coagulation profile (prothrombin time, partial thromboplastin time, platelet count) may be done if the patient has a history of bruising and bleeding. The general preoperative preparation is similar to that described in pages 355 to 363.

Patients facing kidney surgery are apprehensive and usually enter the hospital with pain, fever, hematuria, etc. Thus, it is helpful to encourage the patient to recognize and express any feelings of anxiety. Confidence is reinforced by establishing a relationship of trust and by providing gentle and considerate care. A patient faced with the prospect of losing a kidney may think that he will be an invalid the rest of his life. This is not true in most instances, because normal function may be maintained by a single kidney.

Perioperative Concerns

The operative incisions for renal surgery include the flank approach, the intercostal incision, the lumbodorsal incision, and the transverse abdominal or thoracoabdominal incision (Fig. 43-7). The difficulties in renal surgery are related to difficulty in access to the kidney.

Recent Trends in Renal Surgery. *Extracorporeal renal surgery* (bench surgery, ex vivo surgery) represents a new development in renal surgery. Certain operations on the kidney and ureter are done with considerable risk because of bleeding, difficult exposure, and poor illumination. Because tumor resections and complicated renal reconstructive procedures temporarily interrupt renal circulation for variable lengths of time, there can be subsequent damage to renal function after 20 to 30 minutes of ischemia.

(At normal body temperature, the kidney will sustain permanent functional damage after 30 minutes.) Recently, it has become possible to correct several pathologic conditions of the renal artery and kidney and to perform reconstructive surgery on the kidney by removing the kidney, placing it on the "bench" (surgical table), repairing the lesion, and reimplanting the kidney. Damage to renal function is prevented by hypothermia of the kidney, which allows renal preservation by depressing renal metabolic activity and preventing ischemic damage. Kidney preservation is achieved during extracorporeal renal surgery by cooling (immersing kidney in a cold salt solution and flushing with a cold perfusate) or by continuous pulsatile perfusion with a kidney preservation machine. This technique is useful in the repair of certain vascular lesions (renal artery stenosis/thrombosis; renal artery aneurysm) and for the removal of renal neoplasms, especially in a solitary kidney.

Percutaneous nephrostomy is the insertion of a tube through the skin into the renal collecting system. It is done to provide external drainage of urine from an obstructed ureter, to provide a route for insertion of an ureteral stent,

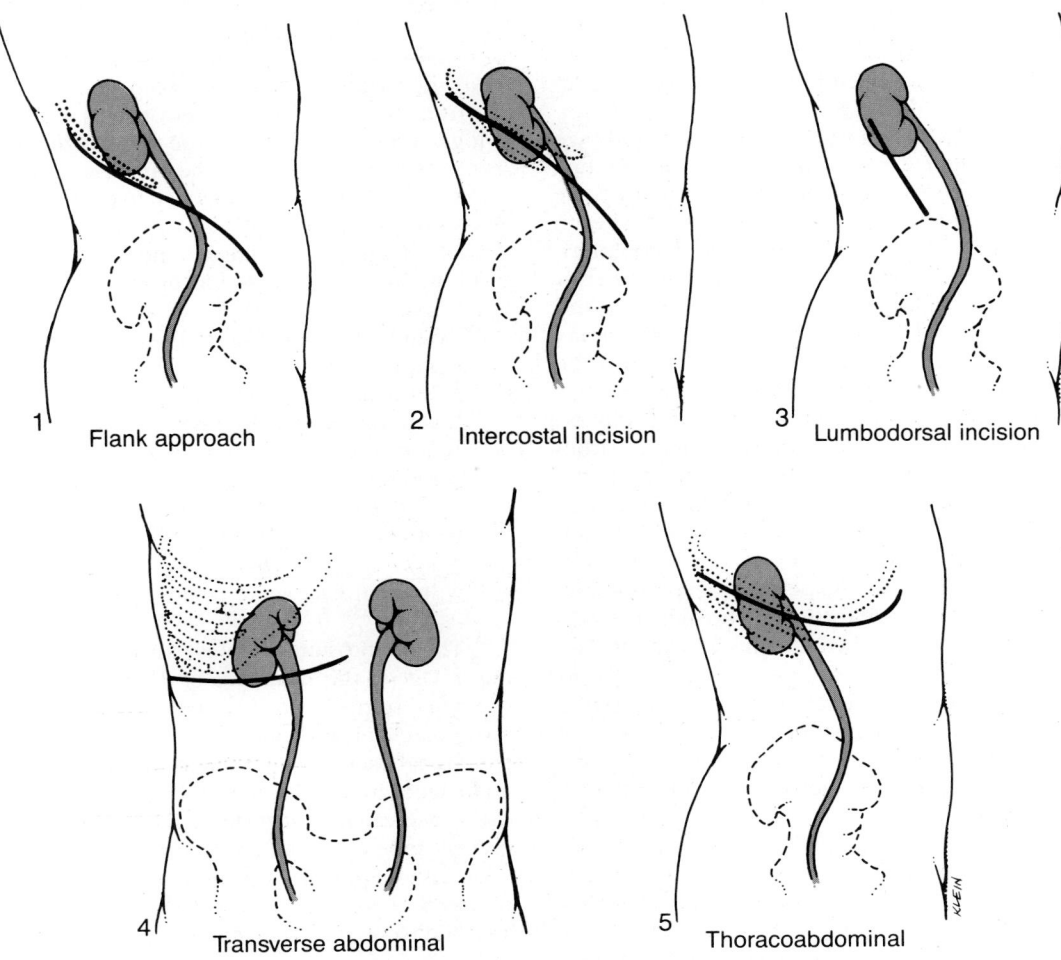

1   Flank approach

2   Intercostal incision

3   Lumbodorsal incision

4   Transverse abdominal

5   Thoracoabdominal

Figure 43-7. Standard incisions for urologic operation.

to dissolve renal calculi (see p. 1010), to dilate strictures, to close fistulas, to administer drugs, to allow insertion of a brush biopsy instrument and nephroscope, and to perform selected surgical procedures.

The skin site is prepared and anesthetized, and the patient is asked to hold his breath while a spinal needle is advanced into the renal pelvis. Urine is aspirated for culture, and contrast material may be injected into the pyelocalyceal system. An angiographic catheter guidewire is introduced through the needle to the kidney. The needle is withdrawn and the tract dilated by the passage of tubes or guidewires. Then the nephrostomy tube is introduced and positioned within the kidney or ureter, fixed by skin sutures, and connected to a closed drainage system.

Postoperative Management and Nursing Implementation

Based on the clinical manifestations and diagnostic assessment data, the patient's postoperative nursing diagnoses include pain and discomfort related to the surgical procedure and presence of drainage tubes/catheters; and potential for complications related to the site of incision and nature of the surgery.

The patient's goals include (1) relief of pain and discomfort, and (2) avoidance of complications. The postoperative nursing goal is to reduce factors that contribute to postoperative complications.

Since the kidney is such a vascular organ, hemorrhage and shock are the chief dangers following renal surgery. Assessment of blood pressure, pulse, and respiration are essential in patient monitoring. The surgical approaches to the kidney predispose the patient to respiratory complications and paralytic ileus. Also, with a subcostal or posterior incision, the patient may have severe pain on breathing and coughing. If the pleura has been opened, pneumothorax may be a problem. The incision is generally close to the diaphragm, and with a substernal incision, the nerves may be stretched and bruised. Pain is also caused from distention of the renal capsule (tumor, blood clot), ischemia (from occlusion of blood vessels), and stretching of the intrarenal blood vessels. The patient requires careful postoperative pain control, as he will tend to splint his chest while deep breathing and turning. If the narcotic is given at proper intervals, the patient will be able to perform deep-breathing and coughing exercises more effectively. The incentive spirometer may be used to help maximize lung inflation. The patient is encouraged to cough after each deep breath to loosen secretions. The patient may also complain of muscular aches and pains resulting from the position assumed on the operating table, which places anatomical and physiologic stresses on the body. Massage, moist heat, and analgesic medications provide relief.

Abdominal distention and paralytic ileus are fairly common following operations on the kidney and ureter, and are thought to be due to a reflex paralysis of intestinal peristalsis and to manipulation of the colon or duodenum in gaining access to the kidney during surgery. Assessment is made by listening to the abdomen with a stethoscope. Oral fluids are avoided until auscultation reveals active bowel sounds or until the passage of flatus is noted. Fluids and electrolytes are replaced intravenously. For relief of abdominal disten-

tion, decompression via a nasogastric tube gives rapid relief. (See p. 837 for treatment of paralytic ileus.) Urine output is monitored to ensure adequate renal functioning.

Drug Therapy. Antibiotics are given as necessary on the basis of culture identification of the causative organism. The toxic manifestations of these agents must be kept in mind when assessing the patient. Subcutaneous therapy with low doses of heparin has been shown to prevent thromboembolism in urologic patients.

Management of Drainage Tubes

Almost all postoperative kidney and urologic patients have drains, tubes, or catheters. Following operations such as nephrostomy, pyelotomy, and ureterotomy, drainage tubes may be placed directly in the kidney, pelvis, or ureter in order to divert the urine and keep the wound dry. All catheters and tubes must remain functioning (e.g., draining) to prevent obstruction by blood clots, which can cause infection. Pain similar to renal colic is caused by the passage of clotted blood down the ureter.

Nephrostomy Drainage. A nephrostomy tube is inserted directly into the kidney for temporary or permanent urinary diversion either by open operation or percutaneously (see p. 989). This may be accomplished by a single tube or by a self-retaining U-loop or circular nephrostomy tube. The purposes of nephrostomy drainage are to provide drainage from the kidney after surgery, conserve and permit physiologic restoration of renal tissue traumatized by obstruction, and provide drainage when the ureter is no longer draining. The nephrostomy tube is attached to closed gravity drainage or to a urostomy appliance. The patient and tubing are observed for signs of bleeding (immediate or delayed), urinary sand, stone formation, and fistulae.

- Evaluate for bleeding at the nephrostomy site (main complication).
- Ensure that the nephrostomy catheter is draining freely. Any plugging of the tube causes pain, trauma, bursting of the suture lines, and infection. If the tube is inadvertently dislodged, it must be immediately replaced by the surgeon, since the nephrostomy opening will contract, making it difficult to reinsert the tube.
- A *nephrostomy tube is not clamped,* as such an action will precipitate acute pyelonephritis.

The nephrostomy tube is irrigated only upon direct request. Due to the small size of the renal pelvis, only 10 ml of warm, sterile saline is used for irrigation purposes to avoid mechanical damage to the kidney or infection from pyelorenal backflow. Fluid intake is encouraged to produce good mechanical flushing and to dilute urinary elements that cause calculus formation. The urine is kept acidic to prevent tube encrustation by urinary sediments. If the patient has a nephrostomy tube in each kidney, separate output records for each catheter are kept. The catheters are attached to leg urinals when the patient becomes ambulatory.

Postpercutaneous Nephrostomy Tube Management. Following percutaneous tube insertion, the patient is also monitored for signs and symptoms of bleeding and infection, as these are the most significant complications. Transient hematuria for 24 to 48 hours may be expected. The amount and color of the urine are noted. Other problems include urine leakage around the nephrostomy tube and tube dislodgment.

Ureteral Stents

A *ureteral stent* is a tubular device designed for placement within the ureter to maintain ureteral flow in patients with ureteral obstruction (from edema, stricture, fibrosis, advanced malignancy), to restore kidney function, to divert urine, to promote healing, and to maintain the caliber/patency of the ureter after surgery (Fig. 43-8).

The stent, usually of soft, flexible silicone, may be temporary or permanent. It may be inserted endoscopically (via cystoscope), percutaneously (also through the nephrostomy tube), or by open operation. Complications include infection from a foreign body in the genitourinary tract, tube encrustation, bleeding or clot obstruction within the stent, and dislodgment of the stent.

Newer stent designs avoid some of these problems. The double-J ureteral stent has a "J"-shaped curve molded into each end, which prevents upward or downward migration. This stent can be used in place of a nephrostomy or pyelostomy for short- or long-term urinary drainage. The double-pigtail ureteral stent has a pigtail coil at each end of the stent, which permits placement of the upper coil (pigtail) in the renal pelvis, with the lower coil at the ureteral orifice. The coils prevent stent migration while allowing free body movement.

The nursing approach is to monitor for bleeding; observe and measure output; evaluate for purulent drainage at the stent's insertion site (if percutaneous) or in the drainage bag; and monitor for stent dislodgment, which is noted by colicky pain and a decrease in urine output.

An indwelling stent usually induces local ureteral reaction, including mucosal edema, which can cause transient ureteral obstruction.

Indwelling Urethral Catheter. Make sure the indwelling urethral catheter is dependent and draining. (See p. 972.)

Patient Education

Prior to discharge, the patient should be informed about the elements of posthospital care. If drainage tubes are still in place, the patient and a family member should be instructed about the care of the tubes and management of the dressings.

The patient is encouraged to continue a liberal intake of fluids. He should know the signs and symptoms of urinary infection. He is advised to take frequent, short rest periods and to increase activity gradually in order to facilitate his return to strength.

Evaluation
Expected Outcomes

1. Experiences relief of pain and discomfort
   a. Reports progressive decrease in pain
   b. Requires analgesics at less frequent intervals
   c. Ambulates with progressive tolerance

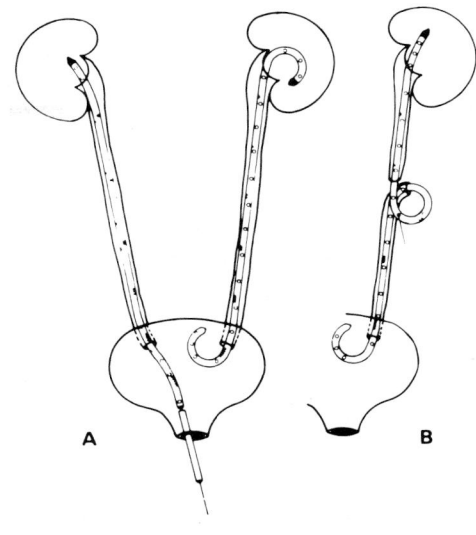

Figure 43-8. (*A*) Retrograde passage of ureteral stent. The Double-J ureteral stent is shaped to resist migration. The proximal J hooks into the lower calix or renal pelvis, and the distal J curves into the bladder. (*B*) Open surgical placement of Double-J stent prior to an ureteral anastomosis. (Courtesy of Medical Engineering Corporation, Racine, Wisconsin.)

2. Experiences no complications
   a. Maintains blood pressure, pulse, respiration, and temperature within preoperative ranges
   b. Maintains clear breath sounds
   c. Uses incentive spirometer as directed
   d. Performs deep-breathing and leg exercises
   e. Attains/maintains active bowel sounds
   f. Maintains fluid and electrolyte balance

▷ Bibliography

Books

Alken C–E, Sokeland J, and Engel RME. Urology. Guide for Diagnosis and Therapy. New York, Thieme, 1982.

Blandy J. Lecture Notes on Urology. Boston, Blackwell Scientific Publications. 1982.

Brenner BM and Rector FC Jr. The Kidney, Vols 1 and 2, 2nd ed. Philadelphia, WB Saunders, 1981.

Cockett ATK and Koshiba K. Manual of Urologic Surgery. New York, Springer–Verlag, 1979.

Ehrlich RM. Urologic Surgery. Mt Kisco, Futura, 1980.

Horsley JA et al. Closed Urinary Drainage Systems. New York, Grune & Stratton, 1981.

Kaufman JJ. Current Urologic Therapy. Philadelphia, WB Saunders, 1980.

Lerner J and Khan Z. Mosby's Manual of Urologic Nursing. St Louis, CV Mosby, 1982.

McConnell EA and Zimmerman MF. Care of Patients with Urologic Problems. Philadelphia, JB Lippincott, 1982.

Mitchell JP. Endoscopic Operative Urology. Boston, Wright PSG, 1981.

Novick AC and Straffon RA. Vascular Problems in Urologic Surgery. Philadelphia, WB Saunders, 1982.

Nursing Photobook: Implementing Urologic Procedures. Horsham, Pennsylvania, Intermed Communications, 1981.

Schrier RW. Manual of Nephrology. Boston, Little, Brown & Co, 1981.

Articles
General

Boh DM and VanSon AR. The water-load test. Am J Nurs 1982 Jan; 82(1):112–113.

Orr ML. Drugs and renal disease. Am J Nurs 1981 May; 81(5):969–971.

Toner M. Urinary tract obstruction: The hidden threats in treatment. RN 1982 May; 45(5):58–61.

Catheterization

Bates P. A troubleshooter's guide to indwelling catheters. RN 1981 Mar; 44(3):62–68.

Blandy JP. How to catheterize the bladder. Br J Hosp Med 1981 July; 26(1):58–60.

Burke JP et al. Prevention of catheter-associated urinary tract infections. Am J Med 1981 Mar; 70(3):655–658.

Christensen PB and Kronborg O. Suprapubic bladder drainage in colorectal surgery. Br J Surg 1981 May; 68(5):348–349.

From the NIH: Urinary catheter care may increase risk of infection. JAMA 1981 July 3; 246(1):30.

Harper WES. An appraisal of 12 solutions used for bladder irrigation or instillation. Br J Urol 1981 Oct; 53(5):433–438.

Killion A. Reducing the risk of infection from indwelling urethral catheters. Nursing '82 1982 May; 12(5):84–88.

Turck M and Stamm W. Nosocomial infection of the urinary tract. Am J Med 1981 Mar; 70(3):651–654.

Warren JW et al. Sequelae and management of urinary infection in the patient requiring chronic catheterization. J Urol 1981 Jan; 125(1):1–8.

Wong ES and Hooton TM. Guidelines for prevention of catheter-associated urinary tract infections. Infection Control 1981 Mar–Apr; 9(2):125–130.

Chronic Hemodialysis

Alcherson E. Home hemodialysis and the spouse assistant. AANNT J 1981 Aug; 8(4):29–34.

Bauer D. Preventing the spread of hepatitis B in dialysis units. Am J Nurs 1980 Feb; 80(2):260–261.

Bulgen RH. Comparative costs of various dialysis treatments. Bull Peri Dial 1981 Sept; 1(6):88–91.

Chambers JK. Assessing the dialysis patient at home. Am J Nurs 1981 Apr; 81(4):750–753.

Clough DH and Higgins PG. Discrepancies in estimating blood loss. Am J Nurs 1981 Feb; 81(2):331–333.

Ostrow LS. Air embolism and central venous lines. Am J Nurs 1981 Nov; 81(11):2036–2038.

Reed SB. Giving more than dialysis. Nursing '82 1982 Apr; 12(4):58–63.

Schlebusch L and Levin A. Can poor compliance in hemodialysis patients be predicted? Dial Transplant 1982 July; 11(7):601–604.

Sokn KA et al. Rescind the risks in administering anticoagulants. Nursing '81 1981 Oct; 11(10):34–41.

Thompson DA. Teaching the client about anticoagulants. Am J Nurs 1982 Feb; 82(2):278–281.

Walser M. Nutritional therapy of renal failure: Current status, future directions. Postgrad Med 1982 Feb; 71(2):9–11, 14.

Intermittent Peritoneal Dialysis

Chan MK et al. Hyperlipidemia in patients on maintenance hemodialysis and peritoneal dialysis: The relative pathogenetic roles of triglyceride production and triglyceride removal. Clin Nephrol 1982 Apr; 17(4):183–190.

Gastaldi L et al. Low flow clearances on peritoneal dialysis in acute renal failure. Nephron 1981; 29(1–2):101–102.

Goodman W, Gallagher N, and Sherrard DJ. Peritoneal dialysis fluid as a source of hepatitis antigen. Nephron 1981; 29(3–4):107–109.

Johnson RS. Home dialysis: The competition between CAPD and hemo. JAMA 1981 Apr; 245(15):1511–1514.

Karanicolas S and Thompson D. Intermittent peritoneal dialysis in the treatment of diabetes with end-stage renal disease. Peritoneal Dialysis Bull [Suppl] 1982 Apr–June; 2(2):515–516.

Kliger AS. Current concepts in peritoneal dialysis. Nephron 1981; 27(4–5):209–214.

LaGreca G, Biasiali S, and Chearamonte S. Acid–base balance on peritoneal dialysis Clin Nephrol 1981 July; 16(1):1–7.

Palmer AP. As it was in the beginning: A history of peritoneal dialysis. Bull Peri Dial 1982 Jan–Mar; 2(1):16–23.

Roxe DM et al. Hemodialysis vs peritoneal dialysis: Results of a 3-year prospective controlled study. Kidney Int 1981 Feb; 19(2):341–348.

Steiner RW, Vas SI, and Stephen I. What are the indications for removal of the permanent peritoneal catheter? Bull Peri Dial 1981 Dec; 1(7):145.

Continuous Ambulatory Peritoneal Dialysis

Amair P et al. Continuous ambulatory peritoneal dialysis in diabetics with end-stage renal disease. N Engl J Med 1982 Mar; 306(11):625–630.

Arenz R. Do it yourself dialysis. RN 1981 July; 44(7):56–60.

Blumenkrantz MJ et al. Retrograde menstruation in women undergoing chronic peritoneal dialysis. Obstet Gynecol 1981 May; 57(5):667–670.

Blumenkrantz MJ et al. Metabolic balance studies and dietary protein requirements in patients undergoing continuous ambulatory peritoneal dialysis. Kidney Int 1982 June; 21:849–861.

Bond WW, Peterson NJ, and Cravelle CR. Hepatitis B virus in peritoneal dialysis fluid: A potential hazard. Dial Transplant 1982 July; 11(7):592, 596–597, 600.

Denniston DJ and Burns KT. Home peritoneal dialysis. Am J Nurs 1980 Nov; 80(11):2022–2026.

Editorial: Ambulatory peritonitis. Lancet 1982 May 15; 1(8281):1104–1105.

Fenton SSA. Selection criteria for CAPD. Bull Peri Dial 1982 Jan–Mar; 81(6):1144–1146.

Handa SP and Greer S. Pseudomembranous colitis and cloudy drainage in patients on peritoneal dialysis. Dial Transplant 1982 Oct; 11(10):910–911.

Irwin BC. Now—peritoneal dialysis for chronic patients too. RN 1981 July; 44(6):49–52.

Johnson BM. Ambulatory health care in the 80's: Decade of dilemmas. Am J Nurs 1980 Jan; 80(1):76–79.

Knowles RD. Managing angry feelings. Am J Nurs 1982 Feb; 82(2):299.

McMarram ME. The manipulative patient. Am J Nurs 1981 June; 81(6):1188–1190.

Oreopoulos DG, Khanna R, and Williams P. Continuous ambulatory peritoneal dialysis—1981. Nephron 1982; 30(4):293–303.

Perras ST and Zappocosta AR. The application of Orem's theory in promoting self-care in a peritoneal dialysis facility. AANNT J 1982 June; 9(3):37–39, 55.

Prowant B and Fruto LV. The continuous ambulatory peritoneal dialysis (CAPD) home training program. AANNT J 1981 Dec; 8(6):18–19.

Rubin J et al. Peritoneal abnormalities during infectious episode of CAPD. Nephron 1981; 29(3–4):124–127.

Schelkewaert R, Bogaerts Y, and Pauwels R. Management of a massive hydrothorax in a CAPD patient: A case report and a review of the literature. Bull Peri Dial 1982 June; 2(2):69–71.

Stanitis MA and Ryan J. Noncompliance—an unacceptable diagnosis? Am J Nurs 1982 June; 82(6):941–942.

Waugh WW. Retrospective appraisal of daily equilibrium peritoneal dialysis and a presage for maintenance dialysis. Dial Transplant 1982 Aug; 11(8):712–713.

Winchester JF et al. Pulmonary function and peritoneal dialysis. Int J Artif Organs 1981 Nov; 4(6):267–269.

Yoos Y. Compliance: Philosophical and ethical considerations. Nurs Pract 1981 Sept/Oct; 6(5):27–30, 34.

Zappacosta AR, Caro J, and Erslen A. Normalization of hematocrit in patients with end-stage renal disease on CAPD: The role of erythropoietin. Am J Med 1982 Jan; 72(1):53–57.

Kidney Surgery

Bigongiari LR et al. Percutaneous ureteral stent placement for stricture management and internal urinary drainage. AJR 1979 Nov; 133(5):865–868.

Cain L and Bigongiari LR. The percutaneous nephrostomy tube. Am J Nurs 1982 Feb; 82(2):296–298.

Cheema P and Pranikoff K. Placement of nephrostomy tube into nondilated system. Urology 1982 Mar; 19(3):312–313.

Cope C and Zeit RM. Pseudoaneurysms after nephrostomy. AJR 1982 Aug; 139(2):255–261.

Hinkle MT and Bowditch RR. The great stent mystery. Nursing '81 1981 Apr; 11(4):94–95.

Kaplan JO et al. Dilatation of a surgically ligated ureter through a percutaneous nephrostomy. AJR 1982 July; 139(1):188–189.

Lawson RK. Extracorporeal renal surgery. J Urol 1980 Mar; 123(3):301–305.

Levine RS, Pollack HM, and Banner MP. Transient ureteral obstruction after ureteral stenting. AJR 1982 Feb; 138(2):323–327.

Pinter J, Szokoly V, and Szabo Z. Local hypothermia in surgery on poorly functioning kidneys. Int Urol Nephrol 1981 13(1):15–24.

Segal AJ and Spitzer RM. Simplified procedure for percutaneous nephrostomy. AJR 1981 Nov; 137(5):1078–1079.

Stables DP. Percutaneous nephrostomy: Techniques, indications and results. Urol Clin North Am 1982 Feb; 9(1):15–29.

Agencies
Governmental

National Institute of Arthritis, Metabolism and Digestive Diseases, National Institutes of Health, Bethesda, Maryland 20205

Voluntary

National Association of Patients on Hemodialysis and Transplantation, 505 Northern Blvd., Great Neck, New York 11021

National Kidney Foundation, 116 E. 27th St., New York, New York 10016

United Ostomy Association, 1111 Wilshire Blvd., Los Angeles, California 90017

44

Management of Patients With Renal and Urinary Disorders

▷ Acute Renal Failure

Pathophysiology

Acute renal failure (ARF) is a sudden and almost complete loss of kidney function caused by failure of the renal circulation or by glomerular or tubular change. Renal failure results when the kidneys are unable to remove the body's metabolic wastes or perform their homeostatic function (*e.g.,* the maintenance of a stable internal environment). The substances normally eliminated in the urine accumulate in the body fluids as a result of impaired renal excretion and lead to a disruption in homeostatic, endocrine, and metabolic functions. Renal failure is a total body disease and is a final common pathway of many different kidney and urinary tract diseases. Each year an estimated 42,000 Americans die of irreversible kidney failure.

Causes. Acute renal failure is manifested by sudden oliguria (less than 500 ml of urine per day), high-output acute renal failure, or anuria (less than 50 ml of urine per day), and a daily rise in serum creatinine and certain other metabolic waste products from the kidney following a variety of insults. Any condition that causes reduction in renal blood flow, such as volume depletion, hypotension, or shock, leads to a reduction in glomerular filtration, renal ischemia, and tubular damage. Renal failure may also result from the adverse effects of burns, crushing injuries, and infection as well as from nephrotoxic agents that cause tubular necrosis and temporary cessation of renal function. Severe transfusion reactions may also cause renal failure as the hemoglobin, which filters through the kidney glomeruli, becomes concentrated in the kidney tubules to such a degree that precipitation occurs, halting the excretion of urine. Following these events, the kidneys become swollen and edematous, and the epithelial cells in the tubules may undergo necrosis (Chart 44-1).

Exact pathogenesis is open to considerable debate with a variety of possible mechanisms for renal failure and oliguria. In many instances, there is a clear-cut underlying disease, mechanical blockage of the urinary tract by calculi or tumor, or renal artery obstruction.

Causes of increased BUN and oliguria, which may be reversible, are: (1) hypovolemia; (2) hypotension due to any cause; (3) congestive heart failure; (4) obstruction, tumor, etc.; and (5) bilateral renal artery or vein obstruction.

In summary, risk factors for renal failure include hypovolemic hypotension (oligemic shock, hemorrhage, dehydration, burns), sepsis, nephrotoxic drugs, trauma, multiple blood transfusions, cardiopulmonary bypass, surgery of the aorta or renal vessels, obstructive jaundice, surgery of the biliary tree, and extensive surgery in the elderly.

Prevention and Health Maintenance

In caring for any patient, the nurse will be alerted by a careful history that reveals whether or not the patient has been taking potentially nephrotoxic antimicrobial agents. The kidneys are especially susceptible to the adverse effects of drugs because they receive such a large blood flow (25% of the cardiac output at rest). The nephrons are thus exposed to high concentrations of antimicrobials as a result of glomerular filtration and tubular secretion and reabsorption. Also, since the kidney is a major excretory pathway for many antimicrobials, it is more likely to suffer toxic effects from drugs. Therefore, in people taking potentially nephrotoxic drugs (aminoglycosides, gentamicin, tobramycin, colistimethate, polymyxin B, amphotericin B, vancomycin, amikacin, capreomycin) renal function should be monitored by BUN and serum creatinine evaluations within 24 hours following initiation of drug therapy and at least twice weekly while the patient is receiving therapy. Any agent that reduces renal blood flow (*i.e.,* chronic analgesic abuse) may cause renal deterioration. Chronic analgesic abuse causes interstitial nephritis and papillary necrosis as the result of a complicated metabolic insult.

Other precautionary measures taken to avoid renal complications include the following:

- Adequate hydration procedures must be initiated before, during, and after operative measures.
- Shock, in any clinical situation, must be prevented or treated promptly with blood and fluid replacement.
- Critically ill patients should be monitored by means of central venous pressure readings and hourly urinary output measurements to detect the onset of renal failure at the earliest possible moment.
- Hypertension states require prompt therapy.
- Persons undergoing intensive diagnostic studies requiring dehydration (barium enema, intravenous pyelogram, etc.) should have "rest days," especially elderly patients who may not have adequate renal reserve. Avoid dehydration.
- All precautions must be taken to ensure that the correct person receives the appropriate blood in order to avoid severe transfusion reactions, which can precipitate renal complications.
- Infections, which may produce progressive renal damage, must be controlled and avoided.
- Special attention must be paid to draining wounds, burns, and other causes of sepsis, etc., which may lead to septicemia.
- Meticulous care must be given to patients with indwelling catheters to prevent ascending infections. Catheters should be removed as soon as possible.

Chart 44-1
Causes of Acute Renal Failure

1. Ischemia (severe hemorrhagic shock, open heart surgery, cross clamping of the aorta)
2. Septic shock
3. Pigment
   a. Hemoglobin (transfusion reaction, blackwater fever, hemolytic anemia due to G-6-PD deficiency)
   b. Myoglobin (crush injury, exercise, electrical shock, seizures, diabetes)
4. Nephrotoxins
   a. Aminoglycosides
   b. Antibiotics
   c. Streptomycin
   d. Arsenic
   e. Mercury
   f. Certain other heavy materials

▶ **Assessment**

Almost every part of the body suffers when there is failure of the normal renal regulatory mechanism. The patient appears critically ill and is lethargic with persistent nausea, vomiting, and diarrhea. The skin and mucous membranes are dry from dehydration, and the breath may have the odor of urine. Drowsiness, headache, muscle twitching, and convulsions are the central nervous system manifestations that are present in varying degrees. The urinary output is scanty, may be bloody, and has a low specific gravity (1.010 compared to 1.025 normally). There is a steady daily rise in serum creatinine with the rate of rise dependent upon the degree of catabolism present.

There are three clinical phases of acute renal failure: the period of oliguria, a period of diuresis, and a period of recovery. The *period of oliguria* (urinary volume less than 400–600 ml/24 hours) is accompanied by a rise in the serum concentration of the elements usually excreted by the kidneys (urea, creatinine, uric acid, organic acids, and the intracellular cations—potassium and magnesium). The oliguria phase lasts approximately 10 days.

In some patients, there can be a decrease in renal function with increasing nitrogen retention, yet the patient is actually excreting 2 or more liters of urine daily. This is the so-called "high-output failure" or nonoliguric form of renal failure and occurs predominantly after nephrotoxic antibiotics are administered to the patient; it also results from burns, traumatic injury, and halogenated anesthesia.

In the second phase, the *period of diuresis,* the patient experiences a gradually increasing urinary output, which signals that glomerular filtration has started to recover. Although the urinary output may reach normal or elevated levels, renal function may be markedly abnormal in the diuretic phase.

The *period of recovery* signals the improvement of renal function and may take from 3 to 12 months. Usually, there is a permanent partial reduction in the glomerular filtration rate and concentrating ability.

Patient Problems/Nursing Diagnoses

Based on the clinical manifestations, the nursing history, and the diagnostic assessment data, the patient's major nursing problems include retention of metabolic wastes related to impaired renal function; fluid and electrolyte imbalance related to impaired renal function; and alterations in sensorium related to cerebral irritability.

▶ Planning and Implementation

Goals

The major goals of the patient include:

1. Excretion of metabolic wastes
2. Fluid and electrolyte balance
3. Normalcy of sensorium

The kidney has a remarkable ability to recover from insult. Therefore, the objective of treatment of acute renal failure is to restore the normal homeostatic environment so that repair of renal tissue and restoration of renal function can take place. A search is made to treat and eliminate any possible cause.

Early dialysis is indicated to prevent serious complications of uremia, such as pericarditis, seizures, etc. Dialysis produces a more sustained correction of biochemical abnormalities; allows for liberalization of fluid, protein, and sodium intake; diminishes bleeding tendencies; and may help wound healing. Peritoneal dialysis (see p. 977) or hemodialysis (see p. 981) may be carried out.

Maintenance of Fluid and Electrolyte Balance. Every effort is made to maintain fluid and electrolyte balance and to prevent acidosis. Guides to establishing fluid balance include daily body weight, serial measurements of central venous pressure, serum and urine concentrations, fluid losses, blood pressure, and the clinical status of the patient. These parameters should be kept on a flow chart to indicate the rate and trend of biochemical deterioration or improvement. Fluids that are given to replace the daily losses usually amount to 400 ml to 500 ml per 24 hours (the balance of insensible loss [1000 ml] and water gained by metabolism [400 ml–600 ml] plus measured fluid losses during the oliguric phase). The input and output are measured, including urine, gastric drainage, stools, wound drainage, and perspiration. The patient is weighed daily and can be expected to lose 0.2 kg to 0.5 kg (½–1 lb) daily. This occurs if the patient is in negative nitrogen balance (*i.e.,* receiving inadequate caloric support). This weight loss represents obligatory tissue breakdown. If the patient fails to lose weight or develops hypertension, this indicates fluid retention. Fluid excesses can be evaluated by the clinical findings of dyspnea, tachycardia, and distended neck veins. The lungs are auscultated for signs of moist crackles (rales). Since pulmonary edema may be precipitated by excessive administration of parenteral fluids, the presacral and pretibial areas must be examined for edema several times daily.

Sodium losses are measured (serum and urine sodium levels) and replaced. Additionally, there may be large losses of sodium from the gastrointestinal tract from diarrhea and vomiting. Patients with acute oliguria cannot eliminate the daily metabolic load produced by the normal metabolic processes. This is reflected by a fall in the blood carbon dioxide combining power and blood *p*H. Thus, progressive acidosis accompanies renal failure. When severe acidosis is present, the arterial blood gases must be monitored and appropriate ventilatory measures instituted if respiratory problems develop. The patient may require sodium bicarbonate therapy or dialysis.

A patient with renal disease in which the glomerular filtration rate is reduced has a decreased ability to excrete potassium. Protein catabolism (breakdown) results in the release of cellular potassium into the body fluids, causing serious potassium intoxication. High serum potassium levels are dangerous and lead to cardiac arrhythmias and arrest. Sources of potassium are tissue breakdown; dietary intake; blood anywhere outside the vascular system, such as in the gastrointestinal tract; or blood transfusion and other sources (intravenous infusions, potassium penicillin, and extracellular shift in response to metabolic acidosis). Thus, a continuing patient assessment for hyperkalemia (potassium intoxication) is conducted by evaluating serum electrolyte determinations (potassium value above 6.0 mEq/liter), ECG assessment (peaked T waves), and patient evaluation. The elevated potassium levels may be reduced by giving ion exchange resins (sodium polystyrene sulfonate [Kayexalate]) orally or by retention enema. The drug's action depends on the ability to move resin through the intestinal tract. Sorbitol induces water loss in the gastrointestinal tract and may be given orally or as an enema with Kayexalate. The patient should be watched for the development of fecal impaction. If a retention enema is given (the colon is the major site for potassium exchange), a catheter with a balloon may be used to facilitate retention if necessary. The patient should retain the resin 30 to 45 minutes to remove potassium.

- A patient with a high and rising level of serum potassium requires immediate peritoneal dialysis or hemodialysis.
- Intravenous glucose and insulin or calcium gluconate is sometimes used as an emergency and temporary measure for potassium intoxication.
- Sodium bicarbonate may be given to promote an elevation of plasma *p*H. Sodium bicarbonate increases the *p*H, which causes potassium to move into the cell, and the result is lowering of potassium in the plasma. This is short-term therapy and is used with other long-term measures.

There may be an increase in serum phosphate concentrations. This problem may be controlled with phosphate-binding agents (aluminum hydroxide) to keep phosphate from being absorbed into the bloodstream and to help prevent a continuing rise in serum phosphate levels.

Serum calcium levels may be low in response to decreased absorption of calcium from the intestine and in association with an elevation of serum phosphate levels.

Adequate blood flow to the kidneys in some patients may be restored by intravenous fluids and medications. Mannitol or furosemide or ethacrynic acid may be prescribed to initiate a diuresis and prevent or minimize subsequent renal failure.

- Observe for signs of dehydration or hypovolemia during the diuretic phase.
- When hypovolemia is associated with hypoproteinemia, an infusion of albumin may be given. Shock, if present, is controlled, and any infection is treated.

Dietary proteins are limited to approximately 1 g per kg of body weight during the oliguric phase to minimize protein breakdown and to prevent accumulation of toxic end products. Caloric requirements are met with high carbohydrate feedings, as carbohydrates have a protein-sparing power. Foods and fluids containing potassium and phosphorus (bananas, citrus fruits and juices, coffee) are restricted. Potassium intake is usually restricted to 40 mEq/day to 60 mEq/day, and sodium is usually restricted to 2 g/day. The patient may require hyperalimentation (see p. 780).

Anemia inevitably accompanies acute renal failure due to multiple causes: blood loss due to uremic gastrointestinal lesions, reduced red cell life span, and reduced erythropoietin production.

The oliguric phase of acute renal failure may last from 10 to 20 days and is followed by the diuretic phase, at which time urinary output begins to increase, signaling that glomerular filtration is taking place. Blood chemistry evaluations are made to determine the amounts of sodium, potassium, and water needed for replacement along with assessment for overhydration or underhydration abnormalities.

- Be alert for urinary tract infection, which is common and potentially dangerous in the diuretic phase.

After the diuretic phase, the patient is placed on a high-protein, high-caloric diet and is encouraged to resume activities gradually since muscle weakness will be present from excessive catabolism.

▶ **Evaluation**

Expected Outcomes

1. Excretes metabolic wastes
   a. Attains normal values of the following chemicals in the blood: urea, creatinine, uric acid, phosphate, potassium, and magnesium
2. Attains/maintains fluid and electrolyte balance
   a. Attains/maintains central venous pressure within normal ranges
   b. Attains/maintains blood pressure within normal ranges
   c. Exhibits absence of circulatory overload: absence of dyspnea, tachycardia, distended neck veins, presacral edema, pretibial edema
   d. Attains/maintains serum sodium within normal ranges
   e. Attains/maintains CO_2 combining power within normal ranges
   f. Attains/maintains serum calcium level within normal ranges
3. Demonstrates normalcy of sensorium
   a. Is oriented to person, place, and time
   b. Responds to sensory stimuli appropriately
   c. Has normal attention span
   d. Denies presence of headache
   e. Experiences no convulsions

▷ **Chronic Renal Failure (Uremia)**

Chronic renal failure is a progressive deterioration in renal function in which the body's homeostatic mechanisms fail, resulting fatally in uremia (an excess of urea and other nitrogenous wastes in the blood) unless dialysis or a kidney transplantation is performed. It may be caused by chronic glomerulonephritis; pyelonephritis; uncontrolled hypertension; hereditary lesions, such as in polycystic kidney disease; vascular disorders; obstructive uropathy; renal disease secondary to systemic disease; renal disease secondary to drugs or toxic agents; infections; etc.

Pathophysiology. As renal function declines, the products of protein metabolism (which forms the constituents of urine) accumulate in the blood. There are imbalances in the body chemistry and in the cardiovascular, hematologic, gastrointestinal, neurologic and skeletal systems. Skin and reproductive changes are also seen.

With the decrease in glomerular filtration, there is a decrease in filtered phosphorus, which will cause serum phosphate to rise. This results in a decrease in ionizable calcium. Serum calcium is reduced mainly due to decreased intestinal absorption of calcium. Consequently, there is an increase in parathyroid release (secondary hyperparathyroidism). The latter normally increases the excretion of phosphate and raises the serum calcium level, but in renal failure, phosphate excretion falls below normal and the major effect of parathyroid hormone is to remove calcium from the bone. Uremic bone disease (renal osteodystrophy) develops from changes in calcium phosphate and parathyroid balance. Also, the active metabolite of vitamin D (1,25-dihydroxycholecalciferol) is manufactured by the kidney, and the availability of this metabolite decreases with the progression of renal disease. On the other hand, the calcification process in the bone may fail, resulting in osteomalacia. The serum magnesium may rise from the inability of the kidney to excrete magnesium.

The patient may be unable to excrete sodium and water loads, causing both sodium and water to be retained. This is one factor that paves the way for edema formation, congestive heart failure, and hypertension. Hypertension may also result from activation of the renin–angiotensin axis and concomitant increased aldosterone secretion.

Some patients have a tendency to lose salt and run the risk of hypotension and hypovolemia. Episodes of vomiting and diarrhea may produce sodium and water depletion, which worsens the uremic state. Metabolic acidosis occurs due to the reduced ability of the kidney to excrete hydrogen ions, produce ammonia, and conserve bicarbonate.

Anemia, which is considered inevitable, develops due to inadequate erythropoietin production, the shortened life span of red cells, and the uremic patient's tendency to bleed, particularly from the gastrointestinal tract.

Neurologic complications of renal failure may occur from renal failure itself, severe hypertension, electrolyte imbalance, water intoxication, and drug effects. Such manifestations include altered mental function, changes in personality and behavior, convulsions, and coma.

A decrease in libido, impotence, and amenorrhea are sexual and menstrual changes that occur. Skin changes include pruritus (in part from calcium/phosphate imbalance), which adds to the patient's distress.

Clinical Manifestations.   Although at times the onset of chronic renal failure is sudden, in the majority of patients it begins with one or more of a group of symptoms—mild fatigue and lethargy, headache, general weakness, gastrointestinal symptoms (anorexia, nausea, vomiting, diarrhea), bleeding tendencies, and mental confusion. There is decreased salivary flow, thirst, a metallic taste in the mouth, loss of smell and taste, and parotitis or stomatitis. If active treatment is begun early, the symptoms may disappear. Otherwise, these symptoms become more marked, and others appear because the metabolic abnormalities of uremia affect virtually every body system.

The patient gradually becomes more and more drowsy; the respiration becomes Kussmaul in character; and a deep coma develops, often with convulsions, which may occur as muscle twitchings or severe spasms (myoclonic jerks) quite similar to those of epilepsy. A white, powdery substance, "uremic frost," composed chiefly of urates, appears on the skin. Unless treatment is successful, death soon follows.

Management.   The aim of management is to help the diseased kidneys to maintain homeostasis for as long as possible. All factors that contribute to the problem (obstructive uropathy, etc.) must be searched for and treated.

With the deterioration of renal function, dietary intervention is necessary with careful regulation of protein intake, fluid intake to balance fluid losses, sodium intake to balance sodium losses, and some restriction of potassium. At the same time, adequate caloric intake and vitamin supplementation must be ensured. There is some restriction of protein since urea, creatinine, uric acid and organic acids—the breakdown products of dietary and tissue proteins—will accumulate rapidly in the blood when there is impaired renal clearance. The allowed protein must be of high biological value (dairy products, eggs, meat) to provide the essential amino acids. Minimally, 25 g of high biological value protein (preferably 40 g/day) should be provided prior to the necessity for dialytic intervention. Usually, the fluid allowance is 500 ml to 600 ml of fluid more than the 24-hour urine output.

Sodium and potassium regulation is determined by measurements of these electrolytes in the serum and urine. If a patient has a tendency to lose sodium, appropriate supplementation is given. Aluminum hydroxide antacids are given because they bind phosphorus in the intestinal tract, resulting in a lowering of serum phosphorus. (These should be given when food is in the intestinal tract.) Calories are supplied by carbohydrates and fat to prevent wasting. Vitamin supplementation is necessary, as a protein-restricted diet does not give the necessary complement of vitamins. (Also, the patient on dialysis may lose water-soluble vitamins from the blood during the dialysis treatment.)

Hypertension is managed by intravascular volume control and a variety of antihypertensive medications. Usually, the metabolic acidosis of chronic renal failure is asymptomatic and may require no treatment; however, sodium bicarbonate supplements or dialysis may be needed to correct the acidosis.

The patient should be observed for early evidence of cerebral abnormalities. These may vary from slight twitching, headache, or delirium. The patient must be protected from self-injury during involuntary movements; thus, it is advisable to pad the side rails. The onset of convulsions is recorded as well as their type, duration, and general effect on the patient. The physician is to be notified immediately. Intravenous diazepam (Valium) or phenytoin (Dilantin) is usually given to control convulsive seizures. (The nursing management of the patient having convulsions is discussed on p. 1360.) Heart failure, infection, and volume depletion may also require treatment.

Ideally, the patient is referred to a dialysis and transplantation center early in the course of progressive renal disease (see p. 976 and below for a discussion of dialysis and transplantation). Dialysis is usually begun when the patient cannot maintain a reasonable life-style with conservative treatment. Unfortunately, not all patients are candidates for dialysis or transplantation because of severe psychological problems or terminal illness.

▷ Kidney Transplantation

Kidney transplantation involves transplanting a kidney from a living donor or human cadaver to a recipient who has end-stage renal failure and requires dialysis in order to maintain life. Transplantation is less expensive than dialysis and provides the patient with a more normal life-style. Selected patients who have irreversible end-stage renal failure may be considered for kidney transplantation. Kidney transplants from well-matched living donors who are related to the patient (those with compatible ABO and HLA antigens) are more successful than those from cadaver donors.

The patient's kidneys, which are nonfunctioning, may or may not be removed, and a dialysis program is instituted until a kidney from a suitable donor is obtained. The donor kidney is transplanted extraperitoneally in either iliac fossa. The ureter of the newly transplanted kidney is transplanted into the bladder or anastomosed to the ureter of the recipient (Fig. 44-1).

Preoperative Management.   The preoperative goal of management is to bring the patient's metabolic state to a level as close to normal as possible. Tissue typing is done to determine histocompatibility of the donor and recipient. Antibody screening is also carried out. Immunosuppressive drugs (azathioprine [Imuran] and prednisone) are given to suppress or overcome the body's immunologic defense mechanism. Hemodialysis is usually done the day before the scheduled transplant. The patient must be free of infection at the time of renal transplantation. The mouth must be treated for gingival disease and dental caries. The lower urinary tract is studied to assess bladder neck function and to detect ureteral reflux. Other aspects of preoperative management are essentially the same as for patients undergoing renal and vascular surgery. Most transplant patients have been on dialysis programs for many months while awaiting

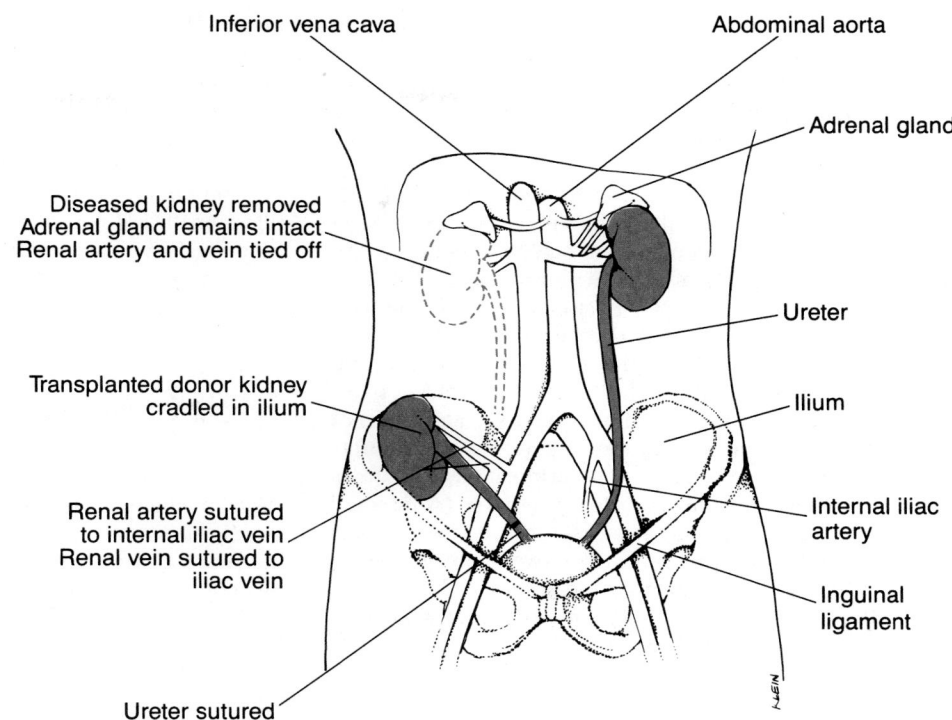

Inferior vena cava

Abdominal aorta

Adrenal gland

Diseased kidney removed
Adrenal gland remains intact
Renal artery and vein tied off

Ureter

Transplanted donor kidney
cradled in ilium

Ilium

Renal artery sutured
to internal iliac vein
Renal vein sutured to
iliac vein

Internal iliac
artery

Inguinal
ligament

Figure 44-1. Renal homotransplantation.

Ureter sutured

a cadaver kidney. The patient may have experienced considerable discouragement, depression, and anxiety. Dealing with these concerns are part of the preoperative management.

Postoperative Management. The goal of care is to maintain homeostasis until the kidney transplant is functioning well. The major limiting factor of this procedure is the body's immunologic response that leads to rejection of the transplanted kidney. The recipient's body recognizes the new kidney as a foreign tissue and attempts to destroy it. The survival of a transplanted kidney depends on the success of techniques that can suppress this immunologic reaction. In order to overcome or minimize the body's defense mechanism, immunosuppressive drugs (azathioprine [Imuran]) and corticosteroids [prednisone]) are given. Plasmaleukapheresis (PLP), lymph drainage, antilymphocytic globulin (ALG), cyclophosphamide, and cyclosporin A are other immunosuppressive agents that may be used. The doses are gradually tapered over a period of several weeks, depending on the patient's immunologic response to the transplant. This therapy is continued indefinitely.

- Following a kidney transplant, the patient must be assessed for signs and symptoms of threatened graft rejection: oliguria, edema, fever, increasing blood pressure, apprehension, weight gain, and swelling or tenderness over the graft. Blood chemistry tests are monitored for abnormalities, and leukocyte and platelet counts are scrutinized, since immunosuppression depresses the formation of leukocytes and platelets.

Renal graft failure may occur early (24 to 72 hours) or within a few days (3 to 14 days) or later (after 3 weeks). Ultrasound may be used to detect enlargement of the kidney, while renal biopsy and radiographic techniques are used to evaluate a failing renal transplant. When severe, intractable rejection occurs or when excessive immunosuppression is required to maintain the kidney, the transplanted kidney is removed (graft nephrectomy) and the patient is returned to maintenance dialysis.

The patient is constantly monitored for infection since the kidney recipient is susceptible to faulty healing and infection due to both immunosuppressive therapy and complications of renal failure.

- A distinction must be made between infection and rejection since impaired renal function and fever are evidence of both infection and rejection.

Immunosuppressive drugs render the transplant patient more vulnerable to opportunistic infections (moniliasis, cytomegalic viral disease, *Pneumocystis carinii* pneumonia) and other relatively nonpathogenic viruses, fungi, and protozoa, which can be a major hazard. Protective isolation may be carried out with health team members wearing masks until immunosuppressive drug dosages are lowered. Septicemia (bacteremia or fungemia) in renal transplant patients is responsible for a significant number of the deaths.

- Clinical manifestations of septicemia include shaking chills, fever, tachycardia, tachypnea, and leukocytosis or leukopenia.

The portal of entry for septicemia may be the urinary tract, the lung, the operative site, and other sources. Urine cultures are done frequently in view of the high incidence of bacteriuria during both the early and late stages of transplant. Any type of wound drainage should be viewed as a potential source of infection since drainage is an excellent culture medium for bacteria. Catheter and drain tips are cultured on removal by cutting off the tip of the catheter or drain (using aseptic technique) and placing it in a sterile container for laboratory culture.

The vascular access for hemodialysis is monitored to ensure patency and to evaluate for evidence of infection. It should be noted, however, that following a successful renal transplant the vascular access usually clots. This may result from improved coagulation with the return of renal function. Hemodialysis may be necessary postoperatively to maintain homeostasis until the transplanted kidney is functioning well. A few donor kidneys function immediately after grafting and may produce large quantities of dilute urine. A cadaver kidney may or may not undergo tubular necrosis and may not function for 2 or 3 weeks. The kidney may produce amounts of urine varying from extremes of no urine to large volumes of urine. The output from the urinary catheter (connected to a closed drainage system) is measured every 30 minutes to an hour. After the catheter is removed, the patient is instructed to void frequently to avoid stressing the bladder closure. Intravenous fluids are given in accordance with urine volume and serum electrolyte levels.

Gastrointestinal ulceration and bleeding (steroid induced) may occur. Fungal colonization of the gastrointestinal tract (especially the mouth) and urinary bladder may occur secondary to steroid and antibiotic administration.

Psychological Considerations.   The rejection of a transplanted kidney remains a matter of concern to the patient, the patient's family, and the supporting health care team for many months. The fears of kidney rejection and the complications of immunosuppressive therapy (Cushingoid facies, diabetes, capillary fragility, osteoporosis, glaucoma, cataracts, acne) place tremendous psychological stresses on the patient. An additional problem is possible tumor growth, since patients on long-term immunosuppressive therapy have been found to develop malignancies more frequently than the general population. This requires understanding and the expert management of emotional crises by all concerned with the person's care.

Patient Education.   The patient is advised that follow-up care after transplantation is a life-long necessity. He receives individual and written instructions concerning diet, medication, fluids, daily weight, daily measurement of urine, management of intake and output, prevention of infection, and resumption of activity and avoidance of strenuous sports.

The patient is instructed to report to the physician immediately if any of the following occur: decrease in urinary output; weight gain; malaise; fever; respiratory distress; tenderness over graft; anxiety; depression; changes in eating, drinking, or other habit patterns; and changes in blood pressure readings. The National Association of Patients on Hemodialysis and Transplantation, Inc.* is a nonprofit organization that serves the needs of kidney patients. Its quarterly publication, *NAPHT News,* has many helpful suggestions.

Organ Donation.   For those interested in donating a kidney, the National Kidney Foundation* will provide a

* See bibliography at end of chapter for address.

folder describing the organ donation program and a card specifying the organ to be donated in the event of death. The card is signed by the donor and two witnesses and is to be carried by the donor at all times. Procurement of an adquate number of kidneys for potential recipients is still a major problem.

Research is being devoted to solving the problem of rejection in kidney transplants. Tissue typing (identifying individuals with similar tissue characteristics) and drugs to suppress the body's natural defense mechanism are the major means of combating rejection.

▷ Acute Glomerulonephritis

Acute glomerulonephritis refers to a group of kidney diseases in which there is an inflammatory reaction in the glomeruli. It is not an infection of the kidney *per se* but rather the result of untoward side-effects of the defense mechanism of the body. In most types of glomerulonephritis, IgG (the major immunoglobulin found in the serum of humans) is demonstrable in the glomerular capillary walls. As a result of an antigen–antibody reaction, aggregates of molecules (complexes) are formed and circulate throughout the body. Some of these complexes lodge in the glomeruli, the filtering bed of the kidney, and induce an inflammatory response.

In most cases, the stimulus of the reaction is group A streptococcus infection of the throat, which ordinarily precedes the onset of nephritis by an interval of 2 to 3 weeks. The streptococcal product, acting as an antigen, generates circulating antibodies and results in an interaction capable of depositing the complexes in the glomeruli and injuring the kidney. Glomerulonephritis may also follow scarlet fever and impetigo. There are many forms of glomerulonephritis: proliferative, membranous, membranoproliferative, focal proliferative, rapidly progressive, etc., the immunopathology of which remains to be defined more satisfactorily.

Pathophysiology.   Cellular proliferation, infiltration of the glomerulus by leukocytes, and thickening of the glomerular filtration membrane (basement membrane) result in scarring and loss of filtering surface. In acute glomerulonephritis, the kidneys become large, swollen, and congested. All the renal tissues—glomeruli, tubules, blood vessels, and stroma—are affected in every form of glomerulonephritis, but in each form, the tissues are involved in varying degrees. In some patients, antigens outside the body (bacteria, viruses) initiate the process, resulting in the complexes being deposited in the glomerulus. In other patients, the membrane tissue of the kidney becomes altered by disease and serves as the inciting antigen. With electron-microscopy and immunofluorescent identification of the immune mechanism, the nature of the lesion can be studied.

Clinical Manifestations.   The disease may be so mild that it is discovered accidentally through a routine urinalysis, or the history may reveal a preceding episode of pharyngitis or tonsillitis with fever. In the more severe form of the disease, the patient presents with headache, malaise, facial edema, and flank pain. Mild to severe hypertension is seen, and tenderness over the costovertebral angle is common.

Acute glomerulonephritis is predominantly a disease of youth. Some cases that develop later are acute exacerbations of a quiescent glomerulonephritis already present.

Laboratory Assessment.   The urine is scanty and bloody; there may even be no urine (anuria) for one or more days. Usually, early in the disease, the patient voids from 50 ml to 200 ml daily of a cola-colored urine, with a specific gravity between 1.020 and 1.025 and with a thick sediment of red blood cells, leukocytes, and all kinds of casts. (RBC casts mean glomerular injury.) The urine contains large amounts of protein. A large percentage of patients have an increased antistreptolysin titre due to a reaction to the streptococcal organism. Usually, there are rising values in blood urea nitrogen and serum creatinine. The patient may be anemic because of loss of the red blood cells into the urine and changes in the hemopoietic mechanism of the body.

As the patient improves, the amount of urine increases, while the urinary protein and urinary sediment diminish. Usually, greater than 90% of children recover. The percentage of recovery for adults is not well established, but is probably about 70%. Some patients become severely uremic and progress to a fatal termination within weeks or months despite every form of therapy that can be offered. Others, after a period of apparent recovery, insidiously develop chronic glomerulonephritis.

Management.   The goals of management are to protect the patient's poorly functioning kidneys and to recognize and treat complications promptly. If residual streptococcal infection is suspected, penicillin is given. Bed rest is encouraged during the acute phase until the urine clears and the BUN, creatinine, and blood pressure normalize. Rest also facilitates diuresis. The urine of the patient may serve as a guide to the duration of bed rest, as increasing activity may increase proteinuria and hematuria.

Dietary protein is restricted when there is evidence of renal insufficiency and nitrogen retention (elevated BUN). Sodium is restricted when hypertension, edema, and congestive heart failure are present. Carbohydrates are given liberally to provide energy and reduce the catabolism of protein.

Fluids are given according to the patient's fluid losses and daily body weight. Insensible fluid loss through respiration and feces is estimated at 500 ml to 1000 ml. Therefore, the intake and output are measured and recorded. Usually, diuresis starts 1 to 2 weeks after the onset of symptoms. Edema decreases and hypertension lessens. However, proteinuria and microscopic hematuria may persist for many months. In some patients, the disease may progress to chronic glomerulonephritis. Complications include hypertensive encephalopathy, congestive heart failure, and pulmonary edema. Hypertensive encephalopathy is considered a medical emergency, and therapy is directed toward reducing the blood pressure without impairing renal function.

Patient Education.   Instructions to the patient include explanations and scheduling for follow-up evaluations of (1) blood pressure, (2) urinalysis for protein, and (3) blood for BUN and creatinine studies to determine if there is exacerbation of disease activity. The patient is cautioned to

call the physician if symptoms of renal failure occur (fatigue, nausea, vomiting, diminishing urinary output, etc.). Any infection must be treated promptly.

▷ Chronic Glomerulonephritis

Pathophysiology.   Chronic glomerulonephritis may have its onset as acute glomerulonephritis or may represent a milder type of antigen–antibody reaction, one so mild that it can be overlooked easily. After repeated occurrences of these reactions, the kidneys are reduced to as little as one fifth their normal size, consisting largely of fibrous tissue. The cortex shrinks to a layer of 1 mm to 2 mm in thickness, and in some areas, it is gone entirely. The surface of the kidney is rough because the renal tissue disappears in irregular patches, and bands of scar tissue distort the remaining cortex. The glomeruli are badly damaged. Many glomeruli and their convoluted tubes become scarred as well. The branches of the renal artery are thickened.

Clinical Manifestations.   The symptoms of chronic glomerulonephritis are variable. Some patients with severe grades of this disease have no symptoms at all for a long time. They may discover their condition as the result of an application for life insurance, from a blood test, or when their blood pressure is found to be elevated. It may be suggested during a routine eye examination, when vascular changes or hemorrhages are found. The first indication of disease may be a sudden, severe nosebleed; a stroke; or a uremic convulsion. Many patients merely notice that their feet are slightly swollen at night, but never markedly so, unless an acute exacerbation of the nephritis is in progress. The majority of all patients also have such general symptoms as loss of weight and strength, increasing irritability, and nocturia. Headaches, dizziness, and digestive disturbances are common.

Physical examination may show a poorly nourished patient with a yellow–gray pigmentation of the skin, and periorbital and peripheral (dependent) edema. Blood pressure may be normal or severely elevated. Retinal findings include hemorrhage, exudate, narrowed tortuous arterioles and papilledema. Mucous membranes are pale due to anemia.

The neck veins may be distended due to fluid overload. Cardiomegaly, a gallop rhythm, and other signs of congestive heart failure may be present. Crackles can be heard in the lungs. Peripheral neuropathy manifested by depressed deep tendon reflexes and neurosensory changes occur late in the illness. When frank uremia occurs, the patient becomes confused and his attention span will be limited. An additional late finding includes evidence of pericarditis with a cardiac friction rub and pulsus paradoxus.

A number of laboratory abnormalities occur. Urinalysis reveals a fixed specific gravity of 1.010, variable proteinuria, and urine sediment changes. As glomerular filtration becomes depressed, the creatinine disturbances include hyperkalemia and decreased serum bicarbonate (metabolic acidosis). Fatal hypermagnesemia may develop when magnesium-containing antacids are given to patients with renal failure. Anemia secondary to decreased erythropoiesis and shortened red cell survival time, hypoalbuminemia with associated pitting edema, and depressed serum calcium with increased serum phosphorus occur as renal failure progresses. Impaired nerve conduction velocity develops in about 50% of patients once the glomerular filtration rate decreases below 50 ml/min. Chest x-ray may show cardiac enlargement and pulmonary edema. About 30% of patients with advanced renal failure have a pericardial effusion demonstrated by echocardiography. Electrocardiography may be normal but may also reflect hypertension with left ventricular hypertrophy and electrolyte disturbances, such as hyperkalemia and spiked T waves.

Management.   The treatment of the ambulatory patient with chronic nephritis is entirely nonspecific and symptomatic, depending on the situation that presents itself at any given time. Thus, if hypertension is present, treatment is directed toward readjusting the diet and fluid intake in an effort to maintain as normal a metabolic situation as possible. Protein intake (of high biologic value) is adjusted according to the response of the patient with adequate calories to prevent protein from being utilized for energy. If there is a urinary tract infection, a possible factor in producing further renal damage, steps should be taken to diagnose it and to treat it.

- Treatment of patients with marked edema presents many difficulties. The patient is elevated in bed and made as comfortable as possible. Daily weights are checked. Water and sodium intake should be adjusted to the patient's ability to excrete water and sodium in the urine. Diuretics may be necessary when symptoms of fluid overload occur. The nurse should watch for all symptoms that suggest renal failure.

▷ Nephrotic Syndrome

The *nephrotic syndrome* is a clinical disorder characterized by (1) marked proteinuria, (2) hypoalbuminemia, (3) edema, and (4) hypercholesterolemia. It is seen in any condition that seriously damages the glomerular capillary membrane. Causes include chronic glomerulonephritis, diabetes mellitus with intercapillary glomerulosclerosis, amyloidosis of the kidney, systemic lupus erythematosus, and renal vein thrombosis. The pathophysiology of nephrotic syndrome is discussed on page 960.

Clinical Manifestations.   There is an insidious onset of fluid retention that progresses to pitting edema. The patient loses protein in the urine (proteinuria), leading to depletion of body proteins (hypoalbuminemia). In addition, the blood cholesterol level is high. The diagnosis is made on assessment of the patient's signs and symptoms, physical examination, renal function tests, measurement of 24-hour urine protein, and serum electrolyte evaluations. Urinalysis shows microscopic hematuria, urinary casts, and other abnormalities. Needle biopsy of the kidney is done for histologic examination of renal tissue to confirm the diagnosis.

Causes of Nephrotic Syndrome.   Causes of nephrotic syndrome fall into five main categories:

1. Glomerulonephritis (idiopathic nephrotic syndrome, intrinsic renal disease, primary renal disease)
2. Systemic illnesses (including allergic manifestations)
3. Circulatory or mechanical causes
4. Certain infections
5. Miscellaneous

Management.   The objective of management is to preserve renal function. It may be necessary to keep the patient on bed rest a few days to mobilize the edema. A high-protein diet is given to replenish wasted tissues and restore body proteins. If the edema is severe, the patient is placed on a low-sodium diet. Diuretics are given in severe edematous states, and adrenocorticosteroids (prednisone) may be used to reduce proteinuria.

In the early stages, the nursing management is similar to that of the patient with acute glomerulonephritis, but as the disease worsens, management is more in accordance with the care of the patient with chronic renal failure (see preceding discussion).

▷ Nephrosclerosis

Nephrosclerosis is hardening or sclerosis of the arteries of the kidney and is usually seen in association with hypertension. It is the renal manifestation of generalized arteriosclerosis.

Malignant nephrosclerosis, as opposed to benign nephrosclerosis, though different in degree, merely represents the situation presented in the section on chronic glomerulonephritis. Patients with the malignant type progress rapidly to a fatal termination through the stages of proteinuria, increasing hypertension, failing renal function, and eyeground changes. They usually die within several months. The factor responsible for this termination may be uremia, congestive heart failure due to hypertensive heart disease, or a cerebral vascular accident. It occurs most commonly among people from the third to the fifth decade of life. It is thought to be a generalized vascular disease that starts in the kidney and finally involves the entire vascular tree.

Patients who develop benign nephrosclerosis are most apt to be found in older age groups. These individuals rarely complain of renal symptoms, although for years the urine has a low and fixed specific gravity and contains a small amount of protein and an occasional hyaline or granular cast. Only late in the disease does renal insufficiency appear.

▷ Hydronephrosis

Hydronephrosis is dilatation of the pelvis and calyces of one or both kidneys with resulting thinning of the renal parenchyma due to obstruction of urinary flow. Obstruction to the normal flow of urine causes the urine to "dam up," resulting in back pressure on the kidney. If the obstruction is in the urethra or the bladder, the back pressure affects both kidneys, but if the obstruction is in the ureter, due to a stone or kink, only one kidney is damaged.

The pelvis of the kidney (including the calyces) is the wide sac into which the urine is poured from the pyramids. As it narrows to a small tube, it becomes the ureter. The pelvis has thin walls whose inner surface is lined with the same type of mucous membrane as the ureter and the bladder.

The pelvis of the kidney and its calyces are distended by the partly dammed-up urine when the ureter is somewhat obstructed. If in such a case no inflammation is present and the fluid is clear, the condition is called *hydronephrosis*. In order to cause dilatation of the pelvis of the kidney, the obstruction of urine is gradual, partial, or intermittent.

Partial or intermittent obstruction may be caused by a renal stone that has formed in the renal pelvis but has dropped into the ureter and blocked it. Or the obstruction may be due to a tumor of some other abdominal or pelvic organ pressing on the ureter, or to bands of scar tissue resulting from an abscess or inflammation near the ureter that pinches it. The disorder may be due to an odd angle at which the ureter leaves the renal pelvis or to an unusual position of the kidney, favoring a ureteral twist or kink. In elderly males, the most common cause is urethral obstruction at the bladder outlet by an enlarged prostate.

Whatever the cause, if the fluid accumulates intermittently in the renal pelvis, it distends the pelvis and its calyces. If the obstructions are frequent, and the pressure that develops is high, in time atrophy of the kidney results, which causes the kidney to spread out into a thin, cystlike shell. As one kidney undergoes gradual destruction, the contralateral kidney gradually enlarges (compensatory hypertrophy). Ultimately, there is impairment of renal function.

Clinical Manifestations.   The onset is often insidious and the patient is asymptomatic. Acute obstruction may produce aching in the flank and back. If infection is present, there are symptoms of bladder irritability (dysuria) and chills, fever, tenderness and pyuria. The hydronephritic kidney may bleed from congestion, causing hematuria. Signs and symptoms of uremia develop when the condition is advanced.

Management.   The goals of management are to discover and remove (if possible) the cause of the obstruction, to treat infection, and to restore and conserve renal function.

To relieve the obstruction, the urine may have to be diverted by nephrostomy (see p. 990) or other types of diversion. The infection is treated with antimicrobials since residual urine in the calyces produces infection and pyelonephritis. The patient is prepared for surgical removal of obstructive lesions (calculus, tumor, obstruction of the ureter). Operations to improve the drainage of the kidney may be done. If one kidney is severely damaged and its function is nil, nephrectomy (removal of the kidney) is performed. (See Management of the Patient Undergoing Renal Surgery, p. 988.)

▷ Infections of the Urinary Tract

Urinary tract infections (UTI) are a group of infections caused by the presence of pathogenic microorganisms in the urinary tract, with or without signs and symptoms. Infection may predominate at the bladder (cystitis), urethra (urethritis), prostate (prostatitis), or kidney (pyelonephritis). The normal urinary tract is sterile except near the urethral orifice.

Bacteriuria refers to the presence of bacteria in the urine. A colony count of at least 100,000 colonies/ml of urine on a clean-catch midstream or catheterized specimen implies infection. Unfortunately, infections in any part of the urinary tract may persist for months or years without symptoms.

The bacteria most commonly responsible for urinary tract infections are *Escherichia coli* (80%–90%); *Proteus mirabilis;* one or more species of *Klebsiella, Enterobacter, Proteus,* and *Pseudomonas;* and the various enterococci. All these are normally found in the fecal flora.

Factors Contributing to Urinary Tract Infection.   (See Fig. 44-2.) It is now believed that the majority of urinary tract infections arise by ascent of bowel organisms from the perineum to the urethra and become established in the bladder (especially in the presence of residual urine) and then travel to the kidneys. Women are more prone to develop bladder infections because of the shortness of the female urethra and its anatomical proximity to the vagina, periurethral glands, and rectum. In the male, the length of the urethra and the antibacterial properties of the prostatic secretions tend to ward off ascending urethral infections. Adult males who develop urinary tract infections should be examined for urinary obstruction, prostatic infection, renal stones, or systemic disease.

Urethrovesical reflux refers to the reflux (flowing back) of urine from the bladder into the urethra. It is caused by an increase in intrabladder pressure (coughing, sneezing), which may squeeze the urine out of the bladder into the urethra. When the pressure returns to normal, the urine flows back into the urethra, bringing back into the bladder the bacteria from the anterior portions of the urethra. Urethrovesical reflux is also caused by dysfunction of the bladder neck or urethra.

Vesicoureteral reflux (or ureterovesical reflux) refers to the reflux (flowing back) of urine from the bladder into one or both ureters. In the normal person, the ureterovesical junction prevents urine from traveling back into the ureter, particularly at the time of voiding. When the ureterovesical valve is incompetent (congenital causes, ureteral abnormalities), the bacteria may reach the kidneys and there may be subsequent dilatation of the ureter, renal pelvis, and calyces with ultimate kidney destruction.

Fecal soiling of the urethral meatus is another common way in which bacteria are introduced into the urinary tract. *Sexual intercourse* plays a role in the ascent of organisms from the perineum into the bladder in women. *Instrumentation* (from catheterization, cystoscopic examinations) is also implicated in producing infections. *Stasis of urine in the bladder* may lead to infection, which may ultimately spread through the entire urinary system. Any *obstruction* to urinary flow renders the kidney more susceptible to infection. Common causes of urinary tract obstruction are congenital anomalies, urethral strictures, contracture of the bladder neck, bladder tumors, ureteral stones, compression of the ureters, and neurologic abnormalities. Urinary tract infection may also be from *hematogenous* (blood) or *lymphogenous* spread. *Metabolic disorders* (diabetes mellitus) predispose to urinary tract infections.

▶ Assessment
Clinical Manifestations.   Signs and symptoms of urinary tract infections cover a broad range. Frequently, the patient is asymptomatic and is found to have bacteriuria

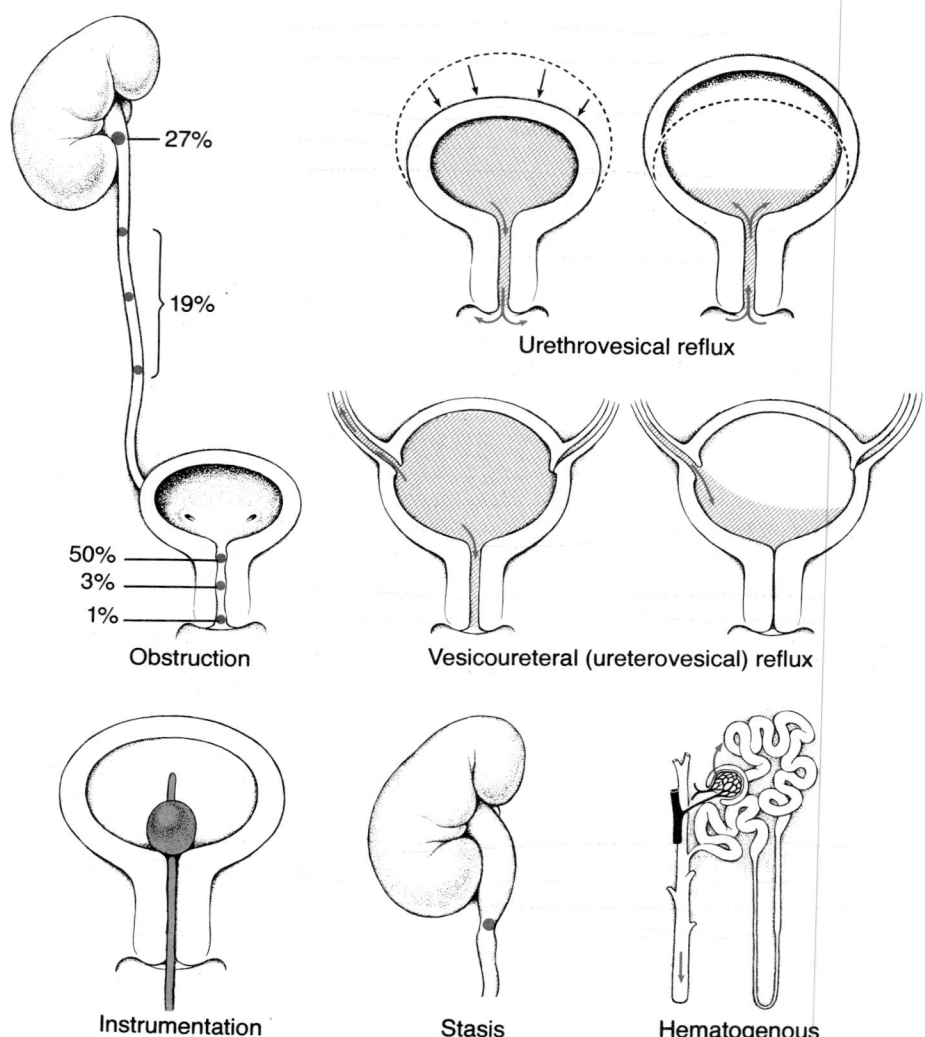

Figure 44-2. Causes of urinary tract and kidney infections.

while undergoing a periodic health checkup. Signs and symptoms of lower urinary tract infection (cystitis) include frequent painful and burning urination, sometimes accompanied by bearing-down sensations and spasms in the region of the bladder and suprapubic area. Hematuria and back pain may also be present. Signs and symptoms of upper urinary tract infection (pyelonephritis) include fever, chills, flank pain, and painful urination. Upon examination there is costovertebral angle pain and tenderness. Symptoms of renal failure may be present: nausea, vomiting, pruritus, weight loss, edema, and shortness of breath. Acute flareups of urinary tract infection may be silent.

Diagnostic Evaluation. It is necessary to demonstrate bacteria in significant numbers in the urine that is collected by a midstream clean-catch technique. As noted earlier, a bacterial count of 100,000 organisms (colonies) per milliliter of urine indicates a urinary infection. Successive urine cultures are also used to find bacterial species present. In the male, a culture is made of prostatic fluid or urine voided after prostatic massage. In persons at high risk of having complicated infections, evaluation studies are done to de-

termine if the infection is secondary to a functional or structural abnormality (intravenous urogram [IVP] and cystoscopy).

Cystitis (Lower Urinary Tract Infection)

Cystitis is an inflammation of the urinary bladder that is most often caused by an ascending infection from the urethra. It may be caused by urethrovesical reflux (flowing back of urine from the urethra into the bladder), fecal contamination, or the use of various instruments such as a catheter or cystoscope.

Cystitis is seen more commonly in women because of the shortness of the urethra and its anatomical proximity to the vagina and periurethral glands and rectum. The distal portion of the urethra is frequently colonized with bacterial flora. In women with recurrent urinary tract infections, bacterial colonization often occurs in the vaginal vestibule. There may be some defect of the mucosa of the urethra, vagina or external genitalia of these patients that allows enteric organisms to adhere and colonize at periurethral sites and to invade the bladder. Acute infections of women are usually caused by *Escherichia coli.* Cystitis may also occur in women following sexual intercourse, which implicates the ascending urethral pathway in its pathogenesis.

About half of the female patients who present with symptoms of acute cystitis (frequency, dysuria) without bacteriuria have *acute urethral syndrome* (symptoms suggesting urinary tract infection but occurring in the presence of sterile urine).

Males have a much lower incidence of cystitis, probably due to the longer length of the urethra and the antibacterial properties of prostatic secretion. Therefore, cystitis in men is secondary to some other factor—infected prostate; epididymitis by reflux of urine along the vas or perivesical lymphatics, as from an infected prostate; or bladder stones.

The patient complains of urgency, frequency, burning and pain on urination, nocturia, and a bearing-down sensation in the region of the bladder and suprapubic area. There is pus, bacteria, and often red cells in the urine.

Patient Problems/Nursing Diagnoses

The patient's nursing diagnosis includes pain, urgency, dysuria, and fever related to infection, and potential for recurring infection.

▶ Planning and Implementation

The patient's goals are relief of pain, urgency, dysuria, and fever and prevention of recurrences. The goals of medical management are to eradicate the causative pathogens, to decrease morbidity, and to prevent recurrences. The specific treatment depends on the cause and location of the infection. A urine specimen is obtained for smears and culture so that the appropriate drug may be selected.

Medical Management.   For an uncomplicated, nonobstructed lower urinary tract infection, the female patient may be treated with single-dose or short-term therapy with an antimicrobial agent to which the organisms are susceptible, especially if the bacteria are not antibody-coated. These infections usually respond favorably to antimicrobials that result in high urinary drug levels. Amoxicillin, sulfonamide, nitrofurantoin, trimethoprim-sulfamethoxazole, and tetracycline derivatives have been used successfully. A potentially effective drug should *rapidly* sterilize the urine and relieve the patient's symptoms. The urine is reexamined 24 hours to 3 days after initiation of treatment to determine if the urine is free of bacteria. In the male patient, prostatitis may require prolonged antimicrobial therapy.

There is a propensity for these infections to recur. Recurrences are of two types: (1) reinfection with a new and different organism, and (2) relapse with the original organism. Patients with recurring infections should undergo periodic urine cultures since most are from new infections with different organisms. Patients with frequent and closely spaced recurrent infections may require long-term, low-dose antimicrobial prophylaxis. It is usually given at bedtime. The rationale is that bacterial activity is maintained in the bladder urine/periurethral zone, thus blocking reinfection. Periodic urine cultures are done to be certain that prophylaxis is effective.

Further diagnostic studies are carried out in patients with suspected complicated infections (obstruction, calculi) or with infections secondary to repeated lack of response to antmicrobial therapy.

The effectiveness of certain antimicrobial drugs is affected by the reaction (pH) of the urine. Aminoglycoside antibiotics (streptomycin, kanamycin, neomycin, and gentamicin) are more active when the urine is alkaline. Sodium bicarbonate may be given to alkalize the urine. The tetracyclines, methenamine mandelate, and nitrofurantoin are more active when the urinary pH is acidic, and ascorbic acid may be given to acidify the urine.

The patient is encouraged to drink liberal amounts of fluids to promote renal blood flow and to flush the bacteria from the urinary tract. Frequent voiding (every 2–3 hours) is encouraged to empty the bladder completely since this can significantly lower urine bacterial counts, reduce urine stasis, and prevent reinfection. Infrequent voiding overstretches the bladder wall, leading to hypoxia of the bladder mucosa, which is then susceptible to bladder invasion. Antispasmodic drugs may be useful in relieving bladder irritability and pain. Aspirin, heat to the perineum, and hot tub baths help relieve urgency, discomfort, and spasm.

Prevention and Patient Education.   Since there is a marked tendency for infection to recur, follow-up urine studies are recommended for at least 2 years or more to determine if asymptomatic infection is present. It is especially important to have follow-up studies if urinary tract infections occurred during pregnancy. Women who have repeated urinary tract infections should receive detailed instructions on the following points:

1. Reduce at the vaginal introitus concentrations of pathogens by hygienic measures:
   a. Shower rather than bathe in a tub, since bacteria in the bath water may gain entrance into the urethra.
   b. Cleanse around the perineum and urethral meatus (cleansing from the front to the back) after each bowel movement.
2. Drink liberal amounts of fluid during the day to flush out bacteria.
3. Void every 2 to 3 hours during the day and completely empty the bladder.
4. If sexual intercourse is the initiating event for development of bacteriuria:
   a. Void immediately after sexual intercourse.
   b. Take the prescribed single dose of an oral antimicrobial agent following sexual intercourse.
5. If bacteria continue to appear in the urine, long-term antimicrobial therapy may be required to prevent colonization of the periurethral area and recurrence of infection. The drug should be taken after emptying the bladder just before going to bed to ensure adequate concentration of the drug during the overnight period.

The patient is taught self-monitoring and testing of the urine for bacteria with dipslides (Microstix) as follows:

1. Wash around the urethral meatus several times, using different washcloths.
2. Collect a midstream specimen.
3. Remove a slide from its container, dip it into the urine sample, and return it to the container.

4. Incubate the slide at room temperature according to product directives.
5. Read the results by comparing the slide with the colony density chart that comes with the product.

Follow-up cultures are required for all patients with urinary tract infections, as many will have recurrent infections within a year. If burning on urination is noted, the physician or clinic is to be notified.

▶ **Evaluation**

Expected Outcomes

1. Experiences relief of pain, urgency, dysuria, and fever
   a. Takes antimicrobial agent as prescribed
   b. Takes analgesics and hot tub baths for discomfort
   c. Drinks 8 to 10 glasses of fluids daily
   d. Voids every 2 to 3 hours
   e. Voids urine that is clear and free from odor
2. Prevents recurrences of urinary tract infection
   a. Uses dipslides to monitor for infection
   b. Takes single-dose antimicrobial following sexual activity as directed
   c. Notifies physician promptly of recurring symptoms

Pyelonephritis (Upper Urinary Tract Infection)

Pyelonephritis is a bacterial infection (acute or chronic) of the renal pelvis, tubules, and interstitial tissue of one or both kidneys. Bacteria may gain access to the bladder via the urethra and ascend to the kidney or may reach the kidney through the bloodstream. Pyelonephritis is frequently secondary to ureterovesical reflux in which an incompetent ureterovesical valve allows the urine to regurgitate into the ureters, usually at the time of voiding (see Fig. 44-2). Urinary tract obstruction (which renders the kidneys more susceptible to infection) and renal diseases are among other causes.

Clinical Manifestations and Pathophysiology. Acute pyelonephritis is an active infection that presents with chills and fever, flank pain, costovertebral angle tenderness, leukocytosis, bacteria and pus in the urine, and frequently symptoms of lower urinary tract involvement, such as dysuria and frequency. Upper urinary tract infection is associated with antibody coating of the bacteria in the urine. (Antibodies coat the bacteria in the renal medulla; when excreted in the urine, the immunofluorescent test can detect the antibody coating.)

There are areas of inflammation in the kidney with interstitial infiltrations of inflammatory cells which in time may produce tubular destruction and abscess formation. Low-grade interstitial inflammation may result in atrophy and destruction of tubules and in hyalinization of the glomeruli. Eventually, when pyelonephritis becomes chronic, the kidneys become scarred, contracted, and of little functional value.

Management. An intravenous urogram and other diagnostic tests are carried out to locate any obstruction in the urinary tract. The relief of obstruction is essential to save the kidney from destruction. The treatment is essentially the same as that of cystitis (preceding discussion).

Culture and sensitivity tests are done on the urine since the choice of antimicrobial is determined by the causative organism. Medication should produce sustained antibacterial concentration of the drugs within the renal parenchyma. The antimicrobial drug must be given for a long enough period to prevent reseeding of a residual foci of infection.

A possible problem in treatment is chronic or recurring infections persisting for months or years without symptoms. After the initial antimicrobial regimen, the patient is kept on continuous antimicrobial treatment until there is no evidence of infection, all causative factors have been treated or controlled, and kidney function is stabilized. Serial urine cultures and other evaluation studies must be continued indefinitely. The patient is also monitored with serum creatinine determinations and blood counts for the duration of the long-term therapy.

Chronic Pyelonephritis (Chronic Interstitial Nephritis)

Repeated bouts of acute pyelonephritis may lead to chronic pyelonephritis (chronic interstitial nephritis).

The patient with chronic pyelonephritis (persistent presence of bacteria in the urine) usually has no symptoms of infection unless an acute exacerbation occurs. Noticeable signs may include fatigue, headache, poor appetite, polyuria, excessive thirst, and weight loss. The persistent and recurring infection may produce progressive scarring of the kidney with ultimate kidney atrophy and failure.

Complications of chronic pyelonephritis include uremia (from progressive loss of nephrons secondary to chronic inflammation and scarring), hypertension, and renal lithiasis (from chronic infection with urea-splitting organisms, resulting in stone formation).

Management. The extent of the disease is determined by intravenous urogram and measurements of urea nitrogen, creatinine levels, and creatinine clearance. Sterilization of the urine is undertaken if significant bacteria are present. The choice of an antimicrobial is based on culture identification of the pathogen. If the urine cannot be made bacteria-free, nitrofurantoin or a combination of sulfamethoxazole and trimethoprim may be tried to suppress bacterial growth. The treatment of uremia is discussed on page 997. Hypertension is also carefully controlled.

Carbuncle of the Kidney

Carbuncle of the kidney is an infection of hematogenous origin that is caused usually by the staphylococcus. It usually follows a cutaneous boil or carbuncle and is characterized by fever, malaise, and dull pain in the region of the kidney. This type of infection, if recognized, usually subsides with chemotherapy and penicillin. Recently, carbuncles of the kidney from gram-negative bacteria have increased in incidence.

Perinephric Abscess

Perinephric abscess is an abscess in the fatty tissue about the kidney that may arise secondary to an infection of the kidney or as a hematogenous infection originating in foci elsewhere in the body. It may be secondary to a staphylococcal infection of the kidney or to the spread of infection from adjacent areas, such as from diverticulitis, appendicitis, etc. The symptoms often are acute in onset, with chills, fever, leukocytosis, and other signs of suppuration. Locally, there is flank or abdominal tenderness or pain. The patient usually appears seriously ill.

Management.   The treatment consists of administration of the appropriate antimicrobial agent and incision and drainage of the abscess. Drains are usually inserted and left in the perinephric space until all significant drainage has ceased. Because the drainage often is profuse, frequent changes of the outer dressings may be necessary. As in the treatment of an abscess in any site, the patient is monitored for sepsis, fluid input and output, and general response to treatment.

Tuberculosis of the Kidney and the Genitourinary Tract
Pathophysiology and Clinical Manifestations.   Tuberculosis of the kidney and urinary tract is caused by the organism *Mycobacterium tuberculosis* and usually disseminates from the lungs via the bloodstream to the kidneys and to other organs of the genitourinary tract. At first the symptoms are mild; there is usually a slight afternoon fever and a loss of weight and appetite. The process of tuberculosis generally starts in one of the renal pyramids; ulceration into the kidney pelvis follows; the organisms are carried down with the urine into the bladder so that the bladder is likely to become infected.

Tuberculosis of the lower genitourinary tract is always secondary to renal tuberculosis, the infection having been propagated downward. In the male, the prostate and epididymis may become infected.

Tuberculosis of the urinary bladder is practically never a primary infection but an extension of tuberculosis of a kidney. This disease gives rise to several small ulcers, the majority of them near the trigone. The symptoms of bladder tuberculosis are those of cystitis in general but with an unusual degree of bladder irritability. Suggestive early symptoms of this disease are an increased urinary output that contains considerable pus and yet is acid in reaction (in nearly all other pyurias the urine is alkaline), and hematuria (either microscopic or gross). The symptoms of pain, dysuria, and urinary frequency, when they occur, are due to bladder infection. Symptoms of bladder irritability (frequency of urination, nocturia) are a later manifestation of the disease.

Management.   A search for tuberculosis elsewhere in the body must be conducted when tuberculosis of the kidney or urinary tract is found. Inquiry is made to determine if the patient has been in previous contact with tuberculosis. At least three clean-voided first morning urine specimens are concentrated and cultured for *M. tuberculosis* for the diagnosis of urinary tract tuberculosis.

The objective of treatment is to eradicate the offending organism. A multiple-drug regimen appears to delay the emergence of resistant organisms. Combinations of ethambutol, isoniazid, and rifampin are among the drugs used (see p. 1509). Shorter-course chemotherapy (4 months) has been proven effective in sterilizing the urine and in penetrating renal tissue. Since renal tuberculosis is a manifestation of a systemic disease, all measures to promote the

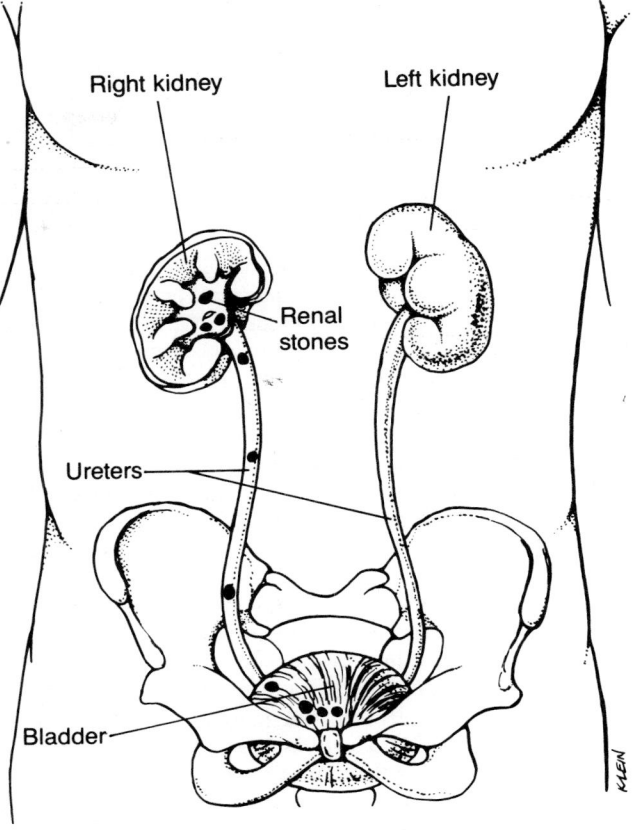

Figure 44-3.   Illustration showing different sites of calculous disease of the urinary tract (urolithiasis).

general health of the person are used. Surgical intervention may be necessary to prevent obstructive problems and to remove an extensively diseased kidney. The patient must realize the need for follow-up examinations (urine cultures, excretory urograms) usually for a period of a year.

Treatment will need to be reinstituted if a relapse occurs and the tubercle bacilli again invade the genitourinary tract. Ureteral stenosis or bladder contractures are complications that may develop during the healing process.

▷ Urolithiasis

Urolithiasis refers to the presence of stones in the urinary system. Stones are formed in the urinary tract by the deposit of crystalline substances (calcium oxalate, calcium phosphate, uric acid) excreted in the urine. They may be found anywhere from the kidney to the bladder and vary in size from mere granular deposits, called sand or gravel, to bladder stones the size of an orange (Fig. 44-3).

Certain factors favor the formation of stones, including infection, urinary stasis, and periods of immobility (produces slowing of renal drainage and altered calcium metabolism). Hypercalcemia (abnormally high concentration of blood calcium compounds) and hypercalciuria (abnormally large amounts of calcium in the urine) may be caused by hyper-parathyroidism, renal tubular acidosis, excessive intake of vitamin D, excessive intake of milk and alkali, and certain myeloproliferative diseases (leukemia, polycythemia vera) which produce an unusual proliferation of blood cells derived from bone marrow. Some stones are caused by an excessive excretion of uric acid, which is the end product of purine metabolism. Urinary stone formation is also a sequela of bowel disease occurring in patients with inflammatory bowel disease and in those with an ileostomy or bowel resection, particularly of the small bowel since these persons absorb more oxalate. Vitamin A deficiency may be another cause. In most patients, no cause may be found.

The problem occurs predominantly in the third to fifth decades, affecting men more than women. Persons who have had two stones tend to have recurrences. The majority of stones contain calcium or magnesium in combination with phosphorus or oxalate. Most stones are radiopaque and can be detected by roentgenography.

▶ Assessment

Clinical Manifestations. The clinical manifestations depend on the presence of obstruction, infection, and edema. When the stones block the flow of urine, obstruction develops, and the constant irritation of the stone may be followed by a secondary infection that causes pyelonephritis and cystitis with chills, fever, and dysuria. Renal parenchymal stones usually produce few symptoms. Renal pelvic stones may be associated with intense, deep ache in the loin and with voiding of increased amounts of urine containing blood and pus cells. A renal stone produces an increase in hydrostatic pressure and distends the renal pelvis and proximal ureter. Thus, painful afferent sensations are initiated. Pain originating in the renal area radiates anteriorly and downward toward the bladder in the female and toward the testicle in the male. If the pain suddenly becomes acute, the loin exquisitely tender, and nausea and vomiting appear, the patient has an attack of *renal colic.* Diarrhea and abdominal discomfort may accompany the attack. These gastrointestinal symptoms are due to renointestinal reflexes and the anatomical relation of the kidneys to the stomach, pancreas, colon, etc.

When stones lodge in the ureter, acute, excruciating, colicky pain is experienced, radiating down the thigh and to the genitalia. The pain usually comes in waves. There is usually a frequent desire to void, but very little urine is passed, and it usually contains blood because of the abrasive action of the stone as urine is passed. This group of symptoms is called *ureteral colic.* In general, the patient will spontaneously pass stones 0.5 cm to 1 cm in diameter. Those over 1 cm in diameter usually must be removed. When stones lodge in the bladder, they usually produce irritative symptoms and may be associated with urinary tract infection and hematuria. If the stone obstructs the bladder neck, there will by urinary retention.

The diagnosis is confirmed by intravenous urogram or retrograde pyelography. Blood studies and a 24-hour urine test for measurement of calcium, uric acid, creatinine, sodium, pH, and total volume are part of the diagnostic workup. A dietary and drug history is also made.

Patient Problems/Nursing Diagnoses

Based on the clinical manifestations and diagnostic assessment data, the patient's nursing diagnosis includes pain related to obstruction, bleeding, and infection, and potential for infection and for nonadherence to the therapeutic program related to dietary restrictions.

▶ Planning and Implementation

Goals

The patient's goals are:

1. Relief of pain
2. Avoidance of infection
3. Adherence to the therapeutic program

The basic goals underlying the management of the patient are to eradicate the stone, to determine the stone type, to prevent nephron destruction, to control infection, and to relieve any obstruction that may be present. Infection and back pressure of obstructed urine can destroy the renal parenchyma.

Active treatment must be instituted for renal and ureteral colic. The immediate objective of treatment is to relieve the pain until its cause can be removed; morphine or meperidine hydrochloride helps allay the pain. Hot baths or moist heat to the flank areas is also useful. Unless the patient is vomiting, fluids are encouraged, as this treatment tends to increase the hydrostatic pressure behind the stone and thus assists it in its downward passage. A high round-the-clock fluid intake reduces the concentration of urinary crystalloids and ensures a high urinary output. Encouraging fluids also lowers the specific gravity of the urine.

No time should be lost in carrying out these treatments, because at times the pain suffered by these patients is so excruciating that shock and syncope result. A patient will be grateful for any relief.

Cystoscopic examination and passage of a small ureteral catheter to dislodge the obstructive stone (when possible) immediately relieves back pressure on the kidney and alleviates the intense pain.

The nursing care of patients with calculi requires constant observation to detect the spontaneous passage of a stone. All urine should be strained through gauze, since uric acid stones may crumble. Any blood clots passed in the urine should be crushed and the sides of the urinal and bedpan inspected for clinging stones.

When stones are recovered, crystallographic analysis is carried out to establish the type of stone formation, since treatment is based on the composition of the stone. For example, calcium oxalate or calcium phosphate stones usually indicate disorders of oxalate or calcium metabolism, while urate stones suggest a disturbance in uric acid metabolism. Struvite stones (infection stones) account for 15% to 20% of urinary calculi. Specific antibacterial agents are administered if infection is present.

Diet Therapy. Diet therapy is most effective when stones are caused by metabolic abnormalities resulting in increased excretion of stone constituents (hypercalciuria) or altered physiochemical properties of the urine (urine acidity). Most stones contain calcium combined with phosphate or other substances. For these patients, the diet selected is moderately reduced in calcium and phosphorus content (Chart 44-2). The urine is acidified. Sometimes stones will cease growing simply by ensuring an adequate fluid intake and limiting certain foods in the diet that make up the main ingredient of the stone (*e.g.*, calcium).

In renal hypercalciuria, thiazide therapy may be beneficial in reducing the calcium loss in the urine and lowering the elevated parathyroid hormone levels.

Patients who are inclined to develop phosphatic calculi should ingest only a limited amount of phosphorus. To offset excess phosphorus, aluminum hydroxide gel often is prescribed, since it combines with the excess phosphorus, causing it to be excreted through the intestinal tract rather than in the urinary system.

For uric acid stones, the patient is placed on a low-purine diet to reduce the output of uric acid in the urine.

Allopurinol (Zyloprim) may be given to reduce serum uric acid and urinary uric acid excretion. The urine is alkalized. For cystine lithiasis, a low-protein diet is given, the urine is alkalized, and penicillamine is given to reduce the amount of cystine in the urine.

For oxalate stones, a dilute urine is maintained and the intake of oxalate is lowered. This means avoiding green, leafy vegetables; beans; celery; beets; rhubarb; chocolate; tea; coffee; and peanuts.

Open Operation. Surgical intervention is indicated if the stone is causing obstruction, unremitting pain, infection that does not respond to treatment, or progressive renal damage. Surgery is also done to correct any anatomical abnormalities within the kidney to improve urinary drainage.

If the stone is in the kidney, the operation performed may be a *nephrolithotomy* (incision into the kidney with removal of the stone) or a *nephrectomy,* if the kidney is functionless due to infection or hydronephrosis. (See p.

Chart 44-2
Moderately Calcium- and Phosphorus-Restricted Diet Plan*

Foods Used

Milk
  Limited to 1 cup (½ pint) a day. Cream may be substituted for part of the milk.
Cheese
  Pot or cottage cheese only; limited to 2 oz
Fats
  As desired
Eggs
  Limited to 1 a day; egg whites as desired
Meat, fish, fowl
  Limited to 4 oz daily of beef, lamb, pork, veal, chicken, turkey, fish. See those to be avoided.
Soups and broths
  All; cream soups made with milk allowance only
Vegetables
  At least 3 servings besides potato. One or 2 servings of deep green or deep yellow vegetables to be included daily. See list of those to be avoided.
Fruits
  All except rhubarb. Include citrus fruit daily.
Breads, cereals, Italian pastas
  White, enriched bread, rolls, and crackers except those made from self-rising white flour; farina (not enriched); cornflakes; corn meal; hominy grits; rice; Rice Krispies; Puffed Rice; macaroni; spaghetti; noodles
Desserts
  Fruit pies, fruit cobblers, fruit ices, gelatin, puddings made with allowed milk and egg, angel food cake (Do not use packaged mixes.)

Beverages
  Coffee, Postum, Sanka, tea, ginger ale
Condiments
  Sugar, jellies, honey, salt, pepper, spices

Foods to Be Avoided

Cheese
  All except pot or cottage cheese
Meat, fish, fowl
  Brains, heart, liver, kidney, sweetbreads, game (pheasant, rabbit, deer, grouse), sardines, fish roe
Vegetables
  Beet greens, chard, collards, mustard greens, spinach, turnip greens, dried beans, peas, lentils, soybeans
Fruits
  Rhubarb
Breads, cereals, Italian pastas
  Whole-grain breads, cereals, and crackers, rye bread; all breads made with self-rising flour; oatmeal; brown and wild rice; bran; Bran Flakes; wheat germ; all dry cereals except those allowed
Desserts
  All except those allowed
Beverages
  Carbonated "soft" drinks, cocoa
Miscellaneous
  Nuts, peanut butter, chocolate, cocoa, condiments having a calcium or a phosphate base (Read labels.)

* This diet will contain from 500 mg to 700 mg of calcium and from 1000 mg to 1200 mg of phosphorus.
(From Anderson L et al. Nutrition in Health and Disease, 17th ed. Philadelphia, JB Lippincott Co, 1982.)

990 for the nursing management of the patient following kidney surgery.) Stones in the kidney pelvis are removed by a *pyelolithotomy,* in the ureter by *ureterolithotomy,* and in the bladder by *cystotomy.* Sometimes an instrument is inserted through the urethra into the bladder, and the stone is crushed in the jaws of this instrument. Such an operation is called a *cystolitholapaxy.*

In prolonged operations for the removal of branched or multiple renal calculi, extracorporeal surgery allows better visualization and provides access for irrigation to remove stone fragments (see p. 989). The postoperative nursing management following kidney surgery is on page 990.

Endourologic Methods of Stone Removal.   The emerging field of endourology integrates the skills of the radiologist and urologist to extract renal calculi without major surgery. A percutaneous nephrostomy is performed (see p. 989), and a nephroscope is introduced through the dilated percutaneous tract into the renal parenchyma. Depending on the size, the stone may be extracted with forceps or by a stone basket. Or an ultrasound probe is introduced through the nephrostomy tube and ultrasonic waves used to pulverize the stone. Small stone fragments and stone dust are irrigated and suctioned out the collecting system. Larger stones may be further reduced by ultrasonic disintegration and then removed with forceps or stone basket. Using a similar method, an electrical discharge is used to create a hydraulic shock wave to crack the stone (electrohydraulic lithotripsy). A probe is passed through the cystoscope, and the tip of the lithotriptor is placed near the stone. The strength of the discharge and pulse frequency can be varied. This procedure is performed under topical anesthesia.

After stone extraction, the percutaneous nephrostomy tube is left in place for a time to ensure that the ureter is not obstructed from edema or blood clots. The most common complications are hemorrhage, infection, and urinary extravasation. Only a very small skin incision is required to remove the stone, a shorter hospital stay is required, and postoperative morbidity is minimal. After tube removal, the nephrostomy tract closes spontaneously.

Stone Dissolution.   Infusions of chemolytic solutions (alkylating agents, acidifying agents, etc.) for the purpose of stone dissolution may be done as an alternative to surgery in patients who are poor risks or have easily dissolved (struvite) stones. Usually, a percutaneous nephrostomy is performed (see p. 989) and the warm irrigating solution is allowed to flow continuously onto the stone. The irrigating solution leaves the renal collecting system via the ureter or the nephrostomy tube. The pressure inside the renal pelvis is monitored during the procedure.

Patient Education and Prevention of Urolithiasis.   Because it is known that urinary calculi may recur after the first stone is found, the patient should be so informed and encouraged to follow a regimen of prophylaxis. One facet of prevention is to *maintain a high fluid intake* since stones form more readily in a concentrated urine. A patient who has shown a tendency to form stones should drink enough to excrete about 3000 ml to 4000 ml of urine every 24 hours, should adhere to the prescribed diet, and should avoid sudden increases in environmental temperatures, which may cause a fall in urinary volume. Occupations and sports that produce excessive sweating can lead to severe temporary

dehydration; fluid intake should be increased. Sufficient fluids should be taken in the evening to prevent urine from becoming too concentrated at night. Urine cultures are done every 1 to 2 months the first year and periodically thereafter. Recurrent urinary infection must be treated vigorously.

Since prolonged immobilization slows renal drainage and alters calcium metabolism, ambulation is to be encouraged whenever possible. In addition, excessive ingestion of vitamins (especially vitamin D) and minerals should be discouraged.

▶ **Evaluation**

Expected Outcomes

1. Experiences relief of pain
   a. Passes stone
   b. Excretes urine freely
   c. Attains/maintains urine free of red blood cells
   d. Ambulates progressively
2. Experiences no infection
   a. Is free of fever
   b. Excretes clear urine
   c. Verbalizes that occurrence of fever, chills, flank pain, and hematuria are to be reported immediately
3. Adheres to the therapeutic program
   a. Drinks prescribed fluid intake
   b. Attains/maintains dilute urine
   c. Takes medication to control stone formation
   d. Monitors urinary *p*H
   e. Recalls the foods permitted on prescribed diet and reasons for dietary control

▷ Renal Tumors

Renal tumors may arise from the renal capsule, parenchyma (renal cell carcinomas), connective tissue (sarcomas), or fatty tissue or may be neurogenic or vascular in origin. Adenocarcinomas constitute 86% to 89% of all renal tumors. These tumors occur more frequently in males and may metastasize early to the lungs, bone, liver, brain, and contralateral kidney. Approximately one quarter to one half of patients will have metastatic disease at the time of diagnosis.

Clinical Manifestations.   Many renal lesions produce no symptoms and are discovered on a routine physical examination as a palpable abdominal mass. The classic triad, occurring late in the course of the disease, is hematuria, pain, and a mass in the flank. *The usual sign that first calls attention to the tumor is painless hematuria,* which may be intermittent, microscopic, or gross. There may be a dull pain in the back from back pressure produced by ureteral compression, perirenal extension, or hemorrhage into the substance of the kidney. Colicky pains occur if a clot or mass of tumor cells passes down the ureter. Symptoms from metastasis may be the first manifestation of renal tumor: unexplained weight loss, increasing weakness, anemia.

A battery of tests is useful in the diagnosis of renal neoplasms: excretion urography, drip infusion nephrotomography, sonography, and selective renal angiography.

Management.   The goal of management is to eradicate the tumor before metastasis occurs. A radical nephrectomy is the preferred treatment if the tumor can be removed. This includes removal of the kidney (and tumor), adrenal gland, surrounding perinephric fat and Gerota's fascia, and lymph nodes. In patients with a solitary kidney or with bilateral renal tumors, extracorporeal renal surgery allows a meticulous dissection and separation of the tumor from surrounding normal renal tissue (see p. 989). (See p. 990 for nursing management following renal surgery.) Radiation therapy may be used adjunctively with surgery. Chemotherapy or hormonal therapy may be tried. Immunotherapy may be helpful.

Renal Artery Embolization. In patients with metastatic renal carcinoma, embolization of the renal artery is being performed. Several days after completion of angiographic studies, a catheter is advanced into the renal artery, and embolizing materials (Gelfoam, autologous blood clot, steel coils) are injected into the artery and carried with the arterial blood flow to mechanically occlude the tumor vessels. This decreases tumor vascularity, making the subsequent nephrectomy technically easier to perform, and theoretically stimulates an immune response. This is based on the concept that infarction of the renal cell carcinoma will release tumor-associated antigens that will enhance the patient's response to metastatic lesions. The procedure is also purported to reduce the number of tumor cells entering the venous circulation during surgical manipulation.

Following renal artery embolization and tumor infarction, a characteristic symptom complex labeled "postinfarction syndrome" occurs, lasting 2 to 3 days. The patient has pain localized to the flank and abdomen, temperature elevation, and gastrointestinal complaints. Pain is treated with parenteral analgesics, while aspirin controls the fever; antiemetics, restriction of oral intake, and maintenance with intravenous fluids are used to treat the gastrointestinal complaints.

Follow-up and Health Teaching. The patient who has had surgery for renal carcinoma should undergo a yearly physical and roentgen examination of the chest throughout life, since late metastases are not uncommon. All subsequent complaints should be evaluated with possible metastases in mind.

Renal Cysts

Cysts of the kidney may be multiple (polycystic) or single. Polycystic disease of the adult is inherited as an autosomal dominant trait and usually involves both kidneys. The patient presents with abdominal or lumbar pain, hematuria, hypertension, palpable renal masses, and recurrent urinary tract infections. Renal insufficiency and failure usually develop in the terminal stages. Polycystic renal disease is also associated with cystic diseases of other organs (liver, pancreas, spleen) and aneurysms of the cerebral arteries. It is characteristically seen in midlife.

Management. As there is no specific treatment for polycystic renal disease, care of the patient is directed toward relief of symptoms and complications. Hypertension and urinary tract infections are treated aggressively. Hemodialysis appears to be effective when the patient reaches end-stage renal disease. Genetic counseling is part of patient education since polycystic kidney disease is a hereditary disease. The patient is advised to avoid sports and occupations that present a risk of trauma to the kidney.

Simple cysts of the kidney usually occur unilaterally

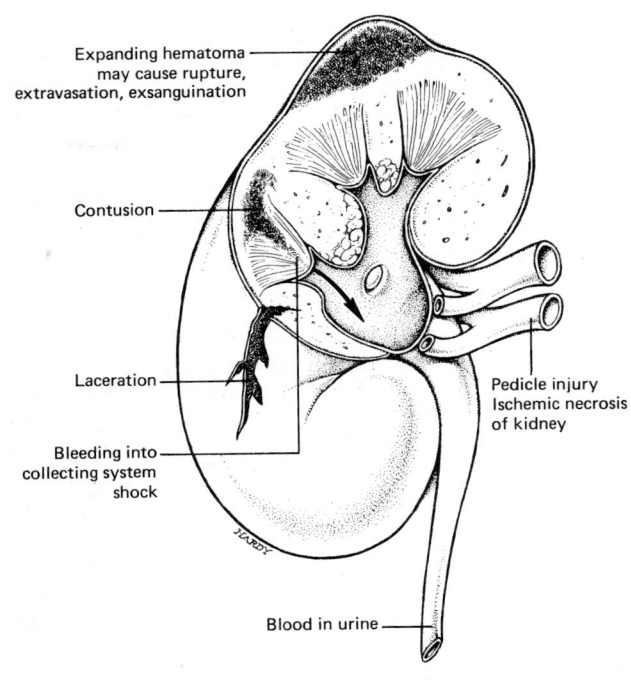

Figure 44-4. Pathophysiologic effect of renal trauma.

and differ clinically and pathophysiologically from polycystic kidney disease. The cyst may be punctured percutaneously.

▷ Congenital Anomalies

Congenital anomalies of the kidney are not uncommon. Occasionally, there is fusion of the two kidneys, forming what is called a *horseshoe kidney*. One kidney may be small and deformed and often is nonfunctioning. Not infrequently there may be a double ureter or congenital stricture of the ureter. The treatment of these anomalies is necessary only if they cause symptoms, but it goes without saying that before renal surgery is attempted, it is important to know that the other kidney is present and functioning.

▷ Renal Trauma

Various types of injuries of the flank, back, or upper abdomen may result in bruising, lacerations or rupture of the kidney, or pedicle injury (Fig. 44-4). The kidneys are protected by the musculature of the back posteriorly and by a cushion of abdominal wall and viscera anteriorly. They are highly mobile and are "fixed" only at the renal pedicle. With traumatic injury, the kidney can be thrust against the lower ribs, resulting in contusion and rupture. Rib fractures occurring with renal displacement or a fracture of the transverse process of the upper lumbar vertebrae may be associated with renal contusion or laceration. Injuries may be blunt (auto and motorcycle accidents, falls, athletic injuries) or penetrating (gunshot wounds, stabbings). Renal trauma is frequently associated with other injuries.

The most common renal injuries are contusions, laceration, rupture, and renal pedicle injuries or small internal laceration of the kidney. The kidneys receive half of the blood flow from the abdominal aorta; therefore, a fairly small renal laceration can produce massive bleeding.

Clinical Manifestations. The clinical manifestations include pain, renal colic (due to clots/fragments obstructing the collecting system), hematuria, flank mass, ecchymoses, and entrance wounds of the lateral abdomen and flank.

Management. The goals of management are to control hemorrhage, pain, and infection; to preserve and restore renal function; and to maintain urinary drainage.

Hematuria is the most common manifestation of renal trauma; therefore, the appearance of blood in the urine following an injury to the loin indicates the possibility of renal injury. There is no correlation between the degree of hematuria and the degree of injury. Hematuria may be absent or noticeable only on microscopic examination. Therefore, all urine is saved and sent to the laboratory for analysis to detect the presence of red cells and to follow the course of bleeding. The time the urine is voided and the volume should be recorded. Serial hematocrit and hemoglobin determinations are done to assess the degree of anemia, as progressive anemia indicates hemorrhage.

The patient is monitored for signs of oligemic shock since a pedicle injury or shattered kidney can lead to rapid exsanguination. An expanding hematoma may cause rupture of the kidney capsule. To detect the presence of hematoma, the area around the lower ribs, upper lumbar vertebrae, flank, and abdomen is palpated for tenderness. A palpable flank or abdominal mass with local tenderness, swelling, and ecchymosis suggests renal hemorrhage or extravasation. The area of the original mass can be outlined with a marking pencil so that the observer can evaluate the area for change. Skin abrasions, lacerations, and entry and exit wounds in the muscles of the upper abdomen, flank, and lower thoracic regions are important signs to check. Severe flank or costovertebral pain may signal a pedicle injury, which can cause ischemic necrosis of the kidney. It is important to remember that renal trauma is associated with other injuries to the abdominal organs (liver, colon, small intestines).

In minor injuries to the kidney, healing may take place with conservative measures. The patient is kept on bed rest until hematuria clears. Intravenous infusions may be necessary, because retroperitoneal bleeding may produce a reflex ileus.

Antimicrobials may be given to discourage infection from perirenal hematoma or urinoma (a cyst containing urine). Patients with retroperitoneal hematomas will have a low-grade fever as absorption of the clot takes place.

The patient should be evaluated frequently during the first few days following injury in order to detect flank and abdominal pain, muscle spasm, and swelling over the flank.

- Watch for any *sudden* change in the patient's condition that may indicate hemorrhage and require surgical intervention. The vital signs are monitored to detect evidences of bleeding. Narcotic analgesia is avoided as this may mask accompanying abdominal symptoms.

- Prepare for surgical exploration if the patient has an increasing pulse rate, hypotension, and impending shock.

Most penetrating injuries require surgical exploration because of the high incidence of other organ system involvement and serious complications if untreated. The damaged kidney may have to be removed (nephrectomy), although on occasion it is possible to repair it.

The postoperative management is discussed on page 990. Early complications (within 6 months) include rebleeding, abscess, sepsis, urine extravasation, and fistula formation.

Follow-up: Patient Education. Follow-up care includes monitoring the blood pressure to detect hypertension that may occur on a renovascular basis. Other complications include stone formation, infection, cysts, vascular aneurysms, and loss of renal function. Activity is usually restricted for 1 month following trauma to minimize the incidence of delayed or secondary bleeding.

▷ Bladder Injuries

Injury to the bladder may occur with pelvic fractures and multiple trauma or from a blow to the lower abdomen when the bladder is full. Blunt trauma may result in contusion (an ecchymosis involving a segment of the bladder wall) or in rupture of the bladder, extraperitoneally, intraperitoneally, or a combination of both. Complications from these injuries (hemorrhage, shock, sepsis, and extravasation) must be treated promptly.

A retrograde urethrogram is done first to evaluate for urethral injury. The patient is catheterized after the urethrogram is done.

Management. Treatment for traumatic rupture of the bladder involves immediate surgical exploration and repair of the laceration, with suprapubic drainage of the bladder and the perivesical space (around the bladder) along with insertion of an urethral indwelling catheter.

In addition to the usual postoperative care following urologic surgery (see p. 990), the drainage systems (suprapubic, indwelling urethral catheter, and perivesical drains) are observed to ensure adequate drainage until healing takes place. The patient with a ruptured bladder may have gross bleeding for several days after repair. Complications of urethral injuries include stricture, incontinence, and impotence.

▷ Cancer of the Bladder

Cancer of the urinary bladder is seen more frequently in persons from age 50 onward and affects men more than women (3:1). Statistics indicate that these tumors make up approximately 2% of all cancers in the body and are on the increase. The most common type is transitional cell cancer.

Risk factors for cancer of the bladder include cigarette smoking and carcinogens in the work environment, such as dyes, rubber, leather, ink, or paint. There may be a relationship between coffee drinking and bladder cancer.

Chronic schistosomiasis (parasitic infection that irritates the bladder) is also a risk factor. Cancers arising from the prostate, colon, and rectum in males and from the lower gynecologic tract in females may metastasize to the bladder.

Clinical Manifestations. These tumors usually arise at the base of the bladder and involve the ureteral orifices and bladder neck. Gross, painless hematuria is the most common symptom of bladder tumor, particularly cancer of the bladder. Infection of the urinary tract is a common complication, producing frequency, urgency, and dysuria. However, any disturbance of micturition or change in the urine may indicate cancer of the bladder. Pelvic or back pain may be due to distant metastasis.

The diagnostic evaluation includes excretory urography, cystoscopy, and bimanual examination under anesthesia. Biopsies of the tumor and mucosa adjacent to the tumor are the definitive diagnostic procedures.

Histologic grade transitional cell carcinomas and carcinomas in-situ shed recognizable cancer cells. Cytologic examination of fresh urine and saline bladder washings provide prognostic information in patient evaluation, especially for those at high risk for recurrence of primary bladder tumors. Computed tomography and angiography of the pelvic vessels may be carried out to evaluate the stage of tumor invasion.

Management. Treatment of bladder cancer depends on the grade of the tumor (based on the degree of cellular differentiation), the stage of growth (the degree of local invasion and the presence or absence of metastasis), and the multicentricity (having many centers) of the tumor. The patient's age and physical, mental, and emotional status are considered in determining treatment modalities.

Transurethral resection or fulguration may be done for simple papillomas, although aggressive malignancies may develop from these tumors. One of the greatest challenges is the management of patients with superficial bladder cancers, as it is now known that there are widespread abnormalities in the bladder mucosa of these patients. The entire urothelium is at risk, as carcinomatous changes are not only found in the mucosa of the bladder but also in that of the renal pelvis, ureter, and urethra. Recurrences are a serious problem and approximately 60% of superficial bladder tumors recur after transurethral resection or fulguration. Even persons with benign papillomas should be followed with cytology and cystoscopy periodically for the rest of their lives.

Topical chemotherapy (intravesical chemotherapy) is considered when there is high risk of recurrences, when cancer in-situ is present, or when tumor resection has been incomplete. Topical chemotherapy delivers a high concentration of drug (thiotepa, Adriamycin, 5-fluorouracil) to the tumor to promote tumor destruction. Fluid intake may be limited during instillation of the drug to prevent the need to void during the procedure, which takes approximately 2 hours. At the conclusion, the patient is encouraged to void and drink liberal amounts of fluid to flush the drug from the bladder.

Sometimes the tumor is irradiated preoperatively to reduce microextension of the neoplasm and viability of tumor cells, thus reducing the chances of recurrence for local implantation or hematogenous/lymphatic dissemination. Radiation is also used in combination with surgery or to control the disease in the inoperable patient.

A simple cystectomy (removal of the bladder) or a radical cystectomy is done for invasive or multifocal bladder cancer. Radical cystectomy in the male involves removal of the bladder, prostate, and seminal vesicles and immediate adjacent perivesical tissues. In the female, radical cystectomy involves removal of the bladder, lower ureter, uterus, tubes, ovaries, anterior vagina, and urethra. It may or may not include a pelvic lymphadenectomy. Removal of the bladder requires a urinary diversion procedure (see below).

The transitional cell variety of bladder cancer is poorly responsive to chemotherapy. Cisplatin, Adriamycin, and cyclophosphamide have been administered in various doses and schedules and appear most effective.

Bladder cancer may also be treated by direct infusion of the cytotoxic agent through the arterial supply of the involved organ. Thus, a higher concentration of the chemotherapeutic agent can be achieved with lessened toxicity to the system. For more advanced bladder cancer or for patients with intractable hematuria (especially following radiation therapy), a water-filled balloon placed within the bladder produces tumor necrosis by reducing the blood circulating in the bladder wall (hydrostatic therapy). The instillation of formalin, phenol, or silver nitrate has achieved relief of hematuria and strangury (slow and painful discharge of urine) in some patients.

▷ Urinary Diversion

Urinary diversion refers to a means of diverting the urinary stream from the bladder so that it exits via a new avenue. This is done primarily when a large or invasive bladder tumor requires that the entire bladder be removed. Other conditions requiring urinary diversion include pelvic malignancy, birth defects, strictures and trauma to ureters and urethra, neurogenic bladder, and chronic infection causing severe ureteral and renal damage.

There is controversy concerning the best means of establishing permanent diversion of the urinary tract. The age of the patient, condition of the bladder, body build, degree of obesity, intelligence, degree of ureteral dilation, and state of renal function are all taken into consideration.

The most common methods of urinary diversion are:

1. *Ileal conduit:* transplanting the ureters to an isolated section of the terminal ileum and bringing one end to the abdominal wall as an ileostomy (Fig. 44-5 A). The ureter may also be transplanted into the transverse colon (colon conduit) or proximal jejunum (jejunal conduit).
2. *Ureterosigmoidostomy:* introducing the ureter into the sigmoid, thereby allowing urine to flow through the colon and out of the rectum (Fig. 44-5 B)
3. *Cutaneous ureterostomy:* bringing the detached ureter through the abdominal wall and attaching it to an opening in the skin (Fig. 44-5 C)

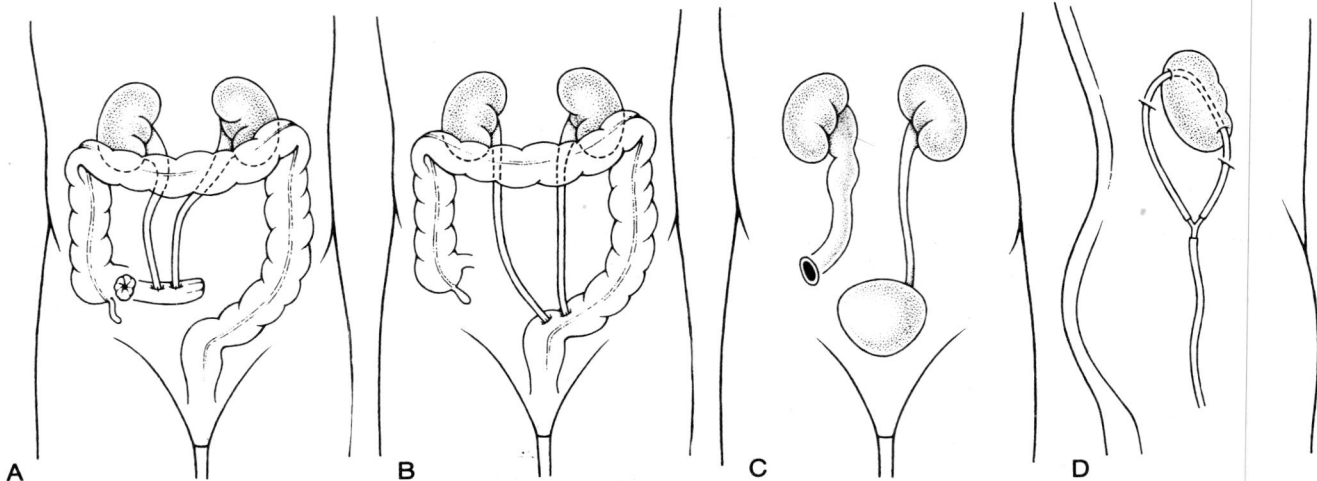

Figure 44-5. Methods of urinary diversion. (*A*) Ileal conduit. (*B*) Ureterosigmoidostomy. (*C*) Cutaneous ureterostomy. (*D*) Nephrostomy tube drainage.

4. *Suprapubic cystostomy* (or *vesicostomy*): draining the bladder through an abdominal wound
5. *Nephrostomy:* inserting a catheter into the renal pelvis via an incision into the flank or by percutaneous catheter placement into the kidney (Fig. 44-5 *D*)

Management

The patient's major nursing diagnosis is potential for morbidity and dependency related to the management of the urinary stoma, and potential complications related to prolonged operation and nature of the surgery.

Preoperative Management. A careful preoperative assessment of cardiopulmonary function is done since patients undergoing cystectomy are usually older people who may not fare well in a lengthy complex procedure. As part of preoperative management, the bowel is cleansed (to minimize fecal stasis, to decompress the bowel, and to minimize postoperative ileus), a low-residue diet is prescribed, and antimicrobial drugs are administered for bowel disinfection to reduce pathogenic flora and to lessen potential complications of wound infection and sepsis. Adequate preoperative hydration is imperative to ensure urine flow during surgery and to prevent hypovolemia during the prolonged operative procedure. Sometimes patients with urogenital tract cancer have severe problems with malnutrition because of increased tumor mass and decreased food intake. Enteral or intravenous hyperalimentation can be used to support the patient, minimize toxicity, promote healing, and improve response to treatment.

An enterostomal therapist is invaluable for preoperative teaching. Explanations of the surgical procedure and the reasons for wearing a collection device postoperatively are given to the patient and the family. The stoma site is planned preoperatively with the patient standing, sitting, and lying in order to locate the stoma away from bony prominences, skin creases, and fat folds. *The patient should be able to see the site for ease of self-care.* The optimum site is marked with indelible ink for intraoperative location. It is desirable to have the patient practice wearing the appliance partially filled with water before surgery.

Psychological Assessment and Support

The threat of bladder removal and cancer initiates fear related to losses—loss of love, body image, and security. In addition to problems in adapting to an external appliance, a stoma, and a scar, the patient must also adapt to alterations in toileting habits, and the male patient must also adapt to sexual impotency. (A penile implant is considered if the patient is a candidate for the procedure.) Women face the fear of loss of appearance because of changed body image. A supportive approach is needed that includes physical, psychological, and psychosocial support. It involves taking a personal interest in the patient, observing the patient's concept and perception of self and the manner in which he responds to stress and loss, and helping him to maintain his usual life-style and independence with as few modifications as possible. The family is included, from the beginning, in the teaching program and in caring for the patient. Allow for verbalization of fear and anxiety. A visitor from the "Ostomy Visitation Program" of the American Cancer Society can give emotional support and make adaptation easier both before and after surgery.

If the disease progresses and death is inevitable, the mourning process begins and the patient moves through the phases of denial, loss, anger (directed toward family, health care personnel, society), depression, and withdrawal. Psychosocial counseling has been found to enhance the quality of the patient's remaining days. The nurse's role is not to lose sight of the human being undergoing this hard experience and to support him through the mourning process to the stage of final resolution and acceptance.

Postoperative Planning and Implementation

The patient's goals are to accomplish the highest level of self-care possible and to avoid complications. The objectives of postoperative nursing management are to preserve renal function and to assist the patient in adapting to an altered body image.

The main focus of management is directed at the urinary and intestinal tract and ileal stoma as well as those elements of care given to a patient who has undergone intestinal surgery (see p. 839). A nasogastric tube is inserted during surgery to allow for decompression and to relieve pressure on the intestinal anastomosis. It is usually kept in place until the 4th to 7th day after surgery. As soon as bowel function resumes, as manifested by bowel sounds, the passage of flatus, and a soft abdomen, the patient is given fluids by mouth. Until that time, fluids and electrolytes are given intravenously. The patient is ambulated as soon as possible. (The remainder of the postoperative management is discussed under the specific urinary diversion procedure.)

Ileal Conduit Urinary Diversion (Ileal Loop)

In an *ileal conduit*, the urine is diverted by implanting the ureter into a loop of ileum that is led out through the abdominal wall as an ileostomy. This loop of ileum is a simple conduit (passageway) for urine from the ureters to the surface. A loop of the sigmoid colon may also be used. An ileostomy bag is used to collect the urine. The bowel continuity is obtained by anastomosis of the remaining ileum.

After surgery, a skin barrier and a transparent, disposable urinary drainage bag are applied around the conduit and connected to drainage. A temporary appliance is used until the edema subsides and the stoma shrinks to normal size. The clear bag allows visualization of the stoma and monitoring of output and stent patency. The ileal bag drains urine constantly, but not feces. The appliance (bag) usually remains in place as long as it is watertight. Then it is changed.

Nursing Interventions.
Urine volumes are checked hourly, as an output below 30 ml/hour may indicate an obstruction in the ileal conduit with possible backflow or leakage from the ureteroileal anastomosis. A catheter may be inserted through the urinary conduit to check for possible stasis or residual urine from a tight stoma.

The stoma is inspected frequently for bleeding. Minimal bleeding may be seen and implies good blood supply. Watch for a change in color from a normal pink to red color to a dark purplish color, which suggests that the vascular supply may be compromised. If congestion and cyanosis persist, surgical intervention may be required.

The stoma is insensitive to touch, but the skin around the stoma is exquisitely sensitive if it becomes irritated by urine or the appliance. The skin is inspected for (1) signs of irritation, bleeding, and friability of the stomal mucosa; (2) alkaline encrustation with peristomal dermatitis (from alkaline urine coming in contact with exposed skin); and (3) wound infections.

The odor of urine around the patient should alert the nursing personnel to the possibility of leakage from the appliance, the presence of an infection, or a problem in hygienic management. Since severe alkaline encrustation can accumulate rapidly around the stoma, the urine *p*H is kept below 6.5. Urine *p*H can be determined by testing the

urine dribbling from the stoma, not from the collecting appliance. A properly fitted appliance is a must to prevent the peristomal skin from being exposed to urine. If the urine is foul smelling, the stoma may be catheterized in order to obtain a specimen for culture and sensitivity or to determine stomal patency and detect the presence of residual urine. Scarring of the stoma can interfere with urine drainage.

A high-fluid diet is encouraged, in order to flush the ileal conduit and prevent mucus from congealing. The patient may excrete a fairly large amount of mucus with the urine as a result of the urine irritating the intestine. To relieve anxiety in this regard, the patient should be reassured that this is a normal occurrence following an ileal conduit.

Complications following this method of urinary diversion include wound infection or wound dehiscence, urinary extravasation, ureteral obstruction, small bowel obstruction, and stomal gangrene. Delayed complications include ureteral obstruction, stomal stenosis, pyelonephritis, and renal calculi.

Patient Education and Rehabilitation

Appliance Selection.
The urinary appliance may consist of one or two pieces and may be temporary/disposable (applied once and discarded) or semidisposable (reusable). The choice of appliance is determined by the location of the stoma and the patient's normal activity, body build, and economic status. A reusable appliance has a faceplate that is attached to the body with cement or adhesive. A semidisposable appliance has a reusable faceplate to which disposable pouches are attached. Disposable appliances are discarded after each use. They have the advantage of having a surface that is already prepared and of being lightweight and easy to conceal.

Determining the Stoma Size.
As the postoperative edema subsides, the stoma opening is recalibrated every 3 to 6 weeks for the first few months postoperatively. The correct appliance size is determined by measuring the widest part of the stoma with a ruler. The permanent appliance should not be more than $\frac{1}{16}$ of an inch larger than the diameter of the stoma to prevent skin reaction to the urine.

Changing the Appliance; Skin Care

- The appliance should be changed at a time that will be most convenient to the patient. Early in the morning, before drinking fluids, when urinary output is lower, is the time chosen by many ostomates. Ideally, the collecting appliance is changed every 5 to 7 days.
- Prepare the new appliance according to the manufacturer's directions. (The center opening is tailored to the individual stomal opening.)
- Moisten the edge of the faceplate with water or adhesive solvent, or soap and water, and gently remove it. Adhesive solvent is not used if skin barriers are used.
- Instruct the patient to bend over quickly and remain in that position a minute to allow the conduit to empty before the skin is washed and dried.

- Clean all cement from the skin with warm water or adhesive solvent, using a soft cloth. Wash the skin with a noncream-based soap and water. Rinse well, as a soap film will prevent appliance adherence. Pat dry. *The skin must be dry or the appliance will not adhere.*
  1. Insert a tampon or gauze or tissue wick at the stoma opening to absorb the urine and keep the skin dry while the appliance is being changed.
  2. Inspect the skin for signs of irritation. Keep the skin free from direct contact with urine.
  3. Apply a skin protector or barrier if required. Center the appliance directly over the stoma and apply it carefully. Apply gentle pressure around the appliance to remove air bubbles and creases so that it will adhere securely.
- Apply hypoallergenic tape in a picture-frame effect around the pouch. The skin under the appliance may be dusted with pure talcum powder. An appliance cover may be used to absorb perspiration and eliminate warmth from the appliance.
- The use of a belt is optional, but the manufacturer's directions should be followed, since a poorly fitting belt may cause abrasion of the stoma.

Since stomal protrusion is not the same in all patients, there are various accessories and custom-made appliances to solve individual problems.

Odor Control. The patient should be advised to avoid foods and medications that give the urine a strong odor. A few drops of liquid deodorizer or diluted white vinegar may be introduced through the drain spout into the bottom of the pouch with a syringe or eyedropper. Taking ascorbic acid by mouth helps acidify the urine and suppresses urine odor problems. Also, the patient should be reminded that the pouch will develop an odor if it is worn too long and not cared for properly.

Managing the Ostomy Appliance. The pouch is emptied by a drain valve when it is one third to one half full, since the weight of the urine may cause it to separate from the skin. Some patients prefer wearing a leg bag attached with an adaptor to the drainage apparatus. To assure uninterrupted sleep, the collecting bottle and tubing (one unit) are snapped onto an adaptor that screws into the ileal appliance. A small amount of urine is left in the bag when the adaptor is screwed on to prevent the bag from collapsing against itself. The tubing may be threaded down the pajama leg to prevent kinking.

Cleaning and Deodorizing the Appliance. Usually, the reusable appliance is rinsed in warm water and soaked in a solution of water and white vinegar or a commercial deodorizing solution for 30 minutes. Then it is rinsed and air-dried away from direct sunlight. After drying, the appliance may be powdered with cornstarch and stored. Two appliances are necessary; one to be worn while the other is air-drying.

The patient is encouraged to contact the local ostomy association for visits, reassurance, and practical information.*

* See bibliography at end of chapter for address.

Evaluation
Expected Outcomes

1. Accomplishes high level of self-care
   a. Acknowledges anatomical deviation due to surgery
   b. Verbalizes acceptance of urinary stoma and appliance
   c. Observes transparent appliance periodically to see that urine is draining
   d. Cares for skin
   e. Changes appliance correctly
   f. Recalls three methods of odor control
   g. Revises daily routine to accommodate urostomy management
   h. Has telephone number of resource person
   i. Has name, address, and telephone number of surgical supply house/pharmacy for ostomy supplies
   j. Verbalizes plans to resume normal activities of daily living
2. Experiences no complications
   a. Progresses to active bowel sounds
   b. Has soft abdomen
   c. Excretes urine freely in appliance
   d. Attains/maintains clear urine
   e. Maintains negative urine culture
   f. Maintains healthy-appearing stoma without evidence of retraction or stenosis
   g. Is free of wound infection or dehiscence

Ureterosigmoidostomy

Ureterosigmoidostomy is an implantation of the ureters into the sigmoid colon. It is usually done for the patient who has had extensive pelvic irradiation, previous small bowel resection, or coexisting small bowel disease. In addition to the usual preoperative regimen, the patient may be placed on a liquid diet for several days preoperatively to keep the colon clean. Antimicrobial agents (neomycin; kanamycin) are administered for bowel disinfection. Ureterosigmoidostomy requires a competent anal sphincter, adequate renal function, and active ureteral peristalsis. The degree of anal sphincter control may be determined by assessing the patient's ability to retain enemas.

The patient will be informed that following surgery voiding will occur from the rectum for the rest of his life and that an adjustment in life-style will be necessary because of urinary frequency (as often as every 2 hours), which will have a consistency equivalent to a watery diarrhea. There will be some degree of nocturia. Activities will have to be planned around the frequent need to urinate, which in turn may restrict the patient's social life. However, the patient has the advantage of urinary control without having to wear an external appliance.

Postoperatively, a catheter is placed in the rectum to drain the urine and prevent reflux of urine into the ureters and kidneys. The tube is taped to the buttocks and special skin care given around the anus to prevent excoriation. Irrigations of the rectal tube may be requested, but force should not be used because of the danger of introducing an infection into the newly implanted ureters.

In this operation, larger areas of the bowel mucosa are exposed to urine and electrolyte reabsorption, so that electrolyte imbalance and acidosis may result. Potassium and magnesium imbalances may occur from the presence of urine in the bowel, which simulates diarrhea. Fluid and electrolyte balance is maintained in the immediate postoperative period by serum chemical determinations and appropriate intravenous infusions. Acidosis may be prevented by placing the patient on a low-chloride diet supplemented with sodium potassium citrate. The patient should be instructed never to wait longer than 3 hours before emptying urine from the intestine in order to keep rectal pressure low and to minimize absorption of urinary constituents from the colon.

After the rectal catheter is removed, the patient learns to control the anal sphincter through special sphincteric exercises. At first urination is frequent. With reassurance and encouragement and the passage of time, the patient will gain greater control and will learn to differentiate between the need to void and the need to defecate.

Pyelonephritis (upper urinary tract infection due to reflux of bacteria from the colon) is fairly common in some patients who may have to take prophylactic antimicrobial therapy for the rest of their lives.

Specific diet instructions include avoidance of gas-forming foods, since flatus can cause stress incontinence and socially embarrassing offensive odors. Other ways to avoid gas are to avoid chewing gum, smoking, and any other activity that involves swallowing air. Salt intake may be restricted to prevent hyperchloremic acidosis. Potassium intake is increased through foods and medication since potassium may be lost in acidosis. A late complication is adenocarcinoma of the sigmoid colon, possibly due to the exposure of colonic mucosa to urine, leading to cellular changes.

Cutaneous Ureterostomy (Cutaneous Urinary Conduit)

A *cutaneous ureterostomy* is accomplished by bringing the detached ureters through the abdominal wall and attaching them to an opening in the skin. This procedure is used in selected patients with ureteral obstruction (advanced pelvic cancer); for poor-risk patients, as it requires less time than other urinary diversion procedures; and for patients who have had previous abdominal irradiation.

A urinary appliance is fitted immediately following surgery. The management of the patient with a cutaneous ureterostomy is very similar to the care of the patient with an ileal conduit (see p. 1015).

Cystostomy

An infrequently used method of urinary diversion is the *suprapubic cystostomy,* which is accomplished by inserting a special catheter through the abdomen into the bladder either through an incision in the lower abdominal wall or by a trochar punch technique. It is usually done under local anesthesia. Generally, a cystostomy is done on the patient with an obstruction below the bladder (prostatic obstruction) when it is not possible to insert a urethral catheter. A cystostomy may be temporary (until corrective surgery can be done) or permanent.

The patient with a cystostomy requires liberal amounts of fluid to prevent encrustation around the catheter. Other problems encountered include the formation of bladder stones, acute and chronic infections, and problems in collecting urine. The advice and assistance of an enterostomal therapist is needed in choosing the most suitable urine collection bag and to instruct the patient in its use.

▷ Urethral Conditions

Caruncle

A *caruncle* is a small, red, extremely vascular polypoid growth situated just within, and protruding from, the external urethral meatus of women. On rare occasions, it causes no subjective symptoms. However, it may be acutely sensitive, causing a local burning pain exaggerated by exertion and frequency of urination, which is exquisitely painful. Local excision of the caruncle will relieve the troublesome symptoms.

Urethritis

Urethritis, inflammation of the urethra, is usually an ascending infection and may be classified as gonococcal (see p. 1494) or nongonococcal. However, both conditions may be present in the same patient. Urethritis not associated with *Neisseria gonorrhoeae* is usually caused by *Chlamydia trachomatis* or *Ureaplasma urealyticum.* If the male patient is symptomatic, he will complain of mild to severe dysuria and a scanty to moderate urethral discharge. Nongonococcal urethritis requires prompt antimicrobial treatment with tetracycline or doxycycline, or in those patients who do not respond or are allergic to the tetracyclines, erythromycin may be substituted. Follow-up care is necessary to make certain that a cure is achieved. All persons who are sexual partners of patients with nongonococcal urethritis must be examined for sexually transmitted disease and treated.

Gonorrheal Urethritis. Gonorrheal urethritis is caused by *Neisseria gonorrhoeae* and is transmitted by sexual contact. In the male, inflammation of the meatal orifice occurs with burning on urination. A purulent urethral discharge appears 3 to 14 days (or longer) after sexual exposure. However, the disease may be asymptomatic. In the female, there is not always a urethral discharge present, and the disease is often essentially asymptomatic. Therefore, gonorrhea in the female is frequently not reported and diagnosed.

In the male, the infection involves the tissues around the urethra, causing periurethritis, prostatitis, epididymitis, and urethral stricture. Sterility may occur due to vasoepididymal obstruction. Treatment of gonorrhea is discussed on page 1497 and patient education on page 1497.

Urethral Strictures

An urethral stricture is a narrowing of the lumen of the urethra due to scar tissue and contraction. Strictures result from urethral injury (urethral instrumentation for transurethral surgery, indwelling catheters, cystoscopic procedures), straddle injuries and automobile accidents, untreated gonorrheal urethritis, and congenital abnormalities.

There is diminution in the force and size of the urinary stream, along with symptoms of urinary infection and retention. Stricture produces back pressure with resulting cystitis, prostatitis, and pyelonephritis. An important element of prevention is to treat all urethral infections promptly. Prolonged urethral catheter drainage is to be avoided and utmost care taken in any type of urethral instrumentation, including catheterization.

Management. The treatment may be palliative (gradual dilatation of the narrowed area with metal sounds or bougies) or operation under direct vision (internal urethrotomy). If the stricture has become so small as to prevent the passage of a catheter, the urologist uses several small filiform bougies in search of the opening. When one bougie passes beyond the stricture into the bladder, it is fixed in place, and urine will drain from the bladder. The stricture then can be dilated to larger size by the passage of a larger sound (a dilating instrument) following behind the filiform as a guide. Following dilatation, hot sitz baths and nonnarcotic analgesics are given to control the pain. Antimicrobials are given for several days after dilatation to minimize the infectious reaction, thus lessening discomfort.

Surgical excision or urethroplasty may be necessary for severe cases. Sometimes a suprapubic cystostomy must be performed. The postoperative treatment for cystostomy is described on page 973.

▷ Bibliography
Books

Al-Askari S, Golimbu M, and Morales P. Essentials of Basic Sciences in Urology. New York, Grune & Stratton, 1981.

Alken C-E, Sokeland J, and Engel RME. Urology. Guide for Diagnosis and Therapy. New York, Thieme, 1982.

Anderson RJ and Schrier RW (eds). Clinical Use of Drugs in Patients with Kidney and Liver Disease. Philadelphia, WB Saunders, 1981.

Asscher AW. The Challenge of Urinary Tract Infections. New York, Grune & Stratton, 1980.

Barnes RW, Bergman RT, and Hadley HL. Urology. Garden City, New York, Medical Examination, 1980.

Blaisdell FW and Trunkey DD. Trauma Management. New York, Thieme-Stratton, 1982.

Blandy J. Lecture Notes on Urology. Boston, Blackwell Scientific Publications, 1982.

Bookstein JJ and Clark RL. Renal Microvascular Disease. Boston, Little, Brown & Co, 1980.

Brenner BM and Rector FC Jr. The Kidney, Vols 1 and 2, 2nd ed. Philadelphia, WB Saunders, 1981.

Brown RB. Clinical Urology Illustrated. New York, Adis Press, 1982.

Brundage DJ. Nursing Management of Renal Problems, 2nd ed. St Louis, CV Mosby, 1980.

Castro JE (ed) The Treatment of Renal Failure. Lancaster, MTP Press, 1982.

Catto GRD and Smith JAR. Clinical Aspects of Renal Physiology. London, Bailliere Tindall, 1981.

Chatterjee SN (ed). Renal Transplantation. New York, Raven Press, 1980.

Crawford ED and Borden TA (eds). Genitourinary Cancer Surgery. Philadelphia, Lea & Febiger, 1982.

Denis L, Smith PH, and Pavone-Macaluso M. Clinical Bladder Cancer. New York, Plenum Press, 1980.

DeVita VT Jr, Hellman S, and Rosenberg SA. Cancer. Principles and Practice of Oncology. Philadelphia, JB Lippincott, 1982.

Earle DP et al. Manual of Clinical Nephrology. Philadelphia, WB Saunders, 1982.

First MR. Chronic Renal Failure. Garden City, Medical Examination, 1982.

Flamenbaum WF and Hamburger RJ (eds). Nephrology: An Approach to the Patient with Renal Disease. Philadelphia, JB Lippincott, 1982.

Hamburger J et al. Renal Transplantation: Theory and Practice, 2nd ed. Baltimore, Williams & Wilkins, 1981.

Johnson DE and Boileau MA. Genitourinary Tumors. New York, Grune & Stratton, 1982.

Kaufman JJ. Current Urologic Therapy. Philadelphia, WB Saunders, 1980.

Kenner CV, Guzzetta CE, and Dossey BM. Critical Care Nursing, Body—Mind—Spirit. Boston, Little, Brown & Co, 1981.

Klahr S, Nolph KD, and Luke RG. End-State Renal Disease: Pathophysiology, Dialysis and Transplantation. Washington, DC, US Dept of Health and Human Services, 1981.

Larson E, Lindbloom L, and Davis KB. Development of the Clinical Nephrology Practitioner. St Louis, CV Mosby, 1982.

Lerner J and Khan Z. Mosby's Manual of Urologic Nursing. St Louis, CV Mosby, 1982.

Levy NB. Psychonephrology. 1. Psychological Factors in Hemodialysis and Transplantation. New York, Plenum, 1981.

McConnell EA and Zimmerman MF. Care of Patients with Urologic Problems. Philadelphia, JB Lippincott, 1982.

Nardi GL and Zuidema GD. Surgery: Essentials of Clinical Practice, 4th ed. Boston, Little, Brown & Co, 1982.

Schrier RW. Renal and Electrolyte Disorders, 2nd ed. Boston, Little, Brown & Co, 1980.

Smith DR. General Urology, 10th ed. Los Altos, Lange, 1981.

Smith LH, Robertson WG, and Finlayson B. Urolithiasis, Clinical and Basic Research. New York, Plenum Press, 1981.

Stamey TA. Pathogenesis and Treatment of Urinary Tract Infections. Baltimore, Williams & Wilkins, 1980.

Stanton SL and Tanagho EA. Surgery of Female Incontinence. New York, Springer-Verlag, 1980.

Tilney NL and Lazarus JM. Surgical Care of the Patient with Renal Failure. Philadelphia, WB Saunders, 1982.

Articles
General Articles

Cass AS. Immediate radiologic and surgical management of renal injuries. J Trauma 1982 May; 22(5):361–363.

Chester AC et al. Early diagnosis of polycystic kidney disease. Am Fam Physician 1981 Mar; 23(3):175–181.

Editorial: Adult polycystic disease of the kidneys. Br Med J 1981 Apr 4; 282(6270):1097–1098.

Lockwood CM and Peters DK. Plasma exchange in glomerulonephritis and related vasculitides. Annu Rev Med 1980; 31:167–179.

McDougal WS and Persky L. Traumatic injuries of the genitourinary system. International Perspectives in Urology 1981; 1:1–135 (entire volume).

Peters DK. The major glomerulopathies. Hosp Pract 1981 Oct; 16(10):117–122, 124, 129–133.

Rosen S et al. Glomerular disease. Hum Pathol 1981 Nov; 12(11):964–977.

Acute Renal Failure

Ali AS, Amir AS, and Baig FN. Hepatorenal syndrome. Am Fam Physician 1982 June; 25(6):127–131.

Bambauer R and Jutzler GA. Transcutaneous insertion of the Shaldon catheter through the internal jugular vein as access for acute hemodialysis. Dial Transplant 1982 Sept; 11(9):766–773.

Curry RW Jr, Robinson JD, and Seighrue MJ. Acute renal failure with acetaminophen ingestion. JAMA 1982 Feb 19; 247(7):1012–1014.

Doyle JE. Treating renovascular hypertension: Bypass graft surgery. Am J Nurs 1982 Oct; 82(10):1559.

Doyle JE and Sequeera JC. Renal artery dilation. Am J Nurs 1982 Oct; 82(10):1563–1564.

Fink M. Are diuretics useful in the treatment or prevention of acute renal failure? South Med J 1982 Mar; 75(3):329–334.

Friedman FB. Why not use a Foley? RN 1982 Nov; 45(11):71–76.

Habel M. What you need to know about infusing plasma expanders. RN 1980 Aug; 43(8):30–33.

Hargiss CO and Larson E. How to collect specimens and evaluate results. Am J Nurs 1981 Dec; 81(12):2166–2174.

Hinkle MT and Bowditch RR. The great stent mystery. Can you solve it? Nursing '81 1981 Apr; 11(4):94–95.

Kelber MB Sr. Plasma renin activity. Nursing '82 1982 Apr; 12(4):140–144.

Lane G and Peirce AG. When persistence pays off: Resolving the mystery of unexplained electrolyte imbalance. Nursing '82 1982 Jan; 12(1):44–47.

Levitan D. Effects of drug abuse on the kidney. Dial Transplant 1982 Oct; 11(10):885–888.

Mather DG. Ideal conduit surgery: How to help a terrified patient. RN 1981 Oct; 44(10):29–31.

McCarthy JA. Diabetic nephropathy. Am J Nurs 1981 Nov; 81(11):2030–2034.

McConnell EA. Urinalysis: A common test but never routine. Nursing '82 1982 Feb; 12(2):108–111.

Metheny N. Renal stones and urinary pH. Am J Nurs 1982 Sept; 82(9):1372–1375.

Nemchik R. Diabetes today. A startling new body of knowledge. RN 1982 Oct; 45(10):31–37.

Oken DE. On the differential diagnosis of acute renal failure. Am J Med 1981 Dec; 71(6):916–920.

Orr ML. Drugs and renal disease. Am J Nurs 1981 May; 81(5):969–971.

Porter GA and Bennett WM. Nephrotoxic acute renal failure due to common drugs. Am J Physiol 1981 July; 241(1):F1–8.

Richman AV, Narayan JL, and Huschfield JS. Acute interstitial nephritis and acute renal failure associated with cimetidine therapy. Am J Med 1981 June; 70(6):1272–1274.

Schreir RW. Acute renal failure: Pathogenesis, diagnosis and management. Hosp Pract 1981 Mar; 16(3):93–98, 101–105, 109.

Schulmeister L. Vascular access grafts in cancer chemotherapy. Am J Nurs 1982 Sept; 82(9):1388–1389.

Tower M. Urinary obstruction: The hidden threats in treatment. RN 1982 May; 45(5):58–63.

Wright TR and Murray M. Potassium problems: Which patient's in danger? RN 1982 June; 45(6):56–61.

Cancer of the Kidney

Funch RB. Therapeutic embolization for palliation of an inoperable renal carcinoma. J Maine Med Assoc 1980 Oct; 71(10):305–307, 311.

Javadpour N (ed). Recent advances in urologic cancer. International Perspectives in Urology 1982: 2:1–312 (entire volume).

McDonald MW. Current therapy for renal cell carcinoma. J Urol 1982 Feb; 127(2):211–217.

Poster DS et al. Current status of chemotherapy, hormonal therapy and immunotherapy in the treatment of renal cell carcinoma. American Journal of Clinical Oncology 1982 Feb; 5(1):53–60.

Swanson DA, Wallace S, and Johnson DE. The role of embolization and nephrectomy in the treatment of metastatic renal carcinoma. Urol Clin North Am 1980 Oct; 7(3):719–730.

Wallace S et al. Embolization of renal carcinoma. Radiology 1981 Mar; 138(3):563–570.

Whitehead ED. Management of renal carcinoma. NY State J Med 1981 May; 81(6):911–914.

Kidney Transplantation

Cardella CJ, Tom PYW, and Walker JF. Renal transplantation in diabetes mellitus. Peritoneal Dialysis Bulletin [Suppl] 1982 Apr–June; 2(2):S17–S19.

Cianci J and Lamb J. Organ transplantation: Matching donors and recipients. Am J Nurs 1981 Mar; 81(3):544–545.

Cianci J, Lamb J, and Ryan RK. Renal transplantation. Am J Nurs 1981 Feb; 81(2):354–355.

Gokal R et al. Renal transplantation in CAPD. Proc Eur Dial Transplant Assoc 1981; 18:222–227.

Gotch F and Miller P. Teaching patients about adrenal corticosteroids. Am J Nurs 1981 Jan; 81(1):78–81.

Isaacson JJ. Surgery may be the easiest part. Nephrol Nurse 1981 Nov–Dec; 3(6):18–23.

Lamb J. Organ transplantation. Am J Nurs 1980 Sept; 80(9):1600–1601.

Morris PJ. Kidney transplantation. Transplant Proc 1981 Mar; 13(1):26–32.

Najarian JS. Immunologic aspects of organ transplantation. Hosp Pract 1982 Oct; 17(10):61–67.

Reckling JB. Safeguarding the renal transplant patient. Nursing '82 1982 Feb; 12(2):46–49.

Rubin RH et al. Infection in the renal transplant recipient. Am J Med 1981 Feb; 70(2):405–411.

Sachs BL (ed). Special issue on transplantation. AANNT J 1981 Feb; 8(1):9–59 (entire volume).

Sommer BG, Sutherland DER, and Simmons RL. Risk factor analysis in renal transplantation. Dial Transplant 1982 Apr; 11(4):301–304.

Urolithiasis

Ball TP Jr. Endoscopic and percutaneous manipulation in stone disease. Urol Clin North Am 1981 June; 8(2):277–298.

Boyce WH. Calculous disease. J Urol 1982 May; 127(5):859.

Coe FL and Favus MJ. Treatment of renal calculi. Adv Intern Med 1980; 26:373–392.

Cummings NB. Urolithiasis research: Progress and trends. Adv Exp Med Biol 1980; 128:473–481.

Hinman F and Cattolica EV. Branched calculi: Shapes and operative approaches. J Urol 1981 Sept; 126(3):291–294.

Lyles KW and Drezner MK. An overview of calcium homeostasis in humans. Urol Clin North Am 1981 June; 8(2):209–226.

Menon M and Mahle CJ. Oxalate metabolism and renal calculi. J Urol 1982 Jan; 127(1):148–151.

Metheny N. Renal stones and urinary pH. Am J Nurs 1982 Sept; 82(9):1372–1375.

Newhouse JH and Pfister RC. Therapy for renal calculi via percutaneous nephrostomy: Dissolution and extraction. Urol Radiol 1981; 2(3):165–170.

Paxton HM. Percutaneous nephrostomy—technique. Urol Radiol 1981; 2(3):131–139.

Segura JW et al. Percutaneous removal of kidney stones. Mayo Clin Proc 1982 Oct; 57(10):615–619.

Sheldon CA and Smith AD. Chemolysis of calculi. Urol Clin North Am 1982 Feb; 9(1):121–130.

Wickham JEA and Kellet MJ. Percutaneous nephrolithotomy. Br Med J 1981 Dec 12; 283(6306):1571–1572.

Williams HE. Prevention of renal stone disease. Clinical and Experimental Dialysis and Apheresis. 1981; 5(1-2):163–172.

Zuniga–Castaneda WR, Miller RP, and Amplatz K. Percutaneous removal of kidney stones. Urol Clin North Am 1982 Feb; 9(1):113–119.

Bladder Cancer/Urinary Diversion

Barrett N. Cancer of the bladder: A case history. Am J Nurs 1981 Dec; 81(12):2192–2195.

Bonney WW and Prout GR. Bladder Cancer. American Urological Association Monographs 1982; 1:5–357 (entire volume).

Cain L and Bigongiari LR. The percutaneous nephrostomy tube. Am J Nurs 1982 Feb; 82(2):296–298.

Chiang MS et al. Carcinoma in a colon conduit urinary diversion. J Urol 1982 June; 127(6):1185–1187.

Connolly JG (ed). Carcinoma of the bladder. Progress in Cancer Research and Therapy 1981; 18:1–283 (entire volume).

Droller MJ. Bladder Cancer. Curr Probl Surg 1981 Apr; 28(4):209–278.

Johnston S and Patt YZ. Caring for the patient on intraarterial chemotherapy . . . are you ready? Nursing '81 1981 Nov; 11(11):108–112.

Lower GM Jr. Concepts in causality: Chemically induced human urinary bladder cancer. Cancer 1982 Mar 1; 45(5):1056–1066.

Lutzeyer W, Rubben H, and Dahm H. Prognostic parameters in superficial bladder cancer: An analysis of 315 cases. J Urol 1982 Feb; 127(2):250–252.

Mather DG. Ileal conduit surgery: How to help a terrified patient. RN 1981 Oct; 44(10):29–31.

Mathur VK, Krahn HP, and Ramsey EW. Total cystectomy for bladder cancer. J Urol 1981 June; 125(6):784–786.

McFadden DD and Himal HS. Colonic adenocarcinoma: A late complication of ureterosigmoidostomy. Can Med Assoc J 1982 Apr; 126(7):827.

Orr JW. Urinary diversion in patients undergoing pelvic exenteration. Am J Obstet Gynecol 1982 Apr 1; 142(7):883–889.

Skinner DG. Tehnique of radical cystectomy. Urol Clin North Am 1981 June; 8(2):353–366.

Skrabanek P and Walsh A. Workshop on bladder cancer. UICC Tech Report Series 1981; 60(13):11–192.

Smith AD et al. Percutaneous circle-tube nephroureterostomy. J Urol 1982 Jan; 127(1):29–30.

Smith JA et al. Preoperative irradiation and cystectomy for bladder cancer. Cancer 1982 Mar 1; 49(5):869–873.

Smith JA Jr and Whitmore WF Jr. Regional lymph node metastasis from bladder cancer. J Urol 1981 Nov; 126(5):591–595.

Wallace S et al. Transcatheter intraarterial infusion of chemotherapy in advanced bladder cancer. Cancer 1982 Feb 15; 49(4):640–645.

Whitehead ED. Management of bladder carcinoma. NY State J Med 1981 July; 81(8):1201–1206.

Zincke H. Cystectomy and urinary diversion in patients eighty years old or older. Urology 1982 Feb; 19(2):139–142.

Urinary Tract Infections

Andriole V. Advances in the treatment of urinary infections. J Antimicrob Chemother 1982 Jan; 9(Suppl A):163–172.

Belman AB. Urinary tract infection and reflux. JAMA 1981 July 3; 246(1):74.

Buckwold FJ et al. Therapy for acute cystitis in adult women. JAMA 1982 Apr 2; 247(13):1839–1842.

Dudley MN and Barriere SL. Antimicrobial irrigations in the prevention and treatment of catheter-related urinary tract infections. Am J Hosp Pharm 1981 Jan; 38(1):59–65.

Gow JG. The management of genitourinary tuberculosis. Recent Advances in Urology/Andrology 1981; 3:91–105.

Hanson LA et al. Biology and pathology of urinary tract infections. J Clin Pathol 1981 July; 34(7):695–700.

Kunin CM. Urinary tract infections. Surg Clin North Am 1980 Feb; 60(1):223–231.

Kunin CM. Duration of treatment of urinary tract infections. Am J Med 1981 Nov; 71(5):849–854,

Massoud N. Update on the treatment of bacterial urinary tract infections. Drug Intell Clin Pharm 1981 Oct; 14(10):738–750.

Sabath LD and Charles D. Urinary tract infections in the female. Obstet Gynecol 1980 May; 55(5 Suppl):162S–170S.

Saiki J, Vaziri ND, and Barton C. Perinephric and intranephric abscesses: A review of the literature. West J Med 1982 Feb; 136(2):95–102.

Thomas VL and Forland M. Antibody-coated bacteria in urinary tract infections. Kidney Int 1982 Jan; 21(1):1–7.

Turck M. New concepts in genitourinary tract infections. JAMA 1981 Nov 6; 246(18):2019–2023.

Agencies
Governmental

National Institute of Arthritis, Diabetes, Digestive and Kidney Diseases. Division of Kidney, Urologic, and Hematologic Diseases, National Institutes of Health, Bethesda, Maryland 20205

Voluntary

American Society for Artificial Internal Organs, P.O. Box 777, Boca Raton, Florida 33432

Committee on Donor Enlistment, 2022 Lee Rd., Cleveland Heights, Ohio 44118

Medic-Alert Organ Donor Program, 1000 North Palm St., Turlock, California 95380

National Association of Patients on Hemodialysis and Transplantation, 505 Northern Blvd., Great Neck, New York 11021

National Kidney Foundation, 116 E. 27th St., New York, New York 10016

United Ostomy Association, 1111 Wilshire Blvd., Los Angeles, California 90017

Unit XII

Sexual and Reproductive Problems

45

Management During the Reproductive Cycle

▷ Health Maintenance

Over the last decade increased interest has been focused on women's health problems and health maintenance. This interest has been a direct result of the women's movement. Biological as well as psychosocial changes that have a direct bearing on the health of women continue to be studied from conception to death.

As women have moved into the labor market, they have faced changes in life-style, such as new family patterns; competition; exposure to environmental hazards; and greater participation in damaging health patterns, such as smoking and drinking. Greater responsibility for one's personal health (self-care) is being assessed. Delaying the time of having children until well after a career is established is a common practice. The use of the "pill" and IUD (intrauterine device) has become more popular than use of the diaphragm and other contraceptive methods. Physical exercise and competitive sports that once were considered nonfeminine are now popular. Stress-related illnesses have increased, and programs to control stress are common in women's circles.

Nurses are becoming more knowledgeable about preventive care for women, particularly with regard to their unique needs. The nurse encourages female clients to determine their own goals and behaviors. This can be facilitated by assessing health and illness manifestations; offering intervention strategies; and providing support, counseling, and ongoing monitoring as women move toward their health goals.

Hygienic Features: Client/Patient Education

The nurse is in a key position to teach and to advise girls and women about the principles of good health and personal hygiene, especially principles dealing with feminine hygiene related to those parts of the female body concerned with reproduction. The reproductive system, like any other part of the anatomy, will function well if the body has adequate nutrition, exercise, rest, and elimination. Aside from teaching female patients about these general aspects of care, the nurse should provide instruction about sexually transmitted diseases and prenatal and postnatal care.

It is important to recognize that concepts of feminine hygiene vary greatly with different cultures. What may be considered appropriate care for a European woman may be viewed very differently by an American or Japanese woman. In some societies, an emphasis on cleanliness and neatness may be considered unnecessary, while in others, climate and local customs may affect the habits practiced. Even members of the same family may have different opinions about personal tidiness.

Nurses need to understand the variations in attitudes and practices of hygiene and their relation to sexual function. Because many methods of feminine hygiene are empirical, it is necessary to apply common sense. Douching of the vagina has come down from certain old cultures as a traditional practice of feminine hygiene. However, modern studies of vaginal physiology make clear that it has no health virtue; indeed, many douches that were once considered to be necessary may irritate the vaginal mucosa or reduce the normal mechanisms of resistance to infection.

Contrary to popular opinion, genital odor rarely arises from the vagina, but is of external origin, arising from the interaction of oil secreted by the vulvar skin with surface bacteria. Occasionally, old menstrual blood or seminal fluid ejaculated in coitus will give some vaginal odor. A simple, low-pressure, warm water irrigation or, at most, a douche of a solution of 30 ml of white vinegar to a liter of water is appropriate. Significant malodor from the vagina can result from a retained tampon or some other foreign body or from a pathologic condition, indicating the need for examination. In general, a soap and water scrub and a sprinkle of a simple powder maintains cleanliness.

Sex Education. (See Chap. 13, p. 205.)

▷ Assessment

Health History

Complications of gynecologic disturbances can be prevented if proper medical attention and supervision are available. The nurse is in a unique position to acquaint the lay person with the normal physiologic processes of menstruation and menopause. Many difficulties encountered by the young girl or the middle-aged woman usually can be corrected quite easily; if allowed to go untreated, they may cause irreparable damage.

- *Danger signals that every woman should report to her physician are spotting, irregular or excessive bleeding, or any bleeding after menopause.*

Persistent painful menstruation, leukorrhea, and urinary disturbances also should be investigated. Many of these early signs can be corrected simply and permanently. An annual pelvic examination is especially important for women who are past 30 years of age or for those who are sexually active, regardless of age.

"Do-it-yourself" kits, whereby a woman can obtain her own cervical and vaginal smears and mail the slides to a

laboratory, are being studied to determine their effectiveness. Such methods are inexpensive, but accuracy may be lower than desired; the danger is the possible oversight of other problems that could have been detected during a visit to a health professional.

The gynecologic patient often requires more understanding than other patients, because of the emotional as well as physical considerations that govern the situation. A female patient may resent any reference to her genitourinary system, feeling that she is suspected of questionable social or sexual habits. Or she may have a real fear of disturbance of the reproductive process. Perhaps an explanation of the anatomy involved and the proposed treatment will clarify the situation. Any intention of sterilization must be explained carefully to the patient and her partner by the physician. Perhaps religious belief is more important to a patient than physical treatment. The decision rests with the patient, and, when it is made, it must be respected and supported.

Psychic factors may present themselves during the menopausal period. The loss of the reproductive capacity may cause disappointment if the woman has had no children. For a woman with a grown family, it may mean that she feels that she is no longer useful. Leisure time may hang heavily on her hands. Circumstances affect the problems of each patient and must be considered on an individual basis.

Because gynecologic conditions often are of such a personal and private nature, the nurse is expected to respect the confidentiality of any knowledge of the patient's problems. This information is shared only with those directly involved in professional patient care.

For details on the gynecologic examination, see Chapter 5, pp. 83–86.

Tests Performed During the Gynecologic Examination
Cytologic Test for Cancer (Papanicolaou Test; Pap Test). This test is done in order to detect cervical cancer. Vaginal secretions are aspirated or scraped from the posterior fornix, and a smear is transferred to a glass slide (Fig. 45-1). The secretion usually is "fixed" immediately by immersing the slide in equal parts of 95% alcohol and ether. The patient should be instructed not to douche before this examination, since such cleansing will wash away cellular deposits.

The pathologist examines and interprets the cytologic smear. The classification for cytologic findings as suggested by Papanicolaou is as follows:

Class 1: Absence of atypical or abnormal cells
Class 2: Atypical cytology, but no evidence of malignancy
Class 3: Cytology suggestive of, but not conclusive for, malignancy
Class 4: Cytology strongly suggestive of malignancy
Class 5: Cytology conclusive for malignancy

The finding of an abnormal smear (with the exception of Class 5) does not necessarily mean that the patient has cancer, but points out that additional procedures, such as biopsies or a dilatation and curettage, are indicated. The patient will be grateful for this explanation.

Endometrial (Aspiration) Smears and Biopsy. A smear obtained directly from the endometrium provides an even

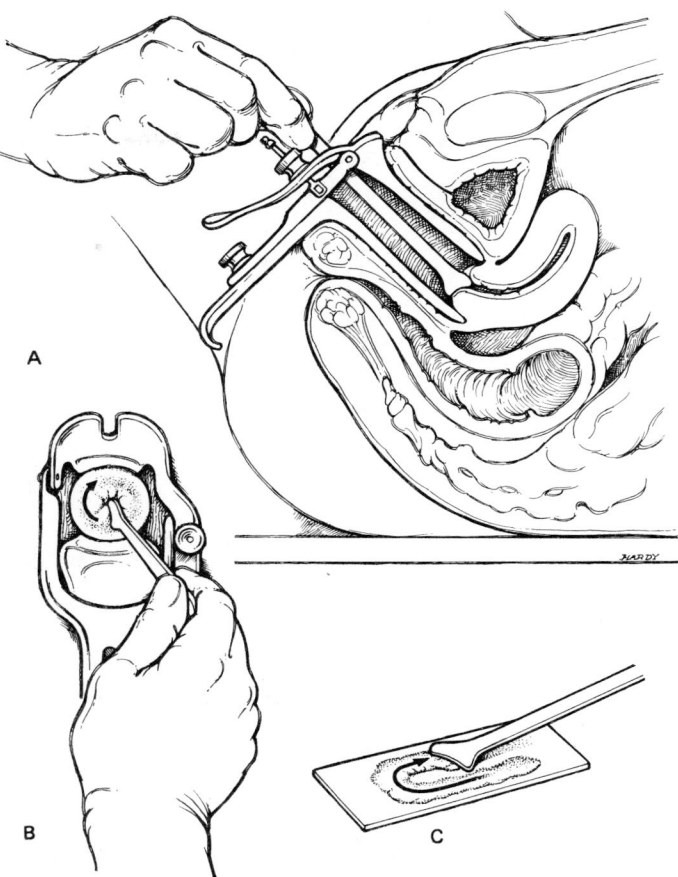

Figure 45-1. Method of using a wooden Ayre spatula to obtain cervical secretions for cytology. (*A*) Shows the speculum in place and the Ayre spatula in position at the cervical os. (*B*) By rotation of the spatula, a representative sample is obtained. (*C*) Cervical secretions are transferred from wooden spatula to glass slide in a single circular motion.

more accurate method of cytologic diagnosis. A cannula is inserted into the endometrial cavity, and tissue is obtained by simple aspiration through a syringe. The *Gravlee Jet Washer* (Fig. 45-2) is a disposable examination unit that is safe, simple to use, and economical for screening patients for endometrial cancer. The unit consists of an intrauterine washing device that employs negative pressure to bathe the endometrium with isotonic solution, so as to dislodge cells and small tissue fragments. The use of negative pressure eliminates the possibility of flushing potentially malignant cells into the uterine (fallopian) tubes.

Another similar diagnostic technique is that of *uterine aspiration* (suction curettage), in which a metal cannula 21 cm long and 3 mm in diameter is inserted through the cervical canal into the uterine cavity. The distal tip is slightly curved and open-ended on the concave surface. Pressure-equalizing holes are located near the proximal end of the cannula, enabling the examiner to maintain negative pressure by closing the holes with the fingertips. The proximal end is attached to a receptacle in which aspirated tissue is gathered and to a suction pump that generates negative pressure. Tissue is placed in a fixative solution and sent to the laboratory for histologic analysis. This is a diagnostic test designed to detect early endometrial malignancy.

Endometrial Biopsy. The procedures described above (endometrial smears) appear useful in screening high-risk

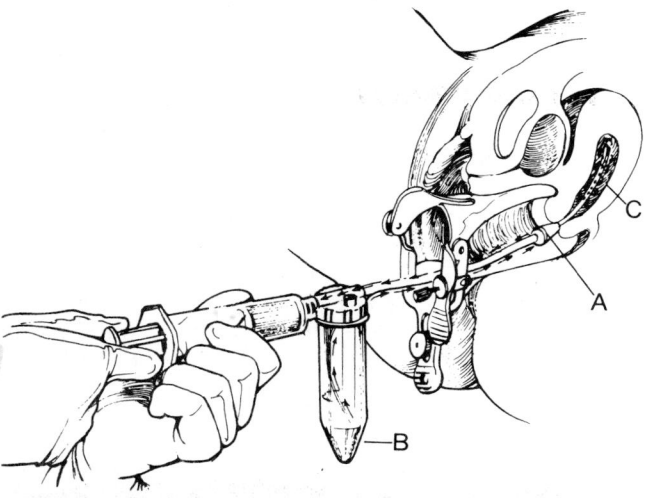

Figure 45-2. The Gravlee Jet Washer. To obtain a specimen, the distal tip of the cannula is inserted into the uterine cavity to a point where a preset rubber stopper (*A*) makes a firm seal with the cervical os. Isotonic saline is in the vertical reservoir (*B*) and is drawn into the uterus (*C*). The saline flows back to a connecting syringe. This fluid specimen is transferred into a vial with a fixative and sent to the laboratory for cytologic examination. (From Patient Care, January 1, 1973. Copyright © 1973, Miller and Fink Corporation, Darien, Conn. All rights reserved.)

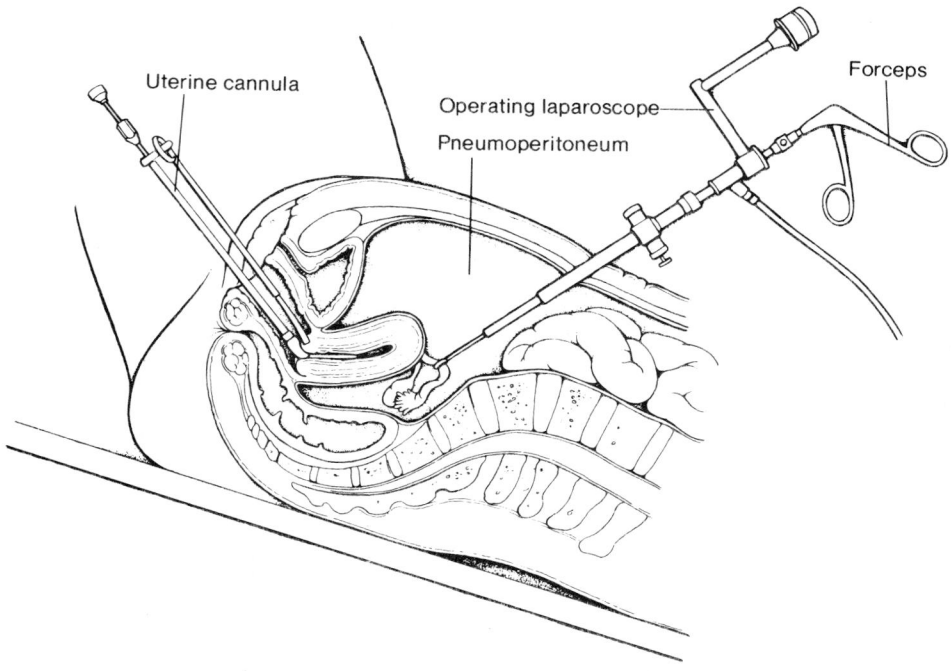

Figure 45-3. Laparoscopy.

patients. However, many physicians prefer endometrial biopsy, claiming that it is more efficient in diagnosing, provides greater patient comfort, and is cost effective. Endometrial biopsy is done as an office procedure during the gynecologic pelvic examination. Following a small amount of intrauterine lidocaine anesthetic, a sound is inserted into the uterus, followed by a thin, hollow curette. Suction (Vabra aspirator) is applied, and endometrial tissue is retrieved for laboratory analysis.

Schiller's Iodine Test. With the patient in the lithotomy position (cervix exposed by speculum), a long cotton applicator is used to paint the cervix with Schiller's iodine solution.* The appearance of a mahogany-brown color covering the entire surface indicates a reaction between the iodine and the glycogen of normal cells. Such a reaction is considered negative. If the cervix is abnormal, immature cells are present and tissues are not stained brown, indicating that the test is positive. The absence of staining directs attention to the sites requiring additional study (*i.e.,* biopsy).

Cervical Biopsy

The type and extent of biopsy of the cervix vary according to the abnormality or to the results of an abnormal Pap smear. When a lesion is clearly visible or can be seen with a magnifying instrument called a *colposcope,* one or more punch biopsies may be done as an office procedure without anesthesia. However, when no lesion is visible, but the Pap smear is "suspicious," biopsy excision of an inverted cone

---

* Aqueous iodine, 1 part; potassium iodide, 2 parts; water, 300 parts. This solution should be stored in a brown bottle to combat photosensitivity and rapid deterioration. The solution should be replaced every 4 to 6 weeks.

of tissue is usually needed. This requires anesthesia and operating room facilities.

Cauterization. The application of a cautery is useful in controlling minor bleeding from small biopsies of the cervix and in treating superficial forms of chronic cervicitis.

Postbiopsy Patient Instruction. The patient is advised to rest for 24 hours after a biopsy and to leave the packing or tampon in place for the recommended time—usually 8 to 24 hours. Any excess bleeding is to be reported. Sexual intercourse is delayed until the physician indicates that it is permissible.

Pelvic Endoscopy

Culdoscopy. With this procedure, it is possible to visualize directly the uterus, uterine tubes, broad ligaments, uterosacral ligaments, rectal wall, sigmoid colon, and small intestine. This diagnostic procedure is done in the operating room with the patient in a knee–chest position. An incision is made in the posterior vaginal cul-de-sac to admit the *culdoscope* (a tubular, lighted instrument). The patient is prepared as for a vaginal operation, and anesthesia may be local, regional, or general.

Culdoscopy is indicated in suspected ectopic pregnancy, in unexplained pelvic pain, and in the presence of undetermined pelvic masses. Following this examination, the scope is withdrawn, and the patient is returned to her room. The incision through the posterior vaginal septum heals easily without sutures. Until healing takes place, the patient is instructed not to douche or have intercourse for about 2 weeks.

Laparoscopy (Pelvic Peritoneoscopy). A laparoscopy is carried out by inserting a scope into the peritoneal cavity through a 2-cm (¾-inch) subumbilical incision (Fig. 45-3).

Indications for laparoscopy are similar to those for culdoscopy. It is also possible to perform minor operative procedures, such as tubal sterilization, ovarian biopsy, and lysis of peritubal adhesions, by means of laparoscopy. A dilatation and curettage (D & C) precedes this procedure, not only because it affords additional information, but also because a surgical instrument (intrauterine sound or cannula) may be positioned to permit manipulation of the uterus during laparoscopy, affording better visualization. A better view of the pelvis, lower abdomen, and visceral contents is also facilitated by the injection of a prescribed amount of carbon dioxide intraperitoneally into the cavity. This separates the intestines from the pelvic organs. The tubes are electrocoagulated, and a segment may be removed for histologic verification. After the purpose of the laparoscopy has been accomplished, the scope is withdrawn, and carbon dioxide is allowed to escape through the outer cannula. The skin incision is closed with stitches and covered with a Band-Aid.

The patient is carefully observed for several hours to detect any untoward signs indicating bleeding, injury, or burns from the coagulator. These rarely occur.

Hysteroscopy. This procedure allows direct visualization of all parts of the uterine cavity by means of a lighted optical instrument. Hysteroscopy is best performed about 5 days after completion of menstruation (estrogenic phase of the menstrual cycle). The vagina and vulva are cleansed, and a pericervical anesthetic block is done. The instrument used for the procedure, a *hysteroscope,* is passed into the cervical canal and advanced under direct vision about 1 cm or 2 cm; uterine-distending fluid (saline or 5% dextrose) is passed through the instrument to dilate the uterine cavity and provide better visualization.

Hysteroscopy is most commonly indicated as a diagnostic procedure in complex situations: infertility, unexplained bleeding, and retained IUD. Hysteroscopy is contraindicated in patients with cervical or endometrial carcinoma.

Colposcopy and Colpomicroscopy. The *colposcope* (magnification, 10 to 25 times) and *colpomicroscope* (magnification to 400 times) are optical instruments designed to permit three-dimensional views of stained or unstained cervical epithelium *in situ.* These instruments provide visual access to suspicious tissue areas, but biopsy of the tissue is required for accurate diagnosis in many instances.

Roentgenogram Studies
Hysterosalpingogram (Uterotubogram).
A *uterotubogram* is an x-ray study of the uterus and the uterine (fallopian) tubes after the injection of a contrast medium. The diagnostic procedure is done to study sterility problems, to evaluate tubal patency, and to determine the presence of pathology in the uterine cavity.

The patient is placed in the lithotomy position, and the cervix is exposed with a bivalved speculum. A cannula is inserted into the cervix, and radiopaque dye is injected into the uterine cavity and the tubes. X-ray films are taken to show the path and the distribution of the contrast materials.

In preparation for a salpingogram, the intestinal tract is prepared by a cathartic and an enema so that gas shadows do not distort the roentgenograms. An analgesic is prescribed for comfort, since some patients experience nausea, vomiting, cramps, and faintness. Following the test, it may be advisable for the patient to apply a perineal pad for several hours, because the radiopaque medium may stain clothing.

Arteriography, Venography, and Radioisotope Scanning. These procedures are also used as required. Since the uterus and adnexa are in close proximity to the kidneys, ureter, and bladder, urologic diagnostic aids, such as the KUB (kidney, ureter, and bladder) and pyelogram, are frequently used.

Ultrasonography. *Ultrasonography* employs a simple procedure based on transmission of sound waves similar to the sonar detection used in submarines. Diagnostic ultrasonic scanning equipment uses pulsed ultrasound waves of a frequency exceeding 20,000 cycles per second; the pelvis and abdomen are scanned in linear fashion. The transducer, which is placed in contact with the abdomen, converts mechanical energy into electrical impulses, which in turn are amplified and recorded on an oscilloscope screen. (A photograph is taken of the pattern.) The entire procedure takes about 10 minutes. The findings of this test, in combination with other diagnostic tools, provide useful adjuncts, particularly in the obstetric patient and the obese patient in whom pelvic examination and x-ray studies may have been unsatisfactory. A definite advantage of ultrasound scanning is that exposure to ionizing radiation is avoided. Patients will appreciate knowing this fact.

▷ Nursing Interventions for Patients With Gynecologic Conditions

Douches are common therapeutic measures in the treatment of patients with gynecologic diseases. They are used both before and after operation and are of two types: vulvar and vaginal.

Vaginal irrigations are used therapeutically to cleanse or disinfect the vagina and adjacent parts, both before and after operation. They also serve to soothe inflamed tissues and to stimulate relaxed tissues. Occasionally, hot or cold douches are indicated in the treatment of oozing.

The patient is placed on the bedpan in the dorsal position with the knees apart and the labia separated. Prevent undue exposure of the patient. Protect the bed by placing a plastic sheet under the bedpan. Commonly used solutions include sterile water, normal saline, and antiseptic solutions.

Douches should be given at a temperature of 43.3° C (110° F) or as prescribed. To give the douche, the patient is placed in the dorsal position on the bedpan and is covered to prevent chilling. The tube leading from the douche bag is clamped, and the end of the tube with the douche nozzle is inserted into the reservoir, which then is hung not more than 60 cm (2 feet) above the level of the patient's hips. The nurse then puts on sterile gloves, and, separating the labia with the thumb and the forefinger of the left hand, cleans the vaginal orifice and inserts the douche nozzle gently into the vagina for a distance of 5 cm (2 inches), the tip being directed toward the hollow of the sacrum. The clamp then is removed from the tube, and the solution is allowed to flow. Pressure should be avoided to prevent the douche fluid from refluxing through the uterus and the tubes. The solution can be allowed to flow intermittently until at least 1 liter of solution has been used.

The treatment should not be done hastily if therapeutic benefits are to be achieved; it should take from 20 to 30 minutes. After the solution has been instilled, the nozzle may be removed, and the patient should be asked to strain as if trying to move the bowels. This act tends to expel the fluid remaining in the vagina. Then, the bedpan is removed, and the perineum is dried with cotton. The patient is instructed to remain recumbent for at least an hour following a warm douche.

After the douche has been completed, the apparatus is cleansed and sterilized again (if not disposable), including the bedpan. When douching is done at home, the patient usually lies in the bathtub and follows the same principles just described.

Vulvar irrigations are indicated chiefly after operations on the perineum. They should be given after each urination or bowel movement in an effort to keep the incision free from infection. The patient is prepared for a vulvar irrigation in the same manner as for a vaginal douche. Warm, sterile water then is poured gently over the vulva from a sterile container. The area is dried with sterile gauze or cotton, and a sterile dressing or pad is applied and held in place with a T-binder.

Vaginal antiseptic jellies are another form of medication that the patient can apply herself by means of an applicator. Creams or jellies can be used before and after operation, and in many instances they are substituted for the therapeutic and cleansing douche. It may be necessary for the patient to wear a perineal pad following application of medication.

▷ Menstruation

Physiologic Overview

The *gonads* are the organs that produce either the egg cells (ova) or the sperm cells of an organism. In the female, the gonads are called *ovaries* and are located in the abdomen. In the male, the gonads are the *testes* and are contained within the scrotum. In addition to their reproductive function, the gonads are important endocrine glands.

Ovarian Hormones. The ovaries produce steroid hormones, predominantly *estrogens* and *progesterone.* Several different estrogens are produced by the ovarian follicle, which consists of the developing ovum and its surrounding cells. The most important of the ovarian estrogens is *estradiol.* Estrogens are responsible for the development and maintenance of the female reproductive organs and the secondary sexual characteristics associated with the adult female. Estrogens have an important role in breast development and in the cyclic changes of the uterus that occur monthly.

Progesterone is also important in regulating the changes that occur in the uterus during the menstrual cycle. It is secreted by the *corpus luteum,* which consists of the ovarian follicle after the ovum has been released. Progesterone is the most important hormone for conditioning the lining of the uterus (endometrium) in preparation for implantation of the fertilized ovum. If pregnancy occurs, the secretion of progesterone becomes largely a function of the placenta.

This secretion is important for the maintenance of normal pregnancy. In addition, progesterone, working in concert with estrogen, prepares the breast for production and secretion of milk.

Androgens are also produced by the ovaries, but only in very small amounts. Very little is known concerning the function of androgens in the female.

Regulation of Ovarian Hormone Secretion. *Follicle-stimulating hormone (FSH)* secreted by the pituitary is primarily responsible for stimulating estrogen secretion. *Luteinizing hormone (LH)* is primarily responsible for stimulating the production of progesterone. Feedback mechanisms in part regulate FSH and LH secretion. Increased estrogen levels in the blood inhibit FSH secretion, but promote LH secretion. Elevated progesterone levels inhibit LH secretion. In addition, stimuli from the hypothalamus (releasing factors) affect the rate of gonadotropin (FSH and LH) release.

Menstrual Cycle. In the female, secretion of ovarian hormones follows a cyclic pattern that results in changes of the uterine endometrium (the inner lining of the uterus) and in menstruation (Fig. 45-4). At the beginning of the cycle (just after menstruation), FSH output is increased and estrogen secretion is stimulated. This causes the endometrium to thicken and become more vascular. Near the middle portion of the cycle, LH output increases and progesterone secretion is stimulated. It is at this time that ovulation occurs. Under the combined stimulus of estrogen and progesterone, the endometrium reaches its peak of thickening and vascularization. If the ovum has been fertilized, estrogen and progesterone levels remain high, and the complex hormonal changes of pregnancy follow. If fertilization has not occurred, the output of FSH and LH diminishes; secretion of estrogen and progesterone falls rapidly; and the vascularized, thickened endometrium is sloughed, with resultant vaginal bleeding (menstruation). The cycle then begins again.

Psychosocial Considerations

The girl between the ages of 11 and 14 who is approaching the *menarche,* or onset of menstruation, should be instructed about this normal process. Psychologically, it is more healthy to refer to this event as "my period" rather than as "being sick" or "having the curse." With adequate nutrition, rest, exercise, and good posture, there will be little discomfort. Some girls do experience breast tenderness and a feeling of fullness a day or two before the onset of menstruation. There may be a greater tendency to fatigue and some discomfort of the lower back, legs, and pelvis on the first day; temperament and mood changes may be apparent. Slight deviations from the usual healthy pattern of daily living is considered normal, but signs of excessive deviations may require investigation. The perineal pad is a widely used method of disposing of menstrual discharge; powder, cream, and spray deodorants for pads are available. Tampons are also used extensively; usually, there is no significant evidence of untoward effects from their use, providing there is no difficulty in inserting them.* Should the "tail" string break and difficulty be encountered in removing the tampon, the

---

* See Toxic Shock Syndrome, page 1048.

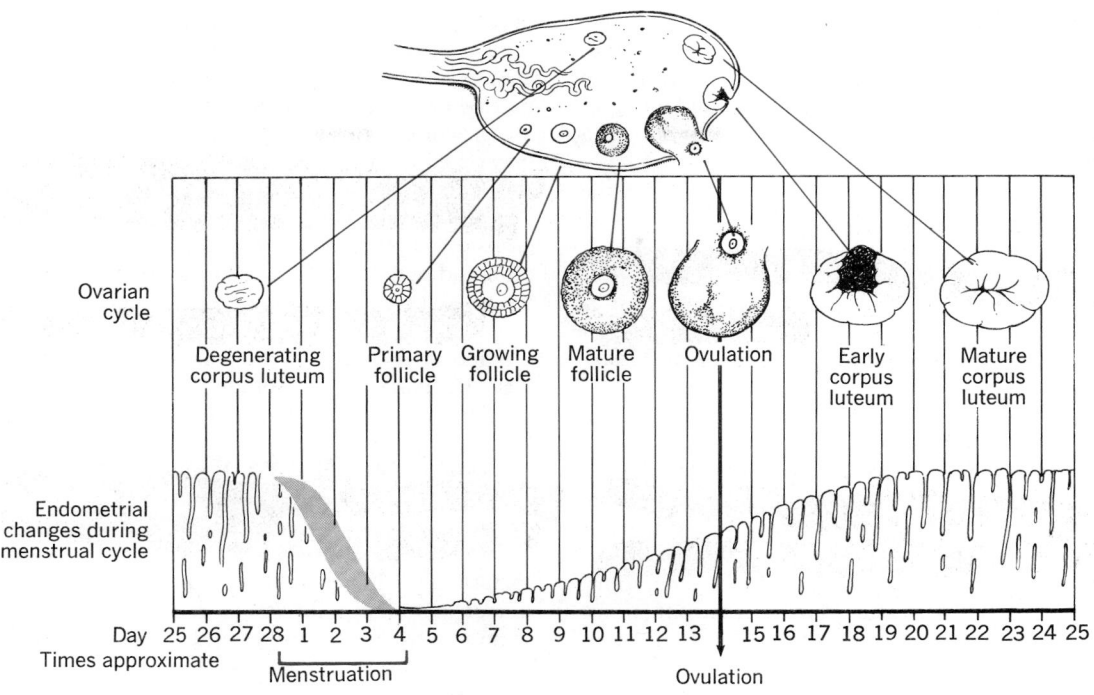

Times approximate

Phase	Menstrual	Follicular	Ovulation	Luteal	Premenstrual
DAYS	1 2 3 4 5 6 7 8 9 10	11 12 13 14 15	16 17 18 19	20 21 22 23 24 25	26 27 28 1 2
Ovary	Degenerating corpus luteum; Beginning follicular development	Growth and maturation of follicle	Ovulation	Active corpus luteum	Degenerating corpus luteum
Estrogen production	Low	Increasing	High	Declining, then a secondary rise	Decreasing
Progesterone production	None	None	Low	Increasing	Decreasing
FSH production	Increasing	High, then declining	Low	Low	Increasing
LH production	Low	Low, then increasing	High	High	Decreasing
Endometrium	Degeneration and shedding of superficial layer. Coiled arteries dilate, then constrict again	Reorganization and proliferation of superficial layer	Continued growth	Active secretion and glandular dilatation; highly vascular; edematous	Vasoconstriction of coiled arteries; beginning degeneration

Figure 45-4. Correlation of hormonal activities with ovarian and uterine changes. (Adapted from Chaffee EE and Greisheimer EM: Basic Physiology and Anatomy, 3rd ed. Philadelphia, JB Lippincott.)

woman's physician should be consulted. A third type of protection is the internal rubber cup, but this is used less frequently.

As mentioned earlier, menstruation may be handled differently in different cultures. Some women believe that it is detrimental to change a pad (or tampon) too frequently; they believe that by allowing the discharge to accumulate, an increased flow is stimulated, which is considered desirable. For the nurse to insist that a pad be changed before

the time the patient believes proper may cause conflict. These differences must be carefully reconciled so that proper understanding develops.

Other psychosocial aspects may need to be considered, such as the vulnerability of the female to illness during menstruation. Many believe it is detrimental to swim, take a cold shower, receive a "permanent wave," get teeth filled, or eat certain foods during one's period. Such myths need to be recognized and corrected. Many other examples of misunderstanding could be listed; however, the objective is to alert the nurse to these unexpressed, deep-rooted beliefs. Aspects of gynecologic problems cannot always be expressed easily. The nurse needs to convey confidence and trust, as well as offer sound advice, in order to set up a communication exchange.

Disturbances of Menstruation

There is a definite interrelation between the hormonal secretions of the ovary, the thyroid, and the pituitary glands. A disturbance of this relationship by an increased or decreased function of one or more of these glands may influence the menstrual function.

Premenstrual Tension

Premenstrual tension is a combination of symptoms prior to the onset of menstruation: low back pain, engorged or painful breasts, feeling of abdominal fullness, and general irritability. Retained fluid, including cerebral edema and weight gain, is believed to account for these symptoms. While diuretics may be administered in extreme situations, the fact that this is a temporary condition makes it more tolerable for most women.

Dysmenorrhea (Primary or Essential)

Dysmenorrhea is painful menstruation. It usually occurs within a few years of the menarche, and in the absence of any organic pelvic pathology is a common condition, occurring in approximately 35% of all older adolescent girls, 25% of female college students, and 60% to 70% of older single women in their 30s. Primary dysmenorrhea accompanies ovulation, since the painful cramps are the result of the effects of progesterone, which causes increased myometrial contractility and arteriolar vasospasm. Psychologic factors, such as anxiety, tension, and dependency, may also contribute to dysmenorrhea.

Assessment and Clinical Manifestations.   The symptoms are mild cramps that begin 12 to 24 hours preceding the onset of flow and become more acute with the flow, lasting an additional 12 to 24 hours. The pain is crampy, is located in the lower midabdomen, and may be associated with chills, nausea, vomiting, headache, irritability, and low backache.

Management.   A complete physical examination is done to rule out possible abnormalities, such as strictures of the cervix or vagina or an imperforate hymen. The reason for the discomfort is explained, and the patient is assured that menstruation is a normal function of the reproductive tract. If the patient is a young girl and is accompanied by her mother, then the mother too can be reassured. Many daughters are conditioned to expect dysmenorrhea because their mothers experienced it. The pain, which is real, can be treated once worry and concern over its possible significance are dispelled through accurate understanding. Symptoms subside in a few years or with normal sexual function and childbearing.

More specific methods of affording relief are as follows. Urge the patient to carry on her usual activities, since mind-occupying functions and physical exercise provide a neurophysiologic basis for relief. Advise simple analgesics before cramps start, in anticipation of discomfort. Aspirin or Empirin may be taken at recommended doses every 4 hours. If necessary, antiemetics, antispasmodics, and mild tranquilizers may be effective. Prostaglandins have been cited as causing dysmenorrhea, so prostaglandin inhibitors appear helpful (Ibuprofen [Motrin]; naproxen [Naprosyn]; mefanamic acid [Ponstel]; napoxin sodium [Anaprox]). Some physicians recommend oral contraceptives to produce anovular cycles to relieve dysmenorrhea.

Dilatation and curettage is usually not indicated as a method of therapy. Psychosomatic evaluation and therapy may be required if the problem appears to be psychosomatic or if a more serious psychiatric problem is suspected.

Amenorrhea (Absence of Menstrual Flow)

Primary amenorrhea (delayed menarche) refers to those instances when a young woman over age 17 has not yet begun to menstruate but otherwise shows evidence of sexual maturation. This may be of considerable concern to the person as well as to her mother, but is more than likely due to minor variations in body build, heredity, and environment, as well as in physical, mental, and emotional development.

The understanding nurse will provide an opportunity for the girl to express her concerns and anxiety about this problem, since she may feel that she is not like her peers and that she may not be able to fulfill her role as a woman. A complete physical examination, careful history, and simple laboratory studies will assist in excluding physiologic disorders, metabolic or endocrine difficulties, and other systemic diseases. Treatment is directed toward correction of any anomalies.

Secondary amenorrhea (at least 6 to 12 months in duration) occurs after a normal menarche and during pregnancy and lactation. In the adolescent, the most common cause is a minor emotional upset related to being away from home, attending college, tension from school work, or interpersonal problems. Since the second most common cause is pregnancy, this possibility should always be investigated.

Secondary nutritional disturbances may also be apparent, such as weight loss or weight gain. This psychogenic or hypothalamic amenorrhea may last for a few years. On occasion there may be a pituitary or thyroid dysfunction that may be helped by appropriate measures. At any rate, consultation with a physician is necessary.

Menorrhagia, Metrorrhagia

Menorrhagia and metrorrhagia refer to abnormal uterine bleeding. In *menorrhagia* (hypermenorrhea) the bleeding is profuse or prolonged at the time of the period, while in *metrorrhagia* the bleeding is irregular. For a more detailed discussion of these disorders see page 1052.

▷ Menopause

Menopause is described as the physiologic cessation of menses associated with failing ovarian function; it is often diagnosed in retrospect when a year has passed with no menses.

The *climacteric* period is the transition period in the life of a woman during which the reproductive function gradually diminishes and is lost.

Physiologic Overview

The menopausal period of a woman's life marks the end of her active reproductive life. It usually occurs between the ages of 49 and 52, but may occur in some women as early as 42 or as late as 55. Menstruation then ceases, and as a result of the complete cessation of activity on the part of the ovaries, the reproductive organs and the mammary glands atrophy. No more ova mature; therefore, no ovarian hormones are produced. A similar situation prevails earlier if the ovaries are removed or destroyed by irradiation, producing an artificial menopause.

Menopause is not a pathologic phenomenon; in addition to estrogen deficiency, there are multifaceted psychological and physiologic changes, including neuroendocrinologic changes related to the aging process.

Assessment and Clinical Manifestations

Usually, symptoms of menopause can be classified according to cause, as arising from (1) endocrine changes due to a lack of estrogen, or (2) psychological changes. The process starts gradually and is recognized by the change in menstruation. The monthly flow becomes smaller in amount, then irregular, and finally ceases. Often, the time between periods gets longer—there may be a lapse of several months between them. Any prolonged menstrual flow or bleeding between periods should be reported promptly to the physician. Hot or warm flashes and other vascular disturbances are also endocrinologic in origin.

Additional physical manifestations may include atrophic changes, suggestion of stress incontinence, sagging structures, senile vaginitis, skin dryness, weight gain, and signs of calcium deficiency (shrinking in stature—osteoporosis).

Psychological Assessment

Symptoms of a more psychological type may occur before or during these changes in the monthly periods (*e.g.,* dizziness, weakness, nervousness, insomnia, headaches, and inability to concentrate). This often is the time in a woman's life when the children have grown up and left home; thus, she may no longer feel needed. This realization, added to an acute awareness of the aging process, can have an effect on symptoms expressed. Fear of growing old may trigger feelings of depression. However, many women have very mild symptoms, and some have none. With a few, the discomfort is very severe.

The menopause is not a complete change of life. The normal sexual urges remain, and women retain their usual reaction to sex long after menopause. There is nothing abnormal about the change of life, and nothing unusual about the continuation of happy marital relations afterward. Many women enjoy better health after the menopause than they have had for years. This is especially true with persons who have always suffered pain during their menstrual periods.

Education of the Woman About Menopause

The majority of patients will respond to a program of education, reassurance, modification of their living habits, and an improved regimen of health. In some patients, mild sedatives and tranquilizers are necessary to control nervousness and to counteract depression, which is not at all unusual at this time. Sometimes even simple, everyday problems are too much to handle.

Persistent and severe hot flashes require treatment by estrogen therapy with diethylstilbestrol, Premarin, or ethinyl estradiol (Estinyl) given on a cyclic basis. The dosage is regulated by the physician according to a desired schedule, such as taking the medication each day except the first 5 days of every month. Close medical supervision is required, and any uterine bleeding is reported. Gradually, estrogen therapy is withdrawn.

Continued use of estrogen therapy to prevent widespread degenerative changes, including physical aging, is still controversial. Most authorities are conservative and prescribe estrogen replacement on an individual basis for acute estrogen deprivation or annoying signs of estrogen deficiency, such as atrophic vaginitis or osteoporosis. Restraint in prescribing estrogens for all menopausal women arises from concern that protracted treatment will induce neoplastic changes in estrogen-sensitive aging tissue. Unopposed long-term use of Premarin has recently been linked to carcinoma of the endometrium. It is believed that addition of progesterone may prevent these changes.

The physician and the nurse should take the time to explain to the patient that the cessation of the menses is a normal physiologic function that is not necessarily accompanied by extreme nervous symptoms and illness. Measures should be taken to promote her general health.

Since many patients are in the menopausal age group, the following factors should be stressed in patient teaching:

1. The climacteric period is normal and self-limiting.
2. Overfatigue and environmental problems exaggerate the symptoms.
3. A nutritious diet and weight control will improve the physical condition.
4. An exercise program in keeping with the patient's needs promotes vitality.
5. Interest and participation in outside activities help to absorb anxiety and to lessen tension.
6. Grown children should be treated as adults, since they are no longer children.
7. Old friendships should be revived, new friendships sought, and self-fulfillment provided.
8. This is an excellent time for intellectual growth and the stimulation of new ideas and experiences.
9. Menopause does not mean a termination of the patient's sex life.
10. An annual physical examination is essential to the maintenance of continuing good health.

The current expected life span after menopause for the average woman is 30 to 35 years. This is an optimistic thought, since it encompasses as many years as the childbearing phase of her life.

Another effect of aging is a tendency to gain weight, particularly around the hips, thighs, and abdomen. Paying increased attention to good grooming tends to give the woman a lift when it is most needed. The individual woman's evaluation of herself and her worth, now and in the future, certainly affects her emotional reaction to this change in her life.

▷ Conception Control

Control of human reproduction has been practiced for various reasons since ancient times. Many methods exist and their acceptance has fluctuated. An ideal method has not been developed; all have advantages and disadvantages. Most methods apply to the female. For the male, only the condom has been acceptable; however, much research continues in an attempt to develop additional contraceptives. According to Mishell, the problems regarding male contraception include (1) difficulty in separating suppression of the major testicular functions, spermatogenesis and androgen production; (2) the long period from initiation of treatment until the elimination of sperm from the ejaculate, usually about 3 months; (3) the problems of reversibility, including a variable delay in the time required for restoration of fertility, as well as the possibility that abnormal sperm may be produced initially; and (4) the lack of motivation of most men to use a contraceptive, as the male is not the member of the couple who becomes pregnant.

The most common types of contraception include:

Family planning—limiting or spacing the number of children born. In preventing unwanted or unplanned births, the means described below are available

Natural planning—the utilization of any natural means of pregnancy prevention to the exclusion of chemical or mechanical means

Contraception—a means of temporarily avoiding pregnancy

Sterilization—a means of permanently preventing pregnancy

Induced abortion—the voluntary evacuation of the fetus before it becomes viable

Natural Methods

The advantages of natural methods of contraception include (1) they are not hazardous to a person's health, (2) they are inexpensive, and (3) they are preferred by some religions. The disadvantages are that they require discipline by the couple and periods of abstinence. Also, they are less effective than other methods. *Abstinence or celibacy* is the only completely effective means of preventing pregnancy. *Coitus interruptus* is the withdrawal of the penis from the vagina before ejaculation, which requires strong willpower. The uncertainty in this method is due to the presence of sperm in the preejaculatory fluid.

Rhythm Method. The *rhythm method* of contraception, to be sure, can be difficult to use because it is based on the woman's ability to determine her time of ovulation and on the avoidance of intercourse during the fertile period. The fertile phase (which requires sexual continence) is estimated to occur about 14 days before menstruation, although it may occur between the 10th and 17th day. It is assumed that spermatozoa can fertilize an ovum up to 72 hours after intercourse and that the ovum can be fertilized for about 24 hours after it leaves the ovary. Studies reveal that of 100 women practicing the rhythm method, up to 40 will conceive during a year.

According to some researchers, if a woman carefully determines her "safe period," based on precise recording of her menstrual dates for at least 1 year, and follows a carefully worked out formula, she may achieve 80% protection. However, it requires a long period of abstinence during each cycle. New methods of detecting ovulation (ovulimeter, etc.) have improved statistics.

Diaphragm

The *diaphragm* is an effective contraceptive device. It is a ring made of flexible spring (approximately 7.5 cm [3 inches] in diameter) which is covered with a domelike rubber cup. A spermicidal jelly or cream is used to coat the concavity of the diaphragm before it is inserted deep into the vagina. The combination of a diaphragm and spermicide prevents spermatozoa from entering the cervical canal. The diaphragm presents no discomfort, since it is lodged against the back wall of the vagina and anteriorly against the edge of the pubic bone. Since women vary in size, diaphragms are designed to fit the client; therefore, it is necessary for the woman to be fitted for the proper size by a physician or a nurse practitioner.

Each time the diaphragm is used, it must be examined carefully by holding it up to a bright light and making sure it has no pinpoint holes, cracks, or tears. Contraceptive jelly or cream is applied in a prescribed manner to the dome of the diaphragm. If it is applied more than 2 hours before intercourse, it must be reapplied. The diaphragm is then positioned to cover the cervix completely (Fig. 45-5). The diaphragm is left in place at least 8 hours after coitus; upon removal it is cleansed thoroughly with mild soap and water, rinsed, and dried before it is stored in its original container.

Intrauterine Devices (IUDs)

Intrauterine devices (IUDs) in principle are not new; however, the modern pioneer was a German physician, Ernst Graefenberg, who, around 1928, inserted silkworm gut and later silver or gold wire coils into the uterine cavity as a means of preventing conception.*

In its current form, the intrauterine device is a plastic or metal piece of varying shapes, usually 2.5 cm × 2 cm (1″ × ¾″), that is inserted through the cervix into the endometrial cavity to prevent pregnancy. The method by which the IUD prevents contraception is thought to be due to a local inflammatory reaction caused by the presence of a foreign body in the uterus. This appears to be toxic to sperm and blastocytes.

---

* Sometimes referred to as IUCD—intrauterine contraceptive device.

Preparing for insertion

Urinate, then wash your hands before inserting the diaphragm. Place 1 to 2 teaspoonsful of contraceptive jelly or cream into the dome of the diaphragm. (Refer to package directions.) Spread the spermicide around the inner surface of the dome, and also a small amount around the rim.

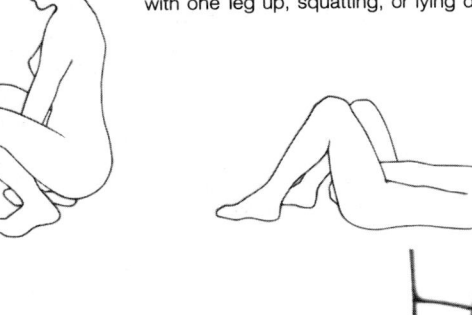

Positions

You can insert the diaphragm while you are standing with one leg up, squatting, or lying down.

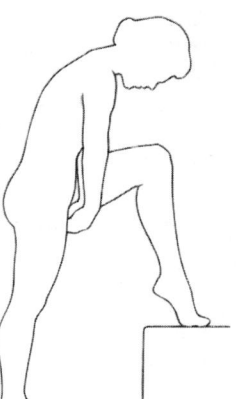

Inserting the diaphragm

Hold the diaphragm with the dome down (spermicide up) and press the opposite sides of the rim together between your thumb and third finger (1). The diaphragm can be held from above or below.

Spread the lips of your vagina with your free hand. Hold the compressed diaphragm dome down (spermicide up) and push it gently inward along the rear wall of the vagina as far as it can go (2).

1

2

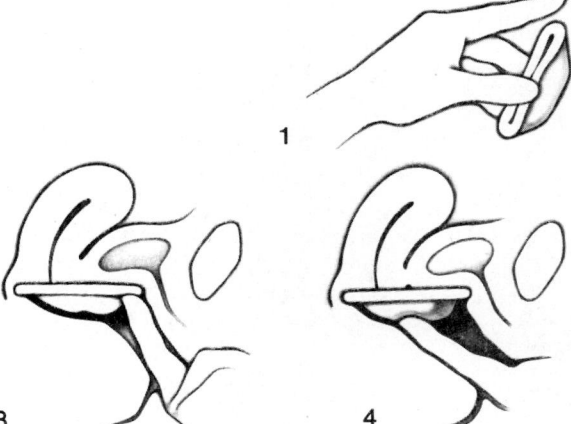

3   4

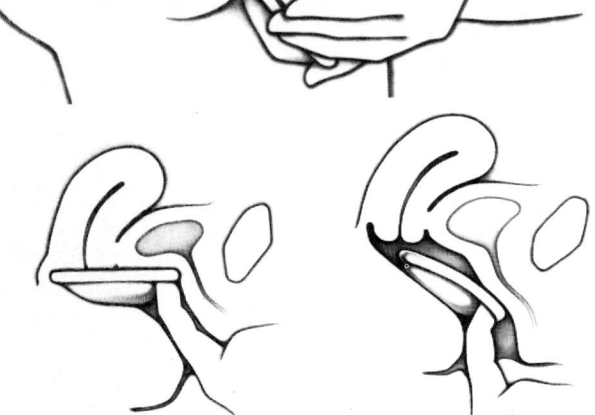

With your index finger, push the front rim of the diaphragm up until it is locked into place just above the pubic bone (3).

Check with your index finger to be sure the diaphragm is in place (4). It is important that the diaphragm be locked in place between the upper edge of the pubic bone and the rear wall of the vagina. You should be able to feel your cervix through the rubber shield.

Removing the diaphragm

To remove the diaphragm, put your index finger behind the front rim. Pull the diaphragm down and out. Bearing down may facilitate its removal. If you get up before it is time to remove the diaphragm and there is a discharge of cream or jelly, you may use a tampon or sanitary napkin.

Figure 45-5. Insertion of a diaphragm. (Material published by Ortho Pharmaceutical Corporation. Used by permission.)

A satisfactory IUD is easy to insert; remains in place; is an effective contraceptive device; causes no problems, such as pain or bleeding; rarely needs to be removed; and is economical. Several types of intrauterine devices are currently in use: double coil, copper T, loop, copper 7, and progesterone-releasing IUDs (Fig. 45-6). Copper and some other metals enhance the effectiveness of an IUD; however, the long-term safety of copper IUDs has still not been established. The IUD is positioned in a narrow, straight stylet that is introduced through the cervical os. The device is then forced into the uterine cavity by means of a plunger. Most devices have nylon-thread tails that are used to remove the IUD and to help indicate that it is still in the uterus. Because the copper component dissolves over a period of time, copper IUDs must be replaced approximately every 4 years; beyond that time, the effectiveness is lost. A plastic IUD is not changed unless there is increased bleeding after it has been in place beyond a year. Progesterone-releasing IUDs need to be replaced annually because the supply of progesterone is gradually depleted.

The advantages of this method are that it is effective, has no systemic effects, and reduces the factor of patient error. The disadvantages are that such a device may cause excessive bleeding, become displaced, perforate the cervix and uterus, and may cause infection. There is also the risk of pregnancy-related complications, such as congenital anomalies, spontaneous or septic abortion, and ectopic pregnancy. However, now that the shield-type IUD is off the market, the safety and popularity of the IUD have been enhanced. It is a desirable method for women who have completed their families but do not prefer sterilization. It is also an alternative for older women who may be at risk by taking steroid contraceptives.

Oral Steroids—The "Pill"

Physiologic Basis. Oral synthetic steroid preparations of estrogen and progesterone tend to block the stimulation of the ovary by the central nervous system by preventing the release of the follicle-stimulating hormone (FSH) from the anterior pituitary. In the absence of FSH, a follicle does not ripen and ovulation does not take place; this is the basis of operation of oral contraceptives. A single pill is taken on the fifth day of menstruation and each day thereafter for 20 or 21 days; this is repeated on the fifth day of each ensuing menstrual period. Some companies provide 28 pills in a convenient case; 7 to 8 are placebos. This means the woman takes a pill each day.

There are two kinds of therapy: "combined" and "gestagen only." The difference lies in the dosage of progestogens. In the *combined therapy,* estrogen and progestogen are present in every pill. The majority of women taking oral contraceptives take this type. Progestogen interferes with cervical mucus production and prevents uterine endometrium from fully developing to receive the fertilized ovum, resulting in a lighter-than-normal menstrual flow. Progestogen *gestagen only* in a smaller dose given daily is the other major kind of oral contraceptive. A small percentage of women take this type.

Side-effects. In a small percentage of patients, side-effects may be noted, such as nausea, pelvic discomfort, backache, irritability, depression, headache, weight gain, leg cramps, breast soreness, hirsutism, and acne. Usually, these disappear after 3 or 4 months. Because such symptoms are related to sodium and water retention caused by estrogen, a smaller dose of the hormone and salt reduction in the diet may alleviate the problem.

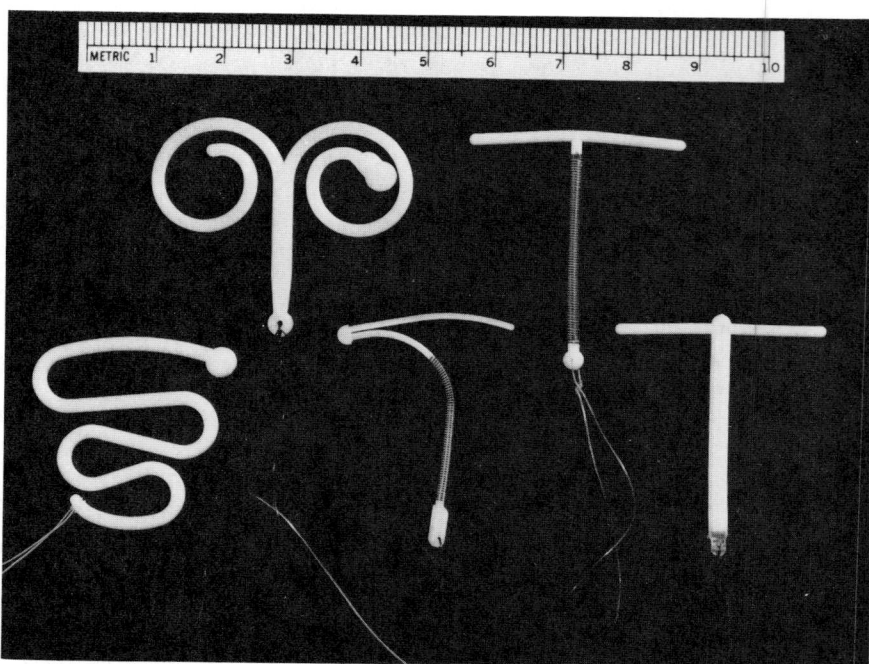

Figure 45-6. IUDs currently approved for use in the United States. (*Top row*) Double coil and copper T. (*Bottom row*) Loop, copper 7, and progesterone-releasing IUD. (From Danforth DN et al (eds): Obstetrics and Gynecology, 4th ed. Philadelphia, Harper & Row, 1982.)

Other problems encountered are the occurrence of thromboembolic disorders, more rapid growth of uterine fibroids, and jaundice. Therefore, these drugs should not be used by women who have had thromboembolic disorders, uterine fibroids, diabetes, or liver or gallbladder disease. Noted also is an increased incidence of heart attack in smokers over the age of 35 who are on the pill. Occasionally, neuro-ocular complications arise, but a cause-and-effect relationship is unknown at present. Should visual disturbances occur, the drug should be terminated. An increased incidence of candidal vulvovaginitis has also been reported.

Certain nutritional side-effects have been noted, such as folic acid deficiency and an increased need for vitamin C and vitamin B_{12}. However, the consequences of metabolic and nutritional effects of the pill are not definitely established. Nutritional counseling must be done on an individual basis. Women with good dietary habits may be able to satisfy nutritional needs; however, women with depleted or limited nutritional resources may require vitamin and mineral supplements.

Women with scanty or irregular periods are strongly advised to use another method of contraception. If they use oral contraceptives, they may have difficulty becoming pregnant or may fail to have menstrual periods after discontinuing the pill. With respect to how soon fertility returns after taking oral contraceptives, resumption of fertility is delayed 2 to 3 months in approximately 20% of users. For some women it is longer; since ovulation may be delayed for varying periods, it is probably helpful (for calculating expected delivery date) for the woman desiring to become pregnant to use a mechanical contraceptive barrier for the first month.

It is generally accepted that no definite long-term undesirable effects following prolonged use of oral contraceptives have been observed so far. Fetal anomalies do not appear to be a concern, and normal reproductive tract function and fertility are restored (although somewhat delayed, as was indicated above) following discontinuance of the pill. Meanwhile, research and experimentation continue toward the development of a single monthly pill or injection that would be safe as well as effective (Chart 45-1).

Interception (Postcoital Conception Control)

A properly timed administration of an adequate dosage of estrogen following intercourse will prevent pregnancy. Such a "morning after" pill is not applicable for use in long-term contraceptive control, but is of real value in emergency situations such as rape, defective or torn condom or diaphragm, or other "accidental" intercourse. Such medication given immediately after fertilization and before the occurrence of implantation is effective. Usually, the therapy is continued over 5 days using diethylstilbestrol or ethinyl estradiol. Nausea can be minimized by taking the medication with meals and with an antiemetic drug. Other side-effects may be experienced, such as breast soreness and irregular menses, but these are transient.

"Permanent" Conception Control

Sterilization is becoming increasingly popular; by the middle of the 1970s, almost one in three married couples were

---

Chart 45-1
Risk Factors and Patient Monitoring

Absolute Contraindications to the Use of Oral Contraceptives (FDA)

1. Known or suspected estrogen-dependent neoplasia
2. Known or suspected cancer of the breast
3. Thrombophlebitis or thromboembolic disease
4. A history of thrombophlebitis, thromboembolism, or thrombotic disease
5. Cerebrovascular and coronary artery disease
6. Abnormal uterine bleeding from an unknown cause
7. Known or suspected pregnancy

Other Contraindications

Hypertension, congenital hyperlipidemia, diabetes mellitus, liver disease, cholestatic jaundice, amenorrhea, migraine headache, leiomyoma of the uterus, heavy cigarette smoking

Oral contraceptives are mainly recommended for young women; systemic disease and the mortality risk in using the pill both increase with age.

---

using this method. It is a preferred method for couples who no longer desire to have children. Sterilization may be achieved by hysterectomy, oophorectomy, or tubal ligation in the female, and by vasectomy in the male. With increasing research, ligations may be reversible; however, they are still considered a permanent means of sterilization.

Tubal sterilization (ligation or electrocoagulation of uterine tubes) terminates a woman's ability to have children without affecting her ovulatory or menstrual function. The number of total ligations is increasing each year, and the most common indications are hypertensive cardiovascular disease, two or more cesarean sections, and multiparity. Various surgical techniques have been developed utilizing the abdominal or vaginal approach.

Laparoscopy is a relatively new technique of sterilization (see p. 1026).

For a discussion of vasectomy in male sterilization, see page 1100.

Investigational Conception Control

Antipregnancy Vaccine. The *human chorionic gonadotropin molecule (HCG)* is the hormone released by a freshly fertilized egg; it stimulates the release of progesterone, which halts menstruation. A vaccine has been produced that stimulates the formation of antibodies that are capable of neutralizing HCG, thereby blocking its signal. The next menses occurs as usual, thereby removing the ovum.

A "Pill" for Males. A drug has been developed that cuts production of male hormones, thereby reducing sperm output. The drug is given with a monthly injection of testosterone (to ensure normal sexual drive) and has shown encouraging results.

Patient Education

Much has been written about family planning and the availability and use of contraceptive devices. The nurse is in a strong position to help patients understand the options available. Religious groups have made clear their teaching and dogma regarding birth control, and these need to be respected and understood as each couple makes its decision. Research is changing the methods used in fertility control, and more acceptable and longer-lasting types are sought. The nurse should be familiar with the information as it becomes available. A valuable source of information is the American College of Obstetrics and Gynecology, 1 E. Wacker, Chicago, Illinois 60601.

▷ Pregnancy Termination

Interruption of pregnancy or expulsion of the contents of the pregnant uterus before the fetus is viable (up to 20 weeks) is called *abortion;* interruption between 20 to 28 weeks is commonly referred to as *miscarriage.* The viability of the fetus is usually considered to be any time after the sixth month of gestation; however, legal periods of viability vary in different states in the United States.

The aborted fetus weighs less than 1000 gm; beyond this weight, the fetus is usually viable, and the term *premature labor* is used, instead of *abortion,* to describe the situation. It is estimated that one out of every five or ten conceptions results in abortion. Most of these occur because of an abnormality in the fetus, so that abortion is nature's method of rejecting a defective conception. Other causes may be due to systemic diseases, hormonal imbalance, or anatomical abnormalities.

Spontaneous Abortion

Spontaneous abortion occurs most commonly in the second or third month of gestation, probably due to a defective ovum and subsequent developmental defects of the fetus and placenta.

There are various kinds of spontaneous abortion, depending on the nature of the process (threatened, inevitable, incomplete, and complete). Uterine bleeding and pain (uterine contractions) are suggestive of an abortion in a woman of childbearing age. In such a *threatened abortion,* the cervix does not dilate; with bed rest and conservative treatment, it can be prevented. If it cannot be prevented, an *inevitable abortion* is imminent. If some of the tissue, but not all, is passed, the abortion is referred to as *incomplete;* however, if the fetus and all related tissue are expressed (removed), the abortion is *complete.*

Habitual Abortion

Habitual abortion is successive, (three) repeated abortions of unknown cause; immunologic rejection is suspected. Ultraconservative measures are employed in an attempt to save the pregnancy, such as complete bed rest, administration of progesterone to prevent sloughing of the endometrium, thyroid extract therapy, and psychotherapy.

In the condition known as "incompetent cervical os," the cervix dilates painlessly in the second trimester of pregnancy, resulting in spontaneous abortion. A surgical procedure called the Shirodkar operation (cervical cerclage) is designed to prevent the cervix from dilating prematurely. A purse-string suture of fascia, polyethylene, or dermal graft strip obtained from the patient's lower abdominal skin is tied snugly around the cervix at the level of the internal os. It is most important that the patient and the nurses attending her, including those in community health agencies and industry, be informed that such a suture is in place. As soon as labor occurs, the physician should be notified immediately so that the suture can be cut and labor allowed to proceed; otherwise, the uterus may possibly rupture. Usually, delivery is by cesarean section.

Therapeutic Abortion

Under certain circumstances, the physician may consider terminating a pregnancy; such a termination is called a *therapeutic abortion,* and is performed by skilled medical personnel. On January 22, 1973, the United States Supreme Court handed down its ruling on abortions, which in effect states the following:

1. In the first trimester of pregnancy, the abortion decision is to be left to the woman and her physician.
2. During the second trimester, the state may not prohibit abortion, but may regulate its practice in the interest of protecting the woman's health. (Permissible regulations could determine who are qualified to do abortions and where they might be done.)
3. During the final weeks of pregnancy, the state may choose to protect the potential life of the fetus by prohibiting abortion, except where necessary to preserve the life or health of the woman.

Even though the liberalization of abortion laws makes many abortions legally permissible, the religious beliefs of the individual involved must be respected. Baptism of all stillborn and aborted fetuses is required by the Roman Catholic faith.

Management. Usually, the opinions of two or more physicians are documented to identify the reasons for performing a therapeutic abortion. Appropriate informed permission is obtained from the patient.

Vacuum aspiration of uterine contents within 14 days of a missed menstrual period may be performed in a physician's office; this is called *menstrual regulation,* or *menstrual extraction.*

Therapeutic abortions may be carried out in the following ways, usually in the operating room:

1. *Dilatation and curettage* (see p. 1053)
2. *Dilatation and evacuation (suction curettage):* The cervix is dilated, and a uterine aspirator is introduced. Suction from a pump is applied, and fetal tissue is removed from the uterus. This method is not used if the pregnancy has advanced beyond 12 weeks, since the fetus at this stage is supposedly too firm. More recently,

some clinics have extended the period to 16 weeks and even beyond.

3. *Intra-amniotic injection of hypertonic saline:* This procedure is used beyond the 14th week of pregnancy. Under local anesthesia, a needle is inserted in the mid-abdomen, and an amniocentesis is performed. Over 200 ml of fluid are withdrawn and replaced by hypertonic saline. In some clinics, after 6 hours, oxytocin is administered intravenously, with lactated Ringer's solution, to initiate labor. If no oxytocics are administered, labor will usually begin spontaneously within 8 to 20 hours, but may be delayed for several days. Subsequent curettage may be necessary to completely remove any remaining placental and residual tissue. The dangers of this procedure, such as accidental intravenous injection of saline, cerebral convulsion, and acute renal failure, need to be realized.

4. *Prostaglandins:* Intra-amniotic instillation of natural or synthetic prostaglandins produces strong uterine contractions, causing cervical dilatation and expulsion of the fetus and placenta within 24 hours. This method appears safer than utilizing hypertonic saline, because it avoids the complication of DIC (disseminated intravascular coagulation) and hypernatremia.

   Prostaglandins continue to be studied; side-effects such as nausea, vomiting, diarrhea, and painful uterine cramping may occur, although the incidence and frequency of such problems vary according to the medication, dosage, and technique of administration. Transvaginal extra-amniotic administration is used to initiate uterine contractions, as are vaginal suppositories and intramuscular prostaglandins. The latter methods are noninvasive with decreased morbidity and ease of administration.

5. *Laminaria:* An age-old method of cervical dilatation is being revived in medical practice. *Laminaria* tents are made from a species of seaweed that grows in cold ocean waters; the stem is dried and cut into lengths of about 6 cm to 8 cm (2.4–3.1 inches) and shaped into cylindrical (tampon-shaped) forms for sizing, from 2 mm to 4 mm, 4 mm to 6 mm, 6 mm to 8 mm, and 8 mm to 10 mm in diameter. A string is looped through one end. When placed in a moist environment, the tent, which is highly hygroscopic, swells to three or five times its original diameter. The tent may be placed in the cervix in order to dilate it. The greatest amount of swelling occurs in 4 to 5 hours; however, additional dilatation may be expected over the next few hours.

   Tents are used prior to the insertion of IUDs, for first- or second-trimester abortions, and for other medical procedures requiring dilatation.

   Advantages of *Laminaria* tents over metal-instrument dilators are many: tents cause limited cervical trauma, hold little risk of other serious complications, and are readily accepted and tolerated by patients. Disadvantages include the following: there is some discomfort and slight uterine cramping immediately after insertion, and mild-to-severe intermittent cramps may be experienced in some women for several hours. There is also risk of low-grade endometritis. Removal of the tent is difficult at times, and on occasion has resulted in the tent's slipping into the uterus. Tents are sterilized in gamma radiation or ethylene oxide gas.

   When it is desirable to insert a tent overnight, hospitalization may be required. In such instances, the nurse needs to know that a tent is in place (string will be noticed in the vagina). Many physicians, however, prefer to use *Laminaria* for just 3 to 4 hours, followed by metal dilatation.

6. *Hysterotomy:* This is a "miniature" cesarean section; usually, this method is reserved for women who also want to be sterilized at the same time. The patient remains in the hospital for 3 to 6 days; care is essentially the same as for an abdominal operation patient.

Septic Abortion

When unskilled attempts to end a pregnancy are made, the methods usually include administering large amounts of drugs (effects are toxic and never really evacuate the uterus) or performing a curettage, with an associated high risk of rupture of the uterus, hemorrhage, or infection.

Although this has been a major problem in the past, with the widespread dissemination of birth control information and the liberalization of abortion laws, a decline in septic abortion will be apparent.

If a woman who has had a simple, uncomplicated septic abortion receives proper medical attention early enough, the prognosis is excellent with treatment with broad-spectrum antibiotics. Fluid and blood replacement is required before very careful attempts are made to evacuate the uterus.

For the treatment of septic abortion complicated by impending shock, see the discussions of shock (p. 402) and pelvic inflammatory disease (p. 1062).

Management of Abortion Patients

Signs of a threatening abortion are vaginal discharge or bleeding and abdominal cramps. The woman is encouraged to see a physician, who will probably recommend bed rest, light diet, and no straining on defecation. According to some estimates, when first seen, less than 30% of patients who are actually threatening to abort have viable fetuses, and 80% or more will proceed to abortion regardless of management.[*]

All tissue passed vaginally is saved for examination by the physician. Sedation or tranquilizers may be prescribed, and if infection is suspected, antibiotics may be given. In the hospital, all personnel caring for the patient are alerted to save the contents of the bedpan for possible placenta tissue or fetus. If there is much bleeding, the patient may require transfusions and fluid replacement. An estimate of the amount of bleeding can be determined by recording the number of perineal pads and the nature of saturation per 24 hours. For an incomplete abortion, oxytocin may be prescribed to contract the fundus prior to the woman's having a dilatation and evacuation (D & E), or suctioning of the uterus. A patient with such an *evacuation of retained se-*

---

[*] Green TH Jr. Gynecology, 2nd ed. Boston, Little, Brown & Co, 1977.

Chart 45-2
Patient Education: Post-therapeutic Abortion

1. Note that bleeding similar to menstruation will continue for 7 days or less.
   - Report: If bleeding is heavier than usual menstrual flow
     If bleeding is followed by severe cramps, backache, nausea
2. During bleeding:
   - Do not take tub baths; showers or sponge baths are permitted.
   - Do not douche or go swimming.
   - Do not use tampons—use sanitary pads. (Tampons may be used during your next period.)
   - Do not have intercourse; preferably, wait until you have one normal period.
   - Avoid strenuous exercise for at least 1 week, since it may cause further bleeding.
3. Medication for bleeding:
   - If medication has been prescribed to prevent bleeding, expect a few cramps or clots.
4. Take your temperature for 5 to 7 days.
   - Report: If it is elevated for 24 to 48 hours
     If it is elevated and accompanied by symptoms mentioned in 1.
5. Normal expected signs due to hormonal changes (these will pass):
   - Some women experience depression.
   - Breasts may be sore and perhaps leak. To combat this, wear a supportive brassiere, and restrict fluids.
6. Follow-up:
   - In about a month (or when requested), report to your physician or clinic for a checkup.

(Adapted from Easterbrook B and Rust B: Abortion counseling. Can Nurse 73:30, Jan 1977.)

cretions (ERS) requires the same nursing care as a person having a dilatation and curettage (see p. 1053).

Since this person often experiences a severe emotional reaction, the component of "caring" for her is an important aspect of nursing. The cause of the abortion colors the problem and the patient's reaction. The response of the woman who desperately wants the baby is quite different from that of the woman who does not want to be pregnant but may be frightened of the possible consequences of an abortion. The nurse must not overlook the fact that in many instances, particularly for the woman having a spontaneous abortion, there is a grieving period that must be handled. Such grieving may be delayed or unresolved, resulting in other problems until the grief reaction has been worked out. There are many reasons for delayed grief reaction: friends may not have known the woman was pregnant; the woman may not have seen the lost fetus and can only imagine the sex, size, etc. of the person who never developed; there is no burial service; those who know about the abortion (family, friends, care-givers) encourage denial and rarely encourage crying and talking about the loss.

In any event, providing opportunities for the patient to talk and vent her emotions will not only help her, but will also provide clues for the nurse in planning more specific care. Encourage those persons closest to the woman to hug her and allow her to talk and cry. If grief is unresolved, it may manifest itself by persistent vivid memories of the events surrounding the time of loss, persistent sadness or anger, and frequent flooding of emotion when recalling the loss. Signs of pathologic grief may require the assistance of a therapist skilled in grief work (also see Chart 45-2).

It is well to remember that the incidence of complications and death is higher for abortion than for other methods of contraception. Because of this, contraception and sterilization are preferred to prevent unwanted pregnancy. Only when these fail, should therapeutic abortion be considered.

▷ Infertility

Infertility is defined as the inability to conceive, and is usually designated as a problem when the couple fails to conceive after a year or more of normal marital contact. However, should the condition persist, it is referred to as *sterility*. In the United States, 15% of married couples (3.5 million couples) are childless because of infertility; it is a major medical and social problem. Both husband and wife are urged to seek medical attention for complete examinations and evaluation. Careful evaluation includes not only anatomical and endocrinologic investigation, but also consideration of psychosocial factors. Often more than one factor may be responsible for the problem. Such tests may require the services of a urologist, gynecologist, endocrinologist, and internist.

Possible causative factors include uterine displacement, tumors, congenital anomalies, and inflammation. For an ovum to become fertilized, the vagina, cervix, and uterus must be patent, and the mucosal secretions must be receptive to the sperm. Semen is alkaline, as is cervical secretion; normal vaginal secretion is acid. Proceeding from this assumption, five types of factors are considered basic to the infertility: for the female, (1) ovarian, (2) tubal, (3) cervical, or (4) uterine conditions, and for the male, (5) seminal. A composite estimate of the relative frequency of these factors as the major cause of infertility is as follows: ovarian, 20%; tubal, 30%; cervical, 18%; seminal, 30%.

Diagnostic Approach. A complete history, physical examination, and laboratory examination are done on both partners to rule out such causative factors as previous sexually transmitted disease, anomalies, injuries, tuberculosis, mumps orchitis, abortions, and psychosocial disorders.

Ovarian Factor. Tests are done to determine whether there is regular ovulation and a progestational endometrium adequate for implantation. This includes keeping a basal body temperature chart for at least four cycles, taking an endometrial biopsy, and performing other tests for ovulation and progesterone production.

Tubal Factor (Tubal Insufflation or Rubin's Test). To determine tubal patency, carbon dioxide is introduced through a sterile cannula into the uterus and the uterine tubes, and then into the peritoneal cavity. By listening with a stethoscope on the abdomen, the physician may hear gas swishing into the abdomen, indicating that the tubes are open. Another positive indication of tubal patency is the feeling by the patient of referred pain under the scapula or shoulder on the side of the patent tube. This suggests that the gas is under the diaphragm, exerting pressure on the phrenic nerve. If normal patency is present, there is a rise in pressure of 80 mm to 120 mm, with a sudden drop to 50 mm to 70 mm as gas passes into the peritoneal cavity. If the gas pressure gauge reaches 200 mm, the test is considered negative, indicating an occlusion.

Hysterosalpingography (see p. 1027) is an x-ray study that is useful when tubal occlusion is apparent since other abnormalities may be found.

Culdoscopy or laparoscopy (see p. 1026) permits direct visualization of the tubes and adnexa, including the status of ovarian function.

Cervical Factor.
Cervical mucus can be examined to determine whether proper changes occur at ovulation time that are favorable to sperm penetration, survival, and growth.

A postcoital cervical mucous test (Sims–Huhner or P–K test) is done between 6 and 12 hours after intercourse. The physician aspirates cervical secretions, using a medicine dropper or special cannula. The woman has been instructed not to void, bathe, or douche between coitus and the examination; a perineal pad is worn until she is placed in a lithotomy position in the examination room. Aspirated material is placed on a slide and examined under the microscope for presence and viability of sperm cells.

Uterine Factor.
Fibroids, polyps, and congenital malformations are possible problems in this category. Their presence may be determined by pelvic examination or by hysterosalpingography.

Seminal Factor.
After 4 or 5 days of sexual abstinence, the sperm specimen is collected in a clean, dry glass container; kept at or below room temperature; and examined within 2 to 4 hours for volume, sperm motility, morphology, and cell count. About 3 ml to 5 ml of viscid alkaline semen is normal; a normal count is 60 to 100 million per ml.

Miscellaneous Factors, Including Immunologic Factors.
These are currently being investigated.

Management.
Sterility may be difficult to treat, since it often is due to a combination of several factors. A total study program should be conducted, including a general physical as well as psychosocial evaluation of both mates. Statistics show that many couples undergoing study conceive without the cause of infertility coming to light; likewise, although some couples undergo all tests, the cause of the problem may remain undiscovered. Between these extremes, many problems, simple as well as complex, can be discovered and corrected, to the happy benefit of the couple. Between 25% and 50% of all infertile couples can be cured.

Therapy may require correction of faulty coital technique, surgery to correct a malfunction or anomaly, hormonal supplements, attention to proper timing, and recognition and correction of psychological or emotional factors.

Note: Additional information may be obtained from the American Fertility Society, 1801 Ninth Ave., South, Birmingham, Alabama 35205.

Artificial Insemination

Artificial insemination is the deposition or introduction of semen into the female genital tract by artificial means. If the sperm cannot penetrate the cervical canal normally, consideration may be given to *artificial insemination,* using the husband's semen (AIH). In the event of azospermia (lack of sperm in the semen), semen from carefully selected donors may be used (AID).

Two indications for using artificial insemination are (1) inability of the male to deposit semen in the vagina; this may be due to premature ejaculation, pronounced hypospadias, or dyspareunia (painful intercourse experienced by the female), and (2) inability of semen to be transported from the vagina to the uterine cavity; this is usually due to faulty chemical conditions, such as may be produced with an abnormal cervical discharge. The latter may be corrected with chemotherapeutic agents.

Husband's Semen.
Certain conditions need to be established before semen is transferred to the vagina. The wife must have no abnormalities of the genital system, the tubes must be patent, and ova must be available. In the husband, sperm need to be normal in shape, amount, motility, and endurance. The time of ovulation in the female should be determined as accurately as possible, so that the 2 or 3 days during which fertilization is possible each month can be utilized. Fertilization seldom occurs from a single insemination. Usually, insemination is attempted between the 10th and 17th day of the cycle; three different attempts are made. Semen is collected in a wide-mouth, 2-ounce jar following masturbation or withdrawal.

Donor's Semen.
A donor may be utilized when the husband's sperm is defective or absent, or when, for hereditary reasons, it is feared that an undesirable disease may be transmitted. Safeguards need to be set up to prevent legal, ethical, emotional, and religious problems. Written consent may protect the wife, donor, donor's wife, and legal status of the child.

The donor is selected on the basis of close resemblance to the husband, both physically and intellectually; there should be no family history of epilepsy, diabetes, or known genetic defects, and a negative Wassermann or Kahn reaction should be obtained.* Preferably, precautions should be taken so that the donor is not known to the recipient, and vice versa.

Insemination Procedure.
The recipient is placed in the lithotomy position on the examining table, a speculum is inserted, and the vagina and cervix are swabbed clean with a cotton applicator. Semen is drawn into a sterile syringe, and a cannula is attached. The semen is then directed to the external os. If this is contraindicated, the semen may be inserted directly into the cervical canal. Following the careful withdrawal of the syringe, the patient is to lie flat on the examining table for a half hour. Thereafter, there is no restriction on the activities of the woman.

The success rate for artificial insemination is about 50%. About three to six inseminations are required over a 2- to 4-month period. Since this procedure is opposed by the

---

* There are commercial firms that bank sperm in Chicago, New York City, Los Angeles, and St. Paul.

Roman Catholic Church, this method should not be suggested to members of this faith.

▷ Ectopic Pregnancy

Ectopic pregnancy is a pregnancy in which the fertilized ovum does not reach the cavity of the uterus, but becomes caught and implanted on any tissue other than the lining of the uterine cavity, such as the uterine tube or, occasionally, in the ovary or the abdomen, or even the cervix of the uterus (Fig. 45-7). As the fertilized ovum increases in size, the tube becomes more and more distended, until finally, about 4 to 6 weeks after conception, rupture takes place, and the ovum is discharged into the abdominal cavity.

Etiology and Incidence.   Precipitating causes of ectopic pregnancy may be salpingitis, endometriosis, pelvic inflammatory disease, chemotherapy for pelvic tuberculosis, congenital anomalies of the tubes, or spasm of the tubes with muscular insufficiency. Factors inherent in the embryo (embryonic abnormalities) may also predispose to ectopic gestation. The Centers for Disease Control report that increasing use of fertility-control measures, such as tubal ligation and abortion, has been directly associated with ectopic pregnancy. Studies have shown the incidence to vary from 1 in 300 pregnancies to 1 in 100.

Assessment and Clinical Manifestations.   Delay in menstruation from 1 to 2 weeks followed by slight (spotting) bleeding may suggest the problem of an ectopic pregnancy. Or amenorrhea may continue several weeks. Symptoms may start with vague soreness on the side affected; frequently the patient experiences sharp, colicky pain at times. When tubal rupture occurs, there is agonizing pain, dizziness, faintness, and some nausea and vomiting (see Fig. 45-7 for nursing assessment). These symptoms are related to peritoneal reaction to blood escaping from the tube. Air hunger and symptoms of shock indicate that the patient is desperately ill; all the signs of hemorrhage—rapid, thready pulse; subnormal temperature; restlessness; pallor; sweating—are in evidence. Later the pain becomes generalized in the abdomen and radiates to the shoulder and neck because of irritation to the diaphragm. By vaginal examination, the surgeon is able to feel a large mass of clotted blood that has collected in the pelvis behind the uterus.

Diagnostic Evaluation.   Usually, the clinical picture makes the diagnosis relatively simple; however, when it is questionable, other aids are of value. Pelvic aspiration from the cul-de-sac of Douglas (culdocentesis) may be useful. Laparoscopy is especially helpful because the physician can visually note an unruptured ectopic pregnancy, thereby circumventing the risks to the patient of a tubal rupture. Ultrasonography may be effective when used with other diagnostic aids.

Because the signs and symptoms of tubal pregnancy are often confused with other problems (pelvic inflammatory disease, ovarian cyst with twisted pedicle, problems with an IUD), careful history taking and monitoring of the patient are essential.

Management.   The goal of treatment is the surgical removal of the ectopic pregnancy, since it is a life-threatening problem; the woman is then relieved of pain and discomfort.

When the operation is performed early, practically all patients recover with remarkable rapidity, but without operation, the mortality is 60% to 70%. The type of surgery is determined by the size and extent of local tubal damage; surgery ranges from conservative to more extensive. Very

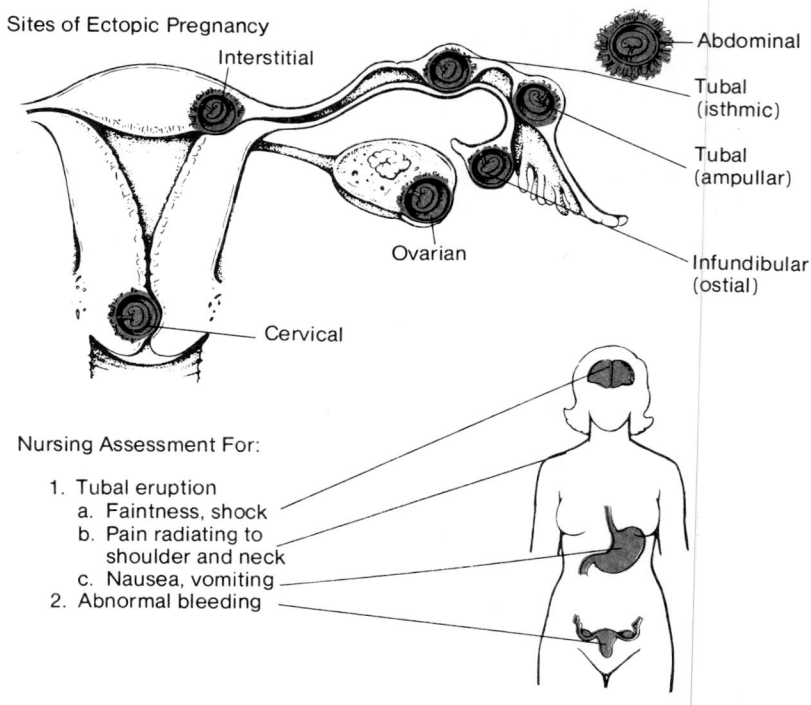

Figure 45-7. Ectopic pregnancy.

conservative surgery would include "milking" an ectopic pregnancy from the tube. Perhaps a resection of the involved tube with end-to-end anastomosis may be effective. Some surgeons today perform a salpingostomy, which involves opening and evacuating the tube, controlling bleeding, and resuturing the tube to preserve it. More radical surgery includes salpingectomy or salpingo-oophorectomy. Depending on the amount of blood lost, blood transfusions and treatment for shock may be necessary preoperatively and operatively. Postoperative care is similar to that for any laparotomy. The pregnancy rate following treatment is about 50%; the expectancy of another ectopic pregnancy is about 10%.

▷ Bibliography

Books

Beacham DW and Beacham WD. Synopsis of Gynecology, 10th ed. St Louis, CV Mosby, 1982.

Danforth DN. Obstetrics and Gynecology, 4th ed. Philadelphia, JB Lippincott, 1982.

Edelman DA et al. Intrauterine Devices and Their Complications. Boston, GK Hall, 1979.

Fogel CI and Wood NF. Health Care of Women. A Nursing Perspective. St Louis, CV Mosby, 1981.

Hawkins JW and Higgins LP. Health Care of Women. Gynecological Assessment. Belmont, California, Wadsworth Health Science Division, 1982.

Hawkins JW and Higgins LP. Maternity and Gynecological Nursing, Philadelphia, JB Lippincott, 1981.

Hogan R. Human Sexuality: A Nursing Perspective. New York, Appleton–Century–Crofts, 1980.

Jones HW and Jones GS. Novak's Textbook of Gynecology. Baltimore, Williams & Wilkins, 1981.

Nursing Photobook. Attending Ob/Gyn Patients. Springhouse, Pennsylvania, Intermed Publications, 1982.

Romney SL et al. Gynecology and Obstetrics, 2nd ed. New York, McGraw–Hill, 1981.

Shain R and Paverstein CJ. Fertility Control. New York, Harper & Row, 1980.

Warner CG. Rape and Sexual Assault: Management and Intervention. Gaithersburg, Maryland, Aspen Systems, 1980.

Willson JR, Carrington ER, and Ledger WJ. Obstetrics and Gynecology, 7th ed. St Louis, CV Mosby, 1983.

Articles
Women's Health Care

Edlund BJ and McKenzie CA. Symposium on women's health issues. Nurs Clin North Am 1982 Mar; 17(1):111–185.

Finley B. Nursing process with the battered woman. Nurse Pract 1981 July-Aug; 6(4):11–13.

Huffman JW. Gynecologic disorders in the geriatric patient. Postgrad Med 1982 Jan; 71(1):39–51.

Latta W and Wiesmeier E. Effects of an educational gynecological exam on women's attitudes. JOGN Nurs 1982 July/Aug; 11(4):242–245.

Peters L. Women's health care. Approaches in delivery to physically disabled women. Nurse Pract 1982 Jan; 7(1):34–35, 48.

Women's health risk expected to increase. AORN J 1981 May; 33(6):1181.

Menstruation and Menopause

Budoff PW. Zomepirac sodium in the treatment of primary dysmenorrhea syndrome. N Engl J Med 1982 Sept 16; 307(12):714–719.

Gaines F. Diagnostic protocol: Secondary amenorrhea, Part 1. Nurse Pract 1981 July/Aug; 6(4):17–29.

Hanna J. Premenstrual syndrome; defeating the curse of the calendar. Nurs Mirror 1980 Oct 2; 151(14):36–37.

Most AF et al. Distress associated with menstruation among Israeli women. Int J Nurs Stud 1981 Jan; 18(1):61–71.

Pearson L. Climacteric. Am J Nurs 1982 July; 82(7):1098–1102.

Woods NF, Most E, and Dery GK. Prevalence of perimenstrual symptoms. Am J Public Health 1982 Nov; 72(11):1257–1264.

Fertility/Infertility

Archer DF and Thomas RL. The fallacy of the postpill amenorrhea syndrome. Clin Obstet Gynecol 1981 Sept; 24(3):943–950.

Beck WW. Complications and contraindications of oral contraception. Clin Obstet Gynecol 1981 Sept; 24(3):893–901.

Bolton GC. Adolescent contraception. Clin Obstet Gynecol 1981 Sept; 24(3):977–986.

Friedman BM. Infertility workup. Am J Nurs 1981 Nov; 81(11):2040–2046.

IngHsuWu D and Langer A. Ectopic pregnancy. Am Fam Physician 1982 Oct; 26(4):161–166.

IUD's: An appropriate contraceptive for many women. Popul Report [B] 1982 July; 10(4):B101–B135.

Keith LG, Berger GS, and Jackson MA. Effective use of vaginal contraception—a method for the 1980's. Contemp Ob/Gyn 1982 June; 19(6):64–85.

Lahteenmaki P et al. Coagulation factors in women using oral contraceptives or intrauterine contraceptive devices immediately after abortion. Am J Obstet Gynecol 1981 Sept 15; 141(2):175–179.

McCusker MP. The subfertile couple. JOGN Nurs 1982 May/June; 11(3):157–162.

Ortho-novum 10/11—a new "bi-phasic" oral contraceptive. The Medical Letter 1982 Oct 15; 24(620):93–94.

Sondheimer S. Metabolic effects of the birth control pill. Clin Obstet Gynecol 1981 Sept; 24(3):927–941.

White LD and White PF. Midtrimester abortion patients. AORN J 1981 Oct; 34(4):756–768.

46

Management of Patients With Gynecologic Disorders

▷ Conditions of the Vulva

The *vulva* (external female genitalia) is made up of the mons veneris, labia majora, labia minora, clitoris, vestibule, and accessory glands (Bartholin's, Skene's).

Inflammatory Conditions (Vulvitis)

Vulvitis, an inflammation of the vulva, usually occurs in conjunction with other local or systemic disorders, such as a dermatologic problem, poor local hygiene, or sexually transmitted disease, or it may be secondary to a specific vaginitis.

Common related conditions include vulvovaginitis (*e.g.,* moniliasis [candidiasis]), trichomoniasis (see p. 1046), sexually transmitted diseases (see p. 1491), neurodermatitis, and "idiopathic pruritus vulvae." This latter problem may be a psychosomatic disorder resulting from precipitating stress factors (*e.g.,* job frustration, marital difficulties). Other problems may include pyoderma, pediculosis, herpes, and lichen sclerosus.

Assessment and Clinical Manifestations. Before therapy can be recommended, a complete physical examination is required, with pelvic evaluation as well as laboratory studies, including vaginal smears, cultures, and blood studies to determine the possibility of diabetes. Symptoms may include complaints of itching and burning pain that is worse during urination and defecation. Genitalia may become red and edematous, and a discharge may be noticed.

Factors that may be involved should be assessed: (1) physical and chemical factors, such as increased perspiration plus decreased evaporation, antiperspirants, perfumes and powders, perineal soil, contraceptive jellies, and vaginal discharges; (2) medical and endocrine factors, such as a predisposition for vulvar involvement in the diabetic, geriatric, or chronically ill patient; (3) anatomical factors, such as the nature of mucocutaneous tissue, and nerve and secretory functions; and (4) psychogenic factors.

Management. The goal is to eliminate the inflammation. The assessment may reveal a specific problem. In addition, the patient should be instructed to avoid too frequent washing and scrubbing, particularly with detergent soaps, and to keep the area clean, dry, and free from irritation (*i.e.,* away from things that may rub against the inflamed area, and from synthetic fabrics that may cause an allergic reaction).

Tight-fitting panty hose, pant suits, and slacks have caused an increase in vulvar and vaginal irritation due to fabric dyes, as well as restricted ventilation. Scratching should be avoided, since it compounds the problem. Talcum powder may be used sparingly to avoid irritation. Soothing compresses alternating with colloidal baths are helpful. Steroid cream may be prescribed; other medications are usually withheld until the specific cause has been determined. Then the medication is specifically directed to treating the cause.

Benign Cysts

A cyst of the greater vestibular gland is a cystic dilation of the duct of the Bartholin's gland resulting from obstruction. This is the most common of vulvar tumors and is located in the posterior third of the vulva, near the vestibule. A simple cyst may be asymptomatic. Infection may be due to the gonococcus organism, *Escherichia coli,* or *Staphylococcus aureus* and can cause an abscess with or without inguinal adenopathy. Incision and drainage, plus antibiotics, are the best treatment.

Potentially Premalignant Lesions

Epithelial Dystrophies. *Lichen sclerosus et atrophicus,* often mistaken for *leukoplakia,* is noted as very slightly raised whitish papules or macules of the vulvar dermis. Symptoms are usually mild or absent, in contrast to the intense pruritus of leukoplakia. It is believed that at least 10% of patients with cancer of the vulva have an associated lichen sclerosus, with or without leukoplakia. Biopsy and a careful follow-up program are definitely recommended. If cancer cells are detected on biopsy, a simple vulvectomy is performed, with continued follow-up.

Cancer of the Vulva

Preinvasive Cancer. Three types of intraepithelial cancers have been recognized: (1) Bowen's disease, (2) Paget's disease, and (3) squamous cell carcinoma *in situ.* The predominant symptoms in at least two thirds of the patients is pruritus, but pain or soreness may be present. *Any vulvar lesion that is ulcerated or does not heal quickly with proper therapy should be biopsied.*

Treatment of *in situ* carcinoma of the vulva varies from superficial to complete vulvectomy without lymphadenectomy, depending on the nature of the lesion. (With invasive carcinoma, the surgery is vulvectomy with lymphadenectomy). The perineum, it must be remembered, is also a potential site for melanoma; up to 8% of melanomas occur here.

Invasive Cancer. Primary cancer of the vulva represents 3% to 4% of all gynecologic malignancies and is seen mostly in elderly women.

▶ **Assessment**

Clinical Manifestations. Long-standing pruritus is the most common symptom. Bleeding, foul-smelling discharge, and pain may also be present. The nurse is in a unique position to encourage a woman with this disease to seek help, since this is one of the most curable of all malignant conditions: it is visible and accessible, and grows relatively slowly. Although it begins on the skin surface and is easily noticed as a small ulcer that becomes infected and causes pain, women so affected seem reluctant to seek medical attention. Procrastination causes more extensive involvement, jeopardizing cure.

Diagnostic Evaluation. In addition to biopsy, which can verify the diagnosis, the Collin's test can assist in determining the extent of the lesion and whether other dystrophic lesions are present. This test is accomplished by staining the vulva with toluidine blue (a nuclear stain) solution, allowing it to dry, and then washing the dye off with 1% acetic acid. Dystrophic and other abnormal lesions take up the stain (have nuclear hyperactivity) and can be identified.

Patient Problems/Nursing Diagnoses

Based on the clinical manifestations and diagnostic evaluation data, the patient's potential problems include reluctance to seek medical attention related to the slow growth of the lesion and the false hope that the problem will disappear with time; anxiety and emotional stress related to fear of cancer and the disruption of the patient's life-style; impairment of skin integrity related to the spread of lesions; disrupted sexual life related to pruritus and dyspareunia; potential development of infection related to the proximity of excretory functions; and potential development of complications related to surgical repair.

▶ **Planning and Nursing Implementation**

Goals

The major goals for the patient include:

1. Control of and possibly elimination of pruritus and dyspareunia
2. Toleration of a surgical experience that causes the least inconvenience
3. Absence of complications
4. Absence of spread of the disease process
5. Psychosocial adjustment to the vulvar problem

Management. Vulvectomy is preferred to radiation therapy. The extensiveness of the vulvectomy depends on the extent of the malignancy. For example, leukoplakic changes call for simple vulvectomy; carcinoma *in situ* requires a total vulvectomy; and invasive carcinoma necessitates a wide radical vulvectomy with pelvic and groin lymph node dissection. Occasionally, even a part of the urethra, vagina, and rectum may have to be removed. With such extensive surgery (pelvic exenteration) there have been encouraging recovery rates.

This patient must be allowed time to talk and ask questions. Fear of mutilation and loss of function is lessened when a woman of childbearing age learns that the possibility of having sexual relations is good and that pregnancy is possible following a simple vulvectomy. Of course, the nurse must know what the physician has told the patient in this regard. Radical vulvectomy is more extensive and may require a second trip to the operating room for skin grafting.

In addition to the nursing care described on page 349, wide preparation of the skin may include scrubbing the lower abdomen, inguinal areas, upper thighs, and vulva with a detergent germicide for several days prior to the operation. The extent of surgery is dependent upon the extent of the spread; more extensive lesions require deep pelvic node dissection. Antibiotic and heparin prophylaxis may be prescribed preoperatively and continued postoperatively.

When the patient returns from the operating room, perineal dressings are more likely to remain in place and be comfortable if a T-binder is used. Groin wounds may be exposed, or covered with simple dressings. Pressure dressings may be placed over the wounds to aid in preventing the accumulation of lymph and serum. Many surgeons insert plastic tubes through stab wounds in each inguinal area with attachment to portable suction. This arrangement facilitates apposition of tissue flaps and prevents accumulation of serum.

Since stitches may be taut because of the surgeon's attempt to approximate tissues, comfortable positioning is required. Perhaps a low Fowler's position, or occasionally a pillow placed under the knees, will relieve tension on the incision. An air mattress or "egg crate" pad or mattress can assist in distributing weight and relieving pressure points. Turning is important, and comfort may be achieved with a pillow placed strategically between the legs and against the lumbar region. Moving from one position to another requires time and patience on the part of both patient and nurse. An overbed trapeze bar helps the patient to move herself. Ambulation may be attempted on the second day.

The wound is cleansed daily with detergent soap solution, dilute hydrogen peroxide, warm saline, or half-strength povidone–iodine solution. After a *gentle* cleansing, a warm-water spray is pleasant and nontraumatizing and enhances circulation. The wound should be exposed to the air at frequent intervals to decrease moisture and maceration of the incision site. While stitches are in, some physicians prefer dry heat from a heating lamp or hair dryer, and later, perineal packs or soaks. Plastic tubes are removed around the fifth day.

A low-residue diet will prevent straining on defecation and wound contamination. Of particular concern is urethral and catheter care, inasmuch as an indwelling catheter is usually in place. The incidence of infection is high, which emphasizes the need for the best in nursing intervention. Many nursing researchers frown on the use of sitz baths for vulvectomy patients because of the likelihood of reinfecting the wound.

Analgesics are given as required for comfort. Since primary healing rarely occurs, debridement is usually performed to provide satisfactory conditions for healing by secondary intention. Because the healing process is slow and the nature of the surgery is often disquieting to a female patient, she is apt to be discouraged. The nurse must be aware of the patient's uneasiness about being "caught" unduly exposed when visitors arrive or someone enters the room. She will tend to be sensitive and apologetic about odors. Thus, cleanliness, deodorant sprays, immediate removal of soiled dressings, and adequate ventilation contribute to a more pleasant environment.

Posthospital care requires giving complete instructions to the community nurse or family member who will care for this patient at home. Gradual resumption of physical and social activities is to be encouraged. The cure rate of properly treated vulvar carcinoma is 50% to 60%. In the absence of lymph node metastasis, the cure rate is around 85% to 90%.

▶ Evaluation

Expected Outcomes

1. Establishes control over and possible elimination of pruritus and dyspareunia
   a. Accepts the surgical therapeutic plan
   b. Maintains cleanliness of the perineum
   c. Utilizes the assistance of prescribed medications when necessary
   d. Explains the process of gradual weaning from prescribed medications
   e. Relates the necessity of following medical directives regarding sexual relations
2. Tolerates surgery with the least inconvenience and a minimum of complications
   a. Takes prescribed medications for discomfort and preoperative relaxation
   b. Participates in cleansing the perineal area
   c. Utilizes available resources in coping with and alleviating emotional stress
   d. Asks questions relating to postoperative expectations
3. Is free of complications
   a. Reports undue discomfort along incision line, as well as general discomfort
   b. Begins to move with a minimum of discomfort
   c. Becomes increasingly active physically, as required to enhance circulation
   d. Maintains cleanliness of site following micturition or defecation
   e. Verbalizes feelings of self-assurance
   f. Forecasts her ability to become self-sufficient
4. Is able to avoid spread of the disease process
   a. Relates accurately the signs and symptoms of infection
   b. Practices clean technique following perineal toilet requirements
   c. Demonstrates the procedure of taking a sitz bath (if prescribed)
   d. Identifies the kinds of garments to avoid or to wear and the rationale for this
   e. Keeps follow-up appointments

5. Adjusts psychosocially to the vulvar problem
    a. Participates in self-care activities
    b. Demonstrates interest in appearance
    c. Applies own cosmetics
    d. Selects garments according to personal preference
    e. Expresses happiness when mate visits
    f. Asks about sexual relations: time, type, possible problems
    g. Identifies signs and symptoms of possible problems and to whom these are to be reported

▷ Conditions of the Vagina

Fistulas of the Vagina

A *fistula* is an abnormal, winding opening between two internal hollow organs or between an internal hollow organ and the exterior of the body. The name of the fistula indicates the two areas that are connected abnormally: a *ureterovaginal fistula* is an opening between the ureter and vagina; a *vesicovaginal fistula,* an opening between the bladder and the vagina; and a *rectovaginal fistula,* an opening between the rectum and the vagina (Fig. 46-1). Fistulas may occur congenitally, but in the adult, breakdown often occurs because of tissue damage resulting from an invasive carcinoma.

Assessment and Clinical Manifestations. A fistula may develop inadvertently following vaginal surgery. It is not common, but the signs are important to detect. The immediate problem becomes one of infection and resulting excoriation. For example, the patient who has a vesicovaginal fistula has a continuous trickling of urine into the vagina. With a rectovaginal fistula, there is fecal incontinence, and flatus is discharged through the vagina. When such a discharge combines with a leukorrhea, a malodorous condition develops that is difficult to control.

Methylene blue dye can be used to delineate the course of the fistula. In vesicovaginal fistula, the dye is instilled into the bladder and appears in the vagina. Following a negative methylene blue test, indigo carmine is injected intravenously; if the dye appears in the vagina, a ureterovaginal fistula is indicated.

Management. The goal is to eliminate the fistula, thereby also controlling infection and excoriation. Frequently, a fistula will heal without surgical intervention. Healing of the tissues is promoted by proper nutrition with an increase in vitamin C and protein, by local cleanliness through douching and enemas, by rest, and by intestinal antibiotics. A rectovaginal fistula will heal faster if the patient is placed on a low-residue diet and if proper drainage of affected tissues is initiated. Sometimes a temporary colostomy is required to keep the site relatively clean; also, a surgical repair of the fistula may be performed, if necessary. If the person is older, more rest is required than in most postoperative patients because of a higher incidence of debilitation and the delicate as well as sensitive nature of the tissues. Warm perineal irrigations and controlled heat-lamp treatments are effective in stimulating the healing process.

For the patient who has had repair of a vesicovaginal fistula, an indwelling catheter is usually inserted. Drainage from the catheter is observed carefully, and care is taken to ensure that the catheter is functioning properly. If the catheter becomes clogged, urine may collect in the bladder, causing pressure that may damage the repaired tissue. Bladder irrigation and vaginal irrigations are done gently, with minimal pressure.

Effective measures to assist the woman whose fistula cannot be repaired must be planned on an individual basis. Cleanliness, frequent sitz baths, and deodorizing douches are required, as well as the use of perineal pads and protective undergarments. Particular attention to skin care is necessary to prevent excoriation. Bland creams or a light dusting of cornstarch may be soothing. Morale boosters and

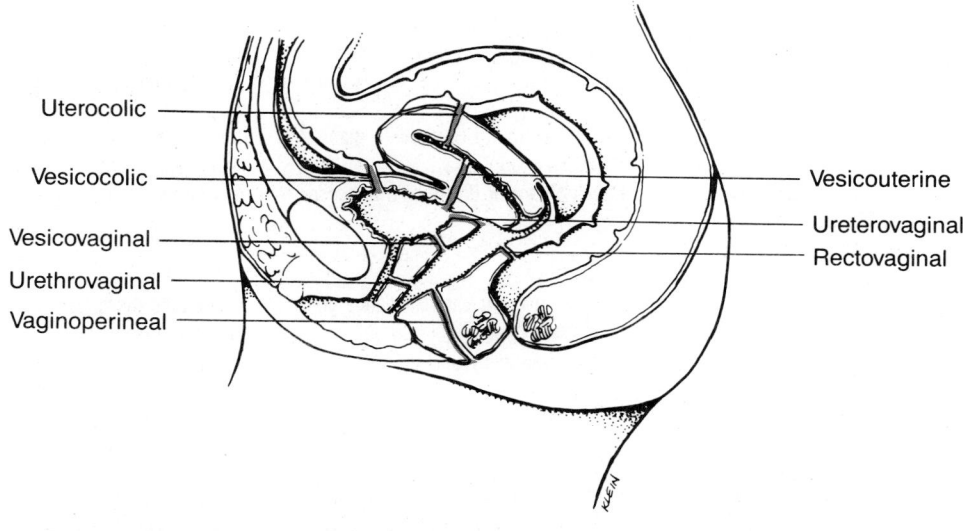

Figure 46-1. Common sites for fistulas.

attention to the social and psychological needs of this patient are essential components of effective care.

Vaginal Infection

See Table 46-1 (below).

Leukorrhea and Simple Vaginitis. *Leukorrhea* is a whitish vaginal discharge; in slight amount it is considered normal at the time of ovulation, just prior to the menarche or onset of menstruation. The vagina is protected from infection by its acid secretion (*p*H 3.5 to 4.5) and the presence of Döderlein's bacilli. If the resistance of the patient is lowered and organisms such as *Escherichia coli,* staphylococci, and streptococci invade the vagina, a more profuse and yellowish mucoid discharge is present, and a simple *vaginitis* or inflammation of the lining of the vaginal wall develops. Often vaginitis is accompanied by urethritis because of the proximity of the urethra to the vagina. The discharge may cause itching, redness, burning, and edema, which may be aggravated by voiding and defecation.

Treatment may be directed toward enhancing the natural flora of the vagina. This can be accomplished by a weak acid douche, 15 ml of vinegar to 1 liter of warm water (1 tablespoon of white vinegar to 1 quart of warm water). In addition, beta lactose, a sugar, can be administered as a vaginal suppository. Upon insertion into the vagina, the suppository dissolves with body heat; the sugar then stimulates the growth of Döderlein's bacilli. An additional objective is to initiate chemotherapy. Local intravaginal applications may be dispensed from a tube with an applicator. The applicator is inserted into the vagina, and medication is expressed in the desired amount. Hydrocortisone vulvar ointment or cream may be applied locally after douching or sitz baths, as prescribed for symptomatic relief of itching. Cleanliness after voiding and defecation is stressed. During menstrual periods, tampons are preferred, since pads often cause chafing.

Trichomoniasis (Trichomonas Vaginitis). *Trichomonas vaginalis* is a protozoan that is a common inhabitant of the vaginal tract. In some instances, however, when the normal *p*H, secretions, or mucosa are altered, an overgrowth of this

Table 46-1
Vaginal Infections

Condition	Cause	Assessment and Clinical Manifestations	Management Goals
Trichomoniasis	*Trichomonas vaginalis* (protozoan)	Inflammation of vaginal epithelium, producing burning and itching Frothy yellowish white or yellowish brown vaginal discharge	To remove exudate, relieve inflammation, restore acidity, and reestablish normal bacterial flora; oral Flagyl For stubborn infections; oral plus vaginal Flagyl For recurrence: repeat treatment, and include sexual partner Some prefer vinegar douche followed by Floraquin vaginal tablets
Monilial infection	*Candida albicans* (fungus)	Inflammation of vaginal epithelium producing itching, reddish irritation White, cheeselike discharge clinging to epithelium	To eradicate the fungus: local applications of gentian violet; Mycostatin vaginal suppositories To relieve other causative factors: stop antibiotic therapy; determine if diabetes or other systemic disease is present
Infection of Bartholin's gland (greater vestibular gland)	*Escherichia coli* *Trichomonas vaginalis* Staphylococcus Streptococcus Gonococcus	Erythema around Bartholin's gland Swelling and edema Development of Bartholin's abscess	To drain the abscess: antibiotic therapy; surgical drainage; excision of gland in patients with chronic bartholinitis
Cervicitis—acute and chronic	Gonorrhea Streptococcus Many pathogenic bacteria	Profuse purulent vaginal discharge Backache Urinary frequency and urgency	To determine the cause: cytologic examination of cervical smear To eradicate the gonococcus, if present: penicillin (as directed) or spectinomycin or tetracycline, if patient is allergic to penicillin To eradicate other causes: cervical cauterization
Postmenopausal vaginitis (atrophic vaginitis)	Lack of estrogen effects	Loss of redness, tissue folds, and epithelial covering of the vagina Itching and burning	To provide estrogen therapy for vaginal epithelialization: topical estrogen therapy; improve nutrition

organism occurs. If trichomoniasis is transferred sexually, the male may be the asymptomatic carrier who harbors the organisms in his urogenital tract and causes reinfection of his partner. The vaginal discharge is thin, frothy yellow to yellow–brown, malodorous, and very irritating. An accompanying vulvitis may result, with intense vulvovaginal burning and itching. In some women, the problem tends to become chronic. It is diagnosed by microscopic detection of the pear-shaped, mobile, flagellate organisms.

The most effective treatment appears to be metronidazole (Flagyl), given as a tablet orally three times a day with meals for 7 days. For stubborn infections, oral therapy is combined with a vaginal insert of the same medication. Some clinics suggest treating the patient and her sexual partner in 1 day by giving them one or two concentrated doses of Flagyl, under physician supervision. Some patients complain of an unpleasant but temporary metallic taste when taking metronidazole. Also, some note nausea and vomiting, as well as a hot and flushed feeling when this medication is taken in combination with an alcoholic beverage. In view of these possible side-effects, the patient should be advised not to take alcohol while on the drug. Because of the tumor-causing potential of metronidazole (this aspect is under investigation), this drug is not recommended for women who are pregnant.

Moniliasis (Candidiasis). *Monilial vaginitis* is a fungal infection caused by *Candida albicans*. It is seen commonly in patients with poorly controlled diabetes mellitus, which supports the fact that this fungus thrives in an environment rich in carbohydrate. *Candida (Monilia)* is also found in patients who have been on antibiotic or steroid therapy for a while, since these medications probably reduce the number of natural protective organisms usually present in the vaginal tract.

In a recent study, Miles found that if *C. albicans* was cultured from the vagina, it was *always* found in the stool. Conversely, if it was not isolated from the stool, it was *never* found in the vagina. This strong correlation suggests that elimination of vaginitis cannot be achieved on a permanent basis unless special attention is directed to the gastrointestinal tract.

The vaginal discharge is irritating, watery, and tenacious, and may contain white, cheesy particles. The discharge causes itching and sometimes severe vaginitis. White material may be noted adhering to the vaginal walls.

Management. The goal is to eliminate this infection. Assessment of the patient includes identifying any underlying factors that may contribute to the overgrowth of monilial organisms, such as pregnancy, diabetes, or estrogenic or oral contraceptive medications. In most cases, this organism can also be cultured from the intestinal tract. The patient should be informed that excessive moisture and chafing (such as may result from perspiration and tight garments, panty hose, etc.) may contribute to the problem.

The medication of choice is nystatin (Mycostatin). Since antifungal medications are not absorbed from the intestinal tract, vaginal nystatin suppositories are usually prescribed twice daily for 10 to 14 days. Antiseptic medications, such as Propion Gel, which contains calcium and sodium propionate, are also useful. Since clinical manifestations frequently disappear early in the course of treatment, it is desirable to do a follow-up culture 4 to 6 weeks after treatment is discontinued. A few patients have annoying recurrences. In some instances, a male sex partner is found to have symptomatic balanitis. By treating this, and extending the length of treatment of nystatin, the infection may be cleared. For the diabetic patient, efforts are directed toward controlling the diabetes.

Atrophic Vaginitis. A common postmenopausal occurrence is atrophy of the vaginal mucosa, which then becomes more prone to infection. An annoying vaginal discharge causes itching and burning. Treatment is similar to that of simple vaginitis. In addition, estrogenic hormones, taken orally or applied locally as an ointment, are effective in restoring epithelium.

Herpes Virus Type 2 Infection (Herpes Genitalis, Herpes Simplex Virus [HSV])

Herpes genitalis is a viral infection that causes herpetic (blisters) lesions on the cervix, vagina, and external genitalia; it is a sexually transmitted disease (STD).

This form of herpes is receiving considerable attention from health care providers and consumers because of its increasing prevalence (about 400,000–500,000 new cases each year). Not only is the infection painful, but it can recur and affect future well-being. There is no cure at present; nevertheless, the condition requires accurate diagnosis, effective care, and specific measures to prevent possible complications.

Etiology. Of the known herpes viruses, five affect humans: herpes simplex type 1 (HSV-1), herpes simplex type 2 (HSV-2), varicella zoster, Epstein–Barr, and cytomegalovirus. Herpes simplex type 2 appears to be the causative virus in over 80% of genital and perineal lesions; about 20% are HSV-1. Close human contact, skin to skin, seems necessary to acquire the infection.

▶ **Assessment**

Clinical Manifestations. The nursing history, including sexual history, a physical examination, and laboratory tests are essential for adequate assessment. At first, the vesicular state may appear as a pimple, which later coalesces, ulcerates, and encrustates. Itching and pain accompany the process as the area becomes red and edematous. In the female, the cervix is the usual primary site, and then possibly the labia, vulva, vagina, and perianal skin. The male is affected on the glans penis, foreskin, and penile shaft. Inguinal lymphadenopathy, temperature elevation, malaise, headache, and dysuria are noted. In the female, secondary bacterial infection may be evident as leukorrhea becomes a purulent discharge.

Within 1 to 4 weeks the lesions disappear, but the virus remains in the body, making recurrences common. Symptoms at this stage for the female are leukorrhea, abnormal bleeding, vaginal pain, and dyspareunia.

▶ **Planning and Nursing Implementation**

The goals of treatment are to prevent the spread of infection, make the patient comfortable, decrease potential health risks, be supportive, and initiate a counseling and education program.

It is significant to note that cervical cancer is higher in women who have had cervical herpes. For the pregnant woman, babies delivered vaginally may become infected with the virus; there is significant fetal morbidity and mortality.

Initial intervention is primarily supportive and directed toward symptomatic relief. By the patient taking frequent sitz baths, the lesions are kept clean. A topical anesthetic such as lidocaine cream or jelly is effective. A gel of 2-deoxy-D-glucose has been effective in providing relief of pain and dysuria in 12–72 hours. Acyclovir (Zovirax*) is a new drug that, while not curative, appears to reduce the healing time of painful blisters and shortens the infectious stage. Antibacterial agents assist in combating secondary infections.

If there is considerable pain and malaise, bed rest may be required. It is necessary to assess the fluid intake of the patient, the presence of bladder distention, and the frequency of voiding. Adequate fluid intake is encouraged; voiding is assisted by pouring warm water over the vulva. Such measures will help in preventing urinary retention and infection.

Patient Education.   Counseling and health education are an essential part of care for the individual with herpes genitalis. She should have an understanding of the nature of the virus and its transmission in order to avoid spreading the infection. Recurrence varies from once a month to once every 6 months. It is recommended that sexual contact be avoided during prodromal symptoms (itching, burning, pain) and until a week to 10 days after the lesions heal.

Because of a higher incidence of female patients showing cervical dysplasia and carcinoma, routine Pap smears should be done every 6 months to 1 year.

The patient's mate may wish to be included in counseling sessions. Keeping up with the latest information is stressed since much research is being directed to this condition. Additional resources include the American Social Health Association (ASHA), P.O. Box 100, Palo Alto, California 94302. Quarterly newsletter: The Helper. Telephone hot line: 1–800–227–8922 (24 hours).

The DES (Diethylstilbestrol) Syndrome

Prior to 1970, carcinoma of the vagina was considered to be a condition that occurred predominantly in the postmenopausal woman. However, in the early 1970s a research study revealed that seven adolescent women had developed adenocarcinoma of the vagina. Further investigation revealed that a common factor existed in such instances—maternal ingestion of diethylstilbestrol (DES). Subsequent studies of a large number of female offspring of women who had received DES during pregnancy showed that characteristic benign genital tract abnormalities had occurred in the majority of those young women who were exposed *in utero*. Follow-up studies continue in an effort to determine whether the benign changes noted represent premalignant lesions, and what percentage of such exposed young women are at risk

for developing malignancies. As part of this ongoing research, daughters of women who took DES are encouraged to have regular vaginal and rectal examinations and possibly culposcopy. Confirmation of the history of exposure to DES is sought through pharmacy and medical records. Pap smears are recommended every 6 months until several are negative, then they are done annually. Young women with dysfunctional bleeding should be checked for possible vaginal malignancy. In many instances, dysplasia noted in one examination had disappeared when the patient was examined subsequently. These women are to be advised to minimize their intake of estrogen preparations.

Although oral contraceptives and DES preparations, taken as lactation suppressives or "morning-after" pills, are not contraindicated, a special task force of the United States Department of Health and Human Services suggests that "the decision to use them should be made only after careful consideration of alternate methods of contraception, patient preference and medical judgment." The task force also recommended that administration of postmenopausal or perimenopausal replacement estrogens should be discouraged and that these substances should be given only to women who have "severe symptoms of the menopausal syndrome that cannot be controlled by other means, for the minimal duration necessary."†

Toxic Shock Syndrome

Toxic shock syndrome (TSS) is a condition caused by a bacterial toxin (*Staphylococcus aureus*); it is usually associated with women under age 30 who are menstruating and use tampons. However, it has occurred less frequently in nonmenstruating women and in men. First identified about 1975, TSS claimed national attention in 1980.

▶ **Assessment**
Clinical Manifestations.   In an otherwise healthy individual, the onset of TSS occurs with a sudden fever up to 38.9° C (102° F), vomiting, diarrhea, myalgia, hypotension, and signs suggesting the onset of shock. An erythematous macular rash often develops. In some patients, this rash makes its first appearance on the body, and in others, it first appears on the hands (palms and fingers) and feet (soles and toes); it may then desquamate in a week to 10 days.

Urine output is decreased and urea nitrogen becomes elevated; such urinary dysfunction may initiate disorientation. Respiratory distress syndrome or signs of "shock lung" have been reported due to pulmonary edema. Hyperemia of mucous membranes may also occur. Blood studies indicate leukocytosis and elevated bilirubin, urea nitrogen, and creatine phosphokinase.

Patient Problems/Nursing Diagnoses

Based on the clinical manifestations, the nursing history, and the diagnostic assessment data, the patient's major nursing problems include acute illness related to sudden onset,

---

* Burroughs Wellcome Company.

† DHEW, FDA Drug Bulletin 8:31, Oct–Nov 1978.

high fever, and rapid progression toward shock; dehydration related to fever and loss of fluids (diarrhea and vomiting); respiratory impairment related to the possibility of shock lung and bronchopneumonia; toxicity (sepsis) related to bacterial infection; anxiety and emotional stress related to sudden onset of acute illnes; and potential development of complications.

▶ **Planning and Nursing Implementation**

Goals

The major goals for the patient include:

1. Recovery from disorientation
2. Respiratory comfort and ease of breathing
3. Absence of fever
4. Control of infection
5. Reduction of anxiety and emotional stress
6. Absence of complications
7. Avoidance of a repetition of this experience

To assist the patient in meeting these goals, the major objectives of therapy are to (1) assess accurately and document the rapidly changing vital signs and symptoms, (2) treat shock, (3) alleviate respiratory embarrassment, (4) control the infection, (5) rehydrate the patient, (6) reduce emotional stressors, (7) educate the patient concerning potential toxic practices (careful use of intracavitary [vaginal] absorbent agents).

Nursing Interventions. Adequate ventilation is necessary for life, therefore, sufficient oxygenation and adequate lung function may require intubation and ventilation. Blood gases, vital signs, and the monitoring of fluid and ventilatory therapy is necessary throughout the acute phase of this illness.

Careful observation and documentation of skin changes, as well as fluid intake and loss, are required. It is also essential to understand the meaning of laboratory results since these can suggest improvement or worsening of infection, dehydration, and kidney and respiratory function. Cultures are taken of all body excretions and of the nose, throat, vagina, and cervix. The result of these will assist the physician in prescribing appropriate antibiotic therapy.

Since disseminated intravascular coagulation (DIC) has been observed in patients with TSS, it is essential for the nurse to be observant for hematomas; petechiae; oozing from needle puncture sites; cyanosis; and coolness of the nose, finger tips, and toes.

Patient Education. Since the use of tampons during menstruation has been linked with TSS, it is recommended that super-absorbent tampons not be used. If tampons are used, alternate their use with pads. Change tampons frequently and do not leave in place longer than 8 hours. Insert tampons carefully to avoid abrasions; some applicators have rough edges, which are to be avoided. All incidents of TSS are to be reported to the Centers for Disease Control.*

---

* Attention: Special Pathogens Branch, Bacterial Diseases Bureau of Epidemiology, Atlanta, Georgia 30333. Phone: (404) 329–3687.

▶ **Evaluation**

Expected Outcomes

1. Recovers from disorientation
   a. Has no subjective complaint of confusion or disorientation
   b. Verbalizes where she is (identifies the hospital and unit)
   c. Responds appropriately when addressed
   d. Carries out directives and answers questions as expected of one under normal conditions
2. Experiences respiratory comfort and ease of breathing
   a. Has respirations within normal limits
   b. Is free of dyspnea
   c. Exhibits nailbeds and general color indicative of normal tissue oxygenation
3. Has no fever
   a. Has normal temperature
   b. Does not have flushed skin or perspiration
4. Has no infection
   a. Is free of hyperemia of mucous membranes
   b. Is free of purulent vaginal discharge
   c. Exhibits temperature within normal range
   d. Has white blood cell count within normal limits
5. Experiences a reduction of anxiety and emotional stress
   a. Expresses happiness about recovering and feeling better
   b. Relaxes comfortably with radio, music, or a good book; requests that her family be informed that she is "allright"
   c. Exhibits interest in dress and makeup
   d. Smiles easily and engages in pleasant talk
6. Is free of complications
   a. Has normal respiratory rate, rhythm, depth, and effort
   b. Eats a well-balanced diet
   c. Experiences little or no pain
   d. Exhibits vital signs within normal limits
   e. Has laboratory values that are within normal limits
   f. Is at ease, psychosocially
   g. Expresses desire to leave the hospital
   h. Complies with therapeutic regimen

▷ # Relaxation of Pelvic Muscles

Cystocele, Rectocele, Enterocele, and Laceration of the Perineum

Cystocele is a downward displacement of the bladder toward the vaginal orifice (Fig. 46-2). Occasionally, it is caused by tissue weakness, but most often it is a result of injuries received during childbirth. The condition appears some years later when genital atrophy associated with aging takes place.

Rectocele and lacerations of the perineum may occur as injuries to the muscles and the tissues of the pelvic floor and may happen at the time of childbirth. Because of tears in muscles below the vagina, the rectum may pouch upward, pushing the posterior wall of the vagina in front of it. This

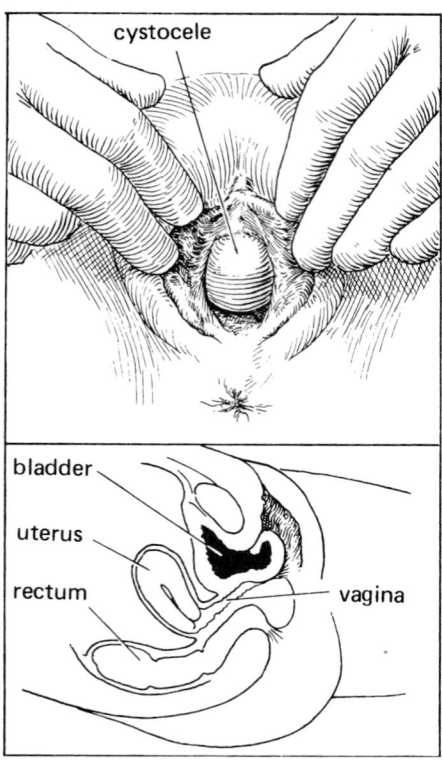

Figure 46-2. Cystocele. Relaxation of the anterior vaginal wall permits downward bulge of bladder on straining.

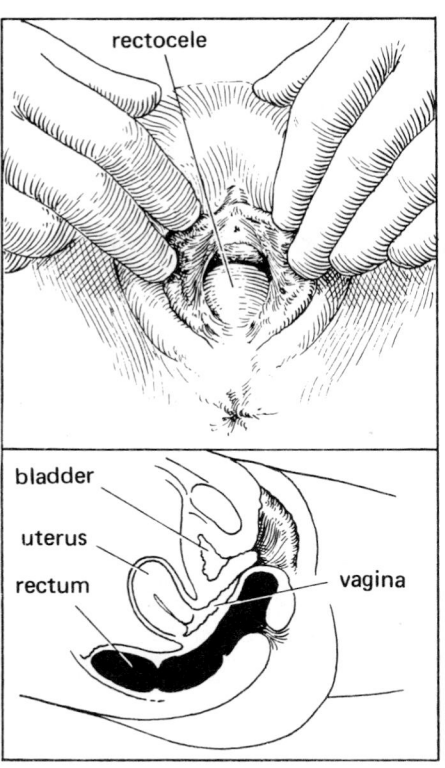

Figure 46-3. Rectocele. Relaxation of the posterior vaginal wall permits bulging of the rectum into the vagina on straining.

condition is termed a *rectocele* (Fig. 46-3). At times, the lacerations may extend to such a degree as to sever completely the fibers of the anal sphincter (complete tear). An *enterocele* is a protrusion of intestinal wall into the vagina.

▶ Assessment

Cystocele occurs as a bulging downward of the anterior vaginal wall that causes a sense of pelvic pressure, easy fatigue, and often such urinary symptoms as incontinence, frequency, and urgency of urination.

The symptoms of rectocele are similar to those given for cystocele, with one exception—instead of urinary symptoms, the patient experiences constipation and incontinence of gas and liquid feces when complete tears have occurred.

Patient Problems/Nursing Diagnoses

Based on the clinical manifestations and diagnostic evaluation data, the patient's potential problems include a tendency to procrastinate being examined by a gynecologist related to an expectation that in time the condition will take care of itself and to a belief that this is a natural and acceptable consequence of childbearing; psychosocial problems, including disrupted sex life related to annoying symptoms such as incontinence, frequency, etc.; and potential development of complications related to failure in seeking professional assistance.

▶ Planning and Nursing Implementation

Goals

The major goals for the patient include:

1. Elimination of uncomfortable and annoying problems due to relaxed pelvic muscles
2. Acceptance of and preparation for surgical intervention, if indicated
3. Relief of disturbing symptoms and discomfort
4. Absence of complications
5. Improvement in psychosocial experiences.

The chief problem is to encourage women with these problems to see a gynecologist. There is a tendency to procrastinate, to feel embarrassed, to expect that in time the condition will take care of itself, or to even believe that this is a natural consequence of childbearing that has to be accepted. Women need to know that the condition can become more restrictive; it cannot cure itself, but can lead to such complications as infections, cervical ulceration, cystitis, hemorrhoids, and other problems.

Surgical Treatment. The treatment of cystocele is surgical, the operation for the repair of the anterior vaginal wall being termed *anterior colporrhaphy*. Perineal exercises are sometimes prescribed and help to strengthen the weakened muscles. These are more effective in the early stages of a cystocele. If surgery is contraindicated, or refused, a pessary may be used. Such a device may be prescribed for mild problems.

A *pessary* is a device inserted in the upper vagina and positioned to assist in keeping an organ, such as the bladder, uterus, or intestine, in proper alignment. It is usually shaped as a ring or doughnut and is made of a variety of materials, such as rubber or plastic. The size and type of pessary are selected and fitted by the gynecologist. The patient can be taught to remove the pessary at bedtime and to reinsert it in the morning. If it remains in place and is not removed by the patient, she should have it removed, checked, and cleaned by the physician or nurse practitioner periodically. At this time, tissues need to be inspected for pressure points or signs of irritation. Normally, there is no pain, discomfort, or discharge with its use. Douching may be recommended if there is a discharge.

The operation for the repair of rectocele and lacerations of the perineum is called a *perineorrhaphy* or a *posterior colporrhaphy*.

Preoperative Management.   Before vaginal surgery, the patient needs to know the extent of the proposed surgery, the expectations for the postoperative period, and the effect of surgery on future sexual functions. Often, a clean, voided specimen is required. If so, the patient is asked to clean her perineum, spread the labia, and void into a sterile bedpan. The specimen is then transferred to a sterile bottle.

In the operating room, special attention is given to placing both of the patient's legs in and out of stirrups simultaneously in order to prevent muscular strain and excess pressure on the legs and thighs. Other preoperative details are similar to that described on page 349.

Postoperative Nursing Management and Rehabilitation. In the postoperative period, the immediate goals are to prevent infection and pressure on the suture line. This will require perineal care and may preclude the use of dressings. The patient is always urged to void within a few hours after operations for cystocele and complete tear. If the patient does not void within this period, feels uncomfortable, or has pain in the region of the bladder after 6 hours, catheterization is performed. Some physicians prefer to have an indwelling catheter in place for 2 to 4 days. There are various other methods of bladder care, as described in Chapter 43.

After each urination or bowel movement, the perineum is irrigated with warm sterile saline (see vulvar douche, p. 1028) and the area blotted dry with sterile cotton.

There are several methods used in caring for the sutures. In one method, the sutures are left alone until healing occurs (*i.e.,* for 5 to 10 days). Thereafter, daily vaginal douches of sterile saline are given during the period of convalescence. In another method—the wet method—small douches of sterile saline are given twice daily, beginning on the day after operation and continuing throughout convalescence. Of course, the method to be used depends on the preference of the surgeon.

A heat lamp may be used to help dry the area and enhance the healing process. Commercially available sprays containing a combination of antiseptic and anesthetic so-

lutions are soothing and effective. An ice pack applied locally may relieve discomfort. For effective relief of this type, a plastic bag can be filled with ice chips. However, the weight of the bag must rest on the bed, and not on the patient.

The routine postoperative care is much like that for an abdominal operation. The patient is placed in bed, with the head and the knees elevated slightly. A liquid diet (many surgeons omit milk) is given on the first day, and then a full diet as soon as desired.

After an operation for a complete perineal laceration (through the rectal sphincter), special care and attention are required. The bladder is emptied by catheterization if the patient is experiencing discomfort. She should be kept flat in bed, with the head raised on a pillow. Most surgeons prefer that the patient have no bowel movements for 5 to 7 days to prevent strain on the incision site. A rectal tube should not be introduced during this period, and enemas are restricted. Liquid diet without milk is given, and medication to reduce peristalsis and inhibit bowel function may be prescribed. On the sixth or seventh day, 30 ml (1 ounce) of mineral oil are given, followed, at the first inclination for a bowel movement, by a small oil enema, 90 ml to 120 ml (3 or 4 ounces), which should be retained for a few minutes.

Throughout the convalescence of all patients who have had plastic surgery, liquid petrolatum or another stool-softening agent is given each night after the patient is permitted a soft diet. Instructions are given regarding douching and when to return to see the gynecologist.

Perineal exercises may be recommended to assist in strengthening muscles. The patient is instructed as follows: tense the perineal muscles by pressing the buttocks together; hold this position; relax. This exercise, done 10 to 20 times each hour, can be performed while the person is sitting or standing.

▶ Evaluation

Expected Outcomes

1. Obtains help to eliminate uncomfortable and annoying problems due to relaxed pelvic muscles
   a. Makes appointment with a gynecologist to diagnose specifically the problem and to plan possible treatment
   b. Participates willingly in providing information for her health history
   c. Relates to her mate the hope that the planned surgical repair will help their relations
   d. Practices perineal exercises
   e. Accepts plan for surgical correction
2. Accepts and prepares for surgical intervention
   a. Verbalizes the need for an operation
   b. Participates in preoperative preparation
   c. Accepts medications prescribed preoperatively
   d. Describes the kinds of exercises she is expected to do postoperatively
   e. Asks questions relating to postoperative care
3. Obtains relief of disturbing symptoms and discomfort
   a. Experiences no discomfort and pain
   b. Has no need for p.r.n. analgesics

c. Controls urination
d. Experiences no limitation in physical activity
e. Practices perineal exercises to strengthen muscles
4. Is free of complications
   a. Moves with minimal discomfort
   b. Practices proper cleansing techniques following urination and defecation
   c. Becomes increasingly active physically
   d. Recounts the signs and symptoms that may suggest the beginning of a complication which need to be reported to a health care person
5. Recounts an improvement in psychosocial experiences
   a. Participates in self-care activities
   b. Asks questions relative to resuming sexual relations with mate
   c. Takes time for attractive grooming (hairstyle, cosmetics, clothes)
   d. Talks positively to her husband about future plans

Displacements of the Uterus

The uterus lies normally with the cervix at right angles to the long axis of the vagina and with the body of the uterus inclined slightly forward. However, it is freely movable, due to the requirements of pregnancy. The strain of this physiologic function, the formation of adhesions, or a weakening of its natural supports may produce changes in the normal position of the uterus that usually cause no severe problems to the patient, but may give rise to many troublesome symptoms.

Backward Displacements.   (See Fig. 46-4.) Backward displacements (*retroversion* and *retroflexion*) of the uterus may give rise to such symptoms as backache, a sense of pelvic pressure, easy fatigue, and leukorrheal discharge. Most retrograde displacements are asymptomatic.

Surgery for backward displacements of the uterus is

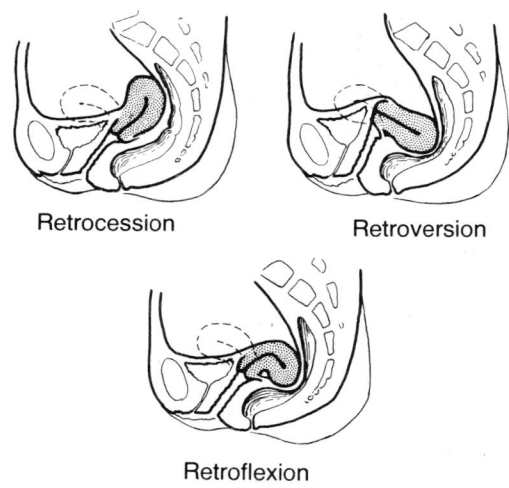

Retrocession   Retroversion

Retroflexion

Figure 46-4.   Retrodisplacements of the uterus. (From Hardy JD: Rhoads Textbook of Surgery. Philadelphia, JB Lippincott.)

carried out only if the condition is incapacitating. An abdominal incision allows access to the uterus, which is brought forward into its normal position and is then maintained there by shortening its ligaments. Some patients with retroversion may be treated by the use of *pessaries*. These are instruments of hard rubber or crystal-clear Plexiglas that maintain the uterus in a forward position by exerting pressure on ligaments attached to the posterior wall of the cervix (Fig. 46-5). They are of great value as a test of the patient's symptoms, and often effect a cure. Pessaries must be removed and cleaned at frequent intervals.

Prolapse and Procidentia.   (See Fig. 46-6.) Due to the weakening of the supports of the uterus, most often brought about by childbirth, the uterus may work its way down the vaginal canal (*prolapse*) and even appear outside the vaginal orifice (*procidentia*).

In its descent, the uterus pulls with it the vaginal walls and even the bladder and the rectum. The symptoms caused are similar to those mentioned for backward displacements, plus urinary symptoms (incontinence and retention) from displacement of the bladder. These symptoms are aggravated when the woman coughs, lifts a heavy object, or stands for a long while. Normal activities are troublesome tasks; even walking up the steps may aggravate the problem. The nurse can encourage women who have such difficulties to seek medical attention, because time is not likely to correct the problem.

The best treatment is operative. The uterus is sutured back into place, and repair work is done to strengthen and tighten muscle bands. In postmenopausal women, the uterus may be removed (hysterectomy). For elderly women or those who are too ill to stand the strain of surgery, pessaries may be the treatment of choice.

▷ Conditions of the Uterus

Abnormal Uterine Bleeding

Menorrhagia.   *Menorrhagia* is excessive bleeding at the time of the regular menstrual flow. In early life, it may be due to endocrine disturbances, but with increase in duration of the menstrual periods in later life, it is usually due to inflammatory disturbances or tumors of the uterus. Emotional disturbance may also affect bleeding.

A woman with menorrhagia is encouraged to see her gynecologist and relate the nature of the excessive bleeding. Although difficult to measure, an estimate might be given in terms of numbers of pads or tampons used in excess of those used for the regular flow.

Metrorrhagia.   *Metrorrhagia* is the appearance of blood from the uterus between the regular menstrual periods or after menopause. It is always the symptom of some disease, often cancer or benign tumors of the uterus; therefore, it merits early diagnosis and treatment. Metrorrhagia is probably the most significant form of menstrual dysfunction; the amount of blood loss is not important, but the fact that it occurs warrants further investigation.

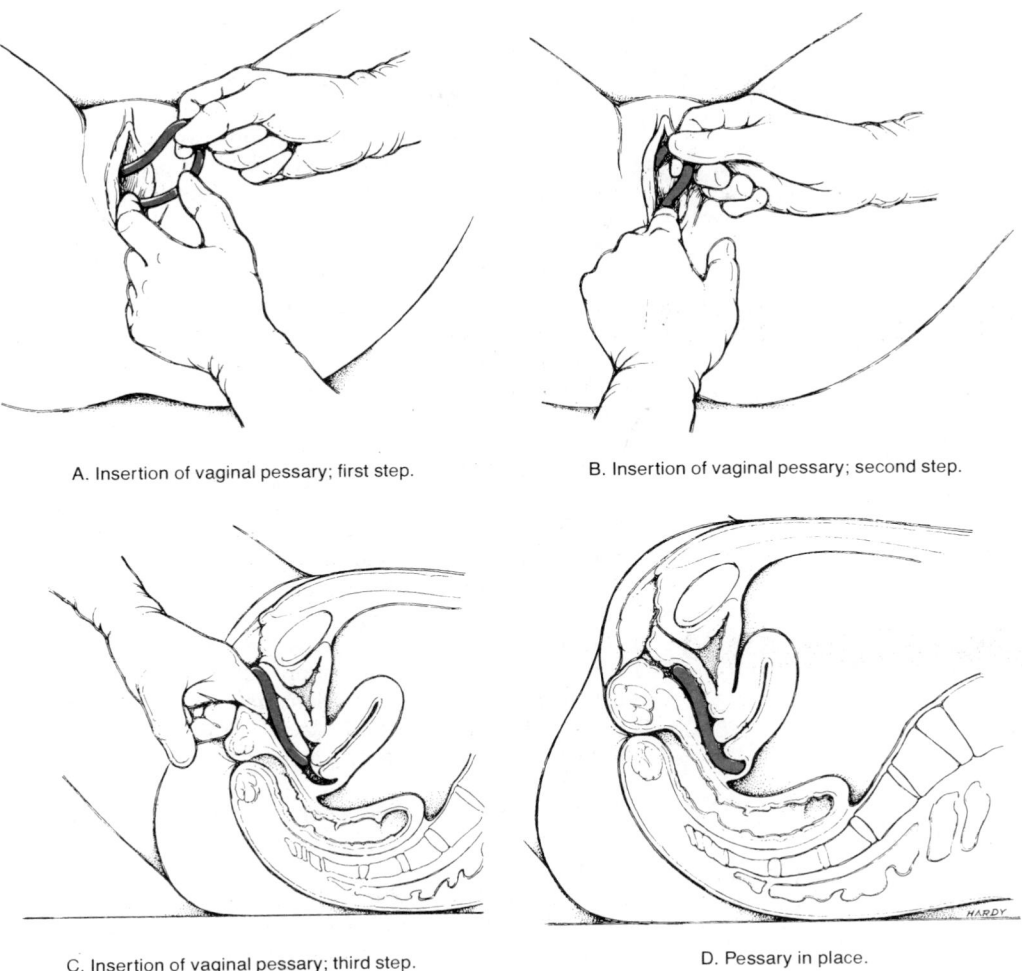

A. Insertion of vaginal pessary; first step.

B. Insertion of vaginal pessary; second step.

C. Insertion of vaginal pessary; third step.

D. Pessary in place.

Figure 46-5. Method of inserting a vaginal pessary. (Redrawn from Greenhill JB: Office Gynecology, 9th ed. Chicago, Year Book Medical Publishers, 1971. Used by permission.)

Lacerations of the Cervix

Lacerations of the cervix may occur as a result of childbirth. When healing takes place, a considerable portion of the mucous membrane, which normally lies in the cervical canal, is everted. It practically always becomes infected and causes an annoying leukorrhea. Most surgeons believe that cervical lacerations predispose to cancer of the cervix, and for this reason these lacerations should be repaired, particularly when the patient is in her 50s, when cancer is most likely to occur.

Dilatation and Curettage

A *dilatation and curettage* (D & C) is the widening of the cervical canal with a dilator and the scraping of the uterine endometrium with a curette. It is done to secure endometrial or endocervical tissue for cytologic examination, to control abnormal uterine bleeding, and as a therapeutic measure for incomplete abortion.

Since this procedure usually is carried out under anesthesia and requires surgical asepsis, it is performed in the operating room. Many gynecologists perform D & Cs under local anesthesia, supplemented with Valium or Demerol. Explanations as well as psychological and physical preparations are done by the nurse. The patient has a right to know what the procedure will involve (usually explained by her gynecologist) and what to expect in the way of postoperative discomfort, drainage, or incapacity. Many physicians do not require perineal shaving, but voiding and evacuation of the intestinal tract by a small enema are usually desired.

In the operating room, the patient is placed in the lithotomy position, the cervix is dilated with an instrument, and scrapings of the endometrium are obtained by means of a curette. Tissue for biopsy also may be obtained with an electric needle or a punch biopsy forceps. A cone of tissue may be obtained with a cautery or scalpel. Packing is placed in the cervical and vaginal canal, and a sterile perineal pad is placed over the perineum.

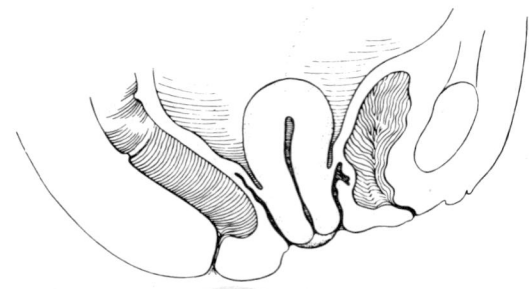

A. First-degree prolapse (cervix comes down to introitus)

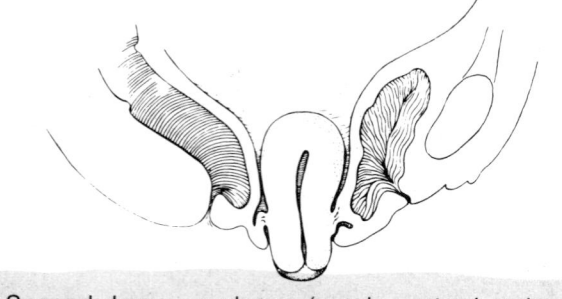

B. Second-degree prolapse (cervix protrudes through introitus)

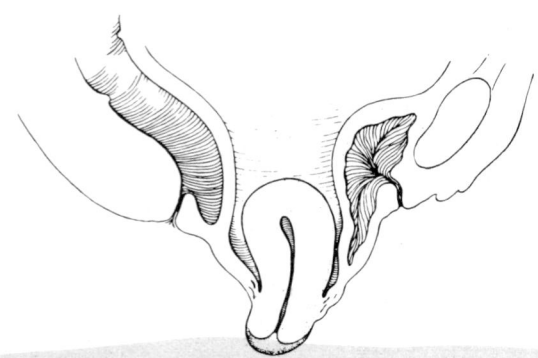

C. Third-degree prolapse—total procidentia (uterus protrudes through introitus)

Figure 46-6. Prolapse of the uterus and the vagina. (Adapted from Gray LA: Postgrad Med 30:209.)

After the operation, a sanitary belt is used to hold the pad in place. When the pad must be changed while the packing is still in place (usually 24 hours), it is replaced with a sterile pad. Evidence of excessive bleeding is reported. Following the operation, the patient remains in bed for the remainder of the day, although she may get up to go to the bathroom. No restrictions are placed on dietary intake. If pelvic discomfort or low back pain occurs, mild analgesics will usually suffice.

Endocervicitis

Endocervicitis is an inflammation of the mucosa and the glands of the cervix. It is a fairly common problem that may occur when organisms gain access to the cervical glands after abortion, intrauterine manipulation, or delivery. It is an infection that, if untreated, may extend into the uterus, tubes, and pelvic cavity. In the majority of patients, the inflammation is caused by the ordinary pyogenic organisms, but gonorrheal infection of the glands can occur.

Inflammation can cause erosion of the cervical tissue, resulting in spotting or bleeding. The chief symptom is leukorrheal discharge, at times associated with sacral backache, low abdominal pain, and urinary and menstrual disturbances.

Management.   Treatment should be preventive as well as curative. Prevention of gonorrhea will reduce the incidence of endocervicitis. Proper obstetric care can also prevent the occurrence of this condition. Delivery ought not to be attempted until the cervix completely dilates spontaneously; cervical lacerations should be repaired immediately.

Palliative treatment consists of douches and the application of antiseptics to the cervix, but often a cure is effected only after the cervical glands are destroyed with a cautery or after the diseased tissue is excised. Anesthesia may or may not be required since cauterization is a painless procedure. Following cauterization, the patient should rest more than usual for the next few days. The nature of vaginal discharge is explained to the patient so that she can expect a grayish green, malodorous discharge for up to 3 weeks, because of sloughing cervical tissue. A follow-up visit is recommended by the gynecologist in 2 to 3 weeks, when the cervix is checked for possible stenosis, which may require dilatation. Usually, 6 to 8 weeks are required for healing. Sexual relations are resumed upon recommendation of the physician.

For more severe chronic cervicitis, conization may be done, which may require overnight hospitalization. Anesthesia is optional. In the operating room, the tip of an electric instrument is inserted into the external os of the cervix and rotated to cut and coagulate a cone of tissue. Aftercare may require packing, but otherwise it is similar to that following electric cauterization. The patient should note any excess bleeding and report it to her physician.

Tumors of the Uterus

Leiomyomas ("Fibroids," Myomas, or Fibromyomas)

Myomatous or *fibroid tumors* of the uterus are benign tumors arising from the muscle tissue of the uterus. They are very common, occurring in about 30% to 40% of all women. They develop slowly between the ages of 25 and 40, and often become large in size after this period. There are instances in which such a tumor causes no symptoms. The most common symptom is menorrhagia. Other symptoms are due to pressure on the surrounding organs—pain, backache, constipation, and urinary symptoms. In addition, such tumors often cause metrorrhagia and even sterility.

Management.   The treatment of uterine fibroids depends to a large extent on their size and location. The patient with minor symptoms is watched closely. If she wishes to have children, treatment is as conservative as possible. As a rule, large tumors that produce pressure symptoms should be removed. Usually, the uterus is removed (hysterectomy), while the ovaries are preserved, if possible. If the tumor is small, it may be removed (myomectomy); the wound in the uterus is then closed. This is the procedure of choice in young women. If the tumor is producing excessive bleeding, the uterus and the tumor are removed (hysteromyomectomy).

Principles of nursing management of the patient having a hysterectomy are on page 1057.

Malignant Tumors of the Uterus

Incidence and Patient Education. Malignant tumors of the female reproductive system (excluding the breast) rank as the second cause of death in the United States, accounting for approximately 10,000 deaths yearly (uterine corpus and endometrium, 3,000; cervix, 7,000). By incidence, uterine cancer is the fourth leading cancer in women (after skin, breast, colon and rectum cancer). However, the death rate for uterine cancer has shown a steady decline in recent years because more women are being educated to seek annual checkups that include the Papanicolaou test. However, when it is realized that a significant number of women in the U.S. over the age of 20 have never had a Pap test, it is obvious that much remains to be done.

Why a woman who knows about the Papanicolaou test does not have it done is a question to be explored by all those concerned with community health. Are women who feel and look healthy afraid to "look for trouble?" Is getting to the clinic or physician inconvenient because of hours, transportation, or babysitting difficulties? Not only is the continued dissemination of information necessary, but it may be necessary for health personnel to "go more than halfway" in order to ensure the broadest possible application of this test. Perhaps a routine Papanicolaou test could be a required part of preemployment examinations, applications for marriage license, admissions to a hospital, and applications for insurance. Whatever measures are followed, an increase in the number of women having this simple, painless test will save lives that otherwise would be claimed by cancer.

There are two main types of primary uterine cancer—carcinoma of the cervix, which is predominantly epidermoid cancer, and carcinoma of the endometrium (corpus and body of the uterus). The incidence ratio of carcinoma of the cervix to carcinoma of the endometrium is 3 to 1.

Cancer of the Cervix

Cancer of the cervix is the most common cancer of the reproductive system in women. Although it rarely occurs before the age of 20, it is most common between the ages of 30 to 50. Statistics indicate that sexual activity has some relationship to the incidence of cancer of the cervix; before age 25, it is more prevalent in those who have had many sex partners and several pregnancies. Studies made on the incidence of cervical cancer among prostitutes also tend toward this conclusion.

Patient Education. Cervical cancer is almost always curable in its preinvasive state. Therefore, in an effort to discover the disease early, every woman over 20 years of age should have a complete gynecologic examination yearly. For the young woman under 20 who is sexually active, an annual Pap test is justified.

Although herpes simplex viral infection of the female genital tract has been tentatively linked to cervical carcinoma, this relationship has not been proven. Regular Pap smears will detect premalignant cervical dysplasia, so that women who have this type of infection and a positive Pap smear for premalignant cervical dysplasia are advised to have a subsequent checkup within 6 months.

Assessment and Clinical Manifestations. Early cancer of the cervix is usually asymptomatic. The two chief symptoms of early carcinoma of the cervix are leukorrhea and irregular vaginal bleeding or spotting. For a long time, leukorrhea may be the only abnormal symptom. The discharge increases gradually in amount and becomes watery and, finally, dark and foul-smelling because of necrosis and infection of the tumor mass. The bleeding occurs at irregular intervals, between periods (metrorrhagia) or after menopause. It may be very slight, just enough to spot the undergarments, and it is noted usually after some form of trauma (intercourse, douching, or defecation). As the disease continues, the bleeding may become constant and may increase in amount.

Chronic infections and erosions of the cervix seem to play a significant part in the development of cervical cancer. Such pathology becomes evident as a large cauliflowerlike growth or a deep, ulcerating crater before giving any symptoms of its presence.

As the cancer advances, the tissues outside the cervix may be invaded, including the lymph glands anterior to the sacrum. In one third of patients with invasive cervical cancer, the disease involves the fundus. The nerves in this region become involved, producing excruciating pain in the back and the legs that is relieved only by large doses of narcotics. The final picture, when untreated, is one of extreme emaciation and anemia, often with irregular fever due to secondary infection and abscesses in the ulcerating mass.

Surgical Management. Radiation is the most frequent form of treatment for invasive cervical cancer; however, radical pelvic surgical procedures may be required for the more advanced lesions. The method selected depends on the stage of the lesion (Table 46-2) and on the judgment and skill of the physician. Radical surgery is advocated by some authorities, especially when a patient is unable to withstand the effects of radiation or has a radiation-resistant cancer. Surgical procedures commonly carried out include the following:

Radical hysterectomy (Wertheim): An abdominal incision is made, and the uterus, adnexa, proximal vaginal, and bilateral lymph nodes are removed en masse.

Radical vaginal hysterectomy (Schauta): A vaginal approach is used to remove the uterus, adnexa, and proximal vagina.

Note: "Radical" used before each of the above procedures means that an extensive area of the paravaginal, paracervical, parametrial, and uterosacral tissues is removed with the uterus.

Bilateral pelvic lymphadenectomy: This is accomplished by removing the common iliac, external iliac, hypogastric, and obturator lymphatics and nodes.

Pelvic exenteration: See below.

Table 46-2

International Classification of Carcinoma of the Uterine Cervix

Stage of Lesion	Area	Description	Possible Therapy	Approximate Recovery Rate
Stage 0	Carcinoma *in situ*	Cancer limited to epithelial layer; no evidence of invasion	Conization—fertility is preserved Hysterectomy, when fertility is not a consideration	95%–100%
Stage I	Carcinoma strictly confined to cervix	Size is not a criterion		70%–85%
Stage IA		Microinvasive	Radiation therapy or surgery (depending on depth of invasion)	
Stage IB		Clinically obvious Stage I	Radiation therapy or surgery (depending on depth of invasion) Wertheim abdominal hysterectomy and pelvic lymphadenectomy or radical Schauta vaginal hysterectomy	
Stage II	Vaginal cancer	Lesion has spread beyond cervix to involve vagina (not lower third) or paracervical region on one or both sides		
Stage IIA		Vaginal extension only	Primary radiation therapy or primary radical therapy	65%–75%
Stage IIB		Paracervical extension with or without vaginal involvement	Primary radiation therapy; if this fails, pelvic exenteration may be required	50%–65%
Stage III	Cancer involves lower third of vagina or has extended to one or both pelvic walls	Unequivocal palpable lymph node disease on the pelvic wall IV pyelogram shows one or both ureters obstructed by the tumor	Primary treatment by radiation If bilateral obstruction exists and renal function is compromised, preliminary nephrostomy may be required	20%–30%
Stage IIIA		Extends to lower third of vagina only		
Stage IIIB		Isolated carcinomatous metastases are palpable on the pelvic wall		
Stage IV	Bladder extension	Evidence that carcinoma involves the bladder seen in cystoscopic examination or by presence of vesicovaginal fistula	Chance of cure by radiation is less than 5% Radical surgery (anterior, posterior, or total pelvic exenteration) may achieve a cure rate of 20%–25%	5%–10%
	Rectal extension Distant spread	Carcinoma spreads outside true pelvis to other organs		

Cancer of the Endometrium

Cancer of the endometrium (fundus or corpus) of the uterus has increased in incidence partly because of extended longevity and more accurate reporting. In the past, the ratio of cervical to endometrial cancer was about 8 to 1; now it is closer to 3 to 1. About 50% of all patients with postmenopausal bleeding have cancer of the fundus. Its progress is slow, metastasis occurs later, and the symptom of irregular vaginal bleeding often appears early enough in the disease to allow cure by removal of the uterus. In late metastasis, radium and roentgen rays are the usual therapeutic measures.

Heretofore, dilatation and curettage was the only means of early diagnosis. The Pap smear is inadequate because it alerts the physician only to about 25% of endometrial lesions; consequently, diagnosis is made only after the development of overt symptoms. Endometrial smears (see p. 1024) are more accurate and relatively inexpensive.

Not all patients qualify for the use of these diagnostic aids because of complicating factors, such as pelvic infection, stenosed cervix, or lack of cooperation on the part of the patient. However, they are helpful for those women who are unable to take the time to enter a hospital for a D & C, those for whom general anesthesia is not advisable, and those for whom a D & C must be repeated or has been unsuccessful.

The major emphasis for the nurse is to encourage all women over age 20 to have annual checkups that include a gynecologic examination. More detailed nursing care following surgery or radiation therapy is found below and on page 1059.

Estrogen and Uterine Cancer. According to recent studies, menopausal and postmenopausal women who take estrogens have an increased risk of acquiring endometrial cancer. The Federal Drug Administration strongly supports warnings that advise health professionals and female patients that the risk is much lower if estrogens are taken in the lowest possible doses. The increased risk of endometrial cancer in estrogen users is proportional to the length of time during which the estrogens are taken (particularly 5 years or longer). It is recommended that estrogens not be given when they are not medically effective, such as in treating simple nervousness and depression during menopause or in helping women to feel and look younger. Estrogens are effective for the vasomotor symptoms of menopause if doses are kept low and treatment is limited to less than a year.

Hysterectomy

A *hysterectomy* is the surgical removal of the uterus. When the ovaries are removed along with the uterus, the procedure is referred to as a *total abdominal hysterectomy* and *bilateral salpingo-oophorectomy* (TAH–BSO).

Patient Problems/Nursing Diagnoses

The major nursing problems of patients undergoing a hysterectomy include inadequate knowledge of the surgical procedures and postoperative course; potential development of complications; and potential nonadherence with the therapeutic regimen.

▶ **Planning and Implementation**

Goals

The major goals for the patient include:

1. Understanding of the surgical procedure and postoperative course
2. Absence of complications
3. Compliance with the therapeutic regimen

Psychological Considerations and Physical Preparation. The psychosocial problems faced by women undergoing gynecologic surgery are similar to those discussed on page 1024. Moreover, when hormonal balances are upset, as often occurs in disturbances of the reproductive system, the patient may exhibit depression and heightened emotional sensitivity to people and situations. Each patient must be understood in the light of such factors and be approached and evaluated individually. This understanding must be shared by the family as well as the health care providers. The nurse who exhibits interest, concern, and willingness to listen to the patient's fears will add immeasurably to the patient's progress throughout the surgical experience, however temporary or prolonged that may be.

Physical preparation differs little from the details described for the preparation of a patient undergoing a laparotomy. The lower half of the abdomen and the pubic and perineal regions usually are carefully shaved and cleansed with soap and water (some clinics do not require shaving). The intestinal tract and the bladder are empty before the patient is sent to the operating room. This is most important to prevent contamination and accidental injury to the bladder or intestinal tract.

Postoperative Nursing Strategies. After operation, the principles of general postoperative care for abdominal surgery apply (see p. 384). In addition, because of the proximity of the surgical intervention to the bladder, problems of voiding may be expected; edema or nerve trauma may cause temporary atony, and an indwelling catheter may be used. If no catheter is in place, catheterization may be necessary if the patient has not voided after 8 hours. If the catheter is in place, it is usually removed on the third or fourth day. Bladder infection may result from the pooling of residual urine; therefore, the patient is catheterized after each voiding.

To combat the discomfort of abdominal distention, a nasogastric tube may be inserted before the patient leaves the operating room, especially if the surgeon realizes that excessive handling of viscera has taken place. If a large tumor was present, its excision could cause edema because of the sudden release of pressure. In the postoperative period, fluids and food may be restricted for a day or two. If there is abdominal flatus, a rectal tube may be prescribed, as well as heat to the abdomen. When peristalsis begins, the patient is served additional fluids and a soft diet. Ambulation facilitates the return to normal.

Vascular disorders, such as phlebitis, thrombosis, or edema, must be guarded against. Frequent changes of position and avoidance of high Fowler's position and pressure under the knees will minimize stasis and pooling of blood. The nurse must be particularly alert if the patient has varicose veins in her legs. Special leg exercises to promote circulation and the application of elastic stockings or bandages can be helpful.

In patients who are anemic because of loss of blood due to a tumor, convalescence may be hastened by a high-protein diet supplemented by iron salts. If the tumor was large enough to produce marked relaxation of the abdominal walls, the patient may be advised to wear an abdominal support or a girdle for a time after the operation. In the immediate postoperative period, the surgeon may have applied an abdominal binder to be worn until support is obtained.

In anticipation of posthospital care, the nurse provides opportunities for the patient to ask questions. The patient should be aware of the nature of her surgery and the immediate and long-range limitations, if any, imposed by it. Hormonal replacement may be prescribed by the physician. The patient needs to know when sexual relations and her usual physical activities can be resumed. Annual or more frequent physical examinations, including gynecologic evaluation, are imperative for maintaining peace of mind and detecting early evidence of pathology.

Vaginal Hysterectomy.   In some women, and especially in women in whom prolapse has occurred, the uterus may be removed through the vagina. Entry via the abdomen is avoided, since in a *vaginal hysterectomy,* the entire procedure is carried out through the vagina. Either the uterus alone is removed or the uterus, the uterine tubes, and the ovaries are taken out. Postoperative care of such patients is similar to that of patients who have undergone plastic surgical procedures (see p. 1051).

Physically, the patient recovers more quickly because there is no abdominal incision. However, she does require psychosocial support to help her adjust to the unnerving sensations triggered by occasional abdominal cramps that occur even though the uterus has been removed. There may also be a loss of vaginal sensation that can last for months. The patient should be assured that these paradoxic feelings will gradually disappear.

▶ **Evaluation**

Expected Outcomes

1. Understands the surgical procedure and postoperative course
    a. Expresses interest in the anesthetic agent to be used
    b. Asks specific questions regarding the effects of this operation on menstruation, procreation, sexual relations, and cancer
    c. Discusses the surgical procedure and postoperative course
    d. Practices deep breathing, turning, and leg exercises
2. Is free of complications
    a. Is afebrile for 24 hours prior to discharge; vital signs stable
    b. Is free of pain with minimum discomfort
    c. Exhibits a clean wound and minimal or no dressing
    d. Increases activity and ambulation daily
    e. Reports adequate fluid intake and adequate urinary output
    f. Ambulates early; no evidence of calf pain, redness, tenderness, or swelling in extremities
3. Adheres to therapeutic regimen
    a. Verbalizes understanding of health needs
    b. Alternates periods of rest with activity
    c. Keeps follow-up clinic or physician appointments
    d. Relates the kind of hormonal replacement she is being prescribed and its purpose

Pelvic Exenteration

Radical Pelvic Surgery.   Pelvic exenteration, or evisceration, may be performed when other forms of therapy prove to be ineffective in checking the spread of cancer.

When this therapy is contemplated, patients are selected carefully on the basis of their likelihood to survive the surgery as well as their ability to adjust to and accept the imposed limitations.

Anterior pelvic exenteration is the removal of the bladder and lower part of the ureters. In addition, in women, the vagina, the adnexa, the pelvic lymph nodes, and the pelvic peritoneum are removed. The ureters are implanted in the colon or the small intestines.

Posterior pelvic exenteration is the removal of the colon and the rectum. In addition, in women, the uterus, the vagina, and the adnexa are removed. The pelvic lymph nodes may or may not be excised.

Total pelvic exenteration is the removal of the rectum, the distal sigmoid colon, the urinary bladder, the distal portion of the ureters, and the internal iliac artery and vein. In addition, in women, all pelvic reproductive organs, lymph nodes, and the entire pelvic floor, including the pelvic peritoneum, levator muscles, and perineum, are removed. Both urinary and fecal diversion are necessary in this procedure; hence, the patient will have a colostomy. A substitute bladder will be made from a segment of ileum.

Nursing Management.   Although the following discussion considers pelvic exenteration from the perspective of the female patient, similar considerations apply to male patients who have undergone similar procedures. This patient has probably faced surgery before and is aware of most of the physical preparation required before going to the operating room. However, the most important preparation is psychological. This patient needs support as she realizes what is about to happen, and fortitude to be able to accept it. Consent to have the operation may have been given without question, since it may be clearly evident that this is a life-saving procedure.

The preoperative period is the time when a careful assessment of psychological, sociologic, and economic needs is made. The patient's spouse or immediate family can be of valuable assistance in providing hope and reason to live, even with an altered body structure. Communication lines between the patient and professional staff must be open to be effective. Strengths and weaknesses of the patient need to be identified, modified, and utilized so that the operation and postoperative phases will be approached in a positive way.

However, the full impact of adjustment may come several days after the operation. The patient may express feelings that will give direction to subsequent care. Usually, this reaction takes one of three courses: (1) she may adjust very well without any abnormal complications; (2) she may become depressed and listless and may wish to die (this reaction may be altered with antidepressant medications; meanwhile, the nurse continues to emphasize the *positive* features of the patient's future); and (3) there may be an insidious reaction in which the patient exalts her disfigurement, assuming an almost martyrlike pose. As she becomes preoccupied with herself and centers her attention on her disability, she may show pettiness, make selfish demands, and withdraw interest from her family. The nurse's hope in this instance is to try to turn the patient's thoughts from herself to others and to help the patient to see her body in its proper perspective, focusing attention on those parts that are intact.

This patient requires intensive care following the operation. Because satisfactory body function depends on adequate fluid balance, particular attention is given to an accurate intake and output record. Proper functioning of the gastrointestinal tract may not return for several days. (See colostomy and ileostomy care on pp. 829 and 819). Likewise, following radical surgery there is a greater risk of complications; therefore, the nurse must be aware of the signs and the symptoms of postoperative complications as well as the ways and means of avoiding such problems.

Patient education and rehabilitation are continuous in the care of the patient with a pelvic exenteration, moving gradually from the simple to the complex. The family is included as the convalescence of the patient continues. The patient's reactions and day-by-day progress are observed carefully; encouragement and understanding go a long way in helping her to achieve as many goals as possible.

▷ Radiation Therapy

(Also see Chap. 18, p. 324.)

Radiation therapy plays a pivotal role in the treatment of gynecologic malignancy. In the treatment of squamous cell carcinoma of the cervix, it is frequently the procedure of choice. In the management of uterine and ovarian cancers, it is usually employed as an adjunct to surgery. In the definitive treatment of cervical disease by irradiation, a combination of external pelvic irradiation and internal intracavitary irradiation is used. Only in the earliest microinvasive carcinomas of the cervix is internal (intracavitary) irradiation used alone. Cure rates of 85% or greater can be expected with cervical cancer that is limited to the cervix alone. As the disease extends into the parametrium, the cure rate drops to approximately 65%. However, once the disease extends to the pelvic sidewalls, perhaps only one third of the patients will be cured, although many more will benefit from the palliative effects of irradiation as a result of the reduction in tumor bulk and the control of infection, pain, and bleeding.

External pelvic irradiation delivered by supervoltage equipment usually extends over 4 to 6 weeks. Thereafter, intracavitary radiation is performed. This sequence may be reversed, depending on anatomical considerations. The cervix and uterus lend themselves naturally to internal irradiation since they act as a receptacle for radioactive sources. Radium and cesium are two isotopes that are the mainstays of intracavitary irradiation.

External Beam Therapy. Betatrons, linear accelerators, and cobalt 60 units are capable of delivering high doses of well collimated irradiation deep within the pelvis to the site of the tumor. Radiation side-effects are cumulative and tend to express themselves as the total dose exceeds the body's natural capacity to repair the radiation effect. Radiation enteritis, expressed by diarrhea and abdominal cramping, and radiation cystitis, manifested by frequency, urgency, and dysuria, may ensue. This clearly does not indicate an overdosage. It is a natural manifestation of the normal tissues'

response to the radiotherapy program. The radiation therapist and nurse inform the patient in advance of these possible side-effects and employ a variety of measures to modify their impact when they occur. These measures include dietary control (by restricting the amount of fiber and roughage), the maintenance of fluid intake, and the use of antispasmodic drugs. On occasion, severe reactions will require that treatment be suspended briefly until the normal tissues repair themselves.

Internal (Intracavitary) Irradiation. In the operating room, an examination is performed under anesthesia, after which specially prepared applicators are inserted into the endometrial cavity and vagina. These devices are not loaded with radioactive material until the patient has returned to her room. X-rays are obtained to determine the precise relationship of the applicator to the normal pelvic anatomy and to the tumor. Only when this study is completed does the radiation therapist load the applicators with predetermined amounts of radioactive material. This is called *afterloading* and allows for precise control of the radiation exposure received by the patient, with minimal exposure of the physician and the nursing and health care team. A patient undergoing internal radiation treatment is placed in a private unit until the application is completed (Chart 46-1).

Various applicators have been developed for intracavitary treatment. Some are inserted into the endometrial cavity and endocervical canal as multiple small irradiators (for example, Heyman's capsules). Others consist of a central tube (tandem or intrauterine "stem") placed through the dilated endocervical canal into the uterine cavity, which remains in fixed relationship with irradiators placed in the upper vagina on each side of the cervix (vaginal ovoids) (Fig. 46-7). The Fletcher-Suit applicator is a well known afterloading form of this classic tandem and ovoid pattern.

At the time of insertion of the applicator, an indwelling bladder catheter is inserted. The applicator is secured in place with vaginal packing. The objective of the internal treatment is to maintain the distribution of internal radiation at a fixed dosage throughout the application. Such applications usually last 24 to 72 hours, depending on dose calculations made by the radiation therapist and the radiation physicist.

Nursing Management During Cesium Treatment

During the application, diligent nursing care must be given. The patient is carefully observed and attended, though the nursing staff must try to reduce as much as possible the radiation exposure to themselves. Nurses should stay in the immediate vicinity of the patient no longer than is necessary to give proper care and attention, and no nurse should attend the patient more than a half hour per day (see Chart 46-1). Of course, a pregnant nurse should not be involved in the immediate care of such patients. Visits to the patient should not be aimless; nurse–patient contacts provide a good opportunity for the patient to talk about her anxiety and fear. To minimize radiation exposure, the nurse may stay at the foot of the bed or at the entrance to the room.

During the application, the patient will be on absolute bed rest. She may move from side to side with her back supported by a pillow, and the head of the bed may be

Chart 46-1
Nursing Care of Patients Undergoing Treatment With Encapsulated Radioactive Sources

_____ is being treated with _____ mg Ra Eq
                    (name)

of radioactive _____   _____ at
                            (cesium, iridium seeds, etc.)   (date)

_____ m. The type of application or implantation is _____
        (time)

_____

Precautions for hospital personnel to observe when handling patients who are undergoing treatment with encapsulated radioactive materials:
1. The PATIENT must be placed in a single room.
2. PREGNANT NURSES SHOULD NOT CARE FOR THESE PATIENTS.
3. NURSES should not stay in the immediate vicinity of the patient longer than is necessary (less than ½ hour per day) to give proper care and attention.
4. VISITORS should stay at least six (6) feet from the bed and limit the visit to less than 1 hour per day. Children under age 18 and pregnant women may not visit.
5. If a radioactive source or applicator becomes dislodged from the patient, pick up the source with the long forceps provided and place it in the lead container located in the patient's room. NOTIFY THE RADIOTHERAPIST IMMEDIATELY. NEVER PICK UP A RADIOACTIVE SOURCE WITH YOUR HANDS.
6. Save all dressings, bed linens, etc. Do not vacuum the floor. Save floor sweepings in the room. Dishes, trays, and eating utensils can leave the room. Do not save any of the patient's excreta or body fluids unless requested to do so by the radiotherapist.
7. Before the patient is discharged, a radiation survey will be made to assure that no radiation hazard remains. The Radiation Therapy Department will then NOTIFY THE HEAD NURSE THAT USED LINENS AND DRESSINGS CAN BE REMOVED.

NOTIFY THE RADIOTHERAPY DEPARTMENT IMMEDIATELY:
1. In case of any doubt as to safe procedure
2. In case of any emergency
3. If any unexpected complications arise
4. In case of death:
   Before postmortem care is given
   Before an autopsy is performed
   Before the body is released
During the day, call the Radiation Therapy Department
During the night, call the Page Operator and request the physician on call be contacted either by telephone or beeper.

(A form similar to that used at American Oncologic Hospital, Fox Chase Cancer Center, Philadelphia, Pennsylvania)

raised to 45 degrees. The patient should be encouraged to practice deep-breathing and cough exercises and to vigorously flex and extend the feet to stretch the calf muscles in order to promote venous return. Back care is much appreciated by the patient, but adequate care is given within the minimum amount of time at the bedside.

Usually, the patient is on a low-residue diet to prevent frequent bowel movements. One is less concerned here with dislodging the radium applicator than with the social and physical discomforts that the patient may experience. The nurse should inspect the catheter frequently to make sure that it is draining properly. The chief hazard of improper drainage is that the bladder may become distended. Although perineal care is omitted at this time, any profuse discharge should be reported immediately to the radiation therapist or gynecologic surgeon.

The patient is observed for evidence of temperature elevation, nausea, and vomiting. These symptoms should be reported, since they may be indicative of infection or perforation. Finally, the radiation therapist takes steps to secure the internal applicator in place. Nursing personnel need not be preoccupied with the fear that the applicator will be prematurely extruded. However, one should check from time to time to see that the applicator or the radioactive sources have not been dislodged. Should this happen, the radioactive source is grasped with a long forceps and held at arm's length and returned to the lead container located in the patient's room. Radioactive sources should never be grasped with the bare hand. The radiotherapist should be notified immediately.

Cesium Removal. The radiation therapist calculates precisely the radiation dose delivered. At the end of the

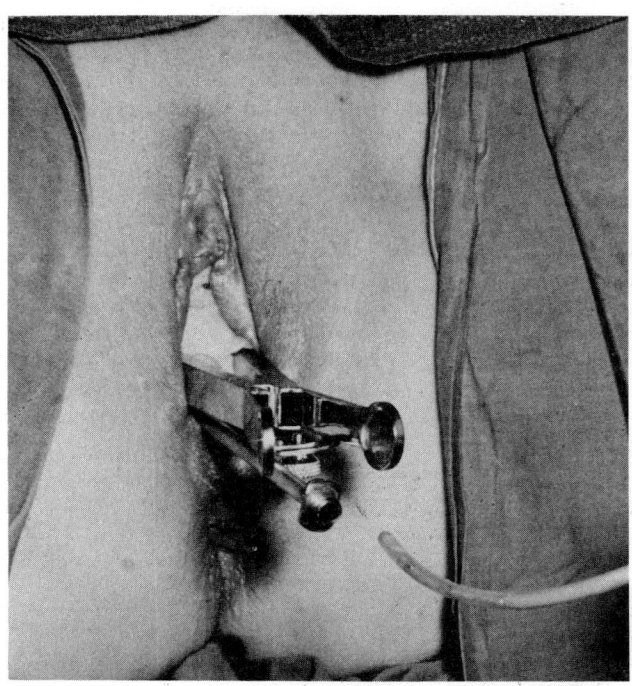

Figure 46-7. Applicator in position ready to be loaded. (From Hilkemeyer N: Nursing care in radium therapy. Nurs Clin North Am.)

prescribed period, the nurse may be requested to assist the physician in removing the applicator. As the sources are "afterloaded," they can be removed by the physician in the same manner as they were inserted. This does not require local or general anesthesia and is done in the patient's room. Medication with a mild sedative may be required before radium is removed.

Postinsertion Care. Slow, progressive ambulation is recommended after the period of enforced bed rest. The patient may shower as soon as she wishes; a vinegar or dilute saline douche may be prescribed. Diet may be advanced as tolerated.

▷ Conditions of the Ovaries and the Pelvic Cavity

Ovarian Cysts and Tumors

Pathophysiology. The ovary is a frequent site for the development of cysts. These may be simply pathologic enlargements of normal ovarian constituents, the graafian follicle or corpus luteum, or they may arise from abnormal growth of the ovarian epithelium. They are considered benign tumors with a possibility of becoming malignant.

Dermoid cysts are tumors that are believed to arise from parts of the ovum that disappear normally as ripening (maturation) takes place. Since their origin is undefined, all that can be said is that they are tumors made up of undifferentiated embryonal cells. They grow slowly and at operation are found to contain a thick, yellow, sebaceous material arising from a skin lining. Hair, teeth, bone, brain, eyes, and many other tissues often are found in a rudimentary state within these cysts.

Clinically, cysts are manifested by their obvious presence as an ovarian mass. There may be lower abdominal pain that may be acute or chronic. Rupture may occur and simulate a variety of acute abdominal emergencies, such as appendicitis or ectopic pregnancy. Larger cysts may produce abdominal swelling and pressure on adjacent abdominal organs.

Ovarian cancer is a particularly frustrating cancer for several reasons: it is difficult to diagnose, and is unique in that it may give rise to many primary cancers and may be the recipient of metastases from other cancers. It carries an annual mortality rate of over 11,500—the sixth most prevalent cancer in women. Therefore, every effort should be made to diagnose this problem early.

Assessment and Clinical Manifestations. Because early signs and symptoms are similar to those of functional ovarian cysts or endometriosis, other means of differentiating benign from potentially malignant growths must be utilized. Manifestations include irregular menses, increasing premenstrual tension, menorrhagia with breast tenderness, and an early menopause. Before puberty and after menopause there may be precocious breast development and uterine bleeding. Virilization may be noted. Ovarian malignancy may be observed more frequently in women who are infertile, nulliparous, anovulatory, or habitual aborters. In addition to a long history of ovarian dysfunction or malfunction, persistent gastrointestinal symptoms in a woman aged 40 or over that cannot be definitely diagnosed should raise a suspicion of ovarian malignancy. Early and insidious symptoms include vague abdominal discomfort, dyspepsia, flatulence, eructations, and a feeling of fullness after a light meal.

The combination of two major clues—(1) a long history of ovarian dysfunction, and (2) vague, undiagnosed, persistent gastrointestinal symptoms in the woman over 40—should alert the nurse to the possibility of early malignancy. Other high-risk signs include a progressively enlarging tumor or indications of a solid mass, as opposed to a cystlike growth.

Management. The treatment of ovarian cysts is surgical removal. However, if malignant degeneration has taken place, with invasion of the abdomen and general emaciation (general carcinomatosis), operation is of little benefit. The patient may be given roentgen therapy and testosterone. The abdomen may be tapped to relieve distention from ascites. The postoperative nursing care after cystectomy is similar to that for abdominal surgery, with one exception. The marked decrease in intra-abdominal pressure incidental to the removal of a large cyst often leads to considerable abdominal distention. This complication may be prevented to some extent by the application of a snug-fitting abdominal binder.

For ovarian cancer, surgical removal is the goal. Because of high morbidity and mortality, every effort is made to stage the tumor as accurately as possible and to direct medical treatment accordingly. Anticipatory nursing can include the liberal use of hyperalimentation, antibiotics, Swan–Ganz catheter monitoring, aggressive surgery, and chemotherapy.

Cisplatin (Platinol) is an intravenous drug that may be combined with doxorubicin (Adriamycin) to treat ovarian cancer.

Endometriosis

Pathophysiology. *Endometriosis* is a benign lesion in which cells similar to those lining the uterus are found growing aberrantly in the pelvic cavity outside of the uterus. It is characteristically found in the young, nulliparous female. A similar condition affecting the uterine lining in older, multiparous patients is referred to as *adenomyosis*. At present, these two conditions, which at one time were thought to be related, are now considered separate entities.

In order of frequency, pelvic endometriosis attacks the ovary, uterosacral ligaments, cul-de-sac, ureterovesical peritoneum, cervix, umbilicus, laparotomy scars, hernial sacs, and appendix. The misplaced endometrium responds to ovarian hormonal stimulation and, indeed, depends on this for survival. When the uterus goes through the process of menstruation, this ectopic tissue bleeds—mostly into areas having no outlet—which then causes pain and adhesions. At surgery, these lesions are typically small, puckered, and brown or blue–black, indicating concealed bleeding. If the endometrial tissue is within an ovarian cyst, there is no outlet for the bleeding and the formation is referred to as a *chocolate cyst*. Symptoms vary and may be misleading, since extensive endometriosis may cause few symptoms, whereas an isolated lesion may produce considerable symptomatology.

Incidence and Etiology.   Endometriosis has been on the increase in the past several decades. There is a high incidence among patients who marry later, bear children later, and have fewer children. In countries such as India, where tradition favors early marriage and early childbearing, endometriosis is rare.

Several theories have been advanced regarding the origin of these lesions: (1) retrograde (reflux) menstruation, or the backflow of menses, causes endometrial tissue to be transported to ectopic sites through the uterine tubes; (2) during surgery, endometrial tissue inadvertently may be transferred by way of instruments; (3) such tissue may possibly be spread by lymphatic or venous channels; and (4) tissue that covers the pelvic peritoneum and ovaries is a remnant of embryonic tissue. A combination of such factors may be responsible.

Pelvic endometriosis, rarely encountered in the black race, occurs in about 25% to 30% of women. It is thought to be the cause of 30% to 40% of all cases of infertility. Upon bimanual examination, fixed tender nodules may be detected, and the uterus may be restricted in motility, indicating adhesion formation.

Assessment and Clinical Manifestations.   The chief symptom is a type of dysmenorrhea, unlike typical uterine cramps. The patient complains of a deep-seated aching in the lower abdomen, vagina, posterior pelvis, and back that occurs a day or two before the menstrual cycle and lasts 2 or 3 days. Some patients, however, have no pain. Abnormal uterine bleeding and dyspareunia (painful intercourse) may also be evident. Infertility is another possible effect.

Conservative Therapy and Nursing Considerations.
Management depends on the severity of the symptoms and the age of the patient. Laparoscopy is useful in evaluating minimal disease. Medical management is initiated with hormonal therapy that blocks ovulation. This relieves dysmenorrhea and postpones surgical intervention. When the function of childbearing is to be considered, conservative therapy is preferred, preserving as much of the reproductive tract as possible. Procedures of choice are resection of cysts, lysis (cutting) of adhesions, and suspension of the uterus. The likelihood of recurrence of endometriosis is high; however, the desire for and possibility of pregnancy takes priority. In women aged 35 to 45 years, ovarian tissue is saved when possible; after the menopause, atrophy occurs and the problem is solved.

Atrophy of the endometrium and subsequent amenorrhea may be produced by a synthetic androgen (danazol [Danocrine]). However, it is an expensive drug with unknown long-term effects. It probably acts by inhibiting release of gonadotropins from the pituitary gland, leading to atrophic changes in intrauterine and ectopic endometrial tissue. Endometriosis tends to recur when medication is stopped. Side-effects to be watched for include weight gain, mild acne, edema, hot flushes, menstrual dysfunction, decrease in breast size, and atrophic vagina.

The nurse's role in patient education is to dispel myths, such as a causative relationship between the use of tampons and endometriosis, which is not true. In order to combat the upward statistical trend of endometriosis, women should be encouraged to have regular physical examinations. Unusual menstrual bleeding patterns should be reported and investigated.

Adenomyosis.   In this condition, endometriosis involves the uterine wall; the incidence is highest in women from 40 to 50 years of age. Symptoms are hypermenorrhea (excessive and prolonged bleeding), acquired dysmenorrhea, polymenorrhea (abnormally frequent bleeding), and premenstrual staining. On physical examination, the uterus is felt to be enlarged, firm, and tender. Treatment depends on the severity of bleeding and pain; hysterectomy offers greater relief than more conservative forms of therapy.

Pelvic Infection (Pelvic Inflammatory Disease)

Pathophysiology.   Pelvic infection is an inflammatory condition of the pelvic cavity that may involve the uterine tubes (salpingitis), ovaries (oophoritis), pelvic peritoneum, or pelvic vascular system. This disease may be acute or chronic and may be caused by the gram-negative bacteria, staphylococcus and streptococcus, or by sexually transmitted disease organisms.

Usually, the site of infection and the method of spread serve to identify two types of infection: gonococcal and mixed infection. The gonococcal infection affects the urethra, cervix, or rectum. The disease may be self-limiting if it is properly treated and if reinfection is avoided. However, frequently the woman is reinfected and the secondary causative organisms (streptococcus, staphylococcus, *E. coli*) flourish, causing a chronic problem. This infection spreads by way of the uterine canal into the tube and fimbria.

The largest group of infections result from pelvic cellulitis, for instance, endometritis resulting from a complication of pregnancy or an intrauterine device. Pathogens spread by way of the lymphatics and blood vessels. Such a cellulitis tends to be unilateral, whereas gonorrheal infection is a bilateral infection. These pathogenic organisms usually are introduced from the outside and pass through the cervical canal and the uterus into the pelvis by way of lymphatic channels, uterine veins, or uterine tubes. When pelvic infection is caused by tubercle bacillus, it is usually conveyed by way of the bloodstream from the lungs.

Management.   The main goal of care is to keep the infection from spreading to other parts of the patient's system or to other people coming in contact with the patient. In order to give effective care, the nurse must know the cause, signs, and symptoms of pelvic infections, as well as methods of spread. This dissemination of infection to others can be controlled in many ways: (1) perineal pads should be handled carefully with an instrument or gloves, and the soiled pad should be deposited in a paper bag for proper disposal; (2) hands should be washed carefully with a good germicidal soap; and (3) all items that come in contact with the patient (utensils, bedpans, toilet seats, and linens) should be properly disinfected by the correct procedure for controlling the specific organisms responsible for the infection. The patient must be informed of the need for these precautions and encouraged to take part in plans to prevent contamination of others as well as protect herself from reinfection.

If reinfection or spread of infection occurs, symptoms may include abdominal pain, nausea and vomiting, elevation of temperature, malaise, malodorous purulent vaginal discharge, and leukocytosis. The patient assumes the semi-Fowler position (dependent drainage). Catheterization and the use of tampons are avoided. In addition, the patient is supported nutritionally and with selective antibiotic therapy.

For comfort, heat can be applied to the abdomen externally and warm douches may be prescribed to improve circulation. Proper recording of vital signs, the patient's physical and mental response to treatment, and the nature and amount of vaginal discharge are necessary to guide the physician in future therapy.

If untreated, pelvic inflammatory disease can lead to chronic pelvic discomfort. Scar tissue may close the uterine tubes, resulting in sterility. Ectopic pregnancy could occur if a fertilized egg is unable to pass the stricture. Adhesions are a common development that eventually may require removal of the uterus, tubes, and ovaries.

The "caring" for the patient with pelvic infection is just as important as the "curing." This infection may be very distressing, both physically and mentally. Such a patient may feel well one day and develop vague symptoms and discomfort the next; she suffers from constipation and menstrual difficulties. These patients are frequently unjustly labeled "neurotic." The nurse must also keep in mind the social aspects of sexually transmitted diseases, which may cause pelvic inflammatory disease (see pp. 1491–1494).

▷ **Bibliography**

Books

Barber HRK. Manual of Gynecologic Oncology. Philadelphia, JB Lippincott, 1980.

Barwin NB and Belisk S. Adolescent Gynecology and Sexuality. New York, Masson, 1982.

Beacham DW and Beacham WD. Synopsis of Gynecology, 10th ed. St Louis, CV Mosby, 1982.

Blaustein A (ed). Pathology of the Female Genital Tract, 2nd ed. New York, Springer–Verlag, 1981.

Bush RS. Malignancies of the Ovary, Uterus and Cervix. Chicago, Year Book Medical Publishers, 1980.

Danforth DN. Obstetrics and Gynecology, 4th ed. Philadelphia, JB Lippincott, 1982.

Delgado G and Smith JP. Management of Complications in Gynecologic Oncology. New York, John Wiley & Sons, 1982.

Hawkins DF. Gynecological Therapeutics. New York, Macmillan, 1981.

Hawkins JW and Higgins LP. Maternity and Gynecological Nursing. Philadelphia, JB Lippincott, 1981.

Jones HW and Jones GS. Novak's Textbook of Gynecology. Baltimore, Williams & Wilkins, 1981.

Nursing Photobook. Attending Ob/Gyn Patients. Springhouse, Pennsylvania, Intermed Publications, 1982.

Ridley JH. Gynecologic Surgery, 2nd ed. Baltimore, Williams & Wilkins, 1981.

Romney S et al. Gynecology and Obstetrics, 2nd ed. New York, McGraw–Hill, 1981.

Sabbagha BE. Diagnostic Ultrasound Applied to Obstetrics and Gynecology. New York, Harper & Row, 1980.

Some Questions and Answers About . . . Herpes. Palo Alto, American Social Health Association, 1980.

Warner CG. Rape and Sexual Assault: Management and Intervention. Gaithersburg, Maryland, Aspen Systems Corp, 1980.

Wren B. Handbook of Obstetrics and Gynecology. New York, Macmillan, 1980.

Wynn RM. Obstetrics and Gynecology. New York, Appleton–Century–Crofts, 1982.

Articles

Diagnostic Studies and Preoperative Care

Koeckeritz JL. Assessing the genitalia. RN 1983 Jan; 46(1):53–59.

Paritzky JF and Overby BA. Preoperative teaching on a gynecology unit. JOGN Nurs 1982 Nov/Dec; 11(6):384–386.

Patterson JE. Colposcopy. JOGN Nurs 1983 Jan/Feb; 12(1):11–15.

Vaginal Conditions

Amstey MS and Jones AP. Preparation of the vagina for surgery. A comparison of povidone iodine and saline solution. JAMA 1981 Feb 27; 245(8):839–841.

Cibley LJ. *Trichomonas vaginalis* vaginitis. Human Sexuality 1980 Mar; 14(3):53–54.

Clough DH and Higgins PG. Discrepancies in estimating blood loss. Am J Nurs 1981 Feb; 81(2):331–333.

Comer JB. Amphotericin B: Ten common questions. Am J Nurs 1981 June; 81(6):1166–1167.

Ervin CT et al. Behavioral factors and vaginitis. Nurse Pract 1982 Feb; 7(2):20–21.

Fleury FJ. Adult vaginitis. Clin Obstet Gynecol 1981 June; 24(2):407–438.

Gever LN. Flagyl I.V. Nursing '81 1981 Aug; 11(8):79.

Goldberg MI et al. Surgical management of invasive carcinoma of the vulva utilizing a lower abdominal midline incision. Gynecol Oncol 1979 June; 7(3):296–308.

Goldberg MI et al. Radical vulvectomy. Contemp Ob/Gyn 1982 June; 19(6):232–245.

Herbst AL. DES update. CA—A Cancer J for Clinicians 1980 Nov/Dec; 30(6):326–332.

Huggins GR. Vaginal odors and secretions. Clin Obstet Gynecol 1981 June; 24(2):355–377.

Metronidozole HCl (Flagyl). The Medical Letter 1981 Feb 20; 23(4):13–14.

Miles MR et al. Recurrent vaginal candidiasis. JAMA 1977 Oct 24; 238(17):1836–1837.

Ostergard DR. DES-related vaginal lesions. Clin Obstet Gynecol 1981 June; 24(2):379–394.

Rees PL and Dixon DM. Opportunistic mycosis. Am J Nurs 1981 June; 81(6):1160–1165.

Robertson WH. A concentrated therapeutic regimen for vulvovaginal candidiasis. JAMA 1980 Dec 5; 244(22):2549–2550.

Vontver LA and Eschenbach DA. The role of Gardnerella vaginalis in nonspecific vaginitis. Clin Obstet Gynecol 1981 June; 24(2):439–460.

Herpes Genitalis

Acyclovir for genital and other herpes virus infections. Am J Nurs 1982 July; 82(7):1124.

Adam E et al. Asymptomatic virus shedding after herpes genitalis. Am J Obstet Gynecol 1980 Aug 1; 137(7):827–830.

Baker DA. Prospects for treating herpes. Contemp Ob/Gyn 1982 Jan; 19(1):179–185.

Bettoli EJ. Herpes: Facts and fallacies. Am J Nurs 1982 June 82(6):924–929.

Fuimara NJ. Scabies and genital herpes: A problem in management. Am Fam Physician 1982 Jan; 25(1):125–129.

Gruman ME et al. The course of untreated recurrent genital herpes simplex infection in 27 women. N Engl J Med 1981 Mar 26; 304(13):759–763.

Haverkos HW and Curran JW. The current outbreak of Karposi's sarcoma and opportunistic infections. CA—A Cancer Journal for Clinicians 1982 Nov/Dec; 32(6):330–339.

Kellum MD and Loucks A. Genital herpes infections: Diagnosis and management. Nurse Pract 1982 Feb; 7(2):14–17, 21.

Raggozino MW. Risk of cancer after herpes zoster; a population-based study. N Engl J Med 1982 Aug 12; 307(7):393–397.

Treatment of sexually transmitted diseases. The Medical Letter 1982 Mar 19; 24(605):29–34.

Toxic Shock Syndrome

Center for Disease Control. Follow-up on toxic shock syndrome—United States. MMWR 1980 June 27; 29(25):297–299.

Center for Disease Control. Follow-up on toxic shock syndrome—United States. MMWR 1980 Sept 19; 29(37):441–445.

Cohen ML and Falkow S. Protein antigens from *Staphylococcus aureus* strains associated with toxic shock syndrome. Science 1981 Feb 20; 211(4484):842–844.

Friedrich EG. Tampon effects on vaginal health. Clin Obstet Gynecol 1981 June; 24(2):395–406.

Gold M. Toxic shock. Science 1980 Dec; 1(8):10.

Norton MM. Toxic shock syndrome. Nurs Forum 1980; 19(4):364–371.

Toxic shock syndrome. . . . Am J Nurs 1981 Aug; 81(8):1451.

Wroblewski SS. Toxic shock syndrome. Am J Nurs 1981 Jan; 81(1)82–85.

Uterus

Andrews WC. Medical versus surgical treatment of endometriosis. Clin Obstet Gynecol 1980 Sept; 23(3):917–924.

Ranney B. Endometriosis: Pathogenesis, symptoms, and findings. Clin Obstet Gynecol 1980 Sept; 23(3):865–874.

Ranney B. Etiology, prevention and inhibition of endometriosis. Clin Obstet Gynecol 1980 Sept; 23(3):875–883.

Richardson AC and Lyon JB. The prevention of postoperative infection in abdominal hysterectomy. Clin Obstet Gynecol 1981 Dec; 24(4):1259–1266.

Riddick DH. Drug therapy of endometriosis. Drug Therapy 1982 May; 12(5):225–230.

Schwarz BE. Does estrogen cause adenocarcinoma of the endometrium? Clin Obstet Gynecol 1981 Mar; 24(1):243–251.

Thompson JD and Birch HW. Indications for hysterectomy. Clin Obstet Gynecol 1981 Dec; 24(4):1245–1258.

Vaughn TC and Hammond CB. Estrogen replacement therapy. Clin Obstet Gynecol 1981 Mar; 24(1):253–283.

Pelvic Inflammatory Disease

Brown ST and Wiesner PJ. Problems and approaches to the control and surveillance of sexually transmitted agents associated with PID in the U.S. Am J Obstet Gynecol 1980 Dec 1; 138(7):1096–1100.

Curran JW. Economic consequences of PID in the U.S. Am J Obstet Gynecol 1980 Dec 1; 138(7):848–851.

Grimes DA. Nongonococcal pelvic inflammatory disease. Clin Obstet Gynecol 1981 Dec; 24(4):1227–1243.

Jones OG et al. Frequency and distribution of salpingitis and pelvic inflammatory disease in short-stay hospitals in the United States. Am J Obstet Gynecol 1980 Dec 1; 138(7):905–908.

Potterat JJ et al. Gonococcal pelvic inflammatory disease: Case-finding observations. Am J Obstet Gynecol 1980 Dec 1; 138(7):1101–1104.

Cancer

Barber HRK. Ovarian cancer, Part I. CA—A Cancer Journal for Clinicians 1979; 29(6):341–351.

Barber HRK. Ovarian cancer, Part II. CA—A Cancer Journal for Clinicians 1979; 30(1):2–15.

Gever LN. Cisplatin. Nursing '80 1980 Dec; 10(12):53.

Gusberg SB. An approach to the control of carcinoma of the endometrium. CA—A Cancer Journal for Clinicians 1980 Jan/Feb; 30(1):16–22.

Hulka BD et al. Protection against endometrial carcinoma by combination-product oral contraceptives. JAMA 1982 Jan 22–29; 247(4):475–477.

Israel MJ and Mood DW. Three media presentations for patients receiving radiation therapy. Cancer Nurs 1982 Feb; 5(1):57–63.

Jusenius K. Sexuality and gynecologic cancer. Cancer Nurs 1981 Dec; 4(6):479–484.

Kaempfer SH. The effects of cancer chemotherapy on reproduction: A review of the literature. Oncol Nurs Forum 1981 Winter; 8(1):11–18.

Krouse HJ and Krouse JH. Cancer as a crisis: The critical elements of adjustment. Nurs Res 1982 Mar/Apr; 31(2):96–101.

Smith WG. Invasive cancer of the vagina. Clin Obstet Gynecol 1981 June; 4(2):503–515.

Winer WK. Laser treatment of cervical neoplasia. Am J Nurs 1982 Sept; 82(9):1384–1387.

Woodruff JD. Carcinoma in situ of the vagina. Clin Obstet Gynecol 1981 June; 24(2):485–501.

47

Assessment and Management of Patients With Breast Disorders

▷ Physiology of Breast Development

Up to the time of puberty, no microscopic difference can be found in the breasts of the two sexes. At puberty, some slight swelling appears in the male breast. At the same time, a pronounced increase in size occurs in the female organ. This begins around the 10th year and increases rapidly up to the 14th and 16th years. The development of the mammary gland is a result of hormonal action that begins with puberty in the female. At this time, the nipple takes on its natural protruding form. In the male, contrary to some statements, breast tissue always exists and may grow.

The breast is a glandular organ with many lobules; its secretion passes through collecting ducts to the nipple. In some women, there is a cyclic engorgement of the breasts, associated with tingling and tenderness; this is hormonal in origin. The symptoms begin usually in the latter part of the menstrual cycle and disappear when menstruation occurs. During pregnancy, about 8 weeks after a woman conceives, her breasts enlarge greatly, the nipples become more prominent and sensitive, and the breasts are prepared to nourish the infant. When pregnancy is over and lactation has ceased, the breasts shrink, lose their excessive fat, and often become flabby and flattened.

Psychosocial Implications

In Western cultures, the breast is considered a significant component of feminine beauty. Shapeliness is a quality much desired and is emphasized in a woman's choice of clothing. Particularly in the United States, the social value placed upon looking young has led to consumer demands for brassieres that further contribute to a trim, fit look. Thus, a woman's reaction to any actual or suspected disease or injury affecting her breast tends to reflect the prevailing societal view of the female breast. Not only do social values play a significant role in the rehabilitation of a patient who has undergone radical breast surgery, but the fear of disfigurement may prevent a woman from seeking immediate medical attention after she has detected suspicious signs or changes in her breast.

A major objective of the health professions is to spread sound advice regarding the prevention of illness and the detection of disease in its early stages. Every woman should be alerted to the early signs of breast pathology and should be well informed about what to do about suspicious changes. The nurse has a major responsibility in the area of the prevention and early detection of breast diseases and in handling the concomitant psychosocial concerns of the patient. The nurse's association with industry, diagnostic clinics, and community health agencies offers opportunities to teach and disseminate information, particularly concerning the value of breast self-examination.

> Incidence of Breast Disease

Although most of the disorders of the female breast are benign in character, the breast is one of the two female organs that are most frequently the primary site of cancer. The breast normally changes during menstruation, pregnancy, lactation, and menopause, and these variations must be differentiated from pathologic changes. Although the breast is fairly accessible to examination, the detection and accurate diagnosis of breast disease can be difficult.

About one fourth of all women have irregular areas in their breasts at some time. Just before menstruation, irregularities produced by hyperplasia and involution occur. These irregularities, which feel granular or finely nodular, usually occur in the upper outer quadrants. Some women have persistently irregular breast tissue that feels shotlike or plaquelike between periods. Such masses are not considered true masses because they usually are bilateral and neither increase in size nor consolidate. On the other hand, true masses do not fluctuate in size and are usually unilateral.

In both females and males, benign lesions of the breast occur more frequently than malignant lesions (70% benign vs. 30% malignant). Of the malignant tumors, 99% occur in females. Benign lesions occur frequently in premenopausal women.

The benign lesions, presented according to order of frequency and the common ages at which they occur, are fibrocystic disease (20 to 45 years), fibroadenoma (20 to 39 years), and intraductal papilloma (35 to 45 years). By way of contrast, cancer of the breast is manifested chiefly in the menopausal and postmenopausal years, the incidence increasing progressively as the woman gets older. Approximately 75% of breast cancers occur in patients over the age of 40; less than 2% occur before the age of 30.

According to the latest statistics reported by the American Cancer Society, approximately 112,000 new cases of malignant breast tumors were discovered, and approximately 37,000 women died from the disease.

▷ Assessment

Breast Examination

Breast examination by palpation should be included in the annual complete physical examination of all women. (The examination procedure is described on p. 69). A breast examination should be done twice a year in women who have a family history of breast cancer.

Self-examination of the Breast (BSE). Because 95% of breast cancers and 65% of early minimal breast cancers are detected by women themselves, top priority must be given to teaching all women how and when to examine their breasts. It is estimated that only a minority (25% to 30%) perform BSE on a monthly basis. Even among women who perform breast self-examination, there often are delays in seeking medical attention. The reasons for this must continue to be explored; among them are economic factors, lack of education, reluctance to do anything if there is no pain, psychological factors, fear (predominant deterrent), false modesty, and depression. Whatever the reason, the nurse is in a unique position in all contacts with women to inform and educate. The nurse can offer advice and arrange for showings of the film *Breast Self-examination,* available from local chapters of the American Cancer Society. The method of BSE, which should be performed monthly, is shown in Figure 47-1.

The importance of this examination should be stressed, especially in the light of recent findings related to the occurrence of "interval cancers" (cancer that may develop after a negative screening visit and prior to the subsequent examination in the physician's office). Breast self-examination is essential in detecting these "interval cancers."

Some cancers grow very rapidly, whereas others grow very slowly. It has been reported that the course of a cancer from its inception to the death of the patient can be as short as 120 days; conversely, a chronic breast cancer has been known to last for 23 years without treatment.

Mammography

Mammography is a roentgenographic examination of the breast that does not require the injection of a contrast medium. The procedure takes about 20 minutes, can be done at most health centers, and is painless. (A balloon attachment may be used as a comfort measure when pressure is applied to flatten the breast while the pictures are being taken.) Usually, two views are taken of each breast: a craniocaudal view, taken from above while the patient is seated, and a mediolateral view.

With mammography, breast cancer may be diagnosed before the appearance of any clinical manifestations. However, a skilled roentgenologist is required to interpret the findings. At the same time, it should be noted that this form of diagnostic examination has limitations, since some carcinomas noted on clinical examination are not detectable by mammography. In addition, mammography is not as effective in studying very small breasts as it is for "fatty" breasts. More recently, certain architectural patterns of the breast have been distinguished, making it possible to identify patients who are at high risk for developing breast cancer.

At present, there is evidence to suggest that a threshold dose level exists beyond which radiation could induce breast cancer. (Many authorities agree that a patient can have approximately 20 mammograms in her lifetime before the incidence increases from 1 in 13 to 1 in 12.) Because of this, guidelines have been set up by the National Cancer Institute

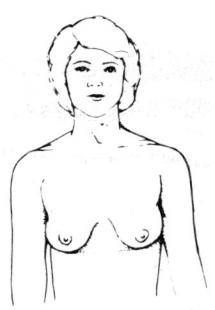

(1)   Sit or stand in front of your mirror, with your arms relaxed at your sides, and examine your breasts carefully for any changes in size and shape.   Look for any puckering or dimpling of the skin, and for any discharge or change in the nipples.

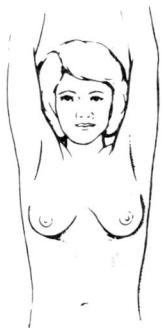

(2)   Raise both arms over your head, and look for exactly the same things.   See if there has been any change since you last examined your breasts.

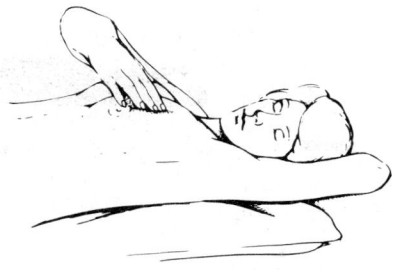

(3)   Lie down on your bed, put a pillow or a bath towel under your left shoulder, and place your left hand under your head. (From this step through Step 8, you should feel for a lump or thickening.) Holding your right hand flat, with fingers together, press gently but firmly with small circular motions to feel the inner upper quarter of your left breast, starting at your breastbone and going outward toward the nipple line.   Also feel the area around the nipple.

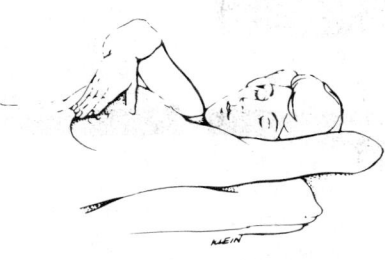

(4)   With the same gentle pressure, feel the lower inner part of your breast.   Incidentally, in this area you will feel a ridge of firm tissue or flesh.   Don't be alarmed.   This is perfectly normal.

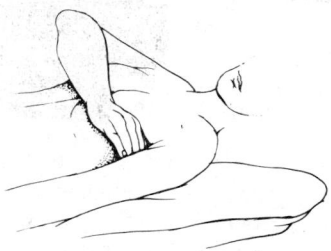

(5)   Now bring your left arm down to your side, and still using the flat part of your fingers, feel under your armpit.

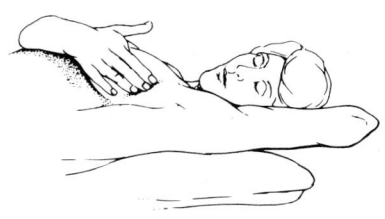

(6)   Use the same gentle pressure to feel the upper, outer quarter of your breast from the nipple line to where your arm is resting.

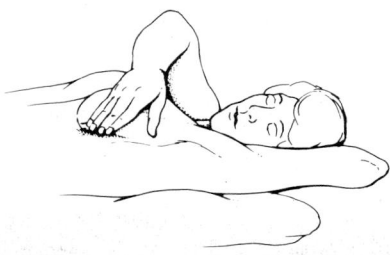

(7)   Finally, feel the lower outer section of your breast, going from the outer part to the nipple.

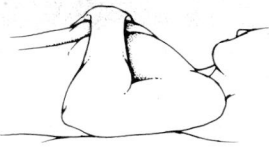

(8)   Repeat the entire procedure, as described, on the right breast.

Figure 47-1.   Self-examination of the breast. (Courtesy, American Cancer Society, Inc.)

to control exposure to x-rays in women, especially those under age 50:

1. Women over 50 should have mammography screening available to them.
2. Women between the ages of 40 and 49:
   a. Who have a family history of cancer or who themselves have had the disease should have mammography performed.
   b. Who are asymptomatic should have a physical examination of the breast annually, and a mammography should be performed at intervals of 1 to 2 years.
3. Mammography should never be used to screen women under age 35.
4. Mammography should be used for any aged woman with a suspected breast neoplasm.
5. Thermography should be dropped from the program.

Nurses as health teachers should inform patients and women with whom they come in contact of the advantages and risks of mammography and the recent decisions about its use.

Thermography and Xerography

Thermography is a diagnostic procedure that provides a picture of the surface temperature of the skin area of the breast. Abnormal circulatory signs may be detected by infrared photography. Signals are electronically converted to an oscilloscopic display. Following patient preparation and instruction similar to those for mammography, the patient is placed in a room under basal conditions (*i.e.,* the room has been cooled to 21° C, or 70° F) for 20 to 30 minutes. By means of a sophisticated heat-sensing apparatus, it is possible to detect minute amounts of heat generated in and around areas of increased blood supply, indicating the existence of pathology. The method requires a well trained radiologist to interpret abnormal patterns. A diagnosis is made only within the context of a thorough history and complete physical examination. However, as was indicated previously, this procedure is no longer advocated as a diagnostic method for breast cancer.

Xerography provides an x-ray of the soft tissue of the breast, using a very limited amount of radiation. In this procedure, a selenium-coated plate is subjected to an electrical charge, the x-ray exposure is made, and the plate is then developed by a special process under careful monitoring. The result is a xerogram in which all tissues of the breast, including the skin, are portrayed in a bas-relief effect.

Biopsy: Aspiration Cytology

This procedure, which involves obtaining tissue specimens for examination, can be done in the hospital outpatient department or the physician's office. Following the injection of a local anesthetic, a No. 22 needle is directed into the site to be sampled. Suction is applied to a syringe, and tissue is drawn into the needle. This material is spread on an albuminized glass slide and stained before being sent to the laboratory. Approximately 98% of lesions can be accurately diagnosed by this technique.

Incisional vs. Excisional Biopsy. Biopsies may be done in the operating room under general anesthesia or as an outpatient procedure under local anesthesia. A biopsy may comprise the entire lesion (excisional) or a piece of the specimen (incisional). Tissue may be sent to the laboratory to be frozen for subsequent study or it may be examined as quickly as possible if a 24-hour report is requested. Very thin slices containing a good cross section of tissue are stained with a dye to facilitate microscopic observation.

▷ Conditions Affecting the Nipple

Fissure of the Nipple. A *fissure of the nipple* is a longitudinal ulcer that tends to develop in any woman who is nursing a baby. The ulcer is irritated constantly by the baby's sucking and causes the mother considerable pain, often associated with bleeding of the nipple. Prophylactic treatment, cleanliness, and washing and drying of the nipple after each nursing usually prevent the occurrence of this condition. In the prenatal period, the woman can wash, dry, and lubricate the nipples in preparation for nursing, in order to help prevent fissure development. If a fissure develops, it should be washed at frequent intervals with sterile saline solution, and nursing should continue only with the use of an artificial nipple. If healing does not occur promptly, or if the case is severe and painful, nursing should be stopped and a breast pump used instead. Persistent ulceration suggests carcinoma or a primary syphilitic lesion.

Bleeding or Bloody Discharge From the Nipple (Intraductal Papilloma). At times, a bloody discharge may seep from the nipple and stain the clothes. Often, there may be one area at the edge of the areola where pressure produces the discharge. Although a bloody nipple discharge may be caused by malignancy, it is most commonly due to a wartlike papilloma growing in one of the larger collecting ducts just at the edge of the areola, or in an area of cystic disease. This bleeds on trauma, and the blood collects in the duct until it is pressed out at the nipple. The duct can be identified in the nipple and traced down, so that the duct and the papilloma can be excised.

Paget's Disease of the Breast. This disease of the nipple is seen most frequently in women over 45; usually, it is unilateral. Most often, it begins as a mild eczematoid condition of the nipple that may spread over the areola and even part of the breast; later, it may become ulcerated or eroded. In the more advanced stages, retraction of the nipple may occur. This is a true carcinoma of the ducts of the breast that converge at the nipple.

When any lesion of the nipple has not healed after a few weeks of treatment by simple cleansing and protective measures, a suspicion of Paget's disease should be confirmed by biopsy examination. This disease demands early and total removal of the breast.

▷ Breast Infection

Lactational Mastitis. Lactational mastitis may occur at the beginning or the end of lactation. Mastitis may result from the transfer of microorganisms to the breast by the hands of the patient or those of the personnel caring for her. The baby with an oral, eye, or skin infection may be a source of infection. Mastitis may be caused by blood-borne organisms. An infection of the ducts results, causing stagnation of milk in one or more lobules. The breast becomes tough or doughy, and the patient complains of dull pain in the region affected. A nipple that is discharging pus, serum, or blood demands investigation.

Treatment consists of taking the baby off the breast temporarily. A broad-spectrum antibiotic may be given to the mother for 7 to 10 days. Progesterone has been found to reduce breast congestion, which in turn relieves the pain. The patient should wear a firm breast support and follow good habits of personal hygiene.

Lactational Mammary Abscess.   A breast abscess usually develops as a sequela of an acute mastitis, although it may occur independently of lactation. The area affected becomes very tender and dusky red, and pus may be expressed from the nipple. Nursing is stopped and adequate support is provided for the breasts. Chemotherapy and antibiotic therapy are prescribed; however, incision and drainage may be performed when fluctuation indicates the presence of pus. Hot, wet dressings increase the drainage and hasten resolution.

▷ Benign Cysts and Tumors of the Breast

- Every growth within the breast should be viewed with suspicion and should be removed unless there is a contraindication.

Cystic Disease of the Breast.   In this condition of the breast, many small cysts are produced due to an overgrowth of fibrous tissue in the area of the ducts. The disease occurs most commonly between the ages of 30 and 50. These cysts are labile, that is, they may develop quickly to a considerable size in a few days and also decrease in size just as rapidly. They may be noted as lumps, which may be either painless or tender when palpated or pressed, particularly before menstruation. Occasionally, shooting pains may be felt. For tenderness, a supporting brassiere worn day and night may be helpful. The cyst itself rarely has any malignant potential, although breasts containing cysts may be more prone to developing cancer than normal breasts. Most cysts can be treated by simple aspiration of the fluid under local anesthesia. Usually, the fluid will not reaccumulate. If the fluid is uncharacteristic on aspiration, biopsy may be recommended.

When pain and tenderness are more severe (enough to warrant suppression of ovarian function), danazol (Danocrine*) may be prescribed. By inhibiting secretion of FSH and LH, ovarian production of estrogen is suppressed. This hypoestrogenic effect may be the reason for a decrease in breast pain and nodularity. Possible side-effects are fluid retention and hepatic disturbance.

_____
* Winthrop Laboratories

Fibroadenomata (Adenofibroma).   _Fibroadenomata_ are firm, round, movable, benign tumors of the breast, usually appearing in the breasts of girls in their late teens and early 20s. They cause no pain and are not tender. They can be removed through a small incision and have no malignant potential.

Nursing Interventions.   The psychological and physical needs of the woman with benign breast problems determine the kind of teaching and assistance that is required. This is ascertained on an individual basis. Obviously, there is greater risk of additional breast problems, including precancerous manifestations. The nurse can emphasize the need for monthly breast self-examination. Comfort measures that can be suggested are as follows: for tenderness and pain, wear a well-supporting bra 24 hours a day; make a determination as to whether warm or cool appliances are effective (warm compresses, heating pad, cool compresses, ice bag); use mild analgesics, such as aspirin or acetaminophen; reduce or eliminate methylxanthines (coffee, tea, cola, theophylline) since this appears to reduce fibrocystic masses; adhere to a low-salt diet, especially the 2 weeks before menstruation (diuretics may be helpful); and reduce fear and anxiety through education, reassurance, and follow-up support.

▷ Breast Carcinoma

Incidence.   The incidence of breast cancer has continued to rise over the past 35 to 40 years, whereas the mortality rate has changed very little. This appears to be a hopeful sign in the battle against this disease and undoubtedly means that a higher proportion of women are being treated earlier and that the methods of treatment have improved. Mortality continues to increase with age except during the menopause, at which time there is a slight decrease in incidence (the reason is unknown). The highest incidence is found in the unmarried female, and the lowest incidence occurs among those who have had multiple pregnancies or those who gave birth to their first child before the age of 27. Low incidence is also noted in women who have had an early artificial menopause. Racial differences have been noted, but no explanation is offered as to why, for example, the women of Japan have the lowest incidence. Upon migrating to the United States, these women adopt our culture; interestingly, their mortality rate from breast cancer then increases (Chart 47-1).

Etiology.   The cause of breast carcinoma is not known; however, several factors appear to influence its occurrence. The strongest factor is genetic; women of succeeding generations are not only predisposed to develop breast cancer, but they develop it 10 to 12 years earlier than women without a family history of breast cancer. Women who have more menstrual periods are more prone to have breast cancer, whereas women with more children have a lower incidence of it. Obviously, bearing children reduces the number of menstrual periods. Breast feeding also appears to protect against breast cancer. The factor of a milk virus being transmitted by nursing mothers has been noted with mice, but studies are insufficient in humans at present.

Chart 47-1
Women at High Risk for Breast Cancer (*High Risk Factors*)

Women over age 40 (North American, West European)
Familial history of breast cancer
Nulliparous women or those whose first parity occurred after age 30
Natural menopause occurring after age 50
Exposure to carcinogens
Chronic psychological stress
Presence of other cancer, such as endometrial, colon-rectum, salivary gland, ovarian

---

The question continues regarding the effect of estrogens in promoting breast cancer. This uncertainty has a bearing on the use of the "pill" for contraceptive purposes. Although the long-range effects of using the "pill" are incomplete, there is reason to suggest that other means of contraception should be used by women who have a family history of breast cancer or by those who have gross cystic disease, multiple breast papilloma, or cancer in one breast.

Pathophysiology.   Basically, breast cancer is a disease of breast tissue. It begins as an atypical area, progresses to a carcinoma *in situ* (either ductal or lobular), and then enters a minimally invasive stage (up to 5 mm [$\frac{3}{16}$ inch]). Once the carcinoma passes this stage, there is a higher likelihood of its invading the lymph nodes and the systemic circulation. Because the same factors affect both breasts, the opposite breast must be carefully watched for the development of a second carcinoma.

The tumor is located most frequently in the upper outer quadrant of the breast. As it grows, it becomes attached to the chest wall or the overlying skin. If no treatment is given, the tumor invades the surrounding tissues and extends to the lymph glands of the adjacent axilla. When the tumor arises in the medial half of the breast, its extension may involve the lymph nodes within the chest along the internal mammary artery (Fig. 47-2). Metastases may occur in the lungs, bone, brain, or liver. In untreated cases, death usually results in 2 or 3 years.

Clinical Classification (Before Treatment)*

Symbols

T—primary tumor

T_1—up to 2 cm ($\frac{3}{4}$ inch), skin uninvolved
T_2—2 cm to 5 cm ($\frac{3}{4}$ inch to 2 inches), skin dimpled

$\left. \begin{array}{l} T_3 \\ T_4 \end{array} \right\}$ varies between International and American classifications

---

* International classification that is used most commonly in the United States.

N—regional lymph nodes
N_0—no palpable lymph nodes
N_1—clinically palpable

$\left. \begin{array}{l} N_2 \\ N_3 \end{array} \right\}$ varies

M—distant metastasis
M_0—no distant metastasis
M_1—evidence of metastasis

Staging
(See Fig. 47-3.)
Classification by T, N, and M in a more precise grouping
Ex. Stage I: $T_1N_0M_0$
Stage III: $T_3 N_2 M_0$
Stage IV: Any TN symbol + M_1

▶ **Assessment**

Clinical Manifestations.   The symptoms of the disease, unfortunately, are insidious. A nontender lump, which may be movable, appears in the breast, usually in the upper outer quadrant. Pain is usually absent, except in the very late stages. Eventually, dimpling or "orange peel" appearance of the skin may be observed. On examination in the mirror, the patient may note asymmetry and an elevation of the affected breast. Nipple retraction may be evident. Later, the breast becomes more or less fixed on the chest wall, and nodules appear in the axilla. Finally, ulceration occurs and malnutrition and general ill health become prominent.

Inflammatory carcinoma is a rare type of breast cancer (1%–2%) that produces symptoms different from those of other breast cancers. The localized tumor is tender and painful; the breast is abnormally firm and enlarged. The skin over it is red and dusky in color. Often edema and nipple retraction occur. These symptoms rapidly increase in severity and usually prompt the woman to seek medical help sooner than the ordinary breast cancer patient.

Prognosis.   Breast cancer is more unpredictable than most other cancers because of hormone dependence, immune response, host resistance, and other variable factors. If the lymph nodes have not been involved, the prognosis is better than in those instances when cancer cells are found in the nodes. In clinical assessment, the absence of palpable nodes does not necessarily mean absence of malignancy (the growth may be microscopic). However, the presence of a palpable node, even a large node, may reflect an inflammation rather than a tumor. Tumor spread at the time of treatment appears to be more significant in prognosis than the type of treatment.

▶ **Planning and Implementation**

Goals

Major goals for the patient include the following:

1. Reduction of emotional stress and anxiety, and ability to cope with the problem
2. Acceptance of and compliance with prescribed treatment plan
3. Absence of or minimal complications
4. Adaptation to a changed life-style and possibly continued supervision and therapy

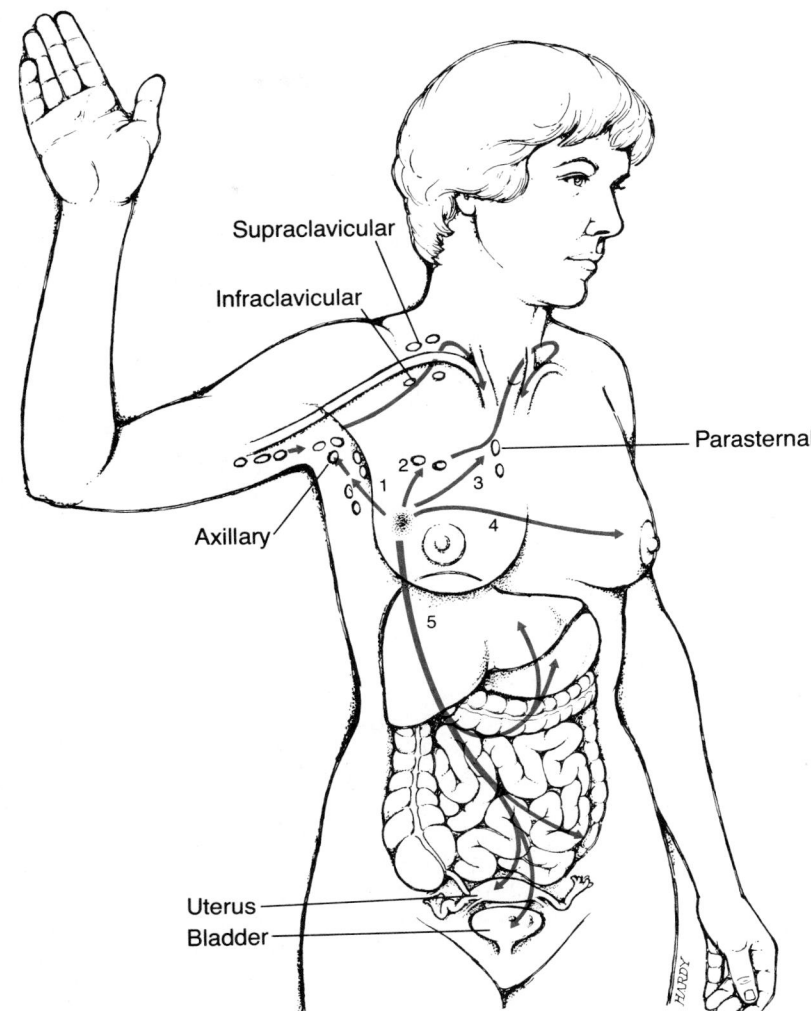

Figure 47-2. Lymphatic drainage of the mammary gland. Metastases from cancer of the mammary gland may follow several lymphatic pathways: 1. Upper outer quadrant to axillary, infraclavicular, supraclavicular nodes, etc. 2. Upper inner quadrant to intercostal and parasternal nodes. 3. Upper inner quadrant directly to parasternal nodes. 4. Directly across midline to opposite breast. 5. Lower quadrants, particularly inner aspect, through pectoralis major, external oblique, and linea alba to subperitoneal lymphatic plexus, followed by abdominal and pelvic spread.

To assist the patient in meeting these goals, the major objectives of therapy are:

1. To prepare the patient for various diagnostic tests
2. To recognize the patient's concerns, provide support, and solicit additional psychosocial–spiritual resources as required; these relate to comfort and coping measures, physical restoration, and cosmetic results as it relates to her sexuality
3. To prepare the patient physiologically, physically, and psychologically for surgery
4. To minimize/prevent postoperative complications
   a. Achieve proper drainage of wound
   b. Avoid injury
   c. Initiate an exercise program (to avoid shoulder dysfunction, lymphedema of arm)
5. To teach patient to adjust to and accept a modified lifestyle if required
   a. Optimal functioning
   b. Early detection of recurrent disease
   c. Proper outlook on life
   d. Reintegration with family, loved ones, and friends

Management

The approach to treating breast cancer has altered during the last decade, reflecting the basic premise that *this disease is not local but systemic in nature.* Because of this assumption, not only is the local cancer treated, but the micrometastatic cancer, which may have disseminated throughout the body or may be present within the surrounding breast tissue, is also treated. More specifically, surgery combined with adjuvant chemotherapy is more effective than surgery alone for certain groups of patients. Studies are being conducted to determine the best strategy, correct combination of chemotherapeutic agents, and optimum timing in the multidisciplinary approach.

One of these approaches includes the use of hormonal manipulation, which is greatly influenced by the index of estrogen and progesterone receptors as determined by an assay done on 1 g of tumor taken at the original biopsy. Early studies suggest a 70% to 80% chance of favorable response to hormone manipulation if the receptor studies are positive.

More recently, combinations of drugs have become an important step in sequential chemotherapy as an adjuvant

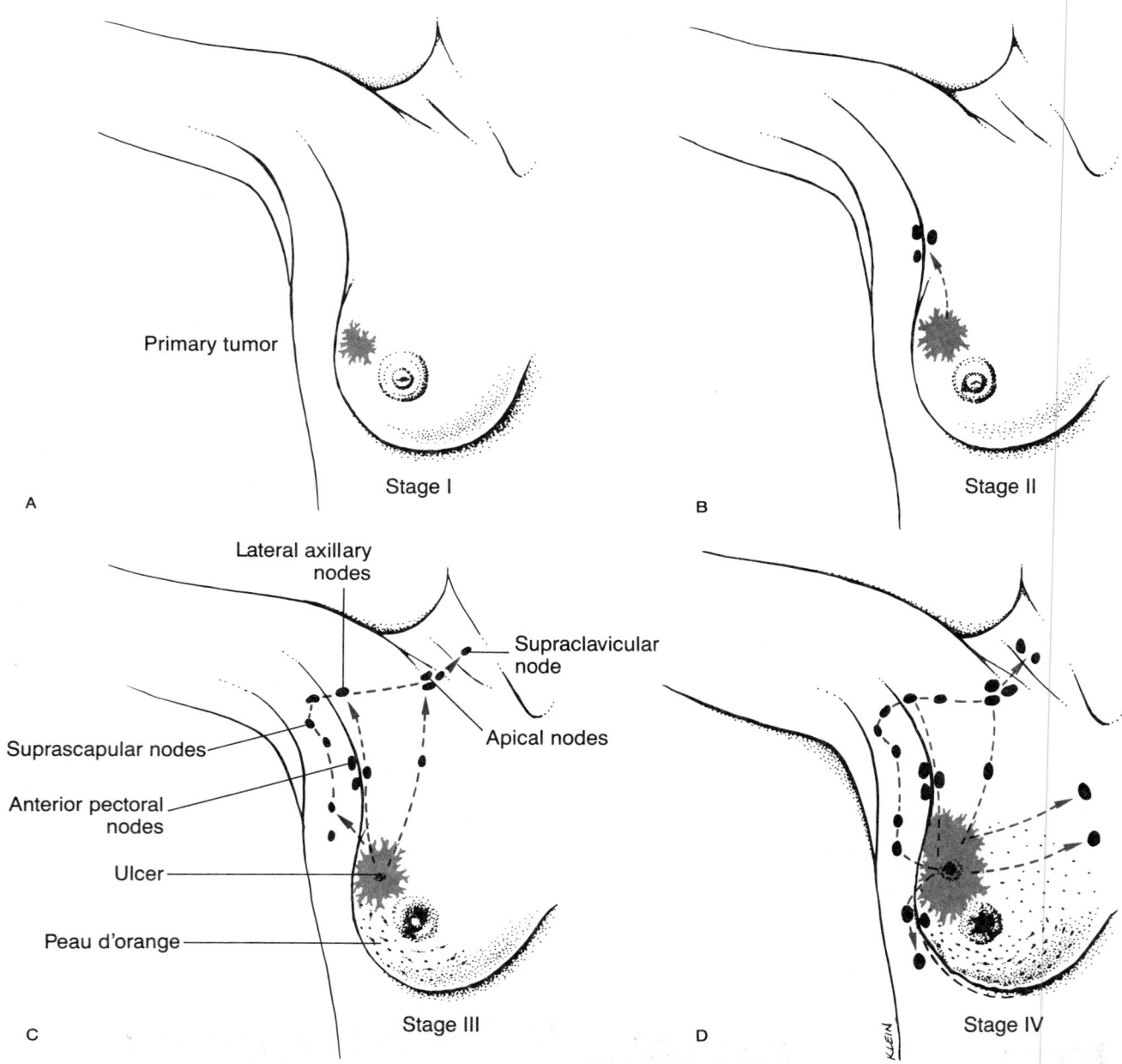

Figure 47-3. Clinical staging of patients with carcinoma of the breast. Staging is determined by the extent of the spread. (*A*) Stage I. Carcinoma is confined to the mammary lobules; no evidence in the regional nodes. (*B*) Stage II. Extension evident outside the lobules with tethering to the skin; axillary nodes clearly contain metastases. (*C*) Stage III. Tumor has infiltrated the skin and may have caused ulceration, or it has invaded the lymphatics and produced peau d'orange over the tumor site. Penetration extends to the deep fascia and perhaps the pectoralis major. Metastases over axillary nodes have extended beyond the capsules. (*D*) Skin is grossly ulcerated, peau d'orange appears over the whole breast, and deep fixation has occurred to the ribs. There is distant metastasis. (Adapted from McCredie JA (ed): Basic Surgery. New York, Macmillan, 1977.)

to surgery. Particularly useful is CMF (Cytoxan, methotrexate, and fluorouracil). This may also be used with nonspecific immunotherapy, such as BCG (bacille Calmette-Guérin).

Adjuvant Chemotherapy of Breast Cancer. *Adjuvant chemotherapy of breast cancer* is the use of cytotoxic drugs following primary excisional therapy; the purpose is to eliminate occult or micrometastatic spread of the disease. When assessing its values, it is important to weigh the efficacy of this form of therapy against its toxic effects.*

* Common chemotherapeutic agents: CMF—three chemicals: cyclophosphamide, methotrexate, 5-Fluorouracil; CMF–VP—five chemicals: cyclophosphamide, methotrexate, 5-Fluorouracil, plus vincristine and prednisone; CAF—cyclophosphamide, Adriamycin, fluouracil.

Following mastectomy, premenopausal patients with histologic evidence of lymph nodal metastases have shown improvement when receiving established combined chemotherapeutic agents. Such survival benefits seem to outweigh the problems of early toxicity. Other problems that should be considered are the increased financial burden and the interruptions in family life and occupations.

Adjuvant chemotherapy for the patient with stage 1 breast malignancy (negative axillary lymph nodes) is not recommended at present. Research is in progress to determine which of these patients are at high risk of relapse after initial surgical therapy; these may then qualify for adjuvant chemotherapy.

Key considerations in determining whether this form of therapeutic intervention is desirable are the involvement of the axillary lymph nodes, menopausal status, and estrogen receptor levels. Also, the nature of drug toxicity, both acute and remote, must be appreciated. As additional research results emerge, more definitive treatment options will be determined. (See also Chap. 17, p. 308.)

Surgical Management.   The usual treatment of carcinoma of the breast is removal or destruction of the whole tumor. It is evident that complete removal of the tumor can be accomplished most surely when the cancer is still confined to the breast. This is borne out by clinical experience, which shows a rate of cure better than 80% if the tumor is confined to the breast. When cancer cells have spread to the nodes of the axilla, the cure rate falls to 40%.

Types of surgical intervention include the following*:

1. Simple excision (lumpectomy or tumorectomy) followed by radiation of unremoved breast tissue and axillary nodes
2. Quadrantectomy: resection of the involved breast quadrant (usually upper outer quadrant), dissection of axillary lymph nodes, and radiotherapy to the ipsilateral residual breast tissue
3. Simple mastectomy followed by radiation of unremoved axillary nodes plus radiation boost to the scar area
4. Modified radical mastectomy: entire breast and axillary lymph nodes removed, with or without pectoral muscle (Fig. 47-4)
5. Radical mastectomy: entire breast, axillary lymph nodes, and both pectoral muscles removed
6. Extended radical mastectomy: same as radical mastectomy, plus other lymph nodes (parasternal) are removed

Some specialists recommend that unless distant metastasis is evident or the disease is highly malignant, radical or modified mastectomy produces the best therapeutic results. However, a great deal of controversy surrounds the choice of treatment.

There continues to be a progressive development of more conservative procedures. This is due to several factors: (1) assessment techniques such as mammography are revealing cancers of smaller dimensions; (2) patients are requesting less mutilative approaches; and (3) it is believed that more conservative treatment will encourage women to do breast self-examination and seek medical advice at the first evidence of a breast lump.

Psychosocial Preparation.   (See Chart 47-2.) Emotional preparation of the patient begins at the moment she is told that hospitalization and biopsy, and possibly other surgery, may be required. Actually, all women, when informed of possible breast disorders, should be prepared to follow through on suspicious findings. Upon admission to a hospital for a questionable tumor of the breast, most women have a real fear of cancer. Unfortunately, many times this fear has made them delay seeking treatment until the tumor has

*"Prophylactic mastectomy"—a total mastectomy for benign disease with removal of the entire breast, including the nipple and areola. This has been requested by women with a positive family history of having had one breast removed for cancer. However, this is a controversial procedure.

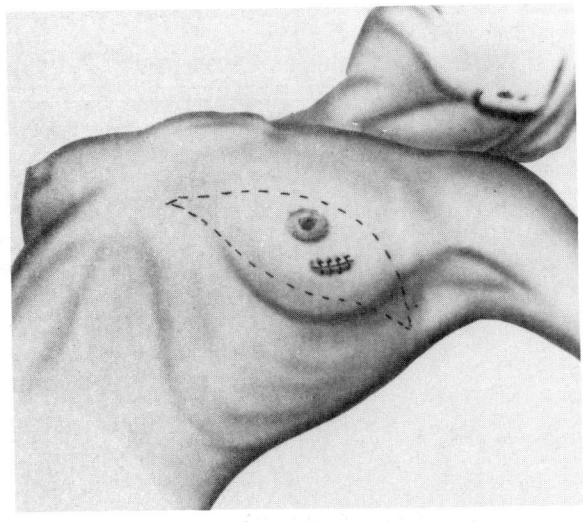

A

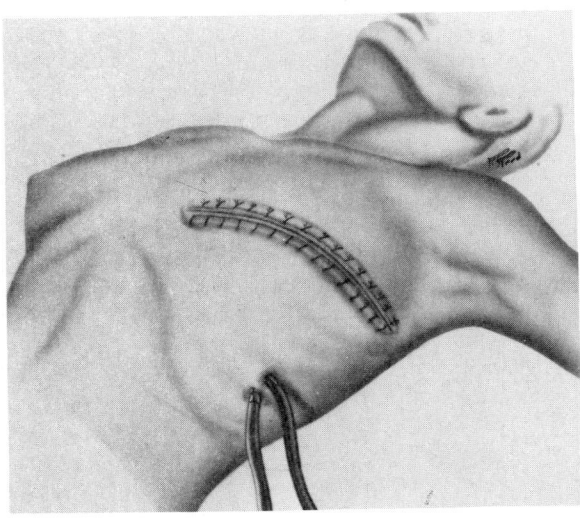

B

Figure 47-4. (*A*) Incision line for a modified radical mastectomy. Note the advantage of a transverse incision—scar is kept below the axilla (lower border of axillary hairline) and remains within the area covered by a brassiere). (*B*) Incision has been closed and suction catheters for postoperative drainage are in place. A light dressing will be placed. (From Hermann and Steiger: Modified radical mastectomy. SCNA, 58:743, Aug 1978.)

(Text continues on page 1079)

Chart 47-2
Psychosocial Problems Faced by the Patient With Breast Cancer

This model is designed as a conceptual tool to assist in the development of a nursing care plan or in analyzing the needs of individual patients with breast cancer. The diagrams reflect most of the major critical events and psychosocial problems associated with breast cancer as well as the usual kinds of responses of patients and their families to those problems and events. Each patient and each patient's family requires a unique assessment and intervention plan, since needs and experiences are as distinctive as they are individual. *This framework is designed to guide in the development of nursing interventions intended to alleviate stress, enhance coping abilities, and improve the patient's and family's chances for emotional recovery.*

I. The Prodromal Profile

By assessing the personal characteristics of the patient, the nurse can anticipate ways in which the patient will respond to or cope with illness.

How does she typically approach problems?

What are her attitudes toward her own health maintenance? toward physicians and seeking medical attention?

How flexible or rigid is she in making adjustments, accepting crisis situations?

What is her intellectual capability to make and accept decisions?

What is her physical condition?

What is her relation to her family? How supportive are they?

What has been the patient's personal experience with illness? with cancer?

How informed is she about breast cancer? about her own illness?

II. The Prediagnostic Period

Usually, shock is part of the reaction of discovering a sign or symptoms of a breast abnormality: a lump, dimpling of the skin, nipple discharge, or pronouncement by the physician of seeing a shadow on the mammogram. Then follow confusion and fear, withdrawal, and even avoidance of care (delay in seeking treatment). The family is usually unable to provide the hoped-for support, which finally forces the patient to seek medical attention and a clarification of the nature of the problem. Therefore, from a state of disorganization, the patient moves to seek more accurate information, which in turn will affect the next step in her ability to cope.

Adapted from Thomas SG: Breast cancer; the psychosocial issues. Cancer Nursing 1:53-60, Feb 1978. Copyright by Masson Publishing USA, Inc., New York.)

I. Prodromal Period

Patient Experience

1. History of prior serious illness, especially cancer
2. Experience with health care system
3. Information about breast cancer
4. Relationship with breast or other cancer patient

Patient Variables	*Family Variables*
1. Personality	1. Stability
2. Coping patterns	2. Number and age of members
3. Health beliefs and practices	3. Proximity and intimacy
4. Affective state	4. Interdependence
5. Intellectual and cognitive abilities	5. Resources
6. Biographical data	6. Roles and responsibilities
7. Attitudes toward breast cancer	7. Cultural/ethnic background
8. Self-concept	

Purpose:

Help toward formulation of planned interventions as patient and family go through critical events

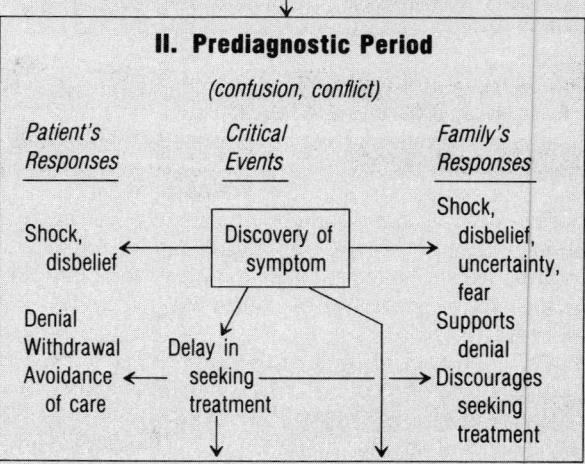

II. Prediagnostic Period

(confusion, conflict)

Patient's Responses	*Critical Events*	*Family's Responses*
Shock, disbelief	Discovery of symptom	Shock, disbelief, uncertainty, fear
Denial Withdrawal Avoidance of care	Delay in seeking treatment	Supports denial Discourages seeking treatment

(continued)

Chart 47-2
Psychosocial Problems Faced by the Patient With Breast Cancer (continued)

III. The Diagnostic Period

The family is usually excluded during this time. The patient is likely to be fearful about test outcomes and even embarrassed in undergoing some of the procedures. Unless there is confirmation of a benign process, she is usually directed to a biopsy or other surgical treatment alternative.

IV. The Preoperative Period

This is a confused time for the patient and her family. The patient usually feels well but realizes she cannot obtain bona fide reassurance from those caring for her. Her care and control are slipping to others, causing her to feel confused. She may feel threatened because decisions are being made by others. The family reflects her confusion.

III. Diagnostic Period

(coping)

Patient		*Family*
Active problem solving		Feels excluded
Seeks reassurance when denial fails	1. Seeks medical advice: x-rays 2. Referral to surgeon 3. Needle biopsy	Encourages patient to seek information
Fearful of outcome		Fearful of result
Anxious about techniques, procedures		

IV. Preoperative Period

(contradictory responses)

Patient		*Family*
↑ Fear of unknown		Confused and uncertain
Ambivalent toward health-care personnel		Tries to be supportive
Fears loss of control over destiny	Decides about biopsy or mastectomy	Feels left out of decision-making process
Fearful of treatment alternatives		
↓ Self-esteem		
Feels alone, confused		

(continued)

V. The Operative Period

The peak of anxiety is felt by the patient and her family. The mastectomy may either immediately follow the biopsy, or an interval of time may separate the two procedures. In some instances, the separation of time may permit the patient to develop coping mechanisms. For other women, this interval may be agonizing. If the patient is part of the decision-making process, her adjustment is improved.

VI. The Immediate Postoperative Period

Again the patient's feelings and responses may be ambivalent. On the one hand, there is relief that the operative phase is over and that she lived through it, but she may be angered about the loss of her breast. Even ambivalence toward herself may be apparent, as is indicated by self-blame for her delay in seeking treatment. This may result in sleeplessness and depression. Her thoughts drift to her family, her relationship with her husband or lover, her job, or her future. Again, the family's reactions may parallel hers.

At home, the patient often feels lonely, isolated, and useless since she is unable to accept her former full role in the household or return to work, and other members of the family may express resentment over their extra work.

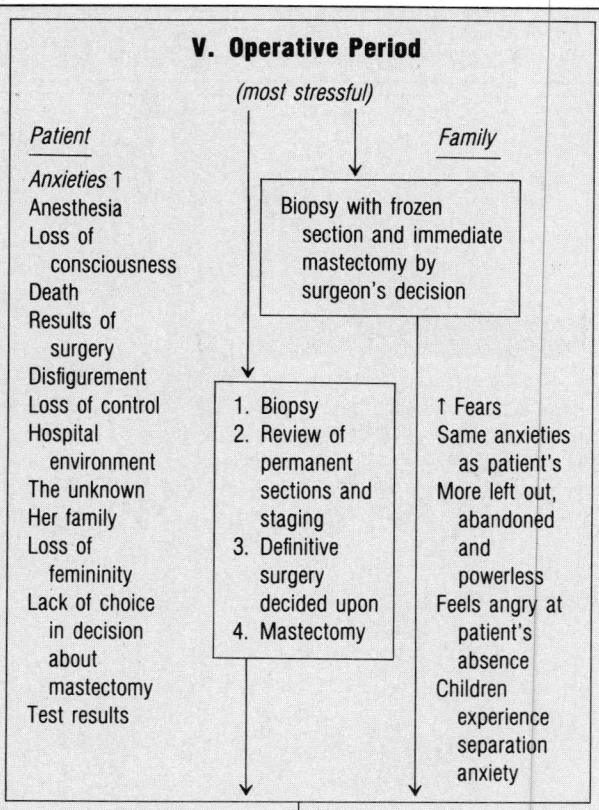

V. Operative Period

(most stressful)

Patient

Anxieties ↑
Anesthesia
Loss of
  consciousness
Death
Results of
  surgery
Disfigurement
Loss of control
Hospital
  environment
The unknown
Her family
Loss of
  femininity
Lack of choice
  in decision
  about
  mastectomy
Test results

Biopsy with frozen section and immediate mastectomy by surgeon's decision

1. Biopsy
2. Review of permanent sections and staging
3. Definitive surgery decided upon
4. Mastectomy

Family

↑ Fears
Same anxieties
  as patient's
More left out,
  abandoned
  and
  powerless
Feels angry at
  patient's
  absence
Children
  experience
  separation
  anxiety

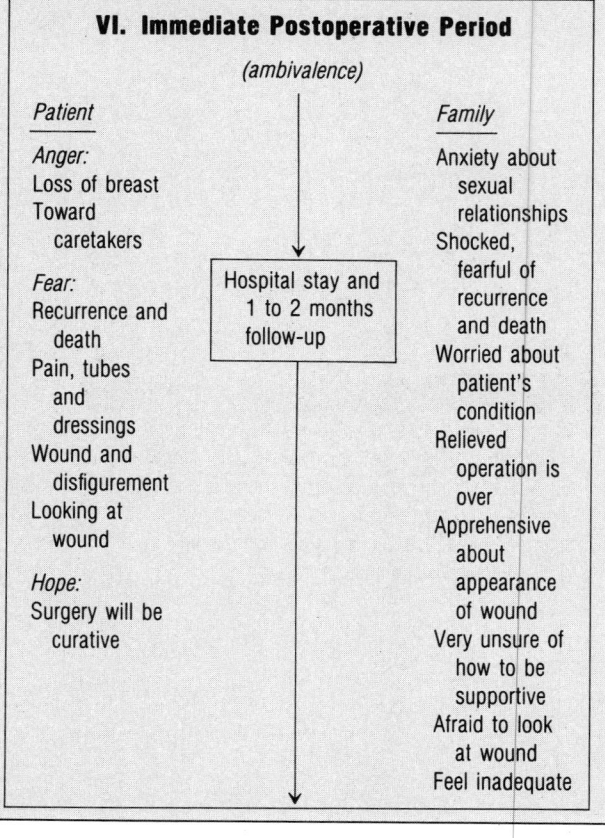

VI. Immediate Postoperative Period

(ambivalence)

Patient

Anger:
Loss of breast
Toward
  caretakers

Fear:
Recurrence and
  death
Pain, tubes
  and
  dressings
Wound and
  disfigurement
Looking at
  wound

Hope:
Surgery will be
  curative

Hospital stay and 1 to 2 months follow-up

Family

Anxiety about
  sexual
  relationships
Shocked,
  fearful of
  recurrence
  and death
Worried about
  patient's
  condition
Relieved
  operation is
  over
Apprehensive
  about
  appearance
  of wound
Very unsure of
  how to be
  supportive
Afraid to look
  at wound
Feel inadequate

VII. The Extended Postoperative Period

The patient and her family are now moving into a period that they hope will bear some resemblance to the more normal time. There is less support and there are greater stresses. The family's responses appear no longer confused, and they may find it difficult to empathize with the patient during this period. Angers are often expressed.

   The patient now faces the ordeal of being fitted for her prosthesis. This can be a trying time.

VIII. The Adjuvant Period

This may not apply to all patients, but it is a difficult adjustment period for those who do experience it. Toxic side-effects, inconvenience of treatments, and length of time involved contribute to making this a distressing time for many patients. For some patients, however, it represents a time of potentiating the positive over the negative. The termination of this period marks the beginning of the most affirmative phase.

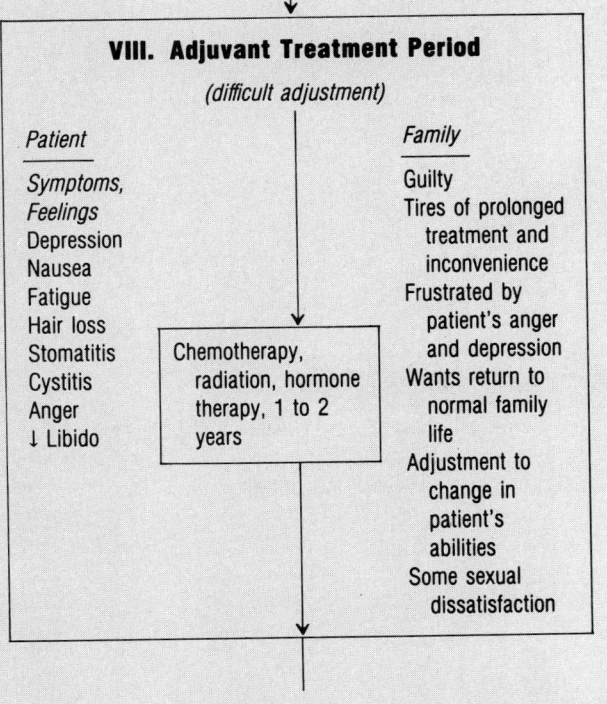

VII. Extended Postoperative Period

(less ambivalence, breakdown of denial, ↑ anger)

Patient		Family
Symptoms, feelings: Guilt Anger Depression Insomnia	Emotional and physical convalescence 2 to 6 months	Tries to forget about illness, represses fears of recurrence and death ↓ Support Anxiety about resuming sexual relations Children more demanding
Fear of death and recurrence, wound or prosthesis ↓ Self-esteem Loss of femininity	Obtaining the first prosthesis	
Stronger Hopeful	No evidence of disease: ←-- follow-up	

VIII. Adjuvant Treatment Period

(difficult adjustment)

Patient		Family
Symptoms, Feelings Depression Nausea Fatigue Hair loss Stomatitis Cystitis Anger ↓ Libido	Chemotherapy, radiation, hormone therapy, 1 to 2 years	Guilty Tires of prolonged treatment and inconvenience Frustrated by patient's anger and depression Wants return to normal family life Adjustment to change in patient's abilities Some sexual dissatisfaction

(continued)

Chart 47-2
Psychosocial Problems Faced by the Patient With Breast Cancer (continued)

IX. The Recovery Period

This is a time of more positive responses and the reordering of values and priorities. The possibility of mammoplasty may be considered by some women. Realistic optimism is increasingly evident.

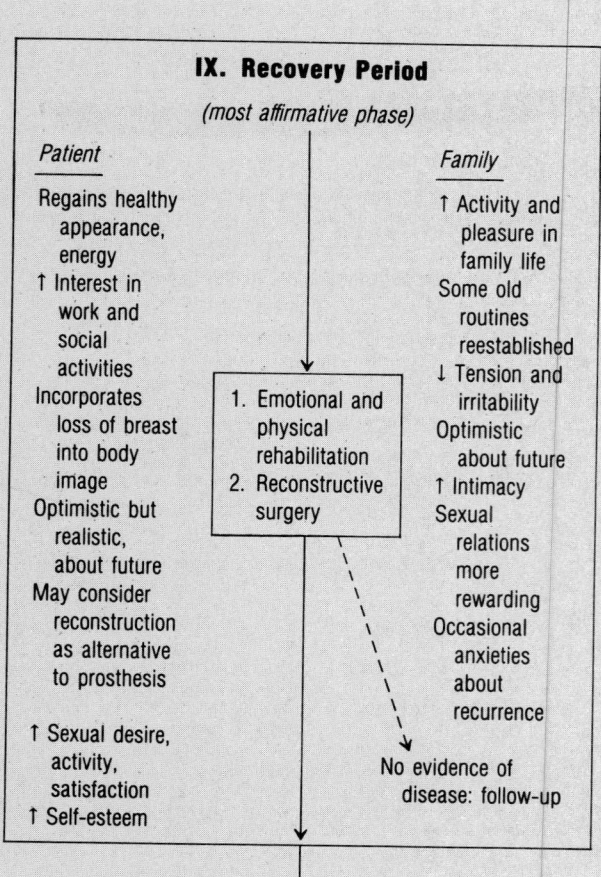

IX. Recovery Period

(most affirmative phase)

Patient		Family
Regains healthy appearance, energy		↑ Activity and pleasure in family life
↑ Interest in work and social activities		Some old routines reestablished
Incorporates loss of breast into body image	1. Emotional and physical rehabilitation 2. Reconstructive surgery	↓ Tension and irritability Optimistic about future
Optimistic but realistic, about future		↑ Intimacy Sexual relations more rewarding
May consider reconstruction as alternative to prosthesis		Occasional anxieties about recurrence
↑ Sexual desire, activity, satisfaction		No evidence of disease: follow-up
↑ Self-esteem		

X. The Terminal Period

For the person whose disease is terminal, the stages described by Kübler-Ross are usually experienced. The quality of life before death overtakes the actual fact of dying.

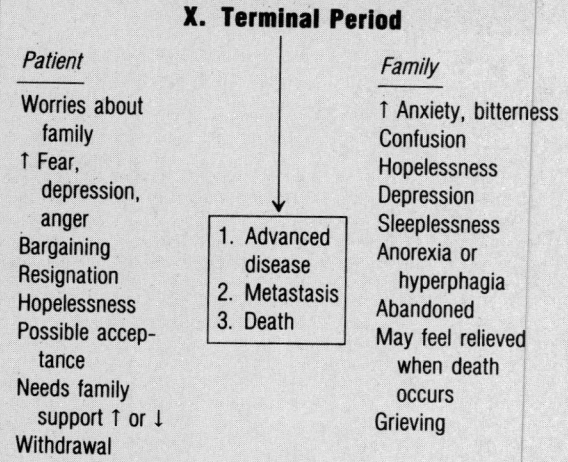

X. Terminal Period

Patient		Family
Worries about family		↑ Anxiety, bitterness
↑ Fear, depression, anger		Confusion Hopelessness Depression
Bargaining Resignation Hopelessness	1. Advanced disease 2. Metastasis 3. Death	Sleeplessness Anorexia or hyperphagia
Possible acceptance		Abandoned
Needs family support ↑ or ↓		May feel relieved when death occurs
Withdrawal		Grieving

metastasized. Fear also stems from the emotional trauma of knowing that the breast may be removed.

It must be recognized that a mastectomy is a significant threat to a women's feeling of femininity. Because of this, the nurse must be available to listen to and support the patient. One way to promote a positive attitude is to point out that loss of a breast, compared to loss of life, is a small price to pay. The availability of well-fitted prostheses means that a woman can dress just as fashionably as she did prior to surgery. Even swimsuits can be worn in attractive styles by the postmastectomy patient.

However, deep-seated concerns may not only stem from problems of physical adjustment, but may be related to other worries. "Will I be as attractive to my husband?" "Will he continue to love me?" "Will I be able to function as a wife?" "Will my children reject me?" These are the types of questions that plague many mastectomy patients. Because of such emotional concerns, the husband should be brought into selected planning sessions intended to prepare the woman for surgery. If he is properly prepared, his support, devotion, and understanding can be of tremendous importance to his wife. A good relationship can soften the impact of surgery, lessen the possibilities of complications, and provide an easier adjustment to her altered image. The nurse is in a position to be most helpful in applying effective mental health principles as part of the patient's preparation for surgery.

Preoperative and Perioperative Management

After proper preoperative staging, nothing should delay the operation except the necessary check of the physical and nutritional needs of the patient. If radical surgery is anticipated, in which there may be fluid and blood loss, blood replacement must be available. The patient is told by the surgeon that there is a possibility of radical surgery, if it is indicated. No patient should go to the operating room anticipating a half-inch incision for a tumor excision and return having had a radical mastectomy. Because the emotional factor is a significant one, encouragement and reassurance must be given all along the way.

A hypnotic is administered and the usual physical preoperative preparation is carried out. Skin preparation should be extensive enough to meet the maximal possible surgery. If it is known that radical surgery, including a skin graft, is to be done, the donor skin area (usually the anterior aspect of the thigh) must be shaved and cleaned.

Surgical Procedure. After receiving general anesthesia, the patient is placed in the supine position on the operating table. The arm of the affected side is positioned upward to expose the axilla. If a biopsy and frozen section are planned, the biopsy is done first. Then the entire field is redraped and a new set of instruments is used so that the possibility of transferring cancer cells from the biopsy site to the other areas of the wound is avoided. A *simple mastectomy* involves removal of a breast without lymph node dissection or with removal of only a few low nodes. A *radical mastectomy* includes removal of the breast and the underlying muscles down to the chest wall after the breast lymphatics in the axilla have been removed. Such a radical operation removes the tumor and the areas of possible lymphatic spread.

Bleeding points are ligated, and the skin is closed as well as possible over the chest wall. Skin grafting is done if the skin flaps are not of sufficient size to close the wound. Nonadhering dressing (Adaptic) permits serum and blood to escape between the strips. Pressure dressings may then be applied. Two drainage tubes are usually placed in the axilla and beneath the superior skin flap; portable suction may be preferred by some surgeons. Final dressings may be held in place by wide elastic bandages. A blood transfusion may be given during the operation to compensate for blood loss, if necessary.

Functional Considerations. The objective in this regard is to restore normal function to the hand, arm, and shoulder girdle on the affected side. Before surgery is performed, the surgeon plans an incision that will provide maximum opportunity to excise the tumor and the affected nodes. At the same time, the patient's life-style should be considered, and efforts should be made to avoid a scar that will be visible and restrictive. Skin flaps and tissue are handled meticulously to ensure proper viability, hemostasis, and drainage. A valuable technique involves injecting fluorescein dye into the peripheral vein at the time of surgical closure and actually inspecting the blood supply to the flaps with a Wood's lamp. When the light is turned off, the manner in which the blood has been distributed to the flaps can be assessed.

▶ Nursing Interventions

Usually, a general anesthetic is chosen for a simple mastectomy, a modified radical mastectomy, or a radical mastectomy. Postoperative care is given with special attention to pulse and blood pressure, since they are valuable indices in detecting shock and hemorrhage. Dressings must be inspected for bleeding, especially under the axilla and in the area on which the patient is lying. At the same time, tube drainage is monitored at close intervals.

After the patient has recovered from the anesthesia, analgesics are given for the relief of pain, and the patient is encouraged to turn and take deep breaths to avert pulmonary complications. The dressing usually is fairly snug; however, it should not be so tight that lung expansion is restricted. Some surgeons prefer to include the arm (flexed at the elbow) in the dressing to give added pressure. In other instances, gauze fluffs or foam rubber sponge may be added to the dressing within the binder to provide pressure.

In many patients, a drainage catheter is inserted through a stab wound into the axilla; this catheter is then attached to a suction machine and drained into a trap bottle. By this means, any serum and blood that collect are aspirated rapidly, and the skinflap is held tightly against the chest wall. Thus, collection of serum and formation of hematomas are avoided. Some surgeons eliminate pressure dressings early in the postoperative period and use portable suction instead. Dressings over incision and donor graft areas are changed according to the surgeon's preference.

Care of Incision Site. When dressings are changed, the nature of the incision, the way it looks and feels, and how it will gradually change are explained. The patient needs to know that sensation in the newly healed area may have lessened because nerves have been severed; however, the area should be bathed gently and blotted dry to avoid injury. Signs of irritation and possible infection should be described, so that if they occur, the patient will recognize them and report them to her physician. When talking about the incision, the nurse should use the term "incision" rather than "scar," since scarring connotes defect, deformity, and ugliness in the minds of many persons.

Gentle massage of the healed incision with cocoa butter helps to increase the elasticity of the skin and encourages circulation.

Positioning of the patient depends on the dressing; a semi-Fowler position is usually desirable. If free, the arm should be elevated with each joint positioned higher than the more proximal joint. Thus, gravity helps to remove the fluid via the lymphatic and venous pathways. Whether the arm is flexed or extended depends on the preference of the physician. Elevation of the arm helps to prevent lymphedema, which may occur after surgery because of interference with the circulatory and lymphatic systems (especially following true radical mastectomy). Whether or not there will be satisfactory postmastectomy lymph drainage depends on how many collateral lymphatic avenues were not destroyed during surgery.

The patient is usually allowed out of bed on the first or the second day after operation; the arm on the affected side may be held in a sling for a time to prevent tension on the wound. Assistance is given only when it is needed; the nurse supports the patient from the unoperated side. A normal diet may be given unless nausea is a symptom. If a drainage tube has been inserted, it is removed usually when the drainage has decreased markedly or has stopped.

Radiotherapy may be prescribed after the operation as a means of destroying any cancer cells that may have escaped removal at operation (if the tumor was central or medial, or if the tumor was very large, or if axillary nodes were involved). Radiation therapy is usually initiated 3 or 4 weeks after surgery. Anorexia, nausea, and vomiting can occur after irradiation; abstinence from eating and drinking for 3 hours before and after these treatments often helps. (See also Chap. 18.)

Psychosocial Considerations.   (See Chart 47-2.) The full impact of the meaning of a mastectomy may not be felt by the patient until several days or even weeks after surgery. Meanwhile, it is frequently helpful if the nurse takes the time to talk or listen to the patient whenever the patient expresses the need for this kind of support. Frequently asked questions include: Is it normal to drain so much? Will the swelling of my arm go down? How will my husband react to my deformity? Will my appearance be changed? Will I be able to wear a regular swimsuit? Will I be able to swim, play tennis, drive a car? The nurse should be able to respond to these questions with empathy and in a way that will help the patient to find the answers she seeks.

A woman's real sexual concern is fear of rejection by her husband or sex partner. Frequently, a postmastectomy patient envisions herself as mutilated and repulsive. This often results in her partner feeling rejected, and a cycle of misunderstanding results. By encouraging the couple to re-

late their concerns to each other, better understanding can result. A personal, caring manner is imperative; this patient needs someone with whom she can share her troubled thoughts.

A real problem may arise if the patient is reluctant to look at the incision site. Although the presence of the scar must eventually be faced, the patient should not be forced at this time to look at her chest area. Her psychological defenses may require that she be spared this added shock at this time. It is sometimes helpful to direct the patient to acceptance by first drawing a picture of the incision line on a piece of paper. Then at a later time, when the dressings are being changed, the patient may show signs of being willing to look at her chest. However, the nurse must explore this area in a very gentle manner. Any resistance on the part of the patient must be sensed and respected. Each woman must work her way to acceptance on the basis of her own individual psychological needs.

Rehabilitation

A carefully orchestrated program for rehabilitation should be a part of the treatment plan for every woman who has breast cancer. Rehabilitation is a team effort that embraces psychosocial, physical, and functional (including vocational) considerations.

Some breast cancers grow and spread rapidly, whereas others may take years to extend. Some cancers may not be excised completely but can be controlled over long periods of time. Thus, the rehabilitative management is geared to patients who have been cured and those whose disease is under control.

Clothing

Hospital Attire.   Since bulky dressings and drainage equipment must be accommodated, the patient's usual attire is the hospital gown or an opaque, full-gathered nightgown with wide sleeves and probably a ribbon drawstring at the neck. The patient and her family should realize the need for this type of gown. Additional special clothing may include a temporary brassiere with an insert, which may be obtained through the hospital or the American Cancer Society's "Reach to Recovery" program, or from a local department store. Usually, the garment can be laundered easily and has a pocket on the mastectomy side to accommodate a filler. (See below, Prosthesis.)

Attire at Home.   Some surgeons use no dressings after the first day, and the patient is encouraged to wear her normal clothing as soon as possible. Cotton wads or a rolled-up stocking may be placed in the brassiere as a temporary prosthesis. If dressings are still in place when the patient is discharged, loose-fitting clothing from the patient's wardrobe is usually satisfactory. The temporary "bra" is worn before the permanent prosthesis is prescribed. The incision must be healed before the surgeon's opinion is obtained regarding the kind of prosthesis needed and when it can be used. Garments that may present problems because of buttons or zippers should be avoided at first. Later, the exercise involved in manipulating buttons and zippers, especially for the arm on the affected side, is desirable. Zipper "pulls" are helpful when dresses with zippers in the back are worn.

Literature from "Reach to Recovery" (American Cancer

Society) offers suggestions for special clothing, such as night clothes, swimsuits, and evening wear. Most large department stores have mastectomy boutiques and personnel who can assist the woman who has had a mastectomy.

Prosthesis.   When a prosthesis is prescribed, its effect on the incision site should be observed. To offset irritation, a layer of lamb's wool is effective when pressure is exerted. The kind of prosthesis suitable for the patient is suggested on an individual basis by the surgeon. Skilled fitters from reliable companies are available, and they usually have many helpful suggestions, literature, and an optimistic, understanding approach that is most encouraging to postmastectomy patients.

In preparation for an individualized prosthesis, a temporary makeshift padded brassiere can be designed with the patient's participation. Loose cotton covered with gauze can be stitched loosely into the patient's own brassiere; snaps can be used in making a pocket to fit the "falsie." Ingenuity and resourcefulness can fashion effective padding from sanitary pads, nylon stockings, and shredded foam rubber.

There are many types of breast prostheses available: foam rubber, air-filled, fluid-filled, fluffed cotton, lamb's wool, plastic, synthetic, and cloth, either ready-made or custommade. A properly fitted brassiere is essential to a well-fitted prosthesis. Breasts readily follow the law of gravity and change their contour and position with every body motion. Therefore, the most satisfactory prostheses are those filled with a slow-flowing, thick fluid. Often when a patient knows that such appliances are available, her fear of disfigurement is greatly reduced.*

When the final prosthesis is to be obtained, consultants are available to assist the patient in selecting the one best suited for her with respect to specific need, cost, and use. Suggestions are given to avoid imbalance, "riding up," and discomfort, along with hints on wearing short-sleeved or sleeveless garments, evening gowns, and swimsuits. With this guidance, the woman should find a fair degree of comfort.

For some patients, reconstruction with a permanent prosthesis may be an alternative, depending on a number of factors (see p. 1087).

Arm Exercises

After 24 hours, the arm on the affected side should be engaged in active exercise. This activity can be increased each day as the patient is encouraged to do more for herself by brushing her teeth, washing her face, and combing her hair with the hand on the affected side. Failure to encourage such exercises as "climbing the wall with the fingers" may prolong the disuse of the arm and promote the development of a contracture. Exercise should not be accompanied by pain; if the patient has had a skin graft or if the incision was closed with considerable tension, such exercises are greatly limited and must be done very gradually.

Many hospitals promote classes for the postmastectomy patient; this provides encouragement for women who would

otherwise remain passive and inactive in their own rooms. At the bedside, pulley-type ropes from the over-bed or curtain frame can be used for one kind of exercise. Turning a jump rope that is attached to the doorknob can be arranged easily (see muscle-training exercises, Fig. 47-5). In all exercises, it is important to emphasize bilateral activity. Likewise, the value of proper posture must be emphasized; if the patient hunches over and favors the affected side as she combs her hair, the purpose of the exercise will be defeated.

Naturally, difficulty with arm movement is much greater in the patient who has undergone the classic radical mastectomy. Limitation of motion after simple and modified radical mastectomy is unusual, and the patient is encouraged to use the arm to the point of complete mobility almost immediately.

Lymphedema and Exercise.   Edema of the arm is a complication that occasionally plagues a woman who has had a radical mastectomy. Although the cause of lymphedema is not known, it will result if the number of properly functioning lymphatic channels is insufficient to ensure a return flow of lymph into the general circulation. Though edema may affect only the upper arm, often the entire arm on the operated side is involved. Such swelling can occur immediately following operation (postoperative surgical edema) or may occur many months or years after surgery (secondary surgical edema). The immediate postoperative edema "can be avoided only by meticulous surgical technique which achieves perfect wound healing . . . a factor in achieving perfect wound healing is skin grafting of the operative wound to avoid the triad of tension on the skin flaps, necrosis and infection."†

When axillary nodes and the lymphatic system have been removed, a collateral system for lymphatic drainage from the hand and arm must be developed (Fig. 47-6). This is done within a month and is facilitated by exercise. Although nine out of ten postmastectomy patients escape massive lymphedema, this complication would occur even less frequently if the nurse impressed upon patients the importance of elevating, massaging, and exercising the affected arm for 3 or 4 months following the operation.

For marked lymphedema, the arm should be elevated, *but not in adduction* since this position is uncomfortable and constricts the axilla. The elbow is elevated on a pillow so that the elbow is higher than the shoulder. The hand is further elevated on another pillow so that the hand is higher than the elbow. Elastic bandages are not recommended at this time since they may interfere with the formation of collateral lymphatic pathways.

One must not rule out the possibility of infection in the presence of significant lymphedema. Recurrent lymphangitis and cellulitis may be secondary to streptococcal infection. Warm packs and antimicrobial therapy are effective. Upon general assessment of the patient, the nurse may recognize that a general weight-reduction plan may be indicated. A diuretic may also help.

When acute infection has subsided, some physicians recommend the use of intermittent pneumatic compression

---

* A valuable guide that describes the various types of prostheses available may be found in the following consumer report article: After mastectomy: Finding the right prosthesis. Nov 1975. Consumer's Union, Orangeburg, New York 10962.

† Haagensen CD. Diseases of the Breast, 2nd ed. Philadelphia, WB Saunders.

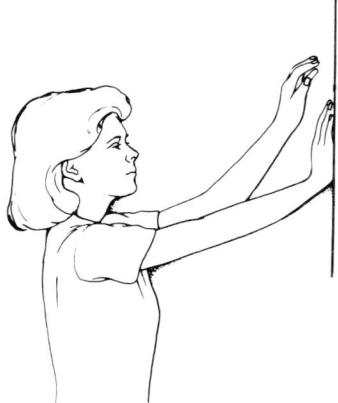

A. *Wall handclimbing.* Stand facing the wall, with the toes as close to the wall as possible—feet apart. With elbows somewhat bent, place the palms on the wall at shoulder level. By flexing the fingers, work hands up the wall until arms are fully extended. Work hands down to starting point.

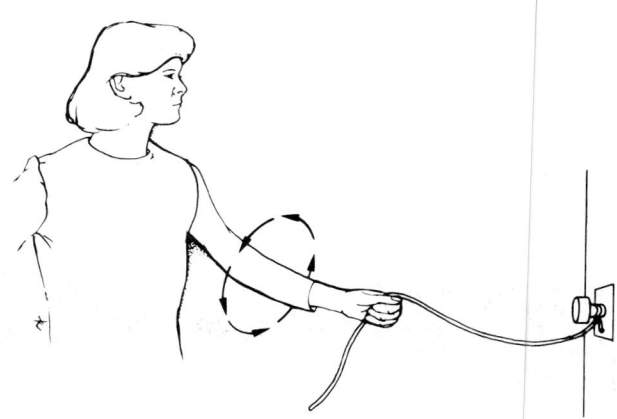

B. *Rope turning.* Stand facing the door. Take free end of light rope in hand of the operated side. Place other hand on hip. With arm extended and held away from the body—nearly parallel with the floor—turn rope, making as wide swings as possible. Slow at first—speed up later.

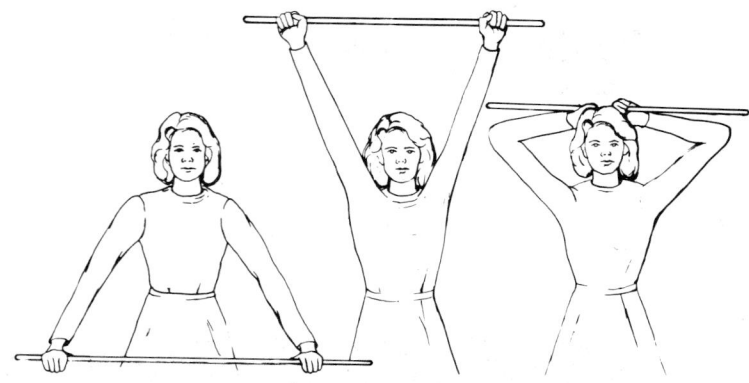

C. *Rod or Broom.* Grasp rod with both hands, held about 2 feet apart. With arms straight, raise rod over the head. Bend elbows lowering rod behind the head. Reverse maneuver, raising rod above the head, then to starting position.

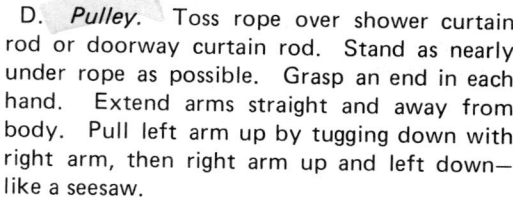

D. *Pulley.* Toss rope over shower curtain rod or doorway curtain rod. Stand as nearly under rope as possible. Grasp an end in each hand. Extend arms straight and away from body. Pull left arm up by tugging down with right arm, then right arm up and left down—like a seesaw.

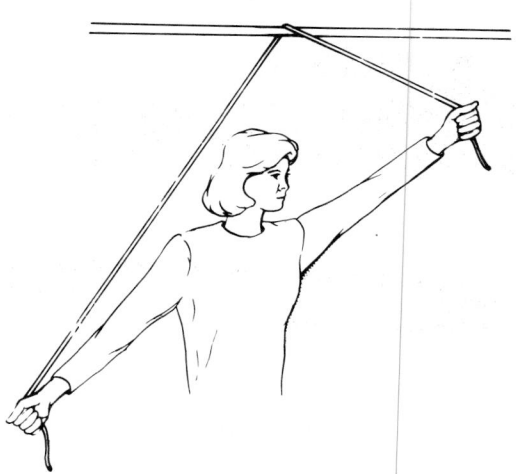

Figure 47-5. The purpose of the exercise program is to secure a complete range of motion of the affected shoulder joint. (Adapted from Radler: A Handbook for Your Recovery. New York, The Society of Memorial Center.)

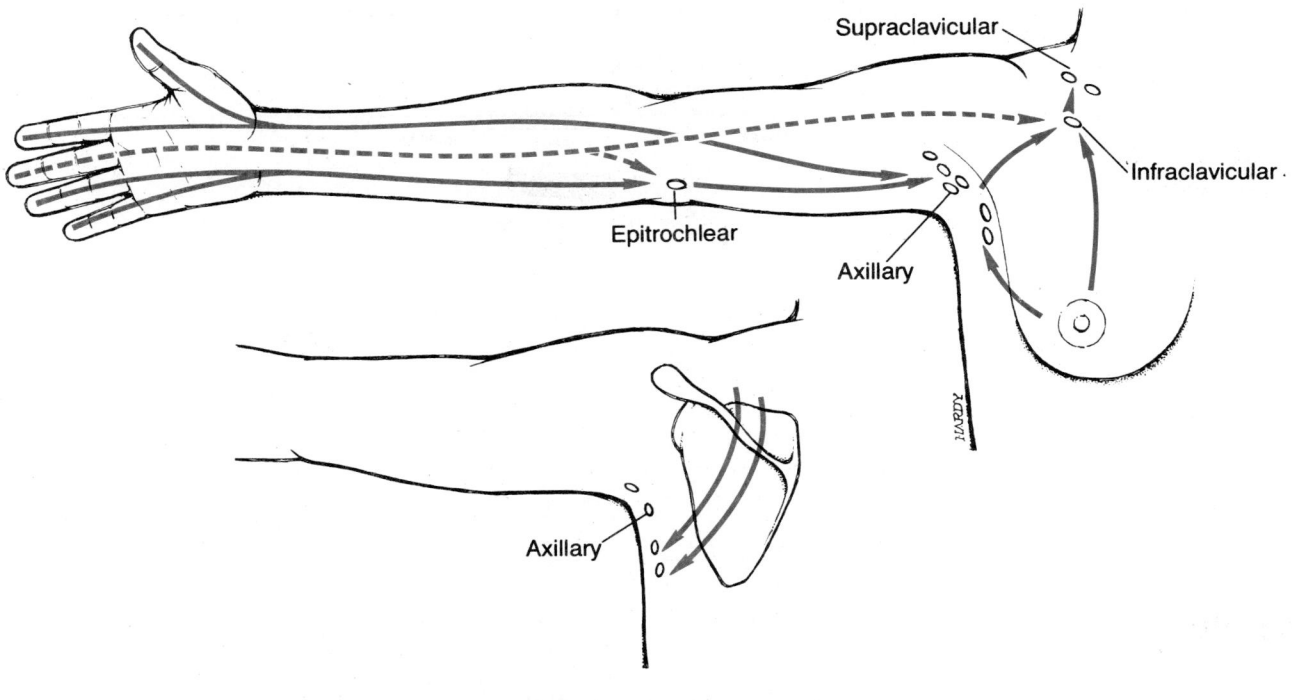

Figure 47-6. Lymphatic drainage of the upper extremity. The lymphatic vessels draining the fingers and the hand converge on the dorsum of the hand. From here the lymphatic drainage pursues three courses. The lymph vessels draining the ulnar aspect (little finger and ring finger) accompany the basilic vein and drain into the epitrochlear nodes and thence into the axillary nodes. The lymph vessels draining the thumb and the index fingers bypass the epitrochlear nodes and go directly to the axillary nodes. The lymph vessels draining the middle fingers may drain into the epitrochlear or the axillary, or may bypass both of these groups of nodes to drain directly into the infraclavicular, and thence into the supraclavicular, and finally into the bloodstream. The axillary nodes also receive lymph from the posterior scapular region (insert).

of the arm, but many doubt its value. For the chronic stage, the patient may wear an elastic sleeve (custom-made) from the wrist to the shoulder during the day when she is up and about.

Since secondary surgical edema may occur much later, one of the most important teaching points to emphasize with the patient is that for months and years she must take extra precautions to avoid cuts, bruises, and infection of the hand and arm on the side of her operation. Even pushing the cuticles back and injuring finger tissue may provide the portal of entry for infection, which in turn may trigger the development of lymphedema. Other precautions are listed in Chart 47-3.

The exercises done in the hospital and illustrated in Figure 47-5 can be related to household activities. Putting dishes on a shelf, dusting window sashes, typing, and piano playing are activities that promote and maintain muscle tone. Other suggestions are to swing the arm while walking; wear loose or nonconstricting clothing; keep the mastectomy site, underarm, and arm scrupulously clean; and avoid injury to the hand and arm.

Follow-up visits are very important for the evaluation of incision healing, mental outlook, general physical condition, and any evidence of recurrence. If there is a need

for consultation with a community nurse, the availability of such a service should be pointed out to the patient.

It should be emphasized that the incidence of primary and secondary lymphedema is markedly reduced in patients who have had modified radical mastectomy instead of the classic radical procedure.

▶ **Evaluation**

Expected Outcomes

1. Experiences a reduction of emotional stress and anxiety, and exhibits an ability to cope with the problem
   a. Is aware that husband or "significant other" has been apprised and prepared with regard to his role in providing support
   b. Recognizes that the loss of a breast is a small price to pay for life
   c. Understands the resources available for prosthetic use and style maintenance
   d. Is acquainted with resources of such organizations as "Reach to Recovery"
   e. Accepts social support of family, friends, or women who have had mastectomies as a significant aid in coping with a stressful experience

Chart 47-3
Special Hand and Arm Care on the Side of the Operation
(*For the Woman Who Has Had a Radical Mastectomy*)

Avoid	**Do**
Cuts, bruises, insect bites, burns	Protect the hand and arm on the operated side.
Injury to cuticles or hangnails	Apply lanolin hand cream several times daily.
Strong detergents	Use a thimble when sewing.
Working near thorny bushes	Stay out of the strong sun.
Digging in the garden	Wear a Medical-Alert tag engraved as follows: *Caution—*
Holding a cigarette	*lymphedema arm—no tests—no needle injections.*
Reaching into a hot oven	See physician if the arm gets red or swollen or becomes
Having blood drawn; injections	unusually hard.
Having a blood pressure cuff applied	
Wearing jewelry or a wrist watch	
Carrying heavy bags or purse	

2. Accepts and adheres to the prescribed treatment plan
   a. Recognizes the possibility of radical surgery following a biopsy
   b. Understands the possibility of grafting skin to the operative site from a donor area
   c. Knows that fluid and blood transfusions are not indicative of a worsening condition, but are necessary for fluid and electrolyte balance
   d. Appreciates the long-term benefits of chemotherapy or radiation (if prescribed), even though there may be uncomfortable side-effects
   e. Understands the nature and importance of proper exercises
3. Experiences little or no complications
   a. Is afebrile 48 hours prior to discharge
   b. Experiences no pain in operative area
   c. Has drainage-free incision site
   d. Has satisfactory wound healing; knows to report signs of redness, heat, pain
4. Adapts to a changed life-style and possibly continued supervision/therapy
   a. Accepts altered body image
   b. Understands what signs and symptoms are reportable and suggestive of complications
   c. Aware of side-effects of chemotherapeutic agents; understands what measures to take in minimizing these effects
   d. Avoids cuts, bruises, infection, and excess stress on hand and arm of operative side
   e. Promises to see her physician for follow-up visits
   f. Has taken initial steps in obtaining a recommended prosthesis

Care of the Patient With Advanced Breast Cancer

Following a radical mastectomy, the woman is asked to adhere to a schedule of follow-up visits to her physician. Usually, visits take place every 3 months for 2 or 3 years, every 6 months for 5 years, and then annually. The hope is that the patient will be free from disease as long as possible.

Unfortunately, many women have recurrences of the tumor or metastatic spread. Likewise, many women who seek medical assistance have a primary cancer that is so far advanced as to be inoperable. Advanced breast cancer may indicate extensive spread within the breast or to adjacent tissues, or even metastasis to other parts of the body. The status of dissemination can be determined by a metastatic x-ray series (chest, skull, long bones, and pelvis); liver chemistries; a mammogram of the other breast; and radioactive scans of the bone, liver, and brain.

Of the patients who have recurrences, almost half show evidence of recurrence locally and in regional lymph nodes; over a quarter have visceral involvement; and a similar percentage have bone involvement of the spine, rib, hips, or pelvis.

Nursing Interventions. Regression or abatement of symptoms for as long as possible is the goal for nursing intervention. However, individual differences make its attainment unpredictable. The emphasis is on improving the quality of survival.

The nurse is challenged to utilize many skills in assessing the physical as well as the psychosocial condition of the patient. Information about changes in behavioral patterns can be elicited from the patient's family. The nurse can also assist the physician in determining the specific kind of palliation suitable for the individual patient. Such therapy is designed to keep the woman as comfortable as possible, although it may not arrest the disease.

A wide range of treatment is available, depending on the specifics of the patient's condition. For a detailed outline of the various treatment modalities that are frequently used, see Table 47-1.

▷ # Reconstructive and Plastic Surgery of the Breast

Hypertrophy of the Breast

The breasts are such an important part of the female figure that abnormalities often lead to requests for surgical man-

Table 47-1
Treatment Modalities for the Patient With Advanced Cancer of the Breast

Palliative Therapy	Objectives of Therapy	Concomitant Effects	Essential Nursing Intervention
Hypophysectomy Method: 1. Major craniotomy 2. Transnasal implantation of radioactive Yttrium (Y^{90}) 3. Transsphenoidal excision of pituitary 4. Stereotactic cryohypophysectomy 5. Stereotactic radio frequency to destroy pituitary	Removes source of adrenocorticotropic hormone (ACTH) as well as hormones that seem to stimulate the breast directly	May cause salt wastage ———→ Following hypophysectomy, diabetes insipidus may occur (inability to conserve body water because of absence of posterior pituitary and its secretion, antidiuretic hormone, ADH). In 4–6 weeks, hypothalamus takes over function of antidiuretic hormone	→Replace adrenal salt-regulating hormone fludrocortisone acetate (Florinef). Many patients do not require this. Recognize need for additional steroid replacement during stress periods, such as minor illness, infection, injury, serious vomiting, surgery. Otherwise, adrenal insufficiency results (symptoms similar to crises described above). For transsphenoidal hypophysectomy: Frequent oral care is required. Observe for hemorrhage, especially after nasal packing is removed. Clear nasal drip and patient swallowing constantly may indicate cerebrospinal leak. Keep patient in Fowler's position to facilitate cerebrospinal fluid drainage. Advise patient to wear Medic Alert bracelet with operation and the name of replacement medication.

Note: Medical adrenalectomy: When it is impossible to do an adrenalectomy or hypophysectomy (because of age, patient refusal, poor condition), administer high doses of cortisone to achieve adrenal suppression.
This is combined with 5-Fluorouracil (5-FU).

Palliative Therapy	Objectives of Therapy	Concomitant Effects	Essential Nursing Intervention
Chemotherapy 1. Antimetabolites 5-Fluorouracil (5-FU) combined with adrenalectomy (See p. 308, chemotherapy.)	Permits a satisfactory mode of palliation and allows return to normal activity	Toxic effects: stomatitis nausea and vomiting diarrhea, alopecia burning sensation in mouth from acid foods	Provide frequent mouth care. Use topical anesthesia for mouth before meals. Administer antiemetics. Change narcotics as tolerance for each develops.
2. Alkylating agents	When above no longer effective, switch to other chemotherapeutic agents: cyclophosphamide (Cytoxan); triethylene thiophosphoramide (Thiotepa).	Bone marrow depression Cystitis Alopecia Jaundice	
3. Corticosteroids (Prednisone)	Suppresses estrogen production by the adrenals and decreases urinary estrogenic metabolites	Does not bring about hypercalcemia as does androgen or estrogen therapy It is a good hormonal treatment for brain metastasis. Induces some degree of Cushing syndrome: fullness of face, gain in body weight, and edema of lower extremities	(See p. 939, steroid therapy.)

(continued)

Table 47-1
Treatment Modalities for the Patient With Advanced Cancer of the Breast (continued)

Palliative Therapy	Objectives of Therapy	Concomitant Effects	Essential Nursing Intervention
Chemotherapy (continued)			
4. Antiestrogen Tamoxifen citrate (Nolvadex)	Effective in palliative treatment in postmenopausal women with positive assays for estrogen receptors May permit delay or avoidance of adrenalectomy or hypophysectomy	Adverse effects usually transient: thrombocytopenia, leukopenia Appears less toxic than other agents	Expect nausea, vomiting, hot flashes. May cause weight gain, vaginal bleeding and discharge, skin rashes, thrombophlebitis, hypercalcemia.
5. Enzyme antagonist (Aminogluthemide [AG])	Inhibition of estrogen synthesis with enzyme antagonists	Adrenal inhibitor	

Radiation (See p. 333.)	Effective in relieving pain
	More effective in skeletal metastasis; less effective in visceral metastasis
		Depends on area affected:
		Chest: esophagitis
		    pneumonitis
		    shortness of
		      breath
		    slight cough
		Abdomen: affects digestion
		Body: general lethargy
			Administer pain-relieving medication as required until effects of radiation lessen the need for such drugs.
			Recognize that fatigue and weakness often result from radiation.
			When pain is controlled, instruct patient to take extra precautions in order to avoid pathologic fractures: avoid lifting heavy packages and children, and strenuous arm movements, such as those used in sweeping.

Oophorectomy	Castration removes cyclic hormone stimulation of the tumor.		(See p. 1061 for surgical care.)

(continued)

agement. The variations most often encountered are in size: breasts are too large or too small. Those that are too large are said to be *hypertrophied;* when the condition occurs in early life, it is called *virginal breast hypertrophy.* The condition is usually bilateral, but may occur on only one side. The hypertrophied breasts that occur in later life are always bilateral.

Symptoms of Breast Hypertrophy.   Patients with breast hypertrophy complain of tender breasts, diffuse pains, and fatigue. The tenderness and pain is particularly marked at the time of the menstrual period. The weight of the breasts causes a dragging sensation on the shoulders, and efforts to support these tremendous breasts with brassieres are futile. Most patients with virginal hypertrophy have deep grooves in the shoulder tissue caused by pressure from brassiere straps.

Not only are physical symptoms present, but psychological difficulties develop, especially in girls and younger women. They become too embarrassed to wear bathing suits, sweaters, or evening gowns. Their social life is restricted, and they become introverts, avoiding social contacts and even marriage. Because they think that they are unattractive, married women with this condition develop a sense of insecurity, fearing the loss of their husband's affection and, possibly, divorce. These are very real difficulties, which cause emotional repercussions that may be very serious.

Mammoplasty.   The operation performed to reduce the size of the breasts is termed a *reduction mammoplasty.* In this operation, the surgeon makes one incision beneath the breast and a similar curved incision in the skin of the anterior breast. The nipple is transplanted to a new location after the redundant tissue is cut away. The remaining skin edges are approximated with sutures, and the nipple is sutured to its new location. Drains are placed in the incision and remain for only a day or two. Simple gauze dressings are used without pressure.

Table 47-1
Treatment Modalities for the Patient With Advanced Cancer of the Breast (continued)

Palliative Therapy	Objectives of Therapy	Concomitant Effects	Essential Nursing Intervention
Oophorectomy (continued)	Preferred for premenopausal women: 1. Surgical ———→Immediate estrogen withdrawal 2. Radiation ———→Estrogen withdrawal takes 4–6 weeks. If breast cancer is localized to breast, oophorectomy may or may not be advised.		
Hormonal Therapy	Androgens, fluoxymesterone (Halotestin) for premenopausal women Estrogens (diethylstilbestrol) for postmenopausal patients	Masculinization ———— Fluid retention Cholestatic jaundice Hypercalcemia —————	→Watch for signs of increased libido, deepening voice, facial hirsutism. →Note serum calcium levels. Observe for signs of: lethargy, insomnia, thirst, nausea, vomiting, thickened speech, fluid retention, collapse, coma. Assist with treatment: Moderately high doses of corticosteroids, vigorous hydration, low-calcium diet
Adrenalectomy, bilateral posterior (flank), or anterior with oophorectomy	Removes another source of endogenous estrogens Effective for metastasis to viscera or bone	Removes a hormone essential to life ————————	→Replace cortisone daily for rest of patient's life. Otherwise, adrenal crisis results.
Adrenalectomy			Symptoms: Hypotension, diarrhea, nausea and vomiting, elevated temperature, weakness, abdominal pain

Postoperative Nursing Intervention. Following mammoplasty, nursing intervention is relatively basic. These patients sit up in bed the day after operation and may be out of bed and eating a normal diet thereafter. The results of these plastic operations are good for both relief of symptoms and appearance. There is no recurrence of the hypertrophy, and the operation is not a serious one. The new transplanted nipple may turn black and be covered by a dry scab. This is to be expected, but the scab will come away after a week or two as the nipple regains a blood supply in its new location. It must be accepted that the breast cannot function for lactation after such an operation.

Usually, these patients are euphoric about the results, but it is not uncommon for some patients to experience negative psychological reactions related to the loss of a part of the body. The patient may feel anxious about this reaction, but it helps to let her know that these feelings occur frequently.

Operations to Enlarge or Uplift the Female Breast

Operations to enlarge or uplift the breast are requested fairly frequently. Although padded brassieres and other devices are available, they do not always give the desired result. The operations are performed through an incision along the undermargin of the breast (circumareolar). The breast is elevated, and a pocket is formed between the breast and the chest wall, into which are inserted various types of plastic and synthetic materials intended to enlarge and uplift the breast. This procedure is called an *augmentation mammoplasty* and may be done on an outpatient basis with local anesthesia by an experienced plastic surgeon. These operations are not serious, but complications do occur occasionally, in some instances requiring the removal of the inserted substance.

Restoration Following Mastectomy. A more recent innovation is restoration of the female breast following mastectomy in patients who have an early stage cancer and favorable prognosis. Findings over the last decade indicate that the skin–subcutaneous complex is far looser and more supple than was previously thought, and that the blood supply is usually sufficient to withstand wide undermining as well as the compromising effects of a tightly compressed prosthesis. Immediate reconstruction is usually not advised because of possible metastatic axillary involvement, and also, there is a higher incidence of prosthetic slough when reconstruction is not delayed. An implant constructed of silicone gel in a molded shape buttressed by internal compartmentalization appears to be an effective device, as are the saline-filled prostheses.

A transverse incision is made in what will become the inframammary fold. Through this incision, the skin and subcutaneous fat of the chest wall are undermined, and the implant is placed in the created pocket. The wound is drained via portable suction and is closed. A few months later, a nipple–areola complex may be reconstructed, the areola being created from a graft of the labia majora or minora, whereas the nipple is constructed from a transplanted portion of the opposite nipple or a portion of earlobe (Fig. 47-7).

Postmastectomy patients are carefully selected by the surgeon in order to ensure effective results. Criteria for ineligibility include the need for large skin grafts, exposure to excessive radiation, and skin that is too tight or thin. The matter of tumor recurrence continues to be raised, but does not appear to be too significant when compared with the psychological and physical advantages of this type of surgery.

After the operation, the patient is instructed to wear a brassiere during the day and night for at least a month. She is instructed to limit arm movement for a period of time to permit the tissues to heal. Usually, this means keeping arms at the side with flexing at the elbows only. The patient should not sleep on her abdomen and should not lift anything weighing more than 13.6 kg (30 lbs) for the first 4 to 6 weeks.

With some very early tumors, there has been a great deal of interest in primary reconstruction at the time of initial surgery. Long-term risks and benefits of restoration must still be evaluated.

▷ Diseases of the Male Breast

In the male, *gynecomastia* (hypertrophy of the breast) is the lesion that most frequently affects the breast. Fibroadenoma is rarely seen in the male. Ninety-nine percent of malignant lesions occur in the female. Gynecomastia may occur in the prepubertal or adolescent boy; is usually unilateral; and presents as a firm, circular, tender mass beneath the areola. In the adult male, diffuse gynecomastia may occur and may be related to certain drugs the patient is taking,

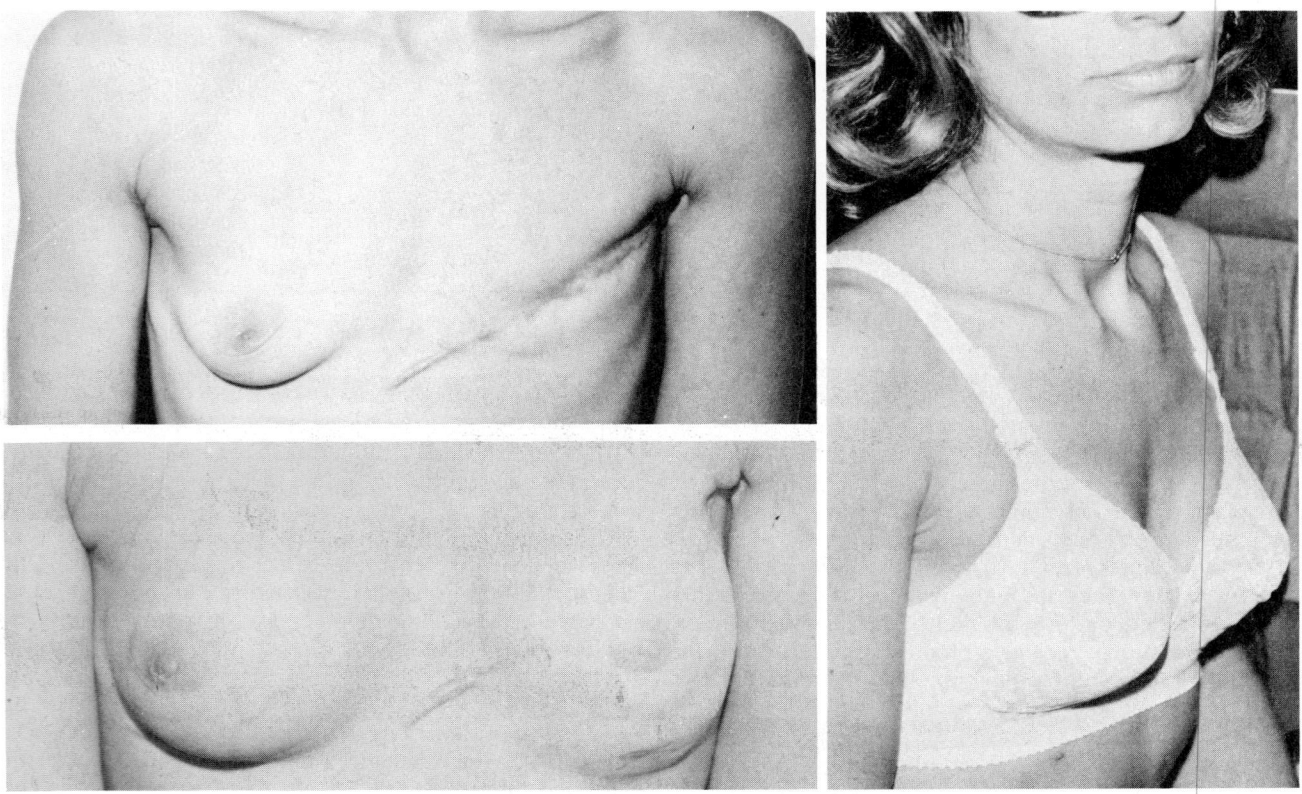

Figure 47-7.   Reconstruction of left breast and augmentation of right breast. (From Guthrie RH Jr: The case for breast reconstruction after mastectomy. CA—A Cancer J for Clinicians, July–Aug 1978.)

such as digitalis. Pain and tenderness are initial symptoms. The enlarged mammary gland is often removed through a small periareolar incision.

▷ Bibliography

Books

Gant TD and Vasconez LO. Post-Mastectomy Reconstruction. Baltimore, Williams & Wilkins, 1981.

Graham J. In the Company of Others. New York, Harcourt Brace Jovanovich, 1982.

Haagensen CD, Bodian C, and Haagensen DE Jr. Breast Carcinoma, Philadelphia, WB Saunders, 1981.

Haagensen CD, Haagensen BE, and Bodian C. Risk and Detection of Breast Carcinoma. Philadelphia, WB Saunders, 1981.

Hawkins JW and Higgins LP. Maternity and Gynecological Nursing, Women's Health Care. Philadelphia, JB Lippincott, 1981.

Kushner R. If You've Thought About Breast Cancer. Rockville, Maryland, Women's Breast Cancer Advisory Center, 1980.

Lewison E (ed). Diagnosis and Treatment of Breast Cancer, Baltimore, Williams & Wilkins, 1981.

Shapiro L and Goodman AA. Never Say Die: A Doctor and Patient Talk About Breast Cancer. New York, Appleton–Century–Crofts, 1980.

Weatherley–White RCA. Plastic Surgery of the Female Breast. New York, Harper & Row, 1980.

Woods NF. Human Sexuality in Health and Illness, 2nd ed. St Louis, CV Mosby, 1979.

Articles
Diagnostic Procedures/Assessment

Baker LH. Breast cancer detection demonstration project. Five-year summary report. CA—A Cancer Journal for Clinicians 1982 July/Aug; 32(4):194–255.

Bennett SE et al. Profile of women practicing breast self-examination. JAMA 1983 Jan 28; 249(4):488–491.

Broadbent RV and Reid MH. Mammography—misunderstood and underutilized. Postgrad Med 1981 Dec; 70(6):93–101.

Hallal JC. The relationship of health beliefs, health locus of control, and self-concept to the practice of breast self-examination in adult women. Nurs Res 1982 May/June; 31(3):137–142.

Mammography 1982: A statement of the American Cancer Society. CA—A Cancer Journal for Clinicians 1982 July/Aug; 32(4):226–230.

Mammography screening for breast cancer. The Medical Letter 1980 June 27; 22(13):53–54.

Margolese RG. Response: The case for the two-step biopsy procedure for breast cancer. Ca—A Cancer Journal for Clinicians 1982 Jan/Feb; 36(1):51–57.

McLendon MS, Fulk CH, and Starnes DC. Effectiveness of breast self-examination teaching to women of low socioeconomic class. JOGN Nurs 1982 Jan/Feb; 11(1):7–10.

Michalek AM et al. Report on a BSE educational program conducted for lay audiences conducted by nurse health educators. Cancer Nurs 1981 Oct; 4(5):385–388.

Nyirjesy I. Breast thermography. Clin Obstet Gynecol 1982 June; 25(2):401–408.

Stromberg M. Screening for early detection. Am J Nurs 1981 Sept; 81(9):1652–1657.

Tallent DD and Halter SA. Cytologic examination of the breast. Postgrad Med 1981 Feb; 69(2):91–98.

Trotta P. Breast self-examination: Factors influencing compliance. Oncol Nurs Forum 1980 Summer; 7(3):13–17.

Wiley KR. Postbiopsy care. Am J Nurs 1981 Sept; 81(9):1660–1662.

Breast Conditions

Danazol for fibrocystic disease of the breast. The Medical Letter 1981 Jan; 27:23(2):5–6.

Greenblatt RB, Vasquez J, and Samaras C. Fibrocystic breast disease. Postgrad Med 1982 Mar; 71(3):159–168.

Greenblatt RB et al. Fibrocystic disease of the breast. Clin Obstet Gynecol 1982 June; 25(2):365–371.

Kinne DW and DeCosse JJ. New developments in the management of breast disease. In Nyhus LM. Surgery Annual, Vol 13, pp 163–183. New York, Appleton–Century–Crofts, 1981.

Koch SJ. Augmentation mammoplasty. Am J Nurs 1980 Aug; 80(8):1480–1484.

Marszalek EJ and Solomon JS. A breast counseling service. Am J Nurs 1981 Sept; 81(9):1658–1659.

Northouse LL. Mastectomy patients and the fear of cancer recurrence. Cancer Nurs 1981 June; 4(3):213–220.

Schwartz GF. Benign neoplasms and "inflammations" of the breast. Clin Obstet Gynecol 1982 June; 25(2):373–385.

Schwartz SI (ed). The breast, Chap. 11. In The Year Book of Surgery 1981. Chicago, Year Book Medical Publishers, 1981.

Small EC. Psychosocial issues in breast diseases. Clin Obstet Gynecol 1982 June; 25(2):447–454.

Townsend CM Jr. Breast lumps. Clin Symp 1980; 32(2):3–32.

Wilcox PM. Benign breast disorders. Am J Nurs 1981 Sept; 81(9):1644–1651.

Breast Cancer

Adjuvant chemotherapy of breast cancer. NIH Consensus Development Conference's Summary, Vol 3, No 3. Oncol Nurs Forum 1981 Winter; 8(1):7–9.

Breast Cancer. Clinics in Oncology. 1982 Nov; entire issue.

Breast cancer: The rush to treatment. Patient Care 1982 Oct 15; 16(17):187–227.

Breast CA treatment trend is conservative. Hosp Pract 1980 Feb; 15(2):44–51.

Carbone PP. Options in breast cancer therapy. Hosp Pract 1981 Feb; 16(4):53–61.

Carino–Pereira J, Costa FO, and Henriques E. Chemotherapy of advanced breast cancer. CA 1981 Oct 1; 48(7):1517–1521.

Costanza ME. The medical management of breast cancer. Clin Obstet Gynecol 1982 June; 25(2):433–441.

Dulcey MP. Addressing breast cancer's assault on female sexuality. Top Clin Nurs 1980 Jan; 1(4):61–68.

Fisher B and Wolmark N. The current status of systemic adjuvant therapy in the management of primary breast cancer. Surg Clin North Am 1981 Dec; 61(6):1347–1360.

Fisher B et al. Treatment of primary breast cancer and chemotherapy and tamoxifen. N Engl J Med 1981 July 2; 305(1):1–6.

Fleagle JM. Helping the patient with breast cancer adjust to teletherapy. Nursing '80 1980 Apr; 10(4):60–61.

Holland JF. Adjuvant chemotherapy for breast cancer. Surg Clin North Am 1981 Dec; 61(6):1361–1370.

Homer MJ. Mammographic detection of breast cancer. Clin Obstet Gynecol 1982 June; 25(2):393–400.

Hunt KE, Fry DE, and Bland KI. Breast carcinoma in the elderly patient: An assessment of operative risk, morbidity and mortality. Am J Surg 1980 Sept; 140(3):330–341.

Kaufman RJ. Advanced breast cancer: Additive hormonal therapy. Ca—A Cancer Journal for Clinicians 1981 July/Aug; 31(4):194–203.

Kinne DW. Opinion: The case for the one-step biopsy procedure for breast cancer. Ca—A Cancer Journal for Clinicians 1982 Jan/Feb; 32(1):46–49.

Lefall LD Jr. Breast cancer in black women. Ca—A Cancer Journal for Clinicians 1981 July/Aug; 31(4):208–218.

Marino LB. Morbidity and quality of life in clients with breast cancer, Chap 24. In Cancer Nursing. St Louis, CV Mosby, 1981.

Nichols DH. Primary treatment of breast cancer. Clin Obstet Gynecol 1982 June; 25(2):425–431.

Patterson P. Experts stymied by mysteries of breast cancer. AORN J 1981 Mar; 33(4):770–774.

Reich SD. Tanoxifen: A brief review. Can Nurs 1981 Oct; 4(5):319–320.

Rose MA et al. Husbands as health educators for their wives: A pilot study in breast cancer education. Oncol Nurs Forum 1980 Summer; 7(3):18–20.

Santen RJ et al. A randomized trial comparing surgical adrenalectomy with aminoglutethimide plus hydrocortisone in women with advanced breast cancer. N Engl J Med 1981 Sept 3; 305(10):545–551.

Scott DW. Quality of life following the diagnosis of breast cancer. Top Clin Nurs 1983 Jan; 4(4):20–37.

Veronesi U et al. Comparing radical mastectomy with quadrantectomy, axillary dissection and radiotherapy in patients with small cancers of the breast. N Engl J Med 1981 July 2; 305(1):6–11.

Welch DA. Spinal metastasis from cancer of the breast. Nurs Pract 1980 July/Aug; 5(4):8–10.

Rehabilitation, Reconstructive Surgery, Breast Prosthesis

Albo RJ, Gruber R, and Kahn R. Immediate breast reconstruction after modified mastectomy for carcinoma of the breast. Am J Surg 1980 July; 140(1):131–136.

Dresen SE. Student experience in surgical day care. (See Reduction and Augmentation Mammoplasty.) Am J Nurs 1982 Jan; 82(1):106.

Frank DI. Sexual counseling to a mastectomy patient. Nursing '81 1981 Jan; 11(1):64–67.

Gohn MK and Goin JM. Midlife reactions to mastectomy and subsequent breast reconstruction. Arch Gen Psychiatry 1980 Mar; 38(3):225–227.

Goldwyn RM. Breast reconstruction. Clin Obstet Gynecol 1982 June; 25(2):443–446.

Kennedy BJ. The encouraging outlook for breast cancer patients. Drug Ther 1980 May; 10(5):63–73.

Kennedy BL. Life after a mastectomy. Drug Ther 1980 May; 10(5):78–80.

Levinger GE. Working through recovery after mastectomy. Am J Nurs 1980 June; 80(6):1118–1120.

Life after a mastectomy (A Drug Therapy Patient Guide). Drug Ther 1980 May; 10(5):78–80.

Lindsey AM et al. Social support and health outcomes in postmastectomy women: A review. Cancer Nurs 1981 Oct; 4(5):377–383.

Mauldin B. Breast reconstruction after mastectomy. AORN J 1980 Mar; 31(4):612–617.

Ruetschi MS. Breast reconstruction after mastectomy. Clin Bull 1980; 10(2):53–61.

Sanger CK and Reznikoff M. A comparison of the psychological effects of breast-saving procedures with the modified radical mastectomy. CA 1981 Nov 15; 48(8):2341–2346.

Thomas SG and Yates MM. Breast reconstruction after mastectomy. Am J Nurs 1977 Sept; 77(9):1438–1442.

48

Management of the Male Patient With Disorders Related to the Reproductive System

In the male, several organs serve as parts of both the urinary tract and the reproductive system. Disease of these organs may produce functional abnormalities of either or both systems. For this reason, diseases of the entire reproductive system in the male usually are treated by the urologist.

▷ Physiologic Overview

The structures included in the male reproductive system are the testes, the vas deferens and the seminal vesicles, the penis, and certain accessory glands, such as the prostate gland and Cowper's gland (Fig. 48-1). The testes are formed in embryonal life within the abdominal cavity near the kidney. During the last month of fetal life, they descend posterior to the peritoneum, to pierce the abdominal wall in the groin. Later they progress along the inguinal canal into the scrotum. In this descent, they are accompanied by blood vessels, lymphatics, nerves, and ducts, which, along with supporting and investing tissue, make up the spermatic cord. This cord extends from the internal inguinal ring through the abdominal wall and the inguinal canal to the scrotum. As the testes descend into the scrotum, a tubular process of peritoneum accompanies them. This normally is obliterated, the only remaining portion being that which covers the testes, the *tunica vaginalis.* (When this peritoneal process is not obliterated but remains open into the abdominal cavity, a potential sac remains, into which abdominal contents may enter to form an indirect inguinal hernia.)

The testes proper consist of numerous seminiferous tubules in which are formed the male reproductive elements, the spermatozoa. These are transmitted by a system of collecting tubules into the epididymis, which is a hoodlike structure lying on the testes and containing tortuous ducts that lead into the vas deferens. This firm tubular structure passes upward through the inguinal canal to enter the abdominal cavity behind the peritoneum and then extends downward toward the base of the bladder. An outpouching from this structure is the seminal vesicle, which acts as a

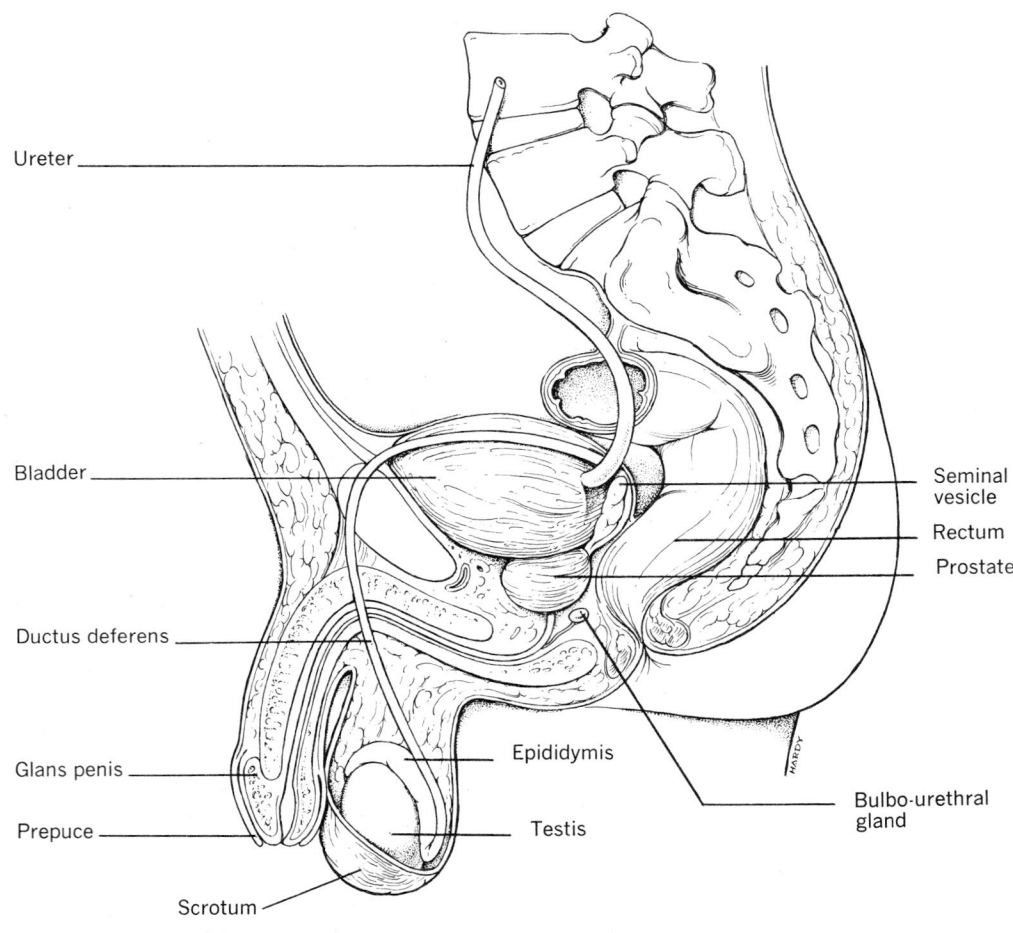

Figure 48-1. Organs of the male reproductive system. (From Chaffee EE and Greisheimer EM: Basic Physiology and Anatomy, 3rd ed. Philadelphia, JB Lippincott.)

reservoir for the secretion of the testes. The tract is continued as the ejaculatory duct, which then passes through the prostate gland to enter the urethra. The secretion of the testes is carried by this pathway to the end of the penis in the reproductive act.

The testes have a dual function. The primary function is reproduction—the formation of spermatozoa from the germinal cells of the seminiferous tubules. However, the testes are also important glands of internal secretion. This secretion is produced by the so-called interstitial cells and is called the male sex hormone, or testosterone, which induces and preserves the male sex qualities.

The prostate gland lies just below the neck of the bladder. It surrounds the urethra posteriorly and laterally and is traversed by the ejaculatory duct, the continuation of the vas deferens. This gland produces a secretion that is chemically and physiologically suitable to the needs of the spermatozoa in their passage from the genital glands.

The penis has a dual function of being the organ of copulation and of urination. Anatomically, it consists of a glans penis, a body, and a root. The glans penis is the soft, rounded portion at the end that retains its soft structure even when erect. The urethra opens at the extremity of the glans. The glans normally is covered or protected by an elongation of the skin of the penis—the foreskin—which may be retracted to expose the glans. The body of the penis is composed of erectile tissues that contain numerous blood vessels that may become distended during sexual excitement. Through it passes the urethra, which extends from the bladder through the prostate to the end of the penis.

Congenital Malformations.   Of the many disturbances of normal growth that may occur, the most common is a failure of the testes to descend into the scrotum. This condition is called *cryptorchidism.*

Failure of the urethra to form normally in the penis can result in hypospadias or epispadias. *Hypospadias* occurs when the urethral opening is on the dorsum of the penis; when the urethral opening is a groove on its ventral surface, the condition is called *epispadias.* These anatomical abnormalities may be repaired by various types of plastic surgery. (The reader is referred to a pediatric textbook for a complete discussion of these conditions.)

▷ Conditions of the Prostate

Benign Prostatic Hyperplasia

In many patients over 50 years of age, the prostate gland enlarges, extending upward into the bladder and obstructing the outflow of urine by encroaching on the vesical orifice. This condition is known as enlargement of the prostate. The etiology is uncertain, but evidence suggests a hormonal cause as initiating hyperplasia of the supporting stromal tissue and of glandular elements in the prostate.

Since enlargement of the prostate gland produces an obstruction to flow of urine, a gradual dilatation of the ureters (hydroureter) and kidneys (hydronephrosis) results. The hypertrophied lobes may obstruct the vesical neck or prostatic urethra and thus cause incomplete emptying and urinary retention. Urinary tract infection may result from urinary stasis.

The symptom complex (referred to as *prostatism*) includes increasing frequency of urination, nocturia, hesitancy in starting urination, diminution in size and force of urinary stream, interruption of urinary stream, terminal dribbling, a sensation of incomplete emptying of the bladder, and acute urinary retention.

A battery of diagnostic examinations may be carried out to determine the degree of prostatic enlargement, the presence of any bladder wall changes, and the efficiency of renal function.

Management. The plan of treatment depends on the cause, the severity of the obstruction, and the condition of the patient. If a patient is admitted as an emergency because he is unable to void, he is immediately catheterized. The ordinary catheter frequently will be too soft and pliable to pass through the urethra into the bladder. A thin wire, called a stylet, is introduced (by a urologist) into the catheter in order to prevent the catheter from collapsing when it encounters resistance. In severe cases, metal catheters with a pronounced *prostatic curve* may be used. Sometimes a suprapubic cystostomy is necessary to give adequate drainage.

Surgery is usually necessary when treatment is required because of obstruction. Complete removal of the hyperplastic prostatic tissue, without removal of the surgical capsule of the prostate, is usually done. (A discussion of nursing management following prostatic surgery follows.)

Prostatitis

Prostatitis is an inflammation of the prostatic gland. It may be caused by bacterial invasion, by other infectious agents (fungi, mycoplasma), or by a variety of other problems (urethral stricture, prostatic hyperplasia, etc.). Microorganisms usually are carried to the prostate from the urethra. The symptoms of prostatitis are many and include perineal discomfort, burning, urgency, frequency, etc. Prostatitis may be classified as bacterial or abacterial depending on the presence or absence of microorganisms in the prostatic fluid.

Prostatodynia or perineal myalgia is manifested by voiding pain or perineal pain symptoms, but there is no evidence of inflammation or bacterial growth in the prostatic fluid.

Acute bacterial prostatitis may produce a sudden onset of fever and chills and perineal, rectal, or back pain. Urinary symptoms of burning, frequency, urgency, nocturia, and terminal dysuria may be evident. Some patients, however, are asymptomatic.

Diagnosis requires a careful history, culture of prostatic fluid or tissue, and, occasionally, a histologic examination of tissue. In order to locate the source of the lower genitourinary infection (bladder neck, urethra, prostate), it is necessary to collect a divided urinary specimen. After the patient cleanses the glans penis and retracts the foreskin (if present), he voids 10 ml to 15 ml of urine into the first container. This represents urethral urine. A second voiding of 50 ml to 75 ml of urine is then collected in a second container without interruption; this represents bladder urine. If the patient does not have acute prostatitis, the physician immediately performs a prostatic massage, and any prostatic fluid that is expressed is collected by gravity drainage into a third container. If it is not possible to collect prostatic fluid, the patient voids a small quantity of urine. This specimen may contain the bacteria present in the prostatic fluid.

Management. The goal of management is to avoid the complications of abscess formation and septicemia. A broad-spectrum antimicrobial (to which the organism causing the infection is susceptible) is given for a period of 10 to 14 days. Intravenous administration of the drug may be necessary to achieve high serum and tissue levels. The patient is encouraged to remain on bed rest as this will alleviate symptoms rapidly. Comfort is promoted with analgesics (pain relief), antispasmodics and bladder sedatives (relieves bladder irritability), sitz baths (relieves pain and spasm), and stool softeners (prevent straining at stool, which increases pain).

Swelling of the gland may produce urinary retention. Other complications include epididymitis, bacteremia or septicemia, and pyelonephritis.

Chronic bacterial prostatitis is a major source of relapsing urinary tract infection in men. The treatment of chronic prostatitis is difficult, because of poor diffusion of most antimicrobials from the plasma into the prostatic fluid. Antimicrobials (trimethoprim-sulfamethoxazole, minocycline, doxycycline) may be given. Continuous suppressive treatment with low-dose antimicrobial drugs may be indicated. The patient is advised of the possibility of relapsing infection. Comfort is promoted with antispasmodics (to relieve bladder irritability), sitz baths, and stool softeners.

The treatment of *nonbacterial prostatitis* is directed toward symptomatic relief: sitz baths, analgesics, etc. The sexual partner should be investigated because of the possibility of cross infection.

Patient Education. Instruct the patient to take the prescribed antibiotic for the full time period. Hot sitz baths (10–20 minutes) may be taken several times daily. Fluids are encouraged to satisfy thirst, but avoid "forcing fluids," as an effective drug level must be maintained in the urine. Foods and drink that have diuretic action or increase prostatic secretions should be avoided: alcohol, coffee, tea, chocolate, cola, and spices. During periods of acute inflammation, sexual arousal and intercourse should be avoided. Sexual intercourse may be beneficial in the treatment of chronic prostatitis. The patient should avoid sitting for long periods of time. Medical follow-up is necessary for at least 6 months to 1 year since recurrence of prostatitis due to the same or different organisms can occur.

The Patient Undergoing Prostatectomy

The preoperative objectives prior to prostatectomy are to assess the patient's general health status and to establish optimum kidney function. The operation should be done before the development of acute urinary retention and infection and certainly before the upper urinary tract and collecting system are damaged. An indwelling catheter is introduced if the patient has continuing urinary retention or if there is evidence of azotemia (accumulation of nitrogenous waste products in the blood). It may be desirable to decompress the bladder gradually over a period of several days, especially if the patient is elderly and hypertensive and has diminished renal function or an excessive amount of urinary retention that has existed for many weeks. *The blood pressure may fluctuate and renal function declines the first few days after bladder drainage is instituted.* If the patient cannot tolerate a urethral catheter, cystostomy drainage is employed (see p. 973). Frequently, the patient is dehydrated from self-limitation of fluids because of urinary frequency. If the patient's cardiac reserve is adequate, a liberal fluid intake (2500 ml–3000 ml daily) is encouraged to help overcome azotemia. The intake and output and daily weight are monitored.

Table 48-1
Comparison of Surgical Approaches for Prostatectomy

The operation of choice depends on (1) the size of the gland, (2) the severity of the obstruction, (3) the age of the patient, (4) the condition of patient and (5) the presence of associated diseases.

Surgical Approach	Advantages	Disadvantages	Nursing Implications
Transurethral (removal of prostatic tissue by instrument introduced through urethra)	Safer for surgical-risk patient Shorter period of hospitalization and convalescence Lower morbidity rate Avoids abdominal incision Causes less pain	Requires highly skilled operator Recurrent obstruction, urethral trauma, and stricture may develop Delayed bleeding may occur	Watch for evidence of hemorrhage (drainage in bag). Observe for symptoms of urethral stricture (dysuria, straining, small urinary stream).
Open Surgical Removal			
Suprapubic	Technically simple Offers wider area of exploration Permits exploration for cancerous lymph nodes Allows more complete removal of obstructing gland Permits treatment of associated lesions in bladder	Requires surgical approach through the bladder Control of hemorrhage difficult Urinary leakage around suprapubic tube Convalescence more prolonged and uncomfortable	Watch for indications of hemorrhage and shock. Give meticulous aseptic attention to area around suprapubic tube.
Perineal	Offers direct anatomical approach Permits gravity drainage Particularly efficacious for radical cancer therapy Allows hemostasis under direct vision Low mortality rate Less incidence of shock Ideal for very old, feeble, and poor-risk patient with large prostate	Higher postoperative incidence of impotency and urinary incontinency Problem of damage to rectum and external sphincter Restricted operative field	Avoid rectal tubes, rectal thermometers, and enemas after perineal surgery. Use drainage pads to absorb excess urinary drainage. Secure foam rubber ring for patient comfort. May be urinary leakage around wound for several days after catheter removal.
Retropubic	Most versatile procedure; affords direct visualization Avoids incision in the bladder Permits easier visualization and control of bleeders Shorter period of convalescence	Cannot treat associated pathology in bladder Increased incidence of hemorrhage from prostatic venous plexus; osteitis pubis	Watch for evidences of hemorrhage. Posturinary leakage may occur for several days after catheter is removed.

► Assessment

Renal function studies are carried out to determine if there is renal impairment from prostatic back pressure and to evaluate renal reserve. All measures are taken to ensure that the patient is in the best possible condition for surgery, since older persons have diminishing reserves of vital-organ function. A complete hematologic investigation is done. Since hemorrhage is a major postoperative complication, all clotting defects must be corrected. A high percentage of these patients have cardiac or respiratory complications, or both. The patient's mode of life during the past few months should also be noted. Has he been reasonably active? Can he raise himself out of bed and return to bed without assistance? This assessment may help determine how quickly the patient will be returned to his normal activities following prostatectomy. He should stop smoking at least 2 days before surgery, especially if he has pulmonary emphysema.

Antiembolism stockings are applied before the operation and are particularly important if the patient is placed in a lithotomy position during surgery. The preoperative enema may prevent straining, which can induce postoperative bleeding.

Patient Problems/Nursing Diagnoses

Based on the clinical manifestations, the nursing history, and the diagnostic assessment data, the major nursing problems of a patient undergoing a prostatectomy include possible inadequate knowledge of the surgical procedures and postoperative course; potential development of complications; and potential nonadherence to the therapeutic regimen.

Surgical Management

Four different approaches are possible in removing the hypertrophied fibroadenomatous portion of the prostate gland (Table 48-1). In all four techniques, all hyperplastic tissue is removed, leaving behind the surgical capsule of the prostate. The transurethral approach is closed, while the other three are open surgical procedures.

A *transurethral resection* of the prostate is the most common procedure and can be carried out by means of an endoscopic instrument that has ocular and operating systems. The instrument is introduced directly through the urethra to the prostate, which can be viewed directly. The gland is then removed in small chips with an electrical cutting loop (Fig. 48-2). The real advantage of this method is the absence of an incision. It may be used for glands of varying size (urologists differ on how large the prostate must be before considering an open procedure), and it is ideal for most poor-risk patients with small glands. This approach means a shorter hospital stay; however, strictures are more frequent, and repeat operations may be necessary.

Suprapubic prostatectomy is one method of removing the gland through an abdominal wound. An opening is made into the bladder, and the gland is removed from above (Fig. 48-3). Such an approach can be used for a gland of any size, and few complications occur, although blood loss may be greater than with other methods. Another disadvantage is the need for an abdominal incision with the concomitant hazards of any major surgical procedure.

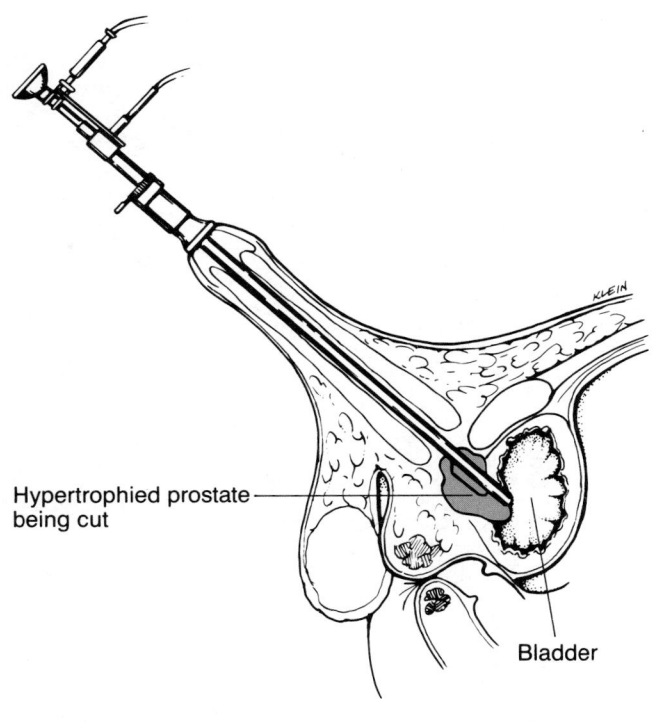

Figure 48-2. Transurethral prostatectomy. A loop of wire connected with a cutting current is rotated in the cystoscope to remove shavings of prostate at the bladder orifice.

Hypertrophied prostate being cut

Bladder

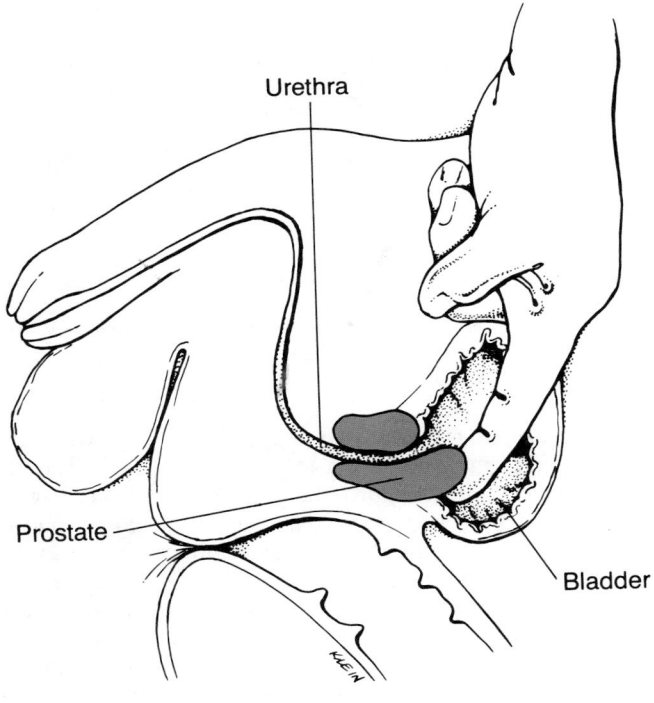

Figure 48-3. Suprapubic prostatectomy. Diagrammatic drawing shows how the prostate is shelled out of its bed with the finger.

Urethra

Prostate

Bladder

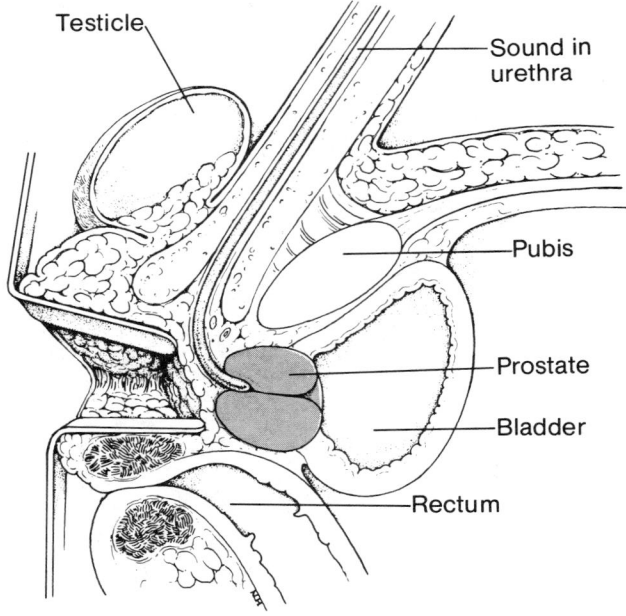

Figure 48-4.   Perineal prostatectomy.

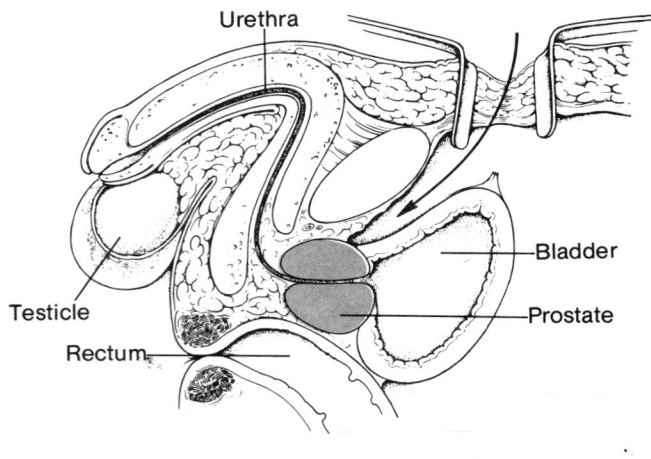

Figure 48-5.   Retropubic prostatectomy.

In *perineal prostatectomy,* the gland is removed through an incision in the perineum (Fig. 48-4). This approach is practical when other approaches are blocked. It is a useful procedure when open biopsy is needed. In the postoperative period, the wound may become contaminated rather easily because of the location of the incision. Incontinence, impotence, or rectal injury are more likely sequelae when this approach is used.

Another technique that is rapidly becoming more popular than the suprapubic approach is *retropubic prostatectomy.* A low abdominal incision is made, and the prostate gland is approached between the pubic arch and the bladder (without entering the bladder) (Fig. 48-5). This procedure

is suitable for large glands located high in the pelvis. Blood loss is controlled more easily and there is better visualization. However, infections can readily start in the retropubic space.

▶ Postoperative Planning and Nursing Implementation

Goals

The major goals for the patient include:

1. Understanding of the surgical procedure and postoperative course
2. Absence of complications such as bleeding, blockage of the catheter, pain, infection, and thromboembolism
3. Adherence to the therapeutic regimen

Bleeding.   Since a hyperplastic prostate gland is very vascular, the immediate dangers following a prostatectomy are bleeding and shock. Bleeding may occur from the bed of the prostate. Bleeding may also result in the formation of clots, which then obstruct the flow of urine. The drainage may be reddish pink and begins to clear to a light pink within 24 hours after operation.

- Bright red bleeding with increased viscosity and numerous clots usually indicates arterial bleeding. Venous bleeding appears darker and less viscous.
- Arterial hemorrhage usually requires surgical intervention (*e.g.,* suturing of bleeders or transurethral coagulation of bleeders), while venous bleeding may be controlled by applying traction to the catheter so that the balloon applies pressure to the prostatic fossa.

Catheter Blockage.   Following a transurethral prostatic resection, *the catheter must drain well;* a blocked catheter will produce distention of the prostatic capsule with resultant hemorrhage. Sometimes the patient is given furosemide to initiate postoperative diuresis, thereby helping to keep the catheter patent.

- Watch and palpate the lower abdomen to see that no blockage of the catheter is occurring. An overdistended bladder presents a distinct rounded swelling above the pubis.
- Check the drainage bag, dressings, and incision site for evidence of bleeding.
- Monitor the blood pressure, pulse, and respirations, and compare with the preoperative vital signs to assess for hypotension. Observe the patient for restlessness; cold, sweating skin; pallor; fall in blood pressure; and an increasing pulse rate.

Drainage of the bladder may be accomplished by gravity through a closed sterile system of drainage. A three-way system is useful in cleansing the bladder and preventing clot formation. Some urologists prefer to leave an indwelling catheter attached to dependent drainage. The catheter can be gently irrigated with a plunger syringe to remove any obstructing clots.

- If the patient complains of pain, check the tubing and irrigate the system, thereby correcting any obstruction, before administering an analgesic. Usually, the catheter is irrigated with 50 ml of irrigating fluid at a time, making sure that the same amount is recovered in the drainage bag.

- Avoid overdistending the bladder, which can produce secondary hemorrhage by stretching the coagulated vessels in the prostatic capsule.
- Maintain an input and output record, including the amount of fluid used for irrigation.

The drainage tube (not the catheter) is taped to the shaved inner thigh to prevent traction on the bladder. If a cystostomy catheter is in place, it is taped to the abdomen. Reexplain to the patient the purpose of the catheter. Assure him that the urge to void is from the presence of the catheter, and bladder spasms. Caution him not to pull on the catheter, since this causes bleeding, subsequent plugging of the tubing, and urinary retention.

Pain.   Usually, the patient is kept on bed rest for the first 24 hours following a prostatectomy. If pain occurs, the patient may strain from bladder irritability, causing an increase in venous pressure, which can initiate bleeding and result in clot retention. Before the prescribed analgesic is given, the patient's blood pressure should be evaluated. Fluids (orally or intravenously) are given in adequate amounts unless contraindicated by congestive heart failure. When the patient is ambulatory, he is encouraged to walk but not to sit for prolonged periods, since this increases intra-abdominal pressure and increases the possibility of bleeding. The bowel movements are kept soft (prune juice, stool softeners) to prevent excessive straining. If an enema is prescribed, it is administered with caution to avoid possible rectal perforation.

Perineal Prostatectomy.   Following perineal prostatectomy, the urologist changes the dressing on the first postoperative day; after that it may become the nurse's responsibility. Careful aseptic technique is practiced, since the possibility of infection is great. Dressings can be held in place by a double-tailed T-binder bandage or a padded athletic supporter. The tails cross over the incision to give double thickness, and then each tail is drawn up on either side of the scrotum to the waistline and is fastened.

Rectal temperatures, rectal tubes, and enemas are to be avoided because of the danger of causing trauma and bleeding in the prostatic fossa. After the perineal sutures are removed, the perineum is cleansed as requested. A heat lamp may be directed to the perineal area to promote healing. The scrotum is protected with a towel while the heat lamp is in use. Sitz baths are also used to encourage healing.

Infection and Thrombosis.   In addition to hemorrhage, urinary tract infections and epididymitis are possible complications following prostatectomy. A vasectomy may be performed at the time of prostatic resection to prevent retrograde spread of infection from the prostatic urethra through the vas and into the epididymis. If epididymitis occurs, it is treated as discussed on page 1099.

Patients undergoing prostatectomy (with the exception of transurethral resection) have a high incidence of deepvein thrombosis and pulmonary embolism. Low-dose heparin therapy may be given prophylactically.

Catheter Removal.   After the catheter is removed (usually when the urine clears), urinary leakage may occur around the wound for several days in patients who have undergone perineal, suprapubic, and retropubic surgery. The cystostomy tube may be removed before or after the urethral catheter is removed. Some urinary incontinence may occur after the catheter is removed. Reassure the patient that this will probably disappear in time.

Rehabilitation and Patient Education
As the days pass and drainage tubes are removed, the patient often shows signs of discouragement and depression because he is not able to regain bladder control immediately. Urinary frequency and burning may occur after the catheter is removed. The following exercises are helpful for regaining urinary control:

- Tense the perineal muscles by pressing the buttocks together; hold this position; relax. This exercise, done 10 to 20 times each hour, can be performed while sitting or standing.
- Try to shut off the urinary stream after starting to void; wait a few seconds and then continue to void.

Perineal exercises are continued until full urinary control is gained. The patient should be instructed to urinate as soon as the *first* desire to do so is felt. It is important for the patient to know that regaining urinary control is a gradual process, and that even though he may continue to "dribble" after being discharged from the hospital, the dribbling should gradually diminish (up to 1 year). The urine may be cloudy for several weeks, but should clear as the prostate area heals.

While the prostatic fossa is healing (6 to 8 weeks), the patient should not engage in any Valsalva efforts (straining at stool, heavy lifting), since this increases venous pressure and may produce hematuria. He should avoid long automobile rides and strenuous exercise, which increase the tendency to bleed. The patient is cautioned to drink enough fluids to avoid dehydration, which increases the tendency for a clot to form and obstruct the flow of urine. Any bleeding or decrease in the size of the urinary stream is to be reported to the physician.

A prostatectomy does not usually cause impotence. (Perineal prostatectomy may cause impotence due to unavoidable damage of the pudendal nerves.) In most instances, sexual activity may be resumed in 6 to 8 weeks, the time required for the prostatic fossa to heal. Following ejaculation, the seminal fluid will go into the bladder and is excreted with the urine. (The anatomical changes in the posterior urethra lead to retrograde ejaculation.)

After total prostatectomy (usually for cancer), impotence is almost always expected. For the younger patient who does not desire to give up sexual activity, a plastic insert may be used to make the penis rigid for sexual intercourse.

▶ **Evaluation**

Expected Outcomes

1. Understands the surgical procedure and postoperative course
   a. Expresses concerns about surgery
   b. Discusses feelings about surgery with health team members and family

c. Discusses the surgical procedure and expected postoperative course

d. Discusses the possible complications of surgery

e. Practices perineal muscle exercises and other techniques used to facilitate control of bladder function

2. Experiences no complications

a. Progresses from red urine to light pink urine 24 hours postoperatively

b. Progresses from light pink urine to amber urine 3 days postoperatively

c. Maintains urinary output within normal ranges and consistent with intake

d. Maintains negative urine cultures

e. Maintains vital signs within normal ranges

f. Increases activity and ambulation daily

g. Utilizes perineal exercises and interruption to urinary stream to promote bladder control

h. Exhibits no signs of venous thrombosis and pulmonary embolism

3. Adheres to therapeutic regimen

a. Copes with urinary incontinence

b. Utilizes perineal exercises as prescribed after discharge

c. Avoids strenuous exercise and activity after discharge

d. Reports changes in urinary function to physician

e. Keeps follow-up clinic/physician appointments

Cancer of the Prostate

Cancer of the prostate is the second most common cause of cancer and the second most common cause of cancer deaths in American males over 55 years of age.

Assessment

Clinical Manifestations.   Early cancer of the prostate does not usually produce symptoms. The obstructive symptoms occur late in the disease. This cancer tends to be variable in its course. If the neoplasm is large enough to encroach on the bladder neck and cause obstruction of urine, there are symptoms and signs of obstruction, namely, difficulty and frequency of urination, urinary retention, and diminution in size and force of the urinary stream. Prostatic cancer commonly metastasizes to bone, lymph nodes, brain, and lungs. Symptoms due to metastases are backache, hip pain, perineal and rectal discomfort, anemia, weight loss, weakness, nausea, and oliguria. Hematuria may be present from urethral or bladder invasion, or both.

Early Detection.   Every male over 40 should have a rectal examination as part of his annual health checkup. Earlier detection is the clue to a higher cure rate. Routine repeated rectal palpation of the gland (preferably by the same examiner) is important because early cancer may be felt as a nodule within the substance of the gland or as a diffuse induration in the posterior lobe.

Diagnostic Evaluation.   On rectal examination, there is an area of increased firmness within the prostate. The more advanced lesion is "stony hard" and fixed. The diagnosis is made on histologic examination of tissue removed surgically by transurethral resection, open prostatectomy, or needle biopsy (perineal or transrectal). The serum acid

phosphatase is frequently increased when cancer extends outside the prostatic capsule. (Acid phosphatase is seen in most body tissues, but is 1000 times more concentrated in the prostate gland.) Smaller amounts of acid phosphatase can be detected with radioimmunoassay. Serum alkaline phosphatase, although elevated in patients with bone or liver metastasis from any tumor, may increase when there is bone metastases.

Other tests include bone scans to detect metastatic bone disease, skeletal x-rays to reveal osteoblastic metastases, excretory urograms to demonstrate changes from ureteral obstruction, and renal-function tests and lymphangiography to seek evidence of metastases to the pelvic nodes.

Management

Treatment selection is based on the stage of the disease and on the patient's age and symptoms. A radical prostatectomy (removal of the prostate and seminal vesicles) still remains the standard operative procedure for patients who have potentially curable disease, and a life expectancy of 10 years or more. This procedure may be followed by bilateral orchiectomy. Sexual impotency follows radical prostatectomy, and 5% to 10% of the patients have various degrees of urinary incontinence. (See p. 1096 for care of the patient following a prostatectomy.)

If the cancer is found in the early stage, the treatment may be curative radiation therapy, either using teletherapy with a linear accelerator or interstitial radiation (implantation of radioactive iodine or gold combined with pelvic lymphadenectomy). Radiation therapy is also used for palliation in patients with late stage disease. Side-effects, which usually are transitory, include proctitis (inflammation of the rectum) and cystitis due to the radiation doses and the proximity of the bladder and rectum. There is better preservation of sexual potency with radiation therapy; therefore, younger patients may prefer this treatment modality.

Since approximately half of the patients have locally advanced tumors or evidence of metastatic disease at the time they present for treatment, palliative measures are indicated. Hormonal therapy may be selected to suppress all androgenic stimuli to the prostate. This is accomplished by either orchiectomy or administration of estrogens (see below). Hormonal therapy is a method of control rather than cure, since adenocarcinoma of the prostate is hormone-dependent. The rationale underlying hormone treatment is that prostatic epithelium becomes atrophied or inactivated when androgen hormones are greatly reduced or inactivated.

Orchiectomy (removal of the testes) lowers plasma testosterone, since 93% of circulating testosterone is of testicular origin. This results in completely removing the testicular stimulus required for continued prostatic growth. Prostatic atrophy occurs after this procedure. Orchiectomy is preferred over hormonal therapy by many urologists because the potential side-effects of estrogen therapy are lacking. However, castration in the male carries a significant emotional impact. The administration of *estrogen* is thought to inhibit the gonadotropins (responsible for testicular androgenic activity), thus removing the androgenic hormone, upon which the growth of the malignancy depends. Diethylstilbestrol is the most widely used estrogen at this time.

Diethylstilbestrol gives symptomatic control, lessens tumor size, lessens pain from metastatic nodules, and imparts an improved sense of well-being. However, there is now evidence that giving higher doses of diethylstilbestrol carries a significant risk of death from cardiovascular disease, especially from thromboembolic phenomena. Gynecomastia (enlargement of breasts in the male) is an annoying complications of estrogen therapy that may be lessened by pretreatment radiation of breast tissue. Impotence almost always occurs following estrogen therapy.

Cryosurgery of the prostate gland has been advocated by some for the poor-risk patient. Chemotherapy may also be tried. Doxorubicin, cisplatin, and cyclophosphamide are under investigation.

For patients failing to respond to conventional therapy, estramustine phosphate (Emcyt), a conjugate of estradiol and nitrogen mustard, has shown to be promising in giving rapid pain relief. It is based on the premise that a hormone can be used as a carrier to bring a chemotherapeutic agent (nitrogen mustard) to hormone-sensitive tissues (prostate). The drug is available in capsule form. Side-effects include nausea, vomiting, and occasionally diarrhea.

To maintain patency of the urethral passage, repeated transurethral resections may have to be performed. When this is impractical, catheter drainage is instituted by way of the suprapubic or transurethral route.

Patients with recurring symptoms are treated symptomatically. Corticosteroids may give relief but do not affect the tumor.

Blood transfusions are given to maintain adequate hemoglobin levels when bone marrow is replaced by tumor. Radiation therapy to skeletal lesions can palliate bone pain. Pain may be controlled by estrogens and narcotics and, if necessary, by severing spinal cord pain fibers via neurosurgery. (See also p. 285, The Nursing Management of the Patient With Pain, and p. 320, The Care of the Patient With Advanced Cancer.)

▷ Conditions Affecting the Testes and Adjacent Structures

Undescended Testis (Cryptorchidism)

Cryptorchidism is the absence of one or both testes from the scrotum. The testes may be located in the abdominal cavity or inguinal canal. If the testis does not descend, hormone therapy or surgery (orchiopexy) are employed to secure proper positioning.

In orchiopexy, an incision is made over the inguinal canal, and the testis is brought down and placed in the scrotum. To maintain proper position of the testis, traction may be applied to the thigh by means of a suture drawn from the lower end of the scrotum.

Epididymitis

Epididymitis is an infection of the epididymis that usually descends from an infected prostate or urinary tract. It may also develop as a complication of gonorrhea. In men under 35 years of age, the major cause of epididymitis is *Chlamydia*

trachomatis. The infection passes upward through the urethra and the ejaculatory duct, and thence along the vas deferens to the epididymis.

The patient complains of pain and soreness in the inguinal canal along the course of the vas deferens, and then develops pain and swelling in the scrotum and the groin. The epididymis becomes swollen and extremely painful; the temperature is elevated. The patient may experience pyuria and bacteriuria with resulting chills and fever.

Management. The patient is placed on bed rest with the scrotum elevated with a scrotal bridge or folded towel to prevent traction on the spermatic cord and to improve venous drainage and relieve pain. Antimicrobials may be given until all evidence of the acute inflammatory reaction has subsided. If the patient is seen within the first 24 hours after onset, the spermatic cord may be infiltrated with a local anesthetic agent to relieve pain. If the epididymitis is chlamydial in origin, the patient's sexual partners must also be treated with antibiotics.

Intermittent cold compresses to the scrotum may help ease the pain. Local heat or sitz baths later in the infection may hasten resolution of the inflammatory process. Analgesics are given for pain relief. The patient is observed for abscess formation. If no improvement occurs within 2 weeks, an underlying testis tumor should be considered. An epididymectomy (excision of the epididymis from the testicle) may be performed for patients with recurrent, incapacitating episodes or for those with chronic, painful conditions.

Patient Education. The patient should avoid straining (lifting) and sexual excitement until the infection is under control. It may take 4 weeks or longer for the epididymis to return to normal.

Tumors of the Testes (Cancer)

Testicular cancer accounts for only 1% of all malignant tumors, but it ranks first in cancer deaths among males in the 20 to 35 age group. The etiology of testicular tumors is unknown, but cryptorchidism, infections, and genetic and endocrine factors appear to play a part in their development. These tumors are usually malignant and tend to metastasize early. Tumors of germinal cell origin comprise the majority of these neoplasms.

Assessment and Clinical Manifestations. The symptoms appear very gradually with a mass in the scrotum and painless enlargement of the testis. The patient may complain of heaviness in the scrotum. Backache (from retroperitoneal node extension), pain in the abdomen, loss of weight, and general weakness may be from metastatic disease. Gynecomastia (enlargement of the breasts) due to elaboration of chorionic gonadotropins produced by the testicular tumor is considered a serious prognostic sign. The metastatic growth may be more marked than the local testicular one. The enlargement of the testicle without pain is a significant diagnostic finding.

Diagnostic Evaluation. Alpha-fetoprotein (AFP) and human chorionic gonadotropin (HCG) are tumor markers that may be elevated in patients with testicular cancer. (Tumor markers are substances synthesized by the tumor cells and released into the circulation in abnormal amounts.) Newer immunocytochemical techniques have made possible the identification of the cells that apparently produce these markers. Other diagnostic tests include an intravenous urogram to detect ureteral deviation secondary to tumor mass, lymphangiography to assess extent of lymphatic spread of the tumor, and computed tomography to identify lesions in the retroperitoneum.

Management. The goals of management are to eradicate the disease and achieve a cure. Treatment selection is based on the cell type and the anatomical extent of the disease. The testicle is removed (orchiectomy) through an inguinal incision with a high ligation of the spermatic cord. Retroperitoneal lymphadenectomy to prevent lymphatic spread may be employed after orchiectomy. Postoperative irradiation to the lymphatic drainage pathways is usually done and is the treatment of choice in pure seminoma. A possible postoperative complication after retroperitoneal lymphadenectomy is dry ejaculation (no seminal fluid emitted during intercourse). Normal libido and orgasm are usually unimpaired, but the patient will not be fertile. Sperm banking before surgery may be considered for the young man as a "hedge" against sterility after surgery. A gel-filled prosthesis can be implanted to offset the absence of one testis.

Testicular carcinomas are highly responsive to drug therapy. Multiple chemotherapy using cisplatin with other agents (vinblastine, bleomycin, dactinomycin, cyclophosphamide) gives a high percentage of complete remission. The program of therapy is probably best prescribed by those trained in oncology, as these regimens are toxic and require intensive therapeutic support. Good results may be obtained by combining different types of treatment, including surgery, radiotherapy, and chemotherapy. Disseminated testicular cancer is regarded as a treatable and probably curable disease.

Patient Education and Support. The patient may have difficulty in accepting his condition. He needs encouragement to maintain a positive attitude during what may be a long course of therapy. Radiotherapy does not necessarily prevent the patient from fathering children, nor will unilateral excision of a tumor necessarily lessen virility.

A patient with a history of one tumor of the testes has a greater chance of developing another. Follow-up evaluation includes chest x-rays, excretory urography, radioimmunoassay of human chorionic gonadotropins and alpha-fetoprotein, and examination of lymph nodes to detect recurrence of malignancy.

Self-examination for testicular tumor is as important for men (especially those between 15 and 35 years, which are the tumor-prone years) as is self-examination for breast cancer by women.

The testis is easily accessible for self-examination, and most tumors are palpable. The patient should conduct the examination monthly, while showering or bathing. The following are guidelines for self-examination for testicular tumor:

1. Use both hands to feel for any abnormalities and to feel differences in weight between the testicles. Examine the contents of the scrotum.
2. Locate the epididymis, which is the cordlike structure

at the back of the testis. This is important in order to avoid confusing the epididymis with an abnormality.
3. Feel each testis between the thumb and first two fingers of each hand. The testes lie freely in the scrotum; are oval in shape; have a spongy, uniform texture; and measure 4 cm to 5 cm in length, 3 cm in width, and about 2 cm in thickness.
4. Note the size and shape, and the presence, of any abnormal tenderness. An abnormality may be felt as a firm area on the front or on the side of the testis.
5. Stand in front of the mirror and look for changes in the size and shape of the scrotum. Tumors tend to involve only one side.

Hydrocele and Varicocele

Hydrocele. A *hydrocele* is a collection of fluid generally in the tunica vaginalis of the testicle, although it may also occur within the spermatic cord. The tunica vaginalis becomes widely distended with fluid. Hydrocele may be acute or chronic and is differentiated from a hernia by the fact that a hydrocele transmits light when transilluminated.

Acute hydrocele occurs in association with acute infectious diseases of the epididymis or as a result of local trauma or systemic infectious diseases, such as mumps. The cause of chronic hydrocele is unknown.

Usually, therapy is not required. Treatment is necessary only if the hydrocele becomes tense and compromises testicular circulation or if the scrotal mass becomes large, uncomfortable, or embarrassing.

In the surgical treatment of hydrocele, an incision is made through the wall of the scrotum down to the distended tunica vaginalis. The sac is resected or, after being opened, is sutured together to collapse the wall. In the postoperative care of these patients, an athletic supporter is worn for comfort and support. The major complication is the formation of a hematoma in the loose tissues of the scrotum. The nursing management is the same as for a varicocele.

Varicocele. A *varicocele* is an abnormal dilation of the veins of the pampiniform venous plexus in the scrotum (network of veins from the testicle and the epididymis, constituting part of the spermatic cord). Varicoceles occur most frequently in the veins on the left side in adults. In some men, a varicocele has been associated with infertility. Very few, if any, subjective symptoms may be produced by the enlargement of the spermatic vein, and as a rule, no treatment is required unless fertility is a matter of concern. Symptomatic varicocele (pain, tenderness, and discomfort in the inguinal region) is corrected surgically by ligating the external spermatic vein at the inguinal area. An ice bag may be applied to the scrotum for the first few hours after operation to relieve edema. The patient then wears a scrotal support.

Vasectomy

A *vasectomy* is the ligation and transection of a section of the vas deferens, with or without removal of a segment of the vas. The severed ends are occluded with ligatures or clips, or the lumen of each vas is coagulated. A bilateral vasectomy may be done as a sterilization procedure, since it interrupts the transportation of the sperm. (The sperm, which are manufactured in the testicle, are unable to travel up the vas deferens because of surgical interruption.)

Seminal fluid is mostly manufactured in the seminal vesicles and prostate gland, which are unaffected by vasectomy. Thus, there will be no noticeable decrease in the amount of ejaculated fluid, except that it contains no sperm. Because the sperm cells have no exit, they are reabsorbed into the body. The procedure has no effect on sexual potency, erection, ejaculation, or production of male hormones.

Two behavioral responses seem to be common after vasectomy. Individuals who were anxious about intercourse because of fear of pregnancy due to contraceptive failure often report a decrease in anxiety and an increase in spontaneous sexual arousal. Some men adopt stereotyped masculine behavior, supposedly to allay concerns that the surgery has decreased their masculinity. Concise and factual preoperative discussion may minimize or avoid the latter behavior. Some studies purport that vasectomy can lead to autoimmune disorders, in that antibodies that agglutinate the patient's own sperm may form and persist for many years after the procedure. However, an increased incidence of autoimmune disorders following vasectomy has not yet been clinically proven, and the implications are not yet clear.

The patient is advised that he will be sterile, but that potency will not be altered following a bilateral vasectomy. The procedure does not prevent sexually transmitted disease. On rare occasions, a spontaneous reanastomosis of the vas deferens occurs, which may result in pregnancy of the partner. A legal consent form (usually signed by both the man and his partner) must be obtained before the procedure is carried out.

Postoperative Considerations.   Ice bags are applied intermittently to the scrotum for several hours after surgery to reduce swelling and relieve discomfort. The patient is advised to wear cotton jockey-type undershorts for added comfort and support. He may become greatly concerned about the discoloration of the scrotal skin and superficial swelling. This occurs frequently after vasectomy and responds to sitz baths. Complications of vasectomy include scrotal ecchymoses and swelling, superficial wound infection, vasitis (inflammation of the vas deferens), epididymitis or epididymo-orchitis, hematomas, and sperm granuloma. A *sperm granuloma* is an inflammatory response to the collection of sperm in the scrotum due to leakage from the severed end of the proximal vas. This can initiate recanalization of the vas, leading to possible pregnancy of the partner.

Patient Education.   Sexual intercourse may be resumed as desired by the patient, although he should be informed that he will still be fertile for a varying length of time after vasectomy until the sperm that are stored distal to the point of interruption of the vas have been evacuated.

Contraceptives should be used until the patient is declared infertile. This declaration is made upon examination of ejaculate. Some physicians examine a sperm specimen 4 weeks after the vasectomy to determine sterility; others use two consecutive specimens 1 month apart, and still others consider a patient sterile after 36 ejaculations.

Vasovasostomy (Sterilization Reversal).   Microsurgical techniques are being used for vasectomy reversal (vasovasostomy), which restores patency to the vas deferens. However, the success rate of this procedure is still under investigation.

Sperm Banking.   Storage of fertile semen in a sperm bank *before* a vasectomy is a possibility should unforeseen life events cause a desire in the patient to father a child. The success rate in achieving pregnancy with frozen sperm is uncertain.

▷ Impotence

Impotence is the alteration of a man's sexual capability either to achieve or maintain an erection sufficient to accomplish intercourse. Impotence can either be erectile or ejaculatory. Erectile impotence has both psychogenic and organic causes. Causes of psychogenic impotence include anxiety, fatigue, depression, and cultural pressure to perform sexually. Research suggests, however, that organic impotence may account for a larger percentage of cases of impotence than previously realized. Organic causes include occlusive vascular disease, endocrine disease (*diabetes,* pituitary tumors, hypogonadism), genitourinary conditions (radical pelvic cancer surgery), hematologic conditions (Hodgkin's disease, leukemia), neurologic disorders (neuropathies, parkinsonism), trauma to the pelvic or genital area, and drugs (alcohol, psychoactive drugs, anticholinergics, drugs of abuse).

Diagnosis of impotence includes a sexual and medical history, an analysis of presenting symptoms, physical examination, and various laboratory studies. The advent of sleep laboratories have made the nocturnal penile tumescence test (NPT) possible. Research revealed that normal males have nocturnal penile erections closely paralleling rapid eye movement sleep (REM) in their occurrence and duration. Organically impotent men show inadequate sleep-related erections that correspond to their waking performance. Changes in penile circumference are monitored (using a mercury strain gauge placed around the penis) and recorded. The NPT test is a means of determining whether erectile impotence has organic or psychogenic etiology.

Arterial blood flow to the penis is measured with the Doppler probe. Nerve conduction tests and psychological evaluation of the patient are part of the diagnostic workup.

Management.   Treatment, which depends to some extent on the cause, can be medical, surgical, or a combination of both. A patient's response to nonsurgical therapy, such as treatment of alcoholism and readjustment of hypertensive agents or other medications, is examined. Impotence secondary to hypothalamic–pituitary–gonadal dysfunction may be reversible with endocrine therapy. Insufficient penile blood flow may be treated with recently developed vascular surgery. Patients with impotence from psychogenic causes are directed to a professional specializing in sex therapy (see p. 220). Patients with impotence secondary to organic causes are considered candidates for penile implants.

Two basic types of penile implants are available: the semirigid rod and the inflatable prosthesis. The semirigid rod, such as the Small–Carrion prosthesis, has no moving parts, unlike the inflatable prosthesis, which simulates natural erections and natural flaccidity. Complications following implant procedures include infection, erosion of the prosthesis through the skin, and persistent pain, which may require removal of the implant.

Impotence, regardless of its cause, has vast psychological and psychosocial implications for most men. Therefore, the nurse must listen and be supportive to both the patient and his significant other.

▷ Conditions Affecting the Penis

Infections

Gonorrhea.   Gonorrhea occurs as a result of an infection due to the gonococcus, which penetrates the tissues of the urethra as a result of sexual exposure. (This condition is discussed in Chap. 63, p. 1494.)

Penile Ulceration.   Several types of penile ulcerations may occur, but because of the danger of chancre (syphilis), all lesions are considered to be syphilitic until proven otherwise. Diagnosis is made by a combination of the history of the disease, a microscopic examination of a darkfield specimen removed from the lesions, and a blood serology examination. The treatment of penile ulceration varies greatly, depending on the cause of the ulceration. Treatment is not started until the diagnosis is made.

Chancre is a venereal ulceration caused by *Treponema pallidum* and is the primary lesion of syphilis. It occurs as a result of sexual exposure. Local treatment is usually unnecessary, other than a mild antiseptic and a protective dressing, the main portion of the treatment being confined to systemic measures that usually result in a rapid healing of the local lesion. Penicillin results in rapid cure.

Chancroid is a sexually transmitted disease caused by *Haemophilus ducreyi.* On a worldwide basis, chancroid may be more prevalent than syphilis. Usually, one or several penile ulcers are present with enlarged lymph nodes. It is more commonly seen in hot climates among those with poor hygiene. Treatment consists of a sulfonamide or tetracycline. Local treatment includes regular cleaning with bland soap and water. Antibiotic cream may be applied to minimize secondary infection.

Genital herpes (Herpes simplex virus [HSV]) is a sexually transmitted disease that produces multiple bilaterally distributed vesicles on or near the penis. The vesicles become pustular and coalesce into ulcers that gradually heal. There may be accompanying urethritis and enlarged, tender inguinal nodes. The lesions of the primary attack take 2 to 4 weeks to heal, while recurrent lesions heal in less time. Recurrent symptomatic sores often occur in the genital area monthly for extended periods of time.

Phimosis

Phimosis is a condition in which the foreskin is constricted so that it cannot be retracted over the glans. There has been a recent trend away from routine circumcision of newborns. Therefore, the child and adult will require early instruction in cleansing of the prepuce. In the adult, when the cleansing of the preputial area is neglected or no longer possible, the accumulation of normal secretions and subsequent inflammation (*balanitis*) occur. This causes adhesions and scarring. The thickened secretions become encrusted with urinary salts and calcifies, forming preputial concretions. In the aged, penile carcinoma may develop. Phimosis is corrected by circumcision (see below). The patient is instructed in proper hygienic care of the foreskin.

Paraphimosis is a condition in which the foreskin is retracted behind the glans and, because of narrowness and subsequent edema, cannot be reduced back to its usual position (covering the glans). It is treated by manual reduction (compressing the glans firmly, to reduce its size, and then pushing the glans back as the prepuce is moved forward). Circumcision is usually indicated once the inflammation and edema subside.

Circumcision

Circumcision is the excision of the foreskin (prepuce) of the glans penis. It is usually done in infancy for hygienic purposes. In adults, it is indicated for phimosis, paraphimosis, recurrent infections of the glans and foreskin, and personal desire of the patient.

Postoperatively, the patient is watched for bleeding. The petrolatum (Vaseline) gauze dressing is changed as indicated. Since the adult male may experience a considerable amount of pain following circumcision, analgesics are given when needed. *Circumcision is an important preventive measure against carcinoma of the penis.*

Carcinoma

Cancer of the penis occurs in the skin of the penis and rarely in circumcised individuals. It appears as a painless, wartlike growth or ulcer on the glans or coronal sulcus under the prepuce and represents about 1% of malignancies in men in the U.S. Smaller lesions involving only the skin may be controlled by excisional biopsy, while penectomy (partial or total) is indicated when the tumor is not amenable to conservative treatment. Radiation therapy may be used as treatment for small squamous cell carcinomas of the penis or for palliation in advanced tumors or lymph node metastasis.

Patient Education.   Circumcision in infancy almost eliminates penile cancer, as chronic irritation and inflammation of the glans penis predisposes to penile tumors. Personal hygiene is an important preventive measure in uncircumcised males.

Priapism

Priapism is an uncontrolled, persistent erection of the penis that causes the penis to become very large, hard, and often painful. It occurs from either neural or vascular causes, including sickle cell thrombosis, spinal cord tumors, and tumor invasion of the penis or its vessels. This condition may result in gangrene and often results in impotence, whether treated or not.

This condition is considered a urologic emergency. The goal of therapy is to improve venous drainage of the corpora cavernosa to prevent ischemia, fibrosis, and impotence. Initially, treatment is directed at relieving the erection and includes bed rest and sedation. The corpora may be irrigated with an anticoagulant which allows aspiration of stagnant blood. Shunting procedures to divert the blood from the turgid corpora cavernosa to the venous system (corpora cavernosa–saphenous vein shunt) or into the corpus spongiosum–glans penis compartment may be tried.

▷ Bibliography

Books

Alken C-E, Sokeland DJ, and Engel RME. Urology, Guide for Diagnosis and Therapy. New York, Georg Thieme, 1982.

Blandy J. Lecture Notes on Urology, 3rd ed. Oxford, Blackwell Scientific, 1982.

Brown RB. Clinical Urology Illustrated. New York, ADIS Press, 1982.

Burger H and DeKretser D. The Testis. New York, Raven Press, 1981.

Cohen J, Cullen JW, and Martin LR. Psychosocial Aspects of Cancer. New York, Raven Press, 1982.

Crawford ED and Borden TA. Genitourinary Cancer Surgery. Philadelphia, Lea & Febiger, 1982.

Finkbeiner AE, Barbour GL, and Bissada NK. Pharmacology of the Urinary Tract and Male Reproductive System. New York, Appleton-Century-Crofts, 1982.

Kaufman JL. Current Urologic Therapy. Philadelphia, WB Saunders, 1980.

Lerner J and Khan Z. Mosby's Manual of Urologic Nursing. St Louis, CV Mosby, 1982.

McConnell EA and Zimmerman MF. Care of Patients with Urologic Problems. Philadelphia, JB Lippincott, 1982.

Mitchell JP. Endoscopic Operative Urology. Boston, Wright PSG, 1981.

Noble RC. Sexually Transmitted Diseases, 2nd ed. Garden City, Medical Examination, 1982.

Report of a WHO Scientific Group. Nongonococcal urethritis and other sexually transmitted diseases of public health importance. World Health Organization Technical Report Series, 1981.

Smith DR. General Urology, 10th ed. Los Altos, Lange Medical Publishers, 1981.

Thin RN. Lecture Notes on Sexually Transmitted Diseases. Boston, Blackwell Scientific, 1982.

von Eschenbach AC and Rodriquez DB. Sexual Rehabilitation of the Urologic Cancer Patient. Boston, GK Hall Medical Publishers, 1981.

Articles
Male Sexual Dysfunction

Allen RP. Erectile impotence: Objective diagnosis from sleep-related erections (nocturnal penile tumescence). J Urol 1981 Sept; 126(3):353.

Ankenman GJ et al. Penile prosthesis for organic impotence. Can J Surg 1981 Nov; 24(6):628–629, 633.

Beaser RS et al. Experience with penile prostheses in the treatment of impotence in diabetic men. JAMA 1982 Aug 27; 248(8):943–948.

Deeths HJ. New concepts in penile prostheses. Nebr Med J 1982 Mar; 67(3):54–55.

Federman DD. Impotence: Etiology and management. Hosp Pract 1982 Mar; 17(3):155–159.

Furlow WL (ed). Symposium on male sexual dysfunction. Urol Clin North Am 1981 Feb; 8(1):1–202 (entire volume).

Godec CJ and Cass AS. Impotence. Evaluation and treatment. Minn Med 1981 July; 64(7):405–409.

Morgan RJ and Pryor JP. The investigation of organic impotence. Br J Urol 1980 Dec; 52(6):571–574.

Smith AD and Lange PH. Impotence. Pathogenesis and evaluation. Minn Med 1980 Oct; 63(10):701–705.

Prostatic Conditions

Abrams PH et al. Blood loss during transurethral resection of the prostate. Anaesthesia 1982 Jan; 37(1):71–73.

Bonney WW et al. Cryosurgery in prostatic cancer: Survival. Urology 1982 Jan; 19(1):37–42.

Droller MJ. Adenocarcinoma of the prostate: An overview. Urol Clin North Am 1980 Oct; 7(3):731–733.

Hoeft RT and Jones AG. Cancer of the prostate: Treating metastasis with estramustine phosphate. Am J Nurs 1982 May; 82(5):828–830.

Jones AG and Hoeft RT. Cancer of the prostate. Am J Nurs 1982 May; 82(5):826–828.

Loprinzi CL. Prostatic cancer. South Med J 1982 Feb; 75(2):193–196.

Meares EM Jr. Prostatitis. Kidney Int 1981 Aug; 20(2):289–298.

Sandberg AA and Karr JP (eds). Symposium on prostatic cancer. Prostate [Suppl] 1981 1:1–136.

Testicular Conditions

Drasga RE, Einhorn LH, and Williams SD. The chemotherapy of testicular cancer. CA—A Cancer Journal for Clinicians 1982 Mar-Apr; 32(2):66–77.

Gault PL. Taking your part in the fight against testicular cancer. Nursing '81 1981 May; 11(5):47–50.

Hussey HH. Vasectomy—a note of concern: Reprise. JAMA 1981 June 12; 245(22):2333.

Li FP, Connelly RR, and Myers M. Improved survival rates among testis cancer patients in the United States. JAMA 1982 Feb 12; 247(6):825–826.

Martin DC. Microsurgical reversal of vasectomy. Am J Surg 1981 July; 142(1):48–50.

Paulson DF. Testicular carcinoma. Curr Probl Cancer 1982 May; 6(11):3–44.

Petitti DB. A survey of personal habits, symptoms of illness and histories of disease in men with and without vasectomies. Am J Public Health 1982 May; 72(5):476–480.

Sotolongo JR Jr. Immunological effects of vasectomy. J Urol 1982 June; 127(6):1063–1066.

Walker AM et al. Hospitalization rates in vasectomized men. JAMA 1981 June 12; 245(22):2315–2317.

Zufall RL. Vasectomy: Five to ten-year follow-up of 200 cases. Urology 1980 Mar; 15(3):278–279.

Other Conditions

Droller MJ. Carcinoma of the penis: An overview. Urol Clin North Am 1980 Oct; 7(3):783–784.

Felmany YM and Nikitas JA. Nongonococcal urethritis. JAMA 1981 Jan 23–30; 245(4):381–386.

Sagalowsky AI. Priapism. Urol Clin North Am 1982 June; 9(2):255–257.

Unit XIII

Immunologic-Related Problems

49

The Immune System and Immunopathology

"Immunity" refers to the body's specific protective response to an invading foreign agent or organism. However, pathological developments within this system lead to certain disease manifestations. Therefore, the term "immunopathology" is used to describe the study of diseases caused by the immune reaction—that protective response which the body initiates but which paradoxically turns on the body and causes tissue damage and disease. However, to understand immunopathology we must first understand how the body's immune system normally functions.

▷ The Immune System

General Immune Responses

When the body is attacked by bacteria or viruses, it has three means of defending itself—the phagocytic immune response, the humoral or antibody immune response, and the cellular immune response.

The first line of defense, the *phagocytic immune response,* involves the white blood cells (granulocytes and macrophages), which actually have the ability to ingest foreign particles. These cells can move to the point of attack to engulf and destroy the foreign agents.

The second protective response, the *humoral or antibody response,* begins with the lymphocyte cells, which can transform themselves into plasma cells that manufacture antibodies. It is the antibodies, which are highly specific proteins, that are transported in the bloodstream and have the ability to disable the invaders.

A third mechanism of defense, the *cellular immune response,* also involves the lymphocytes, which, besides transforming themselves into plasma cells, can also turn into special killer T cells that can attack the microbes themselves.

Of the three modes of immune response, the formation of antibodies constitutes the major protective device employed by the immune system.

Antigens and Antibodies

The part of the attacking organism that is responsible for stimulating the production of an antibody is called an *antigen*. In strict molecular terms, an antigen is a small patch of proteins on the outer surface of the microorganism. A single bacterium, even a single large molecule, such as a toxin (diphtheria or tetanus toxin), may have several such antigens or "markers" on its surface and can therefore induce the body to produce a number of different antibodies. Once an antibody is produced, it is released into the bloodstream and carried to the attacking organism, where it combines with the antigen on its surface, coupling with it like a complementary piece of a jigsaw puzzle (Fig. 49-1).

Stages of the Immune System Response

There are four well-defined stages in an immune response: recognition, proliferation, response, and the effector stage.

Recognition

The basis of any immune reaction is, first and foremost, recognition. It is our immune system's ability to recognize antigens on materials as "foreign," or "nonself," that is the initiating event in the mounting of any immune reaction. The body must first recognize invaders as "foreign" before it can react to them.

Surveillance by Lymph Nodes and Lymphocytes. The body accomplishes its surveillance in two ways. First, instead of being localized centrally in one large organ far away from the obvious points of microbial attack, such as the skin, mouth, eyes and throat, the immune system is widely dispersed—distributed close to all of the body's surfaces, internal as well as external, in the form of tiny organs called lymph nodes. Second, a steady succession of sentries in the form of small lymphocytes is continuously being discharged

from lymph nodes into the bloodstream, where they patrol the tissues and vessels that drain the areas served by that node. Basically, it is the lymphocytes and lymph nodes that make up our immune system.

Lymphocytes.   There are two kinds of lymphocytes, those in the lymph nodes themselves and those that circulate. Figure 49-2 shows the path taken by the recirculating lymphocytes. Taken in aggregate, the total number of lymphocytes in the body adds up to a mass of cells of impressive size. Radioactive labeling of circulating lymphocytes has shown that these cells have no particular fate but to simply recirculate from the blood to lymph nodes—and from their lymph nodes back into the bloodstream again in a neverending series of patrols. Rather astonishingly, these circulating lymphocytes can survive for decades. Some of these small, hardy cells maintain their solitary circuits for the lifetime of the person.

The exact way in which circulating lymphocytes recognize antigens on foreign surfaces is not known. At present, the accepted theory is that recognition depends on specific receptor sites on the surface of the lymphocytes. It appears that macrophages, a type of granulocyte found in the tissues of the body, play an important though as yet undefined role in helping these circulating lymphocytes to process the antigens. Foreign materials enter the body, and a circulating lymphocyte comes into physical contact with the surfaces of these materials. Upon contact, the lymphocyte, with the help of macrophages, either removes the antigen from the surface or in some way picks up an imprint of its structure. For example, during a streptococcal throat infection, the streptococcal organism gains access to the mucous membranes of the throat, and a circulating lymphocyte moving through the tissues of the neck bumps up against the organism. The lymphocyte familiar with the surface markers on the cells of its own body recognizes the antigens on the microbe as being different (nonself) and the streptococcus

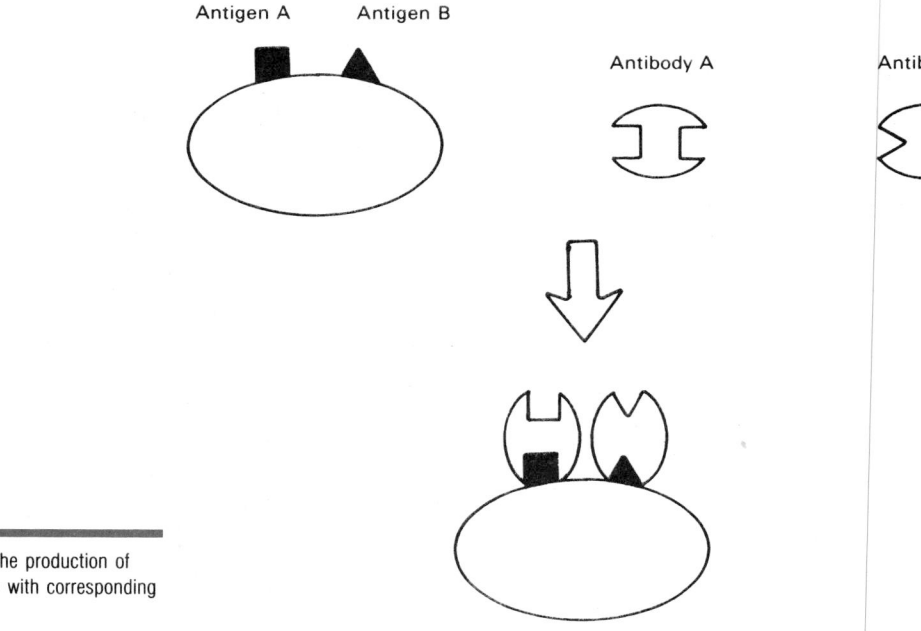

Figure 49-1. Antigens A and B cause the production of specific antibodies A and B, which couple with corresponding antigens.

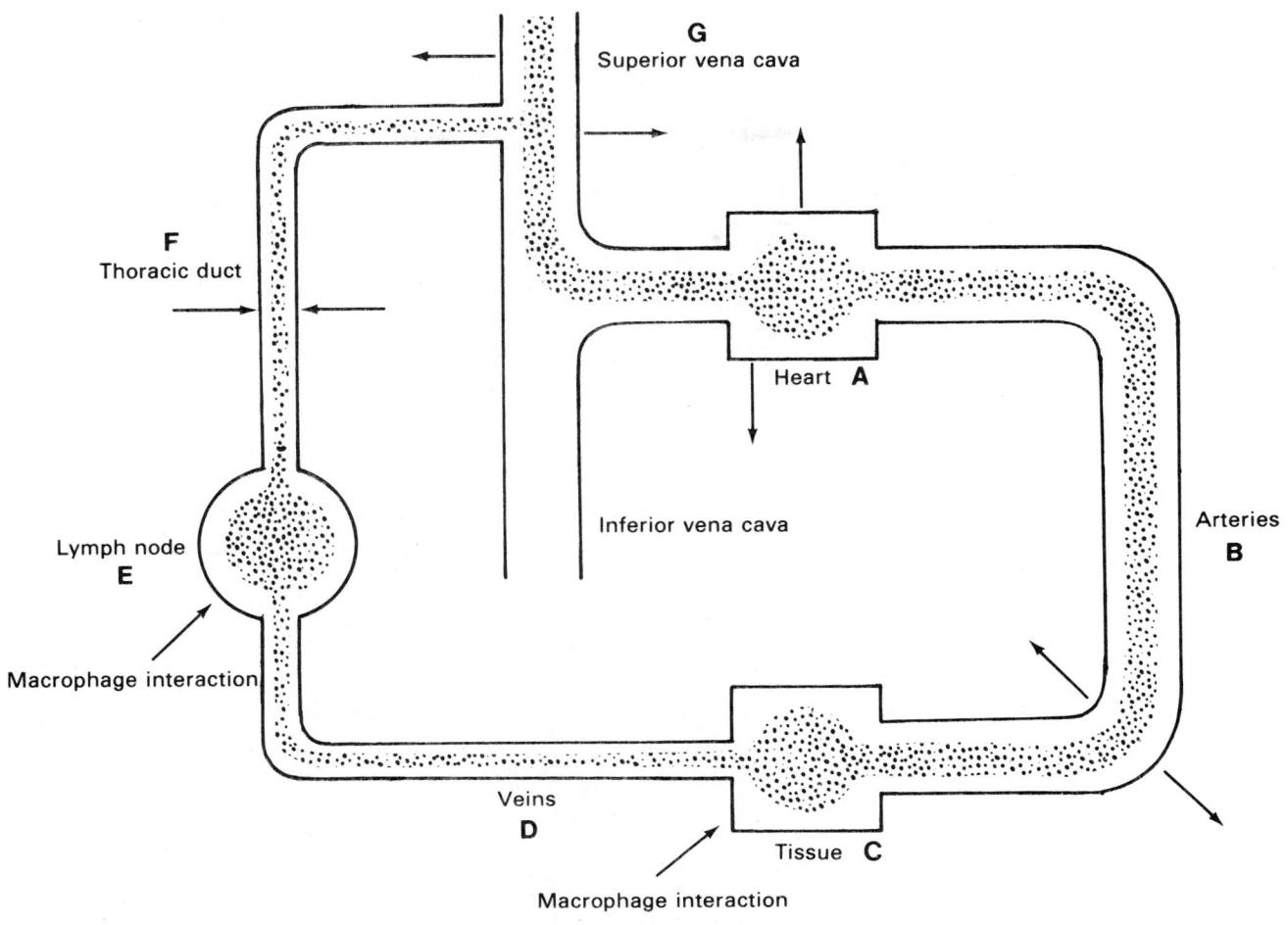

Figure 49-2. Recirculation of small lymphocytes is depicted schematically. For convenience, we shall begin the lymphocyte circuit in the heart (A). From A, the lymphocytes tumble into the aorta and from the aorta into the arteries (B) and eventually out into the tissues of the body (C). Cells then enter the veins (D) and from there move into the nearest lymph node (E). The cells moving through the lymph node leave the node via the lymphatic drainage, eventually entering the thoracic duct (F), through which they enter the superior vena cava (G) via the large veins of the neck. The superior vena cava then takes the cells back to the heart to begin another circuit, which will take the circulating lymphocyte to another part of the body.

as being antigenic (foreign). This triggers the second phase, the immune response—proliferation.

The Proliferation Stage

The circulating lymphocyte containing the antigenic message returns to the nearest lymph node. Once in the node, these "sensitized" lymphocytes stimulate certain of the dormant lymphocytes residing there first to enlarge, divide, and proliferate, and finally to differentiate into antibody-producing plasma cells. Swelling of the lymph nodes in the neck in conjunction with a sore throat is one example of the immune response.

The Response Stage

In the response stage, the changed lymphocytes will function in either a humoral or cellular fashion.

Humoral.   The production of antibodies to a specific antigen is called a humoral response, humoral referring to the fact that the antibodies are released into the bloodstream and so reside in the plasma or fluid fraction of the blood, one of the classical four "humors" of the body. (An explanation of antibody function can be found on p. 1111.)

Cellular.   The exact mechanism of the cellular response is not yet known. It is thought that the returning sensitized lymphocytes probably migrate to areas of the lymph node (other than those areas containing lymphocytes programmed to become plasma cells), where they stimulate the residing lymphocytes to become cells that upon being released back into the circulation will attack microbes personally rather than through the production of antibodies (Fig. 49-3).

These transformed lymphocytes have been given the descriptive name *killer T cells.* The *T* stands for the fact that

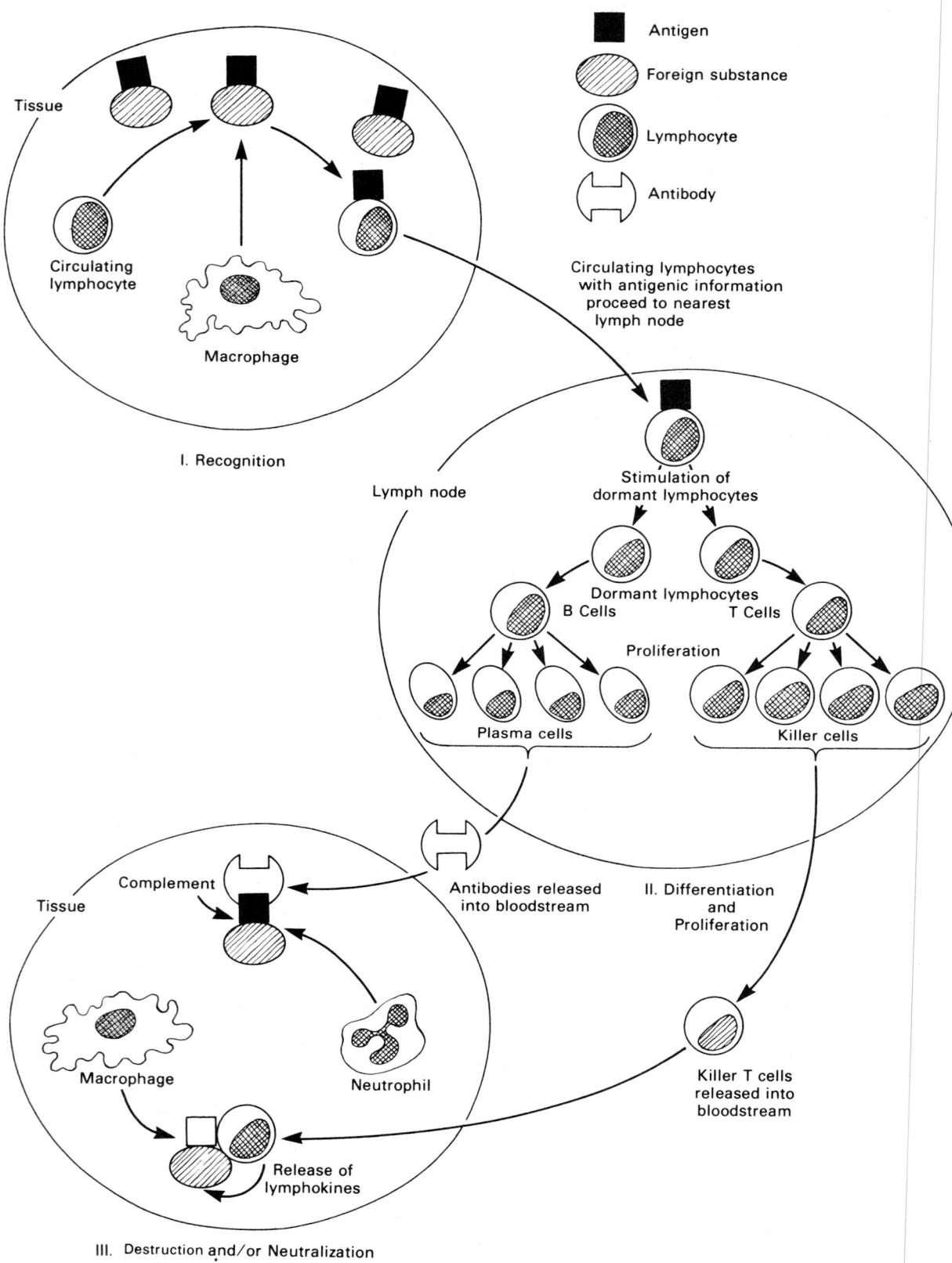

Figure 49-3. Cellular response.

during the embryologic development of the immune system, these lymphocytes spent some time in the thymus of the developing fetus, during which time they were genetically programmed to become (under the direction of an antigenically sensitized circulating lymphocyte) killer T cells rather than plasma cells. Viral rather than bacterial antigens induce a cellular response. This response is manifested by the increasing number of lymphocytes seen in the blood smears of people with viral illnesses, for instance, in the lymphocytosis occurring in infectious mononucleosis.

Most immune reactions to antigens involve both humoral and cellular responses, though usually one predominates. During transplantation rejections, the cellular reaction predominates, whereas in the bacterial pneumonias and sepsis it is the humoral response that plays the dominant protective role (Table 49-1).

The Effector Stage

In the effector stage, the antibody of the humoral response or the killer T cell of the cellular response reaches and couples with the antigen on the surface of the foreign object. The coupling initiates a series of events that in the majority of instances results in the total destruction of the invading microbes or the complete neutralization of the toxin. The events involve an interplay of antibodies, complement, and action by the killer T cells.

Antibodies.   To understand how the production of antibodies can protect the body, we must understand what an antibody looks like and how it works. Figure 49-4 is a schematic representation of an antibody molecule. The various parts have been designated as the Fab fragments and the Fc end.

It is important here to define the "Ig" designation of antibodies. *Ig* refers to the term immunoglobulin. Early in

Table 49-1
Comparison of Cellular and Humoral Immunologic Response

Cell-Mediated Immune Responses	Humoral-Mediated Immune Responses
Transplant rejection	Bacterial phagocytosis and lysis
Delayed hypersensitivity— tuberculin reaction	Viral and toxin neutralization
Contact dermatitis	Anaphylaxis
Graft-vs.-host reactions	Allergic hay fever and asthma
Tumor surveillance or destruction	Immune complex disease
Intracellular infections	

the study of the types and kinds of proteins circulating in blood, machines were developed that could separate blood proteins by the electronic changes on their surfaces. Antibodies were found to be contained in a class of circulating proteins migrating through the electronic field at a rate different from those of the other blood proteins, such as hemoglobins or the clotting factors.

These antibody proteins, defined solely by how they migrated through the charged field, were listed as globulins because of other physical and chemical properties that showed they belonged to the general class of proteins called globulins. They were also given the name immunoglobulins, since they were globulins involved in the immune response. We now know that the body produces five different kinds of globulin antibodies arbitrarily designed as IgA, IgM, IgG, IgD, and IgE, each type differing in size and amino acid composition (Table 49-2). The most common antibodies,

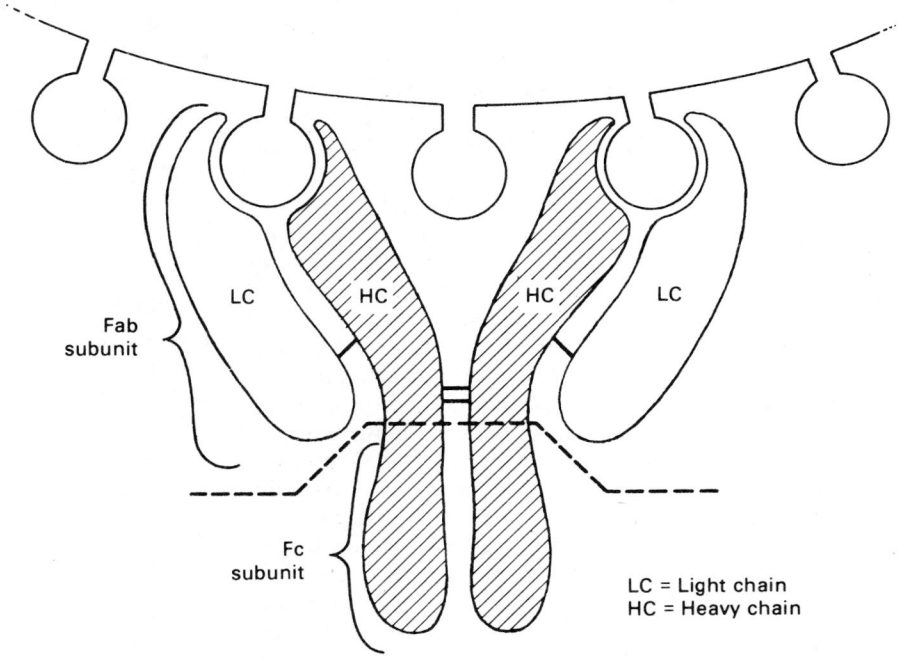

Figure 49-4.   Antibody molecule.

Table 49-2
Classes of Immunoglobulins

Protein	Species	Amino Acid Chain Length	Protein Molecular Weights
IgG (IgG$_1$, IgG$_2$, IgG$_3$, IgG$_4$) $\triangle$	Human	450	150,000
IgA (IgA$_1$, IgA$_2$) $\square$	Human	470	58,000
IgM	Human	575	950,000
IgD	Human	—	175,000
IgE	Human	550	77,000

$\triangle$ Subclasses of IgG molecules
$\square$ Subclasses of IgA molecules

however, are those of the IgG class. Each antibody molecule made against a particular antigen has a slightly different configuration from those of the amino acids making up its Fab (antigen-binding) fragments, so that each Fab fragment fits specifically onto the antigen it was made against (see Fig. 49-4) and onto no other antigen. The Fab part of the molecule can be considered to be the "recognition" end of the antibody. Once the Fab segments couple with its antigen, the Fc fragment, through a change in the antibody's configuration, becomes available to the circulation; that is, it becomes exposed to the blood passing by, and this exposure allows it to interact with the first of a series of 20 circulating proteins, called the complement system.

Complement. The term "complement" refers to a number of circulating plasma proteins made in the liver that can be activated when an antibody couples with its antigen. Once activated, these unique proteins cause alterations of the cell membranes on which antigen and antibody complex form, permitting fluid to enter the cell and leading eventually to cell lysis and death (Fig. 49-5). In addition, activated complement molecules attract macrophages and granulocytes to areas of antigen–antibody reactions. These cells continue the body's defense by devouring the antibody-coated microbes and by releasing bacterial agents.

It is important to realize that antibodies coupling to an antigen do not damage the membrane or surface. Destruction is caused by activation of complement, the arrival of killer T cells, or the attraction of macrophages.

Classical Complement Activation. There are two ways of activating the complement system; one, termed the classical pathway, because it was the first method discovered, involves the reaction of the first of the circulating complement proteins (C$_1$) with the receptor site of the Fc portion of an antibody molecule following coupling of the antibody with the antigen. The activation of the first complement component then activates all the other components in the sequence in which the other components were discovered, namely C$_1$, C$_4$, C$_2$, C$_3$, C$_5$, up to C$_9$ respectively. According to the order of reaction, the C components are designated as follows: C$_{1\,qrs}$, C$_4$, C$_2$, C$_3$, C$_5$, C$_6$, C$_7$, C$_8$, and C$_9$. C$_4$ is

the second reactant in sequence, rather than C$_2$, the first four complement components having been numbered before their reaction sequence was known.[*]

Alternate Pathway of Complement Activation. The alternative method of complement activation occurs without the formation of antigen–antibody complexes. This alternate pathway can be initiated by bacterial products, thus bypassing the requirement for antibody production or antigen–antibody coupling. Whatever the method of activation, however, once activated, the complement can and does destroy cells.

This destruction is not only therapeutic but lifesaving, if the cell attacked by the complement system is a true foreign invader, such as a streptococcus or staphylococcus. However, if that cell is in reality part of the person—a cell of his brain or liver, the tissue lining his blood vessels, or the cells of a donor organ—the result can be devastating disease and even death. The result of the immune response—the implacableness of its attack on any material read as foreign, the deadliness of the struggle—is obvious in the pus (the remains of microbes, granulocytes, and macrophages, circulating and killer T-cell lymphocytes, plasma proteins, complement, and antibodies) that accumulates in wound infections and abscesses.

Killer T Cells and K Cells. It is not only the complement system that can destroy foreign cells, but also sensitized lymphocytes and killer T cells. Cellular rather than humoral destruction is carried out when killer T cells coming into contact with antigenically foreign cells release their own chemical mediators called lymphokines. The various lymphokines have been given names to denote their specific biological effects (Table 49-3). Upon contact with an antigen, killer lymphocytes release low molecular weight factors that attract, hold, and activate other uncommitted circulating lymphocytes and macrophages. One sensitized killer lymphocyte can, through its release of lymphokines, quickly recruit a large number of other cells into the area of antigenically foreign cells, amassing in a short time a large number of effector cells to protect the body. Unfortunately, as with complement activation, such cellular activation can cause tissue injury and disease if the supposedly "foreign" cell under attack is in reality part of the person.

In addition to the T cells, there are effector lymphocytes called K cells that, unlike killer T cells, only attack antigens already coated with antibody. Like molecules of complement, they have special Fc receptor sites on their surfaces that allow them to couple to the Fc end of antibodies.

Suppressor and Helper T Cells

It is now known that the cellular and humoral arms of the immune response are not separate entities. The most recent advances in the field of immunology have shown the artificial nature of dividing immunopathology into either antibody or cellular responses. While the six types of immune reactions are helpful in a schematic way to clarify what one sees clinically in the hospital or in the outpatient departments, immunologic reactions cannot be so neatly separated (Chart 49-1). The cellular and humoral arms of the immune

[*] Austen KF et al. Nomenclature of complements. Int Arch Allerg 1970; 37:661.

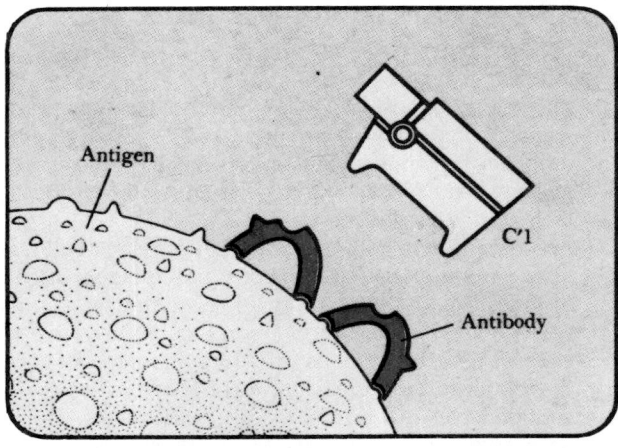

Initiating the sequence is the combination of antigen and complement-fixing antibody. It is hypothesized that under certain conditions, complement binding sites are then exposed.

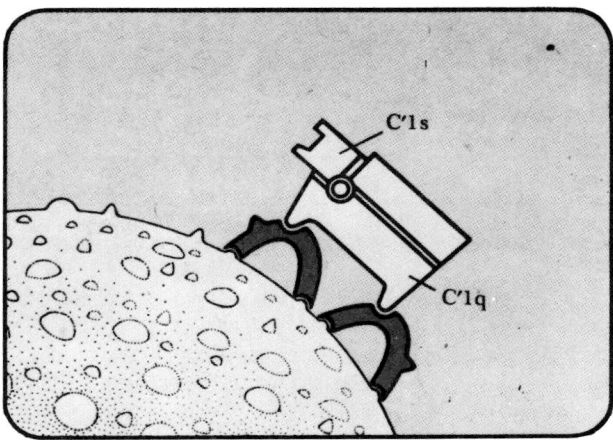

C'1 combines with these sites, with C'1q (a gamma globulin) attaching to the antibody. Enzymatic site (at C'1s) capable of acting with next component is converted to its active form.

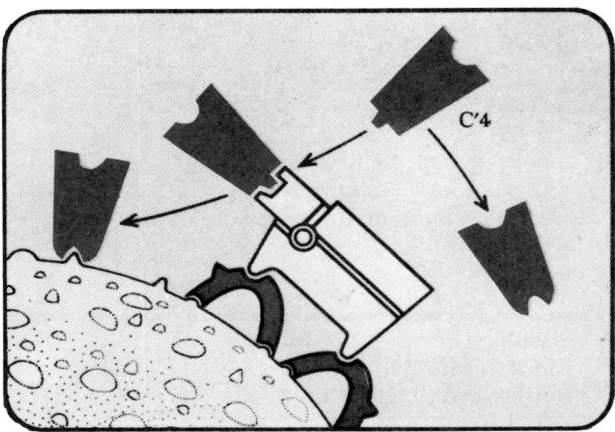

Next in order of appearance is C'4, which is acted upon by C'1s, exposing site for binding C'4 to the surface of the antigen or to the antibody. If unbound, C'4 cannot function in hemolysis.

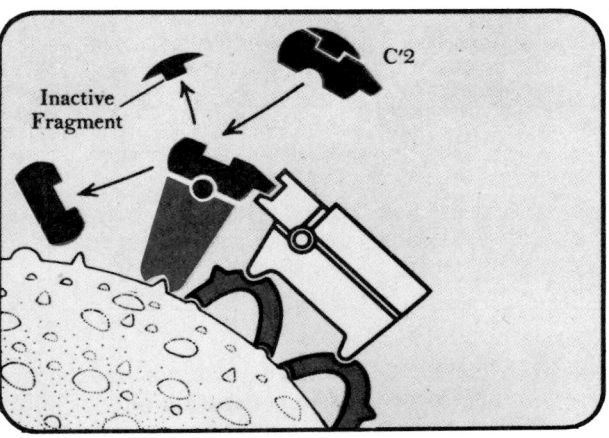

C'2 also interacts with C'1. An inactive fragment is cleaved out, preparing activated C'4-C'2 complex to act on next component. Magnesium is needed for integrity of this complex.

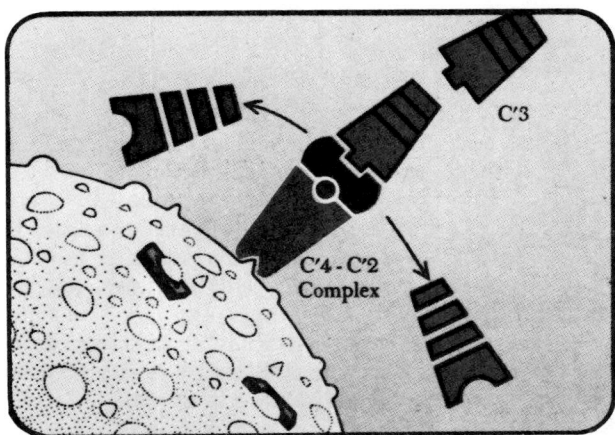

If C'3 appears during the few minutes the C'4-C'2 complex is active, it may be cleaved into at least four parts, one of which may become bound to the surface of the cell.

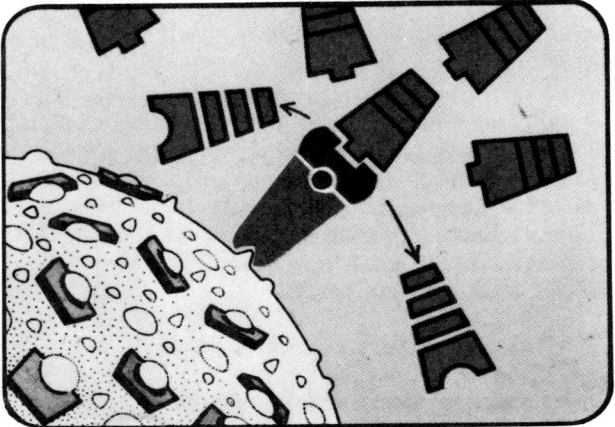

Each C4-C'2 complex can apparently mobilize hundreds of C'3 molecules, thus providing tremendous amplification of immunologic functions served by C'3 and perhaps later C' components.

Figure 49-5. The complement sequence of activation. C'1, the first component of complement, is made up of three subunits called C'1q, C'1s, and C'1r. Activation mechanisms are explained under each individual panel. (Drawings by Irving Geis from Gewurz H: The immunologic role of complement. *Hospital Practice,* Vol. 2, No. 9, Sept 1967, and Good RA and Fisher DW (eds): Immunobiology. Sinauer Associates, Inc., Sunderland, Mass. Reprinted with permission.)

Table 49-3
Lymphocytes and Their Effects

Lymphokine	Effect
Permeability factor	Increases vascular permeability, allowing white cells into area
Interferon	Interferes with viral growth, stopping the spread of viral infection
Migration inhibitory factor	Suppresses movement of macrophages, keeping macrophage in area of foreign cells
Skin reactive factor	Induces inflammatory response
Cytotoxic factor	Kills certain antigenic cells
Macrophage chemotatic factor	Attracts macrophages into the area
Lymphocyte blastogenic factor	Stimulates more lymphocytes, recruiting additional lymphocytes into the area
Macrophage aggregation factor	Causes clumping of macrophages and lymphocytes
Macrophage activation factor	Causes macrophages to adhere to surfaces more readily
Proliferation inhibitor factor	Inhibits growth of certain antigenic cells
Cytophilic antibody	A factor that binds to an Fc receptor on macrophages that permits them to bind to antigens

response can and do affect each other. Elegant experiments have shown that T cells are comprised not only of killer cells and K cells, but of helper and suppressor cells. If one examines a population of T cells with special antibodies, the various populations can be readily identified. T cells that react with IgM antibody to OX erythrocytes have the ability to act on other B cells to enhance antibody production as well as increase killer and K cell differentiation. This subpopulation of cells is called *helper T cells.* Those T cells that bind to another IgG antibody to OX erythrocytes suppress such responses and are called *suppressor T cells.* Helper and suppressor T cells modulate the immune response holding the degree of immune reactivity down to a level compatible with health, at the same time giving the individual the ability to adequately fight infection. In addition, antibodies may themselves feed back to affect the T cell system, influencing further antibody production.

▷ Basis of Immunopathology

It is now generally agreed that the differences in the protective nature of the immune response and its disease-causing potential lies in:

1. The system's mistaken identification of a normal constituent of the body as foreign. An example is the condition myasthenia gravis, in which the body mistakenly makes antibodies against the normal receptors of nerve endings.

2. The passive deposition of immune complexes in vessels where complement is activated and organs injured as innocent bystanders. This is the mechanism involved in many of the vasculitides and in some types of immune-mediated kidney diseases.

3. Abnormalities in helper T cell or suppressor T cell function. As noted in a later chapter on collagen vascular diseases, page 1150, systemic lupus erythematosus may well be a disease of suppressor T cells, in which abnormalities of these cells lead to poor control of B cell function with abnormal production of a vast array of antibodies against normal bodily constituents.

An exact knowledge of how the cells of the immune system "talk to each other" is essential not only to an understanding of the nature of immune-mediated diseases, but to the development of effective and precise methods of intervention.

▷ Treatment

At the present time, the treatment of immune-mediated diseases falls into two categories: (1) removal of offending antigens, and (2) immunosuppression.

Chart 49-1
**Adverse Effects of
Antibody–Antigen Interactions**

The difference between the protective nature of the immune response and its disease-causing potential starts with recognition of what is foreign and what is not. If the antigen is truly foreign, we are protected; if not, autoimmune (self-immune) disease results. Antibody–antigen interactions can cause bodily damage in six ways:

1. Antibodies binding to and neutralizing normally biologically active molecules (neutralization)
2. Antibodies destroying normal cells (cytotoxicity)
3. Deposition of the antibody–antigen complexes in tissues and the activation of complements, as well as the attraction of granulocytes and K cells to the area of the immune complexes (circulating immune complexes)
4. Destruction of tissues by sensitized lymphoid cells, killer T cells, due to direct infiltration of the tissues by the lymphoid cells (delayed hypersensitivity)
5. Accumulation of large masses of cells in an area where the antigen is not easily removed or destroyed (granulomatous reactions)
6. Combination of an antigen with an antibody; that is, mast cell destruction, causing the immediate release of pharmacologic agents (anaphylactoid reactions)

Unfortunately, the vast majority of antigens that cause immune disease have not as yet been recognized or, if recognized, cannot be removed from the body because they constitute normal cellular elements. Immunosuppression has become the major method of dealing with immune reactions.

Since the mounting of an immune response depends on the rapid division of the various subgroups of T cells as well as the proliferation of B cells, it appeared both reasonable and theoretically sound for immunologists, in their efforts to blunt immune reactions, to turn to drugs known to interfere with cellular division. These drugs, referred to as antimetabolites, were first used by cancer specialists in the treatment of malignancies. These drugs kill rapidly dividing cells. They affect all cells, but their greatest effect is on proliferating cells. In malignancies, these are the cancerous cells; in immunology, they are the dividing T and B cells.

Antimetabolites

Cyclophosphamide (Cytoxan) and Chlorambucil. Cyclophosphamide (Cytoxan) and chlorambucil are alkylating agents. These drugs enter the dividing cell, forming energy-rich compounds called *free radicals,* which specifically damage DNA, the control substance within the nucleus of cells. T cells are affected more than B cells. Indeed, within days of starting these medications, there can be a significant drop in the numbers of circulating T cells.

Azathioprine (Imuran) and 6-Mercaptopurine. These drugs act to interfere with DNA replication not by the production of free radicals, but by presenting to the nuclear enzymes that duplicate DNA an abnormal purine molecule, leading to the production of defective DNA molecules. Both types of drugs affect cellular DNA, resulting in decreased cellular division and decreased cellular function.

The major complications with the use of the antimetabolites are (1) increased risk of infections, and (2) the development of second malignancies in cancer patients and primary malignancies in immunosuppressed patients. An increased incidence of acute leukemia, nonHodgkin's lymphoma, and skin and bladder cancers has been reported with the use of chlorambucil, azathioprine (Imuran), 6-Mercaptopurine, and cyclophosphamide.

Steroids (Prednisone and Hydrocortisone)

Unlike antimetabolites, steroids affect the immune response without predisposing the patient to an increased risk of malignancies, though they do increase susceptibility to infections. The precise mechanism by which steroids interfere with the mounting of an immune response is not yet known, although it has been established that steroids do affect T cell differentiation.

Recent investigation has shown that steroids selectively diminish the population of suppressor T cells, having little effect on the numbers of helper T cells. Steroids also interfere with the effector arm of the immune response, inhibiting the liberation or action of the biologically active mediators released by neutrophils and macrophages. Steroids do not appear to affect antibody synthesis in general, but they do seem to selectively affect the production of autoantibodies as well as enhance the removal of such antibodies from the circulation via the reticular–endothelial system. Unfortunately, in addition to causing an increased risk of infection, steroids can cause hypertension, diabetes, gastrointestinal bleeding, cataracts, changes of body habitus, and psychosis

In view of the serious and at times life-threatening complications from the use of antimetabolites as well as the various steroid preparations, the benefits of using these medications must be carefully weighed against the potential risks. When used appropriately, however, these drugs have proven to be beneficial and at times lifesaving.

▷ Bibliography

Books

Annals of the New York Academy of Sciences. Immunological Tolerance to Self and Non-Self, Volume 392, 1982.

Bach J (ed). Immunology, 2nd ed. New York, John Wiley & Sons, 1981.

Barrett JT. Basic Immunology and Its Medical Application, 2nd ed. St Louis, CV Mosby, 1980.

Benacerraf B (ed). Immunogenetics and Immune Regulations. New York, Masson, 1982.

Dolby AE et al. Introduction to Oral Immunology. London, Arnold, 1981.

Eisen HN. Immunology, 2nd ed. New York, Harper & Row, 1980.

Franklin E (ed). Clinical Immunology Update 1983. New York, Elsevier, 1983.

Fudenberg HH et al (eds). Basic and Clinical Immunology, 3rd ed. Los Altos, California, Lange, 1980.

Glasser RJ. The Body is the Hero. New York, Random House, 1976.

Parker CW. Clinical Immunology. Philadelphia, WB Saunders, 1980.

Richter M. Clinical Immunology, 2nd ed. Baltimore, Williams & Wilkins, 1981.

Saunders JP et al (eds). Fundamental Mechanisms in Human Cancer Immunology. New York, Elsevier/North-Holland, 1981.

Sell S. Immunology, Immunopathology, and Immunity, 3rd ed. New York, Harper & Row, 1981.

Stites D et al. Basic and Clinical Immunology, 4th ed. Los Altos, California, Lange, 1982.

Twomey J (ed). Pathophysiology of Human Immunologic Disorders. Baltimore, Urban and Schwarzenberg, 1982.

Yoshitsugi H and Nakamura RM. Immunology and Immunopathology: Basic Concepts. Boston, Little, Brown & Co, 1982.

Articles

Allen J et al. The new epidemic: Immune deficiency, opportunistic infection, and Kaposi's sarcoma. Am J Nurs 1982 Nov; 82(11):1718–1722.

Berk PH et al. Increased incidence of acute leukemia in polycythemia vera associated with chlorambucil therapy. N Engl J Med 1971 Feb 19; 308(8):441–447.

Cameron S. Chlorambucil and leukemia. N Engl J Med 1977 May 5; 296(18):1065.

Coral FS. Immunologic approaches to the diagnosis and treatment of malignant diseases. NITA 1982 July–Aug; 5(4):256–261.

Croft CL. BCG administration and nursing implications. Am J Nurs 1979 Feb; 79(2):315–319.

Dodd MJ. Theoretical bases of immunotherapy. Am J Nurs 1979 Feb; 79(2):309–314.

Donley DL. Nursing the patient who is immunosuppressed. Am J Nurs 1976 Oct; 76(10):1619–1625.

Dwyer JM. Immunologic advances: The promise of HL-A markers. Consultant 1981 June; 21(6):111+.

Good RA. Harnessing the immunity system: From potential to reality. CA—A Cancer Journal for Clinicians 1975 July–Aug; 25(4):178–186.

Herberman RB. Natural killer cells. Hosp Pract 1982 Apr; 4(17):93–103.

Kinlen LJ et al. Collaborative United Kingdom–Australian study of cancer patients treated with immunosuppressive drugs. Br Med J 1979 Dec 8; 2(6203):1461–1466.

Lamers MC. Factors influencing the development of immune-complex diseases. Allergy 1981 Nov; 36(8):527–535.

Leyden JJ. More than skin deep. Emergency Medicine 1982 Sept 30; 14(16):126–130+.

Mandell FL. Immune system defects: How to evaluate them. Consultant 1981 Mar; 21(3):55+.

McKann C. Cancer immunotherapy: A realistic appraisal. CA—A Cancer Journal for Clinicians 1980 Oct; 30(5):286–293.

Sell S. Immunopathology. Teaching monograph. Am J Pathol 1978 Jan; 90(1):211–279.

Sullivan BP. Patient responses to BCG therapy for malignant melanoma. Am J Nurs 1979 Feb; 79(2):320–324.

Weksler ME. The senescence of the immune system. Hosp Pract. 1981 Oct; 16(10):53–64.

Winchester RJ and Kunkel HG. The human Ia system. Adv Immunol 1979; 28:221–292.

50

Assessment and Management of Patients With Allergic Disorders

The human body is menaced by a host of potential invaders—for the most part, microbial organisms—that are constantly threatening its surface defenses. Having penetrated those defenses, these agents compete with the body for its nutrients and, if allowed to flourish unimpeded, disrupt its enzyme systems and destroy its vital tissues. Against these agents, the body is equipped with an elaborate blockade system. The first line of defense consists of the epithelial cells that coat the skin and make up the lining of the respiratory, gastrointestinal, and genitourinary tracts. The structure and continuity of these surfaces and the resistance to penetration are initial deterrents to invaders.

One of the most effective of the body's defense mechanisms is its capacity to equip itself rapidly with weapons (antibodies) individually designed to meet each new invader, namely, specific protein *antigens*. Antibodies react with antigens in a variety of ways: (1) by coating their surface if they are particular substances, (2) by neutralizing them if they are toxic, or (3) by precipitating them out of solution if they are dissolved. In any event, the antibodies prepare the antigen for handling by the phagocytic cells of the blood and the tissues.

▷ Allergic Reaction: Physiologic Overview

Immunity

Some people are born with the ability to resist invasion by certain types of foreign agents. Most persons, however, acquire resistance by actually fighting off the invader. It is also possible to acquire resistance by two other methods:

1. By *actively acquired immunization,* whereby an antigenic substance (one that has lost its ability to produce illness, but is able to stimulate antibody formation) is injected into the body (*e.g.,* virus vaccine and tetanus toxoid)

2. By *passively acquired immunization,* whereby resistance is brought about by the transfer of antibody-containing serum from a sensitized donor to a normal recipient (*e.g.,* human gamma globulin)

Allergic Reaction

The term *allergy* has historically been defined as "altered reactivity"—that is, the body's response to a substance is different from its original response when initially exposed to that substance. Although such a definition proved to be fairly workable during the first half of this century, concepts and definitions have changed somewhat as a result of a better understanding of the events that take place when the body recognizes "foreignness." Thus, the definition of allergy has changed.

We have come to think of an *allergic reaction* as a manifestation of tissue injury resulting from an immunologic process (an interaction between an antigen and an antibody). When the host is invaded by the antigen, usually a protein that is recognized as foreign, a series of events takes place designed to render the invader harmless and to expel it. If white blood corpuscles of the lymphocyte series respond to such an invasion, antibodies may be produced by these cells.

An *antigen,* then, is any substance that, in the course of repeated contacts with the body, stimulates the body to produce another substance called an *antibody,* capable of combining with it in a very specific manner. This antibody may circulate freely in the blood as globulins or may be "fixed" in the tissues. Ordinarily, the net effect is one of protection of the host, in which case immunity results, and the stimulus is then defined as *immunogen* (Fig. 50-1 *A*). If, on the other hand, tissue injury results from the body's attempt to become immune, the stimulus is then defined as an *allergen* (Fig. 50-1 *B*).

Exposure to the specific allergen causes the release of *mediators* (active chemical substances) (Fig. 50-2). These act directly or indirectly on the muscles and glands of the tracheobronchial tree to produce bronchial constriction, excess mucus, and edema. Such chemical mediators include histamine and kinins: serotonin, bradykinin, SRS-A (slow-reacting substance of anaphylaxis), and acetylcholine.

Immunogens and allergens are usually protein in nature, but occasionally large-molecular-weight carbohydrates may also stimulate the initiation of an immune response. Many small-molecular-weight molecules may unite firmly with a tissue protein, the resultant combination then being recognized as foreign. These small molecules, which form a union with proteins, are called *haptens.* The metal nickel and many drugs, such as penicillin, are examples of haptens.

Immunoglobulins

Antibodies that are formed by lymphocytes and plasma cells in response to an immunogenic stimulus comprise a group of serum proteins called *immunoglobulins.* These can be found in the lymph nodes, tonsils, appendix, and Peyer's patches of the intestinal tract, or they may be found circulating in the blood and lymph. These antibodies combine with antigens in a very special way, which has been likened to keys fitting into a lock. Antigens (keys) only fit certain antibodies (locks); hence, the term *specificity* has been coined in relation to the specific reaction of an antibody to an antigen. There are many variations and complexities in these patterns.

Antibody molecules are *bivalent,* which means that they have two combining sites. Because of this, the antibody easily becomes a crosslink between two antigen groups, causing them to clump together (agglutination). By this action, invaders in the bloodstream are cleared. Agglutination is the means of determining blood group in laboratory tests.

There are five classes of immunoglobulins, designated as follows: IgG, IgA, IgM, IgD, and IgE. Antibodies of the IgM, IgG, and IgA classes have definite and well-established protective functions. These include neutralization of toxins and viruses, and precipitation, agglutination, or lysis of bacteria and other foreign cellular material.

IgM ("gamma-M") is the largest molecule, which tends to stay in the bloodstream and is thus primarily engaged in defense in the intravascular compartment, such as in bloodstream infections. If it occurs in a pregnant woman, it will not cross the placenta from the mother to the fetus. Thus, the finding of a high concentration of IgM in the newborn circulation is suggestive of an intrauterine infection.

IgG ("gamma-G"), the most abundant of the immunoglobulins, is one of the smallest immunoglobulins and thus can diffuse readily into the tissue spaces to assist in combating tissue toxins or infections. IgG has the property of crossing the placenta, so that antibodies of this family provide the baby with temporary immunity to many common diseases.

IgA ("gamma-A") circulates in the blood, but its role in that compartment of the body is uncertain. It is distinct

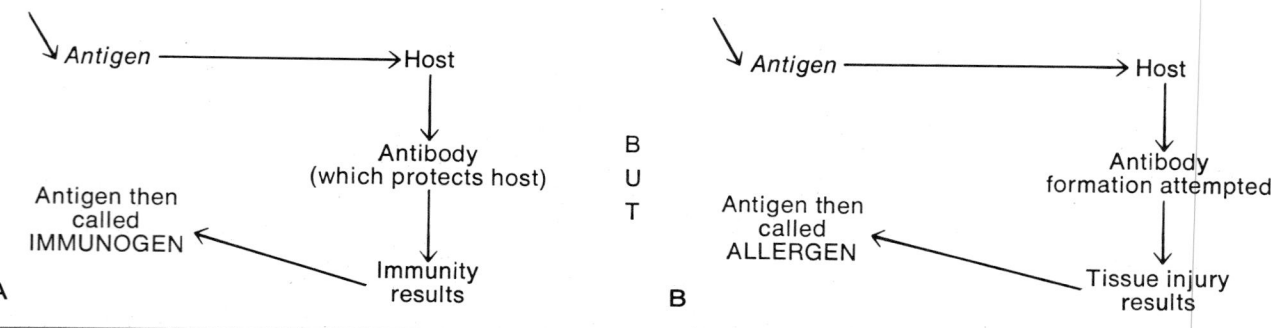

Figure 50-1. (*A*) Diagram describes the effect of an immunogen. (*B*) Diagram describes the effect of an allergen.

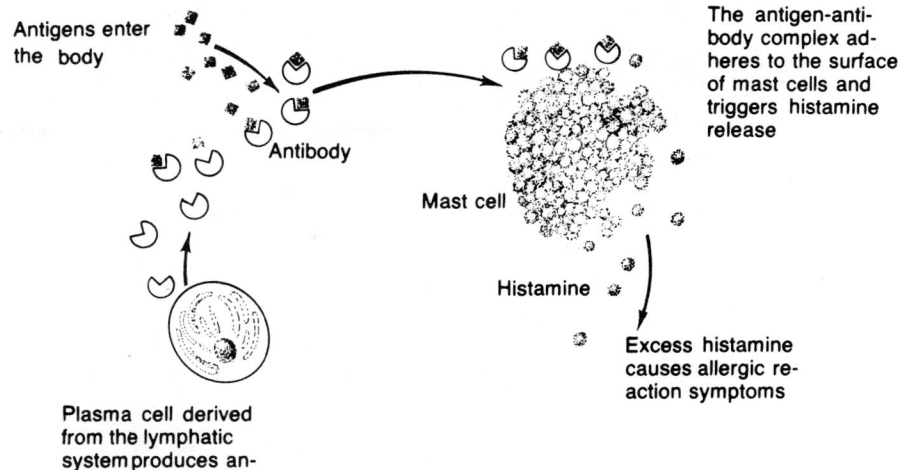

Figure 50-2. How allergic reactions begin. (From Patient Care, Sept. 15, 1973. Copyright © 1973, Miller and Fink Corp., Darien, Conn. All rights reserved.)

in that it is produced in the external secretion, where it provides a primary defense mechanism. IgA is found in saliva, tears, and the respiratory, genitourinary, and gastrointestinal tracts.

The function of *IgD* ("gamma-D") has not yet been determined. It is small, like IgG, and has a molecular pattern distinct from the other known immunoglobulins.

IgE ("gamma-E"), the most recently described immunoglobulin, is responsible for most of the immediate types of allergic reactions, which will be discussed later. It is present only in minute amounts in the blood serum. (In the normal person, 1 of 5000 immunoglobulin molecules are of this class.) The unique feature of IgE is its great affinity for attaching to human epithelium.

A protective role for IgE has not yet been established, but it has been postulated that antibodies in this class may play a role in ridding the host of certain parasites. Deficiency of IgE has been associated with increased susceptibility to infection. The most important aspect regarding IgE is its association with immediate allergic reactions of the anaphylactic type. These reactions appear within minutes of an injection of antigen into a person having anaphylactic antibodies (or after 2 hours, if precipitin antibodies are present).

Delayed Hypersensitivity

The above reaction is in contrast to *delayed hypersensitivity,* which occurs when an antigen is brought into contact with the skin surface of a sensitized individual, with the inflammatory reaction reaching its peak within 24 to 48 hours. The reaction consists of erythema and induration.

Delayed hypersensitivity is mediated not by circulating immunoglobulins (described above), but rather by sensitized "T" (thymus-dependent) lymphocytes. Such lymphocytes, when stimulated on a second or subsequent occasion, elaborate a variety of factors that enhance the host's defense mechanism. The tuberculin skin test is an example of a delayed hypersensitivity reaction, and advantage is taken of this action for diagnostic purposes. Also, contact dermatitis (dermatitis venenata), such as poison ivy, detergent allergy, and skin reactions to a variety of chemicals, including med-

ications, is an example of tissue injury resulting from reexposure of a sensitized individual.

▷ Atopic Disorders

Atopic disorders (allergic rhinitis, bronchial asthma, allergic dermatoses) are allergic manifestations that occur in persons who are genetically predisposed to forming *reagin,* a special antibody of the IgE class, when exposed to a variety of environmental allergens. Such allergens include various plant pollens, mole spores, domestic animal danders, and some foods. An estimated 7% to 10% of the population are subject to atopic disorders. The family history of related allergies can usually be elicited, but this is not always the case. There is recent evidence to show that the immune response gene resides near the HLA (tissue-type) locus on the chromosome. (HLA stands for histocompatibility locus antigen and pertains to compatibility of tissue, that is, whether the recipient can tolerate a particular graft.)

If a sensitized individual is reexposed to an allergen to which he has become sensitive, there is a release of histamine and other mediators that have a prompt and profound effect upon the tissues of the affected organ. These include dilatation of the walls of small blood vessels with loss of fluid from the blood into the tissue, causing swelling. There is also constriction of the smooth muscles surrounding the bronchi and the gastrointestinal tract. While clinical manifestations of atopy are most frequently caused by antigen–antibody interactions, some are initiated by other mechanisms. Nonspecific factors such as autonomic nervous system imbalance, hormonal disturbances, psychic factors, exertion, and changes in barometric pressure may result in tissue changes that mimic allergic reactions.

Assessment

The chief problems for the nurse are to get the patient to avoid medications or attitudes that can aggravate his condition. The nurse must understand the patient with an allergy, offering necessary services and lending an interested, friendly ear, as well as showing empathy for his problems. In the

(*Text continues on page 1122*)

Chart 50-1
Allergy Assessment Sheet

Name _____ Age _____ Sex _____ Date _____

I. Chief complaint:

II. Present illness:

III. Collateral allergic symptoms:

Eyes: Pruritus _____ Burning _____ Lacrimation _____

Swelling _____ Injection _____ Discharge _____

Ears: Pruritus _____ Fullness _____ Popping _____

Frequent infections _____

Nose: Sneezing _____ Rhinorrhea _____ Obstruction _____

Pruritus _____ Mouth-breathing _____

Purulent discharge _____

Throat: Soreness _____ Postnasal discharge _____

Palatal pruritus _____ Mucus in the morning _____

Chest: Cough _____ Pain _____ Wheezing _____

Sputum _____ Dyspnea _____

Color _____ Rest _____

Amount _____ Exertion _____

Skin: Dermatitis _____ Eczema _____ Urticaria _____

IV. Family allergies:

V. Previous allergic treatment or testing:

Prior skin testing:

Drugs: Antihistamines   Improved _____ Unimproved _____

Bronchodilators   Improved _____ Unimproved _____

Nose drops   Improved _____ Unimproved _____

Hyposensitization Improved _____ Unimproved _____

Duration _____

Antigens _____

Reactions _____

Antibiotics   Improved _____ Unimproved _____

Steroids   Improved _____ Unimproved _____

VI. Physical agents and habits:

Bothered by:

Tobacco for _____ years   Alcohol _____ Air cond. _____

Cigarettes _____ packs/day Heat _____ Muggy weath. _____

Cigars _____ per day   Cold _____ Weath. chngs. _____

Pipe _____ per day   Perfumes _____ Chemicals _____

Never smoked _____   Paints _____ Hair spray _____

Bothered by smoke _____   Insecticides _____ Newspapers _____

Cosmetics _____

VII. When symptoms occur:

Time and circumstances of 1st episode:

Prior health:

(continued)

Chart 50-1
Allergy Assessment Sheet (continued)

Course of illness over decades: progressing _____ regressing _____

Time of year: Exact dates

Perennial _____

Seasonal _____

Seasonally exacerbated _____

Monthly variations (menses, occupation):

Time of week (weekends vs. weekdays):

Time of day or night:

After insect stings:

VIII. Where symptoms occur:

Living where at onset:

Living where since onset:

Effect of vacation or major geographic change:

Symptoms better indoors or outdoors:

Effect of school or work:

Effect of staying elsewhere nearby:

Effect of hospitalization:

Effect of specific environments:

Do symptoms occur around:

old leaves _____ hay _____ lakeside _____ barns _____

summer homes _____ damp basement _____ dry attic _____

lawnmowing _____ animals _____ other _____

Do symptoms occur after eating:

cheese _____ mushrooms _____ beer _____ melons _____

bananas _____ fish _____ nuts _____ citrus fruits _____

other foods (list) _____

Home: city _____ rural _____

house _____ age _____

apartment _____ basement _____ damp _____ dry _____

heating system _____

pets (how long) _____ dog _____ cat _____ other _____

Bedroom:	Type	Age	*Living room:*	Type	Age
Pillow	_____	_____	Rug	_____	_____
Mattress	_____	_____	Matting	_____	_____
Blankets	_____	_____	Furniture	_____	_____
Quilts	_____	_____			
Furniture	_____	_____			

Anywhere in home symptoms are worse: _____

IX. What does patient think makes him worse: _____

X. Under what circumstances is he free of symptoms _____

XI. Summary and additional comments:

(From Patterson R: Allergic Diseases, Philadelphia, JB Lippincott.)

many contacts with the patient, the nurse gathers enough data and impressions to characterize the patient fairly accurately from the psychological standpoint, to discern with clarity the environment in which he habitually dwells, and to discover what factors are most important from the standpoint of "triggering" attacks. An assessment sheet such as is presented in Chart 50-1 is effective in providing this information.

The nurse must be prepared to meet the dangerous emergency that allergy creates on occasion in the form of anaphylactic shock or fulminating asthma, when swift and effective countermeasures may spell the difference between life and death (see Anaphylaxis, p. 1135).

Allergic Rhinitis ("Hay Fever," Chronic Allergic Rhinitis, Pollinosis)

Allergic rhinitis is the most common form of respiratory allergy. It affects approximately 8% to 10% of the U.S. population. When untreated, many complications may result, such as allergic asthma, chronic nasal obstruction, chronic otitis media with hearing loss, anosmia (absence of the sense of smell), and, in children, orofacial dental deformities. Consequently, early diagnosis and adequate treatment are strongly recommended.

Since allergic rhinitis is induced by airborne pollens, it is characterized by seasonal occurrences (see also Table 50-1):

Time	Source	Example
Early spring	Tree pollen	Oak, elm, poplar
Early summer ("rose fever")	Grass pollen	Timothy, red top
Early fall	Weed pollen	Ragweed

Each year the attacks begin and end approximately on the same dates.

Pathophysiology. Antibodies of IgE coating the mucosa of the nose and conjunctiva and specific for a given pollen (antigen) combine with the pollen. As a result, cell injury occurs (causing copious secretions, edema, sneezing, local itching). When the offending pollen is blown away, the allergic condition ceases.

Assessment

Clinical Manifestations. Usually, the rhinitis starts in the mucous membrane of the nose, which may become so edematous and swollen that the nostrils are closed completely. The nasal mucous membrane itches, burns, and secretes a thin, irritating discharge. Violent paroxysms of sneezing are the rule. The eyes are usually involved, becoming red, burning, and lacrimating. During the "off season," a nasal examination reveals normal findings.

Management

The goal of therapy is to provide relief from the annoying symptoms just described. Therapy usually takes one or all of the following tracks:

1. Removal of offending pollen (by moving to another locale as dictated by seasons, air conditioning)
2. Hyposensitization by repeated injections of the offending pollens in low concentration
3. Administration of antihistamines, that is, substances protecting cells against the effects of histamine
4. Suppression of the immune response by means of corticosteroids

Nasal sprays containing ephedrine help some persons. Sinusitis or other nasal lesions that may be present should be treated thoroughly during the free seasons. Various eye-washes relieve the conjunctivitis.

The patient's hypersensitivity to the pollens that induce the attacks can usually be confirmed by proper skin, conjunctival, or intradermal tests. These reactions are not necessarily specific, since a positive skin test does not necessarily mean that symptoms are due to that antigen. When properly performed and interpreted, these tests are quite specific in demonstrating reagin to the antigen in question. Accurate identification of the offending antigen, of course, depends on close correlation with the patient's history.

Pharmacotherapy

Underlying Principle. Histamine is found in all body tissue and fluid and is concentrated in skin, lung, and gastrointestinal tissue. An enzyme, histidine decarboxylase, catalyzes histamine biosynthesis from histidine (a precursor amino acid). Histamine is concentrated in mast cells and basophils. When these are degranulated (histamine has been discharged) by certain agents, an anaphylacticlike reaction occurs. Hence, the mast cell is considered the major target cell in acute allergic reactions.

Antihistamines. The basic structure of antihistamines is a substituted ethylamine. Examples are:

- Ethanolamine (Benadryl, Decapryn, Clistin)
- Ethylenediamine (Pyribenzamine, Histadyl)
- Alkylamine (Chlor-Trimeton, Dimetane, Polaramine, Actidil)

Antihistamines given orally are readily absorbed. They are most effective when given at the first sign of symptoms, since they prevent the development of new symptoms by preventing further histamine release. In actual practice, the effectiveness of these drugs is limited to certain patients with hay fever, vasomotor rhinitis, urticaria, and mild asthma; they are rarely effective in other conditions or in severe conditions of any sort. Side-effects vary with the individual; therefore, individualization of dosage is required. Of the side-effects, the most common are dryness of the mouth, dizziness, irritability, drowsiness, and gastrointestinal upset. These are often mild and temporary. Steroid hormones frequently are very helpful in ameliorating manifestations of allergy.

Sympathomimetic Drugs. The sympathomimetic drugs simulate the effects of the sympathetic nervous system. The major agents are norepinephrine (Noradrenaline) and epinephrine (Adrenalin). There are synthetic sympathomimetic drugs that have more specific actions, act longer, and may be taken orally—for example, isoproterenol (Isuprel) and

Table 50-1
Approximate Time of Appearance of Major Pollens and Molds in Various Regions of the U.S.*

Region	Jan.	Feb.	Mar.	Apr.	May	June	July	Aug.	Sept.	Oct.	Nov.	Dec.
Northeast				Elm Maple	Oak	Grass	Alternaria †Hormod.	Ragweed Alternaria Hormod.	Ragweed Alternaria Hormod.	Alternaria Hormod.		
Southeast		Elm	Ash Maple	Oak Sycamore	Pecan Oak Bermuda grass	Bermuda grass Hormod.	Alternaria Hormod.	Ragweed Alternaria Hormod.	Ragweed Alternaria Hormod.	Ragweed Alternaria Hormod.	Hormod.	
North Central				Elm Maple	Oak	Grass Hormod.	Alternaria Hormod.	Ragweed Alternaria Hormod.	Ragweed Alternaria Hormod.	Alternaria Hormod.		
South Central		Elm	Oak Maple Sycamore	Pecan Alternaria	Bermuda grass Alternaria Hormod.	Bermuda grass Alternaria Hormod.	Alternaria Hormod.	Alternaria Hormod.	Ragweed Alternaria Hormod.	Ragweed Alternaria		
Plains			Maple	Cottonwood		Grass Hormod.	Russian thistle Kochia Hormod.	Ragweed Russian thistle Kochia Hormod. Alternaria	Ragweed Sagebrush			
Southwest	Alternaria	Alternaria Cottonwood	Alternaria Ash Mountain cedar	Alternaria Bermuda grass False ragweed	Bermuda grass	Bermuda grass Hormod.		Alternaria Russian thistle Kochia	Alternaria Russian thistle Kochia	Alternaria		
Intermountain Basin			Elm	Cottonwood	Sycamore	Grass		Russian thistle Kochia	Sagebrush			
Pacific Coast North			Alder	Maple Oak	Grass	Grass Plantain	Grass					
Pacific Coast South	Alternaria		Oak Walnut	Oak Walnut Olive	Bermuda grass	Bermuda grass	Bermuda grass	Various ‡Compos.	Elm Compos.	Elm Compos. Alternaria	Alternaria	Alternaria

* There is some variation from year to year. Locations in the northern part of the region usually lag behind locations in the southern parts. Small amounts of the various pollens and molds often are present before and after the season indicated in the table. Bermuda grass, which flourishes in the South, contains different antigens from the northern grasses, but the two regions overlap somewhat. There are may aero-allergens which are not listed which occur in small amounts or in restricted locations.
† Hormod.: Hormodendrum
‡ Compos.: Compositae
(From Asthma, A Practical Guide for Physicians. American Lung Association in cooperation with the Allergy Foundation of America, 1973.)

Naldecon (chlorpheniramine, phenyltoloxamine, phenyl-propanolamine, phenylephrine). The major agents mentioned cannot be taken orally, since they are destroyed in the gastrointestinal tract.

Sympathomimetic drugs cause constriction of smooth muscle in skin, viscera, and mucous membranes and induce dilatation of muscular vasculature, bronchodilatation, and cardiac stimulation. Consequently, they reduce edema of the nasal mucous membrane, but they may induce nervousness and insomnia when given in large doses. Therefore, their use is recommended with caution in patients who have hypertension, heart disease, and hyperthyroidism.

The nurse must be aware of the effects caused by overuse of sympathomimetic agents in nose drops or sprays. A condition referred to as "rhinitis medicamentosa" may result. After topical application of the drug, a rebound period may occur in which the nasal mucous membranes become more edematous and congested than they were before the medication was used. Such a reaction encourages the use of more drug. A circular pattern of activity results much like a "cat chasing its tail." The topical agent must be discontinued immediately in order to correct this problem.

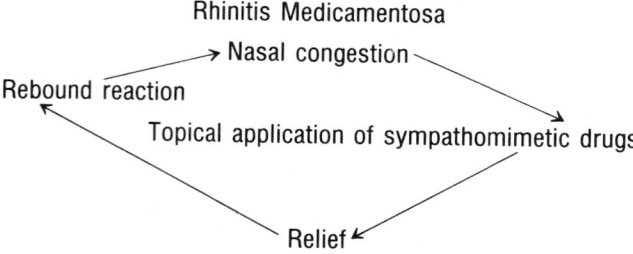

Systemic sympathomimetic drugs may be substituted. These agents must be used with caution in patients with hypertension, cardiovascular disease, diabetes, and thyroid disease.

Immunologic Management

Allergic reactions are triggered by the release of chemical mediators following the reaction of a specific antigen (*e.g.,* ragweed, house dust) with its specific antibody. To prevent this reaction, two methods of approach are possible: (1) avoidance of any exposure to the antigen (avoidance therapy), and (2) immunotherapy, or hyposensitization, which is an attempt to elevate the threshold level of the appearance of symptoms.

Avoidance Therapy

In avoidance therapy, every attempt is made to remove those allergens that act as precipitating factors. For example, allergy due to animal dander would require that the pet be removed from the home environment and that a feather pillow be replaced with a hypoallergenic Dacron pillow.

Aeroallergens are most difficult to avoid, since they are so widely distributed; however, the immediate surroundings may be altered. For example, irritating pollens, dusts, and molds can be avoided by remaining in a building that has central air conditioning with an electrostatic precipitating filter. The limitation here is that one cannot remain indoors all the time. Without such a controlled environment, the rooms where the person spends most of his time can be modified. Mattress and box springs should be encased in elastic fabric casings; upholstered furniture, stuffed toys, chenille bedspreads, etc. should be removed from the bedroom.

Another method is to travel to areas where the offending allergen is absent during certain times of the year. This method is becoming less effective (as well as expensive), since the atmosphere is becoming increasingly filled with allergens.

Sensitivity Tests and Immunotherapy (Hyposensitization)

A knowledge of the general concepts regarding assessment and therapy in allergic diseases is important, since the nurse is very apt to be an active participant in the treatment of these disorders and will almost certainly be in the position to advise patients who are potential candidates for one or another of these procedures.

Skin Tests. The most common method of treatment is the serial injection of one or more antigens that are selected in each particular case on the basis of *skin tests.* Skin testing (Fig. 50-3) entails the simultaneous intradermal inoculation (or superficial application), at separate sites, of several solutions containing individual antigens that comprise an assortment of those allergens deemed most likely to be implicated in the patient's disease. A positive reaction, evidenced by the appearance of an urticarial wheal (Fig. 50-4) or by localized erythema in the area of inoculation or contact, is regarded as evidence of sensitivity to the corresponding antigen.

Skin tests lend important weight to other evidence obtained from the patient's history, indicating which of several antigens are most likely to provoke symptoms and providing some clue to the intensity of the patient's sensitization.

The dosage of the pollen injected is important also; the majority of patients are hypersensitive not to one but to several pollens, and under testing conditions, they may not react to the specific pollens that induce their attacks, but they usually do. Ragweed seems to be the most potent of

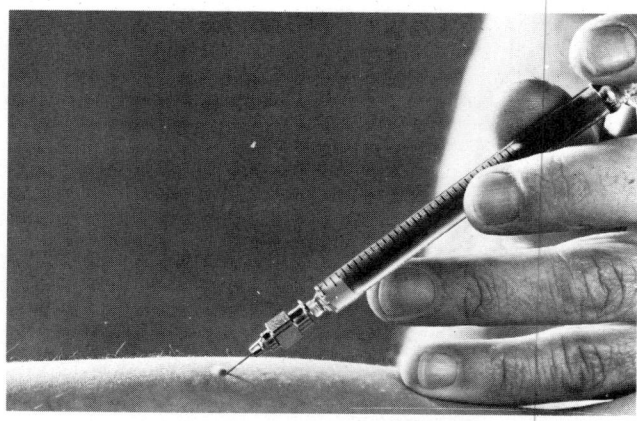

Figure 50-3. Intradermal testing. Cleanse the testing site with alcohol or ether. Tests are made on the volar surface of the lower arm and the outer surface of upper arm, omitting the antecubital space. Intradermal tests are limited to 10 or 20 at most. (Courtesy, Hollister-Stier Laboratories.)

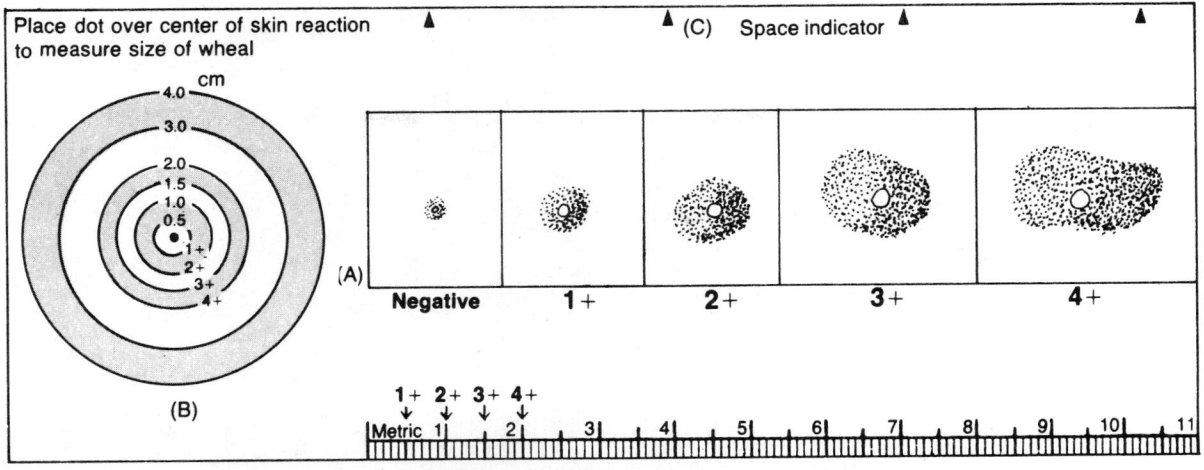

Figure 50-4. (A) These series of reactions indicate the sizes of wheals when the allergist refers to them as 1+, 2+, etc. A negative reaction is shown at the left. (B) The target wheal guide can be traced on a transparent sheet (acetate or x-ray film) and then placed over the wheal to measure the size in centimeters or according to plus-size. The relationship between the two is indicated on the lower metric scale. (C) Showing placement of test sites spaced uniformly. (From Patient Care, Sept. 15, 1973. Copyright © 1973, Miller and Fink Corp., Darien, Conn. All rights reserved.)

all. If there is any doubt about the validity of the skin tests, a RAST (see below) may be done, or a provocative challenge of the suspected antigen to the shock organ tissue can be carried out. An example is applying the antigen to an affected organ, such as the conjunctiva, nasal or bronchial mucosa, or gastrointestinal tract, and observing the response that follows.

Immunotherapy. Correlation of a positive skin test with a positive history is an indication for immunotherapy *if* the allergen cannot be avoided. The value of such injections has been fairly well established in those instances of allergic rhinitis and bronchial asthma that are clearly due to sensitivity to one of the common pollens or molds or to house dust. Although referred to as a "hyposensitization" procedure, the effects are most likely attributable to the opposite process (*i.e.,* immunization), for it appears to stimulate the production of a new antibody with the capacity of neutralizing the allergy-provoking properties of the responsible allergen.

Immunotherapy, while helpful in a majority of patients, does not cure the condition. Before such a program is launched, the physician discusses with the patient what may be expected from immunotherapy and why it is important to continue the therapy for several years. When skin tests are done, they are to be correlated with clinical manifestations; the treatment is based on the patient's needs rather than on the skin tests.

Specific treatment consists of injecting extracts of the pollens or mold spores that cause symptoms in a particular patient. Injections begin with very small amounts and are gradually increased, usually at weekly intervals, until a maximum tolerated dose is attained. Maintenance "booster" injections are then given at 2- to 4-week intervals, frequently for a period of several years, before maximum benefit is achieved.

There are three methods of injection therapy: coseasonal, preseasonal, and perennial. When treatment is given on a *coseasonal basis,* it is initiated during the season when the patient experiences symptoms. This method has been used less widely in recent years; it is not an effective form of therapy, and there is increased risk of systemic reactions. *Preseasonal therapy* injections are given 2 to 3 months before symptoms appear, allowing time for hyposensitization to take place. This treatment is discontinued after the season. *Perennial therapy* is administered all year round, usually on a monthly basis, and is the preferred method because of more effective, longer-lasting results.

Precautions. Since there is a possibility that the injection of an allergen may induce systemic reactions, it is only given in a physician's office where epinephrine is immediately available. Because of the dangers involved, injections ought not to be given by a lay person or by the patient himself. The patient is to remain in the physician's office for a minimum of 20 to 30 minutes and is observed for the possible development of systemic symptoms. If a large, local swelling develops, the next dose should not be increased, since this may be a warning of a possible systemic reaction.

Complications. A systemic reaction is a serious complication that ranges from mild hives to an acute asthmatic attack, hypotension, or even anaphylactic shock. Emergency treatment is presented on page 1135.

RAST. The *radioallergosorbent test* (RAST) is a technique for the laboratory determination of the presence of IgE antibodies in serum. The sensitivity of this procedure correlates very well with carefully conducted skin tests in the detection of immediate-type hypersensitivity. The RAST is probably no more specific than direct skin testing, but may be used to corroborate skin-test findings, especially in questionable cases. The RAST may also substitute for skin testing when the latter may be considered hazardous or when a generalized dermatitis may preclude direct skin testing.

Allergic Dermatoses

Contact Dermatitis

Contact dermatitis (dermatitis venenata) is an inflammatory, often eczematous, condition caused by a skin reaction to a variety of irritating or allergenic materials. Almost any substance can produce contact dermatitis. Poison ivy is probably the most common and best example; cosmetics, soaps, detergents, and industrial chemicals are frequent offenders. The skin sensitivity may develop after brief or prolonged periods of exposure, and a clinical picture may appear hours or weeks after the sensitized skin has been exposed.

The symptoms include itching, burning, erythema, vesiculation, and edema, followed by weeping, crusting, and finally a drying up and peeling of the skin. In very severe responses, hemorrhagic bullae may develop. Repeated reactions may be accompanied by the development of thickening of the skin and pigmentary changes.

Secondary invasion by bacteria may develop in skin abraded by rubbing or scratching. Usually, there are no systemic symptoms unless the eruption is widespread.

Diagnosis may sometimes be made easily on the basis of the location of the eruption and history of exposure. But in cases of obscure irritants or an unobservant patient, diagnosis may be extremely difficult, and many trial-and-error procedures may be involved before the etiology is correctly determined. Patch tests on the skin with suspected offending agents may clarify the picture.

The most important aspect of treatment is to remove the patient from further contact with the irritant or allergen. Burow's solution soaks (aluminum acetate) soothe the blistered erythematous skin and may be followed by corticosteroid ointments or creams. Antimicrobials are given if secondary invasion is present.

Atopic Dermatitis. *Atopic dermatitis* is chronic, pruritic, and familial in nature. It principally involves the skin of the neck, the face, and the flexural creases (Fig. 50-5) and will wax and wane in activity. It has a more prolonged course than simple contact dermatitis. It is frequently associated with allergic respiratory disorders, but the true cause remains unknown. Family history is usually positive for allergies such as allergic rhinitis, asthma, or eczema. Drying of the skin is an aggravating factor; wool and lanolin commonly compound the skin irritation of these patients. Allergy to foods has probably been overstressed but is, nonetheless, a factor. Emotional stress and nervousness aggravate the condition. The principles of treatment are the same as for contact dermatitis.

Drug Reactions (Dermatitis Medicamentosa)

Dermatitis medicamentosa is the term applied to skin rashes induced by the internal administration of certain drugs. While, as a rule, certain drugs tend to induce eruptions of similar types, individuals react differently to each of them.

In general, it may be said that drug rashes appear suddenly, have a particularly vivid color, present characteristics that are more spectacular than the somewhat similar eruptions of infectious origin, and, with the exception of the bromide and the iodide rashes, disappear rapidly after the drug is withdrawn. Some drug rashes are accompanied by constitutional symptoms. Upon discovery of a drug allergy, the patient is warned that he has an idiosyncrasy to a par-

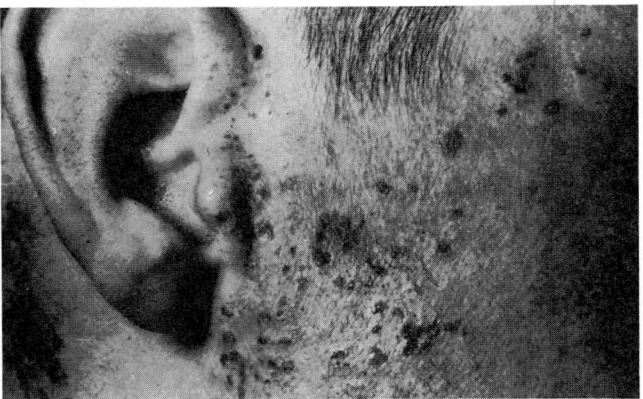
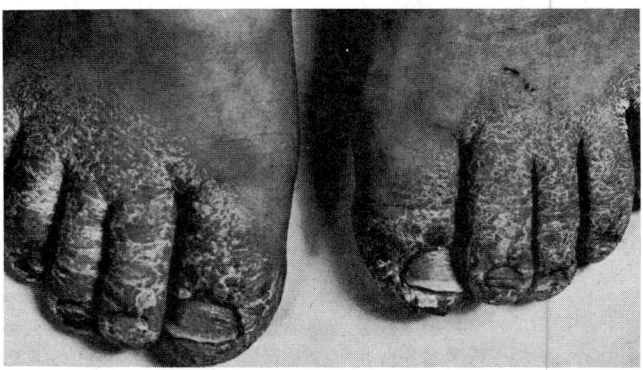

Figure 50-5. Atopic eczema. (From Sauer GC: Manual of Skin Diseases. Philadelphia, JB Lippincott.)

ticular drug and is advised not to take it again. The nurse has an important responsibility in relation to drug eruptions, for these lesions suggest more serious idiosyncrasies. By being in a primary position of initial contact with the patient, the nurse is able to report the appearance of the eruption so that early treatment is initiated.

Urticaria and Angioneurotic Edema

Urticaria (hives) is an allergic affection of the skin characterized by the sudden appearance of pinkish edematous elevations, which vary in size and shape, and itch and smart. They may involve any part of the body, including the mucous membranes, especially those of the mouth, the larynx (occasionally with serious respiratory complications), and the gastrointestinal tract. Each hive remains for a period varying from a few minutes to several hours, then disappears. For hours or days, crops of these lesions may come, go, and return, in a most capricious manner. If this sequence continues indefinitely, the condition is called *chronic urticaria*.

The swellings of *angioneurotic edema* involve the deeper layers of the skin, resulting in more diffuse swelling, rather than the discrete lesions characteristic of hives. On occasion, one may be seen that covers the entire back. The skin over it may appear normal, but often it has a reddish hue. It does not pit on pressure, as ordinary edema does. The regions most often involved are lips, eyelids, cheeks, hands, feet, genitalia, and tongue; also, the mucous membranes of the larynx, the bronchi, and the gastrointestinal canal may be affected, particularly in cases of the hereditary type. An eye may be completely closed; one lip may become so large that eating is impossible; one hand may become so huge that the fingers cannot be flexed. These swellings may appear suddenly; in a few seconds or minutes; or slowly, in 1 or 2 hours. In the latter case, their appearance often is preceded by itching or burning sensations. Seldom does more than a single swelling appear at one time, although one may develop while another is disappearing. Only infrequently do they recur in the same region. The individual lesions usually last from 24 to 36 hours. On rare occasions, they recur with a remarkable periodicity at intervals of 3 or 4 weeks.

The swellings of angioneurotic edema along the gastrointestinal canal may cause acute crises of pain with vomiting, which suggest acute appendicitis, acute cholecystitis, renal colic, or intussusception; those in the throat (edema of the glottis) are especially critical because they may result in sudden suffocation.

Management.   Many patients get relief from antihistamine drugs; others require injections of epinephrine. Corticosteroids usually give rapid resolution. Tracheostomy becomes necessary if laryngeal edema threatens to obstruct the glottis.

Hereditary Angioedema

Hereditary angioedema, although not an immunologic disorder in the usual sense, is included in this section because of its resemblance to allergic angioedema and because of the seriousness of this condition. Symptoms are due to edema of the skin, the respiratory tract, or the digestive tract. Attacks may be precipitated by trauma or may seem to occur spontaneously.

When the skin is involved, the swelling is usually rather diffuse, does not itch, and usually is not accompanied by urticaria. Gastrointestinal edema may cause abdominal pain severe enough to suggest the need for surgery. Edema of the upper respiratory tract may cause marked swelling of the uvula and of the larynx, resulting in suffocation. Acute laryngeal edema is the most serious manifestation of this disorder and has resulted in death due to asphyxiation in nearly 20% of these patients. Attacks usually subside within 3 to 4 days, but during this time the patient should be observed carefully for signs of laryngeal obstruction, which may necessitate tracheostomy as a lifesaving measure. Epinephrine, antihistamines, and corticosteroids are usually employed in treatment, but the success of these agents is limited.

Gastrointestinal Allergy

To a few persons, certain common foods are veritable poisons. There are those who cannot eat strawberries or shellfish without an attack of urticaria. Some people cannot eat pork or cheese, no matter how well disguised these foods may be. They vomit immediately or have diarrhea, often accompanied by considerable pain (due, it is surmised, to urticarial lesions along the gastrointestinal mucosa). Often asthma and urticaria result as well.

Bronchial Asthma

Asthma is a reversible form of airway dysfunction induced by any one of several stimuli, including allergy, inhaled irritants, environmental gases, exercise, and infection (usually viral). The obstruction is caused by one or more of three developments: (1) contraction of muscles surrounding the bronchi, which narrows the air passageway; (2) swelling of membranes that line the bronchi; and (3) filling of the bronchi with thick mucus. A hereditary tendency seems to be present in two thirds of all patients, affecting more males than females. Attacks of allergic rhinitis in about 50% of all patients end as asthma. This condition is generally classified as either extrinsic (related to allergy) or intrinsic.

▶ **Assessment**

Clinical Manifestations.   It is interesting to note that cough may be the only symptom in some patients. In others, in addition to contraction of smooth muscles, there is also edema of the bronchial mucosa and production of excess mucus.

The asthmatic attack starts suddenly with coughing and a sensation of tightness in the chest. Then slow, laborious, wheezy breathing begins. Expiration is always much more strenuous and prolonged than inspiration, which forces the patient to sit upright and use every accessory muscle of respiration. Obstructed airflow creates the sensation of dyspnea. The person becomes blue from hypoxia and breaks out into a profuse sweat; the pulse is weak; the extremities are cold; and there may be fever, and, occasionally, pain, nausea, vomiting, and diarrhea. The cough at first is tight and dry, but it soon becomes more violent; a distinctive sputum of thin mucus containing small, round, gelatinous masses is coughed up with much difficulty. The gelatinous masses are the ''pearls of Laennec,'' which are molds of the smaller bronchi and contain Curschmann's spirals. The attack may last from one half hour to several hours. Under certain circumstances, the attack may subside spontaneously, but this should not be counted on. Such attacks are rarely fatal. However, occasionally ''status asthmaticus'' occurs, in which therapeutic measures fail and the patient has repeated attacks or continuous asthma. This condition is life-threatening (see p. 1132).

Related Reactions.   Allergic reactions related to asthma include eczema (present at some time during life in 75% of asthma patients), urticaria, and angioneurotic edema (present in 50% of patients). Emotional stress may bring on an attack in those who are susceptible, just as any other organ system in the body may be stimulated by psychic factors.

Nursing History and Diagnostic Assessment.   The most important precipitants of asthmatic attacks are respiratory infections of nonbacterial origin, exercise, irritants (environmental, occupational), and drugs.

A clear history of hypersensitivity (at home or at work) to some known substance that may be inhaled or ingested, such as a pollen, a particular type of food, feathers, animal hair, face powder, etc., or a history suggesting the probability of such a sensitivity is very important in determining the type and cause of asthma present in any given patient. The close association of the attacks with allergic rhinitis, together with the discovery, during the attack, of marked pallor and swelling of the nasal mucous membrane, aids in establishing the case as one of extrinsic allergic asthma (Table 50-2).

Table 50-2
Comparison of Extrinsic and Intrinsic Asthma

	Extrinsic (Allergic)	Intrinsic (Infectious)
Age at Onset	3 to 35	Under 3, over 35 or 40
Symptoms	Season or perennial, frequently pollen- and mold-related	Worse in winter, exacerbated by cold air, air pollution, and primarily by infection
Mucus	Clear and foamy	Thick and white or discolored
Family History of Atopy	Positive	No greater than in general population
Skin Tests	Positive and correlating	Negative or positive noncorrelating
Serum IgE	High or normal	Normal
Response to Therapy	Good response to immunotherapy and bronchodilators	Poor response to bronchodilators; no response to immunotherapy

(From Patterson R (ed). Allergic Diseases, 2nd ed, p. 256. Philadelphia, JB Lippincott, 1980.)

The finding of an abnormally high count of eosinophilic cells in the blood or the sputum tends to confirm this diagnostic impression. Blood gas evaluation and simple spirometry are useful in evaluating gas exchange and providing baseline data that assist in identifying dangerous hypoxemia and respiratory acidosis.

Physical exertion may induce acute bronchospasm in most asthmatic patients. The key factor appears to be heat loss from the respiratory tract induced by hyperventilation. Inhalation of cold air during exercise rapidly increases bronchoconstriction, whereas warm, humid air does not.

With more industries releasing chemical irritants at work or into the environment, the asthmogenic result is increasingly apparent. Common air pollutants can depress pulmonary function. Individuals exposed to grains and wood dusts often show symptoms of respiratory irritation and allergic reaction. Certain drugs, such as aspirin, indomethacin, and related anti-inflammatory agents, may trigger asthmatic attacks.

However, "all that wheezes is not asthma," and it is important to be able to rule out congestive cardiac failure or bronchial obstruction due to a foreign body or a tumor as the underlying cause or precipitating factor that may explain the attack. Hence, in every case of doubtful origin, there is the necessity for careful radiologic and, often, bronchoscopic examination.

In individuals who do not have obvious clinical manifestations, testing in a pulmonary function laboratory can usually provide objective evidence of airway obstruction. An office spirometer is less expensive, as is a peak flowmeter (used widely in Great Britain), in determining the presence of asthma. The peak expiratory flow rate (PEFR) measures the maximum flow at the outset of forced expiration.

In an acute asthmatic attack, initial assessment is directed toward answering the following questions:

- How long has acute wheezing taken place? (If several days, the treatment will probably require hospitalization.)
- What is the cough like? Does the patient bring up phlegm, or was the cough dry?
- Was there any other discomfort?
- When did the wheezing start and how long did it last?
- Has he had this experience before? What time of day?
- Can the patient use long sentences in responding to a question, or does he reply in short phrases as he tries to get his breath? Can he speak at all?

Usually, the cough is dry, but later some phelgm is brought up. Chest tightness and resistance to antitussive medications strongly suggest a diagnosis of asthma.

Often a diagnosis is confirmed by instructing the patient to inhale (during a coughing episode) a trial aerosol bronchodilator. If the wheezing is caused by bronchitis, the cough is not relieved; if the underlying cause is asthma, the cough is relieved. An even more effective diagnostic aid is the monitoring of PEFRs. Since this is a simple test, the patient can be instructed to monitor his own flow rates. It has been found that patients are far more accurate in assessing their own PEFR than are health providers. In addition, patients are quite accurate in judging whether the obstruction is better or worse from day to day. Also symptoms as cough and chest tightness must be evaluated.

Patient Problems/Nursing Diagnoses

Based on the clinical manifestations, the nursing history, and the diagnostic assessment data, the patient's major nursing problems include acute episode of respiratory distress related to bronchial obstruction and resultant hypoxia; anxiety related to chronicity of the condition, susceptibility to acute asthmatic attacks, and need for life-style adaptations; and potential nonadherence to continuous regimen of medication therapy related to inadequate knowledge base.

▶ **Planning and Implementation**

Goals

The major goals for the patient include the following:

1. Relief of respiratory distress
2. Utilization of appropriate coping mechanisms to control anxiety about the condition and to prevent acute asthmatic attacks
3. Adherence to continuous regimen of medication therapy that meets his specific needs

Medications. Available pharmacotherapy covers several drugs, including epinephrine and theophylline. Epinephrine (Adrenalin) is a potent bronchodilator that acts rapidly. Theophylline acts primarily as a bronchodilator, pulmonary vasodilator, and smooth muscle relaxant. (See Table 50-3 for pharmacotherapy of asthma.)

Antibiotics, sedatives, and tranquilizers are also part of the pharmacotherapeutic program. Antibiotics are given when infection is present; mild sedatives and tranquilizers are occasionally judiciously prescribed (Table 50-4).

Relieving Anxiety. It should be remembered that asthma is a syndrome that may be produced by many widely different factors. However, the emotional response is more generalized. The hypoxic patient is understandably very anxious, and it is necessary that those who are in attendance relieve the patient's anxiety by acting calmly and confidently and, most importantly, by correcting the hypoxic state. It is thus necessary to relieve the obstruction and to supply sufficient supplementary oxygen to relieve the oxygen deficit.

Respiratory efficiency may be improved and comfort increased during an acute asthmatic attack by elevating the head of the bed and by strapping the pillows in a supporting position. The patient is likely to be most comfortable leaning forward, with arms supported on a pillow-upholstered over-bed table. Every opportunity for sleep and rest should be fostered after an acute asthmatic attack.

These patients are inclined to perspire excessively; therefore, they must be protected against chilling. Covers made of cotton are preferred, and frequent changes of bedclothes are carried out as needed.

Insofar as possible, exposure to offending antigens should be reduced. Bronchial asthma is a chronic disease with a potential for exacerbations that produce symptoms.

Management Beyond the Acute Phase: Health Teaching.
A person recovering from an asthma attack should be encouraged to increase fluid intake in order to maintain liquefied intrabronchial secretions (bronchial hygiene). Otherwise, thickened, retained secretions cause bronchial obstruction and atelectasis. Some authorities disagree with the emphasis on enforced hydration, believing that it may create cardiovascular and pulmonary stress if done to excess.

Detailed and accurate instructions are to be provided the patient with regard to (1) oral medications, injections, or aerosol inhalations to be administered at home (Chart 50-2 and Fig. 50-6); (2) the types of contact that are considered potentially provocative of asthmatic attacks and are therefore to be avoided; (3) scheduling of return visits for observations during and following convalescence (the social worker may assist in securing new employment if a change of occupation is desirable); and (4) permissible activities and contraindicated activities, as follows:

Recommended Activities (Permissible). Air conditioning may be helpful, although occasionally it aggravates symptoms in individual patients. Humidity kept at 30% to 50% is comfortable. Instruct the patient as follows:

- Remain indoors during high-pollution days.
- Maintain adequate hydration and rest.
- Use an oral bronchodilator 15 to 30 minutes before exercise.
- Practice breathing exercises if they help expiratory function. However, explain to the patient that it is not known how effective such a practice really is.
- Promote practices recommended for allergy management, such as environmental controls, particularly in relation to dust, dander, and mold. Radiant heating systems are preferred to those that circulate air.

Contraindicated Activities

- Warn the patient that cigarette smoking enhances the development of bacterial bronchial infection by impairing ciliary movement.
- Instruct the patient *not* to use the hand nebulizer for more than four to six inhalation treatments per day. Overuse has deleterious effects and should be discouraged.

Intrinsic Asthma and Aspirin-Sensitive Asthma. Management is provided primarily through drug therapy. In the latter situation, it is important to avoid aspirin and aspirin-containing drugs to which the patient is sensitive.

Prevention. In every patient with recurrent asthma, evidence should be sought that might implicate a foreign protein to which the patient is hypersensitive and which might precipitate the attacks. If attacks chiefly occur at night, when the patient is in bed, skin tests should be conducted with material from the mattress and pillows. If the test results are positive, then a mattress and pillow made from other materials should be substituted. If attacks appear to be associated with the presence of a particular species of animal, such as a horse or a cat, similar skin tests should be made with an antigen composed of hair or skin scrapings from the animal concerned. The examiner should search for foci of bacterial infection (*e.g.*, of chronically infected sinuses or teeth) because their eradication may be strikingly beneficial in certain patients. A seasonal incidence of attacks in a patient suggest an air-borne allergen as the chief etiologic agent. In such cases, therapy may be attemptd with pollen extracts. Air conditioning offers possibilities in the prevention

(*Text continues on page 1132*)

Table 50-3
Medications for Patients With Asthma

Medication	How Administered	Action	Nursing Intervention

1. *Spasmolytics* (Methyl Xanthines)
a. Aminophylline
b. Theophylline
c. Theophylline (Bronkodyl, Elixophyllin)
d. Aminophylline (Phyllocontin)
e. Theophylline (Sustaire, Theolair SR, Theo-Dur)
	IV for severe bronchospasm
	Oral short-acting (4 hours)
	
	Oral sustained-release (8–12 hours)
		Bronchodilator reverses airway obstruction by relaxing bronchial smooth muscle (inhibits phosphodiesterase) and preventing breakdown of cyclic adenosine monophosphate (relaxes smooth muscle).
		Plasma concentrations should be monitored; optimal range is between 10 μg/ml and 20 μg/ml.
			1. Space drug administration equally over 24-hour period in order to ensure properly spaced coverage.
			2. Administer oral medications with antacid, milk, or crackers to avoid gastric irritation.
			3. Be aware of blood levels (serum theophylline) to prevent toxicity.
			4. Observe for adverse reactions and report:
			  a. Gastrointestinal: nausea, vomiting, hematemesis, diarrhea
			  b. Cardiovascular: palpitation, tachycardia, extrasystoles, hypotension
			  c. Neurologic: headache, insomnia, restlessness, irritability
			5. Recognize the effect of other medications and other conditions on methylxanthines:
			  a. Cimetidine, erythromycin—action prolonged
			  b. Smoking—shortens action
			  c. Liver disease and congestive heart failure—prolong action

2. *Adrenergics* (Sympathomimetics)
a. Metaproterenol (Alupent, Metaprel)
b. Terbutaline (Brethine, Bricanyl)
c. Isoetharine (Bronkosol, Bronkometer)
d. Albuterol, Salbutamol (Proventil, Ventolin)
	Oral: inhaler (metered-dose)
	
	Oral
	
	Inhalant solution; metered-dose inhaler
	Metered-dose inhaler; inhalant solution
		Bronchodilator
		Stimulates beta$_2$ receptors (by increasing cyclic adenosine monophosphate, thus relaxing smooth muscle
		Vasoconstriction (alpha receptors)
		Cardiac stimulation (beta$_1$ receptors)
			1. Space drug administration; when given with a methylxanthine, sandwich one between doses of the other for more even bronchodilation and for less side-effects.
			2. Demonstrate and have patient redemonstrate use and cleaning of the metered-dose inhaler.
			3. Observe for side-effects:
			  a. Overuse: tachycardia, palpitations, heartburn, insomnia, restlessness, dizziness
			  b. Terbutaline: Tremors, shakiness
			  c. Albuterol: Tremor is most common adverse effect

e. Fenoterol (Berotec)	Similar to albuterol (available in Canada and Europe, but not in U.S.A.)		
f. Isoproterenol (Isuprel, Medihaler-Iso, Vapo-Iso)	Metered-dose inhaler; inhalant solution	Stimulates beta$_1$ and beta$_2$ receptors	

(continued)

Table 50-3
Medications for Patients With Asthma (continued)

Medication	How Administered	Action	Nursing Intervention

2. Adrenergics (*continued*)
  g. Epinephrine
    (1) Adrenalin, Medihaler-Epi
    (2) Bronkaid Mist, Primatine Mist
	Subcutaneous; may be repeated in 15–20 min if required
	
	Inhalant
		Stimulates alpha, beta$_1$, and beta$_2$ receptors: their action is short	Observe for side-effects: headache, vomiting, agitation, hypertension, tachycardia, and arrhythmias
			Both Bronkaid Mist and Primatine Mist are over-the-counter drugs. These contain epinephrine. Patient is to be advised of the possible side-effects of tachycardia and palpitations.

3. *Adrenal corticosteroids* a. Prednisone (Deltasone, Paracort)	Oral	Anti-inflammatory; enhances formation of cyclic adenosine monophosphate	1. Recognize these are prescribed only when other more conservative medications fail. 2. Take entire daily dose at one time, preferably in morning with food/antacid. 3. Observe for side-effects: depression, gastric irritation, hypernatremia, hypokalemia, ecchymosis, muscle weakness. 4. Never discontinue abruptly for fear of acute adrenal crisis. 5. Do not inhale steroids during an asthmatic attack. 6. Following an inhaled dose, gargle with water to prevent systemic absorption and possible fungal infection; if this occurs, treat with antifungal preparations. 7. Report stressful experiences. (See p. 940 for long-term side-effects and precautions.)
4. *Cromolyn Sodium* (Aarane, Intal)	Inhaled by turbo inhaler provided with medication	*Prevents,* rather than treats, bronchospasm Prevents the release of histamine and other mediators (after an antigen–antibody reaction) that are responsible for bronchial constriction	1. Use patience in teaching the patient how to use and clean the turbo inhaler. 2. Ask for return demonstrations and follow-up to assure correct technique by the patient. 3. Recognize that this drug does not treat an acute attack; it is prescribed exclusively for prophylaxis. It appears effective in allergic asthma and exercise-induced asthma. Cost may be a factor to consider. 4. If mild throat irritation, cough, or hoarseness occur, this can be relieved by a bronchodilating aerosol. 5. If cromolyn provides no significant help after being used for a month, discontinue slowly to avoid a severe asthma attack. 6. May be used to spare reliance on steroids.

Table 50-4
Medications to be Avoided by Patients With Asthma

Type of Asthma	Drug	Rationale
Acute or chronic	Antihistamines	Dry pulmonary secretions.
	Anticholinergics	Dry pulmonary secretions
	Propranolol	May cause bronchospasm
	Monoamine oxidase inhibitors	Initiate hypertensive crises when they combine with adrenergic drugs
	Cough suppressants	Interfere with clearance of secretions; use only for persistent cough or interruption of sleep
Status asthmaticus	Morphine Meperidine Sedatives Tranquilizers	May suppress respiration

of attacks, depending on the extent to which the patient can restrict his life to air-conditioned rooms during the asthma season. A complete change of climatic environment to a locality with different flora during that period is the most satisfactory solution, when feasible.

Exercise-induced asthma (EIA) can be prevented by inspiring air at 37° C (body temperature) and 100% relative humidity. Covering the nose and mouth with a mask necessitates rebreathing expired air that has been warmed and moistened by its passage through the respiratory tract. A simple face mask is an inexpensive, practical method for asthmatic ball players, runners, and skiers.

Associated Psychotherapeutic Modalities. It is important to remember that asthmatic attacks, once started, may indicate that the patient will be susceptible to repeated attacks. In some patients, attacks may be induced by suggestion alone. Good general physical and mental health is most important.

Complications of Asthma. The acute asthmatic attack per se is seldom serious, although occasionally it does prove to be fatal through respiratory exhaustion, which is particularly possible if sedatives are administered too freely.

Complications of asthma include a ruptured bleb, causing pneumothorax; mediastinal or subcutaneous emphysema; chronic and recurrent acute bronchitis; bronchiectasis; pulmonary hypertension; and hypertrophy of the right side of the heart with right-heart failure (pulmonary heart disease) (Fig. 50-7). Chronic hypoxia due to these complications leads to symptoms and personality changes.

▶ **Evaluation**

Expected Outcomes

1. Obtains relief of acute respiratory distress
   a. Exhibits no signs of cough, chest tightness, excessive expiratory effort, and cyanosis

   b. Has strong, regular pulse of normal rate
   c. Exhibits clear breath sounds—no wheezing
   d. Has arterial blood gases within pre-episode baseline range
2. Utilizes appropriate coping mechanisms to control anxiety about condition and to prevent acute asthmatic attacks
   a. Utilizes appropriate measures to prevent acute asthmatic attacks (*e.g.,* avoids allergens, stress-provoking stimuli)
   b. Describes progress made toward coping with chronic illness
   c. Elicits support from family to alter life-style as appropriate
   d. Seeks services of health team members as appropriate to accomplish necessary life-style changes
   e. Describes proper utilization of medications to prevent and treat acute asthmatic attacks
   f. Keeps follow-up appointments with clinic/physician
3. Adheres to continuous medication therapy regimen
   a. Takes medications as prescribed
   b. Describes the necessity for continuation of medication therapy
   c. Identifies dosage-controlled means for preventing side-effects of medications
   d. Keeps appointments with clinic/physician for monitoring of response to medication therapy
   e. Utilizes antibiotic therapy as prescribed for infections
   f. Family member/significant other, demonstrates knowledge and skill in administration of injectable medicines, if appropriate

Status Asthmaticus

Status asthmaticus is severe asthma that is unresponsive to conventional therapy with epinephrine and theophylline and lasts longer than 24 hours. A vicious self-perpetuating cycle may occur as a result of infection, anxiety, overuse of tranquilizers, nebulizer abuse, dehydration, increased beta-adrenergic block, and nonspecific irritants. An acute episode sometimes may be precipitated by hypersensitivity to aspirin.

Pathophysiology. A combination of factors, including constriction of the bronchiolar smooth muscle, swelling of bronchial mucosa, or thickened (inspissated) secretions, contribute to one pathologic problem—a decrease in the diameter of the bronchi. Another problem is the ventilation–perfusion abnormality that results from hypoxemia and respiratory acidosis or alkalosis. Therefore, blood gas determinations are an important guide to the severity of the condition and offer a reliable method of checking the patient's response to therapy.

There is a reduced arterial PO_2 and an initial respiratory alkalosis with a decreased PCO_2 and an increased pH. As the severity of status asthmaticus increases, the PCO_2 increases and the pH falls—reflecting respiratory acidosis. The rising PCO_2 suggests progressive pulmonary failure and requires aggressive drug intervention and other therapeutic measures to prevent death from respiratory failure.

Assessment and Clinical Manifestations. Breathing is labored, with a greater effort made on exhalation. The neck and even face veins become engorged. Expelled air escapes

Chart 50-2
How to Use an Inhaler (Nebulizer)

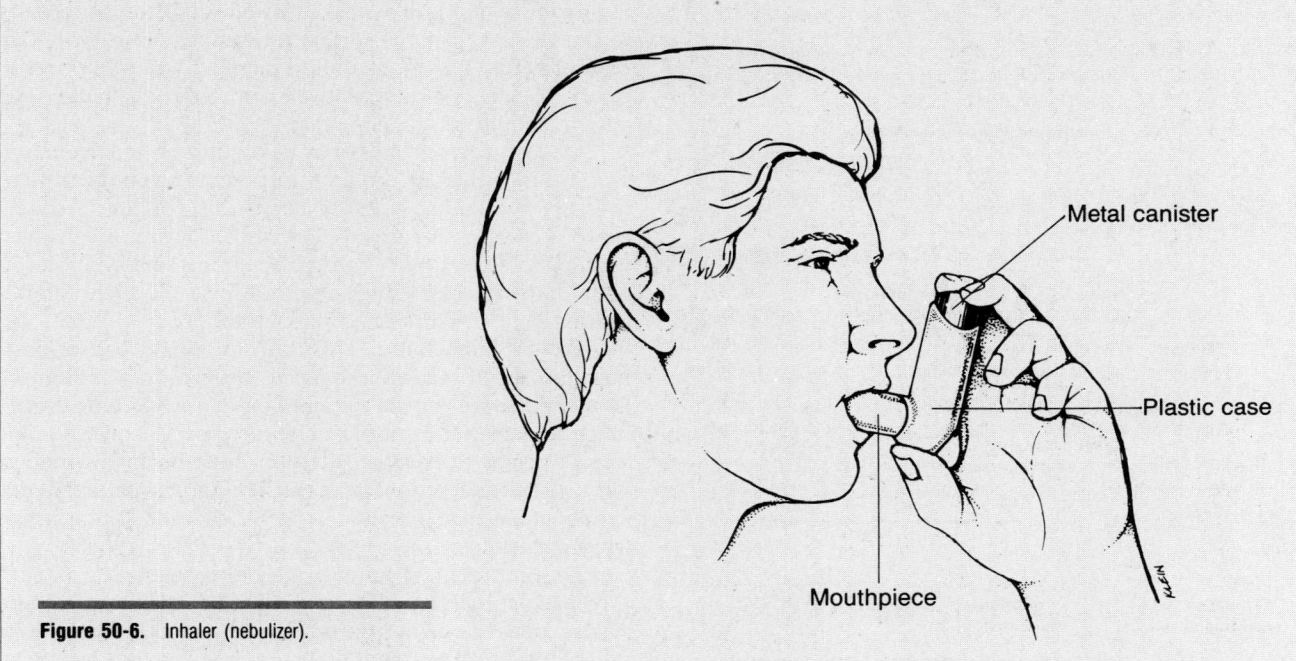

Figure 50-6.   Inhaler (nebulizer).

Action	*Rationale/Amplification*
1. Shake inhaler (canister) thoroughly immediately before using.	1. To loosen particles of medication.
2. Remove cap from mouthpiece.	2. To provide outlet for medication.
3. Exhale fully and steadily, expelling as much air from the lungs as possible.	3. This is in preparation for tissue acceptance of medication.
4. Place mouthpiece fully into mouth (check with insert directions; some types require 1-inch placement from open mouth). Keep inhaler in upright position.	
5. Inhale deeply and steadily in a slow, deep inhalation. At the same time, completely depress tip of inhaler's metal canister with index finger.	
6. Hold breath as long as possible (10 seconds).	6. This will provide maximum benefit of medication.
7. Before exhaling, remove inhaler from mouth. Also, release finger from canister to prevent loss of medication.	
8. Recap mouthpiece.	
9. Clean inhaler frequently. Remove metal canister and cap.	
10. Rinse plastic case and cap thoroughly in warm water.	10. To prevent inhaler from becoming a reservoir for bacteria; these can later be transmitted to the bronchi and lungs.

NOTE: 1. Undue use or abuse of the inhaler carries the potential for tachycardia and for iatrogenic-induced or inhaled adrenergic-induced proximal airway disease. 2. Use only the prescribed number of inhalations in the prescribed time.

---

with a wheeze; however, the amount of wheezing does not correlate with the severity of the attack. With greater obstruction, the wheeze may disappear.

Management and Nursing Intervention.   Treatment is best given in a pulmonary intensive care unit where clinical management is in the hands of the allergist, pulmonary disease specialist, and anesthesiologist, as well as a nurse clinician.

Signs of dehydration are assessed by checking skin turgor and the tongue. Dehydration is one of the primary problems to be corrected, usually through the administration of intravenous fluids up to 3000 ml/day to 4000 ml/day. Fluid

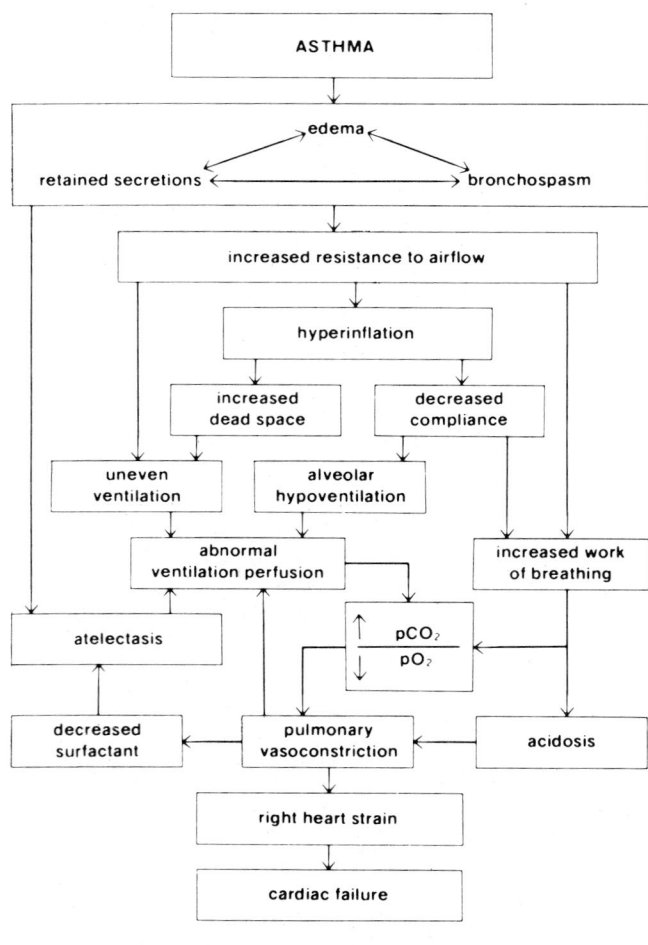

Figure 50-7. Diagrammatic representation of what can happen when asthma gets out of hand. (From Richards W and Siegel SC: Emergency Medicine, 6:299, Feb. 1974.)

intake is essential to combat dehydration, loosen secretions, and to facilitate expectoration. Frequent serum electrolyte determinations are made to suggest proper electrolyte therapy. Aminophylline is administered intravenously or at 6-hour intervals until adequate theophylline levels in the blood serum are reached.

To treat dyspnea, cyanosis, and hypoxemia, oxygen therapy is initiated on low-flow humidified oxygen, either by venturi mask or nasal catheter. The amount is determined following blood gas determinations. Arterial PO_2 is kept between 65 mm Hg and 85 mm Hg.

Corticosteroids are also prescribed to restore bronchial reactivity. Mucolytic agents, such as acetylcysteine (Mucomyst), are effective after bronchodilation. Cough suppressants and sedatives are avoided. If symptoms suggest the presence of an infection, antibiotics are given. The drugs of choice (if the patient is not sensitive to them) are tetracycline, cephalothin, and ampicillin. Appropriate agents are determined following gram-stain sputum studies. Epinephrine may be administered every 4 hours subcutaneously

for acute dyspnea; however, little or no effect is noted in the first 24 hours.

Constant monitoring of the patient by the nurse is important for the first 12 to 24 hours, or until status asthmaticus is broken. When it is necessary to question the patient, try to phase the questions so that he can answer in only one or two words. The room should be quiet and free of respiratory irritants, including flowers and cigarette smoke. The patient should have a nonallergenic pillow.

Mechanical assistance may be required when maximum medical therapy fails. Volume respirators are preferable to pressure ventilators, because large tidal volumes are necessary to overcome airway resistance. During mechanical ventilation, the patient's cardiac function and blood gas volumes must be carefully monitored to avoid such complications as heart failure and pneumothorax.

Patient Education. This is an important part of post-hospital care if recurrences are to be kept to a minimum. Bronchodilators may be required on an "around-the-clock" basis. Certain medications can be increased when asthmatic attacks occur. Adequate hydration must be maintained at home to keep secretions from thickening. The patient needs to recognize that infection is to be avoided, since it can trigger an attack.

In some clinics, patients are being instructed in self-care protocol designed with goals of (1) aborting severe attacks, and (2) giving the asthmatic patient a measure of independence. Included in this regimen is the institution of theophylline with a long-acting oral preparation. This is regulated within the narrow therapeutic ratio with careful instructions on the hazards of overuse. The patient gets a hand-held metered-dose inhaler that utilizes a beta$_2$ selective adrenergic, such as metaproterenol or albuterol. This also is used within prescribed limitations. Should these bronchodilators fail, the patient is further instructed on beginning a corticosteroid pulse (short, high dose), usually prednisone, at a prescribed dosage. He notifies the physician or nurse clinician of his progress.

▷ Serum Sickness

The illness known as *serum sickness* traditionally has resulted from the administration of therapeutic antisera of animal sources for the treatment or prevention of infectious diseases such as tetanus, pneumonia, rabies, diphtheria, and botulism and for bites of venomous snakes and black-widow spiders. However, with the advent of human antitetanus serum and antibiotics, true serum sickness is much less common now than in previous years. However, a variety of drugs, chief of which is penicillin, is now the main cause of a syndrome identical to that caused by foreign sera.

Clinical Manifestations. The symptoms are due to a reaction and immunologic attack upon the serum or the drug. Antibodies appear chiefly to be of the IgE and IgM classes. Early manifestations, beginning 6 to 10 days after the administration of the drug, include an inflammatory reaction at the site of injection of the drug, followed by regional and generalized lymphadenopathy. There is nearly always a skin rash, which may be urticarial or purpuric, and joints are frequently tender and swollen. Vasculitis may occur in any organ, but is most commonly observed in the kidney, resulting in proteinuria and, occasionally, casts. Cardiac involvement, mild to severe in nature, may occur. Peripheral neuritis may cause temporary paralysis of the upper extremities or may be widespread, causing the Guillain-Barré syndrome.

The usual untreated course lasts for several days to a few weeks, but ordinarily responds promptly and completely if treated with antihistamines and corticosteroids.

▷ Anaphylaxis

Anaphylaxis is an immediate, shocklike (life-threatening) allergic reaction following exposure to a substance to which the person is exquisitely sensitive. Drugs, such as foreign sera and penicillin; insect stings; and allergenic extracts used in immunotherapy for extrinsic allergic conditions are the most common causes of anaphylaxis. Iodinated contrast media occasionally present the same clinical picture and are similarly treated.

Assessment and Clinical Manifestations. Initial symptoms may include a generalized feeling of warmth, itching of the palms and soles, itching around the eyes, itching in the ears, hoarseness, dysphagia, a sense of constriction in the throat, and a feeling of impending doom. The patient may experience tightness in the chest, with an audible expiratory wheeze. Fright may be evident, and pruritus severe. Hives may be localized and progress to massive facial angioedema, suggestive of upper respiratory edema. Death may occur within minutes to several hours due to respiratory failure brought on by laryngeal edema or bronchospasm, but if recovery occurs, it is usually complete and without sequelae.

Prevention. A careful history should be taken before the administration of any drug, to be certain that there is no known hypersensitivity to it. Any person who is known to be susceptible to anaphylaxis should carry an identification tag.*

Anyone who is endangered by the sting of Hymenoptera (bees, wasps, hornets, yellow jackets) should carry an emergency kit (during spring and summer) containing parenteral epinephrine. An ANA-Kit (Hollister–Stier), which is available commercially, contains a prefilled syringe with epinephrine and the equipment required for self-administration.

If animal serum is to be given, it is mandatory that careful skin testing be carried out prior to injection of therapeutic doses. (Horse serum, for example, is still used for patients needing snake antivenom and antilymphocyte serum.)

The injection of any drug should, whenever possible, be given sufficiently distal on an extremity so that a tourniquet may be applied proximally in order to retard the absorption of the drug into the circulation.

* Medic Alert Foundation, 1000 North Palm, Turlock, California 05380

In the presence of a positive skin test for a drug that must be given, a procedure of "desensitization" may be carried out. This is done by giving a minute amount of diluted drug or serum, followed by gradually increasing doses every 10 to 15 minutes, until a full therapeutic dose has been achieved. When carefully done, this is a fairly safe procedure but does not obviate the later development of a serum-sicknesslike reaction (described above).

Management and Nursing Intervention. Help should be summoned immediately, but the person suffering the attack should not be left unattended. Immediate assessment of vital functions is done to determine the status of respiration and heart beat. If these have stopped, closed-chest massage or mouth-to-mouth resuscitation is initiated.

Epinephrine (Adrenalin) is the most effective treatment of an acute allergic reaction. An intramuscular injection of 0.1 ml/kg up to 0.3 ml epinephrine 1:1000 is given immediately into the upper arm, and the area is massaged. A tourniquet is then applied, if possible, proximal to the site of injection of the allergen. An additional 0.01 ml/kg up to 0.2 ml of epinephrine is injected into the site of the allergen injection to assist in the reduction of antigen into the system. Routine measures for shock, including assuring an adequate airway, establishing the shock position, providing supplementary oxygen, and giving intravenous fluids, are also indicated. It is not necessary to wait for blood gas determinations to administer oxygen, since it directly relieves hypoxemia and alveolar hypoxia.

Later, on the basis of individual clinical assessment, the following may be required:

For anaphylaxis: diphenhydramine

For bronchospasm: intravenous aminophylline; intravenous fluids; intravenous corticosteroids

For hypotension: volume expanders, vasopressors, isoproterenol

For laryngeal obstruction: tracheostomy and oxygen therapy

For respiratory arrest: intubation, oxygen therapy

For cardiac arrest: cardiopulmonary resuscitation, sodium bicarbonte

▷ Bibliography

Books

Eagle R. Eating and Allergy. Garden City, New York, Doubleday, 1981.

Frazer CA. Insect Allergy. St Louis, Warren H. Green, 1982.

Frost P. Principles of Cosmetics for the Dermatologist. St Louis, CV Mosby, 1982.

Gershwin ME. Bronchial Asthma. New York, Grune & Stratton, 1981.

Johnson F. Immunology and Medical Treatment. Vol. 1: Allergy. Chicago, Year Book Medical Publishers, 1979.

Johnson F. Immunology and Medical Treatment. Vol. 2: Including IgE in Diagnosis and Treatment. Chicago, Year Book Medical Publishers, 1979.

Lawlor GJ Jr and Fischer TJ. Manual of Allergy and Immunology. Boston, Little, Brown & Co, 1981.

Lieberman PL and Crawford LV. Management of the Allergic Patient. New York, Appleton–Century–Crofts, 1982.

Middleton E Jr, Reed CE, and Ellis EF. Allergy: Principles and Practice. St Louis, CV Mosby, 1978.

Patterson R. Allergic Diseases, 2nd ed. Philadelphia, JB Lippincott, 1980.

Speer F. Handbook of Clinical Allergy. Littleton, Massachusetts Wright–ISG, 1982.

Articles

General

Allergic disorders, Chap 4. In Hollister LE (ed.) The Year Book of Drug Therapy 1981. Chicago, Year Book Medical Publishers, 1981.

Allergies, Part I. Harvard Medical School Health Letter 1981 June; 6(8):1–2.

Allergies, Part II. Harvard Medical School Health Letter 1981 July; 6(9):1–2, 5.

Atarax (hydroxyzine) for itching. The Medical Letter 1980 Jan; 22(1):4.

Baker G, Collett P, and Allen D. Bronchospasm induced by metabisulfite-containing foods and drugs. Med J Aust 1981 Nov 18; 2:614–617 (see also Am J Nurs 1982 Aug; 812[8]:1265).

Berquist W et al. Effect of theophylline on gastroesophageal reflux in normal adults. J Allergy Clin Immunol 1981 May; 67(5):407–411.

Dolan B. A rapid desensitization. Am J Nurs 1982 Oct; 82(10):1532–1534.

Elenhaas RM. Anaphylactic shock. Crit Care Q 1980 Mar; 2(4):77–84.

Golbert TM. Current concepts in food allergy. Am Fam Physician 1980 Aug; 22(2):95–96.

Harmon AL and Harmon DC. Anaphylaxis sudden death anytime. Nursing '80 1980 Oct; 10(10):40–43.

Hudgel DW and Madsen LA. Acute and chronic asthma: A guide to intervention. Am J Nurs 1980 Oct; 80(10):1791–1795.

Mullarkey MF. Allergic and non-allergic rhinitis. Postgrad Med 1979 Apr; 65(4):97–107.

Nalebuff DJ and Fadal RG. IgE screening for allergy. Resident and Staff Physician 1980 June; 26(6):61–67.

Parker C. Food allergies. Am J Nurs 1980 Feb; 80(2):262–265.

Slavin RG. Diagnostic tests in clinical allergy. Postgrad Med 1980 Mar; 67(3):72–81.

Swan GF. Management of monosodium glutamate toxicity. J Asthma 1982; 19(2):105–110.

When the patient has allergic rhinitis. Patient Care 1982 Aug 15; 16(14):103–126.

Zeroing in on systemic fungal disease. Patient Care 1982 Aug 15; 16(14):129–161.

Bronchial Asthma

Albuterol. The Medical Letter 1981 Sept 18; 23(19):81–82.

Asthma Roundtable. Confirming asthma by tests and trials. Patient Care 1981 Aug 15; 15(14):89–131.

Asthma Roundtable. Probing asthma's semantics and origins. Patient Care 1981 Aug 15; 15(14):31–52.

Asthma Roundtable. Weighing diagnostic clues to asthma. Patient Care 1981 Aug 15; 15(14):53–84.

Asthma Roundtable. When asthma causes "moderate" trouble. Patient Care 1981 Nov 15; 15(19):143–186.

Asthma Roundtable. When your patient's asthma is mild. Patient Care 1981 Nov 15; 15(19):115–139.

Asthma Roundtable. When your patient's asthma is severe. Patient Care 1981 Nov 30; 15(20):59–97.

Baker G, Collett P, and Allen D. Bronchospasm induced by meta-

bisulfite-containing foods and drugs. Med J Aust 1981 Nov 28; (see reference in Am J Nurs 1982 Aug; 82[8]:1265).

Brenner AM et al. Effectiveness of a portable face mask in attenuating exercise-induced asthma. JAMA 1980 Nov 14; 224(19):2196–2198.

Bronsky EA. Acceptability and efficacy of a new theophylline dosage form: Quibron-T. J Asthma 1982; 19(1):43–46.

Corrao WW, Braman FS, and Irwin RS. Chronic cough as the sole presenting manifestation of bronchial asthma. N Engl J Med 1979 Mar 22; 300(12):633–637.

Drugs for asthma. The Medical Letter 1982 Sept 17; 24(618):83–86.

Fischl MA, Pritchenik A, and Gardner LB. An index predicting relapse and need for hospitalization in patients with acute bronchial asthma. N Engl J Med 1981 Oct; 305(14):783–789.

Goyeche JRM, Abo Y, and Ikemi Y. Asthma: The Yoga Perspective. Part II. Yoga therapy in the treatment of asthma. J Asthma 1982; 19(3):189–201.

Hydgel DW and Madsen LA. Acute and chronic asthma; A guide to intervention. Am J Nurs 1980 Oct; 80(10):1791–1795.

Iredale B. Growing up with "intractable" asthma and growing out of it. J Asthma 1982; 19(3):203–209.

Kirilloff LH and Tibbals SC. Drugs for asthma. A complete guide. Am J Nurs 1983 Jan; 83(1):55–61.

Martin L. Asthma: Current concepts in outpatient management. Hosp Med 1981 Feb; 17(2):22–37.

Newth CJ and Isles AF. Comparison of steady state of sustained-release theophylline tablets and capsules. J Asthma 1982; 19(3):145–149.

Rodman MJ. The drug interactions we all overlook (asthma). RN 1980 Nov; 43(11):41–43.

Rogers TR. Clinical problems in the adult with asthma. Hosp Pract 1981 June; 16(2):293–297.

Scoggin CH. Asthma: Changing concepts and therapies. Modern Medicine 1980 Nov 15–30; 48(19):26–33.

Sly RM. Management of exercise induced asthma. Drug Ther 1982 Mar; 12(3):95–102.

Tinkelman D. Theophylline: The concept of sustained action. J Asthma 1981 Jan; 18(1):35–37.

Tuft L. Guidelines for choosing an antiasthmatic. Drug Ther 1982 Aug; 12(8):199–212.

Webber–Jones JE and Brant MK. Over-the-counter bronchodilators. Nursing '80 1980 Jan; 10(1):34–39.

Williams MH. Expiratory flow rates: Their role in asthma therapy. Hosp Pract 1982 Oct; 17(10):95–110.

Wilson J, Sutherland D, and Thomas A. Has the change to beta-agonists combined with oral theophylline increased cases of fatal asthma? Lancet 1981 June 6; 1(8232):1235–1237.

Status Asthmaticus

Nursing Grand Rounds: Fighting the frustrations of status asthmaticus. Nursing '82 1982 Mar; 12(3):58–63.

Raffen T and Roberts P. The prevention and treatment of status asthmaticus. Hosp Pract 1982 Feb; 17(2):80a–80z·6.

Seaman–Bates LJ. Emergency management of status asthmaticus. J Emerg Nurs 1980 Sept/Oct; 6(5):9–12.

Agencies

American Academy of Allergy, 225 East Michigan Street, Milwaukee, Wisconsin 53202

Asthma and Allergy Foundation of America, 19 W. 44th Street, New York, New York 10036

National Institute of Allergy and Infectious Disease, National Institutes of Health, Bethesda, Maryland 20205

51

Management of Patients With Connective Tissue Disorders

The study of connective tissue disease (CTD) has received its greatest attention during the past decade. Over 100 types of CTD affect more than 32 million people in the U.S. The study of this group of diseases is the major component of *rheumatology*, or the study of rheumatic disease. Simply stated, a *rheumatic disease* is a diffuse disorder in which skeletal muscles, bones, and joints are primarily affected. Most rheumatic diseases are connective tissue diseases and are grouped together because of a common symptomatology.

Connective tissue disease is the newer, more accurate term for collagen disease. These disorders not only affect the collagen portion of connective tissue, but involve other protein components as well. Most CTDs are chronic in nature and are characterized by spontaneous remissions and exacerbations. Disease onset may be acute or insidious.

▷ Physiologic Overview

Connective tissue is distributed throughout the body in the form of three protein types: *collagen,* the most abundant type; *elastin,* providing the elastic properties of tissue; and *reticulin,* closely related to collagen in structure. Bone, skin, muscle, blood vessels, adipose tissue, serous organ coverings, cartilage, tendons, and ligaments are examples of specific connective tissues. Functions include mechanical support, warmth, structure, and movement.

Due to the wide distribution of connective tissue, the clinical manifestations of dysfunction are numerous and vary from person to person even within the same disease. This presents a challenge to nurses assessing and managing these multisystem conditions.

▷ Assessment

Management of CTD begins with a complete and accurate assessment of the patient's signs and symptoms. Vital data can be obtained from the patient history and physical assessment.

Patient History. The patient history is the most valuable diagnostic aid to the physical assessment. In instances of suspected connective tissue disease, it is particularly important to elicit information regarding the patient's complaint of pain. Pain is the symptom that most commonly causes an individual to seek medical attention. Other common complaints include joint swelling, limited movement, stiffness, weakness, and fatigue.

General Appearance. Inspection of the patient's general appearance occurs during the initial contact with the patient. Gait, posture, and general musculoskeletal size and structure are observed. Gross deformities and abnormalities in movement are noted. Deviations away from the body midline are called *varus* deformities (*e.g.,* bow legs); deviations toward the midline are called *valgus* deformities (*e.g.,* knock knees). The symmetry, size, and contour of other connective tissues, such as the skin and adipose tissue, are also noted and recorded.

Since connective tissue is found in nearly all body systems, a complete physical assessment is performed. Special attention is given to the examination of each joint and its adjacent structures. The procedure for musculoskeletal assessment is found in the discussion of rheumatoid arthritis (see p. 1140).

Diagnostic Tests. In addition to the history and physical assessment, a battery of diagnostic studies is utilized to confirm or support a tentative diagnosis.

X-rays are important in evaluating patients with musculoskeletal conditions. Bone films determine bone density, texture, erosion, and changes in bone relationships. X-rays of the bone cortex detect widening, narrowing, and signs of irregularity. Joint x-rays reveal the presence of fluid excess, irregularity, bony overgrowth, narrowing, and changes in the joint structure.

Arthrography is the injection of a radiopaque substance or air into the joint cavity, especially the knee or shoulder, in order to outline the contour of the joint. The joint is passively ranged while a series of x-rays is taken. After the test, the patient should be reassured that the radiopaque substance will be systemically absorbed, and joint swelling will consequently subside. No special post-test precautions are necessary, but the patient should be observed for signs of infection and hemarthrosis (bleeding into the joint).

Myelography, the injection of a radiopaque substance or air into the subarachnoid space of the lumbar or cervical spine, is performed to confirm a diagnosis of degenerative joint disease of the spinal column. Early stages of this CTD may not be detected by this procedure (see p. 1287).

A *bone scan* reflects the degree to which the crystal lattice of bone "takes up" a bone-seeking radioactive isotope that is injected into the system, such as technetium-99. The degree of uptake of isotope is seen in skeletal involvement related to connective tissue disease.

A *joint scan* procedure is similar to that of the bone scan and allows determination of joint damage throughout the body. It is the most sensitive study for the detection of early disease.

In general, *serum laboratory studies* in rheumatology rely on the theory that most connective tissue diseases are autoimmune. While many of the tests are highly complex and technical, no one test *sufficiently* supports a diagnosis of CTD. In Table 51-1, some of the most common serum studies are listed with corresponding normal value ranges and primary indications. Since many of the tests are relatively new and rather costly, they may not be utilized in every health care facility.

An *arthrocentesis* is performed to obtain synovial fluid, especially from the knee or shoulder, for the purpose of examination. The joint is anesthetized locally, and a large-bore needle is inserted into the joint space for aspiration of a fluid specimen. Since this procedure has the potential for introducing bacteria into the joint, aseptic technique must be followed. Following aspiration, no special precautions are necessary, but the patient should be observed for signs of infection and hemarthrosis.

Normally, synovial fluid is clear, pale, straw-colored, and scanty in volume with few cells. The fluid is examined for volume, viscosity, and formation of mucin clot. It is examined microscopically for cell count, cell identification, Gram's stain, and formed elements. In inflammatory joint disease, the fluid often becomes cloudy, milky, or dark yellow and contains numerous inflammatory cells, such as leukocytes and complement. Copious amounts of fluid may also be present in inflammatory disease. Blood in the fluid specimen suggests trauma or a tendency to bleed.

Arthroscopy is an endoscopic procedure that allows direct visualization of a joint, especially the knee (see p. 1393). Although it is performed primarily to detect trauma or lesions, it may be used to obtain a biopsy of synovial tissue for microscopic examination. A synovial biopsy may also be obtained by needle or surgical incision.

Electromyography and *muscle biopsy* may be performed when skeletal muscle is directly affected by connective tissue disease to determine the presence of muscle inflammation or degeneration. A muscle biopsy is carried out for microscopic examination of skeletal muscle. The procedure may be performed in the operating room under local or general anesthesia. A surgical incision is made, and the desired specimen is obtained. A pressure dressing is applied, and the affected extremity is immobilized for 12 to 24 hours. A less invasive type of biopsy, the needle biopsy, may be chosen as an alternative to the incisional procedure.

Arterial biopsy is carried out to examine a specimen of an arterial vessel wall. Most frequently, the temporal artery is selected, but other arteries may be biopsied as indicated. The procedure is similar to that for the incisional muscle biopsy, but is generally performed under local anesthesia in the operating room. Arterial biopsy most often confirms inflammation of the vessel wall, or arteritis, a type of vasculitis.

A *skin biopsy* may be performed to confirm inflammatory connective tissue diseases, such as lupus erythematosus or progressive systemic sclerosis (scleroderma). A specimen may be lightly scraped from the patient's skin without discomfort. Deeper skin biopsies may need to be carried out when scraping is not sufficient.

Thermography measures the degree of heat radiating from the skin surface. It is used to investigate the pathophysiology of inflamed joints and to assess the patient's response to anti-inflammatory drug therapy.

Table 51-1
Common Serum Laboratory Diagnostic Studies for Connective Tissue Disorders

Name	Description	Normal Value	Significance
Rheumatoid factor (RF)	1. Determines the presence of abnormal antibodies seen in CTD 2. Usually measured by two laboratory techniques: Rose–Waaler Latex (bentonite)	Rose = <1:160 (or neg) Latex = <1:80 (or neg)	1. Not a sensitive test for RF, but if positive, usually suggests rheumatoid arthritis (RA) 2. Not specific for RA, but is a sensitive test for determining the presence of rheumatoid factor 3. Positive RF may also suggest SLE, Sjögren's syndrome, or mixed CTD. 4. The higher the titer (number at the right of colon), the greater the degree of inflammation
Antinuclear antibody (ANA)	1. Measures the presence of antibodies that react with a variety of nuclear antigens (as seen in CTD) 2. If antibodies are present, further testing determines the type of ANA circulating in the blood (*e.g.,* anti-DNA, anti-RNA) 3. May be called FANA, as fluorescent lab technique often utilized	<1:10 (neg) **Note:** A small number of healthy adults have a positive ANA.	1. Positive test associated with SLE, RA, PSS, Sjögren's syndrome, necrotizing arteritis 2. The higher the titer, the greater the degree of inflammation
LE prep (LE test)	1. Essentially, a type of ANA (anti-DNP) 2. Not a very specific or sensitive test 3. Often not used, since ANA studies have been developed	<1:10 (neg)	1. Positive in 75% to 80% of patients with SLE 2. Positive results may also be associated with RA and PSS
Complement (C' or CH50)	1. Measures the amount of free-floating complement circulating in the blood 2. *Complement* is a protein substance that binds with antigen–antibody complexes for the purpose of lysis 3. When the number of complexes increases markedly, complement is used for lysis, thus depleting the amount available in the blood	Varies greatly according to the lab test used Look for a *decrease*	1. Decrease may be seen in RA (with extra-articular manifestations), SLE, and necrotizing arteritis (systemic) 2. Decrease indicates severe autoimmune and inflammatory activity
Erythrocyte sedimentation rate (ESR or sed rate)	1. Measures the rate at which RBCs settle out of unclotted blood in 1 hour 2. An increase indicates increased inflammation (as in CTD) or bacterial infection 3. Two most common lab techniques used are Westergren and Wintrobe 4. Westergren is considered the most accurate for measurements > 60 mm/hr	Westergren = Men 0–15 mm/hr Women 0–20 mm/hr Wintrobe = Men 0–9 mm/hr Women 0–15 mm/hr	1. Increase often seen in any inflammatory CTD 2. The higher the sed rate, the greater the inflammatory activity

▷ Rheumatoid Arthritis

The word "arthritis" is often used interchangeably with connective tissue disease or rheumatic disease; however, this usage is not accurate. Arthritis is merely a symptom of CTD, meaning inflammation of a joint. Rheumatoid arthritis and degenerative joint disease (osteoarthritis) are the two main types of CTD in which arthritis is the major manifestation. Due to the chronic nature of these diseases, billions of dollars in work productivity are lost each year; an additional 1 billion dollars is spent on disability benefits.

Pathophysiology

Rheumatoid arthritis is a chronic, systemic, progressive disease of unknown etiology characterized primarily by inflammation of the synovial joints. It affects people of any age, but most often *begins* in women (3:1 over men) between 25 and 35 years of age. Exacerbations of this disease are frequently associated with periods of increased physical or emotional stress.

To understand the pathophysiology of rheumatoid arthritis, the normal anatomy and physiology of joints are reviewed. A joint is an area of the body where two or more bones meet and is primarily comprised of connective tissue. Joints are of three main types: (1) synarthrodial, or immovable (*e.g.,* the joints between the cranial bones); (2) amphiarthrodial, or slightly movable (*e.g.,* the joints between the vertebrae); and (3) diarthrodial, or freely movable (*e.g.,* the knee joint). The *diarthrodial* or *synovial* joint is most commonly affected by inflammation and degeneration as seen in rheumatoid arthritis.

Synovial joints are classified further according to the shapes of the bone surfaces that meet. The *ball and socket* type, or spheroidal joint, best exemplified by the hip and shoulder, permits full freedom of movement. *Hinge* joints, such as the elbow, permit motion in one plane, flexion, and extension. A *condylar* joint, such as the knee, is similar to the hinge, but additionally allows a small degree of rotation. The carpal (wrist) joints are examples of the *plane,* or biaxial joints, and permit only gliding movement. The *pivot* joint is characterized by the articulation between the radius and ulna in the forearm; it permits rotation only.

Articular cartilage covers the bone end of a joint and provides a smooth, resilient surface for movement. Since the cartilage has no vascular supply, it cannot regenerate. Once the cartilage is damaged, it cannot be repaired.

The space between the bone ends is maintained by a sheath of fibrous tissue, the *joint capsule.* The joint capsule is strengthened by bands of connective tissue, or *ligaments,* which help to keep the bones in proper relationship to each other. Ligaments are located both along the outside of the joint capsule and also within the capsule, where they bridge the gap between the bones. *Synovial membrane* lines the inner surface of the fibrous capsule and secretes fluid into the space between the bones. This *synovial fluid* functions as a shock absorber, as well as a lubricant, to allow the joint to move freely in the appropriate direction.

Rheumatoid arthritis is thought to be due to an autoimmunologic response that is centered in the synovial joints.

The pathologic changes are seen first as inflammation occurring in the synovial tissue, or synovitis (Fig. 51-1).

Each of the synovial joints may be the sight of inflammation, with swelling and pain, edema, and infiltration with lymphocytes and plasma cells. The lymphocytes and plasma cells begin to form IgG, IgA, or IgM antiglobulin antibodies (rheumatoid factors) that react with antigen (IgG) to form immune complexes. These generate inflammatory reactions characterized by release of lysomal enzymes and lymphokines, as described in Chapter 49. There is an increase of phagocytic cells to remove the debris. Phagocytic cells produce enzymes that create more destruction—hyperemia, edema, swelling, and thickening of the synovial lining continue. Granulation tissue covers the articular cartilage (pannus), gradually replacing it with fibrous connective tissue. As the process spreads, the joint is destroyed as the articular cartilage becomes eroded, exposing the bone in the joint. Destruction of the joint produces ankylosis and deformity. The muscles are affected as the muscle fibers undergo degenerative changes with loss of muscle elasticity and contractile power.

Major organs or systems of the body may also be affected in rheumatoid arthritis. In addition to the synovial joints, the immune complexes lodge in body organs or in blood vessels supplying these organs. Inflammatory reactions occur, causing destruction, necrosis, and finally impairment or dysfunction.

▶ Assessment

Musculoskeletal Assessment.   In rheumatoid arthritis, a complete physical assessment is performed with special focus on the musculoskeletal system. Joint and skeletal muscle assessments are done concurrently; however, they are discussed separately to enhance understanding of the techniques involved. A systematic approach to assessment is the easiest way of obtaining information about musculoskeletal function. The nurse usually begins with the joints of the upper extremities and proceeds to the joints of the trunk and lower extremities. The patient should be comfortable and relaxed during the physical assessment.

Inspection, palpation, and range of motion comprise the three basic techniques utilized in joint assessment. Special care is taken to prevent increased pain when examining a severely inflamed or painful joint. Other factors, such as age and weight, are considered when performing a joint examination.

The nurse inspects pairs of joints, such as both shoulders, simultaneously to check for symmetry. Then, each joint is observed for size, shape, skin color, and general appearance. Size and shape may be altered by swelling; joint swelling may be due to fluid accumulation, hypertrophied synovium, or bony overgrowth. A severely swollen joint, particularly in the hand, appears taut and shiny, causing the normal "wrinkles" of the skin to disappear. Redness of the skin often indicates inflammation, while pallor or cyanosis indicates lack of blood supply. A prolonged decrease in vascular supply may cause skin ulcerations or vascular skin lesions.

After the joint is inspected, it is palpated anteriorly, posteriorly, and laterally for skin temperature, joint swelling,

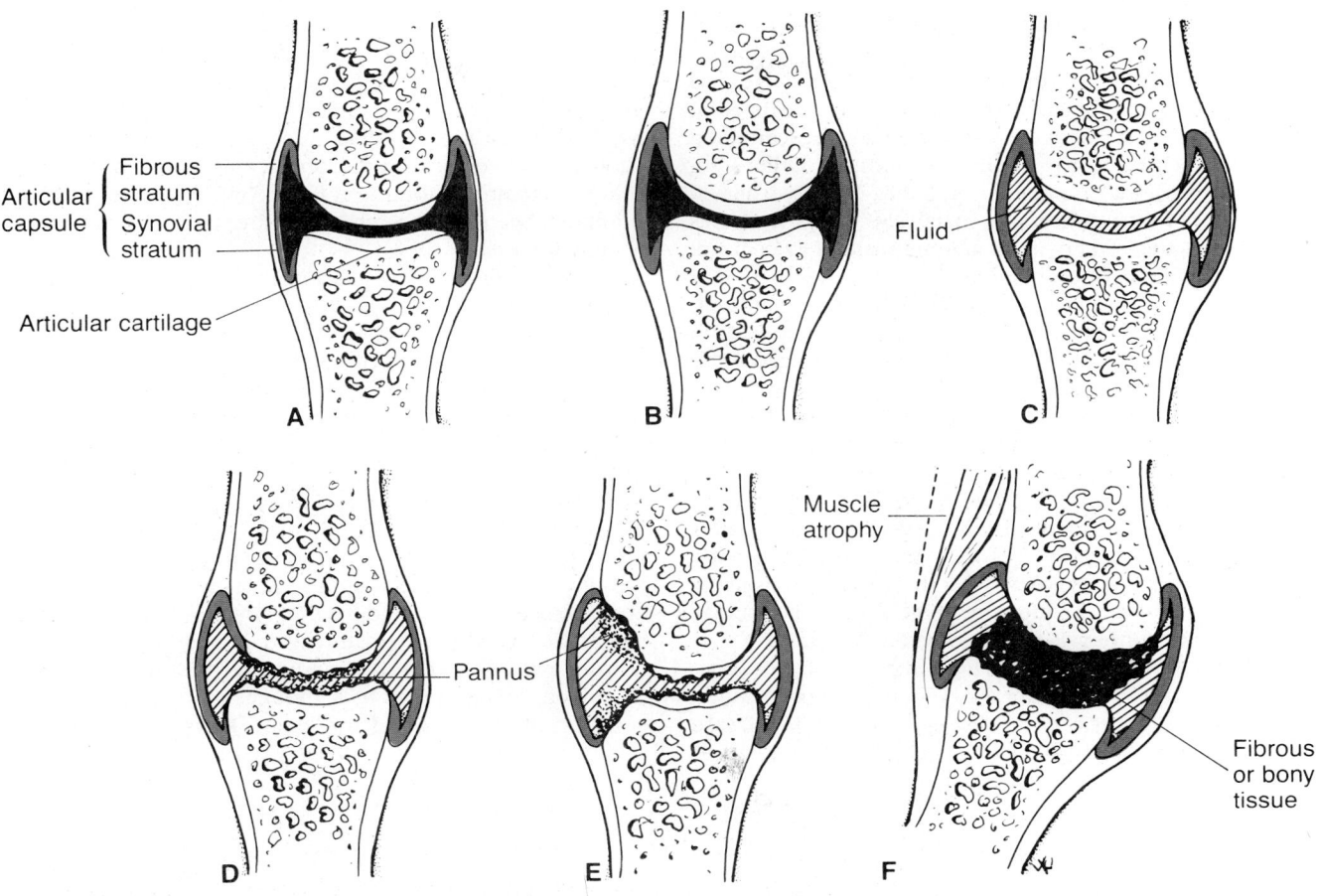

Figure 51-1. Pathophysiology of rheumatoid arthritis. (*A*) Normal. (*B*) Synovial swelling. (*C*) Fluid collects in joint. (*D*) Pannus. (*E*) Eroded articular cartilage. (*F*) Ankylosis and muscle atrophy.

tenderness, and irregularity. A warm, swollen, and tender joint usually indicates inflammation, as seen in rheumatoid arthritis. A cool joint suggests a decrease in blood supply.

Joint swelling may feel spongy, as in synovitis; hard, as in bony enlargement; or soft, as in fluid accumulation (effusion). Often, swelling occurs as a result of the presence of two or more of these conditions; therefore, it may be difficult to ascertain the exact nature of the swollen joint.

The patient may not complain of musculoskeletal pain, but during joint palpation, the patient may experience tenderness. Tenderness is often associated with joint swelling as nerve endings are compressed by excess fluid, synovium, or bone. Percussion over the joint may also elicit tenderness or determine the presence of fluid. Other maneuvers may be utilized to detect fluid, but they are usually performed by specialists in rheumatology.

During the palpation process, the nurse may wish to check peripheral pulses, particularly when vascular supply deficits are suspected. When edema is present, the amount and location are recorded.

Following inspection and palpation, joints are evaluated for their passive range of motion. The nurse should become familiar with the normal range of motion for synovial joints. Range of motion is recorded in approximate degrees of

deviation from a defined neutral zero point for each joint. Normal range may be compromised in the elderly or obese patient in the absence of actual joint pathology. Joint movement that is significantly *greater* than the normal range of motion is also recorded.

The presence of crepitation, or *crepitus,* is noted. Crepitus is the audible, grating sound produced by irregularities of the bony surfaces within a joint. It may also be heard on auscultation of the joint.

During the range of motion process, information is elicited regarding pain and tenderness. Each joint is supported by the nurse during evaluation. If a joint is severely inflamed or painful, it is not fully ranged, as inflammation and pain may increase.

At the time of the joint examination, the adjacent skin and muscles are inspected and palpated. Swelling may occur in areas around the joint in the form of generalized edema or nodules. The subcutaneous nodules of rheumatoid arthritis, for example, are soft and spongy.

Skeletal muscle is inspected for contour and size. A bilateral inspection provides comparison of symmetry in size and shape. Hypertrophy or atrophy is noted; muscle tone, tenderness, and pain on palpation are recorded. Disuse atrophy is seen frequently in patients who have joint pain and limited joint movement due to a disease such as rheumatoid arthritis.

Muscle strength may also be tested. The patient is asked to perform a number of voluntary tasks, for example, picking up a book. Actual strength measurement may be ascertained by devices such as the grip or pinch manometer. Otherwise, muscle strength may be graded on a 0-to-5 scale, where 0 represents no muscle strength (paralysis) and 5 indicates normal strength. Other types of grading scales may be used, but the parameters of each are similar.

If impairments of joint and muscle functions are present, an assessment of the patient's mobility is determined. The desired mobility level is one that allows the patient to be independent in activities of daily living (ADLs). The patient is questioned about his ability to feed, dress, bathe, and ambulate. Precise tools are available to provide a numerical index of the patient's ability to perform these tasks.

Some patients may be asked to perform certain tasks while the examiner observes ability level. One such task is to ask the patient to walk 15.24 meters (50 feet) as quickly as possible. The time it takes to walk the prescribed distance is recorded and used as a measure of mobility. This test may be performed at intervals to assess patient progress.

Clinical Manifestations.   The clinical picture of rheumatoid arthritis is variable, but may generally be determined by the stage and severity of the disease process. The disease usually begins with unusual fatigue, generalized weakness, and anorexia. Signs of joint inflammation (redness, swelling, warmth, pain) begin most commonly in the fingers, particularly involving the proximal interphalangeal joints (PIPs) and metacarpophalangeal joints (MCPs) bilaterally and symmetrically. Additional joints, such as the wrists, elbows, shoulders, knees, and hips, soon become involved, and mobility is impaired. Morning stiffness (lasting longer than 30 minutes after rising) is characteristic, but subsides when activity increases.

Fixed deformities of the hands and feet are common in rheumatoid arthritis (Fig. 51-2). In severe cases, the temporomandibular joints (jaws) and spinal column may also be involved. In approximately 25% of patients, rheumatoid nodules are present. When occurring in the subcutaneous tissue adjacent to joints, they are movable and "spongy." They may also occur in major organs, particularly the heart and lungs.

Cardiac, renal, and pleural involvement resulting from vasculitis or direct immune complex invasion may be fatal. Other problems seen in late or severe stages of rheumatoid arthritis include severe weight loss, fever, anemia, muscle atrophy, osteoporosis, and Sjögren's syndrome. Sjögren's is a condition in which the patient has dry, "gritty" eyes (keratoconjunctivitis sicca); dry mouth (xerostomia); and liver or spleen enlargement. It is thought to be the result of secretory duct and gland infiltration by lymphocytes and immune complexes.

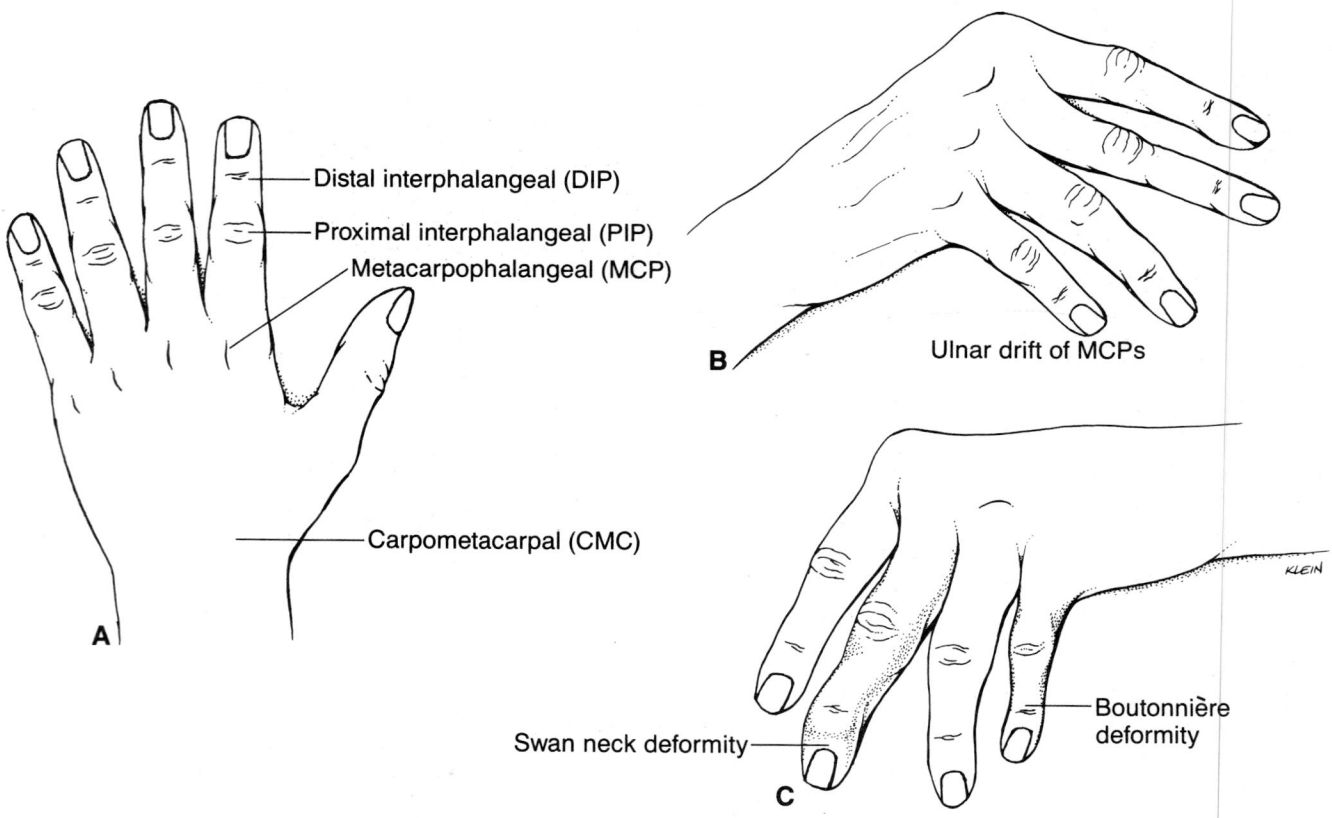

Figure 51-2.   (*A*) Common reference points for rheumatoid arthritis of the hand. (*B* and *C*) Types of rheumatoid arthritis.

Patient Problems/Nursing Diagnoses

Based on the clinical manifestations, the nursing history, and the diagnostic assessment data, the patient's major nursing problems may include alteration in comfort—pain and stiffness related to joint and muscle inflammation and degeneration; impaired physical mobility related to pain or deformity; self-care deficit related to fatigue, pain, or deformity; disturbances in self-concept related to alteration in body image or dependence; alteration in nutrition related to anorexia, weight loss, and anemia; and knowledge deficit related to incongruency between societal myths and professional expertise.

Accompanying these major nursing problems may be fear, ineffective individual or family coping, sexual dysfunction, anticipatory grieving, impaired home maintenance management, noncompliance with treatment plan, and sleep pattern disturbances.

▶ **Planning and Implementation**

Goals

The goals for patients with rheumatoid arthritis vary according to each patient's nursing diagnoses. However, broad goals related to the above-mentioned nursing problems are presented to represent a typical patient situation. The major goals are:

1. Relief of pain and discomfort
2. Increased mobility and muscle strength
3. Optimal independence in ADLs
4. A positive self-concept
5. Attainment or maintenance of optimal nutrition
6. Participation in an ongoing educational program

An interdisciplinary approach to planning patient care should be taken to include other members of the health team (such as physical therapists, occupational therapists).

Relief of Pain and Discomfort

Hot and Cold Applications.   Heat applications are often helpful in relieving pain, stiffness, inflammation, and muscle spasm. Superficial heat may be supplied in the form of warm tub baths and warm, moist compresses. Paraffin baths (dips) offer concentrated heat and are helpful to patients with wrist and small joint involvement. Therapeutic exercises can be carried out more comfortably and effectively after heat has been applied. However, in some patients, heat may actually increase pain, muscle spasm, and synovial fluid volume. If the inflammatory process is acute, cold applications may be tried in the form of moist packs or an ice bag. Both heat and cold are analgesic to nerve pain receptors and relax muscle spasms.

Rest.   Rest also helps to allay pain. Since rheumatoid arthritis is a systemic disease, the whole patient—not merely the joints—must be treated. The amount of rest required is indicated by the amount of inflammatory involvement and the feelings of the patient. When in bed, the patient should lie flat on a firm mattress with only one pillow under the head because of the risk of dorsal kyphosis. (At no time should a pillow be placed under the knees, as this promotes flexion contractures of those joints.)

Frequent periods of bed rest during the day take the weight off the joints and relieve fatigue. If joint inflammation is severe, the patient may be placed on complete bedrest for a brief period. (Nevertheless, range of motion exercises should still be carried out.) At bedrest, the patient should lie flat with feet propped against a footboard. All joints should be supported in a position of optimum function.

Positioning and Movement.   The patient should lie on the abdomen several times daily to prevent flexion deformities. As joint stiffness and tenderness diminish and function improves, the patient is encouraged to perform more out-of-bed activities. Pain can be anticipated in the knees and hips when rising from a chair. The nurse should select a straight-back chair with a seat that is high enough to permit the patient to keep the feet flat on the floor (or stool) while the hips and shoulders are resting against the back of the chair. Toilet seats can be raised by attaching built-up seats to standard toilet fixtures.

A cervical collar to prevent cervical motion may help if the patient has a painful neck. Stretch gloves may control hand and finger pain by providing a mild splinting action and presumably by reducing joint swelling and stasis of blood.

Foot Wear.   When the foot is involved, pain is due to synovial proliferation, distention of the joint capsule, and lax supporting ligaments, which contribute to mechanical deformities. Pain around the metatarsal areas of the forefoot may be relieved by placing a metatarsal bar proximal to the point of impact on the metatarsal heads in order to relieve weight bearing. Pads may be placed in strategic places to relieve stress and irritation. These may be fitted to standard shoes by an expert shoemaker. When there are significant deformities of the feet, custom-made shoes molded to the contours of the feet will permit more comfortable walking. The patient is advised that the foot may continue to change shape and that modifications will need to be made on the shoes. In many instances, corrective surgery can restore function and relieve pain.

Pharmacotherapy.   Drug therapy is used to relieve inflammation and pain and arrest the progress of the disease (Table 51-2). The salicylates (aspirin), when used in full dosage, have an anti-inflammatory as well as analgesic and antipyretic action in the treatment of rheumatoid arthritis. They often provide an effective and inexpensive relief of pain and stiffness. Salicylates reach their peak level in the blood approximately 2 hours after oral ingestion and then gradually decline. To be most effective, the patient should take aspirin every 3 to 4 hours, beginning from the moment he awakens in the morning and regularly throughout the day. The serum salicylate level is kept at 20 mg/100 ml to 30 mg/100 ml, which usually requires 12 to 20 aspirin tablets daily. There are sustained-released salicylate preparations for bedtime usage to maintain a therapeutic blood level at night, but the short-acting aspirin is used most often. Because heavy and continual use of aspirin can produce side-effects, such as the presence of occult gastrointestinal bleeding, the patient is advised to have periodic hematocrit determinations. However, he should be assured that chronic use of aspirin does not lead to tolerance or addiction.

If aspirin is not successful in relieving pain and inflam-

(Text continues on page 1146)

Table 51-2
Drugs Used in Connective Tissue Disease

Drug	Action	Nursing Implications and Assessment for Drug Intolerance
Anti-inflammatory Agents *Salicylates*		
Aspirin (may be buffered or enteric coated)	Aspirin is the cornerstone of treatment, especially in early phase of diseases such as rheumatoid arthritis Has anti-inflammatory, antipyretic, and analgesic effects Optimum dosage will produce blood salicylate levels of 20–30 mg/100 ml Can be used in combination with other analgesics and anti-inflammatory agents	Take salicylates with antacid or milk to protect against gastric irritation. Watch for complaints of tinnitus, gastric intolerance, or GI bleeding and purpuric tendencies.
Nonsteroidal Anti-inflammatory Agents		
Ibuprofen (Motrin)	Anti-inflammatory action, particularly in joints	Gastrointestinal irritation and hemorrhagic erosions but less frequently than aspirin Used in patients who cannot tolerate or who do not respond to aspirin
Fenoprofen (Nalfon)	Mechanism of action may be related to inhibition of prostaglandin synthetase (prostaglandins have a role in inflammatory process, pain, and fever)	Variation among patients in response to these drugs
Naproxen (Naprosyn)	Longer half-life, thus permits less frequent administration	Dosage individualized for each patient
Tolmetin (Tolectin)		
Sulindac (Clinoril)	Anti-inflammatory, analgesic, antipyretic properties	Peptic ulceration and gastrointestinal bleeding have been reported.
Piroxicam (Feldene)	Very long half-life requiring one dose per day	
Other Anti-inflammatory Agents		
Indomethacin (Indocin)	Used for short-term treatment of active synovitis	Can produce significant side-effects: gastrointestinal effects; CNS effects.

Phenylbutazone (Butazolidin)
Oxyphenbutazone (Tandearil)
	Nonsteroidal antirheumatic agents for adjunctive treatment of rheumatoid arthritis
	Exerts analgesic, antipyretic, anti-inflammatory action
	Sometimes remarkably effective in control of articular symptoms
	Patient should be under close medical supervision
	Can cause salt and water retention.
	Usually used only for short periods
		Observe for untoward effects:
		  Gastrointestinal effects:
		    Nausea, vomiting, epigastric distress, precipitation and reactivation of peptic ulcer
		  Hematologic:
		    Bone marrow depression, anemia, leukopenia, agranulocytosis, thrombocytopenia purpura
		    Irreversible blood element depression may occur rapidly despite careful supervision and frequent testing.

Antimalarial Compounds		
Hydroxychloroquine sulfate (Plaquenil)	Appears to be no rational basis for the comparative success of these drugs at this time Used primarily in discoid lupus and rheumatoid arthritis	Useful for severe and destructive forms of arthritis. Stress that patient should have regular ophthalmologic examination every 4–6 months; *drug has potential retinal effects.* Toxic effects: Headache, dizziness, GI complaints, ocular toxicity, and retinopathy.

(continued)

Table 51-2
Drugs Used in Connective Tissue Disease (continued)

Drug	Action	Nursing Implications and Assessment for Drug Intolerance
Gold Therapy (Chrysotherapy)		

Gold sodium thiomalate (Myochrysine) (water-based)	Gold salts may be useful when rheumatoid activity is uncontrolled by nonsteroidal therapy	Toxic effects:
		  Dermatitis, stomatitis, nephropathy, blood dyscrasias.
		  Blood count and urine check for protein performed before each injection.

Aurothioglucose (Solganal) (oil-based)	Gold therapy is cumulative with slow onset of beneficial effects	Question patient at each visit concerning pruritus, rash, sores in mouth, metallic taste.
Note: Oral form of gold being made available	Mechanism of action unknown; exerts an inflammatory-suppressive effect Can produce a long-sustained remission when treatment continued indefinitely Induces remission; 8–14 weeks may pass before benefit is noted Gradual decrease in administration intervals from weekly through monthly	Read package insert before drug administration. Administer deep IM into the ventrogluteal area to avoid local irritation or necrosis of nerves, a potential lethal complication of injection.

Corticosteroids
Prednisone (Deltasone)
Prednisolone
	Corticosteroids used in treatment of incapacitating active rheumatoid arthritis, systemic lupus erythematosus, progressive systemic sclerosis, necrotizing arteritis
	Use of corticosteroids for long periods has wide range of adverse effects
	Steroids should be used with caution and should be tapered to minimal maintenance dose if possible
		Toxic effects:
		  Osteoporosis, fractures, avascular necrosis
		  Gastric ulcers, psychiatric problems, infection susceptibility
		  Hirsutism, acne, moon facies, abnormal fat deposition, edema, emotional disorders, menstrual disorders
		  Hyperglycemia, hypokalemia
		  Hypertension
		  Cataracts and glaucoma

Intra-articular Corticosteroid Injections	Given when arthritic reaction has been suppressed and one or two joints are not responding to treatment Given when only one or two joints affected Given to patient with extremely painful joints so he can undergo physical therapy Relieves pain; benefit may last from weeks to months	An inflamed joint may respond to local injection when it has failed to come under control with other general systemic measures. Joints most amenable to corticosteroid injections are ankles, knees, hips, shoulders, and hands.

Immunosuppressive Drugs
Cyclophosphamide (Cytoxan)
Azathioprine (Imuran)
	Mechanisms underlying action of these drugs not known; thought to affect the production of antibodies at the cellular level
	Suppress auto-immune mechanism
	Used in advanced rheumatoid arthritis or systemic lupus erythematosus that is unresponsive to conventional therapy
	These drugs have teratogenic potential
		Highly toxic:
		  Bone marrow depression, GI ulcerations
		  Skin rashes, alopecia
		  Bladder toxicity
		  Reduces patient's resistance to infections
		Patient must be monitored with weekly blood evaluation and urinalysis.
		Advise patient of contraceptive measures.

Chart 51-1
Patient Education Guidelines for Joint Protection and Energy Conservation in Rheumatoid Arthritis

1. Simplify all activities.
2. Pace yourself when doing activities.
3. Delegate jobs to others when possible.
4. Perform any activity lasting more than ten minutes in a seated position.
5. Organize and arrange materials, utensils, and tools so that they are easy to reach.
6. If any activity does not have to be done, eliminate it.
7. Use correct body mechanics.
8. Avoid rushing.
9. Slide objects instead of lifting and carrying them.
10. If you *must* lift an object, scoop it up in both hands with palms upward.
11. Always use the large joints to perform activities.
12. Use your entire body to move heavy objects.
13. Make work easier with correct counter or table height.
14. Avoid bending or stooping.
15. Avoid prolonged periods of holding the same position.
16. Work with fingers extended to avoid increasing flexion deformities.
17. Always turn hand toward thumb side to prevent ulnar deviation (as when turning a doorknob).
18. Avoid fatigue—rest frequently.
19. Respect pain—do on "good" days, don't do on "bad" days.

mation, other anti-inflammatory drugs are used with salicylate therapy. Nonsteroidal anti-inflammatory drugs (NSAIDs) include a large variety of drugs that not only decrease inflammation, but have an analgesic action as well. Examples are ibuprofen (Motrin), naproxen (Naprosyn), indomethacin (Indocin), and fenoprofen (Nalfon). NSAIDs and aspirin have similar toxic effects.

Additional analgesia may be prescribed for periods of extreme pain. Care should be taken to avoid narcotic analgesics, as the patient may become dependent due to the chronic need for pain relief.

If significant inflammation persists, gold therapy (anti-inflammatory action) may be tried. The patient should be advised of possible dermatologic, hematologic, and renal complications resulting from this therapy.

Penicillamine, an oral chelating agent, may be used as an alternative to gold therapy. Its anti-inflammatory action is not understood, but it has been useful in suppressing the progress of rheumatoid arthritis in some patients. Its adverse effects are similar to those of gold.

Systemic therapy with one of the corticosteroids (such as prednisone) does not alter the course of rheumatoid arthritis, but reduces inflammation and pain and suppresses the production of lymphocytes (part of the immune system). Corticosteroids are used when the patient has a rapid downhill course or when extra-articular manifestations occur. Corticosteroid therapy has undesirable side-effects, including

sodium and water retention, potassium depletion, hypertension, hyperglycemia, menstrual irregularities, and other features of the Cushing syndrome, as well as cataracts, osteoporosis, psychosis, and psychological dependency.

When the disease does not respond sufficiently to daily administration of oral steroids, high doses of intravenous steroids may be administered as "pulse therapy." This consists of a single dose or a series of daily doses for a specified length of time or until inflammation decreases.

Joints that are severely inflamed and fail to respond promptly to the measures outlined above may be treated by the local injection of a corticosteroid. This maneuver suppresses local inflammation and provides temporary relief from pain and disability.

Immunosuppressive drugs that are thought to affect the production of antibodies at the cellular level are reserved for the treatment of severe rheumatoid arthritis. These include methotrexate, cyclophosphamide (Cytoxan), and azathioprine (Imuran). However, these drugs are highly toxic and can produce bone marrow depression, anemia, gastrointestinal disturbances, and skin rashes.

Table 51-2 summarizes the drugs used in the treatment of rheumatoid arthritis. By decreasing inflammation and pain, these drugs can help relieve discomfort. It is important that the nurse, either in a hospital or community setting, be familiar with the side-effects and potential toxicity of these drugs. Patients who take three or more anti-inflammatory drugs concurrently should receive additional monitoring. All patients on drug therapy should be thoroughly instructed regarding drug type, purpose, dosage, side-effects, and toxic effects.

Increased Mobility and Muscle Strength. Inflammation, scarring, or other structural damage to joint structures results in pain and disability. The patient, in an effort to avoid pain, tends to immobilize the affected joints, and muscular spasm further limits their motion. If acutely inflamed, these joints should be rested by applying splints, bivalved casts, or other mechanical devices that will maintain them in functional positions. Simple splints provide rest, support the joint in optimal position to relieve pain and spasm, and help prevent deformity. Above all, the joints should not be permitted to "freeze" in positions of flexion, which is their natural tendency because of the predominant strength of flexor muscles. The knee is splinted at full extension, and the wrist at slight dorsiflexion. Splints may need to be modified when changes occur in joint structure.

Joints may lose their normal range of motion due to deformity and atrophy of the muscles. This loss can be prevented to a large extent by systematic range of motion and specific muscle-strengthening exercises. If activity is painful, the nurse may help the patient (with active, assisted exercises) to perform the required motions. Emphasis must be placed on the need to carry out a regular exercise routine on a daily basis in order to increase muscle strength. These are essential in restoring joint mobility and strengthening the muscles that support the joints. Isometric muscle exercises are especially valuable as the joint is kept at rest during these exercises.

Excess stress and strain of affected joints should be avoided. Guidelines for joint protection and energy conservation are listed in Chart 51-1.

Independence in Activities of Daily Living. In order for the patient to become independent, he must be instructed and supervised by the nurse and others of the rehabilitation team in ADLs. It is important that the nurse work with the patient to achieve the goals of self-care and independence.

The patient with rheumatoid arthritis should be allowed to perform as much of his ADLs as possible, even though additional time might be needed to complete them. Manual assistance from the nurse should be given only when absolutely necessary. Often the patient has the greatest difficulty with fine, delicate movements, such as those required for fastening items of clothing and opening small packages. The nurse should work together with the occupational or physical therapists to teach the patient ways to perform these difficult tasks. There are many self-help devices available to assist with dressing, bathing, grooming, and eating when the patient cannot perform these himself (Fig. 51-3; also see Chap. 14).

When there is difficulty in ambulation, canes or walkers may be prescribed as assistive devices to reduce the amount of weight bearing on the joints of the lower extremities. Well-fitted, supportive shoes should be worn when walking to protect joints and prevent falls. Custom-made corrective shoes may be used to prevent further foot deformity and provide support.

When physical mobility is severely impaired and relief of pain by conventional drug therapy fails, reconstructive joint surgery may restore some function and reduce pain. Many patients receive total joint replacements to achieve pain control and increased mobility (see p. 1409).

A Positive Self-concept. Patients with arthritis show the same fundamental psychological responses to their disease as persons with other chronic diseases: fear, anxiety, depression, anger, and loss. The unpredictability and uncertainty of the course of the disease frequently causes the patient to react in an angry, bitter, and hostile manner.

All aspects of the patient's life, including work role, social life, sexual function, and financial status, may be altered. Body image changes may cause social isolation and depression. The resulting strain on the patient and his family contributes to the often negative attitude of the patient. Such behavior should not be reciprocated with an equally negative response by the nurse. It is better for the patient to express hostility or depression than to suppress it and to ultimately stop trying to communicate with the health care team. Failure of communication also leads to deterioration of interfamily relationships.

The nurse and the family should try to understand the patient's personality and his emotional reactions to the disease. Presenting a realistic but optimistic view by pointing out that only a small percentage of patients become totally disabled can help reassure the patient. At the same time, the favorable outcome must be linked to a faithful adherence to the rehabilitation program that is designed to improve functioning. Social workers, psychiatric liaison nurses, sex counselors, and clergy may serve as valuable resources for reassurance and promotion of a patient's positive self-concept.

Attainment of Optimum Nutrition. Patients with rheumatoid arthritis frequently experience anorexia, weight loss, and anemia. A dietary history should be taken on each patient to determine usual eating habits and food preferences. The patient should be instructed on how to select foods to include the daily requirements from the basic four food groups, with

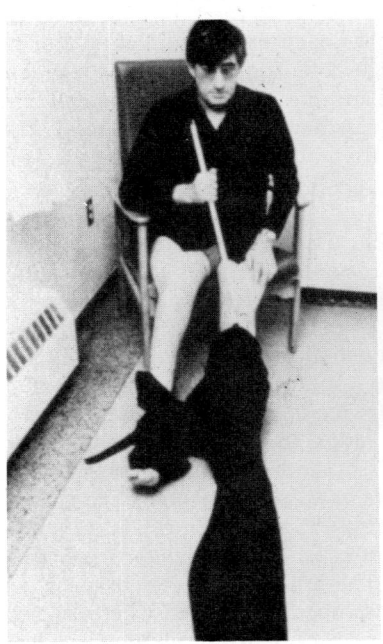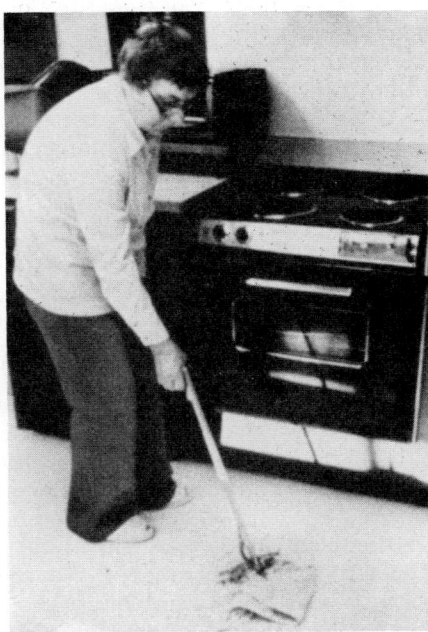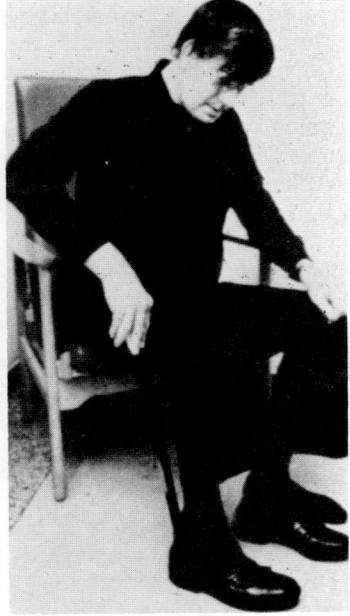

Figure 51-3. Assistive devices with extended handles to promote self-care. (From the AHP Arthritis Teaching Slide Collection, copyright 1980. Used by permission of the Arthritis Foundation.)

emphasis on foods high in vitamins, protein, and iron for tissue building and repair. For the extremely anorexic patient, small, frequent feedings with increased protein supplements may be prescribed.

Care must be taken to prevent obesity. Excess weight causes increased stress on weight-bearing joints, creating further joint damage. If obesity is already present, a weight-reduction diet is prescribed.

Participation in an Ongoing Educational Program. The nurse should assess the patient's knowledge regarding his disease, signs of exacerbations, treatment plan, and drug therapy. If a knowledge deficit exists, the nurse teaches the patient and his family and reinforces the teaching as necessary. This is an integral part of discharge planning. The community health nurse or outpatient department nurse should continue with the teaching plan as outlined.

Another important aspect of patient education is concerned with the quackery of arthritis. More than 1 billion dollars is spent each year on unproven remedies and widely advertised "cures." Patients should be taught that there is no cure for rheumatoid arthritis and should be reminded to check with their physician or nurse before digressing from their treatment regimens. Many so-called remedies can cause potentially fatal health complications.

▶ Evaluation

Specific outcome criteria for evaluation are derived from the broad goals as outlined. Sample outcome criteria that are observable and measurable are included here.

Expected Outcomes

1. Achieves relief of pain and discomfort
   a. Exhibits no signs (redness, warmth, swelling) of joint inflammation
   b. Shows improvement in joint movement
   c. Experiences less pain with use of p.r.n. medication
2. Demonstrates increased mobility and muscle strength
   a. Moves from bed to chair (and vice versa) without manual assistance (may use assistive device, elevated seat, or handrail)
   b. Ambulates without manual assistance inside and outside of home environment (may use cane or walker)
   c. Manipulates steps (at least one flight)
   d. Performs daily tasks of dressing, grooming, bathing, and eating without manual assistance (assistive or adaptive devices may be used)
   e. Shows no signs of disuse muscle atrophy (or no further atrophy after treatment plan initiated)
3. Achieves independence in activities of daily living
   a. Feeds self without assistance
   b. Bathes self without assistance
   c. Grooms self without assistance
   d. Dresses self without assistance
   e. Transports self outside of home environment (by taxi, bus, car, etc.) for purpose of shopping, banking, physician visits, socialization
4. Develops a positive self-concept
   a. Expresses feelings to family
   b. Expresses feelings to health team members
   c. Socializes (conversation) with family members, friends, peers
   d. Participates in social activities, such as bingo, clubs
   e. Demonstrates active interest and participation in hobby or diversional activity (*e.g.,* television, knitting, sewing, bowling)
5. Attains or maintains optimum nutrition
   a. Eats at least three well-balanced meals per day
   b. Includes foods high in protein, iron, and vitamin C in diet
   c. Keeps body weight between ideal and less than 10% over ideal weight
6. Participates in ongoing educational program
   a. Describes disease pathophysiology
   b. Describes treatment plan and its purpose
   c. Is knowledgable about drug therapy (state names, action, dosage, side-effects, toxic effects)
   d. Complies with treatment plan, including drug therapy
   e. Does not participate in "remedies," "cures," and quackery
   f. Keep follow-up clinic or physician appointments

Although there is no specific "cure" for rheumatoid arthritis, much can be done to alleviate suffering and prevent crippling by applying specific therapeutic measures. For the program to be effective, the patient must be wholeheartedly involved in this long-term project. The federal government has established arthritis centers across the U.S. to carry out research and apprise patients and medical personnel of the newest advances in arthritis therapy.

▷ Degenerative Joint Disease

Degenerative joint disease (DJD) is the most common type of connective tissue disease in the U.S., affecting nearly 16 million people. It has been estimated that 80% of people over 55 years of age have some degree of degeneration. Unlike rheumatoid arthritis, DJD is not a systemic, inflammatory disease process. For this reason, the term "osteoarthritis," frequently used interchangably with DJD, is not an accurate synonym.

Pathophysiology

Degenerative joint disease is a "wear and tear" process in which there is degeneration of articular cartilage with resultant formation of osteophytes (irregular bony overgrowths). Most frequently seen in weight-bearing joints, it is thought to be the result of prolonged mechanical stress. DJD affects women twice as often as men and tends to have a familial tendency. Although seen most often in the elderly, the disease may be associated with athletics, obesity, previous trauma, or strenuous physical labor in any age group.

As a joint undergoes repeated mechanical stress, the elasticity of the joint capsule, articular cartilage, and ligaments is reduced. The articular plate is thinned, and its function as a shock absorber is decreased. There is narrowing of the joint space and loss of stability. When the articular plate disappears, bony spurs form at the edges of the joint surfaces, and the capsule and synovial membranes thicken.

The joint cartilage degenerates and atrophies, the bones harden and hypertrophy at their articular surfaces, and the ligaments calcify. As a result, sterile joint effusions and secondary synovitis may be present, particularly in the knees.

▶ Assessment

Musculoskeletal Assessment.   The nurse inspects joints for swelling, indicative of secondary synovitis, effusion, or bony enlargement. Alterations in alignment are also noted. Palpation may elicit tenderness in early degeneration or severe pain in advanced degeneration.

Although DJD occurs most often in weight-bearing joints (hips and knees), finger joints are frequently involved. Unlike rheumatoid arthritis, which affects PIPs and MCPs, degenerative joint disease is seen in the distal interphalangeal joints (DIPs) and the proximal interphalangeals. Characteristic bony nodules may be present, which on inspection and palpation may be painful and inflamed. When present on the DIPs, the nodules are called *Heberden's nodes;* when present on the PIPs, they are called *Bouchard's nodes.* Both are bony enlargements that appear in a bilateral, symmetrical pattern (Fig. 51-4).

Following inspection and palpation, joints are evaluated for range of motion. In severe disease, joint movement is markedly compromised. The vertebral column should also be assessed, as it is commonly involved in patients with degenerative disease. Limitations in movement of the cervical and lumbar areas with an accompanying increase in pain are indicative of spinal involvement. A detailed discussion of the technique for joint assessment is found in the discussion of rheumatoid arthritis.

Clinical Manifestations.   The most common symptom of DJD is pain, which tends to worsen with activity and improve after rest. This is quite different from the pattern of pain and stiffness in rheumatoid arthritis. The rheumatoid patient usually feels better with activity and becomes stiffer after periods of rest. Morning stiffness may occur in DJD, but most often lasts less than 30 minutes after rising.

Upon joint movement, crepitus may be felt or heard. Physical mobility may be impaired, particularly ambulation and gait. Muscle spasm is often present.

Diagnostic Evaluation.   Radiographic examination of degenerating joints demonstrate bony hypertrophy and spur formation, and gross irregularities of the joint structures. Other diagnostic tests are not useful in this disorder. Occasionally, local synovitis may cause a slight elevation in the sedimentation rate.

Patient Problems/Nursing Diagnoses

Based on the clinical manifestations, the nursing history, and the diagnostic assessment data, the patient's major nursing problems include alteration in comfort—pain related to joint degeneration and muscle spasm; impaired physical mobility related to pain and limited joint movement; and self-care deficit related to pain and limited joint movement. Accompanying these major problems may be ineffective individual or family coping, knowledge deficit, sexual dysfunction, impaired home maintenance management, and sleep pattern disturbances.

▶ Planning and Implementation

Goals

The broad goals related to the identified nursing problems are:

1. Relief of pain and discomfort
2. Increased physical mobility and muscle strength
3. Independence in ADLs

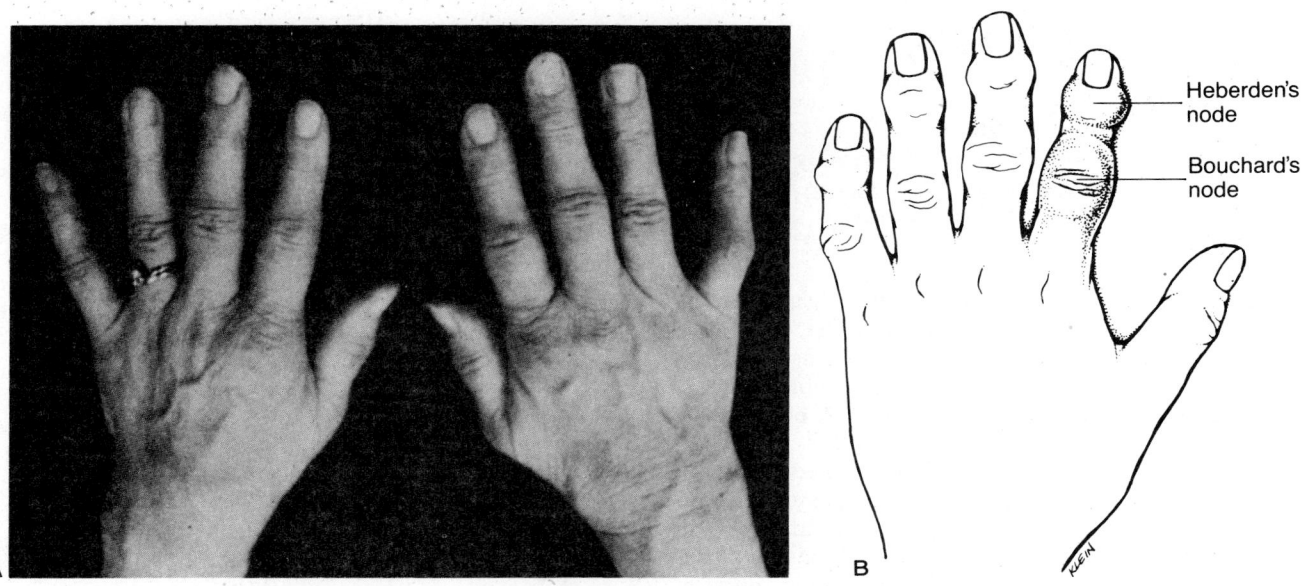

Figure 51-4.   Hand deformities commonly seen in osteoarthritis. (Part A from the Arthritis Foundation Teaching Collection, copyright 1972. Used by permission of the Arthritis Foundation.)

As in rheumatoid arthritis, an interdisciplinary approach should be taken in caring for patients with degenerative disease.

Relief of Pain and Discomfort. Measures for relief of pain, stiffness, and muscle spasm are generally the same as those used in rheumatoid arthritis: rest with alternating periods of activity, an exercise program, heat application, splinting, and joint protection. In addition, a weight-reduction diet may be required to reduce stress on weight-bearing joints.

Unlike rheumatoid arthritis, drug therapy is primarily helpful for its analgesic effect. Although nonsteroidal anti-inflammatory drugs, such as ibuprofen (Motrin), naproxen (Naprosyn), or piroxicam (Feldene) may be prescribed, their anti-inflammatory action may not be helpful in a degenerative process. For long-term relief of pain, however, these drugs are preferred over the chronic use of more potent analgesics. Intra-articular corticosteroids may provide temporary relief of pain in severely affected joints.

When symptomatic treatment is ineffective, total joint replacement surgery is utilized for relief of pain (see p. 1409). Multiple joints, particularly hips and knees, may need to be replaced.

Increased Physical Mobility and Muscle Strength and Independence in Activities of Daily Living. Nursing interventions for promoting mobility and independence are the same as those employed for patients with rheumatoid arthritis. Although gross deformity is not usually present in DJD, joint pain and muscle spasm decrease joint movement and the individual's ability to care for himself.

▶ Evaluation

Specific outcome criteria for evaluation of nursing interventions are similar to those outlined in the discussion of rheumatoid arthritis.

▷ Lupus Erythematosus

Lupus erythematosus, meaning "red wolf," was formerly considered a rare disease. With the advance of better diagnostic techniques, it can now be more readily diagnosed. Although the disease may be fatal, its prognosis is markedly improved with early diagnosis and treatment.

Pathophysiology

There are two major types of lupus erythematosus: systemic (SLE) and discoid (DLE). Most individuals with the condition have the systemic type. SLE may be defined as a chronic, systemic, inflammatory disease involving multiple body systems. DLE affects the skin only, but may later become systemic.

Like rheumatoid arthritis, lupus is classified as autoimmune with a genetic predisposition to the disease. It is characterized by spontaneous remissions and exacerbations and has a variable progressive course. Exacerbations, or "flare-ups," are initiated by sunlight; ultraviolet light; physical stress, such as pregnancy; and emotional stress.

Although there are two major types of lupus erythematosus, it should be noted that certain drugs, such as hydralazine (Apresoline) and procainamide (Pronestyl), may cause a lupuslike syndrome often referred to as drug-induced lupus. In these patients, discontinuation of the offending drug usually resolves the condition.

It is estimated that lupus occurs in 1 out of every 700 persons, with a predominance in nonwhites. Young women of childbearing age are affected 6:1 over men, with an average onset at 30 years of age.

▶ Assessment

The nurse performs a thorough, systematic physical assessment of the patient with lupus. Major body organs and systems are involved due to invasion by immune complexes; systemic inflammation results.

Musculoskeletal Assessment. Most patients with SLE have joint inflammation, or arthritis. As in rheumatoid arthritis, lupus arthritis can be deforming. Therefore, the nurse conducts a total joint assessment as described in the discussion of rheumatoid arthritis. Muscle strength is also evaluated.

Clinical Manifestations. The onset of SLE may be insidious or acute. If insidious (as are most cases), the symptoms may be mild and vague. For this reason, the patient with lupus may be undiagnosed for many years. Initially, the patient may experience extreme fatigue, generalized weakness, and anorexia. Weight loss, fever, rash, and signs of joint inflammation alert the physician toward the suspected diagnosis of lupus. The characteristic "butterfly rash" of the face occurs in less than one half of lupus patients, but other cutaneous lesions may be present on the trunk or extremities. Typically, the rash is either a diffuse, flat pattern or in raised, scaly patches (Fig. 51-5).

Polymyositis (inflammation of skeletal muscle), alopecia, and photosensitivity are common manifestations. (Polymyositis may occur as a separate connective tissue disease.) Life-threatening vasculitis (inflammation of vessel walls) decreases the blood supply to major organs, causing necrosis and dysfunction. Renal, central nervous system (brain), and cardiac complications often lead to death. Gastrointestinal problems, such as nausea and vomiting, esophagitis, and abdominal pain, are common. Pneumonitis, chronic obstructive lung disease, and interstitial fibrosis are typical when lung involvement occurs. Hypertension and peripheral vascular disease result from peripheral vasculitis.

Raynaud's phenomenon is common in lupus erythematosus and results from vasospasm of smaller vessels in the hands and feet. On exposure to cold, the vessels constrict, resulting in the characteristic white to blue to red color changes. These "attacks" of vasoconstriction are painful and may lead to necrosis with eventual distal digit autoamputation.

Diagnostic Evaluation. Serum testing reveals moderate to severe anemia, thrombocytopenia, and leukocytosis or leukopenia. Other diagnostic immunologic tests support, but often do not confirm, the diagnosis. When major body organs are affected, appropriate diagnostic assessments should be incorporated.

Patient Problems/Nursing Diagnoses

Based on the clinical manifestations, nursing history, and the diagnostic assessment data, the patient's major nursing problems may include alteration in skin integrity related to rash and vasculitic lesions; alteration in metabolism related to fever, fatigue, and anorexia; disturbances in self-concept related to skin rash, fatigue, or joint deformity; alteration in comfort—pain and stiffness related to joint and muscle inflammation and degeneration; anticipatory grieving related to unpredictability of chronic, potentially fatal disease; self-care deficit related to fatigue, weakness, pain, or joint deformity; and alteration in nutrition related to anorexia, weight loss, and anemia.

Accompanying these nursing problems may be fear, ineffective individual or family coping, sexual dysfunction, alteration in cardic output, alteration in urinary or bowel patterns, alteration in consciousness (due to CNS involvement), and sleep pattern disturbances.

▶ Planning and Implementation

Goals

The goals for patients with lupus erythematosus vary according to each patient's disease process and subsequent nursing problems. However, broad goals related to the previously identified nursing problems are discussed to represent a typical lupus erythematosus patient. The major goals are:

1. Maintenance of skin integrity
2. Decreased fatigue and weakness
3. A positive self-concept
4. Relief of pain and discomfort
5. Promotion of the grieving process
6. Independence in ADLs
7. Attainment or maintenance of optimum nutrition

Maintenance of Skin Integrity.   The skin rash of DLE or SLE is often scaly and itchy. Cool baths may decrease discomfort and scaliness. The skin should be kept clean and void of powders or other irritants. Topical corticosteroid creams or ointments may be prescribed to decrease inflammation. In some cases, an antimalarial drug, such as hydroxychloroquine (Plaquenil), is given to reduce the inflammatory response of the skin. Its main side-effects and toxic effects include nausea and vomiting, rash, and diminished visual acuity (from retinal damage).

Sunlight and ultraviolet lights (such as fluorescent lighting) must be avoided. Long-sleeved clothing, wide-brim hats, and long pants should be worn to protect the skin. A sunscreen with the maximum solar protection factor rating should be applied to uncovered skin areas, and sunglasses should be worn to decrease photosensitivity.

The nurse monitors superficial vasculitic lesions for frequency and appearance. Appropriate skin hygiene measures, such as keeping the skin clean and dry, but moisturized, help to prevent skin breakdown.

To prevent oral lesions or when oral lesions are present, meticulous mouth care is given. Care is taken when brushing the teeth to prevent gum irritation with subsequent bleeding. Antifungal mouth rinses or tablets may be prescribed for secondary oral yeast infections.

Decreased Fatigue and Weakness.   The patient with SLE often complains of severe fatigue and generalized weak-

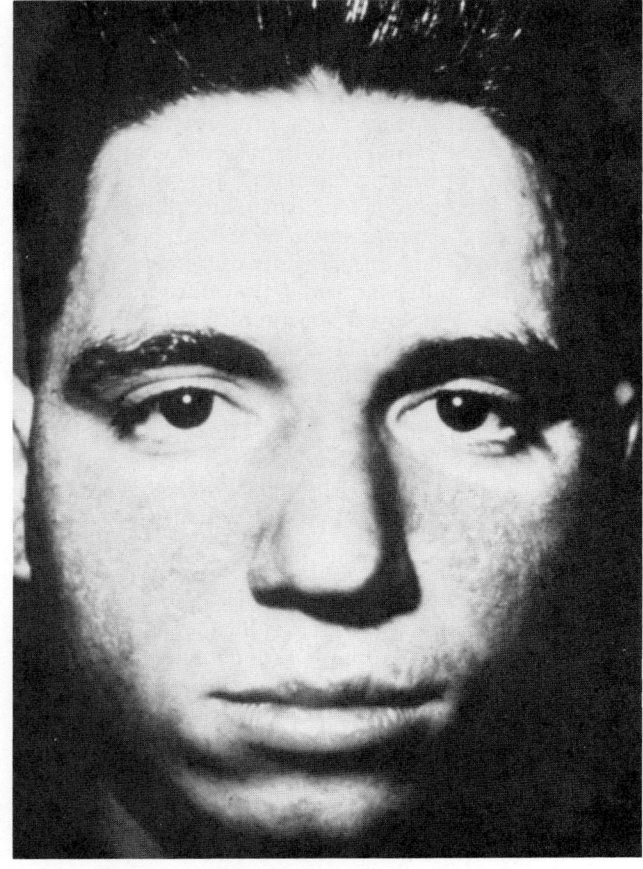

Figure 51-5. Butterfly rash of systemic lupus erythematosus. (From the AHP Arthritis Teaching Slide Collection, copyright 1980. Used by permission of the Arthritis Foundation.)

ness. Frequent rest periods combined with a 10- to 12-hour sleep each night is usually helpful in decreasing fatigue. Principles of energy conservation must be followed to compensate for the weakness experienced by these patients.

A Positive Self-concept.   One of the major changes in body image is the presence of the erythematous rash on the face and other parts of the body. Even when the disease is in remission, the rash may not disappear. Lupus patients, particularly young women, are usually very concerned about the disfigurement caused by the rash. Cosmetologists who specialize in skin disorders may be able to help the patient select appropriate cosmetics to cover the rash and make it less noticeable.

In addition to the skin abnormalities, joint deformity, severe fatigue and weakness, and the unpredictability of the disease contribute to a poor self-concept. The nurse and the family should try to understand this reaction and approach the patient in a realistic but optimistic manner. Further discussion of this goal is found in the section on rheumatoid arthritis.

Relief of Pain and Discomfort.   Drug therapy for the patient with SLE may relieve joint pain and discomfort, but is primarily aimed at decreasing the inflammatory response in the entire body. Patients with mild disease may be controlled by salicylate therapy or NSAIDs, but most patients also require steroid therapy, often in massive doses. (Discoid patients are not usually given systemic steroids.) When the patient does not respond to this drug regimen, immunosuppressive agents or pulse therapy (see p. 1146) may be utilized. Plasmapheresis, a technique in which immune complexes are removed from the patient's blood, is gaining more popularity in the treatment of SLE.

In addition to anti-inflammatory drugs for the relief of joint pain, other relief measures, previously described in this chapter, are employed. An interdisciplinary approach is helpful in managing lupus arthritis.

Promotion of the Grieving Process.   As in rheumatoid arthritis, patients with lupus erythematosus respond to their disease as persons with other chronic diseases. In addition, the SLE patient must face the possibility of severe, life-threatening complications. The nurse and other members of the health team must support the patient and help him through each stage of the grieving process. Hopefully, acceptance will be achieved.

Independence in ADLs.   Joint involvement combined with fatigue, weakness, and muscle inflammation may alter a patient's ability to perform ADLs independently. Nursing interventions for meeting this goal are discussed in the section on rheumtoid arthritis.

Attainment of Optimum Nutrition.   Anorexia may be compounded by dysphagia from esophagitis. Food selection for the dysphagic patient should include foods of soft, bolus-type consistency, such as mashed potatoes and gelatin. Liquids and hard, brittle foods are the most difficult to swallow for a dysphagic patient. Foods high in protein, vitamins, and iron should be encouraged with supplemental feedings as necessary to maintain weight.

▶ Evaluation

Specific outcome criteria for evaluation of nursing interventions are derived from the broad goals as outlined. Sample outcome criteria that are observable and measurable are included here.

Expected Outcomes

1. Maintains skin integrity
   a. Demonstrates no scaliness or itching of skin rash
   b. Achieves a decrease in erythema of skin rash
   c. Is free of skin ulceration
   d. Limits exposure time to sun or fluorescent lighting
   e. Is free of oral lesions
2. Experiences a decrease in fatigue and weakness
   a. Sleeps 10 to 12 hours each night
   b. Takes 2 to 3 naps (½ hour) each day
   c. Follows energy conservation principles
   d. Uses proper body mechanics
3. Develops positive self-concept
   a. Uses cosmetics as necessary to diminish the appearance of the skin rash
   b. Employs meticulous skin hygiene measures
   c. Expresses feelings to family
   d. Expresses feelings to health team members
   e. Socializes (conversation) with family members, friends, peers
   f. Participates in social activities, such as parties, clubs
   g. Demonstrates active interest and participation in hobby or diversional activity (*e.g.,* television, reading, sewing)
4. Achieves relief of pain and discomfort
   a. Has no observable signs of joint inflammation
   b. Experiences no limitation in joint movement
   c. Offers no subjective complaint of joint pain
   d. Does not request p.r.n. analgesic to supplement drug therapy regimen
5. Progresses through the grieving process
   a. Expresses feelings to family, significant others, and health team members
   b. Reaches acceptance stage of the grieving process
6. Achieves independence in activities of daily living
   a. Feeds, bathes, grooms, and dresses self without assistance
   b. Transports self outside of home environment without assistance
7. Attains or maintains optimum nutrition
   a. Eats at least three well-balanced meals per day
   b. Includes foods high in protein, iron, and vitamins in diet each day
   c. Keeps body weight at ideal or no less than 10% below ideal weight

▷ Progressive Systemic Sclerosis

Progressive systemic sclerosis (PSS) is the more accurate term for what is sometimes called "scleroderma." *Scleroderma* means hardening of the skin and is but one manifestation of a systemic, inflammatory disease in which there is chronic hardening and thickening of connective tissue throughout the body.

Pathophysiology

As the name implies, PSS is a progressive disease of connective tissue characterized by inflammatory, fibrotic, and degenerative changes. It is thought to be an autoimmune disease that affects women (of all races) two to three times more often than men. The first symptoms usually appear between the ages of 30 and 50. Like lupus erythematosus, PSS has a variable course with remissions and exacerbations; its prognosis, however, is not as optimistic as that for lupus.

The disease often begins with skin involvement. Initially, the inflammatory response causes edema formation with a resulting taut, smooth, and shiny skin appearance. The skin then undergoes fibrotic changes leading to loss of elasticity and movement. Eventually, the tissue degenerates and is not functional. This chain of events—from inflammation to degeneration—also occurs in blood vessels (vasculitis) and major organs and body systems, often resulting in death.

Assessment

Musculoskeletal Assessment.   Pain and stiffness of synovial joints are common in a patient with PSS. In some cases, polyarthritis like that seen in rheumatoid arthritis is present. Frequently associated with these findings is polymyositis, manifested by severe muscle weakness. The nurse assesses the joints and muscles as described in the discussion of rheumatoid arthritis.

Clinical Manifestations.   The disease starts insidiously on the face and hands, where the skin acquires a tense, wrinkle-free, bound-down appearance. The skin and the subcutaneous tissues become increasingly hard and rigid and cannot be pinched up from the underlying structures (hidebound). Wrinkles and lines are obliterated. The skin is dry since sweat secretion over the involved region is suppressed.

The face appears masklike, immobile, and expressionless, and the mouth becomes rigid. The buccal mucous membrane likewise may be affected. For years these changes may remain localized in the hands and the feet, but the condition spreads slowly. The extremities become stiff and immobile; the fingers semiflexed, immobile, and useless; the hands, clawlike.

The changes within the body, while not visible directly, are vastly more important than the visible changes. The heart muscle becomes fibrotic, causing dyspnea; the esophagus is hardened, interfering with swallowing; the lungs are scarred, impeding respiration; digestive disturbances occur due to hardening of the intestine; progressive renal failure may occur. A variety of other disturbances develop, including Raynaud's phenomenon (see p. 676), calcinosis (calcium deposits in tissues), and telangiectasis (small, red skin lesions caused by vessel dilation).

The patient with PSS is often referred to as a C-R-E-S-Ter, meaning that *c*alcinosis, *R*aynaud's phenomenon, *e*sophagitis, *s*clerodactyly (scleroderma of digits), and *te*langiectasias are all present. The occurrence of esophagitis indicates a poor prognosis.

Planning, Implementation, and Evaluation

Unfortunately, PSS does not usually respond to anti-inflammatory drug therapy as well as patients with rheumatoid arthritis or lupus erythematosus. Steroids and immunosuppressive agents are those most commonly used. The planning, implementation, and evaluation of nursing care for a patient with PSS is very similar to the care for a patient with lupus erythematosus. A discussion of nursing care is found in the discussion of systemic lupus erythematosus.

▷ Gout

Unlike the previously described connective tissue diseases, the cause and treatment of gout have been well established for many years. If treated appropriately, the pathologic changes resulting from gout may be halted and the disorder may be permanently controlled.

Pathophysiology

Gout is a disease manifested by joint inflammation and is caused by the deposit of uric acid crystals in joints and connective tissues. Uric acid is the end product of purine

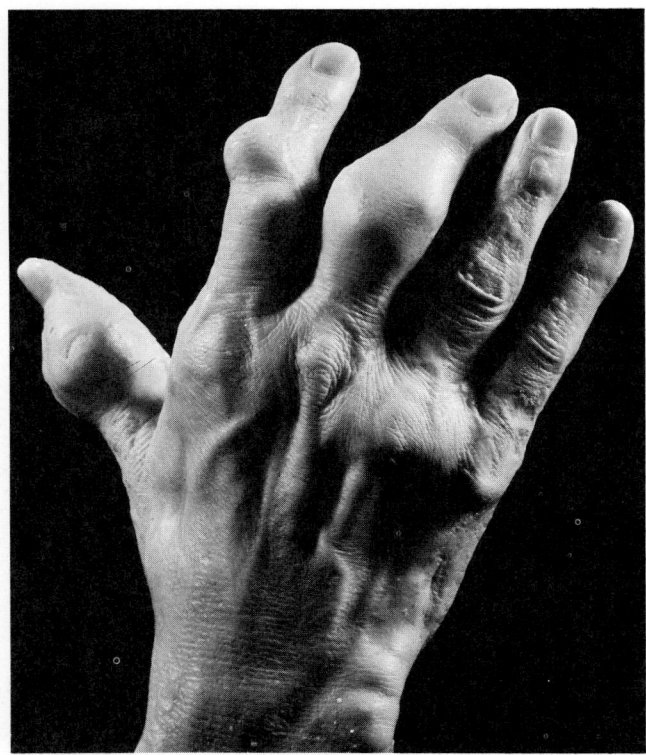

Figure 51-6. Accumulation of uric acid crystals on the knuckles of a patient with gout. (Photo courtesy of National Institute of Arthritis, Metabolism and Digestive Diseases.)

metabolism. Hyperuricemia, the persistent elevation of urates in the blood, is usually found in gout and is caused by *overproduction* or *underexcretion* of uric acid.

Primary gout may be due to a genetic defect of purine metabolism or a renal defect resulting in decreased excretion of uric acid. This disorder occurs most frequently in male patients, usually in their 40s.

In secondary gout (an acquired disease), hyperuricemia occurs in conditions in which there is an increase in cell turnover (leukemia, multiple myeloma, psoriasis) and an increase in cell breakdown. Or it may occur because renal excretion of uric acid is somehow blocked. Other causes of hyperuricemia and gout include prolonged ingestion of certain diuretic agents (thiazides) and aspirin, trauma, or the treatment of myeloproliferative disease.

Because of its low solubility, uric acid tends to precipitate and form deposits at various sites where blood flow is least active, including cartilaginous tissue. These masses of sodium urate crystals, called *tophi,* are deposited in the vicinity of the joints, particularly the great toe, on the knuckles (Fig. 51-6), and in the ears. Tophi may cause pressure symptoms, deformity, or ulceration of overlying skin and are generally considered to be a late sign.

In some patients, renal urate lithiasis (kidney stones) may be the earliest manifestation of gout. Chronic renal disease secondary to urate deposition may develop.

▶ **Assessment**

Musculoskeletal Assessment. The findings from the joint assessment of a patient with gout will depend on the phase of the disease process. During an acute gouty "attack," the patient displays *severe* joint inflammation, particularly in the great toe (podagra), ankle, and knee, causing extreme pain. The patient with acute gout cannot tolerate light touch to an inflamed joint.

During the intercurrent, or intercritical, phase, the patient is usually asymptomatic and no abnormalities are noted on physical assessment. In late stage or chronic gout, the patient presents with tophi, which may be palpable near joints and in the ears or may be internal. Joint deformity may also be present.

Clinical Manifestations. An attack of acute gout usually begins with sudden onset of severe pain in one or more of the peripheral joints, which may be accompanied by intense inflammation, swelling, and tenderness. The first joint of the great toe is most often affected; large joints may also be affected. Sometimes fever is present. An untreated attack of gout subsides in about 1 week. Gouty attacks may be precipitated by starvation, alcohol, fad diets, stress, and certain medications such as aspirin and thiazide diuretics.

The attacks usually recur at irregular intervals. After repeated acute attacks, gout may become chronic, leaving certain joints (particularly those of the hands) permanently disabled, deformed, and painful. Diagnosis is based on the presence of urate crystals noted in fluid aspirated from a joint cavity. Subcutaneous deposits of urates (tophi) are considered to be positive signs of gout. Roentgenograms of the joints reveal tophi and urate deposits.

Almost one half of chronic gout patients have renal involvement secondary to the development of urate kidney stones. Renal function tests are conducted to determine the extent of kidney involvement (see p. 968).

Patient Problems/Nursing Diagnoses

Based on the clinical manifestations, nursing history, and the diagnostic assessment data, the patient's major nursing problems may include alteration in comfort—severe pain related to joint inflammation; alteration in skin integrity related to tophi formation; and alteration in pattern of urinary elimination related to renal failure.

▶ **Planning and Implementation**

Goals

The goals for patients with gout include:

1. Relief of joint pain
2. Maintenance of skin integrity
3. Promotion of adequate renal function

Relief of Joint Pain. The treatment of the acute attack is directed toward relieving pain and inflammation by means of nonsteroidal anti-inflammatory drugs and colchicine (see Table 51-2). Colchicine, given early in the attack, often provides dramatic relief. A response to colchicine is regarded as diagnostic evidence of the disorder. Colchicine has no effect on uric acid metabolism. An initial dose of colchicine

is given and followed by doses every 1 to 2 hours until the pain is relieved or the patient develops symptoms of gastrointestinal irritability: diarrhea, nausea, and vomiting. The drug is then stopped temporarily. Joint pain and swelling start to subside in 6 to 12 hours after therapy is started.

Narcotics or analgesics may be needed for severe pain until specific therapy is effective. The patient is encouraged to rest in bed or a chair, with the affected limb protected (by a bed cradle) and elevated. Weight bearing is avoided until the attack subsides, since early ambulation may precipitate a recurrence. If joints in the hand, wrist, or elbow are involved, a splint may be worn to immobilize the hot and tender joint. Cold applications to the joint may be helpful.

For patients in whom there is an overproduction of uric acid or those who have nephrolithiasis or renal impairment, allopurinol (Zyloprim) may be given. Allopurinol is a xanthine-oxidase inhibitor that interferes with the conversion of the products of purine metabolism to uric acid. Thus, it inhibits uric acid synthesis. The administration of allopurinol generally produces a prompt fall in both serum and urinary uric acid. It is also used prophylactically during chemotherapy for myeloproliferative disorders.

Many persons with chronic gout have been relieved of their joint pain and have experienced increased joint mobility. Tophaceous deposits cease to form and draining urate sinuses tend to heal on this regimen. The dosage is based on serum urate determinations.

Agents that lower uric acid are used for long-term management to prevent complications (destructive joint disease, nephropathy) and to reduce the occurrence of acute attacks. Such a drug inhibits the reabsorption of uric acid by the renal tubules, thus resulting in increased excretion of uric acid, thereby lowering the serum urate level. In time, the size of tophi is reduced, and the formation of new tophi is prevented.

One such drug is probenecid (Benemid), which apparently has no more significant side-effects than an occasional mild gastrointestinal upset and a tendency to constipation. However, this drug is not to be given in conjunction with aspirin or any other salicylate, because each tends to offset the action of the other. Another useful uricosuric drug is sulfinpyrazone (Anturane), which acts similarly to probenecid. Anturane and salicylates are also mutually antagonistic and should not be administered together. Once uricosuric drug therapy is initiated, the urinary concentration of urates may rise to such heights that crystals may precipitate out of solution, causing urolithiasis and renal complications. To avoid this complication, a large fluid intake (at least 8 glasses) is encouraged, to assure a high 24-hour urinary volume.

Maintenance of Skin Integrity. Tophi may become ulcerated and infected due to irritation by clothing and subsequent draining. Care should be taken to provide meticulous skin hygiene measures and to prevent injury to tophaceous areas. Draining tophi should be covered and topical antibiotic ointment applied.

Promotion of Renal Function. In all phases of gout, unless otherwise contraindicated, fluids should be encouraged to promote the excretion of excess uric acid, which could deposit as stones. Intake and output are carefully monitored.

Foods high in purines should be avoided in the diet; sardines, anchovies, shellfish, and organ meats are particularly high in purine content. The physician may prescribe a protein-restricted diet in an attempt to decrease purine intake.

It is more difficult for uric acid to precipitate as urate crystals in the presence of alkaline urine. Therefore, the patient is instructed to eat alkaline-ash foods, such as milk, potatoes, and citrus fruits. Sodium bicarbonate or citrate solution may be given to maintain a high urine pH.

▶ Evaluation

Specific outcome criteria for evaluation of nursing interventions are derived from the broad goals as outlined. Sample outcome criteria that are observable and measurable are included here.

Expected Outcomes

1. Achieves relief of joint pain
   a. Experiences no future attacks of acute gout
   b. Exhibits no joint inflammation or deformity
   c. Continues drug regimen in the absence of acute attacks
2. Maintains skin integrity
   a. Experiences a decrease in the presence of tophi
   b. Exhibits no skin ulceration over tophaceous areas
   c. Is free of infection of tophi
3. Demonstrates adequate renal function
   a. Increases fluid intake to at least 2000 ml per day
   b. Avoids foods high in purine content
   c. Eats foods high in alkaline-ash content to maintain a urine pH of 7 or higher
   d. Maintains a urine output of at least 50 ml per hour
   e. Avoids fad diets, starvation, alcohol, stress, and drugs that interfere with uric acid excretion

▷ Other Connective Tissue Diseases

There are approximately 100 known kinds of connective tissue disease. While the most common disorders have been presented in this chapter, several other diseases will be described in lesser detail. The appropriate nursing care may be extracted from the previous discussion.

Reiter's Syndrome.   Reiter's syndrome affects young adult males and is characterized primarily by urethritis, arthritis, and conjunctivitis. Dermatitis and ulcerations of the mouth and penis may also be present. Treatment includes salicylates, nonsteroidal anti-inflammatory agents, and corticosteroids.

Ankylosing Spondylitis (Marie-Strümpell Disease).
Ankylosing spondylitis is a systemic inflammatory disease of the cartilaginous joints of the spine and surrounding tissues. As the disease progresses, the entire spine may become ankylosed, causing respiratory compromise and complications. Extra-articular manifestations such as iritis and cardiac conduction disturbances may also occur. The drugs of choice are salicylates and NSAIDs.

Psoriatic Arthritis.   Psoriatic arthritis, as the name implies, is associated with a skin disorder known as psoriasis (see p. 1178). Corticosteroids often produce marked improvement in both the skin and joint symptoms.

Necrotizing Arteritis.   *Arteritis* is a term referring to a group of disorders in which vasculitis (particularly the arteries) is the major manifestation. Vital organs and body systems are deprived of blood supply due to arterial wall inflammation. Examples of these disorders are periarteritis nodosa (polyarteritis), giant cell arteritis (such as temporal arteritis), and Takayasu's (aortic) arteritis. In most cases, corticosteroid therapy is the treatment of choice, but immunosuppressants may also be given.

▷ Bibliography

Books

Bates B. A Guide to Physical Examination. Philadelphia, JB Lippincott, 1983.

Bluestone R. Rheumatology. Boston, Houghton Mifflin, 1980.

Burns KR and Johnson PJ. Health Assessment in Clinical Practice. Englewood Cliffs, New Jersey, Prentice-Hall, 1980.

Ehrlich GE. Rehabilitation Management of Rheumatic Conditions. Baltimore, Williams & Wilkins, 1980.

Cohen AS. Rheumatology and Immunology. New York, Grune & Stratton, 1979.

Currey HLF (ed). Mason and Currey's Clinical Rheumatology. Philadelphia, JB Lippincott, 1980.

Fischbach FT. A Manual of Laboratory Diagnostic Tests. Philadelphia, JB Lippincott, 1980.

Giansiracusa DF and Kantrowitz FG. Rheumatic and Metabolic Bone Diseases in the Elderly. Lexington, Massachusetts, DC Heath, 1982.

Golding DN. A Synopsis of Rheumatic Diseases. Littleton, Massachusetts, John Wright-PSG, 1982.

Gordon DA (ed). Rheumatoid Arthritis. Garden City, New York, Medical Examination, 1981.

Hughes GRV. Connective Tissue Diseases. Oxford, Blackwell Scientific, 1979.

Kelley WN et al. Textbook of Rheumatology, Vols 1 & 2. Philadelphia, WB Saunders, 1981.

Malasanos L et al. Health Assessment. St Louis, CV Mosby, 1981.

McCarty DJ (ed). Arthritis and Allied Conditions. Philadelphia, Lea & Febiger, 1979.

Nurse's Guide to Drugs. Horsham, Pennsylvania, Intermed Communications, 1980.

Price SA and Wilson LM. Pathophysiology: Clinical Concepts of Disease Processes. New York, McGraw-Hill, 1982.

Spitell JA Jr. Clinical Medicine. Hagerstown, Maryland, Harper & Row, 1980.

Swinson DR and Swinburn WR. Rheumatology. New York, John Wiley & Sons, 1980.

Thompson JM and Bowers AC. Clinical Manual of Health Assessment. St Louis, CV Mosby, 1980.

Thompson RA (ed). Recent Advances in Clinical Immunology. London, Churchill Livingstone, 1980.

Articles

Bunch TW and Duffy JD. Disease-modifying drugs for progressive rheumatoid arthritis. Mayo Clin Proc 1980 Mar; 55(1):161–179.

Fries JF et al. Measurement of patient outcome in arthritis. Arthritis Rheum 1980 Feb; 23(2):137–145.

Gibson T et al. Renal impairment and gout. Ann Rheum Dis 1980 Oct; 39(5):417–423.

Gotch PM. Teaching patients about adrenal corticosteroids. Am J Nurs 1981 Jan; 81(1):78–81.

Hunder GG and Bunch TW. Treatment of rheumatoid arthritis. Bull Rheum Dis 1982; 32(1):1–6.

Jette AM. Functional capacity evaluation, an empirical approach. Arch Phys Med Rehabil 1980 Feb; 61(2):85–89.

Lanham J and Hughes GRV. The place of antimalarials in rheumatology. Ann Rheum Dis 1981 June; 40(3):323–324.

Meenan RF, Gertman PM, and Mason JH. Measuring health status in arthritis, the arthritis impact measurement scales. Arthritis Rheum 1980 Feb; 23(2):146–152.

Parry HF. Plasma exchange in systemic lupus erythematosus. Ann Rheum Dis 1981 June; 40(3):224–228.

Programmed Instruction: Patient assessment: Examining joints of the upper and lower extremities. Am J Nurs 1981 Apr; 81(4):763–786.

Schwarz HA et al. Muscle biopsy in polymyositis and dermatomyositis: A clinicopathological study. Ann Rheum Dis 1980 Oct; 39(5):500–507.

Strand V and Tatal N. Advances in the diagnosis and concept of Sjögren's syndrome. Bull Rheum Dis 1980; 39(9):1046–1050.

Agencies*
Governmental

National Institute of Arthritis, Diabetes, and Digestive and Kidney Diseases, National Institutes of Health, Bethesda, Maryland 20205

Voluntary

American Occupational Therapy Association, 1383 Piccard Drive, Suite 301, Rockville, Maryland 20850

American Physical Therapy Association, 1156 15th St., N.W., Washington, D.C. 20005

Arthritis Foundation, 3400 Peachtree Rd., N.E., Suite 1101, Atlanta, Georgia 30326

National Easter Seal Society for Crippled Children and Adults, 2023 W. Ogden Ave., Chicago, Illinois 60612

* See also Rehabilitation Agencies, Chapter 14.

Unit XIV

Integumentary Problems

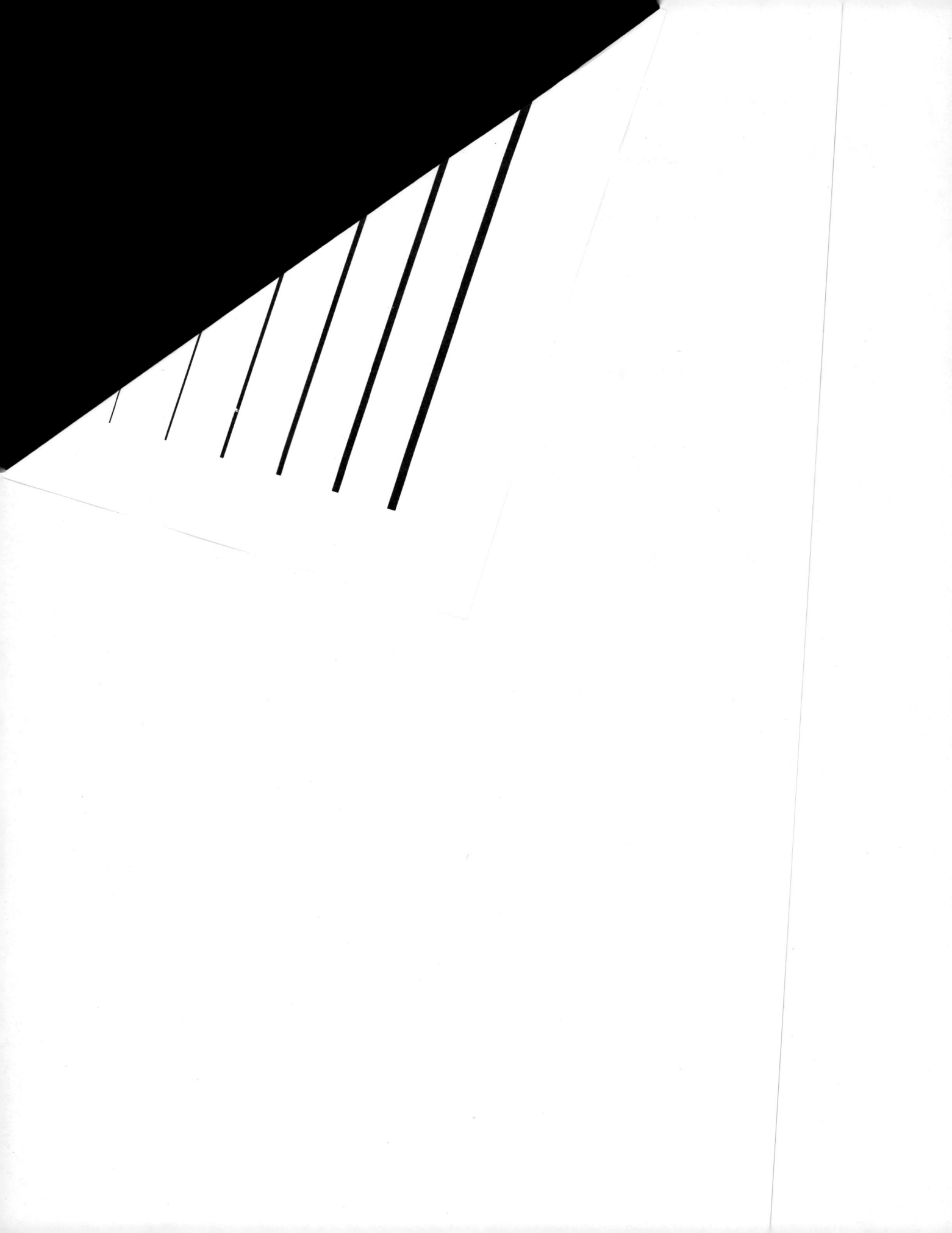

52

Management of Patients With Dermatologic Problems

▷ Physiologic Overview

The skin is a structure that is indispensable for human life. It forms a barrier between the internal organs and the external environment and participates in many vital functions of the body. The skin is continuous with the mucous membrane at the external openings of the organs of the digestive, respiratory, and urogenital systems. Because disorders of the skin are readily visible, dermatologic complaints are frequently the primary reason for patient visits.

Anatomy of the Skin

The skin is composed of two layers of tissue, the *epidermis*, an outer layer, in contact with the environment, and a deeper layer called the *dermis*. The epidermis consists of live, continuously dividing epithelial cells covered on the surface by dead cells that were originally deeper and were pushed upward by newly developing cells underneath. The dead cells are constantly flaking off from the skin, frequently in irregular patches. These dead cells contain large amounts of *keratin,* an insoluble, fibrous protein that forms the outer barrier of the skin. The epidermis is devoid of blood vessels and has few nerve endings. The superficial layers of the epidermis can be shaved from the body without pain or blood loss. The epidermis is modified in different areas of the body. Over the palms of the hands and the soles of the feet it is thickened and contains increased amounts of keratin, in contrast to the thin epidermis over most of the rest of the body. The thickness of the epidermis can increase with use, as is the case, for example, with the hands of a laborer.

The dermis is a broad layer of connective tissue that underlies the epidermal layer. It is composed of collagen and elastic fibers and contains blood and lymph vessels, nerves, sweat and sebaceous glands, and hair roots. Interdigitation between dermis and epidermis produces ripples on the surface of the skin. On the fingertips, these ripples are called *fingerprints.* They are perhaps a person's most individualistic characteristic and they almost never change.

With aging, the number of elastic fibers in the dermis progressively decreases, and the skin becomes wrinkled.

The color of the skin is determined by the pigment called *melanin,* which is produced by cells in the epidermis called *melanocytes.* The skin of black persons and the darker areas of the skin on white persons (for example, the nipple) contain large amounts of this pigment. Production of melanin by melanocytes is largely under the control of a hormone secreted from the hypothalamus of the brain, called melanocyte-stimulating hormone (MSH). Increased production of melanin occurs on exposure to ultraviolet light, such as occurs with suntanning.

The skin is anchored to the muscles and bones underneath by subcutaneous tissue composed of connective tissue interlaced with fat. Fat is deposited and distributed according to the person's sex and in part accounts for the difference in body shape between men and women. Overeating results in increased deposition of fat beneath the skin.

Hair. Hair is present over the entire body except for the palms of the hands and soles of the feet. The hair consists of a root formed in the dermis and a hair shaft that projects beyond the skin. It grows in a cavity called a *hair follicle.* The proliferation of cells in the bulb of the hair causes the hair to form. Hairs in different parts of the body serve different functions. The hairs of the eyes (eyebrows and lashes), nose, and ears screen dust, bugs, and airborne debris. Hair of the skin serves as thermal insulation in lower animals. This function is enhanced during cold or fright by piloerection (hairs "standing on end") caused by contraction of the tiny arrector muscles attached to the hair follicle. The piloerector response that occurs in humans is probably vestigial. The color of hair is due to the presence of varying amounts of melanin within the hair shaft. Gray or white hair is the result of loss of pigment. Growth of hair in certain locations on the body is under the control of sex hormones. The best examples are the hair on the face (beard and mustache) and on the body trunk that are controlled by the presence of the male hormones (androgens).

Nails. On the dorsal surface of the fingers and toes, a hard, transparent plate of keratin, called the *nail,* overlies the skin. The nail grows from its root, which lies under a thin fold of skin called the *cuticle.* The nail helps to protect the fingers and toes, in order to preserve their highly developed sensory function, and aids in the performance of certain fine functions of the fingers, such as picking up small objects.

Glands of the Skin. Sebaceous glands are associated with hair follicles. The ducts of the sebaceous glands empty an oily secretion onto the space between the hair follicle and the hair shaft. For each hair there is a sebaceous gland, whose secretions oil the hair and render the skin soft and pliable.

Sweat glands are found in the skin over most of the body surface. They are heavily concentrated on the palms of the hands and soles of the feet. Only the glans penis, the margins of the lips, the external ear, and the nail bed are devoid of sweat glands. Sweat glands are subclassified into two categories: *eccrine* and *apocrine.* The eccrine sweat glands are found in all areas of the skin. Their ducts open directly onto the skin surface. The apocrine sweat glands

are larger, and in contrast to that of the eccrine glands, their secretion contains parts of the secretory cells. They are located in the axillae, anal region, scrotum, and labia majora. Their ducts generally open onto hair follicles. The apocrine glands become active at the time of puberty. In the female, they enlarge and recede with each menstrual cycle.

Apocrine glands produce a milky sweat that is broken down by bacteria to produce the characteristic underarm odor. Specialized apocrine glands called *cerumenous glands* are found in the external ear, where they produce wax (*cerumen*).

The thin, watery secretion called *sweat* is produced in the basal coiled portion of the eccrine gland and is released into its narrow duct. Sweat is composed predominantly of water and contains about half of the salt content of the blood plasma. Sweat is released from eccrine glands in response to elevated ambient temperature. The rate of sweat secretion is under the control of the sympathetic nervous system. Excessive sweating of the palms and soles, axillae, forehead, and other areas may occur in response to pain and stress.

Functions of the Skin
Protective Function. The skin protects the body against invasion by bacteria and foreign matter. The thickened skin of the palms and soles provides the tough covering necessary for the constant trauma occurring in these areas.

The epidermis is relatively impermeable to most chemical substances. It is this property of skin that allows it to be an effective barrier for protection. Some substances slowly pass through the skin, however, including gases such as oxygen, nitrogen, and carbon dioxide. Lipid-soluble substances tend to move more easily through the skin than do electrolytes and other nonlipid-soluble substances. Their route of penetration into the skin is probably through the follicular orifice and the sebaceous glands. The rate of absorption of a topical medication will depend on how rapidly its suspending vehicle can penetrate the skin.

Sensory Function. Stimulation of the receptor endings of nerves in the skin allows us to constantly monitor the conditions of our immediate environment. The primary functions of the receptors in the skin are to sense temperature, pain, light touch, and pressure (or heavy touch). Different nerve endings are responsible for responding to each of the different stimuli. Although the nerve endings are distributed over the entire body, they are more concentrated in some areas than in others. For example, the fingertips are much more densely innervated than the skin of the back.

Water Balance. Skin forms a barrier that prevents loss of water and electrolytes from the internal environment and also prevents the subcutaneous tissues from drying out. When skin is damaged, such as occurs with a severe burn, for example, large quantities of fluids and electrolytes can be rapidly lost, possibly leading to circulatory collapse, shock, and death. On the other hand, the skin is not completely impermeable to water. Small amounts of water continuously evaporate from the skin surface. This evaporation, called *insensible perspiration,* amounts to approximately 500 ml per day for a normal adult. Insensible water loss may vary with the body temperature, and in the presence of fever, these losses can increase. During immersion in water, the skin can accumulate water up to approximately three or four times its normal weight. A common example of this is the swelling of the skin after prolonged bathing.

Temperature Regulation.   The body continuously produces heat as a result of the metabolism of foodstuffs to produce energy. This heat is dissipated primarily through the skin. Three major physical processes are involved in loss of heat from the body to the environment. The first process, *radiation,* is the ability of a body to give off its heat to another object of lower temperature situated at a distance. The second process, *conduction,* is the transfer of heat from the body to a cooler object in contact with it. Heat transferred by conduction to the air surrounding the body is removed by the third process, *convection,* which consists of bulk movement of warm air molecules away from the body. Evaporation from the skin aids the process of heat loss by conduction. Heat is conducted through the skin into water molecules on its surface, causing the water to evaporate. The source of the water on the skin surface may be insensible perspiration, sweat, or water from the environment. Normally, all of these mechanisms for heat loss are utilized. However, when the ambient temperature is very high, radiation and convection are not effective and evaporation from the skin constitutes the only means for heat loss.

Under normal conditions, metabolic heat production is exactly balanced by heat loss, and the internal temperature of the body is maintained constant at approximately 37° C (98.6° F). The rate of heat loss depends primarily on the surface temperature of the skin, which is in turn a function of the skin blood flow. Skin is richly supplied with blood vessels that carry heat to the skin from the core of the body. Blood flow through these vessels is controlled primarily by the sympathetic nervous system. Increased blood flow to the skin results in delivery of more heat to the skin and a greater rate of heat loss from the body. On the other hand, decreased skin blood flow decreases the skin temperature and helps conserve heat for the body. When the temperature of the body begins to fall, such as occurs on a cold day, the blood vessels of the skin constrict and reduce heat loss from the body. This can be demonstrated by immersing the hand in cold water.

Sweating is another process by which the body can regulate the rate of heat loss. Sweating is increased when body temperature starts to rise. In extremely hot environments, the rate of sweat production may be as high as 1 liter per hour. Under some circumstances, for example, with emotional stress, sweating may occur on a reflex basis unrelated to the necessity to lose heat from the body.

Wheal and Flare Reaction.   Stroking the skin with sufficient firmness to cause local injury results in local reddening. This is followed within a few minutes by localized swelling and more diffuse redness around the injury site. The combination of the swelling (called a *wheal*) and the diffuse redness (called a *flare*) constitutes a normal reaction of the skin to injury. These responses are due to local edema secondary to increased capillary permeability and dilatation of the surrounding arterioles. The wheal and flare reaction is due to the action of locally released hormones, such as histamine and kinins, upon the local blood vessels.

▷ General Approach to Care

▶ Assessment

Skin problems are commonly encountered, and skin-related complaints account for about 7% of all ambulatory patient visits in this country. Many systemic conditions may be accompanied by dermatologic manifestations. Any patient hospitalized with a medical or surgical condition may suddenly develop itching and a rash. Many systemic conditions (hepatitis, cancer) may first announce themselves with dermatologic manifestations.

Nursing History.   The data base that constitutes the basis of the nursing history may be obtained by asking the following questions:

- When did you first notice this skin problem?
- Has it occurred previously?
- Are there any other symptoms besides the rash?
- What site was first affected?
- What did the rash/lesion look like when it first appeared?
- Where and how fast did it spread?
- Are there itching, burning, tingling, or crawling sensations? loss of sensation?
- Is it worse at a particular time? season?
- Do you have any idea how it started?
- Do you have a history of hay fever, asthma, hives, eczema, allergies?
- Does anyone in your family have skin problems or rashes?
- Did the eruptions appear after certain foods were eaten?
- Was there a relationship between a specific event and the outbreak of the rash/lesion?
- What medications are you taking?
- What medication (ointment, cream, salve) have you put on the lesion? (Include over-the-counter medications.)
- What is your occupation?
- What in your immediate environment (plants, animals, chemicals, infections) might be precipitating this problem? Anything new or any changes in the environment?
- Does anything touching your skin cause a rash?
- Is there anything else you wish to talk about in regard to this problem?

Assessment of Skin Lesions.   Assessment of the skin involves the entire skin area, including the mucous membranes, scalp, and nails. *Inspection,* along with *palpation,* constitutes the chief procedure used in examining the skin and requires that the room be well lighted, as well as warm. The patient should completely disrobe and should be adequately draped.

Examine the general appearance of the skin, observing color, temperature, moisture, dryness, skin texture (rough or smooth), and the condition of the hair and nails. Skin turgor and elasticity are also determined by palpation.

A preliminary look at the eruption or lesion should help to identify the type of dermatosis (abnormal skin condition) and indicate whether the lesion is primary or secondary. At the same time, the anatomical distribution of the eruption should be noted, since certain diseases tend to affect certain sites of the body and are distributed in characteristic patterns and shapes. To determine the extent of the distribution, the left and right sides of the body should be compared while the color and shape of the lesion are noted. Following observation, the lesions are palpated to determine their texture, shape, and border and to see if they are soft or filled with fluid, or hard and fixed to the surrounding tissue.

A metric ruler is used to measure the size of the lesions so that any further extension can be compared with this initial baseline measurement. The dermatosis is then documented on the patient's record; it should be described clearly and in detail, using precise terminology.

Types of Skin Lesions. Skin lesions can be described as *primary* (caused directly by the disease process and are characteristic) or *secondary* (result from external causes, such as scratching, trauma, infections, or changes caused by

healing), depending on the stage of development. They are further divided according to type and appearance, as indicated in the following definitions (Fig. 52-1):

Primary Lesions (Initial Lesions)

Macule—a nonelevated discoloration of the skin of various shapes and colors
Papule—a solid, elevated, palpable lesion less than 1 cm (0.4 inch) in diameter
Nodule—a raised, solid lesion that is larger and deeper than a papule
Vesicle—a small elevation of the skin that is filled with clear fluid

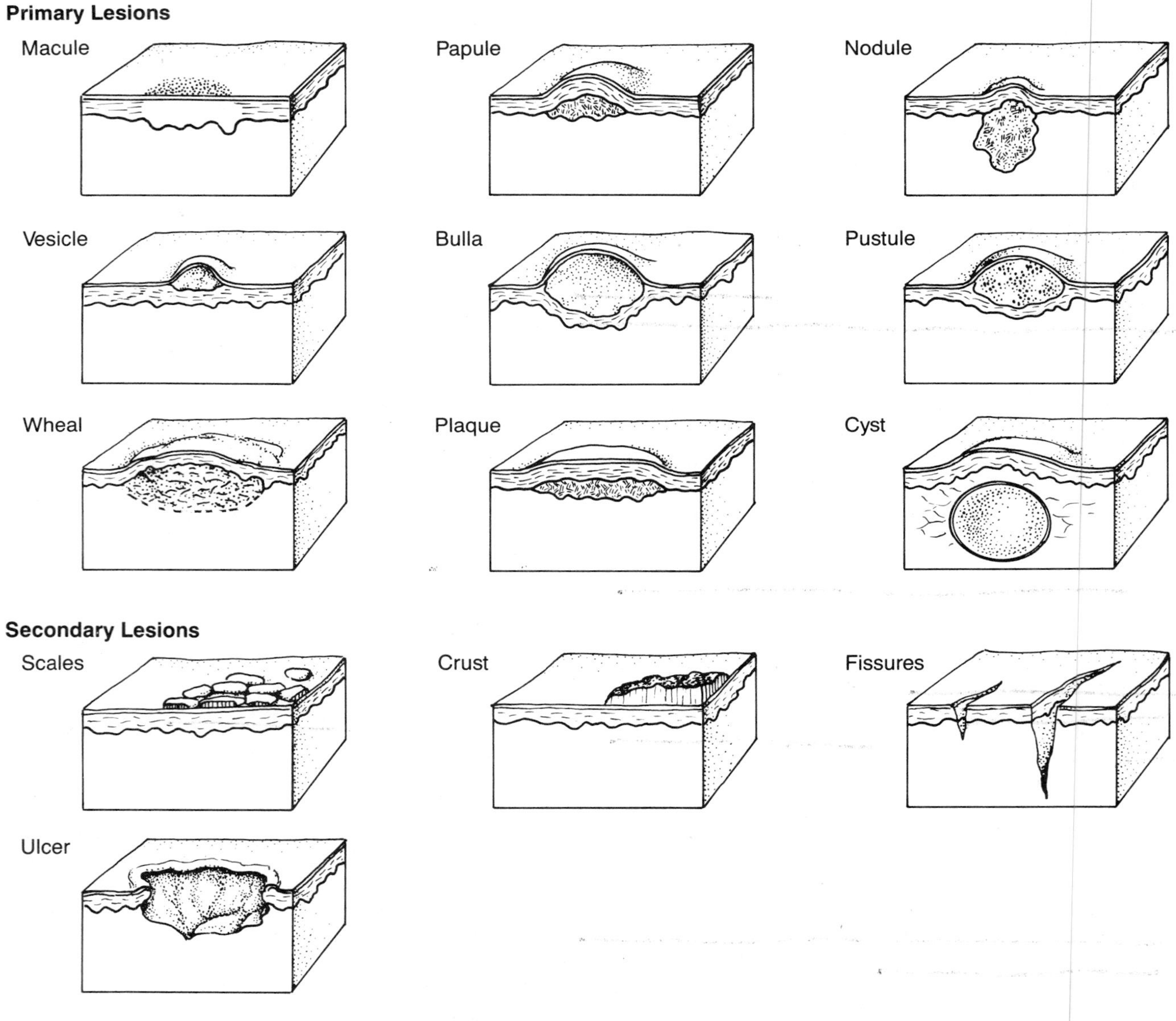

Primary Lesions

Secondary Lesions

Figure 52-1. Types of skin lesions. (From Lindberg J, Hunter M, and Kruszewski A: Introduction to Person-Centered Nursing. Philadelphia, JB Lippincott, 1983.)

Bulla—a large vesicle or blister larger than 1 cm (0.4 inch) in diameter

Pustule—a lesion that contains pus; may form as a result of purulent changes in a vesicle

Wheal—transient elevation of the skin caused by edema of the dermis and surrounding capillary dilatation

Plaque—a solid, elevated lesion on the skin or mucous membrane, greater than 1 cm (0.4 inch) in its largest diameter

Cyst—a tumor that contains semisolid or liquid material

Secondary Lesions.   As the term implies, these are the changes that take place in primary lesions and possibly modify them; they include:

Scales—heaped-up, horny layers of dead epidermis; may develop as a result of inflammatory changes

Crusts—a covering formed from serum, blood, or pus drying on the skin

Excoriations—linear scratch marks or traumatized area of skin

Fissures—cracks in the skin, usually from marked drying and long-standing inflammation

Ulcers—lesions formed by local destruction of the epidermis and part or all of the underlying dermis

Lichenification—thickening of skin accompanied by accentuation of skin markings

Scar—a fibrotic change in the skin following a destructive process

Atrophy—loss of substance

Documentation.   After the characteristic distribution of the lesion has been determined, the following information should be obtained and described clearly and in detail:

- What is (are) the color(s) of the lesion?
- Is there redness, heat, pain, or swelling?
- How large an area is involved? Where is it?
- Is the eruption macular, papular, scaling, oozing, discrete, confluent?
- What is the distribution of the lesion—symmetrical, linear, circular?

Chart 52-1 presents the terms commonly used in dermatology.

Diagnostic Tests.   Skin biopsies, immunologic testing, patch testing, and cultures and smears are used to diagnose skin conditions.

Assessing Patients With Dark or Black Skin

The gradations of color that occur in dark-skinned persons are largely determined by genetic transmission; they may be described as light, medium, or dark. In dark-skinned persons, melanin is produced at a faster rate and in larger quantities than in lighter-skinned persons. Healthy, dark skin has a reddish base or undertone. The buccal mucosa, tongue, lips, and nails normally appear pink.

In examining the dark-skinned or black patient, it is important to have good lighting and to look at the skin and the nail beds as well as in the mouth. All suspicious areas should be palpated.

Chart 52-1
Definition of Terms Commonly Used in Dermatology

Annular—ring shaped
Arcuate—in the form of an arc
Circinate—circular
Confluent—lesions run together or join
Discoid—disc-shaped
Discrete—lesions remain separate
Eczematoid or eczematous—inflammation with a tendency to thicken, scale, vesiculate, crust, or weep
Erythema—red
Generalized—widespread eruption
Grouped—lesions clustered together
Guttate—droplike
Gyrate—twisted spiral
Herpetiform—grouped vesicles
Iris—circle within a circle
Keratosis—circumscribed horny thickening
Keratotic—horny thickening
Linear—in lines
Moniliform—beaded
Multiform—more than one kind of skin lesion
Polymorphous—more than one kind of skin lesion
Serpiginous—snakelike, creeping
Telangiectasia—relatively permanent dilatation of superficial vessels
Universal—entire skin affected
Zosteriform—linear arrangement along a nerve

(Adapted from Lewis GM and Wheeler CE: Practical Dermatology. Philadelphia, WB Saunders.)

Erythema.   Because there is a tendency for black skin to assume a purplish–grayish cast when an inflammatory process is present, it may be difficult to detect erythema. To determine possible inflammation, the skin should be palpated for increased warmth or for signs of smoothness (edema) or hardness. The adjacent lymph nodes are also palpated.

Rash.   In instances of itching, the patient should be asked to indicate what areas of the body are involved. The skin is then stretched gently to decrease the reddish tone and make the rash stand out. The differences in skin texture are then palpated by running the tips of the fingers lightly over the skin. Usually, the borders of the rash can be felt. Included in the examination are the patient's mouth and ears. (Sometimes rubeola will cause a red cast to appear on the tip of the ears.) Finally, the patient's temperature is checked and the lymph nodes are palpated.

Cyanosis.   When a person with black skin goes into shock, the skin usually assumes a grayish cast. To determine signs of cyanosis, the area around the mouth, lips, and over the cheekbones and earlobes should be checked. Other indicative signs to check include a cold, clammy skin; a rapid, thready pulse; and rapid, shallow respirations. When the palpebral conjunctivae are checked for petechiae, it is important to realize that deposits of melanin may normally appear in this area and should not be misinterpreted as petechiae.

Skin Problems in the Black Race.   Because changes in skin color can occur in the black race, these changes are noticeable and cause great distress to the patient. For example, hypopigmentation (loss or decrease in skin color), which may be due to vitiligo (a condition characterized by destruction of melanocytes in small or large skin areas), may cause more concern in the dark-skinned person since it is so readily visible. Hyperpigmentation (increase in color) may occur after disease or injury to the skin. However, pigmented streaks in the nails are considered to be normal. On the other hand, a pigmented nasal crease below the eye may be an external sign of allergy.

In general, persons with black skin suffer from the same skin conditions as those with white skin, although they are less apt to have skin cancer. On the other hand, members of the black race and other dark-skinned persons have a greater propensity for keloid formation, and for disorders of follicular occlusion.

Patient Problems/Nursing Diagnoses

Based on the patient's clinical manifestations and diagnostic assessment data, the patient's major problems include alteration in comfort (itching and discomfort) related to skin condition; alteration in skin integrity (inflammation, oozing, and crusting) related to scratching, trauma, and infection; and anxiety or depression related to altered body image.

▶ **Planning and Implementation**

Goals

The patient's goals include:

1. Relief of itching and discomfort
2. Control of inflammation, oozing, and crusting
3. Mobilization of psychological resources to cope with anxiety/depression

The major objectives of therapy are to (1) prevent damage to the healthy skin, (2) prevent secondary infection, (3) reverse the inflammatory process, and (4) relieve the symptoms.

Preventing Damage to Healthy Skin.   Some skin problems are markedly aggravated by soap and water. Therefore, bathing routines are modified according to the condition being treated.

Denuded skin, whether the area of desquamation is large or small, is excessively prone to damage by chemicals and trauma. The friction of a towel, if applied with vigor, is sufficient to excite a brisk inflammatory response that causes any existing lesion to flare up and increase in extent. Thus, the essence of skin care and protection in bathing a patient with abnormal skin is to use a mild superfatted soap or soap substitute and to ensure the complete removal of the soap when rinsing, before blotting the area dry with a soft cloth. Deodorant soaps should be avoided in these patients.

Pledgets saturated with oil will aid in loosening crusts, removing exudates, or freeing an adherent dry dressing. The dressing also may be saturated with sterile physiologic salt solution or dilute (3%) hydrogen peroxide, which softens it and permits it to be pulled away gently.

Preventing Secondary Infection.   Potentially infectious skin lesions should be regarded strictly as such, and proper precautions should be observed until the diagnosis is established (see Wound and Skin Precautions, p. 1488). Some lesions with pus contain infectious material. Others, such as occur in acne, have no infectious material. Although some genital lesions are suspect, most are minor irritations.

- If the condition is infectious, disposable gloves are worn by the nurse and the physician. Dressings removed from infected skin should be wrapped in paper and burned as soon as possible.

Reversing the Inflammatory Process.   The type of skin lesion (oozing, infected, or dry) usually dictates the local medication or treatment that is prescribed. As a rule, if the skin is acutely inflamed (hot, red, and swollen) and is oozing, it is best to apply wet dressings and soothing lotions. In chronic conditions in which the skin surface is dry and scaly, water-soluble emulsions, creams, ointments, and pastes are used. The therapy must be changed as the response indicates. Explain to the patient that he must contact the physician or clinic if the medication or compresses seem to irritate the dermatosis. Success or failure of skin therapy rests upon adequate instruction and motivation of the patient and the interest and support of the health personnel.

For a general outline of nursing management of the patient with a dermatosis, see Chart 52-2.

▶ **Evaluation**

Expected Outcomes

1. Achieves relief of itching and discomfort
   a. Avoids use of soap and hot water
   b. Avoids external heat
   c. Keeps environment cool and humidified
   d. Uses bath oils/prescribed emollients
   e. Avoids mechanical irritants and rough clothing
2. Performs self-care measures to control inflammation, oozing, and crusting
   a. Applies wet dressings as prescribed
   b. Takes prescribed therapeutic baths
   c. Applies topical medications
   d. Performs own dermatologic treatments
3. Mobilizes psychological resources
   a. Uses progressive muscle relaxation techniques
   b. Improves personal grooming
   c. Reflects on accomplishments
   d. Identifies intellectual/artistic pursuits for ego strengthening
   e. Voices realistic expectations

Psychosocial Aspects of Dermatologic Problems

Because patients with skin conditions (1 in 20 persons) can see and feel their problems, they are more apt to be disturbed by their ailments than are patients with other conditions.

Chart 52-2
The Patient With a Dermatosis

Goals and Interventions of Nursing Management

Goals

- To control itching and relieve pain
- To reverse the inflammatory process
- To control oozing and prevent crust formation
- To avoid skin damage
- To ensure efficacy of topical applications

Interventions

A. To control itching and relieve pain:
   1. Examine area of involvement.
      a. Attempt to discover the cause of discomfort.
      b. Record observations in detail, using descriptive terminology.
      c. Be aware that *sudden* onset of a generalized rash may be from a drug allergy.
   2. Advise patient to employ measures that produce vasoconstriction.
      a. Maintain cool environment.
      b. Remove excess clothing or bedding.
      c. Provide tepid, cooling baths.
      d. Apply cool, wet dressings.
   3. Treat dryness (xerosis) with lubricating creams or lotions applied after bathing and before drying to enhance hydration.
   4. Apply prescribed lotions or ointments.
   5. Supply analgesic and antipruritic medications as indicated.
   6. Administer tranquilizing agents or sedative drugs, as necessary.
   7. Instruct patient to refrain from self-medication with salves or lotions that are commercially advertised.
   8. Assist the anxious patient to identify and cope with his problems.

B. To reverse the inflammatory process:
   1. Apply continuous or intermittent wet dressings to reduce intensity of inflammation.

2. Remove crusts and scales before applying topical medications.
3. Use topical applications containing corticosteroid drugs, as indicated.
   a. Rub topical medicaments well into skin to enhance penetration.
   b. Observe lesion periodically for changes in response to therapy.
   c. Instruct patients of possible ill effects of long-term use of fluorinated topical steroids (especially on the face, eyelids, and genitalia).

C. To control oozing and prevent crust formation:
   1. Provide tub baths and wet dressings to loosen exudates and scales.
   2. Remove medications with mineral oil before reapplying.
   3. Use mildly astringent solutions to precipitate proteins and decrease oozing.
   4. Supply a high-protein diet if oozing is voluminous and serum loss substantial.
   5. Administer antibiotics as indicated.

D. To avoid damage to skin:
   1. Protect healthy skin from maceration when applying wet dressings.
   2. Remove moisture from skin by blotting gently and avoiding friction.
   3. Guard carefully against risk of thermal trauma from excessively hot, wet dressings.
   4. Advise patient to use sunscreening agents to prevent actinic damage (tissue changes from ultraviolet light).

E. To ensure efficacy of topical applications:
   1. Use occlusive dressings, as needed, to retain medication in constant contact with affected skin.
   2. Elicit the patient's cooperation in performing his own dermatologic treatments.
   3. Instruct patient clearly and in detail to ensure that treatments are carried out as prescribed.

Skin conditions can lead to cosmetic disfigurement, social isolation, and economic hardship. In some instances, they are often erroneously associated with immorality and contagion. Some conditions can cost the patient his job, with devastating effects on the person's life. Others may subject the patient to a protracted course of illness, leading to feelings of depression, frustration, self-consciousness, and rejection. Itching and skin irritation may also be a constant annoyance—in fact, they are common features of most skin diseases. The result of these discomforts may be loss of sleep, anxiety, and depression, all of which reinforce the general distress and fatigue that so frequently accompany skin disorders.

Patients suffering from such physical and psychological discomforts require understanding, nursing support, unending patience, and continual encouragement. It takes time to help patients gain insight into their problems and work out their difficulties. It becomes imperative, therefore, to overcome any aversion that might be felt when caring for patients with unattractive skin disorders. There must be no sign of hesitancy when approaching these patients. Such behavior would only reinforce the psychological trauma of the disorder. Since very few skin conditions are contagious, there is no need to fear touching the patient. In fact, touching the patient reduces his sense of isolation, and conveys human warmth and compassion.

Whenever possible, the patient should be given a chance to express any feelings of anger, ambivalence, and depression. An overall optimistic approach by the nursing personnel will help to alleviate these negative feelings and promote a sense of security and confidence.

▷ Dermatologic Therapeutic Modalities

Wet Dressings

Wet dressings (wet compresses applied to areas of the skin) are usually used for acute, weeping, inflammatory lesions. They may be either sterile or unsterile depending on the condition being treated. The purposes of wet dressings are (1) to reduce inflammation by producing vasoconstriction (thus decreasing vasodilatation and the local blood flow in inflammation); (2) to cleanse the skin of exudates, crusts, and scales; and (3) to maintain drainage of infected areas. Before these dressings are applied, the hands should be washed thoroughly.

Wet dressings are used for vesicular, bullous, pustular, and ulcerative disorders, as well as for acute inflammatory disorders, erosions, and exudative, crusted surfaces.

The solutions generally consist of room-temperature tap water or physiologic saline. Other agents may be used to precipitate protein, thus acting as mild astringents and antibacterials. Medication may be applied after wet dressings.

Although some dressings must be covered to prevent evaporation, most are allowed to remain open. The *open dressing* requires frequent changes because evaporation is rapid. The *closed dressing* is changed less frequently. However, there is always a danger that it will cause not only softening, but actual maceration of the underlying skin.

Areas of normal skin that may be exposed to moisture for any extended period should first be coated with petrolatum jelly, a silicone oil, or zinc oxide paste to avoid skin maceration.

Smooth muslin or cotton materials in the form of old bedding, diapers, etc. can be cut and folded to make dressings that are two to four layers thick. The dressing is saturated with the prescribed solution before it is applied. Usually, wet dressings are kept cool or at room temperature. Compresses are removed, wrung out of the solution, and reapplied every 5 to 10 minutes, since compresses reach body temperature in that period of time. Wet dressings are usually applied for 15- to 30-minute intervals every 2 to 3 hours unless otherwise prescribed. Medications applied to moist skin immediately after treatment with compresses are absorbed better than when applied to dry skin. If extensive areas are to be treated with wet compresses, the patient must be kept warm and not more than one third of the body treated at one time.

If warm compresses are prescribed, the area must be watched carefully, since the skin may be burned. If a closed dressing is used, it may be covered with sterile towels to hold the dressing in place and further protected with a plastic film. In this way, the temperature can be maintained for a longer period.

Dressing materials should be laundered or discarded every 24 hours. Usually, the acute stage of dermatitis subsides after 48 to 72 hours of treatment. Wet dressings continued beyond this point can lead to dryness.

Therapeutic Baths (Balneotherapy)

Baths are useful as a means of applying medications to large areas of the skin, removing crusts and scales and old medications, and relieving the inflammation and itching that accompany acute dermatoses. The temperature of the water should be comfortable, and the bath should last from 15 to 30 minutes, although the water should not be allowed to cool excessively. For the different types of therapeutic baths and their uses, see Table 52-1.

Topical Medications

Medications in the form of lotions, creams, ointments, and powders are frequently used to treat skin lesions. In general, wet dressings, with or without medication, are used in the acute stage; lotions and creams are reserved for the subacute stage, whereas ointments are used when inflammation has become chronic and the skin is dry with scaling and lichenification (leathery thickening of the skin).

Lotions exert a cooling action through water evaporation; they also have a protective effect, are antipruritic and drying, and may act as sunscreens. Lotions are applied easily with a soft paintbrush, cotton gauze, or by hand, and are not usually washed off between applications.

Powders usually have a talc, zinc oxide, bentonite, or cornstarch base and are dusted on the skin with a shaker or with cotton sponges. Although their medical action is brief, powders act as hygroscopic agents, absorbing moisture and reducing friction between skin surfaces and between the skin and bedding.

Creams are suspensions of oil and water, are easily applied, and usually are the most cosmetically acceptable to the patient. Creams are generally rubbed into the skin by hand.

Gels are semisolid emulsions that become liquid when applied to the skin. They are cosmetically acceptable to the patient as they vanish after application, and are greaseless and nonstaining. Most topical steroids are prescribed in gel form as the gel appears to penetrate more effectively than other skin preparations.

Pastes are mixtures of powders and ointments and are used in inflammatory conditions. They adhere best to the skin and may need to be removed with mineral or olive oil.

Ointments retard water loss, lubricate and protect the skin, and are preferred in the more chronic or localized skin conditions. Both pastes and ointments are applied with a wooden tongue depressor or by hand, with gloves if necessary.

Sprays and aerosols may be used on extensive lesions. They are seldom necessary.

In all of the aforementioned types of topical medications, the patient should be taught to apply the medication gently but thoroughly. It may also be necessary to cover these medications with a dressing to prevent soiling of clothing.

Table 52-1
Types of Therapeutic Baths

Bath Solution and Medication	Desired Effect	Nursing Action
Water	Same effects as wet dressings	Fill the tub half full.
Saline	Used for widely disseminated lesions	Keep the water at a comfortable temperature.
Colloidal—Oatmeal or Aveeno	Antipruritic and drying	
Sodium bicarbonate	Cooling	Do not allow the water to cool excessively.
Starch		Use a bath mat—*medications may cause tub to be slippery.*
Medicated tars (follow package directions) Alma-Tar, Balnetar	Tar baths are used for psoriasis and chronic eczematous conditions.	Apply a lubricating agent to wet skin after bath if emollient action is desired—increases hydration. Since tars are volatile, the bath area should be well ventilated. Dry by blotting with a towel.
Bath oils Alpha-Keri, Lubath, Nutraderm Bath Oil	Bath oils are used for antipruritic and emollient actions. Used for acute and subacute eczematous eruptions.	Keep room warm to minimize temperature fluctuations. May be applied to wet skin after bathing. Encourage patient to wear light, loose clothing after the bath.

Corticosteroids are being widely used in the treatment of many dermatologic conditions. Topical steroids frequently are used to suppress inflammation, thus relieving pain and itching. The patient should be instructed to use only small quantities of steroid cream and to rub it in thoroughly. Topical corticosteroids are frequently used with occlusive dressings to enhance skin penetration and potency. (See below.) When steroids are applied around the eyes, a great deal of caution is required, as chronic use around the eyes may cause glaucoma, cataracts, and viral and fungal infections. Also, when strong (fluorinated) steroids are put on the face, precautions must be taken, because they may produce an acne-like dermatitis (perioral dermatitis), steroid-induced rosacea, and hypertrichosis (excessive hair growth).

Intralesional therapy consists of the injection of a sterile suspension of medication (usually a corticosteroid) into or just below a lesion. Although this treatment may have an anti-inflammatory effect, local atrophy may result if the injection is made into subcutaneous fat. Skin lesions treated with intralesional therapy include psoriasis, keloids, and cystic acne. Occasionally, immunotherapeutic and antifungal agents are given by intralesional therapy.

Systemic medications are also given for skin conditions. These include the corticosteroids, antibiotics, antifungals, antihistamines, sedatives and tranquilizers, analgesics, and antineoplastics.

Dressings for Skin Conditions

Skin dressings are used to keep topical medication in place and to allay itching and pain. One very effective type of dressing is the occlusive dressing, which increases the local skin temperature and hydration and enhances the absorption of topically applied medications. Occlusive dressings also promote the retention of moisture, which keeps the medication from evaporating and reduces the expense of topical corticosteroid treatment. An airtight plastic film, such as Saran Wrap, is applied to cover the medicated skin. Plastic film is advantageous because it is thin and adapts itself readily to anatomical structures of all sizes and shapes. Plastic surgical tape containing corticosteroid in the adhesive layer can be cut to size and applied to individual lesions. For areas that are difficult to cover, occlusive appliances of thin, clear plastic can be constructed with dental materials. Plastic wrap should generally be used no more than 10 to 12 hours a day. The patient is given the following instructions: (1) wash the area, then pat dry; (2) rub the medication into the lesion while the skin is moist; (3) cover with plastic wrap (Saran Wrap, vinyl gloves, plastic bags, etc.); and (4) cover with an ace bandage, stocking, dressing, or paper tape to seal the edges.

It is important to remember that prolonged use of occlusive dressings may cause local skin atrophy, striae, telangiectasia, folliculitis, nonhealing ulceration or erythema, and systemic absorption of corticosteroids. Dressings should be removed for 12 out of 24 hours to prevent some of these complications.

There are other forms of dressings that can be used to cover topical medications. The best material is soft cotton cloth. Stretchable cotton dressings (Surgitube, Tubegauze) can be used for fingers, toes, and extremities. The hands can be covered with disposable polyethylene or vinyl gloves, sealed at the wrists, while the feet can be wrapped in plastic bags covered by cotton socks. When large areas of the body need to be covered, cotton cloth covered with tubular material can be used. Disposable diapers or cloth folded diaper-fashion are also useful as dressings for the groin and the perineal areas. Sanitary napkins manufactured with an adhesive strip may be used for draining lesions in hairy areas, where tape can cause difficulty. Axillary dressings can be made of cotton cloth taped in place or held by dress shields. A turban or plastic shower cap is useful for holding dressings on the scalp. A face mask may be made from gauze with holes cut out for the eyes, nose, and mouth and held in place with gauze ties looped through holes cut in the four corners of the mask.

▷ Pruritus

Pruritus (itching) is one of the most common complaints in dermatologic disorders. Although it is most frequently due to primary skin disease, it may also reflect systemic disease. Thus, it may be the first indication of an internal disease such as diabetes mellitus, blood disorders, or cancer. Itching may also accompany renal, hepatic, and thyroid diseases. Pruritus may be caused by certain oral medications; by the external application of certain drugs, soaps, and chemicals; by prickly heat (miliaria); and by contact with woolen garments. It may also occur in the elderly as a result of dry skin. Itching may also be caused by psychological factors.

Because pruritus usually leads to scratching, the secondary effects include excoriations, erythema, wheals, infections of the skin, and changes in pigmentation. Severe itching is debilitating.

The cause of pruritus, if known, should be removed. In general, washing with soap and hot water is avoided. The application of a cold agent to the skin for its vasoconstrictive effect may be helpful. Bath oils (Lubath, Alpha-Keri bath oil) containing a surfactant that makes the oil mix with water in the bath may be sufficient for cleansing. (However, an elderly patient should not add oil to the bath because of the danger of slipping in the bathtub.) Soothing baths containing starch or water-soluble tar derivatives may be prescribed. Tepid water is used for such baths. The patient can be instructed to shake off the excess water and to blot between intertriginous areas with a towel. Rubbing vigorously with the towel is avoided since this overstimulates the skin, causing more itching. It also removes water from the stratum corneum. Immediately after bathing, the skin should be lubricated with an emollient that traps moisture.

Topical steroids may prove useful not only for their emollient effect, but also for their anti-inflammatory effect, which may decrease itching. Inability to sleep causes an increased awareness of nighttime itching. Therefore, wearing cotton clothes next to the skin may be helpful. Excessive warmth should be avoided, and the room should be kept cool and humidified. The fingernails can be trimmed to prevent injury from scratching while asleep.

Pruritus of the anal and the genital regions may be caused by poor hygiene; local irritants, such as scabies and lice; local lesions, such as hemorrhoids; infection with certain fungi and yeasts; and pinworm infestation. It occurs also in postmenopausal women and in conditions such as diabetes mellitus, the anemias, hyperthyroidism, and pregnancy. The treatment is removal of the local cause, discontinuation of home and over-the-counter remedies, and following proper anal hygiene after bowel movement. The patient is instructed to rinse the perianal area with lukewarm water and blot the area dry with cotton balls.

Patient Education.   As part of health teaching, the patient is instructed to avoid both bathing in water that is too hot and using bubble baths, sodium bicarbonate, or detergent soaps, all of which aggravate dryness. He should avoid vasodilating agents or stimulants that increase emotional tension (alcohol, coffee) and mechanical irritants, such as rough or woolen clothing. Increasing the humidity with a room humidifier may be useful.

▷ Secretory Disorders

The main secretory function of the skin is performed by the sweat glands, which help to regulate body temperature. These glands excrete a fluid, perspiration, which evaporates and thus cools the body. The sweat glands are located in various parts of the body and respond to different stimuli; those on the trunk generally respond to thermal stimulation; those on the palms and soles respond to nervous stimulation; and those in the axillae and forehead respond to both kinds of stimulation.

As a rule, moist skin is warm, and dry skin is apt to be cool. However, this is not a hard and fast rule. It is not unusual to observe cold sweats; warm, dry skin in a dehydrated patient; and very hot, dry skin peculiar to some febrile states.

Seborrheic Dermatoses

Seborrhea is excessive production of sebum (secretion of sebaceous glands) in those areas where glands are normally found in large numbers (face, scalp, eyebrows, eyelids, nasolabial folds, malar region, ears, axillae, under the breasts, groin, gluteal crease).

Seborrheic dermatitis is a chronic inflammatory disease of the skin with a predilection for areas that are well supplied with sebaceous glands or lie between folds of the skin, where the bacterial count is high.

The characteristic lesions are remarkably variable, but this is a dermatitis of the *seborrheic* areas. It may start in childhood with fine scaling of the scalp and may continue throughout life. The scales may be dry, moist, or greasy. There may be patches of sallow, greasy-appearing skin, with or without scaling; slight erythema, predominantly on the forehead, nasolabial fold, and scalp; and intertriginous regions of the axillae, groin, and breasts.

The dry, flaky desquamation of the scalp with a profuse amount of fine, powdery scales is commonly called *dandruff.* The mild forms of the disease are asymptomatic. When scaling is present, it is often accompanied by pruritus, which may lead to scratching and result in secondary complications, such as infections and excoriations.

Seborrheic dermatitis has a genetic predisposition; hormones, nutritional status, infection, and emotional stress influence its course. There are remissions and exacerbations of this condition, which should be explained to the patient.

Management.   Since there is no known cure for seborrhea, the objective of therapy is to control the disorder and allow the skin to repair itself. The person is advised to remove external irritants and avoid excess heat and perspiration, since rubbing and scratching the skin will prolong the disorder. Seborrheic dermatitis of the body and face may respond to a topically applied corticosteroid cream, which allays the secondary inflammatory response. However, this medication should be used with extreme caution on the eyelids, since it can induce glaucoma in predisposed individuals. A secondary moniliasis (yeast infection) may occur in body creases or folds. To avoid this, patients should be advised to ensure maximum aeration of the skin and to cleanse intertriginous areas carefully. Patients with persistent moniliasis should be evaluated for diabetes.

For control of dandruff, the scalp may be shampooed with selenium sulfide suspension two to three times weekly for 5 to 10 minutes each time. The patient is advised to follow the directions on the container. Other useful antiseborrheic shampoos are zinc pyrithione shampoos, salicylic acid sulfur shampoos, and tar shampoos that contain sulfur and salicylic acid.

Patient Education.   Patients should also be encouraged to avoid systemically aggravating factors, such as overwork, lack of sleep, infection, and emotional stress. Sunlight may be beneficial for this chronic dermatitis.

Acne Vulgaris

Acne vulgaris is a common disorder of the sebaceous (oil) glands and their hair follicles (pilosebaceous follicles) characterized by the presence of closed comedones (white heads), open comedones (black heads), papules, pustules, nodules, and cysts. The sebaceous follicles are more numerous on the face, but are also found on the upper back and shoulders. Acne usually appears in the teenage years but may begin as early as 8 to 10 years of age. It becomes more marked at puberty and during adolescence, perhaps because at this age certain endocrine glands of the body that influence the secretion of the sebaceous glands are functioning at peak activity. It may persist well into adulthood. The etiology of acne appears to be multiple, reflecting an interplay of genetic, hormonal, and bacterial factors.

Pathogenesis of Acne.   During childhood, the sebaceous glands are small and virtually nonfunctioning. These glands are under endocrine control, especially the androgens. During puberty, the presence of androgen stimulates the sebaceous glands, causing them to enlarge and to secrete a natural oil, sebum, which rises to the top of the hair follicle and flows out onto the skin surface. In adolescents who develop acne, androgenic stimulation produces a heightened response in the sebaceous glands. Acne occurs when the pilosebaceous ducts through which the sebum flows become plugged.

▶ **Assessment**

The initial lesions of acne are comedones. *Closed comedones* ("white heads") are obstructive lesions formed from im-

pacted lipids and keratin that plug the dilated follicle. Whiteheads are small, whitish papules with minute follicular openings that generally cannot be seen. These closed comedones may evolve into *open comedones,* in which the contents of the ducts are in open communication with the external environment. Open comedones are termed "black heads." The color of the blackhead is *not* due to dirt, but to lipid with melanin pigment within the mass of horny cells.

Although the exact cause is not known, some closed comedones may rupture and result in an inflammatory reaction due to the leakage of follicular contents (sebum, keratin, bacteria) into the dermis. This inflammatory response may result from the action of certan skin bacteria, such as *Propionibacterium acnes* (formerly called *Corynebacterium acnes*) that live in the hair follicles and break down the triglycerides of the sebum into free fatty acids and glycerin. The resulting inflammation is seen clinically as papules, pustules, nodules, cysts, or abscesses.

Patient Problems/Nursing Diagnoses

Based on the clinical manifestations, the patient's potential problems include anxiety and distress related to unsightly skin appearance, and possible nonadherence with the treatment regimen related to the length of treatment time.

▶ **Planning and Implementation**

Goals

The patient goals are:

1. Relief of anxiety about his appearance
2. Adherence with the prescribed treatment in order to achieve the best appearance possible

The objectives of management are to reduce colonization by the bacteria, prevent follicular obstruction, reduce inflammation, combat secondary infection, minimize scarring, and eliminate factors that may predispose to acne. The therapeutic regimen depends on the type of lesion (comedonal, papular, pustular, cystic). A combination of therapies may be tried.

Before treatment is initiated, the patient is counseled and assured that the problem is not related to uncleanliness, dietary indiscretions, masturbation, sexual activity, etc., all of which are popular misconceptions. When treatment is instituted, it usually takes 4 to 6 weeks or longer for results to be seen. It is of great importance that the problems be taken seriously and that the teenager be given understanding, reassurance, and support. All facets of the emotional factors involved must be taken into account, including the possibility that acne can become a power struggle between teenager and parents.

The patient is instructed to wash his face with mild soap and water twice a day to remove the surface oils and prevent obstruction of the oil glands. Mild abrasive soaps and drying agents are prescribed to eliminate the oily feeling that troubles many patients. However, excessive abrasion is to be avoided since it only makes acne worse. It is also important to realize that soap itself can be irritating to the skin. The use of a polyester sponge pad (Buf-Puf) provides mechanical removal of superficial skin cells (epidermabrasion) and may be helpful in some patients. The hair is shampooed nightly or twice weekly with a medicated shampoo. Blackheads are removed manually with a comedone extractor to relieve the patient of unsightly lesions.

Topical Therapy.   Benzoyl peroxide is useful for more severe involvement. It has an antibacterial effect, suppressing *Propionibacterium acnes,* is thought to act as a depressant of sebum production, and is comedolytic. Initially, benzoyl peroxide causes redness and scaling, but usually the skin accommodates rapidly to its use. Usually, the patient applies a gel preparation of benzoyl peroxide once daily. In many instances, this will be the only treatment needed.

For the patient with more severe involvement, topical agents are used to clear the keratin plugs from the pilosebaceous ducts. One such treatment calls for the application of topical vitamin A acid (tretinoin[Retin-A]), which speeds up the cellular turnover and forces out the comedones and prevents occurrence of new comedones. Thus, it is effective in the treatment of comedonal acne. However, the patient should be informed that symptoms may worsen during the early weeks of therapy, because the underlying noninflammatory lesions convert to inflammatory pustules prior to desquamation. Erythema and peeling are also a frequent result. Improvement may take 8 to 12 weeks. Vitamin A acid may be used alone or with other topical agents. The following instructions are given to the patient when topical vitamin A acid is prescribed for acne:

1. Read the product information brochure.
2. Apply vitamin A acid to thoroughly dry skin, as wet skin increases the potential for irritation.
3. Keep medication away from eyes, nasolabial folds, and corners of the mouth, as it is likely to pool in those areas, causing local irritation.
4. Apply vitamin A acid as tolerated. The concentration of the preparation used and the frequency of its application are adjusted according to the reactivity of the skin to vitamin A acid.
5. Wash hands thoroughly after applying vitamin A acid.
6. Be cautious about exposure to the sun or to sunlamps, since susceptibility to sunburn is increased by the medication.
7. Avoid other irritants, such as strong soaps.

Topical Antibiotics.   Topically applied antibiotics for the treatment of acne has become widely practiced. Topical antibiotics suppress the growth of *P. acnes;* reduce skin-surface free fatty acid levels; decrease comedones, papules, and pustules; and do not have systemic side-effects. Topical tetracycline, meclocycline sulfosalicylate, clindamycin phosphate, and erythromycin are available.

Systemic Antibiotics.   Oral antibiotics given in small doses over a long period are very effective in the treatment of patients with moderate and severe acne, especially when the acne is inflammatory and results in pustules, abscesses, and scarring. They appear to decrease the bacterial count of *P. acnes* and to reduce fatty acids on the skin surface. Thus, inflammation is decreased. Tetracycline, erythromycin, or minocycline is given and adjusted according to the re-

sponse of the patient. Therapy may be continued for months to years. The patient is advised to take tetracycline at least 1 hour before or 2 hours after meals, since the drug is poorly absorbed with food. Side-effects of tetracyclines include photosensitivity, nausea, diarrhea, and moniliasis (vaginitis is seen in women, and cutaneous infection in either sex).

Oral Retinoids.   Synthetic vitamin A compounds (termed "retinoids") are being used with dramatic results in patients with severe nodular cystic acne. These drugs appear to have an inhibitory effect on the sebaceous glands and a marked anti-inflammatory effect. Side-effects include cheilitis; hair loss; dry mucosa of eyes, mouth, and nose; and dermatitis.

Hormone Therapy.   Estrogen therapy (progesterone–estrogen preparations) has been found to suppress sebum production and reduce skin oiliness. It is usually reserved for young women when the acne begins somewhat later than usual and tends to flare at certain times in the menstrual cycle, which is often irregular. Estrogen in the form of estrogen-dominant oral contraceptive compounds may be given on a prescribed cyclic regimen. Estrogen is not given to males because of undesirable side-effects.

Surgical Treatment.   Surgical treatment of acne consists of comedo extraction, injections of intralesional steroids into the inflamed lesions, and incision and drainage of large, fluctuant, nodular cystic lesions. Cryosurgery (freezing with liquid nitrogen) may be used for nodular and cystic forms of acne. Patients with deep scars may be treated with deep abrasive therapy (dermabrasion, p. 1195) in which the epidermis and some superficial dermis are removed down to the level of the scars.

Comedo Extraction.   Comedones may be removed with a comedo extractor. The site is first wiped with an alcohol sponge. The comedo is nicked with an 18-gauge needle or scalpel blade to incise the follicular opening in order to widen the port and facilitate the removal of the comedo. The opening of the extractor is then placed over the lesion, and direct pressure is applied to cause extrusion of the plug through the expressor.

Removal of comedones will leave areas of erythema, which may take several weeks to subside. Recurrence of comedones after extraction is common. The procedure must be performed by a prepared person, although sometimes patients are taught to use the comedo extractor.

Patient Education.   The patient is instructed to keep his hands away from his face and not to squeeze pimples or blackheads. Squeezing merely worsens the problem, since a portion of the blackhead is pushed down into the skin by squeezing, possibly causing the follicle to rupture.

The patient should be cautioned to avoid scrubbing the face constantly, since acne is not caused by dirt and cannot be washed away. All forms of friction and trauma are to be avoided: propping the hands against the face, rubbing the face, and wearing tight collars and helmets. Since cosmetics, shaving creams, and lotion can aggravate acne, these are best avoided unless the patient is advised otherwise. Hair should be kept off the face and shampooed daily if necessary. Treatment is to be continued even though the skin clears. In general, a nutritious diet should be followed.

▶ Evaluation

Expected Outcomes

1. Achieves relief of anxiety about appearance
   a. Reviews drawings of obstructive and inflammatory lesions of acne
   b. Reads patient education brochures on acne
   c. Avoids mirror gazing
   d. Verbalizes that picking and squeezing blemishes and lesions will worsen his condition and may cause scarring
   e. Identifies someone with whom he can talk over his problems
   f. Expresses optimism about outcome of treatment
2. Adheres to the prescribed therapy
   a. States he will make a major commitment to required treatment that may take months or years
   b. Verbalizes that he must continue with the treatment when the skin clears
   c. Follows cleansing program
   d. Avoids overcleansing
   e. Reads the product information brochure of his prescribed medications

▷ Infections and Infestations of the Skin

Bacterial Infections (Pyodermas)

Bacterial infections of the skin may be primary, originating in previously normal-appearing skin and usually caused by a single organism, or secondary, arising from a preexistng skin disorder in which several microorganisms may be implicated. The most common primary bacterial skin infections are impetigo and folliculitis. Folliculitis may lead to furuncles or carbuncles.

Impetigo

Impetigo is a superficial infection of the skin caused by streptococci, staphylococci, or multiple bacteria. The lesions begin as small, red macules, which rapidly become discrete, thin-walled vesicles that soon rupture and become covered with a loosely adherent honey-yellow crust (Fig. 52-2). These crusts are easily removed and reveal smooth, red, moist surfaces on which new crusts soon develop. The exposed areas of the body, face, hands, neck, and extremities are most frequently involved. Impetigo is contagious and may spread to other parts of the patient's skin or to other members of the family who touch the patient or use towels that are soiled with the exudate of the lesions.

Although impetigo is seen at all ages, it is particularly common among children living in poor hygienic conditions. Often it appears secondary to pediculosis capitis, scabies, herpes simplex, insect bites, poison ivy, or eczema. In adults, ill health, poor hygiene, and malnutrition may predispose to impetigo.

Bullous impetigo, a superficial infection of the skin caused by *Staphylococcus aureus,* is characterized by the

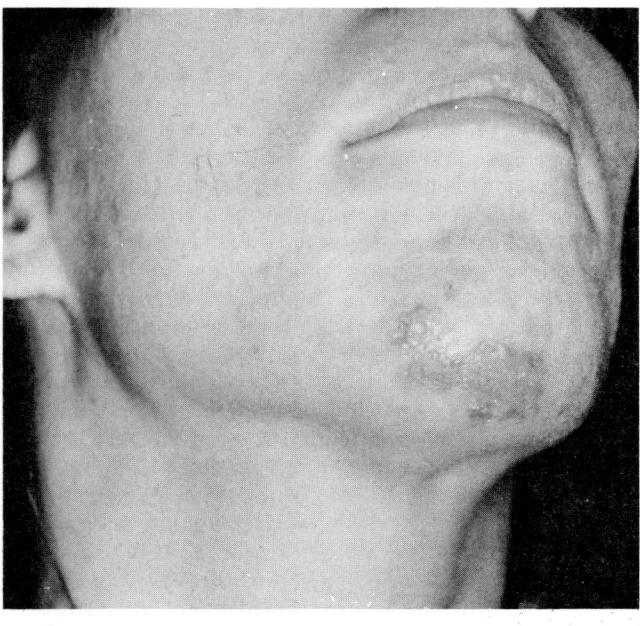

Figure 52-2. Impetigo of the chin. (Courtesy, Mervyn L. Elgart, M.D.)

formation of bullae from original vesicles. The bullae rupture, leaving a raw, red area.

Management. Systemic antibiotic therapy is the usual treatment. In nonbullous impetigo, benzathine penicillin or oral penicillin may be given. Bullous impetigo is treated with a penicillinase-resistant penicillin (oxacillin, cloxacillin, dicloxacillin).

The lesions are soaked or washed with soap solution to remove the loci of bacterial growth and to give the topical antibiotic an opportunity to reach the infected site. After the crusts are removed, a topical medication (neomycin; bacitracin, etc.) is applied. Topical treatment must be done several times a day. (Watch for contact dermatitis.) Gloves should be worn when care is given to these patients.

Patient Education. The patient and family should bathe at least once daily with bactericidal soap. Cleanliness and good hygienic practices help prevent the spread of the lesions from one skin area to another and from one person to another. Each person should have a separate towel and washcloth. Since impetigo is a contagious disorder, an infected child should be kept away from other children.

Folliculitis, Furuncles, and Carbuncles

Folliculitis refers to a staphylococcal infection that arises within the hair follicles. Lesions may be superficial or deep. Single or multiple papules or pustules appear close to the hair follicles. Folliculitis is commonly seen in the beard area of men who shave and on women's legs.

Pseudofolliculitis barbae ("shaving bumps") is an inflammatory reaction on the face of curly haired males caused by ingrowing hairs that pierce the skin and cause an irritative reaction. Curly hair has a curved root that grows at a more acute angle. This is a common problem in black males but may occur in others. The initial treatment is to avoid shaving and grow a beard. If this is not possible, a handbrush may be used over the facial area to mechanically dislodge the hairs. If the patient must shave, a depilatory cream may be useful.

A *furuncle* (boil) is an acute inflammation arising *deep* in one or more hair follicles and spreading into the surrounding dermis. It is a deeper form of folliculitis. (*Furunculosis* refers to multiple or recurrent lesions.) Furuncles may occur anywhere on the body but are more prevalent in areas subjected to irritation, pressure, friction, and excessive perspiration, such as the back of the neck, the axillae, or the buttocks.

A furuncle may start as a small, red, raised, painful "pimple." Frequently, the infection may progress and involve the skin and subcutaneous fatty tissue, causing tenderness, pain, and surrounding cellulitis. The area of redness and induration represents an effort of the body to keep the infection localized. The bacteria (usually staphylococcus) produce necrosis of the invaded tissues, followed in a few days by the characteristic pointing of a boil. When this occurs, the center becomes yellow or black, and the boil popularly is said to have "come to a head."

A *carbuncle* is an abscess of the skin and subcutaneous tissue representing an extension of a furuncle that has invaded several follicles and is larger and more deep-seated. It is usually caused by a staphylococcal infection. Carbuncles appear most commonly in areas in which the skin is thick and inelastic. The back of the neck and the buttocks are common sites. In carbuncles, the extensive inflammation frequently is not associated with a complete walling off of the infection, so that absorption occurs, resulting in high fever, pain, leukocytosis, and even extension of the infection to the bloodstream.

Furuncles and carbuncles are more apt to occur in patients with underlying systemic diseases, such as diabetes or hematologic malignancies, and those receiving immunosuppressive therapy for other diseases.

Management.   In the treatment of staphylococcal infections it is important not to rupture or destroy the protective wall of induration that has localized the infection. Therefore, the boil or pimple should never be squeezed.

The follicular disorders (folliculitis, furuncles, carbuncles) are usually caused by staphylococci. If the immune system is impaired, the causative organisms may be gram-negative bacilli.

Systemic antibiotic therapy, selected by sensitivity study, is generally indicated. Intravenous infusions, fever sponges, and other supportive modalities are indicated for the very ill and toxic patient. Warm, moist compresses increase vascularization and hasten resolution of the furuncle or carbuncle. The surrounding skin is cleansed gently with antibacterial soap, and an antibacterial ointment is applied to prevent spillage and seeding of the bacteria in the event the lesion ruptures or is incised.

When the pus has localized and is fluctuant (moving in palpable waves), a small incision with a scalpel will speed resolution by relieving the tension and ensuring a direct evacuation of the pus and slough. The patient is instructed to keep the draining lesion covered with a dressing. Soiled dressings should be wrapped in paper and burned. Nursing

personnel should carefully follow isolation precautions in order to avoid becoming staphylococcus carriers. Disposable gloves should be worn when caring for these patients.

Special precautions must be taken with boils on the face, for the skin area drains directly into the cranial venous sinuses. Sinus thrombosis, with fatal pyemia, has been known to develop after manipulation of a boil in this location.

Bed rest is advised for patients who have boils on the perineum or about the anal region, and a course of systemic antibiotic therapy is indicated to control the spread of the infection.

Patient Education.   To prevent and control staphylococcal skin infections (boils, carbuncles), the staphylococcus must be eliminated from the skin and environment. Efforts must be made to increase the patient's resistance and provide a hygienic environment. If lesions are actively draining, the mattress and pillow should be covered with plastic material and wiped off with disinfectant daily; the bed linens, towels, and clothing should be laundered after each use; the patient should shower and shampoo with an antibacterial soap and shampoo for an indefinite period. The prescribed antibiotic should be taken for the full length of time as directed.

Infections of the Hand
Superficial Infections.   Trivial accidents in daily living often result in cuts, pricks, and abrasions of the skin, particularly of the hands and fingers. Although these wounds are potentially infected, they rarely become seats of infection if ordinary precautions are taken. Mechanical cleansing with soap and tap water and protection with a Band-Aid or other form of dressing are usually all that is required to permit healing without infection. Antiseptics may be used if desired, but their role in preventing infection is much less important than is ordinary washing with soap and water.

Infections of the fingers and the hand are of extreme importance to the nurse, not only because one must know how to take care of these lesions, but also because frequent accidents in nursing may lead to the development of such infections in the nurse. Therefore, it is important to know the cause and, especially, the prophylactic treatment of these infections, because they may lead to serious disability if not to fatal consequences.

Since almost all inflammations of the hand and finger are due to infection, it is important to identify the organism and to determine its sensitivity to antibiotics. In the treatment of these infections, the appropriate antibiotic properly administered will quickly alleviate the inflammatory process; it may abort the infection in some cases, and in well-established infections it hastens resolution of the infection.

Paronychia.   *Paronychia* ("runaround") is a common pyogenic infection involving the tissues around the fingernail. The infection extends between the soft tissues and the nail on the dorsum of the fingertip and forms a tense, painful, throbbing area of inflammation at the side of the nail. If the infection is allowed to go untreated, it may progress underneath the eponychium (cuticle) and then invade the space underneath the base of the nail. Hence the common name of the infection—runaround.

Cleanliness of the hands and careful care of the nails are the best prophylaxis against paronychia. If the infection does occur, it is treated by warm soaks and by lifting up the soft tissues from the edge of the nail with forceps to allow the pus to drain. A small gauze wick may be inserted into the cavity. Once the pus is evacuated, the inflammation usually subsides. The discharge is cultured, and appropriate antibiotics may be given. If the infection is due to monilia, amphotericin B (Fungizone) lotion or cream, miconazole, or clotrimazole is applied locally. Occasionally, ketoconazole (Nizoral) is used orally in candidal infections.

Infections of the Pulp of the Fingertip. These infections usually are the result of a puncture wound or the stick of a pin or a needle, in which bacteria are carried into the layers of the skin or into the fatty tissues underlying it. This lesion is diagnosed easily, because it forms a small, tender, blisterlike mound at the site of the pinprick. Puncture and removal of the overlying skin may be carried out without anesthesia, exposing the true skin below. In workmen and in others in whom the surface skin is thick, the infection may not progress to the surface so readily and, instead, may perforate through the true skin and invade the subcutaneous fatty tissues. This process is known as a *collar-button abscess,* one abscess cavity lying between layers of the skin connected by a narrow tract with a second abscess lying below the skin. In the treatment of such abscesses, it is important that both the superficial and the deep collection be drained by incision.

Felon (Distal Closed Space Infection). The most common and serious type of infection of the fingertip occurs in the pulp of the finger and is caused by the streptococcus. There usually is a history of needleprick, pinprick, or some other form of puncture, followed several days later by throbbing pain, which may be intense enough to prevent sleep. The swelling and the edema produced by the infection may be sufficient to impair or shut off completely the arterial supply to the soft tissue, so that rapid necrosis and even invasion of the bone may ocur. The resulting disability often is great because of the extreme importance of the fingertips in the use of the hand and fingers.

Management. Early incision and drainage prevent the necrosis from progressing; therefore, wide incision often is practiced for what may appear to be a relatively small area of infection.

After incision, the wound is held open by a rubber dam or gauze drain and immobilized by an appropriate splint. Warm, moist dressings are used until the area of slough has separated entirely, after which time healing may be permitted to take place.

Prevention. To prevent infection of the fingertip, any prick of the finger with a needle or pin should be reported. Occasionally, a slight enlargement of the incision or cauterization of the needle puncture with phenol may abort a serious infection. If throbbing pain becomes a prominent symptom, no time should be wasted before consulting a surgeon. The appropriate antibiotic must be administered.

Viral Infections

Herpes Zoster (Shingles)

Herpes zoster (shingles) is an inflammatory condition in which the virus produces a painful vesicular eruption along the distribution of the nerves from one or more posterior ganglia. It is caused by the varicella virus, commonly known as varicella-zoster virus, which is a member of a group of DNA viruses. (The viruses of chicken pox and zoster are indistinguishable, hence the name varicella-zoster). It is assumed that herpes zoster represents a reactivation of latent varicella (chicken pox) virus and reflects a lowered immunity. After a case of chicken pox runs its course, it is believed that the varicella-zoster viruses responsible for the outbreak lie dormant inside nerve cells near the brain and spinal cord. Later, when these sleeping viruses are reactivated, they traverse via the peripheral nerves to the skin. There, the viruses multiply, creating a red rash of small fluid-filled blisters. About 10% of adults get shingles during their lifetime, usually after the age of 50. There is an increased frequency of herpes zoster in patients with weakened immune systems and malignancies, especially the leukemias and the lymphomas.

Clinical Manifestations. The eruption is generally accompanied or preceded by itching, tenderness, and pain, which may radiate over the entire region supplied by the nerves. The pain may be burning, lancinating, stabbing, or aching. In some cases, pain is absent. Malaise and gastrointestinal disturbances may also precede the eruption.

The patches of grouped vesicles appear on the erythematous and edematous skin. The early vesicles contain serum and later become purulent, rupture, and form crusts. The inflammation is usually unilateral, involving the thoracic, cervical, or cranial nerves in a bandlike configuration. The blisters are usually confined to a narrow region of the face or trunk. The clinical course varies from 1 to 3 weeks. If an ophthalmic nerve is involved, the patient may have a painful eye. Inflammation and a rash on the trunk may cause pain at the slightest touch. The healing time varies between 7 and 26 days.

Management. The objectives of management are to relieve the pain and to reduce or avoid complications. These include infection, scarring, and postherpetic neuralgia and eye complications.

Systemic corticosteroids may be given to prevent postherpetic neuralgia in patients over 60. If the eye is involved, the patient is referred to an ophthalmologist, as keratitis, uveitis, corneal ulceration, and blindness may occur.

The pain is controlled with analgesics, although postherpetic neuralgia does not respond well to analgesics and is a major problem in patient management. Antihistamines are given to control the itching.

Herpes zoster in healthy adults is usually localized and benign. However, in immunosuppressed patients, the disease may be severe and the clinical course acutely disabling.

Mycotic (Fungal) Infections

The fungi, tiny representatives of the plant kingdom that feed on organic matter, are responsible for a variety of common skin infections. In some cases, they affect only the skin and its appendages (*i.e.,* hair and nails), but in others, the internal organs are involved. In the latter instance, fungal disease may be so serious as to constitute a threat to life. Superficial infections, on the other hand, rarely cause temporary disability and respond readily to treatment. Secondary infection with bacteria or *Candida* or both may occur.

To obtain material for diagnosis, the lesion is cleaned and a scalpel is used to remove scales from the margin of the lesion. The scales are dropped onto a slide to which potassium hydroxide has been added. The diagnosis is made by examining the infected scales microscopically and by isolating the organism in culture.

Wood's light (a special ultraviolet light with maximum output in the 363-nm range) induces fluorescence of a specimen of infected hair and may be helpful in diagnosing some cases of tinea capitis.

Tinea Pedis (Athlete's Foot)

Tinea pedis, the most common fungal infection, is a superficial infection that manifests itself as an acute, inflammatory, vesicular process, or as a chronic, scaling, dusky, erythematous rash involving the soles of the feet or the interdigital web spaces. The toenails may or may not be affected; if involved, they are apt to be discolored, brittle, and heaped-up. As a rule, there is moderate to severe itching. Lymphangitis and cellulitis may be seen occasionally when bacterial superinfection occurs. Sometimes a mixed fungal, bacterial, and yeast infection occurs.

Management.   During the acute (vesicular) phase, soaks of Burow's solution, saline, or potassium permanganate are used to remove the crusts, scales, and debris and to reduce the inflammation. Topical antifungals (miconazole; clotrimazole) are applied to the infected areas. Topical therapy is continued for several weeks, as there is a high rate of recurrence. There should be clinical and mycologic examinations to confirm a cure. An antifungal agent, griseofulvin, is given orally if there is an extension of the infection or resistance to topical therapy. The patient is encouraged to rest in bed or elevate his feet frequently if secondary bacterial infection is present.

Preventive Measures and Patient Education.   Since footwear provides a hospitable environment for fungi, the causative fungi may be in the shoes and socks. Because moisture encourages the growth of fungi, the patient is instructed to keep his feet as dry as possible, including the areas between the toes. Small pieces of cotton can be placed between the toes at night to absorb moisture. Socks should be made of absorbent cotton, and hosiery should have cotton feet, since synthetic material does not absorb perspiration as well as cotton. For individuals whose feet perspire excessively, perforated shoes permit better aeration of the feet. Plastic or rubber-soled footwear should be avoided. Talcum powder or antifungal powder (Tinactin) applied twice daily helps to keep the feet dry. The shoes should be alternated so that they may dry completely before they are worn again.

Tinea Capitis (Ringworm of the Scalp)

Ringworm of the scalp is a contagious fungal disease and a common cause of hair loss in children. *Microsporum* and *Trichophyton* species are the dermatophytes (cutaneous fungi) that infect hair. Clinically, one or several round patches of redness and scaling are present. Small pustules or papules may be seen at the edges of such patches. As the hairs in the affected areas are invaded by the fungi, they become brittle and often break off at or near the surface of the scalp, resulting in areas of baldness. Most cases of tinea

capitis heal without scarring, hence the hair loss is only temporary. Sometimes a boggy swelling resembling a furuncle occurs in an area of involvement; this lesion is known as a *kerion*.

In recent years, a second form of ringworm caused by *Trichophyton tonsurans* has become prominent in the inner city. It presents as a scaling dermatitis, similar to seborrhea. The skin may be slightly red and scaly, and there are broken-off hairs. In this condition, diagnosis is made by examining the hair, since fluorescence is not present.

Management.   Griseofulvin, an antifungal antibiotic, is given to patients with tinea capitis. Side-effects of griseofulvin include headache, skin eruptions, and gastrointestinal disturbances. Topical agents are not effective as a cure, since the infection occurs within the hairshaft and below the surface of the scalp. However, topical agents are often used to inactivate organisms already on the hair. This diminishes contagiousness and eliminates the need to clip the hair, which is cosmetically unappealing and only adds to the patient's embarrassment. Infected hairs break off anyway, and noninfected ones may be left in place. The hair should be shampooed two to three times weekly, and a topical antifungal preparation should be applied to reduce dissemination of the organisms.

Patient Education.   Because the disease is contagious, the patient and family should be advised to set up a hygienic regimen for home use. Each person should have his own comb and brush and should avoid exchanging headgear. All infected members of the family and household pets must be examined since familial infections are relatively common.

Tinea Corporis

Tinea corporis or *tinea circinata* is ringworm of the body. Initially, an erythematous macule appears and develops into a ring of vesicles or scale with a clear center that appears alone or in a few areas, usually on the exposed areas of the body—face, arms, shoulders—possibly extending to the scalp. As a rule, there is an elevated border consisting of small papules or vesicles. Coalescence of individual rings may result in large patches with bizarre scalloped borders. Ringworm of the body may cause intense itching. A frequent cause of tinea circinata is the presence of an infected pet in the home.

Management.   Topical antifungal medication may be applied to small areas. Griseofulvin is used in extensive cases. Side-effects of griseofulvin include photosensitivity, skin rashes, headache, and nausea. Ketoconazole, a new antifungal agent, shows real promise in patients with chronic dermatophyte infections, including those resistant to griseofulvin.

Patient Education.   The patient is instructed to use a clean towel and washcloth daily. All areas and skin folds that retain moisture must be dried thoroughly, since fungal infections are fostered by heat and moisture. Clean cotton clothing should be worn next to the skin.

Tinea Cruris.   *Tinea cruris* ("jock itch") is ringworm infection of the groin, which may extend to the inner thighs and buttock area. It is commonly associated with tinea pedis. It occurs most frequently in young joggers, obese individuals, and those who wear tight underclothing. The infection starts with small, red, scaly patches and extends to form circinate (circular) plaques with elevated scaly or vesicular borders. Itching is usually present.

Mild infections may be treated with topical medication such as clotrimazole, miconazole, or haloprogin for at least 3 to 4 weeks to ensure complete eradication of the infection. Oral griseofulvin may be required for more severe infections.

Patient Education.   Heat, friction, and maceration (from sweating) predispose to the infection. The patient is instructed to avoid as far as possible excessive heat and humidity, nylon underwear, tight-fitting clothing, and the prolonged wearing of a wet bathing suit. Concomitant tinea pedis must be treated to minimize reinfection. The groin area should be cleansed, dried thoroughly, and dusted with a topical antifungal agent (tolnaftate [Tinactin]) as a preventive measure, since the infection is apt to recur.

Tinea Unguium (Onychomycosis)

Tinea unguium (ringworm of the nails) is a chronic fungal infection of the toenails or, less commonly, the fingernails and is usually caused by Trichophyton (*T. rubrum, T. mentagrophytes*) as well as *Candida albicans.* It is usually associated with long-standing fungal infections of the feet. The nails become thickened, friable (easily crumbled), and lusterless. In time, debris accumulates under the free edge of the nail, and ultimately the nail plate becomes separated (Fig. 52-3). The nail may be destroyed.

Management.   Griseofulvin is usually given orally for 6 months to a year when the fingernails are involved. Of course, griseofulvin is not of value in treating candidal infections; these infections must be treated topically with amphotericin B lotion, miconazole, clotrimazole, nystatin, or preparations such as thymol 4% in chloroform. These products penetrate poorly, and the infections are difficult to treat. Response to griseofulvin in fungal infections of the toenails is poor at best. Toenails are such slow-growing organs, with growth from the matrix of the nail to its free edge taking 130 to 160 days. Therefore, medications have to be used for a year or more with only a limited chance of cure. Frequently, when the treatment is stopped, the infection returns.

▷ Parasitic Skin Diseases

Pediculosis (Infestation by Lice)

Lice infestation affects persons of all ages. Three varieties of lice infest humans: *Pediculus humanus capitis* (head louse); *Pediculus humanus corporis* (body louse); and *Phthirus pubis* (pubic, or "crab," louse). Lice are termed ectoparasites because they live on the outside of the host's body. Thus, they depend on another host for their nourishment, feeding on human blood approximately five times a day. They inject their digestive juices and excrement into the skin, which causes very itchy bites.

Pediculosis Capitis

Pediculosis capitis is an infestation of the scalp by the head louse, *Pediculus humanus capitis.* The female head louse lays her eggs (nits) close to the scalp. The nits become

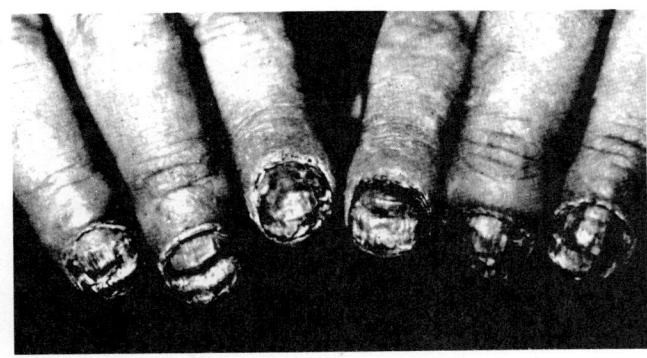

Figure 52-3.   Fungal infection of the fingernails. Note that the disease has spread and involved the nail plate. The nails are hyperkeratotic and cracked. The patient may complain of discomfort from the pressure of the diseased nails. (Courtesy, Ralph E. McDonnell, M.D., New Haven.)

firmly attached to the hair shafts with a tenacious cement bond. The young lice hatch in about 10 days and reach maturity in 2 weeks. Head lice are found most commonly over the back of the head and behind the ears. The eggs are visible to the naked eye as silvery, glistening oval bodies that are difficult to remove from the hair. The bite of the insect causes *intense itching* and the resultant scratching often leads to secondary bacterial infection with pustules, crusts, matted hair, and impetigo and furunculosis. The infestation is more common in children and people with long hair. Head lice may be transmitted by direct physical contact or indirectly by the use of infested combs, brushes, wigs, hats, and bedding.

Management.   Treatment involves washing the hair with a shampoo containing lindane (Kwell) or pyrethrin compounds with piperonyl butoxide (RID). The patient should be instructed to shampoo the scalp and hair according to the product directives. After the hair is rinsed thoroughly, it is combed with a fine-toothed comb that is dipped in vinegar to remove any remaining nits or nit shells freed from the hair shafts. These are extremely difficult to remove and may have to be picked off by the fingernails, one by one. (Thus, the term "nit picking.") All articles, clothing, towels, and bedding that might have lice or nits should be washed in hot water (at least 130° F) or dry-cleaned to prevent reinfestation. Upholstered furniture, rugs, and floors should be vacuumed frequently. Combs and brushes are also disinfected with the shampoo. All family members and close contacts are treated.

Complications such as severe pruritis, pyoderma (pus-forming infection of the skin), and dermatitis are treated with antipruritics, systemic antibiotics, and topical corticosteroids.

Patient Education.   The patient is reassured that head lice infestation may happen to anyone and is not a sign of uncleanliness. This condition spreads rapidly. Therefore, treatment must be started immediately. Control of school epidemics may be helped by having all of the students shampoo their hair on the same night. Students should be warned not to share combs, brushes, or hats. Each family member should be inspected for head lice daily for at least

2 weeks. The patient should be instructed that Kwell may be toxic when not used properly.

Pediculosis Corporis

Pediculosis corporis is an infestation of the body by the body louse, *Pediculus humanus corporis.* This is a disease of the unwashed, usually "street people" who do not change their clothing. The body louse lives chiefly in the seams of underwear and clothing, to which it clings as it pierces the skin with its proboscis. Its bites cause characteristic minute hemorrhagic points. Widespread excoriations may appear on the back and shoulders. Among the secondary lesions produced are hyperemia, parallel linear scratches, and a slight degree of eczema. In long-standing cases, the skin may become thickened, dry, and scaly, with dark pigmented areas. The areas of the skin chiefly involved are those that come in closest contact with the underclothing (*i.e.*, the neck, trunk, and thighs). The lice may be seen in the seams of the clothing. Therefore, the clothing and bedding must be laundered or dry-cleaned to destroy the parasite and its eggs. A shower should be taken and precautionary methods followed to prevent reinfestation.

Complications, such as severe pruritus, pyoderma (pyogenic infection of the skin), and dermatitis are treated with antipruritics, systemic antibiotics, and topical corticosteroids. One must keep in mind that body lice are vectors for rickettsial disease (epidemic typhus, relapsing fever, and trench fever). The causative organism may be in the gastrointestinal tract of the insect and may be excreted on the skin surface of the infested person.

Pediculosis pubis, infestation by *Phthirus pubis* ("crab louse"), is an extremely common problem that is generally localized in the genital region and transmitted chiefly by sexual contact.

Reddish brown "dust" from the excretion of the insects may be found in underclothing. Lice may also infest the hairs of the chest, axillary hair, beard, and eyelashes. Gray-blue macules may sometimes be seen on the trunk, thighs, and axillae as a result either of the reaction of the insects' saliva with bilirubin (converting it to biliverdin) or an excretion produced by the salivary glands of the louse. Examine the pubic crease with a magnifying glass for the presence of *Phthirus pubis* crawling down a hair shaft, or nits cemented to the hair or at the junction with the skin. Itching is the most common symptom, particularly at night. Infestation by pubic lice may coexist with other sexually transmitted diseases (gonorrhea, candidiasis, syphilis).

Management and Patient Education.   The patient is instructed to bathe with soap and water. Then lindane (Kwell) cream, lotion, or shampoo is applied to affected areas of the skin and to hairy areas, according to the product information directives. An alternate topical therapy is a pyrethrin-based pediculicide (RID, which is an over-the-counter preparation) or 0.03% copper oleate (Cuprex). Kwell is not applied to the eyebrows or eyelashes. Nits may be removed manually from the eyebrows and eyelashes with cotton-tipped applicators after physostigmine ophthalmic ointment has been applied.

All sexual contacts and family members must be treated.

The patient and his partner(s) must also be scheduled for a workup for coexisting sexually transmitted disease. All clothing and bedding should be machine washed or dry-cleaned.

Scabies

Scabies is an infestation of the skin by the itch mite, *Sarcoptes scabiei.* There has been a progressive increase in scabies during the past several years. The disease may be found in poor persons living under substandard hygienic conditions, but it is also common in very clean individuals. It is often found among the sexually active. However, infestations are not dependent on sexual activity since the mites frequently involve the fingers, and hand contact may produce infection. In children, overnight stays with friends or the exchange of clothes may be a source of infection. Health care personnel who have prolonged "hands on" physical contact with an infected patient may likewise become infected.

The adult female burrows into the superficial layer of the skin after fertilization has occurred on the skin surface. With her jaws and the sharp edges of the joints of her forelegs, the mite extends the burrow, laying three to four eggs daily for up to 2 months. She then dies. The larvae hatch in about 6 days, go through several molts, and then migrate to the skin surface, where they reach maturity in 2 to 3 weeks. It takes approximately 4 weeks from the time of contact for symptoms to appear.

Assessment and Clinical Manifestations.   The patient complains of severe itching. During examination, the patient should be asked where the itch is most severe. A magnifying glass and a penlight are held at an oblique angle to the skin while a search is made for the small, raised burrows. The burrows may be multiple straight or wavy, brown or black, threadlike lesions, most commonly observed between the fingers, the extensor surfaces of the elbows, knees, outer borders of feet, points of elbows, around the nipples, in axillary folds, under pendulous breasts, and in or near the groin or gluteal fold, penis, or scrotum. Red pruritic eruptions usually appear in intertriginous areas. The burrow, however, is not always seen. Any patient with a rash may have scabies.

One classic sign of scabies is the increased itching that occurs at night, perhaps because the increased warmth of the skin has a stimulating effect on the parasite. Also, hypersensitivity to the organism and its products of excretion may contribute to the itching. If the infection has spread, other members of the family and close friends will also complain of itching about a month later.

Secondary lesions are quite common and include vesicles, papules, pustules, excoriations, and crusts. Bacterial superinfection may result from constant excoriation of the burrows and papules.

To obtain skin scrapings for laboratory testing for the mite causing scabies, a drop of oil is placed over a lesion to prevent the specimen from being lost. A sample of superficial epidermis is scraped off with a small scalpel blade. The scrapings are placed on a microscope slide and examined by low-powered microscope to demonstrate the presence of the mite and its products—eggs, fecal concretions.

Management and Patient Education. The patient is instructed to take a warm, soapy bath or shower to remove scaling debris from the crusts and then to thoroughly dry himself and allow the skin to cool. Then a scabicide, such as lindane (Kwell) or crotamiton (Eurax cream and lotion) is applied in a thin layer to dry skin and rubbed in thoroughly. The entire body is covered with the cream, from the neck down. The medication is left on for 8 to 12 hours, after which the patient is instructed to wash thoroughly. One application is usually curative. The patient should wear clean clothing and sleep between freshly laundered bed linens. All bedding and clothing should be washed in very hot water.

After the treatment is completed, a bland ointment may be applied, because the solution may be irritating to the skin. The hypersensitivity state does not cease upon destruction of the mites. Itching may remain a troublesome problem for a few days or weeks, probably because the dead mites are retained within the epidermis for a few weeks until they are exfoliated. However, this is not a sign that the treatment has failed. The patient is instructed *not* to apply more scabicide (as this will cause more irritation and increased itching) and *not* to take frequent hot showers (as this dries the skin and produces itching).

All family members and close contacts should be treated simultaneously to eliminate the mites. If scabies is sexually transmitted, the patient may require treatment for coexisting sexually transmitted disease. Scabies may also coexist with pediculosis.

Bedbug Infestation

Two species of bedbugs, *Cimex lectularius* and *Cimex hemipterus,* invade human habitations, particularly in older and poorer sections of cities. The female leaves eggs in the cracks of floors and furniture. After the nymphs hatch, they can survive for a month or two without food. Then the mature bug emerges at night to feed on the blood of a sleeping victim. The bites are grouped in a straight line and consist of hemorrhagic spots associated with papular or wheal-like lesions. There may be tiny red points marking the original size of the bites. The legs, particularly the ankles, are most frequently bitten, and the patient experiences variable degrees of itching, burning, pain, and urticaria, depending on the degree of previous sensitization. The patient may find his night clothing and bedding stained with blood. Secondary infection and pyoderma may occur. There is recent evidence that the *Cimex* may act in the transmission of type B hepatitis.

Patient Education and Management. In general, lesions require no treatment. An antipruritic lotion may be applied to small local areas of bites. Antihistamines may be given for intense itching. The insects may be eliminated if all crevices in furniture, walls, floors, mattresses, and beds are sprayed with an insecticide.

▷ Contact Dermatitis

Contact dermatitis (dermatitis venenata) is a common inflammatory, often eczematous, condition caused by a skin reaction to contact with a variety of irritating or allergenic materials. The epidermis is damaged by repeated physical and chemical insults. Contact dermatitis may be of the primary irritant type in which a nonallergic reaction results from exposure to an irritating substance, or it may be allergic in nature (allergic contact dermatitis) resulting from exposure of sensitized individuals to contact allergens. (Allergic dermatoses are discussed in Chap. 50.) Common causes of irritant contact dermatitis are soaps, detergents, scouring compounds, industrial chemicals, etc. Predisposing factors include extremes of heat and cold, frequent immersion in soap and water, and a preexisting skin disease.

Clinical Manifestations. The eruptions begin at the point at which the causative agent contacts the skin. The first reactions include itching, burning, and erythema, followed soon by edema, papules, vesicles, and oozing or weeping. In the subacute phase, these vesicular changes are less marked and alternate with crusting, drying, fissuring, and peeling. If repeated reactions occur or if the patient continually scratches the skin, thickening of the skin (lichenification) and pigmentation (coloration) occur. Secondary bacterial invasion may follow.

Management. The objectives of management are to rest the involved skin and to protect it from further damage. The distribution pattern of the reaction is determined in order to differentiate between allergic contact dermatitis and the irritant type. A detailed history is obtained. Then the offending irritant is identified and removed. Local irritation should be avoided, and soap is not generally used until healing occurs.

There are innumerable preparations advocated for the relief of dermatitis. In general, a bland, unmedicated lotion is used for small patches of erythema. Cool, wet dressings also are applied over small areas of vesicular dermatitis. Finely cracked ice added to the water often enhances its antipruritic affect. Wet dressings usually dry the oozing eczematous lesions. Then a thin layer of cream or ointment containing one of the steroids may be used. Medicated baths at room temperature are prescribed for larger areas of dermatitis. (See also, The Patient With a Dermatosis, p. 1165.)

Systemic administration of sedatives and antihistamines may be required to relieve the intense burning and itching, whereas systemic antibiotics will be necessary if secondary bacterial infection is present.

In more widespread conditions, a short course of systemic steroids may be prescribed. This can diminish the course of a severe disease considerably.

Patient Education. The patient is instructed as follows:

1. Avoid heat, soap, and rubbing; all of these are external irritants.
2. Avoid topical medications except when specifically prescribed.
3. Wash the skin thoroughly immediately after exposure to irritants or antigens.
4. When gloves are used for washing dishes, use cotton-lined gloves, but do not wear them more than 15 to 20 minutes at a time.
5. The instructions should be followed for at least 4 months after the skin appears to be completely healed, since the resistance of the skin is lowered.

▷ Noninfectious Inflammatory Dermatoses

Psoriasis

Psoriasis is a chronic inflammatory disease of the skin in which epidermal proliferation (too rapid turnover of cells in the epidermis) occurs. In psoriasis, the production of the epidermis occurs at a rate that is approximately six to nine times faster than normal. The cells in the basal layer of the skin divide too quickly and the newly formed cells move so rapidly to the skin surface that they become evident as profuse scales or plaques of epidermal tissue. The psoriatic epidermal cell may travel from the basal cell layer of the epidermis to the stratum corneum (skin surface) and be cast off in 3 to 4 days, which is in sharp contrast to the normal 26 to 28 days. As a result of the increased number of basal cells and rapid cell passage, the normal events of cell maturation and keratinization cannot take place. This abnormal process does not allow formation of the normal protective layers of the skin.

Psoriasis is one of the most common skin diseases, with about 2 out of every 100 Americans having this condition. There appears to be a hereditary defect that causes an overproduction of keratin. A combination of specific genetic makeup and environmental stimuli may trigger the onset of disease. More recent data indicate that the immune system may be very important in the pathogenesis of psoriasis. Periods of emotional stress and anxiety aggravate the condition, and trauma, infections, and seasonal and hormonal changes are trigger factors. The onset may occur at any age, but is most common between the ages of 10 to 35 years. Psoriasis has a tendency to improve and then recur throughout life.

▶ Assessment

Clinical Manifestations.   The lesions produced by epidermal hyperplasia and accelerated epidermal turnover appear as circular patches of all sizes that are sharply defined against the normal skin and covered with heavy, dry, silvery scales (Fig. 52-4). If the scales are scraped away, the dark red base of the lesion is exposed, producing multiple bleed-

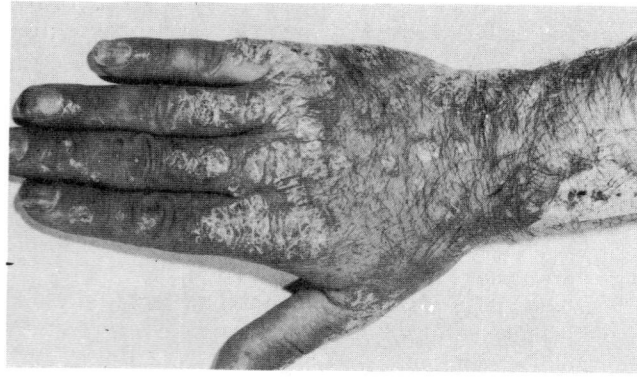

Figure 52-4.   Psoriasis of the hand. (From Sauer GC: Manual of Skin Diseases. Philadelphia, JB Lippincott.)

ing points. These patches are not moist and may or may not itch. The lesions may remain small, giving rise to the term "guttate psoriasis." Usually, the lesions enlarge slowly, but after many months they coalesce, forming extensive irregularly shaped patches. Psoriasis may range from a cosmetic source of annoyance to a physically disabling and disfiguring affliction. Particular sites of the body tend to be affected by this ailment; they include the scalp, the area over the elbows and knees, the lower part of the back, and genitalia.

Psoriasis appears most often on the extensor surfaces of the arms and legs, on the scalp and ears, and over the sacrum and intergluteal fold. Bilateral symmetry is a feature of psoriasis. In approximately one quarter to one half of the patients, the nails are involved, with pitting, discoloration, crumbling beneath the free edges, and separation of the nail plate. When psoriasis occurs on the palms and soles, it can cause pustular lesions. The disease may be associated with arthritis of multiple joints, causing a crippling disability. The relationship between arthritis and psoriasis is not understood. Another complication is an exfoliative psoriatic state in which the disease progresses to involve the total body surface.

Psychological Considerations.   The "heartbreak of psoriasis" is the outcome of a chronic disease that leads to frustration and despair on the part of the patient and a tendency on the part of other people to stare, comment, ask embarrassing questions, or even avoid the person. The disease can eventually exhaust the patient's resources, interfere with his job, and make life miserable in general. Teenagers are especially vulnerable to the psychological effects of this ailment. Many a teenager's personality has been scarred by the occurrence of such a disfiguring disease at a stage of life when appearance is all-important. The family, too, is affected, since time-consuming treatments, messy salves, and constant shedding of scales disrupt home life and cause resentment. In many cases, the patient's frustrations are expressed through hostility directed at the health care personnel.

Patient Problems/Nursing Diagnoses

Based on the clinical manifestations and diagnostic assessment data, the patient's major nursing problems include anxiety related to cosmetically embarrassing appearance, and potential nonadherence with the therapeutic regimen related to long-term treatment that is messy and time-consuming.

▶ Planning and Nursing Intervention

Goals

The patient's goals are:

1. Relief of anxiety about his appearance
2. Adherence to the therapeutic regimen

The goals of management are to reduce the rapid turnover of epidermis and to promote resolution of the psoriatic lesions. Thus, the goal is limited to control of the problem, since there is no known cure.

Management.   The therapeutic approach should be one that the patient understands; it should be cosmetically acceptable and not too disruptive of life-style, and it will involve the commitment of time and effort by the patient and those caring for him.

First, any precipitating or aggravating factors are removed. Then an assessment is made of life-style, since psoriasis is significantly affected by stress. The patient must also be advised that treatment is time-consuming, expensive, and esthetically unappealing at times.

Therapy may be divided into three types: topical, intralesional, and systemic.

Topical Therapy.   Topically applied agents are given to slow down the overactive epidermis without affecting other tissues. Such medications include tar preparations, anthralin, salicylic acid, corticosteroids, etc. These therapies seem to act by suppressing epidermopoiesis. Tar is formulated as lotions, ointments, pastes, creams, and shampoos. Tar baths or tar preparations may retard and inhibit the rapid growth of psoriatic tissue. This aspect of therapy may be combined with carefully graded doses of ultraviolet radiation. The tar is partially removed prior to ultraviolet light exposure to allow maximum transmission of light. During this phase of treatment, the patient is advised to wear goggles and to protect the eyes. Using a timer will prevent the danger of severe burns due to overexposure to the light rays. A daily tar shampoo followed by an application of steroid lotion may be used for scalp lesions. The patient is also taught to remove excess scales by scrubbing with a soft brush while bathing.

Anthralin preparations (a distillate of crude coal tar) are useful for thick and resistant psoriatic plaques. The patient is instructed to apply anthralin medication with a tongue blade or gloved fingers, taking special care not to cover normal skin. The hands must be washed after the medication is handled, because a chemical conjunctivitis can be produced if the patient touches his eyes while medication is still on his hands. Anthralin stains badly and should be covered in some way (gauze dressings, stockinette, old pajamas) when applied. The preparation is left on the skin for 8 to 12 hours.

Topical Steroids.   Topical steroids may be applied for their anti-inflammatory activity and covered with an occlusive plastic film dressing to enhance drug penetration and soften the scaly plaques. Steroid-impregnated tape may be used in patients with relatively few but resistant psoriatic plaques. However, once the steroid treatment is stopped, the psoriasis may quickly reappear (rebound phenomenon) and, in some instances, be more extensive than the original lesions.

Occlusive Dressings.   Some patients will require occlusive dressings over the entire body. For the hospitalized patient, large plastic bags may be used—one for the upper body (with holes cut out for the head and arms) and one for the lower part (with holes for the legs). This leaves only the extremities to wrap. In some dermatologic units, large rolls of tubular plastic are used (such as the kind that dry-cleaners place over clean clothes). However, when these substances are used, *it is important to check for flammability.* Some of these thin, plastic films will burn slowly (if touched by a lighted cigarette), whereas others will burst rapidly into flame and may cause severe injury. The patient should be cautioned not to smoke while wrapped in these dressings.

In patients being treated at home, a plastic vinyl jogging suit may be purchased. The medication is applied and the suit simply put over it. The hands can be wrapped in gloves, the feet in plastic bags, and the head in a shower cap. The suit can be machine washed, making a difficult task much easier.

Intralesional Therapy.   Intralesional injections of triamcinolone acetonide directly into highly visible or isolated patches of psoriasis are highly effective and seldom produce side-effects.

Systemic Therapy.   Systemic cytotoxic preparations, such as methotrexate, have been used in treating extensive psoriasis that fails to respond to other forms of therapy. Methotrexate appears to function by inhibiting DNA synthesis in epidermal cells, therefore reducing the turnover time of the psoriatic epidermis. However, the drug can be very toxic, especially to the liver, which can suffer irreversible damage. Thus, laboratory studies must be monitored to ensure that the hepatic, hematopoietic, and renal systems are functioning adequately.

The patient should avoid drinking alcohol while on methotrexate, since this increases the possibility of liver damage. The drug is teratogenic (producing physical defects in the fetus) in pregnant women.

Oral Retinoids.   Oral retinoids (synthetic derivatives of vitamin A and its metabolite, vitamin A acid) modulate the growth and differentiation of epithelial tissue and thus show great promise in treating the patient with severe psoriasis.

Another drug currently being used is hydroxyurea (Hydrea), which inhibits cell replication by affecting DNA synthesis. The patient is monitored for signs and symptoms of bone marrow depression.

Photochemotherapy (PUVA Therapy).   A new and promising treatment for severely debilitating psoriasis is PUVA (psoralen, and ultraviolet A) therapy. PUVA requires the combined effects of an orally administered phototoxic substance and irradiation with a long-wave ultraviolet light. The 8-methoxypsoralen molecule absorbs the light energy and becomes an active molecule that binds to the DNA of the cell nucleus. It is thought that psoralen, after being modified in the skin by the absorbed light, slows down the growth of psoriatic cells. However, PUVA is not without its hazards, as investigators are concerned with increased occurrence of skin cancers, possible long-term effects of PUVA on the immune system, and a potential risk of cataracts.

PUVA therapy requires that psoralen be taken orally, followed in 2 hours by irradiation with high-intensity long-wave ultraviolet light (UVA). (Ultraviolet light is the portion of the electromagnetic spectrum containing wave lengths from 180 nm to 400 nm.) The PUVA unit consists of a light cabinet containing high-output blacklight lamps and an external reflectance system. The exposure time is calibrated according to the specific unit in use and the anticipated tolerance of the patient's skin. The patient is usually treated two to three times a week until the psoriasis clears. An interim period of 48 hours between treatments is necessary, because it takes this long for any PUVA burns to become evident. The patient is then placed on a maintenance program. Once little or no disease is present, less potent therapies are used to keep minor flare-ups under control.

Patient Education.   PUVA treatment produces photo-sensitization, which means that the patient is sensitive to the sun until methoxsalen has been excreted from the body (about 6 to 8 hours). Therefore, exposure to the sun must be avoided at this time. If exposure is unavoidable, the skin must be protected with sunscreen and clothing. Gray- or green-tinted wraparound sunglasses should be worn to protect the eyes during and after treatment. Ophthalmologic examinations are carried out on a regular basis. Nausea, which may be a problem in some patients, is lessened when Methoxsalen is taken with food. Lubricants and bath oils may be used to help remove scales and prevent excess dryness. No other creams or oils are to be used except on areas that have been shielded from ultraviolet light. Contraceptives should be used while the patient is on this regimen. The patient must remain under constant and careful supervision and is encouraged to look for unusual changes in his skin.

▶ **Evaluation**

Expected Outcomes

1. Achieves relief of anxiety about skin condition
   a. Verbalizes feelings about changes in his life-style imposed by treatment
   b. Engages in activities (hobbies) to divert attention
   c. Takes prescribed antianxiety medication
   d. Verbalizes that trauma, infection, seasonal changes, and emotional stress may be trigger factors
2. Adheres to therapeutic regimen
   a. Keeps skin lubricated
   b. Demonstrates how to apply prescribed topical medication
   c. Can recall three side-effects of prescribed drug therapy

Exfoliative Dermatitis

Exfoliative dermatitis is a serious condition characterized by a progressive inflammation in which erythema and scaling often occur in a more or less generalized distribution. It may be associated with chills, fever, prostration, severe toxicity, and an itchy scaling of the skin. There is a profound loss of stratum corneum (outermost layer of the skin), which causes capillary leakage, hypoproteinemia, and negative nitrogen balance. The iron loss from the skin produces anemia. Thus, exfoliative dermatitis has a marked effect on the entire body.

It may develop as a primary condition, or it may arise secondary to other chronic skin diseases, such as eczema and psoriasis, particularly if these are treated with irritating ointments over a long period of time. Exfoliative dermatitis may appear as a part of the lymphoma group of diseases and may actually precede the appearance of lymphoma. It also appears as a severe reaction to a wide number of drugs, including penicillin and phenylbutazone. Thus, there is a multiplicity of causes.

This condition starts acutely as either a patchy or generalized erythematous eruption accompanied by fever, malaise, and, occasionally, gastrointestinal symptoms. The skin color changes from pink to dark red; then, after a week, the characteristic exfoliation (scaling) begins, usually in the form of thin flakes that leave the underlying skin smooth and red, new scales forming as the older ones exfoliate (cast off). Hair loss may accompany this disorder. Relapses are the rule. The systemic effects include high-output congestive failure, enteropathy, gynecomastia, hyperuricemia, and thermoregulatory disturbances.

Management.   The objectives of management are to maintain fluid and electrolyte balance and to prevent intercurrent or cutaneous infection. The treatment is individualized and supportive and depends on the cause. The patient is hospitalized and placed on bed rest. All drugs that may be implicated are stopped. A comfortable room temperature should be maintained, since the patient does not have normal thermoregulatory control because of fluctuations in temperature due to vasodilatation and evaporative water loss. The fluid and electrolyte balance must be maintained, since there is considerable water and protein loss from the skin surface. Plasma expanders may be indicated.

Continual nursing assessment is carried out to detect intercurrent and cutaneous infection. The erythematous, moist skin is receptive to infection and becomes colonized with pathogenic organisms, which produce more inflammation. Antibiotics are given if infection is present and are selected on the basis of culture and sensitivity.

- Watch for signs and symptoms of congestive heart failure, since hyperemia and increased cutaneous blood flow can produce a cardiac failure of high output origin.

Hypothermia may also occur as increased skin blood flow, coupled with increases in water loss through the skin, leads to heat loss by radiation, conduction, and evaporation.

As in any acute dermatitis, topical therapy is used to give symptomatic relief. Soothing baths, compresses, and lubrication with emollients are used to treat the extensive dermatitis. The patient is likely to be extremely irritable because of the severe itching. Oral or parenteral steroids may be given when the disease is not controlled by more conservative therapy. When a specific cause is known, more specific therapy may be used.

Patient Education.   The patient is advised to avoid all irritants in the future, particularly drugs.

Pemphigus Vulgaris

Pemphigus vulgaris is a serious disease of the skin characterized by the appearance of bullae (blisters) of various sizes (1 cm–10 cm) on apparently normal skin (Fig. 52-5) and mucous membranes (mouth, vagina).

▶ **Assessment**

Clinical Manifestations.   The majority of patients initially present with oral lesions. The skin bullae enlarge; rupture; and leave large, eroded areas that are accompanied by crusting and oozing. There is blistering or sloughing of uninvolved skin when minimal pressure is applied (Nikolsky's sign). The eroded skin heals slowly, so that eventually huge areas of the body are involved. Bacterial superinfection is common. In the mouth, there are irregularly shaped erosions that are painful, bleed easily, and heal slowly.

Since patients with pemphigus are invariably hospitalized at one time or another during exacerbations of the disease, the nurse soon discovers that pemphigus is perhaps the most debilitating skin disease of all. The constant misery of the patient and the foul smell of the lesions makes effective nursing a real challenge.

Available evidence indicates that pemphigus is an autoimmune disease. (See Chap. 49.) Genetic factors may also play a role in its development. The disorder usually occurs in middle and late adult life.

A biopsy specimen from a blister will demonstrate acantholysis (separation of epidermal cells from one another). Circulating antibodies (pemphigus antibodies) may be demonstrated by indirect immunofluorescence in the sera of nearly all patients with pemphigus during the course of the disease.

Patient Problems/Nursing Diagnoses

Based on the clinical manifestations and diagnostic assessment data, the patient's major nursing problems include painful lesions in the mouth related to eroding bullae; raw and denuded areas of the skin related to ruptured bullae; potential fluid and electrolyte imbalance related to loss of tissue fluids; and potential for infection related to loss of skin integrity.

▶ Planning and Nursing Intervention

Goals

The goals of the patient are:

1. Freedom from pain of the oral lesions
2. Relief of skin discomfort
3. Attainment of fluid and electrolyte balance
4. Avoidance of infection

The objectives of therapy are to bring the disease under control as rapidly as possible, to prevent loss of serum and the development of secondary infection, and to promote re-epithelialization of the skin.

Management. Corticosteroids (prednisone) are administered in large doses to control the disease and keep the skin free of blisters. The high dosage level is maintained until remission is apparent. Prednisone is given with or immediately after a meal and may be accompanied by an antacid as prophylaxis against gastric complications. Essential to the patient's therapeutic management are daily evaluations of body weight, measurement of blood pressure, testing of urine for glucose, and recording of fluid balance. (High-dosage corticosteroid therapy has its own serious toxic effects, including psychotic episodes.) Immunosuppressive agents (methotrexate, cyclophosphamide, gold) may be given to help control the disease and reduce the maintenance dose of steroids.

The nursing management has been likened to that required for a patient with an extensive burn. Particular attention is given to assessing the patient for signs of local and systemic infection, maintaining protein and electrolyte balance, and keeping the nutrition and hematologic status at physiologic levels. The patient is given a high-protein, high-calorie diet. There is a significant loss, through the

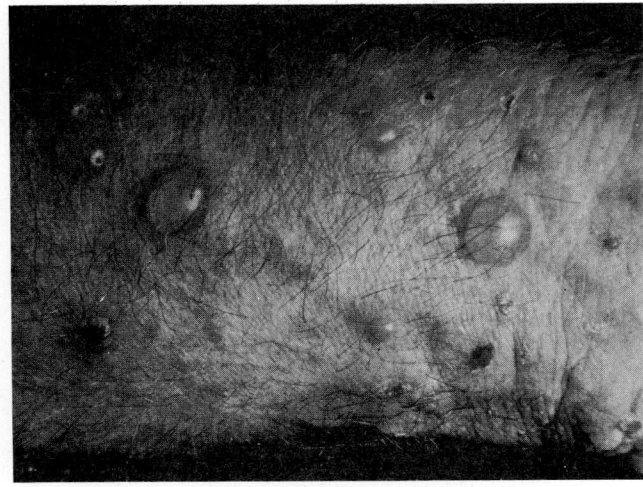

Figure 52-5. Pemphigus vulgaris bullae on the wrist. (From Sauer GC: Manual of Skin Diseases, Philadelphia, JB Lippincott.)

skin, of tissue fluids and, therefore, of sodium chloride. This salt loss is responsible for many of the constitutional symptoms associated with the disease and is combated with administration of adequate saline, parenterally or otherwise.

A large amount of protein and blood is lost from the denuded skin areas. Blood or component therapy (packed red cells, plasma) may be used to maintain the blood volume as well as the hemoglobin and plasma protein concentrations. The patient is susceptible to infection because the barrier function of the skin is compromised. Bullae are also susceptible to infection, and septicemia may follow. Systemic antibiotics are often indicated. Infection is the leading cause of death in these patients.

Cool, wet dressings or baths are protective and soothing. Patients with large areas of blistering have a characteristic odor that is lessened when secondary infection is controlled. Potassium permanganate baths help keep the areas from becoming infected and to some extent precipitate some of the protein that oozes through the open skin. It also has deodorant properties. The potassium permanganate crystals should be thoroughly dissolved, as undissolved crystals can burn the skin. Following the bath, the patient is dried carefully and covered with talcum powder, which enables the patient to move freely in bed. Fairly large amounts are necessary to keep the patient from sticking to the sheets. Tape should never be used on the skin, since it may produce more blisters. Meticulous oral hygiene is important, since lesions in the mouth are common in pemphigus and add greatly to the patient's misery. Thus, mouthwashes should be offered frequently to soothe these ulcerative areas, and the patient is encouraged to drink fluids. Since the patient is usually depressed, the nurse should strive to provide the small but important "extras" that serve to lift the morale.

▶ Evaluation

Expected Outcomes

1. Achieves relief of pain of oral lesions
   a. Identifies therapies that reduce pain

b. Uses mouthwashes and anesthetic–antiseptic aerosol mouth spray

c. Drinks chilled fluids at 2-hour intervals

2. Achieves relief of skin discomfort
   a. States purpose of therapeutic regimen
   b. Cooperates with soaks/bath regimen
   c. Reminds personnel to use liberal amounts of powder on sheets

3. Attains fluid and electrolyte balance
   a. Keeps input record to assure adequate fluid intake
   b. Verbalizes an understanding of necessity of intravenous infusion therapy
   c. Reports that urine output is within normal limit
   d. Has serum chemistries within normal limits

4. Is free of infection
   a. Cultures from bullae, skin, and orifices negative for pathogenic organisms
   b. Shows signs that skin is clearing

Toxic Epidermal Necrolysis (TEN)

Toxic epidermal necrolysis (TEN) is a severe, potentially fatal skin disease most commonly related to drug exposure in adults, although it is occasionally induced by staphylococcus. It is characterized by fever; erythema, involving much of the skin surface; development of large, flaccid bullae; skin necrosis; and widespread sheetlike peeling and denudation of the skin. The skin is excruciatingly tender, and the loss of the superficial layer leaves a weeping surface similar to a second-degree burn. The drugs most commonly implicated are the sulfonamides, phenytoin, phenylbutazone, salicylates, penicillins, and barbiturates, although almost 100 drugs have been suspected. Frozen histologic studies of peeled skin from a fresh lesion of TEN and cytodiagnosis of collections of cellular material from a freshly denuded area are diagnostic procedures used to differentiate the drug-induced from the staphylococcus-induced form of the disease.

Management.   The major nursing goals are control of fluid and electrolyte balance and prevention of death from infection of large areas of raw skin.

All nonessential drugs are stopped immediately, and aggressive treatment similar to that for a severe burn is initiated. The patient is placed in strict isolation to reduce the chances of a secondary infection. Cultures are taken of the nasopharynx, eyes, ears, blood, urine, skin, and unruptured bullae to determine the presence of pathogenic organisms. As there is loss of interstitial fluids, an intravenous infusion is started to maintain fluid and electrolyte balance. However, an indwelling intravenous catheter may result in septicemia, and fluid replacement is carried out by mouth or nasogastric tube as soon as possible. Moderate- to high-dose parenteral steroids may be given in drug-induced TEN to abort widespread skin necrosis and denudation. The local care of the skin is a nursing challenge. Secondary infection can be introduced through the damaged skin surface. Warm compresses of aqueous silver nitrate may be applied gently to the raw areas to reduce the bacterial population. Placing the patient on a circular turning frame facilitates handling him. The room must be kept humidified and warm to prevent heat loss. Meticulous oral hygiene is essential to prevent acute parotitis. Other aspects of treatment are similar to that for a severe burn (see p. 1203).

▷ Ulcers and Tumors of the Skin

Ulcerations

The superficial loss of surface tissue due to death of the cells is called an *ulceration*. A simple ulcer, such as is found in a small, superficial, second-degree burn, tends to heal by granulation if kept clean and protected from injury. If exposed to the air, the serum that escapes from it will dry and form a scab, under which the epithelial cells will grow and cover the surface completely. Certain diseases cause characteristic ulcers—tuberculous ulcers and syphilitic ulcers are examples.

Ulcers Due to a Deficient Arterial Circulation.   These ulcers are seen in patients with peripheral vascular disease, arteriosclerosis, Raynaud's disease, and frostbite. In these patients, the treatment of the ulceration must be carried out in conjunction with the treatment of the arterial disease. The danger is from secondary infection. Frequently, amputation of the part is the only effective therapy.

Decubitus Ulcers.   These skin ulcers, more commonly referred to as *pressure sores*, result from continuous pressure on a particular area of the skin. One of the main objectives in the nursing management of any bedridden patient is to avoid the development of pressure sores (see p. 232).

Tumors of the Skin

Cysts

Cysts of the skin are epithelium-lined cavities containing fluid or solid material.

Epidermal cysts (epidermoid) occur frequently and may be described as slow-growing, firm, elevated tumors found most frequently on the face, neck, upper chest, and back. Removal of the cysts provides cure.

Pilar cysts (trichilemmal cysts), originally called sebaceous cysts, are most frequently found on the scalp. They apparently originate from the middle portion of the hair follicle and from the cells of the outer root sheath. The treatment is surgical removal.

Benign Tumors

Seborrheic Keratoses.   These tumors are benign, wartlike lesions of varying size and color, ranging from light tan to black. They are usually located on the face, shoulders, chest, and back and are the most common skin tumors seen in middle-aged and elderly persons. They may be cosmetically unacceptable to the patient, and a black keratosis may be erroneously diagnosed as malignant melanoma. The treatment is removal of the tumor tissue by excision, electrodesiccation and curettage, or the application of carbon dioxide or liquid nitrogen.

Actinic keratoses are premalignant skin lesions that develop in chronic sun-exposed areas of the body. They appear as rough, scaly patches with underlying erythema. An estimated 10% to 20% of these lesions gradually transform into invasive squamous cell carcinoma.

Verrucae (Warts). *Warts* are common benign skin tumors caused by infection with the human papilloma virus that belongs to the DNA virus group. All age groups may be affected, but the condition occurs most frequently between the ages of 12 and 16. Warts come in many varieties.

As a rule, warts are asymptomatic, except when they occur on weight-bearing areas, such as the soles of the feet. They may be treated with locally applied liquid nitrogen, salicylic acid plasters, electrodesiccation, or the application of cantharidin.

Venereal Warts. Warts occurring on the genitalia and perianal areas are known as *condyloma acuminata* and have been shown to be sexually transmitted. These are treated with podophyllin in tincture of benzoin, which is applied to the wart and washed off later. Other treatment modalities include liquid nitrogen, cryosurgery, electrosurgery, and curettage.

Angiomas (Birthmarks). *Birthmarks* are benign vascular tumors involving the skin and the subcutaneous tissues. They may occur as flat, violet-red patches (port-wine angiomas) or as raised, bright red nodular lesions (strawberry angiomas). The latter have a tendency to involute spontaneously. Port-wine angiomas, on the other hand, usually persist indefinitely and are not easily treated. Most patients use masking cosmetics (Covermark) to camouflage the defect.

Pigmented Nevi (Moles). *Moles* are common skin tumors of various sizes and shades, ranging from yellowish brown to black. They may be flat, macular lesions or elevated papules or nodules that occasionally contain hair. The great majority of pigmented nevi are harmless lesions. However, in rare cases, malignant changes supervene and a melanoma develops at the site of the nevus. Some authorities feel that all congenital moles should be removed, since these may have a higher incidence of malignant change. Nevi that show change in color or size or become symptomatic (itch) or develop notch borders should be removed to determine if malignant changes have occurred. Moles that occur in unusual places should be examined carefully for any irregularity and for notching of the border and variation in color. (Early melanomas may frequently show some redness and irritation and areas of bluish pigmentation where the pigment-containing cells have become deeper in the skin.) Nevi over 1 cm should be examined carefully. Excised nevi should be examined histologically.

Keloids. *Keloids* are benign overgrowths of fibrous tissue at the site of a scar or trauma. They appear to be more prevalent among the black race. Keloids are asymptomatic but may cause disfigurement and cosmetic concern. The treatment, which is not always satisfactory, consists of surgical excision, intralesional corticosteroid therapy, and radiation.

Dermatofibroma. A *dermatofibroma* is a common benign tumor of connective tissue that occurs predominantly on the extremities. It is a firm, dome-shaped papule or nodule that may be skin-colored or a pinkish-brown hue. Excisional biopsy is the recommended method of treatment.

Neurofibromatosis (von Recklinghausen's Disease). This disorder is a hereditary condition manifested by pig-mented patches (café au lait macules), axillary freckling, and cutaneous neurofibromas that vary in size. Developmental changes may occur also in the nervous system, muscles, and bone. Malignant degeneration of the neurofibromas is found in 2% to 5% of the patients.

▷ Cancer of the Skin

Skin cancer is the most common form of cancer in the U.S. If it continues at the present rate, an estimated one of seven Americans will develop skin cancer. Because the skin is accessible to direct visualization, skin cancer is readily detected and is the most successfully treated type of cancer.

Causes and Prevention

The sun is the leading cause of skin cancer; incidence is related to the total amount of exposure to the sun. Sun damage is cumulative, and harmful effects may be severe by the age of 20. The increase in skin cancer is probably due to changing life-styles and emphasis on sunbathing, etc. Therefore, protective measures should be started in childhood and carried on throughout life. Persons who do not produce sufficient melanin pigment in the skin to give protection to underlying tissue are very susceptible to sun damage: those at greatest risk are fair, blue-eyed, red-haired persons of Celtic ancestry or those with ruddy or light complexions, as well as those who suffer prolonged sunburn and do not tan. Others at risk are outdoor workers, such as farmers, sailors, fishermen, and people who are exposed to the sun over a period of time. Elderly persons with sun-damaged skin are also at risk, as are persons who have had a history of x-ray treatment (in years past) for acne or benign skin lesions. Workers exposed to certain chemical agents (*arsenic*, nitrates, coal, tar and pitch, oils and paraffins) are also included in the risk group. People who have scars due to severe burns may develop skin cancer 20 to 40 years later. Squamous cell cancer can develop in areas of chronic draining osteomyelitis. Also, neoplastic changes can develop in chronic fistulae. Chronic ulcers of the lower extremity may be the site of origin of skin cancer. In fact, any condition causing scarring or chronic irritation may lead to cancer. Immunosuppressed patients have an increased incidence of malignant skin tumors. Genetic factors are also involved.

Types of Skin Cancer

Skin cancer is diagnosed by biopsy and histologic evaluation. The most common types of skin cancer are *basal cell carcinoma, squamous cell (epidermoid) carcinoma,* and *malignant melanoma.*

Basal Cell Carcinoma (Epithelioma). Basal cell carcinomas arise from the basal cell layer of the epidermis or the hair follicles. This is the most common type of skin cancer.

It generally appears on the sun-exposed areas of the body and is more prevalent in regions where the population is subjected to intense and extensive exposure to the sun. The incidence is proportional to the age of the patient (av-

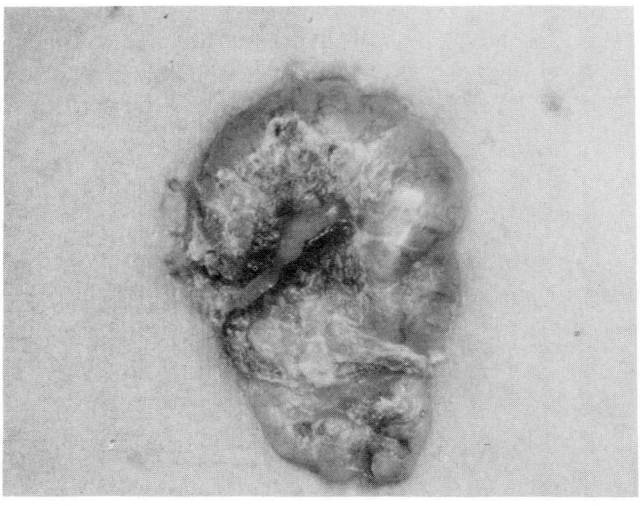

Figure 52-6.   Basal cell carcinoma. (Courtesy, Mervyn L. Elgart, M.D.)

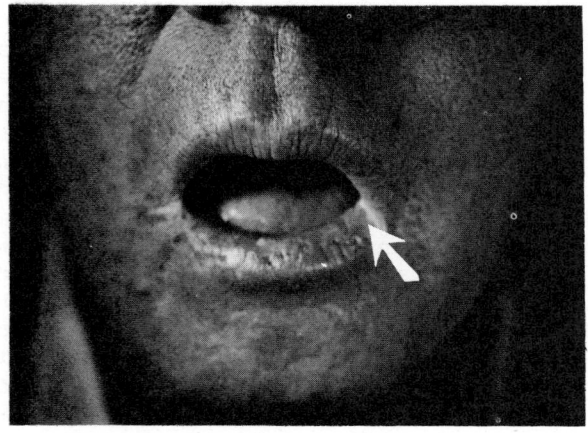

Figure 52-7.   Leukoplakia on the lower lip. Progression to squamous cell carcinoma occurs in 20% to 30% of persons with chronic lesions. (Courtesy, Armed Forces Institute of Pathology, Negative No. 53–19363.)

erage age of 60) and the total amount of sun exposure and is inversely proportional to the amount of melanin pigment in the skin.

It usually presents as a small, waxy nodule with rolled, translucent, pearly borders with telangiectatic (dilation of end-blood vessels) vessels on the surface. As it grows, it undergoes central ulceration and sometimes crusting (Fig. 52-6). The tumors appear most frequently on the face between the hairline and the upper lip. Basal cell carcinoma is characterized by invasion and erosion of contiguous (adjoining) tissues, but it rarely metastasizes. However, a neglected basal cell carcinoma can account for the loss of a nose, an ear, or a lip. Other lesions of this disease may appear as shiny, flat, gray, or yellowish plaques.

Squamous cell carcinoma of the skin is a malignant proliferation arising from the epidermis, usually on sun-damaged skin. However, it may arise from normal skin or

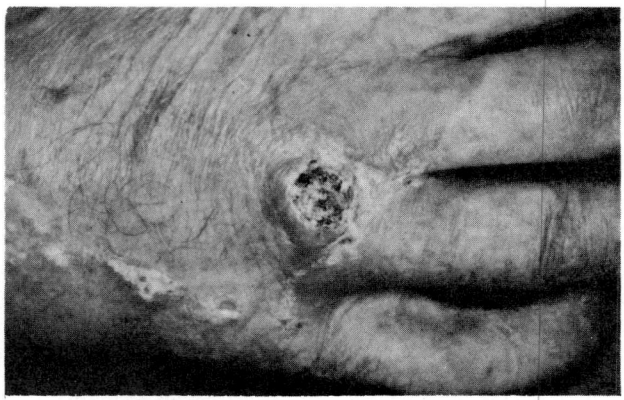

Figure 52-8.   Squamous cell carcinoma. (Courtesy, Mervyn L. Elgart, M.D.)

from preexisting skin lesions. It is of greater concern than basal cell carcinoma because it is a truly invasive carcinoma. The lesions may be primary, arising both on the skin and mucous membranes, or may develop from a precancerous condition, such as actinic keratosis (lesions occurring in sun-exposed areas), leukoplakia (premalignant lesion of the mucous membrane) (Fig. 52-7), or scarred or ulcerated lesions. It appears as a rough, thickened, scaly tumor that may be asymptomatic or may involve bleeding (Fig. 52-8). The border of the lesion may be wider, more infiltrated, and more inflammatory than that of basal cell carcinoma. Secondary infection can occur. Exposed areas, especially of the upper extremities and of the face, lower lip, ears, nose, and forehead, are common sites.

The incidence of metastases is related to the histologic type and the level or depth of invasion. Usually, tumors arising in sun-damaged areas are less invasive and rarely cause death, whereas squamous cell carcinoma arising without a history of sun or arsenic exposure or scar formation appears to have a greater chance of metastatic spread. The patient should be subsequently evaluated for regional lymph node metastases.

Management.   The goal of treatment is to eradicate or completely destroy all the tumor. The method of treatment depends on the tumor location, cell type (location and depth), cosmetic desires of the patient, history of previous treatment, whether or not the tumor is invasive, and if metastatic nodes are present.

The usual method of treatment of both basal cell carcinoma and squamous cell carcinoma is curettage followed by electrodesiccation and surgical excision. Unusual and extensive tumors are treated by chemotherapy.

Curettage Followed by Electrodesiccation.   Curettage is carried out by excising the skin tumor by scraping its surface with a curette; electrodesiccation is then applied to achieve hemostasis and to destroy any viable malignant cells at the base of the wound or along its edges. It is useful for small lesions (less than 1 cm–2 cm [0.4–0.8 inch] in diameter). This method takes advantage of the fact that the tumor in each instance is softer than surrounding skin and therefore can be outlined by a curette, which "feels" the extent of the tumor. The tumor is removed and the base cauterized. The process is repeated three times. Usually, healing occurs within a month.

Surgical Excision.   Wide surgical excision may be necessary. The adequacy of excision is verified by microscopic study of sections of the specimen. Such a histologic study of excised tissue shows whether or not the margins are free of tumor. Skin grafting may be necessary if primary closure is not possible.

Radiation Therapy.   Radiation therapy is frequently done for cancer of the eyelid, the tip of the nose, and areas in or near vital structures (facial nerve). It is reserved for older patients, because x-ray changes may be seen after 5 to 10 years and malignant changes in scars may be induced by x-rays 15 to 30 years later.

The patient should be informed that the skin may become red and blistered. A bland skin ointment (prescribed by the physician) may be applied to relieve discomfort. The patient should also be cautioned against exposure to the sun.

Cryosurgery.   Cryosurgery employs deep freezing to selectively destroy the tumor tissue. A thermocouple apparatus for deep freezing is inserted into the base of the tumor. Liquid nitrogen is sprayed onto the tumor until a temperature of −40° C is reached at the tumor base. The tumor tissue is frozen at this temperature, allowed to thaw, and then refrozen. The site thaws naturally and then becomes gelatinous and heals spontaneously.

Microscopically Controlled Surgery (Chemosurgery). Chemosurgery combines the use of topically applied chemicals and serial surgical excisions of tumors layer by layer. Immediate microscopic examination is made of frozen sections for evidence of cancer cells. This procedure may be repeated until the specimens are cancer-free and all peripheral extensions of the tumor are eradicated. Chemosurgery is useful for recurrent tumors or for infiltrating tumors whose margins cannot be determined.

Topical chemotherapy is the application of a topical antitumor agent (fluorouracil) to destroy cancer cells. The tumors are treated for a period of 3 to 4 weeks. The patient can expect some erythema and discomfort with this treatment. This therapy is only useful for the most superficial tumors.

Patient Education.   The follow-up treatment should be regular, including palpation of the adjacent nodes. The following points of emphasis should be made by way of patient education:

1. Avoid unnecessary exposure to the sun, especially during times when ultraviolet radiation light is most intense (10 AM to 3 PM).
2. *Do not become sunburned.*
3. Apply a protective sunscreen if you must be in the sun; sunscreens block out harmful sunrays.
   a. Sunscreens are rated in strengths from 5 (weakest) to 15 (strongest). This number is called SPF (solar protection factor) and is printed on the bottle.
   b. Sunscreens that contain Para-Aminobenzoic Acid in 55%–70% alcohol do not come off easily; some other sunscreens must be repeatedly applied after perspiration or swimming.

4. Do not use sun lamps for indoor tanning; avoid commercial tanning booths.
5. Wear appropriate protective clothing (*e.g.,* broad-brimmed hat, long-sleeved clothing, etc.). (These do not provide complete protection from ultraviolet rays, as these can pass through a T-shirt, nylon stockings, etc.)
6. Have moles treated that are accessible to repeated friction and irritation.
7. Watch for indications of potential malignancy in moles (*e.g.,* increase in size, ulceration, bleeding, or serous exudation).
8. Have follow-up evaluation throughout lifetime. Watch for development of new lesions. (There is also an incidence of internal malignancy associated with squamous cell cancer.)
9. Caution your children and grandchildren, especially those with fair skin, to avoid excessive exposure to the sun and to use sunscreen so as to prevent later skin cancers.

Malignant Melanoma

A *malignant melanoma* is a tumor of melanocytes (pigment cells) that can occur in one of several forms: superficial spreading melanoma, lentigo-maligna melanoma, nodular melanoma, and acral-lentiginous melanoma. These types have certain clinical and histologic features as well as different biological behaviors. The incidence of melanoma has doubled during the last few decades, probably related to changes in clothing habits and recreational sun exposure.

Melanoma has a higher mortality rate than any other form of skin cancer, but higher percentages of patients are now being cured. Many melanomas appear in preexisting nevi in the skin or develop in the uveal tract of the eye. Melanomas frequently appear simultaneously with cancer of other organs.

The *superficial spreading melanoma* occurs anywhere on the body and is the most common form of melanoma. It usually affects persons of middle age and occurs most frequently on the trunk and lower extremities. The lesion tends to be circular with irregular outer portions. The margins of the lesion may be flat or elevated and palpable (Fig. 52-9). This type of melanoma may appear in a combination of colors, with hues of tan, brown, and black mixed with gray, bluish-black, or white. Sometimes there is a dull pink-rose color in a small area within the lesion.

The *lentigo-maligna melanomas* are slowly evolving pigmented lesions that occur on exposed skin areas, especially of the head and neck, in elderly people. They first appear as tan, flat lesions, which in time undergo changes in size and color.

The *nodular melanoma* is a spherical blueberrylike nodule with a relatively smooth surface and relatively uniform blue-black color (Fig. 52-9). It may be dome-shaped with a smooth surface or rose-gray or black in color and is present as an elevated irregular plaque. The patient may describe this as a "blood blister" that fails to resolve. A nodular melanoma invades directly into subjacent dermis (vertical growth) and hence has a poorer prognosis.

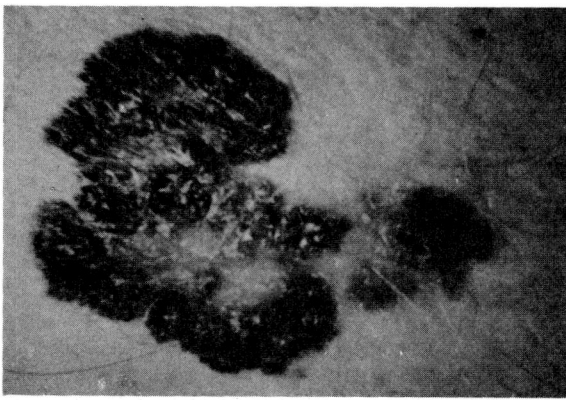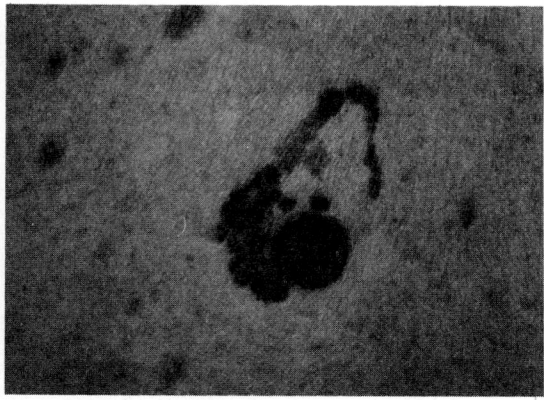

Figure 52-9.   Malignant melanoma: (*Left*) Superficial melanoma. (*Right*) Nodular melanoma. (Courtesy, Mervyn L. Elgart, M.D.)

Acral-lentiginous melanoma is a form of melanoma that occurs in areas not excessively exposed to sunlight and where hair follicles are absent. They are found on the palms of the hands, soles, nail beds, and mucous membranes in blacks and other dark-skinned persons. These melanomas appear as irregular pigmented macules, which develop nodules. They may become invasive early.

Prognosis.   The prognosis is related to the depth of dermal invasion and the thickness of the lesion. The deeper and thicker the melanoma, the greater the likelihood of metastases. If the melanoma is growing radially (horizontally) and is characterized by peripheral growth with minimal or absent dermal invasion, the prognosis is favorable. As the melanoma progresses to the vertical growth phase (dermal invasion), the prognosis is poor. The presence of ulceration correlates with a poor prognosis. Malignant melanoma can spread both through the bloodstream and the lymphatic routes and can metastasize to every organ of the body.

Malignant melanomas most frequently occur on the upper back (men), legs (women), head, neck, and trunk. About one tenth of melanomas occur in the eye. Melanomas of the trunk appear to have a poorer prognosis than those of other sites, perhaps because of the network of lymphatics in the trunk permitting metastasis to regional nodes. In the black race, melanomas are most apt to occur in the less pigmented sites: palms, soles, subungual areas, and mucous membranes.

Causes and Persons at Risk.   The etiology is unknown, but ultraviolet rays are strongly suspected. Epidemiologic evidence indicates that the incidence and mortality rate of malignant melanoma has been increasing. In general, at greatest risk are patients with fair complexions, blue eyes, red or blonde hair, and freckles. These persons synthesize melanin more slowly. Persons of Celtic or Scandinavian origin are at greater risk. Persons who burn and do not tan are also at risk. In areas where sunlight is intense, there is a disproportionate increase in incidence. Older Americans retiring to the Southwestern sunbelt appear to have a higher incidence.

Up to 10% of melanoma patients are members of melanoma-prone families who have unusual (dysplastic) moles

that are susceptible to malignant transformation. Individuals with *dysplastic nevus syndrome* have been found to have unusual moles, larger and more numerous moles, lesions with irregular outlines, and pigmentation located all over the skin. Microscopic examination of dysplastic moles show disordered, faulty growth.

▶ **Assessment**

Clinical Manifestations.   Use a magnifying lens with good lighting. A new or preexisting mole should be checked for irregular color, irregular border, irregular topography, and satellite lesions (lesions situated near the mole). Signs of *variegated* color should also be checked. Colors that may indicate malignancy in a brown or black lesion are shades of red, white, and blue. Shades of blue are considered ominous. White areas in a pigmented lesion are suspicious. Some malignant melanomas are not variegated but are uniformly colored; either bluish-black, bluish-gray, or bluish-red.

If the mole has an *irregular border,* it should be checked for any angular indentation or a notch in the border. However, some melanomas have a smooth surface.

Patient Problems/Nursing Diagnoses

Based on the clinical manifestations and diagnostic assessment data, the patient's major nursing problems include a lesion potentially related to injury by solar radiation; fear and depression related to possible life-threatening consequences of melanoma; and nonadherence to preventive measures related to knowledge deficit.

Management

An excision biopsy specimen is taken to gain histologic information. The therapeutic approach depends on the depth and stage of the lesion.

Surgery.   Small superficial lesions are treated by simple excision, while a wide excision with skin grafting may be necessary depending on the depth of invasion or thickness of the lesion. A regional lymph node dissection may be done. The width of the excision and the need for node dissection are concepts that are undergoing revision at this time.

Microscopically Controlled Surgery (Mohs' Chemosurgery). This is the serial excision of the cutaneous tumor followed by histopathologic examination until the skin is free of malignancy. This technique is useful in the treatment of certain melanomas, since the chance of dislodging melanoma cells is minimized and an extra margin of surface skin can be removed. At the completion of treatment, defects may be treated with a skin graft or flap.

Regional Perfusion. If the lesion is anatomically accessible (*e.g.,* on an extremity), regional perfusion chemotherapy is promising. A specific area is isolated by mechanically controlling its arterial inflow and venous outflow. This allows a high concentration of cytotoxic drugs to be delivered with less systemic toxicity.

Immunotherapy. Immunotherapy involves the use of immune adjuvants to stimulate the patient's immune system (see Chap. 49.) Bacillus Calmette–Guérin (BCG) administered intralesionally, intradermally, orally, or by scarification may limit the growth of the tumor as well as recurrence and may prolong the patient's life. At this time, the role of immunotherapy in the treatment of malignant melanoma has not been firmly established, but there is a suggestion that melanoma may be responsive to immune manipulation.

Chemotherapy. Chemotherapy is generally used when there is recurrence of metastatic disease. New drugs appear frequently, and treatment is usually under the direction of a chemotherapist. The management of the patient undergoing chemotherapy is found in Chapter 17.

▶ **Planning and Implementation**

Goals

The patient's goals are:

1. Eradication of the lesion
2. Relief of anxiety and depression
3. Prevention of recurrence of malignant melanoma

The nursing goals are to support the patient during treatment and to educate him about the importance of follow-up to detect recurrence.

Interventions. Supporting the patient includes allowing him to express his feelings about the seriousness of this cutaneous neoplasm, understanding his anger and sadness, and conveying understanding of these feelings. During the period the diagnosis is being made and the tumor is classified to type and depth, the nurse answers the patient's questions, clarifies information, and helps clear up misconceptions. Learning that he has a melanoma can cause the patient considerable fear and anguish. Pointing out the patient's resources, his past effective coping mechanisms, and social support system helps him to cope with the problems associated with diagnosis, treatment, and continuing follow-up.

The surgical removal of melanoma in different locations (head and neck, eye, trunk, abdomen, extremities, central nervous system) presents different challenges, taking into consideration the removal of the primary melanoma, the intervening lymphatics, and the lymph nodes to which me-

tastases may occur. The nursing management of the patient having surgery of these regions is discussed in the appropriate chapters.

The nursing intervention following malignant melanoma surgery centers on promoting comfort, since wide excision surgery may be necessary. A split-thickness skin graft is done when large defects are created by surgical removal of a melanoma. Anticipating the need for and giving appropriate analgesic medication are part of the nursing function. Psychological support is essential when mutilative surgery is done.

Patient Education. Educating the patient about follow-up care includes explaining the necessity of periodic physical examinations with careful monitoring of nodes at risk for regional spread, chest films, hemogram, and serum chemistry profiles.

The best hope of controlling the disease lies in the education of patients regarding the *early* signs of melanoma. The importance of examining and checking moles or new lesions should be emphasized repeatedly. The patient should report to the physician immediately moles that change color, enlarge, become raised or thicker, or itch. Treatment must be started immediately.

▶ **Evaluation**

Expected Outcomes

1. Experiences eradication of lesion
   a. Is free of fever
   b. Exhibits surgical scar healing with no evidence of heat, redness, or swelling
2. Achieves relief of anxiety and depression
   a. Ventilates fears and fantasies
   b. Asks questions about condition
   c. Requests repetition of facts about melanoma
   d. Identifies interests/hobbies to divert stress
   e. Identifies significant others for positive reinforcement
3. Has no recurrence of malignant melanoma
   a. Recalls several measures to protect self from sun
   b. Reads literature on sunscreen preparations
   c. Verbalizes the following danger signals of melanoma: change in size of mole, color of mole, mole surface, shape or outline of mole, or skin around mole
   d. Demonstrates how to conduct self-examination of skin on a monthly basis to detect mole changes early
   e. Uses a mirror to inspect hard-to-see areas

Metastatic Skin Tumors

The skin is an important, although not common, site of metastatic cancer. All types of cancer may metastasize to the skin, but carcinoma of the breast is the primary source of cutaneous metastases in women. Cancer of the large intestine, ovaries, and lungs are other sources. In men, the primary site is most commonly the lungs, large intestine, oral cavity, kidneys, or stomach. Skin metastases from melanomas are found in both sexes. The clinical appearance of metastatic skin lesions is not distinctive except, perhaps, in some cases of breast cancer where diffuse, brawny hardening of the skin of the involved breast is seen ("cancer en cuirasse"). In most instances, metastatic lesions occur as multiple cutaneous or subcutaneous nodules of varying size that may be skin-colored or show different shades of red.

▷ Dermatologic and Plastic Reconstructive Surgery

The word "plastic" comes from a Greek word meaning "to form." In dermatologic reconstruction surgery, the "forming" is done by transplanting or shifting tissues. Often the terms *plastic* and *reconstructive* are used interchangeably. The goals for this kind of surgery are to repair extravisceral defects and malformations, both congenital and acquired; to restore function; and to prevent further loss of function. Frequently, plastic surgery is done primarily for aesthetic and cosmetic improvement; it is applicable to many parts of the body and to numerous structures, such as bone, cartilage, fat, fascia, mucous membrane, muscle, nerve, and cutaneous structures. Bone inlays and transplants for deformities and nonunion can be done; muscle can be transferred; nerves can be reconstructed and spliced; and cartilage can be replaced. Lastly, but as important as any of these measures, is the reconstruction of the cutaneous tissues around the neck and the face; this is usually referred to as *aesthetic* or *cosmetic surgery*.

Grafts.   Living tissue may be transferred from one part of the body to another or from one person to another. A *graft* is a piece of tissue separated completely from its normal and original position and transferred to another position by one or more stages to correct a distant defect. Transfers or transplants from the same person are termed *autografts;* those from a different person are called *allografts*. The autograft, after a "take," is permanent. The allograft, except in the case of identical twins (*isografts*), is temporary and lasts only a few days or weeks. Some transplant tissues may have been stored in "banks," including bone, fascia, collagen, and corneas of eyes. At times, tissue may be used from animal sources (*xenograft*).

Alloplastic Implants.   These are biologically inert materials used to replace or augment soft tissue and osseous defects. Inert substances have long been used in plastic surgery. Such materials must not irritate the tissues of the recipient, nor must they alter in shape or consistency. On the other hand, the substance ought to match the quality of the part being replaced and provide proper function and cosmetic appeal. In the fascinating history of plastic surgery, a variety of substances have been used, such as metal, ivory, boiled inert bone, rubber, and wax. More recently, silicone and inert plastic materials, such as Teflon and Dacron, have been used with increasingly successful results.

Transplants.   Over the past several decades, kidney, lung, liver, and heart transplants have been performed with varying degrees of success. With all transplants, the recipient reacts to the new tissue as to a foreign invader; the graft acts as an antigen, causing the host to produce antibodies. The autoimmune reaction of the body is not fully understood, but attempts are made to avert such a reaction by immunosuppressive drugs. This has proved to be successful.

Availability of Facilities.   The field of reconstructive and plastic surgery has been expanded to such an extent that often the problem requires the team work of several specialists. For example, in the case of a severed extremity, an orthopedist, a neurosurgeon, and a plastic surgeon combine their talents to replace the extremity. For maxillofacial reconstruction, the work of an oral surgeon; a reconstructive surgeon; and an ear, nose, and throat specialist is required. In addition to the nurse, the services of a sociologist, psychologist, psychiatrist, and chaplain may be required.

The patient in need of plastic or reconstructive surgery may not know that such help is available. In this situation, the nurse, particularly the community health nurse, may be in a position to disseminate information. Parents who have a congenitally deformed child often delay in seeking assistance either because of guilty feelings, conviction that they must bear their own burden, false beliefs that perhaps the child will outgrow his handicap, or ignorance about what can be done.

Children and individuals (up to the age of 21) with congenital defects are eligible for financial support to meet the costs of plastic or reconstructive surgery. Plans for medical care of crippled children are available in each state; these, in turn, are partially supported by the Children's Bureau of the United States.

Assessment.   As in any other form of treatment, it is necessary to assess the status of the patient as a whole person and to view his problem in its entirety. Aside from the basic task of identifying the patient's problem, other aspects of the situation should be assessed: Is his defect a threat to his position or security among his daily contacts? Does the defect affect his interpersonal relations? Are personality changes out of proportion to the size or the nature of his physical problem?

The emotional reaction of the patient to his disfigurement or abnormality is most significant and must be understood if the repair process is to be progressive. The status of an adolescent girl may be threatened if she does not "look like" most of the other girls. The young man's scars may lead him to feel "inferior" to the other members of his class. Such feelings affect the personality, which in turn may affect the individual's level of performance and adjustment to the meaningful experiences of life. Feeling withdrawn and threatened, this person may lash out against his family, friends, and society. Some individuals have long blamed a history of disappointments, limited achievement, and unhappiness on a deformity or disfigurement and believe surgical repair will rechannel the future into a more wonderful course. The personality of the patient and his expectations must be clearly understood and guided, sometimes with professional assistance. The best possible results are obtained when the patient, nurse, and surgeon all follow the same plan of therapy in a cooperative effort.

Presurgical Preparation and Patient Instruction.   Before the operation, the patient's physical state is assessed. Nutritional status is evaluated to see if increased vitamin and protein intake is needed to facilitate tissue healing.

Hemoglobin and clotting time are also noted because their levels can affect the healing process. It is important that the tissues concerned are free of infection, and that other conditions, such as diabetes mellitus, are under control. The general condition of the patient with regard to nutrition, age, and morale should be at an optimal level.

Donor and recipient sites are prepared as for any surgical incision. The patient needs to know those aspects of postoperative care that can contribute significantly to a smooth recovery. The fact that the wound may appear unattractive, red, distorted, and puffy at first does not mean that the incision will not change. The fact that the size of the bandages (such as used with pressure dressings) may be voluminous does not mean that the surgery was correspondingly serious. Whether mirrors in the room should be removed depends on the circumstances. Of course, the family is prepared for the postoperative appearance of the patient so that their surprised or disturbed expressions will not be conveyed to him on the first postoperative visit. Their genuine encour-

agement and support can mean a great deal to the apprehensive patient.

Wound Closure.   Primary approximation of the skin and subcutaneous tissues is the ideal type of wound closure. Fine "hairline" scars can be achieved if the incision lines are parallel to skin lines of minimal tension, such as the "wrinkle lines" or lines of facial expression. If these cannot be followed, incision lines are placed at the junction of dissimilar tissues, such as the hairline of the scalp and face, or the areolar and skin margins of the breast. If a lesion is to be excised, an elliptical incision parallel to skin lines where tension is minimal will give the best result. If sufficient tissue is not available, the next best cosmetic results can be achieved by using skin grafts or pedicle flaps.

Skin Grafts

Prior to the removal of a graft of skin, the donor area is prepared by shaving it free of hairs and cleansing it thor-

Table 52-2
Kinds of Grafts

Type of Graft	Uses	Rationale	Advantages	Disadvantages
Thin split-thickness	Infected wounds and those with poor vascularization	Thicker grafts do not take as well.	Donor site heals readily	Contracture is great Little resistance to trauma Cosmetically poor
Thick split-thickness	Large, superficial face wounds Noninfected wounds on a flexor area	Thickest graft available	Less contracture than thin split-thickness and more resistant to trauma	Survives transplanting less well than thin split-thickness Donor site heals slowly
Full-thickness	Small, superficial facial wounds	Best cosmetic effect	Most similar to normal skin Minimal contracture Sensation good and cosmetically very good	Donor sites are less available Survives transplantation least well
Pedicle	Nasal tip Avulsed wounds with exposed nerves and tendons Good on avascular sites, such as exposed cortical bone or cartilage, or wounds from a deep x-ray "burn"	Repair requires more skin than split- or full-thickness plus an additional blood supply. Free grafts will not survive on avascular surfaces.	Very little contraction Good sensation Good resistance to trauma Often helpful cosmetically if surgeon is adept	Requires a high degree of technical skill Usually, requires several operative procedures
Free flap	Resurfaces a variety of wounds Covers exposed tendons, bones, or major blood vessels Closes wounds with deficient blood supply (*i.e.,* irradiation ulcers)	It can bring a large supply of tissue to a deficient area.	A large area can be covered completely more rapidly than with other types of grafts.	This requires skill in technique of anastomosing arteries and veins (microsurgery). Long periods of immobilization of recipient site may be required.

oughly with a detergent germicide. If the graft is to be successful, the area to be covered must be free of infection and sloughs, because grafts "take" or grow only on a clean "granulating" surface.

Kinds of Grafts

(See Table 52-2.)

Grafts are usually classified as *free* or *pedicle grafts*. *Free grafts* are completely separated from their donor sites, which means that their blood supply is completely interrupted. Thus, the survival of this graft depends on the vascularization of the bed from the recipient site. *Pedicle grafts* are attached to the donor site or to an intermediate transfer site; they carry their own blood supply and therefore do not depend on recipient sites for survival. Free grafts are usually split-thickness or full-thickness grafts, whereas pedicle grafts are usually full-thickness grafts. Split-thickness grafts may be thin, intermediate, or thick (Fig. 52-10). Using standard donor areas, such as the back or buttocks, these grafts will measure approximately as follows:

Thick: 0.010 inch–0.012 inch
Intermediate: 0.016 inch–0.018 inch
Thin: 0.022 inch–0.024 inch

With the advent of microsurgery, a free flap may be used; this is a composite flap that can be taken, completely free of its donor site, and attached to the recipient site by the anastomosis of arteries and veins.

A graft is obtained by using a variety of instruments: razor blade, skin-graft knives, or dermatomes of the manually operated or power-driven variety. Skin is obtained by suction or by adhering it to a drum. The skill of the operator, the nature of the donor site, and the fine adjustment of the instrument are all factors in obtaining the desired graft for the particular need.

Application of the Graft

The graft, when applied to the recipient site may or may not be sutured in place and may or may not be covered with dressings. It may be slit and spread apart for greater area coverage (Fig. 52-11). The exact size of the graft, the correct thickness, and the proper condition of the recipient site all affect how well a graft "takes." When dressings are used, the initial covering often is a single layer of fine mesh gauze impregnated with an ointment to make it nonadherent. This is covered with several thicknesses of gauze cut to the exact size of the area; fluffy dressings are placed on top of this and secured with a wraparound dressing for pressure.

Conditions Required for a Satisfactory "Take"

For a graft to survive and be effective, certain conditions must be met: (1) the recipient bed must be adequately vas-

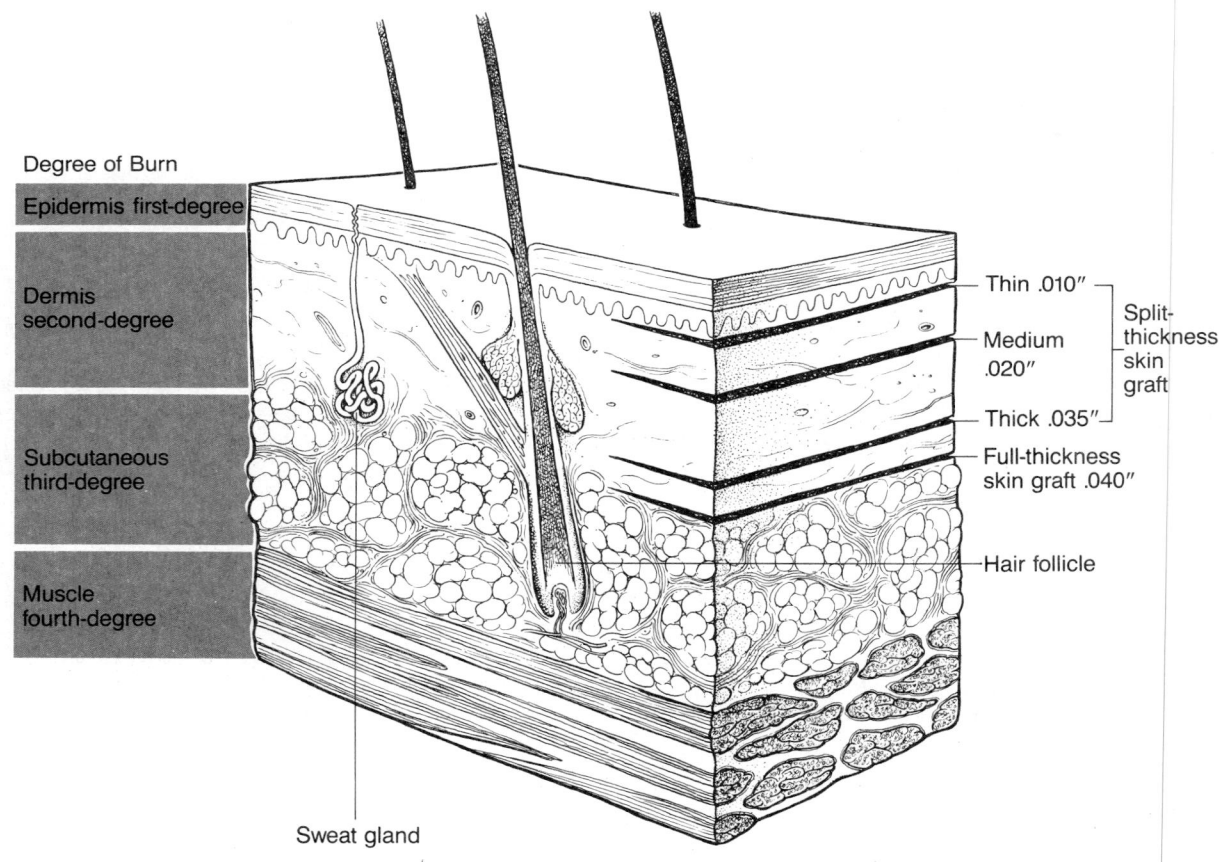

Figure 52-10.   Layers of skin showing split-thickness graft.

cularized, (2) the graft must be in complete contact with the bed, (3) immobilization must be assured, and (4) the area must be free from infection. If infection is present in a wound before it is grafted, local saline compresses, local and systemic antibiotics, and careful debridement may provide an adequate recipient area of clean granulating tissue.

If the above conditions are obtained, skin graft dressings may be left undisturbed for 5 to 7 days. Otherwise, the dressing is changed within 24 to 48 hours and the graft inspected. Any fluid, pus, blood, or serum that has collected is gently evacuated and necrotic tissue carefully debrided before the site is redressed.

Donor Site
Selection Criteria.   The donor site is selected with several criteria in mind: (1) to obtain the closest color match in keeping with the amount of skin graft required, (2) to match the texture and hair-bearing qualities, (3) to obtain the thickest skin graft without jeopardizing the healing process of the donor site (Fig. 52-12), and (4) to consider the cosmetic effects of the donor site on healing, so that it is in an inconspicuous location.

Donor Site Care.   Detailed attention to the donor site is just as important as the care of the recipient area. Usually, a single layer of nonadherent fine mesh gauze is placed directly over the donor site. Absorbent gauze dressings are then placed on top before being taped by pressure bandage.

The dressings are checked in 24 hours to see if the blood that has oozed from the site has been absorbed. If the oozing has stopped, the dressings on top of the nonadherent single layer are left off. If oozing continues, fresh, sterile dressings are applied for another 24 hours. With epithelialization, the nonadherent dressing separates and is gradually trimmed

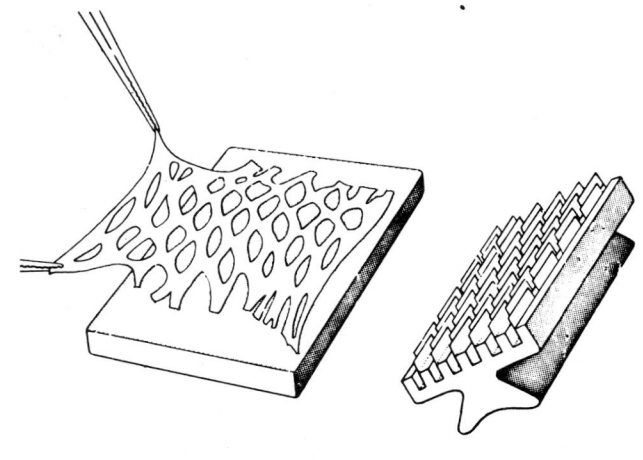

Figure 52-11.   Expansile graft. (Adapted from Feller I and Archambeault C: Nursing the Burned Patient. Ann Arbor, Michigan, The Institute of Burn Medicine.)

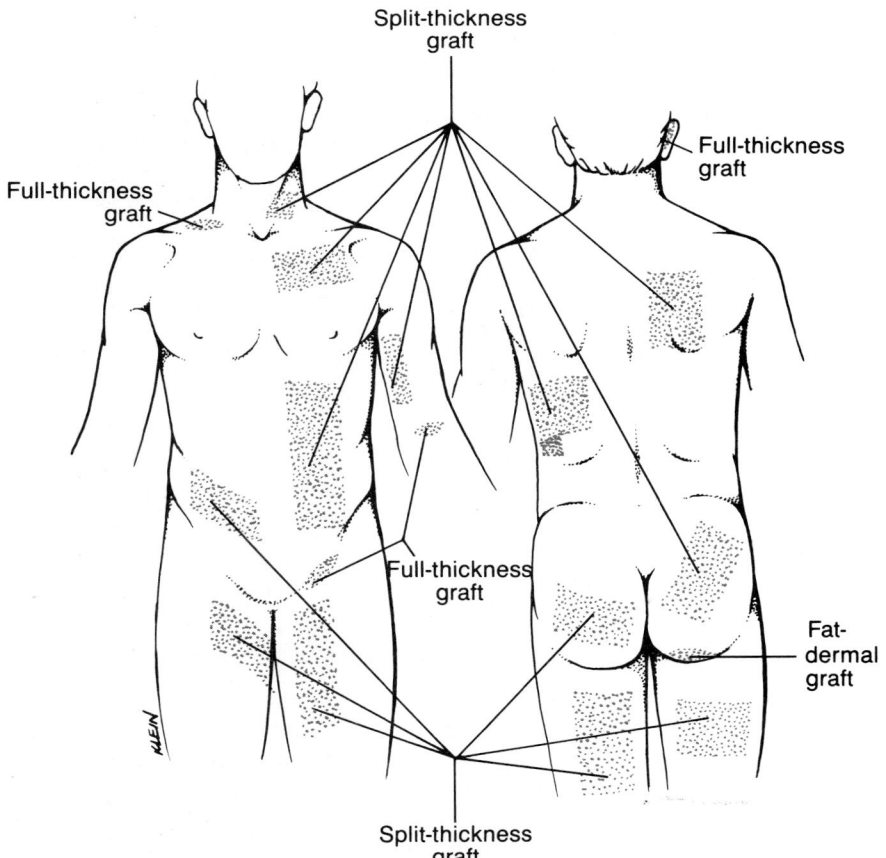

Figure 52-12.   Commonly employed sites for donor areas of skin grafts. (From Converse JM and Brauer RA: Reconstructive Plastic Surgery. Philadelphia, WB Saunders.)

away by the surgeon when the healing process is checked each day.

Pedicle Flaps

A *pedicle flap* is made by raising a section of skin and subcutaneous tissue from one site and moving it to another. However, a segment of skin always remains attached to its donor site. Pedicle flaps include a layer of subcutaneous adipose tissue beneath the skin along with nutrient vessels that must remain attached through the pedicle base in order to provide nourishment. The pedicle is far too thick to absorb its nourishment by osmosis from the wound surface; this is in contrast to the process followed in split- or full-thickness grafts. Newer work in microvascular anastomosis techniques (mainly investigational) may furnish a means of transferring thick pedicles without an attached base.

Types of Pedicle Flaps.   Pedicle flaps may be local or distant, depending on how close they are to the recipient site. They also may be attached at one or more points, depending on the number of attaching points. Pedicle grafts may be classified according to the manner in which skin is moved. This varies with the nature of the tissue and amount of skin desired. The various types of pedicle flaps include advancement flaps, transposed flaps, rotation flaps, tube pedicles (Fig. 52-13), island pedicles, and Z-plasty grafts.

Fascial, Cartilage, and Bone Transplants

Fascial transplants have numerous uses. They are obtained generally from the fascia lata of the thigh and are adaptable for use as suture material, for repair of hernia defects, and for replacement of tendon loss. Cartilage transplantation may be immediate and direct, taken from the costal cartilages and transferred to the nose. Bone grafts demand careful aseptic technique and rigid fixation in their new site. They may be taken from the crest of the tibia, the upper border of the iliac bone, or a rib. All donor areas should receive the same careful treatment given any other surgical wound.

Management of the Patient With Maxillofacial Problems

The face is a part of the body that every person desires to keep at its best. Many individuals try to improve on nature by using cosmetics or adopting their very own hairstyle. When the face becomes disfigured, an emotional reaction

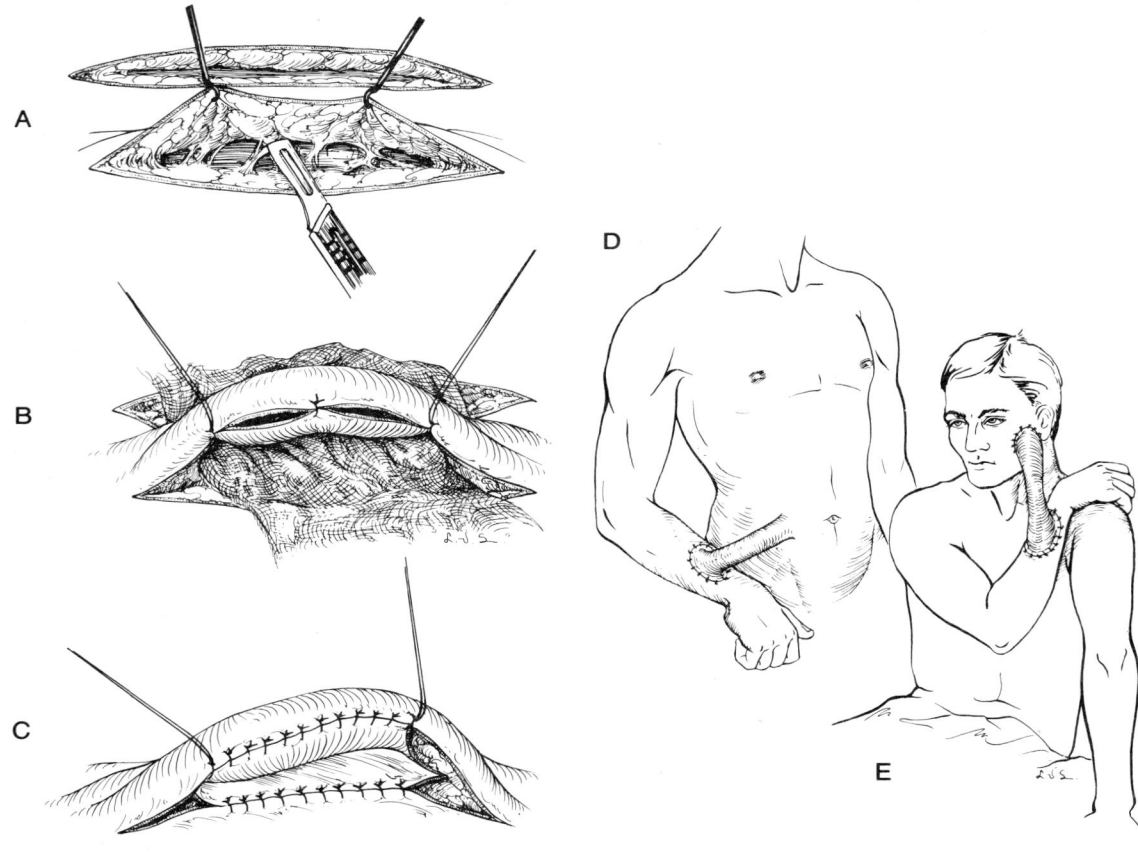

Figure 52-13.   Tube pedicle. The skin and adjacent adipose layer between two parallel incisions are rolled and sutured together (*A, B*). The closed flaps are suitable for transfer to a distant recipient site (*C*). *D* and *E* show the transfer of pedicle graft via wrist carriers. (Reproduced, with permission, from Dunphy JE and Way LW: Current Surgical Diagnosis and Treatment, 3rd ed., 1977. Copyright 1977 by Lange Medical Publications, Los Altos, California.)

occurs. Consequently, an accident victim whose face is injured presents a problem that demands the utmost in understanding and care by the nurse.

The manner in which the person reacts to the medical and nursing personnel is indicative of his inner feelings and is most significant if appropriate measures are to be taken to help him.

Proper management of maxillofacial injuries or fractures depends on knowledge of how the injury occurred and on careful assessment of how extensive the injury is. Initial care includes maintenance of an airway and treatment for shock.

Presurgical Nursing Management

The nurse is in a better position to prepare the patient for the operation when the physician has fully informed the patient about the surgical procedure, the functional defects that may result, the possibility of a prosthesis, the necessity for additional surgery, and the possible need for a tracheostomy.

For any kind of maxillofacial surgery, whether due to injury or cancer, the involved tissues must be thoroughly cleansed if the wound is to heal properly. All wounds are cleansed with soap and water to remove clots, crusts, and foreign material and are then irrigated with normal saline solution. Damaged tissue that appears nonviable should be debrided.

Since the surgery is directed at the maxillofacial area, the patient's mouth is made as clean as possible to lessen the danger of wound infection. The goals of administering preoperative medication are for the purpose of relaxing the patient, diminishing pain, and reducing mouth secretions. If the person is male, the skin of the face is shaved closely and cleansed thoroughly with soap and water. Shaving of face, scalp, etc. is done as requested by the physician. If the entire head is to be shaved, it is best to obtain the patient's written permission.

▶ Postoperative Assessment

Following maxillofacial surgery, the nurse should assess the following parameters: adequacy of the airway, vital signs, wound drainage, severity and duration of pain, fluid and nutritional needs, ability to communicate, and self-image.

Patient Problems/Nursing Diagnoses

Based on the clinical manifestations, nursing history, and diagnostic assessment data, the patient's nursing diagnoses include potential airway obstruction related to laryngeal edema or accumulation of tracheobronchial secretions; potential hemorrhage related to inadequate hemostasis at the surgical site; pain related to surgical trauma; potential nutrient deficit related to impairment of mastication; alteration in ability to communicate related to injury; and alteration in self-image related to disfigurement.

▶ Planning and Implementation

Goals

The major goals for the patient include:

1. Patency of airway
2. Absence of hemorrhage
3. Relief of pain
4. Attainment/maintenance of adequate nutritional status
5. Adequacy of communication
6. Positive self-image

Airway. The main concern of immediate postoperative care is maintenance of an adequate airway. One sign of insufficient oxygen intake, air hunger, or anoxia is restlessness. Thus, if the patient shows signs of restlessness, the airway should be carefully inspected to see if there is laryngeal edema or accumulation of tracheobronchial mucus. Since signs of restlessness can alert the nursing staff to problems of anoxia, sedatives or narcotics should not be administered to the patient without the physician's permission.

Positioning. The position of the patient is determined by the nature of the surgery. If venous return is desired, the patient's head may be elevated. However, if hypotensive medications have been given, the patient should remain recumbent in the immediate postoperative period.

Suctioning. To avoid frequent change of dressings, portable wound suction may be used. Such suction is maintained at 40 mm Hg to 60 mm Hg and must be checked frequently to assure proper functioning.

Complications. Vital signs must be monitored regularly to maintain a check on possible complications.

Early *hemorrhage* may result from inadequate hemostasis, requiring simple aspiration or the removal of a hematoma. Bleeding may be controlled by inserting a gauze pad in the mouth and pressing it against the bleeding part of the jaw. The mouth can then be closed so that the lower teeth exert pressure against the gauze pad. If the patient is conscious, he can cooperate by biting on the pad. Should hemorrhage occur after the first week, it usually indicates infection and must be controlled immediately via direct digital pressure until suturing can be done in the operating room.

Venous congestion may give the face a purplish appearance and may be relieved by elevating the head of the bed to 30 degrees. Note the color of the extremities in order to be certain that discoloration is not due to inadequate circulation. Edema of the face also may be noted in some patients but usually subsides after the fifth day.

Pain. This is more likely to follow operations involving the jaw bones than the soft tissues alone. For postoperative pain, an icebag may offer relief. Whatever measures work best for the individual patient are employed. Analgesics ranging from aspirin to morphine may be required.

Pain may be more severe if secondary infection occurs, a complication that can be minimized if frequent oral hygiene is practiced. To avoid infection, the mouth is cleansed after each feeding. Mouthwash alone is not sufficient. A more effective method is to frequently swab the gums and the teeth with cotton-tipped applicators soaked in hydrogen peroxide. The exact location of sutures in the mouth are noted so that they are not accidentally disturbed during the cleansing procedures. Cold compresses may help to reduce edema.

Fluid and Nutritional Needs. Patients who have undergone maxillofacial surgery need not be denied fluids for any length of time after operation, as may be the case after abdominal operations. The patient may be given cracked ice or water as soon as postanesthetic nausea is over, and a liquid diet may be started as soon as the individual has a desire for food. Very often, soft diet is offered the day after surgery, if tolerated.

In many patients, particularly those with fractures of the jaws, the upper and lower teeth must be fastened together for weeks; hence only liquid food can be taken. Others are able to take soft food, but are unable to masticate. To meet optimum nutritional requirements, it often is necessary to utilize a nasogastric tube, cervical pharyngostomy, or gastrostomy. Blenderized foods are given to meet caloric needs, and water is given for optimum hydration. The patient and perhaps the family may have to be taught to use these special techniques in feeding, particularly if the patient is discharged while still using a feeding tube.

Communication.   Communication problems can present a major difficulty. The patient will find it easier to communicate if he can use gestures or respond to questions with a simple "yes" or "no" answer. The magic slate or pad and pencil can also be useful. Whatever the method of communication, patience and an empathetic understanding of the patient's problems are most helpful.

Psychological Support.   The nurse is in a unique position to help these patients accept their many experiences more easily. Rehabilitation is often a combination of both physical and psychological considerations; it depends not only on eradication of a physical scar, but also on the relief of psychic trauma that can be markedly influenced by the patient's social and emotional background.

If prosthetic devices are to be used, the patient must be taught how to use and care for them so as to gain a greater sense of independence. He needs to be able to accept his new self and adjust to his family and community. Later follow-up visits at a health center are urged.

Many times, the ultimate goal requires a number of operations separated by long intervals of time. Patience is a real factor. Recreational, occupational, and spiritual therapies need to be explored fully, always keeping the interests of the individual patient intact.

Often, the kinds of dressings that have to be worn, the unusual positions that have to be maintained, and the temporary incapacities that must be experienced can be very upsetting to the most stable person. The nurse must be able to offer hope and encouragement and to combine this with a wholesome sense of humor. Tact, patience, and attention to small details will make the nurse an invaluable colleague as the patient regains self-assurance and more normal usefulness and appearance.

▶ **Evaluation**

Expected Outcomes

1. Maintains patent airway
   a. Has respiratory rate within normal limits
   b. Is oriented to time, place, and person
   c. Rests comfortably
   d. Has normal breath sounds
   e. Expectorates mucus easily

2. Experiences no hemorrhage
   a. Has vital signs within normal limits
   b. Is free of bright red bleeding from wound
3. Experiences relief of pain
   a. Verbalizes relief of pain after use of analgesic
   b. Requires progressively less analgesic to relieve pain
   c. Uses icebag to reduce pain
   d. Adheres to oral hygiene regimen to prevent infection and subsequent pain
4. Attains/maintains adequate nutritional status
   a. Drinks liquids as prescribed
   b. Meets basic nutritional requirements through intake of liquid or soft diet
5. Communicates effectively
   a. Uses appropriate aids to enhance communication
   b. Interacts effectively with health team members and family/support persons
6. Develops positive self-image
   a. Demonstrates independence in performing activities of daily living
   b. Assumes responsibility for therapeutic procedures (*e.g.,* oral hygiene, dressing changes, etc.)
   c. Uses prosthetic devices independently (when appropriate)
   d. Plans for resumption of pre-illness activities (*e.g.,* work, recreational, and home activities)
   e. Involves family/support persons in plans for resumption of activities

Chemical Planing

Chemical planing (face peeling, chemabrasion, chemosurgery, chemical face-lifting) is the application of a cauterant (any caustic application) for the purpose of causing superficial destruction of the epidermis and upper layers of the dermis. It is used to treat fine wrinkles, abnormal pigmentation, freckles, and acne scarring on the face. This procedure should be done by someone qualified in reconstructive surgery. A phenol-based chemical in an oil–water emulsion is most frequently used; other agents are salicylic acid and trichloroacetic acid. Prior to the treatment, the skin is cleansed thoroughly with soap and water followed by diethyl ether to remove oily residue. Precautions are taken to avoid the eyes and to prevent the patient from inhaling the ether vapor. Pretreatment medication (analgesic and tranquilizer) is designed to control apprehension.

Chemical Application.   The chemical is carefully applied in a systematic manner to the entire face with cotton-tipped applicators. Following this, a mask of waterproof adhesive tape is applied directly to the skin. This is molded closely, but not too tightly. In 30 to 45 minutes following application of this medication, a burning sensation is experienced. It varies in intensity from person to person; some require additional pain medication.

Postchemical Application.   After 6 or 8 hours, the face becomes edematous. No movement or facial activity is permitted for 48 hours except for bathroom privileges. Liquids are administered by straw to maintain nutrition and hydration. By the second day, the patient may feel moisture under the dressings as the chemically treated skin begins to weep.

Surgical Planing (Dermabrasion)

Dermabrasion (scraping, sandpapering, brushing of the skin) is done in selected patients with facial disfigurements from scars resulting from acne, burns, trauma, a tattoo, nevi, hemangiomas, freckles, and chickenpox or smallpox. Contraindications are keloids, wide scars, deep burn scars, and artistic tattoos. The procedure involves the removal of the epidermis and some superficial dermis while preserving enough of the dermis to allow reepithelialization of the dermabraded areas (Fig. 52-14). Results are best in the face, because it is rich in intradermal epithelial elements. Planing is performed either manually with coarse abrasive paper, or mechanically with an abrader or a rapidly rotating wire brush.

Patient Instruction and Preparation. The primary reason for undergoing dermabrasion is to improve appearance. The surgeon explains to the patient what can be expected from dermabrasion. The patient should also be informed about the nature of the postoperative dressing, what discomfort may be experienced, and how long it will be before the tissues look normal. The extent of the surface to be planed determines whether the procedure takes place in

Second Day. Following sedation of the patient, dressings are removed after 48 hours, exposing skin similar to a second-degree burn. As the dressing is pulled away, the skin is pushed from the dressing with a sterile cotton applicator. Meperidine hydrochloride is administered to relieve pain. Thymol iodide powder, a bacteriostatic medication, is then applied with a cotton-tipped applicator to the entire surface three or four times during the next 24 hours. Color changes occur; the skin becoming dark brown and crusty. The crust remains for several days and then is covered with an ointment such as petrolatum (or vitamin A or D ointment); this is applied to hasten the separation of the crust. In another 24 hours, the face may be washed with plain water. Crusting separates gradually, revealing bright pink epidermis. Any remaining crusts are not removed forcibly.

Discharge Planning. The patient is ready for discharge at the discretion of the physician. For the next 2 to 3 weeks, the skin has a granular appearance. Treatment is limited to washing with clear water and applying a bland ointment. At the end of 3 weeks, cosmetics may be applied. Exposure to the sun is not permitted for 3 to 6 months because melanin (the natural protective mechanism against the sun) in the basal layer of the epidermis is diminished.

Patients are carefully selected for chemical peeling and should realize that 3 to 4 weeks of social isolation is required

and that they may have prolonged facial redness for several weeks.

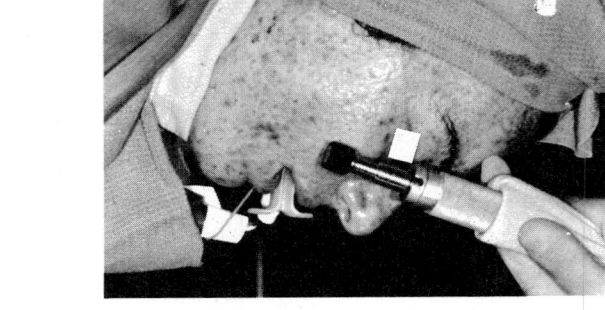

(A) The patient with acne before the dermabrasion procedure.

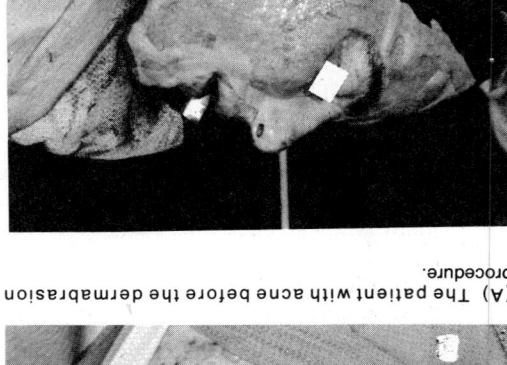

(B) The appearance of the skin after bleeding is controlled by pressure. Upper lip, eyelids, and nostril rims have not yet been abraded.

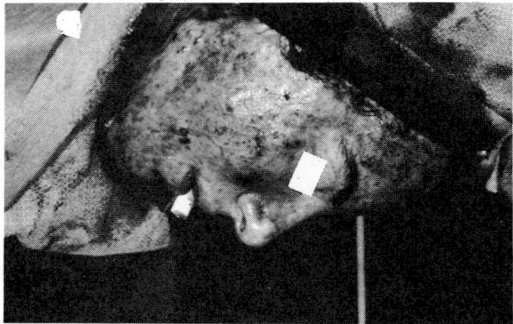

(C) A layer of petrolatum dressing is applied.

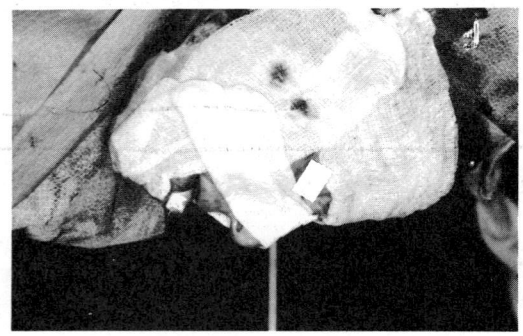

(D) Saline compresses are applied over the petrolatum dressing. This is done to absorb oozing and clotting, which are subject to infection.

Figure 52-14. Dermabrasion procedures. The saline compresses are discontinued after 12 to 24 hours, and the petrolatum dressing is allowed to air dry in place. It is removed in 3 to 5 days. The skin will remain red for 6 to 8 weeks.

the surgeon's office, the clinic, or the hospital. Most often a general anesthetic is used, and the patient is hospitalized. The skin is thoroughly cleansed with pHisoHex for several days before surgery. Shaving is not necessary in the female; however, the male shaves the morning of surgery. In addition to general anesthesia, the use of a topical spray anesthetic (such as Frigiderm) for stabilizing and stiffening the skin may be desirable. The depth of planing can be readily gauged, and the anesthetized area is momentarily bloodless.

During and after planing, copious saline irrigations remove debris and allow for inspection.

Postoperative and Convalescent Management. Usually, petrolatum gauze or perforated plastic-faced ('Telfa') bandages are applied. Pressure dressings may or may not be used, depending on physician preference.

Edema occurs during the first postoperative day and may cause the eyes to close. The patient should be informed that edema will subside; erythema may occur.

Chart 52-3
Lesions Amenable to Argon Laser Treatment

Cutaneous Vascular Lesions
Port-wine hemangiomas
Capillary-cavernous hemangiomas
Strawberry mark (of infancy)
Telangiectasia
Acne rosacea
Campbell-DeMorgan senile angiomas

Inflammatory Lesions
Pyogenic granuloma

Nevoid Lesions
Seborrheic keratosis
Café au lait spots
Giant, hairy nevus
Nevus

Tattoo
Decorative
Traumatic

Miscellaneous
Nevus of Ota
Rhinophyma
Granuloma faciale
Fibrous papule
"Liver spots"

(From Apfelberg DB et al. The argon laser for cutaneous lesions. JAMA 1981; 245(20):2074. Copyright 1981, American Medical Association.)

After about 48 hours, dressings are removed and the sensation is that of a recent sunburn. When the crust forms, lanolin, cocoa butter, or hypoallergenic cream relieves the sensation of tightness. When no dressings are used, oozing may be noticed. In some clinics, the drying process is facilitated by using a hair dryer turned to the warm setting and allowing the air to flow gently over the area. Within 14 days the crusts have separated, and although the skin is still red, most of the scars are gone. The patient is advised to avoid direct sunlight for 3 to 4 months and to use a sunscreen. Repeat treatments are usually advocated. The patient's chief complaint is that the procedure is more annoying than discomforting. The effects produced are well worth the inconvenience in those who are carefully selected for the procedure.

Argon Laser Treatment of Cutaneous Lesions

The argon laser is a nonionizing blue-green (argon laser) light that is absorbed by pigment (e.g., melanin, hemoglobin, pigment of tatoos, foreign body particle) in the dermis; it is then converted to heat followed by selective destruction of specific cutaneous lesions. This treatment spares adjacent dermal tissues, such as sweat glands and hair follicles; the wound subsequently heals with minimal scarring. Lesions amenable to argon laser treatment are listed in Chart 52-3.

Aesthetic (Cosmetic) Surgery

Cosmetic surgery is performed to improve the self-image; it affects mental health, which is as important as physical health. Cosmetic surgery may be done to correct deformities or visible scars, or to compensate for the aging process. Table 52-3 lists the common cosmetic operations.

Rhytidoplasty (Face Lift)

A *rhytidoplasty* is an operation on the face in which excess skin resulting from elastosis is removed and remaining skin is tightened; it is done for cosmetic purposes.

Preoperative Management. The face is cleansed thoroughly with a detergent germicide for 3 days prior to surgery, and the hair is shampooed the night before surgery. Once the patient reaches the operating room, the hair along the incision line is clipped slightly. After anesthesia has been induced, part of the skin is undermined and then stretched to give tension. Excess skin is excised.

Psychological preparation requires that the person recognize the limitations of surgery and understand that it will not necessarily solve all emotional problems. The patient also needs to know that when the dressings are removed after the operation, tissues will still be edematous and will give the face an unpleasant appearance. Several days are required for the edema to subside. Final results depend on the condition of the patient's skin and the skill of the surgeon.

Postoperative Management. The patient is encouraged to rest quietly for the first 2 days until dressings are removed. Relative quiet is recommended, since hematomas are most likely to form during this time if there is too much movement. Thus, excessive talking should be discouraged. The head

Table 52-3
Common Cosmetic Plastic Operations

Operation	Purpose	Surgery	Postoperative Expectations
Rhinoplasty (nose)	To improve the shape of the nose in relation to the rest of the face	1 to 1½ hours. Excess bone or cartilage is removed; nose is reshaped.	Nasal splint; soft intranasal packing; foam rubber dressings
Mentoplasty (chin)	To improve the profile, such as is necessary with a receding chin	Incision approach is within the mouth. Silicone or plastic implant is positioned.	Healing is complete in a week.
Rhytidoplasty (face life)	To remove wrinkles caused by loose skin and to tighten fatty tissues	Incision line is anterior to ear; facial skin is undermined and drawn taut.	Improvement lasts from 5 to 10 years.
Glabellar rhytidoplasty	To remove two vertical furrows between eyebrows	Dermabrasion and excision; skin graft may be required.	
Otoplasty (ear)	To correct deformed, flattened, or protruding ears	1 to 1½ hours. Silicone or plastic implant may be used.	Ear is bandaged for a week; protection during sleep is required for 3 weeks.
Blepharoplasty (eyelid)	To remove wrinkles and bulges caused by aging or inheritance	1 to 1½ hours. Two incisions; one on upper lid and one on lower lid.	Swelling and discoloration subsides in about 10 days.

and upper body may be elevated at least 30 degrees to lower venous pressure. A liquid diet may be given by means of straws; some surgeons will permit a soft diet.

If suction drains are used, it is important to maintain their patency. Although drugs may have to be prescribed for pain, the pain itself is not significant. Antibiotic therapy is usually prescribed to combat infection. A tranquilizer may be given to allay apprehension and maintain a relative degree of quietness.

Pressure dressings are left in place up to 48 hours. No dressings are reapplied; however, the matted hair may be gently combed out with a large-tooth comb dipped in soapy water. At this time, the skin may be gently cleansed of caked blood and other debris.

Since there is edema, ecchymosis, and distortion of the tissues for the first few days, it is preferable that the patient not look into a mirror during this time.

When the patient is discharged, he is treated in the physician's office thereafter. Activities are gradually increased. Sutures are removed on the fifth postoperative day in preauricular incisions, and several days later for post-auricular or temporal sutures. When all sutures are removed, the hair may be shampooed. Hair may be set and dried with warm, not hot, air.

A face lift will last for several years if the person has good skin tone and is between 45 and 55 years of age. It will not last as long for those in the older age group. Rhytidoplasty has been performed two or three times in some patients.

Rhinoplasty

Rhinoplasty is an operation to improve the shape of the nose. A deformed nose resulting from a fracture or a congenital malformation (a large hump, a bulbous nose, or a

drooping tip) may be a source of sensitivity to a young man or woman. Cosmetic nasal reconstruction is suggested when the patient's nose is mature—at about 16 or 17 years of age. The operation is done through intranasal incisions, usually under local anesthesia. Hospitalization is brief, but postoperative edema and periorbital ecchymosis may be in evidence for several postoperative days.

Rhinoplasty is the most widely performed cosmetic surgical operation. If a nose problem is also associated with a receding chin, a *mentoplasty* may be done.

▷ **Bibliography**

Books

Binnick SA. Skin Diseases: Diagnosis and Management in Clinical Practice. Menlo Park, Addison–Wesley, 1982.

Callen JP. Cutaneous Aspects of Internal Disease. Chicago, Year Book Medical Publishers, 1981.

Callen JP, Stawiski MA, and Vorhees JA. Manual of Dermatology. Chicago, Year Book Medical Publishers, 1980.

Chang WHJ (ed). Fundamentals of Plastic and Reconstructive Surgery. Baltimore, Williams & Wilkins, 1980.

Converse JM (ed). Reconstructive Plastic Surgery, 2nd ed. Philadelphia, WB Saunders, 1977.

Cronin E. Contact Dermatitis. New York, Churchill Livingstone, 1980.

Domonkos AN, Arnold HL Jr, and Odom RB. Andrews' Diseases of the Skin. Philadelphia, WB Saunders, 1982.

Fleischmajer R. Progress in Disease of the Skin, Vol 1. New York, Grune & Stratton, 1981.

Frost P and Horwitz SN. Principles of Cosmetics for the Dermatologist. St Louis, CV Mosby, 1982.

Korting GW. Geriatric Dermatology. Philadelphia, WB Saunders, 1980.

Korting GW. Practical Dermatology of the Genital Region. Philadelphia, WB Saunders, 1981.

Lazarus GS, Goldsmith LA, and Tharp MD. Diagnosis of Skin Disease. Philadelphia, FA Davis, 1980.

Maddin S (ed). Current Dermatologic Therapy. Philadelphia, WB Saunders, 1982.

Marks R (ed). Investigative Techniques in Dermatology. Oxford, Blackwell Scientific, 1979.

Marks R. Psoriasis. New York, Arco, 1980.

Marks R and Christophers E (eds). The Epidermis in Disease. Philadelphia, JB Lippincott, 1981.

Roenigk HH Jr. Office Dermatology. Baltimore, Williams & Wilkins, 1981.

Rosen T and Martin S. Atlas of Black Dermatology. Boston, Little, Brown & Co, 1981.

Rosenthal S. Cosmetic Surgery: A Consumer's Guide. Philadelphia, JB Lippincott, 1977.

Safai B and Good RA. Immunodermatology. New York, Plenum, 1981.

Samitz MH. Cutaneous Disorders of the Lower Extremities, 2nd ed. Philadelphia, JB Lippincott, 1981.

Sauer GC. Manual of Skin Diseases, 4th ed. Philadelphia, JB Lippincott, 1980.

Seville RH and Martin E. Dermatological Nursing and Therapy. Oxford, Blackwell Scientific, 1981.

Articles
Acne

Diamant F. Polyester sponge adjunct in acne management. Clin Ther 1980; 3(4):250–253.

Eady EA, Holland KT, and Cuniffe WJ. Topical antibiotics in acne therapy. J Am Acad Dermatol 1981 Oct; 5(4):455–459.

Gun JD. The role of *Propionibacterium acnes* in the pathogenesis of acne. Int J Dermatol 1981 Apr; 20(3):172–173.

Jones H, Cunliffe WJ, and Blanc D. 13-cis-retinoic acid and acne. Lancet 1980 Nov 15; 2(8203):1048–1049.

McKenzie MW et al. Topical clindamycin formulations for the treatment of acne vulgaris. Arch Dermatol 1981 Oct; 117(10):630–634.

Millikan LE and Ameln R. Use of Buf-Puf and benzoyl peroxide in the treatment of acne. Cutis 1981 Aug; 28(2):201–205.

Myslibroski JA and Lumpkin LR. Therapy for acne vulgaris. Compr Ther 1981 Jan; 7(1):13–16.

New topical antibiotics for acne. Med Lett Drugs Ther 1980 Dec 12; 22(25):107–108.

Padilla RS, McCabe JM, and Becker LE. Topical tetracycline hydrochloride vs. topical clindamycin phosphate in the treatment of acne: A comparative study. Int J Dermatol 1981 July–Aug; 20(6):445–448.

Plewig G and Wagner A. Anti-inflammatory effects of 13-Cis-retinoic acid. Arch Dermatol Res 1981; 270(1):89–94.

Plewig G et al. Acne. Acta Derm Venerol [Suppl] (Stockh) 1980; 89:9–95 (entire volume).

Popovich NG. Topical antibiotic therapy for acne. Am Pharm 1981 May; 21(5):55–58.

Quan MA, Rodney WM, and Strick RA. Treatment of acne vulgaris. J Fam Pract 1980 Dec; 11(7):1041–1050.

Vorhees JJ and Orfanos CE. Oral retinoids. Broad spectrum dermatologic therapy for the 1980s. Arch Dermatol 1981 July; 117(7):418–421.

Assessment and Therapy

Anders JE. Topicals: What to use, how to apply. RN 1982 Sept; 45(9):32–42.

Brown ME. Introduction to assessment of the skin. Occup Health Nurs 1980 Aug; 28(8):8–12.

Burton JL. The logic of dermatologic diagnosis. Clin Exp Dermatol 1981 Jan; 6(1):1–21.

Cataldo MF et al. Behavior therapy techniques in treatment of exfoliative dermatitis. Arch Dermatol 1980 Aug; 116(8):919–922.

Flaxman BA. Pruritis. Postgrad Med 1981 May; 69(5):177–188.

Malkiewicz J. The integumentary system. RN 1981 Dec; 44(12):54–60.

Richardson DP. Seborrheic dermatitis and rosacea. Compr Ther 1981 Jan; 7(1):57–60.

Rose R and Mills JM. Look alike lesions. RN 1981 Mar; 44(3):52–53.

Simons HM. Acute life-threatening dermatologic disorders. Med Clin North Am 1981 Jan; 65(1):227–243.

Witkowski JA and Parish LC. The touching question. Int J Dermatol 1981 July–Aug; 20(6):426.

Blistering Diseases

Ahmed AR et al. Pemphigus: Current concepts. Ann Intern Med 1980 Mar; 92(3):396–405.

Artnak KE, Moore LF, and Clements CA. Epidermolysis bullosa: An inherited skin disorder. Am J Nurs 1981 Oct; 81(10):1837–1840.

Barclay WR. Epidermolysis Bullosa Research Association. JAMA 1981 Nov 13; 246(19):2194.

Bauer EA and Cooper TW. Therapeutic considerations in recessive dystrophic epidermolysis bullosa. Arch Dermatol 1981 Sept; 117(9):529–530.

Bean SF and Cox GF. Bullous diseases in the elderly. Geriatrics 1980 June; 35(6):95–99.

Callen JP. Internal disorders associated with bullous disease of the skin. A critical review. J Am Acad Dermatol 1980 Aug; 3(2):107–119.

Editorial: Drug induced bullous eruptions. Br Med J 1981 Feb 7; 282(6262):421–422.

Fine JD et al. Adult scalded skin syndrome totally complicated by mixed gram-negative sepsis and cellulitis. Cutis 1981 Feb; 27(2):162–164, 166–167.

Goodnough LT. Bullous pemphigoid as a manifestation of chronic lymphocytic leukemia. Arch Intern Med 1980 Nov; 140(11):1526–1527.

Hodge L et al. Bullous pemphigoid: The frequency of mucosal involvement and concurrent malignancy related to indirect immunofluorescence findings. Br J Dermatol 1981 July; 105(1):65–69.

Laskaris G. Oral pemphigus vulgaris: An immunofluorescent study of fifty-eight cases. Oral Surg 1981 June; 51(6):626–631.

Laskaris G and Nicolis G. Immunopathology of oral mucosa in bullous pemphigoid. Oral Surg 1980 Oct; 50(4):340–345.

Lyell A. Toxic epidermal necrolysis (the scalded skin syndrome): A reappraisal. Br J Dermatol 1979 Jan; 100(1):69–84.

Matsuoka LY. Pemphigus and pemphigoid. Am Fam Physician 1981 Aug; 24(2):113–115.

Michel B and Schiltz J. Pemphigus. Facts, unanswered questions and speculations. Am J Dermatopathol 1980 Spring; 2(1):65–67.

Pegram PS Jr, Mountz JD, and O'Bar PR. Ethambutol-induced toxic epidermal necrolysis. Arch Intern Med 1981 Nov; 141(12):1677–1678.

Rodriguez AR. L-asparaginase toxic epidermal necrolysis. J Med Assoc Ga 1980 May; 69(5):355, 357.

Thiers BH. Pemphigus. J Am Acad Dermatol 1981 May; 4(5):603–605.

Wilson BD et al. Epidermolysis bullosa acquisita: A clinical disorder of varied etiologies. J Am Acad Dermatol 1980 Sept; 3(3):280–291.

Infection; Infestation

Brem J. Effective topical method of therapy for onychomycosis. Cutis 1981 Jan; 27(1):69–76.

Crissey JT. Bedbugs: An old problem with a new dimension. Int J Dermatol 1981 July–Aug; 20(6):411–414.

Felman YM and Nikitas JA. Pediculosis pubis. Cutis 1980 May; 25(5):482, 487–489.

Heel RC et al. Ketoconazole: A review of its therapeutic efficacy in superficial and systemic fungal infections. Drugs 1982 Jan–Feb; 23(1–2):1–36.

Hernandez AD. An approach to the diagnosis and therapy of dermatophytosis. Int J Dermatol 1980 Dec; 19(10):540–547.

Jones HE, Simpson JG, and Artis WM. Oral ketoconazole. An effective and safe treatment for dermatophytosis. Arch Dermatol 1981 Mar; 117(3):129–134.

Ketoconazole (Nizoral): A new antifungal agent. Med Lett Drugs Ther 1981 Oct 2; 23(20):85–87.

Minster J. Nursing management of patients with scabies and lice. Nurs Clin North Am 1980 Dec; 15(4):747–756.

Rasmussen JE. The problem of lindane. J Am Acad Dermatol 1981 Nov; 5(5):507–516.

Rider JC. Cutaneous fungal infections. Compr Ther 1981 Jan; 7(1):26–30.

Robertson MH et al. Ketaconazole in griseofulvin-resistant dermatophytosis. J Am Acad Dermatol 1982 Feb; 6(2):224–229.

Scott MJ Jr and Scott MJ. Nits or not? Pseudonitis—simple office diagnosis. JAMA 1980 June 13; 243(22):2325–2326.

Shacter B. Treatment of scabies and pediculosis with lindane preparations: an evaluation J Am Acad Dermatol 1981 Nov; 5(5):517–527.

Sher AM. Viral infections of the skin. Compr Ther 1981 Jan; 7(1):35–43.

Smith DE and Walsh J. Treatment of pubic lice infestation: A comparison of two agents. Cutis 1980 Dec; 26(6):618–619.

Taplin D et al. Malathion for treatment of *Pediculus humanus* var *capitis* infestation. JAMA 1982 June 11; 247(22):3103–3105.

Thiers B. Herpes-varicella-zoster. J Am Acad Dermatol 1980 May; 2(5):443–447.

Treatment of head lice. Med Lett Drugs Ther 1980 Aug 8; 22(16):66–68.

Weingeist TA. Herpes zoster and the aging eye. Geriatrics 1981 Jan; 36(1):81–90.

Whitley RJ and Alford CA. Antiviral agents: Clinical status report. Hosp Pract 1981 July; 16(27):109–121.

Psoriasis

Bond CA, Grant K, and Boh L. Photochemotherapy of psoriasis with methoxsalen and longwave ultraviolet light (PUVA). Am J Hosp Pharm 1981 July; 38(7):990–995.

Bryant BG. Treatment of psoriasis. Am J Hosp Pharm 1980 June; 37(6):814–820.

Champion RH. Psoriasis and its treatment. Br Med J 1981 Jan 31; 282(6261):343–346.

Cormane RH. Immunopathology of psoriasis. Arch Dermatol Res 1981; 270(2):201–215.

Cornell RC and Stoughton RB. Use of glucocorticosteroids in psoriasis. Pharmacol Ther 1980; 11(3):497–508.

Cram DL. Psoriasis: Current advances in etiology and treatment. J Am Acad Dermatol 1981 Jan; 4(1):1–14.

Heckel P. Teaching patients to cope with psoriasis: The unshared disease. Nursing '81 1981 June; 11(6):49–51.

Mordovtsev VN, Sergeyev AS, and Alieva PM. Genetic factors in psoriasis. Int J Dermatol 1981 Mar; 20(2):99–101.

Moschella SL. Psoriasis. Pharmacol Ther 1980; 10(1):161–169.

Parrish JA et al. Oral methoxsalen photochemotherapy of psoriasis and mycosis fungoides. Int J Dermatol 1980 Sept; 19(7):379–386.

Wahba A. Immunological alterations in psoriasis. Int J Dermatol 1980 Apr; 19(3):124–129.

Tumors/Malignant Melanoma

Barton FE Jr, Cottel WI, and Walker B. The principle of chemosurgery and delayed primary reconstruction in the management of difficult basal cell carcinomas. Plast Reconstr Surg 1981 Nov; 68(5):746–752.

Bechtel MA, Callen JP, and Owen LG. Etiologic agents in the development of skin cancer. Clin Plast Surg 1980 July; 7(3):265–275.

Beretta G. Medical treatment of malignant melanoma. Oncology 1980; 37(Suppl 1):88–91.

Elder DE et al. Dysplastic nevus syndrome—a phenotypic association of sporadic cutaneous melanoma. Cancer 1980 Oct 15; 46(8):1787–1794.

Fisher RI et al. Adjuvant immunotherapy or chemotherapy for malignant melanoma. Surg Clin North Am 1981 Dec; 61(6):1267–1277.

Freidenbergs I. Psychosocial management of patients with cutaneous cancers. J Dermatol Surg Oncol 1981 Oct; 7(10):828–830.

Goldman LI. Decision in the management of cutaneous malignant melanoma. Semin Oncol 1980 Dec; 7(4):370–375.

Kaiser LR, Burk MW, and Morton DL. Adjuvant therapy for malignant melanoma. Surg Clin North Am 1981 Dec; 61(6):1249–1257.

Levene A. On the histological diagnosis and prognosis of malignant melanoma. J Clin Pathol 1980 Feb; 33(2):101–124.

Mandel MA. Malignant melanoma: An update. Clin Plast Surg 1980 July; 7(3):379–396.

Milton GW. Malignant melanoma. Br J Hosp Med 1980 Jan; 23(1):84–87.

Mysliborski JA. Early recognition of cutaneous neoplasms. Compr Ther 1981 Jan; 7(1):61–65.

Pinsky CM and Oettgen HF. Surgical adjuvant therapy for malignant melanoma. Surg Clin North Am 1981 Dec; 61(6):1259–1266.

Retsas S. The treatment of advanced malignant melanoma. Practitioner 1980 Oct; 224(1348):1019–1021.

Robinson KJ. Mohs' surgery for skin cancer. Am J Nurs 1982. Feb; 82(2):282–283.

Schreiber MM. Primary malignant melanoma of the skin: Factors in predicting prognosis and in determining initial surgical treatment. Cutis 1981 May; 27(5):494–498.

Schulmeister L. Screening for skin cancer: A necessary part of your assessment routine. Nursing '81 1981 Oct; 11(10):42–45.

Stahl D and Veien NK. Cutaneous metastases simulating other dermatoses. Cutis 1980 Sept; 26(3):282–284.

Stehlin JS Jr. Treatment of the primary lesion in melanoma. Surg Gynecol Obstet 1981 Apr; 152(4):499–500.

Plastic Reconstructive Surgery

Acres C and Kraft ER. Skin transplantation. Am J Nurs 1981 Aug; 81(8):1466–1467.

Apfelberg DB et al. The argon laser for cutaneous lesions. JAMA 1981 May 22/29; 245(20):2073–2075.

Beekhuis GJ. Blepharoplasty. Otolaryngol Clin North Am 1982 Feb; 15(1):179–193.

Cameron RR. Rhytidoplasty. Otolaryngol Clin North Am 1982 Feb; 15(1):195–207.

Conlee D. Cosmetic surgery patients. Nursing '81 1981 Nov; 11(11):90–95.

Goldberg BW. Ah, youth! The Pennsylvania Gazette 1982 Apr; 80(6):25–28.

Hallock G. The art and surgery of tatoos. Contemporary Surgery 1982 May; 20(5):65–72.

Hamaker RC and Singer MI. Regional flaps in head and neck reconstruction. Otolaryngol Clin North Am 1982 Feb; 15(1):99–110.

Hien NT, Prawer SE, and Katz HI. Mohs' chemosurgery: A highly effective and reliable method of treatment for skin cancer. Minn Med 1981 Mar; 64(3):135–138.

Hirokawa RH et al. Skin grafts. Otolaryngol Clin North Am 1982 Feb; 15(1):133–145.

Horvath PN. Dermatologic management of facial lesions. Otolaryngol Clin North Am 1982 Feb; 15(1):49–54.

Kornblut AD et al. The role of autografts, homografts, heterografts, and alloplastic implants in reconstructive head and neck surgery. Otolaryngol Clin North Am 1982 Feb; 15(1):147–160.

Kukich E. Rinse procedure simplifies graft preparation. AORN J 1982 Apr; 35(5):899–902.

Lyons RJ. Promoting healing of skin flaps and grafts. AORN J 1982 May; 35(6):1174–1183.

McGregor IA. Local skin flaps in facial reconstruction. Otolaryngol Clin North Am 1982 Feb; 15(1):77–98.

Mohs FE. Chemosurgical techniques. Otolaryngol Clin North Am 1982 Feb; 15(1):209–224.

Reconstruction is the leading edge in plastic surgery. AORN J 1982 Jan; 35(1):86.

Saxe AW and Cocke WM. Simplified method of applying skin grafts. Surg Gynec Obstet 1980 Jan; 150(1):91–92.

Semipermeable membrane dressings. Am J Nurs 1982 Oct; 82(10):1590.

Skin expander helps implant insertions. AORN J 1982 Sept; 36(3):494.

Webster RC, Fanous N, and Smith RC. Male and female face-lift incisions. Arch Otolaryngol 1982 May; 108(5):299–302.

Transplantation

Carpenter CB and Strom TB. Transplantation: Immunogenetic and clinical aspects—Part I. Hosp Pract 1982 Dec; 17(12):125–134.

Najarian JS. Immunologic aspects of organ transplantation. Hosp Pract 1982 Oct; 17(10):61–71.

Penn I. Transplantation. In Liechty RD and Soper RT. Synopsis of Surgery, 4th ed, pp 389–401. St Louis, CV Mosby, 1980.

Strom TB and Carpenter CB. Transplantation: Immunogenetic and clinical aspects—Part II. Hosp Pract 1983 Jan; 18(1):135–150.

Agencies

American Academy of Dermatology, 820 Davis St., Suite 380, Evanston, Illinois 60201

American Academy of Facial Plastic and Reconstructive Surgery, 70 West Hubbard St., Suite 202, Chicago, Illinois 60610

American Cancer Society, 777 Third Ave., New York, New York 10017

National Neurofibromatosis Foundation, Inc., Room 21H, 340 East 80th St., New York, New York 10021

National Psoriasis Foundation, Suite 250, 6415 S.W. Canyon Court, Portland, Oregon 97221

Skin Cancer Foundation, 575 Park Ave., South, New York, New York 10016

53

Management of the Burn Patient

Approximately 12,000 persons die of burns each year in the United States. An additional 2 million experience pain, disability, and disfigurement as a result of burns. Some authorities estimate that reasonable caution and adherence to well-known safety measures could prevent 75% of all burn injuries. By taking advantage of opportunities to teach and to promote legislation for safety practices, the nurse can play an active part in preventing fires and burns.

Four major goals relating to human burns are:

1. Prevention
2. Institution of life-saving measures for the severely burned person
3. Prevention of disability and disfigurement through early specialized, individual treatment
4. Rehabilitation of the individual through reconstructive surgery and rehabilitative programs

▷ Emergency Management

- Once a burn has been sustained, the application of cold is the best first-aid measure. Soaking the burn area intermittently in ice water or applying cold towels gives immediate and striking relief from pain and restricts local tissue edema and damage. However, one should avoid applying ice directly to the burn; such a procedure may worsen the lesion and lead to hypothermia in patients with large burns.
- The burn should also be covered as quickly as possible to minimize bacterial contamination and decrease pain by preventing air from coming into contact with the injured surface. Sterile dressings are best, but any clean, dry cloth can be used as an emergency dressing.
- Ointments and salves are not used. In fact, other than the dressing, no medication or material should be applied to the lesion.
- *Chemical burns,* which result from contact with a corrosive material, are irrigated immediately. Most chemical laboratories have a high-pressure shower for such emer-

gencies; if such an injury occurs at home, all areas of the body that have come in contact with the chemical should be rinsed for several minutes in a shower or other source of continuously running water.

- If a chemical gets in or near the eyes, then the eyes should be flushed with cool, clean water for a period of 15 to 20 minutes. Following this, two or three drops of mild oil (mineral or olive) are instilled, and a physician is promptly consulted.
- *When clothes catch on fire,* the flames can be extinguished if the victim falls to the floor or ground and rolls ("drop and roll"); anything available to smother the flames, such as a blanket, rug, or coat, may be used. Standing still would force the victim to breathe flames and smoke, and running would fan the flames.

After the flames are extinguished, the burned area and adherent clothing are soaked with cold water. The victim is transported to the nearest emergency department. The hospital and physician are alerted that the victim is on the way. Thus, life-saving measures can be initiated immediately by a trained team, with no time lost.

Prehospital Management. A burn victim awaiting transportation to the hospital should remain lying down; no attempt should be made to remove clothing. Exposed burned surfaces can be covered with the cleanest material available to prevent exposure to air and contamination; covering the person with a blanket will prevent loss of body heat. The victim should be kept warm during transportation to the treatment center.

Prevention of Shock.   Prevention of shock in a person with a major burn is imperative. If the hospital cannot be reached within an hour, the physician may initiate fluid therapy intravenously.

- In rare instances in which definitive care is markedly delayed, an effective first-aid measure would be to give the conscious patient fluids to drink, if he can tolerate them. To a quart of water (1 liter), add 1 teaspoon (3 g) of salt and a half teaspoon (1.5 g) of soda bicarbonate. (Salt provides sodium, and soda bicarbonate helps to combat acidosis.)
- Under ordinary circumstances, *nothing* should be given by mouth, and the patient should be placed in a position that will prevent aspiration of vomitus, since nausea and vomiting often occur as a result of paralytic ileus resulting from the stress of injury.

Usually, an emergency medical technician (EMT) or ambulance or fire personnel will take steps to cool the wound, establish an airway, supply oxygen, and perhaps start an intravenous line. The victim is sent directly to the hospital; usually, no pain medication is given before the victim reaches the hospital, where his condition can be assessed.

▷ Pathophysiology of Burns

Burns are wounds produced by various kinds of thermal, electrical, radioactive, or chemical agents, which kill cells by changing the protein substance of the cell. Because these agents attack the organism within its environment, the tissues in direct contact with that environment (*e.g.,* the skin and mucosa of the respiratory tract and the upper alimentary tract) are the first to be damaged.

The depth of the injury depends on the temperature of the burning agent and the duration of contact with the agent. For example, in the case of scald burns, hot tap water at a temperature of 68.9° C (156° F) may result in a burn that destroys both epidermis and dermis (full-thickness injury) in 1 second. Within 15 seconds of exposure to hot water at 56.1° C (133° F), a similar full-thickness injury will occur.

The first effect a burn has is to produce a dilatation of the capillaries and small vessels in the area of the burn, thus increasing capillary permeability. Plasma seeps out into the surrounding tissues, producing blisters and edema. The type, the duration, and the intensity of the burn affect the amount and duration of the fluid loss.

Generally, the fluid leak occurs in greatest magnitude over the first 24 to 36 hours postburn, peaking by 12 hours postinjury. In major burns, capillary leaking continues in small amounts for several weeks. This capillary leak is not confined to the burn area alone in the individual with burns over 30% of the body surface. Rather, edema occurs throughout the body.

- One of the first steps in the management of burns is to provide fluid replacement therapy.

Fluid loss reduces the blood volume, so that the blood becomes thicker; that is, the volume of the cellular elements of the blood increases in relation to the volume of fluid (plasma) of the blood. This change reduces the efficiency of the circulation.

The loss of fluid volume is reflected in the fall of the blood pressure, causing shock. The relative increase in cell volume is reflected in the increasing hematocrit, which is a fairly accurate and reliable measure of the systemic effect of the burn.

As the capillaries begin to regain their integrity, fluid returns to the vascular compartment. With good cardiovascular and renal function, much urine will begin to be excreted beginning about 2 to 5 days after injury and continuing for 2 weeks or more. The patient, however, may develop signs of fluid overload and requires cardiotonic drugs and diuretics to support circulatory function during this period.

Pulmonary Pathophysiology.   Pulmonary pathophysiology related to burn injury is frequent and falls into four categories: carbon monoxide poisoning, smoke inhalation, upper airway injury, and restrictive defects. Carbon monoxide intoxication and smoke inhalation are considered to be the leading causes of death in fire victims. It is estimated that at least 50% of these deaths could have been prevented by such devices as smoke detectors.

Carbon monoxide is a prominent cause of inhalation injury. The pathophysiologic effects are due to tissue hypoxia. Carbon monoxide combines with hemoglobin to form carboxyhemoglobin, which competes with oxygen for available hemoglobin-binding sites. The affinity of hemoglobin for carbon monoxide is 200 times greater than for oxygen. Potentiating factors that enhance carbon monoxide poisoning are decreased oxygen in the burning area and added effects of smoke poisoning.

Smoke inhalation injury results from noxious chemicals formed in the burning process (particularly organic compounds such as plastics); these chemicals include hydrogen cyanide, hydrochloric acid, sulfuric acid, halogens, and benzene.

Smoke inhalation causes loss of ciliary action and severe mucosal edema. Congestion results in atelectasis. Expectoration of carbonaceous sputum may occur. In a few hours, sloughing of the tracheobronchial mucosa occurs, and the patient coughs up mucopurulent material.

Upper airway injury occurs from the effects of heated air or steam and noxious chemical gases on the structures of the upper airway. These cause an inflammatory reaction and edema, which may result in airway obstruction at any time during the first 48 hours postinjury.

Circumferential full-thickness burns of the neck and thorax result in edema of great magnitude. Extrinsic edema may compress the trachea and occlude the airway. Chest excursion may be greatly restricted, resulting in a decreased tidal volume. Fluid shifts from the vascular compartment to the interstitial tissue affect the lung parenchyma and may result in decreased lung compliance, noncardiogenic pulmonary edema, and signs and symptoms of adult respiratory distress syndrome.

Stages of Burn Pathophysiology.   The pathophysiology and management of a burn may be divided into three stages. Although these stages overlap, in general they may be identified as described in Chart 53-1.

▷ Postburn Patient Care

Stage I

▶ Assessment
The general condition and state of health of a burn victim, his approximate age, and when and how he was burned are important factors that may modify treatment. The elderly and very young are more likely to die than the young adult with the same percentage burn. The case of a debilitated 60-year-old man who fell asleep with a lighted cigarette that ignited the sofa would present a pathophysiologic and survival problem different from that of a 38-year-old man whose clothing caught fire while he was burning leaves. Associated trauma or preexisting endocrine or pulmonary diseases, allergy, metabolic disease, a drug history, or joint limitations compound the problem and must be considered in planning care. The nurse has the responsibility to learn as much as possible about the patient, including his preburn weight and state of health, from his relatives and friends.

Additional information includes the place where the accident happened and the type of first-aid measures taken.

Extent of Surface Area Burned (Rule of Nine).   An estimation of the total body surface area (BSA) involved as a result of a burn is simplified by dividing the body into multiples of nine (Rule of Nine—Figs. 53-1 and 53-2). The initial evaluation should be revised on the second and third postburn days, since the demarcation usually is not clear until then.

Depth of Burn.   It is often difficult to immediately determine the depth of a burn. In such instances, assessment remains a clinical judgment, so that often the depth is assessed after the fact—that is, if it healed, it was partial thickness. However, classification of burns by degrees is helpful for description and identification (Table 53-1).

First-degree burns are not serious unless large areas of the body are involved. They produce pain and redness in the burned area.

Second-degree burns are those associated with blister formation (vesicles) in which the superficial layers of skin are destroyed, but the deeper layers escape injury. Patients with large areas of second-degree burns require hospitalization. Skin healing can take place from the deeper skin cells that have remained viable.

Chart 53-1
Stages of Burn Care

Stage	Duration	Priorities
I	From onset of injury to completion of fluid resuscitation	• First Aid • Prevention of shock • Prevention of respiratory distress • Wound assessment and initial care • Detection and treatment of concomitant injuries
II	From beginning of diuresis to near completion of wound closure	• Wound care and closure • Prevention and treatment of complications, including infection • Nutritional support
III	From major wound closure to return to individual's optimal level of physical and psychosocial adjustment	• Prevention of scars and contractures • Physical, occupational, and vocational rehabilitation • Functional and cosmetic reconstruction • Psychosocial counseling

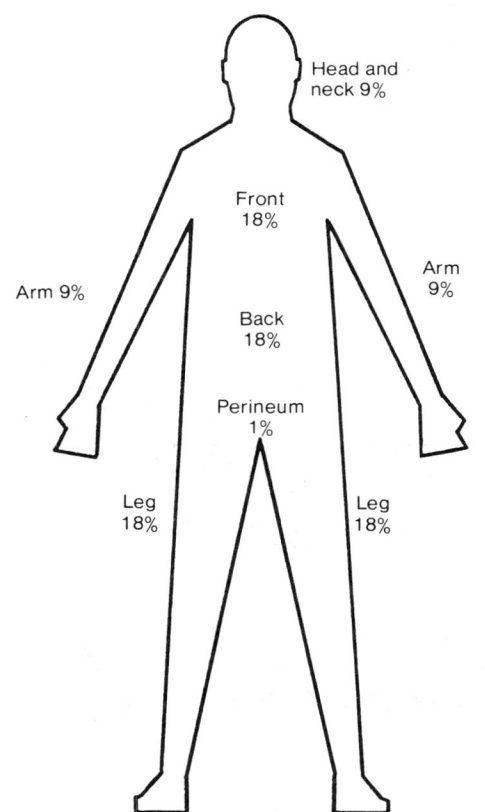

Third-degree burns imply destruction of the full thickness of the skin and often of the underlying fat, muscles, and even bone. Rapid transportation to the hospital is important.

In determining the depth of a burn, it is important that the following be known: (1) the causative agent, such as flame, a scalding liquid, etc.; (2) the duration of exposure; and (3) the thickness of the skin. Hematuria and high plasma hemoglobin suggest deep burns. (See Table 53-2, Types of Burn Injury and Recommended Treatment Sites.)

Survival Prediction.   The best survival expectancy is obtained in children and young adults, ages 5 to 40 years. In this group, burns of about 60% of the body are associated with a 50% mortality. A burn of over 20% of the body endangers life. Table 53-3 gives a clear picture of the effect of age and the percent of the body burned on survival rate.

Prognosis depends on the depth and extent of the burn as well as on the condition and age of the patient. Problems encountered are shock, infection, respiratory distress, cardiovascular and renal disturbances, fluid and electrolyte imbalance, and psychiatric derangements. Such difficulties may occur simultaneously or in sequence. Consequently, instead of thinking of patient care in terms of a "one-system" approach, it is necessary to consider this patient in terms of a "one-body" approach, which includes all systems.

Figure 53-1. "Rule of Nine" chart for calculating percent of body burns in the adult. (Actual values have been modified for practical purposes.)

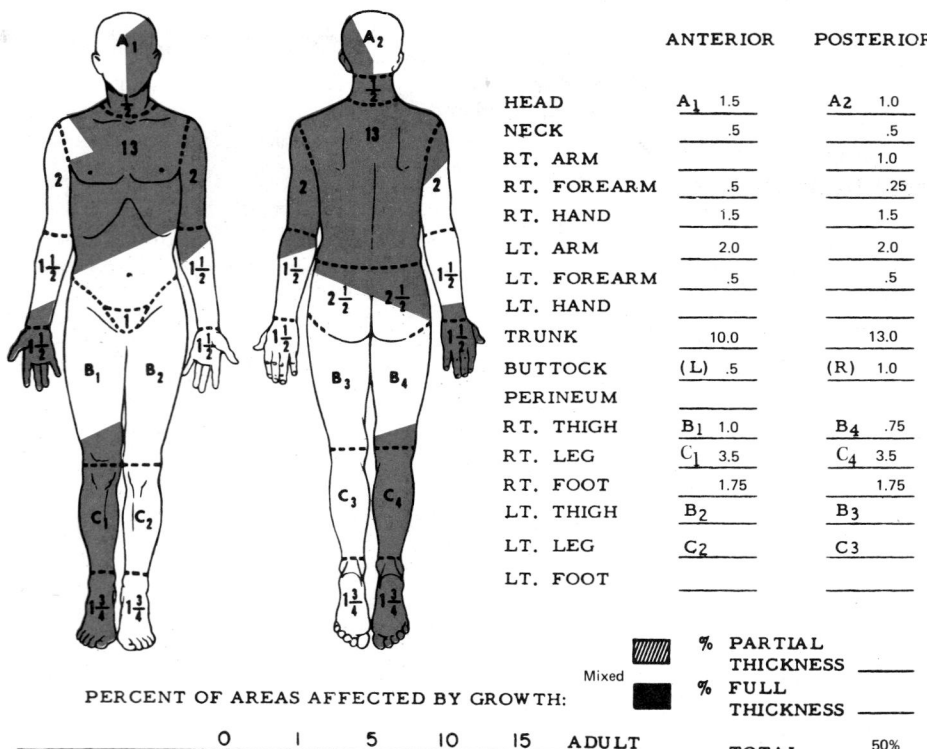

	ANTERIOR	POSTERIOR
HEAD	A_1 1.5	A_2 1.0
NECK	.5	.5
RT. ARM		1.0
RT. FOREARM	.5	.25
RT. HAND	1.5	1.5
LT. ARM	2.0	2.0
LT. FOREARM	.5	.5
LT. HAND		
TRUNK	10.0	13.0
BUTTOCK	(L) .5	(R) 1.0
PERINEUM		
RT. THIGH	B_1 1.0	B_4 .75
RT. LEG	C_1 3.5	C_4 3.5
RT. FOOT	1.75	1.75
LT. THIGH	B_2	B_3
LT. LEG	C_2	C_3
LT. FOOT		

Mixed

	% PARTIAL THICKNESS	_____
	% FULL THICKNESS	_____
	TOTAL	50%

PERCENT OF AREAS AFFECTED BY GROWTH:

		0	1	5	10	15	ADULT
A = ½	HEAD	9½	8½	6½	5½	4½	3½
B = ½	ONE THIGH	2¾	3¼	4	4¼	4½	4¾
C = ½	ONE LEG	2½	2½	2¾	3	3¼	3½

Figure 53-2. Burn Evaluation Chart— estimation percent body burns. (Crozer–Chester Medical Center.)

Clinical Manifestations

Although the local effects of a burn are most evident, the systemic effects pose a greater threat to life. Therefore, it is important to remember the ABCs of all trauma care during the early postburn period: *A*irway, *B*reathing, and *C*irculation.

Pulmonary Function. Breathing must be assessed and a patent airway established during the initial minutes of emergency care. Many burn victims sustain some degree of concomitant pulmonary dysfunction, as previously described.

Criteria that suggest postburn pulmonary damage include the following: (1) a history indicating that the burn occurred in an enclosed area; (2) burns of the face, neck, or circumoral area; (3) singed nasal hair; (4) hoarseness, voice change, dry cough, sooty sputum; (5) bloody sputum, labored respiration, erythema, and blisters of the oral or pharyngeal mucosa.

Arterial blood gas values are obtained to serve as a baseline against which comparisons are later made in order to

Table 53-1
Evaluation of Depth of a Burn

Degree	Cause of Burn	Skin Involvement	Symptoms	Appearance	Course
Superficial (First)	Sunburn Low-intensity flash	Epidermis	Tingling Hyperesthesia Painful Soothed by cooling	Reddened; blanches with pressure Minimal or no edema	Complete recovery within a week Peeling
Partial thickness (Second)	Scalds Flash flame	Epidermis and part of dermis	Painful Hyperesthesia Sensitive to cold air	Blistered, mottled red base; broken epidermis; weeping surface Edema	Recovery in 2 to 3 weeks Some scarring and depigmentation Infection may convert to third-degree
Full thickness (Third)	Fire Prolonged exposure to hot liquids	Epidermis, entire dermis, and sometimes subcutaneous tissue	Painless Symptoms of shock Hematuria and hemolysis of blood likely	Dry; pale white or charred Broken skin with fat exposed Edema	Eschar sloughs Grafting necessary Scarring and loss of contour and function

Table 53-2
Types of Burn Injury and Recommended Treatment Sites

Type of Injury	Major Burn Injury	Moderate Uncomplicated Burn Injury	Minor Burn Injury
Definition	2nd-degree burns > 25% 3rd-degree burns > 10% Smaller burns at extremes of age (<2 or >60) Burns involving face, hands, feet, perineum Burns with inhalation injury Electrical burns Burns with other trauma or illness	2nd-degree burns 15–25% adults 10–20% children or elderly 3rd-degree burns < 10% • no complications • no extremes of age • no inhalation injury • no critical body areas • no other accompanying trauma or illness	2nd-degree < 15% adults <10% children 3rd-degree < 2%
Recommended treatment site	Burn Unit/Center A (Advanced Level)	Burn Program or Burn Unit/Center I (Intermediate Level)	Hospital Emergency Dept. B (Basic Level)

(From Specific Optimal Criteria for Hospital Resources for Care of Patients With Burn Injury. American Burn Association.)

Table 53-3
Survival Rate in Relation to Age and Percentage of Burn

Age	Percent of Body Burned	Survival	Mortality
5 and under	50%	66%	34%
5–40	50%	80%	20%
40–60	50%	51%	49%
Over 60	50%	9%	91%

determine if there has been a lowering of oxygen tension, indicating possible pulmonary injury.

Important considerations in assessment of the chest include auscultation for breath sounds, looking for the appearance of stridor, and a chest x-ray. Observe for symptoms of carbon monoxide poisoning, including headache, mental confusion, decreased vision, weakness, nausea, central nervous system irritability, and ECG changes.

Circulation.   The circulatory system must also be quickly assessed. Apical pulse and blood pressure should be monitored frequently. Tachycardia and slight hypotension are expected in the untreated patient early postburn.

Cardiac monitoring is useful if there is a history of cardiac disease, electrical injury, or respiratory problems, or if the pulse is dysrrhythmic and the rate is abnormally slow or rapid. Peripheral pulses should also be checked hourly on burned extremities. As edema increases in circumferential burns, pressure on small blood vessels and nerves in distal extremities causes obstruction to blood flow and ischemia. The physician may need to perform an escharotomy to relieve the constricting effect of the burned tissue.

Urine output is usually an excellent indicator of circulatory status and should be monitored constantly and measured hourly. Urine specific gravity, pH, glucose, acetone, protein, and hemoglobin should also be assessed periodically.

Central venous pressure measurements may also be helpful in determining hypovolemia and shock. Other invasive methods, including arterial pressure monitoring and pulmonary artery catheters (measurement of pulmonary wedge pressures), are useful. However, due to the increased risk of infection associated with their use, these devices are utilized only when other parameters fail to provide a satisfactory assessment of the individual's hemodynamic status.

Temperature.   Hypothermia frequently accompanies large burn injuries, because the victim has lost the skin's microcirculatory regulation of body temperature. Rectal temperature should be checked hourly for several hours and then two to four times per tour of duty.

GI Function.   Because of the sympathetic nervous system's response to burn trauma, gastric motility is decreased and paralytic ileus may ensue. Nursing assessment of bowel sounds periodically will serve to determine when normal gastrointestinal function has returned and when the patient can begin oral intake.

Lab Data.   The stress response also causes an increase in blood glucose, which may be ascertained by periodic

blood sampling. Other significant laboratory data that should be obtained in the early postburn period include serum electrolytes, BUN, creatinine, and a complete blood count.

Pain.   Victims of partial-thickness burn injury frequently have a good deal of pain. An important part of the nursing assessment of that pain is differentiating symptoms of pain from symptoms of hypoxia. Restlessness and anxiety may be caused by air-hunger. Prior to the administration of analgesics, adequate ventilation should be assured.

Patient Problems/Nursing Diagnoses

Based on the clinical manifestations, nursing assessment, and other diagnostic data, the patient's major nursing problems include potential compromised airway and altered respiratory function related to intrinsic and extrinsic edema; hypovolemia and electrolyte imbalance related to fluid loss and shift; decreased resistance to infection related to loss of skin barrier and altered immune response; pain and anxiety related to nerve injury, exposure, and stress; hypothermia related to loss of skin microcirculation; decreased gastric function due to stress response; presence of associated injuries or manifestations of chronic illness; and potential development of complications related to the severity of the burn injury.

▶ Planning and Implementation

Goals

The major goals for the patient include:

1. Maintenance of a patent airway, adequate ventilation, and tissue oxygenation
2. Optimal fluid and electrolyte balance and perfusion of vital organs
3. Absence of invasion by pathogenic organisms
4. Relief of pain and anxiety
5. Normal body temperature
6. Prevention of gastric distention and vomiting
7. Detection and treatment of associated injuries and illnesses
8. Absence or reduction of potential complications

Overview of Immediate Patient Care

When the patient is admitted to the hospital, his clothes are carefully removed, his weight and height are recorded, and he is placed on or between sterile sheets. Since this patient is usually frightened and may be in emotional shock, those in attendance should demonstrate concern for his care. Encouragement is offered and explanations are given when necessary. Should the patient express the desire to see a spiritual advisor, one should be notified.

Careful attention must be given to aseptic technique. Attending personnel must wear masks, caps, and gowns; sterile gloves are worn when the burn area is handled. The physician evaluates the patient's general condition, assesses the burn, determines the priorities, and directs the individualized plan of treatment, which is divided into systemic management and local care of the burned area.

Photographs should be taken of the burn areas at this time and periodically throughout the treatment. In this way, the progress of healing may be determined quickly. Such evidence is invaluable in insurance claims and courts of law.

Room Preparation. When a bed is prepared for a burn patient, the mattress is completely covered with a plastic sheet, which is covered in turn with a sterile bottom sheet. Sterile Microdon sheeting (3M Co.) atop this bedding prevents the patient from sticking to the sheets as a result of the exudate's oozing from the burn. Caps, masks, and sterile gowns and gloves are available for those attending the patient. The equipment most likely to be required should be in the room, including intravenous therapy equipment, with polyethylene central venous catheters and fluids (*i.e.,* plasmanate and Ringer's lactate solution); blood withdrawal syringes, needles, and tubes; catheterization tray and drainage equipment; urine testing devices; tracheostomy set; intubation equipment; venesection set; suction and oxygen therapy equipment; fresh, pathogen-free linens; overbed cradle; and side rails. The particular procedure to be followed in wound care determines additional needs.

In some clinics, patients with severe burns of the trunk are placed in circular beds and rotated from prone to supine position every 3 hours. The Stryker frame also may be used if it meets the individual patient's needs. An air-fluidized bed or an "egg crate" pad or mattress may also be helpful.

Management of Respiratory Status

- Immediate therapy is directed toward establishing an airway, possibly through oropharyngeal suctioning followed by the administration of 100% oxygen. Such a high concentration of oxygen may not be available under emergency conditions; however, oxygen by mask or nasal prongs is given initially.

In mild cases, inspired air is humidified and the patient is encouraged to cough so that secretions can be suctioned. For more severe situations, it is necessary to remove secretions by bronchial suctioning and administer bronchial dilators and mucolytic agents.

- When oropharyngeal edema is present, it may be necessary to intubate the patient. Hyperinflation hourly with an Ambu-bag helps to prevent atelectasis. Continuous positive airway pressure and mechanical ventilation may also be required.
- Arterial blood gases are evaluated (Swan–Ganz catheter may be required to monitor pulmonary artery wedge pressure) and urine output is checked.

Authorities differ on the administration of antibiotics. Gram stains of the sputum will help in determining antibiotic use; if gram-positive organisms and large numbers of neutrophils are present, penicillin or penicillinase-resistant antibiotics are given. Usually, steroids are not given because disadvantages outweigh advantages. Meticulous aseptic technique in all aspects of tracheal care is required in this infection-prone patient.

Management of Fluid Derangement (Plasma-to-Interstitial Fluid Shift) and Shock

Next to handling respiratory difficulties, the most urgent need is to replace lost fluid and to prevent irreversible shock. In extensive burns (more than 20% of the body surface), a

Table 53-4

Water and Electrolyte Changes in the First 48 Hours of Major Burns

Fluid Accumulation Phase (Shock Phase)
Plasma → Interstitial Fluid (Edema at Burn Site)

Observation	Explanation
1. Generalized dehydration	Plasma leaks through damaged capillaries
2. Reduction of blood volume	Brought about by plasma loss, fall of blood pressure, and diminished cardiac output
3. Decreased urinary output	Secondary to: Fluid loss Decreased renal blood flow Sodium and water retention caused by increased adrenocortical activity (Hemolysis of red blood cells, causing hemoglobinuria and myonecrosis or myoglobinuria)
4. Potassium excess	Massive cellular trauma causes release of K^+ into extracellular fluid (ordinarily, most K^+ is intracellular)
5. Sodium deficit	Large amount of Na^+ is lost in trapped edema fluid and exudate and by shift into cells (ordinarily, most Na^+ is extracellular)
6. Metabolic acidosis (base bicarbonate deficit)	Loss of bicarbonate ions accompanies sodium loss
7. Hemoconcentration (elevated hematocrit)	Liquid blood component lost into extravascular space

(Adapted from Metheny NM and Snively WD: Nurses' Handbook of Fluid Balance. Philadelphia, JB Lippincott.)

dangerous systemic derangement of fluid balance occurs. This begins with the loss of fluid into the tissues surrounding the burn area and loss of fluid by exudation and evaporation from the surface of the burn. The result is a decrease in the circulating fluid of the entire body. Extravasation of fluid into the tissue begins within an hour and reaches its peak in 4 to 6 hours; fluid loss continues into the tissues up to 48 hours postburn (Table 53-4). The result is hemoconcentration—a relative increase in the ratio of blood cells to plasma. An increase in the hematocrit, a less efficient circulation, and a fall in the blood pressure result from the cumulative effects of these processes. In addition to signs of restlessness and disorientation, determination of vital signs may reveal an accelerated heartbeat (tachycardia).

- A pulse rate in excess of 110 beats/minute should be reported immediately, because it means that the heart is attempting to compensate for decreased blood volume.

Because of generalized cellular dehydration, the patient often exhibits extreme thirst. Shock is likely to occur, and the patient is seriously ill.

Therefore, immediate management of the burn patient includes the following:

- An intravenous route via an indwelling catheter is established, preferably through an unburned area.
- Blood specimens are drawn for hematocrit, electrolyte, and blood gas determinations, and for typing and cross matching. These parameters must be followed closely in the resuscitation period.
- An indwelling urinary catheter is inserted so that urine volume and specific gravity can be monitored hourly. The amount of urine first obtained is recorded, since it may assist in determining the extent of renal function. It should also be tested for hemoglobin. Urine volumes of less than 30 ml per hour (10 ml in children) are reported.
- The patient's vital signs are monitored at frequent intervals: temperatures over 38.3° C (101° F) or below 36.1° C (97° F) are reported.

Fluid Replacement.   There is no known way to stop the outpouring of fluids, but replacement of fluids is possible. The physician calculates the projected fluid requirements for the first 24 hours by evaluating the patient's burn injury (see p. 1203). Some combination of fluid categories may be appropriate: (1) colloids: whole blood, plasma, and plasma expanders; and (2) electrolytes: physiologic sodium chloride, Ringer's solution, Hartmann's solution.

Formulas have been evolved for estimating fluid loss based on the estimated percentage of body surface area burned and the weight of the patient. These are modified by physicians and individualized to meet the requirements of each patient.

The Evans Formula

1. Colloids (blood, plasma, dextran): 1 ml × percent burn × kg body weight
2. Electrolytes (saline): 1 ml × percent burn × kg body weight
3. Glucose (5%) in water, 2000 ml (for insensible losses)

Second- to third-degree burns totaling over 50% are calculated on the basis of 50%. In any event, 10,000 ml of total fluids is the maximal amount to be given in a 24-hour period. One half of the calculated fluid is given in the first 8 hours postburn; the remainder is spread evenly over the next 16 hours.

On the second postburn day, the patient receives one half of the colloid, one half of electrolyte, and all of the insensible replacement.

The Brooke Army Hospital Formula.   This formula differs from the Evans formula only in that the colloid fraction is reduced from 1 ml to 0.5 ml and the electrolyte fraction is increased from 1 ml to 1.5 ml. Instead of saline, the electrolyte preferred is lactated Ringer's solution because of its lower chloride content.

On the second postburn day, the patient receives one half of the colloid, one half of the electrolyte, and all of the insensible replacement.

The Parkland or Baxter Formula.   The patient is given 4 ml of Ringer's lactate solution per percent burn, per kilogram body weight. One third is given in the first 8 hours and the rest over the next 16 hours. No fluids are calculated for the second postburn day.

Hypertonic Saline.   This method utilizes concentrated solutions of sodium chloride and lactate so that the resulting solution has a concentration of 300 mEq of sodium. It is administered at a rate sufficient to maintain a desired urinary output. The rate is *not* usually increased during the first 8 hours postburn. The major therapeutic effects are a result of the sustained hypernatremia and the increase in serum osmolality that occurs. Edema is reduced and lung complications from fluid loading are decreased.

The Consensus Formula.   Although each of the above formulas may be used by individual practitioners when confronted by a burn patient, the most popular formula currently is that derived at the NIH Consensus Development Conference in Supportive Therapy in Burn Care in November 1978. It was agreed that salt and water are essential requirements of burn patients, but that colloid may or may not be useful during the first 24 to 48 hours postburn.

The consensus formula provides for the volume of balanced salt solution to be administered in the first 24 hours in a range of 2 to 4 ml per kilogram per percent burn. The volume should be started at the lower level of this range, as the overall goal of fluid therapy is to maintain vital organ function at the least immediate or delayed physiologic cost.

Generally, 2 ml per kilogram per percent burn of lactated Ringer's solution may be used for adults, while children may require 3 ml per kilogram per percent burn. As with the other formulas, half of the calculated total should be given over the first 8 hours postburn and the other half given over the next 16 hours. The rate and volume of the infusion must be regulated according to the patient's response.

Recent studies have demonstrated that with large burns there is a failure of the sodium–potassium pump at the cellular level. Thus, individuals with very large burns may be expected to need proportionately more milliliters of fluid per percent burn than those with smaller burns.

Fluid Replacement Example
70 kg patient with 50% body surface area (BSA) burn

1. Consensus Formula: 2 to 4 ml/kg/% BSA
2. Calculate 2 × 50 × 70 = 7000 ml/24 hours
3. Plan to administer: First 8 hours = 3500 ml = 437 ml/hour; Next 16 hours = 3500 ml = 219 ml/hour

REMEMBER: Formulas are a guide. Patient response is the primary determinant of actual fluid therapy and must be assessed at least hourly.

Fluid Therapy

- The amount and speed of fluid given through an indwelling plastic vein cannula is gauged by the urinary output and the blood pressure and pulse rate. Urine flow from an indwelling catheter should be maintained at 30 ml to 70 ml per hour or 0.5 ml to 1 ml/kg for children. This means that the flow from the indwelling catheter must be collected, measured, and recorded every hour. Pulse should be less than 110 per minute.

These parameters are far more important in resuscitation than any formula. Indeed the patient's individual response *is* the "formula."

- The following observations must be reported:
  1. The presence of hematuria
  2. Urine output below 30 ml per hour—this suggests an inadequate rate of fluid resuscitation
  3. Urine output above 100 ml per hour, which may presage pulmonary edema or imminent water intoxication (suggested by the following signs: tremor, twitching, nausea, diarrhea, salivation, and disorientation)
  4. Blood pressure below 90/60.

If all extremities are burned, blood pressure determination may become difficult. A sterile dressing applied under the blood pressure cuff will protect the wound from contamination. A Doppler (ultrasound), electronic blood pressure device, or other noninvasive means of monitoring may be helpful. An arterial catheter for blood pressure measurement and accessibility for collection of specimens for blood gases may also be indicated.

The Doppler is a useful tool in monitoring peripheral pulses. A more sophisticated method of determining tissue pressure levels to permit early intervention in the event of compartment syndrome is the use of the Wick catheter, connected to a transducer.

Additonal gauges of the fluid requirements include hematocrit and hemoglobin determinations. Blood samples for these examinations and for the determination of electrolytes are withdrawn at frequent intervals. If the hematocrit and hemoglobin determinations decrease, or if the urinary output is more than 50 ml of urine per hour, the speed of flow of the intravenous solution may be decreased as shown in the 24-hour flow chart in Figure 53-3.

Antibiotics may be given by "piggy-back" if required. If nausea or vomiting occurs, a nasogastric tube is introduced into the stomach and attached to a suction apparatus.

The nurse needs to know the maximal amount of fluid the patient is allowed to have; usually, fluids are given intravenously. Infusion pumps and rate controllers are a useful adjunct to the correct delivery of a complex regimen of prescribed fluids. With the addition of piggy-back IVs for

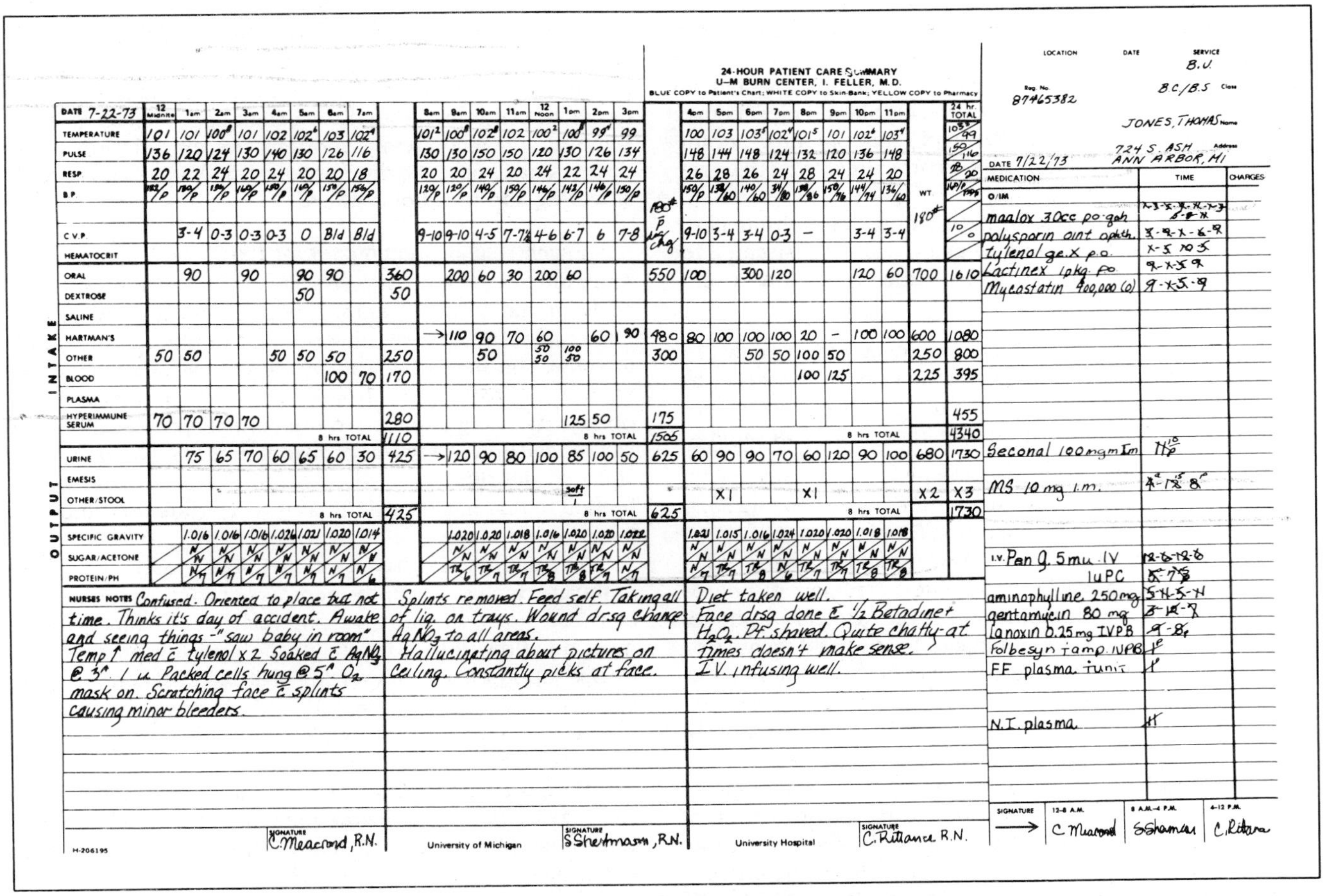

24-HOUR PATIENT CARE SUMMARY
U–M BURN CENTER, I. FELLER, M.D.
BLUE COPY to Patient's Chart; WHITE COPY to Skin-Bank; YELLOW COPY to Pharmacy

LOCATION — DATE — SERVICE B.U.
Reg. No. 87465382 — Class B.C./B.S
Name JONES, THOMAS
Address 724 S. ASH ANN ARBOR, MI

DATE 7-22-73	12 Midnite	1am	2am	3am	4am	5am	6am	7am	
TEMPERATURE	101	101	100^8	101	102	102^6	103	102^4	
PULSE	136	120	124	130	140	130	126	116	
RESP	20	22	24	20	24	20	20	18	
B.P.	182/P	180/P	136/P	160/P	150/P	160/P	150/P	156/P	
C.V.P.		3-4	0-3	0-3	0-3	0	Bld	Bld	
HEMATOCRIT									
ORAL		90		90		90	90		360
DEXTROSE						50			50
SALINE									
HARTMAN'S									
OTHER	50	50			50	50	50		250
BLOOD							100	70	170
PLASMA									
HYPERIMMUNE SERUM	70	70	70	70					280
								8 hrs TOTAL	1110
URINE		75	65	70	60	65	60	30	425
EMESIS									
OTHER/STOOL									
								8 hrs TOTAL	425
SPECIFIC GRAVITY		1.016	1.016	1.016	1.024	1.021	1.020	1.014	
SUGAR/ACETONE		N/N	N/N	N/N	N/N	N/N	N/N	N/N	
PROTEIN/PH		N/7	N/7	N/7	N/7	N/7	N/7	N/6	

	8am	9am	10am	11am	12 Noon	1pm	2pm	3pm	
TEMPERATURE	101^2	100^8	102^8	102	100^2	100^8	99^4	99	
PULSE	130	130	150	150	120	130	126	134	
RESP	20	20	24	20	24	22	24	24	
B.P.	120/P	120/P	140/P	150/P	146/P	142/P	146/P	150/P	
									180# $\bar{p}$ wt chg
C.V.P.	9-10	9-10	4-5	7-7½	4-6	6-7	6	7-8	
HEMATOCRIT									
ORAL		200	60	30	200	60			550
DEXTROSE									
SALINE									
HARTMAN'S	→	110	90	70	60		60	90	480
OTHER			50		50/50	100/50			300
BLOOD									
PLASMA									
HYPERIMMUNE SERUM						125	50		175
								8 hrs TOTAL	1505
URINE	→	120	90	80	100	85	100	50	625
EMESIS									
OTHER/STOOL						soft/1			
								8 hrs TOTAL	625
SPECIFIC GRAVITY		1.020	1.020	1.018	1.016	1.020	1.020	1.022	
SUGAR/ACETONE		N/N	N/N	N/N	N/N	N/N	N/N	N/N	
PROTEIN/PH		TR/6	TR/7	TR/7	TR/8	TR/8	TR/7	N/7	

	4pm	5pm	6pm	7pm	8pm	9pm	10pm	11pm	WT	24 hr. TOTAL
TEMPERATURE	100	103	103^5	102^4	101^5	101	102^6	103^4		103^5/99
PULSE	148	144	148	124	132	120	136	148		150/116
RESP	26	28	26	24	28	24	24	20		28/20
B.P.	150/P	138/60	140/60	34/80	130/86	150/76	144/74	136/60		160/P / [illegible]
									180#	
C.V.P.	9-10	3-4	3-4	0-3	–		3-4	3-4		10/0
HEMATOCRIT										
ORAL	100		300	120			120	60	700	1610
DEXTROSE										
SALINE										
HARTMAN'S	80	100	100	100	20	–	100	100	600	1080
OTHER			50	50	100	50			250	800
BLOOD					100	125			225	395
PLASMA										
HYPERIMMUNE SERUM										455
								8 hrs TOTAL		4340
URINE	60	90	90	70	60	120	90	100	680	1730
EMESIS										
OTHER/STOOL		X1			X1				X2	X3
								8 hrs TOTAL		1730
SPECIFIC GRAVITY	1.021	1.015	1.016	1.024	1.020	1.020	1.018	1.018		
SUGAR/ACETONE	N/N	N/N	N/N	N/N	N/N	N/N	N/N	N/N		
PROTEIN/PH	N/7	TR/7	TR/8	N/6	TR/7	TR/7	TR/8	TR/8		

NURSES NOTES Confused. Oriented to place but not time. Thinks it's day of accident. Awake and seeing things–"saw baby in room" Temp ↑ med c̄ tylenol x 2 Soaked c̄ $AgNO_3$ @ 3^A. 1 u. Packed cells hung @ 5^A. O_2 mask on. Scratching face c̄ splints causing minor bleeders.

Splints removed. Feed self. Taking all of liq. on trays. Wound drsg change $AgNO_3$ to all areas. Hallucinating about pictures on ceiling. Constantly picks at face.

Diet taken well. Face drsg done c̄ ½ Betadine + H_2O_2. Pt. shaved. Quite chatty–at times doesn't make sense. I.V. infusing well.

SIGNATURE C. Meacrond, R.N. — University of Michigan — SIGNATURE S. Shedmann, R.N. — University Hospital — SIGNATURE C. Rittance R.N.

DATE 7/22/73

MEDICATION	TIME	CHARGES
O/IM		
maalox 30cc po q2h	[illegible]	
polysporin oint ophth.	[illegible]	
tylenol gr. x p.o.	[illegible]	
Lactinex 1pkg. po	[illegible]	
Mycostatin 400,000 (o)	[illegible]	
Seconal 100 mgm Im	11^{10}_P	
MS 10 mg i.m.	4^2-12^{15} 8^P	
I.V. Pen G. 5mu. IV	12-6-12-6	
1uPC	[illegible]	
aminophylline 250mg	5-11-5-11	
gentamycin 80 mg	[illegible]	
lanoxin 0.25mg IVPB	[illegible]	
Folbesyn 1amp. IVPB	[illegible]	
FF plasma 1unit	[illegible]	
N.I. plasma	[illegible]	

SIGNATURE	12-8 A.M.	8 A.M.–4 P.M.	4–12 P.M.
→	C Meacrond	S Shamas	C. Ritara

H-206195

Figure 53-3. A 24-hour flow chart including vital signs, medications, CVP, intake, output, and nurse's notations. Note vital sign fluctuations, reported mental confusion, and attempt to stabilize fluid balance. The hourly recordings give a vivid picture of an unstable condition kept under control. (From Feller I and Archambeault C: Nursing the Burned Patient. Ann Arbor, Michigan, The Institute for Burn Medicine.)

antibiotic infusion and hyperalimentation, monitoring intravenous therapy is a major nursing responsibility.

Continued Assessment. Significant changes in the patient's condition must be reported promptly. The recording of patient problems and suggested means of solution are modified as the patient's condition changes. A progressive assessment is required of the patient's appearance and reactions, significant signs and symptoms, intake and output, and all therapies and treatments. Thus, constant surveillance is required.

Preventing Infection

Aside from monitoring fluid requirements and providing constant care, the nurse is responsible for providing a clean and safe environment and for closely scrutinizing the wound in order to detect early manifestations of infection. Wound care includes cleansing and debridement, as well as application of topical or subeschar antimicrobial agents and perhaps physiologic dressings (see p. 1214).

Recent evidence suggests that the primary source of bacterial infection appears to be the patient's own intestinal tract. A major secondary source is the environment. Antibiotics seldom are given prophylactically today because of the tendency to promote resistant strains—except in patients with suspected respiratory injury. Sensitivity to antibiotics should be determined prior to administration. The choice of antibiotics for sepsis is based on the strains present in the patient's unit. The antibiotics chosen should be effective against *Staphylococcus aureus* and *Pseudomonas*. Serum antibiotic levels are monitored for maximal effectiveness and minimal toxicity.

Localized infection must be identified and eliminated. A prime nursing objective is to guard against resistance to antibiotics by maintaining strict isolation precautions. Combination drug regimens may be helpful.

- Ordinarily, a mask and sterile gloves are worn while caring for the patient with extensive burns, in order to prevent infection. Aseptic technique, with cap and gown, may be used when caring directly for burn wounds.

Wound cleansing and debridement are performed by the physician or a specially trained nurse. Warm, bland soap solution or a detergent may be used for cleansing, at which time debridement may also be done. Hexachlorophene soaps are usually avoided because of limited evidence of neurotoxicity associated with absorption of the hexachlorophene.

Because burns are contaminated wounds, adequate tetanus prophylaxis is given. If the patient has been immunized or has had no booster dose in the preceding 4 years, a booster dose of adsorbed tetanus toxoid is administered. If the patient has never had immunizing toxoid, then tetanus immune globulin (TIG) should be given. The amount given depends on the extent of the burn and the environment in which the injury occurred. If the patient was rolled on the earth or has been lying on the earth, the danger of tetanus is increased, hence larger doses of antitoxin are used.

Pain Relief

Intravenous morphine is usually prescribed to relieve pain in the burn patient. Subcutaneous or intramuscular routes are dangerous because of impaired circulation. For individuals with burns of the head and neck, morphine, which can depress respiration, is given in smaller dosages intravenously.

- It should be emphasized that, in the presence of anemia, shock, and hypovolemia, (especially in children) narcotics may cause cardiac arrest! For this reason, it is wise to give very small doses at short intervals (*e.g.*, every 30–60 minutes) in the early, acute phase.

Pain is more severe in second-degree burns than in third-degree burns, because the nerve endings are destroyed in a third-degree burn. Exposed nerve endings are sensitive to cool, moving air; therefore, a sterile covering can help to reduce pain. Fright, hysteria, and severe pain can later cause neurogenic shock.

- Symptoms of restlessness and anxiety, often attributed to pain, may actually be due to hypoxia. Therefore, careful respiratory assessment is essential before giving analgesics in the early postburn period. Intravenous morphine or other narcotics are prescribed as needed, but large doses are avoided because of the danger of respiratory depression and the possibility of masking other symptoms.

Burn patients are prone to chilling. Cotton blankets, ceiling-mounted heat lamps or heat shields, or aluminum-coated "space" blankets are helpful in maintaining the patient's body temperature. An efficient approach to dressing removal and wound care shortens the time during which patients are exposed to the ambient temperature, and reduces shivering and metabolic stress.

Psychosocial Components of Care

Assessment of the emotional status of the patient often reveals an initial state of emotional stress manifested by confusion, fear for survival, uncontrolled emotions, and sleeplessness. This stage can be alleviated somewhat by the nurse's assuring the patient that these reactions are normal and temporary. By being attentive to the patient's needs, the nurse can relieve him of any fear of abandonment. Should he show signs of delirium or disorientation, he should be gently helped to understand where he is, what time it is, and who is caring for him.

The patient may have sustained many losses as a result of the fire, including family members or friends, and a home or possessions, as well as a potential loss of function. He must be allowed to go through the grieving process with caring support from the nursing staff. A consistent, firm approach based on truthful answers to any questions will help the patient develop trust in the staff and will foster the rehabilitative process.

Burn patients are often sensitive about their appearance and may be deeply concerned about disfigurement. Attendants need to remember that any indication of revulsion or shock on their part is noticed by the patient.

Gastrointestinal Disturbances

Gastric dilatation and paralytic ileus occur frequently and are indicated by vomiting and distention; therefore, a nasogastric tube is passed early in the treatment. When oral alimentation is initiated, oral fluids should be administered *slowly*. The patient's tolerance is noted, and if bowel sounds are present, and vomiting, distention, or diarrhea do not occur, fluids may be slowly increased. High-calorie and high-protein or tube feedings (milk and egg) are initiated if the patient is intubated or unable to swallow or requires large amounts of calories.

▶ Evaluation

Expected Outcomes

(See also Chart 53-2.)

1. Maintains patent airway, adequate ventilation, and oxygenation
2. Regains optimal fluid and electrolyte balance and perfusion of vital organs
3. Is free of pathogenic organisms
4. Experiences minimal pain
5. Demonstrates normal body temperature
6. Achieves proper gastric function
7. Is free of associated injuries and illnesses
8. Exhibits no complications

Early Stage II

Physiologic Considerations

Following the shock period, the patient moves into the fluid mobilization phase (48 to 72 hours) (Table 53-5). At this time, the patient's response shifts from a position of defense and emergency to one of repair of damages and mobilization for recovery.

- During this period (second to fifth day), fluid is reabsorbed from the interstitial tissue and moves into the bloodstream, increasing the blood volume. An extra strain is placed on the heart, urinary output is greatly increased, and circulatory fluid overload may cause pulmonary edema. Any such changes should be reported immediately because it is imperative that fluid intake be restricted (particularly intravenous fluid intake).
- Of particular significance are signs of respiratory distress—moist crackles, coughing of frothy liquid, and cyanosis; they may herald a fatal pulmonary edema.

Fluid, Electrolyte, and Blood Needs

Evaporative fluid loss through the burn wound may reach 3 liters to 5 liters or more per 24-hour period. Water replacement can be measured by monitoring serum sodium and potassium; a sodium reading higher than 140 mEq/liter to 144 mEq/liter (normal) would suggest the need for water. More frequently, serum hyponatremia (sodium below 132 mEq/liter) occurs between the third and the tenth day with rapid fluid mobilization from the burned area.

Hypokalemia may occur at this time unless adequate oral intake of food and fluids is possible; the patient may need as much as 80 mEq to 100 mEq per day of potassium. Other indications helpful in determining water replacement are urinary output and weight loss, which should not exceed 1 kg per day. If the patient is not able to stand on a scale at the bedside, a bed scale might be used.

On the second or third postburn day, blood transfusions may be necessary to combat anemia. At this time, the patient should be observed for a possible transfusion reaction.

Wound Closure Stage

This stage of a burn is the period when the tissue killed by the burn (eschar) separates from the underlying viable tissue by a process of liquefaction called *slough formation*. The result is a large open wound that is usually infected, first by gram-positive organisms, then by gram-negative organisms, and finally by fungi.

The infection reveals itself by a gradually increasing fever and local tenderness, by tachycardia, and often by lymphangitis.

- Because infection is almost always a factor in burn treatment, the burn wound is closed as soon as possible and antibiotics are usually added to the intravenous solutions from the beginning.

Cultures are made, sensitivity tests are carried out, and the appropriate antibiotic is selected. The closure of a burn may be divided into two phases: (1) repair of the burned area, and (2) systemic repair. The repair of a large wound left by a burn cannot begin until the area is free of sloughing tissue. In some cases, the death of skin tissue may not have included deeper epithelial elements, so that some degree of epithelialization may occur from these remaining skin cells. When the entire thickness of the skin has been destroyed by the burn, repair must begin at the edges of the wound. This takes a long time in large burns, and permits an overgrowth of granulation tissue to occur.

To minimize this excessive overgrowth of granulation, the burn wound is covered with skin grafts, which also allows earlier healing. Sometimes the burn wound may be covered with cadaver skin (also called *homografts* or *allografts*) preserved in graft banks; this provides an excellent temporary covering but must be replaced by grafts of the patient's own skin. *Xenografts,* also called *heterografts* (pig skin), provide another method of temporary coverage. This biologic dressing is changed every 1 to 3 days and is used to cover the wound temporarily and prepare it for autografting.

Systemic repair includes such measures as blood transfusions to overcome the anemia that always develops in the later stages of large burns, and a high-calorie, high-protein diet. The purpose of this diet is to aid in replacing the nutritional elements lost from the draining wound and to make up for the decreased food intake during the early phases of burn treatment. Extra calories are also needed because of the hypermetabolism experienced by the victim due to stress, an endogenous inability to metabolize carbohydrate, and the work required to evaporate large quantities of surface water. At times, particularly in large burns, the technique of intravenous hyperalimentation is needed in order to supply enough calories (see p. 780).

▶ Assessment

Clinical Manifestations. Because of the lengthy time during which the burn patient is susceptible to infection and is in a catabolic state, he is prone to many complications, including wound infection; septicemia; nutritional deficien-

Chart 53-2
Guidelines for Nursing Implementation of the Patient With Thermal Injury—Stage I

Major Problems/Nursing Diagnoses

1. Potential compromised airway and altered respiratory function
2. Fluid and electrolyte losses and shifts
3. Decreased resistance to infection
4. Pain and anxiety
5. Hypothermia
6. Decreased gastric function
7. Associated injuries or illnesses
8. Potential development of complications

Nursing Goals and Interventions

1. Assure patent airway and adequate respiratory function.
   a. Maintain patent airway through proper positioning, removal of secretions, and artificial airway if indicated.
   b. Provide humidified oxygen through appropriate mode.
   c. Assess breath sounds and respiratory rate, rhythm, and depth.
   d. Monitor patient on mechanical ventilation; check settings and patient responses as determined by arterial blood gases.
   e. Observe for signs of respiratory distress or carbon monoxide poisoning.

2. Monitor fluid and electrolyte losses and shifts; replace as prescribed.
   a. Observe vital signs, urine output, and sensorium for signs of hypovolemia or fluid overload.
   b. Maintain IV lines and regulate fluids at appropriate rates.
   c. Observe for symptoms of deficiency or excess serum sodium, potassium, calcium, phosphorus, and bicarbonate.
   d. Note results of laboratory tests, and report abnormal values to physician.
   e. Document intake and output.
   f. Weigh patient daily.

3. Protect from pathogenic organisms.
   a. Use aseptic technique for wound care and invasive procedures.
   b. Support immune response through prevention of shock.
   c. Reduce reservoirs of infection.

   d. Recognize self as potential source of cross contamination.
   e. Utilize appropriate barrier gowns, gloves, etc.
   f. Administer antimicrobial drugs as prescribed topically, orally, or parenterally.
   g. Administer tetanus immune globulin or tetanus toxoid.

4. Reduce pain and anxiety.
   a. Assess pain, and differentiate from hypoxia.
   b. Administer narcotic analgesics intravenously.
   c. Introduce relaxation techniques, self-administered nitrous oxide, or other adjuncts to analgesics.
   d. Provide emotional support and reassurance.
   e. Give honest information regarding status and medical care required for optimal response.

5. Maintain adequate body temperature.
   a. Provide a warm environment through use of heat shield, space blanket, heat lights, blankets, or thick dressings.
   b. When wounds must be exposed for wound care, work quickly to minimize heat loss.
   c. Monitor rectal temperature.

6. Support gastrointestinal function; prevent nausea and vomiting.
   a. Maintain nasogastric tube on low intermittent suction until bowel sounds return.
   b. Auscultate for bowel sounds every 4 hours.
   c. Begin oral fluids when bowel sounds return; add foods slowly.
   d. Prior to tube feedings, aspirate stomach contents to check for residual amount and pH of gastric contents.
   e. Administer antacid as prescribed for low gastric pH.

7. Detect and treat other injuries or illnesses.
   a. Obtain complete nursing data base on events surrounding the burn injury, as well as past health/illness history.
   b. Complete and document detailed physical assessment and required radiologic and laboratory tests.
   c. Suspect fractures, possible spinal injury, head injury, or internal organ damage in victims of electrical burns or explosions or in those with a history of falling or jumping from fire area.

(continued)

cies; gastrointestinal bleeding; decreased range of motion in body joints; loss of muscle mass; and hazards of immobility, such as pneumonia, venous thrombosis, and pulmonary emboli. Mental changes from fluid and electrolyte imbalance, sensory overload or deprivation, disorientation, and cerebral hypoxia may also be manifested.

The nurse must perform a thorough head-to-toe assessment of the burn patient every tour of duty at least until major wounds are closed. Data should include mental status, vital signs, breath sounds, bowel sounds, motor ability, presence and character of pain, intake and output, weight pattern, and observation of burn wounds and grafts and donor sites.

Chart 53-2
Guidelines for Nursing Implementation of the Patient With Thermal Injury—Stage I (continued)

Nursing Goals and Interventions (continued)

    d. Obtain ophthalmology consultation for any patient with facial burns.

    e. Observe for heightened manifestation of chronic illnesses due to stress of burn injury.

8. Prevent and treat potential complications early.

    a. Assess for cardiac arrhythmias; obtain 12-lead ECG.

    b. Assess peripheral pulses hourly on extremities with circumferential burns.

    c. Report signs of decreased peripheral circulation or nerve or muscle ischemia to physician.

    d. Observe and test urine output for hemoglobin.

    e. Measure urine output hourly; report amount less than expected.

    f. Test urine for glucose, ketones, protein, and pH every 4 hours.

    g. Elevate extremities and head of bed to decrease edema and promote maximal circulatory and respiratory function.

Evaluation

Expected Outcomes

1. Maintains patent airway, adequate ventilation, and oxygenation

    a. Breathes spontaneously

    b. Is free of dyspnea or shortness of breath

    c. Exhibits respiratory rate between 12 and 20

    d. Has pulmonary function parameters within normal limits

    e. Shows lungs clear on auscultation

    f. Is free of cerebral effects of hypoxia

    g. Has arterial blood gases within normal limits

    h. Exhibits respiratory secretions that are minimal, colorless, and thin

2. Regains optimal fluid and electrolyte balance and perfusion of vital organs

    a. Shows intake, output, and body weight that correlate with pattern of physiologic pathology and expected results of therapy

    b. Has serum electrolytes within normal limits

    c. Exhibits urine output between 0.5 ml/kg/hour and 1.0 ml/kg/hour

    d. Has blood pressure greater than 90/60

    e. Shows heart rate less than 110/minute

    f. Exhibits clear sensorium

    g. Is free of thirst

    h. Shows normal reflexes and muscle tone indicative of electrolyte balance

3. Is free of pathogenic organisms

    a. Is free of signs of local or systemic infection

    b. Has negative blood cultures

    c. Has negative wound, sputum, and urine cultures

4. Experiences minimal pain

    a. Shows that patient comfort level permits adequate rest and active participation in required activities

    b. Requires analgesics primarily prior to dressing changes and potentially painful treatments

5. Demonstrates normal body temperature

    Has body temperature in range of 36.1° C (97° F) to 38.3° C (101° F)

6. Achieves proper gastric function

    a. Exhibits bowel sounds

    b. Shows normal gastric aspirate; no bleeding

    c. Tolerates oral or nasogastric feedings

    d. Has negative stools for occult blood

7. Is free of associated injuries and illnesses

    a. Is diagnosed and treated

    b. Has detailed physical assessment completed

    c. Has appropriate radiologic and laboratory studies completed; results noted

    d. Has past medical history obtained and documented

    e. Has treatment for specific associated injuries and illnesses incorporated in plan of care (*i.e.,* fractures immobilized)

8. Exhibits no complications

    a. Shows normal sinus rhythm or slight tachycardia

    b. Has normal serum BUN and creatinine

    c. Exhibits normal visceral organ function

    d. Has normal peripheral pulses

    e. Is free of paresthesias or symptoms of ischemia of nerves and muscles (compartment syndrome)

    f. Has clear, yellow urine; protein, sugar, ketones, pH, and specific gravity within normal limits

    g. Shows normal hemoglobin and hematocrit

    h. Exhibits normal neurology assessment

Purulent drainage, abnormal color, foul odor, redness or swelling in surrounding normal skin, or presence of healing should be noted. Changes in these parameters from one tour of duty to another or from day to day make further investigation and problem solving a necessity. Early signs of septicemia, including tachypnea, a cloudy sensorium, and decreased gastric motility, should be reported to the physician immediately.

Patient Problems/Nursing Diagnoses

Based on the clinical manifestations, the nursing assessment, and other diagnostic data, the patient's major nursing prob-

Table 53-5

Water and Electrolyte Changes Beginning 48 Hours After Major Burns

Fluid Remobilization Phase (State of Diuresis) Interstitial Fluid → Plasma

Observation	Explanation
1. Hemodilution (decreased hematocrit)	Blood cell concentration is diluted as fluid enters the vascular compartment; loss of red blood cells destroyed at burn site
2. Increased urinary output	Fluid shift into intravascular compartment increases renal blood flow and causes increased urine formation
3. Sodium deficit	With diuresis, sodium is lost with water; existing serum sodium is diluted by water influx
4. Potassium deficit (occurs occasionally in this phase)	Beginning on the fourth or fifth postburn day, K^+ shifts from extracellular fluid into cells
5. Metabolic acidosis	Loss of sodium depletes fixed base; relative carbon dioxide content increases

(Adapted from Metheny NM and Snively WD: Nurses' Handbook of Fluid Balance. Philadelphia, JB Lippincott.)

lems include probable wound infection related to loss of skin barrier and colonization of pathogens; aggressive wound care and support of wound healing related to the goal of wound closure; pain related to wound care regimen; need for aggressive nutritional support related to hypermetabolism support of immune system; emotional manifestations related to altered body image; flexion contractures in burned joints related to tendency to maintain position of comfort (i.e., flexors are stronger than extensors); inadequate knowledge of surgical procedures and postoperative course related to inexperience with burn injury; and potential complications related to stress, immobility, systemic infection, and long-term intravenous and antibiotic use.

Planning and Implementation

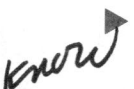

Goals

The major goals for the patient include:

1. Small, open wounds clean and healing
2. Major wounds closed
3. Relief of pain
4. In anabolic state; weight gain
5. Adaptation and adjustment to alterations in body image and life-style (including vocation)
6. Compliance with required participation in care
7. Increased range of joint motion
8. Absence of complications

Local Care of the Burn

Conscientious management of the burned area is of vital importance. When nonviable loose skin is removed, aseptic conditions must be established. Borderline normal skin near the burn wound is shaved to prevent possible contamination from hair follicles. A photograph is taken of all burned areas prior to initiation of treatment; this is filed on the patient's chart.

Infection is the major cause of death in patients who have survived the first few days following extensive burns. The infection begins within the burn site and then is carried into the bloodstream. Because of the danger of infection, cultures are taken of the burn wound on admission and twice weekly to monitor colonization of the wound by microbial organisms. Plastic liners are used in hydrotherapy equipment to prevent cross infection.

A few of the bacteria ever present in our environment contaminate the wound. Bacteria such as staphylococci, Proteus, Pseudomonas, Escherichia coli, and Klebsiella enterobacteria find optimal conditions for growth within the burn. The burn eschar is a nonviable crust with no blood supply, so that polymorphonuclear leukocytes and antibodies, even systemic antibiotics, cannot reach the area. Phenomenal numbers of bacteria—over one billion per gram of tissue—may appear and subsequently spread to the bloodstream or release their toxins, which reach distant sites.

During the time when the burn wound is healing through spontaneous reepithelialization or being prepared for skin grafting, it must be protected from burn wound sepsis. Burn wound sepsis is characterized by:

1. 10^5 bacteria/gram of tissue
2. Inflammation
3. Sludging and thrombosis of dermal blood vessels
4. Clinical symptoms of sepsis

Throughout the years, various approaches have been devised to combat these problems—exposure, occlusive dressings, open method with topical chemotherapy, and excision. All have advantages and disadvantages.

Wound Cleansing

An essential step in wound care is wound cleansing. Wound care in many institutions includes immersing the patient in an electrolyte, soapy, or germicidal bath. A walk-in type bath, a tub, or a whirlpool may be used. The agitation in the whirlpool aids in cleansing and gently massaging the tissues. The temperature of the bath is maintained at 37.8° C (100° F), and the temperature of the room should be between 26.6° C and 29.4° C (80° F to 85° F).

During the bath, the patient should be encouraged to carry out as much activity as possible. Hydrotherapy provides an excellent medium for exercising the extremities and cleaning the entire body. When the patient is removed from the tub following the bath, any residue adhering to the body can be washed away with a spray or shower of clear water.

As the crusts of second-degree burns give way to tender, new pink skin, an active physical therapy program is instituted to recondition muscles and stimulate circulation.

After a week or two, the burned tissue tends to separate

from the remaining normal tissue. The eschar can be separated from the underlying viable tissue (debridement), leaving a granulating, painful, bleeding wound. Physiologic dressings are used until the site is ready for autografting. Many of these wounds, which appear to be very deep, will be found to have some epithelium still remaining in them, and healing can take place from these islands of skin. In other areas where the skin is completely destroyed, nature must have some help to heal the tremendous wounds left by the burn. It is in these patients that skin grafts are more effective.

The burned area is frequently prepared for skin grafts through daily hydrotherapy. The patient may be immersed in the tank for 20 to 30 minutes while the burned areas are washed gently to remove the debris and devitalized skin that is attached to them.

Scissors and forceps may be employed to trim loose eschar and unroof potential abcesses.

As soon as the burn wound becomes a red, granulating area without slough, skin grafts may be used. While giving care to the patient in the bath, the nurse should wear a gown, cap, mask, and sterile gloves in order not to infect the burned area. Since tubbing is metabolically stressful, the nurse should constantly assess the patient for signs of chilling, fatigue, changes in vital signs, and pain unrelieved by pretub analgesics.

Following tubbing, wounds can be gently patted dry with sterile towels, and the prescribed method of wound care employed. Physician preferences; the skill level of nursing staff; and resources in terms of number of personnel, supplies, and time must be considered in choosing the best method for a given patient situation. Whatever the method, the goal is to protect the wound from overwhelming proliferation of pathogenic organisms and invasion of deeper tissues until either spontaneous healing or skin grafting can be achieved. Patient comfort and the ability to participate in the prescribed method of treatment are also important considerations.

Exposure Method

The objective of this method is to control bacterial colonization by exposing the wound to light and maintaining a cool environment. This method is most frequently used to treat burns of the face, neck, perineum, and extensive areas of the trunk. Exposing a burn to the drying effect of air allows the exudate to dry and form a hard crust in about 3 days; this protects the wound. In a second-degree burn, regeneration of skin beneath the crust takes 2 to 3 weeks, at which time the eschar falls off. In a third-degree burn, no epithelialization occurs beneath the eschar. In the untreated burn, the eschar usually separates in 2 to 3 weeks. When full-thickness burns occur circumferentially on the extremities or trunk, the eschar causes a tourniquet effect, compromising distal circulation and chest expansion.

The success of the exposed method depends on keeping the immediate environment free of organisms. Some practitioners maintain that everything coming in contact with the patient must be sterile. Linens are sterile; those who come in direct contact with the patient wear masks, sterile gowns, and gloves; visitors are instructed to wear gowns and masks and not to touch the bed or hand the patient anything. Some practitioners maintain a clean environment and rely on the amazing efficiency of the topical antibacterial agents to limit burn wound infection.

A cradle may be placed over the patient to prevent sheets from coming in contact with the burn area, to minimize the effects of air currents to which a burn patient is unusually sensitive, and to provide some form of covering. (Some persons are sensitive to being unduly exposed.) Heat shields or lamps may be required to maintain the patient's body temperature, since a loss of the microcirculation in the burned areas decreases the patient's ability to maintain body heat.

The use of a sterile "burn pack" facilitates the care of this patient; it may contain sheets, pillowcases, washcloth, bath blanket, loin cloth, halter, and perhaps a gown and mask for the attendant.

The room should be kept scrupulously clean; windows should have screens to keep out flies and other insects. Damp dusting and mopping are preferable to dry dusting and sweeping. Regulation of the room temperature and humidity is necessary for the patient's comfort and for optimal crust development. The patient is acutely aware of temperature changes and is most comfortable when the room is kept within the range of 34° C ± 2° (93° F ± 4°). The most important characteristic of environmental conditions is that the ambient air temperature should be warmer than that of the burned skin.

The room temperature can be adjusted according to the patient's needs. A temperature that is too warm may cause fluid loss through perspiration and, in addition, may promote bacterial growth. If the temperature is too cool, a blanket may be spread over the cradle, or small light bulbs may be placed in the tent. When these lights are used, the patient may want to wear sunglasses or an eyeshade.

The preferred range of humidity in the room is between 40% and 50%. A room that is drier will cause burn eschar to crack and cause pain, whereas a room that is too moist will encourage softening and premature separation of eschar. Portable electric humidifiers or dehumidifiers are effective in controlling humidity.

A light sprinkling of sterile cornstarch on the lower sheet helps to prevent a burn area from sticking to the sheet. Alternatively, one may use Microdon sheeting (3M Co.) or aluminum foil, such as Reynolds Wrap.

When linens are changed, care must be taken not to pull on those parts of the sheet that are adhering to the burn area. Sterile saline may be used to wet the area so that the sheet may be freed gently. Turning is encouraged to prevent pneumonia and contractures and to promote circulation. The patient may prefer to do this without assistance; if help is required, the nurse should don sterile gloves to handle nonburn areas. Even more importantly, the patient should be ambulated as soon as possible—even on the first day— and should be encouraged to use his arms, hands, fingers, and legs.

The advantages of the exposure method are (1) there are no painful dressing changes; (2) less equipment is used;

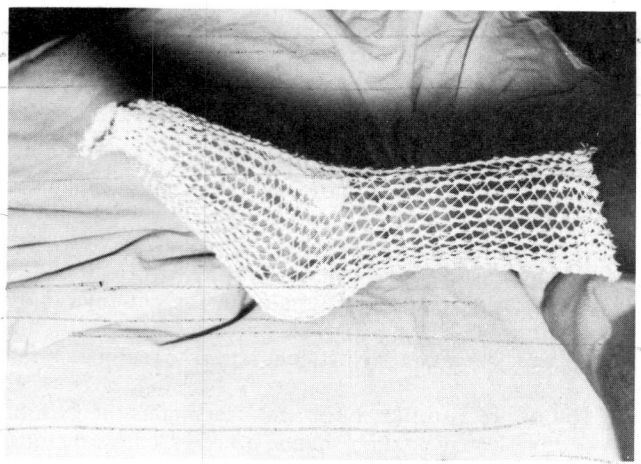

Figure 53-4. Use of tubular mesh overdressing to hold gauze covering in place. Once a wound has been cleansed and debrided, a fine gauze impregnated with a topical antibacterial cream (silver sulfadiazine or mafenide) is applied in one layer. The gauze is cut to fit the wounds only and does not overlap onto unburned skin. The tubular overdressing, holding the gauze in place, is available in several sizes and is elasticized in order to facilitate application to all parts of the body. (Courtesy, Shriners Hospitals for Crippled Children, Burns Institute, Galveston, Texas.)

(3) infection can be detected early; and (4) large numbers of patients can be treated, making this method particularly suitable for disaster situations.

Disadvantages of this method are (1) it is often not suitable for burns of the hands and feet because proper alignment and elevation are difficult to maintain; (2) it is unsuitable when the patient must be transported any distance, as from a battlefront to a base hospital; (3) it is less effective when other injuries exist that require the patient to be turned frequently; and (4) it may cause additional metabolic stress unless the patient's body temperature can be adequately maintained by controlling the immediate environment. Bandaging would be preferable in these instances.

Occlusive (Pressure) Dressings

Occlusive dressings are used primarily for burns of the feet and hands. Fine mesh gauze impregnated with a topical antimicrobial agent is applied lightly to the cleansed burn area and an appropriate dressing is applied. The dressing may consist of sterile, absorptive, fluffed or washed gauze placed in such a way that the material does not clump together.

Precautions are taken to prevent two body surfaces from touching, such as fingers or toes, ear and scalp, the areas under the breast, any point of flexion, or between the genital folds. Functional body alignment positions are maintained; thus, the fingers and thumb curve over fluffed gauze or a bandage roll, the foot is positioned to avoid pronation and dropfoot, and support is placed under the knees.

Some physicians fix the loose gauze in place with an elastic bandage or stockinette; others apply abdominal pads before applying the conforming bandage. Another fixation

bandage is elastic, tubular, woven netting, which is a light, conforming overdressing available in many sizes (Fig. 53-4). Evenly distributed pressure is desired with no constriction to hinder circulation. Circulation may be checked every 3 or 4 hours by noting pulse, color, warmth, and symptoms of paresthesia. Having the tips of fingers or toes exposed provides areas where circulation can be easily checked.

Removal of Soiled Dressings. Dressings are changed in the patient's unit following the administration of an analgesic (20 minutes previously) or in the operating room with the patient anesthetized. If possible, dressings should be changed following or during hydrotherapy, which facilitates the procedure and keeps the patient more comfortable. Otherwise, wetting the dressings (with warm saline, 2 parts to 1 part of 2% hydrogen peroxide) facilitates their removal by softening the exudate and eschar. If exudate stain is noted, indicating moisture, the wet dressings are replaced to encourage drying and to prevent the growth of microorganisms.

- Signs of infection are increased pulse, elevated temperature, and possibly odor, or greenish or yellowish coloring on the dressings.

Occasionally, with bacteremia from *Proteus* or *Pseudomonas,* the urine will become brownish to green in color.

To change the dressing, the nurse dons a mask and gloves, slits the outer dressings with blunt scissors, and spreads the dressing open. The extremity is carefully lifted to withdraw the soiled dressings, and the part is lowered onto a sterile towel. The remaining dressings are carefully removed with forceps and the gloved hand. Loose eschar is then debrided.

Debridement. Since the eschar is dead tissue, it can be cut safely up to the point of bleeding or pain. Using sterile gloves, a smooth forceps, and surgical scissors, the physician or specially trained nurse may debride the eschar. If there is bleeding from a torn small blood vessel, oxidized cellulose (Oxycel) or pressure may be applied for hemostasis. Medication and dressings are reapplied gently and smoothly. The area should be watched for further bleeding, which may require ligation.

Redressing of the Burn. The prescribed topical antibacterial agent is applied according to the preference of the surgeon.

Burns of the extremities are elevated, usually on pillows, to prevent edema. In the case of a hand burn, a bucket-handle suspension device may be improvised.

Open Method and Topical Chemotherapy

The open method, the most popular method of treating burns, consists of a combination of the exposure method and the application of a topical agent. With this method, wound assessment is simpler, physical therapy occurs at an earlier point, and temperature is easier to control. However, there is a delay in eschar separation, as well as a risk of sepsis and patient discomfort due to body chilling.

Bacteriologic cultures are required to monitor the effect of topical medications. Swab cultures or surface cultures (gauze capillarity) may be used. The procedures are non-invasive, simple, and painless but are limited to the area sampled. Wound biopsy cultures (invasive) may be required for quantitative sampling. Systemic antibiotics are used sparingly but are essential for pulmonary or other concomitant infections.

Criteria for topical agents include the following: (1) the agent is effective against gram-negative organisms, *Pseudomonas aeruginosa, Staphylococcus aureus,* and even fungi; (2) it is clinically effective; (3) it penetrates the eschar but is not systemically toxic; (4) it does not lose its effectiveness, thereby permitting another infection to develop; (5) it is cost-effective, available, and acceptable to the patient; and (6) it is inexpensive and easy to apply, minimizing nursing care time.

Silver Sulfadiazine (Silvadene)

Silver sulfadiazine, a popular topical medication used in this method of burn treatment, is synthesized by reacting silver nitrate with sodium sulfadiazine. It is available as a water-soluble cream in concentrations of 1% and is highly effective against gram-negative bacteria. It is more effective when the total burn area involves less than 60% of the body surface area.

Evidence indicates that the *Pseudomonas* cells may split the agent so that silver is bound but sulfadiazine is released. This binding action may account for the potent inhibition of bacterial growth.

Compared with mafenide acetate and other antibacterial agents, silver sulfadiazine is more effective in controlling infection; causes no pain on application; does not disturb acid–base balance, electrolytes, or renal function; allows regeneration of epithelium to progress unhindered; and does not stain. Liberal amounts are applied topically with a gloved hand or on impregnated gauze rolls.

The medicated burn area can be left open or covered with a dressing. When silver sulfadiazine is applied to dermal burns, a proteinaceous gel (several millimeters thick) forms on the wound surface; after 72 hours, this pseudoeschar can be removed easily.

Recently it has been reported that a significant number of gram-negative bacilli can become highly resistant to sulfadiazine as a result of protracted use of this agent.

Silver Sulfadiazine–Cerium Nitrate. Cerium (a lanthanide element) has recently been incorporated into silver sulfadiazine to enhance its clinical effectiveness. A combination of just under 1% of silver sulfadiazine and 2.2% of cerium nitrate provides a thin cream that can be applied topically. It appears to be most effective against gram-negative bacteria and has been credited with lowering mortality rates. Occasionally, a case of methemoglobinemia has been noted; however, on the whole it seems most effective and safe.

Cerium Nitrate Solution. Cerium nitrate solution (1.74%) can be used alone or in conjunction with the combination silver sulfadiazine–cerium nitrate cream as a wet soak to enhance the effectiveness of the antibacterial action of these agents. It must be rewet every 4 hours and applied with a bulky dressing for maximal effectiveness and to assist in maintaining the patient's body temperature at optimal levels. A dry top covering, such as a bandaging layer of stockinette, helps to reduce heat evaporation.

Silver Nitrate Solution (0.5% Aqueous Solution)

Silver nitrate is an effective agent in preventing eschar contamination, particularly in burn injuries involving up to 40% or 50% of the body surface area. However, since the drug is unable to penetrate the eschar, infection can occur in the subeschar region. Because of this possibility, it is necessary to inspect the wound frequently and debride as necessary.

Disagreement still exists about whether the high mortality rate from extensive burns results from toxins produced by the burn or from inanition and overwhelming infection of the burn surface as well as evaporation of body heat from the burn surface. Those who support the latter theory note that covering the burn with continuous wet dressings of 0.5% silver nitrate solution effectively controls the infection. According to this thinking, the bactericidal action of the silver nitrate solution on burn wounds is so effective that cross infection does not occur, therefore, isolation technique is not necessary. Caps, masks, and gowns are not worn routinely, and relatives are permitted to visit freely and even feed the patient. However, cleanliness and handwashing are stressed. Clean (not sterile) strips of gauze are cut from large rolls and used as dressings. Further, masks and sterile gloves are used by personnel when they directly handle the patient.

The treatment begins soon after the patient reaches the hospital. The patient is placed in a sterile bath of warmed Locke's solution,* and all greases and ointments are carefully removed from the burn area; this facet of the treatment may take up to an hour. The burns are then covered with gauze dressings thoroughly soaked with 0.5% silver nitrate solution. Concentrations above 1% produce tissue necrosis, whereas those below 0.5% are ineffective antiseptically.

These dressings are kept wet with the silver nitrate solution, which is applied by means of bulb syringes. The best dressings are composed of six to eight layers of four-ply gauze applied wet and held in place with bandages of bias-cut wide stockinette. The gauze of the dressing *should not contain cotton between the layers,* because this interferes with the efficient action of the silver nitrate solution and causes the dressing to stick to the wound. Catheters may be incorporated into the thick dressings to permit saturation every 2 to 4 hours. The dressings are changed two or three times daily. The patient is covered with one or two dry sheets and a dry cotton blanket. These dry layers prevent or reduce the heat loss produced by vaporization from the wet dressings and from the burned surface. When the coverings become moist, they are changed. The patient is turned frequently to provide pressure and wetness to all areas. For

---

* Modified Locke's solution for the sterile bath for the burned patient is a combination of various salts. It is best prepared from two stock solutions that are mixed at the time that the bath is prepared.

Solution A—g/liter		*Solution B—g/liter*	
NaCl	175.5	NaHCO$_3$	73.3
KCl	9.0	NaH$_2$PO$_4 \cdot$ H$_2$O	3.8
CaCl$_2 \cdot$ 2 H$_2$O	11.1		
MgCl$_2 \cdot$ 6 H$_2$O	9.13		

Add 1 volume of Solution A, followed by 1 volume of B, to 23 volumes of water.

the severely burned patient, the Stryker frame or circular bed may be used.

The use of 0.5% silver nitrate solution dressings is not without danger, because electrolytes, especially sodium and potassium, are withdrawn from the body fluids and pass into the dressings impregnated with silver nitrate solution. The withdrawal of sodium may occur very rapidly, especially in patients with extensive burns and in children, producing an acute electrolyte imbalance.

- In the early phases of the burn treatment, blood must be drawn at frequent intervals—every 2 to 4 hours—to determine sodium, chloride, potassium, and calcium levels. These electrolytes must be replaced, usually by the intravenous administration of Ringer's lactate solution.

Once the patient can take a normal diet, salt is added to the diet. Calcium depression is treated by the addition of calcium lactate or gluconate to the diet (usually within a few days postburn) and potassium depression by the administration of potassium gluconate elixir. Deficits in these constituents of the blood electrolytes naturally are more marked in more extensive burns (comprising 50% to 80% of the body surface).

The silver nitrate solution has the disadvantage of turning black in the sunlight. This means that everything touched by the solution is stained black, including clothes, hands, floors, and other objects. The nurse attending a patient being treated with silver nitrate solution must wear rubber gloves, as a protection against the silver nitrate stains. (Such stains may be prevented by applying an organic iodine preparation, such as Wescodyne or Betadine solutions, to objects that have come in contact with the silver solution and then rinsing them in water.) Stain-resistant floor and wall coverings are available, but such materials increase the cost of care.

Mafenide Acetate (Sulfamylon Acetate)

Mafenide acetate (10%) in cream form with a hydrophilic base diffuses rapidly through the burned skin and eschar and is effective against a broad range of gram-positive and gram-negative organisms in the subeschar area. It is limited in use to the treatment of localized invasive burn wound sepsis caused by organisms sensitive to this agent.

The cream is applied in a thick layer, 3 mm to 4 mm (Fig. 53-5), once or twice daily; a fine mesh gauze may be applied in strips directly to the burn and changed daily or washed off in a whirlpool bath.

Although it is relatively nontoxic, mafenide acetate is a strong carbonic anhydrase inhibitor and may adversely affect the blood pH level, causing a reduction of the renal tubular buffering mechanism. With continued use, severe metabolic acidosis may occur, making is necessary to discontinue mafenide and monitor the respiratory rate, blood gases, and pH. Chest x-rays also may be justified because of possible pulmonary failure.

Another disadvantage of this form of treatment is the burning pain experienced by the patient for a few minutes following application of the cream. Thus, analgesics may be required before the ointment is applied. Another problem is that eschar separates very slowly, thereby delaying skin grafting unless the eschar is aggressively debrided.

Other Topical Agents

Povidone–iodine is commercially available as a brown water-miscible cream for topical use in which the iodine content is 1%. More information is needed in order to recommend its use.

Gentamicin sulfate is a bactericidal aminoglycoside available in a 0.1% cream for topical use. It is useful for short periods of time in small areas of invasive infection. Superinfection with resistant bacterial strains have been reported, indicating the need for very careful monitoring when it is used.

Skin Grafting

Partial-thickness wounds may spontaneously reepithelialize over a period of 10 days to several weeks or even months. With full-thickness burns greater than 2 cm in diameter or

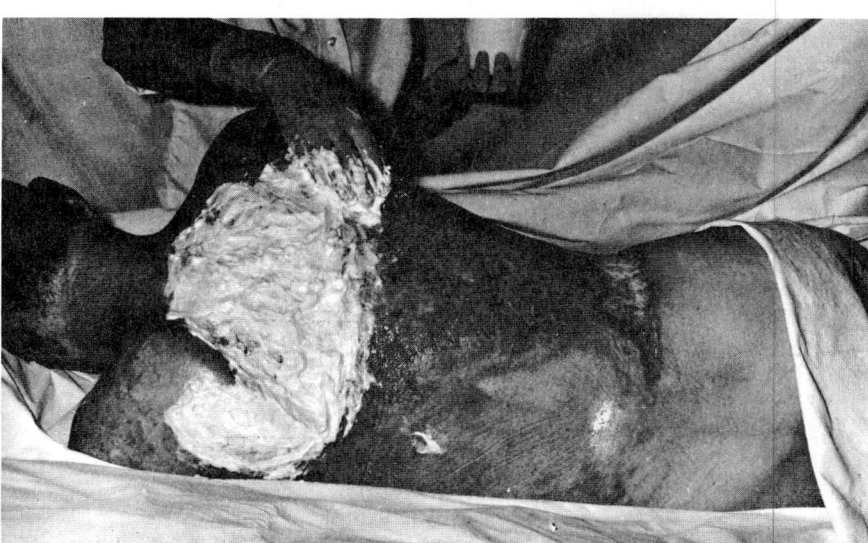

Figure 53-5. Photograph of back of patient with deep second-degree burn being treated with Sulfamylon. The Sulfamylon cream is put on in a thick layer with the gloved hand. (From Artz CP and Mancrief VA: The Treatment of Burns, Philadelphia, WB Saunders.)

in deep partial-thickness wounds, which are likely to take many weeks to heal, skin grafting is usually required. With daily wound cleansing and eschar removal, a base of granulation tissue gradually forms to provide a vascular base for the graft. A more aggressive approach to wound closure, usually used for small areas, such as the hands, employs excisional therapy.

Split-Thickness Grafts. The split-thickness type of skin graft is most often used to cover the area left after the eschar is removed. (See p. 1190 for skin grafting management.) The hands, face, feet, and joints are high-priority areas for grafting.

Nursing care is most important in adjusting the part to its most comfortable position and preventing the skin graft from being dislodged. Skin loss in areas such as the neck, the elbow, etc. produces scars that contract and cause marked deformities. It is in these areas especially that early skin grafting is most efficacious.

Large areas of burn often require hospitalization for a considerable time to permit healing. This is a trying period for the patient, and diversional therapy is most helpful. Occupational therapy and other types of diversion that take the patient's mind away from his troubles are very helpful. Television or radio at eye level and within the patient's control are most useful.

Excisional Therapy

When excisional therapy is the treatment of choice, all nonviable tissue is removed down to a viable base. This relatively new method of treating burns carries less danger of sepsis, creates less metabolic stress, and allows for earlier as well as quicker rehabilitation. When the excisional procedures are carried out, the patient's blood volume must be supported and adequate nutrition must be supplied. Expansion grafting techniques are used, and specific topical antimicrobial agents are selected.

A cold knife or laser scalpel is used to excise tissue. The laser is favored since it involves a minimal amount of blood loss. Usually, the excision is done between the second and fifth postburn days, but it can be done in selected patients after that time. After the nonviable tissue is removed (not more than 25% of total body surface is excised at one time), the excised wounds are closed with expanded autografts or skin substitutes.

Temporary Wound Closure. As soon as nonviable tissue is removed, it is essential that the fresh wound be closed immediately. Sheet autografts are preferred. If the wound is large, involving over 50% of the total body surface, biological dressings (allografts) are the preferred temporary skin substitutes until sufficient autografts are available. The same donor site can be used every 2 to 3 weeks if healing is optimal and autograft skin can be meshed to increase the area that it will cover. (See p. 1190 for skin grafting.)

Broad adherent and barrier dressings are being tried experimentally and appear to hold promise as the preferred method for providing temporary wound closure. Hydron (polyhydroxymethylmethacrylate) is an example of a barrier dressing that is sprayed on a fresh burn or excised burn wound. When incorporated with polyethylene glycol, this compound is converted into an adherent pliable membrane that discourages bacterial penetration. Hydron forms a bond to the underlying wound, is flexible, and permits the patient to engage in physical therapy.

Another excellent source is a skin bank in which cadaver skin (homograft) is stored in liquid nitrogen. Such skin is typed and when needed can be thawed, washed in saline, and made ready for use in less than an hour.

Semipermeable, clear polyurethane film dressings (Op-Site) have been helpful in the care of small, clean wounds and donor sites. A major advantage is that patients report markedly decreased pain compared to other types of dressing materials. Reepithelialization is enhanced, and visual inspection of the healing wound is allowed. Another synthetic alternative is Biobrane.* Early studies have indicated that it compares favorably with the human allograft and porcine heterograft in control of pain and infection, and in adherence to the wound.

A very interesting recent development in burn care is the use of artificial skin, developed by John F. Burke and Ioannis V. Yannis in Boston. Like natural skin, this man-made version is composed of two layers. The innermost (dermal) layer is a mixture of protein from cowhide and carbohydrate from shark cartilage. The epidermal layer is prepared by bonding plastic onto the cowhide–shark layer. When placed on a burn wound, the artificial skin protects the wound. As new natural tissue forms, the dermal layer breaks down and the plastic layer peels off. Although still experimental, this advent is being followed with much interest by burn care specialists.

Permanent Wound Closure. Skin grafts are acquired in a variety of sizes and thicknesses by means of a dermatome designed for this purpose. Meshing devices are available to provide for even expansion of sheet grafts. Skin expanded to the usual ratio of 3:1 makes it possible to cover greater surface areas; such grafts become adherent in approximately 3 to 4 days. Other types of grafts may be required, including rotation flaps, pedicle flaps, or free grafts (see p. 1189).

Postgrafting Wound Care. The success of a graft depends on applying the graft at the optimum time in the optimum way (following original skin lines) and with maximum control over infection. Thereafter, a multidisciplinary effort, including the surgeon, nurse, psychiatrist, physical and occupational therapists, social worker, and family, is required in order to carry out a planned rehabilitative program. Splints and braces may have to be worn to prevent contractures of burned joints. Elastic garments may be used to maintain the position of the tissue on the graft site and to reduce hypertrophic scarring. These devices may be worn for the first year. Massaging the scar area with topical steroids (or injections of steroid locally) may be required to reduce hypertrophic scar formation. Clear, plastic splints are effective in maintaining positions and permitting visualization of pressure points.

An aggressive exercise program with physical and occupational therapy conducted on an outpatient basis, plus conscientious lubrication of the skin and protection from trauma is the kind of continuing care required for successful rehabilitation.

* Hospitex, Pennsauken, New Jersey

Nutritional Support

As soon as gastrointestinal function returns after resuscitation has been established, nutritional support must begin. The enteral route is preferred, and many burn patients will tolerate oral fluids and food. In patients with large burns, tube feeding may be employed to assure a certain number of calories per day. In this case, a meal tray and high-protein, high-calorie snacks may be offered as a supplement to the essential tube feedings.

High-protein drinks are offered and provide an excellent means of supplementing the diet. A diet containing more solid food is usually begun toward the end of the first week, when the patient's tolerance for food improves. The catabolic response of the body is great, as is reflected in calorie expenditures of 5000 to 6000 calories a day. This means that, to meet nutritional demands, the patient must build up nutritional intake to a similar number of calories; he needs approximately 3 g of protein per kilogram of body weight, 20% of the needed calories in the form of fats and the remainder in carbohydrates.

Patients lose a great deal of weight in the process of recovering from severe burns. Reserve fat desposits are tapped during the recovery, fluids have been lost, and calorie intake may have been limited. Because of low resistance to infection and disease, the patient's nutritional state must be improved even though he has a poor appetite and is still weak. Semisolid and then a regular diet are offered on the third or fourth day postburn as tolerated. Encouraging him, catering to his preferences, and offering protein and vitamin supplement snacks are ways of tempting the patient to gradually increase his intake from 3000 to as many as 6000 calories a day. As a general rule, he should be permitted to eat what he likes—as much as he likes, as often as he likes—and then encouraged to eat more. A 70-kg patient with a 50% burn must take in at least 4200 calories per day to maintain weight.

Parenteral hyperalimentation is utilized for patients who are unable to tolerate the required volume of enteral feedings. The risk of infection of the central catheter required by this method must be considered. While solutions commonly used may provide 1000 or more calories per liter, they are deficient in fatty acids. Therefore, intravenous fat solutions will also have to be given periodically.

The incidence of *gastrointestinal tract ulcer* (Curling's ulcer) is in proportion to the extent of the burn area. This condition is manifested by hemorrhage, detected in bloody contents from nasogastric suction or in the stool. A sudden drop in hemoglobin concentration may be diagnostic even before the hemorrhage is evident. Gastric surgery may be indicated. This is not an uncommon complication. For this reason, frequent small feedings (e.g., six or more daily meals) or incorporation of milk and antacid in the diet is a part of proper management.

Proper Positioning and Mobilization

The prevention of pneumonia, the control of edema, and the prevention of pressure sores and contractures are guiding objectives in this facet of management. Deep breathing, turning, and proper repositioning are essential nursing practices modified to meet individual needs. Early ambulation may be encouraged according to the capability of the patient.

Whenever the lower extremities are involved in the burn, Ace bandages should be applied before the patient is placed in an upright position. Both passive and active range of motion exercises are initiated from the day of admission and are continued after grafting within certain limitations.

Psychosocial Response

Throughout the course of treatment, the patient is subjected to a painful and distressing experience. Following the traumatic events related to the fire, the patient's life-style has been dramatically changed from one of independence to one of dependence—within a strange and frightening environment where physical activity is limited, pain is prevalent, and life seems to hang in the balance, while the patient lies helpless, totally dependent on the care of strange people and equipment.

In such a situation, communication is of the utmost importance. Explanations must be given clearly and often repeatedly, so that the patient becomes involved and understands what is being done to, for, and with him. A major responsibility of the nurse is to constantly assess the patient's psychosocial reactions. Why is he fearful? Is he afraid of losing control of his bodily care, of his very sanity? Is he fearful of rejection by his family and loved ones? Is he fearful of being unable to cope with pain, the appearance of his body? Is he concerned about sexual function? Being aware of the patient's anxieties and understanding the basis of his fears will enable the nurse to provide support and to cooperate with other members of the health team in developing a plan of intervention to help the patient handle these feelings. Such measures may include providing medication for adequate sleep, rest, and relief from pain and anxiety; including the patient in planning day-to-day care; soliciting the support of family members and collaborating with other personnel involved in providing burn care.

Aside from showing signs of fear, the patient frequently gives vent to angry feelings. At times the anger may be directed inward because of a sense of guilt—perhaps for causing the fire or even for surviving when loved ones perished; or the anger may reach outward toward those who escaped unharmed or even to those who are now providing care. One way to help the patient handle these emotions is to find someone to whom the patient can vent his feelings without fear of retaliation. A nurse, social worker, clergyman, or family member may fill this role successfully.

When feelings of guilt and depression are pronounced, the patient may need to be helped through the grieving process (see p. 194), since he may frequently be faced with a sense of loss resulting from disfigurement and the possible death of loved ones. In some instances, it may help to provide diversion and physical activity, so that he is involved in more than just his own care.

If the patient becomes delirious, possibly because of psychosis or infection, efforts should be made to orient him to reality. People entering the unit should identify themselves; a clock, calendar, and radio can be used as points of reference for time and events; efforts can be made to give a sense of the hour of the day by placing the patient near a window. During this period of mental disequilibrium, no new personnel should attend to the patient. Familiar faces and voices will give the patient a sense of security and orientation.

Before the patient improves, there may be a period of regression during which he may become very dependent and even pessimistic about his recovery. He needs nursing support, honesty, candor, understanding, and firmness in setting reasonable goals of expectation. The family, too, will need guidance at this time so that they will understand the patient's emotional status. Of course, the family will have been prepared to accept infection-control precautions and the appearance of the patient—the burn itself and its concomitant edema can cause disfiguring distortions, bandaging can appear voluminous, and certain treatments, such as silver nitrate, are most unattractive. Visitors must be instructed to conceal their own shocked reactions from the patient.

As the burn victim progresses, he becomes aware of daily improvement and begins to exhibit basic concerns: Will I be disfigured? How long will I have to be in the hospital? What about my job and family? Will I ever be independent again? How can I pay for my care? Was this the result of my carelessness? As he expresses his concerns, the nurse should take time to listen and to encourage him.

▶ **Evaluation**

Expected Outcomes

(See also Chart 53-3.)

1. Exhibits small open wounds that are clean
2. Demonstrates that majority of wounds are closed
3. Obtains relief of pain
4. Demonstrates optimal nutritional status
5. Has realistic concept of changes in body image and alterations in daily activities as a result of burn injury

(Text continues on page 1224.)

Chart 53-3
Guidelines for Nursing Implementation of the Patient With Thermal Injury—Stage II

Major Problems/Nursing Diagnoses

1. Burn wound sepsis
2. Potential for inadequate wound healing.
3. Pain
4. Hypermetabolism
5. Emotional manifestations of altered body image
6. Potential for development of flexion contractures and muscle atrophy
7. Inadequate knowledge of surgical procedures and postoperative course.
8. Potential complications

Nursing Goals and Interventions

1. Prevent burn wound sepsis.
   a. Wash hands prior to all patient contact.
   b. Prevent shock.
   c. Prevent pressure on wounds.
   d. Apply topical antibacterials as prescribed.
   e. Prevent cross contamination.
   f. Remove possible reservoirs of infection.
   g. Utilize barrier gowns, gloves, masks, and hair covers when wounds are exposed or when in direct contact with patient or bed.
2. Promote adequate wound healing.
   a. Cleanse wound and rest of body, including hair; daily.
   b. Apply topical antibacterial agents and dressing as prescribed.
   c. Prevent pressure, infection, and mobilization of autografts.
   d. Provide donor site care.
   e. Observe and report any signs of poor graft take or loss of skin integrity after healing.
   f. Provide adequate nutritional support.

3. Minimize pain.
   a. Assess patient's pain carefully.
   b. Offer analgesics and relaxation breathing, transcutaneous nerve stimulator, self-administered nitrous oxide, or other appropriate measures.
   c. Assess and document patient's response to interventions.
   d. Assist patient with appropriate means of expressing pain.
   e. Educate patient about the usual pain trajectory in burn recovery.

4. Provide adequate nutritional support.
   a. Provide high-calorie, high-protein diet by appropriate route.
   b. Administer parenteral hyperalimentation according to hospital protocol.
   c. Give supplemental vitamins and minerals as prescribed.
   d. Weigh patient daily; record in graphic form.
   e. Report intolerance manifested by abdominal distention, diarrhea, osmotic diuresis, dehydration.

5. Promote adaptation to and acceptance of altered body image or life-style resulting from burn injury.
   a. Determine patient's readiness to express feelings regarding alteration in body image or life-style.
   b. Provide opportunity for expression of thoughts and feelings.
   c. Maintain positive but honest approach in responding to questions.
   d. Utilize significant others, counselors, and appropriate resource persons to help patient cope.
   e. Support effective premorbid coping mechanisms.

(continued)

Chart 53-3
Guidelines for Nursing Implementation of the Patient With Thermal Injury—Stage II (continued)

Nursing Goals and Interventions (continued)

6. Prevent flexion contractures and muscle atrophy.
   a. Position patient carefully to prevent flexed position in burned areas.
   b. Implement range of motion exercises several times daily.
   c. Assist with ambulation.
   d. Utilize splints and exercise devices recommended by occupational and physical therapists.
   e. Encourage self-feeding and turning and moving in bed.
   f. Provide required assistive devices.

7. Reduce fears and anxiety and promote participation in perioperative care.
   a. Review surgical procedures and postoperative course with patient and family.
   b. Explore patient's previous experience with hospitalization and surgery.
   c. Tailor information given to patient's questions and nonverbal cues to anxiety level.
   d. Define expectations of required patient participation for optimal results.

8. Prevent complications.
   a. Turn every 2 hours from side to side.
   b. Encourage coughing, incentive spirometry, deep breathing (or hyperinflation with Ambu-bag for artificial airway) hourly.
   c. Do chest physical therapy and postural drainage as prescribed.
   d. Maintain adequate fluid intake.
   e. Inspect skin carefully for signs of pressure and breakdown.
   f. Utilize aseptic technique for sterile and invasive procedures.
   g. Administer systemic antibiotics as prescribed.
   h. Maintain closed system and adequate drainage for urinary catheter.
   i. Observe for and treat fungal infections.
   j. Change all IV catheters every 48 hours; change IV tubing every 24 hours.
   k. Observe for and report signs of thrombophlebitis or catheter-induced infections.

Evaluation

Expected Outcomes

1. Exhibits clean small, open wounds
   a. Exhibits open wound areas that are pink, reepithelializing, and free of infection
   b. Shows clean reepithelializing donor sites

2. Demonstrates that majority of wounds are closed
   a. Has completed or nearly completed skin grafting
   b. Shows over 80% of body covered with intact skin

3. Obtains relief of pain
   a. Requests analgesics only occasionally and specifically for muscle and joint pain
   b. Verbally reports minimal pain
   c. Is free of physiologic and nonverbal indicators of moderate or severe pain

4. Demonstrates optimal nutritional status
   a. Demonstrates daily weight gain (by weight curve)
   b. Is free of signs of protein, vitamin, or mineral deficiency
   c. Has increasing energy level
   d. Meets required nutritional needs by oral intake entirely
   e. Exhibits normal serum protein levels

5. Has realistic concept of changes in body image and alterations required in daily activities as a result of burn injury
   a. Verbalizes an accurate description of alterations in body image postburn
   b. Discusses changes in life-style and daily activities that may be required postdischarge
   c. Demonstrates interest in resources that may be able to positively affect cosmetic and functional results of injury
   d. Is free of withdrawal and depression

6. Demonstrates range of joint motion that approaches preburn range
   a. Shows joint motion that permits activities of daily living
   b. Improves range of motion of contracted joints daily
   c. Is free of periarticular calcification

7. Verbalizes understanding of treatments and surgical procedures and participates appropriately in care
   a. Expresses concerns about surgery and treatments with health team and family
   b. Describes surgical procedures, and treatments accurately
   c. Cooperates with required positioning

8. Is free of complications
   a. Has heart rate between 60 and 100 beats per minute
   b. Shows respiratory rate between 12 and 20 breaths per minute
   c. Exhibits blood pressure within normal preburn range
   d. Breathes spontaneously without ventilatory assistance or artificial airway
   e. Demonstrates clear breath sounds
   f. Has normal hemoglobin and hematocrit
   g. Shows body temperature between 36.1° C (97° F) and 38.3° C (101° F)
   h. Has serum osmolarity and electrolytes within normal range
   i. Exhibits adequate fluid intake and urine output
   j. Demonstrates normal pattern of bowel movements

Chart 53-4
Guidelines of Nursing Implementation for the Patient With Thermal Injury—Stage III

Major Problems/Nursing Diagnoses

1. Potential for development of emotional and physical dependence on health team
2. Skin tightness, dryness, and itching
3. Pain on exercise
4. Fatigue and low endurance with activity
5. Small, open wounds
6. Flexion contractures
7. Lack of knowledge for self-care
8. Hypertrophic scarring
9. Grieving and depression

Nursing Goals and Interventions

1. Promote emotional and physical independence.
   a. Be alert for verbal and nonverbal cues of patient concerns regarding rehabilitation and adaptation to altered self-image.
   b. Assist patient to set achievable short-term goals for increased independence in activities of daily living.
   c. Provide positive feedback and support as patient progresses toward independence.
   d. Consult with appropriate health team members for assistance with regressive behavior.
   e. Assist with physical and occupational therapy as outlined by physical medicine staff.
2. Promote soft, lubricated, comfortable skin.
   a. Assist patient with application of cocoa butter, Nivea, or other lubricating cream to healed wounds several times daily.
   b. Use mild soap for daily bathing.
   c. Maintain cool, comfortable environment.
   d. Administer antipruritic medication.
   e. Recommend white, cotton underwear under street clothing.
3. Relieve pain.
   a. Assess pain and document.
   b. Utilize analgesics, transcutaneous nerve stimulator, relaxation therapy, or other appropriate nursing interventions prior to exercise periods.
4. Increase activity tolerance and endurance.
   a. Collaborate with physical and occupational therapists to plan for exercises requiring gradually increasing energy levels.
   b. Plan daily activities to maximize energy required for specific treatments in which patient must actively participate.
   c. Plan care to provide rest period during day and 8 hours sleep during night.
5. Foster healing of remaining wounds.
   a. Continue topical therapy and dressings as prescribed after daily wound cleansing.
   b. Protect newly healed skin from trauma or pressure.

c. Keep fingernails cut short.
   d. Promote high-protein, high-calorie diet.
6. Promote full range of joint motion.
   a. Encourage patient to follow exercise schedule planned by physical therapist.
   b. Apply splints as prescribed to reduce contractures.
   c. Administer analgesics if required prior to major physical therapy treatments.
   d. Utilize creative approaches to encourage patient to move joints in activities of daily living and self-care activities.
7. Educate patient and family or significant others for the required posthospital care.
   a. Teach care of wounds and plan for a return demonstration.
   b. Teach use of splints and pressure garments.
   c. Demonstrate exercises.
   d. Emphasize importance of high-protein diet.
   e. Teach importance of protection of healed wounds from sunlight, pressure, and trauma.
   f. Teach importance of skin lubrication.
   g. Review expected activity and emotional behaviors postdischarge.
   h. Provide a list of resources or referral agencies and people if specific problems arise.
   i. Provide written instruction on all of the above.
8. Prevent hypertrophic scarring.
   a. Apply elastic bandages or pressure garments over healed areas prone to scarring.
   b. Instruct patient in proper use and care of elastic garments for optimal results.
9. Reduce depressed affect.
   a. Employ concepts of psychiatric nursing to explore and improve depressed affect.
   b. Help patient employ short-term goals and a "one day at a time" philosophy.
   c. Recognize need for grieving over losses.
   d. Have patient talk with other patients who are making good progress after similar injury.
   e. Obtain psychiatric consultation and administer prescribed mood elevators if depression lasts abnormally long.
   f. Explain that depression is a normal sequela of major trauma, but is relieved with general improvement in health.

Evaluation

Expected Outcomes

1. Achieves emotional and physical independence
   a. Participates fully in activities of daily living
   b. Is equipped with and knowledgeable in use of prostheses or assistive devices

(continued)

Chart 53-4
Guidelines of Nursing Implementation for the Patient With Thermal Injury—Stage III (continued)

Evaluation (continued)

Expected Outcomes (continued)

    c. Verbalizes realistic view of self and plans for the future
    d. Reports ability to participate in family, social, and vocational spheres

2. Exhibits soft, comfortable, lubricated skin
    a. Demonstrates no evidence of scratching of skin
    b. Is able to sleep without being disturbed by itching
    c. Reports minimal or no itching
    d. Skin feels soft and smooth
    e. Demonstrates no scales, dryness

3. Exhibits no pain
    a. Requests no analgesics
    b. Reports no pain on exercise
    c. Is able to sleep without being disturbed by pain

4. Achieves activity tolerance and endurance consistent with desired levels
    a. Participates in activities of daily living as desired
    b. Has stamina required for usual activities

5. Exhibits intact skin with normal coloration
    a. Shows all wounds completely healed
    b. Has skin free of infection, signs of pressure, or trauma
    c. Exhibits pigmentation near normal preburn color

6. Obtains optimal joint mobility
    Has normal range of motion in all joints

7. Is knowledgeable in required self-care and follow-up
    a. Verbalizes plan for follow-up care
    b. Demonstrates ability to do wound care and exercises
    c. Returns for clinic and physical therapy appointments as scheduled
    d. Lists resource people and agencies to contact for specific problems

8. Achieves optimal cosmetic results
    a. Adapts to and accepts appearance
    b. Utilizes cosmetics, wigs, prostheses as desired to achieve acceptable appearance
    c. Has met plastic surgery goals

9. Returns to preburn level or better level of social and vocational functioning
    a. Socializes with significant others, peers, usual social group
    b. Is able to seek and gain employment or return to role in school or community as contributing member of the group
    c. Has adapted to and resolved grief over losses resulting from burn injury and circumstances surrounding the injury (*i.e.*, death of others involved; damage to house, other property)
    d. Has hopeful attitude toward the future

6. Demonstrates range of joint motion that approaches preburn range
7. Verbalizes understanding of treatments and surgical procedures and participates appropriately in care
8. Is free of complications

The Rehabilitation Phase—Stage III

The burn wound is in a dynamic state for a year or more after wound closure. During this time, aggressive efforts must be made to prevent contracture and hypertrophic scarring of the wound area. A program including elastic pressure garments, splints, and exercise under the supervision of an experienced physiatrist and physical and occupational therapy team is recommended for optimal functional and cosmetic results. As the in-patient phase of burn recovery gets shorter and shorter, much of the rehabilitation of the burn patient takes place on an outpatient basis or in a rehabilitation center.

In the aftermath of the acute stages of illness, the burn victim now increasingly focuses on the changes in his self-image and the alterations in his life-style that may be required. Reconstructive surgery to improve cosmetic and functional results may be required. Counseling, both psychological and vocational, may be valuable. Significant others will also need support and guidance in assisting the patient in returning to optimal health.

Follow-up care planned by a surgeon, physiatrist, or, optimally, the entire burn team will be necessary. In the case of children, such follow-up care is needed for many years. Preparations for this reality should begin during the earlier stages of care. It is a great challenge to the health care team to prepare an individual for independent functioning after such a major traumatic event in his life.

▶ **Assessment**
Clinical Manifestations.   During the rehabilitation phase, the patient may be aware of unusual sensations, numbness, tingling, tightness, itching, heat sensitivity, and fatigue. Though such sensations are to be expected, they may be annoying. It helps to assure the patient that these feelings are not disabling and will subside with time. Before the patient is discharged, he and his family must be instructed in the care of small, unhealed wounds; the general care of healed areas; and the method of carrying out the exercise and splinting program. The patient is encouraged to think about returning to work, school, and normal activities.

Psychosocial rehabilitation is addressed as a continuing process. Adjustments have to be made, and bouts of depression and hostility need to be expressed by the patient, but patience, firmness, and goal-setting must be continually practiced by the nursing staff and those on the rehabilitation team. Well-planned family conferences are most effective in addressing problems of the patient prior to discharge from the hospital.

A possible complication that may occur a few weeks after a burn is the formation of heterotopic bone (a development of calcium deposits near tendons around joints). An early manifestation of beginning ossification is loss of joint function. Laboratory tests that may indicate such calcification are elevated alkaline phosphatase and decreased serum calcium. When x-ray confirms the presence of bone formation, and new formation appears to be halted, surgery may be performed. This is usually not sooner than 6 months after the initial burn injury. Afterward, splinting, hydrotherapy, and exercise may be required to regain functional activity of the part.

Patient Problems/Nursing Diagnoses

The major nursing problems presented during the final stage of recovery from burn injury include reducing emotional and physical dependence on the health team; skin tightness and dryness; itching of healing wounds; pain on exercise; low level of activity tolerance and endurance; small, open wounds and flexion contractures; lack of knowledge of patient and family concerning required care postdischarge; hypertrophic scarring; and depression.

▶ Planning and Nursing Implementation

Goals

The major goals for the patient during rehabilitation include:

1. Emotional and physical independence
2. Optimal mobility of all areas
3. Optimal cosmetic results
4. Ability to resume desired level of social functioning
5. Ability to resume desired vocation
6. Intact skin
7. Knowledge of self-care postdischarge
8. Participation in planned follow-up care
9. Relief of pain and itching

Rehabilitation

The objective of rehabilitation is to return the patient to a productive place in society with the best possible emotional, cosmetic, and functional results. Emotional support is given throughout the postburn period. When passive exercises followed by active exercises are initiated, a team approach ensures that the nurse and the physical and occupational therapists are working toward the same goals.

Rehabilitative efforts may be concentrated in a particular division of the hospital. The patient is transferred to this unit when he is able to assume more and more responsibility for his own care. This is done gradually with continual daily assessment of his progress.

Table 53-6
Water and Electrolyte Changes in Later Stage II

Observation	Explanation
1. Calcium deficit	Since calcium may be immobilized at the burn site in the slough and early granulation phase of burns, symptoms of calcium deficit may occur rarely
2. Potassium deficit	Extracellular K^+ moves into the cells, leaving a deficit of K^+ in the extracellular fluid
3. Negative nitrogen balance (present for several weeks following burns)	Secondary to: Stress reaction Immobilization Inadequate protein intake Protein losses in exudate Direct destruction of protein at burn site
4. Sodium deficit	

(Adapted from Metheny NM and Snively WD: Nurses' Handbook of Fluid Balance. Philadelphia, JB Lippincott.)

Dressings continue to need changing, and special attention is given to healed areas, since tissue is tender at this stage. Padding is applied to areas that may be injured easily. Lubricating cream or lotion is applied to soften crusts.

Splints or functional devices may be applied to extremities for contracture control. The principles of care described on page 230 are applicable to prevent damage to nerves and blood vessels.

At this stage of recovery, attempts are made to establish positive nitrogen balance or anabolism to promote healing (Table 53-6). Such a balance is achieved with a high-calorie, high-protein diet. Activities of daily living and principles of rehabilitation outlined in Chapter 14 are pursued. If reconstructive surgery is required, principles presented on pages 1188–1189 are applicable.

▷ Bibliography
Books

Artz CP, Moncrief JA, and Pruitt BA. Burns: A Team Approach. Philadelphia, WB Saunders, 1979.

Bowden ML, Jones CA, and Feller I. Psycho-Social Aspects of a Severe Burn: A Review of the Literature. Ann Arbor, National Institute for Burn Medicine, 1979.

Braen GR. Minor Burns. Evaluation and Treatment. American College of Emergency Physicians. Kansas City, Marion Laboratories, 1979.

Feller I and Grabb VC. Reconstruction and Rehabilitation of the Burned Patient. Ann Arbor, National Institute for Burn Medicine, 1981.

Hummel RP Jr. Burn Therapy. Littleton, Massachusetts, PSG, 1981.

Johnson CL, O'Shaughnessy EJ, and Ostergren G. Burn Management. New York, Raven Press, 1981.

MacMillan B. Surgical and Medical Support for Burn Patients. Littleton, Massachusetts, PSG, 1981.

Wagner MM (ed). Care of the Burn-Injured Patient. Littleton, Massachusetts, PSG, 1981.

Articles*

Acres C and Kraft ER. Skin transplantation. Am J Nurs 1981 Aug; 81(8):1466–1467.

Andressen MJC et al. Management of emotional reactions in seriously burned adults. N Engl J Med 1979 Jan 13; 286(2):65–69.

Archambeault–Jones C and Feller I. Burn nursing is nursing. Crit Care Q 1978 Dec; 1(3):77–92.

Bayley EW and Moore DA. Group meetings for families of burn victims. Top Clin Nurs 1980 July; 2(2):67–76.

Brandenburg J. Inhalation injury; Carbon monoxide poisoning. Am J Nurs 1980 Jan; 80(1):98–100.

Christopher KL. The use of a model for hemodynamic balance to describe burn shock. Nurs Clin North Am 1980 Sept; 15(3):617–627.

Dolph JL et al. Amnion; A useful biological dressing. Contemp Surg 1980 Aug; 17(2):65–66.

Gaston SF and Schumann LL. Inhalation injury: Smoke inhalation. Am J Nurs 1980 Jan; 80(1):94–97.

Kinzie V. What to do for the severely burned. RN 1980 Apr; 43(4):47–51, 104–110.

Labson LH. Burn therapy—Here's my idea of best burn care. Patient Care 1981 Oct 15; 15(17):12–83.

MacMillan BG. Closing the burn wound. Surg Clin North Am 1978 Dec; 58(6):1205–1231.

Oss SV. Emergency burn care. RN 1981 Oct; 42(10):44–49.

Pierson CL. Infection control in burn care facilities. Crit Care Q 1981 Dec; 3(4):81–92.

Proceedings of the NIH Consensus Development Conference in Supportive Therapy in Burn Care. J Trauma (Suppl) 1979 Nov; 19(11):entire issue.

Pruit BA and McManus WF. Surgical management of burns. Contemp Surg 1980 May; 16(5):11–16.

Psychiatric nurse works with burn patients. Am J Nurs 1980 Jan; 80(1):124–125.

Second Conference on Supportive Therapy in Burn Care. J Trauma (Suppl) 1981 Aug; 21(8):entire issue.

Severely burned patients: Anticipating their emotional needs. Nursing '80 1980 Sept; 10(9):47–50.

Specific Optimal Criteria for Hospital Resources for Care of Patients with Burn Injury. Am Burn Assoc 1976 Apr (leaflet).

Wagner MM. Emergency care of the burned patient. Am J Nurs 1977 Nov; 77(11):1788–1791.

Wooldridge M and Surveyor JA. Skin grafting for full-thickness burn injury. Am J Nurs 1980 Nov; 80(11):2000–2004.

* Note: Also see all issues of *Journal of Burn Care and Rehabilitation.*

Unit XV

Sensorineural Problems

54

Assessment and Management of Patients With Vision Problems and Eye Disorders

▷ Physiologic Overview

The eyeball is a spherical organ situated in a bony cavity called the *orbit*. It is rotated easily in all the necessary directions by six muscles attached to its outer surface (Fig. 54-1); these muscles act in a manner similar to the reins on a team of horses. Four of the muscles are located on each side of the eye and on the top and the bottom of the eye. Each of these four muscles, the *rectus* muscles, leads back to the apex of the orbit and turns the eye in or out, up or down. The other two muscles of the eye, the *oblique* muscles, run from the globe toward the medial wall of the orbit.

For the purpose of study, the eyeball may be divided into three coats or tunics. The dense, white, fibrous outer coat is called the *sclera*. Anteriorly, the sclera becomes continuous with the *cornea*, the translucent structure that bulges forward slightly from the general contour of the eye. Posteriorly, the sclera has an opening through which the optic nerve passes into the eyeball. The nerve spreads out over the posterior two thirds of the inner surface of the globe in a thin layer called the *retina*. In it are situated the tiny nerve endings, which, when properly stimulated, transmit visual impulses to the brain that are interpreted as sight.

Between the sclera and the retina is the pigmented middle coat known as the *uveal tract*. This tract is composed of three parts. The posterior part, the *choroid*, contains most of the blood vessels that nourish the eye. The anterior part is a pigmented muscular structure, the *iris*, which gives the characteristic color to the eye (blue, brown, and so forth). The circular opening at its center, the *pupil*, dilates or contracts according to the intensity of light. These reactions are controlled by two sets of muscle fibers. Contraction of the circular fibers constricts the pupil; the radial fibers enlarge it. Between the iris and the choroid is the third portion of the uveal tract, a muscular body known as the *ciliary body*. It is composed of radial processes arising from a triangular-shaped muscle (ciliary muscle). Between these processes, and to them, are attached delicate ligaments that pass cen-

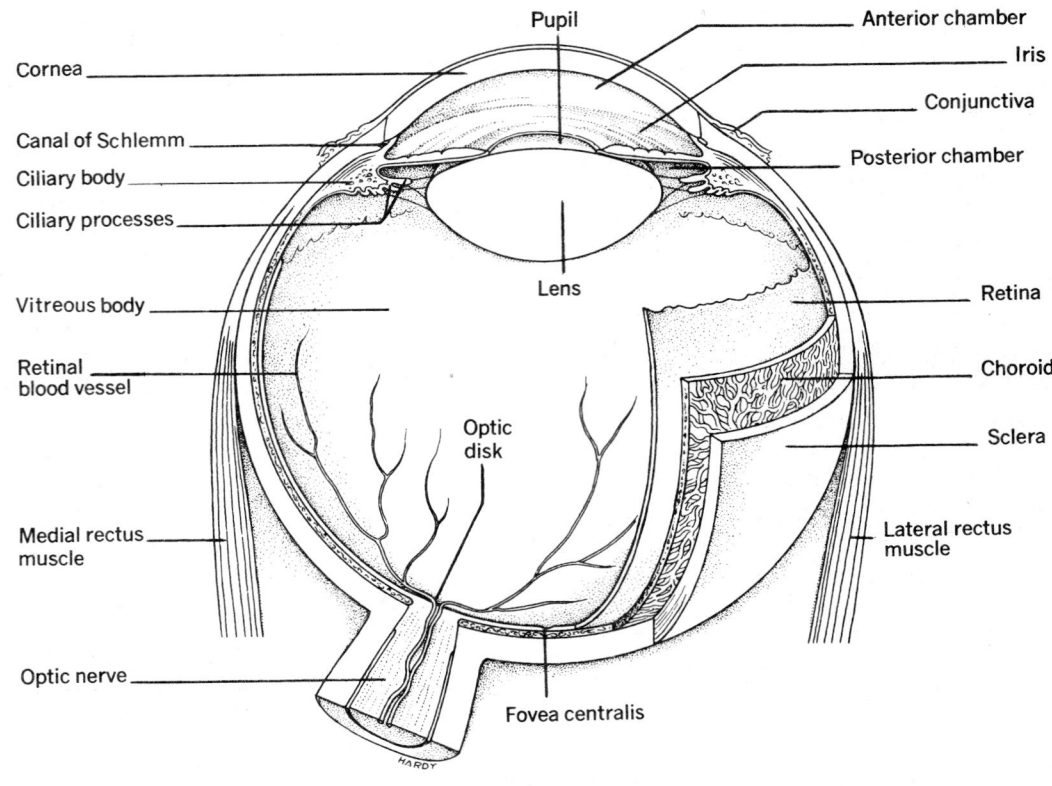

Figure 54-1.   Transverse section of eye. (From Chaffee EE and Greisheimer EM: Basic Physiology and Anatomy. Philadelphia, JB Lippincott.)

trally and become inserted in the capsule of the crystalline lens.

The *lens* is a semisolid body enclosed in a transparent elastic capsule. It is capable of being modified to varying degrees of convexity by the contraction and the relaxation of the ciliary muscle, thus changing the focus of the eye as it looks from one object to another.

The cavity within the eye is divided by the lens into two parts. The posterior part contains a jellylike, translucent substance called the *vitreous humor,* which is the chief factor in maintaining the form of the eyeball. The anterior part contains a clear, watery fluid, the *aqueous humor,* which is secreted by the ciliary processes. It bathes the anterior surface of the lens, escapes at the pupil, and enters the space between the iris and the cornea, known as the *anterior chamber.* Finally, it is drained from the eye through lymph channels (the canal of Schlemm) located at the junction of the iris and the sclera.

Appendages.   The *eyelids* are the protective coverings of the eye. Lining the lids and entirely covering the anterior part of the eye is a highly sensitive membrane, the *conjunctiva,* the surface of which is kept moist by a constant flow of lacrimal fluid tears. This fluid is excreted from the *lacrimal gland,* which is located in the upper and outer part of the orbit. It flows downward and inward across the eye and drains into tiny channels (lacrimal puncta). These channels conduct the fluid to the lacrimal sac and duct, which pass downward, and outward and open into the nasal cavity beneath the inferior turbinate bone.

▷ Eye Care Specialists

The importance of adequate eye examinations cannot be emphasized too strongly. Too often we find patients using a pair of glasses that belonged to a relative or was purchased at the local variety store.

The care of the eye is undertaken by four groups of specialists:

1. The *oculist,* the *ophthalmologist,* or the *ophthalmic physician* is a medical doctor who is skilled in the treatment of all conditions and diseases of the eye. Training and experience enable this physician to make a more thorough and complete examination of the eye for refractive errors and other changes.
2. The *optician* is not a physician, but is concerned with grinding, mounting, and dispensing lenses.
3. The *optometrist* is licensed to examine the eyes and related structures to determine the presence of vision problems, eye diseases, or other abnormalities, and to prescribe and adapt lenses or other optical aids.
4. The *ocularist* is a technician who makes artificial eyes and other prostheses used in ophthalmology.

▷ Assessment of Vision

(See also Chap. 5, Physical Assessment, pp. 58–62.)

Letter Chart/Microprocessor

The most widely accepted method of screening for visual problems is the *letter chart* (Snellen). However, its accuracy is limited. Other devices are available, including a BVAT microprocessor, echography, and endothelial cell counter. In automated visual acuity testing, a *BVAT (Mentor) microprocessor* produces an E of 30 different sizes on a television monitor. A computer monitors the responses the patient makes with a hand-held response box. A computer printout provides the mean visual acuity and standard deviation computed from 20 trials. The time required is about 8 minutes.

Echography

In *echography* (ultrasound, ultrasonography), high-frequency pulses of ultrasound are emitted from a small probe placed on the eye. After striking the ocular tissues, the sound energy is reflected to the probe, which, in turn, is displayed on an oscilloscope. Two primary types of ultrasound are used in ophthalmology:

A-scan—Oscilloscopic reflection is a vertical deflection from the baseline (one-dimensional).

B-scan—Oscilloscopic reflections are lines or dots (two-dimensional).

When used jointly, over 100 lesions or groups of lesions may be detected and differentiated in the orbital and periorbital region. Measurements for intraocular lenses can be done by ultrasound and analyzed by computer; this enables the surgeon to determine lens power for an implant and postoperative refractive power.

This procedure is painless but requires the instillation of topical anesthetic eyedrops. After the examination, the patient is cautioned not to rub his eyes, since corneal lesions may occur.

Endothelial Cell Counter

An *endothelial cell counter* is a photographic instrument that produces very high resolution, revealing subtle details of endothelial cell morphology: cell size, shape, cell population density, nature of cell boundary, and presence of intercellular bodies and pathology. This is a valuable test preoperatively, because if a compromised endothelium is observed, it may suggest an increased risk of postoperative complications.

Refractive Errors

Vision is made possible by the passage of rays of light from an object through the cornea, the aqueous humor, the lens, and the vitreous humor to the retina. In the normal eye, rays coming from an object at a distance of 6 meters or more are brought to a focus on the retina by the lens while perfectly at rest.

Due to abnormalities in the eye structure or in the lens structure, defective vision may occur because objects are not focused correctly on the retina. If the rays of light are brought to a focus in front of the retina, the condition is spoken of as *myopia* (nearsightedness); if the rays are focused behind the retina, the condition is called *hyperopia* (farsightedness). In such conditions, glass lenses are prescribed. These, in association with the lenses of the eye, will correct the fault and restore a normal focus at the retina.

Rays from objects situated at shorter distances (less than 6 meters) require a "stronger" lens to focus them on the retina. This is brought about by a contraction of the ciliary muscle that relaxes the lens capsule and causes the lens to become more convex. This function is called *accommodation*. By means of accommodation, objects at different distances from the eye may be seen distinctly. With increasing age, the elasticity of the lens decreases, so that accommodation for near vision is not complete, a condition called *presbyopia*. This explains why it is so common to see older people reading a paper while holding it at arm's length. "Reading glasses" may be prescribed for these patients to enable them to focus rays from near objects to the retina.

In the case of presbyopia, two different types of lenses may be used (bifocals), one for far distance and one for near vision and reading. Trifocal lenses are also available; these add a third dimension that gives sharp focus in the 68-cm to 127-cm (27-inch to 50-inch) range. Lenses are prescribed for use in eyeglasses, or the lens may be applied directly to the surface of the eye (contact lens).

Astigmatism results from uneven curvature of the cornea—instead of curving equally in all directions, the cornea is shaped somewhat like the bowl of a spoon. Two foci thus occur instead of one, and, as a consequence, the patient is unable to focus horizontal and vertical rays on the retina at the same time. These defects may be corrected with lenses called cylinder lenses. A patient may be myopic or hyperopic and also have astigmatism. In such a situation, a compound spherocylinder lens is prescribed by the optician.

The strength and type of lens that will overcome refractive errors are determined by means of a *retinoscope*, which measures the refractive error. On the basis of this examination, an appropriate corrective lens is selected and then further refined by having the patient read letters on the Snellen chart through several different lenses.

Automated refractors, which rely on photoelectric devices sensitive to light, may also be used. The patient sits in front of the instrument and is instructed to look steadily at a target. A printout on a card or graph indicates the refractive error to be corrected. Other types of automated refractors require the patient to make focusing adjustments by turning a knob. Such equipment is expensive, and although many can be operated by technicians, they need further evaluation to justify their replacing conventional refraction methods. (See Chart 54-1.)

Contact Lenses

More and more people are wearing contact lenses as a means of correcting refractive errors. Better techniques for measuring the eye and improved methods for supervising and instructing those who wish to wear the lenses have increased the appeal of such lenses. They are particularly effective in certain occupations and are desirable for cosmetic reasons. However, not everyone can wear contact lenses; therefore,

Chart 54-1
Abbreviations and Terms Used in Ophthalmology

OD or RE (*oculus dexter*)—right eye
OS or LE (*oculus sinister*)—left eye
OU or O₂ (*oculi uterque*)—both eyes together
D (diopter)—unit of measurement of strength or refractive
        power of lenses. (A 1-diopter lens brings parallel light
        rays to a focus at 1 meter from the lens.)
EOM—extraocular muscles
H (hyperopia, hypermetropia)—farsightedness
HT (hypertropia)—upward deviation of one eye
ST (esotropia)—inward deviation of one eye
XT (exotropia)—outward deviation of one eye
+—plus or convex
−—minus or concave
Diplopia—seeing one object as two ("double vision")
Ectropion—turning out (eversion) of eyelid
Entropion—turning in of eyelid
Ptosis—drooping of upper lid
Epiphora—excessive production of tears
Hemianopia—blindness of one half the field of vision
Photophobia—abnormal sensitivity to light
Presbyopia—lessening of power of accommodation due to
        aging process

all potential candidates should be thoroughly screened by an ophthalmologist.

Medical conditions in which corneal lenses are recommended include absence of lens (aphakia), absence of iris (aniridia), congenital absence of pigment, myopia and hyperopia, some types of astigmatism, cone-shaped deformity of the cornea (keratoconus), and turned-in eyelashes. Contraindications include allergic and inflammatory conditions (such as chronic blepharoconjunctivitis, corneal infection, iritis, uveitis), epiphora (abnormal overflow of tears), severe exophthalmus, pterygium, or local neoplasm.

Contact lenses are usually not recommended for people who do not require full-time visual correction or lack sufficient manual dexterity to insert and remove lenses. Contact lenses are available in either hard or soft form. The hard lens was introduced in the early 1960s, the soft lens in the late 1960s. The most recent innovation has been a lens made of silicone rubber.

Hard Contact Lenses.   The corneal lens is made of lightweight, paper-thin polymethylmethacrylate and is about 10 mm or less in diameter. When properly fitted, contact lenses "float" on the fluid layer of the eyeball and are held loosely in place by the capillary attraction of the tears and the upper lid. The lens moves with the eye and is centered over the cornea.

Hard contact lenses have many advantages over framed lenses: they do not steam up when the wearer goes from the cold outside to a warm room; they are automatically cleaned with each blink of the eyelid; they can be worn

safely during sports; they eliminate the need for less attractive lenses; they provide increased peripheral vision; and they do not break easily.

However, there are certain disadvantages and dangers in wearing contact lenses: contact lenses are more expensive than framed lenses; solutions used to clean the lenses are costly; the adjustment period in learning to use them properly is longer; contact lenses can be lost easily, such as down the sink drain or in a swimming pool; and in the event of a chemical splash to the eye, the chemical agent may seep beneath the lens to cause extensive damage before the contact lens can be removed.

Soft Contact Lenses.   Soft contact lenses are made of polymer gel, although new formulations are being tested as soft lenses grow in popularity. They are brittle when dehydrated, but when immersed in saline or impregnated with tears, they absorb water and become flexible.

When fitting hard lenses, the ophthalmologist usually instills fluorescein into the eye in order to identify changes that occur in the formation of tear film as the lid blinks. However, fluorescein cannot be used with soft lenses because the dye stains the lenses permanently. To offset microbial contamination, special procedures are used to disinfect soft lenses while they are stored during the night.

Soft lenses have certain advantages over hard lenses. They are comfortable from the start and can be worn up to 18 hours a day. They are less easily displaced during wearing than hard lenses and therefore are less likely to drop from the eye. They appear to be superior to hard lenses for those who participate in sports, except for swimming. Since these lenses absorb pool chemicals and ocean salt, they should not be worn while swimming unless goggles and a mask are used. If they are worn only occasionally, rather than daily, the wearer will not lose his tolerance to them, as is the case with hard lenses. Finally, it is easier to switch from soft lenses to eyeglasses than from hard lenses to eyeglasses.

Soft lenses are inserted by placing the lens on the inferior conjunctiva while drawing the lower lid downward. With the release of the lid, the wearer then rolls his eye around or massages the eye through the closed lid to position the lens on the cornea. To remove, the lens is grasped between the clean thumb and forefinger.

Extended-Wear Contact Lenses.   These highly permeable plastic lenses are thinner and more pliable than ordinary soft or hard contact lenses and can be worn continuously for weeks or months. They are more expensive than the usual soft contact lenses and are not completely trouble-free. Extra fitting time is necessary. In addition, other conditions may develop that may require discontinuing their use: microprotein accumulation on the anterior lens surface (soft lens spoilage) and corneal revascularization.

Spoilage or deterioration of soft contact lenses is due to extraneous deposits, physical and chemical changes in the lens material, and microbial invasion. This includes soft lens of acrylic origin, vinyl origin, and silicone. Removal of encrusted deposits leaves surface irregularities and matrix defects; these lenses should be discarded. At present, no soft contact lenses are completely "safe" for extended wear.

Complications.   The improper use of contact lenses (both hard and soft) can cause corneal abrasions and ulcerations, which result from poorly fitted lenses, improper

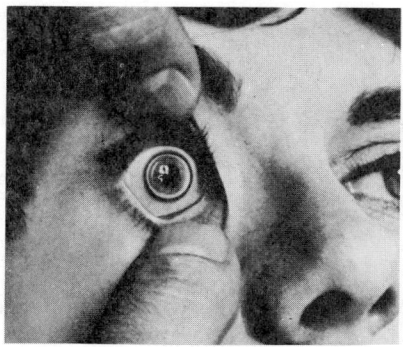 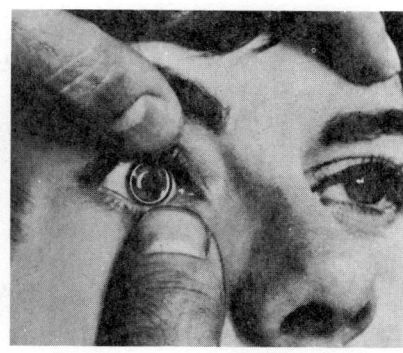 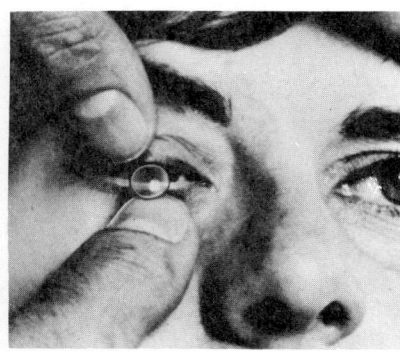

(A) After the eyelids have been separated and the corneal contact lens has been correctly positioned over the cornea, you widen the eyelid margins beyond the top and bottom edges of lens (as shown).

(B) After the lower eyelid margin has been moved near the edge of the bottom of the lens and then the upper eyelid margin has been moved near the edge of the top of the lens, you are ready to move under the bottom edge of the lens by pressing slightly harder on the lower eyelid while moving it upward.

(C) After the lens has tipped slightly, you move the eyelids toward one another and thereby cause the lens to slide out between the eyelids (as shown).

Figure 54-2. Emergency removal of hard contact lenses. (Reprinted with permission of the American Optometric Association.)

technique in applying or removing the lenses, and insufficient tear circulation under the lenses.

Patient Education

Although the advantages outweigh the disadvantages, precautions and safeguards must be understood by the nurse, the wearer, and his employer. The contact lens must be regarded as a medical prosthesis, not a cosmetic device.

Care and precaution must be given to any medical prosthesis and certainly with contact lenses:

1. Wash hands thoroughly before touching the lenses, whether applying them or removing them.
2. Cleanse lenses only with the recommended sterile solution (noncaustic).*
3. Keep the storage kit clean.
4. Do not wear lenses beyond the prescribed time.
5. Do not sleep with contact lenses in place; to do so may cause abrasion and erosion of the corneal epithelium.
6. Do not wet lenses with saliva before insertion; this can cause infection.
7. Restrict the wearing of contact lenses, in order to avoid potential corneal abrasions, if the following signs are present: photophobia, dryness, excessive burning, tearing.
8. Follow the physician's recommendations concerning eye makeup. Some ophthalmologists discourage patients from wearing eye makeup. Some advise applying mascara after lenses are in position.
9. Keep chemicals such as soaps, lotions, and creams away from lenses, since they may adversely affect the lens;

* Some individuals are sensitive to thimerosal, a preservative in cleaning solutions that causes the eyes to sting when the lenses are inserted. Recommendation: Soak lenses in distilled water OR use Pliagel (USA), a thimerosal-free solution, or Solusol (Canada).

instruct the wearer to keep his eyes tightly closed when applying hair perfume and deodorant sprays. Stay away from areas where household sprays are used.
10. Have an ophthalmologic examination every 6 months to ensure proper fit and to check corneal integrity.

Emergency Removal of Contact Lenses

Contact lenses are designed to be worn only while the person is awake and fully conscious (exception: extended-wear lenses). They should be removed as a safety measure if the wearer is incapacitated due to accident, sickness, or other cause. In emergency situations, the following directives should be followed:

1. Determine whether or not the patient is wearing contact lenses. If he is conscious or semiconscious, ask him directly, since he may be able to indicate that he is wearing contact lenses. He may even be able to remove the lenses by himself or with assistance, depending, of course, on his condition. If the patient is unconscious, check "Medic-Alert" tag (bracelet, necklace, keychain, etc.), driver's license, and other identification cards that may reveal that the patient wears contact lenses. Look for observable indications that contact lenses are being worn by gently separating the patient's eyelids. Shining a light—preferably a small penlight—on the eye from the side will help.
2. Remove the patient's contact lenses if he cannot do so himself. With clean hands, position one thumb on the upper eyelid and one thumb on the lower eyelid, with thumbs near the margin of each eyelid. Separate the eyelids. A visible lens should slide easily with a gentle movement of the eyelids (Fig. 54-2). If the lens does not drop out easily, observe for possible lens position and follow instructions given in Figure 54-3 for removal

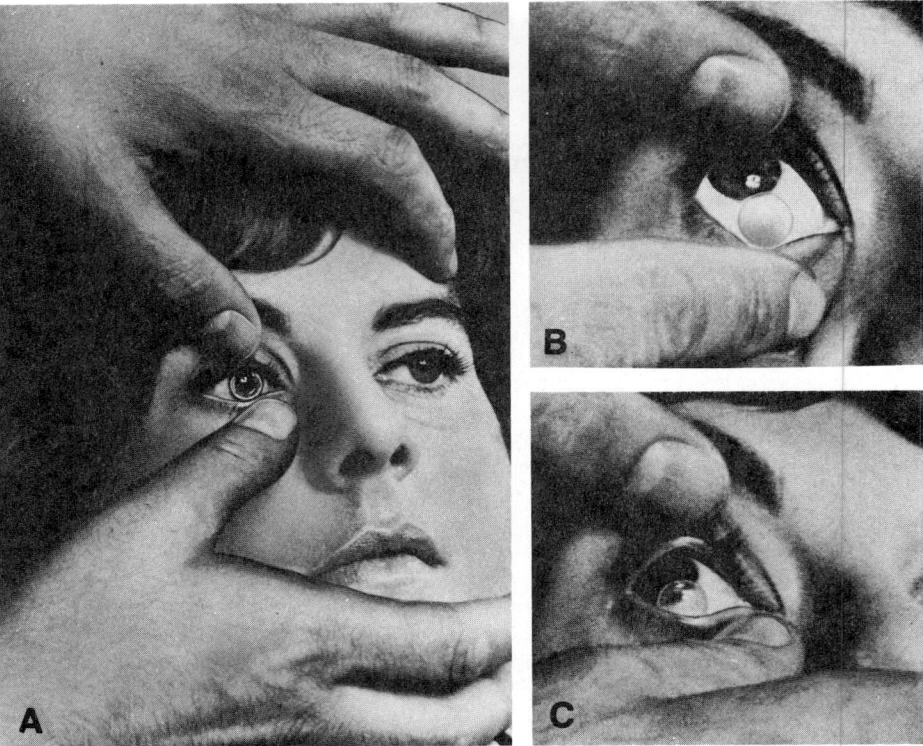

Figure 54-3. Emergency removal of hard contact lens, which is (*A*) in normal position, (*B*) on the sclera, or (*C*) on both the cornea and the sclera. (Reprinted with permission of the American Optometric Association.)

of the lens. Remember that force should not be used. If the lens is seen but cannot be removed, gently slide it onto the sclera, where it can remain with relative safety until experienced help is available.

If the patient is wearing soft contact lenses, it is best to wait until someone experienced in removing these types of lenses is available to lend assistance. If flexible lenses are left in place for many hours, they will do little harm. However, if the emergency is such that they must be removed, then the steps described in Figure 54-4 should be followed.

▷ General Management of Patients With Eye Disorders

It is well to remember that a patient with an eye problem may have other problems as well. Often other physical conditions are primary and affect the eye as a consequence. The appearance of the eye can alert the patient, the nurse, and the physician to difficulties or some disturbances in other parts of the body even before other symptoms present themselves. The mental anxiety frequently experienced by the ophthalmic patient requires as much consideration as his physical condition.

Psychosocial Consideration

One's dependence on sight is emphasized when one faces a temporary or possible permanent loss of this vital sense. Worry, fear, and depression are common reactions in addition to tension, resentment, anger, and rejection. By encouraging the patient to express his feelings, the nurse may discover the basic problems involved and can then take steps to alleviate them.

Sensory Deprivation.   Many patients with eye disorders face unusual problems resulting from loss of sight. Such is the case of the postoperative patient whose eyes are bandaged and who suffers distortions in perception, such as "eye-patch delirium," inappropriate behavior, loss of position sense in bed, and a sensation of floating. Often these problems are magnified and become frightening and upsetting. One way to assist the patient in overcoming these unsettling feelings is to reorient him constantly to reality and offer reassurance, explanations, and understanding.

Other helpful approaches may be followed: Anyone entering the patient's room should speak and identify himself so as not to startle the patient. If the patient is bothered by the restraint on his movements more than by an eye patch, a soothing back rub may offer relaxation.

When permissible, the radio and occupational therapy may be used to keep the patient's mind occupied. While it is important not to be oversolicitous, showing interest, empathy, and understanding enhances the patient's sense of well-being. Because of differences of personality, the approaches in overcoming the anxiety of individual patients vary. When permanent blindness is apparent, re-education may be done by specially trained personnel or similarly afflicted persons.

Daily Care

The daily care of ophthalmic patients should be the same as for other patients. The patient is encouraged to carry out as much self-care as possible in order to promote a feeling

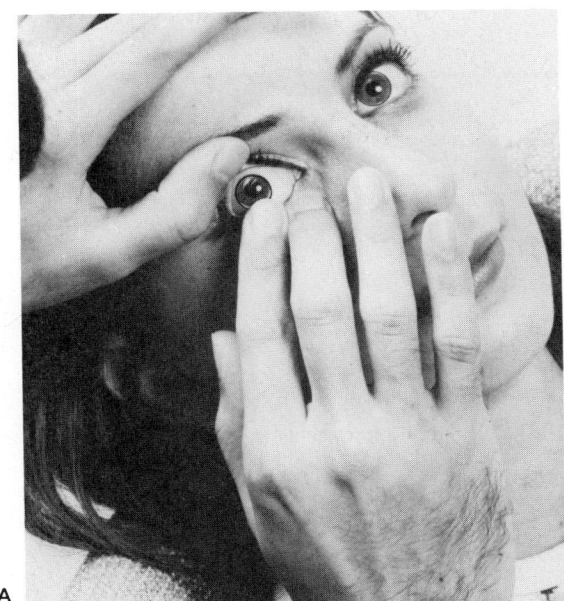
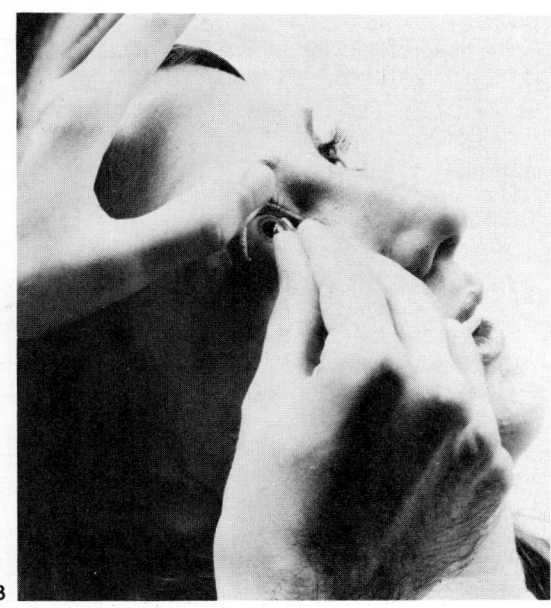

Figure 54-4. Removal of soft contact lens. 1. With clean hands, pull down the lower lid with the middle finger and place the index fingertip on the lower edge of the lens (*A*). 2. Slide the lens down to the white part of the eye. 3. Compress the lens lightly between the thumb and index finger. 4. Bring thumb and index finger together in a "pinching" motion, causing the lens to double up between fingers, allowing air underneath (*B*). 5. Remove the lens from the eye. CAUTION: Inadequate tearing caused by severe injury or shock may cause the lens to adhere to the eye. If the lens resists removal, flush the eye with normal saline solution, wait several minutes, then follow the above five steps for removal. (Reprinted with permission of the American Optometric Association.)

of self-sufficiency. Nursing assistance is given as needed. A patient who cannot see is assisted with eating, but if he is accustomed to feeding himself, he is encouraged to do so. Proper elimination is promoted by proper diet, stool softeners, or enemas, as prescribed. Ambulatory patients are to have a daily rest period in the afternoon. Ophthalmic patients are not to read, smoke, or shave unless given permission by the physician. They must be cautioned against rubbing their eyes or wiping them with a soiled handkerchief. All patients receiving atropine should wear dark glasses.

Reduction of Light. Because light causes pain in many conditions of the eye, and because the eyes should be rested as much as possible before and after undergoing an operation, it is best to maintain subdued lighting in the room. If those assisting the patient need light to carry out their duties, then dimmed artificial lights may be used.

Eyedrops

Various drug solutions are inserted into the eyes in the treatment of nearly every kind of eye disorder (Table 54-1).

Before drops are instilled, it is important to see that the correct drug is being given. Some drugs (*e.g.,* miotics and mydriatics) act in exactly opposite ways (Fig. 54-5, p. 1239). Therefore, if one of these drugs is indicated in the treatment of a certain eye disease, the other is contraindicated. It may seem needless to emphasize this warning, but experience has taught how easy it is to pick up the wrong bottle from a tray containing similar vials when the room is dimly lighted.

In addition, the solution should be checked for color changes or sedimentation, which indicates that the solution

is decomposing. If this is so, the solution should be discarded and a fresh one prescribed and sterilized for use. Patients especially are warned to avoid using medication of any kind if it has been in the medicine cabinet at home for months or years. Of course, the use of small, sterile, disposable containers has helped reduce this problem and has also eliminated the need for a separate dropper.

Instillation.   Before the medication is instilled into the eyes (Fig. 54-6*A,* p. 1239), the lids and the lashes are cleansed. Then the head of the patient is tilted backward and inclined slightly to the side, so that the solution will run away from the tear duct. This latter precaution is especially necessary when toxic solutions, such as atropine, are employed, because absorption of the excess drug by way of the nose and the pharynx may lead to toxic symptoms. In most patients, it is well to press the inner angle of the eye after instilling the drops to prevent the excess solution from entering the nose.

- The lower lid is depressed with the fingers of the left hand, the patient is told to look upward, and the solution is dropped on the everted lower lid.
- *Care must be taken that the pipette does not touch any part of the eye or the lids to guard against contamination of the dropper and injury to the eye.*
- After the drops (one or two at most) are placed in the eye, the lid is released, and any excess fluid is sponged gently from the lids and the cheeks with sterile cotton.
- After the medication is instilled, the patient is instructed to close his eyes gently; patients often have a tendency

(*Text continues on page 1238*)

Table 54-1
Medications Used Frequently in Eye Conditions

Medication	Action
Local Anesthetics	
Tetracaine hydrochloride (Pontocaine), 0.25%	Commonly used topical anesthetic Anesthesia produced in 1 to 2 minutes
Proparacaine hydrochloride (Ophthaine, Alcaine, 0.5%)	More rapid in action Less discomfort during instillation
Procaine hydrochloride, 1% and 2%	Commonly used for injection in eye surgery Lasts about 45 minutes
Lidocaine hydrochloride (Xylocaine), 2%	Some favor this over procaine because its action is more rapid and it lasts longer.
Antimicrobial and Chemotherapeutic Agents	
Neomycin sulfate with polymyxin and bacitracin (Neosporin)	Broad-spectrum, ointment or solution Only disadvantage is its allergenic nature (allergy is to neomycin)
Penicillin	Primarily used in newborns in ointment form Occasionally used for intraocular infection Primarily reserved for systemic use
Sodium methicillin (Staphcillin)	Used for penicillinase-producing organisms
Bacitracin, 500 units/g ointment	Good as a penicillin substitute for local eye uses against gram-positive organisms
Erythromycin, 1% ointment	Effective as a penicillin substitute against resistant staphylococcal organisms

Sulfonamides:
  Sulfisoxazole (Gantrisin), 4% solution or ointment
  Sulfacetamide sodium (Sulamyd Sodium)
	Used in treatment of conjunctivitis; sometimes effective against larger viruses

Dyes	
(For corneal staining to detect superficial abrasions)	
Fluorescein sodium	**NOTE:** Because *Pseudomonas aeruginosa*, highly pathogenic for corneal tissues, grows well in fluorescein solutions, the sterile single-dose containers or sterile Kimura fluorescein papers are recommended.
Rose Bengal, 1% and 2%	Selective dye to stain conjunctiva; mucous shreds stain more brilliantly than with fluorescein
Carbonic Anhydrase Inhibitor	
(Carbonic anhydrase is an enzyme present in body tissues. In the ciliary body, it is directly involved in the production of aqueous humor.)	
Acetazolamide (Diamox)	A sulfonamide used as a diuretic and also effective in decreasing production of aqueous humor by ciliary body in glaucoma
Dichlorphenamide (Daranide)	Because of side-effects (gastric distress, shortness of breath, acidosis, tingling of extremities, dermatitis, ureteral stones), it is prescribed cautiously for selected patients.

(continued)

Table 54-1
Medications Used Frequently in Eye Conditions (continued)

Medication	Action
Sympathomimetic Drugs	
(Used primarily for mydriasis and occasionally as vasoconstrictors)	
Phenylephrine hydrochloride (Neo-Synephrine), 2.5% to 10%	Action lasts 3 hours
Hydroxyamphetamine hydrobromide ophthalmic solution (Paredrine), 1%	Action lasts 3 hours; useful in those with allergy toward phenylephrine
Epinephrine hydrochloride (Adrenalin), 1:1,000; (Glaucon) 0.5%, 1%, and 2%	Lowers intraocular pressure in open-angle glaucoma (inhibits aqueous production)
Parasympathomimetic Drugs	
(Used as miotics for controlling intraocular pressure in glaucoma)	
Group I—Act Directly on Myoneural Junction	
Pilocarpine hydrochloride, 0.5%, 1%, 2%, 3%, 4%, and 6%	Drug of choice in glaucoma Action lasts 6 to 8 hours
Carbachol (Carbacel) 1.5% to 3%	Used if pilocarpine is ineffective
Group II—Cholinesterase Inhibitors	
Physostigmine salicylate (Eserine), 0.25% and 0.5%	Action lasts 6 to 8 hours Because it is allergenic, unstable, and short in its action, it is gradually being replaced by Phospholine.
Echothiophate iodide (Phospholine Iodide), 0.06%, 0.125%, and 0.25%	Water-soluble Causes less local irritation
Isoflurophate (diisopropyl fluorophosphate) (DFP) (Floropryl), 0.025% ophthalmic ointment; 0.1%—ophthalmic solution	Oil-soluble miotic May produce side-effects; watch for vomiting, diarrhea, tenesmus
Parasympatholytic Medications	
(Used as mydriatics to facilitate ophthalmoscopic examination and for mydriasis and cycloplegia in refraction and in treatment of uveitis)	
Mydriatics	
Epinephrine (Epitrate), 1% to 2%	Action lasts 12 hours
Eucatropine hydrochloride (Euphthalmine), 5%	Short-lived action Can dilate pupil without affecting accommodation
Cycloplegics	
Homatropine hydrobromide, 2% and 5%	A popular drug for cycloplegic refraction Action lasts 24 to 36 hours Allergic reactions rare
Scopolamine hydrobromide (Isopto Hyoscine), 0.2% to 0.5%	Used in children's refraction Used in treating uveitis Because of low allergic reaction, it is preferred to atropine May cause dizziness and disorientation in older persons

(continued)

Table 54-1
Medications Used Frequently in Eye Conditions (continued)

Medication	Action
Parasympatholytic Medications *(continued)*	
Atropine sulfate, 0.25%, 0.5%, 1%, and 2%	Most powerful of this group
	Action lasts 10 to 14 days, during which eyes must be protected from bright light
	Used in treating uveitis
	Used in refraction of children
	Contraindicated in narrow-angle glaucoma
	5% of persons are sensitive to it (symptoms: difficulty in swallowing; dizziness; flushed skin with circumoral pallor; rapid, full pulse; delirium)
Cyclopentolate hydrochloride (Cyclogyl), 0.5% and 1%	Action is less than 24 hours
	Very popular drug for cycloplegic refraction
Tropicamide (Mydriacyl), 0.5% and 1%	Newer, shorter acting—lasts 6 hours
Adrenal Corticosteroids	
(Effective in treating inflammatory conditions of the eye: uveitis, episcleritis, chemical burns. Decreases vascularization and scarring following burns, trauma, and severe inflammation.)	
Cortisone acetate, 0.5% to 2.5%—suspension; 1.5%—ointment	Least expensive
Hydrocortisone, 0.5% to 2.5%—suspension; 1.5%—ointment	Greater potency than cortisone, so it can be used in lower concentrations
Prednisone, prednisolone, dexamethasone, and betamethasone	These are thought to be more potent than hydrocortisone.

NOTE: These are highly dangerous when used in the presence of herpes simplex keratitis. The patient should definitely be under the care of an ophthalmologist with these medications. All steroids are now known to produce glaucoma in certain predisposed patients. Use of steroids locally or systemically must be carefully supervised.

to "squeeze" their eyes closed, thereby expelling the medication.

- If the dropper has not been contaminated, it may be replaced in the bottle, but is to be used only for this patient.

Ointments

Ointments of various kinds are used frequently in the treatment of inflammatory diseases of the lids, the conjunctiva, and the cornea. Those prescribed most commonly are sulfonamides, bacitracin, neomycin, chloramphenicol, steroids, and various combinations.

Ointments are applied best by gently pulling down the lower lid and expressing a small amount of the ointment from the tube onto the conjunctiva of the lower lid. Care is taken not to touch the eye or the eyelid with the tube. The lid then may be massaged gently in such a way as to distribute the drug over the eyeball (Fig. 54-6B).

Ocular Irrigations

Ocular irrigations are indicated in treating various inflammations of the conjunctiva, in preparing the patient for eye surgery, and in removing inflammatory secretions. They are also used for their antiseptic effect. The fluid to be employed depends on the condition present and is warmed before being used. The irrigating apparatus is simple, consisting of a commercially prepared irrigating bottle containing sterile ophthalmic solution (Blinx, Dacriose) and a small, curved basin and cotton for catching the fluid and the secretions. Each patient should have his own solutions in a plastic dispenser with a cap.

- The patient lies flat on his back or sits with the head tilted backward and inclined slightly toward the side to be treated. The basin may be held by the patient, if he is sitting, or so placed that when he is lying down it will catch the fluid as it runs from the eye. The nurse stands in front of the patient.
- After the lids are carefully cleansed to remove dust, secretions, and crusts, the lids are held open with the thumb and the fingers of one hand and the eye flushed gently, directing the stream way from the nose. The fluid is never directed toward the nose, because of the danger that it may spill over into the other eye. The procedure is continued until the eye is entirely free of secretions.
- It must be remembered that very little force is to be used, because of the danger of injury. For the same

reason, and to prevent contamination, no part of the irrigator should touch the eye, the lid, or the lashes.

- When the irrigation has been completed, the eye and the cheek are dried gently with cotton.

Continuous Irrigation of the Eye. Continuous irrigation is indicated in chemical burns, resistant corneal ulcers, uveitis, socket infections after enucleation, or conditions in which constant medication or debridement is indicated. Prior to irrigation, Ophthaine is instilled as a local anesthetic.

Hot Compresses

Heat relieves pain and increases the circulation, thereby promoting absorption and reducing tension in the eye. It is especially valuable for conjunctivitis accompanied by excessive secretions. Heat is best applied in the form of compresses composed of seven or eight layers of gauze or cotton just large enough to cover the eye.

- The patient is moved to the side of the bed, and a towel is used to cover the chest. The skin of the lids and the adjacent cheek may be anointed with cold cream or petrolatum.
- The compresses then are moistened in a basin of water or any other prescribed solution that has been heated.
- The fluid, which should be kept at a temperature between 46° C to 49° C (115° F–120° F), is expressed or squeezed from the pad, and the compress, after being tested for temperature on the back of the hand, is placed gently over the closed lids.
- The pads are changed every 30 to 60 seconds for 10 to 15 minutes, and the application is repeated every 2 or 3 hours.

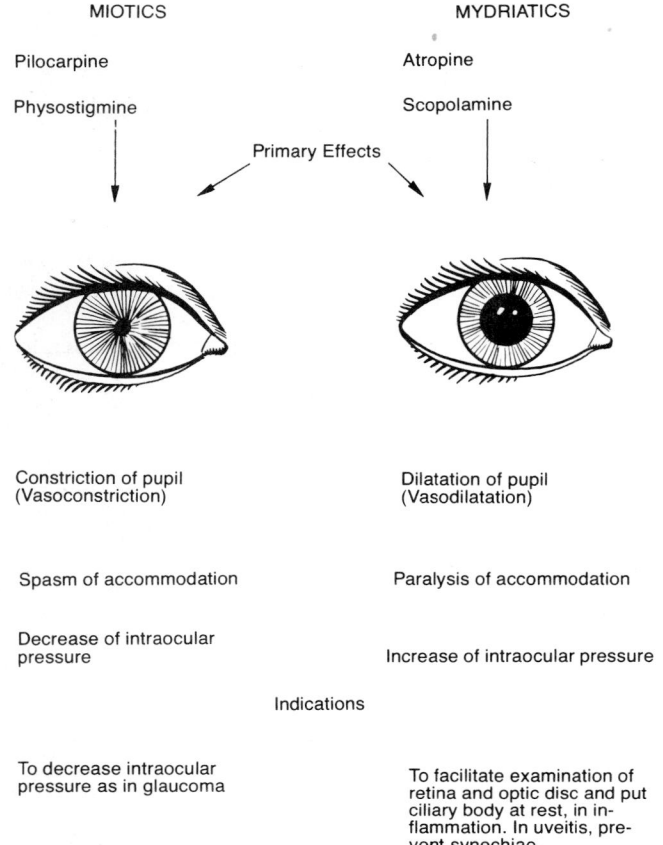

MIOTICS	MYDRIATICS
Pilocarpine	Atropine
Physostigmine	Scopolamine

Primary Effects

Constriction of pupil (Vasoconstriction)	Dilatation of pupil (Vasodilatation)
Spasm of accommodation	Paralysis of accommodation
Decrease of intraocular pressure	Increase of intraocular pressure

Indications

| To decrease intraocular pressure as in glaucoma | To facilitate examination of retina and optic disc and put ciliary body at rest, in inflammation. In uveitis, prevent synechiae. |

Figure 54-5. Effects and indications of miotics and mydriatics.

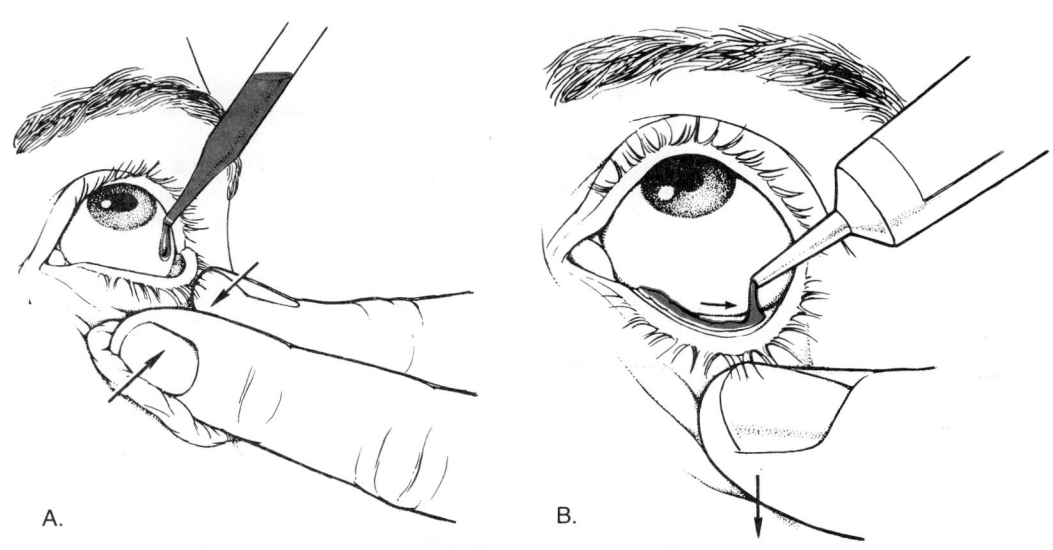

A. B.

Figure 54-6. (*A*) When instilling eye drops, instruct the patient to look upward, then lightly pinch the lower lid to form a receptacle for the dropped medication. (*B*) In applying ointment, instruct the patient to look upward, then depress the lower lid and gently squeeze ointment along the everted lid, beginning at the inner canthus (close to the nose) and then moving outward.

- At the completion of the period of application, the lids are dried gently with cotton.
- New pads are used for each application and, if the eyes have a purulent secretion, the compresses are applied to one eye at a time, the solution and the basin being changed between applications in order not to carry infection from one eye to the other.

Cold Compresses

Cold causes a capillary constriction that tends to reduce the amount of secretion and relieve pain during the early stages of acute inflammatory conditions of the conjunctiva. Cold compresses are useful in relieving itching due to allergic conjunctivitis.

The patient is prepared in the same manner as for the application of hot compresses. The pads are moistened in boric acid solution and placed in rows on a block of ice suspended by a gauze sling over a basin. They are applied to the closed lids and are changed every 15 to 30 seconds, for a period of 5 to 15 minutes each hour.

- Cold compresses are never used in the treatment of inflammations of the eye (iritis, keratitis), because cold, by constricting the capillaries, interferes with the nutrition of the cornea.

▷ Trauma to the Eye

The prevention of eye injuries is a phase of child and adult education that cannot be emphasized too strongly. Children need to be reminded frequently of the dangers of sticks, arrows, darts, BB guns, "sparklers," sling shots, rubber bands, and even harmless-looking toys. Precautions that should be taken when power tools are used need to be explained, along with the reasons protection is necessary from very bright lights, the sun shining on the snow, chemical fumes, sprays, and flying chips of wood. The use of goggles gives protection against most foreign bodies, but specially designed safety goggles or glasses with impact-resistant lenses are preferable if there is danger of flying metal or wood objects that may break the glass. Elderly persons or those unsure of their footing need safeguards where there is a possibility of injury.

General measures in caring for patients with eye injuries may include the following:

- Obtain a history of the injury first, then consult with an ophthalmologist immediately.
- Irrigate the eye with saline solution; however, note that irrigations may be dangerous in the instance of a penetrating eye injury.
- Stain the front surface of the eye with sterile fluorescein paper (Fluor-I-Strip), which uses the yellowish green dye to detect abrasions and ulcers.
- Irrigate the eye again.
- Evaluate the injury and manage as prescribed.
- Employ follow-up care.

Foreign Bodies

Foreign bodies (dust, cinders, and so forth) frequently cause considerable discomfort by irritating the sensitive conjunc-

tiva. If the foreign body has been in the eye only a short time, it may be removed by a nurse. One way to detect foreign particles in the eye is to have the patient close his eyes, then darken the room and gently place a penlight on the lid. The foreign particle will show up as a black shadow. The lower lid is everted, the patient instructed to look up, and the lower half of the conjunctival sac examined. If the particle is not found, the upper eye is examined by everting the upper lid. The examiner stands in front of the patient and instructs him to look down at his feet. The lashes are grasped between the thumb and fingers of one hand, and a matchstick, an applicator, or a toothpick is placed across the upper part of the lid. The lashes are pulled downward and forward, away from the eye, as the applicator is pressed downward, gently. The foreign body may be removed by touching it gently with a small applicator tipped with cotton and moistened in saline solution.

If this method is unsuccessful, or if the offending particle has been in the eye for a considerable time, no attempt should be made to remove it. It may have become embedded in the cornea, and there is considerable danger of serious injury if removal is attempted by unskilled hands. The ophthalmologist usually requires local anesthesia, a hand lens, fluorescein, an eye spud, normal saline for irrigating the eye, and, as a prophylaxis against infection, an antibiotic solution to instill after the offending particle is removed. If the particle is known to be a metal, the physician may use a magnet to remove it.

Acid and Alkali Burns

Careless use of hair sprays and other spray-on products has increased the incidence of chemical burns of the eye.

- Whenever acid or alkali gets on the lids or in the eye, an emergency exists, requiring that immediate action be taken. *In such an instance, the lids, the conjunctiva, and the cornea must be flushed copiously.*

The easiest and quickest way to flush the eye is to have the patient hold his head under a faucet and allow the water to run over the eye and wash it out. However, it is more satisfactory to flush the eye with a syringe, if available, taking care not to contaminate the other eye if it has not already been contaminated. Continuous flushing for at least 15 minutes is desirable. Plain tap water is adequate under such circumstances.

Actinic Trauma

Ultraviolet rays may damage the cornea as a result of excessive sunlight, snow blindness, and the use of a welder's arc ("welder's flash") or a sun lamp. Treatment consists of instilling anesthetic drops and patching both eyes.

Contusions and Hematoma ("Black Eye")

Trauma to the eye frequently results in hemorrhage. The bleeding that enters the loose tissues of the orbit spreads rapidly, discoloring the lids and surrounding skin. In itself, the injury is not too serious, but frequently it is frightening to patients because the discoloration and swelling is so prominent. The bleeding usually stops spontaneously, but it may be reduced and the swelling lessened by the application of cold compresses. Absorption of the blood may be hastened after the first 24 hours by the use of hot compresses applied 15 minutes at a time, at intervals throughout the day. Drugs are now available to help hasten absorption of hematomas.

Corneal Abrasions

Lacerations of the cornea can be detected after being stained with sodium fluorescein (Fluor-I-Strip). A blue penlight more clearly identifies the abrasion than a white light.

Usually, a local anesthetic and antibacterial drops are administered, and an eye patch is applied for 24 to 36 hours. Self-administration of local anesthetic is discouraged, since it may delay the diagnosis of complications and may even lead to further injury. The patient is instructed to keep the eyes at rest to promote comfort and facilitate the healing process. The danger to be guarded against with an abrasion is the development of a corneal ulcer. Therefore, if there is no improvement after 24 hours, an ophthalmic consultation is desirable.

Lacerations

Lacerations of the eyelids are serious because the lids become scarred and are unable to close. Injuries to the lids are treated in the same way as any other wound, but an ophthalmologist usually is requested to care for them.

Lacerations of the eyeball are more serious because visual defects may result. Since more extensive injuries may endanger the entire eye, such injuries are referred invariably to the ophthalmologist for appropriate care. Injuries of this type may entail transplantation of conjunctival flaps to prevent leakage of ocular fluids, excision of the prolapsed iris, and in severe injuries, even removal of the eye.

▷ Conditions of the Eyelids

(See Table 54-2.)

Blepharitis. This common disorder of the lids (inflammation of the eyelids) can be controlled through cleanliness and the prevention of excessive dryness. Since blepharitis is frequently associated with seborrhea, attempts are made to keep the scalp clean. Daily cleaning of the eyelids by rubbing them gently with a clean, wet washcloth helps to remove scales. Usually, an anti-infective ointment is prescribed, such as steroid-sulfa drops, to be applied to the lid margin twice a day. For pure staphylococcal blepharitis, local antibiotic solutions and application of moist heat are helpful.

Table 54-2
Assessment of Acute Eye Conditions

	Acute Conjunctivitis	Acute Iritis (Anterior Uveitis)	Acute Glaucoma (Closed-Angle)	Corneal Ulcer or Trauma
Incidence	Very common	Common	Not common	Common
Vision	Normal	Some blurring	Marked blurring	Blurred (usually)
Pain	None	Moderate	Severe	May have pain
Intraocular Pressure	Normal	Normal or low	Elevated	Normal
Cornea	Clear	Clear	Steamy	May have abrasion, foreign body, or ulcer
Ocular Discharge	Moderate to copious	None	None	Watery and perhaps purulent
Pupillary Response to Light	Normal	Weak	Weak	Normal
Pupil Size	Normal	Small	Dilated	Normal or small
Conjunctival Vessels Dilated	Yes	Mostly circumcorneal	Yes	Yes
Prognosis	Self-limited; 3 to 5 days	Good with treatment	Without proper treatment: Poor	Poor

Table 54-3

Comparison Between Granulomatous and Nongranulomatous Uveitis

	Granulomatous	Nongranulomatous
Location	Any portion of uveal tract, but predilection for posterior part	Anterior portion; iris, ciliary body
Onset	Insidious	Acute
Pain	None or minimal	Marked
Circumcorneal Flush	Slight	Present
Photophobia	Slight	Marked
Course	Chronic	Acute
Prognosis	Fair to poor	Good
Recurrence	Sometimes	Common

Sty (External Hordeolum). A *sty* is an infection of the Zeis glands or Moll's glands that empty at the free edge of the eyelid. When a sty develops, this area becomes swollen, red, tender, and painful. Frequently, an eyelash will be found in the center of the yellow point that appears. Warm compresses applied in the early stage hasten the pointing of the abscess. Removal of the central lash often is followed by drainage of pus, but incision is necessary if resolution does not begin within 48 hours. Antibiotic therapy hastens control of the infection; this is instilled into the conjunctival sac.

Chalazia. A *chalazion* is a cyst of the meibomian glands. It appears as a small, hard, painless lump in the lid and usually occurs secondary to infection of the gland, which results when the opening on the lid margin becomes plugged. Occasionally, such a cyst may become infected. When this occurs, hot compresses are used; an incision and drainage also may be necessary. Incision and drainage (or excision of the cyst) are indicated if the mass distorts vision, causes astigmatism, or becomes a cosmetic blemish. A new method of treatment being used by some ophthalmologists is to inject steroids directly into the chalazion.

Trachoma. This chronic, highly communicable disease of the eyelids is one of the most common diseases of man and affects about 15% of the world's population (5 million). It is the greatest single cause for progressive loss of sight in the world. Trachoma is common in Asian countries and in countries around the Mediterranean Sea, particularly Egypt. In the United States, it is rare except among American Indians and Mexicans in the southwest.

Assessment and Clinical Manifestations. The principal symptoms are mild itching and irritation. After an acute inflammatory process, follicles appear on the conjunctiva. Blurring of vision and increasing discomfort occur. The upper palpebral conjunctiva is affected.

The progress of the disease has been classified into four stages: in stage I (incipient trachoma), immature follicles are present, especially in the upper tarsal conjunctiva. At the top of the cornea there is incipient pannus (abnormal vascularization). Stage II (established trachoma) consists of two types—type A and type B. In type A, follicular hypertrophy is predominant, while in type B, papillary hypertrophy is predominant ("acute trachoma"). In stage III, early conjunctival scarring is observed as fine, white lines; corneal pannus also increases. In stage IV, smooth scarring of the tarsal conjunctiva occurs, and vascular pannus becomes inactive. Secondary bacterial conjunctivitis increases the hazard of corneal ulceration, and this in turn leads to blindness.

Management. Trachoma is spread by direct contact; therefore, personal cleanliness is a key factor in prevention. Isolating known cases and initiating antibiotic therapy early may help control the disease. If untreated, it will last for months or years. Medical treatment consists of a 3-week course of oral sulfonamide (trisulfapyrimidines), during which time the patient is closely observed for signs of toxicity. Should this occur, tetracycline is substituted for the sulfa drugs. The World Health Organization is making great strides in eliminating this curable disease, especially in Japan and the Philippines.

▷ Inflammations of the Eye

Conjunctivitis. *Conjunctivitis* may result from bacterial, viral, and rickettsial infections, or from allergy, trauma, or chemical injury.

No matter what the cause, the symptoms are similar: redness, pain, swelling, and lacrimation. The amount and the nature of discharge depend on the offending organisms; for instance, the pneumococcus and the gonococcus cause an abundant purulent discharge.

Frequent saline irrigations are required to remove the discharge. Warm compresses are recommended, to be applied for 15 minutes three or four times a day. Ointments such as sulfacetamide, gentamicin, or chloramphenicol drops or ointment may be instilled to clear the infection in 1 to 3 days. Untreated, the infection usually subsides in a week to 10 days. Precautions must be taken to prevent dissemination of infection to the other eye, as well as to other persons. Hands should be kept clean when treating the eye; individual clean washcloths and towels should be used.

Uveitis. *Uveitis* is a general term for inflammatory conditions of the uveal tract (iris, ciliary body, choroid), which may be due to a number of causative agents. *Anterior uveitis* refers to *choroiditis* and *chorioretinitis; panuveitis* involves the entire uveal tract. Uveitis (iritis) is usually unilateral and is characterized by pain, photophobia, blurring of vision, redness (circumcorneal flush), and a constricted pupil.

Some authorities prefer to classify the various forms of uveitis as granulomatous and nongranulomatous. In some aspects, the two forms are similar, but in others there occurs a significant difference (Table 54-3).

Complications and sequelae may result, should uveitis go untreated. Adhesions may result, impeding aqueous outflow at the anterior chamber angle and causing glaucoma. If adhesions hinder the flow of aqueous humor from the posterior to the anterior chamber, cataracts may develop. Even retinal detachment may occur as a result of traction exerted on the retina by vitreous strands.

Management. Because the ophthalmologist can differentiate among the various forms of uveitis, treatment is directed to the specific type of involvement. For granulomatous uveitis, atropine is used to reduce the likelihood of adhesions. Anti-infective chemotherapy may be initiated, and if the response is not favorable, it is followed with corticosteroids. Medications for comfort and relief of pain are also prescribed.

Nongranulomatous uveitis is also treated with atropine to keep the pupil dilated. Local, and possibly systemic, steroids may be required.

Nongranulomatous uveitis subsides with treatment in a few weeks. Granulomatous uveitis may last months and even years in spite of treatment.

Sympathetic Ophthalmia. This is a severe granulomatous bilateral uveitis that may occur from 1 week to several years after an eye injury. Fortunately, this is a rare condition, but it may be suspected when there is a history of a penetrating eye injury in one eye (exciting eye) and the patient complains of photophobia, blurring vision, and infection in the other eye (sympathizing eye).

Medical management is directed in one of two directions: corticosteroids are administered both locally and systemically, while atropine is given locally. This treatment has been proven effective. The other, more radical procedure is to suggest preventive enucleation of the severely injured eye before sympathetic ophthalmia develops. This decision is a difficult one; often, a patient can think more clearly and reach a satisfactory decision if he has the time and opportunity to express his thoughts and feelings about the operation. In such a case, it helps to understand the nature of the problem, the patient's ability and condition, and the desired goals of the ophthalmologist. Untreated, the disease progresses to bilateral blindness.

Pterygium. *Pterygium* is an abnormal triangular fold of membrane that extends onto the cornea from the white of the eye; it always occurs toward the nose. It is thought to be caused by chronic irritation, as from dust or wind. Surgical intervention prevents its growth and protects against loss of vision. In some eye clinics, surgery is followed by beta-radiation therapy, which helps to prevent recurrence of pterygium. Patients often erroneously refer to pterygium as a cataract.

▷ The Patient Undergoing Eye Surgery

Preoperative Nursing Management. The preparation of the patient for an ophthalmic operation must be carried out with the most scrupulous care. The lower bowel is evacuated the morning of the operation, and only a liquid diet is given after that. The hair of female patients is so arranged that it will remain in place for several days with bandages applied over it. Before the eyes are prepared for operation, the patient's head should be covered with a stockinette cap. This is followed by a normal cleansing of the face. Chloramphenicol or gentamicin (Garamycin Ophthalmic Solution) is usually instilled as prescribed, prior to surgery, while the patient is awake.

Postoperative Nursing Considerations. Following surgery, the patient is placed in bed in a supine position with a small pillow under his head. Pillows are placed on each side of the head to keep it still, and side rails are set in place to give the patient a sense of security. The patient is provided with a nurse-call system and instructed to ask for help rather than move or strain in an attempt to be self-sufficient. If a local anesthesia is used during the operation, the patient is usually ambulatory in a few hours after surgery.

The ophthalmologist is notified immediately if the patient has excessive pain or if the dressings are disturbed.

- Morphine is never given to ophthalmic patients unless it is certain that vomiting will not injure the eye.

Diversional or recreational therapy is important, but should be of such a nature that the eyes are not fatigued in any way. Even the patient's environment is an important consideration. The walls and the ceiling should be painted in soft, pastel shades. Light should be regulated so that it is not bright and does not produce a glare.

Prior to discharge, the patient is informed thoroughly regarding medications, eye aids (glasses), the type of work allowed, and follow-up visits.

▷ Strabismus (Squint)

Strabismus, or *squint,* is a condition in which one eye deviates from the object at which the person is looking (lay term, "cross-eyed"). The deviating eye may turn in (*esotropia*—ST), or out (*exotropia*—XT), or up (*hypertropia*—HT). It may result from paralysis of the nerves supplying the extraocular muscles, due to injury or disease. Double vision or diplopia results.

A condition frequently associated with strabismus is *amblyopia,* a deficient acuity of central vision without apparent cause. (*Amblyopia ex anopsia* is amblyopia resulting from disuse.)

The following test may be used to determine whether strabismus is present. The patient fixes his vision on a light about 32.5 cm (13 inches) from him. The reflex light is then observed to see if it falls in the center of each pupil (Fig. 54-7).

In children, a strabismus due to ocular defects often develops. It is characterized by single vision, usually because the image seen by the nonfixing eye is suppressed involuntarily. The strabismus in children often may be corrected by properly fitted glasses.

Orthoptic training for muscle disturbances is successful in some instances, without operation. It consists of a series of muscle exercises carried out by means of various instruments, cards, and test objects. Patients with a marked degree of squint usually undergo operation after having had some training; after the eyes are straightened, the exercises are

Orthophoria

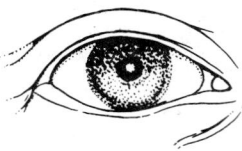
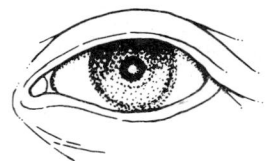

Right esotropia

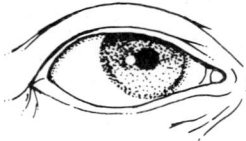
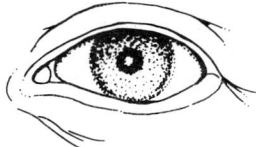

Right exotropia

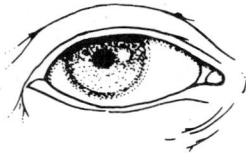
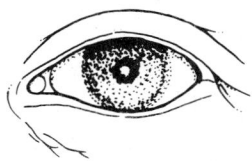

Right hypertropia

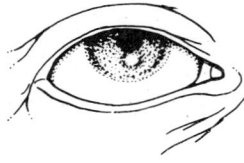
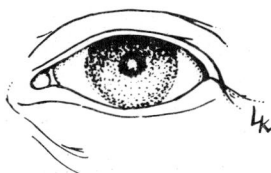

O = Corneal light reflex

Figure 54-7. The Hirschberg Corneal Reflex Test. This is done by having the patient fix his vision on a light about 13 inches away from him. The reflex light is then observed to see where it falls on the pupil. Note where the light falls on the right eye in each of the above conditions.

employed again. Early detection and immediate medical consultation are to be encouraged if the defect is to be corrected satisfactorily.

▷ Corneal Disorders

Corneal Ulcers

Inflammation of the cornea (*keratitis*) with loss of substance results in corneal ulcer. The inflammatory reaction often spreads deeper to the iris (*iritis*), resulting in the formation

of pus, which collects as a white or yellow deposit behind the cornea (*hypopyon*). If the ulceration perforates, the iris may prolapse through the cornea, or other serious complications may follow.

Because the cornea is so important to vision, any ulceration must be considered a most serious condition. Scarring or perforation due to corneal ulceration is a major cause of blindness; 10% of all blindness is caused by corneal ulcers (6% in the U.S.). The healing of all but the most superficial ulcers is attended with some degree of opacity of the cornea and, therefore, with some diminution of vision.

The symptoms of corneal ulceration are pain, marked photophobia, and increased lacrimation. The eye usually appears somewhat injected or "bloodshot."

Management.   Prevention is much simpler and easier than cure. Therefore, prompt removal of foreign bodies and early treatment of infections may prevent the occurrence of a corneal ulcer.

Dark glasses are provided to relieve the photophobia. Mydriatics are given at frequent intervals. Optical anesthetics may be used to relieve pain. Fluorescein generally is used to outline the ulcers before the healing solutions are applied. Antibiotic solutions and chemotherapeutic agents are prescribed for the specific type of infection, since the microorganism may be bacterial, viral, or fungal.

Corneal Transplantation (Keratoplasty)

A keratoplasty may be done to repair a corneal opacity (scar), keratoconus, or chemical burn of the eye. The circular segment of cornea removed from the patient must be exactly matched and replaced by a similar segment of cornea from a donor eye (Fig. 54-8). For best results, the graft should be removed within 5 or 6 hours following the death of the donor (to prevent softening of the cornea), and transplanted within 2 days.*

The graft may be a *penetrating graft* (including all layers of the cornea) or a *lamellar graft* (involving only the outer layers of the cornea) (Fig. 54-8). The lamellar graft, popular in the past, is gradually being replaced by the penetrating graft.

Preoperative and Intraoperative Management.   Since keratoplasty is elective surgery, the patient is probably aware of the nature of the operation and is no doubt optimistic about the likelihood of improved vision. The nurse, nevertheless, must allow time for the expression of concerns or questions that the patient may still have. Psychological and cultural concerns regarding the disability may have to be explored before the patient is in optimal condition for surgery. Physically, the patient should be free from respiratory or eye infections in order to promote postoperative healing.

Usually, a transplant is done under local anesthesia and takes about an hour. A trephining instrument, having an end similar to that of a cookie cutter but the size of the cornea,

* The national eye bank (Eye-Bank for Sight Restoration, Inc., 210 E. 64th St., New York, N.Y. 10021) was founded in 1945. Eyes have been donated from persons all over the country and distributed to qualified ophthalmologists throughout the United States.

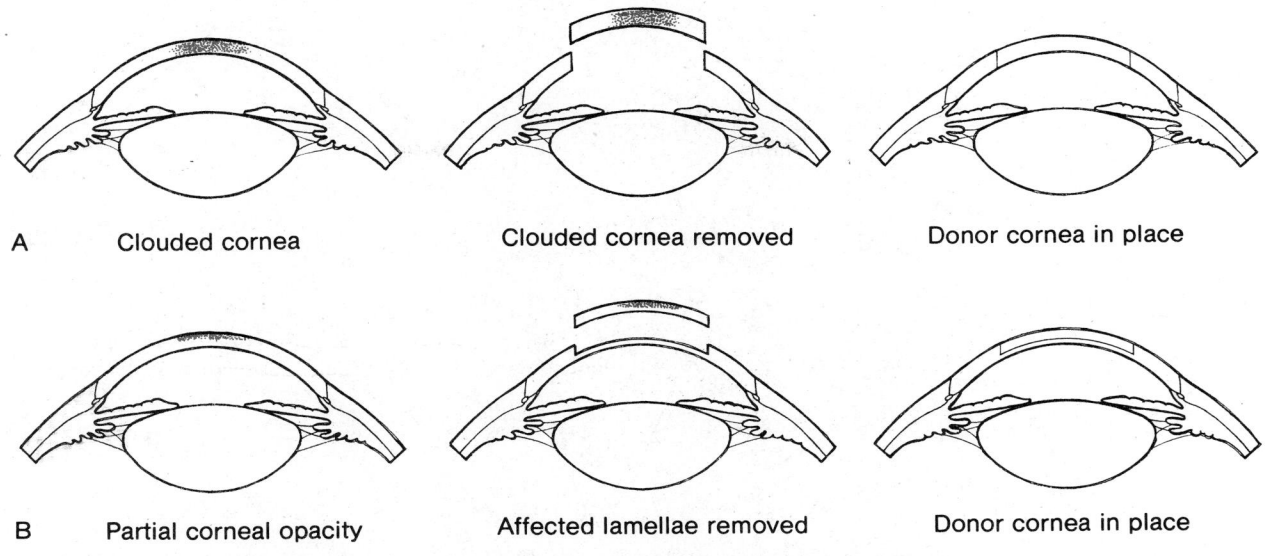

A   Clouded cornea   Clouded cornea removed   Donor cornea in place

B   Partial corneal opacity   Affected lamellae removed   Donor cornea in place

Figure 54-8. (*A*) Penetrating keratoplasty: a full-thickness (7-mm–8-mm) disc is removed from the host and replaced with a matching full-thickness button from the donor. (*B*) Lamellar keratoplasty: a thin layer of corneal tissue is excised from the host eye. Stroma and entire endothelium are spared.

is placed over the opacity, and the cornea is removed. The same instrument is used to remove the donor cornea so that the graft is a perfect fit. Ultrafine sutures are placed evenly to create a tight seal; this is done via an operating microscope.

Postoperative Management. Goals of postoperative patient care are (1) to avoid elevated intraocular pressure, as well as pressure on the operated eye; (2) to provide rest for the eye so that healing progresses smoothly; and (3) to employ measures that will prevent infection of the eye.

Elevated intraocular pressure constricts the vascular supply and can cause retinal atrophy or damage to the graft. To prevent pressure from increasing within the eye, the nurse must be cognizant of those activities that can elevate pressure (see p. 1253). Loss of aqueous humor through the suture line by increased pressure could cause dislocation of the newly transplanted cornea, prolapse of the iris, adhesions of the iris to the cornea, or malformation of the anterior chamber. To avoid these problems, when the patient is transferred from the operating table to the bed or stretcher, adequate personnel are required to move him horizontally in one smooth shift, giving adequate support to his head. Intraocular pressure can be measured by sensitive electronic applanation tonometers. If the pressure is elevated, pharmacologic control can be achieved with such drugs as acetazolamide, which inhibits aqueous production.

Both eyes may be covered to provide rest and to enhance healing. If one eye is uncovered, its movement will affect the operated eye because the two eyes move in unison. Healing is slow because the cornea is avascular, which also increases the possibility of infection. Thus, meticulous sterile technique is followed in dressing changes to protect the susceptible corneal epithelium from infection. Another means of reducing the chance for infection is to provide the patient with soft contact lenses, which protect the suture line. This is particularly effective in patients who have chemical burns. To prevent herpes simplex infection, the administration of antiviral agents may be indicated.

Graft rejection is controlled by topically applied corticosteroids; however, these are to be given only for short periods of time, since they retard healing. Even with the use of corticosteroids, graft rejection still occurs in about 20% of patients.

With this regimen of medical care, it is possible for the patient with a penetrating type of corneal transplant to have bathroom privileges the day of surgery and to be ambulatory the next day. The eye is unpatched on the third day, and the patient may be discharged in a few days. Within a short time, normal activities may be resumed. The very fine sutures are well tolerated and need not be removed until 7 or 8 months after operation, when maximal healing has taken place. Periodic visits to the ophthalmologist will ensure that the patient is progressing as expected.

▷ Radial Keratotomy

Radial keratotomy is a controversial procedure designed to correct myopia. It involves making cuts (usually 8 or 16) into the cornea from the edge toward the center in a pattern that resembles "bicycle spokes" (Fig. 54-9). Incisions are ¾ of the thickness of the cornea. Pressure from the intraocular fluid stretches the radial cuts to distort the cornea into a flatter shape, thereby improving the myopia. The surgery usually takes about 30 minutes and can be performed on an outpatient basis.

This procedure is being studied to determine short-term and long-term effects.

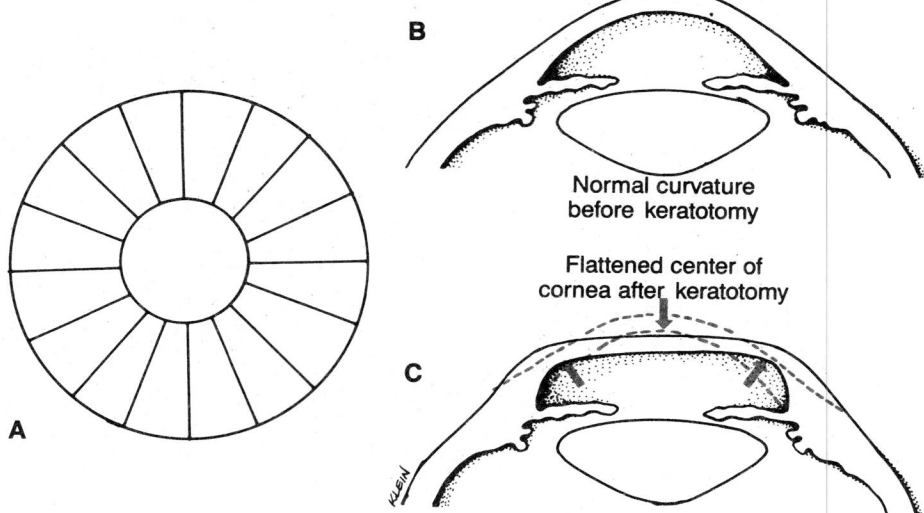

Figure 54-9. Technique for keratotomy. (*A*) Incisions (8 or 16) are made from the edge of the cornea toward its center. (*B*) Lateral view of the cornea, showing its shape in a patient with myopia. (*C*) Following keratotomy, the cornea is flatter.

▷ Detached Retina

A *retinal detachment* occurs when the sensory retina separates from the pigment epithelium of the retina. The retina is that layer of the eye which perceives light and transmits impulses from its nerve cells to the optic nerve. When a tear occurs in the retina, vitreous humor and transudate seep out between the retinal layers, causing detachment. Tears or holes in the retina may occur suddenly or slowly, as a result of trauma or degeneration. It may also result from hemorrhage, exudation, or tumor in front of or behind the retina. Studies have shown that approximately 6% of the population have small holes or tears in the retina. Aging weakens these spots.

Assessment and Clinical Manifestations. The usual symptoms include flashes of light and blurred or "sooty" vision, sudden in onset; the patient may have the sensation of particles moving in his line of vision. These floating particles consist of retinal cells and blood that are released at the time of the tear and cast shadows on the retina as they drift by. Definite areas of vision may be blank (Fig. 54-10), and in a few days the patient may have the sensation of a veil coming up or down in front of the eye, finally resulting in loss of vision.

The suddenness of the incapacity creates confusion and apprehension in most patients, as well as a fear of blindness. Usually, it means that the person must abandon his business or activity, with little or no time to make plans.

Conservative Management. The patient is treated with rest immediately. The eye is bandaged in the hope that the retina will fall back into place as much as possible before surgery.

The patient should be positioned so that the area of detachment will be in the dependent position. For example, a patient with a superior temporal detachment (the most common form) in the right eye should be supine, with the head turned to the right. For a left inferior nasal detachment of the retina, the patient should sit up, with the head turned to the right. Sedation and tranquilizing drugs keep the patient comfortable and quiet.

Surgical Intervention

The objective in surgical treatment is to create a scar that seals the retina to the choroid as it heals. Such treatment may be accomplished in one of several ways: photocoagulation, cryosurgery, electrodiathermy, or scleral buckling.

Photocoagulation makes use of a strong beam of light (from a carbon-arc source) that is directed through the dilated pupil to form a small burn, causing a choroid retinal inflammatory exudate. The *laser beam* (light amplification by stimulated emission of radiation) can be used in photocoagulation. This method of treatment is used for limited retinal detachments and also may be used after operation to reattach small areas.

In *cryosurgery,* a supercooled probe is applied to the sclera, causing minimal damage; the choroid and retina adhere as a result of the scarring. The advantage of this method over the use of diathermy is the reduced damage to the sclera.

In *electrodiathermy,* an electrode needle is passed through the sclera, allowing the subretinal collection of fluid to escape. Because an exudate forms from the choroid, the torn retina adheres to the choroid, which in turn adheres to the sclera. This method is being replaced by cryosurgery.

In *scleral buckling,* the idea is to shorten the sclera to enhance contact between the choroid and retina. After the subretinal fluid is withdrawn, the detachment is treated by one of the methods described above. The treated area is then indented to "buckle" inward toward the vitreous humor (Fig. 54-11).

Postoperative Management

Both eyes are bandaged, and the patient is kept in bed for several days. This routine varies with the surgical procedure; patients with scleral buckling operations are permitted out of bed much sooner than those who have undergone diathermy. Precautions are taken to prevent the patient from bumping his head. After a gradual resumption of function, the patient may resume usual activities in 3 to 5 weeks.

The psychological nursing care of this patient is of major importance. Diversion that is relaxing is desirable, such as

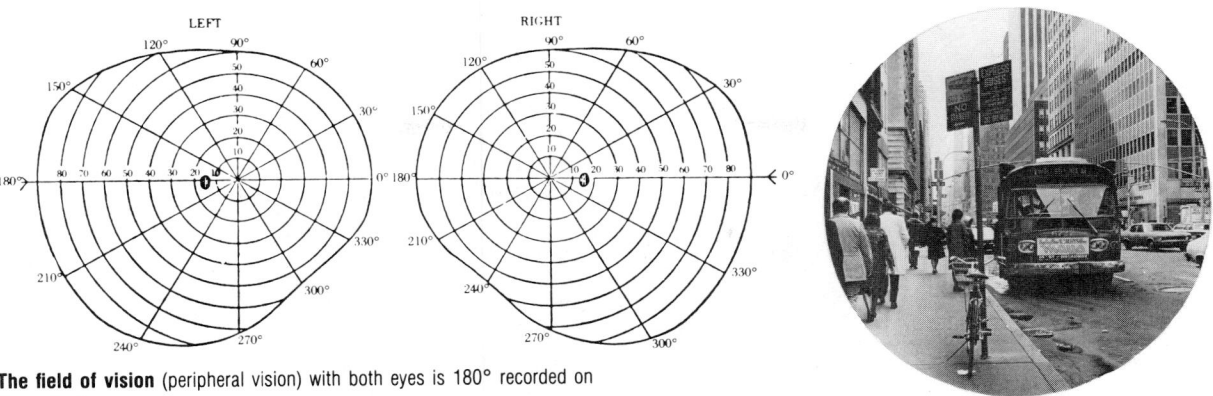

The field of vision (peripheral vision) with both eyes is 180° recorded on these charts.

Normal vision A person with normal or 20/20 vision sees this street scene.

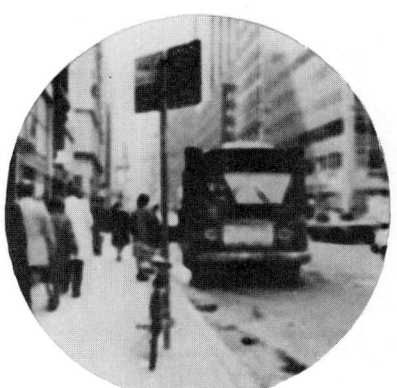

Cataract Diminished acuity from an opacity of the lens. The field of vision is unaffected. There is no scotoma, but the person has an overall haziness of the view, particularly in glaring light conditions.

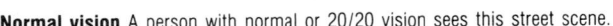

Glaucoma Advanced glaucoma involves loss of peripheral vision but the individual still retains most of his central vision.

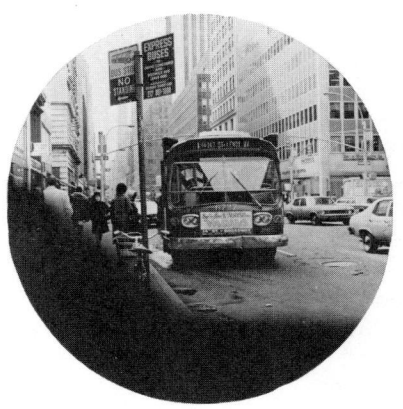

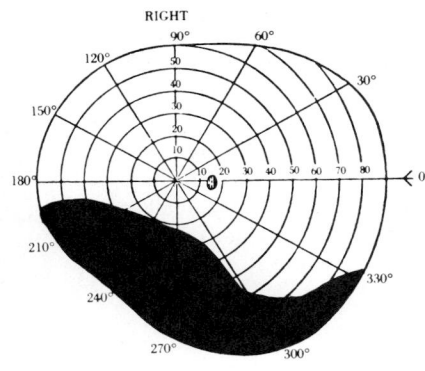

Retinal detachment shown here in the active stage. There are many causes for detachment, but the hole or tear allows fluid to lift the retina from its normal position. This elevated retina causes a field or vision defect, seen as a dark shadow in the peripheral field. It may be above, or below as illustrated.

Figure 54-10. Photographs representing the eye diseases are done as if the camera were the right eye. The accompanying visual-field chart showing the area of visual loss also represents the right eye. (Photo courtesy The Lighthouse, The New York Association for the Blind.)

conversation, listening to music, having someone read a favorite book, and so forth.* These patients become depressed easily; therefore, every attempt should be made to prevent this reaction.

At the time of discharge, the nurse should be sure that

---

* Recordings of books may be obtained from the public library or local association for the blind.

the patient understands all instructions for posthospital care and follow-up visits.

Prognosis. The prognosis for untreated retinal detachment is increasing detachment and eventual blindness. About 90% of patients can be cured with treatment. Some patients may require a second operation, which may be performed about 10 to 14 days after the first one. Twenty percent of all detachments are or will become bilateral.

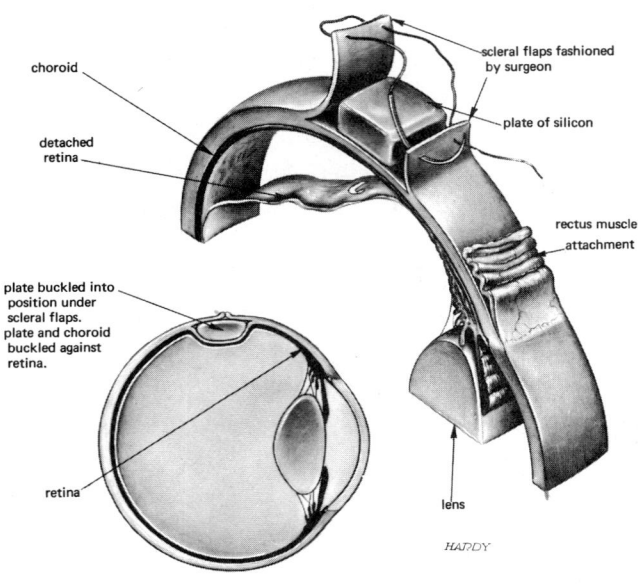

Figure 54-11. Scleral buckling for detached retina. (Ethicon, Inc.)

▷ Senile Macular Degeneration

Senile macular degeneration (SMD) is a retinal disease that may be (1) dry or atrophic, or (2) neovascular or exudative. It is a major cause of blindness among the elderly, but can now be postponed and even prevented by laser treatment.

Pathophysiology. In the "dry" form, deterioration of the macula proceeds very slowly, and most patients can retain their ability to read. In the neovascular type, sight impairment is more severe and can progress rapidly. The membrane between the retina and underlying layer of blood vessels deteriorates. Newly formed branches of vessels move toward the macula. If blood or fluid leaks into the macula, vision cells are destroyed.

Management. Light rays from an argon laser are focused on the tiny involved area of the retina (away from the macula) to seal abnormal blood vessels and a very small retinal area, thereby preventing further fluid leakage (photocoagulation). The success rate is remarkable in patients who are treated early.

▷ Cataracts

A *cataract* is an opacity of the crystalline lens or its capsule. Occasionally, it occurs at birth (congenital cataract) or in younger people as a result of trauma or disease, but most commonly it occurs in adults past middle age (senile cataract).

Pathophysiology. The normal lens is a clear, transparent, buttonlike structure lying in back of the iris; it possesses strong refractive powers. Physical and chemical changes may produce a loss of transparency of the lens. Swelling fibers, for example, cause a distortion of the image. A chemical change in lens protein may cause coagulation, thereby producing a cloudy appearance. Metabolic changes

that result in a reduction of vitamins C and B_{12} in the lens also contribute to the formation of opacities. Although cataracts can be produced in the laboratory in many ways, the real cause of senile cataracts is still unknown.

▶ Assessment

Diagnostic Evaluation. In addition to the usual eye tests, A-scan ultrasound (echography) and endothelial cell counter are particularly useful diagnostic tools. With an endothelial cell count of 2000 cells/mm², the patient is a good candidate for phacoemulsification and insertion of an intraocular lens.

Clinical Manifestations. Because the rays of light entering the eye must pass through the pupil and the lens to reach the retina, any opacity in the lens behind the pupil will produce alterations in vision. Objects may seem distorted, blurred, or hazy (see Fig. 54-10). In bright light, a cataract tends to scatter the light, causing an unpleasant glare. The patient experiences no pain, and visual loss is gradual. In time, the degenerative processes cause more opacification of the lens until the opacity becomes complete. Ordinarily, the lens is not visible; however, when a cataract develops, the pupil, which is normally black, becomes gray, and later milky white. The cataract can be cured only by operation.

Patient Problems/Nursing Diagnoses

Based on the clinical manifestations and diagnostic assessment data, the patient's potential nursing problems include impaired physical mobility related to vision deficit; psychosocial problems related to acceptance of visual deficit; fear related to surgical outcome if surgery is the only alternative; distress related to indecision about the type of surgery to choose; and depression related to the general deterioration process of aging.

▶ Planning and Implementation

Goals

The major goals for the patient include:

1. Acceptance of the progressive nature of cataract development and the need to submit to treatment
2. Adaptation to the requirements of immediate postcataract surgical care
3. Adjustment to alterations in visual–sensory function
4. Adherence to the physical requirements following cataract extraction
5. Ability to cope with psychosocial adjustments following cataract extraction

Surgical Management. In patients with uncomplicated senile cataracts, about 95% will regain satisfactory vision with surgery. Cataract surgery is done at the convenience of the patient and is usually requested when the sight in the better eye causes problems. There are three methods of restoring useful vision after cataract surgery: eyeglasses, contact lenses, and intraocular lenses.

Because this particular surgery can be performed safely on elderly patients, even those in their 90s, the nurse is in a position to dispel the belief that the patient may be "too old" for the procedure. Improvement of a visual defect may make a person more independent and happier.

The patient is oriented to his room so that he will be familiar with his environment when his eyes are bandaged after the operation. The room is also arranged in such a way that the patient's personal needs are considered. For example, the nurse could place the bedside table on the side where the eye with better vision is. The patient can then see his belongings with minimal head movement. Preoperative teaching stresses those activities and restrictions he will experience after the operation, as well as what position he will be expected to maintain if he is kept in bed.

Preoperative Preparation.   Some clinics recommend a facial scrub the evening before and the morning of surgery in order to reduce pathogens and postoperative infection. Prophylactic antimicrobial eye drops may also be administered.

The patient is informed that a local anesthetic will be given in the operating room and that the injection may be uncomfortable at first, but that this discomfort will abate quickly. The surgeon may converse with him during the procedure.

Usually, a sedative is prescribed the night before surgery, and a clear liquid breakfast is given the morning of the operation, depending on the time of day that the operation is scheduled. Preoperative medications in step-up fashion may be given in the morning, including a sedative, narcotic, and tranquilizer. Eye medications may include a topical mydriatic (which facilitates removal of the cataract when the pupil is dilated) and cycloplegics (to paralyze muscles of accommodation).

Surgical Procedures.   Two general types of lens extraction may be performed: extracapsular and intracapsular. *Extracapsular extraction* is more often performed for congenital and traumatic cataracts than for senile cataracts. An incision is made through the sclera, barely outside of the cornea; the lens capsule is excised, and the lens is expressed by pressure exerted on the eye from below with a metal spoon. It is more conservative and simple to perform than the intracapsular extraction; however, in about 30% of patients, a secondary membrane forms that requires *discission* (a needling, or dividing, of the membrane).

The *intracapsular extraction* consists of removing the lens and the capsule that encases it.

Intraoperative Management.   The eyelids are held apart with a speculum (self-retaining retractor) placed inside the lids. Guidelines and traction sutures are placed before the conjunctival incision is made at the 12 o'clock position; this incision is then extended to the 3 o'clock and 9 o'clock positions. The lens capsule is grasped, the cataract is delivered, and final suturing is done. If necessary, the surgeon reforms the anterior chamber with an injection of a balanced salt solution. Usually, an iridectomy is performed at the time of cataract extraction.

When difficulty is expected in freeing the capsule of its zonules, a fibrinolytic and proteolytic enzyme, α-Chymotrypsin, is injected into the anterior chamber under the iris. The lytic action is completed in 2 or 3 minutes and allows the lens to be extracted more easily.

Cryosurgery, a surgical technique in which freezing temperatures are used, is another method for extracting cataracts. All cryosurgical instruments operate on the principle that a cold metal adheres to a moist object. A thin, pencil-like instrument with a metal-probe tip (straight or curved) is activated so that the temperature of the tip ranges from $-30°$ C to $-40°$ C. The conjunctival flap is prepared and dissected as for a regular intracapsular extraction, after which the cryosurgical instrument is placed directly on the lens capsule. An ice ball forms in seconds, causing the capsule to adhere to the probe. A gentle upward and then sideward force frees and delivers the lens. The corneal flap is sutured back in place.

Cryoextraction is indicated for hypermature cataracts, which have a high incidence of capsular rupture, and in patients in whom a capsular rupture may exacerbate a glaucoma or uveitis. Nursing implications both before and after operation are the same as for the conventional intracapsular extraction.

Phacoemulsification is extracapsular removal of a lens by a mechanized instrument that is composed of three systems: irrigation, ultrasonic vibration, and aspiration. As the titanium tip of the instrument vibrates 40,000 times per second, the lens is broken up into minute particles, which are then aspirated. The procedure is generally done under local anesthesia with the use of a microscope. Following surgery, glycerin drops, an eye pad, and an eye shield are applied; the next morning, the dressing is removed, and the patient is discharged. Home care consists of instillation of cycloplegic and corticosteroid medications and a protective eye shield to be worn at night. The patient is permitted full activity with no restrictions.

An advantage for phacoemulsification over planned extracapsular or intracapsular extraction is that the cataract can be removed through a 2½-mm to 3-mm corneoscleral incision. The small incision requires closure with only one or two sutures and thus allows the patient a much more rapid return to usual activities.

An *intraocular implant* (IOL) is a prosthetic lens made of inert polymethylmethacrylate (Perspex, Plexiglas) with "wings" attached to the outer edges that permit the device to be attached to the iris in an anatomically correct position in the eye. This implant can be inserted following any type of cataract extraction.

The chief advantage of this procedure is the minimal distortion in the size or shape of the image. The ideal patient is one who is over 65 and possibly handicapped with arthritis, tremors, etc. (and who is therefore unable to manage spectacles or contact lenses).

Intraocular implants are not recommended for persons under 60 years of age, for a patient who already has an IOL and has developed a reaction, or for a patient who has cataracts in both eyes and is able to use eye glasses or contact lenses. The risk of infection is slightly higher than in simple cataract extraction. When there is extreme pupillary dilatation following lens implant, the implant may slip out of position.

Because existing safety data on the use of IOL are not currently available, the FDA published a regulation specifying the following clinical investigational procedures (applicable to physicians and manufacturers of intraocular lenses): (1) the sponsor of an IOL clinical investigation must receive prior approval from FDA (receiving an IDE—Investigational Device Exemption); (2) written informed-consent agreements must be signed by all prospective patients; and (3) all investigations are to be reviewed by Institutional Review

Boards of each medical facility involved. These regulations are not designed to disrupt research or present difficulties that might impede the availability and benefits of IOLs.

Postoperative care for the patient with an IOL is similar to the care for the cataract patient, described below. Constricting eyedrops are given to the patient having an iris-plane implant, to prevent it from dislodging. Steroid and antimicrobial eyedrops may be required. When the patient goes home, an eye patch or dark glasses must be worn for about a month if the eyes are sensitive to light and are watering. Length of stay in the hospital following cataract surgery may range from 24 hours to 10 days, depending on the type of surgery performed (*e.g.,* phacoemulsification,

intraocular implant, or extracapsular or intracapsular extraction).

For an overall view of the care of the patient undergoing cataract surgery, see Chart 54-2.

Postoperative Management. Major goals of postoperative care of the cataract patient (excluding phacoemulsification) are to prevent hemorrhage and stress on the sutures. The eye is kept bandaged for 1 day and an eye shield is worn over the dressing to protect the eye from injury. Only the operated eye is covered.

The patient is permitted a low, firm pillow immediately after operation and may have the head of the bed raised 30 to 45 degrees. Any strain felt by the patient may be relieved

---

Chart 54-2
Guidelines of Nursing Implementation for the Patient Undergoing Cataract Surgery

Major Goals for the Patient

1. Acceptance of the progressive nature of cataract development and the need to submit to treatment
2. Adaptation to the requirements of the immediate postcataract surgical care
3. Adjustment to alterations in visual-sensory function
4. Adherence to the physical requirements following cataract extraction
5. Coping with psychosocial adjustments following cataract extraction

Nursing Goals and Interventions

A. To prepare the patient for cataract surgery:
  1. Orient the patient to his new environment.
     a. Walk with the patient around the unit.
     b. Explain the plan of care.
     c. Provide side rails on bed if patient is elderly.
  2. Begin rehabilitation measures as soon after admission as possible.
     a. Teach patient to turn to side of the unaffected eye only.
     b. Instruct the patient how to close his eyes slowly without squeezing the lids.
  3. Reduce the conjunctival bacterial count.
     a. Obtain a conjunctival culture, if prescribed.
     b. Use local broad-spectrum antibiotics as prescribed.
     c. Use aseptic technique when doing eye treatments and procedures.
  4. Prepare the affected eye for surgery.
     a. Identify beyond a doubt the proper eye to be operated on.
     b. Instill local mydriatic if prescribed.
     c. Determine whether the pupil is dilated after the instillation of a mydriatic is completed.

B. To give optimal nursing care after the operation:
  1. Reorient the patient to his surroundings.

2. Prevent increased intraocular pressure and stress on the suture line.
     a. Instruct the patient not to cough, sneeze, or move too rapidly.
     b. Position the patient on his back and unoperated side.
     c. Elevate the head of the bed 30 to 45 degrees for comfort.
     d. Keep the eye shield on the operated eye to protect it from injury.
  3. Promote the comfort of the patient.
     a. Position him to relieve back pain.
     b. Give mild analgesics to control pain.
     c. Maintain a quiet and relaxed environment.
     d. Inform the patient when you enter the room.
  4. Observe and treat for complications of hemorrhage or pain.
     a. Notify physician immediately if patient complains of sudden pain in eye.
     b. Observe for, and try to allay, restlessness.

C. To promote the rehabilitation of the patient:
  1. Encourage the patient to become independent.
     a. Teach him to increase his activities gradually.
     b. Walk with him when he gets out of bed.
  2. Instruct the patient and his family about the use of eyedrops.
  3. Refer the patient to proper agencies if home assistance is needed.
  4. Assist the patient to participate in a program of diversional activities during the convalescent period.
  5. Inform the patient that:
     a. Dark glasses may be used after the eye dressing is removed.
     b. Temporary corrective lenses may be prescribed during the convalescent period.
     c. Permanent lenses will be prescribed 6 to 8 weeks after surgery, unless the patient has intraocular implant(s).

somewhat by placing pillows under the knees for short intervals and a small pillow under the small of the back. Later in the day, he may be allowed out of bed, depending on his condition and the physician's preference. However, he is advised to move cautiously and slowly and to avoid straining for at least 3 weeks. For example, he ought not to stoop, pick up objects from the floor, or lift anything. Slip-in slippers will avoid the necessity to bend to tie laces. Even if the patient has vision in one eye, he should not walk through corridors alone; this will prevent his being bumped because of an inability to see objects or persons on the operated side.

Pain usually is slight after cataract extraction, but should it become severe, the surgeon is to be notified at once since it may be the symptom of a serious complication, such as hemorrhage.

Liquid diet is supplemented with custards, junkets, and gelatin. Soft or regular diet is resumed when desired.

Atropine may be instilled 1 hour after operation by the surgeon to relieve pain. Dressings are changed twice daily by the physician for 3 to 5 days.

The effects of sensory deprivation can be minimized if the patient is kept interested in diversional activities, such as the radio, "talking books," or visitors. He is discharged the day after surgery if no complications arise.

Patient Instruction.   Patient instruction includes instillation of eye drops as prescribed, application of moist compresses, and use of a plastic shield at night to protect the operated eye. The eyelids are not to be squeezed together, since this may injure the suture line or cause hemorrhage.

For the patient who is to have eyeglasses, about 3 weeks after the operation, the aphakic (without lens) patient receives a temporary pair of thick biconvex glasses. Adjustment to these is gradual. The sides curve inward, the bottom curves upward, and the top curves downward. Only through the center of the glass will the patient have clear vision. He must learn to turn his head to bring an object into central vision. The patient needs practice in judging distances, such as when climbing stairs or pouring liquids. Objects appear one third larger than they really are. Contact lenses reduce this size discrepancy and allow adjustment to binocular vision more readily. However, not all individuals can adjust to contact lenses. In about 8 weeks, permanent lenses are ordered. By this time, the patient should be making a satisfactory psychological, physical, and visual adjustment (see Chart 54-2).

Behavioral Disturbances in Patients Having Cataract Surgery.   Modern advances in cataract extraction that permit early mobilization, permitting one eye and in some instances both eyes to be uncovered, and a short hospital stay have reduced the incidence of postoperative psychosis to less than 1%. That sensory deprivation is the cause of psychoses following cataract extraction has been refuted. Rather, it appears more likely that postoperative behavioral disturbances represent an acute form of senile psychosis due to psychologic stress.

The elderly depressed patient frequently has experienced a series of frustrations—loneliness; retirement with little activity to replace his former busy life; sensing a feeling of uselessness; a perceptible, steady deterioration of physical and mental abilities; reduced income; a feeling of being rejected by his children, who probably live a distance from him; and the death of a spouse or close friends. As a result of these stresses, this person's basic personality emerges and can be detected by the nurse as depressed, hypochondriacal, flighty, suspicious, or rambling. When such stress becomes overpowering, contact with reality ceases, and the patient becomes psychotic (senile psychosis).

Patterns of behavioral disturbances emerge, such as disorientation, psychomotor disturbances, paranoid delusions, hallucinations, elation, somatic complaints, and anxiety. Some authorities believe that a relationship exists within tissues that have common embryonal origins: in this event, cataracts occur along with other organic brain disease, such as alopecia totalis, and degenerative changes in the cerebral cortex. This may account for many behavioral disturbances.

Another cause of disturbed behavioral manifestations often results from the effects of sedative drugs on patients with organic brain disease. On the whole, it is acceded that degenerative processes in the cerebral cortex are difficult to diagnose; the varying effects of stress depends basically on the patient's emotional reserve.

Symptoms of postoperative behavioral disturbances are usually classified in two major groups: depression and excitement. Both forms are attempts to deny vision loss and helplessness. In summary, one can predict postoperative problems in those persons who have a history of marginal social adjustment (drinking heavily, getting into fights), are excessively frail, and have chronic disabling illness, a language barrier, or a low self-esteem, or any of the problems discussed in this section.

Prophylaxis and Nursing Intervention.   A very effective way to handle postoperative behavioral disturbances is to provide opportunities for the patient to verbalize his anxieties and concerns. If he is praised for his cooperation, even more worries may be elicited, which permits the nurse to target nursing intervention.

Placing the patient in a unit in which there is a stable or well-adjusted roommate can be effective. Permitting a close friend to stay with the patient the day before surgery is helpful. Tranquilizers, his customary evening cocktail, or a night light are all helpful the evening prior to surgery.

Following surgery, compatible and optimistic persons in contact with the patient will reinforce his "good" thoughts. Antianxiety medication may be prescribed. Friendly visitors are helpful, as are pleasant radio and TV programs. If depression occurs, antidepressant drugs may be required.

▶ Evaluation

Expected Outcomes

1. Accepts the progressive nature of cataract development and the need to submit to treatment
   a. Discusses his condition and the need for surgery
   b. Selects surgical correction best suited to his condition
   c. Asks direct questions relating to mobility during the postoperative phase
   d. Inquires as to the kind of anesthetic agent to be used

e. Expresses concern about experiencing pain post-operatively
2. Adapts to the requirements of immediate postcataract surgery
   a. Calls nurse when getting out of bed for first time (because he may experience possible hypotension with some medications)
   b. Describes pain when it is experienced (caused by spasm of the ciliary muscle)
   c. Keeps fingers and tissue-wipes away from eye (it is expected that eye will tear, blur, or itch because of reaction to sutures)
   d. Asks for sunglasses when eye patch is removed (because of sensitivity to light)
3. Adjusts to alterations in visual-sensory function
   a. Indicates the range of vision possibilities with his "new lens"
   b. Describes the widened scope of activities that he can now pursue
   c. Recites the precautions he must take to ensure optimum vision
4. Adheres to the physical requirements following cataract extraction
   a. Adapts to the changes required, such as using eye-glasses or contact lenses
   b. Washes hands before and after treating eye
   c. Instills eyedrops as prescribed
   d. Demonstrates effective technique in keeping peri-orbital area clean, including eyelashes
   e. Makes notations regarding follow-up visits with his family physician as well as ophthalmologist
5. Copes with psychosocial adjustment required following cataract extraction
   a. Describes his new life-style, which will permit activities he was unable to do immediately before surgery
   b. Enumerates stress-relieving experiences, such as listening to music; participates in pleasurable activities
   c. Relates a positive attitude that reveals optimistic thinking
   d. Decries his former attitudes that led to depression and antisocialism

▷ Glaucoma

Glaucoma is a disease characterized by increased tension or pressure within the eye and progressive loss of visual field (see Fig. 54-10). It ordinarily occurs in individuals past 40 and may be classified as primary or secondary:

Primary
1. Chronic simple glaucoma (open-angle)
2. Congestive glaucoma (closed-angle)
   a. Acute
   b. Chronic

Secondary
Many types secondary to such conditions as trauma, aphakia, iritis, tumor, hemorrhage, etc.

Primary Glaucoma

The cause of primary glaucoma is unknown. Some evidence indicates that chronic simple glaucoma, the most common form, is inherited. This disorder is the second most common cause of blindness in the United States. In view of the fact that about 1 million Americans have undiagnosed glaucoma, health professionals have a responsibility to encourage annual eye checkups, because *early detection could substantially reduce the incidence of blindness from glaucoma.*

Pathophysiology. Intraocular pressure increases when the patient exerts energy, as in running, climbing the stairs, bending over to pick up an object, sneezing, or turning the head suddenly. It also occurs in relation to emotional upsets (*e.g.,* apprehension about the nature and prognosis of surgery may cause an increase in pressure). Apparently, both physical and emotional factors are involved in increasing pressure within the eye. The underlying mechanism is episcleral venous pressure engorgement transmitted by the Valsalva phenomenon. The total volume and pressure of intraocular fluid is regulated by the balance between formation and reabsorption of aqueous humor. Ordinarily, the pressure-regulating mechanism maintains an almost constant balance throughout life. The exact operation of this mechanism is not known; however, pathologic changes at the iridocorneal angle usually increase intraocular pressure. Early detection of increased ocular pressure (22 mm Hg–30 mm Hg) does not necessarily mean the patient will develop frank glaucoma.

▶ **Assessment**

Clinical Manifestations. Symptoms are insidious and develop slowly. The patient may have mild discomfort, such as a tired feeling in the eye. Impairment of peripheral vision occurs long before any effects are noted on central vision. The patient may become aware of peripheral visual impairment by bumping into things that he did not see at his side; driving a car may be a hazard to others, because he may not be able to see pedestrians or vehicles approaching laterally. The patient may also note halos around lights.

Diagnostic Assessment and Measurement of Intraocular Pressure. An increase in intraocular pressure or hardening of the eyeball may be noted with the fingers, but more accurately it is measured by means of tonometry, tonography, and peripheral vision testing. *Tonometry* is a simple and painless test in which the patient tilts his head back and looks to the ceiling (Fig. 54-12). The cornea of the eye is anesthetized with a drop of 0.5% Ophthaine. The sterile footplate of the tonometer is placed on the cornea; a small pressure is applied to the central plunger, causing the central cornea to be displaced inward. Pressure within the eye exerts a force that moves an indicator. A normal reading is 11 mm Hg to 22 mm Hg.

Electronic tonometry can be done (applanation, air), but it involves expensive equipment. Tonography units provide a graphic presentation of intraocular pressure for a 4-minute test period. This is a valuable index that assists the physician in determining movement in the aqueous humor. Peripheral vision testing is done to test side vision, since impaired side vision is a sign of glaucoma. Gonioscopy is done to determine the angle between the iris and cornea.

Patient Problems/Nursing Diagnoses

Based on the clinical manifestations and diagnostic assessment data, the patient's potential nursing problems include increasingly impaired vision related to inadequate drainage of aqueous humor; depression related to progressive visual sensory deficit; anxiety related to ability to perform required medicine instillations; concern about controlling emotional and physical activities that aggravate or increase eye pressure; and concern about interruption of life-style related to impact of the glaucoma condition.

▶ Planning and Implementation

Goals

The major goals for the patient include

1. Control of the progressive nature of glaucoma
2. Learning as much about glaucoma as possible
3. Acceptance of surgery to control glaucoma if pharmacotherapy fails
4. Improvement of the quality of life-style
5. Reduction of anxiety and depression

The goal of management is to provide the optimum method in controlling the progression of glaucoma.

Management.   Treatment depends on the stage of the condition, the degree of the reduced angle between the iris and cornea, the response to medication, and the reliability of the patient in adhering to the regimen. In general, pharmacotherapy can keep the condition under control; however, there are alternate options (surgery), including laser treatment.

Pharmacotherapy and Surgical Management.   Primary (open-angle) glaucoma often is treated by one or a combination of the following medications: (1) miotics, such as pilocarpine or carbachol, to increase outflow of aqueous humor; (2) carbonic anhydrase inhibitors, such as acetazolamide (Diamox) or dichlorphenamide (Daranide), to decrease the production of aqueous humor; (3) anticholinesterase, such as echothiophate iodide (Phospholine Iodide) or demecarium bromide (Humorsol), to facilitate the outflow of aqueous humor; and (4) epinephrine drops, to decrease production of aqueous humor and promote its outflow from the eye.

Timolol maleate (Timoptic), a beta-adrenergic receptor blocking agent, is popular for the treatment of primary open-angle glaucoma, aphakic glaucoma, and, in selected patients, secondary glaucoma. It appears to be better tolerated than previously used drugs. When applied topically, timolol decreases production of aqueous humor and reduces intraocular pressure for as long as 24 hours. Pupillary size is not changed nor is the tone of the ciliary body altered; hence, this medication does not interfere with vision.

Drug dosage of timolol is usually one drop twice a day. Occasionally, mild eye irritation or brief blurred vision occurs with timolol. This medication is prescribed with caution for

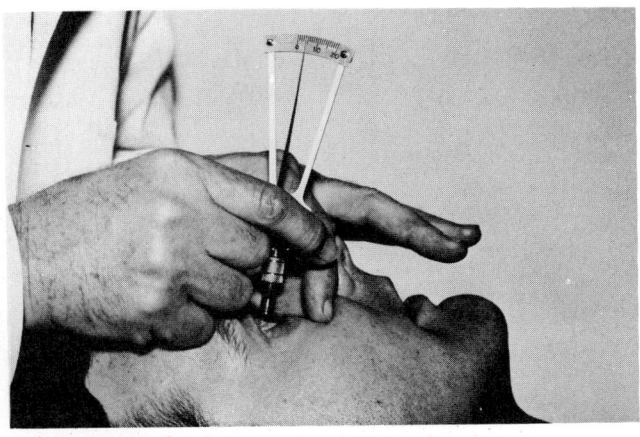

Figure 54-12.   After a local anesthetic is instilled into the eye, the Schiøtz tonometer is gently rested on the eyeball; the indicator measures in mm Hg the ocular tension. (Courtesy, F. H. Roy, M.D.)

patients who may have adverse effects from systemic use of beta-adrenergic receptor blocking agents (such as patients with asthma, heart block, or heart failure).

Remissions may occur, but if there is no improvement, surgery may be done. In the preoperative treatment of these patients, irrigations of both eyes are often prescribed, and weaker solutions of pilocarpine are instilled in the unaffected eye.

The goal in treatment is to decrease the buildup of fluid or increase the rate of drainage through the canal of Schlemm. The surgeon makes a small opening with a circular knife at the junction of the cornea and the sclera. This operation, called *corneal trephining,* leaves a permanent opening through which aqueous humor may drain. Usually, it is covered by a flap of conjunctiva. *Laser trabeculectomy* is growing in popularity; this also achieves the same goals. (Trabeculectomy is the removal of a section of trabecular meshwork, permitting fluid to drain freely.)

Postoperative Management.   After the operation, the patient is kept flat and relatively quiet for 24 hours in order to prevent prolapse of the iris through the incision. He may turn to the unoperated side. Straining, coughing, squeezing the eyelid, and any other activity that can raise intraocular pressure is to be avoided. A liquid diet is permitted. Narcotics or sedatives may be given if necessary. After the first dressing is changed, the patient is allowed more freedom. The hospital stay usually lasts 3 days. Regular visits to the ophthalmologist are required, since glaucoma is a condition that must be followed periodically.

Acute (Closed-Angle) Glaucoma

(See Fig. 54-13.)

Clinical Manifestations.   When pressure increases rapidly, severe pain occurs in and around the eye. Artificial lights appear to have a rainbow around them, and vision becomes cloudy or blurred. The eye is red and the cornea

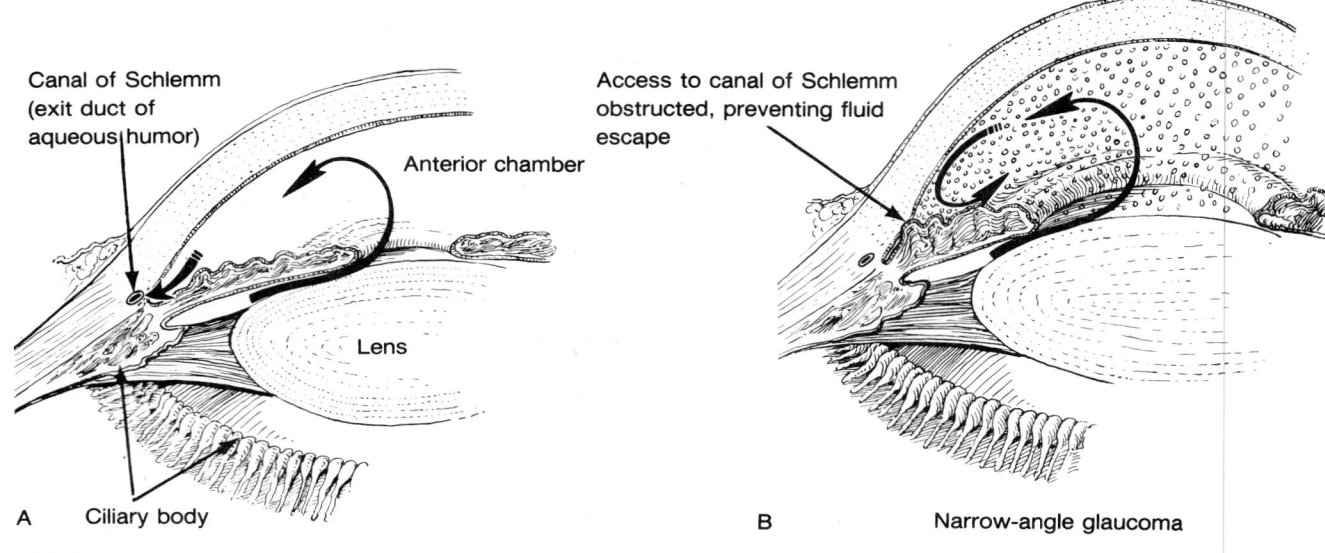

Figure 54-13. (A) Normal flow of aqueous fluid through Canal of Schlemm. (B) Obstruction to the flow of fluid, causing closed-angle glaucoma. (From Lechliger M and Moya F: Introduction to the Practice of Anesthesia, 2nd ed. New York, Harper & Row, 1978.)

is steamy; nausea and vomiting, as well as pupil dilatation, also may be noted. Intraocular pressure is elevated. This is an emergency situation, which, if left untreated, may lead to blindness.

> **NOTE:** Acute closed-angle glaucoma may be precipitated in individuals who have narrow anterior chamber angles by administering anticholinergic drugs, such as atropine and scopolamine.

Management.   Management consists of pharmacotherapy and surgical interventions.

Pharmacotherapy.   Miotic drugs will cause the pupil to contract and the iris to draw away from the cornea, thus allowing the aqueous humor to drain through the lymph spaces into the canal of Schlemm. Pilocarpine, physostigmine (Eserine), or DFP (diisopropyl fluorophosphate) are the drugs employed. Dosage and frequency of drops are regulated to meet the individual requirements.

Another kind of medication (carbonic anhydrase inhibitor) restricts the action of the enzyme that is necessary to produce aqueous humor. Diamox is an example of such an agent. This aids in getting some patients in better condition for surgery and may control tension in other patients to such an extent that surgery is not necessary.

Ordinary U.S.P. glycerin (oral) reduces intraocular pressure through the mechanism of osmotic balance exchange. Glycerin has a high osmotic pressure; it withdraws fluid from the eye through the membrane, and lowers pressure. Mannitol (20%) intravenously may also be used.

Surgical Intervention.   In acute closed-angle glaucoma, an incision is made through the cornea so that a portion of the iris may be drawn out and excised (*iridectomy*). This may be peripheral or sector (keyhole) iridectomy. An iridectomy prevents the iris from bulging forward to crowd the chamber angle and permits drainage of aqueous humor

from the anterior chamber, thereby reducing intraocular tension. Other operations on the iris (*iridencleisis*) are modifications having the same goal, that is, the escape of fluid.

Patient Education.   Although glaucoma cannot be cured, it can be controlled to a great extent. Whether the patient has had surgery or not, certain limitations must be set.

Activities that may increase intraocular pressure and should be avoided are:

1. Excessive fluid intake
2. Use of antihistamines or sympathomimetic medications without proper medical management

A *recommended activity* is carrying a card or "dog tag" indicating that the individual has glaucoma.

▶ **Evaluation**

Expected Outcomes

1. Achieves control of progressive nature of glaucoma
   a. Keeps regular appointments with ophthalmologist
   b. Tells other health care professionals the name of the glaucoma medication he is taking (*e.g.*, tells dentist, etc.)
   c. Lists side-effects of medications to be reported if experienced
   d. Adheres to self-care instillation of eye drops
   e. Avoids emotionally upsetting encounters
2. Learns as much about glaucoma as possible
   a. Participates in group classes arranged for glaucoma patients
   b. Reads the pamphlets on glaucoma provided by the nurse
   c. Asks questions about his particular symptoms

d. Joins a glaucoma group to exchange ideas

e. Relates to spouse what he has learned about his condition

f. Encourages family members to have regular eye checks, since glaucoma tends to run in families

3. Accepts surgery to control glaucoma if pharmacotherapy fails

a. Asks questions relating to type of anesthetic agent he will receive

b. Queries about length of time to be in bed postoperatively

c. Relates description of actual surgical procedure after talking with ophthalmologist

d. Tells spouse of his willing acceptance of surgery, since the alternative is too risky

e. Talks of future plans when he is discharged from hospital

4. Demonstrates improvement in the quality of life-style

a. Visits ophthalmologist regularly, even if no symptoms present

b. Carries an identification card stating he is being treated for glaucoma

c. Establishes regular times to self-administer eye medications

d. Relates his enjoyment of a balanced recreational program: some eye-demanding, some ear-demanding (TV and radio)

5. Copes with anxiety and depression

a. Communicates feelings about glaucoma

b. Tells of specific fears—pain, blindness

c. Indicates his willingness to give up driving "because my side vision is impaired"

d. Identifies support systems in times of crisis

e. Relates the various ways of treating glaucoma, thereby dispelling "fear of the unknown"

f. Tells of importance of having periodic eye pressure checks

▷ Blindness or Near Blindness

Telescopic eyeglasses and magnifying glasses are easily accessible aids that can be recommended by the nurse for those who have exhausted conventional prescribed lenses.

Mobility aids are probably the most basic need for the visually impaired. One needs reassurance that he can move safely from one place to the next. Only about 1% of the blind use guide dogs—probably the reason is that most sightless persons are over age 65, and they are less trusting of dogs and may even have difficulty keeping up with them. The most useful aid is a long, lightweight cane that very subtly provides accurate information by simple maneuvers and assures that the next step is safe in a small, limited area. Overhead hazards are not detected, however.

Other aids are available to supplement the cane in enlarging the world of the visually impaired person. A flashlight eye sonar device (Morvat Sensor*) emits ultrasound waves that bounce back from objects up to 3.66 meters (4 yards). A Sonicguide* has its transmitter and receivers built into an

eyeglass frame. An earphone piece converts sound into a different pitch, loudness, and tone. The lower the pitch, the closer the object. Quality of tone enables the wearer to distinguish surface characteristics—glass, concrete, or wooden walls. Interpretation can be a problem. Recent research is attempting to use the sonar focusing element in the Polaroid camera into a mobility device that minimizes sonic confusion.

Laser canes are also available. A particular model sends out three beams: straight ahead, at head level, and in front of the feet. When an object crosses a beam, the user is warned by hearing a buzzing sound. Such sophisticated devices unfortunately are expensive at present.

For reading (work, study, leisure), a portable electronic magnifying system is available. In this system, one moves a small hand-held camera across the page and then views on a display screen a bright magnified image of the text (Viewscan by Wormald).

Additional aids are telescopic lenses (Honey Bee lens†), a bug-eyed arrangement, glasses combined with mirrors, nightscopes, closed-circuit TV cameras, and fiber-optic systems. By being aware of these possibilities, the nurse is able to recommend invaluable aids to the person with such a need.

▷ Enucleation

Removal of the eyeball, *enucleation,* is necessitated by a variety of factors, including trauma that forces the contents of the globe to escape, infections, and other injuries that threaten to lead to sympathetic ophthalmia (see p. 1243). During the removal of the eye, muscles are cut as close to the globe as possible. These muscles are approximated with sutures over a plastic prosthesis, thereby providing the means for coordinated motion of the prosthesis with the patient's real eye. A plastic, gold, or Teflon ball is placed in the area of the removed eyeball to form a stump on which the ocularist fixes the prosthesis (artificial eye). This prosthesis is colored to match the patient's eye. In successful cases, it is difficult to distinguish the prosthesis from the normal eye.

In certain cases, the sclera can be retained and the rest of the contents of the eye "scooped" out; this procedure is known as *evisceration.* The main advantage of evisceration is that it provides better motion to the artificial eye. The disadvantage is that sympathetic ophthalmia may occur.

Exenteration is usually performed in advanced malignancy or severe war injuries. In this procedure, the eyelids, the eyeball, and all contents of the orbit are removed, down to the bone. This operation is *very* disfiguring, and although the ocularist may attempt to build a prosthesis, it very often appears rather poor and unlifelike. These patients usually wear a black patch.

▷ The Newly Blind

The number of blind people in the world is estimated at 40 million, or approximately 1% of the population; in some

---

* Sensory Aids Corporation, Bensenville, Illinois.

† Vision, New York, New York.

areas, this figure approaches 4%. Between 15 and 25 million of these people have preventable or easily curable blindness. There are about 1,000,000 blind persons in America, and each year nearly 50,000 more go blind. Of these newly blind cases, approximately half could have been prevented with our present knowledge.

When an individual has marked visual impairment or is newly blind, he needs a great deal of help in making a healthy adjustment. For the most part, this help is entrusted to those skilled in such rehabilitation. However, a nurse can follow certain practices when caring for such a person.

The nurse recognizes that there are stages through which this person moves:

1. Denial—Do not deny this phase of the sightless person's experience, since it is a stage through which the person must go.
2. Value changes—adapting to aids that he thought he would never use
3. Independence–dependence conflict—attempting to accept his place without becoming completely dependent
4. Coping with stigma—This person must adjust to unfortunate stigma that is so prevalent among the sighted toward the sightless, such as they are "helpless," "unemployable," "completely dependent," "depressed."
5. Learning to communicate in social settings without visual cues

Goals and Interventions.   The major goals for the patient are to accept the sightless/nearly sightless condition:

1. Adaptation to the use of auxiliary aids.
2. Acceptance of his new visual role without becoming completely dependent
3. Continuing with physical self-care
4. Coping with the social climate and stigmata that are prevalent
5. Learning to communicate without visual clues
6. Adherence to the prescribed therapeutic regimen

The nurse is able to assist the patient in several ways: (1) patient teaching, (2) patient support, (3) patient care, and (4) collaboration with the physician.

Patient teaching is done to familiarize the patient with the anatomy of the eye and its function. By monitoring what the physician has told the patient relative to diagnosis, anticipated treatment, and prognosis, the nurse is able to reinforce this information, answer questions, provide support, and relay back to the ophthalmologist the reaction of the patient and his family. If information is withheld, such as little hope for recovery of vision, this will interfere with the patient's adjustment and rehabilitation. The nurse is often helpful in determining when the time is right for conveying such information. Fears are to be described because they can unearth misinformation. Frequently, self-imposed limitations are more restricting than physical disabilities, such as blindness. Even attitudes and beliefs of the nurse can have a direct or indirect effect on the patient. Such attitudes need to be confronted so that only genuine feelings are transmitted. A positive attitude by those who care for patients will affect the patient's self-esteem and body image in a beneficial way.

A blind person should always be treated with the dignity accorded any other human being. Avoid expressions of pity. Keep the patient from becoming discouraged by seeing to it that he has someone with whom he can talk or that he has some other form of diversion, such as a radio. Help him to overcome his feeling of awkwardness as he performs simple activities.

If he is allowed out of bed, the blind person should survey his room by walking around and touching the furniture. Thereafter, the nurse should be sure that the furniture remains in the same position. Never leave a door half open; it should be either open or shut. When walking with a blind person, allow him to follow you by lightly touching your elbow; do not push him ahead of you. When he walks alone, he should learn to use a lightweight walking stick to warn him of obstacles.

Personal appearance is a significant part of the patient's care. He should be allowed to dress by himself; a woman even can learn to fix her hair and use cosmetics. Table etiquette, writing, etc., are activities that can be acquired with practice.

Familiarity with resources that are available is a nursing responsibility. When a patient is declared legally blind, he should be referred to the state blindness agency. A directory of agencies serving the visually handicapped in the United States is available from the American Foundation for the Blind.* In most states, the only way to obtain rehabilitation training is through a state agency for the blind. Other resources are "Seeing Eye," and state libraries for the blind, which provide prerecorded magazines and books, Talking Book machines, and cassettes.

Interesting and effective aids are devices that "talk"— clocks, calculators, thermometers, scales, etc. There also is an optical scanner that when passed over lines of text in a book, send signals to a computer (programmed to recognize letters) that turns them into words and pronounces them. Another similar device scans words that records the shape of letters, which are then converted into vibrations felt by the fingertips of the user.

Technology continues to provide devices that are becoming available and useful in expanding the world of the sightless.

▷ # Bibliography
Books

Ernest J (ed). Yearbook of Ophthalmology. Chicago, Year Book Medical Publishers, 1980.

Jaffe NS. Cataract Surgery and Its Complications. St Louis, CV Mosby, 1981.

Michels RG. Vitreous Surgery. St Louis, CV Mosby, 1981.

Newell F. Ophthalmology, 5th ed. St Louis, CV Mosby, 1982.

Roth HW and Roth–Wittig M. Contact Lenses. A Handbook for Patients. Hagerstown, Maryland, Harper & Row, 1980.

Shields M. Study Guide for Glaucoma. Baltimore, Williams & Wilkins, 1982.

* 15 West 16th St., New York, New York 10011.

Smith JF and Nachazel DP Jr. Ophthalmological Nursing. New York, Little, Brown & Co, 1980.

Vaughan D and Asbury T. General Ophthalmology. Los Altos, Lange, 1980.

Wingate RB. An Atlas of Ophthalmic Surgery, 3rd ed. Philadelphia, JB Lippincott, 1981.

Articles
Assessment

Au YK and Henkind P. Pain elicited by consensual pupillary reflex: A diagnostic test for acute iritis. Lancet 1981 Dec 5; 2(8258):1254–1255.

Bodis–Wollner I. Test your eyes in 7 minutes. American Health 1982 Nov/Dec; 1(5):52–53.

Byrne SF and Saclarides EE. Standardized ophthalmological echography and the health care professional. Journal of Ophthalmic Nursing and Technology 1982 May; 1(1):19–27.

Howes DH. The concept of vision. Journal of Ophthalmic Nursing and Technology 1982 May; 1(1):7–11.

Jones M and Tippett T. Assessment of the red eye. Nurse Pract 1980 Jan–Feb; 5(1):10–15.

Norman S. The pupil check. Am J Nurs 1982 Apr; 82(4):588–591.

Sagaties MJ. Screening for strabismus and amblyopia. Nurse Pract 1982 Apr; 7(4):19–23.

Sekuler R and Mulvanny P. 20/20 is not enough. American Health 1982 Nov/Dec; 1(5):50–56.

Eye Conditions

Adverse systemic effects from ophthalmic drugs. The Medical Letter 1982 May 28; 24(610):53–54.

Alexander W. Systemic side effects with eye drops. Br J Med 1981 Apr 25; 282(1):1359.

Blackburn DR and Peterson LK. Oculoplethysmography. Nursing '82 1982; 12(10):76–78.

Economou E et al. Handling ophthalmic epidemics with a focus on acute hemorrhagic conjunctivitis. Journal of Ophthalmic Nursing and Technology 1982 Aug; 1(2):9–15.

Gallagher MA. Corneal transplantation. Am J Nurs 1981 Oct; 81(10):1845.

Gaston NC. Kerato refractive surgery; new horizons. AORN J 1981 May; 33(6):1068–1074.

Havron D. How lasers save sight. Science Digest 1981 Oct; 89(9):42–45.

Institute, keratotomists don't see eye to eye (re: keratotomy). Science 1981 July 24; 213(4506):423–424.

Johnson L. Retrolental fibroplasia: A new look at an unsolved problem. Hosp Pract 1981 May; 16(5):109–121.

Johnson L. Laser permits new techniques in eye surgery. AORN J 1982 Jan; 35(1):78–79.

Moore CR. Scleral buckling for retinal detachment. AORN J 1982 Sept; 36(3):495–506.

Norman S. The pupil check. Am J Nurs 1982 Apr; 82(4):588–591.

Phenylephrine eye drops and beta-blockers. The Medical Letter 1982 July 23; 24(614):70.

Sagaties MJ. Screening for strabismus and amblyopia. Nurse Pract 1982 Apr; 7(4):19–27.

Schneeman YT and Taylor JA. A technical look at vitrectomy. AORN J 1981 Apr; 33(5):867–872.

Sekuler R and Mulvanny P. 20/20 is not enough. Am Health 1982 Nov/Dec; 1(5):50–55.

Senile macular degeneration. Test yourself. Am J Nurs 1982 Aug; 82(8):1217.

Contact Lenses

Rakow PL. Perspective on contact lenses. Journal of Ophthalmic Nursing and Technology 1982 May; 1(1):44–45.

Rakow PL. Rethinking the refitting of rigid contact lenses. Journal of Ophthalmic Nursing and Technology 1982 Aug; 1(2):32–35.

Rietschel RL and Wilson LA. Ocular inflammation in patients using soft contact lenses. Arch Dermatol 1982 Mar; 118(3):147–149.

Cataract

Hill BJ. Sensory information, behavioral instructions and coping with sensory alteration surgery (cataract). Nurs Res 1982 Jan/Feb; 31(1):17–21.

Glaucoma

Katz IM and Soll DB. Beta blockers and glaucoma. Am Fam Physician 1980 Apr; 21(4):150–151.

Saclarides EE. Fundamentals in focus: Glaucoma. Journal of Ophthalmic Nursing and Technology 1982 May; 1(1):38–42.

Vision Loss

Oehler JW. The role of the ophthalmic nurse in helping the patient adapt to loss of vision. Journal of Ophthalmic Nursing and Technology 1982 May; 1(1):28–32.

Steeton D Jr. Coping with blindness. N Engl J Med 1981; 305(8):458–460.

Agencies

American Association of Ophthalmology, 1100 17th St., NW, Washington, D.C. 20036

American Council of the Blind, 501 N. Douglas Ave., Oklahoma City, Oklahoma 73106

American Foundation for the Blind, 15 W 16th St., New York, New York 10011

Contact Lens Society of America, 301 First National Bldg., Lexington, Kentucky 40507

Eye-Bank Association of America, 3195 Maplewood Ave., Winston–Salem, North Carolina 27103

Large Print Ltd., 505 Pearl St., Buffalo New York 14204

Leader Dogs for the Blind, 1039 Rochester Rd., Rochester, Michigan 48063

National Society for the Prevention of Blindness, 79 Madison Ave., New York, New York 10016

The Seeing Eye, Morristown, New Jersey 07960

55

Assessment and Management of Patients With Hearing Problems and Ear Disorders

The ear is a very complex sense organ with a dual function—hearing and the maintenance of equilibrium (Fig. 55-1). The early detection and the accurate diagnosis of ear and hearing disorders are important in both children and adults. Among those who take an important part in the diagnosis of auditory disorders are pediatricians, otolaryngologists, psychiatrists, neurologists, psychologists, speech pathologists, educators, and audiologists. Before a child can speak, he must first be able to hear, then to interpret what he hears, and, lastly, to express himself in speech. Disorders due to birth injury, bacterial and viral infections in childhood, toxic drug effects, damage to the ear by noise, and changes in the ear as the result of aging are only a few of the problems that require assessment, treatment, and rehabilitation.

▷ Noise and Its Effect on Hearing

One of the waste products of the 20th century is noise (unwanted and unavoidable sound). The sheer volume of noise that surrounds us daily has grown from a simple annoyance into a potentially dangerous source of physical and psychological damage.

In terms of physical impact, loud, persistent noise can cause constriction of peripheral blood vessels, alterations in blood pressure and heart rate (because of increased output of adrenalin), disturbances in equilibrium, and increased gastrointestinal activity. Additional research is required to answer many questions regarding the overall effects of noise on the human body. However, one thing seems beyond dispute—a quiet environment is more conducive to peace of mind; in the hospital, patients are happier and less upset when noise is kept to a minimum.

Sound Intensity and Frequency. Scientists measure sound *intensity* (pressure exerted by sound) in decibels (dB). For example, the shuffling of papers in quiet surroundings represents about 15 dB; a low conversation, 40 dB; and a jet plane 100 feet away about 140 dB. Sound above 80 dB begins to grate harshly upon the human ear.

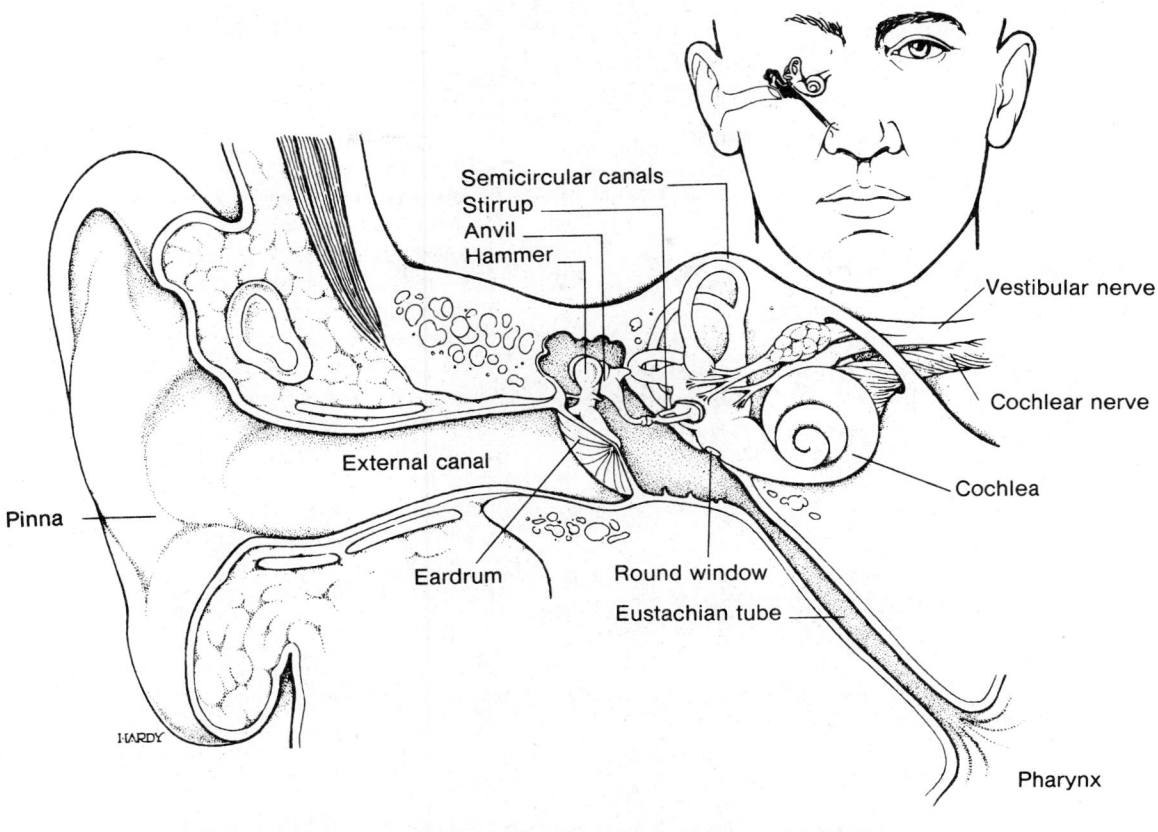

Figure 55-1. Anatomy of the ear.

Over the last several decades, the loudest sounds to which humans are exposed have grown from 120 dB (the roar of a small, two-engine prop plane) to 150 dB (the blast of a giant, four-engine jet). Experiments have shown that 160 dB are lethal for small fur-bearing animals. Research at many universities shows that exposure to noise of 90 dB or more can cause the skin to flush, the stomach muscles to constrict, and tempers to be short.

Frequency refers to the number of sound waves emanating from a source per second—cycles per second (cps or Hz). *Pitch* is the term used to describe frequency; a tone with 100 cps is considered low pitch; a tone of 10,000 cps is considered high pitch. Generally, a young adult can distinguish frequencies from 16 cps to 20,000 cps.

▷ Hearing Loss

Psychosocial Considerations

Impairment of hearing may cause changes in personality and attitude, in the ability to communicate, in the awareness of surroundings, and even in the ability to protect oneself. In a classroom, a student with impaired hearing may show disinterest, inattention, and failing grades. A woman at home may think the "world is dead" because she no longer can hear the clock chime, the refrigerator hum, the birds sing, or the traffic pass. A pedestrian may attempt to cross the street at the wrong time because of failure to hear an approaching car. The person with a hearing loss may miss parts of a conversation and may feel that people are talking about him. Many individuals are not even aware that their hearing is gradually becoming impaired.

More than 20 million persons in the United States suffer from some form of hearing loss. Approximately 90% of these people can be helped through medical or surgical measures or with a hearing aid. The nurse and the family physician play a major role in diagnosing hearing loss and guiding patients toward some type of assistance. Although some hearing difficulty may be due to impacted cerumen (wax), which is readily treated, proper assessment is best done by an otologist.*

Not infrequently, a person with a hearing loss refuses to seek medical attention, because of fear that hearing loss is a sign of advancing age; many people refuse to wear a hearing aid for this reason. Others feel self-conscious when they do wear an aid. These attitudes and behaviors should be taken into account when counseling patients who need hearing assistance.

* The *otologist* is a physician who specializes in the diagnosis and treatment of problems of the ear. An *otolaryngologist* is a physician who specializes in problems relating to the ear, nose, and throat. An *audiologist* is a person who specializes in nonmedical evaluation and rehabilitation of hearing disorders; educational preparation usually includes an M.A. or Ph.D. degree.

Manifestations of Hearing Loss

The symptoms of hearing loss are varied, complex, and often subtle, as is indicated in the danger signals listed in Chart 55-1.

The signs of significant ear disease that require referral to an otolaryngologist have been identified by the National Hearing Aid Society (NHAS)*:

1. Visible congenital or traumatic deformity of the ear
2. Active drainage from the ear within the previous 90 days
3. Sudden or rapidly progressive hearing loss
4. Acute or chronic dizziness or tinnitus
5. Unilateral hearing loss of sudden or recent onset
6. Significant air-bone gap (which can be recognized only from hearing tests)
7. Visible evidence of cerumen accumulation or a foreign body in the ear canal
8. Pain or discomfort in the ear

▷ Assessment of Hearing Ability

Some of the easiest methods of assessing hearing ability is to determine how well a person can detect a whisper or a spoken sound, the ticking of a watch, and the vibrations from a tuning fork. These assessment tools yield qualitative evaluations (see Chap. 5, pp. 62–63). More significant quantitative determinations are made with an electrically calibrated audiometer. Hearing tests not only help to determine the particular type of hearing defect present, but also establish the potential of the patient's hearing.

Audiogram

In the detection of deafness, the audiometer is the single most important diagnostic instrument. Audiometric testing is of two kinds: (1) *pure-tone audiometry,* in which the sound stimulus consists of a pure or musical tone (the louder the tone before the patient perceives it, the greater the hearing loss; the unit of measure of loudness or intensity of sound is the decibel); and (2) *speech audiometry,* in which the spoken word is used to determine the ability to understand and discriminate sounds.

For accuracy, audiometric tests should be done in a soundproof room. The patient wears earphones and is instructed to signal when he hears the tone and again when he no longer hears it. When the tone is applied directly over the external auditory opening, air conduction is measured. When the stimulus is applied to the mastoid bone, thereby bypassing the conductive mechanism, nerve conduction is tested.

The normal human ear perceives sounds ranging from about 20 cps to 20,000 cps; however, only the frequencies from 500 cps to 2000 cps are important in understanding everyday speech. Clinically, this range is referred to as *speech range.* The critical level of loudness is around 30 dB. In

* National Hearing Aid Society, 20361 Middlebelt, Livonia, Michigan 48152

Chart 55-1
Symptoms of Hearing Loss

Speech Deterioration—If a person slurs his words or drops word endings, or if speech is "flat" sounding, he may not be hearing correctly! The ears guide the voice, both in loudness and pronunciation.

Fatigue—If a person tires easily when listening to conversation or to a speech, fatigue may be the result of straining to hear. Under these circumstances, he may become irritable or "touchy" very easily.

Indifference—It is easy for a person to become depressed and disinterested in life in general when he can't hear what others are saying.

Social withdrawal—Not being able to hear what is going on around him causes the hard of hearing person to withdraw from situations which might prove embarrassing.

Insecurity—Lack of self-confidence and fear of mistakes create a feeling of insecurity in many hard of hearing persons. No one likes to "say the wrong thing" or do something that might tend to make him look foolish.

Indecision—Procrastination—Loss of self-confidence makes it increasingly difficult for hard of hearing persons to make decisions.

Suspiciousness—Because he often hears only part of what is being said, the hard of hearing person may suspect that others are talking about him or that portions of the conversation relating to him are deliberately spoken softly so that he will not hear them!

False pride—The hard of hearing individual wants to conceal his hearing loss. Consequently, he often pretends he is hearing when he actually isn't.

Loneliness and unhappiness—Though everyone wishes for quiet now and then, *enforced* silence can be boring and even somewhat frightening. Persons with a hearing loss often feel "left out of things."

Tendency to "hog" the conversation—Many hard of hearing people tend to dominate the conversation, knowing that so long as it is centered on them and they can control it they are not so likely to be embarrassed by some mistake.

(Courtesy of Maico Hearing Instruments.)

---

treating patients surgically to improve hearing loss, the aim is to improve the hearing level to 30 dB or better within the speech frequencies (Figs. 55-2 and 55-3).

▷ Classification of Hearing Loss

Conductive Loss. Conductive loss results from an impairment of the outer ear, middle ear, or both. The inner ear is not involved in this type of loss; it can analyze clearly the sounds that come to it. Correction of the problem may

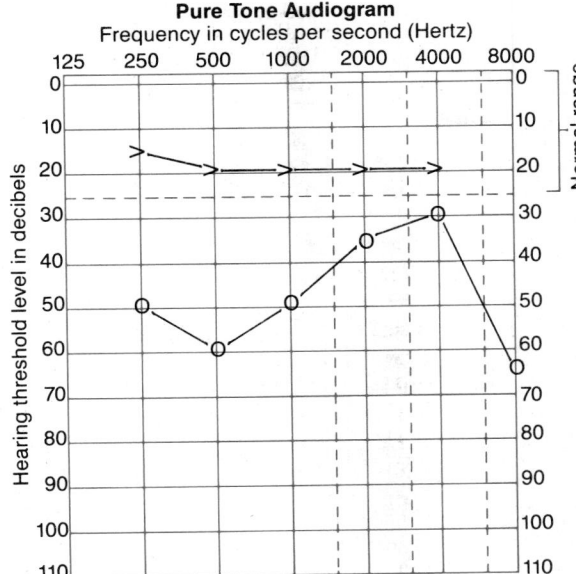

Pure Tone Audiogram
Frequency in cycles per second (Hertz)

Audiogram Code

Ear	Air		Bone	
	Un-masked	Masked	Un-masked	Masked
R	O---O	Δ---Δ	]---]	>--->
L	x---x	□---□	[---[	<---<

Figure 55-2. An audiogram presents a graphic outline of the individual's hearing as measured by tones of different pitches ranging from 125 through 8000 cycles per second (cps or Hz). This audiogram of the right ear shows a sensorineural loss. Thresholds for these different tones as heard by air and bone conduction are plotted. The information is important for determining the type of hearing loss. Also, by testing through the critical speech range (approximately 300 cps to 3000 cps), one can predict how much difficulty there may be in hearing and understanding speech. The code box to the right indicates the signs used on the chart. (From Dayal VS: Clinical Otolaryngology. Philadelphia, JB Lippincott, 1981.)

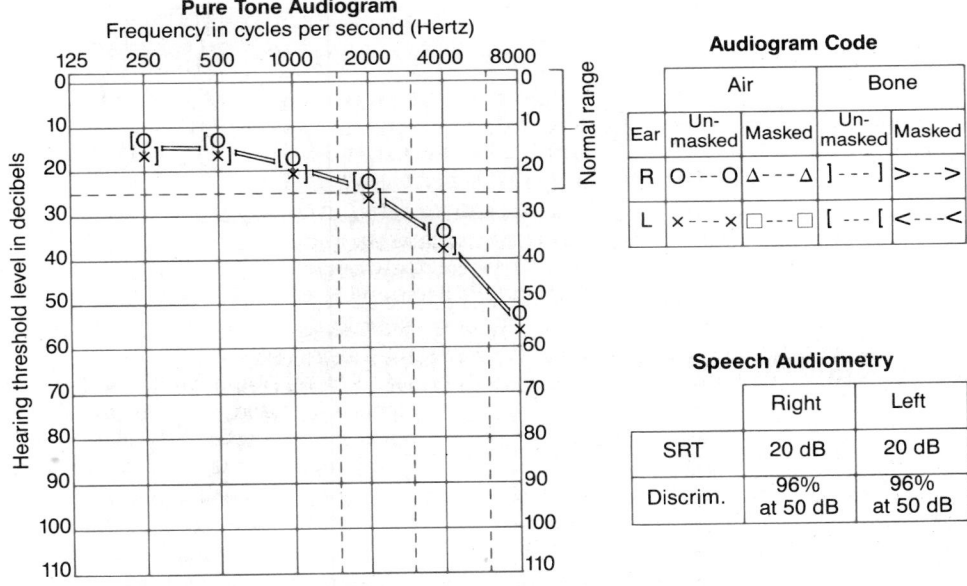

Pure Tone Audiogram
Frequency in cycles per second (Hertz)

Audiogram Code

Ear	Air		Bone	
	Un-masked	Masked	Un-masked	Masked
R	O---O	Δ---Δ	]---]	>--->
L	x---x	□---□	[---[	<---<

Speech Audiometry

	Right	Left
SRT	20 dB	20 dB
Discrim.	96% at 50 dB	96% at 50 dB

Figure 55-3. Audiogram of right ear shows a conductive hearing loss. In this audiogram, speech tests used are speech reception threshold (SRT) and speech discrimination. If the ability of this patient to understand speech is poor, a hearing aid will be of little or no benefit to him, nor will he benefit from reconstructive surgery to correct the conductive hearing loss. (From Dayal VS: Clinical Otolaryngology. Philadelphia, JB Lippincott, 1981.)

be all that is necessary to treat and improve this type of impairment (see pp. 1262–1271). If the problem cannot be corrected (Fig. 55-4), these individuals benefit greatly from hearing aids, because in most instances they require only amplification of sounds.

Sensorineural (Perceptive) Loss.   A disease of the inner ear or nerve pathways produces a type of hearing loss in which sensitivity to and discrimination of sounds are im-

paired. Sounds may be conducted properly through the external and middle ear but are not analyzed correctly in the inner ear. Because of poor sensitivity to sound, hearing aids are not as helpful as they are to those with conductive loss. However, a hearing aid should not be ruled out until the patient's hearing is evaluated in relation to hearing aids, that is, until a variety of aids are tested against the patient's hearing loss.

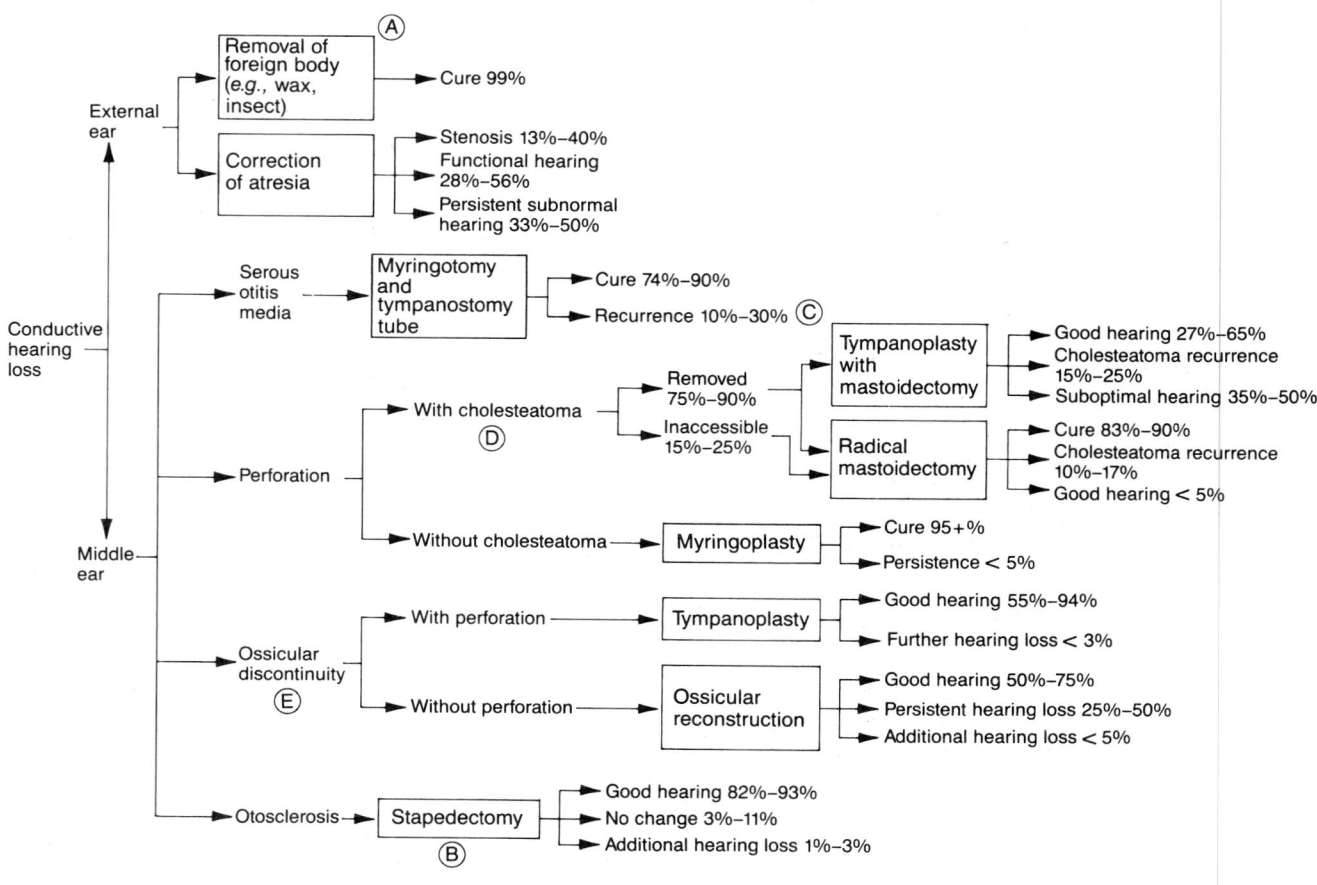

Figure 55-4. Conductive hearing loss. When a patient presents with this problem, the above flow chart indicates how the diagnosis determines the management of the patient and further predicts the outcome. (From Jafek BW and Balkany TJ: Conductive hearing loss. In Eiseman B: Prognosis of Surgical Disease. Philadelphia, WB Saunders, 1980.)

Combined Hearing Loss. A combined hearing loss indicates that the patient has both a conductive and a sensorineural loss.

Psychogenic Hearing Loss (Nonorganic, Functional). Hearing loss of this type is unrelated to detectable structural changes in the hearing mechanisms. Usually, it is a manifestation of an emotional disturbance, and the loss is frequently total. *Malingering* is similar to psychogenic hearing loss, except that in this instance the patient really does hear.

▷ Rehabilitation

It is important to classify the kinds of hearing impairment so that rehabilitative efforts can be directed at meeting a particular need. The Conference of Executives of American Schools for the Deaf* proposed the following classification based on (1) time of onset of hearing loss and (2) functional status of hearing:

* Saunders WH et al. Nursing Care in Eye, Ear, Nose, and Throat Disorders, 4th ed. St Louis, CV Mosby, 1979.

1. The deaf—those in whom the sense of hearing is non-functional for ordinary purposes of life. This general group is made up of two distinct classes:
   a. The congenitally deaf—those who lose hearing before speech is developed
   b. The adventitiously deaf—those who are born with normal hearing but then suffer some illness or accident that causes their hearing to become nonfunctional
2. The hard of hearing—those in whom hearing, although defective, is serviceable with or without a hearing aid

Hearing Aids

A *hearing aid* is an instrument through which sounds, both speech and environmental, are received by a microphone, converted into electrical signals, amplified, and reconverted to acoustical signals. A hearing aid is not a new ear. It is as its name implies, only an aid to hearing. Many aids available for nerve deafness depress the low tones and give better hearing for the high tones. Whether an individual would benefit by a hearing aid can best be determined by an otologist in conjunction with an audiologist. When the hearing loss is more than 30 dB in the range of 500 cps to 2000 cps in the better ear, a patient may benefit (but not with certainty) from a hearing aid. A variety of aids are available; the problem is to select the best aid for the individual patient (Table 55-1). Even this does not ensure optimal benefit from such an instrument. Psychological factors, such as vanity, may be involved, as well as other types of sensitivity.

The patient needs to know that the aid will not restore hearing to the level of the person with normal hearing, but will improve it in the range of 300 cps to 3500 cps (range of primary speech).

A hearing aid makes speech louder, but it does not always make it clear enough for the deaf person to understand what is said. The wearer must experiment and adjust the controls for optimal results. He needs to recognize that he will never hear what others cannot hear, nor will he hear as well as one who has no hearing impairment. It may be necessary to receive auditory training and lessons in speech reading (lip reading) in order to make the new hearing aid effective. With such assistance, this person can learn to interpret sounds and use advantageously whatever hearing remains. Speech reading can help fill in the gaps of those words that might be missed. In auditory training, speech discrimination and listening skills are emphasized. The otologist, nurse clinician, or the hearing center can direct the patient to such classes.

A problem with most hearing aids is that background noise is also amplified, which may be distressing to the wearer. Binaural aids (*i.e.,* one for each ear) may be indicated. Such aids can be concealed in the arms of specially made eyeglasses, as may a single aid.

FDA Regulations. In August 1977, the Food and Drug Administration (FDA) established regulations on hearing aids to protect the health and safety of individuals with hearing impairments:

1. A medical evaluation of the impairment by a licensed physician (preferably one specializing in diseases of the ear) must be obtained within 6 months prior to the purchase of a hearing aid.

   a. Such a written statement from a physician, however, may be waived by the client (a fully informed adult 18 years of age or older) upon signing a document.
   b. Children must be evaluated by a physician.
2. Hearing aid dispensers are required to refer prospective users to physicians if any of the eight specified otologic conditions are evident (see Chart 55-1).
3. A *User Instructional Brochure* is to accompany every hearing aid device. In this brochure, the following information is presented:
   a. Proper use and maintenance of the device are described.
   b. Good health practice requires a medical evaluation before purchasing a hearing aid.
   c. Any of the designated otologic conditions should be investigated by a physician before client purchases an aid.
4. Medical evaluation is required to ensure appropriate medical diagnosis and care.

Care of a Hearing Aid. A hearing aid must be cared for carefully. The ear mold, which is the only part of the instrument that may be washed, is washed in soap and water every day, and the cannula is cleansed with a small applicator or pipe cleaner. The mold must be dry before it is snapped into the receiver. The transmitter usually is worn off the body—behind the ear or in the frame of eyeglasses. A spare battery and cord should be carried by the wearer at all times. (This is suggested, but most patients do not do it.)

When a hearing aid is not functioning properly, the following steps should be taken: (1) note whether the on-off switch is on; (2) check the positioning of the batteries; (3) try a new battery; (4) examine the cord for breaks and whether it is plugged in correctly; and (5) examine the ear mold for cleanliness (see Chart 55-2). If the aid still will not work, notify the local service agency. Meanwhile, if the unit requires days to repair, the agency from whom it was purchased may lend an aid, or one may be borrowed from the local Chapter of the American Hearing Society.

Table 55-1
Types of Hearing Aids

Site/Range of Hearing Loss	Advantages	Disadvantages
Body (40 dB–110 dB)	Separation of receiver and microphone prevents acoustic feedback, allowing high amplification	Bulky; requires long wire, which may be cosmetically displeasing; some loss of high-frequency response
Behind the ear (25 dB–80 dB)	Cosmetically good because easily hidden by hair; comfortable; no long wires	Proximity of microphone and receiver limits the amount of amplification because of feedback
In the ear (25 dB–55 dB)	Smallest; most easily concealed	Very close proximity of amplifier and microphone and size limitations on power make aid suitable only for mild to moderate losses
Eyeglasses (25 dB–70 dB; greater range with special modifications)	Conceals most of the aid with frame of glasses; allows wires separating microphone and receiver to be hidden within glasses	Requires wearing glasses, usually with bulky, stylistically limited frame

(From Sataloff RT: Choosing the right hearing aid. Hosp Pract 1981 May; 16(5):32E.)

Chart 55-2
Hearing Aid Problems

Whistling Noise

Loose ear mold:
    Improperly made
    Improperly worn
    Worn out
Improper aid selection:
    Too much power required in aid with inadequate separation between microphone and receiver
    Open mold used inappropriately

Inadequate Amplification

Dead batteries
Wax in ear
Wax or other material in mold
Wires or tubing disconnected from aid
Aid turned off or volume too low
Improper mold
Improper aid for degree of loss

Pain From Mold

Improperly fitted mold
Ear skin or cartilage infection
Middle-ear infection
Ear tumor
Unrelated causes:
    Temporomandibular joint
    Throat or larynx
    Other

(From Sataloff RT: Choosing the right hearing aid. Hosp Pract 1981 May; 16(5):32A.)

Hearing Guide Dogs

Specially trained dogs are available to assist the person with hearing loss.* At home, the dog reacts to the sound of a telephone, a doorbell, an alarm clock, a baby's cry, a knock at the door, a smoke alarm, or an intruder. The dog does not bark, but jumps on the person, thereby alerting him; the dog then runs to the source of the noise. In public, the dog positions himself between the person with a hearing problem and any potential hazard that the person cannot hear, such as an oncoming vehicle or a hostile person.

The dog wears an orange collar, and the person carries a certification card that reads: "The dog has been professionally trained by Hearing Dog Inc. in auditory awareness to serve its hearing-impaired master. Therefore, as with guide dogs for the blind, this dog shall accompany its master at all times."

In many states, a hard of hearing person with a certified hearing guide dog is legally permitted access to public transportation, public eating places, and stores, including grocery markets.

Communication With a Person Who Has a Hearing Impairment

Terry and coworkers offer the following suggestions for better communication with deaf persons whose speech is difficult to understand†:

1. Devote full attention to what the person is saying. Look and listen—do not try to give attention to another task while listening.
2. Engage him in conversation when it is possible for you to anticipate his replies. This will enable you to become accustomed to any peculiarities in speech patterns.
3. Try to catch the essential context of what is being said; you can often fill in the details from context.
4. Do not try to appear as if you understand when you do not.
5. If you cannot understand at all or have serious doubt about your ability to understand what is being said, have the person write his message rather than risk misunderstanding. Having him repeat his message in speech, after you know its content, will also aid you in becoming accustomed to his pattern of speech.

Suggestions for better communication with a deaf person who lip-reads are as follows:

1. When speaking, always face the person as directly as possible.
2. Make sure your face is as clearly visible as possible; locate yourself so that your face is well-lighted; avoid being silhouetted against strong light; do not obscure that person's view of your mouth in any way; avoid talking with any object held in your mouth.
3. Be sure the patient knows the topic or subject of your verbal expression before going ahead with what you plan to say—this will enable him to use contextual clues in his lip-reading.
4. Speak slowly and distinctly, pausing more frequently than you would normally.
5. If you question whether the patient has understood some important direction or instruction, check to be certain that he has the full meaning of your message.
6. If for any reason your mouth must be covered (as with a mask) and you must direct or instruct the patient, there is no alternative but to write the message for him.

▷ Problems of the External Ear

The auricle or external ear, which varies in size, shape, and position on the head, aids in the collection of sound waves

---

* International Hearing Dog Inc., Henderson, Colorado, provides trained dogs after 3 months of training. Only persons who live alone are eligible to apply for such a dog.

† Terry FJ et al. Rehabilitation Nursing. St Louis, CV Mosby

and their passage into the external auditory canal. The *external auditory canal* is a skin-lined tube that ends at a disc-like structure, which is also lined with skin, tympanic membrane (eardrum). The skin of the canal contains highly specialized glands that secrete a brown waxlike substance, cerumen (earwax). This material serves as a protection for the skin. Hair follicles and sweat glands are also present.

Infections (External Otitis)

Bacterial or fungal infections may result from an abrasion of the ear canal or from swimming in contaminated water; they appear more commonly during the summer. Such infections are painful.

The goals of management are directed toward relieving the discomfort, reducing the swelling in the ear canal, and eradicating the infection. Even touching or moving the auricle increases pain. (In a middle ear infection, movement of the auricle does not increase pain.) Aspirin, codeine, and applications of heat provide comfort. If the tissues are edematous, it may be necessary to insert a wick of cotton gently through the canal to the eardrum so that liquid medications (such as Burow's solution [5% aluminum acetate] or antibiotics) may be introduced. Later, these medications may be given by dropper at room temperature. Such medications usually are combinations of antibiotics and agents to soothe the inflamed membranes. Systemic antibiotic therapy may also be required. The patient is cautioned to avoid swimming or allowing water to enter the ear when shampooing or showering.

Patients prone to "swimmer's ear" (otitis externa) should wear specially fitted ear plugs that are made from instant plastic material molded to exact measure. The patients should also be reminded to avoid self-cleansing of the ear (Q-tips are not to be used).

The chronic form of external otitis is often due to a dermatosis such as psoriasis or seborrheic dermatitis. Even allergic reactions to hair spray, hair dye, and permanent wave lotions can cause dermatitis, which clears when the offending agent is removed.

Furuncle of the External Canal

Infections of the skin and the subcutaneous tissue of the external canal usually result in a great deal of pain in the affected ear. There may be fever, severe headache, and enlargement of the local lymph nodes. This disorder may be mistaken for mastoid infection. The early administration of antibiotics and application of hot packs usually result in resolution of the furuncle. Incision and drainage are rarely done since such measures may result in perichondritis or chondritis. It is better for the furuncle to localize (point) and open spontaneously or resolve by itself.

Cerumen in the Ear Canal

Earwax normally accumulates in the ear in varying degrees and color. While it does not ordinarily need to be removed, on occasion it may become impacted, causing *otalgia* (earache) and hearing difficulties. Attempts to clear the external auditory canal with matches, hair pins, and other implements are dangerous, since trauma to the skin may result in infection or damage to the eardrum.

Management. Wax deposits may be softened by instilling a few drops of warmed glycerin, mineral oil, or acetic acid (0.5%) solution. Other ceruminolytic agents, such as peroxide in glyceryl (Debrox), are available. However, these compounds may cause an allergic reaction in the form of a dermatitis. If the wax deposits cannot be dislodged by this method, the cerumen may be removed with a cerumen spoon used under magnification. As a last resort, the ear canal may be irrigated, although this mode of treatment is the least preferred because (1) it may cause discomfort; (2) it is messy; (3) it may cause vertigo if the temperature of the solution is higher or lower than room temperature; (4) it tends to macerate the skin, increasing the possibility of an external otitis; and (5) it could permit fluid to enter and contaminate the middle ear if the tympanic membrane is perforated.

Foreign Bodies in the External Canal

Small objects are at times inserted into the ear, usually by young children. Such objects may be nonirritating and remain for years without symptoms.

An insect in the ear may be disturbing, but can be easily managed by instilling oil drops that smother the insect and allow it to be floated or flushed out. *However, vegetable foreign bodies have a tendency to swell, so irrigation is contraindicated.* Attempts at removal may be dangerous in unskilled hands, because the object may be pushed completely into the bony portion of the canal, lacerating the skin of the canal and perforating the eardrum. Serious infections of the middle ear and the mastoid, with ensuing deafness, may result. When such an object is trapped in the ear of a very young child, it should be removed with a special instrument under general anesthesia; when this procedure is skillfully performed, there are no sequelae.

Earlobe Piercing

Women, and particularly young girls, often have their earlobes pierced so that they can wear certain types of earrings without fear of losing them. However, piercing of the ears is contraindicated in persons having diabetes, skin disease, or keloids. When ear piercing is permissible, it is suggested that a physician perform the procedure. A large (18-gauge), straight needle with a sterilized and flexible gold or plastic wire is inserted into the bevel and then inside the needle. After a little local anesthesia is applied, the needle is inserted through the back of the earlobe, then withdrawn, leaving the wire in the ear. The wire is tied loosely in place—serving as a type of primitive earring—and is removed 10 days to 2 weeks later. During this time, the area is cleansed daily with soap and water or alcohol followed by a mild antiseptic ointment, and the wire is removed from time to time to ensure patency of the opening in the earlobe. Hair should be kept away from the lobes; hair and perfume spray, bleach, or dye should be avoided for 3 weeks. Swimming also is avoided until the ears have healed.

Some difficulties have been experienced with all types of ear-piercing procedures, among them premature closing of the puncture, hemorrhage into the earlobe, secondary infection, and keloid formation. Many individuals develop contact dermatitis and are sensitive to alloy metals. For this reason, it is recommended that only 14-K gold posts be worn. Any early sign of pain, redness, swelling, or tightness should be reported to the physician.

Irrigation of the External Auditory Canal

Irrigation of the ear canal is used less frequently today than in the past. When it is used, the purposes are (1) to carry out the caloric test for labyrinthine function, (2) to facilitate surgery on the external ear, and (3) to remove impacted cerumen (done by the physician).

The solutions for irrigating the ear should be at a temperature of about 40.6° C to 43.3° C (105° F–110° F). Solutions that are too hot or too cold or are used with too much force may cause pain or dizziness. The patient may sit or lie with his head tilted toward the side of the affected ear. The curved basin can be supported under the ear to catch the solution. To be effective, the fluids must reach the eardrum. To achieve this end, the auricle is pulled upward and backward in order to straighten the external auditory canal. (In children, this canal may be straightened by pulling the auricle down and back.) Extreme gentleness is used, and care must be taken that the fluid has free exit so that it is not driven into the middle ear. After the irrigation, the external opening is plugged lightly with sterile cotton, which is changed when necessary. After the procedure, the patient is instructed to lie on the affected ear so that gravity facilitates drainage.

- **Note:** *If injury to the tympanic membrane is suspected, irrigation should not be performed.*

▷ Problems of the Middle Ear

The middle ear, with its ossicles and ligaments and their connection to the eardrum, is vitally concerned with the function of hearing. The middle ear connects with the posterior portion of the nose by means of the eustachian tube; thus, equal air pressure is maintained on both sides of the eardrum. The tube, which is normally closed, opens by action of the muscles of the palate on yawning or swallowing. The tube serves as a drainage channel for normal and abnormal secretions of the middle ear and equalizes pressure in the middle ear to that of the atmosphere. When the membrane of this tube is inflamed, it offers an easy passage for infection into the middle ear.

Sound waves transmitted by the drum to the ossicles of the middle ear are transferred to the *cochlea,* the organ of hearing, lodged in the labyrinth or inner ear. An important ossicle is the stapes, which rocks on its posterior portion, not unlike a piston, and sets up vibrations in fluids contained in the labyrinth. The fluid waves cause the basilar membrane in which the hair cells of the organ of Corti rest to move in a wavelike manner. The waves set up electrical currents which stimulate the various areas of the cochlea. The hair cell sets up a neural impulse that is encoded and then transferred through the auditory cortex in the brain, where it is decoded into a sound message.

Trauma to the Tympanic Membrane (Perforation)

Permanent perforation of the tympanic membrane occurs most frequently as a result of auto accidents with skull frac-

ture. The next most frequent cause is infection; perforations of the eardrum membrane that fail to heal are often the end result of acute or chronic suppurative otitis media. Traumatic damage may also result from the blast effects of high explosives or from intense compression caused by a severe blow on the ear, which can rupture the eardrum. The eardrum may also be burned by a spark (red-hot slag) from a welder's equipment.

Less frequently, perforation is caused by foreign objects, water, burns of the face that include the external ear and the eardrum membrane, postmyringotomy defects, scuba diving, and accidental or deliberate blows to the face. Perforations may also occur when people use cotton-tipped applicators to clean their ears. A person may insert one into the external ear and inadvertently turn around, jamming the applicator deeper into the ear. Or the tip may be bumped and pushed into the canal. Either occurrence may result in severe destruction of the eardrum, ossicles, and even the inner ear. Thus, all attempts to clean the ear with applicator sticks must be discouraged.

Management.   Most accidental perforations of the drum membrane heal spontaneously. Some persist because of the growth of scar tissue over the edges of the perforation, thus preventing extension of the epithelial areas across the margins and final healing.

- In suspected traumatic perforations, warn the patient against irrigating the ear. Cleanse the outer ear carefully with sterile cotton, but leave the ear canal alone until an otologist can aspirate blood and inspect the eardrum for evidence of perforation.

If the patient has sustained a head injury, he is kept under observation to detect any evidence of cerebrospinal otorrhea, such as clear, watery drainage. Such fluid can be checked in the laboratory to determine whether its source is the cerebrospinal canal.

Middle Ear Effusion (Serous Otitis Media)

Secretory Otitis Media.   Since this condition is found primarily in children, the reader is directed to pediatric nursing texts.

Aerotitis Media.   *Aerotitis media* is a form of serous otitis media in which fluid or air is trapped in the middle ear due to sudden descent in an airplane (barotrauma). The condition usually lasts a short time, but it may continue for days. For this reason, many people avoid flying when they have an upper respiratory infection. Preventive measures to be taken by flight passengers are to chew gum, suck on hard candy, yawn, or swallow several times during the descent of the plane. Those flying should be taught to inflate their ears by the so-called Valsalva method. In this technique, the nostrils are held tightly, and the ears are inflated by vigorous blowing; thus, pressure in the middle ear is equalized to relieve annoying symptoms.

Acute Otitis Media (Infection of the Middle Ear)

Acute otitis media is an acute infection (or abscess) of the middle ear (Table 55-2). The essential cause of acute otitis media is the entrance of pathogenic bacteria into the normally sterile middle ear when the resistance is lowered or when the virulence of the organism is great enough to pro-

Table 55-2
Clinical Features of Acute Diffuse External Otitis and Acute Otitis Media

Feature	External Otitis	Otitis Media
Pain	Persistent Aggravated by moving jaw	Subsides in 6 to 9 hours Relieved immediately if tympanic membrane ruptures Aggravated by swallow, belch
Tenderness	Prominent	Absent
Systemic symptoms	Usually absent	Fever, rhinitis, sore throat
Hearing loss	Conductive type	Conductive type
Swelling of ear canal	Prominent	Absent
Discharge	Foul odor Blue pus, never profuse	No odor
Tympanic membrane	Inflamed but intact No middle ear fluid	May be perforated Fluid in middle ear

(From Farmer HS: A guide for the treatment of external otitis. Am Fam Physician 1980 June; 21(6):98. Published by the American Academy of Family Physicians.)

duce inflammation. Bacteria commonly found, in the order of importance, are the *Streptococcus pneumoniae,* the staphylococcus, and the *Haemophilus influenzae.* The mode of entry of the bacteria in most patients is spread by way of the auditory canal or the eustachian tube during the indiscriminate use of nose drops or nasal douching, forcible blowing of the nose, or sneezing; in rare cases, infection may enter after fracture of the skull.

Assessment and Clinical Manifestations. The symptoms may vary with the severity of the infection and may be either very mild and transient or very severe and fraught with serious complications. Pain in and about the ear is the first symptom. It may be intense and is relieved after spontaneous perforation of the drum or after myringotomy (see below). Fever varies and in severe cases may range between 40.0° C and 40.6° C (104° F–105° F). Deafness, ear noises, headache, loss of appetite, nausea, and vomiting are other symptoms.

Management. The end results of otitis media depend on the virulence of the bacteria, the efficiency of the therapy, and the resistance of the patient. With early and appropriate wide-spectrum antibiotic therapy, otitis media may clear with healing, with no serious sequelae.

It is important to note that symptoms may be masked by the antibiotic therapy and that during the course of treatment of an acute middle ear infection, symptoms such as headache, slow pulse, vomiting, and vertigo are all significant

and should be recorded for evaluation by the otologist. The appropriate antibiotic, often determined by culture and sensitivity tests, is important to the prognosis for eventual cure.

The condition may become subacute, with persistent purulent discharge from the ear. Healing may take place with permanent deafness.

Perforation as the result of rupture of the eardrum may persist and develop into a chronic form of otitis media. Secondary complications, with involvement of the mastoid, and other serious intracranial complications, such as meningitis or brain abscess, may result.

Myringotomy. In a *myringotomy,* an incision is made into the posterior or inferior aspect of the tympanic membrane for draining purposes in order to relieve pressure and drain pus from middle ear infection. In mild cases treated early, myringotomy may not be necessary. However, if pain persists, this procedure is important for promoting surgical drainage. It also offers a ready means of identifying the type of organism present to test its sensitivity to chemotherapeutic agents.

An incision is made in the posterior inferior aspect of the tympanic membrane. Even though a sweeping incision is made to relieve pressure and pus from a middle ear infection, the incision heals rapidly and hearing is not impaired. This procedure is now performed much less frequently than it was before the advent of antibiotic therapy. Usually, when myringotomy is done, a plastic tube is inserted through the eardrum.

Chronic Otitis Media

Chronic otitis media results from repeated attacks of otitis media causing persistent perforation of the drum. It is due to particular virulence of the infecting organism or to bacterial resistance to antibiotic therapy. The chronically infected ear is characterizted by persistent or recurrent purulent discharge, with or without pain, and varying degrees of deafness, usually conductive or mixed. Most chronic otitis media begins in childhood and may persist to adult life.

Classification. Chronic suppurative middle ear infection has been classified into five groupings, as indicated in Table 55-3.

Assessment. The symptoms of chronic otitis media may be minimal, with varying degrees of deafness and the presence of a persistent or intermittent foul-smelling discharge of variable quantity. Pain may or may not be present. Symptoms such as sudden facial paralysis, unusually profound deafness or dizziness, onset of headache with dizziness, and stiff neck may herald a beginning meningitis or brain abscess or erosion into the semicircular canals. The diagnosis is corroborated by the physical findings, but, in addition, roentgenograms of the mastoids usually show pathologic changes.

Management. Local treatment consists of (1) careful cleansing of the ear, (2) instillation of antibiotic drops, (3) application of antibiotic powders, and (4) x-ray study. Tympanoplastic procedures may be required early to prevent further damage to hearing and more serious complications.

Mastoiditis and Mastoidectomy

Mastoiditis is an inflammation of the mastoid, resulting from an infection of the middle ear; if untreated, osteomyelitis

Table 55-3
Classification of Chronic Otitis Media

Type	Specific Condition	Involvement	Manifestation
I	Chronic otitis media simplex	Central perforation of the tympanic membrane	Mucoid serous discharge
II	Chronic otitis media with cholesteatoma*	Usually, attic perforation (posterior superior part of eardrum) With or without perforation	Usually, odorous discharge
III	Chronic adhesive otitis media	Marked retraction of tympanic membrane	No discharge Marked hearing loss
IV	Chronic otitis media with tympanosclerosis	Tympanosclerosis, a degenerative process in eardrum and middle ear Plaque of amorphous connective tissue	Severe hearing loss No discharge
V	Chronic serous otitis media	If untreated or neglected, may result in severe deafness, chronic adhesive otitis media, cholesteatoma,* or tympanosclerosis	Repeated bout of serous or fluid ear

(By Woodrow D. Schlesser, M.D., personnel communication.)

* *Cholesteatoma* is due to the ingrowth of the skin of the external ear canal (squamous epithelium) into the middle ear. The skin from the external canal forms the outer sac, which fills with degenerated skin and sebaceous material. The sac is attached to the structures of the middle ear and mastoid and produces changes by pressure necrosis.

may occur. Symptoms are pain and tenderness behind the ear, discharge from the middle ear, and swelling of the mastoid. Usually, this is successfully treated with antibiotics and occasionally myringotomy.

When there is recurrent or persistent tenderness, fever, headache, and discharge from the ear, it may be necessary to remove the mastoid process (mastoidectomy).

Preoperative Management. Aside from general preoperative preparation of the patient, the postauricular or endaural area (whichever is selected as the incision site) is cleansed thoroughly. To keep hair out of the operative field, a water-soluble jelly (KY jelly) may be applied to the hairline in the operating room, or a commercially available plastic drape with a small, central hole to expose the operative site may be used. (The edge of the hole adheres to the skin with adhesive.)

During the operation, the infection is removed completely from the mastoid process by removing the mastoid cells, and the middle ear is drained (myringotomy), thus preventing spread of the infection to surrounding structures. The middle ear can be saved from further damage, and possible permanent hearing loss can be prevented.

Postoperative Management. Sedatives usually are indicated after the operation and during the first postoperative days to control pain and restlessness. Fluids are given freely when the anesthetic reaction clears. The mastoid is drained by means of a small Teflon drain. The small patch dressing is changed in about 4 or 5 days. Antibiotics are continued for several days.

A possible complication after mastoidectomy is facial paralysis due to possible erosion of the bone that protects the facial nerve. The nurse may be the first to note this serious indication of facial nerve inflammation or injury. The

patient shows immobility of the side affected, so that the eye cannot be closed and the mouth droops. He is unable to drink without water dripping from the mouth, and he is unable to whistle. When the patient attempts to speak or grimace, the facial paralysis is more pronounced, due to the immobility of the paralyzed side. Any evidence of facial paralysis is reported immediately to the otologist. The patient may be taken back to the operating room, the wound opened, and repair of the facial nerve done at once. Other possible complications are meningitis or brain abscess (see p. 1341).

Tympanoplasty

Tympanoplasty denotes a number of reconstructive operations on middle ear structures that have become diseased or are congenitally deformed (Table 55-4). Utilizing an illuminated binocular microscope, the otologist is able to visualize and reconstruct defective conductive mechanisms to maintain or improve hearing. Chemotherapy or antibiotics maintain an infection-free area so that healing is promoted.

Physiologic Principles Underlying Sound Conduction. The conductive function of the eardrum and the ossicles transforms sound waves from airborne vibrations to mechanical stimulation of the endolymphatic fluids. The prevailing physiologic concept holds that the ratio of the large tympanic membrane to the smaller oval window, combined with the lever action of the ossicles, transforms stimuli from the ear to the inner ear fluids with great increase in force.*

* Weaver and Lawrence (*Physiological Acoustics,* Princeton University Press) indicate that an actual ratio is 21:1, but an effective ratio is 14:1 (23 dB). Since ordinarily sound-transfer from air to liquid sustains a loss of 30 dB, this is compensated for by the action of the tympanic membrane and the ossicles (up to 23–25 dB).

Table 55-4
Tympanoplastic Procedures

Type	Damage of Middle Ear	Methods of Repair
I	Perforated tympanic membrane with normal ossicular chain	Closure of perforation; same as myringoplasty
II	Perforation of tympanic membrane with erosion of malleus	Closure with graft against incus or remains of malleus
III	Destruction of tympanic membrane and ossicular chain *but with* intact and mobile stapes	Graft contacts normal stapes; also gives sound protection to round window
IV	Similar to type III, but head, neck, and crura of stapes missing; footplate mobile	Mobile footplate left exposed; air pocket between round window and graft provides sound protection for round window
V	Similar to type IV plus *fixed* footplate	Fenestra in horizontal semicircular canal; graft seals off middle ear to give sound protection for round window

(From DeWeese DD and Saunders WH: Textbook of Otolaryngology, 6th ed. St Louis, CV Mosby, 1982.)

Obviously, defects in the tympanic membrane or interruption of the ossicular chain will disturb that mass relationship to the oval window and will cause a loss of the sound–pressure ratio, resulting in hearing loss.

The functional physiology of the round and oval windows plays an important role as well. The oval window is bordered by the annular ligament, and the unimpeded motility of the stapedial footplate receives impulses transmitted by the incus and the malleus from the eardrum membrane. The round window, opening on the opposite side of the cochlear duct, permits motion of the endolymphatic fluids with sound-wave stimulation. With the normally intact eardrum membrane, sound waves stimulate the oval window first, and a lag occurs before the terminal effect of the stimulus reaches the round window. This phase lag, normally present with an intact eardrum, is changed by a perforation of the eardrum that is large enough to allow sound waves to impinge on both the round and oval windows simultaneously. This effect cancels the lag and prevents the maximal effect of labyrinth fluid motility and its subsequent effect in stimulating the hair cells in the organ of Corti. The result is a reduction in hearing ability.

Pathophysiology. Pathologic sequelae vary after otitis media, with minimal or large defects remaining in the tympanic membrane. In protracted or virulent infections, necrotic involvement of the ossicles may occur. Involvement

of motility may result with fibrosis or necrosis of all or part of the ossicular chain. The malleus commonly is involved, the handle being lost by osteonecrosis as the perforation in the eardrum enlarges. The lenticular process of the incus often is involved because of its tenuous blood supply. Osteonecrosis may involve the entire ossicular chain, so that the stapedial footplate is the only portion remaining. The oval and round windows may be impeded functionally by granuloma, polyps, and fibrous or bony plaques. Otosclerosis may exist along with the pathologic sequelae of otitis media. Obstruction of the tympanic orifice of the eustachian tube by pathologic tissue deposits or fibrotic stenosis may result in dysfunction of this structure.

Procedures.   Tympanoplasty is performed to reestablish two functions of the middle ear: (1) the transformer action, and (2) sound protection for the round window.

Originally, five types of tympanoplastic procedures were described (see Table 55-4). Since then, modifications and innovations have been devised. In the original procedures of types I, II, and III, both of the above objectives were achieved; however, with types IV and V, only sound protection was provided for the round window. Variations of these operations are being done with the following innovations: incus interposition and prosthetic replacement.

Incus interposition is a procedure in which the incus is detached from the malleus, diseased segments of the incus are removed, and the remains of the incus are balanced on the head of the stapes; the contact is maintained with pieces of Gelfoam.

Homologous tympanic membrane, including annulus and malleus, may be taken from a cadaver and used in place of a fascial graft. Other prostheses may include tragal cartilage or a piece of shaped cortical bone from the patient's own mastoid.

Tympanoplasty, Type I (Myringoplasty)
Indications and Management.   *Myringoplasty* is a plastic-surgical procedure designed to close perforations of the tympanic membrane. The operation has dual goals: (1) to create a closed middle ear cavity by graft over the perforation, and (2) to improve hearing.

The most important advantage of the closed tympanic membrane is the avoidance of the risk of contamination of the middle ear during bathing, swimming, or diving. Thus, the reactivation of a chronic otitis media or mastoiditis may be prevented. Dramatic improvement in hearing may result from closure of a perforation if there is no involvement of the ossicles. The probability of improved hearing after closure of the eardrum membrane can be prognosticated to some degree by an audiometric study with evaluation of the air–bone conduction levels. Preoperative testing, with and without a patch prosthesis over the perforation, usually provides a fairly accurate estimate of the degree of hearing levels. Temporary patching of the defect with glazed paper, latex, or a cotton collodium disc should be a routine maneuver during the preliminary examination of the patient. When the patching of a perforation of the eardrum is not followed by audiometric improvement, one must consider involvement of the ossicular chain. During the surgical repair of a perforation, a careful inspection of the middle ear contents, with particular attention to the continuity of the ossicles, is important.

Contraindications. Medical or surgical closure of perforations of the eardrum in the presence of an active infection usually is contraindicated. In chronic disease of the middle ear with malfunction of the eustachian tube, and therefore inadequate drainage from the middle ear (the only avenue for egress of discharges), surgery is contraindicated. Involvement of the nasopharynx because of chronic infectious discharge from sinusitis or allergy, plus a history of acute exacerbations of otitis media, is an obvious contraindication.

Postoperative Management. An antibiotic is administered routinely for at least 5 days after surgery. The dressing is left undisturbed except for the external bandage, which may be changed if it becomes soiled from bleeding. The gauze strip is removed from the canal on the seventh day; the Gelfoam is left undisturbed. No suction or probing is carried out at this time.

On the 20th day, capillary suction can be used carefully to remove the Gelfoam or crusted debris. Gentle inflation may be carried out to test the efficiency of the closure of the perforation by the graft.

The patient is seen at 5-day intervals and is instructed to avoid contaminating the ear by shampooing or showering. Antibiotics are given for 1 week, but may be continued if there is evidence of complicating respiratory infection. An antihistamine with an ephedrine derivative is used routinely for 1 month postoperatively. In those patients with known seasonal or perennial rhinologic allergy, an antihistamine is continued.

Tympanoplasty, Types II to V and Modified Versions

Tympanoplasty may be done by various techniques. Either the postauricular or endaural approach is used. Skin grafts have been replaced by fascial grafts. The operation may be done in one or two stages. When done in two stages, the first is performed to clear the infection or remove cholesteatoma, and the second stage is directed to mechanical correction of the deficient sound-transmission system.

Preoperative Care. The bacterial flora in all patients is studied by culture and sensitivity tests. In those whose treatment is accompanied by the parenteral administration of an appropriate antibiotic, the postoperative morbidity is reduced. Topical and systemic antibiotic treatment should precede surgery when the patient's ear is continuously or frequently discharging.

Operative Procedure. Part of the tympanoplastic procedure includes restoring the continuity of the sound mechanism, when it is involved. Ossicular interruption is most frequent in otitis media, but problems of reconstruction occur with malformations of the middle ear and ossicular dislocations due to head injuries.

Polyethylene tubing, stainless steel wire, bone, and cartilage have been used as replacements, either to utilize the remaining parts of the ossicles or to create a columella (little column) effect for the transmission of impulses from the tympanic graft to the oval window.

A two-stage procedure may be necessary—the first for the surgical eradication of all pathology and the establishment of a healed, dry middle ear, and the second for the reconstructive process. The ear should remain dry for 2 or

3 months before the second stage for the exploration of the window niches and the restoration of a conductive mechanism. Remaining parts of the ossicular chain may be repositioned to establish impulse transmission to the oval window.

Postoperative Care. Outer dressings may be reinforced if soiled with blood or drainage, but the inner dressing is undisturbed. The patient is hospitalized for 3 or 4 days.

The patient must be assisted the first time out of bed since dizziness and nystagmus are typical reactions. Medications to combat vertigo and nausea may be prescribed. The patient is cautioned to avoid blowing his nose or wetting the dressings during bathing. Eventually, he will be permitted to resume showering and swimming.

Clinical Results. Patients with a lengthy history of disease may regain as much hearing as those with less protracted infections. In patients whose otitis media has been healed and whose ear has remained dry for a lengthy period, hearing improvement may be marked after tympanoplasty. Younger patients achieve better results than older patients. The simpler the surgery, the better the chance for hearing gain; this, of course, relates directly to the functional integrity of the ossicular chain and the efficiency of the newly created tympanic covering.

Continued research is being done to improve tympanoplasty procedures. In some instances, clinical failures have been due to infection, poor technique, and tissue rejection of graft or prosthesis.

Otosclerosis

Otosclerosis or otospongiosis is the term applied to a form of progressive deafness caused by the formation of new, spongy bone in the labyrinth that locks the shape in a fixed position (clinical otosclerosis) and prevents sound transmission by the vibrating ossicles to the inner ear fluids.

The cause of this condition is unknown, but it occurs most commonly in women, beginning after puberty, and it has a hereditary basis. The condition, which usually involves both ears about equally, begins with insidious loss of hearing and a ringing or buzzing in the ears. The patient gives a history of slowly progressive hearing loss without middle ear infection.

Assessment. The diagnosis is evident from the findings of the audiometer test. Sound transmission by air as tested with a tuning fork is markedly reduced, while intensification of sound is noted by placing the tuning-fork handle over the mastoid and recording the marked difference in hearing between air and bone. The bone conduction is far better than air conduction, which is the reverse of normal. There is no known medical treatment for this form of deafness other than the help offered by amplification with an electric hearing aid or, preferably, a stapedectomy.

Stapedectomy

A *stapedectomy* involves removing the otosclerotic lesion at the footplate of the stapes and creating a suitable tissue implant with a prosthesis to replace this portion of the conductive mechanism.

Indications. As a consequence of the increasing numbers of regressions that occurred after stapes mobilization, stapedectomy was employed as a secondary operative technique to salvage the failures of initial mobilization attempts. With the initial success of this operation, the indications have extended to all classes of otosclerosis; and in some clinics where this technique is carried out, virtually all patients with otosclerosis are treated by a routine stapedectomy. Others use the procedure only after failure of a stapes mobilization (seldom done today since stapedectomy is the operation of choice).

Microsurgery. The otologic binocular microscope is of distinct value in this operation. To bridge the gap between the incus and the inner ear, Schuknecht uses steel wire and fat implant, whereas House's technique employs Gelfoam and prefabricated stainless steel wire (two popular procedures). Kos uses wire and a segment of a vein as a plug in the oval window, and Shea advocates a vein graft with polyethylene tubing (Fig. 55-5). In any case, the prosthetic device is fashioned and ready prior to the removal of the stapedial footplate.*

Postoperative Management. The position that the patient assumes in bed in the immediate 24-hour postoperative period varies with the preference of the physician. Some prefer the patient to lie on the operated ear to facilitate drainage; others desire the operated ear to be uppermost in order to prevent graft displacement. Still others allow the patient to choose the most comfortable position and one that does not cause vertigo. If dizziness is noted, the patient is instructed to change from one position to another slowly; diphenhydramine (Benadryl) or diazepam (Valium) may also be prescribed. The patient can be prevented from falling by keeping side rails up when he is in bed and assisting him when he gets out of bed. This precaution is mandatory if the patient is dizzy.

Unusual symptoms such as fever, headache, vertigo, or ear pain are to be noted, and the patient is instructed to avoid blowing his nose or sneezing. If he must do so, he should take care to avoid violent head movements. In addition, smoking should be stopped.

Any subjective symptoms, such as pain, taste changes, a "sloshy" feeling in the ear, or unusual sensations, are noted and reported.

Patient Education. The patient is discharged in 3 to 4 days and may be depressed because his hearing has not improved appreciably. Since initial hearing gain at the time of operation is masked by ear packing and subsequent edema of the tissues, the patient should be reassured that hearing gain may be noted from 1 to several weeks after surgery. Packing is removed about the fifth or sixth day in the physician's office.

Before leaving the hospital, the patient is instructed as follows:

- Avoid sudden head movements and risks of infections.
- Do not wet head (in showers or by swimming) for about 6 weeks.
- Postpone washing hair for 2 weeks; after this time, when washing hair, be careful to avoid getting water into the ear for an additional 4 weeks.
- Avoid flying for several months, and stay away from people who have upper respiratory infections.

---

* Most surgeons use a tissue graft and wire prosthesis. Most commonly used are vein grafts or fat grafts.

▷ Problems of the Inner Ear

Body balance is maintained by the cooperation of muscles, joints, tendons, visceral senses, eyes, and inner ear or vestibular apparatus. The last is the most important in this function. The inner apparatus of the ear provides feedback regarding the movements and the position of the head in space, coordinates all body muscles, and positions the eyes during rapid motion or head movement.

The vestibular apparatus consists of the utricle, the saccule, and the semicircular canals, of which there are three in each ear. Each canal lies in a plane at right angles to the others, with the entire apparatus grouped in working pairs for this complex function. The mechanism of action of the semicircular canals may be likened to the cochlea or organ of hearing. Here, also, fluids are set in motion by head or body movement, which in turn stimulate extremely delicate nerve fibers that transmit messages as electric impulses along the nerve to centers in the brain, where they are interpreted.

Motion Sickness

Motion sickness is a disturbance of equilibrium caused by constant motion, such as occurs aboard ship on the ocean, riding on a merry-go-round or swing, or even riding a distance in the back seat of a car. Symptoms are dizziness, nausea, and frequently vomiting. These manifestations may persist several hours after the stimulation stops. Dimenhydrinate (Dramamine), scopolamine, and other antivertiginous (against dizziness and motion sickness) drugs are helpful in providing some relief. Some side-effects may be experienced, such as dry mouth, cycloplegia, and drowsiness. These complications are reduced by using a disc (Transderm-V)† in which scopolamine has been incorporated. The disc is applied to the skin, usually the posterior earlobe, for 4 to 16 hours before embarking on a long trip and left there for 3 days, if necessary. Dry mouth may develop, which can be relieved with lozenges.

Hydrops of the Labyrinth (Meniere's Syndrome)

Meniere's disease or *syndrome* is an inner ear problem stemming from a labyrinthine dysfunction, the cause of which has not been definitely established. Many theories have been advanced, such as an increase in pressure in the endolymph; sodium retention; vasomotor changes, causing a spasm of the internal auditory artery; an emotional or endocrine disturbance; or an allergic reaction. Some attribute impairment of the microvasculature of the inner ear to abnormal metabolites (sugar, insulin, triglycerides, and cholesterol) in the bloodstream.

▶ Assessment
Clinical Manifestations. Meniere's syndrome is characterized by the presence of a triad of symptoms: paroxysmal whirling vertigo, tinnitus, and sensorineural hearing loss.

---

† Alza Corp., Pasadena, California.

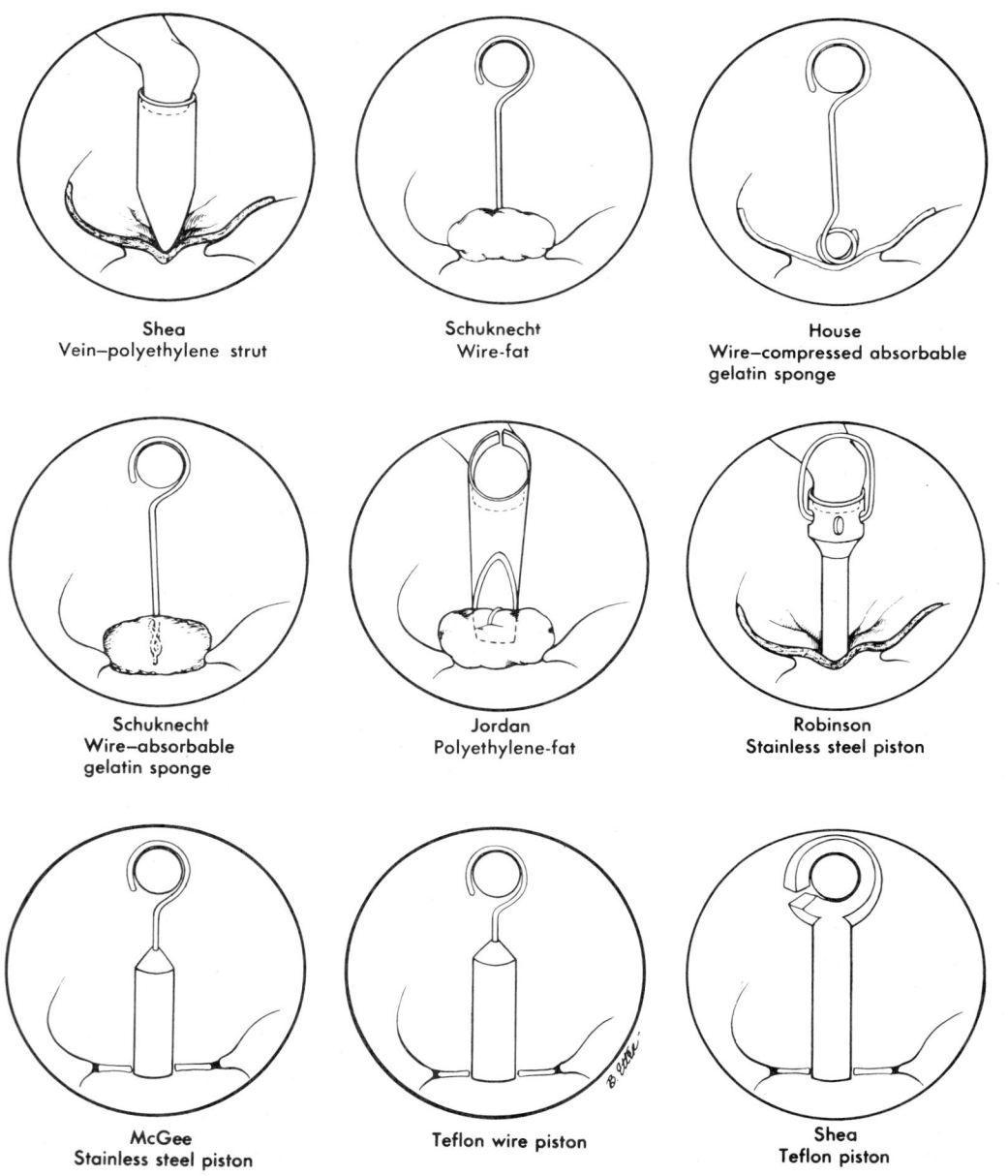

Shea
Vein–polyethylene strut

Schuknecht
Wire-fat

House
Wire–compressed absorbable
gelatin sponge

Schuknecht
Wire–absorbable
gelatin sponge

Jordan
Polyethylene-fat

Robinson
Stainless steel piston

McGee
Stainless steel piston

Teflon wire piston

Shea
Teflon piston

Figure 55-5.   Stapedectomy prostheses. Top three diagrams and middle three diagrams show various prostheses used after footplate has been removed. Bottom three diagrams indicate that the footplate has been "drilled" to precisely accept a prefabricated piston. (From Saunders WH, Paparella MM, and Miglets AW: Atlas of Ear Surgery, 3rd ed. St Louis, CV Mosby, 1980.)

At the onset of the condition, perhaps only one or two of these symptoms are manifested; however, the disease is not diagnosed as Meniere's syndrome until all three signs are present (Fig. 55-6).

Vertigo, the outstanding symptom of Meniere's disease, occurs as a sudden attack, appearing at irregular intervals and possibly persisting for several hours. Early in this condition, weeks or months pass between attacks, but the time is gradually reduced so that they may be experienced every 2 to 3 days. Usually, only one ear is involved.

Some patients experience an aura or some warning sign, such as a sense of pressure or fullness in the ear, that tells

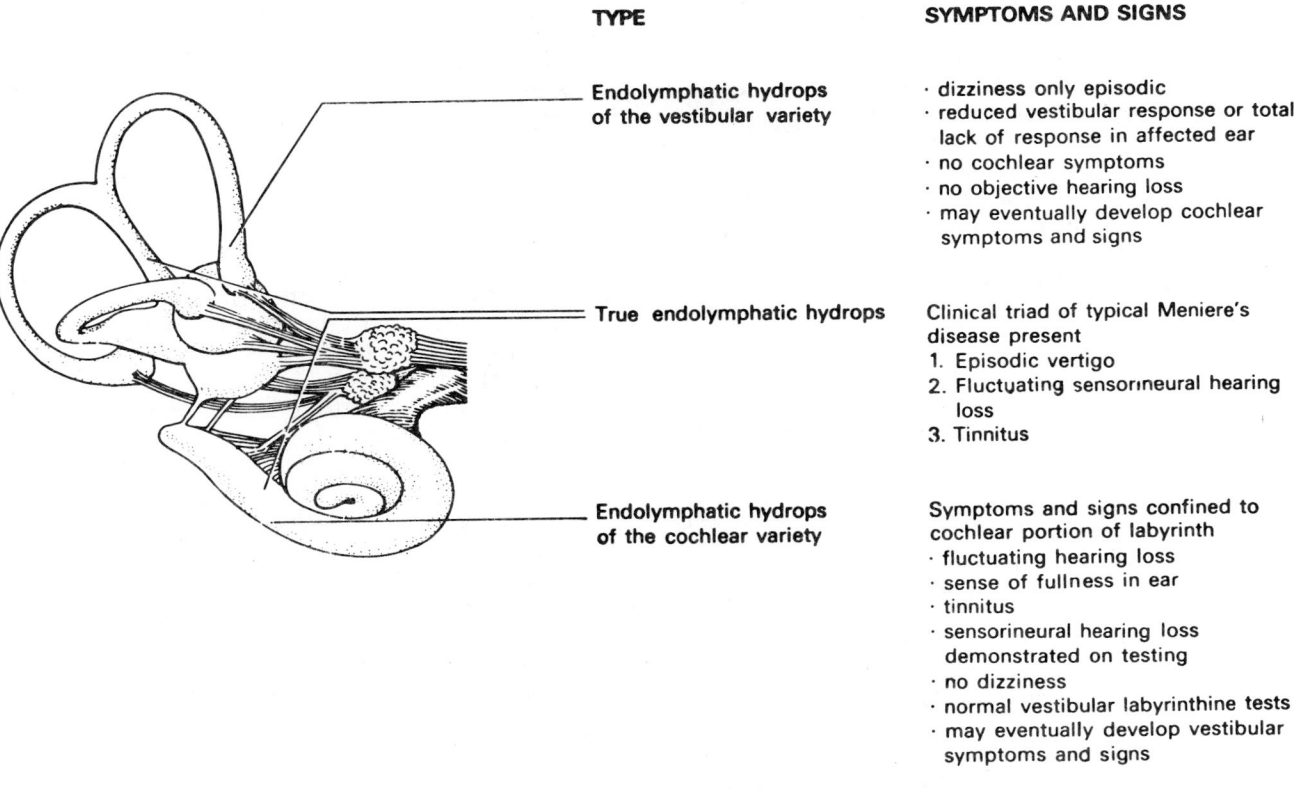

TYPE	SYMPTOMS AND SIGNS
Endolymphatic hydrops of the vestibular variety	· dizziness only episodic · reduced vestibular response or total lack of response in affected ear · no cochlear symptoms · no objective hearing loss · may eventually develop cochlear symptoms and signs
True endolymphatic hydrops	Clinical triad of typical Meniere's disease present 1. Episodic vertigo 2. Fluctuating sensorineural hearing loss 3. Tinnitus
Endolymphatic hydrops of the cochlear variety	Symptoms and signs confined to cochlear portion of labyrinth · fluctuating hearing loss · sense of fullness in ear · tinnitus · sensorineural hearing loss demonstrated on testing · no dizziness · normal vestibular labyrinthine tests · may eventually develop vestibular symptoms and signs

Figure 55-6. A practical classification of Meniere's disease.

them an attack is coming on. This gives them time to lie down, stop the car, etc. Each attack lasts from a few minutes to several hours or all day, and the patient complains of the room appearing to spin around him. Any sudden motion of the head may induce vomiting. This symptom complex often occurs in persons who have had previous ear trouble and allergic symptoms, especially vasomotor rhinitis. When vasospasm of the blood vessels occurs, the muscous membrane of the cochlea becomes swollen and congested, the fluid increases in quantity, and the resultant pressure on the labyrinth produces the symptoms of Meniere's syndrome. This patient may also complain of headache, nausea, vomiting, and incoordination; however, there is no pain or loss of consciousness. The patient generally prefers to lie quietly with his eyes shut.

Between attacks, the patient works or proceeds normally and complains only of tinnitus or hearing impairment. *Tinnitus* is characteristically a low, fluctuating, buzzing sound in the ears. It is often louder preceding and during an attack. Sensorineural loss applies to low tones and usually occurs in only one ear. It gets progressively worse and may cause severe cochlear damage if untreated.

Diagnostic Evaluation. Because Meniere's disease simulates signs and symptoms of acoustic neuroma and other cerebellopontine angle tumors, careful diagnostic evaluation is required, including an audiogram, head scan, and allergy evaluation. Early in the condition, patients are evaluated for

glucose tolerance and for abnormal insulin levels. With abnormal results, these individuals are regarded as prediabetic and are managed by a controlled-carbohydrate weight-reduction diet.

A caloric test is not done during an acute attack, but performed when the patient is in remission and free of vertigo. It is important to check to make sure the patient is not taking an antihistamine or tranquilizer, since this modifies the test. Electronystagmography (ENG) is the preferred test; it measures the electropotential of the eye movements when nystagmus is produced, and provides a graphic record of labyrinthine function.

The patient with Meniere's disease has a normal or hyperactive response early in the disease. As the disease becomes chronic and the hearing decreases, the responses become hypoactive or absent. In acoustic neuroma, the labyrinthine response is hypoactive or absent. If the nystagmus is not present with water at 30° C (86° F), ice water is used. If there is no response to 15 ml of ice water, the labyrinth is considered nonresponsive.

In suspected acoustic tumors or intracranial lesions, the Hallpike bithermal (hot and cold water) test is used to study the directional preponderance and to localize a lesion. In Meniere's disease with a nonfunctioning labyrinth and severe hearing loss, compensation is already occurring and the opposite ear is taking over. In situations of this type, patients are candidates for total labyrinthectomy.

Patient Problems/Nursing Diagnoses

Based on the clinical manifestations and diagnostic assessment data, the patient's major nursing problems include bouts of dizziness, ringing in the ears, and hearing loss related to labyrinthine dysfunction; psychosocial problems related to the sudden attacks of vertigo; and concerns and worries related to the possibility of losing completely the ability to hear with the involved ear.

▶ **Planning and Implementation**

Goals

The patient's goals include:

1. Control and preferably elimination of "rotational" dizziness and ringing in the ears
2. Relief of nausea, vomiting, and headaches
3. Ability to return to usual lifestyle with a positive self-concept
4. Retention of as much of the ability to hear as possible
5. Adherence to the therapeutic regimen

Management. The goals of treatment are to eliminate vertigo and improve or stabilize the patient's hearing. This is accomplished by a combination of methods done early in the disease in order to avoid severe hearing loss. For an acute attack, the patient is permitted to assume whatever position is most comfortable. Usually, an intravenous line is started to permit the administration of medications such as diazepam (Valium), which is given slowly to control vertigo. Vital signs and the patient's condition are monitored. On occasion, a rectal suppository of dimenhydrinate (Dramamine) may be prescribed. Other oral antivertiginous drugs may be prescribed.

Three quarters of the patients respond to the treatment of a salt-free diet (Chart 55-3) and ammonium chloride. If there is an immediate favorable reaction to this regimen, it is continued for 2 or 3 months before the amount of ammonium chloride is gradually decreased. The patient, however, never returns to the full use of salt. Food allergy is investigated and may require that certain elements be eliminated from the diet.

Vasodilating drugs, such as nicotinic acid, tolazoline hydrochloride (Priscoline), and methantheline bromide (Banthine), improve tinnitus.

For patients with a history of allergy (about 5% of these patients), relief may be obtained from dimenhydrinate (Benadryl and Dramamine). Phenobarbital may be prescribed to relieve the tension factor. Antivertiginous drugs are effective for prolonged control. Alcohol is contraindicated, and smoking is discouraged because of the vasospastic action of nicotine.

Nursing Interventions. The nursing approach to the individual who has vertigo attacks is two-fold. First, the patient needs understanding and encouragement, because many find it difficult to define a problem that has subjective symptoms. The patient looks well enough to work, but he does not feel well. Secondly, he needs assistance in slowing down his movements so that he does not precipitate an attack. This need for self-protection is extended when an

attack takes place; the best place for him is lying in a bed equipped with side rails, but, if he is standing, he needs help to avoid injury from a possible fall. The patient is taught to lie down, to avoid sudden motion, and, if driving, to pull off the road and stop the car. The life-style of the individual with excessive work habits needs to be investigated and perhaps adjusted.

Surgical Management. A variety of medical and surgical treatments exist for Meniere's disease, one of which

---

Chart 55-3
Diet for Meniere's Disease (Fürstenberg Diet)

1. Fluids not restricted; however, excessive quantities of water discouraged
2. Proteins unrestricted or forced; calories permitted as indicated; sodium allowance low
3. All foods to be prepared and served without salt
4. The following foods to be eaten daily:
   Eggs, meat, fish, and fowl as desired
   Bread as desired
   Cereal, one of the following: farina, oatmeal, rice, puffed rice, or puffed wheat
   Potato and at least one of the following: macaroni, spaghetti, rice, corn, plums, prunes, or cranberries
   Any fruit and any vegetable not listed below
   Milk as desired
   Butter, cream, honey, jellies, jam, sugar, and candy (except chocolate) as desired
5. The following foods are to be avoided at all times:
   Salted meats and fish
   Bread, crackers, and butter prepared with salt

Carrots	Cheese
Spinach	Condensed milk
Endive	Olives
Cow peas	Raisins
Clams	Caviar
Oysters	

6. The following foods may be taken no more than twice weekly:

Chard	Limes
Kohlrabi	Peaches
Pumpkin	Figs
Watercress	Dates
Beets	Muskmelon
Cauliflower	Dried currants
Turnips	Dried coconut
Rutabagas	Buttermilk
Radishes	Peanuts
Celery	Horseradish
Cantaloupe	Mustard
Strawberries	

(From DeWeese DD and Saunders WH: Textbook of Otolaryngology, 6th ed. St Louis, CV Mosby, 1982.)

may give a particular patient the relief he needs. Research continues in an effort to find the cause of this syndrome, which will more clearly suggest definitive therapy.

Total labyrinthectomy (destruction of the membranous labyrinth—inner ear) is probably the most helpful technique when medical management fails (in about 10%–20% of cases) and the patient has had progressive hearing loss and experiences severe vertigo attacks (loss of hearing, 60 dB, loss of nerve response, and poor discrimination). This is done through the ear canal in the same manner as a stapedectomy. The stapes is removed and the endolabyrinth is aspirated with suction. The inner ear is packed with streptomycin.

An *endolymphatic subarachnoid shunt* is a procedure favored by many otolaryngologists. The procedure is successful in two thirds of patients in providing relief without destroying function. It involves decompressing the endolymphatic sac and sectioning the vestibular nerve.

Cryosurgery is a surgical approach in which a postauricular incision is made and the horizontal semicircular canal is approached through a simple mastoidectomy. The cryogenic probe (−160° C) is applied for a total of 6 minutes. Fascia and skin are then closed. Postoperatively, the patient is moderately dizzy for about 2 days; unsteadiness may persist for 2 or 3 weeks. The patient is hospitalized for 6 or 7 days. Within a month of discharge he may resume work.

Ultrasonic surgery is still another technique that has been tried. A mastoidectomy incision is made to gain access to the horizontal semicircular canal. Ultrasonic energy is then applied directly to the bone in the canal by means of a probe. Proponents claim that hearing is preserved while vertigo is eliminated.

Postoperatively, the patient who has had surgical destruction of the labyrinth may experience vertigo for up to 48 hours, after which it gradually subsides and permits him to get out of bed. Some unsteadiness and vertigo may persist as long as 3 to 6 weeks, but this may be controlled if the patient moves easily.

As for ultrasonic surgery, the destructive efforts of ultrasonic vibrations last for 3 to 5 days. Usually, the patient is able to be up and about in 2 to 3 days, leaves the hospital in a week, and returns to work in 3 weeks.

Bell's palsy (a peripheral facial weakness attended by aching pain near the angle of the jaw or behind the ear) may be a postoperative complication, but this clears between 2 weeks and 3 months. The patient should be forewarned about the possibility of this sequelae.

▶ Evaluation

Expected Outcomes

1. Controls and preferably eliminates "rotational" dizziness and ringing in the ears
   a. Tells of the aura prior to a sudden attack of vertigo
   b. Takes antivertiginous medications as prescribed
   c. Lies down and remains quiet immediately before an attack
   d. Queries the physician about his condition
   e. Submits to various diagnostic tests cooperatively
   f. Provides a health history that includes allergy sensitivities

g. Relates the components of a "safe" environment so that injury is minimized during an attack
2. Obtains relief from nausea, vomiting, and headaches
   a. Describes the aura prior to an attack; relates the prescribed drugs to take, such as an antiemetic, an antivertiginous drug, or Tylenol
   b. Tells how he tries to minimize subsequent symptoms of an attack: lying down, remaining quiet, turning or moving slowly
   c. Stops smoking to avoid vasospasm and vasoconstriction
   d. Indicates what relaxing activities help him: back rub; listening to records; moist, cool cloths to his forehead
3. Returns to his usual life-style with a positive self-concept
   a. Takes mild sedatives to help overcome the anxiety between attacks
   b. Expresses appreciation for the support of the health team and family
   c. Develops menus indicative of his understanding of the necessity of a salt-free diet
   d. Recites the nature of prescribed medications, as well as the purpose, dosage, and possible side-effects
4. Salvages as much as possible the ability to hear
   a. Accepts all phases of the prescribed medical therapeutic regimen
   b. Conducts a dialogue with the otologist to develop an understanding of surgical options in the event that medical intervention is unsuccessful
   c. Learns to read lips "just in case"
   d. Accepts surgical intervention that the physician suggests is best for relief of his symptoms
5. Adheres to the therapeutic regimen
   a. Moves and turns slowly when an aura is recognized
   b. Takes medications as prescribed; tells which medication is to be taken immediately when aura is apparent
   c. Explains why it is important to have a low-sodium or salt-free diet
   d. Participates in lip reading/hearing therapy classes
   e. Talks with family about plans for "adapting" to a more normal life-style with present hearing deficit

▷ **Bibliography**

Books

Adams GL, Boies LR, and Paparella MM. Boies' Fundamentals of Otolaryngology, 5th ed. Philadelphia, WB Saunders, 1978.

Ballantyne J and Groves J (eds). Scott Brown's Diseases of the Ear, Nose and Throat, Vol 2, The Ear, 4th ed. London, Butterworths, 1979.

Bradford LJ and Hardy WG. Hearing and Hearing Impairment. New York, Grune & Stratton, 1979.

Dayal VS. Clinical Otolaryngology. Philadelphia, JB Lippincott, 1981.

DeWeese DD and Saunders WH. Textbook of Otolaryngology, 6th ed. Philadelphia, WB Saunders, 1982.

English GM. Otolaryngology: A Textbook. Hagerstown, Maryland, Harper & Row, 1976.

Goodhill V. Ear Diseases, Deafness, and Dizziness. Hagerstown, Maryland, Harper & Row, 1979.

Hurvitz J and Carmen R. Special Devices for Hard of Hearing, Deaf and Deaf-Blind Persons. Boston, Little, Brown & Co, 1981.

Maurer JF and Rupp RR. Hearing and Aging: Tactics for Intervention. New York, Grune & Stratton, 1979.

Rosenblum EH. Fundamentals of Hearing for the Health Professionals. Boston, Little, Brown & Co, 1979.

Sataloff J, Sataloff RT, and Vassallo LA. Hearing Loss. Philadelphia, JB Lippincott, 1980.

Saunders WH et al. Nursing Care in Eye, Ear, Nose and Throat Disorders, 4th ed. St Louis, CV Mosby, 1979.

Snow JB. Controversy in Otolaryngology. Philadelphia, WB Saunders, 1980.

Articles
Hearing and Hearing Loss

Browning GG, Swan IRC, and Gatehouse S. Hearing loss in minor head injury. Arch Otolaryngol 1982 Aug; 108(8):475–477.

Curry JL. The hearing-impaired patient: Stranger in a strange land. Ethicon Point of View 1980; 17(4):18–20.

Jafek BW and Balkany TJ. Conductive hearing loss. In Eiseman B. Prognosis of Surgical Disease, pp 70–72. Philadelphia, WB Saunders, 1980.

Harrison RJ. Current concepts in the management of hearing loss. Am Fam Physician 1979 Jan; 19(1):135–142.

LeBuffe FP and LeBuffe LA. Psychiatric aspects of deafness. Primary Care 1979 June; 6(2):295–310.

Miller RR. Deafness due to plain and long-acting aspirin tablets. J Clin Pharmacol 1978 Oct; 18(10):468–471.

Raafat JR and Adams CT. American sign language. Md Nurse 1980 Aug; 37

Sataloff RT and Vassallo LA. Choosing the right hearing aid. Hosp Pract 1981 May; 16(5):32A–32S.

Schiff M and Cohen IJ. What every otolaryngologist should know about hearing aids. The Laryngoscope 1978 June; 88(6):932–945.

Hearing Devices

Maurer and Rupp. Hearing and Aging, pp 269–274 (Learning to Hear Again, Appendix C). New York, Grune & Stratton, 1979. (Excellent guidelines for the new hearing aid wearer)

Salatoff RT and Vassallo LA. Choosing the right hearing aid. Hosp Pract 1981 May; 16(5):32A–32S.

Schiff M and Cohen IJ. What every otolaryngologist should know about hearing aids. The Laryngoscope 1978 June; 88(6):932–945.

Ear Problems

Antimicrobial agents for acute otitis media. The Medical Letter 1981 Oct 30; 23(22):93–95.

Black FO et al. Easing proneness to motion sickness. Patient Care 1980 Mar 30; 14(6):114–128.

Brennman AK, Meltzer CR, and Milner R. Myringotomy and tube ventilation in adults. Am Fam Physician 1982 Oct; 26(4):181–184.

Clark JL. Otalgia: Identifying the source. Postgrad Med 1981 Oct; 70(4):99–103.

Duvall AJ and Lowell SH. The "chronic" ear: How to manage mild to severe otitis. Postgrad Med 1979 Aug; 66(2):94–101.

Farmer HS. A guide for the treatment of external otitis. Am Fam Physician 1980 June; 21(6):96–101.

Middle ear infections. The Harvard Medical School Health Letter 1982 May; 7(6):1, 2, 5.

Luotonen J. Equipment for aspirating middle ear fluid samples. Laryngoscope 1981 Oct; 92(10):1196–1197.

Marshall L and Gossman MA. Management of ear-canal collapse. Arch Otolaryngol 1982 June; 108(6):357–361.

McNicoll WD. Eustachian tube dysfunction in submariners and divers. Arch Otolaryngol 1982 May; 108(5):279–283.

Meade RH III. Complications of earache. Hosp Pract 1979 Aug; 14(8):78–81.

Newman RK and Johnson JT. Unresponsive unilateral serous otitis. Postgrad Med 1980 Mar; 67(3):143–149.

Otalgia: Identifying the source. Postgrad Med 1981 Oct; 70(4):99–103.

Otitis media. The Medical Letter 1981 Oct 30; 23(22):93–95.

Price N et al. Transdermal scopolamine in the prevention of motion sickness at sea. Clin Pharmacol Ther 1981 Mar; 29(3):414–419.

Pulec JL. Meniere's syndrome. Hospital Medicine 1980 May; 16(5):46–47.

Schwartz RH. New concepts in otitis media. Am Fam Physician 1979 May; 19(5):91–98.

Schwartz RH. Myringotomy: A neglected office procedure. Am Fam Physician 1979 Dec; 20(6):102–108.

Stewart TW. Common otolaryngologic problems of flying. Am Fam Physician 1979 Feb; 19(2):113–119.

Strauss MB, Groner-Strauss W, and Cantrell RW. Swimmer's ear. Physician and Sport's Medicine 1979 June; 7(8):101–105.

Treating Meniere's disease nonsurgically. Am Fam Physician 1980 Dec; 22(6):136.

Agencies

Alexander Graham Bell Association for the Deaf, Inc., 3417 Volta Place, N.W., Washington, D.C. 20007

American Speech–Language–Hearing Association, 10801 Rockville Pike, Rockville, Maryland 20852

American Tinnitus Association, P.O. Box #5, Portland, Oregon 97207

National Association for Hearing and Speech Action, Suite #1000, 6110 Executive Blvd., Rockville, Maryland 20852

National Association for the Deaf, Suite 301, 814 Thayer Ave., Silver Spring, Maryland 20910

National Hearing Association, Suite 308, 1010 Jorie Blvd., Oak Brook, Illinois 60521

The Deafness Research Foundation, 55 East 34th St., New York, New York 10016

Self-Help for Hard of Hearing People, Inc., P.O. Box 34889, Bethesda, Maryland 20034

Hearing Aid Helpline: Toll free number for information about hearing aids and hearing health (sponsored by National Hearing Aid Society): 1-800-521-4247 (all states except Michigan) 9 AM–4 PM EST, Mon. through Fri.

Collect Call Hotline: 301-897-8682 to Kresge Hearing Research Laboratory of the South in New Orleans—for "ultra-audiometric" problems (capacity to hear, but only at extremely high frequencies)

56

Assessment of Neurologic Function

▷ Physiologic Overview

The nervous system is comprised of the brain and the spinal cord together with all extensions therefrom and neural connections thereto. Its function is to control and to coordinate cellular activities throughout the body. The signaling device that it employs involves the transmission of electrical impulses, a system that permits each stimulus to be placed accurately in the area that is intended to receive it. These impulses are routed by way of nerve fibers, pathways that are direct and continuous, and the responses that these elicit are practically instantaneous because changes in electrical potential transmit the signals.

The Brain

The brain is divided into the cerebrum, brain stem, and cerebellum. It is enclosed in a rigid, bony box—the skull or cranium. At the base of this box is the *foramen magnum,* an opening through which the spinal cord forms a continuous connection with the brain (Fig. 56-1). The brain has three coverings: (1) the *dura,* the outer covering of dense fibrous tissue that closely hugs the inner wall of the skull; (2) the *arachnoid;* and (3) the *pia mater,* which adheres closely to the brain and the spinal cord.

The *brain stem* consists, from top down, of midbrain, pons, and medulla oblongata.

The *cerebrum* is divided into two hemispheres and consists of four lobes: frontal, parietal, temporal, and occipital (Fig. 56-2). The cerebrum is the largest part of the brain, and on its surface or cortex are located the "centers" from which motor impulses are carried to the muscles, and to which sensory impulses come from the various sensory nerves.

The *midbrain* connects the pons and the cerebellum with the cerebral hemispheres. The *cerebellum* is located below and behind the cerebrum. Its function is the control or the coordination of muscles and equilibration.

The *pons* is situated in front of the cerebellum between the midbrain and the medulla and is a bridge between the

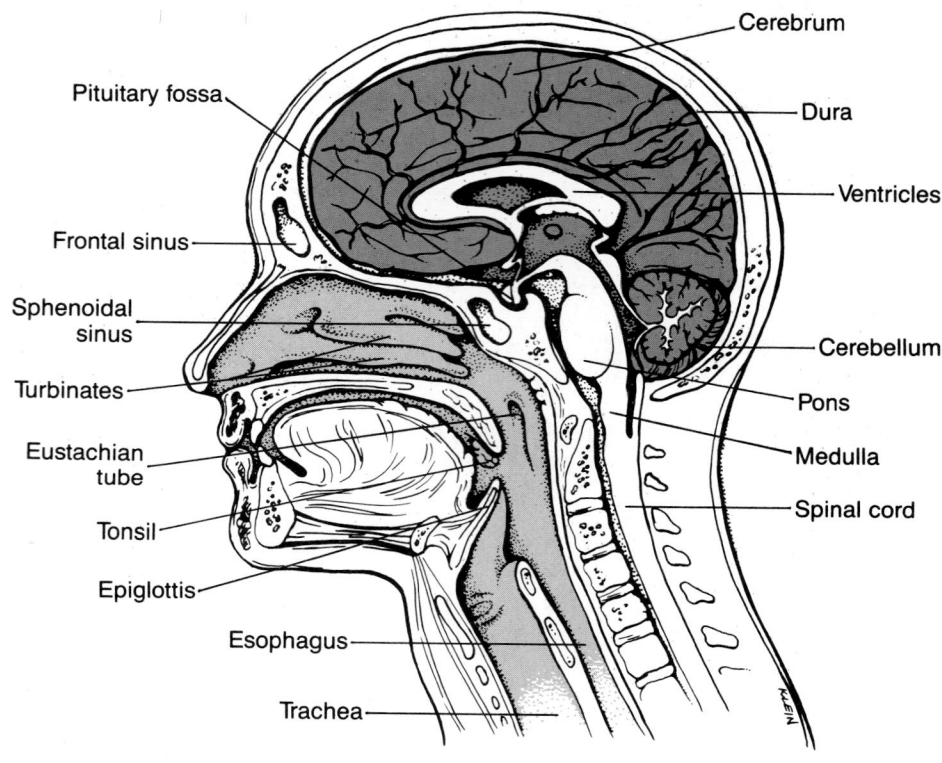

Figure 56-1. Cross-sectional view showing the anatomical position and the relation of structures of the head and the neck.

two halves of the cerebellum as well as between the medulla and the cerebrum.

The *medulla oblongata* transmits motor fibers from the brain to the spinal cord and sensory fibers from the spinal cord to the brain. The majority of these fibers decussate at this level. The pons also contains important centers controlling heart, respiration, and blood pressure, and gives origin to the fifth, sixth, seventh, and eighth cranial nerves.

There are two glands present in the brain: the pituitary and the pineal. The pituitary gland is frequently approached surgically. It lies at the base of the brain in a bony fossa termed the sella turcica, just posterior to the optic chiasm, upon which it may press when the gland is enlarged.

Cerebral Cortex.   While the cells in the cerebral cortex are quite similar in appearance, their functions vary widely, depending on their geographic location. Figure 56-2 depicts the topography of the cortex in relation to certain of its specific functions. The posterior portion of each hemisphere (*i.e.,* the occipital lobe) is devoted to all aspects of visual perception; the lateral region, or temporal lobe, incorporates the auditory center. The mid-central zone, or parietal zone, posterior to the fissure of Rolandi, is concerned with sensation; the anterior portion is concerned with voluntary muscle movements. The large, uncharted area beneath the forehead (*i.e.,* the frontal lobes) contains the association pathways that determine emotional attitudes and responses and contributes to the formation of thought processes. Damage to the frontal lobes as a result of trauma or disease is by no means incapacitating from the standpoint of muscular control

or coordination, but has decided effect on the personality of the individual, as reflected by basic attitudes, sense of humor and propriety, self-restraint, and motivations.

Internal Capsule, Pons, and Medulla.   Nerve fibers from all portions of the cortex converge in each hemisphere and make their exit in the form of tight bundles known as the "internal capsule." Having entered the pons and the medulla, each bundle crosses the corresponding bundle from the opposite side. Some of these axons make connections with axons from the cerebellum, basal ganglia, thalamus, and hypothalamus; some connect with the cranial nerve cells. Other fibers from the cortex and the subcortical centers are channeled through the pons and the medulla into the spinal cord.

The Spinal Cord and Its Connections

The *spinal cord,* a direct continuation of the medulla oblongata, is that part of the nervous system contained within the vertebral column (Fig. 56-3). It is a cord about 45 cm (18 inches) long and approximately the thickness of a finger, extending from the foramen magnum of the skull, where it is continuous with the medulla oblongata, to the first lumbar vertebra, where it tapers off into a fine thread of tissue. The spinal cord is an important center of reflex action for the body and contains the conducting pathways to and from the higher centers in the cord and the brain. Like the brain, it consists of gray and white matter, but, although in the brain the gray matter is external and the white internal, in the cord the gray matter is in the center and is surrounded on

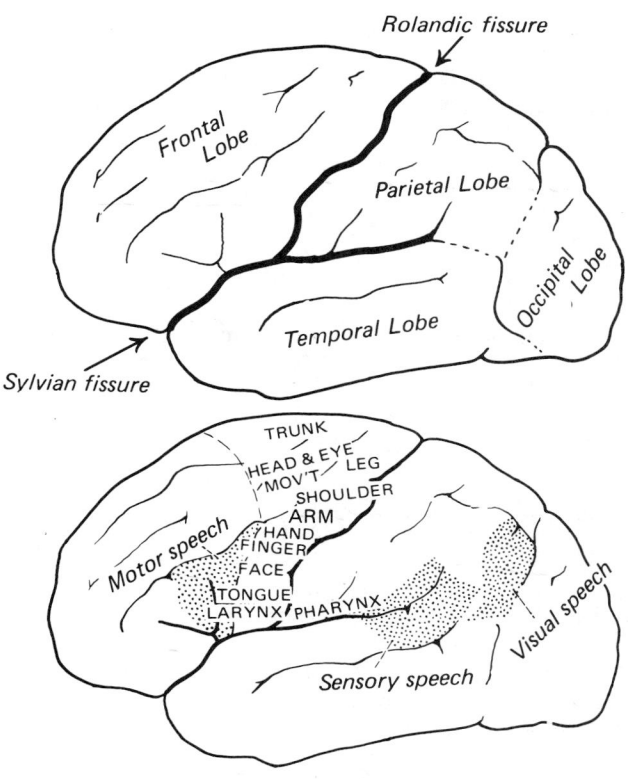

Figure 56-2. (*Top*) Diagrammatic representation of the cerebrum, showing relative locations of various lobes of the brain and the principal fissures. (*Bottom*) Diagrammatic representation of cerebral localization for motor movements of various portions of the body.

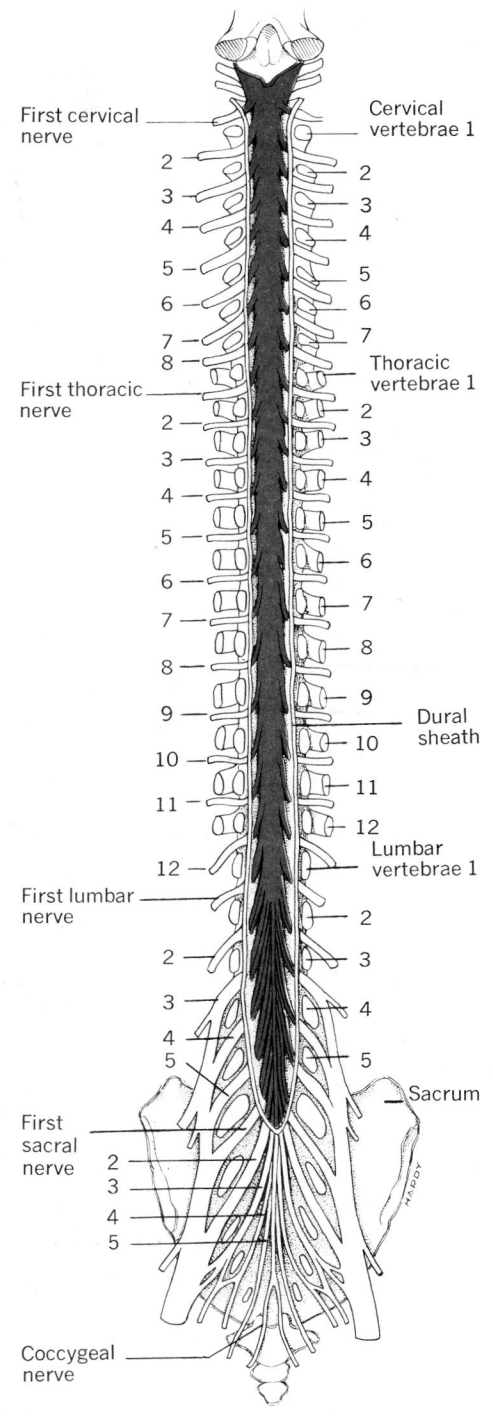

Figure 56-3. Spinal cord lying within the vertebral canal; spinous processes and laminae have been removed; dura and arachnoid have been opened. Spinal nerves are numbered on the left side; vertebrae are numbered on the right side. (From Chaffee EE and Greisheimer EM: Basic Physiology and Anatomy, 4th ed. Philadelphia, JB Lippincott, 1979.)

all sides by the white fibers, both those of sensory tracts running up to the brain and those of motor fibers coming down from the brain.

Gray Matter.   The gray matter is shaped like two pairs of horns, the anterior horn and the posterior horn. The cord gives off 31 pairs of spinal nerves. Each is formed by the union of two roots, an anterior or motor root and a posterior or sensory root on which is the sensory ganglion. These two roots unite to form one spinal nerve. As a result, all the spinal nerves are mixed. Those leaving the right side of the cord supply the muscles, the skin, and the organs on the right side of the body; those of the left side supply the corresponding muscles on that side of the body.

Cerebrospinal Fluid

Within each cerebral hemisphere is a central cavity, the lateral ventricle, which is filled with clear *cerebrospinal fluid.* This fluid is extracted from the blood as it circulates through the capillaries of the choroid plexus. It then passes through well-defined channels from the lateral ventricles through narrow, tubular openings to the third and the fourth ventricles. From this narrow cavity it escapes to the subarachnoid space to bathe the entire surface of the brain and the spinal cord. The cerebrospinal fluid normally is absorbed by the large venous channels of the skull and along the spinal and the cranial nerves.

The spinal fluid is clear and colorless, having a specific gravity of 1.007. The average patient's ventricular and subarachnoid systems contain about 150 ml of this fluid. The organic and inorganic contents of the cerebrospinal fluid are very similar to that of the plasma; however, their concentration is somewhat different.

Disease produces changes in the composition of the cerebrospinal fluid. Determinations of the protein content and the quantity of glucose and chloride present constitute the chief chemical examinations. In a state of health, there are a minimal number of white cells and no red cells in the spinal fluid. Cerebrospinal fluid is also tested for immunoglobulins.

By replacing cerebrospinal fluid with air, the radiologist is able to visualize with x-rays the size, shape, and position of the ventricles. Any interference or distortion may be suggestive of a space-occupying lesion.

▷ Pathophysiology

Vision and Cortical Blindness

There is a definite area in the rear of each hemisphere where the fibers of the corresponding optic nerve end. It is by means of these receiving cells that vision is possible. The eyes may be normal and the optic nerve perfect, but if these cells in one hemisphere are diseased, the person is half-blind and has *cortical blindness*. He cannot see to one side of the midline. He sees only half of any object. This is known as *hemianopsia* (half-blindness).

Cortical blindness of one optic area (*i.e.,* of the posterior tip of one cerebral hemisphere) always affects both eyes equally. Total blindness in one eye may be due to disease of that eye itself or to disease of its optic nerve. Just behind the two eyes, however, the two optic nerves become confluent (the chiasm), then again become separate and continue to the brain as two optic tracts.

In each of these tracts is just half of each optic nerve, so that if one tract is injured, there is complete blindness of exactly one half of each retina. For example, if the right tract is injured, the patient is blind on the right half of each retina, so that with either eye he can see nothing to his left but will see perfectly to his right. If the cortical optical area of the hemisphere to which that tract runs is destroyed, this same form of hemianopsia occurs.

The pituitary gland is located just beneath the chiasm; a tumor of this gland often disturbs the chiasm and produces blindness of both inner halves of the retinas, since it is only the fibers in the nasal halves of the optic nerves that cross. In many cases of blindness, it is thus possible to locate the disorder.

Motor Controls: Paralysis and Dyskinesia

A vertical band of cortex on each cerebral hemisphere governs the voluntary movements of the body. This region, known as the "motor cortex," can be located accurately.

We know the exact location of the cells in which originate the voluntary movements of the muscles of the face, the thumb, the hands, the arm, the trunk, or the leg. Before a person can move a muscle, these particular cells must send the stimulus down along their fibers. If these cells are stimulated with an electric current, the muscles they control will contract.

En route to the pons, as described previously, the motor fibers converge into a tight bundle known as the *capsule*. A comparatively small injury to the capsule causes paralysis in more muscles than does a much larger injury to the cortex itself.

The brain is like a telephone station, in which one blow of an axe can sever all the wires at the point where they leave the building, but a similar blow on the switchboard would sever only a few.

The ordinary cause of a stroke, followed by paralysis of one half of the body (hemiplegia), is usually a small hemorrhage from a blood vessel in the capsule. A much larger hemorrhage nearer to or in the cortex might paralyze one limb, but hardly half of the body. Hemiplegia may be due to the rupture of a microaneurysm of a tiny artery running to the internal capsule or to the plugging of this artery by a thrombus or an embolus, and the subsequent death of the fibers that it supplies with blood.

Immediately after a stroke, one half of the body, as a rule, is paralyzed. Then, gradually, the person recovers the use of certain muscles, usually those of the leg, often those of the upper arm, least often those of the hand. Although the hemorrhage actually destroys the fibers of only a few nerves, it temporarily injures all those in its neighborhood, perhaps by the pressure of the escaped blood or by the edema that surrounds it. As the swelling from the hemorrhage diminishes, these latter fibers resume their function, but those actually destroyed never do.

Within the medulla, the motor axons from the cortex form two well-defined bands known as the *corticospinal* or *pyramidal tracts*. Here the majority of these fibers cross (or decussate) to the opposite side, continuing thereafter as the "crossed pyramidal tract." The remaining fibers then enter the spinal cord on the original side as the "direct pyramidal tract," each fiber in this tract finally crossing to the opposite side of the cord near the point of termination and coming to an end within the gray matter comprising the anterior horn on that side, in close proximity to a motor nerve cell. Fibers of the crossed pyramidal tract terminate within the anterior horn and make connections with anterior horn cells on the same side. All of the motor fibers of the spinal nerves represent extensions of these anterior horn cells, with each of these fibers communicating with only one particular muscle fiber.

Thus, each muscle fiber is under voluntary control through a combination of two nerve cells. One is located in the motor cortex, its fiber in the direct or crossed pyramidal tract, and the other is located in the anterior horn of the spinal cord, its fiber running to the muscle. The former is referred to as the upper motor neuron; the latter, as the lower motor neuron. Every motor nerve serving a muscle is a bundle comprised of several thousand lower motor neurons.

Several motor nerve tracts, other than the corticospinal, are contained in the spinal cord. Some represent the pathways of the so-called "extrapyramidal system," establishing connections between the anterior horn cells and the automatic control centers located in the basal ganglia and the cerebellum. Others are components of reflex arcs, forming synaptic connections between anterior horn cells and sensory fibers that have entered adjacent or neighboring segments of the cord.

Motor Paralysis.   Paralysis of a muscle may be due to pathologic changes in either the upper or the lower motor neuron. If a motor nerve is cut somewhere between the muscle and the spinal cord, the muscle becomes paralyzed, and the individual is not able to move it. Furthermore, it takes no part in reflex movements. Moreover, this muscle becomes limp and wastes away; that is, it atrophies due to disuse. The injury to the spinal nerve trunk may heal, and the patient may regain the use of the muscles that it supplies. But if the anterior horn motor nerve cells are destroyed, the nerve cannot regenerate, and that muscle never will be useful again. This is exactly what occurs in anterior poliomyelitis.

If the upper motor neuron is destroyed, a different condition exists in the muscle. It is paralyzed as far as voluntary movement is concerned, but not necessarily for reflex (involuntary) movements, because these originate in the nerve cells in the cord or the medulla. The muscle does not atrophy, and it will not become limp; on the contrary, it remains permanently more tense than normal. This paralysis seldom affects a part of one muscle, one single muscle, or only a few muscles; it usually affects a whole extremity, both extremities, or an entire half of the body (hemiplegia).

A good illustration of this form of paralysis is the spastic (stiff) paralysis of those infants who during birth receive some mechanical injury that may have caused the rupture of a subdural blood vessel. The long-continued pressure of the escaped blood may injure large areas of cortex; hence, these children are frequently mentally retarded. Many have convulsions. When such a child begins to walk, the legs and the arms are stiff. During life, movements are awkward, stiff, and weak. Since those muscles that draw the feet and the knees toward each other (the adductor muscles) are naturally stronger than those that spread those limbs apart (the abductor muscles), these persons walk by a cross-legged progression, called also the *scissors gait;* that is, in each step the leg is moved not only forward but is swung round across the front of the other. When both legs are paralyzed, the condition is called *paraplegia;* and when the arm and the leg on the same side are paralyzed, the term *hemiplegia* is used. Paralysis of all four extremities is *quadriplegia.*

A common illustration of upper motor neuron paralysis is hemiplegia. If a hemorrhage, an embolus, or a thrombus destroys the fibers from the motor area in the internal capsule, the arm and the leg of the opposite side promptly become stiff and more or less paralyzed, and the reflexes are exaggerated. Another illustration of upper neuron disease is seen in adults with spastic paraplegia, a chronic stiffness of both legs due to a gradual degeneration of the fibers in the pyramidal tract. The person so afflicted walks stiffly, as though wading through water, the knees always touching each other and the feet scarcely raised from the ground (the spastic gait).

Both an upper and a lower motor neuron paralysis may result from an injury that crushes the spinal cord, a type of injury that is all too common. A person diving into too-shallow water, for example, strikes his head and "breaks" his neck. That is, at one point the vertebrae are no longer in line, and the cord is badly crushed at the point of the dislocation. Knuckling of the backbone due to tuberculosis may accomplish the same thing, only more slowly. The result of such crushing of the cord leads to a rigid paralysis on both sides of all muscles whose nerves leave the cord below the crushed spot. Flaccid paralysis also occurs in those muscles whose motor nerve fibers come from cells in the crushed area. There also will be insensibility of the skin below the crushed area, since the sensory fibers from below the injury no longer reach the brain. Tumors of the cord ultimately cause this same picture. At first, only that part of the cord directly involved is disturbed, but as the tumor grows, it may completely crush the cord.

Extrapyramidal Motor Controls.   The smoothness, the accuracy, and the strength that characterize the muscular movements of a normal individual are attributable to the influence of the cerebellum and the basal ganglia.

The cerebellum (see Fig. 55-1), nestled beneath the posterior lobe of the cerebrum, chief assistant to the higher motor centers in the cerebral cortex, is responsible for coordinating, balancing, timing, and synergizing with precision all muscular movements that originate in those centers. Through the agency of the cerebellum, the contractions of opposing muscle groups are adjusted in relation to each other to maximal mechanical advantage; muscular contractions can be sustained evenly at the desired tension and without significant fluctuation, and reciprocal movements can be reproduced at high and constant speed, in stereotyped fashion, and with relatively little effort.

The basal ganglia are masses of gray matter in the midbrain beneath the cerebral hemispheres. These border or project into the lateral ventricles and lie in close apposition to the internal capsule. It is their function to control habitual or automatic acts and to maintain a "postural background" against which voluntary movements are performed. These ganglia, aided by their connections with the organs of special sense, keep the contractile tone of every muscle in the trunk and the extremities in a constant state of adjustment, so that an individual is able to keep his balance regardless of the posture of his body, in darkness as well as in light and irrespective of the status underfoot. Moreover, thanks to this control station, the individual is equipped to react swiftly, appropriately, and automatically to any smell, sight, or sound that demands an immediate response.

Dyskinesias.   Loss of cerebellar function, which may occur as a result of intracranial injury, hemorrhage, abscess, or tumor, results in muscular flabbiness, weakness, and fatigue. The patient exhibits a coarse involuntary tremor that increases in intensity in association with voluntary movements. He is unable to control his movements accurately or to coordinate his muscles efficiently or smoothly, every act being performed in disjointed fashion, according to stages, or "by the numbers." He is incapable of performing alternating movements with speed or uniformity, a characteristic of cerebellar disease called "adiadochokinesis." When he walks, he staggers, lurching from side to side as though intoxicated, feet wide apart, but steps short and not stamping (*i.e.,* with the vertiginous, reeling gait of cerebellar ataxia).

Destruction or dysfunction of the basal ganglia does not lead to paralysis but to muscular rigidity, with consequent disturbances of posture and movement. Such patients are afflicted by a tendency to display involuntary movements. These may take the form of coarse tremors, characterized by approximately six oscillations per second; *athetosis,* namely, movements of a slow, squirming, writhing, twisting type; or *chorea,* marked by spasmodic, purposeless, and grotesque motions of the trunk and the extremities, and facial grimacing. Clinical syndromes based on lesions involving the basal ganglia include parkinsonism (see p. 1346); Huntington's disease (see p. 1349); Wilson's disease, or "hepatolenticular degeneration"; and spasmodic torticollis.

Sensory Pathways and Disturbances

The Thalamus.   The *thalamus,* a major receiving and communication center for the afferent sensory nerves, is a large and complicated structure located in the midbrain. It lies in close relation to the third ventricle, forming its lateral wall, and to the lateral ventricle, forming its floor, and is in close proximity to the basal ganglia and adjacent to the internal capsule. To the thalamus may be attributed the vague awareness of sensations described as "feelings" of pleasure, discomfort, or pain. Moreover, it is responsible for the routing of all sensory stimuli to their many destinations, including the cerebral cortex, which receives them and translates them automatically into appropriate responses.

Sensory Pathways.   The transmission of sensory impulses from their points of origin to their cerebral destinations involves three neuron relays; moreover, there are three major pathways by which they may be routed, depending on the type of sensation that is registered. Specific knowledge regarding these paths is of great importance from the standpoint of neurologic diagnoses, being indispensable for the accurate localization of brain and cord lesions in many patients.

The axon of the nerve in which the sensory impulse originates enters the spinal cord by way of the posterior root. Axons conveying sensations of heat, cold, and pain immediately enter the posterior gray column of the cord, where they make connections with the cells of secondary neurons. Pain and temperature fibers cross immediately to the opposite side of the cord and course upward to the thalamus. Fibers carrying sensations of touch, light pressure, and localization do not connect immediately with the second neuron but ascend the cord for a variable distance before entering the gray matter and completing this connection. The axon of the secondary neuron crosses the cord and proceeds upward to the thalamus.

The third category of sensation, produced by stimuli arising from muscles, joints, and bones, includes position sense and vibratory sense. These stimuli are conveyed, uncrossed, all the way to the brain stem by the axon of the primary neuron. In the medulla, synaptic connections are made with cells of the secondary neurons, whose axons then cross to the opposite side and proceed to the thalamus.

Sensory Losses.   Severance of a sensory nerve results in total loss of sensation in its area of distribution. Transection of the spinal cord yields complete anesthesia below the level of injury. Selective destruction or degeneration of the posterior columns of the spinal cord, a characteristic of combined system disease, is responsible for a loss of position sense in segments distal to the lesion, unaccompanied by loss of touch, pain, or temperature perception. Such individuals, unless they look, cannot tell where their feet are or in what direction they are pointing. Moreover, they cannot perceive vibrations in the affected area. A lesion, such as a cyst, in the center of the cord causes dissociation of sensation, that is, loss of pain at the level of the lesion. This is explainable on the basis of the fact that the fibers carrying pain and temperature cross the cord immediately upon entering; thus, any lesion that divides the cord longitudinally divides these fibers likewise. Other sensory fibers ascend the cord for variable distances, some even to the medulla itself, before crossing, thereby bypassing the lesion and avoiding destruction.

Dysesthesias.   Irritative lesions affecting the posterior spinal nerve roots may cause intermittent severe pains that are referred to their areas of distribution. This phenomenon explains the pains of tabes dorsalis. The sensation of tingling of the fingers and the toes constitutes a prominent symptom of combined systems disease, presumably due to degenerative changes in the sensory fibers that extend to the thalamus (*i.e.,* belonging to the spinothalamic tract).

Autonomic Nervous System

The contractions of muscles that are not under voluntary control, including the heart muscle, the secretions of all digestive and sweat glands, and the activity of certain endocrine organs as well, are controlled by a major component of the nervous system known as the *autonomic nervous system.* The term "autonomic" refers to the fact that the operations of this system are independent of the desires and the intentions of the individual. It is not subject to his will; that is, it is in a sense autonomous.

To the extent that it is not subject to regulation by the cerebral cortex, the autonomic nervous system resembles the extrapyramidal systems that are centered in the cerebellum and the basal ganglia. However, in other respects it is unique. First, its regulatory effects are exerted not on individual cells but on large expanses of tissue and on entire organs. Second, the responses that it elicits do not appear instantaneously, but only after a lag period, and they are sustained far longer than other neurogenic responses, a type of response that is calculated to ensure maximal functional efficiency on the part of receptor organs, such as the blood vessels and the hollow viscera.

The quality of these responses is explained by the fact that the autonomic nervous system transmits its impulses only partly by way of nerve pathways, the remainder of the route being serviced by chemical mediators, resembling in this respect the endocrine system. Electrical impulses, conducted through nerve fibers, stimulate the formation of specific chemical agents at strategic locations within the muscle mass, the diffusion of these chemicals being responsible for the contraction.

The Hypothalamus.   Overall supervision of the autonomic nervous system is considered a function of the hypothalamus. The *hypothalamus* is a portion of the diencephalon (interbrain) located immediately beneath and lateral to the lower portion of the wall of the third ventricle. It includes among its components the optic chiasm; the tuber cinereum; the pituitary stalk, which originates from the latter; and the pituitary gland itself. Large cell groups in adjacent portions of the hypothalamus have been assigned the role of the probable centers of autonomic regulation. These centers are richly endowed with connections linking the autonomic system with the thalamus, the cortex, the olfactory apparatus, and the pituitary gland. Here reside the mechanisms for the control of visceral and somatic reactions that were designed originally for defense or attack, but in man these are associated with his emotional states (*i.e.,* his fears, anger, anxiety); for the control of metabolic processes, including fat, carbohydrate, and water metabolism; for the regulation of body temperature, arterial pressure, and all muscular and glandular activities of the gastrointestinal tract; the genital functions; and the sleep rhythm. The close proximity, histologic similarity, and multiple connections between the pituitary gland, master gland of the endocrines, and this portion of the brain suggest that here may be located the supreme headquarters of the endocrine and autonomic nervous systems, commanding all vital processes.

Sympathetic and Parasympathetic Nervous Systems

The *autonomic nervous system* comprises two divisions that are anatomically and functionally distinct, referred to as the sympathetic and the parasympathetic nervous systems. The majority of the tissues and the organs under autonomic control are innervated by both systems. Sympathetic stimuli are mediated by norepinephrine, and parasympathetic impulses by acetylcholine. These chemicals produce opposing and mutually antagonistic effects, as indicated in Table 56-1.

Sympathetic Nervous System. Sympathetic neurons are located in the thoracic and the lumbar segments of the spinal cord; their axons, called *preganglionic fibers,* emerge by way of all anterior nerve roots from the eighth cervical or first thoracic segment to the second or third lumbar segment, inclusive. A short distance from the cord these fibers diverge to join a chain composed of 22 linked ganglia that extends the entire length of the spinal column, flanking the vertebral bodies on both sides. Some form multiple synapses with nerve cells within the chain. Others traverse the chain without making connections or losing continuity to join large "prevertebral" ganglia in the thorax, the abdomen, or the pelvis, or one of the "terminal" ganglia in the vicinity of an organ, such as the bladder or the rectum. Postganglionic nerve fibers originating in the sympathetic chain rejoin the spinal nerves that supply the extremities and are distributed to blood vessels, sweat glands, and smooth muscle tissue in the skin. Postganglionic fibers from the prevertebral plexuses (*i.e.,* the cardiac, pulmonary, splanchnic, and pelvic plexuses) supply structures in the head and the neck, the thorax, the abdomen, and the pelvis, respectively, having been joined in these plexuses by fibers from the parasympathetic division.

The adrenals, the kidneys, the liver, the spleen, the stomach, and the duodenum are under the control of the giant celiac plexus, familiarly known as the "solar plexus." This receives its sympathetic nerve components by way of the three splanchnic nerves, composed of preganglionic fibers from nine segments of the spinal cord (*i.e.,* T4 to L1),

Table 56-1
Comparison of Parasympathetic and Sympathetic Effects on Specific Organs and Tissues

Organ or Tissue	Parasympathetic Effects	Sympathetic Effects
Vessels:		
Cutaneous	—	Constriction
Muscular	—	Variable
Coronary	Constriction	Dilatation
Salivary gland	Dilatation	Constriction
Buccal mucosa	—	Dilatation
Pulmonary	Variable	Variable
Cerebral	Dilatation	Constriction
Of abdominal and pelvic viscera	—	Constriction
Of external genitalia	Dilatation	Constriction
Heart	Inhibition	Acceleration
Eye:		
Iris	Constriction	Dilatation
Ciliary muscle	Contraction	Relaxation
Smooth muscle of orbit and upper lid	—	Contraction
Bronchi	Constriction	Dilatation
Glands:		
Sweat	—	Secretion
Salivary	Secretion	Secretion
Gastric	Secretion	Inhibition? Secretion of mucus
Pancreatic		
Acini	Secretion	—
Islets	Secretion	—
Liver	—	Glycogenolysis
Adrenal medulla	—	Secretion
Smooth muscle:		
Of skin	—	Contraction
Of stomach wall	Contraction (predominantly)	Inhibition (predominantly)
Of small intestine	Increased tone and motility	Inhibition
Of large intestine	Increased tone and motility	Inhibition
Of bladder wall (detrusor muscle)	Contraction	Inhibition
Of trigone and sphincter	Inhibition	Contraction
Of uterus, pregnant	None	Contraction
Of uterus, nonpregnant	None	Inhibition

(From Best CH and Taylor NB: Physiological Basis of Medical Practice, 6th ed. Baltimore, Williams & Wilkins.)

and is joined by the vagus nerve, representing the parasympathetic division. From the celiac plexus, fibers of both divisions travel along the course of blood vessels to their target organs.

Parasympathetic System.   The preganglionic nerve cells of the sympathetic division, as described above, are consolidated in consecutive segments of the cord, from C7 to L1 or L2. Those of the parasympathetic system, on the other hand, are located in two sections, one in the brain stem and the other from spinal segments below L2. On this account, the parasympathetic system is referred to as the "craniosacral" division, as distinct from the "thoracolumbar" division of the autonomic nervous system.

The cranial parasympathetics arise from the midbrain and the medulla oblongata. Fibers from cells in the midbrain travel with the third oculomotor nerve to the ciliary ganglia, whence postganglionic fibers of this division are joined by those of the sympathetic system. Forming the ciliary nerve, these channel to the ciliary muscles of the eye to control the caliber of the pupil. Parasympathetic fibers from the medulla travel with the seventh (facial), ninth (glossopharyngeal), and tenth (vagus) cranial nerves. Those from the facial nerve end in the splenopalatine ganglion, whence emanate the fibers that innervate the lacrimal glands, the ciliary muscle, and the sphincter of the pupil. Those from the glossopharyngeal nerve innervate the parotid gland. The vagus nerve carries preganglionic parasympathetic fibers without interruption to the organs that it innervates, joining ganglion cells within the myocardium and within the walls of the esophagus, the stomach, and the intestine.

Preganglionic parasympathetic fibers from the anterior roots of the sacral nerves coalesce to become the pelvic nerves, consolidate and regroup in the pelvic plexus, and terminate around ganglion cells in the musculature of the pelvic organs. These innervate the colon, the rectum, and the bladder, inhibiting the muscular tone of the anal and the bladder sphincters and dilating the blood vessels of the bladder, the rectum, and the genitalia.

The vagus, splanchnic, pelvic, and other autonomic nerves carry impulses generated in the viscera to the dorsal nucleus of the vagus, where connections are made with efferent parasympathetic neurons, forming a series of reflex arcs. These provide the basis for self-regulation, a cardinal feature of the autonomic nervous system, and one reason for "autonomy."

Autonomic Functions and Dysfunctions.   A detailed listing of the effects produced by the two divisions of the autonomic nervous system is supplied in Table 56-1. This listing provides impressive evidence of the scope and the importance of autonomic activity in relation to all bodily functions and from the standpoint of survival itself. Both sympathetic and parasympathetic divisions are in a constant state of activity, the activity of each relative to the other being one of controlled opposition, with a delicate balance maintained between the two at all times.

Sympathetic Syndromes.   Certain syndromes are distinctive of diseases of the sympathetic nerve trunks. Among these are dilatation of the pupil of the eye on the same side as a penetrating wound of the neck (evidence of disturbance of the cervical sympathetic cord); temporary paralysis of the bowel (indicated by the absence of peristaltic waves and the distention of the intestine by gas) following fracture of any one of the lower dorsal or upper lumbar vertebrae with hemorrhage into the base of the mesentery; and the marked variations in pulse rate and rhythm that often follow compression fractures of the upper six thoracic vertebrae.

▷ General Assessment

The nurse's observations relative to all systems of the body may be of great assistance in establishing the diagnosis of many neurologic disorders.

- Of utmost importance are changes in muscle strength and disturbances of sensation.
- The appearance of pain, its type, and its location, should be noted with care.
- Oliguria and incontinence should be reported as well as any episode of vomiting with a full description of when and how it occurred (whether or not it was accompanied by nausea, what its relationship to the preceding meal was, and the nature of the vomitus).
- Mental and nervous symptoms should be observed and studied analytically, because their complete description is likely to be of value in the diagnosis and the therapeutic management of the patient. The general attitude of the patient may reveal depression or euphoria; the mood swings may run the gamut of irritability, apprehension, anger, and elation.
- Disturbances of vision, hearing, speech, smell, taste, touch, pressure, or pain may be elicited in the course of patient management, possibly indicating a new development in the patient's neurologic status.

Diagnostic Assessment*

The purposes of the neurologic examination are to determine if the patient has a neurologic dysfunction and if a lesion is present, and if so, where it is located. In addition to the usually complete history and physical examination, every patient suspected of having a neurologic disorder, and every neurosurgical patient, is subjected to a systematic and detailed neurologic examination. Mental status is assessed, including state of responsiveness, intelligence, orientation, and the ability of the patient to express himself and understand speech.

Examination of the peripheral motor and the sensory systems also is done. Motor tests include observation of posture and gait, reflex tests, coordination observations, etc. Sensory tests determine skin sensation and deeper tissue sensation, as well as the ability to recognize objects by the sense of touch.

For an overview of general neurologic assessment pertaining to levels off consciousness, cranial nerve function, reflex actions, muscle strength, sensory perception, mental status, etc., see pages 86–91 of Chapter 5, Physical Assessment.

---

* See also Neurologic Examination, pages 86–91.

Cranial Nerve Tests.   Cerebral lesions affect the cranial nerves by producing a variety of dysfunctions, such as loss of vision in one eye, pupillary inequality or differences in eye movement, unilateral weakness of masseter muscle, disturbances of smell and taste, facial paralysis, loss of hearing, swallowing dysfunction, hoarseness, and difficulty in elevating the shoulders and turning the head. Identifying the presence of such lesions involves the testing of each cranial nerve in the manner specified in Chapter 5. Maximal cooperation of the patient is essential for the proper conduct of this diagnostic routine and can be elicited only if he understands what he is expected to do. All equipment for these tests should be available in one place.

Skull X-rays.   Skull x-rays are generally taken for the diagnostic assessment of patients with neurologic problems. They reveal configuration, density, vascular markings, and intracranial calcification and tumor.

Computed Tomography (Computed Axial Tomography; CT Scanning)

Computed tomography makes use of a narrow beam of x-ray to scan the head in successive layers. The images that are produced provide cross-sectional views of the brain, with distinguishing differences in tissue densities of the skull, cortex, subcortical structures, and ventricles. A computer printout is obtained of the absorption values of the tissues in the plane that is being scanned. The data are transformed into an image through a series of complex equations. Therefore, the brightness of each portion or "slice" of brain in the final image is proportional to the degree to which it absorbs x-ray. The image is displayed on an oscilloscope or TV monitor and is photographed (Fig. 56-4).

Lesions within the brain are seen as variations in tissue density differing from the surrounding normal brain tissue.

Abnormalities of tissue density indicate possible tumor masses, brain infarction, displacement of the ventricles, cortical atrophy, etc.

Computed tomography is usually done first without contrast material and then with intravenous contrast enhancement. The patient lies on an adjustable table, with his head held in a fixed position, while the scanning system rotates around the head. (The patient is used as the axis, and the machine is rotated around this axis, resulting in a cross-cut image). The patient must lie with the head held perfectly still, and with a careful effort not to talk or move the face, as head motion causes considerable artifact.

Computed tomography is the most revolutionary development in neurologic diagnosis in this century. It is noninvasive, painless, and has a high degree of sensitivity for detecting lesions.

Positron Emission Tomography (PET).   *Positron emission tomography* is a computer-based nuclear imaging technique that can produce pictures of actual organ functioning (Fig. 56-5). The patient either inhales a radioactive gas or is injected with a radioactive substance that emits positively charged particles. When these positrons combine with negatively charged electrons (normally found in the body's

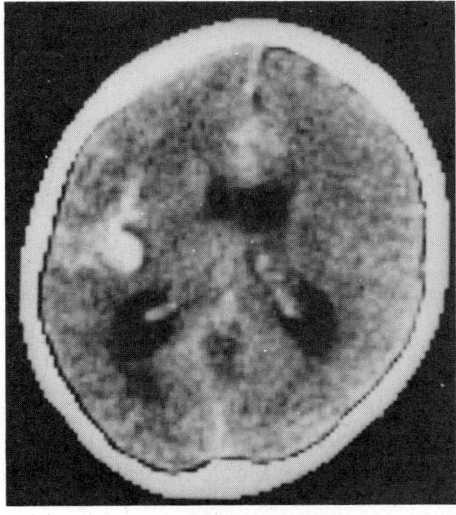

Figure 56-4.   CT scan of the brain. A dense clot can be seen in the left sylvian and interhemispheric fissures. Note the peripheral zone of edema around the left sylvian clot. (Scan courtesy of Toronto General Hospital) (See also Fig. 18-5.)

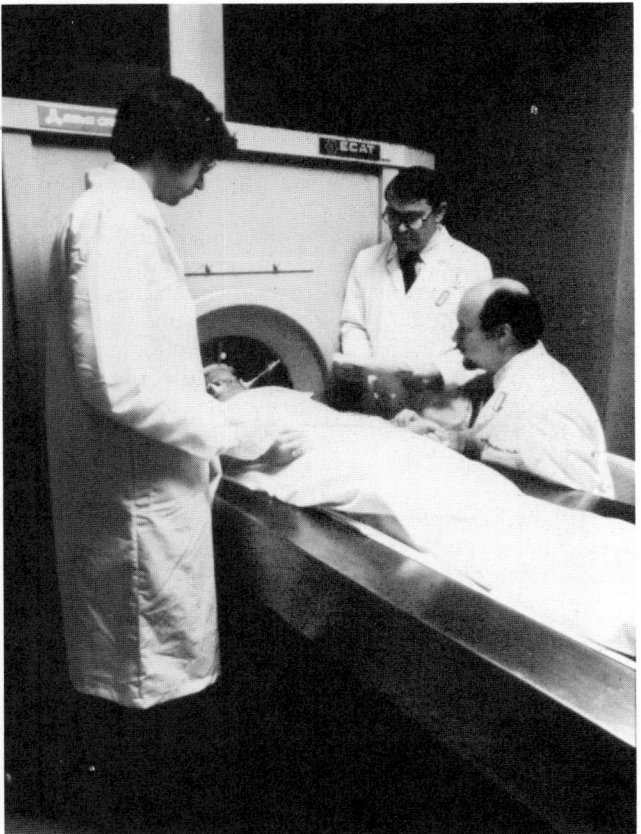

Figure 56-5.   The Neuro-ECAT Scanner is an analytical instrument for positron emission tomography which can study the dynamic processes of the brain in stroke and other disorders. (Courtesy, National Institute of Neurological and Communicative Disorders and Stroke.)

cells), the resultant gamma rays can be detected by a scanning device. This study permits the measurement of blood flow, tissue composition, and brain metabolism. With PET, researchers can "watch" what happens to radioactively tagged substances such as oxygen and glucose inside the living nerve cells deep within the brain. At the present time, it is regarded as a clinical research tool that has exciting potential in the area of neurologic and psychiatric diagnosis.

Nuclear Magnetic Resonance. *Nuclear magnetic resonance* devices are being developed that produce high-resolution views of the cerebrum and brain stem, which are obtained without exposure to radiation. Brain tumors undetected by CT have been spotted with nuclear magnetic resonance scans. (See also Chap. 18, p. 340.)

Air Studies

The cerebrospinal fluid spaces in and around the brain may be seen in x-ray examination when the fluid is replaced with a gas. This is based on the principle that gas, replacing the fluid within the ventricular and subarachnoid systems, serves as a contrast medium, because air is less dense than fluid to roentgen rays. The cerebrospinal fluid may be partially replaced with air through *pneumoencephalography* and *ventriculography*.

Pneumoencephalography is a diagnostic procedure in which air or gas is instilled through a lumbar puncture as a means of demonstrating the ventricular system and subarachnoid space overlying the hemispheres and basal cisterns. A small amount of cerebrospinal fluid is removed and an equal amount of air injected. A special chair allows the patient to be rotated in all directions so that air may be placed selectively in the desired cavities. Films are then taken and studied.

This procedure is usually done under local or neuroleptic anesthesia and may be accompanied and followed by unpleasant side-effects, including severe headache associated with nausea, vomiting, photophobia, diaphoresis, pallor, restlessness, and syncope. Adequate personnel should be available to treat the complications. The patient may be informed that the air inserted into the spine can be felt rising up to the ventricles and that a "sloshing sound" may be heard as a result of the air in the ventricles as the head is repositioned.

Although used less frequently since the advent of computed tomography, pneumoencephalography is useful in demonstrating lesions in the pituitary region and in assessing intraventricular and brainstem lesions.

A *ventriculogram* is an x-ray taken of the lateral ventricles following withdrawal of cerebrospinal fluid and injection of air or gas into the lateral ventricles through openings in the skull. This procedure is usually done under local anesthesia with the patient sitting in a special chair. The posterior half of the head is prepared and draped. Trephines (burr holes) are made through scalp incisions, and the ventricles are punctured by a special needle or thin, plastic catheter. The fluid is replaced with air, the cannulae are withdrawn, and the scalp wounds are closed. If a lesion is present, there is a change in size, shape, or position of the ventricular, subarachnoid, or cisternal spaces.

During this procedure, the patient develops a mild headache, may become nauseated, may retch, and very rarely may have a convulsive seizure. The reaction to this procedure is usually milder than that attending pneumoencephalography.

Preparation of the Patient. The night before pneumoencephalography or ventriculography, the patient should have a good rest. On the morning of the test, breakfast is withheld in order to avoid post-test nausea and vomiting (side-effects of these procedures).

Appropriate sedatives and analgesics are administered before the patient is taken to the operating room or x-ray department. The back of the head should be shaved before ventriculography. The entire head is shaved if craniotomy is to follow. All hairpins should be removed; however, long hair should *not* be braided before pneumoencephalography, since braids cast shadows on the x-ray films. As with other surgical procedures, dentures are removed.

Postprocedure Assessment. The patient is observed for signs of increased or decreased intracranial pressure (see p. 1293) or shock. Disturbances of intracranial pressure may cause downward herniation of the supratentorial and posterior fossa contents. If this occurs, preparations should be made for a ventricular tap and prompt decompression. Special care must be taken to see that the patient does not aspirate any vomitus. Vital signs are taken frequently until they are stabilized, and neurologic checks, especially level of responsiveness, are made. Parenteral fluids may be necessary for the first 24 hours.

Since a pounding headache is the major complaint following these procedures, an ice cap may be placed on the head and adequate analgesics given while the headache lasts. The duration of the headache depends on how quickly the intracranial air is absorbed. Since these discomforts are related to the amount of air used, the instillation of smaller amounts of air has reduced the frequency, severity, and duration of the symptoms.

Isotope Cisternography. *Isotope cisternography* uses a radioactive tracer injected into the lumbar subarachnoid space. It is useful in studying cerebrospinal fluid circulation, to locate cerebrospinal fluid leaks, and to evaluate hydrocephalus.

Cerebral Angiography

Cerebral angiography is an x-ray study of the cerebral circulation following injection of contrast material into a selected artery.

Cerebral angiography is the primary investigative tool for intracranial aneurysm, arteriovenous malformation, cerebral vascular occlusive disease, and study of collateral blood flow. It also has value in localizing mass lesions and may aid in preoperative diagnosis. It is frequently done prior to craniotomy.

The majority of cerebral angiograms are done by the transfemoral route, but the procedure may be accomplished by direct puncture of the carotid/vertebral artery or by retrograde injection of contrast medium into the brachial artery.

Patient Preparation. The patient should be well-hydrated, and clear liquids are usually permitted up to the time of the study. Before going to the radiology department, the patient is requested to void. A felt-tip pen may be used to mark the appropriate peripheral pulses. The patient is informed that he should try to remain immobile during the film sequence and that a brief feeling of warmth in the face, behind the eyes, or in the jaw, teeth, tongue, and lips, and a metallic taste are likely to be expected.

After the groin is shaved and prepared, a local anesthetic is used for patient comfort and for reduction of arterial spasm. A catheter is introduced into the femoral artery, flushed with heparinized saline, and filled with contrast material. Under fluoroscopic guidance, it is advanced to the appropriate vessel(s). During injection of the contrast medium, x-rays are made of the arterial and venous phases of circulation through the brain.

Postprocedure Management.   In some instances, patients may experience major or minor arterial block due to embolism, thrombosis, or hemorrhage, producing a neurologic deficit. Signs of such an occurrence include alterations in the level of responsiveness and consciousness, weakness on one side of the body, motor or sensory deficits, or speech disturbances. It is necessary to observe the patient repeatedly for these signs and to report them immediately if they occur.

The injection site is observed for hematoma formation, and an ice cap may be applied intermittently to the puncture site to relieve swelling and discomfort. Since a hematoma at the puncture site or embolization to a distant artery will affect the peripheral pulses, these signs are monitored frequently. The color and temperature of the involved extremity are also noted as a means of detecting possible embolism.

Myelography

A *myelogram* is an x-ray of the spinal subarachnoid space taken after an opaque medium or air is injected into the spinal subarachnoid space through a spinal puncture. It outlines the spinal subarachnoid space and shows any distortion of the spinal cord or spinal dural sac caused by tumors, cysts, herniated intervertebral discs, or other lesions.

After the contrast medium is injected, the head of the table is tilted down and the course of the contrast medium is observed radioscopically.

The newer water-soluble contrast medium used in myelography, metrizamide (Amipaque), is absorbed by the body and excreted by the kidneys. It does not have to be removed via the needle route from the spinal canal because it is highly soluble and clears relatively quickly from the cerebrospinal fluid. Side-effects include headache, which is most probably due to irritation of the central nervous system by the metrizamide.

If iophendylate (Pantopaque), an oil-based iodine compound, is used for myelography, the radiologist may remove it by syringe and needle aspiration. The patient may complain of sharp pain down the leg during aspiration if a nerve root is affected. This is remedied by rotating the needle point or adjusting the depth of the needle.

Nursing Management.   Since most patients have some misconceptions about this procedure, the nurse can answer questions and clarify the explanation offered by the physician. The patient should be aware that the x-ray table may be tilted in varying positions during the study. The meal that would normally be eaten prior to the procedure is omitted. The patient may be given a light sedative to help cope with a rather lengthy test.

Following myelography, when a water-soluble medium has been used, the patient lies in bed with the head of the bed elevated 15 to 30 degrees to reduce the rate of upward dispersion of the medium. The patient may be ambulatory or remain in bed per the physician's request.

Following a procedure in which Pantopaque has been used, the patient should lie in a recumbent position for the amount of time specified by the physician (usually 12–24 hours) to reduce cerebrospinal fluid leakage and decrease the frequence of headache. Usually, he is permitted to turn from side to side.

The patient is encouraged to drink liberal amounts of fluid for rehydration and replacement of cerebrospinal fluid and to decrease the incidence of postlumbar puncture headache. The blood pressure, pulse, respiratory rate, and temperature are monitored, as well as the patient's ability to void. Other untoward signs to watch for include fever, stiff neck, photophobia, or signs of chemical or bacterial meningitis.

Other X-ray Procedures

Lumbar Epidural Venography.   In this procedure, a catheter is inserted percutaneously into the femoral vein and guided into the ascending lumbar vein or internal iliac veins. The contrast medium is injected to fill the epidural veins overlying the disc spaces and to opacify the epidural venous plexus. The procedure may be useful in the diagnosis of herniated lumbar discs that are not demonstrated by myelography. It reveals deviation or compression of the epidural veins due to a herniated disc or tumor. The procedure is relatively easy to perform, well tolerated, fairly painless, and not associated with arachnoiditis. Lumbar epidural venography and myelography may be done as complementary diagnostic studies.

Following the test, the site is observed for evidence of hematoma formation.

Discography.   *Discography* is the injection of a radiopaque substance directly into the intervertebral disc, followed by x-ray studies. While this procedure may be done in suspected instances of herniated discs, it is infrequently used.

Lumbar Puncture

A *lumbar puncture* is carried out by inserting a needle into the lumbar subarachnoid space in order to withdraw cerebrospinal fluid for diagnostic and therapeutic purposes. The purposes are to obtain spinal fluid for examination, to measure and relieve spinal fluid pressure, to determine the presence or absence of blood in the spinal fluid, to detect spinal subarachnoid block, and to administer antibiotics intrathecally in certain cases of infection.

The needle is usually inserted into the subarachnoid space between the third and fourth lumbar spinous interspace. Since the spinal cord divides into a sheaf of nerves at the first lumbar vertebra, the needle is inserted below the level of the third lumbar vertebra (Fig. 56-6) to prevent the spinal cord from being punctured.

A successful lumbar puncture requires that the patient be relaxed, since an anxious patient may become tense, thereby causing an increase in the pressure reading. The normal range of spinal fluid pressure with the patient in a lateral position is 70 mm to 180 mm of water. Pressures over

200 mm of water are considered abnormal. A lumbar puncture may be quite dangerous in the presence of an intracranial mass lesion, because when pressure is released, the intracranial contents may herniate.

Lumbar Manometric Test (Queckenstedt Test).

This test is done when a spinal subarachnoid block (by tumor, vertebral fracture, or dislocation) is suspected. Pressure may be applied manually by pressing firmly and simultaneously upon the jugular veins on each side of the neck for a period of 10 seconds. Or a blood pressure cuff may be placed around the patient's neck and inflated to a pressure of 20 mm Hg. The increase in the pressure caused by the compression is noted. Then the pressure is released and pressure readings are made at 10-second intervals. In normal persons, the cerebrospinal fluid pressure rises rapidly in response to compression of the jugular veins and returns quickly to normal when the compression is released. A slow rise and fall in pressure indicates a partial block due to a lesion compressing the spinal subarachnoid pathways. If there is no pressure change, a complete block is indicated. This test is not done if an intracranial lesion is suspected.

Nursing Support.

During the initial explanations, the patient should be assured that inserting a needle into the spine will not result in paralysis. Prior to the lumbar puncture, the bladder and bowel should be emptied. The patient is placed on his side with his back toward the physician. The thighs and head are flexed as much as possible to increase the space between the spinous processes of the vertebrae and afford easier entry into the subarachnoid space. A pillow fixed between the legs will prevent the upper leg from rolling forward. A small pillow is placed under the patient's head so that the spine is maintained in a horizontal position. The nurse may assist the patient to maintain the position in order to avoid sudden movement, which can produce a traumatic (bloody) tap. During the procedure, the patient is instructed to breathe normally since hyperventilation may lower an elevated pressure. Following the procedure, the patient is to lie flat for 6 to 12 hours. A liberal fluid intake is encouraged.

Examination of the Cerebrospinal Fluid.

Spinal fluid should be clear and colorless. Bloody spinal fluid may indicate cerebral contusion, laceration, or subarachnoid hemorrhage. Usually, specimens are sent to the laboratory for cell count, culture, and chemical analysis. The specimens should be sent immediately, since changes will take place and alter the result if the specimens are allowed to stand. (See Appendix for the normal values of cerebrospinal fluid.)

Postlumbar Puncture Headache.

A postlumbar puncture headache, ranging from mild to severe, may appear in a few hours to several days following the procedure. It is a throbbing bifrontal or occipital headache, dull and deep in character, that is particularly severe when the patient sits or stands upright, but lessens or disappears when he lies down in a horizontal position.

The cause of this unpleasant complication is the leakage of spinal fluid at the puncture site. The fluid continues to escape into the tissues by way of the needle tract from the spinal canal. It is then absorbed promptly by the lymphatics, never having accumulated in sufficient volume to be detected. As a result of this leak, the supply of cerebrospinal fluid in the cranium is depleted to a point at which it is insufficient to maintain proper mechanical stabilization of the brain. This leakage of spinal fluid allows settling of the brain when the patient assumes an upright position. This produces tension and stretching of venous sinuses and pain-sensitive structures. Both traction and pain are lessened and the leakage reduced when the patient lies down.

If the postpuncture headache persists, the *epidural blood patch* technique may be used. Blood is withdrawn from the patient's antecubital vein and injected into the epidural space, usually via the site of the previous spinal puncture. The rationale is that the blood acts as a gelatinous plug to seal the hole in the dura, thus preventing continuing loss of cerebrospinal fluid.

The lumbar puncture headache may be avoided if a needle with a small gauge is used and if the patient is encouraged to remain recumbent for 6 to 12 hours following the procedure. When large volumes of fluid are collected (>20 ml), the patient is positioned prone for 2 hours, then flat in a side-lying position for 2 hours, and then supine or prone for 6 more hours. Keeping the patient flat overnight may reduce the incidence of headaches.

Other complications of a spinal puncture include herniation of the intracranial contents, spinal epidural abscess, spinal epidural hematoma, and meningitis.

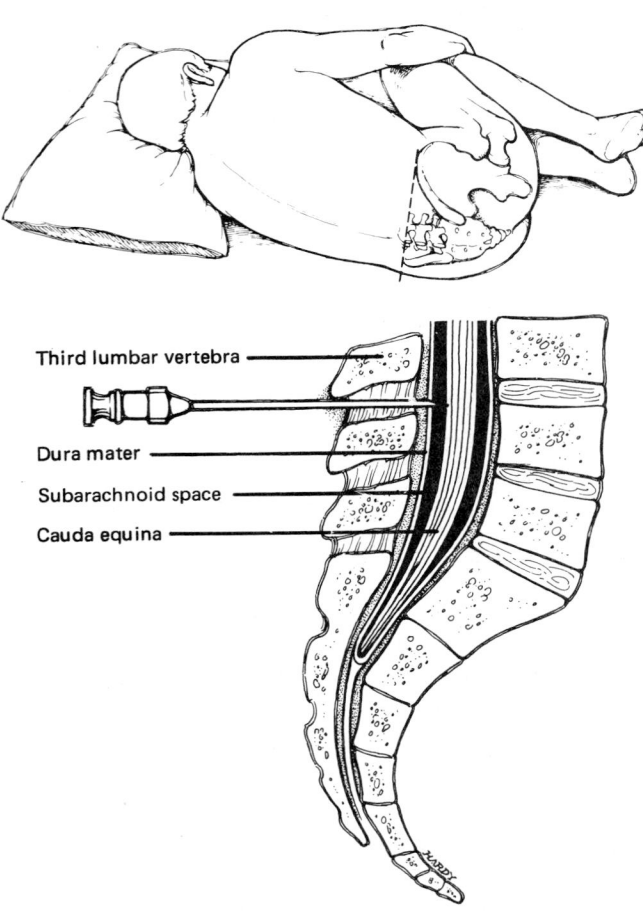

Third lumbar vertebra

Dura mater

Subarachnoid space

Cauda equina

Figure 56-6. Technique of lumbar puncture. The interspaces between the spines of L3 and L5 are just below the line joining the anterosuperior iliac spines.

Electroencephalography (EEG)

An *electroencephalogram* represents a record of the electrical activity generated in the brain and obtained through electrodes applied on the scalp surface or through microelectrodes placed within the brain tissue. It provides physiologic assessment of cerebral activity. EEG is a useful test for diagnosing seizure disorders such as the epilepsies, and is a screening procedure for coma or organic brain syndrome. It also serves as an indicator of brain death. Tumors, abscesses, brain scars, blood clots, and infection may cause electric changes to differ from normal patterns of rhythm and rate.

Electrodes are arranged on the scalp to record the electrical activity in various regions of the head (Fig. 56-7). The amplified activity of the neurons is recorded on a continuously moving paper sheet. For a baseline recording, the patient lies quietly with his eyes closed. Then he may be asked to hyperventilate for 3 to 4 minutes and then to look at a bright, flashing light for photic stimulation. These are activation procedures done to evoke abnormal electrical discharges, especially seizure potentials. A sleep EEG may be recorded following sedation because some abnormal brain waves are seen only when the patient is asleep. If the epileptogenic area is inaccessible to the conventional scalp electrodes, nasopharyngeal electrodes may be used.

Depth recording of EEG is done by introducing electrodes stereotactically into a target area of the brain as dictated by the patient's seizure pattern and scalp EEG. It is used to select patients who may benefit from surgical excision of epileptogenic foci.

Evoked potential studies involve the changes and responses in brain waves recorded from scalp electrodes that are evoked by the introduction of an external stimulus—a light, a click, or a slight shock. These evoked changes are detected with the aid of computerized devices that extract the signal, display it on an oscilloscope, and store the data on magnetic tape or disc. In clinical practice, the systems most often used for evoked potential studies are the *visual* (strobe light flash), *auditory* (click), and *somatosensory* (external stimulus) systems. These studies are based on the concept that any insult or dysfunction that can alter neuronal metabolism or disturb membrane function may change evoked responses in brain waves.

Patient Preparation.   Tranquilizers and stimulants may be withheld 24 to 48 hours before an EEG, since these medications can alter the EEG wave patterns or mask the abnormal wave patterns of seizure disorders. Coffee, tea, or cola drinks are omitted in the meal before the test because of their stimulating effect. However, the meal is not omitted because an altered blood sugar level can also cause changes in the brain wave patterns.

The patient is informed that the EEG will take approximately 45 to 60 minutes, or longer if a sleep EEG is performed. At the same time, the patient is assured that the procedure will not cause an electric shock and that the EEG is a test, not a form of treatment.

Electromyography (EMG)

An *electromyogram* is obtained by introducing needle electrodes into the skeletal muscles in order to study changes in the electrical potential of the muscles and the nerves leading to them. The electrical potentials are shown on an oscilloscope and amplified by a loudspeaker so that both the sound and the appearance of the waves can be analyzed and compared simultaneously. EMGs are useful in determining the presence of a neuromuscular disorder and myopathies. They help to distinguish weakness due to neuropathy (functional or pathologic changes in the peripheral nervous system) from weakness due to other causes.

No special patient preparation is required. The patient is told that he will experience a sensation similar to that of an intramuscular injection as the needle is inserted into the

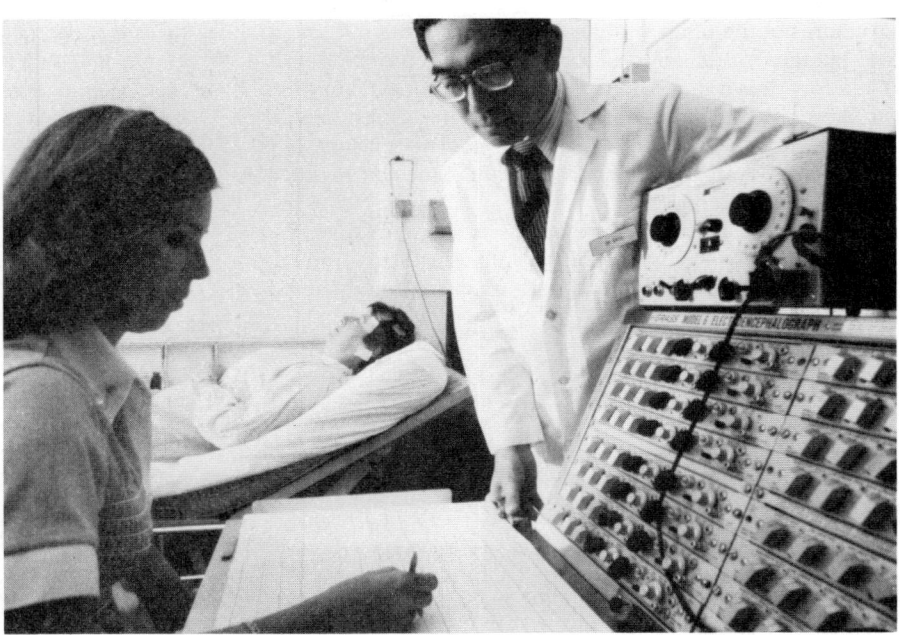

Figure 56-7. Neurologist and EEG technician checking the patient's electroencephalograph, which is a valuable diagnostic instrument in epilepsy and other neurologic disorders. (Courtesy, National Institute of Neurological and Communicative Disorders and Stroke.)

muscle. The muscles examined may ache for a short time following the procedure.

Nerve conduction studies are performed by stimulating a peripheral nerve at several points along its course and recording the muscle action potential or the sensory action potential that results. Surface or needle electrodes are placed on the skin over the nerve to stimulate the nerve fibers.

Radionuclide Imaging Studies (Brain Scan)

In this procedure, the patient is given an intravenous injection of a radiopharmaceutical. The radioactivity subsequently transmitted through the skull is traced by a scanner which prints out a picture based on the number of counts received from the brain as it is scanned. Or a gamma camera is used to monitor the passage of the radiopharmaceutical through the cerebral circulation to gain information about cerebral blood flow. (See Chap. 18, p. 339.)

This test is based on the principle that a radiopharmaceutical may diffuse through a disrupted blood–brain barrier into abnormal cerebral tissue or in areas where there is new vascularization. (Normal brain tissue is relatively impermeable.) There is an increased uptake of radioactive material at the site of pathology.

Brain scanning is particularly useful in evaluating vascular lesions of the brain and meninges and in locating vascular neoplasms and brain tumors. It is useful in the early detection and evaluation of stroke, abscess, and follow-up of surgical or radiation therapy of the brain. Newer techniques permit the evaluation of cerebral circulation during the brain scan. However, CT scanning is replacing traditional radioisotope scanning.

Echoencephalography

Echoencephalography is the recording of echoes from the deep structures within the skull by means of ultrasound (high-frequency sound waves). Ultrasonic transducers are positioned over specified areas of the head, while echoes are transcribed into images. Echoencephalography is a rapid and useful technique to determine the position of midline structures of the brain and the distance from the midline to the lateral ventricular wall or the third ventricular wall. Therefore, it is done to detect a shift of the cerebral midline structures caused by subdural hematoma, intracerebral hemorrhage, massive cerebral infarction, and neoplasms. It is useful in the evaluation of hydrocephalus, since it can detect dilation of the ventricles.

The nurse may explain that this is a noninvasive test, and that some type of water-soluble jelly is used to eliminate the air gap between the hand-held transducer and the patient's head.

▷ Bibliography

Books

Adams RD and Victor M. Principles of Neurology, 2nd ed. New York, McGraw–Hill, 1981.

Balla JI. Pathways in Neurological Diagnosis. London, Edward Arnold, 1980.

Bickerstaff ER. Neurological Examination in Clinical Practice. Boston, Blackwell Scientific, 1980.

Black RB, Herman BP, and Shope JT. Nursing Management of Epilepsy. Rockville, Maryland, Aspen, 1982.

Boller F and Frank E. Sexual Dysfunction in Neurological Disorders. New York, Raven Press, 1982.

Calenoff L (ed). Radiology of Spinal Cord Injury. St Louis, CV Mosby, 1981.

Collins R. Illustrated Manual of Neurological Diagnosis, 2nd ed. Philadelphia, JB Lippincott, 1982.

Guyton AC. Basic Human Neurophysiology, 3rd ed. Philadelphia, WB Saunders, 1981.

Hayward R. Essentials of Neurosurgery. Oxford, Blackwell Scientific, 1980.

Hickey J. The Clinical Practice of Neurological and Neurosurgical Nursing. Philadelphia, JB Lippincott, 1981.

Kaufman DM. Clinical Neurology for Psychiatrists. New York, Grune & Stratton, 1981.

Magee KR and Saper JR. Clinical and Basic Neurology for Health Professionals. Chicago, Year Book Medical Publishers, 1981.

Mayo Clinic and Mayo Foundation. Clinical Examinations in Neurology. Philadelphia, WB Saunders, 1981.

Meyer JS and Shaw T. Diagnosis and Management of Stroke and TIAs. Menlo Park, Addison–Wesley, 1982.

Omer GE and Spinner M. Management of Peripheral Nerve Problems. Philadelphia, WB Saunders, 1980.

Osborn AG. Introduction to Cerebral Angiography. Hagerstown, Harper & Row, 1981.

Pryse–Phillips W and Murray TJ. Essential Neurology, 2nd ed. Garden City, New York, Medical Examination, 1982.

Rosenberg RN (ed). Neurology. New York, Grune & Stratton, 1980.

Scheinberg P. Modern Practical Neurology, 2nd ed. New York, Raven Press, 1981.

Smith RR. Essentials of Neurosurgery. Philadelphia, JB Lippincott, 1980.

Sutherland JM. Fundamentals of Neurology. New York, ADIS Press, 1981.

Taylor JW and Ballenger S. Neurological Dysfunctions and Nursing Interventions. New York, McGraw–Hill, 1980.

Youmans JR (ed). Neurological Surgery, Vols 1, 2, 3, 4, 5, 6, 2nd ed. Philadelphia, WB Saunders, 1982.

Articles

Bubb D. Neurodiagnostic studies: Pre- and post-procedure care. RN 1981 Nov; 44(11):64–65.

Evoked potential emerging as valuable medical tool. JAMA 1981 Sept 18; 246(12):1287–1291.

Goodwin PN. Recent developments in instrumentation for emission computed tomography. Semin Nucl Med 1980 Oct; 10(4):322–334.

Greenberg RP and Ducker TB. Evoked potentials in the clinical neurosciences. J Neurosurg 1982 Jan; 56(1):1–18.

National Institute of Neurological and Communicative Disorders and Strokes. Computed tomographic scanning of the brain. JAMA 1982 Apr 9; 247(14):1955–1958.

Olendorf WH. Nuclear medicine in clinical neurology: An update. Ann Neurol 1981 Sept; 10(3):207–213.

Raichle ME. Measurement of local cerebral blood flow and metabolism in man with positron emission tomography. Fed Proc 1981 June; 40(8):2331–2334.

Rimel RW and Tyson GW. The neurologic examination in patients with central nervous system trauma. J Neurosurg Nurs 1979 Sept; 11(3):148–155.

Yamamoto YL et al. Positron emission tomography for measurement of regional cerebral blood flow. Adv Neurol 1981; 30:41–53.

57

Management of Patients With Neurologic Dysfunction

▷ Scope of Neurologic Nursing

Many disorders of the nervous system are chronic conditions resulting in impaired function and long-term disability. Recovery from organic disease of the nervous system is not always followed by complete restoration of function. The rehabilitation needs of these patients are usually complex.

Through optimism, nursing ability, and concern for the patient as a person, the nurse can help to ease many of the difficulties experienced by the patient and family. Patients with neurologic dysfunction often display behavioral signs and symptoms. Upon realizing that the behavior and the personality of a person can be affected markedly by organic lesions of the brain, one is less inclined to think of a patient as being uncooperative or having a foul disposition; instead he becomes a person who needs help and understanding. His reactions may be beyond his control; anyone caring for these patients must realize this.

The many interesting diagnostic tests in which the nurse participates are much like solving a puzzle. But the diagnosis is not the end; it is merely a steppingstone to the removal of the cause. Surgery must be done accurately, otherwise the penalty may be the death of the patient or the reduction of his mental or physical abilities to the level of mere existence. Although surgery has many successful outcomes, there are patients in which an injury is too great to repair, or a tumor too extensive to remove, and the patient's prognosis is hopeless.

Sensitive awareness and skilled attention to the patient's needs are the nursing focus. The goal for the patient is to achieve the highest level of functioning and comfort that is possible.

▷ Special Problems of Neurologic Patients

Skin Care.   Special nursing problems arise from paralyses, sensory disturbances, psychosis, and coma. Patients with chronic neurologic conditions usually have some physical deficit and are at high risk for pressure sores. Eternal vigilance is essential for their prevention. See pages 232 to 242 for prevention of pressure sores.

Nutritional Needs. Nutritional problems arise if there is any disturbance connected with the swallowing reflex. Such problems may be overcome by homogenizing the patient's meals in a food blender and feeding him through a tube. Vitamin preparations usually are added to the feeding. The blenderized meal is tolerated well, since the patient's gastrointestinal tract is accustomed to this type of diet, and there is less incidence of diarrhea. Plastic drinking tubes should be used by patients who are subject to convulsions, and dentures, of course, are removed from the mouths of such patients, as well as from those in coma.

Oral Hygiene. The condition of the patient's mouth should be checked often, because the buccal structures tend to become exceedingly dry after a short period of mouth breathing. The lips, the tongue, and the gums should be lubricated systematically, and the hydration of the patient should be maintained at an adequate level.

Eye Care. When facial palsy, from any cause, makes it impossible to shut the eyes, special eye care must be given, such as irrigating the eyes with sterile ophthalmic solution and instilling sterile mineral oil to prevent drying and injury to the cornea. These procedures should be carried out several times each day, and the eyes should be inspected regularly for signs of inflammation. An eye shield should be worn at night. Patients who are conscious and cooperative can administer their own eye care with proper instruction and supervision.

The Incontinent Patient. Many patients with diseases of the central nervous system initially or eventually, temporarily or permanently, exhibit urinary and fecal incontinence. The hygienic care of patients with incontinence is an important nursing priority.

The management of bladder disturbances due to a lesion of the nervous system is discussed on page 975. The management of urinary incontinence from other causes is discussed on page 251. Promotion of a bowel training program is described on page 251.

Prevention of Deformities. Any paralyzed extremity deserves careful attention. Care must be taken lest a patient lie on it, or circulation to the part becomes impeded in any way. Footboards or cradles prevent pressure from weighty bed linens.

To prevent contractures, the nurse must see that the patient is positioned correctly, and that the joints are moved, either actively or passively, through their range of motion several times daily. When the condition of the patient permits, active exercises (bathing, walking, therapeutic exercises) are desirable. Massage may be instituted and perhaps later supplemented by electrical stimulation. Passive exercises and, as soon as possible, active motions are prescribed for the purpose of developing strength.

Fatigue may appear early, because patients with progressive disorders may have lost part of the normal neuronal reserve. In general, encourage the maximum activity of which the patient is capable.

Psychological Considerations. Patients with neurologic dysfunctions are faced with multiple stresses; serious and often unpredictable outcomes; assault of self image; and in many instances, a long-term illness. The patient and his family experience reactive responses to the crisis of diagnosis and prolonged treatment. The patient may react to these stresses with a mix of psychological responses, including regression, depression, anger, denial, and anxiety.

The family faces the disruption of illness, which means an alteration in life-style, role changes, and possible intrafamilial conflicts. Denial or nonacceptance by the family can produce enormous strains on its individual members. The family will require time to deal with their feelings of powerlessness, ambivalence, anger, and guilt. They should be included and educated about the patient's therapy, understand the nature of the neurologic dysfunction and the meaning of remissions and exacerbations, and have some awareness of present and future changes.

The nursing goal is to help the patient to adapt to his dysfunction and continue with his life in as meaningful a way as possible. Nursing support includes knowing and accepting the patient's self-protective responses, providing information, answering questions, helping the patient set concrete goals, offering reassurance, and reinforcing positive coping skills. The health care personnel have a constructive influence, as the patient and family can be increasingly receptive even during a time of disequilibrium.

▷ Increased Intracranial Pressure

Pathophysiology

The rigid cranial vault contains brain (1400 g), blood (75 ml), and cerebrospinal fluid (75 ml), which are normally in a state of pressure and volume equilibrium. Since there is limited space for expansion within the skull, an increase of any one of these components necessitates a reciprocal change in the volume of the other, either by displacement or shift of cerebrospinal fluid, increased cerebrospinal fluid absorption, or decreased cerebral blood volume. Under normal circumstances, there are minor changes in blood and cerebrospinal fluid volumes occurring constantly, with changes in intrathoracic pressure (coughing, sneezing, straining), postural and blood pressure changes, and fluctuations in arterial blood gases.

Pathologic conditions such as head injury, cerebrovascular accident, inflammatory lesions, brain tumor, or intracranial surgery can influence intracranial volume–pressure relationships in a negative manner. Increased intracranial pressure may significantly reduce cerebral blood flow, and the resultant ischemia stimulates the vasomotor center, leading to a rise in systemic pressure. The brain is very vulnerable to ischemia and generally will not recover function if it is subjected to more than 3 to 5 minutes of complete ischemia.

The concentration of CO_2 in the blood and brain tissues also has a role in the regulation of cerebral blood flow. A rise in PCO_2 produces dilatation of the cerebral blood vessels, causing increased cerebral blood flow and increased intracranial pressure, while a fall in PCO_2 has a vasoconstrictor effect. Decreased venous outflow may also increase cerebral blood volume, thus raising intracranial pressure. Thus, increased intracranial pressure is the summation of a number of physiologic processes. Increased intracranial pressure from any cause affects cerebral perfusion and causes distortion and shift of brain tissues.

▶ **Assessment**

Clinical Manifestations.   When intracranial pressure increases to the point where compensatory limits have been reached, neural function is impaired and may be expressed by changes in the level of consciousness and by abnormal respiratory and vasomotor responses.

1. Changes in the Levels of Responsiveness or Consciousness.   The level of responsiveness/consciousness is the most important measure of the patient's condition.

* The earliest sign of increasing intracranial pressure is *lethargy*. Watch for slowing of speech and a delay in response to verbal suggestions.

Any sudden change in condition, such as shifting from quietness to restlessness (without apparent cause), from orientation to confusion, or increasing drowsiness, has neurologic significance. These signs may result from compression of the brain due to either swelling from hemorrhage or edema or an expanding intracranial lesion (hematoma or tumor) or a combination of both.

As pressure increases, the patient may react only to loud auditory or painful stimuli. At this stage, serious impairment of brain circulation is probably taking place, and immediate surgical intervention may be required. If the stupor deepens, the patient responds to painful stimuli by moaning but may not attempt to withdraw. As the condition worsens, the extremities become flaccid and reflexes are absent. The jaw sags and the tongue becomes flaccid, producing inadequate respiratory exchange. When the coma is profound, with the pupils dilated and fixed and the respirations impaired, a fatal outcome is usually inevitable.

Nursing Assessment.   The nursing assessment for determining the patient's level of responsiveness can be organized on these levels: (1) eye opening, (2) verbal performance, and (3) observation of motor responses. In order to provide all health care personnel with information on the baseline condition and the patient's present status, a neurologic observation record is kept of the following points of assessment:

1. Eye opening
   a. Opens eyes spontaneously
   b. Opens eyes when spoken to
   c. Opens eyes when painful stimulus is applied
   d. Does not respond
2. Verbal response: response to commands
   a. Answers questions readily and correctly; can perform a requested maneuver
   b. Shows delayed response
   c. Engages in confused conversation and inappropriate speech
   d. Responds only to loud voice
   e. Does not respond
3. Observation of motor responses (to painful stimuli)
   a. Obeys verbal commands; changes position
   b. Localizes pain
   c. Withdraws from pain by means of flexion

   d. Exhibits abnormal flexion
   e. Exhibits abnormal extension
   f. Does not respond

2. Subtle Changes.   Restlessness, headache, forced breathing, purposeless movements, and mental cloudiness may be early clinical indications of rising intracranial pressure.

3. Changes in Vital Signs.   Alterations in vital signs may be a late sign of increased intracranial pressure.

* As the pressure increases, the pulse rate and respiratory rate are slowed and the blood pressure and temperature rise. Special signs to look for are arterial hypertension, bradycardia, and respiratory irregularity; the development of any of these signs warrants further investigation. (Cheyne–Stokes or Kussmaul breathing are the respiratory irregularities frequently seen.)

The body signs compensate as long as the major circulation of the brain is preserved. If, as a result of brain compression, the major circulation begins to fail, the pulse and respirations become rapid, and the temperature usually rises but does not follow a consistent pattern. The pulse pressure (the difference between the systolic and diastolic pressure) widens; this is considered a serious development. Immediately preceding this reversal of clinical responses, there is usually a period of rapid fluctuations in pulse, varying from a slow rate to a rapid one. Surgical intervention is indicated or death will ensue.

* The vital signs may not always be altered, even in the event of increased intracranial pressure. The patient is assessed for changes in the level of responsiveness and for the presence of shock (Table 57-1), to aid in evaluation.

4. Headache.   The headache is constant, increasing in intensity, and aggravated by movement or straining.

5. Pupillary Changes.   Increasing pressure or an expanding clot can displace the brain against the oculomotor or optic nerves, producing pupillary changes.

* The pupils are periodically inspected with a flashlight to evaluate size, configuration, and reaction to light. Both eyes are compared for similarities or differences.
* Gaze is evaluated as to whether it is conjugate (paired; working together) or dysconjugate.
* The ability of the eyes to abduct (cranial nerve function) and adduct (cranial nerve function) is assessed.
* The retina and optic nerve are inspected for hemorrhage and papilledema.

6. Vomiting.   Vomiting is recurrent and may be projectile.

Clinical assessment is not always a reliable guide in recognizing increased intracranial pressure, especially in comatose patients. In certain situations, intracranial pressure monitoring is an essential part of management (see p. 1295).

Patient Problems/Nursing Diagnoses

Based on the clinical manifestations and diagnostic assessment data, the patient's nursing diagnoses include altered

Table 57-1
Comparison of Manifestations of Increased Intracranial Pressure and Shock

	The Patient With Increased Intracranial Pressure	The Patient With Shock
Levels of Responsiveness	Variable: Alert and active Lethargic → drowsy Stuporous → comatose	Alert → coma
Pulse	Slowing rate to 60 or below Increasing rate to 100 or above	Rapid
Respiration	Slowing of rate with lengthening periods of apnea Irregular respirations may occur, with Cheyne–Stokes or Kussmaul breathing	Rapid and shallow
Blood Pressure	Falling diastolic pressure Widening pulse pressure	Falling
Temperature	Moderately elevated Does not usually rise until brain compression is quite extensive	Subnormal
Skin Temperature (by Palpation)	Normal until hyperthermia develops	Cold, moist, and clammy, unless hyperthermia develops

level of consciousness related to increased intracranial pressure; and potential for complications related to neurologic deficit.

▶ **Planning and Implementation**

Goals

The patient's goals are:

1. Attainment and maintenance of consciousness
2. Avoidance of complications

The nursing goals are to assist in reducing intracranial pressure and to use nursing surveillance and nursing strategies to protect the patient from the consequences of increased intracranial pressure.

Interventions

- Increased intracranial pressure constitutes a true emergency and must be treated promptly. As pressure rises, the brain substance is compressed. Secondary phenomena caused by circulatory impairment and edema may lead to death.

The immediate management for relief of increased intracranial pressure is based on the principle of reducing the volume of the extracellular compartment. This goal is accomplished by administration of osmotic diuretics, drainage of cerebrospinal fluid, administration of steroids, hyperventilating the patient, controlling fever, and reducing cellular metabolic demands.

Osmotic diuretics (mannitol) may be given to dehydrate the brain and reduce cerebral edema. They act by displacing extracellular brain water into the vascular system and then into the kidneys. Since hyperosmolar solutions produce diuresis when administered parenterally, an indwelling urethral catheter is usually inserted.

Cerebrospinal fluid drainage is frequently employed since the removal of even 1 ml or 2 ml of cerebrospinal fluid may dramatically reduce intracranial pressure.

Steroids (such as dexamethasone) produce clinical improvement of the edema surrounding brain tumors when a brain tumor is the cause of increased intracranial pressure.

Ventilatory management must be instituted to prevent hypercapnia and hypoxia (see Chap. 25). Therefore, the patient may be hyperventilated with a volume ventilator to reduce the blood volume in the brain by promoting constriction of cerebral vasculature, which in turn decreases intracranial pressure.

Temperature control is aimed at preventing an elevation of temperature, since fever increases cerebral metabolism and the rate at which cerebral edema forms. Cardiac output is monitored if measures are taken to reduce the patient's temperature.

Reducing cellular metabolic demands may also be accomplished through the administration of high doses of barbiturates when the patient is not responsive to conventional treatment. The mechanism by which barbiturates decrease intracranial pressure and protect the brain is uncertain, but the resultant comatose state is thought to reduce metabolic requirements of the brain, thus giving it some protection.

- The patient receiving high-dose barbiturates experiences loss of all neurologic clinical parameters. Barbiturates are significant cardiorespiratory depressants. Thus, prolonged barbiturate anesthesia requires a high level of nursing surveillance and support, as the patient is totally dependent and vulnerable to many complications. Nursing surveillance includes monitoring of intracranial pressure, EEG, arterial pressures, and blood and serum barbiturate levels.

Other Nursing Strategies.   Certain positions and activities are to be avoided in instances of increased intracranial pressure:

- The prone position, extreme rotation of the head, flexion of the neck, and extreme hip flexion should be avoided.
- Slight head elevation should be maintained to aid in venous drainage unless otherwise prescribed.
- The Valsalva maneuver, which can be produced by straining at defecation or even moving in bed, is to be avoided. The patient can be instructed to exhale (which opens the glottis) while being moved or turned passively by the nurse.
- Stool softeners may be prescribed to prevent straining, but enemas and cathartics are avoided if possible.
- Isometric muscle contractions are also contraindicated, since they raise the systemic blood pressure and hence the intracranial pressure.
- If monitoring parameters demonstrate that turning the patient raises his intracranial pressure, place him on an alternating pressure mattress or other device to prevent pressure sores.
- Frequent arousal from sleep and emotional stress are to be avoided. A calm atmosphere must be maintained.
- Nursing activities such as turning, suctioning, etc. should not be clustered in the same time period. Nursing activities are to be spaced, and uninterrupted periods of rest permitted.

A neurologic observation record (see p. 1367) is kept, and all observations are made from the baseline condition of the patient. Repeated assessments of the patient are made (sometimes minute by minute) so that improvement or deterioration may be noted immediately. If the patient's condition deteriorates, preparations are made for surgical intervention (see p. 1320).

▶ Evaluation

Expected Outcomes

1. Attains and maintains consciousness
   a. Becomes increasingly more oriented to time, place, person, and situation
   b. Demonstrates equal and reactive pupils
   c. Follows verbal commands; answers questions readily and correctly
   d. Moves extremities in a purposeful manner
   e. Is able to do problem solving; can count by 3s, 4s, and 5s
2. Avoids complications
   a. Changes position when requested to do so
   b. Maintains vital signs within normal range
   c. Reveals no lung congestion upon auscultation

Monitoring Intracranial Pressure

Intracranial pressure (ICP) monitoring is the recording of the pressure exerted within the skull by the brain, cerebral blood, and cerebrospinal fluid. The volume of any of these elements can expand as a result of tumor, trauma, edema, bleeding, cerebral vessel dilatation, etc. ICP monitoring provides a continuous reflection of the intracranial state.

The purposes of ICP monitoring are to (1) identify increased pressure early in its course (before cerebral damage occurs), (2) quantitate the degree of abnormality, (3) initiate

appropriate treatment, (4) have access to cerebrospinal fluid for sampling and drainage, and (5) evaluate the effectiveness of treatment.

ICP is not in a steady state, but fluctuates as indicated by waves of high pressure and troughs of relatively normal pressure. These waves have been classified as A waves (plateau waves), B waves, and C waves. The *plateau waves (A waves)* are transient, paroxysmal, recurring elevations of ICP that may last from 5 to 20 minutes and range in amplitude between 50 mm Hg to 100 mm Hg. Plateau waves have clinical significance and are usually related to cerebral dysfunction caused by brain shift or distortion. They may increase in amplitude and frequency, reflecting cerebral ischemia and brain damage that can occur before overt signs and symptoms of raised ICP are seen clinically. This is especially true in the unconscious patient. Rapid variations of pressure waves may also indicate a potentially serious intracranial situation. Therefore, ICP monitoring provides a more objective evaluation of early or changing trends of ICP than other forms of observation.

B waves are of shorter duration (½ to 2 minutes) with smaller amplitude (up to 50 mm Hg). They have less clinical significance and appear to be related to Cheyne–Stokes respiration.

C waves are small, rhythmic oscillations with frequencies of approximately six per minute. They appear to be related to rhythmic variations of the systemic arterial blood pressure.

There are a large number of devices available that monitor ICP by means of sensors or transducers that are either connected to an intraventricular catheter or implanted in the skull (Fig. 57-1). The three main types are the ventricular catheter, subarachnoid screw, and epidural transducer.

Ventricular Catheter Monitoring. *Ventricular catheter monitoring* consists of placing a fine catheter into the frontal horn of a lateral ventricle via a burr hole or twist drill hole. The intraventricular catheter is connected to an external pressure monitor by means of tubing filled with normal saline. The transducer transmits the impulses, and the pressures are recorded. The device can be mounted on a stand located beside the bed at the level of the patient's foramen of Monro (the reference point). Or a smaller transducer can be fixed on the patient's head. The output from the pressure transducer is amplified and displayed on a chart recorder. In addition to obtaining continuous pressure recordings, the ventricular catheter allows for drainage of cerebrospinal fluid, particularly during acute rises in pressure.

This method of monitoring is useful in patients with infratentorial brain tumors and aneurysms. Also, continuous drainage of ventricular fluid under pressure control is an effective method of treating intracranial hypertension. Another advantage of an indwelling ventricular catheter is the route it provides for the intraventricular administration of drugs and the instillation of air or contrast medium for ventriculography. Complications include ventricular infection, meningitis, ventricular collapse, and problems with the monitoring system.

Subarachnoid Screw. (See Fig. 57-1.) The *subarachnoid screw* is a hollow screw that is bolted into the calvarium (dome of skull) to record ICP over the brain cavities. It has

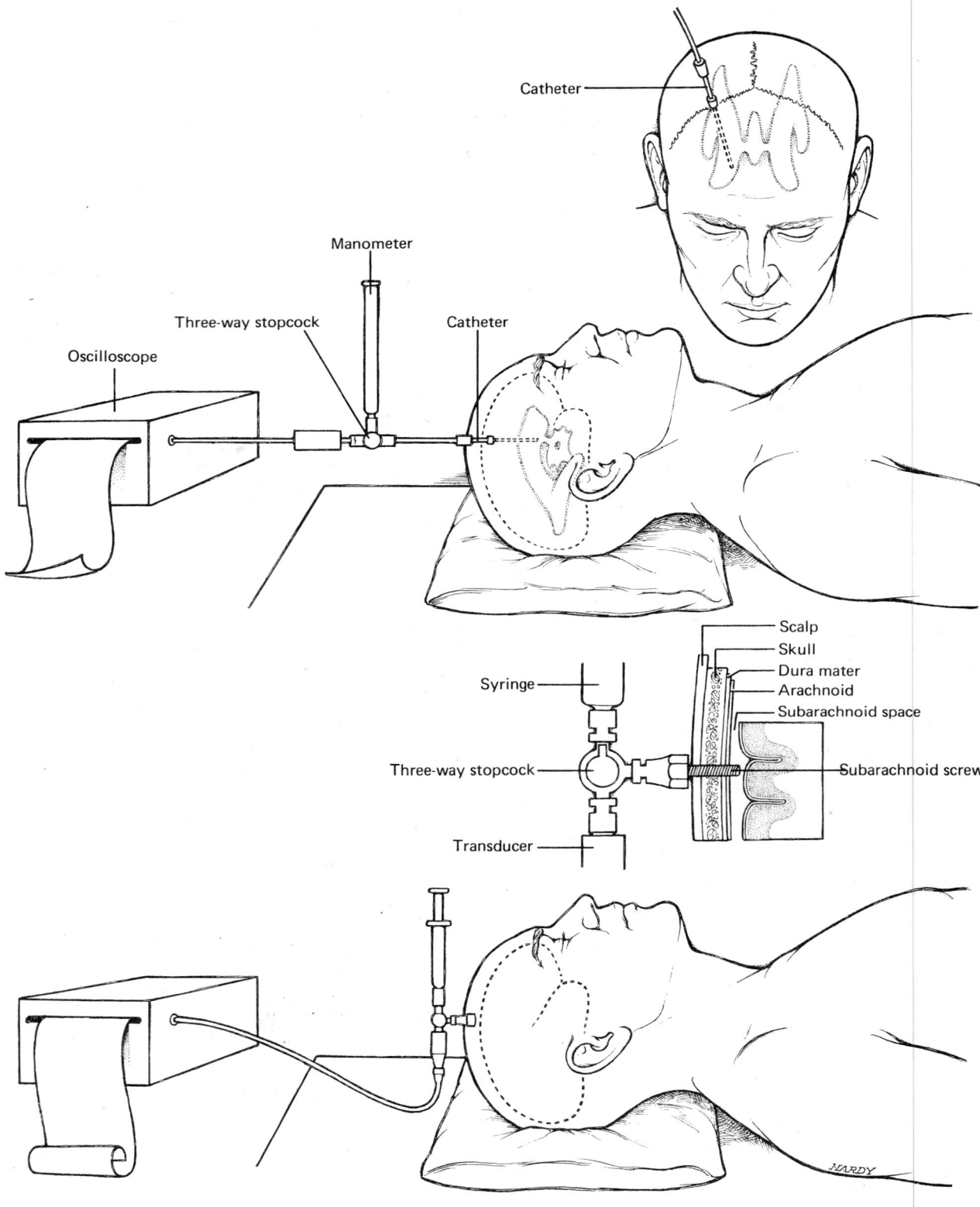

Figure 57-1. Intracranial pressure monitoring. (*Top*) Ventricular catheter. (*Center*) Subarachnoid or hollow screw. (*Bottom*) Monitoring system connected to pressure transducer and display system.

the advantage of not requiring a ventricular puncture. The subarachnoid screw is inserted through a small twist drill hole in the skull under local anesthesia; it is attached to a pressure transducer, and the output is recorded on an oscilloscope for continuous monitoring. The hollow screw technique is useful in patients with head trauma and those with supratentorial brain tumors. It has the additional advantage of avoiding complications from brain shift and small ventricle size. Complications include blockage of the screw from high ICP levels, and bleeding, which may occur when the dura and arachnoid are opened.

A disposable stopcock network is used for both the ventricular catheter and hollow screw monitoring systems to connect the patient to a pressure transducer and display system. The network contains a three-way stopcock attached to the screw or ventricular catheter, a nondistensible saline-filled tubing leading from one outlet of the three-way stopcock to a manifold containing the pressure transducer. The pressure transducer transmits a wave form through the electrical circuitry to a display system for continuous monitoring. The system is flushed with sterile saline at varying time intervals (*e.g.,* every 6 hours) to keep the device patent.

Another method of monitoring is by *epidural* implantation of a miniature pressure sensor and transmitter in the epidural space, usually through a burr hole in the skull.

Implications.   The measurement of ICP is only one parameter of patient assessment. ICP is expressed by ventricular fluid pressures, which normally fluctuate in the range of 110 mm H_2O to 140 mm H_2O or 0 to 10 mm Hg. Pressures above 200 mm H_2O or 15 mm Hg are considered abnormal.

▷ Hyperthermia

Because of damage to the heat-regulating center in the brain or severe intracranial infection, neurologic and neurosurgical patients often develop very high temperatures. Such temperature elevations must be controlled, because the increased metabolic demands by the brain will overburden brain circulation and oxygenation, resulting in cerebral deterioration. Persistent hyperthermia is indicative of brain stem damage and has a poor prognosis. It has been shown that body temperatures well below normal decrease cerebral edema, reduce the quantity of oxygen and metabolites required by the brain, and protect the brain from continued ischemia. Also, the collateral circulation in the brain may be able to provide an adequate blood supply to the brain if the body metabolism can be lowered.

The induction and maintenance of hypothermia is a major clinical procedure and requires knowledge and skilled nursing observation and management. It is desirable to begin treatment before the patient's temperature gets too high.

- All bedding over the patient should be removed (with the possible exception of a light sheet or loin cloth).
- Repeated doses of aspirin or acetaminophen may be given.

- Alcohol or cool water sponging and an electric fan blowing over the patient to increase surface cooling are also helpful.
- Chlorpromazine may be given to control shivering.

At the present time, the use of the hypothermia blanket and equipment is usually effective in controlling neurogenic hyperthermia.

▷ The Unconscious Patient

Unconsciousness is a condition in which there is a depression of cerebral function, ranging from stupor to coma. In stupor, the patient shows symptoms of annoyance when stimulated by something unpleasant, such as a pinprick, loud clapping of hands, etc. He may draw back or make facial grimaces or unintelligible sounds. In a deep coma, the patient does not respond appropriately to any stimuli, and reflexes are absent.

Unconsciousness may be associated with brain injury from trauma, stroke, hypotension and disorders of metabolism (hepatic or renal failure), drug overdose, or alcohol ingestion.

▶ Assessment

Clinical Manifestations.   The level of responsiveness (consciousness) is assessed by evaluating eye opening, verbal responses, and motor responses to a command or painful stimulus. These measurements are assessed and graded using the Glasgow coma scale rating (see p. 1367). The pupils are evaluated as to size, equality, and reaction to light. In addition, the movement of the eyes is noted. Facial symmetry, swallowing reflexes, and deep tendon reflexes are elicited. Important signs to evaluate in assessing the unconscious patient are noted in Chart 57-1 and on page 1364, the assessment of the patient with a head injury.

Patient Problems/Nursing Diagnoses

Based on the clinical manifestations and diagnostic assessment data, the patient's problems/nursing diagnoses include ineffective airway clearance related to accumulation of secretions; nutritional alteration (less than body requirements) related to inability to ingest food and fluids; alteration in bladder and bowel elimination (incontinence) related to the unconscious state; potential impairment of skin integrity related to impaired mobility; and self-care deficits (oral hygiene, bathing, feeding, toileting) related to the unconscious state.

▶ Planning and Implementation

Goals

The goals of care include

1. Maintenance of a clear airway
2. Adequate nutritional status
3. Bladder and bowel continence
4. Absence of skin breakdown

Chart 57-1
Nursing Assessment of the Unconscious Patient

Examination	Clinical Assessment	Clinical Significance
Level of responsiveness or consciousness	See page 1293.	
Respirations	Cheyne–Stokes	Lesions deep in both hemispheres, area of basal ganglia and upper brain stem
	Hyperventilation	Systemic acidosis
	Ataxic respiration with irregularity in depth and rate	Grave sign of imminent failure of medullary centers
Eyes: Pupils	Progressive dilatation	Indicates increased cranial pressure
	Equal or unequal diameter	Localizing sign

Size

Equality

Examination	Clinical Assessment	Clinical Significance
Reaction to light	Pupils react or do not react to light	Localizing sign
Eye movements	Eyes move from side to side	Absent in lesions of brain stem or pons
Corneal reflex	When cornea is touched with a wisp of clean cotton, blink response is normal	Absent in deep coma Tests cranial nerves V and VII Localizing sign if unilateral

Examination	Clinical Assessment	Clinical Significance
Facial symmetry	Asymmetry (sagging; decrease in wrinkles)	Sign of paralysis
Swallowing reflex	Drooling versus spontaneous swallowing	Absent in coma Paralysis of cranial nerves X and XII
Neck	Stiff neck	Subarachnoid hemorrhage; meningitis
	Absence of spontaneous neck movement	Fracture or dislocation of cervical spine
Response of extremity to pain	Firm pressure on a joint of the upper and lower extremity	Asymmetrical response in paralysis Absent in deep coma

(continued)

Chart 57-1
Nursing Assessment of the Unconscious Patient (continued)

Examination (continued)	Clinical Assessment (continued)	Clinical Significance (continued)
Deep tendon reflexes	Tap patellar and biceps tendons	Brisk response may have localizing value Asymmetrical response in paralysis Absent in deep coma
Pathologic reflexes 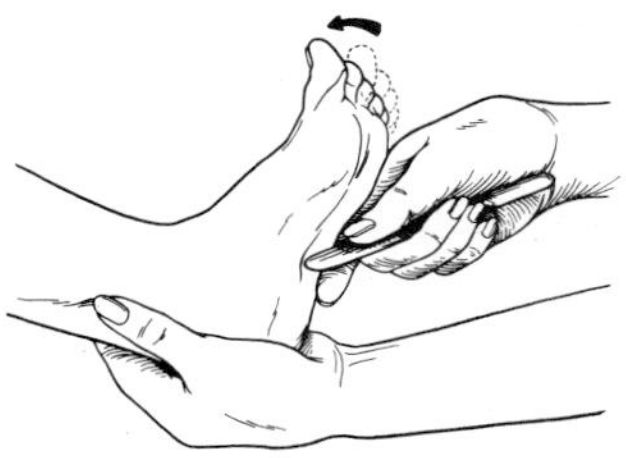	Firm pressure with blunt object on sole of foot moving along lateral margin and crossing to the ball of foot	Flexion of the toes, especially the great toe, is normal except in newborn Dorsiflexion of toes (especially great toe) indicates contralateral pathology of corticospinal tract (Babinski reflex) Localizing signs
Pathologic posturing	Decerebrate rigidity (*left, below*) Decorticate rigidity (*right, below*)	Implies brain stem pathology; poor prognostic sign Seen with cerebral hemisphere pathology

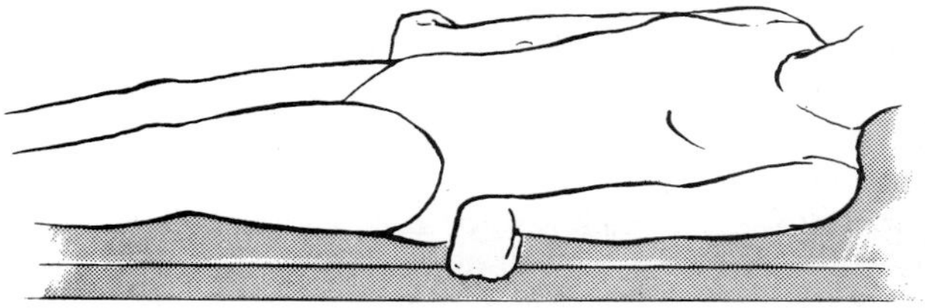

Decerebrate rigidity 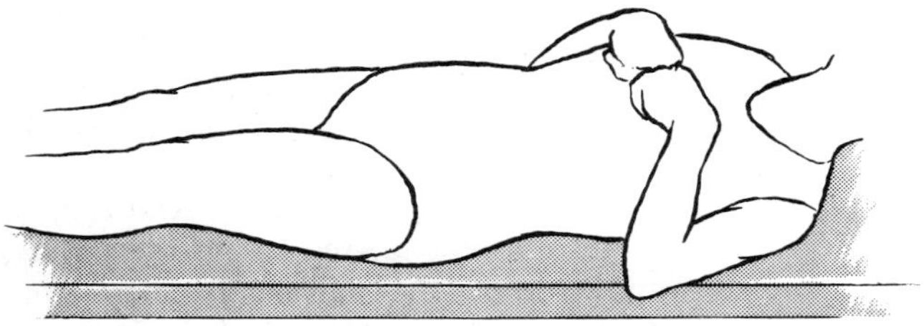   Decorticate rigidity

Muscle tone	Flexor or extensor rigidity or limb flaccidity	Indicates paralysis

The quality of nursing care given an unconscious patient may literally mean the difference between life and death, since the patient's protective reflexes are impaired. The nurse must assume responsibility for the patient until the basic reflexes return (coughing, blinking, and swallowing) and the patient becomes conscious and oriented. Thus, the major nursing goal is to assume these protective reflexes for the patient until he is aware of himself and can function consciously. This includes establishing and maintaining an adequate airway, assessing the level of responsiveness/consciousness, maintaining fluid and nutritional balance, and giving continuing nursing support (to maintain bladder and bowel elimination, provide skin care and positioning, maintain temperature control, attend to eye care, be alert for cerebrospinal fluid seepage, provide safety, and assist in promoting self-care). In addition, the needs of the family must be addressed.

Maintaining a Clear Airway. The most important consideration in the management of the unconscious patient is to establish and maintain the airway. The unconscious patient is at risk for an obstructed airway from the tongue falling back in the oropharynx.

- The patient is positioned in a lateral or semiprone position to facilitate drainage of respiratory secretions. (*Never allow an unconscious patient to remain on his back.*)

The accumulation of secretions in the pharynx presents a serious problem that demands intelligent and conscientious management. Since the patient is unable to swallow and lacks pharyngeal reflexes, these secretions must be removed to eliminate the danger of aspiration.

- Suction is employed to remove secretions from the posterior pharynx and upper trachea.

With the suction turned *off,* a whistle-tip catheter is lubricated with a water-soluble lubricant and maneuvered to the desired level. Then the suction is turned on (negative pressure) while the aspirating catheter is withdrawn with a twisting motion of the thumb and forefinger. This twisting maneuver prevents the suctioning end of the catheter from irritating the tracheal or pharyngeal mucosa, since irritation merely increases secretions and produces mucosal bleeding. The suction catheter should be kept meticulously clean. (If the patient has a tracheostomy, it should be kept sterile.) The frequency of suctioning is determined by the amount of secretions present.

The mouth of the unconscious patient is an area that needs conscientious care. The mouth should be cleansed with a gauze-covered tongue blade or a washcloth and rinsed carefully. A soothing lubricant within the mouth and on the lips prevents drying and the formation of encrustations.

Assessing the Level of Responsiveness.   Evaluating the level of responsiveness/consciousness is done by assessing eye-opening and motor and verbal responses (see p. 1293). Vital signs, pupils, eye movements, and motor power are also assessed. The use of the Glasgow coma scale (see p. 1367) is a reliable tool in grading the patient's responses and in following trends in his progress.

Maintaining Fluid and Nutritional Balance.   The nutritional needs of this patient are initially met by giving the required fluids intravenously and then by nasogastric or gastrostomy feedings.

- Intravenous solutions and blood transfusions for patients with intracranial conditions must run in slowly. If given too rapidly, they may increase the ICP. The quantity of fluids administered may be limited to minimize the possibility of producing cerebral edema.
- Never give fluids by mouth to the patient who cannot swallow. One way of testing to see whether the patient is able to swallow without choking is to give him a wet swab to suck.
- A nasogastric tube may be passed, and the patient can be given liquid and blenderized feedings (see p. 773).

Bladder and Bowel Elimination.   The bladder is palpated to determine if urinary retention is present, as a full bladder may be the overlooked cause of incontinence. Urinary incontinence may be managed by inserting a three-way catheter attached to continuous drainage or by instituting tidal drainage. This is important if diuretics are used. Clamping the catheter at intervals helps to prevent contracture of the bladder, as this procedure more closely approximates normal functioning.

Abdominal distention is evaluated by listening for bowel sounds and measuring the girth of the abdomen with a tape measure. Enemas may be administered every second or third day to eliminate fecal incontinence or reduce the frequency of involuntary stools. Frequent loose stools are an indication of fecal impaction. Methods of regaining control of bladder and bowel function are described on page 251.

Skin Care and Positioning.   Special attention is given to unconscious patients because they are insensitive to external stimuli. They must be turned frequently and positioned properly. Turning also provides kinesthetic, proprioceptive, and vestibular stimulation as well as relief of pressure. (See pp. 238–242 for prevention of pressure sores.)

Maintaining correct body position is important; equally important is passive exercise of the extremities, so that contractures are prevented. The use of a footboard aids in the prevention of footdrop and eliminates the pressure of bedding on the toes. Trochanter rolls supporting the hip joints keep the legs in good position (see p. 238, Fig. 14-1). The arm should be in abduction, the fingers lightly flexed, and the hand in a position of slight supination.

Temperature Control.   The temperature of the environment is determined by the patient's condition. An elevated temperature would call for a minimum amount of bed clothing—a sheet or perhaps only a loin cloth.

The room may be cooled to 18.3° C (65° F). However, if the patient is older and does not have an elevation of temperature, a warmer atmosphere is needed. Regardless of the temperature, the air should be fresh and free from odors.

- The body temperature of an unconscious patient never is taken by mouth. Rectal temperature is preferred to the less accurate axillary temperature.

Eye Care.   Because there are occasions when the corneal reflex is absent, the cornea is likely to become irritated or scratched, leading to keratitis and corneal ulcers. It may be necessary to irrigate the eyes with normal saline solution and to lubricate them with sterile mineral oil. Often, periocular edema occurs following head surgery. Cold compresses may be used, and care must be exerted to avoid contact with the cornea.

Fluid Seepage.   If there is ear or nasal bleeding, or oozing of cerebrospinal fluid, the physician should be notified immediately. A small, sterile, cotton pledget may be placed loosely in the nostril or ears, but no attempt to clean them should be made until the patient is further evaluated.

Safety.   For the protection of the patient, padded side-rails should be provided. Every measure that is available and appropriate for calming and quieting the disturbed patient should be carried out. Any form of restraint is likely to be countered by resistance, whether the patient is fully conscious or not, and fury so incited may lead to self-injury or to a dangerous increase in ICP.

Attaining Self-care.   The unconscious patient is dependent on the nursing staff for all his activities of daily living. As soon as consciousness returns, the nurse begins to teach, support, encourage, and supervise in these activities until the patient gains independence. (See Activities of Daily Living, p. 242.)

Family of Unconscious Patient.   The family of the unconscious patient may be thrown into a sudden state of crisis and go through the process of high anxiety, denial, anger, remorse, grief, and reconciliation. In order to assist family members to mobilize their own adaptive capacities, the nursing personnel can reinforce and clarify information about the patient's condition, permit the family to be involved in the care of their loved one, and listen and encourage ventilation of feelings and concerns while supporting them in their decision-making process concerning posthospitalization management and placement.

A summary of the nursing management of the unconscious patient is found in Chart 57-2.

(Text continues on page 1305)

Chart 57-2
Nursing Management of the Unconscious Patient

Goals, Nursing Strategies, and Rationale of Care
The basic nursing principles underlying the care of an unconscious patient are applicable to any unconscious patient, regardless of the clinical cause. There are two major threats to the patient; (1) the disease or trauma that produced unconsciousness, and (2) the threat of the unconscious state. The primary problem is that the patient's normal protective reflexes are impaired. The nursing goal is to assume these protective mechanisms for the patient until he is aware of himself and can function in his environment.

Goals and Interventions	*Rationale/Amplification*
A. To establish and maintain an adequate airway, respiratory exchange, and circulation	Inadequate respiratory exchange promotes CO_2 retention, which can produce diffuse cerebral edema. Airway obstruction will aggravate cerebral swelling and may be a cause of continuing or deepening unconsciousness.
1. Place the patient in a three-quarters prone position or a lateral position with his head turned to one side. (In the event of increased intracranial pressure, the head of the bed may be elevated as prescribed.)	1. This position prevents the tongue from obstructing the airway and encourages drainage of respiratory secretions, thus preventing aspiration and promoting oxygen and carbon dioxide exchange.
2. Insert oral airway if tongue is paralyzed or is obstructing airway.	2. *A noisy airway is an obstructed airway.* (An obstructed airway increases intracranial pressure.) The use of an oropharyngeal airway is considered a short-term measure.
3. Prepare for insertion of cuffed endotracheal tube if patient's condition requires (inefficient cough reflex, respiratory failure).	3. Endotracheal intubation is more effective in permitting positive-pressure ventilation. The cuffed tube seals off the digestive tract, thus preventing aspiration, and allows efficient removal of tracheobronchial secretions.
4. Utilize humidified oxygen therapy, positive-pressure assisted breathing techniques, or mechanical ventilation with a ventilator when there is indication of impending respiratory failure.	4. When arterial blood gas measurements reveal the patient has insufficient ventilation and gas exchange, respiratory failure may ensue.
5. Keep the airway free of secretions with efficient suctioning.	5. With the absence of the cough and swallowing reflexes, secretions rapidly accumulate in the posterior pharynx and upper trachea and can pave the way to fatal respiratory complications.
a. Attach open-end catheter to Y-tube.	
b. Keep one end of Y-tube open while inserting the catheter.	
c. When catheter is at desired level, close the open-end of Y with finger.	
d. Turn the suction *on* and slowly withdraw catheter with a twisting motion of the thumb and forefinger.	d. Negative pressure (suction on) is applied only as the catheter is withdrawn. The twisting motion of the suction catheter reduces prolonged contact with the pharyngeal mucosa. Forceful suction irritates the mucosa, increases the amount of secretions, produces mucosal bleeding, and can precipitate infection.
e. Gently turn the head from side to side while suctioning. (1) Limit tracheal aspiration to intervals of a few seconds. (2) Allow patient to rest between aspirations. (3) Oxygenate the patient between aspirations as required.	

(continued)

Chart 57-2
Nursing Management of the Unconscious Patient (continued)

Goals and Interventions *(continued)*	**Rationale/Amplification** *(continued)*
6. Evaluate pulses (radial, carotid, apical, pedal); measure blood pressure.	6. These are a measure of circulatory adequacy/inadequacy.
7. Carry out periodic determinations of arterial PO_2 and PCO_2.	7. These evaluations determine adequacy of treatment.
8. Assist with passage of a gastric tube.	8. A gastric tube permits aspiration (suctioning) of stomach contents and provides a route for oral feeding.

9. Prepare for tracheostomy if coma is deepening and if there is evidence of inadequate respiratory exchange.
  a. Keep tracheostomy tube meticulously clean.
    (1) Carefully inject 3 ml to 5 ml saline solution through trachea stoma and then suction.
	(1) The dryness of the respiratory tract produces rapid formation of mucous plugs, which are difficult to remove. The careful washing (3 ml–5 ml of saline) of the trachea also stimulates the cough reflex, which helps to clear the tracheobronchial tree.

b. Wear sterile gloves and use a sterile catheter each time the tracheostomy is aspirated. c. Suction trachea around cannula and through tube.	c. Keeping the upper respiratory tract clean and free of mucous plugs and dried secretions lessens subsequent pulmonary complications.
d. Have adequate humidification. 10. Assess cardiac function. 11. Give antibiotics as per schedule.	11. A screen of broad-spectrum antibiotics may be given to the unconscious patient to prevent infectious and pulmonary complications.
12. Assist with diagnostic tests (blood, urine, nasogastric aspirate).	12. Blood is drawn to determine if there is a metabolic cause for coma (*e.g.,* hypoglycemia).
B. To assess the level of responsiveness 1. Maintain a constant assessment of the patient's level of consciousness and changes in responsiveness.	1. The level of consciousness is the most important measure of the patient's condition. Unconscious patients may deteriorate rapidly from numerous clinical causes.
2. Record the patient's *exact reactions:* eye opening, verbal response, movements, and quality of speech. Describe the patient's responses and the stimuli required to elicit them (see p. 1293).	2. An unconscious patient is unable to obey commands or utter recognizable words.
3. Examine pupils of eyes for size, shape, and reaction to light. 4. Assess movement of extremities in response to verbal commands or painful stimulus.	4. No response or a delayed or unequal response is an unfavorable clinical sign.
C. To evaluate the progression of vital signs 1. Know the patient's base-line (initial) vital signs, and alert the physician if there are significant fluctuations of blood pressure and instability of the pulse and respiratory cycles.	1. Fluctuations of vital signs indicate a change in intracranial homeostasis. Monitoring of vital signs is also essential to detect hidden bleeding.
2. Take blood pressure readings, pulse and respiratory rate and pattern, and temperature at frequently specified intervals until there is clinical evidence of stabilization.	2. Taking and recording of temperature is mandatory since temperature-regulating mechanisms may be disturbed. Hyperthermia is an unfavorable prognostic sign. The systolic blood pressure must be adequate to maintain cerebral perfusion pressure. A slow pulse, rising blood pressure, and slowing respiration are associated with cerebral compromise.

(continued)

Chart 57-2
Nursing Management of the Unconscious Patient (continued)

Goals and Interventions *(continued)*

D. To maintain fluid and electrolyte balance

    1. Give intravenous fluids as indicated.

    2. Or use hyperalimentation feedings.
    3. Or initiate nasogastric feedings.

       a. Insert small gastric tube through nose into stomach.
       b. Aspirate stomach before each feeding.

       c. Elevate patient's head and thorax and give 100 ml to 150 ml blenderized formula slowly. Give small amount at first and gradually increase until 400 ml to 500 ml are given at each feeding.
       d. Give 2000 ml to 2500 ml of fluid through tube daily.

       e. Rinse the tube with water or cranberry juice after each feeding.
       f. Keep tube feeding refrigerated.
       g. Measure urinary output and specific gravity.
       h. Prepare for gastrostomy if patient's condition indicates.

E. To give nursing support as the patient's changing condition indicates

    1. Be aware of the varying phases of restlessness.

       a. Have adequate lighting in the room to prevent hallucinations in the patient who is regaining consciousness.
       b. Pad side rails, apply mitts or boxing gloves on hands, or use other devices to protect patient.
       c. Avoid oversedating the patient.

Rationale/Amplification *(continued)*

1. Serial laboratory electrolyte evaluations are made when the patient is maintained on intravenous fluids to ensure proper balance.
2. See page 780.
3. Feeding through a gastric tube ensures better nutrition than does intravenous feeding. Electrolyte and protein balance is maintained by selective absorption. Also, paralytic ileus is fairly frequent in the unconscious patient, and a nasogastric tube assists in gastric decompression.

    b. If aspirated residual exceeds 50 ml, the patient may be developing an ileus. Gastric distention and vomiting may result.
    c. Elevation of the patient's head before, during, and after feeding reduces likelihood of esophageal reflux regurgitation and aspiration.

    d. An unconscious patient requires adequate fluids daily. High-protein feedings can produce a solute diuresis, which will produce dehydration and hyperosmolar coma unless an adequate fluid intake is ensured. Fever, excessive sweating, or fluid loss elsewhere in the body increases the fluid requirements.

    h. Prolonged nasogastric intubation can cause esophagitis (from gastric reflux) and erosion of the nasal septum.

1. A certain degree of restlessness may be favorable, as it may indicate the patient is regaining consciousness. However, restlessness is quite common in cerebral hypoxia or when there is a partially obstructed airway, distended bladder, overlooked bleeding, or fracture; it may be a manifestation of brain injury.

    c. Sedatives and narcotics depress the level of responsiveness, which is a guide to clinical assessment. Certain drugs affect pupillary size and reaction, which are important signs.

(continued)

Chart 57-2
Nursing Management of the Unconscious Patient (continued)

Goals and Interventions (continued)	*Rationale/Amplification (continued)*
d. Avoid restraints if at all possible.	
e. Speak softly to the patient, calling him by name.	
f. Touch him as gently as possible.	
2. Keep the skin clean, dry, and free of pressure.	2. Comatose patients are susceptible to the formation of pressure sores. All these activities are to prevent the formation of pressure sores on pressure-sensitive areas.
a. Lubricate skin with emollient lotions to prevent sheet irritation, dryness, chafing, and cracking.	a. See pages 238 to 242 for other preventive measures for pressure sores.
b. Inspect pressure areas for evidence of skin redness and breakdown.	
c. Clip patient's nails to prevent skin excoriation.	
3. Put all extremities through range of motion exercises four times daily.	3. Contracture deformities develop early in unconscious patients.
4. Turn the patient from side to side at regular intervals. Carry out chest physical therapy as indicated.	4. Turning relieves pressure areas and helps keep lungs clear by mobilizing secretions. Prolonged pressure on extremities produces nerve palsies and pressure sores.
5. Observe the patient for indications of an overdistended bladder.	
a. Utilize external sheath catheter (condom catheter) for male patient.	a. Involuntary voiding indicates an impaired state of consciousness.
b. If patient is unable to void, insert three-way indwelling catheter with continuous drainage.	b. Infection invariably follows prolonged use of an indwelling catheter that is attached to straight drainage.
6. Watch for constipation and diarrhea.	6. Constipation results from immobilization and lack of dietary fiber. Diarrhea occurs from infection, antibiotics, hyperosmolar feedings, and fecal impaction.
7. Carry out meticulous oral care.	
8. Protect the eye from corneal irritation.	
a. Make sure patient's eye is not rubbing against the bedding.	a. The cornea functions as a shield. If the eyes remain open for long periods, corneal drying, irritation, and ulceration are apt to result.
b. Routinely inspect size of pupils and condition of eyes using a flashlight.	
c. Remove contact lenses if worn.	
d. Irrigate eyes with sterile prescribed solution and instill ophthalmic ointment in each eye.	d. This removes discharge and helps prevent glazing and corneal ulceration.
e. Prepare for temporary tarsorrhaphy (suturing of eyelids in closed position) if unconscious state is prolonged.	
9. Protect the patient during seizures (see p. 1360).	9. A patient with head trauma is a potential candidate for seizures.
a. Protect the patient from self-injury.	
b. Observe the patient during the seizure and record observations.	
c. Give prescribed anticonvulsant medications via the nasogastric tube.	

(continued)

Chart 57-2
Nursing Management of the Unconscious Patient (continued)

Goals and Interventions (continued)	*Rationale/Amplification* (continued)

10. Be alert for complications.
   a. Respiratory complications (infection, aspiration, obstruction, atelectasis)
   b. Fluid and electrolyte imbalance
   c. Infection (urinary, pressure sores, central nervous system)
   d. Bladder and gastrointestinal distention
   e. Seizures
   f. Gastrointestinal bleeding	

11. Provide for environmental enrichment and social contacts.
   a. Direct conversation to the patient; encourage family to talk to the patient.
   b. Arouse patient; touch him; stimulate his senses.
   c. Introduce sounds from the patient's home and work environment via a tape recorder to "normalize" the environment.
	11. Introducing meaningful sounds stimulates the cortical levels.
	   a. Attempt to stimulate the patient's senses to overcome sensory deprivation.
	
	   c. Know the patient's preferences in music, radio, TV, and patterns of daily living.

12. Give the patient an explanation of what has happened during period of unconsciousness. Permit him to question and talk about the experience of unconsciousness.	12. This will help the patient to cope with anxieties, mobilize psychological defenses, and promote psychological recovery.

▶ **Evaluation**

Expected Outcomes

1. Maintains clear airway
   a. Coughs up secretions
   b. Turns from side to side
   c. Has no crackles on lung auscultation
   d. Responds to appropriate stimuli
2. Attains/maintains adequate nutritional status
   a. Demonstrates swallowing reflexes
   b. Has no clinical signs of dehydration
   c. Demonstrates normal range of serum electrolytes
   d. Reveals bowel sounds upon auscultation
   e. Shows minimal weight loss
3. Attains bladder and bowel control
   a. Experiences no bladder or bowel distention
   b. Tries to void at specified intervals
   c. Takes active part in bowel rehabilitation program
4. Is free from skin breakdown
   a. Turns from side to side
   b. Uses sheepskin to lie on
5. Attains self-care
   a. Helps with oral hygiene
   b. Performs part of bath
   c. Tries to feed self

   d. Signals when bedpan/urinal is needed
   e. Participates actively in muscle strengthening exercises

▷ **Aphasia**

Aphasia is a disturbance of language function resulting from injury or disease of the brain centers. It may involve impairment of the ability to read and write as well as to speak, listen, calculate, comprehend, and understand gestures (Chart 57-3). Nearly 1 to 1 and a half million adults in this country have a chronic disabling aphasia. The major causes are stroke, head injury, and brain tumor.

The cortical area that is responsible for integrating the myriad association pathways required for the comprehension and formulation of language measures little more than a square inch in extent (marked "Motor speech" in Fig. 56-2). The principal speech center, called *Broca's area,* is located in a convolution adjoining the middle cerebral artery. Here are stored the combinations of muscular movements necessary to speak each word. They are not the cells that govern the muscles of speech; these cells are in the motor area itself. Each word requires for its utterance a combination or sequence of combinations of muscular contractions. Not

---

Chart 57-3
Glossary of Selected Terms Relating to Aphasia*

Acalculia; dyscalculia—difficulty in dealing with mathematical processes or numerical symbols in general

Agnosia—failure to recognize familiar objects perceived by the senses

   Auditory agnosia—inability to recognize significance of sounds

   Color agnosia—inability to recognize differences in color

   Tactile agnosia—inability to recognize familiar objects by touch or feel

   Visual object agnosia—inability to recognize objects; visual acuity may or may not be intact

Agraphia; dysgraphia—disturbances in writing intelligible words

Alexia; dyslexia—difficulty in reading

Anomia; dysnomia—difficulty in selecting appropriate words, particularly nouns

Apraxia—inability to perform previously learned purposeful motor acts on a voluntary basis

   Verbal apraxia—difficulty in forming and organizing intelligible words although the musculature is intact

Dysarthria—defects of articulation due to neurologic causes

Hemianopia—blindness for one half of the field of vision in one or both eyes

Paraphasia—a frequently observed characteristic in many aphasic patients; uses wrong words, word substitutions, grammatical errors, faults in word usage; may be observed in both oral and written language

Perseveration—continued and automatic repetition of an activity or word or phrase that is no longer appropriate

---

* The prefix *a* means "without" or "absence." The prefix *dys* refers to "difficulty" or "disordered." These prefixes are frequently used interchangeably in these conditions.

---

only must the muscles of the vocal cords contract, but also those of the throat, the tongue, the soft palate, the lips, and the chest wall. These combinations are stored in the cells of Broca's convolution. They direct the cells of the motor area, which make the muscles contract at the proper time and with the proper force.

Broca's area is so near the left motor area that a disturbance in the motor area often affects the speech area. This is the reason that so many persons paralyzed on the right side (due to a lesion of the left hemisphere) are unable to speak, whereas in those paralyzed on the left side, speech disturbances are less common. Some patients are not affected, but these usually are left-handed persons whose speech area is located on the right hemisphere.

Aphasic Syndromes

There are a wide range of language dysfunctions and differing classifications, depending on whose school of thought is being read. One method of classifying asphasias is to divide them into *nonfluent* and *fluent* types. The type of aphasia is determined by listening to the speech output. In general, people with nonfluent aphasia have lesions located in the anterior part of the brain, while those with fluent aphasias have lesions in the posterior area.

Nonfluent Aphasia (Broca's Aphasia, Motor Aphasia, Expressive Aphasia). This type of aphasia is manifested as a difficulty in producing language, characterized by sparse verbal output that is produced with effort. The patient understands most of what is said to him; he knows the words he wants to say; he may be able to write them and read them; but he cannot produce the sequence of movements necessary to utter them, and, if he tries, he makes an unintelligible noise. He is conscious of this defect (verbal apraxia), and it distresses him greatly. The destruction of Broca's convolution by stroke or tumor results in this type of motor aphasia. To cause a permanent motor aphasia, the lesion must (and usually does) affect the white matter beneath this convolution where the fibers are going to and coming from other parts of the brain. When only the gray matter of Broca's convolution is destroyed, the aphasia may be transitory.

Global aphasia is characterized by severe, almost complete loss of function distributed across all language modalities, including inability to speak, comprehend, and repeat or name. This is the most severe aphasic syndrome and may result from destruction of both Broca's and Wernicke's areas.

Fluent Aphasia. In this type of aphasia, there is difficulty in comprehension of language; this includes Wernicke's aphasia, conduction aphasia, and anomic aphasia.

In *Wernicke's (sensory) aphasia,* the patient speaks readily, but his speech lacks clear content, information, and direction and at times is incomprehensible ("jargon"). The area affected is the posterior part of the left superior temporal gyrus (Wernicke's area), but lesions can extend beyond this area. This type of aphasia is seen in about 15% of the aphasic population and increases with age.

In *conduction aphasia,* the patient can comprehend almost everything that is said but has difficulty in uttering the correct sounds and in repeating phrases or sentences. This type is seen in up to 10% of aphasic patients.

In *anomic or amnesic aphasia,* the speech is almost normal but marred by word-finding difficulty. It is seen in about 5% of the patients with aphasia.

Nursing Management

There are a variety of symptoms and disorders underlying aphasia. The treatment is individualized and is based on the patient's background and interest. Recovery depends on the extent of brain damage, the patient's personality, and the support system available (family and friends). The potential for recovery is assessed by the speech pathologist or therapist in cooperation with the neurologist. Some patients with extensive brain damage never regain speech.

Assessment of the aphasic patient includes *listening* to him, asking him to follow simple directions (*i.e.,* "pick up the book''), tests of naming objects, repetition of spoken language, and writing.

The goal is to increase auditory stimulation and to restore speech communication.

Positive Self-image. A patient with aphasia should be given as much psychological security as possible. The same manner is used with this patient as with a young child learning to speak. At the same time, the patient is treated as an adult. A kind, unhurried manner combined with encouragement, patience, and a willingness to invest time are required. Relearning speech and language skills may take several years.

Accept the patient's behavior, relieve his embarrassment, and give support by assuring him that there is nothing wrong with his intelligence and that you realize he knows what he wants to say. The environment should be relaxed and permissive, and the patient should be encouraged to socialize with family and friends. The typical aphasic individual has almost an obsession with orderliness. Thus, nurses and family members should return items in the room to their proper place.

Increasing Auditory Stimulation. First the patient is encouraged to *listen.* Speaking is thinking out loud, and the emphasis is on *thinking.* The patient must think and sort out incoming messages and formulate a response. Listening requires mental effort, yet the patient must struggle against mental inertia and needs time to organize an answer.

In working with the aphasic patient, the nurse must remember to *talk* to the patient while caring for him. This provides social contact for the patient.

It is best to face the patient and establish eye contact, at the same time speaking in a normal manner but in short phrases, pausing between phrases. The emphasis here is on ensuring that the patient understands what is being said. Conversation should be confined to practical and concrete matters, and supplemented with gestures, pictures, and objects. As the patient handles and uses the object, the word should be stated; it helps when words are matched with actions. Consistency is important and the same wording and gestures are used each time instructions are given and questions are asked. Since the patient is easily fatigued and distracted, extraneous noises and sounds must be kept at a minimum since the patient cannot sort out messages when there is too much noise and confusion in the environment.

Restoring Speech. When the patient attempts to communicate, the nurse should make a real effort to understand him and to treat him as an intelligent adult. It is important to behave in a way that shows acceptance of the patient as a worthwhile human being. The patient should never be forced to correct his mistakes since this merely adds to his tension. Nor should the nurse rush to finish sentences for him. During periods of emotional liability, the patient should be approached in a calm, accepting, and deliberate manner since frustration and depression are frequent reactions to the inability to communicate. Because speech that is motivated by emotions usually comes first (*i.e.,* swearing), the content of this speech should be ignored by the nursing personnel.

Patients with aphasia must be stimulated both internally and externally to action. Therapy is based on a recognition of the patient's needs, *previous* interests, drives, and motivation. If the patient's speech is unintelligible or filled with jargon, his gestures may offer a clue to his intent. Continue to listen to him. Nod and make neutral statements occasionally. When appropriate, shift the topic to gain another point of interest and frame of reference.

The environment should provide sensory input, with auditory stimulation supplemented with visual stimulation. Reading is encouraged for a few minutes at a time, and the patient can look at pictures while another person talks about them. Games stimulate the mind and help organize the thoughts. Try to elicit responses from the patient, asking him to nod his head if he understands. Reinforce every correct response. For more relaxed forms of communication, the television, radio, and tape recorder can be used.

Family Support. The attitude of the family is an important factor in helping the patient adjust to this deficit. They are encouraged to act naturally and treat the patient in the same manner as before his illness. They should be aware that the patient's ability to speak may vary from day to day and that fatigue will have an adverse effect on speech. They should also be aware that the patient may strike out verbally when his emotional controls are lowered. Support groups such as Stroke Clubs and group therapy for aphasic persons can help in the socialization and motivation of the patient as well as aid in the relief of anxiety and tension. The strain of the constant adjustment to the patient's illness, demands, and needs, as well as the financial drain and the change in life-style, can produce explosive pressures on the family. In addition to the family learning as much as possible about the support of the patient with aphasia, they should also be counseled to continue a life of their own and to seek the aid of a social worker, clergyman, or psychologist if they need additional help in dealing with their frustrations and pressures.

▷ Neurologic Deficits Due to Stroke

Cerebrovascular disease is the third ranking cause of death in the United States and strikes over 400,000 persons in this country every year. Two thirds of those who survive have some permanent disability. Thus, 2 and a half million persons in this country are disabled by stroke.

Pathophysiology. Cerebrovascular disease refers to any functional abnormality of the central nervous system caused by interference with the normal blood supply to the brain. The pathology may involve an artery, a vein, or both, when the cerebral circulation becomes impaired as a result of partial or complete occlusion of a blood vessel or hemorrhage resulting from a tear in the vessel wall. The blood vessel most frequently associated with cerebrovascular disease is the internal carotid artery.

Vascular disease of the central nervous system may be caused by arteriosclerosis (most common), hypertensive changes, arteriovenous malformations, vasospasm, inflammation, arteritis, or embolism. As a result of vascular disease, blood vessels lose their elasticity, become hardened, and develop atheromatous deposits, or plaques, which may be the source of an embolus. The lumen of the vessel may gradually close, causing impairment of cerebral circulation and ischemia of the brain. If cerebral ischemia is transient, there is usually no lasting neurologic deficit. However, occlusion of a large vessel produces cerebral infarction (Fig. 57-2). The vessel may rupture and produce hemorrhage.

Stroke (Cerebrovascular Accident)

A *stroke* is a sudden loss of brain function resulting from a disruption of the blood supply to a part of the brain. Frequently, it is the culmination of cerebrovascular disease of many years standing.

A stroke is usually brought on by one of four events: (1) thrombosis (a blood clot within a blood vessel of the brain or neck), (2) cerebral embolism (a blood clot or other material carried to the brain from another part of the body), (3) ischemia (decrease of blood flow to an area of the brain), and (4) cerebral hemorrhage (rupture of a cerebral blood vessel with bleeding or pressure into the brain substance). The result is an interruption in the blood supply to the brain, causing temporary or permanent loss of movement, thought, memory, speech, or sensation.

Risk Factors and Prevention of Stroke

Prevention of stroke is the best possible approach; steps are taken to alter those factors and human conditions that predispose certain people to stroke or increase their risk of having a stroke.

- The most important risk factors are advanced age, hypertension, and preexisting heart disease.
- The person at risk must be identified and assisted in managing the underlying condition that predisposes them to stroke. This is especially true of patients with hypertension, since this disease is highly correlated with stroke. Diabetes mellitus and hypercholesterolemia are significant risk factors.
- The prevalence of transient ischemic attacks among the elderly seems to be related to the occurrence of cerebral

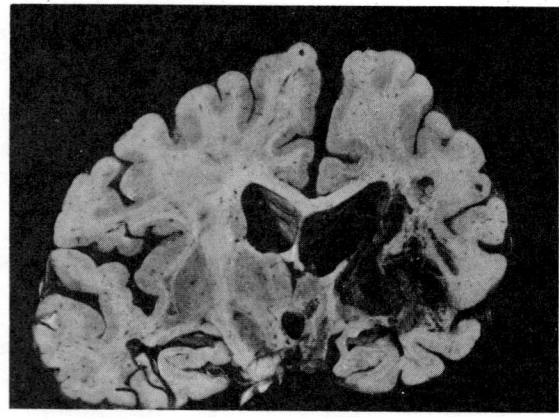

Figure 57-2. Impairment of cerebral circulation leading to a stroke. Note the area of cerebral infarction. (Armed Forces Institute of Pathology: Neg. No. 55–13956)

vascular accident in this patient population. Signs of transient ischemic attacks (TIA) include weakness or transient paralysis of an extremity, loss of or change in speech, visual problems, light-headedness, dizziness, or blackouts (see below). Stroke in people with these manifestations may be prevented with surgery or drugs.

- Persons receiving oral anticoagulants should be monitored to assure that their prothrombin times are kept within the range necessary to prevent intracerebral bleeding.
- Patients with cardiac disease (atherosclerotic/valvular heart disease), those with abnormalities of heart rhythm and heart sounds, and those with electrocardiogram abnormalities should be under medical treatment, since cerebral embolism of cardiac origin is a cause of stroke.
- Oral contraceptives are still considered to be a risk factor by some researchers in light of the number of strokes that have been documented in young women who were taking these drugs, yet had no evidence of other risk factors.
- An excessive or prolonged fall of blood pressure following shock, hemorrhage, surgery, diagnostic procedures, and ingestion of certain drugs may cause general cerebral ischemia. In these instances, the patient requires careful monitoring.
- Drug abuse is a cause of stroke, particularly in adolescents and young adults.
- In younger persons, attention should be directed at controlling blood lipids (particularly cholesterol), blood pressure, cigarette smoking, and obesity.

Transient Ischemic Attacks (Little Strokes)

A *transient ischemic attack* (TIA) is a transient or temporary episode of neurologic dysfunction commonly manifested by a sudden loss of motor, sensory, or visual function, lasting a few seconds or minutes but no longer than 24 hours. Complete recovery usually occurs between attacks. As was indicated above, a TIA may serve as a warning of impending stroke. The cause of this clinical entity is a temporary impairment of blood flow to a specific region of the brain due to a variety of reasons, including atherosclerosis of the vessels supplying the brain, obstruction of cerebral microcirculation by a small embolus, a fall in cerebral perfusion pressure, cardiac arrhythmias, etc.

The most common sites of atherosclerosis in the extracranial arteries are located at the bifurcation of the common carotid and at the origin of the vertebral arteries. Among the intracranial arteries, the middle cerebral artery is the most common location of atherosclerosis. If the ischemia arises in the carotid system, the patient may experience hemiparesis, blindness in one eye, aphasia, or confusion. If the ischemia occurs in the vertebral basilar system, vertigo, blindness, disturbances of consciousness, and various signs of motor and sensory impairments may occur.

Diagnostic Evaluation. A *bruit* (abnormal sound heard on auscultation) may be heard over the carotid artery. There are diminished or absent carotid pulsations in the neck.

Carotid phonoangiography may be done, which provides auscultation, direct visualization, and photographic recording of carotid bruits. *Oculoplethysmography* (OPG) measures pulsation in blood flow through the ophthalmic artery. *Carotid arteriography* visualizes intracranial and cervical vessels.

Management of TIA. Some patients are treated by reconstructive vascular procedures, such as carotid endarterectomy or extracranial/intracranial bypass graft.

Carotid Endarterectomy. A *carotid endarterectomy* is the removal of atherosclerotic plaque(s) or thrombus from the carotid artery to prevent a stroke in persons with extracranial occlusive disease. A temporary bypass shunt is made to give the brain maximum protection during the surgical procedure. The artery is occluded below and above the lesion. The atheromatous lesion or thrombus and a portion of the artery are then removed.

- Following endarterectomy, a neurologic flow sheet is kept to maintain close assessment of the neurologic status. The neurosurgeon must be notified immediately if the patient develops any motor or sensory deficits. The primary complications of carotid endarterectomy are neurologic deficits (stroke), infection/hematoma of a wound, and carotid artery disruption.
- Watch for respiratory insufficiency resulting from edema due to operative manipulation or hematoma at the operative site.
- It is important to maintain adequate blood pressure levels in the immediate postoperative period. Hypotension is avoided to prevent cerebral ischemia and thrombosis.
- Excessive hypertension may precipitate cerebral hemorrhage. Edema, hemorrhage in the operative wound, or disruption of the arterial reconstruction may also result from excessive hypertension. Rapid-acting antihypertensive drugs (trimethaphan [Arfonad]) are used when necessary.
- Long-term complications include recurrent cerebrovascular disease and myocardial infarction.

Extracranial/Intracranial Bypass Grafting. In patients with extracranial and intracranial lesions, a relatively new procedure may be done to prevent stroke. Microvascular techniques are used to help establish an anastomosis of the superficial temporal artery to the middle cerebral artery or one of its branches in order to augment the collateral blood supply to the ischemic areas of the brain.

Postoperative assessment includes monitoring the blood pressure and measuring the central venous pressure. Blood pressure and blood volume are maintained with infusions of colloid, pressors, or nitroprusside. When the patient becomes ambulatory, the blood pressure is controlled with oral agents. To keep the graft patent, aspirin and dipyridamole may be given twice daily for 6 months.

Drug Therapy. Patients who are not candidates for surgical intervention may be placed on anticoagulant therapy (Coumadin) in order to prevent future attacks and a possible massive cerebral infarction. Antiplatelet aggregation drugs (particularly aspirin) are very useful in decreasing the occurrence of cerebral infarction in patients who have experienced multiple TIAs.

Thrombosis, Embolism, and Hemorrhage as Causes of Stroke

Cerebral Thrombosis. Cerebral arteriosclerosis and slowing of the cerebral circulation are major causes of cerebral thrombosis, which is the most common cause of stroke.

Headache is rather uncommon at the onset of cerebral thrombosis. Some patients may experience dizziness, mental disturbances, or convulsions, and some may have an onset indistinguishable from that of intracerebral hemorrhage or cerebral embolism. In general, cerebral thrombosis does not develop abruptly, and a transient loss of speech, hemiplegia, or paresthesias in one half of the body may precede the onset of a severe paralysis by a few hours or days.

Cerebral Embolism. Pathologic abnormalities of the left heart, such as infective endocarditis, rheumatic heart disease, and myocardial infarction, as well as pulmonary infections, are the sites where emboli originate. It is possible that the insertion of a prosthetic heart valve may precipitate a stroke since there seems to be an increased incidence of embolism following this procedure. The incidence of stroke following this procedure can probably be reduced with postoperative anticoagulant therapy. Pacemaker failure, atrial fibrillation, and cardioversion for atrial fibrillation are other possible causes of cerebral emboli and stroke.

The embolus usually lodges in the middle cerebral artery or its branches, where it disrupts the cerebral circulation.

- Sudden onset of hemiparesis or hemiplegia with or without aphasia or loss of consciousness in a patient with cardiac or pulmonary disease is characteristic of cerebral embolism.

Although endarterectomies of the intracranial arteries are being performed, the treatment of cerebral thrombosis and embolism consists chiefly of medical and nursing management similar to that given patients with intracerebral hemorrhage.

Hemorrhage as a Cause of Stroke

In the Framingham Study on Heart Disease and Stroke, which covered 24 years of study, hemorrhage was found to be the mechanism of stroke in 15% of the patients. Hemorrhage may occur outside the dura mater (extradural hemorrhage), beneath the dura matter (subdural hemorrhage), in the subarachnoid space (subarachnoid hemorrhage), or within the brain substance (intracerebral hemorrhage).

Extradural Hemorrhage. *Extradural hemorrhage* (epidural hemorrhage) is a neurosurgical emergency that requires urgent care. It usually follows skull fracture with a tear of the middle artery or other meningeal artery. If the patient is not treated within hours following the accident, he has very little chance of survival. (This is discussed under head injuries on p. 1362.)

Subdural Hemorrhage. This type of hemorrhage (excluding the acute subdural) is basically the same as an epidural hemorrhage, except that in *subdural hematoma* usually a bridging vein is torn. Thus, a longer period of time (longer lucid interval) is required for the hematoma to form and cause pressure on the brain. (This is discussed under head injuries on p. 1363.)

Subarachnoid Hemorrhage.   *Subarachnoid hemorrhage* (hemorrhage occurring in the subarachnoid space) may occur as a result of trauma or hypertension, but the most common cause is a leaking aneurysm in the area of the circle of Willis and congenital arteriovenous malformations of the brain. Any artery within the brain can be the site of an aneurysm. The treatment of intracranial aneurysms is discussed on page 1340.

Intracerebral Hemorrhage.   Hemorrhage or bleeding into the brain substance is most common in patients with hypertension and cerebral atherosclerosis, since degenerative changes due to these diseases usually cause rupture of the vessel. The bleeding is usually arterial and occurs particularly around the basal ganglia. *Intracerebral hemorrhage* is occasionally due to hemorrhagic disorders, such as leukemia or thrombocytopenia, or may be a complication of anticoagulant therapy. The clinical picture and the prognosis depend mainly on the degree of hemorrhage and brain damage. Occasionally, the bleeding ruptures the wall of the lateral ventricle and causes intraventricular hemorrhage, which is frequently fatal.

Usually, the onset is abrupt, with severe headache. As the hematoma enlarges, a more pronounced neurologic deficit occurs in the form of decreased alertness and abnormalities in the vital signs. If the bleeding is limited or develops gradually, there may be no significant pressure effects. On the other hand, the full deficit may evolve in a matter of hours. A marked reduction in consciousness (stupor/coma) in the early phase of the bleeding episode usually has an ominous prognosis.

The treatment of intracerebral hemorrhage is controversial. If the hemorrhage is small, the patient is treated conservatively and symptomatically.

- The blood pressure is carefully lowered with antihypertensive drugs. The patient's neurologic deficit may worsen if the blood pressure is dropped too low or lowered too rapidly. The most effective form of treatment is the prevention of hypertensive vascular disease.

Other Causes of Stroke
Cavernous Sinus Thrombosis.   Infections of the upper half of the face, orbit, and nasal sinuses may extend into the cavernous sinus and, by causing thrombosis, interrupt the venous drainage of the eye and other veins that drain the brain. Initially, edema, congestion, proptosis (bulging of the eyeball), and pain occur in the homolateral eye, and later in the contralateral eye as well because of extension of the infection to the other cavernous sinus. These patients are treated by antibiotic and anticoagulant medications and occasionally by surgical intervention.

Sagittal Sinus Thrombosis.   Infective processes involving the frontal or nasal sinuses and osteomyelitis of the skull may extend into the sagittal sinus and disturb the cerebral venous drainage, producing cerebral congestion and edema. Usually, there are no localizing signs, but symptoms and signs of increased ICP may develop.

Cerebral Arteriovenous Malformation.   There are two types of congenital cerebral arteriovenous (A–V) malformation: (1) the cryptic type, which usually occurs mainly in the brain stem, and (2) the large type, which is usually located on or near the surface of the cerebral hemisphere, particularly in the parietal region. They commonly produce either spontaneous subarachnoid or intracerebral hemorrhage or focal seizures. The treatment consists of anticonvulsive medications or surgical removal of the A–V malformation.

Carotid Cavernous Fistula.   This condition is usually post-traumatic, occurring either from a small tear in the intracavernous portion of the internal carotid artery, or from disruption of one of its branches in this location. Through this abnormal communication, the high-pressure carotid flow enters the cavernous sinus and disturbs the sinus drainage.

The clinical manifestations consist of headaches, noise in the head, congestion of the eye (chemosis), proptosis, papilledema, and bruit in the homolateral eye. Carotid angiography demonstrates the arterial flow into the cavernous sinus.

Management consists of one of the several surgical procedures designed to obliterate the fistula.

▶ Assessment
Clinical Manifestations.   A stroke or cerebral vascular accident can produce an array of neurologic deficits that require extensive and careful nursing management from onset through rehabilitation.

Motor Loss.   *Stroke* is a disease of the upper motor neurons and results in loss of voluntary control over motor movements. Since the upper motor neurons decussate, a disturbance of voluntary motor control on one side of the body may reflect damage to the upper motor neurons on the opposite side of the brain. The most common residual effect is *hemiplegia* (paralysis on one side of the body).

In the early stage of stroke, the initial clinical feature may be flaccid paralysis and loss or decrease in the deep tendon reflexes. When these deep reflexes reappear (usually by 48 hours), increased tone is observed along with spasticity (resistance to motion) of the extremities on the affected side. In the hemiplegic patient, the greatest amount of neurologic recovery occurs in the first 4 to 8 weeks.

Communication Loss.   Other brain functions affected by stroke are language and communication. Dysfunction in these areas may be manifested by *dysarthria* (difficulty in speaking), as demonstrated by poorly intelligible speech caused by paralysis of the muscles responsible for producing speech; *dysphasia* or *aphasia* (defective speech or loss of speech), which is mainly expressive or receptive in nature (see p. 1305); or *apraxia* (inability to perform a previously learned action), as may be seen when a patient picks up a fork and attempts to comb his hair with it. (The nursing management of aphasia is discussed on p. 1306.)

Visual Field Loss.   *Homonymous hemianopia* (loss of half of the visual field) may occur from stroke and may be temporary or permanent. In such instances, the patient will not be able to see food on half of the tray; only half of the room will be visible.

To assess for hemianopia, request the patient to look at your face. Place the examining finger about 28 cm (12 inches) from the patient's ear on the unaffected side and move it inward toward his field of vision. Inability to detect movement on one or both sides suggests visual neglect and hemianopia. This decreased field of vision must be kept in mind during all rehabilitation procedures. Personnel should approach the patient on the side where visual perception is intact. All visual stimuli (clock, calendar, television) should be placed on this side. The patient can be taught to turn his head in the direction of the defective visual field in order to compensate for this loss.

If there is a disturbance in *visual perception* (seen more frequently in left hemiplegia), the patient will have problems in performing those tasks involving spatial analysis and perceptual organization.

Sensory Loss.   Sensory losses from stroke may take the form of slight impairment of touch or be more severe with loss of position sense or hemianesthesia, loss of awareness of half of the body.

Bladder Impairment.   Occasionally, following a stroke the bladder becomes atonic with impaired sensation in response to bladder filling. Sometimes control of the external urinary sphincter is lost or diminished. During this period, intermittent catheterization with sterile technique is carried out. When muscle tone increases and deep tendon reflexes return, bladder tone increases and spasticity of the bladder may develop. Because the patient's sense of awareness is clouded, persistent urinary incontinence or urinary retention may be symptomatic of bilateral brain damage. Continuing bladder and bowel incontinence may reflect extensive neurologic damage.

Impairment of Mental Activity and Psychological Effects. If damage has occurred to the frontal lobe, then learning capacity, memory, or other higher cortical intellectual functions may be impaired. Such dysfunction may be reflected in a limited attention span, difficulties in comprehension, forgetfulness, and a lack of motivation, which cause these patients to encounter frustrating problems in their rehabilitation programs. Depression is a natural response to such a catastrophic illness. Other psychological problems are myriad and are manifested by emotional lability, hostility, frustration, resentment, and noncooperation.

Patient Problems/Nursing Diagnoses

Based on the clinical manifestations and diagnostic assessment data, the patient's major nursing problems include impaired communication related to the location of the lesion in the brain; impaired motor activity related to loss of movement, balance, and spasticity of the affected side; impaired sensory function related to the brain lesion; impaired cognitive functioning related to brain damage; self-care deficits (hygiene, toileting, transfers) related to stroke sequelae; altered self-concept related to the crisis of stroke; and chronic disability and alterations in bladder and bowel elimination related to the stroke process.

▶ Planning and Implementation: Acute Phase

A patient who is in a deep coma on admission to the hospital is considered to have a poor prognosis. Conversely, a fully conscious patient faces a more favorable outcome.

Goals

The nursing goals in the acute phase of management are to keep the patient alive and to minimize cerebral damage by providing adequately oxygenated blood to the brain. Skilled nursing is required while the patient is unconscious. (The principles underlying the management of the unconscious patient are summarized on pp. 1301–1305.)

- A patent airway and circulation to the brain are maintained.
- Adequate oxygenation of blood to the brain is necessary to minimize cerebral damage. Brain function is absolutely dependent on available oxygen being delivered to the neuronal tissues. During the acute stage, the cerebral vessels involved are maximally dilated due to tissue acidosis and ischemia. The blood pressure and cardiac output must be maintained to sustain cerebral blood flow, and hydration (intravenous fluids) must be ensured to reduce blood viscosity and improve cerebral blood flow. Oxygen therapy, if necessary, should be given at an adequate perfusion pressure.
- The patient is placed in a lateral or semiprone position with the head of the bed slightly elevated to lower cerebral venous pressure.
- Endotracheal intubation and mechanical ventilation are necessary for patients with massive stroke since respiratory arrest is usually the life-threatening factor in this situation.
- If stertorous respirations are present, an artificial airway should be inserted. The negative pressure produced by the stertorous respirations causes an increase in the amount of secretions.
- If oropharyngeal suctioning is indicated, the catheter should be lubricated with water, "pinched off," and inserted through the nose to the epiglottis. This initiates the cough reflex and serves to make the suctioning procedure more efficient. Repeated irritation to the mucous membrane by suctioning produces an increase of secretions, which is the direct opposite of its purpose. Suctioning may also cause an increase in intracranial pressure and therefore could be dangerous in the presence of brain hemorrhage.
- Evaluate the heart for abnormalities in size, rhythm, and signs of congestive heart failure.
  a. An arrhythmia may have caused a cerebral embolus and must be corrected.
  b. Cerebral embolism may occur following myocardial infarction or atrial fibrillation, or may originate from a prosthetic heart valve.
  c. If the patient is hypertensive, the blood pressure is brought under control.
  d. The blood pressure should not be allowed to drop precipitously, as brain ischemia or myocardial ischemia may result.

A neurologic flow sheet is maintained to reflect the following significant observations:

1. A change in the level of responsiveness as evidenced by movement, resistance to changes of position, and

response to stimulation; orientation to time, place, and person

2. Presence or absence of voluntary or involuntary movements of the extremities; the tone of the muscles; the body posture and the position of the head

3. Stiffness or flaccidity of the neck

4. Eye opening, the comparative size of the pupils and pupillary reactions to light, and ocular position

5. The color of the face and the extremities; the temperature and the moisture of the skin

6. The quality and the rates of pulse and respiration; the body temperature and the arterial pressure

7. The ability to speak

8. The volume of fluids ingested or administered, and the volume of urine excreted each 24 hours

9. Arterial blood gas measurements

Medical treatment for acute stroke may include antiedema therapy, (steroids, dehydrating agents), anticoagulation and antiplatelet aggregation drugs, and treatment to improve cerebral blood flow and metabolism.

When the patient begins to regain consciousness, signs of extreme fatigue and confusion will be apparent as a result of the cerebral edema that follows a stroke. To offset any anxiety, efforts should be made at frequent intervals to orient the patient to time and place and to reassure him that he has not lost his mind. Some aphasia can be expected to accompany right-sided hemiplegia. (See nursing support of the patient with aphasia, p. 1306.)

Sterile intermittent catheterization is usually discontinued, and the patient is placed on a bladder and bowel training program.

▶ **Planning and Implementation: Rehabilitation Phase**

Although rehabilitation begins on the day the patient has the stroke, the process is intensified during the convalescent phase and requires a coordinated team effort. The team has to know about the patient before this catastrophic illness: what he was able to do, his mental and emotional state, behavioral characteristics, and activities of daily living.

Goals

The patient's goals include:

1. Avoidance of deformities
2. Improved mobility
3. Improved self-concept and self-care
4. Improved cognitive function
5. Bladder and bowel continence

The *immediate nursing goals* are (1) to prevent deformities, (2) to retrain the affected arm and leg, (3) to mobilize the patient, (4) to help the patient gain independence in self-care, (5) to help the patient adapt and adjust to his residual function, and (6) to provide health education to the patient and his family.

Preventing Deformities

A hemiplegic patient has unilateral paralysis. When control of the voluntary muscles is lost, the strong flexor muscles

exert control over the extensors. The arm tends to adduct (adductor muscles are stronger than abductors) and to rotate internally. The elbow and the wrist tend to flex, the affected leg tends to rotate externally at the hip joint and flex at the knee, while the foot at the ankle joint supinates and tends toward plantar flexion (Fig. 57-3).

Positioning. Correct positioning in bed is of prime importance (Fig. 57-4) in order to prevent contractures, relieve pressure, assist in maintaining good body alignment, and prevent compressive neuropathies, especially of the ulnar and peroneal nerves. A bed board under the mattress provides firm support for the body. The patient should remain flat in bed except when engaged in activities of daily living. Maintaining the upright position in bed for extended periods of time is one of the greatest contributors to hip flexion deformity. A footboard may be used at intervals to keep the feet at right angles to the legs when the patient is in a supine (dorsal) position. This prevents footdrop and the heel cord from shortening as a result of contracture of the gastrocnemius muscle. However, many therapists feel that the continuous use of the footboard will stimulate the plantar surfaces of the feet, producing plantar flexion. If the affected extremity is spastic, a bed cradle is used to keep the bedding off the extremity.

Because flexor muscles are stronger than extensor muscles, it may be necessary to apply a posterior splint at night to prevent flexion of the affected extremity. If such a splint is not available, it may be improvised by applying a cast to the affected extremity, bivalving it and padding the posterior portion. The heel portion should be well padded with foam rubber or lamb's wool. The leg is positioned in the cast and wrapped with an elastic bandage to keep it in an extended position. The posterior splint is used only at night to maintain correct positioning while the patient is sleeping.

To prevent external rotation at the hip joint, a trochanter roll is used, extending from the crest of the ilium to the midthigh, since the hip joint lies between these two points (Fig. 57-4 *B*). Sandbags applied laterally to the leg will not prevent external rotation inasmuch as this motion originates in the ball and socket joint of the hip. The knee has no such rotating function. The trochanter roll acts as a mechanical wedge under the projection of the greater trochanter and prevents the femur from rolling.

To prevent adduction of the affected shoulder, a pillow is placed in the axilla (Fig. 57-4 *A*). This keeps the arm away from the chest. A pillow is placed under the arm, and the arm is placed in a neutral (slightly flexed) position, with each joint positioned higher than the preceding one. Thus, the elbow is higher than the shoulder, and the wrist is higher than the elbow. The elevation of the arm helps to prevent edema and the resultant fibrosis that will prevent normal range of motion if the patient regains control of the arm.

The fingers are positioned so that they are barely flexed. The hand is placed in slight supination, which is its most functional (*i.e.,* useful) position. If the upper extremity is flaccid, a volar resting splint can be used to support the wrist and hand in a functional position (Fig. 57-4 *C*). If the upper extremity is spastic, a hand roll is *not* desirable, as it stimulates the grasp reflex. In this instance, a dorsal splint is useful in allowing the palm to be free of pressure.

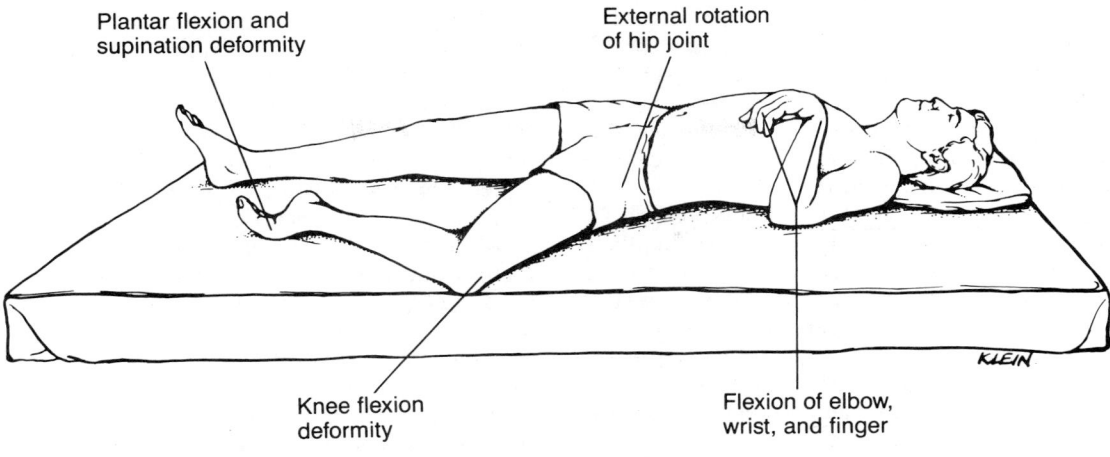

Plantar flexion and
supination deformity

External rotation
of hip joint

Knee flexion
deformity

Flexion of elbow,
wrist, and finger

Figure 57-3. Hemiplegic deformities. The involved leg immediately falls into external rotation. The knee almost invariably flexes. As soon as knee flexion occurs, abduction of the upper leg follows. The foot falls into plantar flexion, so that there is always a footdrop and a shortening of the Achilles tendon. This position of the leg is assumed whether the leg is flaccid or spastic.

   The arm of the affected side is held against the body. Often, a flail arm is placed across the body for convenience in handling the patient, but if spastic, the elbow flexes to about 90 degrees. With the arm across the body, the wrist is dropped. If the arm is spastic, the fingers curl into a fist, with the thumb adducted and flexed under the fingers. (After Covalt NK: Preventive technics of rehabilitation for hemiplegic patients. GP 17:131)

Figure 57-4 A. Positioning for a patient following a stroke. (Dark side of pajamas represents affected or hemiplegic side.) A pillow is placed in the axilla to prevent adduction of the affected shoulder. Pillows are placed under the arm, which is in a slightly flexed position with each joint positioned higher than the preceding one.

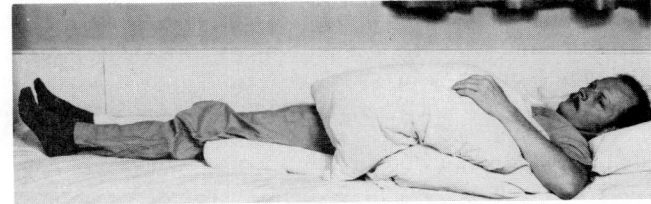

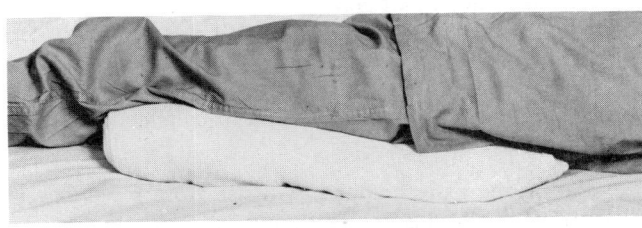

B. The trochanter roll should extend from the crest of the ilium to the midthigh, since the hip joint lies between these two points. The trochanter roll acts as a mechanical wedge under the projection of the greater trochanter and prevents the femur from rolling.

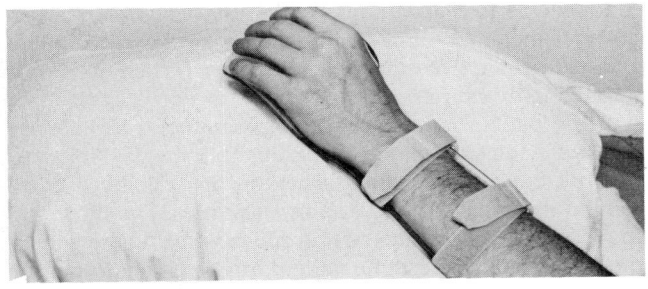

C. A volar resting splint may be used to support the wrist and hand if the upper extremity is flaccid.

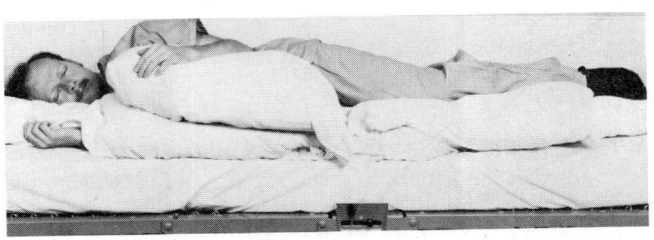

D. Lateral or side-lying position. The patient should be turned on his unaffected side. The upper thigh should not be acutely flexed.

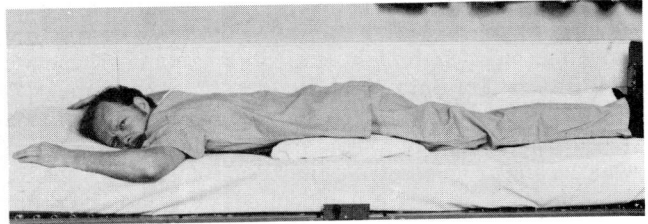

E. Prone position. A pillow is placed under the pelvis to help promote hyperextension of the hip joints, which is essential for normal gait. Note position of arms.

Changing Positions.   The patient's position should be changed every 2 hours. To place a patient in a lateral (side-lying) position, a pillow is placed between the legs before the patient is turned. The patient may be turned from side to side, but the amount of time spent on the affected side should be limited because of impaired sensation. The upper thigh should not be acutely flexed (Fig. 57-4 *D*).

The patient should be placed in a prone position for 15 minutes to a half hour several times a day. A small pillow or a support is placed under the pelvis, extending from the level of the umbilicus to the upper third of the thigh (Fig. 57-4 *E*). This helps to promote hyperextension of the hip joints, which is essential for normal gait and helps prevent knee and hip flexion contractures. The prone position also helps to drain bronchial secretions and prevents contractural deformities of the shoulders and knees.

Retraining the Affected Extremities
Exercise.   The affected extremities are exercised passively and put through a full range of motion four to five times a day to prevent contracture development in the paralyzed extremity, to prevent further deterioration of the neuromuscular system, to stretch soft tissues, and to enhance circulation. Exercise is helpful in the prevention of venous stasis, which may predispose to thrombosis and pulmonary embolus.

Repetition of an activity forms new pathways in the central nervous system and therefore encourages new patterns of motion. At first, the extremities are usually flaccid. If tightness occurs in any area, the range of motion exercises should be done more frequently. (See pp. 232–237 for techniques of range of motion exercises.) Signs to watch for include shortness of breath, chest pain, cyanosis, and increasing pulse rate during the exercise period.

Frequent short periods of exercise always are preferred to longer periods at infrequent intervals. *Regularity* in exercise is most important. Improvement in muscle strength and maintenance of range of motion can be achieved only through daily exercise.

The patient is encouraged and reminded to exercise the unaffected side at intervals throughout the day. It is well to work out a written time schedule that can be used to remind the patient of the exercise activities. The nurse has the responsibility of supervising and supporting the patient during these activities. The patient can be taught to put the unaffected leg under the affected one to move it when turning and exercising. Flexibility, strengthening, coordination, endurance, and balancing exercises prepare the patient for ambulation and give the patient a goal. Quadriceps muscle setting and gluteal setting exercises are started early to improve the muscle strength needed for walking. These are done at least five times daily for 10 minutes at a time.

Quadriceps Setting.   Instruct the patient to contract the quadriceps muscle (on the anterior portion of the thigh) while raising the heel and pushing the popliteal space against the mattress. The muscle contracture is held until the count of 5, then relaxed until the count of 5. Repeat. This exercise is performed by each extremity.

Gluteal Setting.   Contract or "pinch" the buttocks together until the count of 5. Then relax until the count of 5. Repeat.

Electromyographic biofeedback is being used in neuromuscular re-education for improving muscle strength and reducing spasticity.

Care of Affected Upper Extremity.   If the patient's arm is paralyzed completely, subluxation (incomplete dislocation) at the shoulder can occur from the weight of the paralyzed arm. A sling will prevent this complication and will help the patient maintain balance when ambulating. Subluxation can be avoided when the patient is seated by placing a pillow under the arm for support or resting the arm on the arm of the chair. The sling is discarded when spasticity develops, because spasticity of the shoulder muscles will help prevent subluxation.

Shoulder–hand syndrome (painful shoulder and generalized swelling and pain of the hand) can cause "frozen shoulder" and atrophy of subcutaneous tissues. The sling is removed frequently to exercise the affected arm. Instruct the patient to interlace his fingers, placing the palms together, and lift both arms above his head repeatedly throughout the day. A clothesline may be strung through a pulley attached to a door jamb (or over a shower rod) and tied on the affected hand. The patient pulls the rope up and down with the unaffected hand and so exercises the affected arm and shoulder. The combination of sling support and range of motion exercises will prevent painful frozen shoulder and subluxation. If the position of the chair is changed, other shoulder motions may be carried out. The patient is instructed to flex the affected wrist at frequent intervals and to move all the joints of the affected fingers.

Mobilizing the Patient
As soon as possible, the patient is assisted out of bed. Usually, when hemiplegia has resulted from a thrombosis, an active rehabilitation program is started as soon as the patient regains consciousness, whereas a patient who has had a cerebral hemorrhage cannot participate actively until all evidence of bleeding is gone.

Sitting Balance.   A hemiplegic patient tends to lose his sense of balance and needs to learn to maintain balance in a sitting position before learning to balance himself in the standing position.

- Before the patient attempts to rise from a recumbent position, blood pressure should be checked since orthostatic hypotension may occur. A fall in blood pressure may further damage the ischemic area.
- To develop sitting balance, raise the head of the bed to an upright position; instruct the patient to hold the bedrail with his good hand.

The patient is then helped to come to a sitting position on the edge of the bed. This may be achieved in the following manner:

1. Adjust the bed to the low position.
2. Instruct the patient to place the strong leg beneath the weak leg and lift it toward the side of the bed.
3. Instruct the patient to press the strong elbow that is flexed to a 90-degree angle into the mattress and come to a sitting position by transferring weight to the forearm and then to the hand, while lifting the uninvolved leg with the strong leg over the edge of the bed. The force

of gravity, set in motion by pushing against the hand and moving the legs, is sufficient to pivot the patient's torso on the buttocks.

4. Extend the patient's strong arm with his hand flat on the bed behind him to assist in balancing.

5. Stand in front of the patient to observe and, if necessary, help him to maintain this posture.
   - A change in color, shortness of breath, increasing pulse rate, or profuse perspiration is an indication that the patient should be placed in bed again. The sitting time is increased as rapidly as the patient's condition permits.

Standing Balance. As soon as the patient is able to balance while sitting, he is taught standing balance. He should wear walking shoes with a strong shank for all ambulation activities.

- Seat the patient on the edge of the bed, and place a straightback chair on each side of him (Fig. 57-5). If the patient lacks strength to grasp and to push the chair with his affected hand, the hand can be tied to the top of the chair. The stabilization gives the patient greater support.
- Help the patient to come to a standing position by supporting his lower back with your hands and positioning your knees on the outside of the patient's knees. This will give the patient maximum support in the standing position and will prevent his knees from buckling. The

patient should be reminded to lean forward when he comes from a sitting to a standing position. The patient's arms must be left free for balance and support.

- Stand behind the patient and stabilize him at his waist. Place a waistband or a belt (a scultetus binder can serve as a waistband) around the patient's waist and grasp it for patient support.
- Dizziness, pallor, and an increasing pulse rate indicate that the patient should be permitted to rest in a sitting position. If the symptoms continue, the patient should be put back in bed. With repeated effort, the patient will tolerate this activity for longer periods.
- Have the patient practice standing and shifting weight from one leg to another.

If the patient has difficulty in achieving standing balance, a tilt table will help him assume an upright position. There should be frequent periods of standing before walking is started.

Walking. The patient is usually ready to walk as soon as standing balance is achieved. Parallel bars are useful when the patient first starts to walk. A chair or wheelchair should be readily available in the event of sudden fatigue or vertigo. The following method is one way to ambulate the patient:

1. Instruct the patient to stand between the parallel bars or beside one rail with his weight evenly distributed on both feet and his strong arm on the rail 10 cm (about 4 inches) in front of his body.

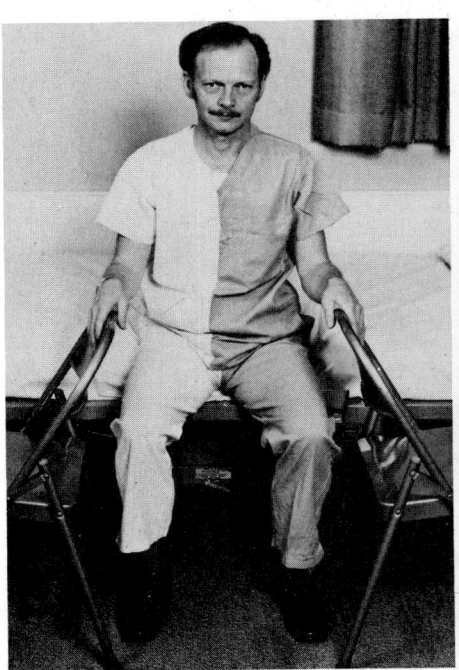 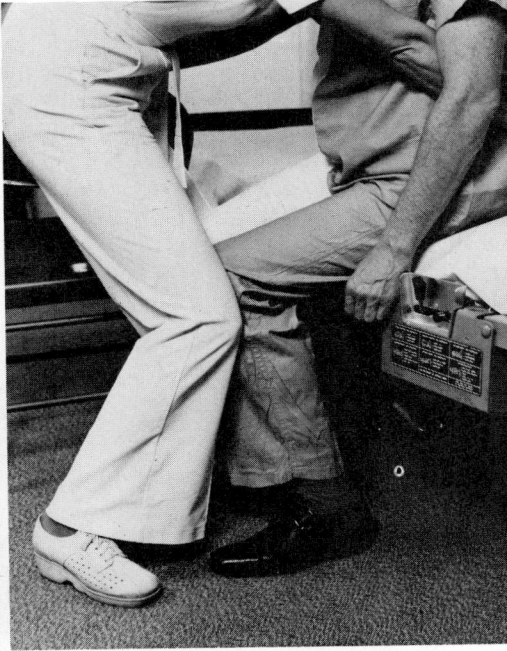 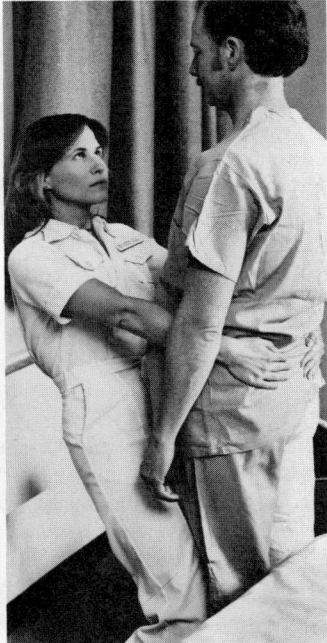

Figure 57-5. Getting the patient out of bed following a stroke. (*Left*) Place the bed in the low position so that the feet are resting on the floor. Observe the patient's reaction and increase the sitting time as rapidly as the patient's condition permits. (*Center*) Getting ready to arise to a standing position. Positioning the nurse's knees on the outside of the patient's knees will prevent the patient's knees from buckling. (*Right*) Stabilizing the patient as he assumes a standing position. Note that the nurse is (1) stabilizing the patient's lower back and knees and (2) assessing his reaction to standing. (Courtesy, Washington Adventist Hospital; Glenn Dalby, photographer.)

2. Have the patient shift the weight to the strong leg and advance the involved leg while pushing *down* on the rail.

3. The patient then shifts the weight to the weak leg. (If the patient has poor muscle tone and cannot advance his involved leg, functional electrical stimulation may be used. Stimulating muscles electrically may increase strength, reverse atrophy, and enhance voluntary control.)

4. Encourage the patient to look at his feet occasionally, as proprioceptive loss may accompany hemiplegia.

The training periods for ambulation should be short and frequent. As the patient gains in strength and confidence, he can begin to walk with an adjustable aluminum cane. Generally a three- or four-prong cane provides a more stable support in the early phases of this training program.

Bracing.   If the patient has a weakened or absent quadriceps muscle, the knee joint may be supported with a splint applied to the back of the knee. Reflex contractures of those muscles used in standing are brought into play by putting on a posterior knee brace and having the patient stand. Temporary splints can be constructed from lightweight thermoplastic material and Velcro straps.

Splinting the extremity and helping the patient to a standing position early in the rehabilitation program offers the following advantages: (1) the muscle tone is maintained through reflex action, (2) the patient develops a better command of balance, and (3) position sense is retained. After a period of time has elapsed, the physician determines whether the patient needs to be fitted with a short- or a long-leg brace.

Wheelchair.   If the patient needs a wheelchair, the folding type with hand brakes is the most practical since it allows the patient to manipulate the chair. The chair should be low enough so that the patient can propel it with the uninvolved foot and narrow enough to permit it to be used in the home. To propel the wheelchair, the patient places the strong hand on the hand rim and the stronger foot on the floor to guide and direct the chair.

When the patient is transferred from the wheelchair, the brakes are applied on both sides of the chair. The technique for transferring from a wheelchair is as follows:

- Place wheelchair on patient's unaffected side.
- The patient lifts the foot pedals out of the way and moves forward in the chair, placing weight on the strong leg.
- Push up with the strong arm and foot.
- Place most of the weight on the strong leg while keeping the weak knee locked.
- Pivot in the direction of the stronger leg; bring weak leg over to stronger leg. Maintain standing position for a few minutes.
- Lower body into wheelchair gradually, using strong arm and leg.

Wheelchair mobility provides greater independence in self-care activities. When a permanent wheelchair is needed, it is ordered with specific instructions for the individual patient.

Self-care and Activities of Daily Living

As soon as the patient is able to sit up, he is encouraged to assist in his personal hygiene. He is helped to set realistic goals and if feasible, a new task is added daily. The first step is to have the patient carry out all self-care activities on the unaffected side. Such activities as combing the hair, brushing the teeth, shaving with an electric razor, bathing, and eating can be carried out with one hand and are suitable for self-care. While the patient may feel awkward at first, the various motor skills can be learned by repetition, and the unaffected side will become stronger with use. Be sure that he does not neglect his affected side. Assistive devices will help make up for some of the patient's deficits.

Dressing Activities.   The patient's morale will improve if ambulatory activities are carried out while he is fully dressed. The family is instructed to bring in clothing that is preferably a size larger than that normally worn. Clothing fitted with front or side fasteners or Velcro closures is the most suitable. The patient has better balance if most of the dressing activities are done in a seated position.

In the early stages, when the patient needs to be helped or supported by the nurse, he should not be permitted to become overfatigued and discouraged. Even with intensive training, not all patients are able to achieve independence in dressing skills.

The following procedure for dressing has been found to be workable for many patients. However, the nurse must use judgment in assisting the patient to work out individual modifications.

Underclothing
Use a flare leg or boxer-type shorts with an elastic waistband.
With the unaffected hand, place the affected ankle in a resting position on top of the unaffected knee.
Place the unaffected hand through the outside opening of the shorts. Thrust the hand through the shorts, grasp the affected foot firmly, and shake the garment off the unaffected hand and well over the affected foot.
While holding the garment, allow the affected foot to rest on the floor. Draw the shorts up the affected leg.
Then put the unaffected leg into the shorts, and pull them up as far as possible.
To complete the procedure of bringing the shorts up over the buttocks, roll to each side and pull up the shorts on the opposite side.

Undershirt
Place the undershirt in the lap, with the back of the shirt facing upward.
Thread the paralyzed arm through the appropriate armhole to above the elbow.
Introduce the normal arm through its armhole.
With the good arm, pull the garment on the affected side up to the shoulder and over the head, and adjust the garment with the normal hand.

Brassiere
Stabilize one end of the garment with the affected arm while fastening it in the front with the unaffected hand.

Slide the garment around the body, so that the fastener is in the back.

Use the unaffected hand to pull the affected arm through the strap and place the strap over the shoulder. Then place the unaffected arm through the other strap.

Shirt, Blouse, or Front-fastening Dress

Button the cuff on the normal side.

Thread the sleeve over the paralyzed arm to the shoulder.

Place the hand and the arm through the other sleeve.

Button the sleeve on the affected side.

It is wise to wear collars a size larger than normal, because buttoning a tight neckband is difficult. Snap-on ties may be worn, or four-in-hand ties may be loosened and slipped over the head without being untied.

Trousers

The use of suspenders makes it easier to pull up the trousers. Trousers are put on in the same manner as shorts. If the patient prefers, he can pull the shorts and the trousers up over the buttocks at the same time. When more balance has been achieved, an over-the-head garment (dress, slip, sweater) is put on in the same manner as is the undershirt. It is suggested that stretchable clothing be used.

Sexuality of Persons Following Stroke. Sexual functioning can be profoundly altered by disability. A stroke is such a catastrophic illness that the patient often experiences loss of self-esteem and loss of value as a sexual being. Although research in this area of stroke management is limited, it appears that poststroke patients believe that sexual function is important, but most experience sexual dysfunction following stroke. (See Sexuality and the Disabled, p. 230.)

Patient and Family Education

The family plays an important role in the patient's recovery. Some type of counseling and support system should be available to them to prevent the care of the patient from taking a significant toll on their health and interfering too radically with their life-style.

The family may have difficulty in accepting the patient's disability and may be unrealistic in their expectations. They must be counseled to avoid doing for the patient those things that he can do for himself. Assure them that their loving and warm interest is part of the patient's therapy. The family needs to be informed that the rehabilitation of the hemiplegic patient requires many months and that progress may be slow. The gains made by the patient during hospitalization must be maintained. All should approach the patient with a supportive and optimistic attitude.

If the patient has some brain damage, he may be emotionally labile. The family should be prepared to expect occasional episodes of emotional instability. The patient may laugh or cry easily. He may be irritable and demanding, or depressed and confused. The patient's behavior may also be related to speech dysfunction. Since a stroke frequently occurs in the late stages of life, there is the possibility of intellectual decline related to dementia. Explain to the family that the patient's laughing does not necessarily mean that

he is glad nor does crying mean that he is sad, and that emotional lability usually improves with time. Advise the family that the patient will tire easily, will become irritable and upset by small events, and is apt to show less interest in things. As progress is made in the rehabilitation program, these problems will diminish. The family can help by supporting the patient and giving honest praise for the progress that is being made.

Usually, the home environment has to be rearranged for the patient's activities and safety. Ramps and widening of doors may be required to accommodate the wheelchair. A shower is more convenient than a tub for the hemiplegic patient, as most patients do not gain sufficient strength to get up and down from a tub. Sitting on a stool of medium height with rubber suction tips will permit him to wash with greater ease. A long-handled bath brush with a soap container is helpful to the patient who has only one functional hand. If a shower is not available, a stool may be placed in the tub and a portable shower hose attached to the faucet. Handrails may be attached beside the bathtub and the toilet. There are numerous self-help devices on the market that can assist the patient in the activities of daily living. Community-based "Stroke Clubs" give the patient a feeling of belonging and fellowship with others who have similar problems.

When feasible, it is best if the patient can return to work or some modification of his former job. The local or the regional branch of the State Office of Vocational Rehabilitation provides individual evaluation and retraining services, depending on the needs of the patient.

All nurses coming in contact with the patient, whether as members of the hospital health team, community health nurses, or office or industrial nurses, should encourage the patient to *keep active,* faithfully adhere to the exercise program, accept the limitations, and yet, confidently continue to remain as self-sufficient as possible.

▶ **Evaluation**

Expected Outcomes

1. Demonstrates improved communication
   a. Makes attempts at communication
   b. Engages in socializing with family
   c. Has appointment for continuation with speech therapy following discharge from hospital
2. Achieves improved mobility
   a. Participates in range of motion and prescribed exercise program
   b. Achieves sitting balance before attempting to stand
   c. Follows demonstrated techniques of using stronger leg for balance and pivoting
   d. Increases sitting and standing intervals daily
   e. Uses unaffected side to compensate for loss of function of hemiplegic side
   f. Uses adaptive equipment (walker, cane)
3. Shows awareness of sensory dysfunction
   a. Watches feet while practicing walking between parallel bars
   b. Works with occupational therapist to stimulate tactile sensation (touches/handles objects)

4. Participates in cognitive improvement program
   a. Has memory aids and stimuli: lists, clock, calendar, TV, radio
   b. Follows written daily schedule
   c. Family cooperates in stimulating patient by reading newspaper, working puzzles, etc.
   d. Family accepts periods of emotional lability in non-judgmental way
5. Strives toward independence in activities of daily living
   Uses adaptive equipment (reaching tongs, built-up utensils) as assistive devices
6. Demonstrates improved self-concept
   a. Verbalizes fears and anxieties of being dependent
   b. Sets short-term goals
   c. Takes active part in rehabilitation
   d. Family shows positive attitude toward patient's coping mechanisms
   e. Family encourages patient to do things for self
7. Attains/maintains bladder and bowel continence
   Participates in bladder and bowel retraining program
   (see p. 251)

▷ Neurosurgical Treatment of Pain

The management of long-term pain requires a multidisciplinary approach. (The reader is referred to Chap. 16 for a discussion of the basic theories of the psychophysiology of pain and its management.)

Intractable pain refers to pain that cannot be relieved satisfactorily by drugs without causing drug addiction or incapacitating sedation. Such pain usually is the result of malignancy (especially of the cervix, bladder, prostate, and lower bowel), but it does occur in many other conditions, such as postherpetic neuralgia, trigeminal neuralgia, spinal cord arachnoiditis, and uncontrollable ischemia and other forms of tissue destruction. Surgical intervention should be considered before narcotic addiction and debilitation become problems.

The objective of neurosurgical procedures for the management of intractable pain is to interrupt the pathways by which painful sensations are perceived. Pain-conducting fibers can be interrupted at any point from their origin to the cerebral cortex. The challenge is to select the appropriate level. The range of diverse surgical techniques points to the fact that the ultimate treatment of pain has not yet been found. With surgery there is destruction of some part of the nervous system, which can result in varying amounts of neurologic deficit and incapacity. In time, pain usually returns as a result of either regeneration of axonal fibers or the development of alternate pain pathways.

Rhizotomy

A posterior or spinal *rhizotomy* is the surgical interruption of selected posterior spinal nerve roots between the ganglion and the cord. This results in permanent loss of sensation and may be done at any spinal level. In the head or torso, the resultant numbness is not troublesome. In the extremities, however, the extremity is useless (even though muscle strength is intact), as there is loss of positional feedback to the spinal cord and cerebellum.

Rhizotomy is used in controlling the severe chest pain that may be experienced in lung cancer and is used to give pain relief in head and neck malignancies.

The length of the incision for rhizotomy varies directly with the number of nerves that are to be cut. This requires a fairly extensive laminectomy, and the patient should be in condition to tolerate a major operative procedure.

Since many patients with metastatic malignancies may not be able to tolerate an open rhizotomy, a *percutaneous rhizotomy* may be done, whereby a radiofrequency current is used to selectively coagulate the pain fibers, while the fibers concerned with touch and proprioception are preserved.

A *chemical rhizotomy* is one in which alcohol, phenol, or a mixture of drugs is injected into the subarachnoid space. The medication is maneuvered over the affected nerve roots by tilting the patient to the desired level. This renders the sensory nerve roots functionless. The patient's perception of pain is absent, but the motor nerve roots are usually not affected.

Cordotomy and Sympathectomy

Cordotomy. An *open cordotomy* is the surgical division of the anterolateral columns of the spinal pain fibers high in the thoracic or cervical region. This procedure interrupts or destroys conduction of pain and temperature sense, while touch and position sense are preserved. The cord is exposed by laminectomy. Cordotomy is used most frequently in controlling the severe pain of terminal cancer, especially of the thorax, abdomen, or lower extremities. Since a significant percentage of cordotomies lose their effectiveness in 1 to 5 years, the procedure is used for pain associated with conditions in which survival time is limited.

Postoperative Nursing Management. The principles of nursing management following a laminectomy are applicable in the postoperative and rehabilitation requirements of this patient (see p. 1376). Following a cordotomy, the patient may be kept flat for the prescribed time period, because there is less tension on the incision when this position is assumed. A patient with a thoracic cordotomy may be turned to the prone position. In instances of a cervical incision, pillows should not be used when the patient is in a supine position. Trauma to the surgical site is eliminated when the neck is kept in a neutral position. The patient is turned as a unit ("log" fashion) by two persons using a turning sheet to avoid twisting the body and putting pressure on the incision.

Assessment for Complications. The patient is watched for respiratory complications, as well as for signs of fatigue and weakening of the voice. The patient may ventilate adequately while awake but may experience progressive hypercarbia and hypoxia while asleep. Therefore, arterial blood gases are monitored, and assisted mechanical ventilation initiated when required.

Since hemorrhage may result in motor and sensory loss, the motion, strength, and sensation of each extremity must be tested every few hours (or more frequently if necessary) during the first 48 hours postoperatively. If hemorrhage is indicated, immediate surgical intervention is imperative. Because the patient has no sense of temperature, the skin should be felt at intervals to ascertain any changes in temperature. Since pressure sores may develop without the patient realizing it, the patient should be taught to inspect his skin using a hand mirror to view the hard-to-see places.

Urinary retention is usually transient. If there is permanent loss of motor control from a high cervical procedure, a bladder training program is carried out (see p. 251).

Percutaneous Cordotomy. The *percutaneous approach* (which is a simplified form of surgical cordotomy) uses radiofrequency currents to produce lesions in the anterolateral spinal cord. Under local anesthesia, a needle is inserted into the neck below and behind the mastoid process. It is guided into the spinal cord under x-ray control and then an electrode is inserted through it. By means of radiofrequency currents, a lesion is made at the desired spinal cord level.

Verification of electrode placement is determined by the patient's response to stimulation. The procedure is tolerated by wasted and debilitated patients and gives complete relief of pain in approximately 80% of patients. Percutaneous cordotomy is replacing open cordotomy as the procedure of choice.

Patient and Family Education. Since temperature sense is permanently lost, the patient is instructed concerning external temperature changes. Bath water should be tested by a family member before the patient gets into the tub. Because frostbite and sunburn can occur without any sense of discomfort, protection must be taken against temperature variations. Warn the patient of the danger of impaired circulation and the need to avoid constricting clothing, such as tightly tied shoes. Sexual function is usually impaired in males.

Sympathectomy. *Sympathectomy* is the interruption of afferent pathways in the sympathetic division of the autonomic nervous system. It is used to control the pain in patients with vascular insufficiency, particularly Raynaud's disease. The operation eliminates vasospasm and improves peripheral blood supply. A sympathectomy may be done to relieve visceral pain, as this procedure destroys the visceral afferents that accompany the sympathetic fibers to the viscera.

Psychosurgical Approaches

The purpose of these procedures is to alter the patient's response to pain. A *thalamotomy* is the destruction (either unilateral or bilateral) of the specific cell groups within the thalamus. Burr holes are made in the skull, electrodes are placed in the target area by stereotaxic techniques, and a radiofrequency current is then directed through the electrodes to create the lesion. This procedure represents the highest level in the central nervous system in which pain pathways can be interrupted and is usually done for malignancy of the head and neck.

Cingulumotomy is a unilateral or bilateral interruption of the anterior cingulate bundle in the frontal lobe of the brain. It is accomplished either by an open or stereotaxic approach. It tends to modify the patient's affective reaction to pain.

Electrical Stimulation for the Control of Pain (Neuromodulation)

Electrical stimulation or *neuromodulation* is a method of suppressing pain by applying an electronic device that stimulates the different parts of the nervous system for pain relief. This therapy is based on the gate control theory (see p. 282), which explains how nondestructive stimuli can interfere with the transmission of pain within the central nervous system. The neural mechanism in the dorsal horns of the spinal cord acts like a gate, which can increase or decrease the flow to the central nervous system. Electrical stimulation is thought to relieve pain by preventing messages from reaching the brain. It is accomplished through electrodes applied to the skin, by stimulation of the peripheral nerves or peripheral nerve plexuses, by stimulation of the anterior and posterior surfaces of the spinal cord, or by implants into selected areas within the brain. Currently, flexible electrodes are being implanted into the spinal epidural space percutaneously to stimulate the spinal cord. This newer procedure eliminates a major operation. At the present time, transcutaneous electrical stimulation and dorsal column stimulation are the procedures most frequently done. In addition, there are also brain stimulators in which stimulating electrodes are implanted in the periventricular area of the posterior third ventricle. It allows self-stimulation of the periventricular gray area to produce analgesia.

These are nondestructive means of relieving pain and are now replacing their more destructive surgical counterparts (rhizotomy, cordotomy, thalamotomy) in many instances. Indeed, electrical-stimulation techniques may be the wave of the future in the management of severe pain.

Transcutaneous Electric Nerve Stimulation

Transcutaneous electric nerve stimulation (TENS) is the passage of small electrical currents through the skin for the purpose of controlling pain. The stimulating electrodes are placed over the site of pain or along the course of the major peripheral nerves innervating the area or over the peripheral plexus. The patient operates the amplitude control until stimulation, detected by a buzzing or tingling sensation, is felt. The amplitude is increased until the sensation is strong but not uncomfortable. The patient controls the amplitude, frequency, and duration of stimulation. It appears to be very useful in highly motivated patients with long-term pain problems related to nervous system damage.

Patient Education. The skin is cleansed and electrode gel is applied to the electrodes, which are then placed over the nerves that serve the painful area. The electrodes are secured with nonallergenic tape. The patient is given the instruction booklet provided by the manufacturing company that explains care of the skin, electrodes, and generator. The major problems of transcutaneous nerve stimulation are irritation or soreness of the skin under the electrode, and the inability of some patients to learn to use the device.

Dorsal Column Stimulation (DCS)

Dorsal column stimulation (DCS) is a technique used for the relief of chronic intractable pain in which a surgically implanted device allows the patient to apply pulsed electrical stimulation to the dorsal aspect of the spinal cord to block pain impulses. It is hypothesized that electrical stimulation of larger peripheral nerve fibers causes a negative feedback to "close the gate" in the spinal cord, preventing the transmission of pain sensation to the brain. Some researchers feel that the mechanism of peripheral nerve stimulation is actually a blockade of the nerve. The explanation for pain relief from electrical stimulation is not yet available.

The dorsal column stimulation unit consists of a radio-frequency stimulation transmitter, a transmitter antenna, a radio-frequency receiver, and a stimulation electrode. The battery-powered transmitter and antenna are worn externally while the receiver and electrode are implanted. A laminectomy is performed above the highest level of pain input, and the electrode is placed in the epidural space over the posterior column of the spinal cord. (The placement of the stimulating systems is varied.) The subcutaneous pocket is constructed over the clavicular area or some other site for placement of the receiver. The two are connected by a subcutaneous tunnel.

Postoperative Nursing Management. The postoperative nursing management is similar to that following a laminectomy. The patient is assessed for evidences of paraplegia, quadriplegia, and urinary incontinence. The extremities are evaluated for movement. Leakage of cerebrospinal fluid at the laminectomy site is also checked since the dura is opened during surgery. The implant site is checked for signs of infection. As soon as the patient is fully alert, the dorsal column stimulation system may be tested, although initial testing may not be accurate because a bandage may cover the receiver site. Complications include infection, cord trauma, cerebrospinal fluid leakage, and pain around the implantation site.

Patient Education. The patient is given the manufacturer's booklet to become acquainted with the system. Proper skin care is taught as well as the method for attaching the antenna to the skin, connecting the transmitter, and adjusting the settings. Different stimulation frequencies should be tried to determine which one gives the best pain relief. A record is to be kept of the stimulation used. The patient is also instructed to keep several batteries in reserve. (Battery life depends on the extent of use.) The transmitter and antenna are cleaned according to the manufacturer's directions.

Percutaneous Epidural Neurostimulation

Percutaneous epidural neurostimulation is a method of neurostimulation in which electrodes are inserted percutaneously into the spinal epidural space. It appears effective in treating arachnoiditis and postamputation neuroma.

▷ The Patient Undergoing Intracranial Surgery

In recent years, certain technological advances have helped to refine existing neurologic procedures and develop newer ones. Superior neuroradiologic techniques have made it possible to localize intracranial lesions, while microsurgical instruments with improved illumination and magnification have made it possible to obtain a three-dimensional view of the field of operation (Fig. 57-6).

It is now possible to coagulate vessels adjacent to structures without causing injury to the structures themselves.

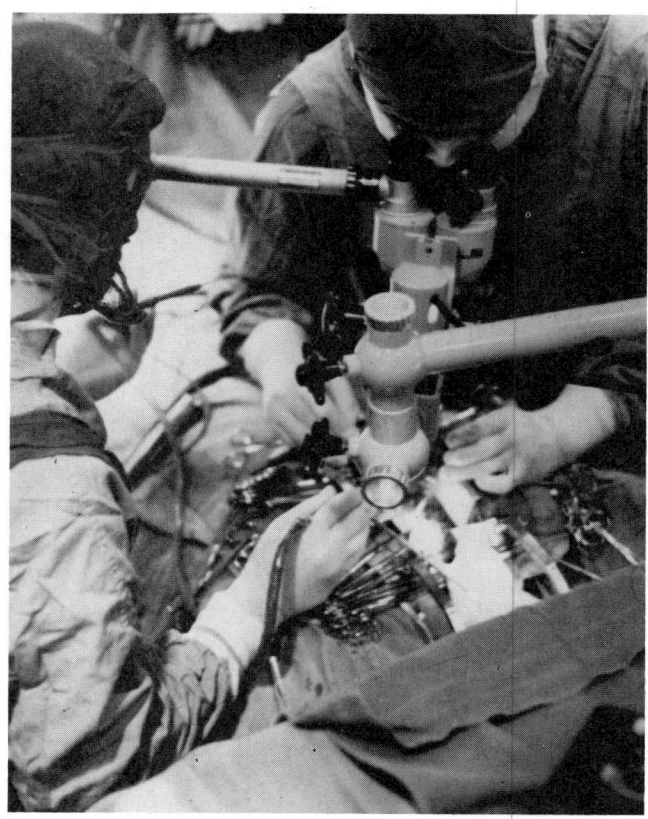

Figure 57-6. Intracranial surgery.

Microsurgical instruments (miniaturized probes, hooks, clamps, needle holders) allow delicate tissue to be separated without trauma. Suture material smaller than a strand of human hair permits very small nerves and vessels to be sutured and anastomosed.

Surgical Approaches

A *craniotomy* is the surgical opening of the skull to gain access to intracranial structures. This procedure is done to remove a tumor, relieve intracranial pressure, evacuate a blood clot, and control hemorrhage. The skull is opened by making a bony flap that is replaced following surgery and fixed in position by periosteal or wire sutures. In general, two approaches are used: (1) above the tentorium (supratentorial craniotomy) into the supratentorial compartment and (2) below the tentorium into the infratentorial (posterior fossa) compartment.

The intracranial structures may be approached through *burr holes* (Fig. 57-7), which are circular openings made in the skull by either a hand drill or an automatic craniotome (which has a self-controlled system to stop the drill when the bone is penetrated). Burr holes are made for exploration or diagnosis. They may be used to determine the level of brain tension and the size and position of the ventricles. They are also a means of evacuating an intracranial hematoma or abscess, making a bone flap in the skull and allowing

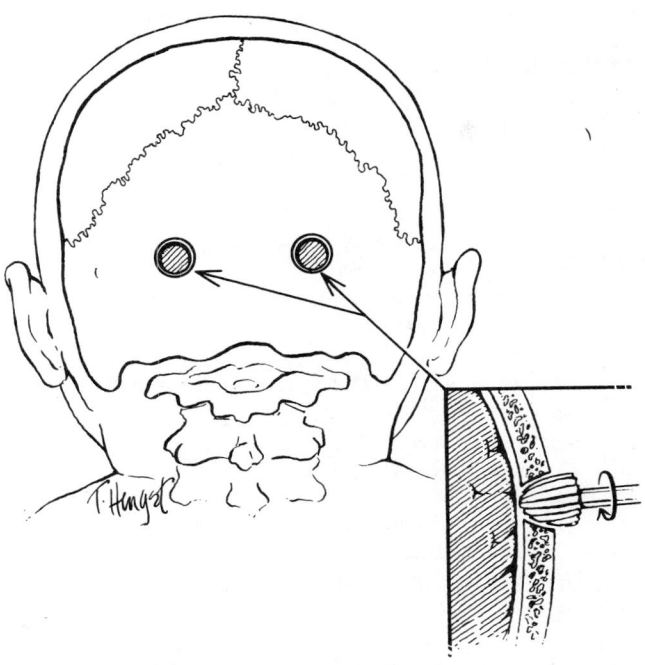

Figure 57-7. (*Posterior view*) Burr holes in intracranial surgery.

access to the ventricles for decompression purposes, ventriculography, or shunting procedures.

Other cranial procedures include *craniectomy* (an excision of a portion of the skull) and *cranioplasty* (repair of a cranial defect by means of a plastic or metal plate).

▶ Preoperative Assessment

Proper assessment of the postoperative status of the patient requires an awareness of the patient's signs and symptoms so that a comparison may be made between the preoperative and postoperative conditions. Included in this assessment are evaluation of the level of responsiveness/consciousness and the presence of any neurologic deficits. Observations of paralysis, visual dysfunction, alterations in personality or speech, and bladder and bowel disturbances are made. Motor function of the hands can be tested by the hand grip. Observations of leg movement should be especially noted if the patient is not ambulatory.

If there is paralysis of the extremities, trochanter rolls should be applied to both extremities, and the feet positioned against a footboard. Patients who have speech difficulties, failing vision, and hearing loss are a challenge to the nurse's ingenuity. If the patient is aphasic, writing materials or picture and word cards showing the bedpan, glass of water, blanket, etc., may be supplied to help improve communication. If the patient is able to ambulate, he should be encouraged to do so in a quiet, unhurried way.

The emotional preparation of the patient is also important, including informing him of postoperative expectations. The large head dressing applied following surgery may impair his hearing ability temporarily. He will have difficulty seeing if his eyes are swollen shut. If he has a tracheostomy or endotracheal tube, he will be unable to

talk. Thus, an alternate method of communication should be developed before surgery. The patient may not realize that he is about to undergo surgery. Even so, encouragement and attention to his needs usually will reinforce his confidence. Whatever the state of awareness of the patient, the family needs reassurance and consideration, since they recognize the seriousness of a brain operation.

Immediate Preparation for Operation. The scalp is shaved immediately prior to surgery so that any resultant superficial abrasions will not have time to become infected. Most patients find this alteration in their appearance very distressing. Reassuring the patient that his head will be covered with a head dressing after surgery will help him cope. He may be given diazepam preoperatively to allay anxiety. Patients at risk for postoperative epilepsy are usually given phenytoin (Dilantin).

Other preoperative *anticipatory* measures include giving preoperative steroids when steroid deficiency is anticipated, and intravenous infusions of hyperosmotic agents to decrease cerebrospinal fluid, and inserting an indwelling urethral catheter to assess urinary volume during the dehydrating operative period.

Patient Problems/Nursing Diagnoses

Based on his clinical problems, nursing history, and assessment, the patient's major postoperative problems include impairment of neurologic status related to intracranial surgery; sensory deprivation related to impaired hearing due to head dressing, impaired vision due to swollen eyes, and possibly impaired speech due to an endotracheal tube; and alteration in fluid and electrolyte balance related to possible metabolic/hormonal dysfunction.

▶ Planning and Implementation

Goals

Following an intracranial operation, the major goals of the patient include:

1. Improved neurologic status
2. Ability to cope with temporary sensory deprivation
3. Maintenance of fluid and electrolyte balance

The nursing goals are to maintain an adequate airway and assure brain oxygenation, to assist in controlling postoperative cerebral edema, to perform supportive measures until the patient can care for himself, to watch for life-threatening complications, and to assist in the rehabilitation and patient education program to restore impaired function.

Nursing assessment and management will affect the patient's clinical course. Since the patient will be unconscious during the initial postoperative period, the reader is referred to the nursing management of the unconscious patient outlined in Chart 57-2. The nursing management of a patient undergoing an intracranial operation is summarized in Chart 57-4.

Maintaining an Adequate Airway and Assuring Brain Oxygenation. Attention to the respiratory status is essential, as small degrees of hypoxia can aggravate cerebral ischemia (Chart 57-4).

(*Text continues on page 1324*)

Chart 57-4
Summary: Nursing Management of the Patient Having Intracranial Surgery

Goals, Nursing Strategies, and Rationale of Care

Preoperative Care

Goal: To determine the precise location of the lesion (clot, tumor, aneurysm)

1. Assist the patient undergoing diagnostic tests and frequent neurologic examinations.
2. Evaluate and record patient's symptoms and signs before the operation in order to make postoperative comparisons.
3. Support the patient with motor and sensory defects.
   a. Position paralyzed extremities correctly to prevent contracture deformities.
   b. Familiarize the blind patient with his environment.
      (1) Personnel entering the room should announce themselves—helps the patient understand incoming stimuli.
      (2) Help the patient to assume an active role in his care.
   c. Assist the aphasic patient to communicate by means of picture cards, writing materials, gestures, etc.
   d. Protect the confused patient.
      (1) Remove disturbing environmental stimuli.
      (2) Keep the patient oriented to time and place; place wall calendar and clock where he can see them.
   e. Instruct and encourage the patient and his family about the impending surgery.
4. Prepare the patient physically for surgery.
   a. Clip and shampoo the hair with bacteriostatic shampoo; shaving the operative area is usually done immediately prior to surgery.
   b. Report any evidence of scalp infection.
   c. Give enemas only as directed—straining upon defecation raises intracranial pressure.
   d. Give medications and treatments as indicated.
      (1) Steroids—to decrease brain edema
      (2) Anticonvulsants—to prevent seizures
      (3) Indwelling spinal catheter connected to a stopcock—to decrease brain edema. Lumbar drainage can be stopped and started as required during procedure.
      (4) Indwelling urethral catheter—to assess urinary volume during dehydrating operative period
      (5) Parietal burr holes may be made immediately prior to posterior fossa surgery to facilitate ventricular cannulation for cerebrospinal fluid drainage.

Postoperative Management

Goals:

1. To watch for life-threatening complications, namely increasing intracranial pressure from edema and bleeding
2. To improve the functional status of the patient

1. Establish proper respiratory exchange and adequate brain oxygenation to eliminate systemic hypercarbia and hypoxia, which increase cerebral edema.
   a. Keep the patient in a lateral or a semiprone position to facilitate respiratory exchange.
   b. Employ tracheopharyngeal aspiration cautiously to remove secretions; suctioning can raise intracranial pressure.
   c. Carry out arterial blood gas studies to determine respiratory adequacy.
   d. Check eye opening (spontaneous, to sound, to pain) and reaction of pupils to light.
   e. Elevate the head of the bed 30.5 cm (12 inches) after patient is conscious to aid venous drainage of the brain.
   f. See that the patient has nothing by mouth until an active coughing and swallowing reflex is demonstrated.

2. Assess patient's level of responsiveness:
   a. Response to commands
      (1) Answers questions readily and correctly
      (2) Can perform a complex maneuver
      (3) Responds to simple command
      (4) Shows delayed or unequal response
      (5) Reacts only to loud voice
      (6) Does not respond
   b. Assessment of spinal motor reflexes (pinch Achilles tendon, arm, or other body site):
      (1) Prompt, purposeful withdrawal
      (2) Sluggish or nonpurposeful movement of extremities
      (3) Facial grimace
      (4) Involuntary voiding
      (5) No response
   c. Observation of patient's spontaneous activity:
      (1) Verbal or other communication
      (2) Changes in posture (frequency)
      (3) Breathing pattern
      (4) Retching, vomiting
      (5) Restlessness, twitching, tremors, convulsions

3. Keep the patient normothermic during the postoperative period, since temperature control may be lost in certain neurologic states and a higher temperature increases the metabolic demands of the brain.
   a. Take rectal temperature at specified intervals.
      Extremities may be cold and dry due to paralysis of heat-losing mechanisms (vasodilation and sweating).
   b. Employ measures to reduce excessive fever when present.
      (1) Remove blankets; place loincloth over patient.
      (2) Give aspirin if indicated.

(continued)

Chart 57-4
Summary: Nursing Management of the Patient Having Intracranial Surgery (continued)

Postoperative Management *(continued)*

   (3) Apply ice bags to axillae and groin—application of cold over large, superficial vessels helps lower body temperature.
   (4) Give tepid water or alcohol sponge.
   (5) Place a fan so that it will blow on patient and increase surface cooling.
   (6) Use hypothermia blanket.
   (7) Give chlorpromazine (IM) to prevent shivering.
   (8) Utilize ECG monitoring to detect arrhythmias during hypothermia procedures.

4. Evaluate for signs and symptoms of increasing intracranial pressure.
   a. Assess patient (minute by minute, hour by hour) for:
      (1) Diminished response to stimuli
      (2) Fluctuations of vital signs
      (3) Restlessness
      (4) Weakness and paralysis of extremities
      (5) Increasing headache
      (6) Changes or disturbances of vision; pupillary changes
   b. Control postoperative cerebral edema.
      (1) Give steroids, osmotic dehydrating agents, and glycerol when prescribed in postoperative period to reduce brain swelling.
      (2) Keep patient *slightly* underhydrated to combat cerebral edema.
      (3) Record urinary specific gravity at intervals—especially indicated for surgery of the pituitary and hypothalamus.
      (4) Evaluate electrolyte status.
         (a) Early postoperative gain indicates fluid retention; a greater than estimated weight loss indicates negative water balance.
         (b) Loss of sodium and chlorides will produce weakness, lethargy, and coma.
         (c) Low potassium will cause confusion and decreased level of responsiveness.
      (5) Institute hypothermia procedures (see above) to decrease brain metabolism.
      (6) Employ hyperventilation when prescribed to reduce cerebral blood flow.
      (7) Elevate head of bed 20 to 30 degrees to reduce intracranial pressure and facilitate respirations.

5. Perform supportive measures until the patient is able to care for himself.
   a. Change the position frequently, since pain and pressure responses are variable.
   b. Give analgesics that do not mask the level of responsiveness (codeine, aspirin).
   c. Support the patient if convulsive seizures occur (see p. 1360).

   d. Relieve signs of periocular edema.
      (1) Lubricate eyelids and around eyes with petrolatum.
      (2) Apply light, cold compresses in pliofilm (taped over eye) at specified intervals.
      (3) Watch for signs of keratitis if cornea has no sensation.
   e. Put extremities through range of motion exercises.
   f. Use aseptic measures in management of indwelling three-way urethral catheter (see p. 972).
   g. Evaluate and support patient during episodes of restlessness.
      (1) Evaluate for airway obstruction, distended bladder, meningeal irritation from bloody cerebrospinal fluid.
      (2) Pad patient's hands and bedrails—to protect from injury.
   h. Watch for leakage of cerebrospinal fluid, since there is an ever-present danger of meningitis.
      (1) Differentiate between cerebrospinal fluid and mucus.
         (a) Collect fluid on Dextrostix; if cerebrospinal fluid is present, the indicator will have a positive reaction since cerebrospinal fluid contains sugar.
         (b) Assess for moderate elevation of temperature and mild neck rigidity.
      (2) Keep cerebrospinal pressure low.
         (a) Periodic lumbar punctures—to reduce cerebrospinal fluid pressure and decrease its force against the wound
         (b) Ventricular catheters may be inserted in patient undergoing surgery of posterior fossa (ventriculostomy); catheter(s) connected to a closed reservoir system.
         (c) Elevate head of bed as prescribed.
         (d) Give antibiotics as indicated.
   i. Reinforce blood-stained dressings with sterile dressing; blood-soaked dressings act as a culture medium for bacteria.
   j. Evaluate patient with hypophysectomy (surgery on pituitary) for diabetes insipidus.
      (1) Weigh daily.
      (2) Keep input and output record.

6. Assess for complications.
   a. Intracranial hemorrhage (Postoperative bleeding may be intraventricular, intracerebral, intracerebellar, subdural, or extradural.)
      (1) Watch for progressive impairment of state of responsiveness, signs of increasing intracranial pressure.
      (2) Prepare patient for cerebral angiography; CT scan.

(continued)

Chart 57-4
Summary: Nursing Management of the Patient Having Intracranial Surgery (continued)

Postoperative Management (*continued*)

    (3) Prepare patient for reoperation and evacuation of
        hematoma.
  b. Brain edema
  c. Postoperative meningitis; infection
  d. Wound infections (scalp, bone flap)—wound may have
     to be reopened.

  e. Pulmonary complications
  f. Epilepsy (There is a greater risk of epilepsy with
     supratentorial operations.)
     (1) Give anticonvulsants on a long-term basis.
     (2) Watch for status epilepticus, which may occur
         after any intracranial operation.
  g. Gastrointestinal ulceration (signs and symptoms of
     hemorrhage and perforation or both).

(Brunner LS and Suddarth DS. The Lippincott Manual of Nursing Practice, 3rd ed. Philadelphia, JB Lippincott, 1982.)

Controlling Postoperative Cerebral Edema.   Postoperative edema may be controlled through drug therapy and by monitoring for drainage from ventricular catheters and maintaining fluid and electrolyte balance.

Drug Therapy.   Some degree of edema of the brain occurs following brain surgery, which tends to be maximal 24 to 36 hours postoperatively. This is why there may be a slump in the patient's level of responsiveness on the second postoperative day. Cerebral edema may be treated with the intravenous administration of dehydrating agents (mannitol, dexamethasone, oral glycerol). Antacids are given with steroids to protect the gastric mucosa. (See p. 1294 for treatment of increased ICP.)

Sometimes external decompression is achieved by removing the bone flap.

Drainage.   Ventricular catheters are frequently inserted in patients undergoing surgery for tumors of the posterior fossa. These catheters are connected to an external drainage bottle. The patency of the catheter can be noted by the pulsations of the fluid in the tubing. In addition, the degree of ICP can be determined by the height of the fluid level in the tube above the level of the ventricle. The catheter is removed when the ventricular pressure is normal and no further fluid is draining (usually, within 2 or 3 days). The neurosurgeon should be notified if at any time the catheter appears to be obstructed. A more recent innovation is the use of ventriculoatrial shunts to lower ICP before certain operations, particularly in patients with posterior fossa tumors.

When drainage catheters are not used, a hematoma frequently forms under the scalp and spreads down to the orbit, producing an area of ecchymosis (black eye). Sometimes the eyes cannot be opened for a few days due to edema of the eyelids.

Fluid and Electrolyte Balance.   Electrolyte imbalance, particularly sodium imbalance, may contribute to the development of postoperative brain edema. Sodium retention is observed in the immediate postoperative period. Serum and urine electrolytes, BUN, blood glucose, weight, and clinical status are evaluated. The input and output are measured in view of the losses incurred from fever, respiration, and ventricular/spinal drainage. Fluids may need to be restricted. The postoperative fluid regimen is calculated on an individual basis, and the volume and composition are adjusted according to daily electrolyte determinations. Fluid overload is scrupulously avoided.

Performing Supportive Measures.   Such measures include proper positioning of the patient, dressing changes, and control of headache.

Postoperative Positioning.   The head-up position promotes venous drainage. Extreme head rotation is avoided, as this raises ICP. Following a supratentorial operation, the patient is placed on his side (unoperated side if a large lesion was removed) with one pillow under his head. The head of the bed may be elevated 15 to 45 degrees according to the level of the ICP and the neurosurgeon's directives. (Usually, the patient is kept in relatively the same position as during the operation.) Following a posterior fossa operation (infratentorial), the patient is kept flat on his side (off his back) with his head on a small, firm pillow. He may be turned on either side, but his head should not be flexed on his chest. When the patient is being turned, his body should be turned as a unit to prevent strain on the wound and possible tearing of the sutures.

The patient's position is changed every 2 hours and skin care is given frequently. If the position is changed too frequently, the intracranial monitoring equipment will be disrupted. A turning sheet from the head to the mid-thigh level will make it easier to move the patient.

Dressings.   The dressing is often stained with blood in the immediate postoperative period. It is important to reinforce the dressing with sterile pads so that contamination and infection may be avoided. (Blood is an excellent culture medium for bacteria.) If the dressing is heavily stained or displaced, it should be reported immediately. A drain is sometimes placed in the craniotomy wound to facilitate drainage.

Following suboccipital operations, cerebrospinal fluid may leak through the wound. This complication is dangerous because of the possibility of meningitis. Any sudden discharge of fluid from a cranial or spinal wound should be reported at once.

Patients with suboccipital surgery are sometimes dressed with firm adhesive strappings to prevent movement of the head and the neck.

Control of Headache.   There will be a certain amount of headache following craniotomy, which is mostly attributed to stretching or irritation of the nerves of the scalp that occurs during operation. Codeine, given parenterally, is usually sufficient to relieve headache. Anticonvulsant medication (diazepam, phenytoin) is given to patients who have undergone supratentorial craniotomy because of the high risk of epilepsy following supratentorial neurosurgical procedures.

Postoperative Complications. Complications that may develop within hours following surgery include intracranial bleeding, cerebral edema, and water intoxication.

- A drop in blood pressure, a fast pulse and respiration, and a pale and cold body are usually manifestations of hypovolemic shock following long operations. This type of shock is best treated by blood transfusion.
- Conversely, an increase in blood pressure and decrease in pulse with respiratory failure may indicate increased ICP.

Aside from the immediate postoperative complications, other complications may occur during the first 2 weeks or later and may endanger the patient's recovery. The most important of these are pulmonary infection, pressure sores, urinary infection, and thrombophlebitis. The majority of these complications may be avoided by frequent change of position, nasopharyngeal suctioning, observation and auscultation for pulmonary complications, and urinary bladder and skin care as is described in the care of patients with cerebrovascular disease.

Status epilepticus (occurrence of prolonged seizures without recovery of consciousness in the intervals between seizures) may occur after craniotomy as a result of the intracranial lesion. Intravenous phenobarbital, phenytoin (Dilantin), or diazepam (Valium) may relieve the seizures. Sometimes general anesthesia is necessary to halt the seizures. Other complications are summarized on page 1323.

Rehabilitation and Patient Education. The convalescence of a neurosurgical patient depends on the extent of trauma and the success with which treatment was carried out. When a benign tumor is removed successfully, it is most gratifying to help the patient toward recovery. Good nursing management eliminates untoward complications and permits the major emphasis to be placed on regaining function. Helping the patient to gradually exercise his arms and legs, get out of bed, and feed himself are methods by which the nurse can encourage self-care. Doing everything for the patient hinders successful rehabilitation. However, he should be accompanied when he is walking, because sudden attacks of dizziness or unconsciousness may occur.

Close cooperation between the nurse and the physical therapist helps the patient to achieve good muscle function. If the patient is aphasic, speech therapy may be necessary. This is likely to become a long-term and time-consuming project—one demanding great patience and continual encouragement on the part of the nurse (see p. 1306).

The family must be aware of the limitations of the patient, but should be informed of his progress and how they can help to promote his recovery.

When tumor, injury, or disease is of such a nature that the prognosis is poor, care is directed toward making the patient as comfortable as possible.

With return of the tumor or cerebral compression, the patient becomes less alert and aware. Other possible sequelae include paralysis, blindness, or seizures. When the family is kept informed of the progress of the patient by the surgeon, many times the real expression of their emotions takes place after the physician leaves. It is then that the nurse must help them to work out their feelings.

Often the care of this patient is transferred to some member of the family. Whoever is responsible must have proper instruction regarding the physical and emotional care of the patient. If a family member is not able to give this care, perhaps some arrangements can be made for a community health nurse to assume part care as needed. The medical social worker may be consulted in making financial arrangements or in helping to place the patient in an extended-care facility.

▶ **Evaluation**

Expected Outcomes

1. Exhibits improved neurologic status
   a. Opens eyes on request
   b. Utters recognizable words, progressing to normal speech
   c. Shows increasing alertness
   d. Obeys commands with appropriate motor responses
   e. Participates in program of graded exercises
   f. Gradually participates in self-care activities
2. Copes with temporary sensory deprivation
      Uses alternate method of communication (finger tapping or head nodding)
3. Attains fluid and electrolyte balance
   a. Demonstrates serum chemistries within acceptable limits for patient undergoing intracranial surgery
   b. Becomes less drowsy after 36 hours postoperatively
   c. Exhibits ECG within normal limits
   d. Gradually regains alertness
   e. Complies with fluid restriction

Transsphenoidal Surgery

Pituitary tumors (which comprise 10% of all intracranial tumors) may be treated by surgery or radiation. Surgical removal may be carried out through an open craniotomy (usually transfrontal) or through the transsphenoidal approach. The choice is determined by anatomical considerations and the extent and nature of the pathologic process.

Tumor located within the sella turcica (intrasellar) and small adenomas of the pituitary can be removed by way of the nasal sphenoid sinus (transsphenoidal approach), usually via the sublabial transseptal method or intranasal transseptal approach. This approach, which is being used with greater frequency, offers direct access to the sella with minimal risk of trauma and hemorrhage. It avoids many of the risks of craniotomy and the postoperative discomfort is similar to that of other transnasal operations. It is also used for hypophysectomy for endocrine ablation in the treatment of metastatic breast cancer, prostatic cancer, and diabetic retinopathy.

The preoperative workup includes a series of endocrine tests, rhinologic evaluation (to assess status of the sinuses and nasal cavity), and neuroradiologic studies. Funduscopic examination and visual field determinations are done, as the most serious effect of pituitary tumor is localized pressure on the optic nerve or chiasm. In addition, the nasopharyngeal secretions are cultured. Cortisone may be given preoperatively and postoperatively (as the source of ACTH is removed). Antibiotics may or may not be administered prophylactically. Deep-breathing is taught preoperatively. The patient is instructed that vigorous coughing and sneezing may cause a cerebrospinal fluid leak after surgery. Instruct him to apply pressure on the inner aspect of both sides of the nose to control sneezing.

While the initial opening may be made by an otorhinolaryngologist, the neurosurgeon completes the opening into the sphenoid sinus and exposes the floor of the sella. Microsurgical techniques provide improved illumination, magnification, and visualization so that nearby vital structures can be avoided.

Postoperative Management.   The vital signs are monitored. Visual acuity is checked. The intake and output are measured as a guide to fluid and electrolyte replacement, and the urinary specific gravity is measured after each voiding. Fluids are given when nausea ceases, and the patient progresses to a regular diet in 24 to 48 hours. Medications include antimicrobials, which are continued until the nasal packing is removed; cortisone; analgesics; and agents for the control of diabetes insipidus (pitressin). The head of the bed is raised to a 30-degree angle to decrease pressure on the sella turcica, and to alleviate headache.

The major discomfort of the patient is related to the nasal packing and to mouth dryness and thirst from mouth breathing. Usually, toothbrushing is avoided until the incision above the teeth has healed. The use of mouthwash, dental floss, and a mist mask is helpful.

The nasal packing is generally removed on the fourth to fifth postoperative day. The patient is cautioned against blowing his nose or engaging in any activity that raises ICP, such as bending over or straining during urination or defecation.

The patient may be given a protective external aluminum nasal mold and tape and instructed to apply this mold at bedtime for a prescribed time period.

Manipulation of the posterior pituitary gland during operation may produce transient diabetes insipidus of several days duration, which is treated with pitressin. Occasionally, there is permanent diabetes insipidus. Another complication is hypopituitarism, which can lead to addisonian crisis. The patient is monitored for weakness, lethargy, orthostatic hypotension, dizziness, fever, and nausea. Other complications include transient cerebrospinal fluid leakage and postoperative meningitis.

▷ **Bibliography**

Books

Adams RD and Victor M. Principles of Neurology, 2nd ed. New York, McGraw-Hill, 1981.

Aurelia JC. Aphasia Therapy Manual. Danville, Illinois, Interstate Printers and Publisher, 1980.

Bakay L and Glasauer FE. Head Injury. Boston, Little, Brown & Co, 1980.

Boller F and Frank E. Sexual Dysfunction in Neurological Disorders. New York, Raven Press, 1982.

Boullin DJ. Cerebral Vasospasm. New York, John Wiley & Sons, 1980.

Campkin TV and Turner JM. Neurosurgical Anaesthesia and Intensive Care. Boston, Butterworths, 1980.

Conway-Rutkowski BL: Carini and Owens' Neurological and Neurosurgical Nursing, 8th ed. St Louis, Mosby, 1982.

Dalessio DJ (ed). Wolff's Headache and Other Head Pain. New York, Oxford University Press, 1980.

Hayward R. Essentials of Neurosurgery. Oxford, Blackwell Scientific, 1980.

Hickey J. The Clinical Practice of Neurological and Neurosurgical Nursing. Philadelphia, JB Lippincott, 1981.

Kaufman DM. Clinical Neurology for Psychiatrists. New York, Grune & Stratton, 1981.

Litel GR, Mahoney PE, and Keen J. Neurosurgery and the Clinical Team. New York, Springer, 1980.

Logigian MK (ed). Adult Rehabilitation: A Team Approach for Therapists. Boston, Little, Brown & Co, 1982.

Magee KR and Saper JR. Clinical and Basic Neurology for Health Professionals. Chicago, Year Book Medical Publishers, 1981.

Meyer JS and Shaw T. Diagnosis and Management of Stroke and TIAs. Menlo Park, Addison-Wesley, 1982.

Pasztor E. Concise Neurosurgery. New York, S Karger, 1980.

Pryse-Phillips W and Murray TJ. Essential Neurology, 2nd ed. Garden City, New York, Medical Examination, 1982.

Rosenberg RN (ed). Neurology. New York, Grune & Stratton, 1980.

Salcman M (ed). Neurologic Emergencies: Recognition and Management. New York, Raven Press, 1980.

Scheinberg P. Modern Practical Neurology, 2nd ed. New York, Raven Press, 1981.

Smith RR. Essentials of Neurosurgery. Philadelphia, JB Lippincott, 1980.

Snyder M and Jackle M. Neurologic Problems: A Critical Care Nursing Focus. Bowie, Robert J. Brady, 1981.

Steefel JS. Dysphagia Rehabilitation for Neurologically Impaired Adults. Springfield, Illinois, Charles C Thomas, 1981.

Sutherland JM. Fundamentals of Neurology. New York, ADIS Press, 1981.

Taylor JW and Ballenger S. Neurological Dysfunctions and Nursing Interventions. New York, McGraw-Hill, 1980.

Thompson RA and Green JR (eds). Critical Care of Neurologic and Neurosurgical Emergencies. New York, Raven Press, 1979.

Weiner WJ (ed). Respiratory Dysfunction in Neurologic Disease. Mt Kisco, Futura, 1980.

Youmans JR (ed). Neurological Surgery, Vols. 1, 2, 3, 4, 5, 6, 2nd ed. Philadelphia, WB Saunders, 1982.

Articles

Aphasia

Enderby P. A nurse's guide to managing the patient with speech handicap following a stroke or head injury. Nurs Times 1980 Nov 27; 76(48):2114–2115.

Eslinger JP and Damasio AR. Age and type of aphasia in patients with stroke. J Neurol Neurosurg Psychiatry 1981 May; 44(5):377–381.

Louis MC and Povse SM. Aphasia and endurance: Considerations in the assessment and care of the stroke patient. Nurs Clin North Am 1980 June; 15(2):265–282.

Sarno MT and Levita E. Some variations on the nature of recovery in global aphasia after stroke. Brain Lang 1981 May; 13(1):1–12.

Thrush J. Communicating with patients with a language problem. Br Med J 1981 Mar 14; 282(6267):878–879.

Weinhouse I. Speaking to the needs of your aphasic patient. Nursing '81 1981 Mar; 11(3):34–36.

Headache

Barrett–Griesemer P, Meisel S, and Rate R. A guide to headaches—and how to relieve their pain. Nursing '81 1981 Apr; 11(4):50–57.

Caviness VS and O'Brien P. Current concepts: Headache. N Engl J Med 1980 Feb 21; 302(8):446–450.

Conway-Rutkowski B. Getting to the cause of headaches. Am J Nurs 1981 Oct; 81(10):1846–1849.

Diamond S and Medina JL. Newer drug therapies for headache. Postgrad Med 1980 July; 68(1):125–140.

Diehr P et al. Acute headaches: Presenting symptoms and diagnostic rules to identify patients with tension and migraine headaches. J Chronic Dis 1981; 34(4):147–158.

Editorial: Biofeedback and tension headache. Lancet 1980 Oct 25; 2(8200):898–899.

Huston KA and Hunder GG. Giant cell (cranial) arteritis: A clinical review. Am Heart J 1980 July; 100(1):99–105.

Kunkel RS. Evaluating the headache patient: History and workup. Headache 1979 Apr; 19(3):122–126.

Larson EB, Omenn GS, and Lewis H. Diagnostic evaluation of headache. JAMA 1980 Jan 25; 243(4):359–362.

Packard RC. What does the headache patient want? Headache 1979 Nov; 19(7):370–374.

Robb DA and Ongkiko CM. The differential diagnosis of headache and its nursing management. J Neurosurg Nurs 1980 Dec; 12(4):214–216.

Schramm VL. A guide to diagnosing and treating facial pain and headache. Geriatrics 1980 Aug; 33(8):78–80, 82–95, passim.

Intracranial Pressure Monitoring

Budassi SA. Intracranial pressure monitoring. JEN 1979 May–June; 5(3):45–46.

Burchiel KJ, Steege D, and Wyler AR. Intracranial pressure changes in brain-injured patients requiring positive end-expiratory pressure ventilation. Neurosurgery 1981 Apr; 8(4):443–449.

Haller J. Intracranial pressure monitoring in Reye's syndrome. Hosp Pract 1980 Feb; 15(2):101–108.

Harvey J. Intracranial pressure monitoring (intraventricular monitoring and drainage). In Hirsch J and Hannock L. Mosby's Manual of Clinical Nursing Procedures, pp. 259–264. St Louis, CV Mosby, 1981.

Harvey J. Intracranial pressure monitoring (subarachnoid or subdural screw). In Hirsch J and Hannock L. Mosby's Manual of Clinical Nursing Procedures, pp 265–267. St Louis, CV Mosby, 1981.

Healy TEJ, Pathakji GS, and Weston PAM. Intracranial pressure measurements in patients suffering head injury managed in a non-neurosurgical unit. Injury 1980 Sept; 12(2):96–100.

Mitchell PH. Intracranial hypertension: Implications of research for nursing care. J Neurosurg Nurs 1980 Sept; 12(3):145–154.

Mitchell PH, Ozuna J, and Lipe HP. Moving the patient in bed: Effects on intracranial pressure. Nurs Res 1981 July–Aug; 30(4):212–218.

Reed M. High-dose barbiturate therapy for severe head injury—is it justifiable? Headache 1980 Nov; 20(6):341–343.

Ricci MM. Intracranial hypertension: Barbiturate therapy and the role of the nurse. J Neurosurg Nurs 1979 Dec; 11(4):247–252.

Riley JM. Intracranial pressure monitoring made easy. RN 1981 Sept; 44(9):53–57.

Young MS. Understanding the signs of intracranial pressure. A bedside guide. Nursing '81 1981 Feb; 11(2):59–62.

Neurosurgery

Allen MB, El Grammal T, and Nathan MD. Transsphenoidal surgery on the pituitary. Am Surg 1981 July; 47(7):291–306.

Camunas C. Transsphenoidal hypophysectomy. Crit Care Update 1981 June; 8(6):22–27.

D'Angelo CM and Whistler WW. The neurosurgical patient. In Goldin MD. Intensive Care of the Surgical Patient, 2nd ed, pp 421–439. Chicago, Year Book Medical Publishers, 1981.

Gumprecht TF and Jafek BW. Transsphenoidal hypophysectomy. Ear Nose Throat J 1980 July; 59(7):281–288.

Kenan PD. Surgical approaches for pituitary tumors. Clin Obstet Gynecol 1980 June; 23(2):413–423.

Laws ER Jr, Abboud CF, and Kern EB. Perioperative management of patients with pituitary microadenoma. Neurosurgery 1980 Dec; 7(6):566–570.

May M. Management of cranial nerves I through VII following skull base surgery. Otolaryngol Head Neck Surg 1980 Sept–Oct; 88(5):560–575.

Nabarro JDN. Pituitary surgery for endocrine disorders. Clin Endocrinol (Oxf) 1980 Sept; 13(3):285–298.

Puckett CL et al. The transnasal–transsphenoidal approach for pituitary surgery. Plast Reconstr Surg 1980 Dec; 66(6):821–825.

Spooner TR, Grin OD, and Herz DA. Transseptal transsphenoidal hypophysectomy. Otolaryngol Head Neck Surg 1980 Nov–Dec; 88(6):721–725.

Pain

Bates JAV and Nathan PW. Transcutaneous electrical nerve stimulation for chronic pain. Anaesthesia 1980 Aug; 35(8):817–822.

Blazer D. Chronic pain: A multiaxial approach to psychosocial assessment and prevention. South Med J 1981 Feb; 74(2):203–207; 214.

Fields H. Pain II: New approaches to management. Ann Neurol 1981 Feb; 9(2):101–106.

Stroke

Andrews K and Stewart J. Stroke recovery: He can but does he? Rheumatol Rehabil 1979 Feb; 18(1):43–48.

Boller F. Stroke and behavior: Disorders of higher cortical functions. Current Concepts in Cerebrovascular Disease and Stroke 1981 Jan–Feb; 16(1):1–4.

Bray GP, DeFrank RS, and Wolfe TL. Sexual functioning in stroke survivors. Arch Phys Med Rehabil 1981 June; 62(6):286–288.

Brocklehurst JC et al. Social effects of stroke. Soc Sci Med [A] 1981 Jan; 15A(1):35–39.

Chaudhuri G. Rehabilitation of the stroke patient. Geriatrics 1980 Oct; 35(10):45–46, 49–50, 54.

Czaplinski R, Gardner M, and Hurley CL. Test your knowledge of caring for the stroke patient. Nursing '80 1980 Sept; 10(9):68–71.

Feigenson JS. Stroke rehabilitation. Current Concepts in Cerebrovascular Disease and Stroke 1980 Nov–Dec; 15(6):21–26.

Garraway WM. Management of acute stroke in the elderly: Follow-up of a controlled trial. Br Med J 1980 Sept 27; 281(6244):827–829.

Hewer RL. How does arm movement recover? Practitioner 1979 Dec; 223(1338):800–803.

Johnston K and Olson E. Application of Bobath principles for nursing care of hemiplegic patient. ARN J 1980 Mar–Apr; 5(2):8–11.

Medcalf TE and Vandiver RL. Stroke forum. Phys Ther 1980 July; 60(7):905.

Millikan CH and McDowell FH. Treatment of progressive stroke. Prog Cardiovasc Dis 1980 May–June; 22(6):397–414.

Redford JB and Harris JD. Rehabilitation of the elderly stroke patient. Am Fam Physician 1980 Sept; 22(3):153–160.

Reinisch ES. Quick assessment of hemiplegics' functioning Am J Nurs 1981 Jan; 81(1):102–104.

Ripeckyj A and Lazarus LW. Family guide to the problems of the stroke patient. Geriatrics 1980 Oct; 35(10):47–48.

Rogers EJ. Goals in hemiplegia care. J Am Geriatr Soc 1980 Nov; 28(11):497–498.

Rusinski PS. Neurological assessment of the hemiplegic patient. Nurs Pract 1979 May–June; 4(3):26–27, 30–32.

Stonnington HH. Rehabilitation in cerebrovascular diseases. Primary Care 1980 Mar; 7(1):87–106.

Wallace JD and Levy LL. Blood pressure after stroke. JAMA 1981 Nov 13; 246(19):2177–2180.

Warren M. Relationship of constructional apraxia and body scheme disorders in dressing performance in adult CVA. Am J Occup Ther 1981 July; 35(7):431–437.

Williamson–Kirkland TE and Berni R. Neurological aspects of rehabilitation. Part 1: Brain injury. ARN J 1980 May–June; 5(3):10–12, 20.

Wolf SL, Baker MP, and Kelly JL. EMG biofeedback in stroke: A 1-year follow-up on the effect of patient characteristics. Arch Phys Med Rehabil 1980 Aug; 61(8):351–355.

Yatsu FM. Acute medical therapy of strokes. Current Concepts in Cerebrovascular Disease and Stroke 1982 Jan–Feb; 17(1):1–4.

Unconscious Patient

Horton JM. Use of anesthesia. Care of the unconscious. Br Med J 1980 July 5; 281(6232):38–40.

Jennett B and Teasdale G. Aspects of coma after severe head injury. Lancet 1977 Apr 23; 1(8017):878–881.

LeWinn EB. The coma arousal team. R Soc Health J 1980 Feb; 100(1):19–21.

Loen M and Snyder M. Psycho-social aspects of care of the long-term comatose patient. J Neurosurg Nurs 1979 Dec; 11(4):235–237.

Loen M and Snyder M. Care of the long-term comatose patient: A pilot study. J Neurosurg Nurs 1980 Sept; 12(3):134–137.

Miller M. Emergency management of the unconscious patient. Nurs Clin North Am 1981 Mar; 16(1):59–73.

Myco F and McGilloway FA. Care of the unconscious patient: A complementary perspective. J Adv Nurs 1980 May; 5(3):273–278.

Agencies

Governmental

Division for the Blind and Physically Handicapped, Library of Congress, Washington, D.C. 20542

National Institute of Neurological and Communicative Disorders and Stroke, National Institutes of Health, Bethesda, Maryland 20205

Voluntary

American Heart Association (Stroke), 7320 Greenville Avenue, Dallas, Texas 75231

American Speech–Language–Hearing Association, 10801 Rockville Pike, Rockville, Maryland 20852

National Committee on the Treatment of Intractable Pain, P.O. Box 34571, Washington, D.C. 20034

National Easter Seal Society, Inc., 2023 West Ogden Avenue, Chicago, Illinois 60612

National Migraine Foundation, 5214 North Western Avenue, Chicago, Illinois 60625

The Stroke Foundation, Inc., 898 Park Avenue, New York, New York 10021

58

Management of Patients With Neurologic Disorders

▷ Cranial, Spinal, and Peripheral Neuropathies

First Cranial (Olfactory) Nerve

Disturbances of the olfactory bulbs due to intracranial diseases reveal themselves when the sense of smell is lost (anosmia) or altered (perversions).

Anosmia.   Loss of smell follows fractures of the base of the skull that cause lacerations of the olfactory nerves (fine filaments that pass from the bulb to the olfactory mucous membrane through small holes in the cribriform plate of the ethmoid bone). Falls or blows on the back of the head that merely jar the skull but cause contusion of these filaments may also produce temporary anosmia. The nerve may be damaged by tumor (*i.e.*, meningioma in the region of the olfactory groove).

Second Cranial (Optic) Nerve

Diseases of and injuries to the optic nerves, whatever their nature, cause reduction in the acuity of vision and contraction of the visual fields—symptoms that may progress to complete blindness.

Papilledema or Choked Disc.   Edematous swelling of the head of the optic nerve appears in all conditions that increase the intracranial pressure, such as brain tumors, abscess, and acute hemorrhage into the brain.

Secondary Optic Atrophy.   Optic atrophy is the outcome of prolonged severe choking of the optic disc, neuritis of the optic nerve, closure of its central artery, pressure against it by brain tumors, and fractures of the base of the skull that involve the optic foramen (through which the optic nerve leaves the skull). Optic atrophy is also an important early sign of multiple sclerosis. It is one of the manifestations of central nervous system syphilis and an effect of methanol poisoning.

Third, Fourth, and Sixth Cranial (Oculomotor, Trochlear, and Abducens) Nerves

The *oculomotor nerve* supplies all but two of the muscles that move the eyeball. One of these two, the superior oblique,

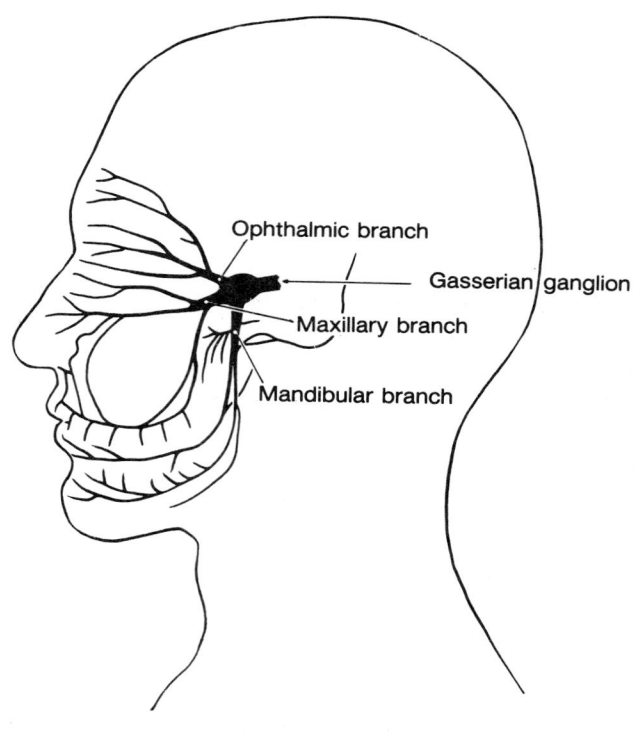

Figure 58-1. The main divisions of the trigeminal nerve are the ophthalmic, maxillary, and mandibular branches. Sensory root fibers arise in the Gasserian ganglion.

is innervated by the fourth cranial (*trochlear*) nerve; the other, the external rectus muscle, which rotates the eyeball outward, is innervated by the sixth cranial (*abducens*) nerve. Paralysis of any one of these three nerves produces a particular type of strabismus (squint) (depending on the muscle paralyzed). Paralysis of the third nerve produces ptosis and dilation of the pupils as well. Such paralysis may be caused by tumors, aneurysms, and stroke. A new onset of third-nerve palsy in the neurologic patient may indicate impending herniation of the uncus.

Fifth Cranial (Trigeminal) Nerve

The *trigeminal nerve* supplies all the sensory fibers to the skin of the face (except the angle of the jaw and the anterior half of the scalp), the teeth, the conjunctivae, the mucous membrane covering the inside of the mouth, the nose, the paranasal sinuses, and the greater part of the tongue. The lowest branch of this nerve also contains the motor fibers that control the muscles of mastication (Fig. 58-1).

One, two, or all three branches of this nerve (ophthalmic, maxillary, and mandibular) may be affected by disease and by trauma, and the disturbances that follow always correspond exactly to the areas of distribution of the branch affected. Severe injury to one of these nerves, such as contusions over the supraorbital notch or the intraorbital foramen, may be followed by anesthesia of the area it supplies. If the trauma merely irritates or compresses the nerve, then pain follows. If, however, the trauma causes bleeding into the tissue in the area of the nerve, the scar tissue that forms afterward may so compress its fibers that months later localized pain appears in the forehead or the cheek. This pain may continue indefinitely.

Other Causes of Facial Pain.   Facial pain related to the trigeminal nerve may result from lesions that directly irritate the trigeminal nerve or its ganglion or from diseases of other organs that refer their pains to the area distributed by the trigeminal nerve. Among such lesions are inflammatory processes and neoplasms in the soft tissues and the bones of the face; paranasal sinus infections; infected teeth; unerupted third molar teeth; tumors and aneurysms about the base of the skull; venous sinus thrombosis; basilar meningitis; tumors of the Gasserion ganglion; diseases of the sphenopalatine ganglion, the middle ear, and the orbit of the eye; such conditions as migraine, and multiple sclerosis; and occasionally syphilis, diabetes, nephritis, and malaria. Facial pain for which no cause can be demonstrated is referred to as atypical facial pain. A very specific type of facial pain is trigeminal neuralgia or tic douloureux (see below).

Trigeminal Neuralgia (Tic Douloureux)

Trigeminal neuralgia is a condition of the fifth cranial nerve characterized by an explosive onset of pain similar to an electric shock or a lancinating burning sensation in the area distributed by one or more branches of the trigeminal nerve. The pain ends as abruptly as it starts. Each pain episode can be described as stabbing and explosive and produces contraction of some of the facial muscles, such as a sudden closing of the eye or a twitch of the mouth; hence the name *tic douloureux* (painful twitch). The etiology is not known, but some investigators believe that it may be due to vascular pressure from structural abnormalities (loop of an artery) encroaching upon the trigeminal nerve, Gasserian ganglion, or root entry zone. Early attacks, appearing most often in the fifth decade of life, are usually mild and brief. Pain-free intervals may be measured in terms of minutes, hours, days, or longer. With advancing years, the painful episodes tend to become more and more frequent and agonizing.

The pain of this neuralgia is felt in the skin, not in the deeper structures, but it is more severe at the peripheral areas of distribution of the affected nerve, notably over the lip, the chin, and the ala nasi, and in the teeth. Paroxysms are aroused by any stimulation of the terminals of the affected branches, such as washing the face, shaving, brushing the teeth, eating, and drinking. A draft of cold air and direct pressure against the nerve trunk may also cause pain. Certain areas are called *trigger points,* since the slightest touch immediately starts a paroxysm. To avoid stimulating these areas, patients with trigeminal neuralgia try not to touch or wash their faces, shave, chew, or do anything else that might cause an attack. Behavior of this type is a clue to diagnosis.

Management.   The antiepileptic drugs carbamazepine (Tegretol) and phenytoin (Dilantin) will relieve pain in most patients. Carbamazepine is taken with meals, in gradually increased dosages until relief is obtained. Side-effects include nausea, dizziness, drowsiness, and hepatic dysfunction. The patient's blood is monitored for bone marrow depression. Phenytoin also produces such side-effects as nausea, dizziness, somnolence, ataxia, and skin allergies.

Alcohol injection of the Gasserian ganglion and peripheral branches of the trigeminal nerve will relieve pain for several months. However, the pain returns after the nerve regenerates.

Percutaneous Radio-frequency Trigeminal Gangliolysis.

Surgical interruption of the trigeminal system is considered when drugs do not relieve pain without causing considerable side-effects. Percutaneous radio-frequency interruption of the Gasserian ganglion, whereby the small unmyelinated and thinly myelinated fibers that conduct the pain are thermally destroyed, is becoming the procedure of choice.

Under local anesthesia, the needle is introduced through the cheek on the affected side. Under fluoroscopic control, the needle electrode is guided through the foramen ovale into the Gasserian ganglion. The divisions of the Gasserian ganglion (mandibular, maxillary, and ophthalmic) are encountered sequentially. The nerve is stimulated with a small current, while the patient is awake. The patient then reports when a tingling sensation is felt. When the electrode needle is in the desired position, the patient is anesthetized briefly and a radio-frequency current (heating current to destroy the nerve) is passed in a controlled manner to thermally injure the trigeminal ganglion and rootlets (Fig. 58-2). The patient is then awakened from the anesthetic and examined for sensory deficits. Repeat lesions may be produced until the desired effect is achieved. The operative procedure takes less than 1 hour and gives permanent pain relief in most patients. Touch and proprioceptive functions are left intact.

Microvascular Decompression of the Trigeminal Nerve.

An intracranial approach (retromastoid craniectomy) can be used to decompress the trigeminal nerve since tic douloureux may be caused by vascular compression of the entry zone of the trigeminal root by an arterial loop and occasionally by a vein. With the aid of an operating microscope, the artery loop is lifted from the nerve in order to relieve the pressure, and a small prosthetic device is inserted to prevent recurrence of impingement on the nerve. The postoperative management is the same as for any intracranial operation.

Preoperative Management.

Preoperative management of a patient with trigeminal neuralgia includes recognizing that certain factors may aggravate excruciating facial pain, such as food that is too hot or too cold or jarring the bed. Even washing the face, combing the hair, or brushing the teeth may produce acute bouts of pain. The nurse can lessen these discomforts in a variety of ways—by using cotton pads to wash the patient's face, substituting a blunt-tooth comb to comb the hair, etc.

Seventh Cranial (Facial) Nerve

The *facial nerve* is the chief motor nerve of the muscles of the face. Its few sensory fibers are disregarded in this discussion.

Facial Paralysis.

There are three types of facial paralysis: peripheral, nuclear, and upper motor neuron. The peripheral type is produced by interruption or dysfunction of the facial nerve when the trunk of the nerve is involved distal to its exit from the skull or within the temporal bone through which it courses. External lesions are usually the result of direct trauma or a suppurative infection of the par-

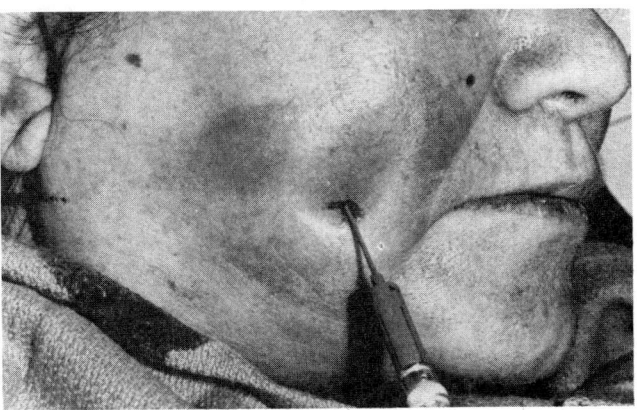

Figure 58-2. Percutaneous radio-frequency rhizotomy for relief of pain from trigeminal neuralgia. The needle electrode has been inserted so that it may be advanced under x-ray control to the area where the heat lesion will be made. This procedure requires only a brief hospital stay without the time, expense, and hazards of an open cranial procedure. (From Silverberg GD: Percutaneous radio-frequency rhizotomy in the treatment of trigeminal neuralgia. Western J Med Aug 1978, p 98.)

otid gland, whereas those occurring within the skull are encountered as complications of mastoiditis, mastoid surgery, or fractures of the skull that involve the temporal bone.

Peripheral facial neuritis is manifested by complete paralysis of the face on the same side as the lesion. As a result, the mouth is drawn toward the normal side, the wrinkles of the forehead and the nasolabial fold are obliterated on the paralyzed side, and the eye remains open, its upper lid drooping and its lower lid slightly everted, allowing the tears to escape over the cheek. The patient cannot puff out the cheek, close the mouth, or show the teeth on the paralyzed side. One form of peripheral paralysis is Bell's palsy.

Bell's Palsy

Bell's palsy (facial paralysis) is due to peripheral involvement of the seventh cranial nerve on one side which results in weakness or paralysis of the facial muscles. The etiology is unknown, although possible causes may include vascular ischemia, viral disease (herpes simplex, herpes zoster), autoimmune disease, or a combination of all of these factors.

Pathophysiology.

Bell's palsy is considered by some to represent a type of pressure paralysis. The inflamed, edematous nerve becomes compressed to the point of damage, or its nutrient vessel is occluded to the point of producing ischemia necrosis of the nerve within its long canal—a channel in which the fit at best is very snug. There is distortion of the face from paralysis of the facial muscles; increased lacrimation (tearing); and painful sensations in the face, behind the ear, and in the eye. The patient may experience speech difficulties and may be unable to eat on the affected side because of relaxation of the facial muscle.

Management.

The objectives of treatment are to maintain the muscle tone of the face and to prevent or minimize denervation. The patient should be reassured that he has not had a stroke and that spontaneous recovery occurs within 3 to 5 weeks in the majority of cases.

Steroid therapy (prednisone) may be given to reduce inflammation and edema, which in turn reduces vascular compression and permits restoration of blood circulation to the nerve. Early administration of the drug appears to diminish the severity of the disease, relieve the pain, and help prevent or minimize denervation.

While the paralysis lasts, the involved eye must be protected. Frequently, the patient's eye does not close completely, and the blink reflex is diminished so that the eye is vulnerable to dust and foreign particles. Corneal irritation and ulceration are a major threat to this patient. Sometimes there is an overflow of tears down the cheek (epiphora) from keratitis caused by drying of the cornea and lack of the blink reflex. The laxity of the lower lid alters the proper drainage of tears. To counter these problems, the eye should be covered with a protective shield at night. However, the eye patch may abrade the cornea, since there is some difficulty in keeping the partially paralyzed eyelids closed. The application of eye ointment at bedtime will cause the eyelids to adhere to one another and remain closed during sleep. If this approach does not work, the eyelids may have to be temporarily sutured together. Wraparound sunglasses or goggles are worn to decrease normal evaporation from the eye.

Face pain is controlled with analgesics. Heat may be applied to the involved side of the face to promote comfort and the flow of blood through the muscles. If the nerve is not too sensitive, the face may be massaged several times daily to maintain muscle tone. The technique is to massage the face with a gentle upward motion. Facial exercises, such as wrinkling the forehead, blowing out the cheeks, and whistling, may be performed with the aid of a mirror and are intended to prevent muscle atrophy. The face should be kept warm.

Electrical stimulation may be applied to the face to prevent atrophy of the muscle until reinnervation occurs.

In selected patients, surgical decompression of the facial nerve has been recommended to allow the edematous facial nerve to expand into the stylomastoid foramen. The decision as to which patient should be treated surgically is a difficult one and is made on the basis of the patient's clinical status, electrical testing of the facial muscles, and the physician's clinical experience. Although most patients recover with conservative treatment (80%–90%), surgical intervention is necessary in some patients to help regain maximum function of the facial nerve and to avoid and minimize the complications of degeneration and regeneration.

Other forms of facial paralysis include nuclear facial paralysis and upper motor neuron facial paralysis:

Nuclear Facial Paralysis.   The nuclear type of facial palsy is caused by destruction of the nuclei from which the fibers of the seventh nerve originate. Neoplastic, vascular, or degenerative lesions in the pons are usually responsible for this form of facial palsy.

Upper Motor Neuron Facial Paralysis.   If this type of paralysis is due to lesions (such as tumors, abscesses, depressed skull fractures, etc.) that injure the motor cortical area governing the face, only the muscles of the lower half of the face become paralyzed. The muscles around the eyes and the forehead escape because they are bilaterally inner-vated from the cortex. The paralysis occurs on the side opposite that of the lesion. Patients with facial palsy of the upper motor neuron type cannot force a smile, no matter how hard they try, but they do smile involuntarily when amused. Their seventh nerve connections to the cortex are severed, but the nerve itself is intact, and the subcortical centers are in sole control.

Eighth Cranial (Auditory–Vestibular) Nerve

Each eighth cranial nerve has two divisions: the auditory (cochlear) and the vestibular portions (the nerve to the semicircular canal system). Disturbances of the auditory nerve impair hearing; disturbances of the vestibular nerve produce vertigo (sensations of turning or falling) and nystagmus. Meniere's disease, a disease of the eighth cranial nerve, is discussed in Chapter 55.

Ninth Cranial (Glossopharyngeal) Nerve

Glossopharyngeal Paralysis.   This paralysis (usually in association with disturbances of the vagus nerve) results in difficulty in swallowing, anesthesia of the upper portion of the pharynx, and loss of taste over the posterior third of the tongue on the same side as the lesion. It most often is due to brain diseases—such as tumors.

Glossopharyngeal Neuralgia.   Neuropathy of the ninth nerve causes glossopharyngeal neuralgia, which is characterized by severe pain radiating from the base of the tongue to deep in the ear. There is also an increase in salivation. Resection of this nerve may cure the problem.

Tenth Cranial (Vagus) Nerve

The *vagus nerve* is the motor nerve of the voluntary muscles of the throat and the larynx, and is the nerve that slows the rate of heartbeat and supplies the parasympathetic nerves to the lungs, the stomach, the esophagus, and other abdominal organs.

Neuritis.   Neuritis of this nerve occasionally occurs in such acute infections as pneumonia and influenza and results from the action of such poisons as alcohol, lead, and arsenic. The vagus nerve (usually in association with the glossopharyngeal nerve) frequently is injured by lesions of the pons and the base of the skull.

Paralysis.   Paralysis of one vagus nerve causes unilateral paralysis of the larynx, with resultant impairment of speech, difficulty in swallowing, temporary changes in the heart rate and rhythm, and occasionally, vomiting, abdominal pain, and anorexia. Complete paralysis of both vagi is followed by permanent tachycardia, since the accelerator nerves of the heart (sympathetic fibers) then lack the normal inhibition of the vagi.

The recurrent laryngeal branch of this nerve, because of its position, is injured easily. The result is paralysis of the larynx and, therefore, hoarseness. This may be caused by the pressure of mediastinal tumors, masses of enlarged lymph nodes in the mediastinum or the neck, aneurysms of the aorta or the subclavian artery, and malignant growths of the thyroid gland or adjacent structures. This nerve is occasionally severed by wounds and operations on the neck, such as thyroidectomy.

Eleventh Cranial (Spinal Accessory) Nerve

The *spinal accessory nerve,* entirely motor in nature, supplies the sternomastoid muscle and the upper portion of the trapezius muscles. Injuries to and diseases of this nerve, therefore, weaken the power to rotate the head to the side opposite the lesion and cause a slight drooping of the shoulder on the side of the lesion. Such paralysis may result from penetrating wounds and operations on the neck, fractures of the skull, injuries to and diseases of the cervical vertebrae, unilateral poliomyelitis, and all diseases that involve the upper portion of the cervical cord.

Twelfth Cranial (Hypoglossal) Nerve

The *hypoglossal nerves,* entirely motor in character, innervate the muscles of the tongue only. Injury to one of these nerves, with resultant paralysis of that side of the tongue, is rare but can occur from deep, penetrating wounds; abscesses and tumors of the neck; and trauma to and tuberculosis of the first cervical vertebra. Much more frequently, this paralysis is evidence of brain disease.

The tongue, when paralyzed on one side, will deviate toward the weak side when it protrudes from the mouth. When both hypoglossal nerves are paralyzed, the tongue cannot be moved; hence, speech, mastication, and swallowing cannot be performed properly.

The Brachial Plexus

Paralysis of the brachial plexus and the nerves arising from it occasionally follows violent movements of the shoulder, the head, and the arm, which overstretch or even tear the root of this plexus. The brachial plexus (and also its roots) occasionally suffers from the pressure of local tumors, aneurysms, and masses of enlarged lymph nodes in the neck or the axilla.

Cervical Ribs.   A *cervical rib* is one or a pair of extra ribs attached usually to the seventh cervical vertebra. If a pair is present, one only may produce symptoms. They are found more frequently in women than in men, occasionally in several members of the same family, and usually in association with other anatomical anomalies.

A cervical rib is a lifelong hazard to the brachial plexus. Because of its presence, the plexus may be crushed by accidents that suddenly force or pull the shoulder down; this trauma is followed by pain and numbness, felt first in the fingers and gradually extending up the forearm, and later by weakness, followed by atrophy of the muscles of that hand and arm. The continuous pressure of a cervical rib on the brachial plexus (the symptoms of which seldom appear before middle life) affects first its sympathetic nerve fibers, as shown by such vasomotor signs as cyanosis, coldness, paleness, and edema (a syndrome that at first may suggest Raynaud's disease). Later this pressure causes disturbances of sensation and finally atrophy of the muscles of the arm and the hand.

Since the presence of a cervical rib frequently produces developmental abnormalities in the pattern of the brachial plexus, the findings on physical examination often are puzzling. Thus, various muscles and skin areas of the arm and the hand seem to be supplied by the wrong nerves; the arteries of the shoulder region may lie in an unusual position

or be abnormal in their relative size; and often the pulse volume of the radial artery of that arm is unusually small and the blood pressure low. Cervical ribs are not always visible on x-ray films, since some constitute merely fibrous bands. However, they exert pressures just as serious as those produced by bone.

The Nerves of the Arms

Radial Nerve Paralysis.   This paralysis, causing *wrist-drop,* may be the result of pressure against the trunk of the radial nerve as it lies in the axilla. Such pressure may be caused by a crutch or the back of a bench, over which the arm is thrown. It also follows blows against the outer aspect of the upper arm, where this nerve lies in an unprotected position. The same type of paralysis also may be caused by a tourniquet that is applied to the arm too tightly or allowed to remain on for too long a time. Late radial paralysis, appearing 3 to 4 weeks following fracture of the humerus, results from the gradual compression of this nerve by either excessive callus formation or—more often—by contracting scar tissue formed in tissues infiltrated by blood.

Ulnar Nerve.   The ulnar nerve is often traumatized at the elbow, where it lies in an exposed position. To hit the "crazy bone" really is to strike the ulnar nerve. Even the simple act of reclining on the elbow may cause a pressure paralysis of several weeks' duration in the muscles that this nerve supplies. Dislocation of the elbow and fracture of the bones near this joint may stretch or compress this nerve, causing immediate paralysis of the same muscles or weakness of muscles supplied by the nerves.

The Intercostal Nerves

The intercostal nerves may be injured by trauma to the chest wall and fracture of the ribs, causing pain in their areas of distribution. Anesthesia never results if only a single nerve is injured, because of the overlapping of the areas supplied by the two adjacent nerves.

Neuritis.   Intercostal neuritis is usually due to disease of the nerve proper (as in herpes zoster) or of the nerve roots in the spinal canal (as in exostoses of the vertebrae in hypertrophic osteoarthritis or in metastatic malignancy of the vertebrae). The sensation is generally described as a sore, burning, or shooting "electric" pain.

The Lumbar and Sacral Plexuses

The Lumbar Plexus.   Tumors of the vertebrae, retroperitoneal neoplasms, enlarged inflamed pelvic lymph nodes, and psoas abscesses occasionally cause enough pressure on the lumbar plexus to cause weakness or paralysis of the anterior thigh muscles that are supplied by the femoral nerve.

The Sacral Plexus.   The sacral plexus may be torn by fractures of the lower lumbar vertebrae and the sacrum, or it may be subjected to pressure from large fibroid tumors of the uterus and malignant growths within the pelvis. It may also be traumatized during difficult labor. The chief symptom produced is spasmodic or continuous pain, often called *sciatica.*

Sciatica.   The term *sciatica* refers to any condition in which the most prominent symptom is pain along the course of the sciatic nerve. Its etiology in many instances is uncertain. Some patients give a past history of sprain of the lumbosacral or the sacroiliac joints. In other instances, spondylitis, spondylolisthesis, or a ruptured intervertebral disc pressing on the cauda equina may be responsible.

Peripheral Neuropathies

A *peripheral neuropathy* is a disorder affecting the peripheral motor, sensory, or autonomic nerves. Peripheral nerves, by connecting the spinal cord and brain to all other body organs, transmit motor impulses outward and relay back sensory impulses to encode sensation in the brain. If one nerve is affected, it is considered a *mononeuropathy,* if several nerves are involved, the pattern is characterized as *polyneuropathy.* The involvement of multiple single peripheral nerves or their branches is termed *mononeuritis multiplex.*

The most common causes of peripheral neuropathy are diabetes, alcoholism, and occlusive vascular disease. Many bacterial and metabolic toxins and exogenous poisons also affect the structure and function of the peripheral nerves. Due to the growing use of chemicals in industry, agriculture, and medicine, the number of substances known to cause peripheral neuropathies is increasing. In the developing countries, leprosy is a major cause of severe nerve disease.

The major symptoms of peripheral nerve deficit are loss of sensation, muscle atrophy, weakness, diminished reflexes, and pain and paresthesia (tingling, prickling) of the extremities. The patient frequently describes some part of the extremity as "numb." Autonomic features include decreased or reduced sweating, nocturnal diarrhea, tachycardia, impotence, and atrophic skin and nail changes.

Mononeuropathy. Mononeuropathy is limited to a single peripheral nerve and its branches. It arises when the trunk of the nerve is *traumatized,* as when bruised by a blow; *overstretched,* as in cases of dislocation of a joint; *compressed,* as by a tumor, a cervical rib, a crutch, or bony exostoses (*e.g.,* in that type of arthritis that narrows the apertures between adjacent vertebrae through which the spinal nerves pass); *punctured* by a needle used to inject a drug or poisoned by the drugs thus injected; or *inflamed* because of the extension to its trunk of an adjacent infectious process. Mononeuropathy is frequently seen in the diabetic patient.

One type of mononeuropathy appears many months after an injury that caused considerable bleeding into the tissues surrounding a nerve. In tissues thus infiltrated with blood, considerable scar tissue forms, which contracts and slowly compresses the nerve. Similarly, delayed nerve paralysis follows the healing of an abscess, the encapsulation of a foreign body or sequestra of bone, and the healing of fractured bone. In this last case, however, the nerve trunk is caught in the callus.

Pain is seldom a conspicuous symptom of mononeuropathy due to trauma, but in patients with complicating inflammatory conditions, such as arthritis, this feature is prominent. Such pain is increased by all body movements that tend to stretch, strain, or cause pressure on the injured nerve, and by all sudden jars of the body, such as those incident to coughing and sneezing. The skin in the areas supplied by nerves that are injured or diseased may become reddened and glossy; its subcutaneous tissue may become edematous, and the nutrition of the nails and the hair in this area, defective. Chemical injuries to a nerve trunk, such as those caused by drugs injected into or near it, often are permanent.

Management. The objective of treatment of mononeuropathy is to remove the cause if possible, such as by freeing the compressed nerve. The pain may be relieved by aspirin or codeine, and the function of the muscles may be maintained by weak galvanic currents.

Causalgia. *Causalgia* (Greek words for heat and pain) refers to the group of symptoms and signs that follow peripheral nerve injuries. The nerves most often affected, in order of frequency, are the median, the ulnar, the radial, and the internal and external popliteals.

The chief symptom of causalgia is severe burning pain along the course of the injured nerve. The pain may be described as "hot," "burning," "stabbing," or "crushing." This is more or less persistent, but becomes severe following such physical stimuli as the contact of clothes. The skin over the affected extremity becomes hot, shiny, and, at times, swollen; it shows abnormalities in sweating and eventually undergoes atrophic changes involving also the nails. The patient holds the extremity quiet, since each movement tends to increase the pain. Sympathetic nerve blocks, repair of local nerve lesions, and aggressive physical therapy are part of the treatment program. Experience with battle casualties revealed that active and passive exercises with very early mobilization appeared to reduce the incidence of causalgia following wounds of the extremities.

Polyradiculitis. *Polyradiculitis (Guillain-Barré syndrome)* is a clinical syndrome of unknown cause involving the nervous system and characterized by varying degrees of motor and sensory disturbances. In the majority of patients, the syndrome is preceded by an infection (respiratory or gastrointestinal), but in some instances it has occurred following vaccination and surgery. It may be due to a primary viral infection, an immune reaction, some other process, or a combination of processes. One hypothesis is that a viral infection induces an autoimmune reaction that attacks the myelin of the peripheral nerves.

Proximal portions of the nerves tend to be affected most often, and the nerve roots within the subarachnoid space are commonly involved. Autopsy findings have revealed inflammatory edema and demyelination with some lymphocytic infiltration that is especially prominent in the spinal nerve roots.

Clinical Manifestations. There is variation in the mode of onset. The initial neurologic symptoms are paresthesia (tingling and numbness) and muscle weakness of the legs, which may progress to the upper extremities, trunk, and facial muscles. Muscle weakness may be followed quickly by complete paralysis. The cranial nerves are frequently involved, resulting in marked difficulty in swallowing, talking, and chewing. Sensory disturbances include loss of sensation and sphincter disturbances of the bladder and rectum. There may be back pain, muscle soreness, and loss of position sense, as well as diminished or absent tendon reflexes. Spinal fluid shows elevation in total protein with no increase in cell count.

Management. Since the cause of the disease is unknown, there is no specific therapy. The treatment is supportive. A course of corticosteroid therapy may be beneficial in the early phase of the disease, but its role is controversial.

- *Careful and continued assessment of respiratory function is necessary since respiratory insufficiency and failure may develop quickly.* Since respiratory failure is the main cause of death, vital capacity should be monitored. Signs to watch for are breathlessness while talking, shallow and irregular breathing, increasing pulse rate, use of accessory muscles while breathing, and any *change* in the respiratory pattern. If difficulties develop, the patient may require tracheostomy and mechanical ventilation.

When bulbar nerves are involved, the airway must be protected against the hazards of regurgitation and vomiting. If the patient is unable to swallow, nasogastric tube feedings are instituted.

- The heart is monitored for arrhythmias since cardiac arrest may occur if the vagus nerve becomes affected.

Urinary retention may be encountered during the acute phase of the disease. The paralyzed extremities are supported in functional positions and given passive range of motion exercises at least twice daily. The prevention of contracture deformities (see p. 230) and pressure sores (see p. 238) is a major nursing challenge. For severely paralyzed patients, the principles of nursing management of the unconscious patient (see p. 1297) may be applied, although these patients are in full possession of their mental faculties.

Because of paralysis, tracheostomy, and intubation, the patient is unable to talk, laugh, or cry and thus has no outlet for emotional expression. These problems are compounded by boredom, dependency, isolation, and frustration. To establish some form of communication, lip reading and the use of picture cards, combined with a system of blinking the eyes to indicate "yes" or "no," may be tried. Diversional therapy (television, radio, visits from the family) can alleviate some of the frustrations encountered by these patients.

Patients with polyradiculitis are dependent on quality medical and nursing management for recovery. Unless there is fatal respiratory failure, the rate of recovery is usually related to the degree of involvement and may take many months for some patients. However, full recovery is seen in the majority of patients.

▷ Headache

Possibly the most common of all human afflictions is headache or *cephalgia* ("condition of head pain"). Headache may arise from a variety of sources due to a variety of mechanisms, such as vascular spasms caused by muscle contraction or inflammation of pain-sensitive structures inside or outside the skull. Most headaches are not caused by structural diseases but are a symptom of the patient's problems in coping or adapting to a life situation.

Assessment

When data are obtained for the nursing history, the patient should be given a chance to describe his headache *in his own words* as related to the following questions:

- What is the location? Is it unilateral or bilateral?
- What is the quality—dull, aching, steady, boring, burning, intermittent, continuous, paroxysmal?
- What are the number of headaches during a given time?
- Are there any precipitating factors (environmental, such as sunlight and weather change; foods; exertion; etc.)?
- What makes the headache worse (coughing, straining)?
- What time (day/night) does it occur?
- Are there any associated symptoms (facial pain, lacrimation, scotomas (blind spots in field of vision)?
- What usually relieves the headache (aspirin, ergot preparation, food, heat, rest, neck massage)?
- Is there nausea, vomiting, weakness, numbness in the extremities?
- Are there any allergies?
- Does the patient have insomnia, poor appetite, loss of energy
- Is there a family history of headache? "sick" headache?
- What is the relationship of the headache to the lifestyle: physical/emotional stress?
- What is the patient's medication history?

The patient's goals are to prevent or obtain relief of the headache.

The physical examination includes a careful history, physical assessment of the head and neck, a neurologic examination of the cranial nerves, evaluation of the size and reactions of the pupils, a funduscopic examination of the eyes, and a test of motor and sensory systems. For patients with abnormalities on the neurologic examination, computed tomography and other types of diagnostic tests are employed if a mass lesion is suspected.

Tension Headache (Muscle Contraction Headache)

Emotional or physical stress may cause contraction of the muscles in the neck and scalp, resulting in tension headache. The headache may be characterized by a steady, pressing ache, which usually begins in the forehead, the temple, or the back of the neck. It is often bandlike and is located at the base of the skull. Tension headaches tend to be more chronic than severe and are probably the most common type of headaches. The patient needs reassurance that his headache is not due to a brain tumor. This is a common unspoken fear. A discussion of the patient's problems (instead of his headache) can be very helpful. To obtain long-term relief, the person needs to understand the source of any emotional conflicts and attempt to change or adapt to stressful and anxiety-producing situations. This requires supportive counseling and education, including biofeedback, relaxation techniques, and behavioral therapy.

Various pharmacologic agents are used in the treatment of severe tension headache, including nonnarcotic analgesics, nonsteroidal anti-inflammatory medications, muscle relaxants, tranquilizing agents, and antidepressant drugs.

Vascular Headaches

Migraine.   Migraine is a symptom-complex character-ized by unilateral (or generalized) periodic attacks of severe headache. The cause of migraine has not been clearly dem-onstrated, but it is primarily a vascular disturbance that occurs more commonly in women. A positive family history is pres-ent in 65% of patients with migraine.

A "preheadache" phase or an "aura" (warning sign) may occur, forewarning the patient of an impending attack and providing enough time to take the prescribed medication in order to avert a full-blown attack. The aura may be in the form of visual, sensory, or motor symptoms. These sensations preceding the headache are described at times as "scintil-lating scotomata" or "visual field defects" and are attributed to vasoconstriction and ischemia within the cerebral cortex and possibly also in the retina. Other neurologic phenomena preceding the attacks include paresis of an extremity, aphasia, or confusion.

Pathophysiology and Clinical Manifestations.

The ce-rebral symptoms and signs of migraine are the results of cortical ischemia of varying degree. The typical attack begins with vasoconstriction affecting the arteries of the scalp and certain cerebral or retinal vessels. The patient appears pale and may experience sensory, motor, and mood disturbances. Extracranial and intracranial blood vessels dilate, causing pain and discomfort. Studies suggest that the dilated artery becomes hyperpermeable and that sterile local inflammatory reactions occur in the vicinity of the painful, dilated arteries. It is proposed that vasoactive substances (histamine, sero-tonin, plasmokinins) participate in this sterile inflammatory reaction.

The pain begins in the supraorbital, retro-orbital, or temporal areas on one side and increases in such intensity that the patient is prostrated, frequently with nausea and vomiting. The attack may last 2 hours to several days. Sleep tends to relieve the symptoms.

Prevention.

The first step in assessing the problem is to obtain a careful medical and neurologic evaluation as well as a survey of social, environmental, and personality factors. Although there is a wide variation in the personality types of those who are subject to migraine, there is evidence that the hard-driving, somewhat compulsive perfectionist is most vulnerable to this condition.

The patient can be helped to develop insight into his feelings, behavior, and conflicts and to make the necessary modifications in life-style on the basis of these analyses. Regular periods of exercise and relaxation are suggested, and any offending or provoking factors (allergens, fatigue, foods, environmental stresses) are removed or reduced in order to obtain relief. A record may be kept of the circum-stances surrounding the attacks (activities, food, feelings) to determine if there is a pattern to the migraine episodes. If so, a change in the pattern may help to avoid the attacks.

Management of Acute Attack.

The objective of man-agement during an acute attack is to prevent the painful dilation of cranial vessels. Ergotamine preparations (taken orally, sublingually, intramuscularly, by rectum, or inhaled) may be effective in aborting the headache if taken *early* in the migraine process. Ergotamine tartrate acts on smooth muscle, causing prolonged constriction of the cranial blood vessels. Each patient's dosage is titrated according to indi-vidual needs. Side-effects include aching muscles, pares-thesias, nausea, and vomiting. During the acute attack, the patient may find relief by lying quietly in a darkened room with the head slightly elevated. Drinking black coffee may also be helpful in counteracting the attack. Symptomatic therapy for migraine includes analgesics, sedatives, and an-tianxiety agents.

Management Between Attacks.

Methysergide maleate (Sansert) is an effective prophylactic agent in preventing frequent and severe migraine attacks. Troublesome side-effects include abdominal discomfort, muscle cramps, edema, numbness, tingling of extremities, and depression. There should be a medication-free interval after every 6-month course of treatment because of the potential com-plication of retroperitoneal fibrosis and pleuropulmonary and cardiac fibrosis.

It has been found that migraine headaches may dis-appear in patients who are taking propranolol hydrochloride (Inderal) for coexisting heart problems. In selected patients, this drug is being used with varying success for the treatment of migraine. Cyproheptadine hydrochloride (Periactin), which is an antagonist to serotonin and histamine, reduces the severity of pain in some patients and also affords head-ache prophylaxis.

Antidepressants, barbiturates, and tranquilizers may help the patient to cope with stress. Because of the diversity of treatment for migraine, the patient must be treated on an individual basis and followed closely.

Cluster Headache.   *Cluster headaches* are another form of vascular headache and are considered by some to be a variant of migraine. They are seen most frequently in men. The attacks come in "clusters" or groups with severe and excruciating pain localized in the eye and orbit that radiates to the facial and temporal regions. The pain is ac-companied by watering of the eye and nasal congestion. The duration of the pain is quite short, lasting less than an hour. One theory is that this type of headache is due to dilatation of orbital and nearby extracranial arteries. Cluster headaches may be precipitated by alcohol, nitrates, vaso-dilators, and histamines. Eliminating these factors helps in preventing the headaches. Cluster headache responds to vasoconstricting agents (ergotamine tartrate) or the serotonin antagonist methysergide (Sansert) may give relief. Chlor-promazine may also be effective.

Cranial Arteritis.   Inflammation of the cranial arteries is characterized by a severe headache localized to the region of the temporal arteries. It may be generalized, in which cranial arteritis is part of a vascular disease, or of a focal type, in which only the cranial arteries are involved. Cranial arteritis is a disease of the elderly.

Often the disease begins with constitutional manifes-tations, such as fatigue, malaise, weight loss, and fever. Clin-ical manifestations associated with inflammation (heat, red-ness, swelling, tenderness or pain over the involved artery) are usually present. Sometimes a tender, swollen, or nodular temporal artery is visible. Visual problems are caused by ischemia of the involved structures.

Cranial arteritis is thought to represent an immune vas-culitis in which immune complexes are deposited within the walls of affected blood vessels, producing vascular injury and inflammation.

Treatment consists of early administration of a corticosteroid drug to prevent the possibility of loss of vision due to vascular occlusion or rupture of the involved artery. Analgesic agents are given for comfort. The temporal artery is usually biopsied.

Other Types of Headaches

Headache in Brain Tumor. Headache is a common sign of brain tumor, particularly a rapidly expanding tumor that produces traction on pain-sensitive structures of the head. If the tumor is slow growing, the headache may be mild or transitory. In about one third of the patients, the headache occurs in the area overlying the tumor. *If the patient has not had a previous history of headaches, a headache of recent onset is significant.* The headache is usually accompanied or overshadowed by other complaints: weakness, visual loss, or seizures.

Headache in Meningitis. Inflammation and stretching of the meninges and blood vessels are the cause of headache in meningitis. The headache is rapid in onset, usually generalized and accompanied by a stiff neck. A slight movement of the head may markedly aggravate the headache. Photophobia and fever are common.

Headache in Subarachnoid Hemorrhage. This headache is severe and sudden in onset and has been described as a "violent bursting sensation in my head." It is commonly located in the occipital region but becomes generalized rather quickly. If the hemorrhage is severe, there is almost immediate loss of consciousness followed rapidly by death. More often, consciousness is lost for a short interval. Vomiting frequently accompanies the early stage, and within an hour or so there is neck stiffness and a positive Kernig's sign, indicating meningeal irritation. The severe, constant, and generalized headache gradually subsides and is usually amenable to analgesics such as codeine. (Subarachnoid hemorrhage is discussed on p. 1339.)

Hypertensive Headache. This type of headache may take any form, but it is typically a dull, pounding, occipital headache that is present upon awakening in the morning and tends to wear off during the day. The precise mechanism of the headache is not certain, but it is thought to emanate from overly stretched extra- and intra-cranial arteries. The headache is relieved by antihypertensive therapy (see p. 679).

▷ Brain Tumors

A brain tumor is a localized intracranial lesion that occupies space within the skull and tends to cause a rise in intracranial pressure.

In 95% of patients with tumors of the brain, the tumor originates in the brain (including the roots of the cranial nerves and the meninges). The remaining 5% are either metastases from primary growths elsewhere in the body or malignancies of the skull that have ulcerated through into the cranial cavity. (In the adult, the highest incidence of intracranial tumors occurs between the ages of 55 and 70 years, and the majority of these are supratentorial.) Brain

---

Chart 58-1
Classification of Brain Tumors

Tumors originating in the brain tissue
  Gliomas; infiltrating tumors that may invade any portion of the brain; most common type of brain tumor
    Astrocytomas
      (grades 1 and 2)
    Glioblastomas (grades 3 and ⎫
      4 astrocytomas)   ⎬ Subclassified according
    Ependymomas   ⎪ to cell type
    Medulloblastomas   ⎪
    Oligodendrogliomas   ⎪
    Colloid cysts   ⎭

Tumors arising from covering of brain
  Meningioma; encapsulated, well-defined, growing outside the brain tissue; compresses rather than invades brain

Tumors developing in or on the cranial nerves
  Acoustic neuroma; derived from sheath of acoustic nerve
  Optic nerve spongioblastoma polare

Metastatic lesions (most commonly from lung and breast)

Tumors of the ductless glands
  Pituitary
  Pineal

Blood vessel tumors
  Hemangioblastoma
  Angioma

Congenital tumors

---

tumors rarely metastasize outside the central nervous system but cause death by impairing vital functions either by direct involvement or by increasing intracranial pressure.

Classification

Brain tumors may be classified into several groups: (1) those arising from the coverings of the brain, such as the dural meningioma; (2) those developing in or on the cranial nerves, best exemplified by the acoustic neuroma and the optic nerve spongioblastoma polare; (3) those originating in the brain tissue, such as the various gliomas; and (4) metastatic lesions originating elsewhere in the body (see also Chart 58-1). The major concern is tumor localization and its histological character. Tumors may be benign or malignant. However, because a benign tumor may occur in a vital area, it may have effects as serious as those of a malignant tumor.

Specific Tumors

Gliomas. The malignant glioma is the most frequently seen brain neoplasm. Usually, these tumors cannot be totally removed because they spread by infiltrating into the surrounding neural tissue.

Pituitary Adenomas.   The *pituitary gland* is a small, olive-shaped body located in a small pocket just below the optic nerves. The activity of this gland may be increased or decreased by the presence of a tumor. Adenomas originating from the anterior lobe of the pituitary cause signs of endocrine dysfunction (generally secretory overactivity), signs of an expanding mass (usually, suprasellar extension with visual impairment), or a combination of these. Increased function (hyperpituitarism) accelerates growth, which in children results in gigantism. In adults, the face becomes coarse and the hands large, a condition called *acromegaly.* Hyperfunction of the gland may cause other conditions, such as Cushing's disease, lactation, etc.

A decrease in function leads to hypopituitarism, characterized by changes in skin pigmentation, anemia, and loss of sexual characteristics. In addition to these disturbances of function, the tumor, by exerting pressure on the optic nerves, causes a progressive loss of vision that results in blindness.

The majority of pituitary adenomas are treated by transsphenoidal microsurgical removal (see p. 1325), while the remainder of tumors that cannot be completely removed are treated by radiation.

Angiomas.   Brain angiomas (masses composed largely of abnormal blood vessels) are found either in or on the surface of the brain. Some persist throughout life without causing symptoms; others give rise to symptoms of brain tumor. Occasionally, the diagnosis is suggested by the presence of another angioma somewhere in the head or by a bruit audible over the skull. Since the walls of the blood vessels in angiomas are thin, a cerebral vascular accident frequently occurs. In fact, cerebral hemorrhage in persons under 40 years of age should suggest the possibility of an angioma.

Acoustic Neuroma.   An *acoustic neuroma* is a tumor of the eighth cranial nerve, the nerve of hearing and balance. It usually arises just within the internal auditory meatus where it frequently expands before filling the cerebellopontine recess.

An acoustic neuroma may grow slowly and attain a considerable size before it is correctly diagnosed. The patient usually experiences loss of hearing, tinnitus, and episodes of vertigo and staggering. As the tumor becomes larger, painful sensations of the face may occur on the same side, as a result of the tumor's compressing the fifth cranial nerve.

With improved radiologic techniques and the use of the operating microscope and microsurgical instrumentation, even large tumors can be removed through a relatively small craniotomy.

Clinical Manifestations

Brain tumors produce clinical manifestations when they cause increased intracranial pressure or produce localizing symptoms and signs due to local effects of the tumor's interference with specific regions of the brain.

Increased Intracranial Pressure.   These symptoms are caused by a gradual compression of the brain due to the growth of the tumor. The effect is to disrupt the equilibrium that exists between the brain, the cerebrospinal fluid, and the cerebral blood—all located within the skull. As the tumor grows, compensation may occur through compression of intracranial veins, through reduction of cerebrospinal fluid volume (by increased absorption or decreased production), by a modest decrease of cerebral blood flow, and through reduction of intra- and extra-cellular brain tissue mass. When these compensatory mechanisms fail, the patient develops signs and symptoms.

The most common symptoms produced by increased intracranial pressure are headache, vomiting, papilledema (choked disc) with associated blurring of vision and diplopia, and stupor. Headache, though not always present, is most common in the early morning and is made worse by coughing, straining, or sudden movement.

Headaches are usually described as deep or expanding or as dull but unrelenting. Frontal tumors usually produce a bilateral frontal headache; pituitary gland tumors produce pain radiating between the two temples (bitemporal), whereas in cerebellar tumors the headache may be located in the suboccipital region.

Vomiting, usually unrelated to food intake, is usually due to irritation of the vagal centers in the medulla. If the vomiting is of the forceful type, it is described as "projectile" vomiting.

Papilledema (edema of the optic nerve) is present in a large percentage of patients.

Localizing Symptoms.   Localizing symptoms occur when specific regions of the brain are disrupted, resulting in locally referable signs, such as sensory and motor abnormalities, visual alterations, and convulsive seizures.

Because the functions of the different parts of the brain are known, the location of the tumor can be determined, in part, by identifying those functions that are affected by the presence of the tumor. For example, a tumor of the motor cortex manifests itself by causing convulsive movements localized to one side of the body, spoken of as "Jacksonian seizures." Tumors of the occipital lobe cause blindness in half of each eye (hemianopsia) by involving the centers of the tracts for vision of one side of the brain. Tumors of the cerebellum cause dizziness and a staggering gait, with a tendency to fall toward the side of the lesion, and marked muscle incoordination and nystagmus (rhythmical vibration of the eyeballs). Tumors of the frontal lobe frequently produce personality disorders, changes in the emotional state and behavior, and a disinterested mental attitude. The patient often becomes extremely untidy and careless and may use obscene speech.

Tumors of the cerebellopontine angle usually originate in the sheath of the acoustic nerve and give rise to a sequence of symptoms that is the most characteristic of all brain tumors. First, tinnitus and vertigo appear, soon followed by progressive nerve deafness (eighth nerve dysfunction); next, there is numbness and tingling of the face and the tongue (due to involvement of the fifth nerve); still later, weakness or paralysis of the face develops (seventh nerve involvement); and finally, since the enlarging tumor presses on the cerebellum, abnormalities in motor control may be present.

Many tumors are not so easily localized, because they lie in the so-called silent areas of the brain (*i.e.,* areas where functions are not definitely determined).

The *progression* of the signs and symptoms is important, because it indicates tumor growth and expansion.

Diagnostic Evaluation

The history of the illness and the manner in which the symptoms evolved is important. A neurologic examination indicates the areas of the central nervous system involved. To assist in the precise localization of the lesion, a battery of tests is performed. Computed tomography (CT) will give specific information concerning the number, size, and density of the lesion(s) and the extent of secondary cerebral edema. It also provides information about the ventricular system. The use of CT has resulted in the detection of smaller lesions. Cerebral angiography provides visualization of cerebral blood vessels and can localize most cerebral tumors.

A brain scan may be valuable, since an abnormal amount of radioactive material will accumulate in the area of the tumor and can be localized with a scintillation counter. An electroencephalogram can detect abnormal brain waves in regions occupied by the tumor and can evaluate temporal lobe seizures. Echoencephalography can show whether certain structures have been displaced from the midline by a lesion in one hemisphere. Pneumoencephalography provides critical information in selected patients.

Cytologic studies of the cerebrospinal fluid may be done to detect malignant cells.

Management

An untreated brain tumor ultimately leads to death, either from progressively increasing intracranial pressure or from primary brain damage. Patients with possible brain tumor should be investigated and treated as soon as possible before irreversible damage occurs.

The objective of management is to remove as much or all of the tumor as possible without increasing the neurologic deficit (paralysis, blindness) or to achieve palliation by partial tumor removal and by decompression, radiation, or chemotherapy, or a combination of these. The majority of patients with brain tumors undergo a neurosurgical procedure, when possible, followed by radiation therapy or chemotherapy when indicated. Corticosteroids are highly effective in combating cerebral edema, thus allowing for a thorough diagnostic workup and a carefully planned surgical approach. (Also, appropriate dosages of corticosteroids treat postoperative swelling and facilitate a smoother, more rapid recovery.) In general, patients with meningiomas, acoustic neuromas, cystic astrocytomas of the cerebellum, colloid cyst of the third ventricle, congenital tumors such as dermoid cyst, and some of the granulomas can be cured by surgical removal of the tumor. A complete extirpation of the infiltrating gliomas is not possible. In these patients, the treatment consists of biopsy, to establish the diagnosis; partial removal; decompression, if necessary; and radiation therapy. Certain chemotherapeutic agents combined with radiation therapy are also being used. More recently, deep-seated brain tumors have been removed using the carbon dioxide laser with CT scanning and stereotactic techniques. Newer drugs are continually being evaluated, and there is hope that these will be more successful in the future. Sometimes a bypass operation is performed to relieve obstructive hydrocephalus.

See page 1320 for care of the patient undergoing intracranial surgery.

Cerebral Metastases

A significant number of patients (20% in one cancer institute) suffer central nervous system complications as a result of systemic cancer and neurologic symptoms caused by cerebral metastases. Cancer of the lung commonly metastasizes to the brain, as do tumors of the breast, kidney, gastrointestinal tract, prostate gland, uterus, thyroid, and skin (melanoma). Neurologic symptoms include headache, personality changes, mental changes (memory loss and confusion), focal weakness, paralysis, aphasia, and seizures. These problems may be devastating to the patient and his family.

The treatment is palliative and involves eliminating or reducing serious symptomatology. Bear in mind that even when palliation is the goal, distressing signs and symptoms can be resolved, thereby improving the quality of life that remains. Patients with intracerebral metastases who are not treated have a steady downhill course with a very limited survival time.

The therapeutic approach includes surgery (usually for a single intracranial metastasis), radiation therapy, and chemotherapy, or a combination of these methods. Adrenocorticosteroid hormones may be helpful in relieving headache and alterations of consciousness. It is thought that adrenocorticosteroids (dexamethasone, prednisone) reduce inflammatory reaction around the metastatic deposits and decrease the edema surrounding them. Other drugs include osmotic agents (mannitol, glycerol), which are useful because of their ability to reduce intracranial pressure. (It has also been found that infusions of mannitol can increase the amount of chemotherapeutic drugs by the brain.) Anticonvulsant drugs (phenytoin) are used to prevent and treat seizures.

Radiation to the whole brain is the foundation of treatment of intracerebral metastases (although surgical removal may be appropriate for a single metastatic brain tumor). With the advent of nitrosourea derivatives that cross the blood–brain barrier, there have been encouraging results with the use of chemotherapy. (See also the care of the patient undergoing radiotherapy, p. 335; chemotherapy, p. 308; and the care of the patient with advanced cancer, p. 320).

▷ # Intracranial Aneurysms (Rupture of Intracranial Aneurysm With Subarachnoid Hemorrhage)

An *intracranial (cerebral) aneurysm* is a dilation of the walls of a cerebral artery (Fig. 58-3). An aneurysm may be due to atherosclerosis, reflecting an acquired defect in the vessel wall with subsequent weakness of the wall; a congenital defect of the vessel wall; hypertensive vascular disease; head trauma; or advancing age. An aneurysm is most commonly located on the internal carotid, anterior cerebral, anterior communicating, and middle cerebral arteries. A small percentage develop in the vertebrobasilar territory. Multiple cerebral aneurysms are not uncommon.

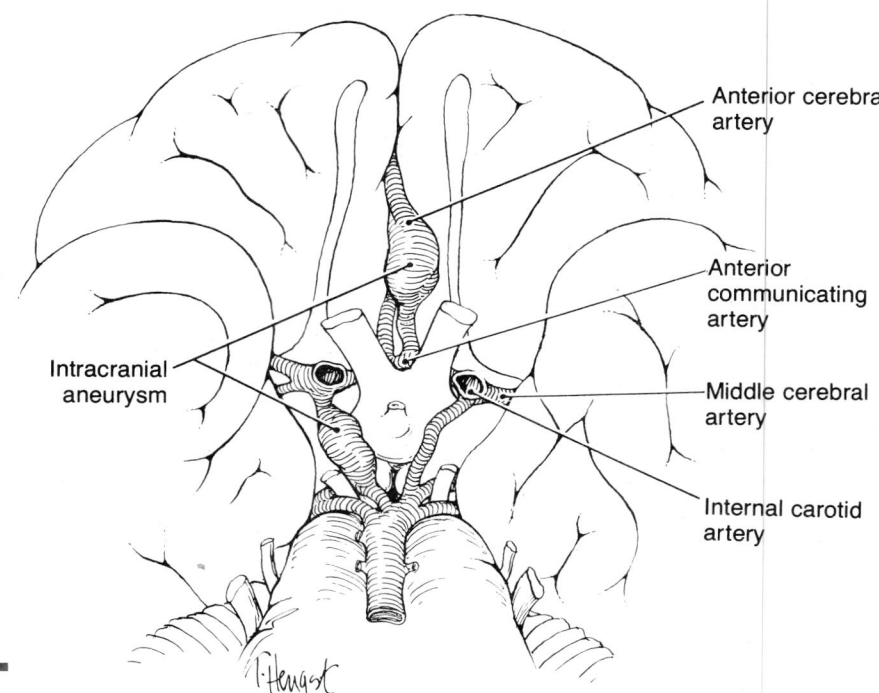

Figure 58-3. Intracranial aneurysm.

Clinical Manifestations

Symptoms are produced when the aneurysm enlarges and presses on nearby cranial nerves or brain substance or, more drastically, when the aneurysm ruptures, causing *subarachnoid hemorrhage*. Rupture of the aneurysm usually produces a *sudden* severe, localized headache with a stiff neck and often loss of consciousness for a variable period of time. (Other causes of subarachnoid hemorrhage include arteriovenous malformation, tumors, trauma, and blood dyscrasias.) There may be pain and rigidity in the back of the neck and spine due to meningeal irritation. Visual disturbances (visual loss, diplopia, ptosis) occur when the aneurysm is adjacent to the oculomotor nerve. Tinnitus, dizziness, and hemiparesis may also occur. The diagnosis is confirmed by CT scanning, lumbar puncture (confirms blood in cerebrospinal fluid), and cerebral angiography.

At times, an aneurysm will ''leak'' blood, leading to the formation of a clot that seals the site of rupture. In this instance, the patient may show little neurologic deficit. Or there may be severe bleeding, resulting in coma followed rapidly by death.

Aneurysms that produce subarachnoid hemorrhage in adults occur most frequently in middle life. The mortality rate corresponds to the level of consciousness and neurologic deficit, but there is a high *immediate* mortality rate. The patient who lives to reach the hospital faces two major complications: rebleeding and ischemic complications from cerebral vasospasm.

Management

The goals of management are to support the patient through the critical period immediately following the subarachnoid bleeding, and to prepare him for subsequent surgery.

The patient is placed on immediate and strict bed rest, since activity and stress may potentiate bleeding. Any activities that increase the blood pressure or obstruct venous return are to be avoided. These include the Valsalva maneuver, straining, sneezing, pulling up in bed, acute flexion or rotation of the head and neck (compromises jugular veins), and cigarette smoking. Any activity requiring exertion is contraindicated. Because of this consideration, stool softeners are given to prevent straining. The head of the bed may be elevated 30 to 45 degrees to promote venous drainage, although some neurologists prefer that it remain flat to increase cerebral perfusion and thus reduce hypoxia.

The patient is monitored constantly to recognize neurologic deterioration from recurrent bleeding, increased intracranial pressure (see p. 1293), or vasospasm and to determine the best time for surgical intervention. Barbiturates may be administered to avoid emotional upset and consequent hypertension. Anticonvulsants are administered to prevent seizures.

Antifibrinolytic medication (aminocaproic acid [Amicar]) may be given to decrease fibrinolysis (dissolution of the fibrin plug) at the site of the aneurysmal rupture that causes the early recurrent hemorrhages, and thus reduce the incidence of rebleeding.

- Periodic observations are made to assess for signs of a decrease in mental alertness, an increase in headache, and alteration in the size of the pupils. Any of these changes are reported immediately, since they usually signify additional bleeding. Quick action is necessary if a fatal hemorrhage is to be prevented.

Antihypertensive medication (propranolol, hydralazine) may be given to reduce the systolic arterial thrust on the weakened arterial wall as well as to reduce the chance of bleeding. A precipitous drop in blood pressure, which can produce brain ischemia, is to be avoided.

Mannitol and other osmotic diuretics are used to reduce intracranial pressure. Oxygen may be necessary to reduce hypoxia.

Cerebral vasospasm (constriction of intracranial blood vessels) that may be due to a morphologic change in the arterial wall is a serious complication of subarachnoid hemorrhage and often is correlated with a poor clinical condition and prognosis. The mechanism responsible for vasospasm is not clear. The spasm initially occurs immediately after the bleed, which probably exerts a protective effect on the affected artery. Spasm frequently recurs during the fourth to tenth day following initial hemorrhage. It is also during this time that the clot undergoes the lytic process (dissolves) and increases the chances of rebleeding. The major vessels at the base of the brain may be affected, thereby compromising the blood flow in the area. Hemiparesis, visual field defects, seizures, mental clouding, and paralysis may occur. An Aminophylline–Isuprel regimen is one method of treatment currently being used in an attempt to modify vasospasm and increase blood flow through the cerebral vessels. Also, the patient's blood volume may be expanded to increase perfusion through spastic cerebral vessels.

Other complications following subarachnoid hemorrhage from a ruptured aneurysm include epilepsy, hydrocephalus, and psychiatric and psychological problems. Anxiety and depressive states may be complicating factors.

Surgical Approach

There is considerable controversy concerning the timing of surgery for the low-risk patient. A patient severely affected by massive hemorrhage is usually not a candidate for surgery. Since the advent of the operative microscope and microsurgical techniques, there has been a decreased morbidity and mortality in low-risk patients. Magnified vision and improved lighting allow the neurosurgeon to see the details of the vascular relationships and identify aneurysms deep in the brain.

The objecive of surgery is to protect the patient from further hemorrhage. This is done by isolating the aneurysm from its circulation or by strengthening its wall. An aneurysm may be treated by excluding it from the circulation by means of a ligature or a clip across its neck (Fig. 58-4). If this is not anatomically possible, the aneurysm can be reinforced by wrapping it with plastic, muscle, or some other substance. An extracranial–intracranial arterial bypass may be done to establish collateral blood supply in order to allow surgery on the aneurysm. Or, an extracranial method may be used, whereby the carotid artery is occluded in the neck in order to reduce pressure within the blood vessel (carotid endarterectomy, see p. 1309). Following ligation of the carotid artery, there is some risk of cerebral ischemia and sudden hemiplegia, because during the operative procedure there is a temporary occlusion to the blood supply to the brain (unless a temporary inlying bypass shunt is used). In anticipation of these complications, measurements of cerebral blood flow and internal carotid pressure may be taken in order to identify those patients who are at risk for postoperative ischemic episodes.

Other postoperative complications include the appearance of psychological symptoms (disorientation, amnesia, Korsakoff's syndrome, personality impairment), intraoperative embolization, postoperative internal artery occlusion, water and electrolyte disturbances (from dysfunction of the neurohypophyseal system), and gastrointestinal bleeding. (The management of the patient following intracranial surgery is discussed on pp. 1322–1325.)

▷ ## Intracranial Infection— Brain Abscess

True *brain abscesses* are collections of pus within the substance of the brain itself. They may occur by *direct invasion of the brain* from intracranial trauma or surgery; by *spread of infection from nearby sites* (paranasal sinus infections, otitis media, or mastoiditis); or by *spread of infection from other organs* (lung infections, infective endocarditis). As a

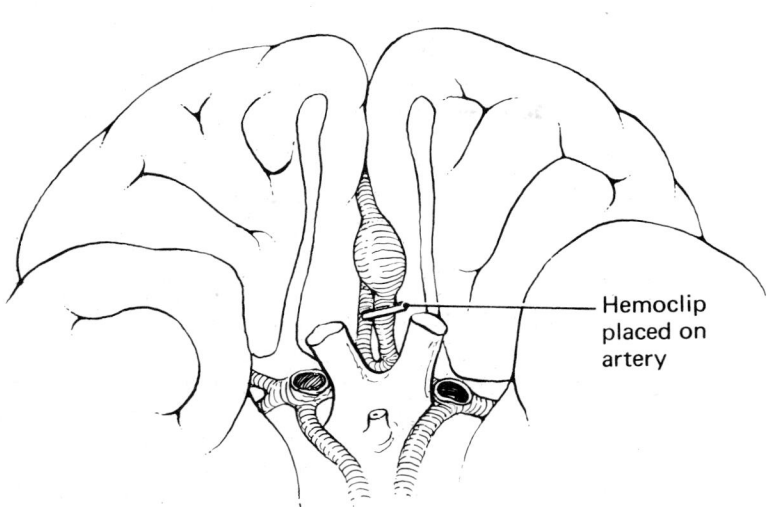

Hemoclip placed on artery

Figure 58-4. Cerebral aneurysm isolated by means of a hemoclip.

preventive measure, otitis media, mastoiditis, sinusitis, and systemic infections should be promptly treated to prevent brain abscesses.

Clinical Manifestations.   The clinical manifestations result from alterations in intracranial mass dynamics (edema, brain shift), infection, or the location of the abscess. Headache, usually worse in the morning, is the patient's most constant symptom. Vomiting is also common. Focal neurologic signs (weakness of an extremity, decreasing vision, seizures) may occur, depending on the site of the abscess.

Any localizing symptoms that occur are not as typical as those seen in patients with brain tumor. When they do occur, they usually indicate pathology in either the temporal lobe or the cerebellum, since so many abscesses are aural in origin. There may be a change in the patient's mental alertness as reflected in lethargic, confused, or disoriented behavior. Although fever is a constant presenting feature, a thick-walled abscess may cause a subnormal temperature.

Repeated neurologic examinations and continuing nursing assessment of the patient are necessary to determine accurately the location of the abscess. Computed tomography is invaluable in showing the site of the abscess and following the evolution and resolution of suppurative lesions and to determine the optimum time for surgical intervention.

Management.   The goal of management is to eliminate the abscess.

- A neurologic flow chart is maintained and the patient is monitored frequently for signs and symptoms of increased intracranial pressure (see p. 1293), which may result suddenly from cerebral edema caused by a rapidly growing abscess. Secondary compression of the midbrain and brain stem can quickly lead to coma and death.

Cerebral edema may be treated with dexamethasone, although use of this drug is controversial since steroids reduce resistance to infection. Antimicrobial therapy is given to eliminate the causative organism or reduce its virulence. Large doses are necessary to penetrate the abscess cavity until it becomes encapsulated and ready for surgical intervention. Anticonvulsant medications (phenytoin, phenobarbital) may be given as a prophylaxis against seizures. Multiple abscesses may be treated with appropriate antimicrobial therapy alone, with the patient closely followed by computer-assisted tomography.

The definitive treatment of a brain abscess is surgical intervention, either aspiration or excision. Pus may be evacuated by a needle or catheter that is placed through burr holes into the abscess cavity. Or a craniotomy with elevation of bone flap and excision of the abscess is carried out. (See the care of the patient undergoing intracranial surgery, p. 1320.)

Postoperative Management

- Following surgery, drainage may be copious. Dressings are reinforced as soon as they become moist, and strict aseptic technique is maintained. The patient should lie on the operative side to promote drainage.
- The antimicrobial agents are administered on an exact time schedule because *meningitis is an ever-present danger.* These patients must be watched carefully for

retraction of the head, stiffness of the neck, headache, chill, sweats, etc.—symptoms suggestive of a postoperative meningitis.

- It is important that the patient be maintained on a high-calorie diet.

Serial computerized tomographic examinations are carried out to see if the infection has been eradicated. The mortality rate is fairly high and relapse is common. Neurologic deficits following treatment of brain abscess include hemiparesis, seizures, visual defects, and cranial nerve palsies.

Patient Education.   Antimicrobial agents may be continued for 3 to 4 weeks or longer after the brain abscess is excised or drained. It is important that the patient remember to take the prescribed anticonvulsant medication daily for an indefinite period of time.

▷ Multiple Sclerosis

Pathophysiology.   *Multiple sclerosis* (MS) is a chronic, frequently progressive disease of the central nervous system, characterized by the occurrence of small patches of demyelination in the brain and spinal cord. (*Demyelination* refers to the destruction of myelin, the fatty and protein material that ensheathes certain nerve fibers and forms the white matter of the brain and spinal cord.) In this disease, the demyelination is scattered irregularly throughout the central nervous system with relative sparing of the axon (Fig. 58-5). In time, myelin peels off the axis cylinders, and the axons themselves degenerate. The plaques or patches in the involved areas become sclerosed, interrupting the flow of nerve impulses and resulting in a variety of manifestations, depending on which nerves are affected. The areas most frequently affected are the optic nerve and chiasm; the margins of the lateral, third, and fourth ventricles; the pons; medulla and cerebellar peduncles; and the spinal cord.

This is one of the most disabling neurologic diseases of the young adults (20–40 years of age) in this country. Its occurrence among the young maximizes the medical, psychological, social, and economic problems encountered by the patient and the family.

Causes and Epidemiology.   The cause of multiple sclerosis is not known. Research evidence suggests that the plaques and subsequent scars that damage the brain and spinal cord are precipitated by an autoimmune response. Certain individuals with a particular genetic makeup (having certain tissue antigen types) may be more susceptible to the disease. It may be that this defective immune response developed in relation to a persistent viral infection of the nervous system. There has been a great deal of interest in the role of a slow virus in causing the disease. Although the initiating mechanism may stem from some form of viral infection, a defective immune response probably plays a major role in the pathogenesis of multiple sclerosis.

Epidemiologic factors have been the subject of much research. Findings indicate that this disease is rare in tropical countries. It is aggravated by extremes of temperature, especially heat. Relapses are often associated with periods of emotional and physical stress (illness, injuries, inoculations).

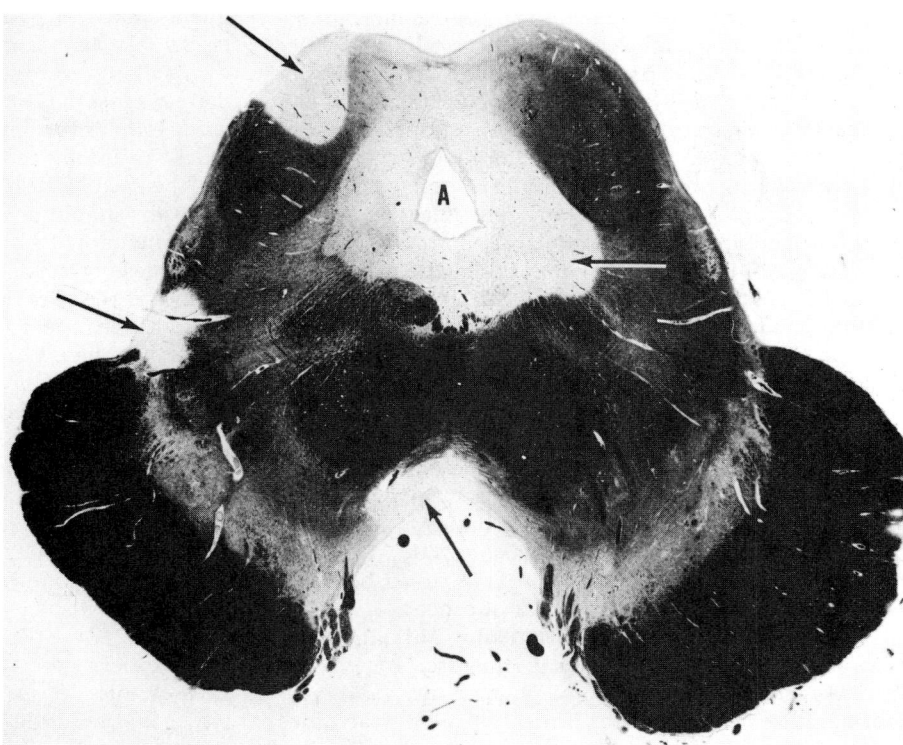

Figure 58-5. Cross section from the midbrain (enlarged approximately three times) of a patient with chronic MS. Specimen stained to show myelin (black). The four white areas indicated by the arrows are typical plaques in which the myelin has been destroyed. The plaque to the right of the aqueduct (*A*) impinges upon periaqueductal gray matter. The nerve fibers in these plaques have lost their myelin sheaths, and as a consequence, conduction of stimuli in these areas would be impeded or lost. (Courtesy of Cedric S. Raine, M.D., Professor of Pathology [Neuropathology] and Neuroscience. Albert Einstein College of Medicine of Yeshiva University.)

▶ Assessment

Clinical Manifestations. The signs and symptoms of MS involve sensory, motor, and coordinative dysfunctions. They are varied and multiple, reflecting the location of the demyelination within the central nervous system.

Early symptoms of MS can be easily mistaken for neurosis, peripheral neuropathy, or spinal lesions, since many systems or parts of the body are involved. Symptoms include visual disturbances due to lesions in the optic nerves or their connections; nystagmus; transient diplopia; blurring of vision; patchy blindness (scotoma); or total blindness. Speech impairment may be manifested by "scanning" speech (slow, monotonous, and slurred). Gait and extremity ataxia may be present due to involvement of the cerebellum. Motor dysfunction with loss of muscle tone and tremor is encountered. Spastic weakness of the extremities and loss of the abdominal reflexes are due to involvement of the main motor pathways (pyramidal tracts) of the spinal cord. Emotional hyperexcitability and inappropriate euphoria result from loss of the control connections between the cortex and the basal ganglia. Vertigo, with nausea and vomiting, may occur if the vestibular nuclei or their connections are diseased; bladder, rectal, and sexual problems also occur if the process involves the cord pathways connected with the sacral plexus. The most common group of symptoms includes spastic paraplegia with slight speech disturbance and nystagmus.

The disease is characterized by remissions and exacerbations or steady progression. However, as evidenced by CT scanning, many plaques do not produce serious symptoms and many patients are not seriously incapacitated, hav-

ing periods of remissions between episodes. The prognosis for a fairly prolonged life is good.

Diagnostic Assessment. Diagnosis is based on clinical judgment, results of tests to determine alteration in color vision, and the cerebrospinal fluid examination, which may reveal a significant elevation of IgG and oligoclonal bands. In some instances, CT scans and evoked potential studies are helpful. Nuclear magnetic resonance scans, where available, have become a primary diagnostic tool for showing white–gray differentiation in the brain.

Patient Problems/Nursing Diagnoses

Based on the clinical manifestations and diagnostic assessment data, the patient's potential nursing problems include alterations in sensory function, impaired physical mobility, and impaired bladder function related to the demyelination process; self-care deficits related to effects of the disease, and psychosocial problems related to coping with MS and social isolation.

▶ Planning and Implementation

Goals

The major goals for the patient include:

1. Coping with alterations in sensory function
2. Adaption to impaired physical mobility
3. Improvement in bladder function
4. Participation in self-care activities
5. Coping with psychological problems

The goals of nursing are *to keep the patient functional* and in as good physical condition as possible, to manage symptoms caused by demyelination, to combat muscle dysfunction and contracture deformities, to establish bladder and bowel training, to prevent complications (urinary infections, pressure sores), and to improve the quality of life. The nursing framework also centers on the person faced with chronic demyelinating disease, and focuses on social and psychological problems of chronic disease. An individualized program of physical therapy, rehabilitation, and education is combined with emotional support.

Relieving the Symptoms.
At this time, there is no cure for MS, but an individualized, organized, and rational treatment program can relieve the patient's symptoms and provide him with continuing support. Since there are possible immune mechanisms in the pathogenesis of MS, immunosuppressive drugs (corticosteroids, alkylating agents, and antimetabolites) are being evaluated in selected patients. ACTH may be beneficial in shortening the duration of the acute attack, possibly due to the drug's anti-inflammatory and antiedema properties, which may improve nerve conduction. Alkylating agents (cyclophosphamide) and antimetabolites (azathioprine) may control symptoms, but long-term treatment may increase the risk of cancer.

Promoting Functional Improvement.
Although rehabilitation measures will not alter the disease process, it is the aim of the rehabilitation program to bring about functional improvement, so that the patient can perform activities of daily living whether he is ambulatory, in a wheelchair, or confined to bed. If the patient's disease is not progressing too rapidly, the goal is to return the patient to satisfying employment or to keep him happily engaged in his present employment. An individualized therapeutic program is established after an appraisal has been made of the extent of disability and muscle strength.

Sometimes the patient presents the clinical picture of hemiplegia, although more commonly he may have the same disabilities as the patient with paraplegia. Any one extremity or combination of extremities may be involved. Therefore, the principles of rehabilitation of these conditions can be used for the patient who has similar problems due to MS (see p. 1312).

Combating Muscle Dysfunction.
Daily exercises for muscle stretching are prescribed to minimize joint contractures. Special attention is given to hamstrings, gastrocnemius muscles, hip adductors, biceps, and wrist and finger flexors. Muscle spasticity is common and interferes with normal function. A stretch–hold–relax routine is helpful for relaxing and treating muscle spasticity. Swimming and stationary bicycling are useful, while progressive weight bearing will relieve spasticity in the legs. Baclofen (Lioresal) may be given for spasticity.

Patients with severe spasticity and contractures may require surgical intervention to prevent further disability.

Relaxation and coordination exercises promote muscle efficiency. Progressive resistive exercises are used to strengthen weak muscles since diminishing muscle power is a significant problem. The patient is encouraged to work up to the point just short of fatigue. However, prolonged exercise that fatigues an extremity may cause paresis, numbness, or incoordination. The patient is advised to take frequent short rest periods, preferably lying down. Extreme fatigue may be a contributing factor in exacerbation.

Walking exercises improve the gait, paticularly when there is a loss of position sense of the legs. If certain muscle groups are irreversibly affected, other muscles can be trained to take over their action. Warm packs and muscle relaxants may be beneficial if painful muscle spasm is present, but hot baths should be avoided.

If motor dysfunction causes problems of incoordination, clumsiness or ataxia may be apparent. To overcome this disability, the patient can be taught to walk with his feet wide apart in order to widen the base of support and increase walking stability. A cane or walker affords additional support. If incoordination and intention tremor of the upper extremities occur, weighted bracelets or wrist cuffs are helpful. The patient is trained in transfer activities and activities of daily living to promote as much independence as possible.

Progressive Dysfunction.
Exacerbation of the disease may reflect some internal or external environmental change. During periods of exacerbation of the disease, the patient is encouraged to reduce activity or remain resting in a chair or on bedrest since continued activity appears to worsen the attack. Any aspects of the patient's life-style that might cause exacerbation—exposure to heat/cold, psychologic stresses, infections (particularly urinary), trauma, and electrolyte and water disturbances—should be avoided.

As the patient's disease progresses, self-help devices that include feeding devices, handrails, canes, braces, wheelchairs, and ramps are utilized to maintain independence for as long as possible. Corrective action is taken as each new problem arises. Creative nursing calls for inventiveness, adaptation, and modification of equipment that can be used for self-help devices so that the patient will not lose ground.

Bladder and Bowel Training.
Management of bladder and bowel control are among the patient's most difficult problems if sphincter control is impaired. Bladder dysfunction may lead to progressive renal failure. A high level of fluid input helps to reduce the urinary bacterial count and minimizes precipitation of urinary crystals and subsequent stone formation. Ascorbic acid may be given to acidify the urine.

The patient with urinary frequency, urgency, or incontinence requires special support. Drugs to treat bladder dysfunction (oxybutynin) may be helpful to relieve bladder spasticity and allow the patient greater independence. The sensation of the need to void must be heeded immediately, hence the bedpan or urinal should be readily available. A voiding time schedule should be set up (every 1½–2 hours initially, with gradually lengthening time intervals). The patient is instructed to drink a measured amount of fluid every 2 hours and then attempts to void 30 minutes after drinking. An alarm clock may be set for the patient with diminished warning sensation.

If the female patient has permanent urinary incontinence, a urinary diversion procedure (ileal conduit) may have to be performed. The male patient may wear a condom appliance for urine collection. Intermittent self-catheterization may be utilized.

Bowel problems include constipation, fecal impaction, and incontinence. A bowel-training program is effective for these problems (see p. 251).

Sensory Impairment.   Measures may be taken if optic and speech defects occur (the cranial nerves relating to sight and speech are affected by MS). An eye patch or an eyeglass occluder may be used to block visual impulses of one eye when the patient has diplopia (double vision). Prism glasses may be helpful for the bedridden patient. When the vision begins to fail, painting the cane tip and shoe tips with fluorescent paint helps. Persons with any physical limitations preventing them from reading regular print materials are eligible for the free talking book services of the Library of Congress (address at end of chapter).

When the cranial nerves controlling the mechanisms of speech are involved, dysarthrias (defects of articulation) marked by slurring, low volume of speech, and difficulties in phonation are seen. There are problems with shallow breathing and low breath pressure. A speech pathologist may recommend therapy to alleviate these problems.

Since sensory loss may occur in addition to motor loss, pressure sores are a continuing threat to skin integrity. Confinement to a wheelchair compounds the threat. (See pp. 238–242 for a discussion of the prevention and treatment of pressure sores.)

Sexuality and Multiple Sclerosis.   MS patients (and their partners) face problems that interfere with sexual activity: easy fatigability, conflicts arising from dependency and depression, emotional lability, and loss of self-esteem and self-worth. All of these affect sexual relationships. Difficulties with sustaining an erection and impotence in males, and adductor spasms of the thigh muscles in females, can make intercourse difficult or impossible. Bladder and bowel incontinence and urinary tract infections compound the problem.

Through sharing and communicating feelings, planning for sexual activity (to counteract fatigue), exercising different sexual options, and demonstrating a willingness to experiment may open up a wide range of sexual enjoyment and experiences. The booklet *Sexuality and Multiple Sclerosis* by Michael Barrett, published by the Multiple Sclerosis Society of Canada, contains practical information as well as suggested readings.

Psychological Support and Patient Education.   MS imposes numerous stresses on the patient and the family. Embarrassing and humiliating symptoms may result in "inappropriate" responses by the patient. As there may be organic changes in the brain, MS patients may be forgetful and easily distracted and may show emotional instability. Patients adapt to illness in a variety of ways—denial (with euphoria), depression, withdrawal, and hostility. Compassion and significant emotional support are required to help the patient adapt to a new identity as a handicapped person (a new self-image) and cope with the disruption in his life. Help the patient set meaningful and realistic short-term goals to achieve a sense of purpose. The patient should be encouraged to remain in the mainstream of life as much as possible and to keep up social interests and activities. Hobbies help the patient's morale and provide satisfying interests when the disease has progressed to the stage in which normal activities cannot be pursued.

The nurse has the responsibility of emphasizing to the patient and the family the importance of a regular program of exercise, work, and recreation. Once certain abilities are lost, they are almost impossible to regain. Physical abilities may vary from day to day. Modifications that allow continuance of self-care activities should be sought (raised toilet seat, bathing helps, telephone modifications, long-handled comb, tongs, modified clothing). Physical and emotional stresses should be avoided as much as possible, since these worsen symptoms and impair performance. Exposure to heat appears to increase fatigue, and fatigue lessens motor power. Air-conditioning in at least one room is recommended. Exposure to extreme cold may increase spasticity. The patient must remain under continuing medical supervision.

Encourage the patient to contact the local chapter of the National Multiple Sclerosis Society for services, publications, and contact with other MS patients. Local chapters give direct services to patients. Through group participation, the patient has an opportunity to identify with others having similar problems, gain relief and release, and learn self-help methods in a social environment.

▶ Evaluation

Expected Outcomes

1. Adjusts to alterations in sensory function
   a. Participates in gait-training program
   b. Inspects skin twice daily for evidence of pressure sores
   c. Uses eye patch or occluder attached to eyeglasses during periods of diplopia
   d. Watches hands while performing tasks to compensate for decreased sense of touch/position sense
   e. Uses large-print books from public library
   f. Verbalizes that "talking books" are available
2. Adapts to impaired physical mobility
   a. Establishes balanced program of rest and exercise
   b. Arranges schedule to accommodate periods of high energy levels
   c. Avoids exposure to infection
   d. Avoids heat
   e. Is able to ask for help
   f. Identifies measures designed to conserve energy
   g. Reads about work-simplification techniques
   h. Uses assistive devices when necessary
3. Attains/maintains improved bladder function
   a. Maintains 2000 ml to 3000 ml fluid intake/24 hours (if urinary retention is not a problem)
   b. Tests urinary pH daily
   c. Performs bacteriologic test on urine; identifies necessity for calling physician at the first sign of infection
   d. Monitors self for urine retention
   e. Employs self-catheterization as needed
4. Participates in self-care activities
   a. Uses assistive devices
   b. Reports to occupational therapist/physical therapist

for evaluation of function and instruction in adapting to changing function

5. Copes with psychological problems
   a. Allows self to grieve for change in life-style and altered self-image
   b. Makes plans to redesign life-style
   c. Makes lists to compensate for memory losses
   d. Discusses problems with trusted advisor/friend
   e. Substitutes new activities for those that have to be given up
   f. Has joined MS support group
   g. Contacts Vocational Office of Rehabilitation

▷ Parkinson's Disease

Parkinson's disease is a progressive neurologic disorder affecting the brain centers that are responsible for control and regulation of movement. It is characterized by bradykinesia (slowness of movement), tremor, and muscle stiffness or rigidity.

Pathophysiology.   The major lesion appears to result in a loss of pigmented neurons, particularly those in the substantia nigra of the brain. (The *substantia nigra* is a collection of midbrain nuclei that project fibers to the corpus striatum). One of the major neurotransmitters in this area of the brain, and in other parts of the central nervous system, is dopamine, which has an important inhibiting function in the central control of movement. Although dopamine normally exists in high concentration in certain parts of the brain, in Parkinson's disease it is depleted in the substantia nigra and the corpus striatum. Depletion of dopamine levels in the basal ganglia is associated with bradykinesia, rigidity, and tremors.

In the majority of patients, the cause of the disease is unknown. Arteriosclerotic parkinsonism is seen more frequently in older age groups. It may follow encephalitis, poisoning or toxicity (manganese, carbon monoxide) or hypoxia, or may be drug-induced.

The disease most frequently attacks persons in their 50s and 60s and is the second most common neurologic disorder of the elderly.

▶ Assessment
Clinical Manifestations.   The chief manifestations of Parkinson's disease are impaired movement, muscular rigidity, tremor, muscle weakness, and loss of postural reflexes. Early signs include a stiffening of the extremities and a wax-like rigidity in the performance of all movements. The patient has difficulty in initiating, maintaining, and performing motor activities, and experiences some delay in carrying out normal activity. As the disease progresses, the tremor begins, frequently in one hand and arm, then the other, and later in the head, although the tremor may remain unilateral (Fig. 58-6).

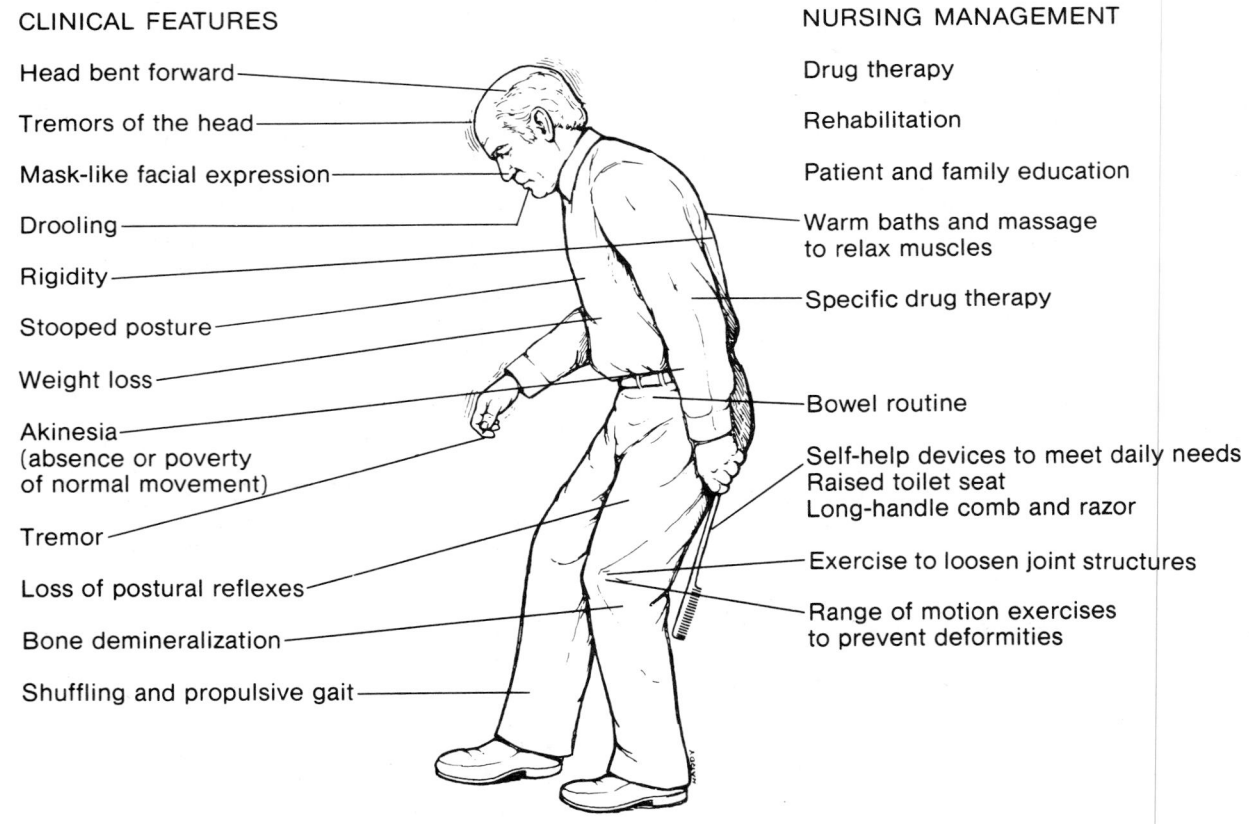

CLINICAL FEATURES

Head bent forward
Tremors of the head
Mask-like facial expression
Drooling
Rigidity
Stooped posture
Weight loss
Akinesia
(absence or poverty
of normal movement)
Tremor
Loss of postural reflexes
Bone demineralization
Shuffling and propulsive gait

NURSING MANAGEMENT

Drug therapy
Rehabilitation
Patient and family education
Warm baths and massage
to relax muscles
Specific drug therapy
Bowel routine
Self-help devices to meet daily needs
Raised toilet seat
Long-handle comb and razor
Exercise to loosen joint structures
Range of motion exercises
to prevent deformities

Figure 58-6.   Clinical manifestations and nursing management of the patient with parkinsonism.

The tremor is characteristic; it is a slow, turning motion (pronation–supination) of the forearm and the hand, and a motion of the thumb against the fingers, as if rolling a pill between the fingers. If the patient gets excited, the tremor becomes worse; when he makes a voluntary motion, it ceases, allowing him to perform the most delicate acts, such as picking up a pin.

Other characteristics of the disease affect the face, stature, and gait. There is loss of normal arm swing. Eventually, the rigid limbs become definitely weaker. Since there is limited movement in the muscles, the face has so little expression that it is said to be masklike (with infrequency of blinking), a feature that can be recognized at a glance.

There is a loss of postural reflexes, and the patient stands with his head bent forward and walks as if in danger of falling on his face. Difficulty in pivoting and loss of balance (either forward or backward) may lead to frequent falls.

Frequently, these patients show signs of depression, and it has not been established whether the depression is reactive or related to a biochemical abnormality. Mental manifestations may appear in the form of cognitive, perceptual, and memory deficits. Mental confusion may be a feature of the disease as well as a side-effect of drug treatment.

Patient Problems/Nursing Diagnoses

Based on the clinical manifestations and diagnostic assessment data, the patient's major nursing problems include impaired mobility related to muscle rigidity and weakness; potential for injury (falling) related to displaced center of gravity; self-care deficits (feeding, hygiene, dressing, toileting) related to motor dysfunction and tremors; and depression related to dysfunction from progression of disease.

▶ **Planning and Implementation**

Goals

The major goals for the patient include:

1. Improved mobility
2. Absence of falling
3. Independence in activities of daily living
4. Improved emotional outlook
5. Adherence to the therapeutic regimen

The nursing goal is to *keep the patient functionally useful and productive for as long as possible.* This is done with appropriate drug therapy, physical therapy, rehabilitation techniques, and patient and family education.

Pharmacotherapy

Drug therapy for persons with Parkinson's disease is aimed at restoring the deficiency of dopaminergic activities and includes antihistamines, anticholinergics, amantadine, and levodopa.

Antihistamine Drugs. Antihistamine drugs (diphenhydramine [Benadryl], orphenadrine [Disipal] have mild central anticholinergic and sedative effects, and may be helpful in allaying tremors.

Anticholinergic Therapy. Anticholinergic drugs, such as trihexyphenidyl (Artane), cycrimine (Pagitane), procyclidine (Kemadrin), and benztropine mesylate (Cogentin) continue to be useful for patients who have a mild disability or those who respond poorly to levodopa or are sensitive to it. These anticholinergic drugs may also be used in combination with levodopa. They counteract the action of acetylcholine in the central nervous system. (Relative cholinergic dominance appears to play a role in symptomatology.) With the administration of anticholinergics there is some degree of impairment of mental acuity, ranging from mild difficulty in concentration and recall to confusion and hallucinations. Other side-effects include dry mouth, blurred vision, flushing, rash, constipation, and urinary hesitancy. Patients with prostatic hyperplasia as well as Parkinson's disease must be monitored for urinary retention, which may result from a combined effect of the enlarged prostate and the drug treatment for parkinsonism.

Amantadine Hydrochloride. *Amantadine hydrochloride* (Symmetrel), an antiviral agent, is used in the early treatment of Parkinson's disease and is thought to enhance the release of endogenous stores of dopamine from the presynaptic neuron. It has been shown to reduce rigidity, tremor, and bradykinesia with a low risk of adverse reactions.

Levodopa Therapy. Levodopa (Dopar, Larodopa), constitutes an important facet of treatment and is useful in the treatment of moderate parkinsonism. Early efforts to replace dopamine were unsuccessful, since dopamine would not cross the blood–brain barrier (a protective biochemical mechanism that screens substances passing from the blood into the cells of the central nervous system). However, levodopa (a precursor of dopamine) was found to be effective because it traverses the blood–brain barrier. Levodopa is not a cure for parkinsonism but is effective in controlling symptoms, particularly bradykinesia and rigidity, for a period of time. However, levodopa must be given in large enough doses and for a long enough period of time to build up an effective and stable blood level. The dosage is increased gradually until side-effects begin to appear, including nausea, vomiting, anorexia, postural hypotension, mental changes (confusion, agitation, mood alterations), cardiac arrhythmias, and twitching.

The beneficial effects of levodopa are most pronounced in the first few years of treatment. Benefits to the patient begin to wane and adverse side-effects become more severe with the passage of time. Confusion, hallucinations, depression, and sleep alterations are associated with prolonged use of the drug. The patient may experience an "on–off" reaction in which he has sudden periods of near immobility ("off effect") lasting minutes to hours followed by sudden return of effectiveness ("on effect"). Dyskinesias (involuntary movements) are fairly common side-effects of levodopa therapy.

Levodopa is now usually given in combination with a decarboxylase inhibitor, carbidopa, which slows down the peripheral metabolism of dopa. The administration of carbidopa with levodopa makes more levodopa available for transport to the brain. Sinemet (a combination of carbidopa and levodopa) potentiates the therapeutic effects of levodopa by blocking extracerebral metabolism of levodopa, thus permitting a reduction in the dosage level and incidence of side-effects.

Dopamine Agonists. These drugs mimic the action of dopamine by directly affecting the postsynaptic receptors in the striatum. They bypass the enzymatic conversion of levodopa to dopamine. Bromocriptine and lergotrile are ergot alkaloids that have been shown to give improvement.

Antidepressant Drugs. *Antidepressant drugs* (imipramine [Tofranil], amitriptyline [Elavil]) are given to alleviate depression.

Surgical Intervention. In some selected patients, surgery may be effective in providing some relief of tremor and rigidity that encompasses one side of the body. The purpose of the surgery is to destroy a part of the thalamus (stereotaxic thalamotomy) in order to relieve certain types of excessive muscle contraction.

The stereotaxic technique allows the neurosurgeon to precisely position and localize a small target deep within the brain. Special guiding instruments and rapid x-rays are used to place an electrode or freezing probe with pinpoint precision in the target area of the brain. A lesion is then created at that point.

Although this procedure provides a certain amount of relief, it does not alter the course of Parkinson's disease, nor does it assure permanent improvement.

Measures to Improve Mobility and Activities of Daily Living

Exercise. A progressive program of daily exercise will increase muscle strength, improve coordination and dexterity, reduce muscular rigidity, and prevent contractures that occur when muscles are not used. Walking, riding a stationary bicycle, swimming, and gardening are all exercises that help maintain joint mobility. Stretching exercises (stretch–hold–relax) will help loosen the joint structures. Postural exercises are important to counter the tendency of the head and neck to be drawn forward and down. Special walking techniques must also be learned to offset the shuffling gait and the tendency to lean forward. There are defective balancing reflexes. The patient may also walk off balance because of the rigidity of his arms. (Arm swinging is necessary in normal walking.) The patient is taught early in the course of the disease to concentrate on walking erect, to keep his eyes on the horizon and to use a broad-based gait (*i.e.*, walking with the feet separated). A conscious effort must be made to swing the arms and raise the feet while walking and to use a heel–toe, heel–toe gait in fairly long strides. Breathing exercises while walking help to mobilize the rib cage. Frequent rest periods are important during the training period to avoid fatigue and frustration.

Warm baths and massages in addition to passive and active exercises help relax muscles and relieve painful muscle spasms that accompany rigidity.

Environmental modifications are necessary to compensate for functional disabilities. These patients have difficulty turning in bed and getting in and out of bed. Bedside rails or a rope tied to the foot of the bed will provide assistance in pulling up without help. A bedside commode is important.

Speech. The low-pitched, monotonous, soft speech of the patient with parkinsonism requires that he make a real effort to speak slowly with deliberate effort and attention. Remind the patient to face the listener, exaggerate the pronunciation of words, and speak in short sentences. A speech–language pathologist may be helpful in designing speech-improvement exercises. A small, electronic amplifier (such as that used by the laryngectomee) is useful if the patient has a weak voice.

Bowel Routine. A patient with parkinsonism has severe problems with constipation. Among the factors causing this condition are weakness of the muscles used in defecation, lack of exercise, an inadequate fluid intake, and decreased autonomic nervous system activity. The drugs used for the treatment of the disease also inhibit normal intestinal secretions. A regular bowel routine may be established by encouraging the patient to follow a regular habit time, consciously increase fluid intake, and eat foods with a moderate fiber content. A raised toilet seat is a useful device to facilitate toilet activities, since the patient has difficulty in changing from a standing to a sitting position.

Nutritional Considerations. The patient also has a problem in keeping his weight up. He becomes embarrassed by his slowness and untidiness in eating. His mouth is dry from the medications, and he experiences difficulty in chewing and swallowing. (This last factor can result in aspiration pneumonia, which occurs fairly commonly in this disease.) Some patients have saliva buildup due to a slow rate of swallowing. Because of problems in eating, the patient in time suffers a considerable weight loss. Demineralization starts in the bones as a result of malnutrition. Thus, there is the added threat of fractures occurring should the patient fall. Supplementary feedings will keep calorie intake up, and an electrical warming tray will keep food hot and permit the patient to rest during the prolonged time that it takes to eat. A stabilized plate, nonspill cup, and built-up eating utensils are useful self-help devices. Teach the patient to place the food on his tongue, close his lips and teeth, and lift the tongue up, then back, and swallow.

Promoting Psychological Well-being and Self-care

Help the patient set achievable goals (*e.g.*, improvement of mobility). Since parkinsonism tends to lead to withdrawal and depression, the patient must be an *active* participant in his therapeutic program, including social and recreational events. There should be a planned program of activity throughout the day to prevent too much daytime sleeping as well as disinterest and apathy.

Every effort should be made to encourage the patient to carry out his own daily needs and to retain his independence. "Doing things" for the patient merely to save time runs contrary to this basic goal of management.

Faithful adherence to an exercise and walking program helps to delay the progress of the disease. Encouragement and reassurance can be given by praising the patient for his perseverance and pointing out that his activities are being maintained through active participation. A combination of physiotherapy, psychotherapy, drug therapy, and sociotherapy may be necessary to help combat the depression that so often accompanies this condition.

Patient Education. It is important that the patient understand this ailment and that every effort be made to explain the nature of the disease in order to offset anxieties and fears that may be as disabling as the disease. The disease may be described as one that affects a small motor control station at the base of the brain. Although it progresses in severity, it does so very slowly, with lengthy periods of 5 to 15 years occurring between stages in the progression of symptoms. The American Parkinson's Disease Foundation publishes illustrated booklets and a newsletter for patient education (see discussion under Exercise, Speech, Bowel Routine, Nutritional Considerations for other aspects of patient education).

▶ **Evaluation**

Expected Outcomes

1. Strives toward improved mobility
   a. Participates in therapeutic exercise program *daily*
   b. Demonstrates techniques of muscle relaxation
   c. Identifies necessity of reporting for joint range evaluation at specified intervals
   d. Has information about availability of catapult spring seats, self-help devices
2. Uses mobility techniques to avoid falls
   a. Sits on side of bed for a time before standing
   b. Walks with a wide base of support, feet about 10 inches apart, and with a lengthened stride
   c. Consciously raises his feet when walking
   d. Exaggerates normal arm swing when walking
   e. Practices "marching" to music
3. Progresses toward independence in activities of daily living
   a. Uses self-help devices and environmental aids for hygiene
   b. Uses modified clothing for self-help in dressing
   c. Plans activities to avoid rushing
4. Strives toward improved emotional outlook
   a. Sets realistic goals
   b. Undertakes a planned program of daily activities
   c. Schedules frequent rest periods to avoid frustration
   d. Verbalizes his feelings about his life-style changes
   e. Discusses with family ways to maintain normal life-style
5. Adheres to therapeutic regimen
   a. Takes medication as prescribed
   b. Verbalizes that he understands the importance of a well-balanced diet with moderate fiber content

▷ **Huntington's Disease**

Huntington's disease is a chronic progressive neurologic disease of hereditary origin that affects men and women of all races. Because it is transmitted as an autosomal dominant genetic disorder, each child of a parent with Huntington's disease has a 50% risk of inheriting the illness.

The basic pathology involves an unexplained loss of cells in the basal ganglia and portions of the cerebral cortex. Research suggests that the disease may be related to a lack of important brain chemicals (gamma-aminobutyric acid [GABA] and acetylcholine [ACh]) that inhibit nerve action. Onset usually occurs between the ages of 35 and 45; the patient slowly progresses toward death in 10 to 20 years. Approximately 10% of victims are children. There is at present no means of detecting the Huntington's disease gene before symptoms appear.

Assessment and Clinical Manifestations

The most prominent clinical features of the disease are abnormal involuntary movements (chorea), intellectual decline, and, often, emotional disturbance. As the disease progresses, a constant writhing, twisting, uncontrollable movement may involve the entire body. These motions are devoid of purpose or rhythm, although patients may try to turn them into purposeful movement. All of the body musculature is involved. Facial movements produce tics and grimaces. Speech is affected, becoming slurred, hesitant, often explosive, and eventually unintelligible. Chewing and swallowing are difficult and there is a constant danger of choking and aspiration. Like speech, the gait becomes disorganized to the point that ambulation eventually is impossible. Although independent ambulation should be encouraged for as long as possible, a wheelchair is usually necessary at some point (eventually, the patient is confined to bed, as the chorea interferes with walking, sitting, and all activities). Bladder and bowel control is lost. The sensorium likewise is usually involved. There is progressive intellectual impairment, although the patient is generally aware that the disease is responsible for the myriad dysfunctions he experiences.

The mental and emotional changes may be more devastating to the patient and family than the abnormal movements. Patients may be nervous, clumsy, irritable, or impatient. Particularly in the early stages of the illness, patients are subject to uncontrollable fits of anger; profound, often suicidal depression; apathy; or euphoria. Judgment and memory are impaired. Hallucinations, delusions, and paranoid thinking may even precede the appearance of disjointed movements. Emotional symptoms often become less acute as the disease progresses, although dementia eventually ensues. Despite a ravenous appetite, often for sweets, patients usually become emaciated and exhausted. Eventually, patients succumb from heart failure, pneumonia, or infection, or die as a result of a fall or choking.

Management

Although no treatment halts or reverses the underlying process, several methods of management have fairly good palliative action. The phenothiazine or butyrophenone antipsychotic drugs improve the chorea in many cases. Haloperidol (Haldol), fluphenazine (Prolixin), mesoridazine (Serentil), trifluoperazine (Stelazine), chlorpromazine (Thorazine), and perphenazine (Triavil, Trilafon) are being used in this country. The patient's motor signs must be assessed and evaluated on a continuing basis so that optimal therapeutic drug levels may be reached. Akathisia (motor restlessness) in the overmedicated patient is a danger since it may be mistaken for the restless fidgetiness of the illness and consequently be overlooked.

In certain types of the disease in which hypokinetic motor impairment resembles parkinsonism, some benefit may be obtained from antiparkinsonism therapy (see p. 1347). Patients who have emotional disturbances, particularly depression, may be helped by antidepressant medications. Psychotic symptoms usually respond to antipsychotic drugs. Psychotherapy aimed at allaying anxiety and reducing stress may be beneficial. It is imperative that nurses look beyond the disease to focus on the patient's needs and capabilities (Chart 58-2).

A program combining medical, psychological, social, occupational, speech, and physical rehabilitation services is needed to help the patient and family cope with this severely disabling illness. More than most disorders, Huntington's disease exacts enormous emotional, physical, social, and financial tolls on every member of the patient's family. Since there is no test to determine the carriers of the disease, entire families often live under a heavy burden of uncertainty, anxiety, and guilt. Not only is genetic counseling crucial, but patients and their families also require access to long-term psychological counseling, marriage counseling, and emotional, financial, and legal support. Some form of home care assistance, work and recreation day centers, respite care, and eventually skilled long-term care is necessary to help the patient and family cope with the constant strain of the illness. Although nothing can stop the relentless progress of the disease, families who have had good care have benefited tremendously.

Voluntary Health Organizations.   Voluntary health organizations are major aids to families and have been largely responsible for bringing the illness to national attention. The Committee to Combat Huntington's Disease and the National Huntington's Disease Association are oriented toward helping patients and their families by providing information, referrals, family and public education, and support for research.

▷ Neuromuscular Diseases

Myasthenia Gravis

Myasthenia gravis is a disorder affecting the neuromuscular transmission of the voluntary muscles of the body; it is char-

---

Chart 58-2
The Challenges of a Patient With Huntington's Disease

Nursing Goal: To develop creative approaches until the complex needs of the patient are met

Problem	*Nursing Approach*
Constant movement	Pad the sides and head of the bed.
	Use lamb's wool padding for heel and elbow protection.
Skin excoriation	Keep the skin meticulously clean.
Abrasions or pressure sores	Apply emollient cleansing agent and skin lotion frequently.
	Use *soft* sheets and bedding.
Falls	Encourage ambulation with assistance to maintain muscle tone. Tie the patient (only if absolutely necessary) in bed or chair with padded protective devices, making sure that they are loosened frequently.
Feeding*	
Constant movement	Give phenothiazines before meals; appears to calm some patients.
Difficulty in chewing or swallowing	Talk to the patient before mealtime to help him relax; use mealtime for social
Choking/Aspiration	interaction. Give your undivided attention.
Malnutrition	Learn the position that is best for *this* patient. Keep patient as close to upright as
Dehydration	possible while feeding. Stabilize patient's head gently with one hand while feeding.
Emaciation	Encircle patient with one arm and get as close as possible to provide stability and support. Use pillows and wedges for additional support.
	Do not interpret stiffness, turning away, or sudden turning of head as rejection; these are uncontrollable choreiform movements.
	Use a long-handled spoon (iced-tea spoon). Place spoon on middle of tongue and exert slight pressure.
	Place bite-size food between teeth. Serve stews, casseroles, thick liquids; avoid too many milk drinks (produces mucus).
	Use dysphagia therapy.
	Disregard "messiness." Treat the person with dignity.
	Wait for patient to chew and swallow before introducing another spoonful. Make sure that bite-sized food is small.

(continued)

acterized by excessive fatigability of muscle function. It affects younger women; men who develop the disease do so later in life.

Pathophysiology. The basic abnormality in myasthenia gravis is a defect in the transmission of impulses from nerve to muscle cells due to loss of available or normal receptors on the postsynaptic side of the neuromuscular junction. Myasthenia gravis is considered an autoimmune disease in which antibodies directed against acetylcholine receptor (AChR) impair neuromuscular transmission.

Assessment
Clinical Manifestations. The disease is characterized by *extreme muscular weakness* and easy fatigability, which generally is worse after effort and is relieved by rest. Patients with this disease tire on such slight exertion as combing the hair, chewing, and talking, and must stop for rest. Symptoms vary according to the muscles affected. Symmetrical muscles are involved, first and foremost those innervated by cranial nerves. Because of the involvement of the ocular

muscles, diplopia (double vision) and ptosis (drooping) of the eyelids are early symptoms. The patient has a sleepy, masklike expression because the facial muscles are affected. Weakness of the laryngeal and pharyngeal muscles causes the voice to be weak and presents a danger of choking and aspiration of food. *Progressive weakness of the diaphragm and intercostal muscles may produce respiratory distress or myasthenic crisis, which is an acute emergency.*

Diagnostic Assessment. The signs and symptoms of myasthenia gravis are sometimes so striking that a presumptive diagnosis can be made on the basis of the patient's history and physical examination. An injection of edrophonium (Tensilon), a drug that facilitates the transmission of nerve–muscle messages, is used to confirm the diagnosis. Within 30 seconds of an intravenous injection of edrophonium, most patients will improve substantially, but only temporarily. Improvement in muscle strength following administration of this agent usually confirms the diagnosis of myasthenia. Measurement of the anti-AChR antibody in the serum is a reliable adjunct to the edrophonium (Tensilon)

Chart 58-2
The Challenges of a Patient With Huntington's Disease (continued)

Problem (continued)	Nursing Approach (continued)
	Give between-meal feedings. Constant movement burns more calories. Patients are often voracious, particularly for sweets.
	Use *blenderized meals* if patient cannot chew; do not give the same strained baby foods.
	For swallowing difficulties:
	Rub fingers in circles on patient's cheeks.
	Rub fingers simultaneously down each side of patient's throat.
	Know the Heimlich maneuver (to be used in the event of choking).

Psychological support and communication
  Grimacing
  Unintelligible speech
	Respect the patient as a fellow human being with rights and needs.
	Use eye contact. Touch the patient.
	Talk, even though the patient may not be able to answer.
	Read to the patient.
	Employ biofeedback and relaxation therapy to reduce stress.
	Use speech and language therapy to help maintain and prolong communication abilities.
	Try to devise a communication system, perhaps using cards with words or pictures of familiar objects, before verbal communication becomes too difficult.
	Patients can indicate correct card by hitting it with hand, grunting, or blinking the eyes.
	Learn how this particular patient expresses needs and wants; particularly nonverbal messages (widening of eyes, responses).
	Patient can understand even if he cannot speak. Do not isolate patient by ceasing to communicate with him.

Progressive intellectual impairment and emotional disturbance	Have a clock, calendar, and wall posters in view. Interact with the patient in a *creative* manner. Use every opportunity for one-to-one contact. Use music for relaxation. Keep patient in the social mainstream. Recruit and train volunteers for social interaction. Set a good example. Do not abandon a patient because the disease is eventually terminal. Patients are *living* until the end.

* (Adapted from Perske R et al: Mealtimes for Severely and Profoundly Handicapped Persons, Baltimore, University Park Press, 1977.)

test. Electromyography (EMG) is used to measure the electrical potential of muscle cells.

Management

The patient's goals are to improve strength and endurance, and in addition, the therapeutic aim is to achieve permanent remission. The management is based on (1) improvement of remaining function by anticholinesterase medications, (2) reduction of antibodies, and (3) removal of circulating antibodies.

Anticholinesterase drugs are given to increase the response of the muscles to nerve impulses and to improve strength.

Drugs in current use include pryridostigmine bromide (Mestinon), ambenonium chloride (Mytelase), and neostigmine bromide (Prostigmin). Most patients prefer pyridostigmine because it produces less marked side-effects. The dosage is increased gradually until maximal benefits are obtained (additional strength, less fatigue), although normal muscle strength may not be achieved, and the patient may have to adapt to some disability. Anticholinesterase medications are given with milk, crackers, or other buffering substances. Their side-effects include abdominal cramps, nausea, and vomiting. Small doses of atropine, given once or twice daily, may ameliorate or prevent these side-effects. Other side-effects of anticholinesterase therapy include adverse effects on skeletal muscles, such as fasciculations (fine twitching), spasm, and weakness. The effects on the central nervous system include irritability, anxiety, insomnia, headache, dysarthria, syncope, convulsions, and coma. Increased salivation and lacrimation, increased bronchial secretions, and moist skin may also be noted.

- The nursing (and patient) priority is to give the drug prescribed according to an exact time schedule in order to control the patient's symptoms. *Any delay in drug administration may result in the patient's losing his ability to swallow.* Watch for an increase in muscle weakness within 1 hour after the patient takes the anticholinesterase drug, and be particularly alert for signs of respiratory distress.

After the initial medication doses have been adjusted, the patient learns to take the medication according to his needs and time plan. Further adjustments may be necessary in the presence of physical or emotional stress and intercurrent infection. Timespan Mestinon is sometimes taken at bedtime for its prolonged effect.

Immunosuppressive Therapy.

Immunosuppressive therapy is directed toward reducing the production of antireceptor antibody or its direct removal by plasmapheresis. Included in immunosuppressive therapy are corticosteroids, cytotoxic agents, plasmapheresis, and thymectomy. Corticosteroid therapy may benefit the patient with severe generalized myasthenia. Steroids exert their effect by suppressing the patient's immune response, thus decreasing the amount of blocking antibody. The anticholinesterase dosage is lowered while the patient's ability to maintain effective respirations and to swallow is monitored. The steroid dosage is gradually increased and the anticholinesterase medication is slowly reduced. Prednisone, taken on alternate days because of lower incidence of side-effects, appears to be suc-

cessful in suppressing the disease. Sometimes the patient will show a marked decrease in muscle strength right after steroid therapy is started, but this is usually only temporary. He is given a tap bell to use in emergency situations.

Cytotoxic agents (cyclophosphamide, azathioprine, methotrexate) are used to reduce antibodies to acetylcholine receptors.

Thymectomy.

In some patients, histologic abnormalities have been identified in the thymus gland. Thymectomy (surgical removal of the thymus) causes substantial remission of the disease, especially in patients with tumor or hyperplasia of the thymus gland. Thymectomy is carried out through the transsternal (sternal-splitting) approach since the entire thymus must be removed.

It is now felt that thymectomy *early* in the course of the disease is specific therapy, as it prevents formation of antireceptor antibodies. Following surgery, the patient is monitored in an intensive care unit; special attention is given to ventilatory function.

Plasmapheresis.

Removal of the plasma containing the IgG antibodies (plasmapheresis) to lower antibody levels may improve muscle strength in patients who do not respond to anticholinesterase therapy, corticosteroids, and thymectomy and are in crisis. This process is combined with prednisone or a cytotoxic agent and has caused remarkable improvement in some patients, but does not treat the underlying abnormality (production of antireceptor antibody) over the long term.

Myasthenic Crisis

Myasthenic crisis is the sudden onset of muscular weakness in patients with myasthenia. It may be manifested by sudden respiratory distress and an inability to swallow or speak. Weakness of respiratory, laryngeal, pharyngeal, and bulbar musculature causes respiratory depression and airway obstruction as well as cerebral hypoxia with its attendant sequelae of central nervous system injury and death.

Myasthenic crisis may result from progression of the disease, emotional upset, upper respiratory infection, certain drugs, surgery, or trauma, or it may be brought about by ACTH therapy.

Cholinergic crisis occurs from overmedication with anticholinesterase drugs which release too much acetylcholine at the neuromuscular junction. *Brittle crisis* occurs when the receptors at the neuromuscular junction become insensitive to anticholinesterase medication. It is not controlled by increasing or decreasing anticholinesterase therapy.

Recognition and Intervention for Myasthenic Crisis.

Respiratory distress combined with varying signs of dysphagia (difficulty in swallowing), dysarthria (difficulty in speaking), eyelid ptosis, and diplopia are symptoms of impending crisis.

- Providing adequate ventilatory assistance takes precedence in the immediate management of the patient with myasthenic crisis.
- The patient is suctioned, since aspiration is a common problem. Arterial blood is drawn for arterial blood gas analysis. Endotracheal intubation and mechanical ventilation may be needed (see Chap. 25). The patient is placed in an intensive care unit for constant monitoring,

since this condition is marked by intense and sudden fluctuations.

Intravenous edrophonium (Tensilon) is given to differentiate the type of crisis. It improves the condition of the patient in myasthenic crisis, temporarily worsens that of the patient in cholinergic crisis, and is unpredictable in brittle crisis. If the patient is in true myasthenic crisis, neostigmine methylsulfate (Prostigmin) is administered intramuscularly or intravenously.

If the edrophonium (Tensilon) test is uncertain or there is increasing respiratory weakness, all anticholinesterase drugs are withdrawn and atropine sulfate is given to reduce excessive secretions.

Other supportive measures include:

- Monitoring arterial blood gases, serum electrolytes, input and output, and daily weight
- Establishing postural drainage by elevating the foot of the bed for 20 minutes each hour, followed by turning and suctioning the patient
- Feeding the patient via nasogastric tube (200 ml at a time) if he is unable to swallow (Postural drainage should not be done for one half hour after feeding.)
- Avoiding use of sedatives and tranquilizing drugs, since these agents aggravate hypoxia and hypercapnia and can cause respiratory and cardiac depression
- Establishing a method of maintaining communication: hand bell, picture cards, hand signals, etc.
- Reassuring patient that the crisis should pass and that he will not be left alone

Patient Education.   To be a participant in his treatment the patient should learn the basic facts about anticholinergic drugs: their action, timing, dosage adjustment, symptoms of overdose, and toxic effects. Stress the importance of taking the medication on time. Anticholinesterase drugs are not to be taken with morphine, ether, quinine (commercial cold products), procainamide, and certain antibiotics. Novocain may not be well tolerated, and the patient's dentist should be so advised.

Mealtimes should coincide with the peak effects of anticholinesterase if the patient has difficulty in swallowing. If choking occurs frequently, blenderized food may be easier to swallow. Standby suction should be available at home.

If diplopia occurs, wearing an eye patch over one eye (alternating from side to side) is useful.

Certain factors may increase weakness and precipitate a myasthenic crisis: emotional upset, infections (particularly respiratory infections), vigorous physical activity, and exposure to heat (hot baths, sun bathing) and cold. These situations should be avoided. To avoid the risk of fatigue, it is best to rest *before* becoming too tired. A cervical collar is useful for patients with weak neck muscles. Adaptive or self-help devices are available and are useful in helping the patient handle the disease more effectively, enabling him to live as full a life as possible.

Amyotrophic Lateral Sclerosis

Amyotrophic lateral sclerosis (ALS, Lou Gehrig's disease) is a disease of unknown cause in which there is a loss of motor neurons (nerve cells controlling muscles) in the anterior horns of the spinal cord and the motor nuclei of the lower brain stem. As these cells die, the muscle fibers that they supply undergo atrophic changes. The degeneration of the neurons may occur in both the upper and lower motor neuron systems.

ALS affects more men than women, with onset occurring usually in the fifth or sixth decade. In this country, it is often referred to as "Lou Gehrig's disease" after the famous ballplayer who died from it.

Assessment
Clinical Manifestations.   The chief symptoms are fatigue, muscle weakness, atrophy, and fasciculations (twitching). The clinical picture depends on the location of the affected motor neurons, since specific neurons activate specific muscle fibers. Loss of motor neurons in the anterior horns of the spinal cord will result in progressive weakness and atrophy of the muscles of the arms, trunk, or legs. Spasticity is usually present and the stretch reflexes become brisk and overactive. Usually, the anal and bladder sphincters are not affected. When bulbar muscles are affected, there is progressive difficulty in speaking and swallowing, and choking becomes a problem. The voice assumes a nasal sound and speech articulations become so disrupted that the patient is unintelligible. Some emotional lability may be present, but intellectual function usually is not impaired. The prognosis generally is based on the area involved and the speed with which the disease progresses. Usually, the patient dies from a secondary cause, such as pneumonia or infection. While 50% of patients with ALS die in approximately 3 years, 20% survive beyond 5 years, 10% survive beyond 10 years, and up to 20% experience plateaus for extended periods, and the disease may arrest permanently.

ALS is a progressively incapacitating disease. The patient and family facing this cruel affliction need compassionate and caring support. It is often agonizing to discuss this disease with the patient and his family. When all voluntary movement becomes impossible, the patient is helpless— unable to feed himself or even turn or move in bed. Yet he is alert and aware of his plight. Weakness of the posterior tongue and palate impairs the ability to laugh, cough, or even blow the nose. Sometimes the patient cannot swallow. Eventually, respiratory function is compromised. Understandably the patient is depressed and frustrated by the relentlessly progressive course of the disease.

Management
No specific treatment is available. Symptomatic treatment and rehabilitative measures are employed to support the patient and improve the quality of life. The nursing care plan is revised and adaptations are made as the patient's condition changes. The patient should remain active as long as possible without tiring the involved muscles. Active exercises and range of motion exercises help to strengthen uninvolved muscles and maintain muscle power at optimum levels. Stretching exercises (stretch, hold, relax) are beneficial. Exercise is stopped short of fatigue. Such devices as ankle–foot orthoses for patients with weak dorsiflexors, which impair dorsiflexion of the ankle, help keep the patient mobile. Hand splints can provide a stronger grip and more

effective use of the hand, while other devices to support weakened extremities or neck muscles can maintain optimum joint position.

Baclofen (Lioresal) or diazepam (Valium) may be useful for patients troubled by spasticity, as spasticity causes pain and interferes with self-care. Quinine therapy may be prescribed for painful muscle cramps. If the patient has severe hip adduction, adduction blocks may be tried.

As the muscles grow weaker, the patient may use a wheelchair for activities outside of the house. Assistive devices are used to help the patient function independently for as long as possible. He should be instructed in energy conservation and work-simplification methods. When the illness has progressed to the point where the patient is confined to a wheelchair, an electrically powered model can be used. At this stage, the prevention of contractures is important. When the patient becomes dependent, a mechanical lift for bed, toilet, and tub transfers will be needed, and special instructions will have to be given to the family concerning the best way to position the patient for the greatest comfort. (See p. 238 for prevention of pressure sores.)

Nutrition is very important, especially in the patient with bulbar symptoms (choking, difficulty in swallowing and speaking). Aspiration is a constant danger. Standby suction should be available. The patient is placed in an upright position with his neck slightly flexed to facilitate swallowing. Foods with consistency (soft foods in gravy) seem to be more easily swallowed than liquids. A soft cervical collar is useful if the patient has difficulty holding his head up. In time, nasogastric or gastrostomy feedings may be considered.

The patient requires a communication system when speech is lost. If the patient can use his hands, small computers are available with artificial speech articulation. A pointer held in the teeth may be used with a picture or word chart. A predetermined code using eye blinks for "yes" or "no" may be the patient's only means of communication.

The most serious complication in the later stages of the disease is respiratory dysfunction, since all muscles involved in breathing may be affected. Techniques to enhance pulmonary function (breathing exercises, suctioning of excess secretions, chest physical therapy, incentive spirometry, ventilator therapy) usually are necessary when this occurs. The treatment of respiratory failure is discussed in Chapter 25.

The Muscular Dystrophies

The *muscular dystrophies* are a group of chronic muscle disorders characterized by progressive weakening and wasting of the skeletal or voluntary muscles. Most of these diseases are inherited.

The pathologic features include muscle fiber necrosis, variation in muscle fiber size, cellular reaction, increased internal nuclei, and replacement of muscle tissue by connective tissue.

The common characteristics of these diseases include varying degrees of muscle wasting and weakness; abnormal elevation in serum creatine phosphokinase, indicating a leakage of muscle enzymes; a myopathic electromyographic pattern; and myopathic findings on muscle biopsy. The differences center around the pattern of inheritance, the muscles involved, the age of onset, and the rate of progression.

Management

There is no specific treatment at this time for the muscular dystrophies. The objectives of supportive management are to keep the patient as active and normal as possible and to minimize functional deterioration. A therapeutic exercise program is prescribed for the individual patient to prevent muscle tightness, contractures, and disuse atrophy. Night splints and stretching exercises are used to delay contractures of the joints, especially the ankles, knees, and hips. Braces may compensate for muscle weakness. If the patient becomes confined to a wheelchair, he is fitted with a Silastic jacket, or a spinal fusion is done to prevent collapse of the trunk. Other surgical procedures may be carried out to correct deformities. Self-help devices can assist in achieving a greater degree of independence. Additional self-help devices become necessary as more muscle groups become affected.

Intercurrent illnesses, upper respiratory infections, and fractures from falls must be vigorously treated in such a way as to minimize immobilization, since joint contractures will become worse if the patient's activities are restricted more than usual. Aside from muscle weakness and contractures, a variety of other difficulties may be manifested in relation to the underlying disease. Dental and speech problems may result from weakness of the facial muscles, which makes it difficult to attend to dental hygiene and to speak coherently. Additional problems affect the gastrointestinal tract, resulting in gastric dilatation, rectal prolapse, and fecal impaction. Finally, cardiomyopathy appears to be a common complication in all forms of muscular dystrophy.

Because of the genetic nature of this disease, parents and siblings of the patient are advised to seek genetic counseling. The Muscular Dystrophy Association works to combat neuromuscular disease through scientific research, programs of patient services and clinical care, and professional and public education.

▷ Convulsive Disorders

Seizures

Seizures are episodes of abnormal motor, sensory, autonomic, or psychic activity (or a combination of these) as a consequence of sudden excessive discharge from cerebral neurons. A part or all of the brain may be involved. The seizures are usually sudden and transient.

The causes are varied and are classified as idiopathic (genetic, developmental defects) and acquired. Among the causes of acquired seizures are hypoxemia of any cause, including vascular insufficiency, fever (childhood), head injury, hypertension, central nervous system infections, metabolic and toxic conditions (renal failure, hyponatremia, hypocalcemia, hypoglycemia, pesticides, etc.), brain tumor, drug withdrawal, and allergies. Often there is memory loss for the convulsive episode and for a short time thereafter. Brain damage may occur when seizures are severe or prolonged. The patient is at risk for hypoxia, vomiting, and pulmonary aspiration or persistent metabolic abnormalities.

The immediate therapeutic objective is to control the seizure, and the long-term goal is to seek out and control the cause. See below for a discussion of epilepsy (the most common clinical syndrome of recurrent seizures) and the nursing management of the patient with seizures.

The Epilepsies

The *epilepsies* are a symptom-complex of several disorders of brain function characterized by recurring seizures. There may be associated loss of consciousness, excess or loss of muscle tone or movement, and disturbances of behavior, mood, sensation, and perception. Thus, epilepsy is not a disease, but a symptom.

The basic problem is thought to be an electrical disturbance (dysrhythmia) in the nerve cells in one section of the brain that give off abnormal, recurring, uncontrolled electrical discharges. The characteristic epileptic seizure is a manifestation of this excessive neuronal discharge.

Incidence.   An estimated 1% of the population (more than 2 million) in the United States have epilepsy at an annual cost of 3 billion dollars. There has been an increasing incidence of this condition, probably due to a number of factors. Improved obstetric and pediatric care salvages babies who previously would have succumbed from cerebral birth defects; these persons are predisposed to intermittent seizures. The improved medical, surgical, and nursing management of patients with head injuries, brain tumors, meningitis, and encephalitis saves those whose conditions may produce cerebral changes with resultant seizures. Also, advances in electroencephalography have aided in the identification of patients with epilepsy. Education has served to enlighten the general public and has lessened the stigmata associated with the condition, so that more persons are more willing to admit that they have epilepsy.

Altered Physiology.   Messages from the body are carried by the neurons (nerve cells) of the brain by means of discharges of electrochemical energy that sweep along them. These impulses occur in bursts whenever a nerve cell has a task to perform. Sometimes certain of these cells or groups of cells continue firing after a task is finished. It is as if a switch sticks in the "on" position until the power source runs down, then closes to allow recharge. During the period of unwanted discharges, parts of the body controlled by the errant cells may perform erratically. Resultant discomfort and dysfunction range from mild to incapacitating and usually cause unconsciousness. When these uncontrolled, abnormal discharges happen repeatedly, a person is said to have epilepsy. The erratic physical movements are called "seizures."*

Causes.   No one knows what makes brain cells in some people cause epilepsy. Scientists have produced seizures in experimental animals through surgical injury or chemical or electrical stimulation. Epilepsies often follow birth trauma, and asphyxia neonatorum, head injuries, some infectious diseases (bacterial, viral, parasitic), toxicity (carbon monoxide and lead poisoning), fever, metabolic and nutritional disorders, and drug or alcohol intoxication. They are also

* Adapted from a report of the National Institute of Neurological Disease and Stroke.

associated with brain tumors, abscesses, and congenital malformations. In many instances the epilepsies are termed "idiopathic" (cause unknown). There is evidence that susceptibility to some types may be inherited. Epilepsy strikes before the age of 20 in more than 75% of patients.

The epilepsies have little to do with intelligence in most cases. If the person with epilepsy does not have other brain or nervous system disabilities, he will fall within the same intelligence ranges as the overall population. Epilepsy is not synonymous with mental retardation or illness. However, many who are retarded because they have serious neurologic damage often have epilepsy too, thus pulling the mean IQ for all epilepsy victims below that of the so-called normal range.

Prevention of Epilepsy.   A full-scale attack incorporating a wide range of measures must be mounted for the prevention of epilepsy. Since the infants of epileptic mothers who take certain antiepileptic medications are at risk, these women need to be monitored carefully, including blood studies to detect the level of antiepileptic drugs taken throughout pregnancy. High-risk mothers (teenagers, women with histories of difficult deliveries, drug addicts, those with diabetes and hypertension) should be identified and supervised closely during pregnancy since brain lesions or injury that ultimately causes epilepsy may occur to the fetus during pregnancy and delivery.

Childhood infections (measles, mumps, bacterial meningitis) should be controlled with appropriate vaccination. Lead poisoning is another preventable cause of epilepsy. Parents with a child who has had a febrile convulsion should be taught fever-regulating techniques (cool sponging, antipyretic medications).

Head injury is one of the main causes that can be prevented. Through highway safety programs and occupational safety precautions, not only can lives be saved, but the possible development of epilepsy from head injury can be prevented.

Screening programs to detect children with seizure disorders at an early age and seizure prevention programs with the judicious use of antiepileptic medications and modification of life-style are part of this prevention plan.

▶ **Assessment**

Diagnostic Assessment.   The diagnostic assessment is aimed at determining the *type* of seizures, their frequency and severity, and the factors that precipitate them. A developmental history is taken, including events of pregnancy and childbirth, to seek evidence of preexisting injury. A search is made for illnesses or head injuries that may have affected the brain. In addition to a physical and neurologic examination, diagnostic examinations include biochemical, hematologic, and serologic studies. Computed tomography may be used to determine whether a tumor or other abnormality is present in the brain.

Of all the tests now available, the most illuminating is the *electroencephalogram* (EEG), which furnishes diagnostic evidence in a substantial proportion of epileptic patients and aids in classifying the type of seizure. Abnormalities in the electroencephalogram usually continue to be apparent between attacks, or, if concealed, may be brought

---

Chart 58-3
International Classification of Epileptic Seizures

  I. Partial seizures (seizures beginning locally)
   A. Partial seizures with elementary symptomatology (generally without impairment of consciousness)
     1. With motor symptoms (*includes Jacksonian seizures*)
     2. With special sensory or somatosensory symptoms
     3. With autonomic symptoms
     4. Compound forms
   B. Partial seizures with complex symptomatology (generally with impairment of consciousness) (*temporal lobe or psychomotor seizures*)
     1. With impairment of consciousness only
     2. With cognitive symptomatology
     3. With affective symptomatology
     4. With "psychosensory" symptomatology
     5. With "psychomotor" symptomatology (automatisms)
     6. Compound forms
   C. Partial seizures secondarily generalized
 II. Generalized seizures (bilaterally symmetrical and without local onset)
     1. Absences (*petit mal*)
     2. Bilateral massive epileptic myoclonus
     3. Infantile spasms
     4. Clonic seizures
     5. Tonic seizures
     6. Tonic–clonic seizures (*grand mal*)
     7. Atomic seizures
     8. Akinetic seizures
III. Unilateral seizures (or predominantly)
 IV. Unclassified epileptic seizures (due to incomplete data)

(Abstracted from Gastaut H: Clinical and electroencephalographical classification of epileptic seizures. Epilepsia 11:102–113.)

Clinical Manifestations. Depending on the location of the discharging neurons, seizures may range from a simple staring spell to prolonged convulsive movements with loss of consciousness. The variations in seizures have been classified internationally based upon clinical and electroencephalographic criteria as partial (simple and complex), generalized, unilateral, and unclassified. (Chart 58-3). Chart 58-4 provides a further breakdown in definition.

The initial pattern of the seizures indicates the region of the brain in which the attack originates. Also, it is important to determine if the patient has had an *aura* (premonitory or warning sensation before an epileptic seizure), which may indicate the origin of the seizure (*e.g.,* seeing a flashing light may indicate the seizure originated in the occipital lobe).

In *simple partial* seizures, only a finger or hand may shake, or the mouth may jerk uncontrollably. The person may speak nonsense, may be dizzy, and may experience unusual or unpleasant sights, sounds, odors, or tastes, but without loss of consciousness.

In *complex partial* seizures, the person either remains motionless or moves automatically but inappropriately for time and place. Or he may experience excessive emotions of fear, anger, elation, or irritability. Whatever the manifestations, the person does not remember the episode when it is over.

Generalized seizures, more commonly referred to as *grand mal seizures,* involve both hemispheres of the brain, causing both sides of the body to react. There may be intense rigidity of the entire body followed by jerky alternations of muscle relaxation and contraction (generalized tonic–clonic contraction). Often the tongue is chewed, and stools and urine may be passed involuntarily. After 1 or 2 minutes, the convulsive movements begin to subside; the patient relaxes and lies in deep coma, breathing noisily. The respirations at this point are chiefly abdominal. In the postseizure state,

---

Chart 58-4
Glossary

Generalized seizure (formerly termed *grand mal*)—a seizure characterized by loss of consciousness and tonic spasms of the trunk and extremities, rapidly followed by repetitive generalized clonic jerking

Partial seizures (formerly termed *petit mal*)—attacks of brief impairment of consciousness often associated with flickering of eyelids and slight twitching of the mouth

Psychomotor seizures—attacks characterized clinically by impairment of consciousness and amnesia for the episode; may be accompanied by motor and psychic activity that is irrelevant for time and place

Focal seizures—seizures beginning with a focal disturbance of cerebral function

Jacksonian seizures—focal motor or sensory convulsions

---

out by hyperventilation or during sleep. In addition, microelectrodes can be inserted deep in the brain to probe the action of single brain cells. It should be noted, however, that some persons with seizures may have normal EEGs, whereas persons who have never had seizures may have abnormal EEGs. Telemetering and computer equipment developed by space technology are used to take and store electroencephalographic readings on computer tapes while patients pursue their normal activities. Videorecording of seizures taken simultaneously with EEG telemetry is useful in determining the type of seizure as well as its duration and magnitude. This type of intensive monitoring is revolutionizing the treatment of severe epilepsy in this country.

the patient may be confused and suffer from headache, malaise, and nausea.

Included under general seizures are those that affect only infants (infantile spasms) and those that cause muscle flabbiness (atonic); muscle rigidity (tonic); muscle spasms (clonic); rapid, rhythmic muscle jerks (myoclonic); and complete muscle collapse (akinetic).

Patient Problems/Nursing Diagnoses

Based on the clinical manifestations and diagnostic evaluation data, the patient's potential problems include seizures related to abnormal nerve cell activity in the brain; impaired psychosocial functioning (denial of employment opportunities) related to socioeconomic stigma; and negative emotional reactions (depression, frustration, low self-esteem) related to the stresses imposed by epilepsy.

▶ Planning and Implementation

The management of epilepsy is planned according to a long-range program, one that is tailored to meet the special needs of each patient and not just to manage and prevent seizures. There is no simple solution, since some forms of epilepsy arise from brain damage and others depend on alterations of brain chemistry.

Goals

The major goals for the patient are to:

1. Maintain control of the seizures
2. Improve psychosocial adjustment
3. Cope with emotional problems

The nursing goals are to help the patient maintain control of seizures, provide health instruction to assist the patient to adjust his life-style accordingly, and provide psychosocial support to enable the patient to cope with the emotional and psychological effects related to potential seizures.

Life-style Adjustments. The patient must learn to adapt to his disease and control its manifestations. The patient's life-style and environment should be examined to determine whether certain factors precipitate the seizures: emotional disturbances, fever, new environmental stresses, onset of menstruation. The patient is encouraged to follow a regular and moderate routine in life-style, diet, exercise, and rest. (Sleep deprivation may lower the patient's threshold to seizures.) Moderate activity is good therapy, but excessive expenditure of energy is to be avoided, as is emotional overstimulation, such as watching late night television. Since seizures are known to follow alcoholic intake, alcoholic beverages are restricted. All in all, the best therapy is to follow the therapeutic program.

Drug Therapy. Many antiepileptic drugs are available to control seizures, although the mechanisms of their actions are still unknown. The objective of drug therapy is to achieve seizure control with minimal side-effects. Drug therapy is a form of control, not cure. The drug is selected according to the type of seizure being treated and the effectiveness and safety of the drug. If properly prescribed and taken, these drugs will result in control of 50% to 60% of patients with recurring seizures, and will partially control another

15% to 35%. The condition of approximately 15% to 35% of patients will not be improved by any currently available drugs.

Usually, treatment is started with a single drug. The starting dose and the rate at which the dosage is increased depend on whether or not side-effects develop. The drug levels are monitored in the blood, since the rate of drug absorption varies among people. Multiple-drug therapy or changing to another drug may be necessary if seizure control is not achieved or when toxicity interferes with further drug increase. The drug may have to be adjusted because of intercurrent illness, weight gain, or increases in stress. Sudden withdrawal of antiepileptic medication can cause seizures to occur with greater frequency or can precipitate the development of status epilepticus.

The side-effects of these medications may be divided into three groups: (1) idiosyncratic or allergic disorders, which present primarily as skin reactions; (2) acute toxicity, which may be manifested when the drug is initially prescribed; or (3) chronic toxicity, which occurs late in the course of drug therapy. The manifestations of drug toxicity are variable and any organ system may be involved. Periodic physical examinations and laboratory tests are done on patients receiving drugs known to have toxic effects on the hematopoietic, genitourinary, or hepatic systems. Table 58-1 summarizes the antiepileptic drugs in current use.

One of the most significant advancements in the treatment of epilepsy has been the development of an accurate method for measuring levels of antiepileptic drugs in the blood. Through the use of serum-level monitoring, the drug dosage can be adjusted more precisely and drug levels can be monitored to determine if the patient is taking the medication. It is of special value to researchers studying the effectiveness of old or new drugs.

Surgery for Epilepsy. Surgery is indicated for patients whose epilepsy results from intracranial tumors, abscess, cysts, or vascular anomalies.

Some patients have intractable seizure disorders and do not respond to drug therapy. There may be a focal atrophic process secondary to trauma, inflammation, stroke, or anoxemia. If the seizures originate in a reasonably well circumscribed area of the brain that can be excised without producing significant neurologic deficits, the removal of the epileptogenic focus generating the seizures seems to give long-term control and improvement. This type of neurosurgery has been aided by several modern advances, including microsurgical techniques, depth electroencephalography, improved illumination and hemostasis, and the introduction of neuroleptanesthetic drugs (droperidol and fentanyl). These techniques, combined with local infiltration of scalp incisions, enable the neurosurgeon to perform surgery on an alert and cooperative patient. With special testing devices, electrocortical mapping, and the patient's response to stimulation, the boundaries of the epileptogenic focus are determined. Any abnormal epileptogenic cortex (*i.e.,* abnormal area of the brain) is then removed.

Other neurosurgical techniques that are considered promising but still experimental are stereotaxic surgery, disconnection surgery, cerebellar stimulation, and cerebral cooling.

Table 58-1
Antiepileptic Drugs*

Generic Name	Trade Name	Side-effects
Carbamazepine	Tegretol	Nausea, vomiting, anorexia, blood dyscrasias, headache
Clonazepam	Clonopin	Drowsiness, ataxia, behavioral problems, anorexia
Diazepam	Valium	Drowsiness, fatigue, ataxia, depression, headache, tremor
Ethosuximide	Zarontin	Nausea, skin rash, blood dyscrasias, drowsiness, hiccups
Ethotoin	Peganone	Dizziness, fatigue, skin rash, insomnia, diplopia
Mephenytoin	Mesantoin	Nervousness, ataxia, nystagmus, pancytopenia, exfoliative dermatitis, drowsiness
Mephobarbital	Mebaral	Dizziness, headache, nausea, facial edema, skin rash
Metharbital	Gemonil	Drowsiness, dizziness, gastric distress, irritability, skin rash
Methsuximide	Celontin	Nausea, vomiting, anorexia, ataxia, rash, drowsiness, dizziness, blood dyscrasias
Paramethadione	Paradione	Nausea, anorexia, insomnia, diplopia, skin rash, bleeding gums, blood dyscrasias
Phenacemide	Phenurone	Gastrointestinal disturbances, anorexia, drowsiness, insomnia, paresthesias, psychic changes, hepatitis, blood dyscrasias, skin rash, nephritis
Phenobarbital	Luminal	Drowsiness, dermatitis
Phensuximide	Milontin	Nausea, ataxia, dizziness, drowsiness, skin eruptions, blood dyscrasias, hematuria
Phenytoin	Dilantin	Skin eruptions, ataxia, slurred speech, nystagmus, mental confusion, motor twitching, nausea, gingival hyperplasia, hirsutism
Primidone	Mysoline	Ataxia, vertigo, anorexia, fatigue, hyperirritability, drowsiness
Trimethadione	Tridione	Bone marrow depression, pancytopenia, exfoliative dermatitis, photophobia, nephrosis, hepatitis
Valproic acid	Depakene	Gastrointestinal disturbances, vomiting, drowsiness, weight gain, transient alopecia, hypersalivation, altered bleeding time, liver toxicity

* Side-effects and sensitivity to antiepileptic drugs vary among patients and at different times in the same patient. The dose for each patient is based on the patient's clinical response (free of seizures and side-effects).
(Adapted from Official Names of Antiepileptic Drugs. Epilepsia, 18:123, 1977.)

Psychosocial Considerations.*   It has been noted that the social, psychological, and behavioral problems frequently accompanying epilepsy can be more of a "handicap" than the actual seizures. Epilepsy imposes feelings of fear, alienation, depression, and uncertainty. The patient must cope with the ever-present fear of a seizure and its embarrassing consequences. Children with epilepsy may be ostracized and excluded from school and peer activities. These problems are compounded in the teen years and add to the

challenges of dating, not being able to drive, and "being different." Adults face all of these problems plus the burden of finding employment and decisions concerning marriage and childbearing, noninsurability, stigma of all kinds, and legal barriers. Alcohol may complicate matters. The burden on the family is great, and family problems run the gamut of outright rejection to overprotection. As a result of all these factors, many persons with epilepsy have psychological and behavioral problems.

Counseling is a must for helping the individual and the family to understand the condition and the limitations imposed by it. Social and recreational opportunities are necessary for good mental health. Some persons are not able

* Commission for the Control of Epilepsy and Its Consequences: Plan for Nationwide Action on Epilepsy. Vol. 1, DHEW Pub. No. (NIH) 78–276.

to cope with epilepsy; others have psychological problems resulting from brain damage. Those with seizures originating in the temporal lobes of the brain (areas controlling thought and emotions) have particular mental problems. Symptoms of schizophrenia, hyposexuality, and impulsive or irritable behavior may be due to brain damage associated with temporal lobe seizures. These patients require comprehensive mental health services.

Patient and Family Education

The complete cooperation of the patient and family is of the utmost importance. They must have confidence in the value of the regimen that is prescribed. It must be emphasized that the prescribed antiepileptic drug must be taken on a continuing basis and that the medicine is not a habit-forming "dope." It may be taken without fear, for many years if necessary, if the patient is under medical supervision and following instructions faithfully.

Of all the services that are contributed by the nurse in the care of the person with epilepsy, perhaps the most valuable are efforts to reorient the attitude of the patient and family to the disease itself. Concepts that reflect all of the ignorance and brutality that might be associated with the Middle Ages still prevail regarding epilepsy. For other patients, public sympathy and support abound; for the epileptic, common responses are abhorrence, rejection, and unemployment.

For the average person, an epileptic seizure is a terrifying or a repulsive spectacle; thus, for the individual who experiences them, every seizure is inevitably a source of humiliation and shame, which in turn breeds anxiety, depression, hostility, secrecy, and deceit, to which the public reacts with abhorrence, etc., and the vicious cycle is complete. The reaction of shame and the recourse to deceit are not confined merely to persons with epilepsy, but extends to their families as well.

In order to escape from this vicious cycle, patients who have epilepsy, their families, and the public at large need facts. These are the facts: Epilepsy is not a mysterious disease; it does not reflect the supernatural. It is not a stigma. Epilepsy is no more disgraceful than diabetes, pernicious anemia, or hyperthyroidism. It is not a form of insanity. It does not tend to get worse with time. It can be controlled effectively. It should not prevent the child from completing his schooling or keep the adult from work. *Activity tends to inhibit, not stimulate, epileptic seizures.* Some 50% to 60% of patients with epilepsy now may have their symptoms controlled.

Enlightenment of the public will give new hope to those facing centuries-old prejudices. Continuing encouragement should be given patients to mobilize their inner resources to overcome feelings of inferiority and self-consciousness resulting from seizures.

The hereditary transmission of epilepsy has not been proved. The matter of marriage and children must be decided on an individual basis, but this right should not be denied to the person with epilepsy merely because he has the disease. However, genetic counseling is advised.

Services to Patients. Since epilepsy is a long-term disorder, the continuous use of expensive medications may present a sizable burden to the patient and his family. The Epilepsy Foundation of America offers a low-cost pharmacy service. A prescription, authorized and signed by the patient's physician, is filled by registered pharmacists and sent by mail to the patient. Life insurance protection is also available through this organization. The licensing of persons with epilepsy to drive automobiles varies from state to state. The patients with epilepsy should carry an Emergency Medical Identification card in his wallet or have an identification bracelet around the wrist.

For many, employment problems still remain the greatest handicap of epilepsy. Studies have demonstrated that the person with epilepsy who is properly placed in his work has a satisfactory job performance. The director of each State Vocational Rehabilitation agency can provide information about vocational rehabilitation. If the individual's seizures are not well controlled, information about workshop opportunities may be obtained. Counseling and job training are provided for qualified persons through the Veterans' Administration. The U.S. Civil Service Commission now grants government jobs to individuals if seizures are controlled and the person is otherwise qualified. The Rehabilitation Act helped to end job discrimination of the handicapped. Private firms are becoming enlightened, and the number of employers who knowingly hire persons with epilepsy is increasing.

The Commission for the Control of Epilepsy and Its Consequences makes recommendations covering all aspects of the problem of epilepsy in the U.S.—social, legal, scientific, economic, and humanitarian.

▶ Evaluation

Expected Outcomes

1. Maintains control of seizures
   a. Complies with drug regimen
   b. Verbalizes the need to take prescribed antiepileptic drug; can relate the hazards of drug stoppage
   c. Recalls the side-effects of drugs
   d. Has laboratory appointment following hospital discharge for serum level determination of antiepileptic drug
   e. Avoids factors/situations he knows that may precipitate his seizures (flickering light, hyperventilation)
   f. Follows a healthful life-style by:
      (1) Getting enough sleep
      (2) Eating meals at regular times to avoid hypoglycemia
   g. Reads pamphlets, etc., about epilepsy
   h. Correctly answers a majority of questions about epilepsy
   i. Wears an identification bracelet
2. Strives to achieve improved psychosocial adjustment
   a. Relates his rights under Federal Law and verbalizes that he cannot be denied access to education/recreation, etc., on the basis of a history of seizures
   b. Informs his employer that he has epilepsy and is taking medication
   c. States he knows that job counseling and job-placement services are available for persons with epilepsy

3. Copes satisfactorily with emotional problems
   a. Identifies friend/family member with whom he can talk
   b. Is able to discuss current feelings
   c. Identifies two ways of constructively coping with anger/frustration
   d. Acknowledges that he has seizures
   e. Verbalizes the desire to enroll in a stress-management class

Nursing Management During a Seizure

During a convulsive seizure, the nursing goal is to prevent injury to the patient. This includes not only physical support, but psychological support as well.

- Provide privacy and protect the patient from curious onlookers. (The patient who has an *aura* [warning of an impending seizure] may have time to seek a safe place.)
- Ease the patient to the floor, if there is enough time.
- Protect the head with a pad to prevent injury (from striking a hard surface).
- Loosen constrictive clothing.
- Push aside any furniture that may be struck by the patient during the attack.
- If the patient is in bed, remove the pillows.
- If an aura precedes the seizure, insert a handkerchief between the teeth to reduce the possibility of the tongue or cheek being bitten. *Do not attempt to pry open jaws that are clenched in a spasm to insert a mouth gag.* Broken teeth and injury to the lips and tongue may result from such an action.
- No attempt should be made to restrain the patient during the seizure, since muscular contractions are strong and restraint can produce a fracture.
- If possible, place the patient on his side, because he is unable to swallow during a convulsive episode, and a lateral position facilitates drainage of mucus and saliva.
- After the seizure, keep the patient turned on his side to prevent aspiration. Make sure he has an adequate airway.
- There is usually a period of confusion following epileptic attacks.
- When the patient awakens, reorient him to his environment.
- If the patient experiences severe excitement following a seizure (postictal), try to handle him with calm persuasion and gentle restraint.

Nursing Assessment During a Seizure.

A major responsibility of the nurse is to observe and to record the sequence of symptoms. The nature of the seizure usually indicates the type of treatment that is employed. Before and during an attack, the following should be noted:

1. Description of the circumstances before the attack (visual stimuli, auditory stimuli, olfactory stimuli, tactile stimuli, emotional or psychic disturbances, sleep, hyperventilation)
2. The first thing the patient does in an attack—where the movements or the stiffness starts, position of the eyeballs and the head at the beginning of the attack. This information gives clues as to the location of the epileptogenic focus in the brain. (In recording, always state whether or not the beginning of the attack was observed.)
3. The type of movements of the part involved
4. The parts involved (Turn back bed covers and expose patient.)
5. The size of both pupils. Are the eyes open? Did the eyes/head turn to one side?
6. Whether or not automatisms (involuntary motor activity such as lip smacking or repeated swallowing) were observed
7. Incontinence of urine or feces
8. Duration of each phase of the attack
9. Unconsciousness, if present, and its duration
10. Any obvious paralysis or weakness of arms or legs after the attack
11. Inability to speak after the attack
12. Movements at the end of the seizure
13. Whether or not the patient sleeps afterward
14. Whether or not the patient was confused following the attack

Status Epilepticus

Status epilepticus (acute prolonged seizure activity) is a series of generalized convulsions that occur without recovery of consciousness between attacks. The term has been broadened to include continuous clinical or electrical seizures lasting at least 30 minutes, even without impairment of consciousness. It is considered a major medical emergency. Status epilepticus produces cumulative effects. There is some respiratory arrest at the height of each seizure that produces venous congestion and hypoxia of the brain. Repeated episodes of cerebral anoxia and swelling may lead to irreversible and fatal brain damage.

Common factors that precipitate status epilepticus include withdrawal of antiepileptic medication, fever, and intercurrent infection.

The objectives of treatment are to stop the seizures as quickly as possible, to ensure adequate cerebral oxygenation, and to maintain the patient in a seizure-free state. An airway and adequate oxygenation are established. Intravenous diazepam (Valium) is given slowly intravenously in an attempt to halt seizures immediately. Sometimes it is necessary to anesthetize the patient with one of the volatile anesthetic drugs.

Other antiepileptic drugs (phenytoin, phenobarbital) are given after diazepam is administered to maintain a seizure-free state. An intravenous line is established and kept open to monitor electrolytes, blood urea, and glucose. EEG monitoring may be useful in determining the nature of epileptogenic activity. Of course, vital and neurologic signs are monitored on a continuing basis. An intravenous infusion of dextrose is given if hypoglycemia caused the seizure. As soon as control of seizures is achieved, serum concentration of the antiepileptic drug is measured, since a low level will suggest that the patient was not taking the medication or that the dosage was too low. Patients recovering from status epilepticus may die within a few days from cardiac involvement or respiratory depression. There is also the potential for postictal (after a seizure) cerebral swelling.

▷ Head Injuries

Injuries to the head encompass trauma to the scalp, skull, and intracranial contents. Head injuries are among the most frequent and serious neurologic disorders and have reached epidemic proportions as a result of traffic accidents. In 1 year an estimated 422,000 Americans were admitted to hospitals with head injuries, and 15- to 24-year-old males incurred more new head injuries than any other age group.

The most important consideration in any head injury is whether or not the brain has been injured. The brain dies when its blood supply is interrupted for only a few minutes; there is no regeneration of damaged neurons. *Injuries to the cervical spine frequently coexist with head injuries.* The patient may also be in shock from scalp lacerations or other body injuries.

If a person has suffered a head injury and is to be transported from the scene of the accident, he should be placed on a board or stretcher with his head and neck maintained in alignment with the axis of the body. Slight traction should be maintained on the head.

Scalp Injury

Because of the many blood vessels, the scalp can bleed profusely when injured, causing the patient to go into shock. Scalp wounds are also a portal of entry for intracranial infections. Trauma may result in an abrasion ("brush wound"), contusion, laceration, or avulsion. An injection of procaine makes it easier for the wound to be cleaned and treated. The area is irrigated to remove foreign material and minimize the chance of infection before lacerations are closed. If the patient is unconscious and showing evidence of shock, this type of wound is the last to receive attention except to stop the bleeding and apply a sterile dressing.

Skull Injury—Fracture of the Skull

Fracture of the skull is treated as a neurosurgical condition, because the fracture in itself is of less importance than the possibility of a brain injury (Fig. 58-7). For this reason, every patient with head injury, even though it appears to be slight, should be under constant observation for several days. If a depressed fracture has occurred, then increased intracranial pressure may be likely and should be watched for.

- All patients with fractures of the skull should be suspected of having brain injury until proven otherwise.

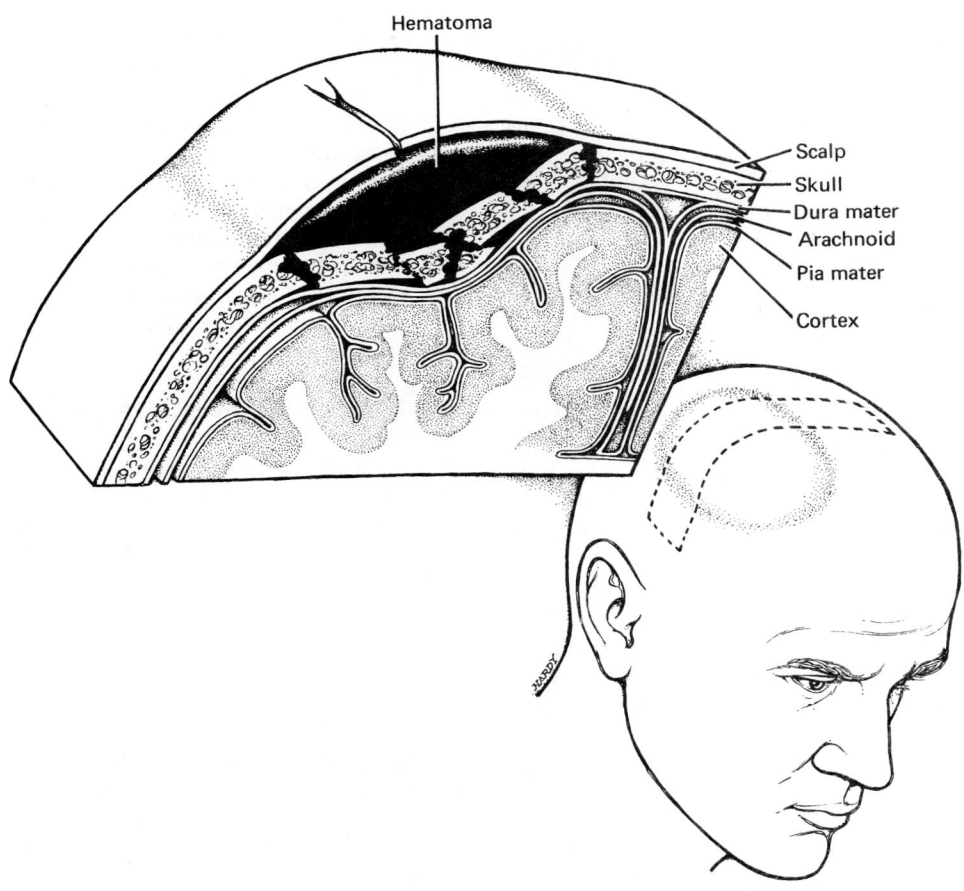

Figure 58-7. Depressed fracture of the skull.

It is possible that the patient may have other injuries that are masked by the head injury.

Clinical Manifestations.   The symptoms, besides those of the local injury, depend on the amount and the distribution of brain injury. Pain, persistent or localized, suggests that a fracture is usually present. Fractures of the vault produce swelling in the region of the fracture, and for this reason an accurate diagnosis cannot be made without a roentgenogram. Fractures of the base of the skull frequently produce hemorrhage from the nose, the pharynx, or the ears, and blood may appear under the conjunctivae. An area of ecchymosis may be seen over the mastoid. The escape of cerebrospinal fluid from the ears (otorrhea) and the nose (rhinorrhea) suggests skull fracture. Bloody spinal fluid, if present, suggests brain laceration or contusion.

Diagnostic Evaluation.   Although a rapid physical examination and evaluation of the neurologic status will reveal the more obvious brain injuries, the less apparent abnormalities found in head injuries may be detected by cranial computed tomography, which can differentiate subtle changes in the degree to which the soft tissue absorbs x-ray. It is accurate and safe in determining the presence, nature, location, and extent of the lesion as well as detecting cerebral edema, contusion, intracerebral or extracerebral hematoma, subarachnoid and intraventricular hemorrhage, and late traumatic changes (infarct, hydrocephalus).

If computed tomography is not available, cerebral angiography will demonstrate the presence of supratentorial, extracerebral, and intracerebral hematomas and cerebral contusion. Lateral and anteroposterior views of the skull are obtained.

Management.   In general, nondepressed skull fractures usually do not require surgical treatment, but close observation of the patient is essential. However, for depressed skull fractures, surgery is indicated. The scalp is shaved and cleansed and the fracture exposed. The skull fragments are elevated and the area is debrided. Closure of the dura is carried out if possible, and the wound is closed. Large defects in the skull can later be repaired with metallic or plastic plates if necessary. In instances of a clean wound and an intact dura, the elevated fragments can be replaced, making a later cranioplasty unnecessary. Penetrating wounds require surgical debridement to remove foreign bodies and devitalized brain tissue and to control hemorrhage. Antibiotic treatment is immediately instituted and blood transfusions are made available.

Fractures of the base of the skull are serious because they are usually open (involving the paranasal sinuses or middle or external ear) and are therefore a possible source of intracranial infection. The nasopharynx and the external ear should be kept clean, and usually a plug of sterile cotton is placed in the ear to absorb discharges.

Brain Injury

Serious brain injury may occur following blows or injuries to the head, with or without fracture of the skull.

A cerebral *concussion* may occur following a head injury in which there is neither structural damage nor persistent neurologic deficit. The jarring of the brain may be so slight as to cause only dizziness and spots before the eyes (spoken of as "seeing stars"), or there may be complete loss of consciousness for a time. If the brain tissue in the frontal lobe is affected, the patient may exhibit bizarre irrational behavior, whereas disruption of brain tissue in the temporal lobe can produce temporary amnesia or disorientation. Continuing amnesia is regarded as a severe concussion.

The treatment of concussion is to observe the patient for headache, dizziness, and nervous instability (postconcussional syndrome), which may follow this type of injury. Giving the patient information, explanations, and encouragement may reduce some of the problems of postconcussional syndrome.

A *cerebral contusion* is a more marked cerebral injury in which the brain is bruised, with possible surface hemorrhage. The patient will be unconscious for a considerable period. The symptoms, as would be expected, are more marked. The patient may lie motionless; the pulse will be feeble, the respiration shallow, and the skin cold and pale. Often there is involuntary evacuation of the bowels and the bladder. The patient may be aroused with effort but soon slips back into unconsciousness. The blood pressure and the temperature are subnormal, and the picture is somewhat similar to that of shock.

In general, persons with diffuse injury who have abnormal motor function, abnormal eye movements, and raised intracranial pressure have a poor outcome. On the other hand, the patient may recover consciousness completely and perhaps pass into a stage of cerebral irritability.

In the stage of cerebral irritability, the patient is no longer unconscious. On the contrary, he is easily disturbed by any form of stimulation, noises, light, and voices, and may become hyperactive at times. Gradually, the pulse, the respiration, the temperature, and the other body functions return to normal. However, recovery is not complete at once. Residual headache and vertigo are common, and often impaired mentality or epilepsy occurs as a result of irreparable cerebral damage.

Epidural, Subdural, and Intracerebral Hemorrhage

The most serious injuries are caused by hematomas that develop within the cranial vault (Fig. 58-8). The hematoma may be epidural, subdural, or intracerebral, depending on the location. *The signs and symptoms of brain ischemia resulting from clot compression are variable and depend on the speed with which vital areas are encroached upon.* In general, a small hematoma that develops rapidly may be fatal, whereas the patient may adapt to a more massive hematoma if it develops slowly.

Epidural Hematoma (Extradural Hematoma or Hemorrhage)

Following a head injury, bleeding may occur in the epidural (extradural) space between the skull and the dura. This often results from fractures of the skull that cause rupture or laceration of the middle meningeal artery which runs between the dura and the skull; hemorrhage from this artery causes pressure on the brain.

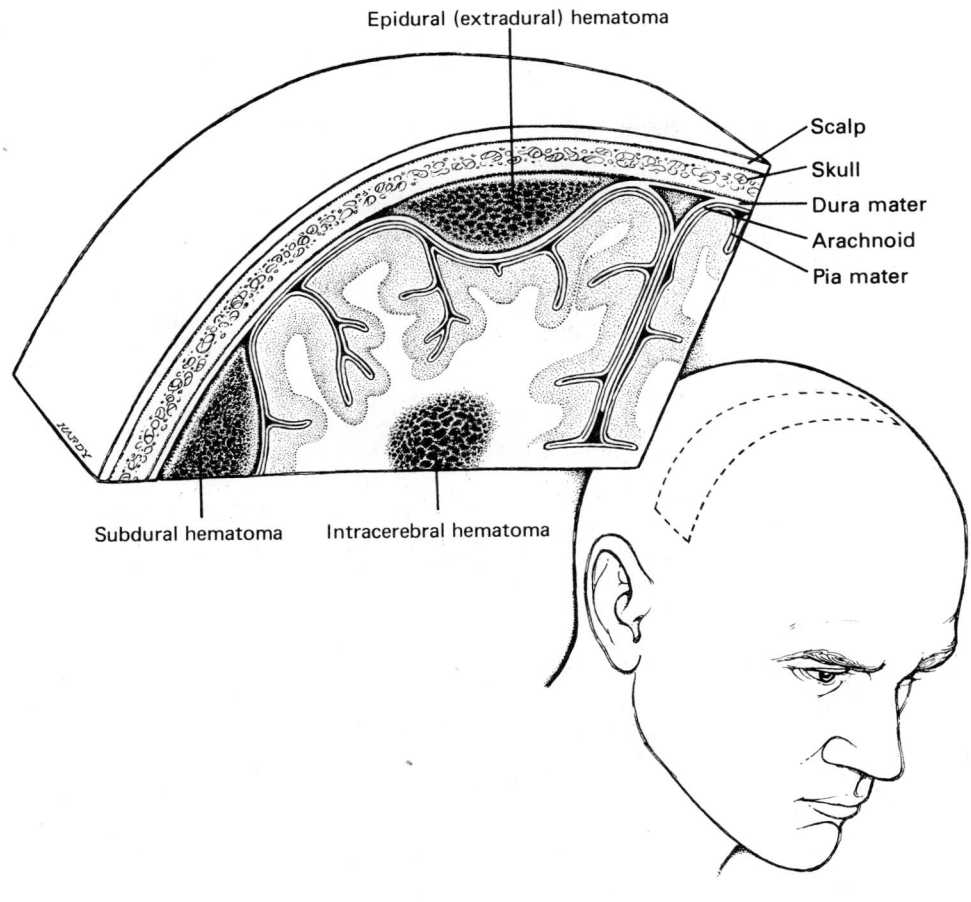

Epidural (extradural) hematoma

Scalp
Skull
Dura mater
Arachnoid
Pia mater

Subdural hematoma   Intracerebral hematoma

Figure 58-8. Diagrammatic views showing epidural, subdural, and intracerebral hematomas.

More frequently, bleeding sites along the fracture line produce acute hematomas. Epidural hematomas most frequently occur in the temporal area.

The symptoms are caused by the expanding hematoma. There is usually a momentary loss of consciousness at the time of injury followed by an interval of apparent recovery (lucid interval). However, a lucid interval is not always present with an epidural hematoma, although it may occur with a subdural hematoma. During the lucid interval, compensation for the expanding hematoma takes place by rapid absorption of cerebrospinal fluid and decreased intravascular volume, which maintains a normal intracranial pressure. But when these mechanisms can no longer compensate, even a small increase in the volume of the blood clot will produce a marked elevation of intracranial pressure. Then, often suddenly, signs of compression appear, usually deterioration of consciousness and signs of focal neurologic deficits (dilation and fixation of a pupil, paralysis of an extremity), and the patient will deteriorate rapidly.

Management. An epidural hematoma is considered an extreme emergency, since marked neurologic deficit or even cessation of breathing may occur within minutes. The treatment consists of making openings through the skull (burr holes), removing the clot, and controlling the bleeding point.

Subdural Hematoma

Not infrequently, either with or without injury, hemorrhage may take place over the surface of the brain underneath the dura. It may arise from a laceration of a superficially located cortical artery. A subdural hemorrhage is more frequently venous in origin, and the blood spreads over the brain surface. A subdural hematoma may be either acute, subacute, or chronic, depending on the size of the involved vessel and the amount of bleeding present. Usually, the patient is comatose, and the clinical signs are similar to those of epidural hematoma. A rising blood pressure with slowing of pulse and respirations indicates a rapidly increasing hematoma.

The mortality rate for patients with acute subdural hematomas is high, as there is frequently concomitant cortical contusion, laceration, and brain stem injury.

If the patient can be rapidly transported to the hospital, an immediate craniotomy is performed to open the dura, allowing for the solid, subdural clot to be evacuated. Successful outcome also depends on the control of intracranial pressure and careful monitoring of respiratory function (see The Patient Undergoing Intracranial Surgery, p. 1320).

Chronic subdural hematoma imitates other conditions and may be mistaken for a stroke. In fact, it has been termed "the great imitator." The bleeding is less profuse and there is compression of the intracranial contents. The blood within the brain changes in character in 2 to 4 days, becoming thicker and darker. In a few weeks the clot breaks down and has the color and consistency of motor oil. Eventually, calcification or ossification of the clot takes place. The brain adapts to this foreign body invasion, and the patient's clinical signs and symptoms fluctuate. There may be severe headache, which tends to come and go; alternating focal neurologic signs; personality changes; mental deterioration; and focal convulsions. Unfortunately, the patient may be labeled "neurotic" or "psychotic" if the cause of the symptoms is overlooked.

The treatment of chronic subdural hematoma consists of surgically evacuating the clot by suctioning or irrigating the area. The procedure may be carried out through multiple burr holes, or a craniotomy may be performed in which the dura is opened and the blood evacuated, along with the membranes, if necessary.

Intracerebral Hematoma

Intracerebral hemorrhages are more frequently seen in the elderly and occur after a fall. In severe injuries to the brain, scattered petechial hemorrhages or a large parenchymal hematoma may occur. The neurologic signs and symptoms may be masked by coma and confusion. The clot may be evacuated by means of a craniotomy, but the associated mortality rate is high.

General Approach to Care

▶ Assessment

When the patient is admitted to the Emergency Department, an initial assessment is done to evaluate the seriousness of injury, to determine the level of brain function, and to help predict the outcome. A head injury may be obscured if the patient is under the influence of alcohol or drugs, as this diminishes his responses, thus complicating assessment. Attention may be diverted from a head injury because of serious trauma elsewhere in the body.

The following observations are significant:

- Does the patient open his eyes? To what stimulus?
- Does he utter recognizable words?
- Does he follow commands?
- Does he move his extremities equally on both sides of his body?
- Are his pupils equal? Reactive to light?
- Is there bleeding from the orifices? eyes? ears? nose? mouth?
- Is there ecchymosis behind the ear, overlying the mastoid (Battle's sign)?
- Are there any focal neurologic signs? (unilateral fixed pupil? hemiparesis?)

- Are there any signs of increased intracranial pressure? (decreasing level of consciousness? bradycardia? irregular respirations? See p. 1293.)

Any observers of the accident should be interviewed. The following questions are significant:

- What caused the injury? a high velocity missile? an object striking the head? a fall? What was the direction and force of the blow?
- Was there a loss of consciousness? What was the duration of the unconscious period? Could the patient be aroused? (A history of amnesia and unconsciousness after a head injury indicates a significant degree of cerebral dysfunction.)
- Did seizures occur?

Monitoring Vital Signs. Although deterioration of the patient's level of consciousness is the most sensitive neurologic indication of impending danger, vital signs are monitored at frequent intervals to assess the intracranial state.

- Signs of rapidly increasing intracranial pressure include slowing of the pulse and respirations and a rapid increase in blood pressure and temperature.
- If brain compression encroaches upon cerebral circulation, the vital signs tend to be reversed—the pulse and respiration become rapid, and the blood pressure may fall. This is an ominous development, as is a rapid fluctuation of vital signs.
- A rapid rise in body temperature is regarded unfavorably because hyperthermia increases the metabolic demands of the brain.

However, a temperature of up to 38.5° C (101° F) is fairly common following head trauma. Look for evidence of infection (chest, urinary tract, wounds) if fever persists. (The nursing management of the patient with hyperthermia is discussed on p. 1297.)

As the damaged brain swells with edema, a rise in intracranial pressure can be expected and requires aggressive treatment. Increased intracranial pressure is managed by avoiding hypoxia; administering mannitol, which reduces brain water by osmotic dehydration; hyperventilation; the use of steroids; a head-up position in bed; intracranial pressure monitoring; and possible neurosurgical intervention. If these modalities fail to reduce an elevated intracranial pressure, high-dose barbiturate therapy (pentobarbital) is given to reduce cerebral edema. (See p. 1294 for management of the patient with increased intracranial pressure). The use of high-dose barbiturate therapy requires constant nursing surveillance.

Patient Problems/Nursing Diagnoses

Based on the clinical manifestations and diagnostic assessment data, the patient's potential nursing problems include ineffective airway clearance, ventilation, and brain oxygenation related to hypoxia; alterations in nutrition, impaired skin integrity, and impaired physical mobility related to disturbances of consciousness; self-care deficits related to unconsciousness and neurologic deficits; and impaired mental status related to the results of head injury.

▶ **Planning and Implementation**

Goals

The patient's goals are:

1. Effective airway clearance, ventilation, and brain oxygenation
2. Adequate nutritional status
3. Maintenance of skin integrity
4. Improved physical mobility
5. Participation in self-care
6. Improved mental status

The major nursing goals include: (1) to assure adequate ventilation, (2) to carry out ongoing evaluations of the patient's level of responsiveness/consciousness, (3) to monitor vital signs and to carry out continuous assessment, (4) to maintain adequate nutritional support and fluid and electrolyte balance, (5) to prevent further brain damage and other complications from secondary processes (physical, physiologic, and metabolic abnormalities), and (6) to initiate and carry out health teaching and nursing rehabilitation procedures. As soon as the initial assessment and diagnostic tests are made, a neurologic flow record is started and maintained (see p. 1367). Figure 58-9 summarizes ongoing nursing assessments, priorities of nursing management, and anticipatory and rehabilitation nursing of the patient with a head injury.

Assuring Adequate Ventilation.   One of the most important nursing goals in the management of the patient with a head injury is to establish and maintain an adequate airway. The brain is extremely sensitive to hypoxia, and a neurologic deficit can worsen if the patient is hypoxic. Therapy is directed toward maintenance of adequately oxygenated circulation so that there will be a supply of oxygenated blood to the brain to preserve cerebral function. An obstructed airway causes CO_2 retention and hypoventilation, which produce cerebral engorgement and increases intracranial pressure.

Therapeutic and nursing activities to ensure an adequate exchange of air are summarized on pages 1301 to 1302 and include the following:

- Monitoring arterial blood gases to assess adequacy of ventilation (The goal is to keep blood gases within normal range to ensure adequate cerebral blood flow.)
- Providing for endotracheal intubation with mechanical ventilation to treat hypoxia
- Establishing effective suctioning procedures (Pulmonary secretions produce coughing and straining, which increase intracranial pressure.)
- Guarding against aspiration and respiratory insufficiency
- Keeping the unconscious patient in a semiprone or prone position with the head of the bed elevated about 30 degrees to decrease intracranial venous pressure

Evaluating Level of Responsiveness.   An equally important nursing objective is constant assessment of the level of responsiveness, since irreversible changes occur rapidly. This nursing priority, discussed in detail on pages 1293 and 1297, includes:

- Determining the orientation of the patient, his reaction to auditory and painful stimuli, response to commands
- Determining his motor responses to stimuli (Abnormal responses carry a worse prognosis.)
- Determining the presence or absence of paralysis as well as observations of spontaneous activity
- Noting any change or variation, no matter how subtle, in the patient's level of responsiveness (Deterioration of the patient's condition may be due to an expanding intracranial hematoma and progressive brain engorgement or edema.)
- Noting any localizing neurologic signs

Neurologic Observation Record (Glasgow Coma Scale).   In order to achieve a clear and objective evaluation of the patient's neurologic status, the *Glasgow Coma Scale* can be used as an effective assessment tool. Three aspects of the patient's behavior are observed and recorded: eye opening, verbal responses, and motor response to a verbal command or painful stimulus. These assessments are further subdivided into different levels of responses, and the best responses the patient makes to predetermined stimuli are recorded as follows:

Eyes Open:	
Spontaneously	4
To speech	3
To pain	2
No response	1
Best Motor Response:	
Obeys	6
Localizes pain	5
Withdraws	4
Abnormal flexion	3
Extends	2
Nil	1
Verbal Response:	
Oriented	5
Confused conversation	4
Inappropriate words	3
Incomprehensible sounds	2
Nil	1
	Total: 3–15

Each response is given a number (high for normal and low for impaired), and the summation of these figures gives an indication of the severity of coma and a possible prediction of outcome. The lowest score is 3, and the highest is 15. In general, a score of 4 or 5 indicates the patient is deeply comatose, a score of 6 to 10 shows intermediate disturbance of consciousness, and a score of more than 10 approaches a more conscious state.

Figure 58-10 shows a chart incorporating the Glascow Coma Scale, vital signs, pupillary size and reactivity, and

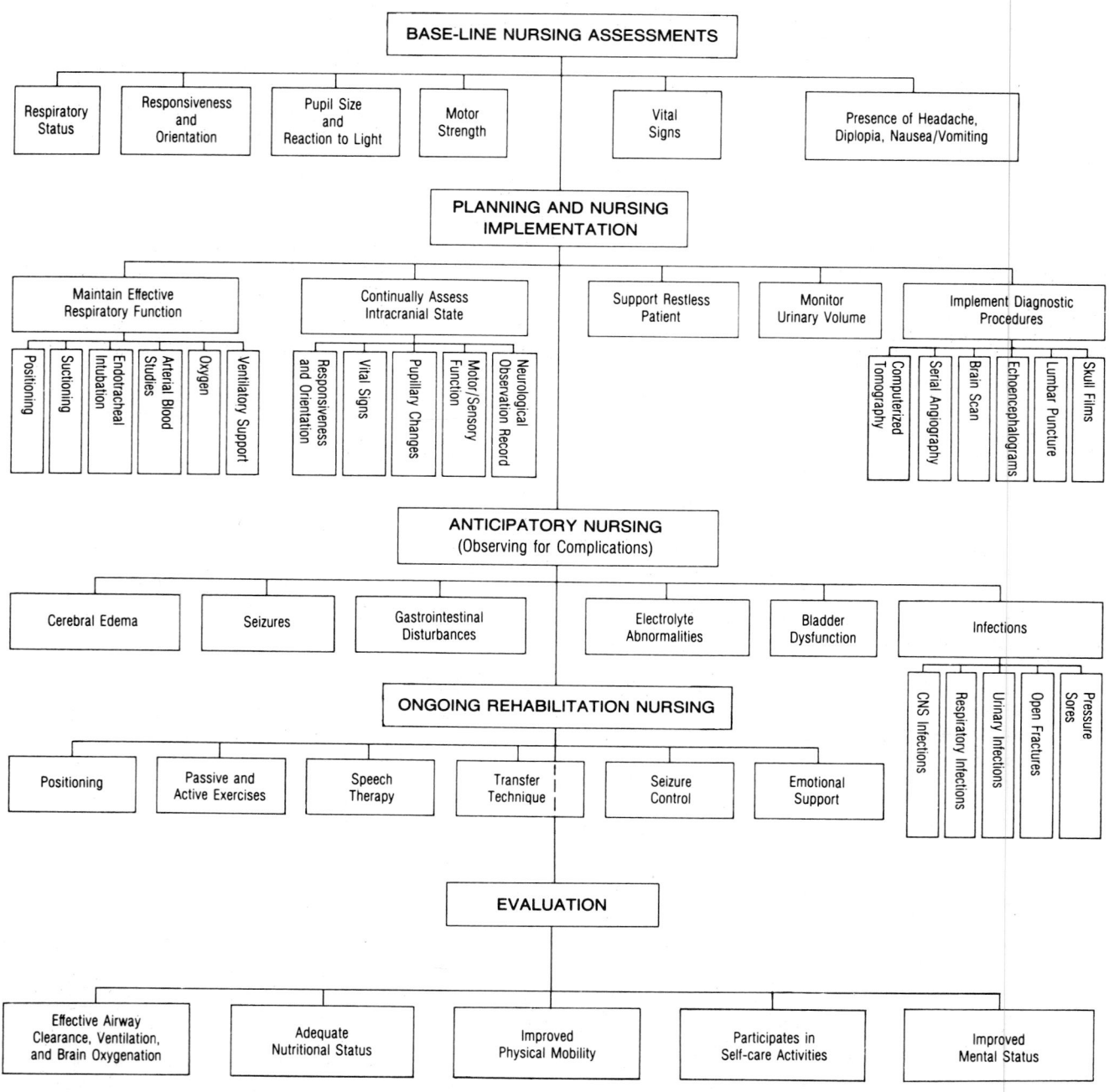

Figure 58-9. The patient with a head injury.

extremity movement and strength, which is a comprehensive record of the patient's neurologic status at any given point in time.

Continuing Assessment

- Assess if the patient is opening his eyes.
- The size of the pupils and their reaction to light are evaluated. A unilaterally dilated and poorly responding pupil may indicate a developing hematoma with subsequent pressure on the third cranial nerve due to shifting of the brain. If both pupils become fixed and dilated,

overwhelming injury and intrinsic damage to the upper brain stem usually are indicated.
- Assess verbal responses.

Motor Function.   Motor function is checked frequently by observing the patient's spontaneous movements, requesting him to raise and lower the extremities, and comparing the power of his hand grip. Notice whether he moves one extremity less frequently than the other. Also, determine the patient's ability to speak and note the quality of the speech.

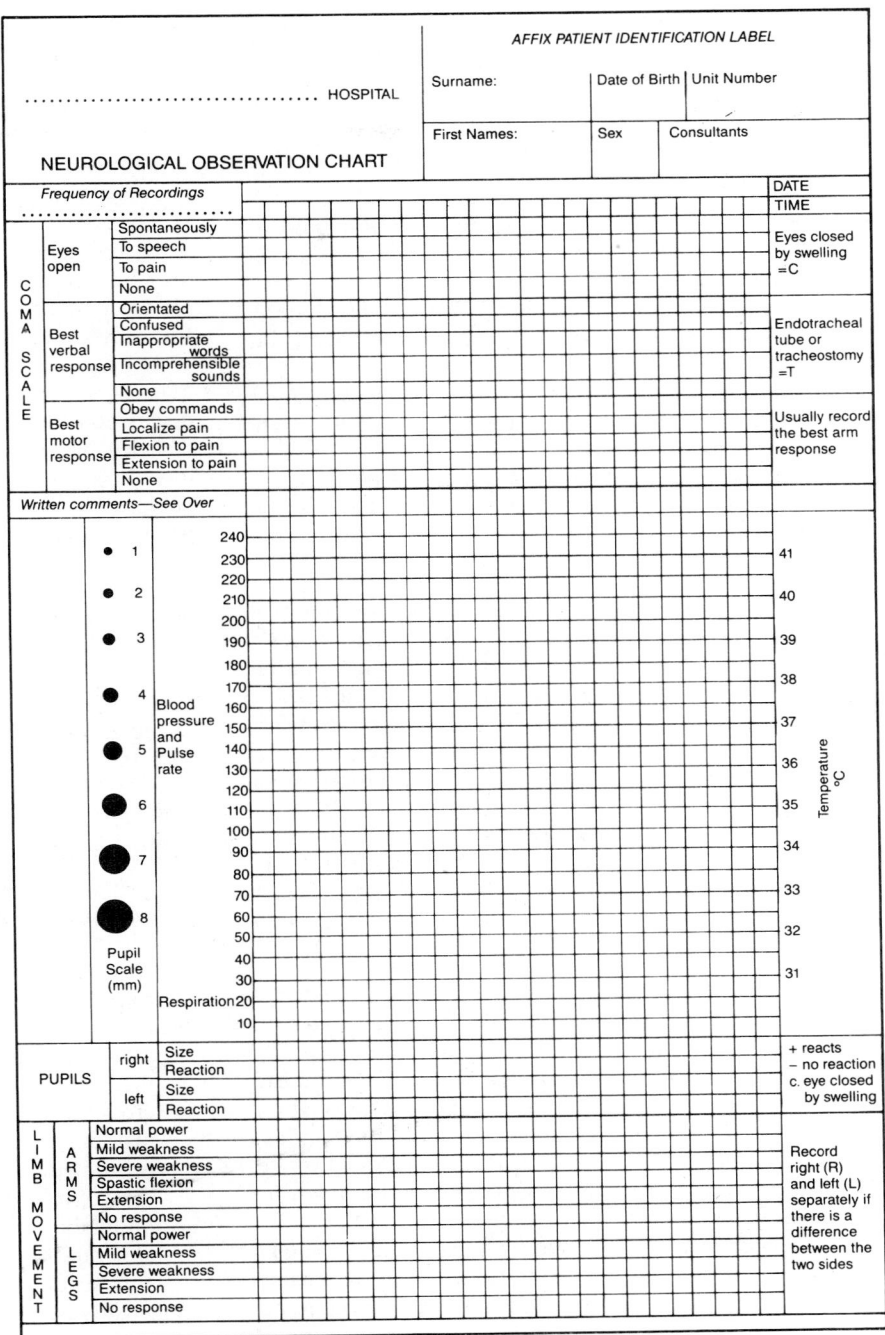

Figure 58-10. Example of observation chart that includes the Glasgow Coma Scale. (Reproduced by courtesy of Butterworth and Company, London, from Campkin and Turner, Neurosurgical Anaesthesia and Intensive Care.)

Cerebrospinal Fluid (CSF) Discharge. The orifices (eyes, ears, nose, mouth) require careful scrutiny.

- To determine whether a fluid discharge is spinal fluid otorrhea or rhinorrhea, blot the area with sterile gauze. If the discharge is bloody (which is readily observed), a red spot forms on the gauze, but if the discharge also contains cerebrospinal fluid, a clear, wet halo encircles the bloody spot.
- Cerebrospinal fluid may also be differentiated from mucus by means of a Dextrostix (used to measure blood

sugar). If the indicator turns blue, sugar is present—cerebrospinal fluid contains sugar; mucus does not.

- Drainage of cerebrospinal fluid from the nose or ears indicates a basal skull fracture. If the patient is conscious, caution him against sneezing or blowing his nose.
- A sterile, cotton pad may be taped loosely against the ear or under the nose to collect the draining fluid.
- The head is usually elevated approximately 30 degrees to reduce intracranial pressure and promote spontaneous closure of the leak. However, some neurosurgeons prefer that the bed be kept flat. Persistence of spinal fluid

otorrhea or rhinorrhea usually requires surgical intervention. Also, cerebrospinal fluid leakage may mask the usual clinical signs of an expanding intracranial hematoma by preventing brain compression.

Fluids and Electrolytes.
Brain damage can produce metabolic and hormonal dysfunctions.

- Serial studies of blood and urine electrolyte and osmolality are carried out, since head injuries may be accompanied by disorders of sodium regulation. Sodium retention may last several days followed by sodium diuresis. Watch for lethargy, confusion, and convulsions due to electrolyte imbalance.
- Endocrine dysfunctions are evaluated by measurements of serum electrolytes, glucose values, and input and output records.
- Urine is tested regularly for sugar and acetone.
- A record of daily weight is kept, especially if the patient has hypothalamic involvement and must be watched for the development of diabetes insipidus.

Nutritional Management.
After 3 to 4 days of parenteral fluids, nasogastric feedings may be started. Small, frequent feedings lessen the possibility of diarrhea and vomiting. Elevating the head of the bed and aspirating the tube before feeding (for evidences of residual feeding in the stomach) are measures used to prevent distention, regurgitation, and aspiration pneumonia. (The principles and technique of nasogastric feeding are discussed on p. 773.)

Restlessness.
Restlessness may be due to hypoxia, fever, pain, or a full bladder. It may indicate injury to the brain, but it is also a sign that the unconscious patient is regaining consciousness. (Some restlessness may be beneficial.)

- Make sure that the patient's airway is adequate and the bladder is not distended. Likewise, bandages and casts should be checked for constriction.
- It is not wise to treat restlessness with opiates and narcotics, because these substances depress respiration, constrict the pupils, and alter the level of the patient's responsiveness. However, small doses of chloral hydrate, paraldehyde, or tranquilizing drugs may be given for restlessness.
- To keep the patient from hurting himself and dislodging body tubes, siderails are padded and the patient's hands are wrapped in mitts. Restraints should be avoided because straining against them can increase intracranial pressure.
- Lubricate the skin with oil or emollient lotion to prevent irritation from rubbing against the sheet.
- If incontinence is a problem, an external sheath catheter may be used on the male patient. Since prolonged use of an indwelling catheter inevitably produces infection, the patient may be placed on an intermittent catheterization schedule.

Complications.
Head injury producing coma results in death in roughly 30% to 50% of patients. Complications following traumatic head injury include focal nerve palsies (anosmia [lack of sense of smell], extraocular movement abnormalities), focal neurologic deficits (aphasia, memory defect, post-traumatic epilepsy), pneumonia, cerebral edema, infection, and vascular complications. After-effects of head injury, usually directly related to the severity of the trauma, include headache, dizziness and vertigo, emotional instability or irritability, brain damage, and post-traumatic neuroses and psychoses.

Seizures.
Seizures following head injury (post-traumatic epilepsy) may occur from bruising of the cortex or may be associated with intracranial hemorrhage. Marked elevation of intracranial pressure may occur during seizures. Intravenous diazepam (Valium) is used to control seizures, and phenytoin (Dilantin) is given after control is obtained. (The nursing management of the patient during seizures is discussed on p. 1360.)

Rehabilitation.
Rehabilitative techniques are employed, including range of motion exercises, correct positioning to prevent contractures, proper skin management to prevent pressure sores, and a graded program of exercises. The patient is kept oriented to time, place, and person, especially if he is emerging from an unconscious state. Adequate lighting may prevent visual hallucinations.

Shock.
Although the presence of shock is rarely the result of a head injury, it is apt to occur in the patient who has associated injuries. Fracture of the extremities, fractured vertebrae, chest wounds, ruptured internal organs, etc., may be extracranial causes of shock in the patient with multiple injuries. Since the presence of shock is life-threatening, its immediate treatment has first priority. Table 57-1 gives comparative data to assist in the clinical assessment of the patient.

- *A brain-injured patient who is in shock is not placed in a head-low position, because this would increase the likelihood of cerebral edema and hemorrhage.* The extremities may be elevated to increase return of blood to the heart.
- Shock is treated with volume replacement using plasma and whole blood. (Plasma and blood tend to stay within the intravascular compartment, while crystalloids can cross the damaged blood–brain barrier if cerebral contusion, laceration, or hemorrhage are present.)
- An indwelling catheter is inserted to measure hourly urinary volume, which indicates adequacy of perfusion.
- An intake and output record is maintained. Monitoring of central venous pressure is useful in determining adequate amounts of fluid intake. The patient may be kept slightly dehydrated to reduce extracellular fluid volume.

Patient and Family Education.
The patient is encouraged to continue on his rehabilitation program following discharge, since improvement in status may continue up to 3 or more years following injury. Headache may be the most reliable guide to recovery. A second pillow or backrest at night may be helpful to alleviate some head discomfort.

Since post-traumatic seizures occur frequently, anticonvulsants may be prescribed for 1 to 2 years following injury. The patient is encouraged to return gradually to his usual activities. Since there may be brain damage, the family needs to understand and set limits in coping with outbursts of anger, crying, etc., and in realistically evaluating the patient's capabilities. It is difficult to understand and accept alterations in a loved one's behavior. The family requires support and respite, including work and social relationships.

If the patient is discharged from the hospital in a relatively short time after a head injury, the family is instructed to look for the following signs and to notify the physician or clinic or bring the patient back to the Emergency Department if they occur: difficulty in awakening, difficulty in speaking, confusion, severe headache, vomiting, pulse change, development of unequal pupils, or weakness of one side of the body.

▶ **Evaluation**

(See also The Unconscious Patient, p. 1297.)

Expected Outcomes

1. Attains/maintains effective airway clearance, ventilation, and brain oxygenation
   a. Achieves the following parameters:
      (1) Arterial blood gases within normal limits
      (2) Normal breath sounds on auscultation
   b. Coughs up secretions
2. Attains/maintains adequate nutritional status
   a. Has less than 50 ml of aspirate in stomach before each tube feeding
   b. Is free of gastric distention and vomiting
   c. Attains/maintains fluid intake and output in balance and within normal ranges
   d. Shows minimal weight loss
3. Attains/maintains skin in healthy condition
   Shows no evidence of skin breakdown or pressure sores
4. Shows improvement in physical mobility
   a. Adheres to turning schedule
   b. Gives no evidence of contractures, external rotation of hip, or plantar flexion
   c. Reveals no stiffening of joints during passive range of motion exercises
5. Participates in self-care activities
   Tries to care for self and participate in activities of daily living as level of responsiveness improves and confusion lessens
6. Shows progress in improved mental status
   a. Shows less confusion
   b. Verbalizes concerns about behavior during period of unconsciousness
   c. Participates in memory retraining
   d. Verbalizes realistic plans for returning to work
   e. Understands importance of taking phenytoin daily

▷ **Spinal Cord Injury**

Spinal cord injury is a major health problem affecting about 200,000 persons in this country, with an estimated 10,000 new injuries occurring each year. Half of these injuries result from motor vehicle accidents, whereas most of the others occur from falls, sporting and industrial accidents, and gunshot wounds. Two thirds of the victims are 30 years of age or younger. The estimated total annual cost of these injuries exceeds $2 billion a year. There is a high frequency of as-

sociated injuries and medical complications. The vertebrae most frequently involved in spinal cord injuries are the fifth, sixth, and seventh cervical (neck); the twelfth thoracic; and the first lumbar vertebrae. These vertebrae are the most susceptible because there is a greater range of mobility in the vertebral column in these areas.

Prevention. To prevent this devastating and catastrophic injury, the following steps should be taken: (1) reduction in driving speed, (2) use of seat belts, (3) wearing of helmets by motorcyclists, (4) educational programs directed against driving while intoxicated, (5) water safety instruction, (6) prevention of falls, and (7) the use of protective devices in sports and proper coaching techniques. Paramedical personnel are taught the importance of properly removing a car-crash victim from a motor vehicle and of following proper methods in transporting the victim to the Emergency Department in order to avoid further and possibly permanent damage to the spinal cord.

Pathogenesis of Spinal Cord Injury. Damage to the spinal cord ranges from transient concussion (from which the patient fully recovers) to contusion, laceration, and compression of the cord substance (either alone or in combination), to complete transection of the cord (which renders the patient paralyzed below the level of the injury). When hemorrhage occurs in the area of the spinal cord, the blood may seep into the extradural, subdural, or subarachnoid spaces of the spinal canal. Immediately after injury (contusion or tear), the nerve fibers begin to swell and disintegrate. Blood circulation to the gray matter of the spinal cord is curtailed. Not only is there injury to the spinal cord vasculature, but there also appears to be a pathogenic process responsible for the progressive damage of acute spinal cord injury. A secondary chain of events produces ischemia, hypoxia, edema, and hemorrhagic lesions, which in turn result in destruction of myelin and axons.

These secondary reactions, believed to be the principal causes of spinal cord degeneration at the level of injury, are now thought to be reversible 4 to 6 hours after injury. Therefore, if the cord has not suffered irreparable damage, some method of *early* treatment is needed to prevent partial damage from developing into total and permanent damage. Dexamethasone, given as an anti-inflammatory agent; mannitol, given to decrease edema; and dextran, given to prevent the blood pressure from dropping and to improve capillary blood flow are being investigated. The effectiveness of using cooling techniques or hypothermia perfusion on the injured area of the spinal cord to counteract the autodestructive forces that follow this type of injury is being studied. The use of high-dosage steroids to maintain the vascular integrity of the cord following acute injury is viewed as promising by researchers.

Emergency Management

The immediate management of the patient at the scene of the accident is critical, because improper handling can cause further damage and loss of neurologic function. Any victim of a motor vehicle or diving accident, a contact sport injury, falls, or any direct trauma to the head and neck should be suspected of having a spinal cord injury until such an injury is ruled out.

- At the scene of the accident, the victim should be immobilized on a spinal (back) board with his head and neck in a neutral position to prevent an incomplete injury from becoming complete.
- One member of the team should assume control of the patient's head to prevent flexion, rotation, or extension.
- Place each hand on either side of the head about the ear to maintain traction and alignment while a spinal board or cervical immobilizing orthosis is applied.

At least four persons should slide the victim carefully onto a board for transfer to the hospital. Any twisting movement may irreversibly damage the spinal cord by causing a bony fragment of the vertebra to cut into, crush, or sever the cord completely. It is desirable that the patient be referred to a regional spinal injury or trauma center because of the multidisciplinary personnel and support services required to counteract destructive changes that occur in the first few hours after injury.

Transferring the Patient.   During treatment in the emergency and x-ray departments, the patient is kept on the transfer board. The transfer of the patient to a bed presents a definite nursing problem:

- The patient always must be maintained in an extended position. No part of the body should be twisted or turned, nor should the patient be allowed to assume a sitting position.

The patient should be placed on a Stryker frame when he is to be transferred to a bed. Later, if it is proved that there is no cord injury, the patient always can be moved to a conventional bed without harm; the reverse, however, is not true. If a Stryker frame is not available, the patient should be placed on a firm mattress with a bedboard under it. The patient may be transferred from the board to the Stryker frame in the following manner:

- The board on which the patient is strapped is placed directly on the posterior frame.
- Unstrap the patient from the board, but do not remove the head strappings.
- Place a blanket roll between the legs.
- Place the anterior frame in position, and secure the frame straps.
- Turn the frame so that the patient is in the prone position.
- Remove the frame straps and the posterior frame. Remove the head strapping with care. Then remove the transfer board.

Assessment and Clinical Manifestations

The consequences of spinal cord injury depend on the level of injury of the cord. There is total sensory loss and motor paralysis below the level of injury, loss of bladder and bowel control (usually urinary retention and bladder distention), loss of sweating and vasomotor tone below the level of the cord injury, and marked reduction of blood pressure from loss of peripheral vascular resistance.

If the patient is conscious, he will probably complain of acute local pain which may radiate peripherally along the involved nerve. Often he will say that he is afraid he has broken his neck or back.

A neurologic examination is carried out repeatedly, with special attention given to function distal to the level of injury. Note evidence of improvement or deterioration.

Respiratory Function

Breathing Pattern
- The breathing pattern must be noted, since respiratory problems are frequently seen in patients with cervical spine injuries because of possible paralysis of the intercostal and abdominal muscles. (The C-4 segment provides the major innervation to the diaphragm by the phrenic nerve.)
- The strength of cough is assessed.
- Vital capacity, which is a guide to respiratory inefficiency, is measured.
- Nasal oxygen is started to maintain a high arterial PO_2, especially in the presence of respiratory compromise.
- Electrical stimulation of the phrenic nerves to pace the diaphragm is being done on selected patients with respiratory paralysis associated with quadriplegia.
- If endotracheal intubation is necessary, every attempt is made to accomplish this without moving the head backward.

Motor and Sensory Function
(The level of spinal cord injury is described as the lowest spinal cord segment with intact motor and sensory function.)

- As soon as possible, the patient is evaluated for motor and sensory changes below the level of injury. It is necessary to record these findings so that changes or progression from the baseline neurologic status can be evaluated accurately.
- Motor ability is tested by requesting the patient to spread his fingers, squeeze the examiner's hand, and move his toes or turn his feet.
- Sensation is evaluated by pinching the skin or pricking it with a pin, starting at the shoulder level and working down both sides of the extremities. The patient is asked where he feels the sensation. The presence or absence of sweating is also noted, since perspiration does not occur on paralyzed areas.
- Edema of the spinal cord may occur with any severe cord injury and may further compromise spinal function. Therefore, the patient is watched constantly for any changes in motor or sensory loss and symptoms of progressive neurologic damage (Fig. 58-11). These, of course, are reported immediately. It may be impossible in the early stages of injury to determine whether the cord has been transected, since signs and symptoms of cord transection are indistinguishable from those of cord edema.

Spinal Shock
- It is important to evaluate for spinal shock (see p. 1373.)

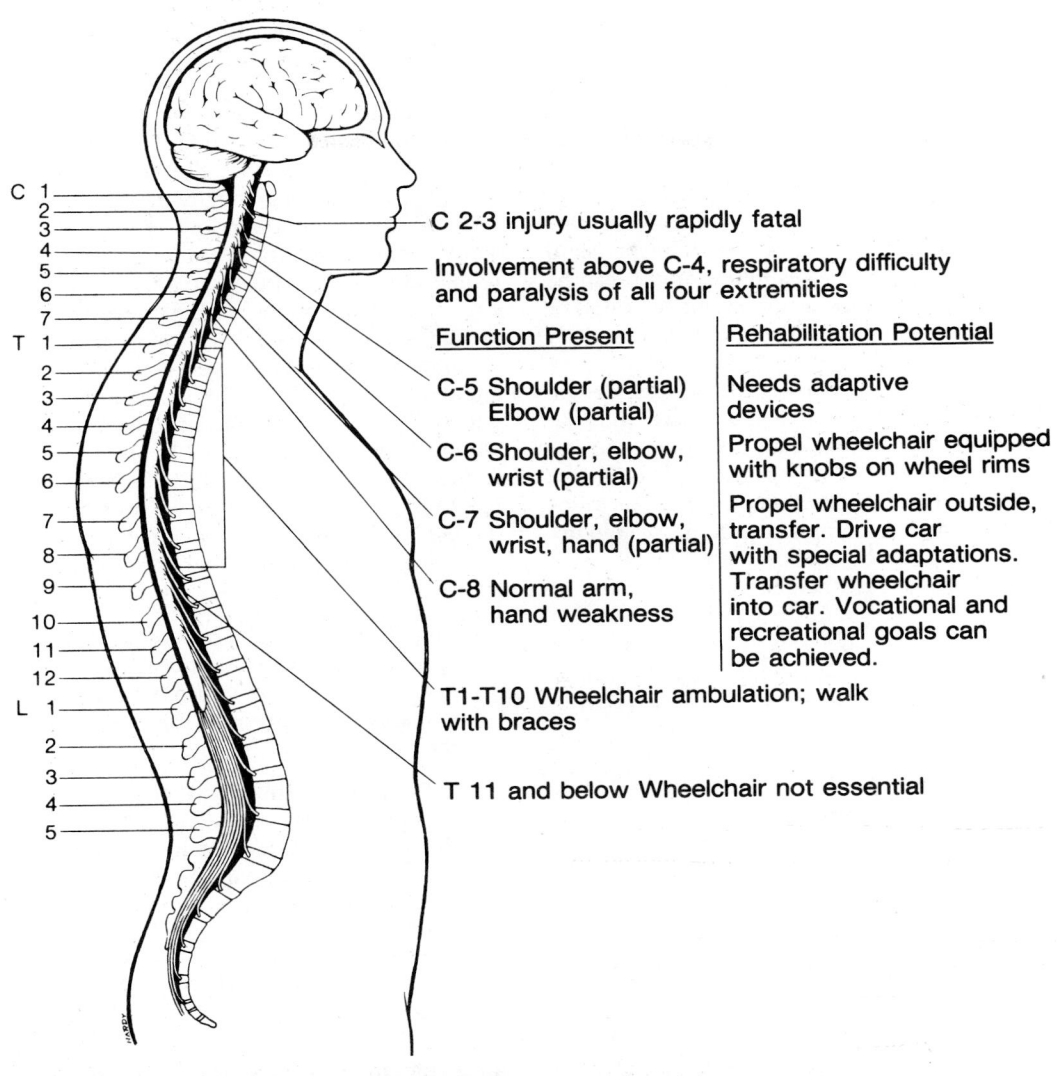

C 2-3 injury usually rapidly fatal

Involvement above C-4, respiratory difficulty
and paralysis of all four extremities

Function Present	Rehabilitation Potential
C-5 Shoulder (partial) Elbow (partial)	Needs adaptive devices
C-6 Shoulder, elbow, wrist (partial)	Propel wheelchair equipped with knobs on wheel rims
C-7 Shoulder, elbow, wrist, hand (partial)	Propel wheelchair outside, transfer. Drive car with special adaptations.
C-8 Normal arm, hand weakness	Transfer wheelchair into car. Vocational and recreational goals can be achieved.

T1-T10 Wheelchair ambulation; walk
with braces

T 11 and below Wheelchair not essential

Figure 58-11. Sequelae of spinal cord injury and rehabilitation challenges. (The vertebrae are numbered on the left side of the drawing and the spinal nerves are numbered on the right.)

Bladder Function

- Immediately after a spinal cord injury, the urinary bladder becomes atonic and cannot contract by reflex activity. Since the patient has no sensation of bladder distention, damage to the urinary tract may occur from overstretching of the bladder. The treatment of choice is intermittent catheterization to avoid overstretching and infection. If this is not feasible, an indwelling catheter is inserted.

Gastric Function

- Gastric intubation and suction are initiated to reduce gastric distention and prevent vomiting and aspiration.

Sexual Function

- Most spinal cord injury patients have sexual concerns. Health care personnel can "permit" early acceptance and verbalization of these concerns, and acknowledge to the patient and his partner that this part of their lives is not over (see p. 1379).

Definitive Management

The goals of management are to prevent further spinal cord injury and to observe for symptoms of progressive neurologic damage.

As soon as the patient is resuscitated and there is stabilization of the spine, mannitol may be administered to reduce cord edema. Steroids (dexamethasone) may also be given.

Management of a cervical spinal injury requires *immobilization, early reduction, and stabilization.*

Cervical Traction. To reduce the fracture dislocation and maintain alignment of the cervical spine fracture, some form of skeletal traction with halo cast or halo vest or one of a variety of skeletal tongs or calipers is used. The patient may require open reduction (surgery). However, measures will still be required to maintain reduction.

Halo Traction. Halo skeletal traction for cervical spine injuries offers some advantages over skull-tong traction. Not only is it relatively simple to apply and comfortable to the patient, but hospitalization time is markedly reduced. Halo traction devices consist of a stainless steel "halo ring" that fits around the head and is attached to the skull by four skull pins inserted through threaded holes in the ring. It can be connected to a plaster body cast or to a plastic halo vest or girdle that suspends the weight of the unit circumferentially around the chest.

The patient may experience a slight headache or discomfort around the skull pins for several days after the pins are inserted. Initially, the patient may not appreciate the rather startling appearance of this apparatus, but he can readily adapt to it because of the comfort the device provides to the unstable neck. He may complain of being "caged in" and of noise created by any object coming in contact with the steel frame, but he should be reassured that he will adapt to this.

The hair around the pin tracts is shaved to facilitate assessment and prevent infection. Some drainage around the pin site is anticipated. These areas are cleansed daily and observed for redness, drainage, and pain. A torque screwdriver should be readily available in case the screws on the frame need tightening. If one of the pins becomes detached, stabilize the patient's head in a neutral position while another person notifies the neurosurgeon.

Skeletal Tongs. A number of skeletal tongs are available, including the Crutchfield (Fig. 58-12), Barton, and Vinke tongs, all of which need to be inserted into the skull. These are usually placed in the outer table of the skull through holes made with a special drill under local anesthesia. The Gardner–Wells tongs require no predrilled holes, and the pins are tightened by hand to the proper depth. These procedures are usually done in the Emergency Department under local anesthesia.

Traction is applied to the tongs by weights, the amount depending on the patient's size and the degree of displacement. (New tongs have been designed that avoid problems such as pulling out when excess weight is applied, etc.) The traction force is exerted along the longitudinal axis of the vertebral bodies with the neck in a neutral position. Then the traction is gradually increased by the addition of more weights. As the amount of traction is increased, the spaces between the intervertebral discs widen, and the vertebrae slip back into position. Reduction usually takes place after correct alignment has been regained. Once reduction is achieved, as verified by cervical spine films and neurologic examination, the weights are gradually removed until the amount of weight needed to maintain the alignment is obtained. The weights should hang free so as not to interfere with the traction. The patient is placed on a turning frame if one is available. (See p. 1370 for a method of transfer to the turning frame.) Some neurosurgeons do not advocate the use of the circOlectric bed for spinal injuries because excessive pressure is placed on the fracture when the patient is turned in a vertical fashion.

- The patient's skull is assessed for signs of infection, including drainage around the tongs. The back of the head is checked periodically for signs of pressure and is massaged at intervals, care being taken not to move the neck.

Surgical Intervention. If the patient's lesion cannot be managed conservatively (*i.e.,* traction), or if there are displaced vertebral bone fragments, or if the injury is likely to cause further nerve damage, surgery may be needed to decompress the cord or to reduce the spinal fracture or dislocation.

A laminectomy may be indicated in the instance of an ascending neurologic lesion, suspicion of epidural hematoma, and penetrating wounds that require surgical debridement. Or, surgery may be done to permit direct visualization and exploration of the cord. (The care of the patient following a laminectomy is discussed on p. 1376.)

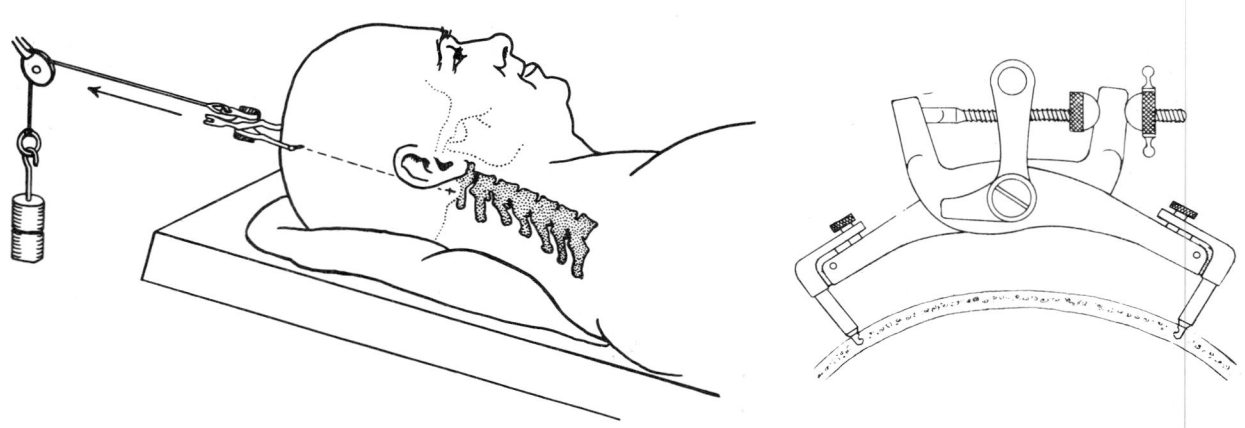

Figure 58-12. Diagrammatic drawing shows the method of application of skull traction. Note that the pegs extend through the outer layer of the skull and thus produce direct skeletal traction. (Courtesy, University of Virginia.)

Other Aspects of Management

Spinal Shock. Spinal shock represents a sudden depression of reflex activity in the spinal cord (arreflexia) below the level of injury. In this condition, the muscles innervated by the part of the cord segment situated below the level of the lesion become completely paralyzed and flaccid, and the reflexes are absent. The blood pressure falls, and the parts of the body below the level of the cord lesion are paralyzed and without sensation. With injuries to the cervical and upper thoracic spinal cord, the innervation to the major accessory muscles of respiration is lost and respiratory problems develop: decreased vital capacity, retention of secretions, increased PCO_2, decreased PO_2, hypoxia, respiratory failure, and pulmonary edema. The reflexes that initiate bladder and bowel function likewise are affected. (The management of the patient with a neurogenic bladder— *i.e.,* a bladder disturbance due to a lesion of the central nervous system—is discussed on p. 975.) Bowel distention and paralytic ileus caused by depression of the reflexes may be treated with intestinal decompression. The patient does not perspire on the paralyzed portions of his body, since sympathetic activity is blocked. Therefore, he must be watched carefully for an abrupt onset of fever. (Hyperthermia is treated as outlined on p. 1297.)

- The patient's body defenses are supported and maintained until spinal shock abates and the system has recovered from the traumatic insult (3–6 weeks). Special attention must also be directed to the respiratory system. There may not be enough intrathoracic pressure for the patient to cough effectively. Chest physical therapy is used to help clear pulmonary secretions.
- During spinal shock and subsequent periods of immobilization, the patient is assessed for signs of venous thrombosis since pulmonary embolism is a major cause of death in the first few weeks after injury. Subcutaneous low-dose heparin may be started.

Usually, the acute period of spinal shock is transient, but residual results may linger for a much longer time. If the injury is incomplete, the prognosis is uncertain.

Prevention of Pressure Sores. Because a patient with a spinal cord injury is immobilized for a period of time, there is an ever-present, life-endangering threat of pressure sores. In areas of local tissue ischemia where there is continuous pressure and where the peripheral circulation is inadequate as a result of the spinal shock and recumbency, pressure sores have been known to develop within 6 hours.

- Turning not only aids in the prevention of pressure sores, but also prevents the pooling of blood and tissue fluid in the dependent areas.
- Frequent skin assessments are essential. Check the skin over the pressure points for redness.
- Avoid tight clothing and material that does not absorb moisture.
- Every few hours the patient's skin should be washed with a mild soap, rinsed well, and *blotted* dry. Sacrum, trochanters, ischia, iliac spines, knees, and heels are especially susceptible to pressure. These areas should be kept soft and well lubricated with bland cream or lotion. Massage should be done gently with a circular motion. The linen under the patient is kept dry.
- The patient must know the danger of pressure sores and accept coresponsibility for prevention. (See p. 238 for other aspects of prevention of pressure sores.)

Positioning. The patient must be maintained in proper alignment at all times. Usually, he is turned every 2 hours. If the patient is not on a turning frame, he should not be turned unless the physician has indicated so. (Directives for turning a patient not on a Stryker frame are found in Chart 58-5.) The patient is placed in a dorsal or supine position as follows:

The feet are positioned against a padded footboard to prevent footdrop. There should be a space between the end of the mattress and the footboard to allow free suspension of the heels. A wooden block on either end of the mattress prevents the mattress from pushing against the footboard.

Chart 58-5
Turning the Patient With Crutchfield Tongs (Not on Stryker Frame)

If Crutchfield tongs are used and the patient is not on a Stryker frame, a directive from the physician must be obtained before the patient is turned. The patient's head *never should be flexed,* neither forward nor laterally, and at all times should be kept in a direct line with the axis of the cervical spine.

To Turn the Patient

The nurse supporting the head gives the commands for turning. Place a pillow between the legs of the patient to prevent the upper leg from slipping forward and jarring the patient's head.

Place a pillow longitudinally on the chest, with the patient's upper arm resting on it. The pillow prevents the shoulder from sagging and pulling on the neck as the patient is turned.

Three persons should turn the patient in a logrolling fashion, making sure that the shoulder turns with the head and the neck. One nurse should support the head; the second nurse or attendant, the shoulders; and the third person, the hips and the legs.

As the patient is turned, the traction should be moved carefully to keep it in direct line with the cervical spine. The patient's position should be adjusted so that the traction, the patient's head, and the cervical spine are in correct alignment.

While the nurse still supports the head in the lateral position, a small pillow is placed under the head to maintain cervical alignment.

Trochanter rolls are applied from the crest of the ilium to the midthigh of both extremities to prevent external rotation of the hip joints.

Exercising. Atrophy of the extremities will result from disuse. To avoid this complication, the physician may direct that passive range of motion exercises be started on the affected extremities within 48 to 72 hours after injury. These exercises preserve joint motion and stimulate circulation. A joint that is immobilized too long becomes fixed as a result of tendon and capsule contracture. Toes, metatarsals, ankles, knees, and hips should be put through a full range of motion at least four, and ideally five, times daily. Range of motion exercises can prevent many complications.

Complications. Pulmonary complications, including atelectasis followed by pneumonia related to decreased ventilation, ineffective cough, excessive secretions, aspiration of secretions and abdominal contents, etc., are a common cause of death. Kidney and bladder complications (infection, calcification, renal failure) and autonomic hyperreflexia may also occur. These problems are discussed elsewhere in the text: for kidney and bladder complications, see page 975; for autonomic hyperreflexia, see page 1379.

Ambulation. After a period of absolute immobilization (either by halo traction or skeletal tongs), the duration of which depends on the severity and mechanism of injury, the patient may be allowed to gradually assume an erect position. The patient will require bracing to reduce movement of the cervical spine and to allow bone healing. The commonly used orthoses are either a two-poster firm brace placed under the chin and the subocciput with a chest extension, or a four-poster cervical brace with chest extension. For the patient with a cervical fracture without neurologic deficit, reduction in traction followed by rigid immobilization for 16 weeks will restore skeletal function in most patients. (The rehabilitation of the patient with a permanent spinal cord injury, *i.e.,* the paraplegic patient, is discussed on p. 1377.)

Herniation or Rupture of an Intervertebral Disc

The *intervertebral disc* is a cartilaginous plate that forms a cushion between the vertebral bodies. This tough gristlelike material is incorporated in a capsule. A ball-like condensation in the disc is called the *nucleus pulposus*. In *herniation of the intervertebral disc* (ruptured disc), the nucleus of the disc protrudes into the annulus (the fibrous ring around the disc) with subsequent nerve compression. Protrusion or rupture of the nucleus pulposus is usually preceded by degenerative changes. The development of radiating cracks in the annulus weakens resistance to nucleus herniation. Following trauma (falls, accidents, and repeated minor stresses, such as lifting), the cartilage may be injured.

In most patients, the immediate symptoms of trauma are short-lived, and those resulting from injury to the disc do not appear for months or years. Then with degeneration in the disc, the capsule pushes back into the spinal canal, or it may rupture and allow the nucleus pulposus to be pushed back against the dural sac or against a spinal nerve as it emerges from the spinal column (Fig. 58-13). This

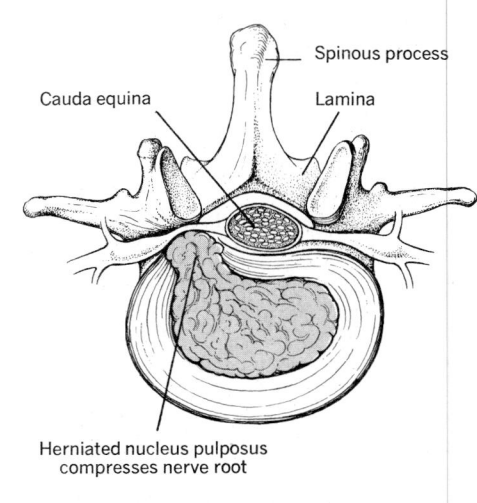

Figure 58-13. Ruptured vertebral disc. (From Chaffee EE and Greisheimer EM: Basic Physiology and Anatomy, 3rd ed. Philadelphia, JB Lippincott.)

sequence produces pain due to pressure in the area of distribution of the involved nerve. Continued pressure may produce degenerative changes in the involved nerve, such as changes in sensation and reflex action.

Assessment
Clinical Manifestations. A herniated disc with accompanying pain may occur in any portion of the spine: cervical, thoracic (rare), or lumbar. The clinical manifestations depend on the location, the rate of development (acute or chronic), and the effect on the surrounding structures.

A *cervical disc herniation* usually occurs at the C5–C6 and C6–C7 interspaces. Pain and stiffness may occur in the neck, the top of the shoulders, and the region of the scapulae. At times, the patient may interpret these signs as symptoms of heart trouble or bursitis. Pain may also occur in the upper extremities and head, accompanied by paresthesia and numbness of the upper extremities. The diagnosis is usually confirmed by cervical myelography.

The majority of *lumbar disc herniations* occur at the L4–L5 or the L5–S1 interspaces. A lumbar disc produces low back pain accompanied by varying degrees of sensory and motor impairment. The patient complains of low back pain with muscle spasms, which is followed by radiation of the pain into one hip and down into the leg (sciatica). Pain is aggravated by actions that increase intraspinal fluid pressure (bending, lifting, straining, as in sneezing or coughing) and is usually relieved by bed rest. There is usually some type of postural deformity, since pain causes an alteration of the normal spinal mechanics. If the patient lies on his back and attempts to raise his leg in a straight position, pain will radiate into the leg because this maneuver (straight-leg raising test) stretches the sciatic nerve. Additional signs include muscle weakness, alterations in tendon reflexes, and sensory loss.

Diagnostic Assessment. A myelogram usually demonstrates the area of pressure and localizes the herniation of the disc. The newer water-soluble compounds (metrizamide) make myelography more acceptable to the patient. Computed tomography scans may be indicated. A neurologic examination is carried out to determine if there is reflex, sensory, or motor impairment from root compression. Electromyography may be used to localize the specific spinal nerve roots involved.

The nursing process is similar to that for low back pain (see p. 1454).

Management: Cervical Disc Herniation

The goals of treatment are (1) to rest and immobilize the cervical spine to give the soft tissues time to heal, and (2) to reduce inflammation in the supporting tissues and the affected nerve roots in the cervical spine. Bed rest (usually 2 weeks) is important since it eliminates the stress of gravity and frees the cervical spine from having to support the weight of the head. It also reduces inflammation and edema in soft tissues around the disc, relieving pressure on the nerve roots. Proper positioning on a firm mattress may bring dramatic relief from pain.

The cervical spine may be rested and immobilized by a cervical collar, cervical traction, or a brace. A collar allows maximal opening of the intervertebral foramina and holds the head in a neutral or slightly flexed position. The patient may have to wear the collar 24 hours a day during the acute phase. The skin site under the collar is inspected for irritation. When the patient is free of pain, cervical isometric exercises are started to strengthen the muscles in the neck.

Cervical traction is accomplished by means of a head halter attached to a pulley and weight. It increases vertebral separation and thus relieves pressure on the nerve roots. The head of the bed is elevated to provide countertraction. If the skin becomes irritated, the halter can be padded. Experience has shown that a male patient may suffer more skin irritation if he shaves; the beard offers a natural form of padding.

Hot, moist compresses (10–20 minutes) applied to the back of the neck several times daily will increase blood flow to the muscles and help to relax the spastic muscles, as well as the patient. Analgesics are given during the acute phase to relieve pain, and sedatives may be administered to control the anxiety often associated with cervical disc disease. Muscle relaxants are administered to interrupt the cycle of muscle spasm and to allow for patient comfort. Anti-inflammatory drugs (aspirin, phenylbutazone [Butazolidin], oxyphenbutazone [Tandearil]) or steroids are given to treat the inflammatory response that usually occurs in the supporting tissues and affected nerve roots. Occasionally, an injection of a corticosteroid drug into the epidural space may be tried as a means of relieving radicular pain. Food and antacids are given with anti-inflammatory agents to prevent gastrointestinal irritation. Periodic blood evaluations should be carried out to detect the development of blood dyscrasias.

Surgical excision of the herniated disc may be necessary when there is a significant neurologic deficit, progression of a neurologic deficit, signs of cord compression, or no improvement or worsening of pain. In the cervical area, an anterior or posterior discectomy may be done (see p. 1376).

Patient Education. The patient must be cautioned against flexing, extending, or rotating the neck in any extreme manner while working. When sleeping, the patient should avoid the prone position and should keep his head in a neutral position, using a feather or down-filled pillow. The patient should be cautioned not to prop himself up in bed with several pillows, since this produces neck flexion.

Long automobile rides during the acute phase should be avoided, because vibration associated with such trips has an adverse effect on the spine. It may take up to 6 weeks to recuperate from a significant disc herniation.

Management: Herniated Lumbar Disc

The objectives of treatment are to relieve the pain and slow the progression of the disease and to increase the functional ability of the patient. Bed rest on a firm mattress (to limit spinal flexion) is encouraged to reduce the weight load and gravitational forces, thereby freeing the disc from stress. The patient is allowed to assume a comfortable position; usually, a semi-Fowler's position with moderate hip and knee flexion is most satisfactory.

Since muscle spasm is prominent during the acute phase, muscle relaxants are used. Anti-inflammatory drugs and systemic steroids may be administered to counter the inflammation that usually occurs in the supporting tissues and the affected nerve roots. Moist heat and massage help to relax spastic muscles and produce a sedating effect on the patient.

Chemonucleolysis. *Chemonucleolysis* (nonoperative chemical removal of displaced lumbar disc material) is a method of treating a protruding lumbar disc accompanied by root irritation. The procedure consists of injecting chymopapain (Discase) into the diseased disc. Chymopapain is an enzyme derived from the papaya plant; it has a proteolytic action that dissolves all or part of the nucleus pulposus, reducing the pressure on the adjacent nerve roots and thus alleviating pain.

This technique is regarded as the last step in the conservative treatment of lumbar disc herniation and not as an alternative to surgical removal of a free disc fragment in the spinal canal. An anaphylactoid reaction is possible with this drug.

Surgical Intervention. Muscle weakness and atrophy, loss of sensory and motor function, and unrelieved acute pain are indications of a significant neurologic deficit. When these manifestations occur, surgical intervention (hemilaminectomy with exposure of the nerve root involved and removal of the disc fragment) is undertaken. If more than one disc is involved, pain and disability tend to recur, requiring another operation. In this event, a spinal fusion may be done (see p. 1376).

Patient Education and Rehabilitation. The patient with a lumbar disc can begin to ambulate gradually when the inflammatory reaction and edema from the disc herniation have subsided. For patients with weak abdominal muscles, a corset or brace may be necessary to help pull the abdomen in and alter the lumbar sacral curve, so as to relieve the strain on the ligaments.

To correct underlying mechanical problems that commonly contribute to painful derangements of the low back, an exercise program is designed to strengthen the abdominal muscles, and gentle stretching exercises are prescribed to improve the suppleness and elasticity of the paraspinal muscles and ligaments. The patient is instructed as follows:

1. Lie on the floor, knees bent, with feet flat on the floor and arms folded across the chest.
2. Slowly elevate the head and shoulders; relax. Continue several times and increase daily.
3. Slowly flex the trunk; relax.
4. Continue the exercises daily for an indefinite period of time.
5. Discontinue the exercises if pain worsens.

The patient is taught to sleep on his side with the knees and hips in a position of flexion (pillow between the legs). Caution him not to sleep in a prone position since this hyperextends the spine. Encourage correct posture while standing, sitting, walking, and working. He should be taught to lift correctly by bending the knees and keeping the back straight and to avoid lifting anything above the elbows. The obese person with a protruding abdomen and lordotic posture has chronic back strain and is encouraged to carry out a weight-control program. (See also, Patient Education, Low Back Strain, p. 1457.)

Disc Surgery

Surgical excision of a herniated disc is done when there is evidence of a progressing neurologic deficit (muscle weakness and atrophy, loss of sensory and motor function, loss of sphincter control) and continuing pain and sciatica. The objective of surgical treatment is to relieve pressure on the nerve root in order to relieve pain. Microsurgical techniques are making possible the precise removal of diseased tissue through a small incision while better preserving the integrity of normal tissue and imposing less trauma on the body. During these procedures, spinal cord function can be monitored electrophysiologically.

To achieve the goal of pain relief, several operative techniques are employed, depending on the type of disc herniation, operative morbidity, and overall results of surgery:

Discectomy—removal of herniated disc tissue and related matter
Laminectomy—removal of the lamina to expose the neural elements in the spinal canal; allows inspection of the spinal canal and identification and removal of pathology and compression from the cord and roots
Laminotomy—division of the lamina of a vertebra
Discectomy with fusion—a bone graft (from iliac crest/bone bank) is used to fuse the vertebral spinous process; the object of spinal fusion is to bridge over the defective disc to stabilize the spine

In the cervical area, an anterior approach may be used through a transverse incision in the neck to remove disc material that has herniated into the spinal canal and foramina. Or a posterior approach may be used at the desired level of the cervical spine. In the lumbar region, the surgical treatment is excision through a posterolateral laminotomy.

Preoperative Management. Most patients fear surgery on any part of the spine and therefore need assurance (that surgery will not "weaken" the back) and explanations all along the way. When data are being collected for the nursing history, any complaints of pain, paresthesia, and muscle spasm are recorded in order to have a baseline for comparison after surgery. Preoperative assessment should also include an evaluation of movement in the extremities as well as bladder and bowel function. To facilitate the postoperative turning procedure, the patient is taught to turn himself as a unit (logrolling) as part of the preoperative preparation. Other facets of the postoperative regimen that should be practiced before the operation are deep-breathing, coughing, and muscle-setting exercises, which will help maintain muscle tone.

Cervical Disc: Postoperative Management. Throughout the postoperative period, vital signs are monitored frequently to detect any signs of respiratory difficulty. Occasionally, during surgery the recurrent laryngeal nerve may be injured by retractors, resulting in hoarseness and inability to cough effectively. The elimination of pulmonary secretions then becomes a problem requiring chest physical therapy. Usually, the major complaint of the patient is a sore throat, which can be relieved by throat sprays (Chloraseptic spray). Throat sprays or lozenges that numb the throat are avoided since the numbness may result in choking. The patient may complain of dysphagia, which is probably due to edema of the esophagus. In this event, a blenderized, soft diet may be given. One sign to watch for following an anterior cervical discectomy is a sudden return of radicular pain, which may indicate that the spine has become unstable.

Lumbar Disc Excision: Postoperative Management. Following surgery, the vital signs are checked frequently and the wound is inspected for evidence of hemorrhage, as vascular injury is a complication of disc surgery. Since postoperative neurologic deficits may occur from nerve root injury, the sensation and motor power of the lower extremities are evaluated at specified intervals, along with the color and temperature of the legs and sensation of the toes. Another important sign to check is possible urinary retention.

To position the patient, a pillow is placed under his head, and the knee rest is elevated slightly since slight knee flexion relaxes the muscles of the back. However, when the patient is lying on his side, extreme knee flexion must be avoided. The patient is encouraged to move from side to side to relieve pressure. But first he is reassured that no injury will result from moving. When the patient is about to be turned, the bed is placed in a flat position and a pillow is placed between his legs. He is then turned as a unit (logrolling) without twisting the back.

Following surgery, the patient may experience varying degrees of pain and sensory manifestations in the legs and may worry about these sensations. Usually, they represent a temporary manifestation due to inflammatory changes, edema, and swelling of the compressed nerve. Occasionally, they may be caused by the presence of disc material adjacent to a nerve root. Narcotics and sedatives are given during the early postoperative period to relieve pain and anxiety.

Early ambulation is encouraged. To assist the patient out of bed, the head of the bed is raised while the patient lies on his side. The patient's head and shoulders are supported while he pushes himself up to a sitting position. At the same time, another person eases the patient's legs over the side of the bed. Coming to a sitting or standing posture should be accomplished by one long, smooth motion.

In cases requiring discectomy with fusion, the patient will have an additional wound if bone fragments are taken from the iliac crest or fibula to serve as wedges in the spine. Therefore, the leg wound must be attended to after surgery, and attention must be given to moving the leg that was operated on. Pillows must be adjusted for support and comfort, and care must be taken to avoid sudden flexion and extension at the knee, which will cause pain. The recovery period is somewhat slower than in those patients who have undergone removal of the ruptured portion of the disc without a spinal fusion, because bony union must take place.

Complications of Disc Surgery. A person having a disc procedure at one level may have degenerative processes at other levels of the vertebral column. A herniation relapse may occur at the same level or elsewhere, so that the patient is apt to become a candidate for another disc procedure. Arachnoiditis may occur after operation (and after myelography) in which there is an insidious onset of diffuse, frequently burning pain in the lower back, radiating into the buttocks. Disc excision can leave adhesions and scarring around the spinal nerves and dura, which then produce inflammatory changes that can create chronic neuritis and neurofibrosis. Disc surgery may relieve pressure on the spinal nerves, but it does not reverse the effects of neural injury and scarring and the pain that ensues.

"Failed disc syndrome" (recurrence of sciatica after lumbar discectomy) remains a common cause of disability.

Patient Education. The patient is advised that since it takes up to 6 weeks for the ligaments of the muscles to heal, activity is to be gradually increased up to the point of tolerance. Activities that produce flexion strain on the spine (driving a car) should be avoided until healing has taken place. Heat may be applied to the back to soothe and relax muscle spasm and help absorb exudates in the tissues. Scheduled rest periods are important. Usually, the patient is advised to avoid heavy work for 2 to 3 months after surgery. Exercises are prescribed to strengthen the abdominal and erector spinal muscles. A back brace or corset may be necessary if back pain persists. (See also Patient Education, low back pain, p. 1457.)

Spinal Cord Tumors

Tumors that occur within the spinal cord or exert pressure on it cause symptoms ranging from weakness and loss of reflexes above the tumor level and localized or shooting pains, to progressive loss of motor function and paralysis. Usually, sharp pain occurs in the area that is innervated by the spinal roots that arise from the cord in the region of the tumor. In addition, increasing paralysis develops below the level of the lesion. The level of the tumor usually may be determined by a neurologic examination; however, myelography is necessary for exact localization.

Surgical Management. The removal of the tumor is usually desired but not always feasible (if the tumor is at-

tached to the spinal cord). However, microsurgical techniques have improved the prognosis for surgical treatment of intramedullary tumors. The nursing management is similar to that following disc surgery (see p. 1376). Other treatment modalities include subtotal removal of the tumor, decompression of the spinal cord, chemotherapy, and radiation therapy.

If the patient has epidural spinal cord compression from metastatic cancer (from breast, prostate, lung), high-dose dexamethasone combined with radiation therapy appears to be effective in relieving pain.

▷ The Paraplegic Patient*

Paraplegia (loss of motion and sensation in lower extremities) most frequently follows trauma due to accidents and gunshot wounds, but may be the result of spinal cord lesions (intervertebral disc, tumor, vascular lesions), multiple sclerosis, infections and abscesses of the spinal cord, and congenital defects. The patient requires extensive rehabilitation, which will be less difficult if appropriate nursing management has been carried out during the acute phase of the injury or illness. (See the management of spinal cord injuries, p. 1369.) The nursing care is one of the determining factors in the success of the rehabilitation program.

Psychological Support

It is usually some time before the patient comprehends the magnitude of the disability. He may go through stages of adjustment, including shock and disbelief, denial, depression, grief, and acceptance. During the acute phase of the injury, denial can be a protective mechanism to shield the patient from the overwhelming reality of what has happened. As he realizes the finality of paraplegia (or quadriplegia), the grieving process may be prolonged by the awareness of "what will never be." A period of depression follows as the patient experiences a loss of self-esteem in areas of self-identity, sexual functioning, and social and emotional roles. Self-esteem is related to being strong, loved, and lovable— all of which are threatened by the injury. To be able to work through this depression, the patient must be able to see some hope for relief in the future. Thus, he is guided toward a sense of confidence in his ability to achieve self-care and relative independence. The role of the nurse ranges from caretaker during the acute phase to teacher, counselor, and facilitator as the patient gains mobility and independence.

Adjustment to the disability leads to the development of realistic goals for the future, making the best of those abilities that are left intact. Rejection of the disability will cause self-destructive neglect and noncompliance with the therapeutic program. This leads to more frustration and depression. The family usually requires counseling, social

---

* *Quadriplegia* (tetraplegia) is loss of motion and sensation involving both upper and lower extremities. These patients require the same meticulous nursing management to prevent complications that are given patients with paraplegia. Their rehabilitation problems and procedures are more complex. Therefore, patients with quadriplegia are treated in rehabilitation centers with personnel and facilities that can meet their special needs.

services and other support systems to help them cope with the changes that will be made in their life-style and socio-economic status. (The psychological implications of a disability are discussed also on p. 229.)

Weight-bearing Activities

A patient with complete severance of the cord can begin weight bearing early, because no further damage can be incurred. The sooner muscles are strengthened, the less chance they will atrophy (disuse atrophy). The earlier the patient is brought to a standing position, the less opportunity there will be for osteoporotic changes to take place in the long bones. Weight bearing also diminishes urinary infections and the formation of renal calculi and enhances many other metabolic processes.

Postural Hypotension. Because vasomotor tone is lacking in the lower extremities, the patient may become hypotensive when placed in an upright position. Profound postural hypotension is seen in all patients with lesions above the midthoracic level. Postural hypotension results because the reflex arcs that normally produce vasoconstriction in the upright position have been interrupted. There is pooling of blood in the peripheral veins and splanchnic bed from lack of muscle tone and poor skin turgor. There is reduced venous return to the heart, orthostatic hypotension, and decreased cerebral blood flow.

To counteract this problem, a tilt table may be used to help the patient overcome vasomotor instability and tolerate the upright posture. Other possible measures include wearing elastic stockings to facilitate venous return in the legs and applying an abdominal binder to alleviate the pooling of blood in the abdominal area.

When a tilt table is used, the patient is gradually elevated to an upright position. At first he may be able to tolerate only an elevation of 45 degrees (or less), but gradually the angle of elevation is increased. The patient should be observed closely for signs of intolerance, including nausea, perspiration, pallor, dizziness, and syncope. The patient's blood pressure is taken before he is allowed up and as soon as he is positioned on the tilt table, since periods of recumbency also favor the development of orthostatic hypotension.

If no tilt table is available, a high-back reclining wheelchair with extension leg rests may be used. To overcome the effects of hypotension, the backrest is raised slowly and the leg rests are lowered gradually over a period of 7 to 10 days. While in the wheelchair, the patient may experience dizziness, tachycardia, hypotension, and blackouts. If he becomes dizzy, the brakes should be placed in the "on" position and the wheelchair tilted back for several minutes. If hypotension is prolonged, cerebral anoxia with the possibility of a cerebrovascular accident is a distinct threat and must be avoided.

Bowel Training Program

The objective of a bowel training program is to establish bowel evacuation through reflex conditioning. This technique is described on page 251. If a cord injury occurs above the sacral segments or nerve roots and there is reflex activity, the anal sphincter may be massaged to stimulate defecation. (If the cord lesion involves the sacral segment

or nerve roots, anal massage is not done, because the anus may be relaxed and lack tone. Massage is also contraindicated if there is spasticity of the anal sphincter.) The anal sphincter is massaged by inserting a gloved finger (which has been adequately lubricated) 2.5 cm to 3.7 cm (1–1½ inches) into the rectum and moving it in a circular motion or from side to side. It will soon become apparent which area triggers the defecation response. This procedure should be done at the same time (usually every 48 hours) after a meal and at a time that will be convenient for the patient when he returns home. The patient is also taught the symptoms of impaction (frequent loose stools; constipation) and cautioned to watch for the development of hemorrhoids. A diet with sufficient bulk is essential to a bowel training program.

Muscle Exercises

The diet for a paraplegic patient usually is high in protein, vitamins, and calories. The unaffected parts of the body are built up to optimal strength to enable the patient to ambulate with braces and crutches. The muscles of the hands, arms, shoulders, chest, spine, abdomen, and neck must be strengthened, since the patient must bear full weight on these muscles. The triceps and the latissimus dorsi are important muscles used in crutch walking. The muscles of the abdomen and the back also are necessary for balance and the maintenance of the upright position.

To strengthen these muscles, the patient can do "push-ups" when he is in a prone position and "sit-ups" while he is in a sitting position. Extending the arms while he holds weights (traction weights can be used) also develops muscle strength. Squeezing rubber balls or crumpling newspaper promotes hand strength.

Through the encouragement of all of the members of the rehabilitation team, the patient develops the increased exercise tolerance needed for gait training and ambulation activities.

Mobilization

When the spine is stable enough to allow the patient to assume an upright posture, mobilization activities are initiated. A brace or vest may be used, depending on the level of the lesion. Braces and crutches enable some patients to ambulate for short distances and even to drive manually operated automobiles. Crutch ambulation in paraplegics requires high energy expenditure. Modern technological developments such as motorized wheelchairs and specially equipped vans, are contributing to the greater independence and mobility of patients with high-level spinal cord injuries.

A major goal of nursing management is to help the patient overcome his sense of futility and to encourage him in the emotional adjustment that must be made before he is willing to venture into the "outside world." To achieve this goal, it is important to realize that an excessively sympathetic attitude may cause the patient to develop an overdependence that defeats the purpose of the entire rehabilitation program.

Teach and help when necessary, but do not take over activities that the patient can do for himself with a little effort. This type of nursing care more than repays itself in the satisfaction of seeing a completely demoralized and helpless patient begin to find meaning in his newly emerging life-style.

Complications

Autonomic dysreflexia (autonomic hyperreflexia) is an acute emergency that occurs as a result of exaggerated autonomic responses to stimuli. This syndrome is characterized by a severe, pounding headache with paroxysmal hypertension, profuse sweating (most often of the forehead), nasal congestion, and bradycardia. It occurs among patients with cord lesions above the T6 level (the sympathetic splanchnic visceral outflow). The sudden rise in blood pressure may cause a rupture of one or more cerebral blood vessels or lead to an increase in intracranial pressure. A number of stimuli may trigger this reflex: distended bladder (the most common cause), distended bowel, stimulation of the skin (tactile, pain, thermal stimuli), or distention or contraction of the visceral organs, especially the bowel (constipation, impaction). Since this is an emergency situation, the objective is to remove the triggering stimulus and to avoid the possible serious complications.

- Place the patient in a sitting position to lower the blood pressure.
- Drain the bladder via the catheter. If the catheter is not patent, irrigate it with a small amount of irrigating solution or insert another catheter.
- After the symptoms subside, the rectum is examined for a fecal mass. If one is present, Dibucaine ointment is applied 10 to 15 minutes before the mass is removed, since visceral distention or contraction can cause autonomic dysreflexia.
- Any other stimulus that can be the triggering event, such as an object on the skin or a draft of cold air, must be removed.
- If these measures do not relieve the patient's hypertension and excruciating headache, a ganglionic blocking agent (hydralazine hydrochloride [Apresoline]) is given slowly by vein.
- The patient's chart should be tagged with an allergic marker.

Any patient with a lesion above the T6 segment should be informed that such an episode is possible and may even occur many years after the initial injury.

Other Complications. Other complications of paraplegia include bladder and kidney infections, which are discussed under neurogenic bladder (see p. 975), pressure sores (see p. 238), and depression (see pp. 229 and 1377). Heterotropic ossification (overgrowth of bone) occurs in 20% to 40% of spinal cord injury patients in the hips, knees, shoulders, and elbows. This complication can produce a loss of range of motion. Disodium etidronate is used investigationally to prevent formation and retard the development of this complication.

Sexuality of the Paraplegic Patient. Most patients with cord injury can have some form of meaningful sexual relationship, although some modifications will have to be made to cope with anxiety. The patient and his partner will benefit from counseling on the range of sexual expression, special techniques, positions, exploration of body sensations offering sensual feelings, and urinary and bowel hygiene as related to sexual activity. Penile prostheses are available for men with erectile failure. Sexual education and counseling services are being included in the rehabilitation services at spinal centers. Small group meetings in which the patients can share their feelings, receive information, and discuss sexual concerns and practical aspects are helpful in producing effective attitudes and adjustments.

Home Care: Continuing Medical and Rehabilitation Care

The patient with a spinal injury is at risk the first few weeks after his return home. Urinary infections, pressure sores, and deconditioning resulting in contractures may appear and may require rehospitalization. To avoid these complications, a family member is taught skin care, catheter care, range of motion exercises, etc., while the patient is still in the hospital. The community health nurse provides follow-up evaluation to reinforce previous teaching and to answer questions. The local counselor for the Division of Vocational Rehabilitation works with the patient with respect to job placement or additional educational or vocational training.

The patient requires continuing lifelong follow-up by the physician, physical therapist, and other rehabilitation team members, because the neurologic deficit is permanent and new problems can erupt that require prompt attention before they take their toll in additional physical impairment, time, morale, and money.

▷ Bibliography

Books

Adams RD and Victor M. Principles of Neurology, 2nd ed. New York, McGraw–Hill, 1981.

Bakay L and Glasauer FE. Head Injury. Boston, Little, Brown & Co, 1980.

Barbeau A (ed). Disorders of Movement. Philadelphia, JB Lippincott, 1981.

Black RB, Hermann BP, and Shope JT. Nursing Management of Epilepsy. Rockville, Maryland, Aspen Systems, 1982.

Boller F and Frank E. Sexual Dysfunction in Neurological Disorders. New York, Raven Press, 1982.

Boullin DJ. Cerebral Vasospasm. New York, John Wiley & Sons, 1980.

Calenoff L (ed). Radiology of Spinal Cord Injury. St Louis, CV Mosby, 1981.

Cline MJ and Haskell CM. Cancer Chemotherapy, 3rd ed. Philadelphia, WB Saunders, 1980.

Dam M, Gram L, and Penry JK. Advances in Epileptology. The XIIth Epilepsy International Symposium. New York, Raven Press, 1980.

Dorros S. Parkinson's Disease: A Patient's View. Cabin John, Maryland, Seven Locks Press, 1981.

Forsythe E. Living with Multiple Sclerosis. Boston, Faber & Faber, 1979.

Hayward R. Essentials of Neurosurgery. Oxford, Blackwell Scientific, 1980.

Hermann BP (ed). A Multidisciplinary Handbook of Epilepsy. Springfield, Illinois, Charles C Thomas, 1980.

Hickey J. The Clinical Practice of Neurological and Neurosurgical Nursing. Philadelphia, JB Lippincott, 1981.

Hopkins A. Epilepsy. The Facts. New York, Oxford University Press, 1981.

Hopkins LN and Long DM. Clinical Management of Intracranial Aneurysms. New York, Raven Press, 1982.

Johnson RT. Viral Infections of the Nervous System. New York, Raven Press, 1982.

Kaufman DM. Clinical Neurology for Psychiatrists. New York, Grune & Stratton, 1981.

Litel GR, Mahoney PE, and Keen J. Neurosurgery and the Clinical Team. New York, Springer, 1980.

Logigian MK (ed). Adult Rehabilitation: A Team Approach for Therapists. Boston, Little, Brown & Co, 1982.

Magee KR and Saper JR. Clinical and Basic Neurology for Health Professionals. Chicago, Year Book Medical Publishers, 1981.

Meyer JS and Shaw T. Diagnosis and Management of Stroke and TIAs. Menlo Park, Addison–Wesley, 1982.

Mulder DW (ed). The Diagnosis and Treatment of Amyotrophic Lateral Sclerosis. Boston, Houghton Mifflin, 1980.

Nogen AG. Epilepsy. Dallas, Taylor, 1980.

Omer GE and Spinner M. Management of Peripheral Nerve Problems. Philadelphia, WB Saunders, 1980.

Perske R et al. Mealtimes for Severely and Profoundly Handicapped Persons. Baltimore, University Park Press, 1977.

Pryse–Phillips W and Murray TJ. Essential Neurology, 2nd ed. Garden City, New York, Medical Examination, 1982.

Reynolds EH and Trimble MR. Epilepsy and Psychiatry. New York, Churchill–Livingstone, 1981.

Rose FC and Capildeo R. Research Progress in Parkinson's Disease. Kent, Pitman Medical, 1981.

Rosenberg RN (ed). Neurology. New York, Grune & Stratton, 1980.

Salcman M (ed). Neurologic Emergencies: Recognition and Management. New York, Raven Press, 1980.

Scheinberg P. Modern Practical Neurology, 2nd ed. New York, Raven Press, 1981.

Seiden MR. Practical Management of Chronic Neurologic Problems. New York, Appleton–Century–Crofts, 1981.

Sha'ked A. Human Sexuality in Rehabilitation Medicine. Baltimore, Williams & Wilkins, 1981.

Smith RR. Essentials of Neurosurgery. Philadelphia, JB Lippincott, 1980.

Snyder M and Jackle M. Neurologic Problems: A Critical Care Nursing Focus. Bowie, Maryland, Robert J Brady, 1981.

Sutherland JM. Fundamentals of Neurology. New York, ADIS Press, 1981.

Tator CH (ed). Early Management of Acute Spinal Cord Injury. New York, Raven Press, 1982.

Taylor JW and Ballenger S. Neurological Dysfunctions and Nursing Interventions. New York, McGraw-Hill, 1980.

Thompson RA and Green JR (ed). Critical Care of Neurologic and Neurosurgical Emergencies. New York, Raven Press, 1979.

Weiner WJ (ed). Respiratory Dysfunction in Neurologic Disease. Mt Kisco, New York, Futura, 1980.

Wilder BJ and Bruni J. Seizure Disorders. A Pharmacological Approach to Treatment. New York, Raven Press, 1981.

Woodbury DM, Penry JK, and Pippenger CE. Antiepileptic Drugs, 2nd ed. New York, Raven Press, 1982.

Youmans JR (ed). Neurological Surgery. Vols 1, 2, 3, 4, 5, 6, 2nd ed. Philadelphia, WB Saunders, 1982.

Articles
Amyotrophic Lateral Sclerosis

Amico LL and Antel JP. Amyotrophic lateral sclerosis. Postgrad Med 1981 Aug; 70(2):50–56, 58–61.

Bartels EJ. Amyotrophic lateral sclerosis. Helping the patient with Lou Gehrig's disease. RN 1979 Dec; 42(12):48–50, 79–82.

Blount M, Bratton C, and Luttrell N. Management of the patient with amyotrophic lateral sclerosis. Nurs Clin North Am 1979 Mar; 14(1):157–171.

DeLisa JA et al. Amyotrophic lateral sclerosis: Comprehensive management. Am Fam Physician 1979 Mar; 19(3):137–142.

Hartley FD. A nurses's view: Amyotrophic lateral sclerosis. J Neurosurg Nurs 1981 Apr; 13(2):89–96.

Lehner WE et al. Home care utilizing a ventilator in a patient with amyotrophic lateral sclerosis. J Fam Pract 1980 Jan; 10(1):39–42.

Mikulik MA, DeLisa JA, and Miller RM. Rehabilitate the patient with ALS? ARN Journal 1979 Nov–Dec; 4(6):4–7.

Rasmussen DJ. Amyotrophic lateral sclerosis. Am J Nurs 1980 Nov; 80(11):2050–2052.

Aneurysms/Brain Tumor

Adams HP. Current status of antifibrinolytic therapy for patients with aneurysmal subarachnoid hemorrhage. Current Concepts of Cerebrovascular Disease and Stroke 1981 Sept–Oct; 16(5):23–27.

Guidetti B and Spallone A. The role of antifibrinolytic therapy in the preoperative management of recently ruptured intracranial aneurysms. Surg Neurol 1981 Apr; 15(4):239–248.

Gunby P. Mannitol opens pathway for brain tumor chemotherapy. JAMA 1981 May 8; 245(18):1802.

Hirsh LF. Modern treatment of intracranial aneurysms. Postgrad Med 1980 Mar; 67(3):153–156, 158–160.

Kelly PJ and Alker GJ Jr. A stereotactic approach to deep-seated central nervous system neoplasms using the carbon dioxide laser. Surg Neurol 1981 May; 15(5):331–334.

Larson E. The epidemiology of primary brain tumors. J Neurosurg Nurs 1980 Sept; 12(3):121–127.

Maniglia AJ et al. Intracranial abscesses secondary to ear and paranasal sinus infections. Otolaryngol Head Neck Surg 1980 Nov–Dec; 88(6):670–680.

Sundt TM et al. Correlation of cerebral blood flow and electroencephalographic changes during carotid endarterectomy. Mayo Clin Proc 1981 Sept; 56(9):533–543.

Takaku A et al. Postoperative complications in 1,000 cases of intracranial aneurysms. Surg Neurol 1979 Aug; 12(2):137–144.

Thompson JE. Cerebral protection during carotid endarterectomy. Mayo Clin Proc 1981 Sept; 56(9):576–577.

Wilkins RH. Update—Subarachnoid hemorrhage and saccular intracranial aneurysms. Surg Neurol 1981 Feb; 15(2):92–101.

Epilepsy

Aminoff MJ. Drug treatment of epilepsy. Compr Ther 1981 Apr; 7(4):6–12.

Dam M. Recent advances in the treatment of epilepsy. Acta Neurol Scand [Suppl] 1980; 78:88–102.

Johannessen SI. Antiepileptic drugs: Pharmacokinetic and clinical aspects. Ther Drug Monit 1981; 3(1):17–37.

Norman SE. Surgical treatment of epilepsy. Am J Nurs 1981 May; 81(5):994–996.

Norman SE and Browne TR. Seizure disorders. Am J Nurs 1981 May; 81(5):984–994.

Polkey CE. Surgery for epilepsy. Br J Hosp Med 1981 Jan; 25(1):48–57.

Reynolds EH and Shorvon SD. Single drug or combination therapy for epilepsy. Drugs 1981 May; 21(5):374–382.

So EL and Penry JK. Epilepsy in adults. Ann Neurol 1981 Jan; 9(1):3–16.

Sutula TP et al. Intensive monitoring in refractory epilepsy. Neurology 1981 Mar; 31(3):243–247.

Tucker CA. Complex partial seizures. Am J Nurs 1981 May; 81(5):996–1000.

Head Injury

Burr M. The rehabilitation and long-term management of the adult patient with head injury. Aust Fam Physician 1981 Jan; 10(1):14–16.

Caring for the patient with elevated intracranial pressure (ICP). Nursing '82 1982 Jan; 12(1):48–49.

Fritz CP. Concussion: What to look for and what to do. Nursing '81 1981 Sept; 11(9):84.

Kaktis JV and Pitts LH. Complications associated with use of megadose corticosteroids in head-injured adults. J Neurosurg Nurs 1980 Sept; 12(3):166–171.

Krayenbühl H, Maspes PE, and Sweet WH. Craniocerebral trauma. Progress in Neurological Surgery 1981; 10:1–384 (entire volume).

Kunkel J. Nursing management of the head injured patient. Crit Care Update 1981 Mar; 8(3):22–33.

Maniglia AJ et al. Intracranial abscesses secondary to ear and paranasal sinuses infections. Otolaryngol Head Neck Surg 1980 Nov–Dec; 88(6):670–680.

Mastrian KG. Of course you can manage head trauma patients. RN 1981 Aug; 44(8):44–51.

Miller JD et al. Further experience in the management of severe head injury. J Neurosurg 1981 Mar; 54(3):289–299.

Minderhoud JM et al. Treatment of minor head injuries. Clin Neurol Neurosurg 1980; 82(2):127–140.

Oddy M and Humphrey M. Social recovery during the year following severe head injury. J Neurol Neurosurg Psychiatry 1980 Sept; 43(9):798–802.

Papo I et al. Traumatic cerebral mass lesions: Correlations between clinical, intracranial pressure and computed tomographic data. Neurosurgery 1980 Oct; 7(4):337–346.

Report on the National Head and Spinal Cord Injury Survey Conducted for the National Institute of Neurological and Communicative Disorders and Stroke. Neurosurgery 1980 Nov; (Suppl):S 1–43.

Rimel RW, Jane JA, and Tyson GW. Emergency management of head injuries. Resuscitation 1981 Mar; 9(1):75–97.

Saul TG and Ducker TB. Management of severe head injuries. Md State Med J 1981 Mar; 30(3):45–48.

Huntington's Disease

Anonymous. Confronting Huntington's disease. Am J Nurs 1979 Aug; 79(8):1432–1433.

Chase TN, Wexler NS, and Barbeau A. Huntington's disease. Adv Neurology 1979; 23:1–801 (entire volume).

Folstein S and Folstein M. Diagnosis and treatment of Huntington's disease. Compr Ther 1981 Apr; 7(4):60–66.

Goetz CG and Weiner WJ. Huntington's disease: Current concepts of therapy. J Am Geriatr Soc 1979 Jan; 27(1):23–26.

Kelly J. Nursing care study. Huntington's chorea: A mother shunned by her family. Nurs Mirror 1979 Apr 12; 148(15):45–46.

Shoulson I and Fahn S. Huntington's disease: Clinical care and evaluation (editorial). Neurology 1979 Jan; 29(1):1–3.

Stipe J, White D, and Van Arsale E. Huntington's disease. Am J Nurs 1979 Aug; 79(8):1428–1433.

Intervertebral Disc

Farfan HF (ed). Symposium. The role of spine fusion for low back pain. Spine 1981 May–June; 6(3):277–314.

Lunsford LD et al. Anterior surgery for cervical disc disease. Part 1: Treatment of lateral disc herniation in 253 cases. J Neurosurg 1980 July; 53(1):1–11.

McCulloch JA. Chemonucleolysis for relief of sciatica due to herniated intervertebral disc. Can Med Assoc J 1981 Apr 1; 124(7):879–889.

Mulford EF. Degenerative disease or "slipped disc?" The clues are clear-cut. RN 1981 Feb; 44(2):45–49.

Ravichandran G and Frankel HL. Paraplegia due to intervertebral disc lesions. Paraplegia 1981; 19(3):133–139.

Sussman BJ, Bromley JW, and Gomez JC. Injection of collagenase in the treatment of herniated lumbar disk. JAMA 1981 Feb 20; 245(7):730–732.

Tindall GT. Clinical aspects of lumbar intervertebral disc disease. J Med Assoc Ga 1981 Apr; 70(4):247–253.

Wilson DH and Harbaugh R. Microsurgical and standard removal of the protruded lumbar disc: A comparative study. Neurosurg 1981 Apr; 8(4):422–427.

Multiple Sclerosis

Blaivas JG. Management of bladder dysfunction in multiple sclerosis. Neurology 1980 July; 30(2):12–18.

Catanzaro M. MS: Nursing care of the person with MS. Am J Nurs 1980 Feb; 80(2):286–291.

Catanzaro M. Nursing care of the MS patient. Neurology 1980 July; 30(7, Part 2):44–47.

Davies GM. The problems of nursing patients with advanced multiple sclerosis at home. J Adv Nurs 1979 Nov; 4(6):635–645.

Editorial: Immunological approaches to therapy in multiple sclerosis. Med J Aust 1981 Jan 10; 1(1):1–3.

Editorial: Immunological treatment in multiple sclerosis. Lancet 1980 Nov 1; 2(8201):953–954.

Ellison GW and Myers LW. Immunosuppressive drugs in multiple sclerosis: Pro and con. Neurology 1980 July; 30(7, Part 2):28–32.

Gilman S. The diagnosis of multiple sclerosis. JAMA 1981 Sept 4; 246(10):1122–1123.

Hallpike JF. New treatments for multiple sclerosis. Br J Hosp Med 1980 Jan; 23(1):63–64, 66, 68.

Holland NJ, McDonnell M, and Wiesel–Levison P. Overview of multiple sclerosis and nursing care of the MS patient. J Neurosurg Nurs 1981 Feb; 13(1):28–33.

Illis LS, Sedgwick EM, and Tallis RC. Spinal cord stimulation in multiple sclerosis: Clinical results. J Neurol Neurosurg Psychiatry 1980 Jan; 43(1):1–14.

Kelly–Hayes M. Guidelines for rehabilitation of multiple sclerosis patients. Nurs Clin North Am 1980 June; 15(2):245–256.

Maggs A. Multiple sclerosis, Part 1. Nurs Times 1981 Mar 5; 77(10):414–418.

Maggs A. Multiple sclerosis, Part 2. Nurs Times 1981 Mar 12; 77(11):464–469.

McDonnell M et al. MS: Problem oriented nursing care plans. Am J Nurs 1980 Feb; 80(2):292–297.

Poser CM. Management of multiple sclerosis. Compr Ther 1981 Apr; 7(4):53–59.

Price G. The challenge to the family. Am J Nurs 1980 Feb; 80(2):283–285.

Read DJ, Matthews WB, and Higson RH. The effect of spinal cord stimulation on function in patients with multiple sclerosis. Brain 1980 Dec; 103(4):803–833.

Rose AS. Long-term care of patients with multiple sclerosis: A neurologist's perspective. Neurology 1980 July; 30(7, Part 2):59–60.

Slater RJ and Yearwood AC. MS: Facts, faith, and hope. Am J Nurs 1980 Feb; 80(2):276–281.

Spiegelberg N. Support group improves quality of life. ARN Journal 1980 Nov–Dec; 5(6):9–11.

Myasthenia Gravis

Anchie T. Plasmapheresis as a treatment for myasthenia gravis. J Neurosurg Nurs 1981 Feb; 13(1):23–27.

Barry L. The patient with myasthenia gravis really needs you. Nursing '82 1982 July; 12(7):50–53.

Clark RE et al. Thymectomy for myasthenia gravis in the young adult. J Thorac Cardiovasc Surg 1980 Nov; 80(5):696–701.

Hochman MS. Ocular myasthenia. JAMA 1982 Jan 1; 247(1):62.

Kornfeld P et al. Plasmapheresis in refractory generalized myasthenia gravis. Arch Neurol 1981 Aug; 38(8):478–481.

Rubin JW, Ellison RG, and Moore HV. Thymectomy in myasthenia gravis: The timing of surgery and significance of thymic pathology. Am Surg 1981 Apr; 47(4):152–156.

Scadding GK and Havard CWH. Pathogenesis and treatment of myasthenia gravis. Br Med J 1981 Oct 17; 283(6298):1008–1012.

Tindall RSA. Diagnosis and treatment of myasthenia gravis. Compr Ther 1981 May; 7(5):33–43.

Wechsler AS and Olanow CW. Myasthenia gravis. Surg Clin North Am 1980 Aug; 60(4):931–945.

Parkinson's Disease

Gelbart AO and Hamilton WJ. Parkinson's disease. Am Fam Physician 1981 June; 23(6):182–189.

Gresh C. Helpful tips you can give your patients with Parkinson's disease. Nursing '80 1980 Jan; 10(1):26–33.

Kelly PJ and Gillingham FJ. The long-term results of stereotaxic surgery and L-dopa therapy in patients with Parkinson's disease. A 10-year follow-up study. J Neurosurg 1980 Sept; 53(3):332–337.

McNairn N. Shirley, a success story. Can Nurse 1980 Dec; 76(11):40–41.

Perlik SJ et al. Parkinsonism: Is your treatment appropriate? Geriatrics 1980 Nov; 35(11):65–70, 74.

Stewart RM. Parkinson's disease: New treatments. Compr Ther 1981 Apr; 7(4):38–44.

Spinal Cord Injuries/Spinal Cord Tumors

Albin MS et al. The patient with spinal cord injury. Curr Probl Surg 1980 Apr; 17(4):190–262.

Anderson RU. Nonsterile intermittent catheterization with antibiotic prophylaxis in the acute spinal cord injured male patient. J Urol 1980 Sept; 124(3):392–394.

Bedbrook GM and Sedgley GI. The management of spinal injuries—past and present. Int Rehabil Med 1980; 2(2):45–61.

Britton C et al. Innovative discharge planning—the results may surprise you. Nursing '80 1980 Oct; 10(10):44–49.

Chehrazi B et al. A scale for evaluation of spinal cord injury. J Neurosurg 1981 Mar; 54(3):310–315.

Fischer G and Mansuy L. Total removal of intramedullary ependymomas: Follow-up of 16 cases. Surg Neurol 1980 Oct; 14(4):243–249.

Green BA et al. Kinetic nursing for acute spinal cord injury patients. Paraplegia 1980 June; 18(3):181–186.

Green BA et al. Acute spinal cord injury: Current concepts. Clin Orthop 1981 Jan–Feb; 154:125–135.

Greenberg HS, Kim J–H, and Posner JB. Epidural spinal compression from metastatic tumor: Results with a new treatment protocol. Ann Neurol 1980 Oct; 8(4):361–366.

Gunby P. New focus on spinal cord injury. JAMA 1981 Mar 27; 245(12):1201–1206.

Gunby P. From "regeneration" to prostheses: Research on spinal cord injury. JAMA 1981 Apr 3; 245(13):1293–1301.

King RB and Dudas S. Rehabilitation of the patient with a spinal cord injury. Nurs Clin North Am 1980 June; 15(2):225–243.

Lazure LL. Defusing the dangers of autonomic dysreflexia. Nursing '80 1980 Sept; 10(9):52–53.

Lindan R et al. Incidence and clinical features of autonomic dysreflexia in patients with spinal cord injury. Paraplegia 1980 Oct; 18(5):385–392.

Miller S, Szasz G, and Anderson L. Sexual health care clinician in an acute spinal cord injury unit. Arch Phys Med Rehabil 1981 July; 62(7):315–320.

Murphy MJ, Ogden JA, and Southwick WO. Spinal stabilization in acute spinal injuries. Surg Clin North Am 1980 Oct; 60(5):1035–1047.

Norrell H. The early management of spinal injuries. Clin Neurosurg 1980; 27:385–400.

Report on the National Head and Spinal Cord Injury Survey Conducted for the National Institute of Neurological and Communicable Disorders and Stroke. J Neurosurg 1980 Nov; (Suppl):S 1–43.

Rimel RW et al. Modified skull tongs for cervical traction. J Neurosurg 1981 Nov; 55(5):848–849.

Wagner FC and Chehrazi B. Spinal cord injury: Indications for operative intervention. Surg Clin North Am 1980 Oct; 60(5):1049–1054.

Williams GO. Management of spinal cord injury. J Fam Pract 1981 Feb; 12(2):231–237.

Trigeminal Neuralgia

Burchiel KJ et al. Comparison of percutaneous radiofrequency gangliolysis and microvascular decompression for the surgical management of tic douloureux. Neurosurgery 1981 Aug; 9(2):111–119.

Dalessio DJ. Treatment of trigeminal neuralgia. JAMA 1981 June 26; 245(24):2519–2520.

Ferguson GG et al. Trigeminal neuralgia: A comparison of the result of percutaneous rhizotomy and microvascular decompression. Can J Neurol Sci 1981 Aug; 8(3):207–214.

Mruthyunjaya B and Raju CG. Trigeminal neuralgia: A comparative evaluation of four treatment procedures. Oral Surg 1981 Aug; 52(2):126–132.

Sweeney PJ. Tic douloureux. Am Fam Physician 1981 Feb; 23(2):153–156.

Thomson T et al. Carbamazepine therapy in trigeminal neuralgia. Arch Neurol 1980 Nov; 37(11):699–703.

Voorhies R and Patterson RH. Management of trigeminal neuralgia (tic douloureux). JAMA 1981 June 26; 245(24):2521–2523.

Wilberger J and Velo A. Microneurosurgical treatment of trigeminal neuralgia and hemifacial spasm. South Med J 1981 Sept; 74(9):1124–1126.

Agencies
Governmental

Division for the Blind and Physically Handicapped, Library of Congress, Washington, D.C. 20542

National Institute of Neurological and Communicative Disorders and Stroke, National Institutes of Health, Bethesda, Maryland 20205

Voluntary

ALS Society of America, 15300 Ventura Blvd., Suite 315, Sherman Oaks, California 91403

American Heart Association (stroke), 7320 Greenville Ave., Dallas, Texas 75231

American Parkinson Disease Association, 116 John Street, New York, New York 10038

American Speech–Language–Hearing Association, 10801 Rockville Pike, Rockville, Maryland 20852

Association for Brain Tumor Research, 6232 North Pulaski Road, Suite 200, Chicago, Illinois 60646

Committee to Combat Huntington's Disease, 250 West 57th St., Suite 2016, New York, New York 10019

Epilepsy Foundation of America, 4351 Garden City Dr., Landover, Maryland 20785

Hereditary Disease Foundation, 9701 Wilshire Blvd., Suite 1204, Beverly Hills, California 90212

Muscular Dystrophy Association, Inc., 810 Seventh Ave., New York, New York 10019

Myasthenia Gravis Foundation, Inc., 15 East 26th St., New York, New York 10010

National ALS Foundation, Inc., 185 Madison Ave., New York, New York 10016

National Committee on the Treatment of Intractable Pain, P.O. Box 34571, Washington, D.C. 20034

National Easter Seal Society, Inc., 2023 West Ogden Ave., Chicago, Illinois 60612

National Head Injury Foundation, Inc., 280 Singletary Lane, Framingham, Massachusetts 01701

National Huntington's Disease Association, 128A East 74th St., New York, New York, 10021

National Migraine Foundation, 5214 North Western Ave., Chicago, Illinois 60625

National Multiple Sclerosis Society, 205 East 42nd St., New York, New York 10017

National Parkinson Foundation, 1501 N.W. Ninth Ave., Miami, Florida 31316

National Spinal Cord Injury Association, 369 Elliot St., Newton Upper Falls, Massachusetts 02164

Paralyzed Veterans of America, Inc., 4350 East–West Highway, Suite 900, Bethesda, Maryland 20814

Parkinson's Disease Foundation, William Black Medical Research Building, Columbia University Medical Center, 640 W. 168th St., New York, New York 10032

The Stroke Foundation, Inc., 898 Park Ave., New York, New York 10021

United Parkinson Foundation, 220 S. State St., Chicago, Illinois 60604

Unit XVI

Musculoskeletal and Locomotion Problems

59

Assessment of Musculoskeletal Function

The musculoskeletal system includes the bones, joints, muscles, tendons, ligaments, and bursae of the body. The occurrence of problems associated with these structures is very common and affects all age groups. Problems with the musculoskeletal system are generally not life-threatening, but they have a significant impact on one's productivity and economical status. Problems associated with the musculoskeletal system will be encountered by the nurse practicing in any field of nursing and during daily living experiences.

▷ Physiologic Overview

The musculoskeletal system is collectively the largest organ system in the body. Bony structures and connective tissue account for approximately 25% of the body weight, and muscle accounts for approximately 50% of the body weight. The health and functions of the musculoskeletal system are interdependent with the rest of the body systems.

    The functions of the musculoskeletal system include protection, support, locomotion, mineral storage, hemopoiesis, and heat production. The bony structure provides protection for vital organs, including the brain, heart, and lungs. The bony skeleton supports body structures by providing a strong and sturdy framework. The muscles attached to the skeleton allow the body to move. Calcium, phosphorus, and magnesium are among the minerals deposited and stored in the bone matrix. Not only do they harden the bones; but they are stored there. The red bone marrow located within the bone cavity is responsible for the production of red and white blood cells. Muscle contraction results in mechanical action as well as heat production. The heat production is important for keeping us warm.

The Skeletal System
Anatomy of the Skeletal System. There are 206 bones in the human body, divided into four categories: *long bones* (*e.g.,* the femur), *short bones* (*e.g.,* the tarsals), *flat bones* (*e.g.,* the sternum), and *irregular bones* (*e.g.,* the vertebrae).

Long bones are shaped as rodlike shafts with rounded ends. The shaft, or diaphysis, is made up of compact bone. The ends of the long bones are called epiphyses and are made up of porous, cancellous bone. The epiphyseal plate separates the epiphyses from the diaphysis and is the center for longitudinal growth in children. In the adult, it is calcified. The ends of long bones are covered by articular cartilage at the joints. Long bones are constructed for weight bearing and movement.

Short bones consist of cancellous bone covered by a layer of compact bone.

Flat bones are important sites for hemopoiesis (formation of blood) and frequently provide vital organ protection. They are made of cancellous bone layered between compact bone.

Irregular bones have unique shapes related to their function. Generally, irregular bone makeup is similar to that of flat bones.

Covering the bone is a dense, fibrous membrane known as the *periosteum.* The periosteum functions in nutrition and growth of bone, and provides for attachment of tendons and ligaments. The periosteum contains nerves, blood vessels, and lymphatics. The layer closest to the bone contains osteoblasts, which are bone-forming cells.

Endosteum is a thin, vascular membrane covering the marrow cavity of long bones and the spaces in cancellous bone. *Osteoclasts,* which dissolve away bone to maintain the marrow cavity, are located near the endosteum and in Howship's lacunae (indentations on bone surfaces).

Bone marrow is a vascular tissue located in the shaft cavity of long bones and in flat bones. Red bone marrow is responsible for the production of red and white blood cells. In the adult; the red bone marrow in the long bone cavity is replaced mostly by fatty, yellow marrow. Red bone marrow in the adult is located mainly in the sternum, ileum, vertebrae, and ribs.

Bone tissue is well vascularized. Periosteal vessels connect with bone tissue through minute Volkmann canals. In addition, nutrient arteries penetrate the periosteum and enter the medullary cavity through nutrient foramen. Nutrient arteries supply blood to the marrow and bone. The venous system may accompany arteries or may exit independently.

The osteon or haversian system is the microscopic functioning unit of mature bone. The center of the osteon contains a capillary. Around the capillary are circles of bone matrix called lamellae. Within the lamellae are *osteocytes* (mature, living bone cells). They are nourished by processes extending into tiny canaliculi canals that communicate with the blood vessel. The size of the osteon is limited by the nutritional supply. Bone cells and their nourishing blood vessel must be less than 0.1 mm apart.

Bone Formation.   Bone begins to form long before birth. The process in which hardening minerals are deposited into the bone is known as *ossification.* There are two basic models of ossification: intramembranous and endochondral. Intramembranous ossification, where bone develops within membrane, occurs in the bones of the face and skull. Therefore, when the skull heals, it is by fibrous union. The other kind of bone formation is known as endochondral ossification, in which a cartilage model exists and is resorbed and replaced by bone. Most bones in the body are formed and healed by endochondral ossification. By the age of 21 years, bone growth and maturation are complete.

Bone is composed of cells, protein matrix, and mineral deposits. The cells are of three basic types—*osteoblasts* (involved in the formation of bone matrix), *osteocytes* (located in the osteons and involved in homeostatic bone formation and destruction), and *osteoclasts* (multinuclear cells involved in bone destruction, resorption, and remodeling). The bone matrix is 98% *collagen,* which has been produced by the osteoblasts, and 2% *ground substances* (glucosamine glycans [acid polysaccharides] and proteoglycans). The matrix is a framework for deposition of the inorganic mineral salts.

The exact mechanism by which ossification occurs is unknown. The cell mitochondria probably play a vital role in the formation of microcrystallites, which are deposited in the matrix as precursors of larger mineral deposits. The ground substances may be the stimulus for the deposition of crystals. In addition, a specific charge may occur on the collagen fibers that initiate the crystal formation and electrostatically hold the crystals, once formed, in place. Actively growing bone is electronegative. The majority of crystals are composed of an insoluble calcium and phosphate complex called hydroxyapatite—$Ca_{10}(PO_4)_6(OH)_2$. More than 99% of the total body calcium is present in the bones. Other minerals deposited within the bone matrix include sodium, magnesium, fluoride, and carbonate.

Bone Maintenance.   Bone is a dynamic tissue in a constant state of turnover (resorption and reforming). Calcium in bone in an adult is replaced at the rate of about 18% a year. The important regulating factors that determine the balance between bone formation and bone resorption include local stress, vitamin D, parathyroid hormone, and calcitonin.

Local stress (weight bearing) acts to stimulate local bone resorption and formation and can result in extensive remodeling. In this way, deformed bones may tend to straighten out. This phenomenon also explains why important weight-bearing bones are thick and strong. When weight bearing or stress is prevented, such as in prolonged bed rest, calcium is lost from the bone.

Vitamin D functions to increase the amount of calcium in the blood by promoting absorption of calcium from the gastrointestinal tract and accelerating mobilization of calcium from the bone.

Parathyroid hormone and calcitonin are the major hormonal regulators of calcium homeostasis. Parathyroid hormone regulates the concentration of calcium in the blood, in part by promoting movement of calcium from the bone. Excessive mobilization of calcium due to excess parathyroid hormone results in demineralization of the bone and formation of bone cysts. Calcitonin, from the thyroid gland, increases the production of bone.

The Articular System

The bones of the body are joined together at *joints* or *articulations,* which allow for a variety of movements. Regardless of the amount of movement possible, the junction of two or more bones is called a joint. There are three basic kinds of joints: synarthrosis, amphiarthrosis, and diarthrosis.

Synarthrosis joints are immovable and are exemplified by the skull sutures. Amphiarthrosis joints, such as the vertebral joints and symphysis, allow some limited motion. The bones are separated by fibrous cartilage. Diarthrosis joints, like the elbow, are freely movable joints. Synovial fluid lubricates the movement of diarthroses (or synovial) joints.

At a typical movable joint, the ends of the articulating bones are covered with a smooth hyaline cartilage. The articulating bones are surrounded by a tough, fibrous sheath, the joint capsule. The capsule is lined with a membrane, the synovium, which secretes the lubricating and shock-absorbing synovial fluid into the joint capsule. Therefore, the bone surfaces do not come in direct contact. In some synovial joints, fibrocartilage discs are located between the articular cartilage surfaces. They provide shock absorption. In some joints, such as the knee, interosseous ligaments within the capsule are found and add strength to the joint. *Ligaments* (fibrous connective tissue bands) bind the articulating bones together. Ligaments and muscle tendons, which pass over the joint provide joint stability.

Movable joints are of several different kinds. The *ball and socket joints,* best exemplified by the hip or the shoulder, permit full freedom of movement. *Hinge joints* permit bending in one direction only and are best exemplified by the elbows and knees. A *saddle joint* allows movement in two planes at right angles to each other. The joint at the base of the thumb is a saddle, biaxial joint. The *pivot joint* is characterized by the articulation between the radius and the ulna. It permits rotation for such activities as turning a doorknob. *Gliding joints* allow for limited movement in all directions and are located at the joints of carpal bones in the wrist.

Bursae are additional structures associated with some joints. A bursa is a sac filled with synovial fluid that is located at a point of friction. Bursae are generally found cushioning the movement of tendons, ligaments, and bones at the elbow, shoulder, knee, and other joints. Tennis elbow and bunion are forms of bursitis.

The Skeletal Muscle System

Anatomy of Skeletal Muscles.   Skeletal (striated) muscles are involved in body movement, posture, and heat-production functions. Muscles are attached by tendons (cords of fibrous connective tissue) or aponeuroses (broad, flat sheets of connective tissue) to bones, connective tissue, other muscles, soft tissue, or skin. Muscles contract to bring the two points of attachment (origin—the movable part, and insertion—the immovable part) closer together. Muscles are of various shapes and sizes according to the activity for which they are responsible. Muscles develop and are maintained when actively used. Age and disuse causes loss of muscular function due to fibrotic tissue replacing the contractile muscle tissue.

The muscles of the body are composed of parallel groups of muscle cells (fasciculi) encased in fibrous tissue called epimysium or fascia. The more fasciculi contained in a muscle, the more precise the movements.

The speed of the muscle contraction is variable. Myoglobulin, a hemoglobin-like protein pigment, is present in striated muscle cells and transports oxygen from the blood capillaries to the muscle cell mitochondria for cellular metabolic needs. Muscles containing large quantities of myoglobulin (red muscle) have been observed to contract slowly and powerfully (*e.g.,* respiratory and postural muscles). Muscles containing little myoglobulin (white muscles) contract quickly and for extended periods of time (*e.g.,* extraocular eye muscles). Most body muscles contain both red and white muscle fibers.

Each muscle cell (also referred to as a muscle fiber) contains myofibrils, which in turn are composed of a series of sarcomeres, the actual contractile units of skeletal muscle. The components of the sarcomeres are known as thick and thin filaments. The thin filaments are composed mainly of a protein known as actin. The thick filaments are composed mainly of myosin, another protein material.

Skeletal Muscle Contraction.   Contraction of a muscle is due to the contraction of each of its component sarcomeres. The muscle shortens because each sarcomere shortens. The contraction of a sarcomere is due to interactions between the thick filaments and the thin filaments brought about by a local increase in the calcium ion concentration. The interaction between the actin and the myosin causes the thick and thin filaments to slide across one another. When calcium concentration in the sarcomere subsequently falls, the myosin and actin filaments cease to interact and the sarcomere returns to its original resting length (relaxation). Intracellular metabolic energy stored in the form of adenosine triphosphate (ATP) is required to break the actin and myosin bonds and allow relaxation. Interaction between actin and myosin does not occur in the absence of calcium because of the presence on the thin filaments of the proteins tropomyosin and troponin. In the presence of calcium, the configuration of these inhibitory proteins is altered, and the cross bridges between the myosin and actin filaments can occur.

Muscle fibers contract in response to electrical stimulation. When stimulated, muscle cells generate an action potential in a manner similar to that described for nerve cells. These action potentials propagate along the muscle cell membrane and lead to the release in the muscle cell of calcium ions that are stored in specialized organelles called the *sarcoplasmic reticulum.* The release of calcium allows the interaction of actin and myosin in the sarcomere. Very shortly after the muscle cell membrane is depolarized, it recovers its resting membrane voltage. Calcium is rapidly removed from the sarcomeres by active reaccumulation in the sarcoplasmic reticulum, and the muscle relaxes.

Depolarization of the muscle cells normally occurs in response to a stimulus delivered by a nerve cell. The communication between the nerve cell and the muscle cell takes place at the motor end plate. The neurons that control the activity of skeletal muscle cells are called *lower motor neurons,* which originate in the anterior horn of the spinal cord.

Energy is consumed during muscle contraction and relaxation. The rate of energy utilization by skeletal muscle is variable; it increases markedly during exercise. The source of energy for the muscle cells is ATP that is generated through cellular oxidative metabolism. Creatine phosphate, also present in muscle cells, functions as a second reservoir of metabolic energy: it can be converted to ATP when necessary.

At low levels of activity, the skeletal muscle synthesizes ATP from the oxidation of glucose to water and carbon dioxide. During periods of high activity when sufficient oxygen may not be available, glucose is metabolized primarily to lactic acid. Although ATP is generated during production of lactic acid, the process is inefficient compared with oxidative pathways. Therefore, increased amounts of glucose are required and are supplied by muscle glycogen. Glycogen is a starch that is produced from glucose, stored in the cells during periods of rest, and utilized during periods of activity. Muscle fatigue is thought to be caused by a rapid rate of work of the muscle, resulting in depletion of glycogen and energy stores and accumulation of lactic acid. As a result, the cycle of muscle contraction and relaxation cannot continue.

During muscle contraction, the energy released from ATP is not completely utilized by the contractile apparatus. This excess energy is dissipated in the form of heat. During isometric contraction, almost all the energy is released in the form of heat, while during isotonic contraction some of the energy is expended in mechanical work. In some situations, such as shivering, the need for generation of heat is the primary stimulus for muscle contraction.

Muscle Status. The contraction of muscle fibers can result in either isotonic or isometric contraction of the muscle. In *isometric contraction,* the length of the muscles remains constant, but the force generated by the muscles is increased. An example of this is when one pushes against an immovable wall. *Isotonic contraction,* on the other hand, is characterized by shortening of the muscle with no increase in tension within the muscle. An example of this is flexion of the forearm. In normal activities, many muscle movements are a combination of isometric and isotonic contraction. For example, during walking, isotonic contraction results in shortening of the leg, while during isometric contraction, the stiff leg pushes against the floor.

Relaxed muscles demonstrate a state of readiness to respond to contraction stimuli. This state of readiness is known as muscle tone (tonus) and is due to the maintenance of some of the muscle fibers in a contracted state. Sense organs in the muscles (muscle spindles) monitor the muscle tone, and through central nervous system innervation, the muscle tone is found to be minimal during sleep and increased when anxious. In lower motor neuron destruction (*e.g.,* polio), the denervated muscle becomes *atonic* (soft and flabby) and atrophies. A muscle that has less than normal tonus is known as *flaccid. Spastic* describes the muscle with greater than normal tonus.

Muscle Actions. Muscles accomplish movement only by contraction. They cannot push. Through the coordination of muscle groups, the body is able to perform a wide variety of movement. The prime mover is the muscle that causes a particular motion. The muscles assisting the prime mover are known as synergists. The muscle causing movement opposite to that of the primary mover is known as the antagonist. The antagonist must relax to allow the prime mover to contract, producing motion. For example, contraction of the biceps causes flexion, while contraction of the triceps causes extension of the elbow joint. When the elbow is flexed, the biceps is the prime mover and the triceps is the antagonist. With muscle paralysis, a person may be able to retrain functioning muscles within a synergistic group to coordinate in such a way as to effect the needed movement. Secondary movers then become the primary mover.

The body movements that muscle contractions can effect are many. *Flexion* is characterized by bending at a joint (*e.g.,* elbow). The opposite movement is *extension* or straightening at a joint. *Abduction* is the action of moving away from the midline of the body. To move toward the midline is *adduction. Rotation* is the turning around a specific axis (*e.g.,* shoulder joint). *Circumduction* is the cone-like movement of the thumb. Special body movements include *supination* (turning the palm up), *pronation* (turning the palm down), *inversion* (turning the sole of the foot inward), *eversion* (the opposite of inversion), *protraction* (the jaw is pulled forward), and *retraction* (the jaw is pulled backward).

Exercise, Disuse, and Repair. Muscles need to be exercised to maintain function and strength. When a muscle is repeatedly caused to develop maximum or close to maximum tension over a long period of time, as in regular exercise with weights, the cross-sectional area of the muscle increases. This is due to an increase in the cross-sectional area of each muscle fiber without increase in the number of muscle fibers. This increase in the size of the individual muscle fibers is called *hypertrophy.* Hypertrophy will persist only if the exercise is continued.

The opposite phenomenon occurs with disuse of muscle over a long period of time. The decrease in the size of a muscle is called *atrophy.* Bedrest and immobility will cause loss of muscle mass and strength. When immobility is due to a treatment mode (*e.g.,* casting or traction), the patient can decrease the effects of immobility by isometric exercise of the muscles of the immobilized part. Quadricep exercises (tightening the muscles of the thigh) and gluteal setting exercises (tightening the muscles of the buttocks) help maintain the large muscle groups that are important in ambulation. Active and weight-resistant exercises of uninjured parts of the body prevent degeneration.

When muscles are injured, they need rest and immobilization until tissue repair occurs. The healed muscle then needs progressive exercise to resume its preinjury functional state.

▷ Nursing Assessment

The nursing assessment is not limited to a detailed examination of the musculoskeletal system, because health problems affect the patient's physical, psychological, and social well-being. The nurse needs to assist the patient in identifying and dealing with his health needs through the nursing process. The patient will indicate his primary health concern and thus provide a beginning point for nursing intervention.

In the initial interview, the nurse obtains a general impression of the patient's status. A general inspection of the body will reveal the existence of any gross deformity, asymmetry of contours or size, swelling, edema, bruising, or breaks in the skin. Observing the patient's posture, movement, and gait will provide information concerning alterations in ability to move, the existence of discomfort, or the presence of involuntary movements (fasciculations or twitches). The nurse will also gather information concerning existing concurrent health problems, the patient's perceptions and expectations related to his health problems, and socioeconomic factors that will affect his restoration of well-being. Principles of clinical interviewing are found in Chapter 4.

History

The nurse needs to obtain subjective data from the patient concerning the onset of the problem, and how it has been managed to this point. The existence of other health problems (e.g., diabetes, heart disease, a cold) needs to be noted for consideration when developing the plan of care. A history of medication use and response to pain medication will aid in designing drug management regimens. Allergies need to be noted and should include the type of reaction the patient has experienced. The use of tobacco, alcohol, and other drugs should be assessed in order to evaluate the effects of these habits on the patient's needs. Notation of the patient's ability to learn, his economic status, and current occupation are needed for discharge planning and for rehabilitation. Additions to the initial interview data will be made as the nurse interacts with the patient. Such data allow for adjustment of the individualized plan of care.

Physical Assessment

Much information about the structure and functioning of the musculoskeletal system can be obtained by physical assessment, discussed in Chapter 5. The nurse is interested in identifying the functional abilities of the patient and the effects that any disabilities and medical treatment have on his ability to meet his needs. Any deviations from normal are noted. Much can be learned by observing the patient as he performs activities of daily living. Throughout the initial assessment, the nurse establishes a baseline for noting and evaluating changes in abilities.

Detailed physical assessment of the patient's total musculoskeletal system is generally not done. Specific methods of conducting a detailed evaluation of the musculoskeletal system are outlined in physical assessment texts. Depending on the health care setting, the nurse may need to incorporate a more detailed physical assessment. Generally speaking, the nurse is interested in assessing the integrity of the musculoskeletal system.

Assessment of Bony Skeleton.

The bony skeleton is assessed for deformities and alignment. Shortened limbs, amputations, and body parts out of anatomical alignment are noted. Possible common deformities of the spine that may be noted include *scoliosis* (a lateral curving deviation of the spine), *kyphosis* (a flexion of the thoracic spine), and *lordosis* (swayback; exaggeration of the lumbar spine curve). Abnormal angulation of long bone or motion at points other than joints are frequently indicative of fracture. *Crepitus* (grating sensation) at the point of abnormal motion may also be detected. Movement of fractures must be minimized to avoid additional injury. Abnormal bony growths due to bone tumors might be observed.

Assessment of Articular System.

The articular system is evaluated by noting joint swelling, deformity, stability, and range of motion. Joint swelling might be noted with arthritis, inflammation, or effusion (fluid accumulated in the joint capsule). Joint deformity may indicate contracture (shortening of surrounding joint structures), dislocation (complete separation of joint surfaces), subluxation (partial separation of articular surfaces), or disruption of structures surrounding the joint. Weakness or disruption of joint-supporting structures may result in a joint that is too weak to function as designed and that may therefore require external supporting appliances. Range of motion is evaluated both actively (the joint is moved by the muscles surrounding the joint) and passively (joint is moved by the examiner).

Range of Motion. Restricted range of motion means that the joint cannot be moved within the normal joint range as defined by the American Academy of Orthopedic Surgeons. Precise measurement of range of motion can be made by an instrument known as a goniometer. (A goniometer is a protractor designed for evaluating joint motion.) Limitation in range of motion may be due to skeletal deformity, joint pathology, muscular weakness, contracture of surrounding muscles and tendons, or neurologic denervation.

Feeling the joint while passively moving it will provide information concerning the integrity of the joint. Normally, the joint moves smoothly. A snap or a crack may indicate that a ligament is slipping over a bony prominence. Slightly roughened surfaces, such as in arthritic conditions, will result in *crepitus* as the surfaces of the joint are moved across one another.

Assessment of Muscular System.

The muscular system is assessed by noting the patient's ability to change position, his muscular strength and coordination, and individual muscle size. Muscular weakness of a group of muscles might indicate a variety of conditions, such as polyneuropathy, electrolyte disturbances (particularly potassium and calcium), myasthenia gravis, poliomyelitis, and muscular dystrophy. By palpating the muscle while passively moving the relaxed extremity, the nurse can determine the muscle tone. Muscle strength can be estimated by having the patient perform certain tasks with and without added resistance. For example, the biceps can be tested by requesting the patient to fully extend his arm and then flex it while the nurse applies resistance to prevent the arm from flexing. A simple handshake provides an indication of grasp strength.

Muscle clonus (rhythmic contractions of a muscle) may be elicited in the ankle or wrist. Fasciculations (involuntary twitching of muscle fiber groups) may be observed.

The girth of an extremity must be measured at times to monitor increased swelling due to edema or bleeding into the muscle or to a decrease in size due to atrophy. The unaffected extremity is measured and used as the reference standard. Measurements are to be taken at the maximum circumference of the extremity. It is important that the measurements be at the same extremity location and with the extremity in the same position with the muscle at rest. Distance from a specific anatomical landmark (e.g., 10 cm below the medial aspect of the knee for measurement of the calf muscle) should be indicated in the chart so that subsequent measurements are made at the same point. For ease of serial assessment, the point of measurement can be indicated by marking the skin. Variations in size need to be more than 1 cm to be considered significant.

Assessment of Skin and Peripheral Circulation.

In addition to the musculoskeletal system, the nurse must inspect the skin and assess peripheral circulation. Cuts, bruises, skin color, evidence of decreased circulation, or infection can influence nursing management. Feeling the skin can reveal if any areas are warmer or cooler than others and if edema is present. Assessing peripheral pulses and capillary refill time can demonstrate peripheral circulatory status.

Subjective Assessment Data.   During the interview and physical assessment, the patient may report the presence of pain, tenderness, tightness, and abnormal sensations. This information needs to be noted and assessed.

Pain

Most patients with diseases and traumatic conditions of muscles, bones, and joints experience pain. *Bone pain* is characteristically described as a dull, deep ache that is boring in nature, whereas *muscular pain* is considered sore and aching and is frequently referred to as muscle cramps. *Fracture pain* is sharp and piercing and is relieved by immobilization. Sharp pain may also result from *bone infection* with muscle spasm or pressure on a sensory nerve.

Most musculoskeletal pain is relieved by rest. Pain that increases with activity may indicate joint sprain or muscle strain, while steadily increasing pain points to a progression of an infectious process (osteomyelitis), a malignant tumor, or vascular complications. Radiating pain is seen in conditions in which pressure is exerted on a nerve root. Pain is variable and its assessment and nursing management must be individualized.

Assessment of Pain

- What was the patient doing before he complained of pain?
- Is his body in proper alignment?
- Is there pressure from traction, bed linen, a cast, or other appliances?
- Is he overly tired from lack of sleep, exciting stimuli, or too much activity?
- Can he localize the pain?
- How does he describe it?
- What was the manner of onset?
- Is there radiation of pain? If so, in what direction does it occur?
- Is there pain in any other part of the body?
- What is the character of the pain (sharp, dull, boring, shooting, throbbing, cramping)?
- Is it constant?
- What relieves it?
- What makes it worse?

Pain and discomfort are important to the patient and must be successfully managed. Not only is pain exhausting, but if prolonged it can force the patient to become increasingly preoccupied and dependent.

Altered Sensations

Sensory disturbances are frequently associated with musculoskeletal problems. The patient may describe the presence of *paresthesias* (burning or tingling sensations) and numbness. These sensations may be due to pressure on nerves or circulatory impairment. Soft tissue swelling or direct trauma to these structures can impair their function. Assessment of the neurovascular status of the involved mus-

culoskeletal area provides information for management. Loss of function can result from impaired nerves and circulatory structures located throughout the musculoskeletal system.

Assessment of Neurovascular Integrity

- Is the patient experiencing any abnormal sensations or numbness?
- When did this begin? Is it getting worse?
- Is the patient also experiencing pain?
- What is the color of the part distal to the problem? Pale? Dusky? Cyanotic?
- Is there a pulse present distal to the problem?
- Is there rapid capillary refill based on the blanche test? (Compress patient's nail and release. When pressure is released, the color of the nailbed should quickly assume a pink hue.)
- Is the motor component of the nerve intact? Is the patient able to move the innervated part?
- Is edema present?
- Is any constrictive device or clothing causing the nerve or vascular compression?
- Is it relieved by elevation of the affected part or modification of position?

▷ Diagnostic Assessment

Radiologic Procedures

X-rays are important in evaluating patients with musculoskeletal disorders. Bone films determine bone density, texture, erosion, and changes in bone relationships. Multiple x-ray views are needed to fully assess the structure being examined. X-ray of the cortex of the bone detects widening, narrowing, and any signs of irregularity. Joint x-rays will reveal the presence of fluid, irregularity, spur formation, narrowing, and changes in the joint structure.

Laminography or tomography shows in detail a specific plane of involved bone.

Computed tomography can be useful in orthopedic diagnosis by identifying tumors of the soft tissue or injuries to the ligaments or tendons. It is helpful in identifying the location and extent of fractures in difficult to define areas (*e.g.*, the acetabulum). The technique of computed tomography is discussed on page 331.

Myelography, the injection of contrast medium into the subarachnoid space of the lumbar spine, is carried out to determine disc herniation or the site of a tumor. This technique is discussed on page 1287.

Discography (see p. 1287) is a study of the intervertebral discs in which a contrast medium is injected into the disc and its distribution is noted.

Arteriography is a study of the arterial system. A radiopaque contrast medium is injected into the selected artery, and serial films are taken of the supplied arterial system. It is useful for determining arterial perfusion and aids in determining the amount of extremity that needs to be amputated.

Arthrography is the injection of a radiopaque substance or air into the joint cavity in order to outline soft tissue structures and the contour of the joint. The joint is put through its range of motion while a series of radiographs are taken. Arthrography is useful in identifying acute or chronic tears of the joint capsule or supporting ligaments of the knee, shoulder, ankle, hips, or wrist. (If a tear is present, the contrast medium will leak out of the joint and show on x-ray.)

Other Studies

An *arthrocentesis* is carried out to obtain synovial fluid for purposes of examination. A needle is inserted into the joint, and fluid is then aspirated. Since this procedure has the potential for introducing bacteria into the joint, aseptic techniques must be followed. Following aspiration, no special precautions are necessary.

Normally, synovial fluid is clear, pale, straw-colored, and scanty in volume. The fluid is examined grossly for volume, color, clarity, and viscosity and formation of mucin clot. It is examined microscopically for cell count, cell identification, Gram's stain, and formed elements. Examination of synovial fluid is helpful in the diagnosis of rheumatoid arthritis and other inflammatory arthropathies, and will reveal the presence of hemarthrosis (bleeding into joint cavity), which suggests trauma or a tendency to bleed.

Arthroscopy is an endoscopic procedure that allows direct visualization of a joint, especially the knee. The procedure is carried out in the operating room, under sterile conditions and following infiltration of a local anesthetic agent or a general anesthesia. A large-bore needle is inserted into the suprapatellar pouch, and the joint is distended with saline. The arthroscope is introduced and the knee joint visualized, including the synovium, articular surfaces, and menisci. If an arthrotomy is not indicated, the puncture wound is covered with a sterile Band-Aid and the extremity is wrapped from the mid-thigh to the midcalf with a compressive wrap that is worn for 24 hours for support. The patient may be advised to limit his activities for 3 days. When arthroscopy is combined with arthrography, a high degree of accuracy is achieved in diagnosing lesions and internal derangement of the knee.

A *bone scan* reflects the degree to which the matrix of bone "takes up" a bone-seeking radioactive isotope that is injected into the system. The degree of nuclide uptake is related to the metabolism of the bone. An increased uptake of isotope is seen in primary skeletal disease (osteosarcoma), metastatic bone disease, inflammatory skeletal disease (osteomyelitis), and certain types of fractures.

Thermography measures the degree of heat radiating from the skin surface. It is used to investigate the pathophysiology of inflamed joints (rheumatoid arthritis) and to assess the patient's response to anti-inflammatory drug therapy.

Electromyography provides information on the electric potential of the muscles and nerves leading to them. The purpose of this procedure is to determine any abnormal physiology involving the motor unit. Needle electrodes are inserted into selected muscles, and responses to electrical stimuli are recorded on an oscilloscope.

Laboratory Studies

Examination of the patient's blood and urine can provide information concerning a primary musculoskeletal problem (*e.g.,* Paget's disease), a developing complication (*e.g.,* in-

fection), baseline information for instituting therapy (*e.g.,* anticoagulant therapy), or response to therapy. The complete blood count will provide information concerning the hemoglobin level (frequently lower after bleeding associated with trauma) and the white blood cell count. Prior to surgery, coagulation studies are done to determine bleeding tendencies, because bone is a very vascular tissue. Blood chemistry studies provide data concerning a great variety of musculoskeletal conditions, including osteomalacia and muscle trauma. Urinalysis will reveal changes in calcium levels (*e.g.,* bone tumors) and creatinine levels (*e.g.,* crush injuries).

▷ Nursing Process Considerations

The nursing assessment will enable the nurse to identify the health problems that can be improved by nursing interventions. With the patient, health goals and nursing strategies will be formulated to achieve the goals and resolve the identified problems.

The patient with a musculoskeletal problem will require support and nursing care during the period of examinations and testing. There will be a need for physical and psychological preparation. Prior to the test, patient education (including what is to be done, why it is being done, and what patient participation is expected) will reduce the patient's anxiety and enable him to be an active participant in his care.

The resulting medical diagnosis and treatment regimen will affect the nursing management of the patient. The nursing plan of care will reflect nursing measures that will facilitate the resolution of the patient's problems.

▷ Bibliography

Books

Gartland J. Fundamentals of Orthopedics, 3rd ed. Philadelphia, WB Saunders, 1979.

Heppenstall R (ed). Fracture Treatment and Healing. Philadelphia, WB Saunders, 1980.

Hilt N and Cogburn S. Manual of Orthopedics. St Louis, CV Mosby, 1981.

Kelsey J, Pastides H, and Bisbee G Jr. Musculo-skeletal Disorders: Their Frequency of Occurrence and Their Impact on the Population of the United States. New York, Prodist, 1978.

Malasanos L et al. Health Assessment, 2nd ed. St Louis, CV Mosby, 1981.

Orthopedic Nurses' Association and American Nurses' Association Division on Medical–Surgical Nursing Practice. Standards of Orthopedic Nursing Practice. Kansas City, Missouri, American Nurses' Association, 1975.

Articles

Cohen S and Viellion G. Programmed Instruction: Patient assessment: Examining joints of the upper and lower extremities. Am J Nurs 1981 Apr; 81(4):763–786.

Crelin E. Development of the musculoskeletal system. Clin Symp 1981; 33(1):entire issue.

Farrell J. Bone structure and function: A self study. ONA J 1979 Apr; 6(4):142–150.

Wassel A. Nursing assessment of injuries to the lower extremity. Nurs Clin North Am 1981 Dec; 16(4):739–748.

60

Management Modalities for Patients With Musculoskeletal Dysfunction

▷ General Interventions

Individuals with problems of the musculoskeletal system require nursing measures to ensure their general health, and specific nursing techniques to manage their needs associated with the treatment modalities used.

Promoting Health. The general health measures include assuring systemic homeostasis, monitoring and encouraging optimum nutritional status, and preventing problems related to immobility. Musculoskeletal problems may be due to an acute traumatic injury or may be of a persistent, recurrent, long-term nature. The psychological and social/economic impact of the problem causes a variety of reactions in these individuals. The nurse needs to assist the patient in coping with the problems associated with musculoskeletal dysfunction and the associated therapies.

Psychological Support. Most patients with acute musculoskeletal problems are anxious and have pain. They experience a curious mixture of fear and anticipation before definitive therapy begins. People who have long-term disabilities frequently experience repeated reconstructive operations. They are familiar with the routines of the hospital and are concerned with the ultimate outcome of the procedure. Their patience and hope may be limited. Individuals with musculoskeletal problems need an understanding, supportive nurse.

One way to aid the patient is to prepare him for the anticipated therapeutic modality. If the patient is given information concerning preparatory measures and if he shares in this preparation, he will be more inclined to accept the care given. Information about what he is to expect during and following the therapy will encourage his active participation in his therapeutic regimen. When possible, specific information concerning anticipated equipment (*e.g.,* casts, traction), mobilization aids (*e.g.,* trapeze, walker, crutches), exercises (*e.g.,* quadriceps setting, deep breathing), and medications (*e.g.,* analgesics, antibiotics) should be shared with the patient. Cognitive preparation decreases anxiety and alerts the patient as to what is expected of him and what is usually involved in recovery. At times the patient can practice recuperative activities, such as using a urinal in a recumbent position, before he is immobilized and needs to tend to his basic bodily functions in unusual positions.

Pain Management. Patients who have bone and joint problems frequently experience severe pain. Many times, the person who has undergone surgery to correct a foot condition is much more uncomfortable than one who has had extensive abdominal surgery. Narcotics and other pain-relieving measures are given, taking into consideration the type of musculoskeletal problem and the size and age of the patient. In the long-term patient, drug dependence may occur and poses a considerable problem.

The pain experienced might result from associated problems rather than the primary musculoskeletal problem. Swelling frequently occurs. When it occurs under restrictive bandages or casts, the blood supply may be diminished and excruciating pain results. Distal to the constriction, the patient will have swelling; diminished capillary refill; dusty, pale, or blue color; cool skin; and diminished or altered sensory or motor function. Usually, swelling can be controlled and prevented by elevating the injured part slightly above heart level and intermittently applying an ice pack to the injury.

Prolonged pressure by restrictive devices over bony prominences (*e.g.,* heel, head of fibula, tibial tuberosity) may cause a burning type of pain. Relieving the pressure is necessary to relieve the pain and prevent further tissue damage.

Muscle spasm is another associated cause of pain. When a muscle is injured, the natural response of the muscle is to contract, thereby splinting and protecting the injured area. Prolonged muscle contraction is painful. Relaxation techniques, traction, or medications may be used to reduce pain from muscle spasm.

Additional information and guidelines to nursing management of the patient with pain are presented in Chapter 16.

Rehabilitation. Throughout the treatment period, the nurse is concerned with health maintenance and ultimate restoration of function. The immobility necessitated by some treatment modalities must not result in undue deterioration. Exercise of nonimmobilized muscles and joints helps maintain their strength and function, minimizes cardiovascular deterioration, and prevents disuse osteoporosis. Involvement in activities of daily living (*e.g.,* hygiene, dressing, eating) provides a sense of independence and accomplishment. Coordinating nursing interventions with special therapy approaches (*e.g.,* physical therapy, occupational therapy) makes it easier for the patient to learn and practice the therapeutic regimens. Emphasis is placed on what the patient is able to do within the limits of the medical treatment modalities.

Before the time of discharge, the patient should have explicit instructions that he understands, indicating those activities he may and may not perform. It is not enough to bid him "good-bye, and take it easy." The patient must know any untoward signs and symptoms that should be reported to his physician. He must be aware of the importance of follow-up visits. If he has any difficulties, he ought to know where and how to get help. The nurse has a major part of the responsibility for educating the patient before he leaves the hospital (see Chap. 14, Principles of Rehabilitation).

▷ Management of the Patient in a Cast

A *cast* is a rigid immobilizing device that is molded to the contours of the body to which it is applied. The purpose of a cast is to immobilize a body part in a specific position and to apply uniform pressure on encased soft tissue. It may be used to immobilize a reduced fracture, correct a deformity, apply uniform pressure to underlying soft tissue, or provide support and stability for weakened joints. Generally, casts permit mobilization of the patient while restricting movement of some body part.

Types of Casts. The condition being treated influences the type and thickness of the cast applied. Generally speaking, the joints proximal and distal to the area to be immobilized are included in the cast. Figure 60-1 illustrates some of the common types of cylindrical casts and areas where pressure problems commonly occur.

Short arm cast—extends from below the elbow to the proximal palmar crease

Gauntlet cast—extends from below the elbow to the proximal palmar crease, including the thumb (thumb spica)

Long arm cast—extends from the upper level of the axillary fold to the proximal palmar crease; the elbow usually is immobilized at a right angle

Short leg cast—extends from below the knee to the base of the toes

Long leg cast—extends from the junction of the upper and middle third of the thigh to the base of the toes; the foot is at a right angle in a neutral position

Walking cast—a short- or long-leg cast with a walking device

Body cast—encircles the trunk

Spica cast—incorporates a portion of the trunk and one or two extremities (single or double spica cast)

- *Shoulder spica cast*—a body jacket that encloses the trunk and the shoulder and elbow
- *Hip spica cast*—encloses the trunk and a lower extremity; may be a single or double hip spica cast

Casting Materials

Plaster. The traditional cast is made of plaster. Rolls of crinoline are impregnated with powdered, anhydrous calcium sulfate (gypsum crystals). Elastic bandage plaster rolls may be used next to the body part to ensure even pressure and smooth body molding. When wet, a crystallizing reaction occurs and heat is given off.

- The heat given off during this reaction can be uncomfortable. Therefore, the water used should be cool. The cast needs to be exposed to allow maximum dissipation of the heat. Most casts are cool after about 15 minutes.

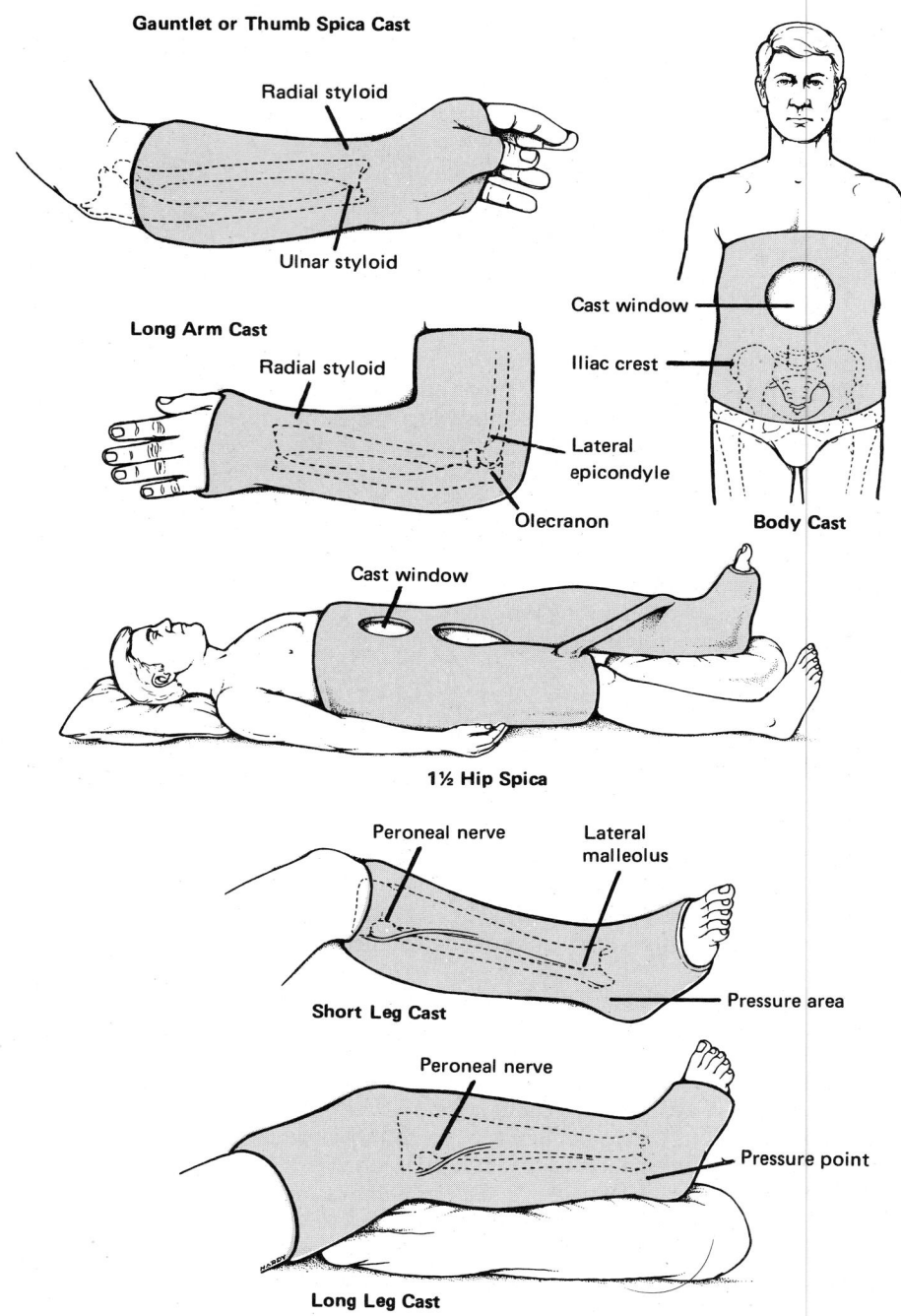

Figure 60-1. Pressure areas in different types of casts.

The crystallization produces a rigid dressing. The speed at which the reaction occurs varies from a few minutes to 15 to 20 minutes. The orthopedist will determine what setting speed is appropriate for the cast being applied.

After the plaster has set, the cast is still wet and somewhat soft. It does not have its full strength until dry. While damp, it can be dented if handled with the fingertips instead of the palms of the hand or if allowed to rest on hard surfaces or sharp edges. These dents produce pressure areas on the skin under the cast. The cast requires 24 to 72 hours to dry, depending on the thickness of the cast and the environmental

drying conditions. A freshly applied cast should be exposed to circulating air to dry. A cast should not be covered, because covers restrict the escape of moisture. A dry cast is white and shiny, resonant, and odorless as well as firm; a wet cast is gray and dull in appearance, is dull to percussion, feels damp, and has a musty odor.

Nonplaster. Newer casting materials are being developed and used. Generally referred to as *fiberglass casts,* these water-activated polyurethane materials have the versatility of plaster and the additional advantages of being of lighter weight and increased strength, water-resistant and radiolucent. They are made of an open-weave, nonabsorbent fabric impregnated with hardners that reach full rigid strength in minutes.

Nonplaster casts are porous and therefore diminish skin problems. They do not soften when wet, which allows for hydrotherapy and bathing. When wet, they are dried with a hair drier on a cool setting. Thorough drying is important to prevent skin breakdown.

Splints. Contoured splints of plaster or pliable thermoplastic materials may be used for conditions that do not require rigid immobilization or for those in which swelling may be anticipated. The splints need to provide for adequate immobilization of adjacent joints. They should be designed to support the body part in a functional position. The splints must be well padded to prevent pressure, skin abrasion, and skin breakdown. In addition, when making plaster splints, in order to prevent burns, use cold water and provide for dissipation of the heat from the exothermic reaction before overwrapping. The splint is overwrapped with an elastic bandage in a spiral fashion. The pressure should be uniform and should not restrict circulation.

Cast Application

It is important to prepare the patient for the application of the cast. The patient needs to know what to expect during application, and that the casted body part will be immobilized following application. The patient is positioned to facilitate casting and is draped to prevent undue exposure and to prevent the plaster materials from coming in contact with other body parts. The body part should be supported adequately when the cast is applied in order to increase the patient's comfort and maintain reduction and alignment.

The part to be casted should be clean and dry. Wiping the skin with povidone-iodine (Betadine) before the cast is applied helps diminish cast odors. Skin abrasions, if present, need to be disinfected and dressed before cast application. When the skin has been prepared, padding is wrapped around the part to minimize pressure and irritation from the cast. Generally, a knitted material (*e.g.,* stockinette) is placed over the part to be casted. This knit material needs to be applied smoothly and in a nonconstrictive manner. Enough material is cut to allow the ends to be folded over the nearly finished cast to provide a smooth, padded edge. Soft, nonwoven, rolled padding is then wrapped smoothly and evenly around the part. Extra padding is placed around bony prominences and at nerve grooves (*e.g.,* peroneal nerve, olecranon process). Nonabsorbent padding materials are used with nonplaster casts.

When adequately padded, the casting material is applied. The plaster and nonplaster materials come in bandaging rolls of various widths to facilitate smooth, contoured application. The bandage is applied evenly on the extremity, turn upon turn, with each turn overlapping the preceding turn by one half the width of the roll. The motion is continuous, without pause, while the bandage is maintained in constant contact with the surface of the extremity. The turns or layers of the bandage are smoothed and rubbed as the cast is applied to form a smooth, solid, and well-contoured cast. Proper shaping of the cast to the body part is required to provide the needed support. At the joints and at points

of anticipated cast stress, additional casting material (splints) are used and incorporated into the cast for additional strength.

During the application, care is given to ensure that the body part is immobilized in the desired position. Improper extremity position can result in contracture or malunion of fractures.

To enhance comfort and the patient's ability to participate in activities, the cast must be "finished" properly. The edges need to be smooth and padded to prevent skin abrasion. Full range of motion of joints adjacent to the immobilized part needs to be assured. If need be, the soft cast can be trimmed and reshaped with a cast knife or manual cutters to allow for full motion and to eliminate any restriction due to the cast.

Plaster materials that have gotten on the skin during application are removed. If not cleaned off, these will loosen, crumble, and slide underneath the cast, causing discomfort and possible skin breakdown.

▶ Assessment

The main concern following the application of a cast is to avoid complications. Experience has taught that any complaint of discomfort must not go unheeded. Two types of complications occur: *constriction of circulation* and *pressure on tissues and bony parts.*

Constriction of Circulation. Trauma or surgery affecting an extremity will produce swelling due to hemorrhage and edema. Unrelieved swelling may result in vascular insufficiency, thereby reducing or obliterating the blood supply to an extremity. If circulation is restricted for too long a period, gangrenous necrosis may occur.

Signs of circulatory impairment are noted by assessing the toes and fingers of a leg or arm that has recently been placed in a cast. The toes and fingers should be pink in color, warm to the touch, and easily moved (wiggled) if the patient is requested to do so. The *blanche test* may be carried out as another means of assessing circulatory sufficiency. The nail beds and pulp of fingers/toes are pressed lightly and then released to check how quickly color returns, thereby indicating return of capillary action. A blue tinge to the toes or fingers suggests venous obstruction, while white and cold fingers or toes suggest arterial obstruction. The temperature of the injured extremity is compared with the uninjured one, as are the pulses. Inability to move the fingers or toes, pain on extension of the hand or foot, and coldness of an extremity are indicative of ischemia. If there is swelling, the cast will seem tight.

- Unrelieved pain, swelling, blanching or discoloration, tingling, numbness, inability to move fingers and toes, or any temperature change must be reported immediately to avoid possible paralysis and necrosis.

Pressure on Tissues or Bony Parts. Any cast that presses on tissues may cause necrosis (tissue death), pressure sores, and nerve palsies or paralysis, such as may occur when a leg cast damages the peroneal nerve. Severe initial pain over bony prominences is a warning symptom of an impending pressure sore. If the pain then disappears, it might very well mean that ulceration has occurred. Those sites most susceptible to pressure on the lower extremity are the heel, malleoli, dorsum of the foot, head of the fibula, and anterior surface of the patella. On the upper extremity, the main pressure sites are located at the medial epicondyl of the humerus and the ulnar styloid (see Fig. 60-1).

- If the patient complains of pain, analgesics should not be given until the cause of the pain is determined. The first step in determining the cause is to ask the patient to indicate the exact site of the pain.

Patient Problems/Nursing Diagnoses

Based on the clinical manifestations, the patient's major nursing problems following application of a cast include potential for development of circulatory impairment related to edema; potential for development of necrosis, pressure sores, and nerve paralysis related to pressure on tissues or bony parts; and potential nonadherence with the therapeutic regimen related to knowledge deficit.

▶ Planning and Implementation

Goals

The major goals for the patient include:

1. Adequate circulation to extremity
2. Absence of necrosis, pressure sores, and nerve paralysis
3. Adherence to therapeutic regimen

Nursing Intervention for Cast Constriction and Pressure. If the patient continues to have pain, the cast may be exerting pressure on a nerve, blood vessel, or bony prominence.

- If constriction of circulation is suspected, the cast may be bivalved to relieve pressure. Bivalving a cast does not disturb the alignment of the fracture.

The procedure for bivalving a cast is as follows:

1. Longitudinally cut the cast into two halves.
2. Cut the underlying padding since blood-soaked padding may shrink and constrict the circulation.
3. Spread the cast sufficiently to relieve constriction.
4. The anterior and posterior parts of the cast may be held together with an elastic compression bandage.
5. After the cast is bivalved, elevate the extremity until the circulation is restored, swelling diminishes, and pain is relieved.

Another method of checking the cause for discomfort or viewing a surgical wound is to cut a *window* in the cast. After the window is opened, a soft pad is inserted and the "window" is replaced with tape to prevent the underlying tissue from swelling through the window and forming pressure areas around its margins.

Nursing Management Following Application of a Cast. Although it takes minutes for a cast to harden, it will take 24 to 72 hours for the cast to dry.

1. Avoid covering the cast with bedding until it is dry.
2. Avoid resting the cast on hard surfaces or sharp edges, which will dent the cast and cause pressure areas.
3. Keep the affected extremity elevated above the heart.

4. Assess the neurovascular status of the involved extremity hourly.
   - Watch for these danger signs (for arm or leg cast): blueness or paleness of toenails or fingernails accompanied by pain and tightness, numbness, cold or tingling sensation.
   - Elevate the affected extremity above the heart and wiggle the toes or fingers. Call the physician if the condition persists.

Exercising the Patient in a Cast. While the patient is in a cast, he should be taught to tense or to contract his muscles without moving the joints. The patient may actually forget how to "will" a motion through the central nervous system pathways to the immobilized muscle. Therefore, isometric muscle contractions (contracting the muscle without moving the part) may be carried out to prevent atrophy and maintain muscle strength.

- If the patient is in a leg cast, place your hand under the knee and instruct the patient to "push down." If the patient has an arm cast, instruct him to "make a fist."

Isometric muscle contractions should be done at least hourly while the patient is awake. He is taught to exercise his fingers and his toes frequently and actively.

Portable electrical muscle stimulators may be attached to the skin over large muscles prior to casting. Muscle contractions are electrically stimulated for about 8 hours a day to prevent the development of disuse atrophy.

Patient Education. When the cast is dry, the patient should be instructed as follows:

1. Move about as normally as possible. Avoid excessive use of the injured extremity.
2. Perform the prescribed exercises faithfully.
3. Elevate the casted extremity above heart level frequently to prevent swelling.
4. Keep the cast dry.
   a. Wetness destroys the hardness of plaster casts.
      (1) Do not cover the cast with plastic or rubber, as this causes condensation and wetting of the cast.
      (2) Avoid walking on wet floors or sidewalks.
   b. Fiberglass casts, after being wet, must be dried thoroughly with a hair drier on a cool setting to avoid skin problems.
5. Cushion rough edges of the cast with tape.
6. Report to the physician if the cast breaks; do not attempt to fix it yourself.
7. To clean a cast:
   a. Remove surface soil with a damp cloth.
   b. Stained areas may be touched up with a thin layer of white shoe polish.
8. Do not attempt to scratch the skin under the cast. This may cause a break in the skin and result in the formation of a cast sore.
9. Note odors about the cast, cast staining areas, and pressure spots, which could indicate pressure sores. Report them to the physician.

Removing a Cast

A cast may be removed with a *cast cutter*—an electric saw with a circular blade that oscillates through the plaster. Before the procedure, the patient should be assured that the cast cutter will cause vibration but will not be painful. The usual method of cutting the cast is to bivalve it. The cast is cut by a series of alternating pressures and linear movements of the blade along the line of the cut (Fig. 60-2). If the saw blade is left against the padding too long, the patient will feel a burning sensation on the skin from the rapidly oscillating blade. Be sure to protect the patient's eyes from flying cast particles during the cast-cutting procedure. As a last step, the padding is cut by scissors.

Management of the Patient After the Cast is Removed.

One of the most important things to remember when a cast has been removed is that the part or parts involved have been immobilized for a considerable period of time. When the support and protection of the cast have been removed, stresses and strains are placed on parts that have been at rest. The patient complains of pain and stiffness, often much different from the original injury, and he may be depressed and discouraged, because the anticipated release from the cast has only added to his problems.

The responsibility of the nurse is to help the patient adjust to this new discomfort. This can be accomplished by supporting the part so that it is maintained in the same position as when in the cast. A small pillow can be used to support the knee, the lumbar spine, etc. The support is then gradually removed. When the extremity is moved, adequate support must be provided and the extremity moved gently. After the cast has been removed, exercises are prescribed to redevelop and to increase strength. If the patient has been doing isometric muscle contractions, he will not have to relearn to contract his muscles and will progress more rapidly with his rehabilitation program.

Once the cast is removed, there will be a considerable amount of desquamated epithelium (dead skin) that may adhere to the underlying skin surface. The skin is washed carefully with detergent or germicidal soap, and blotted dry, and some type of emollient cream is applied. The patient should be cautioned against rubbing or scratching the skin, which could cause a break in the skin.

The skin and the underlying tissues must be handled carefully until normal function is gradually restored. Atrophy of the part may be noted, but this disappears gradually with the return of muscle function. Swelling after a cast is removed

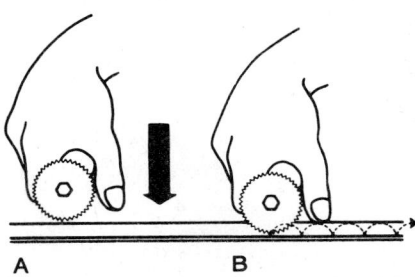

Figure 60-2. Operating a cast cutter. (Courtesy, Stryker Corporation.)

is common and is treated by elevating and supporting the tissues with elastic bandages or an elastic stocking.

If a new cast is to be applied, the patient's skin should be washed and dried carefully. The patient will need to be reminded again of the care of wet casts, needed neurovascular observations, and general cast care instructions.

Patient Education After Cast Removal

1. Cleanse the skin gently with bland soap and water. Blot dry.
2. Apply baby powder, cornstarch, baby oil, or emollient lotion. Avoid scratching the skin.
3. Resume activities and exercise gradually.
4. Control swelling by elevating the extremity above heart level, and use elastic bandages as directed.

▶ Evaluation

Expected Outcomes

1. Maintains adequate circulation to extremity
   a. Is free of pain
   b. Has normal skin color
   c. Demonstrates skin temperature in injured extremity that is similar to that of uninjured extremity
   d. Exhibits pulse in injured extremity that is similar to that of uninjured extremity
   e. Achieves satisfactory capillary refill on testing
   f. Has no swelling, paresthesias, or motor deficits
2. Shows no signs of necrosis, pressure sores, and nerve paralysis
   a. Is free of pain over bony prominence
   b. Demonstrates normal sensory and motor function of injured extremity nerves
   c. Has no musty cast odors, no cast staining, and no warm spots on cast
   d. Exhibits intact skin
3. Adheres to therapeutic regimen
   a. Protects cast during drying
   b. Elevates extremity that is in the cast
   c. Exercises according to instructions
   d. Keeps cast dry
   e. Protects skin from rough cast edges
   f. Reports development of problems
   g. Keeps follow-up clinic or physician appointments

Arm Casts

The patient must readjust to many routine tasks when his arm is immobilized in a cast. The unaffected arm must assume all the upper extremity activities. The patient may experience muscle fatigue due to the additional activities and the weight of the cast. Frequent rest periods are necessary.

To diminish and control swelling when the patient is lying down, the arm is elevated, with each joint positioned higher than the preceding joint (*e.g.,* elbow higher than the shoulder, hand higher than the elbow). When the patient becomes ambulatory, a sling may be used. However, a sling keeps the arm in a dependent position. For adequate drainage, the extremity should be higher than the level of the heart. Thus, the patient should be encouraged to remove the arm from the sling frequently and to extend it above his head.

Slings should be designed to distribute the weight over a large area and not on the cervical neck. Triangular cloth slings, when used, need to be pinned at the sides and not tied with a knot behind the neck, to prevent pressure on cervical spinal nerves.

Circulatory disturbances in the hand may become apparent with signs of cyanosis, swelling, and an inability to move the fingers.

- One serious effect of circulatory constriction in an arm cast is *Volkmann's contracture* (Fig. 60-3), in which contracture of the fingers and wrist occurs as the result of ischemia due to the obstruction of arterial flow to the forearm and hand.

The patient is unable to extend his fingers, describes abnormal sensation, and presents signs of diminished circulation to his hand. This serious complication can be prevented by nursing surveillance and proper care.

The constricting casts need to be removed, and a fasciotomy may be necessary to improve vascular status and prevent permanent damage, which would develop within a few hours.

Leg Casts

The application of a leg cast imposes a degree of immobility on the patient. The leg cast may be a short leg cast, extending to the knee, or a long leg cast, extending to the groin. The fresh cast must be handled in a manner that will not cause denting or disruption.

As with other cast applications, the leg must be assessed for swelling, adequate circulation, and normal nerve function. The leg is supported on soft pillows above heart level to control swelling. Ice packs might be applied over the fracture site for the first day or two. The circulation is assessed by observing the color, temperature, and capillary refill of the exposed toes. Nerve function is assessed by asking the patient to move his toes and by asking about the sensations in the foot. Numbness, tingling, burning, or a cold sensation may be due to peroneal nerve injury from pressure at the head of the fibula.

- Injury to the peroneal nerve as a result of pressure is a common cause of footdrop.

When the cast is dry, the patient is taught how to transfer and ambulate safely with walking aids (*e.g.,* crutches, walker). The gait to be used depends on whether or not the patient's problem allows weight bearing. If the physician plans on weight bearing, the cast will be reinforced to withstand the body weight. A walking heel (a rubber pad) is incorporated into the bottom of the cast, or the patient is given a cast boot to wear over the casted foot (Fig. 60-4). Cast boots are preferred to walking heels because they provide a broader support surface and do not disturb the patient's balance or posture by elevating the injured leg.

After the patient begins to ambulate, he should be encouraged to elevate the cast when he is seated. Several times during the day, he should lie down because a sitting position does not promote complete drainage. If the skin has become irritated at the cast edges, moleskin padding may be used.

Cast Brace

A cast brace is a special type of cast in which hinges are incorporated to allow for joint motion while providing adequate alignment and immobilization (Fig. 60-5). Some cast braces are constructed with hinges at the hip, knee, ankle, elbow, or wrist. Most frequently, cast braces are used when femoral shaft fractures demonstrate some healing and little thigh swelling. Usually, the patient has been in skeletal traction for a few weeks prior to cast brace application.

The application of a cast brace includes the following: A 4-inch elastic bandage may be applied to the knee area to minimize swelling. A circumferential thigh cast and a short leg walking cast are applied. Hinges (metal or polypropylene) are placed on each side of the knee, which will allow flexion movements. They are incorporated into the two casts.

Fracture healing is enhanced with cast braces. Weight bearing (stress) stimulates bone healing. In addition, the cast brace produces hydraulic pressure on the soft tissues, which facilitates fracture healing and minimizes fracture shortening.

The patient managed with a cast brace is better able to maintain physiologic homeostasis. Rehabilitation is pro-

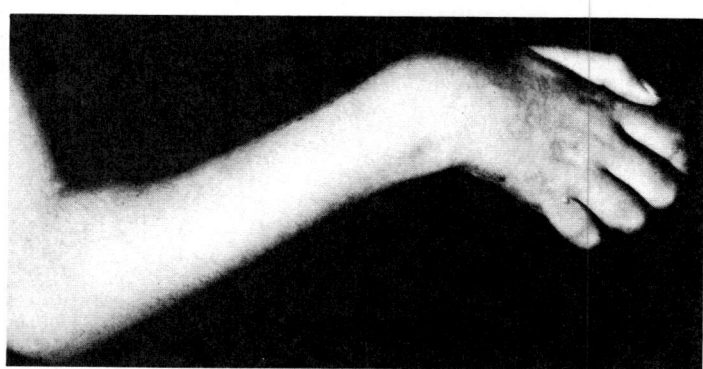

Figure 60-3. Photograph of the forearm and hand of a patient with late Volkmann's ischemic contracture. (From Rockwood CA and Green DP (eds): Fractures, Vol 1. Philadelphia, JB Lippincott.)

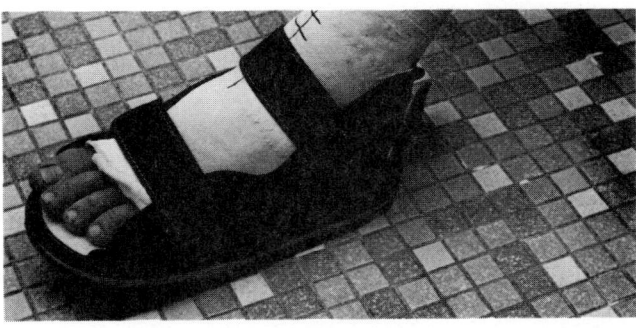

Figure 60-4. Cast boot. (From Farrell J: Illustrated Guide to Orthopedic Nursing, 2nd ed. Philadelphia, JB Lippincott, 1982.)

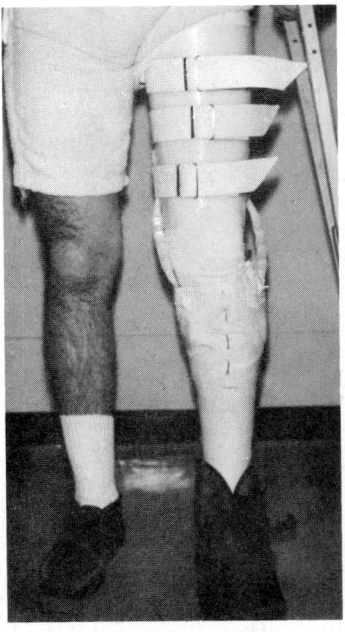

Figure 60-5. Cast brace. A cast brace provides circumferential support to a segment of a fractured extremity while allowing mobility of nearby joints.

moted by maintaining muscle strength and joint mobility. After the cast is dry (about 48 hours for plaster cast braces), the patient can be ambulated with crutches, using a three-point gait (see p. 248) progressing from partial to full weight bearing on the fractured extremity.

Problems that the patient may have after cast brace application include angulation deformity of the fracture site (malalignment of bone resulting in a bend in the bone), edema about the knee, skin breakdown on the thigh as a result of pressure from the edge of the cast, and soiling of the thigh cast. The patient is monitored for excessive swell-

ing, neurovascular problems, and skin breakdown. Since the cast may extend to the groin, measures should be taken to protect this area of the cast from becoming soiled with urine and feces. To promote venous return, the cast brace is elevated when the patient is not walking.

Body or Spica Casts

Casts that encase the trunk (body cast) and portions of the trunk and one or two extremities (spica cast) require special nursing techniques. Examples of these casts are body casts, hip spica casts, 1½ or double hip spica casts, and shoulder spica casts. Body casts may be used in situations requiring spinal immobility. Hip spicas are used for patients following femoral fractures and some hip joint surgeries. Shoulder spica casts are used for some humeral neck fractures. Patient preparation, turning, and skin and hygienic care are the nurse's concern.

Prepare the patient for the casting procedure by explaining the procedure. This will help reduce the patient's apprehension about being encased in a large cast. Often the patient has been immobilized in traction for weeks and anticipates recurrence of pain as he is moved for casting. Also, the fracture table used for large cast application looks like a torture device. Informing the patient that he will be cared for by several people during the application and that support for his injured body will be adequate and as gentle as possible will help to allay his fear. Medications for pain and relaxation administered prior to the procedure will help the patient relax, be comfortable, and cooperate during the procedure. Information concerning the casting procedure will help prepare the patient by knowing what to expect.

Following cast application, the patient needs to be supported by flexible, waterproof pillows until the cast is dry to prevent it from being dented. Inadequate cast support will cause a soft cast to crack or become dented, resulting in subsequent pressure points. The bed receiving the freshly casted patient needs to have firm mattress support. Three pillows placed crosswise on the bed will suffice for the body cast; for a hip spica, one pillow placed crosswise at the waist and two pillows placed lengthwise for the affected leg are necessary. If both legs are involved, two additional pillows are necessary. It is important that the pillows be next to each other, because any spaces in between will allow the damp cast to sag, become weak, and possibly break. It is also important to see that a pillow is not placed under the head and shoulders (of a patient in body cast) while the cast is drying since this causes pressure on the chest.

Patients are turned every 2 hours to relieve pressure and to allow the cast to dry. Sufficient personnel (at least three people) are needed when the patient is turned so that the fresh cast can be adequately supported with the palms of the hands. Vulnerable points in the cast are located at the body joints and need to be supported to prevent the cast from cracking. The patient is encouraged to assist in the repositioning by using the trapeze or bedrail. An abduction bar might be incorporated in spica casts to stabilize cast positioning. This bar is NOT to be used as a turning device. Pillows are readjusted so that support is provided and no pressure areas are present. The patient is turned as a unit toward the uninjured side to prevent stress on the cast and twisting of the body within the cast.

The patient is turned to a prone position twice daily in order to provide postural drainage of the bronchial tree and relieve pressure on the back. A small pillow under the abdomen will be an added comfort measure. Placing a pillow lengthwise under the dorsum of the feet will prevent the toes from being forced into the mattress. Allowing the toes to hang over the edge of the mattress is a welcome change.

Turning the Patient in a Hip Spica Cast

1. The patient is moved with a steady, even, pulling motion to the side of the bed.
2. Pillows are placed along the other side of the bed for cast support.
3. Instruct the patient to assist by using his arm on the involved side to pull his shoulder over when turning.
4. Two nurses are on the side to which the patient is being turned to provide support for the cast while rolling the patient toward them.
5. The third nurse assists in rolling the patient from behind, adjusts the patient's shoulder, and adjusts the pillows.
6. The patient's body should be turned as a unit and positioned comfortably in good alignment.

The skin around the edges of the cast must be inspected frequently for signs of irritation. Some of the area under the cast can be inspected by pulling the skin taut and using a flashlight. Reaching under the cast edges with the fingers allows for removal of cast crumbs and massage of the skin. Accessible skin should be bathed carefully and massaged with an emollient. Turning the patient every 2 to 3 hours is necessary to minimize pressure areas over bony prominences and to mobilize pulmonary secretions.

The area around the perineum needs to be protected from excreta. If the opening in the cast is inadequate for hygienic care, the nurse needs to see that this part of the cast is adjusted. When the cast is dry, the perineum is covered with a towel and the perineal area of the cast is sprayed with a plastic aerosol spray. Clean, dry, plastic sheeting can be inserted under the cast and brought over the cast edge before each elimination to protect the cast from soiling. Fracture bed pans are easier for hip spica patients to use. Good perineal care is essential.

Cast Syndrome

Patients immobilized in large casts may develop psychological and physiologic responses to the confinement. The psychological component of cast syndrome is similar to a claustrophobic reaction. The patient exhibits an acute anxiety reaction characterized by behavioral changes and autonomic responses (*i.e.,* increased respiratory rate, diaphoresis, dilated pupils, increased heart rate, elevated blood pressure). The nurse needs to recognize the anxiety reaction and provide an environment in which the patient feels secure.

The physiologic response to large casts are associated with the imposed immobility. With decreased physical activity, gastrointestinal motility decreases. With accumulation of intestinal gases, pressure increases and actual ileus occurs. The patient has distention, abdominal discomfort, nausea, and vomiting. As with other adynamic ileus situations, the patient is treated conservatively with decompression (nasogastric intubation connected to suction) and intravenous fluid therapy until gastrointestinal motility is restored. If the cast restricts the abdomen, a window needs to be cut in the cast over the abdominal area. Occasionally, the condition will progress to complete obstruction or the bowel may become gangrenous. Then surgical intervention is required.

The nurse needs to be aware of the possible development of cast syndrome in patients with large casts and to provide for its prevention or resolution.

▷ Management of the Patient in Traction

Traction is the application of a pulling force to a part of the body. Traction is used to minimize muscle spasms; to reduce, align, and immobilize fractures; to lessen deformity; and to increase space between opposing surfaces within a joint. Traction must be applied in the desired direction and magnitude to obtain the therapeutic effects. Factors that reduce the effective pull of the traction must be eliminated.

At times, the traction needs to be applied in more than one direction to achieve the desired line of pull. When this is done, part of one of the lines of pull counteracts the other line of pull. These lines of pull are known as the vectors of force. The actual resultant pulling force is somewhere between the two lines of pull (Fig. 60-6). The effects of applied traction are evaluated with x-ray, and adjustments may be necessary. As the muscle and soft tissue relax, the amount of weight used may be changed.

Types of Traction

Straight or *running traction* applies the pulling force in a straight line with the body part resting on the bed. Buck's extension traction (Fig. 60-7) and pelvic traction are examples of straight traction.

Balanced suspension traction (Fig. 60-8) supports the extremity being treated off the bed and allows for some patient mobility without disruption of the line of pull.

Traction may be applied to the skin (*skin traction*) or directly to the bony skeleton (*skeletal traction*). The mode of application is determined by the purpose of the traction.

Traction can be applied with the hands (***manual traction***). This is a very temporary traction that may be used when applying a cast, giving skin care under foam boots, or adjusting traction apparatus.

Principles of Effective Traction

Whenever traction is applied, the *countertraction* must be considered. Countertraction is the force acting in the opposite direction. (Newton's third law of motion states that for every action there is an equal and opposite reaction.) Generally, the patient's body weight supplies the needed countertraction. The bed may be positioned on an angle to supply the needed countertraction.

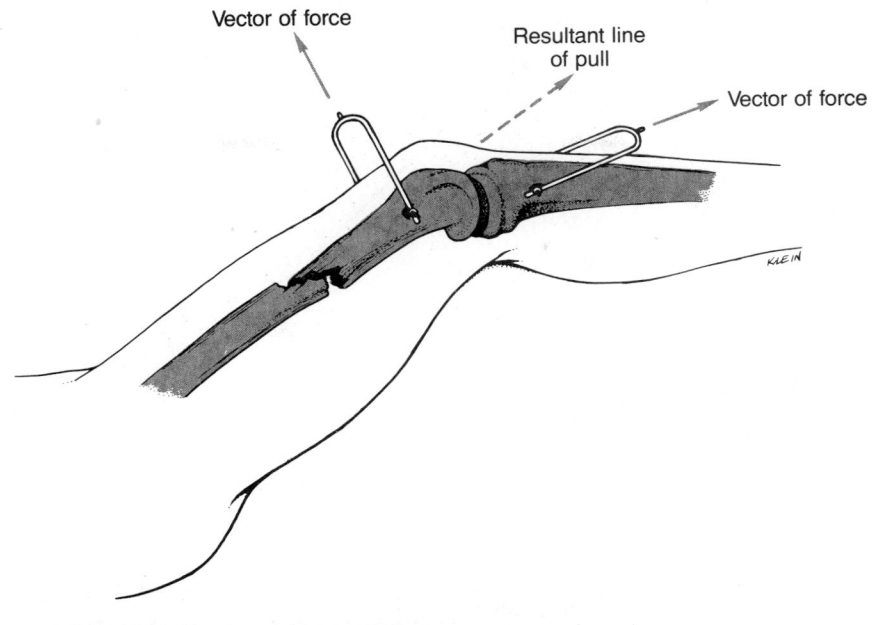

Figure 60-6.   Traction applied in different directions to achieve desired resulting line of pull.

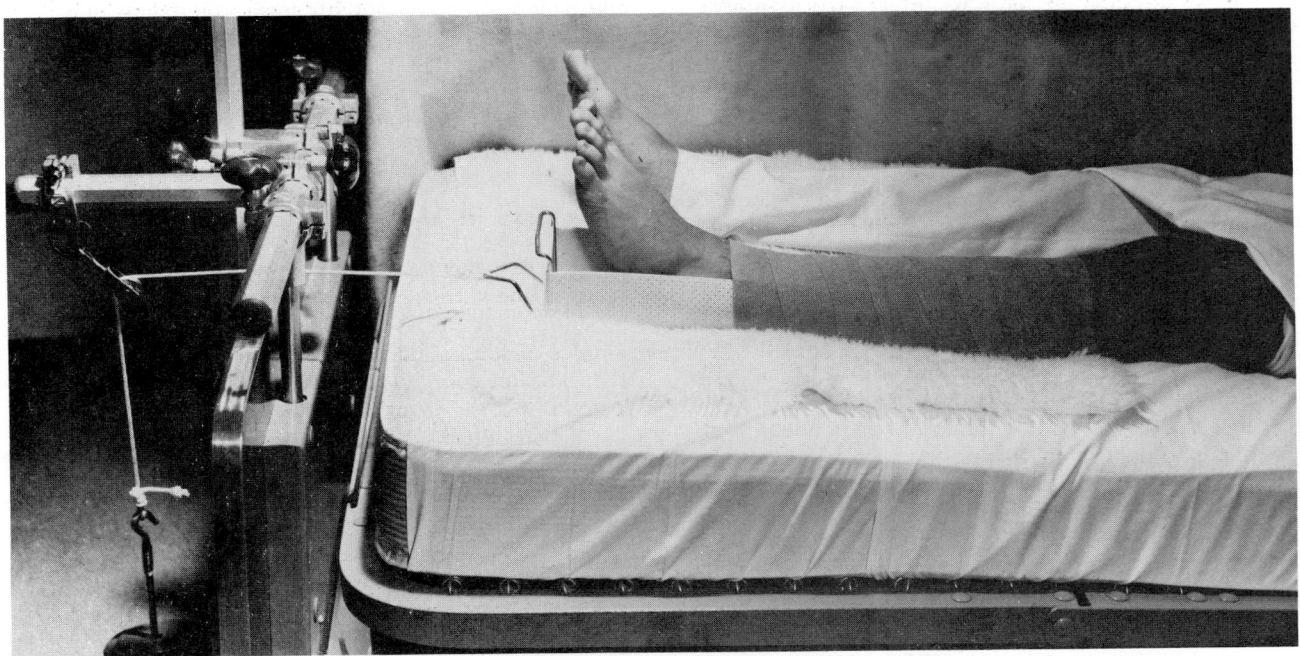

Figure 60-7.   Lower extremity in Buck's extension traction.

- Countertraction must be maintained for effective traction.

For traction to be effective it must also *be continuous.* The physician specifies those traction applications that may be interrupted. Pelvic and cervical skin tractions are fre-

quently used to reduce muscle spasm and are usually prescribed as an intermittent traction.

- Never interrupt skeletal traction.
- Do not remove weights unless the traction is prescribed intermittently.

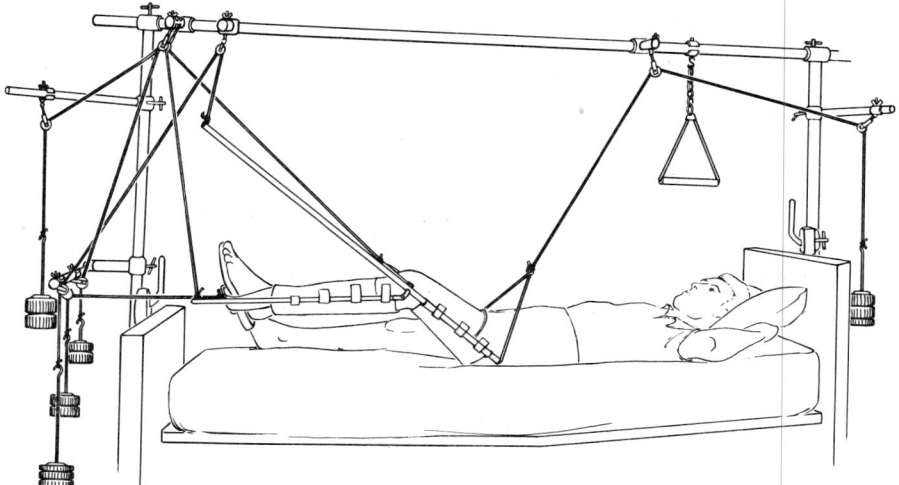

Figure 60-8. Principles of balanced suspension traction with Thomas leg splint. Vertical movement of the patient is permitted as long as longitudinal forces are maintained. Force means to push or pull. Force, as used in traction, means push or pull in a given direction. In the nursing management of the patient in traction, one has to understand the direction in which the force is operating. Study the line drawing carefully. Notice that the force produced by the weights is changed in direction by the pulleys.

Maintain the line of pull. Any factor that might reduce the pull or alter its resultant line of pull must be eliminated.

- The patient is centered in bed and in good bodily alignment when traction is applied.
- Weights should hang free and not rest on the bed or floor.
- Ropes should be unobstructed in straight alignment.
- Knots in the rope or the footplate do not touch the pulley or the foot of the bed.
- The resultant line of pull should be in line with the long axis of the bone.
- The patient must be helped to maintain a position for effective traction.

▶ **Assessment**

Application of traction can be a frightening experience. The equipment looks threatening. Prior to the application of any traction, the patient needs to be informed about the procedure, its purpose, and its implications for him. Talking to the patient about what is being done and why helps allay apprehension.

Since the patient will be immobilized in bed, the mattress needs to be firm and supported with a bed board. If devices to minimize the development of pressure sores (alternating air mattress pads) are to be used, they should be placed on the bed before application of the traction.

- The patient's skin should be examined frequently for evidence of pressure or friction over bony prominences.

During traction therapy, the patient needs to exercise nonimmobilized muscles and joints to diminish the deterioration due to immobilization.

- Active motion of all unaffected joints is encouraged.

The problems associated with immobility that affect other body systems are minimized through active preventive nursing measures.

- Every complaint of the patient in traction is to be investigated immediately.

Patient Problems/Nursing Diagnoses

Based on the clinical manifestations, the patient's major nursing problems when being treated with a traction regimen include potential for disruption of effective traction; potential for development of skin breakdown related to continuous pressure on soft tissues; potential for development of musculoskeletal weakness and diminished flexibility due to disuse; potential for development of other system problems (*i.e.,* respiratory, circulatory, urinary, gastrointestinal) associated with immobility; and potential for nonadherence with therapeutic regimen related to knowledge deficit.

▶ **Planning and Implementation**

Goals

The major goals for the patient include

1. Maintenance of effective traction
2. Psychological adjustment to traction regimen
3. Absence of skin breakdown
4. Absence of muscle weakness and maintenance of normal range of motion
5. Absence of other system problems
6. Adherence to therapeutic regimen

Skin Traction

Skin traction is accomplished by a weight pulling on tape, sponge rubber, or plastic materials that have been attached to the skin. Traction on the skin transmits traction to the musculoskeletal structures. However, only limited traction can be applied with skin traction. No more than 2 kg to 3 kg (4.5–7 pounds) of traction can be used on a part. The amount of weight applied in skin traction must not exceed the tolerance of the skin. Therefore, when prolonged or heavy traction weight is necessary, skeletal traction is used, not skin traction.

This type of traction is used as a temporary measure in adults—Buck's extension for hip fractures and Russell's traction for applying traction to the femoral shaft with the knee flexed.

Buck's extension (unilateral or bilateral) is a form of skin traction in which the pull is exerted in one plane when partial or temporary immobilization is desired (see Fig. 60-7). It is used following injuries to the hip while the patient is awaiting surgical fixation.

Before the traction is applied, the skin is inspected for abrasions and circulatory disturbances, since the skin must be in healthy condition to tolerate the traction. The extremity should be clean and dry before the traction tape or foam boot is applied. Prepadded boots are frequently used (Fig. 60-9). The malleoli and proximal fibula are padded with cast padding to prevent pressure sores and skin necrosis. Foam-rubber padded straps are applied with the foam surface against the skin on each side of the affected leg.

A loop of tape about 10 cm to 15 cm (4–6 inches) is extended beyond the sole of the foot. While one person elevates and supports the extremity under the patient's heel and knee, another person wraps the elastic bandage circumferentially over the traction tape, beginning at the ankle and wrapping up to the tibial tubercle. The elastic bandage helps the tape to adhere to the skin and prevents slipping. A spreader is applied to the distal end of the tape to prevent pressure along the side of the foot. A rope is attached to the spreader and passed over a pulley fastened to the end of the bed. Then a weight is attached to the rope. A sheepskin pad is placed under the leg to reduce the friction of the heel against the bed.

Skin and Nerve Pressure. Skin traction can irritate the skin and cause pressure on peripheral nerves. The circumferential wrappings around the skin tapes should not impair circulation, but must be firm enough to ensure that the tapes will remain in contact with the skin.

- To detect pressure points in skin traction, the area over the traction tapes should be palpated daily. The area over the Achilles tendon should be inspected several times daily since pressure in this region may occur when

skin traction is applied to the leg. Care must be taken to avoid pressure on the peroneal nerve at the point at which it passes around the neck of the fibula just below the knee. Pressure at this point can cause footdrop (see Fig. 60-1).

- When skin traction is applied to the arm, the area around the elbow where the ulnar nerve is located should not be wrapped tight (see Fig. 60-1).

Circulation. Following application, the foot is inspected for circulatory difficulties within a few minutes and then every 2 hours.

- Check peripheral pulses and the color and temperature of the fingers and toes.

Assess for altered sensation, weakness of dorsiflexion or foot movement, and inversion of foot, which might indicate pressure on the common peroneal nerve. Any complaint or burning sensation under the traction bandage is investigated immediately.

- The wrappings applied around the leg should be removed and the skin inspected three times a day.
- A second nurse needs to support the limb in position during skin inspection and care.

To ensure effective traction, observe for wrinkling and slipping of the traction bandage and maintain countertraction. Proper positioning must also be maintained to keep the leg in a neutral position. The patient should not turn from side to side to prevent bony fragments from moving against one another. The patient should have foot supports to prevent footdrop. Special care is given to the back at regular intervals, because the patient maintains a supine position. Check for calf tenderness and for positive Homan's sign for signs of thrombophlebitis.

- Encourage active foot exercise hourly.

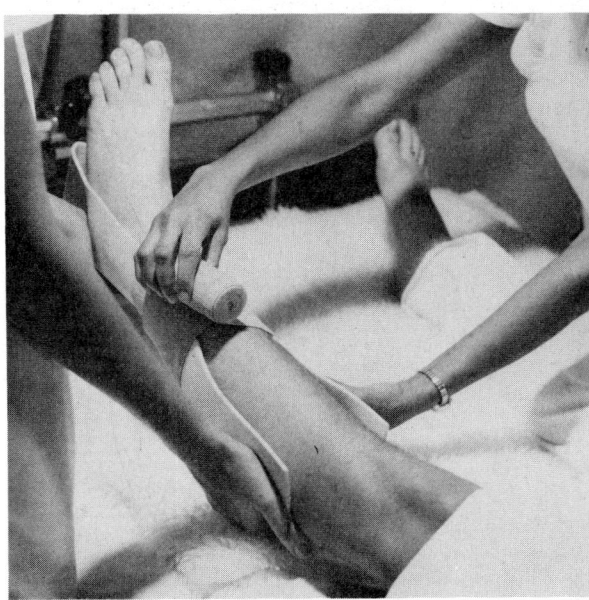

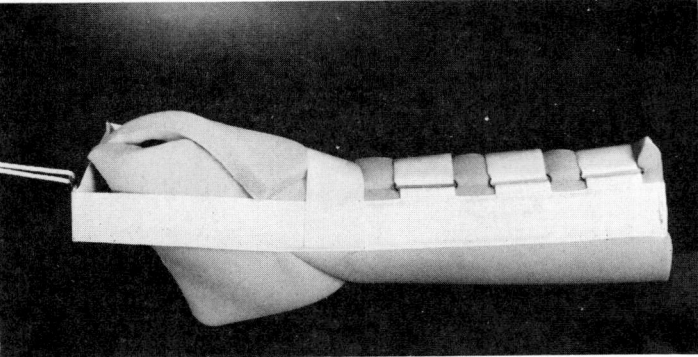

Figure 60-9. (*Left*) Applying elastic bandage for Buck's extension traction. (*Above*) Prepadded boot that may be used in Buck's extension. (Photo of boot courtesy of All Orthopedic Appliances.)

Skeletal Traction

Skeletal traction is applied directly to the bone. This method of traction is used most frequently in the treatment of fractures of the femur, the humerus, the tibia, and the cervical spine. The traction is applied directly to the bones by use of a metal pin or wire (*e.g.,* Kirschner wire, Steinmann's pin) that is inserted through the bone distal to the fracture. Crutchfield or Gardner–Wells head tongs are fixed in the skull to apply traction that immobilizes cervical fractures.

The skeletal traction is applied under surgical asepsis. The insertion site is prepared with surgical scrub, such as povidone-iodine. A local anesthetic is administered at the insertion site. A small skin incision is made, and the sterile pin or wire is drilled through the bone. The patient feels pressure during this procedure and possibly some discomfort when the periosteum is penetrated. Patient preparation contributes to the patient's comfort and cooperation during the pinning procedure. Frequently, the skeletal traction is inserted on the patient care unit and not in the surgical suite.

Following insertion, the pin or wire is attached to the traction bow or caliper. The ends of the wire are covered with corks or tape to prevent injury to the patient. The weights are attached to the bow by a rope–pulley system that exerts the appropriate amount and direction of pull for effective traction. Frequently, the skeletal traction is balanced traction, which supports the affected extremity and facilitates patient independence and nursing care while maintaining effective traction.

The *Thomas splint with the Pearson attachment* is frequently used with skeletal traction in fractures of the femur (see Fig. 60-8). It may be used with skin traction and other balanced suspension apparatus. Because upward traction is required, an overbed frame is utilized. Figure 60-10 shows another type of suspension traction.

The Pin Site.   The wound at the insertion site requires attention. Generally, the site is covered with a sterile dressing. Subsequent care of the pin site is given according to the physician's regimen. The object is to avoid infection and development of an osteomyelitis. Pin care may include applying a sterile cleansing to the site twice a day using povidone-iodine and applying antibiotic or iodine ointment, or sealing of the area with collodion. Regardless of the procedure, the nurse is responsible for inspecting the area for signs of inflammation and infection. Slight serous oozing at the site is to be expected.

- Inspect pin site daily for odor, signs of inflammation, or other evidence of infection.

Circulation.   The skin around the traction is inspected for signs of circulatory impairment. Neurovascular assessment of the immobilized extremity needs to be conducted at least every 2 hours initially and later several times a day.

Pressure.   Specific pressure points need to be checked for redness and skin breakdown. Pressure areas caused by the traction apparatus may include the ischial tuberosity, popliteal space, Achilles tendon, and heel.

Positioning.   The foot should be in a neutral position; rotation inward or outward should be reported. Footdrop is to be avoided, and the patient's foot may be supported in a neutral position by orthopedic devices (*e.g.,* foot supports). Active flexion–extension foot exercises are encouraged.

When traction is being used, the apparatus is checked to see that the ropes are in the wheel groove of the pulleys; that the ropes are not frayed; that the weights hang free, and that the patient has not slipped down in bed; causing ineffective traction. The knots in the rope are tied securely. Figure 60-11 suggests a secure knot tying method.

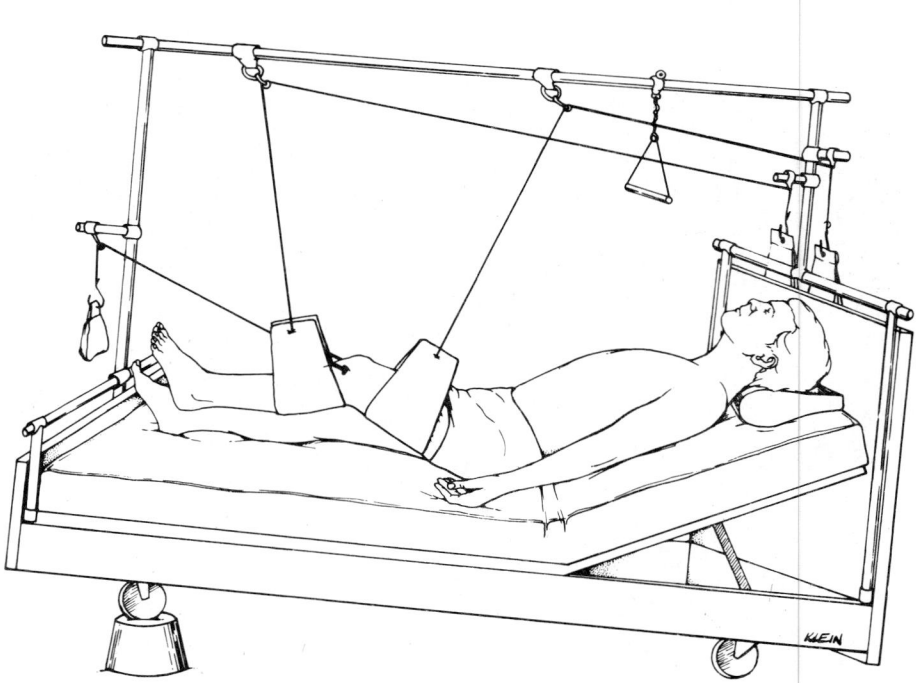

Figure 60-10.   A type of balanced suspension traction for the lower extremity. Patient's leg is supported by weights that balance the injured leg in slings.

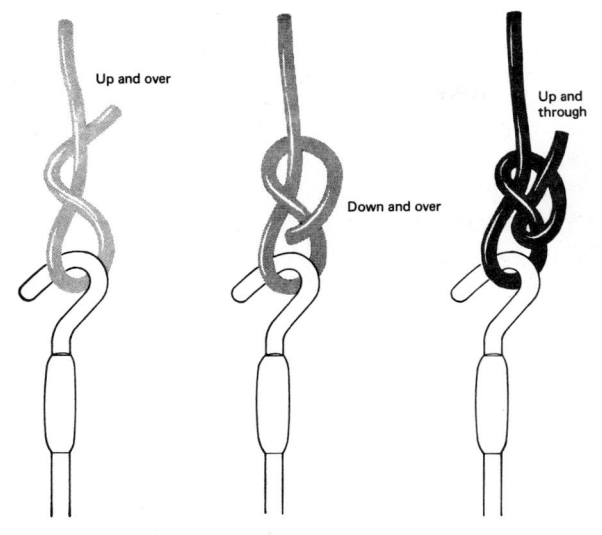

Up and over

Down and over

Up and through

Figure 60-11. Guidelines for traction knot tying. Tying knots correctly is an orthopedic nursing activity essential for the safety of the patient in traction. To save time, follow this simple phrase:

Up and over
Down and over
Up and through

Practice a few times with a traction cord. It is a good idea to secure all knots tightly with adhesive tape. (Courtesy, Zimmer Manufacturing Company.)

Weights.   The weights that are applied initially are sufficient to overcome the shortening spasms of the affected muscles. Skeletal traction frequently uses 7 kg to 15 kg (15–30 pounds) to secure the therapeutic effect. As muscles relax, the traction weight is reduced to prevent fracture distraction and to promote fracture healing.

- *Weights should never be removed from a patient with a fracture unless a life-threatening situation occurs. Weight and pulley traction is applied to secure constant corrective extension. If the weights are removed to move the patient from one department to another, the whole purpose of their use has been defeated.*

Skin Care.   When traction frames are used, a trapeze may be suspended overhead within easy reach of the patient. This apparatus is of great help in assisting the patient to move about in bed and on and off bedpans. It is also a help to the nurse in caring for these patients. When a patient is not permitted to turn on one side or the other or on his abdomen, the nurse must make a special effort to provide good back care and to keep the bed dry and free of crumbs and wrinkles. This can be accomplished by having the patient raise his hips from the bed by holding onto the overhead trapeze. Often a patient uses the heel of his good leg to act as a brace when he raises himself. This digging of the heel into the mattress may cause injury to the tissues; hence, the heel must be massaged and inspected for pressure areas. If the patient is unable to raise himself, the nurse can push down on the mattress with one hand, leaving space for the other hand to massage the skin.

Exercise.   Patient exercises are valuable in maintaining muscle strength and tone and in promoting circulation. Exercises need to be planned within the therapeutic limits of the traction. Active exercise frequently permitted includes pulling up on the trapeze, flexing and extending the feet, and range of motion and weight-resistance exercises for noninvolved joints. The immobilized extremity benefits from isometric exercises. Quadriceps and gluteal setting exercises promote the strength of these muscles, which are important in ambulatory stability. Without bed exercises, the patient will lose much muscle mass and strength, and rehabilitation time will be greatly extended.

Development of thrombophlebitis is a real concern for anyone immobilized for a period of time. Daily assessment for the development of deep vein thrombophlebitis is necessary (see pp. 683–684). Frequently, antiembolic stockings, low-dose subcutaneous heparin, or 600 mg of aspirin twice a day may be prescribed to help prevent thrombus formation. Prompt identification and treatment of thrombophlebitis is essential.

Pin Removal.   After the use of skeletal traction, the pin site wound may heal with a depression scar due to fibrous tissue contraction. This may be prevented by pinching the pin site tissue at the time of pin removal and thereby breaking the fibrous tissue that has formed at the pin site between the skin and periosteum.

Balanced Suspension Traction
Nursing Interventions

1. Following application, assess neurovascular status frequently.
2. The ropes and the pulleys are freely movable, and the traction is applied securely to the leg. The traction must be continuous to be effective.
3. Observe for skin irritation around the traction bandage.
4. Check the patient for signs of odor and infection.
5. Observe for pressure under the sling at the popliteal space and at other common pressure points (ischial tuberosity, popliteal space, heel).
6. Encourage active foot exercises, and use foot supporters as needed.
7. Encourage exercises to minimize deconditioning of the immobilized patient.
8. Involve the patient in his care to help avoid the depression and boredom that frequently accompany weeks of traction therapy.

▶ Evaluation

Expected Outcomes

1. Achieves effective traction
   a. Achieves purpose for which the traction was applied
   b. Maintains line of pull
   c. Maintains countertraction
   d. Uses continuous/intermittent application of traction as prescribed
2. Exhibits psychological adjustment
   a. Participates in therapeutic regimen
   b. Performs activities of daily living

c. Engages in diversional activities
d. Is oriented to time, place, and person
e. Respects self and others

3. Shows no signs of skin breakdown
   a. Exhibits skin free of red pressure areas
   b. Has intact skin
   c. Has skin that is soft, supple, and well hydrated

4. Has no muscle weakness and exhibits normal range of joint motion
   a. Exercises unaffected joints and muscles
   b. Moves self with ease
   c. Achieves normal range of motion

5. Is free of other system problems
   a. Exhibits clear respirations upon auscultation
   b. Has no calf tenderness
   c. Is free of Homans' sign
   d. Shows no orthostatic hypotension
   e. Has clear urine
   f. Is mentally alert
   g. Eats balanced diet
   h. Has normal bowel function

6. Adheres to therapeutic regimen
   a. Understands necessity of traction
   b. Engages in activities within limitations of effective traction
   c. Participates in therapeutic regimen

▷ Orthopedic Surgery

Many patients who have musculoskeletal dysfunction need to undergo surgery to correct the problem. Problems that may be corrected by surgery include impaired function due to unstabilized fracture, deformity, or joint disease; necrotic or infected tissue; impaired circulation (*e.g.,* compartment syndrome); and tumors or growths. Frequent surgical procedures include *open reduction with internal fixation* for fractures; *arthroplasty, meniscectomy,* and *joint replacement* for joint problems; *amputation* for severe extremity problems (*e.g.,* gangrene, massive trauma); *bone graft* for joint stabilization, defect filling, or stimulation of healing; and *tendon transplants* for improvement of motion.

Types of Surgeries

Open reduction—the fracture is reduced and aligned following surgical dissection and exposure of the fracture

Internal fixation—the reduced fracture is stabilized by the use of metal screws, plates, nails, and pins

Bone graft—the placement of bone tissue (autologous or homologous grafts) to promote healing, stabilization, or replacement of diseased bone

Amputation—the removal of a body part

Arthroplasty—the repair of joint problems through the operating arthroscope (an instrument that allows the surgeon to look into a joint without a large incision) or through open joint surgery

Meniscectomy—the excision of damaged knee joint fibrocartilage

Joint replacement—the substitution of joint surfaces with metal or plastic materials

Total joint replacement—the replacement of both articular surfaces within a joint with metal or synthetic materials

Tendon transplant—the movement of tendon insertion to improve function

Fasciotomy—the cutting of the muscle fascia to relieve muscle pressure or to reduce fascia contracture

Preoperative Physical Care.   Whatever the method used in preparing the patient's skin for surgery, the principles remain the same. The procedure usually is more painstaking because of the difficulty in controlling infection in the bone, should that occur. A meticulous nontraumatizing cleansing of the skin with germicidal soap and water is done the day before surgery and is repeated at the time of surgery.

It is known that the number of bacteria on the skin can be reduced by daily washing with a germicidal soap. If the operation is an elective one, the orthopedist may advise the patient to use a germicidal soap for skin cleansing for a period of time before hospital admission.

Permanent disability can result should infection occur within a bone or a joint. In no instance should one rely on the antibiotics to control infection.

Adequate hydration is always an essential objective in orthopedic patients, particularly those immobilized for a long period of time. This prevents the occurrence of stones, infection, and kidney complications. Notice should be taken of urinary output.

It should be determined if the patient has had previous therapy with corticosteroids the year prior to surgery, especially the person with rheumatoid arthritis. Steroid therapy, whether current or past, may adversely affect his response to anesthesia. The prescribed dose of steroid should be given preoperatively to cover the anticipated stress of surgery.

Postoperative Considerations.   In major orthopedic surgery, *shock* may be a problem, especially since orthopedic wounds have a tendency to ooze and bleed more than other surgical wounds. As a result, the nurse must be on the alert for the symptoms of shock. A rising pulse rate or slowly falling blood pressure indicates persistent bleeding or the development of a state of shock. Changes in the respiratory rate or in the patient's color indicate obstruction of respiratory exchange, and pulmonary or cardiac complications. Fat embolus (see p. 1425) and thrombophlebitis (see p. 681) are other complications of orthopedic surgery.

Bone does not mend as rapidly as soft tissues. Therefore, even though the skin incision is well-healed, bony structures underneath still need time to repair. This is especially important to remember in surgery of the lower extremities, for in addition to normal movement, bone must be able to bear weight in ambulation. Metal pins, screws, rods, and plates used in internal fixations are not strong enough to support the body weight and will bend and break if stressed. The stability of the fracture and the bone healing are the important considerations in determining the amount of weight bearing a reduced fracture can tolerate.

Other complications that may occur are similar to those of general surgical patients. They are abdominal distention, wound infection, and pulmonary and circulatory problems. In addition, elderly men usually have some degree of prostatism and may have difficulty in voiding. Thus, it is important to watch the urinary output.

The patient is placed on a normal diet as soon as possible. However, large amounts of milk should not be given to orthopedic patients who are on bed rest, since this only adds to the calcium pool in the body and requires that more calcium be excreted by the kidneys that favors formation of urinary calculi.

Orthopedic operations may require prolonged periods in bed. Hence, the development of pressure sores are a constant threat. Turning, washing, drying, and massaging the skin frequently are necessary to avoid this complication. Well-balanced diets with adequate protein and vitamins are needed for maintenance of healthy tissue and wound healing.

Reconstructive Joint Surgery

At times, the impact of joint disease or deformity will necessitate surgical interventions to relieve pain, improve stability, and improve function. Surgical therapies used for joint disease include excision of damaged and diseased tissue, repair of damaged structures (*e.g.,* ruptured tendon), removal of loose bodies (debridement), immobilizing fusion of a joint (arthrodesis), and replacement of all or part of the joint surfaces (*e.g.,* arthroplasty, prosthesis, total joint). Table 60-1 summarizes some of these procedures.

The procedure is selected according to the patient's underlying problem(s), general physical health, impact of joint disability on life, and age. Timing of these procedures is important for gaining maximum function. Surgery should be performed before surrounding muscles become contracted and atrophied and serious structural abnormalities occur. The total patient must be evaluated so that the procedure with the best chance of success and best long-range benefits is selected. Young patients (under 60 years) may not be selected for total hip replacement due to the limited life of the prosthesis.

Total Joint Replacement

Patients with severe pain and disability associated with the joint may be selected for total joint replacement. Conditions contributing to joint degeneration include rheumatoid arthritis, osteoarthritis (degenerative joint disease), trauma, and congenital deformity. At times, total joint replacement is a salvage procedure due to disruption of the blood supply and subsequent avascular necrosis. Joints frequently replaced include the hip, knee, shoulder, and finger joints (Fig. 60-12). Less frequently, more complex joints (elbow, wrist, and ankle) are replaced.

Most joint replacements consist of metal and high-density polyethylene components. Finger prostheses are generally silastic. The joint implants are cemented in the prepared bone with methyl methacrylate (a bone-bonding agent), which has properties similar to bone. Loosening of the bond in 5 to 15 years is the most common reason for prosthesis failure. Porous, coated, cementless, artificial joint components that allow the patient's bone to grow into and securely fix the prosthesis are being evaluated. It is hoped that they will last several times longer than current cemented components. Accurate fitting and healthy bone stock with adequate blood supply is important in the use of cementless components.

With total joint replacement, excellent pain relief is obtained in 85% to 90% of patients. Return of motion and function depends on the preoperative soft tissue condition, soft tissue reactions, and general muscle strength. Total joint replacements can be expected to last about 10 to 15 years, and early failure is associated with higher levels of activity and prereplacement joint pathology. (Components in patients with osteoarthritis loosen more often than those in patients with rheumatoid arthritis.)

Infection is a major concern because there is no good salvage procedure after prosthesis infection and failure. Strict surgical asepsis and surgical environment controls are used to diminish surgical infection. Keeping the patient optimally free from infection is assured prior to surgery through careful patient assessment. Prophylactic perioperative antibiotics are used. Infection occurs nearly twice as often in patients with rheumatoid arthritis as in those with osteoarthritis. (This may be associated with a deficit in polymorphonuclear leukocyte function observed in many rheumatoid arthritis patients.)

Total Hip Replacement

Total hip replacement is the replacement of a severely damaged hip with an artificial joint. Although a large number of implants are available, most consist of a metal femoral component topped by a spherical ball fitted into a plastic acetabular socket and held in the bone with methyl methacrylate (bone cement) (see Fig. 60-12). Following a successful operation, the hip is free or nearly free of pain, has good motion, is more stable, and usually permits normal or near normal ambulation.

The operation is usually reserved for patients over 60 with unremitting pain or irreversibly damaged hip joints. The following conditions are amenable to this type of surgery: arthritis (degenerative joint disease, rheumatoid arthritis), complications of femoral neck fractures, failure of previous reconstructive surgery (osteotomy, cup arthroplasty, femoral head replacement), and problems resulting from congenital hip disease. More recently, selected patients with pathologic fractures from metastatic cancer have benefitted from total hip-joint replacement.

The procedure is generally an elective one. Full patient status assessment and preoperative management are aimed at establishing the patient in an optimal condition for surgery. Any infection 2 to 4 weeks prior to planned surgery may result in postponement of surgery or the use of antibiotics to prevent a possible source for seeding a joint infection.

▶ Preoperative Planning and Implementation

Goals

The major goals for the patient being prepared for total hip replacement include:

1. An understanding of the expectations related to the surgery, hospitalization, and rehabilitation
2. Modifications of home environment to meet convalescent needs
3. Optimal physiologic status for surgery

Table 60-1
Surgical Procedures on Joints

Underlying Considerations:

1. Surgical intervention is advocated before joints are destroyed and surrounding musculature becomes contracted and atrophied.
2. Surgery is done to prevent further joint destruction. Priority is given to weight-bearing joints.
3. The total patient is considered in selecting a procedure.
4. Evaluation of adjacent joints is important.

Objectives:

1. To keep the patient functional by restoring motion and stability
2. To relieve pain

Type of Surgery	Description	Indications	Nursing Implications
Articular Surgery			
Arthroplasty (Total joint replacement, cup arthroplasty, endoprosthesis)	Reconstruction of a joint with metal and high-density poly-ethylene components	Relief of pain Restore movement and stability Correct deformity	Surveillance for postoperative infection Special emphasis placed on positioning Support patient with exercise program
Arthrodesis	Fusion of a bone to eliminate a joint; results in loss of joint motion	Performed to obtain a stable, painless joint Especially effective in the wrist knee, and foot Permits heavy labor	Maintain immobilization of fused joint Observe for infection
Girdlestone procedure	Removal of acetabular and femoral components after failed infected total hip arthroplasty	Infected, failed total hip arthroplasty	Observe for infection Minimize movement of extremity until scar tissue develops Extremity shortens Eventually, patient able to walk with ambulatory aid Scar tissue acts as cushion between bone ends
Para-articular Surgery			
Osteotomy	Surgical cutting of bones that changes the alignment, with or without bone removal	Osteotomy of tibia or femur corrects valgus or varus deformities of the knee joint Displaces point of maximum stress	Maintain extremity immobilized in position of correction Observe for infection
Tendon Surgery			
Tenorrhaphy	Repair of ruptured tendon; diseased synovium invades tendon and interferes with its nutrition, leading to necrosis and rupture	Restore function Rupture of extensor tendons fairly common in arthritis, causing difficulty in extending part	Repair of tendons does not usually give full extension postoperatively
Tenosynovectomy	Excision of thickened tendon sheath and other tissue surrounding tendon		Institute early joint motion to prevent stiffness and adhesions of flexor tendons
Tendon transfer	Redirecting an intact tendon from one position to another	Done to replace or help muscle function lost from nerve damage, rupture of tendon	
Neurolysis			
Surgical procedure in which entrapped nerve is relieved from pressure by diseased synovium	Surgical decompression for carpal tunnel syndrome (compression of median nerve within the carpal tunnel)	Nerve entrapment can produce loss of motor and nerve function	Encourage patient to exercise hand postoperatively to prevent adhesions and loss of function
	Surgical decompression of ulnar nerve entrapment (excision and release of synovial tissue)	Entrapment of deep peroneal nerve, posterior tibial nerve (tarsal tunnel syndrome) also occurs	Nerve entrapment syndromes characterized by disturbances of sensation, painful tingling, and weakness

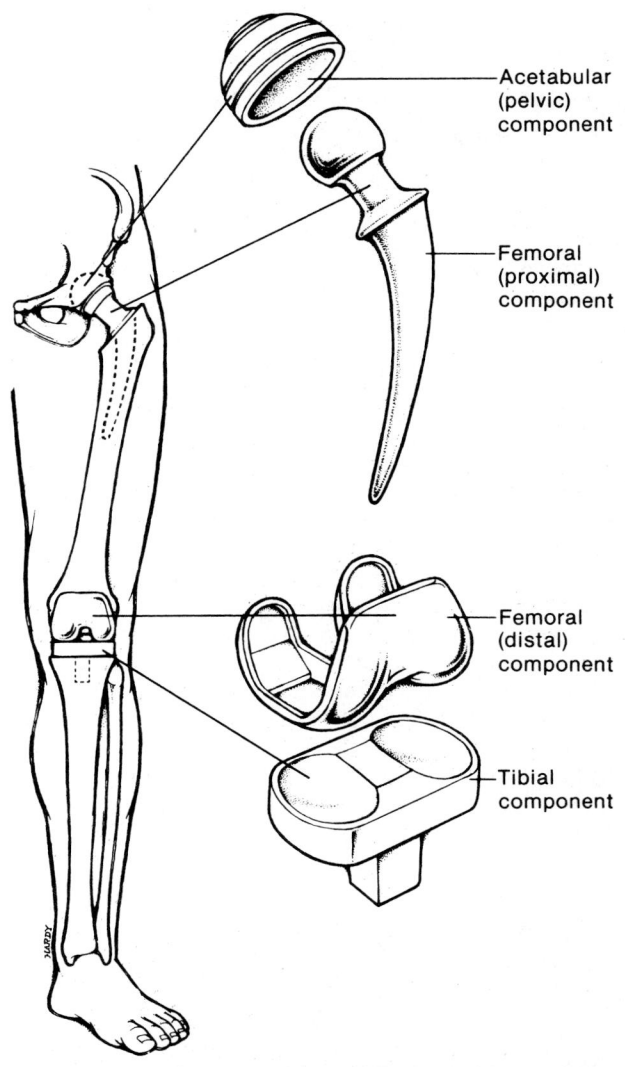

Acetabular
(pelvic)
component

Femoral
(proximal)
component

Femoral
(distal)
component

Tibial
component

Figure 60-12. Hip and knee replacement.

4. Preoperative practice of pulmonary toilet, muscle exercises, positioning, turning, and transfer techniques to be used postoperatively
5. Adherence to the preoperative regimen

Interventions. The patient and the physician have agreed that total hip replacement is the treatment regimen of choice, but the patient and family may have some questions related to the procedure and hospitalization. During the patient interview, the nurse may clarify what the patient can reasonably expect from the surgery, during hospitalization, and during rehabilitation. Early establishment of a rapport will assist the patient in becoming an active participant in his care.

The home environment is assessed early. Stair climbing and stooping are to be avoided during the first 3 months following surgery and kept to a minimum for the next 3 months. Modifications of the home environment may need to be made before the patient gets home.

Assessment. A complete preoperative evaluation is carried out with emphasis on cardiovascular, respiratory, renal, and hepatic function since this surgery is done on the older age group. Every effort is made to prevent pulmonary embolism, as this is the most common cause of postoperative mortality. Obesity, preoperative leg edema, history of deep vein thrombosis, varicose veins, and osteoarthritis increase the risk of postoperative pulmonary embolism. The patient is typed and crossmatched for blood replacement as needed.

Infection is the most feared complication, because it generally means that the implant unit must be removed. A search is made before the operation for any possible source of infection, since an untreated infection anywhere in the body precludes surgery. Preoperative urine cultures are taken since urinary tract infection is a likely portal of entry for bacteria. Research suggests that the majority of deep infections are caused by bacteria that are implanted into the wound at the time of surgery, mostly from airborne sources. During operation, there is strict adherence to aseptic principles, including double gloves, double masks, special gowns with waterproof fronts and sleeves, and devices used to make the operating area as bacteria-free as possible. The operative area is scrubbed twice daily preoperatively, as microorganisms on the skin can cause latent infection.

Preoperatively, the nurse needs to assess the patient's physiologic parameters and the neurovascular status of the lower extremities. Postoperative assessment data are compared with preoperative data to identify deficits and changes. Nerve palsy can occur during surgery. Absence of peripheral pulses postoperatively may be of concern unless the pulse was absent preoperatively also.

Patient Teaching. Patient education in relation to pulmonary toilet, muscle exercises, positioning, turning, and transfer techniques is necessary. Coughing and deep-breathing regimens need to be reviewed and practiced with the patient. The pulmonary complications of atelectasis and pneumonia are frequently seen and can be related to the patient's age, preexisting pulmonary disease, deep anesthesia, minimal activity, and pain medications. Learning how to use the incentive spirometer and intermittent positive pressure breathing equipment before surgery is helpful in maximizing the patient's benefits from these devices and therapy. Calf pumping (isometric contraction of calf muscle) and foot and ankle exercises are taught to prevent thrombophlebitis.

The patient is taught about positioning of the leg in abduction to prevent prosthesis dislocation. The use of abduction splints, wedge pillows, or two to three pillows between the legs is demonstrated. The patient is made aware of his responsibility in maintaining abduction. The limits for hip flexion (45–60 degrees) are also explained and demonstrated.

The patient is taught upper extremity strengthening and isometric exercises of the quadriceps and gluteal muscles. He is fitted with crutches or a walker and is instructed in a nonweight-bearing gait (no weight bearing on the affected extremity) to facilitate postoperative ambulation. The patient is taught how to transfer from the bed to the wheelchair without flexing the hip joints beyond the prescribed limits. Semireclining wheelchairs may be used to help avoid excessive flexion. The use of the overhead frame and trapeze is practiced. When using the fracture bed pan, the patient flexes the unoperated hip and knee and uses the trapeze to lift the pelvis onto the pan. He is instructed not to bear down on the operated hip in flexion when getting on the bed pan.

The more familiar the patient is with what will be expected of him postoperatively, the better the chances of his compliance. Practicing activities before surgery facilitates his ability to do it postoperatively, when he is less agile.

Infection Control. The preoperative care includes adequate skin preparation to reduce the chance of infection. Antibiotics may be administered in loading-dose fashion just prior to surgery or started intraoperatively. (Culture of the hip joint during surgery may be important in identifying and treating subsequent infections. Therefore, antibiotics may not be started until after the culture is obtained.)

The on-call preoperative medications are injected into an uninvolved area. Absorption and tissue response are better in untraumatized areas.

▶ Evaluation

Expected Outcomes

1. Describes expectations related to surgery, hospitalization, and rehabilitation
   a. Describes anticipated surgery in own words
   b. Participates in preoperative regimen
   c. Clarifies participation in rehabilitation activities
2. Arranges for modifications of home environment to meet convalescent needs
   a. Explores with professionals and family the modifications necessary in home for convalescence
   b. Arranges for posthospital assistance with care at home
   c. Considers transportation needs
3. Achieves optimal physiologic status for surgery
   a. Participates in preoperative testing
   b. Consumes balanced high-protein diet
4. Practices pulmonary toilet, muscle exercises, positioning, turning, and transfer techniques to be used postoperatively
   a. States reason for exercises
   b. Participates in practice sessions
5. Adheres to preoperative regimen
   a. Participates in preoperative care activities
   b. Maintains fasting status immediately prior to surgery as prescribed
   c. Refrains from smoking

▶ Postoperative Planning and Implementation

Following the total hip surgery, the patient's major nursing problems include pain related to surgery; potential homeostatic problems related to surgery and inactivity; potential infection related to surgery and inactivity; potential dislocation of hip prosthesis; and potential limitation of mobility.

Goals

The major goals for the patient include:

1. Comfort
2. Homeostasis
3. Absence of infection

4. Stabilization of area in which prosthesis is located
5. Adherence to therapeutic regimen

Interventions. In preparation for the postoperative patient with total hip surgery, the bed should be equipped with a firm mattress and an overbed traction frame and trapeze. A turning sheet will prove useful. An adequate supply of pillows is needed for successful patient positioning and comfort.

Positioning. Following surgery, the patient usually is positioned flat in bed with the affected extremity held in abduction by either an abduction splint or pillows to prevent dislocation of the prosthesis. Usually, the patient is not turned until the physician so indicates. At first the patient is turned only 45 degrees on the unoperated side with the hip kept fully abducted and the entire length of the leg supported by pillows. As the patient becomes familiar with the turning routine, he is encouraged to assist by using the overbed trapeze. He is also instructed not to adduct or flex the operated hip. The head of the bed should not be elevated more than 45 degrees to prevent acute flexion of the hip.

Exercise. On the day following surgery, specific exercises are begun and supervised by the physical therapist. A knee sling may be placed on the extremity to begin active flexion and extension of the knee, hip, and foot (Fig. 60-13) when permitted. The exercises are carried out to increase range of motion and muscle strength in the operative hip and to work toward the goal of independence in ambulation.

Ambulation. When the patient is helped out of bed, usually on the second postoperative day, an abduction splint

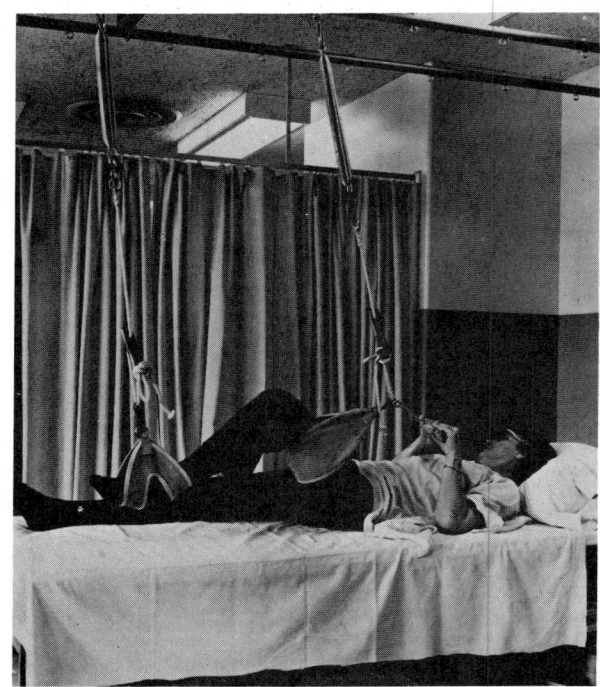

Figure 60-13. A proximal knee sling is used on this patient with a total hip replacement. Hip and knee flexion is assisted by a handle fastened to the proximal knee sling. (Reprinted with permission of Physical Therapy, 52:826, 1972.)

or pillows are kept between the legs. Once the patient is out of bed, the hip is kept at maximum extension. The procedure for assisting the patient out of bed consists of instructing the patient to pivot on the unaffected extremity while the nurse supports the extremity that has the implant. An aged or weakened patient may need to be lifted into a chair by several persons. Active participation of the patient is always encouraged. Frequent short periods of time out of bed are preferred to occasional long periods of sitting.

At first the patient may merely be able to stand because of weakness or light-headedness from orthostatic hypotension. When he is ready to ambulate, he is taught to use a walker by first advancing the walker and then advancing the involved extremity to the walker, bearing most of his weight on his hands. After he has mastered ambulating with the walker, he progresses to crutch walking at which time he is taught the three-point gait, which requires that he lead with the uninvolved extremity while simultaneously moving the involved extremity and the crutches together.

Patient Education. A program of patient education involves teaching the patient how important it is that the hip be maintained in abduction at all times and that stooping be avoided. The patient should also be reminded that until otherwise instructed he should use a pillow between his knees when lying in a supine or side-lying position and when turning. This prevents possible dislocation of the affected hip before the soft tissue has had a chance to heal and adequate muscle control has been restored. He is not to sleep on the operated side until directed to do so by the surgeon, and he should keep the operated leg elevated when he is seated. At no time should he cross his legs.

Postoperative Complications

Dislocation of the Hip Prosthesis. This problem needs to be recognized and reduced early so that circulatory and nerve damage to the leg does not occur. Dislocation may occur with major moves several days postoperatively or through positioning that exceeds the limits of the prosthesis. The indicators of dislocation are shortening of the leg, inability to move it, malalignment, abnormal rotation, and increased discomfort. As the muscles and joint capsule heal, the chance of dislocation diminishes. Stresses to the new hip joint should be minimal for the first 3 to 6 months.

Positioning and activities that will ensure positioning of the femoral head component in the acetabular cup are essential.

Pain. Pain in the immediate postoperative period is controlled by parenteral narcotics. Injection sites should be rotated, and the operative hip and thigh are avoided. Muscle spasm may contribute to the pain experienced. At times the patient will indicate that the degree of postoperative pain is less than that experienced preoperatively, and only moderate amounts of analgesics are needed. By the second or third postoperative day, the pain has generally decreased to a point where oral analgesics provide relief. Planned administration of an analgesic a half hour prior to exercise sessions may allow increased participation due to increased comfort. Surgical edema and fluid collection are controlled, reducing the discomfort associated with increased fluid pressure. An ice pack may be prescribed to the operative site to reduce edema and bleeding. Portable suction of the wound will decrease fluid accumulation and hematoma formation, which could be a focus of infection. Drainage of 200 ml to 500 ml in the first 24 hours is expected; by 48 hours postoperatively, the total drainage in 8 hours has decreased to 30 ml or less, and the suction device is then removed.

Thromboembolism. Monitoring for homeostasis following total joint surgery is important. Respiratory complications are a common problem in the elderly. Lowered arterial blood gas values are common for 4 days following total hip replacement. The overall incidence of clinical and subclinical pulmonary emboli is about 5% of all total hip operations.

Prophylactic aspirin, low-weight dextran, or low-dose heparin or warfarin may be used to minimize the occurrence of thromboembolic disease. Men are more sensitive to the anticoagulant effects of aspirin and need about half the dose women need (men—600 mg b.i.d.; women—600 mg q.i.d.). Fatal pulmonary emboli occur in approximately 2% of patients with total hip operations who have not received prophylactic anticoagulants. Other measures that help reduce the incidence of thrombosis include exercising the ankles and legs (to accelerate blood flow and prevent venous stasis), applying elastic stockings, and assuring adequate hydration. The extremities are checked daily for calf edema and tenderness.

Hematoma. The circulation in the operated extremity is assessed by checking the sensation, pulses, color, and temperature of the leg. These signs are compared with the unoperated extremity. A sudden onset of pain in the extremity may be due to hematoma, especially if the patient is on anticoagulation therapy.

Infection. Deep infection is the most serious complication following total hip replacement. Deep infection may occur as late as 8 years after operation and almost always requires removal of the implant. It may result from bacteria introduced at the time of operation or from a transient septicemia. Classic signs of infection may be present or the patient may at some time months to years after surgery indicate return of discomfort in the hip, which could mean a late infection. The infection rate of patients having total hip surgery with rheumatoid arthritis is greater than those with osteoarthritis. This may be due to the fact that rheumatoid arthritis is a systemic disease, resulting in an overall lower level of health and resistance. In addition, rheumatoid arthritis patients frequently have a defect in their polymorphonuclear leukocyte function that may increase their risk for postoperative infection.

Because total joint infections are so disastrous, all efforts are undertaken to minimize their occurrence. Potential sources of infection are avoided if at all possible. If an indwelling urinary catheter or portable wound suction is used, it is removed as soon as possible to avoid retrograde infections. Antibiotic therapy is continued for 7 to 10 days. If a large surgical hematoma develops, the antibiotic course will probably be extended. Prophylactic antibiotics may be advised if the patient needs any future surgical instrumentation, such as tooth extraction or cystoscopy.

Temperature. Monitoring the patient's temperature can provide good clues to the source of the problem. Temperature elevations within the first 48 hours are frequently related to atelectasis or other respiratory problems. Temperature elevations during the next few days are associated with urinary tract infections. Superficial wound infections take about 5 to 9 days to develop. Phlebitis-associated temperature elevations occur during the second and third week.

Other Complications.   Other complications include those associated with immobility, loosening of the prosthesis, heterotrophic ossification (formation of bone in the periprosthetic space), avascular necrosis, and dead bone caused by loss of blood supply. Because of the potential problem of prosthesis loosening, patient selection is important. Currently, total hip joint replacements last 10 to 15 years because of loosening of the methyl methacrylate. Young, active patients and those with rheumatoid arthritis experience earlier component loosening. Revision operations are difficult.

Discharge Planning

Before the patient prepares to leave the acute care setting, patient education to assist continuation of the therapeutic regimen and full rehabilitation is needed. The patient must accept the responsibility for being his own primary rehabilitative resource.

The patient is advised to be faithful in the daily exercise program in order to maintain the functional motion of the hip joint and strengthen the abductor muscles of the hip. It will take time to strengthen and reeducate the muscles.

Ambulatory aids, crutches, walker, or cane, are used for a period of time. When sufficient muscle tone has developed to permit a normal gait without discomfort, the cane may be abandoned. Walking efficiency after total hip replacement is improved because of the acquired painless normal gait. In general, by 3 months the patient is able to resume all routine daily living activities. Frequent walks, swimming, and use of a high rocking chair are excellent for hip exercises. Sexual activities can be resumed in the dependent position for 3 to 6 months to avoid adduction and flexion of the new hip.

At no time should the patient cross his legs or assume positions of acute flexion, more than 90 degrees. He may need assistance in putting on shoes and socks. Low chairs are avoided as well as sitting for more than 30 minutes at a time to minimize hip flexion and the risk of prosthetic dislocation and to prevent hip stiffness and flexion contracture. Traveling long distances is to be avoided unless frequent changes in position are possible. Other activities to avoid include overexertion, lifting heavy loads, and excessive bending and twisting (lifting, shoveling snow, forceful turning).

▶ Evaluation

Expected Outcomes

1. Achieves comfort
   Experiences no discomfort at rest or with activities of daily living
2. Achieves homeostasis
   a. Exhibits temperature within normal range
   b. Demonstrates respiratory rate within normal range
   c. Has pulse rate within normal range
   d. Shows blood screening values within normal range
   e. Is free of Homans' sign
3. Is free of infection
   a. Has temperature within normal range
   b. Shows incision healed without redness, swelling, or drainage
   c. Has normal operative area skin temperature
   d. Is free of residual or recurrence of pain
4. Demonstrates stabilized prosthesis location
   a. Demonstrates normal length and alignment of leg
   b. Exhibits improved range of motion
   c. Has neurovascular status within normal limits
   d. Avoids excessive hip stressors
5. Adheres to therapeutic regimen
   a. Performs graded exercises daily
   b. Uses ambulatory aids until healing occurs
   c. Walks daily
   d. Avoids positions of flexion and adduction
   e. Avoids activities that would stress the hip joint
   f. Keeps follow-up medical appointments

Total Knee Replacement

Total knee replacement is an implant procedure in which both the tibial and femoral joints are replaced because of destroyed knee joint(s). There are over 300 different knee prostheses in use, but most fall into two classifications: the hinge variety (Young or Walldius prosthesis) or the unattached variety in which the tibial and femoral components are cemented in place and articulate with one another, but are unattached; instead they are held together by muscle action (geometric or polycentric knee). Frequently, these patients are hemophiliacs.

Patient Problems/Nursing Diagnoses

The major nursing problems of the patient who undergoes total knee replacement include: severe, incapacitating joint pain related to pathophysiology; restricted motion with marked instability related to pathophysiology; diminished quality of life related to pain and limited mobility; and potential nonadherence to therapeutic regimen.

▶ Planning and Implementation

Goals

The major goals for the patient include:

1. Comfort
2. Increased mobility with improved stability
3. Improved quality of life
4. Adherence to therapeutic regimen

Preoperative Management.   Since thromboembolism is a complication following surgery for total knee replacement, the patient may be given low-weight dextran or warfarin to prevent thromboembolism and pulmonary embolism. Before surgery, every effort is made to eradicate any foci of infection, with prophylactic antibiotic therapy given before and after the operation. The same principles for the prevention of infection are observed as those carried out for total hip replacement (see p. 1411).

Postoperative Management. Following surgery, the knee is bandaged with a firm compression bandage. The leg may be elevated on pillows above the level of the heart, and the foot of the bed may be elevated to decrease the possibility of postoperative thrombophlebitis. The head of the bed is not elevated except while meals are eaten. Ice packs may be applied to the operative area to minimize swelling.

The operative area is checked for excessive drainage. A suction catheter is in place to provide constant drainage of the knee to remove excessive accumulation of blood. Suction drainage should not exceed 300 ml in 8 hours and should decrease to 25 ml to 30 ml by 48 hours postoperatively.

Quadriceps setting exercises are generally started on the first postoperative day, and flexion and extension of the feet and hips are encouraged. An inability to flex the foot could indicate peroneal nerve palsy due to pressure exerted by the dressing at the Achilles tendon or at the head of the fibula.

Usually, 3 to 7 days postoperatively, the physical therapist starts gentle knee flexion exercises which may then be actively carried out with the aid of a pulley and sling exerciser. Ambulation with crutches or a walker is allowed when the patient can perform straight leg raising and flex and extend the knee adequately. Full weight bearing is usually not tolerated for 6 weeks to allow time for repair of those tissues damaged at the site of the bone–cement interface. If the patient is not able to flex the knee satisfactorily (60 degrees of flexion by the 14th postoperative day), gentle manipulation may be carried out under general anesthesia.

Early complications of total knee replacement are infection, thromboembolism, and peroneal nerve palsy. Deep infection, loosening of the prosthetic components, dislocation and wearing of the implant, as well as fatigue fracture of the tibial plateau are late complications. A resting splint may be prescribed for nighttime use for several weeks to maintain the knee at extension.

Patient Education. The patient is instructed to continue the exercise program until at least 1 year after surgery. A stationary bicycle is helpful in improving range of motion and strengthening the muscles. The patient is instructed to lift weights with the affected leg, starting with one half pound and increasing the weight per physician's directions. Because there is a large implant present and the development of deep infection can be catastrophic, some orthopedists advocate preventive antibiotic therapy if the patient needs any type of subsequent surgical instrumentation, such as tooth extraction or cystoscopy.

▶ **Evaluation**

Expected Outcomes

1. Achieves comfort
   a. Experiences no discomfort at rest or with activities of daily living
   b. Experiences no discomfort when walking

c. Does not use pain medications or other pain-relieving devices
2. Demonstrates increased mobility with improved stability
   Achieves satisfactory range of motion and joint stability
3. Achieves an improved quality of life
   a. Participates in activities of daily living
   b. Participates in family and community activities
   c. Enjoys increased activity level
   d. Experiences less fatigue
4. Adheres to therapeutic regimen
   a. Exercises according to prescribed regimen
   b. Keeps follow-up medical appointments
   c. Informs physician of development of symptoms promptly

▷ **Bibliography**
Books

Benjamin A and Helal B. Surgical Repair and Reconstruction in Rheumatoid Disease. New York, John Wiley & Sons, 1980.
Brantley P and Analla M. The Nurse and Orthopedic Surgery. Altanta, Orthopedic Nurses' Association, 1980.
Brooker A and Schmeisser G. The Orthopaedic Traction Manual. Baltimore, Williams & Wilkins, 1980.
Donahoo C and Spickler L (eds). Core Curriculum of Orthopedic Nursing. Atlanta, Orthopedic Nurses' Association, 1980.
Farrell J. Illustrated Guide to Orthopedic Nursing, 2nd ed. Philadelphia, JB Lippincott, 1982.
Gartland J. Fundamentals of Orthopedics, 3rd ed. Philadelphia, WB Saunders, 1979.
Heppenstall R (ed). Fracture Treatment and Healing. Philadelphia, WB Saunders, 1980.
Hilt N and Cogburn S. Manual of Orthopedics. St Louis, CV Mosby, 1981.
Larson C and Gould M. Orthopedic Nursing, 9th ed. St Louis, CV Mosby, 1978.
Mourad L. Nursing Care of Adults with Orthopedic Conditions. New York, John Wiley & Sons, 1980.
Powell M. Orthopaedic Nursing and Rehabilitation. New York, Churchill–Livingstone, 1982.
Roaf R and Hodkinson L. Textbook of Orthopaedic Nursing, 3rd ed. Oxford, Blackwell Scientific, 1980.

Articles
General

Anderson M. Keeping up with the best in casting. Patient Care 1979 July; 13(13):24–27.
Cohen S and Viellion G. Programmed Instruction: Nursing care of a patient in traction. Am J Nurs 1979 Oct; 79(10):1771–1798.
Douglas G, Rang M, and Clements N. The prevention of depressed scars after the use of skeletal traction. J Bone Joint Surg [Am] 1980 Mar; 62-A(3):307.
Fleming L, Miller K, and Marshall S. Clinical experience with a new casting tape. South Med J 1980 May; 73(5):569–571.
Hardy A and Braddeley S. Pressures generated in the thigh muscles and under the thigh cast of an uninjured subject wearing a cast-brace. J Bone Joint Surg [Am] 1979 Apr; 61-A(4):362–364.
Kaplan S. Burns following application of plaster splint dressing. J Bone Joint Surg [Am] 1981 Apr; 63-A(4):670–672.
Laualette R et al. Setting temperatures of plaster casts. J Bone Joint Surg [Am] 1982 July; 64-A(6):907–911.

Lentz M. Selected aspects of deconditioning secondary to immobilization. Nurs Clin North Am 1981 Dec; 16(4):729–737.

Love–Mignogna S. Taping and splinting. Nursing 80 1980 Apr; 10(4):88–92.

Mahon R. Lighter cast bracing. ONA J 1978 Sept; 5(9):20–22.

Milazzo V. An exercise class for patients in traction. Am J Nurs 1981 Oct; 81(10):1842–1844.

Miller L. Orthopedic patients in an ambulatory surgery facility. Nurs Clin North Am 1981 Dec; 16(4):749–758.

Product Review. Orthopedic Nurs 1982 July–Aug; 1(4):44.

Symposium on Orthopedic Nursing. Nurs Clin North Am 1981 Dec; 16(4):707–766.

Reconstructive Joint Surgery

Brause B. Infected total knee replacement. Orthop Clin North Am 1982 Jan; 13(1):103–122.

Buchanan R and Kraag G. Is there a lower incidence of deep venous thrombosis after joint replacement in rheumatoid arthritis? J Rheumatol 1980 July–Aug; 7(4):551–554.

Chamberlain S. Low-dose heparin therapy. Am J Nurs 1980 June; 80(6):1115–1117.

Dorr L et al. Pulmonary emboli following total hip arthroplasty: Incidence study. J Bone Joint Surg [Am] 1979 July; 61-A(7):1083–1087.

Fox J. Revision arthroplasty of the hip. Nurs Times 1980 Oct 30; 76(44):1930.

Fuller E (ed). Surgical options in OA management. Patient Care 1981 May; 15(9):121–142.

Gallagher L. When your patient has a shoulder arthroplasty. Nursing '80 1980 July; 10(7):46–49.

Glante J. Causes of fractures of the femoral component in total hip replacement. J Bone Joint Surg [Am] 1980 Apr; 62-A(4):670–673.

Head W. Wagner surface replacement arthroplasty of the hip. J Bone Joint Surg [Am] 1981 Mar; 63-A(3):420–426.

Hungerford D et al. The porous coated anatomical total knee. Orthop Clin North Am 1982 Jan; 13(1):103–122.

Johnson B et al. A dynamic splint for use after total wrist arthroplasty. Am J Occup Ther 1981 Mar; 35(3):179–184.

Kegel–Szerejko M. Host factors and prosthetic joint infection. Am J Infect Control 1981 May; 9(2):43–49.

McBeath A et al. Walking efficiency before and after total hip replacement as determined by oxygen consumption. J Bone Joint Surg [Am] 1980 July; 62-A(7):807–810.

Meuli H. Arthroplasty of the wrist. Clin Orthop 1980 June; 149:118–125.

Morrey B. Total elbow arthroplasty. J Bone Joint Surg [Am] 1981 Sept; 63-A(9):1050–1063.

Mulligan R. Late infections in patients with prostheses for total replacement of joints: Implications for the dental practitioner. J Am Dent Assoc 1980 July; 101(1):44–46.

Murray M et al. Joint function after total hip arthroplasty. Clin Orthop 1981 June; 157:119–124.

Scott W (ed). Symposium on total knee arthroplasty. Orthop Clin North Am 1982 Jan; 13(1):entire issue.

Smith C. Physical therapy management of patients with total ankle replacement. Phys Ther 1980 Mar; 60(3):303–306.

Swanson A. Reconstructive surgery in the arthritic hand and foot. Clin Symp 1979; 31(6):2–32.

Tobiason S. The arthritis patient comes to surgery. AORN J 1980 Oct; 32(10):608–613.

61

Management of Patients With Musculoskeletal Trauma

▷ Musculoskeletal Trauma

Injury to one part of the system usually produces injury or dysfunction of adjacent structures and to structures enclosed or supported by them. If the bones are broken, the muscles cannot function; if the nerves do not send impulses to the muscles, as in paralysis, the bones cannot move; if the joint surfaces do not articulate normally, neither the bones nor the muscles can function properly. Thus, although a fracture primarily affects the bone, it may also produce injury to the muscles surrounding the injured bone and to the blood vessels and the nerves in the vicinity of the fracture.

In the treatment of injury to the musculoskeletal system, support is provided for the injured part until nature has time to heal it. Support may be accomplished by bandages, adhesive strapping, splints, or casts, applied externally. Support may be applied directly to the bone in the form of pins or plates. At times traction must be applied to correct deformity or shortening.

After the immediate and the painful effects of the injury have passed, consideration must be given to the prevention of fibrosis and the resulting stiffness in the injured muscles and the joint structures. *Active function by the patient is the best form of treatment to guard against this disability.* In some cases, the support applied may permit active function almost from the start. In other cases, the nature of the injury may not permit function, and even in those instances in which partial function is possible, nature may be aided in the healing process and recovery of function may be hastened by various forms of physical therapy.

▷ Contusions, Sprains, and Dislocations

Contusions

A *contusion* is an injury to the soft tissues, produced by blunt force (a blow, kick, fall, etc.). There is always some hemorrhage into the injured part (ecchymosis), due to the rupture of many small vessels. This produces the well-known discoloration of the skin (bruising), which gradually turns to brown and then to yellow, and finally disappears as absorption becomes complete. When the hemorrhage is sufficient to cause an appreciable collection of blood, it is called *hematoma*. The local symptoms (pain, swelling, and discoloration) are easily explained.

Management. Treatment consists of elevating the affected part and applying moist or dry cold for the first 24 hours to produce vasoconstriction, which results in decreased hemorrhage and edema. Application of cold should be continued for 20 to 30 minutes. In the recovery phase, moist heat is applied for 20 minutes at a time to promote vasodilatation, absorption, and repair. Elastic bandage wrapped over the contused area aids in controlling bleeding and in reducing associated swelling.

Strains

A *strain* is a "muscle pull" due to overuse, overstretching, or excessive stress. Strains are microscopic, incomplete muscle tears with some bleeding into the tissue. The patient experiences sudden pain and then local tenderness. Pain is experienced with muscle use and isometric contraction.

Management. The injured muscle must be allowed to rest and repair itself. Intermittent ice compresses for the first day followed by intermittent heat provides both comfort and increased circulation to the injured muscle, promoting healing. Elevation and an elastic pressure bandage control any associated edema. Patient education needs to emphasize minimal exercise until healing has taken place and then gradual progression of activity. Too much exercise too soon will cause restrain and delayed recovery.

Sprains

A *sprain* is an injury to the ligamentous structures surrounding a joint, caused by a wrench or a twist. The function of a ligament is to maintain stability while permitting mobility. A torn ligament loses its stabilizing ability. As is the case with contusions, blood vessels are ruptured, resulting in rapid swelling due to the extravasation of blood within the tissues. The movement of the joint becomes painful. Actually, the degree of disability and pain increase during the first 2 to 3 hours after the injury because of the associated swelling and bleeding. To be certain that there is no bone injury, these patients should have an x-ray examination. *Avulsion fracture* (a bone fragment is pulled away by a ligament or tendon) may be associated with sprains.

Management. Sprains are treated with thermal therapy (intermittent cold initially, and later heat), elevation, splinting, or immobilization. The application of cold reduces the associated pain and causes vasoconstriction, which retards extravasation of blood and the development of edema. The part should be elevated and rested. Sometimes additional support is provided with either temporary splinting or elastic bandages to reduce swelling and edema.

After 24 hours, mild heat may be applied (15 to 30 minutes, four times daily) to promote absorption. If the sprain is severe (torn muscle fibers and disrupted ligaments), surgical repair or cast immobilization is necessary so that the joint will not lose its stability. A severe sprain will take about a month to heal. Active exercise can begin gradually when the sprain has healed.

Joint Dislocations

A *dislocation* of a joint is a condition in which the articular surfaces of the bones forming the joint are no longer in anatomical contact. The bones are literally "out of joint." Traumatic dislocations are orthopedic emergencies, because the associated joint structures, blood supply, and nerves are distorted and severely stressed. Avascular necrosis (tissue death due to anoxia and diminished blood supply) and nerve palsy may occur.

Dislocations may be (1) congenital (present at birth, due to some maldevelopment, most often noted at the hip); (2) spontaneous or pathologic, due to disease of the articular or the periarticular structures; and (3) traumatic, due to injury, such as the application of force in such a manner as to produce disruption of the joint.

The signs and symptoms of a traumatic dislocation are (1) pain, (2) change in contour of the joint, (3) change in the length of the extremity, (4) loss of normal mobility, and (5) change in the axis of the dislocated bones.

Roentgenograms confirm the diagnosis and should be made in every case, because frequently there is an associated fracture.

Management. The part is immobilized while the patient is transported to the emergency department, x-ray department, or clinical unit. The dislocation is reduced (*i.e.,* displaced parts brought into normal position), usually under anesthesia. The head of the dislocated bone is manipulated back into the joint cavity, and the joint is immobilized by bandages and splints and kept immobile in a stable position until healing takes place.

The nursing management following reduction of a dislocation is essentially the same as that following the reduction of fractures. The part must be kept immobilized for a sufficient time to permit the ligamentous structures about the joint to heal. Therefore, splints and casts are the usual dressings. Complications that are common with such appliances must be watched for, including cyanosis, pain, and the disturbance or the loss of sensation or movement, which are familiar signs of circulatory or nerve impairment due to tight dressings. Attention must be paid to the slightest complaint by the patient. Signs of pressure both within and outside the immobilization dressing must be assessed regularly.

▷ Fractures

A *fracture* is a break in the continuity of bone and is defined according to type and extent (Fig. 61-1). Fractures occur when the bone is subjected to stress greater than it can absorb. Fractures can be caused by direct blow, crushing forces, sudden twisting motion, and even by extreme muscle contraction.

While the bone is the part most directly affected, other structures also may be involved, resulting in soft tissue edema, hemorrhage into the muscles and joints, joint dislocations, ruptured tendons, severed nerves, and damaged blood vessels. Body organs may be injured by the force that caused the fracture or by the fracture fragments.

Types of Fractures

A *complete* fracture involves a break across the entire cross section of the bone and is frequently displaced (removed from normal position). In an *incomplete* fracture, the break occurs only through part of the cross section of the bone and is usually undisplaced.

An *open* fracture is one that extends through the skin or mucous membrane. In a *closed* fracture, the fracture does not communicate with the outside area.

Fractures may also be described according to anatomical placement of fragments—*displaced/nondisplaced* fracture. The following are specific types of fractures (Fig. 61-1):

Greenstick—a fracture in which one side of a bone is broken and the other side is bent

Transverse—a fracture that is straight across the bone

Oblique—a fracture occurring at an angle across the bone (less stable than transverse)

Spiral—a fracture twisting around the shaft of the bone

Comminuted—a fracture in which bone has splintered into several fragments

Depressed—a fracture in which fragment(s) is (are) indriven (seen frequently in fractures of skull and facial bones)

Compression—a fracture in which the fractured bone has been compressed by another bone(s) (seen in vertebral fractures)

Pathologic—a fracture that occurs through an area of diseased bone (bone cyst, Paget's disease, bony metastasis, tumor)

Avulsion—fragment of bone pulled away by ligament or tendon and its attachment

Epiphyseal—separation of the epiphysis from the rest of the bone

Clinical Manifestations

The clinical manifestations of a fracture are pain, loss of function, false motion, deformity, shortening, crepitation, local swelling, and discoloration. In an open fracture, the bone penetrates through the skin.

1. The *pain* is of a continuous type and increases in severity until the bone fragments are immobilized.
2. Following the break, the part cannot be used and tends to move unnaturally (false motion) instead of remaining rigid as it normally would. The displacement of the fragments in a fracture of the arm or leg causes a deformity (either visible or palpable) of the extremity when it is compared to the normal extremity. The extremity cannot function properly because normal function of the muscles depends upon the integrity of the bones to which they are attached.
3. In fractures of long bones, there is actually shortening of the extremity because of the contraction of the muscles that are attached above and below the site of the fracture. The fragments may often overlap as much as an inch or two. The muscle spasm that accompanies fracture is natural splinting to minimize further movement of the fracture fragments.
4. When the extremity is examined with the hands, a grating sensation, called *crepitus,* can be felt due to the rubbing of the fragments one upon the other. (Testing for crepitation can produce further tissue damage.)
5. Localized swelling and discoloration of the skin occur as a result of trauma and hemorrhage that follow a fracture. These signs may not develop for several hours or days following the injury.

All of these signs and symptoms are not necessarily present in every fracture. When there is a linear or fissure fracture, or in cases where the fractured surfaces are driven together (impacted fractures), many of these symptoms do not occur.

The diagnosis of a fracture depends on the symptoms of the patient, the physical signs, and x-ray examination. Usually, there is a history of injury.

Emergency Management

When the patient is transported to the hospital, the fractured extremity is rendered as immobile as possible *before the patient is moved.* If an injured patient must be removed from a vehicle before splints can be applied, the extremity is supported above and below the fracture site, and traction is applied in accordance with the line of the long axis of the bone to prevent rotation as well as angular motion. Movement of fracture fragments will cause additional pain, soft tissue damage, and additional hemorrhage.

Immobilization is established by applying temporary well-padded splints, which are then firmly bandaged over the clothing. Adequate splinting is essential to prevent the soft tissue from being damaged by the bony fragments. Immobilization of the long bones of the lower extremities may also be accomplished by bandaging the extremities together, with the sound extremity serving as a splint for the injured one. In an upper extremity injury, the arm may be bandaged to the chest, or an injured forearm may be placed in a sling. It must be remembered that the pain associated with a fractured bone is severe, and the surest way to decrease pain and hemorrhage and prevent possible shock is by fixing the bone so that the joints above and below the fracture are immobilized. The peripheral pulses distal to the injury should be palpated to assure that circulation has not been hampered.

In an *open fracture,* the wound is covered with a clean (sterile) dressing to prevent contamination of deeper tissues. No attempt is made to reduce the fracture, even if one of the bone fragments is protruding through the wound. Splints should be applied as described above.

Immediately following injury, a patient who is in a state of confusion may not be aware that he has a fracture (*i.e.,* he may walk on a fractured extremity). Therefore, it is important to immobilize that part of the body immediately when a fracture is suspected.

When a patient comes to a hospital suffering from a fracture, a narcotic sufficient to relieve the pain should be given provided there is no head injury. The intravenous route allows smaller dosage and prompt action and is effective in a patient in shock.

Then with care and gentleness the clothes are removed, first from the uninjured side of the body, and then from the injured side. Sometimes the patient's clothing must be cut away on the injured side. The fractured extremity is moved as little as possible to avoid causing more damage.

▷ Physiology of Bone Healing

When the bone is injured, the healing process results in restoration of bone as it was prior to injury. The bone fragments are not merely patched together with scar tissue. The bone regenerates itself.

There are several stages in fracture healing: (1) *inflammation*, (2) *cellular proliferation*, (3) *callus formation*, (4) *callus ossification*, and (5) *consolidation* and *remodeling* into mature bone.

Inflammation. With a fracture, the body response is similar to that of injury elsewhere in the body. There is bleeding, extravasation of blood, and fracture hematoma

Closed fracture—No open wound

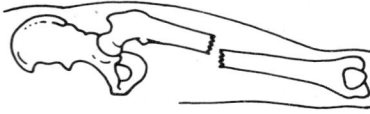

Longitudinal fracture—Break runs parallel with bone

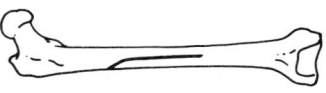

Greenstick fracture—Bone broken, bent but still securely hinged at one side

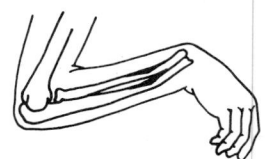

Open fracture—Wound in skin communicates with fracture

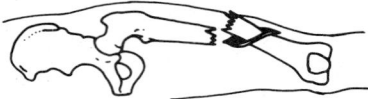

Transverse fracture—Break runs across bone

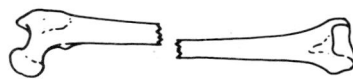

Impacted fracture—Bone broken and wedged into other break

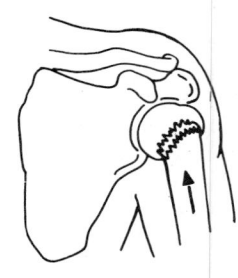

Extracapsular fracture—Bone broken outside joint

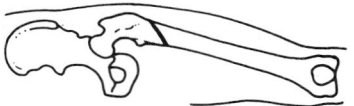

Oblique fracture—Break runs in slanting direction on bone

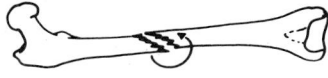

Fracture dislocation—Break complicated by bone out of joint

Intracapsular fracture—Bone broken inside joint

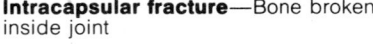
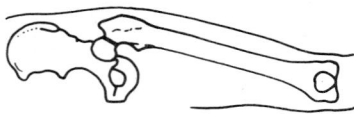

Spiral fracture—Break coils around bone

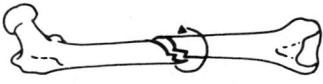

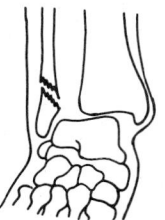

Comminuted fracture—Bone splintered into fragments

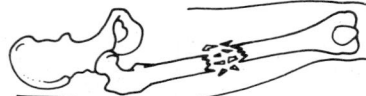

Pathologic fracture—Break is at site of bone disease

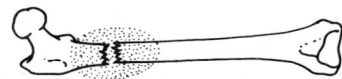

Depressed fracture—Broken skull bone driven inward

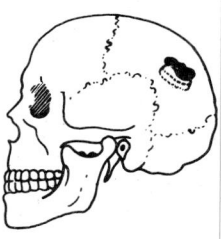

Figure 61-1. Types of fractures. (Courtesy, Ethicon, Inc.)

formation. The area exhibits edema, swelling, inflammation, and pain. The clot undergoes organization, and fibrin strands form within the clot. The fracture fragment ends become devitalized because of the interrupted blood supply. Within a few days tissue repair and healing will progress from adjacent viable tissue. The injured area is invaded by macrophages (large, white blood cells), which debride the area. The inflammatory stage lasts a couple of days, and resolution of the inflammatory response is characterized by a decrease in pain and swelling.

Cellular Proliferation. Within 48 to 72 hours following fracture, adjacent tissue cells modify and invade the fracture site. Fibroblasts and osteoblasts (developed from osteocytes, endosteal cells, and periosteal cells) produce collagen and proteoglycans for a collagen matrix at the fracture. Cartilage and fibrous connective tissue develop. From the periosteum, a collar of growth is evidenced, which is the beginning of an external cartilaginous callus. Capillaries develop in the proliferating tissue and provide nourishment to the forming tissue. Actively growing bone exhibits electronegative potentials.

Callus Formation. Tissue growth continues and the cartilage collar from each bone fragment grows toward each other until the fracture gap is bridged. The fracture fragments are joined. An internal callus also develops and invades the remaining blood clot. The shape of the callus and the volume of tissue required to bridge the defect are directly proportional to the amount of bone damage and displacement. It takes 3 to 4 weeks for fracture fragments to be united by cartilage or fibrous tissue. Clinically, the fragments are no longer easily moved.

Ossification. Ossification of the developed callus begins within 2 to 3 weeks postfracture. The repair cartilage is replaced through the process of endochondral ossification (see Chap. 59—Bone Formation). The mineral deposition continues and produces a firmly reunited bone. The callus surface continues to be electronegative. With major adult long bone fractures, ossification takes 3 to 4 months.

Consolidation and Remodeling. The final stage of fracture repair consists of removal of any remaining devitalized tissue and reorganization of the new bone into its former structural arrangement. Bone architecture is related to its function. Compact and cancellous bone develop according to functional stress subjected to the healing bone. Depending on the extent of bone modification needed, remodeling may take months to years. When remodeling is complete, the fracture surface charge is no longer negative.

Bone Healing With Fragments Firmly Approximated. When fractures are treated with open fixation techniques, the bony fragments can be placed in close direct contact. In this situation, the stages of bone healing are modified. Hematoma formation is not essential and is not observed. Little or no external cartilaginous callus develops. Immature bone develops from the endosteum. There is an intensive regeneration of new osteons. The new osteons develop in the fracture line by a process similar to normal bone maintenance. Fracture strength is obtained when the new osteons have become established. With rigid internal fixation, new bone is established in 5 to 6 weeks.

The progress of bone healing is monitored by serial x-rays. Adequate immobilization is essential until there is

Table 61-1
Approximate Immobilization Time Necessary for Union

Fracture Site	Number of Weeks
Phalanx	3–5
Metacarpal	6
Carpal	6
Scaphoid	10
	(or until x-ray shows union)
Radius and ulna	10–12
Humerus:	
Supracondylar	8
Midshaft	8–12
Proximal (impacted)	3
Proximal (displaced)	6–8
Clavicle	6–10
Vertebra	16
Pelvis	6
Femur:	
Intracapsular	24
Intratrochanteric	10–12
Shaft	18
Supracondylar	12–15
Tibia:	
Proximal	8–10
Shaft	14–20
Malleolus	6
Calcaneus	12–16
Metatarsal	6
Toes	3

(From Compere EL et al: Pictorial Handbook of Fracture Treatment, 5th ed. Chicago, Year Book Medical Publishers.)

radiologic evidence of callus. Progression of the therapeutic regimen (*i.e.,* application of a cast brace to a patient who has had a femur fracture reduced and immobilized by skeletal traction) depends on data indicating fracture healing.

Healing Time of Fractures

Many factors influence the speed with which healing occurs. The reduction of the displaced fracture fragments must be accurate and successfully maintained to assure healing. The affected bone must have an adequate blood supply. In addition, the age of the patient and the type of fracture affect healing time. In general, fractures of flat bones (pelvis, scapula) heal quite rapidly. Fractures at the ends of long bones where the bone is more vascular and cancellous heal more quickly than do fractures in areas where the bone is dense and less vascular (midshaft). Weight bearing will stimulate fracture healing of stabilized lower extremity long bone fractures. In addition, activity minimizes the development of immobility-related osteoporosis (a reduction of total bone mass producing porous and fragile bones due to imbalance in homeostatic bone turnover). Table 61-1 shows the approximate immobilization times necessary for union of the most common types of fractures.

Chart 61-1
The Treatment of Fractures

Principles of Care in Treating Fractures

1. Restore fracture fragments to their normal anatomical position (reduction).
2. Maintain reduction in place until healing occurs (immobilization).
3. Regain normal function and strength of the affected part (rehabilitation).

Methods Used to Obtain Fracture Reduction

1. Closed reduction
2. Traction
3. Open reduction

Methods Used to Maintain Fracture Reduction (Fixation)

1. Cast or cast brace
2. Splints
3. Continuous traction
4. Pin and plaster technique
5. Internal fixation devices
      a. Nails   c. Screws   e. Rods
      b. Plates   d. Wires
6. External fixation devices
7. Endoprosthetic replacements

If the fracture healing is disrupted, the bone union time may be delayed or stopped completely. Factors that may interrupt fracture healing include loss of fracture hematoma by debridement, adjacent tissue devitalized by inadequate blood supply, extensive space between bone fragments, soft tissue interposed between bone ends, inadequate fracture immobilization, infection, treatment regimen complications, and metabolic problems.

▷ Principles of Fracture Management

The principles of fracture treatment include reduction, immobilization, and regaining of normal function and strength (rehabilitation) (Chart 61-1).

Fracture Reduction

Reduction of a fracture ("setting" the bone) refers to restoration of the fracture fragments into anatomical rotation and alignment as nearly as possible. This is accomplished by closed or open manipulation.

Before fracture reduction, the patient should be prepared for the procedure. Medications for pain relief are administered. The extremity that is to be manipulated should be handled gently to avoid additional damage, elevated to minimize swelling, and gently cleaned before being dressed in a cast or splint.

In treating a fracture, the most important objectives are (1) to regain the function of the involved part, (2) to regain and maintain the correct position and alignment and, (3) to return the patient to his usual activities in the shortest time.

Methods to Obtain Fracture Reduction

Several methods may be used to obtain reduction of a fracture; the method selected depends on the nature of the fracture. Variations of these methods are carried out, but the underlying principles are the same. Usually, fractures are reduced as soon as possible inasmuch as tissues may lose their elasticity if infiltrated by edema or hemorrhage. In most cases, fracture reduction becomes more difficult as the injury begins healing.

Closed Reduction. In most instances, closed reduction is accomplished by bringing the bone fragments into apposition (ends in contact) by *manipulation* and *manual traction.*

Following the manipulation, x-ray films are taken to determine that the bone fragments are in correct alignment. A cast is usually applied to immobilize the extremity and maintain the reduction. A second person may maintain traction on the affected extremity while it is being encased in plaster. Anesthesia may be given to relieve the patient's pain and to relax the muscles.

Traction. Traction may be used to effect fracture reduction and immobilization. Adjustments of the magnitude of traction are made as muscle spasm is overcome. X-rays are used to monitor the fracture reduction and bony fragment approximation. As the fracture heals, evidence of callus formation is noted radiologically. When the callus is well established, a cast is frequently used for the immobilization technique. Traction therapy and the nursing management of a patient in traction are discussed more fully on page 1404.

Open Reduction or Open Operation. Some fractures require an operation or open reduction. This necessitates an incision in order that the bone fragments be replaced under direct visualization. Internal fixation devices in the form of metallic pins, wires, screws, plates, nails, or rods may be used to hold the bone fragments in position until solid bone healing occurs. Internal fixation devices may be attached to the sides of bone or inserted through the bony fragments or directly into the medullary cavity of the bone (Fig. 61-2). These devices assure better maintenance of alignment of the fracture fragment.

After closure of the wound, external immobilization of the fracture by cast or traction may be used. Most frequently, the internal fixation will allow early mobilization of the patient. The actual stability of the fracture fixation determines the amount of movement and stress the extremity can withstand. The surgeon can estimate the degree of stability he was able to obtain.

Internal fixation devices may be removed after bony union has taken place, but for the majority of patients it is not removed unless it produces symptoms. Pain and decreased function are the prime problem indicators. Problems that may develop with internal fixation devices include mechanical failure (inadequate insertion and stabilization); material failure (faulty or damaged internal fixation devices); corrosion of the device, causing local inflammation; allergic response to metallic alloy used; and osteoporotic remodeling adjacent to the fixation device (stress needed for bone strength is carried by the device, causing a disuse osteoporosis).

Nursing Management Following Open Reduction. During the immediate postoperative period following open reduction, the nursing management is the same as for any other major surgical procedure (see Chap. 21). If the patient is to be immobilized in traction following surgery, the traction may be applied immediately following surgery in the operating room. Regardless of the need for traction, an overhead trapeze facilitates postoperative patient care. The affected part is elevated, and the circulation of the part evaluated at frequent intervals, by comparing the affected extremity with the unaffected one for color and skin temperature.

- Symptoms of pain, pallor, pulselessness, paresthesia, and paralysis (the five Ps), or coolness, indicate abnormal circulatory changes or neurologic disturbances.
- The orthopedist should be notified immediately so that the dressings may be loosened or the cast bivalved in order to relieve pressure (see p. 1398). Hematoma drainage or fasciotomy may be needed. Dressings should be inspected at regular intervals.

The assessment and management of postoperative pain is an individualized problem. Remember that upon awakening, the patient is susceptible to suggestion. Reassure him that the operative procedure is over and that someone is with him. During the immediate postoperative period, narcotics may be necessary. In general, an elderly patient requires less narcotic than a younger patient. As soon as possible, oral nonnarcotic analgesics should be given, since patients who have undergone orthopedic operations may have prolonged musculoskeletal complaints. Restlessness, anxiety, and general discomfort may be relieved by appropriate nursing measures, reassurance, physical therapy, and other forms of treatment.

Orthopedic wounds have a tendency to ooze more than other surgical wounds. External muscle dissection frequently produces wounds in which hemostasis is poor. Wounds that are closed while under tourniquet control may bleed when the tourniquet is released in the postoperative period.

Maintenance of good aseptic technique is essential when caring for patients having bone surgery. *Osteomyelitis* (bone inflammation) is difficult to treat, and prevention is the objective. Aseptic wound dressing technique is necessary. Prevention of wound infections will eliminate that source for subsequent osteomyelitis. In addition, drains (portable wound suction and Penrose drains) should function in the early postoperative days so that blood accumulations do not become sites for infection.

Fracture Immobilization

After the fracture has been reduced, bone fragments must be immobilized or held in position until union has had time to take place. Immobilization may be accomplished by external or internal fixation. Methods of external fixation include bandages, casts, splints, continuous traction, pin and

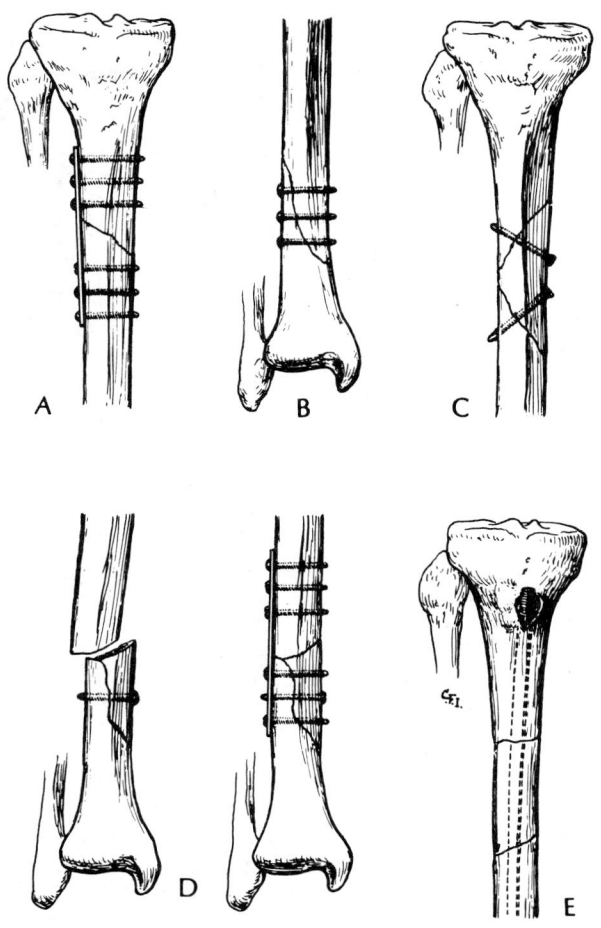

Figure 61-2. Techniques of internal fixation. (*A*) Plate and six screws for a transverse or short oblique fracture. (*B*) Screws for a long oblique or spiral fracture. (*C*) Screws for a long butterfly fragment. (*D*) Plate and six screws for a short butterfly fragment. (*E*) Medullary nail for a segmental fracture. (From Smith H: Fractures. In Crenshaw AH (ed): Campbell's Operative Orthopaedics, Vol 1. St Louis, CV Mosby.)

plaster technique, or external fixators. Internal fixation devices (metal implants) include nails, plates, screws, wires, and rods. These serve as internal splints to hold the fractured bones in alignment while healing takes place.

Bandages of muslin or elastic are used commonly to immobilize certain fractures. The *Velpeau* bandage is used for fractures of the scapula, clavicle, and humerus (Fig. 61-3). Fractured vertebrae may be splinted with an elastic back-supporting girdle. Splints (plastic or plaster) may be used for temporary or permanent immobilization, especially for fractures of the upper extremity. Air splints are quite commonly used by emergency paramedical personnel. Any splint that does not fit the curve of the extremity should be well-padded to prevent pressure.

Management of Open Fractures

In an *open* fracture (one associated with an open wound extending throughout the skin surface and down to the area

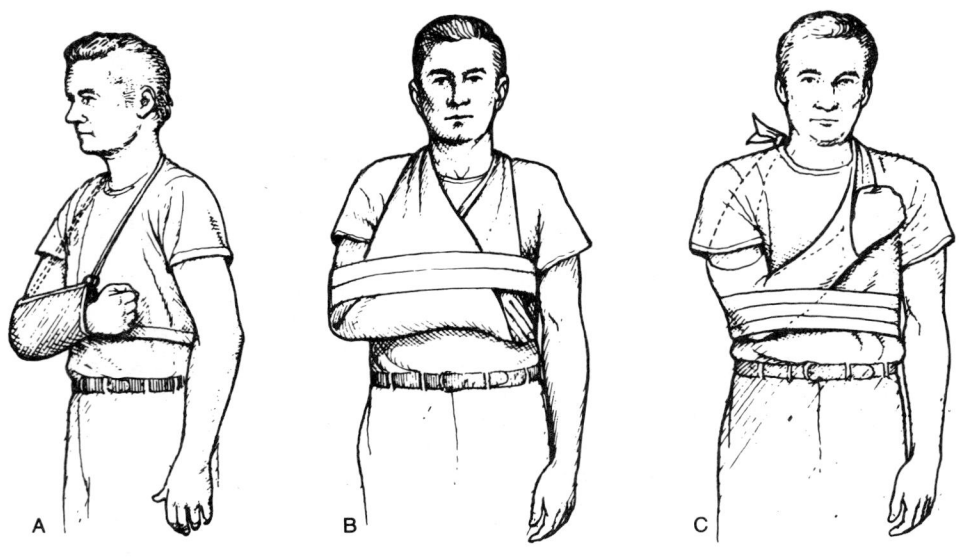

Figure 61-3. The types of immobilizing dressings used for upper humeral fractures. (*A*) A commercial sling and swathe, which permits easy removal of the arm for exercises and is comfortable on the neck. (*B*) A conventional sling and swathe. (*C*) A stockinette Velpeau and swathe used when there is an unstable surgical neck component, because this position relaxes the pectoralis major. (From Rockwood CA and Green DP: Fractures. Philadelphia, JB Lippincott.)

of bone injury) there is risk of *infection*—osteomyelitis, gas gangrene, and tetanus. The objectives of management are to minimize the chance of infection of the wound, soft tissue, and bone and to promote healing of soft tissue and bone.

The patient is taken to the operating room where the wound is cleansed, debrided (foreign matter and devitalized tissue removed), and irrigated. Swabs are taken for culture and sensitivity studies. Devitalized bone fragments are usually removed. The fracture is carefully reduced and stabilized by external fixation. Repair of damage to blood vessels, soft tissue, muscles, nerves, and tendons is usually carried out. A heavily contaminated wound may be left open, dressed with sterile gauze, and not closed until it is clear that infection has been aborted or overcome. Later the wounds may be closed by suture or by autogenous skin or flap grafts. Tetanus prophylaxis is given. Usually, intravenous antibiotics are started to prevent or treat serious infection.

When the patient returns from the operating room, he is observed for signs of shock since considerable loss of blood usually occurs during surgery. The extremity is elevated to minimize the development of edema. The distal pulses are palpated and the extremity observed for evidence of ischemia. The temperature is taken at regular intervals, and the patient is observed for signs that indicate infection.

External Fixators

The use of external fixation devices to manage open fractures has become common (Fig. 61-4). These devices provide stable support for severe comminuted fractures and allow active treatment of soft tissue damage. Complicated fractures of the humerus, forearm, femur, tibia, and pelvis are managed with external skeletal fixators. The fracture is reduced, aligned, and immobilized by a series of pins inserted in the

bone fragments. The pins are maintained in position through attachment to a portable frame. The fixators facilitate patient comfort, early mobility, active exercise of adjacent uninvolved joints, and shorter hospitalization. The patients are frequently discharged from the hospital after soft tissue heals and danger of infection has passed. When the bone has healed, the fixator is removed.

Psychological preparation for application of the external fixator is important. The apparatus looks clumsy and foreign to the patient. Reassurance that the device does not hurt after it is in and that early mobility is anticipated aids in the acceptance of the device. Following application, involvement of the patient in the care associated with the fixator will also help.

Following application of the external fixator, the extremity is elevated to reduce swelling. The neurovascular status of the extremity is monitored frequently. The injured area and pin sites are checked for signs of infection. Some serous drainage from the pin sites is to be expected. Assess each pin site for redness, drainage, tenderness, pain, and loosening of the pin. Twice a day the pin sites need to be cleaned with hydrogen peroxide and saline followed by the application of an antimicrobial agent as prescribed. Aseptic technique using sterile applicators is important so that pin tract infections do not occur.

- NEVER adjust the clamps on the external fixator frame.

Isometric and active exercise is encouraged within the limits of tissue damage. When the swelling has subsided, the patient is mobilized within the limits of his other injuries. If a tibia is being treated with an external fixator, the patient is ambulated with crutches. Weight-bearing limits need to be prescribed. Healing and treatment of complex open frac-

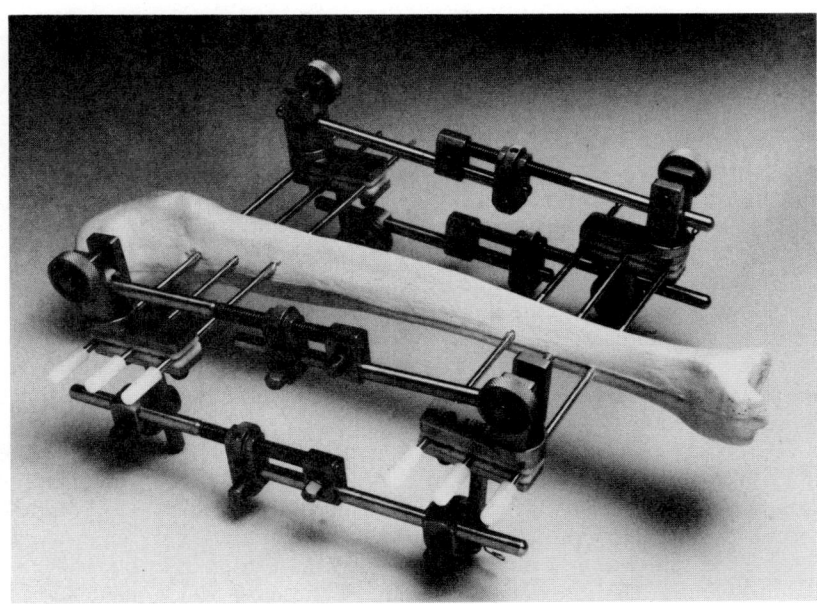

Figure 61-4. External fixation device. Pins are inserted into bone fragments. The fracture is reduced and aligned. The reduction is stabilized by attaching the pins to a rigid portable frame. The device facilitates treatment of soft tissue damaged in complex fracture situations. (Courtesy, Ace Orthopedic Company, Inc.)

tures are enhanced through the use of external fixation devices. In addition, disuse-related and immobility-related complications are minimized.

▷ Complications of Fractures

The immediate complications following fracture are *shock,* which may be fatal within a few hours after injury; *fat embolism,* which may occur within 48 hours or longer; *compartment syndrome,* which may result in permanent loss of extremity function; *infection; thromboembolism* (pulmonary embolism), which may cause death several weeks after injury; and *disseminated intravascular coagulation.*

Shock

Hypovolemic or traumatic shock, resulting from hemorrhage (both external and nonvisible blood loss) and loss of extracellular fluid into damaged tissues, may occur in fractures of the extremities, thorax, pelvis, and spine. Because the bone is very vascular, large quantities of blood may be lost as a result of trauma, especially in femoral and pelvic fractures.

Treatment consists of replacing the depleted blood volume, relieving the patient's pain, providing adequate splinting, and protecting the patient from further injury.

Fat Embolism Syndrome

Following fracture of long bones, pelvis, or multiple fractures, fat emboli may develop, especially in the young adult (20–30 years old) and in the 60 to 70 age group. At the time of fracture, innumerable fat globules may move into the blood, because the marrow pressure is greater than the capillary pressure, or catecholamines elevated by the patient's stress reaction cause mobilization of fatty acids and the development of fat globules in the bloodstream. The fat glob-

ules combine with platelets to form emboli, which then occlude the small blood vessels that supply the brain, lungs, kidneys, and other organs. The onset of symptoms may occur as early as a few hours after injury to a week after injury, but usually about 48 hours after injury. The onset of symptoms is rapid.

The presenting feature is usually cerebral disturbance manifested by bizarre mental symptoms varying from mild agitation and confusion to delirium and coma that occur in response to hypoxia, which results from fat emboli lodging in the brain.

The respiratory response includes tachypnea, dyspnea, crackles, wheezes, and large amounts of thick, white sputum. Blood gases reveal PO_2 below 60 mm Hg. The chest x-ray exhibits a typical "snow storm" infiltrate.

With systemic embolization, petechiae are noted in the buccal membranes and conjunctival sacs, on the hard palate, on the fundus of the eye, and over the chest and anterior axillary folds. Free fat may be found in the urine when emboli reach the kidneys.

- Personality changes, restlessness, irritability, or confusion in a patient who has sustained a fracture is an indication that immediate blood gas studies should be done. Occlusion of a large number of small vessels causes the pulmonary pressure to rise, possibly resulting in acute right heart failure. Edema and hemorrhages in the alveoli impair oxygen transport, leading to hypoxia. There is an increase in respiratory rate, precordial chest pain, cough, dyspnea, and acute pulmonary edema.

Management.   The objectives of management are to support the respiratory system and to correct homeostatic disturbances. Arterial blood gas analysis is done to determine the degree of respiratory impairment, as respiratory failure is the most common cause of death. Respiratory support is provided with oxygen given in high concentrations. Controlled volume ventilation with positive end-expiratory pressure (PEEP) may be employed to decrease and inhibit the formation of pulmonary edema. Steroids to treat the inflammatory lung reaction and to control cerebral edema may be given. Low molecular weight dextran may improve pulmonary and capillary flow because of its desludging effect. Heparin may be used for its lipolytic action (break down fat globules), but its anticoagulant effect may cause hemorrhage at the fracture site.

To allay apprehension, decrease pain, and depress the respiratory center, morphine might be administered to patients on the ventilator.

Fat emboli are a major cause of death in fracture patients. Respiratory support needs to be instituted early. Response to therapy frequently occurs within 48 hours.

Compartment Syndrome

Compartment syndrome is a problem that develops when the muscle vascular perfusion is compromised by increasing edema pressure within a muscle or due to cast-restricted tissue swelling. The forearm and the leg are the most frequently involved. Permanent function can be lost if the situation continues more than 6 to 8 hours (Volkmann's ischemic contracture [Fig. 61-5] results from compression or damage to the brachial artery.)

Venous drainage is stopped by tissue edema, and arterial inflow continues, increasing the tissue pressure. The patient complains of excessive pain, which is not controlled by narcotics. He will possibly exhibit pulselessness, diminished capillary refill or cyanotic nail beds, paralysis, or paresthesia. Palpation of the muscle, if it is possible, will reveal it to be swollen and hard. Passive stretching movement of the muscle will cause acute pain. If it does not, the patient's complaint of pain may be due to nerve compression. The actual tissue pressures can be monitored by inserting a needle into the suspected compartment and determining the pressure via a mercury manometer or through a pressure monitoring setup similar to that used for hemodynamic pressure monitoring. (Normal pressure is up to 20 mm Hg.) Nerve and muscle tissues deteriorate as compartment pressures increase.

Management.   Compartment syndrome can be prevented by consistent elevation of the extremity above heart level and by application of ice after injury. If it occurs, restrictive dressings must be released, and fasciotomy may be needed if conservative measures have not restored tissue perfusion and relieved pain within an hour.

Other Complications

Thromboembolism (discussed on p. 681), *infection* (all open fractures are considered to be contaminated—(see p. 1423), and *disseminated intravascular coagulation* (*DIC*) are other possible complications of fractures. DIC includes a group of bleeding disorders with diverse causes, including massive tissue trauma. Manifestations include ecchymoses, unexpected bleeding after surgery, and bleeding from the mucous membranes, venipuncture sites, and gastrointestinal and urinary tract. The treatment of DIC is discussed on page 718.

Delayed Complications of Fractures

Avascular Necrosis of Bone.   Avascular necrosis occurs when the bone loses its blood supply and dies. It may follow a fracture (especially of the femoral neck), dislocations, prolonged high-dosage steroid therapy, chronic renal disease, sickle cell anemia, and other diseases. The devitalized bone may collapse or reabsorb and be replaced by new bone. The patient develops limitation of movement and pain. X-ray demonstrates calcium loss and structural collapse. Treatment generally consists of attempts to revitalize the bone with bone grafts, prosthetic replacement, or arthrodesis (joint fusion).

Delayed Union and Nonunion.   Delayed union occurs when healing does not advance at a normal rate for the location and type of fracture. *Nonunion* results from failure of the ends of a fractured bone to unite. Delayed union and nonunion are caused by infection at the fracture site; tissue becoming interposed between the bone ends; inadequate immobilization or manipulation, which disrupts callus formation; and a combination of limited bone contact and restricted blood supply. If union does not result by adequate immobilization, the fracture is said to be *ununited.*

In nonunion, only fibrous tissue exists between the bone fragments; no bone salts have been deposited. In such instances, a false joint (pseudoarthrosis) often develops at the site of the fracture. When such an unfortunate result occurs, braces may be used to make the extremity useful. An operation may be performed by which the ends of the bone are freshened, and an attempt is made to unite them by means of a graft removed from another bone, which is placed in position to span the fragments. Fractures of the middle third of the humerus, of the neck of the femur in elderly people, and of the lower third of the tibia most frequently result in nonunion.

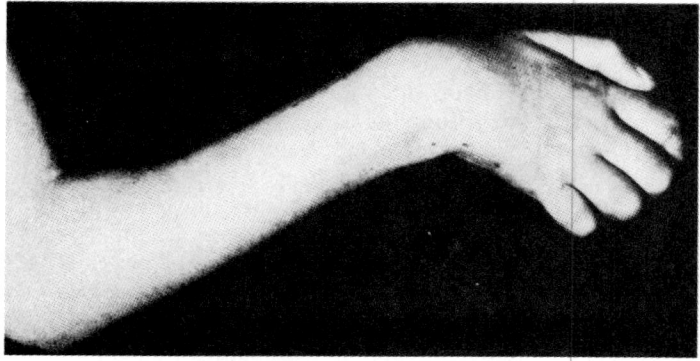

Figure 61-5.   Photograph of the forearm and hand of a patient with late Volkmann's ischemic contracture. (From Rockwood CA and Green DP (eds): Fractures, Vol 1. Philadelphia, JB Lippincott.)

Electrical Stimulation of Osteogenesis.   Methods of stimulating bone growth without bone grafting in situations where delayed union or nonunion exist have been developed. The tissue environment is modified by the electrical stimulation that enhances mineral deposition and bone formation. In some situations, pins that act as cathodes are inserted percutaneously directly into the fracture site, and direct current is continuously passed over the fracture. Another method is noninvasive and pulsing electromagnetic fields (PEMFs) that are delivered for 10 to 12 hours a day to the fracture by an electromagnetic coil implanted in the dressing over the nonunion site (Fig. 61-6). Both approaches appear effective, and the ultimate union rates are similar to those obtained by bone grafting. In addition, there seems to be resolution of low-grade infections that exist in the area. During the electrical stimulation treatment period, the fracture continues to be immobilized.

▷ Fractures of Specific Sites

Management of a patient with a fracture requires an understanding of the extent of the fracture, the therapeutic aim, and the management to accomplish this aim, as well as the care required through convalescence. The overall objective is to restore the function of the affected part to as near normal as possible.

An injury to the skeletal structure may vary from a simple linear fracture to a severe crushing injury. The therapeutic program is determined by the type and location of the fracture and the degree of involvement of surrounding structures.

Chart 61-2 outlines the basic nursing care plan for the patient who has sustained a simple fracture. Fractures of the skull and cervical spine have been considered in Chapter 58 on the management of patients with neurologic disorders. Fracture of the mandible is discussed in Chapter 34.

Clavicle (Collar Bone) Fractures

Fracture of the collar bone is a common fracture that results from a fall on the extended arm or a direct blow to the shoulder. The clavicle helps to hold the shoulder upward, outward, and backward from the thorax. Therefore, when

(Text continues on page 1430)

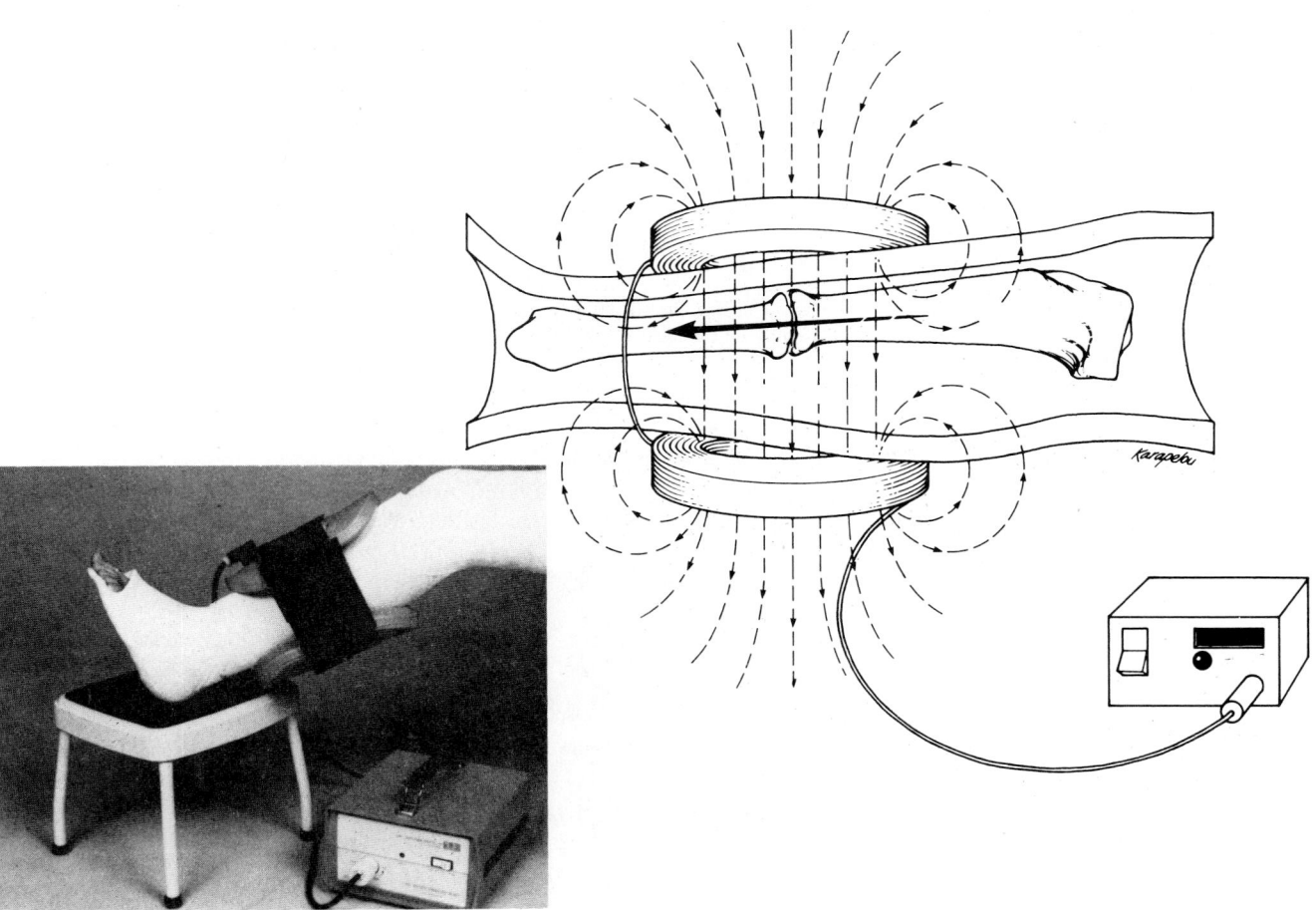

Figure 61-6.   Electrical stimulation for bone healing by the application of electromagnetic fields over the fracture site. (Courtesy, EBI Medical Systems, Inc.)

Chart 61-2
Nursing Process Guidelines for the Patient Who Has Sustained a Simple Fracture

Based on the clinical manifestations and nursing assessment, the patient with a fracture experiences certain problems requiring nursing interventions to assist in the resolution of these problems.

Major Patient Goals
1. Comfort
2. Adherence to therapeutic regimen
3. Identification of development of potential problems during treatment and seeking of prompt aid to minimize adverse effects
4. Participation in activities of daily living during healing
5. Resumption of previous level of activity without residual deficits

Major Patient Problems	Nursing Interventions	Expected Outcomes
1. Pain and tenderness related to fracture and soft tissue damage	Encourage patient to describe type and location of discomfort.	Verbalizes existence of pain
	Describe physiologic basis for discomfort.	Verbalizes reason for acute discomfort
	Splint injured area. Provide immobilization of fracture and adjacent joints.	Minimizes movement of injured part
	Implement nursing measures that will modify pain experience.	Utilizes pain perception modification techniques
	Assess for changes in pain intensity.	Relates decreasing discomfort with fracture and soft tissue healing
		Relates minimal discomfort experienced at fracture site
	Assess patient for behavior that is characteristic of comfort.	Expresses comfort
		Appears relaxed and moves without excessive guarding behavior
2. Emotional stress related to injury, treatment modality, and other problems associated with the injury	Encourage patient to express concerns and to discuss injury and problems associated with injury. Listen actively.	Discusses injury and impact on life
	Recognize and support use of coping mechanisms.	Utilizes available resources and coping mechanisms to modify emotional stress
	Involve significant others and support services as needed and appropriate.	
	Engage patient in development of treatment regimen.	Participates in development of health care plan
	Explain various facets of treatment regimen and his participation.	
	Encourage active participation in activities of daily living within therapeutic limits.	Participates in activities of daily living
3. Swelling related to edema and bleeding in traumatized tissue	Describe the physiologic basis for swelling.	Verbalizes presence of swelling
	Monitor neurovascular status of injured extremity.	Moves uninvolved parts distal to injury
	Encourage active and passive range of motion exercise for nonimmobilized parts distal to injury.	Experiences normal sensations in body parts distal to injury
	Assess nerve status in body part distal to injury.	

(continued)

Chart 61-2
Nursing Process Guidelines for the Patient Who Has Sustained a Simple Fracture (continued)

Major Patient Problems (continued)	Nursing Interventions (continued)	Expected Outcomes (continued)
	Elevate part above heart level. Support injured part in therapeutic position. Apply ice to injury for first 48 hours. Minimize time injured extremity is in dependent position.	Controls swelling
4. Muscle spasm related to bodily responses to injury and immobilization	Explain the physiologic basis for muscle spasm.	Describes the existence of muscle spasm
	Provide nursing care that diminishes spasms: Splint injured part. Make gentle position changes. Minimize spasm-producing procedures. Suggest relaxation techniques. Give muscle relaxants as prescribed.	Utilizes relaxation therapies
		Achieves relaxation and comfort
5. Ecchymosis related to bleeding into soft tissues surrounding fracture	Explain the physiologic basis for ecchymosis related to fractures.	Verbalizes the discomfort related to ecchymosis
	Elevate affected part.	Elevates affected part
	Apply cold to area for first 48 hours after injury, then intermittent heat.	Utilizes thermal therapies
		Achieves normal skin color and texture
6. Potential complications of simple fractures and treatment regimens		
Neurovascular compromise	Assess for the development of neurovascular compromise: Increasing pain Cool skin temperature Increasing swelling Decreased motor abilities Abnormal sensations Diminished capillary refill Teach the signs and symptoms of neurovascular compromise.	Describes signs and symptoms of neurovascular compromise
Skin breakdown	Assess for the development of skin breakdown: Skin abrasion Cast "hot spots" Drainage Irritation sensations Teach the signs and symptoms of skin breakdown.	Describes signs and symptoms of skin breakdown
Diminished muscle function	Encourage active exercise and range of motion of body parts not immobilized. Encourage isometric exercises of immobilized muscles.	Participates in activities that will minimize diminished muscle function
7. Potential injury related to unsafe use of treatment modalities and mobilization aids	Teach safe use of treatment modalities and mobilization aids. Supervise use of treatment modality and mobilization aids to assure safety.	Uses treatment modality and mobilization aids safely

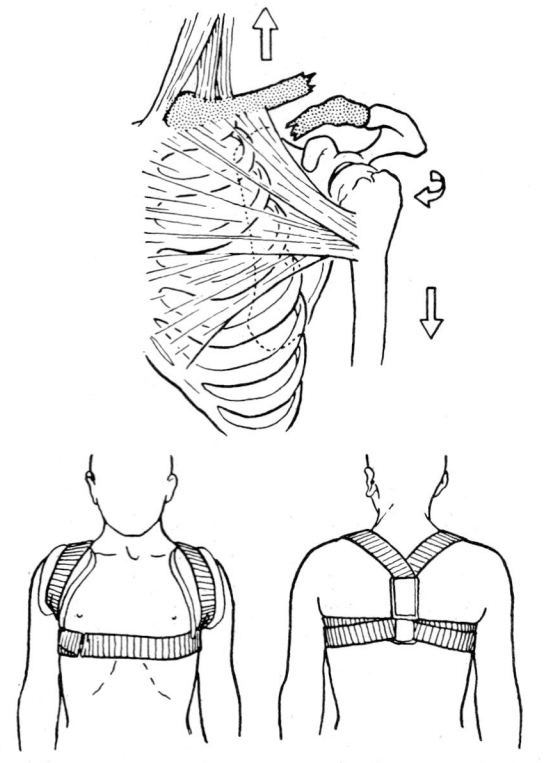

Figure 61-7. Fracture of the clavicle. (*Top*) Anteroposterior view, showing typical displacement of midclavicle fracture. (*Bottom*) Method of immobilization with a clavicular strap. (From Hardy JD: Rhoads Textbook of Surgery. Philadelphia, JB Lippincott.)

the clavicle is fractured, the objective of management is to hold the shoulder in its normal position by means of closed reduction and immobilization with external splinting in the form of a clavicular strap, sling, figure-of-8 bandage or T-splint.

More than 80% of the fractures occur in the middle or inner two thirds of the clavicle, and a figure-of-8 bandage or a commercially available clavicular strap (Fig. 61-7) may be used to pull the shoulders back and hold them in that position. When a clavicular strap is used, the axillae are well padded to prevent a compression injury to the brachial plexus and axillary artery. There should be no restriction of circulatory or nerve function in either arm.

Fracture of the distal third without displacement and ligament disruption are treated with a sling and restricted use of the arm. When the fracture occurs in the distal third of the clavicle with a disrupted coracoclavicular ligament, there is displacement and it is more difficult to obtain healing. Open reduction and internal fixation with a Kirshner wire is recommended. Immobilization of the shoulder with a Velpeau dressing or a shoulder spica is necessary to assure reduction with anatomical alignment.

Complications of clavicular fractures include trauma to the nerves of the brachial plexus or injury to the subclavian vein or artery from a bony fragment.

Patient Education. The patient is cautioned not to elevate his arm above shoulder level until the fracture has united, about 6 weeks. He is also encouraged to exercise the elbow, wrist, and fingers as soon as possible. When the patient is able, shoulder exercises (Fig. 61-8) are prescribed to obtain full shoulder motion. Heavy activity is limited for 3 months.

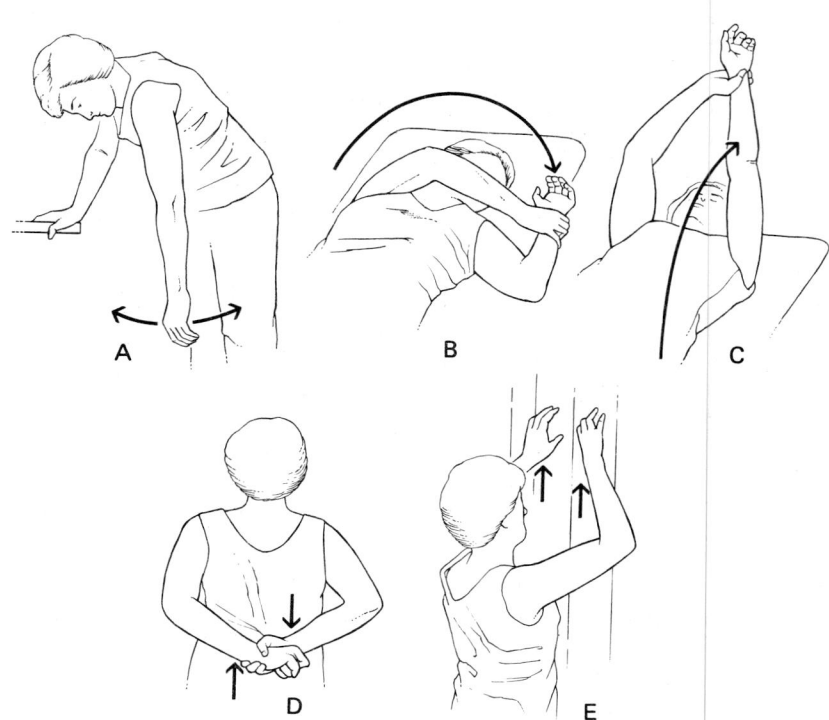

Figure 61-8. Exercises to develop range of motion of shoulder. (*A*) Pendulum exercise. (*B*) External rotation. (*C*) Elevation. (*D*) Internal rotation. In all of these, the unaffected arm is used for power. (*E*) Wall climbing.

Rib Fractures

Uncomplicated fractures of the ribs occur frequently and usually unite with no resultant impairment of function. However, fractures of the ribs produce painful respirations. Thus, the patient tends to decrease his respiratory excursions and refrains from coughing. As a result, tracheobronchial secretions are not coughed up, aeration of the lung is diminished, and a predisposition to pneumonia and atelectasis is created. Intercostal nerve blocks with procaine are done to relieve respiratory pain and permit productive coughing.

Chest strapping to immobilize the rib fracture is not usually used, because decreased chest expansion may result in respiratory complications of pneumonia and atelectasis. The pain associated with rib fracture diminishes significantly in 3 or 4 days, and the fracture is healed by 6 weeks.

Other serious problems may result from rib fractures. Multiple rib fractures may lead to a flail chest (see p. 538), while severe rib fractures may result in puncture of the lung with the escape of air into the pleural space (pneumothorax) or of blood into the pleural space (hemothorax). The management of these patients is discussed on page 539.

Upper Extremity Fractures

Fractures of the Humeral Neck

Fractures of the neck of the humerus may occur through either the surgical or the anatomical neck. The most common fracture in the upper arm and the shoulder is that of the surgical neck of the humerus. It is most frequently seen in the older female. Such a fracture occurs most often from a person falling and striking the ground with his outstretched arm (impacted fracture). The patient comes for aid with the affected arm hanging limp at the side and supported by the uninjured hand.

Neurovascular assessment of the involved extremity is essential to fully evaluate the extent of injury and possible involvement of the neurovascular bundle.

Many of the impacted fractures of the surgical neck of the humerus do not require reduction. The arm is supported by a sling supplemented by a modified Velpeau bandage. When this type of "sling" is used, a soft pad is placed in the axilla to prevent skin maceration.

In any fracture of the arm, limitation of motion and stiffness of the shoulder occur from disuse. Therefore, pendulum exercises are begun as soon as tolerated by the patient. (In pendulum or circumduction exercises, the patient is instructed to lean forward and to allow the affected arm to abduct and rotate [see Fig. 61-8]). Early motion of the joint does not displace the fragments if motion is carried out within the limits imposed by pain.

When a surgical neck fracture is displaced, treatment consists of closed reduction under x-ray control, open reduction, or replacement of the humeral head with a prosthesis. In this type of fracture, there must be a specified period of immobilization before exercises are started.

Patient Education. If the fracture is not displaced, active motion of the shoulder joint is started *early* to prevent limitation of motion and stiffness of the shoulder. These fractures require 6 to 8 weeks to heal, and the patient should avoid vigorous activity, such as tennis, for an additional 4 weeks.

Fractures of the Shaft of the Humerus

Fractures of the shaft of the humerus are most frequently caused by (1) direct violence that results in a transverse, oblique, or comminuted fracture, or (2) an indirect twisting force that results in a spiral fracture. The radial nerve may be injured in this fracture because it lies immediately adjacent to the midportion of the humerus in the musculospiral groove. Initial neurovascular assessment is essential to differentiate trauma nerve injury and treatment nerve injury.

Frequently, the weight of the arm helps to correct any displacement so that surgery is not required. A hanging cast may be applied to an oblique, spiral, or displaced fracture that has resulted in shortening of the humeral shaft. A hanging cast must be dependent (allowed to hang free without support) since the weight of the cast is the means by which continuous traction is applied to the long axis of the arm. The patient is advised to sleep in a fairly upright position so that traction is maintained constantly. Finger exercises are started as soon as the cast is applied, while pendulum exercises are done as directed to provide active movement of the shoulder, thereby preventing adhesions of the shoulder joint capsule. After the cast is removed, a sling is applied and exercises of the shoulder, elbow, and wrist are begun. It requires about 10 weeks for humeral fractures to heal when treated with hanging casts. Problems encountered with this mode of therapy are fracture distraction (pulling fracture fragments too far apart) due to the weight of the cast, and fracture angulation due to excessive fracture motion.

Functional bracing is being used for these fractures. A hanging cast is applied for about 1 week, and then a contoured thermoplastic sleeve is secured in place with Velcro closures around the upper arm. As swelling decreases, the Velcro is tightened, applying uniform pressure and stability to the fracture. Functional bracing allows active use of muscles, shoulder and elbow motion, and good approximation of fracture fragments. The callus that develops is substantial, and the sleeve can be discontinued in about 9 weeks.

Open fractures of the humeral shaft are frequently treated by external fixators (see p. 1424). Open reduction of these fractures is necessary with evidence of nerve palsy and pathologic fractures.

Supracondylar Fractures of the Humerus (Above the Elbow)

This fracture occurs close to the median nerve and brachial artery. Therefore, the most serious complication of a supracondylar fracture of the humerus is Volkmann's ischemic contracture, which results from compression or damage to the brachial artery (see Fig. 61-5). Antecubital swelling is a major concern with these fractures since neurovascular compression may occur.

The treatment for this type of fracture varies. If possible, the bones are aligned by manipulation under general anesthesia. After reduction, the bone fragments are maintained in alignment by keeping the elbow in a 90-degree to 110-degree flexion long arm cast. The cast may be windowed over the antecubital fossa, or a posterior splint may be used to permit tissue swelling without neurovascular compression.

For more severe injuries, skeletal traction is applied with the arm suspended over the face (Fig. 61-9) or in a side-arm position (Fig. 61-10). The traction is established from a Kirschner wire placed through the olecranon process. These methods serve to maintain traction, keep the fracture reduced, decrease edema, and aid the circulation, thereby reducing the risk of Volkmann's contracture.

The traction is replaced with a long arm cast. After about 8 weeks, the cast can be replaced with a splint and gentle range of motion exercise to the elbow is begun with the splint reapplied after each exercise session. The supracondylar fractures require about 12 weeks to heal.

Sometimes open reduction and pin or screw fixation may be necessary.

An important nursing function when managing the patient with a supracondylar fracture of the humerus is to assess for signs of impaired circulation in the forearm and hand.

- Observe the hand for swelling, skin color (blueness and blanching of the nailbeds), and temperature, comparing it with the unaffected hand.
- Evaluate the amplitude of the radial pulse. If it weakens or disappears, the orthopedic surgeon must be informed *immediately* since irreversible ischemia may result. Fasciotomy may become necessary.
- Assess for paresthesias (prickling and burning sensations) in the hand, since such signs may indicate nerve injury or impending ischemia. Early treatment is indicated to restore circulation before irreparable damage occurs.
- Encourage the patient to move his fingers frequently.

Fractures at the Elbow

Intercondylar fractures at the elbow result from automobile accidents, falls on the elbow or with the elbow flexed, or by direct blow. If the fracture is not displaced, the arm is immobilized in a cast with the elbow at 45 to 90 degrees of flexion; or the elbow may be supported with a pressure dressing and a sling.

A displaced fracture is usually treated by open reduction and internal fixation. Sometimes the bone fragments are excised. Additional external support with a plaster splint is then applied.

This type of fracture may result in nerve damage from injury to the median, radial, or ulnar nerves. The patient is evaluated for paresthesias and also for signs of compromised circulation in the forearm and hand.

Increasingly, gentle range of motion exercise of the injured joint is begun about 1 week after internal fixation and after 4 weeks with closed reduction. Motion aids healing of injured joints by movement of synovial fluid into the articular cartilage. Active exercise of the elbow is carried out when prescribed, as limitation of motion is common unless an intensive rehabilitation program is done.

Radius and Ulna Fractures
Head and Neck of the Radius. These fractures are usually produced by a fall on the outstretched hand with the elbow in extension. If blood has collected in the elbow joint (hemarthrosis), it is aspirated to relieve pain and allow early range of motion. Immobilization is accomplished by a sling.

If the fracture is displaced, an open operation is required, with excision of the radial head when necessary.

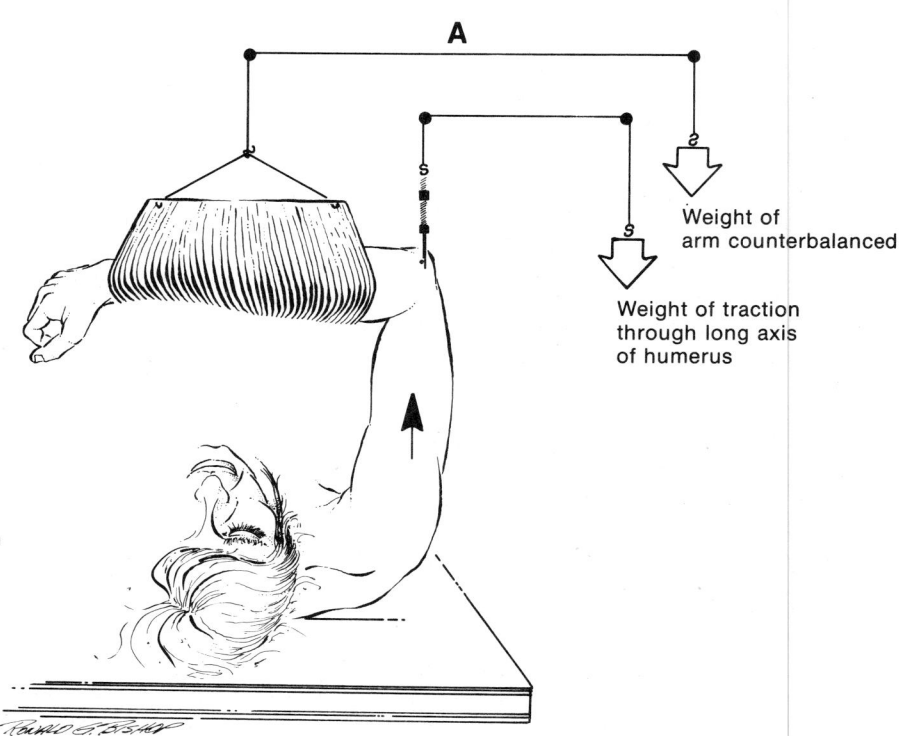

Figure 61-9. Treatment of supracondylar fracture: over-the-face traction is useful when swelling is great enough to compromise circulation. This type of traction reduces swelling by creating a very effective elevation of the extremity. (From Lewis RC: Handbook of Traction, Casting and Splinting Techniques, Philadelphia, JB Lippincott.)

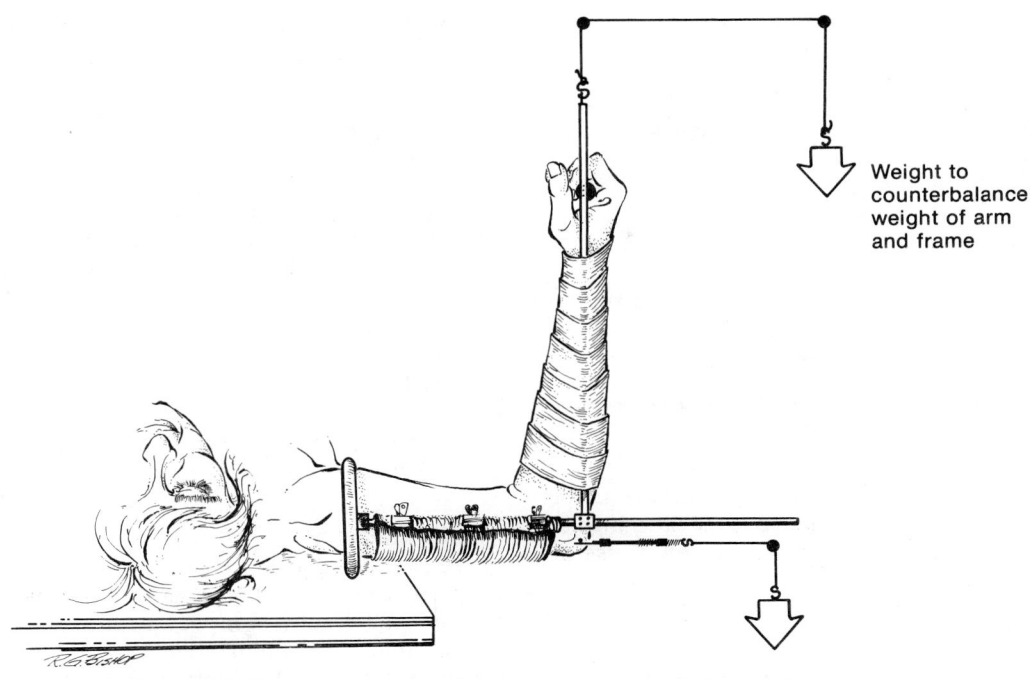

Figure 61-10. Balanced side-arm traction. The arm is passed through the ring, which is then passed up so that it encompasses the shoulder. The upright attachment for the forearm may be moved in either direction to accommodate the length of the humerus. A cloth sling is placed on the horizontal segment to provide a surface on which the arm may rest. The olecranon extends just past the vertical extremity, so that the pin drilled through the olecranon will be clear and allow unimpeded traction. The forearm is placed between the two upright supports, and is usually held there with a circumferentially applied elastic bandage. A rope is attached to the vertical section and is passed through pulleys. A weight is attached to exactly counterbalance the weight of the arm and the frame. Skeletal traction is then applied in the desired amount through the pin in the olecranon. The entire extremity is counterbalanced so that a balanced traction system is created. (From Lewis RC: Handbook of Traction, Casting and Splinting Techniques. Philadelphia, JB Lippincott.)

Postoperatively the arm is immobilized in a posterior plaster splint and sling. The patient is encouraged to carry out a program of active motion of the elbow and forearm when prescribed.

Fractures of the Shafts of the Radius and Ulna. Fractures of the shaft of the bones of the forearm occur frequently in children and are not uncommon in adults. Either the radius or the ulna alone or both bones may be broken at any level. The forearm has the unique functions of pronation and supination and those motions must be preserved by good anatomical position and alignment. The ulna has a relatively poor blood supply, and unfortunately nonunion of this fracture occurs at times.

If the fragments are not displaced, the fracture is treated by closed reduction with a long arm cast applied from the upper arm to the proximal palmar crease. A wire loop may be incorporated in the cast near the elbow and a sling pulled through it to prevent the cast from sagging against the forearm. The fracture is immobilized for about 12 weeks; the last 6 weeks the arm may be in a functional forearm brace that allows exercise of wrist and elbow.

The circulation and motion of the hand is assessed after the cast is applied. The arm is elevated to control edema. Frequent finger flexion and extension are encouraged to reduce edema. Active motion of the involved shoulder is essential.

For displaced fractures, open operation is frequently done with internal fixation obtained by applying a compression plate with screws or inserting some other fixation device (intramedullary nails, Rush rods, pins in plaster). The arm is usually immobilized in plaster splints or a cast until there is evidence of healing.

Fractures of the Wrist and Hand
Fractures of the Wrist. A fracture of the distal radius (Colles' fracture) is a common fracture and is usually the result of a fall on an open hand. It is frequently seen in an elderly person whose bones are osteoporotic.

Treatment usually consists of closed reduction and immobilization with a cast, or plaster-and-pin fixation to assure stabilized reduction. For more severe fractures, traction may be used to maintain length or a Kirschner wire may be inserted through the distal fragments to maintain reduction.

The wrist and forearm are elevated for 48 hours after reduction. Swelling of the fingers (from decreased venous and lymph return) is watched for and actively treated. Constricting casts and bandages must be released promptly. The median nerve is assessed for function (assess sensation by

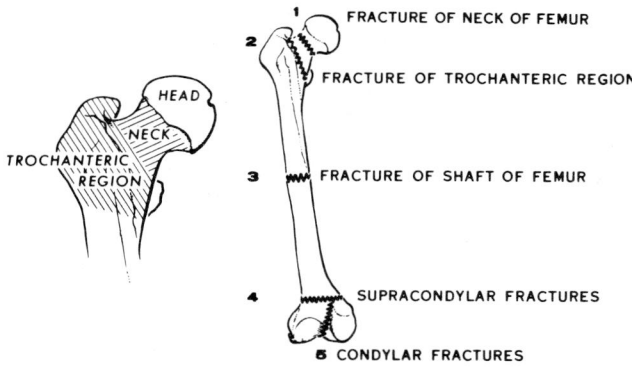

Figure 61-11. Sites of fracture of the femur.

pricking the distal aspect of the index finger, and the motor function by the ability to touch the thumb to the little finger). Active motion of the fingers is essential as well as use of the shoulder and elbow.

The patient is taught to do the following finger exercises to reduce swelling and prevent stiffness:

1. Hold the hand above the level of the heart.
2. Move the fingers from full extension to flexion. Hold and release.
   (Repeat above at least 10 times every half hour when awake.)
3. Use hand in functional activities.
4. Actively exercise the shoulder and elbow.

Fractures of the Hand. Since trauma to the hand can be such a complex problem, one requiring extensive reconstructive surgery, the reader is referred to specialized books on the hand. The objective of treatment is always to regain maximum function of the hand.

For an undisplaced fracture of the distal phalanx (finger bone), the finger is splinted to the adjoining finger to relieve pain and to protect the fingertip from further trauma. Boxing glove dressings are useful in those hand injuries that may cause swelling. Open fractures may be reduced by means of Kirschner wires.

Lower Extremity Fractures

The objectives of management of a fracture of the lower extremity are (1) to obtain adequate bony union with full length and normal alignment and without rotational or angular deformity, (2) to restore muscle power and joint motion, and (3) to restore the preinjury ambulatory status of the patient.

Special Rehabilitation Nursing Measures

- A fractured lower extremity is not to be placed in a dependent position for prolonged periods since *edema is a common problem* following all injuries of the lower extremities.
- The patient is encouraged to exercise regularly all joints that do not move the bone fragments.
- The extremity is elevated intermittently when the patient

becomes ambulatory to minimize recurrence of edema. It is best for the patient to lie down when elevating the cast.

- After the cast is removed, elastic stockings can be worn to support venous circulation, thus reducing the problem of edema.

Since practically all fractures of the lower extremity require the use of crutches, walker, or cane during convalescence, adjustable equipment should be acquired for the patient. The safe use of these ambulatory aids is discussed in Chapter 14.

Femur Fractures

Fractures of the femur can occur at several sites (Fig. 61-11). When the head, neck, or trochanteric region of the femur is involved, a hip fracture results.

Hip Fractures

There is a high incidence of hip fractures among elderly people because their bones are brittle from osteoporosis and they fall readily from weakness of the quadriceps as well as from general frailty due to age and a sedentary existence. Falls in the elderly also occur because of conditions that produce a decrease in cerebral arterial perfusion (transient ischemic attacks, anemia, emboli, cardiovascular disease, drug effects). Their therapeutic and nursing management is further complicated by associated medical diseases (cardiovascular, pulmonary, renal, and endocrine disorders). Hip fractures are the most frequent cause of traumatic death after the age of 75, occurring more frequently in women, often after insignificant injuries. A hip fracture is viewed by the patient and the family as a catastrophic event that will make a negative impact on the patient's life-style.

Classification. There are two major types of hip fractures. *Intracapsular fractures* are fractures of the neck of the femur. *Extracapsular fractures* are fractures of the trochanteric region (between the base of the neck and the lesser trochanter of the femur) and subtrochanteric fractures.

Fractures of the neck of the femur are more difficult to heal than those of the trochanteric region, because the vascular system supplying blood to the head and neck of the femur may be easily damaged with the fracture. The nutrient vessels within the bone may be interrupted and the bone cells may die. For this reason, nonunion or aseptic necrosis is common in patients with these types of fractures.

Extracapsular intertrochanteric fractures have an excellent blood supply and heal readily.

Clinical Manifestations. Because of the fracture, the leg is shortened and externally rotated. The patient may complain of slight pain in the groin or in the medial side of the knee. With most fractures of the femoral neck, the patient is in pain, is unable to move the leg without significant increase in pain, and is able to achieve some comfort with the leg slightly flexed in external rotation. Impacted femoral neck fractures cause moderate discomfort even with movement, may allow the patient to bear weight, and may not demonstrate obvious shortening or rotational changes. With extracapsular femoral fractures, the extremity is significantly shortened, presents external rotation to a greater degree than intracapsular fractures, exhibits muscle spasm that resists positioning the extremity in a neutral position, and has an associated large hematoma or area of ecchymosis.

The diagnosis of fractured hip is confirmed with roentgenograms.

Management Objectives.   The overall major objective is to return the patient to an active role in society as rapidly as possible. Prolonged immobility is disastrous to the elderly. In addition, because of the age of these patients who experience hip fractures, the incidence of concomitant medical problems exists and must be managed also.

The nursing management goals are:

1. To promote fracture healing
2. To prevent secondary medical problems
3. To prevent physical, psychological, and social dependence
4. To mobilize the patient as early as possible
5. To restore the ambulatory function of the hip joint (if the patient was ambulatory before the fracture)

Preoperative Management.   Surgical intervention is carried out as soon as possible after the injury. The preoperative objective is to ensure that the patient is in as favorable a condition as possible. Displaced femoral neck fractures may be treated as elective emergencies, and reduction and internal fixation are done within 12 to 24 hours after fracture. This is to minimize the effects of diminished blood supply and the development of avascular necrosis.

Temporary skin traction in the form of Buck's extension (see p. 1404) can be applied to relieve pain, or sand bags may be used to control the external rotation.

During the preoperative period, the patient should be assessed as to orientation to time, place, and person. Many of these elderly persons are confused, not only as a result of stress of the trauma, but also because of underlying systemic illness. Confusion that develops in some elderly patients may be due to mild cerebral ischemia. Examination of the legs may reveal edema due to congestive heart failure and absent peripheral pulses due to arteriosclerotic vascular disease. Muscle wasting may be evident.

Additional nursing management is directed toward assessing for possible dehydration, which is frequently seen in elderly patients, and encouraging movement of all but the involved hip and knee, along with deep breathing and coughing exercises to ensure adequate pulmonary ventilation. To prevent thromboembolism, anticoagulation therapy, such as subcutaneous low-dose heparin, warfarin, low-molecular weight dextran, or aspirin, may be given from the time the patient is admitted to the hospital until he or she is fully mobilized.

Operative Treatment.   The goal of surgical treatment of hip fractures is to obtain a satisfactory fixation so that the patient can be mobilized quickly and thereby avoid secondary medical complications. Operative treatment consists of (1) reduction of the fracture and internal fixation or (2) replacement of the femoral head with a prosthesis.

After general or spinal anesthesia, the femoral neck fracture is reduced under radiographic control using an image intensifier. A stable fracture is usually fixed with nails, a nail-and-plate combination, multiple pins, or compression screw devices (Fig. 61-12). The choice of fixation device is determined by the fracture site and the preference of the orthopedic surgeon. Adequate reduction is important for fracture healing. (The better the reduction, the better the healing.)

Replacement of the head of the femur with a prosthesis is usually reserved for a fracture that cannot be satisfactorily reduced or securely nailed. Some orthopedists prefer this method because nonunion and avascular necrosis of the head are common complications of internal fixation techniques. However, it appears that after prosthetic replacement, the morbidity rate (infection and dislocation of the prosthesis) and mortality rates are higher than with reduction by internal fixation. Salvage of the hip is usually preferred to prosthetic replacement. Total hip replacement (see p. 1409) may be used in selected patients who cannot be treated satisfactorily.

Postoperative Management.   The immediate postoperative care of a hip fracture patient is similar in many ways to other major surgery patients. However, additional attention is given to preventing secondary medical problems and early mobilization of the patient so that independent functioning can be restored.

During the first 24 to 48 hours, attention is given to the relief of pain and the prevention of respiratory complications. Activity is encouraged in bed. A pillow is used between the legs to maintain alignment and to provide needed support when turning the patient. Foot flexion (calf-pumping exercises) is encouraged hourly. Intravenous antibiotics are used prophylactically. Hydration, general nutrition, and output are monitored.

Turning.   The patient may be turned on the unaffected extremity by means of the following method:

• A pillow is placed between the legs to keep the affected leg in an abducted position. Then the patient is pulled over gently on his or her side. After initial soreness has gone and the incision is healed, the patient usually may be turned in the same manner on the affected hip.

Exercise.   It is also important that the patient exercise as much as possible by means of the trapeze suspended from the fracture bed. However, despite the use of the trapeze, triceps and shoulder exercises should be continued preparatory to ambulatory activities.

On the second or third postoperative day, the patient is generally fairly comfortable and can transfer to a chair with assistance. On the third day, assisted ambulation can begin. The amount of weight bearing that can be permitted depends on the stability of the fracture reduction and the location of the fracture. The physician will prescribe the amount of weight bearing permitted and the rate at which the patient can progress to full weight bearing. Physical therapists will work with the patient on ambulation and the safe use of walker and crutches.

Patients with hip fractures can anticipate discharge with use of an ambulatory aid in 10 days to 3 weeks following reduction. Some modifications in the home to permit safe use of walkers and crutches and for the patient's continuing care may be needed.

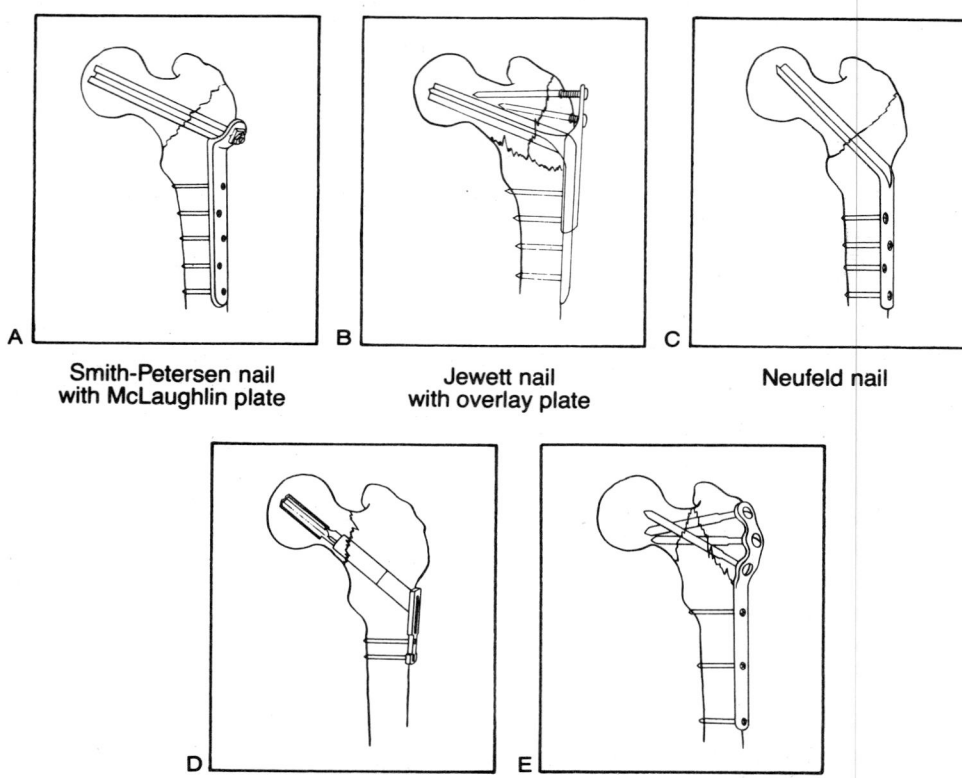

Figure 61-12. Examples of internal fixation for trochanteric fractures. In fractures of the femoral neck and trochanteric region, internal fixation is achieved through the use of nails that are flanged in various configurations for stability inside the bone, and with plates that provide additional stability and fixation. (*A*) Smith–Petersen nail with McLaughlin plate. (*B*) Jewett nail with overlay plate. (*C*) Neufeld nail. (*D*) Massie nail assembly. (*E*) Moe intertrochanteric plate. (Courtesy, Zimmer–USA, Warsaw, Indiana.)

Complications. Elderly persons who suffer hip fractures are particularly prone to develop complications that may require more vigorous treatment than the fracture itself. In some instances, the shock of the injury may prove fatal. In less drastic responses, shock following this traumatic experience may cause bladder incontinence, although urinary control is usually gradually regained. In general, the routine use of an indwelling catheter is to be avoided. Yet urinary problems may occur. Therefore, the color, odor, and volume of urine are monitored to detect problems such as urinary retention, which is common following orthopedic operations, especially in the elderly. To assure proper kidney function, a liberal fluid intake is important.

As in many postoperative situations, thromboembolism is the most common complication. To prevent thromboembolism, preoperative and postoperative prophylactic anticoagulation therapy is frequently used. To detect its occurrence, the patient's legs are checked daily for evidence of thrombophlebitis.

Pulmonary complications are also a threat to elderly patients undergoing hip surgery. Deep-breathing exercises, a change of position at least every 2 hours, and the possible use of an incentive spirometer help to prevent the development of respiratory complications. Breath sounds should be assessed for the development of adventitious or diminished sounds.

Because patients with hip fractures generally have poor circulation and tend to remain in one position, pressure sores frequently develop. Giving proper skin care, especially to the back and heels and under the hips and shoulders, helps relieve the constant pressure. An air or convoluted

foam mattress may provide adequate protection by relieving pressure.

Although the blood supply in a trochanteric fracture is maintained fairly well so that fractures at this site almost always unite, there is a fairly high mortality rate, mainly because the patients are generally older (70 to 85) and are poorer operative risks. Their conditions are further compromised by the degree of soft tissue damage that occurs at the time of injury. Added difficulties can be anticipated when the fracture is comminuted and unstable, as is frequently the case.

Delayed complications of the hip fractures include protrusion of the fixation device through the acetabulum, fixation device fatigue failure, avascular necrosis of the femoral head (particularly with intracapsular fractures), nonunion, and infection. Infection would be suspected if the patient complains of moderate discomfort in the hip and has a mild elevated temperature and a moderately elevated sedimentation rate.

The nursing management of the patient with a hip fracture is summarized in Chart 61-3.

Fractures of the Shaft of the Femur

Considerable force is required to break the shaft of the femur in adults. Most of these fractures are seen in the young male who has been involved in a vehicular accident or has fallen from a height. Frequently, these patients have associated multiple trauma problems.

The patient presents with an enlarged deformed thigh that is tender. The fractures may be transverse, oblique,

(Text continues on page 1440)

Chart 61-3
Nursing Process Guidelines for the Elderly Patient With a Hip Fracture

Based on the clinical manifestations and nursing assessment, the elderly patient with a fractured hip experiences certain problems requiring nursing interventions to assist in the resolution of these problems.

Major Patient Goals
1. Comfort
2. Adherence to therapeutic regimen
3. An uncomplicated recovery
4. Participation in activities of daily living during healing process
5. Resumption of previous level of activity without residual deficits

Nursing Management Goals
1. Promotion of fracture healing
2. Prevention of secondary medical problems
3. Prevention of physical, psychological, and social dependence
4. Mobilization of the patient as early as possible
5. Restoration of the ambulatory function of the hip joint (if the patient was ambulatory before the fracture)

Major Patient Problems	Nursing Interventions	Expected Outcomes
Preoperative		
1. Pain and tenderness related to fracture and soft tissue damage	Encourage patient to describe type and location of pain.	Verbalizes the existence of pain
	Handle the affected extremity gently. Utilize proper positioning techniques. Position for comfort. Apply Buck's traction, or stabilize fracture with sand bags until surgical fixation.	Minimizes movement of part
	Implement nursing measures that will modify pain experience. Give analgesics as patient's condition warrants. Assess patient's response to medications. Assure patient that discomfort will decrease with surgical reduction and fixation.	Relates minimal discomfort
2. Emotional stress related to injury, dependence, and anticipated surgery	Encourage patient to express concerns and to discuss meaning of a fractured hip to self.	Describes feelings concerning fractured hip and implications on life-style
	Recognize and support use of coping mechanisms. Involve significant others and support services as needed. Contact social services, if needed.	Utilizes available resources and coping mechanisms to modify emotional stress
	Explain anticipated treatment regimen to facilitate positive attitude in relation to rehabilitation. Teach exercises—range of motion, respiratory, isometric, and calf-pumping.	Participates in development of health care plan
	Ensure that the patient is in as favorable condition as possible preoperatively: Coordinate studies to assess cardiovascular, pulmonary, renal, and hematologic systems.	Participates in preparations for surgery

(continued)

Chart 61-3
Nursing Process Guidelines for the Elderly Patient With a Hip Fracture (continued)

Major Patient Problems (continued)	Nursing Interventions (continued)	Expected Outcomes (continued)
Preoperative (continued)		
	Avoid taxing cardiac reserve by administering IV fluids slowly.	
	Encourage balanced diet rich in protein and vitamin C.	
	Encourage questions about anticipated surgery.	
	Explain routines and procedures to patient.	
	Encourage active participation in activities of daily living within limits of disability.	Participates in activities of daily living
3. Potential for development of mental confusion related to underlying systemic illness or unfamiliar surroundings	Assess preinjury orientation status.	Demonstrates orientation to time, place, and person
	Encourage use of glasses and hearing aid.	
	Utilize orienting activities and aids (person/time identification, clock, calendar, TV, pictures).	
	Minimize number of staff working with patient.	
	Encourage participation in conversations.	Mental alertness
	Encourage participation in hygiene and nutritional activities.	Participates in activities of self-care
4. Potential problems related to immobility		
Skin breakdown	Reposition patient frequently to relieve pressure areas.	Cooperates with turning and massaging regimen
	Utilize air or convoluted foam mattress to minimize pressure sore development.	
	Inspect and massage pressure areas at bony prominences (heel, sacrum, shoulders, elbows) frequently.	
	Use sheepskin under leg.	
	Keep skin dry to prevent breakdown.	Develops no areas of skin breakdown
Venous stasis/thromboembolism	Elevate foot of bed 30 degrees if possible to promote venous drainage.	
	Teach and encourage calf-pumping exercises.	Performs calf-pumping exercises hourly
	Encourage wearing of antiembolic stockings, except when contraindicated.	Wears prescribed antiembolic stockings
	Inspect legs for development of thrombophlebitis.	
	Administer prescribed low-dose anticoagulants.	
Respiratory problems	Auscultate lungs for adventitious or diminished breath sounds. (Pneumonia is a common cause of death in the elderly.)	Breath sounds clear
	Encourage breathing exercises.	Performs deep-breathing exercises and coughs every 2 hours.
	Encourage fluids.	
Urinary tract problems	Avoid use of indwelling catheter and catheterizations to minimize chance of urinary tract infection.	Maintains adequate urine output

(continued)

Chart 61-3
Nursing Process Guidelines for the Elderly Patient With a Hip Fracture (continued)

Major Patient Problems (continued)	Nursing Interventions (continued)	Expected Outcomes (continued)
Preoperative *(continued)*		
	Encourage use of bedpan/urinal to minimize urine stasis.	
	Promote liberal fluid intake within limits of cardiorenal function.	
	Monitor color, odor, and volume of urinary output.	Exhibits no evidence of urinary tract infection

Postoperative

(Preoperative problems continue into the postoperative period, and nursing management continues to affect resolution of the problems.)

1. Pain/discomfort related to operative procedure and soft tissue damage	Alleviate pain.	Verbalizes the existence of pain
	Encourage patient to use pain medications and other pain relief strategies.	
	Assess response of patient to pain relief measures.	Obtains relief of pain through use of analgesics and other pain relief modalities
	Reposition patient frequently, supporting injured extremity.	Relates a decrease in pain 24–48 hours after surgery
	Use pillow between legs to support leg.	Appears comfortable and relaxed
		Moves with increasing comfort as healing progresses
2. Dependency related to need for assistance in performing basic self-care	Assess patient's need for assistance in hygiene, nutrition, and mobility.	Recognizes need to have assistance in hygiene, nutrition, and mobility
	Provide assistance promptly to minimize frustration related to dependency.	Accepts assistance as needed
	Encourage scheduling of care with patient to optimize patient participation.	Plans with staff for meeting basic self-care needs
	Encourage participation in self-care as condition permits.	Assumes responsibility for increasing amount of self-care as physical condition permits
	Praise patient for efforts and accomplishments.	
	Establish level of independence that promotes fracture healing.	Seeks assistance when needed
	Plan with patient and family for posthospital assistance as needed.	Satisfied with accomplishment in independent self-care and health care
3. Potential for development of inadequate fracture/wound healing	Delineate anticipated plan of care.	States knowledge of therapeutic regimen
	Modify plan with patient to facilitate patient participation.	Plans with nurse the implementation of treatment
	Encourage patient to assist in repositioning activities.	Participates in activities designed to promote fracture healing

	Coach patient in exercises:
	  Calf pumping
	  Range of motion
	  Isometric quadriceps and gluteal sets
	  Deep breathing and coughing	

	Encourage nutritional intake high in protein and vitamins.	

(continued)

Chart 61-3
Nursing Process Guidelines for the Elderly Patient With a Hip Fracture (continued)

Major Patient Problems (continued)	Nursing Interventions (continued)	Expected Outcomes (continued)
Postoperative *(continued)*		
	Remind patient to keep legs abducted with pillow or in neutral position.	
	Elevate leg to promote venous drainage.	
	Utilize elastic stockings to minimize edema by supporting venous circulation.	
	Assess neurovascular status of affected extremity.	
	Monitor wound drainage—amount anticipated to diminish during first 24–48 hours.	
	Monitor patient's vital signs for indication of developing abnormality.	
	Monitor wound healing.	
		Experiences incision healing and fracture ossification
4. Immobility related to fracture and internal fixation	Encourage movement to minimize effects of bed rest.	Moves independently in bed
	Assure cardiovascular adjustment to sitting position before transfer.	Participates in transfer to chair
	Assist patient to wheelchair several times a day as soon as possible (usually 24–72 hours after surgery).	
	Observe limits of weight bearing prescribed by physician and related to stability of reduction (nonweight bearing to partial weight bearing).	

	Supervise and encourage exercises:
	  Gluteal sets
	  Quadriceps
	  Dorsiflexion of foot
	  Knee flexion–extension to prevent contracture
	  Upper extremity strengthening
	Collaborate with physical therapist concerning activity progression
		Exercises to increase endurance, strength, and mobility

	Supervise use of ambulatory aid.	Ambulates with aid of walker, crutches, or cane

(continued)

---

spiral, or comminuted. Frequently, the patient is in impending shock, since the loss of 2 to 3 units of blood into the tissues with this fracture is common. Assessment includes neurovascular status of the extremity, especially circulatory perfusion of the foot. (Check popliteal and pedal pulses and toe capillary refill.) Dislocation of the hip and knee may accompany these fractures.

Treatment is begun with skin traction to immobilize the fracture so that additional soft tissue damage does not occur. Generally, skeletal traction (suspension traction with Thomas splint and Pearson attachment or slings) is used for a while to achieve overdistraction of the fracture fragments (which facilitates the operative procedure) for internal fixation or to achieve reduction and immobilization of the fracture site for subsequent cast bracing (Fig. 61-13).

To preserve muscle strength, the patient should exercise the lower leg, foot, and toes on a regular basis. A common complication following fracture of the femoral shaft is restriction of knee motion. Thus, quadriceps setting exercises should be started early. Active and passive knee exercises

Chart 61-3
Nursing Process Guidelines for the Elderly Patient With a Hip Fracture (continued)

Major Patient Problems (continued)	Nursing Interventions (continued)	Expected Outcomes (continued)
Postoperative (continued)		
	Review safety considerations when using ambulatory aids.	Observes safety factors when using ambulatory aid
	Assess patient's use of ambulatory aid for safety.	
	Assess compliance with weight-bearing prescription.	Complies with weight-bearing prescription
	Evaluate level of mobility prior to discharge.	Mobility adequate to allow independent participation in activities of daily living
	Plan with patient and family for modification needed in posthospital care due to residual immobility.	
		Resumes ambulatory function of hip joint (posthospitalization when fracture has healed)
		Resumes previous level of activity without residual deficits

5. Potential problems related to immobility
    Skin breakdown
    Venous stasis/thromboemboli
    Respiratory problems
    Urinary tract problems
	(See Preoperative Nursing Interventions.)	(See Preoperative Expected Outcomes.)

6. Potential long-term problems related to surgery and fracture Infection	Assess patient for continued moderate discomfort in hip, low-grade fever, and elevated sedimentation rate 2–3 months posthospitalization. Refer for radiologic evaluation of hip.	Shows no indication of deep infection
Nonunion and avascular necrosis	Assess patient for continued discomfort and limited range of motion. Refer for radiologic evaluation of hip.	Exhibits no radiologic evidence of nonunion or avascular necrosis
Internal fixation device failure	Assess patient for changes in alignment, deformity, increased discomfort, and decreased range of motion. Refer for radiologic evaluation of hip.	Has no failure of internal fixation device

are done when healing has occurred. Progressive strengthening exercises for the upper extremities are needed to prepare for ambulation. Continued neurovascular monitoring is needed.

Internal fixation is generally planned 7 to 10 days after injury. Intramedullary nailing using Küntscher rod, Schneider rod, or Sampson rod obtains adequate interal fixation, which allows for early mobilization. The active muscle movement is important for increasing blood supply and increasing generated electrical potentials at the fracture site, which en-

hances healing. Dual compression plates may be used but need external support from a spica cast or cast brace for stability. Also, compression plates need to be removed and resultant osteoporosis needs to be considered when plates are being removed.

A cast brace with mid and distal shaft fractures is commonly used. Two to four weeks after the injury, when pain and swelling have subsided, the patient is removed from skeletal traction and placed in a cast brace (see p. 1400). Minimal partial weight bearing is begun and is progressed

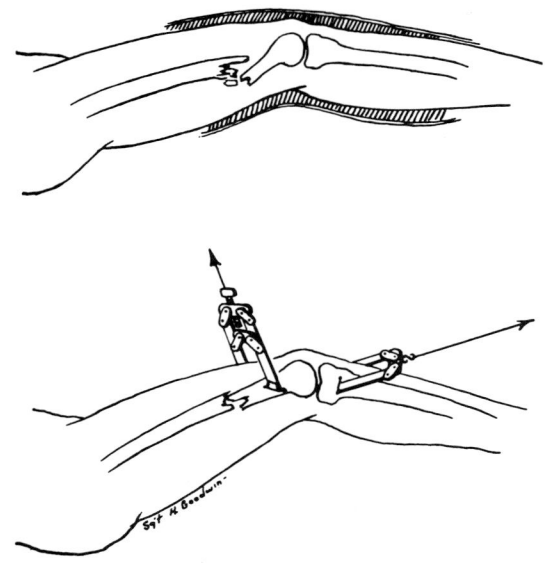

Figure 61-13. Diagrammatic representation of two-wire skeletal traction for fracture of femur in distal third. (*Top*) Deformity on admission to hospital. (*Bottom*) Adequate reduction when additional wire is inserted in lower femoral fragment and vertical lift is secured. (From Hampton OP Jr: Wounds of the Extremities in Military Surgery. St Louis, CV Mosby, p 273.)

to full weight bearing as tolerated. Functional ambulation stimulates fracture healing. The cast brace is worn for 12 to 14 weeks.

Fractures of the Tibia and Fibula

The most common fracture below the knee is a fracture of the lower (distal) one third of the tibia (and fibula) that results from a direct blow or "twisting of the ankle." Fractures of the tibia and fibula frequently occur in association with each other. The patient presents with pain, deformity, obvious hematoma, and considerable edema. Frequently, these fractures have severe soft tissue damage because of little subcutaneous tissue. Peroneal nerve damage needs to be assessed. (The patient is unable to dorsiflex the great toe and has diminished sensation in the first web space.) Tibial artery damage is assessed by capillary refill response. Development of an anterior compartment syndrome could occur. (Symptoms include intense pain, paresthesia, pain on passive movement, and diminished capillary refill.)

Most closed tibial fractures are treated with closed reduction and initial immobilization in a long leg-walking cast. Reduction must be relatively accurate in relation to angulation and rotation. The patient attains full weight bearing in 7 to 10 days. This activity decreases edema, increases circulation, and minimizes displacement because of the cast influence on the distribution of forces to the fracture site. The cast is changed to a short leg cast in 3 to 4 weeks, which allows for knee motion. Fracture healing takes 16 to 24 weeks.

Open and comminuted fractures may be treated with traction (using the Thomas splint or Böhler frame) or with an external fixator. The pins-in-plaster technique is used for those situations in which it is hard to maintain reduction.

The patient is not allowed to bear weight for about 6 weeks. Lottes nails and compression plating may be selected for certain situations.

As with other lower extremity fractures, the leg needs to be elevated to control edema. Continued neurovascular evaluation is needed. The development of an anterior compartment syndrome requires prompt recognition and resolution or there will be a permanent functional deficit.

Fractures of the Thoracolumbar Spine

Injuries to the thoracolumbar spine may involve (1) the vertebral body, (2) the lamina and articulating processes, and (3) the spinous processes or transverse processes. Five percent or less of spinal fractures are associated with neurologic deficits. The fractures are generally due to indirect trauma caused by excessive loading, sudden muscle contraction, or excessive motion beyond physiologic limits. Osteoporosis contributes to vertebral body collapse. The T12 to L2 area of the spine is most vulnerable to fracture.

The patient with a spinal fracture presents with acute tenderness, swelling, paravertebral muscle spasm, and possible change in normal curves or gap between spinous processes. The most important assessment done initially is to determine if there is injury to the spinal cord and if the fracture is stable or unstable. Immobilization is essential until these determinations are made. With a neurologic deficit, immediate spinal cord decompression with laminectomy and fusion is usually performed.

With a stable spinal fracture, only the anterior structural column (vertebral bodies and discs) or the posterior structural column (neural arch, articular processes, ligaments) have been disrupted. Unstable fractures occur with fracture dislocations and exhibit disruption of both anterior and posterior structural columns.

Stable spinal fractures (due to flexion, extension, axial loading, lateral bending, or distraction stresses) are treated conservatively. The patient is placed on bed rest until the acute pain subsides (days to 2–3 weeks). A spinal brace may be used for support during progressive ambulation and resumption of activities. Flexion exercises for the back (*e.g.*, Williams exercises) may be prescribed to enhance flexion of the spine and to strengthen the back and abdominal muscles.

With unstable spinal fractures, the patient is on strict bedrest until open reduction and fixation with spinal fusion and Harrington rod stabilization is accomplished. Ambulation is begun soon after surgery with the patient supported externally with some type of body jacket brace or cast. The conservative alternate is 12 weeks of strict bed rest in good alignment. The immobility-associated problems are apparent.

Patient education emphasizes good posture, good body mechanics, and, when healing is sufficient, back-strengthening exercises.

Pelvic Fractures

Pelvic fractures commonly occur as a result of automobile accidents, crush injuries, and falls from buildings and scaffolds. General symptoms include local swelling, tenderness over the symphysis pubis, anterior iliac spines, iliac crest, sacrum or coccyx, and inability to bear weight without discomfort. In addition, shock and hemorrhage may occur. Pelvic fractures are serious because at least two thirds of these patients have significant and multiple injuries. (The care of the patient with multiple injuries is discussed on p. 1550.) Therefore, a high mortality rate accompanies these fractures. Death may ensue from local hemorrhage in view of the rich blood supply to the pelvis and the possibility of massive and hidden bleeding in the retroperitoneal region. Bleeding also arises from the cancellous surfaces of the fracture fragments and the laceration of veins and arteries by bone spicules. There is also the added danger of intra-abdominal hemorrhage from a torn iliac artery. In addition to hemorrhage, the bladder, the urethra, or the intestines may be ruptured, a condition that can prove to be more serious than the fracture itself.

Management.   The objective of management is to carry out ongoing and continuing nursing assessment for injuries to the bladder, rectum, intestines, and intra-abdominal organs. To check for possible damage to the urinary tract, the patient's urine is examined for blood. A cystourethrogram and intravenous urogram are often done if injury to the urinary tract is suspected. Since hemorrhage is possible in these injuries, the abdomen is examined for evidence of intra-abdominal hemorrhage with peritoneal lavage. The peripheral pulses of both lower extremities are palpated since absence of peripheral pulses may indicate the possibility of a torn iliac artery or one of its branches. The patient is handled carefully and gently to minimize further bleeding and shock. Management of hemorrhage and associated intra-abdominal, thoracic, or cranial injuries have priority over treatment of fractures.

Once the patient has stabilized, the pelvic fracture is treated. Continued assessment of the function of other body systems is appropriate to assure function. Paralytic ileus may accompany pelvic fractures and immobility. Most fractures of the pelvis heal rapidly since the innominate bones are made up mostly of cancellous bone, which has a rich blood supply. Nonoperative treatment consists of bed rest, skeletal traction with a pelvic sling, or the application of a double hip spica cast to immobilize the fracture. The type of immobilization depends on the location of the fracture and the resultant stability of the pelvic ring.

For many patients with fractures of the sacrum and pelvis without disruption of the pelvic ring (Fig. 61-14), bed rest is all that is required. A bedboard is desirable under the mattress to give more stability. The patient is turned as a unit.

For fractures that disrupt the pelvic ring or involve weight-bearing areas, skeletal traction to reduce the displacement, lateral recumbent positioning with spica cast, or an external fixator may be used.

When both sides of the pelvis are fractured, a pelvic sling is used to immobilize the pelvis into a single unit so that the patient can move the rest of his body with less pain. The pelvic sling lifts the weight of the pelvis very slightly from the mattress (Fig. 61-15 *A*) The sling may be folded back over the buttocks in order to permit the patient to use the bedpan. (Some orthopedists permit the sling to be loosened for certain nursing care activities if the patient's condition permits.) Since skin care is a problem, sheep skin may be used to line the sling to prevent excoriation. It is necessary to reach under the sling to give skin care.

If separation of the symphysis pubis has occurred, a compression force must be applied. This is obtained by crossing the ropes from the sling to the weights on the

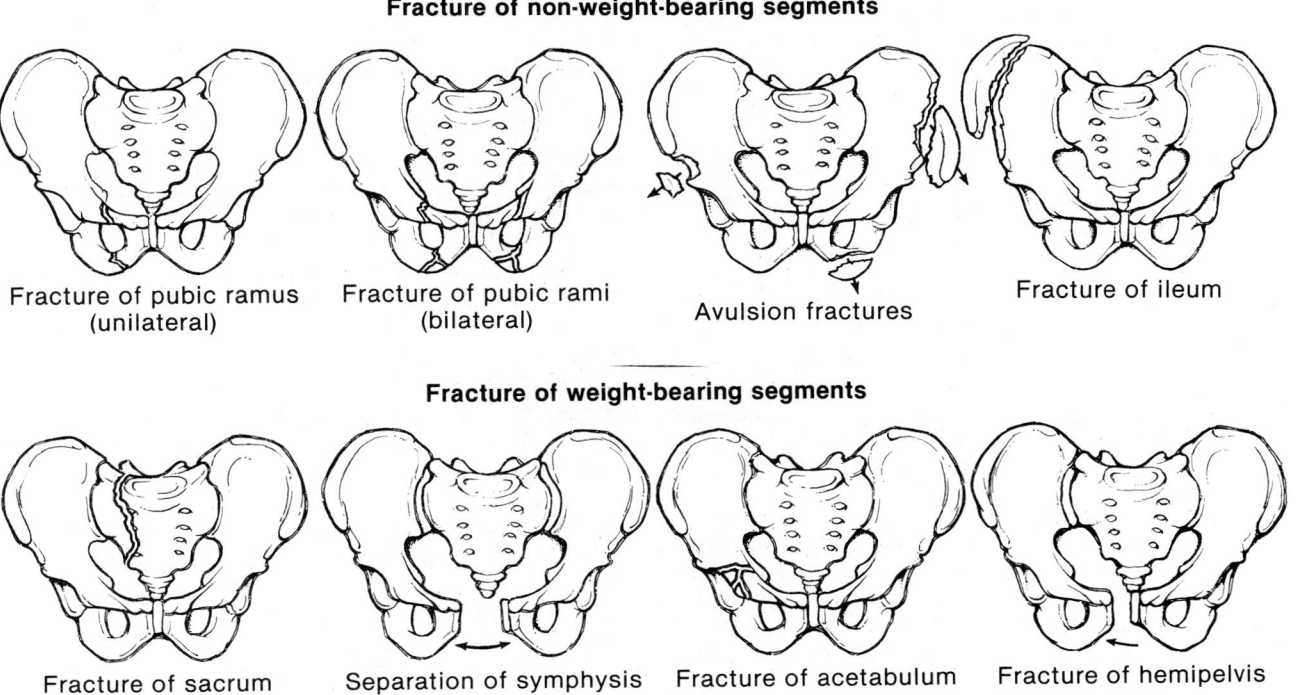

Fracture of non-weight-bearing segments

Fracture of pubic ramus (unilateral)   Fracture of pubic rami (bilateral)   Avulsion fractures   Fracture of ileum

Fracture of weight-bearing segments

Fracture of sacrum   Separation of symphysis   Fracture of acetabulum   Fracture of hemipelvis

Figure 61-14. Fractures of the pelvis.

opposite side (Fig. 61-15 *B*). The pelvic sling is adjusted to exert a compression effect from side to side to correct the separation of bones. Since the sling exerts pressure over the

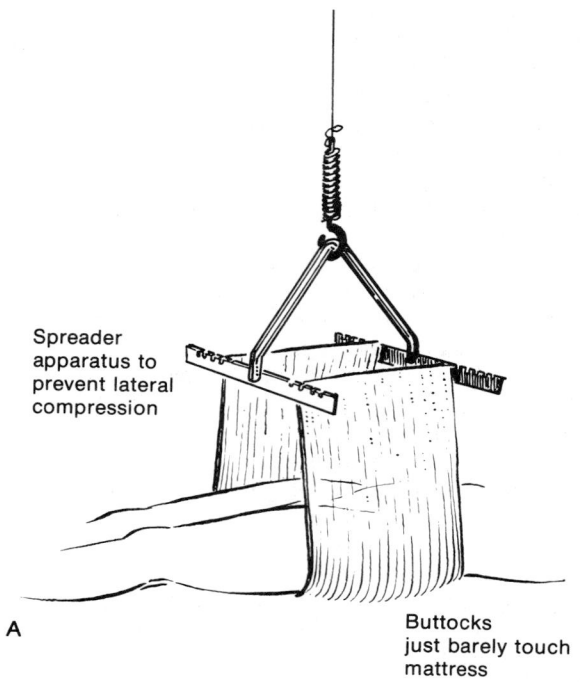

Spreader apparatus to prevent lateral compression

Buttocks just barely touch mattress

A

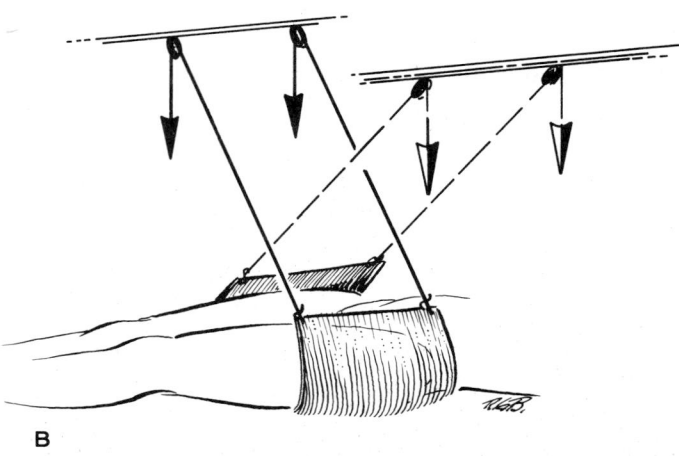

B

Figure 61-15. Pelvic sling suspension for fractures of the pelvis. (*A*) A suspension of the pelvis without an attempt at compression. The sling is suspended by means of a large metal frame, and weight is applied so that the pelvis is largely counterbalanced and becomes, to a certain extent, "weightless." Movement can then occur without moving the pelvic fragments. (*B*) The method for applying compression when there has been separation of the anterior pelvic ring, particularly at the symphysis pubis. The suspension in this type of traction is not as great, but is effective to a certain extent. This suspension compresses the pelvis from side to side to correct any diastasis that may have occurred. Pain developing at pressure points over the trochanters is unavoidable; it will often limit the duration of time that compression traction is useful. (From Lewis RC: Handbook of Traction, Casting and Splinting Techniques. Philadelphia, JB Lippincott.)

trochanteric region, the patient may become quite uncomfortable from soreness over the area.

When acetabular fractures occur, open reduction and fixation with multiple screws or direct lateral skeletal traction by insertion of a large trochanter screw into the femoral head is usually necessary.

During the period of immobility, exercises (leg, respiratory, range of motion, and strengthening), elastic stockings, and elevation of the foot of the bed to aid venous return are appropriate measures to help diminish the effects of prolonged bedrest. When bony healing has taken place in a pelvic fracture, the patient is mobilized with a method of progressive weight bearing, usually with crutches.

Internal Derangement of the Knee

Injury to most joints consists of a tear of the supporting ligaments. In the knee joint, however, there may also be a displacement or tear of the semilunar cartilages, which are two crescent-shaped cartilages attached to the edge of the shallow articulating surface of the head of the tibia. They normally move slightly backward and forward to accommodate the change in the shape of the condyles of the femur when the leg is in flexion or extension. In sports and in certain accidents, the body is often twisted with the foot fixed. Since little torsion movement is normally permitted in the knee joint, either the cartilage is torn from its attachment to the head of the tibia or an actual tear or fracture of the cartilage itself occurs.

These injuries leave a loose cartilage in the knee joint that may slip between the femur and the tibia, preventing full extension of the leg. If this happens when the patient is walking or running, he often describes his disability as his "leg giving way" under him. The patient may hear or feel a click in his knee when he walks, especially when he extends the leg bearing his weight, as in going upstairs. When the cartilage is attached front and back, but torn loose laterally (bucket-handle tear), it may slide between the bones to lie between the condyles and prevent full flexion or extension. As a result, the knee "locks."

These various types of injury are spoken of as internal derangements of the knee joint, and they produce a disturbing disability because the patient never knows when the knee will give him trouble. The treatment of this disability is removal of the injured cartilage. This can be done through an incision into the knee joint or through an operating arthroscope. The joint function can return to normal, and no apparent disability will result from the loss of the cartilage.

Postoperative Nursing Care.   After suture of the wound, a pressure dressing is applied, and at times so is a posterior splint. The leg should be elevated on pillows with a slight bend at the knee. The most common complication is an effusion into the knee joint, which produces marked pain. If this occurs, the physician should be notified. Relief can be obtained by cutting the pressure dressing and reapplying it more loosely. The joint may be aspirated under local anesthesia and pressure relieved by withdrawing the fluid in the joint.

To prevent atrophy of the thigh muscles, these patients are instructed to contract their quadriceps muscles while in bed. After 1 to 2 days, the patient may be up using crutches to bear his weight. In a short time (1 to 2 weeks), full unsupported weight bearing is possible. The knee is supported for another few weeks by an elastic bandage. Additional exercises are given to continue the quadriceps-building program. Full and normal function may be expected in 6 to 8 weeks from the time of surgery. Rehabilitation and recovery time for problems treated through the operating arthroscope are shorter, with the patient resuming some activities as soon as 24 hours postprocedure.

Rupture of the Achilles Tendon

Traumatic rupture of the Achilles tendon is a common occurrence. Sudden contraction of the calf muscle with the foot fixed firmly to the floor may cause snapping of the tendon, generally within the tendon sheath. The patient is acutely aware of his problem due to the pain and inability to plantar flex his foot. Immediate surgical repair usually obtains satisfactory results. Conservative management with a plantar-flexed cast for 6 to 8 weeks can be used.

▷ Amputation

Amputation of an extremity is frequently necessary as a result of peripheral vascular disease, trauma (destruction by crushing injuries, burns, frostbite, electrical burns), congenital deformities, and malignant tumor. Of all these reasons, vascular disease accounts for the majority of amputations of the lower extremities.

Psychological Considerations. Amputation forces anyone to make a major adjustment. Even those patients who have suffered with debilitating and painful diseases due to circulatory problems of the legs must adjust to the loss of an extremity. The way a patient adapts to an amputation depends not only on his physical condition and the ability to use a prosthetic device, but also on his perception of the disability. The change in body image must be integrated so that self-esteem is not lost.

An amputation produces a permanent physical handicap that certainly thwarts some physiologic, psychological, and social needs. The patient must accept these limitations realistically. Physicians, nurses, prosthetists, and physical therapists share the task of helping the amputee make the necessary changes in the pattern of living, with minimal interference in life activities.

▶ Assessment

Clinical Manifestations. Before surgery, the circulatory status of the extremity must be assessed through physical assessment (color, temperature, palpable pulses, responses to positioning) and arteriography. A Doppler (a hand-held ultrasonographic instrument) may be used to evaluate arterial blood flow. The circulatory status of the sound extremity is assessed also. If infection or gangrene exists, the infection is cultured and efforts are directed toward controlling it. The patient's nutritional status is evaluated, and a plan for nutritional care is made when necessary. If the patient has concomitant health problems (dehydration, anemia, cardiac insufficiency, diabetes mellitus), these are treated so that the patient is in the best possible condition to withstand the trauma of surgery.

The patient's psychological status will directly affect his response to amputation and rehabilitation. The victim of traumatic amputation is frequently a young male who has lost the extremity in a vehicular or other accident. These patients need time to work through their feelings about their permanent loss. Their reactions are unpredictable and can range from open, bitter hostility to euphoria. Therapeutic amputations for long-standing problems may relieve a patient of pain, disability, and dependency. These patients have had time to work through some feelings and come to terms with the amputation.

Patient Problems/Nursing Diagnoses

Based on the assessment data and clinical manifestations, the patient's major nursing problems include alteration in body image related to amputation; potential complications associated with amputation surgery; impaired independent life-style related to pathophysiology or amputation; and possible nonadherence to medical regimen related to lack of understanding.

▶ Planning and Implementation

Goals

The major goals for the patient include:

1. Acceptance of altered body image
2. Absence of complications associated with amputation
3. Resumption of independent life-style
4. Adherence to therapeutic regimen

Psychological Preparation. Psychological preparation should not be neglected. Knowing what to expect helps reduce anxiety. Optimism and motivation can be fostered by helping the patient realize that amputation is the first step in the patient's rehabilitation and will make it possible to carry out activities of daily living and be functionally independent.

With a traumatic amputation, there is little opportunity to prepare the patient psychologically. A realistic, supportive approach that actively includes the patient in his care and rehabilitation activities helps the patient to accept his loss.

Throughout the rehabilitation period, the patient needs to be supported as he learns to adjust to life without the extremity. The nurse needs to accept the expressed frustrations and behavior of the patient. He may be depressed and withdrawn. Active participation in self-care activities and mutual establishment of realistic goals helps promote positive feelings. Also, support and acceptance by the family help the patient in his adjustment.

Lower Extremity Amputations

Levels of Amputation. Amputations are usually performed by making soft tissue flaps, which are used to cover the bone end. The site of the amputation is determined by two factors: circulation in the part and the requirements of the prosthesis. For the most part, every attempt is made to preserve as much length as possible and to keep the knee and elbow joints intact. (Fig. 61-16 shows the different levels at which an extremity may be amputated.) Almost any level of amputation can be fitted with a prosthesis. Energy requirements and resultant cardiovascular demands for am-

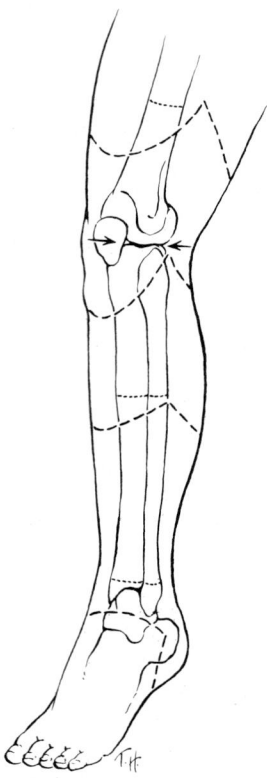

Figure 61-16. Levels of amputation are determined by circulatory adequacy, type of prosthesis, function of the part, and muscle balance.

bulation with a prosthesis increase as the amputation site moves up the leg.

Prosthesis. Some patients may be candidates for a prosthesis. If so, the physician will discuss the possibilities of obtaining and using such a device. Patients who may not qualify include those with infections, delayed healing of the residual limb (amputation stump), and peripheral vascular disease. Other conditions that may limit a patient's ability to walk with a prosthesis include diabetes mellitus, heart disease, stroke, arteriosclerosis obliterans, and advancing age.

Preoperative Physical Conditioning. If the amputation is not an emergency procedure, efforts should be made to strengthen the upper extremities as well as the trunk and the abdominal muscles. The extensor muscles in the arm and the depressor muscles in the shoulder especially need to be strengthened since these muscle groups play an important part in crutch walking. The patient may use traction weights to flex and extend the arms while holding weights. Doing push-ups while in a prone position and sit-ups while seated will strengthen the triceps muscles.

In addition to strengthening the muscles in the arms, the patient should be taught to crutch walk before the surgical procedure in order to prepare for postoperative mobility (see p. 245).

Postoperative Management. During the first 24 hours, especially in older patients, a shocklike state frequently occurs so that the patient does not fully realize that the leg has been amputated. Often the realization may come as a

shock, even though the patient knew before the operation that an amputation was to be performed. Because of the psychological trauma involved, it is important to accept the frustrations and behavior of the patient and to help him modify his self-image after the amputation; it will take time for the patient to make this adjustment.

Potential Complications. Following any surgery, the nurse is concerned with reestablishment of homeostasis and preventing problems related to anesthesia and immobility. Assessment of respiratory function and encouragement of coughing and deep breathing are appropriate. Fluids and balanced nutrition need to be encouraged. Monitoring of excretory function is needed. Repositioning to relieve pressure and general hygiene need to be included in care plans. Surgical pain is located at the incision and can be readily controlled. Amputees also experience *phantom pain* in which the patient describes pain in the part that has been amputated. These pains are real and need to be accepted by the patient and the nurse.

This feeling will eventually disappear, but while it lasts it can have a disquieting effect on the patient. The pathogenesis of phantom limb phenomena is unknown. However, *keeping the patient active* helps decrease the occurrence of phantom limb pain. Phantom limb pain may occur 2 to 3 months after amputation and is seen more frequently in above-knee amputations.

When amputations of the leg have been performed on elderly, debilitated patients, especially those with diabetes and arteriosclerosis, particular care is taken to protect the stump against external infection. Such patients frequently become incontinent of urine and feces, and not infrequently the dressing and the wound of the residual limb may become soiled. In this event, the residual limb is washed with soap and water. Plastic material secured by a wide adhesive strip about the leg above the dressing has proven to be a good method of protecting the residual limb from becoming soiled.

Amputation Dressings

Amputation may be treated with a soft compression dressing or a rigid dressing. Each type of dressing requires a different type of management.

Soft Compression Dressing Approach. The residual limb is wrapped with soft dressings immediately following surgery. The most threatening problem is massive hemorrhage due to a loosened ligature. The patient should be monitored carefully for any signs or symptoms of bleeding. The patient's vital signs need to be monitored and suction drainage observed frequently.

- Immediate postoperative bleeding may develop slowly or take the form of a massive hemorrhage resulting from a loosened ligature.
- A large tourniquet should be in plain sight at the patient's bedside so that if severe bleeding occurs, it can be applied to the residual limb to control the hemorrhage.
- Notify the surgeon promptly in the event of excessive bleeding.

According to the surgeon's preference, the residual limb may be placed in an extended position or elevated for a brief period following surgery.

If the residual limb is to be elevated, the foot of the bed should be raised.

- The residual limb should not be placed on a pillow because a flexion contraction of the hip may result. A contracture of the next joint above the amputation is a frequent complication.

On occasion, especially when the amputation has been done for infection, a guillotine-type operation may be performed without any attempt to suture the skin. In such patients, to prevent the retraction of the skin, traction may be applied and eventual healing brought about. The principles given under Nursing Care of the Patient in Traction (see p. 1402) apply here.

Rigid Dressing Approach.   Immediately following surgery, a rigid plaster dressing is applied and is equipped to attach a prosthetic extension (pylon) and an artificial foot. Following the amputation, a sterilized residual limb sock is applied to the residual limb. Felt pads are placed over pressure-sensitive areas. Starting from the distal end, the residual limb is wrapped with elastic plaster of paris bandages while firm, even pressure is maintained (Fig. 61-17). Care is taken not to constrict circulation. This rigid dressing technique is used as a means for creating a socket for immediate postoperative prosthetic fitting. It controls edema, minimizes pain on movement, and results in improved wound healing and maturation of the residual limb. It seems to be the major advance in early rehabilitation of patients. As soon as the

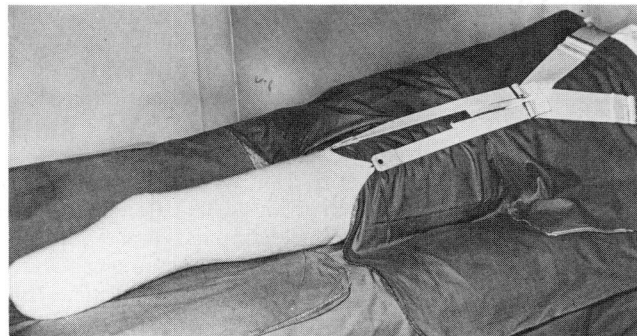

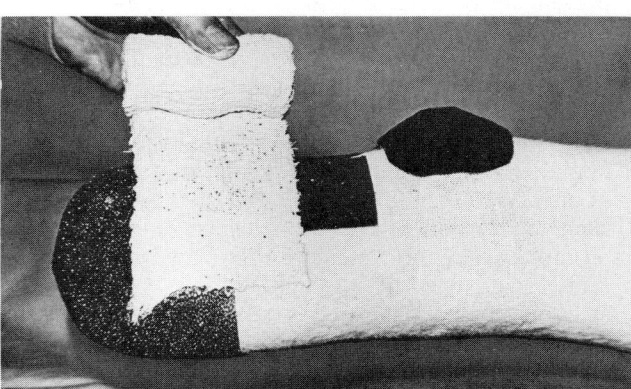

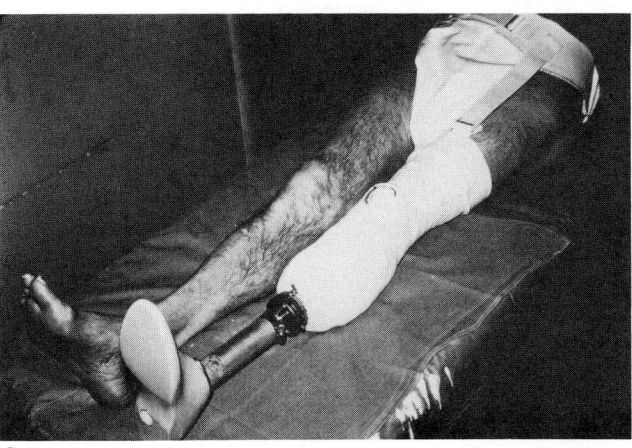

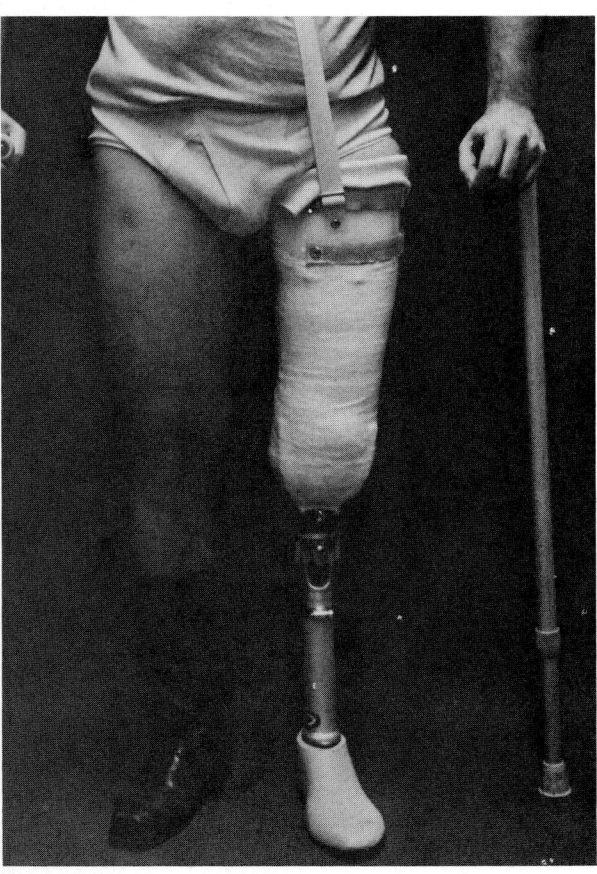

Figure 61-17. Immediate prosthetic fitting after amputation. (*A*) Sterile stocking held under firm tension as the rigid dressing is applied. (*B*) Pressure relief pads and distal polyurethane pad in place prior to application of the plaster of paris rigid dressing. (*C*) Complete assembly of components for the immediate postsurgical prosthetic fitting of the below-knee amputee. (*D*) Immediate postsurgical prosthetic fitting of the above-knee amputee. (Courtesy of the Prosthetics Research Study, Veterans Administration Contract V663P–784.)

rigid dressing has dried, the prosthetic unit, consisting of a prosthetic extension and foot, can be applied. The length of the prosthesis is tailored to the individual patient.

- *A most important consideration is that the residual limb remain in the plaster cast socket during the patient's entire hospitalization.* If the cast inadvertently comes off, the residual limb must be immediately wrapped tightly with an elastic compression bandage and the surgeon notified so that another cast can be applied. Excessive edema will develop in a very short time and will result in a delay in rehabilitation.

Any signs of complications are assessed, including increasing residual limb pain, hematoma, odor emanating from the cast, infection, and residual limb necrosis. If at any time the patient complains of severe pain, the cause is probably undue pressure on the bony prominence. This is relieved by splitting the cast or replacing it. Of course, the surgeon is notified.

Explain to the patient that he may "feel" the amputated foot for a time and that this sensation will help him direct the movement of the artificial foot while he is learning to use the prosthesis. As soon as he is ready, the patient may stand between parallel bars or be raised to an upright position on a tilt table to allow him to extend the foot to the floor with *minimal* weight bearing.

- Excessive pressure is to be avoided since it may compromise wound healing.

At this time, the prosthetist aligns the adjustable prosthetic unit. How soon after surgery the patient is allowed to "touch down" his artificial foot depends on his age and physical status and the condition of the other foot, etc. The rigid dressing is necessary, but early weight bearing is not always feasible. Patients who are debilitated or have severe diabetes or peripheral vascular disease may not be able to tolerate the degree of pressure required to "touch down" the foot and thus must wait a longer period before starting this activity.

Early minimal weight bearing produces surprisingly little pain. In fact, these patients do not complain of the severe pain and phantom limb discomfort that is experienced by patients who are treated by the more conventional method. Usually, only mild opiates are needed to relieve pain during the immediate postoperative period.

The patient usually stands between parallel bars twice daily. As his endurance increases, ambulation is started within the parallel bars, but full weight bearing is not permitted on the amputated side. Crutch walking is started when balance is achieved, but full weight bearing is not permitted until the permanent prosthesis is fitted.

The original cast may be left on for 10 to 14 days unless contraindicated by elevated body temperature, severe pain, loose-fitting cast, etc. A second cast is then applied and changed usually 10 to 14 days after the initial cast change. At this time, the patient may be measured for the definitive prosthesis. A light plaster cast or a tensor bandage is provided to limit edema during the times the patient is not wearing his permanent prosthesis.

Gait training is continued under the supervision of a physical therapist until optimal gait is achieved. Adjustments

of the prosthetic socket are made by the prosthetist to accommodate the residual limb changes that take place during the first 6 months to a year after surgery.

Rehabilitation

The complete rehabilitation of an amputee requires the concerted efforts of the entire rehabilitation team. The orthopedic surgeon, the nurse, the physiatrist, the prosthetist (limb maker), the physical therapist, and the occupational therapist all unite their efforts to condition and train the patient to make a satisfactory adjustment to the prosthesis. The establishment of prosthetic clinics has improved the outlook of amputees. With vocational counseling and job retraining where necessary, many of these patients can return to work.

Effective preprosthetic care is important to assure proper fitting of the prosthesis. The major problems that can delay the prosthetic fitting during this period are (1) flexion deformities, (2) nonshrinkage of the residual limb, and (3) abduction deformities of the hip. These deformities can be avoided.

In a lower extremity amputation, after the first 24 to 48 hours, depending on the physician's preference, the patient should be encouraged to turn from side to side and to assume a prone position to stretch the flexor muscles and to prevent flexion contracture of the hip. A pillow can be placed under the abdomen and the residual limb with the sound foot resting over the edge of the mattress. The legs should remain close together while the patient is in the prone position to prevent an abduction deformity. It is important that the patient recognize the value of moving the residual limb.

The remaining leg and foot are examined daily and protected from injury. The pressure of the bedding should be kept off the foot.

Often during convalescence, while the residual limb muscles are adjusting themselves, twitching and spasms may occur. This discomfort may be alleviated by applying heat, changing the patient's position, or placing a light sandbag on the thigh of the residual limb to counteract the psoas action.

Range of motion exercises (see pp. 232–237) are started early because contracture deformities develop rapidly. Range of motion is carried out to the hip and knee for below-the-knee amputations and to the hip for above-the-knee amputations.

If possible, an overhead trapeze can be used by the patient to change position and strengthen the biceps. However, this set of muscles is not as necessary in crutch walking as are the triceps. The triceps can be strengthened by pressing the palms against the bed while pushing the body upward (push-up exercises). Exercises, such as hyperextension of the residual limb, conducted under the supervision of the physical therapist, also aid in strengthening muscles as well as increasing circulation, reducing edema, and preventing atrophy. When the patient gets out of bed, good posture must be maintained.

The patient should be fairly adept at balancing himself on one leg and walking with crutches before he leaves the hospital. Several weeks or many months may elapse before the patient is fitted with a prosthesis.

Exercises that assist in developing balance are:

1. Arising from a chair and standing
2. Standing on toes while holding on to a chair
3. Bending the knees while holding on to a chair
4. Balancing on one leg without support
5. Hopping on one foot while holding on to a chair

The nurse may stand behind the patient and stabilize him by his waist while he is learning to perform these exercises. While crutch walking, the patient should learn to use a normal gait. The residual limb should move back and forth while the patient is walking with his crutches. The residual limb should not be held up in a flexed position to prevent a permanent flexion deformity from occurring.

Residual Limb Conditioning. After the wound has healed, the residual limb should be bandaged as indicated by the surgeon. The patient or some member of the family can be taught the correct method of bandaging.

The residual limb has to be conditioned if a prosthesis is to be fitted properly. (However, not every patient can be fitted for a prosthetic device.) The residual limb must be shrunk and shaped into a conical form to permit accurate measurement and maximum comfort and fit of the prosthetic device. This is done by applying bandages, an elastic residual limb shrinker, or an air splint. In some instances, a cast (rigid dressing) is applied soon after surgery.

Bandaging supports the soft tissue and minimizes the formation of edematous fluid while the residual limb is in a dependent position. The bandage is applied in such a manner that the remaining muscles required to operate the prosthesis are as firm as possible, while those muscles that are no longer useful will atrophy (Fig. 61-18). An improperly applied elastic bandage contributes to circulatory problems and a poorly-shaped residual limb. A guide to bandaging an amputation residual limb is found in Chart 61-4.

In order to "toughen" the residual limb in preparation for a prosthesis, activities to condition the residual limb are usually prescribed. The patient begins by pushing the residual limb into a soft pillow, then into a firmer pillow, and finally against a hard surface. The patient is taught to massage the residual limb to mobilize the scar, decrease tenderness, and improve vascularity. Massage is usually started when healing takes place and is first done by the physical therapist.

Nonambulatory Amputees. Problems most frequently encountered in rehabilitation are obesity, circulatory insufficiency, and hypertension, which increases with effort. If it is not possible for the patient to use a prosthesis, he can be taught to participate in self-care activities in a wheelchair.

A special wheelchair designed for amputees is advocated for persons who have lost one or both legs. Because of the decreased weight in the front, a regular wheelchair is in danger of tipping-backward when an amputee sits in it. In an amputee wheelchair, the rear axle is set back about 5 cm (2 inches) to compensate for this danger.

Patient Education. Careful skin hygiene is essential to prevent skin irritation, infection, and breakdown. The residual limb should be washed and dried (gently) at least twice daily. The skin needs to be inspected for pressure areas, eczema, and blisters. If present, they must be treated before a major problem develops. Usually, a residual limb sock is worn to absorb perspiration and avoid direct contact between the skin and the prosthetic socket. The residual limb sock is changed daily and must fit smoothly to avoid the irritation caused by wrinkles. The socket of the prosthesis should be washed with a mild detergent, rinsed, and dried thoroughly with a clean cloth. The patient is advised that the socket must be thoroughly dry before the prosthesis is applied.

► Evaluation

Expected Outcomes

1. Accepts altered body image
   a. Uses residual limb to facilitate movement
   b. Uses prosthesis to facilitate movement
   c. Projects self as whole person
   d. Participates in health planning
2. Experiences no complications associated with amputation
   a. Shows no signs of hemorrhage
   b. Demonstrates no signs or symptoms of infection
   c. Exhibits no signs of skin pressure area or skin breakdown
   d. Demonstrates full range of motion
   e. Uses mobility aid safely
   f. Is free of pain
3. Resumes independent life-style
   a. Participates in rehabilitation program
   b. Performs activities of daily living
   c. Recognizes abilities
   d. Seeks assistance when needed
   e. Uses community services and resources as needed
4. Adheres to therapeutic regimen
   a. Exercises according to plan
   b. Carries out residual limb care daily
   c. Reports problems with residual limb, prosthesis, or mobility aid promptly
   d. Keeps follow-up appointments with clinic and physician

Upper Extremity Amputations

The loss of an upper extremity can be a greater catastrophe than the loss of a lower extremity, because the upper limb has such a highly specialized function. The major reasons for upper extremity amputation are severe trauma (acute injury, electrical burns, frostbite), malignant tumors, infection (fulminating gas gangrene, chronic osteomyelitis), and congenital malformations.

If time permits (and it usually does *not* with acute trauma), the patient is able to find out about the available prosthetic replacement and one-handed devices that aid independence. Regardless of what assistive devices are available, psychological support is essential to help the patient adapt to changes that will be made in life-style.

The objective of surgery is to conserve as much limb length as possible, consistent with eradicating the disease process (Fig. 61-19). Following surgery, a rigid plaster dressing with provision for the application of a temporary prosthesis or a compression bandage will be applied. Usually, suction drainage is used to eliminate hematoma and achieve better approximation of tissues. At first, the residual limb may be elevated to prevent edema.

Residual limb exercises (muscle-setting and joint-mobilizing exercises) are started as soon as tolerated to

Chart 61-4
Bandaging an Above-the-Knee Amputation Residual Limb

Purpose: The purpose for bandaging a residual limb is to shrink and to shape it for the application of an artificial leg.

Problems: Improper bandaging will produce:
a. Constriction of the residual limb
b. Delayed healing
c. Skin abrasions
d. Formation of creases or adipose tissue at distal end

Basic Principles: The bandage is applied before the patient gets out of bed after periods of recumbency. The bandage should be maintained continuously and reapplied when tension is lost. Pressure should be applied under moderate tension to the entire residual limb, guarding against any tourniquetlike action at the proximal portion of the residual limb. The residual limb is kept in *hyperextension* while the bandage is applied.

Technique of Applying Bandage

1. Begin the recurrent vertical turns on the anterior surface of the residual limb just inferior to the level of the inguinal ligament (Fig. 61-18 *A*).

   Pass the bandage over the distal end of the residual limb posteriorly to the gluteal fold. The patient assists by holding the recurrents in place.

   Make two additional recurrents over the medial and the lateral aspects of the end of the residual limb.

2. Anchor the recurrents by several horizontal circular turns of the bandage (Fig. 61-18 *B*).

   When anchoring the recurrents, the circular turns begin at the lateral side and run posteriorly to the medial side.

   When the recurrents are firmly secured, bring the bandage down and around the residual limb and up again using oblique turns or a modified figure-of-8.

   Keep the pressure away, up, and out from the distal portion of the residual limb to eliminate creases. Do not use circular turns that are not oblique, since they tend to constrict circulation.

3. Start the hip spica from the anterior medial aspect of the residual limb and bring it laterally across the anterior surface of the residual limb in the inguinal region (Fig. 61-18 *C*). (The hip spica anchors the bandage and covers the tissue high in the groin and the lateral surfaces of the hip, thus eliminating the formation of bulges in this area.)

   Bring the bandage around the body on a level with the iliac crest.

4. Return around the residual limb, making a figure-of-8, and bring the bandage around the pelvis again. Finish the bandaging by making oblique turns on the residual limb.

   Anchor the bandage with safety pins at the lateral or the anterior surface of the residual limb. Fasten where bandage ends and at crossing of spica at the hip (Fig. 61-18 *D*).

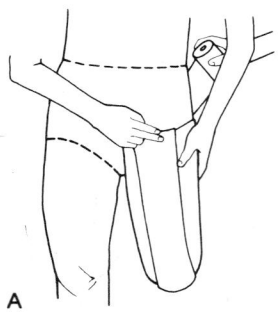 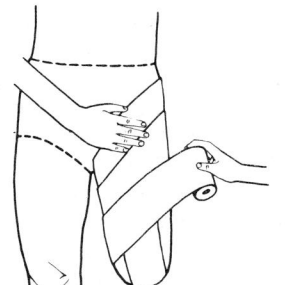 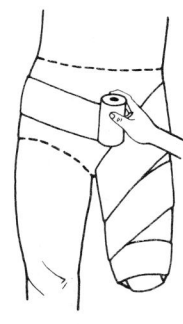 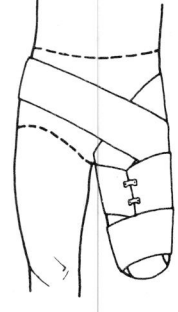

Figure 61-18. Bandaging an above-the-knee amputation residual limb (stump). In applying the elastic bandage, take care to apply it smoothly, with no folds that can produce circulatory problems and skin abrasions.

(Text adapted from Nattress LW Jr: Orthopedic and Prosthetic Appliance Journal.)

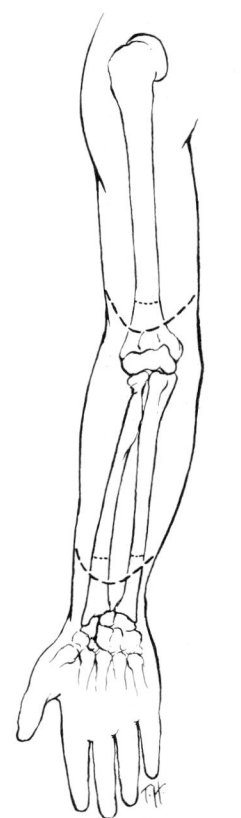

Figure 61-19. Levels of amputation of upper extremity.

strengthen the muscles and mobilize the joints. These exercises are usually done under the supervision of the physical therapist. The muscles of both shoulders are exercised since an upper-extremity amputee uses both shoulders to operate the prosthesis. A patient with an above-the-elbow amputation or shoulder disarticulation is likely to develop a postural abnormality that is caused by loss of weight of the amputated extremity. Thus, postural exercises are helpful.

Usually, the wound is inspected and sutures removed 7 to 10 days after surgery. If the patient is being treated with the rigid dressing, a new plaster socket with a temporary prosthetic device is applied. This type of management enables the patient to practice with the prosthesis and be fitted for a permanent device.

If a compression dressing is used, the residual limb is rewrapped three to four times daily to maintain proper tension in the bandage in order to reduce the edema and shape the residual limb so that a prosthesis may be eventually fitted. The residual limb is kept securely wrapped throughout the 24-hour period except for periods of bathing and exercise.

The fitting of the prosthesis depends on the level of the amputation, the patient's age, and whether or not the joints proximal to the amputation site are weak or have limited range of motion.

Patient Education.   The patient is instructed how to carry out the activities of daily living with one arm. An over-

the-bed trapeze helps in transferring out of bed. The patient is started on one-handed self-care activities as soon as possible. The occupational therapist teaches self-feeding, bathing, grooming, etc.

An upper extremity amputee may wear a cotton T-shirt to prevent contact between the skin and shoulder harness and to promote absorption of perspiration. The prosthetist will advise about cleaning the washable portions of the harness. Periodically, the prosthesis needs to be checked for potential problems.

Complications.   Complications of an upper extremity amputation include the formation of a neuroma (a sensitive tumor of nerve cells growing at the end of severed nerves) and skin problems. Skin problems occur from contact dermatitis that results from irritants in the prosthetic components and from lack of ventilation and poor skin hygiene. Residual limb contracture or residual limb contour problems may develop. Infection, necrosis of the skin edges, and phantom sensations (feeling that the arm is still present) are other complications. Psychological problems (denial, withdrawal) may be influenced by the type of support the patient receives from the rehabilitation team and by how quickly one-handed activities are taught and learned. Knowing the full options and capabilities available in the various prosthetic devices can give the patient a sense of control over the disability. The patient is not fully rehabilitated until he has been fitted with a prosthesis and has learned how to use it. Training of this nature is best accomplished in a specialized rehabilitation unit or center.

▷ Bibliography
Books

Brooker A and Edwards C. External Fixation: The Current State of the Art. Baltimore, Williams & Wilkins, 1979.

Connolly J. DePalma's The Management of Fractures and Dislocations: An Atlas, 3rd ed. Philadelphia, WB Saunders, 1981.

Donahoo C and Spickler L (eds). Core Curriculum of Orthopedic Nursing. Atlanta, Orthopedic Nurses' Association, 1980.

Edmonson A and Crenshaw H (eds). Campbell's Operative Orthopaedics, 6th ed. St Louis, CV Mosby, 1980.

Farrell J. Illustrated Guide to Orthopedic Nursing, 2nd ed. Philadelphia, JB Lippincott, 1982.

Gartland J. Fundamentals of Orthopedics, 3rd ed. Philadelphia, WB Saunders, 1979.

Heppenstall R (ed). Fracture Treatment and Healing. Philadelphia, WB Saunders, 1980.

Hilt N and Cogburn S. Manual of Orthopedics. St Louis, CV Mosby, 1981.

Kerr A. Orthopedic Nursing Procedures, 3rd ed. New York, Springer, 1980.

Mercier L and Pettid F. Practical Orthopedics. Chicago, Year Book Medical Publishers, 1980.

Mourad L. Nursing Care of Adults with Orthopedic Conditions. New York, John Wiley & Sons, 1980.

Powell M. Orthopaedic Nursing and Rehabilitation, 8th ed. New York, Churchill Livingstone, 1982.

Roaf R and Hodkinson L. Textbook of Orthopaedic Nursing, 3rd ed. Oxford, Blackwell Scientific, 1980.

Troup I and Wood M. Total Care of the Lower Limb Amputee. London, Pittman, 1982.

Turek S. Orthopaedics: Principles and Their Application, 4th ed. Philadelphia, JB Lippincott, 1984.

Uhthoff H and Stahl E (eds). Current Concepts of Internal Fixation of Fractures. New York, Springer–Verlag, 1980.

Articles
Fractures

Bassett C et al. Pulsing electromagnetic field treatment in ununited fractures and failed arthrodesis. JAMA 1982 Feb 5; 247(5):623–628.

Borschneck A et al. Sager emergency traction splint: A new splinting device for lower limb fractures. EMT J 1980 Mar; 4(3):42–43.

Brown S. Avoiding postop pitfalls with hip fracture patients. RN 1982 May; 45(5):49–53.

Buckwalter K et al. Pain assessment and management in the patient with a fracture. J Nurs Care 1981 July; 14(7):17–20.

Byrd H et al. The management of open tibial fractures with associated soft-tissue loss: External pin fixation with early flap coverage. Plast Reconstr Surg 1981 July; 68(1):73–82.

Campbell D and Kempson G. Which external fixation device? Injury 1981 Jan; 12(4):291–296.

Compere C (ed). Electromagnetic field and bones. JAMA 1982 Feb 5; 247(5):669.

Crossland S and Deyerle W. Compartmental syndrome. Nursing '80 1980 Nov; 10(11):51–53.

Crow I. Fractures of the hip: A self study. ONA J 1978 Aug; 5(8):12–30.

Dorr L. Treatment of hip fractures in elderly and senile patients. Orthop Clin North Am 1981 Jan; 12(1):153–163.

Duerksen J. Hip fractures: Special considerations for the elderly patient. Orthop Nurs 1982 Jan/Feb; 1(1):11–19.

Dunhery E. Fractured hip: How to position and mobilize patient—without undoing their surgery. RN 1979 June; 42(6):44–57.

Edwards C et al. Management of compound tibial fractures using external fixation. Am Surg 1979 Mar; 45(3):190–203.

Enneking W et al. Autogenous cortical bone grafts in the reconstruction of segmental skeletal defects. J Bone Joint Surg [Am] 1980 July; 62-A(7):1039–1058.

Grossling H and Donohue T. The fat embolism syndrome. JAMA 1979 June 22; 241(25):2740–2742.

Hay B et al. External fixation: Option for fractures. AORN J 1981 Sept; 34(3):417–423.

Hay B et al. A teaching plan for external fixation. AORN J 1981 Sept; 34(3):424–426.

Heilem F. Epidemiology of hip fracture. A review with implications for the physical therapist. Phys Ther 1979 Oct; 59(10):1221–1225.

Jacobs R et al. Internal fixation of intertrochanteric hip fractures: A clinical and biomechanical study. Clin Orthop 1980 Jan–Feb; 146:62–70.

Jewsbury C et al. The hinged long arm cast brace: An alternative to long arm casts. ONA J 1979 July; 6(7):275–280.

Keller C and Laros G. Indications for open reduction of femoral neck fractures. Clin Orthop 1980 Oct; 152:131–137.

Korcok M. Motion, not immobility, advocated for healing synovial joints. JAMA 1981 Nov 6; 246(18):2005–2006.

Kryschyshen P and Fischer D. External fixation for complicated fractures. Am J Nurs 1980 Feb; 80(2):256–259.

Kuska B. Acute onset of compartment syndrome. JEN 1982 Mar/Apr; 8(2):75–79.

Lamb K. Effects of positioning of postoperative fractured-hip patients as related to comfort. Nurs Res 1979 Sep–Oct; 28(5):291–294.

Lawyer R and Lubbers L. Use of Hoffman apparatus in the treatment of unstable tibial fractures. J Bone Joint Surg [Am] 1980 Dec; 62-A(8):1264–1273.

Lentz M. Selected aspects of deconditioning secondary to immobilization. Nurs Clin North Am 1981 Dec; 16(4):729–737.

Lupien A. Head off compartment syndrome before it's too late. RN 1980 Dec; 43(12):38–41, 114.

Mears D and Fu F. Modern concepts of external skeletal fixation of the pelvis. Clin Orthop 1980 Sept; 151:65–72.

Mender J et al. Open fractures of the tibia. Clin Orthop 1981 May; 156:98–104.

Meredith S. Formidable: That's the only word for the external fixation device—and for the care it demands. RN 1979 Dec; 42(12):19–24.

Metcalf R (ed). Symposium on arthroscopic knee surgery. Orthop Clin North Am 1982 Apr; 13(2):entire issue.

Miller L. Orthopedic patients in an ambulatory facility. Nurs Clin North Am 1981 Dec; 16(4):749–758.

Morris G. Prevention of venous thromboembolism. A survey of methods used by orthopedic and general surgeons. Lancet 1980 Sept 13; 2(8194):572–574.

Ross N. Volkmann's ischaemic contracture: A complication following elbow injuries. ONA J 1979 May; 6(5):211–215.

Schöntag H et al. External fixation as an alternative when treating 2nd and 3rd degree open lower leg fractures. Arch Orthop Trauma Surg 1980 Jan; 97(1):13–16.

Spiegel P (ed). Symposium on problems and solutions in the management of fractures. Orthop Clin North Am 1980 July; 11(3):379–679.

Taylor A. External fixation of fractures: A simple method. Injury 1980 Nov; 12(3):213–218.

Uhthoff H. Current concepts of internal fixation of fractures. Can J Surg 1980 May; 23(3):213–214.

Wassel A. Nursing assessment of injuries to the lower extremity. Nurs Clin North Am 1981 Dec; 16(4):739–748.

Williams M et al. Nursing activities and acute confusional states in elderly hip-fractured patients. Nurs Res 1979 Jan–Feb; 28(1):25–35.

Yen P. Fractures and diet—what's the relationship? Geriatr Nurs 1981 Sept/Oct; 2(5):327–328.

Amputations

Beasley R (ed). Symposium on management of upper limb amputations. Orthop Clin North Am 1981 Oct; 12(4):entire issue.

Coleman A. Rehabilitation of the elderly amputee: A review of the literature. ONA J 1979 July; 6(7):281–285.

Curry K et al. Construction of a customized pylon: Simple, quick, and functional . . . allowing trial weight bearing. Phys Ther 1981 July; 61(7):71–72.

Dealing with emergency amputations. Nursing '80 1980 Apr; 10(4):82–83.

Lee B et al. Noninvasive hemodynamic evaluation of amputation level. Surg Gynecol Obstet 1979 Aug; 149(2):241–244.

Malone J. Rehabilitation for lower extremity amputation. Arch Surg 1981 Jan; 116(1):93–98.

Meador R. Learning to live with a new leg. Am J Nurs 1979 Aug; 79(8):1393–1395.

Moore W et al. Prospective use of xenon Xe 133 clearance for amputation level selection. Arch Surg 1981 Jan; 116(1):86–88.

Porter J et al. Lower-extremity amputations for ischemia. Arch Surg 1981 Jan; 116(1):89–92.

Smith A. Common problems of lower extremity amputees. Orthop Clin North Am 1982 July; 13(3):569–578.

Towne N and Condon R. Lower extremity amputations for ischemic disease. Adv Surg 1979; 13:199–227.

Tripses D and Pollak E. Risk factors in healing of below knee amputations. Appraisal of 64 amputations in patients with vascular disease. Am J Surg 1981 June; 141(6):718–720.

Walters J. Coping with a leg amputation. Am J Nurs 1981 July; 81(7):1349–1352.

Wu Y et al. An innovative removable rigid dressing technique for below-the-knee amputation. J Bone Joint Surg [Am] 1979 July; 61-A(5):724–729.

62

Management of Patients With Musculoskeletal Disorders

▷ Low Back Pain

Back pain is a major health problem. An estimated 80% of the population will experience low back pain sometime during their lifetime. Impairments of the back and spine are the third leading cause of disability of people in their employment years. The limitations imposed by low back pain on the individual are severe. The economic cost, in terms of loss of productivity is in the billions of dollars. The number of medical visits resulting from low back pain is second only to upper respiratory illnesses.

Low back pain may be caused by a large variety of conditions. Most low back pain is caused by musculoskeletal problems (*e.g.,* acute lumbosacral strain, unstable lumbosacral ligaments and weak muscles, osteoarthritis of the spine, spinal stenosis, intervertebral disc problems, inequality of leg length). Other causes include kidney disorders, pelvic problems, retroperitoneal tumors, abdominal aneurysms, and psychosomatic problems. Most back pain due to musculoskeletal disturbances is aggravated by activity, whereas pain due to other considerations is not influenced by activity.

Persons with chronic low back pain are frequently obese. They may have problems dealing with stress and exhibit depressed, dependent personalities. Patients with chronic low back pain may develop a dependence on alcohol or analgesics.

Pathophysiology. The spinal column can be considered as an elastic rod constructed of rigid units (vertebrae) and flexible units (intervertebral discs) that are held together by complex facet joints, multiple ligaments, and paravertebral muscles. The unique construction of the back allows for flexibility while providing maximum protection for the spinal cord. The spinal curves absorb vertical shocks from running and jumping. The trunk helps to stabilize the spine. The abdominal and thoracic muscles are important in lifting activities. Disuse weakens these supporting structures. Obesity, postural problems, structural problems, or overstretching of the spinal supports may result in back pain.

The intervertebral discs change in character as the person ages. In the young, the disc is mainly fibrocartilage with a gelatinous matrix. It becomes dense, irregular fibrocartilage in the elderly. Disc degeneration is the most common cause of back pain. Discs L4–5 and L5–S1 are subjected to the greatest mechanical stress and the greatest degenerative changes. Disc protrusion (herniated nucleus pulposa) or facet joint changes can cause pressure on nerve roots that leave the spinal canal and therefore result in radiation nerve pain. About 12% of the people with low back pain have herniated nucleus pulposa. (Management of intervertebral disc disease is discussed on p. 1374.)

▶ Assessment

Clinical Manifestations.   The patient history reveals a complaint of either acute pain (present less than 3 days) or chronic back pain and fatigue. During the initial interview, the location of the pain and whether it radiates along a nerve root (sciatica) needs to be assessed. If the pain is of musculoskeletal origin, the patient will indicate that movement accentuates the pain.

Physical examination may reveal paravertebral muscle spasm (greatly increased muscle tone of the back postural muscles). There is a loss of the normal lumbar lordotic curve and possible spinal deformity. When the patient is examined in a prone position, these muscles relax and any deformity caused by the spasm disappears. The patient's gait, spinal mobility, reflexes, leg length, motor strength, sensory ability, and leg movement (*i.e.,* straight leg raises) are evaluated.

If the patient has some radiculopathy (nerve root problem) or chronic back pain, additional studies may be conducted.

Diagnostic Evaluation.   An x-ray of the spine demonstrates the presence of a fracture, a dislocation, an infection, osteoarthritis, or scoliosis. An electromyogram (EMG) and nerve conduction studies are used to evaluate radiculopathies. A myelogram can indicate disc protrusions and nerve root compression, which could cause the pain. In situations that are difficult to diagnose, a discogram (a small amount of contrast medium is injected into the intervertebral disc) may be used to demonstrate degenerative or ruptured disc. Computed tomography is being used more frequently to identify precisely the underlying problem. Occult soft tissue lesions adjacent to the vertebral column and precise disc problems can be identified with current tomography techniques. Ultrasound may be used to help diagnose narrow spinal canals. Epidural venograms are available to help assess lumbar disc disease as evidenced by displacement of epidural veins.

At times, an organic basis for the back pain cannot be identified. The pain becomes chronic (lasting more than 2 months without improvement) and may be due to a reaction to continuing emotional stresses or secondary gains associated with being incapacitated (*e.g.,* workman's compensation, relaxing role change). Working with these patients is a challenge because major readjustments are coupled with the cure.

Patient Problems/Nursing Diagnoses

Based on the clinical manifestations and diagnostic assessment data, the patient's major nursing problems include pain related to low back pathophysiology and strain on the lumbosacral spine; decreased mobility and flexibility related to muscle spasm or other musculoskeletal alteration; weak back and trunk muscles related to disuse or application of excessive stress; poor posture and body mechanics related to habit; possible obesity related to a caloric intake that is greater than energy expenditure; and a possible nonproductive life-style related to secondary rewards of low back problems.

▶ Planning and Implementation
(See also Chart 62-1.)

Goals

The primary goal of the patient with low back pain is to obtain pain relief. The nurse is able to assist the patient to achieve comfort through physical measures, such as bed rest, thermal modalities, and massage; by administering prescribed medications, such as analgesics, anti-inflammatory agents, and muscle relaxants; and by instructing the patient about exercise activities, body posture, and body mechanics.

Physical Measures.   Since most back pain improves with bed rest and inactivity, the patient is confined to bed on a firm, nonsagging mattress. Acute muscle spasms subside in 3 to 7 days. The best position is a modified supine position with slight lumbar flexion (elevate the head of the bed 30 degrees and have the knees slightly flexed) (Fig. 62-1) or a lateral position with knees and hips flexed. A prone position is avoided because it accentuates lordosis. Bathroom privileges may be allowed, but all other out of bed activities (*e.g.,* answering the phone, checking on the children, general activity due to restlessness) are to be avoided.

Frequently, the patient is unable to comply with a bed rest regimen at home. He is hospitalized for "active conservative management." Pelvic traction with 15 to 30 pounds of weight is prescribed. Traction promotes additional lumbar flexion (Fig. 62-2). The patient feels something is being done to alleviate his back pain and he becomes an active participant in his care by managing the traction. Bed rest with slight lumbar flexion is encouraged. Bed rest does have the associated side-effects of muscle disuse atrophy and circulatory decompensation for which the nurse needs to be alert when patient mobilization is begun.

Physical therapies may be utilized to decrease pain and muscle spasm. Forms of therapy used are thermal modalities (therapeutic cold; infrared radiant heat; hot, moist packs; ultrasound; diathermy; whirlpool). If the patient has had previous episodes of back pain, the history of treatment that was successful previously is valuable for selecting the treatment modality. Each treatment mode is matched with the patient. For example, patients with high blood pressure or rheumatoid arthritis may not tolerate "icing" techniques. Patients with impaired circulation, diminished sensation, and trauma may not be good candidates for hot packs. Whirlpool requires movement of the patient that he may not be

Chart 62-1
Guidelines of Nursing Implementation for the Patient With Low Back Pain

Major Patient Goals

1. Comfort
2. Increased mobility and flexibility
3. Strengthening of weak back and trunk muscles
4. Improvement in posture and use of good body mechanics
5. Ideal weight
6. Resumption of full, productive life-style

Major Patient Problems	Nursing Interventions	Expected Outcomes
1. Pain related to low back pathophysiology or strain on lumbar–sacral spine	Encourage patient to describe the type and location of pain.	Describes the pain
	Encourage bed rest.	Complies with bed rest regimen
	Position patient to minimize lordosis.	
	Encourage use of pelvic traction in Williams position (head of bed elevated 30 to 45 degrees and knees flexed).	Uses pelvic traction, if prescribed and achieves pain relief
	Use physical modalities to assist relief of pain:	Obtains reduction in discomfort through use of physical, pharmaceutical, and psychological measures
	Positioning	
	Limit activities	
	Massage	
	Thermal therapies	
	Use pharmaceuticals according to prescription and patient need:	
	Analgesics	
	Muscle relaxants	
	Anti-inflammatory agents	
	Tranquilizers	
	Use psychological measures to reduce stress.	
	Evaluate patient response to pain reduction modality.	
	Assure patient that discomfort will decrease as muscles relax.	Achieves comfort
2. Decreased mobility and flexibility related to muscle spasm and other musculoskeletal alteration	Plan activity resumption with patient.	Resumes activities gradually
	Limit activities in accordance with return of discomfort.	
	Evaluate resumption of activities according to plan.	Complies with graded activity regimen
	Achieve full mobility and spinal flexibility.	Continues progressive return to full mobility and flexibility
3. Weak back and trunk muscles due to disuse or application of excessive stress	Review general physiology and biophysics of back and trunk muscles.	Verbalizes existence of weakened musculature
	Explain purpose of progressive exercise.	Participates in graded exercise program
	Encourage adherence to exercise regimen.	
	Review current exercise program.	Recognizes the need for long-term exercise
	Evaluate muscle strength and tone.	Has strengthened back and trunk muscles
		Resumes full, productive life-style

(continued)

Chart 62-1
Guidelines of Nursing Implementation for the Patient With Low Back Pain (continued)

Major Patient Problems (continued)	Nursing Interventions (continued)	Expected Outcomes (continued)
4. Poor posture and body mechanics related to habit	Assist patient in analyzing posture and body mechanics. Educate patient as to defensive and protective body mechanics. Teach patient effects of good posture and body mechanics on back health. Involve patient in the development of plan for improvement of posture. Encourage incorporation of good posture and body mechanics into activities of daily living	Compares current posture and body mechanics with that desired Develops plan for improving posture Develops improved body positioning Demonstrates use of good body mechanics
5. Possible obesity related to caloric intake greater than energy expenditure	Explain relationship between excessive weight and back pain. Encourage development of plan to reduce body weight. Monitor patient's compliance and achievement. Praise accomplishment.	Identifies need to lose weight Participates in development of weight-reduction plan Sets realistic goals Complies with weight-reduction regimen Achieves desired weight
6. Possible nonproductive lifestyle related to secondary rewards of low back problems	Encourage resumption of full, productive lifestyle and employment as soon as medically possible. Refer for employment and psychological counseling as appropriate.	Resumes occupation as problem resolves Identifies factors that retard return to full activity Seeks alternate occupation, if necessary

able to manage because it may stress his cardiovascular system due to massive peripheral vasodilatation. Ultrasound produces deep heat, which may increase discomfort due to swelling in the acute stages; therefore, it is contraindicated if the patient has cancer or bleeding disorders. Gentle soft tissue massage is useful to decrease muscle spasm and to increase circulation to the tissues.

Drug Therapy. Acute pain may need to be treated with medications. Narcotic analgesics may be required initially to interrupt the muscle spasm pain cycle and to decrease paraspinal muscle spasm. Anti-inflammatory agents may be used if an associated inflammatory response has occurred.

If the patient exhibits nerve root irritation, short-term corticosteroids may be used to decrease the inflammatory response of the nerves and to prevent the development of neurofibrosis, which results from ischemic changes. Epidural steroid injections may be used for pain relief as well as for diagnostic purposes. Muscle relaxants and tranquilizers will relax the patient and muscles in spasm, thereby providing pain relief. Infiltration of paraspinal muscles with local anesthetics may result in relaxation and pain relief.

Transcutaneous electrical nerve stimulation (TENS) is a portable, noninvasive pain-reduction device that allows the patient to participate in activities comfortably without

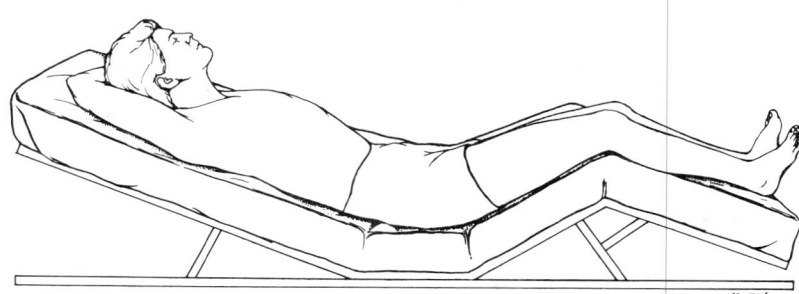

Figure 62-1. Positioning to provide lumbar flexion.

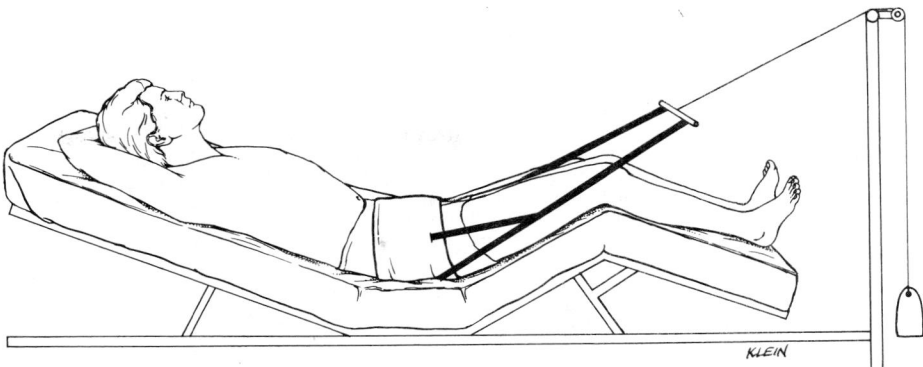

Figure 62-2. Pelvic traction with lumbar flexion to alleviate low back pain.

medication. The unit is thought to afford pain relief through overriding pain input (Gate theory of pain control) and stimulation of endorphins. Since TENS is a relatively new pain relief modality, persons working with the patient need to understand the device and accept its pain relief potential. Electrodes are attached to areas of the body where the patient is able to achieve maximum pain relief. The patient adjusts the stimulator's wave length and intensity to achieve comfort (see also p. 1319). Patients who use cardiac pacemakers should not use TENS. Those who operate machinery need to be aware of the potential for accidental shocks. Generally, the patient uses the device for 1 to 2 months and gradually decreases its use as his pain subsides and his back strengthens through graduated exercises.

Exercise Program. As the patient achieves comfort at rest, activities can be gradually resumed and an exercise program initiated. *The goal is to increase mobility, muscle strength, and flexibility.* Exercises must be done slowly, and the patient begins with relaxation exercises. The goal of many of the exercises is to minimize lumbar lordosis. The exercise program is carried out under the direction of the physical therapist and is adapted to the individual patient. The nurse needs to encourage patient adherence. Erratic exercising is ineffective. For most exercise programs, it is suggested that the person exercise twice a day increasing the number of exercises gradually. Figure 62-3 demonstrates suggested back exercises that increase the strength and flexibility of the back and abdominal muscles. After months of exercises, the patient may become bored with the routine exercises. Recreational activities that the patient enjoys can be allowed. These activities should not cause excessive lumbar strain, twisting, or discomfort. They may be gradually increased as tolerated. Horseback riding and weight lifting should be avoided.

Body Mechanics and Posture. The nurse assesses how the patient moves and stands, and engages in patient teaching as needed. It takes about 6 months for a person to readjust his postural habits. However, good body mechanics and posture are essential to avoid recurrence of back pain. Providing the patient with a list of suggestions will help in making these long-term changes. If the patient wears high heels, low heels are suggested. When sitting, the knees should be level with the hips or higher to minimize lordosis. The feet should be on the floor. If long periods of standing are required, the patient should shift his weight frequently and should rest one foot on a low stool, which decreases lumbar lordosis. He can check his posture by looking in a mirror to see if his chest is up and his stomach is tucked in. Locking the knees when standing is to be avoided. Be sure the patient knows the correct way to lift objects—using the strong quadriceps muscles of the thighs and minimal use of weak back muscles. He should sleep on his side with his knees and hips flexed, or supine with his knees supported in a flexed position. Sleeping prone is to be avoided.

Practicing these protective and defensive postures, positions, and body mechanics results in natural strengthening of the back and diminishes the chance of a recurrence of back pain.

Patient Education

Standing, sitting, lying, and lifting properly are necessary for a healthy back:

Standing
- Avoid prolonged standing and walking.
- When standing for any length of time, rest one foot on a small stool or box to relieve lumbar lordosis.

Sitting
Stress on the back may be greater in the sitting position than in the standing position.

- Avoid sitting for prolonged periods.
- Sit in a straight-back, fairly high-seated chair. Sit with the knees higher than the hips. Use a foot stool.
- Eradicate the hollow of the back by sitting with the buttocks "tucked under."
- Avoid knee and hip extension. When driving a car, have the seat pushed forward as far as possible for comfort. Place a cushion in the small of the back for support.
- Guard against extension strains—reaching, pushing, sitting with legs straight out.
- Alternate periods of sitting with walking.

Lying
- Rest at intervals, as fatigue contributes to spasm of the back muscle.
- Place a firm bedboard under the mattress.
- Avoid sleeping in a prone position.
- When lying on the side, place a pillow under the head and one between the legs, which should be flexed at the hips and knees.

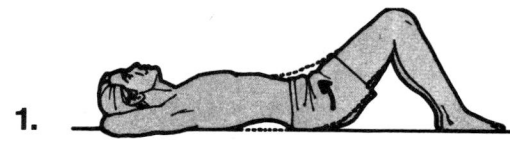

1.

Lie on your back with knees bent and hands clasped behind neck. Feet flat on the floor. Take a deep breath and relax. Press the small of your back against the floor and tighten your stomach and buttock muscles. This should cause the lower end of the pelvis to rotate forward and flatten your back against the floor. Hold for five seconds. Relax.

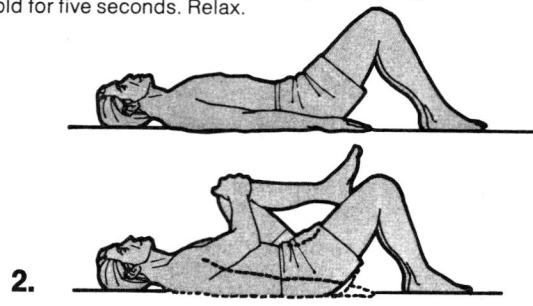

2.

Lie on your back with knees bent. Feet flat on the floor. Take a deep breath and relax. Grasp one knee with both hands and pull as close to your chest as possible. Return to starting position. Straighten leg. Return to starting position. Repeat with alternate leg.

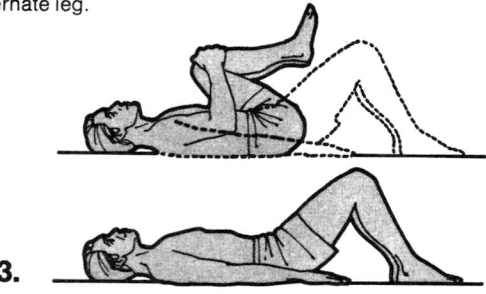

3.

Lie on your back with knees bent. Feet on the floor. Take a deep breath and relax. Grasp *both* knees and pull them as close to your chest as possible. Hold for three seconds, then return to starting position. Straighten legs and relax.

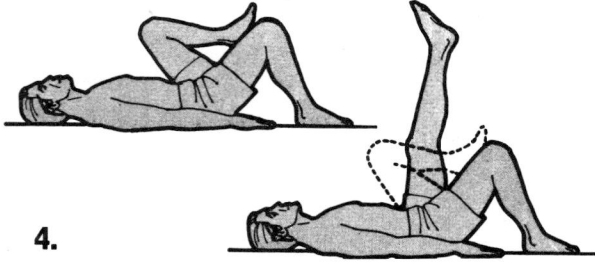

4.

Lie on your back with knees bent. Feet flat on the floor. Take a deep breath and relax. Draw one knee to chest. Then point leg upward as far as possible. Return to starting position. Relax. Repeat with alternate leg.

NOTE: This exercise is useful in stretching tight hamstring muscles, but is not recommended for patients with sciatic pain associated with a herniated disc.

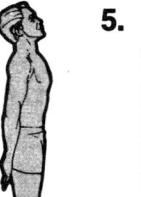

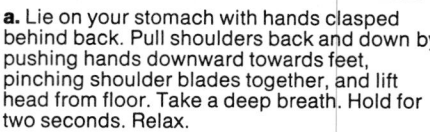

5.

a. Lie on your stomach with hands clasped behind back. Pull shoulders back and down by pushing hands downward towards feet, pinching shoulder blades together, and lift head from floor. Take a deep breath. Hold for two seconds. Relax.

b. Stand erect. With one hand grasp the thumb of other hand behind the back, then pull downwards toward the floor; stand on toes and look at the ceiling while exerting the downward pull. Hold momentarily, then relax. Repeat 10 times at intervals of two hours during the working day. Take an exercise break instead of a coffee break!

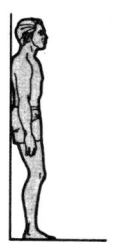
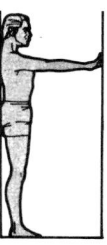

6. Stand with your back against doorway. Place heels four inches away from frame. Take a deep breath and relax. Press the small of your back against doorway. Tighten your stomach and buttock muscles, allowing your knees to bend slightly. This should cause the lower end of the pelvis to rotate forward (as in Exercise 1). Press your neck up against doorway. Press both hands against opposite side of doorway and straighten both knees. Hold for two seconds. Relax.

The following exercises (7, 8, 9) should not be started until you are free of pain and the other exercises have been done for several weeks.

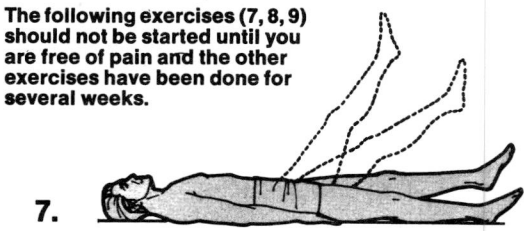

7.

Lie on your back with your legs straight out, knees unbent and arms at your sides. Take a deep breath and relax. Raise legs one at a time as high as is comfortable and lower to floor as slowly as possible. Repeat five times for each leg.

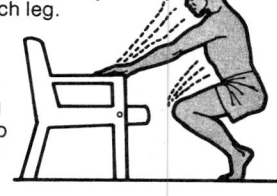

8.

May be done holding onto a chair or table. After squatting, flex head forward, bounce up and down two or three times, then assume erect position.

9.

Lie on your back with knees bent. Feet flat on floor. Take a deep breath and relax. Pull up to a sitting position keeping knees bent. Return to starting position. Relax. Having someone hold your feet down facilitates this exercise.

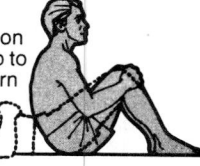

A SERVICE OF RIKER LABORATORIES, INC.   91578 PRINTED IN U.S.A. DECEMBER 1973

Figure 62-3. Back exercises. These exercises have been provided courtesy of Riker Laboratories, Inc. and Everett J. Gordon, M.D., Clinical Associate Professor, Orthopedic Surgery, Georgetown University.

Lifting

- When lifting, keep the back straight and hold the load as close to the body as possible. Lift with the legs, not the back.

- Avoid trunk twisting, lifting above waist level, and reaching up for any length of time.
- Squat down while keeping the back straight when it is necessary to pick something off the floor.

Exercise
- *Daily exercise is important in the prevention of back problems.*
- Walking outdoors with progression in distance and pace is recommended.
- Do prescribed back exercises twice daily.

Additional Therapies.   At times, a patient with low back pain will need to undertake a weight-reduction program. Decreasing the body weight will decrease the stresses on the low back. Incorporating weight reduction into the overall supervised plan is important.

Low back supports and braces may be prescribed to limit spinal motion, to correct posture, and to diminish stress on the lower lumbar spine. (People with jobs that require heavy lifting may wear heavy leather belts [trochanter belts] to decrease the strain on their backs.) When these devices are prescribed, the plan should be geared toward discontinuing these appliances, since they may have the negative effects of promoting disuse muscle atrophy and weakness and decreased muscle elasticity, which in themselves cause low back pain. An individual exercise program is essential so that eventually the needed support can be supplied by the muscles.

Psychological Considerations.   Sometimes low back pain can be a psychosomatic illness or a reaction to environmental and life stresses. Emotional problems resulting from anxiety and stress can evoke muscle spasm, which produces a cycle of anxiety, tension, more spasm, and pain. In some persons, mental conflicts are manifested in physical symptoms. There are psychological components in all illnesses, and chronic pain has an emotional impact. In trying to help the patient, one needs insight into family relationships, environmental variables, and work problems. If the back problem stems from a recent accident, the possibility of pending litigation may be a factor. Psychiatric intervention may be necessary for the patient with chronic depression and low back syndrome.

If the patient has a prolonged recovery and has developed secondary gains associated with the low back disability (*e.g.,* workman's compensation, easier life-style or work load, increased emotional support), a "low back neurosis" may develop. Psychotherapy or counseling may be needed to assist the person in resuming a full, productive life. There are pain centers throughout the country that offer help by teaching the patient the significance of pain and the skills and techniques of coping with it (see p. 293).

▷ # Common Problems of the Upper Extremity

Painful Shoulder Syndrome.   The structures in and about the shoulder are frequently the sites of painful syndromes. With aging, degenerative alterations occur in all joints, including the articulations comprising the shoulder joint (glenohumeral, sternoclavicular, and acromioclavicular). Pain may arise from supraspinatus tendonitis or bicipital tendonitis with the inflammation spreading to the tendon sheaths, other tendons and their sheaths (tenosynovitis), the

bursa, capsule, synovium, cartilage, bone, and surrounding muscles. Frequently encountered syndromes are listed in Table 62-1.

Patient Education.   The following are teaching points to protect the shoulder from further injury:

1. Support the affected arm on pillows while sleeping to keep from rolling over on the shoulder.
2. Avoid working and lifting above the shoulder level or pushing an object against a "locked" shoulder.
3. Do prescribed daily range of motion exercises to strengthen the shoulder girdle and glenohumeral muscle.

"Tennis Elbow".   *"Tennis elbow"* is a painful condition that is due to excessive pronation and supination activities of the forearm (*e.g.,* tennis, sculling, using a screwdriver). The pain characteristically radiates down the extensor surface of the forearm. The forearm is tender. Most times, relief is obtained by resting the arm, moist heat, analgesics, and possibly local injection of a corticosteroid.

Ganglion.   A *ganglion* is a round, firm projection, usually near the wrist. It is a collection of gelatinous material near the tendon sheaths and joints. It is caused by strains, contusions, or a series of repeated minor strains, as a result of which the tissues of the sheath or sac involved have gradually become weakened and distended. As a rule, the ganglion is painless, but the affected joint often is weak and moderately painful secondary to local pressure. A ganglion may be treated by aspiration or excision. Aspiration decompression may need to be repeated since fluid may reaccumulate. Surgical excision may involve surgery to the joint capsule for full removal.

Carpal Tunnel Syndrome.   *Carpal tunnel syndrome* is an entrapment neuropathy caused by pressure from a thickened flexor tendon sheath, skeletal encroachment, or soft tissue mass on the median nerve at the wrist. The patient experiences pain, numbness, paresthesia, and possible weakness along the median nerve (thumb, first and second fingers). Night pain is common. Rest splints, avoidance of work that requires flexion of the wrist, and cortisone injections may relieve the symptoms. Surgical release of the transverse carpal ligament may be necessary.

Dupuytren's Contracture.   *Dupuytren's deformity* is a slowly progressive contracture of the palmar fascia causing flexion of the little finger, the ring finger, and frequently the middle fingers, which renders them more or less useless (Fig. 62-4).

It is a fairly common abnormality, but its cause is unknown. It starts as a thickening of the palmar fascia. The fibrous thickening extends to involve the skin in the distal palm and produces a contracture of the fingers to which the palmar fascia is inserted. This condition always starts in one hand, but eventually both become symmetrically deformed. Plastic surgery, consisting of total excision of the involved palmar fascia, offers excellent relief.

Nursing Management Following Hand/Wrist Surgery.   Following surgery on the hand or wrist, elevation of the hand is important to control swelling. Ice packs may be applied. Neurovascular checks of the exposed fingers are essential. The patient's description of sensations and his

Table 62-1
Painful Shoulder Syndromes

Syndromes	Clinical Features	Clinical Manifestations	Management
Supraspinatus tendonitis Tenosynovitis	Reaction to mechanical stress and strain plus a degenerative process with traumatic inflammation	Pain in shoulder; "catching" sensation Patient grabs affected shoulder with opposite hand Night pain; inability to lie on affected side Painful arc beyond 60-degree abduction (as tendons and cuff impinge under coracoacromial arch)	Intermittent heat/cold applications Pendulum exercises Anti-inflammatory medications—salicylates (aspirin) to tolerance Local injection of steroid or anesthetic agent into shoulder joint
Calcific tendonitis	Calcific deposits develop in tendons; causes reaction in overlying bursa Calcific tendonitis and bursitis often coexist	Occurs in younger and more active persons Abrupt onset of severe aching pain, 1 to 4 days All shoulder and arm movement is painful Acute phase followed by pain relief	Infiltration of subacromial area and aspiration of deposit Analgesics for pain Anti-inflammatory agents (aspirin, phenylbutazone, indomethacin) Applications of heat/cold Injection with local anesthetic agent and steroid Operative treatment may be necessary for excision of calcified deposits
Tears and rupture of rotator cuff	Tears occur at the insertion of rotator cuff into the bone, probably from degenerative changes	Occur most commonly after 50 Abrupt shoulder pain in deltoid area Weakness/inability to abduct shoulder "Clicking" sensation felt in shoulder on abduction/rotation	Partial rupture usually responds to conservative management Infiltration with local anesthetic to relieve pain Confirmation of defect by arthrogram Surgical repair for complete rupture
Bicipital syndromes (lesions on the long head of biceps muscle) Tendonitis Tenosynovitis	Long head of biceps affected by arm and shoulder movement	Chronic pain in anterolateral area of shoulder associated with muscle spasm and pain in trapezius, scalenus, deltoid	Rest of the extremity Gentle exercises within tolerance Salicylates Heat applications to reduce inflammation Avoid movements that put biceps tendon on stretch
Bursitis	Almost all cases of subacromial bursitis have preceding tendonitis and tenosynovitis in the rotator cuff, biceps tendon, and sheath or an inflammatory process in bone or joint; the spread of inflammation to bursa is a secondary event	Deep-seated ache in shoulder Pain upon rotation of the arm	Treatment consists of locating and treating the primary process causing the bursitis

(Adapted from Bateman JE: The Shoulder and Neck. Philadelphia, WB Saunders, 1978.)

ability to move fingers are important data to assess. Generally, the patient is ambulatory and remains hospitalized for only a brief period. Patient education concerning elevation, neurovascular checks, medications (antibiotics and analgesics), and wound care is necessary. Compliance with the medical regimen is emphasized.

▷ Common Foot Problems

Disabilities of the human foot not only develop from poorly fitting shoes but may be the result of hereditary influence. Probably the foot would cause man little pain or disability on its own account if it were not for modern civilization, which disregards the physiology of the foot. Fashion, vanity, and eye appeal, rather than function, are for the most part the determining factors in the design of footwear. The restriction of ill-fitting shoes distorts normal anatomy while inducing deformity and pain.

The discomfort of foot strain can be treated by rest, elevation, physiotherapy, supportive strappings, and orthotic devices. Foot exercises in which active motion occurs will benefit the circulation and help strengthen the feet. Walking is considered the best form of exercise.

Common Foot Ailments

A *corn* is an area of hyperkeratosis (overgrowth of a horny layer of epidermis) produced by pressure from within (the underlying bone is prominent due to congenital or acquired abnormality, commonly arthritis) or from pressure from without (shoes). The usual sites are the lesser toes, mainly the fifth toe, but all toes may be involved.

Corns are treated by soaking and scraping off the horny layer with an instrument, by applying protective shield or pads, or by surgical removal of the underlying offending osseous structure.

Soft corns are located between the toes and are kept soft by moisture and maceration. Treatment consists of drying the affected web spaces and separating the affected toes. Usually, a podiatrist will be needed to treat the underlying cause.

A *callus* is a discretely thickened area of the skin that has been exposed to persistent pressure or friction. Faulty foot mechanics usually precede the formation of a callus. Treatment consists in eliminating the underlying causes and having the callus pared by a podiatrist if it is painful. A keratolytic ointment may be applied and a thin plastic cup worn over the heel if the callus is on this area. Felt padding with adhesive backing is also used to prevent and relieve pressure. Orthotic devices can be made to remove the pressure from the bony protuberance. The protuberance may be excised.

An *ingrown toenail* (onychocryptosis) is a condition in which the free edge of a nail plate has penetrated the surrounding skin, either laterally or anteriorly. It may be accompanied by secondary infection or granulation tissue. This painful condition is caused by improper self-treatment, external pressure (tight shoes or stockings), internal pressure (deformed toes; growth under the nail), trauma, and infection. Trimming the nails properly can prevent this problem. Active treatment consists of relieving the pain by decreasing the pressure on the surrounding soft tissue by the nail plate. A toenail may have to be excised if there is severe infection. If a neoplasm or gangrene is associated with an ingrown toenail, the patient is immediately hospitalized for appropriate care.

Common Deformities of the Foot

(See Fig. 62-5.)

Flatfoot. *Flatfoot* (pes planus) is a common disorder and occurs in various forms. It is most often inherited. Exercises to strengthen the muscles and to improve posture and walking habits are helpful. A number of foot devices are available to give the foot additional support. Severe flat-

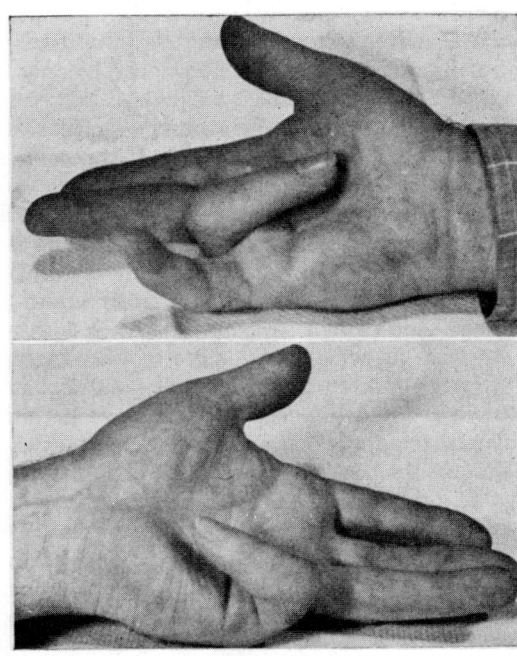

Figure 62-4. Dupuytren's contracture. (From Boyes JH: Bunnell's Surgery of the Hand, 5th ed, p 228. Philadelphia, JB Lippincott.)

foot problems are usually treated by an orthopedic surgeon or a podiatrist.

Hammer Toe. *Hammer toe* is a flexion deformity of the interphalangeal joint and may involve several toes (Fig. 62-5). The condition is usually an acquired deformity. Tight socks or shoes may push an overlying toe back into the line of the other toes. The toes usually are pulled upward, forcing the metatarsal points (ball of foot) downward. Corns develop on top of the toes, and tender calluses under the metatarsal area. The treatment consists of conservative measures: carrying out manipulative exercises, wearing open-toed sandals or shoes that conform to the shape of the foot, and protecting the protruding joints with pads. Surgical correction is necessary for an established deformity.

Hallux Valgus. *Hallux valgus* is a progressive deformity in which the great toe deviates laterally (Fig. 62-5).

Associated with this is a marked prominence of the medial aspect of the first metatarsal–phalangeal joint, with osseous enlargement of the medial side of the first metatarsal head, over which a bursa may form (secondary to pressure and inflammation). This bursa is commonly known as a *bunion.*

Treatment depends on the patient's age, the degree of deformity, and the severity of symptoms. If a bunion deformity is uncomplicated, wearing a shoe that conforms to the shape of the foot or one that is molded to the foot to prevent pressure on the protruding portions may be all the treatment that is needed. If not, surgical removal of the bunion and realignment of the toe may be required.

Postoperatively, the patient may have intense throbbing pain at the operative site, requiring rather liberal doses of analgesic medication. The operated foot is elevated above

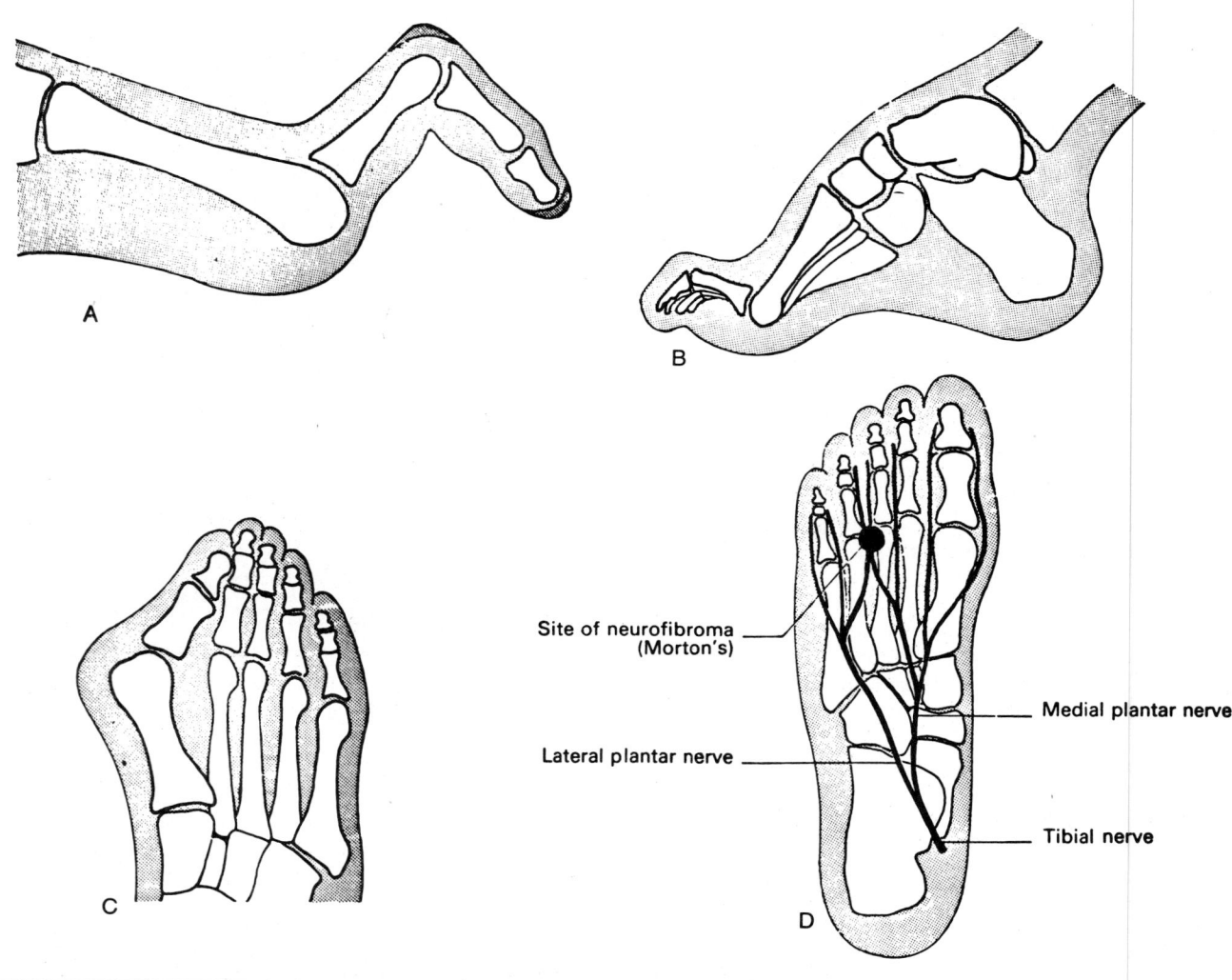

Figure 62-5. Common foot deformities. (*A*) Hammer toe. (*B*) Clawfoot (pes cavus). (*C*) Hallux valgus. (*D*) Sites for Morton's neuroma.

the level of the heart to decrease edema and pain. The great toe is watched for impaired circulation, warmth, color, ability to move the toes, numbness, and tingling. Following surgery, exercises are initiated to flex and extend the toes, since toe flexion is essential in walking. The patient should avoid wearing high heels for prolonged periods because they push the toes into dorsiflexion.

Clawfoot. *Clawfoot* (pes cavus) refers to a foot with an abnormally high arch (Fig. 62-5). This causes shortening of the foot and increased pressure that produces calluses on the metatarsal area and on the dorsum of the foot. Exercises are prescribed to stretch the toe extensors. In severe cases, osteotomies are done to reshape the feet.

Morton's Neuroma. *Morton's neuroma* (plantar neuroma, neurofibroma) is a hypertrophy of the third (lateral) branch of the medial plantar nerve (Fig. 62-5). The third digital nerve, which is located in the third intermetatarsal space, is the most common site involved. Because the fourth metatarsal is not securely anchored at its base, the head of

the metatarsal has a greater degree of motion, which becomes a chronic irritating source on the terminal portion of the third digital nerve.

The result is a throbbing, burning pain in the foot that is usually relieved when the patient rests. Pain sometimes radiates up the leg. Conservative treatment consists of inserting innersoles, metatarsal bars, and pads designed to spread the metatarsal heads and balance the foot posture. Local injections of hydrocortisone and a local anesthetic may give relief. If these fail, surgical intervention is necessary.

Other Foot Problems. Several systemic diseases affect the feet. In the case of rheumatoid arthritis, deformities result. Diabetic persons are prone to develop corns and peripheral neuropathies with diminishing sensation, leading to ulcers over pressure points of the foot. Persons with peripheral vascular disease and arteriosclerosis complain of burning and itching feet with attendant scratching and excoriations. Dermatologic problems commonly affect the feet in the form of fungal infections and plantar warts. The specifics of these problems and others can be found in the discussions of the various dysfunctions covered throughout the text.

▷ Osteoporosis

Osteoporosis is a group of disorders in which there is a reduction of total bone mass without changes in the mineral composition. There is an imbalance in the normal homeostatic bone turnover; the rate of bone resorption is greater than the rate of bone formation, resulting in a reduced total bone mass. The bones become progressively more porous, brittle, and fragile. They fracture easily under stresses that would not break normal bone. Osteoporosis frequently results in compression fractures of the thoracic and lumbar spine, fractures of the femoral neck, and intertrochanteric fractures, and Colles' fractures. Multiple compression fractures of the vertebrae result in skeletal deformity (kyphosis).

Women develop osteoporosis more frequently than men. Black women who have a greater bone mass than white women, and oriental women experience less osteoporosis. More than half of all women over 45 years have evidence of osteoporosis on roentgenogram. By the age of 80, women have lost one third to two thirds of their total bone mass. With the aging of the population, the incidence of fractures associated with osteoporosis is rising.

Causes and Pathogenesis. Involutional or age-related osteoporosis is the most common type of osteoporosis. The withdrawal of estrogens at menopause and with oophorectomy causes an increase in bone resorption that continues to weaken bones significantly for about 20 years. Men do not experience sudden hormonal changes. In addition, the peak bone mass is greater in men and black women, which contributes to their lower incidence of osteoporosis.

Endogenous and exogenous catabolic agents can cause osteoporosis. Excessive corticosteroids, Cushing's syndrome, hyperthyroidism, and hyperparathyroidism contribute to bone loss. The degree of osteoporosis is related to the length of glucocorticoid therapy. When the therapy is discontinued or the metabolic problem is corrected, the progression of osteoporosis is stopped, but restoration of lost bone mass usually does not occur.

Immobility is another common cause of osteoporosis. Bone formation is enhanced by the stress of weight and muscle activity. When immobilized by casts, paralysis, or general inactivity, the bone resorption exceeds bone formation, and osteoporosis occurs.

Nutritional factors contribute to the development of osteoporosis. Dietary calcium and vitamin D need to be adequate to maintain bone remodeling and body functions. Inadequate intake of calcium or vitamin D over a period of years results in lower bone mass and development of osteoporosis. The recommended daily intake of calcium for an adult is 800 mg. The actual estimated average daily intake is 300 mg to 500 mg. To compound the situation, the elderly woman absorbs dietary calcium less efficiently and excretes it more readily through her kidneys. The postmenopausal woman actually needs to consume about 1500 mg of calcium daily. Vitamin D is necessary for calcium absorption and for

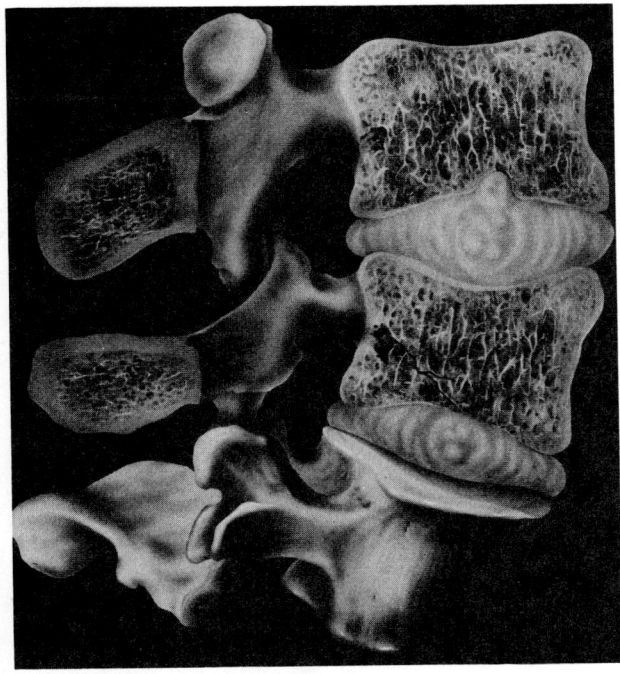

Figure 62-6. Artist's conception of progressive osteoporotic bone loss and compression fractures. (Printed with permission of Ayerst® Laboratories, New York, New York.)

normal bone mineralization. The best source of both calcium and vitamin D is fortified milk.

Other conditions that have been identified as contributing to the development of osteoporosis are cirrhosis, osteogenesis imperfecta, radiation osteonecrosis, and long-term heparin therapy. Osteoporosis is frequently associated with rheumatoid arthritis, chronic obstructive pulmonary disease, juvenile diabetes, and chronic liver disease.

The types of osteoporosis can be differentiated radiographically and biochemically.

▶ Assessment

Clinical Manifestations. The osteoporotic person is asymptomatic until a fracture occurs (Fig. 62-6). Fractures most commonly occur in the mid to lower thoracic and lumbar spine. A sudden severe pain in the low back is the result of a compression fracture of the vertebra. The fracture is usually related to some stress, such as lifting or bending. The pain may be localized or radiate to the abdomen and flanks. Tenderness is experienced over the fracture site. Back motion is painful, and spasm occurs in the paravertebral muscles. A gradual collapse of a vertebra over a period of time may be asymptomatic and be observed as progressive kyphosis.

Fractures of T10 to L2 may result in the development of a mild ileus a couple of days after fracture. It generally resolves itself without specific therapy.

With the development of kyphosis (the dowager's hump), there is an associated loss of height (Fig. 62-7). Some postmenopausal women may lose 2.5 cm to 15 cm

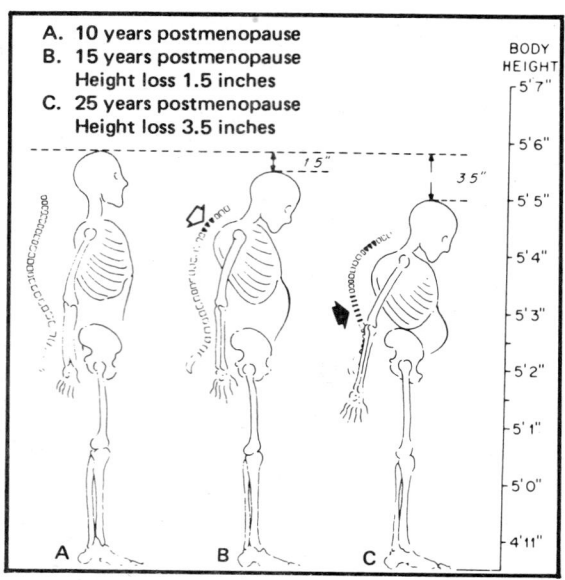

A. 10 years postmenopause
B. 15 years postmenopause
   Height loss 1.5 inches
C. 25 years postmenopause
   Height loss 3.5 inches

BODY HEIGHT

Figure 62-7. Typical loss of height associated with osteoporosis and aging. (Courtesy, Wilson Research Foundation.)

(1–6 inches) in height from vertebral collapse. The postural changes result in relaxation of the abdominal muscles, hence a protruding stomach. The deformity may also produce pulmonary insufficiency. Many patients complain of fatigue.

Diagnostic Evaluation. Laboratory studies (*e.g.,* serum calcium, serum phosphate, alkaline phosphatase, urine calcium excretion, urinary hydroxyproline excretion, hematocrit, erythrocyte sedimentation rate) and roentgenograms may be conducted to exclude other possible medical diagnoses (*e.g.,* multiple myeloma, osteomalacia, hyperparathyroidism, malignancy).

Patient Problems/Nursing Diagnoses

Based on the clinical manifestations, the patient who experiences spontaneous vertebral fracture related to osteoporosis has nursing problems that include pain related to fracture and muscle spasm; potential development of ileus related to immobility; possible development of future vertebral fracture related to porous and fragile bone; decreased physical activity related to age; and nonadherence to the therapeutic regimen related to knowledge deficit.

▶ Planning and Implementation

Goals

The major goals for the patient include:

1. Absence of pain
2. Absence of ileus
3. Absence of additional vertebral fractures
4. Increased level of physical activity
5. Adherence to therapeutic regimen.

Pain relief can be accomplished by bed rest, lying supine or on either side, for several days to a week. The mattress should be firm and nonsagging. Narcotic analgesics may be needed for the first few days. Constipation may develop with the use of narcotics. After a few days, salicylates and other nonnarcotic analgesics afford relief.

If the vertebral collapse involves a T10 to L2 vertebra, the patient may develop an ileus. The nurse therefore monitors the patient's intake and bowel activity.

Compression fractures heal regardless of the treatment regimen. Therapy is directed at diminishing progression of osteoporosis and prevention of additional fractures.

Physical activity is most essential to strengthen muscles, prevent disuse atrophy, and retard progressive bone demineralization. Daily activity, preferably outdoors in the sunshine, is necessary. Isometric exercises can be used to strengthen trunk muscles. Walking, swimming, and stationary bicycle riding are well tolerated. Good body mechanics and posture are to be encouraged. Sudden bending, jarring, and strenuous lifting are to be avoided.

A diet high in calcium, protein, and vitamin D is generally prescribed to slow the rate of bone loss. This would include two or more servings of meat, chicken, or fish or protein equivalent and three glasses of skim or whole milk daily. A calcium preparation (calcium carbonate) is given to add sufficient calcium to the diet, as many older persons frequently suffer from a deficiency in dietary calcium. Vitamin D, necessary for calcium absorption, is frequently added in the form of vitamin D-fortified milk or calcium supplements containing vitamin D.

Estrogen replacement therapy (Premarin) may be given to retard bone loss and prevent occurrence of additional fractures. Estrogens decrease bone resorption as well as bone formation. They do not increase bone mass. Estrogens are not able to diminish the rate of bone loss indefinitely and are of little value in long-term care. During estrogen therapy, the patient must examine her breasts monthly and report for a pelvic examination, including a Pap smear and aspiration of endometrial secretions for histologic examination since estrogens may produce breast and endometrial hyperplasia and cancer. A woman who has had her ovaries removed or has undergone a premature menopause may develop osteoporosis at a fairly young age. Estrogen replacement is considered in this patient.

Calcitonin, a thyroid hormone that decreases bone resorption, has been demonstrated in clinical trials to slow bone loss. Its therapeutic effects, which include increase in bone mass, last for about 18 months. In addition, the use of a fluoride plus calcium regimen is being investigated.

A person with progressive osteoporosis and additional vertebral collapses will develop a *chronic back pain* as kyphosis progresses. Daily intermittent recumbent rest periods relieve the stress of the abnormal posture on the weakened muscles and relieve the discomfort. Participation in activities of daily living with recumbent rest at the onset of discomfort allows these patients to remain productive and independent.

Osteoporosis continues to be a problem in which *prevention through health education* is desirable. Exercise and physical activity are the primary keys to developing bones of high density that are more resistant to becoming osteoporotic. An adequate, balanced dietary intake rich in calcium and vitamin D throughout life with an increased calcium intake beginning in the middle years protects against skeletal demineralization. Encourage outside activities to enhance the body's ability to use sunlight, which aids in producing vitamin D.

▶ Evaluation

Expected Outcomes

1. Is free of pain
   a. Experiences no pain at rest
   b. Experiences no pain during activities of daily living
   c. Demonstrates diminished tenderness at fracture site
2. Avoids ileus
   Demonstrates normal bowel sounds and normal bowel activity
3. Is free of additional vertebral fractures
   a. Maintains good posture
   b. Uses good body mechanics
   c. Experiences no recurrence of sudden back pain due to new fracture
4. Engages in increased level of physical activity
   a. Participates in activities of daily living
   b. Exercises daily within physiologic limits
   c. Walks daily
5. Adheres to therapeutic regimen
   a. Consumes diet high in calcium, protein, and vitamin D
   b. Exercises daily
   c. Rests by lying down a couple of times a day
   d. Participates in outside activities
   e. Prevents falls and minor trauma

▷ Paget's Disease

Paget's disease (osteitis deformans) is a bone disease of unknown cause marked by excessive bone resorption (bone loss) and disordered formation of bone. There is a primary proliferation of osteoclasts that produce bone resorption followed by a compensatory increase in osteoblastic activity that repairs the bone resorbed. This bone destruction and formation (turnover) causes distortion of normal bone anatomy (*e.g.,* enlarged and deformed bones with increasing vascularity). As the bone turnover continues, a classic mosaic pattern of bone matrix develops. The condition affects single bones, most commonly the lumbosacral vertebrae, skull, pelvic bones, femur, and tibia.

The disease occurs slightly more often in men than women. The incidence rises with age and is found in 3% to 4% of the population over 50 years. It is found most commonly in the Anglo–Saxon population, and a familial tendency is frequent.

▶ Assessment

Clinical Manifestations.   The disease is insidious. One third of patients with the disease never know they have it. One third of the patients are asymptomatic but have skeletal deformity and one third have symptomatic problems. The condition is most frequently identified when x-rays have been done at a routine physical examination or in the course of workup for another problem. There are sclerotic changes, skeletal deformities (*e.g.,* bowing of femur and tibia, kyphosis, enlargement of the skull) and cortical thickening of the long bones. Bone scans may detect the disease quite early.

The serum alkaline phosphatase and the level of urinary hydroxyproline excretion are usually increased. In general, the level of alkaline phosphatase correlates with the extent and activity of the disease. The increase in the number, size, and activity of the bone cells is responsible for the biochemical abnormalities of Paget's disease.

Although it may start in any part of the skeleton, it usually begins in the skull, vertebral column, pelvis, or long bones. Pain and tenderness on pressure may be noted in the bones. Such pain, which is wrongly attributed to old age or arthritis by the patient, may precede the skeletal changes by years. There is an increase in skin temperature overlying the bone from increased vascularity of the bone. In the majority of patients, there is deformity involving the skull or long bones. The skull may be thickened and the patient may complain that his hat no longer fits. In well-marked cases of Paget's disease, the cranium is much enlarged, but not the face, which therefore appears small and triangular in shape. Most patients with skull involvement have impaired hearing.

The spine is bent forward and is rigid; the chin rests on the chest. The thorax is compressed and immobile on respiration. The trunk is flexed on the legs to maintain equilibrium; the arms, which are bent outward and forward and appear long in relation to the shortened trunk, give to the patient an apelike appearance; and the legs are greatly bowed, hence the gait is labored and waddling. As a result of the kyphosis and the bowing of the legs, the patient's height may be reduced as much as 30 cm (12 inches). The bones involved are brittle and fractures occur frequently.

Complications.   Associated problems include high output cardiac failure from the increased blood flow to the affected bone, neurologic sequelae secondary to pressure on the brain, cranial nerves and spinal nerve roots by pathologic bone degeneration, and vascular insufficiency and hypercalcemia related to the inability of the kidney to excrete the increased calcium load. Paget's disease in some patients is a precursor of bone tumor, mainly osteogenic sarcoma.

Patient Problems/Nursing Diagnoses

Based on the clinical manifestations and diagnostic assessment data, the symptomatic patient's major nursing problems include bone pain related to abnormal skeletal metabolism; bone deformity and fracture related to the pathologic process; impaired hearing related to skull growth pressing on structures; and potential nonadherence to the therapeutic regimen related to knowledge deficit.

▶ Planning and Implementation

Goals

The major goals for the patient include:

1. Absence of pain
2. Arrest of bone deformities and pathologic fracture

3. Compensated auditory impairment
4. Adherence to therapeutic regimen

Usually, no particular treatment is recommended in the patient without symptoms. The supportive and symptomatic treatment consists of giving aspirin, indomethacin (Indocin), or ibuprofen (Motrin) for pain relief or anti-inflammatory effect.

Patients with a moderate to severe form of the disease may benefit from suppressive therapy. At the present time, there are several agents that are potent inhibitors of bone resorption and under certain conditions may permit replacement of diseased bone with normal lamellar bone: the calcitonins, etidronate disodium (EHDP), and mithramycin. These agents all suppress bone resorption but are mediated by different mechanisms.

Calcitonin therapy can result in remodeling of the pagetoid bone to normal lamellar bone. Calcitonin, a polypeptide hormone, retards bone resorption by decreasing the number and availability of osteoclasts. It is used to relieve bone pain and helps alleviate neurologic and biochemical complications. Three species of calcitonin are available: salmon, porcine, and human. Calcitonin is given by injection, with the subcutaneous route used for self-administration. Flushing of the face and nausea are side-effects. These tend to decrease with time or can be managed by taking the drug before bedtime or concurrently with an antihistamine. Treatment lasts for about 3 months.

Sodium etidronate (EHDP), a diphosphonate compound, produces rapid reduction of bone turnover and relief of pain. It also reduces elevated serum alkaline phosphatase and urinary hydroxyproline levels. It is easy to administer since it can be taken by mouth. Diarrhea may be a side-effect; it is alleviated by spacing the dose. Therapy may continue for up to 6 months.

Mithramycin (Mithracin), a cytotoxic antibiotic, is used to control the disease, since Paget's disease is similar in some ways to a low-grade neoplastic process. This drug has dramatic effects on the serum calcium, alkaline phosphatase, and urinary hydroxyproline levels, possibly due to the fact that mithramycin is toxic to osteoclasts. It is given by intravenous infusion and requires that hepatic, renal, and bone marrow function be monitored during therapy.

Clinical remissions may continue for months after discontinuation of the drugs.

Fractures are managed according to location. Healing does occur if reduction, immobilization, and stability are adequate. Nonunion with femoral neck fractures requires treatment with an endoprosthesis.

Loss of hearing is managed with amplification aids and communication techniques used with the hearing impaired (lip reading, body language, etc.).

▶ **Evaluation**

Expected Outcomes

1. Is free of pain
   a. Experiences no pain
   b. Experiences no tenderness on palpation of bones

2. Achieves arrest of bone deformity and is free of pathologic fracture
   a. Demonstrates no progression of deformities
   b. Exhibits no pathologic fractures
3. Compensates for auditory impairment
   a. Uses auditory aid
   b. Uses lip reading to assist in comprehension of verbal communication
   c. Understands most verbal communications
4. Adheres to therapeutic regimen
   a. Takes prescribed medications
   b. Reports symptoms and problems associated with drugs
   c. Keeps follow-up medical appointments

▷ # Osteomalacia

Osteomalacia is a metabolic bone disease characterized by failure of normal mineralization of bone. (A similar condition in children is called rickets.) In these patients, a large amount of osteoid or remolded bone does not calcify. It is thought that the primary defect is a defective supply of calcium and phosphate from the extracellular fluid to the calcification sites in the bones. As a result of this faulty mineralization, there is softening and weakening of the skeleton, causing pain, tenderness to the touch, and bowing of the bones. In adults, the condition is chronic, and skeletal deformities are not as severe as in children because skeletal growth has been completed.

Pathophysiology.   There are a variety of causes of osteomalacia resulting from a generalized disturbance in mineral metabolism. Risk factors for the development of osteomalacia are dietary deficiencies, malabsorption problems, gastrectomy, chronic renal failure, prolonged drug absorption (phenytoin, phenobarbital), excessive calcium demands of pregnancy and lactation, and insufficient vitamin D (dietary, sunlight).

Osteomalacia may occur as a result of inadequate dietary intake of calcium or phosphate ions, failure of these ions to be absorbed, or excessive loss of these materials from the body.

The malnutrition type (deficiency of vitamin D often associated with poor intake of calcium) is mainly due to poverty, but food faddism and lack of knowledge of nutrition may be factors. It occurs in parts of the world where vitamin D is not added to food and where dietary deficiencies exist and sunlight is scarce.

In the elderly, who are economically and socially deprived, special attention to a nutritious diet is important. Since sunlight is necessary, older people should be encouraged to spend some time in the sun.

Gastrointestinal disorders in which fats are inadequately absorbed are prone to produce osteomalacia through loss of vitamin D (among other fat-soluble vitamins) and calcium, the latter being excreted in the feces in combination with fatty acids. Such disorders include celiac disease, chronic biliary tract obstruction, chronic pancreatitis, and small bowel resections or operative shunts (gastrectomy) that involve the small intestine.

Severe renal insufficiency results in acidosis. The available calcium is used to combat the acidosis, and the parathyroid hormone continues to cause a release of skeletal calcium in an attempt to reestablish a physiologic pH. During this continual drain of skeletal calcium, bony fibrosis occurs and bony cysts form. Chronic glomerulonephritis, obstructive uropathies, and heavy metal poisoning result in a reduced serum phosphate level and demineralization of bone.

In addition, liver and kidney diseases can produce a lack of vitamin D, as these are the organs that convert vitamin D to its active form. Finally, hyperparathyroidism leads to skeletal decalcification, and thus to osteomalacia, through the promotion of phosphate excretion in the urine.

▶ Assessment

Clinical Manifestations.   The most common and distressing symptom of osteomalacia is bone pain and tenderness. As a result of calcium deficiency, there is usually muscle weakness. The patient develops a waddling or limping gait. In the more advanced disease, the legs become bowed (due to body weight and muscle pull). The softened vertebrae become compressed, thus shortening the patient's trunk and deforming the thorax. The sacrum is forced down and forward and the pelvis is compressed laterally. These two deformities explain the characteristic shape of the pelvis that often necessitates cesarean section in pregnant women who are affected with this disease. Weakness and unsteadiness present a danger of falls and fractures.

Patient Problems/Nursing Diagnoses

Based on the clinical data, the patient's major nursing problems include bone pain and tenderness related to mineral metabolic disturbance; loss of calcium from the bone and body related to metabolic disturbance; and possible nonadherence to the therapeutic regimen related to a lack of understanding.

▶ Planning and Implementation

Goals

The major patient goals are:

1. Relief of bone pain and tenderness
2. Mineralization of bone
3. Adherence to therapeutic regimen

Interventions.   Osteomalacia can be treated with gratifying results on an individualized basis. The underlying cause is corrected as far as possible.

Vitamin D is given in the treatment of many forms of osteomalacia. Its various therapeutic actions combine to raise the concentrations of calcium and phosphorus in the extracellular fluid and thus make these ions available for mineralization. If osteomalacia is dietary in origin, a normal diet plus vitamin D is given. If vitamin D deficiency is due to malabsorption, larger doses of vitamin D are required in addition to supplementary doses of calcium. High doses of

vitamin D are toxic and enhance the risk of hypercalcemia. Therefore, the patient's serum calcium is monitored.

With malabsorption the patient may also be treated with ultraviolet irradiation. The patient is encouraged to expose his skin to sunlight, as the ultraviolet portion of sunlight is necessary to transform a cholesterol substance (7-dehydro) present in the skin into vitamin D.

Frequently, skeletal problems associated with osteomalacia resolve themselves when the underlying disease or nutritional deficiency is adequately treated. Some persistent orthopedic deformities may need to be treated with braces or surgery (osteotomy for long bone deformity).

▶ Evaluation

Expected Outcomes

1. Is free of bone pain and tenderness
   a. Exhibits no pain
   b. Experiences no tenderness to touch
2. Shows mineralization of bone
   a. Experiences an arrest of skeletal deformities
   b. Demonstrates radiographic evidence of improvement of bone mineralization
3. Adheres to therapeutic regimen
   a. Consumes therapeutic amounts of calcium
   b. Consumes therapeutic amounts of vitamin D
   c. Exposes self to sunlight
   d. Has serum calcium level monitored throughout therapy
   e. Keeps follow-up medical appointments

▷ Bone and Joint Infections

Osteomyelitis

Osteomyelitis is an infection of the bone. This infection is more difficult to cure than a soft tissue infection. The infection may be due to hematogenous (blood-borne) spread from other foci of infection (*e.g.,* infected tonsils, boils, infected teeth, upper respiratory infections), erosion of adjacent soft tissue infection (*e.g.,* middle ear infection, infected decubitus or vascular ulcers), or direct bone contamination (*e.g.,* open fracture, gun-shot wound, bone surgery). Acute osteomyelitis due to hematogenous spread is seen more frequently in children than adults. Chronic osteomyelitis is seen more frequently in adults. *Staphylococcus aureus* causes 70% to 80% of bone infections. Other pathogenic organisms that cause osteomyelitis include *Proteus, Pseudomonas,* colon bacillus, and *Salmonella.* There has been an increasing incidence of penicillin-resistant, nosocomial, gram-negative, and anaerobic infections.

Pathophysiology.   Osteomyelitis due to hematogenous spread occurs in a bone area where there is lowered resistance, possibly due to subclinical trauma. It often develops in the long bones of children and vertebrae of adults. Regardless of the source of the infective microbe, the initial response is one of inflammation, increased vascularity, and edema. After 2 or 3 days, there is a thrombosis of the blood vessels in the area and a resultant ischemia with bone necrosis due to increasing tissue and medullary pressure. The infection extends into the medullary cavity and under the periosteum. Infective pus may spread the infection into adjacent soft tissues and joint. Unless the infective process is controlled early, bone abscess forms.

In the natural course of events, the abscess may point and drain but, more often, incision and drainage are done by the surgeon. The resulting abscess cavity has in its walls areas of dead tissue, as in any abscess cavity; however, in this case the dead tissue is bone, which cannot liquefy easily and be discharged as pus. This dead bone is called a *sequestrum.* Healing in a bone abscess is more difficult than in an abscess in soft tissue, because the cavity cannot collapse and heal. New bone, the *involucrum,* forms as the body attempts to repair. Often it grows so as to surround a sequestrum. Thus, even though healing appears to take place, a chronically infected sequestrum remains that is prone to produce recurring abscesses throughout the life of the individual. This is the so-called chronic type of osteomyelitis.

Acute Osteomyelitis

▶ Assessment

Clinical Manifestations. When the infection is carried by the blood, the onset is usually sudden, occurring often with a chill, high fever, rapid pulse, and general malaise. In children, in whom the disease usually begins as an acute epiphysitis, these constitutional symptoms at first may overshadow the local signs completely. As the infection extends from the marrow cavity through the cortex of the bone, it involves the periosteum and the soft tissues, with the extremity becoming painful, swollen, and extremely tender. The patient may describe a constant, pulsating pain that intensifies with movement and is due to the pressure of the collecting pus.

When osteomyelitis occurs from spread of adjacent infection or direct contamination, there is no septicemia symptomatology. The area is swollen, warm, painful, and tender to touch.

Diagnostic Evaluation. Early x-rays will show only soft tissue swelling. In about 2 weeks, areas of irregular decalcification, periosteal elevation, and new bone formation will be evident. Blood studies will show elevated leukocytes and an elevated sedimentation rate. Blood cultures and cultures of the abscess are needed for proper antibiotic therapy.

Patient Problems/Nursing Diagnoses

Based on the clinical manifestations and other data, the patient's major nursing problems include infection related to the osteomyelitis process; pain related to infective debris accumulation; decreased body resistance related to the infective process; and possible nonadherence to the therapeutic regimen related to a lack of understanding.

▶ Planning and Implementation

Goals

The major goals of a patient with acute osteomyelitis include:

1. Absence of bone infection
2. Absence of pain
3. Improved body resistance
4. Adherence to therapeutic regimen

Management. The initial objective of therapy is to control and arrest the infective process. Blood cultures and abscess fluid smears and cultures are done to identify the organism and select the best antibiotic. Cultures of other loci of infection may be done if hematogenous spread is suspected. Antibiotic therapy is begun immediately assuming a *Staphylococcus* infection is present that is sensitive to a semisynthetic penicillin. Nafcillin, methicillin, cephalothin, cefazolin, and other similar drugs are used parenterally. A sustained high therapeutic blood level of the antibiotic is important. (A concentration of four to ten times the minimal inhibitory level is necessary.) Around-the-clock dosage administration is necessary. The aim is to control the infection before the blood supply to the infection diminishes as a result of thrombosis. If necessary, when culture results are obtained, the antibiotic can be replaced by one to which the organism is more sensitive. When the infection appears to be controlled, the antibiotic can be administered orally and so continued for 3 to 4 weeks after the patient is afebrile. To enhance absorption of oral antibiotics, they should not be administered with food.

Suspected regions of pus may be evacuated by needle aspiration. If the patient does not respond to treatment, surgery is carried out whereby the involved bone is exposed, the purulent and necrotic material removed, and the area irrigated directly with sterile physiologic saline solution. A high blood level of antibiotic is maintained.

Nursing Interventions. The relief of pain and the promotion of comfort are always goals of nursing.

Osteomyelitis is a disease that demands careful nursing management. The wounds themselves frequently are very painful and must be handled with great care and gentleness. The joints above and below the affected part should be supported and the extremity moved in a smooth manner. The affected part may be immobilized with a splint until the wound has healed. Immobilization decreases pain and muscle spasm.

These patients should be monitored carefully for the development of additional painful areas or sudden rises in temperature. These may indicate the extension of the infection or a secondary infection.

During the acute and convalescent period, the general health and nutrition of the patient needs to be monitored and enhanced. Fluids and a balanced diet high in protein, vitamin C, and vitamin D, are provided. Electrolyte homeostasis and a positive nitrogen balance promote healing.

If there is a draining wound, the patient is isolated and secretion precautions or wound and skin precautions are followed depending on the extent of infection. Careful hand washing is essential because of the possibility of cross infection.

When the patient leaves the acute care setting, adherence to the therapeutic regimen is stressed. Adequate treatment requires appropriate antibiotic therapy and an environment that will enhance bone healing. With early therapy, the infection should be eliminated and bone will heal. If this is not accomplished, chronic osteomyelitis may develop.

▶ **Evaluation**

Expected Outcomes

1. Shows no signs of bone infection
   a. Completes prescribed antibiotic therapy regimen
   b. Exhibits normal body temperature
   c. Shows no signs of purulent drainage
   d. Shows normal blood analysis parameters for infection
2. Is free of pain
   a. Does not complain of pain
   b. Experiences no tenderness in area of previous infection
   c. Experiences no discomfort with movement
   d. Does not need pain relief measures
3. Demonstrates improved body resistance
   a. Consumes balanced diet
   b. Achieves normal blood analysis parameters
   c. Tolerates activity with minimal fatigue
   d. Uses normal precautions to avoid colds and other infections
4. Adheres to therapeutic regimen
   a. Resumes activities gradually
   b. Consumes balanced diet
   c. Reports recurrence of pain or fever promptly
   d. Keeps follow-up clinic or physician appointments

Chronic Osteomyelitis

Assessment and Clinical Manifestations.   The patient with a chronic osteomyelitis presents with a continuously draining sinus or experiences recurrent periods of pain, inflammation, swelling, and drainage. The low-grade infection thrives in the scar tissue with its reduced blood supply. On x-ray, large, irregular cavities; sequestra; or dense bone formations are seen.

Management.   In chronic osteomyelitis, all dead, infected bone and cartilage must be removed before permanent healing takes place. This operation, which is called a *sequestrectomy,* consists of the removal of enough involucrum with mallet and chisel to enable the surgeon to remove the sequestrum. Often sufficient bone is removed to convert a deep cavity into a shallow saucer (saucerization). Antibiotics are used supportively to prevent septicemia and massive local infection. Antibiotics are given preoperatively, intraoperatively, and postoperatively to assure a sterile operative hematoma to optimize eradication of the infection. Antibiotic therapy continues for at least 6 weeks.

The wound is either closed tightly to obliterate the dead space or may be packed to be closed later by granulation or possibly by grafting. A closed suction irrigation system may be used to control the hematoma and remove debris. Physiologic saline solution for 7 to 8 days is usually used. The development of superimposed infection may occur with prolonged irrigation.

Bone and Joint Tuberculosis

Tuberculosis is an infectious disease caused by the tubercle bacillus, *Mycobacterium tuberculosis.* While the lungs are the organs usually invaded directly, involvement of bones and joints is secondary to tuberculosis elsewhere in the body. Therefore, when the bones are affected, a search is made for other active foci of disease. Skeletal tuberculosis is uncommon (3% of all tuberculosis) and occurs most frequently in children. Onset of skeletal pathology is within 2 years of the primary lesion.

Tuberculosis of a bone or joint is usually a low-grade and slowly progressive infection. Characteristically, one joint (monoarticular) or one bone (mono-osseous) is affected. The spine is involved most commonly (Pott's disease), while the hip, the knee, and the ankle may also be affected in some patients. Local symptoms and signs include swelling (caused by synovial inflammation), pain and tenderness, muscle spasm, early stiffness progressing to limitation of active and passive motion (from fibrous ankylosis), slight warmth about the involved site, increased amounts of joint fluid, and muscle atrophy. Constitutional manifestations include fatigue, anorexia, weight loss, and intermittent low-grade fever. Diagnostic evaluation includes skin testing for tuberculosis, x-rays, and synovial biopsy.

The patient who experiences skeletal tuberculosis needs to eradicate the infection, experience comfort, and promote healing of the affected bones and joints through immobilization and nutrition.

Nursing Implementation.   The initial efforts are directed toward controlling and arresting the infection. A combination of antituberculosis drugs is given to eradicate the microbial organisms as rapidly as possible and to minimize the opportunity for the persistence of drug-resistant organisms. (Drug therapy is discussed on p. 1508.) Secondary infection of the bone is treated with the appropriate antimicrobial agent. Orthopedic surgery is indicated when drainage of abscesses, excision of bone, and fixation of a joint are necessary.

When the joint is involved, the cartilage and subchondral bone may be destroyed. In the surgical management of infected joints, the swollen tubercular synovium may be removed.

Spread of the spinal infection can lead to paravertebral (psoas) abscess formation, paraplegia due to abscess or granulation tissue pressure on the spinal cord, or tuberculosis meningitis due to rupture of the abscess through the dura. Skeletal tuberculosis can also result in abscess drainage tracts.

The affected joint must be immobilized to minimize pain and to promote healing. Complete bed rest, plaster casts, spinal braces, and bone fusions may be employed to promote immobilization.

Healing is also promoted through good nutrition and general health measures. Adequate vitamin D is needed for normal bone metabolism.

Other facets of care and patient education are discussed under Management of the Patient With Tuberculosis, p. 1508.

▷ Bone Tumors

Neoplasms of the skeleton are of a variety of types. They may be benign bone tumors, primary malignant sarcomas, or metastatic carcinomas from primary cancers elsewhere in the body. Osteogenic, chondrogenic, fibrogenic, and marrow (reticulum) cell tumors as well as nervous, vascular, and fatty cell tumors may arise in bone. The presence of a tumor in the bone causes the normal bone tissue to react by increasing local osteoclastic reabsorption or by increasing osteoblastic response around the tumor (reactive bone formation). The type of bone tumor, its growth and metastatic characteristics, and the surrounding bone response account for symptomatology and radiographic findings and direct the plan of medical management. Some of the bone tumors are common and some are exceedingly rare. Some present no problem, while others become rapidly life-threatening. Some benign tumors have the potential of undergoing malignant transformation.

Management.   Management of bone tumors includes surgical excision (local excision to amputation and disarticulation), radiation when the tumor is radiosensitive, and chemotherapy for management of metastasis. The possible use of immunotherapy continues to be investigated. Major gains are being made in using wide block excision with restorative grafting technique and chemotherapeutics. Improvement is seen in the quality of life and long-term survival rates.

▶ **Assessment**

Clinical Manifestations.   The patient with a bone tumor presents with a wide range of associated problems. He may be asymptomatic or may have pain (mild and occasional to constant and severe); varying degrees of disability; and at times, obvious bone growth; or he may experience pathologic fracture.

Differential diagnosis is based on the history; physical examination; x-rays, including tomograms, bone scans, arteriography (if appropriate); biochemical assays of the blood and urine; and finally surgical biopsy for histologic identification (Fig. 62-8).

Patient Problems/Nursing Diagnoses

Based on the clinical manifestations and diagnostic assessment data, the patient's major nursing problems include pain and disability related to neoplasm growth; potential pathologic fracture related to structural bone changes; pos-

sible metastasis related to the nature of the neoplasm; potential complications related to the medical therapy regimen; and potential nonadherence to the therapeutic regimen related to a lack of understanding.

Benign Bone Tumors

Benign bone tumors are generally slow growing and well circumscribed, present few symptoms, and are not a cause of death.

Osteochondroma is the most common benign bone tumor and usually occurs as a large projection of bone at the end of long bones (at the knee or shoulder). It develops during growth and then becomes a static bony mass. The cartilage cap of the osteochondroma may undergo malignant transformation following trauma, and a chondrosarcoma may develop.

Enchondroma is a common tumor of the hyaline cartilage that develops during the growing years in the hand, ribs, femur, tibia, humerus, or pelvis. Generally, the only symptom is a mild ache. Pathologic fractures may occur.

A painful tumor that occurs in children and young adults is the *osteoid osteoma*. The neoplastic tissue (nidus) is surrounded by reactive bone formation that assists in its radiologic identification.

Bone cysts are expanding lesions within the bone. *Aneurysmal bone cysts* are seen in young adults and present with a painful, palpable mass of the long bones, vertebrae, or flat bones. *Unicameral bone cysts* occur in children and cause mild discomfort and possible pathologic fractures of the upper humerus and femur. These may heal spontaneously.

Giant cell tumors are benign but may invade local tissue and cause destruction. They occur in young adults and are soft and hemorrhagic. Some giant cell tumors recur or become sarcomas and metastasize.

The general therapeutic approach is to excise completely the tumor tissue and restore the bone continuity with bone grafts. The excised area may be packed with ilium chips to stimulate healing.

▶ **Planning and Implementation**

Goals

The major goals for the patient with a benign bone tumor include:

1. Absence of pain and restoration of function
2. Absence of pathologic fracture
3. Healing of treated bone
4. Absence of postexcision complications
5. Adherence to therapeutic regimen

Interventions.   The nursing care of a patient who has had the excision of a bone tumor is similar in many aspects to other patients who undergo skeletal surgery. The operative part needs to be elevated to control swelling; the neurovascular status of the extremity needs to be assessed. Generally, the area is immobilized by splints, casts, or elastic

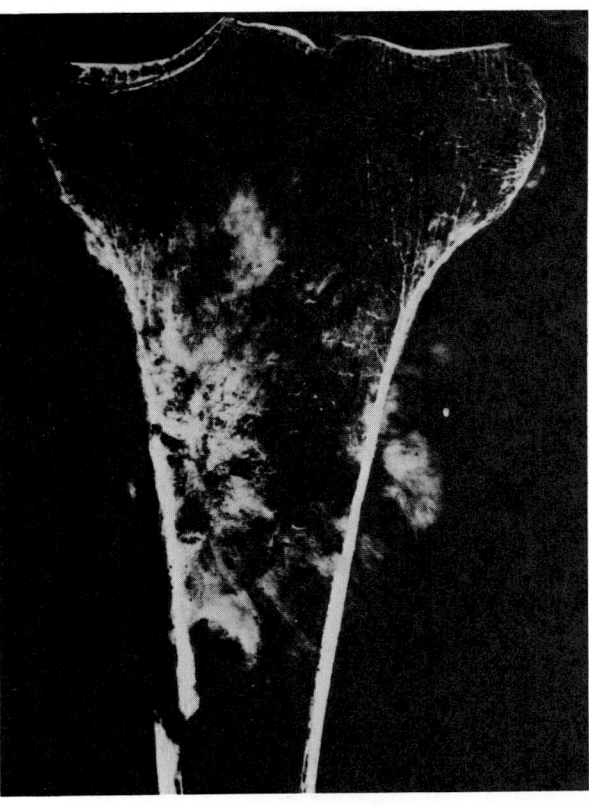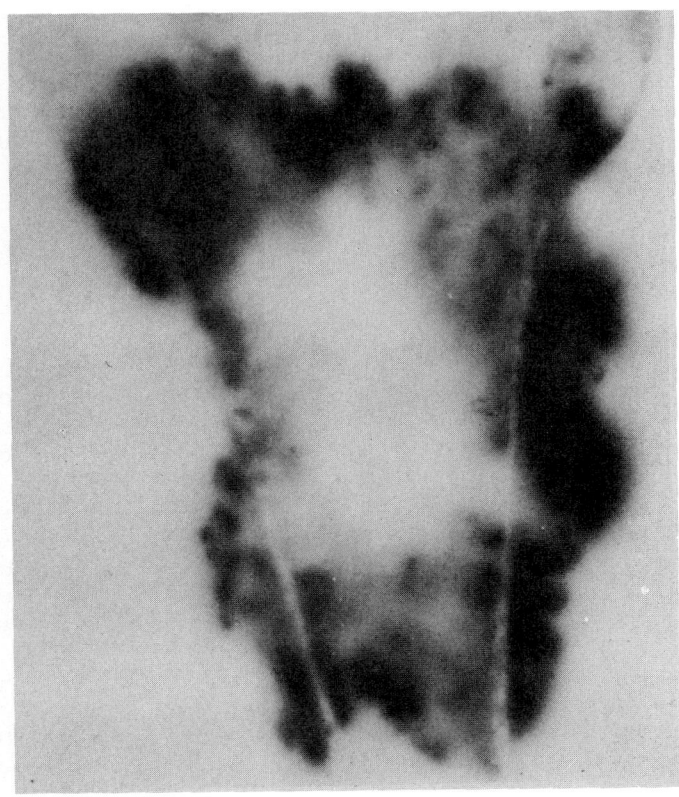

Figure 62-8. (*Left*) X-ray showing osteosarcoma at the proximal end of the tibia. Note the destruction of the normal anatomy of the bone. (*Right*) Contact autoradiograph of the same patient. The patient has received ^{85}Sr intravenously for bone scanning. Note the high uptake (black areas) in the peripheral growing margin and the relative lack of uptake centrally. (Armed Forces Institute of Pathology. Negative numbers 67–4–8, 67–4–9)

bandages until the bone heals. The fluid and electrolyte balance of the patient is monitored. A diet high in protein, with adequate vitamins, especially vitamins C and D, and calcium is encouraged.

Pain is present both at the surgical and graft donor sites. Narcotics are used during the early postoperative period. Later, oral, nonnarcotic analgesics are adequate to control discomfort.

Postexcision complications include those associated with immobility, blood loss, and infection. Osteomyelitis is a concern. Prophylactic antibiotics and strict aseptic dressing techniques are used to diminish the occurrence of this dreaded complication. During healing, other infections (*e.g.,* colds) need to be avoided so that hematogenous spread does not result in an osteomyelitis.

Depending on the site, the use of ambulatory aids might be required. An exercise program is designed to restore function. Active participation in exercises and other rehabilitative activities is encouraged.

As the patient prepares to leave the hospital, patient education concerning continuing care is given. Medications and exercise regimens are reviewed. The nurse encourages needed follow-up medical visits.

▶ **Evaluation**

Expected Outcomes

1. Is free of pain and achieves restoration of function
   a. Experiences no pain at rest or with activity
   b. Exhibits no tenderness at excision site and graft site
   c. Demonstrates normal joint range of motion and normal muscle strength
   d. Achieves normal use of affected bone
   e. Participates in activities of daily living
2. Shows no signs of pathologic fracture
3. Achieves healing of treated bone
4. Experiences no postexcision complications
   a. Exhibits normal temperature, pulse, and respirations
   b. Experiences no calf tenderness or Homans' sign
   c. Shows no evidence of osteomyelitis
   d. Demonstrates normal neurovascular status
5. Adheres to therapeutic regimen
   a. Participates in daily exercise regimen
   b. Accepts activity limitations as prescribed
   c. Takes medications as prescribed
   d. Keeps follow-up physician appointments

Malignant Bone Tumors

Malignant bone tumors may be primary bone tumors arising from bone tissue cells (sarcomas) or bone marrow elements (myeloma) or may be secondary bone tumors (carcinomas) due to metastasis from breast, prostate, kidney, thyroid, or lung cancers. Bone metastasis is frequently to the lungs.

Osteogenic sarcoma (osteosarcoma) is the most frequent and most frequently fatal primary malignant bone tumor. It is characterized by early hematogenous metastasis to the lungs. The tumor carries a high mortality rate since the sarcoma often has spread to the lungs by the time the patient seeks help.

Osteogenic sarcoma appears most frequently in males in the age group between 10 and 25 and in older persons with Paget's disease. It is manifested by pain, swelling, limitation of motion, and weight loss; the latter is considered an ominous finding. The bony mass may be palpable, tender, and fixed with an increase in skin temperature over the mass and venous distention. The primary lesion may involve any bone; the most common sites are the lower end of the femur, the upper end of the tibia, and the upper end of the humerus.

Management. The goal of management is to destroy or remove malignant tissue by the most effective method possible. This requires a multidisciplinary approach, possibly in a cancer treatment center.

Surgical removal of the tumor usually requires that the affected extremity be amputated, with the line of amputation extending through the bone or joint above the bone tumor in order to achieve local control of the primary lesion. (See nursing management of the patient following an amputation, p. 1446.) Some centers are now performing local bone resection without amputation using metallic prosthetics or allografts for bone replacement.

Because of the real danger of metastasis with these tumors, combined chemotherapy is started before and after surgery in an effort to eradicate micrometastatic lesions. The hope is that combined chemotherapy will achieve a greater response at a lower toxicity rate with a minimum amount of resistance to the drugs. Vincristine, high-dose methotrexate with citrovorum factor, doxorubicin, and cyclophosphamide are used in various combinations. Large doses of methotrexate inhibit DNA synthesis and are made more acceptable by the concomitant administration of citrovorum factor, which "rescues" the patient from the excess toxicity of methotrexate. There is an improvement in survival rates.

The nursing management of the patient undergoing chemotherapy can be found on page 308. A patient with a bone tumor requires understanding and support to cope with the disagreeable side-effects of treatment and the uncertain outcome of the disease.

Malignant tumors of the hyaline cartilage are *chondrosarcomas*. These are the second most common primary malignant bone tumors. They are large, bulky, slow-growing tumors that affect adults and affect men more frequently than women. The usual tumor sites include the pelvis, ribs, femur, humerus, spine, scapula, and tibia. Metastasis to the lungs occurs in less than half the patients. If these tumors are well differentiated, large block excision or amputation of the affected extremity results in a good survival rate. These tumors may recur.

▶ **Planning and Implementation**

Goals

The major goals for the patient with malignant bone tumor include:

1. Absence of pain and minimal disability
2. Absence of pathologic fracture
3. Arrest of pathologic process and absence of metastasis
4. No complications of therapeutic regimen
5. Adherence to continuing medical regimen

Interventions. The malignant tumor may be treated by excision or amputation. The nursing care is similar to that for the patient undergoing skeletal surgery or amputation. Observations are made to assess the responses of the treated area.

Pain is controlled by immobilization, gentle handling, narcotics, and nonnarcotic analgesics.

Vital signs and other observations are made to assess for the development of complications: thrombophlebitis, pulmonary emboli, infection, contracture, and disuse atrophy.

Rehabilitative activities are begun early. Active participation in an exercise regimen and activities of daily living are encouraged. The patient and his family need to be supported as they work through the emotional impact of bone cancer.

Surgery is usually combined with chemotherapy. Compliance with medication regimens is encouraged. Long-term follow-up is necessary so that metastasis or recurrence can be identified early.

▶ **Evaluation**

Expected Outcomes

1. Is free of pain and minimal disability
   a. Experiences no pain at rest, during activities, or at surgical sites
   b. Participates in activities of daily living
   c. Exercises daily
   d. Uses ambulatory aids as needed
   e. Uses prosthesis, if needed
2. Is free of pathologic fracture
3. Experiences no pathologic process and metastasis
      Shows no evidence of tumor, pulmonary metastasis, or other metastasis
4. Is free of complications of therapy
   a. Demonstrates vital signs within normal range
   b. Experiences minimal chemotherapy side-effects
   c. Exhibits no evidence of osteomyelitis
5. Adheres to continuing medical regimen
   a. Takes prescribed medications
   b. Keeps physician appointments
   c. Reports recurrence of symptoms

Multiple Myeloma

Multiple myeloma (plasma cell myeloma, plasmacytoma) is a malignant disease of plasma cells that infiltrates bone and soft tissues and occurs characteristically in middle-aged females. This tumor has its origin and principal location in the bone marrow. In later stages, the lymph nodes, liver, spleen, and kidneys may become involved. There is a widespread proliferation of immature plasma cells in the marrow cavity throughout the skeleton. The bones most commonly affected are those that are the site of active hemopoietic marrow—the spine, skull, ribs, sternum, pelvis, and upper ends of the humerus.

▶ **Assessment**

Clinical Manifestations. The patient has constant severe bone pain due to the erosion of the marrow cavity and cortex. Roentgenograms reveal punched-out areas in the bone without sclerosis or reactive bone formation. Skeletal lesions produce swelling, tenderness, pain, and pathologic bone fractures. Low back pain is the most characteristic symptom, and is due to compression fracture of the vertebral body.

Anemia occurs as a result of the marrow being replaced with neoplastic cells. There is a constant threat of hypercalcemia, hypercalciuria, and hyperuricemia due to skeletal destruction. The malignant plasma cells may produce abnormal amounts of an immunoglobulin or parts of immunoglobulin protein (Bence Jones protein) that usually can be detected in the serum or urine by immunoelectrophoresis.

Symptoms of renal failure occur due to the precipitation of the immunoglobulin in the tubules, or to pyelonephritis, hypercalcemia, increased uric acid, infiltration of the kidney with plasma cells (myeloma kidney), and renal vein thrombosis.

A pathologic tendency to bleed is characteristic of myeloma for two major reasons: (1) a numerical deficiency of platelets (thrombocytopenia), due to destruction of the megakaryocytes, their parent cells, in the marrow; and (2) platelet dysfunction, the macroglobulin tending to coat these elements and to interfere with their hemostatic functions.

Diagnosis is made by examination of bone marrow obtained through sternal or iliac crest aspiration.

Patient Problems/Nursing Diagnoses

Based on the clinical manifestations, diagnostic assessment data, and medical management regimen, the patient's major nursing problems include the bone pain related to bone erosion; possible pathologic fractures related to weakening of the skeletal structure; possible acute renal failure related to pathophysiology; possible massive infection without overt symptomatology related to impaired antibody production; hematologic complications related to altered hemopoiesis; and possible nonadherence to the therapeutic regimen related to a lack of understanding.

▶ **Planning and Implementation**

Goals

The major goals for the patient include:

1. Relief of bone pain
2. Arrest of the pathologic process
3. Absence of pathologic fractures
4. Absence of acute renal failure
5. Absence of infection
6. Absence of hematologic complications
7. Adherence to the therapeutic regimen

Management. The major objectives of therapy are to suppress the plasma cell growth and to control the pain. Alkylating agent chemotherapy to reduce the tumor mass is the foundation of treatment. Combination drug therapy appears more effective than single-dose therapy in most patients. Melphalan (Alkeran) and cyclophosphamide (Cytoxan) with or without prednisone are commonly used. Other chemotherapeutic agents are tried when the patient fails to respond to the prescribed regimen. (The care of the patient undergoing chemotherapy is discussed on p. 308.) Allopurinol may be given to control hyperuricemia. Survival depends on the patient's response to chemotherapy.

Interventions. A major problem of the patient is bone pain. To relieve this discomfort, the above-mentioned chemotherapy and steroids are helpful. Radiotherapy is given to relieve bone pain from large lesions (especially from nerve compression and fractures) and to reduce the size of extraskeletal plasma cell tumors. When pain is severe, analgesics and narcotics may be necessary.

It is important that the patient be kept ambulatory as long as possible unless lesions in the spine (extradural plasmacytomas) produce danger of cord compression. If this occurs, the patient may be given radiation therapy to prevent paraplegia, or a laminectomy is done for cord compression or vertebral fractures, since the patient is susceptible to pathologic fractures.

The patient is kept well hydrated (2500 ml–3000 ml urine output daily) to control serum calcium levels and prevent hypercalcemia and hyperuricemia. Dehydration, which can precipitate acute renal failure, must be avoided.

- Thus, patients with multiple myeloma should *not* have their fluids severely restricted prior to x-ray or laboratory tests.

Complications. Because of impaired antibody production, the health care team is on the alert for recurring infection. Infection also occurs because of extensive bone marrow involvement and the effects of chemotherapy, radiotherapy, and steroids, which contribute to leukopenia. The temperature is closely monitored, and signs of respiratory and urinary tract infection are checked. Patients on steroids may not have overt symptoms of infection. Therefore, more subtle signs of apathy and lethargy are to be noted.

In addition to infection, neurologic complications (paraplegia from collapse of supporting structures, infiltration of nerve roots, or cord compression from plasma cell tumors), pathologic fractures, and renal and hematologic complications are ever-present threats to the patient's life. A disordered immune system makes the patient susceptible to multiple tumor involvement.

Compassionate management and supportive care are essential nursing tools, as the disease is ultimately fatal.

A discussion of this disease as it relates to the blood-forming organs is found on page 715.

▶ **Evaluation**

Expected Outcomes

1. Achieves relief of bone pain
   Experiences relief of pain at rest and during activity
2. Demonstrates arrest of the pathologic process
   a. Indicates suppression of plasma cell growth
   b. Experiences improvement of anemic state and hematologic status
   c. Exhibits biochemical assays in normal ranges
3. Is free of pathologic fractures
   Exhibits no symptoms of nerve root compression
4. Is free of acute renal failure
   a. Exhibits improved biochemical urinalysis
   b. Demonstrates adequate urinary output
5. Is free of infection
   a. Achieves temperature in normal range
   b. Is alert and active
6. Is free of hematologic complications
   Experiences no anemia or bleeding tendencies
7. Adheres to therapeutic regimen
   a. Takes medications as prescribed
   b. Keeps follow-up medical appointments
   c. Eats well-balanced diet

Metastatic Bone Cancer

Metastatic bone cancer is more common than any primary malignant bone tumor. Tumors arising from tissues other than the bone may invade the bone, producing localized bone destruction with results that are clinically quite analogous to those occurring in primary bone tumors. Those most frequently metastasizing to bone include carcinomas of the kidney, the prostate, the lung, the breast, the ovary, and the thyroid. Metastatic tumors most frequently attack the skull, spine, pelvis, femur, and humerus. Bone scans are useful in diagnostic workup.

A sign of diagnostic importance in patients with metastatic carcinoma of the prostate is an elevation of the serum acid phosphatase. The first indication of disease in such cases may be a pathologic bone fracture; in later stages, the peripheral blood may show evidence of bone marrow interference. Aspiration or surgical biopsy of the bone tumor can give information as to the primary site if not known.

The treatment of metastatic bone cancer is palliative, and the therapeutic goal is to relieve the patient's discomfort as much as possible. The patient is encouraged to be as independent as possible and function as long as possible. Surgery may be indicated in long bone fractures.

▷ **Bibliography**

Books

Donahoo C and Spickler L (eds). Core Curriculum of Orthopedic Nursing. Atlanta, Orthopedic Nurses' Association, 1980.
Farrell J. Illustrated Guide to Orthopedic Nursing, 2nd ed. Philadelphia, JB Lippincott, 1982.
Fenneson B. Low Back Pain, 2nd ed. Philadelphia, JB Lippincott, 1980.
Gartland J. Fundamentals of Orthopaedics, 3rd ed. Philadelphia, WB Saunders, 1979.
Hilt N and Cogburn S. Manual of Orthopedics. St Louis, CV Mosby, 1981.
Huvos A. Bone Tumors, Diagnosis, Treatment, and Prognosis. Philadelphia, WB Saunders, 1979.
Kelsey J, Pastides H, and Bisbee G Jr. Musculoskeletal Disorders: Their Frequency of Occurrence and Their Impact on the Population of the United States. New York, Prodist, 1978.
LaFreniere J. The Low-Back Patient. New York, Masson, 1979.
Mercier L and Pettid F. Practical Orthopedics. Chicago, Year Book Medical Publishers, 1980.
Mirra J et al. Bone Tumors: Diagnosis and Treatment. Philadelphia, JB Lippincott, 1980.
Mourad L. Nursing Care of Adults with Orthopedic Conditions. New York, John Wiley & Sons, 1980.
Roaf R and Hodkinson L. Textbook of Orthopaedic Nursing, 3rd ed. Oxford, Blackwell Scientific, 1980.

Articles
Low Back Pain

A back and shoulder pain explained . . . scapulocostal syndrome. Emergency Medicine 1980 Oct 15; 12(17):174–175.
Anxiety and the aching back. Emergency Medicine 1980 Feb 15; 12(4):125–126.
Flower A et al. An occupational therapy program for chronic back pain. AJOT 1981 Apr; 35(4):243–248.
Hitch M. Nursing assessment of a patient with low back pain. ONA J 1979 Dec; 6(12):484–488.
Howden L. Basic back care; it doesn't have to hurt. Can Nurs 1981 July/Aug; 77(4):46–50.
Jones A et al. Treating chronic low back pain. Phys Ther 1980 Jan; 60(1):58–63.
Keim H and Kirkaldy-Willis W. Low back pain. Clin Symp 1980; 32(6):entire issue.
Kelsey J et al. The impact of musculoskeletal disorders on the population of the United States. J Bone Joint Surg [Am] 1979 Oct; 61-A(7):959–964.
Krauitz E et al. Paralumbar muscle activity in chronic low back pain. Arch Phys Med Rehabil 1981 Apr; 62(4):172–176.
Lloyd P. Back pain . . . prevention not cure. Nurs Focus 1981 Sept; 3:460–461.
Looking at the low back . . . computed tomography. Emergency Medicine 1981 Apr 30; 13(8):69–71.
Maigne R. Low back pain of thoracolumbar origin. Arch Phys Med Rehabil 1981 Sept; 61(9):389–395.
Mulford E. Degenerative disease or slipped disc? The clues are clear-cut . . . assessment of low back pain. RN 1981 Feb; 44(2):44–49.
Owen B. How to avoid that aching back. Am J Nurs 1980 May; 80(5):894–897.
Pace J. Low back pain. Crit Care Update 1980 Feb; 7(2):8–9.
Selby D. Conservative care of nonspecific low back pain. Orthop Clin North Am 1982 July; 13(3):427–438.
Thomas L et al. Physiological work performance in chronic low back disability. Phys Ther 1980 Apr; 60(4):407–411.
White A et al. Epidural injections for the diagnosis and treatment of low-back pain. Spine 1980 Jan–Feb; 5(1):78–86.

Problems of the Upper Extremity

Berger M and Frolinson A. Hands that hurt: Carpel tunnel syndrome. Am J Nurs 1979 Feb; 79(2):264–266.
Flicker P. The painful shoulder. Primary Care 1980 June; 7(2):271–285.
Miller B. Hands that hurt less. Am J Nurs 1979 Feb; 79(2):266–267.

Neviaser R (ed). Symposium on disorders of the shoulder. Orthop Clin North Am 1980 Apr; 11(2):entire issue.

Osteoporosis/Paget's Disease

Barry H. Orthopedic aspects of Paget's disease of the bone. Arthritis Rheum 1980 Oct; 23(10):1128–1130.

Drugs for postmenopausal osteoporosis. Med Lett Drugs Ther 1980 May 30; 22(11):45–46.

Frost H (ed). Symposium on the osteoporoses. Orthop Clin North Am 1981 July; 12(3):entire issue.

Gordan G. Osteoporosis: Early detection, prevention, and treatment. Consult 1980 Jan; 20(1):64–65.

Ibbertson H et al. Paget's disease of bone: Assessment and management. Drugs 1979 July; 18(1):33–47.

Krane S and Calin A. Osteoporosis and Paget's Disease. Scien Amer Med 1981; 2, Chap. 15:1–12.

Marcus R. Rational management of osteoporosis. Hospital Forum 1981 Mar; 16(3):265–268.

Marx J. Osteoporosis: New help for thinning bones. Science 1980 Feb 8; 207(4431):628–630.

Medical News: Add exercise to calcium in osteoporosis prevention. JAMA 1982 Feb; 247(8):1106.

Raise L. Osteoporosis. Am Geriatr Soc 1982 Jan; 30(2):127–138.

Simons R. Paget's disease in the head and neck. Gerontology 1980 Mar; 26(3):155–159.

Siris E et al. Paget's disease of bone. Bull NY Acad Med 1980 Apr; 56(3):285–304.

Skillman T. Can osteoporosis be prevented? Geriatrics 1980 Feb; 35(2):95–102.

Osteomyelitis

Baum M. Say good bye to lefty . . . facing his second leg amputation. Nursing '79 1979 Dec; 9(12):46–48.

Christianson F. Closed wound irrigation in orthopedics. ONA J Sept 1979; 6(9):359–366.

Ho G and Su E. Therapy for septic arthritis. JAMA 1982 Feb 12; 247(6):797–800.

Kirchner P and Simon M. Radioisotopic evaluation of skeletal disease. J Bone Joint Surg [Am] 1981 Apr; 63-A(4):673–681.

McCarty D. Editorial: Joint sepsis: A chance for cure. JAMA 1982 Feb 12; 247(6):835.

The oral approach to bone infection. Emergency Medicine 1980 Oct 15; 12(17):115–118.

Bone Tumors

Alemany H et al. Femoral allograft. Can Nurs 1979 Oct; 75(10):32–35.

Cores E and Holland J. Adjunctive chemotherapy for primary osteogenic sarcoma. Surg Clin North Am 1981 Dec; 61(6):1391–1404.

Eilber F. Adjunctive treatment of osteosarcoma. Surg Clin North Am 1981 Dec; 61(6):1371–1378.

Enneking W et al. Autogenous cortical bone grafts in the reconstruction of segmental skeletal defects. J Bone Joint Surg [Am] 1980 Oct; 62-A(7):1039–1057.

Goorin A et al. Adjunctive chemotherapy for osteosarcoma: A decade of experience. Surg Clin North Am 1981 Dec; 61(6):1379–1389.

Lewitt D. Multiple myeloma. Am J Nurs 1981 July; 81(7):1345–1347.

Rosenberg S. Treatment of soft tissue and bone sarcomas: Review of studies at the National Cancer Institute. Natl Cancer Inst Monogr 1981 Apr; 56:241–244.

Sim F. Total joint arthroplasty. Applications in the management of bone tumors. Mayo Clin Proc 1979 Sept; 54(9):583–589.

Unit XVII

Other Acute Problems

63

Management of Patients With Infectious Diseases

▷ The Challenge of Infectious Diseases

Infectious diseases are still the major health problem of the vast majority of people inhabiting the earth. In the developing countries, the principal causes of death are infectious and parasitic diseases that drain the capabilities of humans to work and to learn. Thus, the conquering of these diseases is necessary for economic self-sufficiency and national development. In the industrialized countries, the mortality from infectious diseases has declined dramatically, but these diseases represent the most frequent problems requiring professional attention, accounting for a large portion of the cost of health care.

Although many infectious diseases have been conquered, new and emerging problems have been created. Sexually transmitted diseases are among the most common infectious diseases in the U.S. There is an increase in the number of organisms that have developed resistance to a variety of available antimicrobials. Then, too, there is a rapidly growing number of people whose normal host defenses have been compromised by immunosuppressive therapy related to other disorders. Included in this group would be elderly persons with impaired defenses. As a result, they are susceptible to organisms that are considered minimally pathogenic.

On the other hand, the advances in modern medicine have led to the development of more antimicrobial drugs and the ability to cultivate viruses in tissue cultures, as well as an increased knowledge about immunity.

▷ The Infectious Process

Epidemiology is the science concerned with the study of the history and occurrence of a disease, along with those factors that may directly or indirectly favor the development of a disease (Table 63-1).

A chain of events is necessary for the continual spread of an infectious disease, beginning with a *causative agent* or invading organism, which may be bacterial, viral, rickettsial, protozoal, fungal, or helminthic. Infection by each

(Text continues on page 1485)

Table 63-1
Epidemiology, Therapy, and Control of Communicable Infections

Disease	Infective Organism	Infectious Sources	Entry Site	Method of Spread	Incubation Period	Chemotherapy*	Prophylaxis
Amebiasis	*Entamoeba histolytica*	Contaminated water and food	Gastrointestinal tract	Patients and carriers; fecal–oral route; oral and sexual contact	Variable	Metronidazole; emetine; chloroquine; iodoquinol; chlortetracycline	Detection of carriers and their removal from food handling; plumbing safeguards
Bacillary dysentery (Shigellosis)	*Shigella* group	Contaminated water and food	Gastrointestinal tract	Patients and carriers; fecal–oral route	24–48 hours	Ampicillin; chloramphenicol; tetracycline; Sulfa-trimethoprim	Detection and control of carriers; inspection of food handlers; decontamination of water supplies
Brucellosis	*Brucella melitensis* and related organisms	Milk, meat, tissues, blood, and absorbed fetuses and placentas from infected cattle, goats, horses, and pigs	Gastrointestinal tract	Ingestion of or contact with infective material	5–30 days (variable)	Tetracycline and streptomycin or chloramphenicol	Milk pasteurization; control of infection in animals
Chancroid	*Haemophilus ducreyi*	Human cases and carriers	Genitalia	Direct sexual contact	3–5 days	Sulfonamides; streptomycin; tetracycline	Effective case-finding and treatment of infection
Chickenpox (Varicella)	Virus	Human cases	Probably nasopharynx	Probably respiratory droplets	14–16 days	None	Varicella-zoster immune globulin (VZIG) to high-risk susceptible children exposed to varicella zoster within 72 hours
Diphtheria	*Corynebacterium diphtheriae*	Human cases and carriers; fomites; raw milk	Nasopharynx	Nasal and oral secretions; respiratory droplets	2–5 days	Diphtheria antitoxin; penicillin; erythromycin	Active immunization with diphtheria toxoid
Encephalitis, epidemic (eastern and western equine)	Viruses	Chicken and wild-bird mites; horses; hibernating garter snakes	Skin	Mosquitoes	Variable	None	Eastern equine encephalitis vaccine, dried

(continued)

Table 63-1
Epidemiology, Therapy, and Control of Communicable Infections (continued)

Disease	Infective Organism	Infectious Sources	Entry Site	Method of Spread	Incubation Period	Chemotherapy*	Prophylaxis
Gonorrhea	*Neisseria gonorrhoeae*	Urethral and vaginal secretions	Urethral or vaginal mucosa; pharynx; rectum	Sexual activity	2–7 days	Aqueous Procaine Penicillin G, preceded by probenecid or alternative regimen outlined by Public Health Service	Examination culture; treatment of sexual partners
Granuloma inguinale	*Calymmatobacterium granulomatis*	Infectious exudate	External genitalia; cervix	Sexual intercourse	Unknown, presumably 8–80 days	Tetracyclines; trimethoprim–sulfamethoxazole	Chemotherapy of carriers and contacts; case-finding and treatment of patients
Infectious mononucleosis	Epstein–Barr virus	Human cases and carriers	Mouth	Probably oral–pharyngeal route; via blood transfusion in susceptible recipients	2–6 weeks	None	None
Influenza	Virus	Human cases	Respiratory tract	Respiratory	24–72 hours	Amantadine; rimantadine	Specific virus vaccine
Lymphogranuloma venereum	*Chlamydia trachomatis*	Human cases	External genitalia; urethral or vaginal mucosa	Sexual intercourse; indirect contact with contaminated articles/clothing	5–21 days	Tetracyclines	Case-finding and treatment of infection
Malaria	*Plasmodium vivax, falciparum, malariae,* and *ovale*	Human cases	Skin	Mosquitoes (*Anopheles*)	Variable, depending on strain	Chloroquine; primaquine; amodiaquine; quinine; proguanil	Coordinated measures for wide-scale mosquito control; prompt detection and effective treatment of cases; suppressive drugs in malarious areas
Measles	Virus	Human cases	Respiratory mucosa	Nasopharyngeal secretions	8–13 days	None	Measles vaccine

(continued)

Table 63-1
Epidemiology, Therapy, and Control of Communicable Infections (continued)

Disease	Infective Organism	Infectious Sources	Entry Site	Method of Spread	Incubation Period	Chemotherapy*	Prophylaxis
Meningococcal meningitis	*Neisseria meningitidis*	Human cases and carriers	Nasopharynx; tonsils	Respiratory droplets	2–10 days	Penicillin; chloramphenicol	Meningococcal polysaccharide vaccine to persons at risk; rifampin/sulfadiazine for carriers or contacts
Mumps	Virus	Human cases (early)	Upper respiratory tract	Respiratory droplets	12–26 days (avg. 18 days)	None	Live mumps vaccine
Paratyphoid fever	*Salmonella paratyphi A and B* and related organisms	Contaminated food, milk, water; rectal tubes; barium enemas	Gastrointestinal tract	Infected urine and feces	7–24 days	Chloramphenicol; ampicillin; sulfatrimethoprim	Control of public water sources, food vendors, food handlers; treatment of carriers
Pneumococcal pneumonia	*Streptococcus pneumoniae*	Human carriers; patient's own pharynx	Respiratory mucosa	Respiratory droplets	Variable	Penicillin	Polyvalent pneumococcal vaccine; control of upper respiratory infections; avoidance of alcoholic intoxication
Poliomyelitis	Polioviruses (types I, II, III)	Human cases and carriers	Gastrointestinal tract	Infected feces; pharyngeal secretions	7–12 days	None	Oral polio vaccine (OPV), the live attenuated vaccine containing all three strains of poliovirus—produces long-lasting immunity in most recipients
Rocky Mountain spotted fever	*Rickettsia rickettsii*	Infected wild rodents, dogs, wood ticks, dog ticks	Skin	Tick bites	3–10 days	Tetracyclines; chloramphenicol	Avoidance of tick-infected areas, or wearing of protective clothing in such areas; frequent search for, and prompt removal of, ticks from body; specific vaccination of exposed persons

(continued)

Table 63-1
Epidemiology, Therapy, and Control of Communicable Infections (continued)

Disease	Infective Organism	Infectious Sources	Entry Site	Method of Spread	Incubation Period	Chemotherapy*	Prophylaxis
Rubella (german measles)	Virus	Human cases	Respiratory mucosa	Nasopharyngeal secretions	14–21 days	None	Rubella virus vaccine; immune serum globulin (human) given to contacts of rubella; rubella in early stages of pregnancy legally recognized as indication for abortion
Scarlet fever	Group A streptococcus	Human cases; infected food	Pharynx	Nasal and oral secretions	3–5 days	Penicillin	Isolation; prophylactic chemotherapy with penicillin; asepsis during obstetric procedures; specific chemoprophylaxis for persons with rheumatic fever
Syphilis	*Treponema pallidum*	Infected exudate or blood	External genitalia; cervix; mucosal surfaces; placenta	Sexual activity; contact with open lesions; blood transfusion; transplacental inoculation	10–70 days	Penicillin; erythromycin; tetracycline	Case-finding by means of routine serologic testing and other methods; adequate treatment of infected individuals
Tetanus	*Clostridium tetani*	Contaminated soil	Penetrating and crush wounds	Horse and cattle feces	4–21 days (avg. 10 days)	Tetanus immune globulin (human) [TIG] and penicillin	Wound debridement; toxoid booster injections for patients previously immunized; tetanus toxoid and tetanus immune globulin (separate sites and separate syringes) for nonimmune persons

(continued)

Table 63-1
Epidemiology, Therapy, and Control of Communicable Infections (continued)

Disease	Infective Organism	Infectious Sources	Entry Site	Method of Spread	Incubation Period	Chemotherapy*	Prophylaxis
Trichinosis	Trichinella spiralis	Infected pigs	Gastrointestinal tract	Ingestion of infected pork, undercooked	2–28 days	Steroids; thiabendazole	Regulation of hog breeders; adequate meat inspection; thorough cooking of pork
Tuberculosis	Mycobacterium tuberculosis	Sputum from human cases; milk from infected cows (rare in U.S.)	Respiratory mucosa	Sputum; respiratory droplets	Variable	Isoniazid; ethambutol; rifampin; streptomycin; pyrazinamide	Early discovery and adequate treatment of active cases; milk pasteurization
Tularemia	Francisella tularensis	Wild rodents and rabbits	Eyes; skin; gastrointestinal tract	Handling infected animals; ingestion of undercooked, infected meat; drinking contaminated water; bites from infected flies, ticks	1–10 days	Streptomycin; tetracyclines; chloramphenicol	Use of rubber gloves when skinning/handling potentially infectious wild animals; avoidance of contact with potentially infected rodents; adequate cooking of wild rabbit dishes; vaccination of hunters, butchers, laboratory workers risking heavy exposure
Typhoid Fever	Salmonella typhi	Contaminated food and water	Gastrointestinal tract	Infected urine and feces	1–3 weeks	Chloramphenicol; ampicillin; sulfa-trimethoprim	Decontamination of water sources; milk pasteurization; individual vaccination of high-risk persons; control of carriers
Typhus, endemic	Rickettsia typhi (mooseri)	Infected rodents	Skin	Flea bites	1–2 weeks	Tetracyclines; chloramphenicol	Delousing procedures; case quarantine
Whooping cough (pertussis)	Bordetella pertussis	Human cases	Respiratory tract	Infected bronchial secretions	Commonly 7 days	Erythromycin; ampicillin	Active immunization with vaccine; case isolation

* Research developments produce changes in drug therapy. The reader is referred to drug brochures and digests to keep abreast of changing dosages and uses.

type of organism gives rise to specific reactions in the infected organism.

The second link in the chain is a *reservoir*—a place for the invading organisms to live and multiply. The reservoir is the environment in which the agent is found, whether it be human, arthropod, plant, soil, or inanimate matter; for example, humans are the reservoir for syphilis, soil is the reservoir for tetanus, and animals are the reservoir for brucellosis. In humans, infectious diseases most often arise from contact with infected persons.

The next link is the *mode of escape* from the reservoir, including various body systems, such as the respiratory tract (most common when the reservoir is a human), intestinal tract, and genitourinary tract; open lesions; or mechanical escape, including the bite of insects.

After the infectious organism has escaped from its reservoir, it is dangerous only if it finds a way of reaching a host. This *mode of transmission* (the next link) may be direct (person-to-person contact, exposure to animal bite, exposure to droplet spray) or indirect (transfer without close contact, usually from an intermediate vehicle, such as water, serum, contaminated fomites). An example of an organism spread by indirect transmission would be the typhoid bacillus, which is able to survive for a long period of time outside the body. Disease may also be transmitted by the vehicle route (contaminated food, water, drugs, blood), by air (droplets), or by vector (arthropod).

The fifth link in the chain is the *mode of entry* of organisms into the human body. These correspond somewhat to the mode of escape and include the respiratory tract, gastrointestinal tract, direct infection of mucous membranes, or infection through a break in the skin.

The sixth link in the chain is a *susceptible host.* The presence of an infectious agent does not inevitably produce disease. Whether or not the person becomes ill following the entrance of infectious organisms into the body depends on numerous factors, including the number of organisms; the duration of the exposure; the person's age and general physical, mental, and emotional health and nutritional state; the status of the hematopoietic system; the absence of immunoglobulins (or the presence of abnormal immunoglobulins); and the number of T-lymphocytes and their ability to function.

Removing one link in the chain of the infectious process controls infections, which is the purpose of all public health measures.

See Chart 63-1 for a glossary of infectious disease terms.

▷ Reporting of Disease

When a communicable disease occurs in the community, the practicing physician has the legal responsibility of reporting its occurrence to the local health department. The method of reporting may be by telephone, telegraph, or a special written form provided for the purpose. The local health department forwards this information to the state health department, which transmits weekly reports to the Centers for Disease Control in Atlanta, Georgia, where data about communicable and chronic disease are compiled and

published in the *Morbidity and Mortality Weekly Report.* This publication provides an up-to-date picture of epidemiologic notes, trends, and reports and feeds back this information to local health departments. Thus, the occurrence of any local communicable disease becomes part of a huge network of health surveillance. The Centers for Disease Control operations include epidemiology and disease surveillance, laboratory methods, health education, organized disease prevention, and control programming and training.

Among the most frequently reported cases of specified notifiable diseases in the United States are gonorrhea, chickenpox, syphilis, measles, tuberculosis, hepatitis A, salmonellosis, mumps, rubella, hepatitis B, and shigellosis.

The World Health Organization receives data about communicable diseases from all countries. Regional epidemiologists keep a careful watch on regional disease trends and disseminate this information to the appropriate individuals and services within the various countries. Computers are used to help in this rapid dissemination of information.

Diseases subject to international health regulation are cholera, yellow fever, plague, and smallpox. Other diseases receiving emphasis in global surveillance include influenza, poliomyelitis, measles, German measles, sexually transmitted diseases, malaria, relapsing fever, and typhus. Health problems vary from country to country, as do the available medical personnel and financial resources necessary to carry out effective surveillance programs. Only through unrelenting vigilance will it be possible to predict outbreaks of disease and take countermeasures for their control.

▷ Assessment

Many early symptoms of infectious diseases are nonspecific. The illness may begin with malaise and all its attendant sequelae—listlessness, light-headedness, headache, anorexia, arthralgia, and weight loss. As the disease progresses, there is usually fever, although elderly people, in general, do not have as vigorous a febrile response as younger people. Nor will patients who have previously received antibiotics or are taking immunosuppressive agents exhibit fever. Fever may be preceded by a chill in certain infections, such as bacterial pneumonia, streptococcal infection, and influenza. Repeated chills may be seen in the course of fevers caused by bacteremias and in certain other infections, such as malaria.

The first step in identifying an infectious disease is to try to find out the *order and progression* of symptoms:

- Has the patient had a local or systemic infection?
- History of travel?
- Any contact with animals or animal products—raw wool, animal hides, blood?
- Has he had an animal or insect bite, cat scratch, exposure to birds?
- In addition, it is important to determine if the patient has a systemic disease that compromises host defenses, such as chronic renal disease or malignant disease (especially the leukemias and lymphomas), or if immunosuppressive agents or steroids are being taken, which increase susceptibility to infection.

Chart 63-1
Glossary of Infectious Disease Terms

Antigen—agent that is capable of producing antibodies when introduced into the body of a susceptible person

Antiserum—a serum containing antibodies given to provide immunity against a specific disease. Usually regarded as temporary protection

Attenuation—the weakening of the toxicity or virulence of an infectious agent

Bacteremia—presence of bacteria in the circulating blood

Bactericidal—lethal or killing to bacteria

Carrier—one who harbors an infectious agent causing a specific disease, although he gives no evidence of having the disease

Case—a particular instance of disease

Communicable—transmissible from person to person, directly or indirectly

Contact—a person known or believed to have been exposed to an infectious disease

Contaminated—persons or objects that have come in contact with infectious agents or materials

Disinfection—destruction (or render inert) of pathogenic organisms by chemical or physical means

Endemic—a disease occurring habitually within a given geographic area

Endogenous infection—infection caused by microbes derived from the host's own flora

Epidemic—a disease attacking many people in a community simultaneously

Exanthem—an eruption on the skin

Exogenous infection—infection caused by microbes derived from outside the host

Fomites—inanimate vehicles other than food, milk, water, and air that may harbor or be the means of transmission of organisms

Immune—protected against disease

Incubation period—the development of an infection from the time it gains entry into the body until the appearance of the first signs and symptoms

Infectious—capable of causing infection or disease

Infestation—invasion of body by arthropods; including insects, mites, mosquitoes, and ticks, and by helminths

In vitro—within the test tube

In vivo—within a living body

Isolation—procedures directed toward separating one patient from persons

Morbidity rate—the number of illnesses compared to the population. The rate may be measured in *incidence* or *prevalence: incidence*—the number of cases occurring in the population in a year; *prevalence*—the average number of cases existing in the population

Mortality rate—the number of deaths compared to the population

Nosocomial infection—infection acquired during hospitalization; not present or incubating at the time of admission to hospital

Pandemic—disease affecting a large portion of the population; extensive epidemic

Pathogenic—disease-producing

Prodromal—symptoms occurring at the beginning stage of the disease

Prophylaxis—measures taken to prevent disease

Surveillance—dynamic system of collecting, tabulating, analyzing, and reporting data on the occurrence and distribution of disease.

Toxin—a poisonous substance produced by bacterial action

Toxoid—a modified toxin capable of stimulating the production of antibodies

Vaccine—a suspension of attenuated or killed microorganisms given to build up an active immunity against an infectious disease

The physical examination helps in identifying infectious diseases, since many physical findings are diagnostic. An inflamed throat and enlarged lymph glands are compatible with a number of infectious diseases. Characteristic skin rashes and lesions may be present and may be pointed out by the patient who complains "Look at this rash!"

Laboratory examination of exudates (pus, sputum, wound swabbings), body fluids (urine, cerebrospinal fluid, synovial fluid), and tissues (blood, bone marrow) is often essential in the diagnosis of infections.

▷ **Principles of Management in Infectious Diseases**

The management of a patient with any of the infectious diseases requires an understanding of the following information:

1. What is the nature of the infecting organism?
2. Where is this organism habored in the host (*i.e.,* the carrier or patient)?
3. How is the pathogen disseminated by the host?
4. What is the principal portal of entry for this organism?
5. How does the infective agent survive outside the host (*i.e.,* under what circumstances), and how long is it likely to survive?
6. How is immunity to this agent acquired or conferred, and how long is it effective?
7. What precautions or isolation techniques are indicated while caring for a patient with this infection?

Isolation Procedures

The purposes of isolation techniques in health care facilities are to prevent the spread of the infectious agent and to protect the patient, personnel, and visitors from infection. A committee of experts of the Centers for Disease Control reviewed the isolation techniques for hospitalized persons with infectious diseases and established recommended procedures for isolating the disease—not the patient (Chart 63-2).

All isolation techniques fall into one of the following categories:

> Strict isolation
> Respiratory isolation
> Protective isolation
> Enteric precautions
> Wound and skin precautions
> Discharge precautions
> Blood precautions

The principles of isolation can be applied in almost any health care facility, including hospitals, extended care fa-cilities, and mental health facilities, although the specific techniques may need to be modified.

Protective (or reverse) isolation is carried out to protect patients with decreased resistance to disease.

- Patients requiring protective isolation include those with agranulocytosis, those receiving immunosuppressive drugs and large doses of radiation, and certain patients with lymphomas and leukemias.

The objective is to maintain a level of asepsis similar to that of the operating room. The patient is placed in a clean single room with bath. All personnel and visitors wear clean caps and sterile masks and gowns in the room. Gloves are worn by all persons having direct contact with the patient. Everything touching the patient should be either clean or

(Text continues on page 1490)

Chart 63-2
Classification of Infectious Diseases Requiring Isolation or Precautions

Strict Isolation

Private room—*necessary;* door must be kept closed
Gowns—must be worn by all persons entering room
Masks—must be worn by all persons entering room
Hands—must be washed on entering and leaving room
Gloves—must be worn by all persons entering room
Articles—must be discarded or wrapped before being sent to Central Supply for disinfection or sterilization

Diseases Requiring Strict Isolation*
1. Anthrax, inhalation
2. Burn wounds (major) infected with *Staphylococcus aureus* or group A streptococcus
3. Congenital rubella syndrome
4. Diphtheria (pharyngeal or cutaneous)
5. Disseminated neonatal *Herpesvirus hominis* infection (herpes simplex)
6. Herpes zoster, disseminated
7. Lassa fever
8. Marburg virus disease
9. Plague, pneumonic
10. Pneumonia, *Staphylococcus aureus*, or group A streptococcus
11. Rabies
12. Skin infection (major) infected with *Staphylococcus aureus* or group A streptococcus
13. Smallpox
14. Vaccinia (generalized and progressive, and eczema vaccinatum)
15. Varicella (chickenpox)

Respiratory Isolation

Private Room—*necessary;* door must be kept closed
Gowns—not necessary

Masks—must be worn by any person entering room unless that person is not susceptible to the disease
Hands—must be washed on entering and leaving room
Gloves—not necessary
Articles—those contaminated with secretions must be disinfected

Diseases Requiring Respiratory Isolation*
1. Measles (rubeola)
2. Meningococcal meningitis
3. Meningococcemia
4. Mumps
5. Pertussis (whooping cough)
6. Rubella (German measles)
7. Tuberculosis, pulmonary—including tuberculosis of the respiratory tract, suspected or sputum-positive (smear)

Protective Isolation

Private room—*necessary;* door must be kept closed
Gowns—must be worn by all persons entering room
Masks—must be worn by all persons entering room
Hands—must be washed on entering and leaving room
Gloves—must be worn by all persons having direct contact with patient
Articles—See *Isolation Techniques for Use in Hospitals.*

Conditions That May Require Protective Isolation*
1. Agranulocytosis
2. Dermatitis; noninfected vesicular, bullous, or eczematous disease, when severe and extensive
3. Extensive, noninfected burns in certain patients
4. Lymphomas and leukemia in certain patients (especially in the late stages of Hodgkin's disease and acute leukemia)

(continued)

Chart 63-2
Classification of Infectious Diseases Requiring Isolation or Precautions (continued)

Enteric Precautions

Private room—*necessary for children only*
Gowns—must be worn by all persons having direct contact with patient
Masks—not necessary
Hands—must be washed on entering and leaving room
Gloves—must be worn by all persons having direct contact with patient or with articles contaminated with fecal material
Articles—special precautions necessary for articles contaminated with urine and feces. Articles must be disinfected or discarded.

Diseases Requiring Enteric Precautions*

1. Cholera
2. Diarrhea, acute illness with suspected infectious etiology
3. Enterocolitis, staphylococcal
4. Gastroenteritis caused by:
   Enteropathogenic or enterotoxic *Escherichia coli*
   Salmonella species
   Shigella species
   Yersinia enterocolitica
5. Hepatitis, viral, type A, B, or unspecified
6. Typhoid fever (*Salmonella typhi*)

Wound and Skin Precautions

Private room—desirable
Gowns—must be worn by all persons having direct contact with patient
Masks—not necessary except during dressing changes
Hands—must be washed on entering and leaving room
Gloves—must be worn by all persons having direct contact with infected area
Articles—special precautions necessary for instruments, dressings, and linen

Diseases Requiring Wound and Skin Precautions*

1. Burns that are infected, except those infected with *Staphylococcus aureus* or group A streptococcus that are not covered or not adequately contained by dressings (see Strict Isolation)
2. Gas gangrene (due to *Clostridium perfringens*)
3. Herpes zoster, localized
4. Melioidosis, extrapulmonary with draining sinuses
5. Plague, bubonic
6. Puerperal sepsis—group A streptococcus, vaginal discharge
7. Wound and skin infections that are not covered by dressings or that have copious purulent drainage that is not contained by dressings, except those infected with *Staphylococcus aureus* or group A streptococcus, which require strict isolation

8. Wound and skin infections that are covered by dressings so that the discharge is adequately contained, including those infected with *Staphylococcus aureus* or group A streptococcus; minor wound infections, such as stitch abscesses, need only secretion precautions

Discharge Precautions

A. Secretion Precautions—Lesions

1. Use a "no-touch" dressing technique (do not touch the wound or dressings with the hands) when changing dressings on these lesions.
2. Employ proper handwashing procedures.
3. Wash hands before and after patient contact; use sterile equipment when changing dressings; double-bag soiled dressings and equipment.
4. These precautions apply only with lesions from which there is a discharge.

Diseases; Duration of Precautions

1. Actinomycosis, draining lesions—for duration of drainage
2. Anthrax, cutaneous—until culture-negative
3. Brucellosis, draining lesions—for duration of drainage
4. Burn, skin, and wound infections, minor—for duration of drainage
5. Candidiasis, mucocutaneous—for duration of illness
6. Coccidioidomycosis, draining lesion—for duration of drainage
7. Conjunctivitis, acute bacterial (including gonococcal)—until 24 hours after start of effective therapy
8. Conjunctivitis, viral—for duration of illness
9. Gonococcal ophthalmia neonatorum—until 24 hours after start of effective therapy
10. Gonorrhea—until 24 hours after start of effective therapy
11. Granuloma inguinale—for duration of illness
12. *Herpesvirus hominis* (herpes simplex), except disseminated neonatal disease—for duration of illness. For disseminated neonatal disease, see Strict Isolation; for oral *H. hominis* disease, see Secretion Precautions, Oral.
13. Keratoconjunctivitis, infectious—for duration of illness
14. Listeriosis—for duration of illness
15. Lymphogranuloma venereum—for duration of illness
16. Nocardiosis, draining lesions—for duration of illness
17. Orf—for duration of illness
18. Syphilis, mucocutaneous—until 24 hours after start of effective therapy
19. Trachoma, acute—for duration of illness
20. Tuberculosis, extrapulmonary draining lesion—for duration of drainage
21. Tularemia, draining lesion—for duration of drainage

(continued)

Chart 63-2
Classification of Infectious Diseases Requiring Isolation or Precautions (continued)

B. Secretion Precautions—Oral

1. The diseases listed in this section can be spread to susceptible persons by contact with oral secretions.
2. Attention should be given to the proper disposal of oral secretions to prevent spread of infection.
3. Instruct the patient to cough or spit into disposable tissues held close to the mouth; discard tissues in an impervious (impenetrable) bag at the bedside.
4. If the patient has nasotracheal suction or tracheostomy, the suction catheter and gloves should be placed in an impervious bag for disposal.
5. Seal the bag before discarding in the trash.

Diseases; Duration of Precautions

1. Herpangina—for duration of hospitalization
2. Herpes oralis—for duration of illness
3. Infectious mononucleosis—for duration of illness
4. Melioidosis, pulmonary—for duration of illness
5. Mycoplasma pneumonia—for duration of illness
6. Pneumonia, bacterial (if not covered elsewhere)—for duration of illness
7. Psittacosis—for duration of illness. (It may be desirable to place patient with acute psittacosis who is coughing and raising sputum in respiratory isolation.)
8. Q fever—for duration of illness
9. Respiratory infectious disease, acute (if not covered elsewhere)—for duration of illness
10. Scarlet fever—until 24 hours after start of effective therapy
11. Streptococcal pharyngitis—until 24 hours after start of effective therapy

C. Excretion Precautions

1. The diseases listed in this section can be spread to susceptible persons through the oral route by contact with fecal excretions from a person infected with the organism.
2. Strict attention should be paid to careful handwashing following any patient contact and especially following contact with excretions.
3. Instruct the patient on the necessity of careful handwashing after defecating.
4. Make sure there is proper sanitary disposal of excretions; a standard sewage system is adequate.

Diseases; Duration of Precautions

1. Amebiasis—for duration of illness
2. *Clostridium perfringens* (*C. welchii*) food poisoning—for duration of illness
3. Enterobiasis—for duration of illness
4. Giardiasis—for duration of illness

5. Hand, foot, and mouth disease—for duration of hospitalization
6. Herpangina—for duration of hospitalization
7. Infectious lymphocytosis—for duration of hospitalization
8. Leptospirosis (urine only)—for duration of hospitalization
9. Meningitis, aseptic—for duration of hospitalization
10. Pleurodynia—for duration of hospitalization
11. Poliomyelitis—for duration of hospitalization
12. Staphylococcal food poisoning—for duration of symptoms
13. Tapeworm disease (only with *Hymenolepsis nana* and *Taenia solium* [pork])—for duration of illness
14. Viral diseases, other (ECHO or Coxsackie gastroenteritis, pericarditis, myocarditis, meningitis)—for duration of hospitalization

D. Blood Precautions

1. The diseases in this category are associated with circulation of the etiologic agent in blood; be aware of the route of transmission.
2. Blood precautions should be taken for the duration of the clinical disease or for as long as the etiologic agent can be demonstrated in the blood. Blood precautions should be taken with anyone who is HB$_s$Ag-positive.
3. Disposable needles and syringes should be used for patients in isolation. They must not be reused.
4. Used needles need not be recapped; they should be placed in a prominently labeled, impervious, puncture-resistant container designated for this purpose. Needles should not be purposefully bent, because accidental needle puncture may occur.
5. Used syringes should be placed in an impervious bag. Both needle and syringe bags should be incinerated or autoclaved before discarding.
6. Rinse reusable needles and syringes thoroughly in cold water after use; place the needle in a puncture-resistant rigid container; wrap syringes and needles using double-bag technique and return to proper department for decontamination and sterilization.
7. These specifications pertain to needle and syringe precautions and to labeling of blood specimens. Label blood specimens with patient's diagnosis (so that necessary precautions will be taken).

Diseases; Duration of Precautions

1. Arthropod-borne viral fever (dengue, etc.)—for duration of hospitalization
2. Hepatitis, viral, type A, B, or unspecified (also listed under Enteric Precautions)—for duration of hospitalization
3. Malaria—for duration of hospitalization

* See *Isolation Techniques for Use in Hospitals* for details and recommended duration of isolation.
(From *Isolation Techniques for Use in Hospitals*, 2nd ed., U.S. Department of Health, Education and Welfare, Center for Disease Control, 1975.)

sterile. A more restricted environment (laminar airflow room), used to reduce colonization and infection in persons at great risk, is available in some areas.

The following considerations are applicable in the care of all patients with infectious diseases.

Handwashing. *Handwashing is the foundation of controlling infectious disease.* Handwashing can markedly reduce or eliminate hand carriage of pathogenic organisms, most of which are transient flora. A vigorous brief wash with soap under a stream of water is recommended to remove most transient flora. Antiseptics (product with antimicrobial activity designed for skin use) may be used for handwashing in isolation rooms, in the care of the newborn, and before invasive procedures.

Personnel should always wash their hands in the following instances: before performing invasive procedures, before and after contact with wounds, before contact with susceptible patients, after contact with a source that is likely to be contaminated with virulent organisms/hospital pathogens, and between patient contacts, especially those in special care units.

Gowns. Gowns are worn by *all* personnel when they enter the room of a patient with a disease that requires strict isolation and protective isolation, and are to be worn by those coming in direct contact with patients who require enteric, wound, and skin precautions. Gowns are to be used once (individual gown technique) and then discarded in an appropriate container before the user leaves the contaminated area. Clean, freshly laundered or disposable gowns should be available outside the isolation area. Sterile gowns are used for patients in protective isolation or for patients with extensive burns or wound infections.

Masks. When masks are used, they should be fabricated to filter out droplet nuclei and molded to fit tightly over the nose and mouth. A mask is discarded when moist and is not worn longer than an hour. Neither should the mask be lowered around the neck and then reused. It is discarded in a receptable before leaving the patient's room. Supplies of clean masks are kept outside of the isolation unit.

Gloves. Disposable (single-use) gloves are worn when the patient requires strict isolation; protective isolation; and enteric, wound, and skin precautions. In some instances, sterile gloves will be necessary. The gloves are changed after direct contact with the patient's excretions or secretions, even if the care of the patient has not been completed.

Dressings, Tissues, and Disposable Items. For the safe disposal of oral and nasal discharges, the patient is supplied with paper tissues and a disposable paper bag at his bedside. Disposable sputum cups with tops are to be provided, and the patient is instructed in their proper use. All disposable supplies, including tissues, sputum cups, and contaminated dressings, as well as disposable drinking cups, dishes, and utensils, and table wastes wrapped in paper, are to be collected at frequent intervals and placed in a large plastic bag (securely sealed) for burning. Burning is the most effective method of destroying organisms.

Urine and Feces. Each patient should have his own bedpan and urinal; disposable ones, which can be placed in a bag and incinerated upon the patient's discharge, are preferable. If the bedpan is not disposable, it is cleaned and *autoclaved* when the patient is discharged. In most institutions, the sanitary facilities permit disposal of all excreta through the public sewage system that serves the hospital. However, in countries where such facilities are not available, all stools, urine, vomitus, and liquid food waste should be pooled in a covered can containing a disinfectant solution, such as 5% chlorinated lime or 5% creosol, and allowed to stand for an hour before they are emptied into the sewage system. Feces should be broken up into fine particles, so that the lime comes in contact with all parts.

Linen. Contaminated bed linen should be collected and enclosed securely in a color-coded bag that is removed from the room and enclosed in a second clean bag marked "contaminated." All contaminated clothing and linen should be sterilized by autoclaving before they are laundered with noninfectious goods. In the home, linens may be thoroughly washed with soap or detergent and *hot* water.

Instruments and Equipment. Objects contaminated with infectious materials or from patients in certain types of isolation should be wrapped in impervious plastic, marked "Contaminated," and sent to Central Supply for decontamination and disinfection or sterilization. This decreases exposure of personnel to infectious organisms. Gas sterilization (ethylene oxide) is used in the sterilization of many items that cannot be autoclaved. Disposable syringes, needles, and other equipment are available commercially and are recommended for use whenever possible. Used needles should be placed in labeled, impervious, puncture-resistant containers. Avoid bending or breaking needles by hand because of the danger of accidental puncture.

Environmental Control. Microorganisms on the floor or other surfaces become air-borne during sweeping, dry mopping, and dusting, and when mechanical buffers and unfiltered vacuum cleaners are used. Such practices should be avoided, and housekeeping personnel should be instructed in the proper methods of maintaining a clean environment. Since bedmaking contributes to the bacteriologic pollution of hospital air, avoid shaking bed linens. Proper ventilation also is essential; the persistence of odors suggests poor ventilation. The patient's door is to be kept closed, and an effective artificial ventilating system used (*i.e.,* one that takes the room air to the outside).

The most effective way to remove dust is to use a damp cloth and a wet vacuum pick-up with a filtered exhaust system for the floor. If mops are used, disposable or freshly laundered and machine-dried mops and cleaning cloths are necessary. The mop head is to be changed at least every 4 hours. A dirty, wet mop merely serves as a brush to paint the floor with live bacteria. When disinfectant is used in the mop bucket, the soil and bacterial load can reach a heavy enough level to inactivate the disinfectant. The water in the mop bucket must be changed frequently, and the bucket disinfected before being refilled. The buckets are not used outside the isolation area. Painted walls and flat surfaces (other than floors) rarely present a contamination problem. A spray bottle of disinfectant should be used instead of a bucket.

Terminal cleaning of the room upon discharge of the patient includes incinerating disposable items, cleaning and bagging equipment for disinfection or sterilization in Central Supply, washing furniture and mattress covers, washing grossly soiled areas on walls, and wet vacuuming or mopping the floors by means of the double-bucket technique.

▷ Immunity

Immunity is the resistance that a person has against disease. Specific immunity to a particular organism implies that an individual either has generated the appropriate antibody in his own body or has received ready-made antibodies from another source. Immunity may be natural (not acquired through previous contact with the infectious agent) or acquired. Not much is known about the processes responsible for natural immunity or resistance. More is known about acquired immunity, which has been identified as being either active or passive.

Active Immunization. *Active immunization* is produced by natural or acquired stimulation, so that the body produces its own antibodies. It may result from clinical or subclinical infection (*e.g.,* the person "gets the disease"). Or it may be produced by administering live or killed microorganisms or their antigens or inactivated vaccines and toxoids.

Active immunization is the most important and effective tool in preventive medicine. It has been most effective with bacterial exotoxins (diphtherial and tetanus toxoids) and with viruses. Most live-virus vaccines produce antibody responses that consist of prompt (but transient) production of specific immunoglobulins (IgM followed by a sustained production of specific IgG). Live-virus vaccines may produce mild clinical illness, with fever and rash appearing in some patients.

Inactivated vaccines and toxoids give a less complete response after a single injection and may have to be administered in repeated doses according to a prescribed schedule for long-lasting IgG response and sustained protection against infection. Following injection with inactivated vaccines and toxoids, there may be a mild local reaction at the site of injection and occasional systemic symptoms of fever, malaise, and headache.

Active immunization agents that are available for adults include tetanus and diphtheria toxoid, adult-type tetanus toxoid, influenza virus vaccines, mumps virus vaccine, poliomyelitis vaccine, measles vaccine, rubella virus vaccine, hepatitis B vaccine, and pneumococcal pneumonia vaccine. Vaccines are also available for plague, rabies, typhoid, typhus, yellow fever, cholera, and smallpox.

Current recommendations for the use of vaccines and other biologicals used in the prevention of disease are available from the Public Health Service Advisory Committee on Immunization Practices, Centers for Disease Control, Atlanta, Georgia 30333. The recommendations are based on an analysis of the scientific evidence, weighing the benefits and the risks of protection against the effects of infectious or communicable diseases.

Passive Immunity. *Passive immunity* provides temporary protection to a disease and is produced by the injection of serum that contains antibodies that have been formed in another host. It is given for immediate but temporary protection against a disease when active immunizing agents are not available (*e.g.,* immune globulin for hepatitis A) or when there is insufficient time to acquire active immunization following exposure to disease. (Passive immunity is not totally satisfactory because of the risk inherent in providing antibodies of one animal to another.)

There are several types of preparations in use for passive immunity: standard immune globulin (for general use), special immune serum globulins with a known antibody content for specific illnesses, and animal serums or antitoxins. Products made with animal serum may cause an anaphylaxislike reaction or serum sickness. Therefore, products made with human serum are given whenever possible.

Immunization Programs. A national immunization program has been supported by federal legislation (Vaccination Assistance Act) to assist states and communities in carrying out intensive vaccination programs against poliomyelitis, diphtheria, pertussis, tetanus, measles, rubella, and other infectious diseases for which a preventive agent is available. Studies show that socially deprived and low-income groups do not receive the protection of immunization programs; this is a challenge to all health care professionals. A person's acceptance of this type of preventive care may help him to accept other medical services. Nurses, using gentle persuasion, can reach out and listen to the fears of the people and teach them the benefits of immunization.

See Chart 63-3 for nursing interventions for the patient with an infectious disease.

▷ Sexually Transmitted Diseases

Sexually transmitted diseases (STD) are spread by sexual activity and include venereal diseases (gonorrhea, syphilis) as well as nonspecific urethral and genital infections. There is also evidence that a new disease, AIDS (acquired immunity deficiency syndrome) may be transmitted in some instances by sexual activities. The term "sexually transmitted diseases" is replacing the phrase "venereal diseases" in most usage. In the United States, there is a virtual epidemic of STD with estimates of incidence ranging from 8.6 to 11.1 million cases annually, the bulk of which go unreported.

While sexually transmitted diseases, particularly gonorrhea and syphilis, have existed for centuries, the incidence of other STDs, such as those caused by *Chlamydia*, herpesvirus, mycoplasmas, and cytomegaloviruses, have greatly increased. More than 15 infectious diseases are now categorized as being sexually transmitted. This is due to the nature of varying sexual relationships (homosexuality; anogenital, oral-genital sexual practices), liberated attitudes, personal mobility, the large number of postwar babies reaching the peak age of sexual activity, the trend toward nonbarrier methods of contraception, and the problem in locating and bringing to treatment the "silent carriers" of these infections. Persons at high risk for acquiring STDs are sexual partners of infected persons, those with multiple sexual partners, and male homosexuals with multiple sex partners.

The problems and complications of these infections are challenging. STD frequently exists in asymptomatic individuals. Many of these diseases affect women without their

---

Chart 63-3
Nursing Summary: The Patient With an Infectious Disease

Goals and Interventions

A. To assist in identifying the etiologic agent and establishing the diagnosis
1. Obtain specimens of blood, urine, stools, sputum, throat swabbings, nasal secretions, and pyogenic exudates for bacteriologic study.
2. Assist in securing smears of blood and other materials for microscopic examination.
3. Assist with aspirations of spinal fluid, bone marrow, and other body fluids or tissues for cytologic, serologic, and bacteriologic tests.
4. Carry out appropriate skin tests for specific diagnostic reactions as directed.

B. To control the infection in the patient
1. Administer the appropriate antimicrobial agents as requested.
2. Assist in administering specific immune therapy, if available, employing immune antiserum, gamma globulin, antitoxin, toxoid, vaccine, or an appropriate mixture of antigen and antibody, depending on the circumstances.
3. Observe patient carefully for evidence of drug or serum sensitivity.

C. To prevent spread of the infection to others
1. Wash hands immediately after contact with each patient and after every contact with material that may be contaminated and potentially infectious.
2. Use gown as required by disease of patient.
   a. Use gown once and discard in proper receptacle.
   b. Collect linen in water-soluble bags; double-bag, and mark "ISOLATION."
3. Use gloves when indicated by the patient's condition.
   a. Disposable single-use gloves are preferable.
   b. Use once and discard in appropriate receptacle.
4. Handle needles and syringes with extreme care.
   a. Avoid breaking or bending the needle by hand after use.

   b. Place used needle/syringes in a labeled impervious puncture-resistant container. Place in a clean bag in the contaminated area and in a second clean bag outside the patient's room.
5. Disinfect and handle wastes with all due precautions.
6. Handle bed linens and fomites with care.
7. Carry out concurrent disinfection of fomites.
8. Control dissemination of infectious droplets.
   a. Encourage patient to cover nose and mouth when coughing or sneezing.
   b. Wrap contaminated tissues and articles in paper before disposal.
9. Control dust.
   a. Avoid creating aerosols and resuspension of dust—for example, shaking bed linens.
   b. Require damp dusting of furniture and wet vacuum cleaning of floors.
   c. Maintain cleanliness of surroundings; wash soil from walls as soon as it appears.
   d. Reduce to a minimum the activity of personnel in the patient's room.
10. Ventilate the patient's room properly with a system that directs room air to the outside.
   Keep the door to the room closed.

D. To protect the patient who is immunosuppressed or immune-incompetent (organ transplant, leukemia, etc.)
1. Use meticulous handwashing technique.
2. Use protective isolation or protective isolation units (life islands, laminar airflow units) if available.
3. Remember that every item in the room is potentially dangerous to the patient.
4. Some authorities suggest that flowers, plants, and water sources be removed from the patient's environment to decrease patient's contacts with bacteria and fungi that are associated with these items.

(continued)

---

knowledge. There is a high incidence of coinfection, and individuals with one STD are at risk for concurrent infection (*i.e.,* gonorrhea and chlamydial infections). Although the organisms causing some of these diseases are sensitive to antimicrobial therapy, there are other pathogens that are demonstrating levels of resistance to treatment. Another problem is that certain drugs used in treatment predispose to superinfection. Diseases that occur in genital mucosal areas may also occur in nongenital mucosal areas (pharynx) that are used for sexual activity.

Genital chlamydial infections (from *Chlamydial trachomatis*) are epidemic, causing nongonococcal urethritis and epididymitis in men, and mucopurulent cervicitis and an alarming increase in pelvic inflammatory disease in

women. Transmitted to the infant from an infected mother, chlamydial infections are a major cause of neonatal conjunctivitis and pneumonia in infants 1 to 3 months old. Chlamydial infections have been linked to infertility in both sexes, and have been associated with many other health problems. The control of these infections has become an important concern.

Genital herpes is among the most common and psychologically distressing STDs, affecting 5 to 10 million Americans with the number growing by nearly 500,000 a year. This condition is discussed on page 1047.

Homosexual males have an infectious disease profile that differs from the population as a whole. In addition to the more common STDs, they encounter a variety of enteric

Chart 63-3
Nursing Summary: The Patient With an Infectious Disease (continued)

Goals and Interventions (continued)

E. To provide physiologic support of the patient
1. Ensure adequate hydration in the face of excessive fluid loss through vomiting, diarrhea, or excessive sweating.
   a. Encourage liberal fluid intake.
   b. Prepare for the administration of intravenous fluids as required.
2. Reduce the fever when indicated.
   a. Administer antipyretic drugs, as prescribed.
   b. Employ tepid sponges cautiously, as indicated.
3. Measure and record body temperature, pulse, and respiratory rates frequently.
4. Measure arterial blood pressure at regular intervals if patient exhibits a tendency to vascular collapse.
5. Weigh patient periodically, preferably at same hour of day on same scale.

F. To provide symptomatic relief
1. Combat generalized aching and malaise.
   a. Utilize warm applications and massage, as indicated.
   b. Apply cold compresses for headache.
   c. Administer analgesic medications as prescribed.
   d. Attend to oral hygiene.
   e. Limit physical activity.
2. Relieve cough.
   a. Humidify inspired air.
   b. Administer warm gargles and throat irrigations.
   c. Supply expectorants or cough depressants as indicated and prescribed.
3. Relieve anxiety and depression.
   a. Employ a nonjudgmental approach to the patient with sexually transmitted disease.
   b. Recognize loneliness of the isolated patient.
   c. Lend strong encouragement to patient faced with prospect of prolonged convalescence.

G. To protect exposed individuals and public at large against infectious illness
1. Make available, facilitate, or perform whatever vaccination procedures are known to be effective and are indicated for the stimulation of active immunity in exposed and susceptible individuals.
2. Furnish specific immune serum (heterologous or human convalescent) or human gamma globulin, if indicated, to provide passive immunity and temporary protection to contacts who are particularly vulnerable.
3. Isolate patients with communicable infections, as well as known carriers and contacts, when required.
4. Educate the public with respect to:
   a. Availability and importance of prophylactic immunizations
   b. Manner in which infectious illnesses are spread and methods of avoiding spread
   c. Importance of seeking medical advice in the event of a febrile illness or skin eruption
   d. Importance of environmental cleanliness and personal hygiene
   e. Importance of adequate housing and nutrition
   f. Means of preventing the contamination of food and water supplies
      (1) Discipline, cleanliness, and inspection of food handlers
      (2) Dangers of "perishable" foods; the identity of foods that tend to promote bacterial growth; and methods of food preservation
      (3) Significance of milk pasteurization
      (4) Indications for, and methods of, sterilizing food by means of heat
      (5) Importance of meat inspection
   g. Knowledge of insect, rodent, and other animal vectors, and reservoirs of human infections, and importance of eliminating them

infections (hepatitis B, shigellosis, amebiasis, giardiasis), venereal warts, herpes virus infection, and gonococcal and nongonococcal urethritis. They also appear to have an increased incidence of acquired immune deficiency syndrome (see p. 1500). Male homosexuals have patterns of sexual behavior that contribute to the epidemiology and pathology of STDs. They tend to be relatively promiscuous, thereby increasing the pool of those susceptible to infection. The anonymous sexual behavior of some prevents identification of sexual contacts. Also, because there is no need to apply birth control devices (such as the condom, which can interfere with the spread of gonorrhea), the risk of acquiring infection is greater. Some do not seek medical care because of anxiety and societal attitudes. However, homosexual men

are beginning to recognize that STDs are their number one health problem.

Kaposi's sarcoma (KS) is a rare malignant neoplasm that is being seen in men with bisexual or homosexual preferences. There may be a prodromal period (weeks to months) of systemic symptoms, including weight loss, general malaise, and lymphadenopathy. Manifestations may start on the lower extremities as nontender purplish macules and papules that progress to plaques or nodular forms. Several of these patients have had severe opportunistic infections (*Pneumocystis carinii* pneumonia), often leading to death. An underlying immune deficiency appears to be the common denominator for the development of these opportunistic infections. Many newly diagnosed patients have a history of prior sexually transmitted diseases, suggesting that previous or concomitant infections may be related to the development of Kaposi's sarcoma in homosexual men.

STDs are a major health problem of women, as most of the severe complications are experienced by women. Genital herpes may be a precursor for cervical dysplasia and cancer. Pelvic inflammatory diseases (refers to diseases caused by acute ascending genital tract infections) are the most important complications of STDs and are now being recognized as having complex microbiology: gonococcus, chlamydia, mycoplasma, and a mixture of aerobic and anaerobic organisms. Although the economic costs have been estimated to be more than 600 million dollars annually, the human costs of infertility, ectopic pregnancy, and chronic pelvic pain produce untold misery. (Pelvic inflammatory disease is discussed on p. 1062.)

To check the transmission of these diseases, Ob–Gyn clinics, outpatient facilities, and emergency departments should be equipped to diagnose and treat these diseases. Women need to be informed that untreated male partners and multiple male sex partners increase the risk of developing these infections. The risk of infertility is greater with each subsequent recurrence of pelvic inflammatory disease. The use of barrier methods of contraception (condoms, diaphragm with spermicides) has a potential prophylactic value against various agents causing STD.

▶ Assessment

A sexual history including dates of exposure, symptoms, location of lesions/discharges, past history of STD, and self-treatment is taken. Discretion and a nonjudgmental approach must be used in inquiring about the patient's sexual orientation and alternative sexual life-styles. Although there are a variety of clinical manifestations, depending on the disease, the most common are dysuria and urethral or vaginal discharge. At the time the patient enters the health care system, every effort is made to learn the names of the patient's sex partners so they can be brought into treatment.

Patient Problems/Nursing Diagnoses

Based on the clinical manifestations, history, and diagnostic assessment data, the patient's major nursing problems include dysuria and urethral or vaginal discharge, rash, and ulcerative lesions related to infection by an STD; complications related to the invasive nature of these diseases; and potential for recurring infection related to nonadherence to the treatment regimen.

▶ Planning and Implementation

Goals

The patient's goals are:

1. Achievement of cure
2. Absence of complications
3. Prevention of recurrence

In addition, the major goal of the health professionals is to break the chain of contagion by removing (treating) all individuals from the infected pool. This means diligence in contact tracing, providing prophylactic treatment of sex contacts, and promoting self-protective behaviors in patients. Management of the major STDs are found in the discussions of gonorrhea and syphilis that follow.

▶ Evaluation

Expected Outcomes

1. Achieves a cure
   a. Adheres to treatment schedule
   b. Is free of dysuria and urethral/vaginal discharge
   c. Reports for follow-up examination for test for cure
2. Is free of complications
   a. Completes entire course of antimicrobial therapy
   b. Verbalizes that relapse may occur if therapy is aborted
   c. Verbalizes that untreated disease will cause complications
   d. Relates that the risk of infertility and complications is greater with each recurrence of acute pelvic infection
3. Actively participates in a program to prevent recurrence
   a. Identifies sexual partners for treatment
   b. Verbalizes that barrier methods of contraception offer some protection against STD
   c. Repeats symptoms of most common STDs
   d. Repeats the risk factors for recurrence: multiple sex partners, exposure with anonymous contacts, anal–oral sexual activity
   e. Inspects self for lesions/rashes
   f. Seeks treatment for genital infections promptly

Gonorrhea

Gonorrhea is an infection involving the mucosal surface of the genitourinary tract, rectum, and pharynx. It is caused by the gonococcus *Neisseria gonorrhoeae* and is an infectious disease that is transmitted sexually, the exception being gonococcal ophthalmia of the newborn. It may be acquired by sexual intercourse and by orogenital or anogenital contacts between members of the opposite sex as well as members of the same sex.

There is a worldwide increase of gonorrhea that continues to rise. In the United States, it is the most common reportable communicable disease. Although during the years 1965 to 1975 the number of reported cases of gonorrhea tripled, there has been no significant increase since 1975, which is due to the massive efforts of patients and health personnel engaged in preventing transmission of this disease.

One factor that contributes to the rapid spread of gonorrhea is its short incubation period. The problem is further compounded by the fact that there is a growing reservoir of asymptomatic silent carriers (both male and female) of gonorrhea and a growing trend toward nonbarrier methods of contraception. Barrier methods (condoms and vaginal spermicides) may prevent the spread of some sexually transmitted diseases. Gonococcal infection among homosexual males is becoming a major health problem (see p. 1492). In addition, gonorrhea frequently coexists with other sexually transmitted diseases.

The highest rate of gonorrhea occurs among persons between the ages of 20 and 24, followed by those between 15 and 19 years of age, with a rapid rise occurring in teenagers less than 15 years of age.

Pathophysiology. The gonococcus (*N. gonorrhoeae*) causes a surface infection, ascending, in almost all cases, by way of the lower genital tract. The primary infection takes place in or near the urethra in males, and in the cervix, urethra, or rectum in females. If drainage is good, it subsides spontaneously and clears in the course of a few days or weeks. However, infection of the prostatic urethra in the male and also of the female urethral and vaginal glands predisposes to chronic infection, with occasionally very serious sequelae. Females are apt to contract secondarily a mixed infection of the endometrium and, thereafter, of the tubes, constituting pelvic infection, with resultant pelvic peritonitis. The upward spread of the infection into the reproductive tract is precipitated by such factors as menstruation, douches, and the trauma associated with sexual intercourse or instrumentation.

▶ **Assessment**

Clinical Manifestations and Complications. In males, the incubation period lasts for 3 to 14 days, after which an acute anterior urethritis occurs, along with painful urination accompanied by mucopurulent urethral discharge. The infection may extend to involve the posterior urethra and spread to the prostate, seminal vesicles, and epididymis, causing prostatitis, inguinal lymphadenitis, pelvic pain, and fever. A major complication in men is urethritis and urethral stricture, with all its attendant problems—difficulty in voiding, delay in emptying the bladder, with subsequent infection, etc. Postgonococcal urethritis develops in one fourth to one third of men treated for gonorrhea. Many cases of nongonococcal urethritis are secondary to chlamydial infections. A particularly serious problem is that men may have asymptomatic infection ("silent clap") and are carriers of gonorrhea. These men are often not discovered by the usual gonorrhea control measures. They remain infected, untreated, and asymptomatic and can conceivably infect their sexual partners.

In females, the infection is very frequently silent, so that a large percentage of women are asymptomatic and unaware that they are infected. A small number have vaginal discharge, urinary frequency, and dysuria. The sites most frequently involved are the urethra and cervix. As the endocervical gonococcal infection spreads upward into the reproductive tract, it causes pelvic infection (pelvic inflammatory disease), with endometritis, salpingitis, or pelvic peritonitis. An estimated 10% to 17% of women infected with the gonococcus develop pelvic infection, as evidenced by abdominal pain, adnexal tenderness, fever, and vaginal discharge. Pelvic infection causes adhesions about the pelvic organs and rectum. This is a major direct cause of infertility. It also leads to ectopic pregnancy and chronic pelvic inflammation, the sequelae of which require surgical intervention.

Other Manifestations of Gonorrhea. *Anal manifestations* consist of anal itching and irritation (from erythema and edema of the anal crypts), a sensation of rectal fullness, rectal bleeding or diarrhea, mucus in the stools, and painful defecation. Anorectal gonorrhea is reported to be present in 28% to 55% of homosexual males attending sexually transmitted disease clinics.

Oral manifestations may be the result of the direct contact of the infecting organisms with the pharynx, or of their transmission to the oral cavity from infection elsewhere in the body. Although the majority of pharyngeal infections are asymptomatic, the following oral manifestations are seen: sore throat; painful, ulcerative inflammation of the lips; reddened, spongy, and tender gingivae; reddened, dry tongue; and redness and edema of the soft palate and uvula. The oropharynx may be covered with vesicles.

Systemic manifestations may become apparent, since secondary foci of infection may develop in any organ system, causing disseminated gonococcal infection (gonococcal bacteremia). Disseminated gonococcal infection occurs when the gonococci invade the bloodstream from one of the primary sites of infection. The patient presents with tenosynovitis of the small joints and hemorrhagic skin rash. Two to three weeks later, untreated patients will develop septic arthritis, exhibiting hot, red, and swollen joints.

Other systemic complications include gonococcal endocarditis, meningitis, and fulminant gonococcemia.

Physical Assessment. The patient is undressed and inspected for lesions; rashes; adenopathy; and urethral, vaginal, and rectal discharge.

Laboratory Evaluation. There are a variety of ways of identifying gonorrhea through laboratory diagnosis. The gram-negative intracellular diplococci may be found in smears or through direct fluorescent antibody tests, or may be cultured with selective media, such as modified Thayer–Martin media (TM), Martin–Lewis media (ML) or New York City media (NCY). The pharyngeal and anal sites should be cultured in persons who engage in oral or rectal sex, and these cultures should be inoculated on separate plates. In the male, specimens may be obtained from the urethra, anal canal, and pharynx depending on the patient's sexual history and orientation. In the female, cultures are collected from the endocervix and anal canal and are inoculated on separate plates. Sterile, disposable gloves are worn by the nurse when obtaining these cultures. (See Chart 63-4.)

To inoculate the culture plates, the cotton swab is rolled in a large "Z" pattern on the selective medium for transfer of organisms (Fig. 63-1). It is cross streaked immediately with a sterile wire loop or the tip of a swab, as streaking with a wire loop isolates colonies of *N. gonorrhoeae* from the few contaminants that occasionally grow on selective medium. The culture plate may be placed in a CO_2-enriched atmosphere (either a candle jar or CO_2 tablet/plastic bag system [Fig. 63-1]), as successful recovery of *N. gonorrhoeae* requires an atmosphere enriched with carbon dioxide. The plates are incubated at 35° C to 36° C (95° F–96.8° F).

Patient Problems/Nursing Diagnoses

Based on the clinical manifestations and diagnostic assessment, the patient's major nursing problems include urethral/vaginal discharge and urinary frequency related to infection by *N. gonorrhoeae;* and potential for complications related to noncompliance with the therapeutic regimen.

Chart 63-4
Obtaining Culture for Diagnosis of Gonorrhea

For Female Patient

Oropharynx Culture

Swab the posterior pharynx and tonsillar crypts with a cotton-tipped applicator.

Cervical Culture

1. Moisten vaginal speculum with warm water. Do not use any other lubricant.
2. Separate labia. Depress the perineum and posterior vaginal wall with the finger of one hand.
3. Gently insert a bivalve vaginal speculum.
4. Remove excessive cervical mucus with a cotton ball held in ring forceps.
5. Insert sterile cotton-tipped swab into endocervical canal (Fig. 63-1A).
   a. Move from side to side in cervix.
   b. Allow 30 seconds for absorption of organisms by the swab.

Anal Canal Culture (Rectal Culture)

1. Obtain anal specimen *after* getting cervical specimen.
2. Insert sterile cotton-tipped swab approximately 2.5 cm (1 inch) into the anal canal (Fig. 63-1B).
3. Move swab from side to side in anal canal.
4. Allow 10 to 30 seconds for absorption of organism by the swab.

For Male Patient

Oropharynx Culture

(Same as in women)

Urethral Culture

Use a sterile bacteriologic wire loop or a sterile calcium alginate urethral swab to obtain a specimen from the anterior urethra by gently scraping the mucosa (Fig. 63-1C). Do not insert loop or swab more than 2 cm

Anal Canal Culture

(Same as in women)

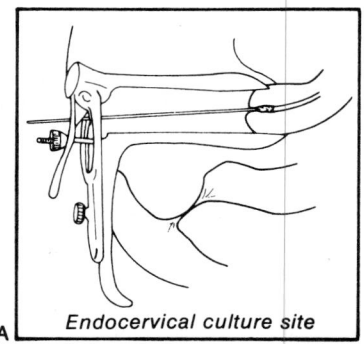

A   *Endocervical culture site*

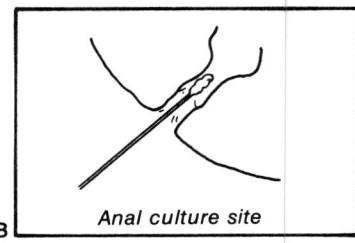

B   *Anal culture site*

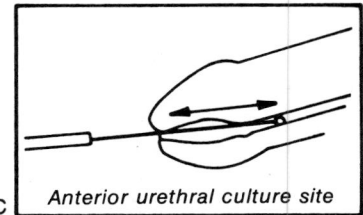

C   *Anterior urethral culture site*

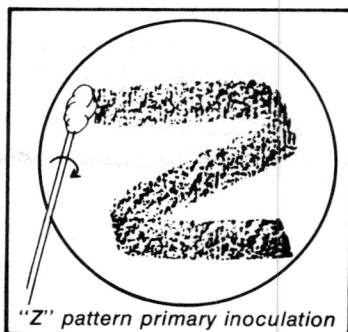

D   *"Z" pattern primary inoculation*

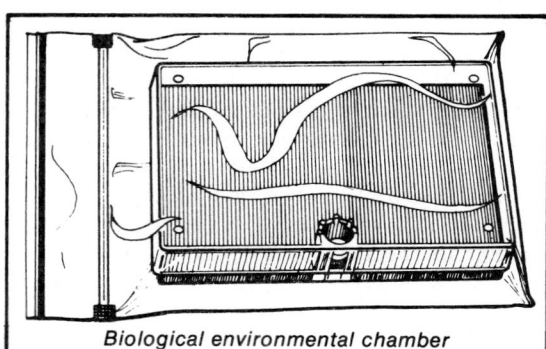

E   *Biological environmental chamber*

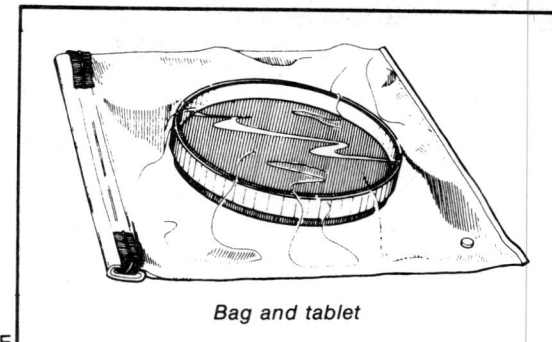

F   *Bag and tablet*

Figure 63-1. Obtaining culture for specimen in diagnosis of gonorrhea. (From Criteria and Techniques for the Diagnosis of Gonorrhea. U.S. Public Health Service, Center for Disease Control.)

► **Planning and Implementation**

Goals

The patient's goals are:

1. Cure of gonococcal infection
2. Prevention of complications

The objectives of treatment are to eradicate the organisms and educate the patient about his condition.

Interventions.   The goal of management is achieved through drug therapy, screening procedures, and patient education. Penicillin is the drug of choice, since it is effective, inexpensive, and will abort incubating syphilis. The patient should wait in the clinic 20 to 30 minutes after penicillin treatment in case of an anaphylactoid reaction. Each year a number of deaths occur from anaphylactic reactions to penicillin. Treatment schedules presently recommended by the Public Health Service are as follows*:

- Tetracycline HCl: 500 mg by mouth four times a day for 7 days, or
- Amoxicillin/ampicillin: Amoxicillin, 3 g, or ampicillin, 3.5 g, either with 1 g probenecid by mouth, or
- Aqueous procaine pencillin G: 4.8 million units injected intramuscularly at two sites, with 1.0 g of probenecid by mouth

Other treatment schedules are used for patients with coexisting chlamydial infection, which has been documented in up to 45% of gonorrhea patients for whom chlamydial cultures are done.

Unfortunately, certain gonococcus strains have become resistant to penicillin. In many areas of the world, including the U.S., pencillinase-producing *N. gonorrhoeae* (PPNG) fail to respond to treatment with any penicillin or ampicillin regimen. Spectinomycin is currently being used by the U.S. Navy for gonococcal infection acquired in the Western Pacific and Far East. Cefoxitin, a cephamycin-derived antimicrobial agent, has been shown to be effective against *N. gonorrhoeae,* including resistant strains. Pharyngeal gonorrhea is treated with a sulfamethoxazole–trimethoprim regimen or with tetracycline or aqueous procaine penicillin.

All patients with gonorrhea should undergo a serologic test for syphilis and be screened for other sexually transmitted diseases at the time of diagnosis. Patients with both gonorrhea and syphilis must be given additional treatment, depending on the stage of the disease. The patient is instructed to avoid reinfection with untreated sexual contacts until they have been treated. It is imperative that follow-up cultures be obtained from appropriate sites 3 to 7 days after completion of treatment, since no therapy is 100% effective. Cultures are also obtained 4 to 6 weeks after treatment to detect reinfection. A positive reculture is most often due to reinfection by infectious contacts. The treatment of complications (endocarditis, bacteremia, etc.) is individualized.

Each patient must be interviewed for the names of contacts. Then the contacts must be investigated and treated within 10 days. Public health programs are geared to trace

---

* Sexually Transmitted Diseases Treatment Guidelines, 1982. MMWR Supplement. Vol. 31 (2S), Aug 20, 1982.

contacts and prevent further spread through reporting, diagnosis, treatment, and follow-up.

Nursing Isolation Procedure.   Use secretion precautions (see p. 1488) for the duration of illness (until lesion stops draining).

Patient Education.   The control of the spread of gonorrhea requires considerable patient involvement, education, and compliance. The following are important points to stress:

1. Venereal disease (VD) is acquired by sexual contact (vaginal sexual intercourse, anal intercourse, oral intercourse) and by close and direct contact with an infected person.
2. A person who thinks that he or she may have VD or who has been exposed to someone who might have it should have a checkup. Immediate treatment should be sought if symptoms develop.
3. Anyone who is sexually active with a number of sexual partners should have regular checkups.
4. Washing the sex organs (before and after sexual contact) and the use of a condom may give limited protection against VD.
5. Birth control pills and IUDs give no protection against VD.
6. Gonorrhea and syphilis are different diseases, caused by different germs; they attack the body in different ways but are spread in the same manner. A person may have both gonorrhea and syphilis as well as other sexually transmitted diseases at the same time.
7. There appears to be no natural or acquired immunity to gonorrhea and syphilis. A person can get gonorrhea and syphilis again and again.
8. Pregnant women may pass an infection of syphilis to an unborn child. Pregnant women may pass gonorrhea to a baby during the birthing process.
9. Bacteria from gonorrhea may enter the bloodstream and affect joints, joint linings, heart valves, etc.
10. The VD National Hotline (800–227–8922 [nationwide]; 800–982–5883 [California]) provides toll-free information and referral services for sexually transmitted diseases.

► **Evaluation**

Expected Outcomes

1. Is cured of gonococcal infection
   a. Reports for treatment
   b. Reports for follow-up cultures for test verifying cure
   c. Is free of urethral/vaginal discharge
   d. Gives names/addresses of sex partners for testing and follow-up
2. Avoids complications
   a. Verbalizes that reinfection can occur
   b. Avoids reinfection with untreated sexual contacts
   c. Uses barrier forms of contraception to lessen chances of infection
   d. Reports for routine gynecologic examinations and cultures for gonorrhea
   e. Returns to VD clinic/physician's office immediately at first sign of urethral discharge, dysuria, or lower abdominal pain

Syphilis (Lues)

Syphilis is an acute and chronic infectious multisystem disease caused by *Treponema pallidum* (a spirochete). It is acquired by sexual contact or may be congenital in origin.

T. pallidum is a threadlike, actively motile spirochete 6 to 20 micra long that always produces its effects locally—never at a distance, as through toxins. It is killed quickly by a few minutes' exposure to drying, heat, or air.

A single initial lesion appears at the point where the treponemata entered the body; widespread transitory cutaneous and visceral manifestations then appear, and, years later, scattered destructive granulomatous lesions develop.

Open, untreated lesions contain spirochetes. These sores and any infected material are capable of transmitting the disease. In the pregnant woman, the fetus is infected from the mother by way of the placenta. The vast majority of cases are contracted through sexual intercourse; the danger of transmission by direct contact is greatest in the first 4 years of the disease.

Syphilitic infection arouses powerful forces of resistance in the recipient, and temporary immunity to further infection develops early in the course of the disease. Probably 10% to 15% of untreated patients with syphilis go on to develop manifestations many years later in the central nervous system, heart, bone, skin, and viscera.

Community and Epidemiologic Aspects

Following the development of penicillin therapy in the 1940s, the incidence of reported cases of syphilis fell dramatically. Relaxation of concern has led to a rising incidence again in recent years, leaving no doubt that the disease is far from being eradicated and that there is still a need for mass screening and strong epidemiologic measures. New cases today are seen particularly among teenage groups, young people, homosexuals, and the lower socioeconomic classes. It is more prevalent in males than females, and more cases are seen in the large urban centers. Each person with syphilis is a potential source for a small outbreak, since each infected individual has an average of 4.6 recent contacts, 2 of whom are infected.

Case reporting of early infectious syphilis is required. Epidemiologic measures are geared to trace the source and spread of the disease by interviewing known patients for sexual contacts. Rapid investigation must be done to identify these contacts within a minimal time period to prevent the further spread of the disease. Then all known contacts must receive preventive treatment.

Assessment

Diagnostic Evaluation.   Since syphilis is the great imitator of many diseases, the clinical history and laboratory evaluation are very important. There are two types of serologic tests:

1. *Nontreponemal* or *reagin tests* are screening tests that detect antibodylike substances called reagin found in the serum of infected patients. The most widely used are the Venereal Disease Research Laboratory (VDRL) slide flocculation test, the rapid plasma reagin (RPR) card tests, and the automated reagin test (ART). These tests are reliable, simple to perform, and inexpensive.

2. *Treponemal tests* are tests to measure specific antibodies to *T. pallidum*. These tests are recommended for patients who have reactive reagin tests and atypical signs of primary or secondary syphilis and for diagnosis of late syphilis. The treponemal tests are the fluorescent treponemal antibody absorption test (FTA–ABS) and the microhemagglutination test (MHA–TP).

Clinical Manifestations.   Syphilis is capable of destroying tissue in almost any organ in the body, so that a wide variety of clinical manifestations are produced. Some of the manifestations of syphilis are designated as early and others as late. The time interval between early and late syphilis is about 4 years, during which period the patient has developed a partial immunity and an altered tissue response to the spirochete.

The incubation period is 10 to 90 days, with an average of 21 days. No symptoms or lesions are noted. However, the patient's blood contains the spirochetes and is infective.

Primary Stage.   During the *primary (early) stage,* the most infectious stage, the chancre, or primary sore, appears at the site where the treponema enters the body—genitalia, anus, rectum, lips, oral cavity, breasts, and fingers (Fig. 63-2)—generally related to the pattern of sexual behavior. The typical primary sore (chancre) is an indurated, painless papule that becomes eroded and heals after 4 to 6 weeks. (The chancres may become painful when the lesions become superinfected with other bacteria.) In some patients, no primary sore can be found. Invariably, the regional lymph nodes become enlarged. Serologic tests usually become positive shortly after the appearance of the chancre. In the untreated patient, the chancre heals within 3 to 6 weeks, but the lymphadenopathy may persist for months.

Even before the chancre appears, and while it is present, the treponema have begun to spread throughout the entire body by way of the lymph system and bloodstream. Some patients become listless, run a slight fever, and lose weight; others show no symptoms during this period of general dissemination.

Secondary Syphilis.   In 6 to 8 weeks following the appearance of the chancre, the so-called secondary symptoms appear. These include cutaneous manifestations (see below), generalized enlarged lymph nodes, and painful joints, as well as enlargement of the spleen and liver. Acute iritis in some patients may be the first and only symptom. Sometimes there is hoarseness and chronic sore throat.

The skin manifestations (which may fail to appear) vary to such a degree that they may simulate practically every known skin disease. However, certain features are more or less common to all variations: the lesions are bilaterally symmetrical in distribution, and the distribution is generalized; the eruptions are usually polymorphous (*i.e.,* almost never are the skin lesions of any one type only, as macules alone, or papules alone); although they last for weeks, they cause no itching and no pain. If untreated, they gradually fade. If treated, they disappear quickly. Concomitantly, the hair often drops out, sometimes in patches, giving the scalp a motheaten appearance.

The macular eruption, which usually appears early, may cover the entire trunk, sparing the face. It may be merely a diffuse rosy blush, rose-colored spots, or an eruption of slightly elevated copper-colored macules. Papular luetic lesions, covered with scales, may appear on the body surface. These papules are prone to become secondarily infected, and the resultant pustular eruption may resemble acne vulgaris or impetigo. Nodular skin lesions—small, bluish red, or brown in color—also may develop. These nodules may persist for years and, on disappearing, leave areas of pigmentation.

The lesions that develop on moist skin surfaces, for example, about the anus or genitalia, take the form of broad wartlike plaques (condylomata), which tend to crack and ulcerate. Those that appear on the mucous membranes of the mouth and the tongue are glistening, slightly elevated, flat, circumscribed patches, usually covered with a white or yellowish exudate. These papules, the so-called mucous patches, are the most characteristic, persistent, and infectious of all syphilitic lesions. Other papules, dry and scaly in character, develop on the palms and the soles. Those on the fingertips occasionally destroy the bed of the nails, which become brittle and fissured.

Late Syphilis.   After the early manifestations disappear (in untreated, or inadequately treated patients), there follows a period of apparent good health. Many patients have no further trouble, with or without treatment. But in some people, after 3 to 10 years or longer, signs of late (formerly called *tertiary*) syphilitic lesions appear. These granulomatous lesions are found mainly in the skin and bones, but may also involve the liver, cardiovascular system, and central nervous system. In fact, any organ of the body may be attacked. The inflammatory reaction may involve the heart and great vessels, with lesions occurring in the aorta, pulmonary artery, or great vessels arising from the aorta. The lesions may result in aortitis and aneurysm. Syphilis invades the central nervous system during the early stage of the infection, but in the absence of treatment, some patients will develop symptomatic neurosyphilis, including meningovascular or parenchymatous syphilis. Meningovascular syphilis results in cerebrovascular occlusion, infarction, and encephalomalacia, while the parenchymatous form includes syphilitic paresis and tabes dorsalis, with personality changes and varying neurologic signs.

The skin lesions of late syphilis produce large, deep, punched-out ulcers on the lower legs; upon healing, these leave characteristic scars, pigmented areolae, and atrophied bases. On the arm, the lesions seen around the elbow consist of peculiar many-layered crusts. The lesions in the mouth, the throat, and the nose ulcerate and perforate the soft palate or the septum and give rise to the "saddle-nose" appearance and the diffuse thickening of the tongue.

Management

The Public Health Service recommends the following treatment schedule, according to the stage of syphilis*:

- *Early syphilis* (primary, secondary, latent syphilis of less than one year's duration): Benzathine penicillin G—2.4 million units total by intramuscular injection at a single session (This is the drug of choice because it provides effective treatment in a single visit.)

* Sexually Transmitted Diseases Treatment Guidelines, 1982. MMWR Supplement Vol 31, No 25, Aug 20, 1982.

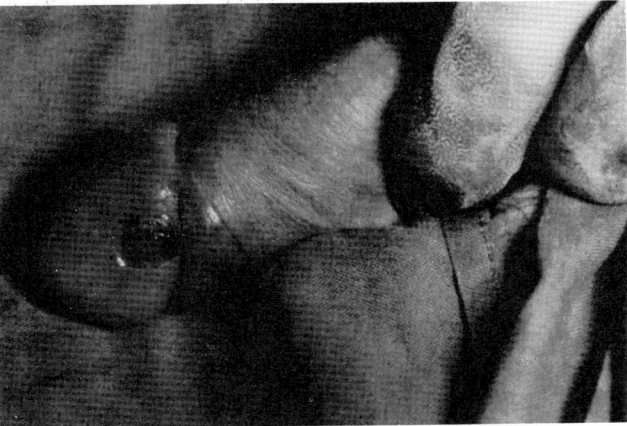
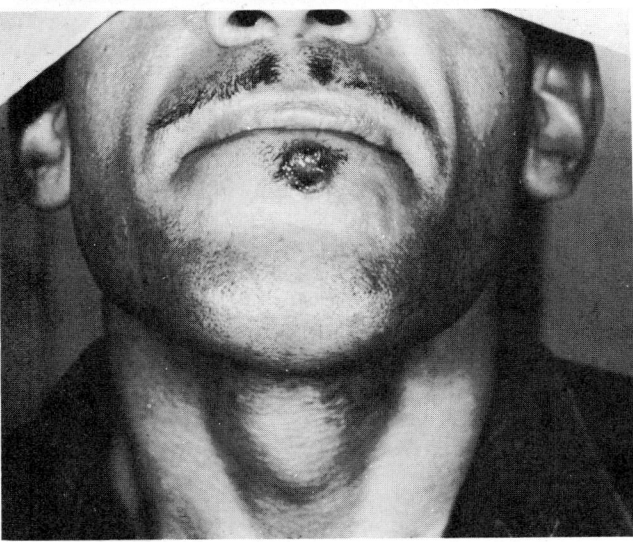

Figure 63-2. (*Top*) Syphilitic chancre on the external surface of the prepuce. (From Elliott H and Rhyz K: Venereal Diseases: Treatment and Nursing. London, Bailliere Tindall, 1972.) (*Bottom*) Primary syphilis. Typical Hunterian chancre on lower lip. (From Syphilis—A Synopsis. U.S. Department of Health, Education and Welfare, Public Health Service.)

- *Penicillin-allergic patients:* Tetracycline HCl—500 mg by mouth, four times a day for 15 days (Patient compliance with this regimen may be difficult, so care should be taken to encourage optimal compliance.)

The optimal treatment schedules for syphilis of greater than 1 year's duration have been less well established than schedules for early syphilis. In general, syphilis of longer duration requires more prolonged therapy.

Although therapy is recommended for established cardiovascular syphilis, antibiotics may not reverse the pathology (loss of elastic tissues in aortic wall) associated with this disease.

Cerebrospinal fluid (CSF) examination is done in patients with suspected symptomatic neurosyphilis and is also desirable in other patients with syphilis greater than 1 year's duration to exclude asymptomatic neurosyphilis. In late syphilis, no treatment can repair structural damage that has already occurred.

The *Jarisch–Herxheimer reaction* is a reaction appearing within hours after initiating therapy for syphilis, particularly in the secondary stage. It consists of transient fever and flulike symptoms of malaise, chills, headache, and myalgia that subside within 24 hours. The reaction is thought to be due to the sudden release of large amounts of treponema antigen with subsequent antigen–antibody reaction in the patient. It is managed with bed rest and aspirin.

Nursing Isolation Procedure.   If the patient has skin and mucous membrane manifestations, secretion precautions (see p. 1488) are carried out until 24 hours after initiation of effective therapy.

Prevention: Patient Education

1. Patients exposed to infectious syphilis within the preceding 3 months should be treated as for early syphilis.
2. All patients with early syphilis should return for repeat nontreponemal tests 3, 6, and 12 months after treatment. Patients with syphilis of more than 1 year's duration should, in addition, have a serologic test 24 months after treatment.
3. Assure the patient infected with primary syphilis that with proper treatment and follow-up, the chancre will disappear (within a week or two) and the blood test should (but not always) become nonreactive within a year.
4. The patient is to be instructed to refrain from sexual contact with previous partners not under treatment.
5. A program of sex education and epidemiologic screening should be ongoing. Mass screening of special groups with a known high incidence of sexually transmitted diseases should be conducted.
6. VD National Hotline: Toll-free telephone numbers are 800–227–8922 (nationwide) and 800–982–5883 (California); provides information and referral services about sexually transmitted diseases.

Acquired Immune Deficiency Syndrome (AIDS)

Acquired immune deficiency syndrome (AIDS) is a condition of unknown etiology, probably viral, that causes a devastation of the body's normal defenses against disease. It is a severe disorder of immunoregulation in which the underlying defect appears to be impairment of cell-mediated immunity (abnormal regulation of the cellular immune response). It involves a weakening of the body's disease-fighting immune system, making the patient vulnerable to opportunistic infections, such as *P. carinii* pneumonia and disseminated cytomegalovirus infections, or to unusual malignant neoplasms (Kaposi's sarcoma).

Etiology.   The cause and mode of the transmission of this new syndrome is unknown, but it seems likely that there is a complex interplay of infection and genetic, environmental, and behavioral factors involved. It is probably transmitted through blood transfusions, semen, and saliva, but this has not been proven. It appears to take 6 months to 2 years to develop.

The high-risk groups are homosexual or bisexual males with multiple sex partners, drug addicts who take drugs by injection, infants and young children who have contact with these groups, blood recipients from a person who has AIDS, and recent Haitian entrants into the US. The common clinical denominator in all of these individuals is a profound immunosuppressed state.

The number of cases of AIDS has been increasing steadily with a high mortality rate and no known cure. An intensive epidemiologic search is being conducted by the Centers for Disease Control to investigate and solve this serious public health problem.

Clinical Manifestations.   The symptoms of AIDS are recurrent infection and fever, swollen lymph glands, anorexia, weight loss, and a general "run-down" feeling. These manifestations worsen during the ensuing weeks and months. Death from severe infection or metastatic tumor occurs in a high number of these patients. By monoclonal antibody analysis, it has been found that patients with AIDS have a selective defect in their T-helper cells and an increase in their T-cytotoxic suppressor cells. There are too few cells that turn on the body's immune response and comparatively too many cells that turn off the process. Thus, there is a reversal in helper cells to the suppressor–cytotoxic cell ratio. (Immunologically healthy people have twice as many helper cells as suppressors, but AIDS patients have the opposite ratio.)

Some patients develop a type of cancer, Kaposi's sarcoma, that has been rare in the U.S. The chief characteristic is the sudden appearance of bluish or brownish lesions, usually on the legs. Other patients contact rampaging opportunistic infections (an opportunistic infection is an illness in individuals whose immune system is temporarily suppressed, such as those receiving organ transplants or those who have such diseases as leukemia). The mortality rate for both these conditions is high.

Management.   The care of patients with AIDS includes careful monitoring of the symptoms as well as supportive therapy for each manifestation. The nurse should be suspicious of AIDS when the symptoms cited above are noted. This is reportable since studies are being made to determine cause and treatment. Safety guidelines have been issued by the Centers for Disease Control on handling patients with AIDS. These are as follows*:

1. Take extraordinary care to avoid accidental wounds from sharp instruments contaminated with potentially infectious material, and avoid contact with open skin lesions with material from AIDS patients.
2. Gloves should be worn when handling blood specimens, blood-soiled items, body fluids, excretions, and secretions, as well as surfaces, materials, and objects exposed to them.
3. Gowns should be worn when clothing may be soiled with body fluids, blood, secretions or excretions.
4. Hands should be washed after removing gowns and gloves and before leaving the rooms of known or suspected AIDS patients. Hands should also be washed thoroughly and immediately if they become contaminated with blood.

* Centers for Disease Control: MMWR. Vol. 31, No. 43, November 5, 1982.

5. Blood and other specimens should be labeled prominently with a special warning, such as "Blood Precautions" or "AIDS Precautions." If the outside of the specimen container is visibly contaminated with blood, use 5.25% sodium hypochlorite (household bleach) with water to clean it. All blood specimens should be placed in a second container, such as an impervious bag, for transport. The container or bag should be examined carefully for leaks or cracks.

6. Blood spills should be cleaned up promptly with a disinfectant solution, such as sodium hypochlorite (see above).

7. Articles soiled with blood should be placed in a impervious bag prominently labeled "AIDS Precaution" or "Blood Precautions" before being sent for reprocessing or disposal. Alternatively, such contaminated items may be placed in plastic bags of a particular color designated solely for the disposal of infectious wastes by the hospital. Disposable items should be incinerated or disposed of in accord with the hospital's policies for disposal of infectious wastes. Reusable items should be reprocessed in accordance with hospital policies for items contaminated with hepatitis V virus. Lensed instruments should be sterilized after use on AIDS patients.

8. Needles should not be bent after use, but should be promptly placed in a puncture-resistant container used solely for such disposal. Needles should not be reinserted into their original sheaths before being discarded into the container, since this is a common cause of needle injury.

9. Disposable syringes and needles are preferred. Only needle-locking syringes or one-piece needle–syringe units should be used to aspirate fluids from patients so that collected fluid can be safely discharged through the needle. If reusable syringes are employed, they should be decontaminated before reprocessing.

10. A private room is indicated for patients who are too ill to use good hygiene, such as those with profuse diarrhea, fecal incontinence, or altered behavior secondary to central nervous system infections.

▷ **Specific Bacterial Infections**

Nosocomial (Hospital-Associated) Infections

A *nosocomial infection* is an infection acquired during hospitalization; it is neither present nor incubating at the time of admission unless it is related to a previous hospitalization.

Approximately 5% of the patients admitted to acute care hospitals in this country acquire an infection. This problem prolongs the hospital stay and leads to over a billion dollars a year in extra direct hospital costs.

Gram-negative Bacterial Infections

The major cause of hospital-associated infections in the United States is gram-negative bacteria; *Escherichia coli* is usually the most frequent etiologic agent, followed by the *Klebsiella–Enterobacter–Serratia* species. *Pseudomonas aeruginosa,* and the *Proteus* and *Providentia* species. In recent years, these organisms have invaded the bloodstreams (bacteremia) of more hospitalized patients than the staphylococcal organisms that were previously responsible for most cases of bacteremia. Such infections arise from the patient's own flora or from opportunistic organisms that colonize patients during hospitalization, or are acquired from other sources. Gram-negative bacilli frequently are responsible for infections of the bloodstream and of the urinary and respiratory tracts. Most gram-negative bacilli are not invasive in normal hosts but become invasive in hospitalized patients who have underlying disease and low resistance, have undergone immunosuppressive therapy, have cardiac prostheses, or invasive diagnostic procedures or monitoring devices.

- These organisms can infect burns or wounds, can be introduced into the bladder by indwelling catheter, inhaled into the lung by contaminated ventilatory equipment (particularly reservoir nebulizers), or transported directly into the bloodstream by intravascular catheters and monitoring devices. Gastrointestinal and biliary surgery, tracheostomies, and contaminated devices account for a significant number of infections.

The risk of developing nosocomial infection parallels the severity of the underlying disease. Gram-negative infections occur in the very young, the elderly, patients with impaired immune systems, blood dyscrasias, burns, trauma, or poorly controlled diabetes, those undergoing prolonged procedures that result in extensive tissue damage, or those in whom a foreign body has been implanted. Potent immunosuppressive and cytotoxic drugs, steroids, radiation, etc., further diminish the patient's defense mechanisms. Antibiotics add to the problem by altering the patient's normal flora and encouraging overgrowth of hospital pathogens that are resistant to antibiotics. Thus, the susceptible patient who is exposed to invasive diagnostic and monitoring equipment is predisposed to develop a gram-negative infection. However, in some patients, the original source of bacteremia cannot be identified.

Table 63-2 shows the site, the precipitating events, and the agents producing the most frequently seen gram-negative infections.

Prevention.   Awareness of the possible risk of infection among hospitalized patients is the first step in preventing such infections.

- Fundamental to the control of infection is correct hand-washing procedures, as well as strict aseptic technique applied to all diagnostic and therapeutic procedures involving the use of catheters, cardiac pacing, intravenous therapy, tracheostomies, tube drainage, and wound care.
- Catheter-associated urinary tract infections are the leading cause of hospital-associated infections. As indicated so many times throughout this text, an indwelling catheter should be used only when absolutely necessary. A patient can be infected with his endogenous bowel flora, by cross contamination with other patients or hospital

Table 63-2
Origin, Precipitating Events, and Etiologic Agents of Bacteremia

Site of Origin	Precipitating Events	Most Frequent Etiologic Agents
Genitourinary tract	Indwelling catheters Instrumentation Obstruction	E. coli Klebsiella–Enterobacter– Serratia Proteus sp. Ps. aeruginosa
Gastrointestinal tract		
Bowel	Obstruction Perforation Abscesses Neoplasia Diverticuli	Bacteroides sp. E. coli Klebsiella–Enterobacter– Serratia Salmonella
Billiary tract	Cholangitis Obstruction (stones) Surgical procedures	E. coli Klebsiella–Enterobacter– Serratia
Reproductive system	Abortion Instrumentation Postpartum	Bacteroides sp. E. coli
Vascular system	Venous cutdowns Intravenous catheters Intracardiac pacemakers Surgical procedures	Ps. aeruginosa Herellea sp. Serratia Erwinia E. cloacae

Skin	Leukemia
	Agranulocytosis
	Immunosuppressive
	  and cancer
	  chemotherapeutic
	  agents
		Ps. aeruginosa
		Herellea
		Serratia

Respiratory tract	Tracheostomy Mechanical ventilatory assistance	Ps. aeruginosa Klebsiella–Enterobacter– Serratia Herellea sp. E. coli
	Aspiration	E. coli Bacteroides sp. Klebsiella–Enterobacter– Serratia

(From McCabe WR: Gram-Negative Bacteremia. Disease-A-Month, Dec, 1973. Copyright © 1973 by Year Book Medical Publishers, Inc. Used by permission.)

flora, or by exposure to contaminated solutions or nonsterile equipment. If possible, avoid the use of indwelling catheters; use an alternate form of drainage, such as condom drainage, suprapubic catheterization, or intermittent catheterization. (See pp. 971–973 for management of patients with catheters.)

Prolonged intravenous therapy should be avoided, and when used, the intravenous catheter should be securely anchored to prevent it from moving in the vein. Scrupulous attention should be paid to inserting the needle properly, protecting the needle site, and observing and caring for the intravenous setup. Intravenous cannulae should be changed at least every 48 to 72 hours.

Great care must be exercised in using and disinfecting respiratory therapy equipment. IPPB therapy should be replaced, when possible, by equally effective and simpler forms of therapy, such as deep breathing or incentive spirometry. Respirator tubing should be changed at least every 24 hours. Every precaution should be taken to reduce the possibility of aspiration.

Transducers are a potential source of nosocomial infection. Reusable transducers and domes must be cleaned and sterilized between use. Personnel should use aseptic technique when handling monitoring equipment.

Every hospital should have infection control personnel to monitor infection control procedures. And every health care provider should use all surveillance methods known to prevent these problems.

▶ **Assessment**

Clinical Manifestations.   Gram-negative bacteremia may be self-limited, transient, intermittent, or continuous. Onset is usually abrupt with a shaking chill and rapid rise in temperature. The fever is often as high as 40° C (105° F–106° F). (Temperature elevation may be blunted in the elderly, debilitated persons, or those receiving corticosteroids.)

As bacilli are destroyed by the host's defense mechanisms, endotoxins are liberated from the bacterial cells. Among the effects that ensue are inadequate perfusion, circulatory insufficiency, increased peripheral resistance, pooling of blood in the microcirculation, and diminished cardiac output and hypoxia. As cerebral blood flow diminishes and shock occurs, the patient becomes confused and disoriented and shows signs of hypotension; tachycardia; weak, thready pulse; cool, clammy skin; peripheral cyanosis; oliguria; and respiratory alkalosis followed by metabolic acidosis. Various abnormalities of intravascular coagulation (disseminated intravascular coagulation, thrombocytopenia) are frequently observed. The development of shock increases the fatality rate of gram-negative bacteremia, with older persons being at increased risk.

Patient Problems/Nursing Diagnoses

Based on the clinical manifestations and diagnostic assessment data, the patient's problems include fever related to bacterial invasion of the bloodstream; and potential for hypotension and shock related to inadequate perfusion, circulatory insufficiency, and diminished cardiac output.

▶ **Planning and Implementation**

Goals

The patient's goals are:

1. Reduction of fever
2. Prevention/recovery from shock through mobilization of his body defenses

The nursing goals are to recognize and implement the treatment for bacteremia, monitor the patient for signs and symptoms of shock and complications, and assist in improvement of perfusion to the vital organs.

Treatment of Bacteremia. The patient is examined to identify the source of sepsis, and the etiologic agent is isolated and identified through blood cultures or cultures of any extravascular sites of infection. Usually, the patient is too ill to await the result of culture and sensitivity tests. Therapy is usually started immediately with agents effective against a broad spectrum of bacteria and with consideration given to the prevalence of resistant strains of bacteria in the hospital. Antibiotics are usually given intravenously to provide high blood, tissue, and body cavity fluid levels.

Any possible source of infection, such as an intravenous or urinary catheter, is removed. Surgical drainage of localized infection is carried out.

Monitoring for Shock and Complications. The nurse monitors the following parameters: state of responsiveness; skin temperature, moisture, color, and turgor; appearance of mucous membranes and nails; respiratory rate; pulse; blood pressure; and intake and urinary output.

Perfusion of Vital Organs. Two or three large intravenous catheters may have to be inserted to provide replacement of fluid and blood to ensure perfusion of vital organs. Central venous pressure measurements provide a gauge for the restoration of the rate and amount of volume replacement. Blood, plasma, low-molecular-weight dextran, or saline may be used to replace fluid volume and to combat vascular collapse. A Swan–Ganz catheter may be inserted to monitor pulmonary artery pressure and to obtain information of the status of left ventricular filling. Blood gas and pH determinations are carried out to assess the patient's need for assisted ventilation. Oxygen is administered to keep the arterial PO_2 at desired levels. Inadequate respiratory exchange is a frequent cause of death in gram-negative shock.

Metabolic acidosis, which appears later, is treated with sodium bicarbonate. Serum electrolytes are monitored. Vasoactive drugs, digitalis, diuretics, and other pharmacologic agents are given as required. Multiple organ failure may result from overwhelming sepsis.

▶ **Evaluation**

Expected Outcomes

1. Reduces fever
   a. Shows progressive decline in temperature over a 3-day interval
   b. Is free from side-effects of antibiotics
   c. Has negative blood cultures
2. Combats shock
   a. Becomes more responsive to environment
   b. Responds to volume replacement by increasing urinary output
   c. Shows progressive increase in blood pressure to normal range
   d. Reveals normalization of skin temperature, turgor, and color
   e. Demonstrates arterial blood gas measurements within normal ranges

Staphylococcus (Staph) Infections

Staphylococci are widely distributed in nature, with humans serving as the predominant reservoir. These bacteria constitute a good part of the common body flora and are found on the skin surface and in the mouth, nose, and throat. It is estimated that 30% to 50% of healthy, nonhospitalized adults carry *Staphylococcus aureus* in their noses. Organisms carried in the nose can be spread to other people or inanimate objects, principally by hand contact. This is frequently how food becomes contaminated by a contaminated food handler who carries the bacteria in the nose, or in skin lesions. (The primary mode of transmission of staphylococci is by direct hand transfer.) Staphylococci are also transmitted through the air (thereby contaminating a wound during dressing changes), via contaminated needles, and through animal sources.

When the continuity of the skin has been disrupted or bypassed (abrasion, wounds, surgical incision, burns, cutaneous viral infection), the patient is a candidate for infection by staphylococci.

Staphylococci are responsible for most human skin infections. The furuncle, or common boil, is almost always a staphylococcal abscess, and the familiar carbuncle on the back of the neck represents a coalition of staphylococcal abscesses. Most staphylococcal abscesses are located in superficial subcutaneous tissues and do not extend beyond the original site. Eventually, their purulent contents, under mounting pressure, perforate the overlying skin and are evacuated externally, leaving the empty cavities to fill in with granulation tissue, close over, and heal.

This common, usually benign, sequence of events might be misconstrued as evidence that the staphylococcus is a relatively innocuous microbe. Far from it! From the standpoint of aggressiveness, destructiveness, tenacity, and talent for survival, this organism has few equals. Although staphylococci cause most superficial infections, they also produce serious infections of the lungs, pleural space, heart valves, bones, kidneys, and surgical wounds. Some strains produce an enterotoxin that is responsible for foodborne disease (staphylococcal food poisoning).

The tendency of the organism to localize in superficial areas of the body merely establishes its potency as an antigen that arouses the defense mechanisms to feverish activity; and the voluminous pus that typifies its lesions demonstrates the lethal effect that it has on tissue cells and defending leukocytes.

Systemic Staphylococcal Infections

If the peripheral defenses are unable to contain the staphylococcus, the infection may spread or invade the bloodstream, attended by profound toxemia. Invasion of the lymphatics may result in axillary, cervical, mediastinal, retroperitoneal, or subdiaphragmatic abscesses. Bloodstream invasion may produce acute bacterial endocarditis, staphylococcal pneumonia, empyema, perinephric abscess, hepatic abscess, staphylococcal enteritis, pyogenic arthritis, meningitis, osteomyelitis, or generalized sepsis. Constitutional symptoms are extremely severe.

Irrespective of location, staphylococcal lesions possess many characteristics in common, including varying degrees of necrosis, a tendency to localize, and a tendency to persist, despite intensive chemotherapy, until the exudate finds an escape route or is evacuated.

Its resistance to therapy is explained in part by the extraordinary ability of the staphylococcus to adapt itself to an unfavorable environment. Resistance to the commonly used antibiotics is frequently observed in strains of staphylococci. Thus, responsiveness to antibiotic chemotherapy, however gratifying at the onset, may diminish to the point of true refractoriness.

Hospital Staphylococcal Infections

Many hospitals throughout the world have experienced serious outbreaks of staphylococcus infections that have been responsible for a number of fatalities.

- Patients who are chronically ill or debilitated, those receiving systemic steroids or cancer chemotherapy, and those undergoing major or prolonged surgery, as well as infants in the nursery, are susceptible and at risk for staphylococcal infections.

Many factors have conspired to produce this situation, among them the capacity of the staphylococcus to develop resistance to most antibiotics, the ability of this organism to penetrate skin and destroy tissue, and the prevalence of the staphylococcus, especially in hospitals, where its presence is ubiquitous.

Control Measures and Prevention.   The major means by which staphylococci are transmitted within the hospital is through person-to-person transmission. The prevention of hospital staphylococcosis requires a working infection control committee, excellent aseptic techniques, and immediate and strict isolation of patients with staphylococcal infections.

Management.   The drug selected for treatment is the one most apt to eradicate the infection rapidly. Penicillinase-resistant penicillins (oxacillin, methicillin, nafcillin) and the cephalosporins (cephalothin) are antistaphylococcal drugs and are selected according to sensitivity studies. Intravenous administration is the route usually selected, because of the large doses required. Serious staphylococcal infections may have to be treated for 4 to 6 weeks to prevent infection of the heart valves.

Nursing Isolation Procedures Required for Staphylococcal Disease (*S. aureus*)

1. Burns—strict isolation, wound and skin precautions, or secretion precautions, depending on extent of infection, for duration of illness (wounds or lesions, until they stop draining)
2. Enterocolitis—enteric precautions until patient is off antibiotics and is culture-negative
3. Gastroenteritis—excretion precautions for duration of illness
4. Lung abscess, draining—strict isolation for duration of illness (until drainage stops)
5. Pneumonia—strict isolation for duration of illness
6. Skin infection—strict isolation, wound and skin precautions, or secretion precautions for duration of illness (depending on extent of infection)

7. Wound infection—strict isolation, wound and skin precautions, or secretion precautions (depending on extent of infection) for duration of illness

Streptococcal Infections

There are many strains of hemolytic streptococci, but group A streptococci accounts for the majority of pathogenic infections in humans. Included in this group are the beta hemolytic streptococci, which gain entrance to the body primarily through the upper respiratory tract from persons with streptococcal infections or those who are asymptomatic carriers. Included in these infections are streptococcal pharyngitis, scarlet fever, sinusitis, otitis media, peritonsillar abscess, pericarditis, pneumonia and empyema, and various wound and skin infections—impetigo, puerperal infections, and erysipelas. Rheumatic fever and acute glomerulonephritis may occur as a sequel of group A streptococci infection.

Streptococcal Pharyngitis

The most common type of streptococcal infection is streptococcal pharyngitis (strep throat) with a group A organism. The organism establishes itself in the lymphoid tissues and produces an abrupt onset of illness, with sore throat, fever (38.2° C [101° F]), chills, and headache. The patient may complain bitterly of throat pain that is aggravated by swallowing or even turning the head. Nasal discharge, cough, and earache may also occur. Upon inspection, the pharynx shows varying degrees of redness and edema and may be covered with an exudate. (A throat culture should be done to confirm the presence of streptococci.) In some patients, a rash appears, starting over the neck and chest and spreading over the skin of the abdomen and extremities. If the rash becomes pronounced, the patient has scarlet fever. (The rash of scarlet fever often disappears in 12 to 18 hours.) Although these are the usual symptoms associated with streptococcal pharyngitis, most patients have some, but not all, of these symptoms.

Management.   Penicillin, in a variety of forms, is the drug of choice in streptococcal infections (except for enterococcal group D infections). If the patient is sensitive to penicillin, one of the cephalosporins, erythromycin, or clindamycin, may be used. Therapy is continued for at least 10 days to eliminate the organisms, reduce the frequency of suppurative complications, prevent the majority of cases of rheumatic fever (and to a lesser extent, acute glomerulonephritis), and help prevent further spread of streptococci.

The patient must understand the importance of *completing* the course of antibiotic treatment in order to prevent the development of complications of this infection, namely, acute rheumatic fever and acute glomerulonephritis.

In addition to penicillin therapy, the therapeutic regimen and nursing support are directed at relieving the patient's symptoms.

Nursing Isolation Procedures

Streptococcal disease (group A)

1. Burns—strict isolation, wound and skin precautions or secretion precautions (depending on extent of infection) until wounds or lesions stop draining

2. Endometritis (puerperal sepsis)—wound and skin precautions until 24 hours after initiation of effective therapy
3. Pharyngitis—secretion precautions until 24 hours after initiation of effective therapy
4. Pneumonia—strict isolation until 24 hours after initiation of effective therapy
5. Scarlet fever—secretion precautions until 24 hours after initiation of effective therapy
6. Skin infection—strict isolation, wound and skin precautions or secretion precautions (depending on extent of infection) until wounds or lesions stop draining
7. Wound infection—strict isolation, wound and skin precautions or secretion precautions (depending on the extent of infection) until wound stops draining
8. Streptococcal disease (not group A) unless covered elsewhere—none

Prevention and Patient Education.   Ongoing health education programs are required to emphasize the relationship of streptococcal infections to heart disease and glomerulonephritis. People with these conditions, especially rheumatic heart disease, are at risk and may require long-term prophylaxis with penicillin. As part of prevention, in other situations, those hospitalized patients who are at risk—and this includes the obstetrical patient—must be protected from personnel or visitors with respiratory or skin infections. For the health of the public at large, food handlers should be instructed about hygienic procedures and closely monitored to assure compliance.

Pulmonary Tuberculosis

Tuberculosis is an infectious disease caused by *Mycobacterium tuberculosis, Mycobacterium bovis,* or rarely *Mycobacterium avium.* It usually involves the lungs, but it also involves and sometimes produces gross lesions in other organs and tissues. The term *Mycobacterium* is descriptive of the organism, which is a bacterium that resembles a fungus. The organisms multiply slowly and are characterized as acid-fast aerobic organisms that can be killed by heat, sunshine, drying, and ultraviolet light.

In contrast with the majority of infectious diseases, the bacillus of tuberculosis, once it has gained a foothold in the body, is likely to remain there, quiescent, for years after the forces of immunity have controlled the original infection. If, during this quiescent period, the resistance of the host is weakened, the germ at once begins to multiply, causing any one of many tuberculous diseases. If the patient's body proves able to recover from this illness, then the tubercle bacilli again become dormant.

Tuberculosis is rapidly becoming a disease of the elderly in the U.S., as many older persons have healed dormant infections due to the prevalence of tuberculosis early in this century. It is also common among certain immigrants from developing countries.

Transmission; Risk Factors.   Tuberculosis is an airborne disease transmitted by droplet nuclei, usually from the respiratory tract of an infected person who expels the organisms during talking, coughing, singing, or sneezing. To acquire the infection, a person must be constantly exposed to the air exhaled by an infected person.

Persons at high risk for acquiring the infection are those whose initial infection was acquired previously; those who harbor live though dormant tuberculous bacilli; those in close contact with someone who has infectious tuberculosis; those whose tuberculin skin tests have been recently converted to a significant reaction; those with lowered resistance because of alcoholism, etc.; elderly persons who live in nursing homes and have healed dormant infections, diabetes, or malignancy or who are on corticosteroid therapy; persons receiving corticosteroid or immunosuppressive therapy; patients with chronic renal failure undergoing maintenance hemodialysis; patients who had had intestinal bypass surgery for obesity; and those with silicosis or diabetes mellitus or who are in a postgastrectomy state.

Crowded living conditions, low incomes, substandard housing, and inadequate health care contribute to the spread of tuberculosis. Tuberculosis is a common infectious disease through the world, as most of the world lives in poverty.

Types of Tuberculosis.   Since tubercle bacilli can establish themselves in almost every type of human tissue, and since there is no organ system that they cannot colonize, the clinical manifestations of tuberculosis are extremely numerous and varied. Most common, by far, of all variants of this infection is pulmonary tuberculosis, in which there is involvement of some portion of the lung parenchyma, together with the bronchi and the bronchioles within it, the mediastinal nodes that drain it, and the pleura that covers it. Lymph nodes, intestine, kidney, brain, meninges, liver, and spleen are commonly involved.

Pathophysiology

Once inhaled by a susceptible host, the tubercle bacilli, in the form of droplet nuclei, pass through the airways and are deposited on the alveolar surface where they begin to multiply.

Tuberculosis is one of the so-called *granulomatous* diseases; that is, when the organism invades normal tissues, the response is the formation of new tissue masses, which are called *infectious granulomas.* The tubercle (little tumor), the characteristic lesion of tuberculosis, is a tiny, spherical infectious granuloma just large enough to be seen with the naked eye.

Another more diffuse and equally characteristic tissue reaction also occurs in response to the tubercle bacillus. Tubercle bacilli, swept along by the lymph and bloodstream, lodge in susceptible tissues in small clumps. The neighboring tissue cells quickly accumulate around each of these "clumps," forming a protective wall that checks their further spread, and may kill them. If immunity is successful, after a long time the germs die, and the tubercle becomes transformed into a tiny mass of fibrous tissue. At the same time, the tissue of the tubercle may become necrotic and transformed into a cheesy mass, a process known as *caseation.* If this occurs, the germs are liberated from the imprisonment and lymph sweeps them into the surrounding tissues, which respond by enclosing these freed germs in new tubercles. In this way, the original miliary (like millet seeds) tubercle grows into larger and larger irregular masses.

The fate of the patient depends on which of these two processes prevails. If the tissue barriers survive, then the imprisoned tubercle bacilli cease to multiply and may die.

Lime salts from the blood are deposited in the dead caseous material, and scar tissue forms around the infected area, which remains throughout life as a healed, calcified mass. However, if the germs survive and are freed from the tubercle, they multiply and are swept along by the lymph stream into the neighboring tissues, and by the bloodstream into other organs, where they lodge and repeat the same process.

Host Defense Mechanisms. Individuals who have experienced a primary tuberculous infection are sensitized or allergic to the chemical constituents of the organism. Henceforth, contact with the bacillus, whether it is alive or killed, produces an acute local tissue inflammation. This is the basis of the tuberculin test, in which a suspension of ground-up killed tubercle bacilli obtained from a culture is injected into the skin. If the patient is allergic—that is, has at one time had a tuberculous infection—a local skin reaction results, whereas if there is no allergy, no reaction is obtained.

A similar inflammatory reaction develops in the lung of a person who has been sensitized previously to the tubercle bacillus if this lung is invaded later by more organisms than the immune processes can handle at the time. In contrast with the relatively bland, silent, primary type of pulmonary tuberculosis, the course of the reinfection type is complicated by necrosis, with resulting ulceration of the infected lung tissue. Clusters of tubercles, as in the primary type of tuberculosis, form at once around the nest of organisms, but now, due to the tissue sensitivity, these become surrounded by zones of inflammatory reaction. The alveoli in the area become filled with exudate; in other words, a tuberculous bronchopneumonia develops. The tuberculous tissue in this area gradually becomes caseous and ulcerates into a bronchus, causing a cavity. At the same time, as the ulcerations heal, considerable scar tissue forms locally, especially around the cavities. The pleura over the infected lobe, more often an upper lobe, becomes inflamed, then thickened and retracted by scar tissue.

This cycle of inflammatory bronchopneumonia proceeds to ulceration with cavitation, followed by scarring. Unless the process can be arrested, it spreads slowly downward toward the hilum and later extends into adjacent lobes. The activity of the process may be very prolonged and characterized by long remissions, when the disease may appear to be arrested, only to be followed by periods of renewed activity.

Depending on whether the predominant pathologic feature of the infection is ulceration or fibrosis, an infection is designated as *chronic ulcerative pulmonary tuberculosis* or *chronic fibroid tuberculosis*. Fibroid tuberculosis is that form of the infection in which the healing process is sufficient to prevent gross caseation of the tuberculous areas, yet cannot halt the infection. The result is a gradual transformation of a lobe, or of the entire lung, into a mass of fibrous tissue. The pleurae become thick and adherent, and the bronchi dilated, their walls pulled apart by the contracting scar tissue in the lung, while the chest on the affected side becomes shrunken, and the spine curved laterally.

According to the Centers for Disease Control, there are 15 million persons in the United States who are infected with the tubercle bacillus. The vast majority of cases arise from the already infected minority of the population.

▶ Assessment

Clinical Manifestations. Chronic pulmonary tuberculosis is insidious in its onset and course. A person with active tuberculosis may have no symptoms until there is extensive disease. The early symptoms seldom suggest the lungs as the seat of the disease. Often the patient notices first that he is losing weight—that, although he feels very well on rising in the morning, he becomes fatigued a little more easily than previously, especially in the afternoon. He becomes a trifle pale, his appetite gradually fails, and he may suffer from "indigestion." He gradually acquires a cough, or at any rate, he "clears his throat" every morning. His temperature, although normal in the morning, may be elevated each afternoon. He may think he has a cold that is just "hanging on."

With the progress of the disease, the anorexia and the "indigestion" may be marked. Abdominal pain or even vomiting may occur after meals. The cough, for weeks passed off as bronchitis or a cigarette cough, gradually becomes more troublesome, and the sputum increases. There is no longer doubt as to the afternoon fever; the patient may have night sweats. Loss of weight and strength is rapid.

Hemoptysis (expectoration of blood or blood-streaked sputum) is common in pulmonary tuberculosis. It may be the first symptom noticed by the patient. These hemorrhages are usually only slight in quantity, but on rare occasions, when an artery ulcerates, the bleeding may be profuse or even fatal. The bleeding occurs unexpectedly and quite independent of exertion or activity. In fact, it may occur during sleep. On the other hand, there may just be slightly blood-streaked sputum.

Diagnostic Assessment. The initial diagnostic evaluation includes a tuberculin skin test, examination of a sputum sample (smear and culture), and an x-ray evaluation of the chest.

Tuberculin Skin Test: Mantoux Test. The Mantoux intracutaneous test is the standard test used to identify the infected person. Tubercle bacillus extract (tuberculin) is inoculated into the intradermal layer of the inner aspect of the forearm. Intermediate strength of purified protein derivative (PPD) is usually used. The tuberculin syringe should be held close to the skin, so that the hub of the needle (26 or 27 gauge) touches it as the needle is introduced, bevel up. This reduces the needle angle at the skin surface and facilitates the injection of tuberculin just beneath the surface of the skin, to form a wheal (Fig. 63-3). The test is read 48 to 72 hours after injection since tuberculin skin tests are tests of delayed hypersensitivity, and this is when the induration is the most evident.

Test reactions should be read in a good light, with the forearm slightly flexed at the elbow. After the area is inspected for the presence of induration (hardening or thickening of tissues), it is lightly palpated across the injection site, from the area of normal skin to the margins of induration. A pencil mark is made where the area of induration is felt. Then the diameter of the induration (*not erythema*) is mea-

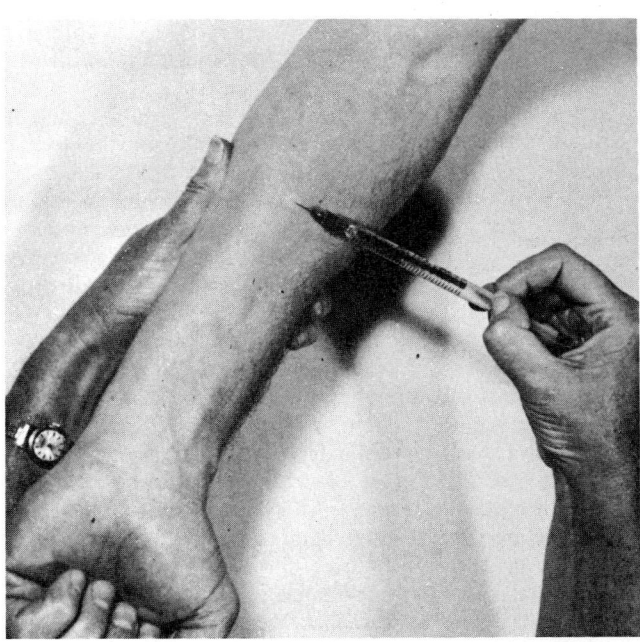

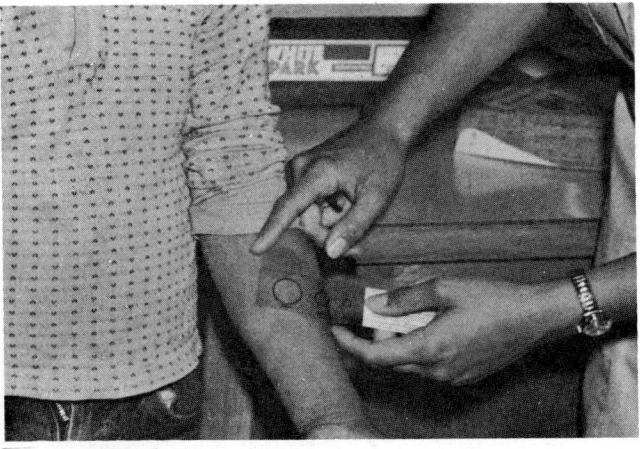

Figure 63-4. Interpretation of Mantoux test. The area of induration is measured most accurately with the aid of a plastic ruler containing concentric circles of specific diameters. (American Lung Association)

Figure 63-3. The Mantoux intracutaneous test. A tuberculin syringe and a subcutaneous needle, with the bevel up, are used to inject tubercle bacillus extract into the skin of the forearm to form a wheal. (American Lung Association)

sured in millimeters, at its widest width (Fig. 63-4). Erythema or redness without induration is generally considered to be of no significance. The size of the induration is documented, as well as the antigen strength, the date the testing was conducted, the date when the reading was taken, and the lot number used, if available.

Interpretation of Skin Test.   An area of *induration* measuring 10 mm or more in diameter is interpreted as significant.

Doubtful reactions measure 5 mm through 9 mm and require that the test be repeated at a different site. (Individuals who are close contacts of persons with active tuberculosis and who have reactions in the 5-mm through 9-mm range should be considered significant reactors and should receive preventive treatment.) Usually, an induration of 0 mm to 4 mm is not considered significant. This shows either a lack of tuberculin sensitivity or low-grade sensitivity that probably is not caused by *M. tuberculosis.*

- *A significant reaction indicates that a patient has had contact with the tubercle bacillus. It does not necessarily mean that active disease is present in the body.* The vast majority (more than 90%) of people who are tuberculin significant reactors will *not* develop clinical tuberculosis. (However, all significant reactors are candidates for active tuberculosis.)

In general, the more intense the reaction, the greater the likelihood of an active infection. A reaction that is not significant is even more valuable diagnostically, for it practically rules out the presence of active tuberculosis, except

in patients with miliary tuberculosis, who may lose their capacity to react to tuberculin, and those who are receiving one of the corticosteroid drugs and may not react in the face of an active infection.

A *tuberculin converter* is a person whose tuberculin reaction changes from less than 10 mm in diameter to more than 10 mm in diameter, with the increase measuring at least 6 mm. (This usually indicates recent infection.)

Other Skin Tests.   Multiple-puncture skin tests are utilized for surveying and screening large groups and are not intended to establish positive diagnosis, since there is no way to standardize the amount of tuberculin introduced. The test introduces tuberculin into the skin (Fig. 63-5) either by puncture with a device with points coated with dried tuberculin or by puncturing through a film of liquid tuberculin. The test is read 48 to 72 hours after administration. If the reaction is in the form of papules, the diameter of the largest single papule or the largest diameter of coalescent induration is measured. If vesiculation is present, the person is sensitive to the tuberculin and is termed a "reactor." However, not all reactors are infected with tuberculosis. All reactors should be retested with the Mantoux test and should have a chest x-ray.

The majority of new cases of active tuberculosis arise from previously quiescent lesions that have become activated. Tuberculin testing serves to identify the group at greatest risk of developing active disease.

Sputum Testing.   Diagnosis is also confirmed by finding the acid-fast bacilli in smears of sputum. Sputum can be coughed up directly or induced by inhaling aerosols, which irritate the trachea and produce coughing. Bronchoscopic aspiration via fiberoptic bronchoscope or transtracheal aspiration are other possible means of obtaining a sputum specimen. An early-morning specimen is more apt to be productive and less contaminated. If the patient is unable to expectorate but has swallowed sputum, then a gastric specimen may be obtained via a nasogastric tube to permit

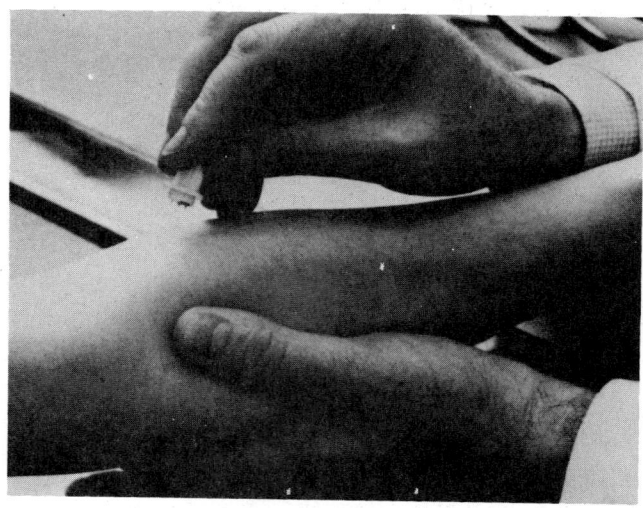

Figure 63-5. This test to detect tuberculosis in humans is easy to apply and is disposable and accurate. Called the Tuberculin Tine Test, it was developed by Lederle Laboratories, a Division of American Cyanamid Company.

study of swallowed sputum. The gastric aspirate is collected early in the morning after the patient has fasted for 8 to 10 hours and preferably when he is still in bed. Tubercle bacilli may also be obtained and cultured from ascitic fluid, pleural fluid, cerebrospinal fluid, urine, and pus that has been aspirated or drained from abscesses. Tissue such as liver, bone marrow, and lymph nodes may also be cultured.

Chest X-ray. Tuberculosis is a possibility in anyone with an abnormal chest x-ray. Abnormal chest x-rays showing pulmonary cavitation or fibrosis may occur before clinical manifestations. Subsequent x-rays are made to determine treatment effectiveness.

Patient Problems/Nursing Diagnoses

Based on the clinical manifestations and diagnostic assessment data, the patient's major nursing problems include abnormalities in respiratory function related to tuberculous infection; and potential nonadherence to the treatment regimen related to knowledge deficit and length of treatment time.

▶ Planning and Implementation

Goals

The patient's goals are:

1. Relief of respiratory symptoms
2. Adherence to the treatment regimen

- Every active case of tuberculosis must be reported to the local health department so that close contacts may be examined and followed. Contacts are usually placed on preventive therapy (usually isoniazid) to prevent the development of active disease.

The objectives of management are (1) to relieve pulmonary and systemic symptoms by eliminating all viable tubercle bacilli; (2) to return the patient to health, work,

and family life as quickly as possible; and (3) to prevent transmission of the infection. The patient may be hospitalized for a more careful and complete diagnostic workup if the infection is serious, if supportive care is required, and if respiratory isolation (see p. 1487) cannot be achieved at home.

Chemotherapy. Active tuberculosis is usually treated with simultaneous administration of two or more drugs to which the organisms are susceptible. Such therapy is carried out until the disease is brought under control. Multiple drug regimens are used to destroy as many viable microbial organisms as quickly as possible and to minimize the emergence of organisms resistant to the various antituberculosis drugs. Although the tubercle bacillus is susceptible to several drugs, there are no drugs to which it cannot develop resistance. Such resistance results from genetic mutations of the organism. Using a variety of drugs enables one agent to destroy those mutants that are resistant to the initial drug.

There are several drug regimens. The drugs in use are combined with one or more of the following: Isoniazid (INH), rifampin (RIF), streptomycin (SM), ethambutol (EMB), and pyrazinamide (PZA). Table 63-3 lists the commonly (and less commonly) used drugs, dosages, and usual side-effects.

Treatment is continued until x-rays demonstrate improvement and negative sputum cultures are obtained. Then the patient is placed on continuing drug therapy for an additional period of time. The total treatment time varies from 9 to 24 months. Recently, it has been found that rifampin and isoniazid are fully bactericidal, highly effective, minimally toxic, and less demanding of the patient, with therapy completed in 9 months. This is much less expensive than older, more prolonged regimens.

Surgical Treatment. Since the advent of chemotherapy, surgical intervention is rarely necessary for tuberculosis. Pulmonary resection may be performed when the possibility of cancer coexists. It may also be carried out for the purpose of eliminating lesions that have ceased to decrease in size after several months of therapy. Such lesions are particularly apt to contain resistant bacilli or to reactivate at a future date. Other indications for surgery may be recurrent or massive hemoptysis and a bronchopleural fistula occurring from tuberculous empyema.

Isolation Procedures. Although tuberculosis is a contagious disease, effective chemotherapy is the most effective means of preventing transmission. However, respiratory isolation (see p. 1487) is advocated until effective therapy puts a stop to infectiousness, as demonstrated when three concentrated sputum specimens are negative for acid-fast bacilli. Usually, appropriate chemotherapy rapidly reduces infection so that after 2 weeks of drug therapy, the risk of transmission is reduced and the patient is permitted to resume normal activity.

If the patient's sputum smears are positive, he is placed in a private room with the flow of air carried to the outside. One of the most important considerations in preventing the spread of tuberculosis is adequate ventilation with fresh air to reduce the number of droplet nuclei in the air. Ultraviolet radiation of the room air is desirable, as it produces a bactericidal effect approximately equal to 30 room changes per hour.

Table 63-3
Commonly Used Drugs in Treating Tuberculosis in Adults and Children

	Dosage*		Most Common Side-effects	Tests for Side-effects*	Remarks*
	Daily	Twice Weekly			
Isoniazid	10–20 mg/kg up to 300 mg PO or IM	15 mg/kg PO or IM	Peripheral neuritis, hepatitis, hypersensitivity	SGOT/SGPT (not as a routine)	Bactericidal. Pyridoxine 10 mg as prophylaxis for neuritis; 50–100 mg as treatment
Ethambutol	15–25 mg/kg PO	50 mg/kg PO	Optic neuritis (reversible with discontinuation of drug; very rare at 15 mg/kg), skin rash	Red-green color discrimination and visual acuity†	Use with caution with renal disease or when eye testing is not feasible
Rifampin	10–20 mg/kg up to 600 mg PO	600 mg PO	Hepatitis, febrile reaction, purpura (rare)	SGOT/SGPT (not as a routine)	Bactericidal. Orange urine color. Affects action of other drugs
Streptomycin	15–20 mg/kg up to 1 g IM	25–30 mg/kg	8th nerve damage, nephrotoxicity	Vestibular function, audiograms; † BUN and creatinine	Use with caution in older patients or those with renal disease
Pyrazinamide	20–40 mg/kg up to 2 g PO		Hyperuricemia, hepatotoxicity	Uric acid, SGOT/ SGPT	Under study as First-Line Drug in short-course regimens

Less Commonly Used Drugs

	Daily	Twice Weekly	Most Common Side-effects	Tests for Side-effects*	Remarks*
Capreomycin	15 mg/kg up to 1 g IM		8th nerve damage, nephrotoxicity	Vestibular function, audiograms; † BUN and creatinine	Use with caution in older patients. Rarely used with renal disease
Kanamycin	15 mg/kg up to 1 g IM		Auditory toxicity, nephrotoxicity, vestibular toxicity (rare)	Vestibular function, audiograms; † BUN and creatinine	Use with caution in older patients. Rarely used with renal disease
Ethionamide	15–30 mg/kg up to 1 g PO		GI disturbance, hepatotoxicity, hypersensitivity	SGOT/SGPT	Divided dose may help GI side-effects
Para-Amino-Salicylic Acid (Aminosalicylic Acid)	200–300 mg/kg up to 12 g PO		GI disturbance, hypersensitivity, hepatotoxicity, sodium load	SGOT/SGPT	GI side-effects very frequent, making cooperation difficult
Cycloserine	10–20 mg/kg up to 1 g PO		Psychosis, personality changes, convulsions, rash	Psychologic testing	Very difficult drug to use. Side-effects may be blocked by pyridoxine, ataractic agents, or anticonvulsant drugs

* Check product labelling for detailed information on dose, contraindications.
† Initial levels should be determined on start of treatment, drug interaction, adverse reactions, and monitoring.
(From Farer LS: Tuberculosis: What the Physician Should Know, p. 11. New York, American Lung Association and American Thoracic Society, 1982.)

The patient is instructed to cover his mouth and nose with double-ply tissue when he coughs or sneezes; these should be discarded in a bag and burned. (Covering the mouth with the bare hand does not stop small droplets.) If the patient refuses to, or cannot, cover his mouth, then he should wear a mask.

Fomites do not constitute a significant infection hazard. Therefore, no special dishwashing or laundering techniques are required. Proper handwashing removes tubercle bacilli from the hands.

Patient Education and Prevention.   Continuing medical and nursing support and supervision are essential. Aspects of the disease should be explained to the patient and any close contacts supervised. Frequent visits to the physician or clinic to determine if the patient is taking the drugs are also important follow-up measures. The American Lung Association has a catalogue of patient teaching aids.

- *A major reason for treatment failure is that patients do not take their medications regularly and for the period of time prescribed.* One of the teaching functions of the community health nurse is to stress the importance of taking the medicine faithfully and exactly as prescribed.

The side-effects of drug therapy are reviewed with the patient, and he is told to report them immediately if they occur. The patient must understand the importance of periodic physical examinations, including roentgenograms of the chest, until drug treatment has been successfully completed.

The patient and family should be instructed carefully in regard to possible complications, including hemorrhage, pleurisy, and other untoward symptoms that are indicative of a possible recurrence of tuberculous activity. Chronic alcoholism is a troublesome complication that makes ambulatory treatment difficult. This patient should be referred to an alcoholic clinic or appropriate health agency.

Usually, the patient can return to his former employment. However, he should avoid exposure to excessive amounts of silicone (dusty jobs in foundry, rock quarry, sand blasting), since silicone dioxide dust may be harmful to the lungs.

Preventive Treatment.   Eradicating tuberculosis depends on prevention, detection, health education, and improved standards of living. Most cases of tuberculosis occur in persons known to be significant tuberculin reactors. These patients are the reservoir from which more than 90% of active disease develops. Infected persons must be identified, and preventive therapy (isoniazid) given to those at risk of developing disease and becoming transmitters. It is recommended that the following be given preventive therapy*:

1. Household members/close associates of newly diagnosed persons
2. Newly infected persons
3. Significant tuberculin skin test reactors with abnormal chest x-rays

---

* American Lung Association; American Thoracic Association. Tuberculosis 1982.

4. Significant tuberculin skin test reactors with special clinical situations (steroids, diabetes, silicosis, gastrectomy)
5. Other significant tuberculin skin test reactors up to age 35
6. Other significant tuberculin skin test reactors over 35 only in special epidemiologic situations

Another means of prevention is the vaccine BCG (bacille Calmette–Guérin), which is considered for persons who are not infected but are likely to become infected. Its use is restricted to persons who are tuberculin negative, because it does not benefit persons who have already been infected. However, BCG vaccination will convert a negative tuberculin reactor to a positive one (for a period of time), thus abolishing the diagnostic value of the tuberculin test. The vaccine is infrequently used in the United States, because the medical and socioeconomic conditions are more favorable here than in some other parts of the world, and there are better methods of control and treatment.

In the developing countries, whose limited resources must be concentrated on the detection and treatment of patients with sputum-positive disease, it has been found that BCG gives substantial protection against tuberculosis. BCG vaccination has been a major tool of the World Health Organization's efforts to control tuberculosis in countries with high rates of transmission.

The American Lung Association is a voluntary, nonprofit health agency dedicated to the prevention and control of lung diseases. The association's official publication is the *Bulletin,* which disseminates information about tuberculosis and respiratory diseases to lay and professional groups. The American Thoracic Society is the medical section of the American Lung Association, and has a monthly publication, *The American Review of Respiratory Diseases,* which is a journal for professional readers.

► Evaluation

Expected Outcomes

1. Obtains relief of respiratory symptoms
   a. Shows no signs of sputum production and cough
   b. Is free of fever
   c. Plans to return to work
2. Adheres to treatment regimen
   a. Encourages his close contacts to report for examination
   b. Takes medication regularly
   c. Marks on calendar when medication has been taken
   d. Reports to provide monthly sputum specimens
   e. Reports for monitoring of SGOT
   f. Recalls three side-effects of drug he is taking
   g. Reports nausea, vomiting, fever, jaundice, or petechiae without delay

Miliary Tuberculosis

Miliary tuberculosis is the result of bloodstream invasion by the tubercle bacillus. It is the most serious form of tuberculosis. The origin of the bacilli that flood the bloodstream is either some chronic focus that has ulcerated into a blood vessel, or multitudes of miliary tubercles lining the inner surface of the thoracic duct. The germs, poured from these foci into the bloodstream, are carried throughout the body and locate throughout all tissues, with myriads of tiny miliary tubercles developing in the lungs, spleen, liver, kidneys, meninges, and other organs.

The clinical course of miliary tuberculosis is varied, depending on which organs are involved earliest and most severely. The usual picture is one of prolonged high, irregular fever, without chills, and intense intoxication. At first, there may be no localizing signs except for splenomegaly, anemia, and leukopenia, or at least the absence of leukocytosis, which distinguishes it from most other bacteremias. Within a few weeks, however, a roentgenogram of the chest reveals small densities scattered diffusely throughout both lung fields; these are the miliary tubercles, which gradually increase in size. Very few physical signs may be elicited on physical examination of the chest, but at this stage the patient suffers from a severe harassing cough, dyspnea, and cyanosis. Treatment is the same as that described for pulmonary tuberculosis.

Atypical Mycobacteria

In recent years, it has been recognized that some bacteria that give a staining reaction similar to that of *M. tuberculosis,* but which have distinctly different growth and cultural characteristics, may produce pulmonary disease clinically similar to tuberculosis. When tuberculosis was a much more common disease than at present, and when more sophisticated bacteriologic techniques were not used, these infections were overlooked or the organisms discarded as contaminants. Today, these strains of mycobacteria, termed *atypical mycobacteria,* are classified more precisely. More than a dozen species of atypical mycobacteria have been identified. Of the nine recognized as human pathogens, *Mycobacterium kansasii* and *Mycobacterium avium–intracellulare* are thought to cause the majority of pulmonary infections. Most of these species are found in a variety of environmental sources, including house dust, tap water, fresh and coastal waters, soil, and milk. There is no evidence of person-to-person transmission.

Antituberculosis drugs are often not effective in treating atypical mycobacterial infections.

Legionnaires' Disease

Legionnaires' disease refers to an acute respiratory infection from a gram-negative bacterium, *Legionella pneumophila.* It is named after an outbreak of the disease that occurred in Philadelphia, in 1976, among persons attending the state convention of the American Legion. While the organism was first isolated in 1977 from autopsy tissues of patients who died from the disease, it is now known that it caused disease as far back as 1965.

Epidemiologic evidence indicates that Legionnaires' disease is transmitted by inhalation of organisms aerosolized in some manner from environmental sources, particularly soil and water. It is proposed that one way in which the aerobic gram-negative bacillus finds its way from the soil into humans is through the cooling towers and evaporative condensers of large air conditioners, where the bacteria multiply and are discharged as an infectious aerosol through fans and exhaust vents. The disease is not considered highly communicable. Persons at risk are the middle-aged and older, especially those who smoke, who drink heavily, and who work on or near construction sites, and those with underlying illness.

Clinical Manifestations. The target organ appears to be the lungs. The earliest symptoms are profound malaise, myalgias, mild headache, and a dry cough. Within a day, the patient experiences a rapidly rising fever and chills. The fever remains high and unremitting 39° C–41° C [102° F–105° F]) until specific therapy is started. Occasionally, diarrhea precedes other symptoms. Associated manifestations include pleuritic pain, confusion, and impaired renal function. A chest x-ray will document evidence of pneumonia. Tachypnea and dyspnea may reflect the extent of the pneumonic process. The diagnosis is made on the basis of an increase in specific serum antibodies and by culture of the organisms on appropriate culture media.

Pathophysiology. Autopsy specimens from tissues of patients with Legionnaires' disease have shown different amounts of lung consolidation in varying distributions. The histologic pattern has been that of an acute fibrinopurulent pneumonia, which resembles a stage of lobar pneumonia. An exudate containing neutrophils, macrophages, and fibrin is found in the alveolar spaces.

Management. Erythromycin (administered early) is the drug of choice in treatment. These patients may be seriously ill. Death may occur from intractable shock and hemodynamic collapse. The nursing management is that described for pneumonia (see p. 514).

Nursing Isolation Procedure. Respiratory isolation is recommended for persons whose illness is strongly suspicious of Legionnaires' disease.

Salmonella Infections (Salmonellosis)

Salmonellosis refers to infections caused by bacteria of the genus *Salmonella*. Clinically, salmonellosis is seen in four forms: gastroenteritis (the most common form), enteric fever (such as typhoid and paratyphoid disease), bacteremia with and without focal extraintestinal infection, and asymptomatic carrier state. Infection caused by *Salmonella typhi* (typhoid fever) is discussed on page 1513. Although approximately 2000 serotypes are known, *Salmonella typhimurium* is the most commonly reported in the U.S.

The diseases resulting from these infections are quite similar, clinically and the infecting organisms are spread in exactly the same manner as the typhoid bacillus. The patient is infected by ingesting the organism in food contaminated by infected feces of man or animal, in whole eggs and egg products, in meat and meat products, in poultry (especially turkey), and in pharmaceuticals of animal origin. There has been a steady increase in the incidence of salmonellosis due to the enormous reservoir of contaminated food products and a changing pattern of mass food processing and distribution. It has been proposed that large numbers of eggs and chickens on the market are contaminated by salmonella microorganisms. Common foods causing salmonella infections include commercially processed meat pies, poultry, sausages, foods containing eggs or egg products, and unpasteurized milk or dairy products. It is also estimated that 0.2% to 5% of persons in the U.S. are chronic carriers of *Salmonella* organisms.

Clinical Manifestations.   Symptoms usually develop within 8 to 48 hours after ingestion of contaminated food. The patient experiences headache, abdominal discomfort, low-grade fever, and watery diarrhea that may contain blood and mucus. Some patients only have a headache and occasional loose stools. The infectious agent may localize and cause necrosis in any body tissue, producing abscesses, cholecystitis, arthritis, endocarditis, meningitis, pericarditis, pneumonia, and pyelonephritis. Petechiae, splenomegaly, and leukopenia may also be manifested.

Diagnosis of *Salmonella* infection is made by isolation of the organism from feces and blood. Later, after acute infection subsides, serologic agglutination tests are useful in establishing the diagnosis.

Management.   The treatment is supportive and includes restriction of food until the abdominal pain, nausea, and vomiting subside. Clear liquids are offered as tolerated. Fluid and electrolyte depletion may have to be corrected intravenously. Antimotility drugs (anticholinergics, paregoric) may be counterproductive, since a slowed peristaltic activity may extend the period of infection by interfering with an effective cleansing mechanism. Enteric precautions are used for the duration of the illness. If a patient has a systemic infection or a focal infection (abscess), treatment is similar to that of typhoid fever (see p. 1513) and a parenteral antibiotic is administered.

Prevention and Patient Education.   There is no active or passive immunization. Raw eggs or egg drinks should not be eaten, nor should dirty or cracked eggs be used, since salmonellae can penetrate cracked eggs. All foods from animal sources, especially fowl, egg products, and meat dishes, should be *thoroughly cooked.* Food service workers should be instructed about food-borne illnesses and given guidelines on avoiding food contamination, storing and preparing food, cleaning of food preparation and service areas (contaminated countertops can serve as a means of transmission), and good personal hygiene. Foods should be refrigerated during storage and protected against insects and rodents. Chickens, ducks, and turtles (as well as other domestic pets) are sources of infection.

The patient must wash his hands after toilet use, particularly during illness and carrier state (several months) to prevent transmission of infection to others. Diarrhea in infants should be investigated promptly since the pediatric population, particularly infants, constitutes the majority of patients affected by *Salmonella* organisms.

Shigellosis (Bacillary Dysentery)

Shigellosis is an acute bacterial disease of the intestinal tract. There are approximately 40 serotypes of shigellae divided into four groups or species: *Shigella dysenteriae, Shigella flexneri, Shigella boydii,* and *Shigella sonnei* (most common serotype isolated in industrialized countries). The source of infection is feces from an infected person, with the route of spread being fecal-oral. *Shigella* species are gaining prevalence as agents of sexually transmitted disease (see p.

1491). Shigellosis may be passed through toilet paper onto the fingers. The bacilli have also been recovered from milk, eggs, cheese, and shrimp.

While encountered in all countries, bacillary dysentery is endemic in the tropics, where serious epidemics are frequently found. It continues to pose a very substantial problem for the citizens of this country, especially those with a substandard environment and those living in a closed-group population—day care centers, military installations, nursing homes, and other resident care centers.

Pathogenesis.   The pathology of shigellosis, in severe cases, consists of organisms reaching the small intestine, where they multiply and release a toxin that initiates secretion of water and electrolytes from the jejunal area. The shigellae are thought to invade the distal ileum and colon, where they establish themselves in epithelial cells, multiply, spread to adjacent cells, and destroy them. The invading pathogens are capable of initiating an intense inflammatory response in the mucosa, followed by small patches of ulceration, which may coalesce to form large ulcers.

Clinical Manifestations.   Initially there is fever, cramping, and abdominal pain. Watery diarrhea soon appears, often followed by frank dysentery, with the passage of varying amounts of blood, mucus, and pus. There may be high fever. At the height of the active infection, the symptoms are severe and the prostration is quite profound. The patient has a constant desire to defecate, and the straining is severe during the attempts. The disease is usually self-limited in healthy adults, and improvement is noted in about 1 week. Some cases last 2 or 3 weeks, and chronic cases last several months, or even years, unless adequately treated. In severe cases, shock, volume depletion, and electrolyte imbalance may supervene.

Management.   The objectives of treatment are to maintain fluid and electrolyte balance and to eliminate the spread of shigellosis to the patient's contacts (*e.g.,* eliminate the carrier state).

The organism may be recovered from the stool, and sensitivity tests done in order to determine the appropriate antibiotic, since the organism may be resistant to certain drugs. Antimotility drugs (Lomotil) are not given, since they may abolish antibiotic effectiveness in reducing diarrhea and positive cultures, thus impeding the body's normal defense mechanisms.

Antibiotics that are absorbed from the intestinal tract and to which the shigellae are sensitive (ampicillin, tetracyclines, sulfamethoxazole-trimethoprim) may shorten the clinical course and decrease the duration of excretion of the organisms.

Intravenous fluids are administered to maintain the electrolyte balance and prevent profound dehydration due to an excessively large loss of water and electrolytes (sodium, potassium, chloride, bicarbonate) in the diarrheic stools. The patient is assessed for weight loss, skin turgor, and dryness of mucous membranes, and his vital signs and urinary volume are monitored. The patient may require supplemental potassium. Clear fluids are offered by mouth during the acute stage.

To eliminate the spread of shigellosis, every patient is questioned about travel to underdeveloped countries, exposure to crowded institutions, swimming in contaminated water, and oral–anal sexual activity. Inquiries are made concerning water supplies and food eaten at home and in restaurants. Local and state authorities are notified.

Nursing Isolation Procedure.   Enteric nursing precautions are carried out until three successive cultures of feces, taken 24 hours apart after cessation of antimicrobial therapy, are negative for the infecting strain.

Prevention and Patient Education.   Dysentery bacilli are spread by drinking water polluted by infected human excreta, by sexual transmission, and by food handled carelessly by shigella carriers, some of whom have the active disease, others being entirely asymptomatic. Thus, the same precautions must be observed, and the same control of water sources and food handling enforced, in the prevention of shigellosis as of typhoid fever. This includes proper handwashing, effective sanitation, adequate sewage disposal, a program of fly control, and the detection of carriers. Untreated sexual partners, particularly those of homosexual men, may reinfect the patient.

Typhoid Fever

Typhoid fever is a bacterial infection transmitted by water, milk, shellfish, or foods contaminated by *S. typhi,* which is harbored in human excreta. This bacillus produces no spores. However, under suitable conditions it can live for months outside the body, and, since it is eliminated in the stools and the urine of patients, it is very likely to find its way into food and water through sewage, flies, and dirty fingers. Today it is spread chiefly by carriers, patients who have recovered from this fever, but whose stools or urine may spread these bacilli for years. Another common source is the ingestion of oysters and shellfish infected from offshore sewage-disposal depots. Typhoid fever, although rare in the U.S., is a serious public health problem in many regions of the world.

Pathophysiology.   The organism enters the body by way of the mouth and invades the walls of the gastrointestinal tract. There, multiplying rapidly, it gives rise to a massive bacteremia that continues for about 10 days. The chief localization of the organism is in the mesenteric lymph nodes and the masses of lymphatic tissue in the mucous membrane of the intestinal wall, which are called *Peyer's patches,* and in small solitary lymph follicles, numerous in the ileum and the colon. The blood vessels of the Peyer's patches become thrombosed, and the swollen mass of lymphatic tissue dies and sloughs away, leaving clean ulcers in the mucous membrane, the floor of which may be the muscularis, or even the peritoneum. If the latter, they may perforate, causing peritonitis. The solitary follicles may or may not ulcerate, but they are so tiny that they do little harm.

Clinical Manifestations.   The distinctive clinical features of typhoid fever consist of prolonged fever, rose-spot rash, enlarged spleen, slow pulse, and leukopenia. The incubation period of typhoid, depending on the size of the infecting dose, is 1 to 3 weeks, with the disease beginning as a subacute illness. Without therapy, the temperature rises steadily, reaching its highest level—usually 40° C to 41° C (104° F–105° F)—in from 3 to 7 days. During this period of rising temperature, most patients suffer with a severe headache and a nonproductive cough. During the second week, if the patient is not treated, the temperature remains consistently high. During the third week, however, it becomes more and more remittent, a little lower each morning and not quite so elevated each afternoon.

The pulse rate may be relatively slow in spite of high fever (fever–pulse dissociation).

Other clinical manifestations are hepatomegaly, splenomegaly, delirium, rose spots (rose-red papules appearing over the abdomen), and intestinal bleeding.

Diagnostic Assessment.   The white blood cell count usually declines below 5000, sometimes to a level as low as 1500 cells per cu mm (leukopenia). The blood and stool cultures are positive for the organism after the first week. Urine cultures, however, may or may not show signs of the organism. The blood serum agglutination test usually becomes positive during the second week.

Complications.   Many structures may become infected in the course of typhoid fever, including the lungs, the pleura, the pericardium, the heart, the kidneys, and the bones. However, the most common of the dangerous complications are intestinal hemorrhage and perforation of the bowel with resultant peritonitis. Since the advent of effective chemotherapy, such incidences have decreased.

Intestinal hemorrhages, from erosion of blood vessels in the ulcerated small intestine and right colon, occur during the third week in about 10% of patients. Some patients have many such hemorrhages. Signs of hemorrhage include apprehension; sweating; pallor; weak, rapid pulse; hypotension; and bloody or tarry stools. During these episodes, food is withheld and blood transfusions given. Operative intervention with resection of the ulcer-bearing segment of the intestine is recommended when bleeding is life-threatening and the patient is not responding to massive transfusion therapy.

Intestinal perforation, the most serious complication, may happen at any time, but most often occurs during the third week. The perforation usually takes place in the lower ileum. It occurs when the ulcer causing the slough involves the entire thickness of the bowel wall. The intestinal contents pour into the abdominal cavity, at once causing peritonitis. The patient usually experiences acute abdominal pain. There is associated abdominal tenderness and rigidity and a silent abdomen. However, the pain may only last a few seconds and then stop, with the patient falling sound asleep within a few minutes. If such signs occur, a nasogastric tube is passed and intravenous fluids started to correct fluid and electrolyte balance. Surgical closure of perforation is usually carried out.

Other complications of typhoid fever include thrombophlebitis, urinary infections, cholecystitis, anemia, and typhoid hepatitis. Cholecystitis, marked by the development of crampy right upper quadrant pain, accompanied by tenderness, nausea, vomiting, and jaundice, may occur from direct infection of the gallbladder by the typhoid bacillus. This is treated conservatively with sedatives, antispasmodics, and parenteral fluids.

Drug Therapy.   Ampicillin, amoxicillin, chloramphenicol, or trimethoprim–sulfonamide combinations are all used in the treatment of typhoid. The fever usually subsides in 3 to 5 days following initiation of antibiotic therapy. However, bacteriologic cure is not achieved in all patients. Relapses have occurred and positive stool cultures have been obtained after one course, and even repeated courses of antibiotic therapy. Thus, while chloramphenicol has reduced the fatality rate of typhoid fever significantly and has curtailed the excretion of typhoid bacilli during convalescence, it has not reduced the frequency of complications or the incidence of the chronic carrier state following typhoid fever.

Nursing Management.   The objectives of nursing management are to give supportive care and to observe for complications such as intestinal perforation.

Delirium is common in the severe form of the disease, and the patient will require special support during this period. He may be drowsy, indifferent to his surroundings, and incontinent of urine and feces. Temperature should be taken by rectum, since the patient may not be able to keep his mouth closed while holding the thermometer. Fever sponges are given for temperatures of 40° C (104° F), and a high fluid intake is encouraged to counteract loss by perspiration. Steroids may be prescribed for toxic or delirious patients.

The patient should be awakened when it is time to turn him; take his temperature; and administer medications, fluid, and food.

Many patients are so toxic that they lose the urge to void, with the result that the bladder becomes distended. Input and output must be measured and recorded in order to obtain quantitative data concerning the status of fluid balance.

Retention of feces, as well as urine, may pose a problem. Low saline enemas are given to relieve this problem. But they are to be given under low pressure, to diminish the chances of intestinal perforation caused by an increase in the pressure or the volume of the fluid within the colon. Distention may be reduced by inserting a rectal tube for short intervals (20 minutes). A high-calorie, low-residue diet is given during the febrile stage.

Nursing Isolation Procedure.   Enteric precautions are used until three consecutive stool cultures taken at least 24 hours apart and not earlier than 1 month after onset (taken after cessation of antimicrobials) are negative for *S. typhi.*

Follow-up.   Since typhoid fever is a very serious disease, the process of recovery may be a slow one. Once a patient has recovered, stools must be checked to see if he has become a carrier, as will be the case in 2% to 5% of typhoid patients. Such carriers harbor the organism and excrete it in their urine and stools. A positive stool or urine culture for a year or more indicates a carrier. Such people must not become food or milk handlers. Carriers may be given ampicillin or amoxicillin with Benemid in an attempt to abolish the carrier state. (Most carriers have biliary infection.) Public health agencies maintain surveillance of carriers, because the occurrence of typhoid fever almost always is traceable to a known or undetected carrier.

Prevention and Patient Education.   The prevention of typhoid fever depends on personal hygiene, cleanliness in food preparation and intake, and proper sewage disposal. Water supplies should be protected and purified. Milk and dairy products require pasteurization and refrigeration. All persons handling food should use proper handwashing techniques. Flies must be controlled by screening and spraying, and their breeding controlled by adequate col-

lection and disposal of garbage. Shellfish should be obtained from an approved source. Patients, convalescents, and carriers must wash their hands after defecation. There is no substitute for good sanitation.

Routine typhoid vaccination is no longer recommended for persons in the United States.

Selective immunization is, however, indicated for the following*:

1. Persons with intimate exposure to a documented typhoid carrier, such as would occur with continued household contact.
2. Travelers to areas where there is a recognized risk of exposure to typhoid because of poor food and water sanitation. It should be emphasized, however, that even after typhoid vaccination, there should be careful selection of foods and water in these areas.

There is no evidence that typhoid vaccine is of value in the United States in controlling common-source outbreaks. Furthermore, there is no reason to use typhoid vaccine for persons in areas of natural disaster, such as floods, or for persons attending rural summer camps.

Primary Immunization.   On the basis of the above recommendations, adults (and children over 10 years old) may be given 0.5 ml of typhoid vaccine subcutaneously on two occasions separated by 4 or more weeks. A booster dose is given at least every 3 years, under conditions of continued or repeated exposure. There is a new, live, attenuated oral vaccine (strain Ty21a oral vaccine) that is being tried successfully in areas of endemic disease.

Meningococcal Meningitis

Meningitis is an inflammation of the meningeal tissues covering the brain, and is caused by bacterial, mycobacterial, or viral agents. The bacteria most frequently encountered in acute bacterial meningitis are *Neisseria meningitidis, Streptococcus pneumoniae* (in adults), and *Haemophilus influenzea* (in children and young adults).

Meningitis is often asymptomatic, but may start as an infection of the nasopharynx or the tonsils, followed by meningococcal septicemia that extends to the meninges of the brain and the upper region of the spinal cord. There are several distinct immunologic strains of the meningococcus, but groups A, B, and C are most important. It can be one of the most fulminating of infectious diseases.

The germ is spread by direct contact, including droplets and discharges from the nose and throat of infected persons and from carriers. Of those exposed to it, the great majority do not develop the infection but become carriers, harboring this organism in the posterior nasopharynx for months.

Meningococcal disease is endemic in the United States and throughout the world, and occurs most frequently in the winter and spring months. Epidemics are most apt to occur when people live in crowded quarters, notably in cities, crowded institutions, military installations, or prisons, but the disease also occurs in rural regions.

* Recommendation of the Public Health Service Advisory Committee on Immunization Practices, 1982.

Pathophysiology.   Predisposing factors include upper respiratory tract infections, otitis media, mastoiditis, sickle cell anemia (or other hemoglobinopathies), recent neurosurgical procedures, head trauma, and immunologic defects. The venous channels serving the posterior nasopharynx, middle ear, and mastoid drain toward the brain and are near the veins draining the meninges. This favors bacterial proliferation.

The meningococci enter the bloodstream and cause an inflammatory reaction in the meninges and underlying cortex, which may result in vasculitis with thromboses and reduced cerebral blood flow. The cerebral tissue is metabolically impaired from the presence of meningeal exudate, vasculitis and underperfusion, and cerebral edema. A purulent exudate may spread over the base of the brain and spinal cord. The inflammation spreads also to the membrane lining the cerebral ventricles. In acute cases, however, the patient dies from the toxin of the bacteria before meningitis develops. In these patients, meningococcemia is overwhelming, with adrenal damage, circulatory collapse, and associated widespread hemorrhages (Waterhouse–Friderichsen syndrome) occurring as a result of endothelial damage and vascular necrosis caused by the meningococci.

Clinical Manifestations.   The onset may be abrupt or insidious. The symptoms result first from the infection, and then from increased intracranial pressure.

During each epidemic, some patients are scarcely ill; others, at once overwhelmed by the toxemia, develop either a high or a subnormal temperature, with purpura on the skin, and die within a few hours of the onset (the fulminant type).

The disease may follow two patterns. Usually, the patient presents with a sudden onset of severe headache, neck pain and stiffness (from spasm of the extensor muscles, due to meningeal irritation), and fever. There is resistance to neck flexion. Other signs of meningeal irritation include:

1. *Positive Kernig's sign:* When the patient is lying with his thigh flexed on the abdomen, he cannot completely extend his leg.
2. *Positive Brudzinski's sign:* When the patient's neck is flexed, flexion of the knees and hips is produced; when passive flexion of the lower extremity of one side is made, a similar movement is seen for the opposite extremity.

Convulsions and vomiting may occur, along with lethargy, and mental confusion. A striking feature is a rash ranging from petechiae to a combination of petechiae and ecchymoses, occurring in about 75% of patients.

In approximately 10% to 20% of the patients, a fulminating infection occurs, with signs of overwhelming septicemia: an abrupt onset of high fever, extensive purpuric lesions (over face and extremities), shock, and signs of intravascular coagulation. Death may occur within a few hours after onset.

Diagnostic Assessment.   Diagnosis is confirmed by finding the meningococci in the cerebrospinal fluid or blood. The cerebrospinal fluid, instead of being clear, contains so much pus that it looks like thin milk; it is under high pressure, and the gram stain of the fluid may reveal the organisms

immediately. On occasion, the cerebrospinal fluid is clear, which may occur as a result of prior therapy with antimicrobial agents active against the particular microorganisms. Counter immunoelectrophoresis is now widely used to detect bacterial antigens in body fluids, particularly cerebrospinal fluid and urine.

Management.   The immediate objective of care is to observe and treat the patient for vasomotor collapse and shock with appropriate fluid replacement and cardiorespiratory support.

The antimicrobial therapy depends on the infecting organism, and the aim is to eradicate the organisms from the subarachnoid space. Antimicrobial agents in current use are penicillin and chloramphenicol. The patient is maintained on large doses of intravenous antibiotics, since most antimicrobials enter the cerebrospinal fluid and central nervous system inefficiently.

- The patient's outcome may depend on the supportive care given. In meningitis of all causes, the patient's clinical status and vital signs are constantly assessed, since altered consciousness may lead to airway obstruction. Arterial blood gas determinations, insertion of a cuffed endotracheal tube (or tracheostomy), and mechanical ventilation may be necessary. Oxygen may be given to maintain the arterial PO$_2$ at desired levels.
- The central venous pressure is monitored to assess for incipient shock, which precedes cardiac or respiratory failure. Generalized vasoconstriction, circumoral cyanosis, and cold extremities may be noted. The high fever must be reduced, to decrease the load on the heart and the brain's oxygen demand.
- Rapid intravenous fluid replacement may be necessary, but care is taken not to overhydrate the patient because of risk of cerebral edema.

The combination of fever, dehydration, decreased fluid intake, and subsequent alkalosis often predispose to convulsive seizures. Airway obstruction, respiratory arrest, or cardiac arrhythmias may follow. Acute cerebral edema may occur. Osmotic diuretics (IV mannitol, urea) are given to decrease cerebral edema. Diazepam (Valium) followed by phenytoin (Dilantin) may be administered to control convulsive seizures. (The care of the patient with seizures is discussed on p. 1360, and the care of the unconscious patient on p. 1301.)

The continuing nursing management requires ongoing assessment of the patient's clinical status, attention to skin and oral hygiene, monitoring of input and output, promotion of comfort, and protection during seizures and while comatose.

Nursing Isolation Procedure.   Use respiratory isolation precautions (see p. 1487) until 24 hours after initiation of effective therapy.

Prevention and Patient Education.   Persons having close contact with the patient should be considered as candidates for antimicrobial prophylaxis (rifampin). Close contacts are observed, and immediately examined if fever or other signs and symptoms of meningitis develop.

Three meningococcal polysaccharide vaccines, monovalent A, monovalent C, and bivalent A–C vaccine, are licensed for selective use in the United States. The monovalent vaccines for the specific serogroup are recommended to control outbreaks of meningococcal disease caused by *N. meningitidis* serogroup A or C. Vaccine may be of benefit for some travelers visiting countries that are experiencing epidemic meningococcal disease. Vaccination should also be considered as an adjunct to antibiotic chemoprophylaxis for anyone living with a patient who has meningococcal disease caused by serogroups A or C. At present, there is no effective vaccine for the prevention of group B meningococcal disease.

Tetanus (Lockjaw)

Tetanus is an acute disease caused by the tetanus bacillus, *Clostridium tetani,* whose spores are introduced into the body when an injury is contaminated with soil, street dust, or animal and human feces. The bacillus is an anaerobe (cannot live in presence of oxygen). It is found most commonly in wounds with small external openings and is also seen in drug addicts. It may occur in any deep wound that is contaminated with soil or harbors foreign bodies. Frequently, the presumed site of infection is a "minor wound." Not infrequently, the wound entrance is so insignificant that it cannot be found. Wounds may be minor injuries, scratches, bee stings, lacerations, frostbite, animal injuries, abortions, circumcision, surgery, and dental and orofacial trauma. The incidence is greater among low-income groups (not receiving immunization) and among women, and the elderly, who never were immunized as children or have lost their immunity.

Pathophysiology. *C. tetani* is known to produce three exotoxins: tetanospasmin, which is a neurotoxin with a special affinity for nervous tissue, especially in the spinal cord and cranial nerves, and which produces intense and severe muscle spasms; nonconvulsive neurotoxin; and tetanolysin, which may have hemolytic and cardiotoxic effects. These neurotoxins are absorbed by the peripheral nerves and carried to the spinal cord, where they produce a reaction that amounts to a stimulation of the nervous tissue. The sensory nerves become sensitive to the slightest stimuli, and the hypersensitive motor nerves carry impulses that produce spasms of the muscles that they supply.

Clinical Manifestations. Early symptoms include irritability, restlessness, headache, low-grade fever, and muscle rigidity. The jaw muscles are the first group affected, making it difficult to open the mouth because of spasms of the masticatory muscles (trismus). This characteristic symptom has given the disease the common name of *lockjaw*. The spasms of the facial muscles produce a distorted grin (risus sardonicus), which is quite characteristic for the disease and persists even during convalescence.

The spasm rapidly involves other groups of muscles, until the whole body is affected with tightness of the chest and rigidity of the abdominal wall, back, and extremities. The spasm is continuous, but the least stimulus—a door banging, or a loud voice—may cause generalized convulsion, with every muscle in violent contraction. In fact, fractures of the vertebral bodies can occur during severe spasms. Because the extensor muscles are stronger than the flexors,

the head is retracted, the feet are extended fully, and the back is arched, so that during a convulsion the whole body may be supported on the back of the head and the feet. This condition is called *opisthotonos.* The patient is alert and in pain from muscle spasms. Death may occur from asphyxia, due to spasms of the respiratory muscles, and from pneumonia.

Management. The goals of management are to provide an airway to prevent respiratory and cardiovascular complications and to neutralize the residual circulating toxins.

For patients with established tetanus, the patient is immediately given human tetanus immune globulin (TIG) 1 to 2 hours before wound debridement so that the neurotoxin released into the circulation during debridement cannot attach to nerve endings. Active immunization with tetanus toxoid is also started at the beginning of treatment since even severe tetanus produces no immunity. When tetanus toxoid and TIG are given concurrently, separate syringes and separate sites should be used.

The wound is debrided, as necrotic tissue favors the growth of tetanus bacillus. The wound is irrigated copiously to wash out tissue fragments and foreign bodies, and may be left open and drainage instituted.

Immune globulin may also be infiltrated into the wound site. Usually, penicillin G (or an alternate antibiotic) is given intravenously or intramuscularly in high doses to eradicate persisting *C. tetani* and other pathogens from the wound.

- In severe tetanus infection, one of the most important nursing objectives and priorities is constant supportive care of the patient to assure respiratory function. Convulsive paroxysms, especially those involving the respiratory muscles, impair pulmonary gas exchange by preventing normal swallowing and by obstructing the airway.
- Tetanic spasms of the larynx, pharynx, and respiratory muscles usually occur during convulsions and can lead to asphyxiation and death. Rigidity and spasm of the trunk muscles also contribute to ventilatory failure. In fact, ventilation ceases during a tetanus convulsion.
- The patient requires expert respiratory management in an intensive care unit, with early endotracheal intubation and mechanical ventilation. Oral secretions are usually constant and heavy, requiring frequent suctioning.

Diazepam is used to reduce restlessness and apprehension (which can induce spasm), for its amnesic effect, and to provide muscle relaxation to treat spasm. Neuromuscular blocking agents (metocurine iodide [Metubine]) is given for treatment of severe tetanus. Curariform drugs may be given for severe convulsions. The nursing management of the patient with convulsions is discussed on page 1360. See Chapter 25 for the management of the patient requiring respiratory intensive care.

Since the slightest stimulation may trigger paroxysmal spasm, sudden stimuli and light must be avoided. The patient is placed in a quiet semidark environment to avoid stimulating reflex spasms. Nursing activities are carried out during the periods when sedation has its maximum effect, so that the patient is disturbed as little as possible, since tactile stimulation often provokes spasms. Usually, a vein is kept open for emergency situations, such as cardiac or respiratory arrest, and for infusions to maintain careful fluid and electrolyte balance. Insensible fluid losses in the form of sweat and saliva are high and result in dehydration, which in the presence of impaired cardiovascular control and overactivity of the sympathetic nervous system can predispose to deep vein thrombosis and pulmonary embolism. Parenteral nutrition may be required as opposed to oral food intake, since aspiration pneumonia is a hazard.

Constant attention is given to the eyes, mouth, skin, and bladder and bowels. The patient is monitored for signs of infection (skin, urinary tract, aspiration pneumonia). Overactivity of the sympathetic nervous system, as manifested by tachycardia, arrhythmias, labile blood pressure, hyperpyrexia, and excessive sweating and salivation, may eventually lead to circulatory failure and death. A significant increase in the heart rate and mean arterial blood pressure may indicate a need for an adrenergic blocking agent (propranolol) to lessen the possibility of catecholamine-induced myocardial damage. Therefore, cardiac monitoring is essential. Phentolamine is used to control hypertensive episodes. Cimetidine may be given to prevent gastrointestinal bleeding, which occurs in many patients with tetanus.

Watch the patient for urinary retention, which occurs when perineal muscles are affected. Pressure sores and contractures can be the outcome of prolonged immobility, and preventive nursing interventions are necessary (see Chap. 14). Even with expert care, the mortality rate of tetanus may be 50% or higher.

Prevention.   Tetanus can be prevented through proper immunization programs, as immunization establishes basal immunity before exposure to the risk of tetanus. For primary immunization of adults, three doses of adult-type tetanus and diphtheria toxoids should be given, followed by a booster dose every 10 years. Every break in the skin must be considered a potential portal of entry for *C. tetani*.

- The most important step in the prevention of tetanus is the thorough washing and cleaning of the wound, with removal of all foreign material and devitalized tissue. This helps eliminate tetanus bacilli from wounds and removes the material that forms a focus in which tetanus spores can develop.

Following injury, the immunization status of the patient will determine whether or not to provide active immunization with tetanus toxoid and passive immunization with tetanus globulin. The nature and age of the wound, the conditions under which it was incurred, and the treatment are considered on an individual basis. Encourage the patient to keep an up-to-date record of his immunization status.

Clostridial Myonecrosis (Gas Gangrene)

Gas gangrene is a severe infection of skeletal muscle caused by several species of gram-positive clostridia that may complicate trauma, compound fractures, contusions, or lacerated wounds by producing exotoxins that destroy tissue. These organisms (*Clostridium perfringens* [also called *Clostridium welchii*], *Clostridium septicum*, *Clostridium histolyticum*, *Clostridium sporogenes*, and others) may produce gas gangrene. They are anaerobes and spore-formers and are found normally in the intestinal tract of man and in soils. Their growth occurs primarily in deep wounds where the oxygen supply is reduced, a situation enhanced by the presence of foreign bodies or necrotic tissue, which leads to further reduction of oxygen tension in wounds.

In contaminated wounds in which the vascular supply may be impaired, the environment is suited for the growth of spores and the production of exotoxins that cause hemolysis, vessel thrombosis, and damage to the myocardium, liver, and kidneys.

Spores formed by anaerobic bacilli are highly resistant to heat, cold, sunlight, drying, and many chemical agents. Because the gas bacillus is an inhabitant of the human intestinal tract, it is likely to be the infecting organism in thigh wounds following amputations, especially if the patient is incontinent. Peripheral vascular disease, gangrene, incontinence, and debility often are combined in patients with diabetes, and it is in the residual limb (amputation stump) of diabetic patients that gas gangrene is most likely to occur.

Clinical Manifestations.   The onset of gas gangrene is usually attended by sudden, severe pain at the site of injury, which is caused by gas and edema in the tissues, usually occurring 1 to 4 days following the injury. The wound is very tender. The surrounding skin initially appears normal, or white and tense, but later becomes bronzed, brown, or even black in color. Vesicles filled with red, watery fluid appear, and crepitus (crackling) produced by gas in the tissue may be felt. Frothy fluid with a foul, sweetish odor may escape from the wound. The gas and edema fluid increase local pressure and impair the blood supply and drainage. The involved muscles become black or reddish purple (necrosis). Amputation of an affected extremity is sometimes necessary. The infection may spread quickly, resulting in systemic toxicity.

The patient is pale, prostrated, and apprehensive, but usually quite alert. Pulse and respirations are rapid, but the temperature usually does not exceed 38.3° C (101° F). Anorexia, diarrhea, vomiting, and vascular collapse may occur. Death from toxemia is frequent.

Prevention.   Gas gangrene may be prevented if all devitalized and infected tissue is excised and debrided, using wide incisions made to render the wound unsuitable for the growth of clostridium.

Management.   Treatment usually involves surgery, antibiotics, and sometimes hyperbaric oxygen. Once infection has developed, extensive incisions in the affected part allow air to inhibit the growth of anaerobic organisms. Antibiotic therapy is combined with prompt surgical debridement of the wound.

Hyperbaric oxygen (oxygen administered under pressure greater than atmospheric) has proven extremely effective in treating gas gangrene. This increases the dissolved oxygen in the arterial system by increasing the partial pressure of oxygen breathed by the patient. Toxin formation and microbial replication (reproduction) may thereby be reduced. With hyperbaric oxygen therapy, it may not be necessary to amputate the extremity or debride as extensive an area. Since gas gangrene produces an intense toxemia, pulmonary capillary wedge pressure, central venous pressure, and urinary output are monitored. Intravenous fluids are given to support the cardiovascular system and to maintain fluid and electrolyte balance. Plasma, albumin, and whole blood may be used to restore protein depletion, which is found in nearly all patients. This is also useful in correcting anemia. Enteral nutrition (see p. 776) is critical in establishing nutritional balance.

Nursing Isolation Procedure. Wound and skin precautions (see p. 1488) are taken until the wound stops draining.

Botulism

Botulism is a type of food poisoning that affects the central nervous system. It is caused by eating food in which the bacterium *Clostridium botulinum* has grown and produced toxins. These toxins are extremely potent and are rapidly absorbed by the GI tract, becoming bound to neural tissue and producing a neuroparalytic syndrome. Human intoxication usually follows ingestion of contaminated foods: home-canned, dried, or smoked foods or poorly processed foods.

Of the eight toxigenic serotypes of *C. botulinum,* types A, B, E, and F have been shown to produce disease in humans.

Clinical Manifestations. The symptoms appear 12 to 36 hours after ingestion of the contaminated food. If the symptoms appear in less than 24 hours after ingestion, a more severe illness and a higher fatality rate are usually encountered.

The toxin causes paralysis of skeletal muscles by interfering with release of acetylcholine. The clinical manifestations begin in the cranial nerve areas and then descend. Cranial nerve symptoms include diplopia, ptosis and blurred vision (extraocular muscle involvement), dysphagia and pharyngeal pain (involvement of pharynx), and dysphonia (involvement of larynx). Paralysis then occurs, slowly descending through the body and affecting all muscle groups, usually in a symmetrical fashion. Throughout the ordeal, the patient's mind remains clear. Almost three fourths of the patients have respiratory problems. In addition, there may be nausea, vomiting, abdominal pain, early diarrhea, dizziness, and, occasionally, urinary retention.

The diagnosis is confirmed by finding the toxin in the serum, gastric contents, stools, and incriminated food. Mouse toxicity tests with antiserum neutralization are considered most useful. There are also characteristic electrophysiologic abnormalities in clinically involved muscle groups. Local, state, and federal public health officials are notified when a case of botulism is diagnosed.

Management. The objectives of treatment are to prevent respiratory failure and to eliminate the toxin and *C. botulinum* from the gastrointestinal tract.

Pentavalent (ABCDE) or trivalent (ABE) botulinal antitoxin may be useful to neutralize any toxin that may be in the circulation. This is available from the Centers for Disease Control. Ventilatory equipment and emergency drugs should be readily available in the event of a life-threatening reaction.

Organisms and unabsorbed toxin are eliminated from the gastrointestinal tract by means of gastric lavage, cathartics, and enemas. In instances of respiratory paralysis or an ileus, these procedures may not be prescribed.

- Since the neurotoxins produced by *C. botulinum* may result in neuroparalytic syndromes, the patient is given respiratory care and support as the basic management to prevent the pulmonary complications that are responsible for most fatalities due to botulism. The patient is prepared for endotracheal intubation and mechanical ventilation. (The respiratory care of the paralyzed patient is discussed in detail in Chap. 25.)

The patient's heart is monitored in order to detect immediately any signs of cardiac arrest. Skin care and positioning are also important facets of management, to prevent pressure sores and musculoskeletal complications.

Guanidine hydrochloride is considered an adjunct to therapy and appears more effective in combating paralysis of eye muscles and extremities than it does in overcoming respiratory paralysis. Superimposed infection is treated with antimicrobials. Recovery from botulism is usually prolonged.

Nursing Isolation Procedure. No precautions are necessary, since botulism is an intoxication, not an infection.

Prevention and Patient Education. Home-processed foods pose a serious danger of *C. botulinum,* because this germ is a spore-bearer and is not killed rapidly at boiling temperature. (Reliable commercial packing houses sterilize their products at 120° C [248° F], which kills all the spores.) Preserved foods in which this germ has been growing look soft, contain gas bubbles, and give off an odor of decay. However, contaminated food items may have a normal appearance and taste. Canned foods should be heated at temperatures over 80° C (176° F) for 30 minutes or boiled for 10 minutes, as these toxins are heat-labile and destroyed by proper cooking of food. Vegetables, including mushrooms, beans, tomatoes, beets, okra, peppers, corn, and asparagus have been implicated, while meats, fish, and poultry have also accounted for some outbreaks.

Home canners should be advised to take care in preparing foods for canning at high altitudes, since it is difficult to provide a temperature high enough to destroy the spores of *C. botulinum.* The use of the pressure cooker method of canning at high altitudes is advised.

Persons are also cautioned not to use punctured and swollen cans or jars with defective seals.

Leprosy (Hansen's Disease)

Leprosy is a chronic infectious disease caused by *Mycobacterium leprae,* a bacillus that produces lesions in the skin tissues and peripheral nerves. This organism resembles the tubercle bacillus in many respects. It is not known exactly how leprosy bacilli enter the body, but transmission may take place by direct personal contact (skin to skin) or by fomites, or the bacilli may enter via the mucous membranes of the nose or mouth. The disease is only mildly contagious, and as much as 90% of the world's population may be immune.

As the bacilli multiply, they invade adjoining skin areas and find their way into the axis cylinders of nerves by way of the axon-plasma filaments (*i.e.*, the ultimate terminals of the nerves supplying the skin). As the infection spreads, organisms break out of the nerves at various points in the skin to produce macules and papules. These are painless, since the bacilli that caused them to form had already destroyed the nerve supply.

Incidence. An estimated 11 to 12 million persons throughout the world suffer from this ancient, feared, and disfiguring disease. It is most prevalent in the third world countries (Africa), which have inadequate manpower and financial resources to cope with leprosy. In the U.S., the influx of immigrants and increasing world travel by U.S. citizens have caused an increase of Hansen's disease in the last 10 years.

Clinical Manifestations. Leprosy chiefly affects the skin and peripheral nerves. The earliest manifestation is a skin lesion, located anywhere on the body. The lesions are either tuberculoid, lepromatous, or borderline. In the tuberculoid type, the lesions are colorless or reddish brown. The earliest sign is usually a loss of feeling in a small area of the skin, as a result of damage to the dermal nerves. Nerve involvement can lead to damage of muscles and bones. In the lepromatous form, the bacillus grows unchecked, with skin lesions (macules, papules, nodules, or plaques) appearing over most of the body. These nodules, resembling skin tumors and sores, may appear anywhere on the body. When the face is involved, the nodules, together with the loss of the eyebrows and eyelashes, give the face a typical leonine appearance. Because the nodules are easily infected, giving rise to deep ulcers that heal slowly, scars deform the face. This process often dissects the nose, fingers, and toes, and destroys sight.

In borderline leprosy, the lesions are variable, falling between the tuberculoid and lepromatous range of the disease.

Diagnosis is made on the basis of the appearance of the lesions and the discovery of the leprosy bacilli, obtained from slit-scrape smears of the skin lesions and smears from nasal mucosa.

Management. The goals of therapy are to give specific chemotherapy until cure is attained and to prevent and treat deformities. Leprosy is best treated with sulfone drugs (related chemically to the sulfonamides), available for oral administration as dapsone (DDS) if the infection is dapsone-sensitive. Effective chemotherapy usually eliminates viable bacilli from skin lesions in a number of months, but treatment must be continued for several years, the length of time depending on the form of leprosy. Multiple drug regimens (rifampin, clofazimine, ethionamide, or prothionamide) are being used to prevent the emergence of resistant mutant strains.

Mucosal lesions respond most readily, disappearing within a few months, resulting in relief of nasal obstruction and clearing of laryngeal lesions. The smaller nodular lesions in the skin shrink and are absorbed, leaving only pigment spots. Larger lesions disperse, with eventual scar formation. However, bacilli can persist following treatment, resulting in relapse at a later date.

Reconstructive surgery and rehabilitation to restore damaged hands, feet, face, etc. require the services of re-constructive and plastic surgeons, physical therapists, orthopedists, and others. Because the disfigurement of leprosy is such a stigma, surgery is absolutely necessary if the patient is to return to society.

To counter the crippling effects of the disease, the patient must realize the importance of maintaining mobility of the affected extremities and preventing fixed deformities. The principles are similar to those stressed in patient education for rheumatoid arthritis (see p. 1143). The patient is encouraged to inspect sites of potential injury (eyes, hands, feet) daily, as these areas are not sensitive and injuries can be neglected. The skin is kept hydrated and an emollient applied to maintain a supple and pliant skin.

The Public Health Service maintains a hospital in Carville, Louisiana (now called National Hansen's Disease Center), that serves as a treatment, research, and training facility. Research is still being conducted in hopes of finding a specific skin test for leprosy. Investigators have succeeded in infecting armadillos with leprosy and are using these microorganisms to produce a vaccine that is to undergo safety trials in the near future.

Nursing Isolation Procedure. No isolation precautions are required, since the infection declines rapidly under chemotherapy. Segregation is no longer required in any state of the U.S.

Ornithosis (Psittacosis)

Ornithosis is an infectious and atypical form of pneumonia or systemic febrile illness transmitted to humans by infected birds. The agents responsible for ornithosis belong to the genus *Chlamydia* (obligate intracellular organisms that were formerly considered viruses but are now classed as bacteria). The chlamydiae cause trachoma, lymphogranuloma venereum, and ornithosis; they may be found in nasal secretions and in the feathers, feces, and blood of sick birds. The organisms, *Chlamydia psittaci,* are transmitted to humans inhaling the etiologic agent from desiccated droppings of infected birds, or directly from infected birds (processing plants), or rarely from person to person. Birds of the parrot family (parakeets, parrots, cockatoos, budgerigars), as well as many other species of birds (canaries, sparrows, pigeons, turkeys), may be infected.

Clinical Manifestations. The illness may appear as a transient, influenzalike illness or a severe pneumonia, or it may be asymptomatic. After an incubation period lasting 4 to 15 days (it may be as long as 6 weeks in man, 6 months in a parrot), the disease begins abruptly, with malaise, headache, photophobia, and chills. Its course is characterized by high fever, great weakness, marked depression, and delirium, with surprisingly slow pulse and respiration. Cough is a prominent symptom. The lungs become involved, with edema, mononuclear cells, and lymphocytes appearing in the alveoli and interstitial areas. Chest x-ray may reveal an interstitial pneumonitis. Convalescence is apt to be prolonged.

Management. Ornithosis responds to the tetracyclines. Supportive therapy includes bed rest, oxygen (when necessary), and measures to reduce the fever. Relapses are common.

Prevention. Persons at risk are those who work in pet shops or around poultry and pigeons, bird fanciers, workers who may handle infected birds in the food processing and marketing business, and veterinarians. Care should be taken to avoid dust from feathers and bird-cage contents. Infected birds should be treated or destroyed. No protective vaccination is available.

Nursing Isolation Procedure. Secretion precautions are necessary for the duration of the illness.

Actinomycosis

Actinomycosis is a chronic, suppurating, granulomatous disease. The usual pathogen in man is an anaerobic, grampositive, branching, filamentous bacterium, *Actinomyces israelii,* a commensal that may be found in the tonsillar crypts, dental caries, and colon of apparently healthy people. Minor trauma, aspiration, or surgical manipulation may initiate the infectious process. Actinomycosis has traditionally been classified as a mycotic or fungal disease because it characteristically resembles the deep mycoses, but the *Actinomyces* are now classified as bacteria.

Clinical Manifestations. The characteristic lesions appear as firm, indurated granulomas that spread slowly to adjacent tissues and break down to form multiple sinus tracts that penetrate to the surface. The exudate from the sinus tracts contains the characteristic sulfur granules that are visible masses of the organism.

Actinomycosis involves three major forms of infection: cervicofacial, abdominal, and thoracic.

Actinomycosis of the head and the neck, the most common locations, starts as a swelling in and around the teeth and extends into the submaxillary region and the neck, producing a flat, hard, painless tumor mass, with a smooth, regular surface and uniform dense consistency, which is fixed firmly to the jawbone. From this mass, a firm, nodular induration extends into the neck, covered by skin that is wrinkled and dusky red in color. Later this granuloma breaks down and becomes riddled with abscesses that perforate externally. The process may extend into the cheek, skull, and brain.

In the abdominal type, any viscera may be affected, including the pelvic organs, especially the ovaries and the tubes, but most commonly the appendix and the cecum. Here, in time, an uneven tumor mass develops, resembling carcinoma. The tumor may spread, involving the abdominal wall and discharging externally through open sinuses.

In the thoracic form, induced by inhaling actinomyces spores, the acute and chronic inflammatory reaction may involve the lungs, pleura, mediastinum, or chest wall, producing chest pain, fever, cough, and hemoptysis.

Management. Actinomycotic lesions respond to penicillin, which is the drug of choice. Large doses are given daily, without interruption for weeks to months. Alternate antibiotics are given if the patient is allergic to penicillin. Surgical drainage and resection of damaged tissues, and excision of sinuses and fistulous tracts, may be required.

Nursing Isolation Procedure. For draining lesions, secretion precautions are necessary until the wound stops draining.

Patient Education. Encourage good dental hygiene to reduce infection around the teeth. There appears to be a relationship between intrauterine device use and colonization or infection of the genital tract with *Actinomyces,* especially when pelvic infection is present.

▷ Viral Infections

Influenza

Influenza is an acute infectious disease caused by an RNA-containing myxovirus. It is characterized by respiratory and constitutional symptoms. It has swept through the entire civilized world approximately every 20 years, attacking as many as 40% of the people in the affected areas. The striking features of these epidemics have been the speed with which they have spread and an extremely high attack rate.

Typical epidemics of influenza have been characterized by three successive waves, separated by brief intermissions. The first wave lasts from 3 to 6 weeks and is explosive in outbreak, widespread, and mild in form in the majority of cases, with few complications. The second wave also is widespread, but lasts longer; the cases are more severe, and the complications are serious. The third wave lasts still longer (from 8 to 10 weeks) and involves fewer persons, but the complications are quite severe. During the years succeeding a major epidemic, there follow scattered local waves of decreasing severity, with sporadic cases of influenza occurring during the intervals.

Etiology. The primary factor in the etiology of influenza is a filtrable virus, of which three major strains have been isolated, designated types A, B, and C. Types A and B have been associated with epidemics. The numerous variants within a given type are called subtypes.

It is difficult to control influenza because the surface antigens of the virus have the capacity to undergo antigenic variation. Major antigenic shifts and new human pandemic influenza strains arise from time to time. Therefore, previously acquired antibodies against earlier influenza strains may not be effective against the new emerging strain, depending on the extent of the surface change. It has been observed that when a new influenza virus strain becomes prevalent throughout the country, the old virus strain disappears.

Transmission is by close contact or by droplets from the respiratory tract of an infected person. The virus is airborne and multiplies in the upper respiratory tract, invading the nasal, tracheal, and bronchial mucosal cells.

Clinical Manifestations. In the majority of patients, influenza begins after a short incubation period (24–72 hours) with an abrupt onset of chills, fever, headache, backache, and malaise. Respiratory features include a dry cough, sore throat, nasal obstruction, and discharge. Other patients start with acute sinusitis, bronchitis, pleurisy, or bronchopneumonia. These symptoms are always abrupt in onset, and prostrating. In still another group, there are gastrointestinal symptoms of nausea, vomiting, abdominal pain, and diarrhea; and finally, in each epidemic, cases develop without local symptoms but with chills or a continuous fever. The patient usually recovers within a week if there are no complications.

Complications. Persons at risk of developing the complications of influenza are the elderly (over 65), persons with chronic pulmonary or cardiac disease (especially rheumatic valve disease), and those with diabetes or other chronic metabolic disorders or chronic renal disease. The influenza virus damages the ciliated epithelium of the tracheobronchial tree, rendering the patient vulnerable to the development of secondary invaders such as pneumococci or staphylococci, *H. influenzae,* various streptococci, and other organisms.

Dyspnea early in the course of the disease points to bronchopneumonia, which is potentially life-threatening. This pneumonia may be viral, mixed viral, or bacterial in origin. Other symptoms include coughing of viscid sputum, tachycardia, and cyanosis. Vigorous supportive care is indicated, including tracheal aspiration, oxygen, and possibly mechanical ventilation. Other complications include myocarditis, myositis, and meningoencephalitis.

Management. The objectives of treatment are to give symptomatic management and to prevent and treat complications. There is no specific treatment for influenza. Usually, the patient will go to bed because of prostration. Antipyretics and analgesics, such as aspirin, will reduce fever and relieve headache and myalgia. Such drugs should be taken regularly to avoid marked swings of temperature with sweating and chills, leading to exhaustion and dehydration. When the patient resumes activities, he should be sure that any sense of well-being and reduction of temperature are not being caused by the aspirin.

Cough syrup may be soothing for a dry, hacking cough. A vaporizer is helpful in reducing irritation of the respiratory mucosa. A liberal fluid intake is advised because of fever.

Prevention and Patient Education. The Immunization Practices Advisory Committee of the Public Health Service recommends annual influenza vaccination for all persons older than 65 and for persons younger than 65 who have chronic underlying illness. However, influenza vaccination has not been recommended as a routine primary procedure because uncomplicated influenza is a self-limited disease with a low mortality rate. The effectiveness of influenza vaccine has been variable, and protection has been relatively brief. Recent vaccine has more antigen than prior products and should give better results.

The National Influenza Immunization Program of 1976 revealed an association of Guillain–Barré Syndrome with influenza vaccination. There is no proof that the currently available vaccine has the same risk, but the possibility exists.

The risk of developing influenza is also related to crowding and close contact of groups of individuals. Therefore, visiting privileges within health care facilities, especially nursing homes, should be restricted during epidemics to minimize any chance of introducing influenza.

Amantadine, an antiviral drug, can prevent clinical infection with influenza A virus. (It blocks an early step in the replication of this virus.) It is given only to certain high-risk patients, since most patients exposed to influenza require no prophylaxis. Amantadine does not protect against endemic influenza or influenza B. Amantadine is also given for the treatment of symptomatic influenza A infection and

may shorten the duration and diminish the severity of illness. Adverse effects, occurring mainly in the elderly, include central nervous system toxicity, confusion, dizziness, slurred speech, headache, sleep disturbances, and visual hallucinations. To be effective, amantadine should be given prior to, and for the duration of, exposure to type A influenza virus. Rimantadine has also been shown to protect against influenza A infection with significantly fewer side-effects.

Nursing Isolation Procedure. No isolation or precautions are necessary for the usual patient. There may be instances when respiratory isolation is indicated, especially if the diagnosis can be made on or soon after admission.

Infectious Mononucleosis

Infectious mononucleosis ("mono") is an acute infectious disease of the lymphatic system caused by the Epstein-Barr virus (EBV), a DNA virus of the herpes virus group. Another virus, cytomegalovirus, can cause virtually identical symptoms. A third infecting organism, *Toxoplasma* (a protozoan), can also produce a similar clinical picture.

The basic pathology is an intense proliferative response of the lymphoid tissue and organs (lymph nodes, spleen, tonsils), but all organs can be affected. Infectious mononucleosis is usually self-limited, but rarely, complications and even death do occur.

Epidemiology. Infectious mononucleosis is encountered most frequently in the 14-to-30 age group. It has been shown that when natural primary infection with EBV develops in childhood, a mild and nonspecific or inapparent illness occurs, and the child has immunity for many years. Infectious mononucleosis only occurs in individuals without antibody to EBV. If natural primary infection does not take place in childhood and a susceptible person (adolescent/young adult) acquires the infection, this event will lead to clinical manifestations of infectious mononucleosis in about 50% of cases. Thus, infectious mononucleosis is more frequently encountered in countries with a high standard of living, whereas in developing countries or among deprived socioeconomic groups, primary infection almost always occurs in early childhood, so that the disease is virtually unknown. In this country, in persons of college age, the rate of clinical attack is three to five times that of the population at large.

Transmission of infectious mononucleosis is by oral contact. The virus may persist in the pharynx for weeks or months. This suggests that a large number of young adults are probably convalescent carriers of this disease. The virus can also be spread by blood transfusion. The incubation period ranges from 30 to 50 days.

Clinical Manifestations. The early clinical manifestations are usually vague and masquerade as those of streptococcal sore throat, leukemia, and hepatitis. The triad of fever, sore throat, and cervical lymph node enlargement suggests infectious mononucleosis. A typical attack begins with fever and chills, anorexia, sore throat, and myalgia. Headache and diarrhea are often seen. On the second or third day, the lymph nodes begin to swell and become tender, usually the posterior cervical group first, and then the anterior groups. This causes pain in the neck. Generalized lymphadenopathy may occur. Early in the course of the disease, supraorbital edema occurs and the spleen enlarges in 50% to 75% of patients. Although hepatomegaly occurs in less than 25% of patients, the majority of patients have abnormal liver function tests. A faint erythematous or maculopapular eruption may appear in the early stage of the disease.

Diagnostic Evaluation.   The diagnosis is made on the basis of the typical picture of clinical illness, as well as such laboratory findings as lymphocytosis with many atypical lymphocytes, abnormal liver function tests, a positive heterophil antibody test, and the persistence of antibody to EBV. In the heterophil test (positive in 90% of cases), heterophil antibodies in a small amount of blood from the patient with infectious mononucleosis will clump red blood cells from sheep or horses. This test can now be done in less than 3 minutes in the physician's office, using a specially prepared slide on which there are sheep or horse red blood cells stabilized by formaldehyde. (Heterophil-negative disease has been reported.) Antibodies to EBV also develop, and a blood test can identify EBV-specific IgM and IgG antibodies.

Management.   The treatment is symptomatic and supportive. The patient is encouraged to remain on bed rest while fever lasts and to rest at intervals during recovery. Aspirin is given for headache and muscle pains. Constipation (which leads to straining and sudden increase in portal venous pressure, which in turn can contribute to splenic rupture) is to be avoided. Steroids may be used when severe or life-threatening complications develop—marked hepatic dysfunction, neurologic manifestations, thrombocytopenia, hemolytic anemia, and airway obstruction. Most patients recover in 1 to 3 weeks.

Patient Education.   Fatigue and increased sleep requirements may remain for a period of time. The enlarged spleen of the patient with infectious mononucleosis is vulnerable to injury and may rupture if subjected to relatively mild trauma. Thus, strenuous physical activity and competitive sports should be avoided until recovery is complete. For the athlete, this may mean up to 6 months. However, the exact length of time is uncertain, since the spleen may rupture after clinical, hematologic, and serologic evidence reveals complete recovery.

The consequences of a ruptured spleen are potentially serious because of the substantial volume of blood that may be lost into the peritoneal cavity. Abdominal pain usually heralds the presence of splenic rupture. The presence of free intraperitoneal blood may irritate the diaphragm and may cause shoulder pain. The treatment is blood transfusions and immediate splenectomy.

Rabies (Hydrophobia)

Rabies is a severe viral infection of the central nervous system communicated to humans from the saliva of infected animals and commonly transmitted by a bite or by contact of the animal's saliva with a mucous membrane or open wound. The disease occurs mainly among wildlife, especially skunks, foxes, raccoons, and bats, and is becoming more prominent. The rabies virus is classified with the rhabdoviruses. The virus is spread from the wound to the peripheral nerves to the central nervous system, where rabies viral encephalitis ensues.

Early signs of rabies in animals include an altered disposition and behavior, fever, loss of appetite, and a change in the tone of bark (in dogs).

Dogs, fortunately, usually present evidence of the disease before becoming infective. The etiologic agent is an ultramicroscopic virus present in the saliva and the central nervous system. Negri bodies (round objects about one quarter the size of red blood corpuscles) are found in the brain tissues so constantly in this disease that their presence is sufficient for diagnosis.

Management of the Biting Animal.   The animal inflicting the bite is captured (if possible) and kept under surveillance by veterinarians or animal control personnel. This may enable the bitten person to avoid undergoing unnecessary rabies vaccination. If the animal remains healthy for about 10 days, it is assumed that it was not infective.

However, if the animal becomes sick, the health department is notified. The animal is humanely killed, and its head is shipped, under refrigeration, to a qualified laboratory where the brain is examined for the characteristic Negri bodies. A wild animal that bites a person without provocation is killed at once, and the brain is sent for examination. If the brain of the animal is negative for rabies, it is assumed that the saliva contained no virus and that the bitten person need not be treated.

Prophylactic Management of the Patient
Local Treatment of the Wound.   The bite wounds should be cleansed immediately with thorough and prolonged (3–4 minutes) washing with soap and water to remove the saliva, to dilute viral exposure, and for the virucidal benefits of soap. Squeezing the wound to make it bleed helps to cleanse it. The patient is then taken immediately for emergency treatment, at which time the wound is again cleansed, debrided as indicated, and again flushed with soap solution and water. Additional protection may be given by applying 70% alcohol to the exposed area. The patient is given tetanus prophylaxis and antimicrobial therapy to counter any other possible infection transmitted by the animal.

Postexposure Prophylaxis.   Postexposure prophylaxis is designed to prevent the development of rabies illness in an exposed person. The decision to give postexposure treatment is made on an individual basis and depends on the type of animal involved (skunk, bat, fox, raccoon), the circumstances surrounding the exposure incident, whether or not the animal was captured, the vaccination status of the animal, and the presence of rabies in the region.

A combination of passive and active immunization is recommended when postexposure treatment is deemed necessary. Two types of immunizing products are used: (1) globulin, providing rapid protection; and (2) vaccine, which induces an active immune response that develops more slowly. As soon as possible, rabies immune globulin (RIG [which is made from the serum of immunized donors and is free of the danger of animal antiserum]) is administered. (Part of the RIG dose is infiltrated around the wound, and the rest is administered intramuscularly in the patient's buttock.) At the same time the single dose of RIG is given, human diploid cell vaccine (HDCV) is given intramuscularly and is followed by four more vaccine doses given at 3, 7, 14, and 28 days. HDCV appears to produce immunity more quickly than previous rabies vaccines and causes substantially fewer side-effects. After the completion of the series of inoculations, a serum specimen for rabies antibody testing is drawn to assure that active immunity has been achieved. Serum antibody testing is arranged through the state health department.

Development of Rabies in Man

Diagnostic Evaluation.   The diagnosis of rabies is made on the basis of the history of exposure (the patient was bitten or exposed to animal saliva), the development of characteristic symptoms, and the demonstration of rabies antibodies in the patient's blood, along with the characteristic Negri bodies in samples of brain tissue taken from the infected animal.

Clinical Course in Man.   The incubation period in humans is extremely variable, depending on the location and severity of the wound and the length of the nerve over which the virus must travel before it reaches the brain. The incubation period may only be 10 days to several weeks for bites around the face, or from 60 to 90 days and up to a year for a bite in another part of the body.

There are several clinical phases of rabies in humans. During the prodromal phase of the illness, there are abnormal sensations around the site of infection, and the individual experiences an uneasy feeling and general anxiety, accompanied by depression and irritability. The patient may have headache, nausea, sore throat, and loss of appetite, or may experience unusual sensitivity to sound, light, and changes in temperature.

Then follows the stage of excitement. There are episodes of irrational excitement alternating with periods of alert calm. During this stage, convulsions occur. Attempting to swallow or even looking at liquids induces such severe and painful spasms of the muscles of swallowing and respiration that the patient writhes, and the ensuing choking may produce apnea. (Hence, the older name for rabies is *hydrophobia,* or fear of water.) Death usually occurs in this stage from cardiac or respiratory failure.

If the patient survives this stage, the muscle spasms and agitation cease. The paralytic phase is one of usually progressive ascending paralysis terminating in coma and death.

Management of Rabies.   There is no specific treatment for rabies, and the care of the patient is supportive. Barbiturates, phenothiazines, and paraldehyde are used symptomatically. The patient is placed in the intensive care unit and receives continuing cardiac and pulmonary monitoring. The room should be quiet and darkened. The outcome is usually fatal.

- Bear in mind that the rabies virus is contained in the saliva of patients with this disease, constituting a distinct hazard to personnel caring for him. All personnel must be on guard against being bitten by such a patient or allowing saliva to contaminate a skin abrasion. If this occurs, personnel must receive the same treatment as the patient, including antirabic serum and rabies vaccine.

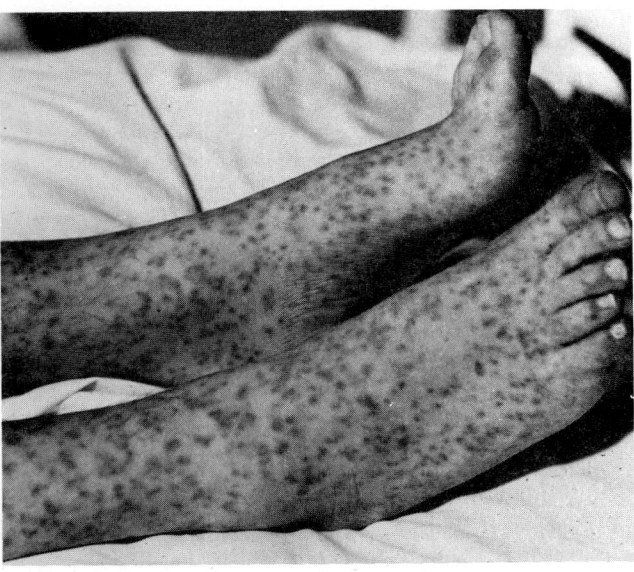

Figure 63-6.   The rash of Rocky Mountain spotted fever. (Armed Forces Institute of Pathology photograph, Neg. No. N–67987-3)

Nursing Isolation Procedure.   Strict isolation precautions are carried out for the duration of the illness.

▷ Rickettsial Infections

Rocky Mountain Spotted Fever

Rocky Mountain spotted fever (tick-borne typhus fever) is characterized by a continuous fever. It is caused by the bite of an infected tick, by an infected tick being crushed on the skin, or by the conjunctiva becoming contaminated with infected tick juice. The organism responsible is the *Rickettsia rickettsii.* The most common vectors for transmitting the disease to man are the wood tick (*Dermacentor andersoni*) and the dog tick (*Dermacentor variabilis*).

Clinical Manifestations.   During infection in humans, *R. rickettsii* organisms localize and proliferate in the vascular endothelium of small vessels, where they produce widespread swelling and degeneration. This generalized vasculitis accounts for the manifestations of the disease, both the cutaneous lesions and visceral disturbances. It may involve virtually every organ.

Early symptoms, appearing several days after an infected tick bite, are severe headache, malaise, anorexia, photophobia, slight fever, and muscle and joint pain. Within a few days, the fever, rash, and edema are quite pronounced. The rash is the most specific manifestation of the infection and consists of rose-colored macules of variable size that appear on the wrists, ankles, soles, and palms, gradually spreading over the entire body. It becomes papular, darker red, and slightly dusky, and after a few days has a petechial or purpuric character (Fig. 63-6). Large subcutaneous hemorrhages may appear. In severe forms of the disease, areas of skin necrosis appear as a result of endarteritis (inflammatory blockage of arterioles). This necrosis may involve the ear lobes, fingers, toes, and scrotum—those areas at the extreme periphery of the vascular system. There may be marked thrombocytopenia due to inflammation of the vessels communicating with the bone marrow. As a result of generalized vascular involvement and resulting escape of serum, generalized edema occurs.

Restlessness, insomnia, and hyperesthesias are distressing symptoms of this disease. Delirium is common at the height of the fever, but convulsions rarely occur. The spleen is large and tender. Gastrointestinal symptoms include abdominal tenderness, pain, and muscular rigidity. There are a slight leukocytosis and a slight secondary anemia. Pneumonia may occur. Mental confusion, deafness, and visual disturbances are common and may last for weeks.

The early diagnosis is important and is almost always made on clinical grounds. Serologic confirmation (complement fixation tests, tests for indirect fluorescent antibodies, indirect hemagglutination, latex agglutination or microagglutination) may not be positive until 10 to 14 days after the onset of illness.

Management.   One of the tetracyclines or chloramphenicol are both specific rickettsiostatic drugs if administered in the *early* stages of the disease. Rocky Mountain spotted fever can run a rapid and fulminating course, and despite the effectiveness of tetracycline or chloramphenicol in treatment, the morbidity and mortality rates are still significant. Because Rocky Mountain spotted fever is an infectious vasculitis, the patient may display marked physiologic disturbances, including circulatory collapse, hypotension, oliguria, azotemia, hypoproteinemia, and edema. Central venous pressure measurements are used to guide fluid and electrolyte replacement. The patient may be given transfusions of packed red blood cells and platelets. Severe coagulation disturbances may be treated with heparin. Supportive nursing measures are used to combat fever, restlessness, and pain, and to promote patient comfort. The majority of patients recover if treated early.

Prevention and Patient Education.   Rocky Mountain spotted fever continues to increase in the United States, with 80% of the cases occurring in the South Atlantic and South Central States. (The disease has almost vanished from its original home in the Rockies.)

As increasing numbers of Americans participate in backpacking and other camping activities, more people will be exposed to this disease. Important aspects of prevention are wearing protective clothing and conscientiously searching for and removing ticks. Persons living in tick-infested areas, or visiting such places, should examine their scalp, skin, and clothing two to three times daily for ticks. This is important, as an infected tick must usually be attached and feeding several hours before it can transmit the disease. Tick repellent should be applied to the exposed parts of the body and clothing, especially socks and trouser cuffs and any openings in the clothing (neck, top of pants, button areas).

Ticks may be removed from the body by grasping the tick with tweezers (or if these are not available, a bent twig or the fingers, covered with paper) and pulling it gently and firmly outward from the body. Care should be taken not to crush the tick, thus avoiding contamination of the broken skin with infectious tick secretions. The tick bite should be disinfected immediately. The hands should be protected with gloves or paper while the tick is being removed and washed thoroughly after tick removal. Other means of removing a tick are to touch it with gasoline or cover it with a thick ointment. Household pets should be examined for ticks on a regular basis.

The Advisory Committee on Immunization Practices recommends vaccine routinely only for those persons with laboratory exposure to *R. rickettsii* (rickettsiologists and their technicians) and those with regular occupational exposure.

▷ Protozoan Infections

Malaria

Malaria is an acute infectious disease caused by protozoa, which are transmitted by way of an intermediate host, the bite of an infective female *Anopheles* mosquito. Malaria has also been transmitted via blood transfusions and from the needles and syringes shared by drug addicts.

Incidence.   Malaria affects approximately 150 to 200 million people in the world. It is claimed that in Africa, one fourth of all adults suffer from malarial fever at one time or other. It causes more disability and a heavier economic burden than any other parasitic disease. International travel and the recent influx of Asian and Middle Eastern immigrants has been responsible for a resurgence in many nontropical countries. In addition, more than 20 species of anopheline mosquitoes have become resistant to commonly used insecticides.

Types of Malaria.   There are four species of malarial parasites, grouped under the generic name *Plasmodium*, each causing a different type of malaria: *Plasmodium falciparum, Plasmodium vivax, Plasmodium malariae,* and *Plasmodium ovale.* Each malarial parasite lives within a red blood corpuscle, utilizing the hemoglobin as food. When full grown, it divides (segments) into 10 to 20 small, young parasites, called *hyalines* (or segments), which burst the cell; this bursting of cells causes chills in the patient. The majority of these hyalines die, but a few find their way into new red cells, and the process described above is repeated.

Assessment

Clinical Manifestations.   The majority of patients present with paroxysms of chills, fever, and sweating. Nausea, fatigue, and dizziness along with intense headache and muscle pains are present. Paroxysms of chills and fever may last about 12 hours, after which the cycle may be repeated daily, every other day, or every third day.

Complications occur most frequently with *P. falciparum.* Patients with severe malaria of any form may become comatose and die (pernicious malaria); they may develop renal failure (due to the precipitation of free hemoglobin in the kidney tubule), a serious gastrointestinal disturbance, or cerebral symptoms (due to an accumulation of the parasites in the blood vessels of the affected organ).

Diagnostic Evaluation.   The patient should be asked where he has been. Travel or residence in an area where malaria is endemic is an important diagnostic clue. The diagnosis is confirmed by the finding of the plasmodium in the patient's blood. The blood should be examined as soon as the patient presents for treatment. More than one blood examination may be required, since the diagnosis can be missed on a routine smear.

Management

The objective of treatment is to destroy the blood trophozoites and schizonts of *Plasmodium* that cause the clinical manifestations and the pathologic effects that characterize the disease.

The use of antimalarial drugs depends on the stage of the life cycle of the parasite that is affected. The species of parasite infecting the patient is determined by way of a blood smear.

Chloroquine is given for infections with *P. malariae* or sensitive *P. falciparum.* This regimen is followed by primaquine phosphate for *P. ovale* and *P. vivax* infections. Quinine is given with either pyrimethamine and sulfadiazine or tetracycline for chloroquine-resistant *P. falciparum* strains.

Other supportive measures include the administration of aspirin, to control fever, muscular aches, and headaches, and the lowering of fever by cool sponges. The fluid balance must be appraised on each patient. Complications are treated as they arise.

Unfortunately, *P. falciparum* is often drug-resistant, and the diagnosis is made when the patient is critically ill. Patients with this type of malaria require hospitalization, as the infection can rapidly overwhelm the patient. In fact, this is considered a medical emergency. If the patient comes from an area known to harbor drug-resistant malaria, the treatment is quinine (orally if possible, or by slow infusion in severely ill patients), pyrimethamine, or one of the sulfonamides. Watch for neurologic toxicity from the quinine infusion—twitching, delirium, confusion, convulsion, and coma.

Oxygen may be given, as tissue anoxia is thought to be common. Jaundice is evaluated and is related to the density of *P. falciparum* parasitemia (presence of malarial parasites in the blood). Abnormalities of hepatic function are common in this type of malaria. The degree of anemia is related to the severity of infection. Abnormal bleeding (nosebleeds, oozing of blood from venipuncture sites, passage of blood in the stool) may be due either to decreased production of clotting factors by a damaged liver or to disseminated intravascular coagulation.

Cerebral malaria, which occurs in about 2% of patients with acute falciparum malaria, is the most feared complication. It produces changes in consciousness, behavioral changes, seizures, and cerebral edema. The patient is monitored closely.

Nursing Isolation Procedures.

Blood precautions should be used for the duration of the patient's hospitalization. A screened room is required for the patient who is ill in a tropical climate.

Prevention and Patient Education.

The essence of malaria control is the eradication of malaria as an endemic disease. In several areas of the world, this goal has been achieved. To escape malaria, one must avoid *Anopheles* mosquitoes that have fed on the blood of patients with malaria about 3 weeks previously. The wearing of long sleeves and trousers after dusk and the application of mosquito repellent to exposed skin decreases the chance of being bitten by anopheline mosquitoes. Other measures include sleeping under a mosquito net, spraying the room, and protecting living quarters with screens.

The Centers for Disease Control publishes *Health Information for International Travel,* which lists the areas of the world where there is risk of infection with malaria, and also the areas with strains of *P. falciparum* that are resistant to chloroquine. Persons planning a visit to endemic malarious areas (in which there is no known chloroquine-resistant strains) are given chloroquine before entry into the area and continue to take the drug for a specified time after returning to the U.S. The Centers for Disease Control will advise of the most recent prophylactic recommendations.

The traveler is advised to seek prompt health care if he develops fever after stopping prophylaxis. Travelers to malarious areas should not donate blood for up to 3 years.

Amebiasis (Amebic Dysentery)

Amebae are protozoa, larger than leukocytes, that move by ameboid action. Only a few amebae infect man. One of the most important of these is *Entamoeba histolytica,* the cause of amebic dysentery. These amebae survive outside the body in resistant encysted forms.

Amebiasis is a worldwide parasitic disease of the large intestine. It is acquired through the ingestion of the cyst stage of *E. histolytica* in food or water contaminated by infected human feces, flies, or the hands of infected food handlers, or by oral–anal or oral–genital sexual contact (both heterosexual and homosexual).

In parts of the world where there is lack of hygiene and sanitation, infection rates of 50% or more occur. In the United States, about 5% of the population is infected. Persons at risk in this country are immigrants and visitors from developing countries, travelers returning from these areas, and sexually active male homosexuals.

Pathophysiology.   The amebae burrow their way into the intestinal mucosa, where they feed mainly on bacteria. Pus pockets may form, with only a small orifice opening into the bowel from which numerous burrows extend for considerable distances in all directions under the mucous membrane. Here the amebae live. Abscesses form in the mucous membrane, and eventually slough off, exposing an underlying ulcer that may enlarge to sizes of 1 cm to 2 cm in diameter. The large bowel may be so covered by such ulcers that very little normal mucous membrane is left. Usually, the floor of these ulcers is the muscle wall of the bowel, but they may perforate its entire wall and cause fatal peritonitis.

In the small intestine, the organism may erode intestinal mucosa, invade the bloodstream, and gain access to the liver through the portal vein.

Clinical Manifestations and Course.   The clinical manifestations depend on the site of involvement. Approximately 50% of patients are asymptomatic. Amebiasis may present as an intestinal or extraintestinal disease. If the intestines have been affected, the chief symptoms are diarrhea, with abdominal cramping and pain. Diarrhea may be mild, with loose stools, or there may be severe dysentery with stools containing considerable amounts of blood, exudate, and mucus, the latter swarming with amebae. Persons with chronic disease usually have associated weight loss and anemia. Amebiasis may mimic irritable bowel syndrome. The illness may present as appendicitis, abdominal mass, or partial intestinal obstruction.

The two important features of this disease are its chronicity (one attack of acute dysentery following another, separated by periods of constipation that last for months) and the tendency of the infection to cause liver abscess, as a result of metastases to the liver by way of the portal vein. Complications include peritonitis, abscess formation, hemorrhage, and extraintestinal disease.

The diagnosis is made by finding trophozoites or cysts in a freshly purged stool specimen or on a nonpurged, warm stool specimen. (Moving trophozoites disintegrate at room temperature, and false negative tests can occur.) Rectal biopsy may reveal the organism. Proctosigmoidoscopic examination reveals mild mucosal friability. If the test is suspected as being falsely negative, there are serologic techniques available to detect amebiasis. In intestinal amebiasis, the indirect hemagglutination (IHA) test is considered the most sensitive.

Management.   The objectives of treatment are to eradicate the organism, to give symptomatic relief, and to replace fluids and electrolytes.

There is uncertainty about what constitutes the best treatment, as a significant number of patients require multiple courses of therapy. Drugs used for the treatment of amebiasis include emetine, tetracycline, paromomycin, metronidazole, and the halogenated quinolines (iodoquinol, diloxanide furoate, Furoxone, quinacrine hydrochloride, chloroquine). Usually, two drugs are used—one to rid the intestines of the trophozoites, and the other to dispose of the cysts.

To support the patient's general condition, intravenous infusions are given as required to correct fluid and electrolyte imbalance resulting from severe diarrhea. If diarrhea is acute, the patient remains on bed rest and is offered low-residue, bland foods. Follow-up study of the stools are necessary, since relapses are common.

Control; Patient Education.   Methods of control include sanitary disposal of human feces, protection of the public water supply, and an ongoing program of health education in personal hygiene, including meticulous handwashing after defecation and before preparing and eating food. Contacts of recently diagnosed patients should be examined. Patients should abstain from oral–anal or oral–genital sexual practices while they are under treatment. Intimate sexual partners of infected patients should have a stool examination.

Nursing Isolation Procedure.   Excretion precautions should be observed for the duration of the illness.

Amebic Liver Abscess

Amebic liver abscess represents the most common extraintestinal complication of amebiasis. It occurs when the amebae infiltrate the liver from the portal circulation. It is found in approximately 3% to 9% of patients with amebiasis.

In most patients, the right lobe of the liver is involved, and the abscess may be single or multiple. The major complaints are pain in the right upper abdomen (caused by the liver's enlarging rapidly and stretching of its capsule), right upper chest pain (due to the liver's enlarging in an upward direction), fever, anorexia, and loss of weight. Physical examination reveals an enlarged, tender liver (due to hepatic abscess) and ausculatory abnormalities of the right lung field (from direct extension or rupture of a contiguous liver abscess). If the abscess is in the left lobe of the liver, a tender epigastric mass is noted. There is fever, sweating, weight loss, and pallor. A liver scan suggests the diagnosis and is useful in identifying the site, size, and number of lesions as well as in following the resolution of the abscess. Ultrasonography is used. Immunologic techniques, mainly serologic methods, are also used in diagnosis. One point to be emphasized is that not infrequently the abscesses are found unexpectedly in patients who have had few or no symptoms suggesting amebiasis.

Usually, the patient responds promptly to amebicidal therapy. Metronidazole (Flagyl) has generally been successful, and it may be combined with iodoquinol or other drugs. Needle drainage of the abscess may be necessary if there is concern that the abscess may rupture and cause peritonitis, or after rupture to reduce further spread of infection, or when clinical illness persists after adequate drug therapy. The supportive treatment is that outlined for amebiasis.

▷ Systemic Mycotic Infections (Fungal Infections)

Fungi are primitive organisms that take their nourishment from living plants and animals and decaying organic material. Fungi have the ability to exist as yeasts or as molds and may alternate between the yeast and mold form. The fungi present difficult problems in control because they are so widespread in nature—in soil, decaying vegetation, and bird excreta. Although there are thousands of known species of fungi, 100 or more species are generally recognized as pathogens to man. The three main types of mycoses (fungal infections), as determined by the tissue level at which the fungus settles, are:

1. Systemic or deep mycoses involving primarily the internal organs, usually centering in the lungs
2. Subcutaneous mycoses that involve the skin, subcutaneous tissue, and sometimes the bone
3. Superficial or cutaneous mycoses that grow in the outer layer of skin (epidermis), the hair, and the nails

Persons at Risk.   The systemic mycoses have occurred more frequently in recent years, since they are more common in patients with impaired immunologic resistance and in patients receiving immunosuppressive agents (steroids, antilymphocyte serum, chemotherapy for cancer). Many patients who are receiving such treatment, or who are debilitated or severely ill and have reduced defenses, become prey to invasion by fungi that they could ordinarily withstand.

In addition to those receiving immunosuppressive agents, patients at risk for invasive fungal infections are those with certain immunologic deficiencies, those with advanced malignancies, kidney or other organ-transplant patients, open heart surgery patients, severely burned patients, patients receiving prolonged intravenous feedings, and those with renal failure and diabetes.

Systemic infections are usually acquired by accidental inhalation (spores carried on wind currents), occasionally by traumatic implantation (from contaminated soil or plant materials), or by the pathologic takeover of a normal inhabitant when the resistance of the host is lowered. It is not transmitted person-to-person.

Histoplasmosis is a chronic systemic fungus infection caused by a spore-bearing mold, *Histoplasma capsulatum.* This highly infectious mycosis is transmitted by airborne dust that contains *H. capsulatum* spores. Partially decayed droppings of pigeons, chickens, bats, and birds offer an excellent medium for growth of this fungus.

Clinical Manifestations. The signs and symptoms closely resemble those of pulmonary tuberculosis: fever, cough, dyspnea, anorexia, and loss of weight and strength. Fungal infections mimic symptoms of other diseases, and the patient may present findings of malignant lymphoma, including anemia, thrombocytopenia, splenomegaly, and hepatomegaly.

Management. Most patients do not require treatment. Bed rest and supportive care may be indicated. Amphotericin B has traditionally been the mainstay of treatment for disseminated or acute pulmonary disease, as it has a wide spectrum of activity against fungal infections. It is given intravenously and is reserved for serious infections, as this agent has significant toxicity.

Ketoconazole is a new antifungal agent that is orally absorbable and effective against the etiologic agents of systemic mycoses. It has been associated with hepatic toxicity requiring close patient monitoring.

Health Education. Avoid stirring up dust by raking and sweeping around bird roosting sites. Exposure to dust in a contained, enclosed environment (chicken coop) should be minimized. Spraying the area with water will reduce dust.

Nursing Isolation Procedure. None required (no person-to-person spread of disease).

▷ Helminthic Infestations

Major helminthic (worm) infections are among the most prevalent of the human infectious diseases. There are three major groups of helminths that are intestinal parasites in man: the nematodes (roundworms), the cestides (tapeworms), and the trematodes (flukes).

Trichinosis (Trichinellosis)

Trichinosis is infestation by the parasite *Trichinella spiralis,* one of the roundworms. It is acquired by consuming infected meat, usually pork.

Clinical Manifestations and Course. This is a disease of pigs in the continental U.S. and of bears in Alaska. Tiny embryos of the parasite, *T. spiralis,* become encysted in the muscle fibers of an infected pig. These calcified cysts, barely visible to the naked eye, appear in the meat like tiny grains of sand. If such pork is insufficiently cooked and then eaten, the embryos are set free by the gastric juice and develop in the intestine during the following week into adult worms, about 3 mm to 4 mm in length. These worms make their way into the mucous membrane and there produce myriad embryos. The intestinal phase starts about 24 hours after larval ingestion, causing symptoms of gastrointestinal disturbance: nausea, vomiting, diarrhea, and abdominal pain.

The embryos, carried by the bloodstream and by their own activity, migrate to all parts of the body. The patient's symptoms, arising from muscle invasion (due to an inflammatory process in the muscles), include edema of the eyelids, scleral hemorrhages, pain on eye motion, and generalized pain and soreness of muscles. Trichinosis causes high fever. Peripheral eosinophilia is a constant finding. Occasional heart iregularities (due to trichinae in the heart muscle) may be seen and may be fatal. Difficulties in breathing, masticating, swallowing, or speaking may also occur.

Diagnostic Evaluation. A biopsy specimen taken from a painful muscle (deltoid, biceps, gastrocnemius) reveals the larvae. Serologic tests may be positive, with demonstrable titers 3 to 4 weeks after the infection. Usually, the eosinophil count begins to rise in the second week. A skin test based on an extract of trichinae as the test antigen becomes positive after 16 to 20 days and may be positive for years afterward.

Management. The treatment of trichinosis is symptomatic. Thiabendazole (Mintezol) produces clinical improvement, but its effect on larvae that have migrated to muscles is not conclusive. Side-effects of this drug include nausea, vertigo, headache, and weakness. The patient is kept on bed rest and given analgesics to relieve muscle pain. Corticosteroids may be given during the acute phase to minimize the allergic reaction and relieve the patient's symptoms. Electrocardiograms are taken to determine the evidence of myocarditis.

Prevention; Patient Education. The public should be educated regarding the importance of thoroughly cooking all pork and pork products, especially sausage. There should be no trace of pink in cooked pork. Cooking pork in a microwave oven may fail to kill larvae. Smoking, pickling, seasoning, or spicing does not make pork safe unless it is cooked. Beef hamburger may be contaminated by a meat grinder that has been used for pork.

Garbage intended for hogs should be cooked. And finally, pork should be inspected by regular meat inspectors to determine if the disease is present.

Hookworm Disease (Ancylostomiasis)

Hookworm disease is the result of infestation of the small intestine by one of two quite similar roundworms about 1.2 cm (½ inch) long. Two species are parasitic in the human intestinal tract: *Necator americanus* (predominant U.S. species) and *Ancylostoma duodenale.* The infection is usually acquired by walking barefoot, whereby infected larvae of the worms penetrate the skin.

Incidence. Approximately 700 to 900 million persons are infected with hookworm. It is found mainly in tropical and subtropical regions, notably Asia, the Mediterranean area, South America, Africa, and in most of the western hemisphere. In the U.S., hookworm infections are more prevalent in the southeastern states.

Pathology and Clinical Course. The embryos of this worm, hatched from eggs passed in human feces onto the ground, live in dirt, sand, and clay, and easily infest man. They enter by mouth when food is eaten with dirty hands, or they bore through the skin of bare feet (ground itch). Having gained access to the blood or lymph vessels, they are carried by the bloodstream to the lungs, and migrate from the pulmonary capillaries into the alveolar sacs. The larvae migrate up the bronchi and trachea, pass over the epiglottis and down the esophagus, and into the bowel. The worms attach themselves to the intestinal mucosa and suck the blood of the host. The effect of the blood-sucking and hemorrhages at the attachment sites is iron-deficiency anemia. A patient with heavy infection and with inadequate dietary iron may develop profound anemia. He presents with lassitude, dyspnea, anorexia, and pedal edema. Severe anemia may cause cardiac symptoms. Maturation of the worms in the intestine may cause diarrhea and other gastrointestinal symptoms. A dry cough and dyspnea develop when the larvae rupture through the capillary bed and are spread throughout the bronchial tree.

Management. Mebendazole or pyrantel pamoate (Antiminth) are both effective for hookworm disease. The patient should be placed on a nutritious diet, since hookworm disease occurs in persons suffering from malnutrition. Protein and iron supplementation is administered to aid in the correction of the anemia.

Prevention. The prevention of hookworm disease depends on sanitary disposal of human excreta and the wearing of shoes. Night soil (human excrement used as fertilizer) and sewage affluents should not be used for fertilizer.

Ascariasis (Roundworm Infestation)

Ascariasis is an infection by the nematode *Ascaris lumbricoides* (intestinal roundworm), which may live in the intestine of man. This is the most common worm parasitizing the intestine of man, with an estimated 1 billion infections worldwide. Ascariasis occurs in approximately 1 million Americans and is more common in the southern states.

This disease is usually found in overcrowded areas with poor sanitation. Contamination of the soil by human feces is a factor in its spread. Indiscriminate defecation in the fields, streets, and doorways provides a major source of infective eggs. Man is infected by ingestion of the eggs in contaminated raw vegetables and drinking water. Infection may be contracted from eating raw vegetables when night soil is used for fertilizer. Water pollution may cause water transmission.

Life Cycle and Clinical Features. The eggs are swallowed and pass into the intestine, where they hatch as larvae. The larvae enter the bloodstream and pass through the pulmonary circulation, migrate through the lungs, and return to the gastrointestinal tract, where they grow, mature, and mate. Large numbers of worms may migrate into various organs of the body and cause obstruction to the trachea, bronchi, bile duct, appendix, and pancreatic duct. Masses of worms in the intestine cause gastrointestinal discomfort, severe abdominal pain, and vomiting. Fever, chills, dyspnea, cough, and pneumonia may develop from invasion of the lungs by large numbers of larvae. Adult worms may migrate

into the ampulla of Vater and then to the pancreatic or biliary ducts, causing acute and agonizing pain.

Ascariasis is diagnosed by detecting ova or worms in the feces.

Management. Mebendazole (Vermox) given twice daily for 3 days is currently the drug of choice. Piperazine (Antepar) and pyrantel pamoate (Antiminth) are also effective drugs.

Nursing Isolation Procedures. No isolation or precautions are required.

Prevention. Preventive measures include providing adequate toilet facilities and teaching the importance of personal hygiene. All patients with the infestation should be treated.

Enterobiasis (Oxyuriasis, Pinworm Disease)

Enterobiasis (oxyuriasis) is the most common helminthic infection in the United States with over 42 million infections estimated. The pinworm (*Enterobius vermicularis*) is a small, white, threadlike worm, about half a centimeter long, commonly found in the rectum of children. It is a worldwide infestation, and infections tend to affect groups (families, institutionalized populations). There is an increasing incidence among homosexuals.

The life cycle of the pinworm begins with the mating of the male and female worms in the human intestinal tract (Fig. 63-7). The gravid female migrates down the large intestine to the anus and deposits eggs on the perianal and perineal skin. These eggs are infectious. One pinworm may produce 5,000 to 15,000 eggs. Anal pruritus and scratching promote anal-to-oral transmission by contaminated fingers. Infection may also occur by ingesting eggs in food, dust, and fomites. Others in the household may be contaminated by hands, food, drink, clothing, and bedding since the eggs remain viable for up to 2 weeks.

The chief symptoms are intense nocturnal itching around the anus, restlessness, and nervousness. Vaginitis may occur if the pinworms migrate into the vagina.

Worms may be seen on freshly passed stool or about the anus. Confirmation of the diagnosis can be obtained by securing anal impressions on transparent tape in the morning, before defecation and bathing, since the eggs remain adherent to the skin of that region. The tape is then applied to a slide, where microscopic examination will reveal numerous eggs.

Management. The treatment of choice is mebendazole, given in a single dose and repeated after 2 weeks. Alternative drugs are pyrantel pamoate or piperazine. All members of the family should be treated on the same day, or reinfection is apt to occur.

Prevention of Reinfection; Patient Education. The fingernails should be cut short and nail biting discouraged, since eggs may be retained under the nails of infected persons. Children who bite their nails should be encouraged to wear gloves until the infection has been controlled. Fingernails should be scrubbed with a brush before bedtime. The hands should be washed frequently. The anal area of the patient should be washed upon arising, and salve or ointment applied around the area to prevent the eggs from dispersing. The infected person should wear snug-fitting cotton underpants to discourage hand contact with the perianal region and contamination of the bed linen. The infected person should sleep alone, and bedding and nightwear must be handled carefully. There are a large number of eggs in a contaminated household. The eggs remain viable for two weeks under normal conditions. All potentially contaminated clothing, sheets, and furniture must be cleaned to prevent reinfection. The airborne element makes this a household infection. Pinworm infection does not mean poor hygiene or indifferent housekeeping. The nurse should reassure these patients that it is an infection, and anyone can get it.

Nursing Isolation Procedure. Excretion precautions are required for the duration of illness.

Tapeworms (Cestode Infections)

Beef Tapeworm. *Taenia saginata,* the beef tapeworm, is the most prevalent endemic tapeworm in the U.S. and is acquired by eating insufficiently cooked "measled" beef (*i.e.,* beef containing this worm in its larval form). In the bowel of man, this worm grows to a length of 4.5 meters to 6 meters (15–20 feet). The head, about the size of a common blackheaded pin is provided with suckers only, and the largest links are about ½ cm broad and 1 cm or more long (¼ in broad to ½ in or more long). Broken-off chains of links, full of eggs, often are passed in the stools.

Pork Tapeworm. *Taenia solium,* the pork tapeworm, rare in America, is acquired by eating insufficiently cooked infested pork. It is smaller than the beef tapeworm, being only from 1.8 meters to 3.6 meters long, and has somewhat smaller links. Its head, also smaller, is provided with suckers and hooks. This worm is much more difficult than the beef worm to expel.

Cysticercosis is infection by the larval stage of the tapeworm and is potentially fatal.

If a person swallows an egg instead of the larval form of the pork tapeworm, an embryo will be hatched in the bowel. This penetrates the intestinal mucous membrane and may be carried by the bloodstream to almost any organ of the body (heart, lungs, liver, kidneys, brain). Wherever it settles, it becomes encysted, and in this larval cyst, about 1 cm in diameter, only the head of the tapeworm develops.

The internal organs and the skin of an infested person may contain one or thousands of these cysts. If the cysts are located in the skin or subcutaneous tissues, there may be painless swelling of the area. However, in the eye, cysticeri (larval form of worm) may produce pain and visual symptoms, and in the brain it may cause meningitis, epilepsy, and increased intracranial pressure.

The treatment of these cysts is surgical removal.

Fish Tapeworm. *Diphyllobothrium latum,* a tapeworm common in Europe and the Far East, but comparatively rare in America, is acquired by eating uncooked, infested fish. It may grow to a length of 7.6 meters to 9.1 meters (25–30 feet).

Manifestations and Diagnosis. The beef and pork tapeworms cause few, if any, symptoms, except those suggested by the patient's knowledge that he has the worm. The fish tapeworm, however, occasionally precipitates an

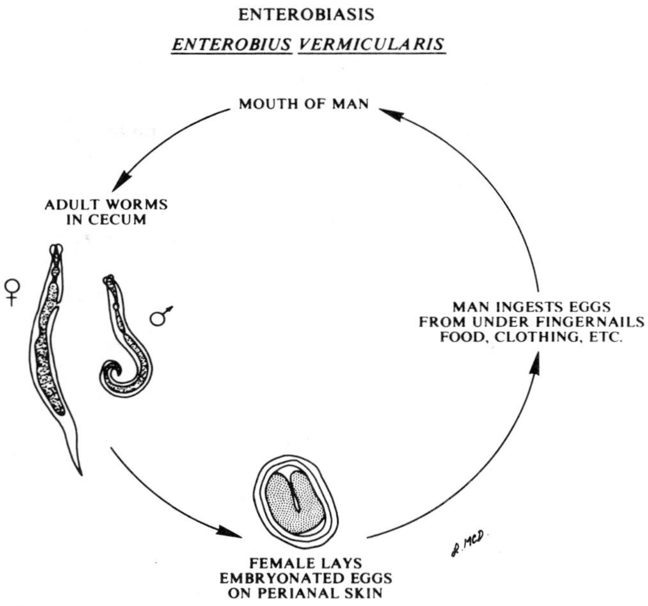

Figure 63-7. Life cycle of *Enterobius vermicularis.* (Armed Forces Institute of Pathology photograph, Neg. No. 75–10881–13)

anemia that scarcely can be distinguished from pernicious anemia.

The diagnosis of all large tapeworms is easy, because their links appear in nearly every stool that the patient passes, and when seen, cannot be mistaken. Ova of the worms may be found on microscopic examination of the stool.

Management. Tapeworm infections may be treated by a single dose of the drug niclosamide. The drug is available through the Parasitic Disease Drug Service of the Centers for Disease Control.

Nursing Isolation Procedures. Excretion precautions are required for patients with pork tapeworm for the duration of the illness. No isolation or precautions are required for persons with the beef tapeworm.

Prevention. There must be adequate inspection, refrigeration, and thorough cooking of fish, beef, and pork products. Other preventive measures include the treatment of human infections and carriers, the proper disposal of human excreta, and good personal hygiene.

▷ Bibliography

Books

Adams ARD and Maegraith BG. Clinical Tropical Diseases. Oxford, Blackwell Scientific, 1980.

Ball AR (ed). Notes on Infectious Diseases. New York, Churchill Livingstone, 1982.

Benenson AS (ed). Control of Communicable Diseases in Man, 13th ed. Washington, DC, American Public Health Association, 1981.

Berquist LM. Microbiology for the Hospital Environment. New York, Harper & Row, 1981.

Braude AI, Davis CE, and Fierer J. Medical and Microbiology and Infectious Diseases. Philadelphia, WB Saunders, 1981.

Brooks SM et al. Handbook of Infectious Disease. Boston, Little, Brown & Co, 1980.

Bruce–Chwatt LJ (ed). Chemotherapy of Malaria. Geneva, World Health Organization, 1981.

Castle M. Hospital Infection Control. New York, John Wiley & Sons, 1980.

Chang RS. Infectious Mononucleosis. Boston, GK Hall, 1980.

Christie AB. Infectious Diseases: Epidemiology and Clinical Practice, 3rd ed. New York, Churchill Livingstone, 1980.

Clark DC and MacMahon B. Preventive and Community Medicine, 2nd ed. Boston, Little, Brown & Co, 1981.

Conte JE Jr and Barriere SL. Manual of Antibiotics and Infectious Diseases. Philadelphia, Lea & Febiger, 1981.

Dixon RE (ed). Nosocomial Infections. New York, Yorke Medical Books, 1981.

Evans AS (ed). Viral Infections of Humans, 2nd ed. New York, Plenum, 1982.

Hoeprich PD (ed). Infectious Diseases, 3rd ed. Philadelphia, Harper & Row, 1983.

Johnson RT. Viral Infections of the Nervous System. New York, Raven Press, 1982.

Kingsley VV. Basic Microbiology for the Health Sciences. Philadelphia, WB Saunders, 1982.

Korting GW. Practical Dermatology of the Genital Region. Philadelphia, WB Saunders, 1981.

Lewis GE Jr and Angel PS (eds). Biomedical Aspects of Botulism. New York, Academic Press, 1981.

Lorian V. Significance of Medical Microbiology in the Care of Patients, 2nd ed. Baltimore, Williams & Wilkins, 1982.

Lowbury EJL et al. Control of Hospital Infection: A Practical Handbook, 2nd ed. Philadelphia, JB Lippincott, 1981.

Mandell GL, Douglas RG, and Bennett JE. Principles and Practice of Infectious Diseases, Vols. 1 and 2. New York, John Wiley & Sons, 1979.

Marr JJ. Infectious Diseases in General Medical Practice. Menlo Park, California, Addison–Wesley, 1982.

Nahmias AJ, Dowdle WR, and Schinazi RF. The Human Herpesviruses. New York, Elsevier, 1980.

Noble RC. Sexually Transmitted Diseases, 2nd ed. Garden City, New York, Medical Examination, 1982.

O'Connell CJ. Laboratory Diagnosis of Infectious Disease, 2nd ed. Garden City, New York, Medical Examination, 1980.

Peterson PK et al. The Management of Infectious Diseases in Clinical Practice. New York, Academic Press, 1982.

Rippon JW. Medical Mycology, 2nd ed. Philadelphia, WB Saunders, 1982.

Rubin RH and Young LS (eds). Clinical Approach to Infection in the Compromised Host. New York, Plenum, 1981.

Sanford JP and Luby JP. Infectious Diseases. New York, Grune & Stratton, 1981.

Wehrle PF and Top FH Sr. Communicable and Infectious Diseases, 9th ed. St Louis, CV Mosby, 1981.

Welsby PD. Infectious Diseases. Lancaster, MTP Press, 1981.

Wenzel RP. Handbook of Hospital Acquired Infections. Boca Raton, Florida, CRC Press, 1981.

World Health Statistics Annual 1981. Vital Statistics and Causes of Death. Geneva, World Health Organization, 1981.

Youmans GP, Paterson PY, and Sommers HM. The Biologic and Clinical Basis of Infectious Diseases. Philadelphia, WB Saunders, 1980.

Articles
Bacterial Infections

Ad Hoc Committee of Scientific Assembly on Tuberculosis. Diagnostic standards and classification of tuberculosis and other mycobacterial diseases. Am Rev Respir Dis 1981 Mar; 123(3):343–358.

American Thoracic Society Executive Committee. The tuberculin skin test. Am Rev Resp Dis 1981 Sept; 124(3):356–363.

Baxley LM. Tetanus is still deadly. Occup Health Nurs 1981 Aug; 29(8):40–42.

Binford CH, Meyers WM, and Walsh GP. Leprosy. JAMA 1982 Apr 23–30; 247(16):2283–2292.

Bolton ME. Hyperbaric oxygen therapy. Am J Nurs 1981 June; 81(6):1199–1201.

Bond GB. Infection control: Seratia—an endemic hospital resident. Am J Nurs 1981 Dec; 81(12):2183–2186.

Budassi SA. A case of tetanus. JEN 1981 Sept–Oct; 7(5):191–194.

Chemoprophylaxis for tuberculosis. Tubercle 1981 Mar; 62(1):69–72.

Chouham MK and Pande SK. Typhoid enteric perforation. Br J Surg 1982 Mar; 69(3):173–175.

Counterimmunoelectrophoresis (CIE) for rapid diagnosis of bacteremias and bacterial meningitis. Med Lett Drugs Ther 1981 May 1; 23(9):43–44.

Curran JW et al. Gonorrhea in the emergency department. JEN 1981 Sept–Oct; 7(5):209–212.

Dasta JF et al. Diazepam infusion in tetanus: Correlation of drug levels with effect. South Med J 1981 Mar; 74(3):278–280.

Davis GS, Winn WC, and Beaty HN. Legionnaires disease. Clin Chest Med 1981 Jan; 2(1):145–166.

Delaney P. Essentials in managing chronic meningitis. Am Fam Physician 1981 Sept; 24(3):175–177.

Drugs for tuberculosis. Med Lett Drugs Ther 1982 Feb 19; 24(603):17–19.

Dutt AK and Stead WW. Short-course chemotherapy. Chest 1981 Dec; 80(6):724–727.

Ellenbogen C. Treatment priorities for septic shock. Am Fam Physician 1982 Feb; 25(2):163–167.

Enna CD and Delgado DD. The surgical management of Hansen's disease: A survey updated. Plast Reconstr Surg 1981 Jan; 27(1):79–93.

Fiumara NJ. Treating gonorrhea. Am Fam Physician 1981 May; 23(5):123–126.

Furste W, Parsons JN, and Cabrera H. Tetanus prevention. Compr Ther 1981 Sept; 7(9):49–57.

Global distribution of penicillinase-producing *Neisseria gonorrhoeae* (PPNG). MMWR 1982 Jan 22; 31(1 & 2):1–3.

Griffin RJ Jr. Newer approaches to an ancient disease: Leprosy. Am Pharm 1981 Sept; 21(9):18–23.

Guidi ML et al. The combined use of hyperbaric oxygen, antibiotics and surgery in the treatment of gas gangrene. Resuscitation 1981 Dec; 9(4):276–273.

Hall KV. Detecting septic shock before it's too late. RN 1981 Sept; 44(9):28–32.

Hamm PT and Jemison–Smith P. Infection control update. Salmonella. Crit Care Update 1982 Jan; 9(1):41–44.

Handsfield HH and Holmes KK. Treatment of uncomplicated gonorrhea with cefotaxime. Sex Transm Dis 1981 July–Sept; 8(3):187–191.

Harrison WO. Prophylaxis against gonorrhea is an ounce of prevention worth the cost. Milit Med 1981 Jan; 146(1):9–13.

Harrison WO. Pharyngeal gonorrhea. JAMA 1981 Dec 11; 246(23):2726–2727.

Huang C L–H. The transmission of leprosy in man. Int J Lepr 1980 Sept; 48(3):309–318.

Hughes JM et al. Clinical features of types A & B food-borne botulism. Ann Intern Med 1981 Oct; 95(4):442–445.

Immunization Practices Advisory Committee. Diphtheria, tetanus and pertussis: Guidelines for vaccine prophylaxis and other preventive measures. Ann Intern Med 1981 Dec; 95(6):723–728.

Imperato PJ. Legionellosis and the indoor environment. Bull NY Acad Med 1981 Dec; 57(10):922–935.

Job CK. Leprosy—the source of infection and its mode of transmission. Lepr Rev 1981 Dec; 52(Suppl 1):69–76.

Kaye W. Catheter- and infusion-related sepsis: The nature of the problem and its prevention. Heart Lung 1982 May–June; 11(3):221–227.

Kerr JH. Insensible fluid losses in severe tetanus. Intensive Care Med 1981; 7(5):209–212.

Kim TC et al. Atypical mycobacterial infections: A clinical study of 92 patients. South Med J 1981 Nov; 74(11):1304–1308.

King JW and White MC. Pulmonary actinomycosis. Arch Intern Med 1981 Aug; 141(9):1234–1235.

Kirby BD. Legionnaires' disease and legionellosis. Compr Ther 1982 Feb; 8(2):8–12.

Koshi G et al. Brain abscess and other protean manifestations of actinomycosis. Am J Trop Med Hyg 1981 Jan; 30(1):139–144.

Kreger BE et al. Gram-negative bacteremia. III. Reassessment of etiology, epidemiology and ecology in 612 patients. Am J Med 1980 Mar; 68(3):332–343.

Kreger BE, Craven DE, and McCabe WR. Gram-negative bacteremia. IV. Re-evaluation of clinical features and treatment in 612 patients. Am J Med 1980 Mar; 68(3):344–355.

Lamb LS. Think you know septic shock? Read this. Nursing '82 1982 Jan; 12(1):34–43.

Levine MM. Bacillary dysentery. Med Clin North Am 1982 May; 66(3):623–638.

Maugh TH. Leprosy vaccine trials to begin soon. Science 1982 Feb 26; 215(4536):1083–1086.

McCormack WM. Clinical spectrum of infection with *Neisseria gonorrhoeae*. Sex Transm Dis 1981 Oct–Dec; 8(4-S):305–307.

McKendrick MW and Geddes AM. Trimethoprim in enteric fever. Br Med J 1981 Jan 31; 282(6261):364.

Melo JC. Typhoid fever. J Ky Med Assoc 1981 Dec; 79(12):791–793.

Moxley GF. Grand Rounds: Psittacosis. Va Med 1981 Apr; 108(4):248–250, 252.

Nebens IA and Jackson BS. A case of acute fulminating meningococcemia. Am J Nurs 1982 Sept; 82(9):1390–1393.

Nelson JD. Antibiotic therapy for Salmonella syndromes. Am J Dis Child 1981 Dec; 135(12):1093–1094.

New drugs for enteric gram-negative bacillary meningitis in adults. Med Lett Drugs Ther 1981 Aug 21; 23(17):73–74.

Orenstein WA et al. Antibiotic treatment of acute Shigellosis: Failure of cefamandole compared with trimethoprim/sulfa-methoxazole and ampicillin. Am J Med Sci 1981 July–Aug; 282(1):27–33.

Palmer SR. Psittacosis in man. J R Soc Med 1982 Apr; 75(4):262–267.

Patten RC. Salmonellosis. Am Fam Physician 1981 Jan; 23(1):112–117.

Potterat JJ and King RD. A new approach to gonorrhea control. The asymptomatic man and incidence reduction. JAMA 1981 Feb 13; 245(6):578–580.

Preheim LC and Sanders WE. Nosocomial pneumonia. Compr Ther 1981 June; 7(6):20–27.

Rahal JJ and Simberkoff MS. Host defense and antimicrobial therapy in adult gram-negative bacillary meningitis. Ann Intern Med 1982 Apr; 96(4):468–474.

Report of the third meeting of the scientific working group on chemotherapy of leprosy (THELEP) of the UNDP/World Bank/WHO special programme for research and training in tropical diseases. Lepr Rev 1981 Dec; 5(4):349–354.

Roderick MA. Botulism. Nursing '82 1982 June; 12(6):59.

Sacks T and McGowan JE. International symposium on nosocomial infection control. Rev Infect Dis 1981 July–Aug; 3(4):640–803.

Sbarbaro JA and Iseman MD. Prophylactic treatment of tuberculosis. Compr Ther 1981 June; 7(6):14–19.

Silber T. Gonorrhea in adolescence: Its impact and consequences. Adolescence 1981 Fall; 16(63):537–541.

Simpson ML et al. Treatment of gonorrhea: Comparison of cefotaxime and penicillin. Antimicrob Agents Chemother 1981 May; 19(5):798–800.

Smith LDS. *Clostridium botulinum:* Characteristics and occurrence. Rev Infect Dis 1979 July–Aug; 1(4):637–641.

Stam WE. Nosocomial infections: Etiologic changes and therapeutic challenges. Hosp Pract 1981 Aug; 16(8):75–88.

Stead WW and Dutt AK. Tuberculosis. Clin Chest Med 1980 May; 1(2):167–284 (entire volume).

Stead WW and Dutt AK. What's new in tuberculosis? Am J Med 1981 July; 71(1):1–4.

Stead WW and Dutt AK. Chemotherapy for tuberculosis today. Am Rev Respir Dis 1982 Mar; 125(3, Part 2):94–101.

Sugerman HJ, Peyton JWR, and Greenfield LJ. Gram-negative sepsis. Curr Probl Surg 1981 July; 18(7):405–475.

Tetanus surveillance and prophylaxis. Br Med J 1982 June 5; 234(6330):1715–1716.

Tice AW Jr and Rodriguez VL. Pharyngeal gonorrhea. JAMA 1981 Dec 11; 246(23):2717–2719.

Vorosmarti J Jr. Hyperbaric oxygen therapy. Am Fam Physician 1981 Jan; 23(1):169–173.

Wahdan MH et al. A controlled field trial of live *Salmonella typhi* strain Ty 212 oral vaccine against typhoid: Three-year results. J Infect Dis 1982 Mar; 145(3):292–295.

Waters MFR. Leprosy. Br Med J 1981 Nov 14; 283(6302):1320–1322.

Welsh F, Matos L, and DeTreville RTP. Medical hyperbaric oxygen therapy: 22 cases. Aviat Space Environ Med 1980 June; 51(6):611–614.

Wiesner PJ. Gonorrhea. Cutis 1981 Mar; 27(3):249–254.

Wig JD et al. Massive lower gastrointestinal bleeding in patients with typhoid fever. Am J Gastroenterol 1981 June; 75(6):445–448.

Williams RA. Penicillinase-producing *Neisseria gonorrhoeae*. Am Fam Physician 1981 Dec; 24(6):117–119.

Woodward TE and Woodward WE. A new oral vaccine against typhoid fever. J Infect Dis 1982 Mar; 145(3):289–291.

Yoshikawa TT and Nagami PH. Adverse drug reactions in TB therapy: Risks and recommendations. Geriatrics 1982 July; 37(7):61–68.

Acquired Immune Deficiency Syndrome

Bardana EJ. A conceptual approach to immunodeficiency. Med Clin North Am 1981 Sept; 65(5):959–976.

Facui AS. The syndrome of Kaposi's sarcoma and opportunistic infections: An epidemiologically restricted disorder of immunoregulation. Ann Intern Med 1982 June; 96(6, Part 1):777–779.

Handsfield HH. Acquired immunodeficiency in homosexual men. AJR 1982 Oct; 139(4):832–833.

Heise ER. Diseases associated with immunosuppression. Environ Health Perspect 1982 Feb; 43:9–19.

Holland GN et al. Ocular disorders associated with a new severe acquired cellular immunodeficiency syndrome. Am J Ophthalmol 1982 Apr; 93(4):393–402.

Masur H et al. Opportunistic infection in previously healthy women. Ann Intern Med 1982 Oct; 97(4):533–539.

News: Acquired immunodeficiency syndrome cause(s) still elusive. JAMA 1982 Sept 24; 248(12):1423–1427; 1431.

Helminthic Infestations

Anderson RM and May RM. Population dynamics of human helminth infections: Control by chemotherapy. Nature 1982 June 17; 297(5867):557–563.

Cline BL. Current drug regimens for the treatment of intestinal helminth infections. Med Clin North Am 1982 May; 66(3):721–742.

Johnson TS. Diagnosis and treatment of five parasites. Drug Intell Clin Pharm 1981 Feb; 15(2):103–110.

Verm RA. Gastrointestinal parasites. Part II. Helminthic infestations. Am Fam Physician 1982 May; 25(5):216–225.

Infection Control

Arking LM and McArthur BJ (eds). Symposium on infection control. Nurs Clin North Am 1980 Dec; 15(4):651–908.

Donaldson JF. Therapy of acute fever: A comparative approach. Hosp Pract 1981 Sept; 16(9):125–138.

Geiderman JM and Baraff LJ. Infectious disease emergencies. Topics in Emergency Medicine 1982 Apr; 4(1):1–94 (entire volume).

Hargiss CO and Larson E. Infection control: How to collect specimens and evaluate results. Am J Nurs 1981 Dec; 81(12):2166–2174.

Hargiss CO and Larson E. Infection control: Guidelines for prevention of hospital acquired infections. Am J Nurs 1981 Dec; 81(12):2175–2183.

Simmons BP, Hooton TM, and Mallison GF. Guidelines for hospital environmental control. Infection Control 1981 Mar–Apr; 2(2):131–146.

Wong ES and Hooton TM. Guidelines for prevention of catheter-associated urinary tract infections. Infection Control 1981 Mar–Apr; 2(2):125–130.

Young LS. Infection in the compromised host. Host Pract 1981 Sept; 16(9):73–84.

Protozoan Infections

Burns TW. Parasitic bowel disease: Three pathogens important in primary care. Postgrad Med 1982 May; 71(5):130–139.

Clift SA and Navab F. Current concepts in amebiasis. J Arkansas Med Soc 1982 Jan; 78(8):339–345.

Eggleston FC, Handa AK, and Verghese M. Amebic peritonitis secondary to amebic liver abscess. Surgery 1982 Jan; 91(1):46–48.

Fitzgerald FT. Malaria: A modern dilemma. West J Med 1982 Mar; 136(3):220–226.

John RL. Giardiasis and amebiasis: symptoms, specimens, the counseling you'll need to do. RN 1981 Apr; 44(4):52–57.

Kapila M et al. Fatal falciparum malaria and the availability of parenteral antimalarial drugs in hospitals. Br Med J 1982 May 22; 284(6328):1547–1548.

Perrin LH, Mackey LJ, and Miescher PA. The hematology of malaria in man. Semin Hematol 1982 Apr; 19(2):70–82.

Taylor DW and Siddiqui WA. Recent advances in malarial immunity. Annu Rev Med 1982; 33:69–96.

Verm RA. Gastrointestinal parasites: Part I. Protozoal infections. Am Fam Physician 1982 Apr; 25(4):170–175.

William DC. Enteric diseases. Cutis 1981 Mar; 27(3):278–285.

Williams GR et al. Delayed diagnosis of malaria. Br Med J 1982 May 29; 284(6329):1616–1617.

Rickettsial Infections

D'Angelo LJ, Bregman DJ, and Winkler WG. Rocky Mountain spotted fever in the United States: Use of age-specific incidence to determine public health policy for a vector-borne disease. South Med J 1982 Jan; 75(1):3–5.

Davis AE and Bradford WD. Abdominal pain resembling acute appendicitis in Rocky Mountain spotted fever. JAMA 1982 May 28; 247(20):2811–2812.

MacCaughelty TC, Ernst G, and Holtz AS. Rocky Mountain spotted fever from St Louis county. Crit Care Med 1982 Feb; 10(2):124–126.

Massey K. Rocky Mountain spotted fever: A national disease. MCN 1982 Mar–Apr; 7(2):104–109.

Smith JD et al. Rocky Mountain spotted fever in Georgia 1975–1980. J Med Assoc Ga 1982 Mar; 71(3):207–211.

Westerman EL. Rocky Mountain spotted fever: A dilemma for the clinician. Arch Intern Med 1982 June; 142(6):1106–1107.

Woodward WE. A petechial rash that came too late. Hosp Pract 1982 May; 17(5):45, 56.

Sexually Transmitted Infections

Burns ST et al. Molluscum contagiosum. Sex Transm Dis 1981 July–Sept; 8(3):227–234.

Campbell CE and Herten RJ. VD to STD: Redefining venereal disease. Am J Nurs 1981 Sept; 81(9):1629–1635.

Corey L. The diagnosis and treatment of genital herpes. JAMA 1982 Sept 3; 248(9):1041–1049.

Council on Scientific Affairs. Health care needs of a homosexual population. JAMA 1982 Aug 13; 248(6):736–739.

Cutler JC. Venereal disease prevention. Cutis 1981 Mar; 27(3):321–327.

Darrow WW et al. The gay report on sexually transmitted diseases. Am J Public Health 1981 Sept; 71(9):1004–1011.

Ellis RE. Chlamydial genital infections: Manifestations and management. South Med J 1981 July; 74(7):809–813.

Felman YM. Sexually-transmitted diseases in women—something can be done. Cutis 1981 Mar; 27(3):298–303.

Felman YM. Approaches to sexually transmitted amebiasis. Bull NY Acad Med 1981 Apr; 57(3):201–206.

Felman YM and Klikatas JA. *Chlamydia trachomatis* in sexually transmitted diseases. A new public health problem. Urology 1981 Oct; 18(4):327–336.

Fuerst ML. How will patients use acyclovir to treat herpes. JAMA 1982 June 11; 247(22):3040–3045.

Handsfield HH, Stamm WE, and Holmes KK. Public health implications and control of sexually transmitted chlamydial infections. Sex Transm Dis 1981 Apr–June; 8(2):85–86.

Hoffman CA. Sexually transmitted diseases. JAMA 1981 Oct 9; 246(15):1709.

Holmes KK. The *Chlamydia* epidemic. JAMA 1981 May 1; 245(17):1718–1723.

Infectious Diseases Society of America. Countering the epidemic of sexually transmitted diseases: A call to action. J Infect Dis 1982 Mar; 145(3):422–426.

Jones RB and Fife KH. Update on sexually transmitted diseases. Medical Times 1982 Apr; 110(4):38S–55S.

Judson FN. Epidemiology of sexually transmitted hepatitis B infections in heterosexuals: A review. Sex Transm Dis 1981 Oct–Dec; 8(4 Suppl):336–343.

Kellum MD and Loucks A. Genital herpes infections: Diagnosis and management. Nurse Pract 1982 Feb; 7(2):14–18, 21.

McCormack WM. Sexually transmitted diseases: Women as victims. JAMA 1982 July 9; 248(2):177–178.

Myskowski PL, Romano JF, and Safai B. Kaposi's sarcoma in young homosexual men. Cutis 1982 Jan; 29(1):31–34.

Rein MF. Recent developments in sexually transmitted chlamydial infections. Med Times 1981 Mar; 109(3):29–35.

Rein MF and McCormack WM. Changing epidemiologic patterns in sexually transmitted diseases: Therapeutic implications. Sex Transm Dis 1981 Apr–June; 8(2 Suppl):93–174 (entire volume).

Sexually transmitted diseases treatment guidelines 1982. MMWR 1982 Aug 20; 31(2 Suppl):35S–60S.

Spirochetal Infections

Felman YM and Nikitas JA. Sexually transmitted diseases. Primary syphilis. Cutis 1982 Feb; 29(2):122–124, 128, 133, 136.

Fitzgerald F. The great imitator, syphilis. West J Med 1981 May; 134(5):424–432.

Fiumara NJ. Treatment of primary and secondary syphilis. JAMA 1980 June 27; 243(24):2500-2502.

Gavin H. Epidemiologic treatment for syphilis and gonorrhea. Sex Transm Dis 1980 July–Sept; 7(3):149–152.

Panconesi E, Zuccati G, and Cantini A. Treatment of syphilis: A short critical review. Sex Transm Dis 1981 Oct–Dec; 8(4 Suppl):321–325.

Rein MF. Treatment of neurosyphilis. JAMA 1981 Dec 4; 246(22):2613.

Sexually transmitted diseases treatment guidelines 1982. MMWR Aug 20; 31(2 Suppl):50S–54S.

Willcox RR. Treatment of syphilis. Bull WHO 1981; 59(5):655–663.

Systemic Mycotic Infections

Comer JB. Amphotericin B: Ten common questions. Am J Nurs 1981 June; 81(6):1166–1167.

Graybill JR and Drutz DJ. Ketoconazole: A major innovation for treatment of fungal disease. Ann Intern Med 1980 Dec; 93(6):921–923.

Rees PL and Dixon DM. Opportunistic mycoses. Am J Nurs 1981 June; 81(6):1160–1165.

Stagno S. Toxoplasmosis. Am J Nurs 1980 Apr; 80(4):720–722.

Watanakunakorn C. Treatment of systemic fungus infections. Compr Ther 1982 Feb; 8(2):35–43.

Viral Infections

Alberty R. Surgical implications in infectious mononucleosis. Am J Surg 1981 May; 141(5):559–561.

Aronson MD et al. Heterophil antibody in adults with severe sore throat. Ann Intern Med 1982 Apr; 96(4):505–508.

Barclay WR. Influenza 1981–1982. JAMA 1981 Sept 25; 246(13):1445.

Barker WH and Mullooly JP. Pneumonia and influenza deaths during epidemics: Implications for prevention. Arch Intern Med 1982 Jan; 142(1):85–89.

Editorial: How does influenza virus pave the way for bacteria? Lancet 1982 Feb 27; 1(8270):485–486.

Evans AS and Niederman JC. EBV-IgA and new heterophil antibody tests in diagnosis of infectious mononucleosis. Am J Clin Pathol 1982 May; 77(5):555–560.

Fekety R. Prevention and treatment of viral infections: Problems and current recommendations. Postgrad Med 1981 Jan; 69(1):133–137, 140–141.

Ferguson CK and Roll LJ. Human rabies. Am J Nurs 1981 June; 81(6):1174–1179.

Glezen WP. Prevention of influenza-related morbidity and mortality. Arch Intern Med 1982 Jan; 142(1):25–26.

Goodman RA et al. Impact of influenza A in a nursing home. JAMA 1982 Mar 12; 247(10):1451–1453.

Krugman S. The newly licensed hepatitis B vaccine. JAMA 1982 Apr 9; 247(14):2012–2015.

Lindtjorn B. Clinical features of rabies in man. Trop Doct 1982 Jan; 12(1):9–12.

Mann JM. Rabies risks: Systematic evaluation and management of animal bites. Compr Ther 1981 Sept; 7(9):58–67.

Morgan EJ et al. Pulmonary function in infectious mononucleosis. Chest 1982 June; 81(6):699–700.

Nicholls ES and Davies JN. Rabies control and management. Can Med Assoc J 1982 June 1; 126(11):1286–1290.

Plotkin SA. Rabies vaccination in the 1980's. Hosp Pract 1980 Nov; 15(11):65–72.

Rosner F and Grunwald HW. Infectious mononucleosis and acute leukemia. JAMA 1981 Oct 16; 246(16):1783–1784.

Scientist discovers white cell protein that speeds up mononucleosis detection. Hospitals 1982 June 16; 56(12):38.

Snydman DR et al. Infectious mononucleosis in an adult progressing to fatal immunoblastic lymphoma. Ann Intern Med 1982 June; 96(6, Part 1):737–742.

Stuart-Harris C. The epidemiology and prevention of influenza. Am Sci 1981 Mar–Apr; 69(2):166–172.

Urman JD and Bobrove AM. Acute polyarthritis and infectious mononucleosis. West J Med 1982 Feb; 136(2):151–153.

Varner MW, McGuiness GA, and Galask RP. Rabies vaccination in pregnancy. Am J Obstet Gynecol 1982 July 15; 143(6):717–718.

Wilkowske CJ. Rabies prevention. Mayo Clin Proc 1981 July; 56(7):459–460.

Agencies
International

World Health Organization (Regional Office for the Americas), Pan American World Health Organization, 525 23rd St., NW, Washington, DC 20037

World Health Organization, Palais de la Sante, Geneva, Switzerland

Governmental

Centers for Disease Control (Center for Prevention Services, Center for Environmental Health, Center for Health Promotion and Education, Center for Infectious Diseases), Atlanta, Georgia 30333

National Institute of Allergy and Infectious Diseases, National Institutes of Health, Bethesda, Maryland 20205

US Department of Health and Human Services, Public Health Service, 200 Independence Ave., SW, Washington, DC 20201

Voluntary

American Lung Association, 1740 Broadway, New York, New York 10019

American Public Health Association, 1015 Fifteenth Street, NW, Washington DC 20005

American Social Health Association, VD National Hotline, 260 Sheridan Ave., Suite 307, Palo Alto, California 94306

American Venereal Disease Association, 4716 Benton Smith Rd., Nashville, Tennessee 37215

64

Emergency Management

▷ Nursing in Emergency Conditions

Emergency management has traditionally referred to the care given to patients with urgent and critical needs. The philosophy of emergency care has broadened to include the concept that an emergency is whatever the patient or his family considers it to be. The staff have an obligation to treat the patient with understanding and to respect the anxiety that he undoubtedly feels. If they downgrade his complaint, the therapeutic process may very well be impaired.

A large number of people seek emergency help for serious life-threatening cardiac conditions, such as myocardial infarction, acute congestive failure and pulmonary edema, and cardiac arrhythmias. The priorities of management of such cardiac conditions together with the ECG patterns evoked by the arrhythmias are discussed in Chapters 28 and 31. This chapter will deal mainly with the emergency management of trauma and other conditions not found elsewhere in this book. *It is assumed that treatment is given under the direction of a physician.*

▷ Psychological Management of Patients and Families in Emergencies and Crisis Situations

Approach to the Patient

Body trauma is an insult to both physiologic and psychological homeostasis and requires both physiologic and psychologic healing. In an emergency situation, one of the objectives is to prevent the patient from becoming psychologically incapacitated.

If the patient is unconscious, he should be treated as if he were conscious—by touching him, calling him by name, and explaining every procedure that is being done. As soon as the patient regains consciousness, a primary concern is to orient him—by stating his name, the date, and the place. If necessary, this basic information should be repeated over and over. The patient is brought back into reality in a calm, reassuring way.

Patients experiencing sudden injury or illness are often overwhelmed by anxiety since they have not had time to mobilize their resources to adapt to the crisis. They experience real and terrifying fear—of death, mutilation, immobilization, and other assaults on their personal identity and body integrity. Those caring for the patient should act confidently and competently to help relieve his excessive anxiety. Personalizing the situation as much as possible and speaking, reacting, and responding to the patient in a warm manner contributes to a sense of security. In addition, explanations should be given on a level that the patient can grasp—an informed patient can cope with psychological and physical stress in a more positive manner. An ongoing human contact helps reduce the panic of the severely injured person, and reassuring words aid in dispelling fear of the unknown. It helps the emotionally distressed patient and family to mobilize their own psychological resources when the emergency department staff conveys optimism and concern for the welfare of the patient in a calm and reassuring manner.

Approach to the Family

In the admitting area, the family is told where the patient is and that he is receiving expert care. When the crisis of trauma, severe disfigurement, and sudden death are confronted, the family goes through several stages, beginning with "unbearable anxiety" and progressing through denial, remorse, grief, anger, and reconciliation. The family members are encouraged to recognize and talk about their feelings of anxiety. The approach here is to tune into the family's thinking and to deal with reality as gently and as quickly as possible. Although denial is an ego-defense mechanism that protects one from recognizing painful and disturbing aspects of reality, it cannot be encouraged or supported, since the family must be prepared for the reality of what has happened (and not for what they wish it could be) and for what may come.

Expressions of remorse and guilt are frequently heard, with members accusing themselves (or each other) of negligence or minor omissions. The nursing approach is to allow expressions of remorse, over and over, if need be until the family realize that there was probably little that they could have done to prevent the accident or illness.

Expressions of anger are common in crisis situations. They are a way of handling the anxiety. The anger is frequently directed at the patient, but it is also expressed toward someone else—the physician, the nurse, the admitting officer. Without condemnation or rejection, the therapeutic approach is to allow the anger to be ventilated in order to help the family identify their feelings of frustration.

Grief is a complex emotional response to anticipated or actual loss. In this stage, the nursing intervention is to help family members work through their grief and to support their usual coping mechanisms, letting them know that it is normal and acceptable for them to cry and feel this way.

The following are guidelines for helping a family deal with sudden death in the emergency department:

- Take the family to a private place.
- Talk to all of the family together.
- Assure the family that everything possible was done; inform them of the treatment rendered.
- Allow the family to talk about the deceased and what he meant to them (permits ventilation of feelings of loss).
- Encourage the family to talk about events preceding admission to the emergency department.
- Encourage the family to support each other and express feelings of loss, anger, helplessness, and disbelief, as well as to shed tears.
- Avoid volunteering unnecessary information (the patient was drinking, etc.).
- Avoid giving sedation to family members, since this may mask or delay the grieving process, which is necessary to achieve emotional equilibrium and prevent prolonged depression.
- Allow the family members to view the body if they wish to do so (helps to integrate the loss); cover mutilated areas. They may need to see that the deceased is "really dead."

▷ Priorities and Principles of Emergency Management

Priorities of Emergency Management

When care is being given to a patient in an emergency situation, many crucial decisions must be made. Such decisions require sound judgment based on an understanding of the condition that produced the emergency and its effect on the person.

The major goals of emergency medical treatment are (1) to preserve life, (2) to prevent deterioration before more definitive treatment can be given, and (3) to restore the patient to useful living.

When the patient is first received into the emergency department, the goal is to determine the extent of injury (illness) and to establish priorities for the initiation of treatment. These priorities are determined by the comparative threat to the person's life. Injuries or conditions interfering with vital physiologic function (obstructed airway, massive bleeding) take precedence. Usually, injuries of the face, neck, and chest that impair respiration command the highest priorities. Every member of the emergency team must be alert to the total problem of the patient since the body cannot be isolated into parts.

Principles of Emergency Management

The following principles are applicable to the emergency management of any patient:

1. Maintain a patent airway and provide adequate ventilation, employing resuscitation measures when necessary. Assess for chest injuries with subsequent airway obstruction.
2. Control hemorrhage and its consequences.
3. Evaluate and restore cardiac output.

4. Prevent and treat shock; maintain or restore effective circulation.
5. Carry out a rapid initial and ongoing physical examination; the clinical course of the injured or seriously ill patient is not static.
6. Assess whether or not the patient can follow commands; evaluate the size and reactivity of the pupils and motor responses.
7. Start ECG monitoring if appropriate.
8. Splint suspected fractures, including fractures of the cervical spine in patients with head injuries.
9. Protect wounds with sterile dressings.
10. Check to see if the patient has a Medic Alert tag or similar identification designating allergies.
11. Start a flow sheet of the patient's vital signs, blood pressure, neurologic status, etc., to guide decision making.

Obtaining Data From the Patient

If possible, a brief history of the accident or illness is taken from the patient or the person accompanying him to the emergency department. As part of the history, the following questions should be answered:

1. What were the circumstances, forces, location, and time of the injury?
2. When did the symptoms appear?
3. How did the patient reach the hospital?
4. What was the health status of the patient before the accident or illness?
5. Is there a past history of illness? of past admissions?
6. Is the patient currently taking any medications: especially hormones, insulin, digitalis, anticoagulants?
7. Does the patient have any allergies?
8. Does the patient have any bleeding tendencies?
9. When was the last meal eaten? (Important if an anesthetic is to be given.)
10. Is the patient under a physician's care? name of physician?
11. What was the date of the patient's most recent tetanus immunization?

Recording of Data

Consent to examine and treat the patient is part of the Emergency Department record. More sophisticated procedures (angiography, lumbar puncture) should be specifically consented to by the patient. If the patient is unconscious and brought to the Emergency Department without family or friends, this fact should be documented. Following treatment, a notation is made on the record concerning the patient's condition on discharge or transfer and the instructions that are given for follow-up care.

▷ Emergency Resuscitation Measures

The first priority in the treatment of any emergency condition is the establishment of the airway. If the airway is obstructed, the ensuing hypoxia will produce permanent brain damage or death within 3 to 5 minutes, depending on the age of the patient.

Complete airway obstruction is readily recognized—the patient is not breathing and is unconscious and in complete collapse.

Partial airway obstruction that interferes with air flow will produce an apprehensive look, inspiratory and expiratory stridor, labored use of accessory muscles (suprasternal and intercostal retraction), flaring nostrils, and progressive anxiety, restlessness, and confusion. Cyanosis of the earlobes and nail beds may be a late sign. Partial obstruction of the airway can produce progressive hypoxia and hypercarbia and can lead to respiratory and cardiac arrest.

Emergency Management

1. Turn the patient on his side or turn his head to one side—to prevent the tongue from occluding the airway.
2. Place your fingers behind the angle of the mandible and pull forward while extending the patient's head at the atlanto-occipital joint.
3. If the patient is still having respiratory distress:
   a. Grasp the tongue and pull forward.
   b. If the jaws are locked, insert the index finger behind the last molar and pry the jaw open; then grip the tongue and pull it forward.
   c. Clear any material from the mouth with a finger of the other hand, or suction if equipment is available.
4. If these maneuvers do not clear the airway and if the patient is still not breathing:
   a. Remove any foreign body obstructing the airway (see below and p. 1538).
   b. Take one of the following steps: (1) insert an oropharyngeal airway (see p. 1537) and start bag-mask resuscitation, (2) insert an esophageal obturator airway (see p. 1537), (3) insert an endotracheal tube (see p. 1540), or (4) perform cricothyroidotomy (see p. 1540).
5. Start artificial ventilation as soon as the upper airway obstruction is cleared.

Artificial Ventilation

Artificial ventilation is instituted on a person who is not breathing. It is accomplished by means of mouth-to-mouth resuscitation or mouth-to-nose resuscitation.

If the patient is unresponsive and there is no palpable carotid or femoral pulse, cardiopulmonary resuscitation (CPR) is initiated immediately. CPR consists of establishing an effective airway and providing artificial ventilation and artificial circulation by external cardiac compression (see p. 599). Advanced CPR involves electrical defibrillation (p. 579), endotracheal intubation (p. 1540), and drug therapy.

Airway management and artificial ventilation are discussed in detail under "Respiratory Insufficiency and Failure," Chapter 24.

Management of Foreign Body Upper Airway Obstruction

Obstruction of the upper airway by food (café coronary) is a cause of sudden death. In adults, a piece of meat is the most common cause of the obstruction. Factors associated with choking on food include alcohol consumption, old age, and poor dentition. In extended care facilities, sedatives and hypnotic drugs and diseases affecting motor coordination (Parkinson's disease) and mental functioning (senility, mental retardation) are risk factors for asphyxiation by food.

The management of foreign body obstruction in the airway is controversial, but limited clinical data suggest a combination of measures (back blows, abdominal thrusts [Heimlich maneuver; Fig. 64–1], chest thrusts [or both]) is preferable to any single maneuver.

Emergency Management

For Partial Obstruction (if Patient is Breathing and Spontaneously Able to Cough)

1. Tell the patient to take a deep breath and cough.
2. If this is unsuccessful, take the patient to the nearest medical facility for instrumental removal of the foreign body under direct visualization.

For Completely Obstructed Airway
See Chart 64-1.

Insertion of Oropharyngeal Airway

An *oropharyngeal airway* is a semicircular-shaped device of plastic, rubber, or metal that is inserted into the lower posterior pharynx over the back of the tongue in a spontaneously breathing patient in order to keep the tongue clear of the airway and permit suctioning of secretions.

Emergency Management

1. Extend the patient's head by placing one hand beneath the neck close to the occiput and gently lifting the neck; simultaneously, with the other hand, tilt the head backward by pressure on the forehead.
2. Insert the airway upside down and rotate through 180 degrees as the airway is introduced over the tongue to the pharynx.

OR

3. Insert from the side of the mouth and rotate into position.

Insertion of Esophageal Obturator Airway (EOA)

The *esophageal obturator airway* (EOA) (Fig. 64-2) is a ventilatory device used in respiratory emergencies for resuscitation. It consists of (1) a face mask to seal off the nose and mouth and anchor the airway; (2) a flexible tube with openings at the level of the pharynx to permit ventilation of the lungs; and (3) a balloon on the distal end of the tube to block the esophagus, thus reducing the possibility of aspirating gastric contents. One type of EOA unit has a central lumen that permits passage of a nasogastric tube. This allows suctioning and decompression of the stomach.

The tube is inserted through the mouth and advanced into the esophagus just below the bifurcation of the trachea. The proximal part of the tube has air holes at the level of the pharynx through which air or oxygen is blown into the lungs.

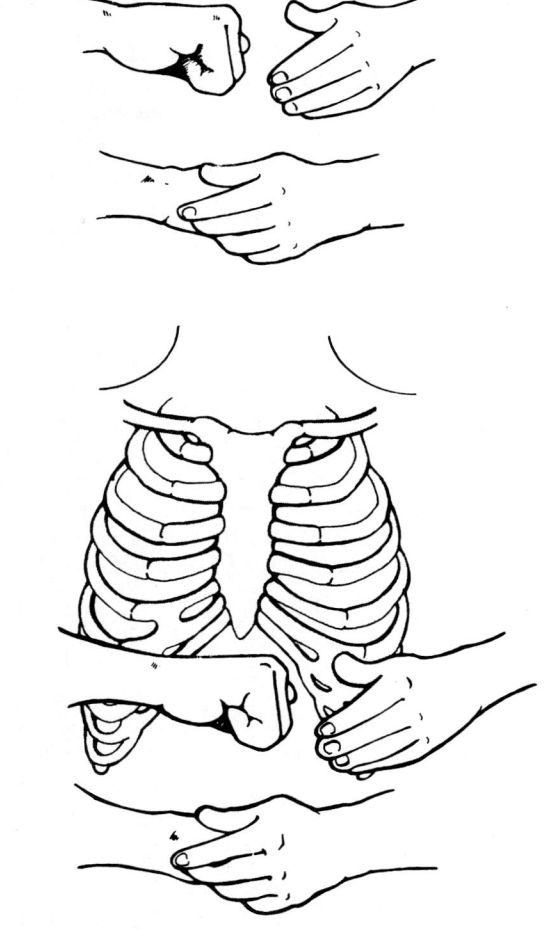

Figure 64-1. Hand placement for abdominal thrusts. (Reprinted from the Supplement to Journal of the American Medical Association, August 1, 1980. Copyright 1980, the American Medical Association. Reprinted with permission from the American Heart Association)

The purpose of the EOA is to ventilate the apneic, unconscious patient; it is an alternative to endotracheal intubation when skilled personnel and special equipment are not available or when intubation cannot be accomplished or is contraindicated.

Equipment
EOA
50-ml syringe
Water-soluble gel
Bag and mask unit

Emergency Management

1. Lubricate the tube and attach the face mask to the tube by the snap lock.
2. Using the left hand, insert the thumb as deeply as possible over the back of the patient's tongue, pulling on it while using the fingers to lift the jaw upward and away from the posterior pharyngeal wall.

Chart 64-1
Guidelines: Management of Foreign Body Airway Obstruction

Assessment of Clinical Manifestations

Weak, ineffective cough; high-pitched noises on inspiration
Respiratory distress
Inability to speak or breathe
Cyanosis; collapse

Action	*Rationale/Amplification*
Carry out a sequence of back blows, manual thrusts, and finger sweeps.	

Back Blows

a. Administer four sharp blows with the heel of the hand over the spine between the shoulder blades while supporting the patient with the other hand on the sternum. Apply the back blows forcefully in rapid succession; they may be administered with the victim sitting, standing, or lying.

        a. A back blow raises pressure in the thorax distal to the obstructing object.

b. If possible, have the patient's head lower than his chest.

Manual Thrusts

a. Abdominal thrust for standing patient:

(1) Stand behind the patient and wrap your arms around his waist. The rescuer's arms should be just above the belt line.

        (1) Manual thrusts to the upper abdomen (abdominal thrust) or lower chest (chest thrust) force air out of the lungs and create an artificial cough intended to remove the foreign body.

(2) Make a fist with one hand and grasp the fist with your other hand. Place the thumb side of your fist against the patient's abdomen between the waist and the rib cage (see Fig. 64-1).

(3) Press your fist four times into the patient's abdomen with a quick inward–upward thrust.

        (3) A combination of back blows and manual thrusts may be effective in removing the obstruction.

(continued)

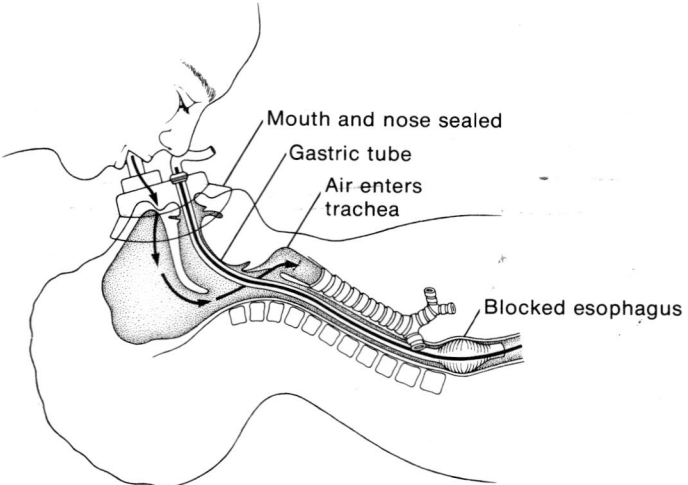

Mouth and nose sealed
Gastric tube
Air enters trachea
Blocked esophagus

3. Insert the EOA into the mouth, carefully guiding the tube over the tongue and past the pharynx; rotate the tube 180 degrees into the esophagus.
4. Stop advancing the tube when the mask reaches the face; press the mask firmly against the face.
5. Ventilate the patient by blowing a few breaths through the tube or by attaching a bag mask to it. IF THE TUBE IS IN THE ESOPHAGUS, THE CHEST WILL RISE.
6. If the chest does not rise, the airway is possibly blocking the trachea; remove airway. Continue ventilating the patient (by bag–mask ventilation) and prepare for and proceed with second attempt at insertion.
7. Auscultate over both lung fields to check that *both* lungs

Figure 64-2.   The Esophageal (Gastric Tube) Airway. (Courtesy of Brunswick Mfg. Co., Inc; Redrawn.)

Chart 64-1
Guidelines: Management of Foreign Body Airway Obstruction (continued)

Action (continued)	**Rationale/Amplification** (continued)
Manual Thrusts (continued)	
b. For lying (unconscious) patient:	
(1) Position the patient on his back.	
(2) Sit astride the patient's hips, facing his head; with one of your hands on top of the other, place the heel of the bottom hand on the patient's abdomen between the waist and rib cage.	(2) Spleen or liver injury may result from a sudden increase of abdominal pressure.
(3) Press into the abdomen with an inward–upward thrust.	
Chest Thrust (An Alternate Technique)	
a. Stand behind the victim with your arms under his axillae and encircling his chest.	
b. Place the thumb side of your fist on the middle of his breast bone. Avoid the xiphoid process and the margins of the rib cage.	
c. Grasp your fist with your other hand and exert four backward thrusts.	c. Each thrust is performed with the intent of relieving the obstruction without having to complete the full series.
Finger Sweep	
a. Open the patient's mouth by grasping both the tongue and lower jaw between your thumb and fingers, and lift the tongue and jaw.	a. This maneuver draws the tongue away from the back of the pharynx and the obstructing foreign body.
b. Sweep your index finger inside the patient's mouth using a hooking action to dislodge and remove the foreign body.	b. The finger probe technique can potentially worsen the situation and should probably be used only under direct visualization or as a last resort.
c. If the patient is still unconscious, attempt to ventilate with mouth-to-mouth ventilation; repeat back blows, manual thrusts, and finger sweep.	

(Adapted from Standards and guidelines for cardiopulmonary resuscitation (CPR) and emergency cardiac care (ECC). JAMA 1980 Aug 1; 244(5):464–467.

are receiving adequate ventilation and that the airway is in the esophagus and *not* in the trachea.

8. Inflate the cuff (balloon) with approximately 30 ml of air. Inflating the cuff results in occlusion of the esophagus, minimizes the incidence of regurgitation, and prevents air leakage.
9. Connect the end of the esophageal obturator to a bag–mask or mechanical ventilator, or continue mouth-to-tube ventilation.
10. Do not remove the EOA until the patient regains consciousness or has a gag reflex *OR* until the endotracheal intubation has been accomplished. The EOA tube must be deflated before it is removed. If the tube is taken out prematurely, regurgitation and aspiration are almost inevitable.
11. This procedure is contraindicated in conscious or semiconscious patients or in those with corrosive poisoning, esophageal disease, or a foreign body in the trachea.

Emergency Endotracheal Procedures
Emergency Endotracheal Intubation
The purpose of endotracheal intubation is to establish and maintain the airway in patients with respiratory insufficiency or hypoxia. Endotracheal intubation is indicated for the following reasons: (1) to establish an airway for patients who cannot be adequately ventilated with an oropharyngeal airway, (2) to bypass an upper airway obstruction, (3) to prevent aspiration, (4) to permit connection of the patient to a resuscitation bag or mechanical ventilator, and (5) to facilitate the removal of tracheobronchial secretions.

Because the procedure requires skill, endotracheal intubation should be done after intensive training in which the technique is practiced on a manikin. It should be done under expert clinical supervision.

Details for emergency endotracheal intubation are outlined in Chart 64-2. Also, see Figure 64-3.

Chart 64-2
Assisting With Emergency Endotracheal Intubation

Clinical Signs for Intubation

1. Respiratory arrest
2. Respiratory insufficiency—marked respiratory effort, substernal retraction, nostril flaring, increasing or decreasing pulse rate, increasing or decreasing respiratory rate, changing color (*cyanosis is a late sign*)
3. Airway obstruction (asphyxia)

Equipment

1. Laryngoscope with curved and straight blades and working light source (Check batteries and bulb periodically.)
2. Endotracheal tubes with low-pressure cuffs (to seal airway) and adapter (to connect tube to ventilator or bag)
3. Stylet to guide endotracheal tube
4. Oral airway (assorted sizes), tongue blade (to keep patient from biting into and occluding endotracheal tube)
5. Adhesive tape   7. Syringes
6. Lubricant jelly   8. Bag–mask unit

Action	*Rationale/Amplification*
1. Remove dental bridgework and plates.	
2. Make sure that the light source of the laryngoscope is working.	
3. Select an endotracheal tube of appropriate size. The average adult will need a tube with an internal diameter of 7.5 mm to 9 mm. Inflate and deflate the cuff to make sure it is intact.	
4. Lubricate the endotracheal tube. Insert a stylet if the tube is very flexible.	

Assist With the Following:

1. If the cervical spine is not injured, place the patient's head in a "sniffing" position, flexed at the junction of the neck and thorax and extended at the junction of the spine and skull.	1. The upper airway is open maximally in this position, and the mouth of the unconscious patient will often open.
2. Ventilate and oxygenate the patient with a resuscitation bag before intubation.	2. This decreases the likelihood of cardiac arrhythmias secondary to hypoxia.
3. Hold the handle of the laryngoscope in the left hand, and hold the patient's mouth open with the right hand by crossing fingers (see Fig. 64-3, *A*).	3. Leverage is improved by crossing the thumb and index fingers when opening the patient's mouth.

(continued)

Crycothyroidotomy or Cricothyroid Membrane Puncture

Crycothyroidotomy is the puncture or incision of the cricothyroid membrane of the larynx with a large-bore needle or a specially designed blade (Fig. 64-4). It is used to establish an airway in situations in which endotracheal intubation cannot be accomplished: airway obstruction from cervical spine injuries, laryngospasm, laryngeal edema (allergic reaction), hemorrhage into neck tissue, or obstruction of the larynx.

Emergency Medical Management

1. Extend the neck.
2. Identify the prominent thyroid cartilage (Adam's apple) and allow your finger to descend in the midline to the depression between the lower border of the thyroid cartilage and the upper border of the cricoid cartilage. This depression represents the cricothyroid membrane.
3. Insert a needle or any sharp instrument at a 10- to 20-degree caudal direction in the midline just above the upper part of the cricoid cartilage.
   a. Listen for air passing back and forth through the needle synchronous with the patient's respiration.
   b. Direct the needle downward and posteriorly.
   c. Tape the needle with adhesive for stability.
4. An alternate method is to make a transverse incision overlying the cricothyroid membrane and a similar incision through the membrane itself. The membrane incision is spread and a tracheotomy tube is advanced caudally into the trachea.

Chart 64-2
Assisting With Emergency Endotracheal Intubation (continued)

Action *(continued)*	Rationale/Amplification *(continued)*
Assist With the Following: *(continued)*	
4. Insert the blade of the laryngoscope along the right side of the tongue, displacing the tongue to the left, and use the right thumb and index finger to pull the patient's lower lip away from his lower teeth (see Fig. 64-3, *B*).	4. Rolling lip away from teeth prevents injury of lip by its being caught between teeth and blade.
5. Lift the laryngoscope forward (toward ceiling) to expose the epiglottis.	
6. Lift the laryngoscope upward and forward at a 45-degree angle to expose the glottis (vocal cords).	6. This stretches the hypoepiglottis ligament, folding the epiglottis upward and exposing the glottis.
7. As the epiglottis is lifted forward (toward the ceiling), the vertical opening of the larynx between the vocal cords will come into view.	7. Do not use your wrist; use your shoulder and arm to lift the epiglottis—to avoid using the teeth as a fulcrum, which could lead to dental damage.
8. Once the vocal cords are visualized, insert the tube into the right corner of the mouth and pass the tube—guided by the blade but keeping the cords in constant view.	8. Make sure you do not insert the tube in the esophagus; the esophageal mucosa is pink and the opening is horizontal rather than vertical.
9. Gently push the tube through the triangular space formed by the vocal cords.	9. If the vocal cords are in spasm (closed), wait a few seconds before passing the tube.
10. Stop the insertion just after the tube cuff has disappeared from view beyond the cords.	10. Advancing the tube further may lead to its entry into a mainstem bronchus (usually the right bronchus), causing collapse of the unventilated lung.
11. Withdraw the laryngoscope, holding the endotracheal tube in place (see Fig. 64-3, *C*).	
12. Inflate the cuff with the minimal amount of air required to occlude the trachea. Attach the tube to a mechanical ventilator or resuscitation bag as required.	12. The amount of air used for cuff inflation depends on the size of the cuff and the diameter of the patient's trachea.
13. Insert an oral airway or bite block.	13. This keeps patient from biting down on the tube and obstructing the airway.
14. Observe the expansion of both sides of the chest by inspection and auscultation of breath sounds.	14. Inspection and auscultation help in determining that the tube remains in position and has not slipped into the right mainstem bronchus and that both lungs are being aerated.
15. Mark the proximal end of the tube with a marking pen or tape.	15. This will allow for detection of any later change in position.
16. Secure the tube with adhesive tape to the patient's face.	16. Taping the tube prevents its expulsion.
17. Take a chest x-ray to verify the tube position.	

5. Prepare for endotracheal intubation. This procedure is usually followed by elective tracheostomy (see p. 491).

Near-drowning

Drowning is one of the three leading causes of accidental death, worldwide, and an estimated 8000 fatalities and 8000 near-drownings occur yearly in the U.S. Factors associated with drowning and near-drowning include alcohol ingestion, inability to swim, diving injuries, hypothermia, and exhaustion. Efforts to save the victim should not be abandoned too soon, since resuscitation has been successful in persons who have been submerged for 10 to 40 minutes.

Following resuscitation, the primary problems of a victim who has nearly drowned are hypoxia, hypercapnia, and respiratory and metabolic acidosis, which will require immediate intervention in the emergency department. The resultant pathophysiologic changes and pulmonary injury following this experience depend on the type of fluid (fresh water or salt water) and the volume of aspiration. When water has been aspirated, alterations of pulmonary function may be anticipated. After a person has survived immersion, secondary drowning (acute adult respiratory distress syndrome) with hypoxia, hypercarbia, and respiratory or metabolic acidosis can occur.

Emergency Management in Emergency Department
The goals are to treat the patient for ventilatory insufficiency, hypoxia, and resultant acidosis.

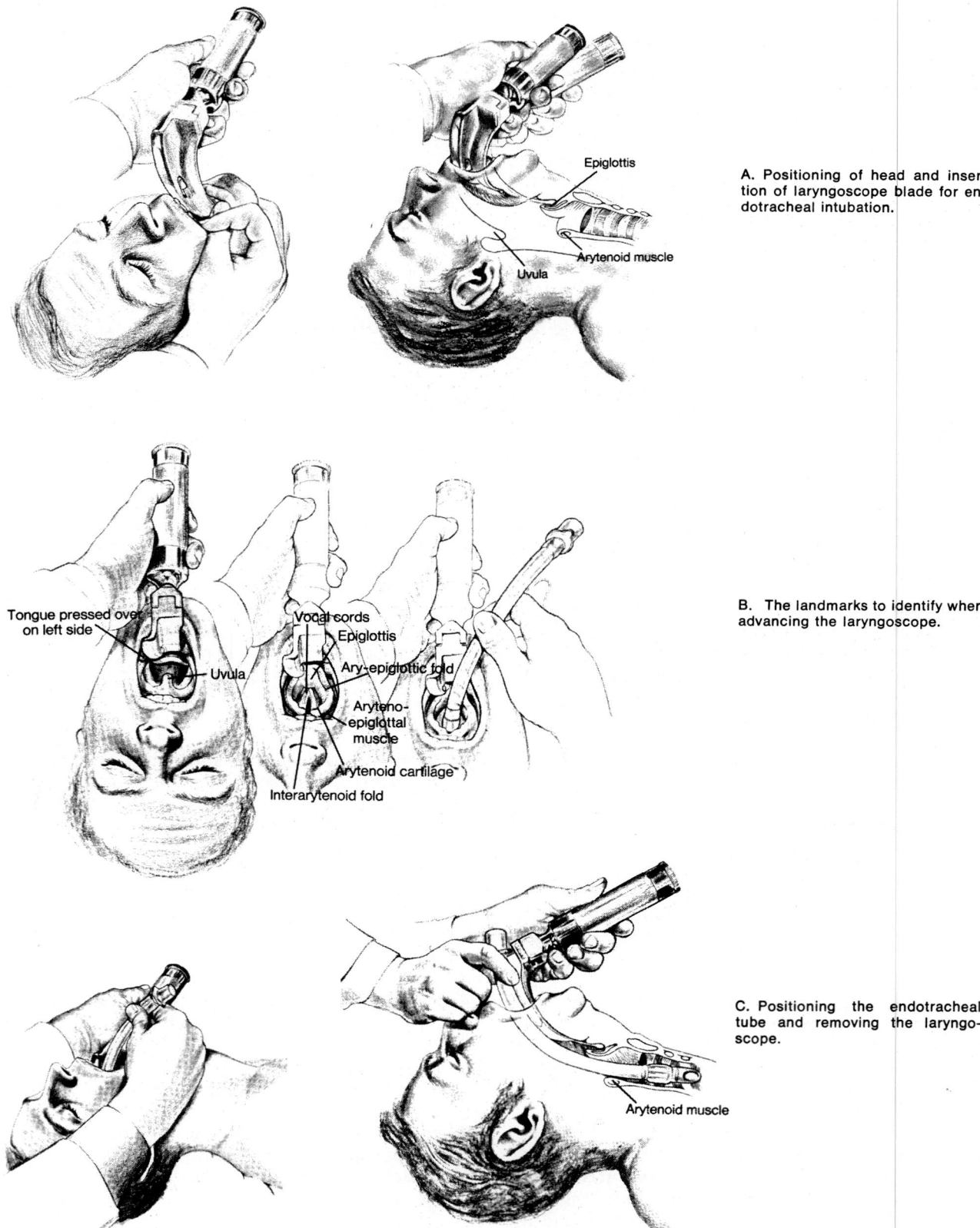

A. Positioning of head and insertion of laryngoscope blade for endotracheal intubation.

Epiglottis

Arytenoid muscle

Uvula

B. The landmarks to identify when advancing the laryngoscope.

Tongue pressed over on left side

Uvula

Vocal cords

Epiglottis

Ary-epiglottic fold

Aryteno-epiglottal muscle

Arytenoid cartilage

Interarytenoid fold

C. Positioning the endotracheal tube and removing the laryngoscope.

Arytenoid muscle

Figure 64-3. Sequence of steps for endotracheal intubation. (Reprinted with permission of Nursing Update, May 1972. Copyright © Miller and Fink Publishing Corporation, Darien, Conn. All rights reserved.)

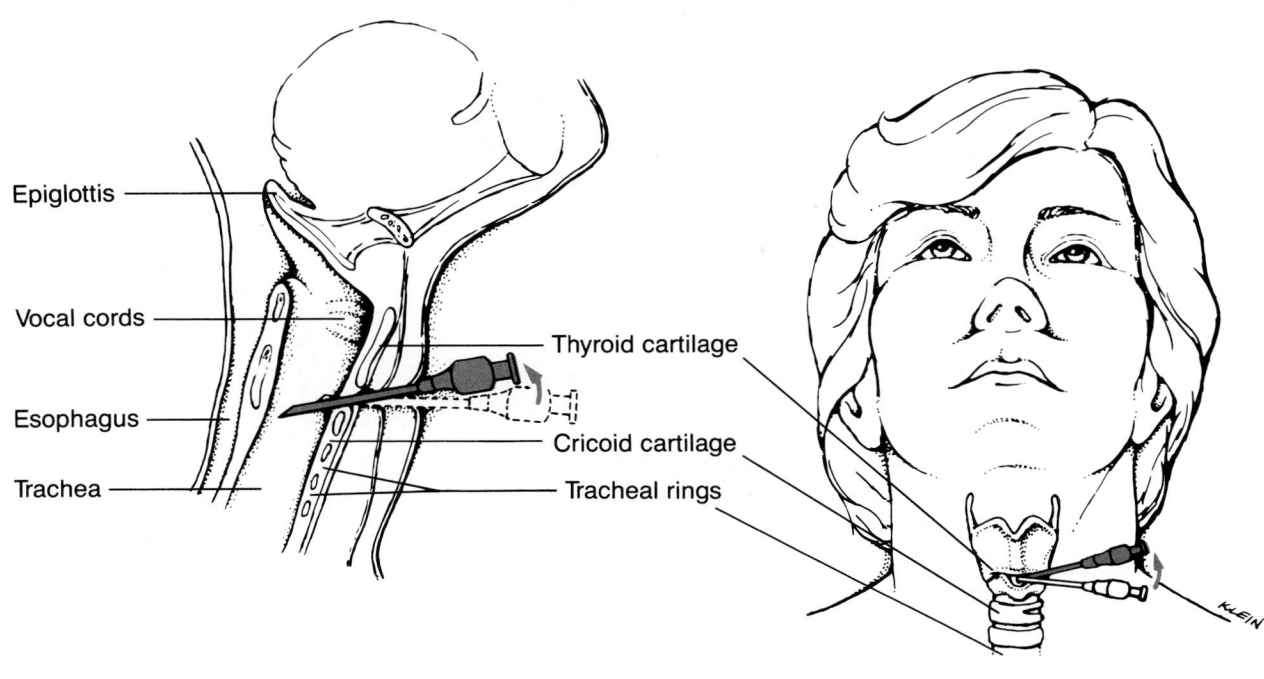

Figure 64-4. Crycothyroidotomy, or cricothyroid membrane puncture.

1. Assess for airway, breathing, circulation, vital signs, and level of responsiveness.
   a. Use a rectal probe to determine the degree of hypothermia if the patient has been submerged in cold water.
   b. Start rewarming procedures (extracorporeal warming; warmed peritoneal dialysis, inhalation of warm aerosolized oxygen, surface warming); these procedures may or may not be indicated.
2. Start an IV line; draw arterial blood to evaluate oxygen and carbon dioxide tensions, pH and bicarbonate levels; these parameters will determine the type of ventilatory support required and the subsequent dosage of sodium bicarbonate to be given.
3. Initiate endotracheal intubation with positive pressure ventilation (with PEEP) to improve oxygenation, to keep alveoli patent, and to correct intrapulmonary shunting and ventilation–perfusion abnormalities (caused by aspiration of water). Continue with 100% oxygen via a mask (if patient is breathing spontaneously) or via an endotracheal tube (if patient is not breathing spontaneously).
4. Assist with nasogastric intubation to empty the stomach to prevent the patient from regurgitating gastric contents.
5. Continue to monitor the patient closely—vital signs, serial arterial blood gas tensions, pH, ECG, intracranial pressure, serum electrolytes, serial chest x-rays.
6. Insert an indwelling catheter to determine urinary output; metabolic acidosis may compromise renal function.
7. Admit the patient to a hospital/ICU; the appearance of the patient may be deceptive. Complications of near-drowning that can lead to death include:

   a. Acute respiratory distress syndrome (see p. 486)
   b. Pulmonary infecton that may be superimposed on a damaged lung
   c. Cerebral swelling and increased intracranial pressure

▷ Control of Hemorrhage Due to Trauma

One of the primary causes of shock is the reduction in circulating blood volume. Only a few conditions, such as obstructed airway or a sucking wound of the chest, take precedence over the immediate control of hemorrhage. "Stop the bleeding" is fundamental to the care and the survival of patients in an emergency or a disaster situation. However, minor bleeding will usually stop spontaneously unless the patient has a bleeding disorder. Most of this type of blood loss will be venous. The objectives of emergency management are to control the bleeding, maintain an adequately circulating blood volume for tissue oxygenation, and prevent shock.

Emergency Management
1. Cut the patient's clothing away quickly to identify the area of hemorrhage, and carry out a rapid physical assessment.
2. Apply direct, firm pressure over the bleeding area or the artery involved (Fig. 64-5). Almost all bleeding can be stopped by direct pressure (except when a major artery has been severed). Unchecked arterial bleeding produces death.

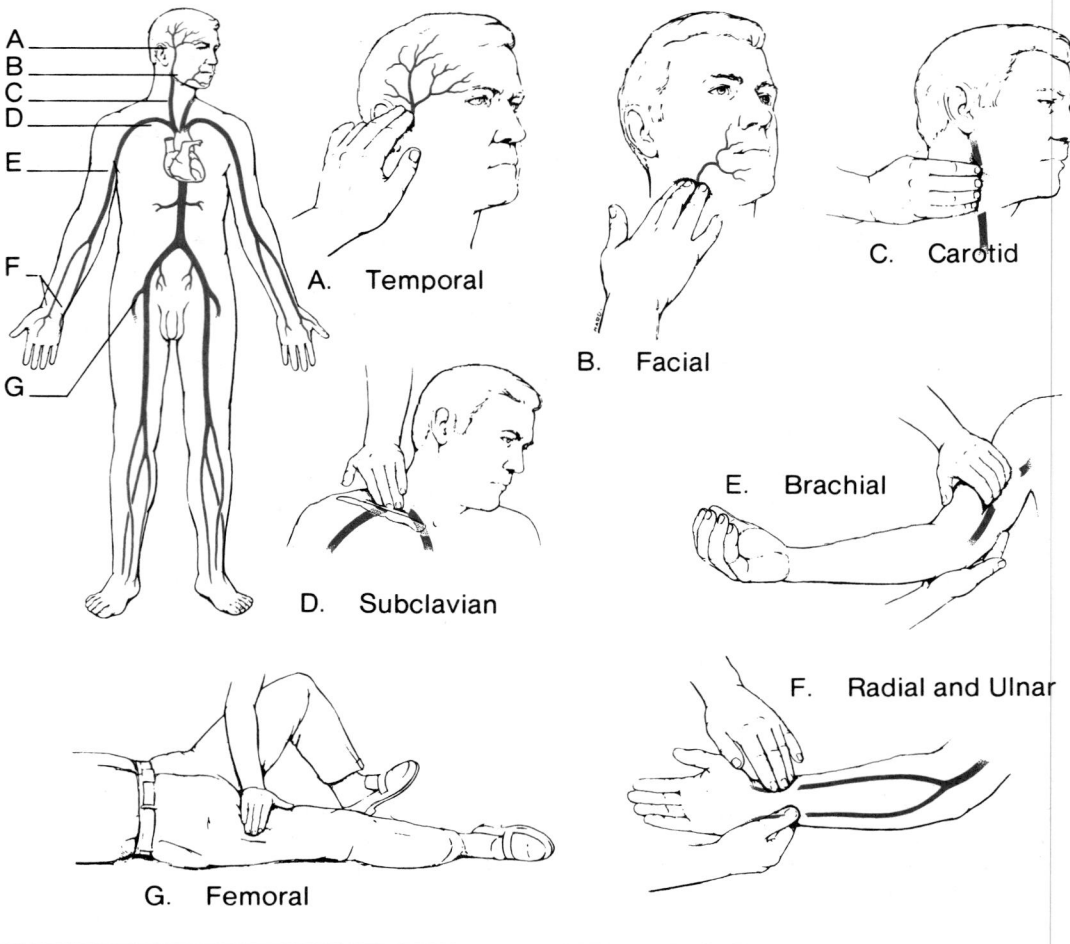

Figure 64-5. Pressure points for control of hemorrhage.

3. Apply a firm pressure dressing. Elevate the injured part to stop venous and capillary bleeding. Immobilize an injured extremity to control blood loss.
4. Insert an intravenous cannula to provide a means of blood replacement.
   a. Withdraw blood samples for analysis, typing, and cross-matching.
   b. Give replacement fluids, including isotonic electrolyte solutions, plasma or plasma protein solution, and blood (depending on clinical estimates of the type and volume of fluid lost).
      (1) Fresh blood is infused when there is massive blood loss to prevent loss of platelets and coagulation factors.
      (2) Additional platelets and clotting factors are given when large amounts of blood are needed, since replacement blood is deficient in clotting factors.
      (3) Warm the blood (commercial warmer or basin of warm water)—massive blood replacement has a cooling effect that can cause cardiac arrest.
   c. The rate of infusion depends on the severity of blood loss and clinical evidence of hypovolemia.
5. Take the following steps for internal bleeding.
   a. Suspect internal bleeding in patients with hypovolemic shock with no external signs of bleeding: rising pulse rate; falling blood pressure; thirst; apprehension; cool, moist skin.
   b. Give whole blood or plasma expanders at the rate of blood loss.
   c. Prepare the patient immediately for surgical intervention.
   d. Apply a wraparound inflatable counterpressure suit ("G" suit, compression suit), if available, to control internal bleeding and to facilitate the blood flow to vital areas (Fig. 64-6)
   e. Obtain blood gas determination; establish central venous pressure monitoring as an index of the amount of fluid the patient can tolerate.
6. Apply a tourniquet only as a *last resort,* when the hemorrhage cannot be controlled by any other method. Anticipate loss of an extremity if a tourniquet is applied.
   a. Apply the tourniquet just proximal to the wound; tie it tightly enough to control the arterial blood flow.
   b. Tag the patient with a skin-marking pencil or on adhesive tape on his forehead with a "T," stating the location of the tourniquet and the time applied.

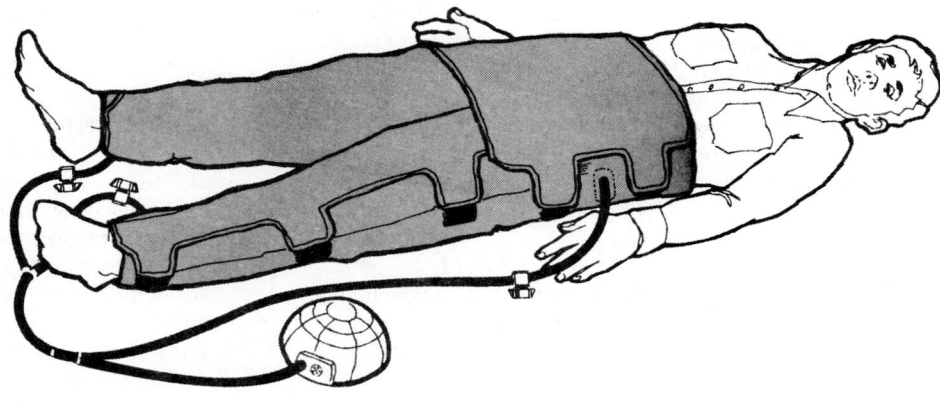

Figure 64-6. The Medical Anti-Shock Trouser (MAST) is a device designed to counteract internal bleeding and hypovolemia by the application of counterpressure around the legs and abdomen, producing an artificial peripheral resistance and ensuring adequate coronary perfusion. MAST is a product of David Clark Company, Inc., 360 Franklin Street, Worcester, Massachusetts 01604. (Courtesy, David Clark Company, Inc.)

   c. Loosen the tourniquet as directed to prevent irreparable vascular or neurologic damage if the patient is in an emergency facility. If there is no arterial bleeding, remove the tourniquet and again try a pressure dressing.

   d. In the event of a traumatic amputation, leave the tourniquet applied until the patient is in the OR.

7. Watch for cardiac arrest; patients who hemorrhage are candidates for cardiac arrest caused by hypovolemia with secondary anoxia.

8. See page 407 for further discussion of hemorrhage.

▷ Control of Hypovolemic Shock*

Shock is a condition in which there is loss of effective circulating blood volume; inadequate organ and tissue perfusion result, ultimately causing cellular metabolic derangements. In any emergency situation, it is wise to anticipate shock before it develops. Any injured person should be assessed immediately to determine the presence of shock. Its underlying cause must be discovered (hypovolemic, cardiogenic, neurogenic, septic shock). Hypovolemia is the most common cause of shock.

The following signs and symptoms, in varying combinations, indicate that the patient is in some degree of shock: decreasing arterial pressure; increasing pulse rate; cold, moist skin; pallor; thirst; diaphoresis; decreased sensorium; oliguria; metabolic acidosis; and hyperpnea. Of these, the most dependable criterion is the level of arterial blood pressure. Start treatment at the first signs of shock.

Emergency Mangement
The objectives of treatment are to restore and maintain tissue perfusion and to correct physiologic abnormalities.

1. Establish and maintain an airway; start resuscitation procedures if necessary. Give oxygen to augment the oxygen-carrying capacity of arterial blood. Give additional ventilatory assistance as required.

2. Restore the circulating blood volume with rapid fluid and blood replacement to correct hypotension and maintain tissue perfusion.

   * See also page 402.

   a. Insert a central venous pressure catheter in or near the right atrium (see p. 596) to serve as a guide for fluid replacement. Continuing central venous pressure (CVP) readings give the direction and degree of change from baseline readings; the catheter also is a vehicle for emergency fluid volume replacement.

   b. Insert large-gauge intravenous needles or catheters into peripheral vein(s); two or more catheters may be necessary for rapid replacement and reversal of hemodynamic instability; the emphasis is on volume replacement.

     (1) Establish IV lines in both upper and lower extremities if there is suspicion that a major vessel in the chest or abdomen has been disrupted.

     (2) Withdraw blood for specimens—arterial blood gases (arterial blood), chemistry studies, typing and cross-matching, and hematocrit.

3. Start intravenous infusion at a rapid rate until CVP rises to a satisfactory level above the baseline measurement or until there is improvement in the patient's clinical condition.

   a. Infusion of lactated Ringer's solution is useful initially to allow time for whole blood typing and crossmatching and to restore circulation and serve as an adjunct to whole blood.

   b. Start transfusion of blood component therapy, especially when blood loss has been severe or when the patient continues to hemorrhage.

   c. Control hemorrhage; hemorrhage will compound the shock state. Carry out serial hematocrit examinations if continued bleeding is suspected.

   d. Maintain the systolic blood pressure at a satisfactory level by administering fluid and blood.

4. Insert an indwelling urinary catheter; record urinary output every 15 to 30 minutes. Urinary volume reveals adequacy of kidney perfusion.

5. Carry out a rapid physical assessment to determine the cause of shock.

6. Maintain ongoing nursing surveillance of the *total patient*—blood pressure, heart and respiratory rates, skin temperature, color, CVP, arterial blood gases, ECG, hematocrit, hemoglobin, coagulation profile, electrolytes, and urinary output—to assess patient response to treat-

ment. Keep a flow sheet of these parameters—trend analysis reveals improvement or deterioration of patient.

7. Elevate the feet slightly to improve cerebral circulation and promote return of venous blood to the heart. (*This position is contraindicated in patients with head injuries.*) Avoid unnecessary movement.

8. Give specific pharmacologic agents (sodium bicarbonate, dopamine, etc.) when indicated by the patient's condition.

9. Support the defense mechanisms of the body.
   a. Reassure and comfort the patient; sedation may be necessary to relieve apprehension.
   b. Relieve pain by *cautious* use of analgesics or narcotics.
   c. Maintain the body temperature.
      (1) Too much heat produces vasodilatation, which counteracts the body's compensatory mechanism of vasoconstriction and also increases fluid loss by perspiration.
      (2) A patient who is in septic shock should be kept cool, since high fever will increase the cellular metabolic effects of shock.

▷ Wounds

Wounds (injury to tissues) vary from minor lacerations to severe crushing injuries. Life-threatening problems, such as airway obstruction, hemorrhage, and shock, must be dealt with before the wound is treated.

Emergency Management
The goals of management are to avoid complications, promote rapid healing, and minimize scarring and prevent deformity.

1. Ask the patient *when* as well as *how* the wound occurred; a delay over 3 hours in treatment increases the risk of infection developing.

2. Inspect the wound, using aseptic technique, to determine the extent of damage to underlying structures.
   a. Shave around the wound (with the exception of eyebrows) only if directed.
   b. Cleanse around the wound with an antimicrobial agent. Do not allow the cleansing solution to get into the wound, since it may be injurious to exposed tissues.
   c. Infiltrate with a local anesthetic intradermally through the wound margins or by regional block.

3. Cleanse and debride the wound.
   a. Irrigate gently and copiously with isotonic sterile saline to remove surface dirt.
   b. Remove devitalized tissue and foreign matter—impairs the wound's ability to resist infection.
   c. Clamp and tie small bleeding vessels (or achieve hemostasis with a cautery).

4. Suture the wound (usually done by physician) if primary closure is indicated (depends on the nature of the wound, the length of time since the injury was sustained, the degree of contamination, and the vascularity of tissues).

   a. Subcutaneous fat is approximated loosely with a few sutures to close off the dead space.
   b. The subcuticular layer is then closed.
   c. The epidermis is closed; sutures are placed close to the wound edge with the skin edges leveled carefully to prevent uneven scar surfaces.
   d. Sterile strips of reinforced microporous tape may be used to close clean, superficial wounds.

5. Apply water-soluble ointment if directed.

6. Apply dressing to protect the wound—may serve as a splint and as a reminder to the patient that he has sustained an injury.

7. For delayed primary closure:
   a. A thin layer of gauze (to ensure drainage and prevent pooling of exudate) covered by an occlusive dressing may be used, or split-thickness cadaver or porcine xenografts may be used to hold the wound apart.
   b. Splint the wound in a position of rest to prevent motion.
   c. Close the wound (with a local anesthetic) when there are no signs of suppuration.

8. Give antimicrobial treatment as directed (depends on how the injury occurred, the age of wound, the presence of soil-infection potential, etc.).

9. Immobilize the site if the wound is contaminated; elevate the site to limit accumulation of fluid in wound interstitial spaces.

10. Give tetanus prophylaxis as indicated.

▷ Intra-abdominal Injuries

Penetrating Abdominal Injuries

Penetrating abdominal injuries (gunshot wounds, stab wounds) are serious and usually require surgery. In penetrating injuries, the most important factor is the velocity with which the missile entered the body. High-velocity missiles (bullets) create extensive tissue damage. Almost all gunshot wounds require surgical exploration. Stab wounds may be managed more conservatively.

Assessment for Abdominal Injuries

- Obtain a history of the mechanism of the injury.
- Assess the patient for progression of distention, involuntary guarding, tenderness, pain, muscular rigidity or rebound tenderness, diminished bowel sounds, hypotension, and shock.
- Auscultate for bowel sounds, as the absence of bowel sounds is an early sign of intraperitoneal involvement. If signs of peritoneal irritation are present, an immediate exploratory celiotomy (surgical incision into abdominal cavity) is usually performed.
- Record all physical signs as the patient is examined.
- Look for chest injuries, which frequently accompany intra-abdominal injuries.

Emergency Management
The objectives of emergency management are to control the bleeding and maintain the blood volume.

1. Keep the patient on the stretcher, since movement may cause fragmentation of a clot in a large vessel and produce massive hemorrhage.
   a. Ensure patency of the airway and stability of the respiratory, circulatory, and nervous systems.
   b. Cut the clothing away from the wound.
   c. Tabulate the number of wounds.
   d. Look for entrance and exit wounds.
   e. If the patient is comatose, splint the neck until after cervical films are made.
2. Assess for signs and symptoms of hemorrhage. *Hemorrhage frequently accompanies abdominal injury,* especially if the liver and spleen have been traumatized.
3. Control the bleeding and maintain the blood volume until surgery can be performed.
   a. Apply compression to external bleeding wounds and occlusion of chest wounds.
   b. Insert indwelling intravenous catheter(s) for rapid fluid replacement to restore circulatory dynamics.
   c. Watch for the occurrence of shock after an initial response to transfusion therapy; this is often the first sign of internal hemorrhage.
4. Aspirate the stomach contents with a nasogastric tube. This procedure also helps detect gastric wounds and prevents lung complications due to aspiration.
5. Cover protruding abdominal viscera with sterile saline dressings to prevent the viscera from drying.
   a. Flex the patient's knees, as this position will prevent further protrusion.
   b. Withhold oral fluids to prevent increased peristalsis and vomiting.
6. Insert an indwelling urethral catheter to ascertain the presence of hematuria and to monitor the urinary output.
7. Keep an ongoing flow sheet of the patient's vital signs, urinary output, central venous pressure readings (when indicated), hematocrit values, and neurologic status.
8. Prepare for paracentesis or peritoneal lavage (Chart 64-3) when there is uncertainty about intraperitoneal bleeding.
9. For stab wounds, prepare for sinography to determine whether there is peritoneal penetration.
   a. A purse-string suture is placed around the wound.
   b. A small catheter is introduced through the wound.
   c. A contrast medium is introduced through the catheter; x-rays are made and will reveal whether or not peritoneal penetration has taken place.
10. Carry out tetanus prophylaxis as directed.
11. Give a broad-spectrum antibiotic to prevent infection, since bacterial contamination is a frequent complication (depending on the history and nature of the wound).
12. Prepare for surgery if the patient shows continuing evidence of shock, blood loss, free air, evisceration, hematuria, etc.

Blunt Abdominal Trauma

Blunt trauma to the abdomen may result from automobile accidents, falls, and blows to the abdomen. These patients are a challenge because of potential hidden injuries that may be difficult to detect. The incidence of delayed trauma-related complications is greater than that associated with penetrating injuries. This is especially true of blunt injuries involving the liver, kidneys, spleen, and pancreas. Blunt abdominal trauma is frequently associated with extra-abdominal injuries to the chest, head, extremities, etc., and the evaluation and treatment of these injuries may take precedence over the abdominal problem.

The clinical manifestations of blunt abdominal trauma include pain (especially on movement), rebound and maximal point tenderness (may indicate peritoneal irritation from blood or gastrointestinal fluid), muscle guarding, and diminishing or absent bowel sounds.

Emergency Management

1. Begin resuscitation procedures and evaluation of the patient simultaneously.
2. Take a detailed history (although this is frequently unobtainable, inaccurate, and misleading). Obtain all possible data about the following:
   a. Method of injury
   b. Time of onset of symptoms
   c. Passenger location; driver frequently sustains rupture of the spleen/liver
   d. Time of last food/fluid intake
   e. Bleeding tendencies
   f. Concurrent disease/medications
   g. Immunization history, with attention to tetanus
   h. Allergies
3. Carry out ongoing physical assessment: inspection, palpation, auscultation, and percussion of the abdomen. The changes noted in subsequent examinations may reveal an undetected abdominal injury.
   a. Avoid moving the patient until the initial assessment is done. Movement may fragment a clot in a large vessel and produce massive hemorrhage
   b. Look for chest injuries, especially for fractures of the lower ribs.
   c. Inspect the front, flanks, and back for bluish discoloration, asymmetry, abrasion, and contusion.
   d. Evaluate for signs and symptoms of hemorrhage, which frequently accompanies abdominal injury, especially if the liver and spleen have been traumatized.
   e. Note tenderness, rebound tenderness, guarding, rigidity, and spasm.
      (1) Press the area of maximal tenderness (let the patient point to the area).
      (2) Remove the fingers quickly; pain at the suspected point indicates peritoneal irritation.
   f. Look for increasing abdominal distention. Measure the abdominal girth at the umbilical level upon admission; this serves as a baseline from which changes can be determined.
   g. Auscultate for bowel sounds; silent abdomen accompanies peritoneal irritation.
   h. Note loss of dullness over the solid organs (liver/spleen)—indicates presence of free air. Dullness over regions normally containing gas indicates presence of blood.

Chart 64-3
Peritoneal Lavage

Peritoneal lavage is a technique of irrigation of the peritoneum and examination of the irrigating fluid in order to evaluate the effects of trauma to the abdomen.

Purposes

1. To test for intra-abdominal bleeding following trauma
2. To look for injuries requiring surgical treatment
3. To test patients with equivocal abdominal findings
4. To avoid unnecessary operation, especially in patients with altered states of consciousness (from head injuries, drugs, alcohol) and when physical findings are unreliable (spinal cord injuries)

Contraindications

1. Multiple abdominal scars
2. Pregnancy

Equipment

Peritoneal dialysis tray
Sterile solution (lactated Ringer's solution, normal saline)
IV tubing, IV pole
Peritoneal dialysis catheter (multiple perforations)
Local skin anesthetic, sterile gloves

Procedure

Nursing Action	*Rationale/Amplification*
Preparatory Phase	
1. Explain the procedure to the patient; see that the consent form has been signed.	
2. Empty the bladder (by catheter if necessary).	2. To prevent puncture of the urinary bladder
3. Prepare the abdomen as for surgery.	3. To minimize or eliminate surface bacteria and decrease the possibility of wound contamination and infection
4. Fill the IV tubing with solution, using aseptic technique.	
Performance Phase (by the Physician)	
1. The skin is infiltrated 2 cm to 3 cm (0.7–1.2 inches) below the umbilicus in the midline with local anesthetic.	1. The midline area is relatively avascular.
2. A vertical incision is made down to the linea alba.	
3. Local pressure is applied to suppress capillary leakage. Bleeding vessels are carefully ligated.	3. Ligation of vessels helps avoid a false positive lavage.

(continued)

4. Assist with rectal or vaginal examination for diagnosis of injury to the pelvis, bladder, and intestinal wall.
5. Avoid giving narcotics during the observation period, since this may mask the clinical picture.
6. Monitor vital signs frequently and carefully. This may be the only clue to intra-abdominal bleeding.
7. Obtain baseline laboratory studies.
   a. Urinalysis—as a guide to possible urinary tract injury (hematuria) and to monitor urinary output

b. Serial hemoglobin and hematocrit levels—their trend reflects the presence or absence of bleeding.
c. CBC—white blood cell count may be elevated with rupture of spleen
d. Serum amylase—rising level may indicate pancreatic injury or trauma to bowel
8. Obtain abdominal and chest x-rays—may reveal free air beneath diaphragm, indicating ruptured hollow viscus.
9. Prepare for peritoneal lavage to test for intraperitoneal

Chart 64-3
Peritoneal Lavage (continued)

Nursing Action (continued)	*Rationale/Amplification (continued)*
Performance Phase (by the Physician) *(continued)*	
4. The peritoneum is opened under direct vision, and a peritoneal dialysis catheter is inserted into the peritoneal cavity.	
5. A syringe is attached to the catheter, and the peritoneal cavity is aspirated.	5. If gross blood is obtained (or bile or intestinal contents), the tap shows positive findings and the patient is prepared for immediate celiotomy (incision into the abdominal cavity).
6. If no blood is present, the catheter is attached to the IV tubing; 500 ml to 1000 ml of solution is infused into the peritoneal cavity through the intravenous tubing attached to the dialysis catheter.	6. If not contraindicated by the patient's condition, he may be turned from side to side to ensure that the solution reaches all parts of the abdominal cavity.
7. Clamp off the IV tubing. Remove the empty IV bottle from the pole and lower the bottle to the floor.	7. Lowering the bottle creates a siphon effect to drain the excess fluid. As much of the fluid as possible is siphoned out of the peritoneal cavity by gravity.
8. Dislodge the air vent from the rubber stopper by removing the IV tubing. Reinsert the IV tubing into the vent hole itself. Unclamp the tubing and allow the fluid to be siphoned from the abdominal cavity.	
9. The fluid recovered from the peritoneal cavity is examined visually and is usually sent to the laboratory for cell counts and microscopic inspection of a spun-down sediment.	
Interpretation of Lavage Fluid	
1. *Gross examination (visual)* Inability to read newsprint through the intravenous tubing usually means that the amount of blood is sufficient to indicate a laparotomy.	1. If the test is positive, a laparotomy is usually done. If the test is negative, the catheter is removed and the wound closed.
2. *Laboratory evaluation (positive tests)* Free aspiration of blood/grossly bloody fluid RBC greater than 100,000/cu mm WBC greater than 500/cu mm Bacteria—pathologic when present Bile—pathologic when present	2. If the test is questionable, the catheter may be left in place and the lavage repeated. If the test is weakly positive, the patient may have echography and arteriography if his condition is stable.
Follow-up Phase	
1. Assess the patient for complications.	1. Complications include wound problems, visceral injury, and inadequate fluid return.
2. Watch the patient closely for any type of deterioration.	2. *Repeated physical examinations* of the abdomen should be carried out when intra-abdominal injury is suspected.

bleeding (see p. 1548); organ laceration or bleeding may be diagnosed by gross and microscopic examination of fluid returned after peritoneal lavage.

10. Assist with insertion of a nasogastric tube to prevent vomiting and subsequent aspiration. It is also helpful in decompressing (removing fluid/air from) the gastrointestinal tract.

11. The patient may be admitted for (1) observation or (2) exploratory laparotomy (especially for refractory hypotension, uncontrollable hemorrhage, viscera extruding from wound, free abdominal air).

Crush Injuries

Crush injuries occur when a person is crushed beneath debris, run over, or compressed by machinery.

The first step is to assess the patient for oligemic shock resulting from the extravasation of blood and plasma into the injured tissues after the compression has been released. The extremity may be paralyzed, erythematous, swollen, tense, and hard, and the skin may be blistered. If the shock persists, prolonged hypotension can cause kidney damage and acute renal insufficiency.

Emergency Management

1. Control shock.
2. Observe carefully for acute renal insufficiency. Injury to the back may cause severe kidney damage.
3. Splint major soft tissue injuries to control bleeding and pain early.
4. Elevate the extremity. Incise fascia if the blood supply is blocked to relieve the pressure of extravasated fluid.
5. Administer medication for pain and anxiety.

Multiple Injuries

The patient with multiple injuries requires a team approach, with one person responsible for coordinating the treatment. Following trauma, there may be general depression of body functions leading to such complications as reduced blood pressure, oxygen deficiency in the bloodstream and primary organ systems, arrhythmias, and respiratory and heart failure. It is thought that the defense mechanism of the body becomes depressed, contributing to total organ failure. Mortality in patients with multiple injuries is related to the severity of the injuries and the number of systems and organs involved.

The goals of treatment are to determine the extent of injuries and to establish priorities of treatment. Obtaining a patent airway and support of respiration and circulation are key priorities. Imperative lifesaving procedures are performed simultaneously by the emergency team. As soon as the patient is resuscitated, the clothes are usually cut off and a rapid physical assessment is done. Critically traumatized patients should not be moved.

Emergency Management

See Figure 64-7. Carry out a *rapid* physical examination to determine if the patient is breathing, bleeding, or in shock; determine the status of his responsiveness and if he has severe wounds or fracture deformities.

1. Establish an open airway.*
   a. Note the character and symmetry of chest wall motion and the pattern of breathing. Auscultate the chest.
   b. Ask the conscious patient if he is having difficulty in breathing. Ask if he has chest pain.
   c. Apply suction to clear the trachea and bronchial tree.
   d. Insert an oropharyngeal airway to prevent occlusion by the tongue.
   e. Ventilate the patient (bag–mask system) to alleviate hypoxia.

---

* Imperative lifesaving procedures are performed simultaneously by the emergency team.

   f. Prepare for endotracheal intubation (see p. 1540) if an adequate airway cannot be maintained.
   g. Suspect serious intrathoracic injuries if respiratory distress continues after an adequate airway has been established. See pages 538 to 541 for management of chest injuries.
2. Assess cardiac function and treat cardiac arrest—hypoxia, metabolic acidosis, and chest trauma may precipitate cardiac arrest.*
   a. For cardiac arrest, start closed chest compression and ventilation (see p. 599).
   b. If the chest wall is unstable (flail chest), emergency thoracotomy and manual compression may be necessary.
   c. Give sodium bicarbonate (IV) to compensate for acidosis if indicated—severely traumatized patients with respiratory and circulatory embarrassment will have some degree of metabolic acidosis.
3. Control hemorrhage.*
   a. Apply pressure over bleeding points if hemorrhage is overt (see p. 1544).
   b. Expect significant blood loss in the patient with a fracture of the shaft of the femur, with multiple fractures, or with major pelvic trauma.
   c. Use tourniquet(s) for massive arterial bleeding from extremities that cannot be halted with pressure.
   d. Prepare for immediate surgical intervention if the patient is bleeding internally.
4. Prevent and treat hypovolemic shock.
   a. Insert at least two (sometimes four) IV lines: one above the diaphragm and one below. Use venous cutdown if necessary.
   b. Draw blood for laboratory studies as directed (typing and crossmatching, baseline CBC, electrolytes, blood urea nitrogen, glucose, prothrombin time).
   c. Introduce a central venous catheter to monitor the patient's response to fluid infusion, to prevent fluid overload, and as a route for fluid infusion.
   d. Start intravenous infusions.
      (1) Balanced saline solution, plasma, or plasma protein fraction is given in a quantity sufficient to maintain blood pressure until blood is available.
      (2) Give blood as directed—massive transfusions have a cooling effect that can cause cardiac irritability and arrest; blood should be warmed.
   e. Give intravenous infusions rapidly enough to keep central venous pressure readings at 5 cm to 15 cm H_2O; monitor the rate and direction of change (important parameters).
   f. Insert an indwelling urethral catheter and monitor urinary output. Do not force the catheter—the patient may have a ruptured urethra.
   g. Monitor the ECG to detect changes.
   h. Carry out ongoing clinical evaluation to observe for improvement or deterioration; improvement in the level of responsiveness, skin warmth, speed of capillary filling, etc., shows a reversal of the shock state.

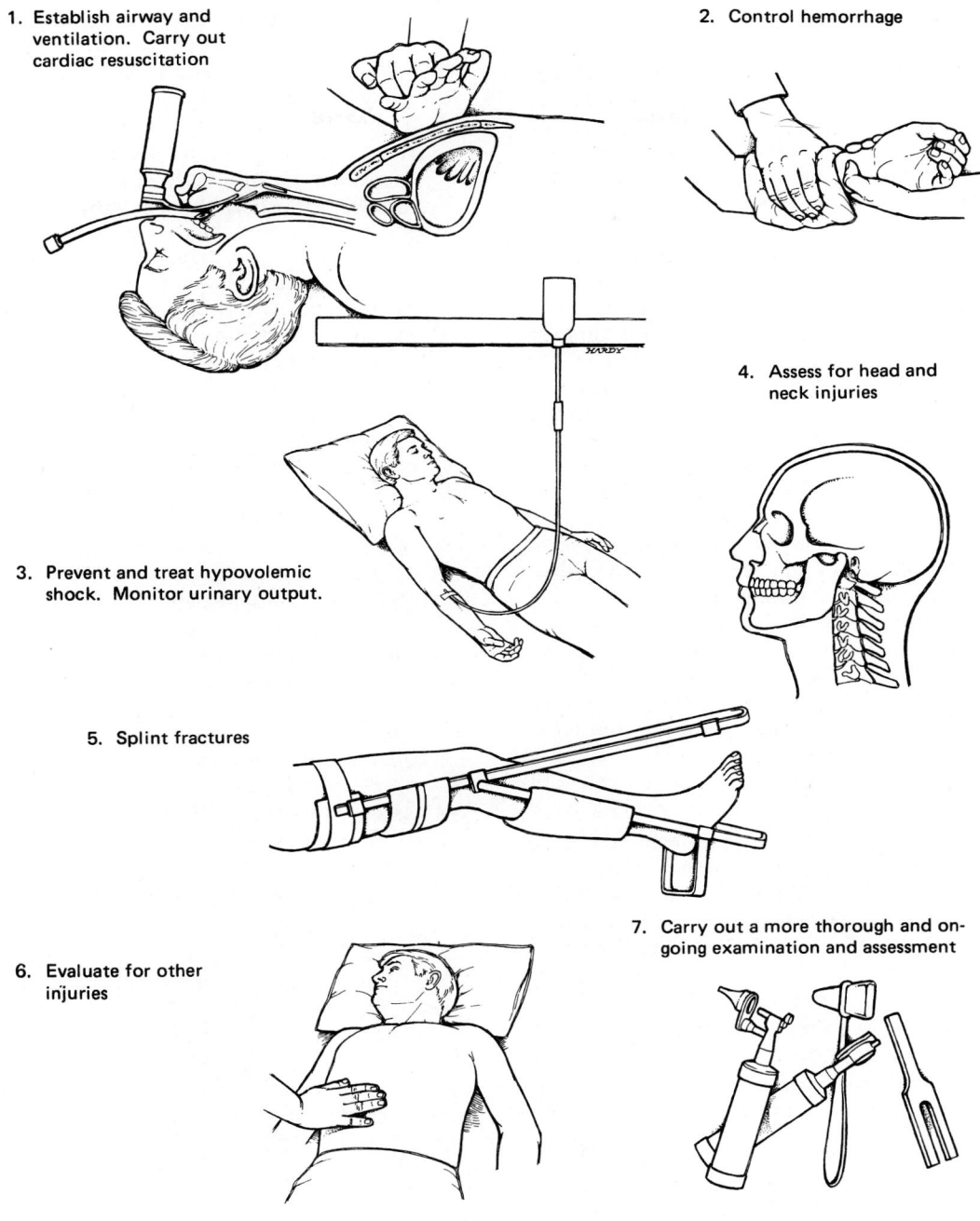

1. Establish airway and ventilation. Carry out cardiac resuscitation

2. Control hemorrhage

3. Prevent and treat hypovolemic shock. Monitor urinary output.

4. Assess for head and neck injuries

5. Splint fractures

6. Evaluate for other injuries

7. Carry out a more thorough and on-going examination and assessment

Figure 64-7. The patient with multiple injuries.

i. Prepare for immediate surgical intervention if the patient does not respond to fluids or blood. Inability to restore blood pressure and circulatory volume in the patient usually indicates major internal bleeding.
5. Assess for head and neck injuries.
   a. Make definite statements concerning the baseline neurologic status of the patient: level of respon-

siveness, size and reactivity of pupils, motor power, reflexes.
   b. Neck (and chest) films may be taken; apply rigid cervical collar until x-rays preclude the possibility of cervical spine injury.
   c. Intracranial pressure monitoring (see p. 1295) may be instituted.

6. Administer dexamethasone as directed—corticosteroids appear to protect pulmonary function in patients with multiple injuries and to help prevent post-traumatic pulmonary insufficiency. (However, this is considered a controversial issue.)
7. Splint fractures to prevent further trauma to soft tissues and blood vessels and to relieve pain; note the presence or absence of pulses in fractured extremities.
8. Assess the patient for gastrointestinal injuries.
   a. Examine the patient repeatedly for abdominal pain, muscular rigidity, tenderness, rebound tenderness, diminished bowel sounds, hypotension, and shock.
   b. Prepare for peritoneal lavage to assess for intraperitoneal bleeding.
   c. Assist with insertion of a nasogastric tube if upper gastrointestinal bleeding is suspected or if gaseous distension of the stomach develops—will decrease the incidence of vomiting and aspiration.
   d. Prepare for laparotomy if the patient shows continuing signs of hemorrhage and deterioration.
9. Continue to monitor urinary output hourly—reflects cardiac output and state of perfusion of visceral organs.
   a. Assess for hematuria and oliguria.
   b. Record measurements on a flow sheet.
10. Evaluate patient for other injuries and institute appropriate treatment, including tetanus immunization.
11. Carry out a more thorough physical examination after resuscitation and management of the above priorities.

▷ Fractures

The immediate management of a fracture may determine the patient's outcome and make the difference between recovery or disability. In examining for fracture, handle the part gently and as little as possible. Cut off clothing to minimize trauma to the part. Evaluate for pain over or near a bone, swelling (from blood, lymph, and exudate infiltrating the tissue), and circulatory disturbance. Look for ecchymosis, tenderness, and crepitation, *Keep in mind that the patient may have multiple fractures accompanied by head, chest, and other serious injuries.*

Emergency Management
A. Give immediate attention to the patient's general condition. If there is any question of multiple injury, the patient needs to be completely undressed, draped, and examined periodically.
   1. Evaluate for respiratory difficulties from edema due to facial and neck injuries, accumulation of secretions in the respiratory tract, etc.
      a. Examine the chest for evidence of sucking chest wounds, pneumothorax, flail chest, etc.
      b. Prepare for tracheal intubation or emergency tracheostomy.
   2. Control hemorrhage.
      a. Control venous bleeding by applying direct pressure along with digital pressure over the artery nearest to the bleeding area.
      b. Suspect internal hemorrhage (pleural, pericardial, or abdominal) in the event of continuing shock and in the presence of injuries to the chest and abdomen.
   3. Treat for shock, which is usually the result of blood loss in patients with fractures.
      a. Assess for falling blood pressure; cold, clammy skin; and rapid, thready pulse.
      b. Keep in mind that a large amount of blood loss may accompany fractures of the femur and pelvis.
      c. Maintain the blood pressure with intravenous infusions, plasma, or plasma expanders.
      d. Give blood transfusion(s) or blood component therapy as soon as blood is available.
      e. Administer oxygen since cardiopulmonary embarrassment causes a decreased oxygen supply to the tissues and circulatory collapse.
      f. Give an analgesic to control pain. (Splinting the extremity and controlling pain are essential in treating shock accompanying fractures.)
      g. Look for evidence of head, chest, and other injuries.
B. Inspect the fractured part(s).
   1. Observe the entire body using a methodical head-to-toe physical examination; inspect for lacerations, swelling, and deformities.
   2. Look for *angulation* (bending), *shortening,* and *rotation.*
   3. Feel the pulse distal to the extremity fracture. Check all peripheral pulses.
   4. Assess for coolness, blanching, decreased sensation and motor function, and diminished or absent pulses; these indicate injury to nerves or the blood supply.
   5. Handle the part gently and as little as possible.
C. Apply the splint before the patient is moved, as splinting relieves pain, improves circulation, prevents further tissue injury, and prevents a closed fracture from becoming an open one.
   1. Immobilize the joint above and below the fracture. Place one hand distal to the fracture and apply some traction while placing the other hand beneath the fracture for support.
   2. Extend the splints well beyond the joints adjacent to the fracture.
      a. Use the patient's clothing for padding (shirt, tie) if nothing else is avilable.
      b. Use newspapers, magazines, pillows, tree limbs, and boards for splints if nothing else is available. Specialized splints are available on ambulances and in hospitals.
      c. Splint joints in functional positions.
   3. Check the vascular status of the extremity after splinting; check color, temperature, pulse, blanching of nail bed.
   4. Evaluate for neurologic deficits caused by the fracture.
   5. Apply a sterile dressing if the fracture is an open one.
D. Investigate any complaint of pain or pressure.

E. Transport the patient carefully and gently.

F. See pages 1427 to 1444 for a complete discussion of the treatment of fractures at specific sites.

▷ Heat Stroke

Heat stroke is an acute medical emergency caused by failure of the heat-regulating mechanisms of the body during extended heat waves, especially with high humidity. Persons at risk are those not acclimatized to heat exposure, those with advanced age, those who are unable to care for themselves, those with chronic and debilitating diseases, and those who are taking certain medications (major tranquilizers, anticholinergics, diuretics, propranolol). Another form of heat stroke, *exertional heat stroke,* is a leading cause of death in athletes in this country.

Heat stroke causes thermal injury at the cellular level and resulting widespread damage to the heart, liver, kidney, and blood coagulation systems. When assessing the patient, note the following: profound central nervous system dysfunction (manifested by confusion, delirium, bizarre behavior, coma); elevated body temperature (40.6° C [105° F] or more); hot, dry skin; and usually absence of sweating.

Emergency Management

The goal of management is to reduce the high temperature as quickly as possible. Mortality is directly related to the duration of hyperthermia.

1. Reduce the core (internal) temperature to 39° C (102° F) rectally as rapidly as possible. Monitor the patient's temperature constantly to avoid hypothermia. If available, monitor the rectal temperature by a rectal thermistor probe left in place. One or more of the following temperature-lowering methods may be used:

   a. Immerse the patient in an ice-water bath. Massage the extremities and skin continuously during immersion (promotes circulation and maintains cutaneous vasodilation).

   b. Sponge the patient continuously with ice-cold water; place an electric fan so that it blows on the patient, since air movement increases evaporation.

   c. Give chilled saline enemas if the temperature does not come down.

2. Monitor the patient carefully; vital signs, ECG, CVP, and level of responsiveness change with rapid alterations in body temperature.

3. Administer oxygen to supply tissue needs exaggerated by the hypermetabolic condition. Intubate the patient with a cuffed endotracheal tube and attach to a ventilator if necessary to support failing cardiorespiratory systems.

4. Start intravenous infusion as directed to replace fluid losses and maintain adequate circulation; give slowly because of the danger of myocardial injury due to high body temperature or poor renal function.

5. Give supportive care as directed:

   a. Dialysis for renal failure

   b. Diuretics (mannitol) to promote diuresis; monitor the blood pressure carefully, as hypotension may be precipitated.

   c. Anticonvulsant agents to control seizures

   d. Potassium for hypokalemia and sodium bicarbonate to correct metabolic acidosis, depending on laboratory results

6. Measure urinary output—acute tubular necrosis is a complication of heat stroke.

7. Continue to monitor ECG for possible ischemia or occult myocardial infarction.

8. Carry out serial testing for bleeding diatheses (disseminated intravascular coagulation) and serum enzymes to estimate thermal hypoxic injury to the liver and muscle.

9. Admit the patient to the intensive care unit—permanent liver, cardiac, and central nervous system damage may occur.

10. *Patient Education:*

    a. Advise the patient to avoid immediate re-exposure to high temperatures; he may remain hypersensitive to high temperatures for a considerable length of time.

    b. Emphasize the importance of maintaining an adequate fluid intake, wearing loose clothing, and reducing activity in hot weather.

    c. Athletes should monitor fluid losses, replace fluids, and use a gradual approach to physical conditioning, allowing sufficient time for acclimatization.

▷ Cold Injuries

Frostbite

Frostbite is trauma due to exposure to freezing temperatures that causes actual freezing of the tissue fluids in the cell and intracellular spaces, resulting in vascular damage. The body parts most frequently affected by frostbite are the feet, hands, nose, and ears. A frozen extremity may be hard, cold, and insensitive to touch and appear white or mottled blue–white. The extent of injury from exposure to cold is not always known when the patient is seen initially.

Emergency Management

The goal of management is to restore normal body temperature.

1. Do not allow the patient to walk if the lower extremities are involved.

2. Remove all constricting clothing.

3. Rewarm the extremity by controlled and rapid rewarming, 38° C to 42° C (100° F to 108° F), usually in a whirlpool, until the tips of the injured part flush (about 20 minutes)—flush indicates that maximum circulatory

flow and vasodilation have been accomplished; early thawing appears to decrease the amount of tissue loss.

 a. Administer an analgesic for pain—the thawing process may be very painful.

 b. Handle the part gently to avoid further mechanical injury.

 c. Protect the thawed part; do not rupture blebs, which develop from 1 hour to a few days after rewarming.

 d. Place sterile gauze/cotton between affected fingers/toes to prevent maceration.

 e. Elevate the part to help control swelling.

 f. Use a foot cradle to prevent contact with bed clothes if the feet are involved.

4. Carry out physical assessment to look for concomitant injury (soft tissue injury, dehydration, alcohol coma, fat embolism).

5. Restore electrolyte balance; dehydration and hypovolemia occur frequently in frostbite victims.

6. Use reverse isolation with sterile technique (sterile sheets; sterile gowns, gloves, masks)—frostbite injuries make the patient susceptible to infection.

7. Give tetanus prophylaxis if indicated by associated trauma.

8. The following may be carried out when appropriate:

 a. Whirlpool bath (with disinfectant) for the affected extremity—to aid circulation, debride dead tissue, and help prevent infection.

 b. Escharotomy—to prevent further tissue damage, allow for normal circulation, and permit joint motion

 c. Fasciotomy—to treat compartment syndrome

 d. Sympathectomy—if the cold injury is severe enough to produce necrosis

9. Encourage hourly active motion of the affected digits to promote maximum restoration of function and to prevent contractures.

10. Prohibit the use of tobacco (because of its vasoconstrictive effect).

Accidental Hypothermia

Accidental hypothermia is a condition in which the core (internal) temperature is less than 35° C (95° F) as a result of exposure to cold.

There is progressive deterioration with apathy, poor judgment, ataxia, dysarthria, drowsiness, and eventually coma. Shivering may be suppressed below a temperature of 32.2° C (90° F). Below this temperature, the body's self-warming mechanisms become ineffective. The heartbeat and the blood pressure may be so weak that the peripheral pulsation becomes undetectable. Cardiac irregularities also may occur. Other physiologic abnormalities include hypoxemia and acidosis.

Emergency Management

Management consists of continuing monitoring, rewarming, and supportive care.

1. Monitor the patient—vital signs, CVP, urinary output, arterial blood gases, blood chemistry determinations (BUN, creatinine, glucose, electrolytes), chest x-ray.

 a. Monitor body temperature with an esophageal or rectal thermistor probe.

 b. Employ continuous ECG monitoring—cold-induced myocardial irritability leads to conduction disturbances, especially ventricular fibrillation.

 c. Maintain an arterial line for recording blood pressure and to facilitate blood sampling.

2. Rewarm the patient: rewarming methods include active core (internal) rewarming, active external rewarming, and passive or spontaneous rewarming. The optimal method is controversial.

3. Supportive care during rewarming includes:

 a. External cardiac massage if indicated

 b. Mechanical ventilation with PEEP and heated humidified oxygen, to maintain tissue oxygenation

 c. IV fluids (warmed)—to correct hypotension and maintain urinary output

 d. Sodium bicarbonate—to correct metabolic acidosis.

 e. Electrical cardioversion of ventricular fibrillation

 f. Antiarrhythmic drugs as necessary

 g. Indwelling urethral catheter—to monitor fluid status

▷ Anaphylactic Reaction

An *anaphylactic reaction* is an acute systemic hypersensitivity reaction that occurs within seconds to minutes after exposure to a variety of foreign substances, namely, foreign sera, drugs, or insect venoms. Repeated administration of parenteral or oral therapeutic agents also may precipitate an anaphylactic reaction.

An anaphylactic reaction is the result of an antigen–antibody interaction in a sensitized individual who, as a consequence of previous exposure, has developed a special type of antibody (immunoglobulin) that is specific for this particular allergen. The antibody immunoglobulin IgE is responsible for the great majority of immediate type of human allergic responses—the individual becomes sensitive to a particular antigen after production of IgE to this antigen.

Anaphylactic reaction produces a wide range of clinical manifestations.

- *Respiratory signs* include (1) possible respiratory distress, which progresses rapidly and is caused by bronchospasm or edema of the larynx; (2) sneezing and coughing; (3) tightness of the chest; and (4) other respiratory difficulties, such as wheezing, dyspnea, and cyanosis.

- *Skin manifestations* appear in the form of flushing with a sense of warmth and diffuse erythema. *Generalized itching over the entire body indicates that a general systemic reaction is developing.* Urticaria (hives) may also appear. When massive facial angioedema develops, upper respiratory edema may occur.

- *Cardiovascular manifestations* include tachycardia or bradycardia and peripheral vascular collapse as indicated by pallor, imperceptible pulse, falling blood pressure, and circulatory failure, leading to coma and death.

- *Gastrointestinal discomforts,* such as nausea, vomiting, and colicky abdominal pains or diarrhea, may contribute to the general sense of malaise.

Emergency Management

1. Establish an airway while another person administers epinephrine.
   a. Turn the face to one side; support the angles of the mandible.
   b. Insert an oropharyngeal or endotracheal tube; apply oropharyngeal suction for excessive secretions.
   c. Employ resuscitative measures (especially for patients with stridor and progressive pulmonary edema).
   d. If glottic edema is present, an incision through the cricothyroid ligament will provide an airway.
   e. Use positive pressure oxygen therapy by mask and compression bag.
   f. Use closed chest cardiac massage if necessary.
2. Give aqueous epinephrine as directed to provide rapid relief of hypersensitivity reaction. This should be done while another person is establishing the airway. Use judgment in choosing the route of administration for epinephrine.
   a. Subcutaneous injection for mild, generalized symptoms.
   b. Intramuscular or sublingual injection when the reaction is more severe and progressive and when there is concern that vascular collapse will inhibit absorption.
   c. Intravenous route (aqueous epinephrine diluted in saline and given *slowly*) given in rare instances in which there is complete loss of consciousness and severe cardiovascular collapse; this method may precipitate cardiac arrhythmias.
3. Apply a tourniquet above the injection site, if an anaphylactic reaction followed the injection or insect sting, to retard antigen absorption.
   a. Infiltrate the injection site with epinephrine as directed.
   b. Loosen the tourniquet at regular intervals to allow adequate circulation to the extremity.
4. Start an intravenous infusion of saline for emergency route and for hypotension.

Additional Treatment as Indicated

5. Give antihistamine drugs, for example, diphenhydramine hydrochloride (Benadryl) (IM)—to block further histamine binding at target cells.
6. Give aminophylline IV *slowly* over a period of time for patients with severe bronchospasm and wheezing. Monitor vital signs.
7. Treat prolonged hypotension with crystalloids or colloids and possibly vasopressors; monitor blood pressure. A patient with reduced cardiac output may respond to an infusion of isoproterenol or dopamine.
8. Administer oxygen if significant respiratory or cardiovascular deficits are present.
9. Watch for arrhythmias and cardiorespiratory arrest.
10. If the patient is convulsing, give an IV injection of short-acting barbiturate or diazepam over a period of several minutes.
11. Administer corticosteroids if the patient is having a prolonged reaction and persistent hypotension or bronchospasm.

Preventive Measures

1. Be aware of the danger of anaphylactic reactions and the early signs of anaphylaxis.
2. Ask about the patient's previous allergies to medications; if positive, do not give medication or injection.
3. Question the patient before giving a foreign serum or other types of antigenic agents to determine whether he has had it at some earlier time.
4. Question the patient concerning previous allergic reactions to food or pollen.
5. Avoid giving drugs to patients with hay fever, asthma, and other allergic disorders unless absolutely necessary.
6. Avoid giving parenteral medications unless absolutely necessary. Anaphylactic reactions are more likely to occur when the agent is given parenterally.
7. Do skin testing before administration of certain materials known to produce anaphylactic reactions, such as horse serum. Skin testing can precipitate anaphylaxis in highly sensitive individuals.
   a. A negative skin test does not always indicate safety.
   b. Have epinephrine, IV infusions, intubation and tracheostomy equipment available as precautionary measures.
8. If the patient is being treated as an outpatient, keep him in the office, hospital, or clinic at least 30 minutes after injection of any agent. Caution the patient to return if symptoms develop.
9. Caution patients who are sensitive to insect bites to carry kits equipped to treat insect stings (tourniquet, epinephrine).
10. Encourage allergic individuals to wear identification tags/bracelet.

▷ Poisoning

Poison is any substance that when ingested, inhaled, absorbed, applied to the skin, or produced within the body in relatively small amounts, causes injury to the body by its chemical action. Poisoning from inhalation and ingestion of toxic materials, both accidental and by design, constitutes a major health hazard. The problem is one of real magnitude, as is reflected in the high number of such patients.

Swallowed Poisons

The goals of emergency treatment are (1) to remove or inactivate the poison before it is absorbed, (2) to give supportive care to maintain vital organ systems, (3) to use the specific antidote to neutralize the poison, and (4) to give treatment to hasten the elimination of the absorbed poison.

General Management

1. Try to discover the product taken, amount, time since ingestion, symptoms, age/weight of the patient, and pertinent health history. Call the poison control center in the area if an unknown toxic agent has been taken, or if it is necessary to identify an antidote for a known toxic agent.
2. Maintain the airway and adequacy of respirations; in the absence of cerebral or renal damage, the patient's prognosis largely depends on successful management of respiratory and circulatory systems.
   a. Give artificial respiration if respiration is depressed. Positive expiratory pressure applied to the airway may help keep the alveoli inflated (bag–mask).
   b. Administer oxygen for respiratory depression, unconsciousness, cyanosis, and shock.
   c. Take arterial blood samples to measure pH and blood gas tensions.
   d. Prevent aspiration of gastric contents by positioning, use of oropharyngeal airway, and suctioning.
   e. Stabilize cardiovascular function.
   f. Insert an indwelling urinary catheter to monitor kidney function.
   g. Assess for central nervous system depression.
3. Give supportive care—there is multisystem involvement from many drugs.
   a. Treat shock appropriately.
   b. Monitor ECG—some agents cause cardiovascular toxicity.
4. Consider gastric lavage or induce emesis as the clinical situation dictates to prevent absorption of orally ingested substances; save gastric aspirate for toxicology screens.
5. Support the patient having convulsions; many poisons excite the central nervous system, or else the patient may convulse from oxygen deprivation.
6. Give specific therapy. Administer a special chemical antidote or specific pharmacologic antagonists as early as possible (if indicated).
7. Monitor central venous pressure as indicated.
8. Monitor for fluid and electrolyte imbalance.
9. Reduce elevated temperature.
10. Give analgesics for pain cautiously; severe pain causes vasomotor collapse and reflex inhibition of normal physiologic functions.
11. Provide constant nursing surveillance and attention to the patient in a coma; coma from poisoning results from interference with brain cell function or metabolism.
12. Assist in carrying out procedures to enhance the removal of the ingested substance—forced diuresis, alteration of urine pH, dialysis.
13. Assist in securing specimens of blood, urine, stomach contents, and vomitus.

Corrosive Poisons

Corrosive poisons include *acid and acidlike substances,* such as sodium acid sulfate (toilet bowl cleaners), acetic acid, sulfuric acid, nitric acid, oxalic acid, hydrofluoric acid (rust removers), iodine, or silver nitrate, and *alkali corrosives,* such as sodium hydroxide (lye, drain cleaners), dish-washer detergents, sodium carbonate (washing soda), ammonia water, and sodium hypochlorite (household bleach).

Patients suspected of swallowing corrosive poisons should be assessed for severe pain and burning sensations in the mouth and throat, pain in swallowing or an inability to swallow, destruction of oral mucosa, vomiting, and drooling.

Emergency Management

1. If the patient can swallow after ingestion of a *corrosive poison,* offer milk as an emollient agent.
2. *Do not induce vomiting if the person has consumed a strong acid, alkali, or other corrosive substance.*

Noncorrosive Poisons

Emergency Management

1. Remove the poison from the patient's stomach immediately by inducing vomiting *Do not induce vomiting if the person has consumed a strong acid, alkali, or other corrosive or hydrocarbon solvent. Do not induce vomiting if patient is in a coma, is unconscious, or is having convulsions.*
   a. Give three to four glasses of milk or water to dilute the poison.
   b. Induce vomiting by giving syrup of ipecac or inserting the index finger or blunt end of a spoon at the back of the patient's throat.
2. Carry out gastric lavage to remove any unabsorbed poison (Chart 64-4). This is *not* done if corrosives or hydrocarbon solvents have been ingested (turpentine, kerosene, gasoline, liquid wax, charcoal lighter fluid, etc.). Persons ingesting hydrocarbons should have a chest film to evaluate for chemical pneumonia.
3. Instruct the family to bring the unused poison to the hospital for identification.
4. Know the poison control center in the area; call the center if an unknown toxic agent has been taken or if it is necessary to identify an antidote for a known toxic agent.

Inhaled Poisons

General Management

1. Carry the patient to fresh air immediately; open all doors and windows.
2. Loosen all tight clothing.
3. Apply artificial respiration if required.
4. Prevent chilling; wrap the patient in blankets.
5. Keep the patient as quiet as possible.
6. Do not give alcohol in any form.

Carbon Monoxide Poisoning

Carbon monoxide poisoning may occur as an industrial or household accident or as an attempted suicide. It causes more deaths than any other toxic agent except alcohol. Carbon monoxide exerts its toxic effect by binding to circulating hemoglobin to reduce the oxygen-carrying capacity of the

Chart 64-4
Assisting With Gastric Lavage

Gastric lavage is the aspiration of the stomach contents and washing out of the stomach by means of a gastric tube.

Gastric lavage may be dangerous after acid or alkali ingestion, in the presence of convulsions, or after ingestion of hydrocarbons or petroleum distillates. It is dangerous after ingestion of strong corrosive agents.

Purposes

1. To remove unabsorbed poison after ingestion of poison
2. To diagnose gastric hemorrhage and to arrest hemorrhage
3. To cleanse the stomach before endoscopic procedures
4. To remove liquid or small particles of material from the stomach

Equipment

Large-bore/orogastric tubes or large-bore Ewald tube
Large irrigating syringe with adapter
Large plastic funnel with adapter to fit stomach tube
Water-soluble lubricant
Tap water or appropriate antidote (milk, saline solution, sodium bicarbonate solution, fruit juice, activated charcoal)
Bucket for aspirate
Mouth gag, nasotracheal or endotracheal tubes with inflatable cuffs
Containers for specimens

Procedure

Action	*Rationale/Amplification*
1. Remove dental appliances and inspect the oral cavity for loose teeth.	1. This will prevent accidental aspiration.
2. Measure the distance between the bridge of the nose and the xiphoid process. Mark the tube with indelible pencil or tape.	2. This distance is a rule-of-thumb measurement of the distance the tube is passed to reach the stomach.
3. Lubricate the tube with water-soluble lubricant.	
4. If the patient is comatose, he is intubated with a cuffed nasotracheal or endotracheal tube.	4. A cuffed endotracheal tube prevents aspiration of gastric contents.
5. Place the patient in a left lateral position with the head, neck, and trunk forming a straight line.	5. This position prevents fluid from running into the trachea and keeps reflux vomitus from being aspirated.
6. Pass the tube via the oral (or nasal) route while keeping the head in a neutral position. Pass the tube to the adhesive marking or about 50 cm (20 inches). After the lavage tube is passed, the head of the table is lowered. Have standby suction available.	6. The depth of insertion of the tube will vary with the height of the patient. If the tube enters the larynx instead of the esophagus, the patient will experience coughing and dyspnea.
7. Submerge the free end of the tube below water level at the moment of the patient's exhalation.	7. If the tube is inadvertently in the lungs, the water will bubble with each exhalation.
8. Aspirate the stomach contents with the syringe attached to the tube before instilling water or an antidote. Save the specimen for analysis.	8. Aspiration is carried out to remove the stomach contents.
9. Remove the syringe. Attach the funnel to the stomach tube, or use a 50-ml syringe to put lavage solution in the gastric tube. The volume of fluid placed in the stomach should be small.	9. Overfilling of the stomach may cause regurgitation and aspiration or force the stomach contents through the pylorus.
10. Elevate the funnel above the patient's head and pour approximately 150 ml to 200 ml of solution into the funnel.	
11. Lower the funnel and siphon the gastric contents into the bucket.	

(continued)

Chart 64-4
Assisting With Gastric Lavage (continued)

Procedure *(continued)*

Action *(continued)*	***Rationale/Amplification*** *(continued)*
12. Save samples of the first two washings.	12. Keep the first washings isolated from other washings for possible analysis.
13. Repeat the lavage procedure until the returns are relatively clear and no particulate matter is seen.	
14. At the completion of lavage:	14.
a. The stomach may be left empty.	
b. An adsorbent (powder form of activated charcoal mixed with water to form slurry, the consistency of thick soup) may be instilled in the tube and allowed to remain in the stomach.	b. An adsorbent limits absorption of the substance ingested.
c. A saline cathartic may be instilled in the tube.	c. A cathartic facilitates the transit of the charcoal and the remains of the ingested drug through the intestinal tract.
15. Pinch off the tube during removal, or maintain suction while the tube is being withdrawn.	15. Pinching off the tube prevents aspiration and the initiation of the gag reflex. Keeping the patient's head lower than the body also gives this protection.
16. Give the patient a cathartic if prescribed.	16. A cathartic may be given if the poison has no corrosive action on the bowel. The cathartic will help remove unabsorbed material from the intestine.

---

blood. The affinity between carbon monoxide and hemoglobin is 200 to 300 times that between oxygen and hemoglobin. (Carbon monoxide combines with hemoglobin to form carboxyhemoglobin.) As a result, there is tissue anoxia.

The central nervous system has a critical need of oxygen and will show signs of carbon monoxide toxicity. A person suffering from carbon monoxide poisoning will appear intoxicated (from cerebral hypoxia). Other symptoms and signs include headache, muscular weakness, palpitation, dizziness, and mental confusion, which can progress rapidly to coma. The skin color is not a reliable sign. Skin color may be pink, cherry red, or cyanotic and pale. History of exposure to carbon monoxide should justify immediate treatment.

Emergency Management
The goals of management are to reverse cerebral and myocardial hypoxia and to hasten carbon monoxide elimination.

1. Give 100% oxygen at atmospheric or hyperbaric pressures to reverse hypoxia and accelerate the elimination of carbon monoxide.
2. Draw blood for carboxyhemoglobin levels—oxygen is administered until the carboxyhemoglobin level is less than 5%.
3. Observe the patient constantly. Psychoses, spastic paralysis, ataxia, visual disturbances, and deterioration of personality may persist following resuscitation and may

be symptoms of permanent central nervous system damage.

Skin Contamination Poisons

Emergency Management
1. Drench the skin with water (shower, hose, faucet).
2. Apply a stream of water to the skin while removing clothing.
3. Cleanse the skin thoroughly with water; rapidity in washing is most important in reducing the extent of injury.

Injected Poisons

Stinging Insects (Bees, Hornets, Yellow Jackets, Wasps)
A person may have an extreme sensitivity to the venoms of the *Hymenoptera* (the stings of bees, hornets, yellow jackets, and wasps). It is thought that insect allergy is an IgE-mediated reaction to venom allergies. This constitutes an acute emergency. Stings of the head and neck are especially serious, although stings in any area of the body can result in anaphylaxis.

The clinical response may range from generalized urticaria, itching, malaise, and anxiety to laryngeal edema, severe bronchospasm, shock, and death. In general, the shorter the time between the sting and the onset of severe symptoms, the worse the prognosis.

Emergency Management

1. Give epinephrine (aqueous) as directed. Massage the site to hasten absorption. If the sting is on an extremity, apply a tourniquet with sufficient compression to occlude venous and lymphatic flow.
2. See page 1555 for treatment of anaphylactic shock.
3. Counsel all persons known to be sensitive to *Hymenoptera* venom to carry a commercially available self-treatment kit containing epinephrine, syringe/needle, capsule containing antihistamine, and ephedrine; the kit is available on prescription.
   a. Instruct the patient to inject epinephrine immediately if he is stung.
   b. Flick the stinger off with a fingernail, or scrape it away with a knife.
   c. Do not squeeze the venom sac; this may cause additional venom to be injected.
   d. Report to the nearest health care facility for further examination.
4. Venom immunotherapy may be considered for a person with this allergy.
5. Instruct the patient to limit exposure to stinging insects by:
   a. Avoiding locales with stinging insects (camp and picnic sites)
   b. Staying away from insect feeding areas—flower beds, ripe fruit orchards, garbage, fields of clover
   c. Not going barefoot outdoors (yellow jackets may nest on the ground)
   d. Avoiding perfumes, scented soaps, and bright colors (attract bees)
   e. Keeping car windows closed
   f. Spraying garbage cans with rapid-acting insecticide
   g. Securing a professional exterminator to dispose of wasp/hornet nests or bee hives in the home area
   h. Remaining motionless if an insect buzzes around you (motion [especially running] increases the likelihood of being stung)
   i. Learning self-injection of epinephrine
6. All allergic individuals should wear medical warning bracelets indicating hypersensitivity.

Food Poisoning

Food poisoning is a sudden, explosive illness that may occur after ingestion of contaminated food or drink. Botulism, a serious form of food poisoning, is discussed on page 1518 since the treatment differs and the patient requires continuing surveillance.

Emergency Management

1. Determine the source and type of food poisoning.
   a. Have the family bring the suspected food to the medical facility.
   b. Take the history:
      (1) How soon after eating did the symptoms occur? Immediate onset suggests chemical, plant, or animal poisoning.
      (2) What was eaten in the previous meal? Did the food have any unusual odor or taste? Most foods causing bacterial poisoning do not have unusual odor or taste.
      (3) Did anyone else eating the same food become ill?
      (4) Did vomiting occur? What was the appearance of the vomitus?
      (5) Did diarrhea occur? Diarrhea is usually absent with botulism, shell-fish, or other fish poisoning.
      (6) Are any neurologic symptoms present? These occur in botulism, chemical, plant, and animal poisoning.
      (7) Does the patient have a fever? Fever is seen in salmonella, favism (ingestion of fava beans), and some fish poisoning.
      (8) What is the patient's appearance?
2. Collect food, gastric contents, vomitus, serum, and feces for examination.
3. Monitor vital signs on a continuing basis.
   a. Assess respiration, blood pressure, sensorium, CVP (if indicated), and muscular activity.
   b. Weigh the patient for future comparisons.
4. Support the respiratory system. Death from respiratory paralysis can occur with botulism, fish poisoning, etc.
5. Maintain fluid and electrolyte balance; severe vomiting produces alkalosis, and severe diarrhea produces acidosis; large amounts of electrolytes and water are lost by vomiting and diarrhea.
   a. Watch for oligemic shock from severe fluid and electrolyte losses.
   b. Evaluate for apathy, rapid pulse, fever, oliguria, anuria, hypotension, and delirium.
   c. Carry out blood electrolyte studies.
6. Correct and control hypoglycemia.
7. Control the nausea.
   a. Give an antiemetic drug parenterally if the patient cannot tolerate fluids or medications by mouth.
   b. Give sips of weak tea, carbonated drinks, or tap water for mild nausea.
   c. Give clear liquids 12 to 24 hours after nausea and vomiting subside.
   d. Graduate to a low-residue, bland diet.

▷ Substance Abuse

Substance abuse includes the use of specific substances that are intended to alter mood or behavior.

Drug Abuse

Drug abuse is the use of drugs for other than legitimate medical purposes. The clinical manifestations may vary with the drug used, but the underlying principles of management are essentially the same. Table 64-1 notes the most commonly abused drugs, listing their clinical manifestations and therapeutic management.

There is a growing tendency among drug users to take a variety of drugs simultaneously, including alcohol, barbiturates, tranquilizers, and sedatives that may have additive effects. The immediate management of a patient suffering from drug intoxication is to support the respiratory and cardiovascular functions and then to give definitive treatment for the drug overdose. In addition, if the patient is unconscious and drug abuse is suspected, he should be undressed and examined for needle marks and antecubital scarring.

Acute Drug Reaction

Emergency Management

1. Assess the presence and adequacy of respirations. Attain control of the airway, ventilation, and oxygenation.

   a. Use a cuffed endotracheal tube and provide assisted ventilation in a severely depressed patient with absent gag or cough reflexes.

   b. Measure arterial blood gases for hypoxia due to hypoventilation and acid–base derangements.

   c. Administer oxygen.

2. Stabilize the cardiovascular system. (This is done simultaneously with airway management.)

   a. Begin external cardiac compression and ventilation in the absence of heartbeat.

   b. Start ECG monitoring.

   c. Draw blood samples for testing glucose, electrolytes, BUN, creatinine, and appropriate toxicologic screen.

   d. Start intravenous fluids.

3. Give a specific drug antagonist if the drug is known; naloxone hydrochloride (Narcan) is frequently used; 50% dextrose in water is also used.

(Text continues on page 1564)

Table 64-1
Emergency Management of Drug Abuses

Drug	Clinical Manifestations	Therapeutic Management

Narcotics
 	
Heroin (most frequently involved)
Opium or paregoric
Morphine, codeine, synthetic
  narcotics (methadone)
	Acute intoxication:
	  Pinpoint pupils
	  Marked respiratory depression
	  Stupor → coma
	  Fresh needle marks along course of any
	    superficial vein
		1. Support respiratory and cardiovascular functions.
		2. Give narcotic antagonist (naloxone hydrochloride [Narcan]) to reverse severe respiratory depression and coma.
		3. Continue to monitor level of responsiveness and respirations, pulse, and BP—duration of action of naloxone hydrochloride is shorter than that of heroin; repeated dosages may be necessary.
		4. Establish an IV line; patient may be given a bolus of glucose to eliminate possibility of hypoglycemia.
		5. Send urine for analysis; opiates can be detected in urine.
		6. Secure blood for chemical and toxicologic analysis for baseline studies.
		7. Secure an ECG.
		8. Do not leave patient unattended—may lapse back into coma rapidly; clinical status may change from minute to minute.
		9. Hemodialysis may be indicated for severe drug intoxication.

	Heroin withdrawal syndrome:
	  Lethargy, yawning
	  Perspiration, lacrimation, runny nose
	  Dilated pupils, poorly reactive to light
	  Gooseflesh, muscular aches
	  Twitching, anorexia, nausea, vomiting, abdominal
	    pain
	  Chills and fever
		1. Methadone may be prescribed if patient is receiving treatment at a methadone center, or substitution therapy should be given in hospital setting.
		2. Give intravenous fluids since patient is dehydrated from vomiting; may progress to toxic delirium.
		3. Assess for concomitant medical problems (hepatitis, pneumonia, severe diarrhea).
		4. Place patient in a protected environment under proper medical supervision.
		5. Make every effort to enroll patient in narcotics treatment program.

(continued)

Table 64-1
Emergency Management of Drug Abuses (continued)

Drug	Clinical Manifestations	Therapeutic Management

Barbiturates
 	
Pentobarbital (Nembutal)
Secobarbital (Seconal)
Amobarbital (Amytal)
	Acute intoxication:
	  Flushed face
	  Decreased pulse rate
	  Increasing nystagmus
	  Depressed tendon reflexes
	  Decreasing mental alertness
	  Difficulty in speaking
	  Poor motor coordination
	  Coma, death
		1. Maintain airway and give respiratory support.
		2. Consider endotracheal intubation or tracheostomy if there is any doubt about the adequacy of airway exchange.
		  a. Check airway frequently.
		  b. Perform *regular* suctioning.
		3. Support cardiovascular and respiratory functions—most deaths result from depression of these systems.
		4. Evacuate stomach with emesis or lavage as soon as possible.
		5. Start intravenous infusion through large-gauge needle or intravenous catheter to support blood pressure—coma and dehydration result in hypotension and respond to infusion of intravenous fluids with elevation of blood pressure.
		6. Sodium bicarbonate may be given to alkalinize urine—increases excretion of phenobarbital.
		7. Assist with hemodialysis—for high blood levels.
		8. Maintain neurologic and vital sign flow sheet.
		9. Patient awakening from overdose may demonstrate hostility; this can stimulate automatic angry response by health personnel. Refer for psychiatric consultation to evaluate suicide potential/drug abuse.

	Withdrawal syndrome:
	  Shakiness, anxiety, muscular irritability,
	    orthostatic hypotension
	  Tachycardia
	  Seizures
	  Withdrawal psychosis
	  Hyperpyrexia
	  Death
		Symptoms of barbiturate withdrawal are serious because of life-threatening nature of abrupt abstinence.
		1. Maintain airway; stimulate depressed respiration.
		2. Administer phenobarbital according to patient's tolerance.
		3. Gradually reduce dosage of barbiturates until drug-free state is achieved.
		4. Carry out gastric lavage to evacuate stomach.
		5. Give oxygen, antibiotics, intravenous fluids as required.
		6. Gradually reduce dosage of barbiturates.
		7. Watch for excessive agitation, confusion, and convulsions.
		8. Consider treatment in residential treatment center.

Amphetamine-Type Drugs (Pep Pills, "Uppers," "Speed")
 	
Amphetamine (Benzedrine)
Dextroamphetamine (Dexedrine)
Methamphetamine (Desoxyn)
	Abrupt or insidious development of behavioral disturbances
	Aggressive type of behavior
	Irritability; insomnia
	Visual misperceptions; auditory hallucinations
	Fearful anxiety/depression; cold, distant hostility
	Hyperactivity; rapid speech; euphoria
		1. Try to communicate with patient—amphetamine paranoid psychosis is frequently seen.
		  a. Patient may have delusions of persecution, ideas of reference, visual and auditory hallucinations, changes in body image, hyperactivity, excitation.
		  b. Maintain verbal contact.

(continued)

Table 64-1
Emergency Management of Drug Abuses (continued)

Drug	Clinical Manifestations	Therapeutic Management

Amphetamine-Type Drugs (Pep Pills, "Uppers," "Speed") *(continued)*

2. Use specific drug therapy to alleviate agitative state, if recommended.
   a. Usually, within 24 hours after last dose of amphetamine, patient will begin to spend increasing amounts of time sleeping.
   b. Keep patient relatively quiet and reassured; patient may become aggressive/assaultive and reach a state of panic.
3. Carry out urine checks for amphetamines.
4. Place patient in protective environment—observe for suicidal attempts.
   a. Use techniques of dealing with acutely paranoid individuals; do not move close to patient or behind him.
   b. Avoid physical and pharmacologic restraints.
   c. Avoid confined spaces; refer to psychiatric nursing textbook.

Hallucinogens or Psychedelic-Type Drugs

Lysergic acid diethylamide (LSD)
Phencyclidine HCl (PCP, "angel dust")
Mescaline, Psilocybin
Jimson weed seeds

Marked confusion bordering on panic
Incoherence; hyperactivity
Hazardous behavior—delirium; mania; self-injury
Hallucinations
Flashback—recurrence of LSD-like state without having taken the drug; may occur weeks or months after drug was taken
Convulsions; coma; circulatory collapse; death

Emergency Management
1. Determine whether patient has ingested hallucinogenic drug or has a toxic psychosis.
2. Try to communicate with the patient—use "vocal anesthesia" to reassure him, except for PCP abusers.
   a. "Talking down" involves understanding the process through which the patient is proceeding and helping him overcome his fears while establishing contact with reality.
   b. Remind the patient that fear is common with this problem.
   c. Reassure the patient that he is not losing his mind—that he is experiencing effect of drugs and that this will wear off.
   d. Instruct the patient to keep his eyes open—reduces intensity of reaction.
   e. *Reduce sensory stimuli*—minimize noise, lights, movement, tactile stimulation.
   f. Do not leave the patient alone.
3. Sedate the patient if his hyperactivity cannot be controlled—diazepam (Valium), or a barbiturate may be given.
4. Search for evidences of trauma—hallucinogen users have a tendency to "act out" their hallucinations.
5. Manage convulsions; place patient in Intensive Care Unit.
6. Watch patient closely—his behavior may become hazardous.
7. Monitor for hypertensive crisis if patient has prolonged psychosis due to drug ingestion.
8. Place patient in a protected environment under proper medical supervision to prevent self-inflicted bodily harm.

(continued)

Table 64-1
Emergency Management of Drug Abuses (continued)

Drug	Clinical Manifestations	Therapeutic Management

Hallucinogens or Psychedelic-Type Drugs (continued)		*Management for Phencyclidine Abusers*
		1. Place patient in a calm, supportive environment to minimize stimuli; protect from self-injury.
		2. Avoid "talking down."
		3. Treat symptoms as they occur.
		   a. Drug effects are unpredictable and prolonged.
		   b. Symptoms are likely to exacerbate; patient becomes out of control.
		4. Refer patient to drug treatment center.

Drugs Producing Sedation, Intoxication, Psychologic and Physical Dependence (Nonbarbiturate Sedatives)
 	
Glutethimide (Doriden)
Methyprylon (Noludar)
Ethchlorvynol (Placidyl)
Ethinamate (Valmid)
Meprobamate (Miltown, Equanil)
Chlordiazepoxide (Librium)
Diazepam (Valium)
Bromides
	Acute intoxication:
	  Decreasing mental alertness
	  Confusion
	  Slurred speech
	  Ataxia
	  Pulmonary edema
	  Coma; death
		Management
		1. Insert endotracheal tube as a precaution; utilize assisted ventilation
		   Watch for sudden apnea and laryngeal spasm (especially in patients habituated to Doriden).
		2. Start ECG monitoring.
		   Watch for cardiovascular instability with arrhythmia.
		3. Assess for hypotension.
		   a. Insert indwelling catheter for comatose patient—decreased urinary volume is an index of reduced renal flow associated with reduced intravascular volume or vascular collapse.
		   b. Start volume expansion with saline, plasma, or dextrose as required.
		4. Assist with gastric lavage.
		5. Use hemodialysis therapy if needed.

Salicylate Poisoning
 	
Aspirin (present in all compound analgesic tablets)
	Abdominal pain, hematemesis (early)
	Late signs and symptoms:
	  Hyperpnea
	  Disturbed acid–base balance
	  Tinnitus and vertigo
	  Mental aberrations
	  Hyperventilation
	  Convulsions; coma
		1. Treat respiratory depression.
		2. Carry out gastric lavage; will remove significant amounts of salicylates up to 10 hours, or give Ipecac.
		3. Give water, milk, or activated charcoal to delay absorption of ingested poison.
		4. Support patient with intravenous infusions to correct electrolyte imbalance and maintain hydration.
		5. Correct acid–base disturbances. Give blood transfusion as indicated.
		6. Prepare for peritoneal dialysis (see p. 977) or hemodialysis for patients with severe intoxication.
		7. Give vitamin K for bleeding; salicylates lower the plasma prothrombin by interfering with vitamin K utilization in the liver.
		8. Monitor electrolytes.

4. Remove the drug from the stomach as soon as possible.
   a. Induce vomiting if the patient is seen early after ingestion; save the vomitus for toxicologic study.
   b. Use gastric lavage if the patient is unconscious or if there is no way to determine when the drug was ingested.

   In patients with absent gag or cough reflexes, carry out this procedure only after intubation with a cuffed endotracheal tube to prevent aspiration of the stomach contents.
   c. Activated charcoal may be a useful adjunct to therapy and is used after emesis or lavage.
   d. Save gastric aspirate for toxicologic analysis.
5. Give supportive care.
   a. Take rectal temperature—extremes of thermoregulation (hyperthermia/hypothermia) must be recognized and treated.
   b. Treat convulsions.
   c. Assist with hemodialysis/peritoneal dialysis for potentially lethal poisoning.
   d. Try to maintain a free urine flow since the drug or metabolites are excreted by the urine.
6. Do a thorough physical examination to rule out insulin shock, meningitis, subdural hematoma, stroke, etc.
   a. Look for needle marks and external evidence of trauma.
   b. Carry out a rapid neurologic survey (level of responsiveness, pupil size and reaction, reflexes, focal neurologic findings).
   c. Keep in mind that many drug users take multiple drugs simultaneously.
   d. Be aware that there is a high incidence of infectious hepatitis among drug users, which is thought to be the result of communal use of unsterile needles and syringes.
   e. Examine the patient's breath for the characteristic odor of alcohol, acetone, etc.
7. Try to obtain a history of the drug experience (from the person accompanying the patient or the patient himself).
   a. Adapt a supportive, empathetic, and realistic relationship with the patient.
   b. Do not leave the patient alone; there is a potential for the patient to harm himself or emergency department staff.
8. Admit the patient to ICU if he remains unconscious; if the patient has deliberately overdosed, psychiatric consultation is necessary.
9. Make every effort to enroll the patient in a drug treatment program (detoxication and rehabilitation) to intervene in a life-style that fosters addiction.

Alcohol Abuse

Acute Alcohol Intoxication

Alcohol is a psychotropic drug affecting mood, judgment, behavior, concentration, and consciousness. There is a high prevalence of alcoholism in emergency patients. Because alcoholic patients return frequently to the emergency department, they are infamous and exasperating, taxing the endurance of the health professionals caring for them. Thus, their management requires patience as well as thoughtful and correct treatment.

Ethanol (alcohol) is a direct multisystem toxin and central nervous system depressant that causes drowsiness, incoordination, slurring of speech or belligerency, grandiosity, and uninhibited behavior. It can cause stupor and coma and even death if taken in excessive amounts.

Emergency Management of Acute Alcohol Intoxication

The treatment involves (1) detoxification of the acute poisoning; (2) recovery, or "drying out"; and (3) rehabilitation.

1. Approach the patient in a nonjudgmental manner, without condemnation or reproach.
   a. Expect the patient to use mechanisms of denial and defensiveness.
   b. Adapt a firm, consistent, accepting, and reasonable attitude.
   c. Speak calmly.
   d. If the patient appears drunk, he is probably drunk even though he denies alcohol intake.
2. Take a blood alcohol test as directed.
3. Allow the drowsy patient to "sleep off" the state of alcoholic intoxication. Acute alcoholic intoxication usually resolves spontaneously within several hours.
   a. Observe for symptoms of central nervous system depression; keep the patient under observation.
   b. Protect the airway.
   c. Undress the patient and cover him with a blanket.
4. Sedate the noisy, belligerent patient as directed.
   a. *Monitor the patient carefully.*
   b. Check vital signs and monitor heart rate and blood pressure.
5. Examine the patient for injuries and organic disease, which can easily be masked by alcoholic intoxication. (Alcoholics suffer more injuries than the general population.)
   a. Assess neurologic status; look for symptoms of head injury.
   b. Assess for alcoholic coma—a medical emergency.
   c. Evaluate for pulmonary infection.
      (1) Pulmonary infections are more common in alcoholic individuals due to an impaired defense system and a tendency toward gastric aspiration.
      (2) The patient may show little increase in temperature or white blood cell count.
   d. Watch for hypoglycemia.
6. Hospitalize the patient if necessary or admit him to a detoxification center; an effort should be made to examine the problems underlying the substance abuse.

Delirium Tremens (Alcoholic Hallucinosis)

Delirium tremens is an acute toxic state that follows a prolonged bout of steady drinking or diminution or withdrawal of alcoholic intake. It may be precipitated by acute injury or infection.

Patients suspected of delirium tremens will show signs of anxiety, uncontrollable fear, tremulousness, irritability, agitation, and insomnia. They will be talkative and preoc-cupied, and will experience visual, tactile, olfactory, and auditory hallucinations that are frequently terrifying. Auto-nomic overactivity will occur and is evidenced by tachycardia, dilated pupils, and profuse perspiration. Usually, all vital signs are elevated in the alcoholic toxic state. Delirium tre-mens is a serious complication and is considered a medical emergency.

Emergency Management

The goals of management are to give proper sedation and support to enable the patient to rest and recover without danger of injury or exhaustion.

1. Take the blood pressure, since the patient's subsequent medication may depend on blood pressure readings.
2. Carry out a physical examination to identify preexisting or contributing illnesses or injuries (head injury, pneu-monia, etc.).
3. Sedate the patient with a sufficient dosage of medication to produce adequate sedation to reduce agitation, pre-vent exhaustion, and promote sleep.
   a. A variety of drugs and combinations of drugs are used—chloral hydrate, diazepam (Valium), hydroxyzine (Vistaril), chlordiazepoxide (Lib-rium), etc.
   b. The dosage is adjusted according to the patient's symptoms (agitation, anxiety) and blood pressure response.
4. Place the patient in a private room and observe closely.
   a. Keep the room lighted to reduce the incidence of visual hallucinations.
   b. Close closet and bathroom doors to eliminate shadows.
   c. Keep the environment calm and nonstressful.
   d. Observe the patient closely—homicidal or suicidal responses may result from hallucinations.
   e. Have someone stay with the patient as much as pos-sible—the presence of another person has a reas-suring and quieting effect and helps the patient maintain contact with reality.
   f. Explain visual misrepresentations (illusions) to strengthen the link with reality.
   g. Explain in detail every procedure being done to the patient.
   h. Shut out loud noises; call the patient by name.
   i. Take the patient to the bathroom if permitted.
   j. Use restraints if necessary, if the patient is not under direct and constant observation.
5. Maintain electrolyte balance and hydration via the oral or intravenous route—fluid losses may be extreme be-cause of profuse perspiration and agitation.
6. Record temperature, pulse, respiration, and blood pres-sure frequently (every 30 minutes in severe forms of delirium) in anticipation of peripheral circulatory col-lapse or hyperthermia (the two most lethal complica-tions).
7. Administer phenytoin (Dilantin) or other anticonvulsant drugs as prescribed to prevent or control alcoholic or epileptic convulsions.

8. Assess the respiratory, hepatic, and cardiovascular status of the patient—pneumonia, liver disease, and cardiac failure are complications.
   a. Hypoglycemia may accompany alcoholic withdrawal, because alcohol depletes liver glycogen stores and impairs gluconeogenesis; also, many alcoholic pa-tients suffer from malnutrition.
   b. Administer parenteral dextrose if the liver glycogen is depleted.
      Give orange juice, Gatorade, or other carbo-hydrates to stabilize the blood sugar and to counteract tremulousness.
9. Give supplemental vitamin therapy and a high-protein diet; these patients are usually vitamin deficient.
10. Refer to an alcoholic treatment center for subsequent follow-up and rehabilitation.

▷ Psychiatric Emergency

A *psychiatric emergency* is an urgent, serious disturbance of behavior, affect, or thought that makes the patient unable to cope with life situations and interpersonal relationships. A patient presenting with a psychiatric emergency may be (1) overactive (or violent), (2) underactive or depressed, or (3) suicidal.

The most important concern of the emergency depart-ment personnel is whether the patient is likely to cause personal harm or injury to others. In general, the aim is to try to maintain the patient's self-esteem (and life, if nec-essary) while carrying out assessment and management. The patient is asked if he is under psychiatric treatment at the current time.

Overactive Patients

Patients in the overactive category will display disturbed, uncooperative, and paranoid behavior, as well as anxiety and paniclike feelings. They may be prone to assaultive and destructive impulses and abnormal social behavior. Intense nervousness, depression, and crying are also evident in some patients. Their disturbed and noisy behavior may be com-pounded by alcohol or drug intoxication.

Emergency Management

1. Determine from the family or another reliable source whether the patient has had past mental illness, hos-pitalizations, injuries, or serious illnesses; uses alcohol or drugs; or has experienced crises in interpersonal relationships or intrapsychic conflicts.
2. Be aware that abnormal thought and behavior may be a manifestation of an underlying physical disorder, such as hypoglycemia, cerebrovascular accident, epilepsy, and drug toxicity, including alcohol toxicity.
3. Try to gain control of the situation.
   a. Approach the patient with a calm, confident, and firm manner—this attitude is therapeutic and will have a calming effect.
   b. Introduce yourself by name.
   c. Tell him, "I am here to help you."
   d. Repeat the patient's name from time to time.

e. Speak in one-thought sentences. Be consistent.

f. Give the patient space. Let him slow down by himself and allow him to become compliant.

g. Be interested in and listen to the patient—encourage him to talk of his thoughts and *feelings*.

h. Offer appropriate explanations. Tell the truth.

4. Give a tranquilizer or psychotropic agent for emergency management of functional psychosis. Chlorpromazine (Thorazine) or haloperidol (Haldol) act specifically against psychotic symptoms of thought fragmentation and perceptual and behavioral aberrations.

a. The initial dosage depends on the patient's body weight and the severity of the symptoms.

b. Observe the patient for 1 hour after the initial dose to determine the degree of change in psychotic behavior.

c. Subsequent dosages depend on the patient's reaction.

d. If the behavior is caused by hallucinogens (LSD, etc.), psychotropic drugs (exerting an effect on the mind) are not used.

5. Use restraints only as a last resort.

6. Admit the patient to a psychiatric unit or arrange for psychiatric outpatient treatment.

The Violent Patient

Violent and aggressive behavior is usually episodic and is a means of expressing feelings of anger, fear, or hopelessness about a situation. Usually, the patient has a history of outbursts of rage, temper tantrums, or generally impulsive behavior. Persons with a tendency to violence frequently lose control when intoxicated with alcohol or drugs. Family members are the most frequent victims of their aggression. Patients with a propensity for violence include those intoxicated by drugs or alcohol; those going through drug or alcohol withdrawal; and those with acute organic brain syndrome, acute psychosis, a paranoid character, a borderline personality, or an antisocial personality.

The goal is to protect the patient and staff from harm. If the interviewer feels anxious or uneasy about the patient's response, security or other health care personnel (or a family member) should be asked to remain in the hall nearby in the event that additional help is needed. A quiet area (special room) with minimal environmental stimulation should be used. Objects that could be used as weapons should not be in sight.

Emergency Management

1. Keep the door of the room open and be in clear view of the staff. Do not block the patient's exit to the door; the patient may feel closed in and threatened.

2. Give the patient space. Do not make any sudden movement. If the patient is carrying a weapon, ask him to place it in a neutral area.

3. Do not leave the patient alone; this can be interpreted as rejection, or the patient may try to harm himself.

4. Adapt a calm, noncritical approach and remain in control of the situation. External calm and structure may help the patient to gain control.

5. Talk and listen to the patient.

a. Crisis intervention is best done with an attitude of interest in the patient's well-being and with an attempt to "tune in" to the patient while at the same time remaining firm.

b. Acknowledge the patient's state of agitation. "I want to work with you to relieve your distress, etc."

c. Give the patient the opportunity to ventilate his anger verbally.

d. Try to hear what the patient is saying.

e. Convey an expectation of appropriate behavior and make him aware that help is available for him to gain control.

(1) Let the patient know that his behavior may be frightening to those around him and that violence is not acceptable.

(2) Describe the help available in crisis situations—clinic, emergency department, mental health facility.

(3) Offer the patient something to eat or drink if talking does not defuse the situation.

6. Allow the security personnel/police to intervene if the patient does not become calm.

a. Offer protection of hospitalization—usually welcomed by the patient who fears losing control or harming himself or others.

b. Offer medication (rapid tranquilization [haloperidol, diazepam, chlorpromazine]) if the above fails to attenuate the patient's tension—to reduce tension, anxiety, and hyperactivity.

c. Use restraints when necessary but with a minimum of force.

(1) Use restraints with verbal intervention to calm the patient and make him more compliant.

(2) Have enough personnel available when applying restraints.

d. Refer the patient for further mental health treatment after combativeness, agitation, and fear have cooled.

Underactive or Depressed Patients

During any given year, 125,000 persons are hospitalized in the United States for depressive symptoms. Another 200,000 depressed people are treated as outpatients. Fifteen percent of all American adults between 18 and 74 will experience some type of depressive episode at some time in their lives. Seventy-five percent of those who attempt suicide suffer from a depressive illness.

The underactive or depressed patient will be fearful, depressed; slow to respond; plagued by feelings of worthlessness, guilt, ambivalence, and indecision; and prone to insomnia, a worsening mood in the morning, sad facial expression, and feelings of isolation.

Emergency Management

1. Listen to the patient in a calm, unhurried manner.

a. The patient will benefit from ventilation of feelings.

b. Give the patient an opportunity to talk about his problems.

c. Anticipate that the patient may be suicidal.

d. Attempt to find out if the patient has thought about or attempted suicide.
   (1) "Have you ever thought about taking your own life?"
   (2) The patient is generally relieved because of the opportunity to discuss his feelings.
e. Find out if there is an illness, perceived or real.
f. Assess whether there has been sudden worsening of depression.
g. Notify relatives about a seriously depressed patient. Do not leave the patient alone, since suicide is usually an act committed in solitude.

2. Give antidepressant and antianxiety agents as prescribed.
3. Point out to the patient that depression is treatable.
4. Be aware of crisis and supportive services in the community: telephone counseling and referral, suicide prevention centers, group therapy, marital and family counseling, befriending programs.
5. Refer the patient for psychiatric consultation or to a psychiatric unit.

Suicidal Patients

Suicide is an act that stems from depression (the loss of a loved one, the loss of body integrity or status, poor self-image) and can be viewed as a cry for help and intervention. Persons at risk include the older person; males; those who are enduring unusual loss or stress, unemployed, divorced, living alone, or showing significant depression (weight loss, sleep disturbances, somatic complaints, suicidal preoccupation); and those who have a history of previous suicidal attempt or who have a psychiatric illness.

Emergency Management
1. Treat the consequences of the suicide attempt (gunshot wound, drug overdose, etc.).
2. Prevent further self-injury—a patient who has made a suicidal gesture may do so again.
3. Employ crisis intervention (a form of brief psychotherapy) to determine suicidal potential; discover areas of depression and conflict; find out about the patient's support system; and determine whether hospitalization, psychiatric referral, etc., are warranted.
4. Admit the patient to ICU (if condition warrants), arrange follow-up care, or admit him to the psychiatric unit, depending on the assessment of suicide potential.

Prevention
1. Have an awareness of persons at risk.
2. Determine whether a person has communicated *suicidal intent:*
   "Tired of living"
   "Put my affairs in order"
   "Better off dead"
   Preoccupied with death
   "Burden to my family"
   Talking of someone else's suicide
3. Determine whether he has ever attempted suicide; risk is much greater.
4. Is there a family history of suicide?
5. Was there loss of a parent at an early age?

▷ Sexual Assault

Legally, *rape* is defined as carnal knowledge of a female by force or the threat of force against her will. It is one of the fastest growing crimes of violence. The feminist movement has focused on the rights and care of rape victims, and law enforcement agencies are becoming increasingly sensitive and aggressive in the management of these crimes. Rape crisis centers offer extensive support and education of victims and help them through the subsequent courtroom experience.

The manner in which the patient is received and treated in the emergency department is important to her future psychological well-being. Crisis intervention should begin when the patient enters the health facility. She should be seen immediately upon entrance into the emergency department. Most hospitals have a written protocol that reflects consideration for the victim's physical and emotional needs as well as concern for meeting requirements for subsequent legal proceedings.

Emergency Management
The goals of management are to give sympathetic support, to reduce the emotional trauma of the patient, and to gather available evidence for possible legal proceedings.

1. Respect the privacy and sensitivity of the patient; be kind and supportive.
   a. Emotional trauma may be present for weeks, months, or years. The patient may go through phases of psychologic reactions:
      (1) Phase of disorganization—fear, guilt, humiliation, anger, self-blame
      (2) Phase of resolution (putting incident into perspective); patient may have sleep disturbances, phobias, sexual fears
   b. Reassure the patient that anxiety is natural and that appropriate support is available from professional and community resources.
   c. Accept the emotional reactions of the patient (hysteria, stoicism, overwhelmed feeling, etc.).
   d. Do not leave the patient alone.
2. Assist with the physical assessment.
   a. Secure informed consent from the patient (or parent/guardian if patient is a minor) for conducting the examination and for taking photographs, if necessary, and for the release of findings to police.
   b. Take a history *only* if the patient has not already talked to a police officer, crisis intervention worker, etc. Do not ask the patient to repeat the history.
   c. Ask if the patient has bathed, douched, brushed her teeth, changed her clothes, or defecated since the attack—may alter interpretation of subsequent findings.
   d. Record the time of admission, time of examination, date and time of the alleged rape, and general appearance of the patient.
      (1) Document any evidence of trauma—discoloration, bruises, lacerations, secretions, evidence of bleeding, torn and bloody clothing.
      (2) Record the patient's emotional state.

e. Assist the patient to undress; drape properly.
 (1) Save clothing; label. Note tears/holes in the clothing and indicate on the label.
 (2) Give to appropriate law enforcement authorities.
3. Assist with physical, pelvic, and rectal examination.
 a. Advise the patient of the nature and necessity of each procedure; give the rationale for each question asked.
 (1) Use a water-moistened vaginal speculum for examination; do not use a lubricant.
 (2) Note the color and consistency of any discharge present.
 b. Assist with securing laboratory specimens.
 (1) Collect vaginal aspirate, which is examined immediately for the presence or absence of motile/nonmotile sperm.
 (2) Use a sterile swab to draw from the vaginal pool for acid phosphatase, blood group antigen of semen, and precipitin test against human sperm and blood.
 (3) Obtain separate smears from the vulva.
 (4) Obtain a culture of body orifices for gonorrhea (see p. 1495).
 (5) Conduct a test for pregnancy if there is a question that the patient may be pregnant.
 (6) Collect foreign material (leaves, grass, dirt) and place in a clean envelope.
 (7) Comb the pubic hairs with a prepackaged clean comb; place in a separate container.
 (8) Inspect the fingers for broken nails and tissue and foreign materials under the nails.
 (9) Label all specimens with the name of the patient, date, and initials of personnel handling specimens to preserve the chain of evidence; give to a pathologist or designated person (forensic laboratory, etc.) and obtain an itemized receipt.
 (10) Photographs are taken by a designated person; the film is usually given to the police for development and printing.
4. Treat associated injuries as indicated.
5. Give the patient the option of prophylaxis against sexually transmitted disease.
 a. Probenecid orally, followed in 30 minutes by IM penicillin
 b. A patient with an allergy to penicillin may receive alternate therapy (see p. 1497) that may not be effective in the treatment of incubating syphilis; the patient should have a serology check in 6 weeks.
6. Antipregnancy measures may be considered if the patient is of childbearing age, is using no contraceptives, and is at high risk in her menstrual cycle.
 a. Postcoital contraceptive drugs may be given after a pregnancy test—ethinyl estradiol (Estinyl) or conjugated estrogens (Premarin).
 b. An antiemetic may be given to decrease discomfort from side-effects.
 c. Inform the patient that if she misses a menstrual period that she has the option of having menstrual extraction or abortion.
7. Offer cleansing douche if the patient desires.

8. Provide for follow-up services:
 a. Make an appointment for follow-up surveillance for pregnancy and sexually transmitted disease.
 b. Encourage the patient to return to the previous level of functioning as soon as possible.
 c. Inform the patient of counseling services to prevent long-term psychologic effects; counseling services should be made available to the family.
 d. The patient should be accompanied by a family member/friend when leaving the health facility.

▷ **Bibliography**

Books

Aguilera DC and Messick JM. Crisis Intervention, Theory and Methodology, 4th ed. St Louis, CV Mosby, 1982.

American College of Surgeons. Committee on Trauma. Early Care of the Injured Patient. Philadelphia, WB Saunders, 1982.

Barber JM and Budassi SA. Mosby's Manual of Emergency Care. St Louis, CV Mosby, 1980.

Blaidsdell FW and Trunkey DD. Trauma Management. Vol 1. Abdominal Trauma. New York, Thieme–Stratton, 1982.

Boswick JA Jr. Emergency Care. Philadelphia, WB Saunders, 1981.

Cohen S. The Substance Abuse Problems. New York, Haworth Press, 1981.

Condon RE and Nyhus LM. Manual of Surgical Therapeutics, 5th ed. Boston, Little, Brown, & Co, 1981.

Cowley RA and Dunham CM. Shock Trauma/Critical Care Manual. Baltimore, University Park Press, 1982.

Delany HM and Jason RS. Abdominal Trauma. New York, Springer–Verlag, 1981.

Eisenberg MS and Copass MK (eds). Emergency Medical Therapy, 2nd ed. Philadelphia, WB Saunders, 1982.

Estes NJ and Heinemann ME. Alcoholism, Development, Consequences and Interventions, 2nd ed. St Louis, CV Mosby, 1982.

Evans R. Emergency Medicine. Boston, Butterworths, 1981.

France K. Crisis Intervention. A Handbook of Immediate Person-to-Person Help. Springfield, Charles C Thomas, 1982.

Goldfrank LR. Toxicologic Emergencies, 2nd ed. New York, Appleton–Century–Crofts, 1982.

Greenberg MI and Roberts JR. (eds). Emergency Medicine: A Clinical Approach to Challenging Problems. Philadelphia, FA Davis, 1982.

Hocutt, JE Jr. Emergency Medicine: A Quick Reference for Primary Care. New York, Arco, 1982.

Kimball CP. Biopsychosocial Approach to the Patient. Baltimore, Williams & Wilkins, 1981.

Kline NS, Lindenmayer J–P. Psychotropic Drugs: Manual for Emergency Management of Overdosage, 2nd ed. Oradell, Medical Economics, 1981.

Lieberman PL and Crawford LV. Management of the Allergic Patient. New York, Appleton–Century–Crofts, 1982.

Lipowski ZJ. Delirium. Springfield, Charles C Thomas, 1980.

Mancini MR and Gale AT. Emergency Care and the Law. Rockville, Maryland, Aspen Systems Corp, 1981.

Margolis OS et al. Acute Grief: Counseling the Bereaved. New York, Columbia University Press, 1981.

McCombie S (ed). The Rape Crisis Intervention Handbook. New York, Plenum Press, 1980.

Miller RH. Textbook of Basic Emergency Medicine, 2nd ed. St Louis, CV Mosby, 1980.

Mitchell JT and Resnik HLP. Emergency Response to Crisis. Bowie, Maryland, RJ Brady, 1981.

Najarian JS and Delaney JP. Emergency Surgery: Trauma, Shock, Sepsis, Burns. Chicago, Year Book Medical Publishers, 1982.

Nursing Photobook. Dealing With Emergencies. Horsham, Pennsylvania, Intermed Communications, 1981.

Odling–Smee W and Crockard A. Trauma Care. New York, Grune & Stratton, 1981.

Pattison EM and Kaufman E (eds). Encyclopedic Handbook of Alcoholism. New York, Gardner Press, 1982.

Proudfoot AT. Diagnosis and Management of Acute Poisoning. Boston, Blackwell Scientific, 1982.

Rund DA. Essentials of Emergency Medicine, New York, Appleton–Century–Crofts, 1982.

Sharp EH. Handbook of General Surgical Emergencies, 2nd ed. Garden City, New York, Medical Examination, 1982.

Simon RR and Koenigsknecht SJ. Orthopedics in Emergency Medicine: The Extremities. New York, Appleton–Century–Crofts, 1982.

Slaby AE, Lieb J, and Tancredi LR. Handbook of Psychiatric Emergencies. Garden City, New York, Medical Examination, 1981.

Swan K and Swan RC. Gunshot Wounds. Littleton, PSG, 1980.

Warner CG. Rape and Sexual Assault. Germantown, Aspen Systems, 1980.

Warner CG (ed). Emergency Care; Assessment and Intervention, 3rd ed. St Louis, CV Mosby, 1983.

Articles
Airway Obstruction and Management

Boster SR and Martinez SA. Acute upper airway obstruction. 2. Causative events. Postgrad Med 1982 Dec; 72(6):61–67.

Brantigan CO and Grow JB. Cricothyroidotomy revisited again. Ear Nose Throat J 1980 July; 59(7):26–38.

Breznen WJ. Common respiratory emergencies of obstruction. Dent Clin North Am 1982 Jan; 26(1):197–208.

Dunkin LJ. How to intubate. Br J Hosp Med 1980 Jan; 23(1):77–80.

Hoffman JR. Treatment of foreign body obstruction of the upper airway. West J Med 1982 Jan; 136(1):11–22.

Kress TD. Cricothyroidotomy. Ann Emerg Med 1982 Apr; 11(4):197–201.

McDowell DE. Cricothyroidotomy for airway access. South Med J 1982 Mar; 75(3):282–284.

Michael TAD. The esophageal obturator airway. JAMA 1981 Sept 4; 246(10):1098–1101.

Mittleman RE and Wetli CV. The fatal cafe coronary. JAMA 1982 Mar 5; 247(9):1285–1288.

Orringer MB. Endotracheal intubation and tracheostomy. Surg Clin North Am 1980 Dec; 60(6):1447–1464.

Schecter WP and Wilson RS. Management of upper airway obstruction in the intensive care unit. Crit Care Med 1981 Aug; 9(8):577–579.

Sumner SM and Grau PE. Emergency! First aid for choking. Nursing '82 1982 July; 12(7):40–49.

Anaphylaxis and Stinging Emergencies

Carlson RW et al. Hypovolemia and permeability pulmonary edema associated with anaphylaxis. Crit Care Med 1981 Dec; 9(12):883–885.

Patterson R and Valentine M. Anaphylaxis and related allergic emergencies including reactions to insect stings. JAMA 1982 Nov 26; 248(20):2632–2636.

Ramirez DA, Summers RJ, and Evans R. The diagnosis of *hymenoptera* hypersensitivity. Ann Allergy 1981 Nov; 47(5, Part 1):303–306.

Rubenstein HS. Bee-sting disease: Who is at risk? What is the treatment? Lancet 1982 Feb 27; 1(8270):496–499.

Schuller DE and Sutton PL. Venom skin testing and alteration of RAST levels. Ann Allergy 1981 Aug; 47(2):84–86.

Zweng DA. Trauma notebook: Bites and stings. JEN 1981 July–Aug; 7(4):179–182.

Emergencies Due to Heat/Cold

Alexy BJ. Problems due to cold. JEN 1980 Jan–Feb; 6(1):22–24.

Boyd LT, Shurett PH, and Coburn C. Heat and heat-related illnesses. Am J Nurs 1981 July; 81(7):1298–1302.

Brown F, Klein S, and Berlin D. Local manifestations of cold injury. J Am Podiatry Assoc 1981 Nov; 71(11):595–598.

Dembert ML. Medical problems from cold exposure. Am Fam Physician 1982 Jan; 25(1):99–106.

Gage AM and Gage AA. Frostbite. Compr Ther 1981 Sept; 7(9):25–30.

Ginsberg BW and Kennedy J. Heat stroke and allied disorders. J Kans Med Soc 1981 May; 82(5):236–239.

Gurkoff JF and Jones RO. Frostbite with main reference to the feet. J Am Podiatry Assoc 1981 Apr; 71(4):219–221.

Hart GR et al. Epidemic classical heat stroke: Clinical characteristics and course of 28 patients. Medicine 1982 May; 61(3):189–197.

Johnson LW. Preventing heat stroke. Am Fam Physician 1982 July; 26(1):137–140.

Kilbourne EM et al. Risk factors for heat stroke. JAMA 1982 June 25; 247(24):3332–3336.

Leecost TBM. Frostbite. Diagnosis and treatment. J Am Podiatry Assoc 1981 Nov; 71(11):599–603.

Treatment of heat stroke. Med Lett Drugs Ther 1981 Aug 21; 23(17):76.

Vanore JV, Rosenthal DC, and Mercado ON. Frostbite. J Am Podiatry Assoc 1980 Dec; 70(12):619–627.

Vaughn PB. Local cold injury—menace to military operations. Milit Med 1980 May; 145(5):305–311.

Yokum RF and Bohler S. Heat stroke. JEN 1981 July–Aug; 7(4):144–147.

Near-drowning

Donahue A. Near-drowning victims. RN 1982 June; 45(6):40–44.

Harries MG. Drowning in man. Crit Care Med 1981 May; 9(5):407–408.

Oakes DD et al. Prognosis and management of victims of near-drowning. J Trauma 1982 July; 22(7):544–549.

Smothers PK. Drowning and near-drowning: An update. JEN 1982 July–Aug; 8(4):176–180.

Stanley RJ and Siegal GP. Death by drowning. An overview. Minn Med 1981 May; 64(5):295–297.

Poisoning/Substance Abuse

Bolton ME. Hyperbaric oxygen therapy. Am J Nurs 1981 June; 81(6):1199–1201.

Elenbaas RM (ed). Poisoning and overdose. Crit Care Quart 1982 Mar; 4(4):1–104 (entire volume).

Holland DJ. Cocaine use and toxicity. JEN 1982 July–Aug; 8(4):166–169.

Leporati NC and Chychula LH. How you can *really* help the drug-abusing patient. Nursing '82 1982 June; 12(6):46–49.

Maull KI. Alcohol abuse: Its implications in trauma care. South Med J 1982 July; 75(7):794–798.

Purdie FRJ et al. The chronic emergency department patient. Ann Emerg Med 1981 July; 10(6):298–301.

Rund DA, Summers WK, and Levin M. Alcohol use and psychiatric illness in emergency patients. JAMA 1981 Mar 27; 245(12):1240–1241.

Wruk KM. Administering emergency antidotes to the acutely poisoned patient. Dimens Crit Care Nurs 1982 July–Aug; 1(4):206–211.

Psychiatric Emergencies

Atkinson JH Jr. Managing the violent patient in the general hospital. Postgrad Med 1982 Jan; 71(1):193–201.

Billings CV. Providing better emergency care when behaviors bar the way. Nursing '82 1982 May; 12(5):57.

Dubin WR. Evaluating and managing the violent patient. Ann Emerg Med 1981 Sept; 10(9):481–484.

Gittleson NL. Psychiatric emergencies. Practitioner 1981 Aug; 225(1358):1144–1149.

Linn L. The treatment of psychiatric emergencies. Curr Psychiatr Ther 1981; 20:177–181.

Perry SW III and Gilmore MM. The disruptive patient or visitor. JAMA 1981 Feb 20; 245(7):755–757.

Pisarcik G. Facing the violent patient. Nursing '81 1981 Sept; 11(9):61–65.

Pisarcik GK. Psychiatric emergencies and crisis intervention. Nurs Clin North Am 1981 Mar; 16(1):85–94.

Slaby AE. Emergency psychiatry: An update. Hosp Community Psychiatry 1981 Oct; 32(10):687–698.

Warner CG and Braen GR. Human violence. Topics in Emergency Room Medicine 1982; 3(4):1–93 (entire volume).

Waxman HM. Geriatric psychiatry in the emergency department: Characteristics of geriatric and non-geriatric admissions. J Am Geriatr Soc 1982 July; 30(7):427–432.

Yoder L and Jones SL. The emergency room nurse and the psychiatric patient. J Psychosoc Nurs Ment Health Serv 1982 June; 20(6):22–28.

Sexual Assault

Binder R. Setting up a rape treatment center. J Am Med Wom Assoc 1980 June; 35(6):145–148.

Danis DM. Aftercare concerns of rape victims. JEN 1982 Jan–Feb; 8(1):42–43.

Gallese LE and Treuting EG. Help for rape victims through group therapy. J Psychosoc Nurs Ment Health Serv 1981 Aug; 19(8):20–21.

Hicks DJ. Rape: Sexual assault. Am J Obstet Gynecol 1980 Aug 15; 137(8):931–935.

Lamphier TA. Rape. Md State Med J 1982 Apr; 31(4):37–43.

Moynihan BA and Duncan JW. The role of the nurse in the care of sexual assault victims. Nurs Clin North Am 1981 Mar; 16(1):95–100.

Shen JTY. Sexual abuse of adolescents. Postgrad Med 1982 June; 71(6):213–219.

Shrier DK. Rape—myths, misconceptions, facts and interventions. J Med Soc NJ 1981 Sept; 78(10):668–672.

Smally AJ. Sperm and acid phosphatase examination of the rape patient: Medicolegal aspects. J Fam Pract 1982 July; 15(1):170–171.

Wertheimer AJ. Examination of the rape victim. Postgrad Med 1982 Mar; 71(3):173–176, 177–180.

Trauma

Cardona VD. Trauma post-op. RN 1982 Mar; 45(3):22–29.

Cayten CG et al. Abdominal stab wounds: A ten-year review of 204 patients. Am Surg 1982 June; 48(6):250–254.

Clutter P. Abdominal trauma and hypovolemic shock. Crit Care Update 1982 Feb; 9(2):5–9.

Ekbom GA et al. Intra-abdominal vascular trauma—a need for prompt operation. J Trauma 1981 Dec; 21(12):1040–1044.

Ensinger C. Multiple emergencies? Don't panic. RN 1981 Aug; 44(8):32–35.

Goldenberger JH et al. Selection of patients with abdominal stab wounds for laparotomy. J Trauma 1982 June; 22(6):476–480.

Gruenberg JC et al. The diagnostic usefulness of peritoneal lavage in penetrating trauma: A prospective evaluation and comparison with blunt trauma. Am Surg 1982 Aug; 48(8):402–407.

Hoffman JR. External counterpressure and the MAST suit: Current and future roles. Ann Emerg Med 1980 Aug; 9(8):419–421.

Kashuk JL et al. Major abdominal vascular trauma—a unified approach. J Trauma 1982 Aug; 22(8):672–679.

Maxwell TM. Resuscitation priorities and assessment of the patient with multiple injuries. Can J Surg 1980 July; 23(4):338–339.

Perdue P. Abdominal injuries and dangerous fractures. RN 1981 July; 44(7):34–37.

Podgorny G and Stanley L. Gunshot victims. RN 1982 Apr; 45(4):46–51, 110–112.

Powell DC, Bivins BA, and Bell RM. Diagnostic peritoneal lavage. Surg Gynecol Obstet 1982 Aug; 155(2):257–264.

Thompson JS and Moore EE. Peritoneal lavage in the evaluation of penetrating abdominal trauma. Surg Gynecol Obstet 1981 Dec; 153(6):861–863.

Trunkey DD (ed). Symposium on trauma. Surg Clin North Am 1982 Feb; 62(1):1–192 (entire volume).

General Articles

Hargreaves AG. Coping with disaster. Am J Nurs 1980 Apr; 80(4):683.

Kucler MA. Discharge dilemma for an ED nurse. Am J Nurs 1981 Nov; 81(11):2010–2012.

Leitzell JD. Emergency medicine: Two points of view. An uncertain future. N Engl J Med 1981 Feb 19; 304(8):477–480.

Riggs LM Jr. Emergency medicine: Two points of view. A vigorous new specialty. N Engl J Med 1981 Feb 19; 304(8):480–483.

Ufema J. Grieving families: Let your heart do the talking. Nursing '81 1981 Nov; 11(11):80–83.

Wells-Mackie JJ. Clinical assessment and priority setting. Nurs Clin North Am 1981 Mar; 16(1):3–12.

Agencies

Governmental

Food and Drug Administration, Poison Surveillance and Epidemiology Branch of the Division of Drug Experience, National Centers for Drugs and Biologics, 5600 Fishers Lane, Room 18B31, Rockville, Maryland 20857

National Institute of Mental Health, National Center for the Prevention and Control of Rape, Parklawn Building, 5600 Fishers Lane, Rockville, Maryland 20857

National Clearinghouse for Mental Health Information, National Rape Information Clearinghouse (above address)

National Institute on Alcohol Abuse and Alcoholism, National Clearinghouse for Alcohol Information (above address)

National Institute on Drug Abuse, National Clearinghouse for Drug Abuse Information (above address)

Voluntary

Alcoholics Anonymous, General Service Board of Alcoholics Anonymous, 468 Park Ave. S, New York, New York 10016

American National Red Cross, 17th and D Sts., NW, Washington, DC 20006

National Council on Alcoholism, Inc., 733 Third Ave., Suite 1405, New York, New York 10017

National Safety Council, 444 North Michigan Ave., Chicago, Illinois 60611

Appendix

Diagnostic Studies and Their Meaning

Table of Abbreviations

kg	= kilogram
g	= gram
mg	= milligram
μg	= microgram
μμg	= micromicrogram
ng	= nanogram
pg	= picogram
L	= liter
dl	= 100 milliliters
ml	= milliliter
cu mm	= cubic millimeter
nM	= nanomolar
mm	= millimeter
μ	= micron or micrometer
mm Hg	= millimeters of mercury
mU	= milliunit
μU	= microunit
mEq	= milliequivalent
IU	= International Unit
mIU	= milliInternational Unit

Normal Values—Hematology*

Determination	Normal Value	Clinical Significance
A_2 hemoglobin	1.90%–3.86%	Increased in certain types of thalassemia
Bleeding time	30 sec–6 min	Prolonged in purpura hemorrhagica, in which platelets are reduced, and in chloroform and phosphorus poisoning
Clotting time	5–10 min	Prolonged in hemorrhagic disease and in various coagulation factor deficiencies
Factor V assay	75%–125%	Pro-accelerin factor
Factor VIII assay (antihemophiliac factor)	50%–150%	Deficient in classical hemophilia
Factor IX assay (plasma thromboplastin component)	75%–125%	Deficient in Christmas disease (pseudohemophilia)
Factor X (Stuart factor)	75%–125%	Stuart clotting defect
Fibrinogen	200–400 mg/dl	Increased in pregnancy, pneumonia, infections accompanied by leukocytosis, and nephrosis. Decreased in acute yellow atrophy of liver, cirrhosis, typhoid fever, chloroform poisoning, abruptio placentae
Fibrinolysins (whole blood clot lysis time)	No lysis in 24 h	Increased activity associated with massive hemorrhage, extensive surgery, and transfusion reactions
Partial thromboplastin time (activated)	20–45 sec	Prolonged in factor VIII, IX, and X deficiency
Prothrombin consumption	Over 20 sec	Impaired in factor VIII, IX, and X deficiency
Prothrombin time	60%–100% of control	Prolonged in factor X deficiency and other hemorrhagic diseases, and in cirrhosis, hepatitis, and acute toxic necrosis of the liver
Erythrocyte count	Males: 4,600,000–6,200,000 per cu mm Females: 4,200,000–5,400,000 per cu mm	Increased in severe diarrhea and dehydration, polycythemia, secondary polycythemia, acute poisoning, pulmonary fibrosis, and Ayerza disease. Decreased in all anemias, in leukemia, and after hemorrhage, when blood volume has been restored.
Erythrocyte indices		
Mean corpuscular volume (MCV)	80–94 (cu microns)	Increased in macrocytic anemias, decreased in microcytic anemia
Mean corpuscular hemoglobin (MCH)	27–32 $\mu\mu$g per cell	Increased in macrocytic anemias, decreased in microcytic anemia
Mean corpuscular hemoglobin concentration (MCHC)	33%–38%	Decreased in severe hypochromic anemia
Reticulocytes	0.5%–1.5% of red cells	Increased with any condition stimulating increase in bone marrow activity, that is, infection, blood loss (acute and chronic); following iron therapy in iron deficiency anemia, polycythemia rubra vera. Decreased with any condition depressing bone marrow activity, acute leukemia, late stage of severe anemias
Erythrocyte sedimentation rate	Males: 0–9 mm/hr Females: 0–20 mm/hr	Increased in tissue destruction, whether inflammatory or degenerative, and during menstruation, pregnancy, and in acute febrile diseases
Hematocrit	Males: 42%–50% Females: 40%–48%	Decreased in severe anemias, anemia of pregnancy, acute massive blood loss. Increased in erythrocytosis of any cause, and in dehydration or hemoconcentration associated with shock
Hemoglobin	Males: 13–16 g/dl Females: 12–14 g/dl	Decreased in various anemias, pregnancy, severe or prolonged hemorrhage, and with excessive fluid intake. Increased in polycythemia, chronic obstructive pulmonary diseases, failure of oxygenation because of congestive heart failure, and normally, in people living at high altitudes

(continued)

Normal Values—Hematology (continued)

Determination	Normal Value	Clinical Significance
Hemoglobin F	Less than 2%	Increased in infants and children, in thalassemia and many anemias
Leukocyte alkaline phosphatase	Score of 40–100	Decreased in chronic myelocytic leukemia and chronic lymphocytic leukemia. Increased in nonleukemic leukocytosis and myeloproliferative diseases
Leukocyte count Neutrophils Eosinophils Basophils Lymphocytes Monocytes	Total: 5,000–10,000 cu mm 60%–70% 1%–4% 0%–0.5% 20%–30% 2%–6%	Elevated in acute infectious diseases—predominantly in the neutrophilic fraction with bacterial diseases, and in the lymphocytic and monocytic fractions in viral diseases. Eosinophils elevated in collagen diseases, allergy, intestinal parasitosis. Elevated in acute leukemia, following menstruation, and following surgery or trauma. Depressed in aplastic anemia, agranulocytosis, and by toxic agents, such as chemotherapeutic agents used in treating malignancy
Osmotic fragility of red cells	Increase if hemolysis occurs in over 0.5% NaCl Decrease if hemolysis is incomplete in 0.3% NaCl	Increased in congenital spherocytosis, idiopathic acquired hemolytic anemia, isoimmune hemolytic disease, ABO hemolytic disease of newborn. Decreased in sickle-cell anemia, thalassemia
Platelet count	200,000–350,000 per cu mm	Increased with chronic granulocytic leukemia, hemoconcentration. Decreased in thrombocytopenic purpura, acute leukemia, aplastic anemia, and during cancer chemotherapy

* Laboratory values vary according to the techniques used in different laboratories.

Normal Chemistries—Serum, Plasma, Whole Blood

Determination	Normal Adult Values	Clinical Significance (Increased)	(Decreased)
Acetoacetate and acetone	0.3–2.0 mg/dl	Diabetic acidosis Fasting Toxemia of pregnancy Carbohydrate-free diet High-fat diet	
Adrenocorticotropic hormone (ACTH) (plasma), RIA*	Less than 100 pg/ml	Pituitary-dependent Cushing's syndrome Ectopic ACTH syndrome Primary adrenal atrophy	Adrenocortical tumor Adrenal insufficiency secondary to hypopituitarism
Aldolase	0.5–3.1 mU/ml	Hepatic necrosis Granulocytic leukemia Myocardial infarction Skeletal muscle disease	
Aldosterone (plasma), RIA	Supine: 3–10 ng/dl Upright: 5–30 ng/dl Adrenal vein: 200–800 ng/dl	Primary (Conn's syndrome) Secondary aldosteronism	Addison's disease
Alpha amino nitrogen	3.0–5.5 mg/dl	Phosphorus, arsenic, chloroform, carbon tetrachloride poisoning Infectious hepatitis Eclampsia	Bacterial pneumonia Administration of anterior pituitary extracts Administration of insulin

* By radioimmunoassay

(continued)

Normal Chemistries—Serum, Plasma, Whole Blood (continued)

Determination	Normal Adult Values	Clinical Significance	
		(Increased)	(Decreased)
Alpha-1-antitrypsin	200–400 mg/dl	Early inflammatory processes Pneumonia Abscess formations Arthritis	Chronic lung disease
Alpha-1-fetoprotein	None detected	Hepatocarcinoma Metastatic carcinoma of liver Germinal cell carcinoma of the testis or ovary	
Alpha-hydroxybutyric dehydrogenase	up to 140 mU/ml	Myocardial infarction Granulocytic leukemia Hemolytic anemias Muscular dystrophy	
Ammonia (plasma)	5–70 μg/dl	Severe liver disease Hepatic decompensation	
Amylase	15–200 units/dl	Acute pancreatitis Mumps Duodenal ulcer Carcinoma of head of pancreas Prolonged elevation with pseudocyst of pancreas	Chronic pancreatitis Pancreatic fibrosis and atrophy Cirrhosis of liver Acute alcoholism Toxemias of pregnancy
Androstenedione, RIA	Females: 0.6–3.0 ng/ml	Increases in many patients with hirsutism and virilization	
Arsenic	6–20 μg/dl	Accidental or intentional poisoning Excessive occupational exposure	
Ascorbic acid (vitamin C)	0.4–1.5 mg/dl	Large doses of ascorbic acid as a prophylactic against the common cold	Rheumatic fever Collagen diseases Deficient vitamin C intake Renal and hepatic disease Congestive heart failure
Bilirubin	Total: 0.1–1.0 mg/dl Direct: 0.1–0.2 mg/dl Indirect: 0.1–0.8 mg/dl	Hemolytic anemia (indirect) Biliary obstruction Hepatocellular damage Pernicious anemia Hemolytic disease of newborn Eclampsia	
Bromsulphalein (BSP)	Less than 5% retention in 45 minutes	Acute hepatic diseases	
Calcitonin	Basal: Nondetectable (below 400 pg/ml)	Medullary carcinoma of the thyroid Some nonthyroid tumors Zollinger–Ellison syndrome Pernicious anemia Chronic renal failure	

(continued)

Normal Chemistries—Serum, Plasma, Whole Blood (continued)

Determination	Normal Adult Values	Clinical Significance (Increased)	(Decreased)
Calcium	8.5–10.5 mg/dl	Tumor or hyperplasia of parathyroid Hyperparathyroidism Hypervitaminosis D Multiple myeloma Nephritis with uremia	Hypoparathyroidism Diarrhea Celiac disease Rickets Osteomalacia Malnutrition Nephrosis After parathyroidectomy
CO_2 content	Adults: 24–32 mEq/liter Infants: 18–24 mEq/liter	Tetany Respiratory disease Intestinal obstruction Vomiting	Acidosis Nephritis Eclampsia Diarrhea Anesthesia
Carcinoembryonic antigen (CEA), RIA	0–2.5 ng/ml	The repeatedly high incidence of this antigen in cancers of the colon, rectum, pancreas, and stomach suggest that CEA levels may be a useful adjunct in the diagnosis of these conditions	
Carotene, beta	70–250 μg/dl	Carotenemia Hypothyroidism Diabetes Hyperlipemia	Malabsorption syndromes Hepatic disease Dietary deficiencies
Catecholamines, plasma, RIA	Recumbent: 200–600 ng/liter Upright: 300–1000 ng/liter	Pheochromocytoma	
Cephalin flocculation	Negative to 1+	Severe liver disease Atypical viral pneumonia Malaria Syphilis Infectious mononucleosis Congestive heart failure	
Ceruloplasmin	Males: 29–80 mg/dl Females: 32–156 mg/dl	Pregnancy Myocardial infarction Hepatic cirrhosis	Wilson's disease (hepatolenticular degeneration)
C_1 Esterase inhibitor	50%–100% of normal control		Hereditary angioneurotic edema Lymphoproliferative disorders
Chloride	95–105 mEq/liter	Nephritis Urinary obstruction Cardiac decompensation Anemia Ether anesthesia	Diabetes Diarrhea Vomiting Pneumonia Heavy metal poisoning Cushing's syndrome Burns Intestinal obstruction Febrile conditions

(continued)

Normal Chemistries—Serum, Plasma, Whole Blood (continued)

Determination	Normal Adult Values	Clinical Significance	
		(Increased)	*(Decreased)*
Cholesterol	150–300 mg/dl	Lipemia Obstructive jaundice Diabetes Hypothyroidism	Pernicious anemia Hemolytic anemia Hyperthyroidism Severe infection Terminal states of debilitating disease
Cholesterol esters	60%–70% of total		The esterified fraction decreases in liver disease
Cholinesterase	Serum: 0.61–1.50 delta pH Red cells: 0.60–1.00 delta pH	Nephrosis Exercise	Nerve gas intoxication (greater effect on red cell activity) Insecticides, organic phosphates (greater effect on plasma activity)
Chorionic gonadotrophin, beta subunit, RIA	0–5 IU/liter	Pregnancy Hydatidiform mole Choriocarcinoma	
Chorionic somatomammotrophin	None detectable	Pregnancy	
Complement, Human C$_3$	Males: 88–252 mg/dl Females: 88–206 mg/dl	Some inflammatory diseases	Acute glomerulonephritis Disseminated lupus erythematosus with renal involvement
Complement, C$_4$	14–51 mg/dl	Some inflammatory diseases	Often decreased in immunological diseases, especially with active SLE Hereditary angioneurotic edema
Complement, total (hemolytic)	90%–94% complement	Some inflammatory diseases	Acute glomerulonephritis Epidemic meningitis Subacute bacterial endocarditis
Congo red	60%–100% retained in bloodstream		Deposits of amyloid in tissue absorb congo red. In amyloid disease, less than 40% of the dye will remain in the plasma. In severe cases, less than 10% is retained.
Copper	70–165 μg/dl	Cirrhosis of liver Pregnancy	Wilson's disease
Cortisol, RIA	8 AM: 7–25 μg/dl 4 PM: 2–9 μg/dl	Stress: infectious disease, surgery, burns, etc. Pregnancy Cushing's syndrome Pancreatitis Eclampsia	Addison's disease Anterior pituitary hypofunction
C-peptide reactivity	1.5–10 ng/ml	Insulinoma	Diabetes
Creatine	0.2–0.8 mg/dl	Biliary obstruction Pregnancy Nephritis Renal destruction Trauma to muscle Pseudohypertrophic muscular dystrophy	

(continued)

Normal Chemistries—Serum, Plasma, Whole Blood (continued)

Determination	Normal Adult Values	Clinical Significance (Increased)	(Decreased)
Creatine phosphokinase (CPK)	Males: 50–325 mU/ml Females: 50–250 mU/ml	Myocardial infarction Skeletal muscle diseases Intramuscular injections Crush syndrome Hypothyroidism Delirium tremens Cerebrovascular disease	
Creatine phosphokinase isoenzymes	MM band present (skeletal muscle): MB band absent (heart muscle)	MB band increased in myocardial infarction	
Creatinine	0.7–1.4 mg/dl	Nephritis Chronic renal disease	
Creatinine clearance	100–150 ml of blood cleared of creatinine/min		Kidney diseases
Cryofibrinogen, qualitative (plasma)	Negative	Neoplasms Acute rheumatic fever Acute glomerulonephritis Ulcerative colitis Thromboembolic states	
Cryoglobulins, qualitative	Negative	Multiple myeloma Chronic lymphocytic leukemia Lymphosarcoma Systemic lupus erythematosus Rheumatoid arthritis Subacute bacterial endocarditis Some malignancies	
Cyclic AMP (plasma), RIA	Males: 17–33 nM/liter Females: 11–27 nM/liter	Has proved valuable in differentiating nephrogenic diabetes insipidus from that of primary hypothalamic diabetes insipidus. Administration of ADH appears to be incapable of eliciting an increase of cyclic AMP in nephrogenic diabetes insipidus.	
11-Desoxycortisol	0–2 μg/dl	Hypertensive form of virilizing adrenal hyperplasia due to an 11-beta hydroxylase defect.	
Dibucaine number	Normal: 70%–85% inhibition Heterozygote: 50%–65% inhibition Homozygote: 16%–25% inhibition		Important in detecting carriers of abnormal cholinesterase activity who are susceptible to succinyldicholine anesthetic shock
Dihydrotestosterone	Males: 50–210 ng/dl Females: None detectable		Testicular feminization syndrome

(continued)

Normal Chemistries—Serum, Plasma, Whole Blood (continued)

Determination	Normal Adult Values	Clinical Significance (Increased)	(Decreased)
Erythropoietin	7–36 milli-immuno-chemical units/ml	Many red blood cell anemias Some cases of "secondary" polycythemia Possible as an early manifestation of kidney transplant rejection	Polycythemia vera Some types of renal disease

Estradiol, RIA	Males: 0.5–5.0 ng/dl
	Females:
	  Menstruation: 1.5–7.5 ng/dl
	  Follicular phase: 2.0–20 ng/dl
	  Midcycle: 12–40 ng/dl
	  Luteal phase: 10–30 ng/dl
	  Postmenopausal: 1.0–5.0 ng/dl
		Pregnancy	Depressed or failure to peak—ovarian failure

Estriol, RIA	Males: less than 0.5 ng/ml
	Nonpregnant females: less than 0.5 ng/ml
	Pregnant females:
	  1st trimester—up to 1.0 ng/ml
	  2nd trimester—0.8–7.0 ng/ml
	  3rd trimester—5.0–25.0 ng/ml
		Pregnancy	Depressed or failure to peak—ovarian failure

Estrogens, total, RIA	Males: 47–74 ng/dl
	Females:
	  Menstrual flow: 43–67 ng/dl
	  Follicular phase: 40–103 ng/dl
	  Ovulation peak: 75–139 ng/dl
	  Luteal phase 47–113 ng/dl
		Pregnancy
		Measured on a daily basis can be used to evaluate response of hypogonadotrophic, hypoestrogenic women to human menopausal or pituitary gonadotropin
			Fetal distress
			Ovarian failure

Estrone, RIA	Females:
	  Day 1–10: 4.3–18.0 ng/dl
	  Day 11–20: 7.5–19.6 ng/dl
	  Day 21–30: 13.0–20.0 ng/dl
	Males: 2.5–7.5 ng/dl
		Pregnancy	Depressed or failure to peak—ovarian failure

Fatty acids	Total: 250–300 mg/dl	Diabetes Anemia Nephrosis Hypothyroidism Nephritis	Hyperthyroidism

(continued)

Normal Chemistries—Serum, Plasma, Whole Blood (continued)

Determination	Normal Adult Values	Clinical Significance	
		(Increased)	*(Decreased)*
Ferritin, RIA	Males: 10–270 ng/ml Females: 5–100 ng/ml	Hemochromatosis Certain neoplastic diseases Acute myelogenous leukemia Multiple myeloma	Iron deficiency
Fibrinogen degradation products (FDP)	Less than 10 μg/ml (negative in the 1:5 dilution)	Thrombotic episodes of any kind, including myocardial infarction, postoperative deep vein thrombosis, and certain pregnancy disorders	
Folic acid, RIA	4–16 ng/ml		Megaloblastic anemias of infancy and pregnancy Inadequate diets Liver disease Malabsorption syndrome Severe hemolytic anemia

Follicle-stimulating hormone (FSH), RIA	Normal Males: 5–25 mIU/ml
	Normal Females:
	  Follicular phase: 5–20 mIU/ml
	  Peak of middle cycle: 12–30 mIU/ml
	  Luteinic phase: 5–15 mIU/ml
	Menopausal Females:
	  40–200 mIU/ml
		Menopause and primary ovarian failure	Pituitary failure

Galactose-1-phosphate uridyl transferase	Above 18 units of activity per gram of hemoglobin 0.05–1.5: Possibly galactosemic 0–0.05: Galactosemic		Galactosemia
Gamma glutamyl transpeptidase	Males: less than 45 IU/liter Females: less than 30 IU/ liter	Hepatobiliary disease Anicteric alcoholics Drug therapy damage	
Gastrin, RIA	Fasting: 50–155 pg/ml liter Postprandial: 80–170 pg/ml Zollinger–Ellison syndrome: 200 to over 2000 pg/ml Pernicious anemia: 130–2260 (mean 912) pg/ml	Zollinger–Ellison syndrome Peptic ulceration of the duodenum Pernicious anemia	
Glucose	Fasting: 60–110 mg/dl Postprandial (2 hr): 65–140 mg/dl	Diabetes Nephritis Hyperthyroidism Early hyperpituitarism Cerebral lesions Infections Pregnancy Uremia	Hyperinsulinism Hypothyroidism Late hyperpituitarism Pernicious vomiting Addison's disease Extensive hepatic damage

(continued)

Normal Chemistries—Serum, Plasma, Whole Blood (continued)

Determination	Normal Adult Values	Clinical Significance	
		(Increased)	*(Decreased)*
Glucose tolerance (oral)	Features of a normal response: 1. Normal fasting between 60–125 mg/dl 2. No sugar in urine 3. The upper limits of normal are: fasting—125 1 hour—190 2 hours—140 3 hours—125	(Flat or inverted curve) Hyperinsulinism Adrenal cortical insufficiency (Addison's disease) Anterior pituitary hypofunction Hypothyroidism Sprue and celiac disease	(High or prolonged curve) Diabetes Hyperthyroidism Primary adrenal cortical tumor or hyperplasia Severe anemia Certain central nervous system disorders
Glucose-6-phosphate dehydrogenase (red cells)	Screening: Decolorization in 20–100 minutes Quantitative: 1.86–2.50 IU/ml RBC		Drug induced hemolytic anemia Hemolytic disease of newborn
Glycoprotein	110–140 mg/dl	Neoplasm Tuberculosis Diabetes complicated by degenerative vascular disease Pregnancy Rheumatoid arthritis Rheumatic fever Infectious liver disease Lupus erythematosus	
Growth hormone, RIA	Males: up to 3 ng/ml Females: up to 5 ng/ml	Acromegaly	Failure to stimulate with arginine or insulin—hypopituitarism
Haptoglobin	50–200 mg/dl	Pregnancy Estrogen therapy Chronic infections Various inflammatory conditions Tissue destruction or necrosis	Hemolytic anemia Hemolytic blood transfusion reaction
Hemoglobin (plasma)	2–7 mg/dl	Transfusion reactions Paroxysmal nocturnal hemoglobinuria Intravascular hemolysis	
Hexosaminidase, total	Controls: 333–375 nM/ml/hr Heterozygotes: 288–644 nM/ml/hr Tay–Sachs disease: 284–1232 nM/ml/hr Diabetics: 567–3560 nM/ml/hr	Diabetes Tay–Sachs disease	
Hexosaminidase A	Controls: 49%–68% of total Heterozygotes: 26%–45% of total Tay–Sachs disease: 0%–4% of total Diabetics: 39%–59% of total		Tay-Sachs disease and heterozygoteses

(continued)

Normal Chemistries—Serum, Plasma, Whole Blood (continued)

		Clinical Significance	
Determination	**Normal Adult Values**	*(Increased)*	*(Decreased)*
High-density lipoprotein Cholesterol (HDL cholesterol)	*Age (years)* *Males (mg/dl)* *Females (mg/dl)* 0–19 30–65 30–70 20–29 35–70 35–75 30–39 30–65 35–80 40–49 30–65 40–85 50–59 30–65 35–85 60–69 30–65 35–85		HDL cholesterol is lower in patients with increased risk for coronary heart disease
17-Hydroxyprogesterone, RIA	Males: 0.4–4.0 ng/ml Females: 0.1–3.3 ng/ml Children: 0.1–0.5 ng/ml	Congenital adrenal hyperplasia Pregnancy Some cases of adrenal or ovarian adenomas	
Icterus index	1–6 units	Biliary obstruction Hemolytic anemias	Secondary anemias
Immunoglobulin A	Adult Males: 60–297 mg/dl Adult Females: 48–295 mg/dl	Gamma A myeloma Wiscott–Aldrich syndrome Autoimmune disease Hepatic cirrhosis	Ataxia telangiectasis Agammaglobulinemia Hypogammaglobulinemia, transient Dysgammaglobulinemia Protein-losing enteropathies
Immunoglobulin D	0–30 mg/dl	IgD multiple myeloma Some patients with chronic infectious diseases	
Immunoglobulin E	20–740 ng/ml	Allergic patients and those with parasitic infestations	
Immunoglobulin G	Adult Males: 635–1400 mg/dl Adult Females: 645–1300 mg/dl	IgG myeloma Following hyperimmunization Autoimmune disease states Chronic infections	Congenital and acquired hypogammaglobulinemia IgA myelomas, Waldenstrom's (IgM) macroglobulinemia Some malabsorption syndromes Extensive protein loss
Immunoglobulin M	Adult Males: 41–248 mg/dl Adult Females: 59–280 mg/dl	Waldenstrom's macroglobulinemia Parasitic infections Hepatitis	Agammaglobulinemias Some IgG and IgA myelomas Chronic lymphatic leukemia
Insulin, RIA	5–25 μU/ml	Insulinoma Acromegaly	Diabetes mellitus
Iodine, protein-bound	4.0–8.0 μg/dl	Hyperthyroidism	Hypothyroidism
Ionized calcium	2.04–2.44 mEq/liter	Ionized calcium is a much more sensitive indicator of disease states than the total calcium. Useful in diagnosing hyperparathyroidism in patients with normal and near normal total calcium levels. Also a necessary protocol in management of hemodialysis patients.	Hypothyroidism

(continued)

Normal Chemistries—Serum, Plasma, Whole Blood (continued)

Determination	Normal Adult Values	Clinical Significance (Increased)	(Decreased)
Iron	65–170 µg/dl	Pernicious anemia Aplastic anemia Hemolytic anemia Hepatitis Hemochromatosis	Iron deficiency anemia
Iron-binding capacity	IBC: 150–235 µg/dl TIBC: 250–420 µg/dl % Saturation: 20–50	Iron deficiency anemia	Chronic infectious diseases
Isocitric dehydrogenase	50–180 units	Hepatitis, cirrhosis Obstructive jaundice Metastatic carcinoma of the liver Megaloblastic anemia	
Lactic acid (whole blood)	9–16 mg/dl	Increased muscular activity Congestive heart failure Hemorrhage Shock Some varieties of metabolic acidosis Some febrile infections May be increased in severe liver disease	
Lactic dehydrogenase (LDH)	100–225 mU/ml	Untreated pernicious anemia Myocardial infarction Pulmonary infarction Liver disease	

Lactic dehydrogenase
  isoenzymes
Total lactic
  dehydrogenase
LDH-1
LDH-2
LDH-3
LDH-4
LDH-5
	100–225 mU/ml
	20%–35%
	25%–40%
	20%–30%
	0%–20%
	0%–25%
		LDH-1 and LDH-2 are increased in
		  myocardial infarction, megaloblastic
		  anemia, and hemolytic anemia.
		LDH-4 and LDH-5 are increased in
		  pulmonary infarction, congestive
		  heart failure, and liver disease.	

Lead (whole blood)	up to 40 µg/dl	Lead poisoning	
Leucine aminopeptidase	1–3 micromoles/hr/ml	Liver or biliary tract diseases Pancreatic disease Metastatic carcinoma of liver and pancreas Biliary obstruction	
Lipase	0.2–1.5 units/ml	Acute and chronic pancreatitis Biliary obstruction Cirrhosis Hepatitis Peptic ulcer	
Lipids, total	400–1000 mg/dl	Hypothyroidism Diabetes Nephrosis Glomerulonephritis	Hyperthyroidism
Lipoprotein phenotype			

(continued)

Normal Chemistries—Serum, Plasma, Whole Blood (continued)
Summary of Findings in the Primary Hyperlipoproteinemias

| Type | Appear-ance | Trigly-ceride | Choles-terol | Lipoprotein Staining | | | | Secondary Causes |
				Beta	Pre-beta	Alpha	Chylo-microns	
Normal	Clear	Normal	Normal	Moderate	Zero to moderate	Moderate	Weak	
I	Creamy	Markedly increased	Normal to moderately increased	Weak	Weak	Weak	Markedly increased	Dysglobulinemia
II	Clear	Normal to slightly increased	Slightly to markedly increased	Strong	Zero to strong	Moderate	Weak	Hypothyroidism, myeloma, hepatic disease, nephrotic syndrome, macroglobulinemia, and high dietary cholesterol
III	Clear, cloudy, or milky	Increased	Increased	Broad intense band	Extends into beta	Moderate	Weak	
IV	Clear, cloudy, or milky	Slightly to markedly increased	Normal to slightly increased	Weak to moderate	Moderate to strong	Weak to moderate	Weak	Hypothyroidism, diabetes mellitus, pancreatitis, glycogen storage diseases, nephrotic syndrome, myeloma, pregnancy, and oral contraceptives
V	Cloudy to creamy	Markedly increased	Increased	Weak	Moderate	Weak	Strong	Diabetes mellitus, pancreatitis, and alcoholism

Types I and II are fat induced; types III and IV are carbohydrate induced; type V is fat and carbohydrate induced.

Lithium	Usual maintenance level: 0.5–1.0 mEq/liter		
Low-density lipoprotein cho-lesterol (LDL cholesterol)	Age (years) mg/dl 0–19 50–170 20–29 60–170 30–39 70–190 40–49 80–190 50–59 80–210	LDL cholesterol is higher in patients with increased risk for coronary heart disease.	
Luteinizing hormone, RIA	Males: 6–30 mIU/ml Females: Follicular Phase: 2–30 mIU/ml Ovulatory Peak: 40–200 mIU/ml Luteal Phase: 0–20 mIU/ml Postmenopausal: 35–120 mIU/ml	Pituitary tumor Ovarian failure	Depressed or failure to peak—pituitary failure
Lysozyme (muramidase)	2.8–8 µg/ml	Certain types of leukemia (acute monocytic leukemia) Inflammatory states and infections	Acute lymphocytic leukemia

(continued)

Normal Chemistries—Serum, Plasma, Whole Blood (continued)

Determination	Normal Adult Values	Clinical Significance	
		(Increased)	*(Decreased)*
Magnesium	1.3–2.4 mEq/liter	Ingestion of Epsom salts Parathyroidectomy	Chronic alcoholism Toxemia of pregnancy Severe renal disease
Manganese	0.08–0.26 μg/dl		Defective growth
Mercury	up to 10 μg/dl	Mercury poisoning	
Myoglobin, RIA	up to 85 ng/ml	Myocardial infarction	
Nonprotein nitrogen	20–35 mg/dl	Acute nephritis Polycystic kidneys Obstructive uropathy Peritonitis Congestive heart failure Pregnancy	
5′ Nucleotidase	3.2–11.6 IU/liter	Hepatobiliary disease	
Osmolality	280–300 milliosmoles/kg	Useful in the study of electrolyte and water balance	Inappropriate secretion of antidiuretic hormone
Oxygen saturation arterial (whole blood)	96%–100%	Polycythemia Anhydremia	Anemia Cardiac decompensation Chronic obstructive pulmonary disease
pCO_2 (whole blood) arterial	35–45 mm Hg	Respiratory acidosis Metabolic alkalosis	Respiratory alkalosis Metabolic acidosis
pH (whole blood) arterial	7.35–7.45	Vomiting Hyperpnea Fever Intestinal obstruction	Uremia Diabetic acidosis Hemorrhage Nephritis
pO_2 (whole blood) arterial	95–100 mm Hg	Directly related to oxygen saturation	
Parathyroid hormone	163–347 pg/ml	Hyperparathyroidism	
Pepsinogen	200–425 units/ml		Conditions that decrease gastric acidity Pernicious anemia Achlorhydria
Phenylalanine	0–6 mg/dl first week 0.7–3.5 mg/dl thereafter	Phenylketonuria Oasthouse urine disease	
Phosphatase, acid, total	0–11 IU/liter	Carcinoma of prostate Advanced Paget's disease Hyperparathyroidism	
Phosphatase, acid, prostatic, RIA	0–10 ng/ml Borderline: 2.5–3.3 IU/liter	Carcinoma of prostate	
Phosphatase, alkaline	Adults: 30–115 mU/ml	Conditions reflecting increased osteoblastic activity of bone Rickets Hyperparathyroidism Liver disease	

(continued)

Normal Chemistries—Serum, Plasma, Whole Blood (continued)

Determination	Normal Adult Values	Clinical Significance	
		(Increased)	*(Decreased)*
Phosphatase, alkaline, thermostable fraction	Thermostable fraction greater than 35%: hepatic disease and combined disease with predominant hepatic component Thermostable fraction between 25%–35%: combined hepatic and skeletal disease Thermostable fraction less than 25%: skeletal disease with increased osteoblastic activity	Hepatic disease	
Phosphohexose isomerase	20–90 IU/liter	Malignancy Diseases of heart, liver, and skeletal muscles	
Phospholipids	125–300 mg/dl	Diabetes Nephritis	
Phosphorus, inorganic	2.5–4.5 mg/dl	Chronic nephritis Hypoparathyroidism	Hyperparathyroidism
Potassium	3.5–5.0 mEq/liter	Addison's disease Oliguria Anuria Tissue breakdown or hemolysis	Diabetic acidosis Diarrhea Vomiting
Progesterone, RIA	Follicular phase: up to 0.8 ng/ml Luteal phase: 10–20 ng/ml End of cycle: less than 1 ng/ml Pregnant: up to 50 ng/ml in 20th week	Useful in evaluation of menstrual disorders and infertility and the evaluation of placental function during pregnancies complicated by toxemia, diabetes mellitus, or threatened miscarriage	
Prolactin, RIA	Males: 7–18 ng/ml Females: 6–24 ng/ml	Pregnancy Functional or structural disorders of the hypothalamus Pituitary stalk section Pituitary tumors Primary hypothyroidism	
Protein, total Albumin Globulin	6.0–8.0 g/dl 3.5–5.0 g/dl 1.5–3.0 g/dl	Hemoconcentration Shock Multiple myeloma (globulin fraction) Chronic infections (globulin fraction) Liver disease (globulin)	Malnutrition Hemorrhage Loss of plasma from burns Proteinuria

(continued)

Normal Chemistries—Serum, Plasma, Whole Blood (continued)

Determination	Normal Adult Values	Clinical Significance	
		(Increased)	*(Decreased)*
Electrophoresis (Cellulose acetate)			
Albumin	3.3–5.0 g/dl		
Alpha$_1$ globulin	0.2–0.4 g/dl		
Alpha$_2$ globulin	0.6–1.0 g/dl		
Beta globulin	0.6–1.2 g/dl		
Gamma globulin	0.7–1.5 g/dl		
Protoporphyrin, erythrocyte (whole blood)	15–100 μg/dl	Lead toxicity Erythropoietic porphyria	
Pyridoxine	3.6–18 ng/ml		A wide spectrum of clinical conditions, such as mental depression, peripheral neuropathy, anemia, neonatal seizures, and reactions to certain drug therapy
Pyruvic acid (whole blood)	0.3–0.7 mg/dl	Diabetes Severe thiamine deficiency Acute phase of some infections, possibly secondary to increased glycogenolysis and glycolysis	

Renin (plasma), RIA	*Normal Diet:*
	  Supine: 0.3–1.9 ng/ml/hr
	  Upright: 0.6–3.6 ng/ml/hr
	Low-Salt Diet:
	  Supine: 0.9–4.5 ng/ml/hr
	  Upright: 4.1–9.1 ng/ml/hr
		Renovascular hypertension
		Malignant hypertension
		Untreated Addison's disease
		Primary salt-losing nephropathy
		Low-salt diet
		Diuretic therapy
		Hemorrhage
			Frank primary aldosteronism
			Increased salt intake
			Salt-retaining steroid therapy
			Antidiuretic hormone therapy
			Blood transfusion

Riboflavin (whole blood)	0.9–1.31 (activity coefficient)		Riboflavin deficiency
Sodium	135–145 mEq/liter	Hemoconcentration Nephritis Pyloric obstruction	Alkali deficit Addison's disease Myxedema
Sulfate	0.5–1.5 mg/dl	Nephritis Nitrogen retention	

Testosterone, RIA	Females: 25–100 ng/dl
	Males: 300–800 ng/dl
		Females:
		  Polycystic ovary
		  Virilizing tumors
			Males: Orchidectomy for neoplastic disease of the prostate or breast
			Estrogen therapy
			Klinefelter's syndrome
			Hypopituitarism
			Hypogonadism
			Hepatic cirrhosis

Thymol turbidity	1–4.5 units/ml	Liver disease Infectious diseases with antibody production	

(continued)

Normal Chemistries—Serum, Plasma, Whole Blood (continued)

Determination	Normal Adult Values	Clinical Significance	
		(Increased)	(Decreased)
T₃ uptake	25%–35%	Hyperthyroidism TBG deficiency Androgens and anabolic steroids	Hypothyroidism Pregnancy TBG excess Estrogens and antiovulatory drugs
T₃, Triiodothyronine (total circulating), RIA	75–200 ng/dl	Pregnancy Hyperthyroidism	Hypothyroidism
T₄, Thyroxine, RIA	4.5–11.5 µg/dl	Hyperthyroidism Thyroiditis Cases of elevated thyroxine-binding proteins caused by oral contraceptives Pregnancy	Primary and pituitary hypothyroidism Idiopathic involvement Cases of diminished thyroxine-binding proteins caused by androgenic and anabolic steroids Hypoproteinemia Nephrotic syndrome
T₄, Thyroxine, free	1.0–2.2 ng/dl	Euthyroid patients with normal free thyroxine levels may have abnormal T₃ and T₄ levels caused by drug preparations	
Thyroid-stimulating hormone (TSH), RIA	0–10 µIU/ml	Primary hypothyroidism	
Thyroid-binding globulin	10–26 µg/dl	Hypothyroidism Pregnancy Estrogen therapy Oral contraceptives Genetic and idiopathic	Androgens and anabolic steroids Nephrotic syndromes Marked hypoproteinemia Hepatic disease
Transaminase (SGOT) (Aspartate aminotransferase)	7–40 mU/ml	Myocardial infarction Skeletal muscle disease Liver disease	
Transaminase (SGPT) (Alanine aminotransferase)	10–40 mU/ml	Same conditions as SGOT, but increase is more marked in liver disease than SGOT	
Transferrin	230–320 mg/dl	Pregnancy Iron-deficiency anemia due to hemorrhaging Acute hepatitis Polycythemia Oral contraceptives	Pernicious anemia in relapse Thalassemic and sickle cell anemia Chromatosis Neoplastic and hepatic diseases
Transketolase (whole blood)	Pentose utilization: 9.66–15.50 micromoles/hr/ml or 1.70–3.04 micromoles/hr/10⁹ red blood cells		Thiamine deficiency
Triglycerides	10–150 mg/dl	See lipoprotein phenotype	
Tryptophan	1.4–3.0 mg/dl		Tryptophan-specific malabsorption syndrome

(continued)

Normal Chemistries—Serum, Plasma, Whole Blood (continued)

Determination	Normal Adult Values	Clinical Significance	
		(Increased)	*(Decreased)*
Tyrosine	0.5–4.0 mg/dl	Hyperthyroidism Tyrosinosis	
Urea nitrogen (BUN)	10–20 mg/dl	Acute glomerulonephritis Obstructive uropathy Mercury poisoning Nephrotic syndrome	Severe hepatic failure Pregnancy
Uric acid	2.5–8.0 mg/dl	Gouty arthritis Acute leukemia Lymphomas treated by chemotherapy Toxemia of pregnancy	Xanthinuria Defective tubular reabsorption
Viscosity	1.4–1.8 relative to water at 37° C (98.6° F)	Patients with marked increases of the gamma globulins	
Vitamin A	50–220 μg/dl	Hypervitaminosis A	Vitamin A deficiency Celiac disease Sprue Obstructive jaundice Cystic fibrosis Giardiasis Parenchymal hepatic disease
Vitamin B$_1$ (thiamine)	1.6–4.0 μg/dl		Anorexia Beriberi Polyneuropathy Cardiomyopathies
Vitamin B$_6$ (pyridoxal phosphate)	3.6–18 ng/ml		Chronic alcoholism Malnutrition Uremia Neonatal seizures Malabsorption, such as celiac syndrome
Vitamin B$_{12}$ RIA	130–785 pg/ml	Hepatic cell damage and in association with the myeloproliferative disorders (the highest levels are encountered in myeloid leukemia)	Strict vegetarianism Alcoholism Pernicious anemia Total or partial gastrectomy Ileal resection Sprue and celiac disease Fish tapeworm infestation
Vitamin E	0.5–2.0 mg/dl		Vitamin E deficiency
Water content	92.6–94.3 g/dl	Useful in the study of electrolyte and water balance	
Xylose absorption test	2 hr 30–50 mg/dl		Malabsorption syndrome
Zinc	55–150 μg/dl	Zinc is essential for the growth and propagation of cell cultures and the functioning of several enzymes	
Zinc turbidity	2–12 units/ml	Same clinical significance as thymol turbidity	

Normal Values—Urine Chemistry

Determination	Normal Value	Clinical Significance (Increased)	(Decreased)
Acetone and acetoacetate	Zero	Uncontrolled diabetes Starvation	
Acid mucopolysaccharides	Negative	Hurler's syndrome Marfan's syndrome Morquio–Ulrich disease	

Aldosterone	*Normal Salt:*
	  Normal: 4–20 µg/24 hr
	  Renovascular: 10–40 µg/24 hr
	  Tumor: 20–100 µg/24 hr
	Low Salt:
	  Normal: 10–40 µg/24 hr
	  Renovascular: 20–100 µg/24 hr
	  Tumor: 20–100 µg/24 hr
		Primary aldosteronism (adrenocortical tumor)
		Secondary aldosteronism
		  Salt depletion
		  Potassium loading
		  ACTH in large doses
		  Cardiac failure
		  Cirrhosis with ascites formation
		  Nephrosis
		  Pregnancy	

Alpha amino nitrogen	64–199 mg/24 hr	Leukemia Diabetes Phenylketonuria Other metabolic diseases	
Amylase	35–260 units excreted/hr	Acute pancreatitis	
Arylsulfatase A	Greater than 2.4 units/ml		Metachromatic leukodystrophy
Bence–Jones protein	None detected	Myeloma	
Bile melanin	Zero	Advanced melanoma Ochronosis	
Calcium	Less than 150 mg/24 hr	Hyperparathyroidism Vitamin D intoxication Fanconi syndrome	Hypoparathyroidism Vitamin D deficiency
Catecholamines	Total: 0–275 µg/24 hr Epinephrine: 10%–40% Norepinephrine: 60%–90%	Pheochromocytoma Neuroblastoma	
Chloride	70–250 mEq/24 hr	Urine chloride levels vary with excretion of sodium, potassium, ammonia, and bicarbonate	
Chorionic gonadotrophin, qualitative (pregnancy test)	Negative	Pregnancy Chorionepithelioma Hydatidiform mole	
Copper	20–70 µg/24 hr	Wilson's disease Cirrhosis Nephrosis	
Coproporphyrin	50–300 µg/24 hr	Poliomyelitis Lead poisoning Porphyria hepatica Porphyria erythropoietica Porphyria cutanea tarda	

(continued)

Normal Values—Urine Chemistry (continued)

Determination	Normal Value	Clinical Significance (Increased)	(Decreased)
Cortisol, free	20–90 μg/24 hr	Cushing's syndrome	
Creatine	0–200 mg/24 hr	Muscular dystrophy Fever Carcinoma of liver Pregnancy Hyperthyroidism Myositis	
Creatinine	0.8–2.0 g/24 hr	Typhoid fever Salmonella infections Tetanus	Muscular atrophy Anemia Advanced degeneration of kidneys Leukemia
Creatinine clearance	100–150 ml of blood cleared of creatinine/min.		Measures glomerular filtration rate Renal diseases
Cystine	10–100 mg/24 hr	Cystinuria	
Delta amino-levulinic acid	0–0.54 mg/dl	Lead poisoning Porphyria hepatica Hepatitis Hepatic carcinoma	
11-Desoxycortisol	20–100 μg/24 hr	Hypertensive form of virilizing adrenal hyperplasia due to an 11-beta hydroxylase defect	
Diagnex blue	Greater than 0.6 mg Presumptive evidence for hypochlorhydria: 0.3–0.6 mg Presumptive evidence for achlorhydria: less than 0.3 mg		Hypochlorhydria Achlorhydria
Estriol (placental)	*Weeks of pregnancy* / *mg/24 hr* 12 / less than 1 16 / 2–7 20 / 4–9 24 / 6–13 28 / 8–22 32 / 12–43 36 / 14–45 40 / 19–46		Decreased values occur with fetal distress of many conditions, including preeclampsia, placental insufficiency, and poorly controlled diabetes mellitus
Estrogens, total (fluorimetric)	Females: Onset of menstruation: 4–25 μg/24 hr Ovulation peak: 28–99 μg/24 hr Luteal peak: 22–105 μg/24 hr Menopausal: 1.4–19.6 μg/24 hr Males: 5–18 μg/24 hr	Hyperestrogenism due to gonadal or adrenal neoplasm	Primary or secondary amenorrhea

(continued)

Normal Values—Urine Chemistry (continued)

Determination	Normal Value	Clinical Significance	
		(Increased)	*(Decreased)*
Etiocholanolone	Males: 1.9–6.0 mg/24 hr Females: 0.5–4.0 mg/24 hr	Adrenogenital syndrome Idiopathic hirsutism	

Follicle-stimulating hormone, RIA	Males: 5–25 IU/24 hr
	Females:
	  Follicular: 5–20 IU/24 hr
	  Luteal: 5–15 IU/24 hr
	  Midcycle: 15–60 IU/24 hr
	  Menopausal: 50–100
	    IU/24 hr
		Menopause and primary ovarian failure	Pituitary failure

Glucose	Negative	Diabetes mellitus Pituitary disorders Intracranial pressure Lesion in floor of fourth ventricle	
Hemoglobin and myoglobin	Negative	Extensive burns Transfusion of incompatible blood Myoglobin increased in severe crushing injuries to muscle	
Homogentisic acid, qualitative	Negative	Alkaptonuria Ochronosis	
Homovanillic acid	Up to 15 mg/24 hr	Neuroblastoma	
17-hydroxycorticosteroids	2–10 mg/24 hr	Cushing's syndrome	Addison's disease Anterior pituitary hypofunction
5-hydroxyindoleacetic acid, qualitative	Negative	Malignant carcinoid tumors	
Hydroxyproline	25–77 mg/24 hr	Paget's disease Fibrous dysplasia Osteomalacia Neoplastic bone disease Hyperparathyroidism	
17-ketosteroids, alpha-beta fractionation	Alpha concentration 85% or more	Adrenal carcinomas (in beta fraction)	
17-ketosteroids, total	Males: 10–22 mg/24 hr Females: 6–16 mg/24 hr	Interstitial cell tumor of testes Simple hirsutism, occasionally Adrenal hyperplasia Cushing's syndrome Adrenal cancer, virilism Arrhenoblastoma	Thyrotoxicosis Female hypogonadism Diabetes mellitus Hypertension Debilitating disease of mild to moderate severity Eunuchoidism Addison's disease Panhypopituitarism Myxedema Nephrosis

Kynurenic and xanthurenic acids	Kynurenic acid: up to 18
	  mg/24 hr
	Xanthurenic acid: up to 4
	  mg/24 hr
		Vitamin B_6 deficiency
		Acute typhoid fever
		Sandfly fever
		Tularemia	

(continued)

Normal Values—Urine Chemistry (continued)

Determination	Normal Value	Clinical Significance (Increased)	Clinical Significance (Decreased)
Lead	up to 150 μg/24 hr	Lead poisoning	
Lipase	0.1–0.75 units/ml	Pancreatitis	

Luteinizing hormone	Males: 5–18 IU/24 hr
	Females:
	  Follicular phase: 2–25 IU/24 hr
	  Ovulatory peak: 30–95 IU/24 hr
	  Luteal phase: 2–20 IU/24 hr
	  Postmenopausal: 40–110 IU/24 hr
		Pituitary tumor
		Ovarian failure
			Depressed or failure to peak—pituitary failure

Metanephrines, total	Less than 1.3 mg/24 hr	Pheochromocytoma, a few patients with pheochromocytoma may have elevated urinary metanephrines but normal catecholamines and VMA	
Osmolality	Males: 390–1090 milliosmoles/kg Females: 300–1090 milliosmoles/kg	Useful in the study of electrolyte and water balance	
Oxalate	up to 40 mg/24 hr	Primary hyperoxaluria	
Phenolphthalein (PSP)	At least 25% excreted in 15 min, 40% by 30 min, and 60% by 120 min	Primarily measures renal tubular function	Delayed in renal diseases Low in nephritis, cystitis, pyelonephritis, congestive heart failure
Phenylpyruvic acid, qualitative	Negative	Phenylketonuria	
Phosphorus, inorganic	0.8–1.3 g/24 hr	Fever Nervous exhaustion Tuberculosis Rickets Chronic lead poisoning	Acute infections Nephritis Chlorosis Pregnancy
Porphobilinogen, qualitative	Negative	Acute porphyria Liver disease	
Porphobilinogen, quantitative	0–0.03 mg/dl	Acute porphyria Liver disease	
Porphyrins, qualitative	Negative	See porphyrins, quantitative	
Porphyrins, quantitative (Coproporphyrin and Uroporphyrin)	Coproporphyrin: 50–300 μg/24 hr Uroporphyrin: up to 50 μg/24 hr	Porphyria hepatica Porphyria erythropoietica Porphyria cutanea tarda Lead poisoning (only coproporphyrin increased)	
Potassium	40–65 mEq/24 hr	Hemolysis	

(continued)

Normal Values—Urine Chemistry (continued)

Determination	Normal Value	Clinical Significance	
		(Increased)	*(Decreased)*

Pregnanediol	Males: 0.1–2.0 mg/24 hr
	Females:
	  Proliferative phase:
	    0.5–1.5 mg/24 hr
	  Luteal phase: 2–7
	    mg/24 hr
	  Menopause: 0.2–1.0
	    mg/24 hr
	
	Pregnancy:
	(Weeks of
	gestation) *mg/24hr*
	  10–12 5–15
	  12–18 5–25
	  18–24 15–33
	  24–28 20–42
	  28–32 27–47
		Corpus luteum cysts
		When placental tissue remains in the
		  uterus following parturition
		Some cases of adrenocortical tumors
		Pregnancy
			Placental dysfunction
			Threatened abortion
			Intrauterine death

Pregnanetriol	0.4 mg/24 hr	Congenital adrenal androgenic hyperplasia	
Protein	up to 100 mg/24 hr	Nephritis Cardiac failure Mercury poisoning Bence–Jones protein in multiple myeloma Febrile states Hematuria Amyloidosis	
Sodium	130–200 mEq/24 hr	Useful in detecting gross changes in water and salt balance	
Titratable acidity	20–40 mEq/24 hr	Metabolic acidosis	Metabolic alkalosis
Urea nitrogen	9–16 g/24 hr	Excessive protein catabolism	Impaired kidney function
Uric acid	250–750 mg/24 hr	Gout	Nephritis

Urobilinogen	Random urine: less than
	  0.25 mg/dl
	24 hr urine: up to 4
	  mg/24 hr
		Liver and biliary tract disease
		Hemolytic anemias
			Complete or nearly complete biliary
			  obstruction
			Diarrhea
			Renal insufficiency

Uroporphyrins	up to 50 μg/24 hr	Porphyria	
Vanillylmandelic acid (VMA)	0.7–6.8 mg/24 hr	Pheochromocytoma Neuroblastoma Coffee, tea, aspirin, bananas, and several different drugs	

Xylose absorption test
  (5 hr)
	16%–33% of ingested
	  xylose
			Malabsorption syndromes

Zinc	0.15–1.2 mg/24 hr	Zinc is an essential nutritional element	

Normal Values—Cerebrospinal Fluid

Determination	Normal Value	Clinical Significance (Increased)	(Decreased)
Albumin	15.5–32.0 mg/dl	Certain neurologic disorders Lesion in the choroid plexus or blockage of the flow of CSF Damage to the blood–CNS barrier	
Cell count	0–5 mononuclear cells/ cu mm	Bacterial meningitis Neurosyphilis Anterior poliomyelitis Encephalitis lethargica	
Chloride	100–130 mEq/liter	Uremia	Acute generalized meningitis Tubercular meningitis
Colloidal gold	0	Acute meningitis Neurosyphilis	
Glucose	50–75 mg/dl	Diabetes mellitus Diabetic coma Epidemic encephalitis Uremia	Acute meningitides Tuberculous meningitis Insulin shock
Glutamine	6–15 mg/dl	Hepatic encephalopathies, including Reye's syndrome Hepatic coma Cirrhosis	
IgG	0–6.6 mg/dl	Damage to the blood–CNS barrier Multiple sclerosis Neurosyphilis Subacute sclerosing panencephalitis Chronic phases of CNS infections	
Lactic acid	Less than 24 mg/dl	Bacterial meningitis Hypocapnia Hydrocephalus Brain abscesses Cerebral ischemia	
Lactic dehydrogenase	One tenth that of serum	CNS disease	

Protein
  Lumbar
  Cisternal
  Ventricular
	
	15–45 mg/dl
	15–25 mg/dl
	5–15 mg/dl
		Acute meningitides
		Tubercular meningitis
		Neurosyphilis
		Poliomyelitis
		Guillain-Barré syndrome	

Protein Electrophoresis
  (Cellulose acetate)
  Prealbumin
  Albumin
  Alpha$_1$ globulin
  Alpha$_2$ globulin
  Beta globulin
  Gamma globulin
	% of total
	
	3–7
	56–74
	2–6.5
	3–12
	8–18.5
	4–14
		An increase in the level of albumin alone can be the result of a lesion in the choroid plexus or a blockage of the flow of CSF. An elevated gamma globulin value with a normal albumin level has been reported in multiple sclerosis, neurosyphilis, subacute sclerosing panencephalitis, and the chronic phase of CNS infections. If the blood–CNS barrier has been severely damaged during the course of these diseases, the CSF albumin level may also be elevated.	

Miscellaneous Values

Determinations	Normal Value	Clinical Significance
Acetaminophen	Zero	Therapeutic level = 10–20 μg/ml
Aminophylline (theophylline)	Zero	Therapeutic level = 10–20 μg/ml
Bromide	Zero	Therapeutic level = 5–50 mg/dl
Carbon monoxide	0%–2%	Symptoms with over 20% saturation
Digitoxin	Zero	Therapeutic level = 5–30 ng/ml
Digoxin	Zero	Therapeutic level = 0.5–2.0 ng/ml
Dilantin (phenytoin)	Zero	Therapeutic level = 10–20 μg/ml
Ethanol	0%–0.01%	Legal intoxication level = 0.10% or above
		0.3%–0.4% = marked intoxication
		0.4%–0.5% = alcoholic stupor
Gentamicin	Zero	Therapeutic level = 4–10 μg/ml
Librium (chlordiazepoxide)	Zero	Therapeutic level = 1–3 μg/ml
Methanol	Zero	May be fatal in concentrations as low as 10 mg/dl
Mysoline (primidone)	Zero	Therapeutic level = 5–12 μg/ml
Phenobarbital	Zero	Therapeutic level = 15–40 μg/ml
Quinidine	Zero	Therapeutic level = 0.2–0.5 mg/dl
Salicylate	Zero	Therapeutic level = 2–25 mg/dl
		Toxic level = over 30 mg/dl
Sulfonamide	Zero	Therapeutic levels:
		Sulfadiazine 8–15 mg/dl
		Sulfaguanidine 3–5 mg/dl
		Sulfamerazine 10–15 mg/dl
		Sulfanilamide 10–15 mg/dl
Valium (diazepam)	Zero	Therapeutic level: 0.5–2.5 μg/dl

Gastric Analysis

	Normal Value	(Increased)	(Decreased)
Free HCl	0–30 mEq/liter	Neuroses	Pernicious anemia
Total acidity	15–45 mEq/liter	Peptic ulcer	Gastric carcinoma
Combined acid	10–15 mEq/liter	Zollinger–Ellison syndrome	Chronic atrophic gastritis
			Decreases normally with age

Index